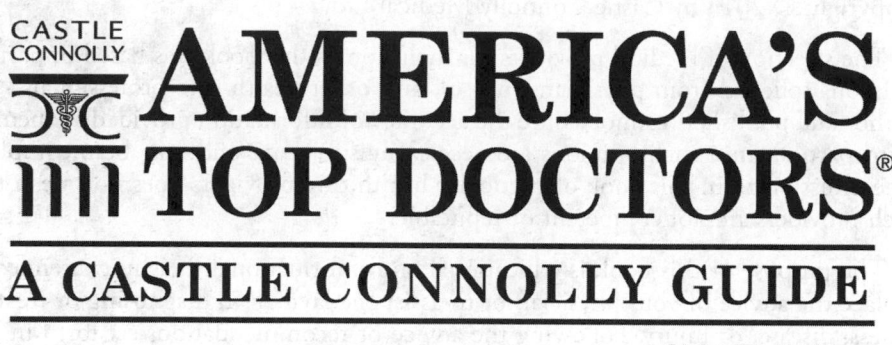

CASTLE CONNOLLY AMERICA'S TOP DOCTORS®

A CASTLE CONNOLLY GUIDE

12th Edition

The Best in American Medicine

America's trusted source for identifying Top Doctors

For more information, please contact:

Castle Connolly Medical Ltd., 42 West 24th St, New York, New York 10010
212-367-8400x110
E-mail: info@castleconnolly.com
Web site: http://www.castleconnolly.com.

Library of Congress Control Number: 2012939940

| ISBN | 1-883769-63-9 | 978-1-883769-63-5 | (paperback) |
| ISBN | 1-883769-62-0 | 978-1-883769-62-8 | (hardcover) |

Printed in the United States of America

Table of Contents

About the Publishers .. xxix

Medical Advisory Board ... xxxi

Foreword .. xxxii

Introduction .. 1

Using This Guide To Find Top Specialists 5

Maximizing Your First Appointment With A Top Doctor 21

Utilizing Special Resources .. 25

How To Use This Guide .. 37

 Locating A Specialist .. 37

 Geographic Regions And States ... 38

Medical Specialties ... 41

 Descriptions And Abbreviations .. 42

The Training Of A Specialist ... 49

Partnership For Excellence Program ... 53

 List Of Participating Hospitals ... 54

 Cleveland Clinic Foundation ... 55

 Continuum Health Partners .. 56

 Dana-Farber/Brigham and Women's Cancer Center 57

 Fox Chase Cancer Center ... 58

 H Lee Moffitt Cancer Center & Research Institute 59

 Hospital for Special Surgery .. 60

 The Johns Hopkins Hospital .. 61

 Keck Medical Center of USC ... 62

 Maimonides Medical Center .. 63

 Mount Sinai Medical Center ... 64

 New York Eye & Ear Infirmary 65

 NewYork-Presbyterian Hospital 66

 North Shore-LIJ Health System 67

 NYU Langone Medical Center 68

 NYU Hassenfeld Pediatric Center 69

Table of Contents

NYU Hospital for Joint Diseases .. 70

NYU Rusk Institute for Rehabilitation ... 71

Penn Medicine .. 72

St. Francis Hospital -The Heart Center .. 73

University Hospitals Case Medical Center 74

Vanderbilt University Medical Center .. 75

Physician Listings .. **77**

Adolescent Medicine .. **79**

New England ... 80

Mid Atlantic .. 80

Midwest ... 81

Great Plains & Mountains .. 81

Southwest .. 82

West Coast & Pacific ... 82

Allergy & Immunology .. **83**

New England ... 84

Mid Atlantic .. 84

Southeast ... 86

Midwest ... 87

Southwest .. 89

West Coast & Pacific ... 90

Cardiovascular Disease...**93**

 Cardiovascular Disease..**94**

 New England...94

 Mid Atlantic...96

 Southeast..103

 Midwest..106

 Great Plains & Mountains..113

 Southwest...113

 West Coast & Pacific...116

 Cardiac Electrophysiology ...**118**

 New England...118

 Mid Atlantic...119

 Southeast..121

 Midwest..122

 Great Plains & Mountains..124

 Southwest...124

 West Coast & Pacific...125

 Interventional Cardiology ...**126**

 New England...126

 Mid Atlantic...127

 Southeast..129

 Midwest..130

 Great Plains & Mountains..132

 Southwest...132

 West Coast & Pacific...133

 Centers of Excellence

 Cleveland Clinic...134

 Continuum Health Partners135

 Maimonides Medical Center136

 Mount Sinai Medical Center137

 NewYork-Presbyterian Hospital138

 NYU Langone Medical Center...............................139-140

 Penn Medicine...141

Table of Contents

St Francis Hospital - The Heart Center142-143

Vanderbilt University Medical Center ...144

Child Neurology..**145**

New England...146

Mid Atlantic...147

Southeast ...149

Midwest..150

Great Plains & Mountains..152

Southwest ..152

West Coast & Pacific..153

Clinical Genetics ...**155**

New England...156

Mid Atlantic...156

Southeast ...158

Midwest..160

Great Plains & Mountains..161

Southwest ..161

West Coast & Pacific..162

Centers of Excellence

Mount Sinai Medical Center...165-166

Colon & Rectal Surgery ...**167**

New England...168

Mid Atlantic...169

Southeast ...171

Midwest..173

Great Plains & Mountains..176

Southwest ..176

West Coast & Pacific..177

Centers of Excellence

Cleveland Clinic...179

NYU Langone Medical Center ..180

Dermatology .. **181**

 New England...182

 Mid Atlantic...184

 Southeast...189

 Midwest...192

 Great Plains & Mountains...196

 Southwest..196

 West Coast & Pacific..198

 Centers of Excellence

 Cleveland Clinic..201

 Mount Sinai Medical Center...202

 NYU Langone Medical Center..203

Endocrinology, Diabetes & Metabolism**205**

 New England...206

 Mid Atlantic...208

 Southeast...213

 Midwest...216

 Great Plains & Mountains...220

 Southwest..220

 West Coast & Pacific..221

 Centers of Excellence

 Cleveland Clinic..225

Gastroenterology...**227**

 New England...228

 Mid Atlantic...230

 Southeast...239

 Midwest...243

 Great Plains & Mountains...249

 Southwest..250

 West Coast & Pacific..253

Table of Contents

Centers of Excellence

Cleveland Clinic ..256

Mount Sinai Medical Center ..257

NewYork-Presbyterian Hospital ...258

NYU Langone Medical Center ...259

Geriatric Medicine ...**261**

New England ..262

Mid Atlantic ...262

Southeast ..263

Midwest ..264

Great Plains & Mountains ..265

Southwest ..266

West Coast & Pacific ...266

Centers of Excellence

Cleveland Clinic ..268

Maimonides Medical Center ...269

Mount Sinai Medical Center ...270

NYU Langone Medical Center ..271

Gynecologic Oncology ..**273**

New England ..274

Mid Atlantic ...275

Southeast ..280

Midwest ..283

Great Plains & Mountains ..286

Southwest ..286

West Coast & Pacific ...289

Centers of Excellence

Cleveland Clinic ..292

Hand Surgery ... **293**

 New England .. 294

 Mid Atlantic .. 295

 Southeast ... 298

 Midwest .. 300

 Great Plains and Mountains .. 302

 Southwest .. 303

 West Coast & Pacific ... 303

 Centers of Excellence

 Cleveland Clinic ... 306

 NYU Hospital for Joint Diseases 307

Hematology & Medical Oncology ... **309**

 Hematology .. **310**

 New England .. 310

 Mid Atlantic .. 311

 Southeast ... 316

 Midwest .. 318

 Great Plains & Mountains ... 322

 Southwest .. 323

 West Coast & Pacific ... 325

 Medical Oncology ... **327**

 New England .. 327

 Mid Atlantic .. 333

 Southeast ... 353

 Midwest .. 364

 Great Plains & Mountains ... 374

 Southwest .. 376

 West Coast & Pacific ... 383

 Centers of Excellence

 Cleveland Clinic ... 393

 Continuum Health Partners .. 394

 H Lee Moffit Cancer Center & Research Institute 395

 Keck Medical Center of USC ... 396

 Maimonides Medical Center ... 397

Table of Contents

Mount Sinai Medical Center...398-399

NewYork-Presbyterian Hospital ..400

NYU Langone Medical Center...401

Penn Medicine...402

Vanderbilt University Medical Center403

Hospice & Palliative Medicine...**405**

New England...406

Mid Atlantic...406

Southeast ..407

Midwest...407

Great Plains & Mountains..407

Southwest..408

West Coast & Pacific...408

Infectious Disease...**409**

New England...410

Mid Atlantic...410

Southeast ..414

Midwest...416

Great Plains & Mountains..418

Southwest..418

West Coast & Pacific...419

Centers of Excellence

Cleveland Clinic...421

NYU Langone Medical Center...422

Internal Medicine...**423**

New England...424

Mid Atlantic...424

Southeast ..424

Midwest...425

Great Plains & Mountains..426

West Coast & Pacific...426

Centers of Excellence

NYU Langone Medical Center...427

Table of Contents

Maternal & Fetal Medicine ... 429
 New England...430
 Mid Atlantic...431
 Southeast..434
 Midwest..435
 Great Plains & Mountains...438
 Southwest...438
 West Coast & Pacific..439
 Centers of Excellence
 Cleveland Clinic..442
 NYU Langone Medical Center...................................443

Neonatal-Perinatal Medicine .. 445
 New England...446
 Mid Atlantic...446
 Southeast..448
 Midwest..450
 Great Plains & Mountains...451
 Southwest...451
 West Coast & Pacific..452
 Centers of Excellence
 NYU Langone Medical Center...................................453

Nephrology ... 455
 New England...456
 Mid Atlantic...456
 Southeast..459
 Midwest..461
 Southwest...463
 West Coast & Pacific..464
 Centers of Excellence
 Cleveland Clinic..467
 Mount Sinai Medical Center.....................................468

Neurological Surgery ... 469
 New England...470

Table of Contents

Mid Atlantic .. 472

Southeast .. 481

Midwest .. 485

Great Plains & Mountains .. 491

Southwest ... 492

West Coast & Pacific .. 495

Centers of Excellence

Cleveland Clinic ... 500

Mount Sinai Medical Center .. 501

North Shore-LIJ Health System ... 502

NYU Langone Medical Center ... 503

Penn Medicine ... 504

Neurology ... **505**

New England .. 506

Mid Atlantic ... 509

Southeast .. 519

Midwest .. 524

Great Plains & Mountains .. 531

Southwest ... 532

West Coast & Pacific .. 535

Centers of Excellence

Cleveland Clinic ... 540

Continuum Health Partners ... 541

Mount Sinai Medical Center .. 542

NewYork-Presbyterian Hospital .. 543

NYU Langone Medical Center ... 544

Penn Medicine ... 545

Nuclear Medicine ... **547**

Mid Atlantic ... 548

Southeast .. 549

Midwest .. 550

Southwest ... 550

West Coast & Pacific .. 551

Table of Contents

Centers of Excellence

Cleveland Clinic ..552

NYU Langone Medical Center553

Obstetrics & Gynecology ...**555**

New England ...556

Mid Atlantic ...556

Southeast ..559

Midwest...560

Great Plains & Mountains ..562

Southwest ...563

West Coast & Pacific...563

Centers of Excellence

Cleveland Clinic ..564

Maimonides Medical Center ..565

Mount Sinai Medical Center566

NYU Langone Medical Center567

Penn Medicine..568

Ophthalmology ...**569**

New England ...570

Mid Atlantic ...571

Southeast ..581

Midwest...587

Great Plains & Mountains ..595

Southwest ...596

West Coast & Pacific...598

Centers of Excellence

Cleveland Clinic ..606

Mount Sinai Medical Center607

New York Eye & Ear Infirmary608

Orthopaedic Surgery ...**609**

New England ...610

Mid Atlantic ...613

Southeast ..627

Table of Contents

Midwest..631

Great Plains & Mountains...638

Southwest...640

West Coast & Pacific...641

Centers of Excellence

Cleveland Clinic...647

Hospital for Special Surgery ...648

Mount Sinai Medical Center ...649

NYU Hospital for Joint Diseases...................................650-651

Penn Medicine..652

Otolaryngology ...**653**

New England...655

Mid Atlantic..657

Southeast..667

Midwest..672

Great Plains & Mountains..679

Southwest..681

West Coast & Pacific..684

Centers of Excellence

Cleveland Clinic..689

Johns Hopkins Hospital ...690

Mount Sinai Medical Center ..691

New York Eye & Ear Infirmary ..692

NYU Langone Medical Center..693

Pain Medicine ...**695**

New England...696

Mid Atlantic..696

Southeast..698

Midwest..699

Great Plains & Mountains..700

Southwest..701

West Coast & Pacific..702

Centers of Excellence

Cleveland Clinic..704

Pathology ... **705**

 New England ... 706

 Mid Atlantic .. 707

 Southeast .. 713

 Midwest .. 714

 Great Plains & Mountains ... 717

 Southwest .. 717

 West Coast & Pacific .. 719

Pediatrics ... **723**

 Pediatrics ... **726**

 New England ... 726

 Mid Atlantic .. 726

 Southeast .. 727

 Midwest .. 727

 Southwest .. 728

 West Coast & Pacific .. 728

 Pediatric Allergy & Immunology .. **729**

 New England ... 729

 Mid Atlantic .. 729

 Southeast .. 730

 Midwest .. 731

 Great Plains & Mountains ... 732

 Southwest .. 732

 West Coast & Pacific .. 733

 Pediatric Cardiology ... **733**

 New England ... 733

 Mid Atlantic .. 734

 Southeast .. 737

 Midwest .. 738

 Great Plains & Mountains ... 739

 Southwest .. 740

 West Coast & Pacific .. 740

 Pediatric Critical Care Medicine ... **741**

 Mid Atlantic .. 741

Table of Contents

Southeast ...741

Midwest ...742

Great Plains & Mountains742

Southwest ..742

West Coast & Pacific ..743

Pediatric Endocrinology**743**

New England ...743

Mid Atlantic ..744

Southeast ...745

Midwest ...746

Great Plains & Mountains748

West Coast & Pacific ..748

Pediatric Gastroenterology**749**

New England ...749

Mid Atlantic ..750

Southeast ...752

Midwest ...752

Great Plains & Mountains754

Southwest ..755

West Coast & Pacific ..755

Pediatric Hematology-Oncology**756**

New England ...756

Mid Atlantic ..758

Southeast ...765

Midwest ...769

Great Plains & Mountains774

Southwest ..775

West Coast & Pacific ..776

Pediatric Infectious Disease**779**

New England ...779

Mid Atlantic ..780

Southeast ...781

Midwest ...782

Southwest ..784

West Coast & Pacific ..784

Pediatric Nephrology ...**785**

 New England...785

 Mid Atlantic...785

 Southeast ...786

 Midwest...787

 West Coast & Pacific ...788

Pediatric Otolaryngology ...**789**

 New England...789

 Mid Atlantic...789

 Southeast ...791

 Midwest...791

 Great Plains & Mountains...792

 Southwest ...792

 West Coast & Pacific ...793

Pediatric Pulmonology ...**794**

 New England...794

 Mid Atlantic...794

 Southeast ...796

 Midwest...796

 Great Plains & Mountains...797

 Southwest ...797

 West Coast & Pacific ...798

Pediatric Rheumatology ...**799**

 New England...799

 Mid Atlantic...799

 Southeast ...800

 Midwest...800

 Southwest ...801

Pediatric Surgery ...**801**

 New England...801

 Mid Atlantic...802

 Southeast ...805

 Midwest...806

 Great Plains & Mountains...808

 Southwest ...809

Table of Contents

West Coast & Pacific ...810

Centers of Excellence

Cleveland Clinic ...812

Maimonides Medical Center ...813

Mount Sinai Medical Center ...814-818

NewYork-Presbyterian Hospital ..819

North Shore-LIJ Health System ...820

NYU Langone Medical Center ..821-831

Vanderbilt University Medical Center832

Physical Medicine & Rehabilitation ...**833**

New England ..834

Mid Atlantic ...834

Southeast ...838

Midwest ...839

Great Plains & Mountains ...842

Southwest ..842

West Coast & Pacific ...843

Centers of Excellence

Cleveland Clinic ...845

Mount Sinai Medical Center ...846

NYU Langone Medical Center ..847

Plastic Surgery ...**849**

New England ..850

Mid Atlantic ...852

Southeast ...860

Midwest ...864

Great Plains & Mountains ...869

Southwest ..869

West Coast & Pacific ...872

Centers of Excellence

Cleveland Clinic ...878

New York Eye & Ear Infirmary ...879

Preventive & Occupational Medicine..**881**

 Occupational Medicine..**882**

 Mid Atlantic..882

 Southwest...882

 Preventive Medicine...**882**

 Mid Atlantic..882

 Centers of Excellence

 NYU Langone Medical Center..............................884-885

Psychiatry...**887**

 Psychiatry...**888**

 New England..888

 Mid Atlantic..890

 Southeast..895

 Midwest..897

 Great Plains & Mountains..898

 Southwest...899

 West Coast & Pacific...900

 Addiction Psychiatry...**904**

 New England..904

 Mid Atlantic..904

 Southeast..905

 Midwest..905

 Great Plains & Mountains..905

 Southwest...906

 West Coast & Pacific...906

 Child & Adolescent Psychiatry..**906**

 New England..906

 Mid Atlantic..907

 Southeast..910

 Midwest..910

 Great Plains & Mountains..911

 Southwest...911

 West Coast & Pacific...912

 Geriatric Psychiatry..**913**

 Mid Atlantic..913

Table of Contents

Southeast..914

Midwest..914

Great Plains & Mountains.......................................914

West Coast & Pacific..915

Centers of Excellence

Cleveland Clinic...916

Mount Sinai Medical Center..................................917

NYU Langone Medical Center......................918-920

Pulmonary Disease..**921**

New England...922

Mid Atlantic..924

Southeast..929

Midwest..933

Great Plains & Mountains.......................................936

Southwest..938

West Coast & Pacific..938

Centers of Excellence

Cleveland Clinic...942

Mount Sinai Medical Center..................................943

NYU Langone Medical Center..............................944

Radiation Oncology..**945**

New England...946

Mid Atlantic..948

Southeast..953

Midwest..958

Great Plains & Mountains.......................................962

Southwest..963

West Coast & Pacific..965

Centers of Excellence

Cleveland Clinic...969

Radiology...**971**

Diagnostic Radiology...**973**

New England...973

Mid Atlantic ...974

Southeast ...978

Midwest..980

Great Plains & Mountains..981

Southwest ..982

West Coast & Pacific ..982

Neuroradiology ...**984**

New England...984

Mid Atlantic ...985

Southeast ...987

Midwest..988

Great Plains & Mountains..990

Southwest ..990

West Coast & Pacific ..990

Vascular & Interventional Radiology ...**992**

New England...992

Mid Atlantic ...992

Southeast ...994

Midwest..995

Great Plains & Mountains..996

Southwest ..997

West Coast & Pacific ..997

Centers of Excellence

Cleveland Clinic...999

Maimonides Medical Center ...100

Mount Sinai Medical Center ...1001

New York-Presbyterian Hospital ...1002

NYU Langone Medical Center...1003

Reproductive Endocrinology ...**1005**

New England...1006

Mid Atlantic ...1008

Southeast ...1011

Midwest..1012

Great Plains & Mountains..1015

Table of Contents

Southwest ...1015

West Coast & Pacific...1016

Centers of Excellence

Cleveland Clinic...1019

NYU Langone Medical Center..1020-1021

Rheumatology...**1023**

New England..1024

Mid Atlantic...1025

Southeast..1029

Midwest..1030

Great Plains & Mountains..1032

Southwest...1032

West Coast & Pacific..1033

Centers of Excellence

Cleveland Clinic...1035

NYU Langone Medical Center..1036-1037

Sports Medicine ..**1039**

New England..1040

Mid Atlantic...1040

Southeast..1042

Midwest..1043

Great Plains & Mountains..1043

Southwest...1044

West Coast & Pacific..1044

Centers of Excellence

Cleveland Clinic...1045

Surgery...**1047**

New England..1048

Mid Atlantic...1053

Southeast..1064

Midwest..1074

Great Plains & Mountains..1085

Southwest...1086

West Coast & Pacific...1093

Centers of Excellence

Cleveland Clinic..1102

Fox Chase Cancer Center...1103

Mount Sinai Medical Center...1104-1105

NYU Langone Medical Center..1106

Penn Medicine...1107

University Hospitals Case Medical Center.............................1108

Thoracic & Cardiac Surgery...**1109**

New England...1110

Mid Atlantic...1113

Southeast...1123

Midwest...1130

Great Plains & Mountains...1136

Southwest..1137

West Coast & Pacific..1140

Centers of Excellence

Mount Sinai Medical Center...1144-1145

NYU Langone Medical Center..1146

Urology ...**1147**

New England...1148

Mid Atlantic...1150

Southeast...1159

Midwest...1165

Great Plains & Mountains...1171

Southwest..1172

West Coast & Pacific..1175

Centers of Excellence

Cleveland Clinic..1180

Mount Sinai Medical Center..1181

NYU Langone Medical Center..1182

Vascular Surgery...**1183**

New England...1184

Table of Contents

Mid Atlantic..1185

Southeast..1189

Midwest..1190

Great Plains & Mountains...1192

Southwest...1192

West Coast & Pacific...1193

Centers of Excellence

Maimonides Medical Center ..1195

NYU Langone Medical Center......................................1196

Appendices

Appendix A: Medical Boards ...1199

Appendix B: Self-Designated Medical Specialties....................1209

Appendix C: Hospital Listings...1213

Appendix D: Selected Resources..1275

Appendix E: Source of Quality Data on Hospitals....................1281

Indices

Subject Index ..1284

Specialty & Special Expertise Index ...1289

Alphabetical Listing of Doctors ..1461

Acknowledgements ...1537

Corporate Products ...1539

 Services for Corporations & Organizations1539

 The New Movers Program ..1540

 Healthcare Solutions ..1541

Strategic Relationships ...1544

 US News & World Report ..1544

 Vitals ...1545

 Everyday Health ..1546

 Empowered Doctor ..1547

 Consumer's Medical Resource (CMR)1548

 Sharecare ...1549

 Grandparents.com ...1550

 DrScore.com ..1551

 Goodworks Health ...1552

Castle Connolly Lifestream MD ...1553

National Physician of the Year Awards ...1555

Castle Connolly and Social Media ...1563

Castle Connolly Top Cosmetic Doctors Online1564

Doctor-Patient Advisor for Individual Consumers1565

Premium Membership at www.CastleConnolly.com1565

Other Products and Services from Castle Connolly1566

The Best in American Medicine
www.CastleConnolly.com

About The Publishers

John K. Castle, the Chairman of Castle Connolly Medical Ltd., has spent much of the last three decades involved with healthcare institutions and issues. Mr. Castle served as Chairman of the Board of New York Medical College for eleven years, an institution where he served on the Board of Trustees for twenty-two years.

Mr. Castle has been extensively involved in other healthcare and voluntary activities as well. He served for five years as a commissioner and officer of the Joint Commission formerly known as (JCAHO), the body which accredits most public and private hospitals throughout the United States. Mr. Castle has also served as a trustee of five different hospitals in the metropolitan New York region, including NewYork Presbyterian Hospital, where he continues to serve.

Mr. Castle has also served as the Chairman of the Columbia Presbyterian Science Advisory Council and as a Director of the Whitehead Institute for Biomedical Research. He is a Fellow of New York Academy of Medicine and has served as a Trustee of the Academy. He was Chairman of the United Hospital Fund of New York's Capital Campaign and continues as Director Emeritus of the United Hospital Fund. He is a Life Member of the MIT Corporation, the governing body of the Massachusetts Institute of Technology.

Mr. Castle received his bachelor's degree from the Massachusetts Institute of Technology, his MBA as a Baker Scholar with High Distinction from Harvard, and two Honorary Doctorate degrees.

Mr. Castle's goal, as is the goal of Dr. John Connolly and all the Castle Connolly team, is to publish *America's Top Doctors®, America's Top Doctors® for Cancer, Top Doctors: New York Metro Area*, and other materials as well as build websites to help the public identify the very best in healthcare resources.

John J. Connolly, Ed.D., - the nation's foremost expert on identifying top physicians, is the President & CEO of Castle Connolly Medical Ltd. publisher of *America's Top Doctors*® and other consumer guides to help people find the best healthcare. He is also Vice-Chairman of Castle Connolly Graduate Medical Ltd., which publishes review manuals to assist resident physicians and fellows in preparing for their board exams.

Dr. Connolly served as President of New York Medical College, the nation's second largest private medical college, for more than ten years. He is a Fellow of the New York Academy of Medicine, a Fellow of the New York Academy of Sciences, a Director of the Northeast Business Group on Health, a member of the President's Council of the United Hospital Fund, and a member of the Board of the American Swiss Foundation.

Dr. Connolly has served as trustee of two hospitals and as Chairman of the Board of one. He is extensively involved in healthcare and community activities and has served on a number of voluntary and corporate boards including the Board of the American Lyme Disease Foundation, of which he is a founder and past chairman, and the Culinary Institute of America for over 20 years where he is now Chairman Emeritus. He also served as a director and Chairman of the Professional Examination Service and is presently on the board of the American Swiss Foundation. His current corporate board service includes: Baker and Taylor; Air Methods Corporation; Dearborn Risk Management and the Advisory Board of the Hudson Group. Past board positions include Morton's of Chicago and Marie Callendar's-Perkins Restaurant Group. He holds a Bachelor of Science degree from Worcester State College, a Master's degree from the University of Connecticut, and a Doctor of Education degree in College and University Administration from Teacher's College, Columbia University, honorary doctorates (LHD) from Mercy College and Worcester State University.

Over the years, Dr. Connolly has served on the boards of, and as an officer of, numerous not-for-profit organizations including: President, Sullivan County Association for Retarded Children; Director and Chairman United Way of Dutchess County; Director and Founding Chairman Dutchess County Industrial Development Agency; Director and Founder Dutchess County Economic Development Association, President, Westchester County Historical Society.

Medical Advisory Board

Castle Connolly Medical Ltd. is pleased to have associated with a distinguished group of medical leaders who offer invaluable advice and wisdom in our efforts to assist consumers in making good healthcare choices. We thank each member of the Medical Advisory Board for their valuable contributions.

Jeremiah A. Barondess, M.D.
President Emeritus
New York Academy of Medicine,
Professor of Clinical Medicine
Emeritus, Weill-Cornell Medical
College

Menard M. Gertler, M.D., D.Sc.
Clinical Professor of Medicine
Cornell University Medical School

Yutaka Kikkawa, M.D.
Professor and Chairman (Emeritus)
Department of Pathology
University of California
Irvine College of Medicine

Edward D. Miller, M.D.
Dean/CEO Emeritus
Johns Hopkins Medicine
Professor of Anesthesiology &
Critical Care Medicine

Ronald Pion, M.D.
Chairman and CEO
Medical Telecommunications
Associates

Leon G. Smith, M.D.
Chairman of Medicine
St. Michael's Medical Center, NJ

Ralph Snyderman, M.D.
Former President and CEO
Duke University Health System

Roger Bulger, M.D.
National Institutes of Health (Ret.)

Leo Hennikoff, M.D.
President and CEO (Ret.)
Rush Presbyterian-St. Luke's
Medical Center

David Paige, M.D.
Professor
Bloomberg School of Public Health
John Hopkins University

Richard L. Reece, M.D.
Editor
Physician Practice Options

Helen Smits, M.D.
Former Deputy Director
Health Care Financing
Administration (HCFA)

Foreword

The challenge of finding the best healthcare is a formidable one for most Americans and for others who seek medical care in the United States. While this country offers the best medical care in the world, many people are overwhelmed by its complexity and bureaucracy.

While most of us are fortunate and never need to venture beyond our local communities to find medical specialists able to meet our healthcare needs, the needs of many patients cannot be met in their local areas. For them, the search for the top specialists can be as important as life itself!

This great nation is fortunate in possessing some of the world's leading medical centers and specialty hospitals where cutting edge research is conducted and innovative new therapies are practiced daily. These health centers employ and train many of the world's most skilled physicians. The organization which I formerly headed, the Association of Academic Health Centers, serves as a forum of exchange for these centers of medical excellence and, therefore, I know them well. However, I also know well the difficulty and challenges that patients and their families face in identifying and locating the tremendous wealth of medical talent and dedication that lies within the walls of these outstanding facilities.

Castle Connolly Medical Ltd. has dedicated extensive time and resources to identify-ing the best healthcare this nation has to offer. They have done this not to serve physicians or hospitals, but to serve healthcare consumers. Their efforts will be vital and important resources to Americans and others who seek the best medical care available in this country—wherever it is being practiced.

Roger Bulger, M.D.
Former President, Association of Academic Health Centers (AAHC)
Washington DC

The Best in American Medicine
www.CastleConnolly.com

The Best in American Medicine
www.CastleConnolly.com

Introduction

There are times in life when the nature of a disease or medical condition that afflicts you or a loved one warrants identifying the top doctor—the very best specialist anywhere in the nation—to diagnose or treat that particular medical problem. At times like these, you need Castle Connolly's *America's Top Doctors*®, the national guide designed to assist you under just these circumstances.

While the overall quality of medical care throughout the United States is generally of very high quality and in many places is superb, there are still those rare, complex or extremely difficult problems that demand resources beyond the ordinary or that require talents that are exceptional.

This guide identifies those top medical specialists throughout the country who possess the skill and experience to address these problems. Top specialists who provide excellent care tend to be located predominantly, although not exclusively, at major medical centers, specialty hospitals and leading teaching hospitals. These exceptional physicians are acknowledged as such by their peers and are recognized for their expertise by the medical profession.

The top specialists we have identified are not the only excellent physicians who are caring for patients in this nation. Since there are more than 720,000 doctors in the United States, we cannot identify every top specialist. Therefore, we have included narrative to assist those using this guide who may not find the specialist they need within its listings. Clearly, there are many primary care physicians and other well-trained specialists in communities and hospitals throughout the United States.

Most physicians in this guide are board certified not only in a specialty, but also in a subspecialty or in multiple subspecialties. Board or subspecialty certification alone, however, does not distinguish them from excellent specialists at hospitals in your community, many of whom are also board certified in both a specialty and a subspecialty.

However, the majority of physicians included in this guide have trained at the top medical centers under medical pioneers who possess state-of-the-art knowledge in a specific disease or problem and have often devised new techniques and therapeutic approaches, many of which are life-saving procedures or cures. These doctors most often practice their science and art at leading hospitals and, more specifically, in programs at hospitals that are recognized for their excellence in a given field. Many others have been trained at leading centers in other nations since the U.S. is not alone in pioneering new medical knowledge, although its position as the leader in "high-tech" medicine is generally acknowledged.

Another major characteristic distinguishing the majority of physicians in this guide from those at local hospitals is their continued focus and training. Rather than practicing at a community hospital (or even at a leading regional hospital) and developing a general, broad-based practice, these physicians continued their training in a particular disease, syndrome or subspecialty to such a degree that they developed extensive knowledge and unique skills in treating that particular problem.

Often that focused, advanced training is accompanied by active involvement in clinical research. This is an additional reason why the physicians listed in this guide are located at only a few hundred of the more than six thousand hospitals in the United States. It is difficult, although not impossible, to conduct important clinical research in isolation or without an environment supportive of research. It takes time, money, residents, research associates, technicians, equipment and more to produce significant clinical research. Certainly there have been individuals who have made important and lasting contributions to research with little or none of this support, but those instances are rare. Today, for the most part, major advances in medicine occur in the labs and on the floors of major medical centers and specialty hospitals, in medical schools and in clinical labs created and financed for that purpose by commercial enterprises.

How Physicians Were Selected For Inclusion In This Guide

Castle Connolly's Top Doctors™ selection process begins with surveys of physicians and healthcare professionals. Each year, Castle Connolly surveys thousands of physicians and other healthcare professionals and asks them to identify excellent doctors in every specialty in their region and throughout the nation. When we began the research for the first edition of America's Top Doctors® 20 years ago, we surveyed over 230,000 of the nation's leading medical specialists, department chairs, residency program directors, vice presidents of medical affairs and presidents of the nation's leading medical centers and specialty hospitals. In addition to mail and online surveys, the Castle Connolly physician-led research team makes thousands of phone calls each year, talking with leading specialists, chairs of clinical departments and vice presidents of medical affairs, seeking to identify top specialists for every disease and procedure.

The Castle Connolly physician-led research team carefully reviews the credentials of every physician being considered for inclusion in Castle Connolly Guides, magazine features and website. The review includes, among other factors, scrutiny of medical education, training, hospital appointments, administrative posts, professional achievements, and malpractice and disciplinary history. Information on outcomes, procedure volume and malpractice is becoming increasingly available, but the public disclosure varies from state to state. Castle Connolly uses its best efforts to gather the information that is available and use it effectively. Ultimately, however, it is the professional judgment of the Castle Connolly editors, the Chief Medical and Research Officer and the research staff, which determines Castle Connolly Top Doctor™ selection.

Physicians may also be removed from the Castle Connolly lists if, in the judgment of the selection team, that is warranted. Some of the reasons physicians are removed include retirement, change in practice (taking a full time administrative post, for example), unavailability to patients, malpractice or disciplinary issues, negative physician or patient feedback, professional demeanor or a change in the "mix" of specialists Castle Connolly will present for a given community. Being removed from a Castle Connolly list does not necessarily indicate something negative about the physician.

Castle Connolly does not claim to identify every excellent physician in the nation or a region; it is impossible to identify them all. Those identified by Castle Connolly are clearly among the very best in the nation. That is why our guides, websites and other distribution channels for this critical information describe a process whereby consumers can identify excellent physicians using their own efforts. Furthermore, there are many excellent physicians on the regional level, especially in primary care, that are not included in this guide. Included in this guide are the nation's top referral specialists and those skilled at treating a specific condition or disease; they are found primarily at teaching hospitals, major medical centers and leading specialty hospitals.

How do we accomplish this enormous task? Over the years, the Castle Connolly physician-led research team developed its extensive database of physicians across the nation through periodic mail, telephone and email surveys. This cumulative database is systematically maintained and continuously updated. Surveyed physicians nominate top doctors in both their own and related specialties – especially those to whom they would refer their own patients. Each year this database is supplemented by further mail surveys and telephone interviews with leaders in the various medical specialties and leading physicians at major medical centers.

To augment our large mail, telephone and online polling process, additional surveys are conducted among the following carefully selected groups: directors of graduate medical programs, directors of clinical services at member hospitals of the Council of Teaching Hospitals (COTH), board members of medical specialty academies, associations and societies and deans and chairs of departments at medical schools

Building on years of prior research, thousands of top doctors included in earlier editions of our guides are invited to offer their nominations for Castle Connolly *America's Top Doctors*®. Beginning in 2011, and moving forward, the nomination process invited every licensed MD and DO across the country to participate. This involved contacting over 50,000 physicians and healthcare executives, a nationwide distribution of nomination notifications via various media channels and partnering with US News and World Report as a means of expanding our process to physicians across the country.

More than 48,000 physicians have been nominated through this process this year. Extensive biographical forms were sent to those physicians most frequently nominated for completion. After careful review of their professional backgrounds, the Castle Connolly research staff conducted further research to check disciplinary, certification and license histories.

We do not intentionally include physicians simply because they have important titles. While a position as a chief of service or a department head at a teaching hospital is an important post, such positions are achieved through a combination of many talents including administrative skills, seniority and factors that are not as important for inclusion in this guide as is skill in clinical care. The same is true of leaders of county medical societies, professional associations or even specialty groups. While these are significant positions and acknowledge a leadership among peers, these titles are not essential to clinical skill recognition.

The same perspective applies to research expertise. Many physicians listed in the Guide are engaged in clinical research and make significant contributions to their fields, with some devoting a substantial portion of their time to research. However, we avoided including those physicians who solely conduct research and who do not provide patient care.

The result of this extensive research effort is a list of outstanding, highly skilled physicians who are recognized as among the best in their specialties and in the nation; a list which consumers/patients can use to find the very best specialists to meet their particular needs.

Lastly, this book differs from the regional Castle Connolly Guides in two important ways. First, Castle Connolly *America's Top Doctors® 12th Edition* is national, not regional, in scope. Second, the regional Guides are based on the generally accurate premise that healthcare is local and most people find their healthcare where they live and work. However, Castle Connolly *America's Top Doctors® 12th Edition* is designed to meet the needs of those people who cannot find the right specialists locally but who can and will travel anywhere in the country to be cared for by a top specialist at an outstanding hospital. This guide will assist readers in that important search and, for that reason, does not include primary care physicians.

Using This Guide To Find
Top Specialists

This guide is organized and planned to be as user-friendly as possible. Still, as with anything as complex as medical specialties, subspecialties and the myriad of diseases and problems that specialists treat, there needs to be a system to organize the physicians' names, the diseases and problems they manage and their special expertise.

To organize the specialists in this guide, we have followed the American Board of Medical Specialties (ABMS) format. The ABMS is the authoritative body for the recognition of medical specialties. Without the ABMS as the official controlling body there would be hundreds of unregulated medical specialties.

The ABMS recognizes twenty-five specialties and more than ninety subspecialties. The listing of ABMS specialties and subspecialties can be found in Appendix A. In addition to ABMS recognized specialties, there are at least one hundred other groups calling themselves "medical specialists" that are not recognized by the ABMS. Some of these groups are working toward recognition and have exams and other standards for membership. Others are organizations of physicians interested in a particular problem or area of medicine that exist to exchange information but have no intention of seeking ABMS recognition. Some groups calling themselves "boards" really have little authority or meaningful standards. Thus, while a physician may state he/she is, for example, a specialist in cosmetic surgery, there is no ABMS recognized specialty by that name. Therefore, you have no idea whether this physician has any special training and expertise or is simply trying to recruit paying patients to a lucrative aspect of surgical practice.

You can get information on a doctor's credentials from the doctor, from the doctor's hospital (Medical Affairs Office) or from your health plan if a doctor is in the network. You can also get this information from numerous Web sites, including www.castleconnolly.com. You can check on a physician's board certification by calling the ABMS at (866) 275-2267 or by logging on to its Web site at www.abms.org.

If you seek a particular type of specialist or subspecialist, turn to the section of this guide covering that medical specialty or subspecialty. There you will be able to further restrict your search to a specific geographic region or, if you prefer, to search throughout the nation.

To make your search easier, we have organized the specialties and subspecialties into the following regions: New England, Mid Atlantic, Midwest, Southeast, Southwest, Great Plains and Mountains, and West Coast and Pacific. To find an outstanding cardiologist in St. Louis, for example, look under Cardiovascular Disease and then under the Midwest region. (See Pages 38-39 for geographical regions and states.)

A second way to use this guide is to look at the Special Expertise Index, which lists the areas of special expertise of included physicians. This list of special expertise indicates more than 2,000 medical topics including diseases, therapeutic approaches and techniques. You can look up the particular disease, problem or technique you are interested in and locate a physician in that manner. We assume that many people using this guide will know what their particular problem is and will begin their exploration with this index. However, we encourage you to read the entire text since it will help you to better understand how to find the right physician for yourself or a family member, especially if one is not found in this guide.

Choosing An Appropriate Specialist

It may seem that choosing the correct specialist to treat a particular medical problem is simply a matter of finding a top doctor in a specific medical specialty. For treatment of a problem with your vision, you would choose an ophthalmologist. A skin or hair problem would require treatment by a dermatologist and a broken bone would need the care of an orthopaedic surgeon.

Sometimes, however, the type of specialist needed may not be obvious. For example, back surgery may be performed by either an orthopaedic surgeon or a neurosurgeon. Different aspects of sports medicine, as another example, are practiced by orthopaedic surgeons who treat sports-related injuries in both adults and children, pediatricians who treat only children or internists and family practitioners whose focus is on prevention of injuries.

In some cases, several specialists with expertise in different areas of medical practice all become involved in treating the same patient's health problem. For example, a person with diabetes might need care from an endocrinologist, a cardiologist and an ophthalmologist. In other situations, doctors trained in different specialties may use varied approaches or differing therapies to manage a disease or condition. Such is the case, for example, with prostate cancer: a patient could be treated by a urologist, a medical oncologist, or a radiation oncologist. The urologist might provide the patient with a surgical treatment option, while the medical oncologist would treat the patient with chemotherapy and the radiotherapist would use radiation therapy and/or radioactive seed implantation. All approaches could be successful, or one might be preferable to another, depending on the patient and his condition. Therefore, a wise patient will thoroughly explore all options before making a choice.

Finding the right specialist is also important in terms of the quality of your care. For example, many orthopaedic surgeons will operate on hands, but it is clearly preferable to have someone trained and certified specifically in hand surgery (a subspecialty of both orthopaedic surgery and plastic surgery) to perform that delicate surgery. Similarly, a dermatologist may indicate that his/her practice includes cosmetic surgery; however, there is no approved ABMS dermatology subspecialty or fellowship training in cosmetic surgery. While many dermatologists do pursue additional training in cosmetic surgery, it should be understood that dermatologic practice is limited to cutaneous procedures ranging from the removal of skin tumors to laser resurfacing. On the other hand, some board certified otolaryngologists have additional training that enables them to perform cosmetic surgery procedures on the head and neck.

Choosing the right type of specialist is as important as selecting the right doctor. For example, the diagnosis of melanoma, a very serious, potentially life threatening form of skin cancer, is missed in many cases. Therefore, if you have a skin lesion that might possibly be melanoma, you should be certain that the pathologist reading your slides is board certified in the subspecialty of dermatopathology.

These examples illustrate this important principle: always seek the best healthcare. Look for the best-trained doctors, not those who simply can do the job. That doesn't mean that you need to consult a doctor listed in this guide every time you have a health problem. It does mean you should be certain that the physicians who care for you, whether in your community or at a world-class medical center, are trained appropriately and are qualified to provide the care you require. Remember, when it comes to healthcare no one wants second best!

Given this complexity, how do you find the right specialist to provide your care? The first and most important person to look to for guidance is your primary care physician. He/she will assess your medical condition, determine the appropriate type of specialist to recommend and perhaps refer you to a specific doctor or doctors. You should always ask your primary care physician why a particular specialist is being recommended, since that specialist may be a colleague in your doctor's medical group or may be the only (or the most conveniently located) specialist of the type in your health plan. Ask how well your primary care physician knows the specialist, whether they have a long-standing professional relationship and if other patients referred to the specialist had successful outcomes. Be sure to ask for several recommendations, if possible, to provide you with some choice among specialists.

If you do not have a primary care doctor, try to learn as much as you can about your medical problem and the type of specialist best suited to treat it. However, keep in mind that many diseases or conditions present with symptoms that often are indistinguishable from those of other diseases or conditions, making them difficult to diagnose precisely even for physicians armed with the results of diagnostic tests.

Judging The Qualifications Of A Physician

The specialists listed in Castle Connolly *America's Top Doctors®* are clearly among the best in the nation and have been identified through a rigorous research process and thorough screening by the Castle Connolly research team. Through our extensive surveys and research we have done much of the work in finding a top referral specialist for you. But how do you judge the qualifications of a physician who may not be listed in this Guide? If you are trying to find a specialist on your own, how should you go about it? How can you tell when a physician has the appropriate training in a specialty and how do you distinguish what is meaningful and what is not from among all those plaques and certificates on a doctor's wall?

The following pages will outline that process for you. In fact, what is written here reflects much of the logic that underlies the selection of physicians for this book.

The following material will help you not only in finding a top specialist in this Guide, but it also should be helpful to you in choosing among the many specialists, primary care doctors and other physicians that you will need to consult throughout your life.

The reality is that few of us see only one doctor in our lifetime. Each of us may be cared for by a primary care physician, an ophthalmologist, an orthopaedic surgeon, a dermatologist, a surgeon or a number of other specialists. The choices can be many and they can be among the most important choices that we make in our lives.

Education

Your review of your prospective doctor's education and training should begin with medical school. While you may feel that the institution at which someone earned a bachelor's degree could be an indication of the quality of the doctor, most people in the medical field do not believe it plays a major role. A degree from a highly selective undergraduate college or university will help an aspiring doctor gain admission to a medical school, but once there, all students are peers. However, the information on undergraduate colleges, if important to you, is available in *The Official ABMS Directory of Board Certified Medical Specialists®* and other medical directories.

American medical schools are highly standardized, at least in terms of basic quality. A group known as the Liaison Committee for Medical Education (LCME) accredits all U.S. medical schools that grant medical degrees (MDs) and osteopathic degrees (DOs). Most also are accredited by the appropriate state agency, if one exists, and by regional accrediting agencies that accredit colleges and universities of all kinds.

Furthermore, U.S. medical schools have universally high standards for admission, including success on the undergraduate level and on the Medical College Admissions Tests (MCATs). Although frequently criticized for being slow to change and for training too many specialists, the system of medical education in the United States has insured high quality in medical practice. One recent positive change is a strong effort in most medical schools to diversify the composition of the student body. While these schools have been less successful in enrolling racial minorities, the number of women in U.S. medical schools has increased to the point that women now make up about 50 percent of most classes. In certain specialties preferred by women medical graduates (pediatrics, for example) it is possible that in coming years the majority of specialists will be female.

Most doctors practicing in the United States are graduates of U.S. medical schools, but there are two other groups of doctors who make up a relatively significant portion of the total physician population. They are (1) foreign nationals who graduated from foreign schools and (2) U.S. nationals who graduated from foreign schools. (Canadian medical schools are not considered foreign). Those two groups comprise almost one-third of physicians in practice in the U.S.

Foreign Medical Graduates

Foreign medical schools vary greatly in quality. Even some of the oldest and finest European schools have become virtually "open door," with huge numbers of unscreened students making teaching and learning difficult. Others are excellent and provided the model for our system of medical education.

The fact that someone graduated from a foreign school does not mean that he/she is a poor doctor. Foreign schools, like U.S. schools, produce good doctors and poor doctors. Foreign medical graduates must pass the same exam taken by U.S. graduates for licensure, but the failure rate for foreign graduates is significantly higher. In the first year of using the new United States Medical Licensing Exam (USMLE), 93 percent of U.S. medical school graduates passed Step II, the clinical exam, as compared with 39 percent of the foreign graduates. It is clear that the quality of foreign schools, if not individual doctors, is not the same as U.S. medical schools, at least as measured by our standards. Nonetheless, many communities and patients have been well served by foreign medical graduates practicing in this country—often in areas where it has been difficult to attract graduates of American schools. In fact, almost one-third of physicians practicing in the U.S. are foreign trained.

In addition, many foreign medical schools and their teaching hospitals are world renowned for their leadership in medical care, research and teaching and many of the technologies and techniques we utilize in the U.S. today have been developed and perfected in foreign countries.

Residency

Most doctors practicing today have at least three years of postgraduate training (following the MD or DO) in an approved residency program. This not only is an important step in the process of becoming a competent doctor, but it is also a requirement for board (specialty) certification. Most people assume that a prospective doctor needs to complete a three-year residency program to obtain a medical license. That is not an accurate assumption! New York State, for example, requires only one postgraduate year. However, since all approved residencies last at least three years and some, such as those in neurosurgery, general surgery, orthopaedic surgery and urology, may extend for five or more years, it is important to know the details of a doctor's training. Licensure alone is not enough of a basis upon which to make a decision.

Without undertaking extensive and detailed research on every residency program, the best assessment you can make of a doctor's residency program is to see if it took place in a large medical center whose name you recognize. The more prestigious institutions tend to attract the best medical students, sometimes regardless of the quality of the individual residency program. If in doubt about a doctor's training, ask the doctor if the residency he/she completed was in the specialty of the practice; if not, ask why not.

It is also important to be certain that a doctor completed a residency that has been approved by the appropriate governing board of the specialty, such as the American Board of Surgery, the American Board of Radiology, or the American Osteopathic Board of Pediatrics. These board groups are listed in Appendix A. If you are really concerned about a doctor's training, you should call the hospital that offered the residency and ask if the residency program was approved by the appropriate specialty group. If still in doubt, consult the publication *Directory of Graduate Medical Education Programs*, often called the "green book," found in medical school or hospital libraries, which lists all approved residencies.

Board Certification

With an MD or DO degree and a license, an individual may practice in any medical specialty with or without additional training. For example, doctors with a license but no special training may call themselves cardiologists, pediatricians or gynecologists. This is why board certification is such an important factor. The American Board of Medical Specialties (ABMS) recognizes 25 specialties and more than 90 subspecialties. Visit www.abms.org or call 866-275-2267 for more information. Eighteen boards certify in 106 specialties under the aegis of the American Osteopathic Association (AOA). Visit www.osteopathic.org or call 800-621-1773 for more information. Doctors who have qualified for such specialization are called board certified; they have completed an approved residency and passed the board's exam. (See Appendix A for the approved ABMS and AOA lists). While many doctors who are not board certified do call themselves "specialists," board certification is the best standard by which to measure competence and training. Throughout this Guide a description of each specialty and subspecialty is provided as an introduction to the listing of physicians in that specialty.

You can be confident that doctors who are board certified have, at a minimum, the proper training in their specialty and have demonstrated their proficiency through supervision and testing. While there are many non-board certified doctors who are highly competent, it is more difficult to assess the level of their training. While board certification alone does not guarantee competence, it is a standard that reflects successful completion of an appropriate training program. If it is impossible to find a doctor in your area who is board certified in a particular subspecialty, for example, geriatric medicine or sports medicine, at least be certain the physician is board certified in a related specialty such as internal medicine or orthopaedic surgery.

Board certified doctors are referred to as Diplomates of the Board. Some of the colleges of medical specialties (e.g., the American College of Radiology, the American College of Surgeons) have multiple levels of recognition. The first is basic membership and the second, more prestigious and difficult to obtain, is status as a Fellow. Fellowship status in the colleges is meaningful and is based on experience, professional achievement and recognition by one's peers, including extensive experience in patient care. It should be viewed as a significant professional qualification.

Board Eligibility

Many doctors who have been more recently trained are waiting to take the boards. They are sometimes described as "board eligible," a common term that the ABMS advocates abandoning because of its ambiguity. Board eligible means that the doctor has completed an approved residency and is qualified to sit for the related board's exam.

Each member board of the ABMS has its own policy regarding the use and recognition of the board eligible term. Therefore, the description "board eligible" should not be viewed as a genuine qualification, especially if a doctor has been out of medical school long enough to have taken the certification exam. To the boards, a doctor is either board certified or not. Furthermore, most of the specialty boards permit unlimited attempts to pass the exam and, in some cases, doctors who have failed the exam twice or even ten times continue to call themselves board eligible. In osteopathic medicine, the board eligible status is recognized only for the first six years after completion of a residency.

In addition to the approved lists of specialties and subspecialties of the ABMS and AOA, there are a wide variety of other doctors and groups of doctors who call themselves specialists. At present there are at least 100 such groups called "self-designated medical specialties." They range from doctors who are working to create a recognized body of knowledge and subspecialty training to less formal groups interested in a particular approach to the practice of medicine. These groups may or may not have standards for membership. There is no way to determine the true extent of their members' training and neither the ABMS or the AOA recognizes them. While you should be cautious of doctors who claim they are specialists in these areas, many do have advanced training and the groups at least offer a listing of people interested in a particular approach to medical care. Rely on board certification to assure yourself of basic competence, and use membership in one of these groups to indicate strong interest and possible additional training in a particular aspect of medicine. A list of these self-designated medical specialties may be found in Appendix B.

Recertification

A relatively new focus of the specialty boards is the area of recertification. Until recently, board certification lasted for an unlimited time. Now, almost all the boards have put time limits on the certification period. For example, in Internal Medicine and Anesthesiology, the time limit is ten years; in Family Practice, six, and under some circumstances, seven years. These more stringent standards reflect an increasing emphasis on recertification by both the medical boards and state agencies responsible for licensing doctors.

Since the policies of the boards vary widely, it is a good procedure to ask a doctor if certification was awarded and when. If the date was seven to ten years ago, ask if he/she has been recertified. Unfortunately, many boards permit "grandfathering," whereby already certified doctors do not have to be recertified, and recertification requirements apply only to newly certified doctors. Appendix A contains a list of the names and addresses of the boards and the certification period for each board specialty. Even if recertification is not required, it is good professional practice for doctors to undertake the process. It assures you, the patient, that they are attempting to stay current.

Many states have a continuing medical education requirement for doctors. These states typically require a minimum number of continuing medical education (CME) credits for a doctor to maintain a medical license. Seven states require 150 CME credits over a three-year period. Osteopathic doctors are required to take 120 hours of CME credits within three years to maintain certification.

Fellowships

The purpose of a fellowship is to provide advanced training in the clinical techniques and research of a particular specialty. Fellowships usually, but not always, are designed to lead to board certification in a subspecialty such as cardiology, which is a subspecialty of internal medicine. Many physicians listed in this Guide have had fellowship training. In the U.S. there are a variety of fellowship programs available to doctors, which fall into two broad categories: approved and unapproved. Approved fellowships are those that are approved by the appropriate medical specialty board (e.g., the American Board of Radiology) and lead to subspecialty certificates. Fellowship programs that are unapproved are often in the same areas of training as those that are approved, but they do not lead to subspecialty certificates. Unfortunately, all too often, an unapproved fellowship exists only to provide relatively inexpensive labor for the research and/or patient care activities of a clinical department in a medical school or hospital. In such cases, the learning that takes place is secondary and may be a good deal less than in an approved fellowship. On the other hand, any fellowship is better than none at all and some unapproved fellowships have that status for a valid reason that should not reflect negatively on the program. For example, the fellowship may have been recently created, with approval being sought. To check that a fellowship is an approved one, call the hospital where the training took place or call the medical board for that specialty.

Some physicians may have completed more than one fellowship and may be boarded in two or more subspecialties. Also, some physicians may pursue fellowship training and subspecialty certification, but then choose to practice in their primary field of certification. For example, a doctor who is board certified in internal medicine also may have obtained board certification in cardiology, but may choose to practice primarily internal medicine rather than cardiology. For the most part, the physicians in this Guide practice in their subspecialties.

Professional Reputation

There are doctors who meet every professional standard on paper, but who are simply not good doctors. In all probability the medical community has ascertained that and, while the individual may still practice medicine, his/her reputation will reflect that collective assessment. There are also doctors who are outstanding leaders in their fields because of research or professional activities but who are not particularly strong, or perhaps even active, in patient care. It is important to distinguish that kind of professional reputation from a reputation as a competent, caring doctor in delivering patient care, or in the case of this Guide, as an outstanding practitioner in a given specialty.

Hospital Appointment

Most doctors are on the medical staff of one or more hospitals and are known as "attendings;" some are not. If a doctor does not have admitting privileges or is not on the attending staff of a hospital, you may wish to consider choosing a different doctor. It can be very difficult to ascertain whether or not the lack of hospital appointment is for a good reason. For example, it is understandable that some doctors who are raising families or heading toward retirement choose not to meet the demands (meetings, committees, etc.) of being an attending. However, if you need care in a hospital, the lack of such an appointment means that another doctor will have to oversee that care. In some specialties, such as dermatology and psychiatry, doctors may conduct their entire practice in the office and a hospital appointment is not as essential, or as good a criterion for assessment, as in other specialties.

While mistakes are made, most hospitals are quite careful about admissions to their medical staffs. The best hospitals are highly selective, so a degree of screening (or "credentialing") has been done for you. In other words, the best doctors practice at the best hospitals. Since caring for a patient in a hospital is often a team effort involving a number of specialists, the reputation of the hospital to which the doctor admits patients carries special weight. Hospital medical staffs review their colleagues' credentials and authorize performance of specific procedures. In addition, they typically review and reappoint their medical staff every two or three years. In effect, this is an additional screening to protect patients. It is especially true of hospitals that have what are known as closed staffs, where it is impossible to obtain admitting privileges unless there is a vacancy that the administration and medical staff deem necessary to fill. If you are having a surgical procedure and are concerned about the doctor's skill or experience, it may be worthwhile to call the Medical Affairs office at the doctor's hospital to see if he/she is authorized to perform that procedure in that hospital.

The reasons for a hospital's selectivity are easy to understand: no hospital wishes to expose itself to liability and every hospital wants to have the best reputation possible in order to attract patients. Obviously, the quality of the medical staff is immensely important in creating that reputation.

Physicians listed in this guide are primarily on the staffs of major medical centers, usually teaching hospitals, and leading specialty hospitals, e.g. children's, cancer, heart, psychiatric, etc. There are many excellent physicians on the staffs of community hospitals that call themselves "medical centers," but they are not physicians who typically attract complex cases and referrals from outside their area.

To learn about a hospital visit its website. It is also useful to review a hospital's accreditation status under the Joint Commission on the Accreditation of Healthcare Organizations at www.JCAHO.com. A new website created by the federal government, www.hospitalcompare.hhs.gov, offers some measures of comparative hospital quality and may be of interest as well. U.S. News & World Report also offers its authoritative guide to the best hospitals in the U.S., which is available at http://health.usnews.com/best-hospitals.

A last and very important reason why a hospital appointment is an essential requirement in your choice of doctor is that some states permit doctors to practice without malpractice insurance. If you are injured as a result of a doctor's poor care, you could be without recourse. However, few hospitals permit doctors to practice in them unless they carry malpractice insurance. This not only protects the hospital, but the patient as well.

Medical School Faculty Appointment

Many doctors have appointments on the faculties of medical schools. There is a range of categories from "straight" appointments, meaning full-time appointment as professor, associate professor, assistant professor or instructor, to clinical ranks that may reflect lesser degrees of involvement in teaching or research. If someone carries what is known as a straight academic rank (i.e. "professor of surgery," without clinical in the title), this usually means that the individual is engaged full-time in medical school research, teaching activities and patient care. The title "clinical professor of surgery" usually indicates a less direct involvement in medical school activities such as teaching and research.

Doctors who are full-time academicians may be in the forefront of new techniques and research, but they are not necessarily better doctors. Nonetheless, you would be assured that they have the support of other faculty, residents and medical students.

When you are seeking a subspecialist, a doctor's relationship to a medical school becomes more meaningful since medical school faculties tend to be made up of subspecialists. You are less likely to find large numbers of general or primary care practitioners engaged full-time on a medical school faculty. The newest approaches and techniques in medicine, for the most part, are explored and developed by medical school faculties in their laboratories and clinical practice settings. This is where they practice their subspecialties, as well as teach and conduct research. Such leading specialists are not necessarily better doctors than community doctors; rather, they are trained to provide a different kind of medical care. Obviously the type of medical care users of this guide are seeking is that different kind of care available primarily from top subspecialists at leading hospitals and medical centers.

Medical Society Membership

Most medical society memberships sound very prestigious and some are; however, there are many societies that are not selective and which virtually any doctor can join. In addition, membership in many of the more prestigious societies is based on research and publication or on leadership in the field and may have little to do with direct patient care. While it is clearly an honor to be invited to join these groups, membership may be less than helpful in discerning whether a doctor can deliver the excellent clinical care you require.

Experience

Experience is difficult to assess. Obviously, in most cases, an older doctor has more experience; on the other hand, a younger doctor has been more recently immersed in the challenge of medical school, residency, or even a fellowship, and may be the most up-to-date. If a doctor is board certified, you may assume that assures at least a minimal amount of experience, but since it could be as little as a year, check the date of graduation from medical school or completion of residency to know precisely how long a doctor has been in practice.

There is a good deal of evidence that there is a positive relationship between quantity of experience and quality of care. It may be that, the more a doctor performs a procedure, the better he/she becomes at it. That is why it is important to ask a doctor about his or her experience with the procedure that you need. Does the doctor see and treat similar cases every day, every week or only rarely? Of course, with some rare diseases, rarely is the only possible answer, but it is relative frequency that is critical. Major metropolitan areas, especially New York and San Francisco, became leaders in the treatment of AIDS because of the number of patients seen in those metropolitan areas. Doctors in the suburbs of New York City (especially in New York's Westchester, Nassau and Suffolk counties) and in Fairfield County, Connecticut became leaders in the research and treatment of Lyme disease because that region is the epicenter of the disease.

In some states, data is available on volume or numbers of certain procedures performed at hospitals. Likewise, The Leapfrog Group (www.leapfroggroup.org) compares hospitals' performance on the national standards of safety, quality and efficiency - areas of healthcare that are most relevant to consumers and this information is later used to improve hospital quality, save healthcare spending and assist hospital employees with purchasing strategies. The federal government has posted outcome data for hospitals, but for a limited number of procedures, on a website www.hospitalcompare.hhs.gov/hospital-search.aspx. There is a good deal of controversy, however, on the validity and usefulness of such data. Opponents cite the fact that some of the data is produced from Medicare patient records only and, thus, is based solely on an elderly population that does not represent the total activity of a hospital or doctor. Proponents of the use of such volume data agree that it is not perfect, but suggest it can be one useful criterion in selecting the best places to receive care for these specific problems. Other helpful sites include www.whynotthebest.org and www.leapfroggroup.org.

The one type of experience you should specifically want to know about is that dealing with any special procedure, particularly a surgical one, that has recently been developed and introduced into practice. For example, in the 1980's many doctors using laparoscopic cholecystectomy, a then new surgical technique for removing gallbladders, experienced a high percentage of problems because they were not properly trained. This prompted the American Board of Surgery to announce new standards for the training of surgeons using this technique. Do not hesitate to ask about your doctor's training in a procedure and how frequently and with what degree of success he/she has performed it. Practice may not lead to perfection, but it does improve skills and enhance the probability of success.

In some cases, relatively young doctors have recently completed residency or fellowship training under recognized leaders who have developed new approaches or techniques for dealing with a particular problem. They may have learned the new techniques from their mentors and may be far ahead of the field (and ahead of more senior and distinguished colleagues) in using those approaches. So age and experience must be considered and weighed along with other factors when choosing a physician.

Second Opinions

Second opinions are a valuable medical tool, too infrequently used in many instances and overused in others. Clearly, you do not want to seek another doctor's opinion on every ailment or problem that you face, but a second opinion should be pursued in the following situations:

• before major surgery

• if the diagnosis is serious or life threatening

• if a rare disease is diagnosed

• if a diagnosis is uncertain

• if the number of tests or procedures recommended might be excessive

• if a test result has serious implications (e.g., a positive Pap smear)

• if the treatment suggested is risky or expensive

• if you are uncomfortable with the diagnosis and/or treatment

• if a course of treatment is not successful

• if you question your doctor's competence

• if your insurance company requires it

Most doctors will be supportive if you request a second opinion and many will recommend it. In many cases, insurance companies will pay for second opinions, but check ahead of time to make sure your insurance plan does cover them. In an HMO you may have to be more assertive because one way HMOs control costs is by limiting second opinions. Often, the opinion of a second doctor will confirm the opinion of the first, but the reassurance may be worth the time and extra cost. On the other hand, if the second opinion differs from the first, you have two alternatives: seek the opinion of a third doctor, or educate yourself as much as possible by talking to both doctors, reading up on the problem, and trusting your instincts about which diagnosis is correct.

Office And Practice Arrangements

Although clearly not as important as training or reputation, a specialist's office and practice arrangements often are of significance to patients. Practice arrangements include office hours, office location, billing procedures and accessibility among the many factors that result in how well the office is run.

Some specialists only will see new patients who are referred to them by another doctor. Therefore, you may need to have your treating physician contact the specialist's office to arrange for your initial visit. Your health plan may also require that your primary care doctor provide a referral.

If English is not your first language, it may be advisable to determine whether someone in the specialist's office speaks your primary language or if a translator can be present during appointments. This will ease communication and assure that all questions, responses and instructions are understood.

Accessibility of the specialist's office may be a concern if you are wheelchair-bound, are elderly or cannot climb stairs or negotiate narrow corridors. Convenient parking may also be important to you.

Other arrangements that may need to be made in advance of your first visit or discussed with the specialist's office staff concern payment. You may wish to ask the following:

- Does the specialist accept your health insurance coverage?

- Is the specialist within your plan's network and will you need to pay a co-payment? Or, is the specialist out-of-network and will you have to pay for your care out-of-pocket, meet a deductible or submit a form for reimbursement?

- Are credit cards an acceptable mode of payment?

- Does the specialist accept Medicare, Medicaid or no-fault insurance? Does the specialist treat workers' compensation cases?

- If you are a non-resident of the United States, will you need to arrange for the transfer or exchange of currency to pay the specialist's fee?

When you are choosing a top specialist, these issues may be of lesser or greater importance, depending on the problem and type of care warranted. If you are traveling a great distance to have a specific procedure performed by a top specialist at a major medical center, continuing long-term monitoring or follow-up care by that physician may not be required or may not be feasible and such things as office practice arrangements are of less importance. On the other hand, if you have a chronic problem that needs to be monitored with follow-up care provided by the same top specialist, then such issues as accessibility of the doctor's office, appointment hours, waiting times and courtesy and professionalism of the staff become more significant.

Personal Chemistry

One element of the doctor-patient relationship that we stress in our guides is chemistry between doctor and patient, a part of which is often referred to as a doctor's "bedside manner." While this factor is of major import in a long-term relationship such as one you would have with your primary care physician, it is of less importance when you see a specialist only once or twice. However, since many people using this book may have chronic conditions that require ongoing care, it is important to give the matter some consideration.

It is vital that there is a sense of mutual trust and respect between patient and doctor; a judgment that individuals must make for themselves. Among the many talented doctors listed in this guide, there are very likely some to whom you would relate well and others with whom you may not feel as comfortable.

Patients prefer doctors who listen, demonstrate concern, are responsive to patient needs and spend sufficient time with them. The qualities of physicians in this regard, even the excellent ones in this guide, vary immensely.

You, the patient, are the only one who can assess these qualities because individuals react differently to various personalities. It is important for you to carefully judge your feelings towards a physician, especially if you are embarking on a long-term relationship. You should feel you can be open, trusting and responsive to your physician and that your relationship will be a positive one. Otherwise, find another doctor, since not doing so could adversely affect your care.

Once you have used this guide to identify the top specialist(s) best suited to treat your condition, there is much you can do to maximize the value of your first visit.

Top Doctors Make a Difference

The Best in American Medicine
www.CastleConnolly.com

Maximizing Your First Appointment With A Top Doctor

After your research is done and you've secured an appointment for an initial consultation with a top doctor known for his/her expertise in the diagnosis or treatment of your particular medical condition, what should you do?

Whether your visit to the specialist's office is a car ride or a plane trip away, there undoubtedly will be arrangements to make before your appointment. You may have to take time off from work, arrange for childcare while you are away and make travel plans and hotel reservations, but there are a number of other important steps to take to assure that you and the specialist make the best use of the time you spend together.

Have you done everything you can to prepare yourself and the specialist for the consultation? The following checklist will help you maximize the value of your visit to the specialist and will go a long way toward focusing you on the task at hand— getting the best advice or treatment for your health problem from one of the top doctors in the medical specialty related to your condition.

Gathering The Facts

- Does the specialist have all the information needed to make a diagnosis of or treatment plan for your condition?

- Have your medical records, test results and X-rays been sent ahead of time to allow for their review by the specialist in advance of your first appointment?

- Have you written out your medical history, including that of your siblings, parents and grandparents, emphasizing the particular problem for which you are visiting this specialist?

- Are you prepared with a written list of questions?

- Do you understand the answers?

A specialist becoming newly involved in your care needs to learn as much as possible about the state of your health in a very limited time. Since top doctors are extremely busy people with many demands on their time, you should make certain that all relevant records and case summaries are obtained and sent to the specialist well in advance of your appointment.

Obtaining Your Records

All healthcare providers, including hospitals, doctors and their staffs, are under legal obligation to maintain the privacy of your medical records. In order to obtain release of those records, you must make a request in writing. If you need to obtain records from a number of providers, you should write one clear and concise letter authorizing release of your records and including your name, address, telephone number, date of birth, identification number and any other identifying information such as a hospital chart number. You then can make photocopies of this letter, but be sure to sign and date each copy as if it were an original. You also may want to specifically name those test results (e.g., pathology slides) or X-ray films (not just written reports or summaries) that must be included in addition to making a general request for your records. It's also a good idea to indicate the date of your appointment so the office staff can respond in a timely manner.

Although state laws require the timely release of medical records, hospital medical records departments and doctors' offices often take several weeks to pull and review patient charts and get them in the mail either to you or to another doctor. In addition to written authorization, you may be asked to pay the costs involved in copying your records, test results and X-ray films because many doctors' offices will not release the originals. Consider placing a call in advance to determine the procedure for releasing your records, how long you can expect it to take and the costs involved so that you can save time by including payment with your release authorization letter. Be sure to allow sufficient time in advance of your consultation appointment for your request to be processed. Since you often must wait several weeks for an appointment with a specialist, allow at least that amount of time to obtain your records.

Even after making your written requests, you should follow up each letter with a telephone call to be sure that your records actually are sent. You should not assume that your request for records will be promptly fulfilled by an often overburdened, although well-intentioned, office staff.

Remember, the more information the specialist has about your condition, the fewer repeat or additional tests or procedures you will need to undergo, the lower the costs of your consultation and, most important, the more expeditiously the specialist will be able to render an opinion.

The Facts And Only The Facts

Be thorough and organized in documenting your personal and familial medical histories, the medications you take and in relaying information about your condition. Even seemingly minor bits of information may provide subtle clues to the nature of your medical problem and the optimal way in which to treat it. It's also advisable to bring a list with you of names, addresses and telephone numbers of all physicians who have cared for you, especially those you have seen regarding your current medical problem.

Even though thoroughness is essential to presenting a clear picture of your medical condition, bear in mind that the specialist needs to get to your core health concerns as quickly as possible. Therefore, if you have a complex medical history, you may want to ask your current doctors to provide treatment summaries in addition to copies of your medical records. Hospital records should include your admission history and physical exam, dictated consultation and operation notes and discharge summaries for all hospitalizations. You may also be able to get a cumulative lab and X-ray summary for your hospital stays.

Unlike X-rays, which can be copied at reasonable cost, original pathology slides must be transported by mail or hand-carried. Your specialist may wish to have the pathologist with whom he/she works speak directly with the pathologist who initially interpreted your slides as part of the process of evaluating your case.

Being Prepared

You are likely to be a bit nervous when you meet with the specialist you have chosen. Anxiety about your health and concern about your future care may cause you to forget information you should provide or miss hearing or understanding important information that the specialist communicates. Therefore, you may want to write down all relevant information so that you do not leave out anything of importance when you meet with the specialist or complete forms in the office. You also may want to write out your questions in advance so you don't forget anything.

To avoid leaving out important details of your condition or past treatment, prepare a concise, chronological summary before your consultation takes place. You may wish to type it and provide a copy to the specialist for inclusion in your chart. Highlight major medical results or significant events in the course of an illness or treatment if these will enlighten the doctor about your condition. Your personal perspective on the state of your health is vital to a full understanding of your medical problem.

It is possible that the specialist will use language that you do not understand or may speak quickly assuming certain knowledge on your part about your condition or its treatment. Don't hesitate to ask for clarification as often or repeatedly as you may need to in order to fully comprehend what you are being told. If you are concerned that you may forget what the doctor tells you, ask the doctor's permission to take notes or ask if you might bring along a tape recorder so you can later replay what was said, especially any instructions you are given. You may prefer to bring along a relative or close friend to serve as a "second set of ears," but, again, seek the doctor's permission to do so in advance of your appointment.

Following this process will assure that you and the specialist you are consulting get the most from your appointment. After all, you both have the same goal: restoring you to optimal health and well being.

What To Do If You Can't Get An Appointment

At times it may be difficult, perhaps even impossible, to secure an appointment with the specific specialist you have identified. There are a number of reasons why this may occur. For example, the specialist may not be taking any new patients or may have such a busy schedule that it takes several weeks or months to get an appointment. He/she may only see patients during very limited hours because of teaching, research or other responsibilities or currently may have other limitations related to the acceptance of new patients.

However, bear in mind that the doctors in this guide are the leaders in their specialties and therefore they work with and train the very best and brightest in their specialties. So, if you are unable to consult with a particular doctor, consider making an appointment with one of his/her outstanding colleagues. You can do this by asking a member of the doctor's office staff to refer you to an associate who is a member of the practice group or to another excellent physician who is specially trained to address your particular medical issue.

You can be comfortable knowing that you will receive high quality care from another specialist who practices in the same top setting.

Utilizing Special Resources

The following information on special resources has been included to meet the needs of healthcare consumers who have extraordinarily difficult or unique health problems, and have been unable to identify the resources to address their problems. These patients and their doctors may need to search for very new, cutting-edge, perhaps even experimental and not yet approved therapies. In such cases the search may lead to clinical trials; tests of new drugs and new medical devices or innovative therapeutic approaches. Fortunately, these situations are rare, but when they do occur, they are critical.

In addition to the outstanding private and public hospitals recognized in this guide, the U.S. government maintains its own unique, expert source of patient care and clinical research at the National Institutes of Health (NIH). In fact, the NIH operates its own hospital at which the care provided is usually related to clinical studies its researchers are undertaking.

In addition to those at the NIH, clinical trials also are conducted at leading medical centers and other organizations throughout the country. These facilities may be testing a new drug therapy, a new use for an existing medication or a medical device to deal with a problem that is not being resolved through the use of more traditional approaches.

This section will guide you in utilizing these special resources.

The Clinical Trial As A Treatment Option

For some patients the best medical treatment may only be available through clinical trials (also called treatment studies), which are designed to develop improved ways to use current medical treatments or to find new medical treatments by studying their effects on humans. Treatments are studied to determine if they are safe, effective and better treatments than conventional or standard therapies. Only if they meet all three of these criteria are they made available to the general public.

Many people are frightened by the term "clinical trial" because it conveys the notion of being a "guinea pig" in an experiment. Contrary to popular belief, however, most new treatments are extensively studied by scientists in the laboratory before they are ever tested by physicians in clinical settings. Among the factors that keep patients from participating in clinical trials are: lack of awareness about clinical trials as a treatment option; fear of side effects or adverse reactions to treatment; refusal of insurance companies to pay for experimental treatments; failure of a physician to inform the patient about clinical trials; difficulty finding suitable clinical trials; unavailability of clinical trials for certain medical problems; distance of the patient from major medical centers conducting clinical trials; disruption of personal and family life; and the decision to stop medical treatment altogether.

Despite these and other obstacles, many people do seek out clinical trials. One of the most pressing reasons to participate is the opportunity to obtain treatment that might not be available otherwise. New medical treatments can offer participants hope for a cure, an extended lifespan, or an improvement in how they feel. Some participants also take comfort in knowing that others may benefit from their contribution to medical knowledge.

Deciding if a clinical trial is the right treatment option for you is no simple matter. Certainly, you will want to talk about it with your doctor(s) and other professionals involved in your care, as well as with family members and friends. But in order to fully benefit from what others have to say — based on either their professional knowledge or personal experience — you need to understand exactly what a clinical trial is and what your role as a volunteer will be.

Understanding Clinical Trials

Clinical trials are conducted for just about every medical condition, including life-threatening diseases such as AIDS or cancer; chronic illnesses such as diabetes and asthma; psychiatric disorders such as depression or anxiety; behavioral problems such as smoking and substance abuse; and even common ailments such as hair loss and acne. Chances are, there is at least one trial (and probably more) that may be appropriate for you.

With more than 100 different types of cancer, it is understandable that a large number of clinical trials are cancer-related. Extensive information about clinical trials for cancer can be found on www.cancer.gov, the Web site of the National Cancer Institute (NCI). NCI is part of the NIH. CenterWatch, an online clinical trials listing service, identifies over 14,000 clinical trials that are actively recruiting patients. Veritas Medicine, another useful online organization, allows individuals to perform personalized searches of its clinical trials database. See Appendix D for "Selected Resources" for more information on clinical trials.

Most clinical trials study new medical treatments, combinations of treatments, or improvements in conventional treatments using drugs, surgery and other medical procedures, medical devices, radiation or other therapies. Newer types of clinical trials, called screening or prevention trials, study how to prevent the incidence or recurrence of disease through the use of medicines, vitamins, minerals or other supplements; and how to screen for disease, especially in its early stages. Another type of trial studies how to improve the quality of life for patients, including both their physical and emotional well-being.

Clinical trials are sponsored both by the federal government (through the National Institutes of Health, the National Cancer Institute and many others) and by private industry through pharmaceutical and biotechnology companies, and through healthcare institutions (hospitals or health maintenance organizations) and community-based physician-investigators. The National Cancer Institute sponsors clinical trials at more than 1000 sites in the United States. Trials are carried out in major medical research centers such as teaching hospitals as well as in community hospitals, specialized medical clinics (for example, those for the treatment of AIDS or Alzheimer's disease) and in doctors' offices.

Though clinical trials often involve hospitalized patients, a fair number of trials are conducted on an outpatient basis. Many trials are part of a cooperative network which may include as few as one or two sites or hundreds of locations, although one center generally assumes responsibility for overall coordination of the research. More than 45 research-oriented institutions, recognized for their scientific excellence, have been designated by the NCI as comprehensive or clinical cancer centers. See Appendix D "Selected Resources" to find out how to locate these centers.

Clinical research is based on a protocol (established rules or procedures) describing who will be studied, how and when medications, procedures and/or treatments will be administered and how long the study will last. Trials that are conducted simultaneously at different sites use the same protocol to ensure that all patients are treated identically and all data are collected uniformly so that study findings can be compared.

Clinical trials generally are conducted in four phases. The first phase begins testing of the treatment on a small group of human subjects after rigorous and successful animal testing has been concluded. Phases Two and Three involve a broader test group and are designed to further evaluate the treatment's safety and more accurately determine appropriate dosage, application methods and side effects. The fourth phase, conducted after the treatment has been approved by the FDA for widespread use, monitors its long-term efficacy and is used to determine if any restrictions should be placed on the population of patients to whom the treatment is administered, or if any adverse effects result from interactions with other medications.

Some clinical trials test one treatment on one group of subjects, while others compare two or more groups of subjects. In such comparison studies participants are divided into two groups: the control group that receives the standard treatment and the experimental or treatment group which receives the new treatment. For example, the control group may undergo a surgical procedure while the experimental or treatment group undergoes a surgical procedure plus radiation to determine which treatment modality is more effective. To ensure that patient characteristics do not unduly influence the study findings, patients may be randomly assigned to either the control or the experimental group, meaning that each patient's assignment is based purely on chance. In cases in which a standard treatment does not exist for a particular disease, the experimental group of patients receives the new treatment and the control group receives no treatment at all, or receives a placebo, an inactive medicine or procedure that has no treatment value and is sometimes called a "dummy" pill or a "sugar" pill. It is important to keep in mind that patients are never put into a control group without any treatment if there is a known treatment that could help them. Also, whether a patient is receiving an investigational drug or a placebo, he/she receives the same level and quality of medical care as those receiving the investigational treatment.

Questions to ask your doctor and the trial's research team if you are considering participating in a clinical trial:

- Who is sponsoring the trial?

- How many patients will be involved?

- Will the trial be testing a single treatment or a combination of treatments?

- Will there be one treatment group or more than one treatment group?

- If more than one treatment group, how are patients assigned to each group?

- Has this treatment been studied in previous clinical trials? What were the findings?

Protecting the Rights of Participants

The safety of those who participate in clinical trials is a serious matter and is the number one priority of medical investigators. All clinical research, regardless of type of sponsorship, is guided by the same ethical and legal codes that govern the medical profession and the practice of medicine. Most clinical research is federally funded or federally regulated (at least in part) with built-in safeguards for patients. According to federal government regulations (and some state laws), every clinical trial in the United States must be approved and monitored by an Institutional Review Board (IRB), which is an independent committee of physicians, statisticians, community advocates and others (representing at least five distinct disciplines) to ensure that the protocol is being followed.

Government regulations require researchers to fully inform participants about all aspects of a clinical trial before they agree to participate through a process called informed consent. To be sure that you understand your role in a clinical trial, you should jot down any questions beforehand so as not to forget them. You should also consider bringing along a friend or family member for support and additional input, and perhaps even tape recording the conversation (after asking permission to do so) to make sure you do not forget or misunderstand anything. Each participant in a clinical trial must be given a written consent form, which should be available in English and other languages. The consent form explains the following:

- Why the research is being done.

- What the researchers hope to accomplish.

- What types of treatment interventions (and other tests or procedures) will be performed.

- How long the study will continue.

- What the expected benefits and the possible risks are.

- What other treatments are available.

- What costs will be covered by the study, by the patient or by third-party payers such as Medicare, Medicaid or private insurance.

Patients also are informed that they may leave the trial, or exclude themselves from any part of it, at any time. Informed consent means exactly what the term implies: you agree to join a clinical trial only after you completely understand exactly what your participation will involve for the duration of the study. By law, each patient must be provided with a copy of the signed consent form, which also must include the name and telephone number of a contact person for questions or additional information. Informed consent is a continuous process, so do not hesitate to ask questions before, during or after the trial.

The investigators must protect the privacy of each participant in a clinical trial by ensuring that all medical records are kept confidential except for inspection by the sponsoring agency, the Food and Drug Administration and other agencies involved in regulating the drug or treatment, and all data are collected anonymously by assigning a numeric code or initials to each individual.

During the course of the trial, participants are regularly seen by members of the research team to monitor their health and well-being. Participants also should be responsible for their own health by following the treatment plan (such as taking the proper dosage of medications on time), keeping all scheduled visits and informing members of the healthcare team about any symptoms that occur. If during the course of the trial, the treatment proves to be ineffective or harmful, the patient is free to leave the study and still obtain conventional care. Conversely, as soon as there is evidence that one treatment modality is better than another, all patients in the trial are given the benefit of the new information.

Questions to ask the sponsors about your rights as a participant in a clinical trial:

- Who is responsible for approving and monitoring this research?
 Is there an IRB?

- Who informs me about the trial process? Do I sign a consent form? Will I receive a copy?

- May I leave the trial at any time? Have previous patients dropped out? Why?

- Whom do I contact if I am experiencing any difficulty with this trial?

Enrolling In Clinical Trials

Each clinical trial has its own guidelines, called eligibility criteria, for determining who can participate. Treatment studies recruit participants who have a disease or other medical condition, while screening and prevention studies generally recruit healthy volunteers. Inclusion criteria (those that allow you to participate in a study) and exclusion criteria (those that keep you from participating in a study) ensure that the study will answer the research questions posed in the research protocol while maintaining the safety of participants. The disease being studied is a primary factor in selecting suitable patients, but other factors such as the patient's gender, age, treatment history and other diagnosed medical conditions may also be important. Unfortunately, eligibility also may depend upon ability to pay. Many health plans do not cover all of the costs associated with clinical trials because they define these trials as experimental procedures. However, trials sometimes pay volunteers for their time and/or reimburse them for travel, childcare, meals and lodging.

To prevent people who qualify from being excluded from clinical trials for financial reasons, agencies such as the National Cancer Institute are working with health plans to find solutions and a growing number of states require insurance companies to pay for all routine patient care costs in cancer trials. To encourage more senior citizens to participate in cancer trials, Medicare plans to revise its payment policy to cover those trials.

When choosing a clinical trial you should determine the factors that are most important to you. For instance, patients generally prefer to participate in trials near their homes so that they can maintain their usual day-to-day activities, be surrounded by family and friends and avoid travel and lodging costs. If travel or temporary relocation becomes necessary, try to find a trial site that is near to some family member or friend or one that is in a locale similar to your own city or town. Many organizations, such as the National Cancer Institute, will work with patients and their families to identify support networks for them wherever they participate.

Questions to ask the trial's sponsor about eligibility criteria:

- What are the inclusion and exclusion criteria for the clinical trial(s) I am considering?

- How can I improve my chances of being accepted?
 Can I change my health plan to one that will cover the trial's costs?
 Can I relocate to another city or state?

- If I am not eligible for one trial, what other trials are being conducted for my condition?

- Will I be paid for my time or reimbursed for my out-of-pocket expenses?

Participating In A Clinical Trial

Clinical trials are conducted by a research team led by a principal investigator (usually a physician) and are comprised of physicians, nurses and other health professionals such as social workers, psychologists and nutritionists. As a participant you may be required to commit a fair amount of time to a clinical trial, often more than with standard treatment. Initially, you will probably be given a physical examination and asked for your medical history. During the trial, you will have regular or periodic visits to the trial site which may include diagnostic and laboratory tests. You also may be asked to follow fixed schedules for medications and other interventions and to keep detailed records of your symptoms and health condition. Generally, clinical trials last from six to twenty-six weeks, though some (called maintenance trials) can last up to a year to determine if a treatment will prevent the relapse of a medical condition.

Participants in clinical trials should remain under the care of their regular physician(s) since clinical trials tend to provide short-term treatment for a specific medical condition and do not generally provide comprehensive primary care. In fact, some trials require that a patient's regular physician sign a consent form before the patient is enrolled. In addition, your regular physician can collaborate with the research team to make sure there are no adverse reactions between your other medications or treatments and the investigational treatment.

Questions to ask the research team or your physician about your role in a clinical trial:

- Who are the members of the health team?
 Who will be in charge of my care?

- How long will the trial last?

- How does treatment in the trial compare with or differ from the standard treatment?

- Will I be hospitalized? How often? For how long a period of time?

- What will occur during each visit?
 What treatments or procedures will I be given?

- Will I still be able to see my regular physician(s)?
 Will my doctor and the research team collaborate?

- Can I be put in touch with other patients who have participated in this trial?

Weighing The Benefits And Risks Of A Clinical Trial

If you are considering participation in a clinical trial, you need to consider the medical, emotional and financial ramifications of participation. Of course, the obvious benefit of a clinical trial is the chance that a new treatment may improve your health and prognosis. You will have access to drugs and other medical interventions before they are widely available to the public and you will obtain expert and specialized medical care at leading healthcare facilities. Many patients receive an added psychological benefit by taking an active role in their treatment.

It is important to bear in mind that some medical interventions used in clinical trials may carry potential risks depending upon the type of treatment and the patient's condition. While many side effects or adverse reactions are temporary (such as hair loss and nausea caused by some anti-cancer drugs), other more serious reactions can be permanent and even life-threatening (for example, heart, liver or kidney damage).

Deciding whether or not to participate in a clinical trial is often a matter of determining if the trial's potential benefits outweigh its possible risks. This is a highly personal decision that may be difficult to make in situations involving experimental treatment in which limited medical information may be available.

Questions to ask the research team about the benefits and risks of a clinical trial:

- What other treatment option(s) do I have at this time?
 Is there any chance that a more promising treatment may be available soon?

- What are the short and long-term benefits and risks as compared with standard treatment?

- Will I experience any known side effects or adverse reactions?
 Will these be temporary, long-term or permanent?
 Relatively minor or perhaps life-threatening?

- If I am harmed in any way by the new treatment, what other treatments will I be entitled to?
 Who will pay for subsequent treatment?

Getting Information On Clinical Trials

The more information you have about a clinical trial, the easier it will be to make a decision about whether or not it is right for you, and the more confident you will be that you made an appropriate decision. In addition to the "Selected Resources" appendix in this guide, the staff at your local public library, community hospital, or major medical center can assist you in locating the information you need from books, consumer organizations and on the Internet.

Learning About The National Institutes Of Health(NIH)

The National Institutes of Health (NIH) comprise one of the world's leading medical research centers and the Federal government's principal agency for biomedical research. An agency of the United States Department of Health, United States Public Health Service, NIH encompasses 25 separate institutions and centers with its main campus located in Bethesda, Maryland. Research is also conducted at several field units across the country and abroad.

Patient Care At The NIH

The Warren Grant Magnuson Clinical Center, NIH's principal medical research center and hospital located in Bethesda, Maryland, provides medical care only to patients participating in clinical research programs. Two categories of patients participate in the Clinical Center studies: children and adults who wish to improve their own health, such as those with newly diagnosed medical problems, ongoing medical problems or family history of disease; and healthy volunteers wishing to advance knowledge about the causes, progress and treatment of disease. The patient's case must fit into an ongoing NIH research project for which the patient has the precise kind or stage of illness under investigation. General diagnostic and treatment services common to community hospitals are not available.

The Magnuson Clinical Center is the world's largest biomedical research hospital and ambulatory care facility, housing 1,600 laboratories conducting basic and clinical research. There are 1,200 tenured physicians, dentists and researchers on staff along with 660 nurses and 570 allied healthcare professionals (dieticians, imaging technologists, medical technologists, medical records and clerical staff, pharmacists and therapists).

The Center's hospital is specially designed for medical research and accommodates 540 carefully selected patients who are participating in clinical research programs. Its 350-bed facility has 24 inpatient care units to which 7,000 patients are admitted annually. The Center also has an Ambulatory Care Research Facility (ACRF) that serves 68,000 outpatient visits each year. A new facility, called the Mark O. Hatfield Clinical Research Center, which began accepting patients in early 2005, has 242 beds for inpatient care and 90 day-hospital stations for outpatient care. The Mark O. Hatfield Center carries out the latest biomedical research that results in new forms of disease diagnosis, prevention and treatment, which is then incorporated into improved methods of patient care.

This is a fine example of Translational Medicine where excellent research discoveries are translated into new and improved methods of clinical treatment. In other words, the laboratory discoveries are brought to the bedside.

The Clinical Center also maintains a Children's Inn for pediatric outpatients and their families. This family-centered residence operates 24 hours a day, 7 days a week, 365 days a year.

In an effort to bring clinical research to the community, NIH supports approximately 80 General Clinical Research Centers (GCRCs) around the country, located within hospitals of major academic medical centers.

It is important to note that, as part of the federal government, the Warren Grant Magnuson Clinical Center provides treatment in clinical trials at no cost to its patients. In some cases, patients receive a stipend to help cover the costs of traveling to Bethesda for treatment and follow-up care. Travel costs for the initial screening visit, however, are not covered.

Areas Of Clinical Study At The NIH

At the Magnuson Clinical Center alone, NIH physician-scientists conduct nearly 1,000 studies each year. Among the areas of study are cancer and related diseases.

Not all of these clinical areas are under investigation at any given time, however. The Patient Recruitment and Public Liaison Office (PRPL) at the NIH Clinical Center assists patients, their families and their physicians in obtaining information about participation in NIH clinical trials. Trained nurses are available to answer questions about the research programs and admission procedures.

Cancer Care At The Warren Grant Magnuson Clinical Center

The National Cancer Institute (NCI) is the largest of the biomedical research institutes and centers at NIH. There, clinical studies are designed to evaluate new and promising ways to prevent, detect, diagnose and treat cancer. The Warren Grant Magnuson Clinical Center provides a separate outpatient division for cancer patients and also has several designated inpatient units.

If you are interested in entering a cancer study at the Magnuson Clinical Center (or at the General Clinical Research Centers), you should first discuss treatment options with a physician. As a general rule, patients interested in participating in clinical studies must be referred by a physician. However, in some instances, self-referral may be permitted.

Patients with medical problems other than cancer or healthy volunteers who wish to participate in a clinical study should contact the particular NIH institute responsible for the clinical area involved.

Cancer Care At The NCI Clinical Centers And Comprehensive Cancer Centers

You may also obtain clinical oncology services (education, screening, diagnosis or treatment) or participate in clinical trials at one of the 22 Cancer Centers or 39 Comprehensive Cancer Centers designated by the NCI for their scientific excellence and extensive resources devoted to cancer and cancer-related problems. Centers are located in 32 states, with the majority of sites in California, New York and Pennsylvania. You can find out about clinical trials at the NCI-designated centers by contacting NCI's Clinical Studies Support Center (CSSC) or by calling each center directly. Information about other cancer-related services at these centers also may be obtained from the center itself. For more information, you can visit the National Cancer Institute's website at www.cancer.gov.

The Best in American Medicine
www.CastleConnolly.com

How To Use This Guide

Locating A Specialist

This guide is organized to make finding the right specialists for you or your loved ones as simple as possible. Physicians' biographies are presented by specialty and are organized by geographic region within each specialty or subspecialty. Thus, you may search for a particular type of specialist or subspecialist in one or more regions or throughout the nation.

A second way to locate the right specialist is to use the **"Specialty & Special Expertise Index"** beginning on page 1285. This index is organized according to diseases, conditions, procedures or techniques as well as the doctor's specialty. For example, you can locate a top specialist for diabetes or for Mohs' surgery by looking for those terms in the **"Specialty & Special Expertise Index."**

If you already know a specialist's name, you can find his/her listing by using the **"Alphabetical Listing of Doctors"** beginning on page 1457.

SAMPLE PHYSICIAN LISTING

Smith, John MD [Ped] - **Spec Exp:** Asthma Allergy; **Hospital:** Children's Hosp (page 120);
Name [Specialty] Special Expertise(s) Admitting Hospital & Hospital
 Information Page

Address: 300 Ridge Road Boston, MA 12345; **Phone:** (617) 555-2343; **Board Cert:** Ped 75;
Office Address Office Phone Board Certification(s)

Med School: Harvard Med Sch 70; **Resid:** Ped, Children's Hosp 73;
Medical School Residency(ies)

Fellow: AM, Children's Hosp 74; **Fac Appt:** Assoc Prof Ped, The Med Sch
Fellowship(s) Faculty Appointment

Geographic Regions And States

To assist you in using Castle Connolly *America's Top Doctors*® in the most efficient and effective manner, the Guide is divided into seven geographic regions. This will help you to locate a specialist in your local or neighboring region. For example, if you live in Mississippi in the Southeast region and you are willing and able to travel to Louisiana in the Southwest region to consult with a specialist in neurology, you can review just those two regions, under the section headed "NEUROLOGY." However, if you prefer to review the information on neurologists throughout the country, you can search the entire neurology section. Or, you can consult the "SPECIAL EXPERTISE INDEX" in the back of this Guide and choose a neurologist who has specific expertise to meet your particular needs.

The geographic regions are as follows:

New England

Mid Atlantic

Southeast

Midwest

Great Plains and Mountains

Southwest

West Coast and Pacific

The states that are included in each region are listed on the following page and a map of the regions is also provided. Please note that not all regions are represented in all specialties. For example, in "Geriatric Psychiatry" there are no listings in the Southwest region.

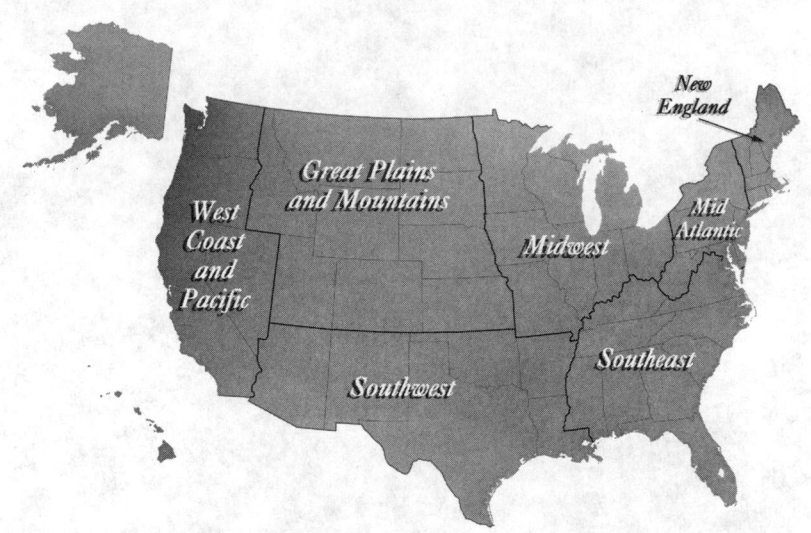

West Coast and Pacific:
Alaska
California
Hawaii
Nevada
Oregon
Washington

**Great Plains and
Mountains:**
Colorado
Idaho
Kansas
Montana
Nebraska
North Dakota
South Dakota
Utah
Wyoming

Southwest:
Arizona
Arkansas
Louisiana
New Mexico
Oklahoma
Texas

Midwest:
Illinois
Indiana
Iowa
Michigan
Minnesota
Missouri
Ohio
Wisconsin

New England:
Connecticut
Maine
Massachusetts
New Hampshire
Rhode Island
Vermont

Mid Atlantic:
Delaware
Maryland
New Jersey
New York
Pennsylvania
Washington, DC
West Virginia

Southeast:
Alabama
Florida
Georgia
Kentucky
Mississippi
North Carolina
South Carolina
Tennessee
Virginia

The Best in American Medicine
www.CastleConnolly.com

Medical Specialties

In the pages that follow, each list of doctors in a medical specialty or subspecialty is preceded by a brief description of that specialty (or subspecialty) and the training required for board certification.

Critical Care Medicine has been excluded because in emergency situations there is neither time nor opportunity for choice. A number of other specialities not relevant to most patients (e.g., Forensic Psychiatry) have not been included as well.

The following descriptions of medical specialties and subspecialties were provided by the American Board of Medical Specialties (ABMS), an organization comprised of the 24 medical specialty boards that provide certification in 25 medical specialties. A complete listing of all specialists certified by the ABMS can be found in *The Official ABMS Directory of Board Certified Medical Specialists*, and is published by *Marquis Who's Who*. It is available (either in a multi-volume directory or on CD-ROM) in most public libraries, hospital libraries, university libraries and medical libraries. The ABMS also operates a toll-free phone line at 1-866-275-2267 and a website at www.abms.org to verify the certification status of individual doctors.

The following important policy statement, approved by the ABMS Assembly on March 19, 1987, remains valid.

The Purpose Of Certification

The intent of the certification process, as defined by the member boards of the American Board of Medical Specialties, is to provide assurance to the public that a certified medical specialist has successfully completed an approved educational program and an evaluation, including an examination process designed to assess the knowledge, experience and skills requisite to the provision of high quality patient care in that specialty.

Medical Specialties

Medical Specialty and Subspecialty Descriptions and Abbreviations

The following medical specialties and subspecialties are indicated in the doctors' listings by their abbreviations. Specialties are indicated in bold, subspecialties in italics, and the four primary care specialties in bold capitals. To review the official American Board of Medical Specialties (ABMS) organization of specialties, refer to Appendix A.

Addiction Psychiatry *AdP*

Deals with habitual psychological and physiological dependence on a substance or practice which is beyond voluntary control.

Adolescent Medicine *AM*

Involves the primary care treatment of adolescents and young adults.

Allergy & Immunology **A&I**

Diagnosis and treatment of allergies, asthma, and skin problems such as hives and contact dermatitis.

Anesthesiology **Anes**

Provides pain relief in maintenance or restoration of a stable condition during and following an operation. Anesthesiologists also diagnose and treat acute and long standing pain problems.

Cardiac Electrophysiology (Clinical) *CE*

Involves complicated technical procedures to evaluate heart rhythms and determine appropriate treatment for them.

Cardiovascular Disease *Cv*

Involves the diagnosis and treatment of disorders of the heart, lungs, and blood vessels.

Child & Adolescent Psychiatry *ChAP*

Deals with the diagnosis and treatment of mental diseases in children and adolescents.

Child Neurology *ChiN*

Diagnosis and medical treatment of disorders of the brain, spinal cord, and nervous system in children.

Clinical Genetics **CG**

Deals with identifying the genetic causes of inherited diseases and ailments and preventing, when possible, their occurrence.

Colon and Rectal Surgery **CRS**

Surgical treatment of diseases of the intestinal tract, colon and rectum, anal canal, and perianal area.

Critical Care Medicine *CCM*

Involves diagnosing and taking immediate action to prevent death or further injury of a patient. Examples of critical injuries include shock, heart attack, drug overdose, and massive bleeding.

Dermatology **D**

Diagnosis and treatment of benign and malignant disorders of the skin, mouth, external genitalia, hair and nails, as well as a number of sexually transmitted diseases.

Diagnostic Radiology *DR*

Involves the study of all modalities of radiant energy in medical diagnoses and therapeutic procedures utilizing radiologic guidance.

Endocrinology, Diabetes & Metabolism *EDM*

Involves the study and treatment of patients suffering from hormonal and chemical disorders.

FAMILY MEDICINE **FP**

Deals with and oversees the total healthcare of individual patients and their family members. Family practitioners are more common in rural areas and may perform procedures more commonly performed by specialists (e.g., minor surgery).

Forensic Psychiatry *FPsy*

Concerns the evaluation of certain diagnostic groups of patients that include those with sexual disorders, antisocial personality disorders, paranoid disorders, and addictive disorders.

Gastroenterology *Ge*

The study, diagnosis and treatment of diseases of the digestive organs including the stomach, bowels, liver, and gallbladder.

Geriatric Medicine *Ger*

Deals with diseases of the elderly and the problems associated with aging.

Geriatric Psychiatry *GerPsy*

Involves the diagnosis, prevention, and treatment of mental illness in the elderly.

Gynecologic Oncology *GO*

Deals with cancers of the female genital tract and reproductive systems.

Hand Surgery *HS*

Involves the treatment of injury to the hand through surgical techniques.

Hematology *Hem*

Involves the diagnosis and treatment of diseases and disorders of the blood, bone marrow, spleen, and lymph glands.

Hospice and Palliative Medicine *H&PM*

Palliative care relieves the suffering and provides the best quality of life to people suffering from serious and severe chronic illness. Hospice care focuses on the palliation of a terminally ill patient's symptoms and also provides passionate support to both the patient and their surrounding loved ones.

Infectious Disease *Inf*

The study and treatment of diseases caused by a bacterium, virus, fungus, or animal parasite.

INTERNAL MEDICINE **IM**

Diagnosis and nonsurgical treatment of diseases, especially those of adults. Internists

may act as primary care specialists, highly trained family doctors, or they may subspecialize in specialties such as cardiology or nephrology.

Maternal & Fetal Medicine

MF

Involves the care of women with high-risk pregnancies and their unborn fetuses.

Medical Oncology

Onc

Refers to the study and treatment of tumors and other cancers.

Neonatal-Perinatal Medicine

NP

Involves the diagnosis and treatments of infants prior to, during, and one month beyond birth.

Nephrology

Nep

Concerned with disorders of the kidneys, high blood pressure, fluid and mineral balance, dialysis of body wastes when the kidneys do not function, and consultation with surgeons about kidney transplantation.

Neurological Surgery

NS

Involves surgery of the brain, spinal cord, and nervous system.

Neurology

N

Diagnosis and medical treatment of disorders of the brain, spinal cord, and nervous system.

Neuroradiology

NRad

Involves the utilization of imaging procedures during diagnosis as they relate to the brain, spine and spinal cord, head, neck, and organs of special sense in adults and children.

Nuclear Medicine

NuM

Evaluation of the functions of all the organs in the body and treatment of thyroid disease, benign and malignant tumors, and radiation exposure through the use of radioactive substances.

Nuclear Radiology

NR

Involves the use of radioactive substances to diagnose and treat certain functions and diseases of the body.

OBSTETRICS & GYNECOLOGY

ObG

Deals with the medical aspects of and intervention in pregnancy and labor and the overall health of the female reproductive system.

Occupational Medicine

OM

Concentrates on the effect of the work environment on the health of employees.

Ophthalmology

Oph

Diagnosis and treatment of diseases of and injuries to the eye.

Orthopaedic Surgery

OrS

Involves operations to correct injuries which interfere with the form and function of the extremities, spine, and associated structures.

Otolaryngology **Oto**

Explores and treats diseases in the interrelated areas of the ears, nose and throat.

Otology/Neurotology *ON*

Concentrates on the management, prevention, cure and care of patients with diseases of the ear and temporal bone, including disorders of hearing and balance.

Pain Medicine *PM*

Involves providing a high level of care for patients experiencing problems with acute or chronic pain in both hospital and ambulatory settings.

Pediatric Cardiology *PCd*

Involves the diagnosis and treatment of heart disease in children.

Pediatric Critical Care Medicine *PCCM*

Involves the care of children who are victims of life threatening disorders such as severe accidents, shock, and diabetes acidosis.

Pediatric Dermatology *PD*

Diagnosis and treatment of benign and malignant disorders of the skin, mouth, external genitalia, hair and nails in children.

Pediatric Endocrinology *PEn*

Involves the study and treatment of children with hormonal and chemical disorders.

Pediatric Gastroenterology *PGe*

The study, diagnosis, and treatment of diseases of the digestive tract in children.

Pediatric Hematology-Oncology *PHO*

The study and treatment of cancers of the blood and blood-forming parts of the body in children.

Pediatric Infectious Disease *PInf*

The study and treatment of diseases caused by a virus, bacterium, fungus, or animal parasite in children.

Pediatric Nephrology *PNep*

Deals with the diagnosis and treatment of disorders of the kidneys in children.

Pediatric Otolaryngology *POto*

Involves the diagnosis and treatment of disorders of the ear, nose, and throat which affect children.

Pediatric Pulmonology *PPul*

Involves the diagnosis and treatment of diseases of the chest, lungs, and chest tissue in children.

Pediatric Radiology *PR*

Involves diagnostic imaging as it pertains to the newborn, infant, child, and adolescent.

Pediatric Rheumatology *PRhu*

Involves the treatment of diseases of the joints and connective tissues in children.

Pediatric Surgery *PS*

Treatment of disease, injury, or deformity in children through surgical techniques.

PEDIATRICS **Ped**

Diagnosis and treatment of diseases of childhood and monitoring of the growth, development, and well-being of preadolescents.

Physical Medicine & Rehabilitation **PMR**

The use of physical therapy and physical agents such as water, heat, light electricity, and mechanical manipulations in the diagnosis, treatment, and prevention of disease and body disorders.

Plastic Surgery **PlS**

Involves reconstructive and cosmetic surgery of the face and other body parts.

Preventive Medicine **PrM**

A specialty focusing on the prevention of illness and on the health of groups rather than individuals.

Psychiatry **Psyc**

Examination, treatment, and prevention of mental illness through the use of psychoanalysis and/or drugs.

Public Health & General Preventive Medicine *PHGPM*

Involves the investigation of the causes of epidemic disease and the prevention of a wide variety of acute and chronic illness.

Pulmonary Disease *Pul*

Involves the diagnosis and treatment of diseases of the chest, lungs, and airways.

Radiation Oncology *RadRo*

Involves the use of radiant energy and isotopes in the study and treatment of disease, especially malignant cancer.

Reproductive Endocrinology *RE*

Deals with the endocrine system (including the pituitary, thyroid, parathyroid, adrenal glands, placenta, ovaries, and testes) and how its failure relates to infertility.

Rheumatology *Rhu*

Involves the treatment of diseases of the joints, muscles, bones and associated structures.

Sleep Medicine *Sleep Med*

Involves the investigation and treatment of patients with sleep disorders.

Spinal Cord Injury Medicine *SpCdInj*

Involves the prevention, diagnosis, treatment and management of traumatic spinal cord injuries.

Sports Medicine *SM*

Refers to the practice of an orthopaedist or other physician who specializes in injuries to the bone or other soft tissues (muscles, tendons, ligaments) caused by participation in athletic activity.

Surgery S

Treatment of disease, injury, and deformity by surgical procedures.

Surgery of the Hand SHd

Involves providing appropriate care for all structures in the upper extremity directly affecting the hand and wrist function.

Surgical Critical Care SCC

Involves specialized care in the management of the critically ill patient, particularly the trauma victim and postoperative patient in the emergency department, intensive care unit, trauma unit, burn unit, and other similar settings.

Thoracic and Cardiac Surgery T&CS

Involves surgery on the heart, lungs, and chest area.

Urology U

Diagnosis and treatment of diseases of the genitals in men and disorders of the urinary tract and bladder in both men and women.

Vascular & Interventional Radiology VIR

Involves diagnosing and treating diseases by percutaneous methods guided by various radiologic imaging modalities.

Vascular Surgery VascS

Involves the operative treatment of disorders of the blood vessels excluding those to the heart, lungs, or brain.

The Best in American Medicine
www.CastleConnolly.com

The Training Of A Specialist

Excerpted from "Which Medical Specialist For You?" American Board of Medical Specialties, Evanston, IL, Revised 2000

Everyone knows that a "medical doctor" is a physician who has had years of training to understand the diagnosis, treatment and prevention of disease. The basic training for a physician specialist includes four years of premedical education in a college or university, four years of medical school, and after receiving the M.D. degree, at least three years of specialty training under supervision (called a "residency"). Training in subspecialties can take an additional one to three years.

Some specialists are primary care doctors such as family physicians, general internists and general pediatricians. Other specialists concentrate on certain body systems, specific age groups, or complex scientific techniques developed to diagnose or treat certain types of disorders. Specialties in medicine developed because of the rapidly expanding body of knowledge about health and illness and the constantly evolving new treatment techniques for disease.

A subspecialist is a physician who has completed training in a general medical specialty and then takes additional training in a more specific area of that specialty called a subspecialty. This training increases the depth of knowledge and expertise of the specialist in that particular field. For example, cardiology is a subspecialty of internal medicine, pediatric surgery is a subspecialty of surgery and pediatrics, and child and adolescent psychiatry is a subspecialty of psychiatry. The training of a subspecialist within a specialty requires an additional one or more years of full-time education.

The training, or residency, of a specialist begins after the doctor has received the M.D. degree from a medical school. Resident physicians dedicate themselves for three to seven years to full-time experience in hospital and/or ambulatory care settings, caring for patients under the supervision of experienced specialists. Educational conferences and research experience are often part of that training. In years past, the first year of post-medical school training was called an internship, but is now called residency.

Licensure

The legal privilege to practice medicine is governed by state law and is not designed to recognize the knowledge and skills of a trained specialist. A physician is licensed to practice general medicine and surgery by a state board of medical examiners after passing a state or national licensure examination. Each state or territory has its own procedures to license physicians and sets the general standards for all physicians in that state or territory.

Who Credentials A Specialist And Subspecialist?

Specialty boards certify physicians as having met certain published standards. There are 24 specialty boards that are recognized by the American Board of Medical Specialties (ABMS) and the American Medical Association (AMA). All of the specialties and subspecialties recognized by the ABMS and the AMA are listed in the brief descriptions that follow. Remember, a subspecialist first must be trained and certified as a specialist.

In order to be certified as a medical specialist by one of these recognized boards a physician must complete certain requirements. Generally, these include:

1 Completion of a course of study leading to the M.D. or D.O. (Doctor of Osteopathy) degree from a recognized school of medicine.

2 Completion of three to seven years of full-time training in an accredited residency program designed to train specialists in the field.

3 Many specialty boards require assessments and documentation of individual performance from the residency training director, or from the chief of service in the hospital where the specialist has practiced.

4 All of the ABMS Member Boards require that a person seeking certification have an unrestricted license to practice medicine in order to take the certification examination.

5 Finally, each candidate for certification must pass a written examination given by the specialty board. Fifteen of the 24 specialty boards also require an oral examination conducted by senior specialists in that field. Candidates who have passed the exams and other requirements are then given the status of "Diplomate" and are certified as specialists. A similar process is followed for specialists who want to become subspecialists.

All of the ABMS Member Boards now, or will soon, issue only time-limited certificates which are valid for six to ten years. In order to retain certification, diplomates must become "recertified," and must periodically go through an additional process involving continuing education in the specialty, review of credentials and further examination. Boards that may not yet require recertification have provided voluntary recertification with similar requirements.

How To Determine If A Physician Is A Certified Specialist

Certified specialists are listed in *The Official ABMS Directory of Board Certified Medical Specialists* published by *Marquis Who's Who*. The ABMS Directory can be found in most public libraries, hospital libraries, university libraries and medical libraries, and is also available on CD-ROM. Alternatively, you could ask for that information from your county medical society, the American Board of Medical Specialties, or one of the specialty boards.

The ABMS operates a toll free number (1-866-275-2267) to verify the certification status of individual physicians. Additionally, information about the ABMS organization and links to an electronic directory of certified specialists can be accessed through the ABMS Web site at www.abms.org.

Almost all board certified specialists also are members of their medical specialty societies. These societies are dedicated to furthering standards, practice and professional and public education within individual medical specialties. Some, such as the American College of Surgeons and the American College of Obstetricians and Gynecologists, require board certification for full membership. A physician who has attained full membership is called a "Fellow" of the society and is entitled to use this designation in all formal communications such as certificates, publications, business cards, stationery and signage. Thus, "John Doe, M.D., F.A.C.S." (Fellow of the American College of Surgeons) is a board certified surgeon. Similarly, F.A.A.D. (Fellow of the American Academy of Dermatology) following the M.D. or D.O. in a physician's title would likely indicate board certification in that specialty.

The Partnership For Excellence Program

Among the more than 6,000 acute care and specialty hospitals in the United States, many have extraordinary capabilities for superior patient care. These hospitals, renowned for their use of state-of-the-art equipment and up-to-the-minute technology, also attract outstanding physicians and other healthcare professionals. Many of their physicians are among those in the listings in this Guide.

To assist you in your search for top specialists and to supplement the information contained in the physician listings that follow, we invited a select group of these fine institutions to profile their services, special programs and centers of excellence in the *Partnership for Excellence* program. This special section contains pages sponsored by the included hospitals. This paid sponsorship program is totally separate from the physician selection process, which is based upon nominations by physicians and a completely independent review by our physician led research team.

The *Partnership for Excellence* program provides an overview of the programs and services offered by the included hospitals with information related to their accreditation and sponsorship. Most also provide their physician referral numbers, should you wish to ask the hospitals for recommendations of doctors not listed in Castle Connolly **America's Top Doctors**® 12th Edition.

In addition to the *Partnership for Excellence* program, profiled hospitals were also invited to highlight their special programs or services that focus on a particular disease or medical condition. These can be found in the "Centers of Excellence" sections that are interspersed throughout this book following the medical specialties and/or subspecialties to which they relate. Sponsored pages in the centers of excellence sections reflect the depth of commitment of these hospitals, which provide the staff, resources and financial support necessary to develop these special programs.

By visiting our website **www.CastleConnolly.com**, you may also link to the websites of these outstanding hospitals for even more detailed information on their cancer programs. We believe you will find this informaton helpful in your search for the best healthcare—from both physicians and hospitals—throughout the United States!

Participating Hospitals

- Cleveland Clinic Foundation

- Continuum Health Partners

- Dana-Farber/Brigham and Women's Cancer Center

- Fox Chase Cancer Center

- H Lee Moffitt Cancer Center & Research Institute

- Hospital for Special Surgery

- The Johns Hopkins Hospital

- Keck Medical Center of USC

- Maimonides Medical Center

- Mount Sinai Medical Center

- New York Eye & Ear Infirmary

- New York-Presbyterian Hospital

- North Shore-LIJ Health System

- NYU Langone Medical Center

- NYU Hassenfeld Pediatric Center

- NYU Hospital for Joint Diseases

- NYU Rusk Institute of Rehabilitation

- Penn Medicine

- St. Francis Hospital -The Heart Center

- University Hospitals Case Medical Center

- Vanderbilt University Medical Center

Cleveland Clinic

Every life deserves world class care.

Cleveland Clinic is one of the largest and busiest health centers in America. Founded in 1921, it integrates clinical and hospital care with research and education in a private, non-profit group practice. Cleveland Clinic is ranked among the top four hospitals in America in *U.S. News & World Report's* annual survey, and is ranked No. 1 in America for heart care, urology and nephrology.

At Cleveland Clinic and Cleveland Clinic Florida, 2,800 full-time salaried physicians representing 120 medical specialties and subspecialties provide for more than 4.6 million outpatient visits and approximately 160,000 hospital admissions a year, for patients from throughout the United States and more than 80 countries. A major inpatient and outpatient surgery center, it performs more than 187,000 cases a year.

The main campus of Cleveland Clinic occupies 46 buildings on 166 acres east of downtown Cleveland, Ohio. Cleveland Clinic also includes a system of eight full-service Community Hospitals, and 18 family health and surgery centers in surrounding communities.

Cleveland Clinic has a growing international presence. It serves patients at Cleveland Clinic Canada, in Toronto and at the Lou Ruvo Center for Brain Health in Las Vegas. It manages Sheikh Kahlifa Medical City, in Abu Dhabi, and is in the process of constructing Cleveland Clinic Abu Dhabi – a comprehensive clinic and hospital in Dubai.

Cleveland Clinic was founded by four physicians who had served in World War I and hoped to replicate the organizational efficiency of military medicine. They established Cleveland Clinic as a not-for-profit group practice with a mission of patient care, research and education. Cleveland Clinic has grown through the years by adhering to that model.

Cleveland Clinic's integrated structure enables it to control costs, measure and improve quality, and provide access to high-quality healthcare services across a broad regional system.

Cleveland Clinic
9500 Euclid Avenue
Cleveland, OH 44195

Offering Same-Day Appointments
Call 800.274.2009.

Treatment Guides
Cleveland Clinic has developed comprehensive treatment guides for many diseases and conditions. To download our free treatment guides, visit clevelandclinic.org/treatmentguides.

Online Medical Second Opinion
Call 216.444.3223 or 800.223.2273 ext. 43223 or email eclevelandclinic@ccf.org.

Out-of-State Patients Assistance
Call 800.223.2273, ext. 55580 or email medicalconcierge@ccf.org.

Visit Us At:
clevelandclinic.org

Follow Us On:
Facebook
www.facebook.com/clevelandclinic

Twitter
@ClevelandClinic

You Tube
www.youtube.com/clevelandclinic

Health Hub
health.clevelandclinic.org

FOX CHASE
CANCER CENTER
TEMPLE HEALTH

333 Cottman Avenue
Philadelphia, PA 19111-2497
Phone: 1-888-FOX CHASE • Fax: 215-728-2702
www.foxchase.org

Sponsorship	Affiliate of Temple Health
Beds	100 licensed beds
Accreditation	The Joint Commission; American Hospital Association; American College of Surgeons Commission on Cancer with commendation; College of American Pathology; American College of Radiology; American Nurses Credentialing Center's Magnet designation

Overview

Fox Chase Cancer Center, part of the Temple University Health System, is one of the leading cancer research and treatment centers in the United States. Founded in 1904 in Philadelphia as one of the nation's first cancer hospitals, Fox Chase was also among the first institutions to be designated a National Cancer Institute Comprehensive Cancer Center in 1974. Fox Chase researchers have won the highest awards in their fields, including two Nobel Prizes. Fox Chase physicians are also routinely recognized in national rankings, and the Center's nursing program has received Magnet status for nursing excellence three consecutive times, having been the first hospital in Pennsylvania and the nation's first cancer hospital to earn this distinction from the American Nurses Credentialing Center. Today, Fox Chase conducts a broad array of nationally competitive basic, translational, and clinical research, with special programs in cancer prevention, detection, survivorship, and community outreach.

- Fox Chase's 100-bed hospital is one of the few in the country devoted entirely to adult cancer care.
- Fox Chase sees more than 8,400 new patients a year. Annual hospital admissions exceed 4,800, and outpatient visits to physicians total more than 88,400 a year.
- Fox Chase's board-certified specialists are recognized nationally and internationally in medical, radiation and surgical oncology, diagnostic imaging, diagnostic pathology, pain management, oncology nursing and oncology social work.
- The staff provides a coordinated approach to meet the treatment needs of each patient. Special multidisciplinary centers provide consultations and treatment recommendations for specific types of cancer.
- The nursing staff of specially trained oncology nurses maintains excellent nurse-to-patient ratios.
- Fox Chase investigators have received numerous awards and honors, including Nobel Prizes in medicine and chemistry, a Kyoto Prize, a Lasker Clinical Research Award, memberships in the National Academy of Sciences and General Motors Cancer Research Foundation Prizes.
- Fox Chase maintains the first known cancer affiliate network in the United States. Established in 1986, Fox Chase Cancer Center Partners is a select group of 19 community hospitals in Pennsylvania and New Jersey with Fox Chase-affiliated cancer programs.
- Fox Chase is a founding member of the National Comprehensive Cancer Network, an alliance of the nation's leading academic cancer centers that is dedicated to improving the quality and effectiveness of cancer care.

MOFFITT CANCER CENTER

BEDS:	206
SPONSORSHIP:	Free-standing cancer center, not-for-profit corporation
ACCREDITATIONS:	JCAHO, American College of Surgeons Commission on Cancer, American College of Radiology and National Accreditation Program for Breast Centers

One of the fastest-growing cancer centers in the United States, Moffitt Cancer Center is the only National Cancer Institute-designated Comprehensive Cancer Center based in Florida. As a private, not-for-profit corporation with more than 2 million square feet dedicated to research and patient care, the center includes a 36-bed blood and marrow transplant unit, an outpatient clinic with a complete digital imaging center, a state-of-the-art radiation therapy department, infusion center, 14 operating rooms, two research buildings, and offsite locations, including a screening center for high-risk patients and a 50,000-square-foot outpatient facility. Moffitt has also created a network of strategic partners within Florida and beyond.

Moffitt collaborates with academic centers, including University of South Florida, University of Florida, Florida Agricultural and Mechanical University, Florida State University, Florida Institute for Human & Machine Cognition, Scripps Florida and University of Central Florida.

Moffitt supports a staff of more than 300 physicians, known as the Moffitt Medical Group. Most are fellowship trained and among the best in their fields. The center's clinical services are organized into disease-oriented interdisciplinary programs with a full complement of services.

Moffitt is at the forefront of personalized medicine with its commitment to Total Cancer Care® – a system of care enabling researchers and treatment teams to identify and meet all of the needs of patients and their families. Total Cancer Care® encompasses all aspects of the disease, including prevention, genetic predisposition, the impact of lifestyle and the use of integrative medicine during treatment.

The foundation of this approach is the Total Cancer Care® research protocol, a longitudinal study that enrolls patients from Moffitt, as well as cancer treatment sites across Florida and nationwide. The partnership among patients, doctors and researchers is designed to advance cancer care by maintaining a repository of human tissue specimens and clinical data. This data will further the discovery of biomarkers that can be used to identify those at high risk, facilitate early detection, improve prognoses, allow drug targeting and toxicity predictions, and match individuals to the best treatment and to the right clinical trials.

REFERRAL INFORMATION: To make an appointment, please call the New Patient Appointment Center at 813-745-3980 or visit MOFFITT.org

MOFFITT CANCER CENTER
12902 MAGNOLIA DRIVE, TAMPA, FL

MOFFITT CANCER CENTER AT INTERNATIONAL PLAZA
4101 JIM WALTER BOULEVARD, TAMPA, FL

H. LEE MOFFITT CANCER CENTER & RESEARCH INSTITUTE
AN NCI COMPREHENSIVE CANCER CENTER | 1-888-MOFFITT

MOFFITT CANCER CENTER

CLOSER TO OUR PATIENTS. CLOSER TO A CURE.®

JOHNS HOPKINS
MEDICINE

www.hopkinsmedicine.org
Baltimore, Maryland

Johns Hopkins Medicine unites physicians and scientists of the Johns Hopkins University School of Medicine with the organizations, health professionals and facilities of the Johns Hopkins Health System, including the world-renowned Johns Hopkins Hospital. All share a single mission: to improve the health of the community and the world by setting the standard of excellence in medical education, research and clinical care.

We heal. The Johns Hopkins Hospital, ranked as America's top Hospital for the 21 years between 1991 and 2011 by *U.S. News & World Report*, as well as our family of hospitals and health care and surgery centers serve as beacons of hope for thousands of patients in our community, in our nation and throughout the world.

We discover. Research is the foundation of clinical care. Johns Hopkins physicians and researchers consistently receive more research grants from the National Institutes of Health than faculty at any other institution. Johns Hopkins is home to four Lasker Awards, 26 National Academy of Sciences members, 58 Institute of Medicine members, and 36 people associated with Johns Hopkins as faculty or trainees have been awarded the Nobel Prize.

We teach. The Johns Hopkins University School of Medicine educates and trains medical students, graduate students and postdoctoral fellows from around the world.

Learn more about innovations happening right now in our specialty centers, including
- Brady Urological Institute
- Comprehensive Transplant Center
- Geriatric Medicine and Gerontology
- Heart and Vascular Institute
- Johns Hopkins Children's Center
- Neurology, Neurosurgery and Neurosciences
- Otolaryngology–Head and Neck Surgery
- Psychiatry
- Rheumatology
- Sidney Kimmel Comprehensive Cancer Center
- Wilmer Eye Institute

To find a physician or make an appointment, call 410-955-5464 (adults) or 410-955-2000 (pediatrics) in Maryland.

For calls outside Maryland, call 855-695-4872.

For calls outside the United States, call +1-410-502-7683.

Keck Medical Center of USC

1500 San Pablo Street
Los Angeles, CA 90033
800.USC.CARE
KeckMedicalCenterofUSC.org

THE NEW NAME IN WORLD-CLASS MEDICINE

The University of Southern California's (USC) renowned doctors and nationally ranked hospitals have a new name: Keck Medical Center of USC. Our new name is a symbol of USC's commitment to change lives through the spark of scientific discovery and the healing power of compassion. This innovative team includes the newly renamed Keck Hospital of USC, USC Norris Cancer Hospital, and over 500 faculty physicians of the Keck School of Medicine of USC. The Keck Medical Center of USC brings hope back to health care, connecting patients with some of the brightest medical minds in the country.

OUR HOSPITALS

Keck Hospital of USC is conveniently located just off the San Bernardino and Golden State freeways near downtown Los Angeles. Among the hospital's advanced services are heart, lung, and vascular care; weight loss and digestive disorders; urology; gynecology; transplantation; orthopedics; and neurology and neurosurgery.

USC Norris Cancer Hospital is one of only a few facilities in Southern California built exclusively for cancer patient care and research. The hospital is part of the nationally recognized USC Norris Comprehensive Cancer Center—one of the original eight comprehensive cancer centers designated by the National Cancer Institute.

HONORS AND RECOGNITION

• *U.S.News & World Report* again named Keck Hospital of USC as one of "America's Best Hospitals" in 2012-13.

• Many USC doctors are cited in "Best Doctors," and extensive polls of medical specialists in the U.S.

• USC hospitals are accredited by The Joint Commission.

SPECIALTIES & RESEARCH

The Keck Medical Center of USC is known throughout the region for expertise and excellence in:

+ Alzheimer's/dementia
+ Bariatric surgery
+ Brain tumor care
+ Breast cancer
+ Cardiovascular medicine and surgery
+ Cardiac arrhythmia
+ Epilepsy surgery
+ Esophageal, digestive, and colorectal diseases
+ Gynecology
+ Hip and knee replacement surgery
+ Liver, pancreatic, and hepatic diseases
+ Lung cancer
+ Neurosurgery
+ Ophthalmology
+ Organ transplantation
+ Orthopedics
+ Plastic and reconstructive surgery
+ Prostate cancer
+ Sports medicine
+ Stroke care
+ Valvular and aortic diseases
+ Women's health

Maimonides Medical Center

4802 Tenth Avenue • Brooklyn, New York 11219
Phone: 718.283.6000
Physician Referral: 888.MMC.DOCS (662.3627)
www.maimonidesmed.org

Maimonides
Medical Center

Sponsorship:	Voluntary, Not-for-Profit
Beds:	705 acute, 70 psychiatric
Accreditation:	The Joint Commission
	American College of Surgeons
	American Council of Graduate Medical Education (ACGME)

Maimonides Medical Center is among the largest independent teaching hospitals in the US and trains more than 450 fellows and residents each year. Widely recognized for major achievements in medical technology and patient safety, Maimonides is a conductor of clinical trials for new treatments and therapies, and cited for clinical excellence by numerous health care evaluation services.

CENTERS OF EXCELLENCE

Cancer Center
The Maimonides Cancer Center offers a fully integrated approach which includes prevention, screening, diagnostics, treatment, palliative care and clinical research. Staffed by leading physicians, nurses and social workers, the Center provides compassionate, patient-centered, state-of-the-art care.

Cardiac Institute
Maimonides is in the top 2% of hospitals in the nation for heart attack outcomes. Its renowned Cardiac Institute includes Catheterization Labs, state-of-the-art hybrid ORs, an electrophysiology lab, two ICUs, a Chest Pain Observation Unit, Advanced Cardiac Care Unit, Congestive Heart Failure Program, and Atrial Fibrillation Center.

Jaffe Stroke Center
The Jaffe Stroke Center at Maimonides received the *Gold Plus Quality Award* from the American Stroke Association. Currently the site of clinical trials for new stroke medications, medical devices and protocols, the Stroke Center offers interventional neuroradiology techniques and telemedicine.

Infants & Children's Hospital
The Maimonides Infants & Children's Hospital of Brooklyn, one of only five accredited children's hospitals in NYC, includes comprehensive inpatient services and more than 30 pediatric subspecialties. The Children's Hospital also has a Child Life Program, Pediatric ICU, Neonatal ICU and Pediatric ER.

Vascular & Endovascular Surgery
The Maimonides Division of Vascular & Endovascular Surgery offers comprehensive services for patients with vascular disease and associated conditions. The accreditation of our Vascular Diagnostics Laboratory assures patients that they are receiving the highest standard of care possible.

Stella & Joseph Payson Birthing Center
Maimonides delivers more babies than any other hospital in New York State. With excellent outcomes, the Payson Birthing Center includes a Perinatal Testing Center, offers the services of doulas, and includes midwifery in a home-like setting – while utilizing the most advanced technology.

Geriatrics Program
Maimonides serves one of the oldest populations in New York City, with one in four patients over the age of 75. The Geriatrics Program is fully equipped to meet the special needs of seniors and encompasses inpatient and outpatient services.

MOUNT SINAI
SCHOOL OF
MEDICINE

THE MOUNT SINAI MEDICAL CENTER
One Gustave L. Levy Place
Fifth Avenue and 100th Street
New York, NY 10029-6574
Physician Referral: 1-800-MD-SINAI (637-4624)
www.mountsinai.org

Sponsorship:	Voluntary Not-for-Profit
Beds:	1,171
Accreditation:	The Joint Commission;
	Commission for Accreditation of Rehabilitation Facilities;
	Magnet Award for Nursing Excellence

For 160 years, The Mount Sinai Medical Center has been a leader in patient care and translational research, with generations of patients benefitting from our teams of physicians and scientists working together to convert research into better medicine.

In 2012, Mount Sinai was again named among America's Best Hospitals, earning a spot on *U.S. News & World Report's* "Honor Roll" and ranking 14th out of 5,000 hospitals nationwide. We also ranked highly in 11 specialties: geriatric care; digestive disorders; cardiology and heart surgery; rehabilitation; diabetes and endocrinology; ear, nose and throat; psychiatry; neurology and neurosurgery; kidney disorders; gynecology; and urology. In addition, our School of Medicine was ranked 18th by the "Best Graduate Schools" edition.

Under the direction of Valentin Fuster, MD, PhD, **Mount Sinai Heart** incorporates world-class resources, innovative thinking and interdisciplinary programs to prevent and treat cardiovascular disease. In a statewide study, our Cardiac Catheterization Laboratory was deemed both the busiest and, with the lowest 30-day risk-adjusted mortality rate, the safest. Building on the expertise of our internationally renowned cardiologists, interventionalists and cardiac surgeon, we provide patients with the most advanced approach to care.

The Tisch Cancer Institute coordinates a full-service diagnostic and treatment program for cancer patients, treating cancer of the liver, breast, prostate, and head and neck, as well as hematological malignancies, such as myeloproliferative disorders. Our **Dubin Breast Center** provides advanced detection and treatment - and addresses every aspect of breast health – all in one centralized location. This year, the **Derald H. Ruttenberg Treatment Center**, our outpatient cancer facility, will double in size upon its move to the new **Leon and Norma Hess Center for Science and Medicine**. In addition, the Hess Center will house two full floors dedicated to cancer research.

The Recanati/Miller Transplantation Institute is one of the few places in the country to provide multi-organ transplantation. We were the first in New York State to perform many combined transplant procedures, including liver and kidney transplantation, pediatric liver transplantation, and living adult-and pediatric-donor liver transplantation.

The Department of Genetics and Genomic Sciences is one of the largest medical genetics centers in the nation, providing expert diagnostic, therapeutic, and counseling services for patients and families with or at risk for genetic disorders or birth defects. The department performs sophisticated diagnostic tests in its state-of-the-art molecular, biochemical, and cytogenetic laboratories, which are New York State and Clinical Laboratory Improvement Amendments (CLIA) licensed, and accredited by the College of American Pathologists (CAP).

NewYork-Presbyterian
The University Hospital of Columbia and Cornell

Affiliated with Columbia University College of Physicians and Surgeons and Weill Cornell Medical College

NewYork-Presbyterian Hospital
Columbia University Medical Center
622 West 168th Street
New York, NY 10032

NewYork-Presbyterian Hospital
Weill Cornell Medical Center
525 East 68th Street
New York, NY 10065

1-877-NYP-WELL (1-877-697-9355) www.nyp.org

Sponsorship:	Voluntary Not-for-Profit
Beds:	2,409
Accreditation:	Joint Commission on Accreditation of Healthcare Organizations (JCAHO), Commission on Accreditation of Rehabilitation Facilities (CARF) and College of American Pathologists (CAP)

The #1 hospital in New York. 12 years running. Once again, we are proud to be named the top-ranked hospital in the New York metro area. NewYork-Presbyterian placed higher on the Honor Roll of 'America's Best Hospitals' than any other hospital in the region. This is the 12th consecutive year that we've been recognized to the Honor Roll by *U.S. News & World Report*™. NewYork-Presbyterian has the most physicians listed in *New York Magazine's* "Best Doctors" issue and is recognized for having more top doctors than any other hospital in the nation.

Overview

NewYork-Presbyterian Hospital, based in New York City, is the nation's largest not-for-profit, non-sectarian hospital, with 2,409 beds. The Hospital has nearly 2 million inpatient and outpatient visits in a year, including 12,797 deliveries and 195,294 visits to its emergency departments. NewYork-Presbyterian's 6,144 affiliated physicians and 19,376 staff provide state-of-the-art inpatient, ambulatory and preventive care in all areas of medicine. The Hospital enjoys a unique affiliation with two of the nation's leading Ivy League medical schools—Columbia University College of Physicians and Surgeons and the Joan and Sanford I. Weill Medical College of Cornell University.

NewYork-Presbyterian Hospital Features Renowned CENTERS OF EXCELLENCE Including:

Morgan Stanley Children's Hospital and the Komansky Center for Children's Health— One of the largest, most comprehensive children's hospitals in the world, providing highly sophisticated pediatric medical, surgical, and intensive care services in a family-friendly, compassionate environment.

NewYork-Presbyterian Cancer Centers—Through a multidisciplinary team approach, we deliver seamless care and offer the latest therapeutic options and clinical trials for all cancer types.

NewYork-Presbyterian Digestive Disease Services—Our collaborative team manages and treats patients with digestive cancers and nonmalignant digestive diseases, such as inflammatory bowel disease, pancreatic and biliary disorders, and colorectal cancer with compassionate care.

NewYork-Presbyterian Heart—Advances in cardiac care—from clinical cardiology, to interventional procedures, to surgical solutions—offer outstanding outcomes to adult and pediatric heart patients.

NewYork-Presbyterian Neuroscience Centers—Expert teams provide the most sophisticated diagnostic and treatment services for Alzheimer's disease, multiple sclerosis, Parkinson's disease, aneurysms, epilepsy, brain tumors, strokes, and other neurological disorders.

NewYork-Presbyterian Psychiatry—NewYork-Presbyterian Hospital's behavioral health and psychiatric services for adults, children, and adolescents offer a full continuum of programs at all levels of care.

NewYork-Presbyterian Transplant Institute—Our experts are internationally known for performing adult and pediatric heart, liver, kidney, pancreas, lung, bone marrow/stem cell, and intestinal and ex vivo transplantation.

NewYork-Presbyterian Vascular Care Center—We provide comprehensive, multidisciplinary preventive, diagnostic, and treatment services for aortic aneurysm, carotid artery disease, blood clots, and peripheral vascular diseases.

William Randolph Hearst Burn Center—NewYork-Presbyterian Hospital is home to the largest and busiest burn center in the nation, caring for more than 900 inpatients and 4,000 outpatients annually.

In addition, we offer extraordinary expertise, comprehensive programs, and specialized resources in the fields of AIDS, reproductive medicine and infertility, trauma care, and women's health.

North Shore-LIJ Health System
Administration Offices
145 Community Drive
Great Neck, New York 11021
www.northshorelij.com
(516) 465-8000

The nation's third-largest, non-profit, secular healthcare system, North Shore-LIJ delivers world-class clinical care throughout the New York metropolitan area. We are pioneering medical research at The Feinstein Institute for Medical Research, and highlighting a visionary approach to medical education through the Hofstra North Shore-LIJ School of Medicine. With nearly $7 billion in revenue and a workforce of more than 44,000, North Shore-LIJ is the largest employer on Long Island and the third-largest private employer in New York City.

North Shore-LIJ cares for people at every stage of life at 16 hospitals including a dedicated children's hospital, long-term care facilities and more than 270 ambulatory care centers throughout the region. North Shore-LIJ's owned hospitals and long-term care facilities house more than 6,000 beds, employ more than 10,000 nurses and have affiliations with more than 9,400 physicians. **In the most recent rankings by** *U.S. News and World Report*, **North Shore-LIJ hospitals were recognized with 57 national and regional designations, more than any other health system in New York.**

In addition to our network of hospitals, our health system delivers clinical care through the North Shore-LIJ Medical Group, the nation's sixth-largest physician group practice with more than 2,400 full-time physicians.

Beyond care delivery, North Shore-LIJ is home to The Feinstein Institute for Medical Research, which ranks among the nation's top five percent of all institutions that receive funding from the National Institutes of Health. At the Feinstein, scientists and investigators are conducting breakthrough research in oncology, immunology, psychiatry, neurology and many other specialties, and are leading more than 1,300 clinical trials involving 12,000 subjects.

North Shore-LIJ Network of Hospitals

- **Five tertiary hospitals**
 - **Lenox Hill Hospital,** Manhattan
 - Manhattan Eye, Ear and Throat Hospital
 - **Long Island Jewish Medical Center,** New Hyde Park - Zuckerberg Pavilion
 - **North Shore University Hospital,** Manhasset
 - **Southside Hospital,** Bay Shore
 - **Staten Island University Hospital,** North

- **Three specialty care hospitals**
 - **South Oaks Hospital,** Amityville
 - **Steven & Alexandra Cohen Children's Medical Center of New York,** New Hyde Park
 - **The Zucker Hillside Hospital,** Glen Oaks

- **Seven community hospitals**
 - **Forest Hills Hospital**
 - **Franklin Hospital,** Valley Stream
 - **Glen Cove Hospital**
 - **Huntington Hospital**
 - **Plainview Hospital**
 - **Staten Island University Hospital,** South
 - **Syosset Hospital**

- **One affiliate hospital**
 - **Nassau University Medical Center,** East Meadow

To find a doctor: **1-888-321-DOCS** or visit **www.northshorelij.com**

550 First Avenue *(at 31st Street)*
New York, NY 10016
www.NYULMC.org
Physician Referral: **888-7-NYU-MED** *(888-769-8633)*

NYU LANGONE MEDICAL CENTER

NYU Langone Medical Center is one of the nation's premier centers of excellence in health care, biomedical research, and medical education. For over 170 years, Medical Center physicians and researchers have made countless contributions to the practice and science of health care.

NYU Langone is comprised of Tisch Hospital, Rusk Institute of Rehabilitation Medicine, Hospital for Joint Diseases, Hassenfeld Pediatric Center, and NYU School of Medicine.

In a culture where treating the whole person and not simply the disease is the norm, NYU Langone Medical Center is renowned for clinical excellence across a wide array of specialties, including cardiology, cardiac and vascular surgery, cancer, musculoskeletal (including orthopaedics and rehabilitation), neurosurgery and children's services.

As an academic medical center, NYU Langone's clinical services are continually informed and enhanced by hundreds of basic and clinical research projects, as well as by major initiatives in translational research that promise to speed the transfer of laboratory discoveries to the patient's bedside.

Areas of Expertise:

Adult Cardiovascular Services
Behavioral Health
Cardiac Surgery
Child and Adolescent Psychiatry
Colon and Rectal Surgery
Dermatology
Gastroenterology
Hematology/Oncology
Infectious Diseases
Internal Medicine
Maternal and Fetal Medicine
Minimally Invasive Surgery
Neonatal-Perinatal Medicine
Obstetrics and Gynecology

Orthopaedic Services
Otolaryngology
Pediatric Subspecialties
Program for IVF Reproductive
Psychiatry
Pulmonology
Radiology
Radiation Oncology
Reconstructive Plastic Surgery
Rheumatology
Thoracic Surgery
Urology
Vascular Surgery

550 First Avenue (*at 31st Street*)
New York, NY 10016
www.NYULMC.org
Children's Services Access Line: **855-NYU-KIDS**

HASSENFELD PEDIATRIC CENTER

The new Hassenfeld Pediatric Center (HPC) is a full-service specialty children's hospital that works as a cohesive team across all children's health services at NYU Langone Medical Center. At HPC, newborns, children, adolescents and young adults receive the most comprehensive and advanced care possible from a team of pediatricians and pediatric specialists across more than 30 medical and surgical disciplines. With more than 150 full-time pediatric specialists, as well as pediatric nurses, child life specialists and social workers, the Hassenfeld Pediatric Center is uniquely equipped to provide innovative pediatric subspecialty care in a highly personalized manner.

About Children's Services at NYU Langone
NYU Langone Medical Center is nationally recognized in many pediatric specialty fields, including craniofacial anomalies, cardiac surgery, orthopaedic surgery, rehabilitation medicine, brain tumors, leukemia, sarcoma, and epilepsy. Our specialists work collaboratively to optimize care for each child, from the operating room and pediatric intensive care unit to the Emergency Department and pediatric inpatient unit.

A Family-Centered Approach
Integral to the care we provide is a myriad of support services for children and their families. We recognize that the best outcomes are achieved when the child's family is actively involved in every step of care. For that reason, our trained specialists address the needs of not just the patient, but of parents and siblings through ongoing education and communication.

The Future Shape of Pediatric Care at HPC
In 2017, a 160,000 square foot pediatric hospital, on the Medical Center's main campus, will become the inpatient centerpiece of the Hassenfeld Pediatric Center. This state-of-the-art facility will enhance the Center's ability to deliver world-class care through all private rooms, a feature that increases patient safety by decreasing exposure to infections, while providing a private, supportive environment for the patients and their families. HPC will be the only pediatric inpatient facility in Manhattan with this amenity, which will also include a "family zone" offering a sleep-in couch, storage, and Web access for each room.

The new pediatric hospital will also include a child-friendly pre-operative unit along with recovery bays where parents can be by the child's bedside during post-operation. Rounding out the new hospital will be a Family Center for orientation activities geared to patients, space for child-life activities and performances, as well as support, education and respite services for families.

HOSPITAL FOR JOINT DISEASES
301 East 17th Street *(at Second Avenue)*
New York, NY 10003
www.NYULMC.org/HJD
212-598-6000 fax: 212-260-1203

HOSPITAL FOR JOINT DISEASES

About the Hospital for Joint Diseases

The Hospital for Joint Diseases at NYU Langone Medical Center (HJD) is one of the nation's leading inpatient orthopaedic and rheumatologic specialty hospitals, and is ranked among the nation's top 10 for both orthopaedics and rheumatology in the 2012-2013 *U.S. News & World Report* annual survey of "Best Hospitals" in America. HJD is dedicated to the prevention and treatment of musculoskeletal diseases, providing some of the most advanced programs in the region for musculoskeletal disorders and the largest pediatric orthopaedic program in New York City. HJD also offers a number of unique and highly specialized services to provide tailored, world-class care to patients with specific musculoskeletal conditions and needs. We specialize in the following areas:

Orthopaedic Surgery

The clinical expertise of our internationally-renowned surgeons represents the full range of subspecialty areas of orthopaedic surgery, including Adult Reconstructive, Sports Medicine, Spine, Shoulder & Elbow, Foot & Ankle, Hand Surgery, Trauma & Fracture, Orthopaedic Oncology, and Pediatric Orthopaedics; additional areas of focus include minimally-invasive hip surgery and robotic-assisted joint replacement.

Rheumatology

HJD houses the Division of Rheumatology's Osteoporosis Center, offering a multidisciplinary approach to the evaluation and treatment of osteoporosis, including a range of advanced drug therapies.

Rehabilitation

Rehabilitation care at HJD is provided by the world-renowned Rusk Rehabilitation. Rusk's CARF-Accredited Brain Injury Rehabilitation Program is a center of innovation and excellence for the treatment of disabling neurological and neurocognitive disorders. HJD also houses Rusk's Orthopaedic Rehabilitation Unit, where an expert multidisciplinary rehabilitation team aids patients in their recovery after orthopaedic surgery or injury.

Neurology – Spine & Nerve

HJD provides a broad range of diagnostic and therapeutic services to patients with neurological disorders. Its outstanding clinical staff includes specialists in pain management, spine and nerve pain, and cerebral palsy.

Radiology

HJD provides complete diagnostic orthopaedic radiology services, including MRI, computed tomography, ultrasonography and conventional radiography, as well as a multitude of musculoskeletal interventional procedures. The medical team includes several internationally-known musculoskeletal radiologists with expertise in all aspects of osteoradiology.

Rusk Rehabilitation
550 First Avenue *(at 31st Street)*
New York, NY 10016
www.NYULMC.org/RUSK
Physician Referral: **888-7-NYU-MED** (888-769-8633)

RUSK INSTITUTE OF REHABILITATION MEDICINE

Rusk Rehabilitation at NYU Langone Medical Center (Rusk) has been ranked the best rehabilitation hospital in New York and among the top ten in the country by *U.S. News & World Report* for 23 consecutive years. Rusk is internationally renowned for the treatment of adults and children with disabilities, providing the full continuum of inpatient and outpatient rehabilitation care at multiple, state-of-the-art NYU Langone facilities and across all specialties: physical, occupational, speech/swallowing and vocational therapy, psychology, music and recreational therapy, nutrition, nursing, and social work.

Rusk's CARF-Accredited Brain Injury Rehabilitation Program is tailored for patients who have medical, physical, cognitive, and behavioral changes as a result of a brain injury or neurological illness.

The Amputee Program provides specialized limb deficiency rehabilitation to patients who have undergone amputations.

The Joan and Joel Smilow Cardiac and Pulmonary Rehabilitation & Prevention Center offers a model of transitional care for patients with cardiac and lung conditions.

Orthopaedic/Musculoskeletal Rehabilitation is offered for patients with back, neck, hip, elbow and shoulder disorders, arthritis-related joint pain, conditions affecting the bones, tendon, ligaments and muscles, and for pre- and post-surgical patients.

The Spinal Cord Injury program offers a comprehensive, patient-centered array of specialized and innovative clinical and educational programs to optimize quality of life.

Sports Injury Rehabilitation addresses the needs of patients with sports-related conditions, including post-operative rehabilitation for patients who require orthopaedic surgery.

Rusk's CARF-Accredited Stroke Program offers an interdisciplinary team with specialized training in the medical, nursing or therapeutic care and treatment of stroke patients.

Vestibular Rehabilitation addresses the evaluation and treatment of patients suffering from dizziness and imbalance.

The Women's Health Program addresses issues that uniquely affect women, including pelvic floor muscle dysfunction/pain, urinary incontinence, cancer rehabilitation and lymphedema, and prenatal and postpartum musculoskeletal conditions.

Chest Physical Therapy cares for individuals with lung congestion, secretion retention or areas of lung collapse.

The Outpatient Rehabilitation Psychology Service provides care to patients with neurological and medical conditions on an outpatient basis.

Speech-Language Pathology & Swallowing is dedicated to patients with communication disorders due to neurological problems as well as diagnosis and management of swallowing and feeding disorders.

Vocational Services provides disabled individuals with the competencies needed to return to school or work and to lead a productive life.

For more than two centuries, Penn physicians and scientists have been committed to the highest standards of patient care, education and research. That commitment has been recognized throughout the Greater Philadelphia region and across the nation.

Penn Medicine received $397 million in research grant funding from the National Institutes of Health in 2011, making Penn the third highest funded medical school in the country. *U.S. News & World Report* also consistently ranks Penn Medicine, the Perelman School of Medicine and the School of Nursing among the nation's best.

What Sets Penn Apart?

Penn's physicians and scientists are united in the health system's mission to expand the frontiers of medicine through new discoveries in the detection, treatment and prevention of human disease. Because they develop and test new treatments through clinical trials, their patients gain access to the very latest advances and future generations will benefit from the work they do today.

Penn continues to lead the way in discovering new treatment methods for diseases once considered incurable, including groundbreaking research in cancer, cardiac, neurosciences, orthopaedics, genetics and imaging. Over the past 30 years, Penn physicians and scientists have participated in many important discoveries, including:

- The first general vaccine against pneumonia.
- The introduction of total intravenous feeding.
- The development of cognitive therapy.
- The development of magnetic resonance imaging and other imaging technologies.
- The development of a treatment for patients with chronic lymphocytic leukemia using genetically engineered versions of their own T-cells.
- The development of techniques to minimize complications associated with Transcatheter Aortic Valve Replacement.
- Pioneering new procedures in robotic-assisted surgery.

Locations

Patients are seen at:

- Hospital of the University of Pennsylvania
- Penn Presbyterian Medical Center
- Pennsylvania Hospital
- Penn Medicine Bucks County
- Penn Medicine Cherry Hill
- Penn Medicine Media
- Penn Medicine Radnor
- Penn Medicine Rittenhouse
- Penn Medicine Valley Forge
- Penn Medicine Woodbury Heights
- Penn's primary care physician network provides services in the local communities in Bucks, Chester, Delaware, Montgomery and Philadelphia counties in Pennsylvania and in Southern New Jersey.
- Hospice and home care services are provided by Penn Home Care and Hospice Services.

On the Web

Visit **PennMedicine.org** for the latest patient education with explanation of surgical procedures and follow-up care, screening tools, drug interactions and descriptions, as well as an encyclopedia of health information.

For more information or to schedule an appointment, call 800.789.PENN (7366) or visit PennMedicine.org.

Hospital of the University of Pennsylvania | Penn Presbyterian Medical Center | Pennsylvania Hospital
Philadelphia, PA | 800.789.PENN | PennMedicine.org

72

Sponsored Page

St. Francis Hospital The Heart Center®
100 Port Washington Blvd.
Roslyn, New York 11576
www.stfrancisheartcenter.com
(516) 562-6000 1-888-HEARTNY

St. Francis Hospital, The Heart Center® is New York State's only specialty designated cardiac center and a nationally recognized leader in cardiac care. Founded in 1922 by the Franciscan Missionaries of Mary, the Hospital is an innovator in the delivery of specialized cardiovascular services in an environment where excellence and compassion are emphasized. St. Francis also offers an outstanding program in non-cardiac surgery, including some of the most advanced technology and minimally invasive techniques available for vascular, prostate, ear-nose-throat (ENT), abdominal, oncologic, gastrointestinal, and orthopedic surgery and procedures.

Cardiac Diagnostics and Treatment
St. Francis Hospital performs one of the highest volumes of cardiac surgical, interventional and arrhythmia procedures in the nation and has been consistently recognized for its outstanding quality of care. In 2012-13, St. Francis Hospital was ranked one of America's best hospitals by *U.S. News & World Report.*

Cardiac surgery: : In 2011, 1,477 open-heart surgeries were performed at St. Francis Hospital. The Hospital's cardiothoracic surgical staff has the combined experience of over 20,000 open-heart procedures in the last 10 years alone and are experts in all types of heart surgery, from conventional, open-heart bypass to off-pump coronary artery bypass (OPCAB) to the newest, minimally invasive valve procedures, including surgical techniques designed to treat certain cardiac arrhythmias or irregular heart rhythms.

Cardiac catheterization: In 2011, St. Francis interventional cardiologists performed 7,959 cardiac catheterizations and 3,046 percutaneous coronary interventions (angioplasty and insertion of stents). The Hospital is also recognized as one of the East Coast's highest volume centers for catheter-based techniques to close atrial septal defects (ASDs) and patent foramen ovale (PFO).

Arrhythmia and Pacemaker Center: St. Francis has a leading national program for pacemaker implantation and the diagnosis and treatment of cardiac rhythm abnormalities. The Center has unparalleled expertise in radiofrequency cardiac ablation, including treatment of atrial fibrillation.

Research and Technology: At the St. Francis Cardiac Research Institute, a team of world-renowned researchers is working with the latest noninvasive imaging technology, including advanced techniques and world-class expertise in cardiac CT angiography, cardiac magnetic resonance imaging (MRI), cardiac PET/CT and three-dimensional echocardiography. This multimodality approach to investigating the heart's function and disease processes is aimed at improving methods of diagnosing heart disease.

Prevention and Education
St. Francis Hospital's satellite campus, The DeMatteis Center for Cardiac Research and Education, in Greenvale, New York, is one of the few freestanding campuses in the U.S. dedicated to the prevention of heart disease. It is the site of community health lectures, as well as the largest medically staffed cardiac fitness and rehabilitation program on Long Island.

Physician referral: **1-888-HEARTNY**

Sponsorship:	Voluntary not-for-profit
Beds:	306
Accreditation:	Awarded accreditation from the Joint Commission.

University Hospitals
Case Medical Center

11100 Euclid Avenue
Cleveland, OH 44106
1-866-UH4-CARE (1-866-844-2273)
UHhospitals.org

Sponsorship: Voluntary Not-for-Profit
Beds: 1,032
Accreditation: Full Joint Commission – ANNS Magnet Status

Overview

Founded in 1866, University Hospitals Case Medical Center, our physicians, nurses, and staff work with a devotion to the UH mission – To Heal. To Teach. To Discover. Ranked among the top hospitals in 12 medical specialties by U.S.News & World Report, UH Case Medical Center is located in Northeast Ohio near the shores of Lake Erie and in the heart of Cleveland's University Circle. University Hospitals Case Medical Center is a 1,032-bed hospital specializing in adult and pediatric medical and surgical specialties.

Shaping the Future of Health Care

As the primary affiliate of Case Western Reserve University School of Medicine, UH Case Medical Center was recognized as a national model for quality care as the recipient of the 2012 American Hospital Association – McKesson Quest for Quality Prize. The prestigious award named UH Case Medical Center the top hospital in the nation for its leadership and innovation in quality improvement and safety.

University Hospitals Seidman Cancer Center is one of only 12 freestanding cancer hospitals designated by the National Cancer Institute as a Comprehensive Cancer Center through our affiliation with Case Western Reserve University School of Medicine and offers more than 300 clinical trials. University Hospitals Rainbow Babies & Children's Hospital is the region's largest group of medical professionals providing care to children and is recognized by U.S.News & World Report as one of America's Best Children's Hospitals. It boasts a Neonatal Intensive Care Unit ranked among the best in the world. University Hospitals MacDonald Women's Hospital is the only hospital in Ohio solely dedicated to women's health specializing in high-risk pregnancy, infertility, gyn-oncology and breast health.

Among the nation's leading academic medical centers, University Hospitals Case Medical Center is the primary affiliate of Case Western Reserve University School of Medicine, a nationally recognized leader in medical research and education.

UH Case Medical Center is the 2012 recipient of the American Hospital Association–McKesson Quest for Quality Prize.

To schedule an appointment with any University Hospitals physician, call **1-866-UH4-CARE (1-866-844-2273)** or visit UHhospitals.org.

VANDERBILT ᴠ UNIVERSITY
MEDICAL CENTER

1211 Medical Center Drive | Nashville, TN 37232 | (615) 322-5000 | VanderbiltHealth.com

Overview

Vanderbilt University Medical Center has built a strong reputation throughout the U.S. as a leader in patient care, research and education over its 137-year history. Vanderbilt specializes in applying new discoveries and innovations into patient care and medical education while offering every patient compassionate, personalized care.

In 2011, Vanderbilt had more than 1.5 million outpatient visits and nearly 52,000 admissions. Our Emergency Department, Level 1 Trauma Center, Burn Center and Lifeflight air ambulance service provide trauma care for a three-state region.

Elite National Rankings

Vanderbilt is consistently ranked among the nation's best by *U.S. News & World Report*'s Best Hospitals listing. In 2012, Vanderbilt was ranked in the top 1% of America's highest performing health care providers. In addition, its Monroe Carell Jr. Children's Hospital at Vanderbilt is listed among the nation's best children's hospitals, ranking in 10 of 10 specialties.

Specialty Programs

Monroe Carell Jr. Children's Hospital at Vanderbilt
Vanderbilt-Ingram Cancer Center
Heart and Vascular Institute
Neurosciences
Orthopaedics
Women's Health

Discovery, Innovation and Collaboration

Vanderbilt thrives on a culture of collaboration that produces world-leading discovery and innovation. Learn more.

Recently our institution has produced:
- One of the nation's most advanced electronic medical records
- Leading programs in personalizing care for heart disease, cancer and other conditions based on each patient's DNA
- A program developing new drugs for schizophrenia, Parkinson's disease and more

My Health at Vanderbilt

Vanderbilt patients can manage their care through our secure, convenient electronic medical record system, My Health at Vanderbilt. This free service is just one of the ways we're making healthcare more efficient and personal.

The Best in American Medicine
www.CastleConnolly.com

Physician
Listings

The Best in American Medicine
www.CastleConnolly.com

Adolescent Medicine

a subspecialty of Pediatrics

An internist or pediatrician who specializes in adolescent medicine is a multidiciplinary healthcare specialist trained in the unique physical, psychological and social characteristics of adolescents, their healthcare problems and needs.

Training Required: Three years in internal medicine OR three years in pediatrics *plus* additional training and examination for certification in adolescent medicine

ADOLESCENT MEDICINE

New England

Emans, Sarah Jean H MD [AM] - **Spec Exp:** Pediatric Gynecology; Adolescent Gynecology; **Hospital:** Children's Hospital - Boston; **Address:** Childrens Hosp, Dept Adolescent Med, 300 Longwood Ave, Boston, MA 02115-5724; **Phone:** 617-355-7170; **Board Cert:** Pediatrics 1993; Adolescent Medicine 2009; **Med School:** Harvard Med Sch 1970; **Resid:** Pediatrics, Chldns Hosp 1973; **Fellow:** Adolescent Medicine, Chldns Hosp 1975; **Fac Appt:** Prof Ped, Harvard Med Sch

Mid Atlantic

Adger Jr, Hoover MD [AM] - **Spec Exp:** Adolescent Medicine; Addiction/Substance Abuse; Parenting Issues; **Hospital:** Johns Hopkins Hosp (page 61); **Address:** Johns Hopkins Harriet Lane Clinic, 200 N Wolfe St, rm 2065, Rubenstein Child Hlth Bldg, Baltimore, MD 21287; **Phone:** 410-955-2910; **Board Cert:** Pediatrics 1986; Adolescent Medicine 2009; **Med School:** Case West Res Univ 1979; **Resid:** Pediatrics, Cincinnati Chldns Hosp Med Ctr 1982; **Fellow:** Adolescent Medicine, UCSF Med Ctr 1984; **Fac Appt:** Prof Ped, Johns Hopkins Univ

Chambers, Christopher V MD [AM] - **Spec Exp:** Metabolic Syndrome; Sexually Transmitted Diseases; **Hospital:** Thomas Jefferson Univ Hosp; **Address:** Jefferson Med Coll, Dept Family Med, 833 Chestnut St E, Ste 301, Philadelphia, PA 19107; **Phone:** 215-955-7190; **Board Cert:** Family Medicine 2008; Adolescent Medicine 2001; **Med School:** Duke Univ 1980; **Resid:** Family Medicine, Thomas Jefferson Univ Hosp 1983; **Fellow:** Adolescent Medicine, UCSF Med Ctr 1985; **Fac Appt:** Prof FMed, Jefferson Med Coll

Diaz, Angela MD [AM] - **Spec Exp:** Adolescent Gynecology; Abuse/Neglect; **Hospital:** Mount Sinai Med Ctr (page 64); **Address:** 320 E 94th St Fl 2, New York, NY 10128-5604; **Phone:** 212-423-2900; **Board Cert:** Pediatrics 1987; **Med School:** Columbia P&S 1981; **Resid:** Pediatrics, Mt Sinai Med Ctr 1984; **Fellow:** Adolescent Medicine, Mt Sinai Med Ctr 1985; **Fac Appt:** Prof Ped, Mount Sinai Sch Med

Ginsburg, Kenneth R MD [AM] - **Spec Exp:** Behavioral Disorders; Adolescent Behavior-High Risk; **Hospital:** Chldns Hosp of Philadelphia; **Address:** 3550 Market St Fl 4, Philadelphia, PA 19104; **Phone:** 215-590-3537; **Board Cert:** Adolescent Medicine 2009; **Med School:** Albert Einstein Coll Med 1987; **Resid:** Pediatrics, Chldns Hosp 1990; **Fac Appt:** Assoc Prof Ped, Univ Pennsylvania

Murray, Pamela J MD [AM] - **Spec Exp:** Adolescent Gynecology; Menstrual Disorders; **Hospital:** Ruby Memorial - WVU Hosp; **Address:** W Virginia Univ Sch Medicine, Dept Pediatrics-Robert C Byrd HSC, PO Box 9214, Morgantown, WV 26505; **Phone:** 304-598-4835; **Board Cert:** Pediatrics 1983; Adolescent Medicine 2009; **Med School:** Med Coll PA 1978; **Resid:** Pediatrics, Chldns Hosp 1981; **Fellow:** Public Health, Univ New South Wales 1987; **Fac Appt:** Prof Ped, W VA Univ

Rudy, Bret J MD [AM] - **Spec Exp:** HIV in Adolescents; AIDS/HIV; **Hospital:** NYU Langone Med Ctr (page 68); **Address:** 227 E 30th St, rm 713, New York, NY 10016; **Phone:** 212-263-6425; **Board Cert:** Pediatrics 1998; Adolescent Medicine 2001; **Med School:** Univ Pittsburgh 1985; **Resid:** Pediatrics, Chldns Hosp of Philadelphia 1989; **Fellow:** Immunology, Chldns Hosp of Philadelphia 1991

Slap, Gail MD [AM] - **Spec Exp:** Chronic Illness; Developmental Disorders; **Hospital:** Chldns Hosp of Philadelphia; **Address:** Childrens Hosp Philadelphia, Main Bldg, 34th St & Civic Center Blvd, Philadelphia, PA 19104; **Phone:** 215-590-5868; **Board Cert:** Internal Medicine 1980; Adolescent Medicine 2004; **Med School:** Univ Pennsylvania 1977; **Resid:** Internal Medicine, Hosp Univ Penn 1980; **Fellow:** Adolescent Medicine, Chldns Hosp 1982; **Fac Appt:** Prof Ped, Univ Pennsylvania

Midwest

Bravender, Terrill D MD [AM] - **Spec Exp:** Eating Disorders; Nutrition; **Hospital:** Nationwide Chldn's Hosp; **Address:** 495 E Main St, Columbus, OH 43215; **Phone:** 614-722-2450; **Board Cert:** Pediatrics 2004; Adolescent Medicine 2007; **Med School:** Univ Mich Med Sch 1992; **Resid:** Pediatrics, Duke Med Ctr 1996; **Fellow:** Adolescent Medicine, Chldns Hosp 1998; **Fac Appt:** Asst Prof Med, Ohio State Univ

Kokotailo, Patricia K MD [AM] - **Spec Exp:** Adolescent Gynecology; Substance Abuse; **Hospital:** Univ WI Hosp & Clins; **Address:** UW Health, Univ Station Clinic, 2880 University Ave, Ste 9010, Madison, WI 53705; **Phone:** 608-263-6421; **Board Cert:** Pediatrics 1987; Adolescent Medicine 2009; **Med School:** Northwestern Univ 1982; **Resid:** Pediatrics, Johns Hopkins Hosp 1985; **Fellow:** Adolescent Medicine, Johns Hopkins Hosp 1989; **Fac Appt:** Prof Ped, Univ Wisc

Singh, Nimi MD [AM] - **Spec Exp:** Anxiety & Depression; Eating Disorders; Nutrition; **Hospital:** Univ Minn Med Ctr, Fairview - Riverside Campus; **Address:** Fairview Chldns Clinic, 2535 University Ave SE, Minneapolis, MN 55414; **Phone:** 612-672-2350; **Board Cert:** Pediatrics 2009; Adolescent Medicine 2005; **Med School:** Mount Sinai Sch Med 1989; **Resid:** Pediatrics, Rainbow Babies & Chldns Hosp 1992; **Fellow:** Adolescent Medicine, Univ Wash Med Ctr 1997; **Fac Appt:** Asst Prof Ped, Univ Minn

Great Plains and Mountains

Bermudez, Ovidio B MD [AM] - **Spec Exp:** Eating Disorders; Obesity; **Address:** Eating Recovery Center, 8140 E Fifth Ave, Lawry, CO 80230; **Phone:** 877-825-8584; **Board Cert:** Pediatrics 2012; Adolescent Medicine 2009; **Med School:** Dominican Republic 1985; **Resid:** Pediatrics, Med Coll Penn Hosp 1988; **Fellow:** Adolescent Medicine, Univ Alabama 1990; **Fac Appt:** Clin Prof Ped, Univ Okla Coll Med

Kaplan, David W MD [AM] - **Spec Exp:** Anxiety Disorders; Adolescent Gynecology; Depression; **Hospital:** Chldn's Hosp - Aurora (CO); **Address:** Chldns Hosp, 13123 E 16th Ave, Aurora, CO 80045; **Phone:** 720-777-6131; **Board Cert:** Pediatrics 1975; Public Health & Genl Preventive Med 1980; Adolescent Medicine 2009; **Med School:** Case West Res Univ 1970; **Resid:** Pediatrics, Univ Colorado Med Ctr 1972; Pediatrics, Chldns Hosp Med Ctr 1975; **Fellow:** Public Health & Genl Preventive Med, Harvard Sch Pub Hlth 1976; **Fac Appt:** Prof Ped, Univ Colorado

Sigel, Eric J MD [AM] - **Spec Exp:** Eating Disorders; **Hospital:** Chldn's Hosp - Aurora (CO); **Address:** Children's Hosp, Adolescent Med Clinic, 13123 E 16th Ave, Aurora, CO 80045; **Phone:** 720-777-6131; **Board Cert:** Pediatrics 2007; Adolescent Medicine 2012; **Med School:** Case West Res Univ 1989; **Resid:** Pediatrics, Rainbow Babies & Chldns Hosp 1992; **Fellow:** Adolescent Medicine, Chldns Hosp 1993; **Fac Appt:** Assoc Prof Ped, Univ Colorado

Southwest

Hergenroeder, Albert C MD [AM] - **Spec Exp:** Pediatric & Adolescent Sports Medicine; Eating Disorders; Adolescent Gynecology; **Hospital:** Texas Chldns Hosp; **Address:** TCH-Adolescent & Sports Med Service, TCH Clinical Care Ctr Fl 11, 6701 Fannin St, Houston, TX 77030; **Phone:** 832-822-4887; **Board Cert:** Pediatrics 1993; Sports Medicine 2004; Adolescent Medicine 2009; **Med School:** Univ Pittsburgh 1980; **Resid:** Pediatrics, Duke Univ Med Ctr 1983; **Fellow:** Adolescent Medicine, Univ Wash Affil Hosp 1985; **Fac Appt:** Assoc Prof Ped, Baylor Coll Med

West Coast and Pacific

Anderson, Martin M MD [AM] - **Hospital:** UCLA Ronald Reagan Med Ctr; **Address:** UCLA Med Ctr, Dept Pediatrics, 10833 Le Conte Ave, 12-358MDCC, Los Angeles, CA 90095; **Phone:** 310-825-9346; **Board Cert:** Pediatrics 1986; Adolescent Medicine 2009; **Med School:** UC Davis 1980; **Resid:** Pediatrics, Mott Chldns Hosp 1983; **Fellow:** Adolescent Medicine, UCSF Med Ctr 1986; UCLA Med Ctr 1998; **Fac Appt:** Prof Ped, UCLA

Irwin Jr, Charles E MD [AM] - **Spec Exp:** Eating Disorders; Adolescent Gynecology; **Hospital:** UCSF Med Ctr; **Address:** UCSF Chldns Hosp, 400 Parnassus Ave Fl 2, Box 0314, San Francisco, CA 94143; **Phone:** 415-353-2002; **Board Cert:** Pediatrics 1993; **Med School:** UCSF 1971; **Resid:** Pediatrics, UCSF Med Ctr 1974; **Fellow:** Adolescent Medicine, UCSF Med Ctr 1977; **Fac Appt:** Prof Ped, UCSF

MacKenzie, Richard G MD [AM] - **Spec Exp:** Eating Disorders; Menstrual Disorders; **Hospital:** Chldns Hosp - Los Angeles; **Address:** 5000 Sunset Blvd, Fl 4, Los Angeles, CA 90027-5861; **Phone:** 323-361-2153; **Med School:** McGill Univ 1966; **Resid:** Internal Medicine, Royal Victoria Hosp-Montreal 1969; **Fellow:** Adolescent Medicine, Chidrens Hosp 1970; **Fac Appt:** Assoc Prof Ped, USC Sch Med

Staggers, Barbara C MD [AM] - **Spec Exp:** Adolescent Behavior-High Risk; **Hospital:** Chldns Hosp - Oakland; **Address:** 5400 Telegraph Ave, Oakland, CA 94618; **Phone:** 510-428-3387; **Board Cert:** Adolescent Medicine 2011; **Med School:** UCSF 1980; **Resid:** Pediatrics, Chldns Hosp 1983; **Fellow:** Adolescent Medicine, UCSF Med Ctr 1985

Allergy & Immunology

An allergist-immunologist is trained in evaluation, physical and laboratory diagnosis and management of disorders involving the immune system. Selected examples of such conditions include asthma, anaphylaxis, rhinitis, eczema and adverse reactions to drugs, foods and insect stings as well as immune deficiency diseases (both acquired and congenital), defects in host defense and problems related to autoimmune disease, organ transplantation or malignancies of the immune system. As our understanding of the immune system develops, the scope of this specialty is widening.

Training programs are available at some medical centers to provide individuals with expertise in both allergy/immunology and adult rheumatology, or in both allergy/immunology and pediatric pulmonology. Such individuals are candidates for dual certification.

Training Required: Two years in allergy/immunology OR prior certification in internal medicine or pediatrics *plus* additional training and examination

ALLERGY & IMMUNOLOGY

New England

Castells, Maria C MD/PhD [A&I] - **Spec Exp:** Drug Allergy; Food Allergy; Anaphylaxis; Mast Cell Diseases; **Hospital:** Brigham and Women's Hosp (page 57); **Address:** Brigham & Women's Hosp, Allergy Div, 850 Boylston St, Ste 540, Chestnut Hill, MA 02467; **Phone:** 617-732-9850; **Board Cert:** Internal Medicine 2004; Allergy & Immunology 2005; **Med School:** Spain 1979; **Resid:** Internal Medicine, Kansas Univ Med Ctr 1988; Allergy & Immunology, Medical Coll Virginia 1990; **Fac Appt:** Assoc Prof Med, Harvard Med Sch

MacLean, James A MD [A&I] - **Spec Exp:** Asthma; Allergy; Urticaria; **Hospital:** Mass Genl Hosp, N Shore Med Ctr - Salem Hosp; **Address:** Mass General Hosp, 55 Fruit St, Cox 201, Boston, MA 02114-2621; **Phone:** 617-726-3850; **Board Cert:** Internal Medicine 1988; Allergy & Immunology 2011; **Med School:** McGill Univ 1985; **Resid:** Internal Medicine, Royal Victoria Hosp 1989; **Fellow:** Allergy & Immunology, Mass Genl Hosp 1991; Immunopathology, Mass Genl Hosp 1994; **Fac Appt:** Asst Prof A&I, Harvard Med Sch

Umetsu, Dale T MD/PhD [A&I] - **Spec Exp:** Asthma; Immune Deficiency; Eczema; Food Allergy; **Hospital:** Children's Hospital - Boston; **Address:** Karp Labs, Rm 10127, 1 Blackfan Cir, Boston, MA 02115; **Phone:** 617-919-2439; **Board Cert:** Pediatrics 1984; Allergy & Immunology 1985; **Med School:** NYU Sch Med 1979; **Resid:** Pediatrics, Chldns Hosp 1982; **Fellow:** Allergy & Immunology, Chldns Hosp 1984; **Fac Appt:** Prof Ped, Harvard Med Sch

Wong, Johnson T MD [A&I] - **Spec Exp:** Asthma; Rhinosinusitis; Urticaria; Immune Deficiency; **Hospital:** Mass Genl Hosp, Newton - Wellesley Hosp; **Address:** 8 Hawthorne Pl, Ste 104, Boston, MA 02114; **Phone:** 617-742-5730; **Board Cert:** Internal Medicine 1983; Allergy & Immunology 1985; **Med School:** UCSF 1980; **Resid:** Internal Medicine, UCLA-Wadsworth VA Hosp 1983; **Fellow:** Allergy & Immunology, Mass Genl Hosp 1986; **Fac Appt:** Asst Prof Med, Harvard Med Sch

Mid Atlantic

Buchbinder, Ellen MD [A&I] - **Spec Exp:** Asthma & Allergy; Rhinitis; Hives; Food & Drug Allergy; **Hospital:** Mount Sinai Med Ctr (page 64); **Address:** 111B E 88th St, New York, NY 10128; **Phone:** 212-410-3246; **Board Cert:** Internal Medicine 1981; Allergy & Immunology 1983; **Med School:** Tulane Univ 1978; **Resid:** Internal Medicine, New England Deaconess Hosp 1981; **Fellow:** Allergy & Immunology, Mass Genl Hosp 1983; **Fac Appt:** Asst Clin Prof Med, Mount Sinai Sch Med

Chandler, Michael MD [A&I] - **Spec Exp:** Asthma; Sinus Disorders; Airway Disorders; **Hospital:** Mount Sinai Med Ctr (page 64); **Address:** 115 E 61st St Fl 12, New York, NY 10065; **Phone:** 212-486-6715; **Board Cert:** Internal Medicine 1984; Allergy & Immunology 1987; **Med School:** Wayne State Univ 1981; **Resid:** Internal Medicine, Northwestern Meml Hosp 1984; **Fellow:** Allergy & Immunology, Northwestern Meml Hosp 1986; **Fac Appt:** Asst Clin Prof Med, Mount Sinai Sch Med

Cunningham-Rundles, Charlotte MD/PhD [A&I] - **Spec Exp:** Immunotherapy; Immunodeficiency Disorders; **Hospital:** Mount Sinai Med Ctr (page 64); **Address:** 5 E 98th St Fl 11, New York, NY 10029; **Phone:** 212-659-9268; **Board Cert:** Internal Medicine 1972; **Med School:** Columbia P&S 1969; **Resid:** Internal Medicine, Bellevue Hosp Ctr 1972; **Fellow:** Allergy & Immunology, NYU Med Ctr 1974; **Fac Appt:** Prof Med, Mount Sinai Sch Med

Ein, Daniel MD [A&I] - **Spec Exp:** Asthma & Allergy; Sinus Disorders; Food Allergy; Immune Deficiency; **Hospital:** G Washington Univ Hosp; **Address:** 2300 M St NW, Fl 2, Ste 200, Washington, DC 20037; **Phone:** 202-741-2770; **Board Cert:** Internal Medicine 1980; Allergy & Immunology 1989; **Med School:** Albert Einstein Coll Med 1964; **Resid:** Internal Medicine, Mass Genl Hosp 1969; **Fellow:** Immunology, Natl Cancer Inst 1968; **Fac Appt:** Clin Prof A&I, Geo Wash Univ

Fishman, Henry J MD [A&I] - **Spec Exp:** Asthma & Allergy; Chemical Exposure; **Hospital:** G Washington Univ Hosp; **Address:** 2141 K St NW, Ste 206, Washington, DC 20037; **Phone:** 202-833-3500; **Board Cert:** Internal Medicine 1982; Allergy & Immunology 1985; **Med School:** Univ Rochester 1979; **Resid:** Internal Medicine, Geo Wash Med Ctr 1982; **Fellow:** Allergy & Immunology, Georgetown Univ Hosp 1984; **Fac Appt:** Asst Clin Prof Med, Georgetown Univ

Kaliner, Michael A MD [A&I] - **Spec Exp:** Asthma & Allergy; Sinusitis; Rhinitis; **Hospital:** Washington Hosp Ctr; **Address:** Institute for Asthma and Allergy, 5454 Wisconsin Ave, Ste 700, Chevy Chase, MD 20815; **Phone:** 301-986-9262; **Board Cert:** Internal Medicine 1974; Allergy & Immunology 1993; **Med School:** Univ MD Sch Med 1967; **Resid:** Internal Medicine, UCSF Med Ctr 1970; **Fellow:** Allergy & Immunology, Harvard Univ 1973; **Fac Appt:** Clin Prof Med, Geo Wash Univ

Mazza, David S MD [A&I] - **Spec Exp:** Asthma; Sinus Disorders; Eczema; **Hospital:** St. Luke's - Roosevelt Hosp Ctr - Roosevelt Div (page 56); **Address:** 7 Lexington Ave, Ste P3, New York, NY 10010-5517; **Phone:** 212-677-7170; **Board Cert:** Pediatrics 1983; Allergy & Immunology 2008; **Med School:** Univ VT Coll Med 1977; **Resid:** Pediatrics, NYU-Bellevue Hosp 1980; **Fellow:** Pediatric Allergy & Immunology, Bellevue Hosp 1982; **Fac Appt:** Assoc Prof Ped, Columbia P&S

Metcalfe, Dean D MD [A&I] - **Spec Exp:** Mast Cell Diseases; Anaphylaxis; **Hospital:** Natl Inst of Hlth - Clin Ctr; **Address:** Natl Inst Allergy & Infectious Disease, Allergic Disease Lab, MS 1881, 10 Center Drive Bldg 10 - rm 11C207, Bethesda, MD 20892-1881; **Phone:** 301-496-2165; **Board Cert:** Internal Medicine 1975; Allergy & Immunology 1977; Rheumatology 1980; **Med School:** Univ Tenn Coll Med 1972; **Resid:** Internal Medicine, Univ Mich Hosps 1974; Allergy & Immunology, Natl Inst Allergy & Infectious Dis-NIH 1977; **Fellow:** Rheumatology, Peter Bent Brigham Hosp 1979

Phillips, S Michael MD [A&I] - **Spec Exp:** Allergy; Autoimmune Disease; Immunodeficiency Disorders; **Hospital:** Penn Presby Med Ctr - UPHS (page 72), Hosp Univ Penn - UPHS (page 72); **Address:** 51 N 39th St, Mutch Bldg - Fl 5, Philadelphia, PA 19104-2640; **Phone:** 215-662-2775; **Board Cert:** Internal Medicine 1974; Allergy & Immunology 1979; **Med School:** Univ Wisc 1966; **Resid:** Internal Medicine, Hosp Univ Penn 1968; **Fellow:** Immunology, Hosp Univ Penn 1969; Immunology, Peter Bent Brigham Hosp 1972; **Fac Appt:** Prof Med, Univ Pennsylvania

Shepherd, Gillian M MD [A&I] - **Spec Exp:** Food & Drug Allergy; Rhinosinusitis & Asthma; Urticaria; Insect Allergies; **Hospital:** NY-Presby/Weill Cornell Med Ctr, NY (page 66); **Address:** 235 E 67th St, Ste 203, New York, NY 10065; **Phone:** 212-288-9300; **Board Cert:** Internal Medicine 1979; Allergy & Immunology 1981; **Med School:** NY Med Coll 1976; **Resid:** Internal Medicine, Lenox Hill Hosp 1979; **Fellow:** Allergy & Immunology, New York Hosp-Cornell 1981; **Fac Appt:** Assoc Clin Prof Med, Cornell Univ-Weill Med Coll

Slankard, Marjorie MD [A&I] - **Spec Exp:** Sinus Disorders; Asthma; Food Allergy; Hereditary Angioedema; **Hospital:** NY-Presby/Columbia Univ Med Ctr, NY (page 66), Valley Hosp; **Address:** 16 E 60th St, Ste 321, New York, NY 10022-1002; **Phone:** 212-326-8410; **Board Cert:** Internal Medicine 1974; Allergy & Immunology 1977; **Med School:** Univ MO-Columbia Sch Med 1971; **Resid:** Internal Medicine, New York Hosp 1974; Internal Medicine, Rockefeller Univ Hosp 1974; **Fellow:** Immunology, New York Hosp-Cornell 1976; Immunology, Mount Sinai Med Ctr 1980; **Fac Appt:** Clin Prof Med, Columbia P&S

Allergy & Immunology

Southeast

Benenati, Susan V MD [A&I] - **Spec Exp:** Asthma; Latex Allergy; Sinus Disorders; Nasal Allergy; **Hospital:** Baptist Hosp of Miami, South Miami Hosp; **Address:** 6705 Red Rd, Ste 318, Coral Gables, FL 33143; **Phone:** 305-665-1623; **Board Cert:** Internal Medicine 1988; Allergy & Immunology 2011; **Med School:** Univ S Fla Coll Med 1984; **Resid:** Internal Medicine, Indiana Univ Med Ctr 1988; **Fellow:** Allergy & Immunology, Johns Hopkins Hosp 1990

Bonner, James R MD [A&I] - **Spec Exp:** Asthma; Urticaria; Food Allergy; Infectious Disease; **Hospital:** Univ of Ala Hosp at Birmingham, Birmingham, Alabama VA Med Ctr; **Address:** Alabama Allergy & Asthma Center, 504 Brookwood Blvd, Birmingham, AL 35209; **Phone:** 205-871-9661; **Board Cert:** Internal Medicine 1974; Infectious Disease 1976; Allergy & Immunology 1979; **Med School:** Univ Mich Med Sch 1971; **Resid:** Internal Medicine, Univ Ala Med Ctr 1974; **Fellow:** Allergy & Immunology, Univ Ala Med Ctr 1977; **Fac Appt:** Prof Med, Univ Alabama

DeShazo, Richard D MD [A&I] - **Spec Exp:** Immunodeficiency Disorders; Allergy; Rheumatology; Pediatric Allergy & Immunology; **Hospital:** Univ Mississippi Med Ctr, G.V. (Sonny) Montgomery VA Med Ctr - Jackson; **Address:** Univ Mississippi Med Ctr, Dept Med, 2500 N State St, Jackson, MS 39216; **Phone:** 601-815-1078; **Board Cert:** Internal Medicine 1974; Allergy & Immunology 1977; Rheumatology 1982; Geriatric Medicine 2005; **Med School:** Univ Alabama 1971; **Resid:** Internal Medicine, Walter Reed Genl Hosp 1974; **Fellow:** Microbiology, Walter Reed Army Inst Rsch 1975; Clinical Immunology, Walter Reed Genl Hosp 1977; **Fac Appt:** Prof Med, Univ Miss

Friedman, Stuart A MD [A&I] - **Spec Exp:** Asthma; Sinus Disorders; Allergy; **Hospital:** Boca Raton Regl Hosp, Delray Med Ctr; **Address:** 5162 Linton Blvd, Ste 201, Delray Beach, FL 33484; **Phone:** 561-495-2580; **Board Cert:** Internal Medicine 1980; Allergy & Immunology 1983; **Med School:** Spain 1976; **Resid:** Internal Medicine, Winthrop Univ Hosp 1980; **Fellow:** Immunology, Univ Cincinnati 1982

Ledford, Dennis K MD [A&I] - **Spec Exp:** Asthma; **Hospital:** Florida Hosp-Tampa, Tampa Genl Hosp; **Address:** Allergy,Asthma & Immunology Assocs, 13801 Bruce B. Downs Blvd, Ste 502, Tampa, FL 33613-4745; **Phone:** 813-971-9743; **Board Cert:** Internal Medicine 1980; Rheumatology 1984; Allergy & Immunology 1985; Clinical & Laboratory Immunology 1986; **Med School:** Univ Tenn Coll Med 1976; **Resid:** Internal Medicine, City of Memphis Hosp 1980; **Fellow:** Rheumatology, NYU Hosp-Bellevue 1982; Allergy & Immunology, Univ S Florida Coll Med 1985; **Fac Appt:** Assoc Prof A&I, Univ S Fla Coll Med

Lieberman, Phillip L MD [A&I] - **Spec Exp:** Asthma; Rhinitis; Anaphylaxis; **Hospital:** Baptist Memorial Hospital-Memphis, Methodist Univ Hosp - Memphis; **Address:** Allergy & Asthma Care, 7205 Wolf River Blvd, Ste 200, Germantown, TN 38138; **Phone:** 901-757-6100; **Board Cert:** Internal Medicine 1970; Allergy & Immunology 2003; **Med School:** Univ Tenn Coll Med 1965; **Resid:** Internal Medicine, Memphis City Hosps 1969; **Fellow:** Allergy & Immunology, Northwestern Univ Affil Hosp 1971; **Fac Appt:** Clin Prof A&I, Univ Tenn Coll Med

Lockey, Richard F MD [A&I] - **Spec Exp:** Asthma & Allergy; Rhinitis; Immune Deficiency; Hereditary Angioedema; **Hospital:** Florida Hosp-Tampa, Tampa Genl Hosp; **Address:** 13801 Bruce B Downs Blvd, Ste 502, Tampa, FL 33613; **Phone:** 813-971-9743; **Board Cert:** Internal Medicine 1970; Allergy & Immunology 1974; **Med School:** Temple Univ 1965; **Resid:** Internal Medicine, Univ Mich Hosp 1968; **Fellow:** Allergy & Immunology, Univ Mich Hosp 1970; **Fac Appt:** Prof Med, Univ S Fla Coll Med

Markert, M Louise MD [A&I] - **Spec Exp:** DiGeorge Syndrome; Immunodeficiency Disorders; **Hospital:** Duke Univ Hosp; **Address:** Research Park 4, 109B, 6 Circuit Drive, Durham, NC 27710; **Phone:** 919-684-6263; **Board Cert:** Allergy & Immunology 1987; Pediatrics 1987; Diagnostic Lab Immunology 1988; **Med School:** Duke Univ 1982; **Resid:** Pediatrics, Duke Univ Med Ctr 1984; **Fellow:** Allergy & Immunology, Duke Univ Med Ctr 1987

Pacin, Michael P MD [A&I] - **Spec Exp:** Insect Allergies; Asthma; Rhinitis; **Hospital:** Baptist Hosp of Miami, South Miami Hosp; **Address:** Florida Ctr Asthma & Allergy, 9035 Sunset Drive, Ste 202, Miami, FL 33173; **Phone:** 305-279-3366; **Board Cert:** Internal Medicine 1974; Allergy & Immunology 1979; **Med School:** Washington Univ, St Louis 1969; **Resid:** Internal Medicine, Jewish Hosp 1971; Internal Medicine, Jackson Meml Hosp 1972; **Fellow:** Allergy & Immunology, Long Beach VA Hosp 1974

Sullivan III, Timothy J MD [A&I] - **Spec Exp:** Drug Allergy; Anaphylaxis; Asthma; Urticaria; **Hospital:** Northside Hosp, St. Joseph's Hosp - Atlanta; **Address:** Atlanta ENT, Sinus & Allergy Assocs, 5555 Peachtree Dunwoody Rd, Ste 125, Atlanta, GA 30342; **Phone:** 404-255-2918; **Board Cert:** Allergy & Immunology 1979; **Med School:** Univ Miami Sch Med 1966; **Resid:** Internal Medicine, Barnes Hosp 1971; **Fellow:** Allergy & Immunology, Washington Univ 1973; **Fac Appt:** Assoc Clin Prof Ped, Med Coll GA

Sundy, John S MD/PhD [A&I] - **Spec Exp:** Asthma; Allergic Rhinitis; Immunotherapy; Gout; **Hospital:** Duke Univ Hosp, Durham Regional Hosp; **Address:** Duke Univ Medical Center, Box 3278, Durham, NC 27710; **Phone:** 919-668-7630; **Board Cert:** Internal Medicine 2006; Allergy & Immunology 2009; Rheumatology 2008; **Med School:** Hahnemann Univ 1991; **Resid:** Internal Medicine, Duke Univ Med Ctr 1993; **Fellow:** Rheumatology, Duke Univ Med Ctr 1996; Allergy & Immunology, Duke Univ Med Ctr 1998; **Fac Appt:** Assoc Prof Med, Duke Univ

Midwest

Baker Jr, James Russell MD [A&I] - **Spec Exp:** Immune Deficiency-Thyroid; **Hospital:** Univ of Michigan Hosp; **Address:** Univ MI Allergy Specialty Clin, 24 Frank Lloyd Wright Drive, Ste H-2100, PO Box 442, Ann Arbor, MI 48106; **Phone:** 734-936-5634; **Board Cert:** Internal Medicine 1981; Allergy & Immunology 1983; Clinical & Laboratory Immunology 1986; **Med School:** Loyola Univ-Stritch Sch Med 1978; **Resid:** Internal Medicine, Walter Reed Army Med Ctr 1981; **Fellow:** Allergy & Immunology, Walter Reed Army Med Ctr/NIAID 1984; **Fac Appt:** Prof A&I, Univ Mich Med Sch

Ballas, Zuhair K MD [A&I] - **Hospital:** Univ Iowa Hosp & Clinics; **Address:** UIHC Dept of Internal Med, 200 Hawkins Drive, Iowa City, IA 52242; **Phone:** 319-356-8133; **Board Cert:** Internal Medicine 1977; Allergy & Immunology 1981; Diagnostic Lab Immunology 1988; **Med School:** Amer Univ Beirut 1974; **Resid:** Internal Medicine, Rutgets Med Sch Affil Hosp 1975; Internal Medicine, Jefferson Univ Hosp 1976; **Fellow:** Allergy & Immunology, Johns Hopkins Univ Hosp 1978; Allergy & Immunology, Fred Hutchinson Cancer Rsch Ctr 1980; **Fac Appt:** Prof A&I, Univ Iowa Coll Med

Bernstein, David Isaac MD [A&I] - **Spec Exp:** Occupational Asthma; Asthma; Rhinosinusitis; **Hospital:** Univ Hosp - Cincinnati; **Address:** 8444 Winton Rd, Cincinnati, OH 45231; **Phone:** 513-931-0775; **Board Cert:** Internal Medicine 1980; Allergy & Immunology 1983; Diagnostic Lab Immunology 1988; **Med School:** Univ Cincinnati 1977; **Resid:** Internal Medicine, Cleveland Clinic 1980; **Fellow:** Allergy & Immunology, Northwestern Univ 1982; **Fac Appt:** Clin Prof Med, Univ Cincinnati

Allergy & Immunology

Bernstein, Jonathan A MD [A&I] - **Spec Exp:** Asthma; Occupational Asthma; Drug Allergy; Eczema; **Hospital:** Univ Hosp - Cincinnati; **Address:** 8444 Winton Rd, Cincinnati, OH 45267-0563; **Phone:** 513-931-0775; **Board Cert:** Internal Medicine 1988; Allergy & Immunology 2011; **Med School:** Univ Cincinnati 1985; **Resid:** Internal Medicine, Cleveland Clinic 1988; **Fellow:** Allergy & Immunology, Northwestern Univ 1990; **Fac Appt:** Assoc Prof Med, Univ Cincinnati

Busse, William W MD [A&I] - **Spec Exp:** Asthma; Autoimmune Disease; Rhinitis; **Hospital:** Univ WI Hosp & Clins; **Address:** CSC Bldg, Ste K4, rm 910, 600 Highland Ave, Madison, WI 53792; **Phone:** 608-263-6180; **Board Cert:** Internal Medicine 1972; Allergy & Immunology 1974; **Med School:** Univ Wisc 1966; **Resid:** Internal Medicine, Cincinnati Genl Hosp 1968; Internal Medicine, Cincinnati Genl Hosp 1971; **Fellow:** Allergy & Immunology, Univ Wisconsin 1973; **Fac Appt:** Prof A&I, Univ Wisc

Grammer, Leslie C MD [A&I] - **Spec Exp:** Asthma; Sinusitis; Drug Allergy; **Hospital:** Northwestern Meml Hosp; **Address:** Northwestern Med Faculty Fdn, Amb Care Ctr, 675 N St Clair, Ste 18-250, Chicago, IL 60611-5975; **Phone:** 312-695-8624; **Board Cert:** Internal Medicine 1979; Allergy & Immunology 1981; Diagnostic Lab Immunology 1986; Occupational Medicine 1989; **Med School:** Northwestern Univ 1976; **Resid:** Internal Medicine, Northwestern Meml Hosp 1979; **Fellow:** Allergy & Immunology, Northwestern Meml Hosp 1981; **Fac Appt:** Prof Med, Northwestern Univ

Greenberger, Paul A MD [A&I] - **Spec Exp:** Asthma; Anaphylaxis; Drug Allergy; Hypersensitivity Pneumonitis; **Hospital:** Northwestern Meml Hosp, Jesse Brown VA Med Ctr; **Address:** Northwestern Med Faculty Fdn, Ambulatory Care Ctr, 675 N St Clair Fl 18 - Ste 18-250, Chicago, IL 60611; **Phone:** 312-695-8624; **Board Cert:** Internal Medicine 1976; Allergy & Immunology 1979; Diagnostic Lab Immunology 1986; **Med School:** Indiana Univ 1973; **Resid:** Internal Medicine, Jewish Hosp 1976; **Fellow:** Allergy & Immunology, Northwestern Meml Hosp 1978; **Fac Appt:** Prof A&I, Northwestern Univ-Feinberg Sch Med

Jost, Barbara Capes MD [A&I] - **Spec Exp:** Sinusitis; Drug Allergy; **Hospital:** St. Luke's Hosp - Chesterfield, MO, Barnes-Jewish Hosp; **Address:** Internal Medicine Assocs, South Medical Bldg, Ste 5009, 224 S Woods Mill Rd, Chesterfield, MO 63017; **Phone:** 314-878-6260; **Board Cert:** Internal Medicine 2011; Allergy & Immunology 2005; **Med School:** St Louis Univ 1998; **Resid:** Internal Medicine, Barnes Jewish Hosp 2001; Allergy & Immunology, Barnes Jewish Hosp 2005

Korenblat, Phillip E MD [A&I] - **Spec Exp:** Allergy; Asthma; Anaphylaxis; Airway Disorders; **Hospital:** Barnes-Jewish West County Hosp, Missouri Baptist Med Ctr; **Address:** 1040 N Mason Rd, Ste 115, St Louis, MO 63141-6361; **Phone:** 314-542-0606; **Board Cert:** Internal Medicine 1971; Allergy & Immunology 1974; **Med School:** Univ Ark 1960; **Resid:** Internal Medicine, Barnes Jewish Hosp 1965; **Fellow:** Allergy & Immunology, Scripps Clin Rsch Fdn 1966; **Fac Appt:** Clin Prof A&I, Washington Univ, St Louis

Li, James Tung-Chieh MD [A&I] - **Spec Exp:** Asthma; Allergy; **Hospital:** St. Mary's Hosp - Rochester MN (Mayo), Rochester Methodist Hosp; **Address:** Mayo Clinic - Division of Allergic Diseases, 200 First St SW, Box W15B, Rochester, MN 55905; **Phone:** 507-284-4966; **Board Cert:** Internal Medicine 1984; Allergy & Immunology 1985; **Med School:** Duke Univ 1981; **Resid:** Internal Medicine, Duke Univ Hosp 1984; **Fellow:** Allergy & Immunology, Mayo Med Ctr&Clin-Rochester 1985

Routes, John M MD [A&I] - **Spec Exp:** Immunodeficiency Disorders; Asthma; Allergy; **Hospital:** Chldns Hosp - Wisconsin; **Address:** Children's Hosp Wisconsin, 9000 W Wisconsin Ave, Ste 440, Milwaukee, WI 53226; **Phone:** 414-266-6840; **Board Cert:** Internal Medicine 1984; Allergy & Immunology 1987; **Med School:** Indiana Univ 1981; **Resid:** Internal Medicine, Univ Utah Affil Hosps 1984; **Fellow:** Allergy & Immunology, Natl Jewish Hosp 1989; Infectious Disease, Natl Jewish Hosp 1990; **Fac Appt:** Prof Ped, Med Coll Wisc

Sanders, Georgiana MD [A&I] - **Spec Exp:** Asthma; Food Allergy & Eczema; Rhinitis; **Hospital:** Univ of Michigan Hosp; **Address:** Univ MI Allergy Specialty Clin, 24 Frank Lloyd Wright Dr, Ste H-2100, PO Box 442, Ann Arbor, MI 48105; **Phone:** 734-936-5634; **Board Cert:** Pediatrics 1982; Allergy & Immunology 1985; **Med School:** Univ Cincinnati 1975; **Resid:** Pediatrics, Chldns Hosp Mich 1978; Pediatrics, Boston City Hosp 1979; **Fellow:** Allergy & Immunology, Univ of Michigan Hosp 1984; **Fac Appt:** Asst Clin Prof Med, Univ Mich Med Sch

Tillinghast, Jeffrey MD [A&I] - **Hospital:** Barnes-Jewish Hosp; **Address:** 1040 N Mason Rd, Ste 115, St Louis, MO 63141; **Phone:** 314-542-0606; **Board Cert:** Internal Medicine 1984; Allergy & Immunology 1987; **Med School:** Washington Univ, St Louis 1980; **Resid:** Internal Medicine, Barnes Hospital 1983; Allergy & Immunology, Natl Inst Health 1985; **Fac Appt:** Assoc Prof Med, Washington Univ, St Louis

Wood, John A MD [A&I] - **Spec Exp:** Asthma; **Hospital:** St. Luke's Hosp - Chesterfield, MO; **Address:** Internal Med Assocs, 224 S Woods Mill Rd, Ste 500 S, Chesterfield, MO 63017; **Phone:** 314-878-6260; **Board Cert:** Internal Medicine 1972; Pulmonary Disease 1978; Allergy & Immunology 1979; **Med School:** Univ Okla Coll Med 1968; **Resid:** Internal Medicine, Univ Hosp 1970; Internal Medicine, Barnes Hosp-Wash Univ Sch Med 1971; **Fellow:** Pulmonary Disease, Wash Univ Sch Med 1977; Allergy & Immunology, Wash Univ Sch Med 1977; **Fac Appt:** Asst Prof Med, Washington Univ, St Louis

Southwest

Freeman, Theodore M MD [A&I] - **Spec Exp:** Insect Allergies; Asthma; Rhinitis; **Hospital:** Methodist Hosp-San Antonio; **Address:** 5282 Medical Drive, Ste 500, San Antonio, TX 78229; **Phone:** 210-614-7594; **Board Cert:** Internal Medicine 1983; Allergy & Immunology 1987; Clinical & Laboratory Immunology 1988; **Med School:** Univ S Fla Coll Med 1980; **Resid:** Internal Medicine, Keesler Med Ctr 1983; **Fellow:** Allergy & Immunology, Wilford Hall Med Ctr 1986; Diagnostic Lab Immunology, Mass Genl Hosp 1987; **Fac Appt:** Assoc Prof Med, Uniformed Srvs Univ, Bethesda

Gruchalla, Rebecca S MD/PhD [A&I] - **Spec Exp:** Asthma & Allergy; Drug Allergy; Immunodeficiency Disorders; **Hospital:** UT Southwestern Med Ctr at Dallas, Chldns Med Ctr of Dallas; **Address:** Div Allergy & Immunology, 5323 Harry Hines Blvd, Dallas, TX 75390-8872; **Phone:** 214-645-2800; **Board Cert:** Internal Medicine 1988; Allergy & Immunology 2001; **Med School:** Univ Tex SW, Dallas 1985; **Resid:** Internal Medicine, Hosp Univ Penn 1988; **Fellow:** Allergy & Immunology, Univ Tex SW Med Ctr 1990; **Fac Appt:** Prof Med, Univ Tex SW, Dallas

Lewis, John C MD [A&I] - **Spec Exp:** Asthma; Rhinosinusitis; Mast Cell Diseases; Eosinophil Disorders; **Hospital:** Mayo Clinic - Scottsdale; **Address:** Mayo Clinic-Div Allergy & Immunology, 13400 E Shea Blvd, Scottsdale, AZ 85259-5404; **Phone:** 480-301-8227; **Board Cert:** Internal Medicine 1985; Allergy & Immunology 2001; **Med School:** Loyola Univ-Stritch Sch Med 1982; **Resid:** Internal Medicine, Wilford Hall USAF Med Ctr 1985; **Fellow:** Allergy & Immunology, Mayo Clinic 1990; **Fac Appt:** Asst Prof Med, Mayo Med Sch

Allergy & Immunology

Schubert, Mark S MD/PhD [A&I] - **Spec Exp:** Asthma & Allergy; Sinus Disorders; **Hospital:** Banner Good Samaritan Regl Med Ctr - Phoenix, St. Joseph's Hosp & Med Ctr - Phoenix; **Address:** Allergy Asthma Clinic, 300 W Clarendon Rd, Ste 120, Phoenix, AZ 85013-2517; **Phone:** 602-277-3337; **Board Cert:** Internal Medicine 1987; Allergy & Immunology 2009; **Med School:** Univ Ariz Coll Med 1983; **Resid:** Neurological Surgery, Barrow Neurological Inst 1985; Internal Medicine, Good Samaritan Med Ctr 1987; **Fellow:** Allergy Immunology & Rheumatology, Stanford Univ Med Ctr 1989; **Fac Appt:** Assoc Clin Prof Med, Univ Ariz Coll Med

Wong, Duane W MD [A&I] - **Spec Exp:** Pediatric Allergy & Immunology; **Hospital:** Phoenix Children's Hosp, Mercy Gilbert Med Ctr; **Address:** Arizona Allergy Assocs, 348 E Virginia Ave, Phoenix, AZ 85004; **Phone:** 480-897-6992; **Board Cert:** Allergy & Immunology 2012; Pediatrics 2010; **Med School:** Northwestern Univ-Feinberg Sch Med 1984; **Resid:** Pediatrics, Children's Hosp/UCLA 1986; Pediatrics, Phoenix Children's Hosp 1987; **Fellow:** Allergy & Immunology, Children's Hosp/UCLA 1989

West Coast and Pacific

Altman, Leonard C MD [A&I] - **Spec Exp:** Urticaria; Asthma; Sinusitis; Allergy; **Hospital:** Univ Wash Med Ctr, Seattle Chldns Hosp; **Address:** 9725 3rd Ave NE, Ste 500, Seattle, WA 98115; **Phone:** 206-527-1200; **Board Cert:** Internal Medicine 1975; Allergy & Immunology 1979; **Med School:** Harvard Med Sch 1969; **Resid:** Internal Medicine, Univ Wash Affil Hosps 1971; Internal Medicine, Univ Wash Affil Hosps 1975; **Fellow:** Allergy & Immunology, Natl Inst Hlth 1974; **Fac Appt:** Clin Prof Med, Univ Wash

Henderson Jr, William R MD [A&I] - **Spec Exp:** Asthma; Allergic Rhinitis; **Hospital:** Univ Wash Med Ctr; **Address:** 1959 NE Pacific St, Box 356166, Seattle, WA 98195-6166; **Phone:** 206-598-4615; **Board Cert:** Internal Medicine 1976; Allergy & Immunology 1979; **Med School:** UCSF 1973; **Resid:** Internal Medicine, Stanford Med Ctr 1975; Internal Medicine, Natl Inst Hlth 1976; **Fellow:** Allergy & Immunology, Natl Inst Hlth 1978; **Fac Appt:** Prof Med, Univ Wash

Meltzer, Eli O MD [A&I] - **Spec Exp:** Asthma & Allergy; Sinus Disorders; Rhinitis; **Hospital:** Rady Children's Hosp - San Diego, Sharp Meml Hosp; **Address:** Allergy & Asthma Medical & Research Ctr, 5776 Ruffin Rd, San Diego, CA 92123; **Phone:** 858-292-1144; **Board Cert:** Pediatrics 1969; Allergy & Immunology 1972; Pediatric Allergy & Immunology 1969; **Med School:** Jefferson Med Coll 1964; **Resid:** Pediatrics, St Christophers Hosp Chldn 1967; **Fellow:** Pediatric Allergy & Immunology, National Jewish Hosp 1969; **Fac Appt:** Clin Prof Ped, UCSD

Montanaro, Anthony MD [A&I] - **Spec Exp:** Asthma; Allergy; Immunodeficiency Disorders; **Hospital:** OR Hlth & Sci Univ; **Address:** OHSU Div Allergy & Clin Immunology, 3181 SW Sam Jackson Park Rd, MC OP-34, Portland, OR 97239-2098; **Phone:** 503-494-4300; **Board Cert:** Internal Medicine 1981; Allergy & Immunology 1993; Rheumatology 1984; **Med School:** Univ Wash 1978; **Resid:** Internal Medicine, Mercy Med Ctr 1981; **Fellow:** Allergy Immunology & Rheumatology, Oregon Hlth Sci Univ 1983; **Fac Appt:** Prof Med, Oregon Hlth & Sci Univ

Ostrom, Nancy K MD [A&I] - **Spec Exp:** Asthma & Allergy; **Hospital:** Rady Children's Hosp - San Diego; **Address:** Allergy/Asthma Med Group & Research Ctr, 5776 Ruffin Rd, San Diego, CA 92123; **Phone:** 858-292-1144; **Board Cert:** Pediatrics 1984; Allergy & Immunology 1987; **Med School:** Mayo Med Sch 1980; **Resid:** Pediatrics, Mayo Clinic 1983; **Fellow:** Allergy & Immunology, Mayo Clinic 1985; **Fac Appt:** Assoc Clin Prof Ped, UCSD

Spector, Sheldon Laurence MD [A&I] - **Spec Exp:** Asthma; Urticaria; **Hospital:** UCLA Ronald Reagan Med Ctr; **Address:** 11645 Wilshire Blvd, Ste 1155, Los Angeles, CA 90025; **Phone:** 310-966-9022; **Board Cert:** Internal Medicine 1974; Allergy & Immunology 1980; **Med School:** Wayne State Univ 1964; **Resid:** Internal Medicine, Mt Sinai Hosp 1965; Internal Medicine, UCLA Med Ctr 1969; **Fellow:** Allergy & Immunology, Natl Jewish Hosp-Rsch Ctr 1971; **Fac Appt:** Clin Prof Med, UCLA

Tamaroff, Marc A MD [A&I] - **Spec Exp:** Sinus Disorders; Asthma; Rhinitis; Immune Deficiency; **Hospital:** Long Beach Meml Med Ctr, Lakewood Reg Med Ctr; **Address:** 3816 Woodruff Ave, Ste 209, Long Beach, CA 90808-2145; **Phone:** 562-496-4749; **Board Cert:** Internal Medicine 1979; Allergy & Immunology 1983; **Med School:** Univ Ariz Coll Med 1974; **Resid:** Internal Medicine, St Mary Med Ctr 1977; **Fellow:** Allergy & Immunology, UCLA Med Ctr 1979; **Fac Appt:** Assoc Clin Prof Med, UCLA

Wasserman, Stephen I MD [A&I] - **Spec Exp:** Asthma; Rhinitis; Sinus Disorders; Urticaria; **Hospital:** UCSD Med Ctr, VA San Diego Hlthcre Sys; **Address:** 9350 Campus Point Drive, Ste 2B, La Jolla, CA 92093-0637; **Phone:** 858-657-8400; **Board Cert:** Internal Medicine 1973; Allergy & Immunology 2008; **Med School:** UCLA 1968; **Resid:** Internal Medicine, Peter Bent Brigham Hosp 1970; **Fellow:** Allergy & Immunology, R Breck-PB Brigham Hosps 1974; **Fac Appt:** Prof Med, UCSD

The Best in American Medicine
www.CastleConnolly.com

Cardiovascular Disease

a subspecialty of Internal Medicine

Cardiovascular Disease: An internist specializing in diseases of the heart, lungs and blood vessels and manages complex cardiac conditions such as heart attacks and life-threatening, abnormal heartbeat rhythms.

Cardiac Electrophysiology: A field of special interest within the subspecialty of cardiovascular disease which involves intricate technical procedures to evaluate heart rhythms and determine appropriate treatment for them.

Interventional Cardiology: An area of medicine within the subspecialty of cardiology which uses specialized imaging and other diagnostic techniques to evaluate blood flow and pressure in the coronary arteries and chambers of the heart, and uses technical procedures and medications to treat abnormalities that impair the function of the heart.

Training Required: Three years in internal medicine *plus* additional training and examination for certification in cardiovascular disease, clinical electrophysiology or interventional cardiology

CARDIOVASCULAR DISEASE

New England

Balady, Gary MD [Cv] - **Spec Exp:** Preventive Cardiology; **Hospital:** Boston Med Ctr; **Address:** Boston Med Ctr, Dept Cardiology, 732 Harrison Ave, Preston Family Bldg Fl 3, Boston, MA 02118; **Phone:** 617-638-7490; **Board Cert:** Internal Medicine 1982; Cardiovascular Disease 1985; **Med School:** UMDNJ-Rutgers Med Sch 1979; **Resid:** Internal Medicine, Boston Univ Med Ctr 1982; **Fellow:** Cardiovascular Disease, Boston Univ Med Ctr 1985; **Fac Appt:** Prof Med, Boston Univ

Cabin, Henry S MD [Cv] - **Spec Exp:** Interventional Cardiology; Cardiac Catheterization; **Hospital:** Yale-New Haven Hosp, Yale Med Group; **Address:** 11 Harrison Ave, Branford, CT 06405; **Phone:** 203-483-8300; **Board Cert:** Internal Medicine 1978; Cardiovascular Disease 1983; **Med School:** Yale Univ 1975; **Resid:** Internal Medicine, Yale-New Haven Hosp 1978; **Fellow:** Internal Medicine, Natl Heart Lung and Blood Inst 1981; Cardiovascular Disease, Yale-New Haven Hosp 1982; **Fac Appt:** Prof Med, Yale Univ

Catherwood, Edward MD [Cv] - **Hospital:** Dartmouth - Hitchcock Med Ctr; **Address:** Dartmouth-Hitchcock Medical Ctr, Div Cardiology, 1 Medical Center Drive, Lebanon, NH 03756; **Phone:** 603-650-7607; **Board Cert:** Internal Medicine 1978; Cardiovascular Disease 1981; Critical Care Medicine 2009; **Med School:** Jefferson Med Coll 1975; **Resid:** Internal Medicine, Hahnemann Univ Hosp 1978; **Fellow:** Cardiovascular Disease, Hahnemann Univ Hosp 1980; **Fac Appt:** Asst Prof Med, Dartmouth Med Sch

DeNofrio, David MD [Cv] - **Spec Exp:** Transplant Medicine-Heart; Heart Failure; **Hospital:** Tufts Med Ctr; **Address:** Tufts Med Ctr, Cardiovascular Div, 800 Washington St, Box 5931, Boston, MA 02111; **Phone:** 617-636-8068; **Board Cert:** Internal Medicine 2011; Cardiovascular Disease 2005; **Med School:** Tufts Univ 1988; **Resid:** Internal Medicine, Barnes Hosp 1991; **Fellow:** Cardiovascular Disease, Duke Univ Med Ctr 1995

Diver, Daniel J MD [Cv] - **Spec Exp:** Angioplasty; Coronary Artery Disease; **Hospital:** St. Francis Hosp & Med Ctr; **Address:** St Francis Hosp - Div Cardiology, 114 Woodland St, Hartford, CT 06105; **Phone:** 860-714-4019; **Board Cert:** Internal Medicine 1984; Cardiovascular Disease 1989; **Med School:** Johns Hopkins Univ 1981; **Resid:** Internal Medicine, Johns Hopkins Hosp 1984; **Fellow:** Cardiovascular Disease, Beth Israel Hosp/Harvard 1987; **Fac Appt:** Prof Med, Univ Conn

Hutter Jr, Adolph M MD [Cv] - **Hospital:** Mass Genl Hosp; **Address:** Mass Genl Hosp, 55 Fruit St, Yawkey Ctr, rm 5B, Boston, MA 02114-3139; **Phone:** 617-726-2884; **Board Cert:** Internal Medicine 1969; Cardiovascular Disease 1971; **Med School:** Univ Wisc 1963; **Resid:** Internal Medicine, Strong Meml Hosp 1968; **Fellow:** Cardiovascular Disease, Mass Genl Hosp 1970; **Fac Appt:** Prof Med, Harvard Med Sch

Johnson, Paula A MD [Cv] - **Spec Exp:** Heart Disease in Women; Women's Health; **Hospital:** Brigham and Women's Hosp (page 57); **Address:** Brigham & Womens Hosp, 75 Francis St, PB5-534, Boston, MA 02115; **Phone:** 857-307-4000; **Board Cert:** Internal Medicine 1988; Cardiovascular Disease 2011; **Med School:** Harvard Med Sch 1985; **Resid:** Internal Medicine, Brigham & Womens Hosp 1988; **Fellow:** Cardiovascular Disease, Brigham & Womens Hosp 1991; **Fac Appt:** Assoc Prof Med, Harvard Med Sch

Kirshenbaum, James M MD [Cv] - **Spec Exp:** Cardiac Catheterization; Coronary Artery Disease; Congestive Heart Failure; **Hospital:** Brigham and Women's Hosp (page 57); **Address:** Brigham & Womens Hosp, Div Cardiology, 75 Francis St, Boston, MA 02115; **Phone:** 857-307-1967; **Board Cert:** Internal Medicine 1982; Cardiovascular Disease 1985; **Med School:** Harvard Med Sch 1979; **Resid:** Internal Medicine, Peter Bent Brigham Hosp 1982; **Fellow:** Cardiovascular Disease, Brigham & Womens Hosp 1985; **Fac Appt:** Assoc Prof Med, Harvard Med Sch

Konstam, Marvin A MD [Cv] - **Spec Exp:** Transplant Medicine-Heart; Heart Failure; Coronary Angioplasty/Stents; **Hospital:** Tufts Med Ctr; **Address:** Tufts Med Ctr, Div Cardiology, 800 Washington St, Box 108, Boston, MA 02111; **Phone:** 617-636-6293; **Board Cert:** Internal Medicine 1979; Cardiovascular Disease 1981; Diagnostic Radiology 1980; Advanced Heart Failure & Transplant Cardiology 2010; **Med School:** Columbia P&S 1975; **Resid:** Diagnostic Radiology, Mass Genl Hosp 1978; Internal Medicine, Mass Genl Hosp 1979; **Fellow:** Cardiovascular Disease, Brigham & Women's Hosp 1981; **Fac Appt:** Prof Med, Tufts Univ

Kuvin, Jeffrey T MD [Cv] - **Spec Exp:** Preventive Cardiology; Congenital Heart Disease; Echocardiography; **Hospital:** Tufts Med Ctr; **Address:** 750 Washington St, Box 315, Boston, MA 02111; **Phone:** 617-636-5846; **Board Cert:** Internal Medicine 2005; Cardiovascular Disease 2009; **Med School:** Emory Univ 1992; **Resid:** Internal Medicine, New England Med Ctr 1996; **Fellow:** Cardiovascular Disease, New England Med Ctr 1999; **Fac Appt:** Assoc Prof Med, Tufts Univ

Liang, Bruce T MD [Cv] - **Spec Exp:** Ischemic Heart Disease; Congestive Heart Failure; **Hospital:** Univ of Conn Hlth Ctr, John Dempsey Hosp; **Address:** 263 Farmington Ave, MS 06030, Cardiopulmonary & Hypertension Service, Farmington, CT 06030-2202; **Phone:** 860-679-3343; **Board Cert:** Internal Medicine 1985; Cardiovascular Disease 1987; **Med School:** Harvard Med Sch 1982; **Resid:** Internal Medicine, Hosp Univ Penn 1985; **Fellow:** Cardiovascular Disease, Brigham & Womens Hosp 1987; **Fac Appt:** Prof Med, Univ Conn

Loscalzo, Joseph MD/PhD [Cv] - **Spec Exp:** Coronary Artery Disease; Peripheral Vascular Disease; **Hospital:** Brigham and Women's Hosp (page 57); **Address:** Brigham & Women's Hosp, Div Cardiology, 75 Francis St, Boston, MA 02115; **Phone:** 617-732-6340; **Board Cert:** Internal Medicine 1981; Cardiovascular Disease 1983; **Med School:** Univ Pennsylvania 1978; **Resid:** Internal Medicine, Peter Bent Brigham Hosp 1981; **Fellow:** Cardiovascular Disease, Brigham & Women's Hosp 1983; **Fac Appt:** Prof Med, Harvard Med Sch

Manning, Warren J MD [Cv] - **Spec Exp:** Heart Valve Disease; Echocardiography; Cardiomyopathy; **Hospital:** Beth Israel Deaconess Med Ctr - Boston; **Address:** Beth Israel Deacones Med Ctr, 330 Brookline Ave, Boston, MA 02215-5400; **Phone:** 617-667-2192; **Board Cert:** Internal Medicine 1986; Cardiovascular Disease 1989; Echocardiography 2006; **Med School:** Harvard Med Sch 1983; **Resid:** Internal Medicine, Beth Israel Hosp 1986; **Fellow:** Cardiovascular Disease, Beth Israel Hosp 1989; **Fac Appt:** Prof Med, Harvard Med Sch

O'Gara, Patrick T MD [Cv] - **Spec Exp:** Heart Valve Disease; Coronary Artery Disease; Aortic Diseases & Dissection; **Hospital:** Brigham and Women's Hosp (page 57); **Address:** Brigham & Womens Hosp, Cardiovascular Div, 75 Francis St, Boston, MA 02115; **Phone:** 857-307-1990; **Board Cert:** Internal Medicine 1981; Cardiovascular Disease 1983; **Med School:** Northwestern Univ 1978; **Resid:** Internal Medicine, Mass Genl Hosp 1981; **Fellow:** Cardiovascular Disease, Mass Genl Hosp 1983; **Fac Appt:** Assoc Prof Med, Harvard Med Sch

Pfeffer, Marc Alan MD [Cv] - **Hospital:** Brigham and Women's Hosp (page 57); **Address:** Brigham & Women's Hosp, 75 Francis St, Boston, MA 02115; **Phone:** 617-732-5681; **Board Cert:** Internal Medicine 1979; Cardiovascular Disease 1981; Advanced Heart Failure & Transplant Cardiology 2010; **Med School:** Univ Okla Coll Med 1976; **Resid:** Internal Medicine, Peter Bent Brigham Hosp 1979; **Fellow:** Cardiovascular Disease, Peter Bent Brigham Hosp 1980; **Fac Appt:** Prof Med, Harvard Med Sch

Cardiovascular Disease

Phillips, Robert A MD/PhD [Cv] - **Spec Exp:** Hypertension; Coronary Artery Disease; Heart Valve Disease; **Hospital:** UMass Memorial Med Ctr; **Address:** UMass Meml Med Ctr-Univ Campus, 55 Lake Ave North, S3-836, Worcester, MA 01655; **Phone:** 508-334-3452; **Board Cert:** Internal Medicine 1983; Cardiovascular Disease 1985; **Med School:** Mount Sinai Sch Med 1980; **Resid:** Internal Medicine, Columbia Presby Med Ctr 1983; **Fellow:** Cardiovascular Disease, Mt Sinai Med Ctr 1985; Hypertension, Mt Sinai Med Ctr 1986; **Fac Appt:** Prof Med, Univ Mass Sch Med

Ridker, Paul M MD [Cv] - **Spec Exp:** Coronary Artery Disease; Preventive Cardiology; Cholesterol/Lipid Disorders; **Hospital:** Brigham and Women's Hosp (page 57); **Address:** Southern Jamaica Plain Health Ctr, 640 Centre St, Jamaica Plains, MA 02130; **Phone:** 617-278-0869; **Board Cert:** Internal Medicine 1989; **Med School:** Harvard Med Sch 1986; **Resid:** Internal Medicine, Brigham & Women's Hosp 1989; **Fellow:** Cardiovascular Disease, Brigham & Women's Hosp 1991; **Fac Appt:** Assoc Prof Med, Harvard Med Sch

Roberts, Barbara H MD [Cv] - **Spec Exp:** Heart Disease in Women; Preventive Cardiology; **Hospital:** Miriam Hosp; **Address:** The Miriam Hosp - Women's Cardiac Ctr, 164 Summit Ave, Fain Med Bldg, Providence, RI 02906; **Phone:** 401-793-5750; **Board Cert:** Internal Medicine 1975; Cardiovascular Disease 1975; **Med School:** Case West Res Univ 1968; **Resid:** Internal Medicine, Yale-New Haven Hosp 1971; **Fellow:** Cardiovascular Disease, PB Brigham Hosp-Harvard 1975; **Fac Appt:** Assoc Clin Prof Med, Brown Univ

Stevenson, Lynne W MD [Cv] - **Spec Exp:** Heart Failure; Transplant Medicine-Heart; **Hospital:** Brigham and Women's Hosp (page 57); **Address:** Brigham & Women's Hospital, 75 Francis St, Boston, MA 02115; **Phone:** 857-307-4000; **Board Cert:** Internal Medicine 1982; Cardiovascular Disease 1985; **Med School:** Stanford Univ 1979; **Resid:** Internal Medicine, UCLA Med Ctr 1982; **Fellow:** Cardiovascular Disease, UCLA Med Ctr 1984; **Fac Appt:** Prof Med, Harvard Med Sch

Zusman, Randall M MD [Cv] - **Spec Exp:** Hypertension; Cholesterol/Lipid Disorders; Atrial Fibrillation; Coronary Artery Disease; **Hospital:** Mass Genl Hosp; **Address:** Mass Genl Hosp, Yawkey Ctr, 55 Fruit St, Ste 5928, Boston, MA 02114; **Phone:** 617-726-7790; **Board Cert:** Internal Medicine 1976; Cardiovascular Disease 1983; **Med School:** Yale Univ 1973; **Resid:** Internal Medicine, Mass General Hosp 1978; Internal Medicine, Natl Heart, Lung, & Blood Inst (NHBLI) 1977; **Fellow:** Cardiovascular Disease, Mass General Hosp 1979; **Fac Appt:** Assoc Prof Med, Harvard Med Sch

Mid Atlantic

Andersen, Holly S MD [Cv] - **Spec Exp:** Preventive Cardiology; Women's Health; Mitral Valve Prolapse; **Hospital:** NY-Presby/Weill Cornell Med Ctr, NY (page 66); **Address:** 425 E 61st St Fl 6, New York, NY 10021; **Phone:** 212-628-6100; **Board Cert:** Internal Medicine 2002; Cardiovascular Disease 2005; **Med School:** Univ Rochester 1989; **Resid:** Internal Medicine, NY Presby-Cornell Med Ctr 1992; **Fellow:** Cardiovascular Disease, NY Presby-Cornell Med Ctr 1995; **Fac Appt:** Assoc Clin Prof Med, Cornell Univ-Weill Med Coll

Blumenthal, David S MD [Cv] - **Spec Exp:** Heart Valve Disease; Preventive Cardiology; Coronary Artery Disease; **Hospital:** NY-Presby/Weill Cornell Med Ctr, NY (page 66); **Address:** 407 E 70th St, Fl 1, New York, NY 10021-5302; **Phone:** 212-861-3222; **Board Cert:** Internal Medicine 1978; Cardiovascular Disease 1981; **Med School:** Cornell Univ-Weill Med Coll 1975; **Resid:** Internal Medicine, NY Hosp 1978; Internal Medicine, NY Hosp 1981; **Fellow:** Cardiovascular Disease, Johns Hopkins Hosp 1980; **Fac Appt:** Clin Prof Med, Cornell Univ-Weill Med Coll

Blumenthal, Roger S MD [Cv] - **Spec Exp:** Preventive Cardiology; Hypertension; Cardiovascular Disease/Young Adult; **Hospital:** Johns Hopkins Hosp (page 61); **Address:** Johns Hopkins Medicine, 601 N Caroline St, Outpatient Center Fl 7, Baltimore, MD 21287; **Phone:** 410-502-0550; **Board Cert:** Internal Medicine 1988; Cardiovascular Disease 2003; **Med School:** Cornell Univ-Weill Med Coll 1985; **Resid:** Internal Medicine, Johns Hopkins Hosp 1988; **Fellow:** Cardiovascular Disease, Johns Hopkins Hosp 1992; **Fac Appt:** Assoc Prof Med, Johns Hopkins Univ

Borer, Jeffrey S MD [Cv] - **Spec Exp:** Heart Valve Disease; Heart Failure; Nuclear Cardiology; **Hospital:** SUNY Downstate Med Ctr (Univ Hosp of Bklyn), NY-Presby/Weill Cornell Med Ctr, NY (page 66); **Address:** SUNY Downstate Med Ctr, Div Cardiology, 445 Lenox Rd, Brooklyn, NY 11226; **Phone:** 212-289-7777; **Board Cert:** Internal Medicine 1973; Cardiovascular Disease 1975; **Med School:** Cornell Univ-Weill Med Coll 1969; **Resid:** Internal Medicine, Mass Genl Hosp 1971; **Fellow:** Cardiovascular Disease, Natl Heart, Lung & Blood Inst 1974; Cardiovascular Disease, Guy's Hosp 1975; **Fac Appt:** Prof Med, SUNY Downstate

Bove, Alfred A MD/PhD [Cv] - **Spec Exp:** Diving Medicine; Heart Failure; Sports Medicine; **Hospital:** Temple Univ Hosp; **Address:** Temple Univ Hosp, Div Cardiology, 3401 N Broad St, Parkinson Pavillon, Fl 9, Philadelphia, PA 19140; **Phone:** 215-707-9259; **Board Cert:** Internal Medicine 1971; Cardiovascular Disease 1983; Undersea & Hyperbaric Medicine 2010; **Med School:** Temple Univ 1966; **Resid:** Internal Medicine, Temple Univ Hosp 1970; **Fellow:** Physiology, Temple Univ Hosp 1970; Physiology, Mayo Clinic 1971; **Fac Appt:** Prof Emeritus Med, Temple Univ

Brozena, Susan C MD [Cv] - **Spec Exp:** Transplant Medicine-Heart; Congestive Heart Failure; Heart Disease in Women; **Hospital:** Hosp Univ Penn - UPHS (page 72); **Address:** 250 King of Prussia Rd, Ste 2G, Radnor, PA 19087; **Phone:** 610-902-2273; **Board Cert:** Internal Medicine 1984; Cardiovascular Disease 2011; Advanced Heart Failure & Transplant Cardiology 2010; **Med School:** Temple Univ 1981; **Resid:** Internal Medicine, Temple Univ Hosp 1984; **Fellow:** Cardiovascular Disease, Temple Univ Hosp 1986; **Fac Appt:** Assoc Prof Med, Univ Pennsylvania

Cohen, Howard A MD [Cv] - **Spec Exp:** Interventional Cardiology; Carotid Artery Stent Placement; **Hospital:** Lenox Hill Hosp (page 67); **Address:** Lenox Hill Hospital, Interventional Cardiology, 130 E 77th St Fl 9, New York, NY 10075; **Phone:** 212-434-2606; **Board Cert:** Internal Medicine 1974; Cardiovascular Disease 1977; **Med School:** NYU Sch Med 1970; **Resid:** Internal Medicine, Bellevue Hosp Ctr 1974; **Fellow:** Cardiovascular Disease, Johns Hopkins Hosp 1976

Coppola, John T MD [Cv] - **Spec Exp:** Cardiac Catheterization; Angioplasty; **Hospital:** NYU Langone Med Ctr (page 68), Bellevue Hosp Ctr; **Address:** 275 7th Ave Fl 3, New York, NY 10001; **Phone:** 646-660-9999; **Board Cert:** Internal Medicine 1981; Cardiovascular Disease 1983; Interventional Cardiology 2009; **Med School:** NY Med Coll 1978; **Resid:** Internal Medicine, St Vincent Catholic Med Ctr 1981; **Fellow:** Cardiovascular Disease, St Vincent Catholic Med Ctr 1983

Devereux, Richard B MD [Cv] - **Spec Exp:** Marfan's Syndrome; **Hospital:** NY-Presby/Weill Cornell Med Ctr, NY (page 66); **Address:** 525 E 68th St, rm K-415, New York, NY 10065; **Phone:** 212-746-4655; **Board Cert:** Internal Medicine 1974; Cardiovascular Disease 1977; **Med School:** Univ Pennsylvania 1971; **Resid:** Internal Medicine, New York Hosp 1974; **Fellow:** Cardiovascular Disease, Hosp Univ Penn 1976; **Fac Appt:** Prof Med, Cornell Univ-Weill Med Coll

Edmundowicz, Daniel MD [Cv] - **Spec Exp:** Preventive Cardiology; Cholesterol/Lipid Disorders; **Hospital:** Jeanes Hosp, Temple University Hosp-Episcopal Campus; **Address:** 3401 N Broad St, Parkinson Pavilion, 9th FL, Philadelphia, PA 19140; **Phone:** 215-707-9259; **Board Cert:** Internal Medicine 2005; Cardiovascular Disease 2009; **Med School:** Hahnemann Univ 1990; **Resid:** Internal Medicine, Temple Univ Hosp 1993; **Fellow:** Cardiovascular Disease, Univ Pittsburgh Med Ctr 1996; **Fac Appt:** Assoc Prof Med, Univ Pittsburgh

Cardiovascular Disease

Eisen, Howard J MD [Cv] - **Spec Exp:** Transplant Medicine-Heart; Congestive Heart Failure; **Hospital:** Hahnemann Univ Hosp; **Address:** Drexel Univ Coll Med, Div Cardiology, 230 N Broad St, Ste 740, Philadelphia, PA 19102; **Phone:** 215-762-3829; **Board Cert:** Internal Medicine 1984; Cardiovascular Disease 1987; Advanced Heart Failure & Transplant Cardiology 2010; **Med School:** Univ Pennsylvania 1981; **Resid:** Internal Medicine, Hosp Univ Penn 1984; **Fellow:** Cardiovascular Disease, Barnes Jewish Hosp 1987; **Fac Appt:** Prof Med, Drexel Univ Coll Med

Follansbee, William P MD [Cv] - **Spec Exp:** Nuclear Cardiology; Amyloid Heart Disease; Rheumatic Heart Disease; Scleroderma; **Hospital:** UPMC Presby, Pittsburgh; **Address:** A429 PUH UPMC Heart & Vascular Inst, 200 Lothrop St, Ste 5B, Pittsburgh, PA 15213; **Phone:** 412-647-3437; **Board Cert:** Internal Medicine 1977; Cardiovascular Disease 1981; **Med School:** Univ Pennsylvania 1974; **Resid:** Internal Medicine, Hosp Univ Penn 1978; **Fellow:** Cardiovascular Disease, Hosp Univ Penn 1980; **Fac Appt:** Prof Med, Univ Pittsburgh

Friedman, Sanford MD [Cv] - **Spec Exp:** Preventive Cardiology; **Hospital:** Mount Sinai Med Ctr (page 64); **Address:** 941 Park Ave, New York, NY 10028; **Phone:** 212-988-3772; **Board Cert:** Internal Medicine 1980; Cardiovascular Disease 1977; **Med School:** Tufts Univ 1971; **Resid:** Internal Medicine, Mt Sinai Med Ctr 1974; **Fellow:** Cardiovascular Disease, Mt Sinai Med Ctr 1976; **Fac Appt:** Assoc Clin Prof Med, Mount Sinai Sch Med

Fuster, Valentin MD/PhD [Cv] - **Spec Exp:** Coronary Artery Disease; Heart Valve Disease; Congenital Heart Disease; Preventive Cardiology; **Hospital:** Mount Sinai Med Ctr (page 64); **Address:** One Gustave Levy Pl, Box 1030, MS 10029, New York, NY 10029-6500; **Phone:** 212-241-7911; **Board Cert:** Internal Medicine 1976; Cardiovascular Disease 1977; **Med School:** Spain 1967; **Resid:** Internal Medicine, Mayo Clin 1972; Cardiovascular Disease, Mayo Clin 1974; **Fellow:** Cardiovascular Disease, Univ Edinburgh 1971; **Fac Appt:** Prof Med, Mount Sinai Sch Med

Gardin, Julius M MD [Cv] - **Spec Exp:** Echocardiography; Geriatric Cardiology; Preventive Cardiology; Cholesterol/Lipid Disorders; **Hospital:** Hackensack Univ Med Ctr; **Address:** Hackensack Univ Med Ctr, Dept Medicine, 30 Prospect Ave, 1 Main, Ste 1647, Hackensack, NJ 07601; **Phone:** 551-996-3500; **Board Cert:** Internal Medicine 1975; Cardiovascular Disease 1977; **Med School:** Univ Mich Med Sch 1972; **Resid:** Internal Medicine, Univ Mich Hosp 1975; **Fellow:** Cardiovascular Disease, Georgetown Univ Hosp 1977; **Fac Appt:** Prof Med, UMDNJ-Univ Med Dent NJ

Gliklich, Jerry MD [Cv] - **Spec Exp:** Heart Valve Disease; Arrhythmias; **Hospital:** NY-Presby/Columbia Univ Med Ctr, NY (page 66); **Address:** 173 Fort Washington Ave, Ste 606, New York, NY 10032; **Phone:** 212-305-5588; **Board Cert:** Internal Medicine 1978; Cardiovascular Disease 1981; **Med School:** Columbia P&S 1975; **Resid:** Internal Medicine, NY Hosp 1978; **Fellow:** Cardiovascular Disease, Columbia-Presby Med Ctr 1981; **Fac Appt:** Clin Prof Med, Columbia P&S

Goldberg, Nieca MD [Cv] - **Spec Exp:** Heart Disease in Women; Preventive Cardiology; Echocardiography; Women's Health; **Hospital:** NYU Langone Med Ctr (page 68), Lenox Hill Hosp (page 67); **Address:** Joan H. Tisch Ctr for Women's Hlth, 207 E 84th St, New York, NY 10028; **Phone:** 212-289-2045; **Board Cert:** Internal Medicine 1987; Cardiovascular Disease 2005; **Med School:** SUNY Downstate 1984; **Resid:** Internal Medicine, St Lukes Roosevelt Hosp Ctr 1987; **Fellow:** Cardiovascular Disease, SUNY Hlth Sci Ctr 1990; **Fac Appt:** Assoc Clin Prof Med, NYU Sch Med

Goodman, Dennis A MD [Cv] - **Spec Exp:** Preventive Cardiology; Cholesterol/Lipid Disorders; Complementary Medicine; **Hospital:** NYU Langone Med Ctr (page 68); **Address:** 635 Madison Ave Fl 3, New York, NY 10022; **Phone:** 212-439-6690; **Board Cert:** Internal Medicine 1984; Cardiovascular Disease 1989; Integrative Medicine 1995; **Med School:** South Africa 1979; **Resid:** Internal Medicine, Montefiore Med Ctr 1984; **Fellow:** Cardiovascular Disease, Baylor Coll Med 1987; **Fac Appt:** Clin Prof Med, NYU Sch Med

Gottdiener, John S MD [Cv] - **Spec Exp:** Echocardiography; **Hospital:** Univ of MD Med Ctr; **Address:** 110 S Paca St Fl 7, Baltimore, MD 21201; **Phone:** 410-328-6072; **Board Cert:** Internal Medicine 1975; Cardiovascular Disease 1979; **Med School:** Georgetown Univ 1970; **Resid:** Internal Medicine, Univ NC Hosp 1972; **Fellow:** Cardiovascular Disease, Georgetown Univ Hosp 1976; **Fac Appt:** Prof Med, Univ MD Sch Med

Gottlieb, Stephen Scott MD [Cv] - **Spec Exp:** Heart Failure; Transplant Medicine-Heart; **Hospital:** Univ of MD Med Ctr; **Address:** Univ Maryland Med Ctr, Cardiology, 419 W Redwood St, Ste 520, Baltimore, MD 21201; **Phone:** 410-328-8788; **Board Cert:** Internal Medicine 1984; Cardiovascular Disease 1987; **Med School:** Brown Univ 1981; **Resid:** Internal Medicine, Univ Chicago Hosps 1984; **Fellow:** Cardiovascular Disease, Mt Sinai Hosp 1985; **Fac Appt:** Prof Med, Univ MD Sch Med

Greenberg, Mark A MD [Cv] - **Spec Exp:** Interventional Cardiology; Cardiac Catheterization; Heart Valve Disease; **Hospital:** Montefiore Med Ctr-Moses Campus, NY; **Address:** 111 E 210th St, Division of Cardiology, Bronx, NY 10467; **Phone:** 718-920-4212; **Board Cert:** Internal Medicine 1976; Cardiovascular Disease 1979; **Med School:** Univ IL Coll Med 1973; **Resid:** Internal Medicine, Montefiore Med Ctr 1976; **Fellow:** Cardiovascular Disease, Montefiore Med Ctr 1978; **Fac Appt:** Clin Prof Med, Albert Einstein Coll Med

Halperin, Jonathan L MD [Cv] - **Spec Exp:** Peripheral Vascular Disease; Atrial Fibrillation; **Hospital:** Mount Sinai Med Ctr (page 64); **Address:** 1190 Fifth Ave, New York, NY 10029; **Phone:** 212-241-7243; **Board Cert:** Internal Medicine 1980; Cardiovascular Disease 1981; **Med School:** Boston Univ 1975; **Resid:** Internal Medicine, Mass Genl Hosp 1977; **Fellow:** Vascular Medicine, Boston Univ Med Ctr 1978; Cardiovascular Disease, Boston Univ Med Ctr 1980; **Fac Appt:** Prof Med, Mount Sinai Sch Med

Herling, Irving M MD [Cv] - **Spec Exp:** Cholesterol/Lipid Disorders; Preventive Cardiology; Heart Valve Disease; **Hospital:** Lankenau Hosp; **Address:** Lankenau Medical Ctr, Medical Office Bldg East, Ste 450, 100 E Lancaster Ave, Wynnewood, PA 19096; **Phone:** 484-572-0112; **Board Cert:** Internal Medicine 1977; Cardiovascular Disease 1979; **Med School:** Univ Pennsylvania 1974; **Resid:** Internal Medicine, Hosp Univ Penn 1977; **Fellow:** Cardiovascular Disease, Hosp Univ Penn 1979

Horn, Evelyn M MD [Cv] - **Spec Exp:** Pulmonary Hypertension; Heart Failure; Ventricular Assist Device (LVAD); Heart Disease-Complex; **Hospital:** NY-Presby/Weill Cornell Med Ctr, NY (page 66); **Address:** 520 E 70th St Starr Bldg Fl 4 - Ste 443, New York, NY 10021; **Phone:** 212-746-2381; **Board Cert:** Internal Medicine 1983; Cardiovascular Disease 1985; Advanced Heart Failure & Transplant Cardiology 2010; **Med School:** Mount Sinai Sch Med 1980; **Resid:** Internal Medicine, Mt Sinai Hosp 1983; **Fellow:** Cardiovascular Disease, Cedars-Sinai Med Ctr 1985; **Fac Appt:** Clin Prof Med, Cornell Univ-Weill Med Coll

Inra, Lawrence A MD [Cv] - **Spec Exp:** Coronary Artery Disease; Preventive Cardiology; Cholesterol/Lipid Disorders; Hypertension; **Hospital:** NY-Presby/Weill Cornell Med Ctr, NY (page 66), Hosp For Special Surgery (page 60); **Address:** 407 E 70th St, New York, NY 10021; **Phone:** 212-249-1011; **Board Cert:** Internal Medicine 1979; Cardiovascular Disease 1981; **Med School:** Johns Hopkins Univ 1976; **Resid:** Internal Medicine, NY Hosp 1979; **Fellow:** Cardiovascular Disease, Mt Sinai Hosp 1981; **Fac Appt:** Assoc Clin Prof Med, Cornell Univ-Weill Med Coll

Cardiovascular Disease

Jessup, Mariell MD [Cv] - **Spec Exp:** Congestive Heart Failure; Transplant Medicine-Heart; **Hospital:** Hosp Univ Penn - UPHS (page 72), Penn Presby Med Ctr - UPHS (page 72); **Address:** 2 East Perelman Pavilion, 3400 Civic Ctr Blvd, Philadelphia, PA 19104; **Phone:** 215-615-0808; **Board Cert:** Internal Medicine 1979; Cardiovascular Disease 1981; Advanced Heart Failure & Transplant Cardiology 2010; **Med School:** Hahnemann Univ 1976; **Resid:** Internal Medicine, Hahnemann Hosp 1979; **Fellow:** Cardiovascular Disease, Hosp Univ Penn 1982; **Fac Appt:** Prof Med, Univ Pennsylvania

Katz, Stuart D MD [Cv] - **Spec Exp:** Heart Failure; Transplant Medicine-Heart; **Hospital:** NYU Langone Med Ctr (page 68); **Address:** NYU Cardiology Assocs, 530 First Ave, Ste 9U, New York, NY 10016; **Phone:** 212-263-7751; **Board Cert:** Internal Medicine 1986; Cardiovascular Disease 1989; Advanced Heart Failure & Transplant Cardiology 2010; **Med School:** SUNY Downstate 1983; **Resid:** Internal Medicine, Francis Scott Key Med Ctr 1986; **Fellow:** Cardiovascular Disease, Montefiore Med Ctr 1989; **Fac Appt:** Prof Med, NYU Sch Med

Kostis, John B MD [Cv] - **Spec Exp:** Hypertension; Coronary Artery Disease; Cholesterol/Lipid Disorders; **Hospital:** Robert Wood Johnson Univ Hosp - New Brunswick; **Address:** 125 Paterson St, CAB Bldg - Fl 5 - Ste 5200, 1 Robert Wood Johnson Pl, New Brunswick, NJ 08901; **Phone:** 732-235-7685; **Board Cert:** Internal Medicine 1973; Cardiovascular Disease 1973; **Med School:** Greece 1960; **Resid:** Internal Medicine, Evanglismos Hosp 1964; Internal Medicine, Cumberland Med Ctr 1967; **Fellow:** Cardiovascular Disease, Philadelphia Genl Hosp 1969; **Fac Appt:** Prof Med, UMDNJ-RW Johnson Med Sch

Landzberg, Joel S MD [Cv] - **Spec Exp:** Preventive Cardiology; Coronary Artery Disease; Heart Failure; Heart Valve Disease; **Hospital:** Hackensack Univ Med Ctr, Valley Hosp; **Address:** 333 Old Hook Rd, Ste 200, Westwood, NJ 07675-3200; **Phone:** 201-664-0201; **Board Cert:** Internal Medicine 1986; Cardiovascular Disease 1989; Interventional Cardiology 2002; **Med School:** Columbia P&S 1983; **Resid:** Internal Medicine, Vanderbilt Univ Hosp 1986; **Fellow:** Cardiology Research, Moffit Hosp 1987; Cardiovascular Disease, Brigham & Womens Hosp 1991; **Fac Appt:** Assoc Clin Prof Med, UMDNJ-NJ Med Sch, Newark

Mather, Paul J MD [Cv] - **Spec Exp:** Heart Failure; Transplant Medicine-Heart; **Hospital:** Thomas Jefferson Univ Hosp; **Address:** Jefferson Heart Inst, 925 Chestnut St Fl Mezzainine, Philadelphia, PA 19107; **Phone:** 215-955-5050; **Board Cert:** Internal Medicine 2002; Cardiovascular Disease 2005; **Med School:** Temple Univ 1988; **Resid:** Internal Medicine, Temple Univ 1991; **Fellow:** Cardiovascular Disease, Temple Univ 1994; **Fac Appt:** Assoc Prof Med, Temple Univ

Meller, Jose MD [Cv] - **Hospital:** Mount Sinai Med Ctr (page 64); **Address:** 941 Park Ave, New York, NY 10028; **Phone:** 212-988-3772; **Board Cert:** Internal Medicine 1973; Cardiovascular Disease 1975; **Med School:** Chile 1969; **Resid:** Internal Medicine, Elmhurst Hosp 1971; Internal Medicine, Mt Sinai Med Ctr 1972; **Fellow:** Cardiovascular Disease, Mt Sinai Med Ctr 1974; **Fac Appt:** Clin Prof Med, Mount Sinai Sch Med

Naccarelli, Gerald V MD [Cv] - **Spec Exp:** Pacemakers; Arrhythmias; **Hospital:** Penn State Milton S Hershey Med Ctr; **Address:** 500 University Drive, UPC Bldg - Fl 1 - Ste 600, PO Box 850, Hershey, PA 17033; **Phone:** 717-531-3907; **Board Cert:** Internal Medicine 1979; Cardiovascular Disease 1981; **Med School:** Penn State Coll Med 1976; **Resid:** Internal Medicine, NC Bapt Hosp 1978; Internal Medicine, Hershey Med Ctr 1979; **Fellow:** Cardiovascular Disease, Indiana Univ Med Ctr 1982; **Fac Appt:** Prof Med, Penn State Coll Med

Parrillo, Joseph E MD [Cv] - **Spec Exp:** Septic Shock; Heart Failure; **Hospital:** Cooper Univ Hosp; **Address:** Cooper Medical Ctr, Div Cardiology, 1 Cooper Plaza, Dorrance Bldg, Ste D384, Camden, NJ 08103; **Phone:** 856-968-8349; **Board Cert:** Internal Medicine 1975; Allergy & Immunology 1977; Cardiovascular Disease 1981; Critical Care Medicine 2005; **Med School:** Cornell Univ-Weill Med Coll 1972; **Resid:** Internal Medicine, Mass Genl Hosp 1975; Allergy & Immunology, Natl Inst Hlth 1978; **Fellow:** Cardiovascular Disease, Mass Genl Hosp 1980; **Fac Appt:** Prof Med, UMDNJ-RW Johnson Med Sch

Poon, Michael MD [Cv] - **Spec Exp:** Coronary Artery Disease; Pulmonary Hypertension; Cardiac CT Angiography; Cardiac Imaging; **Hospital:** Stony Brook Univ Med Ctr, Mount Sinai Med Ctr (page 64); **Address:** Stony Brook Health Science Ctr, Level 4, rm 120, Stony Brook, NY 11794-8460; **Phone:** 631-444-5400; **Board Cert:** Cardiovascular Disease 2007; **Med School:** Mount Sinai Sch Med 1987; **Resid:** Internal Medicine, Mount Sinai Med Ctr 1991; **Fellow:** Cardiovascular Disease, Mount Sinai Med Ctr 1993; **Fac Appt:** Prof Med, SUNY Stony Brook

Reis, Steven E MD [Cv] - **Spec Exp:** Heart Disease in Women; Congestive Heart Failure; Metabolic Syndrome; Preventive Cardiology; **Hospital:** UPMC Presby, Pittsburgh, Magee-Womens Hosp - UPMC; **Address:** UPMC Cardiovascular Inst at Univ Ctr, 120 Lytton Ave, Ste 100B, Pittsburgh, PA 15213; **Phone:** 412-802-3000; **Board Cert:** Internal Medicine 2011; Cardiovascular Disease 2000; **Med School:** Harvard Med Sch 1987; **Resid:** Internal Medicine, Brigham & Womens Hosp 1990; **Fellow:** Cardiovascular Disease, Johns Hopkins Hosp 1994; **Fac Appt:** Assoc Prof Med, Univ Pittsburgh

Russell, Stuart D MD [Cv] - **Spec Exp:** Heart Failure; Transplant Medicine-Heart; **Hospital:** Johns Hopkins Hosp (page 61); **Address:** Johns Hopkins Hospital, 1800 Orleans St Zayed Bldg - rm 7125S, Baltimore, MD 21287; **Phone:** 410-955-5708; **Board Cert:** Internal Medicine 2006; Cardiovascular Disease 2007; Advanced Heart Failure & Transplant Cardiology 2010; **Med School:** Univ Wash 1991; **Resid:** Internal Medicine, Johns Hopkins Hosp 1994; **Fellow:** Cardiovascular Disease, Duke Univ Med Ctr 1997; **Fac Appt:** Assoc Prof Med, Johns Hopkins Univ

Saunders, Elijah MD [Cv] - **Spec Exp:** Hypertension-Complex; Coronary Disease in Black Populations; **Hospital:** Univ of MD Med Ctr; **Address:** Univ MD Med Sch, Div Hypertension, 419 W Redwood St, Ste 620, Baltimore, MD 21201; **Phone:** 410-328-4366; **Med School:** Univ MD Sch Med 1960; **Resid:** Internal Medicine, Univ Maryland Med Ctr; **Fellow:** Cardiovascular Disease, Univ Maryland Med Ctr; **Fac Appt:** Prof Med, Univ MD Sch Med

Schulman, Steven P MD [Cv] - **Hospital:** Johns Hopkins Hosp (page 61); **Address:** Johns Hopkins Medicine, 601 N Caroline St, Outpatient Center Fl 7, Baltimore, MD 21287; **Phone:** 410-502-0550; **Board Cert:** Internal Medicine 1986; Cardiovascular Disease 1989; **Med School:** Johns Hopkins Univ 1981; **Resid:** Internal Medicine, Johns Hopkins Hosp 1984; **Fellow:** Cardiovascular Disease, Johns Hopkins Hosp 1988; **Fac Appt:** Assoc Prof Med, Johns Hopkins Univ

Schwartz, Allan MD [Cv] - **Hospital:** NY-Presby/Columbia Univ Med Ctr, NY (page 66); **Address:** 173 Fort Washington Ave, Ste 4-600C, New York, NY 10032; **Phone:** 212-305-5367; **Board Cert:** Internal Medicine 1977; Cardiovascular Disease 1979; **Med School:** Columbia P&S 1974; **Resid:** Internal Medicine, Columbia-Presby Med Ctr 1976; **Fellow:** Cardiovascular Disease, Mass Genl Hosp 1978; **Fac Appt:** Clin Prof Med, Columbia P&S

Schwartz, William J MD [Cv] - **Spec Exp:** Coronary Artery Disease; Cardiac Catheterization; Congestive Heart Failure; **Hospital:** Mount Sinai Med Ctr (page 64); **Address:** Mt Sinai Multispecialty Physicians, 150 E 77th St, Ste 1E, New York, NY 10075; **Phone:** 212-439-6000; **Board Cert:** Internal Medicine 1978; Cardiovascular Disease 1981; **Med School:** Albert Einstein Coll Med 1975; **Resid:** Internal Medicine, Bronx Municipal Hosp 1978; **Fellow:** Cardiovascular Disease, Bronx Municipal Hosp 1979

Cardiovascular Disease

Shlofmitz, Richard A MD [Cv] - **Spec Exp:** Interventional Cardiology; Cardiac Catheterization; **Hospital:** St. Francis Hosp - The Heart Ctr (page 73); **Address:** 100 Port Washington Blvd, Ste 105, Vizza Pavilion, Roslyn, NY 11576; **Phone:** 516-390-9640; **Board Cert:** Internal Medicine 1984; Cardiovascular Disease 1987; **Med School:** NYU Sch Med 1980; **Resid:** Internal Medicine, North Shore Univ Hosp 1984; **Fellow:** Cardiovascular Disease, Columbia Presby Med Ctr 1987

Silvestry, Frank E MD [Cv] - **Spec Exp:** Heart Valve Disease; Ischemic Heart Disease; Non-Invasive Cardiology; Percutaneous Valve Repair; **Hospital:** Hosp Univ Penn - UPHS (page 72); **Address:** Hosp Univ of Penn, 3400 Spruce St, East Gates Bldg - Fl 9th, rm 9007, Philadelphia, PA 19104; **Phone:** 215-662-3990; **Board Cert:** Cardiovascular Disease 2008; Echocardiography 2003; **Med School:** Univ Pennsylvania 1990; **Resid:** Internal Medicine, Hosp Univ Penn 1994; **Fellow:** Cardiology Research, Hosp Univ Penn 1997; **Fac Appt:** Assoc Prof Med, Univ Pennsylvania

Slater, William R MD [Cv] - **Spec Exp:** Arrhythmias; Heart Valve Disease; Cardiac Electrophysiology; **Hospital:** NYU Langone Med Ctr (page 68); **Address:** NYU Medical Ctr, Div Cardiology, 530 First Ave, Ste 9U, New York, NY 10016; **Phone:** 212-263-7463; **Board Cert:** Internal Medicine 1981; Cardiovascular Disease 1985; Cardiac Electrophysiology 2002; **Med School:** Harvard Med Sch 1978; **Resid:** Internal Medicine, NYU-Bellevue Med Ctr 1981; **Fellow:** Cardiovascular Disease, Mt Sinai Hosp 1984; Cardiovascular Disease, Mass Genl Hosp/Brigham-Womens Hops 1986; **Fac Appt:** Assoc Prof Med, NYU Sch Med

Steingart, Richard M MD [Cv] - **Spec Exp:** Heart Failure; Nuclear Cardiology; Heart Disease in Cancer Patients; Cardiac Effects of Cancer/Cancer Therapy; **Hospital:** Meml Sloan-Kettering Cancer Ctr; **Address:** 1275 York Ave, New York, NY 10065; **Phone:** 212-639-8488; **Board Cert:** Internal Medicine 1977; Cardiovascular Disease 1979; **Med School:** Mount Sinai Sch Med 1974; **Resid:** Internal Medicine, Yale-New Haven Hosp 1977; **Fellow:** Cardiovascular Disease, Mt Sinai Med Ctr 1979; **Fac Appt:** Prof Med, Cornell Univ-Weill Med Coll

Tenenbaum, Joseph MD [Cv] - **Spec Exp:** Heart Valve Disease; Coronary Artery Disease; Atrial Fibrillation; **Hospital:** NY-Presby/Columbia Univ Med Ctr, NY (page 66); **Address:** 161 Ft Washington Ave, Ste 5-520, Irving Pavilion, New York, NY 10032; **Phone:** 212-305-5288; **Board Cert:** Internal Medicine 1977; Cardiovascular Disease 1979; **Med School:** Harvard Med Sch 1974; **Resid:** Internal Medicine, Columbia-Presby Med Ctr 1977; **Fellow:** Cardiovascular Disease, Mt Sinai Hosp 1979; **Fac Appt:** Prof Med, Columbia P&S

Waxman, Harvey L MD [Cv] - **Spec Exp:** Arrhythmias; Cardiac Catheterization; Heart Valve Disease; **Hospital:** Penn Presby Med Ctr - UPHS (page 72); **Address:** Penn Presby Med Ctr, Philadelphia Heart Inst, 51 N 39th St, 4PHI, Philadelphia, PA 19104; **Phone:** 215-662-9000; **Board Cert:** Internal Medicine 1977; Cardiovascular Disease 1979; Cardiac Electrophysiology 2002; **Med School:** Mount Sinai Sch Med 1974; **Resid:** Internal Medicine, Bellevue Hosp 1977; **Fellow:** Cardiovascular Disease, Jackson Meml Hosp 1979; Cardiac Electrophysiology, Hosp Univ Penn 1980; **Fac Appt:** Clin Prof Med, Univ Pennsylvania

Weitz, Howard H MD [Cv] - **Spec Exp:** Preventive Cardiology; **Hospital:** Thomas Jefferson Univ Hosp; **Address:** Jefferson Heart Inst, 925 Chestnut St, Mezzanine Level, Philadelphia, PA 19107; **Phone:** 215-955-5050; **Board Cert:** Internal Medicine 1981; Cardiovascular Disease 1985; **Med School:** Thomas Jefferson Univ 1978; **Resid:** Internal Medicine, Thos Jefferson Univ Hosp 1982; **Fellow:** Cardiovascular Disease, Thos Jefferson Univ Hosp 1984; **Fac Appt:** Prof Med, Thomas Jefferson Univ

Southeast

Bashore, Thomas M MD [Cv] - **Spec Exp:** Heart Valve Disease; Pulmonary Hypertension; Congenital Heart Disease-Adult; **Hospital:** Duke Univ Hosp; **Address:** DUMC, Box 3012, Durham, NC 27710-0001; **Phone:** 919-684-2407; **Board Cert:** Internal Medicine 1975; Cardiovascular Disease 1977; **Med School:** Ohio State Univ 1972; **Resid:** Internal Medicine, NC Meml Hosp 1975; **Fellow:** Cardiovascular Disease, Duke Univ Med Ctr 1977; **Fac Appt:** Prof Med, Duke Univ

Bass, Theodore A MD [Cv] - **Spec Exp:** Interventional Cardiology; Coronary Artery Disease; **Hospital:** Shands Jacksonville Med Ctr; **Address:** Shands Jacksonville Cardiovascular Ctr, 655 W 8th St ACC Bldg Fl 5, Jacksonville, FL 32209; **Phone:** 904-244-2655; **Board Cert:** Internal Medicine 1979; Cardiovascular Disease 1981; Interventional Cardiology 2011; **Med School:** Brown Univ 1976; **Resid:** Internal Medicine, Mayo Clinic 1979; **Fellow:** Cardiovascular Disease, University Hosp 1981; **Fac Appt:** Prof Med, Univ Fla Coll Med

Borzak, Steven L MD [Cv] - **Spec Exp:** Coronary Artery Disease; Arrhythmias; Heart Failure; Cholesterol/Lipid Disorders; **Hospital:** JFK Med Ctr - Atlantis, Bethesda Memorial Hosp; **Address:** Florida Cardiology Group, 110 JFK Drive, Ste 110, Atlantis, FL 33462-1146; **Phone:** 561-641-9541; **Board Cert:** Internal Medicine 1987; Cardiovascular Disease 2011; **Med School:** Univ IL Coll Med 1984; **Resid:** Internal Medicine, Michael Reese Hosp 1988; **Fellow:** Cardiovascular Disease, Brigham & Womens Hosp 1991; **Fac Appt:** Prof Med, Nova SE Univ, Coll Osteo Med

Bourge, Robert C MD [Cv] - **Spec Exp:** Heart Failure; Pulmonary Hypertension; Transplant Medicine - Heart; Nuclear Cardiology; **Hospital:** Univ of Ala Hosp at Birmingham; **Address:** University of Alabama at Birmingham, 1900 University Blvd, 321k, THT Bldg, Birmingham, AL 35294-0001; **Phone:** 205-934-3624; **Board Cert:** Internal Medicine 1982; Cardiovascular Disease 1985; Nuclear Medicine 1987; **Med School:** Louisiana State U, New Orleans 1979; **Resid:** Internal Medicine, Univ Alabama Hosps 1982; Nuclear Medicine, Univ Alabama Hosps 1985; **Fellow:** Cardiovascular Disease, Univ Alabama Hosps 1984; **Fac Appt:** Prof Med, Univ Alabama

Byrd III, Benjamin F MD [Cv] - **Spec Exp:** Congenital Heart Disease; Echocardiography; Heart Valve Disease; **Hospital:** Vanderbilt Univ Med Ctr (page 75); **Address:** Vanderbilt Heart & Vascular Inst, 1215 21st Ave, MCE S Tower, Ste 5209, Nashville, TN 37232; **Phone:** 615-322-2318; **Board Cert:** Internal Medicine 1981; Cardiovascular Disease 1983; **Med School:** Vanderbilt Univ 1977; **Resid:** Psychiatry, Harvard/Mass Mental Hlth 1979; Internal Medicine, Vanderbilt Univ Hosp 1981; **Fellow:** Cardiovascular Disease, Vanderbilt Univ Hosp 1983; Cardiovascular Disease, UCSF Med Ctr 1984; **Fac Appt:** Prof Med, Vanderbilt Univ

Califf, Robert M MD [Cv] - **Spec Exp:** Coronary Artery Disease; Cholesterol/Lipid Disorders; Heart Failure; **Hospital:** Duke Univ Hosp; **Address:** 200 Trent Drive, 1117 Davison Bldg, DUMC 3701, Durham, NC 27710; **Phone:** 919-668-8820; **Board Cert:** Internal Medicine 1984; Cardiovascular Disease 1985; **Med School:** Duke Univ 1978; **Resid:** Internal Medicine, UCSF Med Ctr 1980; **Fellow:** Cardiovascular Disease, Duke Univ Med Ctr 1983; **Fac Appt:** Prof Med, Duke Univ

Chizner, Michael A MD [Cv] - **Spec Exp:** Preventive Cardiology; Coronary Artery Disease; Cardiac Catheterization; Coronary Angioplasty/Stents; **Hospital:** Broward Hlth Med Ctr, Broward Hlth Imperial Point; **Address:** 1625 SE 3rd Ave, Ste 300, Fort Lauderdale, FL 33316; **Phone:** 954-355-5001; **Board Cert:** Internal Medicine 1977; Cardiovascular Disease 1979; **Med School:** Cornell Univ 1974; **Resid:** Internal Medicine, New York Hosp 1977; **Fellow:** Cardiovascular Disease, Georgetown Univ 1979; **Fac Appt:** Clin Prof Med, Univ Miami Sch Med

Clements Jr, Stephen D MD [Cv] - **Spec Exp:** Cardiac Catheterization; Echocardiography; Heart Valve Disease; **Hospital:** Emory Univ Hosp; **Address:** Emory Clinic, 1365A Clifton Rd NE, Ste 2200, Atlanta, GA 30322; **Phone:** 404-778-3468; **Board Cert:** Internal Medicine 1971; Cardiovascular Disease 1975; **Med School:** Med Coll GA 1966; **Resid:** Internal Medicine, Grady Meml Hosp 1970; **Fellow:** Cardiovascular Disease, Emory Univ Hosp 1971; **Fac Appt:** Prof Med, Emory Univ

Corrigan, Victor E MD [Cv] - **Spec Exp:** Cardiac Catheterization; Interventional Cardiology; Transplant Medicine-Heart; **Hospital:** Piedmont Hosp, St. Joseph's Hosp - Atlanta; **Address:** Piedmont Heart Inst, 275 Collier Rd, Ste 300, Atlanta, GA 30309; **Phone:** 404-605-2800; **Board Cert:** Internal Medicine 1986; Cardiovascular Disease 1989; Interventional Cardiology 2009; **Med School:** Med Coll GA 1983; **Resid:** Internal Medicine, Emory Univ Hosp 1986; **Fellow:** Cardiovascular Disease, Emory Univ 1988

Gandy Jr, Winston H MD [Cv] - **Spec Exp:** Echocardiography; Cardiovascular Imaging; Preventive Cardiology; **Hospital:** Piedmont Hosp; **Address:** Piedmont Heart Institute-Perimeter, 1140 Hammond Drive, Ste 300, Atlanta, GA 30328; **Phone:** 404-851-5400; **Board Cert:** Internal Medicine 1989; Cardiovascular Disease 2002; Echocardiography 2008; **Med School:** Howard Univ 1986; **Resid:** Internal Medicine, Emory Univ Affil Hosps 1989; **Fellow:** Cardiovascular Disease, Univ Alabama 1992

Hare, Joshua M MD [Cv] - **Spec Exp:** Heart Failure; Stem Cell Therapy in Heart Failure; **Hospital:** Univ of Miami Hosp; **Address:** University of Miami, 1295 NW 14th St, South Bldg, Ste A, Miami, FL 33125; **Phone:** 305-243-7040; **Board Cert:** Cardiovascular Disease 2006; **Med School:** Johns Hopkins Univ 1988; **Resid:** Internal Medicine, Johns Hopkins Hosp 1991; **Fellow:** Cardiovascular Disease, Brigham & Women's Hosp 1993

Harrison, J Kevin MD [Cv] - **Spec Exp:** Interventional Cardiology; Heart Valve Disease; **Hospital:** Duke Univ Hosp; **Address:** Duke Box 3331, 7624B Hosp North, Durham, NC 27710; **Phone:** 919-681-3763; **Board Cert:** Internal Medicine 1988; Cardiovascular Disease 2001; Interventional Cardiology 2003; **Med School:** NYU Sch Med 1984; **Resid:** Internal Medicine, Johns Hopkins Hosp 1987; **Fellow:** Cardiovascular Disease, Duke Univ Med Ctr 1990; **Fac Appt:** Prof Med, Duke Univ

Iskandrian, Ami E MD [Cv] - **Spec Exp:** Nuclear Cardiology; Coronary Artery Disease; Heart Valve Disease; **Hospital:** Univ of Ala Hosp at Birmingham; **Address:** Univ Alabama-Birmingham, 318 LHRB, 1900 University Blvd, Birmingham, AL 35294-0006; **Phone:** 205-934-0545; **Board Cert:** Internal Medicine 1974; Cardiovascular Disease 1975; Nuclear Cardiology 1999; **Med School:** Iraq 1965; **Resid:** Internal Medicine, Univ Baghdad Affil Hosp 1971; Internal Medicine, Hahnemann Univ Hosp 1973; **Fellow:** Cardiovascular Disease, Hahnemann Univ Hosp 1975; **Fac Appt:** Prof Med, Univ Alabama

Linton, MacRae F MD [Cv] - **Spec Exp:** Cholesterol/Lipid Disorders; Preventive Cardiology; Metabolic Syndrome; **Hospital:** Vanderbilt Univ Med Ctr (page 75); **Address:** Vanderbilt Heart & Vascular Inst, 719 Thompson Ln, Ste 22100, Nashville, TN 37204; **Phone:** 615-322-2318; **Board Cert:** Internal Medicine 1988; **Med School:** Univ Tenn Coll Med 1985; **Resid:** Internal Medicine, Vanderbilt Univ Med Ctr 1988; **Fellow:** Endocrinology, UCSF Med Ctr 1991; **Fac Appt:** Prof Med, Vanderbilt Univ

Myerburg, Robert J MD [Cv] - **Spec Exp:** Arrhythmias; Pacemakers; Heart Attack; **Hospital:** Jackson Meml Hosp, Univ of Miami Hosp; **Address:** Univ Miami Hosp, 1295 NW 14th St South Bldg Fl 2 - Ste A, Miami, FL 33136; **Phone:** 305-585-5523; **Board Cert:** Internal Medicine 1968; Cardiovascular Disease 1970; **Med School:** Univ MD Sch Med 1961; **Resid:** Internal Medicine, Charity Hosp 1966; **Fellow:** Cardiovascular Disease, Grady Meml Hosp 1968; Cardiac Electrophysiology, Columbia P&S 1970; **Fac Appt:** Prof Med, Univ Miami Sch Med

Nocero Jr, Michael A MD [Cv] - **Spec Exp:** Nuclear Cardiology; **Hospital:** Florida Hosp - Orlando; **Address:** Central Florida Cardiology Grp, 1745 N Mills Ave, Orlando, FL 32803; **Phone:** 407-841-7151 x1111; **Board Cert:** Internal Medicine 1972; Cardiovascular Disease 1976; **Med School:** NYU Sch Med 1966; **Resid:** Internal Medicine, Bellevue Hosp Ctr NYU 1971; **Fellow:** Cardiovascular Disease, Bellevue Hosp Ctr NYU 1973

O'Connell Jr, John B MD [Cv] - **Spec Exp:** Congestive Heart Failure; Ventricular Assist Device (LVAD); Transplant Medicine-Heart; **Hospital:** Med Ctr of Central GA; **Address:** 765 First St, Macon, GA 31201; **Phone:** 478-633-1000; **Board Cert:** Internal Medicine 1978; Cardiovascular Disease 2011; Advanced Heart Failure & Transplant Cardiology 2010; **Med School:** Loyola Univ-Stritch Sch Med 1974; **Resid:** Internal Medicine, Loyola Univ McGaw Hosp 1978; **Fellow:** Cardiovascular Disease, Loyola Univ McGaw Hosp 1980

O'Connor, Christopher M MD [Cv] - **Spec Exp:** Heart Failure; **Hospital:** Duke Univ Hosp; **Address:** Duke Univ Med Ctr, Box 3356, Durham, NC 27710; **Phone:** 919-681-6195; **Board Cert:** Internal Medicine 1988; Cardiovascular Disease 1989; **Med School:** Univ MD Sch Med 1983; **Resid:** Internal Medicine, Duke Univ Med Ctr 1986; **Fellow:** Cardiovascular Disease, Duke Univ Med Ctr 1989; **Fac Appt:** Prof Med, Duke Univ

Oparil, Suzanne MD [Cv] - **Spec Exp:** Hypertension; Heart Disease in Women; **Hospital:** Univ of Ala Hosp at Birmingham; **Address:** UAB Cardiology, 1530 3rd Ave S, ZRB 1034, Birmingham, AL 35294; **Phone:** 205-801-7563; **Board Cert:** Internal Medicine 1970; **Med School:** Columbia P&S 1965; **Resid:** Internal Medicine, Columbia Presby Med Ctr 1967; Internal Medicine, Mass Genl Hosp 1968; **Fellow:** Cardiovascular Disease, Mass Genl Hosp 1971; **Fac Appt:** Prof Med, Univ Alabama

Pepine, Carl J MD [Cv] - **Spec Exp:** Coronary Artery Disease; Hypertension; Heart Disease in Women; **Hospital:** Shands at Univ of FL; **Address:** Univ Florida, Div Cardiovascular Med, 7120 NW 11th Pl, Gainesville, FL 32605; **Phone:** 352-265-0139; **Board Cert:** Internal Medicine 1971; Cardiovascular Disease 1973; **Med School:** UMDNJ-NJ Med Sch, Newark 1966; **Resid:** Internal Medicine, Jefferson Univ Hosp 1968; Internal Medicine, Naval Hosp-Thomas Jefferson Univ 1969; **Fellow:** Cardiovascular Disease, Naval Hosp-Thomas Jeff Univ 1971; **Fac Appt:** Prof Med, Univ Fla Coll Med

Phillips III, Harry R MD [Cv] - **Spec Exp:** Cardiac Catheterization; **Hospital:** Duke Univ Hosp; **Address:** Duke Univ Med Ctr, Box 3126, Durham, NC 27710; **Phone:** 919-681-4804; **Board Cert:** Internal Medicine 1978; Cardiovascular Disease 1979; Interventional Cardiology 2001; **Med School:** Duke Univ 1975; **Resid:** Internal Medicine, Mass Genl Hosp 1977; **Fellow:** Cardiovascular Disease, Mass Genl Hosp 1979; **Fac Appt:** Prof Med, Duke Univ

Powers, Eric R MD [Cv] - **Spec Exp:** Heart Valve Disease; Interventional Cardiology; Coronary Artery Disease; **Hospital:** MUSC Med Ctr; **Address:** MUSC Heart & Vascular Ctr, 25 Courtenay Drive, Ashley River Tower Fl 7, Charleston, SC 29425-5920; **Phone:** 843-792-1952; **Board Cert:** Internal Medicine 1977; Cardiovascular Disease 1979; **Med School:** Harvard Med Sch 1974; **Resid:** Internal Medicine, Mass Genl Hosp 1976; **Fellow:** Cardiovascular Disease, Mass Genl Hosp 1979; **Fac Appt:** Prof Med, Med Univ SC

Rogers, Joseph G MD [Cv] - **Spec Exp:** Congestive Heart Failure; Transplant Medicine-Heart; **Hospital:** Duke Univ Hosp; **Address:** DUMC, Box 3034, Durham, NC 27710; **Phone:** 919-681-3398; **Board Cert:** Cardiovascular Disease 2005; **Med School:** Univ Nebr Coll Med 1988; **Resid:** Internal Medicine, Univ Nebraska Med Ctr 1991; **Fellow:** Cardiovascular Disease, Wash Univ Med Ctr 1995; **Fac Appt:** Assoc Prof Med, Duke Univ

Cardiovascular Disease

Smith Jr, Sidney C MD [Cv] - **Spec Exp:** Coronary Artery Disease; Invasive Cardiology; **Hospital:** NC Memorial Hosp - UNC; **Address:** 300 Meadowmont Village Cir, Ste 313, Chapel Hill, NC 27517; **Phone:** 919-966-7244; **Board Cert:** Internal Medicine 1972; Cardiovascular Disease 1973; **Med School:** Yale Univ 1967; **Resid:** Internal Medicine, Peter Bent Brigham Hosp 1969; **Fellow:** Cardiovascular Disease, Peter Bent Brigham Hosp 1971; Research, Harvard Med Sch 1971; **Fac Appt:** Prof Med, Univ NC Sch Med

Vetrovec, George MD [Cv] - **Spec Exp:** Interventional Cardiology; **Hospital:** Med Coll of VA Hosp; **Address:** 1200 E Broad St, rm 607, Box 980036, West Hospital, Richmond, VA 23298; **Phone:** 804-828-8885; **Board Cert:** Internal Medicine 1974; Cardiovascular Disease 1977; Interventional Cardiology 2010; **Med School:** Univ VA Sch Med 1970; **Resid:** Internal Medicine, Med Coll Virginia Hosp 1974; **Fellow:** Cardiovascular Disease, Med Coll Virginia Hosp 1976; **Fac Appt:** Prof Med, Med Coll VA

Vignola, Paul MD [Cv] - **Spec Exp:** Interventional Cardiology; **Hospital:** Watauga Med Ctr; **Address:** The Cardiology Center, Appalachian Regional Healthcare System, 175 Mary St, Boone, NC 28607; **Phone:** 828-264-9664; **Board Cert:** Internal Medicine 1974; Cardiovascular Disease 1977; Interventional Cardiology 2009; **Med School:** Yale Univ 1971; **Resid:** Internal Medicine, Yale-New Haven Hosp 1974; **Fellow:** Cardiovascular Disease, Harvard/Mass Genl Hosp 1976; **Fac Appt:** Assoc Clin Prof Med, Univ Miami Sch Med

Wells, Gretchen L MD/PhD [Cv] - **Spec Exp:** Heart Valve Disease; Congenital Heart Disease-Adult; Heart Disease in Pregnancy; Cardiac Effects of Chemotherapy; **Hospital:** Wake Forest Baptist Med Ctr; **Address:** Wake Forest Baptist Med Ctr, Dept Cardiology, Medical Center Blvd, Winston-Salem, NC 27157-1045; **Phone:** 336-716-6674; **Board Cert:** Cardiovascular Disease 2010; **Med School:** Univ Alabama 1994; **Resid:** Internal Medicine, NC Baptist Hosp 1997; **Fellow:** Cardiovascular Disease, Wake Forest Bapstist Med Ctr 2000; **Fac Appt:** Assoc Prof Med, Wake Forest Univ

Midwest

Bonow, Robert O MD [Cv] - **Spec Exp:** Heart Valve Disease; Coronary Artery Disease; Cardiomyopathy; **Hospital:** Northwestern Meml Hosp; **Address:** Northwestern Bluhm Cardiovascular Inst, 675 N St Clair St, Galter 19-100, Chicago, IL 60611; **Phone:** 312-695-4965; **Board Cert:** Internal Medicine 1976; Cardiovascular Disease 1981; **Med School:** Univ Pennsylvania 1973; **Resid:** Internal Medicine, Hosp Univ Penn 1976; **Fellow:** Cardiovascular Disease, Natl Inst Health-NHLBI 1979; **Fac Appt:** Prof Med, Northwestern Univ

Braverman, Alan C MD [Cv] - **Spec Exp:** Marfan's Syndrome; Aortic Diseases & Dissection; Aneurysm; Heart Valve Disease; **Hospital:** Barnes-Jewish Hosp; **Address:** Wash Univ Med Sch, Div Cardiovascular Disease, 660 S Euclid Ave, Box 8086, St Louis, MO 63110; **Phone:** 314-362-1291; **Board Cert:** Internal Medicine 1988; Cardiovascular Disease 2011; **Med School:** Univ MO-Kansas City 1985; **Resid:** Internal Medicine, Brigham & Womens Hosp 1988; Internal Medicine, Brigham & Womens Hosp 1991; **Fellow:** Cardiovascular Disease, Brigham & Womens Hosp 1990; **Fac Appt:** Prof Med, Washington Univ, St Louis

Burket, Mark W MD [Cv] - **Spec Exp:** Peripheral Vascular Disease; Coronary Artery Disease; Percutaneous Vascular Interventions; **Hospital:** Univ of Toledo Med Ctr; **Address:** 3000 Arlington Ave, Ste 1192, Toledo, OH 43614; **Phone:** 419-383-3697; **Board Cert:** Internal Medicine 1982; Cardiovascular Disease 1985; **Med School:** Ohio State Univ 1979; **Resid:** Internal Medicine, Ohio State Univ 1982; **Fellow:** Cardiovascular Disease, Med Coll Ohio 1985; **Fac Appt:** Prof Med, Med Univ Ohio at Toledo

Cerqueira, Manuel MD [Cv] - **Spec Exp:** Cardiac Imaging; Nuclear Cardiology; Coronary Artery Disease; **Hospital:** Cleveland Clin (page 55); **Address:** Cleveland Clinic, 9500 Euclid Ave, Desk JB3, Cleveland, OH 44195; **Phone:** 216-444-2665; **Board Cert:** Internal Medicine 1981; Nuclear Medicine 1984; Cardiovascular Disease 1989; **Med School:** NYU Sch Med 1976; **Resid:** Internal Medicine, Bellevue Hosp Ctr 1980; Cardiovascular Disease, Yale-New Haven Hosp 1982; **Fellow:** Nuclear Medicine, Yale-New Haven Hosp 1983; **Fac Appt:** Prof Med, Cleveland Cl Coll Med/Case West Res

Chaitman, Bernard R MD [Cv] - **Spec Exp:** Nuclear Cardiology; Echocardiography; **Hospital:** St. Louis Univ Hosp; **Address:** SLUCare, Div Cardiology, Univ Club Tower, 1034 S Brentwood Blvd, Ste 1120, St Louis, MO 63117; **Phone:** 314-977-4663; **Board Cert:** Internal Medicine 1973; Cardiovascular Disease 1975; Echocardiography 2001; Cardiovascular Computed Tomography 2009; **Med School:** McGill Univ 1969; **Resid:** Internal Medicine, Royal Victoria Hosp 1972; **Fellow:** Cardiovascular Disease, Univ Oregon Hosps 1974; Cardiovascular Disease, Univ Montreal 1975; **Fac Appt:** Prof Med, St Louis Univ

Connolly, Heidi M MD [Cv] - **Spec Exp:** Congenital Heart Disease; Heart Disease in Pregnancy; **Hospital:** Mayo Med Ctr & Clin - Rochester; **Address:** Mayo Clin, Div Cardiovasc Disease, 200 First St SW, Rochester, MN 55905; **Phone:** 507-284-1226; **Board Cert:** Internal Medicine 1989; Cardiovascular Disease 2011; **Med School:** Ireland 1986; **Resid:** Internal Medicine, Mayo Clinic 1989; **Fellow:** Cardiovascular Disease, Mayo Clinic 1991; **Fac Appt:** Prof Med, Mayo Med Sch

Cooper, Christopher J MD [Cv] - **Spec Exp:** Interventional Cardiology; **Hospital:** Univ of Toledo Med Ctr; **Address:** University of Toledo, 3000 Arlington Ave, Ste 1192, Toledo, OH 43614; **Phone:** 419-383-3697; **Board Cert:** Internal Medicine 2004; Cardiovascular Disease 2005; Interventional Cardiology 2009; **Med School:** Univ Cincinnati 1988; **Resid:** Internal Medicine, Brigham & Womens Hosp 1991; **Fellow:** Cardiovascular Disease, Brigham & Women's Hosp-Harvard Med Sch 1994; **Fac Appt:** Prof Med, Univ Toledo, Med Univ OH

Davidson, Michael MD [Cv] - **Spec Exp:** Preventive Cardiology; Cholesterol/Lipid Disorders; **Hospital:** Univ of Chicago Med Ctr; **Address:** 150 E Huron St, Avenue Hotel Bldg, Ste 900, Chicago, IL 60611; **Phone:** 773-834-4150; **Board Cert:** Internal Medicine 1984; Cardiovascular Disease 1987; **Med School:** Ohio State Univ 1981; **Resid:** Internal Medicine, Rush Presby-St Lukes Med Ctr 1984; **Fellow:** Cardiovascular Disease, Rush Presby-St Lukes Med Ctr 1986; **Fac Appt:** Clin Prof Med, Univ Chicago-Pritzker Sch Med

Eagle, Kim A MD [Cv] - **Spec Exp:** Aortic Diseases & Dissection; Acute Coronary Syndromes; Heart Attack; Peripheral Vascular Disease; **Hospital:** Univ of Michigan Hosp; **Address:** Dominos Farms, 24 Frank Lloyd Wright Drive, Ann Arbor, MI 48106-0363; **Phone:** 734-998-7400; **Board Cert:** Internal Medicine 1982; Cardiovascular Disease 1987; **Med School:** Tufts Univ 1979; **Resid:** Internal Medicine, Yale New Haven Hosp 1983; **Fellow:** Cardiovascular Disease, Mass Genl Hosp-Harvard 1986; **Fac Appt:** Asst Prof Med, Univ Mich Med Sch

Fintel, Dan MD [Cv] - **Spec Exp:** Coronary Artery Disease; Cholesterol/Lipid Disorders; Nuclear Cardiology; **Hospital:** Northwestern Meml Hosp; **Address:** Bluhm Cardiovascular Inst, 675 N St Clair St, Ste 100, Chicago, IL 60611; **Phone:** 312-695-2745; **Board Cert:** Internal Medicine 1982; Cardiovascular Disease 1985; **Med School:** Harvard Med Sch 1979; **Resid:** Internal Medicine, Mt Sinai Hosp 1982; **Fellow:** Cardiovascular Disease, Johns Hopkins Hosp 1985; **Fac Appt:** Assoc Prof Med, Northwestern Univ

Geltman, Edward M MD [Cv] - **Spec Exp:** Congestive Heart Failure; Transplant Medicine-Heart; Non-Invasive Cardiology; **Hospital:** Barnes-Jewish Hosp, Barnes-Jewish West County Hosp; **Address:** Washington Univ Sch of Med, Cardiovascular Division, 660 S Euclid Ave, Box 8086, St Louis, MO 63110; **Phone:** 314-362-1291; **Board Cert:** Internal Medicine 1974; Cardiovascular Disease 1979; Advanced Heart Failure & Transplant Cardiology 2010; **Med School:** NYU Sch Med 1971; **Resid:** Internal Medicine, Bellevue Hosp 1974; **Fellow:** Cardiovascular Disease, Barnes Jewish Hosp 1978; **Fac Appt:** Prof Med, Washington Univ, St Louis

Gibbons, Raymond J MD [Cv] - **Spec Exp:** Nuclear Cardiology; Heart Attack; **Hospital:** Mayo Med Ctr & Clin - Rochester; **Address:** Mayo Clin, Div Cardiovasc Disease, 200 First St SW, Rochester, MN 55905; **Phone:** 507-284-2541; **Board Cert:** Internal Medicine 1979; Cardiovascular Disease 1981; **Med School:** Harvard Med Sch 1976; **Resid:** Internal Medicine, Mass Genl Hosp 1978; **Fellow:** Cardiovascular Disease, Duke Univ Med Ctr 1981; **Fac Appt:** Prof Med, Mayo Med Sch

Grubb, Blair P MD [Cv] - **Spec Exp:** Autonomic Disorders; **Hospital:** Univ of Toledo Med Ctr, St. Vincent's Mercy Med Ctr - Toledo; **Address:** 3000 Arlington Rd, Ste 1192, Toledo, OH 43614-2598; **Phone:** 419-383-3697; **Board Cert:** Internal Medicine 1985; Cardiovascular Disease 1987; **Med School:** Dominican Republic 1980; **Resid:** Internal Medicine, Grtr Baltimore Med Ctr 1985; **Fellow:** Cardiovascular Disease, MS Hershey Med Ctr/Penn State 1987; Cardiac Electrophysiology, MS Hershey Med Ctr/Penn State 1988; **Fac Appt:** Prof Med, Univ SD Sch Med

Hauptman, Paul J MD [Cv] - **Spec Exp:** Heart Failure; **Hospital:** St. Louis Univ Hosp; **Address:** SLUCare Div Cardiology, Univ Club Tower, 1034 S Brentwood Blvd, Ste 1120, Saint Louis, MO 63117; **Phone:** 314-977-4663; **Board Cert:** Cardiovascular Disease 2003; **Med School:** Cornell Univ 1987; **Resid:** Internal Medicine, Brigham and Women's Hosp 1990; **Fellow:** Cardiovascular Disease, Mount Sinai Med Ctr 1992; Cardiovascular Disease, Brigham and Women's Hosp 1993; **Fac Appt:** Prof Med, St Louis Univ

Hayes, Sharonne N MD [Cv] - **Spec Exp:** Heart Disease in Women; Preventive Cardiology; Cholesterol/Lipid Disorders; Echocardiography; **Hospital:** Mayo Med Ctr & Clin - Rochester; **Address:** Mayo Clin-Women's Heart Clin, 200 First St SW, Rochester, MN 55905; **Phone:** 507-284-3683; **Board Cert:** Internal Medicine 1986; Cardiovascular Disease 1989; **Med School:** Northwestern Univ 1983; **Resid:** Internal Medicine, Mayo Clin 1986; **Fellow:** Cardiovascular Research, Mayo Clin 1987; Cardiovascular Disease, Mayo Clin 1990; **Fac Appt:** Assoc Prof Med, Mayo Med Sch

Heroux, Alain MD [Cv] - **Spec Exp:** Transplant Medicine-Heart; Heart Failure; **Hospital:** Loyola Univ Med Ctr; **Address:** 2160 S 1st Ave Bldg 111, Maywood, IL 60153; **Phone:** 708-327-2738; **Med School:** Canada 1981; **Resid:** Internal Medicine, Laval Univ Med Ctr 1985; Cardiovascular Disease, Royal Victory Hosp 1987; **Fellow:** Univ Virginia Med Coll 1989; **Fac Appt:** Asst Prof Med, Rush Med Coll

Jaffe, Allan S MD [Cv] - **Spec Exp:** Ischemic Heart Disease; Heart Disease & Depression; **Hospital:** Mayo Med Ctr & Clin - Rochester; **Address:** Mayo Clinic, Div Cardiovascular Disease, 200 First St SW, Gonda 5-468, Rochester, MN 55905; **Phone:** 507-284-1648; **Board Cert:** Internal Medicine 1976; Cardiovascular Disease 1979; **Med School:** Univ MD Sch Med 1973; **Resid:** Internal Medicine, Barnes Hosp 1975; Internal Medicine, Wash Univ 1976; **Fellow:** Cardiovascular Disease, Barnes Hosp 1978; **Fac Appt:** Prof Med, Mayo Med Sch

Johnson, Maryl R MD [Cv] - **Spec Exp:** Congestive Heart Failure; Transplant Medicine-Heart; **Hospital:** Univ WI Hosp & Clins, Meriter Hosp; **Address:** Univ Wisconsin Hosp/Clins-Cardio, 600 Highland Ave, MS 5710, Madison, WI 53792-0001; **Phone:** 608-263-0080; **Board Cert:** Internal Medicine 1981; Cardiovascular Disease 1983; **Med School:** Univ Iowa Coll Med 1977; **Resid:** Internal Medicine, Univ Iowa Hosp 1981; **Fellow:** Cardiovascular Disease, Univ Iowa Hosp 1982; **Fac Appt:** Prof Med, Univ Wisc

Kereiakes, Dean J MD [Cv] - **Spec Exp:** Coronary Angioplasty/Stents; Congestive Heart Failure; Interventional Cardiology; **Hospital:** Christ Hosp, The - Cincinnati; **Address:** Ohio Heart & Vascular Center, 2123 Auburn Ave, Ste 136, Cincinnati, OH 45219; **Phone:** 513-721-8881; **Board Cert:** Internal Medicine 1981; Cardiovascular Disease 1985; **Med School:** Univ Cincinnati 1978; **Resid:** Internal Medicine, UCSF Med Ctr 1982; Internal Medicine, Mass Genl Hosp 1981; **Fellow:** Cardiovascular Disease, UCSF Med Ctr 1984; Coronary Angioplasty, Sequoia Hosp 1984; **Fac Appt:** Clin Prof Med, Ohio State Univ

Klein, Lloyd W MD [Cv] - **Spec Exp:** Coronary Artery Disease; Angiography-Coronary; Interventional Cardiology; Coronary Syndrome-Acute; **Hospital:** Gottlieb Meml Hosp, Adv Illinois Masonic Med Ctr; **Address:** Clinical Cardiology Associates, 675 W North Ave, POB Bldg - Fl 4 - Ste 406, Melrose Park, IL 60160; **Phone:** 708-681-7862; **Board Cert:** Internal Medicine 1980; Cardiovascular Disease 1983; Interventional Cardiology 2009; **Med School:** Univ Cincinnati 1977; **Resid:** Internal Medicine, Einstein-Bronx Muni Hosp 1980; **Fellow:** Cardiovascular Disease, Mt Sinai Hosp 1982; **Fac Appt:** Prof Med, Rush Med Coll

Mehlman, David J MD [Cv] - **Spec Exp:** Echocardiography; Heart Valve Disease; Coronary Artery Disease; **Hospital:** Northwestern Meml Hosp; **Address:** Northwestern Cardiovascular Inst, 675 N St Clair St, Galter Bldg Fl 19 - Ste 100, Chicago, IL 60611; **Phone:** 312-695-4965; **Board Cert:** Internal Medicine 1976; Cardiovascular Disease 1979; **Med School:** Johns Hopkins Univ 1973; **Resid:** Internal Medicine, Johns Hopkins Hosp 1976; **Fellow:** Cardiovascular Disease, Univ Chicago Hosps 1978; **Fac Appt:** Assoc Prof Med, Northwestern Univ

Moran, John F MD [Cv] - **Spec Exp:** Coronary Artery Disease; Congestive Heart Failure; Cholesterol/Lipid Disorders; **Hospital:** Loyola Univ Med Ctr; **Address:** 2160 S 1st Ave, EMS Bldg Fl 6, Maywood, IL 60153; **Phone:** 708-327-2784; **Board Cert:** Internal Medicine 1971; Cardiovascular Disease 1973; **Med School:** Loyola Univ-Stritch Sch Med 1964; **Resid:** Internal Medicine, Univ Illinois Med Ctr 1967; **Fellow:** Cardiovascular Disease, Univ Chicago Hosps 1969; **Fac Appt:** Prof Med, Loyola Univ-Stritch Sch Med

Nishimura, Rick A MD [Cv] - **Spec Exp:** Echocardiography; Pericardial Disease; **Hospital:** Mayo Med Ctr & Clin - Rochester, St. Mary's Hosp - Rochester MN (Mayo); **Address:** Mayo Clinic, 200 First St SW, Gonda 5-368, Rochester, MN 55905; **Phone:** 507-284-8342; **Board Cert:** Internal Medicine 1981; Cardiovascular Disease 1983; **Med School:** Rush Med Coll 1978; **Resid:** Internal Medicine, Mayo Clin 1980; **Fellow:** Cardiovascular Disease, Mayo Clin 1983; **Fac Appt:** Prof Med, Mayo Med Sch

Nissen, Steven E MD [Cv] - **Spec Exp:** Cholesterol/Lipid Disorders; Intravascular Ultrasound; Cardiac Intensive Care; **Hospital:** Cleveland Clin (page 55); **Address:** 9500 Euclid Ave, Desk J2-3, Cleveland, OH 44195; **Phone:** 216-445-6852; **Board Cert:** Internal Medicine 1981; Cardiovascular Disease 1983; **Med School:** Univ Mich Med Sch 1978; **Resid:** Internal Medicine, UC Davis Med Ctr 1981; **Fellow:** Cardiovascular Disease, Univ Kentucky-Chandler Med Ctr 1983; **Fac Appt:** Prof Med, Cleveland Cl Coll Med/Case West Res

Cardiovascular Disease

O'Neill, William W MD [Cv] - **Spec Exp:** Interventional Cardiology; Heart Valve Disease; **Hospital:** Henry Ford Hosp; **Address:** Center for Structural Heart Disease, 2799 W Grand Blvd, Ste K-14, Detroit, MI 48202; **Phone:** 313-916-1878; **Board Cert:** Internal Medicine 1980; Cardiovascular Disease 1983; **Med School:** Wayne State Univ 1977; **Resid:** Internal Medicine, Wayne State Univ Affil Hosps 1980; **Fellow:** Cardiovascular Disease, Univ Mich Med Ctr 1982; **Fac Appt:** Assoc Prof Med, Univ Mich Med Sch

Raff, Gilbert L MD [Cv] - **Spec Exp:** Cardiac CT Angiography; Cardiac MRI; **Hospital:** Beaumont Hosp-Royal Oak; **Address:** 3601 W 13 Mile Rd, Royal Oak, MI 48073; **Phone:** 248-898-1767; **Board Cert:** Internal Medicine 1978; Cardiovascular Disease 1981; **Med School:** UC Davis 1975; **Resid:** Internal Medicine, Univ Michigan Hosp 1978; **Fellow:** Cardiovascular Disease, UCSF Med Ctr 1981; **Fac Appt:** Prof Med, Oakland Univ-William Beaumont Med Sch

Rahko, Peter S MD [Cv] - **Spec Exp:** Congestive Heart Failure; Heart Valve Disease; Echocardiography; Echocardiography-Transesophageal; **Hospital:** Univ WI Hosp & Clins, Meriter Hosp; **Address:** 600 Highland Ave, rm G7-343 CSC, MC 3248, Madison, WI 53792-3248; **Phone:** 608-263-1530; **Board Cert:** Internal Medicine 1982; Cardiovascular Disease 1985; **Med School:** Univ Minn 1979; **Resid:** Internal Medicine, Indiana Univ Med Ctr 1982; **Fellow:** Cardiovascular Disease, Univ Pittsburgh Med Ctr 1985; **Fac Appt:** Prof Med, Univ Wisc

Reiss, Craig MD [Cv] - **Spec Exp:** Ischemic Heart Disease; Heart Valve Disease; Preventive Cardiology; Coronary Artery Disease; **Hospital:** Barnes-Jewish Hosp, Barnes-Jewish West County Hosp; **Address:** Wash Univ Med Sch, Div Cardiovascular Disease, 660 S Euclid Ave, Box 8086, St Louis, MO 63110; **Phone:** 314-362-1291; **Board Cert:** Internal Medicine 1986; Cardiovascular Disease 1989; **Med School:** Univ MO-Kansas City 1983; **Resid:** Internal Medicine, Brigham & Women's Hosp 1989; **Fellow:** Cardiovascular Disease, Brigham & Women's Hosp 1988; **Fac Appt:** Prof Med, Washington Univ, St Louis

Rich, Stuart MD [Cv] - **Spec Exp:** Pulmonary Hypertension; Heart Failure; **Hospital:** Univ of Chicago Med Ctr; **Address:** 5841 S Maryland Ave, MC 5403, Chicago, IL 60637; **Phone:** 773-702-6049; **Board Cert:** Internal Medicine 1978; Cardiovascular Disease 1981; **Med School:** Loyola Univ-Stritch Sch Med 1974; **Resid:** Internal Medicine, Barnes-Jewish Hosp 1978; **Fellow:** Cardiovascular Disease, Univ Chicago Hosp 1980; **Fac Appt:** Prof Med, Rush Med Coll

Rihal, Charanjit S MD [Cv] - **Spec Exp:** Acute Coronary Syndromes; Coronary Artery Disease; Interventional Cardiology; **Hospital:** Mayo Med Ctr & Clin - Rochester; **Address:** 200 First St SW, MB 4-506, Rochester, MN 55905; **Phone:** 507-255-2440; **Board Cert:** Internal Medicine 1989; Cardiovascular Disease 2011; Interventional Cardiology 2009; **Med School:** Canada 1985; **Resid:** Internal Medicine, Mayo Clinic 1989; **Fellow:** Cardiovascular Disease, Mayo Clinic 1992; **Fac Appt:** Prof Med, Mayo Med Sch

Rosenbush, Stuart W MD [Cv] - **Spec Exp:** Cardiac Catheterization; Coronary Angioplasty/Stents; Coronary Artery Disease; Heart Failure; **Hospital:** Rush Univ Med Ctr, Skokie/North Shore Univ Htlh Syst; **Address:** Univ Cardiologists, 1725 W Harrison St, Ste 1159, Chicago, IL 60612-3835; **Phone:** 312-942-5020; **Board Cert:** Internal Medicine 1979; Cardiovascular Disease 1981; Interventional Cardiology 2000; **Med School:** Univ IL Coll Med 1976; **Resid:** Internal Medicine, Michael Reese Hosp 1979; **Fellow:** Cardiovascular Disease, Rush Presby-St Lukes Med Ctr 1981; **Fac Appt:** Asst Prof Med, Rush Med Coll

Safian, Robert D MD [Cv] - **Spec Exp:** Interventional Cardiology; **Hospital:** Beaumont Hosp-Royal Oak; **Address:** Beaumont Heart Ctr, 3601 W 13 Mile Rd Fl 3, Royal Oak, MI 48073; **Phone:** 248-898-4163; **Board Cert:** Internal Medicine 1983; Cardiovascular Disease 1987; Interventional Cardiology 2010; **Med School:** Univ Fla Coll Med 1979; **Resid:** Pathology, Univ Miami Med Ctr 1981; Internal Medicine, UCSD Med Ctr 1983; **Fellow:** Cardiovascular Disease, Beth Israel Hosp-Harvard 1987

Sanborn, Timothy MD [Cv] - **Spec Exp:** Interventional Cardiology; Gene Therapy-Cardiac An-giogenesis; Heart Valve Disease; Carotid Artery Stent Placement; **Hospital:** Evanston/North Shore Univ Hlth Sys; **Address:** 2650 Ridge Ave, Walgreen Bldg Fl 3, Evanston, IL 60201; **Phone:** 847-570-2250; **Board Cert:** Internal Medicine 1980; Cardiovascular Disease 2003; Interventional Cardiology 2009; **Med School:** Northwestern Univ 1977; **Resid:** Internal Medicine, Boston City Hosp 1980; **Fellow:** Cardiovascular Disease, Boston Univ Med Ctr 1983; **Fac Appt:** Prof Med, Northwestern Univ

Shapiro, Jerrold MD [Cv] - **Spec Exp:** Echocardiography; Preventive Cardiology; **Address:** 4801 W Peterson Ave, Ste 610, Chicago, IL 60646; **Phone:** 773-283-5900; **Board Cert:** Internal Medicine 1976; Cardiovascular Disease 1977; **Med School:** Univ IL Coll Med 1968; **Resid:** Internal Medicine, Ill Masonic Med Ctr 1972; **Fellow:** Cardiovascular Disease, Northwestern Meml Hosp 1974

Shea, Richard J MD [Cv] - **Spec Exp:** Heart Valve Disease; Echocardiography; Nuclear Cardiology; Echocardiography-Transesophageal; **Hospital:** Franciscan St. Francis Hlth-Indianapolis, Comm Hosp S - Indianapolis; **Address:** Indiana Heart Physicians, 5330 E Stop 11 Road, Indianapolis, IN 46237; **Phone:** 317-893-1664; **Board Cert:** Cardiovascular Disease 2009; **Med School:** Georgetown Univ 1989; **Resid:** Internal Medicine, Fitzsimons Army Med Ctr 1992; **Fellow:** Cardiovascular Disease, Washington Hosp Ctr 1995

Simon, Daniel I MD [Cv] - **Spec Exp:** Interventional Cardiology; **Hospital:** Univ Hosps Case Med Ctr (page 74); **Address:** UH Case Medical Center, 11100 Euclid Ave, Cleveland, OH 44106-5038; **Phone:** 216-368-1145; **Board Cert:** Cardiovascular Disease 2003; Interventional Cardiology 2010; **Med School:** Harvard Med Sch 1987; **Resid:** Internal Medicine, Brigham & Womens Hosp 1989; Interventional Cardiology, Beth Isreal 1995; **Fellow:** Cardiovascular Disease, Brigham & Womens Hosp 1992; **Fac Appt:** Prof Med, Case West Res Univ

Sorrentino, Matthew MD [Cv] **Spec Exp:** Preventive Cardiology; Hypertension; **Hospital:** Univ of Chicago Med Ctr; **Address:** 5841 S Maryland Ave, MC 6080, Chicago, IL 60637; **Phone:** 773-702-9461; **Board Cert:** Internal Medicine 1987; Cardiovascular Disease 2001; **Med School:** Univ Chicago-Pritzker Sch Med 1984; **Resid:** Internal Medicine, Univ Chicago Hosps 1989; **Fellow:** Cardiovascular Disease, Univ Chicago Hosps 1991; **Fac Appt:** Assoc Prof Med, Univ Chicago-Pritzker Sch Med

Stein, James H MD [Cv] - **Spec Exp:** Preventive Cardiology; Echocardiography; Cholesterol/Lipid Disorders; **Hospital:** Univ WI Hosp & Clins; **Address:** UW Heart & Vascular Clin G3/4, 600 Highland Ave, Madison, WI 53792; **Phone:** 608-263-1530; **Board Cert:** Internal Medicine 2003; Cardiovascular Disease 2007; **Med School:** Yale Univ 1990; **Resid:** Internal Medicine, Univ Chicago Hosps 1993; **Fellow:** Cardiovascular Disease, Rush-Presby St Lukes Med Ctr 1996; **Fac Appt:** Prof Med, Univ Wisc

Stewart, William James MD [Cv] - **Spec Exp:** Heart Valve Disease; Echocardiography; **Hospital:** Cleveland Clin (page 55); **Address:** Div Cardiovascular Medicine, 9500 Euclid Ave, Desk J1-5, Cleveland, OH 44195; **Phone:** 216-444-5923; **Board Cert:** Internal Medicine 1980; Cardiovascular Disease 1983; **Med School:** Univ Cincinnati 1977; **Resid:** Internal Medicine, Univ Mich Hosp 1980; **Fellow:** Cardiovascular Disease, Boston Univ Med Ctr 1982; Cardiovascular Disease, Mass Genl Hosp 1984; **Fac Appt:** Prof Med, Cleveland Cl Coll Med/Case West Res

Cardiovascular Disease

Volgman, Annabelle Santos MD [Cv] - **Spec Exp:** Heart Disease in Women; Arrhythmias; Atrial Fibrillation; Preventive Cardiology; **Hospital:** Rush Univ Med Ctr, Rush Oak Park Hosp; **Address:** Rush Heart Ctr for Women, 1725 W Harrison St, Professional Bldg, Ste 1159, Chicago, IL 60612; **Phone:** 312-942-5020; **Board Cert:** Cardiovascular Disease 2006; **Med School:** Columbia P&S 1984; **Resid:** Internal Medicine, Univ Chicago Hosps 1987; **Fellow:** Cardiovascular Disease, Northwestern Meml Hosp 1989; Cardiac Electrophysiology, Northwestern Meml Hosp 1990; **Fac Appt:** Prof Med, Rush Med Coll

von der Lohe, Elisabeth MD [Cv] - **Spec Exp:** Heart Disease in Women; Interventional Cardiology; Pulmonary Hypertension; **Hospital:** IU Health University Hosp, IU Health Methodist Hosp; **Address:** Krannert Inst of Cardiology, 1801 N Senate Blvd, Ste 4000, Indianapolis, IN 46202; **Phone:** 317-962-0500; **Board Cert:** Internal Medicine 2000; Cardiovascular Disease 2011; Interventional Cardiology 2003; **Med School:** Germany 1978; **Resid:** Internal Medicine, Marien Hosp 1981; **Fellow:** Cardiovascular Disease, Klinikum Aachen 1986; **Fac Appt:** Clin Prof Med, Indiana Univ

Wagoner, Lynne E MD [Cv] - **Spec Exp:** Congestive Heart Failure; Heart Disease in Women; Transplant Medicine-Heart; Pulmonary Hypertension; **Hospital:** Mercy Hosp - Fairfield, Christ Hosp, The - Cincinnati; **Address:** 3000 Mack Rd, Ste 100, Fairfield, OH 45014; **Phone:** 513-751-4222; **Board Cert:** Internal Medicine 1989; Cardiovascular Disease 2003; **Med School:** E Carolina Univ 1986; **Resid:** Internal Medicine, Pitt Co Meml Hosp/E Carolina Univ 1989; **Fellow:** Cardiovascular Disease, Univ Utah Affil Hosp 1994

Walsh, Mary N MD [Cv] - **Spec Exp:** Heart Disease in Women; Nuclear Cardiology; Congestive Heart Failure; Transplant Medicine-Heart; **Hospital:** St. Vincent Indianapolis Hosp; **Address:** The Care Group at St Vincent, 8333 Naab Rd, Ste 400, Indianapolis, IN 46260; **Phone:** 317-338-6666; **Board Cert:** Internal Medicine 1986; Cardiovascular Disease 2011; Advanced Heart Failure & Transplant Cardiology 2010; **Med School:** Univ Minn 1983; **Resid:** Internal Medicine, Univ Tex SW Med Ctr 1986; **Fellow:** Cardiovascular Disease, Wash Univ 1989; **Fac Appt:** Asst Clin Prof Med, Indiana Univ

Weaver, W Douglas MD [Cv] - **Spec Exp:** Heart Attack; Angioplasty; Cholesterol/Lipid Disorders; **Hospital:** Henry Ford Hosp, Henry Ford- W Bloomfield Hosp; **Address:** Henry Ford Hosp, One Ford Pl, Ste 4F83A, Detroit, MI 48202-3450; **Phone:** 313-874-4420; **Board Cert:** Internal Medicine 1974; Cardiovascular Disease 1977; **Med School:** Tufts Univ 1971; **Resid:** Internal Medicine, Univ Wash Hosps 1974; **Fellow:** Cardiovascular Disease, Univ Wash Hosps 1976; **Fac Appt:** Prof Med, Wayne State Univ

Webb, Gary D MD [Cv] - **Spec Exp:** Congenital Heart Disease-Adult; **Hospital:** Cincinnati Chldns Hosp Med Ctr; **Address:** The Heart Inst, Cincinatti Chldn's Hosp, 3333 Burnett Ave, MC 2003, Cincinnati, OH 45229; **Phone:** 513-803-7329; **Med School:** McGill Univ 1967; **Resid:** Internal Medicine, Royal Victoria Hosp 1972; **Fellow:** Cardiovascular Disease, Toronto Genl Hosp 1974

Wilkoff, Bruce L MD [Cv] - **Spec Exp:** Defibrillator Cable Extraction; **Hospital:** Cleveland Clin (page 55); **Address:** Cleveland Clinic, 9500 Euclid Ave, Desk J2-2, Cleveland, OH 44195; **Phone:** 216-444-4975; **Board Cert:** Internal Medicine 1982; Cardiovascular Disease 1985; **Med School:** Ohio State Univ 1979; **Resid:** Internal Medicine, Univ Hosps 1982; **Fellow:** Cardiovascular Disease, Univ Hosps 1984; Cerebrovascular Disease, Ohio State Univ 1986

Williams, Eric S MD [Cv] - **Spec Exp:** Ischemic Heart Disease; Acute Coronary Syndromes; Coronary Artery Disease; Cardiomyopathy; **Hospital:** IU Health Methodist Hosp; **Address:** Methodist Hosp, Fairbanks Hall, 340 W 10th St, Ste 6100, Indianapolis, IN 46202; **Phone:** 317-962-0551; **Board Cert:** Internal Medicine 1974; Cardiovascular Disease 1977; **Med School:** Indiana Univ 1971; **Resid:** Internal Medicine, Indiana Univ Hosps 1973; **Fellow:** Cardiovascular Disease, Indiana Univ Hosps 1975; **Fac Appt:** Prof Med, Indiana Univ

Williams Sr, Kim A MD [Cv] - **Spec Exp:** Nuclear Cardiology; Coronary Artery Disease; **Hospital:** Harper Univ Hosp; **Address:** Wayne St Univ Sch Med, Harper Univ Hosp, 3990 John R St, 1 Brush North, Detroit, MI 48201; **Phone:** 313-745-2620; **Board Cert:** Internal Medicine 1982; Cardiovascular Disease 1985; Nuclear Medicine 1986; **Med School:** Univ Chicago-Pritzker Sch Med 1979; **Resid:** Internal Medicine, Emory Univ 1982; **Fellow:** Cardiovascular Disease, Univ Chicago 1984; Nuclear Medicine, Univ Chicago 1986; **Fac Appt:** Prof Med, Wayne State Univ

Young, James B MD [Cv] - **Spec Exp:** Transplant Medicine-Heart; Heart Failure; Ventricular Assist Device (LVAD); Amyloid Heart Disease; **Hospital:** Cleveland Clin (page 55); **Address:** 9500 Euclid Ave, Desk J3-4, Cleveland, OH 44195; **Phone:** 216-444-2333; **Board Cert:** Internal Medicine 1977; Cardiovascular Disease 1979; **Med School:** Baylor Coll Med 1974; **Resid:** Internal Medicine, Baylor Affil Hosp 1977; Internal Medicine, Methodist Hosp 1980; **Fellow:** Cardiovascular Disease, Baylor Affl Hosp 1979; **Fac Appt:** Prof Med, Cleveland Cl Coll Med/Case West Res

Great Plains and Mountains

Anderson, Jeffrey L MD [Cv] - **Spec Exp:** Arrhythmias; Cholesterol/Lipid Disorders; Cardiac MRI; **Hospital:** LDS Hosp, Salt Lake Regional Med Ctr; **Address:** Intermountain Med Ctr, 5121 S Cottonwood St, Murray, UT 84107-5701; **Phone:** 801-507-4757; **Board Cert:** Internal Medicine 1975; Cardiovascular Disease 1979; Cardiac Electrophysiology 2002; **Med School:** Harvard Med Sch 1972; **Resid:** Internal Medicine, Mass Genl Hosp 1974; **Fellow:** Research, Natl Inst Hlth 1976; Cardiovascular Disease, Stanford Univ Med Ctr 1978; **Fac Appt:** Prof Med, Univ Utah

Benjamin, Ivor J MD [Cv] - **Spec Exp:** Arrhythmias; **Hospital:** Univ Utah Hlth Care; **Address:** Div Cardiology, 30 N 1900 E, rm 4A100, Salt Lake City, UT 84132; **Phone:** 801-581-7715; **Board Cert:** Internal Medicine 1985; Cardiovascular Disease 1989; **Med School:** Johns Hopkins Univ 1982; **Resid:** Internal Medicine, Yale-New Haven Hosp 1985; **Fellow:** Cardiology Research, Yale-New Haven Hosp 1988; Echocardiography, Michael Reese Hosp 1989; **Fac Appt:** Prof Med, Univ Utah

Lindenfeld, JoAnn MD [Cv] - **Spec Exp:** Congestive Heart Failure; Transplant Medicine-Heart; Heart Disease in Women; **Hospital:** Univ of CO Hosp - Anschutz Inpatient Pav; **Address:** 12605 E 16th Ave, B120, Aurora, CO 80045; **Phone:** 720-848-5300; **Board Cert:** Internal Medicine 1976; Cardiovascular Disease 2011; Advanced Heart Failure & Transplant Cardiology 2010; **Med School:** Univ Mich Med Sch 1973; **Resid:** Internal Medicine, UCSD Med Ctr 1977; **Fellow:** Cardiovascular Disease, UT Hlth Sci Ctr 1979; **Fac Appt:** Prof Med, Univ Colorado

Southwest

Abi-samra, Freddy M MD [Cv] - **Spec Exp:** Arrhythmias; Atrial Fibrillation; **Hospital:** Ochsner Med Ctr-New Orleans; **Address:** Oschner Med Ctr, Cardiovascular, 1514 Jefferson Hwy Fl 3rd, Clinic Tower, New Orleans, LA 70121; **Phone:** 504-842-4145; **Board Cert:** Internal Medicine 1984; Cardiovascular Disease 1985; **Med School:** Lebanon 1979; **Resid:** Internal Medicine, Amer Univ Med Ctr 1981; Cardiovascular Disease, Metro Genl Hosp 1984; **Fellow:** Hypertension, Cleveland Clin Fdn 1982; Cardiac Electrophysiology, Cleveland Clin Fdn 1986

Alpert, Joseph S MD [Cv] - **Spec Exp:** Coronary Artery Disease; **Hospital:** Univ Arizona Med Ctr-Univ Campus; **Address:** Univ Arizona Sarver Heart Ctr, 1501 N Campbell Ave Fl 6, Tuscon, AZ 85724; **Phone:** 520-626-2763; **Board Cert:** Internal Medicine 1973; Cardiovascular Disease 1975; **Med School:** Harvard Med Sch 1969; **Resid:** Internal Medicine, Brigham-Womens Hosp 1971; **Fellow:** Cardiovascular Disease, Brigham-Womens Hosp 1974

Ballantyne, Christie M MD [Cv] - **Spec Exp:** Preventive Cardiology; Cholesterol/Lipid Disorders; **Hospital:** Methodist Hosp - Houston; **Address:** Methodist Hospital, DeBakey Heart & Vascular Ctr, 6565 Fannin St, Houston, TX 77030; **Phone:** 713-790-5800; **Board Cert:** Internal Medicine 1985; Cardiovascular Disease 1987; **Med School:** Baylor Coll Med 1982; **Resid:** Internal Medicine, Univ Tex SW Med Ctr 1985; **Fellow:** Cardiovascular Disease, Baylor Coll Med 1988; **Fac Appt:** Prof Med, Baylor Coll Med

Carabello, Blase A MD [Cv] - **Spec Exp:** Heart Valve Disease; **Hospital:** DeBakey VA Med Ctr-Houston; **Address:** Houston VA Medical Ctr, 2002 Holcombe Blvd, MS 111MCL, Houston, TX 77030; **Phone:** 713-794-7070; **Board Cert:** Internal Medicine 1977; Cardiovascular Disease 1979; **Med School:** Temple Univ 1973; **Resid:** Internal Medicine, Mass Genl Hosp 1976; **Fellow:** Cardiovascular Disease, Peter Bent Brigham Hosp 1978; **Fac Appt:** Prof Med, Baylor Coll Med

Freeman, Gregory L MD [Cv] - **Spec Exp:** Interventional Cardiology; **Hospital:** Univ Hlth Syst-San Antonio; **Address:** Methodist Cardiology Clinic, 4411 Medical Drive, Ste 300, San Antonio, TX 78229; **Phone:** 210-614-5400; **Board Cert:** Internal Medicine 1979; Cardiovascular Disease 1983; **Med School:** Loyola Univ-Stritch Sch Med 1976; **Resid:** Internal Medicine, Cook County Hosp 1979; **Fellow:** Cardiovascular Disease, Loyola Univ Med Ctr 1981; Research, UCSD Sch Med 1983; **Fac Appt:** Prof Med, Univ Tex, San Antonio

Gould, K Lance MD [Cv] - **Spec Exp:** Preventive Cardiology; PET Imaging; Cholesterol/Lipid Disorders; **Hospital:** Meml Hermann Hosp - Texas Med Ctr; **Address:** Univ Texas - PET Imaging Ctr, 6431 Fannin St, rm 4.256 MSB, Houston, TX 77030-1501; **Phone:** 713-500-6611; **Med School:** Case West Res Univ 1964; **Resid:** Internal Medicine, Univ Wash Med Ctr 1967; Cardiovascular Disease, Univ Wash Med Ctr 1964; **Fellow:** Cardiovascular Disease, Univ Wash Med Ctr 1971; **Fac Appt:** Prof Med, Univ Tex, Houston

Krajcer, Zvonimir MD [Cv] - **Spec Exp:** Peripheral Vascular Disease; Carotid Artery Disease; Aneurysm-Abdominal & Thoracic Aortic; **Hospital:** St. Luke's Episcopal Hosp-Houston; **Address:** 6624 Fannin St, Ste 2780, Houston, TX 77030; **Phone:** 713-790-9401; **Board Cert:** Internal Medicine 1975; Cardiovascular Disease 1977; **Med School:** Slovenia 1970; **Resid:** Internal Medicine, Northwestern Medical Ctr 1974; **Fellow:** Cardiovascular Disease, St Luke's Episcopal Hosp 1977; **Fac Appt:** Clin Prof Med, Baylor Coll Med

Massin, Edward K MD [Cv] - **Spec Exp:** Congestive Heart Failure; Transplant Medicine-Heart; Coronary Artery Disease; **Hospital:** St. Luke's Episcopal Hosp-Houston; **Address:** Cardiology Consultants Houston, 6624 Fannin St, Ste 2310, Houston, TX 77030-2335; **Phone:** 713-796-2668; **Board Cert:** Internal Medicine 1973; Cardiovascular Disease 1973; **Med School:** Washington Univ, St Louis 1965; **Resid:** Internal Medicine, Barnes Hosp 1967; **Fellow:** Cardiovascular Disease, Univ CO Med Ctr 1971; **Fac Appt:** Clin Prof Med, Baylor Coll Med

McPherson, David D MD [Cv] - **Spec Exp:** Echocardiography; Congenital Heart Disease-Adult; Heart Valve Disease; Echocardiography-Transesophageal; **Hospital:** Meml Hermann Hosp - Texas Med Ctr; **Address:** UT Adult Congenital Heart Disease, 6410 Fannin St, Ste 600, Houston, TX 77030; **Phone:** 832-325-7216; **Board Cert:** Internal Medicine 2005; Cardiovascular Disease 2007; **Med School:** Univ Alberta 1978; **Resid:** Internal Medicine, Dalhousie Univ Hosp 1981; **Fellow:** Cardiovascular Disease, Dalhousie Univ 1983; Cardiovascular Disease, Univ Iowa 1984; **Fac Appt:** Prof Med, Univ Tex, Houston

Nagueh, Sherif F MD [Cv] - **Spec Exp:** Echocardiography; Heart Failure; **Hospital:** Methodist Hosp - Houston; **Address:** Methodist DeBakey Heart & Vascular Ctr, 6550 Fannin St, Ste 1901, Smith Tower, Houston, TX 77030; **Phone:** 713-441-1100; **Board Cert:** Internal Medicine 2003; Cardiovascular Disease 2007; **Med School:** Egypt 1986; **Resid:** Internal Medicine, Baylor Coll Med 1993; **Fellow:** Cardiovascular Disease, Baylor Coll Med 1996; **Fac Appt:** Prof Med, Cornell Univ-Weill Med Coll

Quinones, Miguel A MD [Cv] - **Spec Exp:** Echocardiography; Heart Valve Disease; **Hospital:** Methodist Hosp - Houston; **Address:** Methodist DeBakey Heart & Vascular Ctr, 6550 Fannin St, rm 1901, Smith Tower, Houston, TX 77030; **Phone:** 713-441-1100; **Board Cert:** Internal Medicine 1972; Cardiovascular Disease 1974; **Med School:** Puerto Rico 1968; **Resid:** Internal Medicine, Harlem Hosp 1971; **Fellow:** Cardiovascular Disease, Baylor Coll Med 1974; **Fac Appt:** Prof Med, Univ Tex, Houston

Ramee, Stephen R MD [Cv] - **Spec Exp:** Interventional Cardiology; Angioplasty; Carotid Artery Stent Placement; Renovascular Disease; **Hospital:** Ochsner Med Ctr-New Orleans; **Address:** Ochsner Medical Ctr, Cardiovascular, 1514 Jefferson Hwy, Clinic Tower, New Orleans, LA 70121; **Phone:** 504-842-3727; **Board Cert:** Internal Medicine 1983; Cardiovascular Disease 1985; **Med School:** Geo Wash Univ 1980; **Resid:** Internal Medicine, Letterman Army Med Ctr 1983; **Fellow:** Cardiovascular Disease, Letterman Army Med Ctr 1985

Smart, Frank W MD [Cv] - **Spec Exp:** Congestive Heart Failure; Transplant Medicine-Heart; Ventricular Assist Device (LVAD); Pulmonary Hypertension; **Hospital:** Touro Infirmary, Ochsner Baptist Med Ctr; **Address:** LSU Health Care Network, 3700 Saint Charles Ave, New Orleans, LA 70112; **Phone:** 504-412-1366; **Board Cert:** Internal Medicine 1988; Cardiovascular Disease 2001; Advanced Heart Failure & Transplant Cardiology 2010; **Med School:** Louisiana State U, New Orleans 1985; **Resid:** Internal Medicine, Ochsner Fdn Hosp 1988; **Fellow:** Cardiovascular Disease, Baylor Coll Med 1991; **Fac Appt:** Prof Med, Louisiana State U, New Orleans

Stainback III, Raymond F MD [Cv] - **Spec Exp:** Stroke; Coronary Artery Disease; Heart Valve Disease; Echocardiography-Transesophageal; **Hospital:** St. Luke's Episcopal Hosp-Houston; **Address:** Hall-Garcia Cardiology Assoc, 6624 Fannin St Ste 2480, Houston, TX 77030-2309; **Phone:** 713-529-5530; **Board Cert:** Cardiovascular Disease 2007; Echocardiography 2008; **Med School:** Baylor Coll Med 1987; **Resid:** Internal Medicine, Vanderbilt Univ Med Ctr 1990; **Fellow:** Cardiovascular Disease, Vanderbilt Univ Med Ctr 1993; Echocardiography, UCSF Med Ctr 1995; **Fac Appt:** Assoc Clin Prof Med, Baylor Coll Med

Thames, Marc D MD [Cv] - **Spec Exp:** Coronary Artery Disease; Congestive Heart Failure; **Hospital:** Scottsdale Hlthcare - Shea; **Address:** Cardiovascular Consultants, 3805 E Bell Rd, Ste 3100, Phoenix, AZ 85032-3356; **Phone:** 602-867-8644; **Board Cert:** Internal Medicine 1974; Cardiovascular Disease 1979; **Med School:** Med Coll VA 1970; **Resid:** Internal Medicine, Peter Bent Brigham Hosp 1974; **Fellow:** Cardiology Research, Peter Bent Brigham Hosp 1975; Cardiovascular Disease, Mayo Clinic 1977

Wilansky, Susan MD [Cv] - **Spec Exp:** Heart Disease in Women; Heart Disease in Pregnancy; Echocardiography; Heart Valve Disease; **Hospital:** Mayo Clinic - Phoenix; **Address:** Mayo Clinic, Div Cardiology, 13400 E Shea Blvd, Scottsdale, AZ 85259; **Phone:** 480-301-8200; **Board Cert:** Cardiovascular Disease 1989; **Med School:** McMaster Univ 1979; **Resid:** Internal Medicine, Univ Toronto Affil Hosp 1983; **Fellow:** Cardiovascular Disease, Univ Toronto 1985; Echocardiography, Univ Toronto 1986; **Fac Appt:** Assoc Prof Med, Mayo Med Sch

Zoghbi, William A MD [Cv] - **Spec Exp:** Echocardiography; **Hospital:** Methodist Hosp - Houston; **Address:** Methodist DeBakey Heart & Vascular Ctr, 6550 Fannin St, Ste 1901, Smith Tower, Houston, TX 77030; **Phone:** 713-441-1100; **Board Cert:** Internal Medicine 1982; Cardiovascular Disease 1985; **Med School:** Meharry Med Coll 1979; **Resid:** Internal Medicine, Baylor Coll Affil Hosps 1982; **Fellow:** Cardiovascular Disease, Baylor Coll Med 1985

Cardiovascular Disease

West Coast and Pacific

Bairey, Cathleen Noel MD [Cv] - **Spec Exp:** Preventive Cardiology; Heart Disease in Women; **Hospital:** Cedars-Sinai Med Ctr; **Address:** Cedars-Sinai Women's Heart Ctr, 444 S San Vicente Blvd, Ste 600, Los Angeles, CA 90048; **Phone:** 310-423-9680; **Board Cert:** Internal Medicine 1984; Cardiovascular Disease 1987; **Med School:** Harvard Med Sch 1981; **Resid:** Internal Medicine, UCSF Med Ctr 1984; **Fellow:** Cardiovascular Disease, Cedars-Sinai Med Ctr 1986; **Fac Appt:** Assoc Clin Prof Med, UCLA

Blanchard, Daniel G MD [Cv] - **Spec Exp:** Echocardiography; Hypertension; **Hospital:** UCSD Med Ctr; **Address:** 7434 Medical Center Drive, #7241, La Jolla, CA 92037; **Phone:** 858-657-8530; **Board Cert:** Internal Medicine 1988; Cardiovascular Disease 2002; **Med School:** UCSD 1985; **Resid:** Internal Medicine, UCSD Med Ctr 1988; **Fellow:** Cardiovascular Disease, USCD Med Ctr 1991; **Fac Appt:** Prof Med, UCSD

Budoff, Matthew J MD [Cv] - **Spec Exp:** Cholesterol/Lipid Disorders; Preventive Cardiology; Cardiac Imaging; **Hospital:** LAC - Harbor - UCLA Med Ctr, Little Co of Mary-Torrance Hosp; **Address:** 1124 W Carson St, Torrance, CA 90502; **Phone:** 310-222-5101; **Board Cert:** Internal Medicine 2003; Cardiovascular Disease 2007; **Med School:** Geo Wash Univ 1990; **Resid:** Internal Medicine, UCLA/Harbor Med Ctr 1993; **Fellow:** Cardiovascular Disease, UCLA/Harbor Med Ctr 1997; **Fac Appt:** Prof Med, UCLA

Dichek, David A MD [Cv] - **Spec Exp:** Coronary Artery Disease; Gene Therapy; **Hospital:** Univ Wash Med Ctr; **Address:** UWMC-Regl Heart Ctr, 1959 NE Pacific St, Box 356171, Seattle, WA 98195; **Phone:** 206-598-4300; **Board Cert:** Internal Medicine 1987; Cardiovascular Disease 2004; **Med School:** UCLA 1984; **Resid:** Internal Medicine, Mass Genl Hosp 1987; **Fellow:** Cardiovascular Disease, NIH/Johns Hopkins Hosp 1992; **Fac Appt:** Prof Med, Univ Wash

Edelen, John S MD [Cv] - **Spec Exp:** Angioplasty & Stent Placement; Interventional Cardiology; **Hospital:** Alta Bates Summit Med Ctr-Alta Bates Campus; **Address:** Berkeley Cardiovascular Med Grp, 3300 Webster St Fl 4, Oakland, CA 94609; **Phone:** 510-549-4220; **Board Cert:** Internal Medicine 1974; Cardiovascular Disease 1975; Interventional Cardiology 2001; **Med School:** Columbia P&S 1969; **Resid:** Internal Medicine, Columbia-Presby Med Ctr 1971; **Fellow:** Cardiovascular Disease, Pacific Med Center 1975

Elkayam, Uri MD [Cv] - **Spec Exp:** Congestive Heart Failure; Heart Disease in Pregnancy; Heart Valve Disease; Cardiomyopathy; **Hospital:** LAC & USC Med Ctr; **Address:** USC Cardiovascular Medicine, 2020 Zonal Ave, rm 331, Los Angeles, CA 90033; **Phone:** 323-226-7541; **Board Cert:** Internal Medicine 1989; Cardiovascular Disease 2009; **Med School:** Israel 1973; **Resid:** Internal Medicine, Tel Aviv Sowaski Med Ctr 1976; **Fellow:** Cardiovascular Disease, Albert Einstein Hosp 1978; Cardiovascular Disease, Cedars Sinai Med Ctr 1979; **Fac Appt:** Prof Med, USC Sch Med

Fishbein, Daniel P MD [Cv] - **Spec Exp:** Congestive Heart Failure; Transplant Medicine-Heart; **Hospital:** Univ Wash Med Ctr; **Address:** UWMC-Regl Heart Ctr, 1959 NE Pacific St, Box 356171, Seattle, WA 98195; **Phone:** 206-598-4300; **Board Cert:** Internal Medicine 1983; Cardiovascular Disease 1987; **Med School:** Albert Einstein Coll Med 1980; **Resid:** Internal Medicine, Univ Wash Med Ctr 1983; **Fellow:** Cardiovascular Disease, Univ Wash Med Ctr 1987; Interventional Cardiology, Univ Wash Med Ctr 1989; **Fac Appt:** Assoc Prof Med, Univ Wash

Fonarow, Gregg C MD [Cv] - **Spec Exp:** Cardiomyopathy; Congestive Heart Failure; Transplant Medicine-Heart; Preventive Cardiology; **Hospital:** UCLA Ronald Reagan Med Ctr; **Address:** 200 UCLA Medical Plaza, Ste 224, Los Angeles, CA 90095; **Phone:** 310-825-8816; **Board Cert:** Cardiovascular Disease 2003; **Med School:** UCLA 1987; **Resid:** Internal Medicine, UCLA Med Ctr 1990; **Fellow:** Cardiovascular Disease, UCLA Med Ctr 1993; **Fac Appt:** Prof Med, UCLA

French, William J MD [Cv] - **Spec Exp:** Heart Failure; Interventional Cardiology; Coronary Artery Disease; Cholesterol/Lipid Disorders; **Hospital:** LAC - Harbor - UCLA Med Ctr; **Address:** Harbor-UCLA Med Ctr, 1000 W Carson St, Torrance, CA 90509-2004; **Phone:** 310-222-2415; **Board Cert:** Internal Medicine 1973; Cardiovascular Disease 1979; Interventional Cardiology 2002; **Med School:** Univ VT Coll Med 1968; **Resid:** Internal Medicine, Harlem Hosp-Columbia 1971; Nephrology, Grad Hosp Univ Penn 1972; **Fellow:** Critical Care Medicine, Hollywood Pres Hosp-USC 1975; Cardiovascular Disease, Harbor-UCLA Med Ctr 1977; **Fac Appt:** Prof Med, UCLA

Hunt, Sharon Ann MD [Cv] - **Spec Exp:** Transplant Medicine-Heart; **Hospital:** Stanford Univ Hosp & Clinics; **Address:** Stanford Univ Div Cardiovascular Med, 300 Pasteur Drive, CVRB 265, Stanford, CA 94305; **Phone:** 650-498-6605; **Board Cert:** Internal Medicine 1977; Cardiovascular Disease 2011; Advanced Heart Failure & Transplant Cardiology 2010; **Med School:** Stanford Univ 1972; **Resid:** Internal Medicine, Stanford Univ Hosp 1974; **Fellow:** Cardiovascular Disease, Stanford Univ 1976; **Fac Appt:** Prof Med, Stanford Univ

Johnson, Allen D MD [Cv] - **Spec Exp:** Congenital Heart Disease-Adult; Congestive Heart Failure; **Hospital:** Scripps Green Hosp; **Address:** Scripps Clinic-Torrey Pines, 10666 N Torrey Pines Rd, SW 206, La Jolla, CA 92037; **Phone:** 858-554-8836; **Board Cert:** Internal Medicine 1973; Cardiovascular Disease 1973; **Med School:** Johns Hopkins Univ 1965; **Resid:** Internal Medicine, Johns Hopkins Hosp 1970; **Fellow:** Cardiovascular Disease, UCSD Med Ctr 1972; **Fac Appt:** Clin Prof Med, Univ SD Sch Med

Judelson, Debra R MD [Cv] - **Spec Exp:** Hypertension; Cholesterol/Lipid Disorders; Heart Disease in Women; **Hospital:** Cedars-Sinai Med Ctr, Brotman Med Ctr; **Address:** Cardiovascular Med Group Southern CA, 414 N Camden Drive, Ste 1100, Beverly Hills, CA 90210-4532; **Phone:** 310-278-3400 x155; **Board Cert:** Internal Medicine 1979; Cardiovascular Disease 1981; **Med School:** Harvard Med Sch 1976; **Resid:** Internal Medicine, Kaiser Foundation Hosp 1979; **Fellow:** Cardiovascular Disease, Kaiser Foundation Hosp 1981

Kaul, Sanjiv MD [Cv] - **Spec Exp:** Cardiac Imaging; Echocardiography; Coronary Artery Disease; Preventive Cardiology; **Hospital:** OR Hlth & Sci Univ; **Address:** OHSU Cardiovascular Med, 3181 SW Sam Jackson Park Rd, MC UHN62, Portland, OR 97239; **Phone:** 503-494-8750; **Board Cert:** Internal Medicine 1980; Cardiovascular Disease 1983; **Med School:** India 1975; **Resid:** Internal Medicine, Univ Vermont Med Ctr 1980; Cardiovascular Disease, Wadsworth VA Hosp-UCLA 1982; **Fellow:** Cardiovascular Disease, Mass Genl Hosp 1984; **Fac Appt:** Prof Med, Oregon Hlth & Sci Univ

Kobashigawa, Jon A MD [Cv] - **Spec Exp:** Transplant Medicine-Heart; Congestive Heart Failure; Heart Valve Disease; **Hospital:** Cedars-Sinai Med Ctr, UCLA Ronald Reagan Med Ctr; **Address:** California Heart Ctr, 8536 Wilshire Blvd, Ste 302, Beverly Hills, CA 90211; **Phone:** 310-248-8300; **Board Cert:** Internal Medicine 1983; Cardiovascular Disease 1987; **Med School:** Mount Sinai Sch Med 1980; **Resid:** Internal Medicine, UCLA Med Ctr 1983; **Fellow:** Cardiovascular Disease, UCLA Med Ctr 1986; **Fac Appt:** Clin Prof Med, UCLA

Lewis, Sandra J MD [Cv] - **Spec Exp:** Heart Disease in Women; Preventive Cardiology; Congestive Heart Failure; **Hospital:** Legacy Good Samaritan Med Ctr, Legacy Emanuel Hospital; **Address:** Northwest Cardiovascular Inst, 2222 NW Lovejoy St, Ste 606, Portland, OR 97210; **Phone:** 503-229-7554; **Board Cert:** Internal Medicine 1980; Cardiovascular Disease 1985; **Med School:** Stanford Univ 1977; **Resid:** Internal Medicine, Stanford Univ Med Ctr 1980; **Fellow:** Cardiovascular Disease, Stanford Univ Med Ctr 1983; **Fac Appt:** Assoc Clin Prof Med, Oregon Hlth & Sci Univ

Cardiovascular Disease

Redberg, Rita F MD [Cv] - **Spec Exp:** Echocardiography; Heart Disease in Women; Preventive Cardiology; **Hospital:** UCSF Med Ctr; **Address:** UCSF Cardiology, 535 Mission Bay Blvd S, Box 0327, San Francisco, CA 94158; **Phone:** 415-353-2873; **Board Cert:** Internal Medicine 1985; Cardiovascular Disease 1989; **Med School:** Univ Pennsylvania 1982; **Resid:** Internal Medicine, Columbia-Presby Med Ctr 1985; **Fellow:** Cardiovascular Disease, Columbia-Presby Med Ctr 1988; **Fac Appt:** Prof Med, UCSF

Schnittger, Ingela MD [Cv] - **Spec Exp:** Echocardiography; Echocardiography-Transesophageal; **Hospital:** Stanford Univ Hosp & Clinics; **Address:** 300 Pasteur Drive, rm H2157, Stanford, CA 94305-5233; **Phone:** 650-723-5196; **Board Cert:** Internal Medicine 1980; Cardiovascular Disease 1983; **Med School:** Sweden 1975; **Resid:** Internal Medicine, Stanford Univ Hosp 1980; **Fellow:** Cardiovascular Disease, Stanford Univ 1983; **Fac Appt:** Prof Med, Stanford Univ

Shah, Prediman K MD [Cv] - **Spec Exp:** Coronary Artery Disease; Cholesterol/Lipid Disorders; Preventive Cardiology; Heart Valve Disease; **Hospital:** Cedars-Sinai Med Ctr; **Address:** Cedars-Sinai Med Ctr, 8700 Beverly Blvd, Ste 5531, Los Angeles, CA 90048; **Phone:** 310-423-3884; **Board Cert:** Internal Medicine 1975; Cardiovascular Disease 1977; **Med School:** India 1969; **Resid:** Internal Medicine, All India Inst Med Scis 1971; Internal Medicine, Montefiore Hosp 1974; **Fellow:** Cardiovascular Disease, Montefiore Hosp 1976; Research, Cedars Sinai Med Ctr 1977; **Fac Appt:** Prof Med, UCLA

Skolnick, Alan E MD [Cv] - **Spec Exp:** Nuclear Cardiology; **Hospital:** Providence Alaska Med Ctr; **Address:** Alaska Heart Institute, 3841 Piper St, Ste T-100, Anchorage, AK 99508; **Phone:** 907-561-3211; **Board Cert:** Internal Medicine 2002; Cardiovascular Disease 2005; Nuclear Cardiology 1998; **Med School:** Albert Einstein Coll Med 1989; **Resid:** Internal Medicine, Beth Israel Hosp 1992; **Fellow:** Cardiovascular Disease, Boston Univ Med Ctr 1994

Tobis, Jonathan Marvin MD [Cv] - **Spec Exp:** Interventional Cardiology; **Hospital:** UCLA Ronald Reagan Med Ctr; **Address:** 100 UCLA Medical Plaza, Ste 630, Los Angeles, CA 90095; **Phone:** 310-825-9011; **Board Cert:** Internal Medicine 1976; Cardiovascular Disease 1979; Interventional Cardiology 2009; **Med School:** Albert Einstein Coll Med 1973; **Resid:** Internal Medicine, Lincoln Hosp 1975; Internal Medicine, Univ CA Irvine Med Ctr 1976; **Fellow:** Cardiovascular Disease, Univ CA Irvine Med Ctr 1978; **Fac Appt:** Prof Med, UCLA-David Geffen Sch Med

Topol, Eric J MD [Cv] - **Spec Exp:** Genetic Arrhythmias; **Hospital:** Scripps Meml Hosp - La Jolla; **Address:** 3344 N Torrey Pines Ct SGM 300, La Jolla, CA 92037; **Phone:** 858-554-5708; **Board Cert:** Internal Medicine 1982; Cardiovascular Disease 1985; **Med School:** Univ Rochester 1979; **Resid:** Internal Medicine, UCSF Med Ctr 1982; **Fellow:** Cardiovascular Disease, Johns Hopkins Hosp 1985; **Fac Appt:** Prof CG

CARDIAC ELECTROPHYSIOLOGY

New England

Buxton, Alfred E MD [CE] - **Spec Exp:** Arrhythmias; **Hospital:** Beth Israel Deaconess Med Ctr - Boston; **Address:** Beth Israel Deaconess Med Ctr, 330 Brookline Ave, Boston, MA 02215; **Phone:** 617-667-8800; **Board Cert:** Internal Medicine 1977; Cardiovascular Disease 1981; Cardiac Electrophysiology 2002; **Med School:** Univ Pennsylvania 1973; **Resid:** Internal Medicine, Hosp Univ Penn 1977; **Fellow:** Cardiovascular Disease, Hosp Univ Penn 1980; Cardiac Electrophysiology, Hosp Univ Penn 1981

Epstein, Laurence M MD [CE] - **Spec Exp:** Arrhythmias; Defibrillator Cable Extraction; Defibrillaters; Pacemakers; **Hospital:** Brigham and Women's Hosp (page 57); **Address:** Brigham & Women's Hosp, Cardiology, 75 Francis St, Boston, MA 02115; **Phone:** 857-307-4000; **Board Cert:** Internal Medicine 1989; Cardiac Electrophysiology 2002; **Med School:** Univ Chicago-Pritzker Sch Med 1985; **Resid:** Internal Medicine, UCSF Med Ctr 1989; **Fellow:** Cardiovascular Disease, Hosp Univ Penn 1991; Cardiac Electrophysiology, UCSF Med Ctr 1992; **Fac Appt:** Assoc Prof Med, Harvard Med Sch

Estes, N.A. Mark MD [CE] - **Spec Exp:** Arrhythmias; **Hospital:** Tufts Med Ctr; **Address:** Tufts Medical Ctr, Div Cardiology, 800 Washington St, Box 197, Boston, MA 02111; **Phone:** 617-636-6156; **Board Cert:** Internal Medicine 1980; Cardiovascular Disease 1983; Cardiac Electrophysiology 2002; **Med School:** Univ Cincinnati 1977; **Resid:** Internal Medicine, New England Deaconess Hosp 1980; **Fellow:** Cardiovascular Disease, New England Med Ctr 1980; Cardiac Electrophysiology, Mass General Hosp 1983

Link, Mark S MD [CE] - **Spec Exp:** Arrhythmias; Ventricular Tachycardia Ablation; Heart Disease in Athletes; Sudden Death Prevention; **Hospital:** Tufts Med Ctr; **Address:** Tufts Med Ctr, 800 Washington St, Box 197, Boston, MA 02111; **Phone:** 617-636-5902; **Board Cert:** Internal Medicine 1989; Cardiovascular Disease 2007; Cardiac Electrophysiology 2008; **Med School:** Tufts Univ 1986; **Resid:** Internal Medicine, NY Presby Hosp/Columbia 1989; **Fellow:** Cardiovascular Disease, New England Med Ctr 1996; Cardiac Electrophysiology, New England Med Ctr 1997; **Fac Appt:** Prof Med, Tufts Univ

Ruskin, Jeremy N MD [CE] - **Spec Exp:** Arrhythmias; **Hospital:** Mass Genl Hosp; **Address:** Cardiac Arrhythmia Service, Mass General Hosp, 55 Fruit St, Boston, MA 02114; **Phone:** 617-726-8514; **Board Cert:** Internal Medicine 1974; Cardiovascular Disease 1975; Cardiac Electrophysiology 2003; **Med School:** Harvard Med Sch 1971; **Resid:** Internal Medicine, Beth Israel Hosp 1974; Cardiovascular Disease, Mass Genl Hosp 1977; **Fac Appt:** Assoc Prof Med, Harvard Med Sch

Stevenson, William G MD [CE] - **Spec Exp:** Arrhythmias; **Hospital:** Brigham and Women's Hosp (page 57); **Address:** Brigham & Womens Hosp, Cardiovascular Div, 75 Francis St, Boston, MA 02115; **Phone:** 857-307-4040; **Board Cert:** Internal Medicine 1982; Cardiovascular Disease 1985; Cardiac Electrophysiology 2005; **Med School:** Tulane Univ 1979; **Resid:** Internal Medicine, UCLA Med Ctr 1982; **Fellow:** Cardiovascular Disease, UCLA Med Ctr 1984; Cardiac Electrophysiology, UCLA Med Ctr 1985; **Fac Appt:** Prof Med, Harvard Med Sch

Mid Atlantic

Berger, Ronald D MD/PhD [CE] - **Spec Exp:** Catheter Ablation; **Hospital:** Johns Hopkins Hosp (page 61); **Address:** Johns Hopkins Medicine, 601 N Caroline St, Outpatient Center Fl 7, Baltimore, MD 21287; **Phone:** 410-502-0550; **Board Cert:** Cardiovascular Disease 2004; Cardiac Electrophysiology 2006; **Med School:** Harvard Med Sch 1987; **Resid:** Internal Medicine, Brigham & Women's Hosp 1990; **Fellow:** Cardiovascular Disease, Johns Hopkins Hosp 1993; **Fac Appt:** Prof Med, Johns Hopkins Univ

Callans, David J MD [CE] - **Spec Exp:** Arrhythmias; Pacemakers; **Hospital:** Hosp Univ Penn - UPHS (page 72); **Address:** Hosp Univ Penn - Cardiology, 3400 Spruce St Founders Bldg Fl 9, Philadelphia, PA 19104; **Phone:** 215-662-6052; **Board Cert:** Internal Medicine 1989; Cardiovascular Disease 2005; Cardiac Electrophysiology 2005; **Med School:** Johns Hopkins Univ 1986; **Resid:** Internal Medicine, Hosp Univ Penn 1989; **Fellow:** Cardiovascular Disease, Hosp Univ Penn 1993; Cardiac Electrophysiology, Hosp Univ Penn 1994; **Fac Appt:** Prof Med, Univ Pennsylvania

Chinitz, Larry MD [CE] - **Spec Exp:** Arrhythmias; Pacemakers; Defibrillators; Atrial Fibrillation; **Hospital:** NYU Langone Med Ctr (page 68); **Address:** 403 E 34th St, Heart Rhythm Center, 4th Fl, New York, NY 10016-6402; **Phone:** 212-263-7149; **Board Cert:** Internal Medicine 1982; Cardiovascular Disease 1985; **Med School:** NYU Sch Med 1979; **Resid:** Internal Medicine, Bellevue Hosp Ctr 1983; **Fellow:** Cardiovascular Disease, NYU Med Ctr/Bellevue Hosp Ctr 1986; Cardiac Electrophysiology, Montefiore Hosp 1985; **Fac Appt:** Assoc Prof Med, NYU Sch Med

Cohen, Martin B MD [CE] - **Spec Exp:** Arrhythmias; Pacemakers; Defibrillators; Coronary Angioplasty/Stents; **Hospital:** Westchester Med Ctr, White Plains Hosp; **Address:** Westchester Heart & Vascular, 19 Bradhurst Ave Fl 3 - Ste 3850 South, Hawthorne, NY 10532-2140; **Phone:** 914-909-6900; **Board Cert:** Internal Medicine 1983; Cardiovascular Disease 1985; Cardiac Electrophysiology 2006; Interventional Cardiology 2004; **Med School:** SUNY Downstate 1980; **Resid:** Internal Medicine, Univ Hosp 1983; **Fellow:** Cardiovascular Disease, Univ Hosp 1985; Interventional Cardiology, Westchester Co Med Ctr 1986; **Fac Appt:** Assoc Clin Prof Med, NY Med Coll

Curtis, Anne B MD [CE] - **Spec Exp:** Pacemakers; Arrhythmias; Defibrillators; **Hospital:** Buffalo General Hosp; **Address:** 100 High St, Ste D2-76, Buffalo, NY 14203; **Phone:** 716-859-4828; **Board Cert:** Internal Medicine 1982; Cardiovascular Disease 1985; Cardiac Electrophysiology 2002; **Med School:** Columbia P&S 1979; **Resid:** Internal Medicine, Columbia- Presby Hosp 1982; **Fellow:** Cardiovascular Disease, Duke Univ Med Ctr 1985; Cardiac Electrophysiology, Duke Univ Med Ctr 1986; **Fac Appt:** Prof Med, SUNY Buffalo

Epstein, Andrew E MD [CE] - **Spec Exp:** Arrhythmias; Defibrillators; Catheter Ablation; Genetic Arrhythmias; **Hospital:** Hosp Univ Penn - UPHS (page 72), VA Med Ctr - Philadelphia; **Address:** Hosp Univ Penn - Cardiology, 3400 Spruce St, 9 Founders, Philadelphia, PA 19104; **Phone:** 215-615-5455; **Board Cert:** Internal Medicine 1980; Cardiovascular Disease 1983; Cardiac Electrophysiology 2006; **Med School:** Univ Rochester 1977; **Resid:** Internal Medicine, Barnes-Jewish Hosp 1980; **Fellow:** Cardiovascular Disease, Univ Ala Hosp 1982; **Fac Appt:** Prof Med, Univ Pennsylvania

Gomes, J Anthony MD [CE] - **Spec Exp:** Arrhythmias; Heart Attack; Atrial Fibrillation; Pacemakers; **Hospital:** Mount Sinai Med Ctr (page 64); **Address:** Mount Sinai Medical Ctr, One Gustave L Levy Pl, New York, NY 10029-6500; **Phone:** 212-241-7272; **Board Cert:** Internal Medicine 1974; Cardiovascular Disease 1975; **Med School:** India 1970; **Resid:** Internal Medicine, Mt Sinai Med Ctr 1973; **Fellow:** Cardiovascular Disease, Mt Sinai Med Ctr 1975; Cardiac Electrophysiology, USPHS Cardio-Pulmonary Lab 1976; **Fac Appt:** Prof Med, Mount Sinai Sch Med

Halperin, Henry R MD [CE] - **Spec Exp:** Catheter Ablation; Pacemakers; **Hospital:** Johns Hopkins Hosp (page 61); **Address:** Johns Hopkins Medicine, 601 N Caroline St, Outpatient Center Fl 7, Baltimore, MD 21287; **Phone:** 410-502-0550; **Board Cert:** Internal Medicine 1981; Cardiovascular Disease 1983; Cardiac Electrophysiology 2009; **Med School:** Louisiana State U, Shrevport 1977; **Resid:** Internal Medicine, LSU Charity Hosp 1981; **Fellow:** Cardiovascular Disease, Johns Hopkins Hosp 1983; **Fac Appt:** Prof Med, Johns Hopkins Univ

Lerman, Bruce MD [CE] - **Spec Exp:** Catheter Ablation; Atrial Fibrillation; Defibrillators; Arrhythmias; **Hospital:** NY-Presby/Weill Cornell Med Ctr, NY (page 66); **Address:** NY Weill Cornell Med Ctr, 520 E 70th St, Starr 4, New York, NY 10021-9800; **Phone:** 212-746-2169; **Board Cert:** Internal Medicine 1980; Cardiovascular Disease 1985; Cardiac Electrophysiology 2012; **Med School:** Loyola Univ-Stritch Sch Med 1977; **Resid:** Internal Medicine, Northwestern Univ Hosp 1980; Internal Medicine, Univ Michigan Med Ctr 1981; **Fellow:** Cardiovascular Disease, Hosp Univ Penn 1982; Cardiovascular Disease, Johns Hopkins Hosp 1983; **Fac Appt:** Prof Med, Cornell Univ-Weill Med Coll

Levine, Joseph H MD [CE] - **Spec Exp:** Arrhythmias; Sudden Death Prevention; Atrial Fibrillation; Pacemakers; **Hospital:** St. Francis Hosp - The Heart Ctr (page 73); **Address:** 100 Port Washington Blvd, Roslyn, NY 11576; **Phone:** 516-622-1011; **Board Cert:** Internal Medicine 1983; Cardiovascular Disease 1987; Cardiac Electrophysiology 2003; **Med School:** Univ Rochester 1980; **Resid:** Internal Medicine, Yale-New Haven Hosp 1983; **Fellow:** Cardiovascular Disease, Johns Hopkins Hosp 1986; Cardiac Electrophysiology, Hosp Univ Penn 1986

Marchlinski, Francis E MD [CE] - **Spec Exp:** Pacemakers; Arrhythmias; **Hospital:** Hosp Univ Penn - UPHS (page 72); **Address:** Hosp Univ Penn, Div Cardiology, 3400 Spruce St Founders Bldg Fl 9, Philadelphia, PA 19104-4206; **Phone:** 215-662-6005; **Board Cert:** Internal Medicine 1979; Cardiovascular Disease 1981; Cardiac Electrophysiology 2002; **Med School:** Univ Pennsylvania 1976; **Resid:** Internal Medicine, Hosp Univ Penn 1979; **Fellow:** Cardiovascular Disease, Hosp Univ Penn 1982; **Fac Appt:** Prof Med, Univ Pennsylvania

Mehta, Davendra MD/PhD [CE] - **Spec Exp:** Arrhythmias; Congenital Heart Disease-Adult; Atrial Fibrillation; Heart Failure; **Hospital:** Mount Sinai Med Ctr (page 64); **Address:** One Gustave L Levy Pl, Box 1030, New York, NY 10029-6501; **Phone:** 212-241-7272; **Board Cert:** Cardiovascular Disease 2009; Cardiac Electrophysiology 2009; **Med School:** India 1979; **Resid:** Internal Medicine, Leicester Royal Infirmary 1983; **Fellow:** Cardiovascular Disease, Groby Road Hosp 1986; Electrocardiography, St George's Hosp 1989; **Fac Appt:** Prof Med, Mount Sinai Sch Med

Tomaselli, Gordon F MD [CE] - **Spec Exp:** Arrhythmias; Sudden Death Prevention; **Hospital:** Johns Hopkins Hosp (page 61); **Address:** Johns Hopkins Medicine, 601 N Caroline St, Outpatient Center Fl 7, Baltimore, MD 21287; **Phone:** 410-502-0550; **Board Cert:** Internal Medicine 1985; Cardiovascular Disease 1989; Cardiac Electrophysiology 2005; **Med School:** Albert Einstein Coll Med 1982; **Resid:** Internal Medicine, UCSF Med Ctr 1985; **Fellow:** Cardiovascular Disease, Johns Hopkins Hosp 1986; **Fac Appt:** Prof Med, Johns Hopkins Univ

Southeast

DeLurgio, David B MD [CE] - **Spec Exp:** Arrhythmias; Atrial Fibrillation; Sudden Death Prevention; Heart Failure; **Hospital:** Emory Univ Hosp Midtown, Emory Univ Hosp; **Address:** Emory Univ Hosp Midtown, 550 Peachtree St NE Fl 6, Atlanta, GA 30308; **Phone:** 404-686-2504; **Board Cert:** Cardiovascular Disease 2007; Cardiac Electrophysiology 2008; **Med School:** UCLA 1990; **Resid:** Internal Medicine, Emory Univ Med Ctr 1993; **Fellow:** Cardiovascular Disease, UCLA 1995; **Fac Appt:** Assoc Prof Med, Emory Univ

DiMarco, John P MD/PhD [CE] - **Spec Exp:** Arrhythmias; Pacemakers; Defibrillators; **Hospital:** Univ of Virginia Health Sys; **Address:** Univ Virginia Hlth Scis Ctr, PO Box 800158, Charlottesville, VA 22908-0158; **Phone:** 434-924-2031; **Board Cert:** Internal Medicine 1978; Cardiovascular Disease 1981; Cardiac Electrophysiology 2005; **Med School:** Case West Res Univ 1975; **Resid:** Internal Medicine, Mass Genl Hosp 1977; Critical Care Medicine, Case West Res Univ 1978; **Fellow:** Cardiovascular Disease, Mass Genl Hosp 1980; Cardiac Electrophysiology, Mass Genl Hosp 1981; **Fac Appt:** Prof Med, Univ VA Sch Med

Ellenbogen, Kenneth A MD [CE] - **Spec Exp:** Arrhythmias; Pacemakers; Defibrillators; **Hospital:** Med Coll of VA Hosp, Henrico Doctors Hosp; **Address:** Dept Electrophysiology, PO Box 980053, Richmond, VA 23298; **Phone:** 804-828-7565; **Board Cert:** Internal Medicine 1983; Cardiovascular Disease 1985; Cardiac Electrophysiology 2005; **Med School:** Johns Hopkins Univ 1980; **Resid:** Internal Medicine, Johns Hopkins Hosp 1983; **Fellow:** Cardiovascular Disease, Duke Univ Med Ctr 1986; **Fac Appt:** Prof Med, Med Coll VA

Cardiac Electrophysiology

Interian Jr, Alberto MD [CE] - **Spec Exp:** Arrhythmias; **Hospital:** Mercy Hosp, Jackson Meml Hosp; **Address:** Mercy Arrhythmia & Syncope Ctr, 3641 S Miami Ave, Ste 221, Bayside Pavillion Bldg, Miami, FL 33133; **Phone:** 305-285-2642; **Board Cert:** Internal Medicine 1985; Cardiovascular Disease 1987; **Med School:** Univ Miami Sch Med 1982; **Resid:** Internal Medicine, Univ Miami Hosps 1985; **Fellow:** Cardiovascular Disease, Univ Miami Hosps 1988; **Fac Appt:** Prof Med, Univ Miami Sch Med

Kay, G Neal MD [CE] - **Spec Exp:** Arrhythmias; Atrial Fibrillation; Pacemakers; **Hospital:** Univ of Ala Hosp at Birmingham; **Address:** UAB, Div Cardiovascular Disease, 1720 2nd Ave S, FOT 930, Birmingham, AL 35294; **Phone:** 205-934-1335; **Board Cert:** Internal Medicine 1983; Cardiovascular Disease 1989; Cardiac Electrophysiology 2006; **Med School:** Univ Mich Med Sch 1979; **Resid:** Internal Medicine, Univ Alabama Hosp 1983; **Fellow:** Cardiovascular Disease, Duke Univ Med Ctr 1986; **Fac Appt:** Prof Med, Univ Alabama

Onufer, John R MD [CE] - **Spec Exp:** Atrial Fibrillation; Catheter Ablation; Pacemakers; Defibrillators; **Hospital:** Henrico Doctors Hosp; **Address:** Virginia Cardiovascular Specialists, 7611 Forest Ave, Ste 100, Richmond, VA 23229; **Phone:** 804-288-4827; **Board Cert:** Internal Medicine 1987; Cardiovascular Disease 2001; Cardiac Electrophysiology 2002; **Med School:** Washington Univ, St Louis 1984; **Resid:** Internal Medicine, Barnes Jewish Hosp 1987; **Fellow:** Cardiovascular Disease, Washington Univ 1990; Cardiac Electrophysiology, Washington Univ 1991

Sorrentino, Robert A MD [CE] - **Spec Exp:** Arrhythmias; Defibrillators; Pacemakers; Heart Failure; **Hospital:** Med Coll of GA Hosp and Clin (MCG Health Inc); **Address:** Medical College of Georgia, 1120 15th St BBR Bldg - rm 6513B, Augusta, GA 30912-0004; **Phone:** 706-721-4997; **Board Cert:** Internal Medicine 1988; Cardiovascular Disease 2002; Cardiac Electrophysiology 2008; **Med School:** Albany Med Coll 1985; **Resid:** Internal Medicine, Duke Univ Med Ctr 1988; **Fellow:** Cardiovascular Disease, Duke Univ Med Ctr 1991; **Fac Appt:** Prof Med, Med Coll GA

Midwest

Anderson, Mark E MD/PhD [CE] - **Spec Exp:** Arrhythmias; **Hospital:** Univ Iowa Hosp & Clinics; **Address:** 200 Hawkins Drive, GH Bldg, rm SE308 GH, Iowa City, IA 52242-1081; **Phone:** 319-356-2745; **Board Cert:** Internal Medicine 2005; Cardiovascular Disease 2005; **Med School:** Univ Minn 1989; **Resid:** Internal Medicine, Stanford Univ Med Ctr 1991; **Fellow:** Cardiovascular Disease, Stanford Univ Sch Med 1994; Cardiac Electrophysiology, Stanford Univ Sch Med 1996; **Fac Appt:** Prof Med, Univ Iowa Coll Med

Asirvatham, Samuel J MD [CE] - **Spec Exp:** Atrial Fibrillation; **Hospital:** Mayo Med Ctr & Clin - Rochester, Rochester Methodist Hosp; **Address:** 200 1st St SW Mary-Brig Bldg Fl 4 - Ste 523, Rochester, MN 55905; **Phone:** 507-293-3376; **Board Cert:** Internal Medicine 2007; Cardiovascular Disease 2008; Cardiac Electrophysiology 2010; **Med School:** India 1991; **Resid:** Internal Medicine, Univ WI Hosp & Clins 1994; **Fellow:** Cardiovascular Disease, OU Med Ctr 1998; Cardiac Electrophysiology, Mayo Med Ctr & Clin 2000; **Fac Appt:** Prof Med, Mayo Med Sch

Donahue, J Kevin MD [CE] - **Spec Exp:** Arrhythmias; Catheter Ablation; Defibrillators; Ventricular Tachycardia Ablation; **Hospital:** MetroHealth Med Ctr; **Address:** MetroHealth Hosp, 2500 MetroHealth Drive, R-653, Dept Heart & Vascular, Cleveland, OH 44109; **Phone:** 216-778-2328; **Board Cert:** Cardiovascular Disease 2009; Cardiac Electrophysiology 2011; **Med School:** Washington Univ, St Louis 1992; **Resid:** Internal Medicine, Hosp Univ Penn 1994; **Fellow:** Cardiovascular Disease, Johns Hopkins Hosp 1999; Cardiac Electrophysiology, Johns Hopkins Hosp 1999; **Fac Appt:** Prof Med, Case West Res Univ

Faddis, Mitchell N MD/PhD [CE] - **Spec Exp:** Arrhythmias; **Hospital:** Barnes-Jewish Hosp; **Address:** Barnes-Jewish Hosp, Dept Cardiology, Ctr for Avanced Med, 1 Barnes Hosp Pl Fl 8, St Louis, MO 63110; **Phone:** 314-362-1291; **Board Cert:** Internal Medicine 2006; Cardiovascular Disease 2009; Cardiac Electrophysiology 2010; **Med School:** Washington Univ, St Louis 1993; **Resid:** Internal Medicine, Barnes-Jewish Hosp 1995; **Fellow:** Cardiovascular Disease, Barnes-Jewish Hosp 1996; **Fac Appt:** Assoc Prof Med, Washington Univ, St Louis

Hammill, Stephen C MD [CE] - **Spec Exp:** Pacemakers; Arrhythmias; **Hospital:** Mayo Med Ctr & Clin - Rochester; **Address:** Mayo Clinic, 200 First St SW, Rochester, MN 55905; **Phone:** 507-284-2129; **Board Cert:** Internal Medicine 1978; Cardiovascular Disease 1981; Cardiac Electrophysiology 2005; **Med School:** Univ Colorado 1974; **Resid:** Internal Medicine, Univ Colorado Hlth Sci Ctr 1977; **Fellow:** Cardiovascular Disease, Duke Univ Med Ctr 1981; **Fac Appt:** Prof Med, Mayo Med Sch

Hayes, David L MD [CE] - **Spec Exp:** Pacemakers; **Hospital:** Mayo Med Ctr & Clin - Rochester; **Address:** Mayo Clinic, 200 1st St SW, Rochester, MN 55905; **Phone:** 507-284-2511; **Board Cert:** Internal Medicine 1980; Cardiovascular Disease 1981; **Med School:** Univ MO-Kansas City 1977; **Resid:** Internal Medicine, Mayo Clin 1980; **Fellow:** Cardiovascular Disease, Mayo Clin 1982; **Fac Appt:** Prof Med, Mayo Med Sch

Lindsay, Bruce MD [CE] - **Spec Exp:** Arrhythmias; **Hospital:** Cleveland Clin (page 55); **Address:** Cleveland Clinic, 9500 Euclid Ave, Desk J2-2, Cleveland, OH 44195; **Phone:** 216-444-4293; **Board Cert:** Internal Medicine 1980; Cardiovascular Disease 1987; Cardiac Electrophysiology 2002; **Med School:** Jefferson Med Coll 1976; **Resid:** Internal Medicine, Univ Michigan Med Ctr 1980; **Fellow:** Cardiovascular Disease, Barnes-Jewish Hosp 1985; **Fac Appt:** Assoc Prof Med

Love, Charles J MD [CE] - **Spec Exp:** Defibrillator Cable Extraction; Pacemakers; **Hospital:** Ohio St Univ Med Ctr; **Address:** Heart & Lung Inst Fl 2, 473 W 12 Ave, Columbus, OH 43210; **Phone:** 614-293-4947; **Board Cert:** Internal Medicine 1986; Cardiovascular Disease 1989; Cardiac Electrophysiology 2004; **Med School:** Univ Pittsburgh 1983; **Resid:** Internal Medicine, Ohio State Univ Hosp 1986; **Fellow:** Cardiac Electrophysiology, Ohio State Univ Hosp 1988; **Fac Appt:** Prof Med, Ohio State Univ

Miller, John M MD [CE] - **Spec Exp:** Arrhythmias; Catheter Ablation; Atrial Fibrillation; **Hospital:** IU Health Methodist Hosp, IU Health University Hosp; **Address:** Krannert Inst of Cardiology, 1800 N Senate Blvd, MPC 2, Ste 4000, Indianapolis, IN 46202; **Phone:** 317-962-0101; **Board Cert:** Internal Medicine 1982; Cardiovascular Disease 1985; Cardiac Electrophysiology 2003; **Med School:** Penn State Coll Med 1979; **Resid:** Internal Medicine, NC Meml Hosp 1982; **Fellow:** Cardiovascular Disease, Hosp Univ Penn 1985; **Fac Appt:** Prof Med, Indiana Univ

Morady, Fred MD [CE] - **Spec Exp:** Arrhythmias; WPW Syndrome; **Hospital:** Univ of Michigan Hosp; **Address:** Specialty Electrophysiology, 1500 E Med Ctr Drive, SPC 3rd FL 5856, Ann Arbor, MI 48109; **Phone:** 734-647-7321; **Board Cert:** Internal Medicine 1978; Cardiovascular Disease 1981; Cardiac Electrophysiology 2005; **Med School:** UCSF 1975; **Resid:** Internal Medicine, UCSF Med Ctr 1978; **Fellow:** Cardiovascular Disease, UCSF Med Ctr 1980; **Fac Appt:** Prof Med, Univ Mich Med Sch

Prystowsky, Eric N MD [CE] - **Spec Exp:** Arrhythmias; Catheter Ablation; Atrial Fibrillation; **Hospital:** St. Vincent Indianapolis Hosp; **Address:** St Vincent Medical Group, 8333 Naab Rd, Ste 400, Indianapolis, IN 46260; **Phone:** 317-338-6024; **Board Cert:** Internal Medicine 1976; Cardiovascular Disease 1979; Cardiac Electrophysiology 2005; **Med School:** Mount Sinai Sch Med 1973; **Resid:** Internal Medicine, Mt Sinai Hosp 1976; **Fellow:** Cardiovascular Disease, Duke Univ Med Ctr 1979

Schuger, Claudio D MD [CE] - **Spec Exp:** Arrhythmias; Defibrillators; **Hospital:** Henry Ford Hosp; **Address:** Henry Ford Hosp, Div Cardiology, 2799 W Grand Blvd, Ste 322, Detroit, MI 48202; **Phone:** 313-916-2417; **Board Cert:** Cardiac Electrophysiology 2008; Cardiovascular Disease 2007; **Med School:** Argentina 1977; **Resid:** Internal Medicine, Hacarmel Hosp 1982; **Fellow:** Cardiovascular Disease, Bikur Cholim Hosp 1985; Cardiac Electrophysiology, Harper Hosp 1990; **Fac Appt:** Prof Med, Wayne State Univ

Tchou, Patrick J MD [CE] - **Spec Exp:** Arrhythmias; **Hospital:** Cleveland Clin (page 55); **Address:** Dept Cardiology, 9500 Euclid Ave, Desk J2-2, Cleveland, OH 44195; **Phone:** 216-444-6792; **Board Cert:** Internal Medicine 1982; Cardiovascular Disease 1985; Cardiac Electrophysiology 2002; **Med School:** Case West Res Univ 1979; **Resid:** Internal Medicine, Metro Genl Hosp 1982; **Fellow:** Cardiovascular Disease, Metro Genl Hosp 1984; Cardiac Electrophysiology, Mt Sinai Med Ctr 1985; **Fac Appt:** Prof Med, Ohio State Univ

Waldo, Albert Leon MD [CE] - **Spec Exp:** Arrhythmias; Syncope; Long QT Interval Syndrome; Atrial Fibrillation; **Hospital:** Univ Hosps Case Med Ctr (page 74); **Address:** University Hospitals Case Medical Center, 11100 Euclid Ave, MS LKS-5038, Cleveland, OH 44106-1736; **Phone:** 216-844-7690; **Board Cert:** Internal Medicine 1971; Cardiovascular Disease 1975; **Med School:** SUNY Downstate 1962; **Resid:** Internal Medicine, Baltimore City Hosp 1965; Internal Medicine, Kings Co Hosp 1966; **Fellow:** Cardiovascular Disease, Columbia Presby Med Ctr 1968; Cardiac Electrophysiology, Columbia Presby Med Ctr 1969; **Fac Appt:** Prof Med, Case West Res Univ

Wilber, David J MD [CE] - **Spec Exp:** Atrial Fibrillation; Catheter Ablation; Sudden Death Prevention; **Hospital:** Loyola Univ Med Ctr; **Address:** Loyola Univ Med Ctr, Cardiovascular Inst, 2160 S First Ave Bldg 110 - rm 6232, Maywood, IL 60153; **Phone:** 708-216-2642; **Board Cert:** Internal Medicine 1980; Cardiovascular Disease 1985; Cardiac Electrophysiology 2002; **Med School:** Northwestern Univ 1977; **Resid:** Internal Medicine, Northwestern Meml Hosp 1980; **Fellow:** Cardiovascular Disease, Univ Mich Med Sch 1984; Cardiac Electrophysiology, Mass Genl Hosp 1986; **Fac Appt:** Prof Med, Loyola Univ-Stritch Sch Med

Great Plains and Mountains

Lewkowiez, Laurent MD [CE] - **Spec Exp:** Arrhythmias; Ventricular Tachycardia Ablation; Atrial Fibrillation; **Address:** Franklin Medical Offices, 2045 Franklin St, Denver, CO 80205; **Phone:** 303-338-4545; **Board Cert:** Cardiovascular Disease 2010; Cardiac Electrophysiology 2003; **Med School:** Univ SC Sch Med 1992; **Resid:** Internal Medicine, Univ Colorado Affil Hosp 1996; **Fellow:** Nuclear Cardiology, Univ Colorado 1998; Cardiac Electrophysiology, Univ Colorado 2001; **Fac Appt:** Asst Prof Med, Univ Colorado

Southwest

Natale, Andrea MD [CE] - **Spec Exp:** Arrhythmias; Atrial Fibrillation; **Hospital:** St. David's Med Ctr; **Address:** Texas Cardiac Arrhythmia Institute, 3000 N IH 35, Ste 700, Austin, TX 78705; **Phone:** 512-807-3150; **Board Cert:** Cardiovascular Disease 2012; **Med School:** Italy 1985; **Resid:** Internal Medicine, Univ Rome Med Ctr 1989; **Fellow:** Cardiovascular Disease, Univ Western Ontario 1992; Cardiac Electrophysiology, Sinai Samaritan Med Ctr/Univ WI 1994

Shen, Win-Kuang MD [CE] - **Spec Exp:** Arrhythmias; Catheter Ablation; Defibrillators; Autonomic Disorders; **Hospital:** Mayo Clinic - Phoenix; **Address:** 5777 E Mayo Blvd, Pheonix, AZ 85054; **Phone:** 480-342-0348; **Board Cert:** Internal Medicine 1986; Cardiovascular Disease 2011; Cardiac Electrophysiology 2002; **Med School:** NY Med Coll 1983; **Resid:** Internal Medicine, Mayo Clinic-Rochester 1986; **Fellow:** Cardiovascular Disease, Mayo Clinic-Rochester 1988; Cardiac Electrophysiology, Duke Univ 1991; **Fac Appt:** Prof Med, Mayo Med Sch

Snyder, David W MD [CE] - **Hospital:** E Jefferson Genl Hosp; **Address:** East Jefferson Cardiology Consultants, 4200 Houma Blvd Fl 2, Metairie, LA 70002; **Phone:** 504-454-4102; **Board Cert:** Internal Medicine 1978; Cardiovascular Disease 1981; Cardiac Electrophysiology 2002; **Med School:** Duke Univ 1975; **Resid:** Internal Medicine, Barnes-Jewish Hosp 1978; **Fellow:** Cardiovascular Disease, Barnes-Jewish Hosp 1978

West Coast and Pacific

Cannom, David S MD [CE] - **Spec Exp:** Arrhythmias; **Hospital:** Good Samaritan Hosp - LA; **Address:** 1245 Wilshire Blvd, Ste 703, Los Angeles, CA 90017; **Phone:** 213-977-0419; **Board Cert:** Internal Medicine 1980; Cardiovascular Disease 1975; **Med School:** Univ Minn 1967; **Resid:** Internal Medicine, Yale-New Haven Hosp 1969; **Fellow:** Cardiovascular Disease, Stanford Univ 1973; **Fac Appt:** Clin Prof Med, UCLA

Feld, Gregory K MD [CE] - **Hospital:** UCSD Med Ctr; **Address:** 9434 Medical Drive, La Jolla, CA 92037; **Phone:** 858-657-8530; **Board Cert:** Internal Medicine 1980; Cardiovascular Disease 1983; Cardiac Electrophysiology 2002; **Med School:** Dartmouth Med Sch 1977; **Resid:** Internal Medicine, Wadsworth VA Hosp 1981; **Fellow:** Cardiothoracic Research, Wadsworth VA Hosp 1984; **Fac Appt:** Prof Med, UCSD

Gang, Eli S MD [CE] - **Spec Exp:** Arrhythmias; **Hospital:** Cedars-Sinai Med Ctr, Brotman Med Ctr; **Address:** 414 N Camden Drive, Ste 1100, Beverly Hills, CA 90210; **Phone:** 310-278-3400; **Board Cert:** Internal Medicine 1978; Cardiovascular Disease 1981; **Med School:** Columbia P&S 1975; **Resid:** Internal Medicine, Roosevelt Hosp 1978; **Fellow:** Cardiovascular Disease, Columbia Presby Hosp 1979; **Fac Appt:** Clin Prof Med, UCLA

Higgins, Steven MD [CE] - **Spec Exp:** Arrhythmias; Defibrillators; **Hospital:** Scripps Meml Hosp - La Jolla, Tri-City Med Ctr - Oceanside; **Address:** 9850 Genesee Ave, Ste 940, La Jolla, CA 92037; **Phone:** 858-658-0088; **Board Cert:** Internal Medicine 1982; Cardiovascular Disease 1985; Cardiac Electrophysiology 2003; **Med School:** Univ Rochester 1979; **Resid:** Internal Medicine, Univ CO Med Ctr 1982; **Fellow:** Cardiovascular Disease, Univ CO Med Ctr 1985

Swerdlow, Charles D MD [CE] - **Spec Exp:** Defibrillators; Arrhythmias; Pacemakers; WPW Syndrome; **Hospital:** Cedars-Sinai Med Ctr, UCLA Ronald Reagan Med Ctr; **Address:** 414 N Camden Drive, Ste 1100, Beverly Hills, CA 90210; **Phone:** 310-278-3400; **Board Cert:** Internal Medicine 1979; Cardiovascular Disease 1981; Cardiac Electrophysiology 2004; **Med School:** Harvard Med Sch 1976; **Resid:** Internal Medicine, LAC-Harbor Genl Hosp 1979; **Fellow:** Cardiovascular Disease, Stanford Univ Med Ctr 1981; **Fac Appt:** Clin Prof Med, UCLA

Wang, Paul J MD [CE] - **Spec Exp:** Arrhythmias; Atrial Fibrillation; Defibrillators; **Hospital:** Stanford Univ Hosp & Clinics; **Address:** Stanford Univ Cardiovascular Med, 300 Pasteur Drive, rm A260, Stanford, CA 94305; **Phone:** 650-723-7111; **Board Cert:** Internal Medicine 1986; Cardiovascular Disease 1989; Cardiac Electrophysiology 2002; **Med School:** Columbia P&S 1983; **Resid:** Internal Medicine, NY Presby-Columbia Med Ctr 1986; **Fellow:** Cardiovascular Disease, Brigham & Women's Hosp 1989; **Fac Appt:** Prof Med, Stanford Univ

INTERVENTIONAL CARDIOLOGY

New England

Gibson, C Michael MD [IC] - **Spec Exp:** Acute Coronary Syndromes; Clinical Trials; **Hospital:** Beth Israel Deaconess Med Ctr - Boston; **Address:** Beth Israel Deaconess Med Ctr, 185 Pilgrim Rd, Room Deaconess 319, Boston, MA 02215; **Phone:** 617-667-8800; **Board Cert:** Internal Medicine 1989; Cardiovascular Disease 2002; Interventional Cardiology 2002; **Med School:** Univ Chicago-Pritzker Sch Med 1986; **Resid:** Internal Medicine, Brigham & Womens Hosp 1989; Internal Medicine, Brigham & Womens Hosp 1993; **Fellow:** Cardiovascular Disease, Beth Israel Deaconess Med Ctr 1992; **Fac Appt:** Assoc Prof Med, Harvard Med Sch

Jacobs, Alice K MD [IC] - **Spec Exp:** Cardiac Catheterization; Heart Disease in Women; **Hospital:** Boston Med Ctr; **Address:** Boston Univ Med Ctr, Dept Cardiology, 88 E Newton St, rm C822, Boston, MA 02118; **Phone:** 617-638-8707; **Board Cert:** Internal Medicine 1978; Endocrinology 1979; Cardiovascular Disease 1985; **Med School:** St Louis Univ 1975; **Resid:** Internal Medicine, St Louis Univ Hosp 1977; **Fellow:** Endocrinology, UCSD Med Ctr 1980; Cardiovascular Disease, Boston Univ Med Ctr 1982; **Fac Appt:** Prof Med, Boston Univ

Kimmelstiel, Carey D MD [IC] - **Spec Exp:** Cardiac Catheterization; Heart Failure; **Hospital:** Tufts Med Ctr; **Address:** Tufts Medical Center, 800 Washington St, rm 264, Boston, MA 02111-1526; **Phone:** 617-636-5914; **Board Cert:** Cardiovascular Disease 1989; Internal Medicine 1985; Interventional Cardiology 2009; **Med School:** SUNY Downstate 1982; **Resid:** Internal Medicine, Kings Co Hosp/SUNY Downstate 1986; **Fellow:** Cardiovascular Disease, UMass Memorial Med Ctr 1989; Interventional Cardiology, Tufts-New Engl Med Ctr 1990; **Fac Appt:** Assoc Prof Med, Tufts Univ

Laham, Roger MD [IC] - **Spec Exp:** Angioplasty; **Hospital:** Beth Israel Deaconess Med Ctr - Boston; **Address:** Beth Israel Deaconess Med Ctr, 185 Pilgrim Rd, Baker 4, Boston, MA 02215; **Phone:** 617-667-8800; **Board Cert:** Internal Medicine 2004; Cardiovascular Disease 2005; Interventional Cardiology 2010; **Med School:** Amer Univ Beirut 1989; **Resid:** Internal Medicine, Duke Univ Med Ctr 1992; **Fellow:** Cardiovascular Disease, Harvard Med Sch 1995; **Fac Appt:** Assoc Prof Med, Harvard Med Sch

Palacios, Igor F MD [IC] - **Spec Exp:** Interventional Cardiology; **Hospital:** Mass Genl Hosp; **Address:** Mass Genl Hosp, Cardiac Unit, 55 Fruit St, GRB 800, Boston, MA 02114; **Phone:** 617-726-8424; **Board Cert:** Internal Medicine 1979; Cardiovascular Disease 1981; Interventional Cardiology 2009; **Med School:** Venezuela 1969; **Resid:** Cardiovascular Disease, Hosp Univ de Caracas 1973; **Fellow:** Cardiovascular Disease, Mass Genl Hosp-Harvard 1980; **Fac Appt:** Assoc Prof Med, Harvard Med Sch

Rosenfield, Kenneth MD [IC] - **Spec Exp:** Angioplasty & Stent Placement; **Hospital:** Mass Genl Hosp; **Address:** Mass Genl Hosp, 55 Fruit St, Ste GRB800, Boston, MA 02114; **Phone:** 617-724-1935; **Board Cert:** Internal Medicine 1985; Cardiovascular Disease 1989; Interventional Cardiology 2002; **Med School:** Univ Mass Sch Med 1982; **Resid:** Internal Medicine, Kaiser Fdn Hosp 1985; **Fellow:** Cardiovascular Disease, New Eng Med Ctr 1988; Interventional Cardiology, St Elizabeth's Med Ctr 1989

Williams, David O MD [IC] - **Spec Exp:** Cardiac Catheterization; **Hospital:** Brigham and Women's Hosp (page 57); **Address:** Brigham & Women's Hosp, Cardiovascular Div, 1620 Tremont St Fl 3, Boston, MA 02115; **Phone:** 857-307-1987; **Board Cert:** Internal Medicine 1972; Cardiovascular Disease 1975; **Med School:** Hahnemann Univ 1969; **Resid:** Internal Medicine, Hahnemann Univ Hosp 1972; **Fellow:** Cardiovascular Disease, UC Davis Med Ctr 1974; **Fac Appt:** Prof Med, Brown Univ

Zelman, Richard MD [IC] - **Spec Exp:** Angioplasty & Stent Placement; **Hospital:** Cape Cod Hosp; **Address:** 40 Quinlan Way, Ste 104, Hyannis, MA 02601; **Phone:** 508-862-7645; **Board Cert:** Internal Medicine 1986; Cardiovascular Disease 1989; Interventional Cardiology 2009; **Med School:** Univ Tex, San Antonio 1983; **Resid:** Internal Medicine, Brigham & Womens Hosp 1986; **Fellow:** Cardiovascular Disease, Brigham & Womens Hosp 1989

Mid Atlantic

Chang, Gene MD [IC] - **Spec Exp:** Cardiac Catheterization; Angioplasty & Stent Placement; Atrial Septal Defect; **Hospital:** Penn Presby Med Ctr - UPHS (page 72); **Address:** Philadelphia Heart Inst, 51 N 39th St, Fl 4, Ste 400, Philadelphia, PA 19104; **Phone:** 215-662-9000; **Board Cert:** Cardiovascular Disease 2008; Interventional Cardiology 2009; **Med School:** Tufts Univ 1991; **Resid:** Internal Medicine, New England Deaconess Hosp 1994; **Fellow:** Cardiovascular Disease, Hosp U Penn 1998; Interventional Cardiology, Hosp U Penn 1999; **Fac Appt:** Asst Prof Med, Univ Pennsylvania

Gray, William A MD [IC] - **Spec Exp:** Peripheral Vascular Disease; Percutaneous Valve Repair; Coronary Artery Disease; Mitral Valve Surgery; **Hospital:** NY-Presby/Columbia Univ Med Ctr, NY (page 66); **Address:** Ctr for Interventional Vascular Therapy, 161 Fort Washington Ave, Fl 6th, New York, NY 10032; **Phone:** 212-305-7060; **Board Cert:** Internal Medicine 1987; Cardiovascular Disease 2002; Interventional Cardiology 2011; Vascular Medicine 2004; **Med School:** Temple Univ 1984; **Resid:** Internal Medicine, Rhode Island Hosp/Brown Univ 1988; **Fellow:** Cardiovascular Disease, Brown Univ 1992; **Fac Appt:** Assoc Prof Med, Columbia P&S

Herrmann, Howard C MD [IC] - **Spec Exp:** Cardiac Catheterization; Angioplasty & Stent Placement; Heart Valve Disease; Atrial Septal Defect; **Hospital:** Hosp Univ Penn - UPHS (page 72), Penn Presby Med Ctr - UPHS (page 72); **Address:** 3400 Spruce St, 9308 Gates Pavillion Pl, Philadelphia, PA 19104-4283; **Phone:** 215-662-2180; **Board Cert:** Internal Medicine 1984; Cardiovascular Disease 1987; Interventional Cardiology 2009; **Med School:** Harvard Med Sch 1981; **Resid:** Internal Medicine, Mass General Hosp 1984; **Fellow:** Cardiovascular Disease, Mass General Hosp 1987; **Fac Appt:** Prof Med, Univ Pennsylvania

Lee, Joon Sup MD [IC] - **Spec Exp:** Cardiac Catheterization; **Hospital:** UPMC Presby, Pittsburgh; **Address:** UPMC Presbyterian, Div Cardiology, 200 Lothrop St, Ste A333, Pittsburgh, PA 15213; **Phone:** 412-647-1385; **Board Cert:** Internal Medicine 2005; Cardiovascular Disease 2005; Interventional Cardiology 2009; **Med School:** Duke Univ 1988; **Resid:** Internal Medicine, Mass General Hosp 1991; **Fellow:** Cardiovascular Disease, Mass General Hosp 1996; **Fac Appt:** Asst Prof Med, Univ Pittsburgh

Leon, Martin B MD [IC] - **Hospital:** NY-Presby/Columbia Univ Med Ctr, NY (page 66); **Address:** 161 Ft Washington Ave, Irving Pavillion Fl 6 - Ste 607, New York, NY 10032; **Phone:** 212-305-7060; **Board Cert:** Internal Medicine 1979; Cardiovascular Disease 1983; **Med School:** Yale Univ 1975; **Resid:** Internal Medicine, Yale-New Haven Hosp 1978; **Fellow:** Cardiovascular Disease, Yale-New Haven Hosp 1980

Moses, Jeffrey W MD [IC] - **Spec Exp:** Angiography-Coronary; Angioplasty & Stent Placement; Heart Valve Disease; **Hospital:** NY-Presby/Columbia Univ Med Ctr, NY (page 66); **Address:** 161 Ft Washington Ave Fl 6, New York, NY 10032; **Phone:** 212-305-7060; **Board Cert:** Internal Medicine 1977; Cardiovascular Disease 1981; Interventional Cardiology 2009; **Med School:** Univ Pennsylvania 1974; **Resid:** Internal Medicine, Penn Presby Med Ctr 1977; **Fellow:** Cardiovascular Disease, Penn Presby Med Ctr 1980

Parikh, Manish A MD [IC] - **Spec Exp:** Coronary Angioplasty/Stents; **Hospital:** Lenox Hill Hosp (page 67); **Address:** 16 E 60th St, Ste 322, New York, NY 10022; **Phone:** 212-326-8532; **Board Cert:** Cardiovascular Disease 2010; Interventional Cardiology 2010; **Med School:** UMDNJ-NJ Med Sch, Newark 1990; **Resid:** Internal Medicine, New York Hosp 1993; **Fellow:** Cardiovascular Disease, New York Hosp 1997; **Fac Appt:** Asst Prof Med, Cornell Univ-Weill Med Coll

Petrossian, George A MD [IC] - **Spec Exp:** Carotid Artery Stent Placement; Peripheral Vascular Disease; Coronary Angioplasty/Stents; Renovascular Disease; **Hospital:** St. Francis Hosp - The Heart Ctr (page 73), South Nassau Comm Hosp; **Address:** 1405 Old Northern Blvd, 1st Floor, Roslyn, NY 11576-1353; **Phone:** 516-484-6777; **Board Cert:** Internal Medicine 1986; Cardiovascular Disease 1989; Interventional Cardiology 2010; **Med School:** Mount Sinai Sch Med 1983; **Resid:** Internal Medicine, Columbia-Presby Med Ctr 1987; **Fellow:** Cardiovascular Disease, Columbia -Presby Med Ctr 1989; Interventional Cardiology, Mass Genl Hosp 1990

Pichard, Augusto MD [IC] - **Spec Exp:** Angioplasty & Stent Placement; Cardiac Catheterization; **Hospital:** Washington Hosp Ctr; **Address:** 110 Irving St NW, Ste 4B1, Washington, DC 20010; **Phone:** 202-877-5975; **Board Cert:** Internal Medicine 1975; Cardiovascular Disease 1977; Interventional Cardiology 1999; **Med School:** Chile 1969; **Resid:** Internal Medicine, Univ Chile 1970; Internal Medicine, Catholic Univ 1971; **Fellow:** Cardiovascular Disease, Cleveland Clinic 1973; **Fac Appt:** Clin Prof Med, Geo Wash Univ

Reiner, Jonathan S MD [IC] - **Spec Exp:** Angioplasty & Stent Placement; **Hospital:** G Washington Univ Hosp; **Address:** GWU Med Faculty Assocs, 2150 Pennsylvania Ave NW, rm 4-417, Washington, DC 20037; **Phone:** 202-741-3333; **Board Cert:** Internal Medicine 1989; Cardiovascular Disease 2004; Interventional Cardiology 1999; **Med School:** Georgetown Univ 1986; **Resid:** Internal Medicine, North Shore Univ Hosp 1989; **Fellow:** Cardiovascular Disease, George Wash Univ Sch Med 1993; **Fac Appt:** Asst Prof Med, Geo Wash Univ

Resar, Jon R MD [IC] - **Spec Exp:** Percutaneous Coronary Intervention; Percutaneous Valve Repair; Percutaneous ASD/PFO closure; **Hospital:** Johns Hopkins Hosp (page 61); **Address:** Johns Hopkins Hosp, Dept Cardiology, 600 N Wolfe St, Carnegie 568, Baltimore, MD 21287; **Phone:** 410-614-1132; **Board Cert:** Internal Medicine 1988; Cardiovascular Disease 2000; Interventional Cardiology 2009; **Med School:** Med Coll Wisc 1985; **Resid:** Internal Medicine, Johns Hopkins Hosp 1988; **Fellow:** Cardiovascular Disease, Johns Hopkins Hosp 1990; Interventional Cardiology, Johns Hopkins Hosp; **Fac Appt:** Assoc Prof Med, Johns Hopkins Univ

Roubin, Gary MD/PhD [IC] - **Spec Exp:** Coronary Angioplasty/Stents; Carotid Artery Stent Placement; Peripheral Vascular Disease; **Hospital:** St. Luke's - Roosevelt Hosp Ctr - St Luke's Hosp (page 56); **Address:** 1000 10 Ave, Ste 10G, New York, NY 10019; **Phone:** 212-523-7200; **Med School:** Australia 1975; **Resid:** Internal Medicine, Royal Prince Albert Hosp 1979; Cardiovascular Disease, Hallstrom Inst of Cardiology 1981; **Fellow:** Cardiology Research, Natl Heart Fdn 1983; Interventional Cardiology, Emory Univ 1985; **Fac Appt:** Clin Prof Med, NYU Sch Med

Sacchi, Terrence J MD [IC] - **Spec Exp:** Arrhythmias; Cardiac Catheterization; Coronary Angioplasty/Stents; Percutaneous Coronary Intervention; **Hospital:** New York Methodist Hosp; **Address:** NY Methodist Hospital, 506 6th St, Brooklyn, NY 11215; **Phone:** 718-780-7830; **Board Cert:** Internal Medicine 1979; Cardiovascular Disease 1981; Interventional Cardiology 2009; **Med School:** Albany Med Coll 1976; **Resid:** Internal Medicine, St Vincents Hosp 1979; **Fellow:** Cardiovascular Disease, Georgetown Univ Hosp 1981; Interventional Cardiology, Mercy Hosp 1987; **Fac Appt:** Assoc Clin Prof Med, SUNY Downstate

Shani, Jacob MD [IC] - **Spec Exp:** Cardiac Catheterization; Angioplasty & Stent Placement; Percutaneous Valve Repair; **Hospital:** Maimonides Med Ctr (page 63); **Address:** Maimonides Med Ctr, Cardiac Cath Lab, 4802 10th Ave, Brooklyn, NY 11219-2844; **Phone:** 718-283-7480; **Board Cert:** Internal Medicine 1981; Cardiovascular Disease 1983; Interventional Cardiology 2009; **Med School:** Israel 1977; **Resid:** Internal Medicine, Maimonides Med Ctr 1981; **Fellow:** Cardiovascular Disease, Beth Israel Hosp 1983; **Fac Appt:** Prof Med, NYU Sch Med

Sharma, Samin K MD [IC] - **Spec Exp:** Angioplasty & Stent Placement; Heart Valve Disease; **Hospital:** Mount Sinai Med Ctr (page 64); **Address:** One Gustave L Levy Pl, Box 1030, New York, NY 10029; **Phone:** 212-241-4021; **Board Cert:** Internal Medicine 1986; Cardiovascular Disease 1989; **Med School:** India 1978; **Resid:** Internal Medicine, SMS Hosp 1982; Internal Medicine, NYU Downtown Hosp 1986; **Fellow:** Cardiovascular Disease, City Hosp Ctr at Elmhurst 1988; Interventional Cardiology, Mt Sinai Hosp 2000; **Fac Appt:** Prof Med, Mount Sinai Sch Med

Shorofsky, Stephen R MD/PhD [IC] - **Spec Exp:** Arrhythmias; **Hospital:** Univ of MD Med Ctr; **Address:** 22 Greene St, Ste N3W77, Baltimore, MD 21201; **Phone:** 410-328-6056; **Board Cert:** Internal Medicine 1988; Cardiac Electrophysiology 2004; **Med School:** Univ Chicago-Pritzker Sch Med 1985; **Resid:** Internal Medicine, Univ Chicago Hosps 1988; **Fellow:** Cardiovascular Disease, Univ Chicago Hosps 1991; **Fac Appt:** Assoc Prof Med, Univ MD Sch Med

Stone, Gregg W MD [IC] - **Spec Exp:** Angioplasty & Stent Placement; Coronary Artery Disease; **Hospital:** NY-Presby/Columbia Univ Med Ctr, NY (page 66); **Address:** 161 Fort Washington Ave, Irving Pavillion Fl 6 - Ste 607, New York, NY 10032; **Phone:** 212-305-7060; **Board Cert:** Internal Medicine 1985; Cardiovascular Disease 1987; **Med School:** Johns Hopkins Univ 1982; **Resid:** Internal Medicine, NY Hosp-Cornell Medical Ctr 1985; **Fellow:** Cardiovascular Disease, Cedars-Sinai Medical Ctr 1988; Coronary Angioplasty, Mid-America Heart Inst 1989; **Fac Appt:** Prof Med, Columbia P&S

Southeast

Applegate, Robert J MD [IC] - **Spec Exp:** Cardiac Catheterization; Angioplasty; **Hospital:** Wake Forest Baptist Med Ctr; **Address:** Medical Ctr Blvd, Winston-Salem, NC 27157-1045; **Phone:** 336-716-6674; **Board Cert:** Internal Medicine 1983; Cardiovascular Disease 1987; Interventional Cardiology 2009; **Med School:** Univ VA Sch Med 1980; **Resid:** Internal Medicine, Oregon Hlth Sci Univ Hosp 1983; **Fellow:** Pharmacology, Univ Texas Hlth Sci Ctr 1984; Cardiovascular Disease, Univ Texas Hlth Sci Ctr 1986; **Fac Appt:** Prof Med, Wake Forest Univ

Bittl, John A MD [IC] - **Spec Exp:** Cardiac Catheterization; Invasive Cardiology; **Hospital:** Munroe Regional Med Ctr; **Address:** Ocala Heart Inst, 1500 SW 1st Ave, Ocala, FL 34471; **Phone:** 352-351-7206; **Board Cert:** Internal Medicine 1982; Cardiovascular Disease 1985; Interventional Cardiology 2011; **Med School:** Johns Hopkins Univ 1979; **Resid:** Internal Medicine, UCLA Med Ctr 1982; **Fellow:** Cardiovascular Disease, Brigham-Womens Hosp 1984

Douglas Jr, John S MD [IC] - **Spec Exp:** Angioplasty & Stent Placement; Cardiac Catheterization; Coronary Artery Disease; **Hospital:** Emory Univ Hosp; **Address:** Emory Univ Hosp-Div Cardiology, 1364 Clifton Rd, rm F606, Atlanta, GA 30322; **Phone:** 404-727-7040; **Board Cert:** Internal Medicine 1972; Cardiovascular Disease 1975; Interventional Cardiology 2009; **Med School:** Washington Univ, St Louis 1967; **Resid:** Internal Medicine, NC Memorial Hosp 1969; Internal Medicine, Grady Memorial Hosp 1972; **Fellow:** Cardiovascular Disease, Emory Affil Hosps 1974; **Fac Appt:** Prof Med, Emory Univ

Interventional Cardiology

Kandzari, David E MD [IC] - **Spec Exp:** Angioplasty & Stent Placement; Peripheral Vascular Disease; Clinical Trials; **Hospital:** Piedmont Hosp; **Address:** Piedmont Heart Institute, 275 Collier Rd NW, Ste 300, Atlanta, GA 30309; **Phone:** 404-605-2800; **Board Cert:** Cardiovascular Disease 2003; Interventional Cardiology 2005; **Med School:** Duke Univ 1995; **Resid:** Internal Medicine, Johns Hopkins Hosp 1998; **Fellow:** Cardiovascular Disease, Duke Univ 2002; Interventional Cardiology, Duke Univ 2004

Khawaja, Shazib N MD [IC] - **Spec Exp:** Peripheral Vascular Disease; Vascular Medicine; Echocardiography; Nuclear Cardiology; **Hospital:** Tanner Med Ctr; **Address:** 705 Dixie St, Ste 401, Carrollton, GA 30117; **Phone:** 770-836-9326; **Board Cert:** Cardiovascular Disease 2012; Interventional Cardiology 2003; Vascular Medicine 2007; **Med School:** Univ S Ala Coll Med 1995; **Resid:** Internal Medicine, Albany Med Ctr 1998; **Fellow:** Cardiovascular Disease, Dartmouth Hitchcock Med Ctr 2000; Interventional Cardiology, Univ Minnesota Med Ctr 2002; **Fac Appt:** Asst Clin Prof Med, Emory Univ

Knopf, William D MD [IC] - **Spec Exp:** Coronary Angioplasty/Stents; Percutaneous Coronary Intervention; Carotid Artery Stent Placement; Angiogenesis; **Hospital:** Piedmont Hosp; **Address:** Piedmont Heart Inst, 275 Collier Rd, Ste 300, Atlanta, GA 30309; **Phone:** 404-605-2800; **Board Cert:** Internal Medicine 1982; Cardiovascular Disease 1985; Interventional Cardiology 2009; **Med School:** Emory Univ 1979; **Resid:** Internal Medicine, Parkland Hosp 1982; **Fellow:** Cardiovascular Disease, Emory Univ Hosp 1985; **Fac Appt:** Assoc Clin Prof Med, Med Coll GA

Matar, Fadi MD [IC] - **Spec Exp:** Angioplasty; **Hospital:** Tampa Genl Hosp, St. Joseph's Hosp - Tampa; **Address:** 509 S Armenia Ave, Ste 200, Tampa, FL 33609; **Phone:** 813-353-1515; **Board Cert:** Cardiovascular Disease 2007; Interventional Cardiology 2009; **Med School:** Amer Univ Beirut 1987; **Resid:** Internal Medicine, Maryland Genl Hosp 1990; **Fellow:** Cardiovascular Disease, Wash Hosp Ctr 1994; **Fac Appt:** Asst Prof Med, Univ S Fla Coll Med

Morris, Douglas C MD [IC] - **Spec Exp:** Angioplasty; Cardiac Catheterization; Heart Valve Disease; **Hospital:** Emory Univ Hosp, Emory Univ Hosp Midtown; **Address:** Emory Clinic - Cardiology, 1365 Clifton Rd NE, A Bldg Fl 2, Atlanta, GA 30322; **Phone:** 404-778-5299; **Board Cert:** Internal Medicine 1973; Cardiovascular Disease 1975; **Med School:** Baylor Coll Med 1968; **Resid:** Internal Medicine, Vanderbilt Univ Med Ctr 1970; Internal Medicine, Vanderbilt Univ Med Ctr 1973; **Fellow:** Cardiovascular Disease, Emory Univ Hosps 1975; **Fac Appt:** Prof Med, Emory Univ

Reddy, Bhagat K MD [IC] - **Spec Exp:** Angioplasty & Stent Placement; Carotid Artery Stent Placement; Peripheral Vascular Disease; Intravascular Ultrasound; **Hospital:** Piedmont Hosp; **Address:** Piedmont Heart Institute, 275 Collier Rd NW, Ste 300, Atlanta, GA 30309; **Phone:** 404-605-2800; **Board Cert:** Cardiovascular Disease 2002; Interventional Cardiology 2003; Vascular Medicine 2004; **Med School:** India 1995; **Resid:** Internal Medicine, Robert Packer Hosp 1999; **Fellow:** Cardiovascular Disease, Med Coll Ohio 2002; Interventional Cardiology, Vanderbilt Univ 2003

Midwest

Bach, Richard G MD [IC] - **Spec Exp:** Cardiac Catheterization; Acute Coronary Syndromes; Cardiomyopathy-Hypertrophic; **Hospital:** Barnes-Jewish Hosp; **Address:** Washington Univ Sch Med, Cardiovascular Div, 660 S Euclid Ave, Campus Box 8086, St Louis, MO 63110; **Phone:** 314-362-1963; **Board Cert:** Internal Medicine 1987; Cardiovascular Disease 2011; Interventional Cardiology 2011; **Med School:** NYU Sch Med 1984; **Resid:** Internal Medicine, Bellvue Hosp/NYU Med Ctr 1987; **Fellow:** Cardiovascular Disease, Bellvue Hosp/NYU Med Ctr 1990; Interventional Cardiology, NYU Med Ctr 1991; **Fac Appt:** Assoc Prof Med, Washington Univ, St Louis

Dieter, Robert S MD [IC] - **Spec Exp:** Vascular Medicine; Peripheral Vascular Disease; Angioplasty & Stent Placement; Renal Artery Stenosis; **Hospital:** Loyola Univ Med Ctr; **Address:** Loyola Univ MC, Dept Cardiology, 2160 S First Ave EMS Bldg, Maywood, IL 60153; **Phone:** 708-216-4466; **Board Cert:** Internal Medicine 2010; Cardiovascular Disease 2002; Interventional Cardiology 2003; **Med School:** Univ IL Coll Med 1996; **Resid:** Internal Medicine, UIC Med Ctr 1999; Cardiovascular Disease, Univ Wisconsin 2002; **Fellow:** Interventional Cardiology, Univ Wisconsin; Vascular Medicine, Georgetown Univ; **Fac Appt:** Asst Prof Med, Loyola Univ-Stritch Sch Med

Ellis, Stephen G MD [IC] - **Spec Exp:** Angioplasty & Stent Placement; Angiogenesis; **Hospital:** Cleveland Clin (page 55); **Address:** Cleveland Clinic, Dept Cardiology, 9500 Euclid Ave, Desk J2-3, Cleveland, OH 44195; **Phone:** 216-445-6712; **Board Cert:** Internal Medicine 1981; Cardiovascular Disease 1985; Interventional Cardiology 2009; **Med School:** UCLA 1978; **Resid:** Internal Medicine, Cedars-Sinai Med Ctr 1981; **Fellow:** Cardiovascular Disease, Stanford Univ Med Ctr 1985; Interventional Cardiology, Emory Univ Hosp 1986; **Fac Appt:** Prof Med, Cleveland Cl Coll Med/Case West Res

Feldman, Ted E MD [IC] - **Spec Exp:** Angioplasty; **Hospital:** Evanston/North Shore Univ Hlth Sys; **Address:** ENH Med Group, Cardiology, 2650 Ridge Ave Walgreen Bldg Fl 3, Evanston, IL 60201; **Phone:** 847-570-2250; **Board Cert:** Internal Medicine 1981; Cardiovascular Disease 1985; Interventional Cardiology 2009; **Med School:** Indiana Univ 1978; **Resid:** Internal Medicine, Rush-Presby-St Lukes Hosp 1982; **Fellow:** Cardiovascular Disease, Univ Chicago 1985; **Fac Appt:** Prof Med, Northwestern Univ

Henry, Timothy D MD [IC] - **Spec Exp:** Acute Coronary Syndromes; Angiogenesis; **Hospital:** Abbott - Northwestern Hosp; **Address:** 920 E 28th St, Ste 300, MS 33300, Minneapolis, MN 55407; **Phone:** 612-863-3900; **Board Cert:** Internal Medicine 1985; Cardiovascular Disease 1989; **Med School:** UCSF 1982; **Resid:** Internal Medicine, Univ Colorado Hosp 1985; **Fellow:** Cardiovascular Disease, Univ Minnesota 1990; Interventional Cardiology, Univ Minnesota 1991; **Fac Appt:** Prof Med, Univ Minn

Holmes Jr, David R MD [IC] - **Spec Exp:** Heart Attack; Acute Coronary Syndromes; Angioplasty & Restenosis; **Hospital:** Mayo Med Ctr & Clin - Rochester; **Address:** Mayo Clinic, Div Cardiovasc Dis, 200 First St SW, Rochester, MN 55905; **Phone:** 507-255-2504; **Board Cert:** Internal Medicine 1974; Cardiovascular Disease 1977; Interventional Cardiology 2009; **Med School:** Med Coll Wisc 1971; **Resid:** Internal Medicine, Mayo Clinic 1974; **Fellow:** Cardiovascular Disease, Mayo Clinic 1977; **Fac Appt:** Prof Med, Mayo Med Sch

Lasala, John M MD/PhD [IC] - **Spec Exp:** Coronary Artery Disease; Coronary Angioplasty/Stents; Cardiac Catheterization; Aortic Diseases & Dissection; **Hospital:** Barnes-Jewish Hosp; **Address:** Washington Univ Sch Med, 660 S Euclid Ave, Box 8086, St Louis, MO 63110; **Phone:** 314-747-4535; **Board Cert:** Internal Medicine 1986; Cardiovascular Disease 1989; Interventional Cardiology 2009; **Med School:** Univ Conn 1983; **Resid:** Internal Medicine, Barnes-Jewish Hosp 1986; **Fellow:** Cardiovascular Disease, Yale-New Haven Hosp 1989; Interventional Cardiology, Yale-New Haven Hosp 1990; **Fac Appt:** Assoc Prof Med, Washington Univ, St Louis

Schreiber, Theodore L MD [IC] - **Spec Exp:** Coronary Angioplasty/Stents; Carotid Artery Disease; Aortic Diseases & Dissection; **Hospital:** Harper Univ Hosp; **Address:** Harper Univ Hosp, 3990 John R St, Webber Bldg - Ste 9370, Detroit, MI 48201; **Phone:** 313-745-7025; **Board Cert:** Internal Medicine 1981; Cardiovascular Disease 1983; **Med School:** Cornell Univ-Weill Med Coll 1978; **Resid:** Internal Medicine, NY Hosp-Cornell Med Ctr 1981; **Fellow:** Cardiovascular Disease, NY Hosp-Cornell Med Ctr 1983; **Fac Appt:** Assoc Prof Med, Wayne State Univ

Interventional Cardiology

Whitlow, Patrick MD [IC] - **Spec Exp:** Cardiac Catheterization; **Hospital:** Cleveland Clin (page 55); **Address:** Cleveland Clinic, Dept Cardiology, 9500 Euclid Ave, Desk J2-3, Cleveland, OH 44195; **Phone:** 216-444-1746; **Board Cert:** Internal Medicine 1979; Cardiovascular Disease 1981; **Med School:** Duke Univ 1976; **Resid:** Internal Medicine, Parkland Meml Hosp 1979; **Fellow:** Cardiovascular Disease, Univ Alabama Hosp 1979

Great Plains and Mountains

Carroll, John D MD [IC] - **Spec Exp:** Heart Valve Disease; Congenital Heart Disease-Adult; Coronary Artery Disease; **Hospital:** Univ of CO Hosp - Anschutz Inpatient Pav; **Address:** Univ Colorado, Dept Cardiology, 12605 E 16th Ave, MC B120, Denver, CO 80045; **Phone:** 720-848-5300; **Board Cert:** Internal Medicine 1979; Cardiovascular Disease 1981; Interventional Cardiology 2009; **Med School:** Univ Chicago-Pritzker Sch Med 1976; **Resid:** Internal Medicine, Tufts-New Engl Med Ctr 1978; **Fellow:** Cardiovascular Disease, Tufts-New Engl Med Ctr 1981; **Fac Appt:** Prof Med, Univ Colorado

Southwest

Bailey, Steven R MD [IC] - **Spec Exp:** Coronary Artery Disease; Angioplasty & Stent Placement; Congenital Heart Disease; Heart Valve Disease; **Hospital:** Univ Hlth Syst-San Antonio, Christus Santa Rosa Med Ctr Hosp; **Address:** 8300 Floyd Curl Drive Fl 3, San Antonio, TX 78229-3900; **Phone:** 210-567-4601; **Board Cert:** Internal Medicine 1981; Cardiovascular Disease 1983; Interventional Cardiology 2009; **Med School:** Oregon Hlth & Sci Univ 1978; **Resid:** Internal Medicine, Fitzsimmons AMC 1981; **Fellow:** Cardiovascular Disease, Fitzsimmons AMC 1983; **Fac Appt:** Prof Med, Univ Tex, San Antonio

Feldman, Marc D MD [IC] - **Spec Exp:** Cardiac Catheterization; **Hospital:** Univ Hlth Syst-San Antonio; **Address:** UTHSCSA-Cardiology, 7703 Floyd Curl Drive, MS 7872, San Antonio, TX 78229-3900; **Phone:** 210-567-2106; **Board Cert:** Internal Medicine 1984; Cardiovascular Disease 1989; Interventional Cardiology 2010; **Med School:** Univ Pennsylvania 1981; **Resid:** Internal Medicine, Univ Chicago Hosp 1984; **Fellow:** Cardiovascular Disease, Beth Israel Med Ctr 1987; **Fac Appt:** Prof Med, Univ Tex, San Antonio

Kleiman, Neal S MD [IC] - **Spec Exp:** Angioplasty & Stent Placement; **Hospital:** Methodist Hosp - Houston; **Address:** Methodist DeBakey Cardiology Assocs, 6550 Fannin St, Ste 1901, Smith Tower, Houston, TX 77030; **Phone:** 713-441-1100; **Board Cert:** Internal Medicine 1984; Cardiovascular Disease 1987; Interventional Cardiology 2009; **Med School:** Columbia P&S 1981; **Resid:** Internal Medicine, Baylor Affil Hosp 1984; **Fellow:** Interventional Cardiology, Baylor Coll Med 1987; **Fac Appt:** Assoc Prof Med, Cornell Univ-Weill Med Coll

Perin, Emerson C MD/PhD [IC] - **Spec Exp:** Stem Cell Therapy in Heart Failure; Angiogenesis; **Hospital:** St. Luke's Episcopal Hosp-Houston; **Address:** Southwest Cardiology Consultants, 6624 Fannin St, Ste 2220, St Lukes Medical Tower Fl 22, Houston, TX 77030-2334; **Phone:** 713-791-9400; **Board Cert:** Internal Medicine 1988; Cardiovascular Disease 2010; **Med School:** Brazil 1983; **Resid:** Internal Medicine, Jackson Meml Hosp 1988; **Fellow:** Cardiovascular Disease, St Luke's Episcopal Hosp 1991; **Fac Appt:** Asst Prof Med, Baylor Coll Med

Smalling, Richard W MD/PhD [IC] - **Spec Exp:** Coronary Artery Disease; Peripheral Vascular Disease; Heart Valve Disease; Congenital Heart Disease; **Hospital:** Meml Hermann Hosp - Texas Med Ctr; **Address:** 6410 Fannin St, Ste 600, Houston, TX 77030-1501; **Phone:** 832-325-7211; **Board Cert:** Internal Medicine 1978; Cardiovascular Disease 1981; Interventional Cardiology 2009; **Med School:** Univ Tex, Houston 1975; **Resid:** Internal Medicine, UCSD Med Ctr 1978; **Fellow:** Cardiovascular Disease, UCSD Med Ctr 1980; **Fac Appt:** Prof Med, Univ Tex, Houston

West Coast and Pacific

Greene, Robert M MD [IC] - **Spec Exp:** Cardiac Catheterization; Acute Coronary Syndromes; **Hospital:** Alta Bates Summit Med Ctr-Alta Bates Campus, Alta Bates Summit Med Ctr-Oakland; **Address:** Berkeley Cardiovascular Med Grp, 3300 Webster St Fl 4, Oakland, CA 94609; **Phone:** 510-549-4220; **Board Cert:** Internal Medicine 1976; Cardiovascular Disease 1977; Interventional Cardiology 2009; **Med School:** UCSF 1972; **Resid:** Internal Medicine, Wadsworth VA Hosp 1975; **Fellow:** Cardiovascular Disease, UCLA Med Ctr 1977

Mahmud, Ehtisham MD [IC] - **Spec Exp:** Cardiac Catheterization; Carotid Artery Stent Placement; Stem Cell Therapy in Heart Failure; Gene Therapy; **Hospital:** UCSD Med Ctr; **Address:** 9434 Medical Center Drive, SCVC Bldg, MS 7784, La Jolla, CA 92037; **Phone:** 858-657-8030; **Board Cert:** Cardiovascular Disease 2010; Interventional Cardiology 2001; **Med School:** Univ Alberta 1989; **Resid:** Internal Medicine, UC San Diego 1995; **Fellow:** Cardiovascular Disease, UC San Diego 1999; Interventional Cardiology, Emory Univ 2000; **Fac Appt:** Prof Med, UCSD

Teirstein, Paul S MD [IC] - **Spec Exp:** Coronary Angioplasty/Stents; Heart Valve Disease; **Hospital:** Scripps Green Hosp; **Address:** Scripps Clinic, 10666 N Torrey Pines Rd, Mail Drop S1056, La Jolla, CA 92037; **Phone:** 858-554-9905; **Board Cert:** Internal Medicine 1983; Cardiovascular Disease 1987; Interventional Cardiology 2009; **Med School:** Mount Sinai Sch Med 1980; **Resid:** Internal Medicine, Brigham & Womens Hosp 1983; **Fellow:** Cardiovascular Disease, Stanford Univ 1986; Interventional Cardiology, Mid-Amer Heart Inst 1987

Yeung, Alan C MD [IC] - **Spec Exp:** Mitral Valve Surgery; Coronary Artery Disease; **Hospital:** Stanford Univ Hosp & Clinics; **Address:** Stanford Univ Med Ctr, Div Interventional Cardiology, 300 Pasteur Drive, rm H2103, MC 5218, Stanford, CA 94305-5218; **Phone:** 650-723-0180; **Board Cert:** Internal Medicine 1987; Cardiovascular Disease 1989; Interventional Cardiology 2010; **Med School:** Harvard Med Sch 1984; **Resid:** Internal Medicine, Mass Gen Hosp 1987; **Fellow:** Cardiovascular Disease, Brigham & Womens Hosp 1990; **Fac Appt:** Prof Med, Stanford Univ

Cleveland Clinic

Every life deserves world class care.

Cardiovascular Disease

Cleveland Clinic's Sydell and Arnold Miller Family Heart & Vascular Institute is one of the largest and most experienced cardiovascular specialty groups in the world, providing patients with expert medical management and a full range of therapies. Our areas of expertise combine research, education and clinical practice to provide innovative and scientifically based treatments for cardiovascular disease. *U.S. News & World Report* has ranked Cleveland Clinic best in the nation for heart care every year since 1995.

Patients come to the Heart & Vascular Institute from every state in the country and from around the world. In 2010, our staff recorded more than 370,000 patient visits, completed more than 13,000 procedures, performed more than 4,000 open cardiac surgeries and more than 1,300 thoracic surgeries.

Clinical Trials and Research

Our Heart & Vascular Institute is a recognized leader in multicenter and international trials. An outstanding clinical infrastructure and strong commitment to basic science places Cleveland Clinic on the cutting edge of treatment and research in cardiovascular disease. Currently, Cleveland Clinic is conducting more than 200 trials and clinical research projects. Our researchers are investigating new alternative treatment options for patients with severe aortic valve stenosis and are researching non-invasive repair of the mitral and tricuspid valves.

History of Innovations

Cleveland Clinic doctors and researchers have helped define the modern era of cardiovascular care, having pioneered coronary angiography and saphenous vein bypass surgery. Today, our staff continues this proud tradition of innovation and discovery to shape the future of cardiovascular care.

Cleveland Clinic
Heart & Vascular Institute
9500 Euclid Avenue
Cleveland, OH 44195

Offering Same-Day Appointments
Call 800.274.2009.

Treatment Guides
Cleveland Clinic has developed comprehensive treatment guides for many diseases and conditions. To download our free treatment guides, visit clevelandclinic.org/ treatmentguides.

Online Medical Second Opinion
Call 216.444.3223 or 800.223.2273 ext. 43223 or email eclevelandclinic@ccf.org.

Out-of-State Patients Assistance
Call 800.223.2273, ext. 55580 or email medicalconcierge@ccf.org.

Visit Us At:
clevelandclinic.org

Follow Us On:
Facebook
www.facebook.com/clevelandclinic

Twitter
@ClevelandClinic

You Tube
www.youtube.com/clevelandclinic

Health Hub
health.clevelandclinic.org

Continuum
Cardiovascular Services

| Beth Israel Medical Center
Beth Israel Brooklyn
Roosevelt Hospital
St. Luke's Hospital

**Cardiovascular Specialists
Referral Service
800.420.4004**

Continuum Cardiovascular Centers of New York
New Cardiac and Vascular Programs of Excellence

The newly conceived Continuum Cardiovascular Centers of New York, led by the internationally renowned Interventional Cardiologist Gary Roubin, MD, PhD, is moving forward to expand the extensive cardiac and vascular services now offered at St. Luke's and Roosevelt Hospitals and Beth Israel Medical Center. By adding preeminent experts and expanding and upgrading facilities, Continuum Cardiovascular Services will provide the most cutting-edge, patient-oriented, compassionate care in the region.

The first expansion milestone has been reached: the opening of the Al-Sabah Arrhythmia Institute in the fall of 2012. This world-class electrophysiology facility is being directed by nationally celebrated physician leaders in management of complex arrhythmias and ablation therapy. Heralding facility upgrades throughout the Continuum Cardiovascular Centers across New York, the new arrhythmia center is equipped with state-of-the-art technology that enhances both outcomes and patient experience.

The driving force behind the development of the Continuum Cardiovascular Centers of New York is our commitment to excellence. A well-developed integrated clinical care system combines the world's most innovative physicians, gifted researchers, educators, and professional staff. We are building our reality upon a foundation of advanced technology and sophisticated facilities to ensure continued superior clinical outcomes and patient satisfaction.

For a referral to one of the expert cardiovascular specialists at the Continuum Cardiovascular Centers of New York, please call 800.420.4004.

Visit us online:
BethIsraelNY.org
StLukesHospitalNYC.org
RooseveltHospitalNYC.org

Continuum
Health Partners

Beth Israel Medical Center
Beth Israel Brooklyn
Roosevelt Hospital
St. Luke's Hospital
NY Eye and Ear Infirmary

Having pioneered numerous heart care innovations through the years, the Cardiac Institute offers diagnostic studies and therapeutic treatments, procedures and surgeries. It has been ranked by the Centers for Medicare and Medicaid Services among the few hospitals which have achieved excellent ratings in both heart attack and heart failure patient outcomes.

Cardiology
Among the most published and respected in the field, the Maimonides cardiology team continuously sets higher standards for patient care. Edgar Lichstein, MD, Chair of Medicine, has been chief investigator of NIH-sponsored cardiac drug trials, and our Congestive Heart Failure (CHF) Program is among the most effective in the nation.

Interventional Cardiology
Led by Cardiac Institute Chair, Jacob Shani, MD, numerous therapeutic devices have been developed and implemented here. Our Electrophysiology Lab has a superb record of achievement in diagnosing and treating arrhythmias. Close collaboration with the Department of Emergency Medicine ensures that chest pain patients are evaluated immediately and that interventional procedures are used to stop heart attacks in progress whenever necessary.

Cardiothoracic Surgery
The Maimonides Division of Cardiothoracic Surgery has an illustrious history, setting a national standard for advances in cardiothoracic. Under the direction of Greg Ribakove, MD, minimally invasive and robotic heart surgeries, as well as advanced procedures such as LVAD and TAVI, are offered in state-of-the-art facilities, including a hybrid OR. In collaboration with Electrophysiology, Cardiothoracic Surgery has established an Atrial Fibrillation Center of Excellence. Maimonides provides one of the most prestigious cardiothoracic residency programs in the US.

Historic Moments
- In 1967, the first successful human heart transplant in the nation was performed at Maimonides.
- The intra-aortic balloon pump was developed here in 1970.
- Surgical techniques that protect the spine during cardiothoracic surgery were perfected here in 1982.
- Revolutionary cardiac catheterization devices were invented here in 1992 and 1997.
- Maimonides was the first hospital in the US to implement fully automatic external cardiac defibrillators in 2001.

The Centers for Medicare and Medicaid Services, an agency of the federal government, recently published the latest data on 30-day mortality rates for hospitals across the country. Maimonides Medical Center achieved better-than-expected results in all three categories measured – heart attack, heart failure and pneumonia – a distinction only 22 hospitals in the U.S. achieved.

Maimonides Medical Center
Passionate about medicine.
Compassionate about people.

www.maimonidesmed.org/cardiac

THE MOUNT SINAI MEDICAL CENTER
MOUNT SINAI HEART - CARDIOVASCULAR HEALTH

One Gustave L. Levy Place
Fifth Avenue and 100th Street
New York, NY 10029-6574
Physician Referral: 1-800-MD-SINAI (637-4624)
www.mountsinai.org/heart

At **MOUNT SINAI HEART**, our integrated system of care brings together the world's most accomplished physicians, research scientists, and educators who share the common goal of preventing and treating cardiovascular disease. **In 2012, *U.S. News & World Report* ranked our cardiology and heart surgery service 10th in the nation.**

With access to the latest discoveries and a diversity of the most experienced minds, our doctors ensure that patients receive the best individualized care. The rapid translation of innovative research into prevention, diagnosis, and therapy means that patients receive multidisciplinary treatment of unprecedented quality. Our programs treat patients of all ages – from the unborn fetus well into the advanced elderly years.

We specialize in consultative cardiology, cardiac catheterization, heart and lung transplantation, cardiovascular surgery, heart failure, pulmonary hypertension, lipid management, and hypertension, as well as:

Noninvasive diagnostic imaging – We offer state-of-the-art echocardiography, nuclear cardiology, PET, CT, and MRI technology.

Coronary artery disease – We are ranked as New York State's safest and busiest center for coronary angioplasty and other catheter-based procedures. We lead many innovative device trials in the development phase before getting final approval for commercial use.

Cardiac rhythm disturbances – We manage all aspects of heart rhythm disorders under the auspices of pioneers in the field, including atrial fibrillation (AFib), the most common abnormal heart rhythm, and ventricular tachycardias, the most common cause of sudden cardiac death, as well as implantable devices, such as pacemakers and defibrillators.

Valvular heart disease – We deliver medical and surgical options, including a leading valve-repair program and long-term follow-up care. We are one of the few centers in the country to provide both types of percutaneous non-surgical aortic valves.

Aortic diseases – We pioneer and advance techniques for stent-graft repair of thoracic and abdominal aortic aneurysms and for surgical correction of the most complex aortic pathology.

Congenital heart disease – Our cardiologists offer minimally invasive approaches to the correction of congenital heart defects in children and adults.

Cardiac failure and transplantation – We take a multidisciplinary team approach to comprehensive, compassionate care for patients with the most advanced forms of heart failure and cardiomyopathy.

Comprehensive cardiac disease prevention and rehabilitation – Our unique synergy provides unparalleled superior patient care and breakthroughs in cardiovascular disease prevention and treatment, while promoting cardiovascular health globally through six projects around the world.

Vascular medicine and surgery – We offer an interdisciplinary approach to disease management, including medical, surgical, catheter-based, and gene therapy techniques for arterial obstruction, limb salvage, venous, and lymphatic diseases. A pioneer in large-artery stenting, Mount Sinai fostered the development of stenting of abdominal aortic aneurysms.

Mount Sinai's Cardiac Catheterization Laboratory – We study the heart with the most precise technologies available, including diagnostic angiography, angioplasty, and biopsy. In a statewide study, our Cath Lab was found to be the safest, with the lowest 30-day risk-adjusted mortality rate for percutaneous coronary intervention (angioplasty), as well as the busiest.

LEADING SURGEONS, INNOVATIVE TREATMENTS
Under the direction of internationally renowned cardiologist Valentin Fuster, MD, PhD, Mount Sinai Heart is recognized worldwide for expert evaluation, management, and prevention of cardiovascular disease through integrated patient care, education, and research. Mount Sinai Heart encompasses the Zena and Michael A. Wiener Cardiovascular Institute and the Marie-Josée and Henry R. Kravis Center for Cardiovascular Health at Mount Sinai, both preeminent resources for the study and treatment of heart and blood vessel diseases.

NewYork-Presbyterian
The University Hospital of Columbia and Cornell

Affiliated with Columbia University College of Physicians and Surgeons and Weill Cornell Medical College

NewYork-Presbyterian Hospital
Columbia University Medical Center
622 West 168th Street
New York, NY 10032

NewYork-Presbyterian Hospital
Weill Cornell Medical Center
525 East 68th Street
New York, NY 10065

1-877-NYP-WELL (1-877-697-9355) www.nyp.org/heart

NewYork-Presbyterian Heart

In 2012-2013, NewYork-Presbyterian Hospital's heart and heart surgery program was ranked 4th in the nation in the annual 'Best Hospitals' survey conducted by *U.S. News & World Report*™. NewYork-Presbyterian has leading clinical programs for patients with coronary artery disease and a wide range of other heart disorders, with particular expertise in the management of:

- Aortic aneurysms, acute dissections, and trauma, with rapid diagnosis and effective medical and surgical interventions
- Heart failure, featuring a robust mechanical circulatory support program. Patients come from all over the world for placement of ventricular assist devices to be used long-term or as a bridge to transplant. NewYork-Presbyterian Hospital/Columbia University Medical Center is one of the world's leading institutions for heart transplantation and is one of the few centers offering patients a total artificial heart
- Adults with congenital heart disorders: echocardiography, interventional cardiac catheterization, interventional electrophysiology, and surgery. NewYork-Presbyterian's adult congenital heart surgeons are among the world's best for complex congenital heart surgery and cardiac transplantation. Related care is provided by specialists in high-risk pregnancy, genetics, fetal echocardiography, GI and liver disease, pulmonary, and hematology
- Cardiac rhythm abnormalities, with experienced electrophysiologists who diagnose and treat atrial fibrillation and other arrhythmias using pacemakers, implantable cardioverter defibrillators, ablation, and novel approaches to restore normal heart rhythm
- Valve disorders: using minimally invasive surgical approaches whenever possible. NewYork-Presbyterian Hospital investigators led the PARTNER Trial, which in 2011 demonstrated that transcatheter aortic valve replacement (TAVR) was as effective as conventional open-heart surgery for reducing mortality among high-risk patients with aortic stenosis. We've performed more TAVR procedures than any other center in the country. In addition, NewYork-Presbyterian Hospital is participating in the EVEREST II clinical trial, evaluating a new device to repair mitral valve leakage
- Heart disorders in the elderly: NewYork-Presbyterian Hospital surgeons have earned a reputation for performing heart surgery on the very elderly (over age 80), achieving excellent outcomes
- Patients who require surgery may receive treatment using a robotic approach, delivered using the Siemens Artis zeego® medical imaging system. This system provides surgeons with exceptional visualization of blood vessels.

A Reputation for Excellence

At NewYork-Presbyterian Hospital, the optimal care of patients with heart disease is achieved by combining an experienced team of clinicians with the latest advances in technology. Basic science and clinical research efforts are aimed at developing more effective ways to prevent, diagnose, and treat cardiac disorders. NewYork-Presbyterian Hospital features renowned cardiac care programs in the following areas:

- Cardiac diagnostics
- Electrophysiology
- Clinical cardiology
- Interventional cardiology
- Cardiac assist devices
- Cardiothoracic surgery, including transplantation
- Mitral valve repair

NewYork-Presbyterian Hospital is designated by the Society of Chest Pain Centers as an Accredited Chest Pain Center, dedicated to reducing heart-related deaths by improving the response time for the diagnosis and treatment of chest pain.

CARDIAC AND VASCULAR INSTITUTE
550 First Avenue *(at 31st Street)*
New York, NY 10016
www.NYULMC.org
Physician Referral: **888-7-NYU-MED** *(888-769-8633)*

CARDIAC SURGERY

NYU Langone Medical Center is one of the largest cardiac surgery centers in the country, and a nationally recognized leader in advanced treatment for the most complex cases of adult, pediatric and congenital heart disease. World renowned surgeons at the Medical Center pioneered minimally invasive heart surgery and valve repair or replacement, and have since performed over 6,000 minimally invasive procedures. They also perform state-of-the-art surgical procedures for aortic aneurysm disease, coronary artery disease, heart valve disease, and congenital heart disease, while specializing in cardiac surgery for high-risk and elderly patients.

Structural and Valvular Heart Disease Center
Mitral Valve Repair. NYU Langone's heart surgeons introduced mitral valve repair to the U.S. more than 30 years ago, and have since performed more than 4,000 mitral valve repairs, the most in the country.
High Risk Cardiac Surgery. Our cardiac surgery team specializes in the surgical care of high-risk patients, including re-operative surgery in the elderly, coronary bypass surgery, heart valve repair or replacement, surgical repair of the failing heart, and ventricular assist device implantation.
Minimally Invasive Cardiac Surgery. NYU Langone is in the vanguard of minimally invasive cardiac surgery, the benefits of which include reduced pain, lower risk of bleeding and infection, and a faster recovery.

Aortic Disease Center
The Medical Center is committed to a multidisciplinary approach in the treatment of complex aortic disease, and the long-term management of patients with aortic dissection and connective tissue disorders. A wide range of treatment and therapeutic options is offered, including open surgery and stent graft therapy for patients with aortic aneurysms, aortic dissections and genetic diseases of the aorta, like Marfan's syndrome.

Pediatric and Adult Congenital Heart Disease Center
The Division of Pediatric and Adult Congenital Cardiac Surgery treats patients of all ages with inherited and acquired cardiac defects. Our surgeons are experts in reconstructive procedures for complex cardiovascular disorders. The Division maintains a highly experienced team of specialists in pediatric and adult cardiology, neonatal and pediatric cardiac intensive care, pediatric cardiac anesthesiology, nursing, and extracorporeal perfusion.

CARDIAC AND VASCULAR INSTITUTE
550 First Avenue (*at 31st Street*)
New York, NY 10016
www.NYULMC.org
Physician Referral: **888-7-NYU-MED** (*888-769-8633*)

ADULT CARDIOVASCULAR SERVICES

The Cardiac and Vascular Institute (CVI) at NYU Langone Medical Center continues to advance new techniques for repairing heart valves, curing heart rhythm disorders, and treating aortic diseases and congestive heart failure. CVI is consistently ranked among the leading heart and heart surgery centers in U.S. News & World Report's annual 'Best Hospitals.'

Cardiac Catheterization
The Cardiac Catheterization Laboratory offers superior catheter-based diagnosis and evaluation of cardiac health. It provides a full range of procedures to evaluate heart muscle, valves, and coronary arteries and recommends appropriate treatment as needed.

Cardiac Rehabilitation and Prevention
The Joan and Joel Smilow Cardiopulmonary Rehabilitation and Prevention focuses on individualized patient care in a state-of-the-art facility.

Cardiac Surgery
The Division of Cardiac Surgery is a nationally recognized leader with a multidisciplinary approach in performing more than 6,000 minimally invasive heart surgery procedures since pioneering the technique in 1996. Moreover it offers over 30 years experience in mitral valve repairs as well as heart valve replacements and aortic aneurysm repairs.

Cardiology
The Leon H. Charney Division of Cardiology is a leader in cardiovascular patient care, biomedical research, and education. Clinicians and researchers are advancing the field of cardiovascular medicine and contributing to the reputation of NYU Langone Medical Center as a comprehensive cardiovascular center of excellence.

Heart Failure
The cardiologists and surgeons at the Heart Failure Center offer advanced echocardiograms, pacemaker/defibrillator implantations, open heart surgeries and ventricular assist devices.

Nuclear Cardiology/Stress
The Nuclear Cardiology/Stress Laboratory performs a range of tests that assist cardiologists in the assessment and diagnosis of heart disease.

Vascular Surgery
The Division of Vascular and Endovascular Surgery has treated thousands of patients for arterial aneurysms, deep vein thrombosis, carotid stenosis and limb salvage, emphasizing minimally invasive diagnostic and treatment approaches.

Penn Heart and Vascular combines the renowned expertise of clinicians, researchers and educators to provide a better quality of life for patients whose options are limited by conventional medicine.

A National and Regional Referral Center

The Penn Heart and Vascular Center in the Perelman Center for Advanced Medicine brings Penn's expert heart and vascular team together in one location. This provides greater convenience for patients, increases collaboration among caregivers and catalyzes clinical research. Penn's specialists work closely with colleagues and referring physicians to ensure a seamless continuum of care.

Heart Failure and Transplantation:
As one of the nation's top three adult heart transplant centers, Penn performs more adult heart transplants than all other area hospitals combined. Penn also offers the most advanced mechanical assist device options.

Cardiac Arrhythmia Program:
The Hospital of the University of Pennsylvania (HUP) was the first in the region to use implantable devices for patients at risk for recurrent sustained ventricular tachycardia or atrial fibrillation and to improve cardiac function in patients with heart failure. HUP's EP program is the largest on the east coast and one of the two largest in the country.

Valve Disease Program: Penn has the largest valve program in the region with a nationally recognized team of physicians who have performed over 2,500 minimally invasive valve repairs and replacements. Penn is one of the largest valve centers in the U.S. for advanced port access surgery for mitral valve repair or replacement.

World-Class Heart and Vascular Care

As one of the nation's leading cardiovascular programs, Penn provides diagnostic, medical, interventional and surgical treatment options that are not available anywhere else in the region.

- Consultations and second opinions
- Preventive cardiovascular disease
- Electrophysiology
- Heart failure treatment
- Heart transplantation
- Transcatheter Aortic Valve Replacement (TAVR)
- Familial cardiomyopathy
- Pulmonary hypertension
- Complex lipid disease
- Cardiac interventions

- Implantable cardiac defibrillators and pacemakers
- Ablation therapies for heart rhythm disorders
- Minimally invasive mitral and aortic valve repair and replacement
- Endovascular stent graft repair for thoracic aortic aneurysms
- Congenital heart repair
- Mechanical assist devices
- Venous disease

Technology and Research

Among the few surgical institutions in the nation with a fully incorporated research facility, Penn ensures the future progress of cardiovascular research by:

- Pioneering the most advanced techniques and devices, such as ablation therapy for ventricular tachycardia and atrial fibrillation
- Offering a full-range of surgical options including transcatheter, minimally invasive robotic, off-pump, port access and bloodless techniques
- Serving as the lead national site for several clinical trials

See all Penn Heart and Vascular clinical trials: PennMedicine.org/heart/clinicaltrials

Recognized Expertise

- Penn Heart and Vascular at HUP is ranked among the top in the nation and best in the Philadelphia region, for cardiology and heart surgery by *U.S. News & World Report*.
- HUP and Penn Presbyterian Medical Center are recognized Blue Distinction Centers for Cardiac Care by Independence Blue Cross.
- *Best Doctors in America®* lists more doctors from Penn Medicine than any other academic medical center or health system in the Philadelphia region.

For more information or to schedule an appointment, call 800.789.PENN (7366) or visit PennMedicine.org/heart

Hospital of the University of Pennsylvania | Penn Presbyterian Medical Center | Pennsylvania Hospital
Philadelphia, PA | 800.789.PENN | PennMedicine.org

St. Francis Hospital The Heart Center®
100 Port Washington Blvd.
Roslyn, New York 11576
www.stfrancisheartcenter.com
(516) 562-6000 1-888-HEARTNY

A Leader in Cardiac Care

St. Francis Hospital, The Heart Center® is New York State's only specialty designated cardiac center and is one of the busiest heart centers in the nation. Located in Roslyn, New York, on Long Island's North Shore, St. Francis Hospital has been ranked among the best hospitals in the United States by *U.S. News & World Report* for the six consecutive years. In 2012-13, the Hospital was nationally ranked in cardiology and heart surgery, gastroenterology, geriatrics, and neurology and neurosurgery.

St. Francis Hospital:

• Has a highly experienced team of physicians and surgeons with one of the largest volumes in the nation for cardiac surgery, interventional cardiology and arrhythmia procedures

• Offers innovative approaches to cardiac surgery, including minimally invasive procedures and off-pump coronary artery bypass surgery, designed to minimize trauma and reduce surgical complications

• Performs one of the region's highest volumes of catheter-based techniques to correct congenital heart defects such as atrial septal defects (ASDs) and patent foramen ovale (PFO)

• Operates a nationally recognized Arrhythmia and Pacemaker Center staffed with electrophysiologists with over a decade of experience in radiofrequency ablation, a permanent cure for certain arrhythmias, including atrial fibrillation

• Maintains a high volume center for the implantation of cardiac pacemakers and defibrillators

• Offers a world-class program in cardiac imaging that fully integrates all technologies, including advanced methods in cardiac MRI, coronary CT angiography, PET/CT and three-dimensional echocardiography

• Has received the Magnet Award for excellence in nursing services for the second consecutive three-year approval period

• Is a premier center for clinical trials and studies of the application of image-guided methods of diagnosis and treatment of heart disease, such as CoreValve, eValve, CREST, and Symplicity

St. Francis Hospital has near-perfect patient satisfaction ratings, with over 99 percent of patients saying they would recommend the Hospital to family and friends.

"Our large cardiac caseload and our growing research program put us in an excellent position to introduce new techniques that can benefit thousands of people in need each year."

–Alan D. Guerci, M.D.
President and Chief Executive Officer
St. Francis Hospital, The Heart Center®

St. Francis Hospital The Heart Center®
100 Port Washington Blvd.
Roslyn, New York 11576
www.stfrancisheartcenter.com
(516) 562-6000 1-888-HEARTNY

Noninvasive Cardiac Imaging
Using the latest in noninvasive cardiac imaging technology, St. Francis Hospital's physicians can evaluate blood flow, heart muscle strength, anatomy, and coronary artery blockages, allowing them to more effectively guide a patient's course of treatment.

Among the most recent advances in St. Francis Hospital's range of services are:

Coronary CT Angiography
St. Francis Hospital was the first hospital on Long Island to offer Multidetector Computed Tomography (MDCT) for noninvasive coronary artery imaging. Now, with installation of more advanced technology, St. Francis can minimize radiation exposure for every patient.

Cardiac MRI
The only center on Long Island with a dedicated Cardiac MRI program and world-class expertise in cardiac MRI, St. Francis Hospital uses MRI to evaluate heart anatomy, function, blood flow, scarring, and inflammation using advanced techniques on two state-of-the-art scanners. Cardiac MRI allows physicians to evaluate effects of heart attack and coronary artery blockages and non-coronary causes of heart failure to determine whether or not patients will benefit from heart surgery or other therapies. World-renowned cardiac MRI authority Nathaniel Reichek, M.D., leads St. Francis Hospital's clinical and research applications with cardiac MRI.

Three-Dimensional Echocardiography
St. Francis Hospital is an internationally recognized leader in three-dimensional echocardiography for quantifying the effects of heart disease and is the leading center in the New York metropolitan area in this field. By creating three-dimensional reconstructions of the heart and blood flow within it, this technology provides diagnostic information that far surpasses that available with conventional echocardiography in many patients.

Nuclear Imaging
Conventional nuclear imaging involves the injection of nuclear isotopes and imaging by a gamma camera that circles the patient's body, improving the accuracy of stress testing. St. Francis Hospital offers the latest advances in nuclear cardiology, such as positron emission tomography of the heart with CT attenuation correction (PET/CT). The nuclear cardiology laboratory at St. Francis Hospital is also a leader in developing new types of computer analysis to improve the value of all forms of cardiac nuclear imaging, and was among the first facilities in the U.S. to receive accreditation from The Intersocietal Commission for the Accreditation of Nuclear Medicine Laboratories.

Noninvasive Imaging at St. Francis Hospital
Noninvasive imaging services at St. Francis Hospital include:

• Multidetector computed tomographic coronary angiography
• Cardiac MRI
• SPECT/CT nuclear Imaging
• Cardiac PET/CT imaging
• Transesophageal echocardiography
• Three-dimensional echocardiography
• Stress testing with nuclear, echocardiographic or MRI imaging.

St. Francis Hospital's leading-edge noninvasive imaging technology is also being applied in its research programs on cardiovascular disease. Drawing on its depth of experience with various imaging modalities, the Hospital has launched a multi-disciplinary effort at its Cardiac Research Institute to improve methods for the diagnosis and treatment of cardiac disease. Past research efforts at the Hospital include The St. Francis Heart Study – a pioneering effort and the largest study of CT calcium scoring to be conducted at any single center – which supported the use of CT calcium scoring for atherosclerotic plaque detection as a tool in cardiac risk evaluation.

Vanderbilt Heart and Vascular Institute

Medical Center East | 1215 21st Ave. S. | Nashville, TN 37232 | (615) 322-2318 | VanderbiltHeart.com

Overview

Vanderbilt Heart is the top provider of cardiology and heart surgery in Middle Tennessee and southern Kentucky. We are the only program in either state ranked in the nation's top 50 by *U.S. News & World Report.*

We treat patients with many kinds of cardiovascular disease, including very complex cases. We offer a wide range of services at our main Vanderbilt campus in Nashville as well as 23 locations in Tennessee and Kentucky.

Treatment Programs

Vanderbilt Heart offers the latest in heart treatments and programs. These include programs for acquired and inherited heart disease in adults; arrhythmia; atrial fibrillation; cardiac surgery; congestive heart failure; general cardiology; heart transplant; interventional cardiology and radiology; heart disease prevention; valve repair and replacement; vascular surgery; and heart disease in women.

Our Team

Our team of cardiologists, surgeons, nurses and staff is highly skilled and specialized in many areas of heart care. We value a culture of collaboration that ensures each patient receives personalized, compassionate care from a team of experts.

DISCOVERY AND INNOVATION

Our PREDICT program is the first of its kind in a U.S. academic medical center. PREDICT uses genetic tests to find which blood-thinning and cholesterol-lowering drugs will be most effective for each patient. The information goes into our advanced electronic medical record, which allows our doctors to choose the right dose of the right drug, the first time.

We are the only center in Tennessee to study a new way to replace the aortic valve without open-heart surgery. This minimally invasive technique allows for a smaller incision, requires less time to perform and can reduce recovery time. Learn more.

When heart attack patients are on their way to Vanderbilt, we use a proven therapy that cools the body. This prevents brain damage, which can make for a better recovery.

Vanderbilt University Medical Center was the first hospital in the region to offer a novel approach to cardiac surgery that's raising our standard of care. Our Hybrid Operating Room/Catheterization Lab houses equipment and monitoring devices for open-heart surgeries such as coronary bypass as well as less invasive procedures such as angioplasty and stenting. If a patient needs two kinds of heart procedures, they can be done at the same time. This can cut down on complications and costs.

VANDERBILT UNIVERSITY

MEDICAL CENTER

Child Neurology

a subspecialty of Neurology

A neurologist specializes in the diagnosis and treatment of all types of disease or impaired function of the brain, spinal cord, peripheral nerves, muscles and autonomic nervous system, as well as the blood vessels that relate to these structures. A child neurologist has special skills in the diagnosis and management of neurologic disorders of the neonatal period, infancy, early childhood and adolescence.

Training Required: Four years

CHILD NEUROLOGY

New England

Bourgeois, Blaise MD [ChiN] - **Spec Exp:** Epilepsy/Seizure Disorders; **Hospital:** Children's Hospital - Boston; **Address:** Chldn's Hosp-Boston, Fegan 9, 300 Longwood Ave, Boston, MA 02115; **Phone:** 617-355-2413; **Board Cert:** Pediatrics 1981; Child Neurology 1990; Clinical Neurophysiology 2006; **Med School:** Switzerland 1971; **Resid:** Neurology, Washington Univ/Barnes Jewish Hosp 1979; Child Neurology, Washington Univ/Barnes Jewish Hosp 1981; **Fellow:** Neurological Pharmacology, Washington Univ/Barnes Jewish Hosp 1982; **Fac Appt:** Prof N, Harvard Med Sch

Darras, Basil T MD [ChiN] - **Spec Exp:** Neuromuscular Disorders; Cerebral Palsy; **Hospital:** Children's Hospital - Boston; **Address:** Childrens Hosp, Neurology, Fegan 11, 300 Longwood Ave, Boston, MA 02115; **Phone:** 617-355-8235; **Board Cert:** Clinical Genetics 1987; Pediatrics 1988; Child Neurology 1992; Neuromuscular Medicine 2008; **Med School:** Greece 1977; **Resid:** Pediatrics, Nassau County Med Ctr 1982; Child Neurology, Tufts-New England Med Ctr 1985; **Fellow:** Clinical Genetics, Yale Univ Sch Med 1988; **Fac Appt:** Prof N, Harvard Med Sch

Griesemer, David A MD [ChiN] - **Spec Exp:** Epilepsy/Seizure Disorders; Brain Injury; **Hospital:** Tufts Med Ctr, Floating Hosp for Children at Tufts Med Ce; **Address:** Tufts Med Ctr, 800 Washington St, Box 330, Boston, MA 02111; **Phone:** 617-636-8100; **Board Cert:** Child Neurology 1992; **Med School:** Johns Hopkins Univ 1976; **Resid:** Pediatrics, Johns Hopkins Hosp 1978; **Fellow:** Child Neurology, Univ Michigan Hosp 1985; **Fac Appt:** Prof N, Tufts Univ

Holmes, Gregory L MD [ChiN] - **Spec Exp:** Epilepsy/Seizure Disorders; **Hospital:** Dartmouth - Hitchcock Med Ctr; **Address:** Dartmouth-Hitchcock Med Ctr, Dept Neurology, 1 Medical Center Drive, Lebanon, NH 03756; **Phone:** 603-650-4211; **Board Cert:** Pediatrics 1979; Neurology 1980; **Med School:** Univ VA Sch Med 1974; **Resid:** Pediatrics, Yale-New Haven Hosp 1976; **Fellow:** Pediatric Neurology, Univ Virginia 1979; **Fac Appt:** Prof N, Dartmouth Med Sch

Mandelbaum, David E MD/PhD [ChiN] - **Spec Exp:** Epilepsy/Seizure Disorders; Neonatal Neurology; Autism; **Hospital:** Rhode Island Hosp, Women & Infants Hosp of RI; **Address:** Dept of Neurology, 593 Eddy St George Bldg Fl 1, Providence, RI 02903; **Phone:** 401-444-5685; **Board Cert:** Child Neurology 1987; Pediatrics 1987; Clinical Neurophysiology 2003; Neurodevelopmental Disabilities 2011; **Med School:** Columbia P&S 1980; **Resid:** Pediatrics, Yale-New Haven Hosp 1982; Neurology, Neuro Inst-Columbia 1983; **Fellow:** Child Neurology, Neuro Inst-Columbia 1985; **Fac Appt:** Prof Ped, Brown Univ

Pomeroy, Scott L MD/PhD [ChiN] - **Spec Exp:** Neuro-Oncology; Brain Tumors; **Hospital:** Children's Hospital - Boston, Dana-Farber Cancer Inst (page 57); **Address:** Chldns Hosp, Dept Neurology-Fegan 11, 300 Longwood Ave, Boston, MA 02115; **Phone:** 617-355-6386; **Board Cert:** Child Neurology 1988; **Med School:** Univ Cincinnati 1982; **Resid:** Pediatrics, Chldns Hosp 1984; Neurology, St. Louis Chldn's Hosp/Wash Univ 1985; **Fellow:** Neurological Biology, Wash Univ Hosp 1990; Pediatric Neurology, St. Louis Chldn's Hosp/Wash Univ 1990; **Fac Appt:** Prof N, Harvard Med Sch

Shaywitz, Bennett A MD [ChiN] - **Spec Exp:** Learning Disorders; Dyslexia; Headache; **Hospital:** Yale-New Haven Hosp, Yale Med Group; **Address:** Yale Univ Sch Med, Dept Peds, 333 Cedar St, Box 208064, New Haven, CT 06520-8064; **Phone:** 203-785-4641; **Board Cert:** Pediatrics 1968; Child Neurology 1973; **Med School:** Washington Univ, St Louis 1963; **Resid:** Pediatrics, Bronx Muni Hosp Ctr 1967; **Fellow:** Child Neurology, Albert Einstein Coll Med 1970; **Fac Appt:** Prof Ped, Yale Univ

Volpe, Joseph J MD [ChiN] - **Spec Exp:** Neonatal Neurology; Cerebral Palsy; **Hospital:** Children's Hospital - Boston, Mass Genl Hosp; **Address:** Childrens Hosp Boston, 300 Longwood Ave, Fegan 11, Boston, MA 02115-5724; **Phone:** 617-355-8994; **Board Cert:** Pediatrics 1970; Child Neurology 1974; **Med School:** Harvard Med Sch 1964; **Resid:** Pediatrics, Mass Genl Hosp 1966; Neurology, Mass Genl Hosp 1971; **Fellow:** Research, Natl Inst Child Hlth Human Dev 1968; **Fac Appt:** Prof N, Harvard Med Sch

Mid Atlantic

Allen, Jeffrey MD [ChiN] - **Spec Exp:** Neuro-Oncology; Brain Tumors; Neurofibromatosis; **Hospital:** NYU Langone Med Ctr (page 68); **Address:** Hassenfeld Childrens Ctr, 160 E 32nd St Fl 2 - Ste L3, New York, NY 10016; **Phone:** 212-263-9907; **Board Cert:** Child Neurology 1977; **Med School:** Harvard Med Sch 1969; **Resid:** Pediatrics, Montreal Chldns Hosp 1973; Pediatric Neurology, Montreal Neur Inst/McGill 1976; **Fac Appt:** Prof Ped, NYU Sch Med

Bergman, Ira MD/PhD [ChiN] - **Spec Exp:** Complex Diagnosis; Neuro-Oncology; **Hospital:** Chldns Hosp of Pittsburgh - UPMC; **Address:** Chldns Hosp Pittsburgh, 4401 Penn Ave Fl 8, Pittsburgh, PA 15224; **Phone:** 412-692-5520; **Board Cert:** Pediatrics 1981; Child Neurology 1980; **Med School:** Univ Chicago-Pritzker Sch Med 1974; **Resid:** Pediatrics, Mass Genl Hosp 1976; **Fellow:** Neurology, Mass Genl Hosp 1979; **Fac Appt:** Assoc Prof Ped, Univ Pittsburgh

Comi, Anne M MD [ChiN] - **Spec Exp:** Sturge-Weber Syndrome; **Hospital:** Kennedy Krieger Inst, Johns Hopkins Hosp (page 61); **Address:** Kennedy-Krieger Institute, 707 N Broadway, Baltimore, MD 21205; **Phone:** 443-923-9150; **Board Cert:** Child Neurology 2000; **Med School:** SUNY Buffalo 1993; **Resid:** Pediatrics, Childrens Hosp Buffalo 1996; Pediatric Neurology, Johns Hopkins Hospital 1999; **Fac Appt:** Assoc Prof N, Johns Hopkins Univ

Crawford, Thomas O MD [ChiN] - **Spec Exp:** Neuromuscular Disorders; Muscular Dystrophy; Ataxia Telangiectasia; **Hospital:** Johns Hopkins Hosp (page 61); **Address:** Pediatric Neurology, 200 N Wolfe St, Ste 2158, Baltimore, MD 21287; **Phone:** 410-955-4259; **Board Cert:** Pediatrics 1986; Child Neurology 1990; **Med School:** USC Sch Med 1980; **Resid:** Pediatrics, LAC-USC Med Ctr 1984; Child Neurology, Chldns Hosp 1987; **Fellow:** Neuromuscular Medicine, Johns Hopkins Hosp 1988; **Fac Appt:** Assoc Prof N, Johns Hopkins Univ

De Vivo, Darryl C MD [ChiN] - **Spec Exp:** Metabolic Disorders; Neuromuscular Disorders; Spinal Muscular Atrophy (SMA); **Hospital:** NY-Presby/Columbia Univ Med Ctr, NY (page 66); **Address:** Neurological Institute, 710 W 168th St, Ste NI 101, New York, NY 10032; **Phone:** 212-305-5244; **Board Cert:** Child Neurology 1972; **Med School:** Univ VA Sch Med 1964; **Resid:** Pediatrics, Mass Genl Hosp 1966; Neurology, Mass Genl Hosp 1967; **Fellow:** Neurology, Natl Inst Hlth 1969; Child Neurology, Children's Hosp 1970; **Fac Appt:** Prof N, Columbia P&S

Ichord, Rebecca N MD [ChiN] - **Spec Exp:** Stroke in Children; Brain Injury; **Hospital:** Chldns Hosp of Philadelphia; **Address:** Chldn's Hosp Philadelphia, Wood Ctr Fl 6, 34th & Civic Ctr Blvd, Philadelphia, PA 19104-4318; **Phone:** 215-590-4142; **Board Cert:** Pediatrics 1984; Child Neurology 1992; **Med School:** Geo Wash Univ 1979; **Resid:** Pediatrics, Children's Natl Med Ctr 1983; **Fellow:** Developmental-Behavioral Pediatrics, Johns Hopkins Hosp 1985; Child Neurology, Johns Hopkins Hosp 1991; **Fac Appt:** Assoc Prof N, Univ Pennsylvania

Kosofsky, Barry MD/PhD [ChiN] - **Spec Exp:** Developmental Disorders; Autism; Stroke; **Hospital:** NY-Presby/Weill Cornell Med Ctr, NY (page 66); **Address:** NY-Cornell Med Ctr, Dept Pediatrics, 505 E 70th St, Helmsley Tower Fl 3, New York, NY 10021; **Phone:** 212-746-3321; **Board Cert:** Child Neurology 1993; **Med School:** Johns Hopkins Univ 1985; **Resid:** Pediatrics, Chldns Hosp 1987; Child Neurology, Mass Genl Hosp 1990; **Fellow:** Neurological Biology, Mass Genl Hosp 1992; **Fac Appt:** Prof Ped, Cornell Univ-Weill Med Coll

Legido, Agustin MD/PhD [ChiN] - **Spec Exp:** Mitochondrial Disorders; Neonatal Neurology; Epilepsy; **Hospital:** St. Christopher's Hosp for Chldn; **Address:** St Christopher's Hosp, Dept Neurology, 3601 A St, Philadelphia, PA 19134; **Phone:** 215-427-5452; **Board Cert:** Pediatrics 2011; Child Neurology 1991; **Med School:** Spain 1980; **Resid:** Pediatrics, St Christopher's Hosp 1989; Neurology, Hosp Univ Penn 1990; **Fellow:** Child Neurology, Chldns Hosp 1988; **Fac Appt:** Prof Ped, Drexel Univ Coll Med

Maytal, Joseph MD [ChiN] - **Spec Exp:** Epilepsy/Seizure Disorders; Migraine; **Hospital:** Steven & Alexandra Cohen Chldn's Med Ctr of NY (page 67); **Address:** Div Pediatric Neurology, 410 Lakeville Rd, Ste 105, Lake Success, NY 11042; **Phone:** 516-465-5255; **Board Cert:** Pediatrics 1986; Child Neurology 1988; **Med School:** Israel 1979; **Resid:** Pediatrics, Brookdale Hosp 1983; Child Neurology, Montefiore Med Ctr 1986; **Fellow:** Neurological Physiology, Albert Einstein Med Coll 1987; **Fac Appt:** Clin Prof N, Albert Einstein Coll Med

Mink, Jonathan W MD/PhD [ChiN] - **Spec Exp:** Movement Disorders; Tourette's Syndrome; Dystonia; **Hospital:** Univ of Rochester Strong Meml Hosp; **Address:** Univ Rochester, Child Neurology, 601 Elmwood Ave, Box 631, Rochester, NY 14642; **Phone:** 585-275-2808; **Board Cert:** Child Neurology 2007; **Med School:** Washington Univ, St Louis 1989; **Resid:** Pediatrics, St Louis Chldns Hosp 1991; Neurology, Barnes Hosp 1992; **Fellow:** Child Neurology, St Louis Chldns Hosp 1994; **Fac Appt:** Prof N, Univ Rochester

Nass, Ruth D MD [ChiN] - **Spec Exp:** Autism; ADD/ADHD; Learning Disorders; Migraine; **Hospital:** NYU Langone Med Ctr (page 68); **Address:** 1 Park Ave Fl 7, New York, NY 10016; **Phone:** 212-263-6622; **Board Cert:** Pediatrics 1980; Child Neurology 1981; **Med School:** Albert Einstein Coll Med 1975; **Resid:** Pediatrics, NY Hosp 1977; Child Neurology, Columbia-Presby 1980; **Fellow:** Neurology, NY Hosp 1982; **Fac Appt:** Prof N, NYU Sch Med

Packer, Roger J MD [ChiN] - **Spec Exp:** Brain Tumors; Neurofibromatosis; **Hospital:** Chldns Natl Med Ctr; **Address:** 111 Michigan Ave NW, MS 20010, Washington, DC 20010-2978; **Phone:** 202-476-6230; **Board Cert:** Child Neurology 1982; Pediatrics 1982; **Med School:** Northwestern Univ 1976; **Resid:** Pediatrics, Chldns Med Ctr 1978; Neurology, Chldns Hosp-Univ Penn 1981; **Fac Appt:** Prof N, Geo Wash Univ

Phillips, Peter C MD [ChiN] - **Spec Exp:** Brain Tumors; Neuro-Oncology; Neurofibromatosis; **Hospital:** Chldns Hosp of Philadelphia; **Address:** Chldns Hosp Philadelphia, 34th St & Civic Center Blvd, CTRB Bldg - Ste 4027, Philadelphia, PA 19104; **Phone:** 215-590-5188; **Board Cert:** Pediatrics 1985; Child Neurology 1986; **Med School:** Univ Conn 1978; **Resid:** Pediatrics, Chldns Hosp 1980; Pediatric Neurology, Neuro Inst 1983; **Fellow:** Neuro-Oncology, Meml Sloan Kettering Cancer Ctr 1986; **Fac Appt:** Prof N, Univ Pennsylvania

Riviello Jr, James J MD [ChiN] - **Spec Exp:** Epilepsy/Seizure Disorders; Epilepsy in Tuberous Sclerosis; Electrical Status Epilepticus Of Sleep; **Hospital:** NYU Langone Med Ctr (page 68); **Address:** NYU Epilepsy and Neurology Center, 223 E 34th St Fl 1, New York, NY 10016; **Phone:** 646-558-0808; **Board Cert:** Pediatrics 1984; Child Neurology 1985; Clinical Neurophysiology 2006; **Med School:** Tufts Univ 1978; **Resid:** Pediatrics, St Christopher Hosp Chldn 1980; Neurology, Temple Univ Hosp 1983; **Fellow:** Pediatric Neurology, St Christopher Hosp Chldn 1983; **Fac Appt:** Prof N, NYU Sch Med

Santos, Cesar C MD [ChiN] - **Spec Exp:** Epilepsy; Sleep Disorders; Stroke in Children; Clinical Trials; **Hospital:** Georgetown Univ Hosp; **Address:** Georgetown Univ Hosp, Peds-Child Neuro, 3800 Reservoir Rd NW, Pasquerilla Healthcare Ctr, Fl 2, Washington, DC 20007; **Phone:** 202-444-8785; **Board Cert:** Pediatrics 2004; Child Neurology 2004; Clinical Neurophysiology 2005; **Med School:** Philippines 1982; **Resid:** Pediatrics, St Lukes Roosevelt Hosp 1988; **Fellow:** Neurology, Duke Univ Med Ctr 1991; Neurological Physiology, Duke Univ 1992; **Fac Appt:** Prof N, Wake Forest Univ

Shinnar, Shlomo MD/PhD [ChiN] - **Spec Exp:** Epilepsy/Seizure Disorders; Headache; **Hospital:** Montefiore Med Ctr-Moses Campus, NY; **Address:** Montefiore Med Ctr, Dept Neurophsiology, Pediatric Neurology, 111 E 210th St Fl 4, Bronx, NY 10467; **Phone:** 718-920-4378; **Board Cert:** Neurology 1984; Pediatrics 1984; Clinical Neurophysiology 2005; **Med School:** Albert Einstein Coll Med 1978; **Resid:** Pediatrics, Johns Hopkins Hosp 1980; Neurology, Johns Hopkins Hosp 1983; **Fac Appt:** Prof N, Albert Einstein Coll Med

Southeast

Dure, Leon S MD [ChiN] - **Spec Exp:** Huntington's Disease; Tourette's Syndrome; Movement Disorders; **Hospital:** Children's Hospital - Birmingham, Univ of Ala Hosp at Birmingham; **Address:** UAB Pediatric Neurology, 1600 7th Ave S, CHB 314, Birmingham, AL 35233-0011; **Phone:** 205-996-7850; **Board Cert:** Child Neurology 1991; **Med School:** Baylor Coll Med 1984; **Resid:** Pediatrics, Columbia Presby Hosp 1986; Child Neurology, Texas Chldns Hosp 1989; **Fellow:** Child Neurology, Univ Michigan Affil Hosp 1990; **Fac Appt:** Prof N, Univ Alabama

Finkel, Richard S MD [ChiN] - **Spec Exp:** Neuromuscular Disorders; **Hospital:** Nemours Chldns Hosp - Orlando; **Address:** Nemours Chldns Clin-Neurology, 1717 S Orange Ave, Ste 100, Orlando, FL 32806; **Phone:** 407-650-7715; **Board Cert:** Pediatrics 1984; Child Neurology 1986; Neuromuscular Medicine 2008; **Med School:** Washington Univ, St Louis 1978; **Resid:** Pediatrics, Chldn's Hosp 1980; **Fellow:** Neurology, Chldn's Hosp/ Brigham & Women's Hosp 1983; **Fac Appt:** Clin Prof Ped, Univ Pennsylvania

Goldstein, Edward M MD [ChiN] - **Spec Exp:** Neuromuscular Disorders; Headache; Cerebral Palsy; Botox Therapy; **Hospital:** Chldns Hlthcare Atlanta @ Scottish Rite; **Address:** Child Neurology Assocs, 5505 Peachtree Dunwoody Rd, Ste 500, Atlanta, GA 30342; **Phone:** 404-256-3535; **Board Cert:** Child Neurology 1994; **Med School:** Johns Hopkins Univ 1985; **Resid:** Pediatrics, Johns Hopkins Hosp 1987; Neurology, Johns Hopkins Hosp 1990; **Fellow:** Neuromuscular Disease, Emory Univ 1993; **Fac Appt:** Assoc Clin Prof N, Mercer Univ Sch Med

Greenwood, Robert S MD [ChiN] - **Spec Exp:** Neurofibromatosis; Epilepsy; **Hospital:** NC Memorial Hosp - UNC; **Address:** 101 Manning Drive, CB #7025, Chapel Hill, NC 27599; **Phone:** 919-966-2528; **Board Cert:** Pediatrics 1974; Child Neurology 1979; **Med School:** Univ Tex Med Br, Galveston 1968; **Resid:** Pediatrics, Chldns Hosp 1971; Child Neurology, Chldns Hosp 1975; **Fellow:** Child Neurology, Chldns Hosp 1977; **Fac Appt:** Prof N, Univ NC Sch Med

Lavenstein, Bennett L MD [ChiN] - **Spec Exp:** Movement Disorders; Neuromuscular Disorders; **Hospital:** Chldns Natl Med Ctr, Inova Fairfax Hosp for Chldn; **Address:** 8501 Arlington Blvd, Ste 200, Fairfax, VA 22031; **Phone:** 571-226-8368; **Board Cert:** Pediatrics 1977; Child Neurology 1979; **Med School:** Univ MD Sch Med 1974; **Resid:** Pediatrics, Univ of MD Hlth System 1977; Neurology, Georgetown Univ Hosp 1979; **Fellow:** Neuromuscular Medicine, Natl Inst Hlth; **Fac Appt:** Assoc Clin Prof N, Univ VA Sch Med

Tennison, Michael MD [ChiN] - **Spec Exp:** Epilepsy; Headache; Neurophysiology; Neurogenetics; **Hospital:** NC Memorial Hosp - UNC; **Address:** CB 7025 UNC-CH, Campus Box 7025, Chapel Hill, NC 27599-7025; **Phone:** 919-966-2528; **Board Cert:** Pediatrics 1979; Child Neurology 1983; **Med School:** Harvard Med Sch 1975; **Resid:** Pediatrics, UCLA Affil Hosp 1978; Pediatric Neurology, Univ NC Hosp 1981; **Fellow:** Clinical Neurophysiology, Univ NC Hosp; **Fac Appt:** Prof N, Univ NC Sch Med

Child Neurology

Wheless, James W MD [ChiN] - **Spec Exp:** Epilepsy/Seizure Disorders; **Hospital:** Le Bonheur Chldns Med Ctr, St. Jude Children's Research Hosp; **Address:** 50 N Dunlap St, Ste L-400, Memphis, TN 38103; **Phone:** 901-287-5060; **Board Cert:** Pediatrics 1987; Child Neurology 1989; Clinical Neurophysiology 2007; **Med School:** Univ Okla Coll Med 1982; **Resid:** Pediatrics, Univ Oklahoma Med Ctr 1985; **Fellow:** Pediatric Neurology, Chldns Meml Hosp 1988; Epilepsy, Med Coll Georgia Affil Hosp 1989; **Fac Appt:** Prof N, Univ Tenn Coll Med

Midwest

Brunstrom, Janice MD [ChiN] - **Spec Exp:** Cerebral Palsy; **Hospital:** St. Louis Chldns Hosp; **Address:** Washington Univ Sch Med, Dept Ped Neuro, 660 S Euclid Ave, Box 8111, St Louis, MO 63110; **Phone:** 314-454-6120; **Board Cert:** Pediatrics 2003; Child Neurology 2005; **Med School:** Med Coll VA 1987; **Resid:** Neurology, St Louis Chldns Hosp 1989; Neurology, Barnes Jewish Hosp 1990; **Fellow:** Child Neurology, St Louis Chldns Hosp 1995; **Fac Appt:** Asst Prof N, Washington Univ, St Louis

Cohen, Bruce H MD [ChiN] - **Spec Exp:** Brain Tumors; Mitochondrial Disorders; Neurometabolic Disorders; **Hospital:** Akron Children's Hosp; **Address:** 1 Perkins Square, Akron, OH 44308; **Phone:** 330-543-8050; **Board Cert:** Child Neurology 1990; **Med School:** Albert Einstein Coll Med 1982; **Resid:** Pediatrics, Chldns Hosp 1984; Child Neurology, Neurologic Inst-Columbia 1987; **Fellow:** Pediatric Neuro-Oncology, Chldns Hosp 1989; **Fac Appt:** Prof Ped, NE Ohio Univ

Edgar, Terence MD [ChiN] - **Spec Exp:** Neuromuscular Disorders; Cerebral Palsy; Epilepsy; **Hospital:** St. Vincent Hosp - Green Bay; **Address:** Prevea Health, 1821 S Webster Fl 3, Green Bay, WI 54301; **Phone:** 920-272-1270; **Board Cert:** Pediatrics 2010; Child Neurology 2006; **Med School:** South Africa 1984; **Resid:** Pediatrics, Univ Wisconsin Hosp & Clin 1995; Child Neurology, Univ Wisconsin Hosp & Clin 1996; **Fellow:** Neuromuscular Disease, Univ Wisconsin Hosp & Clin 1996; Epilepsy, Mayo Clinic 2010

Epstein, Leon G MD [ChiN] - **Spec Exp:** Migraine; **Hospital:** Lurie Chldn's Hosp-Chicago; **Address:** Chldns Meml Hosp, Div Neurology, 2515 N Clark St Fl 8, Chicago, IL 60614; **Phone:** 773-880-4352; **Board Cert:** Child Neurology 1979; **Med School:** Wayne State Univ 1973; **Resid:** Neurology, St Josephs Mercy Hosp 1974; Neurology, Univ Arizona Med Ctr 1976; **Fellow:** Neurology, Columbia Presby Med Ctr 1978; **Fac Appt:** Prof Ped, Northwestern Univ

Hershey, Andrew D MD/PhD [ChiN] - **Spec Exp:** Headache; Migraine; **Hospital:** Cincinnati Chldns Hosp Med Ctr; **Address:** Children's Hospital, Dept Neurology, 3333 Burnet Ave, Cincinnati, OH 45229; **Phone:** 513-636-4222; **Board Cert:** Child Neurology 2008; **Med School:** Univ Wash 1992; **Resid:** Pediatrics, St Louis Children's Hosp 1995; Neurology, Barnes-Jewish Hosp 1997; **Fellow:** Pediatric Neurology, St Louis Children's Hosp; **Fac Appt:** Prof Ped, Univ Cincinnati

Keating, Gesina F MD [ChiN] - **Spec Exp:** Brain Tumors; Spinal Tumors; Cancer Survivors-Late Effects of Therapy; Chiari's Deformity; **Hospital:** Mayo Med Ctr & Clin - Rochester; **Address:** 200 First St SW, Mayo Clinic, Rochester, MN 55905; **Phone:** 507-284-2511; **Board Cert:** Child Neurology 2008; **Med School:** Mayo Med Sch 1991; **Resid:** Pediatrics, Vanderbilt Univ Med Ctr 1993; Child Neurology, Mayo Clinic 1996; **Fellow:** Pediatric Neuro-Oncology, Beth Israel Med Ctr 1997

Kotagal, Suresh MD [ChiN] - **Spec Exp:** Sleep Disorders/Apnea; **Hospital:** Mayo Med Ctr & Clin - Rochester, St. Mary's Hosp - Rochester MN (Mayo); **Address:** Mayo Clinic, 200 First St SW, Rochester, MN 55905-0002; **Phone:** 507-266-0774; **Board Cert:** Pediatrics 1979; Child Neurology 1982; Sleep Medicine 2009; **Med School:** India 1974; **Resid:** Child Neurology, Chldns Hosp 1976; Pediatrics, St Louis Univ Hosp 1979; **Fellow:** Sleep Medicine, Stanford Univ 1982; **Fac Appt:** Prof N, Mayo Med Sch

Kovnar, Edward H MD [ChiN] - **Spec Exp:** Epilepsy/Seizure Disorders; Neurophysiology; Developmental Disorders; **Hospital:** Chldns Hosp - Wisconsin; **Address:** Advanced Healthcare, SC, 3003 W Good Hope Rd, Milwaukee, WI 53209-0996; **Phone:** 414-352-8828; **Board Cert:** Pediatrics 1984; Child Neurology 1984; Clinical Neurophysiology 2004; Neurodevelopmental Disabilities 2005; **Med School:** Washington Univ, St Louis 1977; **Resid:** Pediatrics, Chldns Hosp 1979; Neurology, Barnes Hosp 1980; **Fellow:** Pediatric Neurology, Chldns Hosp 1982; Clinical Neurophysiology, Chldns Hosp 1991

Noetzel, Michael MD [ChiN] - **Spec Exp:** Cerebral Palsy; Brain Injury; Movement Disorders; **Hospital:** St. Louis Chldns Hosp; **Address:** Washington Univ Ped Neurology Ctr, 660 S Euclid Ave, Box 8111, St Louis, MO 63110; **Phone:** 314-454-6120; **Board Cert:** Child Neurology 1984; Pediatrics 1984; **Med School:** Univ VA Sch Med 1977; **Resid:** Pediatrics, St Louis Chldns Hosp 1979; Neurology, Barnes Hosp 1980; **Fellow:** Child Neurology, St Louis Chldns Hosp 1982; **Fac Appt:** Prof Ped, Washington Univ, St Louis

Patterson, Marc C MD [ChiN] - **Spec Exp:** Neurogenetics; Developmental Disorders; Metabolic Disorders; **Hospital:** Mayo Med Ctr & Clin - Rochester; **Address:** Mayo Clinic, Div Child & Adolescent Neurology, 200 First St SW, Rochester, MN 55905; **Phone:** 507-284-3351; **Board Cert:** Child Neurology 2004; Neurodevelopmental Disabilities 2011; **Med School:** Australia 1981; **Resid:** Neurology, Univ Queenland 1988; Child Neurology, Mayo Clinic 1990; **Fellow:** Metabolic Neurology, Natl Inst Health 1992; Pediatrics, Mayo Cilnic 1993; **Fac Appt:** Prof N, Mayo Med Sch

Scher, Mark S MD [ChiN] - **Spec Exp:** Epilepsy; Neonatal Neurology; **Hospital:** UH Rainbow Babies & Chldns Hosp (page 74), Univ Hosps Case Med Ctr (page 74); **Address:** UH Rainbow Babies & Children's Hospital, Pediatric Neurology, 11100 Euclid Ave, MS 6090, Cleveland, OH 44106; **Phone:** 216-844-3691; **Board Cert:** Pediatrics 1986; Child Neurology 1983; **Med School:** SUNY Downstate 1976; **Resid:** Pediatrics, NY Presby Hosp 1978; **Fellow:** Pediatric Neurology, Univ MN Med Ctr 1980; Epilepsy, Stanford Univ Med Ctr 1983; **Fac Appt:** Prof N, Case West Res Univ

Sivaswamy, Lalitha MD [ChiN] - **Spec Exp:** Headache; Migraine; **Hospital:** Chldns Hosp of Michigan; **Address:** Children's Hosp of Michigan, Dept Neurology, 3901 Beaubien Blvd, Detroit, MI 48201; **Phone:** 313-993-2596; **Board Cert:** Child Neurology 2006; Headache Medicine ; **Med School:** India 1989; **Resid:** Pediatrics, Henry Ford Hosp 1996; **Fellow:** Genetics, Chidren;s Hosp of British Columbia 1998; Child Neurology, Children's Hosp of Michigan 2005; **Fac Appt:** Assoc Prof Ped, Univ Mich Med Sch

Tonsgard, James MD [ChiN] - **Spec Exp:** Epilepsy/Seizure Disorders; Tuberous Sclerosis; **Hospital:** Univ of Chicago Med Ctr; **Address:** Univ Chicago Med Ctr, 5841 S Maryland Ave, MC 3055, Chicago, IL 60637-1463; **Phone:** 773-702-6487; **Board Cert:** Pediatrics 1981; **Med School:** Yale Univ 1975; **Resid:** Pediatrics, Yale-New Haven Hosp 1977; Neurology, Univ Chicago Hosp 1980; **Fellow:** Child Neurology, Univ Chicago Hosp 1981; **Fac Appt:** Assoc Prof Ped, Univ Chicago-Pritzker Sch Med

Tuxhorn, Ingrid E MD [ChiN] - **Spec Exp:** Epilepsy; Gravet Syndrome; **Hospital:** UH Rainbow Babies & Chldns Hosp (page 74), Univ Hosps Case Med Ctr (page 74); **Address:** UH Rainbow Babies & Children's Hospital, Pediatric Epileptology, 11100 Euclid Ave, MS 6009, Cleveland, OH 44106; **Phone:** 216-286-6644; **Board Cert:** Pediatrics 1985; **Med School:** Africa 1975; **Resid:** Pediatrics, Baystate Med Ctr 1982; Pediatrics, Yale-New Haven Hosp 1983; **Fellow:** Pediatric Neurology, U Mass Meml Med Ctr 1990; Neurological Physiology, Cleveland Clinic 1992; **Fac Appt:** Prof N, Case West Res Univ

Child Neurology

Wiznitzer, Max MD [ChiN] - **Hospital:** UH Rainbow Babies & Chldns Hosp (page 74); **Address:** Rainbow Babies & Chldns Hosp, 11100 Euclid Ave, MS RBC6090, Cleveland, OH 44106; **Phone:** 216-844-3691; **Board Cert:** Pediatrics 1982; Child Neurology 1986; Neurodevelopmental Disabilities 2004; **Med School:** Northwestern Univ 1977; **Resid:** Pediatrics, Chldns Hosp Med Ctr 1980; **Fellow:** Developmental-Behavioral Pediatrics, Cincinnati Med Ctr 1981; Pediatric Neurology, Chldns Hosp 1984; **Fac Appt:** Assoc Prof Ped, Case West Res Univ

Wyllie, Elaine MD [ChiN] - **Spec Exp:** Epilepsy/Seizure Disorders; **Hospital:** Cleveland Clin (page 55); **Address:** Cleveland Clinic, Div Ped Neurology, 9500 Euclid Ave, Desk S5-1, Cleveland, OH 44195; **Phone:** 216-444-5559; **Board Cert:** Pediatrics 1982; Child Neurology 1986; **Med School:** Indiana Univ 1978; **Resid:** Pediatrics, Indiana Univ Med Ctr 1980; Pediatrics, Case West Med Ctr 1981; **Fellow:** Child Neurology, Cleveland Clinic 1984; Clinical Neurophysiology, Cleveland Clinic 1985; **Fac Appt:** Prof Ped, Cleveland Cl Coll Med/Case West Res

Yamada, Kelvin MD [ChiN] - **Spec Exp:** Epilepsy; **Hospital:** St. Louis Chldns Hosp; **Address:** Washington Univ Ped Neurology Ctr, 660 S Euclid Ave, Box 8111, Saint Louis, MO 63110; **Phone:** 314-454-6120; **Board Cert:** Pediatrics 2011; Child Neurology 1990; Clinical Neurophysiology 2004; Sleep Medicine 2007; **Med School:** Baylor Coll Med 1983; **Resid:** Pediatrics, Baylor Coll Affil Hosp 1985; Neurology, Barnes-Jewish Hosp 1986; **Fellow:** Child Neurology, St Louis Chldn's Hosp 1990; **Fac Appt:** Prof Ped, Washington Univ, St Louis

Great Plains and Mountains

Bale Jr, James F MD [ChiN] - **Spec Exp:** Infections-Neurologic; Infections-Congenital; **Hospital:** Primary Children's Med Ctr, Univ Utah Hlth Care; **Address:** Primary Chldns Med Ctr, 100 N Mario Capecchi Drive, Salt Lake City, UT 84113; **Phone:** 801-587-7575; **Board Cert:** Pediatrics 2002; Child Neurology 1982; **Med School:** Univ Mich Med Sch 1975; **Resid:** Pediatrics, Univ Utah Hosps 1977; Neurology, Univ Utah Hosps 1980; **Fellow:** Infectious Disease, Univ Utah 1981; Neurovirology, UCSF-VA Med Ctr 1982; **Fac Appt:** Prof N, Univ Utah

Southwest

Filipek, Pauline A MD [ChiN] - **Spec Exp:** Autism; Autism in Infants; Developmental Disorders; **Hospital:** Children's Meml Hermann Hosp; **Address:** Autism Ctr-Childrens Learning Institute, 7000 Fannin St, Ste 2453, Houston, TX 77030; **Phone:** 713-500-3600; **Board Cert:** Pediatrics 1985; Child Neurology 2010; **Med School:** Georgetown Univ 1980; **Resid:** Pediatrics, Univ Mass Med Ctr 1983; Child Neurology, Mass Genl Hosp 1986; **Fellow:** Neuroimaging, Mass Genl Hosp 1987; **Fac Appt:** Prof Ped, Univ Tex, Houston

Iannaccone, Susan T MD [ChiN] - **Spec Exp:** Neuromuscular Disorders; **Hospital:** Chldns Med Ctr of Dallas, UT Southwestern Med Ctr at Dallas; **Address:** 1935 Med District Drive, Ste 5400, Dallas, TX 75207; **Phone:** 214-456-2768; **Board Cert:** Pediatrics 1975; Child Neurology 1976; **Med School:** SUNY Hlth Sci Ctr 1969; **Resid:** Pediatrics, St Louis Chldns Hosp 1972; Neurology, Strong Meml Hosp 1975; **Fellow:** Neurology, Strong Meml Hosp 1975; **Fac Appt:** Prof N, Univ Tex SW, Dallas

Sharp, Gregory B MD [ChiN] - **Spec Exp:** Epilepsy; **Hospital:** UAMS Med Ctr, Arkansas Chldns Hosp; **Address:** 1 Children's Way, Little Rock, AR 72202; **Phone:** 501-364-1850; **Board Cert:** Pediatrics 2011; Child Neurology 1993; **Med School:** Univ Ark 1984; **Resid:** Pediatrics, Univ Ark Chldns Hosp 1987; **Fellow:** Pediatric Neurology, Mayo Clinic 1990; **Fac Appt:** Prof Ped, Univ Ark

West Coast and Pacific

Ashwal, Stephen MD [ChiN] - **Spec Exp:** Metabolic Disorders; **Hospital:** Loma Linda Chldns Hosp; **Address:** Pediatric Neurosciences Ctr, 2195 Club Ctr Drive, Ste A, San Bernadino, CA 92408; **Phone:** 909-835-1810; **Board Cert:** Pediatrics 1975; Child Neurology 1978; **Med School:** NYU Sch Med 1970; **Resid:** Pediatrics, Bellevue Hosp 1973; **Fellow:** Child Neurology, Univ Minn Med Ctr 1976; **Fac Appt:** Prof Ped, Loma Linda Univ

Fisher, Paul G MD [ChiN] - **Spec Exp:** Neuro-Oncology; Brain Tumors; **Hospital:** Lucile Packard Chldn's Hosp; **Address:** Stanford Cancer Ctr-Dept Neurology, 750 Welch Rd, Ste 317, MC 5784, Palo Alto, CA 94304; **Phone:** 650-721-5889; **Board Cert:** Pediatrics 2003; Child Neurology 2008; **Med School:** UCSF 1989; **Resid:** Pediatrics, Johns Hopkins Univ Hosp 1991; Neurology, Johns Hopkins Univ Hosp 1994; **Fellow:** Neuro-Oncology, Children's Hosp 1994; **Fac Appt:** Assoc Prof Ped, Stanford Univ

Gospe Jr, Sidney M MD/PhD [ChiN] - **Spec Exp:** Epilepsy/Seizure Disorders; Neuromuscular Disorders; Neurotoxicology; **Hospital:** Seattle Chldns Hosp; **Address:** Seattle Children's Hospital, 4800 Sand Point Way NE, MS B5552, Seattle, WA 98105; **Phone:** 206-987-2078; **Board Cert:** Pediatrics 2005; Child Neurology 2010; **Med School:** Duke Univ 1981; **Resid:** Pediatrics, Baylor Coll Med 1983; **Fellow:** Child Neurology, Baylor Coll Med 1986; **Fac Appt:** Prof N, Univ Wash

Haas, Richard H MD [ChiN] - **Spec Exp:** Mitochondrial Disorders; Neurometabolic Disorders; **Hospital:** UCSD Med Ctr, Rady Children's Hosp - San Diego; **Address:** UCSD Sch Med, Div Ped Neuro, 9500 Gilman Drive, MC 0935, La Jolla, CA 92093-0935; **Phone:** 858-822-6700; **Board Cert:** Child Neurology 1983; Pediatrics 1985; **Med School:** England, UK 1972; **Resid:** Pediatrics, Univ London 1979; Child Neurology, Univ Colo Hlth Sci Ctr 1981; **Fellow:** Biochemical Mental Retardation, Univ Colo Hlth Sci Ctr 1981; **Fac Appt:** Prof Ped, UCSD

Lott, Ira T MD [ChiN] - **Spec Exp:** Down Syndrome; **Hospital:** Chldns Hosp Orange Co, UC Irvine Med Ctr; **Address:** 1120 W La Veta Ave, Ste 125, Orange, CA 92868; **Phone:** 714-532-7601; **Board Cert:** Pediatrics 1975; Child Neurology 1977; **Med School:** Ohio State Univ 1967; **Resid:** Pediatrics, Mass Genl Hosp 1969; **Fellow:** Research, Natl Inst Hlth 1971; Neurology, Harvard-Mass Genl Hosp 1974; **Fac Appt:** Prof N, UC Irvine

Mitchell, Wendy G MD [ChiN] - **Spec Exp:** Epilepsy/Seizure Disorders; Opsoclonus-Ataxia in Children; Neurodegenerative Disorders; **Hospital:** Chldns Hosp - Los Angeles; **Address:** Chldns Hosp Los Angeles, Dept Neuro, 4650 Sunset Blvd, MS 82, Los Angeles, CA 90027-6062; **Phone:** 323-361-2498; **Board Cert:** Pediatrics 1978; Child Neurology 1983; **Med School:** UCSF 1973; **Resid:** Pediatrics, Moffit Hosp-UCSF 1975; Child Neurology, Univ North Carolina 1981; **Fellow:** Behavioral Pediatrics, Mt Zion Hosp 1976; Univ North Carolina 1978; **Fac Appt:** Prof N, USC Sch Med

Pinter, Joseph David MD [ChiN] - **Spec Exp:** Down Syndrome; Tourette's Syndrome; Epilepsy; **Hospital:** Doernbecher Chldns Hosp/OHSU; **Address:** OHSU, Dept Child Neurology, 707 SW Gaines Rd, MC CDRCP, Portland, OR 97239; **Phone:** 503-494-5856; **Board Cert:** Child Neurology 2008; **Med School:** UCLA 1990; **Resid:** Pediatrics, Univ Washington/Cedars Sinai Med Ctr 1993; Child Neurology, Chldn's Hosp 1996; **Fellow:** Neurological Science, UCSF Med Ctr 1999; **Fac Appt:** Assoc Prof N, Oregon Hlth & Sci Univ

Roddy, Sarah M MD [ChiN] - **Spec Exp:** Tourette's Syndrome; **Hospital:** Loma Linda Chldns Hosp; **Address:** Pediatric Neuroscience Ctr, 2195 Club Ctr Drive, Ste A, San Bernadino, CA 92408; **Phone:** 909-835-1810; **Board Cert:** Child Neurology 1987; Pediatrics 1987; **Med School:** Loma Linda Univ 1980; **Resid:** Pediatrics, Loma Linda Univ Med Ctr 1983; **Fellow:** Pediatric Neurology, Loma Linda Univ Med Ctr 1986; **Fac Appt:** Assoc Prof N, Loma Linda Univ

Child Neurology

Rosser, Tena L MD [ChiN] - **Spec Exp:** Neurocutaneous Disorders; Neurofibromatosis; Tuberous Sclerosis; **Hospital:** Chldns Hosp - Los Angeles; **Address:** Chldns Hosp Los Angeles, Dept Neurology, 4650 Sunset Blvd, MS 82, Los Angeles, CA 90027; **Phone:** 323-361-2498; **Board Cert:** Pediatrics 2007; Child Neurology 2003; **Med School:** Univ NC Sch Med 1996; **Resid:** Pediatrics, Chldn's Natl Med Ctr 1999; **Fellow:** Child Neurology, Chldn's Natl Med Ctr 2003; **Fac Appt:** Asst Prof N, USC-Keck School of Medicine

Sankar, Raman MD/PhD [ChiN] - **Spec Exp:** Epilepsy/Seizure Disorders; Headache; Migraine; **Hospital:** Mattel Chldns Hosp at UCLA, UCLA Ronald Reagan Med Ctr; **Address:** UCLA Sch Med-Div Ped Neurology, 10833` Le Conte Ave, rm 22-474, Los Angeles, CA 90095; **Phone:** 310-825-6196; **Board Cert:** Child Neurology 2005; **Med School:** Tulane Univ 1986; **Resid:** Pediatrics, Chldns Hosp 1988; Neurology, UCLA Med Ctr 1989; **Fellow:** Child Neurology, UCLA Med Ctr 1991; **Fac Appt:** Prof Ped, UCLA

Trauner, Doris A MD [ChiN] - **Spec Exp:** Autism; Speech Disorders; **Hospital:** Rady Children's Hosp - San Diego; **Address:** Rady Chldn's Specialists, 8010 Frost St, Ste 510, San Diego, CA 92123; **Phone:** 858-966-5819; **Board Cert:** Pediatrics 1978; Child Neurology 1979; Neurodevelopmental Disabilities 2011; **Med School:** Med Coll VA 1972; **Resid:** Pediatrics, UCSD Med Ctr 1974; Neurology, UCSD Med Ctr 1975; **Fellow:** Child Neurology, Univ Chicago 1977; **Fac Appt:** Prof Ped, UCSD

Zupanc, Mary L MD [ChiN] - **Spec Exp:** Epilepsy; **Hospital:** Chldns Hosp Orange Co; **Address:** CHOC Childrens Neurology Ctr, 1120 W La Veta Ave, Ste 125, Orange, CA 92868; **Phone:** 714-532-7601; **Board Cert:** Pediatrics 1985; Child Neurology 2010; Clinical Neurophysiology 2006; **Med School:** UCLA 1979; **Resid:** Pediatrics, Univ Wash Med Ctr 1981; Pediatrics, UCLA-Harbor Med Ctr 1982; **Fellow:** Pediatric Neurology, Univ Wisconsin 1985

Clinical Genetics

A specialist trained in diagnostic and therapeutic procedures for patients with genetically-linked diseases. This specialist uses modern cytogenetic, radiologic and biochemical testing to assist in specialized genetic counseling, implements needed therapeutic interventions and provides prevention through prenatal diagnosis.

A clinical geneticist demonstrates competence in providing comprehensive diagnostic, management and counseling services for genetic disorders.

A medical geneticist plans and coordinates large scale screening programs for inborn errors of metabolism, hemoglobinopathies, chromosome abnormalities and neural tube defects.

Training Required: Two or four years

CLINICAL GENETICS

New England

Bale, Allen E MD [CG] - **Spec Exp:** Cancer Genetics; **Hospital:** Yale-New Haven Hosp, Yale Med Group; **Address:** 333 Cedar St, SHM Bldg - rm 1321, New Haven, CT 06519; **Phone:** 203-785-2660; **Board Cert:** Internal Medicine 1983; Clinical Genetics 1987; Clinical Molecular Genetics 2006; **Med School:** Univ Mass Sch Med 1979; **Resid:** Internal Medicine, Western Penn Hosp 1983; **Fellow:** Medical Genetics, Natl Inst of Health 1987; **Fac Appt:** Assoc Prof CG, Yale Univ

Bianchi, Diana MD [CG] - **Spec Exp:** Prenatal Genetic Diagnosis; Fetal Abnormalities; Twin to Twin Transfusion Syndrome (TTTS); **Hospital:** Tufts Med Ctr; **Address:** Tufts Med Ctr/Floating Hosp for Children, Div of Genetics, 800 Washington St, Box 394, Boston, MA 02111; **Phone:** 617-636-1468; **Board Cert:** Pediatrics 1985; Clinical Genetics 1987; Neonatal-Perinatal Medicine 1987; **Med School:** Stanford Univ 1980; **Resid:** Pediatrics, Chldns Hosp 1983; **Fellow:** Neonatology, Chldns Hosp 1986; Clinical Genetics, Harvard Med Sch 1987; **Fac Appt:** Prof Ped, Tufts Univ

Holmes, Lewis B MD [CG] - **Spec Exp:** Birth Defects; Inherited Disorders; Prenatal Diagnosis; **Hospital:** Mass Genl Hosp, Brigham and Women's Hosp (page 57); **Address:** Mass Genl Hosp, Dept Pediatrics, 175 Cambridge St Fl 5 - rm 504, Boston, MA 02114; **Phone:** 617-726-1742; **Board Cert:** Pediatrics 1968; Clinical Genetics 1982; **Med School:** Duke Univ 1963; **Resid:** Pediatrics, Mass Genl Hosp 1965; **Fellow:** Pediatric Endocrinology, Mass Genl Hosp 1966; **Fac Appt:** Prof Ped, Harvard Med Sch

Mahoney, Maurice J MD [CG] - **Spec Exp:** Fetal Therapy; Prenatal Diagnosis; **Hospital:** Yale-New Haven Hosp, Yale Med Group; **Address:** Yale Genetics Consultation Serv, 333 Cedar St, rm WWW330, New Haven, CT 06520-8005; **Phone:** 203-785-2661; **Board Cert:** Pediatrics 1967; Clinical Genetics 1982; Clinical Biochemical Genetics 1982; **Med School:** Univ Pittsburgh 1962; **Resid:** Pediatrics, Johns Hopkins Hosp 1965; Pediatrics, Childrens Hosp 1966; **Fellow:** Clinical Genetics, Yale Univ Sch Med 1970; **Fac Appt:** Prof CG, Yale Univ

Pauker, Susan Perlmutter MD [CG] - **Spec Exp:** Prenatal Diagnosis; Marfan's Syndrome; **Hospital:** Brigham and Women's Hosp (page 57); **Address:** 133 Brookline Ave, Boston, MA 02215-3904; **Phone:** 617-421-3320; **Board Cert:** Pediatrics 1976; Clinical Genetics 1987; **Med School:** Tufts Univ 1971; **Resid:** Pediatrics, Mass Genl Hosp 1973; **Fellow:** Clinical Genetics, Mass Genl Hosp 1975; **Fac Appt:** Assoc Clin Prof Ped, Harvard Med Sch

Seashore, Margretta MD [CG] - **Spec Exp:** Inherited Metabolic Disorders; **Hospital:** Yale-New Haven Hosp, Yale Med Group; **Address:** Yale Univ Sch Med, Dept Genetics, 333 Cedar St, rm 305, Box 208005, New Haven, CT 06520-8005; **Phone:** 203-785-2660; **Board Cert:** Pediatrics 1970; Clinical Biochemical Genetics 1982; Clinical Genetics 1982; **Med School:** Yale Univ 1965; **Resid:** Pediatrics, Yale-New Haven Hosp 1968; **Fellow:** Clinical Genetics, Yale-New Haven Hosp 1970; **Fac Appt:** Prof CG, Yale Univ

Mid Atlantic

Anyane-Yeboa, Kwame MD [CG] - **Spec Exp:** Dysmorphology; Prenatal Diagnosis; **Hospital:** Morgan Stanley Children's Hosp of NY-Presby, NY; **Address:** Morgan Stanley Chldn's Hosp NY, 3959 Broadway, rm 601A, New York, NY 10032; **Phone:** 212-305-6731; **Board Cert:** Pediatrics 1979; Clinical Genetics 1982; **Med School:** Ghana 1972; **Resid:** Pediatrics, Harlem Hosp 1977; **Fellow:** Clinical Genetics, Babies Hosp-Columbia Presby 1980; **Fac Appt:** Assoc Prof Ped, Columbia P&S

Bialer, Martin G MD/PhD [CG] - **Spec Exp:** Marfan's Syndrome; Neurofibromatosis; Metabolic Genetic Disorders; Cancer Genetics; **Hospital:** Steven & Alexandra Cohen Chldn's Med Ctr of NY (page 67), NS-LIJ Hlth Sys (page 67); **Address:** 1554 Northern Blvd, Ste 204, Manhasset, NY 11030; **Phone:** 516-365-3996; **Board Cert:** Pediatrics 1987; Clinical Biochemical Genetics 1990; Clinical Genetics 1990; **Med School:** Med Univ SC 1983; **Resid:** Pediatrics, N Shore Univ Hosp 1986; **Fellow:** Clinical Genetics, Univ VA Hlth Sci Ctr 1989; **Fac Appt:** Clin Prof Ped, NYU Sch Med

Davis, Jessica G MD [CG] - **Spec Exp:** Marfan's Syndrome; Mental Retardation; Neurofibromatosis; Ehlers-Danlos Syndrome; **Hospital:** NY-Presby/Weill Cornell Med Ctr, NY (page 66), Hosp For Special Surgery (page 60); **Address:** 505 E 70th St, Box 128, New York, NY 10065; **Phone:** 646-962-2205; **Board Cert:** Clinical Genetics 1984; **Med School:** Columbia P&S 1959; **Resid:** Pediatrics, St Luke's Hosp 1962; Clinical Genetics, Albert Einstein Coll Med 1965; **Fellow:** Cytogenetics, Albert Einstein Coll Med 1966; Pediatrics, Albert Einstein Col Med 1968; **Fac Appt:** Assoc Clin Prof Ped, Cornell Univ-Weill Med Coll

Desnick, Robert John MD/PhD [CG] - **Spec Exp:** Inherited Metabolic Disorders; Lysosomal Disease; Gaucher Disease; Porphyria; **Hospital:** Mount Sinai Med Ctr (page 64); **Address:** Mount Sinai School of Medicine, Icahn Medical Institute, 1425 Madison Ave, Fl 14, rm 14-34, Box 1498, New York, NY 10029; **Phone:** 212-659-6700; **Board Cert:** Clinical Genetics 1982; Clinical Biochemical Genetics 1982; Clinical Molecular Genetics 2009; **Med School:** Univ Minn 1971; **Resid:** Pediatrics, Univ Minn Hosps 1973; **Fac Appt:** Prof Emeritus CG, Mount Sinai Sch Med

Desposito, Franklin MD [CG] - **Spec Exp:** Birth Defects; Genetic Disorders; **Hospital:** Univ Hosp-UMDNJ—Newark, Saint Barnabas Med Ctr; **Address:** 90 Bergen St, Ste 5400, Newark, NJ 07103; **Phone:** 973-972-3300; **Board Cert:** Pediatrics 1986; Clinical Genetics 1982; Clinical Cytogenetics 1990; Clinical Molecular Genetics 2010; **Med School:** Ros Franklin Univ/Chicago Med Sch 1957; **Resid:** Pediatrics, Long Island Jewish Hosp 1961; **Fellow:** Hematology, Univ Wisc Sch Med 1963; **Fac Appt:** Prof Ped, UMDNJ-NJ Med Sch, Newark

Driscoll, Deborah A MD [CG] - **Spec Exp:** Prenatal Genetic Diagnosis; Fetal Abnormalities; Adolescent Gynecology; **Hospital:** Hosp Univ Penn - UPHS (page 72); **Address:** Hosp Univ Penn, Dept Obstetrics & Gynecology, 3400 Spruce St, Philadelphia, PA 19104; **Phone:** 215-662-3232; **Board Cert:** Obstetrics & Gynecology 2012; Clinical Genetics 1990; **Med School:** NYU Sch Med 1983; **Resid:** Obstetrics & Gynecology, Hosp Univ Penn 1987; **Fellow:** Clinical Genetics, Hosp Univ Penn 1989; **Fac Appt:** Prof ObG, Univ Pennsylvania

Gilbert, Fred MD [CG] - **Spec Exp:** Cancer Genetics; Prenatal Diagnosis; **Hospital:** NY-Presby/Weill Cornell Med Ctr, NY (page 66); **Address:** 240 Willoughby St, Brooklyn, NY 11201; **Phone:** 718-250-6911; **Board Cert:** Clinical Genetics 1982; Clinical Cytogenetics 1982; **Med School:** Albert Einstein Coll Med 1966; **Resid:** Internal Medicine, Barnes Hosp 1968; Internal Medicine, Natl Inst Hlth 1971; **Fellow:** Clinical Genetics, Yale-New Haven Hosp 1974; **Fac Appt:** Assoc Prof Ped, Cornell Univ-Weill Med Coll

Kronn, David F MD [CG] - **Spec Exp:** Bone Disorders-Metabolic; Bone Disorders-Inherited; **Hospital:** Westchester Med Ctr, Children's & Women's Phys.of Westchester; **Address:** Regional Medical Genetics, 503 Grasslands Rd, Ste 200, Valhalla, NY 10595; **Phone:** 914-304-5300; **Board Cert:** Clinical Genetics 2007; Pediatrics 2002; Clinical Biochemical Genetics 1999; **Med School:** Ireland 1989; **Resid:** Pediatrics, NYU Med Ctr 1996; **Fellow:** Clinical Genetics, NYU Med Ctr 1996; **Fac Appt:** CG, NY Med Coll

Clinical Genetics

Marion, Robert W MD [CG] - **Spec Exp:** Spina Bifida; Williams Syndrome; Marfan's Syndrome; Down Syndrome; **Hospital:** Montefiore Med Ctr-Moses Campus, NY, Blythedale Children's Hosp; **Address:** 3415 Bainbridge Ave, Bronx, NY 10467; **Phone:** 718-741-2323; **Board Cert:** Pediatrics 1985; Clinical Genetics 1987; **Med School:** Albert Einstein Coll Med 1979; **Resid:** Pediatrics, Montefiore Med Ctr 1982; **Fellow:** Clinical Genetics, Montefiore Med Ctr 1984; **Fac Appt:** Prof Ped, Albert Einstein Coll Med

Ostrer, Harry MD [CG] - **Spec Exp:** Genetic Disorders; Hereditary Cancer; **Hospital:** Montefiore Med Ctr-Wakefield Campus, NY; **Address:** Albert Einstein College of Medicine, 1300 Morris Park Ave, Ullman Bldg, rm 819, Bronx, NY 10461; **Phone:** 718-430-8605; **Board Cert:** Clinical Genetics 1984; Pediatrics 1985; Clinical Cytogenetics 1990; Clinical Molecular Genetics 2010; **Med School:** Columbia P&S 1976; **Resid:** Pediatrics, Johns Hopkins Hosp 1978; Clinical Genetics, Johns Hopkins Hosp 1984; **Fellow:** Molecular Genetics, Natl Inst Health 1981; **Fac Appt:** Prof Path, Albert Einstein Coll Med

Pyeritz, Reed E MD/PhD [CG] - **Spec Exp:** Marfan's Syndrome; Hereditary Hemorrhagic Telangiectasia; Inherited Disorders; **Hospital:** Hosp Univ Penn - UPHS (page 72), Chldns Hosp of Philadelphia; **Address:** Perelman School of Medicine, 3400 Spruce St, Penn Tower 1115, Philadelphia, PA 19104; **Phone:** 215-662-4740; **Board Cert:** Internal Medicine 1978; Clinical Genetics 2004; **Med School:** Harvard Med Sch 1975; **Resid:** Internal Medicine, Peter Bent Brigham Hosp 1977; Clinical Genetics, Johns Hopkins Hosp 1978; **Fac Appt:** Prof CG, Univ Pennsylvania

Rosenbaum, Kenneth MD [CG] - **Spec Exp:** Birth Defects; **Hospital:** Chldns Natl Med Ctr, Shady Grove Adven Hosp; **Address:** Chldns Natl Med Ctr, Dept Med Genetics, 111 Michigan Ave NW, rm 1950, Washington, DC 20010; **Phone:** 202-476-6287; **Board Cert:** Pediatrics 1976; Clinical Genetics 1982; Clinical Cytogenetics 1982; **Med School:** Univ Louisville Sch Med 1971; **Resid:** Pediatrics, Childrens Natl Med Ctr 1974; **Fellow:** Clinical Genetics, Johns Hopkins Hosp 1977; **Fac Appt:** Assoc Prof Ped, Geo Wash Univ

Shapiro, Lawrence R MD [CG] - **Spec Exp:** Dysmorphology; Prenatal Diagnosis; Hereditary Cancer; **Hospital:** Westchester Med Ctr; **Address:** Regional Medical Genetics, 503 Grasslands Rd, Ste 200, Valhalla, NY 10595; **Phone:** 914-304-5300; **Board Cert:** Pediatrics 1967; Clinical Genetics 1982; Clinical Cytogenetics 1982; **Med School:** NYU Sch Med 1962; **Resid:** Pediatrics, Chldns Hosp 1964; Pediatrics, Bellevue Hosp 1965; **Fellow:** Clinical Genetics, Mount Sinai Med Ctr 1968; **Fac Appt:** Prof Ped, NY Med Coll

Zackai, Elaine MD [CG] - **Spec Exp:** Craniosynostosis; Cytogenetic Disorders; **Hospital:** Chldns Hosp of Philadelphia; **Address:** Chldns Hosp Philadelphia, Dept Clinical Genetics, 34th St & Civic Center Blvd, rm 8C05, Philadelphia, PA 19104; **Phone:** 215-590-2920; **Board Cert:** Pediatrics 1977; Clinical Genetics 1982; Clinical Cytogenetics 1982; **Med School:** NYU Sch Med 1968; **Resid:** Pediatrics, Chldns Hosp 1970; **Fellow:** Clinical Genetics, Chldns Hosp 1971; Clinical Genetics, Yale Univ Med Sch 1972; **Fac Appt:** Prof Ped, Univ Pennsylvania

Southeast

Driscoll, Daniel J MD/PhD [CG] - **Spec Exp:** Prader-Willi Syndrome; Obesity-Pediatric; Angelman Syndrome; **Hospital:** Shands at Univ of FL; **Address:** Pediatric Genetics & Metabolism, Univ FL Hlth Sicence Ctr, PO Box 100296, Gainesville, FL 32610-0296; **Phone:** 352-294-5050; **Board Cert:** Pediatrics 1987; Clinical Genetics 1990; Clinical Cytogenetics 1990; **Med School:** Albany Med Coll 1983; **Resid:** Pediatrics, Johns Hopkins Hosp 1986; **Fellow:** Clinical Genetics, Johns Hopkins Hosp 1989; **Fac Appt:** Prof Ped, Univ Fla Coll Med

Jayakar, Parul MD [CG] - **Spec Exp:** Neuro-Genetics; **Hospital:** Univ of Miami Hosp, Baptist Hosp of Miami; **Address:** Miami Chldn's Hosp, 3100 SW 62nd Ave, Brain Inst Fl 3, Miami, FL 33155-3009; **Phone:** 786-624-4717; **Board Cert:** Clinical Genetics 2004; Pediatrics 2004; Clinical Genetics 2010; Clinical Biochemical Genetics 2005; **Med School:** India 1978; **Resid:** Internal Medicine, Lady Hardinge Med Sch 1980; Clinical Genetics, Jackson Meml Hosp 1992

Korf, Bruce R MD/PhD [CG] - **Spec Exp:** Inherited Disorders; Neuro-Genetics; Neurofibromatosis; **Hospital:** Univ of Ala Hosp at Birmingham; **Address:** UAB Dept Genetics, 720 20th St S, KAUL 230, Birmingham, AL 35294-0024; **Phone:** 205-934-4983; **Board Cert:** Clinical Genetics 1984; Child Neurology 1986; Pediatrics 1988; Clinical Molecular Genetics 2010; **Med School:** Cornell Univ-Weill Med Coll 1980; **Resid:** Pediatrics, Chldns Hosp 1982; Child Neurology, Chldns Hosp 1985; **Fellow:** Clinical Genetics, Chldns Hosp 1985; **Fac Appt:** Prof CG, Univ Alabama

Saul, Robert MD [CG] - **Spec Exp:** Birth Defects; Neurofibromatosis; **Hospital:** Self Regional Healthcare; **Address:** Greenwood Genetic Ctr, 106 Gregor Mendel Cir, Greenwood, SC 29646; **Phone:** 864-941-8119; **Board Cert:** Pediatrics 1981; Clinical Genetics 1982; **Med School:** Univ Colorado 1976; **Resid:** Pediatrics, Duke Med Ctr 1979; **Fellow:** Clinical Genetics, Greenwood Genetics Ctr 1981; **Fac Appt:** Clin Prof Ped, Univ SC Sch Med

Shoffner IV, John M MD [CG] - **Spec Exp:** Mitochondrial Disorders; Angelman Syndrome; Prader-Willi Syndrome; Neurogenetics; **Hospital:** Northside Hosp, Chldns Hlthcare Atlanta @ Scottish Rite; **Address:** Medical Neurogenetics, 5505 Peachtree Dunwoody Rd, Ste 500, Atlanta, GA 30342; **Phone:** 678-225-0222; **Board Cert:** Neurology 1992; Clinical Molecular Genetics 2004; Clinical Biochemical Genetics 2004; **Med School:** Emory Univ 1985; **Resid:** Neurology, Emory Univ Hosp 1989; **Fac Appt:** Assoc Prof CG, Emory Univ

Stevenson, Roger E MD [CG] - **Spec Exp:** Birth Defects; Mental Retardation; **Hospital:** Self Regional Healthcare; **Address:** Greenwood Genetic Ctr, 113 Gregor Mendel Cir, Research Bldg, Greenwood, SC 29646; **Phone:** 864-941-8146; **Board Cert:** Pediatrics 1971; Clinical Genetics 1982; Clinical Cytogenetics 1984; **Med School:** Wake Forest Univ 1966; **Resid:** Pediatrics, Johns Hopkins Hosp 1969; **Fellow:** Clinical Genetics, Johns Hopkins Hosp 1972

Sutphen, Rebecca MD [CG] - **Spec Exp:** Genetic Disorders; Hereditary Cancer; Cancer Risk Assessment; **Hospital:** H Lee Moffitt Cancer Ctr & Research Inst (page 59); **Address:** 3650 Spectrum Blvd, MDC 221, Tampa, FL 33612; **Phone:** 813-396-9234; **Board Cert:** Clinical Molecular Genetics 2010; Clinical Genetics 2010; **Med School:** Temple Univ 1990; **Resid:** Pediatrics, All Children's Hosp 1993; **Fellow:** Clinical Genetics, Univ S Fla Coll Med 1995; **Fac Appt:** Prof CG, Univ S Fla Coll Med

Ward, Jewell C MD/PhD [CG] - **Spec Exp:** Inborn Errors of Metabolism; Metabolic Genetic Disorders; Phenylketonuria (PKU); Reproductive Genetics; **Hospital:** Le Bonheur Chldns Med Ctr; **Address:** Le Bonheur Physicians Medical Bldg, 777 Washington Ave, Ste 400, Memphis, TN 38105; **Phone:** 901-866-8818; **Board Cert:** Clinical Genetics 1982; Clinical Biochemical Genetics 1982; **Med School:** Indiana Univ 1971; **Resid:** Pediatrics, Ohio's Chldns Hosp 1974; **Fellow:** Medical Genetics, Indiana Univ Affil Hosp 1975; Medical Genetics, Johns Hopkins Univ Hosp 1979; **Fac Appt:** Prof Ped, Univ Tenn Coll Med

Clinical Genetics

Midwest

Bartholomew, Dennis W MD [CG] - **Spec Exp:** Genetic Disorders; **Hospital:** Nationwide Chldn's Hosp; **Address:** Nationwide Chldn's Hosp: Timken Hall, 700 Children's Drive Fl Second, Columbus, OH 43205; **Phone:** 614-722-3537; **Board Cert:** Pediatrics 1986; Clinical Biochemical Genetics 1990; Clinical Genetics 1987; **Med School:** Northwestern Univ 1980; **Resid:** Pediatrics, David Grant Med Ctr 1983; **Fellow:** Genetics, Johns Hopkins Hosp 1987; **Fac Appt:** Clin Prof Ped, Ohio State Univ

Burton, Barbara MD [CG] - **Spec Exp:** Marfan's Syndrome; Phenylketonuria (PKU); Lysosomal Diseases; Inborn Errors of Metabolism; **Hospital:** Lurie Chldn's Hosp-Chicago, Northwestern Meml Hosp; **Address:** Chldns Meml Hosp, Dept Genetics, 225 E Chicago Ave, Box 59, Chicago, IL 60611; **Phone:** 773-880-4462; **Board Cert:** Pediatrics 1978; Clinical Genetics 1982; Clinical Biochemical Genetics 1982; **Med School:** Northwestern Univ 1973; **Resid:** Pediatrics, Chldns Meml Hosp 1975; **Fellow:** Clinical Genetics, Chldns Meml Hosp 1977; **Fac Appt:** Prof Ped, Northwestern Univ

Charrow, Joel MD [CG] - **Spec Exp:** Biochemical Genetics; Lysosomal Diseases; Neurofibromatosis; **Hospital:** Lurie Chldn's Hosp-Chicago; **Address:** Chldns Meml Hosp-Div Genetics, 225 E Chicago Ave, Box 59, Chicago, IL 60611; **Phone:** 773-880-4462; **Board Cert:** Pediatrics 1980; Clinical Genetics 1982; Clinical Biochemical Genetics 1987; **Med School:** Mount Sinai Sch Med 1976; **Resid:** Pediatrics, Chldns Meml Hosp 1979; **Fellow:** Clinical Genetics, Chldns Meml Hosp-Northwestern Univ 1981; **Fac Appt:** Prof Ped, Northwestern Univ

Pergament, Eugene MD/PhD [CG] - **Spec Exp:** Prenatal Genetic Diagnosis; Down Syndrome; Genetic Preimplantation Diagnosis; **Hospital:** Northwestern Meml Hosp; **Address:** 680 N Lake Shore Drive, Ste 1230, Chicago, IL 60611; **Phone:** 312-981-4400; **Board Cert:** Clinical Genetics 1982; Clinical Cytogenetics 1984; **Med School:** Univ Chicago-Pritzker Sch Med 1970; **Resid:** Pediatrics, Univ Chicago 1972; **Fac Appt:** Prof ObG, Northwestern Univ

Saal, Howard M MD [CG] - **Spec Exp:** Craniofacial Disorders; Cleft Palate/Lip; Neurofibromatosis; **Hospital:** Cincinnati Chldns Hosp Med Ctr; **Address:** Chldns Hosp Med Ctr, Div Human Genetics, 3333 Burnet Ave Bldg E5 - rm 5430, MC 4006, Cincinnati, OH 45229-3039; **Phone:** 513-636-4760; **Board Cert:** Clinical Genetics 1984; Clinical Cytogenetics 1984; Pediatrics 1985; **Med School:** Wayne State Univ 1979; **Resid:** Pediatrics, Univ Conn Hlth Ctr 1982; **Fellow:** Medical Genetics, Univ Washington 1984; **Fac Appt:** Prof Ped, Univ Cincinnati

Shulman, Lee P MD [CG] - **Spec Exp:** Prenatal Diagnosis; Ovarian Cancer; **Hospital:** Northwestern Meml Hosp; **Address:** 250 E Superior St, rm 05-2174, Division Clinical Genetics, Chicago, IL 60611; **Phone:** 312-472-4683; **Board Cert:** Obstetrics & Gynecology 2011; Clinical Genetics 1990; **Med School:** Cornell Univ 1983; **Resid:** Obstetrics & Gynecology, N Shore Univ Hosp 1987; **Fellow:** Reproductive Genetics, Univ Tenn Med Ctr 1989; **Fac Appt:** Prof ObG, Northwestern Univ

Weaver, David D MD [CG] - **Spec Exp:** Bone Disorders-Inherited; Genetic Disorders; Inherited Disorders; Weaver Syndrome; **Hospital:** Riley Hosp for Children, IU Health North Hosp; **Address:** 975 W Walnut St, rm IB 130, Indianapolis, IN 46202-5251; **Phone:** 317-274-3966; **Board Cert:** Pediatrics 1978; Clinical Genetics 1982; **Med School:** Oregon Hlth & Sci Univ 1966; **Resid:** Pediatrics, Oregon HSU Affil Hosp 1972; **Fellow:** Clinical Genetics, Univ Washington 1974; Metabolic Diseases, Oregon Health Scis Univ 1976; **Fac Appt:** Prof Emeritus CG, Indiana Univ

Whelan, Alison MD [CG] - **Spec Exp:** Gynecologic Cancer Risk; Colon & Rectal Cancer Risk; Hereditary Cancer; **Hospital:** Barnes-Jewish Hosp, St. Louis Chldns Hosp; **Address:** Washington Univ Sch Med, 660 S Euclid Ave, Campus Box 8116, St Louis, MO 63110; **Phone:** 314-454-6093; **Board Cert:** Internal Medicine 1989; Clinical Genetics 2010; **Med School:** Washington Univ, St Louis 1986; **Resid:** Internal Medicine, Barnes Hosp 1989; Pediatrics, Wash Univ Sch Med 1994; **Fellow:** Research, Wash Univ Sch Med 1991; Clinical Genetics, Wash Univ Sch Med 1994; **Fac Appt:** Prof Med, Washington Univ, St Louis

Great Plains and Mountains

Carey, John C MD [CG] - **Spec Exp:** Neurofibromatosis; Birth Defects; Hearing Loss; **Hospital:** Primary Children's Med Ctr, Univ Utah Hlth Care; **Address:** Div Med Genetics, 50 N Med Drive Bldg SOM - rm 2C412, Salt Lake City, UT 84132; **Phone:** 801-581-8943; **Board Cert:** Pediatrics 1979; Clinical Genetics 1982; **Med School:** Georgetown Univ 1972; **Resid:** Pediatrics, UCSF Med Ctr 1975; **Fellow:** Clinical Genetics, UCSF Med Ctr 1979; **Fac Appt:** Prof Ped, Univ Utah

Hoyme, H Eugene MD [CG] - **Spec Exp:** Fetal Alcohol Syndrome; Cytogenetic Disorders; Dysmorphology; **Hospital:** Sanford USD Med Ctr; **Address:** Sanford Children's Specialty Clinic, 1600 W 22nd St, Sioux Falls, SD 57117-5039; **Phone:** 605-312-1000; **Board Cert:** Pediatrics 1980; Clinical Genetics 1984; Clinical Cytogenetics 1987; **Med School:** Univ Chicago-Pritzker Sch Med 1976; **Resid:** Pediatrics, UCSD Med Ctr 1979; **Fellow:** Dysmorphology, UCSD Med Ctr 1981; **Fac Appt:** Prof Ped, Univ SD Sch Med

Southwest

Andersson, Hans C MD [CG] - **Spec Exp:** Pediatric Clinical Genetics; Inherited Metabolic Disorders; **Hospital:** Tulane Med Ctr, Womens & Chldns Hosp-Lafayette; **Address:** Haywood Genetics Ctr SL-31, Tulane Univ Medical School, 1430 Tulane Ave, New Orleans, LA 70112; **Phone:** 504-988-5229; **Board Cert:** Clinical Genetics 1990; Clinical Biochemical Genetics 1990; Pediatrics 1989; **Med School:** Tulane Univ 1984; **Resid:** Pediatrics, Tulane Univ Med Ctr 1987; **Fellow:** Clinical Genetics, NIH 1991; Research, Univ Gottingen 1993; **Fac Appt:** Prof Ped, Tulane Univ

Craigen, William J MD/PhD [CG] - **Spec Exp:** Biochemical Genetics; Mitochondrial Disorders; **Hospital:** Texas Chldns Hosp, Ben Taub Genl Hosp; **Address:** Texas Children's Genetic Clinic, 6701 Fannin St, Fl 16, MC CC 1560, Houston, TX 77030; **Phone:** 832-822-4280; **Board Cert:** Clinical Genetics 2010; Clinical Biochemical Genetics 2010; **Med School:** Baylor Coll Med 1988; **Resid:** Pediatrics, Baylor Coll Med 1990; Pediatrics, Baylor Coll Med 1992; **Fellow:** Clinical Genetics, Baylor Coll Med 1990; **Fac Appt:** Assoc Prof CG, Baylor Coll Med

Cunniff, Christopher M MD [CG] - **Spec Exp:** Genetic Disorders; Developmental Disorders; Sexual Differentiation Disorders; Fetal Alcohol Syndrome; **Hospital:** Univ Arizona Med Ctr-Univ Campus; **Address:** Univ Ariz Dept Pediatric Genetics, 1501 N Campbell Ave, PO Box 245073, Tucson, AZ 85724; **Phone:** 520-626-5175; **Board Cert:** Pediatrics 2010; Clinical Genetics 1990; **Med School:** Univ Alabama 1984; **Resid:** Pediatrics, MC Hosp Vermont 1987; **Fellow:** Clinical Genetics, UCSD 1989; **Fac Appt:** Prof Ped, Univ Ariz Coll Med

Mulvihill, John J MD [CG] - **Spec Exp:** Genetic Disorders; Neurofibromatosis; Fertility in Cancer Survivors; **Hospital:** Chldns Hosp OU Med Ctr; **Address:** Chldn's Hosp-OU Med Ctr, Dept Ped Genetics, Dept Pediatric Genetics, 1200 N Phillips Ave, Ste 12100, Oklahoma City, OK 73104; **Phone:** 405-271-4401; **Board Cert:** Pediatrics 1975; Clinical Genetics 1982; **Med School:** Univ Wash 1969; **Resid:** Pediatrics, Johns Hopkins Hosp 1974; **Fellow:** Research, NCI-Natl Inst Hlth 1972; **Fac Appt:** Prof CG, Univ Okla Coll Med

Clinical Genetics

Northrup, Hope MD [CG] - **Spec Exp:** Biochemical Genetics; Neuro-Genetics; Dysmorphology; **Hospital:** Meml Hermann Hosp - Texas Med Ctr, LBJ General Hosp; **Address:** UT Physicians-Div Med Genetics, 6410 Fannin St, Ste 500, Houston, TX 77030; **Phone:** 713-500-5765; **Board Cert:** Pediatrics 1988; Clinical Genetics 1990; Clinical Biochemical Genetics 1990; **Med School:** Med Univ SC 1983; **Resid:** Pediatrics, Chldns Med Ctr-Univ Tex SW 1986; **Fellow:** Medical Genetics, Inst Molec Gene-Baylor Coll Med 1989; **Fac Appt:** Prof Ped, Univ Tex, Houston

Plon, Sharon E MD/PhD [CG] - **Spec Exp:** Hereditary Cancer; Cancer Risk Assessment; Breast Cancer Risk Assessment; Ovarian Cancer; **Hospital:** Texas Chldns Hosp, St. Luke's Episcopal Hosp-Houston; **Address:** Texas Chldn's Hosp, 1102 Bates St, MC FC1200, Houston, TX 77030; **Phone:** 832-824-4539; **Board Cert:** Clinical Genetics 2010; **Med School:** Harvard Med Sch 1987; **Resid:** Internal Medicine, Univ Washington Affil Hosp 1988; **Fellow:** Molecular Genetics, National Cancer Inst 1990; Medical Genetics, Fred Hutchinson Cancer Research Ctr 1993; **Fac Appt:** Prof CG, Baylor Coll Med

West Coast and Pacific

Boles, Richard G MD [CG] - **Spec Exp:** Mitochondrial Disorders; Vomiting-Cyclic; **Hospital:** Chldns Hosp - Los Angeles; **Address:** 4650 Sunset Blvd, MS 90, Los Angeles, CA 90027; **Phone:** 323-361-2178; **Board Cert:** Clinical Genetics 2010; Clinical Biochemical Genetics 2010; Pediatrics 2009; **Med School:** UCLA 1987; **Resid:** Pediatrics, Harbor-UCLA Med Ctr 1990; **Fellow:** Genetics and Metabolism, Yale Univ 1993; **Fac Appt:** Assoc Prof Ped, USC Sch Med

Cassidy, Suzanne MD [CG] - **Spec Exp:** Prader-Willi Syndrome; Connective Tissue Disorders; Neurocutaneous Disorders; **Hospital:** UCSF Med Ctr; **Address:** 533 Parnassus Ave, rm U-100A, Box 0706, San Francisco, CA 94143; **Phone:** 415-476-2757; **Board Cert:** Pediatrics 1982; Clinical Genetics 1983; **Med School:** Vanderbilt Univ 1976; **Resid:** Pediatrics, Univ Wash Affil Prgms 1979; **Fellow:** Clinical Genetics, Univ Wash 1981; **Fac Appt:** Prof Ped, UC Irvine

Cederbaum, Stephen D MD [CG] - **Spec Exp:** Inborn Errors of Metabolism; Genetic Disorders; **Hospital:** UCLA Ronald Reagan Med Ctr; **Address:** 635 Charles E Young Drive S, rm 347, Los Angeles, CA 90095-7332; **Phone:** 310-825-0402; **Board Cert:** Clinical Genetics 1982; Clinical Biochemical Genetics 1982; **Med School:** NYU Sch Med 1964; **Resid:** Internal Medicine, Barnes-Jewish Hosp 1966; **Fellow:** Clinical Genetics, Univ Wash 1970; **Fac Appt:** Prof Emeritus CG, UCLA

Curry, Cynthia J MD [CG] - **Hospital:** Chldns Hosp Central CA, Comm Regl Med Ctr - Fresno; **Address:** UCSF Fresno, 155 N Fresno St, Fresno, CA 93701; **Phone:** 559-227-4472; **Board Cert:** Pediatrics 1973; Clinical Genetics 1982; **Med School:** Yale Univ 1967; **Resid:** Pediatrics, Univ Wash Orth Chldns Hosp 1969; Pediatrics, Univ Minn Hosp 1970; **Fellow:** Dysmorphology, UCSF Med Ctr 1976; **Fac Appt:** Prof CG, UCSF

Falk, Rena MD [CG] - **Spec Exp:** Prenatal Diagnosis; Mental Retardation; Prenatal Genetic Diagnosis; **Hospital:** Cedars-Sinai Med Ctr; **Address:** 8700 Beverly Blvd, PACT 400, Los Angeles, CA 90048; **Phone:** 310-423-9914; **Board Cert:** Pediatrics 1976; Clinical Genetics 1982; Clinical Cytogenetics 1984; **Med School:** UCLA 1971; **Resid:** Pediatrics, Cedars-Sinai Med Ctr 1973; **Fellow:** Clinical Genetics, UCLA Med Schl 1975; UCLA 1977; **Fac Appt:** Prof Ped, UCLA

Graham Jr, John M MD [CG] - **Spec Exp:** Dysmorphology; Craniofacial Disorders; Mental Retardation; Vascular Malformations; **Hospital:** Cedars-Sinai Med Ctr; **Address:** 8700 Beverly Blvd, PACT-Suite 400, Los Angeles, CA 90048; **Phone:** 310-423-9909; **Board Cert:** Pediatrics 1982; Clinical Genetics 1982; **Med School:** Med Univ SC 1975; **Resid:** Pediatrics, Boston Chldns Hosp-Harvard 1977; **Fellow:** Developmental-Behavioral Pediatrics, Boston Chldns Hosp 1978; Dysmorphology, Univ Wash 1980; **Fac Appt:** Prof Ped, UCLA

Grody, Wayne W MD/PhD [CG] - **Spec Exp:** Genetic Disorders; Hereditary Cancer; **Address:** UCLA School Medicine, Div, Med Genetic & Molecular Pathology, 10833 Le Conte Ave, Los Angeles, CA 90095-1732; **Phone:** 310-206-6581; **Board Cert:** Clinical Genetics 1990; Anatomic & Clinical Pathology 1987; Clinical Biochemical Genetics 1990; Molecular Genetic Pathology 2001; **Med School:** Baylor Coll Med 1977; **Resid:** Pathology, UCLA Med Ctr 1986; **Fellow:** Clinical Genetics, UCLA Med Ctr 1987; **Fac Appt:** Prof CG, UCLA

Hudgins, Louanne MD [CG] - **Spec Exp:** Congenital Anomalies-Limb; Prenatal Diagnosis; **Hospital:** Stanford Univ Hosp & Clinics; **Address:** Stanford Univ Med Ctr, Div Medical Genetics, 300 Pasteur Drive, rm H315, Stanford, CA 94305; **Phone:** 650-723-6858; **Board Cert:** Clinical Genetics 2010; **Med School:** Univ Kansas 1984; **Resid:** Pediatrics, UConn Hlth Science Ctr 1987; **Fellow:** Clinical Genetics, Univ Connecticut 1990; **Fac Appt:** Prof Ped, Stanford Univ

Jonas, Adam J MD [CG] - **Spec Exp:** Inherited Disorders; **Hospital:** LAC - Harbor - UCLA Med Ctr; **Address:** Harbor-UCLA Med Ctr, Div Med Genetics, 1000 W Carson St, Box 17, Torrance, CA 90509-2910; **Phone:** 310-222-2301; **Board Cert:** Pediatrics 1982; Clinical Biochemical Genetics 1987; Clinical Genetics 1990; **Med School:** UCSD 1976; **Resid:** Pediatrics, Chldns Ortho Hosp 1978; Pediatrics, Univ Hosp 1979; **Fellow:** Genetics and Metabolism, UCSD Sch Med 1982; **Fac Appt:** Prof Ped, UCLA

Jones, Marilyn MD [CG] - **Spec Exp:** Dysmorphology; Craniofacial Disorders; **Hospital:** Rady Children's Hosp - San Diego, UCSD Med Ctr; **Address:** 3020 Chldns Way, MC 5031, San Diego, CA 92123-2746; **Phone:** 858-966-5840; **Board Cert:** Pediatrics 1979; Clinical Genetics 1982; **Med School:** Columbia P&S 1974; **Resid:** Internal Medicine, UCSD Med Ctr 1977; Pediatrics, UCSD Med Ctr 1978; **Fellow:** Dysmorphology, UCSD Med Ctr 1979

Morris, Colleen A MD [CG] - **Spec Exp:** Williams Syndrome; Inherited Disorders; Fetal Alcohol Syndrome; **Hospital:** Univ Med Ctr - Las Vegas; **Address:** Univ Nevada Sch Medicine, Dept Pediatrics/Genetics, 2040 W Charleston Blvd, Ste 401, Las Vegas, NV 89102; **Phone:** 702-671-2200; **Board Cert:** Pediatrics 1986; Clinical Genetics 1987; **Med School:** Loyola Univ-Stritch Sch Med 1981; **Resid:** Pediatrics, Phoenix Hosp 1984; **Fellow:** Clinical Genetics, Univ Utah Sch Med 1986; **Fac Appt:** Prof Ped, Univ Nevada

Nussbaum, Robert MD [CG] - **Spec Exp:** Genetic Disorders; **Hospital:** UCSF Med Ctr; **Address:** Inst Human Genetics, 1600 Divisadero St Fl 2, San Francisco, CA 94143; **Phone:** 415-885-7779; **Board Cert:** Internal Medicine 1978; Clinical Genetics 1982; Clinical Molecular Genetics 2004; **Med School:** Harvard Med Sch 1975; **Resid:** Internal Medicine, Barnes Hosp 1978; **Fellow:** Clinical Genetics, Baylor Univ 1983

Randolph, Linda MD [CG] - **Spec Exp:** Dysmorphology; Skeletal Dysplasia; Prenatal Genetic Diagnosis; Neurofibromatosis; **Hospital:** Chldns Hosp - Los Angeles, Van Nuys Comm Hosp; **Address:** 4650 Sunset Blvd, MS 90, Los Angeles, CA 90027; **Phone:** 323-361-2178; **Board Cert:** Pediatrics 1987; Clinical Genetics 1987; Clinical Cytogenetics 1990; **Med School:** Geo Wash Univ 1982; **Resid:** Pediatrics, Chldns Natl Med Ctr 1985; **Fellow:** Clinical Molecular Genetics, Harbor-UCLA Med Ctr/Cedar-Sinai Med Ctr 1989; **Fac Appt:** Asst Prof Ped, USC-Keck School of Medicine

Seaver, Laurie H MD [CG] - **Spec Exp:** Birth Defects; Fetal Alcohol Syndrome; Dysmorphology; Prenatal Diagnosis; **Hospital:** Kapiolani Med Ctr for Women & Chldn, Queen's Med Ctr - Honolulu; **Address:** Hawaii Community Genetics, 1441 Kapiolani Blvd, Ste 1800, Honolulu, HI 96814; **Phone:** 808-973-3403; **Board Cert:** Pediatrics 2005; Clinical Genetics 2010; **Med School:** Univ Ariz Coll Med 1987; **Resid:** Pediatrics, Univ Ariz Med Ctr 1990; **Fellow:** Clinical Genetics, Univ Ariz Coll Med 1993; **Fac Appt:** Assoc Prof Ped, Univ Hawaii JA Burns Sch Med

Clinical Genetics

Weitzel, Jeffrey N MD [CG] - **Spec Exp:** Breast Cancer; Ovarian Cancer; Hereditary Cancer; **Hospital:** City of Hope Natl Med Ctr; **Address:** City of Hope Cancer Ctr, 1500 E Duarte Rd, Duarte, CA 91010; **Phone:** 626-256-8662; **Board Cert:** Internal Medicine 1986; Medical Oncology 1989; Clinical Genetics 2009; **Med School:** Univ Minn 1983; **Resid:** Internal Medicine, Univ Minn Hosps 1986; Hematology, Hammersmith Hosp 1987; **Fellow:** Hematology & Oncology, Tufts-New England Med Ctr 1992; Clinical Genetics, Tufts-New England Med Ctr 1996; **Fac Appt:** Assoc Clin Prof Med, USC Sch Med

Wilcox Jr, William R MD/PhD [CG] - **Spec Exp:** Inborn Errors of Metabolism; Skeletal Dysplasia; Fabry's Disease; Rare Genetic Disorders; **Hospital:** Cedars-Sinai Med Ctr; **Address:** Cedars Sinai Med Ctr, Dept Med Genetics, 8700 Beverly Blvd, PACT 400, Los Angeles, CA 90048; **Phone:** 310-423-9914; **Board Cert:** Clinical Genetics 2010; Clinical Biochemical Genetics 2010; Clinical Molecular Genetics 2010; **Med School:** UCLA 1988; **Resid:** Pediatrics, UCLA Med Ctr 1991; **Fellow:** Clinical Genetics, Cedars-Sinai Med Ctr 1994; **Fac Appt:** Prof Ped, UCLA

THE MOUNT SINAI MEDICAL CENTER
GENETICS AND GENOMIC SCIENCES

One Gustave L. Levy Place
Fifth Avenue and 100th Street
New York, NY 10029-6574
Physician Referral: 212-241-6947
www.mountsinaimedicalgenetics.org

THE DEPARTMENT OF GENETICS AND GENOMIC SCIENCES at The Mount Sinai Medical Center is one of the largest medical genetics centers in the nation, providing expert diagnostic, therapeutic, and counseling services for patients and families with or at risk for genetics disorders or birth defects. The department performs sophisticated diagnostic tests in its state-of-the-art molecular, biochemical, and cytogenetics laboratories, which are New York State and Clinical Laboratory Improvement Amendments (CLIA) licensed, and certified by the College of American Pathologists (CAP).

The department has more than 50 internationally recognized faculty members, including physicians, counselors, and laboratory geneticists who are certified by the American Board of Medical Genetics or the American Board of Genetic Counseling.

Programs and services offered by the department include:

- Clinical Genetic Disorders Program
- Program for Inherited Metabolic Diseases
- Reproductive Genetic Counseling Program
- Cancer Genetic Counseling Program
- Mount Sinai Center for Jewish Genetic Diseases
- International Center for Fabry Disease
- Mount Sinai Comprehensive Gaucher Disease Treatment Center
- Porphyria Comprehensive Diagnostic and Treatment Center
- Congenital Anomalies and Craniofacial Program
- Cardiovascular Genetics Program
- Niemann Pick Disease Center

Advances In Diagnosis And Disease Treatment – In the past several years, Mount Sinai researchers have identified genes responsible for various genetic diseases and developed new treatments for inherited disorders. The following are some examples and results of this important work:

- We have identified genes involved in over a dozen diseases, most recently a debilitating juvenile arthritis, several dystonias, and an inherited form of obesity. The identification of these genes leads to precise diagnosis, understanding disease pathogenesis, and new treatments for these diseases. We have also recently identified a gene linked to prostate cancer.

GROUNDBREAKING RESEARCH AND NEW FORMS OF TREATMENT
There are more than 10,000 known genetic disorders, and current research is identifying the genetic susceptibilities and causative genes for many of these diseases. The faculty of the Department of Genetics and Genomic Sciences at Mount Sinai is performing research to develop new and improved methods for the diagnosis, prevention, and treatment of rare and common diseases. The Human Genome Project, and advances in gene analysis technology and stem cell biology, have accelerated this research.

- Our researchers helped identify eight genes involved in causing Noonan syndrome, a common genetic disorder that causes congenital heart defects. Affected families can now receive early diagnosis and prevention.

- Research pioneered by the Department of Genetics and Genomic Sciences resulted in the development of a safe, effective, FDA-approved treatment for Fabry disease, an inherited metabolic disorder that can cause kidney failure, heart disease, stroke, and premature death.

- Departmental faculty have developed a treatment for Niemann-Pick Type B disease, a hereditary disorder that results in death in childhood or early adulthood.

MOUNT SINAI SCHOOL OF MEDICINE

THE MOUNT SINAI MEDICAL CENTER
GENETICS AND GENOMIC SCIENCES

One Gustave L. Levy Place
Fifth Avenue and 100th Street
New York, NY 10029-6574
Physician Referral: 212-241-6947
www.mountsinaimedicalgenetics.org

THE DEPARTMENT OF GENETICS AND GENOMIC SCIENCES at The Mount Sinai Medical Center is one of the largest medical genetics centers in the nation, providing expert diagnostic, therapeutic, and counseling services for patients and families with or at risk for genetics disorders or birth defects. The department performs sophisticated diagnostic tests in its state-of-the-art molecular, biochemical, and cytogenetics laboratories, which are New York State and Clinical Laboratory Improvement Amendments (CLIA) licensed, and certified by the College of American Pathologists (CAP).

The department has more than 50 internationally recognized faculty members, including physicians, counselors, and laboratory geneticists who are certified by the American Board of Medical Genetics or the American Board of Genetic Counseling.

Programs and services offered by the department include:

- Clinical Genetic Disorders Program
- Program for Inherited Metabolic Diseases
- Reproductive Genetic Counseling Program
- Cancer Genetic Counseling Program
- Mount Sinai Center for Jewish Genetic Diseases
- International Center for Fabry Disease
- Mount Sinai Comprehensive Gaucher Disease Treatment Center
- Porphyria Comprehensive Diagnostic and Treatment Center
- Congenital Anomalies and Craniofacial Program
- Cardiovascular Genetics Program
- Niemann Pick Disease Center

Advances In Diagnosis And Disease Treatment – In the past several years, Mount Sinai researchers have identified genes responsible for various genetic diseases and developed new treatments for inherited disorders. The following are some examples and results of this important work:

- We have identified genes involved in over a dozen diseases, most recently a debilitating juvenile arthritis, several dystonias, and an inherited form of obesity. The identification of these genes leads to precise diagnosis, understanding disease pathogenesis, and new treatments for these diseases. We have also recently identified a gene linked to prostate cancer.

- Our researchers helped identify eight genes involved in causing Noonan syndrome, a common genetic disorder that causes congenital heart defects. Affected families can now receive early diagnosis and prevention.

- Research pioneered by the Department of Genetics and Genomic Sciences resulted in the development of a safe, effective, FDA-approved treatment for Fabry disease, an inherited metabolic disorder that can cause kidney failure, heart disease, stroke, and premature death.

- Departmental faculty have developed a treatment for Niemann-Pick Type B disease, a hereditary disorder that results in death in childhood or early adulthood.

GROUNDBREAKING RESEARCH AND NEW FORMS OF TREATMENT
There are more than 10,000 known genetic disorders, and current research is identifying the genetic susceptibilities and causative genes for many of these diseases. The faculty of the Department of Genetics and Genomic Sciences at Mount Sinai is performing research to develop new and improved methods for the diagnosis, prevention, and treatment of rare and common diseases. The Human Genome Project, and advances in gene analysis technology and stem cell biology, have accelerated this research.

Colon & Rectal Surgery

A colon and rectal surgeon is trained to diagnose and treat various diseases of the intestinal tract, colon, rectum, anal canal and perianal area by medical and surgical means. This specialist also deals with other organs and tissues (such as the liver and gallbladder) involved with primary
intestinal disease.

Colon and rectal surgeons have the expertise to diagnose and often manage anorectal conditions such as hemorrhoids, fissures (painful tears in the anal lining), abscesses and fistulae (infections located around the anus and rectum) in the office setting. They also treat problems of the intestine and colon and perform endoscopic procedures to evaluate and treat problems such as cancer, polyps (precancerous growths) and inflammatory conditions.

Training Required: Six years (including general surgery)

COLON & RECTAL SURGERY

New England

Bleday, Ronald MD [CRS] - **Spec Exp:** Colon & Rectal Cancer; **Hospital:** Brigham and Women's Hosp (page 57), Dana-Farber Cancer Inst (page 57); **Address:** Brigham & Women's Hosp, Dept Surgery, 75 Francis St Fl 3 - Ste A, Boston, MA 02115; **Phone:** 617-732-8460; **Board Cert:** Surgery 2009; Colon & Rectal Surgery 2011; **Med School:** McGill Univ 1982; **Resid:** Surgery, Rhode Island Hosp 1989; Surgical Oncology, Brigham & Womens Hosp 1986; **Fellow:** Endoscopy, Mass Genl Hosp 1990; Colon & Rectal Surgery, Univ Minn 1991; **Fac Appt:** Assoc Prof S, Harvard Med Sch

Hackford, Alan W MD [CRS] - **Hospital:** Steward St Elizabeth's Med Ctr-Boston; **Address:** St Elizabeth's Medical Office, 11 Nevins St MOB Bldg Fl 2 - Ste 201, Boston, MA 02135; **Phone:** 617-789-2442; **Board Cert:** Colon & Rectal Surgery 1985; Surgery 2002; **Med School:** Univ Conn 1977; **Resid:** Surgery, New England Med Ctr 1982; **Fellow:** Colon & Rectal Surgery, Lahey Clinic 1984; **Fac Appt:** Prof S, Tufts Univ

Harnsberger, Jeffrey R MD [CRS] - **Spec Exp:** Colon & Rectal Cancer; Inflammatory Bowel Disease; **Hospital:** Elliot Hosp, Dartmouth - Hitchcock Med Ctr; **Address:** Dartmouth-Hitchcock Manchester, 100 Hitchcock Way, Manchester, NH 03104; **Phone:** 603-695-2840; **Board Cert:** Surgery 2011; Colon & Rectal Surgery 2005; **Med School:** Med Coll OH 1987; **Resid:** Surgery, Dartamouth-Hitchkock Med Ctr 1992; **Fellow:** Colon & Rectal Surgery, St Louis Univ Med Ctr 1993; **Fac Appt:** Asst Prof S, Dartmouth Med Sch

Hyman, Neil H MD [CRS] - **Spec Exp:** Inflammatory Bowel Disease; Colon & Rectal Cancer; **Hospital:** Fletcher Allen Health Care- Med Ctr Campus; **Address:** FAHC 111 Colchester Ave, Burlington, VT 05401; **Phone:** 802-847-3339; **Board Cert:** Surgery 2008; Colon & Rectal Surgery 2011; **Med School:** Univ VT Coll Med 1984; **Resid:** Surgery, Mt Sinai Med Ctr 1989; **Fellow:** Colon & Rectal Surgery, Cleveland Clinic 1990; **Fac Appt:** Prof S, Univ VT Coll Med

Longo, Walter E MD [CRS] - **Spec Exp:** Colon & Rectal Cancer; Gastrointestinal Surgery; Inflammatory Bowel Disease; **Hospital:** Yale-New Haven Hosp, Yale Med Group; **Address:** Dept Surgery/Gastroenterology, 330 Cedar St, rm LH118, Box 208062, New Haven, CT 06520-8062; **Phone:** 203-785-2616; **Board Cert:** Surgery 2001; Colon & Rectal Surgery 2006; **Med School:** NY Med Coll 1984; **Resid:** Surgery, Yale-New Haven Hosp 1990; **Fellow:** Research, Yale-New Haven Hosp 1988; Colon & Rectal Surgery, Cleveland Clinic 1991; **Fac Appt:** Prof S, Yale Univ

Nagle, Deborah A MD [CRS] - **Spec Exp:** Colon & Rectal Cancer; Anal Cancer; Laparoscopic Surgery; **Hospital:** Beth Israel Deaconess Med Ctr - Boston; **Address:** BIDMC - Colon & Rectal Surgery, 330 Brookline Ave, Boston, MA 02215; **Phone:** 617-667-4159; **Board Cert:** Colon & Rectal Surgery 2006; Surgery 2004; **Med School:** Univ Pennsylvania 1988; **Resid:** Surgery, Graduate Hosp 1993; Colon & Rectal Surgery, Thos Jefferson Univ Hosp 1994; **Fac Appt:** Prof CRS, Univ Pennsylvania

Orkin, Bruce A MD [CRS] - **Spec Exp:** Colon & Rectal Cancer; Laparoscopic Surgery; Robotic Surgery; Microsurgery; **Hospital:** Tufts Med Ctr, Floating Hosp for Children at Tufts Med Ce; **Address:** Tufts Medical Center, 800 Washington St, rm 6190, Boston, MA 02111; **Phone:** 617-636-6190; **Board Cert:** Colon & Rectal Surgery 2010; Surgery 2008; **Med School:** Univ Minn 1981; **Resid:** Surgery, UCLA Med Ctr 1983; Surgery, Mayo Clinic 1986; **Fellow:** Surgical Research, Mayo Clinic 1988; Colon & Rectal Surgery, Cleveland Clinic 1989; **Fac Appt:** Prof S, Tufts Univ

Read, Thomas E MD [CRS] - **Spec Exp:** Colon & Rectal Cancer; Inflammatory Bowel Disease; Laparoscopic Surgery; Diverticulitis; **Hospital:** Lahey Clin; **Address:** Lahey Clin, Dept Colon and Rectal Surgery, 41 Mall Rd, Ste 6W-Clin, Burlington, MA 01805; **Phone:** 781-744-8971; **Board Cert:** Surgery 2005; Colon & Rectal Surgery 2008; **Med School:** UCSF 1988; **Resid:** Surgery, UCSF Med Ctr 1995; **Fellow:** Colon & Rectal Surgery, Lahey Clinic 1996; **Fac Appt:** Prof S, Tufts Univ

Roberts, Patricia L MD [CRS] - **Spec Exp:** Diverticulitis; Colon & Rectal Cancer; Inflammatory Bowel Disease; Crohn's Disease; **Hospital:** Lahey Clin; **Address:** Lahey Clinic, 41 Mall Rd, Ste 6W-Clin, Burlington, MA 01805; **Phone:** 781-744-8243; **Board Cert:** Colon & Rectal Surgery 2003; **Med School:** Boston Univ 1981; **Resid:** Surgery, Boston City Hosp 1986; **Fellow:** Colon & Rectal Surgery, Lahey Clinic 1988; **Fac Appt:** Prof S, Tufts Univ

Schoetz Jr, David J MD [CRS] - **Spec Exp:** Inflammatory Bowel Disease/Crohn's; Colon & Rectal Cancer; Incontinence-Fecal; Anorectal Disorders; **Hospital:** Lahey Clin; **Address:** Lahey Clin Med Ctr, Dept Colon & Rectal Surg, 41 Mall Rd, Burlington, MA 01805-0001; **Phone:** 781-744-8889; **Board Cert:** Surgery 2001; Colon & Rectal Surgery 2009; **Med School:** Med Coll Wisc 1974; **Resid:** Surgery, Boston Univ Med Ctr 1981; Surgery, Boston Univ Med Ctr 1978; **Fellow:** Colon & Rectal Surgery, Lahey Clin 1982; **Fac Appt:** Prof S, Tufts Univ

Shah, Nishit S MD [CRS] - **Spec Exp:** Anorectal Disorders; Colon & Rectal Cancer; Inflammatory Bowel Disease; **Hospital:** Rhode Island Hosp, Miriam Hosp; **Address:** University Surgical Associates, 2 Dudley St, Ste 370, Providence, RI 02905; **Phone:** 401-553-8322; **Board Cert:** Surgery 2010; Colon & Rectal Surgery 2004; **Med School:** England, UK 1989; **Resid:** Surgery, Univ Pittsburgh Med Ctr 1995; **Fellow:** Colon & Rectal Surgery, Cleveland Clinic 1996; Colon & Rectal Surgery, Univ Illinois

Shellito, Paul C MD [CRS] - **Spec Exp:** Colon & Rectal Cancer; Ulcerative Colitis; Anorectal Disorders; **Hospital:** Mass Genl Hosp; **Address:** 15 Parkman St, Ste 460, Boston, MA 02114-3117; **Phone:** 617-724-0365; **Board Cert:** Surgery 2002; Colon & Rectal Surgery 1994; **Med School:** Harvard Med Sch 1977; **Resid:** Surgery, Mass Genl Hosp 1983; Surgery, Auckland Univ Med Sch 1981; **Fellow:** Colon & Rectal Surgery, Univ Minn 1985; **Fac Appt:** Asst Prof S, Harvard Med Sch

Mid Atlantic

Efron, Jonathan E MD [CRS] - **Spec Exp:** Colon & Rectal Cancer; Incontinence-Fecal; Inflammatory Bowel Disease; Anorectal Disorders; **Hospital:** Johns Hopkins Hosp (page 61), Johns Hopkins Bayview Med Ctr (page 61); **Address:** Johns Hopkins Hosp, Div Surgery, 600 N Wolfe St, Baltimore, MD 21287; **Phone:** 410-933-1233; **Board Cert:** Surgery 2008; Colon & Rectal Surgery 2009; **Med School:** Univ MD Sch Med 1993; **Resid:** Surgery, LIJ Medical Ctr 1999; **Fellow:** Colon & Rectal Surgery, Cleveland Clinic 2000; Research, Cleveland Clinic 2001; **Fac Appt:** Assoc Prof S, Johns Hopkins Univ

Eisenstat, Theodore E MD [CRS] - **Spec Exp:** Colon Cancer; Inflammatory Bowel Disease; Anorectal Disorders; Hemorrhoids; **Hospital:** Robert Wood Johnson Univ Hosp - New Brunswick, JFK Med Ctr - Edison; **Address:** 3900 Park Ave, Ste 101, Edison, NJ 08820-3032; **Phone:** 732-494-6640; **Board Cert:** Surgery 1974; Colon & Rectal Surgery 1994; **Med School:** NY Med Coll 1968; **Resid:** Surgery, Thomas Jefferson Univ Hosp 1971; Surgery, Pennsylvania Hosp 1973; **Fellow:** Colon & Rectal Surgery, Muhlenberg Med Ctr 1978; **Fac Appt:** Clin Prof S, UMDNJ-RW Johnson Med Sch

Fry, Robert D MD [CRS] - **Spec Exp:** Colon & Rectal Cancer; Rectal Cancer/Sphincter Preservation; Ulcerative Colitis; Anorectal Disorders; **Hospital:** Pennsylvania Hosp-UPHS (page 72), Hosp Univ Penn - UPHS (page 72); **Address:** Pennsylvania Hospital, Div Colon & Rectal Surgery, 700 Spruce St, Ste 305, Philadelphia, PA 19106-4023; **Phone:** 215-662-2078; **Board Cert:** Surgery 2006; Colon & Rectal Surgery 1998; **Med School:** Washington Univ, St Louis 1972; **Resid:** Surgery, Barnes Jewish Hosp 1977; **Fellow:** Colon & Rectal Surgery, Cleveland Clinic 1978; **Fac Appt:** Prof S, Univ Pennsylvania

Gearhart, Susan L MD [CRS] - **Spec Exp:** Colon & Rectal Cancer-Hereditary; Incontinence-Fecal; Inflammatory Bowel Disease/Crohn's; **Hospital:** Johns Hopkins Hosp (page 61); **Address:** Johns Hopkins Hosp, Dept of Surgery, 600 N Wolfe St, Blalock 658, Baltimore, MD 21287; **Phone:** 410-955-7323; **Board Cert:** Surgery 2011; Colon & Rectal Surgery 2003; **Med School:** Loyola Univ-Stritch Sch Med 1993; **Resid:** Surgery, John Hopkins Hospital 2000; **Fellow:** Colon & Rectal Surgery, Cleveland Clin 2002; **Fac Appt:** Asst Prof S, Johns Hopkins Univ

Geisler, Daniel P MD [CRS] - **Spec Exp:** Colon & Rectal Cancer & Surgery; Minimally Invasive Surgery; Rectal Cancer/Sphincter Preservation; Anal Cancer; **Hospital:** Allegheny General Hosp; **Address:** Allegheny Cancer Center, 320 East North Ave, Ste 261, Pittsburgh, PA 15212; **Phone:** 412-359-3901; **Board Cert:** Surgery 2003; Colon & Rectal Surgery 2005; **Med School:** St Louis Univ 1996; **Resid:** Surgery, Univ Oklahoma Affil Hosp 2001; **Fellow:** Colon & Rectal Surgery, Saint Vincent Hosp 2002; Minimally Invasive Surgery, Lankenau Hosp 2003

Goldstein, Scott D MD [CRS] - **Spec Exp:** Colon & Rectal Cancer; Inflammatory Bowel Disease; Laparoscopic Surgery; **Hospital:** Thomas Jefferson Univ Hosp; **Address:** Jefferson Dept Surgery, 1100 Walnut St, Ste 500, Philadelphia, PA 19107; **Phone:** 215-955-5869; **Board Cert:** Surgery 2007; Colon & Rectal Surgery 1985; **Med School:** SUNY Buffalo 1978; **Resid:** Surgery, Lenox Hill Hosp 1983; Colon & Rectal Surgery, UMDNJ Affil Hosps 1984; **Fac Appt:** Assoc Prof S, Thomas Jefferson Univ

Gorfine, Stephen R MD [CRS] - **Spec Exp:** Anal Disorders & Reconstruction; Hemorrhoids; Rectal Cancer; Anal Cancer; **Hospital:** Mount Sinai Med Ctr (page 64), Lenox Hill Hosp (page 67); **Address:** 25 E 69th St, New York, NY 10021-4925; **Phone:** 212-517-8600; **Board Cert:** Internal Medicine 1981; Surgery 2007; Colon & Rectal Surgery 1988; **Med School:** Univ Mass Sch Med 1978; **Resid:** Internal Medicine, Mt Sinai Hosp 1981; Surgery, Mt Sinai Hosp 1985; **Fellow:** Colon & Rectal Surgery, Ferguson Hosp 1987; **Fac Appt:** Clin Prof S, Mount Sinai Sch Med

Guillem, Jose MD [CRS] - **Spec Exp:** Colon & Rectal Cancer; Rectal Cancer/Sphincter Preservation; Colon & Rectal Cancer-Hereditary; Peritoneal Mucinous Carcinomatosis; **Hospital:** Meml Sloan-Kettering Cancer Ctr; **Address:** 1275 York Ave, New York, NY 10065; **Phone:** 212-639-8278; **Board Cert:** Surgery 2004; Colon & Rectal Surgery 2005; **Med School:** Yale Univ 1983; **Resid:** Surgery, Columbia-Presby Med Ctr 1990; **Fellow:** Colon & Rectal Surgery, Lahey Clinic 1991; **Fac Appt:** Prof CRS, Cornell Univ-Weill Med Coll

Medich, David S MD [CRS] - **Spec Exp:** Colon & Rectal Cancer; Ulcerative Colitis; Inflammatory Bowel Disease/Crohn's; **Hospital:** UPMC Passavant-McCandless; **Address:** UPMC Cancer Ctr at UPMC Passavant, Ground FL, South Pavilion, 9100 Babcock Blvd, Pittsburgh, PA 15237; **Phone:** 877-684-7189; **Board Cert:** Surgery 2004; Colon & Rectal Surgery 2006; **Med School:** Ohio State Univ 1987; **Resid:** Surgery, Univ Pittsburgh Med Ctr 1990; **Fellow:** Research, Univ Pittsburgh 1993; Colon & Rectal Surgery, Cleveland Clinic 1994; **Fac Appt:** Assoc Prof CRS, Univ Pittsburgh

Milsom, Jeffrey W MD [CRS] - **Spec Exp:** Inflammatory Bowel Disease; Laparoscopic Surgery; Colon & Rectal Cancer; Crohn's Disease; **Hospital:** NY-Presby/Weill Cornell Med Ctr, NY (page 66); **Address:** NY Cornell Med Ctr, Div Colorectal Surgery, 1315 York Ave Fl 2, New York, NY 10065-5304; **Phone:** 212-746-6030; **Board Cert:** Colon & Rectal Surgery 1986; **Med School:** Univ Pittsburgh 1979; **Resid:** Surgery, Roosevelt Hosp 1981; Surgery, Univ Virginia Med Ctr 1984; **Fellow:** Colon & Rectal Surgery, Ferguson Hosp 1985; **Fac Appt:** Prof S, Cornell Univ-Weill Med Coll

Pello, Mark J MD [CRS] - **Spec Exp:** Colon & Rectal Cancer; Inflammatory Bowel Disease; Laparoscopic Surgery; **Hospital:** Cooper Univ Hosp; **Address:** 3 Cooper Plaza, Ste 411, Camden, NJ 08103; **Phone:** 856-342-2270; **Board Cert:** Surgery 2007; Colon & Rectal Surgery 1980; **Med School:** Jefferson Med Coll 1975; **Resid:** Surgery, Cooper Med Ctr 1979; Colon & Rectal Surgery, Wm Beaumont Hosp 1980; **Fac Appt:** Assoc Prof S, UMDNJ-RW Johnson Med Sch

Procaccino Jr, John A MD [CRS] - **Spec Exp:** Inflammatory Bowel Disease/Crohn's; Colon & Rectal Cancer; Anorectal Disorders; Colon & Rectal Cancer-Familial Polyposis; **Hospital:** N Shore Univ Hosp (page 67), Long Island Jewish Med Ctr (page 67); **Address:** Chief, Division of Colon & Rectal Surg, 900 Northern Blvd, Ste 100, Great Neck, NY 11021; **Phone:** 516-730-2100; **Board Cert:** Surgery 2009; Colon & Rectal Surgery 2011; **Med School:** NYU Sch Med 1984; **Resid:** Surgery, N Shore Univ Hosp 1989; **Fellow:** Colon & Rectal Surgery, Cleveland Clinic 1990; **Fac Appt:** Asst Clin Prof S, Cornell Univ-Weill Med Coll

Stein, David E MD [CRS] - **Spec Exp:** Colon & Rectal Cancer & Surgery; Laparoscopic Surgery; Inflammatory Bowel Disease; Cancer Risk Assessment; **Hospital:** Hahnemann Univ Hosp, St. Francis Hosp; **Address:** 245 N 15th St, NCB Bldg - Fl 7th - Ste 7119, MS 413, #4013, Philadelphia, PA 19102; **Phone:** 215-762-1545; **Board Cert:** Surgery 2003; Colon & Rectal Surgery 2004; **Med School:** SUNY Downstate 1997; **Resid:** Surgery, Thom Jefferson Univ Hosp 2002; **Fellow:** Colon & Rectal Surgery, Cleveland Clin 2003; **Fac Appt:** Assoc Prof S, Drexel Univ Coll Med

Steinhagen, Randolph MD [CRS] - **Spec Exp:** Colostomy Avoidance; Colon & Rectal Cancer; Inflammatory Bowel Disease/Crohn's; Ulcerative Colitis; **Hospital:** Mount Sinai Med Ctr (page 64), St. John's Riverside Hosp-Andrus Pavil; **Address:** Div Colon & Rectal Surgery, 5 E 98th St Fl 14, Box 1259, New York, NY 10029-6501; **Phone:** 212-241-3547; **Board Cert:** Surgery 2002; Colon & Rectal Surgery 1985; **Med School:** Wayne State Univ 1977; **Resid:** Surgery, Mount Sinai Hosp 1982; **Fellow:** Colon & Rectal Surgery, Cleveland Clinic 1983; **Fac Appt:** Prof S, Mount Sinai Sch Med

Whelan, Richard L MD [CRS] - **Spec Exp:** Laparoscopic Surgery; Colon & Rectal Cancer; **Hospital:** St. Luke's - Roosevelt Hosp Ctr - Roosevelt Div (page 56); **Address:** 425 W 59th St, Ste 7B, New York, NY 10019; **Phone:** 212-523-8172; **Board Cert:** Surgery 1997; Colon & Rectal Surgery 1989; **Med School:** Columbia P&S 1982; **Resid:** Surgery, Columbia Presby Hosp 1987; **Fellow:** Colon & Rectal Surgery, Univ Minn Med Ctr 1988; **Fac Appt:** Assoc Clin Prof S, Columbia P&S

Southeast

Beck, Sandra J MD [CRS] - **Hospital:** Univ of Kentucky Albert B. Chandler Hosp; **Address:** Univ Kentucky Chandler Hosp, Dept Surgery, 800 Rose St, Lexington, KY 40536; **Phone:** 859-323-6346 x232; **Board Cert:** Surgery 2011; Colon & Rectal Surgery 2012; **Med School:** Wright State Univ 1995; **Resid:** Surgery, Allegheny Gen Hosp 2001; **Fellow:** Colon & Rectal Surgery, Cleveland Clinic 2002; **Fac Appt:** Assoc Prof S, Univ KY Coll Med

Galandiuk, Susan MD [CRS] - **Spec Exp:** Colon & Rectal Cancer; Inflammatory Bowel Disease/Crohn's; **Hospital:** Univ of Louisville Hosp, Norton Hosp; **Address:** Univ Surgical Assocs, 401 E Chestnut St, Ste 710, Louisville, KY 40202; **Phone:** 502-583-8303; **Board Cert:** Surgery 2008; Colon & Rectal Surgery 2002; **Med School:** Germany 1982; **Resid:** Surgery, Cleveland Clinic Fdn 1988; **Fellow:** Research, Univ Louisville Hosp 1989; Colon & Rectal Surgery, Mayo Clinic 1990; **Fac Appt:** Prof CRS, Univ Louisville Sch Med

Golub, Richard W MD [CRS] - **Spec Exp:** Colon & Rectal Cancer; Laparoscopic Surgery; Hemorrhoids; **Hospital:** Sarasota Meml Hosp, Doctors Hosp - Sarasota; **Address:** Surgical Specialists, 3333 Cattlemen Rd, Ste 206, Sarasota, FL 34232; **Phone:** 941-341-0042; **Board Cert:** Surgery 2000; Colon & Rectal Surgery 2003; **Med School:** Albert Einstein Coll Med 1984; **Resid:** Surgery, Univ Hosp 1990; **Fellow:** Colon & Rectal Surgery, Grant Medical Center 1991

Hartmann, Rene F MD [CRS] - **Spec Exp:** Laparoscopic Surgery; Rectovaginal Fistula; Colon Cancer; Inflammatory Bowel Disease; **Hospital:** Baptist Hosp of Miami, Jackson Meml Hosp; **Address:** JMG Specialty Physicians, 9195 Sunset Drive, Ste 230, Miami, FL 33173; **Phone:** 305-271-0300; **Board Cert:** Colon & Rectal Surgery 1994; **Med School:** Venezuela 1971; **Resid:** Surgery, Jackson Meml Hosp 1976; Surgery, Orange Meml Hosp 1977; **Fellow:** Colon & Rectal Surgery, Grant Hosp 1978; **Fac Appt:** Assoc Clin Prof S, Univ Miami Sch Med

Mantyh, Christopher R MD [CRS] - **Spec Exp:** Colon & Rectal Cancer & Surgery; Rectal Cancer/Sphincter Preservation; Incontinence-Fecal; Colon & Rectal Cancer-Familial Polyposis; **Hospital:** Duke Univ Hosp; **Address:** DUMC, Box 3117, Durham, NC 27710; **Phone:** 919-681-3977; **Board Cert:** Surgery 2008; Colon & Rectal Surgery 2010; **Med School:** Univ Wisc 1991; **Resid:** Surgery, Duke Univ Med Ctr 1998; **Fellow:** Colon & Rectal Surgery, Cleveland Clinic 1999; **Fac Appt:** Assoc Prof CRS, Univ Wisc

Marcet, Jorge E MD [CRS] - **Spec Exp:** Colon & Rectal Cancer; Crohn's Disease; Anal Disorders & Reconstruction; **Hospital:** Tampa Genl Hosp; **Address:** USF Dept Surgery, 1 Tample General Circle, Ste F-145, Tampa, FL 33606; **Phone:** 813-844-4545; **Board Cert:** Surgery 2010; Colon & Rectal Surgery 2013; **Med School:** Cornell Univ-Weill Med Coll 1985; **Resid:** Surgery, St Luke's-Roosevelt Med Ctr 1990; **Fellow:** Colon & Rectal Surgery, Columbia Presby Hosp 1990; Colon & Rectal Surgery, St Luke's-Roosevelt Hosp 1991; **Fac Appt:** Assoc Prof S, Univ S Fla Coll Med

Nogueras, Juan J MD [CRS] - **Spec Exp:** Colon & Rectal Cancer; Inflammatory Bowel Disease/Crohn's; Incontinence-Fecal; Laparoscopic Surgery; **Hospital:** Cleveland Clin - Weston (page 55); **Address:** Cleveland Clinic, Dept Colorectal Surgery, 2950 Cleveland Clinic Blvd, Weston, FL 33331; **Phone:** 954-659-5251; **Board Cert:** Surgery 2007; Colon & Rectal Surgery 2003; **Med School:** Jefferson Med Coll 1982; **Resid:** Surgery, Columbia Presby Med Ctr 1987; **Fellow:** Colon & Rectal Surgery, Univ Minnesota 1991

Sands, Laurence R MD [CRS] - **Spec Exp:** Colon & Rectal Cancer; **Hospital:** Univ of Miami Hosp & Clins/Sylvester Comp Canc Ctr, Jackson N Med Ctr; **Address:** 1475 NW 12th Ave, Rm 3550, Div Colon-Rectal Surgery, Miami, FL 33136; **Phone:** 305-243-9110; **Board Cert:** Colon & Rectal Surgery 2009; Surgery 2004; **Med School:** Northwestern Univ 1990; **Resid:** Surgery, Albert Einstein Med Ctr 1995; **Fellow:** Colon & Rectal Surgery, Cleveland Clin Fla 1996; **Fac Appt:** Asst Clin Prof S, Univ Miami Sch Med

Vernava III, Anthony M MD [CRS] - **Spec Exp:** Colon & Rectal Cancer; Colon & Rectal Cancer-Familial Polyposis; Inflammatory Bowel Disease; Crohn's Disease; **Hospital:** Physicians Regl Hlthcare Med Ctr-Pine Ridge; **Address:** Physicians Regl Med Grp, 6101 Pine Ridge Rd, Naples, FL 34119; **Phone:** 239-348-4531; **Board Cert:** Surgery 2007; Colon & Rectal Surgery 1989; **Med School:** St Louis Univ 1982; **Resid:** Surgery, St Louis Univ Med Ctr 1988; Colon & Rectal Surgery, Univ Minnesota Med Ctr 1989; **Fellow:** Colon & Rectal Surgery, St Marks Hosp 1990; Colon & Rectal Surgery, Natl Cancer Ctr 1989

Wexner, Steven D MD [CRS] - **Spec Exp:** Colon & Rectal Cancer; Inflammatory Bowel Disease/Crohn's; Laparoscopic Surgery; Incontinence-Fecal; **Hospital:** Cleveland Clin - Weston (page 55); **Address:** 2950 Cleveland Clinic Blvd, Weston, FL 33331-3609; **Phone:** 954-659-5251; **Board Cert:** Surgery 2005; Colon & Rectal Surgery 2006; **Med School:** Cornell Univ 1982; **Resid:** Surgery, Roosevelt Hosp 1987; **Fellow:** Colon & Rectal Surgery, Univ Minnesota 1988; **Fac Appt:** Prof S, Ohio State Univ

Midwest

Abcarian, Herand MD [CRS] - **Spec Exp:** Rectal Cancer/Sphincter Preservation; Inflammatory Bowel Disease; Anorectal Disorders; Incontinence-Fecal; **Hospital:** Univ of IL Med Ctr at Chicago, Gottlieb Meml Hosp; **Address:** Univ of IL Med Ctr, Division of Colorectal Surgery, 840 S Wood St, Fl 5, Ste 518, MS 958, Chicago, IL 60612; **Phone:** 312-413-2708; **Board Cert:** Surgery 1972; Colon & Rectal Surgery 1972; **Med School:** Iran 1965; **Resid:** Surgery, Cook County Hosp 1971; Colon & Rectal Surgery, Cook County Hosp 1972; **Fac Appt:** Prof S, Univ IL Coll Med

Birnbaum, Elisa H MD [CRS] - **Spec Exp:** Colon & Rectal Cancer; Inflammatory Bowel Disease/Crohn's; Pelvic Organ Prolapse; Rectovaginal Fistula; **Hospital:** Barnes-Jewish Hosp; **Address:** Washington Univ Sch Med, Div Colorectal Surgery, 660 S Euclid, Box 8109, St Louis, MO 63110; **Phone:** 314-454-7177; **Board Cert:** Surgery 2009; Colon & Rectal Surgery 2011; **Med School:** Univ IL Coll Med 1985; **Resid:** Surgery, LIJ Med Ctr 1990; **Fellow:** Colon & Rectal Surgery, Barnes Jewish Hosp 1991; **Fac Appt:** Prof S, Washington Univ, St Louis

Church, James Michael MD [CRS] - **Spec Exp:** Colon & Rectal Cancer; Colon & Rectal Cancer-Familial Polyposis; Desmoid Tumors; Incontinence-Fecal; **Hospital:** Cleveland Clin (page 55); **Address:** 9500 Euclid Ave, A Bldg - Fl 3, Cleveland, OH 44195; **Phone:** 216-444-6536; **Med School:** New Zealand 1974; **Resid:** Surgery, Aukland Hosps 1980; **Fellow:** Research, Aukland Hosps 1983; Colon & Rectal Surgery, Cleveland Clinic 1984; **Fac Appt:** Prof CRS, Cleveland Cl Coll Med/Case West Res

Delaney, Conor P MD/PhD [CRS] - **Spec Exp:** Laparoscopic Surgery; Colon & Rectal Cancer; Inflammatory Bowel Disease/Crohn's; Rectal Cancer/Sphincter Preservation; **Hospital:** Univ Hosps Case Med Ctr (page 74); **Address:** 11100 Euclid Ave, Univ Hosp-Dept of Surgery, Cleveland, OH 44106-5047; **Phone:** 216-844-8087; **Board Cert:** Surgery 1998; Colon & Rectal Surgery 1998; **Med School:** Ireland 1989; **Resid:** Surgery, Univ Hosp 1993; Surgery, Univ Hosp 1999; **Fellow:** Research, Univ of Pittsburgh 1995; Colon & Rectal Surgery, Cleveland Clinic 2000; **Fac Appt:** Prof S, Cleveland Cl Coll Med/Case West Res

Dietz, David W MD [CRS] - **Spec Exp:** Colon & Rectal Cancer; Anal Cancer; Anorectal Disorders; Pelvic Floor Disorders; **Hospital:** Cleveland Clin (page 55); **Address:** Cleveland Clinic, Colorectal Surgery, 9500 Euclid Ave, Desk A30, Cleveland, OH 44195; **Phone:** 216-445-6597; **Board Cert:** Surgery 2010; Colon & Rectal Surgery 2002; **Med School:** Jefferson Med Coll 1993; **Resid:** Surgery, Cleveland Clinic 1999; Colon & Rectal Surgery, Cleveland Clinic 2001

Fleshman Jr, James W MD [CRS] - **Spec Exp:** Colon & Rectal Cancer; Laparoscopic Surgery; Inflammatory Bowel Disease; **Hospital:** Barnes-Jewish Hosp, Barnes-Jewish West County Hosp; **Address:** Wash Univ Sch Med, Div Colorectal Surgery, 660 S Euclid Ave, Box 8109, St Louis, MO 63110; **Phone:** 314-454-7177; **Board Cert:** Colon & Rectal Surgery 1988; Surgery 2002; **Med School:** Washington Univ, St Louis 1980; **Resid:** Surgery, Jewish Hospital 1986; **Fellow:** Colon & Rectal Surgery, Univ Toronto 1987; **Fac Appt:** Prof S, Washington Univ, St Louis

Foley, Eugene F MD [CRS] - **Spec Exp:** Colon & Rectal Cancer; Ulcerative Colitis; **Hospital:** Univ WI Hosp & Clins; **Address:** Univ WI Hosp & Clins, 600 Highland Ave, Madison, WI 53792-7375; **Phone:** 608-263-2521; **Board Cert:** Surgery 2003; Colon & Rectal Surgery 2005; **Med School:** Harvard Med Sch 1985; **Resid:** Surgery, New England Deaconess Hosp 1991; **Fellow:** Colon & Rectal Surgery, Lahey Clinic 1993; **Fac Appt:** Prof S, Univ Wisc

Kodner, Ira J MD [CRS] - **Spec Exp:** Colon & Rectal Cancer; Inflammatory Bowel Disease/Crohn's; Laparoscopic Surgery; **Hospital:** Barnes-Jewish Hosp; **Address:** Wash Univ Sch Med, Div Colorectal Surgery, 660 S Euclid Ave, Box 8109, St Louis, MO 63110; **Phone:** 314-454-7177; **Board Cert:** Surgery 1975; Colon & Rectal Surgery 1975; **Med School:** Washington Univ, St Louis 1967; **Resid:** Surgery, Barnes-Jewish Hosp 1974; **Fellow:** Colon & Rectal Surgery, Cleveland Clinic 1975; Medical Ethics, Univ Chicago Hosps & Hlth Sys 2004; **Fac Appt:** Prof S, Washington Univ, St Louis

Lavery, Ian C MD [CRS] - **Spec Exp:** Colon & Rectal Cancer; Inflammatory Bowel Disease; Pediatric Gastrointestinal Surgery; **Hospital:** Cleveland Clin (page 55); **Address:** 9500 Euclid Ave, Desk A30, Cleveland, OH 44195; **Phone:** 216-444-6930; **Board Cert:** Colon & Rectal Surgery 1998; **Med School:** Australia 1967; **Resid:** Surgery, Princess Alexandra Hosp 1974; Colon & Rectal Surgery, Cleveland Clinic 1977; **Fac Appt:** Prof S, Case West Res Univ

Lederman, Eric D MD [CRS] - **Spec Exp:** Colon & Rectal Cancer; Anorectal Disorders; Crohn's Disease; Diverticulitis; **Hospital:** Missouri Baptist Med Ctr; **Address:** Suburban Surgical Assocs, 555 N New Ballas Rd, Ste 265, St Louis, MO 63141-6886; **Phone:** 314-991-4644; **Board Cert:** Surgery 2008; Colon & Rectal Surgery 2010; **Med School:** Washington Univ, St Louis 1992; **Resid:** Surgery, Albany Med Ctr 1999; **Fellow:** Colon & Rectal Surgery, St Louis Univ Hosp 2001

Lowry, Ann C MD [CRS] - **Spec Exp:** Anal Sphincter Repair; Rectovaginal Fistula; Inflammatory Bowel Disease; **Hospital:** Abbott - Northwestern Hosp, Fairview Southdale Hosp; **Address:** 1055 W Gate Drive, Ste 190, St Paul, MN 55114; **Phone:** 651-312-1700; **Board Cert:** Colon & Rectal Surgery 1988; **Med School:** Tufts Univ 1977; **Resid:** Surgery, New Eng Med Ctr Hosps 1982; **Fellow:** Colon & Rectal Surgery, Univ Minn Affil Hosps 1987; **Fac Appt:** Clin Prof S, Univ Minn

Ludwig, Kirk A MD [CRS] - **Spec Exp:** Colon & Rectal Cancer & Surgery; Pelvic Organ Prolapse; Rectal Cancer/Sphincter Preservation; Incontinence-Fecal; **Hospital:** Froedtert and Med Ctr of WI; **Address:** 9200 W Wisconsin Ave, Dept Surgery, Milwaukee, WI 53226; **Phone:** 414-805-5783; **Board Cert:** Surgery 2005; Colon & Rectal Surgery 2007; **Med School:** Univ Cincinnati 1988; **Resid:** Surgery, Med Coll Wisc 1994; **Fellow:** Colon & Rectal Surgery, Cleveland Clinic 1996; **Fac Appt:** Assoc Prof S, Med Coll Wisc

Madoff, Robert D MD [CRS] - **Spec Exp:** Colon & Rectal Cancer; Inflammatory Bowel Disease; Incontinence/Pelvic Floor Disorders; **Hospital:** Univ Minn Med Ctr, Fairview - Riverside Campus; **Address:** 420 Delaware St SE, Minneapolis, MN 55455; **Phone:** 612-624-9708; **Board Cert:** Colon & Rectal Surgery 2002; **Med School:** Columbia P&S 1979; **Resid:** Surgery, Univ Minn Hosps 1987; **Fellow:** Colon & Rectal Surgery, Univ Minn Hosps 1988; **Fac Appt:** Prof S, Univ Minn

Mutch, Matthew G MD [CRS] - **Spec Exp:** Colon & Rectal Cancer; Inflammatory Bowel Disease; Incontinence/Pelvic Floor Disorders; Rectovaginal Fistula; **Hospital:** Barnes-Jewish Hosp; **Address:** Washington U Med Sch, Dept Surgery, 660 S Euclid Ave, Ste 14102, Box 8109, St Louis, MO 63110-1010; **Phone:** 314-454-7177; **Board Cert:** Surgery 2002; Colon & Rectal Surgery 2003; **Med School:** Washington Univ, St Louis 1994; **Resid:** Surgery, Barnes Jewish Hosp 2001; **Fellow:** Research, Barnes Jewish Hosp 1998; Colon & Rectal Surgery, Lahey Clinic 2002; **Fac Appt:** Assoc Prof S, Washington Univ, St Louis

Nelson, Heidi MD [CRS] - **Spec Exp:** Colon & Rectal Cancer; Gastrointestinal Cancer; **Hospital:** Mayo Med Ctr & Clin - Rochester, Rochester Methodist Hosp; **Address:** 200 First St SW, Mayo Clinic, Rochester, MN 55905; **Phone:** 507-284-2218; **Board Cert:** Surgery 2007; Colon & Rectal Surgery 1989; **Med School:** Univ Wash 1981; **Resid:** Surgery, Oregon Hlth Sci Univ Hosp 1987; Colon & Rectal Surgery, Oregon Hlth Sci Univ Hosp 1985; **Fellow:** Colon & Rectal Surgery, Mayo Clinic 1988; **Fac Appt:** Prof S, Mayo Med Sch

Pemberton, John H MD [CRS] - **Spec Exp:** Inflammatory Bowel Disease/Crohn's; Colon & Rectal Cancer; **Hospital:** Rochester Methodist Hosp, St. Mary's Hosp - Rochester MN (Mayo); **Address:** Mayo Clinic, Div Colon & Rectal Surg, 200 First St SW, Gonda Bldg - rm 9-205, Rochester, MN 55905; **Phone:** 507-284-2359; **Board Cert:** Surgery 2001; Colon & Rectal Surgery 1985; **Med School:** Tulane Univ 1976; **Resid:** Surgery, Mayo Clinic 1983; **Fellow:** Colon & Rectal Surgery, Mayo Clinic 1984; **Fac Appt:** Prof S, Mayo Med Sch

Rafferty, Janice F MD [CRS] - **Spec Exp:** Colon & Rectal Cancer; Ulcerative Colitis; Crohn's Disease; Anal Disorders & Reconstruction; **Hospital:** Christ Hosp, The - Cincinnati, Univ Hosp - Cincinnati; **Address:** Univ Cincinnati, Colon & Rectal Surgery, 2123 Auburn Ave, Ste 524, Cincinnati, OH 45219; **Phone:** 513-929-0104; **Board Cert:** Surgery 2004; Colon & Rectal Surgery 2008; **Med School:** Ohio State Univ 1988; **Resid:** Surgery, Univ Cincinnati Hosp 1995; Colon & Rectal Surgery, Barnes Jewish Hosp 1996; **Fac Appt:** Prof S, Univ Cincinnati

Remzi, Feza H MD [CRS] - **Spec Exp:** Colon & Rectal Cancer & Surgery; Inflammatory Bowel Disease; Laparoscopic Surgery; **Hospital:** Cleveland Clin (page 55); **Address:** Cleveland Clinic, 9500 Euclid Ave, Dept A30, Cleveland, OH 44195; **Phone:** 216-445-5020; **Board Cert:** Surgery 2006; Colon & Rectal Surgery 2007; **Med School:** Turkey 1989; **Resid:** Colon & Rectal Surgery, Cleveland Clinic 1996; Colon & Rectal Surgery, Cleveland Clinic 1997

Saclarides, Theodore J MD [CRS] - **Spec Exp:** Rectal Cancer/Sphincter Preservation; Laparoscopic Surgery; Inflammatory Bowel Disease; **Hospital:** Loyola Univ Med Ctr; **Address:** Loyola Univ Med Ctr, 2160 S First Ave, Maywood, IL 60153; **Phone:** 708-327-2705; **Board Cert:** Surgery 2007; Colon & Rectal Surgery 1989; **Med School:** Univ Miami Sch Med 1982; **Resid:** Surgery, Rush Univ Med Ctr 1987; **Fellow:** Colon & Rectal Surgery, Mayo Clinic 1988; **Fac Appt:** Prof S, Rush Med Coll

Stryker, Steven J MD [CRS] - **Spec Exp:** Colon & Rectal Cancer; Inflammatory Bowel Disease; Laparoscopic Surgery; **Hospital:** Northwestern Meml Hosp; **Address:** 676 N Saint Clair St, Ste 1525A, Chicago, IL 60611-2862; **Phone:** 312-943-5427; **Board Cert:** Surgery 2004; Colon & Rectal Surgery 1986; **Med School:** Northwestern Univ 1978; **Resid:** Surgery, Northwestern Meml Hosp 1983; **Fellow:** Colon & Rectal Surgery, Mayo Clinic 1985; **Fac Appt:** Clin Prof S, Northwestern Univ

Trudel, Judith L MD [CRS] - **Spec Exp:** Colon & Rectal Cancer; Anorectal Disorders; **Hospital:** St. John's Hosp-Maplewood MN, St. Joseph's Hosp; **Address:** Colon & Rectal Surgery Assocs, 1055 Westgate Drive, Ste 190, St Paul, MN 55114; **Phone:** 651-312-1620; **Board Cert:** Surgery 2007; Colon & Rectal Surgery 2006; **Med School:** Canada 1979; **Resid:** Surgery, Montreal Genl Hosp 1984; **Fellow:** Colon & Rectal Surgery, Cleveland Clin 1986; **Fac Appt:** Assoc Prof S, Univ Minn

Wise, Paul E MD [CRS] - **Spec Exp:** Colon & Rectal Cancer & Surgery; Minimally Invasive Surgery; Colon & Rectal Cancer-Hereditary; Inflammatory Bowel Disease; **Hospital:** Barnes-Jewish Hosp, Barnes-Jewish West County Hosp; **Address:** 660 S Euclid Ave, Box 8109, Saint Louis, MO 63110; **Phone:** 615-454-7177; **Board Cert:** Surgery 2004; Colon & Rectal Surgery 2005; **Med School:** Johns Hopkins Univ 1996; **Resid:** Surgery, Vanderbilt Univ Med Ctr 2003; **Fellow:** Colon & Rectal Surgery, Barnes-Jewish Hosp 2004; **Fac Appt:** Assoc Prof S, Washington Univ, St Louis

Colon & Rectal Surgery

Wolff, Bruce G MD [CRS] - **Spec Exp:** Inflammatory Bowel Disease; Crohn's Disease; Colon & Rectal Cancer; **Hospital:** Mayo Med Ctr & Clin - Rochester; **Address:** Mayo Clinic, Gonda 9 South, 200 First St SW, Rochester, MN 55905; **Phone:** 507-284-2511; **Board Cert:** Surgery 2000; Colon & Rectal Surgery 2001; **Med School:** Duke Univ 1973; **Resid:** Surgery, NY Hosp-Cornell Med Ctr 1981; **Fellow:** Colon & Rectal Surgery, Mayo Clinic 1982; **Fac Appt:** Prof S, Mayo Med Sch

Great Plains and Mountains

Blatchford, Garnet J MD [CRS] - **Spec Exp:** Colon Cancer; Anal Disorders & Reconstruction; **Hospital:** Alegent Hlth - Immanuel Med Ctr; **Address:** 9850 Nicholas St, Ste 110, Omaha, NE 68114; **Phone:** 402-343-1122; **Board Cert:** Colon & Rectal Surgery 2009; **Med School:** Univ Nebr Coll Med 1983; **Resid:** Surgery, Univ Nebraska Med Ctr 1988; Colon & Rectal Surgery, Creighton Univ 1990; **Fac Appt:** Assoc Prof S, Creighton Univ

Schatz, Lisa Shawn MD [CRS] - **Spec Exp:** Gastrointestinal Surgery; **Hospital:** Rose Med Ctr; **Address:** Rocky Mountain Surgical Associates, 4545 E 9th Ave, Ste 460, Denver, CO 80220; **Phone:** 303-388-2922; **Board Cert:** Surgery 2011; Colon & Rectal Surgery 2012; **Med School:** Case West Res Univ 1995; **Resid:** Surgery, Univ Hosps of Cleveland 2000; Colon & Rectal Surgery, Ochsner Clinic 2001; **Fac Appt:** Assoc Clin Prof CRS, Univ Colorado

Thorson, Alan G MD [CRS] - **Spec Exp:** Colon & Rectal Cancer; Rectal Cancer/Sphincter Preservation; Incontinence-Fecal; Laparoscopic Surgery; **Hospital:** Nebraska Meth Hosp, Bergan Mercy Med Ctr-Alegant Hlth; **Address:** 9850 Nicholas St, Ste 100, Ste 100, 9850 Nicholas St, Omaha, NE 68114-2191; **Phone:** 402-343-1122; **Board Cert:** Colon & Rectal Surgery 1999; **Med School:** Univ Nebr Coll Med 1979; **Resid:** Surgery, Univ Nebraska Affil Hosp 1984; Colon & Rectal Surgery, Univ Minn Affil Hosp 1985; **Fac Appt:** Clin Prof S, Creighton Univ

Williams, Shauna Tseu MD [CRS] - **Hospital:** St. Alphonsus Regl Med Ctr; **Address:** 1072 N Liberty St, Ste 201, Boise, ID 83704; **Phone:** 208-377-2273; **Board Cert:** Surgery 2009; Colon & Rectal Surgery 2010; **Med School:** Univ Hawaii JA Burns Sch Med 1984; **Resid:** Surgery, Univ Oregon Hlth Sci Ctr 1990; **Fellow:** Colon & Rectal Surgery, Mayo Clinic 1991

Southwest

Bailey, H Randolph MD [CRS] - **Spec Exp:** Rectal Cancer/Sphincter Preservation; Inflammatory Bowel Disease; Incontinence-Fecal; Endometriosis-Intestine; **Hospital:** Methodist Hosp - Houston, St. Luke's Episcopal Hosp-Houston; **Address:** Colon & Rectal Clinic, Smith Tower, 6550 Fannin St, Ste 2307, Houston, TX 77030-2717; **Phone:** 713-790-9250; **Board Cert:** Surgery 1974; Colon & Rectal Surgery 2004; **Med School:** Univ Tex SW, Dallas 1968; **Resid:** Surgery, Hermann Hosp 1973; **Fellow:** Colon & Rectal Surgery, Ferguson-Droste Hosp 1974; **Fac Appt:** Clin Prof S, Univ Tex, Houston

Beck, David E MD [CRS] - **Spec Exp:** Colon & Rectal Cancer; Minimally Invasive Surgery; Inflammatory Bowel Disease; **Hospital:** Ochsner Med Ctr-New Orleans, Ochsner Med Ctr-Baton Rouge; **Address:** Ochsner Med Ctr, Div Colorectal Surg, 1514 Jefferson Hwy Fl 4, New Orleans, LA 70121-2429; **Phone:** 504-842-4060; **Board Cert:** Colon & Rectal Surgery 1987; **Med School:** Univ Miami Sch Med 1979; **Resid:** Surgery, Wilford Hall USAF Med Ctr 1984; **Fellow:** Colon & Rectal Surgery, Cleveland Clinic Fdn 1986; **Fac Appt:** Assoc Clin Prof S, Louisiana State U, New Orleans

Haas, Eric M MD [CRS] - **Spec Exp:** Laparoscopic Surgery; Colon & Rectal Cancer; Inflammatory Bowel Disease/Crohn's; Incontinence-Fecal; **Hospital:** Methodist Hosp - Houston, St. Luke's Episcopal Hosp-Houston; **Address:** 7900 Fannin St, Ste 2700, Houston, TX 77054; **Phone:** 713-790-0600; **Board Cert:** Surgery 2003; Colon & Rectal Surgery 2004; **Med School:** Univ Tex, Houston 1997; **Resid:** Surgery, St Joseph Hosp 2002; **Fellow:** Colon & Rectal Surgery, Univ Texas 2003

Heppell, Jacques P MD [CRS] - **Spec Exp:** Colon & Rectal Cancer; Inflammatory Bowel Disease; Anorectal Disorders; **Hospital:** Mayo Clinic - Phoenix; **Address:** Mayo Clinic, 5777 E Mayo Blvd, Phoenix, AZ 85054; **Phone:** 480-342-2697; **Board Cert:** Surgery 2004; Colon & Rectal Surgery 1995; **Med School:** Univ Montreal 1974; **Resid:** Surgery, Univ Montreal Affil Hosps 1979; **Fellow:** Colon & Rectal Surgery, Mayo Clinic 1983; **Fac Appt:** Prof S, Mayo Med Sch

Hicks, Terry C MD [CRS] - **Spec Exp:** Colon & Rectal Cancer; **Hospital:** Ochsner Med Ctr-New Orleans; **Address:** Ochsner Med Ctr, Div Colorectal Surg, 1514 Jefferson Hwy Fl 4, New Orleans, LA 70121-2429; **Phone:** 504-842-5884; **Board Cert:** Colon & Rectal Surgery 2002; **Med School:** Univ Tex, San Antonio 1977; **Resid:** Surgery, Univ Louisville Med Ctr 1982; Colon & Rectal Surgery, Ochsner Clinic 1983; **Fac Appt:** Assoc Prof S, Louisiana State U, New Orleans

Huber Jr, Philip J MD [CRS] - **Spec Exp:** Colon & Rectal Cancer; Inflammatory Bowel Disease; **Hospital:** Med City Dallas Hosp, TX Hlth Presby Hosp Dallas; **Address:** 7777 Forest Lane, Ste C-204, Dallas, TX 75230; **Phone:** 972-566-6115; **Board Cert:** Colon & Rectal Surgery 1993; **Med School:** Columbia P&S 1972; **Resid:** Surgery, Parkland Hosp 1977; Colon & Rectal Surgery, Presby Hosp 1978

West Coast and Pacific

Beart Jr, Robert W MD [CRS] - **Spec Exp:** Colon & Rectal Cancer; Rectal Cancer/Sphincter Preservation; **Hospital:** Glendale Mem Hosp & Hlth Ctr; **Address:** Colorectal Surgery Inst, 222 W Eulalia St, Ste 100A, Glendale, CA 91204; **Phone:** 818-244-8161; **Board Cert:** Colon & Rectal Surgery 1995; **Med School:** Harvard Med Sch 1971; **Resid:** Surgery, Univ Colo Med Ctr 1976; Colon & Rectal Surgery, Mayo Clinic 1978; **Fellow:** Transplant Surgery, Univ Colo Med Ctr 1975; **Fac Appt:** Prof Emeritus S, USC Sch Med

Chiu, Yanek S MD [CRS] - **Hospital:** CA Pacific Med Ctr-Pacific Campus; **Address:** 3838 California St, Ste 616, San Francisco, CA 94118; **Phone:** 415-668-0411; **Board Cert:** Colon & Rectal Surgery 1997; **Med School:** Boston Univ 1971; **Resid:** Surgery, Boston Med Ctr 1976; **Fellow:** Colon & Rectal Surgery, Mayo Clinic 1978; **Fac Appt:** Assoc Clin Prof CRS, UCSF

Coutsoftides, Theodore MD [CRS] - **Spec Exp:** Laparoscopic Surgery; Inflammatory Bowel Disease; Anal Sphincter Repair; **Hospital:** St. Joseph's Hosp - Orange; **Address:** 1310 W Stewart Drive, Ste 605, Orange, CA 92868-3857; **Phone:** 714-532-2544; **Board Cert:** Colon & Rectal Surgery 1977; **Med School:** Israel 1970; **Resid:** Surgery, Cleveland Clinic 1973; Surgery, Royal Victoria Hosp 1976; **Fellow:** Colon & Rectal Surgery, Cleveland Clinic 1977; **Fac Appt:** Assoc Prof S, UC Irvine

Lee, Patrick Y H MD [CRS] - **Hospital:** Providence Portland Med Ctr, Legacy Good Samaritan Med Ctr; **Address:** Surgical Specialty Group, Colon & Rectal Clinic, 9155 SW Barnes Rd, Ste 839, Portland, OR 97225; **Phone:** 503-222-1615; **Board Cert:** Surgery 2004; Colon & Rectal Surgery 2007; **Med School:** Northwestern Univ-Feinberg Sch Med 1988; **Resid:** Surgery, Oregon Hlth Sci Ctr 1994; **Fellow:** Colon & Rectal Surgery, Cleveland Clinic 1995

Colon & Rectal Surgery

Ramamoorthy, Sonia L MD [CRS] - **Spec Exp:** Colon & Rectal Cancer; Diverticulitis; Incontinence/Pelvic Floor Disorders; Inflammatory Bowel Disease; **Hospital:** UCSD Med Ctr; **Address:** 3855 Health Sciences Drive, La Jolla, CA 92093; **Phone:** 858-822-6277; **Board Cert:** Surgery 2002; Colon & Rectal Surgery 2005; **Med School:** Boston Univ 1996; **Resid:** Surgery, UCSD Med Ctr 2001; **Fellow:** Colon & Rectal Surgery, Barnes-Jewish Hosp 2002; Research, UCSD Med Ctr 2006; **Fac Appt:** Assoc Prof S, UCSD

Senagore, Anthony MD [CRS] - **Spec Exp:** Laparoscopic Surgery; Colon & Rectal Cancer; Anorectal Disorders; Inflammatory Bowel Disease/Crohn's; **Hospital:** USC Norris Cancer Hosp (page 62); **Address:** USC North Cancer Hosp, 1441 Eastlake Ave, Ste 7418, Los Angeles, CA 90033; **Phone:** 323-865-3690; **Board Cert:** Surgery 2006; Colon & Rectal Surgery 2009; Surgical Critical Care 2006; **Med School:** Mich State Univ 1981; **Resid:** Surgery, Butterworth Hosp 1987; Colon & Rectal Surgery, Ferguson Hosp 1989; **Fac Appt:** Prof S

Sokol, Thomas P MD [CRS] - **Spec Exp:** Colon & Rectal Cancer & Surgery; Incontinence-Fecal; Constipation; Gastrointestinal Motility Disorders; **Hospital:** Cedars-Sinai Med Ctr; **Address:** 8737 Beverly Blvd, Ste 402, Los Angeles, CA 90048-1828; **Phone:** 310-854-3580; **Board Cert:** Colon & Rectal Surgery 2008; **Med School:** Ros Franklin Univ/Chicago Med Sch 1980; **Resid:** Surgery, Habor UCLA Med Ctr 1985; **Fellow:** Colon & Rectal Surgery, Carle Fdn Hosp/Univ Ill 1986; **Fac Appt:** Assoc Clin Prof S, UCLA

Stamos, Michael J MD [CRS] - **Spec Exp:** Rectal Cancer/Sphincter Preservation; Laparoscopic Surgery; Inflammatory Bowel Disease; Colon & Rectal Cancer; **Hospital:** UC Irvine Med Ctr; **Address:** UC Irvine Med Ctr, Div Colon & Rectal Surg, 333 City Blvd W, Ste 700, Orange, CA 92868; **Phone:** 714-456-6262; **Board Cert:** Surgery 2010; Colon & Rectal Surgery 2003; **Med School:** Case West Res Univ 1985; **Resid:** Surgery, Jackson Meml Hosp 1990; Colon & Rectal Surgery, Ochsner Clinic 1991; **Fac Appt:** Prof S, UC Irvine

Varma, Madhulika G MD [CRS] - **Spec Exp:** Colon & Rectal Cancer & Surgery; Inflammatory Bowel Disease; Pelvic Floor Disorders; Laparoscopic Surgery; **Hospital:** UCSF - Mt Zion Med Ctr; **Address:** Center for Colorectal Surgery, 2330 Post St, Ste 260, San Francisco, CA 94115-1799; **Phone:** 415-885-3606; **Board Cert:** Colon & Rectal Surgery 2010; Surgery 2007; **Med School:** Brown Univ 1991; **Resid:** Surgery, UCSF Med Ctr 1998; **Fellow:** Colon & Rectal Surgery, Univ Minnesota Med Ctr 2000; Research, UCSF Med Ctr 2001; **Fac Appt:** Asst Prof S, UCSF

Welton, Mark L MD [CRS] - **Spec Exp:** Ulcerative Colitis; Crohn's Disease; Colon & Rectal Cancer; Anal Cancer; **Hospital:** Stanford Univ Hosp & Clinics; **Address:** The Cancer Ctr, 875 Blake Wilbur Drive, Stanford, CA 94305; **Phone:** 650-723-5461; **Board Cert:** Surgery 2000; Colon & Rectal Surgery 2005; **Med School:** UCLA 1984; **Resid:** Surgery, UCLA Med Ctr 1992; **Fellow:** Colon & Rectal Surgery, Barnes Jewish Hosp 1993; **Fac Appt:** Assoc Prof S, Stanford Univ

Wong, Ronald J MD [CRS] - **Spec Exp:** Laparoscopic Surgery; **Hospital:** Queen's Med Ctr - Honolulu; **Address:** Queen's Physicians' Office Bldg 1, 1380 Lusitana St, rm 614, Honolulu, HI 96813; **Phone:** 808-524-1856; **Board Cert:** Surgery 2008; **Med School:** Univ Hawaii JA Burns Sch Med 1981; **Resid:** Surgery, Univ Hawaii 1985; Surgery, Catholic Med Ctr 1987; **Fellow:** Research, pCornell Univ Med Ctr 1988; Colon & Rectal Surgery, Suburban Hosp 1989; **Fac Appt:** Clin Prof S, Univ Hawaii JA Burns Sch Med

Worsey, Michael J MD [CRS] - **Spec Exp:** Colon & Rectal Cancer; Inflammatory Bowel Disease; **Hospital:** Scripps Meml Hosp - La Jolla; **Address:** Advanced Surgical Assocs, 9834 Genesee Ave, Ste 201, La Jolla, CA 92037; **Phone:** 858-558-2272; **Board Cert:** Surgery 2009; Colon & Rectal Surgery 2008; **Med School:** England, UK 1985; **Resid:** Surgery, Bristol Royal Infirm/Royal Gwent Hosp 1989; Surgery, Univ Pittsburgh Med Ctr 1997; **Fellow:** Colon & Rectal Surgery, Cleveland Clin 1998

 Cleveland Clinic

Every life deserves world class care.

Colorectal Surgery

Cleveland Clinic's Digestive Disease Institute (DDI) is one of the largest digestive programs in the country and is ranked No. 2 in the nation by *U.S. News & World Report*. DDI was the first to fully integrate its departments of Colorectal Surgery, Gastroenterology & Hepatology, General Surgery and Nutrition. Combining these disciplines in one location facilitates unprecedented patient care, multidisciplinary education and collaborative research. In 2011, DDI physicians performed over 16,000 surgical cases and close to 51,000 endoscopic cases. Transplant surgeons completed over 150 digestive disease-related organ transplants, including liver, pancreas and intestinal transplantation, achieving outstanding outcomes.

Highlights of the Department of Colorectal Surgery:

- The first ileoanal pouch for ulcerative colitis was performed at Cleveland Clinic in the 1980s.
- Our colorectal surgeons performed the world's first colon resection entirely through a single incision in the belly button in 2008.
- We performed the world's first single-incision proctocolectomy and ileoanal pouch anastomosis (removing the entire large intestine and rectum) in 2009, leaving only a coin-sized scar in the patient's abdomen.
- We have an international reputation for excellence in inflammatory bowel disease, performing the most Crohn's disease operations, especially the bowel-conserving strictureplasty. We also perform the world's highest volume of J-Pouch surgeries and are the nation's largest referral center for repairing failed pelvic pouches.
- Our team performs more colon and rectal cancer surgeries than any other hospital in Ohio and one of the highest volumes in the nation.
- Led by a team of female physicians, our pelvic floor center treats the entire spectrum of bowel disorders, including fecal incontinence and chronic constipation.

Cleveland Clinic
Digestive Disease Institute
9500 Euclid Avenue
Cleveland, OH 44195

Offering Same-Day Appointments
Call 800.274.2009.

Treatment Guides
Cleveland Clinic has developed comprehensive treatment guides for many diseases and conditions. To download our free treatment guides, visit clevelandclinic.org/treatmentguides.

Online Medical Second Opinion
Call 216.444.3223 or 800.223.2273 ext. 43223 or email eclevelandclinic@ccf.org.

Out-of-State Patients Assistance
Call 800.223.2273, ext. 55580 or email medicalconcierge@ccf.org.

Visit Us At:
clevelandclinic.org

Follow Us On:
Facebook
www.facebook.com/clevelandclinic

Twitter
@ClevelandClinic

You Tube
www.youtube.com/clevelandclinic

Health Hub
health.clevelandclinic.org

NYU Langone
MEDICAL CENTER

550 First Avenue *(at 31st Street)*
New York, NY 10016
www.NYULMC.org
Physician Referral: **888-7-NYU-MED** *(888-769-8633)*

COLON AND RECTAL SURGERY

About the Division of Colon and Rectal Surgery
Colorectal surgeons at NYU Langone perform more than 5,000 outpatient and inpatient procedures each year using laser, laparoscopic, endoscopic and other minimally invasive techniques. Candidates for surgery receive same-day care that includes imaging, radiation and nutritional support. We specialize in cancer, diverticulitis, IBD, anorectal conditions, and bowel disorders.

Adrenalectomies
Our surgeons are skilled at performing adrenalectomies, the surgical removal of one or both of the adrenal glands. This procedure is usually advised for patients with tumors of the adrenal glands, which may be malignant or benign. Adrenalectomy, once performed by conventional (open) surgery, is now routinely done laparoscopically through four very small incisions, which allows patients to usually be discharged within 36 hours.

Colorectal Cancer
We offer the most advanced screening options available for the diagnosis of colon cancer, the second leading cause of cancer death in the U.S. Additionally, we continue to investigate colorectal cancer screenings in special populations such as women, veterans, immigrants, minorities and patients with HIV, and offer the use of virtual colonoscopy for the detection of colorectal polyps and cancer.

Laparoscopic Techniques
Surgeons at NYU Langone use tiny incisions to remove a segment of the colon, which dramatically speeds recovery and reduces the need for pain medication. Laparoscopic techniques are used to treat pancreatic tumors, splenic related conditions, hiatus hernias, small bowel tumors and adrenalectomies.

Liver Lesions
Our surgeons treat liver lesions with painless radiofrequency ablation. Minimally invasive resections and open liver surgery are also routinely performed.

Virtual Colonoscopy
The Medical Center offers the latest developments in colon cancer detection, including virtual colonoscopy. This noninvasive procedure makes use of sophisticated imaging techniques to generate a 3-D reconstruction of the inner surface of the colon, which can then be evaluated for abnormalities by specially trained radiologists.

Dermatology

A dermatologist is trained to diagnose and treat pediatric and adult patients with benign and malignant disorders of the skin, mouth, external genitalia, hair and nails, as well as a number of sexually transmitted diseases. The dermatologist may have additional training and experience in the diagnosis and treatment of skin cancers, melanomas, moles and other tumors of the skin, the management of contact dermatitis and other allergic and nonallergic skin disorders, and in the recognition of the skin manifestations of systemic (including internal malignancy) and infectious diseases. Dermatologists may have special training in dermatopathology and in the surgical techniques used in dermatology. They also have expertise in the management of cosmetic disorders of the skin such as hair loss and scars, and the skin changes associated with aging.

Training Required: Four years.

Certification in the following subspecialties requires additional training and examination.

Dermatopathology: A dermatopathologist has the expertise to diagnose and monitor diseases of the skin including infectious, immunologic, degenerative and neoplastic diseases. This entails the examination and interpretation of specially prepared tissue sections, cellular scrapings and smears of skin lesions by means of routine and special (electron and fluorescent) microscopes.

Pediatric Dermatology: A dermatologist trained to diagnose and treat pediatric patients with dermatologic diseases.

DERMATOLOGY

New England

Anderson, Richard Rox MD [D] - **Spec Exp:** Birthmarks/Hemangiomas; **Hospital:** Mass Genl Hosp; **Address:** Dermatology Laser Center, 50 Staniford St, Ste 250, Boston, MA 02114; **Phone:** 617-724-6960; **Board Cert:** Dermatology 2009; **Med School:** Harvard Med Sch 1984; **Resid:** Dermatology, Mass Genl Hosp 1991; **Fellow:** Dermatologic Research, Mass Genl Hosp 1988; **Fac Appt:** Assoc Prof D, Harvard Med Sch

Arndt, Kenneth MD [D] - **Spec Exp:** Skin Laser Surgery; Cosmetic Dermatology; **Hospital:** Beth Israel Deaconess Med Ctr - Boston, New England Bapt Hosp; **Address:** Skincare Physicians, 1244 Boylston St, Ste 302, Chestnut Hill, MA 02467; **Phone:** 617-731-1600; **Board Cert:** Dermatology 1966; **Med School:** Yale Univ 1961; **Resid:** Dermatology, Mass Genl Hosp 1965; **Fellow:** Dermatology, Harvard Med Sch 1965; **Fac Appt:** Clin Prof D, Harvard Med Sch

Bolognia, Jean L MD [D] - **Spec Exp:** Melanoma; Skin Cancer; **Hospital:** Yale-New Haven Hosp, Yale Med Group; **Address:** 2 Church St S, Ste 305, New Haven, CT 06519; **Phone:** 203-789-1249; **Board Cert:** Dermatology 2009; **Med School:** Yale Univ 1980; **Resid:** Internal Medicine, Yale-New Haven Hosp 1982; Dermatology, Yale-New Haven Hosp 1985; **Fellow:** Dermatology, Yale-New Haven Hosp 1987; **Fac Appt:** Prof D, Yale Univ

Dover, Jeffrey MD [D] - **Spec Exp:** Cosmetic Dermatology; Skin Laser Surgery; **Hospital:** Beth Israel Deaconess Med Ctr - Boston, New England Bapt Hosp; **Address:** Skincare Physicians, 1244 Boylston St, Ste 302, Chestnut Hill, MA 02467; **Phone:** 617-731-1600; **Board Cert:** Dermatology 1985; **Med School:** Univ Ottawa 1981; **Resid:** Dermatology, Univ Toronto 1984; Dermatology, St Johns Hosp 1985; **Fellow:** Dermatology, Mass Genl Hosp-Harvard 1987; **Fac Appt:** Assoc Prof D, Yale Univ

Dufresne, Raymond G MD [D] - **Spec Exp:** Mohs' Surgery; Skin Cancer; **Hospital:** Rhode Island Hosp; **Address:** University Dermatology, 593 Eddy St, APC 10, Providence, RI 02903; **Phone:** 401-444-7024; **Board Cert:** Internal Medicine 1983; Dermatology 1986; **Med School:** Vanderbilt Univ 1980; **Resid:** Internal Medicine, Vanderbilt Univ Med Ctr 1983; Dermatology, Vanderbilt Univ Med Ctr 1986; **Fellow:** Mohs Surgery, Cleveland Clinic 1987; **Fac Appt:** Prof D, Brown Univ

Edelson, Richard L MD [D] - **Spec Exp:** Cutaneous Lymphoma; Immune Deficiency-Skin Disorders; **Hospital:** Yale-New Haven Hosp, Yale Med Group; **Address:** 2 Church St S, Ste 305, New Haven, CT 06519; **Phone:** 203-789-1249; **Board Cert:** Dermatology 1977; **Med School:** Yale Univ 1970; **Resid:** Dermatology, Mass Genl Hosp 1972; Dermatology, Natl Inst Hlth 1975; **Fac Appt:** Prof D, Yale Univ

Falanga, Vincent MD [D] - **Spec Exp:** Wound Healing/Care; Collagen Vascular Diseases; Scleroderma; **Hospital:** Roger Williams Med Ctr; **Address:** Roger Williams Med Ctr, Dept Dermatology, 50 Maude St Elmhurst Bldg Fl 1, Providence, RI 02908; **Phone:** 401-456-2521; **Board Cert:** Internal Medicine 1980; Dermatology 1982; **Med School:** Harvard Med Sch 1977; **Resid:** Internal Medicine, Univ Miami Med Ctr 1980; **Fellow:** Dermatology, Hosp Univ Penn 1982; **Fac Appt:** Prof D, Boston Univ

Fewkes, Jessica L MD [D] - **Spec Exp:** Mohs' Surgery; Skin Cancer-Head & Neck; Melanoma-Head & Neck; Cosmetic Dermatology; **Hospital:** Mass Eye & Ear Infirmary, Mass Genl Hosp; **Address:** Facial & Cosmetic Surgery Center, Mass Eye & Ear Infirmary, 243 Charles St, 9th Fl, Boston, MA 02114; **Phone:** 617-573-3789; **Board Cert:** Dermatology 1982; **Med School:** UCSF 1978; **Resid:** Dermatology, Mass Genl Hosp 1982; **Fellow:** Chemosurgery, Duke Univ Med Ctr 1983; **Fac Appt:** Asst Prof D, Harvard Med Sch

Gellis, Stephen MD [D] - **Spec Exp:** Pediatric Dermatology; Melanoma; Pigmented Lesions; **Hospital:** Children's Hospital - Boston; **Address:** Chldn's Hosp-Boston, 300 Longwood Ave Fegan Bldg Fl 6, Boston, MA 02115; **Phone:** 617-355-6117; **Board Cert:** Pediatrics 1978; Dermatology 1979; Pediatric Dermatology 2006; **Med School:** Harvard Med Sch 1973; **Resid:** Pediatrics, Chldn's Hosp 1976; Dermatology, Mass Genl Hosp 1978; **Fac Appt:** Asst Prof D, Harvard Med Sch

Gilchrest, Barbara MD [D] - **Spec Exp:** Photoaging; Melanoma; Skin Cancer; **Hospital:** Boston Med Ctr; **Address:** Boston Med Ctr- Dermatolgy Dept, 609 Albany St, Ste 105, Doctor's Off Bldg, Boston, MA 02118; **Phone:** 617-638-7420; **Board Cert:** Internal Medicine 1975; Dermatology 1978; **Med School:** Harvard Med Sch 1971; **Resid:** Internal Medicine, Boston City Hosp 1973; Dermatology, Harvard Med Sch 1976; **Fellow:** Photo Biology, Harvard Med Sch 1975; **Fac Appt:** Prof D, Boston Univ

Gottlieb, Alice B MD/PhD [D] - **Spec Exp:** Psoriasis; Psoriatic Arthritis; Atopic Dermatitis; Clinical Trials; **Hospital:** Tufts Med Ctr; **Address:** Tufts Medical Center, 800 Washington St, Box 114, Boston, MA 02111; **Phone:** 617-636-0156; **Board Cert:** Internal Medicine 1982; Dermatology 2011; Rheumatology 1984; **Med School:** Cornell Univ-Weill Med Coll 1980; **Resid:** Internal Medicine, New York Hosp 1982; Dermatology, New York Hosp 1993; **Fellow:** Rheumatology, Hosp Special Surgery 1984; **Fac Appt:** Prof D, Tufts Univ

Kane, Kay S MD [D] - **Spec Exp:** Pediatric Dermatology; **Hospital:** Children's Hospital - Boston; **Address:** Skincare Physicians, 1244 Boylston St, Chestnut Hill, MA 02467; **Phone:** 617-731-1600; **Board Cert:** Dermatology 2005; **Med School:** Harvard Med Sch 1993; **Resid:** Dermatology, Mass General Hosp 1997; **Fac Appt:** Asst Prof D, Harvard Med Sch

Kupper, Thomas S MD [D] - **Spec Exp:** Melanoma; Cutaneous Lymphoma; Skin Cancer; **Hospital:** Brigham and Women's Hosp (page 57), Dana-Farber Cancer Inst (page 57); **Address:** Brigham & Women's Hosp, Dept Dermatology, 77 Avenue Louis Pasteur, Ste 671, Boston, MA 02115; **Phone:** 617-632-6869; **Board Cert:** Dermatology 1989; **Med School:** Yale Univ 1981; **Resid:** Surgery, Yale-New Haven Hosp 1983; Dermatology, Yale-New Haven Hosp 1989; **Fac Appt:** Prof D, Harvard Med Sch

Leffell, David J MD [D] - **Spec Exp:** Mohs' Surgery; Melanoma; Skin Cancer; Skin Laser Surgery; **Hospital:** Yale-New Haven Hosp, Yale Med Group; **Address:** 40 Temple St, Ste 5a, New Haven, CT 06510; **Phone:** 203-785-3466; **Board Cert:** Internal Medicine 1984; Dermatology 2009; **Med School:** McGill Univ 1981; **Resid:** Internal Medicine, New York Hosp 1984; Dermatology, Meml Sloan Kettering Cancer Ctr 1986; **Fellow:** Dermatology, Yale Sch Med 1987; Dermatologic Surgery, Univ Michigan Med Ctr 1988; **Fac Appt:** Prof D, Yale Univ

Maloney, Mary E MD [D] - **Spec Exp:** Mohs' Surgery; Skin Cancer; Dermatologic Surgery; **Hospital:** UMass Memorial Med Ctr; **Address:** UMass Meml Med Ctr-Hahnemann Campus, 281 Lincoln St Fl 4, Worcester, MA 01605; **Phone:** 508-334-5962; **Board Cert:** Dermatology 1982; **Med School:** Univ VT Coll Med 1977; **Resid:** Internal Medicine, Hartford Hospital 1979; Dermatology, Dartmouth-Hitchcock Med Ctr 1982; **Fellow:** Dermatologic Surgery, UCSF Med Ctr 1983; **Fac Appt:** Prof D, Univ Mass Sch Med

Dermatology

Neel, Victor A MD/PhD [D] - **Spec Exp:** Mohs' Surgery; Skin Cancer; Cosmetic Dermatology; **Hospital:** Mass Genl Hosp; **Address:** 50 Staniford St, Ste 270, Boston, MA 02114; **Phone:** 617-726-1869; **Board Cert:** Dermatology 2009; **Med School:** Cornell Univ-Weill Med Coll 1995; **Resid:** Pediatrics, Rhode Island Hosp 1997; Dermatology, Rhode Island Hosp 2000; **Fellow:** Mohs Surgery, UCLA Med Ctr 2001

Olbricht, Suzanne M MD [D] - **Spec Exp:** Skin Cancer; Mohs' Surgery; Muir-Torre Syndrome; **Hospital:** Lahey Clin; **Address:** Lahey Clinic, Dept Dermatology Surgery, 20 Wall St, Burlington, MA 01805; **Phone:** 781-744-8348; **Board Cert:** Internal Medicine 1979; Dermatology 1983; **Med School:** Baylor Coll Med 1976; **Resid:** Internal Medicine, Mass General Hosp 1979; Dermatology, Mass General Hosp 1983; **Fellow:** Mohs Surgery, Mass General Hosp 1991; **Fac Appt:** Assoc Prof D, Harvard Med Sch

Stern, Robert S MD [D] - **Spec Exp:** Psoriasis; Phototherapy; Drug Allergy; Skin Cancer; **Hospital:** Beth Israel Deaconess Med Ctr - Boston; **Address:** Beth Israel Deaconess Med Ctr, Dept Dermatology, 330 Brookline Ave, Boston, MA 02215-5400; **Phone:** 617-667-3689; **Board Cert:** Dermatology 1977; **Med School:** Yale Univ 1970; **Resid:** Dermatology, Mass Genl Hosp 1976; **Fellow:** Epidemiology, NIH 1973; **Fac Appt:** Prof D, Harvard Med Sch

Tsao, Hensin MD/PhD [D] - **Spec Exp:** Melanoma; Melanoma Genetics; Skin Cancer; **Hospital:** Mass Genl Hosp; **Address:** Mass Genl Hosp, Dept Dermatology, 55 Fruit St Edwards Bldg - rm 211, Boston, MA 02114-2543; **Phone:** 617-726-2914; **Board Cert:** Dermatology 2006; **Med School:** Columbia P&S 1993; **Resid:** Dermatology, Brigham & Women's Hosp 1996; **Fellow:** Dermatology, Mass Genl Hosp 1997; **Fac Appt:** Assoc Prof D, Harvard Med Sch

Mid Atlantic

Alster, Tina MD [D] - **Spec Exp:** Skin Laser Surgery; Scar Revision; Birthmarks/Hemangiomas; **Hospital:** Georgetown Univ Hosp; **Address:** 1430 K St NW, Ste 200, Washington Inst of Derm Laser Surgery, Washington, DC 20005; **Phone:** 202-628-8855; **Board Cert:** Dermatology 1990; **Med School:** Duke Univ 1986; **Resid:** Dermatology, Yale Univ 1989; **Fellow:** Dermatologic Laser Surgery, Boston Univ Hosp 1990; **Fac Appt:** Clin Prof D, Georgetown Univ

Anhalt, Grant J MD [D] - **Spec Exp:** Blistering Diseases; Pemphigus; Autoimmune Disease; **Hospital:** Johns Hopkins Hosp (page 61); **Address:** Hopkins at Green Spring Station, 10751 Falls Rd, Ste 304, Lutherville, MD 21093; **Phone:** 410-321-5900; **Board Cert:** Dermatology 2009; Clinical & Laboratory Dematologic Immunology 1987; **Med School:** Canada 1975; **Resid:** Internal Medicine, Hlth Scis Ctr 1977; Dermatology, Univ Mich Med Ctr 1980; **Fellow:** Immunology, Univ Mich Med Ctr 1981; **Fac Appt:** Prof D, Johns Hopkins Univ

Avram, Marc R MD [D] - **Spec Exp:** Hair Restoration/Transplant; Skin Laser Surgery; Cosmetic Dermatology; Botox Therapy; **Hospital:** NY-Presby/Weill Cornell Med Ctr, NY (page 66), SUNY Downstate Med Ctr (Univ Hosp of Bklyn) - LICH; **Address:** 905 5th Ave, MS 10021, New York, NY 10021-2650; **Phone:** 212-734-4007; **Board Cert:** Dermatology 2012; Hair Restoration Surgery 2007; **Med School:** SUNY Downstate 1989; **Resid:** Dermatology, Mass Genl Hosp 1994; **Fac Appt:** Clin Prof D, Cornell Univ-Weill Med Coll

Belsito, Donald V MD [D] - **Spec Exp:** Contact Dermatitis; Cutaneous Lymphoma; Psoriasis; Atopic Dermatitis; **Hospital:** NY-Presby/Columbia Univ Med Ctr, NY (page 66); **Address:** Columbia Doctors Eastside, 16 E 60th St Fl 3 - Ste 300, New York, NY 10022; **Phone:** 212-305-5293; **Board Cert:** Internal Medicine 1979; Dermatology 1983; Clinical & Laboratory Dematologic Immunology 1985; **Med School:** Cornell Univ-Weill Med Coll 1976; **Resid:** Internal Medicine, Case West Res Univ Hosps 1979; Dermatology, NYU Med Ctr 1982; **Fellow:** Dermatologic Research, NYU Med Ctr 1983; **Fac Appt:** Clin Prof D, Columbia P&S

Bernstein, Robert M MD [D] - **Spec Exp:** Hair Restoration/Transplant; Hair Loss in Women; . **Hospital:** NY-Presby/Columbia Univ Med Ctr, NY (page 66); **Address:** 110 E 55th St, Fl 11, New York, NY 10022; **Phone:** 212-826-2400; **Board Cert:** Dermatology 1982; Hair Restoration Surgery 1998; **Med School:** UMDNJ-NJ Med Sch, Newark 1978; **Resid:** Dermatology, Montefiore Med Ctr 1982; **Fac Appt:** Clin Prof D, Columbia P&S

Bickers, David R MD [D] - **Spec Exp:** Skin Cancer; Photodynamic Therapy; Psoriasis; Phototherapy; **Hospital:** NY-Presby/Columbia Univ Med Ctr, NY (page 66); **Address:** 16 E 60th St, Ste 300, New York, NY 10022-1002; **Phone:** 212-326-8465; **Board Cert:** Dermatology 1974; **Med School:** Univ VA Sch Med 1967; **Resid:** Dermatology, NYU Med Ctr 1973; **Fellow:** Pharmacology, Rockefeller Univ Hosp 1974; **Fac Appt:** Prof D, Columbia P&S

Bondi, Edward E MD [D] - **Spec Exp:** Skin Cancer; Melanoma; **Hospital:** Hosp Univ Penn - UPHS (page 72); **Address:** Hospital Univ of Pennsylvania, Rhoads Bldg, 3400 Spruce St Fl 2, Philadelphia, PA 19104; **Phone:** 215-662-2397; **Board Cert:** Dermatology 1978; **Med School:** Hahnemann Univ 1974; **Resid:** Dermatology, Hosp U Penn 1978; **Fac Appt:** Prof D, Univ Pennsylvania

Brandt, Fredric S MD [D] - **Spec Exp:** Botox Therapy; Cosmetic Dermatology; **Address:** Laser & Skin Surgery Ctr, 323 E 34th St Fl 2, New York, NY 10016; **Phone:** 212-889-7096; **Board Cert:** Internal Medicine 1978; Dermatology 1981; **Med School:** Hahnemann Univ 1975; **Resid:** Internal Medicine, VA Hosp 1981; Dermatology, Univ Miami Hosps 1983

Braun III, Martin MD [D] - **Spec Exp:** Mohs' Surgery; Skin Cancer; **Hospital:** G Washington Univ Hosp, Washington Hosp Ctr; **Address:** Braun Dermatology, 2112 F St NW, Ste 701, Washington, DC 20037; **Phone:** 202-293-7618; **Board Cert:** Dermatology 1977; Dermatopathology 1982; **Med School:** Univ MD Sch Med 1970; **Resid:** Dermatology, Univ Mich Med Ctr 1976; **Fellow:** Mohs Surgery, Precept w/ Dr Frederic Mohs 1975; **Fac Appt:** Clin Prof D, Geo Wash Univ

Brodland, David G MD [D] - **Spec Exp:** Mohs' Surgery; Skin Cancer; Reconstructive Surgery-Skin; **Hospital:** UPMC Shadyside; **Address:** Shadyside Medical Bldg, 5200 Centre Ave, Ste 303, Pittsburgh, PA 15232; **Phone:** 412-681-9400; **Board Cert:** Dermatology 1989; **Med School:** Southern IL Univ 1985; **Resid:** Dermatology, Mayo Clinic 1989; **Fellow:** Mohs Surgery, John A Zitelli MD 1990; **Fac Appt:** Asst Prof D, Univ Pittsburgh

Brown, Marc D MD [D] - **Spec Exp:** Skin Cancer; Mohs' Surgery; Melanoma; **Hospital:** Univ of Rochester Strong Meml Hosp; **Address:** University Dermatology Assoc, 601 Elmwood Ave Box 697, Rochester, NY 14642; **Phone:** 585-275-9208; **Board Cert:** Dermatology 2009; **Med School:** Georgetown Univ 1979; **Resid:** Internal Medicine, Strong Meml Hosp/Univ Rochester 1982; Dermatology, Univ Mich Hosps 1987; **Fellow:** Cutaneous Oncology, Univ Mich Hosps 1989

Cohen, Bernard A MD [D] - **Spec Exp:** Pediatric Dermatology; Skin Laser Surgery; Hemangiomas; Vascular Malformations; **Hospital:** Johns Hopkins Hosp (page 61); **Address:** Johns Hopkins Div Ped Dermatology, Rubenstein Child Health Bldg, 200 N Wolfe St Fl 1, Baltimore, MD 21287; **Phone:** 410-955-2049; **Board Cert:** Pediatrics 1982; Dermatology 1984; Pediatric Dermatology 2004; **Med School:** Johns Hopkins Univ 1977; **Resid:** Pediatrics, Johns Hopkins Hosp 1980; Dermatology, Johns Hopkins Hosp 1984; **Fac Appt:** Prof D, Johns Hopkins Univ

Cotsarelis, George MD [D] - **Spec Exp:** Hair Loss; Scalp Disorders; **Hospital:** Hosp Univ Penn - UPHS (page 72); **Address:** Perelman Ctr for Advanced Medicine, 3400 Civic Center Blvd, Ste 330-1 South, Philadelphia, PA 19104; **Phone:** 215-662-2737; **Board Cert:** Dermatology 2010; **Med School:** Univ Pennsylvania 1987; **Resid:** Dermatology, Hosp Univ Penn 1992; **Fellow:** Dermatology, Hosp Univ Penn; **Fac Appt:** Prof D, Univ Pennsylvania

Dermatology

DeLeo, Vincent A MD [D] - **Spec Exp:** Photosensitive Skin Diseases; Contact Dermatitis; Facial Rejuvenation; Eczema; **Hospital:** St. Luke's - Roosevelt Hosp Ctr - Roosevelt Div (page 56), Beth Israel Med Ctr - Petrie Division (page 56); **Address:** 1090 Amsterdam Ave, Fl 11, New York, NY 10025; **Phone:** 212-523-5898; **Board Cert:** Dermatology 2009; **Med School:** Louisiana State U, New Orleans 1969; **Resid:** Dermatology, Columbia-Presby Med Ctr 1976; **Fac Appt:** Clin Prof D, Columbia P&S

Dzubow, Leonard M MD [D] - **Spec Exp:** Mohs' Surgery; Skin Cancer; **Address:** 101 Chesley Drive, Media, PA 19063; **Phone:** 484-621-0082; **Board Cert:** Internal Medicine 1978; Dermatology 2009; **Med School:** Univ Pennsylvania 1975; **Resid:** Internal Medicine, Hosp Univ Penn 1978; Dermatology, NYU-Skin Cancer Unit 1980; **Fellow:** Mohs Surgery, NYU-Skin Cancer Unit 1981

Franks Jr, Andrew G MD [D] - **Spec Exp:** Lupus/SLE; Raynaud's Disease; Scleroderma; Dermatomyositis; **Hospital:** NYU Langone Med Ctr (page 68); **Address:** NYU Dermatologic Assocs, Faculty Practice Tower, 530 First Ave Fl 7 - Ste 7R, New York, NY 10016; **Phone:** 212-263-5889; **Board Cert:** Internal Medicine 1975; Dermatology 1977; Rheumatology 1978; **Med School:** NY Med Coll 1971; **Resid:** Internal Medicine, Beth Israel Med Ctr 1974; Dermatology, Columbia-Presby Med Ctr 1975; **Fellow:** Rheumatology, Columbia-Presby Med Ctr 1977; **Fac Appt:** Prof D, NYU Sch Med

Geronemus, Roy G MD [D] - **Spec Exp:** Skin Laser Surgery; Cosmetic Dermatology; Mohs' Surgery; Skin Cancer; **Hospital:** New York Eye & Ear Infirm (page 65); **Address:** 317 E 34 St, Ste 11N, New York, NY 10016-4974; **Phone:** 212-686-7306; **Board Cert:** Dermatology 1983; **Med School:** Univ Miami Sch Med 1979; **Resid:** Dermatology, NYU-Skin Cancer Unit 1983; **Fellow:** Mohs Surgery, NYU-Skin Cancer Unit 1984; **Fac Appt:** Clin Prof D, NYU Sch Med

Gordon, Marsha MD [D] - **Spec Exp:** Cosmetic Dermatology; Botox Therapy; Facial Rejuvenation; **Hospital:** Mount Sinai Med Ctr (page 64); **Address:** 5 E 98th St Fl 5, New York, NY 10029-6574; **Phone:** 212-241-9728; **Board Cert:** Dermatology 1988; **Med School:** Univ Pennsylvania 1984; **Resid:** Dermatology, Mt Sinai Hosp 1988; **Fac Appt:** Clin Prof D, Mount Sinai Sch Med

Greenbaum, Steven S MD [D] - **Spec Exp:** Mohs' Surgery; Skin Cancer; Cosmetic Dermatology; **Hospital:** Thomas Jefferson Univ Hosp, Hahnemann Univ Hosp; **Address:** 1528 Walnut St Fl 11 - Ste 1101, Philadelphia, PA 19102; **Phone:** 215-735-4994; **Board Cert:** Dermatology 1987; **Med School:** Tulane Univ 1983; **Resid:** Dermatology, Henry Ford Hosp 1987; **Fellow:** Mohs Surgery, UCSF Med Ctr 1988; **Fac Appt:** Clin Prof D, Drexel Univ Coll Med

Grossman, Melanie MD [D] - **Spec Exp:** Skin Laser Surgery; Facial Rejuvenation; Body Contouring; Cosmetic Dermatology; **Hospital:** NY-Presby/Columbia Univ Med Ctr, NY (page 66); **Address:** 161 Madison Ave, Ste 4NW, New York, NY 10016-5405; **Phone:** 212-725-8600; **Board Cert:** Dermatology 2010; **Med School:** NYU Sch Med 1988; **Resid:** Internal Medicine, Yale-New Haven Hosp 1989; Dermatology, Columbia-Presby Med Ctr 1992; **Fellow:** Laser Surgery, Mass Genl Hosp 1995; **Fac Appt:** Asst Clin Prof D, Columbia P&S

Halpern, Allan C MD [D] - **Spec Exp:** Skin Cancer; Melanoma; Melanoma Early Detection/Prevention; **Hospital:** Meml Sloan-Kettering Cancer Ctr; **Address:** 160 E 53rd St Fl 2, New York, NY 10022; **Phone:** 212-610-0766; **Board Cert:** Internal Medicine 1984; Dermatology 1988; **Med School:** Albert Einstein Coll Med 1981; **Resid:** Internal Medicine, Montefiore Hosp 1985; Dermatology, Hosp Univ Penn 1989; **Fellow:** Epidemiology, Hosp Univ Penn 1989; **Fac Appt:** Assoc Prof Med, Cornell Univ-Weill Med Coll

James, William D MD [D] - **Spec Exp:** Contact Dermatitis; Acne; Rosacea; **Hospital:** Hosp Univ Penn - UPHS (page 72); **Address:** Univ Penn Dept Dermatology, 3400 Spruce St, 2 Maloney, Philadelphia, PA 19104; **Phone:** 215-662-4282; **Board Cert:** Dermatology 1981; Diagnostic Lab Immunology 1985; **Med School:** Indiana Univ 1977; **Resid:** Dermatology, Letterman Army Med Ctr 1981; **Fac Appt:** Prof D, Univ Pennsylvania

Kalb, Robert E MD [D] - **Spec Exp:** Psoriasis; Phototherapy; **Hospital:** Buffalo General Hosp; **Address:** Buffalo Med Grp, 325 Essjay Rd, Ste 210, Williamsville, NY 14221; **Phone:** 716-630-1102; **Board Cert:** Dermatology 1986; **Med School:** SUNY Downstate 1982; **Resid:** Dermatology, Columbia Presby Med Ctr 1986; **Fac Appt:** Clin Prof D, SUNY Buffalo

Kress, Douglas W MD [D] - **Spec Exp:** Pediatric Dermatology; **Hospital:** Chldns Hosp of Pittsburgh - UPMC; **Address:** Chldn's Dermatology Ctr, 11279 Perry Hwy, Ste 108, Wexford, PA 15090; **Phone:** 724-933-9190; **Board Cert:** Dermatology 2006; Pediatric Dermatology 2004; **Med School:** Jefferson Med Coll 1992; **Resid:** Dermatology, Univ Pittsburgh Med Ctr 1996; **Fellow:** Pediatric Dermatology, Children's Hosp 2003; **Fac Appt:** Assoc Clin Prof D, Univ Pittsburgh

Kriegel, David MD [D] - **Spec Exp:** Mohs' Surgery; Laser Surgery; Skin Cancer; Cosmetic Surgery; **Hospital:** Mount Sinai Med Ctr (page 64); **Address:** 250 W 57th St, Ste 825, New York, NY 10107-0809; **Phone:** 212-489-6669; **Board Cert:** Dermatology 2003; **Med School:** Boston Univ 1987; **Resid:** Dermatology, New England Med Ctr 1991; **Fellow:** Mohs Surgery, Stony Brook Univ Hosp 1993; **Fac Appt:** Assoc Prof D, Mount Sinai Sch Med

Lebwohl, Mark G MD [D] - **Spec Exp:** Skin Cancer; Psoriasis; Cutaneous Lymphoma; Pseudoxanthoma Elasticum; **Hospital:** Mount Sinai Med Ctr (page 64); **Address:** 5 E 98th St, Fl 5, New York, NY 10029-6501; **Phone:** 212-241-9728; **Board Cert:** Internal Medicine 1981; Dermatology 1983; **Med School:** Harvard Med Sch 1978; **Resid:** Internal Medicine, Mt Sinai Hosp 1981; Dermatology, Mt Sinai Hosp 1983; **Fellow:** Dermatology, Mt Sinai Hosp 1983; **Fac Appt:** Prof D, Mount Sinai Sch Med

Lessin, Stuart R MD [D] - **Spec Exp:** Cutaneous Lymphoma; Skin Cancer; Melanoma Risk Assessment; Mycosis Fungoides; **Hospital:** Bryn Mawr Hosp; **Address:** Bryn Mawr Skin & Cancer Ctr, 919 Conestoga Rd, Bldg 2 - Ste 106, Rosemont, PA 19010; **Phone:** 610-525-5028; **Board Cert:** Dermatology 1986; **Med School:** Temple Univ 1982; **Resid:** Dermatology, Hosp Univ Penn 1986; **Fellow:** Molecular Biology, Wistar Inst 1987; **Fac Appt:** Prof D, Temple Univ

Lowitt, Mark H MD [D] - **Spec Exp:** Skin Cancer; Melanoma; Acne; Eczema; **Hospital:** Greater Baltimore Med Ctr; **Address:** 6565 N Charles St, Ste 315, Baltimore, MD 21204; **Phone:** 410-321-1195; **Board Cert:** Dermatology 2012; **Med School:** Tulane Univ 1987; **Resid:** Internal Medicine, New England Deaconess Hosp 1990; **Fellow:** Dermatology, Univ Maryland 1993; **Fac Appt:** Assoc Clin Prof D, Univ MD Sch Med

Miller, Stanley J MD [D] - **Spec Exp:** Skin Cancer; Mohs' Surgery; Melanoma; **Hospital:** Johns Hopkins Hosp (page 61), Univ of MD Med Ctr; **Address:** Charles Towson Bldg, 1104 Kenilworth Drive, Ste 201, Towson, MD 21204; **Phone:** 443-279-0340; **Board Cert:** Dermatology 2009; **Med School:** Univ VT Coll Med 1984; **Resid:** Dermatology, UCSD Med Ctr 1989; **Fellow:** Dermatologic Surgery, Univ Penn 1991; **Fac Appt:** Assoc Prof D, Johns Hopkins Univ

Nigra, Thomas P MD [D] - **Spec Exp:** Hair Loss; Psoriasis; Skin Cancer; Vitiligo; **Hospital:** Washington Hosp Ctr, Natl Rehab Hosp; **Address:** Dermatology Assocs, 110 Irving St NW, Ste 2B28, Washington, DC 20010; **Phone:** 202-877-6227; **Board Cert:** Dermatology 1973; **Med School:** Univ Pennsylvania 1967; **Resid:** Dermatology, Mass Genl Hosp 1973; Dermatology, Natl Inst of Health 1971; **Fac Appt:** Clin Prof D, Geo Wash Univ

Orlow, Seth J MD/PhD [D] - **Spec Exp:** Pediatric Dermatology; Birthmarks/Hemangiomas; Psoriasis/Eczema; **Hospital:** NYU Langone Med Ctr (page 68); **Address:** 530 1st Ave, Ste 7R, New York, NY 10016-6402; **Phone:** 212-263-5889; **Board Cert:** Dermatology 2009; Pediatric Dermatology 2004; **Med School:** Albert Einstein Coll Med 1986; **Resid:** Pediatrics, Mt Sinai Hosp 1987; Dermatology, Yale-New Haven Hosp 1989; **Fellow:** Pediatric Dermatology, Yale-New Haven Hosp 1990; **Fac Appt:** Prof D, NYU Sch Med

Prioleau, Philip G MD [D] - **Spec Exp:** Melanoma; Skin Cancer; Mohs' Surgery; **Hospital:** NY-Presby/Weill Cornell Med Ctr, NY (page 66); **Address:** 1035 Fifth Ave, Ste C, New York, NY 10028; **Phone:** 212-794-3548; **Board Cert:** Surgery 1973; Anatomic Pathology 1979; Dermatopathology 1980; Dermatology 1983; **Med School:** Med Univ SC 1967; **Resid:** Surgery, Univ Va Hosp 1972; Plastic Surgery, Duke Univ Hosp 1975; **Fellow:** Pathology, Barnes Jewish Hosp 1980; Dermatopathology, NYU Med Ctr 1981; **Fac Appt:** Assoc Prof D, Cornell Univ-Weill Med Coll

Ramsay, David L MD [D] - **Spec Exp:** Cutaneous Lymphoma; Skin Cancer; **Hospital:** NYU Langone Med Ctr (page 68); **Address:** 530 1st Ave, Ste 7G, New York, NY 10016-6402; **Phone:** 212-683-6283; **Board Cert:** Dermatology 1974; **Med School:** Indiana Univ 1969; **Resid:** Dermatology, NYU Med Ctr 1973; **Fellow:** Dermatology, Univ Ill Hosp 1973; **Fac Appt:** Clin Prof D, NYU Sch Med

Ratner, Desiree MD [D] - **Spec Exp:** Mohs' Surgery; Skin Cancer; Dermatologic Surgery; **Hospital:** NY-Presby/Columbia Univ Med Ctr, NY (page 66); **Address:** Columbia Presbyterian Med Ctr, 161 Fort Washington Ave Fl 12, New York, NY 10032; **Phone:** 212-305-3625; **Board Cert:** Dermatology 2003; **Med School:** Johns Hopkins Univ 1989; **Resid:** Dermatology, Univ Michigan Med Ctr 1993; **Fellow:** Mohs Surgery, New England Med Ctr 1994; Mohs Surgery, Lahey Clinic 1995; **Fac Appt:** Prof D, Columbia P&S

Rigel, Darrell S MD [D] - **Spec Exp:** Melanoma; Skin Cancer; Cosmetic Dermatology; **Hospital:** NYU Langone Med Ctr (page 68), Mount Sinai Med Ctr (page 64); **Address:** 35 E 35th Street, Ste 208, New York, NY 10016-3823; **Phone:** 212-684-5964; **Board Cert:** Dermatology 1983; **Med School:** Geo Wash Univ 1978; **Resid:** Dermatology, NYU Med Ctr 1982; **Fellow:** Dermatologic Surgery, NYU Med Ctr 1983; **Fac Appt:** Clin Prof D, NYU Sch Med

Rook, Alain H MD [D] - **Spec Exp:** Cutaneous Lymphoma; Immune Deficiency-Skin Disorders; Mycosis Fungoides; Cutaneous T-cell Lymphoma; **Hospital:** Hosp Univ Penn - UPHS (page 72); **Address:** Dept Dermatology, Perelman Center, Fl 1, Ste 330-S, 3400 Civic Center Blvd, Philadelphia, PA 19104-4283; **Phone:** 215-662-7610; **Board Cert:** Internal Medicine 1979; Nephrology 1980; Dermatology 2011; **Med School:** Univ Mich Med Sch 1975; **Resid:** Internal Medicine, McGill Univ Med Ctr 1977; Dermatology, Hosp Univ Penn 1989; **Fellow:** Nephrology, McGill Univ Med Ctr 1979; Immunology, NIH 1986; **Fac Appt:** Prof D, Univ Pennsylvania

Schultz, Neal MD [D] - **Spec Exp:** Cosmetic Dermatology; Melanoma Early Detection/Prevention; Skin Laser Surgery; Tattoo Removal; **Hospital:** Mount Sinai Med Ctr (page 64); **Address:** 1130 Park Ave, New York, NY 10128; **Phone:** 212-369-9600; **Board Cert:** Dermatology 1978; **Med School:** Columbia P&S 1973; **Resid:** Internal Medicine, Mt Sinai Hosp 1975; Dermatology, Mt Sinai Hosp 1978; **Fac Appt:** Asst Clin Prof D, Mount Sinai Sch Med

Shupack, Jerome L MD [D] - **Spec Exp:** Rare Skin Disorders; Psoriasis; Eczema; Blistering Diseases; **Hospital:** NYU Langone Med Ctr (page 68); **Address:** 530 1st Ave, HCC 7F, New York, NY 10016-6402; **Phone:** 212-263-7344; **Board Cert:** Dermatology 1970; **Med School:** Columbia P&S 1963; **Resid:** Internal Medicine, Mt Sinai Hosp 1965; Dermatology, NYU Med Ctr 1970; **Fac Appt:** Prof D, NYU Sch Med

Soter, Nicholas A MD [D] - **Spec Exp:** Urticaria; Psoriasis; Vasculitis; Phototherapy; **Hospital:** NYU Langone Med Ctr (page 68); **Address:** 240 E 38th St Fl 12, New York, NY 10016-6402; **Phone:** 212-263-5889; **Board Cert:** Dermatology 1970; Diagnostic Lab Immunology 1985; **Med School:** Univ Tex SW, Dallas 1965; **Resid:** Dermatology, Baylor Med Ctr 1968; Dermatology, Mass Genl Hosp 1969; **Fellow:** Immunology, Harvard Med Sch 1973; **Fac Appt:** Prof D, NYU Sch Med

Stanley, John R MD [D] - **Spec Exp:** Blistering Diseases; Pemphigus; **Hospital:** Hosp Univ Penn - UPHS (page 72); **Address:** Perelman Ctr for Advanced Medicine, 3400 Civic Center Blvd, Ste 330 - 1 South, Philadelphia, PA 19104; **Phone:** 215-662-2737; **Board Cert:** Dermatology 1978; Clinical & Laboratory Dematologic Immunology 1985; **Med School:** Harvard Med Sch 1974; **Resid:** Dermatology, NYU Med Ctr 1978; **Fac Appt:** Prof D, Univ Pennsylvania

Werth, Victoria P MD [D] - **Spec Exp:** Autoimmune Disease; Lupus/SLE; Connective Tissue Disorders; Blistering Diseases; **Hospital:** Hosp Univ Penn - UPHS (page 72); **Address:** Perelman Ctr for Advanced Medicine, 3400 Civic Ctr Blvd, Ste 330 - 1 South, Philadelphia, PA 19104; **Phone:** 215-662-2737; **Board Cert:** Internal Medicine 1983; Dermatology 1986; Diagnostic Lab Immunology 1989; **Med School:** Johns Hopkins Univ 1980; **Resid:** Internal Medicine, Northwestern Meml Hosp 1983; Dermatology, NYU Med Ctr 1986; **Fellow:** Immunological Dermatology, NYU 1988; **Fac Appt:** Prof D, Univ Pennsylvania

Yan, Albert C MD [D] - **Spec Exp:** Pediatric Dermatology; Hemangiomas; Genetic Disorders-Skin; Atopic Dermatitis; **Hospital:** Chldns Hosp of Philadelphia, Hosp Univ Penn - UPHS (page 72); **Address:** Chldn's Hosp of Philadelphia, Dept Dermatology, 34th & Civic Ctr Blvd, Philadelphia, PA 19104; **Phone:** 215-590-2169; **Board Cert:** Pediatrics 2004; Dermatology 2008; Pediatric Dermatology 2004; **Med School:** Univ Pennsylvania 1993; **Resid:** Pediatrics, Chldn's Hosp 1996; Dermatology, Hosp Univ Penn 1999; **Fac Appt:** Assoc Prof Ped, Univ Pennsylvania

Zitelli, John MD [D] - **Spec Exp:** Mohs' Surgery; Skin Cancer; Melanoma; Reconstructive Surgery-Skin; **Hospital:** UPMC Shadyside; **Address:** Shadyside Medical Bldg, 5200 Centre Ave, Ste 303, Pittsburgh, PA 15232; **Phone:** 412-681-9400; **Board Cert:** Dermatology 2009; **Med School:** Univ Pittsburgh 1976; **Resid:** Dermatology, Univ Hlth Ctr Hosp 1979; **Fellow:** Mohs Surgery, Univ Wisconsin 1980; **Fac Appt:** Assoc Clin Prof D, Univ Pittsburgh

Southeast

Amonette, Rex A MD [D] - **Spec Exp:** Skin Cancer; Mohs' Surgery; **Address:** Memphis Dermatology Clin, 1455 Union Ave, Memphis, TN 38104-6727; **Phone:** 901-726-6655; **Board Cert:** Dermatology 1974; **Med School:** Univ Ark 1966; **Resid:** Dermatology, Univ Tenn Med Ctr 1971; **Fellow:** Mohs Surgery, NYU Med Ctr 1972; **Fac Appt:** Clin Prof D, Univ Tenn Coll Med

Brody, Harold J MD [D] - **Spec Exp:** Cosmetic Dermatology; Dermatologic Surgery; Facial Rejuvenation; Skin Laser Surgery-Resurfacing; **Hospital:** Emory Univ Hosp Midtown; **Address:** 1218 W Paces Ferry Rd, Ste 200, Atlanta, GA 30327; **Phone:** 404-525-7409; **Board Cert:** Dermatology 1978; **Med School:** Med Univ SC 1974; **Resid:** Dermatology, Emory Affil Hosps 1978; **Fac Appt:** Clin Prof D, Emory Univ

Burton III, Claude S MD [D] - **Spec Exp:** Skin Laser Surgery; **Hospital:** Duke Univ Hosp; **Address:** Duke Univ Med Ctr, Box 3511, Durham, NC 27710; **Phone:** 919-684-3432; **Board Cert:** Internal Medicine 1982; Dermatology 1984; **Med School:** Duke Univ 1979; **Resid:** Internal Medicine, Duke Univ Med Ctr 1982; Dermatology, Duke Univ Med Ctr 1984; **Fac Appt:** Prof D, Duke Univ

Dermatology

Callen, Jeffrey P MD [D] - **Spec Exp:** Lupus/SLE; Dermatomyositis; Vasculitis; Psoriasis; **Hospital:** Univ of Louisville Hosp, Kosair Chldn's Hosp; **Address:** 310 E Broadway, Ste 200, Louisville, KY 40202; **Phone:** 502-583-1749; **Board Cert:** Internal Medicine 1975; Dermatology 2009; **Med School:** Univ Mich Med Sch 1972; **Resid:** Internal Medicine, Univ Mich Med Ctr 1975; Dermatology, Univ Mich Med Ctr 1977; **Fac Appt:** Prof Med, Univ Louisville Sch Med

Camisa, Charles MD [D] - **Spec Exp:** Psoriasis; Oral Dermatology; Lichen Planus; Cutaneous T-cell Lymphoma; **Address:** Riverchase Dermatology, 261 9th St S, Naples, FL 34102; **Phone:** 239-216-4337; **Board Cert:** Dermatology 1981; Clinical & Laboratory Dematologic Immunology 1987; **Med School:** Mount Sinai Sch Med 1977; **Resid:** Dermatology, NYU Med Ctr 1981; **Fac Appt:** Assoc Prof D, Univ S Fla Coll Med

Cohen, Bernard H MD [D] - **Spec Exp:** Hair Restoration/Transplant; Hair Loss; **Address:** The Hair Loss Ctr, 550 Biltmore Way, Ste 870, Coral Gables, FL 33134; **Phone:** 305-443-9977; **Board Cert:** Dermatology 1972; Hair Restoration Surgery ; **Med School:** Columbia P&S 1967; **Resid:** Dermatology, NYU Med Ctr 1971; **Fac Appt:** Clin Prof D, Univ Miami Sch Med

Cook, Jonathan L MD [D] - **Spec Exp:** Skin Cancer; Mohs' Surgery; Reconstructive Surgery-Skin; Skin Laser Surgery; **Hospital:** Duke Univ Hosp; **Address:** DUMC, Box 3915, 5324 McFarland Drive, Ste 400, Durham, NC 27707; **Phone:** 919-419-4945; **Board Cert:** Dermatology 2005; **Med School:** Med Univ SC 1992; **Resid:** Dermatology, Emory Univ Hosp 1996; **Fellow:** Dermatologic Surgery, Hosp Univ Penn 1997; **Fac Appt:** Prof D, Duke Univ

Eichler, Craig J MD [D] - **Spec Exp:** Skin Cancer; Dermatologic Surgery; **Hospital:** Physicians Regl Hlthcare Med Ctr-Pine Ridge; **Address:** 6101 Pine Ridge Rd, Naples, FL 34119; **Phone:** 239-348-4325; **Board Cert:** Dermatology 2003; **Med School:** Univ Fla Coll Med 1989; **Resid:** Dermatology, Univ Texas Med Branch 1993

Elmets, Craig A MD [D] - **Spec Exp:** Psoriasis/Eczema; Phototherapy; Contact Dermatitis; Photodynamic Therapy; **Hospital:** Univ of Ala Hosp at Birmingham, Birmingham, Alabama VA Med Ctr; **Address:** 1530 3rd Ave S, EFH Bldg, rm 414, Birmingham, AL 35294; **Phone:** 205-996-7546; **Board Cert:** Internal Medicine 1978; Dermatology 2009; Clinical & Laboratory Dematologic Immunology 1989; **Med School:** Univ Iowa Coll Med 1975; **Resid:** Internal Medicine, Kansas Med Ctr 1978; Dermatology, Univ Iowa Hosps 1980; **Fellow:** Immunological Dermatology, Univ Texas Hlth Sci Ctr 1982; **Fac Appt:** Prof D, Univ Alabama

Fenske, Neil A MD [D] - **Spec Exp:** Skin Cancer; Melanoma; Psoriasis; **Hospital:** H Lee Moffitt Cancer Ctr & Research Inst (page 59), Tampa Genl Hosp; **Address:** 12901 Bruce B Downs Blvd, MDC-79, Tampa, FL 33612; **Phone:** 813-974-4744; **Board Cert:** Dermatology 1977; Dermatopathology 1984; **Med School:** St Louis Univ 1973; **Resid:** Dermatology, Wisc Hlth Sci Ctr 1977; **Fac Appt:** Prof Med, Univ S Fla Coll Med

Flowers, Franklin P MD [D] - **Spec Exp:** Mohs' Surgery; Dermatopathology; **Hospital:** Malcolm Randall VA Med Ctr; **Address:** Shands Healthcare, PO Box 100383, Gainesville, FL 32608; **Phone:** 352-376-1611; **Board Cert:** Dermatology 1976; Dermatopathology 1981; **Med School:** Univ Fla Coll Med 1971; **Resid:** Dermatology, Ohio State Univ 1975; **Fellow:** Mohs Surgery, Univ Alabama 1993; **Fac Appt:** Prof Med, Univ Fla Coll Med

Garrett, Algin MD [D] - **Spec Exp:** Skin Cancer; Mohs' Surgery; **Hospital:** Med Coll of VA Hosp; **Address:** Stonypoint Medical Park, 9000 Stonypoint Pkwy Fl 2, Richmond, VA 23235; **Phone:** 804-560-8991; **Board Cert:** Dermatology 1983; **Med School:** Penn State Coll Med 1978; **Resid:** Internal Medicine, VA Med Ctr 1980; Dermatology, Med Col VA 1983; **Fellow:** Mohs Surgery, Cleveland Clin Fdn 1988; **Fac Appt:** Prof D, Va Commonwealth Univ Sch Med

Green, Howard A MD [D] - **Spec Exp:** Mohs' Surgery; Skin Cancer; **Hospital:** St. Mary's Med Ctr - W Palm Bch; **Address:** 120 Butler St, Ste A, West Palm Beach, FL 33407-6106; **Phone:** 561-659-1510; **Board Cert:** Internal Medicine 1988; Dermatology 2011; **Med School:** Boston Univ 1985; **Resid:** Internal Medicine, Jefferson Univ Hosp 1988; Dermatology, Harvard Affil Hosps 1992; **Fellow:** Mohs Surgery, Boston Univ Med Ctr 1993

Grichnik, James M MD/PhD [D] - **Spec Exp:** Melanoma; Skin Cancer; Photodynamic Therapy; **Hospital:** Univ of Miami Hosp & Clins/Sylvester Comp Canc Ctr; **Address:** 1501 NW 10th Ave, BRB Bldg, rm 912, Miami, FL 33136; **Phone:** 305-243-6045; **Board Cert:** Dermatology 2003; **Med School:** Harvard Med Sch 1990; **Resid:** Dermatology, Duke Univ Med Ctr 1994; **Fac Appt:** Prof D, Univ Miami Sch Med

Johr, Robert MD [D] - **Spec Exp:** Pigmented Lesions; Melanoma; Pediatric Dermatology; **Hospital:** Boca Raton Regl Hosp, Univ of Miami Hosp & Clins/Sylvester Comp Canc Ctr; **Address:** 1050 NW 15th St, Ste 201A, Boca Raton, FL 33486-1341; **Phone:** 561-368-4545; **Board Cert:** Dermatology 1981; **Med School:** Mexico 1975; **Resid:** Dermatology, Roswell Park Cancer Ctr 1977; Dermatology, Metro Med Ctr 1979; **Fac Appt:** Clin Prof D, Univ Miami Sch Med

Jorizzo, Joseph L MD [D] - **Spec Exp:** Rheumatologic Dermatology; Immune Deficiency-Skin Disorders; Complex Diagnosis; Behcet's Syndrome; **Hospital:** Wake Forest Baptist Med Ctr; **Address:** Wake Forest Univ Sch Med, Dept Derm, 4618 Country Club Rd, Winston-Salem, NC 27104; **Phone:** 336-716-3926; **Board Cert:** Dermatology 1979; **Med School:** Boston Univ 1975; **Resid:** Dermatology, UNC Meml Hosp 1979; **Fellow:** Dermatology, Dermatology Inst 1980; **Fac Appt:** Prof D, Wake Forest Univ

Kirsner, Robert S MD/PhD [D] - **Spec Exp:** Wound Healing/Care; Leg Ulcers; **Hospital:** Univ of Miami Hosp, Jackson Meml Hosp; **Address:** Univ Miami, Dept Dermatology, 1295 NW 14th St South Bldg - Ste M, Miami, FL 33125; **Phone:** 305-243-6704; **Board Cert:** Dermatology 2005; **Med School:** Univ Miami Sch Med 1988; **Resid:** Internal Medicine, Univ Miami-Jackson Meml Hosp 1990; Dermatology, Univ Miami-Jackson Meml Hosp 1995; **Fellow:** Wound Healing, Univ Miami-Jackson Meml Hosp 1992; **Fac Appt:** Prof D, Univ Miami Sch Med

Leshin, Barry MD [D] - **Spec Exp:** Skin Cancer; Mohs' Surgery; **Address:** 1450 Professional Park Drive, Ste 150, Winston-Salem, NC 27103; **Phone:** 336-724-2434; **Board Cert:** Dermatology 2009; **Med School:** Univ Tex, Houston 1981; **Resid:** Dermatology, Univ Iowa Hosp 1985; **Fellow:** Dermatologic Surgery, Univ Iowa Hosp 1986; **Fac Appt:** Clin Prof PlS, Wake Forest Univ

McMichael, Amy J MD [D] - **Spec Exp:** Hair Loss; Ethnic Skin Disorders; Pigmented Lesions; Skin Cancer; **Hospital:** Wake Forest Baptist Med Ctr; **Address:** Wake Forest Univ Baptist Med Ctr, 4618 Country Club Rd, Winston-Salem, NC 27104; **Phone:** 336-716-3926; **Board Cert:** Dermatology 2004; **Med School:** Univ Pennsylvania 1990; **Resid:** Dermatology, Univ Mich Hosps 1994

Nouri, Keyvan MD [D] - **Spec Exp:** Mohs' Surgery; Skin Cancer; **Hospital:** Univ of Miami Hosp & Clins/Sylvester Comp Canc Ctr; **Address:** Univ Miami Hosp, Dept Derm, 1295 NW 14th St South Bldg Fl 2, Miami, FL 33136; **Phone:** 305-243-4183; **Board Cert:** Dermatology 2005; **Med School:** Boston Univ 1993; **Resid:** Dermatology, Univ of Miami Hosp 1997; **Fellow:** Dermatologic Surgery, NYU Med Ctr 1999; **Fac Appt:** Prof D, Univ Miami Sch Med

Olsen, Elise A MD [D] - **Spec Exp:** Cutaneous Lymphoma; Hair Loss; Hirsutism; **Hospital:** Duke Univ Hosp; **Address:** Duke Univ Med Ctr, Box 3294, Durham, NC 27710; **Phone:** 919-684-3432; **Board Cert:** Dermatology 1983; **Med School:** Baylor Coll Med 1978; **Resid:** Internal Medicine, Univ NC Meml Hosp 1980; Dermatology, Duke Univ Med Ctr 1983; **Fac Appt:** Prof D, Duke Univ

Dermatology

Russell, Mark A MD [D] - **Spec Exp:** Skin Cancer; Mohs' Surgery; Dermatofibrosarcoma Protruberans; Microcystic Adnexal Carcinoma; **Hospital:** Univ of Virginia Health Sys; **Address:** 1221 Lee St, PCC Bldg - Fl 3rd, Box 800718, Charlottesville, VA 22908; **Phone:** 434-924-5599; **Board Cert:** Dermatology 2005; Dermatopathology 2001; **Med School:** Ohio State Univ 1993; **Resid:** Dermatology, Vanderbilt Univ Med Ctr 1997; **Fellow:** Mohs Surgery, Vanderbilt Univ Med Ctr 1999; Dermatopathology, Univ Virginia Hlth System 2000; **Fac Appt:** Assoc Prof Med, Univ VA Sch Med

Sherertz, Elizabeth F MD [D] - **Spec Exp:** Eczema; Contact Dermatitis; Occupational Skin Diseases; **Hospital:** Waccamaw Community Hosp; **Address:** Dermatology Assoc of Waccamaw, Waccamaw Medical Park-East, 4033 Highway 17 Bypass, Ste 105, Murrells Inlet, SC 29576; **Phone:** 843-652-8110; **Board Cert:** Dermatology 1982; **Med School:** Univ VA Sch Med 1978; **Resid:** Dermatology, Duke Univ Med Ctr 1982; **Fac Appt:** Clin Prof D, Wake Forest Univ

Sobel, Stuart A MD [D] - **Spec Exp:** Skin Cancer; Cosmetic Dermatology; Pemphigus; Skin Laser Surgery; **Hospital:** Meml Regl Hosp, Joe DiMaggio Chldns Hosp; **Address:** 4340 Sheridan St, Ste 101, Hollywood, FL 33021-3511; **Phone:** 954-983-5533; **Board Cert:** Dermatology 2009; **Med School:** Tufts Univ 1972; **Resid:** Dermatology, Mt Sinai Hosp 1976

Sokoloff, Daniel O MD [D] - **Spec Exp:** Skin Cancer; Cosmetic Dermatology; **Hospital:** Good Sam Med Ctr - W Palm Beach, St. Mary's Med Ctr - W Palm Bch; **Address:** Palm Beach Dermatology, 4475 Medical Center Way, Ste 2, West Palm Beach, FL 33407; **Phone:** 561-863-1000; **Board Cert:** Dermatology 1982; **Med School:** Geo Wash Univ 1977; **Resid:** Dermatology, Baylor Med Ctr 1982

Thiers, Bruce H MD [D] - **Spec Exp:** Cutaneous Lymphoma; Skin Cancer; Psoriasis; **Hospital:** MUSC Med Ctr; **Address:** 135 Rutledge Ave, MS 578, Fl 11, Charleston, SC 29425; **Phone:** 843-792-9784; **Board Cert:** Dermatology 1978; **Med School:** SUNY Buffalo 1974; **Resid:** Dermatology, SUNY Buffalo Med Ctr 1978; **Fac Appt:** Prof D, Med Univ SC

Midwest

Arpey, Christopher J MD [D] - **Spec Exp:** Mohs' Surgery; Skin Cancer; Skin Laser Surgery; Wound Healing/Care; **Hospital:** Mayo Med Ctr & Clin - Rochester; **Address:** Mayo Clinic - Dept Dermatology, 200 First St SW, Rochester, MN 55905; **Phone:** 507-284-2536; **Board Cert:** Dermatology 2011; Internal Medicine 1989; **Med School:** Univ Rochester 1986; **Resid:** Internal Medicine, Univ Iowa Hosps & Clinics 1989; Dermatology, Univ Hosps 1992; **Fellow:** Mohs Surgery, Univ Iowa Hosps & Clinics 1994; **Fac Appt:** Prof D, Mayo Med Sch

Bailin, Philip L MD [D] - **Spec Exp:** Mohs' Surgery; Skin Laser Surgery; Skin Cancer; **Hospital:** Cleveland Clin (page 55); **Address:** 9500 Euclid Ave, MC A-60, Dermatology & Plastic Surg Inst, Cleveland, OH 44195; **Phone:** 216-444-2115; **Board Cert:** Dermatology 1975; **Med School:** Northwestern Univ 1968; **Resid:** Dermatology, Cleveland Clin 1974; **Fellow:** Dermatopathology, Armed Forces Inst Pathology 1975; Mohs Surgery, Univ Wisc Hosp & Clin

Barbosa, Victoria H MD [D] - **Spec Exp:** Ethnic Skin Disorders; Hair Loss; Pigmented Lesions; Acne; **Hospital:** Rush Univ Med Ctr; **Address:** Rush Univ Med Ctr, 30 N Michigan Ave, Ste 1429, Chicago, IL 60602; **Phone:** 312-407-0000; **Board Cert:** Dermatology 2007; **Med School:** Yale Univ 1994; **Resid:** Dermatology, Yale-New Haven Hosp 1998; **Fac Appt:** Asst Prof D, Rush Med Coll

Bayliss, Susan J MD [D] - **Spec Exp:** Pediatric Dermatology; Eczema; Vascular Malformations; Hemangiomas/Birthmarks; **Hospital:** St. Louis Chldns Hosp; **Address:** St Louis Chldns Hosp, 1 Children's Pl, rm 3N48, St Louis, MO 63110; **Phone:** 314-454-6187; **Board Cert:** Dermatology 1982; Pediatric Dermatology 2006; **Med School:** Univ Tex Med Br, Galveston 1977; **Resid:** Pediatrics, St Louis Chldns Hosp 1980; **Fac Appt:** Prof Med, Washington Univ, St Louis

Cornelius, Lynn A MD [D] - **Spec Exp:** Melanoma; **Hospital:** Barnes-Jewish Hosp; **Address:** Washington Univ Dept Dermatology, 4921 Parkview Place, Campus Box 8123, St Louis, MO 63110; **Phone:** 314-362-2643; **Board Cert:** Dermatology 1989; **Med School:** Univ MO-Columbia Sch Med 1984; **Resid:** Dermatology, Barnes Jewish Hosp-Wash Univ 1989; **Fellow:** Immunological Dermatology, Emory Univ Med Ctr 1992; **Fac Appt:** Assoc Prof D, Washington Univ, St Louis

Crutchfield III, Charles Edward MD [D] - **Spec Exp:** Skin Cancer; Psoriasis; Eczema; Cosmetic Dermatology; **Hospital:** Regions Hosp - St Paul; **Address:** Crutchfield Dermatology, 1185 Town Ctr Drive, Ste 101, Eagan, MN 55123; **Phone:** 651-209-3600; **Board Cert:** Dermatology 2008; **Med School:** Mayo Med Sch 1994; **Resid:** Dermatology, Univ Minnesota Affil Hosp 1998; **Fac Appt:** Assoc Clin Prof D, Univ Minn

Fivenson, David P MD [D] - **Spec Exp:** Blistering Diseases; Wound Healing/Care; Lupus/SLE; Behcet's Syndrome; **Hospital:** St. Joseph Mercy Hosp - Ann Arbor; **Address:** 3001 Miller Rd, Ann Arbor, MI 48103; **Phone:** 734-222-9630; **Board Cert:** Dermatology 1989; Clinical & Laboratory Dematologic Immunology 1991; **Med School:** Univ Mich Med Sch 1984; **Resid:** Dermatology, Univ Cincinnati Med Ctr 1989; **Fellow:** Immunological Dermatology, UCSD Med Ctr 1986; **Fac Appt:** Assoc Clin Prof Med, Mich State Univ

Fosko, Scott W MD [D] - **Spec Exp:** Mohs' Surgery; Skin Cancer; Dermatologic Surgery; **Hospital:** St. Louis Univ Hosp; **Address:** 1755 S Grand Blvd, Ste 210, St Louis, MO 63104; **Phone:** 314-256-3420; **Board Cert:** Internal Medicine 1989; Dermatology 2001; **Med School:** Univ MD Sch Med 1986; **Resid:** Internal Medicine, Univ Va Med Ctr 1989; Dermatology, Yale-New Haven Hosp 1992; **Fellow:** Mohs Surgery, Hosp UPenn 1993; **Fac Appt:** Prof D, St Louis Univ

Garden, Jerome M MD [D] - **Spec Exp:** Skin Laser Surgery; Facial Rejuvenation; Vascular Birthmarks; **Hospital:** Northwestern Meml Hosp, Lurie Chldn's Hosp-Chicago; **Address:** 150 E Huron St, Ste 1200, Chicago, IL 60611-2946; **Phone:** 312-280-0890; **Board Cert:** Dermatology 1984; **Med School:** Northwestern Univ 1980; **Resid:** Internal Medicine, Northwestern Univ Affil Hosp 1981; Dermatology, Northwestern Univ Affil Hosp 1984; **Fac Appt:** Prof D, Northwestern Univ

Hanke, C William MD [D] - **Spec Exp:** Mohs' Surgery; Skin Laser Surgery; Cosmetic Dermatology; Photodynamic Therapy; **Hospital:** St. Vincent Carmel Hosp; **Address:** Laser & Skin Surgery Ctr of Indiana, 13400 N Meridian St, Ste 290, Carmel, IN 46032-1486; **Phone:** 317-660-4900; **Board Cert:** Dermatology 2009; Dermatopathology 1982; **Med School:** Univ Iowa Coll Med 1971; **Resid:** Dermatology, Cleveland Clinic 1978; Dermatopathology, Indiana Univ 1982; **Fellow:** Cutaneous Oncology, Cleveland Clinic 1979; **Fac Appt:** Clin Prof D, Indiana Univ

Hruza, George J MD [D] - **Spec Exp:** Skin Laser Surgery; Mohs' Surgery; Cosmetic Surgery; **Hospital:** St. Luke's Hosp - Chesterfield, MO, St. Louis Univ Hosp; **Address:** 1001 Chesterfield Pkwy E, Ste 101, St Louis, MO 63017; **Phone:** 314-878-3839; **Board Cert:** Dermatology 1986; **Med School:** NYU Sch Med 1982; **Resid:** Dermatology, NYU Med Ctr-Skin Cancer Unit 1986; **Fellow:** Laser Surgery, Mass Genl Hosp-Harvard 1987; Mohs Surgery, Univ Wisc Affil Hosp 1988; **Fac Appt:** Clin Prof D, St Louis Univ

Johnson, Timothy M MD [D] - **Spec Exp:** Melanoma; Mohs' Surgery; **Hospital:** Univ of Michigan Hosp; **Address:** Univ Michigan Dermatology, 1500 E Med Ctr Drive, Ste 5918, Ann Arbor, MI 48109-5314; **Phone:** 734-936-6360; **Board Cert:** Dermatology 1988; **Med School:** Univ Tex, Houston 1984; **Resid:** Dermatology, Univ Texas Med Ctr 1988; **Fellow:** Cutaneous Oncology, Univ Mich Med Ctr 1989; Mohs Surgery, Univ Oregon Hlth Sci Ctr 1990; **Fac Appt:** Prof D, Univ Mich Med Sch

Dermatology

Krunic, Aleksandar L MD [D] - **Spec Exp:** Mohs' Surgery; Skin Cancer; Melanoma; Dermatologic Surgery; **Hospital:** Univ of IL Med Ctr at Chicago; **Address:** Univ Illinois Med Ctr, Derm Ctr, 1801 W Taylor St, Ste 3E, Chicago, IL 60612; **Phone:** 312-996-8666; **Board Cert:** Dermatology 2003; **Med School:** Yugoslavia 1988; **Resid:** Dermatology, Univ Chicago Hosp 2003; **Fellow:** Mohs Surgery, Duke Univ Med Ctr 1997; Mohs Surgery, Univ Texas SW Med Ctr 2004; **Fac Appt:** Assoc Clin Prof D, Univ IL Coll Med

Lim, Henry W MD [D] - **Spec Exp:** Phototherapy; Vitiligo; Cutaneous Lymphoma; Skin Cancer; **Hospital:** Henry Ford Hosp; **Address:** Henry Ford Hosp, Dept Derm, 3031 W Grand Blvd, Ste 800, Detroit, MI 48202-3141; **Phone:** 313-916-4060; **Board Cert:** Dermatology 2005; Clinical & Laboratory Dematologic Immunology 1985; **Med School:** SUNY Downstate 1975; **Resid:** Dermatology, NYU Med Ctr 1979; **Fellow:** Immunological Dermatology, NYU Med Ctr 1980; **Fac Appt:** Prof Path, Wayne State Univ

Liu, Vincent MD [D] - **Hospital:** Univ Iowa Hosp & Clinics; **Address:** Univ Iowa Hosp, Dermatology Clin, 200 Hawkins Drive, rm 30 000-PFP, Iowa City, IA 52242; **Phone:** 319-356-7546; **Board Cert:** Dermatology 2009; Dermatopathology 2001; **Med School:** Univ Pennsylvania 1996; **Resid:** Dermatology, Mass Genl Hosp 2000; **Fellow:** Dermatopathology, Mass Genl Hosp 2001; **Fac Appt:** Assoc Clin Prof D, Univ Iowa Coll Med

Lowe, Lori MD [D] - **Spec Exp:** Dermatopathology; Skin Cancer; **Hospital:** Univ of Michigan Hosp; **Address:** Univ Michigan Dept Pathology, 1301 Catherine Rd, M3261-Med Sci I, Ann Arbor, MI 48109-5602; **Phone:** 734-764-4460; **Board Cert:** Dermatology 1990; Dermatopathology 1991; **Med School:** Univ Tex, Houston 1985; **Resid:** Dermatology, Univ Tex Hlth Sci Ctr 1990; **Fellow:** Dermatopathology, Univ Colo Hlth Sci Ctr 1991; **Fac Appt:** Prof D, Univ Mich Med Sch

Lucky, Anne W MD [D] - **Spec Exp:** Pediatric Dermatology; Acne; **Hospital:** Cincinnati Chldns Hosp Med Ctr; **Address:** Dermatology Associates of Cincinnati, 7691 Five Mile Rd, Ste 312, Cincinnati, OH 45230; **Phone:** 513-232-3332; **Board Cert:** Pediatrics 1975; Pediatric Endocrinology 1978; Dermatology 1981; Pediatric Dermatology 2004; **Med School:** Yale Univ 1970; **Resid:** Pediatrics, Boston Chldns Hosp 1973; Dermatology, Yale-New Haven Hosp 1981; **Fellow:** Pediatric Endocrinology, Natl Inst Hlth 1976; **Fac Appt:** Prof D, Univ Cincinnati

Mutasim, Diya F MD [D] - **Spec Exp:** Immune Deficiency-Skin Disorders; Dermatopathology; **Hospital:** Univ Hosp - Cincinnati; **Address:** 222 Piedmont Ave, Ste 5300, Cincinnati, OH 45219; **Phone:** 513-475-7630; **Board Cert:** Dermatology 1990; Immunopathology 1991; Dermatopathology 1993; **Med School:** Lebanon 1979; **Resid:** Dermatology, Johns Hopkins Hosp 1989; **Fellow:** Immunological Dermatology, Johns Hopkins Hosp 1985; **Fac Appt:** Prof D, Univ Cincinnati

Neuburg, Marcelle MD [D] - **Spec Exp:** Mohs' Surgery; Skin Cancer; Pigmented Lesions; **Hospital:** Froedtert and Med Ctr of WI; **Address:** Clinical Cancer Ctr-Dermatology Dept, 9200 W Wisconsin Ave, Milwaukee, WI 53226; **Phone:** 414-805-0080; **Board Cert:** Internal Medicine 1985; Dermatology 1988; **Med School:** Oregon Hlth & Sci Univ 1982; **Resid:** Internal Medicine, Georgetown Univ Hosp 1985; Dermatology, Boston Univ Sch Med Ctr 1988; **Fellow:** Mohs Surgery, Tufts New England Med Ctr 1990; **Fac Appt:** Prof D, Med Coll Wisc

Otley, Clark C MD [D] - **Spec Exp:** Mohs' Surgery; Skin Cancer; Skin Cancer in Transplant Patients; Dermatologic Surgery; **Hospital:** Mayo Med Ctr & Clin - Rochester; **Address:** Mayo Clinic, 200 First St SW, Rochester, MN 55905; **Phone:** 507-284-3579; **Board Cert:** Dermatology 2004; **Med School:** Duke Univ 1991; **Resid:** Dermatology, Mass Genl Hosp 1995; **Fellow:** Dermatologic Surgery, Mayo Clinic 1996; **Fac Appt:** Assoc Prof D, Mayo Med Sch

America's Top Doctors® 12th Edition

Paller, Amy S MD [D] - **Spec Exp:** Genetic Disorders-Skin; Immune Deficiency-Skin Disorders; Atopic Dermatitis; Pediatric Dermatology; **Hospital:** Lurie Chldn's Hosp-Chicago; **Address:** Anne & Robert H. Lurie Children's Hosp, 155 E Superior St, Fl 5th, Chicago, IL 60611; **Phone:** 312-227-6060; **Board Cert:** Pediatrics 1982; Dermatology 2007; Pediatric Dermatology 2004; **Med School:** Stanford Univ 1978; **Resid:** Pediatrics, Chldns Meml Hosp 1981; Dermatology, Northwestern Meml Hosp 1983; **Fellow:** Research, Univ NC Hosp 1984; **Fac Appt:** Prof D, Northwestern Univ

Rhodes, Arthur R MD [D] - **Spec Exp:** Melanoma; Melanoma Risk Assessment; Melanoma Early Detection/Prevention; Pediatric Dermatology; **Hospital:** Rush Univ Med Ctr; **Address:** Rush Univ Dermatology Patient Svcs, 1725 W Harrison St, Ste 264, Chicago, IL 60612; **Phone:** 312-942-2195; **Board Cert:** Internal Medicine 1972; Dermatology 2009; **Med School:** Columbia P&S 1969; **Resid:** Internal Medicine, Beth Israel Hosp 1972; Dermatology, Mass Genl Hosp 1978; **Fac Appt:** Prof D, Rush Med Coll

Shea, Christopher R MD [D] - **Spec Exp:** Melanoma; Cutaneous Lymphoma; Pigmented Lesions; **Hospital:** Univ of Chicago Med Ctr; **Address:** Univ of Chicago Med Ctr, Ctr for Advanced Medicine, 5758 S Maryland Ave, MC 9815, Chicago, IL 60637; **Phone:** 773-702-6559; **Board Cert:** Dermatology 2009; Dermatopathology 1991; Anatomic Pathology 1998; **Med School:** Georgetown Univ 1983; **Resid:** Dermatology, Mass Genl Hosp 1986; Anatomic Pathology, Georgetown Univ Hosp 1981; **Fellow:** Dermatology, Harvard-Mass Genl Hosp 1989; Dermatopathology, NY-Presby/Weill Cornell Med Ctr 1991; **Fac Appt:** Prof Med, Univ Chicago-Pritzker Sch Med

Treadwell, Patricia A MD [D] - **Spec Exp:** Pediatric Dermatology; Vascular Birthmarks; **Hospital:** Riley Hosp for Children, Wishard Hlth Srvs; **Address:** Wishard Hosp Dept Peds, 1001 W 10th St Bryce Bldg - rm B2101, Indianapolis, IN 46202; **Phone:** 317-630-7396; **Board Cert:** Pediatrics 1982; Dermatology 1983; **Med School:** Cornell Univ-Weill Med Coll 1977; **Resid:** Pediatrics, Riley Hosp 1980; Dermatology, Indiana Univ Med Ctr 1983; **Fac Appt:** Prof D, Indiana Univ

Voorhees, John MD [D] - **Spec Exp:** Psoriasis; Photoaging; **Hospital:** Univ of Michigan Hosp; **Address:** Univ Michigan, Dept Dermatology, 1500 E Med Ctr Drive, rm 1910 Taubman Ctr, Ann Arbor, MI 48109-5314; **Phone:** 734-936-4054; **Board Cert:** Dermatology 1970; **Med School:** Univ Mich Med Sch 1963; **Resid:** Dermatology, Univ Mich Hosp 1969; **Fac Appt:** Prof D, Univ Mich Med Sch

Witman, Patricia Mary MD [D] - **Spec Exp:** Pediatric Dermatology; **Hospital:** Nationwide Chldn's Hosp; **Address:** 555 S 18th St, Nationwide Chldn's Hosp, Columbus, OH 43205; **Phone:** 614-722-5777; **Board Cert:** Dermatology 2007; Pediatric Dermatology 2006; **Med School:** Med Coll Wisc 1994; **Resid:** Dermatology, Froedtert Meml Hosp 1998; **Fellow:** Pediatric Dermatology, UCSF Med Ctr 2002; **Fac Appt:** Asst Prof D, Ohio State Univ

Wood, Gary S MD [D] - **Spec Exp:** Cutaneous Lymphoma; Melanoma; Skin Cancer; Parapsoriasis; **Hospital:** Univ WI Hosp & Clins, Wm S Middleton Mem Vet Hosp-Madison; **Address:** Univ Wisconsin Health, Dept Dermatology, 1 S Park St, Fl 7, Madison, WI 53715-1375; **Phone:** 608-287-2620; **Board Cert:** Anatomic Pathology 1983; Dermatology 1986; Dermatopathology 1987; **Med School:** Univ IL Coll Med 1979; **Resid:** Anatomic Pathology, Stanford Univ Med Ctr 1983; Dermatology, Stanford Univ Med Ctr 1985; **Fellow:** Immunopathology, Stanford Univ Med Ctr 1981; **Fac Appt:** Prof D, Univ Wisc

Zelickson, Brian D MD [D] - **Spec Exp:** Skin Laser Surgery; **Hospital:** Abbott - Northwestern Hosp, Fairview Southdale Hosp; **Address:** 825 Nicollet Mall, Med Arts Bldg - Ste 1002, Minneapolis, MN 55402; **Phone:** 612-338-0711; **Board Cert:** Dermatology 2009; **Med School:** Mayo Med Sch 1986; **Resid:** Dermatology, Mayo Clinic 1990; **Fac Appt:** Asst Prof D, Univ Minn

Dermatology

Great Plains and Mountains

Bowen, Glen M MD [D] - **Spec Exp:** Melanoma; Cutaneous Lymphoma; Clinical Trials; Mohs' Surgery; **Hospital:** Univ Utah Hlth Care, Cottonwood Hosp & Med Ctr; **Address:** Huntsman Cancer Inst, 2000 Circle of Hope, Ste 2400, Salt Lake City, UT 84132; **Phone:** 801-585-0197; **Board Cert:** Dermatology 2005; **Med School:** Univ Utah 1990; **Resid:** Dermatology, Univ Michigan Med Ctr 1993; **Fellow:** Immunological Dermatology, Univ Michigan Med Ctr 1995; Mohs Surgery, Univ Utah 2001; **Fac Appt:** Assoc Prof D, Univ Utah

Krueger, Gerald MD [D] - **Spec Exp:** Psoriasis; **Hospital:** Univ Utah Hlth Care; **Address:** Univ Utah Hlth Sci Ctr, Dept Derm, 30 N 1900 E, rm 4A330 SOM, Salt Lake City, UT 84132; **Phone:** 801-581-6465; **Board Cert:** Dermatology 1973; **Med School:** Loma Linda Univ 1966; **Resid:** Dermatology, Univ Colorado Med Ctr 1972; **Fac Appt:** Prof D, Univ Utah

Sontheimer, Richard D MD [D] - **Spec Exp:** Immune Deficiency-Skin Disorders; Lupus/SLE; Dermatomyositis; **Hospital:** Univ Utah Hlth Care; **Address:** Univ Hlth Care, Dept Dermatology, 30 N 1900 E, rm 4A330, Salt Lake City, UT 84132; **Phone:** 801-581-6465; **Board Cert:** Internal Medicine 1976; Dermatology 1979; Clinical & Laboratory Dematologic Immunology 1985; **Med School:** Univ Tex SW, Dallas 1972; **Resid:** Internal Medicine, Univ Utah Affil Hosps 1976; Dermatology, Parkland Meml Hosp 1979; **Fellow:** Research, Southwestern Med Sch 1978; **Fac Appt:** Prof D, Univ Utah

Southwest

Butler, David F MD [D] - **Spec Exp:** Skin Cancer; **Hospital:** Scott & White Mem Hosp; **Address:** Scott White Meml Hosp, Dept Dermatology, 409 W Adams St, Temple, TX 76501; **Phone:** 254-742-3724; **Board Cert:** Dermatology 1985; **Med School:** Univ Tex Med Br, Galveston 1980; **Resid:** Dermatology, Walter Reed Army Med Ctr 1985; **Fac Appt:** Assoc Prof D, Texas Tech Univ

Carney, John M MD [D] - **Spec Exp:** Mohs' Surgery; Skin Cancer; **Hospital:** UAMS Med Ctr; **Address:** Southwest Med Arts Bldg, 11321 Interstate 30, Ste 201, Little Rock, AR 72209; **Phone:** 501-455-4700; **Board Cert:** Dermatology 1984; **Med School:** Northwestern Univ 1979; **Resid:** Dermatology, Univ Hosps 1984; **Fellow:** Physiology, Harvard Med Sch 1985; Dermatologic Surgery, Univ Tenn Med Ctr 1986

Cather, Jennifer Clay MD [D] - **Spec Exp:** Cutaneous Lymphoma; Cutaneous T-cell Lymphoma; Psoriasis; **Hospital:** Baylor Univ Medical Ctr-Dallas; **Address:** Modern Dermatology, 9101 N Central Expy, Ste 160, Dallas, TX 75231; **Phone:** 214-265-1818; **Board Cert:** Dermatology 1999; **Med School:** Univ Tex SW, Dallas 1994; **Resid:** Dermatology, UT Derm Hosp 2000; **Fellow:** Research, MD Anderson Canc Ctr 1997

Cockerell, Clay J MD [D] - **Spec Exp:** Dermatopathology; **Hospital:** UT Southwestern Med Ctr at Dallas; **Address:** Cockerell & Assocs, 2330 Butler St, Ste 115, Dallas, TX 75235; **Phone:** 214-530-5200; **Board Cert:** Dermatology 2008; Dermatopathology 1986; **Med School:** Baylor Coll Med 1981; **Resid:** Dermatology, NYU Langone Med Ctr 1985; **Fellow:** Dermatopathology, NYU Langone Med Ctr 1986; **Fac Appt:** Prof DP, Univ Tex SW, Dallas

Duvic, Madeleine MD [D] - **Spec Exp:** Cutaneous Lymphoma; Skin Cancer; Alopecia Areata; **Hospital:** UT MD Anderson Cancer Ctr; **Address:** Dept Dermatol - MD Anderson Cancer Ctr, 1400 Pressler St - Unit 1452, Houston, TX 77030; **Phone:** 713-745-4615; **Board Cert:** Dermatology 1981; Internal Medicine 1982; **Med School:** Duke Univ 1977; **Resid:** Dermatology, Duke Univ Med Ctr 1980; Internal Medicine, Duke Univ Med Ctr 1982; **Fellow:** Geriatric Medicine, Duke Univ Med Ctr 1984; **Fac Appt:** Prof D, Univ Tex, Houston

Hansen, Ronald C MD [D] - **Spec Exp:** Pediatric Dermatology; **Hospital:** Phoenix Children's Hosp; **Address:** Phoenix Childrens Hosp, Dermatology Clinic F, 1919 E Thomas Rd, Phoenix, AZ 85006; **Phone:** 602-933-0895; **Board Cert:** Pediatrics 1974; Dermatology 1980; **Med School:** Univ Iowa Coll Med 1968; **Resid:** Pediatrics, Childrens Hosp 1970; Pediatrics, Stanford Univ Med Ctr 1972; **Fellow:** Dermatology, Univ Arizona 1980; **Fac Appt:** Prof D, Univ Ariz Coll Med

Levy, Moise L MD [D] - **Spec Exp:** Pediatric Dermatology; Vascular Birthmarks; Genetic Disorders-Skin; Blistering Diseases; **Hospital:** Dell Children's Med Ctr of Central Texas; **Address:** 1301 Barbara Jordan Blvd, Ste 200, Pediatrics Bldg, Ste 200, Austin, TX 78723; **Phone:** 512-628-1920; **Board Cert:** Pediatrics 1985; Dermatology 1986; Pediatric Dermatology 2004; **Med School:** Univ Tex, Houston 1979; **Resid:** Pediatrics, Univ Tex Affil Hosp 1983; Dermatology, Baylor Coll Med 1986; **Fac Appt:** Prof D, Baylor Coll Med

Lim Quan, Katherine K MD [D] - **Spec Exp:** Mohs' Surgery; Skin Cancer; **Hospital:** Chandler Regional Med Ctr; **Address:** Valley Skin Cancer Surgery, 1100 S Dobson Rd, Ste 223, Chandler, AZ 85286; **Phone:** 480-214-0388; **Board Cert:** Dermatology 2006; **Med School:** Northwestern Univ 1992; **Resid:** Dermatology, Mayo Clinic 1996; **Fellow:** Mohs Surgery, Mayo Clinic 1997

Linder, Jennifer L MD [D] - **Spec Exp:** Mohs' Surgery; Skin Cancer; Cosmetic Dermatology; **Address:** Linder Dermatology & Skin Cancer Ctr, 6710 E Camelback Rd, Ste 220, Scottsdale, AZ 85251; **Phone:** 480-946-7939; **Board Cert:** Dermatology 2003; **Med School:** Washington Univ, St Louis 1999; **Resid:** Dermatology, Thomas Jeff Univ Hosp 2003; **Fellow:** Dermatologic Surgery, Mohs College 2004

Menter, M Allan MD [D] - **Spec Exp:** Psoriasis; Cosmetic Dermatology; Eczema; **Hospital:** Baylor Univ Medical Ctr-Dallas, UT Southwestern Med Ctr at Dallas; **Address:** 3900 Junius St, Ste 145, Dallas, TX 75246; **Phone:** 972-386-7546 x400; **Board Cert:** Dermatology 1978; **Med School:** South Africa 1966; **Resid:** Dermatology, Pretoria Genl Hosp 1971; Dermatology, Guys Hosp 1972; **Fellow:** Dermatology, St Johns Hosp 1973; Dermatology, Univ Texas SW 1979; **Fac Appt:** Clin Prof D, Univ Tex SW, Dallas

Orengo, Ida F MD [D] - **Spec Exp:** Mohs' Surgery; Skin Cancer; Melanoma; **Hospital:** Methodist Hosp - Houston, DeBakey VA Med Ctr-Houston; **Address:** Baylor Dermatology, 1977 Butler Blvd, Ste 1425, Houston, TX 77030; **Phone:** 713-798-6925; **Board Cert:** Dermatology 2011; **Med School:** Baylor Coll Med 1987; **Resid:** Dermatology, Baylor Coll Med 1991; **Fellow:** Dermatologic Surgery, Harvard Med Sch/Mass Genl Hosp 1992; **Fac Appt:** Prof D, Baylor Coll Med

Perone, Jennifer Beth MD [D] - **Spec Exp:** Mohs' Surgery; **Hospital:** UT Southwestern Med Ctr at Dallas; **Address:** North TX Prof Building, 2817 S Mayhill Rd, Ste 115, Denton, TX 76208; **Phone:** 940-591-0900; **Board Cert:** Dermatology 2003; **Med School:** NYU Sch Med 1999; **Resid:** Dermatology, Duke Univ Med Ctr 2003; **Fellow:** Mohs Surgery, UT Southwestern Med Ctr-Dalla 2006

Pitts, Jeanette M MD [D] - **Spec Exp:** Mohs' Surgery; Skin Cancer; Melanoma; Skin Laser Surgery; **Hospital:** Univ Arizona Med Ctr-Univ Campus; **Address:** Univ Arizona Cancer Ctr, Nortn Campus, 3838 N Campbell Ave, Tucson, AZ 85719-1454; **Phone:** 520-694-2873; **Board Cert:** Dermatology 2009; **Med School:** Univ Kansas 1996; **Resid:** Dermatology, Emory Univ 1999; **Fellow:** Mohs Surgery, Penn State/Hershey Med Ctr 2000; **Fac Appt:** Assoc Clin Prof Med, Univ Ariz Coll Med

Dermatology

Taylor III, R Stan MD [D] - **Spec Exp:** Mohs' Surgery; Melanoma; Skin Cancer; **Hospital:** UT Southwestern Med Ctr at Dallas, Parkland Hlth & Hosp Sys; **Address:** Univ Tex SW Med Sch, Dept Derm, 5323 Harry Hines Blvd, Dallas, TX 75390-7208; **Phone:** 214-645-8950; **Board Cert:** Dermatology 1989; **Med School:** Univ Tex Med Br, Galveston 1985; **Resid:** Dermatology, Univ Mich Med Ctr 1989; **Fellow:** Immunological Dermatology, Univ Mich Med Ctr 1990; Mohs Surgery, Oregon Hlth Sci Univ 1991; **Fac Appt:** Prof D, Univ Tex SW, Dallas

Wheeland, Ronald G MD [D] - **Spec Exp:** Skin Laser Surgery; Mohs' Surgery; Cosmetic Dermatology; Cutaneous Lymphoma; **Hospital:** Univ Arizona Med Ctr-Univ Campus; **Address:** 12345 E Summer Trail St, Tucson, AZ 85749; **Phone:** 520-404-1516; **Board Cert:** Dermatology 2009; Dermatopathology 1978; **Med School:** Univ Ariz Coll Med 1973; **Resid:** Dermatology, Univ OK Affil Hosp 1977; **Fellow:** Dermatopathology, Univ Oklahoma 1978; Mohs Surgery, Cleveland Clinic 1984; **Fac Appt:** Prof Emeritus D, Univ Ariz Coll Med

West Coast and Pacific

Bennett, Richard G MD [D] - **Spec Exp:** Mohs' Surgery; Skin Cancer; Hidradenitis Suppurativa; Dermatofibrosarcoma Protruberans; **Hospital:** Keck Med Ctr of USC (page 62), UCLA Ronald Reagan Med Ctr; **Address:** 1301 20th St, Ste 570, Santa Monica, CA 90404-2080; **Phone:** 310-315-0171; **Board Cert:** Dermatology 1975; **Med School:** Case West Res Univ 1970; **Resid:** Dermatology, Hosp Univ Penn 1974; **Fellow:** Mohs Surgery, NYU Med Ctr 1977; **Fac Appt:** Clin Prof D, UCLA

Berg, Daniel MD [D] - **Spec Exp:** Skin Cancer; Mohs' Surgery; Skin Laser Surgery; Hair Restoration/Transplant; **Hospital:** Univ Wash Med Ctr; **Address:** 4225 Roosevelt Way NE, Fl 4th, Box 354697, Seattle, WA 98105; **Phone:** 206-598-6647; **Board Cert:** Dermatology 2009; **Med School:** Univ Toronto 1985; **Resid:** Internal Medicine, Sunnybrook Med Ctr 1988; Dermatology, Duke Univ Med Ctr 1991; **Fellow:** Dermatologic Surgery, Univ Toronto 1992; Dermatologic Surgery, Univ British Columbia 1994; **Fac Appt:** Prof D, Univ Wash

Cunningham, Bari Bickel MD [D] - **Spec Exp:** Pediatric Dermatology; Birthmarks/Hemangiomas; Laser Surgery; **Hospital:** Rady Children's Hosp - San Diego; **Address:** 477 N El Camino Real, Ste C204, Encinitas, CA 92024; **Phone:** 760-634-3376; **Board Cert:** Dermatology 2006; Pediatric Dermatology 2006; **Med School:** Emory Univ 1992; **Resid:** Dermatology, Northwestern Meml Hosp 1996; **Fellow:** Pediatric Dermatology, Chldn's Meml Hosp

Eichenfield, Lawrence F MD [D] - **Spec Exp:** Eczema; Acne; Vascular Birthmarks; Pediatric Dermatology; **Hospital:** Rady Children's Hosp - San Diego, UCSD Med Ctr; **Address:** Chldns Hosp, Ped & Adolescent Dermatology, 8010 Frost St, Ste 602, San Diego, CA 92123-4204; **Phone:** 858-966-6795; **Board Cert:** Dermatology 2009; Pediatric Dermatology 2004; **Med School:** Mount Sinai Sch Med 1984; **Resid:** Pediatrics, Chldns Hosp 1987; Dermatology, Hosp Univ Penn 1991; **Fac Appt:** Prof Ped, UCSD

Fitzpatrick, Richard E MD [D] - **Spec Exp:** Cosmetic Dermatology; Skin Laser Surgery-Resurfacing; Hair Restoration/Transplant; **Address:** 9339 Genesee Ave, Ste 300, San Diego, CA 92121; **Phone:** 858-657-1002; **Board Cert:** Dermatology 2003; **Med School:** Emory Univ 1970; **Resid:** Dermatology, UCLA Med Ctr 1978; **Fac Appt:** Assoc Clin Prof D, UCSD

Frieden, Ilona J MD [D] - **Spec Exp:** Pediatric Dermatology; Vascular Birthmarks; Hemangiomas; **Hospital:** UCSF - Mt Zion Med Ctr; **Address:** UCSF, Dept Dermatology, 1701 Divisadero St, Fl 3, Box 0316, San Francisco, CA 94115; **Phone:** 415-353-7800; **Board Cert:** Dermatology 2005; Pediatrics 1983; Pediatric Dermatology 2004; **Med School:** UCSF 1977; **Resid:** Pediatrics, UCSF Med Ctr 1980; Dermatology, UCSF Med Ctr 1983; **Fac Appt:** Clin Prof D, UCSF

Friedlander, Sheila Fallon MD [D] - **Spec Exp:** Pediatric Dermatology; Infectious Disease; Vascular Malformations; Hemangiomas; **Hospital:** Rady Children's Hosp - San Diego, UCSD Med Ctr; **Address:** 8010 Frost St, Ste 602, San Diego, CA 92123; **Phone:** 858-966-6795; **Board Cert:** Pediatrics 1984; Dermatology 1990; Pediatric Dermatology 2004; **Med School:** Univ Chicago-Pritzker Sch Med 1979; **Resid:** Pediatrics, Bronx Municipal Hosp 1983; Dermatology, UCLA Med Ctr 1990; **Fellow:** Infectious Disease, Montefiore Med Ctr 1986; **Fac Appt:** Clin Prof Ped, UCSD

Glogau, Richard G MD [D] - **Spec Exp:** Cosmetic Dermatology; Skin Laser Surgery; Mohs' Surgery; Botox Therapy; **Hospital:** UCSF Med Ctr; **Address:** 350 Parnassus Ave, Ste 400, San Francisco, CA 94117; **Phone:** 415-564-1261; **Board Cert:** Dermatology 2009; Dermatopathology 1982; **Med School:** Harvard Med Sch 1973; **Resid:** Dermatology, UCSF Med Ctr 1977; **Fellow:** Chemosurgery, UCSF Med Ctr 1978; **Fac Appt:** Clin Prof D, UCSF

Greenway Jr, Hubert T MD [D] - **Spec Exp:** Skin Cancer; Mohs' Surgery; Melanoma; **Hospital:** Scripps Green Hosp; **Address:** Scripps Clinic, Div Mohs' Surgery, 10666 N Torrey Pines Rd, La Jolla, CA 92037; **Phone:** 858-554-8646; **Board Cert:** Dermatology 1982; **Med School:** Med Coll GA 1974; **Resid:** Dermatology, Naval Hosp 1982; **Fellow:** Mohs Surgery, Univ Wisconsin Med Ctr 1981

Grimes, Pearl E MD [D] - **Spec Exp:** Pigmented Lesions; Ethnic Skin Disorders; Vitiligo; Cosmetic Dermatology; **Hospital:** UCLA Ronald Reagan Med Ctr; **Address:** 5670 Wilshire Blvd, Ste 650, Los Angeles, CA 90036; **Phone:** 323-467-4389; **Board Cert:** Dermatology 1979; **Med School:** Washington Univ, St Louis 1974; **Resid:** Dermatology, Howard Univ Hosp 1979; **Fac Appt:** Clin Prof D, UCLA

Hanifin, Jon M MD [D] - **Spec Exp:** Atopic Dermatitis; **Hospital:** OR Hlth & Sci Univ; **Address:** OHSU, Dept Dermatology, 3303 SW Bond Ave, MC CH16D, Portland, OR 97239; **Phone:** 503-418-3376; **Board Cert:** Dermatology 1970; **Med School:** Univ Wisc 1965; **Resid:** Dermatology, UCSF Med Ctr 1969; **Fellow:** Clinical & Laboratory Immunology, UCSF Med Ctr; **Fac Appt:** Prof D, Oregon Hlth & Sci Univ

Kilmer, Suzanne L MD [D] - **Spec Exp:** Skin Laser Surgery-Resurfacing; Facial Rejuvenation; Cosmetic Dermatology; **Hospital:** Mercy General Hosp - Sacramento; **Address:** The Laser & Skin Surgery Center, 3835 J St, Sacramento, CA 95816-5520; **Phone:** 916-456-0400; **Board Cert:** Dermatology 2009; **Med School:** UC Davis 1987; **Resid:** Dermatology, UC Davis Med Ctr 1991; **Fellow:** Laser Surgery, Mass Genl Hosp 1992; **Fac Appt:** Asst Clin Prof D, UC Davis

Kim, Youn Hee MD [D] - **Spec Exp:** Cutaneous Lymphoma; Skin Cancer; **Hospital:** Stanford Univ Hosp & Clinics; **Address:** 875 Blake Wilbur Drive, Clinic A, Palo Alto, CA 94304; **Phone:** 650-498-6000; **Board Cert:** Dermatology 1989; **Med School:** Stanford Univ 1984; **Resid:** Dermatology, Metropolitan Hosp 1989

Koo, John Ying Ming MD [D] - **Spec Exp:** Psoriasis/Eczema; Photosensitive Skin Diseases; Phototherapy; Psychodermatology; **Hospital:** UCSF Med Ctr; **Address:** Psoriasis Day Treatment Ctr, 515 Spruce St, San Francisco, CA 94118; **Phone:** 415-476-4701; **Board Cert:** Dermatology 1988; Psychiatry 1988; **Med School:** Harvard Med Sch 1981; **Resid:** Psychiatry, UCLA Neur Psyc Inst 1985; Dermatology, UCSF Med Ctr 1988; **Fac Appt:** Prof D, UCSF

Lask, Gary P MD [D] - **Spec Exp:** Cosmetic Dermatology; Mohs' Surgery; Skin Laser Surgery-Resurfacing; Scar Revision; **Hospital:** UCLA Ronald Reagan Med Ctr; **Address:** 16260 Ventura Blvd, Ste 530, Encino, CA 91436; **Phone:** 818-788-4022; **Board Cert:** Dermatology 1983; **Med School:** Mexico 1977; **Resid:** Dermatology, ML King Jr-Drew Med Ctr 1983; **Fellow:** Mohs Surgery, ML King Jr-Drew Med Ctr 1984; **Fac Appt:** Clin Prof D, UCLA

Nghiem, Paul T MD/PhD [D] - **Spec Exp:** Merkel Cell Carcinoma; Skin Cancer; **Hospital:** Univ Wash Med Ctr; **Address:** Seattle Cancer Care Alliance, 825 Eastlake Ave E, Seattle, WA 98109; **Phone:** 206-288-1024; **Board Cert:** Dermatology 2009; **Med School:** Stanford Univ 1994; **Resid:** Dermatology, Massachusetts General Hosp 1998; **Fellow:** Research, Harvard Univ 2002; **Fac Appt:** Assoc Prof D, Univ Wash

Richardson, Timothy F MD [D] - **Spec Exp:** Mohs' Surgery; Skin Cancer; **Hospital:** Eisenhower Med Ctr; **Address:** 36867 Cook St, Ste 101, Palm Desert, CA 92211; **Phone:** 760-341-1999; **Board Cert:** Internal Medicine 1987; Dermatology 2004; **Med School:** Georgetown Univ 1983; **Resid:** Internal Medicine, Loma Linda Univ Med Ctr 1986; Dermatology, Loma Linda Univ Med Ctr 1994; **Fellow:** Mohs Surgery, Loma Linda Univ Med Ctr 1995

Rubin, Mark G MD [D] - **Spec Exp:** Skin Laser Surgery; Cosmetic Dermatology; **Hospital:** UCSD Med Ctr; **Address:** 153 S Lasky Drive, Ste 1, Beverly Hills, CA 90212; **Phone:** 310-556-0119; **Board Cert:** Dermatology 1985; **Med School:** Jefferson Med Coll 1981; **Resid:** Dermatology, Henry Ford Hosp 1985; **Fac Appt:** Assoc Prof D, UCSD

Swanson, Neil A MD [D] - **Spec Exp:** Skin Cancer; Mohs' Surgery; Reconstructive Surgery-Skin; Cosmetic Dermatology; **Hospital:** OR Hlth & Sci Univ, VA Medical Center - Portland; **Address:** 3303 SW Bond Ave, MC CH-5D, Portland, OR 97239; **Phone:** 503-418-3376; **Board Cert:** Dermatology 1980; **Med School:** Univ Rochester 1976; **Resid:** Dermatology, Univ Michigan Med Ctr 1979; **Fellow:** Dermatology, UCSF Med Ctr 1980; **Fac Appt:** Prof D, Oregon Hlth & Sci Univ

Swetter, Susan M MD [D] - **Spec Exp:** Melanoma; Melanoma Early Detection/Prevention; Skin Cancer; **Hospital:** Stanford Univ Hosp & Clinics, VA Hlth Care Sys - Palo Alto; **Address:** Stanford Univ Med Ctr, Dept Dermatology, 875 Blake Wilbur Dr, Clinic A, MC 5334, Stanford, CA 94305; **Phone:** 650-498-6000; **Board Cert:** Dermatology 2001; **Med School:** Univ Pennsylvania 1990; **Resid:** Dermatology, Stanford Univ Med Ctr 1994; **Fac Appt:** Assoc Prof D, Stanford Univ

Woodley, David T MD [D] - **Spec Exp:** Autoimmune Disease; Blistering Diseases; Pemphigus; Psoriasis; **Hospital:** Keck Med Ctr of USC (page 62); **Address:** USC Dermatology, 1520 San Pablo St, Los Angeles, CA 90033; **Phone:** 323-442-6200; **Board Cert:** Dermatology 1982; Internal Medicine 1976; Clinical & Laboratory Dermatologic Immunology 1993; **Med School:** Univ MO-Columbia Sch Med 1973; **Resid:** Internal Medicine, Univ Nebraska Med Ctr 1976; Dermatology, Univ NC Med Ctr 1978; **Fellow:** Dermatologic Research, Univ Paris 1980; **Fac Appt:** Prof D, USC-Keck School of Medicine

Cleveland Clinic

Every life deserves world class care.

Dermatology

Cleveland Clinic's Department of Dermatology, part of the Dermatology & Plastic Surgery Institute, offers a full array of subspecialized care for adult and pediatric patients. Our physicians diagnose and treat all disorders of the skin, hair and nails, whether primary or related to an underlying systemic illness, including industrial-related conditions.

Volume-Leading Mohs Center

The department offers a full range of procedures in the subspecialty area of dermatologic surgery. These include Mohs micrographic surgery for high-risk skin cancers (including local tissue reconstruction), laser surgery, chemical peels, soft tissue augmentation, Botox® injections, hair transplant and liposuction. We performed more than 2,000 Mohs procedures in the past year alone. Additionally, our Cutaneous Care Center provides outpatient treatment, rather than hospitalization, for patients with extensive, severe or chronic skin diseases utilizing phototherapy and excimer laser treatment. Staff dermatologists and residents are involved in research, either institutionally or through industrial support of clinical trials.

Cleveland Clinic's Department of Dermatology provides expertise in the diagnosis and management of the full spectrum of dermatologic conditions, as well as an extensive range of cosmetic evaluations and surgeries. We continue to meet our community responsibility through active participation in skin cancer screening and other activities related to National Skin Cancer Week. The Department of Dermatology also provides medical missionary assistance in developing countries. We continuously strive to improve outcomes in dermatology, not just for the patients who entrust us with their care today, but for future generations.

Cleveland Clinic
Dermatology & Plastic
Surgery Institute
9500 Euclid Avenue
Cleveland, OH 44195

Offering Same-Day Appointments
Call 800.274.2009.

Treatment Guides
Cleveland Clinic has developed comprehensive treatment guides for many diseases and conditions. To download our free treatment guides, visit clevelandclinic.org/treatmentguides.

Online Medical Second Opinion
Call 216.444.3223 or 800.223.2273 ext. 43223 or email eclevelandclinic@ccf.org.

Out-of-State Patients Assistance
Call 800.223.2273, ext. 55580 or email medicalconcierge@ccf.org.

Visit Us At:
clevelandclinic.org

Follow Us On:
Facebook
www.facebook.com/clevelandclinic

Twitter
@ClevelandClinic

You Tube
www.youtube.com/clevelandclinic

Health Hub
health.clevelandclinic.org

THE MOUNT SINAI DEPARTMENT OF DERMATOLOGY

One Gustave L. Levy Place
Fifth Avenue and 100th Street
New York, NY 10029-6574
Physician Referral: 1-800-MD-SINAI (637-4624)
www.mountsinai.org/dermatology

MOUNT SINAI
SCHOOL OF
MEDICINE

The Mount Sinai Department of Dermatology has one of the most comprehensive programs for skin health and the treatment of skin diseases in the nation. In addition to our offices at Mount Sinai Hospital, the department has satellite offices throughout New York City and in the suburbs.

Skin Cancer
Our department is at the forefront of research in the treatment and prevention of skin cancer. Drs. Hooman Khorasani and David Kriegel perform state-of-the-art surgical treatment and repairs for all types of skin cancer.

Dr. Orit Markowitz uses new imaging techniques for the early diagnosis and prevention of melanoma. We are one of the few dermatology departments with optical coherence tomography (OCT) technology, Molemax technology and Melafind systems. The latter devices are useful for evaluating non-melanoma skin cancers and pigmented lesions and for following and diagnosing melanoma.

Drs. Czernik, Goldenberg, Goldstein, Lamb, Lebwohl, Levitt, Markowitz, Shim-Chang, and Zeichner have expertise in the diagnosis, prevention, and treatment of all skin cancers and have developed many of the treatments currently in use to prevent and treat cancerous and precancerous skin lesions. We also treat one of the largest groups of patients with cutaneous T-cell lymphoma.

General Dermatology
Psoriasis:
Our faculty number among the country's leading experts in psoriasis, including our department chairman, Dr. Mark Lebwohl, and Drs. Norman Goldstein, Gary Goldenberg, Jacob Levitt, Annette Czernik and Angela Lamb. Our center includes a state-of- the-art phototherapy unit, an infusion center for intravenous treatments, and a research center where many new therapies available for psoriasis are tested.

Autoimmune and inflammatory skin diseases:
We have one of the largest centers for inflammatory skin diseases where we treat psoriasis, atopic dermatitis and contact dermatitis. Dr. Emma Guttman is doing clinical research in new targeted therapies for severe atopic dermatitis. Dr. Suhail Hadi is one of the most experienced in the use of the excimer laser for psoriasis and vitiligo. Our faculty also includes three renowned acne experts, Drs. Angela Lamb, Joshua Zeichner, and Susan Bershad.

Our bullous disease center is run by Drs. Jacob Levitt and Annette Czernik. We are one of the few dermatology departments in the nation with its own infusion unit, so patients may be treated either as outpatients in the infusion unit or as inpatients at The Mount Sinai Medical Center.

Pediatric and Adolescent Dermatology
Our faculty treats all ages for skin. Dr. Susan Bershad is a board-certified pediatric and adolescent dermatologist. Dr. Emma Guttman is a trailblazer in research on atopic dermatitis and other forms of eczema.

Cosmetic Dermatology Center
We were one of the first programs in the nation to have a procedural dermatology fellowship, which is run by Drs. David Kriegel and Hooman Khorasani. Along with Drs. Marsha Gordon, Heidi Waldorf, Gary Goldenberg, Joshua Zeichner, and Helen Shim-Chang, our team is renowned for noninvasive skin rejuvenation combining topical regimens, soft tissue fillers, botulinum toxin, photodynamic therapy and laser and radio frequency devices. Members of our faculty perform liposuction, blepharoplasty, microdermabrasion, laser hair removal, sclerotherapy, skin tightening procedures, laser removals of tattoos, and pigmented and vascular lesions as well as laser resurfacing such as fraxel and total Fx.

DERMATOLOGY

About the Ronald O. Perelman Department of Dermatology

The Ronald O. Perelman Department of Dermatology is a national and international leader in dermatology, employing the most advanced science and medicine to diagnose and treat skin disorders. The Department provides dermatologic care for more than 100,000 patients each year, as well as conducting research into some of the most significant dermatologic problems. Services include adult and pediatric medical dermatology, dermatologic/skin cancer surgery and cosmetic dermatology. We specialize in the following areas:

Dermatologic / Skin Cancer Surgery and Cosmetic Dermatology

NYU Langone Medical Center's dermatologists provide specialized care for the treatment of malignant and benign skin lesions and offer cutting-edge therapies for aesthetic and cosmetic concerns.

General Dermatology

Dermatologic associates offer multi-subspecialty dermatology care in private office settings for patients with disorders of the skin, hair, and nails, including inflammatory skin diseases such as psoriasis and lupus, cancers and other skin tumors, hair loss, infections and allergic skin diseases such as eczema, contact dermatitis and hives.

Pediatric and Adolescent Dermatology

The Medical Center also boasts a specialized professional practice dedicated to the treatment of diseases affecting the skin, hair, and nails of infants, children and adolescents. These disorders include acne, atopic dermatitis/eczema, hair loss, hemangiomas, moles, birthmarks, vitiligo and genetic disorders affecting the skin.

Charles C. Harris Skin and Cancer Unit / Dermatology Clinical Trials Unit

The Charles C. Harris Skin and Cancer Unit at Tisch Hospital is an outpatient dermatology teaching center combining unique patient care with superior medical education. Resident and attending physicians provide diagnosis and treatment of skin diseases that include acne, eczema and warts as well as complex medical conditions such as connective tissue disorders, pigmented lesions, skin allergies and skin cancers.

Dermatopathology

Highly trained dermatopathologists at the Medical Center examine skin tissues submitted by physicians from biopsies and surgeries to diagnose skin diseases and malignancies. One of the busiest academic skin pathology units in the country, the Dermatopathology section of the Department also provides consultative services for the review of skin pathology specimens performed elsewhere.

The Best in American Medicine
www.CastleConnolly.com

Endocrinology, Diabetes & Metabolism

a subspecialty of Internal Medicine

An internist who concentrates on disorders of the internal (endocrine) glands such as the thyroid and adrenal glands. This specialist also deals with disorders such as diabetes, metabolic and nutritional disorders, pituitary diseases, menstrual and sexual problems.

Training Required: Three years in internal medicine *plus* additional training and examination for certification in endocrinology, diabetes and metabolism.

ENDOCRINOLOGY, DIABETES & METABOLISM

New England

Abrahamson, Martin J MD [EDM] - **Spec Exp:** Diabetes; **Hospital:** Beth Israel Deaconess Med Ctr - Boston; **Address:** Joslin Diabetes Ctr, 1 Joslin Pl, Ste 260, Boston, MA 02215; **Phone:** 617-309-2501; **Board Cert:** Internal Medicine 2005; Endocrinology, Diabetes & Metabolism 2005; **Med School:** South Africa 1977; **Resid:** Internal Medicine, Groote Schuuer Hosp-Univ Cape Town 1983; **Fellow:** Endocrinology, Diabetes & Metabolism, Groote Schuuer Hosp-Univ Cape Town 1985; Research, Univ Cape Town 1987; **Fac Appt:** Assoc Prof Med, Harvard Med Sch

Axelrod, Lloyd MD [EDM] - **Spec Exp:** Diabetes; Geriatric Endocrinology; **Hospital:** Mass Genl Hosp; **Address:** MGH Diabetes Unit, 50 Staniford St Fl 3 - Ste 340, Boston, MA 02114; **Phone:** 617-726-8722; **Board Cert:** Internal Medicine 1973; Endocrinology, Diabetes & Metabolism 1973; **Med School:** Harvard Med Sch 1967; **Resid:** Internal Medicine, Brigham & Womens Hosp 1969; Internal Medicine, Mass Genl Hosp 1971; **Fellow:** Endocrinology, Diabetes & Metabolism, Brigham & Womens Hosp 1970; Endocrinology, Diabetes & Metabolism, Mass Genl Hosp 1972; **Fac Appt:** Assoc Prof Med, Harvard Med Sch

Beaser, Richard S MD [EDM] - **Spec Exp:** Diabetes; **Hospital:** Beth Israel Deaconess Med Ctr - Boston; **Address:** Joslin Diabetes Ctr, One Joslin Pl, Boston, MA 02215; **Phone:** 617-732-2665; **Board Cert:** Internal Medicine 1980; **Med School:** Boston Univ 1977; **Resid:** Internal Medicine, Univ Mass Med Ctr 1980; **Fellow:** Diabetes, Joslin Clinic 1981; Endocrinology, Lahey Clinic 1982; **Fac Appt:** Assoc Clin Prof Med, Harvard Med Sch

Bhasin, Shalender MD [EDM] - **Spec Exp:** Reproductive Endocrinology; Sexual Dysfunction; **Hospital:** Boston Med Ctr; **Address:** Boston Med Ctr, Div Endocrinology, 670 Albany St, Boston, MA 02118; **Phone:** 617-638-7470; **Board Cert:** Internal Medicine 1981; Endocrinology, Diabetes & Metabolism 2008; **Med School:** India 1976; **Resid:** Internal Medicine, Northwestern Univ Med Ctr 1981; **Fellow:** Endocrinology, Diabetes & Metabolism, Harbor-UCIA Med Ctr 1984; **Fac Appt:** Prof Med, Boston Univ

Biller, Beverly M K MD [EDM] - **Spec Exp:** Pituitary Disorders; Cushing's Syndrome; Acromegaly; **Hospital:** Mass Genl Hosp; **Address:** Neuroendocrine Clinic Center, Zero Emerson Pl, Ste 112, Boston, MA 02114-3117; **Phone:** 617-726-7948; **Board Cert:** Internal Medicine 1986; Endocrinology 1989; **Med School:** Univ Okla Coll Med 1983; **Resid:** Internal Medicine, Beth Israel Deaconness Hosp 1986; **Fellow:** Endocrinology, Diabetes & Metabolism, Mass Genl Hosp 1989; **Fac Appt:** Assoc Prof Med, Harvard Med Sch

Braverman, Lewis E MD [EDM] - **Spec Exp:** Thyroid Disorders; **Hospital:** Boston Med Ctr; **Address:** Boston Med Ctr, Dept Endocrinology, Diabetes & Nutrition, 732 Harrison Ave Fl 2, Boston, MA 02118-2309; **Phone:** 617-638-7470; **Board Cert:** Internal Medicine 1963; Nuclear Medicine 1972; **Med School:** Johns Hopkins Univ 1955; **Resid:** Internal Medicine, Boston City Hosp 1960; **Fellow:** Endocrinology, Thorndike Meml Lab-Harvard 1962; **Fac Appt:** Prof Med, Boston Univ

Comi, Richard J MD [EDM] - **Spec Exp:** Diabetes; Hypoglycemia; Thyroid Disorders; Pituitary Disorders; **Hospital:** Dartmouth - Hitchcock Med Ctr; **Address:** Dartmouth-Hitchcock Med Ctr, Dept Endocrinology, 1 Med Ctr Drive Fl 5C, Lebanon, NH 03756; **Phone:** 603-650-8630; **Board Cert:** Internal Medicine 1983; Endocrinology 1987; **Med School:** Harvard Med Sch 1980; **Resid:** Internal Medicine, Mass Genl Hosp 1983; **Fellow:** Endocrinology & Diabetes, Natl Inst Hlth 1986

Cushing, Gary W MD [EDM] - **Spec Exp:** Thyroid Disorders; **Hospital:** Lahey Clin; **Address:** Lahey Clin, 4 West Endocrinology, 41 Mall Rd, Burlington, MA 01805; **Phone:** 781-744-2088; **Board Cert:** Internal Medicine 1983; Endocrinology 1985; **Med School:** Univ Mass Sch Med 1980; **Resid:** Internal Medicine, St Vincent Hosp 1983; **Fellow:** Endocrinology, Beth Israel Hosp 1985; **Fac Appt:** Assoc Clin Prof Med, Tufts Univ

Daniels, Gilbert H MD [EDM] - **Spec Exp:** Thyroid Disorders; Parathyroid Disease; Adrenal Disorders; Thyroid Cancer; **Hospital:** Mass Genl Hosp; **Address:** 15 Parkman St WACC Bldg - Ste 730, Boston, MA 02114; **Phone:** 617-726-8430; **Board Cert:** Internal Medicine 1972; Endocrinology, Diabetes & Metabolism 1975; **Med School:** Harvard Med Sch 1966; **Resid:** Internal Medicine, Mass Genl Hosp 1972; **Fellow:** Biochemistry, Natl Inst Hlth 1970; Endocrinology, Diabetes & Metabolism, UCSF Med Ctr 1971; **Fac Appt:** Prof Med, Harvard Med Sch

Holick, Michael F MD/PhD [EDM] - **Spec Exp:** Bone Disorders-Metabolic; Osteoporosis; Calcium Disorders; Nutrition; **Hospital:** Boston Med Ctr; **Address:** Boston Univ Sch Med, 732 Harrison Ave Fl 2, Boston, MA 02118; **Phone:** 617-638-7470; **Board Cert:** Internal Medicine 1979; **Med School:** Univ Wisc 1976; **Resid:** Internal Medicine, Mass Genl Hosp 1979; **Fellow:** Endocrinology, Mass Genl Hosp 1980; **Fac Appt:** Prof Med, Boston Univ

Inzucchi, Silvio E MD [EDM] - **Spec Exp:** Diabetes; Pituitary Disorders; Growth Hormone Disorder-Adult; Cholesterol/Lipid Disorders; **Hospital:** Yale-New Haven Hosp, Yale Med Group; **Address:** Yale Diabetes Center, 789 Howard Ave, Dana Clinic Bldg fl 2, New Haven, CT 06520; **Phone:** 203-737-1932; **Board Cert:** Internal Medicine 1988; Endocrinology, Diabetes & Metabolism 2006; **Med School:** Harvard Med Sch 1985; **Resid:** Internal Medicine, Yale-New Haven Hosp 1988; **Fellow:** Endocrinology, Diabetes & Metabolism, Yale-New Haven Hosp 1994; **Fac Appt:** Prof Med, Yale Univ

Kahn, Barbara B MD [EDM] - **Spec Exp:** Obesity; Nutrition; **Hospital:** Beth Israel Deaconess Med Ctr - Boston; **Address:** Beth Israel Deaconess Medical Ctr, 330 Brookline Ave, rm E/CLS747, Boston, MA 02215; **Phone:** 617-735-3324; **Board Cert:** Internal Medicine 1980; Endocrinology, Diabetes & Metabolism 1985; **Med School:** Stanford Univ 1977; **Resid:** Internal Medicine, UC Davis Med Ctr 1980; **Fellow:** Endocrinology, Diabetes & Metabolism, Natl Inst Hlth 1982; **Fac Appt:** Prof Med, Harvard Med Sch

Klibanski, Anne MD [EDM] - **Spec Exp:** Pituitary Disorders; Prolactin Disorders; Acromegaly; **Hospital:** Mass Genl Hosp; **Address:** Neuroendocrine Clinical Center, Zero Emerson Pl Fl 1 - Ste 112, Boston, MA 02114; **Phone:** 617-726-7948; **Board Cert:** Internal Medicine 1978; Endocrinology, Diabetes & Metabolism 1981; **Med School:** NYU Sch Med 1975; **Resid:** Internal Medicine, Bellevue Hosp Ctr 1978; **Fellow:** Endocrinology, Mass Genl Hosp 1981; **Fac Appt:** Prof Med, Harvard Med Sch

Kronenberg, Henry M MD [EDM] - **Spec Exp:** Bone Disorders-Metabolic; Parathyroid Disease; **Hospital:** Mass Genl Hosp; **Address:** Endocrine Associates, 15 Parkman Street, Wang AC 730A, Boston, MA 02114; **Phone:** 617-726-8720; **Board Cert:** Internal Medicine 1973; Endocrinology, Diabetes & Metabolism 1975; **Med School:** Columbia P&S 1970; **Resid:** Internal Medicine, Mass Genl Hosp 1972; **Fellow:** Endocrinology, Mass Genl Hosp 1975; **Fac Appt:** Prof Med, Harvard Med Sch

Larsen, Philip Reed MD [EDM] - **Spec Exp:** Thyroid Disorders; **Hospital:** Brigham and Women's Hosp (page 57); **Address:** 221 Longwood Ave Fl 2, Boston, MA 02115; **Phone:** 617-732-5666; **Board Cert:** Internal Medicine 1970; **Med School:** Columbia P&S 1963; **Resid:** Internal Medicine, NY Presby-Columbia Med Ctr 1965; Internal Medicine, Cincinnati General Hosp 1967; **Fellow:** Endocrinology, NIH 1968; Endocrinology, Cincinnati General Hosp 1969; **Fac Appt:** Prof Med, Harvard Med Sch

LeBoff, Meryl S MD [EDM] - **Spec Exp:** Osteoporosis; Bone Disorders-Metabolic; **Hospital:** Brigham and Women's Hosp (page 57); **Address:** 221 Longwood Ave Fl 2, Boston, MA 02115; **Phone:** 617-732-5666; **Board Cert:** Internal Medicine 1979; Endocrinology, Diabetes & Metabolism 1981; **Med School:** UMDNJ-NJ Med Sch, Newark 1975; **Resid:** Internal Medicine, USC Med Ctr 1979; **Fellow:** Endocrinology, Brigham & Womens Hosp 1982; **Fac Appt:** Assoc Prof Med, Harvard Med Sch

Lechan, Ronald M MD/PhD [EDM] - **Spec Exp:** Pituitary Disorders; Hypothalamic Dysfunction; Endocrine Cancers; Adrenal Disorders; **Hospital:** Tufts Med Ctr; **Address:** Tufts Medical Ctr, 800 Washington St, Box 268, Boston, MA 02111; **Phone:** 617-636-5689; **Board Cert:** Internal Medicine 1979; Endocrinology, Diabetes & Metabolism 1981; **Med School:** Univ VT Coll Med 1976; **Resid:** Internal Medicine, Beth Israel Hosp 1978; **Fellow:** Endocrinology, Diabetes & Metabolism, Tufts-New England Med Ctr 1981; **Fac Appt:** Prof Med, Tufts Univ

Levine, Robert A MD [EDM] - **Spec Exp:** Thyroid Cancer; Thyroid Disorders; Thyroid Ultrasound; **Hospital:** St. Joseph Hosp & Trauma Ctr; **Address:** Thyroid Center of New Hampshire, 5 Coliseum Ave, Ste 209, Nashua, NH 03063; **Phone:** 603-881-7141; **Board Cert:** Internal Medicine 1984; Endocrinology, Diabetes & Metabolism 1987; **Med School:** Univ Conn 1981; **Resid:** Internal Medicine, Mt Auburn Hosp 1984; **Fellow:** Endocrinology, Yale Univ 1987

Nathan, David M MD [EDM] - **Spec Exp:** Diabetes; **Hospital:** Mass Genl Hosp; **Address:** MGH Diabetes Center, 50 Staniford St Fl 3, Box 340, Boston, MA 02114; **Phone:** 617-726-8722; **Board Cert:** Internal Medicine 1978; Endocrinology, Diabetes & Metabolism 1981; **Med School:** Mount Sinai Sch Med 1975; **Resid:** Internal Medicine, Brigham & Women's Hosp 1978; **Fellow:** Endocrinology, Diabetes & Metabolism, Mass Genl Hosp 1980; **Fac Appt:** Prof Med, Harvard Med Sch

Pearce, Elizabeth N MD [EDM] - **Spec Exp:** Thyroid Disorders; **Hospital:** Boston Med Ctr; **Address:** 732 Harrison Ave, Fl 2, Boston, MA 02118; **Phone:** 617-638-7470; **Board Cert:** Endocrinology, Diabetes & Metabolism 2002; **Med School:** Harvard Med Sch 1997; **Resid:** Internal Medicine, Beth Israel Deaconess Med Ctr 2000; **Fellow:** Endocrinology, Diabetes & Metabolism, Boston Med Ctr 2003; **Fac Appt:** Assoc Prof Med, Boston Univ

Ross, Douglas S MD [EDM] - **Spec Exp:** Thyroid Disorders; Thyroid Cancer; **Hospital:** Mass Genl Hosp; **Address:** 15 Parkman St WAC Bldg - Ste 730 S, Boston, MA 02114; **Phone:** 617-726-3872; **Board Cert:** Internal Medicine 1980; Endocrinology, Diabetes & Metabolism 1983; **Med School:** Harvard Med Sch 1977; **Resid:** Internal Medicine, Mass General Hosp 1980; **Fellow:** Endocrinology, Mass General Hosp 1983; **Fac Appt:** Prof Med, Harvard Med Sch

Seely, Ellen Wells MD [EDM] - **Spec Exp:** Pregnancy & Endocrine Disorders; Diabetes in Pregnancy; Diabetes in Women; Thyroid Disorders in Pregnancy; **Hospital:** Brigham and Women's Hosp (page 57); **Address:** Brigham & Womens Hosp, Endocrine Div, 221 Longwood Ave Fl 2, Boston, MA 02115; **Phone:** 617-732-5661; **Board Cert:** Internal Medicine 1984; Endocrinology, Diabetes & Metabolism 1987; **Med School:** Columbia P&S 1981; **Resid:** Internal Medicine, Brigham & Womens Hosp 1984; **Fellow:** Endocrinology, Diabetes & Metabolism, Brigham & Womens Hosp 1987; **Fac Appt:** Prof Med, Harvard Med Sch

Mid Atlantic

Ball, Douglas W MD [EDM] - **Spec Exp:** Thyroid Cancer; **Hospital:** Johns Hopkins Hosp (page 61); **Address:** Sidney Kimmel Cancer Ctr, 1830 E Monument St, Ste 333, Baltimore, MD 21287; **Phone:** 410-955-9270; **Board Cert:** Internal Medicine 1987; **Med School:** Geo Wash Univ 1984; **Resid:** Internal Medicine, Univ Pittsburgh 1987; **Fellow:** Endocrinology, Diabetes & Metabolism, Johns Hopkins Hosp 1991; **Fac Appt:** Assoc Prof Med, Johns Hopkins Univ

Bergman, Donald MD [EDM] - **Spec Exp:** Osteoporosis; Thyroid Disorders; Calcium Disorders; Paget's Disease of Bone; **Hospital:** Mount Sinai Med Ctr (page 64); **Address:** 1199 Park Ave, Ste 1F, New York, NY 10128; **Phone:** 212-876-7333; **Board Cert:** Internal Medicine 1975; Endocrinology, Diabetes & Metabolism 1977; **Med School:** Jefferson Med Coll 1971; **Resid:** Obstetrics & Gynecology, Mt Sinai Hosp 1972; Internal Medicine, Mt Sinai Hosp 1975; **Fellow:** Endocrinology, Diabetes & Metabolism, Mt Sinai Hosp 1977; **Fac Appt:** Clin Prof Med, Mount Sinai Sch Med

Bilezikian, John P MD [EDM] - **Spec Exp:** Osteoporosis; Bone Disorders-Metabolic; Parathyroid Disorders; **Hospital:** NY-Presby/Columbia Univ Med Ctr, NY (page 66); **Address:** Columbia Metabolic Bone Disease Program, Harkness Pavilion, 180 Ft Washington Ave Fl 9 - Ste 904, New York, NY 10032; **Phone:** 212-305-2663; **Board Cert:** Internal Medicine 1975; Endocrinology, Diabetes & Metabolism 1977; **Med School:** Columbia P&S 1969; **Resid:** Internal Medicine, Columbia-Presby Hosp 1975; **Fellow:** Endocrinology, Diabetes & Metabolism, Natl Inst Health 1977; **Fac Appt:** Prof Med, Columbia P&S

Blum, Conrad B MD [EDM] - **Spec Exp:** Cholesterol/Lipid Disorders; Thyroid Disorders; Diabetes; **Hospital:** NY-Presby/Columbia Univ Med Ctr, NY (page 66); **Address:** 16 E 60th St, Ste 320, New York, NY 10022-1002; **Phone:** 212-326-8421; **Board Cert:** Internal Medicine 1976; Endocrinology, Diabetes & Metabolism 1977; **Med School:** Northwestern Univ 1971; **Resid:** Internal Medicine, Brigham Women & Chldn's Hosp 1976; **Fellow:** Endocrinology, Diabetes & Metabolism, Northwestern Univ Med Sch 1977; **Fac Appt:** Clin Prof Med, Columbia P&S

Bockman, Richard S MD/PhD [EDM] - **Spec Exp:** Bone Disorders-Metabolic; Osteoporosis; Parathyroid Disorders; Paget's Disease of Bone; **Hospital:** Hosp For Special Surgery (page 60), NY-Presby/Weill Cornell Med Ctr, NY (page 66); **Address:** 519 E 72nd St, Ste 206, New York, NY 10021; **Phone:** 212-606-1458; **Board Cert:** Internal Medicine 1975; **Med School:** Yale Univ 1968; **Resid:** Internal Medicine, NYU Med Ctr 1975; **Fellow:** Internal Medicine, NY-Cornell Med Ctr 1973; **Fac Appt:** Prof Med, Cornell Univ-Weill Med Coll

Brillon, David J MD [EDM] - **Spec Exp:** Diabetes; Thyroid Disorders; Clinical Trials; **Hospital:** NY-Presby/Weill Cornell Med Ctr, NY (page 66); **Address:** Cornell-Weill Physicians-Endocrinology, 525 E 68th St, Box 136, New York, NY 10065; **Phone:** 212-746-6290; **Board Cert:** Internal Medicine 1983; Endocrinology, Diabetes & Metabolism 1987; **Med School:** Brown Univ 1980; **Resid:** Internal Medicine, Rochester Genl Hosp 1983; **Fellow:** Endocrinology, Rochester Genl Hosp 1986; Endocrinology, Diabetes & Metabolism, UCSD Med Ctr 1988; **Fac Appt:** Clin Prof Med, Cornell Univ-Weill Med Coll

Burman, Kenneth D MD [EDM] - **Spec Exp:** Thyroid Disorders; Thyroid Cancer; **Hospital:** Washington Hosp Ctr; **Address:** Wash Hosp Ctr, Endocrinology Section, 110 Irving St NW, rm 1A-50B, Washington, DC 20010; **Phone:** 202-877-0333; **Board Cert:** Internal Medicine 1973; Endocrinology, Diabetes & Metabolism 1975; **Med School:** Univ MO-Columbia Sch Med 1970; **Resid:** Internal Medicine, Barnes Hosp 1972; **Fellow:** Endocrinology, Diabetes & Metabolism, Walter Reed Hosp 1974; **Fac Appt:** Prof Med, Georgetown Univ

Calvi, Laura M MD [EDM] - **Spec Exp:** Neuroendocrinology; Pituitary Disorders; **Hospital:** Univ of Rochester Strong Meml Hosp; **Address:** 601 Elmwood Ave, Box 693, Rochester, NY 14642; **Phone:** 585-273-2343; **Board Cert:** Endocrinology, Diabetes & Metabolism 2010; **Med School:** Harvard Med Sch 1995; **Resid:** Internal Medicine, Mass Genl Hosp 1998; **Fellow:** Endocrinology, Mass Genl Hosp 2000; **Fac Appt:** Assoc Prof Med, Univ Rochester

Endocrinology, Diabetes & Metabolism

Cooper, David S MD [EDM] - **Spec Exp:** Thyroid Disorders; **Hospital:** Johns Hopkins Hosp (page 61); **Address:** Div Endocrinology & Metabolism, 1830 E Monument St, Ste 333, Baltimore, MD 21287; **Phone:** 410-502-4926; **Board Cert:** Internal Medicine 1987; Endocrinology, Diabetes & Metabolism 2008; **Med School:** Tufts Univ 1973; **Resid:** Internal Medicine, Barnes Hosp 1976; **Fellow:** Endocrinology, Mass Genl Hosp 1978; **Fac Appt:** Prof Med, Johns Hopkins Univ

Davies, Terry F MD [EDM] - **Spec Exp:** Thyroid Disorders in Pregnancy; Graves' Disease; Hashimoto's Disease; Thyroid Cancer; **Hospital:** Mount Sinai Med Ctr (page 64), VA Hudson Valley-FDR/Montrose; **Address:** 5 E 98th St, Box 1055, New York, NY 10029-6500; **Phone:** 212-241-7975; **Med School:** England, UK 1971; **Resid:** Internal Medicine, Univ Newcastle 1975; **Fellow:** Endocrinology, Diabetes & Metabolism, Univ Newcastle 1977; Endocrinology, Diabetes & Metabolism, Natl Inst Hlth 1979; **Fac Appt:** Prof Med, Mount Sinai Sch Med

Dobs, Adrian S MD [EDM] - **Spec Exp:** Hormonal Disorders; Hypogonadism-Male; Metabolic Disorders; Complementary Medicine; **Hospital:** Johns Hopkins Hosp (page 61); **Address:** Johns Hopkins Hosp, 1830 E Monument St Fl 3 - Ste 328, Baltimore, MD 21287; **Phone:** 410-502-4926; **Board Cert:** Internal Medicine 1981; Endocrinology 1987; **Med School:** Albany Med Coll 1978; **Resid:** Internal Medicine, Montefiore Hosp 1982; **Fellow:** Endocrinology, Johns Hopkins Hosp 1984; **Fac Appt:** Prof Med, Johns Hopkins Univ

Donner, Thomas W MD [EDM] - **Spec Exp:** Diabetes; **Hospital:** Johns Hopkins Hosp (page 61); **Address:** Johns Hopkins Comprehensive Diabetes Ctr, 601 N Caroline St, Ste 2008, Baltimore, MD 21287; **Phone:** 410-955-7139; **Board Cert:** Internal Medicine 1989; Endocrinology, Diabetes & Metabolism 2007; **Med School:** Univ VA Sch Med 1986; **Resid:** Internal Medicine, Univ Maryland 1989; **Fellow:** Endocrinology, Diabetes & Metabolism, Univ Maryland 1991; **Fac Appt:** Assoc Prof Med, Johns Hopkins Univ

Greene, Loren Wissner MD [EDM] - **Spec Exp:** Thyroid Disorders; Osteoporosis; Pituitary Disorders; Diabetes; **Hospital:** NYU Langone Med Ctr (page 68), NY Downtown Hosp; **Address:** 650 First Ave Fl 7, New York, NY 10016-6402; **Phone:** 212-263-7449; **Board Cert:** Internal Medicine 1978; Endocrinology, Diabetes & Metabolism 1981; **Med School:** NYU Sch Med 1975; **Resid:** Internal Medicine, Bellevue Hosp Ctr-NYU 1978; **Fellow:** Endocrinology, Bellevue Hosp Ctr-NYU 1980; **Fac Appt:** Assoc Clin Prof Med, NYU Sch Med

Greenspan, Susan L MD [EDM] - **Spec Exp:** Osteoporosis; Osteoporosis in Men; **Hospital:** UPMC Presby, Pittsburgh; **Address:** Univ Pittsburgh, Osteoporosis Ctr, 3471 Fifth Ave, Kaufmann Bldg - Ste 1110, Pittsburgh, PA 15213; **Phone:** 412-692-2220; **Board Cert:** Internal Medicine 1982; Endocrinology, Diabetes & Metabolism 1987; **Med School:** Harvard Med Sch 1979; **Resid:** Internal Medicine, Beth Israel Hosp 1982; **Fellow:** Endocrinology, Mass Genl Hosp 1985; Geriatric Medicine, Beth Israel Hosp 1986; **Fac Appt:** Prof Med, Univ Pittsburgh

Jacobs, Thomas MD [EDM] - **Spec Exp:** Adrenal Disorders; Pituitary Disorders; Calcium Disorders; Thyroid Disorders; **Hospital:** NY-Presby/Columbia Univ Med Ctr, NY (page 66); **Address:** 161 Fort Washington Ave, rm 210, MS 10032, New York, NY 10032-3713; **Phone:** 212-305-5578; **Board Cert:** Internal Medicine 1973; Endocrinology, Diabetes & Metabolism 1975; **Med School:** Johns Hopkins Univ 1968; **Resid:** Internal Medicine, Columbia Presby Hosp 1973; **Fellow:** Endocrinology, Diabetes & Metabolism, Univ Wash Med Ctr 1975; **Fac Appt:** Clin Prof Med, Columbia P&S

Kleinberg, David L MD [EDM] - **Spec Exp:** Pituitary Disorders; Neuroendocrinology; **Hospital:** NYU Langone Med Ctr (page 68); **Address:** 530 1st Ave, Ste 4C, New York, NY 10016; **Phone:** 212-263-6772; **Board Cert:** Internal Medicine 1972; Endocrinology 1975; **Med School:** Univ Miami Sch Med 1966; **Resid:** Internal Medicine, Maimonides Med Ctr 1968; Internal Medicine, Columbia-Presby Med Ctr 1971; **Fellow:** Endocrinology, Diabetes & Metabolism, Columbia-Presby Med Ctr 1970; **Fac Appt:** Prof Med, NYU Sch Med

Korytkowski, Mary T MD [EDM] - **Spec Exp:** Diabetes; Diabetes Clinical Trials; Hormonal Disorders; **Hospital:** UPMC Presby, Pittsburgh; **Address:** Center for Diabetes & Endocrinology, Faulk Medical Bldg, 3601 Fifth Ave, Ste 3B, Pittsburgh, PA 15213-3403; **Phone:** 412-586-9714; **Board Cert:** Internal Medicine 1985; Endocrinology 1989; **Med School:** Univ NC Sch Med 1982; **Resid:** Internal Medicine, Francis Scott Key Med Ctr 1985; **Fellow:** Endocrinology, Diabetes & Metabolism, Sinai Hosp/Johns Hopkins Hosp 1988; **Fac Appt:** Prof Med, Univ Pittsburgh

Ladenson, Paul W MD [EDM] - **Spec Exp:** Thyroid Disorders; Thyroid Cancer; **Hospital:** Johns Hopkins Hosp (page 61); **Address:** Johns Hopkins Hosp, Div Endocrinology & Metabolism, 1830 E Monument St, rm 333, Baltimore, MD 21287; **Phone:** 410-502-4926; **Board Cert:** Internal Medicine 1978; Endocrinology, Diabetes & Metabolism 1981; **Med School:** Harvard Med Sch 1975; **Resid:** Internal Medicine, Mass Genl Hosp 1978; **Fellow:** Endocrinology, Diabetes & Metabolism, Mass Genl Hosp 1980; **Fac Appt:** Prof Med, Johns Hopkins Univ

Lipson, Ace MD [EDM] - **Spec Exp:** Diabetes; Thyroid Disorders; Pituitary Disorders; Adrenal Disorders; **Hospital:** G Washington Univ Hosp; **Address:** 1120 19th St NW, Ste 200, Washington, DC 20036; **Phone:** 202-296-3443; **Board Cert:** Internal Medicine 1976; Endocrinology, Diabetes & Metabolism 1979; **Med School:** Washington Univ, St Louis 1973; **Resid:** Internal Medicine, George Washington Univ Med Ctr 1976; **Fellow:** Endocrinology, Johns Hopkins Hosp 1978; **Fac Appt:** Clin Prof Med, Geo Wash Univ

Mandel, Susan J MD [EDM] - **Spec Exp:** Thyroid Disorders; Thyroid Cancer; Thyroid Disorders in Pregnancy; Thyroid Ultrasound; **Hospital:** Hosp Univ Penn - UPHS (page 72); **Address:** Div Endocrinology, Perelman Ctr for Advanced Medicine, 3400 Civic Ctr Blvd Fl 4-West, Philadelphia, PA 19104; **Phone:** 215-662-2300; **Board Cert:** Internal Medicine 1989; Endocrinology 2011; **Med School:** Columbia P&S 1986; **Resid:** Internal Medicine, Columbia Presby Med Ctr 1989; **Fellow:** Endocrinology, Brigham & Womens Hosp 1992; **Fac Appt:** Prof Med, Univ Pennsylvania

McConnell, Robert J MD [EDM] - **Spec Exp:** Thyroid Disorders; Thyroid Ultrasound; **Hospital:** NY-Presby/Columbia Univ Med Ctr, NY (page 66); **Address:** 161 Fort Washington Ave, Ste 210, New York, NY 10032-3713; **Phone:** 212-305-5579; **Board Cert:** Internal Medicine 1978; Endocrinology, Diabetes & Metabolism 1981; **Med School:** Columbia P&S 1973; **Resid:** Internal Medicine, Barnes Hosp 1975; **Fellow:** Endocrinology, Diabetes & Metabolism, Columbia-Presby Hosp 1978; **Fac Appt:** Clin Prof Med, Columbia P&S

Roberts, Michelle M MD [EDM] - **Spec Exp:** Osteoporosis; **Hospital:** UPMC Presby, Pittsburgh; **Address:** Center for Diabetes & Endocrinology, Faulk Medical Bldg, 3601 Fifth Ave, Ste 3B, Pittsburgh, PA 15213; **Phone:** 412-586-9714; **Board Cert:** Internal Medicine 1986; Endocrinology, Diabetes & Metabolism 1989; **Med School:** Duke Univ 1983; **Resid:** Internal Medicine, Univ Pittsburgh Med Ctr 1986; **Fellow:** Endocrinology, Diabetes & Metabolism, Univ Pittsburgh 1989; **Fac Appt:** Assoc Prof Med, Univ Pittsburgh

Rodbard, Helena W MD [EDM] - **Spec Exp:** Diabetes; Gynecomastia; **Hospital:** Shady Grove Adven Hosp; **Address:** 3200 Tower Oaks Blvd, Ste 250, Rockville, MD 20852; **Phone:** 301-770-7373; **Board Cert:** Internal Medicine 1981; Endocrinology, Diabetes & Metabolism 1983; **Med School:** Brazil 1972; **Resid:** Internal Medicine, Washington Hosp 1981; **Fellow:** Endocrinology, Diabetes & Metabolism, Natl Inst Hlth 1979; Endocrinology, Diabetes & Metabolism, Geo Wash Univ 1982

Schutta, Mark H MD [EDM] - **Spec Exp:** Diabetes; Diabetes Prevention; Hypoglycemia; **Hospital:** Hosp Univ Penn - UPHS (page 72); **Address:** Penn Rodebaugh Diabetes Ctr, Perelman Ctr for Advanced Medicine, 3400 Civic Center Blvd, 4 West, Philadelphia, PA 19104; **Phone:** 215-662-2300; **Board Cert:** Endocrinology, Diabetes & Metabolism 2002; **Med School:** Jefferson Med Coll 1993; **Resid:** Internal Medicine, T Jefferson Univ Hosp 1996; **Fellow:** Endocrinology, Hosp Univ Penn 1999; **Fac Appt:** Assoc Prof Med, Univ Pennsylvania

Schwartz, Stanley S MD [EDM] - **Spec Exp:** Diabetes; Metabolic Syndrome; Thyroid Disorders; **Hospital:** Lankenau Hosp, Bryn Mawr Hosp; **Address:** 233 E Lancaster Ave, Ste 305, Ardmore, PA 19003-2321; **Phone:** 610-642-6800; **Board Cert:** Internal Medicine 1976; Endocrinology, Diabetes & Metabolism 1979; **Med School:** Univ Chicago-Pritzker Sch Med 1973; **Resid:** Internal Medicine, Hosp U Penn 1976; **Fellow:** Endocrinology, Diabetes & Metabolism, Univ Chicago Hosps 1978; **Fac Appt:** Prof Emeritus Med, Univ Pennsylvania

Seplowitz, Alan H MD [EDM] - **Spec Exp:** Thyroid Disorders; Cholesterol/Lipid Disorders; Diabetes; **Hospital:** NY-Presby/Columbia Univ Med Ctr, NY (page 66); **Address:** 161 Fort Washington Ave, Ste 4-422, New York, NY 10032-3729; **Phone:** 212-305-5503; **Board Cert:** Internal Medicine 1975; Endocrinology 1977; **Med School:** Columbia P&S 1972; **Resid:** Internal Medicine, Columbia-Presby Med Ctr 1974; **Fellow:** Lipid Metabolism, Natl Insts Hlth 1976; Endocrinology, Diabetes & Metabolism, Columbia-Presby Med Ctr 1978; **Fac Appt:** Assoc Clin Prof Med, Columbia P&S

Shuldiner, Alan R MD [EDM] - **Spec Exp:** Diabetes; Eating Disorders/Obesity; **Hospital:** Univ of MD Med Ctr; **Address:** Univ MD Sch Med, Div Endocrinology, 660 W Redwood St, rm HH-494, Baltimore, MD 21201; **Phone:** 410-706-1623; **Board Cert:** Internal Medicine 1988; Endocrinology 1989; **Med School:** Harvard Med Sch 1984; **Resid:** Internal Medicine, Columbia-Presby Hosp 1986; **Fellow:** Endocrinology, Diabetes & Metabolism, Natl Inst Hlth 1990; **Fac Appt:** Prof Med, Univ MD Sch Med

Siris, Ethel MD [EDM] - **Spec Exp:** Osteoporosis; Paget's Disease of Bone; Bone Disorders-Metabolic; **Hospital:** NY-Presby/Columbia Univ Med Ctr, NY (page 66); **Address:** 180 Ft Washington Ave, HP Bldg - Fl 9 - Ste 964, New York, NY 10032-3710; **Phone:** 212-305-9531; **Board Cert:** Internal Medicine 1974; Endocrinology, Diabetes & Metabolism 1977; **Med School:** Columbia P&S 1971; **Resid:** Internal Medicine, Columbia-Presby Med Ctr 1974; **Fellow:** Research, Natl Inst Hlth 1976; Endocrinology, Diabetes & Metabolism, Columbia-Presby Med Ctr 1977; **Fac Appt:** Prof Med, Columbia P&S

Snyder, Peter J MD [EDM] - **Spec Exp:** Pituitary Tumors; Reproductive Endocrinology-Male; Neuroendocrine Tumors; **Hospital:** Hosp Univ Penn - UPHS (page 72); **Address:** Perelman Center-Endocrinology, 3400 Civic Ctr Blvd, Ste 4-900, Philadelphia, PA 19104; **Phone:** 215-662-2300; **Board Cert:** Internal Medicine 1972; Endocrinology, Diabetes & Metabolism 1972; **Med School:** Harvard Med Sch 1965; **Resid:** Internal Medicine, Beth Israel Hosp 1967; Internal Medicine, Beth Israel Hosp 1970; **Fellow:** Endocrinology, Diabetes & Metabolism, Hosp Univ Penn 1971; **Fac Appt:** Prof Med, Univ Pennsylvania

Surks, Martin I MD [EDM] - **Spec Exp:** Thyroid Disorders; **Hospital:** Montefiore Med Ctr-Moses Campus, NY, N Central Bronx Hosp; **Address:** 3400 Bainbridge Ave Fl 2, Bronx, NY 10467; **Phone:** 866-633-8255; **Board Cert:** Internal Medicine 1967; Endocrinology, Diabetes & Metabolism 1977; **Med School:** NYU Sch Med 1960; **Resid:** Internal Medicine, Montefiore Hosp Med Ctr 1962; Internal Medicine, VA Hosp 1964; **Fellow:** Research, Natl Inst Arthritis-Metabolic Disease 1964; **Fac Appt:** Prof Med, Albert Einstein Coll Med

Tuttle, R Michael MD [EDM] - **Spec Exp:** Thyroid Cancer; **Hospital:** Meml Sloan-Kettering Cancer Ctr; **Address:** Meml Sloan Kettering Cancer Ctr, 1275 York Ave, New York, NY 10065; **Phone:** 646-888-2716; **Board Cert:** Endocrinology, Diabetes & Metabolism 2004; **Med School:** Univ Louisville Sch Med 1987; **Resid:** Internal Medicine, DD Eisenhower Army Med Ctr 1990; **Fellow:** Endocrinology, Diabetes & Metabolism, Madigan Army Med Ctr 1993; **Fac Appt:** Prof Med, Cornell Univ-Weill Med Coll

Wartofsky, Leonard MD [EDM] - **Spec Exp:** Thyroid Cancer; Thyroid Disorders; **Hospital:** Washington Hosp Ctr; **Address:** 110 Irving St NW, Washington, DC 20010-2975; **Phone:** 202-877-3109; **Board Cert:** Internal Medicine 1971; Endocrinology, Diabetes & Metabolism 1972; **Med School:** Geo Wash Univ 1964; **Resid:** Internal Medicine, Barnes Jewish Hosp 1966; Internal Medicine, Montefiore Med Ctr 1967; **Fellow:** Endocrinology, Diabetes & Metabolism, Boston City Hosp 1969; **Fac Appt:** Prof Med, Georgetown Univ

Wondisford, Frederic E MD [EDM] - **Spec Exp:** Diabetes; **Hospital:** Johns Hopkins Hosp (page 61); **Address:** Johns Hopkins Outpatient Ctr, 601 N Caroline St, Baltimore, MD 21287; **Phone:** 410-955-9270; **Board Cert:** Internal Medicine 1986; Endocrinology, Diabetes & Metabolism 1989; **Med School:** NE Ohio Univ 1983; **Resid:** Internal Medicine, U Hosps/Case Western Res U 1986; **Fellow:** Endocrinology, Natl Inst Health Clin Ctr 1989; **Fac Appt:** Prof Med, Johns Hopkins Univ

Xing, Michael M MD/PhD [EDM] - **Spec Exp:** Thyroid Disorders; Thyroid Cancer; **Hospital:** Johns Hopkins Hosp (page 61); **Address:** Johns Hopkins Hosp, Div Endocrinology & Metabolism, 1830 E Monument St, Ste 333, Baltimore, MD 21287; **Phone:** 410-502-4926; **Board Cert:** Internal Medicine 2000; Endocrinology, Diabetes & Metabolism 2003; **Med School:** China 1984; **Resid:** Internal Medicine, Greater Baltimore Med Ctr 2000; **Fellow:** Endocrinology, Johns Hopkins Hosp 2003; **Fac Appt:** Assoc Prof Med, Johns Hopkins Univ

Young, Iven MD [EDM] - **Spec Exp:** Thyroid Disorders; Osteoporosis; Pituitary Disorders; Cushing's Syndrome; **Hospital:** NYU Langone Med Ctr (page 68); **Address:** 275 W Seventh Ave Fl 2, MS 10001, New York, NY 10001; **Phone:** 212-675-9332; **Board Cert:** Internal Medicine 1966; Endocrinology, Diabetes & Metabolism 1973; **Med School:** NYU Sch Med 1959; **Resid:** Internal Medicine, VA Med Ctr 1963; **Fellow:** Endocrinology, NYU Med Ctr 1966; **Fac Appt:** Assoc Clin Prof Med, NYU Sch Med

Southeast

Ain, Kenneth B MD [EDM] - **Spec Exp:** Thyroid Cancer; Thyroid Disorders; **Hospital:** Univ of Kentucky Albert B. Chandler Hosp, Lexington VA Med Ctr; **Address:** Thyroid Oncology Program, 800 Rose St, rm MN524, Lexington, KY 40536-0298; **Phone:** 859-323-3778; **Board Cert:** Internal Medicine 1984; Endocrinology, Diabetes & Metabolism 1987; **Med School:** Brown Univ 1981; **Resid:** Internal Medicine, Hahnemann Univ Hosp 1984; **Fellow:** Endocrinology, Univ Chicago 1986; Thyroid Oncology, NIDDK, Natl Inst Hlth 1990; **Fac Appt:** Prof Med, Univ KY Coll Med

Barrett, Eugene J MD/PhD [EDM] - **Spec Exp:** Diabetes; Diabetic Vascular Disease Prevention; **Hospital:** Univ of Virginia Health Sys; **Address:** Univ Virginia, Div Endocrinology, PO Box 801410, Charlottesville, VA 22908-1410; **Phone:** 434-924-1825; **Board Cert:** Internal Medicine 1978; **Med School:** Univ Rochester 1975; **Resid:** Internal Medicine, Strong Meml Hosp 1977; **Fellow:** Endocrinology, Diabetes & Metabolism, Yale Univ 1980; **Fac Appt:** Prof Med, Univ VA Sch Med

Bell, David S H MD [EDM] - **Spec Exp:** Diabetes; Thyroid Disorders; Cholesterol/Lipid Disorders; Adrenal Disorders; **Hospital:** Univ of Ala Hosp at Birmingham; **Address:** Southside Endocrinology, 3938 montclair Rd S, Fl 1, rm 130, Birmingham, AL 35213; **Phone:** 205-803-1113; **Board Cert:** Internal Medicine 1987; Endocrinology, Diabetes & Metabolism 1981; **Med School:** Ireland 1970; **Resid:** Internal Medicine, Royal Victoria Hosp 1973; Endocrinology, Diabetes & Metabolism, Univ Saskatchewan Hosp 1975; **Fellow:** Endocrinology, Diabetes & Metabolism, Greater Baltimore Med Ctr 1976

Buse, John B MD/PhD [EDM] - **Spec Exp:** Diabetes; **Hospital:** NC Memorial Hosp - UNC; **Address:** UNC Highgate Specialty Center, 5316 Highgate Drive, Ste 125, Chapel Hill, NC 27513; **Phone:** 919-484-1015; **Board Cert:** Internal Medicine 1989; Endocrinology, Diabetes & Metabolism 2011; **Med School:** Duke Univ 1986; **Resid:** Internal Medicine, Univ Chicago Hosps 1988; **Fellow:** Endocrinology, Diabetes & Metabolism, Univ Chicago Hosps 1991; **Fac Appt:** Prof Med, Univ NC Sch Med

Clore, John N MD [EDM] - **Spec Exp:** Diabetes; Hypoglycemia; Pancreatic Islet Cell Transplant; **Hospital:** Med Coll of VA Hosp; **Address:** VCU Med Ctr - Div Endocrinology, 1200 E Broad St, PO Box 980155, Richmond, VA 23298; **Phone:** 804-828-2161; **Board Cert:** Internal Medicine 1985; Endocrinology, Diabetes & Metabolism 1989; **Med School:** Med Coll VA 1982; **Resid:** Internal Medicine, Med Coll Virginia Hosps 1985; **Fellow:** Endocrinology, Diabetes & Metabolism, Med Coll Virginia 1988; **Fac Appt:** Prof Med, Va Commonwealth Univ Sch Med

Dalkin, Alan C MD [EDM] - **Spec Exp:** Bone Disorders-Metabolic; Osteoporosis; **Hospital:** Univ of Virginia Health Sys; **Address:** Univ Virginia Div Endocrinology, PO Box 800412, Charlottesville, VA 22908; **Phone:** 434-924-1825; **Board Cert:** Internal Medicine 1987; Endocrinology 1989; **Med School:** Univ Mich Med Sch 1984; **Resid:** Internal Medicine, Univ Chicago Hosps 1987; **Fellow:** Endocrinology, Diabetes & Metabolism, Univ Michigan 1990; **Fac Appt:** Prof Med, Univ VA Sch Med

Earp III, H Shelton MD [EDM] - **Spec Exp:** Cancer-Hormonal Influences; **Hospital:** NC Memorial Hosp - UNC; **Address:** UNC Lineberger Comprehensive Cancer Ctr, 450 West Drive, Fl 1 - rm 10-012, Chapel Hill, NC 27599; **Phone:** 919-966-3036; **Board Cert:** Internal Medicine 1976; Endocrinology, Diabetes & Metabolism 1977; **Med School:** Univ NC Sch Med 1970; **Resid:** Internal Medicine, NC Memorial Hosp 1975; **Fellow:** Endocrinology, Diabetes & Metabolism, Univ North Carolina 1977; **Fac Appt:** Prof Med, Univ NC Sch Med

Feinglos, Mark MD [EDM] - **Spec Exp:** Diabetes; Thyroid Disorders; **Hospital:** Duke Univ Hosp; **Address:** DUMC, Box 3921, Durham, NC 27710-0001; **Phone:** 919-684-4005; **Board Cert:** Internal Medicine 1976; Endocrinology, Diabetes & Metabolism 1977; **Med School:** McGill Univ 1973; **Resid:** Internal Medicine, Duke Univ Med Ctr 1975; **Fellow:** Endocrinology, Diabetes & Metabolism, Duke Univ Med Ctr 1978; **Fac Appt:** Prof Med, Duke Univ

Goodman, Neil F MD [EDM] - **Spec Exp:** Reproductive Endocrinology; Polycystic Ovarian Syndrome; Hormonal Disorders; Infertility; **Address:** 9150 SW 87 Ave, Ste 210, Miami, FL 33176-2313; **Phone:** 305-595-6855; **Board Cert:** Internal Medicine 1973; Endocrinology, Diabetes & Metabolism 1975; **Med School:** Columbia P&S 1970; **Resid:** Internal Medicine, Beth Israel Deaconess Med Ctr 1972; **Fellow:** Endocrinology, Mass Genl Hosp 1974; **Fac Appt:** Clin Prof Med, Univ Miami Sch Med

Koch, Christian A MD [EDM] - **Spec Exp:** Endocrine Cancers; Thyroid Cancer; Pituitary Disorders; **Hospital:** Univ Mississippi Med Ctr; **Address:** 2500 N State St, Jackson, MS 39216; **Phone:** 601-984-5495; **Board Cert:** Endocrinology, Diabetes & Metabolism 2011; Internal Medicine 2010; **Med School:** Germany 1991; **Resid:** Internal Medicine, Ohio State Univ Hosp 1997; **Fellow:** Endocrinology, Natl Inst Hlth 2001; **Fac Appt:** Prof Med, Univ Miss

Marshall, John C MD/PhD [EDM] - **Spec Exp:** Pituitary Disorders; Neuroendocrinology; Polycystic Ovarian Syndrome; **Hospital:** Univ of Virginia Health Sys; **Address:** PO Box 800612, OMS Bldg - Fl 5th - Ste 5826, Box 800612, Univ Virginia health Center, Charlottesville, VA 22908-0001; **Phone:** 434-924-2431; **Board Cert:** Internal Medicine 1978; Endocrinology, Diabetes & Metabolism 1981; **Med School:** England, UK 1965; **Resid:** Neurology, Natl Hosp Queen Square 1968; Cardiovascular Disease, Natl Heart Hosp 1969; **Fellow:** Endocrinology, Diabetes & Metabolism, Hammersmith Hosp 1972; Endocrinology, Diabetes & Metabolism, UCLA 1974; **Fac Appt:** Prof Med, Univ VA Sch Med

Nestler, John E MD [EDM] - **Spec Exp:** Polycystic Ovarian Syndrome; Diabetes; **Hospital:** Med Coll of VA Hosp; **Address:** Medical College of Virginia/Department of Internal Medicine, Box 980663, Richmond, VA 23298-0663; **Phone:** 804-828-2161; **Board Cert:** Internal Medicine 1982; Endocrinology 1985; **Med School:** Univ Pennsylvania 1979; **Resid:** Internal Medicine, Med Coll Virginia 1983; **Fellow:** Endocrinology, Hosp Univ Penn 1985; **Fac Appt:** Prof Med, Med Coll VA

Ober, K Patrick MD [EDM] - **Spec Exp:** Diabetes; **Hospital:** Wake Forest Baptist Med Ctr; **Address:** Medical Center Blvd, Winston-Salem, NC 27157; **Phone:** 336-713-7251; **Board Cert:** Internal Medicine 1977; Endocrinology, Diabetes & Metabolism 1979; **Med School:** Univ Fla Coll Med 1974; **Resid:** Internal Medicine, NC Baptist Hosp 1976; **Fellow:** Endocrinology & Metabolism, NC Baptist Hosp 1978; **Fac Appt:** Prof Med, Wake Forest Univ

Ovalle, Fernando MD [EDM] - **Spec Exp:** Diabetes; Diabetes in Women; **Hospital:** Univ of Ala Hosp at Birmingham; **Address:** UAB Kirklin Clinic, 2000 6th Ave S, MCDC Clinic Fl 4, Birmingham, AL 35233; **Phone:** 205-934-4171; **Med School:** Mexico 1989; **Resid:** Internal Medicine, Henry Ford Hosp 1995; **Fellow:** Endocrinology, Diabetes & Metabolism, Barnes Hosp-Wash Univ 1997; **Fac Appt:** Assoc Prof Med, Univ Alabama

Powers, Alvin C MD [EDM] - **Spec Exp:** Diabetes; Thyroid Disorders; **Hospital:** Vanderbilt Univ Med Ctr (page 75); **Address:** Vanderbilt Diabetes Ctr, 1215 21st Ave S, 8210 MCE S Tower, Nashville, TN 37232-0202; **Phone:** 615-343-8332; **Board Cert:** Internal Medicine 1982; Endocrinology, Diabetes & Metabolism 1985; **Med School:** Univ Tenn Coll Med 1979; **Resid:** Internal Medicine, Duke Univ Med Ctr 1982; **Fellow:** Endocrinology, Diabetes & Metabolism, Joslin Diabetes Ctr 1983; Endocrinology, Diabetes & Metabolism, Mass Genl Hosp 1985; **Fac Appt:** Prof Med, Vanderbilt Univ

Quinn, Suzanne L MD [EDM] - **Spec Exp:** Diabetes; Thyroid Disorders; **Hospital:** Shands at Univ of FL, Malcolm Randall VA Med Ctr; **Address:** Shands Univ Florida, Dept Endocrinology, 2000 SW Archer Rd Fl 3, Gainesville, FL 32610; **Phone:** 352-265-8230; **Board Cert:** Internal Medicine 1988; Endocrinology, Diabetes & Metabolism 2003; **Med School:** Univ Fla Coll Med 1985; **Resid:** Internal Medicine, Shands at Univ Fla 1988; **Fellow:** Endocrinology, Diabetes & Metabolism, Univ Fla 1992; **Fac Appt:** Assoc Prof Med, Univ Fla Coll Med

Skyler, Jay S MD [EDM] - **Spec Exp:** Diabetes; **Hospital:** Univ of Miami Hosp, Jackson Meml Hosp; **Address:** Univ Miami Diabetes Research Inst, 1450 NW 10th Ave, Ste 3054, Miami, FL 33136; **Phone:** 305-243-6146; **Board Cert:** Internal Medicine 1972; Endocrinology, Diabetes & Metabolism 1973; **Med School:** Jefferson Med Coll 1969; **Resid:** Internal Medicine, Duke Univ Med Ctr 1971; **Fellow:** Endocrinology, Diabetes & Metabolism, Duke Univ Med Ctr 1973; **Fac Appt:** Prof Med, Univ Miami Sch Med

Thorner, Michael MD [EDM] - **Spec Exp:** Cushing's Syndrome; Growth Hormone Disorder-Adult; Metabolic Syndrome; Pituitary Disorders; **Hospital:** Univ of Virginia Health Sys; **Address:** Univ VA Hlth Sys, PO Box 801411, Charlottesville, VA 22908; **Phone:** 434-982-3297; **Med School:** England, UK 1970; **Resid:** Internal Medicine, Brompton Hosp 1972; **Fellow:** Endocrinology & Metabolism, St Bartholomew's Hosp 1974; **Fac Appt:** Prof Med, Univ VA Sch Med

Vance, Mary Lee MD [EDM] - **Spec Exp:** Pituitary Disorders; Adrenal Disorders; **Hospital:** Univ of Virginia Health Sys; **Address:** Univ Virginia Div Endocrinology, PO Box 800601, Charlottesville, VA 22908-0601; **Phone:** 434-982-3591; **Board Cert:** Internal Medicine 1980; **Med School:** Louisiana State U, New Orleans 1977; **Resid:** Internal Medicine, Baylor Univ Med Ctr 1980; **Fellow:** Endocrinology, Univ Virginia 1983; **Fac Appt:** Prof Med, Univ VA Sch Med

Endocrinology, Diabetes & Metabolism

Weissman, Peter N MD [EDM] - **Spec Exp:** Diabetes; **Hospital:** Baptist Hosp of Miami; **Address:** Endocrinology Associates, 7867 N Kendall Drive, Ste 80, Miami, FL 33156; **Phone:** 305-595-0777; **Board Cert:** Internal Medicine 1972; Endocrinology, Diabetes & Metabolism 1972; **Med School:** NYU Sch Med 1966; **Resid:** Internal Medicine, Barnes Hosp/Wash Univ 1969; **Fellow:** Geriatric Medicine, Gerontology Rsch Ctr 1970; Endocrinology, Diabetes & Metabolism, Univ Mich Hosp 1972; **Fac Appt:** Assoc Clin Prof Med, Univ Miami Sch Med

Midwest

Bahn, Rebecca S MD [EDM] - **Spec Exp:** Graves' Disease; Graves' Disease-Eye; **Hospital:** Mayo Med Ctr & Clin - Rochester; **Address:** Mayo Clin, Div Endocrinology, 200 First St SW, Rochester, MN 55905; **Phone:** 507-284-1600; **Board Cert:** Internal Medicine 1985; Endocrinology, Diabetes & Metabolism 1987; **Med School:** Mayo Med Sch 1981; **Resid:** Internal Medicine, Mayo Clin 1984; **Fellow:** Endocrinology, Diabetes & Metabolism, Mayo Clin 1986; **Fac Appt:** Prof Med, Mayo Med Sch

Brennan, Michael D MD [EDM] - **Spec Exp:** Thyroid Disorders; Diabetes; **Hospital:** Mayo Med Ctr & Clin - Rochester; **Address:** Mayo Clin, Div Endocrinology, 200 First St SW, Rochester, MN 55905; **Phone:** 507-284-1600; **Board Cert:** Internal Medicine 1975; Endocrinology, Diabetes & Metabolism 1977; **Med School:** Ireland 1969; **Resid:** Internal Medicine, Henry Ford Hosp 1972; Internal Medicine, Mayo Clinic 1975; **Fellow:** Endocrinology, Diabetes & Metabolism, Mayo Clinic 1977; **Fac Appt:** Assoc Prof Med, Mayo Med Sch

Broadstone, Vasti Lima MD [EDM] - **Spec Exp:** Diabetes; Weight Management; **Hospital:** Floyd Meml Hosp & Hlth Svcs; **Address:** Floyd Meml-Joslin Diabetes Ctr Affil, 2019 State St, New Albany, IN 47150; **Phone:** 812-949-5700; **Board Cert:** Internal Medicine 1987; Endocrinology, Diabetes & Metabolism 2002; **Med School:** Brazil 1976; **Resid:** Internal Medicine, Wright State Univ Affil Hosps 1981; **Fellow:** Endocrinology, Diabetes & Metabolism, Univ Louisville Affil Hosps 1984

Burmeister, Lynn MD [EDM] - **Spec Exp:** Thyroid Disorders; Hashimoto's Disease; Graves' Disease; **Hospital:** Univ Minn Med Ctr, Fairview - Riverside Campus; **Address:** Univ of Minnesota Physicians, 516 Delaware St SE, Clinic 6A, Minneapolis, MN 55455; **Phone:** 612-625-8690; **Board Cert:** Internal Medicine 1988; **Med School:** Univ Minn 1985; **Resid:** Internal Medicine, Univ Minnesota Med Ctr 1988; **Fellow:** Endocrinology, Univ Minnesota Med Ctr 1989; **Fac Appt:** Assoc Prof Med, Univ Minn

Clutter, William E MD [EDM] - **Spec Exp:** Endocrine Cancers; Calcium Disorders; Bone Disorders-Metabolic; **Hospital:** Barnes-Jewish Hosp, Washington Univ Physicians; **Address:** Washington Univ, Div Endo, Metabolism & Lipid Rsch, 660 S Euclid Ave, Campus Box 8121, St Louis, MO 63110; **Phone:** 314-362-3500; **Board Cert:** Internal Medicine 1978; Endocrinology, Diabetes & Metabolism 1981; **Med School:** Ohio State Univ 1975; **Resid:** Internal Medicine, Barnes Jewish Hosp 1978; **Fellow:** Endocrinology, Diabetes & Metabolism, Barnes Jewish Hosp 1980; **Fac Appt:** Assoc Prof Med, Washington Univ, St Louis

Cohen, Robert M MD [EDM] - **Spec Exp:** Diabetes; Metabolic Disorders; **Hospital:** Univ Hosp - Cincinnati; **Address:** Univ Cincinnati Physicians, 222 Piedmont Ave, Ste 6300, Cincinnati, OH 45219; **Phone:** 513-475-7400; **Board Cert:** Internal Medicine 1981; Endocrinology, Diabetes & Metabolism 1983; **Med School:** Univ Rochester 1978; **Resid:** Internal Medicine, Rush-Presby-St Lukes Hosp 1981; **Fellow:** Endocrinology, Univ Chicago 1984; **Fac Appt:** Prof Med, Univ Cincinnati

Cryer, Philip E MD [EDM] - **Spec Exp:** Diabetes; Hypoglycemia; **Hospital:** Barnes-Jewish Hosp, St. Louis Chldns Hosp; **Address:** Wash Univ Sch Med, Div Endo, Metab & Lipid Rsch, 660 S Euclid Ave, Box 8127, St Louis, MO 63110-1093; **Phone:** 314-362-3500; **Board Cert:** Internal Medicine 1972; Endocrinology, Diabetes & Metabolism 1972; **Med School:** Northwestern Univ 1965; **Resid:** Internal Medicine, Barnes Jewish Hosp 1972; **Fellow:** Endocrinology, Diabetes & Metabolism, Barnes Hosp-Wash Univ 1968; **Fac Appt:** Prof Med, Washington Univ, St Louis

D'Alessio, David A MD [EDM] - **Spec Exp:** Diabetes; **Hospital:** Univ Hosp - Cincinnati; **Address:** Univ Cincinnati Physicians, 222 Piedmont Ave, Ste 6300, Cincinnati, OH 45219; **Phone:** 513-475-7400; **Board Cert:** Internal Medicine 1986; Endocrinology, Diabetes & Metabolism 1989; **Med School:** Univ Wisc 1983; **Resid:** Internal Medicine, Temple Univ Med Ctr 1986; **Fellow:** Endocrinology, Univ Washington 1990; **Fac Appt:** Prof Med, Univ Cincinnati

Econs, Michael J MD [EDM] - **Spec Exp:** Osteoporosis; Paget's Disease of Bone; Bone Disorders-Metabolic; Parathyroid Disease; **Hospital:** IU Health University Hosp; **Address:** 550 University Blvd, Ste 2180, Indianapolis, IN 46202; **Phone:** 317-274-1339; **Board Cert:** Internal Medicine 1986; Endocrinology, Diabetes & Metabolism 1989; **Med School:** UCSF 1983; **Resid:** Internal Medicine, Univ Maryland Hosp 1986; **Fellow:** Endocrinology, Duke Univ Med Ctr 1989; **Fac Appt:** Prof Med, Indiana Univ

Ehrmann, David A MD [EDM] - **Spec Exp:** Polycystic Ovarian Syndrome; Diabetes; **Hospital:** Univ of Chicago Med Ctr; **Address:** Center for Advanced Medicine, 5758 S Maryland Ave, Fl 5 - Ste 5A, Chicago, IL 60637; **Phone:** 773-702-6138; **Board Cert:** Internal Medicine 1985; Endocrinology, Diabetes & Metabolism 1987; **Med School:** Univ Mich Med Sch 1982; **Resid:** Internal Medicine, Univ Mich Med Ctr 1985; **Fellow:** Endocrinology, Diabetes & Metabolism, Univ Chicago Hosps 1987; **Fac Appt:** Assoc Prof Med, Univ Chicago-Pritzker Sch Med

Emanuele, Mary Ann MD [EDM] - **Spec Exp:** Diabetes; Osteoporosis; Thyroid Disorders; Parathyroid Disorders; **Hospital:** Loyola Univ Med Ctr; **Address:** Loyola Outpatient Center, Endocrinology Dept Fl 1, 2160 S First Ave, Maywood, IL 60153-3304; **Phone:** 708-216-0160 x2; **Board Cert:** Internal Medicine 1978; Endocrinology, Diabetes & Metabolism 1983; **Med School:** Loyola Univ-Stritch Sch Med 1975; **Resid:** Internal Medicine, Univ Hawaii Med Ctr 1978; **Fellow:** Endocrinology, Edward Hines Jr VA Hosp 1980; **Fac Appt:** Prof Med, Loyola Univ-Stritch Sch Med

Emanuele, Nicholas V MD [EDM] - **Hospital:** Edward Hines, Jr. VA Hosp; **Address:** Hines VA Hosp Bldg 200 Fl 4, 5000 S 5th Ave, Hines, IL 60141; **Phone:** 708-202-2445; **Board Cert:** Internal Medicine 1975; Endocrinology 1979; **Med School:** Northwestern Univ 1967; **Resid:** Internal Medicine, Hines VA Hosp 1974; **Fellow:** Endocrinology, Northwestern Univ Affil Hosp 1976

Hammer, Gary D MD/PhD [EDM] - **Spec Exp:** Adrenal Cancer; Adrenal Disorders; **Hospital:** Univ of Michigan Hosp; **Address:** Univ Michigan Comprehensive Cancer Ctr, 1500 E Medical Ctr Drive Fl 1 - rm 1127, Ann Arbor, MI 48109-2200; **Phone:** 734-647-8906; **Board Cert:** Endocrinology, Diabetes & Metabolism 2007; **Med School:** Tufts Univ 1992; **Resid:** Internal Medicine, UCSF Med Ctr 1994; **Fellow:** Endocrinology, UCSF 1997; **Fac Appt:** Assoc Prof Med, Univ Mich Med Sch

Herman, William H MD [EDM] - **Spec Exp:** Diabetes; **Hospital:** Univ of Michigan Hosp; **Address:** U-M Metabolism, Endocrinology & Diabetes, East Ann Arbor Health & Geriatrics Ctr, 4260 Plymouth Rd Fl 1, Anne Arbor, MI 48109; **Phone:** 734-764-6831; **Board Cert:** Internal Medicine 1982; Endocrinology, Diabetes & Metabolism 1989; **Med School:** Boston Univ 1979; **Resid:** Internal Medicine, Univ Mich Med Ctr 1982; **Fellow:** Preventive Medicine, Ctrs Dis Control 1985; Endocrinology, Diabetes & Metabolism, Univ Mich Med Ctr 1988; **Fac Appt:** Prof Med, Univ Mich Med Sch

Endocrinology, Diabetes & Metabolism

Jensen, Michael D MD [EDM] - **Spec Exp:** Eating Disorders/Obesity; Nutrition; **Hospital:** Mayo Med Ctr & Clin - Rochester; **Address:** Mayo Clin, Div Endocrinology, 200 First St SW, Rochester, MN 55905; **Phone:** 507-284-1600; **Board Cert:** Internal Medicine 1982; Endocrinology, Diabetes & Metabolism 1985; **Med School:** Univ MO-Kansas City 1979; **Resid:** Internal Medicine, Mayo Clinic 1982; **Fellow:** Endocrinology, Diabetes & Metabolism, Mayo Clinic 1985; **Fac Appt:** Prof Med, Mayo Med Sch

Kennedy, Laurence MD [EDM] - **Spec Exp:** Diabetes; Adrenal Disorders; Acromegaly; Pituitary Disorders; **Hospital:** Cleveland Clin (page 55); **Address:** Cleveland Clinic, 9500 Euclid Ave, MC F20, Cleveland, OH 44195; **Phone:** 216-445-8645; **Med School:** Northern Ireland 1972; **Resid:** Internal Medicine, Queens Univ Affil Hosp 1975; **Fellow:** Endocrinology, Queens Univ Affil Hosp 1978; Endocrinology, Univ Florida 1980

Khosla, Sundeep MD [EDM] - **Spec Exp:** Osteoporosis; Bone Disorders-Metabolic; **Hospital:** Mayo Med Ctr & Clin - Rochester; **Address:** Mayo Clin, Div Endocrinology, 200 First St SW, Rochester, MN 55905; **Phone:** 507-284-1600; **Board Cert:** Internal Medicine 1985; Endocrinology 1987; **Med School:** Harvard Med Sch 1982; **Resid:** Internal Medicine, Mass Genl Hosp 1985; **Fellow:** Endocrinology, Diabetes & Metabolism, Mass Genl Hosp 1988; **Fac Appt:** Asst Prof Med, Mayo Med Sch

Kopp, Peter A MD [EDM] - **Spec Exp:** Thyroid Cancer; Pituitary Disorders; Parathyroid Disease; McCune-Albright Syndrome; **Hospital:** Northwestern Meml Hosp; **Address:** Northwestern Medical Faculty Foundation, 675 N St Clair St, Ste 14-100, Galter Pavillion, Chicago, IL 60611; **Phone:** 312-695-7970; **Board Cert:** Internal Medicine 2003; Endocrinology, Diabetes & Metabolism 2004; **Med School:** Switzerland 1985; **Resid:** Internal Medicine, Regl Hosp 1992; Internal Medicine, Univ Bern 1992; **Fellow:** Endocrinology, Diabetes & Metabolism, Univ Bern 1992; Endocrinology, Diabetes & Metabolism, Northwestern Univ Hosp 1997; **Fac Appt:** Assoc Prof Med, Northwestern Univ-Feinberg Sch Med

Lash, Robert W MD [EDM] - **Spec Exp:** Osteoporosis; Diabetes; Diabetes in Pregnancy; Thyroid Disorders; **Address:** UM Metabolism, Endocrinology, Diabetes, Domino's Farms Lobby C, Ste 1300, 24 Frank Lloyd Wright Drive, Ann Arbor, MI 48106; **Phone:** 734-936-5504; **Board Cert:** Internal Medicine 1987; Endocrinology, Diabetes & Metabolism 1989; **Med School:** Albert Einstein Coll Med 1984; **Resid:** Internal Medicine, UCSF Med Ctr 1987; **Fellow:** Endocrinology, Natl Inst Hlth 1990; **Fac Appt:** Clin Prof Med, Univ Mich Med Sch

Mazzone, Theodore MD [EDM] - **Spec Exp:** Diabetes; Cholesterol/Lipid Disorders; **Hospital:** Evanston/North Shore Univ Hlth Sys; **Address:** Northshore Medical Group, Endocrinology Dept, 1000 Central St, Ste 800, Chicago, IL 60201; **Phone:** 847-663-8540; **Board Cert:** Internal Medicine 1980; Endocrinology 1983; Endocrinology, Diabetes & Metabolism 2011; **Med School:** Northwestern Univ 1977; **Resid:** Internal Medicine, UCLA Med Ctr 1980; **Fellow:** Endocrinology, Diabetes & Metabolism, Univ Wash Med Ctr 1983; **Fac Appt:** Clin Prof Med, Univ IL Coll Med

McGill, Janet B MD [EDM] - **Spec Exp:** Diabetes; Thyroid Disorders; **Hospital:** Barnes-Jewish Hosp; **Address:** Center for Advanced Disease, 4921 Parkview Pl Fl 13 - Ste B, St Louis, MO 63110-1010; **Phone:** 314-747-7300; **Board Cert:** Internal Medicine 1983; Endocrinology, Diabetes & Metabolism 1987; **Med School:** Mich State Univ 1979; **Resid:** Internal Medicine, William Beaumont Hosp 1984; **Fellow:** Endocrinology, Diabetes & Metabolism, William Beaumont Hosp 1985; Diabetes, Washington Univ 1987; **Fac Appt:** Assoc Prof Med, Washington Univ, St Louis

McMahon, M Molly MD [EDM] - **Spec Exp:** Nutrition; Diabetes; **Hospital:** Mayo Med Ctr & Clin - Rochester; **Address:** Mayo Clin, Div Endocrinology, 200 First St SW, Rochester, MN 55905; **Phone:** 507-284-1600; **Board Cert:** Internal Medicine 1985; Endocrinology, Diabetes & Metabolism 1987; **Med School:** Univ Wisc 1981; **Resid:** Internal Medicine, Med Coll Wisconsin 1984; **Fellow:** Endocrinology, Diabetes & Metabolism, Mayo Clinic 1987; Nutrition, New Eng Deaconess Hosp 1988; **Fac Appt:** Prof Med, Mayo Med Sch

Osei, Kwame MD [EDM] - **Spec Exp:** Diabetes; Nutrition; Diabetes in Minority Populations; **Hospital:** Ohio St Univ Med Ctr; **Address:** OSU Dept Medicine, Div Endocrinology, 561 McCampbell Hall, 1581 Dodd Drive, Columbus, OH 43210; **Phone:** 614-685-3333; **Board Cert:** Internal Medicine 1982; Endocrinology, Diabetes & Metabolism 1985; **Med School:** Ghana 1976; **Resid:** Pathology, Hahnemann Hosp 1979; Internal Medicine, Episcopal Hosp 1982; **Fellow:** Endocrinology, Diabetes & Metabolism, Ohio State Univ 1984; **Fac Appt:** Prof Med, Ohio State Univ

Philipson, Louis H MD/PhD [EDM] - **Spec Exp:** Diabetes; **Hospital:** Univ of Chicago Med Ctr; **Address:** Univ Chicago Kovler Diabetes Ctr, 5758 S Maryland Ave DCAM Bldg - Ste 5A, Chicago, IL 60637; **Phone:** 773-702-6138; **Board Cert:** Internal Medicine 1989; Endocrinology, Diabetes & Metabolism 2002; **Med School:** Univ Chicago-Pritzker Sch Med 1986; **Resid:** Internal Medicine, Univ Chicago Med Ctr 1989; **Fellow:** Endocrinology, Diabetes & Metabolism, Univ Chicago Med Ctr 1991; **Fac Appt:** Prof Med, Univ Chicago-Pritzker Sch Med

Semenkovich, Clay F MD [EDM] - **Spec Exp:** Cholesterol/Lipid Disorders; Diabetes; Thyroid Disorders; Adrenal Disorders; **Hospital:** Barnes-Jewish Hosp; **Address:** Center for Advanced Disease, 4921 Parkview Pl Fl 13 - Ste B, St Louis, MO 63110; **Phone:** 314-747-7300; **Board Cert:** Internal Medicine 1984; Endocrinology, Diabetes & Metabolism 1987; **Med School:** Washington Univ, St Louis 1981; **Resid:** Internal Medicine, Barnes-Jewish Hosp 1984; **Fellow:** Endocrinology, Diabetes & Metabolism, Wash Univ Hosp 1986; **Fac Appt:** Prof Med, Washington Univ, St Louis

Smith, Steven A MD [EDM] - **Spec Exp:** Diabetes; **Hospital:** Mayo Med Ctr & Clin - Rochester; **Address:** Mayo Clinic-Endocrinology, 200 1st St SW, Rochester, MN 55905; **Phone:** 507-284-2191; **Board Cert:** Internal Medicine 1981; Endocrinology, Diabetes & Metabolism 1987; **Med School:** Med Coll GA 1978; **Resid:** Internal Medicine, Meml Med Ctr 1981; **Fellow:** Endocrinology, Mayo Clinic 1987; **Fac Appt:** Prof Med, Mayo Med Sch

Sowers, James R MD [EDM] - **Spec Exp:** Diabetes; Hypertension; Cholesterol/Lipid Disorders; **Hospital:** Univ of Missouri Hosp; **Address:** UMC, Dept Internal Med, 1 Hosp Drive, rm D109, Columbia, MO 65212; **Phone:** 573-882-2573; **Board Cert:** Internal Medicine 1974; Endocrinology, Diabetes & Metabolism 1977; **Med School:** Univ MO-Columbia Sch Med 1971; **Resid:** Internal Medicine, St Johns Mercy Med Ctr 1974; **Fellow:** Endocrinology, Wadsworth VA Hosp Ctr-UCLA 1976; **Fac Appt:** Prof Med, Univ MO-Columbia Sch Med

Watts, Nelson B MD [EDM] - **Spec Exp:** Osteoporosis; Bone Disorders-Metabolic; Paget's Disease of Bone; Gorham-Stout Disease; **Hospital:** Jewish Hosp - Kenwood - Cincinnati; **Address:** 4760 E Galbraith Rd, Ste 212, Cincinnati, OH 45236; **Phone:** 513-686-2663; **Board Cert:** Internal Medicine 1972; Endocrinology, Diabetes & Metabolism 2010; **Med School:** Univ NC Sch Med 1969; **Resid:** Internal Medicine, Charlotte Meml Hosp 1972; **Fellow:** Endocrinology, Diabetes & Metabolism, NC Meml Hosp 1971

Weiss, Roy E MD/PhD [EDM] - **Spec Exp:** Cushing's Syndrome; Pituitary Disorders; Thyroid Disorders; **Hospital:** Univ of Chicago Med Ctr; **Address:** Univ Chicago, Sect, Adult/Ped Endo-Diabetes-Metabolism, 5788 S Maryland Ave, Ste 5A, Chicago, IL 60637; **Phone:** 773-702-9266; **Board Cert:** Endocrinology, Diabetes & Metabolism 2011; **Med School:** Israel 1985; **Resid:** Internal Medicine, Univ Chicago Hosp 1988; **Fellow:** Endocrinology, Diabetes & Metabolism, Univ Chicago Hosp 1990; **Fac Appt:** Prof Med, Univ Chicago-Pritzker Sch Med

Endocrinology, Diabetes & Metabolism

Werner, Phillip L MD [EDM] - **Spec Exp:** Diabetes; Thyroid Disorders; **Hospital:** Adv Luth Genl Hosp; **Address:** Advocate Medical Group, Nesset Pavillion-Endocrinology Dept, 1775 W Ballard Rd Fl 2, Park Ridge, IL 60068; **Phone:** 847-318-2400; **Board Cert:** Internal Medicine 1975; Endocrinology 1977; **Med School:** Univ IL Coll Med 1972; **Resid:** Internal Medicine, Univ Illinois Affl Hosp 1975; **Fellow:** Endocrinology, Diabetes & Metabolism, Univ Wash Med Ctr 1977; **Fac Appt:** Assoc Clin Prof Med, Ros Franklin Univ/Chicago Med Sch

Zimmerman, Robert S MD [EDM] - **Spec Exp:** Diabetes; **Hospital:** Cleveland Clin (page 55); **Address:** Cleveland Clinic Diabetes Ctr, 10685 Carnegie Ave, Cleveland, OH 44106; **Phone:** 216-444-9428; **Board Cert:** Internal Medicine 1984; Endocrinology, Diabetes & Metabolism 1987; **Med School:** Johns Hopkins Univ 1981; **Resid:** Internal Medicine, Duke Univ Hosp 1984; **Fellow:** Endocrinology, Mayo Clinic 1987

Great Plains and Mountains

Eckel, Robert H MD [EDM] - **Spec Exp:** Cholesterol/Lipid Disorders; Eating Disorders/Obesity; Diabetes; Cardiovascular Disease; **Hospital:** Univ of CO Hosp - Anschutz Inpatient Pav; **Address:** 12605 E 16th Ave, Ste B120, Anschutz Medical Campus, Aurora, CO 80045; **Phone:** 720-848-5300; **Board Cert:** Internal Medicine 1976; Endocrinology, Diabetes & Metabolism 2008; **Med School:** Univ Cincinnati 1973; **Resid:** Internal Medicine, Univ Wisconsin Hosps 1976; **Fellow:** Endocrinology, Diabetes & Metabolism, Univ Wash Med Ctr 1979; **Fac Appt:** Prof Med, Univ Colorado

Recker, Robert Roy MD [EDM] - **Spec Exp:** Osteoporosis; Diabetes; Endocrinology; **Hospital:** Alegent Creighton Univ Med Ctr, Omaha VA Med Ctr; **Address:** Creighton Univ Med Ctr, Div Endocrinology, 601 N 30th St, Ste 4820, Omaha, NE 68131; **Phone:** 402-280-4470; **Board Cert:** Internal Medicine 1971; **Med School:** Creighton Univ 1963; **Resid:** Internal Medicine, Creighton Affil Hosps 1969; **Fellow:** Endocrinology, Diabetes & Metabolism, Creighton Univ 1971; **Fac Appt:** Prof Med, Creighton Univ

Ridgway, E Chester MD [EDM] - **Spec Exp:** Thyroid Cancer; Thyroid Disorders; Pituitary Disorders; **Hospital:** Univ of CO Hosp - Anschutz Inpatient Pav; **Address:** UCHSC at Fitzsimons, Div Endocrinology, 1635 Aurora Court, Box 6510, MS F732, Aurora, CO 80045; **Phone:** 720-848-2650; **Board Cert:** Internal Medicine 1972; Endocrinology 1973; **Med School:** Univ Colorado 1968; **Resid:** Internal Medicine, Mass Genl Hosp 1970; **Fellow:** Endocrinology, Mass Genl Hosp 1972; **Fac Appt:** Prof Med, Univ Colorado

Southwest

Cunningham, Glenn R MD [EDM] - **Spec Exp:** Diabetes; Hypogonadism; Erectile Dysfunction; **Hospital:** St. Luke's Episcopal Hosp-Houston; **Address:** 6620 Main St, Ste 1225, Houston, TX 77030; **Phone:** 713-798-2500; **Board Cert:** Internal Medicine 1972; Endocrinology, Diabetes & Metabolism 1972; **Med School:** Univ Okla Coll Med 1966; **Resid:** Internal Medicine, Duke Univ Med Ctr 1970; Internal Medicine, VA Hosp 1971; **Fellow:** Endocrinology, Duke Univ Med Ctr 1970; **Fac Appt:** Prof Med, Baylor Coll Med

Gagel, Robert F MD [EDM] - **Spec Exp:** Thyroid Cancer; **Hospital:** UT MD Anderson Cancer Ctr; **Address:** MD Anderson Cancer Ctr, 1515 Holcombe Blvd, Unit 433, Houston, TX 77030; **Phone:** 713-563-4400; **Board Cert:** Internal Medicine 1975; Endocrinology 1977; **Med School:** Ohio State Univ 1971; **Resid:** Internal Medicine, New England Med Ctr 1973; **Fellow:** Endocrinology, New England Med Ctr 1975; Research, Harvard Med Sch 1981; **Fac Appt:** Prof Med, Univ Tex, Houston

Hsueh, Willa A MD [EDM] - **Spec Exp:** Heart Disease in Diabetes Patients; **Hospital:** Methodist Hosp - Houston; **Address:** Methodist Hosp Rsch Inst, 6670 Bertner St, Ste R8-111, Houston, TX 77030; **Phone:** 713-441-2520; **Board Cert:** Internal Medicine 1976; Endocrinology, Diabetes & Metabolism 1977; **Med School:** Ohio State Univ 1973; **Resid:** Internal Medicine, Johns Hopkins Hosp 1975; **Fellow:** Endocrinology, Diabetes & Metabolism, Johns Hopkins Hosp 1976; **Fac Appt:** Prof Med, Cornell Univ-Weill Med Coll

Lavis, Victor R MD [EDM] - **Spec Exp:** Diabetes; **Hospital:** UT MD Anderson Cancer Ctr; **Address:** MD Anderson Cancer Ctr, 1515 Holcombe Blvd, Unit 1461, Houston, TX 77030; **Phone:** 713-792-2841; **Board Cert:** Internal Medicine 1969; Endocrinology, Diabetes & Metabolism 2008; **Med School:** Stanford Univ 1962; **Resid:** Internal Medicine, Boston Cty Hosp 1964; Internal Medicine, UCLA Med Ctr 1967; **Fellow:** Endocrinology, Diabetes & Metabolism, Univ Washington 1970; **Fac Appt:** Prof Med, Univ Tex, Houston

Robbins, Richard J MD [EDM] - **Spec Exp:** Thyroid Cancer; Pituitary Tumors; Pituitary Disorders; **Hospital:** Methodist Hosp - Houston; **Address:** 6550 Fannin St, Ste 1001, Houston, TX 77030; **Phone:** 713-441-6640; **Board Cert:** Internal Medicine 1978; Endocrinology, Diabetes & Metabolism 1983; **Med School:** Creighton Univ 1975; **Resid:** Internal Medicine, New York Hosp 1978; **Fellow:** Endocrinology, New England Med Ctr 1981; **Fac Appt:** Prof Med, Cornell Univ-Weill Med Coll

Rubenfeld, Sheldon MD [EDM] - **Spec Exp:** Thyroid Cancer; Thyroid Disorders; Diabetes; **Hospital:** St. Luke's Episcopal Hosp-Houston, Methodist Hosp - Houston; **Address:** 7515 S Main St, Ste 690, Houston, TX 77030; **Phone:** 713-795-5750; **Board Cert:** Internal Medicine 1976; Endocrinology, Diabetes & Metabolism 1979; **Med School:** Georgetown Univ 1971; **Resid:** Internal Medicine, Baylor Affil Hosps 1976; **Fellow:** Endocrinology, Baylor Affil Hosps 1978; **Fac Appt:** Clin Prof Med, Baylor Coll Med

Sherman, Steven I MD [EDM] - **Spec Exp:** Thyroid Cancer; Endocrine Cancers; **Hospital:** UT MD Anderson Cancer Ctr; **Address:** MD Anderson Cancer Ctr, 1515 Holcombe Blvd, Unit 435, Houston, TX 77030; **Phone:** 713-792-2840; **Board Cert:** Internal Medicine 1988; Endocrinology, Diabetes & Metabolism 2007; **Med School:** Johns Hopkins Univ 1985; **Resid:** Internal Medicine, Johns Hopkins Hosp 1988; **Fellow:** Endocrinology, Diabetes & Metabolism, Johns Hopkins Hosp 1991; **Fac Appt:** Prof Med, Baylor Coll Med

Waguespack, Steven G MD [EDM] - **Spec Exp:** Thyroid Cancer; Pituitary Tumors; Hereditary Endocrine Cancers; **Hospital:** UT MD Anderson Cancer Ctr; **Address:** UT MD Anderson Cancer Center, Dept of Endocrine Neoplasia, 1515 Holcombe Blvd, MS 1461, Houston, TX 77030; **Phone:** 713-563-4400; **Board Cert:** Endocrinology, Diabetes & Metabolism 2002; Pediatric Endocrinology 2011; **Med School:** Univ Tex, Houston 1994; **Resid:** Internal Medicine & Pediatrics, Indiana Univ Hosps 1998; **Fellow:** Endocrinology, Diabetes & Metabolism, Indiana Univ Hosps 2001; Pediatric Endocrinology, Riley Chldns Hosp 2002

West Coast and Pacific

Ahmann, Andrew J MD [EDM] - **Spec Exp:** Diabetes; Clinical Trials; **Hospital:** OR Hlth & Sci Univ; **Address:** OHSU Div Endocrinology, 3181 SW Sam Jackson Park Rd, MC PPV05, Portland, OR 97239; **Phone:** 503-494-3273; **Board Cert:** Internal Medicine 1983; Endocrinology, Diabetes & Metabolism 1987; **Med School:** Univ Colorado 1980; **Resid:** Internal Medicine, Fitzsimons Army Med Ctr 1983; **Fellow:** Endocrinology, Diabetes & Metabolism, Walter Reed Army Med Ctr 1986; **Fac Appt:** Prof Med, Oregon Hlth & Sci Univ

Endocrinology, Diabetes & Metabolism

Akatsu, Haruko MD [EDM] - **Spec Exp:** Thyroid Cancer; Thyroid Disorders; Diabetes; Metabolic Disorders; **Hospital:** Stanford Univ Hosp & Clinics; **Address:** Stanford Univ Div Endocrinology, 300 Pasteur Drive, Ste A-175, Stanford, CA 94305; **Phone:** 650-723-6961; **Board Cert:** Endocrinology, Diabetes & Metabolism 2003; **Med School:** Brown Univ 1994; **Resid:** Internal Medicine, Stanford Univ Med Ctr 1997; **Fellow:** Endocrinology, Stanford Univ 1999; **Fac Appt:** Assoc Clin Prof Med, Stanford Univ

Berkson, Richard A MD [EDM] - **Spec Exp:** Diabetes; Thyroid Disorders; **Hospital:** St. Mary Med Ctr - Long Beach, Long Beach Meml Med Ctr; **Address:** 1868 Pacific Ave, Long Beach, CA 90806-6113; **Phone:** 562-595-4718; **Board Cert:** Internal Medicine 1975; Endocrinology, Diabetes & Metabolism 1977; **Med School:** SUNY Buffalo 1972; **Resid:** Internal Medicine, SUNY Buffalo Affil Hosp 1975; **Fellow:** Endocrinology, Diabetes & Metabolism, Joslin Clin 1976; Endocrinology, Diabetes & Metabolism, UCLA Med Ctr 1977; **Fac Appt:** Assoc Clin Prof Med, UCLA

Braunstein, Glenn D MD [EDM] - **Spec Exp:** Hormonal Disorders; Thyroid Cancer; Reproductive Endocrinology; Endocrine Cancers; **Hospital:** Cedars-Sinai Med Ctr; **Address:** Cedars Sinai Med Ctr, 8700 Beverly Blvd, Ste 2119, Los Angeles, CA 90048; **Phone:** 310-423-5140; **Board Cert:** Internal Medicine 1973; Endocrinology, Diabetes & Metabolism 1975; **Med School:** UCSF 1968; **Resid:** Internal Medicine, Peter Bent Bringham Hosp 1970; **Fellow:** Endocrinology, Diabetes & Metabolism, Natl Inst Hlth-NICHHD 1972; Endocrinology, Diabetes & Metabolism, LAC Harbor Genl Hosp 1973; **Fac Appt:** Prof Med, UCLA

Edelman, Steven V MD [EDM] - **Spec Exp:** Diabetes; **Hospital:** UCSD Med Ctr; **Address:** Perlman Medical Office, 9350 Campus Point Drive Fl 2 - Ste B, La Jolla, CA 92037; **Phone:** 858-657-8440; **Board Cert:** Internal Medicine 1986; Endocrinology, Diabetes & Metabolism 2003; **Med School:** UC Davis 1982; **Resid:** Internal Medicine, UCLA-San Fernando 1985; **Fellow:** Diabetes, The Joslin Clinic 1986; Endocrinology, Diabetes & Metabolism, The Lahey Clinic 1987; **Fac Appt:** Prof Med, UCSD

Fitzgerald, Paul A MD [EDM] - **Spec Exp:** Thyroid Disorders; Diabetes; Pheochromocytoma; Pituitary Tumors; **Hospital:** UCSF Med Ctr; **Address:** 350 Parnassus Ave, Ste 710, San Francisco, CA 94117-3685; **Phone:** 415-665-1136; **Board Cert:** Internal Medicine 1975; Endocrinology, Diabetes & Metabolism 1981; **Med School:** Jefferson Med Coll 1972; **Resid:** Internal Medicine, Presby Med Ctr-Univ Colo 1975; **Fellow:** Endocrinology, Diabetes & Metabolism, UCSF Med Ctr 1978; **Fac Appt:** Clin Prof Med, UCSF

Heber, David MD [EDM] - **Spec Exp:** Nutrition & Cancer Prevention; Nutrition & Disease Prevention/Control; Nutrition & Obesity; **Hospital:** UCLA Ronald Reagan Med Ctr; **Address:** 900 Veteran Ave, Rm 12-217, UCLA Center for Human Nutrition, Los Angeles, CA 90095-1742; **Phone:** 310-206-1987; **Board Cert:** Internal Medicine 1976; Endocrinology, Diabetes & Metabolism 1977; **Med School:** Harvard Med Sch 1973; **Resid:** Internal Medicine, LAC Harbor Genl Hosp 1975; **Fellow:** Endocrinology, Diabetes & Metabolism, LAC Harbor Genl Hosp 1978; **Fac Appt:** Prof Med, UCLA

Hirsch, Irl B MD [EDM] - **Spec Exp:** Diabetes; **Hospital:** Univ Wash Med Ctr; **Address:** Univ Wash Med Ctr, Diabetes Care Ctr, 4225 Roosevelt Way NE, Ste 101, Box 354691, Seattle, WA 98195; **Phone:** 206-598-4882; **Board Cert:** Internal Medicine 1987; Endocrinology, Diabetes & Metabolism 1989; **Med School:** Univ MO-Columbia Sch Med 1984; **Resid:** Internal Medicine, Mt Sinai Med Ctr 1987; **Fellow:** Metabolism, Washington Univ 1989; **Fac Appt:** Prof Med, Univ Wash

Hoffman, Andrew R MD [EDM] - **Spec Exp:** Pituitary Disorders; Pituitary Tumors; Neuroendocrinology; **Hospital:** Stanford Univ Hosp & Clinics, VA Hlth Care Sys - Palo Alto; **Address:** 300 Pasteur Drive, Div of Endocinology, Stanford, CA 94305-5103; **Phone:** 650-723-6961; **Board Cert:** Internal Medicine 1979; Endocrinology 1981; **Med School:** Stanford Univ 1976; **Resid:** Internal Medicine, Mass Genl Hosp 1978; **Fellow:** Endocrinology, Natl Inst Hlth 1980; Endocrinology, Mass Genl Hosp 1982; **Fac Appt:** Prof Med, Stanford Univ

Ipp, Eli MD [EDM] - **Spec Exp:** Diabetes; **Hospital:** LAC - Harbor - UCLA Med Ctr; **Address:** 21840 S Normandy Ave, Ste 600, Torrance, CA 90502; **Phone:** 310-222-5101; **Board Cert:** Internal Medicine 1979; Endocrinology, Diabetes & Metabolism 1981; **Med School:** South Africa 1968; **Resid:** Internal Medicine, Tel Hashomer Hosp 1974; **Fellow:** Endocrinology, Diabetes & Metabolism, Univ Tex SW Med Ctr 1978; **Fac Appt:** Prof Med, UCLA

Kamdar, Vikram V MD [EDM] - **Spec Exp:** Diabetes; Diabetic Leg/Foot; Thyroid Disorders; **Hospital:** Santa Monica - UCLA Med Ctr & Ortho Hosp, UCLA Ronald Reagan Med Ctr; **Address:** 1245 16th St, Ste 309, Santa Monica, CA 90404; **Phone:** 310-828-7172; **Board Cert:** Internal Medicine 1978; Endocrinology, Diabetes & Metabolism 1979; **Med School:** India 1971; **Resid:** Internal Medicine, Lemuel Shattuck Hosp 1972; 1977; **Fellow:** Endocrinology, Diabetes & Metabolism, Cedars-Sinai Med Ctr 1975; Endocrinology, Diabetes & Metabolism, LA Co-USC Med Ctr; **Fac Appt:** Assoc Clin Prof Med, UCLA

Kandeel, Fouad MD/PhD [EDM] - **Spec Exp:** Thyroid Cancer; Endocrine Cancers; Neuroendocrinology; **Hospital:** City of Hope Natl Med Ctr; **Address:** City of Hope, Div Endocrinology, 1500 E Duarte Rd, Duarte, CA 91010; **Phone:** 626-256-4673; **Med School:** Egypt 1969; **Resid:** Internal Medicine, Birmingham & Midland Hosp for Women 1972; **Fellow:** Endocrinology, Diabetes & Metabolism, Queen Elizabeth Hosp 1975; **Fac Appt:** Assoc Clin Prof Med, UCLA

Katznelson, Laurence MD [EDM] - **Spec Exp:** Neuroendocrinology; Pituitary Disorders; Acromegaly; Cushing's Syndrome; **Hospital:** Stanford Univ Hosp & Clinics, Lucile Packard Chldn's Hosp; **Address:** Stanford Comprehensive Cancer Ctr, 875 Blake Wilbur Drive, MC 5826, Stanford, CA 94305; **Phone:** 650-736-2062; **Board Cert:** Internal Medicine 1988; **Med School:** UCLA 1985; **Resid:** Internal Medicine, Hosp Univ Penn 1988; **Fellow:** Endocrinology, Mass Genl Hosp 1991; **Fac Appt:** Assoc Prof Med, Stanford Univ

Klonoff, David C MD [EDM] - **Spec Exp:** Diabetes; **Hospital:** Mills-Peninsula Med Ctr; **Address:** 1720 El Camino Real, Ste 130, Burlingame, CA 94010; **Phone:** 650-697-4345; **Board Cert:** Internal Medicine 1980; Endocrinology, Diabetes & Metabolism 1981; **Med School:** UCSF 1976; **Resid:** Internal Medicine, UCLA Med Ctr 1978; Internal Medicine, UCSF Hosps 1979; **Fellow:** Endocrinology, Diabetes & Metabolism, Metab Rsch Unit-UCSF Med Ctr 1981; **Fac Appt:** Clin Prof Med, UCSF

Melmed, Shlomo MD [EDM] - **Spec Exp:** Pituitary Tumors; Acromegaly; Pituitary Disorders; **Hospital:** Cedars-Sinai Med Ctr; **Address:** Cedars Sinai Med Ctr, 8700 Beverly Blvd, Ste 2015, Los Angeles, CA 90048; **Phone:** 310-423-2830; **Board Cert:** Internal Medicine 1979; Endocrinology, Diabetes & Metabolism 1983; **Med School:** South Africa 1970; **Resid:** Internal Medicine, Sheba Med Ctr 1976; **Fellow:** Endocrinology, Diabetes & Metabolism, Wadsworth VA Hosp 1980; **Fac Appt:** Prof Med, UCLA

Orwoll, Eric S MD [EDM] - **Spec Exp:** Osteoporosis; Osteoporosis in Men; Bone Disorders-Metabolic; **Hospital:** OR Hlth & Sci Univ; **Address:** OHSU, Div Endocrinology, 3181 SW Sam Jackson Park Rd, MC PPV05, Portland, OR 97239; **Phone:** 503-494-3273; **Board Cert:** Internal Medicine 1977; Endocrinology, Diabetes & Metabolism 1979; **Med School:** Univ MD Sch Med 1974; **Resid:** Internal Medicine, Providence Med Ctr 1977; **Fellow:** Endocrinology, Diabetes & Metabolism, Univ Oregon 1979; **Fac Appt:** Prof Med, Oregon Hlth & Sci Univ

Peters, Anne L MD [EDM] - **Spec Exp:** Diabetes; **Hospital:** Keck Med Ctr of USC (page 62); **Address:** USC Westside Center for Diabetes, 150 N Robertson Blvd, Ste 210, Beverly Hills, CA 90211; **Phone:** 310-657-3030; **Board Cert:** Internal Medicine 1986; Endocrinology, Diabetes & Metabolism 2010; **Med School:** Univ Chicago-Pritzker Sch Med 1983; **Resid:** Internal Medicine, Stanford Univ Med Ctr 1985; Internal Medicine, Harbor-UCLA Med Ctr 1986; **Fellow:** Endocrinology, Diabetes & Metabolism, Cedars-Sinai Med Ctr 1988; **Fac Appt:** Prof Med, USC-Keck School of Medicine

Riddle, Matthew C MD [EDM] - **Spec Exp:** Diabetes; Clinical Trials; **Hospital:** OR Hlth & Sci Univ; **Address:** OHSU, Div Endocrinology, 3181 SW Sam Jackson Park Rd, MC PPV05, Portland, OR 97239-3011; **Phone:** 503-494-3273; **Board Cert:** Internal Medicine 1972; Endocrinology, Diabetes & Metabolism 1972; **Med School:** Harvard Med Sch 1964; **Resid:** Internal Medicine, Rush-Presby-St Lukes Hosp 1969; **Fellow:** Endocrinology, Diabetes & Metabolism, Rush Univ 1971; Endocrinology, Diabetes & Metabolism, Univ Washington 1973; **Fac Appt:** Prof Med, Oregon Hlth & Sci Univ

Rushakoff, Robert J MD [EDM] - **Spec Exp:** Diabetes; **Hospital:** UCSF - Mt Zion Med Ctr; **Address:** UCSF-Mt Zion Med Ctr, 1600 Divisadero St, Fl 4, Box 1616, San Francisco, CA 94143-1616; **Phone:** 415-885-3868; **Board Cert:** Internal Medicine 1985; Endocrinology, Diabetes & Metabolism 1989; **Med School:** Med Coll Wisc 1982; **Resid:** Internal Medicine, Mt Zion Hosp Med Ctr 1985; **Fellow:** Endocrinology, Mt Zion Hosp/Cell Biol 1986; Endocrinology, Cedars-Sinai Med Ctr 1987; **Fac Appt:** Prof Med, UCSF

Singer, Peter A MD [EDM] - **Spec Exp:** Thyroid Disorders; Pituitary Disorders; **Hospital:** Keck Med Ctr of USC (page 62); **Address:** 1520 San Pablo St, Ste 1000, Los Angeles, CA 90033; **Phone:** 323-442-5100; **Board Cert:** Internal Medicine 1972; Endocrinology, Diabetes & Metabolism 1973; **Med School:** UCSF 1965; **Resid:** Internal Medicine, LAC-USC Med Ctr 1971; **Fellow:** Endocrinology, Diabetes & Metabolism, LAC-USC Med Ctr 1973; **Fac Appt:** Clin Prof Med, USC Sch Med

Swerdloff, Ronald S MD [EDM] - **Spec Exp:** Reproductive Endocrinology-Male; Pituitary Disorders; **Hospital:** LAC - Harbor - UCLA Med Ctr; **Address:** 1000 W Carson St, Box 446, Torrance, CA 90509-2910; **Phone:** 310-222-1867; **Board Cert:** Internal Medicine 1968; Endocrinology 1972; **Med School:** UCSF 1962; **Resid:** Internal Medicine, Univ Washington Hosp 1964; Internal Medicine, UCLA 1966; **Fellow:** Endocrinology, Diabetes & Metabolism, NIH Gerontology Branch 1968; Endocrinology, Diabetes & Metabolism, Harbor-UCLA Med Ctr 1969; **Fac Appt:** Prof Med, UCLA

Woeber, Kenneth A MD [EDM] - **Spec Exp:** Thyroid Disorders; **Hospital:** UCSF - Mt Zion Med Ctr; **Address:** Endocrine Clinic at Mt. Zion, 2200 Post St, Ste C-432, Campus Box 1640, San Francisco, CA 94143-1640; **Phone:** 415-885-7574; **Board Cert:** Internal Medicine 1980; Endocrinology, Diabetes & Metabolism 1973; **Med School:** South Africa 1957; **Resid:** Internal Medicine, Johannesburg Hosp 1962; **Fellow:** Endocrinology, Diabetes & Metabolism, Harvard/Boston City Hosp 1964; **Fac Appt:** Prof Med, UCSF

Cleveland Clinic

Every life deserves world class care.

Endocrinology, Diabetes and Metabolism

Cleveland Clinic Endocrinology & Metabolism Institute is committed to providing the highest quality healthcare for patients with diabetes, endocrine or metabolic disorders, or obesity. Our staff includes endocrinologists, endocrine surgeons, bariatric and general surgeons, psychologists, bariatricians and a cardiologist, as well as dietitians, nurse practitioners and clinical nurse specialists. We are ranked No. 2 in the nation by *U.S. News & World Report* — the highest ranking in Ohio.

We Offer Specialized Endocrine Clinics

The Endocrinology & Metabolism Institute has an array of disease-specific clinics, including:

- Thyroid/parathyroid disorders
- Pituitary disorders
- Post-pancreas transplant care
- Liver/adrenal tumor care
- Type 1 and Type 2 diabetes
- Calcium disorders
- Preventive cardiology
- Transition endocrine (pediatrics to adult)

Leading Thyroid Center

Our Thyroid Center is designed so that all specialists work together as a team to accurately and proactively diagnose and treat all forms of thyroid disorders, including thyroid cancer. We have been the leader in incorporating fine needle aspirations and ultrasounds into the realm of endocrinology.

We also offer nationally recognized pituitary care and enhanced diabetes care. Cleveland Clinic is one of the top centers in the U.S. for volume of pituitary surgeries at an institution.

Additionally, we take on all of the clinical challenges that chronic disease management continues to offer as we seek to develop healthier communities.

Cleveland Clinic
Endocrine & Metabolism
Institute
9500 Euclid Avenue
Cleveland, OH 44195

Offering Same-Day Appointments
Call 800.274.2009.

Treatment Guides
Cleveland Clinic has developed comprehensive treatment guides for many diseases and conditions. To download our free treatment guides, visit clevelandclinic.org/treatmentguides.

Online Medical Second Opinion
Call 216.444.3223 or
800.223.2273 ext. 43223 or
email eclevelandclinic@ccf.org.

Out-of-State Patients Assistance
Call 800.223.2273, ext. 55580 or
email medicalconcierge@ccf.org.

Visit Us At:
clevelandclinic.org

Follow Us On:
Facebook
www.facebook.com/clevelandclinic

Twitter
@ClevelandClinic

You Tube
www.youtube.com/clevelandclinic

Health Hub
health.clevelandclinic.org

The Best in American Medicine
www.CastleConnolly.com

Gastroenterology
a subspecialty of Internal Medicine

An internist who specializes in diagnosis and treatment of diseases of the digestive organs including the stomach, bowels, liver and gallbladder. This specialist treats conditions such as abdominal pain, ulcers, diarrhea, cancer and jaundice and performs complex diagnostic and therapeutic procedures using endoscopes to see internal organs.

Training Required: Three years in internal medicine *plus* additional training and examination for certification in gastroenterology.

GASTROENTEROLOGY

New England

Aslanian, Harry R MD [Ge] - **Spec Exp:** Endoscopic Ultrasound; Esophageal Cancer; Pancreatic Cancer; Rectal Cancer; **Hospital:** Yale-New Haven Hosp; **Address:** 333 Cedar St, Fl 1080 Imp, Box 208019, Department of Internal Medicine, New Haven, CT 06520-8019; **Phone:** 203-200-5083; **Board Cert:** Gastroenterology 2002; **Med School:** Brown Univ 1996; **Resid:** Internal Medicine, Mayo Clin 1999; **Fellow:** Gastroenterology, Yale Univ Affil Hosp 2002; Endoscopy, Yale Univ Affil Hosp 2003; **Fac Appt:** Assoc Prof Med, Yale Univ

Butterly, Lynn MD [Ge] - **Spec Exp:** Colonoscopy; Endoscopy; Colon & Rectal Cancer Detection; Colon & Rectal Cancer-Familial Polyposis; **Hospital:** Dartmouth - Hitchcock Med Ctr; **Address:** Dartmouth-Hitchcock Med Ctr, Dept Gastro, 1 Med Ctr Drive, Lebanon, NH 03756; **Phone:** 603-650-5261; **Board Cert:** Internal Medicine 1983; Gastroenterology 1985; **Med School:** Harvard Med Sch 1979; **Resid:** Internal Medicine, Mass Genl Hosp 1983; **Fellow:** Gastroenterology, Mass Genl Hosp 1985; **Fac Appt:** Asst Prof Med, Dartmouth Med Sch

Chung, Daniel C MD [Ge] - **Spec Exp:** Colonoscopy; Colon & Rectal Cancer-Familial Polyposis; Pancreatic Cancer(Familial); Pancreatic Endocrine Tumors; **Hospital:** Mass Genl Hosp; **Address:** Gastroenterology Associates, 55 Fruit St Blake Bldg Fl 4, Boston, MA 02114; **Phone:** 617-726-3544; **Board Cert:** Gastroenterology 2003; **Med School:** Harvard Med Sch 1988; **Resid:** Internal Medicine, Mass Genl Hosp 1991; **Fellow:** Gastroenterology, Mass Genl Hosp 1995; **Fac Appt:** Assoc Prof Med, Harvard Med Sch

Chung, Raymond T MD [Ge] - **Spec Exp:** Transplant Medicine-Liver; Liver Disease; Hepatitis C; **Hospital:** Mass Genl Hosp; **Address:** Mass General Hosp, 55 Fruit St, Boston, MA 02114; **Phone:** 617-724-6006; **Board Cert:** Internal Medicine 1989; Gastroenterology 2007; Transplant Hepatology 2008; **Med School:** Yale Univ 1986; **Resid:** Internal Medicine, Johns Hopkins Hosp 1989; **Fac Appt:** Assoc Prof Med, Harvard Med Sch

Dienstag, Jules L MD [Ge] - **Spec Exp:** Liver Disease; Hepatitis; Transplant Medicine-Liver; **Hospital:** Mass Genl Hosp; **Address:** Mass Genl Hosp, GI Unit, 55 Fruit St Warren Bldg Fl 10, Boston, MA 02114-2622; **Phone:** 617-726-7450; **Board Cert:** Internal Medicine 1975; **Med School:** Columbia P&S 1972; **Resid:** Internal Medicine, Univ Chicago-Billings Hosp 1974; **Fellow:** Virology, Natl Inst Hlth 1976; Gastroenterology, Mass Genl Hosp 1978; **Fac Appt:** Prof Med, Harvard Med Sch

Farraye, Francis A MD [Ge] - **Spec Exp:** Endoscopy; Inflammatory Bowel Disease; Colon & Rectal Cancer Detection; Diarrheal Diseases; **Hospital:** Boston Med Ctr; **Address:** Boston Med Ctr, Div Gastroenterology, 830 Harrison Ave Moakley Bldg Fl 2, Boston, MA 02118; **Phone:** 617-638-6525; **Board Cert:** Gastroenterology 1989; Internal Medicine 1985; **Med School:** Albert Einstein Coll Med 1982; **Resid:** Internal Medicine, Beth Israel Hosp 1985; **Fellow:** Gastroenterology, Beth Israel Hosp 1988

Fisher, Rosemarie Louise MD [Ge] - **Spec Exp:** Nutrition; Nutrition in Bowel Disorders; Inflammatory Bowel Disease/Crohn's; Endoscopy; **Hospital:** Yale-New Haven Hosp, St. Mary's Hosp - Waterbury; **Address:** 20 York St, Tompkins Bldg Fl 236, New Haven, CT 06510; **Phone:** 203-688-1449; **Board Cert:** Internal Medicine 1975; Gastroenterology 1977; **Med School:** Tufts Univ 1971; **Resid:** Internal Medicine, Montefiore Med Ctr 1973; **Fellow:** Gastroenterology, Yale-New Haven Hosp 1975; **Fac Appt:** Prof Med, Yale Univ

Friedman, Lawrence S MD [Ge] - **Spec Exp:** Liver Disease; **Hospital:** Newton - Wellesley Hosp, Mass Genl Hosp; **Address:** Newton-Wellesley Hosp, Dept Medicine, 2014 Washington St, Newton, MA 02462; **Phone:** 617-243-5480; **Board Cert:** Internal Medicine 1981; Gastroenterology 2005; **Med School:** Johns Hopkins Univ 1978; **Resid:** Internal Medicine, Johns Hopkins Hosp 1981; **Fellow:** Gastroenterology, Mass Genl Hosp 1984; **Fac Appt:** Prof Med, Harvard Med Sch

Gordon, Stuart R MD [Ge] - **Spec Exp:** Pancreatic & Biliary Disease; Pancreatic/Biliary Endoscopy (ERCP); Endoscopic Ultrasound; **Hospital:** Dartmouth - Hitchcock Med Ctr; **Address:** Dartmouth-Hitchcock Medical Center, Lebaonon, NH 03756, Lebanon, NH 03756; **Phone:** 603-650-5261; **Board Cert:** Internal Medicine 2002; Gastroenterology 2005; **Med School:** Columbia P&S 1988; **Resid:** Internal Medicine, Dartmouth-Hitchcock Med Ctr 1991; **Fellow:** Gastroenterology, Dartmouth-Hitchcock Med Ctr 1994; **Fac Appt:** Assoc Prof Med, Dartmouth Med Sch

Kaplan, Lee M MD/PhD [Ge] - **Spec Exp:** Obesity; Weight Management; Liver Disease; **Hospital:** Mass Genl Hosp; **Address:** Mass Genl Hosp, Dept Gastroenterology, 55 Fruit St Bldg 4, Boston, MA 02114-2517; **Phone:** 617-724-6007; **Board Cert:** Gastroenterology 1987; Internal Medicine 1984; **Med School:** Albert Einstein Coll Med 1981; **Resid:** Internal Medicine, Mass Genl Hosp 1984; **Fellow:** Gastroenterology, Mass Genl Hosp 1987; **Fac Appt:** Assoc Prof Med, Harvard Med Sch

Kelsey, Peter B MD [Ge] - **Spec Exp:** Endoscopy; Pancreatic & Biliary Disease; **Hospital:** Mass Genl Hosp; **Address:** Mass Genl Hosp, 55 Fruit St, Blake Bldg Fl 4, Boston, MA 02114-2621; **Phone:** 617-724-6044; **Board Cert:** Gastroenterology 1985; Internal Medicine 1982; **Med School:** Columbia P&S 1979; **Resid:** Internal Medicine, New York-Presbyterian Hosp 1982; **Fellow:** Gastroenterology, Massachusetts Genl Hosp 1984; **Fac Appt:** Asst Prof Med, Harvard Med Sch

La Mont, J Thomas MD [Ge] - **Spec Exp:** Clostridium Difficile Disease; Inflammatory Bowel Disease; **Hospital:** Beth Israel Deaconess Med Ctr - Boston, Boston Med Ctr; **Address:** BIDMC,Div of Gastroenterology/GI East, 330 Brookline Ave RabbRose Bldg - Ste 101, Boston, MA 02215; **Phone:** 617-667-8377; **Board Cert:** Internal Medicine 1972; Gastroenterology 1975; **Med School:** Univ Rochester 1965; **Resid:** Internal Medicine, UCLA Ronald Reagan Med Ctr 1971; **Fellow:** Gastroenterology, Mass Genl Hosp 1973; **Fac Appt:** Prof Med, Harvard Med Sch

Lichtenstein, David R MD [Ge] - **Spec Exp:** Pancreatic & Biliary Disease; Peptic Acid Disorders; Endoscopic Therapies; **Hospital:** Boston Med Ctr; **Address:** 85 E Concord St, Ste 7717, Boston, MA 02118; **Phone:** 617-638-6525; **Board Cert:** Internal Medicine 1988; Gastroenterology 2004; **Med School:** Univ Pennsylvania 1985; **Resid:** Internal Medicine, Duke Univ Med Ctr 1988; **Fellow:** Gastroenterology, Beth Israel Hosp 1990; Advanced Endoscopy, Duke Univ Med Ctr 1992; **Fac Appt:** Assoc Prof Med, Univ Pennsylvania

Mason, Joel B MD [Ge] - **Spec Exp:** Nutrition in Acute Illness; Nutrition in Bowel Disorders; Nutrition & Cancer Prevention; Inflammatory Bowel Disease; **Hospital:** Tufts Med Ctr; **Address:** Tufts Med Ctr, 800 Washington St, Box 239, Boston, MA 02111-1513; **Phone:** 617-636-5883; **Board Cert:** Internal Medicine 1984; Gastroenterology 1987; **Med School:** Univ Chicago-Pritzker Sch Med 1981; **Resid:** Internal Medicine, Univ Iowa Hosps 1984; **Fellow:** Gastroenterology, Univ Chicago Hosps 1986; Nutrition, Univ Chicago Hosps 1986; **Fac Appt:** Prof Med, Tufts Univ

Nunes, David P MD [Ge] - **Spec Exp:** Liver Disease; Hepatitis; **Hospital:** Boston Med Ctr; **Address:** Boston Med Ctr, Div Gastroenterology, 830 Harrison Ave Mokley Bldg Fl 2, Ste 2100, Boston, MA 02118; **Phone:** 617-638-6525 x3; **Board Cert:** Internal Medicine 2006; Gastroenterology 2007; **Med School:** Ireland 1984; **Resid:** Gastroenterology, Federated Dublin Volunt Hosps 1987; **Fac Appt:** Assoc Prof Med, Boston Univ

Gastroenterology

Proctor, Deborah D MD [Ge] - **Spec Exp:** Inflammatory Bowel Disease; Colon Cancer Screening; Endoscopy; **Hospital:** Yale-New Haven Hosp, Yale Med Group; **Address:** 40 Temple St, Ste 1A, New Haven, CT 06519; **Phone:** 203-785-4138; **Board Cert:** Gastroenterology 2003; **Med School:** Univ Cincinnati 1982; **Resid:** Internal Medicine, Beth Israel Hosp 1990; **Fellow:** Gastroenterology, Beth Israel Hosp 1992; **Fac Appt:** Prof Med, Yale Univ

Rothstein, Richard I MD [Ge] - **Spec Exp:** Gastroesophageal Reflux Disease (GERD); Swallowing Disorders; Barrett's Esophagus; Endoscopy; **Hospital:** Dartmouth - Hitchcock Med Ctr; **Address:** Dartmouth-Hitchcock Med Ctr, Div Gastroenterology, 1 Medical Center Drive, Lebanon, NH 03756; **Phone:** 603-650-5261; **Board Cert:** Internal Medicine 1983; Gastroenterology 1987; **Med School:** Boston Univ 1980; **Resid:** Internal Medicine, Univ Mass Med Ctr 1983; **Fellow:** Gastroenterology, Dartmouth-Hitchcock Med Ctr 1985; **Fac Appt:** Prof Med, Dartmouth Med Sch

Siegel, Corey A MD [Ge] - **Spec Exp:** Ulcerative Colitis; Crohn's Disease; Colonoscopy; Inflammatory Bowel Disease; **Hospital:** Dartmouth - Hitchcock Med Ctr; **Address:** Dartmouth-Hitchcock Med Ctr, Gastroenterology & Hepatology Div, 1 Medical Ctr Drive, Lebanon, NH 03756; **Phone:** 603-650-5261; **Board Cert:** Gastroenterology 2005; **Med School:** Tufts Univ 1998; **Resid:** Internal Medicine, Dartmouth-Hitchcock Med Ctr 2002; **Fellow:** Gastroenterology, Dartmouth-Hitchcock Med Ctr 2004; Inflammatory Bowel Disease, Mass Genl Hosp 2005

Weinstock, Joel V MD [Ge] - **Spec Exp:** Endoscopy; Inflammatory Bowel Disease; **Hospital:** Tufts Med Ctr; **Address:** Tufts Med Ctr, 800 Washington St, Box 233, Boston, MA 02111; **Phone:** 617-636-5883; **Board Cert:** Internal Medicine 1976; Gastroenterology 1979; **Med School:** Wayne State Univ 1973; **Resid:** Internal Medicine, Univ Hosp Michigan 1976; **Fellow:** Gastroenterology, Univ Hosp Michigan 1978; **Fac Appt:** Prof Med, Tufts Univ

Mid Atlantic

Al-Kawas, Firas H MD [Ge] - **Spec Exp:** Pancreatic & Biliary Disease; **Hospital:** Georgetown Univ Hosp; **Address:** GI Division Georgetown Hosp, 3800 Reservoir Rd NW Fl 2 - Ste M2025, Washington, DC 20007; **Phone:** 202-444-1670; **Board Cert:** Internal Medicine 1979; Gastroenterology 1983; **Med School:** Syria 1974; **Resid:** Internal Medicine, Georgetown Univ Hosp 1979; **Fellow:** Gastroenterology, VA Med Ctr 1981; **Fac Appt:** Assoc Prof Med, Georgetown Univ

Albert, Michael B MD [Ge] - **Spec Exp:** Inflammatory Bowel Disease; Ulcerative Colitis; Endoscopy; Colon Cancer Screening; **Hospital:** G Washington Univ Hosp; **Address:** DC Gastroenterology, 2131 K St NW, Ste 800A, Washington, DC 20037; **Phone:** 202-223-5544; **Board Cert:** Internal Medicine 1985; Gastroenterology 1987; **Med School:** Johns Hopkins Univ 1982; **Resid:** Internal Medicine, Mayo Clinic 1984; Internal Medicine, Duke Univ Med Ctr 1985; **Fellow:** Gastroenterology, G Washington Univ Med Ctr 1987; **Fac Appt:** Prof Med, Geo Wash Univ

Aronchick, Craig A MD [Ge] - **Spec Exp:** Colonoscopy; Colon Cancer Screening; **Hospital:** Pennsylvania Hosp-UPHS (page 72); **Address:** Wills Eye Surgery Center, 3340 S Broad St, Philadelphia, PA 19145; **Phone:** 267-354-2632; **Board Cert:** Internal Medicine 1981; Gastroenterology 1983; **Med School:** Temple Univ 1978; **Resid:** Internal Medicine, Temple Univ Hosp 1981; **Fellow:** Gastroenterology, Hosp Univ Penn 1983

Bayless, Theodore MD [Ge] - **Spec Exp:** Inflammatory Bowel Disease/Crohn's; Ulcerative Colitis; Malabsorption Syndrome; Microscopic Colitis; **Hospital:** Johns Hopkins Hosp (page 61); **Address:** Johns Hopkins Hosp, 600 N Wolfe St, Blalock Bldg - Ste 461, Baltimore, MD 21287-0005; **Phone:** 410-955-4916; **Board Cert:** Internal Medicine 1966; **Med School:** Ros Franklin Univ/Chicago Med Sch 1957; **Resid:** Internal Medicine, Cornell-Bellevue Hosp 1958; Internal Medicine, Meml Sloan Kettering Hosp 1960; **Fellow:** Gastroenterology, Johns Hopkins Hosp 1962; **Fac Appt:** Prof Med, Johns Hopkins Univ

Benjamin, Stanley MD [Ge] - **Spec Exp:** Gastrointestinal Motility Disorders; Esophageal Disorders; Gastroesophageal Reflux Disease (GERD); **Hospital:** Georgetown Univ Hosp; **Address:** GUMC - Second Floor, Main Hospital, 3800 Reservoir Rd NW, rm M2210, Washington, DC 20007; **Phone:** 202-444-1669; **Board Cert:** Internal Medicine 1977; Gastroenterology 1979; **Med School:** Univ Pittsburgh 1974; **Resid:** Internal Medicine, Natl Naval Med Ctr 1977; **Fellow:** Gastroenterology, Natl Naval Med Ctr 1979; **Fac Appt:** Prof Med, Georgetown Univ

Borum, Marie L MD [Ge] - **Spec Exp:** Colon Cancer Screening; AIDS/HIV-Gastrointestinal Complications; Women's Health; Liver Disease; **Hospital:** G Washington Univ Hosp; **Address:** MFA Dept Medicine, 2150 Pennsylvania Ave NW Fl 3, Washington, DC 20037; **Phone:** 202-741-3333; **Board Cert:** Internal Medicine 1988; Gastroenterology 2001; **Med School:** UMDNJ-Rutgers Med Sch 1985; **Resid:** Internal Medicine, G Washington Univ Med Ctr 1988; **Fellow:** Gastroenterology, G Washington Univ Med Ctr 1991; **Fac Appt:** Prof Med, Geo Wash Univ

Brandt, Lawrence MD [Ge] - **Spec Exp:** Inflammatory Bowel Disease; Clostridium Difficile Disease; **Hospital:** Montefiore Med Ctr-Moses Campus, NY; **Address:** 3400 Bainbridge Ave Fl 2, Bronx, NY 10467-2401; **Phone:** 866-633-8255; **Board Cert:** Internal Medicine 1972; Gastroenterology 2006; **Med School:** SUNY Downstate 1968; **Resid:** Internal Medicine, Mt Sinai Hosp 1972; **Fellow:** Gastroenterology, Mt Sinai Hosp 1972; **Fac Appt:** Prof Emeritus Med, Albert Einstein Coll Med

Brown Jr, Robert S MD [Ge] - **Spec Exp:** Hepatitis; Liver Disease; Transplant Medicine-Liver; Autoimmune Liver Disease; **Hospital:** NY-Presby/Columbia Univ Med Ctr, NY (page 66), NY-Presby/Weill Cornell Med Ctr, NY (page 66); **Address:** Ctr for Liver Disease & Transplantation, 622 W 168th St, PH Bldg - Fl 14, rm 105, New York, NY 10032; **Phone:** 212-305-1305; **Board Cert:** Internal Medicine 2002; Gastroenterology 2005; Transplant Hepatology 2010; **Med School:** NYU Sch Med 1989; **Resid:** Internal Medicine, Beth Israel Deaconess Med Ctr 1992; **Fellow:** Gastroenterology, UCSF Med Ctr 1994; Hepatology, UCSF Med Ctr 1995; **Fac Appt:** Prof Med, Columbia P&S

Canto, Marcia MD [Ge] - **Spec Exp:** Endoscopy; Endoscopic Ultrasound; Pancreatic Cancer-Early Detection; **Hospital:** Johns Hopkins Hosp (page 61); **Address:** Johns Hopkins Gastroenterology, 10700 Charter Drive, Ste 310, Columbia, MD 21044; **Phone:** 410-715-0350; **Board Cert:** Internal Medicine 1989; Gastroenterology 2008; **Med School:** Philippines 1985; **Resid:** Internal Medicine, SUNY Hlth Sci Ctr 1991; **Fellow:** Gastroenterology, SUNY Hlth Sci Ctr 1993; **Fac Appt:** Prof Med, Johns Hopkins Univ

Carr-Locke, David L MD [Ge] - **Spec Exp:** Pancreatic/Biliary Endoscopy (ERCP); Pancreatic & Biliary Disease; Endoscopy; **Hospital:** Beth Israel Med Ctr - Petrie Division (page 56); **Address:** 1st & 16th St, New York, NY 10003; **Phone:** 212-420-4015; **Board Cert:** Internal Medicine 1974; **Med School:** England, UK 1972; **Resid:** Obstetrics & Gynecology, Orsett Hosp 1974; Internal Medicine, Leicester Hosp 1976; **Fellow:** Gastroenterology, Leicester Hosp 1978; Research, New Eng Baptist Hosp 1979; **Fac Appt:** Assoc Prof Med, Harvard Med Sch

Cohen, Jonathan MD [Ge] - **Spec Exp:** Pancreatic/Biliary Endoscopy (ERCP); Colonoscopy; Barrett's Esophagus; Gastrointestinal Cancer; **Hospital:** NYU Langone Med Ctr (page 68); **Address:** 232 E 30th St, New York, NY 10016-8202; **Phone:** 212-889-5544; **Board Cert:** Gastroenterology 2005; **Med School:** Harvard Med Sch 1990; **Resid:** Internal Medicine, Beth Israel Hosp 1993; **Fellow:** Gastroenterology, UCLA Med Ctr 1995; Endoscopy, Wellesley Hosp 1995; **Fac Appt:** Clin Prof Med, NYU Sch Med

Gastroenterology

Cohen, Lawrence B MD [Ge] - **Spec Exp:** Gastroesophageal Reflux Disease (GERD); Esophageal Disorders; Colon & Rectal Cancer; Endoscopy; **Hospital:** Mount Sinai Med Ctr (page 64); **Address:** 311 E 79th St, Ste 2A, New York, NY 10075; **Phone:** 212-996-6633; **Board Cert:** Internal Medicine 1981; Gastroenterology 1983; **Med School:** Hahnemann Univ 1978; **Resid:** Internal Medicine, Mt Sinai Hosp 1981; **Fellow:** Gastroenterology, Mt Sinai Hosp 1983; **Fac Appt:** Assoc Clin Prof Med, Mount Sinai Sch Med

DeCross, Arthur J MD [Ge] - **Hospital:** Univ of Rochester Strong Meml Hosp; **Address:** 180 Saw Grass Drive, Rochester, NY 14620; **Phone:** 585-758-0209; **Board Cert:** Gastroenterology 2003; **Med School:** Albany Med Coll 1988; **Resid:** Internal Medicine, Strong Meml Hosp 1991; **Fellow:** Gastroenterology, Univ Virginnia Med Ctr 1994; **Fac Appt:** Assoc Prof Med, Univ Rochester

Di Marino Jr, Anthony J MD [Ge] - **Spec Exp:** Celiac Disease; Gastroesophageal Reflux Disease (GERD); Esophageal Disorders; Crohn's Disease; **Hospital:** Thomas Jefferson Univ Hosp; **Address:** 132 S 10th St, Ste 480, Div Gastroenterology, Philadelphia, PA 19107; **Phone:** 215-955-2728; **Board Cert:** Internal Medicine 1977; Gastroenterology 1972; **Med School:** Hahnemann Univ 1968; **Resid:** Internal Medicine, Hahnemann Univ Hosp 1970; Internal Medicine, Hosp Univ Penn 1971; **Fellow:** Gastroenterology, Hosp Univ Penn 1973; **Fac Appt:** Prof Med, Thomas Jefferson Univ

Dieterich, Douglas T MD [Ge] - **Spec Exp:** Hepatitis; AIDS/HIV-Gastrointestinal Complications; Liver Disease; Endoscopy; **Hospital:** Mount Sinai Med Ctr (page 64); **Address:** 5 E 98th St Fl 11, New York, NY 10029; **Phone:** 212-241-7270; **Board Cert:** Internal Medicine 1981; Gastroenterology 1987; **Med School:** NYU Sch Med 1978; **Resid:** Internal Medicine, Bellevue Hosp Ctr-NYU 1981; **Fellow:** Gastroenterology, Bellevue Hosp Ctr-NYU 1983; **Fac Appt:** Prof Med, Mount Sinai Sch Med

Falk, Gary W MD [Ge] - **Spec Exp:** Barrett's Esophagus; Swallowing Disorders; Esophageal Disorders; **Hospital:** Hosp Univ Penn - UPHS (page 72); **Address:** 9 Penn Tower/One Convention Ave, Fl 9, Philadelphia, PA 19104; **Phone:** 215-662-4279; **Board Cert:** Internal Medicine 1983; Gastroenterology 1985; **Med School:** Univ Rochester 1980; **Resid:** Internal Medicine, George Washington Univ Hosp 1983; **Fellow:** Gastroenterology, Univ Michigan Med Ctr 1986; **Fac Appt:** Prof Med, Univ Pennsylvania

Fisher, Robert S MD [Ge] - **Spec Exp:** Gastrointestinal Motility Disorders; Peptic Acid Disorders; Gastrointestinal Functional Disorders; **Hospital:** Temple Univ Hosp; **Address:** 3401 N Broad St, Philadelphia, PA 19140; **Phone:** 215-707-3433; **Board Cert:** Internal Medicine 1971; Gastroenterology 1973; **Med School:** Univ Pennsylvania 1964; **Resid:** Internal Medicine, Temple Univ Med Ctr 1970; **Fellow:** Gastroenterology, Hosp Univ Penn 1972

Freiman, Hal MD [Ge] - **Spec Exp:** Gastroesophageal Reflux Disease (GERD); Biliary Disease; Pancreatic/Biliary Endoscopy (ERCP); Hepatitis; **Hospital:** Beth Israel Med Ctr - Petrie Division (page 56), NYU Langone Med Ctr (page 68); **Address:** 59 W 12th St, Ste 1D, New York, NY 10011-8520; **Phone:** 212-206-0074; **Board Cert:** Internal Medicine 1981; Gastroenterology 1983; **Med School:** Albany Med Coll 1978; **Resid:** Internal Medicine, St Vincent's Hosp 1981; **Fellow:** Gastroenterology, Westchester Co Med Ctr 1983

Gerdes, Hans MD [Ge] - **Spec Exp:** Endoscopy; Endoscopic Ultrasound; Barrett's Esophagus; Gastrointestinal Cancer; **Hospital:** Meml Sloan-Kettering Cancer Ctr; **Address:** 1275 York Avenue, New York, NY 10065; **Phone:** 800-525-2225; **Board Cert:** Internal Medicine 1987; Gastroenterology 1989; **Med School:** Cornell Univ-Weill Med Coll 1983; **Resid:** Internal Medicine, New York Hosp 1986; **Fellow:** Gastroenterology, Meml Sloan Kettering Cancer Ctr 1989

Giardiello, Francis MD [Ge] - **Spec Exp:** Colon Cancer; Colon & Rectal Cancer-Familial Polyposis; Cancer Risk Assessment; **Hospital:** Johns Hopkins Hosp (page 61); **Address:** Johns Hopkins Hosp, Div Gastroenterology, 1830 E Monument St, rm 431, Baltimore, MD 21205; **Phone:** 410-955-2635; **Board Cert:** Internal Medicine 1983; Gastroenterology 1985; **Med School:** Tufts Univ 1980; **Resid:** Internal Medicine, Univ Michigan 1983; **Fellow:** Gastroenterology, Johns Hopkins 1985; **Fac Appt:** Prof Med, Johns Hopkins Univ

Ginsberg, Gregory G MD [Ge] - **Spec Exp:** Pancreatic/Biliary Endoscopy (ERCP); Endoscopy; Endoscopic Ultrasound; Barrett's Esophagus; **Hospital:** Hosp Univ Penn - UPHS (page 72); **Address:** Perelman Ctr for Advanced Medicine, 3400 Civic Center Blvd, South Pavilion, 4th Fl, Philadelphia, PA 19104; **Phone:** 215-349-8222; **Board Cert:** Gastroenterology 2000; **Med School:** Jefferson Med Coll 1987; **Resid:** Internal Medicine, Georgetown Univ Med Ctr 1990; **Fellow:** Gastroenterology, Georgetown Univ 1992; **Fac Appt:** Prof Med, Univ Pennsylvania

Goggins, Michael MD [Ge] - **Spec Exp:** Pancreatic Cancer-Early Detection; **Hospital:** Johns Hopkins Hosp (page 61); **Address:** Johns Hopkins Univ Sch Med, 1550 Orleans St, CRB II, rm 342, Baltimore, MD 21231; **Phone:** 410-933-7495; **Med School:** Ireland 1988; **Resid:** Internal Medicine, St Jame's Hosp 1990; **Fellow:** Gastroenterology, St Jame's Hosp 1992; **Fac Appt:** Assoc Prof Med, Johns Hopkins Univ

Green, Peter H R MD [Ge] - **Spec Exp:** Celiac Disease; Endoscopy; Colonoscopy; Malabsorption Syndrome; **Hospital:** NY-Presby/Columbia Univ Med Ctr, NY (page 66); **Address:** Celiac Disease Ctr, Harkness Bldg, 180 Fort Washington Ave, Ste 936, New York, NY 10032-3713; **Phone:** 212-305-5590; **Med School:** Australia 1970; **Resid:** Internal Medicine, North Shore Med Ctr 1974; **Fellow:** Gastroenterology, North Shore Med Ctr 1976; Gastroenterology, Beth Israel Hosp 1977; **Fac Appt:** Clin Prof Med, Columbia P&S

Greenwald, Bruce D MD [Ge] - **Spec Exp:** Endoscopic Ultrasound; Barrett's Esophagus; Esophageal Cancer; Clinical Trials; **Hospital:** Univ of MD Med Ctr; **Address:** Univ MD Med Ctr Dept Gastroenterology, 22 S Greene St Fl 3 - rm N3W62, Baltimore, MD 21201; **Phone:** 410-328-8731; **Board Cert:** Gastroenterology 2000; **Med School:** Univ MD Sch Med 1987; **Resid:** Internal Medicine, Univ Virginia Hlth Sys 1990; **Fellow:** Gastroenterology, Univ Maryland Med Ctr 1992; **Fac Appt:** Assoc Prof Med, Univ MD Sch Med

Haber, Gregory B MD [Ge] - **Spec Exp:** Endoscopy; Pancreatic/Biliary Endoscopy (ERCP); Endoscopic Ultrasound; Barrett's Esophagus; **Hospital:** Lenox Hill Hosp (page 67); **Address:** 100 E 77th St Fl 2, New York, NY 10075; **Phone:** 212-434-6279; **Med School:** Univ Toronto 1970; **Resid:** Internal Medicine, Univ Toronto Med Ctr 1975; **Fellow:** Gastroenterology, Univ Toronto Med Ctr 1978

Haluszka, Oleh MD [Ge] - **Spec Exp:** Pancreatic/Biliary Endoscopy (ERCP); Gastrointestinal Cancer; Endoscopic Ultrasound; Endoscopic Therapies; **Hospital:** Temple Univ Hosp; **Address:** Temple Univ Div Gastroenterology, 3401 N Broad St, Zone 3, Ste 831, Philadelphia, PA 19140; **Phone:** 215-707-9577; **Board Cert:** Internal Medicine 1987; Gastroenterology 2011; **Med School:** Uniformed Srvs Univ, Bethesda 1982; **Resid:** Internal Medicine, US Naval Hosp 1987; **Fellow:** Gastroenterology, US Naval Hosp 1990; Endoscopy, Med Coll Wisconsin 1993; **Fac Appt:** Assoc Clin Prof Med, Temple Univ

Herrine, Steven K MD [Ge] - **Spec Exp:** Liver Disease; Hepatitis C; Transplant Medicine-Liver; **Hospital:** Thomas Jefferson Univ Hosp; **Address:** 132 S 10th St, Ste 450, Div Gastroenterology & Hepatology, Philadelphia, PA 19107; **Phone:** 215-955-8900; **Board Cert:** Internal Medicine 2003; Gastroenterology 2005; Transplant Hepatology 2006; **Med School:** Jefferson Med Coll 1990; **Resid:** Internal Medicine, Hosp U Penn 1993; **Fellow:** Gastroenterology, Thos Jefferson Univ Hosp 1995; **Fac Appt:** Prof Med, Thomas Jefferson Univ

Gastroenterology

Hoops, Timothy C MD [Ge] - **Spec Exp:** Esophageal Disorders; Endoscopy; Colonoscopy; **Hospital:** Penn Presby Med Ctr - UPHS (page 72); **Address:** Penn Presbyterian Med Ctr, Wright-Saunders, Ste 218, 51 N 39th St, Philadelphia, PA 19104; **Phone:** 215-662-8900; **Board Cert:** Internal Medicine 1984; Gastroenterology 1987; **Med School:** Univ IL Coll Med 1981; **Resid:** Internal Medicine, Univ Colorado Hlth Sci Ctr 1984; **Fellow:** Gastroenterology, Univ Colorado Hlth Sci Ctr 1986; **Fac Appt:** Clin Prof Med, Univ Pennsylvania

Infantolino, Anthony MD [Ge] - **Spec Exp:** Interventional Endoscopy; Gastrointestinal Cancer; Endoscopic Ultrasound; Barrett's Esophagus; **Hospital:** Thomas Jefferson Univ Hosp; **Address:** 132 S 10th St, Main Bldg - Fl 5, MS 19107, Div Gastroenterology & Hepatology, Philadelphia, PA 19107; **Phone:** 215-955-8900; **Board Cert:** Internal Medicine 1988; Gastroenterology 2012; **Med School:** UMDNJ-RW Johnson Med Sch 1985; **Resid:** Internal Medicine, Thom Jefferson Univ Hosp 1988; **Fellow:** Gastroenterology, Graduate Hosp-UPHS 1991; **Fac Appt:** Assoc Prof Med, UMDNJ-Rutgers Med Sch

Itzkowitz, Steven H MD [Ge] - **Spec Exp:** Colon & Rectal Cancer; Colon & Rectal Cancer Detection; Inflammatory Bowel Disease; Hereditary Cancer; **Hospital:** Mount Sinai Med Ctr (page 64); **Address:** 5 E 98th St, Box 1625, New York, NY 10029-6501; **Phone:** 212-241-4299; **Board Cert:** Internal Medicine 1982; Gastroenterology 1985; **Med School:** Mount Sinai Sch Med 1979; **Resid:** Internal Medicine, Bellevue Hosp/NYU Med Ctr 1982; **Fellow:** Gastroenterology, UCSF Med Ctr 1984; **Fac Appt:** Prof Med, Mount Sinai Sch Med

Jacobson, Ira M MD [Ge] - **Spec Exp:** Liver & Biliary Disease; Pancreatic Disease; Hepatitis; Hepatitis C; **Hospital:** NY-Presby/Weill Cornell Med Ctr, NY (page 66); **Address:** 1305 York Ave Fl 4, New York, NY 10021-5016; **Phone:** 646-962-4040; **Board Cert:** Internal Medicine 1982; Gastroenterology 2009; Transplant Hepatology 2006; **Med School:** Columbia P&S 1979; **Resid:** Internal Medicine, UCSF Med Ctr 1982; **Fellow:** Gastroenterology, Mass Genl Hosp 1984; **Fac Appt:** Prof Med, Cornell Univ-Weill Med Coll

Kalloo, Anthony N MD [Ge] - **Spec Exp:** Endoscopy; Pancreatic Disease; **Hospital:** Johns Hopkins Hosp (page 61); **Address:** Johns Hopkins Hosp, Div Gastroenterology, 600 N Wolfe St, Blalock 465, Baltimore, MD 21231; **Phone:** 410-955-9697; **Board Cert:** Internal Medicine 1985; Gastroenterology 1987; **Med School:** Jamaica 1979; **Resid:** Internal Medicine, Howard Univ Hosp 1985; **Fellow:** Gastroenterology, VA Med Ctr/Georgetown Univ Hosp 1987; **Fac Appt:** Assoc Prof Med, Johns Hopkins Univ

Kantsevoy, Sergey V MD/PhD [Ge] - **Spec Exp:** Pancreatic Disease; Endoscopic Ultrasound; Pancreatic/Biliary Endoscopy (ERCP); **Hospital:** Mercy Med Ctr - Baltimore; **Address:** 301 St Paul Pl, Ste 718, Professional Off Bldg, Baltimore, MD 21202; **Phone:** 410-332-9356; **Board Cert:** Gastroenterology 2000; **Med School:** Russia 1983; **Resid:** Internal Medicine, Bronx-Lebanon Hosp Ctr 1995; Internal Medicine, Washington Hosp Ctr 1997; **Fellow:** Gastroenterology, Johns Hopkins Hosp 2000; **Fac Appt:** Asst Prof Med, Johns Hopkins Univ

Kastenberg, David M MD [Ge] - **Spec Exp:** Colon & Rectal Cancer Detection; Capsule Endoscopy; Celiac Disease; Nutrition & Cancer Prevention; **Hospital:** Thomas Jefferson Univ Hosp; **Address:** Jefferson Univ Physicians-Div GI, 132 S 10th St, Main Bldg - Ste 480, Phildelphia, PA 19107; **Phone:** 215-955-8900; **Board Cert:** Internal Medicine 2010; Gastroenterology 2000; **Med School:** NYU Sch Med 1987; **Resid:** Internal Medicine, Temple Univ Hosp 1990; **Fellow:** Gastroenterology, Thomas Jefferson Univ Hosp 1992; **Fac Appt:** Assoc Prof Med, Jefferson Med Coll

Katz, Philip O MD [Ge] - **Spec Exp:** Gastroesophageal Reflux Disease (GERD); Swallowing Disorders; Barrett's Esophagus; Esophageal Disorders; **Hospital:** Albert Einstein Med Ctr; **Address:** 5401 Old York Rd, Klein Bldg - Ste 202, Philadelphia, PA 19141; **Phone:** 215-456-8210; **Board Cert:** Internal Medicine 1981; Gastroenterology 1987; **Med School:** Bowman Gray 1978; **Resid:** Internal Medicine, NC Baptist Hosp 1981; **Fellow:** Gastroenterology, NC Baptist Hosp 1986; **Fac Appt:** Clin Prof Med, Thomas Jefferson Univ

Kochman, Michael L MD [Ge] - **Spec Exp:** Endoscopy; Pancreatic/Biliary Endoscopy (ERCP); Gastrointestinal Cancer; **Hospital:** Hosp Univ Penn - UPHS (page 72); **Address:** Univ Penn Div Gastroenterology, 1 Convention Ave, 9th Fl - Penn Tower, Philadelphia, PA 19104-4206; **Phone:** 215-662-4279; **Board Cert:** Internal Medicine 1989; Gastroenterology 2003; **Med School:** Univ IL Coll Med 1986; **Resid:** Internal Medicine, Univ Illinois Med Ctr 1990; **Fellow:** Gastroenterology, Univ Michigan 1993; **Fac Appt:** Prof Med, Univ Pennsylvania

Korsten, Mark A MD [Ge] - **Spec Exp:** Constipation; Gastrointestinal Motility Disorders; Spinal Cord Injury & Colonic Motility; Liver Disease; **Hospital:** James J. Peters VA Med Ctr-Bronx; **Address:** 130 W Kingsbridge Rd, Ste 3H, Bronx, NY 10468; **Phone:** 718-584-9000 x6753; **Board Cert:** Internal Medicine 1973; Gastroenterology 1975; **Med School:** Yale Univ 1970; **Resid:** Internal Medicine, Mt Sinai Hosp 1973; **Fellow:** Gastroenterology, Mt Sinai Hosp 1975; **Fac Appt:** Prof Med, Mount Sinai Sch Med

Kotler, Donald P MD [Ge] - **Spec Exp:** Esophageal Disorders; Nutrition & AIDS; Hepatitis; **Hospital:** St. Luke's - Roosevelt Hosp Ctr - St Luke's Hosp (page 56); **Address:** 1111 Amsterdam Ave, SR 12, New York, NY 10025; **Phone:** 212-523-3670; **Board Cert:** Internal Medicine 1976; Gastroenterology 1979; **Med School:** Albert Einstein Coll Med 1973; **Resid:** Internal Medicine, Jacobi Med Ctr 1976; **Fellow:** Gastroenterology, Hosp Univ Penn 1978; **Fac Appt:** Prof Med, Columbia P&S

Kowalski, Thomas E MD [Ge] - **Spec Exp:** Pancreatic Disease; Biliary Disease; Pancreatic/Biliary Endoscopy (ERCP); Endoscopic Ultrasound; **Hospital:** Thomas Jefferson Univ Hosp; **Address:** 132 S 10th St Main Bldg - Ste 585, Philadelphia, PA 19107; **Phone:** 215-955-8900; **Board Cert:** Internal Medicine 2003; Gastroenterology 2003; **Med School:** SUNY Buffalo 1988; **Resid:** Internal Medicine, Johns Hopkins Hosp 1991; **Fellow:** Gastroenterology, Hosp Univ Penn 1993; Advanced Endoscopy, Hosp Univ Penn 1994; **Fac Appt:** Assoc Prof Med, Thomas Jefferson Univ

Kurtz, Robert C MD [Ge] - **Spec Exp:** Pancreatic Cancer(Familial); Gastrointestinal Cancer; Endoscopy; Cancer Prevention; **Hospital:** Meml Sloan-Kettering Cancer Ctr; **Address:** 1275 York Ave, New York, NY 10065; **Phone:** 212-639-7620; **Board Cert:** Internal Medicine 1971; Gastroenterology 1977; **Med School:** Jefferson Med Coll 1968; **Resid:** Internal Medicine, NY Hosp/Meml Sloan Kettering Cancer Ctr 1971; **Fellow:** Gastroenterology, Meml Sloan Kettering Cancer Ctr 1973; **Fac Appt:** Prof Med, Cornell Univ-Weill Med Coll

Lebwohl, Oscar MD [Ge] - **Spec Exp:** Endoscopy; Inflammatory Bowel Disease/Crohn's; Ulcerative Colitis; Gastrointestinal Cancer; **Hospital:** NY-Presby/Columbia Univ Med Ctr, NY (page 66); **Address:** 161 Fort Washington Ave, rm 420, New York, NY 10032-3713; **Phone:** 212-305-5363; **Board Cert:** Internal Medicine 1975; Gastroenterology 1977; **Med School:** Harvard Med Sch 1972; **Resid:** Internal Medicine, Mt Sinai Med Ctr 1975; **Fellow:** Gastroenterology, Columbia-Presby Med Ctr 1976; Hepatology, Mt Sinai Med Ctr 1977; **Fac Appt:** Clin Prof Med, Columbia P&S

Lewis, Blair MD [Ge] - **Spec Exp:** Endoscopy; Capsule Endoscopy; **Hospital:** Mount Sinai Med Ctr (page 64); **Address:** 1067 5th Ave, New York, NY 10128-0101; **Phone:** 212-369-6600; **Board Cert:** Internal Medicine 1985; Gastroenterology 1987; **Med School:** Albert Einstein Coll Med 1982; **Resid:** Internal Medicine, Montefiore Med Ctr 1985; **Fellow:** Gastroenterology, Mt Sinai Med Ctr 1987; **Fac Appt:** Clin Prof Med, Mount Sinai Sch Med

Gastroenterology

Lichtenstein, Gary R MD [Ge] - **Spec Exp:** Inflammatory Bowel Disease; Crohn's Disease; Ulcerative Colitis; **Hospital:** Hosp Univ Penn - UPHS (page 72); **Address:** Perelman Ctr for Advanced Medicine, 3400 Civic Center Blvd, South Pavilion, 4th Fl, Philadelphia, PA 19104; **Phone:** 215-349-8222; **Board Cert:** Internal Medicine 1987; Gastroenterology 1989; **Med School:** Mount Sinai Sch Med 1984; **Resid:** Internal Medicine, Duke Univ Med Ctr 1987; **Fellow:** Gastroenterology, Hosp Univ Penn 1990; **Fac Appt:** Prof Med, Univ Pennsylvania

Lightdale, Charles J MD [Ge] - **Spec Exp:** Barrett's Esophagus; Gastrointestinal Cancer; Endoscopic Ultrasound; **Hospital:** NY-Presby/Columbia Univ Med Ctr, NY (page 66); **Address:** Columbia-Presby Med Ctr, Irving Pavilion, 161 Fort Washington Ave, rm 812, New York, NY 10032-3713; **Phone:** 212-305-3423; **Board Cert:** Internal Medicine 1972; Gastroenterology 1973; **Med School:** Columbia P&S 1966; **Resid:** Internal Medicine, Yale-New Haven Hosp 1968; Internal Medicine, NY Hosp-Cornell 1969; **Fellow:** Gastroenterology, NY Hosp-Cornell 1973; **Fac Appt:** Clin Prof Med, Columbia P&S

Lipshutz, William H MD [Ge] - **Spec Exp:** Inflammatory Bowel Disease/Crohn's; Colonoscopy; Esophageal Disorders; Gastroesophageal Reflux Disease (GERD); **Hospital:** Pennsylvania Hosp-UPHS (page 72); **Address:** 230 W Washington Sq, Farm Journal Bldg Fl 4, Philadelphia, PA 19106; **Phone:** 215-829-3561; **Board Cert:** Internal Medicine 1972; Gastroenterology 1973; **Med School:** Univ Pennsylvania 1967; **Resid:** Internal Medicine, Pennsylvania Hosp 1972; **Fellow:** Gastroenterology, Hosp Univ Penn 1971

Magun, Arthur M MD [Ge] - **Spec Exp:** Hepatitis; Ulcerative Colitis; Endoscopy; Crohn's Disease; **Hospital:** NY-Presby/Columbia Univ Med Ctr, NY (page 66); **Address:** 161 Fort Washington Ave, Herbert Irving Pavillion Fl 3 - rm 338, New York, NY 10032-3713; **Phone:** 212-305-5287; **Board Cert:** Internal Medicine 1980; Gastroenterology 1983; **Med School:** Mount Sinai Sch Med 1977; **Resid:** Internal Medicine, Columbia-Presby Med Ctr 1980; **Fellow:** Gastroenterology, Columbia-Presby Med Ctr 1983; **Fac Appt:** Clin Prof Med, Columbia P&S

Markowitz, David D MD [Ge] - **Spec Exp:** Gastroesophageal Reflux Disease (GERD); Esophageal Disorders; **Hospital:** NY-Presby/Columbia Univ Med Ctr, NY (page 66); **Address:** 161 Ft Washington Ave, Ste 853, New York, NY 10032; **Phone:** 212-305-1024; **Board Cert:** Internal Medicine 1988; Gastroenterology 2011; **Med School:** Columbia P&S 1985; **Resid:** Internal Medicine, Columbia-Presby Hosp 1988; **Fellow:** Gastroenterology, Columbia-Presby Hosp 1991; **Fac Appt:** Assoc Prof Med, Columbia P&S

Mayer, Lloyd MD [Ge] - **Spec Exp:** Inflammatory Bowel Disease/Crohn's; Ulcerative Colitis; **Hospital:** Mount Sinai Med Ctr (page 64); **Address:** 1425 Madison Ave, rm 11-20, New York, NY 10029; **Phone:** 212-659-9266; **Board Cert:** Internal Medicine 1979; Gastroenterology 1981; **Med School:** Mount Sinai Sch Med 1976; **Resid:** Internal Medicine, Bellevue Hosp 1979; **Fellow:** Gastroenterology, Mt Sinai Hosp 1981; **Fac Appt:** Prof Med, Mount Sinai Sch Med

Metz, David C MD [Ge] - **Spec Exp:** Peptic Acid Disorders; Neuroendocrine Tumors; Gastroesophageal Reflux Disease (GERD); Gastrointestinal Motility Disorders; **Hospital:** Hosp Univ Penn - UPHS (page 72); **Address:** Hosp Univ Penn, Div Gastroenterology, 1 Convention Ave, 9 Penn Tower, Philadelphia, PA 19104; **Phone:** 215-349-8222; **Board Cert:** Internal Medicine 1989; Gastroenterology 2011; **Med School:** South Africa 1982; **Resid:** Internal Medicine, Albert Einstein Med Ctr 1988; **Fellow:** Gastroenterology, Natl Inst Hlth 1991; **Fac Appt:** Prof Med, Univ Pennsylvania

Miskovitz, Paul MD [Ge] - **Spec Exp:** Endoscopy; Liver Disease; Biliary Disease; **Hospital:** NY-Presby/Weill Cornell Med Ctr, NY (page 66); **Address:** 635 Madison Ave, Fl 17, New York, NY 10022; **Phone:** 212-717-4966; **Board Cert:** Internal Medicine 1978; Gastroenterology 1981; **Med School:** Cornell Univ-Weill Med Coll 1975; **Resid:** Internal Medicine, NY Hosp 1978; **Fellow:** Gastroenterology, NY Hosp 1980; **Fac Appt:** Clin Prof Med, Cornell Univ-Weill Med Coll

Munoz, Santiago J MD [Ge] - **Spec Exp:** Liver Disease; Transplant Medicine-Liver; Hepatitis; **Hospital:** Temple Univ Hosp; **Address:** Temple University Hospital, Div Gasteoenterology & Transplantation, 3401 N Broad St, Philadelphia, PA 19150; **Phone:** 215-707-9900; **Board Cert:** Internal Medicine 1985; Gastroenterology 1989; Transplant Hepatology 2006; **Med School:** Chile 1978; **Resid:** Internal Medicine, Jefferson Hosp 1985; **Fellow:** Pharmacology, Johns Hopkins Hosp 1983; Gastroenterology, Jefferson Hosp 1987; **Fac Appt:** Assoc Prof Med, Temple Univ

Okolo III, Patrick I MD [Ge] - **Spec Exp:** Liver Cancer; Pancreatic Cancer; Gastrointestinal Cancer; Clinical Trials; **Hospital:** Johns Hopkins Hosp (page 61); **Address:** The John Hopkins Hospital, 600 N Wolfe St, Baltimore, MD 21287; **Phone:** 410-933-7495; **Board Cert:** Internal Medicine 2004; Gastroenterology 2008; **Med School:** Nigeria 1988; **Resid:** Internal Medicine, Indiana Univ Med Ctr 1994; **Fellow:** Gastroenterology, John Hopkins Hosp 1997; **Fac Appt:** Assoc Prof Med, Johns Hopkins Univ

Pasricha, P Jay MD [Ge] - **Spec Exp:** Swallowing Disorders-Botox Therapy; Gastrointestinal Motility Disorders; Pancreatic Disease; Gastroparesis; **Hospital:** Stanford Univ Hosp & Clinics; **Address:** Johns Hopkins School of Medicine, Center for Neurogastroenterology, 4940 Eastern Ave, Ste A-505, Baltimore, MD 21224-5309; **Phone:** 410-550-1793; **Board Cert:** Internal Medicine 1988; Gastroenterology 2006; **Med School:** India 1983; **Resid:** Internal Medicine, DC Genl Hosp 1988; **Fellow:** Pulmonary Disease, New England Med Ctr 1990; Gastroenterology, Johns Hopkins Hosp 1992; **Fac Appt:** Prof Med, Stanford Univ

Peikin, Steven MD [Ge] - **Spec Exp:** Endoscopy; **Hospital:** Cooper Univ Hosp; **Address:** Cooper Digestive Health Inst, 501 Fellowship Rd, Ste 101, Mt Laurel, NJ 08054; **Phone:** 856-642-2133; **Board Cert:** Internal Medicine 1977; Gastroenterology 1979; **Med School:** Jefferson Med Coll 1974; **Resid:** Internal Medicine, Moffit Hosps 1977; **Fellow:** Gastroenterology, Mass Genl Hosp 1980; **Fac Appt:** Prof Med

Pezzone, Michael A MD/PhD [Ge] - **Spec Exp:** Irritable Bowel Syndrome; Inflammatory Bowel Disease; Pain-Pelvic; **Hospital:** Washington Hosp, The, UPMC Presby, Pittsburgh; **Address:** Manifold Professional Bldg #3, 86 Wellness Way, Washington, PA 15301; **Phone:** 724-503-4637; **Board Cert:** Internal Medicine 2007; Gastroenterology 2010; **Med School:** Univ Pittsburgh 1994; **Resid:** Internal Medicine, Univ Pittsburgh Med Ctr 1997; **Fellow:** Gastroenterology, Univ Pittsburgh Med Ctr 2000; **Fac Appt:** Assoc Prof Med, Univ Pittsburgh

Pochapin, Mark B MD [Ge] - **Spec Exp:** Pancreatic Cancer; Endoscopic Ultrasound; Colon & Rectal Cancer Detection; Diarrheal Diseases; **Hospital:** NYU Langone Med Ctr (page 68); **Address:** 207 E 84th St Fl 4, 1315 York Ave Fl Ground, New York, NY 10028; **Phone:** 646-501-6760; **Board Cert:** Gastroenterology 2004; **Med School:** Cornell Univ-Weill Med Coll 1988; **Resid:** Internal Medicine, NY Hosp-Cornell Med Ctr 1991; **Fellow:** Gastroenterology, Montefiore Med Ctr 1993; **Fac Appt:** Assoc Clin Prof Med, Cornell Univ-Weill Med Coll

Ravich, William J MD [Ge] - **Spec Exp:** Swallowing Disorders; Gastroesophageal Reflux Disease (GERD); Barrett's Esophagus; Achalasia; **Hospital:** Johns Hopkins Hosp (page 61), Greater Baltimore Med Ctr; **Address:** 10751 Falls Rd, Ste 401, Lutherville, MD 21093; **Phone:** 410-616-2840; **Board Cert:** Internal Medicine 1978; Gastroenterology 1981; **Med School:** Ros Franklin Univ/Chicago Med Sch 1975; **Resid:** Internal Medicine, Montefiore Hosp 1978; **Fellow:** Gastroenterology, Johns Hopkins Hosp 1981; **Fac Appt:** Assoc Prof Med, Johns Hopkins Univ

Reddy, K Rajender MD [Ge] - **Spec Exp:** Liver Disease; Transplant Medicine-Liver; Hepatitis; **Hospital:** Hosp Univ Penn - UPHS (page 72); **Address:** Perelman Ctr for Advanced Medicine, 3400 Civic Center Blvd, South Pavilion, 4th Fl, Philadelphia, PA 19104; **Phone:** 215-349-8222; **Board Cert:** Internal Medicine 1980; Gastroenterology 1983; Transplant Hepatology 2006; **Med School:** India 1972; **Resid:** Internal Medicine, NY Med Coll Hosps 1980; Gastroenterology, Johnson City Hosp 1982; **Fellow:** Hepatology, Univ Miami 1983; **Fac Appt:** Prof Med, Univ Pennsylvania

Gastroenterology

Reynolds, James C MD [Ge] - **Spec Exp:** Gastroesophageal Reflux Disease (GERD); Gastrointestinal Motility Disorders; Barrett's Esophagus; **Hospital:** Hahnemann Univ Hosp; **Address:** Drexel Gastroenterology Assocs, 219 N Broad St Fl 5, Philadelphia, PA 19107; **Phone:** 215-965-6000; **Board Cert:** Internal Medicine 1980; Gastroenterology 1985; **Med School:** Univ Fla Coll Med 1977; **Resid:** Internal Medicine, New York Hosp 1980; **Fellow:** Gastroenterology, Hosp Univ Penn 1983; **Fac Appt:** Prof Med, Drexel Univ Coll Med

Scherl, Ellen MD [Ge] - **Spec Exp:** Inflammatory Bowel Disease; Crohn's Disease; Ulcerative Colitis; **Hospital:** NY-Presby/Weill Cornell Med Ctr, NY (page 66), Beth Israel Med Ctr - Petrie Division (page 56); **Address:** 1315 York Ave, Mezzanine Level, New York, NY 10021; **Phone:** 212-746-5077; **Board Cert:** Internal Medicine 1983; **Med School:** NY Med Coll 1977; **Resid:** Internal Medicine, Beth Israel Med Ctr 1981; **Fellow:** Gastroenterology, Mt Sinai Med Ctr 1983; **Fac Appt:** Asst Prof Med, Cornell Univ-Weill Med Coll

Schiano, Thomas D MD [Ge] - **Spec Exp:** Liver Disease; Transplant Medicine-Liver; Transplant Medicine-Bowel; Hepatitis; **Hospital:** Mount Sinai Med Ctr (page 64); **Address:** 5 E 98th St, Fl 12, Box 1104, MS 10029, New York, NY 10029; **Phone:** 212-241-8035; **Board Cert:** Internal Medicine 2000; Gastroenterology 2005; Transplant Hepatology 2006; **Med School:** Mexico 1987; **Resid:** Internal Medicine, Maimonides Med Ctr 1992; Gastroenterology, Temple Univ 1995; **Fellow:** Nutrition, Meml Sloan-Kettering Cancer Ctr 1993; Hepatology, Mt Sinai Med Ctr 1996; **Fac Appt:** Prof Med, Mount Sinai Sch Med

Shike, Moshe MD [Ge] - **Spec Exp:** Gastrointestinal Cancer; Nutrition & Cancer Prevention; Endoscopy; **Hospital:** Meml Sloan-Kettering Cancer Ctr; **Address:** 1275 York Ave, New York, NY 10065; **Phone:** 212-639-7230; **Board Cert:** Internal Medicine 1977; Gastroenterology 1981; **Med School:** Israel 1975; **Resid:** Internal Medicine, Mt Auburn Hosp 1977; **Fellow:** Gastroenterology, Toronto Genl Hosp 1981; **Fac Appt:** Prof Med, Cornell Univ-Weill Med Coll

Slivka, Adam MD/PhD [Ge] - **Spec Exp:** Pancreatic & Biliary Disease; Pancreatic Cancer; Pancreatic/Biliary Endoscopy (ERCP); **Hospital:** UPMC Presby, Pittsburgh; **Address:** Digestive Disorders Center, 200 Lothrop St, 3rd Fl-PUH D-Wing, Pittsburgh, PA 15213; **Phone:** 412-647-8666; **Board Cert:** Internal Medicine 2002; Gastroenterology 2005; **Med School:** Mount Sinai Sch Med 1988; **Resid:** Internal Medicine, Brigham & Womens Hosp 1991; **Fellow:** Gastroenterology, Brigham & Womens Hosp 1994; **Fac Appt:** Prof Med, Univ Pittsburgh

Tobias, Hillel MD [Ge] - **Spec Exp:** Liver Disease; Hepatitis B & C; Liver & Biliary Disease; **Hospital:** NYU Langone Med Ctr (page 68); **Address:** 232 E 30th St, New York, NY 10016-8202; **Phone:** 212-889-5544; **Board Cert:** Internal Medicine 1967; Gastroenterology 1979; Transplant Hepatology 2006; **Med School:** Washington Univ, St Louis 1960; **Resid:** Internal Medicine, Bellevue Hosp 1963; Hepatology, Royal Free Hosp 1965; **Fellow:** Hepatology, Mount Sinai Hosp 1967; **Fac Appt:** Prof Med, NYU Sch Med

Waye, Jerome D MD [Ge] - **Spec Exp:** Endoscopy; Colon Cancer; Colonoscopy; **Hospital:** Mount Sinai Med Ctr (page 64), Lenox Hill Hosp (page 67); **Address:** 650 Park Ave, New York, NY 10065; **Phone:** 212-439-7779; **Board Cert:** Internal Medicine 1965; Gastroenterology 1970; **Med School:** Boston Univ 1958; **Resid:** Internal Medicine, Mt Sinai Hosp 1961; **Fellow:** Gastroenterology, Mt Sinai Hosp 1962; **Fac Appt:** Clin Prof Med, Mount Sinai Sch Med

Weinberg, David S MD [Ge] - **Spec Exp:** Colonoscopy; Cancer Risk Assessment; Cancer Prevention; Endoscopy; **Hospital:** Fox Chase Cancer Ctr (page 58); **Address:** Fox Chase Cancer Ctr, Dept Medicine, 333 Cottman Ave, Ste P3047, Philadelphia, PA 19111; **Phone:** 215-214-1424; **Board Cert:** Gastroenterology 2006; **Med School:** Cornell Univ 1989; **Resid:** Internal Medicine, Beth Israel Hosp 1992; **Fellow:** Gastroenterology, Hosp Univ Penn 1995; Epidemiology, Hosp Univ Penn 1995; **Fac Appt:** Prof Med, Temple Univ

Southeast

Abreu, Maria T MD [Ge] - **Spec Exp:** Inflammatory Bowel Disease; Ulcerative Colitis; Crohn's Disease; **Hospital:** Univ of Miami Hosp; **Address:** Univ Miami Miller Sch Med, 1475 NW 12th Ave, Miami, FL 33136; **Phone:** 305-243-8644; **Board Cert:** Gastroenterology 2005; **Med School:** Univ Miami Sch Med 1990; **Resid:** Internal Medicine, Brigham & Women's Hosp 1992; **Fellow:** Gastroenterology, UCLA Med Ctr 1995; **Fac Appt:** Prof Med, Univ Miami Sch Med

Baillie, John MD [Ge] - **Spec Exp:** Pancreatic/Biliary Endoscopy(ERCP); **Hospital:** Carteret Genl Hosp; **Address:** 300 Penny Ln, Moorehead, NC 28557; **Phone:** 252-648-8712; **Med School:** Scotland, UK 1977; **Resid:** Internal Medicine, Victoria Infirmary 1981; **Fellow:** Gastroenterology, Univ of Minnesota Med Ctr 1984; Gastroenterology, Middlesex Hospital 1988; **Fac Appt:** Prof Med, Wake Forest Univ

Barkin, Jamie S MD [Ge] - **Spec Exp:** Pancreatic & Biliary Disease; Gastrointestinal Cancer; Endoscopy; **Hospital:** Mount Sinai Med Ctr - Miami, Univ of Miami Hosp & Clins/Sylvester Comp Canc Ctr; **Address:** Mount Sinai Medical Center, Gumenick Bldg, 4300 Alton Rd, Ste 2522, Miami Beach, FL 33140-2800; **Phone:** 305-674-2240; **Board Cert:** Internal Medicine 1973; Gastroenterology 1975; **Med School:** Univ Miami Sch Med 1970; **Resid:** Internal Medicine, Univ Miami Hosp 1973; **Fellow:** Gastroenterology, Univ Miami Hosp 1975; **Fac Appt:** Prof Med, Univ Miami Sch Med

Bloomer, Joseph R MD [Ge] - **Spec Exp:** Porphyria; Liver Disease; Transplant Medicine-Liver; Hepatitis B; **Hospital:** Univ of Ala Hosp at Birmingham, UAB Highlands Hosp; **Address:** UAB Liver Center, 1918 University Blvd, MCLM 284, Birmingham, AL 35294-0005; **Phone:** 205-975-5676; **Board Cert:** Internal Medicine 1972; **Med School:** Case West Res Univ 1966; **Resid:** Internal Medicine, UCSF Med Ctr 1968; **Fellow:** Hepatology, Yale Univ 1972; **Fac Appt:** Prof Med, Univ Alabama

Brazer, Scott R MD [Ge] - **Spec Exp:** Gastroesophageal Reflux Disease (GERD); Colon Cancer Screening; **Hospital:** Durham Regional Hosp; **Address:** 249 E NC 54, Ste 200, Durham, NC 27713; **Phone:** 919-806-8322; **Board Cert:** Internal Medicine 1984; Gastroenterology 1987; **Med School:** Case West Res Univ 1981; **Resid:** Internal Medicine, Duke Univ Med Ctr 1984; Internal Medicine, Duke Univ Med Ctr 1988; **Fellow:** Gastroenterology, Duke Univ 1987

Castell, Donald O MD [Ge] - **Spec Exp:** Esophageal Disorders; Gastroesophageal Reflux Disease (GERD); Gastrointestinal Motility Disorders; **Hospital:** MUSC Med Ctr; **Address:** MUSC Digestive Disease Ctr, 25 Courtenay Drive, ART-7100A, MC CMS290, Charleston, SC 29425; **Phone:** 843-876-4265; **Board Cert:** Internal Medicine 1977; Gastroenterology 1970; **Med School:** Geo Wash Univ 1960; **Resid:** Internal Medicine, US Naval Hosp 1965; **Fellow:** Gastroenterology, Tufts Univ 1969; **Fac Appt:** Prof Med, Univ SC Sch Med

DeVault, Kenneth MD [Ge] - **Spec Exp:** Gastroesophageal Reflux Disease (GERD); **Hospital:** Mayo - Jacksonville; **Address:** Mayo Clinic Davis Bldg Fl 6, 4500 San Pablo Rd S, Jacksonville, FL 32224-1865; **Phone:** 904-953-2254; **Board Cert:** Internal Medicine 1989; Gastroenterology 2003; **Med School:** Bowman Gray 1986; **Resid:** Internal Medicine, Vanderbilt Univ Med Ctr 1989; **Fellow:** Gastroenterology, Thomas Jefferson Univ Med Ctr 1992; **Fac Appt:** Prof Med, Mayo Med Sch

Gastroenterology

Drossman, Douglas A MD [Ge] - **Spec Exp:** Gastrointestinal Motility Disorders; Pain-Abdominal/Functional; Gastrointestinal Functional Disorders; **Hospital:** NC Memorial Hosp - UNC; **Address:** Drossman Gastroenterology, 55 Vilcom Center Drive, Ste 110, Chapel Hill, NC 27514; **Phone:** 919-929-7790; **Board Cert:** Internal Medicine 1973; Gastroenterology 1979; **Med School:** Albert Einstein Coll Med 1970; **Resid:** Internal Medicine, NC Meml Hosp 1972; Internal Medicine, Bellevue Hosp Ctr-NYU 1973; **Fellow:** Psychiatry, Univ Rochester 1976; Gastroenterology, NC Meml Hosp-UNC 1978; **Fac Appt:** Prof Med, Univ NC Sch Med

Elliott, Norman L MD [Ge] - **Spec Exp:** Enteroscopy-Small Bowel; Endoscopy; **Hospital:** Emory Univ Hosp Midtown, Piedmont Hosp; **Address:** Atlanta Gastroenterology Assocs, 550 Peachtree St NE, Ste 1600, Atlanta, GA 30308; **Phone:** 404-881-1094; **Board Cert:** Internal Medicine 1982; Gastroenterology 1985; **Med School:** Yale Univ 1979; **Resid:** Internal Medicine, Emory Univ Hosp 1982; **Fellow:** Gastroenterology, Univ Alabama 1985; **Fac Appt:** Asst Clin Prof Med, Emory Univ

Estores, David S MD [Ge] - **Spec Exp:** Barrett's Esophagus; Swallowing Disorders; Esophageal Cancer; **Hospital:** Tampa Genl Hosp; **Address:** Ctr for Swallowing Disorders, 12901 Bruce B Downs Blvd, MDC 72, Tampa, FL 33612-4742; **Phone:** 813-974-3374; **Board Cert:** Internal Medicine 1989; Gastroenterology 2011; **Med School:** Philippines 1985; **Resid:** Internal Medicine, St Lukes Hosp 1989; **Fellow:** Gastroenterology, Univ Pittsburgh-Presby Hosp 1992

Forsmark, Christopher MD [Ge] - **Spec Exp:** Pancreatic/Biliary Endoscopy (ERCP); Celiac Disease; Pancreatic Disease; Endoscopy; **Hospital:** Shands at Univ of FL; **Address:** University of Florida, 1600 SW Archer Rd, Box 100214, Gainesville, FL 32610; **Phone:** 352-273-9400; **Board Cert:** Internal Medicine 1986; Gastroenterology 2006; **Med School:** Johns Hopkins Univ 1983; **Resid:** Internal Medicine, UCSF Med Ctr 1987; **Fellow:** Gastroenterology, USCF Med Ctr 1990; **Fac Appt:** Prof Med, Univ Fla Coll Med

Fried, Michael W MD [Ge] - **Spec Exp:** Transplant Medicine-Liver; Liver Disease; Hepatitis; **Hospital:** NC Memorial Hosp - UNC; **Address:** 8015A Burnett-Womak Bldg, CB 7584, Chapel Hill, NC 27599; **Phone:** 919-966-2516; **Board Cert:** Internal Medicine 1987; Gastroenterology 1989; **Med School:** Israel 1984; **Resid:** Internal Medicine, SUNY Upstate Med Ctr 1987; **Fellow:** Gastroenterology, SUNY Upstate Med Ctr 1989; **Fac Appt:** Prof Med, Univ NC Sch Med

Hawes, Robert H MD [Ge] - **Spec Exp:** Endoscopic Ultrasound; Pancreatic/Biliary Endoscopy (ERCP); Pancreatic Disease; **Hospital:** Florida Hosp - Orlando; **Address:** 601 E Rollins St, Orlando, FL 32803; **Phone:** 407-303-2570; **Board Cert:** Internal Medicine 1985; Gastroenterology 1987; **Med School:** Indiana Univ 1980; **Resid:** Internal Medicine, Indiana Univ Hosp 1984; **Fellow:** Gastroenterology, Indiana Univ Hosp 1985; Endoscopy, Peter B Cotton/Steve Brown 1986; **Fac Appt:** Prof Med, Med Univ SC

Hoffman, Brenda J MD [Ge] - **Spec Exp:** Endoscopic Ultrasound; Gastrointestinal Cancer; Colon & Rectal Cancer-Familial Polyposis; Endoscopic Therapies; **Hospital:** MUSC Med Ctr, R H Johnson VA Med Ctr - Charleston; **Address:** 25 Courteney Street St ART Bldg Fl 7, ART7100A, Ste 7095, MS 29425, MSC290, Charleston, SC 29425; **Phone:** 843-876-4265; **Board Cert:** Internal Medicine 1986; Gastroenterology 1989; **Med School:** Univ KY Coll Med 1983; **Resid:** Internal Medicine, MUSC Med Ctr 1987; **Fellow:** Gastroenterology, Med Univ SC 1989; **Fac Appt:** Prof Med, Med Univ SC

Isaacs, Kim L MD/PhD [Ge] - **Spec Exp:** Inflammatory Bowel Disease; Crohn's Disease; Ulcerative Colitis; **Hospital:** NC Memorial Hosp - UNC; **Address:** Univ NC, Div Digestive Disease/Nutrition, CB# 7080, Bioinformatics Bldg, 130 Mason Farm Rd Fl 1, Chapel Hill, NC 27599-7080; **Phone:** 919-966-2511; **Board Cert:** Internal Medicine 1987; Gastroenterology 2001; **Med School:** SUNY Stony Brook 1984; **Resid:** Internal Medicine, Univ NC Hosps 1987; **Fellow:** Gastroenterology, Univ NC Hosps 1989; **Fac Appt:** Assoc Prof Med, Univ NC Sch Med

Koch, Kenneth L MD [Ge] - **Spec Exp:** Gastrointestinal Motility Disorders; Gastroparesis; Esophageal Disorders; **Hospital:** Wake Forest Baptist Med Ctr; **Address:** Medical Ctr Blvd, Winston-Salem, NC 27157; **Phone:** 336-713-7777; **Board Cert:** Internal Medicine 1978; Gastroenterology 1983; **Med School:** Univ Iowa Coll Med 1975; **Resid:** Internal Medicine, Penn State Affil Hosp 1978; **Fellow:** Gastroenterology, Univ Florida Affil Hosp 1980; **Fac Appt:** Prof Med, Univ NC Sch Med

Lambiase, Louis R MD [Ge] - **Spec Exp:** Pancreatic Disease; Endoscopic Ultrasound; Pain-Abdominal/Functional; Liver Disease; **Hospital:** Erlanger Med Ctr; **Address:** 979 E 3rd St, Ste C-825, Chattanooga, TN 37403; **Phone:** 423-778-4830; **Board Cert:** Internal Medicine 2002; Gastroenterology 2003; **Med School:** Univ Miami Sch Med 1987; **Resid:** Internal Medicine, Presbyterian/VA Hosps 1990; **Fellow:** Gastroenterology, Univ Fla 1993; **Fac Appt:** Prof Med, Univ Tenn Coll Med

Liddle, Rodger A MD [Ge] - **Spec Exp:** Pancreatic Disease; Hormone Secreting Tumors; **Hospital:** Duke Univ Hosp, Durham VA Med Ctr; **Address:** Duke Box 3913, 303 Sands Bldg, Durham, NC 27710; **Phone:** 919-681-6380; **Board Cert:** Internal Medicine 1981; Gastroenterology 1983; **Med School:** Vanderbilt Univ 1978; **Resid:** Internal Medicine, UCSF Med Ctr 1981; **Fellow:** Gastroenterology, UCSF Med Ctr 1984; **Fac Appt:** Prof Med, Duke Univ

Lind, Christopher D MD [Ge] - **Spec Exp:** Gastroesophageal Reflux Disease (GERD); Swallowing Disorders; Biliary Disease; Gastrointestinal Motility Disorders; **Hospital:** Vanderbilt Univ Med Ctr (page 75); **Address:** 1660 TVC - Digestive Disease Center Vanderbilt University Medical Center, Nashville, TN 37232-5280; **Phone:** 615-322-0128; **Board Cert:** Internal Medicine 1984; Gastroenterology 1987; **Med School:** Vanderbilt Univ 1981; **Resid:** Internal Medicine, Univ Virginia Hosps 1985; **Fellow:** Gastroenterology, Shands/Univ Florida 1986; Gastroenterology, Univ Virginia Hosps 1988; **Fac Appt:** Prof Med, Vanderbilt Univ

Martin, Paul MD [Ge] - **Spec Exp:** Liver Disease; Hepatitis; Transplant Medicine-Liver; **Hospital:** Univ of Miami Hosp, Jackson Meml Hosp; **Address:** University of Miami, 1475 NW 12th Ave, Miami, FL 33136; **Phone:** 305-243-5787; **Board Cert:** Internal Medicine 1984; Gastroenterology 1987; Transplant Hepatology 2006; **Med School:** Ireland 1978; **Resid:** Internal Medicine, St Vincent's Hosp 1982; Internal Medicine, Univ Alberta 1984; **Fellow:** Gastroenterology, Queen Univ 1986; Hepatology, Natl Inst Hlth 1989; **Fac Appt:** Prof Med, Univ Miami Sch Med

Mertz, Howard R MD [Ge] - **Spec Exp:** Endoscopic Ultrasound; Irritable Bowel Syndrome; Inflammatory Bowel Disease; **Hospital:** Saint Thomas Hosp - Nashville; **Address:** Nashville Gastrointestinal Specialists, 4230 Harding Rd, Ste 309W, Nashville, TN 37205; **Phone:** 615-383-0165; **Board Cert:** Internal Medicine 1989; Gastroenterology 2002; **Med School:** Baylor Coll Med 1986; **Resid:** Internal Medicine, Johns Hopkins Hosp 1989; **Fellow:** Gastroenterology, UCLA Med Ctr 1991; **Fac Appt:** Assoc Clin Prof Med, Vanderbilt Univ

Plevy, Scott MD [Ge] - **Spec Exp:** Inflammatory Bowel Disease; Crohn's Disease; Ulcerative Colitis; **Hospital:** NC Memorial Hosp - UNC; **Address:** 4100 Bioinformatics Bldg, 130 Mason Farm Rd, GI Clinic, CB 7080, Chapel Hill, NC 27599; **Phone:** 919-966-2511; **Board Cert:** Gastroenterology 2007; **Med School:** Columbia P&S 1988; **Resid:** Internal Medicine, Brigham-Womens Hosp 1991; **Fellow:** Gastroenterology, UCLA Med Ctr 1992; Inflammatory Bowel Disease, Cedars Sinai Med Ctr 1994; **Fac Appt:** Assoc Prof Med, Univ NC Sch Med

Porayko, Michael K MD [Ge] - **Spec Exp:** Liver Disease; Transplant Medicine-Liver; Liver Cancer; Hepatitis-Chronic; **Hospital:** Vanderbilt Univ Med Ctr (page 75); **Address:** Digestive Disease Center, 1301 Medical Center Drive, Ste 1660, Nashville, TN 37232; **Phone:** 615-322-0128; **Board Cert:** Internal Medicine 1984; Gastroenterology 1987; Transplant Hepatology 2006; **Med School:** Univ IL Coll Med 1981; **Resid:** Internal Medicine, MSU Affil Hosps 1984; **Fellow:** Gastroenterology, Lahey Clinic/New England Deaconess Hosp 1987; Hepatology, Mayo Clinic 1988; **Fac Appt:** Prof Med, Vanderbilt Univ

Gastroenterology

Raiford, David S MD [Ge] - **Spec Exp:** Autoimmune Liver Disease; Steatohepatitis; Transplant Medicine-Liver; **Hospital:** Vanderbilt Univ Med Ctr (page 75); **Address:** Vanderbilt Digestive Disease Center, 1301 Medical Ctr Drive, Ste 1660, Nashville, TN 37232-5280; **Phone:** 615-322-0128; **Board Cert:** Internal Medicine 1989; Gastroenterology 2011; Transplant Hepatology 2006; **Med School:** Johns Hopkins Univ 1985; **Resid:** Internal Medicine, Johns Hopkins Hosp 1988; **Fellow:** Hepatology, Johns Hopkins Hosp 1991; **Fac Appt:** Prof Med, Vanderbilt Univ

Rao, Satish S C MD/PhD [Ge] - **Spec Exp:** Constipation; Incontinence-Fecal; Chest Pain-Non Cardiac; Gastroesophageal Reflux Disease (GERD); **Hospital:** Med Coll of GA Hosp and Clin (MCG Health Inc); **Address:** Med Coll GA Hosp, 1120 15th St, Augusta, GA 30912; **Phone:** 706-721-9522; **Board Cert:** Gastroenterology 2008; **Med School:** India 1978; **Resid:** Internal Medicine, Sunderland Hosps 1982; Internal Medicine, York Dist Hosp 1984; **Fellow:** Royal Hallamshire Hosp 1986; Gastroenterology, Royal Liverpool Hosp 1988; **Fac Appt:** Prof Med, Med Coll GA

Reuben, Adrian MD [Ge] - **Spec Exp:** Liver Disease; **Hospital:** MUSC Med Ctr; **Address:** MUSC GI & Hepatology, 25 Courtenay Drive, ART 7100A, MC MSC 290, Charleston, SC 29403; **Phone:** 843-792-6901; **Med School:** England, UK 1969; **Resid:** Internal Medicine, National Heart 1972; Gastroenterology, Hammersmith Hosps; **Fellow:** Hepatology, Guy's Hosp; **Fac Appt:** Prof Med, Med Univ SC

Sartor, Ryan B MD [Ge] - **Spec Exp:** Inflammatory Bowel Disease; **Hospital:** NC Memorial Hosp - UNC; **Address:** 130 Mason Farm Rd, Bioinformatics Bldg, CB 7080, Chapel Hill, NC 27599; **Phone:** 919-966-2511; **Board Cert:** Internal Medicine 1978; Gastroenterology 1981; **Med School:** Baylor Coll Med 1974; **Resid:** Internal Medicine, Baylor Affil Hosp 1977; **Fellow:** Gastroenterology, Univ NC Hosps 1981; **Fac Appt:** Prof Med, Univ NC Sch Med

Schiff, Eugene R MD [Ge] - **Spec Exp:** Hepatitis C; Liver Disease; **Hospital:** Univ of Miami Hosp, Jackson Meml Hosp; **Address:** Ctr for Liver Disease, 1475 NW 12th Ave, Miami, FL 33136; **Phone:** 305-243-5787; **Board Cert:** Internal Medicine 1980; Gastroenterology 1972; **Med School:** Columbia P&S 1962; **Resid:** Internal Medicine, Cincinnati Genl Hosp 1964; Internal Medicine, Parkland Meml Hosp 1967; **Fellow:** Gastroenterology, Univ Tex SW Med Ctr 1969; **Fac Appt:** Prof Med, Univ Miami Sch Med

Scudera, Peter L MD [Ge] - **Spec Exp:** Colon & Rectal Cancer Detection; Pancreatic/Biliary Endoscopy (ERCP); Hepatitis-Chronic; **Hospital:** Inova Fair Oaks Hosp, Inova Fairfax Hosp; **Address:** 3700 Joseph Siewick Dr, Ste 308, Fairfax, VA 22033; **Phone:** 703-716-8700; **Board Cert:** Internal Medicine 1987; Gastroenterology 1989; **Med School:** Cornell Univ-Weill Med Coll 1984; **Resid:** Internal Medicine, New York Hosp 1987; **Fellow:** Gastroenterology, New York Hosp-Cornell 1989

Seidner, Douglas L MD [Ge] - **Spec Exp:** Nutrition; Malabsorption Syndrome; Nutrition in Bowel Disorders; Endoscopy; **Hospital:** Vanderbilt Univ Med Ctr (page 75); **Address:** Vanderbilt Ctr Human Nutrition, 1211 21st Ave S, Med Arts Bldg - Ste 514, Nashville, TN 37232; **Phone:** 615-936-1288; **Board Cert:** Internal Medicine 1986; Gastroenterology 2000; **Med School:** SUNY Upstate Med Univ 1983; **Resid:** Internal Medicine, Beth Israel Deaconess Med Ctr 1986; **Fellow:** Nutrition & Metabolism, Beth Israel Deaconess Med Ctr 1987; Gastroenterology, George Washington Univ Med Ctr 1989

Shiffman, Mitchell L MD [Ge] - **Spec Exp:** Transplant Medicine-Liver; Hepatitis C; Liver Disease; Liver Cancer; **Hospital:** Bon Secours St Mary's Hosp, Bon Secours Mary Immaculate Hosp; **Address:** 5855 Bremo Rd, Ste 509, 12720 McManus Blvd, Ste 313, Richmond, VA 23226; **Phone:** 804-977-8920; **Board Cert:** Internal Medicine 1986; Gastroenterology 1989; **Med School:** SUNY Upstate Med Univ 1983; **Resid:** Internal Medicine, Med Coll Va Hosp 1986; **Fellow:** Gastroenterology, Med Coll Va Hosp 1988; **Fac Appt:** Clin Prof Med, Eastern VA Med Sch

Smoot, Duane T MD [Ge] - **Spec Exp:** Colon & Rectal Cancer Detection; Gastrointestinal Cancer; Peptic Acid Disorders; **Hospital:** Nashville Genl Hosp; **Address:** Meharry Med Grp, Dept Internal Med, 1005 TB Todd Jr Blvd, Nashville, TN 37208; **Phone:** 615-327-6277; **Board Cert:** Internal Medicine 1987; Gastroenterology 2003; **Med School:** Howard Univ 1983; **Resid:** Internal Medicine, Univ MD Hosp 1986; **Fellow:** Gastroenterology, Univ MD Hosp 1989; **Fac Appt:** Prof Med, Meharry Med Coll

Toskes, Phillip MD [Ge] - **Spec Exp:** Nutrition; Malabsorption Syndrome; Pancreatic Disease; **Hospital:** Shands at Univ of FL; **Address:** Univ Florida, Div Gastroenterolgy, 1600 SW Archer Rd, HD 602, Box 100214, Gainesville, FL 32610-0214; **Phone:** 352-273-9400; **Board Cert:** Internal Medicine 1970; Gastroenterology 1973; **Med School:** Univ MD Sch Med 1965; **Resid:** Internal Medicine, Univ Maryland Hosp 1968; **Fellow:** Gastroenterology, Hosp Univ Penn 1970; **Fac Appt:** Prof Med, Univ Fla Coll Med

Vaezi, Michael F MD/PhD [Ge] - **Spec Exp:** Gastroesophageal Reflux Disease (GERD); Esophageal Disorders; Achalasia; **Hospital:** Vanderbilt Univ Med Ctr (page 75); **Address:** Vanderbilt Digestive Disease Center, 1301 Medical Ctr Drive, Ste 1660, Nashville, TN 37232; **Phone:** 615-322-0128; **Board Cert:** Internal Medicine 2007; Gastroenterology 2009; **Med School:** Univ Alabama 1992; **Resid:** Internal Medicine, Univ AL-Birmingham Med Ctr 1995; **Fellow:** Gastroenterology, Cleveland Clin 1996; **Fac Appt:** Prof Med, Vanderbilt Univ

Wilcox, C Mel MD [Ge] - **Spec Exp:** Pancreatic & Biliary Disease; Zollinger-Ellison Syndrome; Endoscopic Therapies; Pancreatic/Biliary Endoscopy (ERCP); **Hospital:** Univ of Ala Hosp at Birmingham; **Address:** UAB-Div Gastroenterology, 1808 7th Ave South, BDB 380, Birmingham, AL 35294-0007; **Phone:** 205-975 4958; **Board Cert:** Internal Medicine 1986; Gastroenterology 2007; **Med School:** Med Coll GA 1983; **Resid:** Internal Medicine, Univ Alabama Hosps 1986; **Fellow:** Gastroenterology, UCSF 1990; **Fac Appt:** Prof Med, Univ Alabama

Yanda, Randy J MD [Ge] - **Spec Exp:** Endoscopy; Pancreatic/Biliary Endoscopy (ERCP); Colon Cancer Screening; **Hospital:** Piedmont Hosp; **Address:** Digestive Healthcare of Georgia, 95 Collier Rd NW, Ste 4055, Atlanta, GA 30309; **Phone:** 404-355-3200; **Board Cert:** Internal Medicine 1987; Gastroenterology 2011; **Med School:** Univ Iowa Coll Med 1984; **Resid:** Internal Medicine, UCSF Med Ctr 1987; **Fellow:** Gastroenterology, UCSF 1990

Younossi, Zobair MD [Ge] - **Spec Exp:** Liver Disease; **Hospital:** Inova Fairfax Hosp; **Address:** Ctr for Liver Diseases, Fairfax Hosp, 3300 Gallows Rd, Claude Moore Bldg, Falls Church, VA 22042; **Phone:** 703-776-3182; **Board Cert:** Gastroenterology 2005; Transplant Hepatology 2006; **Med School:** Univ Rochester 1989; **Resid:** Gastroenterology, Scripps Clin & Rsch Fdn 1993; **Fellow:** Hepatology, Scripps Clin & Rsch Fdn 1995; **Fac Appt:** Prof Med, Va Commonwealth Univ Sch Med

Midwest

Bacon, Bruce Raymond MD [Ge] - **Spec Exp:** Hepatitis C; Hepatic Iron Metabolism; Liver Disease; **Hospital:** St. Louis Univ Hosp, SSM St Mary's Hlth Ctr - St Louis; **Address:** 3660 Vista Ave, Ste 308, St Louis, MO 63110-2540; **Phone:** 314-577-6000; **Board Cert:** Internal Medicine 1978; Gastroenterology 2008; Transplant Hepatology 2006; **Med School:** Case West Res Univ 1975; **Resid:** Internal Medicine, Metro Genl Hosp 1979; **Fellow:** Gastroenterology, Metro Genl Hosp 1982; **Fac Appt:** Prof Med, St Louis Univ

Gastroenterology

Barnes, David S MD [Ge] - **Spec Exp:** Biliary Disease; Hepatitis; Liver Disease; Transplant Medicine-Liver; **Hospital:** Cleveland Clin (page 55); **Address:** Cleveland Clinic, Div Gastroenterology, 9500 Euclid Ave, Cleveland, OH 44195; **Phone:** 216-444-1764; **Board Cert:** Internal Medicine 1984; Gastroenterology 1987; Transplant Hepatology 2006; **Med School:** Univ NC Sch Med 1981; **Resid:** Internal Medicine, Univ Mass Med Ctr 1984; **Fellow:** Gastroenterology, Case Western Reserve Univ 1985

Baron, Todd H MD [Ge] - **Spec Exp:** Endoscopy; Pancreatic/Biliary Endoscopy (ERCP); **Hospital:** Mayo Med Ctr & Clin - Rochester; **Address:** Mayo Clin-Div Gastroenterology, 200 First St SW Fl 9, Rochester, MN 55905; **Phone:** 507-284-2174; **Board Cert:** Internal Medicine 1989; Gastroenterology 2003; **Med School:** Univ Fla Coll Med 1986; **Resid:** Internal Medicine, Univ Alabama Med Ctr 1990; **Fellow:** Gastroenterology, Univ Alabama Med Ctr 1993; **Fac Appt:** Assoc Prof Med, Univ Ariz Coll Med

Brown, Kimberly A MD [Ge] - **Spec Exp:** Liver Disease; Transplant Medicine-Liver; Hepatitis C; Liver Cancer; **Hospital:** Henry Ford Hosp; **Address:** Henry Ford Hosp, Dept Gastroenterology, 2799 W Grand Blvd Fl K16, Detroit, MI 48202-2608; **Phone:** 313-916-8865; **Board Cert:** Internal Medicine 1988; Gastroenterology 2002; Transplant Hepatology 2006; **Med School:** Wayne State Univ 1985; **Resid:** Internal Medicine, Univ Michigan Med Ctr 1989; **Fellow:** Gastroenterology, Univ Michigan Med Ctr 1992

Chari, Suresh T MD [Ge] - **Spec Exp:** Pancreatic Disease; **Hospital:** Mayo Med Ctr & Clin - Rochester; **Address:** Mayo Clin-Div Gastroenterology, 200 First St SW Fl 9, Rochester, MN 55905; **Phone:** 507-284-2141; **Board Cert:** Gastroenterology 2009; **Med School:** India 1982; **Resid:** Internal Medicine, Univ Arizona Hlth Sci Ctr 1996; **Fellow:** Gastroenterology, Mayo Clinic 1999; **Fac Appt:** Prof Med, Mayo Med Sch

Chey, William D MD [Ge] - **Spec Exp:** Gastrointestinal Motility Disorders; Gastrointestinal Functional Disorders; Peptic Acid Disorders; Gastroesophageal Reflux Disease (GERD); **Hospital:** Univ of Michigan Hosp; **Address:** 3912 Taubman Center, SPC5362, Ann Arbor, MI 48109-5362; **Phone:** 734-936-4775; **Board Cert:** Internal Medicine 1989; Gastroenterology 2003; **Med School:** Emory Univ 1986; **Resid:** Internal Medicine, Emory Univ Med Ctr 1989; **Fellow:** Gastroenterology, Univ Mich Hosps 1993; **Fac Appt:** Prof Med, Univ Mich Med Sch

Cominelli, Fabio MD/PhD [Ge] - **Spec Exp:** Inflammatory Bowel Disease/Crohn's; Ulcerative Colitis; **Hospital:** Univ Hosps Case Med Ctr (page 74), Louis Stokes Cleveland VA Med Ctr-Wade Park Campus; **Address:** Univ Hosps Case Medical Ctr, Div Gastroenterology, 11100 Euclid Ave, Cleveland, OH 44106-5066; **Phone:** 216-844-7344; **Med School:** Italy 1983; **Resid:** Gastroenterology, Careggi Hosp/Univ Italy 1986; **Fellow:** Gastroenterology, Harbor-UCLA Med Ctr 1989; **Fac Appt:** Prof Med, Case West Res Univ

Crippin, Jeffrey S MD [Ge] - **Spec Exp:** Transplant Medicine-Liver; Liver Disease; Liver Failure; Gastrointestinal Cancer; **Hospital:** Barnes-Jewish Hosp; **Address:** Barnes Jewish Hosp, Div Gastroenterology, 660 S Euclid Ave Campus Box 8124, St Louis, MO 63110; **Phone:** 314-454-8160; **Board Cert:** Internal Medicine 1987; Gastroenterology 2011; Transplant Hepatology 2006; **Med School:** Univ Kansas 1984; **Resid:** Internal Medicine, Kansas Univ Med Ctr 1988; **Fellow:** Gastroenterology, Mayo Clinic 1991; **Fac Appt:** Assoc Prof Med, Washington Univ, St Louis

Di Bisceglie, Adrian M MD [Ge] - **Spec Exp:** Hepatitis C; Hepatitis; Liver Cancer; **Hospital:** St. Louis Univ Hosp; **Address:** St Louis Univ, Div Gastroenterology, 1402 S Grand Blvd, St Louis, MO 63110; **Phone:** 314-577-6000; **Board Cert:** Internal Medicine 2002; Gastroenterology 2002; Transplant Hepatology 2010; **Med School:** South Africa 1977; **Resid:** Internal Medicine, Baragwanath Hosp 1984; **Fellow:** Hepatology, Natl Inst Hlth 1988; **Fac Appt:** Prof Med, St Louis Univ

Early, Dayna S MD [Ge] - **Spec Exp:** Colon & Rectal Cancer Detection; Endoscopic Ultrasound; Endoscopic Therapies; **Hospital:** Barnes-Jewish Hosp, Barnes-Jewish West County Hosp; **Address:** Center for Advanced Medicine, 4921 Parkview Pl Fl 8, Saint Louis, MO 63110; **Phone:** 314-747-2066; **Board Cert:** Internal Medicine 2003; Gastroenterology 2005; **Med School:** Univ MO-Columbia Sch Med 1990; **Resid:** Internal Medicine, Vanderbilt Univ Med Ctr 1993; **Fellow:** Gastroenterology, Vanderbilt Univ Med Ctr 1995; **Fac Appt:** Prof Med, Washington Univ, St Louis

Edmundowicz, Steven A MD [Ge] - **Spec Exp:** Endoscopy; Biliary Disease; Pancreatic Disease; Pancreatic Cancer; **Hospital:** Barnes-Jewish Hosp; **Address:** Washington Univ Sch Med, Div Gastroenterology, 660 S Euclid Ave, Box 8124, St Louis, MO 63110; **Phone:** 314-747-2066; **Board Cert:** Internal Medicine 1986; Gastroenterology 1989; **Med School:** Jefferson Med Coll 1983; **Resid:** Internal Medicine, Barnes Hosp 1986; **Fellow:** Gastroenterology, Barnes Hosp/Wash Univ 1989; **Fac Appt:** Prof Med, Washington Univ, St Louis

Elliott, David MD/PhD [Ge] - **Spec Exp:** Celiac Disease; Inflammatory Bowel Disease/Crohn's; Intestinal Parasites; **Hospital:** Univ Iowa Hosp & Clinics; **Address:** UIHC Ctr for Digestive Diseases, 200 Hawkins Drive, rm 4501 JCP, Iowa City, IA 52242; **Phone:** 319-356-4060; **Board Cert:** Internal Medicine 2003; Gastroenterology 2003; **Med School:** Wayne State Univ 1988; **Resid:** Internal Medicine, Johns Hopkins Hosp 1991; **Fellow:** Gastroenterology, Univ Iowa Hosps 1993; **Fac Appt:** Assoc Prof Med, Univ Iowa Coll Med

Elta, Grace H MD [Ge] - **Spec Exp:** Pancreatic & Biliary Disease; **Hospital:** Univ of Michigan Hosp; **Address:** Univ Michigan Hlth Sys, 1500 E Med Ctr Drive, 3912 Taubman Ctr, Ann Arbor, MI 48109-0362; **Phone:** 734-647-5944; **Board Cert:** Internal Medicine 1980; Gastroenterology 1983; **Med School:** Univ Mich Med Sch 1977; **Resid:** Internal Medicine, New England Med Ctr 1980; **Fellow:** Gastroenterology, New England Med Ctr 1982; **Fac Appt:** Prof Med, Univ Mich Med Sch

Gholam, Pierre M MD [Ge] - **Spec Exp:** Liver Disease; Transplant Medicine-Liver; **Hospital:** Univ Hosps Case Med Ctr (page 74); **Address:** UH Case Medical Center, 11100 Euclid Ave, Cleveland, OH 44106; **Phone:** 216-844-5387; **Board Cert:** Gastroenterology 2002; Transplant Hepatology 2006; Internal Medicine 2011; **Med School:** Lebanon 1996; **Resid:** Internal Medicine, St Lukes-Roosevelt Hosp 1999; **Fellow:** Gastroenterology, St Lukes-Roosevelt Hosp 2002; **Fac Appt:** Asst Prof Med, Case West Res Univ

Goldberg, Michael J MD [Ge] - **Spec Exp:** Colon Cancer; Inflammatory Bowel Disease; Pancreatic & Biliary Disease; Pancreatic/Biliary Endoscopy (ERCP); **Hospital:** Evanston/North Shore Univ Hlth Sys, Glenbrook Hosp-NorthShore Univ Hlth Syst; **Address:** 2650 Ridge Ave, Ste G-208, Evanston, IL 60201; **Phone:** 847-657-1900; **Board Cert:** Internal Medicine 1978; Gastroenterology 1981; **Med School:** Univ IL Coll Med 1975; **Resid:** Internal Medicine, Univ Illinois Hosp 1978; **Fellow:** Gastroenterology, Tufts-New England Med Ctr 1980; **Fac Appt:** Assoc Clin Prof Med, Northwestern Univ

Gostout, Christopher MD [Ge] - **Spec Exp:** Endoscopy; **Hospital:** Mayo Med Ctr & Clin - Rochester; **Address:** Mayo Clin, Div Gastroenterology, 200 First St SW Fl 9, Rochester, MN 55905; **Phone:** 507-284-2141; **Board Cert:** Internal Medicine 1979; Gastroenterology 1981; **Med School:** SUNY Downstate 1976; **Resid:** Internal Medicine, Mayo Clin 1979; **Fellow:** Gastroenterology, Mayo Clin 1981

Hanauer, Stephen B MD [Ge] - **Spec Exp:** Inflammatory Bowel Disease; Crohn's Disease; Ulcerative Colitis; Clinical Trials; **Hospital:** Univ of Chicago Med Ctr; **Address:** University of Chicago Medicine, 5841 S Maryland Ave, Chicago, IL 60637-1426; **Phone:** 773-702-1466; **Board Cert:** Internal Medicine 1980; Gastroenterology 2010; **Med School:** Univ IL Coll Med 1977; **Resid:** Internal Medicine, Univ Chicago Hosps 1980; **Fellow:** Gastroenterology, Univ Chicago Hosps 1982; **Fac Appt:** Prof Med, Univ Chicago-Pritzker Sch Med

Jensen, Donald M MD [Ge] - **Spec Exp:** Transplant Medicine-Liver; Hepatitis C; Liver & Biliary Disease; Liver Cancer; **Hospital:** Univ of Chicago Med Ctr; **Address:** Univ of Chicago, Ctr for Liver Disease, 5841 S Maryland Ave, rm M454, MS 7120, Chicago, IL 60637; **Phone:** 773-702-2300; **Board Cert:** Internal Medicine 1975; Gastroenterology 1981; **Med School:** Univ IL Coll Med 1972; **Resid:** Internal Medicine, Rush Presby St Lukes Hosp 1975; Gastroenterology, Rush Presby St Lukes Hosp 1976; **Fellow:** Gastroenterology, King's Coll Hosp 1978; **Fac Appt:** Prof Med, Univ Chicago-Pritzker Sch Med

Jonnalagadda, Sreenivasa S MD [Ge] - **Spec Exp:** Pancreatic/Biliary Endoscopy(ERCP); Endoscopic Ultrasound; Interventional Endoscopy; **Hospital:** St. Luke's Hosp of Kansas City, St. Luke's South; **Address:** St Luke's Hospital, 4401 Wornall Rd, Kansas City, MO 64111; **Phone:** 913-491-9100; **Board Cert:** Internal Medicine 2005; Gastroenterology 2007; **Med School:** India 1990; **Resid:** Internal Medicine, St. Louis Univ Hlth Sci Ctr 1995; **Fellow:** Gastroenterology, Truman Med Ctr 1997; Advanced Endoscopy, Wellesley Hosp 1998; **Fac Appt:** Prof Med, India

Kahrilas, Peter J MD [Ge] - **Spec Exp:** Esophageal Disorders; Swallowing Disorders; **Hospital:** Northwestern Meml Hosp; **Address:** 675 N St Clair, Fl 17, Ste 250, Chicago, IL 60611; **Phone:** 312-695-5620; **Board Cert:** Internal Medicine 1982; Gastroenterology 1987; **Med School:** Univ Rochester 1979; **Resid:** Internal Medicine, Univ Hosp 1982; **Fellow:** Gastroenterology, Northwestern Meml Hosp 1984; Research, Med Coll Wisconsin 1986; **Fac Appt:** Prof Med, Northwestern Univ

Konicek, Frank J MD [Ge] - **Spec Exp:** Endoscopy; Inflammatory Bowel Disease/Crohn's; Pancreatic Disease; Liver Disease; **Hospital:** Swedish Covenant Hosp, Adv Illinois Masonic Med Ctr; **Address:** 3004 N Ashland Ave, Chicago, IL 60657-3012; **Phone:** 773-871-4600; **Board Cert:** Internal Medicine 1977; Gastroenterology 1975; **Med School:** Loyola Univ-Stritch Sch Med 1963; **Resid:** Internal Medicine, St Francis Hosp 1965; Internal Medicine, Hines VA Hosp 1969; **Fellow:** Gastroenterology, Hines VA Hosp 1971; **Fac Appt:** Clin Prof Med, Loyola Univ-Stritch Sch Med

Kwo, Paul Y MD [Ge] - **Spec Exp:** Hepatitis B & C; Transplant Medicine-Liver; Liver Disease; **Hospital:** IU Health University Hosp; **Address:** 975 W Walnut St, IB327, Indianapolis, IN 46202-5181; **Phone:** 317-274-3090; **Board Cert:** Gastroenterology 2005; Transplant Hepatology 2006; **Med School:** Wayne State Univ 1988; **Resid:** Internal Medicine, Univ Maryland Med Ctr 1991; **Fellow:** Gastroenterology, Mayo Clinic 1995; **Fac Appt:** Prof Med, Indiana Univ

La Russo, Nicholas F MD [Ge] - **Spec Exp:** Transplant Medicine-Liver; Liver & Biliary Disease; **Hospital:** St. Mary's Hosp - Rochester MN (Mayo), Rochester Methodist Hosp; **Address:** Mayo Clinic, Div Gastroenterology, 200 First St SW, Guggenheim Bldg Fl 17 - rm 21D, Rochester, MN 55905; **Phone:** 507-284-1006; **Board Cert:** Internal Medicine 1972; Gastroenterology 1979; **Med School:** NY Med Coll 1969; **Resid:** Internal Medicine, Mayo Clinic 1972; **Fellow:** Gastroenterology, Mayo Clinic 1975; **Fac Appt:** Prof Med, Mayo Med Sch

Lashner, Bret A MD [Ge] - **Spec Exp:** Inflammatory Bowel Disease; **Hospital:** Cleveland Clin (page 55); **Address:** 2049 E 100th St Crile Bldg, Desk A-31, Cleveland, OH 44195; **Phone:** 216-444-6536; **Board Cert:** Internal Medicine 1983; Gastroenterology 1985; **Med School:** NYU Sch Med 1980; **Resid:** Internal Medicine, Temple Univ Hosp 1983; **Fellow:** Gastroenterology, Univ Chicago Hosps 1986; **Fac Appt:** Assoc Prof Med, Case West Res Univ

Levy, Michael J MD [Ge] - **Spec Exp:** Pancreatic/Biliary Endoscopy(ERCP); Endoscopic Ultrasound; **Hospital:** Mayo Med Ctr & Clin - Rochester; **Address:** 200 First St SW, Rochester, MN 55905; **Phone:** 507-284-2141; **Board Cert:** Gastroenterology 2009; **Med School:** Univ SC Sch Med 1991; **Resid:** Internal Medicine, New Hanover Reg Med Ctr 1994; **Fellow:** Gastroenterology, Univ of S Alabama Hlth System 1996; **Fac Appt:** Prof Med, Mayo Med Sch

Loftus Jr, Edward V MD [Ge] - **Spec Exp:** Inflammatory Bowel Disease; Crohn's Disease; Ulcerative Colitis; Microscopic Colitis; **Hospital:** Mayo Med Ctr & Clin - Rochester; **Address:** Mayo Clin, Div Gastroenterology, 200 First St SW Fl 9, Rochester, MN 55905; **Phone:** 507-284-2141; **Board Cert:** Internal Medicine 2003; Gastroenterology 2005; **Med School:** Univ Pennsylvania 1988; **Resid:** Internal Medicine, Temple Univ Hosp 1991; **Fellow:** Gastroenterology, Mayo Clinic 1995; **Fac Appt:** Prof Med, Mayo Med Sch

Lucey, Michael R MD [Ge] - **Spec Exp:** Liver Disease; Transplant Medicine-Liver; **Hospital:** Univ WI Hosp & Clins; **Address:** Univ Wisc Hosps & Clins, 1685 Highland Ave, Centennial Bldg Fl 4, Madison, WI 53705-2281; **Phone:** 608-263-7322; **Board Cert:** Gastroenterology 2011; Transplant Hepatology 2006; **Med School:** Ireland 1980; **Resid:** Gastroenterology, St Bartholomews Hosp/Kings Coll Hosp 1983; Hepatology, Kings Coll Hosp 1985; **Fellow:** Gastroenterology, Univ Michigan Med Ctr 1987; **Fac Appt:** Prof Med, Univ Wisc

Meiselman, Mick S MD [Ge] - **Spec Exp:** Pancreatic & Biliary Disease; Barrett's Esophagus; Endoscopic Ultrasound; Colonoscopy; **Hospital:** Evanston/North Shore Univ Hlth Sys, Glenbrook Hosp-NorthShore Univ Hlth Syst; **Address:** Kellogg Cancer Center, 2650 Ridge Ave Fl 2, Evanston, IL 60201; **Phone:** 847-570-2030; **Board Cert:** Internal Medicine 1982; Gastroenterology 1985; **Med School:** Northwestern Univ 1979; **Resid:** Internal Medicine, Cedars-Sinai/UCLA 1982; **Fellow:** Gastroenterology, UCSF Med Ctr 1984; **Fac Appt:** Asst Clin Prof Med, Univ Chicago-Pritzker Sch Med

Murray, Joseph A MD [Ge] - **Spec Exp:** Celiac Disease; Esophageal Disorders; **Hospital:** Mayo Med Ctr & Clin - Rochester; **Address:** Mayo Clin, Div Gastroenterology, 200 First St SW Fl 9, Rochester, MN 55905; **Phone:** 507-284-2141; **Board Cert:** Internal Medicine 2009; Gastroenterology 2010; **Med School:** Ireland 1983; **Resid:** Internal Medicine, St Laurences Hosp 1986; Gastroenterology, Beaumont Hosp 1988; **Fellow:** Gastroenterology, Univ Iowa Hosps & Clins 1990; **Fac Appt:** Prof Med, Mayo Med Sch

Owyang, Chung MD [Ge] - **Spec Exp:** Gastrointestinal Motility Disorders; Digestive Disorders; **Hospital:** Univ of Michigan Hosp; **Address:** Univ Mich, Div Gastroenterology, 1500 E Med Ctr Dr, Rm 3912 Taubman Ctr, Ann Arbor, MI 48109-0362; **Phone:** 734-647-5944; **Board Cert:** Internal Medicine 1976; Gastroenterology 1981; **Med School:** McGill Univ 1972; **Resid:** Internal Medicine, Montreal Genl Hosp 1975; **Fellow:** Gastroenterology, Mayo Grad Med Sch 1978; **Fac Appt:** Prof Med, Univ Mich Med Sch

Pfau, Patrick R MD [Ge] - **Spec Exp:** Barrett's Esophagus; Endoscopy; **Hospital:** Univ WI Hosp & Clins; **Address:** 451 Junction Rd, Madison, WI 53717; **Phone:** 608-265-8528; **Board Cert:** Gastroenterology 2010; **Med School:** Northwestern Univ-Feinberg Sch Med 1994; **Resid:** Internal Medicine, Hosp of The Univ of Pennsylvania 1997; **Fellow:** Gastroenterology, Hosp of The Univ of Pennsylvania 2000; **Fac Appt:** Assoc Prof Med, Univ Wisc

Reichelderfer, Mark MD [Ge] - **Spec Exp:** Endoscopy; Inflammatory Bowel Disease; **Hospital:** Univ WI Hosp & Clins; **Address:** 1685 Highland Ave, Centennial Bldg Fl 4, Madison, WI 53705-2281; **Phone:** 608-263-4033; **Board Cert:** Internal Medicine 1977; Gastroenterology 1979; **Med School:** Columbia P&S 1974; **Resid:** Internal Medicine, Mary Imogene Bassett Hosp 1977; **Fellow:** Gastroenterology, Univ Wisc Hosps & Clin 1979; **Fac Appt:** Prof Med, Univ Wisc

Rex, Douglas K MD [Ge] - **Spec Exp:** Endoscopy; Endoscopic Ultrasound; Colon & Rectal Cancer Detection; Inflammatory Bowel Disease; **Hospital:** IU Health University Hosp; **Address:** IU Health Univ Hosp, 550 N University Blvd, Ste 4100, Indianapolis, IN 46202; **Phone:** 317-948-9763; **Board Cert:** Internal Medicine 1985; Gastroenterology 1987; **Med School:** Indiana Univ 1980; **Resid:** Internal Medicine, Indiana Univ Med Ctr 1982; Internal Medicine, Indiana Univ Hosp 1985; **Fellow:** Gastroenterology, Indiana Univ Med Ctr 1984; **Fac Appt:** Prof Med, Indiana Univ

Gastroenterology

Schulze, Konrad S MD [Ge] - **Spec Exp:** Gastroesophageal Reflux Disease (GERD); Peptic Acid Disorders; Gastroparesis; **Hospital:** Univ Iowa Hosp & Clinics; **Address:** UIHC Ctr for Digestive Diseases, 200 Hawkins Drive, rm 4501 JCP, Iowa City, IA 52242; **Phone:** 319-356-4060; **Board Cert:** Internal Medicine 1987; Gastroenterology 1975; **Med School:** Germany 1968; **Resid:** Psychiatry, Boston City Hosp 1971; Internal Medicine, Montreal Genl Hosp 1974; **Fellow:** Gastroenterology, Univ Iowa 1977; **Fac Appt:** Prof Med, Univ Iowa Coll Med

Semrad, Carol E MD [Ge] - **Spec Exp:** Celiac Disease; Diarrheal Diseases; Malabsorption Syndrome; Nutrition; **Hospital:** Univ of Chicago Med Ctr; **Address:** 5841 S Maryland Ave, rm S401, MC 4080, Chicago, IL 60637; **Phone:** 773-702-6921; **Board Cert:** Internal Medicine 1985; Gastroenterology 1987; **Med School:** Columbia P&S 1982; **Resid:** Internal Medicine, Columbia-Presby Med Ctr 1985; **Fellow:** Gastroenterology, Columbia-Presby Med Ctr 1986; **Fac Appt:** Assoc Prof Med, Univ Chicago-Pritzker Sch Med

Shaker, Reza MD [Ge] - **Spec Exp:** Swallowing Disorders; Gastrointestinal Motility Disorders; Gastroesophageal Reflux Disease (GERD); Pancreatic/Biliary Endoscopy (ERCP); **Hospital:** Froedtert and Med Ctr of WI, Clement J Zablocki VA Med Ctr; **Address:** Med Coll Wisconsin/Gastroenterology, 9200 W Wisconsin Ave, rm E4510, Milwaukee, WI 53226; **Phone:** 414-955-6840; **Med School:** Iran 1975; **Resid:** Internal Medicine, Kingsbrook Jewish Med Ctr 1985; **Fellow:** Gastroenterology, Med Coll Wisconsin 1988; **Fac Appt:** Prof Med, Univ Wisc

Sherman, Stuart MD [Ge] - **Spec Exp:** Pancreatic & Biliary Disease; Endoscopy; Pancreatic/Biliary Endoscopy (ERCP); **Hospital:** IU Health University Hosp; **Address:** Indiana Univ Hosp, rm 4100, 550 N University Blvd, Indianapolis, IN 46202; **Phone:** 317-944-0925; **Board Cert:** Internal Medicine 1985; Gastroenterology 1989; **Med School:** Washington Univ, St Louis 1982; **Resid:** Internal Medicine, Presby Univ Hosp 1985; **Fellow:** Gastroenterology, UCLA Med Ctr 1989; **Fac Appt:** Prof Med, Indiana Univ

Silverman, William B MD [Ge] - **Spec Exp:** Pancreatic/Biliary Endoscopy (ERCP); Liver Disease; **Hospital:** Univ Iowa Hosp & Clinics; **Address:** UIHC Ctr for Digestive Diseases, 200 Hawkins Drive, rm 4501 JCP, Iowa City, IA 52242; **Phone:** 319-356-4060; **Board Cert:** Internal Medicine 1988; Gastroenterology 2008; **Med School:** Belgium 1984; **Resid:** Internal Medicine, Lutheran General Hosp 1987; **Fellow:** Gastroenterology, Case Western Res Univ 1989; Gastroenterology, Indiana Univ Hosp 1990; **Fac Appt:** Prof Med, Univ Iowa Coll Med

Te, Helen MD [Ge] - **Spec Exp:** Liver Disease; Transplant Medicine-Liver; Hepatitis; **Hospital:** Univ of Chicago Med Ctr; **Address:** 5841 S Maryland Ave, Box MC 7120, Chicago, IL 60637; **Phone:** 773-702-2395; **Board Cert:** Internal Medicine 2006; Gastroenterology 2011; Transplant Hepatology 2006; **Med School:** Philippines 1992; **Resid:** Internal Medicine, Rush Presby Hosp 1996; **Fellow:** Gastroenterology, Univ Chicago Hosp 2000; **Fac Appt:** Assoc Prof Med, Univ Chicago-Pritzker Sch Med

Tremaine, William J MD [Ge] - **Spec Exp:** Inflammatory Bowel Disease/Crohn's; Ulcerative Colitis; Irritable Bowel Syndrome; **Hospital:** Mayo Med Ctr & Clin - Rochester, St. Mary's Hosp - Rochester MN (Mayo); **Address:** Mayo Clin, Div Gastroenterology, 200 First St SW, Mayo E-9, Rochester, MN 55905; **Phone:** 507-284-2468; **Board Cert:** Internal Medicine 1979; Gastroenterology 1981; **Med School:** Univ Miss 1976; **Resid:** Internal Medicine, Mayo Clin 1980; **Fellow:** Gastroenterology, Mayo Clin 1981; **Fac Appt:** Prof Med, Mayo Med Sch

Vargo, John J MD [Ge] - **Spec Exp:** Endoscopy; Barrett's Esophagus; Pancreatic/Biliary Endoscopy (ERCP); Pancreatic Disease; **Hospital:** Cleveland Clin (page 55); **Address:** Cleveland Clinic, 2049 E 100th St Crile Bldg, Desk A-31, Cleveland, OH 44195; **Phone:** 216-445-5012; **Board Cert:** Internal Medicine 1988; **Med School:** Univ Rochester 1985; **Resid:** Internal Medicine, Montefiore Hosp 1988; **Fellow:** Gastroenterology, Cleveland Clinic 2000; **Fac Appt:** Assoc Prof Med, Case West Res Univ

Vege, Santhi S MD [Ge] - **Spec Exp:** Pancreatic Disease; **Hospital:** Mayo Med Ctr & Clin - Rochester; **Address:** Mayo Clin-Div Gastroenterology, 200 First St SW Fl 9, Rochester, MN 55905; **Phone:** 507-284-2141; **Board Cert:** Internal Medicine 2007; **Med School:** India 1975; **Resid:** Internal Medicine, Govt Genl Hosp 1978; Internal Medicine, Mayo Clin 1997; **Fellow:** Gastroenterology, Post Grad Inst 1981; Gastroenterology, Mayo Clin 1998; **Fac Appt:** Prof Med, Mayo Med Sch

Wald, Arnold MD [Ge] - **Spec Exp:** Constipation; Gastrointestinal Motility Disorders; Irritable Bowel Syndrome; Incontinence-Fecal; **Hospital:** Univ WI Hosp & Clins; **Address:** 1685 Highland Ave, Centennial Bldg Fl 4, Madison, WI 53705-2281; **Phone:** 608-263-1995; **Board Cert:** Internal Medicine 1972; Gastroenterology 1975; **Med School:** SUNY Downstate 1968; **Resid:** Internal Medicine, SUNY - Downstate Med Ctr 1971; **Fellow:** Gastroenterology, Johns Hopkins Hosp 1975; **Fac Appt:** Prof Med, Univ Wisc

Waxman, Irving MD [Ge] - **Spec Exp:** Gastrointestinal Cancer; Pancreatic Cancer; Endoscopy; Interventional Endoscopy; **Hospital:** Univ of Chicago Med Ctr; **Address:** 5758 S Maryland Ave, MS MC 9028, Chicago, IL 60637; **Phone:** 773-702-1459; **Board Cert:** Internal Medicine 1988; Gastroenterology 2003; **Med School:** Mexico 1985; **Resid:** Internal Medicine, New Eng Deaconess Hosp 1988; **Fellow:** Gastroenterology, Georgetown Univ Med Ctr 1991; Endoscopy, Univ Academic Med Ctr 1991; **Fac Appt:** Prof Med, Univ Chicago-Pritzker Sch Med

Wiesner, Russell H MD [Ge] - **Spec Exp:** Transplant Medicine-Liver; **Hospital:** Mayo Med Ctr & Clin - Rochester; **Address:** Mayo Clin-Div Gastroenterology, 200 First St SW Fl 9, Rochester, MN 55905; **Phone:** 507-284-2141; **Board Cert:** Internal Medicine 1978; Gastroenterology 1981; **Med School:** Med Coll Wisc 1975; **Resid:** Internal Medicine, Mayo Clin 1978

Wolfe, M Michael MD [Ge] - **Hospital:** MetroHealth Med Ctr; **Address:** MetroHealth Med Ctr, Dept Medicine, 2500 MetroHealth Drive, rm G-575, Cleveland, OH 44109; **Phone:** 216-778-8266; **Board Cert:** Internal Medicine 1979; Gastroenterology 1981; **Med School:** Ohio State Univ 1976; **Resid:** Internal Medicine, Med Coll Penn Hosp 1979; **Fellow:** Gastroenterology, Univ Florida Hosps 1982; **Fac Appt:** Prof Med, Case West Res Univ

Great Plains and Mountains

Burt, Randall W MD [Ge] - **Spec Exp:** Colon Cancer; Colon & Rectal Cancer-Familial Polyposis; **Hospital:** Univ Utah Hlth Care; **Address:** Huntsman Cancer Inst, 2000 Circle of Hope, Salt Lake City, UT 84112; **Phone:** 801-585-3281; **Board Cert:** Internal Medicine 1977; Gastroenterology 1979; **Med School:** Univ Utah 1974; **Resid:** Internal Medicine, Barnes Hosp 1977; **Fellow:** Gastroenterology, Univ Utah Med Ctr 1979; **Fac Appt:** Prof Med, Univ Utah

Fang, John C MD [Ge] - **Spec Exp:** Endoscopy; Esophageal Disorders; Irritable Bowel Syndrome; Barrett's Esophagus; **Hospital:** Univ Utah Hlth Care; **Address:** 50 N Med Drive, Clinic 3, Salt Lake City, UT 84132; **Phone:** 801-581-2215; **Board Cert:** Gastroenterology 2008; **Med School:** Washington Univ, St Louis 1989; **Resid:** Internal Medicine, Temple Univ Hosp 1992; **Fellow:** Gastroenterology, Univ VA Hlth Sci Ctr 1995; **Fac Appt:** Assoc Prof Med, Univ Utah

Hunter, Ellen B MD [Ge] - **Spec Exp:** Hepatitis; **Hospital:** St. Luke's Boise Med Ctr; **Address:** Idaho Gastroenterology Assocs, 425 W Vannock St, Boise, ID 83702; **Phone:** 208-343-6458; **Board Cert:** Internal Medicine 1986; Gastroenterology 1989; **Med School:** Georgetown Univ 1983; **Resid:** Internal Medicine, Vanderbilt Univ Med Ctr 1986; **Fellow:** Gastroenterology, Mayo Clinic 1989

Gastroenterology

Levine, Joel B MD [Ge] - **Spec Exp:** Colon & Rectal Cancer Detection; Colonoscopy; Gastroesophageal Reflux Disease (GERD); **Hospital:** Univ of CO Hosp - Anschutz Inpatient Pav; **Address:** 1635 Aurora Ct, Aurora, CO 80045; **Phone:** 720-848-2777; **Board Cert:** Internal Medicine 1973; Gastroenterology 1977; **Med School:** SUNY Downstate 1969; **Resid:** Internal Medicine, Univ Chicago Hosps 1971; Internal Medicine, Mass Genl Hosp 1974; **Fellow:** Gastroenterology, Mass Genl Hosp 1977; **Fac Appt:** Prof Med, Univ Colorado

Shah, Raj J MD [Ge] - **Spec Exp:** Pancreatic/Biliary Endoscopy(ERCP); **Hospital:** Univ of CO Hosp - Anschutz Inpatient Pav; **Address:** Univ CO Hosp, 1635 Aurora Ct, MS F735, Aurora, CO 80045; **Phone:** 720-848-2775; **Board Cert:** Gastroenterology 2010; **Med School:** NE Ohio Univ 1994; **Resid:** Internal Medicine, Univ of Pittsburgh Med Ctr 1997; **Fellow:** Gastroenterology, Univ Hosps of Cincinnati 2000; Advanced Endoscopy, Maine Med Ctr 2001; **Fac Appt:** Assoc Prof Med, Univ Colorado

Sorrell, Michael MD [Ge] - **Spec Exp:** Transplant Medicine-Liver; Hepatitis; Liver Tumors; Liver Disease; **Hospital:** Nebraska Med Ctr; **Address:** 983285 Nebraska Medical Ctr, Omaha, NE 68198-3285; **Phone:** 402-559-7912; **Board Cert:** Internal Medicine 1972; **Med School:** Univ Nebr Coll Med 1959; **Resid:** Internal Medicine, Univ Nebraska Hosp 1968; Gastroenterology, Univ Nebraska Hosp 1969; **Fellow:** Hepatology, New Jersey Coll Med 1971; **Fac Appt:** Prof Med, Univ Nebr Coll Med

Young, Renee L MD [Ge] - **Spec Exp:** Inflammatory Bowel Disease; Crohn's Disease; **Hospital:** Nebraska Med Ctr; **Address:** Univ Nebraska Medical Ctr, 982000 Nebraska Medical Center, Omaha, NE 68198-2000; **Phone:** 404-559-6209; **Board Cert:** Internal Medicine 1986; Gastroenterology 2011; **Med School:** Univ Nebr Coll Med 1983; **Resid:** Internal Medicine, Univ Nebraska Med Ctr 1986; **Fellow:** Gastroenterology, Univ Nebraska Med Ctr 1990; **Fac Appt:** Assoc Prof Med, Univ Nebr Coll Med

Southwest

Anderson, Karl E MD [Ge] - **Spec Exp:** Porphyria; Liver Disease; **Hospital:** UT Med Br at Galveston(Joh Sealy Hosp); **Address:** 301 University Blvd, Galveston, TX 77555-1109; **Phone:** 409-772-4661; **Board Cert:** Internal Medicine 1972; Gastroenterology 1972; **Med School:** Johns Hopkins Univ 1965; **Resid:** Internal Medicine, Vanderbilt Univ Hosp 1967; Internal Medicine, New York Hosp 1968; **Fellow:** Gastroenterology, New York Hosp-Cornell 1970; **Fac Appt:** Prof Med, Univ Tex Med Br, Galveston

Balart Jr, Luis A MD [Ge] - **Spec Exp:** Hepatitis C; Liver Disease; **Hospital:** Tulane Med Ctr; **Address:** Tulane Gastroenterology, 1430 Tulane Ave, Ste SL35, New Orleans, LA 70112; **Phone:** 504-988-5800; **Board Cert:** Internal Medicine 1976; Gastroenterology 1981; **Med School:** Cuba 1973; **Resid:** Internal Medicine, Naval Regl Med Ctr 1976; **Fellow:** Gastroenterology, Ochsner Medical Fdn 1981; Hepatology, Ranchos Amigos Hosp-USC 1982; **Fac Appt:** Prof Med, Tulane Univ

Boland, Clement R MD [Ge] - **Spec Exp:** Colon & Rectal Cancer Detection; Hereditary Cancer; Cancer Genetics; **Hospital:** Baylor Univ Medical Ctr-Dallas; **Address:** GI Cancer Rsch Lab H-250, 3500 Gaston Ave, Ste 250, Dallas, TX 75246; **Phone:** 214-820-2692; **Board Cert:** Internal Medicine 1978; Gastroenterology 1981; **Med School:** Yale Univ 1973; **Resid:** Internal Medicine, USPHS Hosp 1978; **Fellow:** Gastroenterology, UCSF Med Ctr 1981; **Fac Appt:** Clin Prof Med, Univ Tex SW, Dallas

Boyer, Thomas D MD [Ge] - **Spec Exp:** Liver Disease; Hepatitis; Transplant Medicine-Liver; **Hospital:** Univ Arizona Med Ctr-Univ Campus; **Address:** Univ Medical Ctr, Div Gastroenterology, 1501 N Campbell Ave, rm 6309c, PO Box 245136, Tucson, AZ 85724; **Phone:** 520-626-5952; **Board Cert:** Internal Medicine 1975; Gastroenterology 1977; Transplant Hepatology 2008; **Med School:** USC-Keck School of Medicine 1969; **Resid:** Internal Medicine, LAC-USC Med Ctr 1974; **Fellow:** Hepatology, USC 1976; **Fac Appt:** Prof Med, Univ Ariz Coll Med

Bresalier, Robert MD [Ge] - **Spec Exp:** Gastrointestinal Cancer; Peptic Acid Disorders; **Hospital:** UT MD Anderson Cancer Ctr; **Address:** MD Anderson Canc Ctr, GI Med & Nutrition, 1515 Holcombe Blvd - Unit 1466, Houston, TX 77030; **Phone:** 713-745-4340; **Board Cert:** Internal Medicine 1981; Gastroenterology 1983; **Med School:** Univ Chicago-Pritzker Sch Med 1978; **Resid:** Internal Medicine, Barnes Hosp-Washington Univ 1981; **Fellow:** Gastroenterology, UCSF Med Ctr 1983; **Fac Appt:** Prof Med, Univ Tex, Houston

Bulat, Robert S MD [Ge] - **Hospital:** Tulane Med Ctr; **Address:** Tulane Univ Med Ctr, 1430 Tulane Ave, Ste SL35, New Orleans, LA 70112; **Phone:** 504-988-5800; **Board Cert:** Gastroenterology 2010; **Med School:** McMaster Univ 1990; **Resid:** Internal Medicine, Univ Toronto Med Ctr 1993; **Fellow:** Gastroenterology, McMaster Univ 1995; Gastroenterology, McMaster Univ 1997; **Fac Appt:** Prof Med, Tulane Univ

Cunningham, John T MD [Ge] - **Spec Exp:** Pancreatic Cancer; Biliary Disease; Pancreatic/Biliary Endoscopy (ERCP); **Hospital:** Univ Arizona Med Ctr-Univ Campus; **Address:** Univ Medical Ctr, Div Gastroenterology, 1501 N Campbell Ave, rm 6402, PO Box 245028, Tucson, AZ 85724-5028; **Phone:** 520-626-8659; **Board Cert:** Internal Medicine 1975; Gastroenterology 1977; **Med School:** Med Coll VA 1970; **Resid:** Internal Medicine, Med Univ S Carolina 1975; **Fellow:** Gastroenterology, Med Univ S Carolina 1977; **Fac Appt:** Prof Med, Univ Ariz Coll Med

Das, Ananya MD [Ge] - **Spec Exp:** Endoscopy; Endoscopic Ultrasound; Pancreatic/Biliary Endoscopy (ERCP); Gastrointestinal Cancer; **Hospital:** Mercy Gilbert Med Ctr; **Address:** Arizona Ctr for Digestive Health, 2680 S Val Vista Drive Bldg 4 - Ste 116, Gilbert, AZ 85295; **Phone:** 480-507-5678; **Board Cert:** Gastroenterology 2008; **Med School:** India 1987; **Resid:** Internal Medicine, SUNY Downstate Med Ctr 1996; **Fellow:** Gastroenterology, Cleveland Clinic 1998; Endoscopy, Cleveland Clinic 2000; **Fac Appt:** Prof Med, Mayo Med Sch

Davis, Gary L MD [Ge] - **Spec Exp:** Liver Disease; Hepatitis; Transplant Medicine-Liver; **Hospital:** Baylor Univ Medical Ctr-Dallas; **Address:** 3410 Worth St Fl 8 - Ste 860, Transplant Services Dept, Dallas, TX 75246; **Phone:** 214-820-8500; **Board Cert:** Internal Medicine 1979; Gastroenterology 1983; **Med School:** Univ Minn 1976; **Resid:** Internal Medicine, Mayo Clinic 1979; **Fellow:** Gastroenterology, Mayo Clinic 1981; Hepatology, Natl Inst Hlth 1984; **Fac Appt:** Prof Med, Baylor Coll Med

Faigel, Douglas O MD [Ge] - **Spec Exp:** Pancreatic/Biliary Endoscopy (ERCP); Endoscopic Ultrasound; Pancreatic & Biliary Disease; **Hospital:** Mayo Clinic - Scottsdale; **Address:** Mayo Clinic-Gastroenterology, 13400 E Shea Blvd, Scottsdale, AZ 85259; **Phone:** 480-301-6990; **Board Cert:** Internal Medicine 2003; Gastroenterology 2005; **Med School:** Univ Pennsylvania 1990; **Resid:** Internal Medicine, UCSF Med Ctr 1993; **Fellow:** Gastroenterology, Univ Penn Hosp 1995; **Fac Appt:** Assoc Prof Med, Mayo Med Sch

Fallon, Michael B MD [Ge] - **Spec Exp:** Liver Disease; Hepatitis C; **Hospital:** Meml Hermann Hosp - Texas Med Ctr; **Address:** Univ TX Professional Bldg, 6411 Fannin, Ste J400, Houston, TX 77030; **Phone:** 713-704-6800; **Board Cert:** Internal Medicine 1988; Gastroenterology 2011; Transplant Hepatology 2008; **Med School:** Univ VA Sch Med 1984; **Resid:** Internal Medicine, Yale-New Haven Hosp 1988; **Fellow:** Gastroenterology, Yale-New Haven Hosp 1990; **Fac Appt:** Assoc Prof Med, Univ Tex, Houston

Gastroenterology

Fleischer, David E MD [Ge] - **Spec Exp:** Esophageal Cancer; Barrett's Esophagus; **Hospital:** Mayo Clinic - Scottsdale; **Address:** Mayo Clinic-Gastroenterology, 13400 E Shea Blvd, Scottsdale, AZ 85259; **Phone:** 480-301-6990; **Board Cert:** Internal Medicine 1975; Gastroenterology 1977; **Med School:** Vanderbilt Univ 1970; **Resid:** Internal Medicine, Metro Genl Hosp 1975; **Fellow:** Gastroenterology, LA Co Harbor-UCLA Med Ctr 1977; **Fac Appt:** Prof Med, Mayo Med Sch

Galati, Joseph S MD [Ge] - **Spec Exp:** Liver Disease; Transplant Medicine-Liver; Hepatitis C; Liver Cancer; **Hospital:** Methodist Hosp - Houston, St. Luke's Episcopal Hosp-Houston; **Address:** 6624 Fannin St, Ste 1990, Houston, TX 77030; **Phone:** 713-794-0700; **Board Cert:** Gastroenterology 2005; **Med School:** Grenada 1987; **Resid:** Internal Medicine, Kings Co Hosp 1991; **Fellow:** Gastroenterology, Univ Nebraska Med Ctr 1994; Transplant Hepatology, Univ Nebraska Med Ctr 1994; **Fac Appt:** Asst Prof Med, Univ Tex, Houston

Glombicki, Alan P MD [Ge] - **Spec Exp:** Hepatitis; Transplant Medicine-Liver; Digestive Disorders; **Hospital:** Methodist Hosp - Houston, Meml Hermann Hosp - Texas Med Ctr; **Address:** 6550 Fannin St, Ste 2301, Smith Tower, Houston, TX 77030; **Phone:** 713-796-8627; **Board Cert:** Internal Medicine 1986; Gastroenterology 1987; **Med School:** Univ IL Coll Med 1981; **Resid:** Internal Medicine, Baylor Affil Hosp 1984; Hepatology, Baylor Affil HOsp 1987; **Fellow:** Gastroenterology, Baylor Coll Med 1986; **Fac Appt:** Assoc Prof Med, Univ Tex, Houston

Leighton, Jonathan A MD [Ge] - **Spec Exp:** Capsule Endoscopy; Inflammatory Bowel Disease; Ulcerative Colitis; **Hospital:** Mayo Clinic - Scottsdale; **Address:** Mayo Clinic-Gatroenterology Dept, 13400 E Shea Blvd, Scottsdale, AZ 85259; **Phone:** 480-301-6990; **Board Cert:** Internal Medicine 1984; Gastroenterology 2011; **Med School:** Univ Ariz Coll Med 1981; **Resid:** Internal Medicine, UT Affil Hosp 1984; **Fellow:** Gastroenterology & Nutrition, UT San Antonio 1987; Research, UT San Antonio 1991; **Fac Appt:** Assoc Prof Med, Mayo Med Sch

Poordad, Fred F MD [Ge] - **Spec Exp:** Liver Disease; Hepatitis B & C; Transplant Medicine-Liver; **Hospital:** Camden Genl Hosp; **Address:** 607 Camden, San Antonio, TX 78215; **Phone:** 210-253-3422; **Board Cert:** Gastroenterology 2005; Transplant Hepatology 2006; **Med School:** Canada 1990; **Resid:** Internal Medicine, St Thomas Med Ctr/Ohio State Univ Med Ctr 1993; **Fellow:** Gastroenterology, Univ S Carolina Med Ctr 1995; Hepatology, Johns Hopkins Hosp 2005; **Fac Appt:** Assoc Prof Med, UCLA-David Geffen Sch Med

Raju, Gottumukkala S MD [Ge] - **Spec Exp:** Colon Cancer; **Hospital:** UT MD Anderson Cancer Ctr; **Address:** UT MD Anderson Cancer Center, 1515 Holcombe Blvd, Houston, TX 77030; **Phone:** 713-792-2330; **Board Cert:** Gastroenterology 2007; **Med School:** India 1986; **Resid:** Internal Medicine, Cleveland Clin 1995; **Fellow:** Gastroenterology, Univ Iowa Hosp & Clin 1997; Endoscopy, Beth Israel Deaconess Hosp 1998

Schiller, Lawrence R MD [Ge] - **Spec Exp:** Diarrheal Diseases; Gastrointestinal Functional Disorders; Gastrointestinal Motility Disorders; **Hospital:** Baylor Univ Medical Ctr-Dallas; **Address:** Digestive Health Associates of Texas, 712 N Washington Ave, Ste 200, Dallas, TX 75246; **Phone:** 214-545-3990; **Board Cert:** Internal Medicine 1976; Gastroenterology 1981; **Med School:** Jefferson Med Coll 1972; **Resid:** Internal Medicine, Temple Univ Hosp 1976; **Fellow:** Gastroenterology, Univ Texas Hlth Sci Ctr 1980; **Fac Appt:** Clin Prof Med, Univ Tex SW, Dallas

Speeg, Kermit V MD/PhD [Ge] - **Spec Exp:** Transplant Medicine-Liver; **Hospital:** Univ Hlth Syst-San Antonio; **Address:** Dept Gastroenterology, 7703 Floyd Curl Drive, MC 7878, San Antonio, TX 78229-3900; **Phone:** 210-567-4879; **Board Cert:** Internal Medicine 1976; **Med School:** Univ Tex SW, Dallas 1972; **Resid:** Internal Medicine, Vanderbilt Univ Hosp 1974; **Fellow:** Gastroenterology, Vanderbilt Univ Hosp 1977; **Fac Appt:** Prof Med, Univ Tex, San Antonio

Stump, David L MD [Ge] - **Hospital:** Methodist Hosp-San Antonio; **Address:** Gastroenterology Clinic Of San Antonio, 8550 Datapoint Drive, Ste LL100, San Antonio, TX 78229-3436; **Phone:** 210-615-8308; **Board Cert:** Internal Medicine 1983; Gastroenterology 1985; **Med School:** Indiana Univ 1980; **Resid:** Internal Medicine, Indiana Univ Med Ctr 1983; **Fellow:** Gastroenterology, UT San Antonio 1985

Vierling, John M MD [Ge] - **Spec Exp:** Liver Disease; Transplant Medicine-Liver; Autoimmune Liver Disease; Hepatitis B & C; **Hospital:** St. Luke's Episcopal Hosp-Houston; **Address:** Baylor Clinic, 6620 Main St, Ste 1475, Houston, TX 77030; **Phone:** 713-798-8355; **Board Cert:** Internal Medicine 1975; Gastroenterology 1979; Transplant Hepatology 2006; **Med School:** Stanford Univ 1972; **Resid:** Internal Medicine, Strong Meml Hosp 1974; Hepatology, Natl Inst Hlth 1977; **Fellow:** Gastroenterology, UCSF 1978; **Fac Appt:** Prof Med, Baylor Coll Med

West Coast and Pacific

Cello, John P MD [Ge] - **Spec Exp:** Endoscopy; Colonoscopy; Capsule Endoscopy; Pancreatic/Biliary Endoscopy (ERCP); **Hospital:** San Francisco Genl Hosp, UCSF Med Ctr; **Address:** San Francisco Genl Hosp-UCSF, 1001 Potrero Ave, Ste NH3D, San Francisco, CA 94110; **Phone:** 415-206-8822; **Board Cert:** Internal Medicine 1972; Gastroenterology 1977; **Med School:** Harvard Med Sch 1969; **Resid:** Internal Medicine, Peter Bent Brigham Hosp 1972; **Fellow:** Gastroenterology, UCSF Med Ctr 1977; **Fac Appt:** Prof Med, UCSF

Chang, Kenneth J MD [Ge] - **Spec Exp:** Gastrointestinal Cancer; Endoscopic Ultrasound; Interventional Endoscopy; Barrett's Esophagus; **Hospital:** UC Irvine Med Ctr; **Address:** Comprehensive Digestive Disease Ctr, 101 The City Drive South, Bldg 22C, Rt 99 - rm 106, Orange, CA 92868; **Phone:** 714-456-6187; **Board Cert:** Internal Medicine 1988; Gastroenterology 2011; **Med School:** Brown Univ 1985; **Resid:** Internal Medicine, Rhode Island Hosp 1988; **Fellow:** Gastroenterology, UC Irvine Med Ctr 1990; **Fac Appt:** Clin Prof Med, UC Irvine

Dea, Stanley MD [Ge] - **Spec Exp:** Endoscopy; Pancreatic/Biliary Endoscopy (ERCP); Capsule Endoscopy; Endoscopic Ultrasound; **Hospital:** Olive View-UCLA Med Ctr, VA Greater Los Angeles Hthecare Sys; **Address:** 14445 Olive View Drive, rm 2B-182, Sylmar, CA 91342; **Phone:** 818-364-3205; **Board Cert:** Internal Medicine 2004; Gastroenterology 2008; **Med School:** Univ Chicago-Pritzker Sch Med 1990; **Resid:** Internal Medicine, Harbor-UCLA Med Ctr 1993; **Fellow:** Gastroenterology, UCLA Med Ctr 1995; **Fac Appt:** Clin Prof Med, UCLA-David Geffen Sch Med

Eisen, Glenn MD [Ge] - **Spec Exp:** Endoscopy; Liver Disease; Barrett's Esophagus; **Hospital:** Providence St Vincent Med Ctr; **Address:** Peterkort Med Office-West Hills, 9701 SW Barnes Rd, Ste 300 & 310, Portland, OR 97225; **Phone:** 503-297-8081; **Board Cert:** Internal Medicine 2002; Gastroenterology 2006; **Med School:** Albert Einstein Coll Med 1987; **Resid:** Internal Medicine, Mt Sinai Med Ctr 1991; **Fellow:** Gastroenterology, Duke Univ Med Ctr 1996; Epidemiology, Univ NC Hosp 1992; **Fac Appt:** Clin Prof Med, Oregon Hlth & Sci Univ

Ellis, Jonathan C MD [Ge] - **Hospital:** Cedars-Sinai Med Ctr; **Address:** 9090 Wilshire Blvd, Ste 101, Beverly Hills, CA 90211; **Phone:** 310-550-0400; **Board Cert:** Internal Medicine 1985; Gastroenterology 1989; **Med School:** Stanford Univ 1982; **Resid:** Internal Medicine, Cedars Sinai Med Ctr 1986; **Fellow:** Gastroenterology, UCLA 1988; **Fac Appt:** Assoc Prof Med, UCLA

Feldman, Edward Jon MD [Ge] - **Spec Exp:** Inflammatory Bowel Disease; Colonoscopy; Irritable Bowel Syndrome; Gastroesophageal Reflux Disease (GERD); **Hospital:** Cedars-Sinai Med Ctr; **Address:** 8635 W 3rd St, Ste 960W, Los Angeles, CA 90048-6101; **Phone:** 310-652-8031; **Board Cert:** Internal Medicine 1972; Gastroenterology 1977; **Med School:** Indiana Univ 1969; **Resid:** Internal Medicine, LA Co Habor Genl Hosp 1972; Internal Medicine, Hammersmith Hosp 1973; **Fellow:** Gastroenterology, UCLA Med Ctr 1976; **Fac Appt:** Clin Prof Med, UCLA

Gastroenterology

Fennerty, M Brian MD [Ge] - **Spec Exp:** Gastroesophageal Reflux Disease (GERD); **Hospital:** OR Hlth & Sci Univ; **Address:** Digestive Hlth, Ctr for Hlth & Healing, 3303 SW Bond Ave, MC CH6D, Portland, OR 97239; **Phone:** 503-494-4373; **Board Cert:** Internal Medicine 1984; Gastroenterology 2008; **Med School:** Creighton Univ 1980; **Resid:** Internal Medicine, Naval Hospital 1984; **Fellow:** Gastroenterology, Arizona Hlth Sci Ctr 1989; **Fac Appt:** Prof Med, Oregon Hlth & Sci Univ

Gerson, Lauren B MD [Ge] - **Spec Exp:** Gastroesophageal Reflux Disease (GERD); Barrett's Esophagus; Esophageal Disorders; Capsule Endoscopy; **Hospital:** Stanford Univ Hosp & Clinics; **Address:** Stanford Univ Div Gastroenterology, 450 Broadway St, Pavilion C Fl 4, MC 6341, Redwood City, CA 94063; **Phone:** 650-736-5555; **Board Cert:** Gastroenterology 2002; **Med School:** SUNY Buffalo 1990; **Resid:** Internal Medicine, California Pacific Med Ctr 1993; **Fellow:** Gastroenterology, Stanford Univ Med Ctr 1995; **Fac Appt:** Assoc Prof Med, Stanford Univ

Gish, Robert MD [Ge] - **Spec Exp:** Liver Cancer; Transplant Medicine-Liver; Hepatitis; Clinical Trials; **Hospital:** UCSD Med Ctr; **Address:** UCSD Medical Center, 200 W Arbor Drive, Ste 342, MC 8413, San Diego, CA 92103; **Phone:** 619-543-5415; **Board Cert:** Internal Medicine 1984; Gastroenterology 1987; Transplant Hepatology 2006; **Med School:** Univ Kansas 1980; **Resid:** Internal Medicine, UCSD Med Ctr 1983; **Fellow:** Gastroenterology, UCLA Med Ctr 1988; **Fac Appt:** Clin Prof Med, UCSD

Han, Steven-Huy MD [Ge] - **Spec Exp:** Transplant Medicine-Liver; Hepatitis B & C; Liver Disease; **Hospital:** UCLA Ronald Reagan Med Ctr; **Address:** UCLA Medical Ctr, 200 UCLA Medical Plaza, Ste 214, Los Angeles, CA 90095; **Phone:** 310-794-7788; **Board Cert:** Gastroenterology 2008; Transplant Hepatology 2006; **Med School:** Albany Med Coll 1990; **Resid:** Internal Medicine, Santa Clara Valley Med Ctr 1993; **Fellow:** Hepatology, USC 1996; Gastroenterology, UCLA 1998; **Fac Appt:** Assoc Prof Med, UCLA

Kimmey, Michael B MD [Ge] - **Spec Exp:** Pancreatic/Biliary Endoscopy (ERCP); Endoscopy; Endoscopic Ultrasound; Inflammatory Bowel Disease; **Hospital:** St. Joseph Med Ctr - Tacoma, St. Anthony Hosp -Gig Harbor; **Address:** Tacoma Digestive Disease Ctr, 1112 6th Ave, Ste 200, Tacoma, WA 98405; **Phone:** 253-272-8664; **Board Cert:** Internal Medicine 1982; Gastroenterology 1987; **Med School:** Washington Univ, St Louis 1979; **Resid:** Internal Medicine, Univ Wash Med Ctr 1982; **Fellow:** Gastroenterology, Univ Wash 1987; **Fac Appt:** Clin Prof Med, Univ Wash

Kozarek, Richard A MD [Ge] - **Spec Exp:** Pancreatic/Biliary Endoscopy (ERCP); Inflammatory Bowel Disease; Pancreatic Disease; **Hospital:** Virginia Mason Med Ctr; **Address:** 1100 9th Ave, PO Box 24163, Seattle, WA 98101-2756; **Phone:** 206-223-6934; **Board Cert:** Internal Medicine 1977; Gastroenterology 1979; **Med School:** Univ Wisc 1973; **Resid:** Internal Medicine, Good Samaritan Hosp 1976; **Fellow:** Gastroenterology, Univ Arizona/ VA Hosp 1978; **Fac Appt:** Clin Prof Med, Univ Wash

Loomba, Rohit MD [Ge] - **Spec Exp:** Liver Disease; **Hospital:** UCSD Med Ctr; **Address:** 9444 Medical Ctr Dr ECOB Bldg, MC 0956, La Jolla, CA 92023; **Phone:** 858-534-2757; **Board Cert:** Internal Medicine 2004; Gastroenterology 2009; **Med School:** India 1999; **Resid:** Internal Medicine, St Luke's Hosp 2004; **Fellow:** Hepatology, Natl Inst Health 2007; Gastroenterology, UCSD Med Ctr 2009; **Fac Appt:** Asst Prof Med, UCSD

Mittal, Ravinder MD [Ge] - **Spec Exp:** Gastrointestinal Motility Disorders; Esophageal Disorders; Swallowing Disorders; **Hospital:** UCSD Med Ctr; **Address:** 9350 Campus Point Drive, MC 7788, La Jolla, CA 92037; **Phone:** 619-543-6834; **Board Cert:** Internal Medicine 1982; Gastroenterology 1985; **Med School:** India 1978; **Resid:** Internal Medicine, Lincoln Hosp 1982; **Fellow:** Gastroenterology, New Haven Hosp 1985; **Fac Appt:** Prof Med, UCSD

Ostroff, James W MD [Ge] - **Spec Exp:** Pancreatic/Biliary Endoscopy (ERCP); Pancreatic Disease; Colonoscopy; **Hospital:** UCSF Med Ctr, UCSF - Mt Zion Med Ctr; **Address:** 350 Parnassus Ave, Ste 410, San Francisco, CA 94117-3608; **Phone:** 415-502-2112; **Board Cert:** Internal Medicine 1980; Gastroenterology 1983; **Med School:** Cornell Univ-Weill Med Coll 1977; **Resid:** Internal Medicine, NY Hosp-Cornell Med Ctr 1980; **Fellow:** Gastroenterology, UCSF Hosps 1982; **Fac Appt:** Prof Med, UCSF

Petrini, John L MD [Ge] - **Spec Exp:** Endoscopy; **Hospital:** Santa Barbara Cottage Hosp; **Address:** 317 W Pueblo St, Santa Barbara, CA 93105; **Phone:** 805-681-7500; **Board Cert:** Internal Medicine 1980; Gastroenterology 1983; **Med School:** UCSF 1977; **Resid:** Internal Medicine, Emory Univ Affil Hosps 1980; **Fellow:** Gastroenterology, UCLA-Wadsworth VA Hosp 1982; **Fac Appt:** Assoc Clin Prof Med, USC-Keck School of Medicine

Roth, Bennett E MD [Ge] - **Spec Exp:** Gastroesophageal Reflux Disease (GERD); Inflammatory Bowel Disease/Crohn's; Irritable Bowel Syndrome; Esophageal Disorders; **Hospital:** UCLA Ronald Reagan Med Ctr; **Address:** 200 UCLA Med Plaza, Ste 365A, Los Angeles, CA 90095; **Phone:** 310-825-1597; **Board Cert:** Internal Medicine 1972; Gastroenterology 1975; **Med School:** Hahnemann Univ 1968; **Resid:** Internal Medicine, Hosp Univ Penn 1971; **Fellow:** Gastroenterology, UCLA Med Ctr 1974; **Fac Appt:** Prof Med, UCLA

Sandborn, William J MD [Ge] - **Spec Exp:** Inflammatory Bowel Disease/Crohn's; Ulcerative Colitis; Crohn's Disease; **Hospital:** UCSD Med Ctr; **Address:** Perlman Med Office, 9500 Gilman Drive, La Jolla, CA 92093-0063; **Phone:** 858-534-3320; **Board Cert:** Gastroenterology 2003; **Med School:** Loma Linda Univ 1987; **Resid:** Internal Medicine, Loma Linda Univ 1990; **Fellow:** Gastroenterology, Mayo Clinic 1993; **Fac Appt:** Assoc Prof Med, Mayo Med Sch

Savides, Thomas MD [Ge] - **Spec Exp:** Gastrointestinal Cancer; Barrett's Esophagus; Colonoscopy; Endoscopic Ultrasound; **Hospital:** UCSD Med Ctr; **Address:** 9350 Campus Point Drive, San Diego, CA 92103-8413; **Phone:** 619-543-2347; **Board Cert:** Internal Medicine 2003; Gastroenterology 2003; **Med School:** UCSD 1987; **Resid:** Internal Medicine, UCLA Med Ctr 1990; **Fellow:** Gastroenterology, UCLA Med Ctr 1993; Gastroenterology, Indiana Univ Med Ctr 1994; **Fac Appt:** Asst Clin Prof Med, UCSD

Surawicz, Christina MD [Ge] - **Spec Exp:** Clostridium Difficile Disease; Infectious Diarrhea; **Hospital:** Harborview Med Ctr; **Address:** 325 9th Ave, Box 359866, Seattle, WA 98104-2420; **Phone:** 206-744-7070; **Board Cert:** Internal Medicine 1976; Gastroenterology 1979; **Med School:** Univ KY Coll Med 1973; **Resid:** Internal Medicine, Univ Washington Med Ctr 1976; **Fellow:** Gastroenterology, Univ Washington Med Ctr 1979; **Fac Appt:** Prof Med, Univ Wash

Targan, Stephan R MD [Ge] - **Spec Exp:** Inflammatory Bowel Disease; Crohn's Disease; **Hospital:** Cedars-Sinai Med Ctr; **Address:** Cedars-Sinai IBD Ctr, 8730 Alden Drive, Ste 204, Los Angeles, CA 90048; **Phone:** 310-423-4100; **Board Cert:** Internal Medicine 1974; Infectious Disease 1976; Gastroenterology 1979; **Med School:** Johns Hopkins Univ 1971; **Resid:** Internal Medicine, Harbor-UCLA Med Ctr 1976; **Fellow:** Infectious Disease, Harbor-UCLA Med Ctr 1976; Gastroenterology, UCLA Med Ctr 1978; **Fac Appt:** Prof Med, UCLA

Zaman, Atif MD [Ge] - **Spec Exp:** Liver Disease; Hypertension; Hepatitis; **Hospital:** OR Hlth & Sci Univ; **Address:** OHSU, MC CH6D, 3303 SW Bond Ave, Portland, OR 97201; **Phone:** 503-494-4373; **Board Cert:** Gastroenterology 2008; **Med School:** Tufts Univ 1991; **Resid:** Internal Medicine, Baylor Coll Affil Hosp 1994; **Fellow:** Gastroenterology, Oregon Hlth Science Univ 1998; **Fac Appt:** Prof Med, Oregon Hlth & Sci Univ

Cleveland Clinic

Every life deserves world class care.

Cleveland Clinic
Digestive Disease Institute
9500 Euclid Avenue
Cleveland, OH 44195

Gastroenterology

Cleveland Clinic's Digestive Disease Institute (DDI) is one of the largest digestive programs in the country and is ranked No. 2 in the nation by *U.S. News & World Report*. DDI was the first to fully integrate its departments of Colorectal Surgery, Gastroenterology & Hepatology, General Surgery, and Nutrition. Combining these disciplines in one location facilitates unprecedented patient care, multidisciplinary education and collaborative research. In 2011, DDI physicians performed over 16,000 surgical cases and close to 51,000 endoscopic cases. Transplant surgeons completed over 150 digestive disease-related organ transplants, including liver, pancreas and intestinal transplantation, achieving outstanding outcomes.

Highlights of our Department of Gastroenterology:

- We have a state-of-the-art endoscopy facility designed to improve patient satisfaction while emphasizing both safety and quality.
- Our advanced endoscopy team performs a range of endoscopic procedures annually, including endoscopic retrograde cholangiopancreatography, endoscopic ultrasound and percutaneous endoscopic gastrostomy.
- Our Center for Swallowing & Esophageal Disorders offers comprehensive treatment for swallowing and esophageal disorders.
- DDI developed the world's first Pouchitis Clinic.
- A new section of Comprehensive Gastroenterology focuses on typically underserved disorders such as small bowel diseases, including celiac disease.
- Our liver specialists have the experience and expertise to accurately diagnose and treat all forms of liver disease, including viral hepatitis, fatty liver, alcoholic liver disease, autoimmune liver diseases, genetic liver diseases and liver cancer.

Offering Same-Day Appointments
Call 800.274.2009.

Treatment Guides
Cleveland Clinic has developed comprehensive treatment guides for many diseases and conditions. To download our free treatment guides, visit clevelandclinic.org/treatmentguides.

Online Medical Second Opinion
Call 216.444.3223 or 800.223.2273 ext. 43223 or email eclevelandclinic@ccf.org.

Out-of-State Patients Assistance
Call 800.223.2273, ext. 55580 or email medicalconcierge@ccf.org.

Visit Us At:
clevelandclinic.org

Follow Us On:
Facebook
www.facebook.com/clevelandclinic

Twitter
@ClevelandClinic

You Tube
www.youtube.com/clevelandclinic

Health Hub
health.clevelandclinic.org

THE MOUNT SINAI MEDICAL CENTER
GASTROINTESTINAL AND SURGICAL SPECIALTIES
One Gustave L. Levy Place
Fifth Avenue and 100th Street
New York, NY 10029-6574
Physician Referral: 1-800-MD-SINAI (637-4624)
www.mountsinai.org

Mount Sinai's **DIVISIONS OF GASTROENTEROLOGY, COLON AND RECTAL SURGERY, LIVER DISEASES, PEDIATRIC GASTROENTEROLOGY, AND PEDIATRIC HEPATOLOGY** are renowned for their delivery of patient care, research, and education in diseases of the gastrointestinal (GI) tract. In 2000, the National Institutes of Health (NIH) recognized the importance of Mount Sinai as a research center with a grant for GI/Liver fellowship training. Mount Sinai is the only medical school in New York City to earn this prestigious award.

Mount Sinai's Division of Gastroenterology ranks 7th among all institutions in the country, according to the *U.S. News & World Report's* 2012–2013 "Best Hospitals" issue. Successes include breakthroughs in the medical and surgical management of the inflammatory bowel diseases (IBD): ulcerative colitis, and Crohn's disease. Mount Sinai spearheaded novel therapies for treating severe IBD and helped establish the role of colonoscopy in preventing colon cancer by removing precancerous polyps. More recent innovations include employing a tiny camera within a swallowable capsule to capture images in the stomach and intestines. Mount Sinai offers patients advanced comprehensive and interdisciplinary care; newer agents through clinical trials; services of psychologists and nutritionists; and world-class expertise in endoscopic procedures.

Division of Colon and Rectal Surgery — Continuing a long tradition of expertise in gastrointestinal disorders, Mount Sinai surgeons focus on surgical therapies for all diseases involving the colon, rectum, and anus. Highly skilled in the treatment of Crohn's disease (which was first described at Mount Sinai in 1932), ulcerative colitis, colon and rectal cancer, and diverticulitis, they specialize in the most advanced techniques of rectal surgery with an emphasis on colostomy avoidance. They also employ minimally invasive techniques and cutting-edge technologies for the treatment of hemorrhoids, fistulas, rectal tumors, and fecal incontinence.

Division of Liver Diseases — With a program that is among the largest and most successful in the world, Mount Sinai carries out a diverse portfolio of research projects. Featuring both clinical care and scientific investigations, they involve transplantation; diagnosis and treatment of viral hepatitis, including trials for revolutionary new drugs for Hepatitis B and C; treatment of scarring, or fibrosis; management of primary biliary cirrhosis, an autoimmune disease of bile ducts; treatment of liver cancer; and diagnosis and treatment of genetic liver diseases, including Wilson's disease (copper overload) and hemachromatosis (iron overload).

Division of Pediatric Gastroenterology — The division provides consultation and treatment for the full range of children's digestive and nutritional diseases. The Children's IBD Center offers comprehensive, multidisciplinary, family-centered care for pediatric patients with Crohn's disease and ulcerative colitis, and receives referrals from across the country. The division also provides care to families of infants, children, and teens who have the full range of both complex and common digestive disorders, including celiac disease, gastroesophageal reflux disease, and irritable bowel syndrome. Additionally, the division is involved in both basic science and clinical research, allowing physicians to provide state-of-the-art, evidence-based care.

Division of Pediatric Hepatology — The Transplant Program is one of the largest in the nation and was the first program in New York to perform liver transplants and, later, small bowel transplants. The division is active in clinical research in IBD, focusing on issues of genetic factors, psychosocial interactions, and drug trials in liver disease.

GASTROENTEROLOGY

About the Division of Gastroenterology, Department of Medicine
The Division of Gastroenterology at NYU Langone Medical Center is dedicated to the diagnosis and treatment of patients with diseases of the gastrointestinal tract. Physicians draw on their extensive knowledge and experience in the diagnosis and management of inflammatory bowel disease, peptic ulcer disease, esophageal disorders, gastrointestinal cancer, and liver, biliary and pancreatic diseases. We specialize in the following areas:

Colorectal Cancer
The Medical Center offers the most advanced screening options available for the diagnosis of colon cancer. Additionally, physicians continue to investigate colorectal cancer in special populations such as women, veterans, immigrants, minorities and patients with HIV, and offer the use of virtual colonoscopy for the detection of colorectal polyps and cancer.

Esophageal Diseases
The Esophageal Disease Center offers patients state-of-the-art diagnosis and treatment of esophageal disorders. The Center focuses on gastroesophageal reflux disease, esophageal motility disorders, Barrett's esophagus, adenocarcinoma of the esophagus and swallowing disorders. It also offers diagnostic studies on esophageal manometry, impedance testing for swallowing, pH catheter and impedance testing for reflux and BRAVO capsule pH testing, as well as such therapies as Barrett's ablation and esophageal dilations.

Gastrointestinal Cancers
Cancer Institute physicians treat patients with all types of gastrointestinal cancers, including those of the esophagus, stomach, colon/rectum, small intestine, liver, pancreas, gallbladder, and biliary tract. They also treat individuals with complex recurring disease, including those originally treated elsewhere. Patients have the opportunity to participate in numerous clinical trials.

Complex Treatments and Diagnosis
Physicians in the Division of Gastroenterology are highly experienced in the use of enteroscopy and capsule endoscopy for the diagnosis of gastrointestinal bleeding of unknown origin. They have special interest in the diagnosis and treatment of patients with complex pancreatic-biliary disease through the use of ERCP and endoscopic ultrasound.

Virtual Colonoscopy
NYU Langone Medical Center is in the vanguard of advanced colon cancer detection through virtual colonoscopy. The study gives a complete evaluation of the entire surface of the colon and ensures greater accuracy and less patient discomfort.

The Best in American Medicine
www.CastleConnolly.com

Geriatric Medicine

a subspecialty of Internal Medicine
or Family Practice

An internist or family physician with special knowledge of the aging process and special skills in the diagnostic, therapeutic, preventive and rehabilitative aspects of illness in the elderly. This specialist cares for geriatric patients in the patient's home, the office, long-term care settings such as nursing homes and the hospital.

Family Medicine

A family physician is concerned with the total healthcare of the individual and the family, and is trained to diagnose and treat a wide variety of ailments in patients of all ages. The family physician receives a broad range of training that includes internal medicine, pediatrics, obstetrics and gynecology, psychiatry and geriatrics. Special emphasis is placed on prevention and the primary care of entire families, utilizing consultations and community resources when appropriate.

Training Required: Three years in internal medicine or family practice *plus* additional training and examination for certification in geriatric medicine.

GERIATRIC MEDICINE

New England

Cooney Jr, Leo M MD [Ger] - **Spec Exp:** Geriatric Functional Assessment; Rheumatology; Mobility Evaluation & Treatment; **Hospital:** Yale-New Haven Hosp, Yale Med Group; **Address:** Yale-New Haven Hosp, Adler Geriatric Ctr, 20 York St, New Haven, CT 06510; **Phone:** 203-688-2204; **Board Cert:** Internal Medicine 1974; Rheumatology 1978; **Med School:** Yale Univ 1969; **Resid:** Internal Medicine, Boston City Hosp 1971; Internal Medicine, Boston City Hosp 1974; **Fellow:** Rheumatology, Boston Med Ctr 1975; **Fac Appt:** Prof Med, Yale Univ

Lipsitz, Lewis Arnold MD [Ger] - **Spec Exp:** Falls in the Elderly; Hypertension; Hypotension; Syncope; **Hospital:** Beth Israel Deaconess Med Ctr - Boston, Hebrew Senior Life; **Address:** Beth Israel Med Ctr, Gerontology, 110 Francis St, LMOB 1B, Boston, MA 02215; **Phone:** 617-632-8696; **Board Cert:** Internal Medicine 1980; Geriatric Medicine 2009; **Med School:** Univ Pennsylvania 1977; **Resid:** Internal Medicine, Beth Israel Hosp 1980; **Fellow:** Geriatric Medicine, Mass Genl Hosp 1983; **Fac Appt:** Prof Med, Harvard Med Sch

Minaker, Kenneth MD [Ger] - **Spec Exp:** Aging; Neuroendocrinology; Cardiovascular Disease; **Hospital:** Mass Genl Hosp, Brigham and Women's Hosp (page 57); **Address:** Charles River Plaza, Ste 502, 165 Cambridge St, Boston, MA 02114-2723; **Phone:** 617-726-4600; **Med School:** Univ Toronto 1972; **Resid:** Internal Medicine, Univ Toronto 1981; **Fellow:** Geriatric Medicine, Mass Gen Hosp 1983; **Fac Appt:** Assoc Prof Med, Harvard Med Sch

Tinetti, Mary E MD [Ger] - **Spec Exp:** Falls in the Elderly; Geriatric Functional Assessment; **Hospital:** Yale-New Haven Hosp, Yale Med Group; **Address:** Yale-New Haven Hosp, Adler Geriatric Ctr, 20 York St, New Haven, CT 06510; **Phone:** 203-688-6361; **Board Cert:** Internal Medicine 1981; **Med School:** Univ Mich Med Sch 1978; **Resid:** Internal Medicine, Univ Minnesota 1981; **Fellow:** Geriatric Medicine, Univ Rochester 1984; **Fac Appt:** Prof Med, Yale Univ

Mid Atlantic

Bloom, Patricia A MD [Ger] - **Spec Exp:** Complementary Medicine; Dementia; Pain Management; **Hospital:** Mount Sinai Med Ctr (page 64); **Address:** 1440 Madison Ave, New York, NY 10029-6542; **Phone:** 212-659-8552; **Board Cert:** Internal Medicine 1978; Geriatric Medicine 2011; **Med School:** Univ Minn 1975; **Resid:** Internal Medicine, Montefiore Med Ctr 1978; **Fac Appt:** Assoc Prof Med, Mount Sinai Sch Med

Burton, John R MD [Ger] - **Hospital:** Johns Hopkins Bayview Med Ctr (page 61); **Address:** Division of Geriatric Medicine, 5505 Hopkins Bayview Cir, Terrace Level 01, Baltimore, MD 21224; **Phone:** 410-550-0520; **Board Cert:** Internal Medicine 1980; Nephrology 1974; Geriatric Medicine 2005; **Med School:** McGill Univ 1965; **Resid:** Internal Medicine, Baltimore City Hosp 1971; **Fellow:** Nephrology, Mass Genl Hosp 1972; **Fac Appt:** Prof Med, Johns Hopkins Univ

Callahan, Eileen MD [Ger] - **Spec Exp:** Frail Elderly; Preventive Medicine; Dementia; **Hospital:** Mount Sinai Med Ctr (page 64); **Address:** Martha Stewart Ctr for Living, 1440 Madison Ave, New York, NY 10029; **Phone:** 212-659-8552; **Board Cert:** Internal Medicine 2004; Geriatric Medicine 2008; Hospice & Palliative Medicine 2005; **Med School:** UMDNJ-NJ Med Sch, Newark 1991; **Resid:** Internal Medicine, St Vincents Hosp Med Ctr 1994; **Fellow:** Geriatric Medicine, Mount Sinai Hosp 1996; **Fac Appt:** Assoc Prof Med, Mount Sinai Sch Med

Finucane, Thomas E MD [Ger] - **Spec Exp:** Pain Management; Swallowing Disorders; Ethics; Palliative Care; **Hospital:** Johns Hopkins Bayview Med Ctr (page 61), Johns Hopkins Hosp (page 61); **Address:** 5505 Hopkins Bayview Cir, Terrace Level 01, Baltimore, MD 21224; **Phone:** 410-550-0925; **Board Cert:** Internal Medicine 1982; Geriatric Medicine 2008; **Med School:** Emory Univ 1978; **Resid:** Internal Medicine, George Washington Univ Hosp 1982; **Fac Appt:** Prof Med, Johns Hopkins Univ

Gambert, Steven R MD [Ger] - **Spec Exp:** Endocrinology; Osteoporosis; Aging; **Hospital:** Univ of MD Med Ctr; **Address:** Univ Maryland, Dept Med, 22 S Greene St, rm N3E09, Baltimore, MD 21201; **Phone:** 410-328-1143; **Board Cert:** Internal Medicine 1978; **Med School:** Columbia P&S 1975; **Resid:** Internal Medicine, Dartmouth Affl Hosp 1977; **Fellow:** Geriatric Medicine, Beth Israel Hosp-Harvard 1979; Endocrinology, Beth Israel Hosp-Harvard 1979; **Fac Appt:** Prof Med, Univ MD Sch Med

Lachs, Mark S MD [Ger] - **Spec Exp:** Abuse/Neglect; **Hospital:** NY-Presby/Weill Cornell Med Ctr, NY (page 66); **Address:** Irving Sherwood Wright Med Ctr on Aging, 1484 First Ave, New York, NY 10075; **Phone:** 212-746-7000; **Board Cert:** Internal Medicine 1988; Geriatric Medicine 2002; **Med School:** NYU Sch Med 1985; **Resid:** Internal Medicine, Hosp Univ Penn 1988; **Fellow:** Geriatric Medicine, Yale-New Haven Hosp 1990; **Fac Appt:** Prof Med, Cornell Univ-Weill Med Coll

Resnick, Neil M MD [Ger] - **Spec Exp:** Voiding Dysfunction; Incontinence; **Hospital:** UPMC Presby, Pittsburgh, UPMC Shadyside; **Address:** 3471 5th Ave, Kaufmann Bldg, Ste 500, Pittsburgh, PA 15213-3313; **Phone:** 412-692-2364; **Board Cert:** Internal Medicine 1980; Geriatric Medicine 2009; **Med School:** Stanford Univ 1977; **Resid:** Internal Medicine, Beth Israel Hosp 1980; **Fellow:** Geriatric Medicine, Harvard Univ 1982; Urodynamics, Harvard Univ 1984; **Fac Appt:** Prof Med, Univ Pittsburgh

Studenski, Stephanie A MD [Ger] - **Spec Exp:** Balance Disorders; Mobility Evaluation & Treatment; Falls in the Elderly; **Hospital:** UPMC Presby, Pittsburgh; **Address:** 3459 Fifth Ave Fl 4, Pittsburgh, PA 15213; **Phone:** 412-692-4200; **Board Cert:** Internal Medicine 1982; Rheumatology 1984; Geriatric Medicine 2002; **Med School:** Univ Kansas 1979; **Resid:** Internal Medicine, Duke Univ Med Ctr 1982; **Fellow:** Rheumatology, Duke Univ Med Ctr 1984; Geriatric Medicine, Duke Univ Med Ctr 1986; **Fac Appt:** Prof Med, Univ Pittsburgh

Southeast

Allman, Richard M MD [Ger] - **Spec Exp:** Geriatric Rehabilitation; Mobility Evaluation & Treatment; Palliative Care; **Hospital:** Univ of Ala Hosp at Birmingham; **Address:** UAB Center for Aging, 1720 2nd Ave S, CH 19-201, Birmingham, AL 35294-2041; **Phone:** 205-934-9261; **Board Cert:** Internal Medicine 1983; Geriatric Medicine 1998; **Med School:** W VA Univ 1980; **Resid:** Internal Medicine, W Va Univ Hosp 1983; **Fellow:** Internal Medicine, Johns Hopkins Univ 1985; **Fac Appt:** Prof Med, Univ Alabama

Ciocon, Jerry O MD [Ger] - **Spec Exp:** Chronic Fatigue-Elderly; Pain-Musculoskeletal; Memory Disorders; Incontinence; **Hospital:** Cleveland Clin - Weston (page 55); **Address:** Cleveland Clinic, Div Geriatrics, 2950 Cleveland Clinic Blvd, Weston, FL 33331-3609; **Phone:** 954-659-5867; **Board Cert:** Internal Medicine 1985; Geriatric Medicine 2000; **Med School:** Philippines 1980; **Resid:** Internal Medicine, Mercy Hosp 1985; **Fellow:** Geriatric Medicine, LI Jewish Med Ctr 1987

Geriatric Medicine

Greganti, Mac Andrew MD [Ger] - **Spec Exp:** Diagnostic Problems; Dementia; **Hospital:** NC Memorial Hosp - UNC; **Address:** Univ of North Carolina School of Medicine, Chapel Hill, Dept Med, 125 MacNider Bldg CB#7005, Chapel Hill, NC 27599-7005; **Phone:** 919-966-3063; **Board Cert:** Internal Medicine 1987; **Med School:** Univ Miss 1972; **Resid:** Internal Medicine, Strong Meml Hosp 1975; **Fac Appt:** Prof Med, Univ NC Sch Med

Hanson, Laura C MD [Ger] - **Spec Exp:** Frailty Syndrome; Palliative Care; **Hospital:** NC Memorial Hosp - UNC; **Address:** UNC Sch Med, 5003 Old Clinic Bldg, CB 7550, Chapel Hill, NC 27599; **Phone:** 919-966-5945 x251; **Board Cert:** Internal Medicine 1989; Geriatric Medicine 2002; Hospice & Palliative Medicine 2009; **Med School:** Harvard Med Sch 1986; **Resid:** Internal Medicine, Brigham & Womens Hosp 1988; Internal Medicine, Univ North Carolina Hosp 1989; **Fellow:** Geriatric Medicine, Univ North Carolina Hosp 1991; **Fac Appt:** Assoc Prof Med, Univ NC Sch Med

Lyles, Kenneth W MD [Ger] - **Spec Exp:** Bone Disorders-Metabolic; Tumoral Calcinosis; Parathyroid Disease; Osteoporosis; **Hospital:** Duke Univ Hosp, Durham VA Med Ctr; **Address:** Duke Box 3881, 2507 Busse Bldg, Durham, NC 27710; **Phone:** 919-660-7520; **Board Cert:** Internal Medicine 1977; Endocrinology 1979; Geriatric Medicine 2000; **Med School:** Med Coll VA 1974; **Resid:** Internal Medicine, Med Coll VA 1977; **Fellow:** Endocrinology, Diabetes & Metabolism, Duke Univ Med Ctr 1979; Geriatric Medicine, Duke Univ/VA Med Ctr 1981; **Fac Appt:** Prof Med, Duke Univ

Palmer, Robert M MD [Ger] - **Spec Exp:** Geriatric Functional Assessment; Dementia; **Hospital:** Sentara Norfolk Genl Hosp; **Address:** 825 Fairfax Ave Fl 2 - rm 201, Norfolk, VA 23507; **Phone:** 757-446-7040; **Board Cert:** Internal Medicine 1975; Geriatric Medicine 2009; **Med School:** Univ Mich Med Sch 1971; **Resid:** Internal Medicine, LA County Med Ctr 1975; **Fellow:** Geriatric Medicine, UCLA Med Ctr 1986

Midwest

Carr, David B MD [Ger] - **Spec Exp:** Polypharmacology (Excess Medications); Alzheimer's Disease; **Hospital:** Barnes-Jewish Hosp; **Address:** Wash Univ Sch Med, Div Geriatrics, 4488 Forest Park, Ste 160, St Louis, MO 63108; **Phone:** 314-286-1967; **Board Cert:** Internal Medicine 1989; Geriatric Medicine 2000; **Med School:** Univ MO-Columbia Sch Med 1985; **Resid:** Internal Medicine, Mich State Univ Affil Hosps 1988; **Fellow:** Geriatric Medicine, Duke Univ 1990; **Fac Appt:** Prof Med, Washington Univ, St Louis

Dale, Lowell C MD [Ger] - **Spec Exp:** Tobacco Abuse; Nutrition; **Hospital:** Mayo Med Ctr & Clin - Rochester; **Address:** Mayo Clinic, 200 First St SW, Rochester, MN 55905; **Phone:** 507-284-2439; **Board Cert:** Internal Medicine 1984; **Med School:** Univ Minn 1981; **Resid:** Internal Medicine, Mayo Clin 1984; **Fellow:** Internal Medicine, Mayo Clin 1985; **Fac Appt:** Asst Prof Med, Mayo Med Sch

Duthie Jr, Edmund H MD [Ger] - **Spec Exp:** Geriatric Functional Assessment; **Hospital:** Froedtert and Med Ctr of WI, Clement J Zablocki VA Med Ctr; **Address:** 9200 W Wisconsin Ave Fl 5, Milwaukee, WI 53226; **Phone:** 414-805-0728; **Board Cert:** Internal Medicine 1979; Geriatric Medicine 2008; **Med School:** Georgetown Univ 1976; **Resid:** Internal Medicine, Med Coll Wisc Hosps 1979; **Fellow:** Geriatric Medicine, Jewish Inst Geri Care-SUNY 1980; **Fac Appt:** Prof Med, Med Coll Wisc

Flaherty, Joseph MD [Ger] - **Spec Exp:** Drugs & Aging; **Hospital:** St. Louis Univ Hosp; **Address:** 1402 Grand Blvd, rm M238, St Louis, MO 63104; **Phone:** 314-977-8462; **Board Cert:** Internal Medicine 2003; Geriatric Medicine 2006; **Med School:** St Louis Univ 1990; **Resid:** Internal Medicine, Kansas City Univ Med Ctr 1993; **Fellow:** Geriatric Medicine, St Louis Univ 1995; **Fac Appt:** Assoc Prof Med, St Louis Univ

Gorbien, Martin J MD [Ger] - **Spec Exp:** Dementia; Alzheimer's Disease; Geriatric Functional Assessment; Palliative Care; **Hospital:** Rush Univ Med Ctr; **Address:** 1725 W Harrison St, Ste 955, Senior Care, Professional Bldg 3, Chicago, IL 60612; **Phone:** 312-942-7030; **Board Cert:** Geriatric Medicine 2008; Hospice & Palliative Medicine 2008; **Med School:** Mexico 1983; **Resid:** Internal Medicine, Mercy Hosp & Med Ctr 1987; **Fellow:** Geriatric Medicine, UCLA Med Ctr 1989; **Fac Appt:** Assoc Prof Med, Rush Med Coll

Morley, John MD [Ger] - **Spec Exp:** Endocrinology; Menopause-Male; Alzheimer's Disease; Frailty Syndrome; **Hospital:** St. Louis Univ Hosp; **Address:** St Louis Univ Hlth Sci Ctr, Div Ger Med, 3660 Vista Ave, Ste 204, St Louis, MO 63110; **Phone:** 314-977-6157; **Board Cert:** Internal Medicine 1978; Endocrinology, Diabetes & Metabolism 1981; Geriatric Medicine 2008; **Med School:** South Africa 1972; **Resid:** Internal Medicine, Johannesburg Genl Hosp 1974; Internal Medicine, Baragwanath Hosp 1976; **Fellow:** Endocrinology, Diabetes & Metabolism, Wadsworth VA Hosp-UCLA 1979; **Fac Appt:** Prof Med, St Louis Univ

Olson Jr, Jack C MD [Ger] - **Spec Exp:** Dementia; Depression; **Hospital:** Rush Univ Med Ctr; **Address:** Senior Care, Rush Univ Professional Bldg 3, 1725 W Harrison St, Ste 955, Chicago, IL 60612-3836; **Phone:** 312-942-7030; **Board Cert:** Internal Medicine 1987; **Med School:** Univ Mich Med Sch 1984; **Resid:** Internal Medicine, Univ Wisconsin Affil Hosp 1987; **Fellow:** Geriatric Medicine, Univ Wisconsin Affil Hosp 1989; **Fac Appt:** Asst Prof Med, Univ Chicago-Pritzker Sch Med

Sachs, Greg A MD [Ger] - **Spec Exp:** Memory Disorders; Alzheimer's Disease; Palliative Care; **Hospital:** IU Health University Hosp; **Address:** 1050 Wishard Blvd, West Outpatient Bldg, rm M200, Indianapolis, IN 46202; **Phone:** 317-630-2557; **Board Cert:** Internal Medicine 1988; Geriatric Medicine 2010; Hospice & Palliative Medicine 2010; **Med School:** Yale Univ 1985; **Resid:** Internal Medicine, Univ Chicago Hosps 1987; **Fellow:** Geriatric Medicine, Univ Chicago Hosps 1990; **Fac Appt:** Prof Med, Indiana Univ

Thomas, David R MD [Ger] - **Spec Exp:** Wound Healing/Care; Nutrition; Frail Elderly; **Hospital:** St. Louis Univ Hosp, Des Peres Hosp; **Address:** St Louis Univ Sch Med, Div Geri Med, 1402 S Grand Blvd, Ste M238, St Louis, MO 63104; **Phone:** 314-977-8462; **Board Cert:** Internal Medicine 1975; Geriatric Medicine 2009; **Med School:** Univ Miss 1971; **Resid:** Internal Medicine, Univ Miss Med Ctr 1975; **Fellow:** Geriatric Medicine, Johns Hopkins Hosp 1988; **Fac Appt:** Prof Med, Univ MO-Columbia Sch Med

Great Plains and Mountains

Schwartz, Robert S MD [Ger] - **Spec Exp:** Diabetes; Hormonal Disorders; **Hospital:** Univ of CO Hosp - Anschutz Inpatient Pav, VA Eastern CO Health Care Sys-Denver; **Address:** Anschutz Outpatient Pav, 1635 N Aurora Ct Fl 5, MS F750, Aurora, CO 80045; **Phone:** 720-848-3400; **Board Cert:** Internal Medicine 1977; Endocrinology 1981; **Med School:** Ohio State Univ 1974; **Resid:** Internal Medicine, Univ Wash Med Ctr 1977; **Fellow:** Endocrinology, Diabetes & Metabolism, Univ Wash Med Ctr 1980; **Fac Appt:** Prof Med, Univ Colorado

Geriatric Medicine

Supiano, Mark A MD [Ger] - **Spec Exp:** Hypertension; Geriatric Functional Assessment; **Hospital:** Univ Utah Hlth Care; **Address:** Univ Utah, Geriatrics Div, 30 N 1900 E, AB 193 SOM, Salt Lake City, UT 84132; **Phone:** 801-587-9103; **Board Cert:** Internal Medicine 1985; Geriatric Medicine 1998; **Med School:** Univ Wisc 1982; **Resid:** Internal Medicine, Univ Mich Med Ctr 1985; **Fellow:** Geriatric Medicine, Univ Mich Med Ctr 1987; **Fac Appt:** Prof Med, Univ Utah

Southwest

Dyer, Carmel B MD [Ger] - **Spec Exp:** Elder Abuse; Dementia; Delirium; Geriatric Functional Assessment; **Hospital:** Meml Hermann Hosp - Texas Med Ctr, LBJ General Hosp; **Address:** 6431 Fannin St, rm MSB-4.200, Houston, TX 77030; **Phone:** 713-486-5150; **Board Cert:** Geriatric Medicine 2000; **Med School:** Baylor Coll Med 1988; **Resid:** Internal Medicine, Baylor Affil Hosps 1991; **Fellow:** Geriatric Medicine, Baylor Affil Hosps 1993; **Fac Appt:** Prof Med, Univ Tex, Houston

Liem, Pham MD [Ger] - **Spec Exp:** Dementia; Alzheimer's Disease; Delirium; **Hospital:** UAMS Med Ctr, Cent Ark Vet Hlthcare Sys; **Address:** UAMS Thomas A Lyon Longevity Ctr, 4301 W Markham St, Slot 547-13, Little Rock, AR 72205-7101; **Phone:** 501-686-6219; **Board Cert:** Family Medicine 2006; Geriatric Medicine 2008; **Med School:** Vietnam 1973; **Resid:** Family Medicine, Univ Ark Med Sch 1980; **Fellow:** Geriatric Medicine, Univ Ark Med Sch 1982; **Fac Appt:** Prof Med, Univ Ark

Lipschitz, David A MD/PhD [Ger] - **Spec Exp:** Preventive Medicine; Nutrition; **Hospital:** St. Vincent Med Ctr; **Address:** Longevity Center-St Vincent Senior Hlth, One St Vincent Circle, Ste 210, Little Rock, AR 72205; **Phone:** 501-552-4777; **Board Cert:** Internal Medicine 1975; Hematology 1976; **Med School:** South Africa 1966; **Resid:** Internal Medicine, Johannesburg Genl Hosp 1972; **Fellow:** Hematology, Univ Washington 1974; Internal Medicine, Montefiore Hosp 1975; **Fac Appt:** Prof Med, Univ Ark

Raji, Mukaila A MD [Ger] - **Spec Exp:** Memory Disorders; Cognitive Loss in Aging; **Hospital:** UT Med Br at Galveston(Joh Sealy Hosp); **Address:** UTMB-Geriatrics Dept, 400 Harborside Drive, Ste 100, Galveston, TX 77550; **Phone:** 409-772-3373; **Board Cert:** Internal Medicine 2009; Geriatric Medicine 2009; **Med School:** Nigeria 1997; **Resid:** Internal Medicine, Washington Hosp Ctr 1997; **Fellow:** Geriatric Medicine, Duke Univ Med Ctr 1999; **Fac Appt:** Prof Med, Univ Tex Med Br, Galveston

Wei, Jeanne MD/PhD [Ger] - **Spec Exp:** Cardiovascular Disease; **Hospital:** UAMS Med Ctr, John L McClellan VA Med Ctr; **Address:** UAMS Thomas A Lyon Longevity Ctr, 4301 W Markham St, Slot 547-13, Little Rock, AR 72205; **Phone:** 501-686-6219; **Board Cert:** Internal Medicine 1978; Cardiovascular Disease 1979; Geriatric Medicine 2001; **Med School:** Univ IL Coll Med 1975; **Resid:** Internal Medicine, Johns Hopkins Hosp 1977; **Fellow:** Cardiovascular Disease, Johns Hopkins Hosp 1979; Research, Natl Inst Aging 1979; **Fac Appt:** Prof Med, Univ Ark

West Coast and Pacific

Abrass, Itamar B MD [Ger] - **Spec Exp:** Geriatric Endocrinology; Endocrine Disorders; Diabetes; **Hospital:** Harborview Med Ctr, Univ Wash Med Ctr; **Address:** Harborview Medical Ctr, 325 9th Ave, Box 359860, Seattle, WA 98104; **Phone:** 206-744-4191; **Board Cert:** Internal Medicine 1974; Endocrinology, Diabetes & Metabolism 1975; **Med School:** UCSF 1966; **Resid:** Internal Medicine, Columbia-Pesby Med Ctr 1968; **Fellow:** Endocrinology, Diabetes & Metabolism, UCSD Med Ctr 1971; **Fac Appt:** Prof Med, Univ Wash

McCormick, Wayne MD [Ger] - **Spec Exp:** Dementia; AIDS/HIV; **Hospital:** Harborview Med Ctr, Univ Wash Med Ctr; **Address:** Harborview Med Ctr, 325 9th Ave, Box 359755, Seattle, WA 98104; **Phone:** 206-744-4191; **Board Cert:** Internal Medicine 1986; Geriatric Medicine 2002; Public Health & Genl Preventive Med 1992; Hospice & Palliative Medicine 2010; **Med School:** Washington Univ, St Louis 1983; **Resid:** Internal Medicine, Michael Reese Hosp 1987; **Fellow:** Geriatric Medicine, Univ Wash Med Ctr 1990; **Fac Appt:** Asst Prof Med, Univ Wash

Reuben, David B MD [Ger] - **Spec Exp:** Geriatric Functional Assessment; **Hospital:** UCLA Ronald Reagan Med Ctr, Santa Monica - UCLA Med Ctr & Ortho Hosp; **Address:** UCLA Med Ctr, 1245 16th St, Ste 204, Santa Monica, CA 90404; **Phone:** 310-319-4371; **Board Cert:** Internal Medicine 1980; Geriatric Medicine 2005; **Med School:** Emory Univ 1977; **Resid:** Internal Medicine, Rhode Island Hosp 1980; **Fellow:** Geriatric Medicine, UCLA Med Ctr 1987; **Fac Appt:** Prof Med, UCLA

Tenover, Joyce S MD/PhD [Ger] - **Spec Exp:** Polypharmacology; Dementia; Depression; **Hospital:** VA Hlth Care Sys - Palo Alto; **Address:** VA Palo Alto HCS, GRECC (182B), 3801 Miranda Ave, Palo Alto, CA 94304-1290; **Phone:** 650-493-5000 x66946; **Board Cert:** Internal Medicine 1983; Geriatric Medicine 2008; **Med School:** Geo Wash Univ 1980; **Resid:** Internal Medicine, Univ Wash Affil Hosps 1983; Internal Medicine, VA Med Ctr 1984; **Fellow:** Geriatric Medicine, VA Med Ctr 1987; **Fac Appt:** Clin Prof Med, Geo Wash Univ

Cleveland Clinic

Every life deserves world class care.

Cleveland Clinic
Center for Geriatric Medicine
9500 Euclid Avenue
Cleveland, OH 44195

Geriatric Medicine

Cleveland Clinic's Center for Geriatric Medicine, part of the Medicine Institute at Cleveland Clinic, specializes in diagnosing and treating frail, elderly patients with complex medical conditions and social problems.

Our Center for Geriatric Medicine consists of an inter-disciplinary team of healthcare professionals dedicated to creating comprehensive, coordinated care plans for all patients. The center offers several specialized programs to help ensure older patients receive the full scope of care necessary for optimal outcomes.

These programs include:

Geriatric Evaluation and Management Program is the cornerstone of the comprehensive care offered to senior patients and their families. It takes an in-depth look at each patient's physical and psychological health, including the person's medical history, current status, recent changes and special concerns.

Geriatric Falls Clinic provides evaluation and follow-up for the treatment and prevention of falls. The multidisciplinary assessment includes screenings for vision, medical conditions, polypharmacy, nutritional status, mental alertness, physical function, balance and strength.

Geriatric Consultations

One of the special features that Cleveland Clinic offers older adults hospitalized for acute medical or surgical problems is an inpatient geriatrics assessment. These assessments can be requested by the attending physician for specific geriatric concerns, including depression, delirium (acute confusion), dementia, falls and medication issues.

Offering Same-Day Appointments
Call 800.274.2009.

Treatment Guides
Cleveland Clinic has developed comprehensive treatment guides for many diseases and conditions. To download our free treatment guides, visit clevelandclinic.org/treatmentguides.

Online Medical Second Opinion
Call 216.444.3223 or
800.223.2273 ext. 43223 or
email eclevelandclinic@ccf.org.

Out-of-State Patients Assistance
Call 800.223.2273, ext. 55580 or
email medicalconcierge@ccf.org.

Visit Us At:
clevelandclinic.org

Follow Us On:
Facebook
www.facebook.com/clevelandclinic

Twitter
@ClevelandClinic

You Tube
www.youtube.com/clevelandclinic

Health Hub
health.clevelandclinic.org

MOUNT SINAI
SCHOOL OF
MEDICINE

THE MOUNT SINAI MEDICAL CENTER
THE BROOKDALE DEPARTMENT OF
GERIATRICS AND PALLIATIVE MEDICINE
One Gustave L. Levy Place
Fifth Avenue and 100th Street
New York, NY 10029-6574
Physician Referral: 1-800-MD-SINAI (637-4624)
www.mountsinai.org/geriatrics
www.mountsinai.org/palliative

The Best in Clinical Care

In recognition of the care offered to older patients, The Mount Sinai Medical Center's **BROOKDALE DEPARTMENT OF GERIATRICS AND PALLIATIVE MEDICINE** is cited time and time again among the finest in the nation. In 2012, *U.S. News & World Report* ranked our geriatrics specialty #2 and our medical school program #1 in the United States.

We offer a full spectrum of patient care, including a specialized inpatient care team for the elderly to minimize complications sometimes associated with an older person's hospital stay, a primary care geriatrics practice for older adults living in the community, a hospital-based consultation service for patients throughout Mount Sinai, a number of community-linked programs and partnerships, and a palliative care team dedicated to ensuring the highest quality care and support for patients and families facing serious illnesses.

The Martha Stewart Center for Living, a modern facility designed by renowned architect C.C. Pei, provides clinical care and education for patients and serves as a training ground for physicians. Our newly opened Wiener Family Palliative Care Unit, the only one of its kind in Manhattan, provides inpatient care for patients and families facing serious and life-threatening illness.

Groundbreaking Research—Mount Sinai's researchers continue to advance the understanding, prevention, and treatment of age-related disorders. The extensive research on aging conducted by the Brookdale Department of Geriatrics and Palliative Medicine includes studies on health services, medical decision making and ethical dilemmas, palliative care, the neurobiology of aging, and clinical interventions to promote independence in old age. The department's expertise serves as a renowned educational resource for all Mount Sinai affiliates and other institutions in teaching geriatrics and palliative medicine to medical students, medical residents, geriatrics and palliative care fellows, established physicians, and health profession trainees in other disciplines.

History Of Excellence—The Mount Sinai Medical Center is a pioneer in geriatric medicine. In 1909, a Mount Sinai physician coined the term "geriatrics," and in 1914, he wrote the first textbook on medical care for older adults. Today, the Brookdale Department of Geriatrics and Palliative Medicine continues to break new ground, offering comprehensive care, disease prevention, and the promotion of healthy and productive aging. The department's enhanced expertise in assessing and managing patients with dementia greatly complements its established, interdisciplinary approach to patient care, in which medical staff and social workers address each patient's needs as a team. Our newly opened Wiener Family Palliative Care Unit, the only one of its kind in Manhattan, provides inpatient care for patients and families facing serious and life-threatening illness.

THE FIRST FREESTANDING DEPARTMENT OF GERIATRICS AT A U.S. MEDICAL SCHOOL
Mount Sinai's Brookdale Department of Geriatrics and Palliative Medicine was the first freestanding department of geriatrics established by a U.S. medical school, and it continues to be one of the very best. It offers unparalleled inpatient and outpatient care, as well as numerous treatment programs designed to meet the unique needs of older adults. Mount Sinai is also home to world-class researchers dedicated to advancing our understanding of Alzheimer's disease and other common geriatric conditions. At the department's heart are its patients. The geriatricians of The Mount Sinai Medical Center work hard to improve life and longevity for New York's elderly.

GERIATRIC MEDICINE

About the Section of Geriatrics, Division of General Internal Medicine, Department of Medicine
NYU Langone Medical Center has a distinguished history as a federally designated research center and leader in the care of geriatrics. We specialize in the following areas:

Inpatient Geriatrics Services
Using a team approach, a senior geriatrician leads nurses, pharmacists, geropsychiatrists, rehabilitation experts and fellowship trainees in caring for geriatric patients with complex conditions. If screening reveals a hospitalized patient is suffering from a geriatric problem (such as cognitive impairment), special consultation is offered to the patient's health care team.

The Healthy Aging Initiative
A fundamental part of the care provided by geriatricians within NYU Langone Medical Center's faculty group practice is assessing and advising older individuals on how to avoid developing problems like cognitive or functional impairment.

The William and Sylvia Silberstein Aging and Dementia Research Center
The Silberstein Aging and Dementia Research Center is a National Institute on Aging-designated Center of Excellence in Alzheimer's treatment. The facility provides comprehensive diagnostic evaluations to determine if memory loss is "normal" or more serious; a memory enhancement program for age-related memory decline; clinical trials for mild memory loss and for Alzheimer's treatment; state-of-the-art brain imaging techniques; methods to minimize disability in Alzheimer's patients; and comprehensive counseling and support groups for patients, caregivers and family members.

The Pearl Barlow Center for Memory Evaluation and Treatment
The Pearl Barlow Center for Memory Evaluation and Treatment is the clinical care and diagnostic unit of the Silberstein Alzheimer's Institute at NYU Langone Medical Center. The Pearl Barlow Center for Memory Evaluation and Treatment is focused on patients with memory impairments caused by neurological, psychological and physical ailments, as well as memory issues resulting from medication side effects, anxiety, depression and the effects of normal aging, including Alzheimer's disease. This multidisciplinary medical approach, integrated with advanced research capabilities, is the first of its kind in New York City for the treatment of memory disorders.

The Best in American Medicine
www.CastleConnolly.com

Gynecologic Oncology
a subspecialty of
Obstetrics & Gynecology

An obstetrician/gynecologist who provides consultation and comprehensive management of patients with gynecologic cancer, including those diagnostic and therapeutic procedures necessary
for the total care of the patient with gynecologic cancer and resulting complications.

Training Required: Four years *plus* two years in clinical practice before certification in obstetrics and gynecology is complete *plus* additional training and examination in gynecologic oncology.

GYNECOLOGIC ONCOLOGY

New England

Azodi, Masoud MD [GO] - **Spec Exp:** Laparoscopic Surgery; Ovarian Cancer-Early Detection; Uterine Cancer; **Hospital:** Yale-New Haven Hosp, Yale Med Group; **Address:** Smilow Cancer Hosp, 25 Park St, Ste B, New Haven, CT 06519; **Phone:** 203-785-4013; **Board Cert:** Gynecologic Oncology 2009; Obstetrics & Gynecology 2009; **Med School:** Wright State Univ 1992; **Resid:** Obstetrics & Gynecology, Aultman Hospital 1996; **Fellow:** Obstetrics & Gynecology, Yale-New Haven Hosp 1999; **Fac Appt:** Assoc Prof ObG, Yale Univ

Berkowitz, Ross S MD [GO] - **Spec Exp:** Gynecologic Cancer; **Hospital:** Brigham and Women's Hosp (page 57), Dana-Farber Cancer Inst (page 57); **Address:** Brighan & Women's Hospital, Div OB/GYN Oncology, 75 Francis St, Ste A3150, Boston, MA 02115; **Phone:** 617-732-8840; **Board Cert:** Obstetrics & Gynecology 1981; Gynecologic Oncology 1982; **Med School:** Boston Univ 1973; **Resid:** Surgery, Brigham and Women's Hosp 1975; Obstetrics & Gynecology, Brigham and Women's Hosp 1978; **Fellow:** Gynecologic Oncology, Brigham and Women's Hosp 1980; **Fac Appt:** Prof ObG, Harvard Med Sch

Brewer, Molly A MD [GO] - **Spec Exp:** Ovarian Cancer; Gynecologic Cancer; Gynecologic Cancer-Rare; **Hospital:** Univ of Conn Hlth Ctr, John Dempsey Hosp, Hartford Hosp; **Address:** Univ Conn Hlth Ctr, Div Gyn Oncology, 263 Farmington Ave, MC2875, Farmington, CT 06032-2875; **Phone:** 860-679-2100; **Board Cert:** Obstetrics & Gynecology 2009; Gynecologic Oncology 2009; **Med School:** SUNY Upstate Med Univ 1991; **Resid:** Obstetrics & Gynecology, Oregon Hlth Scis Ctr 1995; **Fellow:** Gynecologic Oncology, MD Anderson Cancer Ctr 1997; **Fac Appt:** Prof ObG, Univ Conn

Cain, Joanna M MD [GO] - **Spec Exp:** Ovarian Cancer; Breast Cancer Risk Assessment; Uterine Cancer; Ovarian Cancer-Early Detection; **Hospital:** UMass Memorial Med Ctr; **Address:** Women & Infants Hospital, 101 Dudley St, Worcester, MA 01605; **Phone:** 508-334-1377; **Board Cert:** Obstetrics & Gynecology 2011; Gynecologic Oncology 2011; **Med School:** Creighton Univ 1978; **Resid:** Obstetrics & Gynecology, Univ Washington Med Ctr 1981; **Fellow:** Gynecologic Oncology, Meml Sloan Kettering Cancer Ctr 1983; **Fac Appt:** Prof ObG, Univ Mass Sch Med

DeMars, Leslie R MD [GO] - **Spec Exp:** Gynecologic Cancer; Laparoscopic Surgery; **Hospital:** Dartmouth - Hitchcock Med Ctr; **Address:** Dartmouth-Hitchcock Med Ctr, Gyn-Oncology, 1 Medical Center Drive, Lebanon, NH 03756; **Phone:** 603-653-3530; **Board Cert:** Obstetrics & Gynecology 2009; Gynecologic Oncology 2009; **Med School:** Univ VT Coll Med 1987; **Resid:** Obstetrics & Gynecology, Univ NC Hosp 1991; **Fellow:** Gynecologic Oncology, Univ NC Hosp 1994; **Fac Appt:** Assoc Prof ObG, Dartmouth Med Sch

Granai, Cornelius O MD [GO] - **Spec Exp:** Gynecologic Cancer; Complementary Medicine; International Health; **Hospital:** Women & Infants Hosp of RI, Kent Hosp; **Address:** Women & Infants Hosp, Womens Oncology Program, 101 Dudley St, Providence, RI 02905; **Phone:** 401-453-7520; **Board Cert:** Obstetrics & Gynecology 2011; Gynecologic Oncology 2011; **Med School:** Univ VT Coll Med 1977; **Resid:** Obstetrics & Gynecology, Tufts-New England Med Ctr 1981; **Fellow:** Gynecologic Oncology, Tufts Univ 1983; **Fac Appt:** Prof ObG, Brown Univ

Muto, Michael G MD [GO] - **Spec Exp:** Ovarian Cancer; Cervical Cancer; Vulvar & Vaginal Cancer; Robotic Surgery; **Hospital:** Dana-Farber Cancer Inst (page 57), Brigham and Women's Hosp (page 57); **Address:** Brigham & Womens Hosp, Div Gynecologic Oncology, 75 Francis St, Ste A3173, Boston, MA 02115; **Phone:** 617-732-8843; **Board Cert:** Obstetrics & Gynecology 2011; Gynecologic Oncology 2011; **Med School:** Univ Mass Sch Med 1983; **Resid:** Obstetrics & Gynecology, Brigham & Women's Hosp 1987; **Fellow:** Gynecologic Oncology, Brigham & Women's Hosp 1990; **Fac Appt:** Assoc Prof ObG, Harvard Med Sch

Rutherford, Thomas J MD [GO] - **Spec Exp:** Ovarian Cancer; Uterine Cancer; Ovarian Cancer-Early Detection; Cervical Cancer; **Hospital:** Yale-New Haven Hosp, Yale Med Group; **Address:** Smilow Cancer Hosp, 25 Park St Fl 1, New Haven, CT 06519; **Phone:** 203-200-4176; **Board Cert:** Obstetrics & Gynecology 2011; Gynecologic Oncology 2011; **Med School:** Med Coll OH 1989; **Resid:** Obstetrics & Gynecology, Cooper Hosp 1993; **Fellow:** Gynecologic Oncology, Yale-New Haven Hosp 1995; **Fac Appt:** Assoc Prof ObG, Yale Univ

Santin, Alessandro MD [GO] - **Spec Exp:** Immunotherapy; Ovarian Cancer; Vulvar & Vaginal Cancer; **Hospital:** Yale-New Haven Hosp, Yale Med Group; **Address:** Yale Gynecologic Oncology, 333 Cedar St, PO Box 208063, New Haven, CT 06510; **Phone:** 203-200-4176; **Med School:** Italy 1989; **Resid:** Obstetrics & Gynecology, Univ Brescia Sch Med 1993; **Fellow:** Gynecologic Oncology, UC Irvine 1995; Gynecologic Oncology, UAMS Med Ctr 2000; **Fac Appt:** Prof ObG, Yale Univ

Schorge, John O MD [GO] - **Spec Exp:** Ovarian Cancer; Uterine Cancer; Cervical Cancer; Minimally Invasive Surgery; **Hospital:** Mass Genl Hosp; **Address:** Mass General Hosp, Gillette Ctr for Gynocological Oncology, 55 Fruit St, Ste YAW 9E, Boston, MA 02114; **Phone:** 617-724-6899; **Board Cert:** Obstetrics & Gynecology 2011; Gynecologic Oncology 2011; **Med School:** Vanderbilt Univ 1993; **Resid:** Obstetrics & Gynecology, Brigham & Women's Hosp 1997; **Fellow:** Gynecologic Oncology, Brigham & Women's Hosp 2000; **Fac Appt:** Assoc Prof ObG, Harvard Med Sch

Schwartz, Peter E MD [GO] - **Spec Exp:** Ovarian Cancer; Uterine Cancer; Gynecologic Surgery-Complex; Cervical Cancer; **Hospital:** Yale-New Haven Hosp, Yale Med Group; **Address:** 20 York St, New Haven, CT 06510-3289; **Phone:** 203-785-4014; **Board Cert:** Obstetrics & Gynecology 1973; Gynecologic Oncology 1979; **Med School:** Albert Einstein Coll Med 1966; **Resid:** Obstetrics & Gynecology, Yale-New Haven Hosp 1970; **Fellow:** Gynecologic Oncology, MD Anderson Cancer Ctr 1975; **Fac Appt:** Prof ObG, Yale Univ

Tarraza, Hector M MD [GO] - **Spec Exp:** Gynecologic Cancer; **Hospital:** Maine Med Ctr; **Address:** 100 Campus Drive, rm 116, Scarborough, ME 04074; **Phone:** 207-883-0069; **Board Cert:** Obstetrics & Gynecology 2012; Gynecologic Oncology 2012; **Med School:** Harvard Med Sch 1981; **Resid:** Obstetrics & Gynecology, Mass Genl Hosp 1985; **Fellow:** Gynecologic Oncology, Mass Genl Hosp 1987; **Fac Appt:** Prof ObG, Tufts Univ

Mid Atlantic

Abbas, Fouad M MD [GO] - **Spec Exp:** Gynecologic Cancer; Ovarian Cancer; Cervical Cancer; **Hospital:** Sinai Hosp - Baltimore; **Address:** Sinai Hosp, Div Gyn Onc, 2411 W Belvedere Ave, Ste 206, Baltimore, MD 21215; **Phone:** 410-601-9030; **Board Cert:** Obstetrics & Gynecology 2011; Gynecologic Oncology 2011; **Med School:** Univ MD Sch Med 1986; **Resid:** Obstetrics & Gynecology, Johns Hopkins Hosp 1990; **Fellow:** Gynecologic Oncology, Johns Hopkins Hosp 1992; **Fac Appt:** Asst Prof ObG, Univ MD Sch Med

Gynecologic Oncology

Abu-Rustum, Nadeem R MD [GO] - **Spec Exp:** Ovarian Cancer; Uterine Cancer; Cervical Cancer; Vulvar Disease/Cancer; **Hospital:** Meml Sloan-Kettering Cancer Ctr; **Address:** 1275 York Ave, New York, NY 10065; **Phone:** 212-639-7051; **Board Cert:** Obstetrics & Gynecology 2009; Gynecologic Oncology 2009; **Med School:** Lebanon 1990; **Resid:** Obstetrics & Gynecology, Greater Baltimore Med Ctr 1994; **Fellow:** Gynecologic Oncology, Meml Sloan-Kettering Cancer Ctr 1997; **Fac Appt:** Assoc Prof ObG, Cornell Univ-Weill Med Coll

Barakat, Richard R MD [GO] - **Spec Exp:** Laparoscopic Surgery; Ovarian Cancer; Uterine Cancer; Robotic Surgery; **Hospital:** Meml Sloan-Kettering Cancer Ctr; **Address:** 1275 York Ave, rm H1305, New York, NY 10065; **Phone:** 646-497-9055; **Board Cert:** Obstetrics & Gynecology 2012; Gynecologic Oncology 2012; **Med School:** SUNY Hlth Sci Ctr 1985; **Resid:** Obstetrics & Gynecology, Bellevue Hosp 1989; **Fellow:** Gynecologic Oncology, Meml Sloan Kettering Cancer Ctr 1991; **Fac Appt:** Assoc Prof ObG, Cornell Univ-Weill Med Coll

Barnes, Willard MD [GO] - **Spec Exp:** Pelvic Tumors; Gynecologic Cancer; **Hospital:** Georgetown Univ Hosp; **Address:** Georgetown Univ Hosp, Lombardi Cancer Ctr, Dept Gyn Oncology, 3800 Reservoir Rd NW, Washington, DC 20007-2194; **Phone:** 202-444-2114; **Board Cert:** Obstetrics & Gynecology 2011; Gynecologic Oncology 2011; **Med School:** Univ Miss 1979; **Resid:** Obstetrics & Gynecology, Univ Miss Med Ctr 1983; **Fellow:** Gynecologic Oncology, Georgetown Univ Med Ctr 1985; **Fac Appt:** Assoc Prof ObG, Georgetown Univ

Barter, James MD [GO] - **Spec Exp:** Laparoscopic Surgery; Ovarian Cancer; Gynecologic Cancer; **Hospital:** Holy Cross Hospital - Silver Spring, Suburban Hosp; **Address:** 6301 Executive Blvd, Rockville, MD 20852; **Phone:** 301-770-4967; **Board Cert:** Obstetrics & Gynecology 2011; Gynecologic Oncology 2011; **Med School:** Univ VA Sch Med 1977; **Resid:** Internal Medicine, Univ Kentucky Med Ctr 1979; Obstetrics & Gynecology, Duke Univ Med Ctr 1983; **Fellow:** Gynecologic Oncology, Univ Alabama 1985; **Fac Appt:** Clin Prof ObG, Georgetown Univ

Boice, Charles R MD [GO] - **Spec Exp:** Gynecologic Cancer; Ovarian Cancer; Cervical Cancer; **Hospital:** Washington Hosp Ctr; **Address:** 10301 Georgia Ave, Ste 205, Silver Springs, MD 20902; **Phone:** 301-592-1600; **Board Cert:** Obstetrics & Gynecology 1981; Gynecologic Oncology 1982; **Med School:** Loma Linda Univ 1973; **Resid:** Obstetrics & Gynecology, Los Angeles Med Ctr 1973; Surgery, City Hope Natl Med Ctr 1978; **Fellow:** Oncology, Univ Texas-MD Anderson Cancer Ctr 1980; **Fac Appt:** Assoc Clin Prof ObG, Univ Wash

Burger, Robert Allen MD [GO] - **Spec Exp:** Ovarian Cancer; Uterine Cancer; Cervical Cancer; Gestational Trophoblastic Disease; **Hospital:** Fox Chase Cancer Ctr (page 58); **Address:** Fox Chase Cancer Ctr, Women's Cancer Ctr, 333 Cottman Ave, Philadelphia, PA 19111; **Phone:** 215-728-2570; **Board Cert:** Obstetrics & Gynecology 2008; Gynecologic Oncology 2008; **Med School:** NYU Sch Med 1988; **Resid:** Obstetrics & Gynecology, Hosp U Penn 1992; **Fellow:** Gynecologic Oncology, UC Irvine Med Ctr 1996

Caputo, Thomas A MD [GO] - **Spec Exp:** Cervical Cancer; Ovarian Cancer; Uterine Cancer; Vulvar Disease/Cancer; **Hospital:** NY-Presby/Weill Cornell Med Ctr, NY (page 66); **Address:** NY Presby Hosp-Weill Cornell, 525 E 68th St, Ste J130, New York, NY 10021; **Phone:** 212-746-3179; **Board Cert:** Obstetrics & Gynecology 1993; Gynecologic Oncology 1977; **Med School:** UMDNJ-NJ Med Sch, Newark 1965; **Resid:** Obstetrics & Gynecology, Martland Hosp 1969; **Fellow:** Gynecologic Oncology, Emory Univ Hosp 1974; **Fac Appt:** Clin Prof ObG, Cornell Univ-Weill Med Coll

Carlson Jr, John A MD [GO] - **Spec Exp:** Gynecologic Cancer; Ovarian Cancer; Gynecologic Surgery-Complex; **Hospital:** St. Peter's Univ Hosp; **Address:** St Peter's Univ Hosp, 254 Easton Ave, Cares Bldg, New Brunswick, NJ 08901; **Phone:** 732-937-6003; **Board Cert:** Obstetrics & Gynecology 1981; Gynecologic Oncology 1982; **Med School:** Georgetown Univ 1974; **Resid:** Obstetrics & Gynecology, Hosp Univ Penn 1978; **Fellow:** Gynecologic Oncology, MD Anderson Cancer Ctr 1980; **Fac Appt:** Prof ObG, Drexel Univ Coll Med

Chi, Dennis S MD [GO] - **Spec Exp:** Ovarian Cancer; Uterine Cancer; Cervical Cancer; Gynecologic Surgery-Complex; **Hospital:** Meml Sloan-Kettering Cancer Ctr; **Address:** 1275 York Ave, New York, NY 10065; **Phone:** 212-639-5016; **Board Cert:** Obstetrics & Gynecology 2011; Gynecologic Oncology 2011; **Med School:** NYU Sch Med 1990; **Resid:** Obstetrics & Gynecology, NYU Med Ctr 1994; **Fellow:** Gynecologic Oncology, Meml Sloan Kettering Cancer Ctr 1997; **Fac Appt:** Prof ObG, NYU Sch Med

Cornelison, Terri L MD/PhD [GO] - **Spec Exp:** Gynecologic Cancer; Ovarian Cancer; Clinical Trials; **Hospital:** Johns Hopkins Hosp (page 61); **Address:** Johns Hopkins Kelly Gynecologic Onc Svc, 600 N Wolfe St Phipps Bldg - Ste 281, Baltimore, MD 21287; **Phone:** 410-502-4245; **Board Cert:** Obstetrics & Gynecology 2010; **Med School:** Yale Univ 1985; **Resid:** Obstetrics & Gynecology, Beth Israel Hosp 1989; **Fellow:** Gynecologic Oncology, Roswell Park Cancer Inst 1992; **Fac Appt:** Asst Prof ObG, Johns Hopkins Univ

Cosin, Jonathan A MD [GO] - **Spec Exp:** Gynecologic Cancer; **Hospital:** Washington Hosp Ctr; **Address:** Washington Hosp Ctr-Dept Gyn. Onc., 110 Irving St NW, rm 5B-33, Washington, DC 20010; **Phone:** 202-877-2391; **Board Cert:** Obstetrics & Gynecology 2009; Gynecologic Oncology 2009; **Med School:** Albany Med Coll 1991; **Resid:** Obstetrics & Gynecology, Baystate Med Ctr 1995; **Fellow:** Gynecology, Meml Sloan Kettering Cancer Ctr 1993; Gynecologic Oncology, Univ Minnesota Hosp 1998; **Fac Appt:** Asst Prof ObG, Georgetown Univ

Coukos, George MD/PhD [GO] - **Spec Exp:** Ovarian Cancer; Gynecologic Cancer; Vaccine Therapy; Clinical Trials; **Hospital:** Hosp Univ Penn - UPHS (page 72); **Address:** Jordan Ctr for Gyn Cancer, Perelman Center, 3400 Civic Center Blvd, Fl 3W, Philadelphia, PA 19104; **Phone:** 215-662-3318; **Board Cert:** Obstetrics & Gynecology 2011; Gynecologic Oncology 2011; **Med School:** Italy 1987; **Resid:** Obstetrics & Gynecology, Hosp Univ Penn 1997; **Fellow:** Gynecologic Oncology, Hosp Univ Penn 2000; **Fac Appt:** Prof ObG, Univ Pennsylvania

Curtin, John P MD [GO] - **Spec Exp:** Uterine Cancer; Ovarian Cancer; Laparoscopic Surgery; Gestational Trophoblastic Disease; **Hospital:** NYU Langone Med Ctr (page 68); **Address:** NYU Clin Cancer Ctr, 160 E 34th St Fl 4, New York, NY 10016-6402; **Phone:** 212-731-5345; **Board Cert:** Obstetrics & Gynecology 2011; Gynecologic Oncology 2011; **Med School:** Creighton Univ 1979; **Resid:** Obstetrics & Gynecology, Univ Minn Med Ctr 1984; **Fellow:** Gynecologic Oncology, Meml Sloan-Kettering Cancer Ctr 1988; **Fac Appt:** Prof ObG, NYU Sch Med

Dottino, Peter R MD [GO] - **Spec Exp:** Laparoscopic Surgery; Gynecologic Cancer; **Hospital:** Mount Sinai Med Ctr (page 64); **Address:** 800-A 5th Ave, Ste 405, The Group for Women, New York, NY 10065; **Phone:** 212-888-8439; **Board Cert:** Obstetrics & Gynecology 2007; Gynecologic Oncology 2007; **Med School:** Georgetown Univ 1979; **Resid:** Obstetrics & Gynecology, SUNY Downstate Med Ctr 1983; **Fellow:** Gynecologic Oncology, Mt Sinai Hosp 1985

Dunton, Charles J MD [GO] - **Spec Exp:** Ovarian Cancer; Uterine Cancer; Cervical Cancer; Gynecologic Surgery-Complex; **Hospital:** Lankenau Hosp; **Address:** Main Line Gyn Oncology, 100 E Lancaster Ave, Medical Office Bldg East, Ste 661, Wynnewood, PA 19096; **Phone:** 610-649-8085; **Board Cert:** Obstetrics & Gynecology 2011; Gynecologic Oncology 2011; **Med School:** Jefferson Med Coll 1980; **Resid:** Obstetrics & Gynecology, Lankenau Hosp 1984; **Fellow:** Gynecologic Oncology, Hosp Univ Penn 1989; **Fac Appt:** Prof ObG, Jefferson Med Coll

Edwards, Robert P MD [GO] - **Spec Exp:** Ovarian Cancer; Gynecologic Cancer; Cervical Cancer; Clinical Trials; **Hospital:** Magee-Womens Hosp - UPMC; **Address:** Univ Pittsburgh Physicians, 300 Halket St, Ste 2130, Pittsburgh, PA 15213; **Phone:** 412-641-1153; **Board Cert:** Obstetrics & Gynecology 2011; Gynecologic Oncology 2011; **Med School:** Univ Pittsburgh 1984; **Resid:** Obstetrics & Gynecology, Magee-Womens Hosp 1989; **Fellow:** Gynecologic Oncology, Univ Alabama 1993; **Fac Appt:** Prof ObG, Univ Pittsburgh

Fields, Abbie L MD [GO] - **Spec Exp:** Fertility Preservation in Cancer; Robotic Surgery; Cancer Genetics; Pelvic Reconstruction; **Hospital:** Washington Hosp Ctr; **Address:** Washington Hospital Center, 110 Irving St NW, rm 5B-33B, Washington, DC 20010; **Phone:** 202-877-2391; **Board Cert:** Obstetrics & Gynecology 2011; Gynecologic Oncology 2011; **Med School:** Ohio State Univ 1987; **Resid:** Obstetrics & Gynecology, Northwestern Univ 1991; **Fellow:** Gynecologic Oncology, Johns Hopkins Hosp 1993

Fishman, David A MD [GO] - **Spec Exp:** Gynecologic Cancer; Ovarian Cancer-Early Detection; Minimally Invasive Surgery; Ultrasound; **Hospital:** Mount Sinai Med Ctr (page 64); **Address:** 5 E 98th St, Fl 2, New York, NY 10029; **Phone:** 212-427-9898; **Board Cert:** Obstetrics & Gynecology 2011; Gynecologic Oncology 2011; **Med School:** Texas Tech Univ 1988; **Resid:** Obstetrics & Gynecology, Yale-New Haven Hosp 1992; **Fellow:** Gynecologic Oncology, Yale-New Haven Hosp 1994; **Fac Appt:** Prof ObG, Mount Sinai Sch Med

Giuntoli II, Robert Lawrence MD [GO] - **Spec Exp:** Gynecologic Cancer; Ovarian Cancer; Gestational Trophoblastic Disease; Immunotherapy; **Hospital:** Johns Hopkins Hosp (page 61); **Address:** Johns Hopkins Kelly Gynecologic Onc Svc, 600 N Wolfe St Phipps Bldg - Ste 281, Baltimore, MD 21287-1281; **Phone:** 410-502-4245; **Board Cert:** Obstetrics & Gynecology 2011; Gynecologic Oncology 2011; **Med School:** Univ Pennsylvania 1994; **Resid:** Obstetrics & Gynecology, Duke Univ Med Ctr 1998; **Fellow:** Gynecologic Oncology, Mayo Clin 2002; **Fac Appt:** Asst Prof ObG, Johns Hopkins Univ

Herzog, Thomas J MD [GO] - **Spec Exp:** Cervical Cancer; Gynecologic Cancer; Laparoscopic Surgery; Ovarian Cancer; **Hospital:** NY-Presby/Columbia Univ Med Ctr, NY (page 66); **Address:** Herbert Irving Pavilion, 161 Fort Washington Ave, 8-837, New York, NY 10032; **Phone:** 212-305-3410; **Board Cert:** Obstetrics & Gynecology 2008; Gynecologic Oncology 2008; **Med School:** Univ Cincinnati 1986; **Resid:** Obstetrics & Gynecology, Good Samaritan Hosp 1990; **Fellow:** Gynecologic Oncology, Barnes Jewish Hosp 1993; **Fac Appt:** Prof ObG, Columbia P&S

Kelley III, Joseph L MD [GO] - **Spec Exp:** Breast Cancer; Ovarian Cancer; Cervical Cancer; Gynecologic Cancer; **Hospital:** Magee-Womens Hosp - UPMC; **Address:** Uiv Pittsburgh Physicians, Div Gyn Oncology, 300 Halket St, Ste 1750, Pittsburgh, PA 15213; **Phone:** 412-641-5411; **Board Cert:** Obstetrics & Gynecology 2011; Gynecologic Oncology 2011; **Med School:** St Louis Univ 1985; **Resid:** Obstetrics & Gynecology, Magee-Womens Hosp 1989; **Fellow:** Gynecologic Oncology, MD Anderson Cancer Ctr 1991; **Fac Appt:** Prof ObG, Univ Pittsburgh

King, Stephanie A MD [GO] - **Spec Exp:** Ovarian Cancer; Uterine Cancer; Cervical Cancer; Trophoblastic Tumors; **Hospital:** Fox Chase Cancer Ctr (page 58); **Address:** Fox Chase Cancer Ctr-Div Gyn Oncology, 333 Cottman Ave, Philadelphia, PA 19111; **Phone:** 215-728-5628; **Board Cert:** Obstetrics & Gynecology 2011; Gynecologic Oncology 2011; **Med School:** Univ Pennsylvania 1983; **Resid:** Obstetrics & Gynecology, Hosp Univ Penn 1988; **Fac Appt:** Assoc Prof S, Drexel Univ Coll Med

Koulos, John P MD [GO] - **Spec Exp:** Uterine Cancer; Ovarian Cancer; Cervical Cancer; **Hospital:** Beth Israel Med Ctr - Petrie Division (page 56); **Address:** Beth Israel Hosp Cancer Ctr, 10 Union Square E, Ste 4C, New York, NY 10003; **Phone:** 212-844-5729; **Board Cert:** Obstetrics & Gynecology 2010; Gynecologic Oncology 2010; **Med School:** Northwestern Univ 1978; **Resid:** Obstetrics & Gynecology, Northwestern Univ Med Sch 1982; **Fellow:** Gynecologic Oncology, Meml Sloan Kettering Cancer Ctr 1984; **Fac Appt:** Assoc Prof ObG, Albert Einstein Coll Med

Lele, Shashikant B MD [GO] - **Spec Exp:** Ovarian Cancer; Reconstructive Surgery; Pelvic Surgery-Complex; **Hospital:** Roswell Park Cancer Inst, Buffalo General Hosp; **Address:** Roswell Park Cancer Inst, Elm & Carlton Streets, Buffalo, NY 14263; **Phone:** 716-845-5855; **Board Cert:** Obstetrics & Gynecology 1976; Gynecologic Oncology 1979; **Med School:** India 1968; **Resid:** Obstetrics & Gynecology, JJ Hosp-Grant Med Ctr 1970; Obstetrics & Gynecology, Mt Sinai Hosp 1973; **Fellow:** Gynecologic Oncology, Roswell Park Cancer Inst 1976; **Fac Appt:** Clin Prof ObG, SUNY Buffalo

Lin, Jeffrey Y MD [GO] - **Spec Exp:** Gynecologic Cancer; Cervical Cancer; Ovarian Cancer; **Hospital:** Sibley Mem Hosp, G Washington Univ Hosp; **Address:** Sibley Ctr for GYN Oncology, 5255 Loughboro Rd NW Fl 4, Washington, DC 20016; **Phone:** 202-243-5295; **Board Cert:** Obstetrics & Gynecology 2011; Gynecologic Oncology 2011; **Med School:** Albany Med Coll 1984; **Resid:** Obstetrics & Gynecology, George Washington Med Ctr 1988; Gynecologic Oncology, Univ Rochester Affil Hosp 1991; **Fac Appt:** Prof ObG, Geo Wash Univ

Morgan, Mark A MD [GO] - **Spec Exp:** Laparoscopic Surgery; Gynecologic Surgery-Complex; Gynecologic Cancer; Uro-Gynecology; **Hospital:** Fox Chase Cancer Ctr (page 58); **Address:** Fox Chase Cancer Ctr-Div Gyn Oncology, 333 Cottman Ave, Philadelphia, PA 19111; **Phone:** 215-214-1430; **Board Cert:** Obstetrics & Gynecology 2011; Gynecologic Oncology 2011; **Med School:** SUNY Downstate 1982; **Resid:** Obstetrics & Gynecology, Hosp Univ Penn 1986; **Fellow:** Gynecologic Oncology, Hosp Univ Penn 1988

Odunsi, Adekunle O MD/PhD [GO] - **Spec Exp:** Ovarian Cancer; Gynecologic Cancer; Immunotherapy; Clinical Trials; **Hospital:** Roswell Park Cancer Inst; **Address:** Roswell Park Cancer Inst, Elm and Carlton Streets, Buffalo, NY 14263; **Phone:** 716-845-5855; **Board Cert:** Obstetrics & Gynecology 2011; Gynecologic Oncology 2011; **Med School:** Nigeria 1984; **Resid:** Obstetrics & Gynecology, Rosie Maternity & Addenbrookes Hosps 1990; Obstetrics & Gynecology, Yale-New Haven Hosp 1999; **Fellow:** Gynecologic Oncology, Roswell Park Cancer Inst 2001; **Fac Appt:** Prof ObG, SUNY Buffalo

Randall, Thomas C MD [GO] - **Spec Exp:** Gynecologic Cancer; Robotic Surgery; **Hospital:** Pennsylvania Hosp-UPHS (page 72); **Address:** Penn Gyn Oncology at Pennsylvania Hosp, 801 Spruce St Fl 7, Philadelphia, PA 19107; **Phone:** 215-829-2345; **Board Cert:** Obstetrics & Gynecology 2011; Gynecologic Oncology 2011; **Med School:** Johns Hopkins Univ 1987; **Resid:** Obstetrics & Gynecology, Johns Hopkins Hosp 1991; **Fellow:** Gynecologic Oncology, Hosp Univ Penn 1992; **Fac Appt:** Assoc Clin Prof ObG, Univ Pennsylvania

Rosenblum, Norman G MD/PhD [GO] - **Spec Exp:** Ovarian Cancer; Uterine Cancer; Vulvar Disease/Cancer; **Hospital:** Thomas Jefferson Univ Hosp; **Address:** 925 Chesnut St, Rothman Bldg Fl 3 - Ste 320A, Philadelphia, PA 19107-5127; **Phone:** 215-955-6200; **Board Cert:** Obstetrics & Gynecology 2010; Gynecologic Oncology 2010; **Med School:** Jefferson Med Coll 1978; **Resid:** Obstetrics & Gynecology, Hosp Univ Penn 1982; **Fellow:** Gynecologic Oncology, Hosp Univ Penn 1984; **Fac Appt:** Prof ObG, Jefferson Med Coll

Rubin, Stephen C MD [GO] - **Spec Exp:** Ovarian Cancer; Uterine Cancer; Cervical Cancer; Gynecologic Cancer-Rare; **Hospital:** Hosp Univ Penn - UPHS (page 72); **Address:** 3400 Civic Center Blvd, PCAM Bldg - Fl 3 West, Jordan Ctr for Gynecologic Cancer, Philadelphia, PA 19104-4283; **Phone:** 215-662-3318; **Board Cert:** Obstetrics & Gynecology 2012; Gynecologic Oncology 2012; **Med School:** Univ Pennsylvania 1976; **Resid:** Obstetrics & Gynecology, Hosp Univ Penn 1980; **Fellow:** Gynecologic Oncology, Hosp Univ Penn 1982; **Fac Appt:** Prof, Univ Pennsylvania

Gynecologic Oncology

Southeast

Alvarez, Ronald D MD [GO] - **Spec Exp:** Gynecologic Cancer; Ovarian Cancer; **Hospital:** Univ of Ala Hosp at Birmingham, Brookwood Med Ctr; **Address:** Univ Alabama, Div Gyn Oncology, 619 6th Ave S, Birmingham, AL 35249; **Phone:** 205-934-4986; **Board Cert:** Obstetrics & Gynecology 2007; Gynecologic Oncology 2007; **Med School:** Louisiana State U, New Orleans 1983; **Resid:** Obstetrics & Gynecology, Univ Alabama Hosp 1987; **Fellow:** Gynecologic Oncology, Univ Alabama Hosp 1990; **Fac Appt:** Assoc Prof ObG, Univ Alabama

Berchuck, Andrew MD [GO] - **Spec Exp:** Ovarian Cancer; Uterine Cancer; **Hospital:** Duke Univ Hosp; **Address:** Duke Univ Med Center, DUMC Box 3079, Durham, NC 27710; **Phone:** 919-684-3765; **Board Cert:** Obstetrics & Gynecology 2011; Gynecologic Oncology 2011; **Med School:** Case West Res Univ 1980; **Resid:** Obstetrics & Gynecology, Case Western Reserve Univ Hosp 1984; **Fellow:** Gynecology, UT Southwestern Affil Hosp 1985; Gynecologic Oncology, Meml Sloan-Kettering Cancer Ctr 1987; **Fac Appt:** Prof ObG, Duke Univ

Bicher, Annette MD [GO] - **Spec Exp:** Ovarian Cancer; Laparoscopic Surgery; **Hospital:** Inova Fairfax Hosp; **Address:** Mid-Atlantic Pelvic Surgery Assocs, 3289 Woodburn Rd, Ste 320, Annandale, VA 22003; **Phone:** 703-698-7100; **Board Cert:** Obstetrics & Gynecology 2011; Gynecologic Oncology 2011; **Med School:** Univ Mich Med Sch 1987; **Resid:** Obstetrics & Gynecology, George Washington Univ Med Ctr 1991; **Fellow:** Research, NCI-NIH 1992; Gynecologic Oncology, UT MD Anderson Cancer Ctr 1994

Clarke-Pearson, Daniel L MD [GO] - **Spec Exp:** Gynecologic Surgery-Complex; Gynecologic Cancer; **Hospital:** NC Memorial Hosp - UNC, Wesley Long Comm Hosp; **Address:** NC Women's Hospital, 101 Manning Drive, Chapel Hill, NC 27599; **Phone:** 919-966-5280; **Board Cert:** Obstetrics & Gynecology 2006; Gynecologic Oncology 2006; **Med School:** Case West Res Univ 1975; **Resid:** Obstetrics & Gynecology, Duke Univ Med Ctr 1979; **Fellow:** Gynecologic Oncology, Duke Univ Med Ctr 1981; **Fac Appt:** Prof ObG, Univ NC Sch Med

Creasman, William T MD [GO] - **Spec Exp:** Uterine Cancer; Ovarian Cancer; Gynecologic Cancer-Rare; Clinical Trials; **Hospital:** MUSC Med Ctr; **Address:** MUSC-Dept ObGyn, 96 Jonathan Lucas St CSB 634, Charleston, SC 29425; **Phone:** 843-792-4509; **Board Cert:** Obstetrics & Gynecology 1991; Gynecologic Oncology 1974; **Med School:** Baylor Coll Med 1960; **Resid:** Obstetrics & Gynecology, Rochester Med Ctr 1967; **Fellow:** Gynecologic Oncology, Anderson Hosp Tumor Inst 1969; **Fac Appt:** Prof ObG, Med Univ SC

Currie, John L MD [GO] - **Spec Exp:** Gynecologic Cancer; Pelvic Reconstruction; Gynecologic Problems of Obesity; **Hospital:** Columbus Regl Med Ctr; **Address:** John B Amos Cancer Center, 1831 5th Ave, Columbus, GA 31904; **Phone:** 706-320-8700; **Board Cert:** Obstetrics & Gynecology 1991; Gynecologic Oncology 1982; **Med School:** Univ NC Sch Med 1967; **Resid:** Gynecologic Oncology, Hosp Univ Penn 1972; **Fellow:** Gynecologic Oncology, Duke Univ Med Ctr 1980

DePriest, Paul D MD [GO] - **Spec Exp:** Ovarian Cancer-Early Detection; Cervical Cancer; Pap Smear Abnormalities; **Hospital:** Univ of Kentucky Albert B. Chandler Hosp; **Address:** Markey Cancer Ctr, Div Gyn Onc, Whitney-Hendrickson Bldg, 800 Rose St, rm 331E1, Lexington, KY 40536; **Phone:** 859-323-5277; **Board Cert:** Obstetrics & Gynecology 2011; Gynecologic Oncology 2011; **Med School:** Univ KY Coll Med 1985; **Resid:** Obstetrics & Gynecology, Univ Kentucky Med Ctr 1989; **Fellow:** Gynecologic Oncology, Univ Kentucky 1991; **Fac Appt:** Prof ObG, Univ KY Coll Med

Duska, Linda R MD [GO] - **Spec Exp:** Cervical Cancer; Gynecologic Cancer; Gynecologic Surgery-Complex; Ovarian Cancer; **Hospital:** Univ of Virginia Health Sys; **Address:** Dept of Obstetrics & Gynecology, Division of Gynecologic Oncology, Box 800712, Charlottesville, VA 22908; **Phone:** 434-924-1851; **Board Cert:** Obstetrics & Gynecology 2011; Gynecologic Oncology 2011; **Med School:** NYU Sch Med 1991; **Resid:** Obstetrics & Gynecology, John Hopkins Hosp 1995; **Fellow:** Gynecologic Oncology, MA Gen Hosp 1998; **Fac Appt:** Assoc Prof ObG, Univ VA Sch Med

Finan, Michael A MD [GO] - **Spec Exp:** Ovarian Cancer; Cervical Cancer; Uterine Cancer; **Hospital:** Univ of S AL Med Ctr, Univ of S Alabama Chil and Wom Hosp; **Address:** 1660 Springhill Ave, Mobile, AL 36604; **Phone:** 251-665-8000; **Board Cert:** Obstetrics & Gynecology 2011; Gynecologic Oncology 2011; **Med School:** Louisiana State U, New Orleans 1986; **Resid:** Obstetrics & Gynecology, Univ South Fla Affil Hosps 1990; **Fellow:** Gynecologic Oncology, H Lee Moffitt Cancer Ctr 1992; **Fac Appt:** Prof ObG, Univ S Ala Coll Med

Fiorica, James V MD [GO] - **Spec Exp:** Endometriosis; Breast Cancer; Uterine Cancer; **Hospital:** Sarasota Meml Hosp; **Address:** 1888 Hillview St, Sarasota, FL 34239; **Phone:** 941-917-8383; **Board Cert:** Obstetrics & Gynecology 2010; Gynecologic Oncology 2010; **Med School:** Tufts Univ 1982; **Resid:** Obstetrics & Gynecology, Univ South Fla Affil Hosp 1986; **Fellow:** Gynecologic Oncology, Univ South Fla Affil Hosp 1989; Breast Disease, Tufts Univ 1990; **Fac Appt:** Clin Prof ObG, Univ S Fla Coll Med

Ghamande, Sharad A MD [GO] - **Spec Exp:** Ovarian Cancer; Gynecologic Surgery-Complex; Clinical Trials; **Hospital:** Med Coll of GA Hosp and Clin (MCG Health Inc), Univ HC Sys - Augusta; **Address:** MCG Health Cancer Centr, 1411 Laney Walker Blvd, Augusta, GA 30912; **Phone:** 706-721-6744; **Board Cert:** Obstetrics & Gynecology 2011; Gynecologic Oncology 2011; **Med School:** India 1990; **Resid:** Obstetrics & Gynecology, Boston Univ Hosp 1997; **Fellow:** Gynecologic Oncology, Roswell Park Cancer Inst 2000; **Fac Appt:** Assoc Prof ObG, Med Coll GA

Havrilesky, Laura J MD [GO] - **Spec Exp:** Ovarian Cancer; **Hospital:** Duke Univ Hosp; **Address:** Duke Univ Med Ctr, Gyn Oncology, Box 3079, Durham, NC 27710; **Phone:** 919-684-3765; **Board Cert:** Obstetrics & Gynecology 2011; Gynecologic Oncology 2011; **Med School:** Duke Univ 1995; **Resid:** Obstetrics & Gynecology, Duke Univ Med Ctr 1999; **Fellow:** Gynecologic Oncology, Duke Univ Med Ctr 2002; **Fac Appt:** Assoc Prof ObG, Duke Univ

Horowitz, Ira R MD [GO] - **Spec Exp:** Laparoscopic Surgery; Ovarian Cancer; Cervical Cancer; **Hospital:** Emory Univ Hosp, Emory Univ Hosp Midtown; **Address:** Emory Clinic, 1365A Clifton Rd NE Fl 4, Atlanta, GA 30322; **Phone:** 404-778-3401; **Board Cert:** Obstetrics & Gynecology 2011; Gynecologic Oncology 2011; **Med School:** Baylor Coll Med 1980; **Resid:** Obstetrics & Gynecology, Baylor Affil Hosp 1984; **Fellow:** Gynecologic Oncology, Johns Hopkins Hosp 1987; **Fac Appt:** Prof ObG, Emory Univ

Kohler, Matthew F MD [GO] - **Spec Exp:** Gynecologic Surgery-Complex; Gynecologic Cancer; Gestational Trophoblastic Disease; **Hospital:** MUSC Med Ctr; **Address:** MUSC Med Ctr-Women's Hlth Ob/Gyn, 86 Jonathan Lucas St, MS 957, Charleston, SC 29425; **Phone:** 843-792-9300; **Board Cert:** Obstetrics & Gynecology 2011; Gynecologic Oncology 2011; **Med School:** Duke Univ 1987; **Resid:** Obstetrics & Gynecology, Duke Univ Med Ctr 1991; **Fellow:** Gynecologic Oncology, Duke Univ 1994; **Fac Appt:** Prof ObG, Med Univ SC

Lancaster, Johnathan M MD/PhD [GO] - **Spec Exp:** Ovarian Cancer; Cancer Genetics; Gene Therapy; **Hospital:** H Lee Moffitt Cancer Ctr & Research Inst (page 59); **Address:** H Lee Moffitt Cancer Ctr - Gyn Oncology, 12902 Magnolia Drive, The Ctr for Women's Oncology, Tampa, FL 33612; **Phone:** 888-860-2778; **Board Cert:** Obstetrics & Gynecology 2011; Gynecologic Oncology 2011; **Med School:** Wales, UK 1997; **Resid:** Obstetrics & Gynecology, Duke Univ Med Ctr 2000; **Fellow:** Gynecologic Oncology, Duke Univ Med Ctr 2003; **Fac Appt:** Asst Prof ObG, Univ S Fla Coll Med

Lentz, Samuel S MD [GO] - **Spec Exp:** Gynecologic Cancer; Pelvic Reconstruction; Incontinence; Incontinence-Fecal; **Hospital:** Wake Forest Baptist Med Ctr; **Address:** Wake Forest Univ Sch Med, Div Gyn Oncology, Medical Center Blvd, Winston-Salem, NC 27157; **Phone:** 336-716-6673; **Board Cert:** Obstetrics & Gynecology 2011; Gynecologic Oncology 2011; **Med School:** Wake Forest Univ 1978; **Resid:** Obstetrics & Gynecology, NC Baptist Hosp 1982; **Fellow:** Gynecologic Oncology, Mayo Clinic 1989; **Fac Appt:** Prof ObG, Wake Forest Univ

Lucci, Joseph A MD [GO] - **Spec Exp:** Cervical Cancer; **Hospital:** Univ of Miami Hosp & Clins/Sylvester Comp Canc Ctr, Jackson Meml Hosp; **Address:** UMHC Sylvester Comp Cancer Ctr, 1475 NW 12th Ave, Ste 3500, Miami, FL 33136; **Phone:** 305-243-2233; **Board Cert:** Obstetrics & Gynecology 2007; Gynecologic Oncology 2007; **Med School:** Univ Tex, Houston 1984; **Resid:** Obstetrics & Gynecology, St Josephs Hosp 1988; **Fellow:** Gynecologic Oncology, UC Irvine 1992; **Fac Appt:** Clin Prof ObG, Univ Miami Sch Med

Makhija, Sharmila K MD [GO] - **Spec Exp:** Ovarian Cancer; Cervical Cancer; Uterine Cancer; **Hospital:** Univ of Louisville Hosp, Norton Hosp; **Address:** James Graham Brown Cancer Ctr, 529 S Jackson St Fl 3, Louisville, KY 40202; **Phone:** 502-561-7220; **Board Cert:** Obstetrics & Gynecology 2011; Gynecologic Oncology 2011; **Med School:** Univ Alabama 1992; **Resid:** Obstetrics & Gynecology, Univ Louisville Hosp 1996; **Fellow:** Gynecologic Oncology, Meml Sloan Kettering Cancer Ctr 1999; **Fac Appt:** Prof ObG, Univ Louisville Sch Med

Modesitt, Susan C MD [GO] - **Spec Exp:** Gynecologic Cancer; Ovarian Cancer; Vulvar Disease/Cancer; **Hospital:** Univ of Virginia Health Sys; **Address:** Gynecologic Oncology Division, University of Virginia Health System, P.O. Box 800712, Charlottesville, VA 22908-0712; **Phone:** 434-924-5197; **Board Cert:** Obstetrics & Gynecology 2011; Gynecologic Oncology 2011; **Med School:** Univ VA Sch Med 1995; **Resid:** Obstetrics & Gynecology, Univ NC Hlth Care System 1999; **Fellow:** Gynecologic Oncology, Univ TX- MD Anderson Cancer Ctr 2002; **Fac Appt:** Assoc Prof ObG, Univ VA Sch Med

Orr Jr, James W MD [GO] - **Spec Exp:** Gynecologic Cancer; **Hospital:** Lee Memorial Hlth Systems; **Address:** 8931 Colonial Ctr Drive, Ste 400, Fort Myers, FL 33905; **Phone:** 239-334-6626; **Board Cert:** Obstetrics & Gynecology 2008; Gynecologic Oncology 2008; **Med School:** Univ VA Sch Med 1976; **Resid:** Obstetrics & Gynecology, Univ Ala Med Ctr 1980; **Fellow:** Gynecologic Oncology, Univ Ala Med Ctr 1982; **Fac Appt:** Clin Prof ObG, Univ S Fla Coll Med

Penalver, Manuel A MD [GO] - **Spec Exp:** Gynecologic Cancer; Cervical Cancer; Pelvic Tumors; **Hospital:** Doctors' Hosp - Coral Gables (FL), Baptist Hosp of Miami; **Address:** 5000 University Drive, Ste 3300, Coral Gables, FL 33146; **Phone:** 305-663-7001; **Board Cert:** Obstetrics & Gynecology 2011; Gynecologic Oncology 2011; **Med School:** Univ Miami Sch Med 1977; **Resid:** Obstetrics & Gynecology, ackson Meml Hosp 1982; **Fellow:** Gynecologic Oncology, Jackson Meml Hosp 1984

Poliakoff, Steven R MD [GO] - **Spec Exp:** Ovarian Cancer; Minimally Invasive Surgery; Cancer Genetics; Robotic Surgery; **Hospital:** Mount Sinai Med Ctr - Miami, South Miami Hosp; **Address:** 6280 Sunset Dr, Ste 502, South Miami, FL 33143-4870; **Phone:** 305-596-0870; **Board Cert:** Obstetrics & Gynecology 1983; **Med School:** Univ NC Sch Med 1975; **Resid:** Obstetrics & Gynecology, Johns Hopkins Hosp 1979; **Fellow:** Gynecologic Oncology, Jackson Meml Hosp/Univ Miami 1981

Runowicz, Carolyn MD [GO] - **Spec Exp:** Ovarian Cancer; Cervical Cancer; Breast Cancer; **Hospital:** Jackson N Med Ctr; **Address:** 11200 S W 8th St SW, AHC2 Bldg Fl 6 - Ste 693, Miami, FL 33199; **Phone:** 305-348-4372; **Board Cert:** Obstetrics & Gynecology 2011; Gynecologic Oncology 2011; **Med School:** Jefferson Med Coll 1977; **Resid:** Obstetrics & Gynecology, Mount Sinai Med Ctr 1981; **Fellow:** Gynecologic Oncology, Mount Sinai Med Ctr 1983; **Fac Appt:** Prof ObG, FIU Coll Med

Soper, John T MD [GO] - **Spec Exp:** Gynecologic Cancer; Gynecologic Surgery-Complex; Gestational Trophoblastic Disease; **Hospital:** NC Memorial Hosp - UNC, Rex HlthCare; **Address:** Div Gyn-Onc, Dept OB/GYN, B110 Physicians Office Bldg, 170 Manning Drive, Chapel Hill, NC 27599-7572; **Phone:** 919-966-1195; **Board Cert:** Obstetrics & Gynecology 2011; Gynecologic Oncology 2011; **Med School:** Univ Iowa Coll Med 1978; **Resid:** Obstetrics & Gynecology, Univ Utah Med Ctr 1982; **Fellow:** Obstetrics & Gynecology, Duke Univ Med Ctr 1985; **Fac Appt:** Prof ObG, Univ NC Sch Med

Spann Jr, Cyril O MD [GO] - **Spec Exp:** Gynecologic Cancer; Ovarian Cancer; Robotic Surgery; **Hospital:** Grady Hlth Sys, Emory Univ Hosp Midtown; **Address:** Dept Gynecology & Obstetrics, 69 Jesse Hill Jr Drive, Ste 400, Atlanta, GA 30303; **Phone:** 404-778-3401; **Board Cert:** Obstetrics & Gynecology 2005; Gynecologic Oncology 2005; **Med School:** Meharry Med Coll 1981; **Resid:** Obstetrics & Gynecology, Emory Univ Med Ctr 1985; **Fellow:** Gynecologic Oncology, NC Meml Hosp 1989; **Fac Appt:** Prof ObG, Emory Univ

Valea, Fidel A MD [GO] - **Spec Exp:** Cervical Cancer; Laparoscopic Surgery; **Hospital:** Duke Univ Hosp; **Address:** Duke Univ Med Ctr, Box 3079, Durham, NC 27710; **Phone:** 919-664-3725; **Board Cert:** Obstetrics & Gynecology 2011; Gynecologic Oncology 2011; **Med School:** SUNY Stony Brook 1985; **Resid:** Surgery, Univ NC Hosps 1987; Obstetrics & Gynecology, Univ NC Hosps 1990; **Fellow:** Gynecologic Oncology, Univ NC Hosps 1992; **Fac Appt:** Assoc Prof ObG, Duke Univ

Van Nagell Jr, John R MD [GO] - **Spec Exp:** Ovarian Cancer; Cervical Cancer; **Hospital:** Univ of Kentucky Albert B. Chandler Hosp; **Address:** Markey Cancer Ctr, Div Gyn Onc, Whitney-Hendrickson Bldg, 800 Rose St Fl 3, Lexington, KY 40536; **Phone:** 859-323-5553; **Board Cert:** Obstetrics & Gynecology 1973; Gynecologic Oncology 1976; **Med School:** Univ Pennsylvania 1967; **Resid:** Obstetrics & Gynecology, Univ Kentucky Med Ctr 1971; **Fellow:** Gynecologic Oncology, Univ Kentucky 1973; **Fac Appt:** Prof ObG, Univ KY Coll Med

Midwest

Cliby, William A MD [GO] - **Spec Exp:** Ovarian Cancer; Robotic Surgery; **Hospital:** Mayo Med Ctr & Clin - Rochester; **Address:** Mayo Clinic, 200 First St SW, Rochester, MN 55905; **Phone:** 507-266-9323; **Board Cert:** Obstetrics & Gynecology 2011; Gynecologic Oncology 2011; **Med School:** Univ VT Coll Med 1987; **Resid:** Obstetrics & Gynecology, Duke Univ Med Ctr 1991; **Fellow:** Gynecologic Oncology, Mayo Clinic 1994; Research, Fred Hutchinson Cancer Rsch Ctr 1997; **Fac Appt:** Prof ObG, Mayo Med Sch

Copeland, Larry J MD [GO] - **Spec Exp:** Ovarian Cancer; Uterine Cancer; Gynecologic Cancer; Gynecologic Cancer-Rare; **Hospital:** Arthur G James Cancer Hosp & Research Inst, Ohio St Univ Med Ctr; **Address:** 320 W 10th Ave, Starling L Bldg - Ste M210, Columbus, OH 43210; **Phone:** 614-293-7642; **Board Cert:** Obstetrics & Gynecology 2012; Gynecologic Oncology 2012; **Med School:** Univ Western Ontario 1973; **Resid:** Obstetrics & Gynecology, McMaster Univ Affil Hosps 1977; **Fellow:** Gynecologic Oncology, MD Anderson Cancer Ctr-Univ Tex 1979; **Fac Appt:** Prof ObG, Ohio State Univ

De Geest, Koen MD [GO] - **Spec Exp:** Ovarian Cancer; Uterine Cancer; Clinical Trials; **Hospital:** Univ Iowa Hosp & Clinics; **Address:** Univ Iowa, Div Gynecological Oncology, 200 Hawkins Drive, rm 4630 JCP, Iowa City, IA 52242; **Phone:** 319-356-2015; **Board Cert:** Obstetrics & Gynecology 2011; Gynecologic Oncology 2011; **Med School:** Belgium 1977; **Resid:** Obstetrics & Gynecology, Univ Ghent 1982; **Fellow:** Gynecologic Oncology, Penn State/Hershey Med Ctr 1990; **Fac Appt:** Prof ObG, Univ Iowa Coll Med

Gynecologic Oncology

Del Priore, Giuseppe MD [GO] - **Spec Exp:** Fertility Preservation in Cancer; **Hospital:** IU Health University Hosp; **Address:** Indiana Univ Cancer Pavilion, 535 Barnhill Drive, rm 433, Indianapolis, IN 46202; **Phone:** 317-944-2130; **Board Cert:** Obstetrics & Gynecology 2010; Gynecologic Oncology 2010; **Med School:** SUNY Downstate 1987; **Resid:** Obstetrics & Gynecology, Northwestern Meml Hosp 1991; **Fellow:** Gynecologic Oncology, Univ Rochester-Strong Meml 1995; **Fac Appt:** Prof ObG, Indiana Univ

Fowler, Jeffrey M MD [GO] - **Spec Exp:** Laparoscopic Surgery; Gynecologic Cancer; Robotic Surgery; Pelvic Reconstruction; **Hospital:** Ohio St Univ Med Ctr; **Address:** OSU Gynecologic Oncology, 3651 Ridge Mill Drive, Hilliard, OH 43026; **Phone:** 614-293-3873; **Board Cert:** Obstetrics & Gynecology 2009; Gynecologic Oncology 2009; **Med School:** Northwestern Univ 1985; **Resid:** Obstetrics & Gynecology, Ohio State Univ Hosp 1989; **Fellow:** Gynecologic Oncology, Cedars-Sinai Med Ctr-UCLA 1991; **Fac Appt:** Prof ObG, Ohio State Univ

Gostout, Bobbie S MD [GO] - **Hospital:** Mayo Med Ctr & Clin - Rochester, St. Mary's Hosp - Rochester MN (Mayo); **Address:** 200 First St SW, Ste W4, Rochester, MN 55905; **Phone:** 507-538-8400; **Board Cert:** Obstetrics & Gynecology 2011; Gynecologic Oncology 2011; **Med School:** Mayo Med Sch 1986; **Resid:** Obstetrics & Gynecology, Mayo Med Ctr & Clin 1991; **Fellow:** Research, Mayo Med Ctr & Clin 1993; Gynecologic Oncology, Mayo Med Ctr & Clin 1996; **Fac Appt:** Asst Prof ObG, Mayo Med Sch

Johnston, Carolyn M MD [GO] - **Spec Exp:** Gynecologic Surgery-Complex; Cervical Cancer; **Hospital:** Univ of Michigan Hosp; **Address:** Womens Hosp-Div Gyn Oncology, 1500 E Med Ctr Drive, rm 5902, Ann Arbor, MI 48109-0276; **Phone:** 734-647-8906; **Board Cert:** Obstetrics & Gynecology 2011; Gynecologic Oncology 2011; **Med School:** Yale Univ 1984; **Resid:** Obstetrics & Gynecology, Univ Chicago Hosp 1988; **Fellow:** Gynecologic Oncology, Mount Sinai Hosp 1990; **Fac Appt:** Assoc Clin Prof ObG, Univ Mich Med Sch

Lurain, John R MD [GO] - **Spec Exp:** Gestational Trophoblastic Disease; Uterine Cancer; Ovarian Cancer; Cervical Cancer; **Hospital:** Northwestern Meml Hosp; **Address:** Northwestern Medical Faculty Foundation, 250 E Superior St Fl 4 - rm 420, Chicago, IL 60611-3056; **Phone:** 312-695-0990; **Board Cert:** Obstetrics & Gynecology 1977; Gynecologic Oncology 1981; **Med School:** Univ NC Sch Med 1972; **Resid:** Obstetrics & Gynecology, Univ Pittsburgh Magee-Womens Hosp 1975; **Fellow:** Gynecologic Oncology, Roswell Park Cancer Inst 1979; **Fac Appt:** Prof ObG, Northwestern Univ

Moore, David H MD [GO] - **Spec Exp:** Cervical Cancer; Ovarian Cancer; Clinical Trials; Robotic Surgery; **Hospital:** Franciscan St. Francis Hlth-Indianapolis, Community Hosps - Indianapolis; **Address:** 8111 S Emerson Ave Cancer Bldg - Ste 204, Indianapolis, IN 46237; **Phone:** 317-528-2555; **Board Cert:** Obstetrics & Gynecology 2011; Gynecologic Oncology 2011; **Med School:** Indiana Univ 1982; **Resid:** Obstetrics & Gynecology, Indiana Univ Hosp 1986; **Fellow:** Gynecologic Oncology, Univ N Carolina 1988

Mutch, David G MD [GO] - **Spec Exp:** Gynecologic Cancer; Pelvic Reconstruction; **Hospital:** Barnes-Jewish Hosp; **Address:** 4911 Barnes Jewish Hosp Plaza, CB 8064, St Louis, MO 63110; **Phone:** 314-362-3181; **Board Cert:** Obstetrics & Gynecology 2011; Gynecologic Oncology 2011; **Med School:** Washington Univ, St Louis 1980; **Resid:** Obstetrics & Gynecology, Barnes Hosp-Wash Univ 1984; **Fellow:** Gynecologic Oncology, Duke Univ Med Ctr 1987; **Fac Appt:** Prof ObG, Washington Univ, St Louis

Potkul, Ronald K MD [GO] - **Spec Exp:** Ovarian Cancer; Cervical Cancer; Robotic Surgery; Vulvar & Vaginal Cancer; **Hospital:** Loyola Univ Med Ctr; **Address:** Loyola Univ Med Ctr, 2160 S 1st Ave Bldg 112 - rm 267, Maywood, IL 60153; **Phone:** 708-327-3500; **Board Cert:** Obstetrics & Gynecology 2011; Gynecologic Oncology 2011; **Med School:** Univ Chicago-Pritzker Sch Med 1981; **Resid:** Obstetrics & Gynecology, Univ Chicago Hosps 1985; **Fellow:** Gynecologic Oncology, Georgetown Univ Hosp 1988; **Fac Appt:** Prof ObG, Loyola Univ-Stritch Sch Med

Rader, Janet S MD [GO] - **Spec Exp:** Cervical Cancer; Ovarian Cancer; Uterine Cancer; **Hospital:** Froedtert and Med Ctr of WI; **Address:** Med Coll of Wisconsin, Dept OB/GYN, 9200 W Wisconsin Ave, Milwaukee, WI 53226; **Phone:** 414-805-6606; **Board Cert:** Obstetrics & Gynecology 2011; Gynecologic Oncology 2011; **Med School:** Univ MO-Columbia Sch Med 1983; **Resid:** Obstetrics & Gynecology, Michael Reese Hosp 1987; **Fellow:** Gynecologic Oncology, Johns Hopkins Hosp 1990; **Fac Appt:** Prof ObG, Washington Univ, St Louis

Reynolds, R Kevin MD [GO] - **Hospital:** Univ of Michigan Hosp; **Address:** Women's Hosp, Div Gyn Onc, 1500 E Med Ctr Drive, rm L4510, Ann Arbor, MI 48109-0276; **Phone:** 734-764-9106; **Board Cert:** Obstetrics & Gynecology 2011; Gynecologic Oncology 2011; **Med School:** Univ New Mexico 1982; **Resid:** Obstetrics & Gynecology, Univ Vt Hosp 1986; **Fellow:** Gynecologic Oncology, Univ Mich Med Ctr 1991; **Fac Appt:** Asst Prof ObG, Univ Mich Med Sch

Rice, Laurel W MD [GO] - **Spec Exp:** Ovarian Cancer; Uterine Cancer; Cervical Cancer; **Hospital:** Univ WI Hosp & Clins; **Address:** 600 Highland Ave, Ste H4-636, Madison, WI 53792; **Phone:** 608-263-3194; **Board Cert:** Obstetrics & Gynecology 2011; Gynecologic Oncology 2011; **Med School:** Univ Colorado 1983; **Resid:** Obstetrics & Gynecology, Brigham-Womens Hosp 1987; **Fellow:** Obstetrics & Gynecology, Brigham-Womens Hosp 1989; **Fac Appt:** Assoc Prof ObG, Univ VA Sch Med

Rose, Peter G MD [GO] - **Spec Exp:** Cervical Cancer; Ovarian Cancer; Uterine Cancer; **Hospital:** Cleveland Clin (page 55), MetroHealth Med Ctr; **Address:** Cleveland Clin, 9500 Euclid Ave A-81, Cleveland, OH 44195; **Phone:** 216-444-1712; **Board Cert:** Obstetrics & Gynecology 2011; Gynecologic Oncology 2011; **Med School:** Boston Univ 1981; **Resid:** Surgery, Vanderbilt Univ Med Ctr 1983; Obstetrics & Gynecology, Ohio State Univ Med Ctr 1986; **Fellow:** Gynecologic Oncology, Roswell Park Cancer Inst 1988; **Fac Appt:** Prof ObG, Case West Res Univ

Rotmensch, Jacob MD [GO] - **Spec Exp:** Gynecologic Cancer; Ovarian Cancer; Cervical Cancer; Uterine Cancer; **Hospital:** Rush Univ Med Ctr; **Address:** Univ Gynecologic Oncology Assocs, 1725 W Harrison St, Professional Bldg, Ste 829, Chicago, IL 60612; **Phone:** 312-942-6300; **Board Cert:** Obstetrics & Gynecology 2011; Gynecologic Oncology 2011; **Med School:** Meharry Med Coll 1977; **Resid:** Obstetrics & Gynecology, Johns Hopkins Hosp 1981; **Fellow:** Gynecologic Oncology, Johns Hopkins Hosp 1984; **Fac Appt:** Prof ObG, Rush Med Coll

Schink, Julian C MD [GO] - **Spec Exp:** Ovarian Cancer; **Hospital:** Northwestern Meml Hosp; **Address:** Northwestern Medical Faculty Foundation, 250 E Superior St, Ste 04-420, Chicago, IL 60611; **Phone:** 312-695-0990; **Board Cert:** Obstetrics & Gynecology 2011; Gynecologic Oncology 2011; **Med School:** Univ Tex, San Antonio 1982; **Resid:** Obstetrics & Gynecology, Northwestern Univ Med Sch 1986; **Fellow:** Gynecologic Oncology, UCLA Med Ctr 1988; **Fac Appt:** Prof ObG, Northwestern Univ

Smith, Donna M MD [GO] - **Spec Exp:** Cervical Cancer; Ovarian Cancer; **Hospital:** Loyola Univ Med Ctr; **Address:** Loyola Univ Medical Ctr, 2160 S 1st Ave Bldg 112 - rm 267, Maywood, IL 60153; **Phone:** 708-327-3500; **Board Cert:** Obstetrics & Gynecology 2008; Gynecologic Oncology 2008; **Med School:** Univ MO-Kansas City 1980; **Resid:** Obstetrics & Gynecology, Emory Univ Hosp 1984; **Fellow:** Gynecologic Oncology, Georgetown Univ Med Ctr 1987; **Fac Appt:** Assoc Prof ObG, Loyola Univ-Stritch Sch Med

Gynecologic Oncology

Stehman, Frederick B MD [GO] - **Spec Exp:** Clinical Trials; Gynecologic Cancer; **Hospital:** IU Health University Hosp, Wishard Hlth Srvs; **Address:** Indiana Univ Cancer Pavilion, 535 Barnhill Drive, rm 436, Indianapolis, IN 46202; **Phone:** 317-944-2130; **Board Cert:** Obstetrics & Gynecology 2005; Gynecologic Oncology 2003; **Med School:** Univ Mich Med Sch 1972; **Resid:** Obstetrics & Gynecology, Univ Kansas Med Ctr 1975; Surgery, Univ Kansas Med Ctr 1977; **Fellow:** Gynecologic Oncology, UCLA Med Ctr 1979; **Fac Appt:** Prof Emeritus ObG, Indiana Univ

Waggoner, Steven MD [GO] - **Spec Exp:** Ovarian Cancer; Cervical Cancer; Uterine Cancer; **Hospital:** Univ Hosps Case Med Ctr (page 74); **Address:** Dept Ob/Gyn & Gyn Oncology, 11100 Euclid Ave, rm 7128, UH MacDonald Women's Hospital, Cleveland, OH 44106; **Phone:** 216-844-3954; **Board Cert:** Obstetrics & Gynecology 2011; Gynecologic Oncology 2011; **Med School:** Univ Wash 1984; **Resid:** Obstetrics & Gynecology, Univ Chicago Hosps 1988; **Fellow:** Gynecologic Oncology, Georgetown Univ Med Ctr 1991; **Fac Appt:** Prof ObG, Case West Res Univ

Great Plains and Mountains

Davidson, Susan MD [GO] - **Spec Exp:** Gynecologic Cancer; **Hospital:** Univ of CO Hosp - Anschutz Inpatient Pav; **Address:** Univ Colorado Hosp, Dept OB/GYN, PO Box 6510- F704, 1665 Aurora Ct, Denver, CO 80045; **Phone:** 720-848-0300; **Board Cert:** Obstetrics & Gynecology 2011; Gynecologic Oncology 2011; **Med School:** Univ Tex, San Antonio 1984; **Resid:** Obstetrics & Gynecology, Univ Texas Med Ctr 1988; **Fellow:** Gynecologic Oncology, Meml Sloan Kettering Cancer Ctr 1990; **Fac Appt:** Assoc Prof ObG, Univ Colorado

Remmenga, Steven W MD [GO] - **Spec Exp:** Ovarian Cancer; Cervical Cancer; Gynecologic Cancer; **Hospital:** Nebraska Med Ctr; **Address:** Department of Obsterics nd Gynecology, MS 0, 983255 Nebraska Med Ctr, Omaha, NE 68198-3255; **Phone:** 402-559-5068; **Board Cert:** Obstetrics & Gynecology 2011; Gynecologic Oncology 2011; **Med School:** Univ Nebr Coll Med 1981; **Resid:** Obstetrics & Gynecology, Naval Hospital 1986; **Fellow:** Gynecologic Oncology, Walter Reed Army Med Ctr 1990; **Fac Appt:** Prof ObG, Univ Nebr Coll Med

Soisson, Andrew P MD [GO] - **Spec Exp:** Cervical Cancer; HPV-Human Papilloma Virus; **Hospital:** LDS Hosp, Univ Utah Hlth Care; **Address:** Huntsman Cancer Hosp, 1950 Circle of Hope, Salt Lake City, UT 84112; **Phone:** 801-585-0100; **Board Cert:** Obstetrics & Gynecology 2006; Gynecologic Oncology 2006; **Med School:** Georgetown Univ 1981; **Resid:** Obstetrics & Gynecology, Madigan AMC 1985; **Fellow:** Gynecologic Oncology, Duke Univ Med Ctr 1990; **Fac Appt:** Assoc Prof ObG, Univ Utah

Southwest

Bodurka, Diane C MD [GO] - **Spec Exp:** Ovarian Cancer; Pelvic Surgery-Complex; **Hospital:** UT MD Anderson Cancer Ctr; **Address:** Univ Texas MD Anderson Cancer Ctr, Dept of Gynecologic Oncology, 1155 Herman Pressler, Box 1362, Houston, TX 77030-4000; **Phone:** 713-745-3358; **Board Cert:** Gynecologic Oncology 2011; Obstetrics & Gynecology 2011; **Med School:** Georgetown Univ 1990; **Resid:** Obstetrics & Gynecology, Univ Alabama Hosp 1994; **Fellow:** Gynecologic Oncology, MD Anderson Cancer Ctr 1996; **Fac Appt:** Prof ObG, Univ Tex, Houston

Borst, Matthew P MD [GO] - **Spec Exp:** Ovarian Cancer; **Hospital:** Banner Good Samaritan Regl Med Ctr - Phoenix; **Address:** Phoenix-Biltmore Cancer Ctr, 2222 E Highland Ave, Ste 400, Phoenix, AZ 85016; **Phone:** 602-253-5300; **Board Cert:** Obstetrics & Gynecology 2011; Gynecologic Oncology 2011; **Med School:** Med Coll VA 1984; **Resid:** Obstetrics & Gynecology, Cook Co Hosp 1988; **Fellow:** Gynecologic Oncology, Univ Alabama 1992; **Fac Appt:** Asst Clin Prof ObG, Univ Ariz Coll Med

Braly, Patricia S MD [GO] - **Spec Exp:** Ovarian Cancer; Breast Cancer; **Hospital:** St. Tammany Parish Hosp, E Jefferson Genl Hosp; **Address:** Women's Cancer Care, 606 W 12th Ave, Covington, LA 70433; **Phone:** 985-892-2252; **Board Cert:** Gynecologic Oncology 1985; Obstetrics & Gynecology 1994; **Med School:** UC Irvine 1976; **Resid:** Obstetrics & Gynecology, UC Irvine Med Ctr 1980; **Fellow:** Gynecologic Oncology, UC Irvine Med Ctr 1983

Burke, Thomas W MD [GO] - **Spec Exp:** Uterine Cancer; Vulvar & Vaginal Cancer; **Hospital:** UT MD Anderson Cancer Ctr; **Address:** UT MD Anderson Cancer Ctr, 1400 Pressler Street, Unit 1485, Houston, TX 77030-4009; **Phone:** 713-745-3825; **Board Cert:** Obstetrics & Gynecology 2011; Gynecologic Oncology 2011; **Med School:** Tulane Univ 1978; **Resid:** Obstetrics & Gynecology, Tripler Army Med Ctr 1982; **Fellow:** Gynecologic Oncology, Walter Reed Army Med Ctr 1986; **Fac Appt:** Prof ObG, Univ Tex, Houston

Burnett, Alexander F MD [GO] - **Spec Exp:** Laparoscopic Surgery; Fertility Preservation in Cancer; Gynecologic Cancer; **Hospital:** UAMS Med Ctr; **Address:** 4301 W Markham St, Slot 793, Little Rock, AR 72205; **Phone:** 501-686-8522; **Board Cert:** Obstetrics & Gynecology 2009; Gynecologic Oncology 2009; **Med School:** Georgetown Univ 1986; **Resid:** Obstetrics & Gynecology, Georgetown Univ Affil Hosp 1990; **Fellow:** Gynecologic Oncology, Georgetown Univ Affil Hosp 1993; **Fac Appt:** Assoc Prof ObG, Univ Ark

Chambers, Setsuko K MD [GO] - **Spec Exp:** Gynecologic Cancer; Breast Cancer; Ovarian Cancer; **Hospital:** Univ Arizona Med Ctr-Univ Campus; **Address:** Arizona Cancer Center, 1515 N Campbell Ave, Tucson, AZ 85724; **Phone:** 520-626-9285; **Board Cert:** Obstetrics & Gynecology 2011; Gynecologic Oncology 2011; **Med School:** Brown Univ 1980; **Resid:** Obstetrics & Gynecology, Yale-New Haven Hosp 1984; **Fellow:** Gynecologic Oncology, Yale-New Haven Hosp 1986; **Fac Appt:** Prof ObG, Univ Ariz Coll Med

Fromm, Geri-Lynn MD [GO] - **Spec Exp:** Cervical Cancer; Ovarian Cancer; Gestational Trophoblastic Disease; **Hospital:** St. Luke's Episcopal Hosp-Houston, Woman's Hosp TX; **Address:** 7580 Fanning St, Ste 335, Houston, TX 77054; **Phone:** 713-665-0404; **Board Cert:** Obstetrics & Gynecology 2011; Gynecologic Oncology 2011; **Med School:** Northwestern Univ 1981; **Resid:** Obstetrics & Gynecology, Magee Womens Hosp 1985; **Fellow:** Gynecologic Oncology, MD Anderson Cancer Ctr 1987; **Fac Appt:** Assoc Clin Prof ObG, Baylor Coll Med

Gershenson, David M MD [GO] - **Spec Exp:** Ovarian Rare & Borderline Tumors; Uterine Cancer-Serous Carcinoma; Fertility Preservation in Cancer; Sex Cord-Stromal Tumors; **Hospital:** UT MD Anderson Cancer Ctr, St. Luke's Episcopal Hosp-Houston; **Address:** PO Box 301439, Unit 1362, Houston, TX 77230-1439; **Phone:** 713-745-2565; **Board Cert:** Obstetrics & Gynecology 2012; Gynecologic Oncology 2012; **Med School:** Vanderbilt Univ 1971; **Resid:** Obstetrics & Gynecology, Yale-New Haven Hosp 1975; **Fellow:** Gynecologic Oncology, MD Anderson Cancer Ctr 1979; **Fac Appt:** Prof ObG, Univ Tex, Houston

Hatch, Kenneth D MD [GO] - **Spec Exp:** Cervical Cancer; Uro-Gynecology; Pelvic Organ Prolapse Repair; **Hospital:** Univ Arizona Med Ctr-Univ Campus, NW Med Ctr; **Address:** Arizona Cancer Center, 1515 N Campbell Ave, Tucson, AZ 85724; **Phone:** 520-626-9285; **Board Cert:** Obstetrics & Gynecology 1993; Gynecologic Oncology 1981; **Med School:** Univ Nebr Coll Med 1971; **Resid:** Obstetrics & Gynecology, Univ Alabama Med Ctr 1976; **Fellow:** Gynecologic Oncology, Univ Alabama Med Ctr 1978; **Fac Appt:** Prof ObG, Univ Ariz Coll Med

Kline, Richard C MD [GO] - **Spec Exp:** Ovarian Cancer; Cervical Cancer; Uterine Cancer; Vulvar & Vaginal Cancer; **Hospital:** Ochsner Med Ctr-New Orleans; **Address:** Ochsner Clinic Foundation, 1514 Jefferson Hwy Fl 5, New Orleans, LA 70121; **Phone:** 504-842-4165; **Board Cert:** Obstetrics & Gynecology 2011; Gynecologic Oncology 2011; **Med School:** Louisiana State U, New Orleans 1980; **Resid:** Obstetrics & Gynecology, Ochsner Fdn Hosp 1984; **Fellow:** Gynecologic Oncology, UT MD Anderson Cancer Ctr 1986

Gynecologic Oncology

Levenback, Charles F MD [GO] - **Spec Exp:** Vulvar Disease/Cancer; Cervical Cancer; Gynecologic Cancer; **Hospital:** UT MD Anderson Cancer Ctr; **Address:** 1515 Holcombe Ave, PO Box 301439 - Unit 1362, Houston, TX 77230; **Phone:** 713-745-2563; **Board Cert:** Obstetrics & Gynecology 2011; Gynecologic Oncology 2011; **Med School:** Mount Sinai Sch Med 1983; **Resid:** Obstetrics & Gynecology, Albert Einstein Affil Hosp 1987; **Fellow:** Gynecologic Oncology, Meml Sloan Kettering Cancer Ctr 1989; **Fac Appt:** Prof ObG, Univ Tex, Houston

Lu, Karen H MD [GO] - **Spec Exp:** Ovarian Cancer; Ovarian Cancer-Early Detection; Uterine Cancer; Cancer Genetics; **Hospital:** UT MD Anderson Cancer Ctr; **Address:** Univ of Texas MD Anderson Cancer Ctr, 1515 Holcombe Blvd Unit 1362, Houston, TX 77030; **Phone:** 713-745-8902; **Board Cert:** Obstetrics & Gynecology 2011; Gynecologic Oncology 2011; **Med School:** Yale Univ 1991; **Resid:** Obstetrics & Gynecology, Brigham & Women's Hosp 1994; **Fellow:** Gynecologic Oncology, Brigham & Women's Hosp 1999

Magrina, Javier MD [GO] - **Spec Exp:** Gynecologic Cancer; Endometriosis; Hysterectomy Alternatives; Robotic Surgery; **Hospital:** Mayo Clinic - Phoenix; **Address:** Mayo Clinic Gynecology, 5779 E Mayo Blvd, Phoenix, AZ 85054; **Phone:** 480-342-2668; **Board Cert:** Obstetrics & Gynecology 1994; Gynecologic Oncology 1982; **Med School:** Spain 1972; **Resid:** Obstetrics & Gynecology, Mayo Clinic 1977; **Fellow:** Gynecologic Oncology, Kansas Med Ctr 1980; **Fac Appt:** Prof ObG, Mayo Med Sch

Miller, David S MD [GO] - **Spec Exp:** Gynecologic Cancer; **Hospital:** UT Southwestern Med Ctr at Dallas; **Address:** 5323 Harry Hines Blvd, Dallas, TX 75390-8585; **Phone:** 214-645-4673; **Board Cert:** Obstetrics & Gynecology 2007; Gynecologic Oncology 2007; **Med School:** Univ Okla Coll Med 1977; **Resid:** Obstetrics & Gynecology, Hosp Univ Penn 1981; **Fellow:** Reproductive Endocrinology, UCSD Med Ctr 1982; Gynecologic Oncology, Stanford Hosps & Clins 1985; **Fac Appt:** Prof ObG, Univ Tex SW, Dallas

Siller, Barry MD [GO] - **Spec Exp:** Cervical Cancer; **Hospital:** Meml Hermann Hosp - Texas Med Ctr; **Address:** 915 Gessner Rd, Ste 400, Medical Plaza 3, Houston, TX 77024; **Phone:** 713-242-2575; **Board Cert:** Obstetrics & Gynecology 2011; Gynecologic Oncology 2011; **Med School:** Baylor Coll Med 1988; **Resid:** Obstetrics & Gynecology, UAB Med Ctr 1992; **Fellow:** Gynecologic Oncology, UAB Med Ctr 1994

Singh, Diljeet K MD [GO] - **Spec Exp:** Gynecologic Cancer; Ovarian Cancer; Ovarian Cancer-Early Detection; **Hospital:** Banner Gateway Med Ctr; **Address:** 2946 E Banner Gateway Drive, Gilbert, AZ 85234; **Phone:** 480-256-3609; **Board Cert:** Obstetrics & Gynecology 2011; Gynecologic Oncology 2011; **Med School:** Northwestern Univ-Feinberg Sch Med 1991; **Resid:** Obstetrics & Gynecology, Johns Hopkins Hosp 1996; **Fellow:** Gynecologic Oncology, MD Anderson Cancer Ctr 1999

Sood, Anil K MD [GO] - **Spec Exp:** Gynecologic Cancer; Ovarian Cancer; **Hospital:** UT MD Anderson Cancer Ctr; **Address:** Univ Texas MD Anderson Cancer Ctr, 1515 Holcomb Blvd Unit 1362, Houston, TX 77030-4000; **Phone:** 713-792-8340; **Board Cert:** Obstetrics & Gynecology 2011; Gynecologic Oncology 2011; **Med School:** Univ NC Sch Med 1991; **Resid:** Obstetrics & Gynecology, Univ FL Med Ctr 1995; **Fellow:** Gynecologic Oncology, Univ Iowa Hosps & Clin 1998

Walker, Joan L MD [GO] - **Spec Exp:** Ovarian Cancer; Cervical Cancer; Uterine Cancer; **Hospital:** OU Med Ctr; **Address:** OU Physicians, 800 NE 10th St, rm 5050, Oklahoma City, OK 73104; **Phone:** 405-271-7770; **Board Cert:** Obstetrics & Gynecology 2011; Gynecologic Oncology 2011; **Med School:** UCLA 1982; **Resid:** Obstetrics & Gynecology, Hosp Univ Penn 1986; **Fellow:** Gynecologic Oncology, UC-Irvine 1990; **Fac Appt:** Assoc Prof ObG, Univ Okla Coll Med

West Coast and Pacific

Berek, Jonathan S MD [GO] - **Spec Exp:** Ovarian Cancer; Uterine Cancer; Cervical Cancer; Vulvar & Vaginal Cancer; **Hospital:** Stanford Univ Hosp & Clinics; **Address:** Stanford Cancer Ctr, 900 Blake Wilbur Drive, Stanford, CA 94305; **Phone:** 650-498-6000; **Board Cert:** Obstetrics & Gynecology 2009; Gynecologic Oncology 2009; **Med School:** Johns Hopkins Univ 1975; **Resid:** Obstetrics & Gynecology, Brigham & Womens Hosp 1979; **Fellow:** Gynecologic Oncology, UCLA Sch Med 1981; **Fac Appt:** Prof ObG, Stanford Univ

Berman, Michael L MD [GO] - **Spec Exp:** Gynecologic Cancer; Cervical Cancer; **Hospital:** UC Irvine Med Ctr, Long Beach Meml Med Ctr; **Address:** Cho Family Comprehensive Cancer Ctr, 101 The City Drive S, Orange, CA 92868-3201; **Phone:** 714-456-8000; **Board Cert:** Obstetrics & Gynecology 2005; Gynecologic Oncology 2005; **Med School:** Geo Wash Univ 1967; **Resid:** Obstetrics & Gynecology, GW Univ Hosp 1969; Obstetrics & Gynecology, LAC-Harbor Hosp 1974; **Fellow:** Gynecologic Oncology, UCLA Med Ctr 1976; **Fac Appt:** Prof ObG, UC Irvine

Bristow, Robert E MD [GO] - **Spec Exp:** Ovarian Cancer; Gynecologic Cancer; **Hospital:** UC Irvine Med Ctr; **Address:** UC Irvine Med Ctr, 101 The City Drive S, Orange, CA 92868; **Phone:** 714-456-8000; **Board Cert:** Obstetrics & Gynecology 2011; Gynecologic Oncology 2011; **Med School:** USC Sch Med 1991; **Resid:** Obstetrics & Gynecology, Johns Hopkins Hosp 1995; **Fellow:** Gynecologic Oncology, UCLA Med Ctr 1998; **Fac Appt:** Prof ObG, UC Irvine

Carney, Michael E MD [GO] - **Spec Exp:** Gynecologic Cancer; Pelvic Surgery-Complex; Minimally Invasive Surgery; **Hospital:** Kapiolani Med Ctr for Women & Chldn, Queen's Med Ctr - Honolulu; **Address:** 1319 Punahou St, Ste 640, Honolulu, HI 96826; **Phone:** 808-983-6090; **Board Cert:** Obstetrics & Gynecology 2011; Gynecologic Oncology 2011; **Med School:** Loyola Univ-Stritch Sch Med 1990; **Resid:** Obstetrics & Gynecology, Duke Univ Med Ctr 1994; **Fellow:** Gynecologic Oncology, Duke Univ Med Ctr 1999; **Fac Appt:** Assoc Prof ObG, Univ Hawaii JA Burns Sch Med

Chan, John CK MD [GO] - **Spec Exp:** Ovarian Cancer; Pelvic Surgery-Complex; Gene Therapy; Clinical Trials; **Hospital:** UCSF Med Ctr; **Address:** UCSF Medical Center, 1600 Divisidaro St, rm A747, Box 1702, San Francisco, CA 94143-1702; **Phone:** 415-353-9600; **Board Cert:** Obstetrics & Gynecology 2006; Gynecologic Oncology 2006; **Med School:** UCLA 1995; **Resid:** Obstetrics & Gynecology, UC Irvine Med Ctr 1999; **Fellow:** Gynecologic Oncology, MD Anderson Cancer Ctr 1999; Gynecologic Oncology, UC Irvine 2003; **Fac Appt:** Assoc Prof ObG, UCSF

Di Saia, Philip J MD [GO] - **Spec Exp:** Ovarian Cancer; Gynecologic Cancer; Cervical Cancer; **Hospital:** UC Irvine Med Ctr; **Address:** 101 The City Drive, Bldg 56, rm 800, Orange, CA 92668-3201; **Phone:** 714-456-5220; **Board Cert:** Obstetrics & Gynecology 1983; Gynecologic Oncology 1974; **Med School:** Tufts Univ 1963; **Resid:** Obstetrics & Gynecology, Yale-New Haven Hosp 1967; **Fellow:** Gynecologic Oncology, MD Anderson Hosp 1971; **Fac Appt:** Prof ObG, UC Irvine

Goff, Barbara A MD [GO] - **Spec Exp:** Ovarian Cancer; Uterine Cancer; Cervical Cancer; Gynecologic Surgery-Complex; **Hospital:** Univ Wash Med Ctr; **Address:** Univ Washington, Dept Gyn/Onc, 825 Eastlake Ave E, Seattle, WA 98109; **Phone:** 206-288-2273; **Board Cert:** Obstetrics & Gynecology 2011; Gynecologic Oncology 2011; **Med School:** Univ Pennsylvania 1986; **Resid:** Obstetrics & Gynecology, Mass Genl Hosp/Brigham & Womens Hosp 1990; **Fellow:** Gynecologic Oncology, Mass Genl Hosp 1993; **Fac Appt:** Prof ObG, Univ Wash

Gynecologic Oncology

Greer, Benjamin E MD [GO] - **Spec Exp:** Gynecologic Cancer; **Hospital:** Univ Wash Med Ctr; **Address:** Seattle Cancer Care Alliance, 825 Eastlake Ave E, MS E2102, Seattle, WA 98109; **Phone:** 206-288-2273; **Board Cert:** Obstetrics & Gynecology 2002; Gynecologic Oncology 2002; **Med School:** Univ Pennsylvania 1966; **Resid:** Obstetrics & Gynecology, Univ Colorado Med Ctr 1970; **Fac Appt:** Prof ObG, Univ Wash

Husain, Amreen MD [GO] - **Spec Exp:** Cervical Cancer; Women's Health; **Hospital:** Stanford Univ Hosp & Clinics; **Address:** Stanford Comprehensive Cancer Ctr, 900 Blake Wilbur Drive, Stanford, CA 94305; **Phone:** 650-498-6004; **Board Cert:** Obstetrics & Gynecology 2009; Gynecologic Oncology 2009; **Med School:** NY Med Coll 1991; **Resid:** Obstetrics & Gynecology, Cornell Univ Med Ctr/NY Hosp 1995; **Fellow:** Gynecologic Oncology, Meml Sloan-Kettering Cancer Ctr 2000; **Fac Appt:** Assoc Prof ObG, Stanford Univ

Karlan, Beth Y MD [GO] - **Spec Exp:** Ovarian Cancer; Gynecologic Cancer; **Hospital:** Cedars-Sinai Med Ctr; **Address:** 8700 Beverly Blvd, Ste 290W, Los Angeles, CA 90048; **Phone:** 310-423-3302; **Board Cert:** Obstetrics & Gynecology 1998; Gynecologic Oncology 1998; **Med School:** Harvard Med Sch 1982; **Resid:** Obstetrics & Gynecology, Yale-New Haven Hosp 1986; **Fellow:** Gynecologic Oncology, UCLA 1989; **Fac Appt:** Prof ObG, UCLA

Muntz, Howard G MD [GO] - **Spec Exp:** Robotic Surgery; Ovarian Cancer; Gynecologic Surgery-Complex; Gestational Trophoblastic Disease; **Hospital:** Northwest Hosp - Seattle; **Address:** Women's Cancer Care of Seattle, 1560 N 115th St, Ste 101, Seattle, WA 98133; **Phone:** 206-368-6806; **Board Cert:** Obstetrics & Gynecology 2011; Gynecologic Oncology 2011; **Med School:** Harvard Med Sch 1984; **Resid:** Obstetrics & Gynecology, Brigham & Womens Hosp 1988; **Fellow:** Gynecologic Oncology, Mass General Hosp 1991; **Fac Appt:** Assoc Clin Prof ObG, Univ Wash

Pejovic, Tanja MD/PhD [GO] - **Spec Exp:** Ovarian Cancer; Gynecologic Cancer-Rare; Uterine Cancer; Cervical Cancer; **Hospital:** OR Hlth & Sci Univ; **Address:** Dept of Gyn Oncology, 3181 SW Sam Jackson Park Rd, MC KPV7, Portland, OR 97239; **Phone:** 503-418-4500; **Board Cert:** Obstetrics & Gynecology 2006; Gynecologic Oncology 2006; **Med School:** Yugoslavia 1984; **Resid:** Gynecologic Oncology, Lund Univ Affil Hosp 1995; Obstetrics & Gynecology, Yale/New Haven Hosp 2000; **Fellow:** Gynecologic Oncology, Yale/New Haven Hosp 2003; **Fac Appt:** Assoc Prof ObG, Oregon Hlth & Sci Univ

Plaxe, Steven C MD [GO] - **Spec Exp:** Ovarian Cancer; Uterine Cancer; Gestational Trophoblastic Disease; **Hospital:** UCSD Med Ctr; **Address:** Moores Cancer Center, 3855 Health Sciences Drive, MC 0987, La Jolla, CA 92093-0987; **Phone:** 858-822-6100; **Board Cert:** Obstetrics & Gynecology 2009; Gynecologic Oncology 2009; **Med School:** Mount Sinai Sch Med 1981; **Resid:** Obstetrics & Gynecology, Yale-New Haven Hosp 1985; **Fellow:** Gynecologic Oncology, Mt Sinai Med Ctr 1988; **Fac Appt:** Prof ObG, UCSD

Smith, Lloyd Herbert MD [GO] - **Spec Exp:** Ovarian Cancer; Uterine Cancer; Vulvar Disease/Cancer; Vaginal Cancer; **Hospital:** UC Davis Med Ctr, Sutter Mem Hospital-Sacramento; **Address:** UC Davis Med Ctr, Dept Ob/Gyn, 4860 Y St, Ste 2500, Sacramento, CA 95817-2307; **Phone:** 916-734-6946; **Board Cert:** Obstetrics & Gynecology 2009; Gynecologic Oncology 2009; **Med School:** UC Davis 1981; **Resid:** Obstetrics & Gynecology, UC Davis Med Ctr 1985; **Fellow:** Gynecologic Oncology, Stanford Univ Hosp 1988; **Fac Appt:** Prof ObG, UC Davis

Spirtos, Nicola Michael MD [GO] - **Spec Exp:** Gynecologic Cancer; Ovarian Cancer; **Hospital:** Sunrise Hosp & Med Ctr, Univ Med Ctr - Las Vegas; **Address:** 3131 La Canada St, Ste 241, Las Vegas, NV 89169; **Phone:** 702-693-6870; **Board Cert:** Obstetrics & Gynecology 2009; Gynecologic Oncology 2009; **Med School:** Northwestern Univ 1980; **Resid:** Obstetrics & Gynecology, Women's Hosp LAC-USC Med Ctr 1984; **Fellow:** Gynecologic Oncology, Stanford Univ Affil Hosp 1987; **Fac Appt:** Prof ObG

Stern, Jeffrey L MD [GO] - **Spec Exp:** Laparoscopic Surgery; Vulvar Disease/Cancer; **Hospital:** Alta Bates Summit Med Ctr-Alta Bates Campus; **Address:** Womens Cancer Ctr Northern Calif, 2001 Dwight Way, Berkley, CA 94704; **Phone:** 510-204-5770; **Board Cert:** Obstetrics & Gynecology 1983; Gynecologic Oncology 1984; **Med School:** SUNY Upstate Med Univ 1976; **Resid:** Obstetrics & Gynecology, Johns Hopkins Hosp 1980; **Fellow:** Gynecologic Oncology, USC Med Ctr 1982

Teng, Nelson NH MD/PhD [GO] - **Spec Exp:** Ovarian Cancer; Clinical Trials; **Hospital:** Stanford Univ Hosp & Clinics; **Address:** Dept Gyn Oncology, 900 Blake Wilbur Drive, Palo Alto, CA 94304; **Phone:** 650-498-6004; **Board Cert:** Obstetrics & Gynecology 2003; Gynecologic Oncology 2003; **Med School:** Univ Miami Sch Med 1977; **Resid:** Obstetrics & Gynecology, UCLA Med Ctr 1981; **Fellow:** Gynecologic Oncology, Stanford Univ Sch Med 1984; **Fac Appt:** Assoc Prof ObG, Stanford Univ

Cleveland Clinic

Every life deserves world class care.

Cleveland Clinic
Women's Health Institute
9500 Euclid Avenue
Cleveland, OH 44195

Gynecological Oncology

Cleveland Clinic Ob/Gyn & Women's Health Institute is designed to meet the unique and changing medical needs of women from adolescence to mature adulthood. Our dedicated team offers coordinated and supportive care. *U.S. News & World Report* has ranked our gynecology program No. 3 in the country. Our physicians are nationally and internationally known, and many serve on leadership boards for professional physician societies.

In the Section of Gynecologic Oncology, the staff employs a multidisciplinary approach to comprehensive management of gynecologic malignancies, incorporating surgery, radiation, chemotherapy and biologic therapy. We offer all types of innovative surgery, including robotics and single-port surgery. We also have a popular Gynecologic Oncology fellowship program.

Our oncologists are members of the Gynecologic Oncology Group, a non-profit organization funded by the National Cancer Institute and the only national cooperative study group devoted exclusively to the investigation of gynecologic malignancies. Extensive clinical trials of the most current treatments and techniques are available. The section also encompasses the Familial Ovarian Cancer Registry and provides complete treatment of pre-invasive lower genital tract disease.

Offering Same-Day Appointments
Call 800.274.2009.

Treatment Guides
Cleveland Clinic has developed comprehensive treatment guides for many diseases and conditions. To download our free treatment guides, visit clevelandclinic.org/treatmentguides.

Online Medical Second Opinion
Call 216.444.3223 or
800.223.2273 ext. 43223 or
email eclevelandclinic@ccf.org.

Out-of-State Patients Assistance
Call 800.223.2273, ext. 55580 or
email medicalconcierge@ccf.org.

Visit Us At:
clevelandclinic.org

Follow Us On:
Facebook
www.facebook.com/clevelandclinic

Twitter
@ClevelandClinic

You Tube
www.youtube.com/clevelandclinic

Health Hub
health.clevelandclinic.org

Hand Surgery

a subspecialty of Orthopaedics, Surgery or Plastic Surgery

A specialist trained in the investigation, preservation and restoration by medical, surgical and rehabilitative means of all structures of the upper extremity directly affecting the form and function of the hand and wrist.

For more information about the mentioned specialties or those physicians, see **Orthopaedic Surgery, Surgery** or **Plastic Surgery** section(s).

Training Required: Five years (including general surgery) in orthopaedics *plus* two years in clinical practice before final certification is achieved *plus* additional training and examination in hand surgery OR five to seven years in plastic surgery *plus* additional training and examination in hand surgery.

HAND SURGERY

New England

Belsky, Mark R MD [HS] - **Spec Exp:** Arthritis; Sports Injuries; Elbow Surgery; Dupuytren's Contracture; **Hospital:** Newton - Wellesley Hosp; **Address:** 2000 Washington St Green Bldg - Ste 201, Newton, MA 02462-1629; **Phone:** 617-965-4263; **Board Cert:** Orthopaedic Surgery 1982; Hand Surgery 2011; **Med School:** Tufts Univ 1974; **Resid:** Surgery, Peter Bent Brigham Hosp 1976; Orthopaedic Surgery, Tufts-New England Med Ctr 1979; **Fellow:** Hand Surgery, Roosevelt Hosp 1980; **Fac Appt:** Clin Prof OrS, Tufts Univ

Cassidy, Charles MD [HS] - **Spec Exp:** Hand & Upper Extremity Surgery; Elbow Surgery; Trauma-Upper & Lower Extremity; **Hospital:** Tufts Med Ctr; **Address:** Tufts Medical Ctr, 800 Washington St, Box 306, Boston, MA 02111; **Phone:** 617-636-5150; **Board Cert:** Hand Surgery 2007; Orthopaedic Surgery 2007; **Med School:** Northwestern Univ 1987; **Resid:** Orthopaedic Surgery, New England Med Ctr 1993; **Fellow:** Hand Surgery, Tufts Univ Med Ctr 1995; **Fac Appt:** Assoc Prof OrS, Tufts Univ

Jupiter, Jesse B MD [HS] - **Spec Exp:** Upper Extremity Trauma; Hand Surgery; Fractures-Non Union; **Hospital:** Mass Genl Hosp, Newton - Wellesley Hosp; **Address:** Mass General Hospital, 55 Fruit St, Yawkey Center, Ste 2100, Boston, MA 02114; **Phone:** 617-726-5100; **Board Cert:** Orthopaedic Surgery 1982; **Med School:** Yale Univ 1972; **Resid:** Surgery, Mass Genl Hosp 1976; Orthopaedic Surgery, Mass Genl Hosp 1979; **Fellow:** Hand Surgery, Univ Louisville 1981; Trauma, AO/ASIF 1980; **Fac Appt:** Prof OrS, Harvard Med Sch

Sampson, Christian E MD [HS] - **Spec Exp:** Hand Injuries; Hand & Fingers Vascular Surgery; **Hospital:** Brigham and Women's Hosp (page 57); **Address:** Brigham & Women's Hosp, Div Plastic Surg, 75 Francis St, Boston, MA 02115; **Phone:** 617-732-6297; **Board Cert:** Plastic Surgery 2004; Hand Surgery 2003; **Med School:** Boston Univ 1986; **Resid:** Surgery, Boston Univ Med Ctr 1991; Plastic Surgery, Brigham & Women's Hosp 1993; **Fellow:** Hand Surgery, Roosevelt Hosp 1994

Waters, Peter Michael MD [HS] - **Spec Exp:** Brachial Plexus Palsy; Hand-Congenital Anomaly; **Hospital:** Children's Hospital - Boston; **Address:** Chldns Hosp, Dept Ortho Surgery, 300 Longwood Ave, Hunnewell - 2, Boston, MA 02115-5724; **Phone:** 617-355-6021; **Board Cert:** Orthopaedic Surgery 2012; Hand Surgery 2012; **Med School:** Tufts Univ 1981; **Resid:** Pediatrics, Mass Genl Hosp 1983; Orthopaedic Surgery, Harvard Combined Prog 1988; **Fellow:** Hand Surgery, Brigham/Chldns Hosp 1989; **Fac Appt:** Assoc Prof OrS, Harvard Med Sch

Weiss, Arnold-Peter MD [HS] - **Spec Exp:** Carpal Tunnel Syndrome; Wrist Surgery; Elbow Replacement; **Hospital:** Rhode Island Hosp; **Address:** Univ Orthopedics, 2 Dudley St, Ste 200, Providence, RI 02905-3248; **Phone:** 401-457-1520; **Board Cert:** Orthopaedic Surgery 2004; Hand Surgery 2004; **Med School:** Johns Hopkins Univ 1985; **Resid:** Orthopaedic Surgery, Johns Hopkins Hosp 1990; **Fellow:** Hand Surgery, Indiana Hand Ctr 1991; **Fac Appt:** Prof OrS, Brown Univ

Mid Atlantic

Athanasian, Edward MD [HS] - **Spec Exp:** Bone & Soft Tissue Tumors; Hand & Upper Extremity Tumors; Hand & Upper Extremity Surgery; **Hospital:** Hosp For Special Surgery (page 60), Meml Sloan-Kettering Cancer Ctr; **Address:** Hospital for Special Surgery, 535 E 70th St, New York, NY 10021; **Phone:** 212-606-1962; **Board Cert:** Orthopaedic Surgery 2008; Hand Surgery 2008; **Med School:** Columbia P&S 1988; **Resid:** Surgery, Beth Israel Hosp 1989; Orthopaedic Surgery, Hosp Special Surgery 1993; **Fellow:** Hand Surgery, Mayo Clinic 1994; Orthopaedic Oncology, Meml Sloan Kettering Cancer Ctr 1995; **Fac Appt:** Asst Prof OrS, Cornell Univ-Weill Med Coll

Baratz, Mark E MD [HS] - **Spec Exp:** Hand Surgery; Upper Extremity Surgery; Elbow Reconstruction; **Hospital:** Allegheny General Hosp, St. Clair Hosp; **Address:** 1307 Federal St Fl 2, Pittsburgh, PA 15212; **Phone:** 412-359-4263; **Board Cert:** Orthopaedic Surgery 2004; Hand Surgery 2004; **Med School:** Univ Pittsburgh 1984; **Resid:** Orthopaedic Surgery, Univ Hlth Ctr 1990; **Fellow:** Orthopaedic Surgery, Univ Hlth Ctr 1987; Hand Surgery, Med Coll Penn 1991; **Fac Appt:** Prof OrS, Drexel Univ Coll Med

Beredjiklian, Pedro K MD [HS] - **Spec Exp:** Hand & Wrist Surgery; Arthroscopic Surgery; Elbow Reconstruction; **Hospital:** Riddle Meml Hosp; **Address:** Rothman Institute, 925 Chestnut Ave Fl 5, Philadelphia, PA 19107; **Phone:** 800-321-9999; **Board Cert:** Orthopaedic Sports Medicine 2011; Hand Surgery 2011; **Med School:** Columbia P&S 1992; **Resid:** Orthopaedic Surgery, Hosp U Penn 1997; **Fellow:** Hand & Microvascular Surgery, Hosp Special Surgery 1998; **Fac Appt:** Assoc Prof OrS, Thomas Jefferson Univ

Bozentka, David J MD [HS] - **Spec Exp:** Hand & Upper Extremity Surgery; Elbow Surgery; **Hospital:** Penn Presby Med Ctr - UPHS (page 72); **Address:** Penn Orthopaedic Institute, I Cupp Pavilion, 39th & Market St, Philadelphia, PA 19104; **Phone:** 215-349-5773; **Board Cert:** Orthopaedic Surgery 2006; Hand Surgery 2006; **Med School:** Jefferson Med Coll 1987; **Resid:** Orthopaedic Surgery, W Virgina Univ Hosp 1992; **Fac Appt:** Assoc Prof OrS, Univ Pennsylvania

Brushart, Thomas M MD [HS] - **Spec Exp:** Hand & Upper Extremity Surgery; Peripheral Nerve Surgery; **Hospital:** Johns Hopkins Hosp (page 61); **Address:** 601 N Caroline St, rm 5221, Baltimore, MD 21287-0882; **Phone:** 410-955-9663; **Board Cert:** Orthopaedic Surgery 1985; **Med School:** Harvard Med Sch 1978; **Resid:** Orthopaedic Surgery, Harvard Affil Hosps 1981; **Fellow:** Hand Surgery, Curtis Hand Ctr 1983; **Fac Appt:** Prof OrS, Johns Hopkins Univ

Carlson, Michelle Gerwin MD [HS] - **Spec Exp:** Sports Injuries; Hand & Upper Extremity Surgery; Pediatric Hand/Arm Surgery; Cerebral Palsy; **Hospital:** Hosp For Special Surgery (page 60); **Address:** 523 E 72nd St, Fl 4, rm 439, New York, NY 10021; **Phone:** 212-606-1546; **Board Cert:** Orthopaedic Surgery 2007; Hand Surgery 2007; **Med School:** Cornell Univ-Weill Med Coll 1987; **Resid:** Surgery, Hosp Special Surg 1992; **Fellow:** Hand Surgery, Hosp Special Surg 1993; **Fac Appt:** Assoc Prof OrS, Cornell Univ-Weill Med Coll

Culp, Randall MD [HS] - **Spec Exp:** Microsurgery; Hand & Upper Extremity Surgery; Elbow Surgery; **Hospital:** Thomas Jefferson Univ Hosp, Lankenau Hosp; **Address:** Philadelphia Hand Center, 700 S Henderson Rd, Ste 200, King of Prussia, PA 19406; **Phone:** 610-768-5959; **Board Cert:** Orthopaedic Surgery 2011; Hand Surgery 2011; **Med School:** Penn State Coll Med 1982; **Resid:** Orthopaedic Surgery, Hosp Univ Penn 1987; **Fellow:** Hand Surgery, Hosp Univ Penn 1988; **Fac Appt:** Prof OrS, Jefferson Med Coll

Hand Surgery

Eglseder Jr, W Andrew MD [HS] - **Spec Exp:** Hand & Upper Extremity Surgery; Trauma; Hand Reconstruction; **Hospital:** Univ of MD Med Ctr; **Address:** Univ Maryland Shock Trauma Ctr, 22 S Greene St, Baltimore, MD 21201; **Phone:** 410-328-6284; **Board Cert:** Orthopaedic Surgery 2010; Hand Surgery 2010; **Med School:** Univ MD Sch Med 1982; **Resid:** Orthopaedic Surgery, Univ Maryland Med Ctr 1987; **Fellow:** Hand Surgery, Univ Louisville Med Ctr 1989; **Fac Appt:** Assoc Prof OrS, Univ MD Sch Med

Glickel, Steven Z MD [HS] - **Spec Exp:** Hand & Wrist Surgery; Elbow Surgery; Peripheral Nerve Surgery; **Hospital:** St. Luke's - Roosevelt Hosp Ctr - Roosevelt Div (page 56); **Address:** 1000 10th Ave Fl 3, New York, NY 10019-1147; **Phone:** 212-523-7590; **Board Cert:** Orthopaedic Surgery 1985; Hand Surgery 2010; **Med School:** Harvard Med Sch 1976; **Resid:** Surgery, Columbia Presby Med Ctr 1978; Orthopaedic Surgery, Harvard Comb Ortho 1981; **Fellow:** Hand Surgery, St Luke's-Roosevelt Hosp Ctr 1983; Research, Columbia Presby Med Ctr 1982; **Fac Appt:** Clin Prof OrS, Columbia P&S

Goitz, Robert J MD [HS] - **Spec Exp:** Hand & Upper Extremity Surgery; **Hospital:** UPMC Mercy, Pittsburgh; **Address:** Kaufman Medical Bldg, Ste 1010, 3471 Fifth Ave, Pittsburgh, PA 15213; **Phone:** 412-605-3324; **Board Cert:** Orthopaedic Surgery 2011; **Med School:** Johns Hopkins Univ 1992; **Resid:** Orthopaedic Surgery, Univ Pittsburgh Med Ctr 1997; **Fac Appt:** Assoc Prof OrS, Univ Pittsburgh

Imbriglia, Joseph E MD [HS] - **Spec Exp:** Arthritis; Carpal Tunnel Syndrome; Shoulder Surgery; Rotator Cuff Surgery; **Hospital:** UPMC Passavant-McCandless, UPMC Shadyside; **Address:** 6001 Stonewood Drive, Wexford, PA 15090-7380; **Phone:** 724-933-3850; **Board Cert:** Orthopaedic Surgery 1977; Hand Surgery 2010; **Med School:** Hahnemann Univ 1970; **Resid:** Surgery, Univ Pittsburgh Med Ctr 1972; Orthopaedic Surgery, Columbia Presby Med Ctr 1975; **Fellow:** Hand Surgery, Columbia Presby Med Ctr 1976; **Fac Appt:** Clin Prof OrS, Univ Pittsburgh

Kozin, Scott H MD [HS] - **Spec Exp:** Congenital Hand Deformities; Brachial Plexus Palsy-Pediatric; Spinal Cord Injury-Pediatric; Hand Surgery; **Hospital:** Philadelphia Shriners Hosp; **Address:** Shriners Hosp for Children, 3551 N Broad St, Philadelphia, PA 19140; **Phone:** 215-430-4074; **Board Cert:** Orthopaedic Surgery 2005; Hand Surgery 2005; **Med School:** Hahnemann Univ 1986; **Resid:** Orthopaedic Surgery, Albert Einstein Med Ctr 1991; **Fellow:** Hand Surgery, Mayo Clinic 1992; **Fac Appt:** Assoc Prof OrS, Temple Univ

Kulick, Roy G MD [HS] - **Spec Exp:** Carpal Tunnel Syndrome; Arthritis; Tendon Surgery; Hand & Upper Extremity Surgery; **Hospital:** Montefiore Med Ctr-Einstein Campus, NY; **Address:** Dept Orthopaedic Surgery, 1250 Waters Pl Fl 11, Bronx, NY 10461; **Phone:** 718-920-2060; **Board Cert:** Orthopaedic Surgery 1980; Hand Surgery 2011; **Med School:** Cornell Univ-Weill Med Coll 1973; **Resid:** Surgery, St Lukes-Roosevelt Hosp 1975; Orthopaedic Surgery, NY Presby Hosp/Columbia Univ Med Ctr 1978; **Fellow:** Hand Surgery, Hosp for Special Surgery 1979; **Fac Appt:** Assoc Prof OrS, Albert Einstein Coll Med

Lane, Lewis B MD [HS] - **Spec Exp:** Carpal Tunnel Syndrome; Arthritis; Sports Injuries; Hand Reconstruction; **Hospital:** N Shore Univ Hosp (page 67), St. Francis Hosp - The Heart Ctr (page 73); **Address:** University Orthopaedics, 611 Northern Blvd, Ste 200, Great Neck, NY 11021; **Phone:** 516-723-2663; **Board Cert:** Orthopaedic Surgery 1981; Hand Surgery 2010; **Med School:** Columbia P&S 1974; **Resid:** Surgery, NY Hosp 1975; Orthopaedic Surgery, Hosp for Special Surg 1979; **Fellow:** Research, Hosp for Special Surg 1976; Hand Surgery, St Luke's-Roosevelt Hosp Ctr 1980; **Fac Appt:** Assoc Clin Prof OrS, Albany Med Coll

Lee, W P Andrew MD [HS] - **Spec Exp:** Reconstructive Surgery; Cartilage Damage; Transplant-Hand; Pediatric Hand Surgery; **Hospital:** Johns Hopkins Hosp (page 61); **Address:** Johns Hopkins Outpatient Ctr, 601 N Carolyn St, Ste 8152F, Baltimore, MD 21287; **Phone:** 410-955-9466 x4; **Board Cert:** Hand Surgery 2005; Plastic Surgery 2005; **Med School:** Johns Hopkins Univ 1983; **Resid:** Surgery, Johns Hopkins Hosp 1989; Plastic Surgery, Mass Genl Hosp 1991; **Fellow:** Microsurgery, Johns Hopkins Hosp 1987; Hand Surgery, Indiana Hand Ctr 1993; **Fac Appt:** Prof S, Johns Hopkins Univ

Lubahn, John D MD [HS] - **Spec Exp:** Microsurgery; **Hospital:** UPMC Hamot, St. Vincent Hlth Ctr; **Address:** 300 State St, Ste 205, Erie, PA 16507; **Phone:** 814-456-6022; **Board Cert:** Orthopaedic Surgery 2010; Hand Surgery 2010; **Med School:** Case West Res Univ 1975; **Resid:** Surgery, Univ Rochester Med Ctr 1977; Orthopaedic Surgery, Univ Rochester Med Ctr 1980; **Fellow:** Hand Surgery, Univ Louisville Hosp 1981

Melone Jr, Charles P MD [HS] - **Spec Exp:** Wrist Surgery; Fractures; **Hospital:** Beth Israel Med Ctr - Petrie Division (page 56); **Address:** 321 E 34th St, New York, NY 10016; **Phone:** 212-340-0000; **Board Cert:** Orthopaedic Surgery 1976; Hand Surgery 2004; **Med School:** Georgetown Univ 1969; **Resid:** Surgery, Nassau Co Med Ctr 1971; Orthopaedic Surgery, Nassau Co Med Ctr 1974; **Fellow:** Hand Surgery, NYU Langone Med Ctr 1975; **Fac Appt:** Prof OrS, Albert Einstein Coll Med

Osterman, A Lee MD [HS] - **Spec Exp:** Upper Extremity Surgery; Wrist Surgery; Neuromuscular Disorders; **Hospital:** Thomas Jefferson Univ Hosp; **Address:** Philadelphia Hand Ctr, 700 S Henderson Rd, Ste 200, King of Prussia, PA 19406-4207; **Phone:** 610-265-3135; **Board Cert:** Orthopaedic Surgery 1980; **Med School:** Univ Pennsylvania 1973; **Resid:** Orthopaedic Surgery, Hosp Univ Penn 1978; **Fellow:** Hand Surgery, Hosp Univ Penn 1979; Microvascular Surgery, Duke Univ Med Ctr 1980; **Fac Appt:** Prof OrS, Jefferson Med Coll

Raphael, James S MD [HS] - **Spec Exp:** Reconstructive Microvascular Surgery; Upper Extremity Trauma; Limb Surgery/Reconstruction; **Hospital:** Albert Einstein Med Ctr, Thomas Jefferson Univ Hosp; **Address:** AEMC, Willowcrest Bldg, Fl 4, 5501 Old York Rd, Philadelphia, PA 19141; **Phone:** 215-456-7900; **Board Cert:** Orthopaedic Surgery 2007; Hand Surgery 2007; **Med School:** SUNY Upstate Med Univ 1988; **Resid:** Orthopaedic Surgery, Mt Sinai Hosp 1993; **Fellow:** Hand Surgery, Thomas Jefferson Univ Hosp/Philadelphia Hand Ctr 1994; **Fac Appt:** Assoc Clin Prof OrS, Jefferson Med Coll

Raskin, Keith B MD [HS] - **Spec Exp:** Wrist/Hand Injuries; Arthritis; Carpal Tunnel Syndrome; Elbow Surgery; **Hospital:** NYU Langone Med Ctr (page 68), NYU Hosp For Joint Diseases (page 70); **Address:** 317 E 34th St, Fl 3, New York, NY 10016; **Phone:** 212-263-4263; **Board Cert:** Orthopaedic Surgery 2002; Hand Surgery 2002; **Med School:** Geo Wash Univ 1983; **Resid:** Orthopaedic Surgery, NYU Med Ctr 1988; **Fellow:** Hand Surgery, Union Mem Hosp 1989; **Fac Appt:** Assoc Clin Prof OrS, NYU Sch Med

Rosenwasser, Melvin P MD [HS] - **Spec Exp:** Carpal Tunnel Syndrome; Sports Injuries; Elbow Surgery; Trauma; **Hospital:** NY-Presby/Columbia Univ Med Ctr, NY (page 66); **Address:** New York Orthopedic Hospital Associates, 622 W 168th St, PH 11, rm 1150, New York, NY 10032; **Phone:** 212-305-8036; **Board Cert:** Orthopaedic Surgery 1999; Hand Surgery 2011; **Med School:** Columbia P&S 1976; **Resid:** Surgery, Roosevelt Hosp 1979; Orthopaedic Surgery, Columbia Presby Hosp 1982; **Fellow:** Hand Surgery, Columbia Presby Hosp 1983; **Fac Appt:** Prof OrS, Columbia P&S

Hand Surgery

Sotereanos, Dean G MD [HS] - **Spec Exp:** Hand & Upper Extremity Surgery; Elbow Surgery; **Hospital:** Allegheny General Hosp; **Address:** 1307 Federal St Fl 2, Pittsburgh, PA 15212; **Phone:** 412-359-4263; **Board Cert:** Orthopaedic Surgery 2003; Hand Surgery 2003; **Med School:** Hahnemann Univ 1984; **Resid:** Surgery, Univ Pittsburgh Med Ctr 1986; Orthopaedic Surgery, Univ Pittsburgh Med Ctr 1989; **Fellow:** Hand Surgery, Duke Univ Med Ctr 1990; **Fac Appt:** Assoc Prof OrS, Univ Pittsburgh

Strauch, Robert MD [HS] - **Spec Exp:** Hand Reconstruction; Hand & Elbow Nerve Disorders; Hand & Wrist Surgery; Elbow Surgery; **Hospital:** NY-Presby/Columbia Univ Med Ctr, NY (page 66); **Address:** 622 W 168th St, rm PH-11-1119, New York, NY 10032; **Phone:** 212-305-4272; **Board Cert:** Orthopaedic Surgery 2005; Hand Surgery 2005; **Med School:** Columbia P&S 1986; **Resid:** Orthopaedic Surgery, Columbia-Presby Hosp 1991; **Fellow:** Hand Surgery, Indiana Hand Center 1992; **Fac Appt:** Prof OrS, Columbia P&S

Thoder, Joseph J MD [HS] - **Spec Exp:** Wrist/Hand Injuries; **Hospital:** Temple Univ Hosp; **Address:** Temple Univ Hosp, Dept Orthopaedics, 3509 N Broad St, Philadelphia, PA 19140; **Phone:** 215-707-2111; **Board Cert:** Orthopaedic Surgery 2011; Hand Surgery 2011; **Med School:** Temple Univ 1982; **Resid:** Orthopaedic Surgery, Temple Univ Hosp 1987; **Fellow:** Hand & Microvascular Surgery, Thos Jefferson Univ Hosp 1988; **Fac Appt:** Prof OrS, Temple Univ

Weiland, Andrew J MD [HS] - **Spec Exp:** Wrist/Hand Injuries; Hand Reconstruction; **Hospital:** Hosp For Special Surgery (page 60), NY-Presby/Weill Cornell Med Ctr, NY (page 66); **Address:** Hospital for Special Surgery, 535 E 70th St, New York, NY 10021-4872; **Phone:** 212-606-1575; **Board Cert:** Orthopaedic Surgery 1977; **Med School:** Wake Forest Univ 1968; **Resid:** Surgery, Univ Michigan Med Ctr 1970; Orthopaedic Surgery, Johns Hopkins Hosp 1975; **Fellow:** Hand Surgery, Kleinert Hosp 1975; **Fac Appt:** Prof OrS, Cornell Univ-Weill Med Coll

Wolfe, Scott W MD [HS] - **Spec Exp:** Wrist Surgery; Nerve Disorders/Surgery; Fractures; **Hospital:** Hosp For Special Surgery (page 60); **Address:** Hospital for Special Surgery, 535 E 70 St, New York, NY 10021; **Phone:** 212-606-1529; **Board Cert:** Orthopaedic Surgery 2003; Hand Surgery 2003; **Med School:** Cornell Univ-Weill Med Coll 1984; **Resid:** Surgery, St Luke's Roosevelt Hosp Ctr 1986; Orthopaedic Surgery, Hosp Special Surg 1989; **Fellow:** Hand & Microvascular Surgery, Columbia Presby Med Ctr 1990; **Fac Appt:** Prof OrS, Cornell Univ-Weill Med Coll

Southeast

Badia, Alejandro MD [HS] - **Spec Exp:** Hand & Upper Extremity Surgery; Shoulder Surgery; Elbow Surgery; Wrist Surgery; **Address:** Badia Hand to Shoulder Ctr, 3650 NW 82nd Ave, Ste 103, Doral, FL 33166; **Phone:** 305-227-4263; **Board Cert:** Orthopaedic Surgery 2009; Hand Surgery 2009; **Med School:** NYU Sch Med 1989; **Resid:** Orthopaedic Surgery, NYU Medical Ctr 1995; **Fellow:** Hand Surgery, Allegheny General Hosp 1997; Hand Surgery, Freiberg 1998

Carneiro, Ronaldo D S MD [HS] - **Spec Exp:** Carpal Tunnel Syndrome; Arthritis; Dupuytren's Contracture; Hand & Wrist Surgery; **Hospital:** Physicians Regl Hlthcare Med Ctr-Pine Ridge; **Address:** 8340 Collier Blvd, Ste 303, Naples, FL 34114; **Phone:** 239-348-4040; **Board Cert:** Plastic Surgery 1990; **Med School:** Brazil 1970; **Resid:** Surgery, Union Meml Hosp 1975; Plastic Surgery, Allentown & Sacred Heart Hosp Ctr 1977; **Fellow:** Hand Surgery, Jackson Meml Hosp-Univ Miami Hosp 1977; Plastic Surgery, Univ Miami Sch Med 1978; **Fac Appt:** Assoc Clin Prof PlS, Univ S Fla Coll Med

Cendales, Linda C MD [HS] - **Spec Exp:** Transplant-Hand; Microsurgery; Reconstructive Surgery; Carpal Tunnel Syndrome; **Hospital:** Emory Univ Hosp, Emory Univ Hosp Midtown; **Address:** Emory Transplant Center, 1365 Clifton Rd NE, Bldg B, Fl 6, Atlanta, GA 30322; **Phone:** 404-727-0701; **Med School:** Mexico 1992; **Resid:** Surgery, Hospital General 1996; Hand Surgery, Natl Inst Orthopaedics 1997; **Fellow:** Hand & Microvascular Surgery, Kleinert Inst, Univ Louisville 2001; Transplant Surgery, Natl Inst Hlth 2004; **Fac Appt:** Asst Prof S, Emory Univ

Friedman, David W MD [HS] - **Spec Exp:** Hand Reconstruction; Arthritis; Microsurgery; Sports Injuries; **Hospital:** Cleveland Clin - Weston (page 55); **Address:** Cleveland Clinic Florida, 2950 Cleveland Clinic Blvd, Weston, FL 33331; **Phone:** 954-659-5430; **Board Cert:** Plastic Surgery 2009; Hand Surgery 2008; **Med School:** Univ Tex SW, Dallas 1988; **Resid:** Surgery, UMDNJ Affil Hosp 1994; Plastic Surgery, NYU Med Ctr 1996; **Fellow:** Hand Surgery, NYU Med Ctr 1997

Greene, Thomas L MD [HS] - **Spec Exp:** Arthritis; Peripheral Nerve Surgery; Arthroscopic Surgery; Tendon Surgery; **Hospital:** Tampa Genl Hosp, St. Joseph's Hosp - Tampa; **Address:** 2727 W Dr Martin Luther King Jr Blvd, Ste 560, Tampa, FL 33607-6009; **Phone:** 813-873-0337; **Board Cert:** Orthopaedic Surgery 1983; Hand Surgery 2000; **Med School:** Ohio State Univ 1975; **Resid:** Surgery, Univ Michigan Med Ctr 1977; Orthopaedic Surgery, Univ Michigan Med Ctr 1980; **Fellow:** Hand Surgery, St Vincent's Hosp 1981

Grossman, John A I MD [HS] - **Spec Exp:** Brachial Plexus Palsy; Hand Surgery; Peripheral Nerve Surgery; Congenital Hand Deformities; **Hospital:** Miami Children's Hosp, NYU Hosp For Joint Diseases (page 70); **Address:** 8940 N Kendall Drive, Ste 904E, Miami, FL 33176-2176; **Phone:** 305-666-2004; **Board Cert:** Plastic Surgery 1989; **Med School:** Univ VA Sch Med 1978; **Resid:** Surgery, Cleveland Clinic 1982; Plastic Surgery, E Virginia Affil Hosp 1985; **Fellow:** Hand Surgery, French Hand Inst 1983; **Fac Appt:** Assoc Clin Prof OrS, NYU Sch Med

Hunt III, Thomas R MD [HS] - **Spec Exp:** Hand & Wrist Surgery; Arthritis; Trauma; Hand Reconstruction; **Hospital:** Univ of Ala Hosp at Birmingham; **Address:** UAB Orthopaedic Surgery, 1313 13th St S, Ste 201, Birmingham, AL 35205-5327; **Phone:** 205-930-8339; **Board Cert:** Orthopaedic Surgery 2006; Hand Surgery 2006; **Med School:** Vanderbilt Univ 1986; **Resid:** Orthopaedic Surgery, Univ Kansas Med Ctr 1992; **Fellow:** Hand Surgery, Hosp Univ Penn 1993; **Fac Appt:** Prof S, Univ Alabama

Koman, L Andrew MD [HS] - **Spec Exp:** Pediatric Hand Surgery; Vascular Disease-Upper Extremity; Pain-Nerve Injury; **Hospital:** Wake Forest Baptist Med Ctr; **Address:** 131 Miller St, Winston-Salem, NC 27103; **Phone:** 336-716-8094; **Board Cert:** Orthopaedic Surgery 1981; Hand Surgery 2010; **Med School:** Duke Univ 1974; **Resid:** Surgery, Duke Univ Med Ctr 1975; Orthopaedic Surgery, Duke Univ Med Ctr 1979; **Fellow:** Hand Surgery, Duke Univ Med Ctr 1980; **Fac Appt:** Prof OrS, Wake Forest Univ

Peljovich, Allan E MD [HS] - **Spec Exp:** Brachial Plexus Palsy; Cerebral Palsy; Trauma; Congenital Limb Deformities; **Hospital:** Northside Hosp, Chldns Hlthcare Atlanta @ Scottish Rite; **Address:** Hand & Upper Extremity Center, 980 Johnson Ferry Rd NE, Ste 1020, Atlanta, GA 30342; **Phone:** 404-255-0226; **Board Cert:** Orthopaedic Surgery 2002; Hand Surgery 2003; **Med School:** Univ Pennsylvania 1992; **Resid:** Orthopaedic Surgery, Case Western Reserve Univ Hosp 1998; **Fellow:** Hand Surgery, Brigham & Womens Hosp/Childrens Hosp 1999; Hand Surgery, MetroHealth Med Ctr 2000

Midwest

Bishop, Allen T MD [HS] - **Spec Exp:** Microsurgery; Brachial Plexus Palsy; **Hospital:** Mayo Med Ctr & Clin - Rochester; **Address:** Mayo Clin, Div Hand Surgery, 200 First St SW, Rochester, MN 55905; **Phone:** 507-284-0475; **Board Cert:** Orthopaedic Surgery 2010; Hand Surgery 2010; **Med School:** Mayo Med Sch 1981; **Resid:** Orthopaedic Surgery, Mayo Clin 1986; **Fellow:** Hand Surgery, St Vincent Hosp 1987; **Fac Appt:** Prof OrS, Mayo Med Sch

Carroll IV, Charles MD [HS] - **Spec Exp:** Carpal Tunnel Syndrome; Dupuytren's Contracture; Elbow Surgery; Shoulder Surgery; **Hospital:** NorthShore Univ HlthSys; **Address:** Northshore Orthopaedic Inst, 680 N Lakeshore Drive, Ste 924, Chicago, IL 60611; **Phone:** 312-664-6848; **Board Cert:** Orthopaedic Surgery 2011; Hand Surgery 2011; **Med School:** Univ MD Sch Med 1982; **Resid:** Surgery, Johns Hopkins Hosp 1984; Orthopaedic Surgery, Johns Hopkins Hosp 1987; **Fellow:** Hand Surgery, Indiana Univ Med Ctr 1988; Shoulder Surgery, Univ Western Ontario 1988; **Fac Appt:** Assoc Clin Prof OrS, Northwestern Univ

Chung, Kevin Chi MD [HS] - **Spec Exp:** Reconstructive Surgery; Hand & Microvascular Surgery; Upper Extremity Trauma; Nail Surgery; **Hospital:** Univ of Michigan Hosp; **Address:** 4029 Ave Maria Drive, Ann Arbor, MI 48106; **Phone:** 734-998-6022; **Board Cert:** Hand Surgery 2007; Plastic Surgery 2007; **Med School:** Emory Univ 1987; **Resid:** Plastic Surgery, Univ Michigan Hosp & Hlth Ctr 1994; Hand Surgery, Union Meml Hosp 1995; **Fac Appt:** Assoc Prof S, Univ Mich Med Sch

Cohen, Mark S MD [HS] - **Spec Exp:** Hand Surgery; Wrist Surgery; Elbow Surgery; **Hospital:** Rush Univ Med Ctr; **Address:** Midwest Orthopedics at Rush, 1611 W Harrison St, Ste 400, Chicago, IL 60612; **Phone:** 312-243-4244; **Board Cert:** Orthopaedic Surgery 2006; Hand Surgery 2006; **Med School:** Harvard Med Sch 1986; **Resid:** Orthopaedic Surgery, UCSD Med Ctr 1992; **Fellow:** Hand Surgery, Indiana Hand Ctr 1993; **Fac Appt:** Prof OrS, Rush Med Coll

Derman, Gordon H MD [HS] - **Spec Exp:** Carpal Tunnel Syndrome; Tendon Surgery; Repetitive Motion Injuries; Nerve Disorders/Surgery; **Hospital:** Rush Univ Med Ctr, NorthShore Univ HlthSys; **Address:** 1725 W Harrison St, Ste 740, Chicago, IL 60612; **Phone:** 312-432-9200; **Board Cert:** Plastic Surgery 1984; Hand Surgery 2009; **Med School:** Rush Med Coll 1975; **Resid:** Surgery, Loyola Univ Med Ctr 1981; Plastic Surgery, Univ Mich Hosp 1983; **Fellow:** Microsurgery, Rush/Presby St Luke's Med Ctr 1976; **Fac Appt:** Asst Prof S, Rush Med Coll

DeSilva, Stephen P MD [HS] - **Spec Exp:** Hand Surgery; **Hospital:** Henry Ford Hosp, Henry Ford- W Bloomfield Hosp; **Address:** Henry Ford Hosp, 2799 W Grand Blvd, Ste K12, Detroit, MI 48202; **Phone:** 248-661-7195; **Board Cert:** Orthopaedic Surgery 2012; Hand Surgery 2012; **Med School:** Johns Hopkins Univ 1983; **Resid:** Orthopaedic Surgery, Mayo Clinic 1988; **Fellow:** Hand Surgery, Union Meml Hosp 1989; **Fac Appt:** Prof OrS, Wayne State Univ

Failla, Joseph M MD [HS] - **Spec Exp:** Hand Surgery; Hand Reconstruction; **Hospital:** Providence Hosp - Southfield, Huron Valley-Sinai Hosp; **Address:** Farmbrook Med Complex, One Bldg, Ste 201, 29829 Telegraph Rd, Southfield, MI 48034; **Phone:** 248-352-4263; **Board Cert:** Orthopaedic Surgery 2011; Hand Surgery 2011; **Med School:** SUNY Buffalo 1982; **Resid:** Orthopaedic Surgery, SUNY-Buffalo 1987; **Fellow:** Hand Surgery, Mayo Clinic 1988

Fischer, Thomas J MD [HS] - **Spec Exp:** Microsurgery; Elbow Reconstruction; Fractures-Complex; **Hospital:** St. Vincent Indianapolis Hosp, IU Health University Hosp; **Address:** Indiana Hand to Shoulder Ctr, 8501 Harcourt Rd, Indianapolis, IN 46260; **Phone:** 317-875-9105; **Board Cert:** Orthopaedic Surgery 2010; Hand Surgery 2010; **Med School:** Indiana Univ 1979; **Resid:** Orthopaedic Surgery, Univ Wash Affil Hosp 1984; **Fellow:** Hand Surgery, Hand Surg Assocs 1985; Hand Surgery, Duke Univ Med Ctr 1986; **Fac Appt:** Assoc Clin Prof OrS, Indiana Univ

Gelberman, Richard H MD [HS] - **Spec Exp:** Tendon Surgery; Peripheral Nerve Surgery; **Hospital:** Barnes-Jewish Hosp; **Address:** Wash Univ Sch Med, Dept Orthopaedics, 660 S Euclid Ave, Box 8233, St Louis, MO 63110; **Phone:** 314-747-2500; **Board Cert:** Orthopaedic Surgery 2007; Hand Surgery 2007; **Med School:** Univ Tenn Coll Med 1969; **Resid:** Surgery, Univ Wisc Med Ctr 1975; **Fellow:** Hand Surgery, Duke Univ Med Ctr 1977; Pediatric Orthopaedic Surgery, Chldns Hosp-Harvard 1986; **Fac Appt:** Prof OrS, Washington Univ, St Louis

Graham, Thomas J MD [HS] - **Spec Exp:** Hand & Wrist Surgery; Elbow Surgery; Sports Injuries; Wrist/Hand Injuries; **Hospital:** Cleveland Clin (page 55); **Address:** Cleveland Clin-Dept Orthopedics, MC GCIC-10, 9500 Euclid Ave, Cleveland, OH 44195; **Phone:** 216-444-6260; **Board Cert:** Orthopaedic Surgery 2007; Hand Surgery 2007; **Med School:** Univ Cincinnati 1988; **Resid:** Orthopaedic Surgery, Univ Michigan Med Ctr 1993; **Fellow:** Hand Surgery, Indiana Hand Ctr 1994; Elbow Surgery, Mayo Clinic 1994

Hastings II, Hill MD [HS] - **Spec Exp:** Wrist Surgery; Elbow Reconstruction; Fractures & Tendon Transfers; Arthritis; **Hospital:** St. Vincent Indianapolis Hosp; **Address:** Indiana Hand to Shoulder Ctr, 8501 Harcourt Rd, Indianapolis, IN 46260; **Phone:** 317-875-9105; **Board Cert:** Orthopaedic Surgery 1982; Hand Surgery 2010; **Med School:** USC Sch Med 1974; **Resid:** Surgery, Univ Colorado Med Ctr 1976; Orthopaedic Surgery, Mass Genl Hosp 1980; **Fellow:** Hand Surgery, St Vincent Hosp 1981; **Fac Appt:** Clin Prof OrS, Indiana Univ

Kleinman, William B MD [HS] - **Spec Exp:** Upper Extremity Surgery-Pediatric; Congenital Hand Deformities; Wrist Reconstruction; Hand Reconstruction; **Hospital:** St. Vincent Indianapolis Hosp; **Address:** Indiana Hand to Shoulder Ctr, 8501 Harcourt Rd, Indianapolis, IN 46260; **Phone:** 317-875-9105; **Board Cert:** Orthopaedic Surgery 1979; Hand Surgery 2000; **Med School:** Cornell Univ-Weill Med Coll 1972; **Resid:** Surgery, Univ Colorado Affil Hosp 1974; Orthopaedic Surgery, NY Orthopaedic Hosp 1977; **Fellow:** Hand Surgery, Columbia-Presby Med Ctr 1978; Microvascular Surgery, Duke Univ 1979; **Fac Appt:** Clin Prof OrS, Indiana Univ

Light, Terry R MD [HS] - **Spec Exp:** Hand-Congenital Anomaly; Hand Injuries-Pediatric; Arthritis; Thumb-Absence; **Hospital:** Loyola Univ Med Ctr, Shriners Hosp for Children-Chicago; **Address:** Loyola Univ Med Ctr, Dept Ortho Surg, 2160 S First Ave Maguire Bldg - rm 1700, Maywood, IL 60153-5590; **Phone:** 708-216-4570; **Board Cert:** Orthopaedic Surgery 1979; Hand Surgery 2010; **Med School:** Ros Franklin Univ/Chicago Med Sch 1973; **Resid:** Orthopaedic Surgery, Yale-New Haven Hosp 1977; **Fellow:** Hand Surgery, Hartford Combined Prog 1977; **Fac Appt:** Prof OrS, Loyola Univ-Stritch Sch Med

Mass, Daniel MD [HS] - **Spec Exp:** Tendon Surgery; Shoulder Reconstruction; Elbow Reconstruction; Wrist Surgery; **Hospital:** Univ of Chicago Med Ctr; **Address:** 5841 S Maryland Ave, Chicago, IL 60637; **Phone:** 773-834-3531; **Board Cert:** Orthopaedic Surgery 2007; Hand Surgery 2007; **Med School:** Univ Chicago-Pritzker Sch Med 1975; **Resid:** Orthopaedic Surgery, Univ Chicago Hosp 1979; **Fellow:** Hand Surgery, St Francis Hosp 1980; **Fac Appt:** Prof S, Univ Chicago-Pritzker Sch Med

Mih, Alexander D MD [HS] - **Spec Exp:** Pediatric Hand Surgery; Congenital Hand Deformities; Hand Reconstruction-Pediatric; Microsurgery; **Hospital:** IU Health University Hosp, St. Vincent Indianapolis Hosp; **Address:** Indiana Hand to Shoulder Ctr, 8501 Harcourt Rd, Indianapolis, IN 46260; **Phone:** 317-875-9105; **Board Cert:** Orthopaedic Surgery 2003; Hand Surgery 2003; **Med School:** Johns Hopkins Univ 1984; **Resid:** Orthopaedic Surgery, Mayo Clinic 1989; **Fellow:** Hand Surgery, Indiana Hand Ctr 1990; **Fac Appt:** Assoc Prof OrS, Indiana Univ

Hand Surgery

Nagle, Daniel J MD [HS] - **Spec Exp:** Wrist Surgery; Carpal Tunnel Syndrome; Cubital Tunnel Syndrome; **Hospital:** Northwestern Meml Hosp, Lurie Chldn's Hosp-Chicago; **Address:** Chicago Hand Surgery, 737 N Michigan Ave, Ste 700, Chicago, IL 60611-7108; **Phone:** 312-337-6960; **Board Cert:** Orthopaedic Surgery 2007; Hand Surgery 2007; **Med School:** Belgium 1978; **Resid:** Orthopaedic Surgery, Northwestern Univ Med Sch 1983; **Fellow:** Hand Surgery, Christine Kleinert 1984; **Fac Appt:** Prof OrS, Northwestern Univ

Putnam, Matthew D MD [HS] - **Spec Exp:** Wrist Surgery; Fracture Deformities/Arm; Arthritis; Nerve Disorders/Surgery; **Hospital:** Univ Minn Med Ctr, Fairview - Riverside Campus; **Address:** 2512 S 7th St, rm 102, Minneapolis, MN 55454; **Phone:** 612-273-9400; **Board Cert:** Orthopaedic Surgery 2008; Hand Surgery 2008; **Med School:** Dartmouth Med Sch 1977; **Resid:** Surgery, Roosevelt Hosp 1979; Orthopaedic Surgery, Univ Pittsburgh 1984; **Fellow:** Hand Surgery, NYOH 1985; **Fac Appt:** Prof OrS, Univ Minn

Seitz Jr, William H MD [HS] - **Spec Exp:** Hand & Upper Extremity Surgery; Shoulder Surgery; Elbow Surgery; Wrist Surgery; **Hospital:** Lutheran Med Ctr - Cleveland, Cleveland Clin (page 55); **Address:** 1730 W 25th St, Ste 2C, Cleveland, OH 44113; **Phone:** 216-363-2331; **Board Cert:** Orthopaedic Surgery 2008; Hand Surgery 2008; **Med School:** Columbia P&S 1979; **Resid:** Surgery, St Vincents Med Ctr 1981; Orthopaedic Surgery, Columbia-Presby Med Ctr 1984; **Fellow:** Hand & Microvascular Surgery, Columbia-Presby Med Ctr 1985; **Fac Appt:** Prof OrS, Case West Res Univ

Steinmann, Scott P MD [HS] - **Spec Exp:** Shoulder Surgery; Elbow Surgery; Brachial Plexus Palsy; Reconstructive Microvascular Surgery; **Hospital:** Mayo Med Ctr & Clin - Rochester; **Address:** Mayo Clin, Dept Hand Surgery, 200 1st St SW, Rochester, MN 55905; **Phone:** 507-284-4577; **Board Cert:** Orthopaedic Surgery 2004; Hand Surgery 2004; **Med School:** Cornell Univ-Weill Med Coll 1988; **Resid:** Orthopaedic Surgery, Hosp Special Surgery 1992; **Fellow:** Shoulder Surgery, NY-Presby/Columbia Univ Med Ctr 1995; Hand Surgery, Mayo Clin 1998; **Fac Appt:** Prof OrS, Mayo Med Sch

Stern, Peter J MD [HS] - **Spec Exp:** Hand & Wrist Surgery; Microsurgery; **Hospital:** Good Samaritan Hosp - Cincinnati, Univ Hosp - Cincinnati; **Address:** Hand Surgery Specialists, 538 Oak St, Ste 200, Cincinnati, OH 45219; **Phone:** 513-961-4263; **Board Cert:** Orthopaedic Surgery 2011; Hand Surgery 2011; **Med School:** Washington Univ, St Louis 1970; **Resid:** Surgery, Beth Israel Hosp 1972; Orthopaedic Surgery, Harvard Combined Prgm 1977; **Fellow:** Hand Surgery, Univ Louisville Hosps 1979; **Fac Appt:** Prof OrS, Univ Cincinnati

Great Plains and Mountains

Idler, Richard S MD [HS] - **Spec Exp:** Upper Extremity Surgery; Microsurgery; **Hospital:** Penrose Hosp, St. Francis Med Ctr; **Address:** Colorado Springs Orthopaedic Grp, 3010 N Circle, Ste 100b, Colorado Springs, CO 80909; **Phone:** 719-632-7669; **Board Cert:** Orthopaedic Surgery 1985; Hand Surgery 2010; **Med School:** Dartmouth Med Sch 1975; **Resid:** Surgery, UCLA Med Ctr 1977; Plastic Surgery, UCLA Med Ctr 1978; **Fellow:** Orthopaedic Surgery, Mass Genl Hosp-Harvard 1981; Hand Surgery, St Vincent Hosp 1982; **Fac Appt:** Asst Clin Prof OrS, Indiana Univ

Southwest

Breidenbach III, Warren C MD [HS] - **Spec Exp:** Transplant-Hand; **Hospital:** Univ Arizona Med Ctr-Univ Campus; **Address:** UPH Clin at Alvernon, 707 N Alvernon Way Fl 2 - Ste 201, Tucson, AZ 85711; **Phone:** 520-694-8888; **Board Cert:** Plastic Surgery 1988; Hand Surgery 2003; **Med School:** Univ Calgary 1975; **Resid:** Surgery, McGill Affil Hosp 1979; Plastic Surgery, McGill Affil Hosp 1981; **Fellow:** Microsurgery, Eastern Va Med Sch 1982; Hand Surgery, Kleinert Inst 1984; **Fac Appt:** Prof PlS, Univ Ariz Coll Med

Collins, Evan D MD [HS] - **Spec Exp:** Hand & Upper Extremity Surgery; Wrist/Hand Injuries; Elbow Surgery; Sports Medicine; **Hospital:** Methodist Hosp - Houston; **Address:** Methodist Hospital, Dept Orthopaedics, 6560 Fannin St, Scurlock Twr Fl 4 Ste 410, Houston, TX 77030; **Phone:** 713-441-3535; **Board Cert:** Orthopaedic Surgery 2011; Hand Surgery 2011; **Med School:** SUNY Downstate 1992; **Resid:** Surgery, Baylor Affil Hosp 1997; **Fellow:** Hand Surgery, Baylor College Med 1999

Ezaki, Marybeth MD [HS] - **Spec Exp:** Hand-Congenital Anomaly; Hand Reconstruction-Pediatric; **Hospital:** Texas Scottish Rite Hosp for Chldn; **Address:** 2222 Welborn St, Dallas, TX 75219; **Phone:** 214-559-7842; **Board Cert:** Orthopaedic Surgery 1985; **Med School:** Yale Univ 1977; **Resid:** Orthopaedic Surgery, Univ Tex SW Med Ctr 1982; **Fellow:** Hand Surgery, Weyham Pk Hosp 1982; **Fac Appt:** Assoc Prof OrS, Univ Tex SW, Dallas

Moneim, Moheb S MD [HS] - **Hospital:** Univ Hosp - New Mexico; **Address:** 1101 Medical Arts Rd Bldg 5, Dept Orthopedics, MSC10-5600, Albuquerque, NM 87131; **Phone:** 505-272-4107; **Board Cert:** Orthopaedic Surgery 1998; Hand Surgery 2010; **Med School:** Egypt 1963; **Resid:** Orthopaedic Surgery, Duke Univ Med Ctr 1975; **Fellow:** Hand Surgery, Hosp for Spec Surgery 1976; **Fac Appt:** Prof OrS, Univ New Mexico

Rayan, Ghazi M MD [HS] - **Spec Exp:** Microsurgery; Congenital Limb Deformities; Arthritis; **Hospital:** Integris Baptist Med Ctr - OK, OU Med Ctr; **Address:** 3366 Northwest Expressway D Bldg - Ste 700, Oklahoma City, OK 73112-4439; **Phone:** 405-945-4888; **Board Cert:** Orthopaedic Surgery 2000; **Med School:** Egypt 1973; **Resid:** Surgery, S Baltimore Genl Hosp 1977; Orthopaedic Surgery, Union Meml Hosp 1980; **Fellow:** Hand & Microvascular Surgery, Union Meml Hosp 1980; **Fac Appt:** Clin Prof OrS, Univ Okla Coll Med

West Coast and Pacific

Abrams, Reid A MD [HS] - **Spec Exp:** Hand & Upper Extremity Surgery; Elbow Reconstruction; Fractures & Tendon Transfers; Carpal Tunnel Syndrome; **Hospital:** UCSD Med Ctr; **Address:** UCSD Med Ctr, Dept Orthopaedic Surgery, 200 W Arbor St, San Diego, CA 92103; **Phone:** 858-657-8200; **Board Cert:** Orthopaedic Surgery 2002; Hand Surgery 2002; **Med School:** Univ Colorado 1982; **Resid:** Orthopaedic Surgery, Univ Colo Med Ctr 1987; **Fellow:** Pediatric Orthopaedic Surgery, Chldns Hosp Hlth Ctr 1988; Hand Surgery, Brigham & Womens Hosp 1989; **Fac Appt:** Prof OrS, UCSD

Atkinson, Robert E MD [HS] - **Spec Exp:** Arthritis; Arthroscopic Surgery; Nerve Disorders/Surgery; **Hospital:** Queen's Med Ctr - Honolulu, Kapiolani Med Ctr @ Pali Momi; **Address:** Queen's Physicians' Office Bldg 1, 1380 Lusitana St, Ste 604, Honolulu, HI 96813; **Phone:** 808-521-8128; **Board Cert:** Orthopaedic Surgery 1985; **Med School:** Jefferson Med Coll 1977; **Resid:** Orthopaedic Surgery, Hosp Special Surgery 1982; **Fellow:** Hand Surgery, Mass Genl Hosp 1983; **Fac Appt:** Clin Prof OrS, Univ Hawaii JA Burns Sch Med

Chang, James MD [HS] - **Spec Exp:** Hand & Upper Extremity Surgery; Reconstructive Surgery; Pediatric Hand Surgery; Peripheral Nerve Surgery; **Hospital:** Stanford Univ Hosp & Clinics; **Address:** SUMC Hand & Upper Extremity Surgery, 450 Broadway St, Pavilion A, Fl 2, Redwood City, CA 94063-6120; **Phone:** 650-723-5256; **Board Cert:** Plastic Surgery 2009; Hand Surgery 2011; **Med School:** Yale Univ 1993; **Resid:** Plastic Surgery, Stanford Univ Med Ctr 1998; **Fellow:** Hand Surgery, UCLA Med Ctr 2000; **Fac Appt:** Prof PlS, Stanford Univ

Godzik, Cathleen A MD [HS] - **Spec Exp:** Congenital Hand Deformities; Sports Injuries; Dupuytren's Contracture; Arthritis; **Hospital:** Good Samaritan Hosp - LA, California Hosp Med Ctr; **Address:** 1245 Wilshire Blvd, Ste 611, Los Angeles, CA 90017; **Phone:** 213-482-6100; **Board Cert:** Orthopaedic Surgery 2001; Hand Surgery 2001; **Med School:** NY Med Coll 1981; **Resid:** Surgery, Brown Univ Sch Med 1983; Orthopaedic Surgery, Univ Conn Sch Med 1985; **Fellow:** Hand Surgery, Joseph Boyes Hand Fell-USC 1987

Hanel, Douglas P MD [HS] - **Spec Exp:** Reconstructive Microvascular Surgery; Hand-Congenital Anomaly; Elbow Reconstruction; **Hospital:** Harborview Med Ctr, Seattle Chldns Hosp; **Address:** Harborview Medical Ctr, 325 9th Ave, Fl 6, MS 359798, Seattle, WA 98104-2420; **Phone:** 206-744-3462; **Board Cert:** Orthopaedic Surgery 2007; Hand Surgery 2007; **Med School:** St Louis Univ 1977; **Resid:** Orthopaedic Surgery, St Louis Univ Hosp 1982; **Fellow:** Hand Surgery, Univ Louisville Hosp 1983; Microsurgery, Univ Louisville Hosp 1983; **Fac Appt:** Prof OrS, Univ Wash

Hentz, Vincent R MD [HS] - **Spec Exp:** Hand & Upper Extremity Surgery; Pediatric Hand Surgery; Brachial Plexus Palsy; **Hospital:** Stanford Univ Hosp & Clinics; **Address:** Hand & Upper Extremity Surgery, 450 Broadway St, Pavilion A Fl 2, Redwood City, CA 94063; **Phone:** 650-723-5256; **Board Cert:** Plastic Surgery 2007; Hand Surgery 2002; **Med School:** Univ Fla Coll Med 1968; **Resid:** Plastic Surgery, Stanford Univ Hosp 1974; **Fellow:** Hand Surgery, Roosevelt Hosp 1975; **Fac Appt:** Prof Emeritus S, Stanford Univ

Jones, Neil F MD [HS] - **Spec Exp:** Hand Reconstruction-Pediatric; Nerve Disorders/Surgery; Tendon Surgery; Toe-to-Hand Transfer; **Hospital:** UC Irvine Med Ctr, Chldns Hosp Orange Co; **Address:** 101 The City Drive S, Pavillion 3, Orange, CA 92868; **Phone:** 714-456-7012; **Board Cert:** Plastic Surgery 1985; **Med School:** England, UK 1974; **Resid:** Surgery, Radcliffe Infirmary 1979; Plastic Surgery, Univ Mich Med Ctr 1981; **Fellow:** Plastic Surgery, St Bartholomew's Hosp 1982; Hand & Microvascular Surgery, Mass Gen Hosp 1983; **Fac Appt:** Prof S, UC Irvine

Meals, Roy A MD [HS] - **Spec Exp:** Hand & Wrist Surgery; **Hospital:** UCLA Ronald Reagan Med Ctr; **Address:** 1033 Gayley Ave, Ste 104, Los Angeles, CA 90024; **Phone:** 310-824-1262; **Board Cert:** Orthopaedic Surgery 1980; Hand Surgery 2010; **Med School:** Vanderbilt Univ 1971; **Resid:** Surgery, Johns Hopkins Hosp 1973; Orthopaedic Surgery, Johns Hopkins Hosp 1978; **Fellow:** Hand Surgery, Mass Genl Hosp 1979; **Fac Appt:** Clin Prof S, UCLA

Slutsky, David J MD [HS] - **Spec Exp:** Preiser's Disease; Keinbocks Disease; Microsurgery; Arthroscopic Surgery; **Hospital:** LAC - Harbor - UCLA Med Ctr, Torrance Memorial Med Ctr; **Address:** The Slutsky Hand & Wrist Inst, 2808 Columbia St, Torrance, CA 90503; **Phone:** 310-618-9922; **Board Cert:** Orthopaedic Surgery 2002; Hand Surgery 2002; **Med School:** Univ Manitoba 1981; **Resid:** Orthopaedic Surgery, Univ Manitoba Med Ctr 1987; **Fellow:** Hand & Microvascular Surgery, Loma Linda Univ Med Ctr 1989; **Fac Appt:** Asst Prof OrS, UCLA

Szabo, Robert M MD [HS] - **Spec Exp:** Peripheral Nerve Surgery; Hand Injuries; Hand & Upper Extremity Tumors; **Hospital:** UC Davis Med Ctr, Mercy General Hosp - Sacramento; **Address:** UC Davis, Dept Orthopaedics, 4860 Y St, Ste 1700, Sacramento, CA 95817; **Phone:** 916-734-3678; **Board Cert:** Orthopaedic Surgery 2009; Hand Surgery 2009; **Med School:** SUNY Buffalo 1977; **Resid:** Surgery, Mt Sinai Hosp 1979; Orthopaedic Surgery, Mt Sinai Hosp 1982; **Fellow:** Hand Surgery, UCSD Med Ctr 1983; Epidemiology, UC Berkeley 1995; **Fac Appt:** Prof OrS, UC Davis

Trumble, Thomas MD [HS] - **Spec Exp:** Nerve Disorders/Surgery; Upper Extremity Trauma; **Hospital:** Overlake Hosp Med Ctr; **Address:** Bellevue Bone & Joint, 1632 116th Ave NE, Ste C, Bellevue, WA 98004; **Phone:** 425-458-5543; **Board Cert:** Orthopaedic Surgery 2009; Hand Surgery 2009; **Med School:** Yale Univ 1979; **Resid:** Orthopaedic Surgery, Yale-New Haven Hosp 1984; **Fellow:** Microvascular Surgery, Duke Univ Med Ctr 1984; Hand Surgery, Mass Genl Hosp 1985; **Fac Appt:** Prof S, Univ Wash

Hand Surgery

Cleveland Clinic's Upper Extremity Center, a center within the Department of Orthopaedic Surgery, provides a centralized, comprehensive diagnostic and treatment center for problems affecting the hand, wrist, elbow and shoulder. Since 1992, *U.S. News & World Report* has consistently ranked the Department of Orthopaedic Surgery among the top 10 orthopaedic programs in the nation.

Surgery of the Upper Extremity

Our surgeons are experts in diagnosing and providing the operative care for a wide array of upper extremity disorders. They perform the newest surgical techniques, such as microsurgery and minimally invasive surgery.

Our team focuses on the advancement of treatments and diagnostic insights by valuing education, research and the latest technologies.

Areas our specialists see and treat on a regular basis include:

Shoulder: fractures and dislocations, arthritis, chronic instability, replacement, rotator cuff tears, brachial plexus, injuries (occupational, sport or accidental)

Elbow: fractures and dislocations, tennis and golfer's elbow, arthritis, throwing elbow

Wrist: fractures and nonunions, dislocations, instability, carpal tunnel syndrome, tendonitis, arthritis

Hand: fractures and dislocations, trigger finger

HAND SURGERY

NYU Langone Medical Center's Department of Orthopaedic Surgery provides the full continuum of care for patients with hand and wrist disorders through its specialized Division of Hand Surgery. These include fractures, congenital anomalies, soft tissue and skeletal trauma, degenerative and rheumatoid arthritis, sports-related injuries, vascular disorders, tumors and occupational disorders.

The Hand Division specializes in fractures of the wrist and distal radius and reconstructive hand surgery. Hand surgery experts have particular expertise in post-traumatic injuries, arthritis and congenital, neuromuscular and neoplastic conditions. Offering one of the largest hand programs in the United States, the Division's hand specialists provide extensive care for the many problems that affect the upper extremity, including acute traumatic injuries (fractures, dislocations and tendon, nerve and vascular lacerations), post-traumatic and arthritic deformities, acquired problems (nerve compressions and tumors), congenital deformities and neuromuscular disorders such as cerebral palsy. Board-certified and fellowship-trained orthopaedists perform more than 5,000 procedures on adults and children each year.

After surgery, hand therapy helps surgical patients recover full or partial use of their hands, providing comprehensive rehabilitation for a variety of ailments associated with the hand and upper body. The hand therapy unit, located at NYU Langone's new, state-of-the-art Center for Musculoskeletal Care, specializes in fractures, traumatic injuries, tendonitis, sports injuries, work-related injuries, repetitive stress injuries, carpal tunnel syndrome, tendon and nerve repairs and arthritis. Hand therapy is provided by the expert occupational therapists of Rusk Rehabilitation, who specialize in treatment of the hand and upper extremities.

Research within the Hand Service focuses on a variety of clinical problems including wrist fractures, non-unions of the scaphoid (bone between the hand and the forearm), Kienbock's disease (the death and fracture of bone tissue due to interruption of blood supply), intercarpal subluxations (incomplete or partial dislocation) and neuropathies (disorders of the nerves) of the upper extremities.

Hematology &
Medical Oncology
a subspecialty of Internal Medicine

Hematology: An internist with additional training who specializes in diseases of the blood, spleen and lymph glands. This specialist treats conditions such as anemia, clotting disorders, sickle cell disease, hemophilia, leukemia and lymphoma.

Medical Oncology: An internist who specializes in the diagnosis and treatment of all types of cancer and other benign and malignant tumors. This specialist decides on and administers chemotherapy for malignancy, as well as consulting with surgeons and radiotherapists on other treatments for cancer.

Training Required: Three years in internal medicine *plus* additional training and examination for certification in hematology or medical oncology.

HEMATOLOGY

New England

Anderson, Kenneth C MD [Hem] - **Spec Exp:** Multiple Myeloma; Hematologic Malignancies; **Hospital:** Dana-Farber Cancer Inst (page 57), Brigham and Women's Hosp (page 57); **Address:** Dana Farber Cancer Inst, 450 Brookline Ave, Ste M557, Boston, MA 02215; **Phone:** 617-632-2144; **Board Cert:** Internal Medicine 1980; **Med School:** Johns Hopkins Univ 1977; **Resid:** Internal Medicine, Johns Hopkins Hosp 1980; **Fellow:** Hematology & Oncology, Dana Farber Cancer Inst 1983; **Fac Appt:** Prof Med, Harvard Med Sch

Ballen, Karen K MD [Hem] - **Spec Exp:** Leukemia; Bone Marrow Transplant; **Hospital:** Mass Genl Hosp; **Address:** Mass General Hospital, 55 Fruit St, COX 1, Ste 120, Boston, MA 02114; **Phone:** 617-724-1124; **Board Cert:** Internal Medicine 1989; Medical Oncology 2003; Hematology 2004; **Med School:** Dartmouth Med Sch 1986; **Resid:** Internal Medicine, Beth Israel Deaconess Med Ctr 1989; **Fellow:** Hematology & Oncology, Brigham & Women's Hosp 1992; **Fac Appt:** Assoc Prof Med, Harvard Med Sch

Comenzo, Raymond MD [Hem] - **Spec Exp:** Plasma Cell Disorders; Stem Cell Transplant; Amyloidosis; POEMS Syndrome; **Hospital:** Tufts Med Ctr; **Address:** Tufts Medical Center, 800 Washington St, Box 826, Boston, MA 02111; **Phone:** 617-636-6454; **Board Cert:** Internal Medicine 1989; Hematology 2004; Blood Banking Transfusion Medicine 1992; **Med School:** Boston Univ 1986; **Resid:** Internal Medicine, Boston City Hosp 1989; **Fellow:** Hematology & Oncology, New Engl Med Ctr 1991

Duffy, Thomas P MD [Hem] - **Spec Exp:** Mast Cell Diseases; Leukemia; Lymphoma; Mast Cell Diseases; **Hospital:** Yale-New Haven Hosp, Yale Med Group; **Address:** Yale Univ, Sect Hematology, 35 Park St Fl 7, New Haven, CT 06520-8021; **Phone:** 203-785-4744; **Board Cert:** Internal Medicine 1972; Hematology 1974; **Med School:** Johns Hopkins Univ 1962; **Resid:** Internal Medicine, Johns Hopkins Hosp 1965; **Fellow:** Hematology, Johns Hopkins Hosp 1970; **Fac Appt:** Prof Med, Yale Univ

Klingemann, Hans-Georg MD/PhD [Hem] - **Spec Exp:** Bone Marrow Transplant; Stem Cell Transplant; **Hospital:** Tufts Med Ctr; **Address:** 303 Columbus Ave, Ste 804, Boston, MA 02116; **Phone:** 617-943-7474; **Med School:** Germany 1976; **Resid:** Internal Medicine, Univ Wurzburg Med Sch 1979; **Fellow:** Hematology & Oncology, Fred Hutchinson Cancer Rsch Ctr 1986; **Fac Appt:** Prof Med, Tufts Univ

Marks, Peter W MD/PhD [Hem] - **Spec Exp:** Leukemia; Platelet Disorders; Bleeding/Coagulation Disorders; Hemophilia; **Hospital:** Yale-New Haven Hosp, Yale Med Group; **Address:** Yale Hematology, 333 Cedar St, Box 208302, New Haven, CT 06520; **Phone:** 203-200-4363; **Board Cert:** Internal Medicine 2004; Hematology 2007; Medical Oncology 2007; **Med School:** NYU Sch Med 1991; **Resid:** Internal Medicine, Brigham & Women's Hosp 1994; **Fellow:** Hematology & Oncology, Brigham & Women's Hosp 1996; **Fac Appt:** Assoc Prof Med, Yale Univ

Meehan, Kenneth MD [Hem] - **Spec Exp:** Bone Marrow Transplant; **Hospital:** Dartmouth - Hitchcock Med Ctr; **Address:** Norris Cotton Cancer Ctr, Dartmouth-Hitchcock Med Ctr, 1 Medical Center Drive, Lebanon, NH 03756; **Phone:** 603-650-4628; **Board Cert:** Internal Medicine 1989; Hematology 2004; **Med School:** Georgetown Univ 1986; **Resid:** Internal Medicine, Georgetown Univ 1989; **Fellow:** Hematology & Oncology, Dartmouth-Hitchcock Med Ctr 1992; **Fac Appt:** Assoc Prof Med, Dartmouth Med Sch

Miller, Kenneth B MD [Hem] - **Spec Exp:** Bone Marrow Transplant; Leukemia; Myelodysplastic Syndromes; **Hospital:** Tufts Med Ctr; **Address:** Tufts Med Ctr, Dept Medicine, 800 Washington St, Box 245, Boston, MA 02111; **Phone:** 617-636-2600; **Board Cert:** Internal Medicine 1976; Hematology 1980; **Med School:** NY Med Coll 1972; **Resid:** Internal Medicine, NYU Med Ctr/VA Hosp 1976; Internal Medicine, NYU Med Ctr 1976; **Fellow:** Hematology, New England Med Ctr 1979; **Fac Appt:** Prof Med, Tufts Univ

Richardson, Paul G MD [Hem] - **Spec Exp:** Multiple Myeloma; **Hospital:** Dana-Farber Cancer Inst (page 57), Brigham and Women's Hosp (page 57); **Address:** Dana Farber Cancer Inst, 450 Brookline Ave, Ste 1B30, Boston, MA 02215; **Phone:** 617-632-2127; **Med School:** England, UK 1986; **Resid:** Internal Medicine, Baystate Med Ctr 1994; **Fellow:** Medical Oncology, Dana Farber Cancer Inst 1995; Hematology, Beth Israel Deaconess Med Ctr 1997; **Fac Appt:** Assoc Prof Med, Harvard Med Sch

Schiffman, Fred J MD [Hem] - **Spec Exp:** Hematologic Malignancies; Anemia-Cancer Related; Bleeding/Coagulation Disorders; **Hospital:** Miriam Hosp; **Address:** Comp Cancer Ctr at Miriam Hospital, 164 Summit Ave, Fain-3, Providence, RI 02906; **Phone:** 401-793-2920; **Board Cert:** Internal Medicine 1979; Hematology 1982; Medical Oncology 1987; **Med School:** NYU Sch Med 1973; **Resid:** Internal Medicine, Yale-New Haven Hosp 1975; Internal Medicine, Yale-New Haven Hosp 1979; **Fellow:** Hematology, Yale-New Haven Hosp 1981; **Fac Appt:** Prof Med, Brown Univ

Spitzer, Thomas R MD [Hem] - **Spec Exp:** Bone Marrow Transplant; Leukemia; **Hospital:** Mass Genl Hosp; **Address:** Mass General Hospital, 55 Fruit St, COX 1, Ste 120, Boston, MA 02114; **Phone:** 617-724-1124; **Board Cert:** Internal Medicine 1977; Medical Oncology 1983; Hematology 1984; **Med School:** Univ Rochester 1974; **Resid:** Internal Medicine, NYew York Hosp-Cornell Med Ctr 1977; Internal Medicine, Mem Sloan Kettering Cancer Ctr 1977; **Fellow:** Hematology & Oncology, Case West Res Univ 1983; **Fac Appt:** Prof Onc, Harvard Med Sch

Stone, Richard M MD [Hem] - **Spec Exp:** Leukemia; **Hospital:** Dana-Farber Cancer Inst (page 57), Brigham and Women's Hosp (page 57); **Address:** Dana Farber Cancer Inst, 450 Brookline Ave, Boston, MA 02215; **Phone:** 617-632-1906; **Board Cert:** Internal Medicine 1984; Medical Oncology 2008; Hematology 1988; **Med School:** Harvard Med Sch 1981; **Resid:** Internal Medicine, Brigham & Womens Hosp 1984; **Fellow:** Medical Oncology, Dana-Farber Cancer Inst 1987; **Fac Appt:** Prof Med, Harvard Med Sch

Mid Atlantic

Abrams, Charles S MD [Hem] - **Spec Exp:** Bleeding/Coagulation Disorders; Thrombotic Disorders; **Hospital:** Hosp Univ Penn - UPHS (page 72); **Address:** Perelman Ctr for Advanced Medicine, 3400 Civic Center Blvd, West Pavilion, 2nd Fl, Philadelphia, PA 19104; **Phone:** 215-615-5858; **Board Cert:** Internal Medicine 1987; Medical Oncology 1989; Hematology 2005; **Med School:** Yale Univ 1984; **Resid:** Internal Medicine, Hosp Univ Penn 1987; **Fellow:** Hematology & Oncology, Hosp Univ Penn 1988; **Fac Appt:** Prof Med, Univ Pennsylvania

Allen, Steven Lee MD [Hem] - **Spec Exp:** Bleeding/Coagulation Disorders; Leukemia & Lymphoma; Multiple Myeloma; Gaucher Disease; **Hospital:** N Shore Univ Hosp (page 67), Long Island Jewish Med Ctr (page 67); **Address:** Monter Cancer Ctr, 450 Lakeville Rd, Lake Success, NY 11042; **Phone:** 516-734-8959; **Board Cert:** Internal Medicine 1980; Hematology 1982; Medical Oncology 1983; **Med School:** Johns Hopkins Univ 1977; **Resid:** Internal Medicine, NY Hosp-Cornell 1980; **Fellow:** Hematology & Oncology, NY Hosp-Cornell 1983; **Fac Appt:** Prof Med, Hofstra N Shore-LIJ Sch Med

Baer, Maria R MD [Hem] - **Spec Exp:** Leukemia; Myelodysplastic Syndromes; Myeloproliferative Disorders; **Hospital:** Univ of MD Med Ctr; **Address:** Univ Maryland, Greenebaum Cancer Ctr, 22 S Greene St, Baltimore, MD 21201; **Phone:** 410-328-7904; **Board Cert:** Internal Medicine 1983; Hematology 1984; **Med School:** Johns Hopkins Univ 1979; **Resid:** Internal Medicine, Vanderbilt Univ Hosp 1982; **Fellow:** Hematology, Vanderbilt Univ Hosp 1985; **Fac Appt:** Prof Hem & Onc, Univ MD Sch Med

Brodsky, Robert A MD [Hem] - **Spec Exp:** Hematologic Malignancies; Autoimmune Disease; Graft vs Host Disease; **Hospital:** Johns Hopkins Hosp (page 61); **Address:** Johns Hopkins Div Hematology, 720 Rutland Ave, Ross Bldg, rm 1025, Baltimore, MD 21205; **Phone:** 410-955-8964; **Board Cert:** Internal Medicine 2002; Hematology 2006; **Med School:** Hahnemann Univ 1989; **Resid:** Internal Medicine, Vanderbilt Univ 1991; **Fellow:** Hematology, Vanderbilt Univ Hosp 1994; Medical Oncology, Johns Hopkins Hosp 1997; **Fac Appt:** Prof Med, Johns Hopkins Univ

Cheson, Bruce D MD [Hem] - **Spec Exp:** Leukemia; Hematologic Malignancies; **Hospital:** Georgetown Univ Hosp; **Address:** GUMC-Lombardi Cancer Ctr, 3800 Reservoir Rd NW, Podium A, Washington, DC 20007; **Phone:** 202-444-7932; **Board Cert:** Internal Medicine 1974; Hematology 1976; **Med School:** Tufts Univ 1971; **Resid:** Internal Medicine, Univ Virginia Hosp 1974; **Fellow:** Hematology, New England Med Ctr Hosp 1976

Diuguid, David L MD [Hem] - **Spec Exp:** Bleeding/Coagulation Disorders; **Hospital:** NY-Presby/Columbia Univ Med Ctr, NY (page 66); **Address:** 161 Ft Washington Ave, Irving Bldg Fl 10, New York, NY 10032; **Phone:** 212-305-0527; **Board Cert:** Internal Medicine 1982; Hematology 1986; Medical Oncology 1985; **Med School:** Cornell Univ-Weill Med Coll 1979; **Resid:** Internal Medicine, Boston Univ Med Ctr 1983; **Fellow:** Hematology & Oncology, New England Med Ctr 1986; **Fac Appt:** Assoc Prof Med, Columbia P&S

Filicko-O'Hara, Joanne E MD [Hem] - **Spec Exp:** Hematologic Malignancies; Leukemia & Lymphoma; Bone Marrow Transplant; **Hospital:** Thomas Jefferson Univ Hosp; **Address:** Jefferson Univ Physicians, 925 Chestnut St, Ste 220A, Phildelphia, PA 19107; **Phone:** 215-955-8874; **Board Cert:** Hematology 2009; Medical Oncology 2010; **Med School:** Hahnemann Univ 1992; **Resid:** Internal Medicine, Thomas Jefferson Univ Hosp 1995; **Fellow:** Hematology & Oncology, Thomas Jefferson Univ Hosp 1998; **Fac Appt:** Asst Prof Med, Jefferson Med Coll

Friedman, Alan L MD [Hem] - **Spec Exp:** Leukemia & Lymphoma; Myelodysplastic Syndromes; Multiple Myeloma; **Hospital:** Albert Einstein Med Ctr, Jeanes Hosp; **Address:** Albert Einstein Med Ctr, 5501 Old York Rd Braemer Bldg Fl 2 - Ste 1, Philadelphia, PA 19141; **Phone:** 215-456-3880; **Board Cert:** Internal Medicine 1978; Medical Oncology 1982; Hematology 1981; **Med School:** Hahnemann Univ 1975; **Resid:** Internal Medicine, Albert Einstein Med Ctr 1978; **Fellow:** Medical Oncology, Meml Sloan-Kettering Cancer Ctr 1980; Hematology, Thomas Jefferson Univ Hosp 1981

Fruchtman, Steven M MD [Hem] - **Spec Exp:** Myeloproliferative Disorders; Polycythemia Rubra Vera; **Address:** 1150 Park Ave, Ste Medical, New York, NY 10128; **Phone:** 212-427-7700; **Board Cert:** Internal Medicine 1980; Hematology 1984; **Med School:** NY Med Coll 1977; **Resid:** Internal Medicine, Univ Hosp 1981; **Fellow:** Hematology, Mount Sinai Med Ctr 1984; Hematology, Meml Sloan Kettering Cancer Ctr 1985; **Fac Appt:** Assoc Prof Hem & Onc, NY Med Coll

Goldberg, Jack MD [Hem] - **Spec Exp:** Leukemia; Lymphoma; Multiple Myeloma; Bone Marrow Transplant; **Hospital:** Penn Presby Med Ctr - UPHS (page 72), Hosp Univ Penn - UPHS (page 72); **Address:** Abramson Cancer Ctr at Penn-Presby Hosp, 51 N 39th St, Medical Arts Bldg, Ste 103A, Philadelphia, PA 19104; **Phone:** 215-662-9801; **Board Cert:** Internal Medicine 1976; Hematology 1980; Medical Oncology 1989; **Med School:** SUNY Upstate Med Univ 1973; **Resid:** Internal Medicine, Boston Univ Hosp 1975; **Fellow:** Hematology & Oncology, SUNY Syracuse 1977; **Fac Appt:** Clin Prof Med, Univ Pennsylvania

Isola, Luis M MD [Hem] - **Spec Exp:** Bone Marrow Transplant; Stem Cell Transplant; Myelodysplastic Syndromes; Anemia; **Hospital:** Mount Sinai Med Ctr (page 64); **Address:** 1190 Fifth Ave, New York, NY 10029; **Phone:** 212-241-6021; **Board Cert:** Internal Medicine 1986; Hematology 1988; **Med School:** Argentina 1979; **Resid:** Internal Medicine, Ctr for Med Education 1983; **Fellow:** Hematology, Mt Sinai Med Ctr 1985; **Fac Appt:** Assoc Prof Med, Mount Sinai Sch Med

Kempin, Sanford J MD [Hem] - **Spec Exp:** Bleeding/Coagulation Disorders; Leukemia; Lymphoma; Thrombotic Disorders; **Hospital:** Beth Israel Med Ctr - Petrie Division (page 56); **Address:** 325 W 15th St, New York, NY 10011; **Phone:** 212-604-6010; **Board Cert:** Internal Medicine 1976; Medical Oncology 1977; Hematology 1978; **Med School:** Belgium 1971; **Resid:** Internal Medicine, Lemuel Shattuck Hosp 1972; **Fellow:** Hematology, St Jude Chldns Rsch Hosp 1975; Medical Oncology, Meml Sloan Kettering Cancer Ctr 1976; **Fac Appt:** Asst Prof Hem & Onc, Albert Einstein Coll Med

Kessler, Craig M MD [Hem] - **Spec Exp:** Bleeding/Coagulation Disorders; Hemophilia; Hematologic Malignancies; **Hospital:** Georgetown Univ Hosp; **Address:** GUMC, Lombardi Cancer Ctr, 3800 Reservoir Rd NW, Podium A, Washington, DC 20007; **Phone:** 202-444-8676; **Board Cert:** Internal Medicine 1976; Hematology 1980; **Med School:** Tulane Univ 1973; **Resid:** Internal Medicine, Ochsner Fdn Hosp 1976; **Fellow:** Hematology, Johns Hopkins Hosp 1978; **Fac Appt:** Prof Med, Georgetown Univ

Luger, Selina M MD [Hem] - **Spec Exp:** Myelodysplastic Syndromes; Myeloproliferative Disorders; Bone Marrow Transplant; **Hospital:** Hosp Univ Penn - UPHS (page 72); **Address:** Heme/Onc Perelman Center, 2 W 34th and Civic Ctr Blvd, Philadelphia, PA 19104; **Phone:** 215-662-6348; **Board Cert:** Hematology 1994; **Med School:** Canada 1987; **Resid:** Internal Medicine, Univ Pittsburgh Med Ctr 1990; **Fellow:** Hematology & Oncology, Pennsylvania Hosp-UPHS 1993; **Fac Appt:** Assoc Prof Med, Univ Pennsylvania

Mangan, Kenneth F MD [Hem] - **Spec Exp:** Bone Marrow Transplant; Hematologic Malignancies; Anemia-Aplastic; Paroxysmal Nocturnal Hemoglobinuria; **Hospital:** Temple Univ Hosp, Jeanes Hosp; **Address:** Temple BMT Program, Friends Hall Physicians Bldg, 7604 Central Ave, Lower Level, Philadelphia, PA 19111-2499; **Phone:** 215-214-3129; **Board Cert:** Internal Medicine 1976; Hematology 1978; **Med School:** Geo Wash Univ 1973; **Resid:** Internal Medicine, G Washington Univ Hosps 1976; **Fellow:** Hematology, Tufts-New England Med Ctr 1977

Marks, Stanley M MD [Hem] - **Spec Exp:** Leukemia; Lymphoma; Multiple Myeloma; **Hospital:** UPMC Shadyside, UPMC Presby, Pittsburgh; **Address:** UPMC- Hillman Cancer Ctr, 5115 Centre Ave Fl 3, Pittsburgh, PA 15232; **Phone:** 412-235-1020; **Board Cert:** Internal Medicine 1976; Hematology 1978; **Med School:** Univ Pittsburgh 1973; **Resid:** Internal Medicine, Presby Univ Hosp 1976; **Fellow:** Hematology & Oncology, Brigham Hosp/Dana Farber Cancer Ctr 1978; **Fac Appt:** Clin Prof Med, Univ Pittsburgh

Maslak, Peter G MD [Hem] - **Spec Exp:** Leukemia; Stem Cell Transplant; Myelodysplastic Syndromes; Clinical Trials; **Hospital:** Meml Sloan-Kettering Cancer Ctr; **Address:** 1275 York Avenue, New York, NY 10065; **Phone:** 212-639-5518; **Board Cert:** Internal Medicine 1987; Hematology 2000; Medical Oncology 1989; **Med School:** Mount Sinai Sch Med 1984; **Resid:** Internal Medicine, Univ Michigan Med Ctr 1987; **Fellow:** Hematology & Oncology, Meml Sloan Kettering Cancer Ctr 1990

Mears, John Gregory MD [Hem] - **Spec Exp:** Lymphoma; Leukemia; Multiple Myeloma; **Hospital:** NY-Presby/Columbia Univ Med Ctr, NY (page 66); **Address:** 161 Ft Washington Ave, Ste 923, New York, NY 10032; **Phone:** 212-305-3506; **Board Cert:** Internal Medicine 1976; Hematology 1978; **Med School:** Columbia P&S 1973; **Resid:** Internal Medicine, Boston Univ Med Ctr 1975; **Fellow:** Hematology & Oncology, Columbia-Presby Med Ctr 1978; **Fac Appt:** Clin Prof Med, Columbia P&S

Millenson, Michael M MD [Hem] - **Spec Exp:** Leukemia & Lymphoma; Thromboembolic Disorders; Hematologic Malignancies; **Hospital:** Fox Chase Cancer Ctr (page 58); **Address:** Fox Chase Cancer Center, 333 Cottman Ave, Philadelphia, PA 19111; **Phone:** 215-728-2600; **Board Cert:** Internal Medicine 1987; Medical Oncology 2000; **Med School:** Temple Univ 1984; **Resid:** Internal Medicine, Temple Univ Hosp 1987; **Fellow:** Hematology & Oncology, Beth Israel Hosp 1991

Porter, David L MD [Hem] - **Spec Exp:** Leukemia; Bone Marrow Transplant; Lymphoma; Gene Therapy; **Hospital:** Hosp Univ Penn - UPHS (page 72); **Address:** Perelman Ctr for Advanced Med Fl 2, 3400 Civic Center Blvd, Philadelphia, PA 19104; **Phone:** 215-615-5858; **Board Cert:** Hematology 2006; **Med School:** Brown Univ 1987; **Resid:** Internal Medicine, Univ Hosp 1990; **Fellow:** Hematology & Oncology, Brigham & Womens Hosp 1992; **Fac Appt:** Prof Med, Univ Pennsylvania

Rai, Kanti R MD [Hem] - **Spec Exp:** Leukemia; Lymphoma; Multiple Myeloma; **Hospital:** Long Island Jewish Med Ctr (page 67); **Address:** 410 Lakeville Rd, Ste 212, Long Island Jewish Med Ctr, Div of Hem-Onc, New Hyde Park, NY 10042; **Phone:** 718-470-4050; **Board Cert:** Pediatrics 1959; **Med School:** India 1955; **Resid:** Pediatrics, Lincoln Hosp 1958; Pediatrics, North Shore Univ Hosp 1959; **Fellow:** Hematology, LI Jewish Med Ctr 1960; **Fac Appt:** Prof Med, Albert Einstein Coll Med

Rao, A Koneti MD [Hem] - **Spec Exp:** Bleeding/Coagulation Disorders; Thromboembolic Disorders; Platelet Disorders; Inherited Disorders; **Hospital:** Temple Univ Hosp; **Address:** Temple Univ School of Med-Div Hematology, Old Med Sch Bldg, rm 310, Philadelphia, PA 19140; **Phone:** 215-707-4684; **Board Cert:** Internal Medicine 1977; Hematology 1980; **Med School:** India 1973; **Resid:** Internal Medicine, Thom Jeff Univ Hosp 1977; **Fellow:** Hematology & Oncology, Temple Univ Hosp 1978; Hematology, Thom Jeff Univ Hosp 1979; **Fac Appt:** Prof Hem & Onc, India

Raphael, Bruce Gordon MD [Hem] - **Spec Exp:** Lymphoma; Leukemia; Multiple Myeloma; Anemia; **Hospital:** NYU Langone Med Ctr (page 68), Bellevue Hosp Ctr; **Address:** NYU Clinical Cancer Ctr, 240 E 38th St Fl 19, New York, NY 10016-6402; **Phone:** 212-731-5185; **Board Cert:** Internal Medicine 1978; Hematology 1980; Medical Oncology 1981; **Med School:** McGill Univ 1975; **Resid:** Internal Medicine, Jewish Genl Hosp 1977; **Fellow:** Medical Oncology, Meml Sloan Kettering Cancer Ctr 1978; Hematology, NYU Med Ctr 1980; **Fac Appt:** Clin Prof Med, NYU Sch Med

Rapoport, Aaron P MD [Hem] - **Spec Exp:** Leukemia; Lymphoma; Multiple Myeloma; **Hospital:** Univ of MD Med Ctr; **Address:** Greenebaum Cancer Ctr, 22 S Greene St, Ste N9E12, Baltimore, MD 21201; **Phone:** 410-328-1230; **Board Cert:** Internal Medicine 1989; Hematology 2002; **Med School:** Harvard Med Sch 1986; **Resid:** Internal Medicine, Strong Meml Hosp 1989; **Fellow:** Hematology, Strong Meml Hosp 1989; **Fac Appt:** Prof Med, Univ MD Sch Med

Rowley, Scott D MD [Hem] - **Spec Exp:** Stem Cell Transplant; Bone Marrow Transplant; Graft vs Host Disease; **Hospital:** Hackensack Univ Med Ctr; **Address:** 92 2nd St, Ste 230, Hackensack, NJ 07601; **Phone:** 201-336-8289 x8291; **Board Cert:** Internal Medicine 1981; Medical Oncology 1983; Hematology 1984; **Med School:** Univ Mass Sch Med 1978; **Resid:** Internal Medicine, Rhode Island Hosp 1981; **Fellow:** Hematology & Oncology, Rhode Island Hosp 1984; **Fac Appt:** Assoc Prof Med, UMDNJ-NJ Med Sch, Newark

Savage, David G MD [Hem] - **Spec Exp:** Stem Cell Transplant; Multiple Myeloma; Lymphoma; **Hospital:** NY-Presby/Columbia Univ Med Ctr, NY (page 66); **Address:** 177 Fort Washington Ave, Fl 10, Millstein Bldg - Fl 6, rm 435, New York, NY 10032; **Phone:** 212-305-9783; **Board Cert:** Internal Medicine 1977; Hematology 1982; Medical Oncology 1985; **Med School:** Columbia P&S 1974; **Resid:** Internal Medicine, Harlem Hosp/Columbia Presby Med Ctr 1977; **Fellow:** Hematology & Oncology, Harlem Hosp/Columbia Presby Med Ctr 1982; **Fac Appt:** Prof Med, Columbia P&S

Schuster, Michael W MD [Hem] - **Spec Exp:** Bone Marrow Transplant; Hematologic Malignancies; Myelodysplastic Syndromes; Anemia-Aplastic; **Hospital:** Stony Brook Univ Med Ctr; **Address:** HSC T-15, Room 020, Z-8151, Stony Brook University Medical Center, Stony Brook, NY 11794-7909; **Phone:** 631-444-3577; **Board Cert:** Internal Medicine 1984; Hematology 1986; **Med School:** Dartmouth Med Sch 1980; **Resid:** Internal Medicine, Beth Israel Deaconess Med Ctr 1983; **Fellow:** Hematology & Oncology, Beth Israel Deaconess Med Ctr 1987; **Fac Appt:** Prof Hem & Onc, SUNY Stony Brook

Schuster, Stephen J MD [Hem] - **Spec Exp:** Lymphoma; Bone Marrow Transplant; **Hospital:** Hosp Univ Penn - UPHS (page 72); **Address:** Abramson Cancer Ctr, Perelman Ctr, West Pavilion Fl 2, 3400 Civic Ctr Blvd, Philadelphia, PA 19104; **Phone:** 215-614-1846; **Board Cert:** Internal Medicine 1984; Hematology 1986; Medical Oncology 1989; **Med School:** Jefferson Med Coll 1981; **Resid:** Internal Medicine, Pennsylvania Hosp 1984; **Fellow:** Hematology & Oncology, Thos Jefferson Univ Hosp 1986; **Fac Appt:** Assoc Prof Med, Univ Pennsylvania

Slease, Robert B MD [Hem] - **Spec Exp:** Hematologic Malignancies; Hodgkin's Lymphoma; Stem Cell Transplant; Clinical Trials; **Hospital:** Wilmington Hosp; **Address:** Cristiana Care Hlth Svs, Div Hematology, Medical Pavilion, 4701 Ogletown-Stanton Rd, Ste 4200, Newark, DE 19713; **Phone:** 302-737-7700; **Board Cert:** Internal Medicine 1975; Hematology 1978; **Med School:** Univ Kansas 1972; **Resid:** Internal Medicine, Natl Naval Med Ctr 1975; **Fellow:** Hematology, Natl Naval Med Ctr 1977; **Fac Appt:** Clin Prof Med, Jefferson Med Coll

Soff, Gerald A MD [Hem] - **Spec Exp:** Bleeding/Coagulation Disorders; Thrombotic Disorders; Hematologic Disorders in Cancer Patients; Anemia; **Hospital:** Meml Sloan-Kettering Cancer Ctr; **Address:** MSKCC Div of Hematology, 1275 York Ave Fl 4 - Ste 6, New York, NY 10021; **Phone:** 212-639-2335; **Board Cert:** Internal Medicine 1984; Hematology 1988; **Med School:** Johns Hopkins Univ 1981; **Resid:** Internal Medicine, Med Coll Virginia 1984; **Fellow:** Hematology & Oncology, Beth Israel Med Ctr 1988

Spivak, Jerry L MD [Hem] - **Spec Exp:** Myeloproliferative Disorders; Polycythemia Rubra Vera; Leukemia; Anemia; **Hospital:** Johns Hopkins Hosp (page 61); **Address:** 720 Rutland Ave, Traylor Bldg Fl 9 - Ste 924, Baltimore, MD 21205; **Phone:** 410-955-5454; **Board Cert:** Internal Medicine 1971; Hematology 1974; **Med School:** Cornell Univ-Weill Med Coll 1964; **Resid:** Internal Medicine, Johns Hopkins Hosp 1966; Internal Medicine, Johns Hopkins Hosp 1972; **Fellow:** Hematology, Natl Cancer Inst 1968; Hematology, Johns Hopkins Hosp 1971; **Fac Appt:** Prof Med, Johns Hopkins Univ

Strair, Roger MD/PhD [Hem] - **Spec Exp:** Leukemia; Lymphoma; Bone Marrow Transplant; Multiple Myeloma; **Hospital:** Robert Wood Johnson Univ Hosp - New Brunswick; **Address:** Cancer Inst of NJ, 195 Little Albany St, New Brunswick, NJ 08903; **Phone:** 732-235-7464; **Board Cert:** Internal Medicine 1984; Hematology 1986; Medical Oncology 1987; **Med School:** Albert Einstein Coll Med 1981; **Resid:** Internal Medicine, Brigham & Women's Hosp 1984; **Fellow:** Hematology & Oncology, Brigham & Women's Hosp 1988; **Fac Appt:** Assoc Prof Med, UMDNJ-RW Johnson Med Sch

Streiff, Michael B MD [Hem] - **Spec Exp:** Bleeding/Coagulation Disorders; Polycythemia Rubra Vera; Clinical Trials; **Hospital:** Johns Hopkins Hosp (page 61); **Address:** Johns Hopkins Div Hematology, 1830 E Monument St, Ste 7300, Baltimore, MD 21205; **Phone:** 410-955-3142; **Board Cert:** Internal Medicine 2002; Hematology 2004; **Med School:** Johns Hopkins Univ 1988; **Resid:** Internal Medicine, Shands Hosp-Univ Fla Coll Med 1991; **Fellow:** Hematology & Oncology, Johns Hopkins Univ Hosp 1994; **Fac Appt:** Assoc Prof Med, Johns Hopkins Univ

Hematology

Tallman, Martin S MD [Hem] - **Spec Exp:** Bone Marrow Transplant; Leukemia; Hairy Cell Leukemia; **Hospital:** Meml Sloan-Kettering Cancer Ctr; **Address:** 1275 York Ave, Box 380, Ste 21-100, New York, NY 10065; **Phone:** 212-639-3842; **Board Cert:** Internal Medicine 1983; Medical Oncology 1987; Hematology 1988; **Med School:** Ros Franklin Univ/Chicago Med Sch 1980; **Resid:** Internal Medicine, Evanston Hosp 1983; **Fellow:** Medical Oncology, Fred Hutchinson Cancer Ctr 1987; **Fac Appt:** Prof Med, Cornell Univ-Weill Med Coll

Wisch, Nathaniel MD [Hem] - **Spec Exp:** Lymphoma; Breast Cancer; Leukemia; Anemia-Cancer Related; **Hospital:** Lenox Hill Hosp (page 67), Mount Sinai Med Ctr (page 64); **Address:** Central Park Hematology & Oncology, 12 E 86th St, New York, NY 10028-0506; **Phone:** 212-861-6660; **Board Cert:** Internal Medicine 1965; Hematology 1972; Medical Oncology 1977; **Med School:** Northwestern Univ 1958; **Resid:** Internal Medicine, VA Hosp 1960; Internal Medicine, Montefiore Hosp 1961; **Fellow:** Hematology & Oncology, Mount Sinai Hosp 1962; **Fac Appt:** Clin Prof Med, Mount Sinai Sch Med

Yanovich, Saul MD [Hem] - **Spec Exp:** Bone Marrow Transplant; **Hospital:** Univ of MD Med Ctr; **Address:** 22 S Greene St, rm N9E12, Baltimore, MD 21201; **Phone:** 410-328-1230; **Board Cert:** Internal Medicine 1980; Hematology 1976; Medical Oncology 1981; **Med School:** Colombia 1970; **Resid:** Internal Medicine, Univ Miami-Jackson Meml Hosp 1974; Hematology, Univ Miami-Jackson Meml Hosp 1976; **Fellow:** Oncology, Dana Farber Canc Ctr 1978; **Fac Appt:** Prof Med, Univ MD Sch Med

Southeast

Adams-Graves, Patricia MD [Hem] - **Spec Exp:** Sickle Cell Disease; **Hospital:** Regional Med Ctr - Memphis; **Address:** 880 Madison Ave Fl 5 - Ste 5C01, Sickle Cell Center, Memphis, TN 38103; **Phone:** 901-545-8535; **Board Cert:** Internal Medicine 1989; **Med School:** Univ Louisville Sch Med 1986; **Resid:** Internal Medicine, Univ Louisville Affil Hosp 1989; **Fellow:** Hematology & Oncology, Univ Tennessee Hlth Science Ctr 1993; **Fac Appt:** Prof Med, Univ Tenn Coll Med

Bigelow, Carolyn L MD [Hem] - **Spec Exp:** Bone Marrow Transplant; Sickle Cell Disease; Leukemia; **Hospital:** Univ Mississippi Med Ctr; **Address:** Univ Mississippi Med Ctr-Div Hematology, 2500 N State St, Jackson, MS 39216; **Phone:** 601-984-5615; **Board Cert:** Internal Medicine 1982; Hematology 1988; **Med School:** Univ Miss 1979; **Resid:** Internal Medicine, Univ Mississippi Med Ctr 1982; **Fellow:** Hematology & Oncology, Univ Washington Med Ctr 1987; **Fac Appt:** Prof Med, Univ Miss

Djulbegovic, Benjamin MD/PhD [Hem] - **Spec Exp:** Multiple Myeloma; Lymphoma; Myeloproliferative Disorders; Clinical Trials; **Hospital:** H Lee Moffitt Cancer Ctr & Research Inst (page 59), Tampa Genl Hosp; **Address:** 12901 Bruce B Downs Blvd, MDC 27, Tampa, FL 33612; **Phone:** 813-396-9178; **Board Cert:** Internal Medicine 2002; Hematology 2004; **Med School:** Bosnia 1976; **Resid:** Internal Medicine, Univ Med Ctr 1983; Internal Medicine, Univ Louisville Med Ctr 1988; **Fellow:** Univ Manchester 1985; Hematology & Oncology, Univ Louisville 1990; **Fac Appt:** Prof Med, Univ S Fla Coll Med

Greer, John P MD [Hem] - **Spec Exp:** Leukemia & Lymphoma; Lymphoma-Cutaneous T Cell(CTCL); Stem Cell Transplant; Hematologic Malignancies; **Hospital:** Vanderbilt Univ Med Ctr (page 75); **Address:** Vanderbilt Ingram Cancer Ctr, 1301 Medical Center Drive, Ste 3297, Nashville, TN 37232; **Phone:** 615-936-8422; **Board Cert:** Pediatrics 1985; Internal Medicine 1979; Hematology 1984; Medical Oncology 1985; **Med School:** Vanderbilt Univ 1976; **Resid:** Internal Medicine, Tulane Univ Med Ctr 1979; Pediatrics, Med Coll Virginia Hosps 1981; **Fellow:** Hematology & Oncology, Vanderbilt Univ Med Ctr 1984; **Fac Appt:** Prof Med, Vanderbilt Univ

Komrokji, Rami S MD [Hem] - **Spec Exp:** Myelodysplastic Syndromes; Leukemia-Myeloid; Hodgkin's Lymphoma; Clinical Trials; **Hospital:** H Lee Moffitt Cancer Ctr & Research Inst (page 59); **Address:** H Lee Moffitt Canc Ctr & Rsch Inst, 12902 Magnolia Drive, Tampa, FL 33612; **Phone:** 813-745-8986; **Board Cert:** Hematology 2004; Medical Oncology 2004; **Med School:** Jordan 1996; **Resid:** Internal Medicine, Case Western Univ Affil Hosp 2001; **Fellow:** Hematology, Strong Meml Hosp 2004; **Fac Appt:** Assoc Prof

Laughlin, Mary J MD [Hem] - **Spec Exp:** Bone Marrow Transplant; Stem Cell Transplant; **Hospital:** Univ of Virginia Health Sys; **Address:** Univ Va Hlth, Dept Hematology/Oncology, Bone Marrow & Stem Cell Transplant Prgm, 1240 Lee St, Charlottesville, VA 22908; **Phone:** 434-982-6406; **Board Cert:** Internal Medicine 2003; Hematology 2004; **Med School:** SUNY Buffalo 1988; **Resid:** Internal Medicine, Duke Univ Med Ctr 1991; **Fellow:** Hematology & Oncology, Duke Univ Med Ctr 1992; Bone Marrow Transplant, Rosewell Park Cancer Inst 1994; **Fac Appt:** Assoc Prof Med, Case West Res Univ

Nimer, Stephen D MD [Hem] - **Spec Exp:** Bone Marrow Transplant; Myelodysplastic Syndromes; Leukemia; Stem Cell Transplant; **Hospital:** Univ of Miami Hosp & Clins/Sylvester Comp Canc Ctr; **Address:** 1550 NW 19th Ave, Fox 200 (M867), Miami, FL 33136; **Phone:** 305-243-5302; **Board Cert:** Internal Medicine 1982; Hematology 1986; Medical Oncology 1985; **Med School:** Univ Chicago-Pritzker Sch Med 1979; **Resid:** Internal Medicine, UCLA Med Ctr 1982; **Fellow:** Hematology & Oncology, UCLA Med Ctr 1986; **Fac Appt:** Prof Med, Univ Miami Sch Med

Ortel, Thomas L MD/PhD [Hem] - **Spec Exp:** Bleeding/Coagulation Disorders; Hemophilia; Thrombotic Disorders; **Hospital:** Duke Univ Hosp; **Address:** Duke Box 3422, 0563 Stead Bldg, Durham, NC 27710; **Phone:** 919-684-5350; **Board Cert:** Internal Medicine 1988; Hematology 2002; **Med School:** Indiana Univ 1985; **Resid:** Internal Medicine, Duke Univ Med Ctr 1988; **Fellow:** Hematology & Oncology, Duke Univ Med Ctr 1989; **Fac Appt:** Prof Med, Duke Univ

Powell, Bayard L MD [Hem] - **Spec Exp:** Leukemia; Myelodysplastic Syndromes; **Hospital:** Wake Forest Baptist Med Ctr; **Address:** Wake Forest Univ Baptist Med Ctr, Med Ctr Blvd-Cancer Center, Winston-Salem, NC 27157-1082; **Phone:** 336-716-7970; **Board Cert:** Internal Medicine 1983; Medical Oncology 1985; **Med School:** Univ NC Sch Med 1980; **Resid:** Internal Medicine, NC Baptist Hosp 1983; **Fellow:** Hematology & Oncology, Wake Forest Univ Sch Med 1986; **Fac Appt:** Prof Med, Wake Forest Univ

Rosenblatt, Joseph D MD [Hem] - **Spec Exp:** Lymphoma; Leukemia; Multiple Myeloma; Lymphomas-Rare; **Hospital:** Univ of Miami Hosp & Clins/Sylvester Comp Canc Ctr, Jackson Meml Hosp; **Address:** Sylvester Comprehensive Cancer Ctr, 1475 NW 12th Ave, D8-4, Ste 3300, Miami, FL 33136; **Phone:** 305-243-4860; **Board Cert:** Internal Medicine 1983; Medical Oncology 1985; **Med School:** UCLA 1980; **Resid:** Internal Medicine, UCLA Med Ctr 1983; **Fellow:** Hematology & Oncology, UCLA 1986; **Fac Appt:** Prof Onc, Univ Miami Sch Med

Schwartzberg, Lee S MD [Hem] - **Spec Exp:** Breast Cancer; Lung Cancer; Stem Cell Transplant; **Hospital:** Baptist Memorial Hospital-Memphis; **Address:** The West Clinic, 100 N Humphreys Blvd, Memphis, TN 38120; **Phone:** 901-683-0055; **Board Cert:** Internal Medicine 1983; Medical Oncology 1985; Hematology 1986; **Med School:** NY Med Coll 1980; **Resid:** Internal Medicine, North Shore Univ Hosp 1983; Internal Medicine, Meml Sloan Kettering Cancer Ctr 1985; **Fellow:** Hematology & Oncology, Meml Sloan Kettering Cancer Ctr 1984; Hematology & Oncology, Meml Sloan Kettering Cancer Ctr 1987; **Fac Appt:** Assoc Prof Med, Univ Tenn Coll Med

Hematology

Sokol, Lubomir MD/PhD [Hem] - **Spec Exp:** Lymphoma; Hematologic Malignancies; **Hospital:** H Lee Moffitt Cancer Ctr & Research Inst (page 59); **Address:** H Lee Moffitt Cancer Ctr & Rsch Inst, 12902 Magnolia Drive, MS FOB3-HEME, Tampa, FL 33612; **Phone:** 813-745-8212; **Board Cert:** Internal Medicine 2000; Medical Oncology 2002; Hematology 2003; **Med School:** Czech Republic 1981; **Resid:** Radiation Oncology, Charles Univ 1984; Internal Medicine, LSU Med Ctr 1999; **Fellow:** Radiation Oncology, Charles Univ 1990; Hematology & Oncology, USF Med Ctr 2002

Solberg, Lawrence A MD/PhD [Hem] - **Spec Exp:** Leukemia & Lymphoma; Myelodysplastic Syndromes; Bone Marrow Transplant; Multiple Myeloma; **Hospital:** Mayo - Jacksonville; **Address:** 4500 San Pablo Rd Mayo Bldg Fl 8, Jacksonville, FL 32224; **Phone:** 904-953-7290; **Board Cert:** Internal Medicine 1978; Hematology 1980; **Med School:** St Louis Univ 1975; **Resid:** Internal Medicine, Mayo Clinic 1978; **Fellow:** Hematology, Mayo Clinic 1980; **Fac Appt:** Prof Med, Mayo Med Sch

Telen, Marilyn J MD [Hem] - **Spec Exp:** Sickle Cell Disease; Anemias & Red Cell Disorders; Transfusion Medicine; **Hospital:** Duke Univ Hosp; **Address:** Duke Box 2615, 333 Med Sci Res Bldg, Durham, NC 27710; **Phone:** 919-684-5378; **Board Cert:** Internal Medicine 1980; Hematology 1984; **Med School:** NYU Sch Med 1977; **Resid:** Internal Medicine, Erie Co Med Cr 1980; **Fellow:** Hematology, Duke Univ Med Ctr 1983; **Fac Appt:** Prof Med, Duke Univ

Williams, Michael E MD [Hem] - **Spec Exp:** Lymphoma; Multiple Myeloma; Leukemia; Mantle Cell Lymphoma; **Hospital:** Univ of Virginia Health Sys; **Address:** UVA Hlth Sys, Div Hem/Oncology, Box 800716, Charlottesville, VA 22908-0716; **Phone:** 434-924-9637; **Board Cert:** Internal Medicine 1982; Medical Oncology 1987; Hematology 2009; **Med School:** Univ Cincinnati 1979; **Resid:** Internal Medicine, Univ Virginia Med Ctr 1983; **Fellow:** Hematology & Oncology, Univ Virginia Med Ctr 1986; **Fac Appt:** Prof Med, Univ VA Sch Med

Zuckerman, Kenneth S MD [Hem] - **Spec Exp:** Myeloproliferative Disorders; Leukemia; Myelodysplastic Syndromes; Anemia; **Hospital:** H Lee Moffitt Cancer Ctr & Research Inst (page 59), Tampa Genl Hosp; **Address:** H Lee Moffitt Cancer Center, 12902 USF Magnolia Drive, Tampa, FL 33612-9416; **Phone:** 813-745-8090; **Board Cert:** Internal Medicine 1975; Hematology 1978; **Med School:** Ohio State Univ 1972; **Resid:** Internal Medicine, Ohio State Univ Hosps 1975; **Fellow:** Hematology, Peter Bent Brigham Hosp/Harvard Univ 1978; **Fac Appt:** Prof Med, Univ S Fla Coll Med

Midwest

Baron, Joseph M MD [Hem] - **Spec Exp:** Bleeding/Coagulation Disorders; Lymphoma; Myeloproliferative Disorders; **Hospital:** Univ of Chicago Med Ctr; **Address:** 5841 S Maryland Ave, MC 2115, Chicago, IL 60637-1463; **Phone:** 773-702-6149; **Board Cert:** Internal Medicine 1969; Hematology 1972; Medical Oncology 1975; **Med School:** Univ Chicago-Pritzker Sch Med 1962; **Resid:** Internal Medicine, Univ Chicago Hosps 1964; Internal Medicine, Univ Chicago Hosps 1968; **Fellow:** Hematology, Univ Chicago Hosps 1968; **Fac Appt:** Assoc Prof Med, Univ Chicago-Pritzker Sch Med

Blinder, Morey MD [Hem] - **Spec Exp:** Bleeding/Coagulation Disorders; Anemia; Sickle Cell Disease; **Hospital:** Barnes-Jewish Hosp; **Address:** Washington Univ School of Medicine, Hematology Division, 660 S Euclid Ave, Box 8125, St Louis, MO 63110; **Phone:** 314-362-8814; **Board Cert:** Internal Medicine 1984; Hematology 1988; Medical Oncology 1987; **Med School:** St Louis Univ 1981; **Resid:** Internal Medicine, Univ Illinois Hosp 1984; **Fellow:** Hematology & Oncology, Univ Wash Med Ctr 1986; **Fac Appt:** Assoc Prof Med, Washington Univ, St Louis

Bockenstedt, Paula MD [Hem] - **Spec Exp:** Bleeding/Coagulation Disorders; Leukemia; Von Willebrand's Disease; **Hospital:** Univ of Michigan Hosp; **Address:** Div Hematology, 1500 E Med Ctr Dr, MIB, rm C-344, Ann Arbor, MI 48109-8048; **Phone:** 734-936-6393; **Board Cert:** Internal Medicine 1981; Hematology 1984; **Med School:** Harvard Med Sch 1978; **Resid:** Internal Medicine, Brigham-Womens Hosp 1981; **Fellow:** Hematology, Brigham-Womens Hosp 1984; **Fac Appt:** Assoc Clin Prof Med, Univ Mich Med Sch

Byrd, John C MD [Hem] - **Spec Exp:** Leukemia-Chronic Lymphocytic; **Hospital:** Arthur G James Cancer Hosp & Research Inst; **Address:** 320 W 10th Ave, B302 Starling-Loving Hall, Columbus, OH 43210; **Phone:** 614-293-3196; **Board Cert:** Hematology 2007; **Med School:** Univ Ark 1991; **Resid:** Internal Medicine, Walter Reed AMC 1994; **Fellow:** Hematology & Oncology, Walter Reed AMC 1997; **Fac Appt:** Assoc Prof Med, Ohio State Univ

Copelan, Edward A MD [Hem] - **Spec Exp:** Leukemia; Myelodysplastic Syndromes; Bone Marrow Transplant; Multiple Myeloma; **Hospital:** Cleveland Clin (page 55); **Address:** Cleveland Clinic Fdn, 9500 Euclid Ave, Cleveland, OH 44195; **Phone:** 216-445-5647; **Board Cert:** Internal Medicine 1980; Hematology 1982; Medical Oncology 1983; **Med School:** Tufts Univ 1977; **Resid:** Internal Medicine, Ohio State Univ Hosp 1980; **Fellow:** Hematology & Oncology, Ohio State Univ Hosp 1983; Bone Marrow Transplant, UCLA Med Ctr; **Fac Appt:** Prof Med, Cleveland Cl Coll Med/Case West Res

Di Persio, John F MD/PhD [Hem] - **Spec Exp:** Bone Marrow Transplant; Hematologic Malignancies; Leukemia; **Hospital:** Barnes-Jewish Hosp; **Address:** Wash Univ Sch Med, Sect Bone Marrow Transplant & Leukemia, 660 S Euclid Ave, Box 8007, St Louis, MO 63110; **Phone:** 314-454-8306; **Board Cert:** Internal Medicine 1984; Medical Oncology 1987; Hematology 1988; **Med School:** Univ Rochester 1980; **Resid:** Internal Medicine, Parkland Meml Hosp 1984; **Fellow:** Hematology & Oncology, UCLA Med Ctr 1987; **Fac Appt:** Prof Med, Washington Univ, St Louis

Farag, Sherif S MD/PhD [Hem] - **Spec Exp:** Multiple Myeloma; Leukemia & Lymphoma; Bone Marrow Transplant; Stem Cell Transplant; **Hospital:** IU Health University Hosp; **Address:** Center of Immunobiology, 980 W Walnut St, R3 Bldg, rm C414, Indianapolis, IN 46202; **Phone:** 317-944-0920; **Med School:** Australia 1995; **Resid:** Internal Medicine, Univ Melbourne Med Ctr; **Fellow:** Hematology & Oncology, Roswell Park Cancer Inst; **Fac Appt:** Assoc Prof Med, Indiana Univ

Flynn, Patrick J MD [Hem] - **Spec Exp:** Hematologic Malignancies; Colon & Rectal Cancer; Clinical Trials; Breast Cancer; **Hospital:** Abbott - Northwestern Hosp, Fairview Southdale Hosp; **Address:** 910 E 26th St, Ste 200, Minneapolis, MN 55404; **Phone:** 612-884-6300; **Board Cert:** Internal Medicine 1978; Medical Oncology 1981; Hematology 1982; **Med School:** Univ Minn 1975; **Resid:** Internal Medicine, Hennepin Co Med Ctr 1978; **Fellow:** Hematology & Oncology, Univ Minnesota Hosp 1981

Gertz, Morie A MD [Hem] - **Spec Exp:** Multiple Myeloma; Amyloidosis; Waldenstrom's Macroglobulinemia; Plasma Cell Disorders; **Hospital:** Mayo Med Ctr & Clin - Rochester, Rochester Methodist Hosp; **Address:** 200 SW 1st St, Fl W10, Rochester, MN 55905; **Phone:** 507-284-3725; **Board Cert:** Internal Medicine 1979; Hematology 1982; Medical Oncology 1983; **Med School:** Loyola Univ-Stritch Sch Med 1975; **Resid:** Internal Medicine, St Lukes Hosp 1979; **Fellow:** Hematology & Oncology, Mayo Clin 1982; **Fac Appt:** Prof Hem & Onc, Mayo Med Sch

Gordon, Leo I MD [Hem] - **Spec Exp:** Lymphoma, Non-Hodgkin's; Hodgkin's Lymphoma; Bone Marrow Transplant; **Hospital:** Northwestern Meml Hosp; **Address:** Northwestern Univ-Feinberg Sch Med, Robert H Lurie Comprehensive Cancer Ctr, 676 N St Clair St, Ste 850, Chicago, IL 60611-3124; **Phone:** 312-695-4546; **Board Cert:** Internal Medicine 1976; Hematology 1978; Medical Oncology 1979; **Med School:** Univ Cincinnati 1973; **Resid:** Internal Medicine, Univ Chicago Hosps 1976; **Fellow:** Hematology, Univ Minnesota Hosps 1978; Hematology & Oncology, Univ Chicago Hosps 1979; **Fac Appt:** Prof Med, Univ Chicago-Pritzker Sch Med

Gregory, Stephanie A MD [Hem] - **Spec Exp:** Lymphoma; Leukemia; Plasma Cell Disorders; Multiple Myeloma; **Hospital:** Rush Univ Med Ctr; **Address:** Rush University Medical Center, 1725 W Harrison St, Ste 834, Chicago, IL 60612; **Phone:** 312-942-5982; **Board Cert:** Internal Medicine 1972; Hematology 1972; **Med School:** Med Coll PA Hahnemann 1965; **Resid:** Internal Medicine, Rush/Presby-St Luke's Med Ctr 1969; **Fellow:** Hematology, Rush/Presby-St Luke's Med Ctr 1972; **Fac Appt:** Prof Med, Rush Med Coll

Grever, Michael R MD [Hem] - **Spec Exp:** Hematologic Malignancies; Leukemia; Drug Development; Clinical Trials; **Hospital:** Ohio St Univ Med Ctr; **Address:** 395 W 12th Ave, Rm 392, Doan Tower, Columbus, OH 43210; **Phone:** 614-293-8724; **Board Cert:** Internal Medicine 1975; Medical Oncology 1979; Hematology 1988; **Med School:** Univ Pittsburgh 1971; **Resid:** Internal Medicine, Univ of Pittsburgh 1974; **Fellow:** Hematology & Oncology, Ohio State Univ 1978; **Fac Appt:** Prof Med, Ohio State Univ

Habermann, Thomas M MD [Hem] - **Spec Exp:** Lymphoma; Hodgkin's Lymphoma; Leukemia; **Hospital:** Mayo Med Ctr & Clin - Rochester; **Address:** Mayo Clin, 200 1st St SW, Rochester, MN 55905; **Phone:** 507-284-3159; **Board Cert:** Internal Medicine 1982; Hematology 1984; **Med School:** Creighton Univ 1979; **Resid:** Internal Medicine, Mayo Clinic 1982; **Fellow:** Hematology, Mayo Clinic 1985; **Fac Appt:** Prof Med, Mayo Med Sch

Juckett, Mark B MD [Hem] - **Spec Exp:** Bone Marrow Transplant; **Hospital:** Univ WI Hosp & Clins; **Address:** 600 Highland Ave, Ste H4/534, Madison, WI 53792; **Phone:** 608-265-1700; **Board Cert:** Hematology 2004; Medical Oncology 2005; **Med School:** Univ Louisville Sch Med 1987; **Resid:** Internal Medicine, Univ Minnesota 1990; **Fellow:** Hematology & Oncology, Univ Minnesota 1992; **Fac Appt:** Assoc Prof Med, Univ Wisc

Kraut, Eric H MD [Hem] - **Spec Exp:** Hematologic Malignancies; Leukemia; Drug Development; Clinical Trials; **Hospital:** Ohio St Univ Med Ctr; **Address:** 320 W 10th Ave, A358 SL, Columbus, OH 43210; **Phone:** 614-293-2887; **Board Cert:** Internal Medicine 1975; Medical Oncology 1977; Hematology 1978; **Med School:** Temple Univ 1972; **Resid:** Internal Medicine, Univ Pittsburgh 1975; **Fellow:** Hematology & Oncology, Ohio State Univ Hosp 1977; **Fac Appt:** Prof Med, Ohio State Univ

Kuriakose, Philip MD [Hem] - **Spec Exp:** Leukemia; **Hospital:** Henry Ford Hosp; **Address:** Henry Ford Hosp, Hematology/Oncology, 2799 W Grand Blvd, K13, Detroit, MI 48202; **Phone:** 313-916-1841; **Board Cert:** Internal Medicine 2009; Medical Oncology 2002; Hematology 2002; **Med School:** India 1990; **Resid:** Internal Medicine, Christian Med Coll 1992; Internal Medicine, Henry Ford Hosp 1994; **Fellow:** Hematology & Oncology, Mayo Clinic 1995

Larson, Richard A MD [Hem] - **Spec Exp:** Leukemia & Lymphoma; Bone Marrow Transplant; Myelodysplastic Syndromes; **Hospital:** Univ of Chicago Med Ctr; **Address:** University of Chicago Medical Center, 5841 S Maryland Ave, MS 2115, Chicago, IL 60637; **Phone:** 773-702-6149; **Board Cert:** Internal Medicine 1980; Hematology 1982; Medical Oncology 1983; **Med School:** Stanford Univ 1977; **Resid:** Internal Medicine, Univ Chicago Med Ctr 1980; **Fellow:** Hematology & Oncology, Univ Chicago Med Ctr 1983; **Fac Appt:** Prof Hem & Onc, Univ Chicago-Pritzker Sch Med

Litzow, Mark R MD [Hem] - **Spec Exp:** Bone Marrow Transplant; Leukemia; **Hospital:** Mayo Med Ctr & Clin - Rochester; **Address:** Mayo Clinic, Div Hematology, 200 First St SW, Rochester, MN 55905; **Phone:** 507-284-5362; **Board Cert:** Internal Medicine 1983; Hematology 1988; Medical Oncology 1989; **Med School:** Univ Chicago-Pritzker Sch Med 1980; **Resid:** Internal Medicine, Mayo Clinic 1984; **Fellow:** Medical Oncology, Mayo Clinic 1990; **Fac Appt:** Asst Prof Med, Mayo Med Sch

Maciejewski, Jaroslaw P MD/PhD [Hem] - **Spec Exp:** Anemia-Aplastic; Hematologic Malignancies; Stem Cell Transplant; **Hospital:** Cleveland Clin (page 55); **Address:** Cleveland Clinic, 9500 Euclid Ave, Desk R40, Cleveland, OH 44195; **Phone:** 216-445-5962; **Med School:** Germany 1990; **Resid:** Internal Medicine, Univ Nevada Med Ctr 1997; **Fellow:** Hematology, Natl Inst Hlth 2000; **Fac Appt:** Prof Med, Case West Res Univ

McGlave, Philip B MD [Hem] - **Spec Exp:** Leukemia; Bone Marrow Transplant; **Hospital:** Fairview Lakes Med Ctr; **Address:** Univ Minn, Dept Med, Div Hem/Onc Transplanatation, 420 Delaware St SE, MMC 480, Minneapolis, MN 55455; **Phone:** 612-273-2800; **Board Cert:** Internal Medicine 1977; Hematology 1980; **Med School:** Univ IL Coll Med 1974; **Resid:** Internal Medicine, Univ Minnesota Med Ctr 1977; **Fellow:** Hematology & Oncology, Univ Minnesota Med Ctr 1980; **Fac Appt:** Prof Med, Univ Minn

Milhem, Mohammed M MD [Hem] - **Spec Exp:** Bone Cancer; Bone Marrow Transplant; Sarcoma; Melanoma; **Hospital:** Univ Iowa Hosp & Clinics; **Address:** Univ Iowa Hosp & Clinics, 200 Hawkins Drive, rm C32 GH, Iowa City, IA 52242; **Phone:** 319-356-4200; **Board Cert:** Hematology 2003; Medical Oncology 2003; **Med School:** Jordan 1995; **Resid:** Internal Medicine, Univ IL Med Ctr 2000; **Fellow:** Hematology & Oncology, Univ IL Med Ctr 2003; Bone Marrow Transplant, Univ IL Med Ctr 2004; **Fac Appt:** Asst Clin Prof Hem & Onc, Univ Iowa Coll Med

Nand, Sucha MD [Hem] - **Spec Exp:** Myelodysplastic Syndromes; Myeloproliferative Disorders; Leukemia; Lymphoma, Non-Hodgkin's; **Hospital:** Loyola Univ Med Ctr; **Address:** Loyola University Medical Center, Cardinal Bernardin Cancer Ctr, 2160 S First Ave Bldg 112 - rm 342, Maywood, IL 60153-3304; **Phone:** 708-327-3217; **Board Cert:** Internal Medicine 1979; Medical Oncology 1981; Hematology 1982; **Med School:** India 1971; **Resid:** Physical Medicine & Rehabilitation, Northwestern Meml Hosp 1976; Internal Medicine, North Chicago VA Hosp 1978; **Fellow:** Hematology & Oncology, Northwestern Meml Hosp 1981; **Fac Appt:** Prof Hem & Onc, Loyola Univ-Stritch Sch Med

Palascak, Joseph E MD [Hem] - **Spec Exp:** Hemophilia; Bleeding/Coagulation Disorders; Thrombotic Disorders; **Hospital:** Univ Hosp - Cincinnati; **Address:** Barrett Center, 222 Piedmont Ave Fl 2, Cincinnati, OH 45219; **Phone:** 513-475-8500; **Board Cert:** Internal Medicine 1975; Hematology 1978; **Med School:** Jefferson Med Coll 1968; **Resid:** Internal Medicine, Thomas Jefferson Univ Hosp 1971; **Fellow:** Hematology, Thomas Jefferson Univ Hosp 1972; Hematology, Thomas Jefferson Univ Hosp 1976; **Fac Appt:** Prof Med, Univ Cincinnati

Porcu, Pierluigi MD [Hem] - **Spec Exp:** Lymphoma; Lymphoma, Non-Hodgkin's; Immunotherapy; **Hospital:** Ohio St Univ Med Ctr; **Address:** 320 W 10th Ave, B320 Starling Loving Hall, Columbus, OH 43210; **Phone:** 614-293-9273; **Board Cert:** Medical Oncology 2011; **Med School:** Italy 1987; **Resid:** Internal Medicine, Indiana Univ Hosp 1996; **Fellow:** Hematology & Oncology, Indiana Univ Hosp 1999; **Fac Appt:** Asst Prof Med, Ohio State Univ

Roodman, G David MD/PhD [Hem] - **Spec Exp:** Multiple Myeloma; Hematologic Malignancies; **Hospital:** IU Health University Hosp; **Address:** 980 W Walnut St, R3 Bldg - Fl 3rd - Ste C312, Indianapolis, IN 46202; **Phone:** 317-278-6255; **Board Cert:** Internal Medicine 1978; Hematology 1980; **Med School:** Univ KY Coll Med 1973; **Resid:** Internal Medicine, Univ Minnesota Hosp 1978; **Fellow:** Hematology, Univ Minnesota Hosp 1980; **Fac Appt:** Prof Hem & Onc, Indiana Univ

Singhal, Seema MD [Hem] - **Spec Exp:** Multiple Myeloma; **Hospital:** Northwestern Meml Hosp; **Address:** Northwestern Div Hematology/Oncology, 676 N St Clair St, Ste 2100, Chicago, IL 60611; **Phone:** 312-695-0990; **Board Cert:** Internal Medicine 2005; **Med School:** India 1989; **Resid:** Internal Medicine, King Edward Meml Hosp 1991; Hematology, King Edward Meml Hosp 1991; **Fellow:** Bone Marrow Transplant, Hadassah Univ Hosp 1992; **Fac Appt:** Prof Med, Northwestern Univ

Hematology

Stiff, Patrick J MD [Hem] - **Spec Exp:** Bone Marrow Transplant; Leukemia; Lymphoma, Non-Hodgkin's; Vaccine Therapy; **Hospital:** Loyola Univ Med Ctr, Gottlieb Meml Hosp; **Address:** 2160 S First Ave Bldg 112 - rm 255, Maywood, IL 60153; **Phone:** 708-327-3148; **Board Cert:** Internal Medicine 1978; Medical Oncology 1981; Hematology 1982; **Med School:** Loyola Univ-Stritch Sch Med 1975; **Resid:** Internal Medicine, Cleveland Clinic Fdn 1978; **Fellow:** Hematology & Oncology, Meml Sloan Kettering Cancer Ctr 1981; **Fac Appt:** Prof Hem & Onc, Loyola Univ-Stritch Sch Med

Tefferi, Ayalew MD [Hem] - **Spec Exp:** Myeloproliferative Disorders; Leukemia; **Hospital:** Mayo Med Ctr & Clin - Rochester; **Address:** 200 1st St SW, Rochester, MN 55905; **Phone:** 507-538-1068; **Board Cert:** Internal Medicine 1986; Hematology 1988; **Med School:** Greece 1982; **Resid:** Internal Medicine, St Josephs Hosp 1986; **Fellow:** Hematology, Mayo Clinic 1988; **Fac Appt:** Prof Hem & Onc, Mayo Med Sch

Uberti, Joseph P MD/PhD [Hem] - **Spec Exp:** Bone Marrow Transplant; Stem Cell Transplant; **Hospital:** Barbara Ann Karmanos Cancer Inst; **Address:** Barbara Ann Karmanos Cancer Inst, 4100 John R St, MC HW04H0, Detroit, MI 48201; **Phone:** 313-576-8760; **Board Cert:** Internal Medicine 1986; Medical Oncology 1989; **Med School:** Wayne State Univ 1983; **Resid:** Internal Medicine, Detroit Receiving Hosp 1986; **Fellow:** Hematology & Oncology, Wayne State Univ Hosps 1988; **Fac Appt:** Prof Med, Wayne State Univ

Van Besien, Koen W MD [Hem] - **Spec Exp:** Lymphoma; Stem Cell Transplant; **Hospital:** Univ of Chicago Med Ctr; **Address:** Stem Cell Transplant Program, 5841 S Maryland Ave, Chicago, IL 60637; **Phone:** 773-702-6149; **Board Cert:** Internal Medicine 2005; Medical Oncology 2005; Hematology 2006; **Med School:** Belgium 1984; **Resid:** Internal Medicine, Univ Leuven Med Ctr 1987; **Fellow:** Hematology & Oncology, Indiana Univ Med Ctr 1990; **Fac Appt:** Prof Med, Univ Chicago-Pritzker Sch Med

Winter, Jane N MD [Hem] - **Spec Exp:** Lymphoma, Non-Hodgkin's; Hodgkin's Lymphoma; Bone Marrow Transplant; Langerhans Cell Histiocytosis (LCH); **Hospital:** Northwestern Meml Hosp; **Address:** Northwestern Univ - Div Hem/Oncology, 675 N St Clair St, Ste 21-100, Chicago, IL 60611-2927; **Phone:** 312-695-0990; **Board Cert:** Internal Medicine 1980; Hematology 2008; Medical Oncology 1983; **Med School:** Univ Pennsylvania 1977; **Resid:** Internal Medicine, Univ Chicago Hosps 1980; **Fellow:** Hematology & Oncology, Columbia Presby Hosp 1981; Hematology & Oncology, Northwestern Univ 1983; **Fac Appt:** Prof Hem & Onc, Northwestern Univ

Great Plains and Mountains

Rodgers III, George M MD/PhD [Hem] - **Spec Exp:** Hematopathology; Anemia-Cancer Related; Bleeding/Coagulation Disorders; **Hospital:** Univ Utah Hlth Care; **Address:** Univ Utah Med Ctr - Div Hematology, 30 N 1900 E, rm 5C402, Salt Lake City, UT 84132; **Phone:** 801-585-3229; **Board Cert:** Internal Medicine 1979; Hematology 1982; Pathology 1984; **Med School:** Tulane Univ 1976; **Resid:** Internal Medicine, Baylor Affil Hosps 1979; **Fellow:** Hematology, UCSF Med Ctr 1982; **Fac Appt:** Prof Med, Univ Utah

Vose, Julie M MD [Hem] - **Spec Exp:** Lymphoma; **Hospital:** Nebraska Med Ctr; **Address:** 987630 Nebraska Med Ctr, Emile @ 42nd St, Omaha, NE 68198-7630; **Phone:** 402-559-5600; **Board Cert:** Internal Medicine 1987; Medical Oncology 2011; Hematology 2000; **Med School:** Univ Nebr Coll Med 1984; **Resid:** Internal Medicine, Univ Nebraska Med Ctr 1987; **Fellow:** Hematology & Oncology, Univ Nebraska Med Ctr 1990; **Fac Appt:** Prof Med, Univ Nebr Coll Med

Southwest

Adams, Roberta H MD [Hem] - **Spec Exp:** Bone Marrow Transplant; Stem Cell Transplant; Sarcoma; **Hospital:** Phoenix Children's Hosp, Mayo Clinic - Phoenix; **Address:** Phoenix Chldns Hosp-Hematology/Oncology Dept, 1919 E Thomas Rd, Phoenix, AZ 85016; **Phone:** 602-546-0920; **Board Cert:** Pediatrics 1986; Pediatric Hematology-Oncology 2009; **Med School:** Columbia P&S 1981; **Resid:** Pediatrics, Boston Chldns Hosp 1984; **Fellow:** Pediatric Hematology-Oncology, Univ of Utah Hosp 1990; **Fac Appt:** Asst Prof Med, Mayo Med Sch

Barlogie, Bart MD/PhD [Hem] - **Spec Exp:** Bone Marrow Transplant; Plasma Cell Disorders; Multiple Myeloma; **Hospital:** UAMS Med Ctr; **Address:** UAMS-Myeloma Inst Rsch & Therapy, 4301 West Markham St, Slot 816, Little Rock, AR 72205; **Phone:** 501-686-8230; **Med School:** Germany 1969; **Resid:** Internal Medicine, Univ Muenster Med Sch; **Fellow:** Medical Oncology, MD Anderson Cancer Ctr-Tumor Inst 1976; **Fac Appt:** Prof Med, Univ Ark

Brenner, Malcolm K MD/PhD [Hem] - **Spec Exp:** Gene Therapy; Bone Marrow Transplant; **Hospital:** Methodist Hosp - Houston, Texas Chldns Hosp; **Address:** 1102 Bates St, Ste 1630, Houston, TX 77030; **Phone:** 832-824-4671; **Med School:** England, UK 1975; **Resid:** Internal Medicine, Cambridge Univ Affil Hosp 1979; **Fellow:** Immunology, Clinical Rsch Ctr 1984; Hematology & Oncology, Royal Free Hosp 1986; **Fac Appt:** Prof Med, Baylor Coll Med

Champlin, Richard E MD [Hem] - **Spec Exp:** Bone Marrow Transplant; Stem Cell Transplant; Leukemia & Lymphoma; **Hospital:** UT MD Anderson Cancer Ctr; **Address:** MD Anderson Cancer Ctr, Stem Cell Transplantation Ctr, 1515 Holcombe Blvd, Unit 0423 FC 5.3042, Houston, TX 77030; **Phone:** 713-792-6100; **Board Cert:** Internal Medicine 1978; Hematology 1980; Medical Oncology 1981; **Med School:** Univ Chicago-Pritzker Sch Med 1975; **Resid:** Internal Medicine, LAC Harbor/UCLA Med Ctr 1978; **Fellow:** Hematology & Oncology, LAC Harbor/UCLA Med Ctr 1980; **Fac Appt:** Prof Med, Univ Tex, Houston

Cobos, Everardo MD [Hem] - **Spec Exp:** Bone Marrow Transplant; Bleeding/Coagulation Disorders; **Hospital:** Univ Med Ctr-Lubbock; **Address:** 3601 4th St, MS 9410, SCRTC Dept, Lubbock, TX 79430; **Phone:** 806-743-3155 x222; **Board Cert:** Internal Medicine 1985; Medical Oncology 1987; Hematology 1988; **Med School:** Univ Tex, San Antonio 1981; **Resid:** Internal Medicine, Letterman Army Med Ctr 1985; **Fellow:** Hematology & Oncology, Letterman Army Med Ctr 1988; **Fac Appt:** Prof Hem & Onc, Texas Tech Univ

Cooper, Barry MD [Hem] - **Spec Exp:** Leukemia; Lymphoma; Bleeding/Coagulation Disorders; **Hospital:** Baylor Univ Medical Ctr-Dallas; **Address:** 3410 Worth St, Ste 400, Dallas, TX 75246-2096; **Phone:** 214-370-1002; **Board Cert:** Internal Medicine 1974; Medical Oncology 1977; Hematology 1978; **Med School:** Johns Hopkins Univ 1971; **Resid:** Internal Medicine, Johns Hopkins Hosp 1973; **Fellow:** Metabolism, Natl Inst Health 1975; Hematology, Peter Bent Brigham Hosp 1977; **Fac Appt:** Clin Prof Med, Univ Tex SW, Dallas

Cortes, Jorge E MD [Hem] - **Spec Exp:** Leukemia; Myelodysplastic Syndromes; Myeloproliferative Disorders; **Hospital:** UT MD Anderson Cancer Ctr; **Address:** UT MD Anderson Cancer Center, Leukemia Center, 1515 Holcombe Blvd, Unit 357, Houston, TX 77030; **Phone:** 713-792-8760; **Med School:** Mexico 1986; **Resid:** Internal Medicine, Instituto Nacional de la Nutricion 1989; **Fellow:** Hematology, UT MD Anderson Cancer Ctr 1992; Hematology & Oncology, UT MD Anderson Cancer Ctr 1995; **Fac Appt:** Prof Med, Univ Tex, Houston

Emanuel, Peter D MD [Hem] - **Spec Exp:** Lymphoma; Leukemia; Hodgkin's Lymphoma; Multiple Myeloma; **Hospital:** UAMS Med Ctr; **Address:** 4301 W Markham, Slot 623, Little Rock, AR 72205; **Phone:** 501-526-2272; **Board Cert:** Internal Medicine 1988; **Med School:** Univ Wisc 1985; **Resid:** Internal Medicine, Univ Alabama Hosp 1988; **Fellow:** Hematology & Oncology, Univ Alabama 1991; **Fac Appt:** Prof Med, Univ Ark

Fonseca, Rafael MD [Hem] - **Spec Exp:** Multiple Myeloma; **Hospital:** Mayo Clinic - Scottsdale, Mayo Clinic - Phoenix; **Address:** Mayo Clinic-Hematology Div, 13400 E Shea Blvd, Scottsdale, AZ 85259; **Phone:** 480-301-7085; **Board Cert:** Hematology 2010; **Med School:** Mexico 1991; **Resid:** Internal Medicine, Jackson Meml Med Ctr 1994; **Fellow:** Hematology & Oncology, Mayo Clinic 1998; **Fac Appt:** Assoc Prof Med, Mayo Med Sch

Kantarjian, Hagop M MD [Hem] - **Spec Exp:** Leukemia; **Hospital:** UT MD Anderson Cancer Ctr; **Address:** MD Anderson Cancer Ctr, Dept of Leukemia, Unit 428, 1400 Holcombe Blvd, Houston, TX 77030; **Phone:** 713-792-7026; **Board Cert:** Internal Medicine 1983; Medical Oncology 1985; **Med School:** Amer Univ Beirut 1979; **Resid:** Internal Medicine, Univ Tex MD Anderson Cancer Ctr 1983; **Fellow:** Hematology & Oncology, Univ Tex MD Anderson Cancer Ctr 1983; **Fac Appt:** Prof Med, Univ Tex, Houston

Keating, Michael MD [Hem] - **Spec Exp:** Leukemia-Chronic Lymphocytic; **Hospital:** UT MD Anderson Cancer Ctr; **Address:** MD Anderson Cancer Ctr, 1400 Holcombe Blvd, Unit 428, Houston, TX 77030-4000; **Phone:** 713-745-2376; **Med School:** Australia 1966; **Resid:** Internal Medicine, St Vincents Hosp 1973; **Fellow:** Hematology, MD Anderson Cancer Ctr 1975; **Fac Appt:** Prof Med, Univ Tex, Houston

Lin, Weei-Chin MD/PhD [Hem] - **Spec Exp:** Hematologic Malignancies; Bleeding/Coagulation Disorders; **Hospital:** Ben Taub Genl Hosp; **Address:** One Baylor Plaza, MARB Bldg - rm 410, MS 187, Houston, TX 77030; **Phone:** 713-798-2641; **Med School:** Taiwan 1986; **Resid:** Internal Medicine, Duke Univ Med Ctr 1996; **Fellow:** Hematology & Oncology, Duke Univ Med Ctr 1999; **Fac Appt:** Assoc Prof Hem & Onc, Baylor Coll Med

Lyons, Roger M MD [Hem] - **Spec Exp:** Leukemia & Lymphoma; Multiple Myeloma; Bleeding/Coagulation Disorders; Platelet Disorders; **Hospital:** Methodist Hosp-San Antonio, Methodist Spec & Transpl Hosp; **Address:** 4411 Medical Drive, Ste 100, San Antonio, TX 78229-3325; **Phone:** 210-595-5300; **Board Cert:** Internal Medicine 1981; Hematology 1982; **Med School:** Canada 1967; **Resid:** Internal Medicine, Winnipeg Genl Hosp 1969; Internal Medicine, Barnes-Wohl Hosps 1972; **Fellow:** Hematology, Washington Univ Hosps 1975; **Fac Appt:** Clin Prof Med, Univ Tex, San Antonio

Mesa, Ruben A MD/PhD [Hem] - **Spec Exp:** Myeloproliferative Disorders; Myelodysplastic Syndromes; Leukemia; **Hospital:** Mayo Clinic - Scottsdale, Select Specialty Hosp-Phoenix; **Address:** Mayo Clinic-Hematology Dept, 13400 E Shea Blvd, Scottsdale, AZ 85259; **Phone:** 480-301-8335; **Board Cert:** Internal Medicine 2008; Hematology 2011; Medical Oncology 2002; **Med School:** Mayo Med Sch 1995; **Resid:** Internal Medicine, Mayo Clinic 1998; **Fellow:** Hematology & Oncology, Mayo Clinic 2003; **Fac Appt:** Prof Hem & Onc, Mayo Med Sch

Munker, Reinhold MD [Hem] - **Spec Exp:** Leukemia & Lymphoma; Bone Marrow Transplant; Hematologic Malignancies; **Hospital:** Louisiana State Univ Hosp; **Address:** LSU Health Shreveport, Feist-Weiller Cancer Ctr, 1501 Kings Hwy, Shreveport, LA 71130; **Phone:** 318-813-1016; **Board Cert:** Internal Medicine 2004; Hematology 2006; **Med School:** Germany 1979; **Resid:** Internal Medicine, Univ Clinic of Grosshaden 1989; **Fellow:** Hematology & Oncology, Univ Clinic of Grossharden 1993; Blood Banking, Univ Clinic of Grossharden 1997; **Fac Appt:** Assoc Prof Med, Louisiana State U, Shrevport

Stewart, A Keith MD [Hem] - **Spec Exp:** Multiple Myeloma; **Hospital:** Mayo Clinic - Scottsdale; **Address:** Mayo Clinic-Hematology Div, 13400 E Shea Blvd, Scottsdale, AZ 85259; **Phone:** 480-301-7085; **Med School:** Scotland, UK 1984; **Resid:** Internal Medicine, Kingston Genl Hosp 1988; 1990; **Fellow:** Hematology, Toronto Genl Hosp 1990; Hematology Research, New England Med Ctr 1992; **Fac Appt:** Prof Med, Mayo Med Sch

Strauss, James F MD [Hem] - **Spec Exp:** Bleeding/Coagulation Disorders; Leukemia; Lymphoma; **Hospital:** TX Hlth Presby Hosp Dallas; **Address:** Texas Oncology at Presbyterian, 8220 Walnut Hill Ln Bldg 2 - Ste 700, Dallas, TX 75231; **Phone:** 214-739-4175; **Board Cert:** Internal Medicine 1976; Hematology 1978; Medical Oncology 1981; **Med School:** NYU Sch Med 1972; **Resid:** Internal Medicine, Baylor Univ Medical Ctr 1976; **Fellow:** Hematology, Univ Texas SW Medical Ctr 1977

Yeager, Andrew M MD [Hem] - **Spec Exp:** Bone Marrow & Stem Cell Transplant; Graft vs Host Disease; Leukemia; **Hospital:** Univ Arizona Med Ctr-Univ Campus; **Address:** Arizona Cancer Ctr, 1515 N Campbell Ave, Ste 2956, Tucson, AZ 85724-5024; **Phone:** 520-694-2873; **Board Cert:** Pediatrics 1979; Pediatric Hematology-Oncology 1980; **Med School:** Johns Hopkins Univ 1975; **Resid:** Pediatrics, Johns Hopkins Hosp 1978; Pediatrics, Johns Hopkins Hosp 1982; **Fellow:** Pediatric Hematology-Oncology, Johns Hopkins Hosp 1980; **Fac Appt:** Prof Med, Univ Ariz Coll Med

West Coast and Pacific

Damon, Lloyd E MD [Hem] - **Spec Exp:** Leukemia; Lymphoma; Stem Cell Transplant; **Hospital:** UCSF Med Ctr; **Address:** UCSF Comprehensive Cancer Ctr, 400 Parnassus Ave Fl 5, San Francisco, CA 94143; **Phone:** 415-353-2421; **Board Cert:** Internal Medicine 1985; Medical Oncology 1987; Hematology 1988; **Med School:** Univ Mich Med Sch 1982; **Resid:** Internal Medicine, UCSF Med Ctr 1985; **Fellow:** Hematology & Oncology, UCSF Med Ctr 1988; **Fac Appt:** Prof Med, UCSF

DeLoughery, Thomas MD [Hem] - **Spec Exp:** Thrombotic Disorders; Myeloproliferative Disorders; Bleeding/Coagulation Disorders; Platelet Disorders; **Hospital:** OR Hlth & Sci Univ; **Address:** 3303 SW Bond Ave, MC CH7M, Portland, OR 97239; **Phone:** 503-494-6594; **Board Cert:** Internal Medicine 1988; Blood Banking Transfusion Medicine 1995; Medical Oncology 2011; Hematology 2002; **Med School:** Indiana Univ 1985; **Resid:** Internal Medicine, Oregon Hlth & Science Univ 1988; **Fellow:** Hematology & Oncology, Oregon Hlth & Science Univ 1991; **Fac Appt:** Prof Med, Oregon Hlth & Sci Univ

Forman, Stephen J MD [Hem] - **Spec Exp:** Lymphoma; Leukemia; Bone Marrow Transplant; **Hospital:** City of Hope Natl Med Ctr; **Address:** City Hope Natl Med Ctr, Dept Hematology, 1500 E Duarte Rd, rm 3002, Duarte, CA 91010-3012; **Phone:** 626-256-4673 x62403; **Board Cert:** Internal Medicine 1977; **Med School:** USC Sch Med 1974; **Resid:** Internal Medicine, LAC-Harbor UCLA Med Ctr 1976; **Fellow:** Hematology, LAC-USC Med Ctr 1978; Hematology, City of Hope Med Ctr 1979; **Fac Appt:** Clin Prof Med, USC Sch Med

Heinrich, Michael C MD [Hem] - **Spec Exp:** Hematologic Malignancies; Sarcoma; Gastrointestinal Stromal Tumors; **Hospital:** VA Medical Center - Portland, OR Hlth & Sci Univ; **Address:** 3710 SW US Veteran's Hospital Rd, MC P3RND19, Portland, OR 97239; **Phone:** 503-220-8262 x51169; **Board Cert:** Internal Medicine 1987; Hematology 2010; Medical Oncology 2011; **Med School:** Johns Hopkins Univ 1984; **Resid:** Internal Medicine, Oreg Hlth Scis Univ 1988; **Fellow:** Hematology & Oncology, Oreg Hlth Scis Univ 1991; **Fac Appt:** Prof Med, Oregon Hlth & Sci Univ

Kipps, Thomas J MD/PhD [Hem] - **Spec Exp:** Leukemia; Lymphoma, Non-Hodgkin's; **Hospital:** UCSD Med Ctr; **Address:** Moores UCSD Cancer Ctr, 3855 Health Sciences Drive, MC 0820, La Jolla, CA 92093; **Phone:** 858-822-5635; **Board Cert:** Internal Medicine 1982; Hematology 1984; **Med School:** Harvard Med Sch 1979; **Resid:** Internal Medicine, Stanford Univ Med Ctr 1981; **Fellow:** Hematology & Oncology, Stanford Univ Med Ctr 1984; **Fac Appt:** Prof Med, UCSD

Hematology

Leung, Lawrence L MD [Hem] - **Spec Exp:** Bleeding/Coagulation Disorders; **Hospital:** Stanford Univ Hosp & Clinics, VA Hlth Care Sys - Palo Alto; **Address:** Stanford Cancer Center - Hematology, 875 Blake Wilbur Drive, Palo Alto, CA 94305; **Phone:** 650-498-6000; **Board Cert:** Internal Medicine 1978; Hematology 2009; Medical Oncology 1981; **Med School:** Columbia P&S 1975; **Resid:** Internal Medicine, New York Hosp 1978; **Fellow:** Hematology & Oncology, New York Hosp/Cornell 1981; **Fac Appt:** Prof Med, Stanford Univ

Levine, Alexandra M MD [Hem] - **Spec Exp:** Lymphoma; AIDS Related Cancers; AIDS/HIV; **Hospital:** City of Hope Natl Med Ctr; **Address:** 1500 E Duarte Rd, Needleman 213, Duarte, CA 91010; **Phone:** 626-471-7213; **Med School:** USC Sch Med 1971; **Resid:** Internal Medicine, LAC-USC Med Ctr 1974; **Fellow:** Hematology & Oncology, Grady Meml Hosp-Emory Univ 1975; Hematology, LAC-USC Med Ctr 1978; **Fac Appt:** Prof Med, USC Sch Med

Lill, Michael MD [Hem] - **Spec Exp:** Stem Cell Transplant; Lymphoma; Hematologic Malignancies; **Hospital:** Cedars-Sinai Med Ctr; **Address:** Cedars-Sinai Med Ctr-Outpt Cancer Ctr, 8700 Beverly Blvd, Ste AC 1070, Los Angeles, CA 90048; **Phone:** 310-423-1160; **Med School:** Australia 1982; **Resid:** Internal Medicine, Sir Charles Gairdner Hospital 1985; **Fellow:** Hematology, Royal Perth Hospital 1989; Hematopathology, Sir Charles Gairdner Hosp 1989; **Fac Appt:** Prof Med, UCLA

Linenberger, Michael MD [Hem] - **Spec Exp:** Bone Marrow Transplant; Bleeding/Coagulation Disorders; Multiple Myeloma; Leukemia & Lymphoma; **Hospital:** Univ Wash Med Ctr; **Address:** 825 Eastlake Ave E, MS G4100, Seattle, WA 98109-1023; **Phone:** 206-288-1260; **Board Cert:** Internal Medicine 1985; Hematology 1988; **Med School:** Univ Kansas 1982; **Resid:** Internal Medicine, Rhode Island Hosp 1985; **Fellow:** Hematology, Univ Wash Med Ctr 1989; **Fac Appt:** Assoc Prof Med, Univ Wash

Maziarz, Richard MD [Hem] - **Spec Exp:** Leukemia; Immunotherapy; Bone Marrow Transplant; Lymphoma; **Hospital:** OR Hlth & Sci Univ; **Address:** OHSU Ctr Hematologic Malignancies, 3181 SW Sam Jackson Park Rd, Multnomah Pavilion, MC UHN73A, Portland, OR 97239; **Phone:** 503-494-5058; **Board Cert:** Internal Medicine 1982; Hematology 1988; Medical Oncology 1989; **Med School:** Harvard Med Sch 1979; **Resid:** Internal Medicine, Univ Hosp 1982; **Fellow:** Hematology & Oncology, Brigham & Womens Hosp 1988; **Fac Appt:** Prof Med, Oregon Hlth & Sci Univ

Mitchell, Beverly S MD [Hem] - **Spec Exp:** Hematologic Malignancies; Leukemia; Lymphoma; **Hospital:** Stanford Univ Hosp & Clinics; **Address:** Stanford Cancer Institute, Lorry Lokey Bldg-SIM 1, 265 Campus Drive, Ste G2167, Stanford, CA 94305-5456; **Phone:** 650-736-7716; **Board Cert:** Internal Medicine 1973; Hematology 1978; **Med School:** Harvard Med Sch 1969; **Resid:** Internal Medicine, Univ Washington Med Ctr 1972; **Fellow:** Metabolism, Univ Zurich 1975; Hematology & Oncology, Univ Michigan 1977; **Fac Appt:** Prof Med, Stanford Univ

Nademanee, Auayporn P MD [Hem] - **Spec Exp:** Lymphoma; Hematologic Malignancies; Clinical Trials; **Hospital:** City of Hope Natl Med Ctr; **Address:** City of Hope Med Ctr-Dept Hematology, 1500 Duarte Rd, Duarte, CA 91010; **Phone:** 626-256-4673 x62691; **Board Cert:** Hematology 1982; Medical Oncology 1983; Internal Medicine 1978; **Med School:** Thailand 1973; **Resid:** Internal Medicine, Touro Infirm-Tulane Univ 1978; **Fellow:** Hematology & Oncology, Sepulveda VA Hosp 1980; Hematology & Oncology, USC Med Ctr 1981; **Fac Appt:** Prof Med, UCLA

Negrin, Robert S MD [Hem] - **Spec Exp:** Bone Marrow Transplant; **Hospital:** Stanford Univ Hosp & Clinics; **Address:** BMT Program, 300 Pasteur Drive, rm H0101, MC 5623, Stanford, CA 94305; **Phone:** 650-723-0822; **Board Cert:** Internal Medicine 1987; Hematology 2007; **Med School:** Harvard Med Sch 1984; **Resid:** Internal Medicine, Stanford Univ Hosp 1987; **Fellow:** Hematology, Stanford Univ Hosp 1990; **Fac Appt:** Prof Med, Stanford Univ

O'Donnell, Margaret R MD [Hem] - **Spec Exp:** Leukemia; Clinical Trials; **Hospital:** City of Hope Natl Med Ctr; **Address:** City of Hope National Med Ctr, 1500 E Duarte Rd, MOB-rm 3001, Duarte, CA 91010; **Phone:** 626-359-8111 x62405; **Board Cert:** Internal Medicine 1978; Hematology 1980; Medical Oncology 1979; **Med School:** Med Coll PA 1974; **Resid:** Internal Medicine, Montreal Genl Hosp 1976; Hematology, Royal Victoria Hosp-Montreal 1977; **Fellow:** Hematology & Oncology, Fred Hutchinson Cancer Ctr 1979

Petersdorf, Stephen MD [Hem] - **Spec Exp:** Lymphoma; Myelodysplastic Syndromes; Leukemia; **Hospital:** Univ Wash Med Ctr; **Address:** Seattle Cancer Care Alliance, 825 Eastlake Ave E, MS E2102, Seattle, WA 98109-1023; **Phone:** 206-288-6202; **Board Cert:** Internal Medicine 1986; Hematology 2011; Medical Oncology 2011; **Med School:** Brown Univ 1983; **Resid:** Internal Medicine, Univ Washington Med Ctr 1986; **Fellow:** Hematology & Oncology, Univ Washington Med Ctr 1989; **Fac Appt:** Assoc Prof Med, Univ Wash

Saven, Alan MD [Hem] - **Spec Exp:** Leukemia; Lymphoma; **Hospital:** Scripps Green Hosp; **Address:** Scripps Green Hosp, Hematology, 10666 N Torrey Pines Rd, MS 312, La Jolla, CA 92037; **Phone:** 858-554-9489; **Board Cert:** Internal Medicine 1987; Medical Oncology 1989; **Med School:** South Africa 1982; **Resid:** Internal Medicine, Albert Einstein Med Ctr 1986; **Fellow:** Hematology & Oncology, Scripps Clinic 1987

Schiller, Gary J MD [Hem] - **Spec Exp:** Leukemia; **Hospital:** UCLA Ronald Reagan Med Ctr; **Address:** 10833 Le Conte Ave, rm 42-121 CHS, Los Angeles, CA 90095; **Phone:** 310-206-6745; **Board Cert:** Internal Medicine 1987; Medical Oncology 1989; Hematology 2000; **Med School:** USC Sch Med 1984; **Resid:** Internal Medicine, UCLA Med Ctr 1987; **Fellow:** Hematology & Oncology, UCLA Med Ctr 1990; **Fac Appt:** Prof Med, UCLA

Snyder, David S MD [Hem] - **Spec Exp:** Leukemia; Bone Marrow Transplant; Myeloproliferative Disorders; **Hospital:** City of Hope Natl Med Ctr; **Address:** 1500 E Duarte Rd, rm 1003, Duarte, CA 91010-3012; **Phone:** 626-256-4673 x62691; **Board Cert:** Internal Medicine 1980; Hematology 1984; **Med School:** Harvard Med Sch 1977; **Resid:** Internal Medicine, Beth Israel Deaconess Med Ctr 1980; **Fellow:** Immunology, Harvard Med Sch 1982; Hematology & Oncology, New England Bapt Hosp 1984

MEDICAL ONCOLOGY

New England

Antin, Joseph H MD [Onc] - **Spec Exp:** Bone Marrow Transplant; Stem Cell Transplant; Anemia-Aplastic; Myelodysplastic Syndromes; **Hospital:** Brigham and Women's Hosp (page 57), Dana-Farber Cancer Inst (page 57); **Address:** Dana-Farber Cancer Institute, 450 Brookline Ave, rm D1B30, Boston, MA 02215; **Phone:** 617-632-3245; **Board Cert:** Internal Medicine 1981; Medical Oncology 1983; Hematology 1984; **Med School:** Cornell Univ-Weill Med Coll 1978; **Resid:** Internal Medicine, Peter Bent Brigham Hosp 1981; **Fellow:** Hematology & Oncology, Brigham & Womens Hosp/Dana Farber 1984; **Fac Appt:** Prof Onc, Harvard Med Sch

Birrer, Michael J MD/PhD [Onc] - **Spec Exp:** Ovarian Cancer; Clinical Trials; Gynecologic Cancer; **Hospital:** Mass Genl Hosp; **Address:** Mass General Hospital, 55 Fruit St, Ste YAW 9E, Boston, MA 02114; **Phone:** 617-724-4000; **Board Cert:** Internal Medicine 1985; Medical Oncology 1987; **Med School:** Albert Einstein Coll Med 1982; **Resid:** Internal Medicine, Mass General Hosp 1985; **Fellow:** Medical Oncology, NIH 1987; **Fac Appt:** Prof Med, Harvard Med Sch

Medical Oncology

Bubley, Glenn J MD [Onc] - **Spec Exp:** Prostate Cancer; **Hospital:** Beth Israel Deaconess Med Ctr - Boston; **Address:** BIDMC-Div os Hematology/Onc, 330 Brookline Ave, Shapiro Bldg Fl 9, Boston, MA 02215; **Phone:** 617-735-2062; **Board Cert:** Internal Medicine 1980; Medical Oncology 1983; **Med School:** Mich State Univ 1977; **Resid:** Internal Medicine, St Francis Hosp 1980; **Fellow:** Hematology & Oncology, Beth Israel Deaconess Med Ctr 1983; **Fac Appt:** Assoc Prof Med, Harvard Med Sch

Burstein, Harold J MD [Onc] - **Spec Exp:** Breast Cancer; **Hospital:** Dana-Farber Cancer Inst (page 57), Brigham and Women's Hosp (page 57); **Address:** 450 Brookline Ave, Ste Y1250, Boston, MA 02215; **Phone:** 617-632-4587; **Board Cert:** Medical Oncology 2010; **Med School:** Harvard Med Sch 1994; **Resid:** Internal Medicine, Mass Genl Hosp 1997; **Fellow:** Medical Oncology, Dana Farber Cancer Inst 2000; **Fac Appt:** Assoc Prof Med, Harvard Med Sch

Canellos, George P MD [Onc] - **Spec Exp:** Lymphoma-Second Opinion; Hodgkin's Disease-Second Opinion; **Hospital:** Dana-Farber Cancer Inst (page 57), Brigham and Women's Hosp (page 57); **Address:** Dana Farber Cancer Inst, 450 Brookline Ave, DANA IB-14, Boston, MA 02215; **Phone:** 617-632-3470; **Board Cert:** Internal Medicine 1967; Hematology 1972; Medical Oncology 1973; **Med School:** Columbia P&S 1960; **Resid:** Internal Medicine, Mass Genl Hosp 1963; Internal Medicine, Mass Genl Hosp 1966; **Fellow:** Medical Oncology, Natl Cancer Inst 1965; Hematology, Royal Post Graduate Sch of Med 1967; **Fac Appt:** Prof Med, Harvard Med Sch

Chabner, Bruce A MD [Onc] - **Spec Exp:** Breast Cancer; Colon & Rectal Cancer; **Hospital:** Mass Genl Hosp; **Address:** Mass General Hospital, Hematology/Oncology Assocs, 55 Fruit St, MS LRH 214, Boston, MA 02114; **Phone:** 617-724-3200; **Board Cert:** Internal Medicine 1971; Medical Oncology 1973; **Med School:** Harvard Med Sch 1965; **Resid:** Internal Medicine, Peter Bent Brigham Hosp 1967; Internal Medicine, Yale-New Haven Hosp 1970; **Fellow:** Medical Oncology, Natl Inst Hlth 1969; **Fac Appt:** Prof Med, Harvard Med Sch

Come, Steven E MD [Onc] - **Spec Exp:** Breast Cancer; Hodgkin's Lymphoma; **Hospital:** Beth Israel Deaconess Med Ctr - Boston, Dana-Farber Cancer Inst (page 57); **Address:** Beth Israel Deaconess Hosp, 330 Brookline Ave, Ste CC913, Boston, MA 02215-5400; **Phone:** 617-667-4599; **Board Cert:** Internal Medicine 1975; Medical Oncology 1979; **Med School:** Harvard Med Sch 1972; **Resid:** Internal Medicine, Beth Israel Hosp 1977; **Fellow:** Medical Oncology, Natl Cancer Inst 1976; **Fac Appt:** Assoc Prof Onc, Harvard Med Sch

DeVita Jr, Vincent T MD [Onc] - **Spec Exp:** Lymphoma Consultation; Hodgkin's Disease Consultation; **Hospital:** Yale-New Haven Hosp, Yale Med Group; **Address:** Yale Cancer Ctr, 333 Cedar St, rm FMP117, New Haven, CT 06520-8028; **Phone:** 203-737-1010; **Board Cert:** Internal Medicine 1974; Hematology 1972; Medical Oncology 1973; **Med School:** Geo Wash Univ 1961; **Resid:** Internal Medicine, Geo Wash Hosp 1963; Internal Medicine, Yale-New Haven Hosp 1966; **Fellow:** Medical Oncology, Natl Cancer Inst 1965; **Fac Appt:** Prof Med, Yale Univ

Dizon, Don S MD [Onc] - **Spec Exp:** Gynecologic Cancer; Breast Cancer; Cancer Survivors-Late Effects of Therapy; Sexual Health in Cancer Survivors; **Hospital:** Mass Genl Hosp; **Address:** Mass General Hospital, 55 Fruit St, Yawkey 9E, Boston, MA 02114; **Phone:** 617-724-4000; **Board Cert:** Internal Medicine 2008; Medical Oncology 2002; **Med School:** Univ Rochester 1995; **Resid:** Internal Medicine, Yale-New Haven Hosp 1998; **Fellow:** Oncology, Meml Sloan Kettering Cancer Ctr 2001; **Fac Appt:** Asst Prof Med, Harvard Med Sch

Erban III, John K MD [Onc] - **Spec Exp:** Breast Cancer; Hematologic Malignancies; Stem Cell Transplant; **Hospital:** Tufts Med Ctr; **Address:** 800 Washington St, Box 245, Boston, MA 02111; **Phone:** 617-636-8077; **Board Cert:** Internal Medicine 1984; Medical Oncology 1989; Hematology 2010; **Med School:** Tufts Univ 1981; **Resid:** Internal Medicine, Hosp Univ Penn 1984; **Fellow:** Hematology & Oncology, New England Med Ctr 1990; **Fac Appt:** Prof Onc, Tufts Univ

Ernstoff, Marc Stuart MD [Onc] - **Spec Exp:** Melanoma; Genitourinary Cancer; Skin Cancer; **Hospital:** Dartmouth - Hitchcock Med Ctr; **Address:** 1 Medical Center Drive, Lebanon, NH 03756; **Phone:** 603-650-5534; **Board Cert:** Internal Medicine 1981; Medical Oncology 1989; **Med School:** NYU Sch Med 1978; **Resid:** Internal Medicine, Albert Einstein Coll Med 1981; **Fellow:** Medical Oncology, Yale Univ Affil Hosp 1984; **Fac Appt:** Prof Med, Dartmouth Med Sch

Flaherty, Keith T MD [Onc] - **Spec Exp:** Melanoma-Advanced; Clinical Trials; **Hospital:** Mass Genl Hosp; **Address:** Mass Genl Cancer Ctr, 32 Fruit St, Ste YAW-7, Boston, MA 02114; **Phone:** 617-724-4800; **Board Cert:** Medical Oncology 2003; **Med School:** Johns Hopkins Univ 1997; **Resid:** Internal Medicine, Brigham & Women's Hosp 2000; **Fellow:** Hematology & Oncology, Pennsylvania Hosp-UPHS 2002

Foss, Francine M MD [Onc] - **Spec Exp:** Lymphoma, Cutaneous T Cell (CTCL); Stem Cell Transplant; Graft vs Host Disease; Multiple Myeloma; **Hospital:** Yale-New Haven Hosp, Yale Med Group; **Address:** 35 Park St Fl 7, New Haven, CT 06520-8032; **Phone:** 203-200-4363; **Board Cert:** Internal Medicine 1985; Medical Oncology 1987; **Med School:** Univ Mass Sch Med 1982; **Resid:** Internal Medicine, Brigham & Womens Hosp 1985; **Fellow:** Medical Oncology, Natl Cancer Inst 1988; **Fac Appt:** Prof Med, Yale Univ

Freedman, Arnold S MD [Onc] - **Spec Exp:** Lymphoma; Bone Marrow Transplant; Stem Cell Transplant; **Hospital:** Brigham and Women's Hosp (page 57), Dana-Farber Cancer Inst (page 57); **Address:** Dana-Farber Cancer Inst, 450 Brookline Ave, Dana-1B30, Boston, MA 02115; **Phone:** 617-582-9086; **Board Cert:** Internal Medicine 1982; Medical Oncology 1985; **Med School:** Univ Mass Sch Med 1979; **Resid:** Internal Medicine, Memorial Hosp 1982; **Fellow:** Medical Oncology, Dana Farber Cancer Inst 1985; **Fac Appt:** Assoc Prof Med, Harvard Med Sch

Fuchs, Charles S MD [Onc] - **Spec Exp:** Gastrointestinal Cancer; Esophageal Cancer; **Hospital:** Dana-Farber Cancer Inst (page 57), Brigham and Women's Hosp (page 57); **Address:** Dana Farber Cancer Inst, 450 Brookline Ave, Ste D1220, Boston, MA 02215; **Phone:** 617-632-5840; **Board Cert:** Internal Medicine 1989; Medical Oncology 2002; **Med School:** Harvard Med Sch 1986; **Resid:** Internal Medicine, Brigham & Womens Hosp 1989; **Fellow:** Hematology & Oncology, Dana Farber Cancer Inst 1992; **Fac Appt:** Prof Med, Harvard Med Sch

Garber, Judy E MD [Onc] - **Spec Exp:** Breast Cancer; Breast Cancer Genetics; Cancer Risk Assessment; **Hospital:** Dana-Farber Cancer Inst (page 57), Brigham and Women's Hosp (page 57); **Address:** Dana Farber Cancer Inst, 450 Brookline Ave, Boston, MA 02215; **Phone:** 617-632-5961; **Board Cert:** Internal Medicine 1984; Medical Oncology 1987; Hematology 1988; **Med School:** Yale Univ 1981; **Resid:** Internal Medicine, Brigham & Womens Hosp 1984; **Fellow:** Hematology & Oncology, Brigham & Womens Hosp/Dana Farber Cancer Inst 1988; Cancer Epidemiology, Dana Farber Cancer Inst 1990; **Fac Appt:** Assoc Prof Med, Harvard Med Sch

Garnick, Marc B MD [Onc] - **Spec Exp:** Prostate Cancer; Urologic Cancer; **Hospital:** Beth Israel Deaconess Med Ctr - Boston; **Address:** Beth Israel Deaconess Med Ctr, SCC9, 330 Brookline Ave, Boston, MA 02215; **Phone:** 617-735-2062; **Board Cert:** Internal Medicine 1976; Medical Oncology 1979; **Med School:** Univ Pennsylvania 1972; **Resid:** Internal Medicine, Hosp Univ Penn 1974; **Fellow:** Research, Natl Inst Hlth 1976; Medical Oncology, Dana-Farber Cancer Inst 1978; **Fac Appt:** Clin Prof Med, Harvard Med Sch

George, Suzanne MD [Onc] - **Spec Exp:** Bone Tumors; Sarcoma-Soft Tissue; Gastrointestinal Cancer; **Hospital:** Dana-Farber Cancer Inst (page 57), Brigham and Women's Hosp (page 57); **Address:** Dana-Farber Cancer Inst, 450 Brookline Ave, rm D1212, Boston, MA 02215; **Phone:** 617-632-5122; **Board Cert:** Medical Oncology 2011; **Med School:** Univ Mass Sch Med 1995; **Resid:** Internal Medicine, Univ NC Hlth Sys 1997; **Fellow:** Hematology & Oncology, New England Med Ctr 2001; **Fac Appt:** Asst Prof Med, Harvard Med Sch

Medical Oncology

Grunberg, Steven M MD [Onc] - **Spec Exp:** Lung Cancer; Head & Neck Cancer; Thyroid Cancer; Cancer Risk Assessment; **Hospital:** Fletcher Allen Health Care- Med Ctr Campus; **Address:** FAHC Division of Hematology/Oncology, 89 Beaumont Ave, Given Bldg, E214, Burlington, VT 05405; **Phone:** 802-847-8400; **Board Cert:** Internal Medicine 1978; Medical Oncology 1983; **Med School:** Cornell Univ-Weill Med Coll 1975; **Resid:** Internal Medicine, Mofitt Hosp-U Calif 1978; **Fellow:** Medical Oncology, Sidney Farber Cancer Ctr 1981; **Fac Appt:** Prof Onc, Univ VT Coll Med

Herbst, Roy S MD/PhD [Onc] - **Spec Exp:** Lung Cancer; Thoracic Cancers; Drug Development; Clinical Trials; **Hospital:** Yale-New Haven Hosp; **Address:** Smilow Cancer Hosp, Thoracic Cancer Div, 20 York St Fl 4, New Haven, CT 06504; **Phone:** 203-200-5864; **Board Cert:** Medical Oncology 2007; **Med School:** Cornell Univ-Weill Med Coll 1991; **Resid:** Internal Medicine, Brigham & Women's Hosp 1994; **Fellow:** Medical Oncology, Dana Farber Cancer Inst 1996; **Fac Appt:** Assoc Prof Med, Univ Tex, Houston

Hochberg, Ephraim P MD [Onc] - **Spec Exp:** Lymphoma; Hodgkin's Lymphoma; Lymphomatoid Granulomatosis; **Hospital:** Mass Genl Hosp; **Address:** Mass General Hospital, 55 Fruit St, Ste YAW 7B, Boston, MA 02114; **Phone:** 617-724-4000; **Board Cert:** Medical Oncology 2002; Hematology 2004; **Med School:** Case West Res Univ 1996; **Resid:** Internal Medicine, Brigham & Women's Hosp 1999; **Fellow:** Hematology & Oncology, Dana Farber Cancer Inst 2002

Hochster, Howard S MD [Onc] - **Spec Exp:** Gastrointestinal Cancer; Gynecologic Cancer; Colon & Rectal Cancer; **Hospital:** Yale-New Haven Hosp, Yale Med Group; **Address:** Smilow Cancer Center, 333 Cedar St, Box 208028, New Haven, CT 06520-8028; **Phone:** 203-785-4191; **Board Cert:** Internal Medicine 1983; Medical Oncology 1985; Hematology 1986; **Med School:** Yale Univ 1980; **Resid:** Internal Medicine, NYU Med Ctr 1983; **Fellow:** Hematology & Oncology, NYU Med Ctr 1985; Medical Oncology, Jules Bordet Inst 1986; **Fac Appt:** Prof Med, Yale Univ

Hollister Jr, Dickerman MD [Onc] - **Spec Exp:** Breast Cancer; Lung Cancer; Colon Cancer; Leukemia & Lymphoma; **Hospital:** Greenwich Hosp; **Address:** 77 Lafayette Pl, Ste 260, Greenwich, CT 06830; **Phone:** 203-863-3737; **Board Cert:** Internal Medicine 1978; Hematology 1980; Medical Oncology 1981; **Med School:** Univ VA Sch Med 1975; **Resid:** Internal Medicine, NY Hosp-Cornell Med Ctr 1978; **Fellow:** Hematology & Oncology, NY Hosp-Cornell Med Ctr 1981; **Fac Appt:** Asst Clin Prof Med, Yale Univ

Johnson, Bruce E MD [Onc] - **Spec Exp:** Lung Cancer; Thoracic Cancers; Mesothelioma; Mesothelioma; **Hospital:** Dana-Farber Cancer Inst (page 57), Brigham and Women's Hosp (page 57); **Address:** Dana-Farber Cancer Institute, 450 Brookline Ave, Boston, MA 02215; **Phone:** 617-632-4790; **Board Cert:** Internal Medicine 1982; Medical Oncology 1985; **Med School:** Univ Minn 1979; **Resid:** Internal Medicine, Univ Chicago Hosps 1982; **Fellow:** Medical Oncology, Natl Cancer Inst 1985; **Fac Appt:** Prof Onc, Harvard Med Sch

Kantoff, Philip W MD [Onc] - **Spec Exp:** Genitourinary Cancer; Prostate Cancer; Testicular Cancer; **Hospital:** Dana-Farber Cancer Inst (page 57), Brigham and Women's Hosp (page 57); **Address:** Dana Farber Cancer Inst, 450 Brookline Avenue, Dana 1230, Boston, MA 02215; **Phone:** 617-632-1914; **Board Cert:** Internal Medicine 1982; Medical Oncology 1989; **Med School:** Brown Univ 1979; **Resid:** Internal Medicine, NYU/Bellevue Hosp 1982; **Fellow:** Molecular Genetics, NIH 1986; Hematology & Oncology, Dana Farber Cancer Inst 1988; **Fac Appt:** Prof Onc, Harvard Med Sch

Kaufman, Peter A MD [Onc] - **Spec Exp:** Breast Cancer; Clinical Trials; **Hospital:** Dartmouth - Hitchcock Med Ctr; **Address:** DHMC, Dept Hem-Onc, One Medical Center Drive, Lebanon, NH 03756; **Phone:** 603-653-6181; **Board Cert:** Internal Medicine 1986; Medical Oncology 1989; **Med School:** NYU Sch Med 1983; **Resid:** Internal Medicine, Duke Univ Med Ctr 1986; **Fellow:** Hematology & Oncology, Duke Univ Med Ctr 1989; **Fac Appt:** Assoc Prof Med, Dartmouth Med Sch

Lacy, Jill MD [Onc] - **Spec Exp:** Colon & Rectal Cancer; Gastrointestinal Cancer; Brain Tumors; Pancreatic Cancer; **Hospital:** Yale-New Haven Hosp, Yale Med Group; **Address:** Yale Univ Sch Med-Div Medical Oncology, 333 Cedar St, PO Box 208032, New Haven, CT 06520-8032; **Phone:** 203-785-4191; **Board Cert:** Internal Medicine 1982; Medical Oncology 2005; **Med School:** Yale Univ 1978; **Resid:** Internal Medicine, Yale-New Haven Hosp 1981; **Fellow:** Medical Oncology, Yale-New Haven Hosp 1985; **Fac Appt:** Assoc Prof Onc, Yale Univ

Legare, Robert D MD [Onc] - **Spec Exp:** Breast Cancer; Breast Cancer Risk Assessment; **Hospital:** Women & Infants Hosp of RI; **Address:** Women & Infants Hosp, 101 Dudley St, Providence, RI 02905; **Phone:** 401-453-7540; **Board Cert:** Internal Medicine 2005; Hematology 2006; Medical Oncology 2008; **Med School:** Tufts Univ 1990; **Resid:** Internal Medicine, Yale-New Haven Hosp 1992; **Fellow:** Hematology & Oncology, Brigham & Womens Hosp 1996; **Fac Appt:** Assoc Prof Med, Brown Univ

Lynch Jr, Thomas J MD [Onc] - **Spec Exp:** Lung Cancer; Thoracic Cancers; **Hospital:** Yale-New Haven Hosp, Yale Med Group; **Address:** 35 Park St Fl 4, New Haven, CT 06510; **Phone:** 203-688-5864; **Board Cert:** Internal Medicine 1989; Medical Oncology 2003; **Med School:** Yale Univ 1986; **Resid:** Internal Medicine, Mass Genl Hosp 1989; **Fellow:** Medical Oncology, Dana-Farber Cancer Inst 1991; **Fac Appt:** Assoc Prof Med, Yale Univ

Mathew, Paul MD [Onc] - **Spec Exp:** Prostate Cancer; Genitourinary Cancer; **Hospital:** Tufts Med Ctr; **Address:** Tufts Med Ctr, Div Hematology-Oncology, 800 Washington St, Box 245, Boston, MA 02111; **Phone:** 617-636-8483; **Board Cert:** Hematology 2004; Medical Oncology 2003; **Med School:** Nigeria 1985; **Resid:** Internal Medicine, Cook Co Hosp 1990; **Fellow:** Hematology & Oncology, Mayo Clinic 1994; **Fac Appt:** Assoc Prof Onc, Tufts Univ

Matulonis, Ursula A MD [Onc] - **Spec Exp:** Gynecologic Cancer; Ovarian Cancer; Breast Cancer; Fertility Preservation in Cancer; **Hospital:** Dana-Farber Cancer Inst (page 57); **Address:** Dana Farber Cancer Inst, 450 Brookline Ave Fl 14, Boston, MA 02215; **Phone:** 617-632-2334; **Board Cert:** Medical Oncology 2000; **Med School:** Albany Med Coll 1987; **Resid:** Internal Medicine, Univ Pittsburgh Med Ctr 1990; **Fellow:** Medical Oncology, Dana Farber Cancer Inst 1993; **Fac Appt:** Assoc Prof Med, Harvard Med Sch

Mayer, Robert J MD [Onc] - **Spec Exp:** Colon & Rectal Cancer; Gastrointestinal Cancer; **Hospital:** Dana-Farber Cancer Inst (page 57), Brigham and Women's Hosp (page 57); **Address:** Dana Farber Cancer Inst, 450 Brookline Ave, Boston, MA 02115; **Phone:** 617-632-3474; **Board Cert:** Internal Medicine 1973; Medical Oncology 1975; Hematology 1976; **Med School:** Harvard Med Sch 1969; **Resid:** Internal Medicine, Mt Sinai Hosp 1971; Hematology & Oncology, Natl Cancer Inst 1974; **Fellow:** Dana Farber Cancer Inst 1976; **Fac Appt:** Prof Med, Harvard Med Sch

Petrylak, Daniel P MD [Onc] - **Spec Exp:** Testicular Cancer; Prostate Cancer; Bladder Cancer; Kidney Cancer; **Hospital:** Yale-New Haven Hosp, Greenwich Hosp; **Address:** 333 Cedar St, New Haven, CT 06520; **Phone:** 203-200-4822; **Board Cert:** Internal Medicine 2001; Medical Oncology 2003; **Med School:** Case West Res Univ 1985; **Resid:** Internal Medicine, Jacobi Med Ctr 1988; **Fellow:** Oncology, Meml-Sloan Kettering Cancer Ctr 1991; **Fac Appt:** Prof Onc, Yale Univ

Ryan, David MD [Onc] - **Spec Exp:** Colon Cancer; Pancreatic Cancer; Gastrointestinal Cancer; **Hospital:** Mass Genl Hosp; **Address:** Mass General Hospital, 55 Fruit St, Ste YAW 7E, Boston, MA 02114; **Phone:** 617-724-4000; **Board Cert:** Medical Oncology 2009; **Med School:** Columbia P&S 1992; **Resid:** Internal Medicine, NY-Presby/Columbia Univ Med Ctr 1996; **Fellow:** Hematology & Oncology, Mass Genl Hosp 1998; **Fac Appt:** Asst Prof Med, Harvard Med Sch

Medical Oncology

Saif, M Wasif MD [Onc] - **Spec Exp:** Pancreatic Cancer; Colon & Rectal Cancer; **Hospital:** Tufts Med Ctr; **Address:** Tufts Medical Ctr, 800 Washington St, Box 245, Boston, MA 02111; **Phone:** 617-636-5627; **Med School:** Pakistan 1992; **Resid:** Internal Medicine, Univ Conn Med Ctr 1998; **Fellow:** Medical Oncology, Natl Cancer Inst 2001; Hematology, Natl Heart Lung & Blood Inst; **Fac Appt:** Clin Prof Med, Columbia P&S

Schnipper, Lowell E MD [Onc] - **Spec Exp:** Breast Cancer; **Hospital:** Beth Israel Deaconess Med Ctr - Boston; **Address:** BIDMC-Div of Hematology/Onc, 330 Brookline Ave Shapiro Bldg Fl 9, Boston, MA 02215; **Phone:** 617-667-1921; **Board Cert:** Internal Medicine 1973; Medical Oncology 1983; **Med School:** SUNY Downstate 1968; **Resid:** Internal Medicine, Yale-New Haven Hosp 1970; Medical Oncology, Natl Cancer Inst 1973; **Fellow:** Hematology & Oncology, Barnes Jewish Hosp 1974; **Fac Appt:** Prof Med, Harvard Med Sch

Shulman, Lawrence N MD [Onc] - **Spec Exp:** Breast Cancer; **Hospital:** Dana-Farber Cancer Inst (page 57), Brigham and Women's Hosp (page 57); **Address:** Dana-Farber Cancer Inst, 450 Brookline Ave, DANA 1608, Boston, MA 02215; **Phone:** 617-632-2277; **Board Cert:** Internal Medicine 1978; Medical Oncology 1981; Hematology 1982; **Med School:** Harvard Med Sch 1975; **Resid:** Internal Medicine, Beth Israel Hosp 1977; **Fellow:** Hematology & Oncology, Beth Israel Hosp 1980; **Fac Appt:** Assoc Prof Med, Harvard Med Sch

Smith, Matthew R MD/PhD [Onc] - **Spec Exp:** Prostate Cancer; **Hospital:** Mass Genl Hosp; **Address:** Mass Genl Hosp, Hematology/Oncology, 55 Fruit St, Ste YAW 7E, Boston, MA 02114; **Phone:** 617-724-5257; **Board Cert:** Medical Oncology 2007; **Med School:** Duke Univ 1992; **Resid:** Internal Medicine, Brigham & Women's Hosp 1994; **Fellow:** Medical Oncology, Dana Farber Cancer Inst 1997; **Fac Appt:** Assoc Prof Med, Harvard Med Sch

Soiffer, Robert J MD [Onc] - **Spec Exp:** Stem Cell Transplant; Bone Marrow Transplant; Leukemia; Lymphoma; **Hospital:** Dana-Farber Cancer Inst (page 57), Brigham and Women's Hosp (page 57); **Address:** Dana-Farber Cancer Inst, 450 Brookline Ave Dana Bldg - Ste 1B30, Boston, MA 02215; **Phone:** 617-632-3667; **Board Cert:** Internal Medicine 1986; Medical Oncology 1989; **Med School:** NYU Sch Med 1983; **Resid:** Internal Medicine, Brigham & Women's Hosp 1986; **Fellow:** Medical Oncology, Brigham & Women's Hosp 1989; **Fac Appt:** Prof Med, Harvard Med Sch

Strauss, Gary M MD [Onc] - **Spec Exp:** Lung Cancer; Thoracic Cancers; Melanoma; Breast Cancer; **Hospital:** Tufts Med Ctr; **Address:** Tufts Medical Ctr, Div of Hem/Onc, 800 Washington St, Box 245, Boston, MA 02111; **Phone:** 617-636-5291; **Board Cert:** Internal Medicine 1975; Medical Oncology 1979; Hematology 1980; **Med School:** Yale Univ 1972; **Resid:** Internal Medicine, Boston City Hosp 1974; Internal Medicine, Mass Genl Hosp 1977; **Fellow:** Medical Oncology, Natl Cancer Inst 1976; Hematology & Oncology, Mass General Hosp 1979; **Fac Appt:** Prof Med, Tufts Univ

Strenger, Rochelle MD [Onc] - **Spec Exp:** Breast Cancer; Hematologic Malignancies; Lymphoma; **Hospital:** Miriam Hosp, Rhode Island Hosp; **Address:** Comprehensive Cancer Ctr-Miriam Hosp, 164 Summit Ave, Fain 3, Providence, RI 02906; **Phone:** 401-793-2920; **Board Cert:** Internal Medicine 1986; Medical Oncology 2009; **Med School:** Albert Einstein Coll Med 1982; **Resid:** Internal Medicine, Brigham & Womens Hosp 1985; **Fellow:** Hematology & Oncology, Brigham & Womens Hosp 1988

Sweeney, Christopher J MD [Onc] - **Spec Exp:** Genitourinary Cancer; Prostate Cancer; Testicular Cancer; **Hospital:** Dana-Farber Cancer Inst (page 57); **Address:** Dana Farber Cancer Inst, 450 Brookline Ave, Ste D-1230, Boston, MA 02215; **Phone:** 617-632-4524; **Board Cert:** Medical Oncology 2011; **Med School:** Australia 1993; **Resid:** Internal Medicine, Gundersen Lutheran Med Ctr 1997; **Fellow:** Hematology & Oncology, Indiana Univ Med Ctr 2000; **Fac Appt:** Assoc Prof Med, Harvard Med Sch

Taplin, Mary-Ellen MD [Onc] - **Spec Exp:** Prostate Cancer; Genitourinary Cancer; **Hospital:** Dana-Farber Cancer Inst (page 57), Brigham and Women's Hosp (page 57); **Address:** Dana Farber Cancer Inst, 450 Brookline Ave, Ste D-1230, Boston, MA 02215; **Phone:** 617-632-3237; **Board Cert:** Internal Medicine 1989; Hematology 2006; Medical Oncology 2003; **Med School:** Univ Mass Sch Med 1986; **Resid:** Internal Medicine, Univ Mass Med Ctr 1990; **Fellow:** Hematology & Oncology, Beth Israel Deaconess Med Ctr 1993; **Fac Appt:** Assoc Prof Med, Harvard Med Sch

Verschraegen, Claire F MD [Onc] - **Spec Exp:** Ovarian Cancer; Drug Discovery; Gynecologic Cancer; Sarcoma; **Hospital:** Fletcher Allen Health Care- Med Ctr Campus; **Address:** 89 Beaumont Ave, Ste Given, rm E214, Vermont Cancer Center, Burlington, VT 05405; **Phone:** 802-656-5487; **Board Cert:** Medical Oncology 2000; **Med School:** Belgium 1982; **Resid:** Internal Medicine, Bordet 1985; Internal Medicine, Univ Texas 1991; **Fellow:** Cancer Research, Stehlin Fdn for Cancer Research 1988; Oncology, MD Anderson Cancer Ctr 1994; **Fac Appt:** Prof Med, Univ VT Coll Med

Weisberg, Tracey MD [Onc] - **Spec Exp:** Breast Cancer; **Hospital:** Maine Med Ctr; **Address:** Maine Ctr for Cancer Medicine, 100 Campus Drive, Unit 108, Scarborough, ME 04074; **Phone:** 207-396-7600; **Board Cert:** Internal Medicine 1987; Medical Oncology 1989; **Med School:** SUNY Stony Brook 1983; **Resid:** Internal Medicine, Mount Sinai Hosp 1985; Internal Medicine, Hartford Hosp 1986; **Fellow:** Medical Oncology, Yale Univ Hosp 1988

Winer, Eric P MD [Onc] - **Spec Exp:** Breast Cancer; **Hospital:** Dana-Farber Cancer Inst (page 57), Brigham and Women's Hosp (page 57); **Address:** Dana Farber Cancer Inst, 450 Brookline Ave Yawkey Bldg - Ste 1250, Boston, MA 02215; **Phone:** 617-632-6876; **Board Cert:** Internal Medicine 1987; Medical Oncology 1989; **Med School:** Yale Univ 1983; **Resid:** Internal Medicine, Yale-New Haven Hosp 1987; **Fellow:** Hematology & Oncology, Duke Univ Med Ctr 1989; **Fac Appt:** Prof Med, Harvard Med Sch

Mid Atlantic

Abraham, Jame MD [Onc] - **Spec Exp:** Breast Cancer; Clinical Trials; **Hospital:** Ruby Memorial - WVU Hosp; **Address:** Mary Babb Randolph Cancer Center, MS 9162, W Virginia University, Morgantown, WV 26506; **Phone:** 304-598-4552; **Board Cert:** Internal Medicine 2007; Medical Oncology 2000; **Med School:** India 1991; **Resid:** Internal Medicine, Univ Conn Sch Med 1997; **Fellow:** Medical Oncology, Natl Cancer Inst 1999; Hematology, Natl Heart Lung & Blood Inst; **Fac Appt:** Prof Onc, W VA Univ

Aghajanian, Carol A MD [Onc] - **Spec Exp:** Ovarian Cancer; Gynecologic Cancer; Trophoblastic Tumors; **Hospital:** Meml Sloan-Kettering Cancer Ctr; **Address:** 300 E 66th St, New York, NY 10065; **Phone:** 646-888-4217; **Board Cert:** Internal Medicine 2002; Medical Oncology 2005; **Med School:** SUNY Downstate 1989; **Resid:** Internal Medicine, Mt Sinai Med Ctr 1993; **Fellow:** Medical Oncology, Meml Sloan Kettering Cancer Ctr 1995; **Fac Appt:** Assoc Prof Med, Cornell Univ-Weill Med Coll

Ahlgren, James D MD [Onc] - **Spec Exp:** Gastrointestinal Cancer; Carcinoid Tumors; Neuroendocrine Tumors; **Hospital:** G Washington Univ Hosp; **Address:** 2150 Pennsylvania Ave NW, Ste 1-207, Washington, DC 20037-3201; **Phone:** 202-741-2478; **Board Cert:** Internal Medicine 1980; Medical Oncology 1989; **Med School:** Georgetown Univ 1977; **Resid:** Internal Medicine, Georgetown Univ Hosp 1979; **Fellow:** Medical Oncology, Georgetown Univ Hosp 1981; **Fac Appt:** Prof Med, Geo Wash Univ

Medical Oncology

Aisner, Joseph MD [Onc] - **Spec Exp:** Lung Cancer; Solid Tumors; Thymoma; Mesothelioma; **Hospital:** Robert Wood Johnson Univ Hosp - New Brunswick; **Address:** Cancer Inst of New Jersey, 195 Little Albany St, rm 2006, New Brunswick, NJ 08903-2681; **Phone:** 732-235-6777; **Board Cert:** Internal Medicine 1973; Medical Oncology 1975; **Med School:** Wayne State Univ 1970; **Resid:** Internal Medicine, Georgetown Univ Hosp 1972; **Fellow:** Medical Oncology, Natl Cancer Inst 1975; **Fac Appt:** Prof Med, UMDNJ-RW Johnson Med Sch

Algazy, Kenneth M MD [Onc] - **Spec Exp:** Lung Cancer; Head & Neck Cancer; Hematologic Malignancies; **Hospital:** Hosp Univ Penn - UPHS (page 72), VA Med Ctr - Philadelphia; **Address:** Hosp Univ Pennsylvania, 3400 Convention Ave, The Perelman Ctr, Fl 2, Philadelphia, PA 19104; **Phone:** 215-615-5810; **Board Cert:** Internal Medicine 1972; Hematology 1974; Medical Oncology 1979; **Med School:** Temple Univ 1969; **Resid:** Internal Medicine, Strong Meml Hosp 1972; **Fellow:** Hematology & Oncology, Johns Hopkins Hosp 1974; **Fac Appt:** Clin Prof Onc, Temple Univ

Ambinder, Richard F MD/PhD [Onc] - **Spec Exp:** Lymphoma; Hodgkin's Lymphoma; AIDS Related Cancers; **Hospital:** Johns Hopkins Hosp (page 61); **Address:** Johns Hopkins Hosp, Sidney Kimmel Cancer Ctr, 410 N Broadway, Ste 1343, Baltimore, MD 21231; **Phone:** 410-955-8964; **Board Cert:** Internal Medicine 1982; Medical Oncology 1985; **Med School:** Johns Hopkins Univ 1979; **Resid:** Internal Medicine, Johns Hopkins Hosp 1981; **Fellow:** Internal Medicine, Johns Hopkins Hosp 1982; Medical Oncology, Johns Hopkins Hosp 1985; **Fac Appt:** Prof Med, Johns Hopkins Univ

Arlen, Philip M MD [Onc] - **Spec Exp:** Prostate Cancer-Vaccine Therapy; Vaccine Therapy-Clinical Trials Only; Clinical Trials Only; **Hospital:** Natl Inst of Hlth - Clin Ctr, Natl Naval Med Ctr; **Address:** Natl Cancer Inst-Ctr for Cancer Rsch, Laboratory of Tumor Immunology & Bio, 10 Center Drive Bldg 10 - rm 809, Bethesda, MD 20892-1750; **Phone:** 301-496-4343; **Board Cert:** Medical Oncology 2008; **Med School:** Med Coll GA 1991; **Resid:** Internal Medicine, Georgia Baptist Hlth Care Syst 1994; **Fellow:** Hematology & Oncology, Emory Univ Med Ctr 1997; Oncology Research, Natl Cancer Inst-NIH 1999

Astrow, Alan B MD [Onc] - **Spec Exp:** Ovarian Cancer; Breast Cancer; Lymphoma; **Hospital:** Maimonides Med Ctr (page 63); **Address:** MMC Hematology/Oncology, 6300 8th Ave, Brooklyn, NY 11220; **Phone:** 718-765-2653; **Board Cert:** Internal Medicine 1983; Hematology 1986; Medical Oncology 1987; **Med School:** Yale Univ 1980; **Resid:** Internal Medicine, Boston City Hosp 1983; **Fellow:** Hematology & Oncology, NYU Med Ctr 1986; **Fac Appt:** Assoc Clin Prof Med, NY Med Coll

Atkins, Michael B MD [Onc] - **Spec Exp:** Melanoma; Kidney Cancer; Immunotherapy; **Hospital:** Georgetown Univ Hosp; **Address:** Lombardi Comprehensive Cancer Ctr, 3800 Reservoir Rd NW, Washington, DC 20007; **Phone:** 202-444-2223; **Board Cert:** Internal Medicine 1983; Medical Oncology 1987; **Med School:** Tufts Univ 1980; **Resid:** Internal Medicine, New England Med Ctr 1983; **Fellow:** Hematology & Oncology, New England Med Ctr 1987; **Fac Appt:** Prof Onc, Georgetown Univ

Attas, Lewis MD [Onc] - **Spec Exp:** Breast Cancer; Lymphoma; Bleeding/Coagulation Disorders; Gaucher Disease; **Hospital:** Englewood Hosp & Med Ctr, Holy Name Med Ctr; **Address:** 350 Engle St, Englewood, NJ 07631; **Phone:** 201-568-5250; **Board Cert:** Internal Medicine 1985; Medical Oncology 1987; Hematology 1988; **Med School:** Mount Sinai Sch Med 1982; **Resid:** Internal Medicine, Montefiore Hosp Med Ctr 1985; **Fellow:** Hematology & Oncology, North Shore Univ Hosp 1988; **Fac Appt:** Assoc Clin Prof Med, Mount Sinai Sch Med

Axelrod, Rita S MD [Onc] - **Spec Exp:** Head & Neck Cancer; Lung Cancer; Complementary Medicine; **Hospital:** Thomas Jefferson Univ Hosp; **Address:** 925 Chestnut St Fl 3, Philadelphia, PA 19107; **Phone:** 215-955-8874; **Board Cert:** Internal Medicine 1976; Medical Oncology 1977; Hematology 1978; **Med School:** NYU Sch Med 1970; **Resid:** Internal Medicine, Med Coll Georgia Hosps 1973; **Fellow:** Hematology & Oncology, Hosp Univ Penn 1975; **Fac Appt:** Prof Med, Thomas Jefferson Univ

Azzoli, Christopher MD [Onc] - **Spec Exp:** Lung Cancer; Lung Cancer (advanced); **Hospital:** Meml Sloan-Kettering Cancer Ctr; **Address:** 300 E 66th St, New York, NY 10065; **Phone:** 646-888-4198; **Board Cert:** Internal Medicine 2009; Medical Oncology 2001; **Med School:** Johns Hopkins Univ 1996; **Resid:** Internal Medicine, Johns Hopkins Hosp 1999; **Fellow:** Medical Oncology, Meml Sloan Kettering Cancer Ctr 2002; **Fac Appt:** Asst Prof Med, Cornell Univ-Weill Med Coll

Bajorin, Dean F MD [Onc] - **Spec Exp:** Genitourinary Cancer; Bladder Cancer; Testicular Cancer; **Hospital:** Meml Sloan-Kettering Cancer Ctr; **Address:** 1275 York Avenue, New York, NY 10065; **Phone:** 646-422-4333; **Board Cert:** Internal Medicine 1981; Medical Oncology 1985; **Med School:** NY Med Coll 1978; **Resid:** Internal Medicine, Hartford Hosp 1981; **Fellow:** Medical Oncology, Meml Sloan Kettering Ctr 1986; **Fac Appt:** Prof Med, Cornell Univ-Weill Med Coll

Bashevkin, Michael MD [Onc] - **Spec Exp:** Solid Tumors; Bleeding/Coagulation Disorders; Hematologic Malignancies; **Hospital:** Maimonides Med Ctr (page 63); **Address:** 1660 E 14st St, Ste 501, Brooklyn, NY 11229; **Phone:** 718-382-8500 x501; **Board Cert:** Internal Medicine 1976; Hematology 1978; Medical Oncology 1979; **Med School:** SUNY Downstate 1973; **Resid:** Internal Medicine, VA Med Ctr 1976; **Fellow:** Hematology & Oncology, Maimonides Med Ctr 1979

Belani, Chandra P MD [Onc] - **Spec Exp:** Lung Cancer; Drug Discovery; **Hospital:** Penn State Milton S Hershey Med Ctr; **Address:** Penn State Hershey Cancer Institute, 500 University Drive, PSHCI Bldg, MS CH72, Hershey, PA 17033; **Phone:** 717-531-1078; **Board Cert:** Internal Medicine 1986; Medical Oncology 1987; **Med School:** India 1978; **Resid:** Internal Medicine, SMS Med Hosp 1981; Internal Medicine, Good Samaritan/Univ MD Hosps 1985; **Fellow:** Hematology & Oncology, Univ Maryland Hosp 1987; **Fac Appt:** Prof Med, Penn State Coll Med

Biggs, David D MD [Onc] - **Spec Exp:** Breast Cancer; Kidney Cancer; Melanoma; Skin Cancer; **Hospital:** Christiana Hospital; **Address:** Med Onc/Hem Consultants, 4701 Ogletown-Stanton Rd, Ste 3400, Newark, DE 19713; **Phone:** 302-366-1200; **Board Cert:** Internal Medicine 1988; Hematology 2002; Medical Oncology 2012; **Med School:** Univ Kansas 1984; **Resid:** Internal Medicine, Med Coll Wisconsin 1989; **Fellow:** Hematology & Oncology, Hosp Univ Penn 1991; **Fac Appt:** Asst Clin Prof Med

Bosl, George MD [Onc] - **Spec Exp:** Testicular Cancer; **Hospital:** Meml Sloan-Kettering Cancer Ctr; **Address:** 1275 York Avenue, New York, NY 10065; **Phone:** 212-639-8473; **Board Cert:** Internal Medicine 1976; Medical Oncology 1979; **Med School:** Creighton Univ 1973; **Resid:** Internal Medicine, NY Hosp 1975; Internal Medicine, Meml Sloan-Kettering Cancer Ctr 1977; **Fellow:** Medical Oncology, Univ Minn Hosps 1979; **Fac Appt:** Prof Med, Cornell Univ-Weill Med Coll

Brufsky, Adam M MD/PhD [Onc] - **Spec Exp:** Breast Cancer; **Hospital:** Magee-Womens Hosp - UPMC, UPMC Presby, Pittsburgh; **Address:** 300 Halket St, Ste 4628, Pittsburgh, PA 15213; **Phone:** 412-641-6500; **Board Cert:** Internal Medicine 2004; Medical Oncology 2005; **Med School:** Univ Conn 1990; **Resid:** Internal Medicine, Brigham & Womens Hosp 1992; **Fellow:** Medical Oncology, Dana Farber Cancer Inst 1995; Bone Marrow Transplant, Dana Farber Cancer Inst 1993; **Fac Appt:** Prof Onc, Univ Pittsburgh

Medical Oncology

Carabasi, Matthew H MD [Onc] - **Spec Exp:** Bone Marrow Transplant; Stem Cell Transplant; Leukemia & Lymphoma; **Hospital:** Thomas Jefferson Univ Hosp; **Address:** Jefferson Univ Physicians, Div Medical Oncology, 925 Chestnut St, Ste 420A, Philadelphia, PA 19107; **Phone:** 215-955-8874; **Board Cert:** Internal Medicine 1983; Medical Oncology 1987; **Med School:** Jefferson Med Coll 1980; **Resid:** Internal Medicine, Hahnemann Univ Hosp 1984; **Fellow:** Hematology & Oncology, Meml Sloan-Kettering Cancer Ctr 1988; Research, Meml Sloan-Kettering Cancer Ctr 1989; **Fac Appt:** Assoc Prof Med, Jefferson Med Coll

Carducci, Michael A MD [Onc] - **Spec Exp:** Urologic Cancer; Drug Discovery & Development; Vaccine Therapy; Clinical Trials; **Hospital:** Johns Hopkins Hosp (page 61); **Address:** Johns Hopkins Hosp, Sidney Kimmel Cancer Ctr, 401 N Broadway, Ste 1343, Baltimore, MD 21231; **Phone:** 410-955-8964; **Board Cert:** Internal Medicine 2011; Medical Oncology 2005; **Med School:** Wayne State Univ 1988; **Resid:** Internal Medicine, Univ Colorado Hlth Sci Ctr 1992; **Fellow:** Medical Oncology, Johns Hopkins Hosp 1995; **Fac Appt:** Prof Med, Johns Hopkins Univ

Celano, Paul MD [Onc] - **Spec Exp:** Gynecologic Cancer; Genitourinary Cancer; Breast Cancer; **Hospital:** Greater Baltimore Med Ctr, Johns Hopkins Hosp (page 61); **Address:** GBMC Cancer Ctr, 6569 N Charles St, Ste 201, Baltimore, MD 21204; **Phone:** 443-849-3051; **Board Cert:** Internal Medicine 1984; Medical Oncology 1987; **Med School:** Mount Sinai Sch Med 1981; **Resid:** Internal Medicine, Thos Jefferson Univ Hosp 1984; **Fellow:** Medical Oncology, Johns Hopkins Hosp 1987; **Fac Appt:** Asst Prof Onc, Johns Hopkins Univ

Chachoua, Abraham MD [Onc] - **Spec Exp:** Lung Cancer; Thoracic Cancers; **Hospital:** NYU Langone Med Ctr (page 68); **Address:** NYU Clinical Cancer Ctr, 160 E 34th St Fl 8, New York, NY 10016; **Phone:** 212-731-5388; **Med School:** Australia 1978; **Resid:** Internal Medicine, Alfred Hosp 1982; **Fellow:** Hematology & Oncology, Alfred Hosp 1985; Hematology & Oncology, NYU Med Ctr 1988; **Fac Appt:** Assoc Prof Med, NYU Sch Med

Chapman, Paul B MD [Onc] - **Spec Exp:** Melanoma; Immunotherapy; Clinical Trials; Vaccine Therapy; **Hospital:** Meml Sloan-Kettering Cancer Ctr; **Address:** 1275 York Avenue, New York, NY 10065; **Phone:** 646-888-2378; **Board Cert:** Internal Medicine 1984; Medical Oncology 1987; **Med School:** Cornell Univ-Weill Med Coll 1981; **Resid:** Internal Medicine, Univ Chicago Hosps 1984; **Fellow:** Medical Oncology, Meml Sloan-Kettering Cancer Ctr 1987; **Fac Appt:** Prof Med, Cornell Univ-Weill Med Coll

Chu, Edward MD [Onc] - **Spec Exp:** Colon & Rectal Cancer; Gastrointestinal Cancer; Clinical Trials; **Hospital:** UPMC Shadyside, UPMC Presby, Pittsburgh; **Address:** Univ of Pittsburgh Cancer Institute, 5150 Centre Ave, Fl Fifth, rm 571, Univ of Pittsburgh Cancer Institute, Pittsburgh, PA 15232; **Phone:** 412-648-6589; **Board Cert:** Internal Medicine 1986; Medical Oncology 1989; **Med School:** Brown Univ 1983; **Resid:** Internal Medicine, Roger Williams Hosp 1987; **Fellow:** Medical Oncology, Natl Cancer Inst 1992; **Fac Appt:** Prof Onc, Univ Pittsburgh

Claxton, David F MD [Onc] - **Spec Exp:** Leukemia; Bone Marrow Transplant; Hematologic Malignancies; Anemia-Aplastic; **Hospital:** Penn State Milton S Hershey Med Ctr; **Address:** 500 University Drive, rm T4422, Hershey, PA 17033; **Phone:** 717-531-8678; **Board Cert:** Internal Medicine 1984; Medical Oncology 2004; **Med School:** McGill Univ 1978; **Resid:** Internal Medicine, Royal Victoria Hosp 1984; **Fellow:** Hematology, Royal Victoria Hosp 1986; Medical Oncology, UT-MD Anderson Cancer Ctr 1989; **Fac Appt:** Prof Med

Cohen, Gary I MD [Onc] - **Spec Exp:** Hematologic Malignancies; Stem Cell Transplant; Melanoma; **Hospital:** Greater Baltimore Med Ctr; **Address:** GBMC Sandra & Malcolm Berman Cancer Inst, 6569 N Charles St, Ste 205, Baltimore, MD 21204; **Phone:** 443-849-3051; **Board Cert:** Internal Medicine 1978; Hematology 1982; Medical Oncology 1985; **Med School:** Univ MD Sch Med 1975; **Resid:** Internal Medicine, SUNY Health Sci Ctr 1978; **Fellow:** Hematology & Oncology, Dana Farber Cancer Ctr 1980

Cohen, Philip MD [Onc] - **Spec Exp:** Breast Cancer; **Hospital:** Georgetown Univ Hosp; **Address:** Georgetown Univ Hosp, Lombardi Cancer Ctr, 3800 Reservoir Rd NW, Washington, DC 20007; **Phone:** 202-444-2198; **Board Cert:** Internal Medicine 1973; Medical Oncology 1975; Hematology 1976; **Med School:** Harvard Med Sch 1970; **Resid:** Internal Medicine, Mass Genl Hosp 1972; **Fellow:** Medical Oncology, Natl Cancer Inst 1974; **Fac Appt:** Assoc Prof Med, Geo Wash Univ

Cohen, Roger B MD [Onc] - **Spec Exp:** Head & Neck Cancer; Lung Cancer; Drug Discovery & Development; Clinical Trials; **Hospital:** Hosp Univ Penn - UPHS (page 72); **Address:** Penn Hematology/Oncology, 16 Penn Tower, 3400 Spruce St, Philadelphia, PA 19104; **Phone:** 215-662-4469; **Board Cert:** Internal Medicine 1984; Hematology 1986; Medical Oncology 2005; **Med School:** Harvard Med Sch 1980; **Resid:** Internal Medicine, Mt Sinai Hosp 1982; Hematology, Mt Sinai Hosp 1986; **Fellow:** Research, Sloan Kettering Cancer Inst 1985; Medical Oncology, Natl Cancer Inst 1993; **Fac Appt:** Prof Med, Univ Pennsylvania

Cohen, Seymour M MD [Onc] - **Spec Exp:** Breast Cancer; Melanoma; Lung Cancer; Lymphoma; **Hospital:** Mount Sinai Med Ctr (page 64); **Address:** 1150 5th Ave, New York, NY 10128; **Phone:** 212-249-9141; **Board Cert:** Internal Medicine 1971; Medical Oncology 1973; **Med School:** Univ Pittsburgh 1962; **Resid:** Internal Medicine, Montefiore Med Ctr 1964; Internal Medicine, Mount Sinai Med Ctr 1965; **Fellow:** Hematology, Mount Sinai Med Ctr 1966; Hematology & Oncology, LI Jewish Hosp 1969; **Fac Appt:** Assoc Clin Prof Med, Mount Sinai Sch Med

Coleman, Morton MD [Onc] - **Spec Exp:** Leukemia & Lymphoma; Hodgkin's Lymphoma; Multiple Myeloma; Waldenstrom's Macroglobulinemia; **Hospital:** NY-Presby/Weill Cornell Med Ctr, NY (page 66); **Address:** 407 E 70th St Fl 3, New York, NY 10021-5302; **Phone:** 212-517-5900; **Board Cert:** Internal Medicine 1971; Hematology 1972; Medical Oncology 1973; **Med School:** Med Coll VA 1963; **Resid:** Internal Medicine, Grady Meml Hosp-Emory 1965; Internal Medicine, NY-Presby/Cornell Univ Med Ctr 1968; **Fellow:** Hematology & Oncology, NY-Presby/Cornell Univ Med Ctr 1970; **Fac Appt:** Clin Prof Med, Cornell Univ-Weill Med Coll

Cristofanilli, Massimo MD [Onc] - **Spec Exp:** Breast Cancer; Breast Cancer-Inflammatory; **Hospital:** Fox Chase Cancer Ctr (page 58); **Address:** Fox Chase Cancer Ctr, 333 Cottman Ave, rm C315, Philadelphia, PA 19111; **Phone:** 215-728-2570; **Board Cert:** Medical Oncology 2010; **Med School:** Italy 1986; **Resid:** Internal Medicine, Cabrini 1996; **Fellow:** Medical Oncology, MD Anderson Cancer Ctr 1998; **Fac Appt:** Prof Med, Univ Pennsylvania

Cullen, Kevin MD [Onc] - **Spec Exp:** Head & Neck Cancer; **Hospital:** Univ of MD Med Ctr; **Address:** Greenebaum Cancer Ctr, 22 S Greene St, rm N9E22, Baltimore, MD 21201; **Phone:** 410-328-5506; **Board Cert:** Internal Medicine 1986; Medical Oncology 1989; **Med School:** Harvard Med Sch 1983; **Resid:** Internal Medicine, Beth Israel Hosp 1986; Internal Medicine, Hammersmith Hosp 1985; **Fellow:** Medical Oncology, Natl Cancer Inst 1988

Czuczman, Myron S MD [Onc] - **Spec Exp:** Hodgkin's Lymphoma; Multiple Myeloma; Leukemia-Chronic Lymphocytic; Waldenstrom's Macroglobulinemia; **Hospital:** Roswell Park Cancer Inst, Buffalo General Hosp; **Address:** Roswell Park Cancer Institute, Elm & Carlton Sreets, Buffalo, NY 14263; **Phone:** 716-845-1643; **Board Cert:** Internal Medicine 1988; **Med School:** Penn State Coll Med 1985; **Resid:** Internal Medicine, North Shore Univ Hosp 1988; **Fellow:** Hematology & Oncology, Meml Sloan-Kettering Cancer Ctr 1992; **Fac Appt:** Prof Med, SUNY Buffalo

Daly, Mary B MD/PhD [Onc] - **Spec Exp:** Breast Cancer; Breast Cancer Risk Assessment; Cancer Prevention; Ovarian Cancer Risk Assessment; **Hospital:** Fox Chase Cancer Ctr (page 58); **Address:** Fox Chase Cancer Ctr, 333 Cottman Ave, P1054, Philadelphia, PA 19111; **Phone:** 215-728-2791; **Board Cert:** Internal Medicine 1981; Medical Oncology 1983; **Med School:** Univ NC Sch Med 1978; **Resid:** Internal Medicine, Univ Texas Hlth Sci Ctr 1981; **Fellow:** Medical Oncology, UT San Antonio 1983; **Fac Appt:** Clin Prof Med, Temple Univ

Dang, Chi V MD/PhD [Onc] - **Spec Exp:** Anemia-Aplastic; Bone Marrow Failure Disorders; Myeloproliferative Disorders; **Hospital:** Hosp Univ Penn - UPHS (page 72); **Address:** 399 S 34th St, Penn Tower Bldg - Fl 16 - Ste 1600, Philadelphia, PA 19104; **Phone:** 215-662-3929; **Board Cert:** Internal Medicine 1985; Medical Oncology 1987; **Med School:** Johns Hopkins Univ 1982; **Resid:** Internal Medicine, Johns Hopkins Hosp 1985; **Fellow:** Medical Oncology, UCSF Med Ctr 1987; **Fac Appt:** Prof Med, Johns Hopkins Univ

Dawson, Nancy MD [Onc] - **Spec Exp:** Prostate Cancer; Kidney Cancer; Bladder Cancer; **Hospital:** Georgetown Univ Hosp; **Address:** Lombardi Cancer Ctr, Georgetown Univ Hosp, 3800 Reservoir Rd NW, Washington, DC 20007; **Phone:** 202-444-9094; **Board Cert:** Internal Medicine 1982; Hematology 1984; Medical Oncology 1985; **Med School:** Georgetown Univ 1979; **Resid:** Internal Medicine, Walter Reed AMC 1982; **Fellow:** Hematology & Oncology, Walter Reed AMC 1985; **Fac Appt:** Prof Med, Georgetown Univ

Dickler, Maura N MD [Onc] - **Spec Exp:** Breast Cancer; **Hospital:** Meml Sloan-Kettering Cancer Ctr; **Address:** 1275 York Ave, New York, NY 10065; **Phone:** 646-497-9064; **Board Cert:** Medical Oncology 2008; **Med School:** Univ Chicago-Pritzker Sch Med 1991; **Resid:** Internal Medicine, Univ Chicago Hosps 1994; **Fellow:** Medical Oncology, Meml Sloan Kettering Cancer Ctr 1998; **Fac Appt:** Assoc Prof Med, Cornell Univ-Weill Med Coll

DiPaola, Robert S MD [Onc] - **Spec Exp:** Genitourinary Cancer; Prostate Cancer; Urologic Cancer; **Hospital:** Robert Wood Johnson Univ Hosp - New Brunswick; **Address:** Cancer Inst of New Jersey, 195 Little Albany St, New Brunswick, NJ 08903-2681; **Phone:** 732-235-6777; **Board Cert:** Internal Medicine 2011; Medical Oncology 2005; **Med School:** Univ Utah 1988; **Resid:** Internal Medicine, Duke Univ Med Ctr 1991; **Fellow:** Hematology & Oncology, Univ Penn Hosp 1994; **Fac Appt:** Assoc Prof Med, UMDNJ-RW Johnson Med Sch

Domchek, Susan M MD [Onc] - **Spec Exp:** Breast Cancer; Breast Cancer Genetics; Breast Cancer Risk Assessment; **Hospital:** Hosp Univ Penn - UPHS (page 72); **Address:** Abramson Cancer Ctr, Perelman Ctr, 3 West, 3400 Civic Center Blvd, Philadelphia, PA 19104; **Phone:** 215-615-3341; **Board Cert:** Medical Oncology 2011; **Med School:** Harvard Med Sch 1995; **Resid:** Internal Medicine, Mass Genl Hosp 1998; **Fellow:** Medical Oncology, Dana Farber Cancer Inst 2001; **Fac Appt:** Assoc Prof Med, Univ Pennsylvania

Donehower, Ross Carl MD [Onc] - **Spec Exp:** Pancreatic Cancer; Colon Cancer; Prostate Cancer; **Hospital:** Johns Hopkins Hosp (page 61); **Address:** Johns Hopkins Hosp, Sidney Kimmel Cancer Ctr, 410 N Broadway, Ste 1343, Baltimore, MD 21231; **Phone:** 410-955-8964; **Board Cert:** Internal Medicine 1977; Medical Oncology 1979; **Med School:** Univ Minn 1974; **Resid:** Internal Medicine, Johns Hopkins Hosp 1976; **Fellow:** Medical Oncology, Natl Inst Hlth 1980; **Fac Appt:** Prof Med, Johns Hopkins Univ

Doroshow, James H MD [Onc] - **Spec Exp:** Drug Discovery & Development; Colon Cancer; Breast Cancer; **Hospital:** Natl Inst of Hlth - Clin Ctr; **Address:** National Cancer Inst, Div Cancer Treatment & Diagnosis, 31 Center Dr, Bldg 31-rm 3A44, Bethesda, MD 20892-2440; **Phone:** 301-496-4291; **Board Cert:** Internal Medicine 1976; Medical Oncology 1977; **Med School:** Harvard Med Sch 1973; **Resid:** Internal Medicine, Mass Genl Hosp 1975; **Fellow:** Medical Oncology, Natl Cancer Inst 1978

Dutcher, Janice P MD [Onc] - **Spec Exp:** Kidney Cancer; Melanoma; Breast Cancer; Lymphoma; **Hospital:** St. Luke's - Roosevelt Hosp Ctr - Roosevelt Div (page 56); **Address:** Continuum Cancer Center of NY, 1000 Tenth Ave, Ste 11C-02, New York, NY 10019; **Phone:** 212-636-3334; **Board Cert:** Internal Medicine 1978; Medical Oncology 1983; **Med School:** UC Davis 1975; **Resid:** Internal Medicine, Rush Presbyterian Med Ctr 1978; **Fellow:** Medical Oncology, National Cancer Inst 1981; **Fac Appt:** Prof Med, NY Med Coll

Edelman, Martin J MD [Onc] - **Spec Exp:** Thoracic Cancers; Lung Cancer; Drug Discovery & Development; **Hospital:** Univ of MD Med Ctr; **Address:** Greenebaum Cancer Ctr, 22 S Greene St, rm N9E08, Baltimore, MD 21201; **Phone:** 410-328-2703; **Board Cert:** Internal Medicine 1986; Medical Oncology 1989; **Med School:** Albany Med Coll 1982; **Resid:** Internal Medicine, Naval Hosp 1986; **Fellow:** Hematology & Oncology, Naval Hosp 1990; **Fac Appt:** Prof Med, Univ MD Sch Med

Eisenberger, Mario MD [Onc] - **Spec Exp:** Prostate Cancer; **Hospital:** Johns Hopkins Hosp (page 61); **Address:** Johns Hopkins Hosp, Sidney Kimmel Cancer Ctr, 410 N Broadway, Ste 1343, Baltimore, MD 21231; **Phone:** 410-614-3511; **Board Cert:** Internal Medicine 1976; Medical Oncology 1979; **Med School:** Brazil 1972; **Resid:** Internal Medicine, Michael Reese Hosp 1975; **Fellow:** Hematology, Michael Reese Hosp 1976; Medical Oncology, Jackson Meml Hosp/Univ Miami 1979; **Fac Appt:** Prof Med, Johns Hopkins Univ

Emens, Leisha A MD/PhD [Onc] - **Spec Exp:** Breast Cancer; Immunotherapy; **Hospital:** Johns Hopkins Hosp (page 61); **Address:** Johns Hopkins Hosp, Sidney Kimmel Cancer Ctr, 410 N Broadway, Ste 1343, Baltimore, MD 21231; **Phone:** 410-955-8964; **Board Cert:** Internal Medicine 2008; Medical Oncology 2001; Hematology 2002; **Med School:** Baylor Coll Med 1995; **Resid:** Internal Medicine, Univ TX SW Affil Hosps 1998; **Fellow:** Medical Oncology, Johns Hopkins Hosps 2001; Research, Lab of Bio Chem- NCI 1993; **Fac Appt:** Assoc Prof Med, Johns Hopkins Univ

Engstrom, Paul F MD [Onc] - **Spec Exp:** Neuroendocrine Tumors; Gastrointestinal Cancer; Colon & Rectal Cancer; **Hospital:** Fox Chase Cancer Ctr (page 58); **Address:** Fox Chase Cancer Ctr, Medical Oncology, 333 Cottman Ave, Philadelphia, PA 19111; **Phone:** 215-728-2986; **Board Cert:** Internal Medicine 1969; Medical Oncology 1973; **Med School:** Univ Minn 1962; **Resid:** Internal Medicine, Univ Minn Hosp 1965; **Fac Appt:** Prof Med, Temple Univ

Ettinger, David S MD [Onc] - **Spec Exp:** Lung Cancer; Sarcoma; Clinical Trials; **Hospital:** Johns Hopkins Hosp (page 61); **Address:** Bunting Blaustein Cancer Rsch Bldg, 1650 Orleans St, rm G88, Baltimore, MD 21287-0013; **Phone:** 410-955-8847; **Board Cert:** Internal Medicine 1976; Medical Oncology 1977; **Med School:** Univ Louisville Sch Med 1967; **Resid:** Internal Medicine, Mayo Grad Schl 1971; **Fellow:** Medical Oncology, Johns Hopkins Hosp 1975; **Fac Appt:** Prof Med, Johns Hopkins Univ

Fine, Howard A MD [Onc] - **Spec Exp:** Brain Tumors; Neuro-Oncology; **Hospital:** Natl Inst of Hlth - Clin Ctr; **Address:** National Cancer Inst, 9030 Old Georgetown Rd, Bldg 82, Rm 225, MSC 8202, Bethesda, MD 20892-0001; **Phone:** 301-402-6298; **Board Cert:** Internal Medicine 1987; Medical Oncology 1989; **Med School:** Mount Sinai Sch Med 1984; **Resid:** Internal Medicine, Hosp Univ Penn 1987; **Fellow:** Medical Oncology, Dana Farber Cancer Ctr 1990

Fine, Robert Lance MD [Onc] - **Spec Exp:** Pancreatic Cancer; Drug Development; Neuroendocrine Tumors; Clinical Trials; **Hospital:** NY-Presby/Columbia Univ Med Ctr, NY (page 66); **Address:** 650 W 168th St Fl 20th - Ste BB20-05, New York, NY 10032; **Phone:** 212-305-1168; **Board Cert:** Internal Medicine 1983; Medical Oncology 1985; **Med School:** Univ Chicago-Pritzker Sch Med 1979; **Resid:** Internal Medicine, Stanford Univ Med Ctr 1982; **Fellow:** Medical Oncology, National Cancer Inst 1988; **Fac Appt:** Assoc Prof Med, Columbia P&S

Fisher, Richard I MD [Onc] - **Spec Exp:** Lymphoma; Hodgkin's Lymphoma; **Hospital:** Univ of Rochester Strong Meml Hosp; **Address:** James P Wilmot Cancer Ctr, 601 Elmwood Ave, Box 704, Rochester, NY 14642; **Phone:** 585-275-5823; **Board Cert:** Internal Medicine 1973; Medical Oncology 1977; **Med School:** Harvard Med Sch 1970; **Resid:** Internal Medicine, Mass Genl Hosp 1972; **Fac Appt:** Prof Med, Univ Rochester

Medical Oncology

Flomenberg, Neal MD [Onc] - **Spec Exp:** Bone Marrow Transplant; Stem Cell Transplant; Leukemia & Lymphoma; **Hospital:** Thomas Jefferson Univ Hosp; **Address:** Thomas Jefferson Univ Hosp, 925 Chestnut St Fl 2, Philadelphia, PA 19107; **Phone:** 215-955-8874; **Board Cert:** Internal Medicine 1979; Medical Oncology 1981; Hematology 1982; **Med School:** Jefferson Med Coll 1976; **Resid:** Internal Medicine, Montefiore Med Ctr 1979; **Fellow:** Hematology & Oncology, Meml Sloan Kettering Cancer Ctr 1982; **Fac Appt:** Clin Prof Med, Thomas Jefferson Univ

Forastiere, Arlene A MD [Onc] - **Spec Exp:** Esophageal Cancer; Head & Neck Cancer; **Hospital:** Johns Hopkins Hosp (page 61); **Address:** Johns Hopkins Hosp, Sidney Kimmel Cancer Ctr, 410 N Broadway, Ste 1343, Baltimore, MD 21231; **Phone:** 410-955-8964; **Board Cert:** Internal Medicine 1978; Medical Oncology 1981; **Med School:** NY Med Coll 1975; **Resid:** Internal Medicine, Albert Einstein Med Ctr 1977; Internal Medicine, Univ Conn Health Ctr 1978; **Fellow:** Medical Oncology, Meml Sloan Kettering Cancer Ctr 1980; **Fac Appt:** Prof Med, NY Med Coll

Fox, Kevin R MD [Onc] - **Spec Exp:** Breast Cancer; Lymphedema; **Hospital:** Hosp Univ Penn - UPHS (page 72); **Address:** Penn Hematology/Oncology, 16 Penn Tower, 3400 Spruce St, Philadelphia, PA 19104; **Phone:** 215-662-7469; **Board Cert:** Internal Medicine 1985; Medical Oncology 1987; **Med School:** Johns Hopkins Univ 1981; **Resid:** Internal Medicine, Johns Hopkins Hosp 1984; **Fellow:** Hematology & Oncology, Hosp Univ Penn 1987; **Fac Appt:** Prof Med, Univ Pennsylvania

Friedberg, Jonathan MD [Onc] - **Spec Exp:** Lymphoma; Hodgkin's Lymphoma; Clinical Trials; **Hospital:** Univ of Rochester Strong Meml Hosp; **Address:** James P Wilmot Cancer Ctr, 601 Elmwood Ave, Box 704, Rochester, NY 14642-8704; **Phone:** 585-275-4911; **Board Cert:** Medical Oncology 2000; Hematology 2000; **Med School:** Harvard Med Sch 1994; **Resid:** Internal Medicine, Mass Genl Hosp 1997; Hematology & Oncology, Dana-Farber/Partners Cancer Ctr 1999; **Fac Appt:** Prof Med, Univ Rochester

Gabrilove, Janice MD [Onc] - **Spec Exp:** Myelodysplastic Syndromes; Leukemia; Hematologic Malignancies; Myeloproliferative Disorders; **Hospital:** Mount Sinai Med Ctr (page 64); **Address:** Mount Sinai Med Ctr, One Gustave L Levy Pl, Box 1079, Dept Hem Onc, New York, NY 10029-6574; **Phone:** 212-241-9650; **Board Cert:** Internal Medicine 1980; Medical Oncology 1983; **Med School:** Mount Sinai Sch Med 1977; **Resid:** Internal Medicine, Columbia-Presby Med Ctr 1980; **Fellow:** Hematology & Oncology, Meml Sloan-Kettering Cancer Ctr 1983; **Fac Appt:** Prof Med, Mount Sinai Sch Med

Gelmann, Edward P MD [Onc] - **Spec Exp:** Prostate Cancer; Bladder Cancer; Kidney Cancer; **Hospital:** NY-Presby/Columbia Univ Med Ctr, NY (page 66); **Address:** Columbia Univ Med Ctr, Milstein Hosp Bldg 6-435, 177 Fort Washington Ave, New York, NY 10032; **Phone:** 212-305-8602; **Board Cert:** Internal Medicine 1979; Medical Oncology 1981; **Med School:** Stanford Univ 1976; **Resid:** Internal Medicine, Univ Chicago Hosps 1978; **Fellow:** Medical Oncology, National Cancer Inst 1981; **Fac Appt:** Prof Med, Columbia P&S

Glick, John H MD [Onc] - **Spec Exp:** Breast Cancer; Hodgkin's Lymphoma; Lymphoma, Non-Hodgkin's; **Hospital:** Hosp Univ Penn - UPHS (page 72); **Address:** Abramson Cancer Ctr, 3400 Civic Ctr Blvd, PCAM Bldg Fl 3 - Ste 3-300S, Philadelphia, PA 19104; **Phone:** 215-662-6065; **Board Cert:** Internal Medicine 1973; Medical Oncology 1975; **Med School:** Columbia P&S 1969; **Resid:** Internal Medicine, Presbyterian Hosp 1971; **Fellow:** Medical Oncology, Natl Cancer Inst 1973; Medical Oncology, Stanford Univ 1974; **Fac Appt:** Prof Med, Univ Pennsylvania

Goldstein, Lori J MD [Onc] - **Spec Exp:** Breast Cancer; Breast Cancer-Novel Therapies; **Hospital:** Fox Chase Cancer Ctr (page 58); **Address:** Fox Chase Cancer Ctr, Dept Med Oncology, 333 Cottman Ave, Philadelphia, PA 19111; **Phone:** 215-728-2689; **Board Cert:** Internal Medicine 1985; Medical Oncology 2002; **Med School:** SUNY Upstate Med Univ 1982; **Resid:** Internal Medicine, Presby Univ Hosp 1985; **Fellow:** Medical Oncology, Natl Cancer Inst/NIH 1990; **Fac Appt:** Prof Med, Temple Univ

Goy, Andre MD [Onc] - **Spec Exp:** Lymphoma; Hodgkin's Lymphoma; **Hospital:** Hackensack Univ Med Ctr; **Address:** 92 2nd St, Hackensack, NJ 07601; **Phone:** 201-996-5900; **Med School:** France 1988; **Resid:** Internal Medicine, Grenoble Univ Med Ctr 1992; **Fellow:** Hematology & Oncology, Grenoble Univ Med Ctr 1993

Grana, Generosa MD [Onc] - **Spec Exp:** Breast Cancer; Cancer Genetics; Cancer Prevention; **Hospital:** Cooper Univ Hosp, Lourdes Med Ctr of Burlington Co; **Address:** 900 Centennial Blvd, Ste M, Voorhees, NJ 08043; **Phone:** 856-325-6750; **Board Cert:** Internal Medicine 1988; Medical Oncology 2011; **Med School:** Northwestern Univ 1985; **Resid:** Internal Medicine, Temple Univ Hosp 1988; **Fellow:** Hematology & Oncology, Fox Chase Cancer Ctr 1992; **Fac Appt:** Assoc Prof Med, UMDNJ-RW Johnson Med Sch

Grossbard, Michael L MD [Onc] - **Spec Exp:** Lymphoma; Gastrointestinal Cancer; Breast Cancer; **Hospital:** St. Luke's - Roosevelt Hosp Ctr - Roosevelt Div (page 56), Beth Israel Med Ctr - Petrie Division (page 56); **Address:** 1000 10th Ave, Fl 11, Ste C02, St Luke's-Roosevelt Hospital, New York, NY 10019; **Phone:** 212-523-5419; **Board Cert:** Internal Medicine 1989; Medical Oncology 2011; **Med School:** Yale Univ 1986; **Resid:** Internal Medicine, Mass Genl Hosp 1989; **Fellow:** Medical Oncology, Dana Farber Cancer Inst 1991; **Fac Appt:** Clin Prof Hem & Onc, Columbia P&S

Grossman, Stuart MD [Onc] - **Spec Exp:** Brain Tumors; Neuro-Oncology; Pain-Cancer; **Hospital:** Johns Hopkins Hosp (page 61); **Address:** David Koch Cancer Rsch Bldg, 1550 Orleans St, Ste 1-M16, Baltimore, MD 21287; **Phone:** 410-955-8964; **Board Cert:** Internal Medicine 1976; Medical Oncology 1983; **Med School:** Univ Rochester 1973; **Resid:** Internal Medicine, Strong Meml Hosp 1976; **Fellow:** Medical Oncology, Johns Hopkins Hosp 1981; **Fac Appt:** Prof Med, Johns Hopkins Univ

Gulley, James L MD/PhD [Onc] - **Spec Exp:** Prostate Cancer-Vaccine Therapy; Vaccine Therapy-Clinical Trials Only; Clinical Trials Only; **Hospital:** Natl Inst of Hlth - Clin Ctr; **Address:** NIH Center for Cancer Research, 10 Center Drive, MSC 1750, Bldg 10-rm 13N208, Bethesda, MD 20892; **Phone:** 301-435-2956; **Board Cert:** Medical Oncology 2010; **Med School:** Loma Linda Univ 1995; **Resid:** Internal Medicine, Emory Univ Med Ctr 1998; **Fellow:** Medical Oncology, Natl Cancer Inst-NIH 2000

Haas, Naomi S Balzer MD [Onc] - **Spec Exp:** Genitourinary Cancer; Kidney Cancer; Clinical Trials; Prostate Cancer; **Hospital:** Hosp Univ Penn - UPHS (page 72); **Address:** Penn Hematology/Oncology, 16 Penn Tower, 3400 Spruce St, Philadelphia, PA 19104; **Phone:** 215-662-7402; **Board Cert:** Internal Medicine 1988; Medical Oncology 2005; **Med School:** NE Ohio Univ 1985; **Resid:** Internal Medicine, Abington Meml Hosp 1988; **Fellow:** Hematology & Oncology, Fox Chase Cancer Ctr 1989; **Fac Appt:** Assoc Prof Med, Univ Pennsylvania

Hageboutros, Alexandre MD [Onc] - **Spec Exp:** Gastrointestinal Cancer; Lung Cancer; Colon & Rectal Cancer; **Hospital:** Cooper Univ Hosp; **Address:** 900 Centennial Blvd, Ste M, Voorhees, NJ 08043-4689; **Phone:** 856-325-6750; **Board Cert:** Hematology 2004; Medical Oncology 2005; **Med School:** Lebanon 1987; **Resid:** Internal Medicine, Cooper Hosp 1991; **Fellow:** Hematology & Oncology, Temple Univ Hosp 1992; Hematology & Oncology, Fox Chase Cancer Ctr 1994; **Fac Appt:** Assoc Prof Med, UMDNJ-NJ Med Sch, Newark

Henry, David H MD [Onc] - **Spec Exp:** AIDS Related Cancers; **Hospital:** Pennsylvania Hosp-UPHS (page 72); **Address:** 230 W Washington Square Fl 2, Philadelphia, PA 19106; **Phone:** 215-829-6088; **Board Cert:** Internal Medicine 1978; Hematology 1980; Medical Oncology 1981; **Med School:** Univ Pennsylvania 1975; **Resid:** Internal Medicine, Hosp Univ Penn 1978; **Fellow:** Hematology & Oncology, Hosp Univ Penn 1978; **Fac Appt:** Clin Prof Med, Univ Pennsylvania

Himelstein, Andrew L MD [Onc] - **Spec Exp:** Leukemia & Lymphoma; Palliative Care; **Hospital:** Christiana Hospital; **Address:** Medical Onc/Hem Consultants, 4701 Ogletown-Stanton Rd, Ste West 3400, Helen Graham Cancer Ctr, Newark, DE 19713; **Phone:** 302-366-1200; **Board Cert:** Internal Medicine 1988; Hematology 2010; Medical Oncology 2011; Hospice & Palliative Medicine 2010; **Med School:** Washington Univ, St Louis 1985; **Resid:** Internal Medicine, Mt Sinai Hosp 1988; **Fellow:** Hematology & Oncology, Colum-Presby Univ Hosp 1991; **Fac Appt:** Asst Clin Prof Med, Thomas Jefferson Univ

Hogan, Thomas F MD [Onc] - **Spec Exp:** Urologic Cancer; Kidney Cancer; Genitourinary Cancer; **Hospital:** Ruby Memorial - WVU Hosp; **Address:** Mary Babb Randolph Cancer Ctr, One Medical Ctr Drive, Morgantown, WV 26506-8110; **Phone:** 304-598-4552; **Board Cert:** Internal Medicine 1975; Medical Oncology 1977; Anatomic Pathology 1997; **Med School:** Med Coll VA 1972; **Resid:** Internal Medicine, Thomas Jefferson Univ Hosp 1975; **Fellow:** Medical Oncology, Univ Wisconsin Affil Hosp 1977; **Fac Appt:** Prof Med, W VA Univ

Holcombe, Randall F MD [Onc] - **Spec Exp:** Gastrointestinal Cancer; Liver Cancer; Clinical Trials; **Hospital:** Mount Sinai Med Ctr (page 64); **Address:** The Derald H. Ruttenberg Treatment Ctr, 1190 5th Ave, New York, NY 10029; **Phone:** 212-241-6756; **Board Cert:** Internal Medicine 1986; Medical Oncology 2003; Hematology 2002; **Med School:** UMDNJ-NJ Med Sch, Newark 1983; **Resid:** Internal Medicine, Brigham & Womens Hosp 1986; **Fellow:** Hematology, Harvard Med Sch; **Fac Appt:** Prof Med, Mount Sinai Sch Med

Holland, James F MD [Onc] - **Spec Exp:** Breast Cancer; Colon Cancer; Lung Cancer; Pancreatic Cancer; **Hospital:** Mount Sinai Med Ctr (page 64); **Address:** Mount Sinai Medial Center, 1 Gustave I Levy Pl, Box 1079, New York, NY 10029; **Phone:** 212-241-4495; **Board Cert:** Internal Medicine 1955; **Med School:** Columbia P&S 1947; **Resid:** Internal Medicine, Columbia-Presby Hosp 1949; Internal Medicine, Francis Delafield Hosp 1952; **Fellow:** Medical Oncology, Francis Delafield Hosp 1953; **Fac Appt:** Prof Med, Mount Sinai Sch Med

Horwitz, Steven M MD [Onc] - **Spec Exp:** Lymphoma, Cutaneous T Cell (CTCL); Hodgkin's Lymphoma; Lymphoma, Non-Hodgkin's; **Hospital:** Meml Sloan-Kettering Cancer Ctr; **Address:** Meml Sloan-Kettering Cancer Ctr, 1275 York Ave, New York, NY 10065; **Phone:** 212-639-3045; **Board Cert:** Medical Oncology 2011; **Med School:** Case West Res Univ 1993; **Resid:** Internal Medicine, Strong Memorial Hosp 1996; **Fellow:** Medical Oncology, Stanford Univ Med Ctr 1999

Hudes, Gary R MD [Onc] - **Spec Exp:** Prostate Cancer; Genitourinary Cancer; Kidney Cancer; **Hospital:** Fox Chase Cancer Ctr (page 58); **Address:** 333 Cottman Ave, rm C307, Philadelphia, PA 19111; **Phone:** 215-728-3889; **Board Cert:** Internal Medicine 1982; Hematology 1984; Medical Oncology 1985; **Med School:** SUNY Downstate 1979; **Resid:** Internal Medicine, Graduate Hosp 1982; **Fellow:** Hematology & Oncology, Presby-Univ Penn Med Ctr 1985

Hudis, Clifford A MD [Onc] - **Spec Exp:** Breast Cancer; **Hospital:** Meml Sloan-Kettering Cancer Ctr; **Address:** 1275 York Avenue, New York, NY 10065; **Phone:** 646-888-5449; **Board Cert:** Internal Medicine 1986; Medical Oncology 2001; **Med School:** Med Coll PA Hahnemann 1983; **Resid:** Internal Medicine, Hosp Med Coll Penn 1987; **Fellow:** Medical Oncology, Meml Sloan Kettering Cancer Ctr 1991; **Fac Appt:** Prof Med, Cornell Univ-Weill Med Coll

Ilson, David H MD/PhD [Onc] - **Spec Exp:** Esophageal Cancer; Colon & Rectal Cancer; Mesothelioma; Unknown Primary Cancer; **Hospital:** Meml Sloan-Kettering Cancer Ctr; **Address:** 300 E 66th St, New York, NY 10065; **Phone:** 646-888-4183; **Board Cert:** Internal Medicine 1989; Medical Oncology 2002; **Med School:** NYU Sch Med 1986; **Resid:** Internal Medicine, Bellevue-NYU Sch Med 1989; **Fellow:** Medical Oncology, Meml Sloan Kettering Hosp 1992; **Fac Appt:** Assoc Prof Med, Cornell Univ-Weill Med Coll

Isaacs, Claudine J MD [Onc] - **Spec Exp:** Breast Cancer; Breast Cancer Risk Assessment; **Hospital:** Georgetown Univ Hosp; **Address:** 3800 Reservoir Road Rd NW, Washington, DC 20007; **Phone:** 202-444-3677; **Board Cert:** Internal Medicine 2002; Medical Oncology 2003; **Med School:** McGill Univ 1987; **Resid:** Internal Medicine, Montreal Genl Hosp 1990; Hematology & Oncology, McGill Univ Hosp 1992; **Fellow:** Medical Oncology, Georgetown Univ Med Ctr 1993; **Fac Appt:** Prof Onc, Georgetown Univ

Jurcic, Joseph G MD [Onc] - **Spec Exp:** Leukemia; Myelodysplastic Syndromes; Clinical Trials; **Hospital:** Meml Sloan-Kettering Cancer Ctr; **Address:** 1275 York Avenue, New York, NY 10065; **Phone:** 212-639-2955; **Board Cert:** Internal Medicine 2001; Medical Oncology 2005; Hematology 2008; **Med School:** Univ Pennsylvania 1988; **Resid:** Internal Medicine, Barnes Hosp 1991; **Fellow:** Hematology & Oncology, Meml Sloan Kettering Cancer Ctr 1994; **Fac Appt:** Assoc Prof Med, Cornell Univ-Weill Med Coll

Karp, Judith MD [Onc] - **Spec Exp:** Leukemia; Clinical Trials; Myelodysplastic Syndromes; **Hospital:** Johns Hopkins Hosp (page 61); **Address:** Bunting Blaustein Cancer Rsch Bldg 1, 1650 Orleans St, rm 2M44, Baltimore, MD 21287; **Phone:** 410-502-7726; **Board Cert:** Internal Medicine 1976; **Med School:** Stanford Univ 1971; **Resid:** Internal Medicine, John Hopkins Hosp 1974; **Fellow:** Medical Oncology, John Hopkins Hosp 1977; **Fac Appt:** Prof Med, Johns Hopkins Univ

Kelly, W Kevin DO [Onc] - **Spec Exp:** Prostate Cancer; Urologic Cancer; Solid Tumors; **Hospital:** Thomas Jefferson Univ Hosp; **Address:** Jefferson Medical Oncology, 925 Chestnut St, Ste 220A, Philadelphia, PA 19107; **Phone:** 215-955-8874; **Board Cert:** Medical Oncology 2003; **Med School:** Philadelphia Coll Osteo Med 1986; **Resid:** Internal Medicine, Albert Einstein Med Ctr 1990; **Fellow:** Hematology & Oncology, Meml Sloan Kettering Cancer Ctr 1993; **Fac Appt:** Prof Med, Thomas Jefferson Univ

Kelsen, David Paul MD [Onc] - **Spec Exp:** Gastrointestinal Cancer; Neuroendocrine Tumors; Unknown Primary Cancer; Merkel Cell Carcinoma; **Hospital:** Meml Sloan-Kettering Cancer Ctr; **Address:** 300 E 66th St, New York, NY 10065; **Phone:** 646-888-4179; **Board Cert:** Internal Medicine 1976; Medical Oncology 1979; **Med School:** Hahnemann Univ 1972; **Resid:** Internal Medicine, Temple Univ Hosp 1976; **Fellow:** Medical Oncology, Meml Sloan Kettering Cancer Ctr 1978; **Fac Appt:** Prof Med, Cornell Univ-Weill Med Coll

Kemeny, Nancy MD [Onc] - **Spec Exp:** Colon Cancer; Rectal Cancer; Liver Cancer; **Hospital:** Meml Sloan-Kettering Cancer Ctr; **Address:** 300 E 66th St, New York, NY 10065; **Phone:** 646-888-4180; **Board Cert:** Internal Medicine 1974; Medical Oncology 1981; **Med School:** UMDNJ-NJ Med Sch, Newark 1971; **Resid:** Internal Medicine, St Luke's Hosp 1974; **Fellow:** Medical Oncology, Mem Sloan Kettering Cancer Ctr 1976; **Fac Appt:** Prof Med, Cornell Univ-Weill Med Coll

Kirkwood, John M MD [Onc] - **Spec Exp:** Melanoma; Immunotherapy; **Hospital:** UPMC Shadyside, UPMC Presby, Pittsburgh; **Address:** UPMC Hillman Cancer Center, 5117 Centre Ave, Pittsburgh, PA 15213-1862; **Phone:** 412-623-7707; **Board Cert:** Internal Medicine 1976; Medical Oncology 1981; **Med School:** Yale Univ 1973; **Resid:** Internal Medicine, Yale-New Haven Hosp 1976; **Fellow:** Medical Oncology, Dana Farber Cancer Inst 1979; **Fac Appt:** Prof Med, Univ Pittsburgh

Kohn, Elise C MD [Onc] - **Spec Exp:** Ovarian Cancer; Gynecologic Cancer; Clinical Trials; **Hospital:** Natl Inst of Hlth - Clin Ctr; **Address:** NIH-Medical Oncology Branch, 9000 Rockville Pike Bldg 10 - rm 12N226, Bethesda, MD 20892; **Phone:** 301-451-1228; **Board Cert:** Internal Medicine 1986; Medical Oncology 1989; **Med School:** Univ Mich Med Sch 1983; **Resid:** Internal Medicine, Michigan Hosp & Med Ctr 1986; **Fellow:** Medical Oncology, NCI-NIH Clin Ctr 1989

Kressel, Bruce R MD [Onc] - **Spec Exp:** Lung Cancer; **Hospital:** G Washington Univ Hosp, Sibley Mem Hosp; **Address:** Washington Oncology-Hematology Center, 2141 K St NW, Ste 707, Washington, DC 20037; **Phone:** 202-293-5382; **Board Cert:** Internal Medicine 1976; Medical Oncology 1977; Hematology 1978; **Med School:** Tufts Univ 1973; **Resid:** Internal Medicine, George Washington Univ Med Ctr 1975; **Fellow:** Hematology & Oncology, George Washington Univ Med Ctr 1977; Oncology, George Washington Univ Med Ctr 1978; **Fac Appt:** Clin Prof Hem & Onc, Geo Wash Univ

Kris, Mark G MD [Onc] - **Spec Exp:** Lung Cancer; Mediastinal Tumors; Thymoma; Thoracic Cancers; **Hospital:** Meml Sloan-Kettering Cancer Ctr; **Address:** 300 E 66th St, New York, NY 10065; **Phone:** 646-888-4197; **Board Cert:** Internal Medicine 1980; Medical Oncology 1983; **Med School:** Cornell Univ-Weill Med Coll 1977; **Resid:** Internal Medicine, New York Hosp 1980; **Fellow:** Medical Oncology, Meml Sloan Kettering Cancer Ctr 1983; **Fac Appt:** Prof Med, Cornell Univ-Weill Med Coll

Laheru, Daniel A MD [Onc] - **Spec Exp:** Pancreatic Cancer; Gastrointestinal Cancer; Vaccine Therapy; **Hospital:** Johns Hopkins Hosp (page 61); **Address:** Bunting Blaustein Cancer Rsch Bldg, 1650 Orleans St, rm 4M09, Baltimore, MD 21287-0013; **Phone:** 410-955-8974; **Board Cert:** Medical Oncology 2010; **Med School:** Baylor Coll Med 1995; **Resid:** Internal Medicine, Univ Utah Hosp & Clinics 1998; **Fellow:** Medical Oncology, Johns Hopkins Hosp 1998; **Fac Appt:** Assoc Prof Med, Johns Hopkins Univ

Langer, Corey J MD [Onc] - **Spec Exp:** Lung Cancer; Head & Neck Cancer; Mesothelioma; Thoracic Cancers; **Hospital:** Hosp Univ Penn - UPHS (page 72); **Address:** Penn Hematology/Oncology, 16 Penn Tower, 3400 Spruce St, Philadelphia, PA 19104; **Phone:** 215-615-5121; **Board Cert:** Internal Medicine 1984; Hematology 1986; Medical Oncology 1987; **Med School:** Boston Univ 1981; **Resid:** Internal Medicine, Graduate Hosp 1984; Hematology & Oncology, Presby Hosp 1986; **Fellow:** Medical Oncology, Fox Chase Cancer Ctr 1987; **Fac Appt:** Prof Med, Univ Pennsylvania

Leighton Jr, John C MD [Onc] - **Spec Exp:** Gastrointestinal Cancer; Liver Cancer; Breast Cancer; **Hospital:** Albert Einstein Med Ctr, Jeanes Hosp; **Address:** Albert Einstein Med Ctr, 9880 Bustleton Ave, Ste 208, Philadelphia, PA 19415; **Phone:** 215-827-1570; **Board Cert:** Internal Medicine 2002; Medical Oncology 2005; Hematology 2006; **Med School:** Temple Univ 1989; **Resid:** Internal Medicine, Albert Einstein Med Ctr 1992; **Fellow:** Hematology, Temple Univ Sch Med 1994; Medical Oncology, Fox Chase Cancer Ctr 1995

Levine, Ellis G MD [Onc] - **Spec Exp:** Breast Cancer; Testicular Cancer; Bladder Cancer; Prostate Cancer; **Hospital:** Roswell Park Cancer Inst; **Address:** Roswell Park Cancer Institute, Elm & Carlton Streets, Buffalo, NY 14263-0001; **Phone:** 716-845-8547; **Board Cert:** Internal Medicine 1982; Medical Oncology 1985; **Med School:** Univ Pittsburgh 1979; **Resid:** Internal Medicine, Univ Minn Hosps 1982; **Fellow:** Medical Oncology, Univ Minn Hosps 1984; **Fac Appt:** Assoc Prof Onc, SUNY Buffalo

Levy, Michael H MD/PhD [Onc] - **Spec Exp:** Pain Management; Palliative Care; Pain-Cancer; Ethics; **Hospital:** Fox Chase Cancer Ctr (page 58); **Address:** Fox Chase Cancer Ctr, Dept Med Oncology, Div Pain & Palliative Med, 333 Cottman Ave, Ste C307, Philadelphia, PA 19111; **Phone:** 215-728-3637; **Board Cert:** Internal Medicine 1979; Medical Oncology 1981; Hospice & Palliative Medicine 2008; **Med School:** Jefferson Med Coll 1976; **Resid:** Internal Medicine, Mt Sinai Med Ctr 1978; Internal Medicine, Hosp Univ Penn 1979; **Fellow:** Hematology & Oncology, Hosp Univ Penn 1981

Maki, Robert G MD/PhD [Onc] - **Spec Exp:** Sarcoma-Soft Tissue; Bone Tumors; Gastrointestinal Stromal Tumors; Desmoid Tumors; **Hospital:** Mount Sinai Med Ctr (page 64); **Address:** 1 Gustave L. Levy Pl, 1468 Madison Ave, Box 1208, New York, NY 10029-6574; **Phone:** 212-241-6756; **Board Cert:** Internal Medicine 2005; Medical Oncology 2007; **Med School:** Cornell Univ-Weill Med Coll 1992; **Resid:** Internal Medicine, Brigham & Womens Hosp 1995; **Fellow:** Medical Oncology, Dana-Farber Cancer Inst 1998; **Fac Appt:** Prof Onc, Mount Sinai Sch Med

Markman, Maurie MD [Onc] - **Spec Exp:** Ovarian Cancer; Gynecologic Cancer; Drug Development; Palliative Care; **Hospital:** CTCA at Eastern Regl Med Ctr; **Address:** Cancer Treatment Ctrs of America, at Eastern Regional Med Ctr, 1331 E Wyoming Ave, Philadelphia, PA 19124; **Phone:** 215-537-7502; **Board Cert:** Internal Medicine 1977; Hematology 1982; Medical Oncology 1981; **Med School:** NYU Sch Med 1974; **Resid:** Internal Medicine, Bellevue Hosp Ctr 1978; **Fellow:** Medical Oncology, Johns Hopkins Hosp 1980

Marshall, John L. MD [Onc] - **Spec Exp:** Gastrointestinal Cancer; Drug Development; **Hospital:** Georgetown Univ Hosp; **Address:** Lombardi Cancer Ctr, Podium A, 3800 Reservoir Rd NW, Washington, DC 20007; **Phone:** 202-444-7064; **Board Cert:** Internal Medicine 2001; Medical Oncology 2003; **Med School:** Univ Louisville Sch Med 1988; **Resid:** Internal Medicine, Georgetown Univ Hosp 1991; **Fellow:** Medical Oncology, Georgetown Univ Hosp 1993; **Fac Appt:** Assoc Prof Med, Georgetown Univ

Masters, Gregory A MD [Onc] - **Spec Exp:** Lung Cancer; Esophageal Cancer; Thoracic Cancers; **Hospital:** Christiana Hospital; **Address:** Medical Oncology-Hematology Consultants, Graham Cancer Ctr, 4701 Ogletown-Stanton Rd, Ste 3400, Newark, DE 19713; **Phone:** 302-366-1200; **Board Cert:** Internal Medicine 2003; Medical Oncology 2005; **Med School:** Northwestern Univ 1990; **Resid:** Internal Medicine, Hosp Univ Penn 1993; **Fellow:** Medical Oncology, Univ Chicago Hosps 1995; **Fac Appt:** Assoc Prof Med, Thomas Jefferson Univ

McGuire III, William P MD [Onc] - **Spec Exp:** Gynecologic Cancer; Ovarian Cancer; **Hospital:** Franklin Square Hosp; **Address:** 9103 Franklin Square Drive, Ste 2200, Baltimore, MD 21237; **Phone:** 443-777-7826; **Board Cert:** Internal Medicine 1974; Medical Oncology 1981; **Med School:** Baylor Coll Med 1971; **Resid:** Internal Medicine, Yale-New Haven Hosp 1973; **Fellow:** Medical Oncology, Natl Cancer Inst 1976; **Fac Appt:** Clin Prof Med, Univ MD Sch Med

Mintzer, David M MD [Onc] - **Spec Exp:** Breast Cancer; Gastrointestinal Cancer; Head & Neck Cancer; Palliative Care; **Hospital:** Pennsylvania Hosp-UPHS (page 72); **Address:** Pennsylvania Hematology/Oncology Assocs, 230 W Washington Square Fl 2, Philadelphia, PA 19106; **Phone:** 215-829-6088; **Board Cert:** Internal Medicine 1980; Hematology 1982; Medical Oncology 1983; Hospice & Palliative Medicine 2004; **Med School:** Jefferson Med Coll 1977; **Resid:** Internal Medicine, Pennsylvania Hosp 1980; **Fellow:** Hematology, Jefferson Med Coll 1982; Medical Oncology, Meml Sloan Kettering Cancer Ctr 1984

Moore, Anne MD [Onc] - **Spec Exp:** Breast Cancer; **Hospital:** NY-Presby/Weill Cornell Med Ctr, NY (page 66); **Address:** Weill Cornell Breast Ctr, 425 E 61st St Fl 8, New York, NY 10065; **Phone:** 212-821-0550; **Board Cert:** Internal Medicine 1973; Hematology 1976; Medical Oncology 2008; **Med School:** Columbia P&S 1969; **Resid:** Internal Medicine, Cornell Univ Med Ctr 1973; **Fellow:** Medical Oncology, Rockefeller Univ 1973; **Fac Appt:** Prof Med, Cornell Univ-Weill Med Coll

Morginstin, Mark S DO [Onc] - **Spec Exp:** Hematologic Malignancies; Breast Cancer; **Hospital:** Albert Einstein Med Ctr, Jeanes Hosp; **Address:** Albert Einstein Med Ctr, 5501 Old York Rd Fl 1, Philadelphia, PA 19141; **Phone:** 215-456-3880; **Board Cert:** Internal Medicine 2003; Medical Oncology 2008; Hematology 2009; **Med School:** UMDNJ Sch Osteo Med 1996; **Resid:** Internal Medicine, Albert Einstein Med Ctr 1999; **Fellow:** Hematology & Oncology, Univ of Conn Hlth Ctr, John Dempsey Hosp 2008

Medical Oncology

Motzer, Robert J MD [Onc] - **Spec Exp:** Kidney Cancer; Testicular Cancer; Prostate Cancer; **Hospital:** Meml Sloan-Kettering Cancer Ctr; **Address:** 1275 York Avenue, New York, NY 10065; **Phone:** 646-422-4312; **Board Cert:** Internal Medicine 1984; Medical Oncology 1987; **Med School:** Univ Mich Med Sch 1981; **Resid:** Internal Medicine, Meml Sloan Kettering Cancer Ctr 1984; **Fellow:** Medical Oncology, Meml Sloan Kettering Cancer Ctr 1987; **Fac Appt:** Assoc Prof Med, Cornell Univ-Weill Med Coll

Muggia, Franco M MD [Onc] - **Spec Exp:** Gynecologic Cancer; **Hospital:** NYU Langone Med Ctr (page 68); **Address:** NYU Clinical Cancer Ctr, 160 E 34th St Fl 4, New York, NY 10016; **Phone:** 212-731-5433; **Board Cert:** Internal Medicine 1968; Medical Oncology 1973; Hematology 1974; **Med School:** Cornell Univ-Weill Med Coll 1961; **Resid:** Internal Medicine, Hartford Hosp 1964; Internal Medicine, Francis A Delafield Hosp 1966; **Fac Appt:** Prof Med, NYU Sch Med

Nanus, David M MD [Onc] - **Spec Exp:** Prostate Cancer; Bladder Cancer; Testicular Cancer; Genitourinary Cancer; **Hospital:** NY-Presby/Weill Cornell Med Ctr, NY (page 66); **Address:** NY Hosp-Cornell Med Ctr,Payson Pavillion, 525 E 68th St Fl 3 - Ste 341, New York, NY 10021; **Phone:** 646-962-2072; **Board Cert:** Internal Medicine 1985; Medical Oncology 1987; **Med School:** Univ Hlth Scis, Chicago Med Sch 1982; **Resid:** Internal Medicine, Bronx Muni Hosp 1985; **Fellow:** Medical Oncology, Meml Sloan Kettering Canc Ctr 1989; **Fac Appt:** Prof Med, Cornell Univ-Weill Med Coll

Nissenblatt, Michael J MD [Onc] - **Spec Exp:** Breast Cancer; Colon Cancer; Lung Cancer; Hereditary Cancer; **Hospital:** Robert Wood Johnson Univ Hosp - New Brunswick, St. Peter's Univ Hosp; **Address:** 205 Easton Ave, New Brunswick, NJ 08901-1722; **Phone:** 732-390-7750; **Board Cert:** Internal Medicine 1976; Medical Oncology 1979; **Med School:** Columbia P&S 1973; **Resid:** Internal Medicine, Johns Hopkins Hosp 1976; **Fellow:** Medical Oncology, Johns Hopkins Hosp 1978; **Fac Appt:** Clin Prof Med, UMDNJ-RW Johnson Med Sch

Norton, Larry MD [Onc] - **Spec Exp:** Breast Cancer; **Hospital:** Meml Sloan-Kettering Cancer Ctr; **Address:** 300 E 66th St, BAIC Bldg Fl 9 - Ste 933, New York, NY 10065; **Phone:** 646-888-5438; **Board Cert:** Internal Medicine 1975; Medical Oncology 1977; **Med School:** Columbia P&S 1972; **Resid:** Internal Medicine, Bronx Muni Hosp 1974; **Fellow:** Medical Oncology, Natl Cancer Inst 1977; **Fac Appt:** Prof Med, Cornell Univ-Weill Med Coll

O'Connor, Owen A MD/PhD [Onc] - **Spec Exp:** Hodgkin's Lymphoma; Lymphoma, Non-Hodgkin's; Drug Development; Clinical Trials; **Hospital:** NY-Presby/Columbia Univ Med Ctr, NY (page 66); **Address:** 16 E 60th St, Ste 330, New York, NY 10065; **Phone:** 212-326-5720; **Board Cert:** Internal Medicine 2004; Medical Oncology 2005; **Med School:** UMDNJ-RW Johnson Med Sch 1994; **Resid:** Internal Medicine, NY-Presby/Weill Cornell Univ Med Ctr 1996; **Fellow:** Medical Oncology, Memorial Sloan-Kettering Cancer Ctr 2000; **Fac Appt:** Prof Med, NYU Sch Med

O'Reilly, Eileen M MD [Onc] - **Spec Exp:** Pancreatic Cancer; Liver Cancer; Biliary Cancer; Neuroendocrine Tumors; **Hospital:** Meml Sloan-Kettering Cancer Ctr; **Address:** 300 E 66th St, rm 1021, Memorial Sloan-Kettering Cancer Center, New York, NY 10065; **Phone:** 646-888-4182; **Med School:** Ireland 1990; **Resid:** Internal Medicine, St Vincent's Hosp 1994; **Fellow:** Hematology & Oncology, St Vincent's Hosp 1995; Medical Oncology, Memorial-Sloan Kettering Cancer Ctr 1997; **Fac Appt:** Assoc Prof Onc, Cornell Univ-Weill Med Coll

Offit, Kenneth MD [Onc] - **Spec Exp:** Cancer Genetics; Breast Cancer; Lymphoma; **Hospital:** Meml Sloan-Kettering Cancer Ctr; **Address:** Memorial Sloan-Kettering Cancer Center, 1275 York Ave, New York, NY 10065; **Phone:** 646-888-4050; **Board Cert:** Internal Medicine 1985; Medical Oncology 1987; **Med School:** Harvard Med Sch 1982; **Resid:** Internal Medicine, Lenox Hill Hosp 1985; **Fellow:** Hematology & Oncology, Meml Sloan Kettering Cancer Ctr 1988; **Fac Appt:** Prof Med, Cornell Univ-Weill Med Coll

Oh, William K MD [Onc] - **Spec Exp:** Genitourinary Cancer; Prostate Cancer; Testicular Cancer; Adrenal Cancer; **Hospital:** Mount Sinai Med Ctr (page 64); **Address:** Ruttenberg Treatment Center, 1190 Flfth Ave, New York, NY 10029; **Phone:** 212-659-5429; **Board Cert:** Medical Oncology 2009; **Med School:** NYU Sch Med 1992; **Resid:** Internal Medicine, Brigham & Womens Hosp 1995; **Fellow:** Medical Oncology, Dana-Farber Cancer Inst 1997; **Fac Appt:** Prof Med, Mount Sinai Sch Med

Oratz, Ruth MD [Onc] - **Spec Exp:** Breast Cancer; **Hospital:** NYU Langone Med Ctr (page 68); **Address:** 345 E 37th St, Ste 202, New York, NY 10016; **Phone:** 212-400-4904; **Board Cert:** Internal Medicine 1985; Medical Oncology 1989; **Med School:** Albert Einstein Coll Med 1982; **Resid:** Internal Medicine, NYU Med Ctr 1982; **Fellow:** Medical Oncology, NYU Med Ctr 1985; **Fac Appt:** Assoc Clin Prof Med, NYU Sch Med

Oster, Martin W MD [Onc] - **Spec Exp:** Breast Cancer; Gastrointestinal Cancer; Head & Neck Cancer; **Hospital:** NY-Presby/Columbia Univ Med Ctr, NY (page 66); **Address:** NY Presby Hosp-Columbia University Med Ctr, 161 Fort Washington Ave, New York, NY 10032-3713; **Phone:** 212-305-8231; **Board Cert:** Internal Medicine 1974; Medical Oncology 1975; **Med School:** Columbia P&S 1971; **Resid:** Internal Medicine, Mass Genl Hosp 1973; **Fellow:** Medical Oncology, Natl Cancer Inst/NIH 1976; **Fac Appt:** Assoc Clin Prof Onc, Columbia P&S

Parnes, Howard L MD [Onc] - **Spec Exp:** Cancer Prevention; Prostate Cancer; **Hospital:** Natl Inst of Hlth - Clin Ctr; **Address:** Chief, Prostate & Urologic Cancer Research Group, NCI-Div Cancer Prevention, Ste 2100, 6130 Executive Blvd, MSC-7318, Bethesda, MD 20892; **Phone:** 301-402-3606; **Board Cert:** Internal Medicine 1984; Medical Oncology 1987; **Med School:** UMDNJ-NJ Med Sch, Newark 1981; **Resid:** Internal Medicine, Baltimore City Hosps 1984; **Fellow:** Medical Oncology, Univ Maryland Cancer Ctrs 1987

Pasmantier, Mark W MD [Onc] - **Spec Exp:** Lung Cancer; Ovarian Cancer; Breast Cancer; Lymphoma; **Hospital:** NY-Presby/Weill Cornell Med Ctr, NY (page 66); **Address:** 407 E 70th St Fl 3, New York, NY 10021-5302; **Phone:** 212-517-5900; **Board Cert:** Internal Medicine 1972; Hematology 1974; Medical Oncology 1975; **Med School:** NYU Sch Med 1966; **Resid:** Internal Medicine, Harlem Hosp 1970; **Fellow:** Hematology, Montefiore Med Ctr 1971; Medical Oncology, NY Hosp 1972; **Fac Appt:** Clin Prof Med, Cornell Univ-Weill Med Coll

Pavlick, Anna C MD [Onc] - **Spec Exp:** Melanoma; Skin Cancer; Merkel Cell Carcinoma; **Hospital:** NYU Langone Med Ctr (page 68); **Address:** 160 E 34th St, Fl 9, NYU Cancer Institute, New York, NY 10016; **Phone:** 212-731-5431; **Board Cert:** Medical Oncology 2008; **Med School:** UMDNJ Sch Osteo Med 1990; **Resid:** Internal Medicine, Hackensack Med Ctr 1993; **Fellow:** Hematology & Oncology, Meml Sloan Kettering Cancer Ctr 1996; **Fac Appt:** Assoc Prof Med, NYU Sch Med

Pecora, Andrew L MD [Onc] - **Spec Exp:** Stem Cell Transplant; Myelodysplastic Syndromes; Melanoma; Immunotherapy; **Hospital:** Hackensack Univ Med Ctr; **Address:** The Cancer Ctr-Hackensack Univ Med Ctr, 92 2nd St, Hackensack, NJ 07601; **Phone:** 201-996-5814; **Board Cert:** Internal Medicine 1986; Hematology 1988; Medical Oncology 1989; **Med School:** UMDNJ-NJ Med Sch, Newark 1983; **Resid:** Internal Medicine, New York Hosp 1986; **Fellow:** Hematology & Oncology, Meml Sloan Kettering Cancer Ctr 1988; **Fac Appt:** Prof Med, UMDNJ-NJ Med Sch, Newark

Perry, David J MD [Onc] - **Spec Exp:** Gastrointestinal Cancer; Lung Cancer; Genitourinary Cancer; Clinical Trials; **Hospital:** Washington Hosp Ctr; **Address:** Washington Hosp Ctr-Dept Med Oncology, 110 Irving St NW, rm C-2151, Washington, DC 20010; **Phone:** 202-877-2843; **Board Cert:** Internal Medicine 1979; Medical Oncology 1981; Hematology 1982; **Med School:** Univ Pennsylvania 1974; **Resid:** Internal Medicine, Walter Reed AMC 1979; **Fellow:** Hematology & Oncology, Walter Reed AMC 1979; **Fac Appt:** Assoc Prof Med, Eastern VA Med Sch

Pfister, David G MD [Onc] - **Spec Exp:** Head & Neck Cancer; Laryngeal Cancer; Thyroid Cancer; Skin Cancer; **Hospital:** Meml Sloan-Kettering Cancer Ctr; **Address:** 300 E 66th St, New York, NY 10065; **Phone:** 646-888-4232; **Board Cert:** Internal Medicine 1985; Medical Oncology 1989; **Med School:** Univ Pennsylvania 1982; **Resid:** Internal Medicine, Hosp Univ Penn 1985; **Fellow:** Epidemiology, Yale-New Haven Hosp 1987; Hematology & Oncology, Meml Sloan Kettering Cancer Ctr 1989; **Fac Appt:** Prof Med, Cornell Univ-Weill Med Coll

Posner, Marshall R MD [Onc] - **Spec Exp:** Head & Neck Cancer; Skin Cancer-Head & Neck; **Hospital:** Mount Sinai Med Ctr (page 64); **Address:** Mount Sinai Med Ctr, 1 Gustave L Levy Pl, Box 1128, New York, NY 10029; **Phone:** 212-241-6756; **Board Cert:** Internal Medicine 1978; Medical Oncology 1981; **Med School:** Tufts Univ 1975; **Resid:** Internal Medicine, Boston City Hosp 1978; **Fellow:** Oncology, Dana-Farber Cancer Inst 1981; **Fac Appt:** Assoc Prof Med, Mount Sinai Sch Med

Raptis, George MD [Onc] - **Spec Exp:** Breast Cancer; **Hospital:** Mount Sinai Med Ctr (page 64); **Address:** Ruttenberg Treatment Ctr, 1190 5th Ave, Box 1129, New York, NY 10029; **Phone:** 212-241-6756; **Board Cert:** Medical Oncology 2003; **Med School:** Mount Sinai Sch Med 1987; **Resid:** Internal Medicine, Mt Sinai Med Ctr 1990; **Fellow:** Hematology & Oncology, Meml Sloan-Kettering Canc Ctr 1993; **Fac Appt:** Assoc Prof Med, Mount Sinai Sch Med

Remick, Scot C MD [Onc] - **Spec Exp:** AIDS Related Cancers; Clinical Trials; Drug Development; Thyroid Cancer; **Hospital:** Ruby Memorial - WVU Hosp; **Address:** WVU Mary Babb Randolph Cancer Ctr, 1801 RCB Health Sciences Center S, Box 9300, Morgantown, WV 26506-9300; **Phone:** 304-598-4552; **Board Cert:** Internal Medicine 1985; Medical Oncology 1987; **Med School:** NY Med Coll 1982; **Resid:** Internal Medicine, Johns Hopkins Hosp 1985; **Fellow:** Medical Oncology, Univ Wisconsin Clin Cancer Ctr 1988; **Fac Appt:** Prof Onc, W VA Univ

Ruggiero, Joseph T MD [Onc] - **Spec Exp:** Gastrointestinal Cancer; **Hospital:** NY-Presby/Weill Cornell Med Ctr, NY (page 66); **Address:** 1305 York Ave Fl 12, New York, NY 10021-4635; **Phone:** 646-962-6200; **Board Cert:** Internal Medicine 1980; Hematology 1982; Medical Oncology 1983; **Med School:** NYU Sch Med 1977; **Resid:** Internal Medicine, New York Hosp 1980; **Fellow:** Hematology & Oncology, New York Hosp/Cornell 1983; **Fac Appt:** Assoc Clin Prof Med, Cornell Univ-Weill Med Coll

Saltz, Leonard B MD [Onc] - **Spec Exp:** Colon & Rectal Cancer; Gastrointestinal Cancer & Rare Tumors; Neuroendocrine Tumors; **Hospital:** Meml Sloan-Kettering Cancer Ctr; **Address:** Memorial Sloan Kettering Cancer Center, 300 E 66th St, rm 1049, New York, NY 10065; **Phone:** 646-888-4181; **Board Cert:** Internal Medicine 1986; Hematology 1988; Medical Oncology 1989; **Med School:** Yale Univ 1983; **Resid:** Internal Medicine, New Yor Hosp 1986; **Fellow:** Hematology & Oncology, New York Hosp-Cornell/Rockefeller Univ 1989; **Fac Appt:** Prof Med, Cornell Univ-Weill Med Coll

Scheinberg, David MD/PhD [Onc] - **Spec Exp:** Leukemia; Immunotherapy; Vaccine Therapy; **Hospital:** Meml Sloan-Kettering Cancer Ctr; **Address:** 1275 York Avenue, New York, NY 10065; **Phone:** 646-888-2190; **Board Cert:** Internal Medicine 1986; Medical Oncology 2005; **Med School:** Johns Hopkins Univ 1983; **Resid:** Internal Medicine, NY Hosp-Cornell Med Ctr 1985; **Fellow:** Medical Oncology, Meml Sloan Kettering Cancer Ctr 1987; **Fac Appt:** Prof Med, Cornell Univ-Weill Med Coll

Scher, Howard MD [Onc] - **Spec Exp:** Genitourinary Cancer; Prostate Cancer; Bladder Cancer; **Hospital:** Meml Sloan-Kettering Cancer Ctr; **Address:** 1275 York Avenue, New York, NY 10065; **Phone:** 646-422-4330; **Board Cert:** Internal Medicine 1979; Medical Oncology 1985; **Med School:** NYU Sch Med 1976; **Resid:** Internal Medicine, Bellevue Hosp 1980; **Fellow:** Medical Oncology, Meml Sloan Kettering Cancer Ctr 1983; **Fac Appt:** Prof Med, Cornell Univ-Weill Med Coll

Schilder, Russell J MD [Onc] - **Spec Exp:** Gynecologic Cancer; Cervical Cancer; Ovarian Cancer; Drug Development; **Hospital:** Thomas Jefferson Univ Hosp, Methodist Hosp; **Address:** Jefferson Medical Oncology, 925 Chestnut St, Ste 220A, Philadelphia, PA 19107; **Phone:** 215-955-8874; **Board Cert:** Internal Medicine 1986; Hematology 1988; Medical Oncology 1989; **Med School:** Univ Miami Sch Med 1983; **Resid:** Internal Medicine, Temple Univ Hosp 1986; **Fellow:** Hematology & Oncology, Fox Chase Cancer Ctr 1989; **Fac Appt:** Prof Med, Jefferson Med Coll

Schuchter, Lynn M MD [Onc] - **Spec Exp:** Melanoma; Breast Cancer; Clinical Trials; **Hospital:** Hosp Univ Penn - UPHS (page 72); **Address:** Penn Hematology/Oncology, 16 Penn Tower, 3400 Spruce St, Philadelphia, PA 19104-4206; **Phone:** 215-662-7907; **Board Cert:** Internal Medicine 1985; Medical Oncology 1989; **Med School:** Univ Hlth Scis, Chicago Med Sch 1982; **Resid:** Internal Medicine, Michael Reese Hosp 1985; **Fellow:** Medical Oncology, Johns Hopkins Hosp 1989; **Fac Appt:** Prof Med, Univ Pennsylvania

Sidransky, David MD [Onc] - **Spec Exp:** Head & Neck Cancer; **Hospital:** Johns Hopkins Hosp (page 61); **Address:** David Koch Cancer Rsch Bldg, 1550 Orleans St, Ste 5-N03, Baltimore, MD 21231; **Phone:** 410-502-5153; **Board Cert:** Internal Medicine 1988; **Med School:** Baylor Coll Med 1984; **Resid:** Internal Medicine, Baylor Coll Med 1988; **Fellow:** Medical Oncology, Johns Hopkins Hosp 1992; **Fac Appt:** Prof Oto, Johns Hopkins Univ

Silverman, Lewis R MD [Onc] - **Spec Exp:** Myelodysplastic Syndromes; Leukemia & Lymphoma; Multiple Myeloma; **Hospital:** Mount Sinai Med Ctr (page 64); **Address:** Ruttenberg Treatment Ctr, 1190 5th Ave, Box 1129, New York, NY 10029; **Phone:** 212-241-6756; **Board Cert:** Internal Medicine 1981; Hematology 1986; Medical Oncology 1987; **Med School:** Belgium 1978; **Resid:** Internal Medicine, Metro Hospital 1980; Internal Medicine, Montefiore Med Ctr 1981; **Fellow:** Hematology, Montefiore Med Ctr 1982; Neoplastic Diseases, Mt Sinai Med Ctr 1984; **Fac Appt:** Assoc Prof Med, Mount Sinai Sch Med

Smith, Mitchell R MD/PhD [Onc] - **Spec Exp:** Lymphoma; Leukemia; Hodgkin's Lymphoma; Multiple Myeloma; **Hospital:** Fox Chase Cancer Ctr (page 58); **Address:** Fox Chase Cancer Ctr, 333 Cottman Ave, Ste C307, Philadelphia, PA 19111; **Phone:** 215-728-2674; **Board Cert:** Internal Medicine 1985; Medical Oncology 1987; Hematology 1988; **Med School:** Case West Res Univ 1979; **Resid:** Pathology, Barnes Jewish Hosp 1983; Internal Medicine, Barnes Jewish Hosp 1984; **Fellow:** Medical Oncology, Meml Sloan-Ketter Cancer Ctr 1988

Smith, Thomas Joseph MD [Onc] - **Spec Exp:** Breast Cancer; Palliative Care; **Hospital:** Johns Hopkins Hosp (page 61); **Address:** Johns Hopkins Hosp, Sidney Kimmel Comprehensive Cancer Ctr, 600 N Wolfe St, Blalock 371, Baltimore, MD 21287; **Phone:** 410-955-2091; **Board Cert:** Internal Medicine 1982; Medical Oncology 1987; Hospice & Palliative Medicine 2008; **Med School:** Yale Univ 1979; **Resid:** Internal Medicine, Hosp Univ Penn 1982; **Fellow:** Medical Oncology, Med Coll Virginia 1987; **Fac Appt:** Prof Med, Va Commonwealth Univ Sch Med

Socinski, Mark A MD [Onc] - **Spec Exp:** Lung Cancer; **Hospital:** UPMC Shadyside; **Address:** Hillman Cancer Ctr, 5115 Centre Ave Fl 2, Pittsburgh, PA 15232; **Phone:** 412-692-4724; **Board Cert:** Internal Medicine 1988; Medical Oncology 2002; **Med School:** Univ VT Coll Med 1984; **Resid:** Internal Medicine, Beth Israel Hosp 1986; **Fellow:** Medical Oncology, Dana-Farber Cancer Inst 1989; **Fac Appt:** Prof Med, Univ Pittsburgh

Speyer, James L MD [Onc] - **Spec Exp:** Ovarian Cancer; Breast Cancer; Cardiac Effects in Cancer Therapy; **Hospital:** NYU Langone Med Ctr (page 68); **Address:** 160 E 34th St, Fl 8, New York, NY 10016-4750; **Phone:** 212-731-5432; **Board Cert:** Internal Medicine 1977; Hematology 1978; Medical Oncology 1979; **Med School:** Johns Hopkins Univ 1974; **Resid:** Internal Medicine, Columbia-Presby Med Ctr 1976; Hematology, Columbia-Presby Med Ctr 1977; **Fellow:** Medical Oncology, Natl Cancer Inst 1979; **Fac Appt:** Prof Med, NYU Sch Med

Medical Oncology

Spriggs, David R MD [Onc] - **Spec Exp:** Ovarian Cancer; Drug Development; Uterine Cancer; Gynecologic Cancer; **Hospital:** Meml Sloan-Kettering Cancer Ctr; **Address:** 300 E 66th St, New York, NY 10065; **Phone:** 646-888-4223; **Board Cert:** Internal Medicine 1981; Medical Oncology 2006; **Med School:** Univ Wisc 1977; **Resid:** Internal Medicine, Columbia-Presby Hosp 1981; **Fellow:** Medical Oncology, Dana-Farber Cancer Inst 1985; **Fac Appt:** Prof Med, Cornell Univ-Weill Med Coll

Staddon, Arthur P MD [Onc] - **Spec Exp:** Sarcoma; **Hospital:** Pennsylvania Hosp-UPHS (page 72); **Address:** Pennsylvania Oncology/Hematology Assocs, 230 W Washington Square Fl 2, Philadelphia, PA 19106; **Phone:** 215-829-6088; **Board Cert:** Internal Medicine 1975; Medical Oncology 1979; Hematology 1980; **Med School:** Univ Pennsylvania 1972; **Resid:** Internal Medicine, Univ Penn Hosps 1975; **Fellow:** Hematology & Oncology, Univ Penn Hosps 1980; **Fac Appt:** Assoc Clin Prof Med, Univ Pennsylvania

Stadtmauer, Edward A MD [Onc] - **Spec Exp:** Bone Marrow & Stem Cell Transplant; Leukemia & Lymphoma; Multiple Myeloma; Amyloidosis; **Hospital:** Hosp Univ Penn - UPHS (page 72); **Address:** Abramson Cancer Ctr, Univ of Penn, 2 PCAM, 34th & Civic Ctr Blvd, Philadelphia, PA 19104; **Phone:** 215-662-7910; **Board Cert:** Internal Medicine 1986; Hematology 1988; Medical Oncology 1989; **Med School:** Univ Pennsylvania 1983; **Resid:** Internal Medicine, Bronx Muni Hosp 1986; **Fellow:** Hematology & Oncology, Hosp Univ Penn 1989; **Fac Appt:** Prof Onc, Univ Pennsylvania

Stoopler, Mark Benjamin MD [Onc] - **Spec Exp:** Lung Cancer; Esophageal Cancer; Unknown Primary Cancer; **Hospital:** NY-Presby/Columbia Univ Med Ctr, NY (page 66); **Address:** 161 Fort Washington Ave, Ste 936, New York, NY 10032-3713; **Phone:** 212-305-8230; **Board Cert:** Internal Medicine 1978; Medical Oncology 1981; **Med School:** Cornell Univ-Weill Med Coll 1975; **Resid:** Internal Medicine, North Shore Univ Hosp 1978; Internal Medicine, NY Meml Hosp 1978; **Fellow:** Medical Oncology, Meml-Sloan Kettering Cancer Ctr 1980; **Fac Appt:** Assoc Clin Prof Onc, Columbia P&S

Straus, David J MD [Onc] - **Spec Exp:** Lymphoma; Multiple Myeloma; **Hospital:** Meml Sloan-Kettering Cancer Ctr; **Address:** 1275 York Ave, Box 406, New York, NY 10065; **Phone:** 212-639-8365; **Board Cert:** Internal Medicine 1972; Hematology 1976; Medical Oncology 1977; **Med School:** Marquette Sch Med 1969; **Resid:** Internal Medicine, Montefiore Med Ctr 1972; Medical Oncology, Meml Sloan Kettering Cancer Ctr 1977; **Fellow:** Hematology, Beth Israel Hosp 1973; **Fac Appt:** Prof Onc, Cornell Univ-Weill Med Coll

Sun, Weijing MD [Onc] - **Spec Exp:** Gastrointestinal Cancer; Pancreatic Cancer; Esophageal Cancer; **Hospital:** Hosp Univ Penn - UPHS (page 72); **Address:** Penn Hematology/Oncology, 16 Penn Tower, 3400 Spruce St, Philadelphia, PA 19104; **Phone:** 215-662-6319; **Board Cert:** Medical Oncology 2011; **Med School:** China 1982; **Resid:** Internal Medicine, Loyola Univ Med Ctr 1998; **Fellow:** Hematology & Oncology, Hosp Univ Penn 2001; **Fac Appt:** Assoc Prof Med, Univ Pennsylvania

Swain, Sandra MD [Onc] - **Spec Exp:** Breast Cancer; **Hospital:** Washington Hosp Ctr; **Address:** Washington Cancer Inst, 110 Irving St NW Fl 1 - rm C-2149, Washington, DC 20010; **Phone:** 202-877-8112; **Board Cert:** Internal Medicine 1983; Medical Oncology 1985; **Med School:** Univ Fla Coll Med 1980; **Resid:** Internal Medicine, Vanderbilt Univ Affil Hosp 1983; **Fellow:** Medical Oncology, NIH- Natl Cancer Inst 1986; **Fac Appt:** Assoc Prof Med, Georgetown Univ

Tagawa, Scott T MD [Onc] - **Spec Exp:** Prostate Cancer; Bladder Cancer; Kidney Cancer; Urologic Cancer; **Hospital:** NY-Presby/Weill Cornell Med Ctr, NY (page 66); **Address:** NY Presby-Weill Cornell Med Ctr, 525 E 68th St, Box 403, New York, NY 10065; **Phone:** 646-962-2072; **Board Cert:** Medical Oncology 2005; Hematology 2006; **Med School:** USC-Keck School of Medicine 1998; **Resid:** Internal Medicine, USC Med Ctr 2002; **Fellow:** Hematology & Oncology, USC Med Ctr 2005; **Fac Appt:** Asst Prof Hem & Onc, Cornell Univ-Weill Med Coll

Tester, William MD [Onc] - **Spec Exp:** Lung Cancer; Prostate Cancer; **Hospital:** Albert Einstein Med Ctr; **Address:** Einstein Cancer Center, 5501 Old York Rd, Philadelphia, PA 19141; **Phone:** 215-456-3880; **Board Cert:** Internal Medicine 1980; Medical Oncology 1983; Hematology 1986; **Med School:** Hahnemann Univ 1977; **Resid:** Internal Medicine, Albert Einstein Med Ctr 1980; **Fellow:** Medical Oncology, NIH-Natl Cancer Inst 1982; Hematology, Georgetown Univ 1983; **Fac Appt:** Clin Prof Onc, Thomas Jefferson Univ

Tkaczuk, Katherine H MD [Onc] - **Spec Exp:** Breast Cancer; **Hospital:** Univ of MD Med Ctr; **Address:** Greenebaum Cancer Ctr, 22 S Greene St, rm S9D12, Baltimore, MD 21201; **Phone:** 410-328-7904; **Board Cert:** Medical Oncology 2011; **Med School:** Poland 1984; **Resid:** Internal Medicine, St Agnes Hosp 1989; **Fellow:** Hematology & Oncology, Univ Maryland Cancer Ctr 1992; **Fac Appt:** Assoc Prof Med, Univ MD Sch Med

Toppmeyer, Deborah L MD [Onc] - **Spec Exp:** Breast Cancer; Hereditary Cancer; **Hospital:** Robert Wood Johnson Univ Hosp - New Brunswick; **Address:** Cancer Inst of New Jersey, 195 Little Albany St, New Brunswick, NJ 08903; **Phone:** 732-235-9692; **Board Cert:** Internal Medicine 1988; Medical Oncology 2006; **Med School:** Albany Med Coll 1985; **Resid:** Internal Medicine, Univ Pittsburgh Hlth Ctr Hosp 1988; **Fellow:** Medical Oncology, Dana Farber Cancer Inst 1993; **Fac Appt:** Assoc Prof Med

Trump, Donald L MD [Onc] - **Spec Exp:** Prostate Cancer; Genitourinary Cancer; Drug Discovery & Development; Clinical Trials; **Hospital:** Roswell Park Cancer Inst; **Address:** Roswell Park Cancer Institute, Elm and Carlton Streets, Buffalo, NY 14263; **Phone:** 716-845-2300; **Board Cert:** Internal Medicine 1973; Medical Oncology 1977; **Med School:** Johns Hopkins Univ 1970; **Resid:** Internal Medicine, Johns Hopkins Hosp 1975; **Fellow:** Medical Oncology, Johns Hopkins Hosp 1974; **Fac Appt:** Prof Med, SUNY Buffalo

Vahdat, Linda T MD [Onc] - **Spec Exp:** Breast Cancer; Breast Cancer Novel Therapies; Clinical Trials; **Hospital:** NY-Presby/Weill Cornell Med Ctr, NY (page 66); **Address:** 425 E 61st St Fl 8, New York, NY 10065; **Phone:** 212-821-0644; **Board Cert:** Medical Oncology 2005; **Med School:** Mount Sinai Sch Med 1987; **Resid:** Internal Medicine, Mt Sinai Hosp 1990; **Fellow:** Hematology & Oncology, Meml Sloan Kettering Cancer Ctr 1994; **Fac Appt:** Prof Med, Cornell Univ-Weill Med Coll

Vaughn, David J MD [Onc] - **Spec Exp:** Testicular Cancer; Bladder Cancer; Prostate Cancer; Genitourinary Cancer; **Hospital:** Hosp Univ Penn - UPHS (page 72); **Address:** Penn Hematology/Oncology, 16 Penn Tower, 3400 Spruce St, Philadelphia, PA 19104; **Phone:** 215-349-8498; **Board Cert:** Medical Oncology 2003; **Med School:** Harvard Med Sch 1987; **Resid:** Internal Medicine, New York Hosp 1990; **Fellow:** Hematology & Oncology, Hosp Univ Penn 1993; **Fac Appt:** Prof Med, Univ Pennsylvania

Vinciguerra, Vincent P MD [Onc] - **Spec Exp:** Breast Cancer; Gastrointestinal Cancer; Lung Cancer; Cancer Prevention; **Hospital:** N Shore Univ Hosp (page 67); **Address:** Monter Cancer Ctr, 450 Lakeville Rd, Lake Success, NY 11042; **Phone:** 516-734-8954; **Board Cert:** Internal Medicine 1971; Hematology 1974; Medical Oncology 1975; **Med School:** Georgetown Univ 1966; **Resid:** Internal Medicine, NY Hosp-Cornell 1969; Internal Medicine, N Shore Univ Hosp 1971; **Fellow:** Hematology & Oncology, NY Hosp-Cornell 1970; Hematology & Oncology, N Shore Univ Hosp 1974; **Fac Appt:** Prof Med, NYU Sch Med

Medical Oncology

von Mehren, Margaret MD [Onc] - **Spec Exp:** Sarcoma; Melanoma; Immunotherapy; Gastrointestinal Stromal Tumors; **Hospital:** Fox Chase Cancer Ctr (page 58); **Address:** Fox Chase Cancer Ctr, Dept Med Oncology, 333 Cottman Ave, Philadelphia, PA 19111-2434; **Phone:** 215-728-2814; **Board Cert:** Medical Oncology 2007; **Med School:** Albany Med Coll 1989; **Resid:** Internal Medicine, NYU Med Ctr 1993; **Fellow:** Hematology & Oncology, Fox Chase Cancer Ctr 1996; **Fac Appt:** Assoc Prof Med, Temple Univ

Waintraub, Stanley E MD [Onc] - **Spec Exp:** Breast Cancer; Bleeding/Coagulation Disorders; **Hospital:** Hackensack Univ Med Ctr; **Address:** Regional Cancer Care Associates, 92 Second St, Fl 4, Hackensack, NJ 07601; **Phone:** 201-996-5864; **Board Cert:** Internal Medicine 1980; Hematology 1982; Medical Oncology 1983; **Med School:** NY Med Coll 1977; **Resid:** Internal Medicine, Metropolitan Hosp Ctr 1980; **Fellow:** Hematology, Montefiore Hosp Med Ctr 1982; Medical Oncology, Meml Sloan Kettering Cancer Ctr 1983

Weiner, Louis M MD [Onc] - **Spec Exp:** Gastrointestinal Cancer; Immunotherapy; Liver Cancer; **Hospital:** Georgetown Univ Hosp; **Address:** 3800 Reservoir Rd NW, Washington, DC 20007; **Phone:** 202-444-2198; **Board Cert:** Internal Medicine 1980; Medical Oncology 1985; **Med School:** Mount Sinai Sch Med 1977; **Resid:** Internal Medicine, Med Ctr Hosp Vermont 1981; **Fellow:** Hematology & Oncology, New England Med Ctr 1984; **Fac Appt:** Prof Med, Georgetown Univ

Wetzler, Meir MD [Onc] - **Spec Exp:** Leukemia; Leukemia-Chronic Myeloid; Myelodysplastic Syndromes; Myeloproliferative Disorders; **Hospital:** Roswell Park Cancer Inst; **Address:** Roswell Park Cancer Inst, Elm and Carlton Streets, Buffalo, NY 14263; **Phone:** 716-845-8907; **Board Cert:** Internal Medicine 2011; Medical Oncology 2003; **Med School:** Israel 1980; **Resid:** Internal Medicine, Kaplan Hosp 1986; **Fellow:** Medical Oncology, MD Anderson Cancer Ctr 1992; **Fac Appt:** Prof Med, SUNY Buffalo

Wilson, Wyndham MD [Onc] - **Spec Exp:** Lymphoma; **Hospital:** Natl Inst of Hlth - Clin Ctr; **Address:** National Cancer Inst, 9000 Rockville Pike, Bldg 10 - rm 4N-115, Bethesda, MD 20892; **Phone:** 301-435-2415; **Board Cert:** Internal Medicine 1985; Medical Oncology 1987; **Med School:** Stanford Univ 1981; **Resid:** Internal Medicine, Stanford Univ 1984; **Fellow:** Oncology, Natl Cancer Inst-NIH 1987

Wolchok, Jedd D MD/PhD [Onc] - **Spec Exp:** Melanoma; Immunotherapy; Clinical Trials; Vaccine Therapy; **Hospital:** Meml Sloan-Kettering Cancer Ctr; **Address:** Meml Sloan Kettering Cancer Ctr, 1275 York Ave, New York, NY 10065; **Phone:** 646-888-2395; **Board Cert:** Medical Oncology 2011; **Med School:** NYU Sch Med 1994; **Resid:** Internal Medicine, NYU Med Ctr 1996; **Fellow:** Medical Oncology, Meml Sloan-Kettering Canc Ctr 1997

Wolff, Antonio C MD [Onc] - **Spec Exp:** Breast Cancer; Drug Development; **Hospital:** Johns Hopkins Hosp (page 61); **Address:** 1650 Orleans St, CRB1 Bldg, rm 189, Baltimore, MD 21287; **Phone:** 410-614-4192; **Board Cert:** Medical Oncology 2000; **Med School:** Brazil 1986; **Resid:** Internal Medicine, Mt Sinai Med Ctr 1991; **Fellow:** Hematology & Oncology, Washington Univ Med Ctr 1992; Medical Oncology, Johns Hopkins Hosp 1995; **Fac Appt:** Prof Med, Johns Hopkins Univ

Zelenetz, Andrew D MD/PhD [Onc] - **Spec Exp:** Lymphoma; **Hospital:** Meml Sloan-Kettering Cancer Ctr; **Address:** 205 E 64th St, New York, NY 10065; **Phone:** 212-639-2656; **Board Cert:** Medical Oncology 2009; **Med School:** Harvard Med Sch 1984; **Resid:** Internal Medicine, Stanford Univ Med Ctr 1986; **Fellow:** Medical Oncology, Stanford Univ Med Ctr 1991; **Fac Appt:** Asst Prof Med, Cornell Univ-Weill Med Coll

Southeast

Anthony, Lowell B MD [Onc] - **Spec Exp:** Gastrointestinal Cancer; Carcinoid Tumors; Neuroendocrine Tumors; **Hospital:** UK HealthCare Good Samaritan Hosp; **Address:** UK HealthCare, Markey Cancer Ctr, Whitney Hendrickson Bldg, 800 Rose St Fl 1, Lexington, KY 40536; **Phone:** 866-340-4488; **Board Cert:** Internal Medicine 1983; Medical Oncology 1989; **Med School:** Vanderbilt Univ 1979; **Resid:** Internal Medicine, Vanderbilt Univ Med Ctr 1982; **Fellow:** Medical Oncology, Vanderbilt Univ Med Ctr 1985; **Fac Appt:** Assoc Prof Med, Louisiana State U, New Orleans

Antonia, Scott J MD/PhD [Onc] - **Spec Exp:** Kidney Cancer; Lung Cancer; **Hospital:** H Lee Moffitt Cancer Ctr & Research Inst (page 59); **Address:** H Lee Moffitt Cancer Ctr, 12902 Magnolia Drive, Tampa, FL 33612; **Phone:** 813-979-3883; **Board Cert:** Internal Medicine 2002; Medical Oncology 2006; **Med School:** Univ Conn 1989; **Resid:** Internal Medicine, Yale-New Haven Hosp 1991; **Fellow:** Medical Oncology, Yale-New Haven Hosp 1994; **Fac Appt:** Assoc Prof Med, Univ S Fla Coll Med

Arteaga, Carlos L MD [Onc] - **Spec Exp:** Breast Cancer; **Hospital:** Vanderbilt Univ Med Ctr (page 75); **Address:** Vanderbilt Hematology Oncology, 2220 Pierce Ave, 683 Preston Rsch Bldg, Nashville, TN 37232-6838; **Phone:** 615-322-2064; **Board Cert:** Internal Medicine 1984; Medical Oncology 1989; **Med School:** Ecuador 1980; **Resid:** Internal Medicine, Grady Meml Hosp 1984; **Fellow:** Hematology & Oncology, Univ Texas 1987; **Fac Appt:** Prof Med, Vanderbilt Univ

Balducci, Lodovico MD [Onc] - **Spec Exp:** Genitourinary Cancer; Breast Cancer; **Hospital:** H Lee Moffitt Cancer Ctr & Research Inst (page 59), Tampa Genl Hosp; **Address:** H Lee Moffitt Cancer Ctr, 12902 Magnolia Drive, Tampa, FL 33612; **Phone:** 813-745-8658; **Board Cert:** Internal Medicine 1987; Hematology 1978; Medical Oncology 1979; **Med School:** Italy 1968; **Resid:** Internal Medicine, Univ Miss Med Ctr 1976; Hematology & Oncology, Univ Miss Med Ctr 1979; **Fellow:** Internal Medicine, A Gemelli Genl Hosp 1970; **Fac Appt:** Prof Med, Univ S Fla Coll Med

Benedetto, Pasquale W MD [Onc] - **Spec Exp:** Genitourinary Cancer; Bone Tumors; Gastrointestinal Cancer; Pancreatic Cancer; **Hospital:** Univ of Miami Hosp & Clins/Sylvester Comp Canc Ctr, Jackson Meml Hosp; **Address:** Sylvester Comp Cancer Ctr, Med Oncology, 1475 NW 12th Ave, rm 3310, Miami, FL 33136; **Phone:** 305-243-1000; **Board Cert:** Internal Medicine 1979; Medical Oncology 1981; Hematology 1982; **Med School:** Cornell Univ-Weill Med Coll 1976; **Resid:** Internal Medicine, Johns Hopkins Hosp 1979; **Fellow:** Medical Oncology, Meml Sloan Kettering Cancer Ctr 1981; **Fac Appt:** Prof Med, Univ Miami Sch Med

Berlin, Jordan D MD [Onc] - **Spec Exp:** Gastrointestinal Cancer; Pancreatic Cancer; Liver Cancer; Clinical Trials; **Hospital:** Vanderbilt Univ Med Ctr (page 75); **Address:** Vanderbilt Hematology/Oncology, 2220 Pierce Ave, 777 Preston Rsch Bldg, Nashville, TN 37232-6307; **Phone:** 615-986-8422; **Board Cert:** Internal Medicine 2002; Medical Oncology 2005; **Med School:** Univ IL Coll Med 1989; **Resid:** Internal Medicine, Univ Cincinnati Med Ctr 1992; **Fellow:** Medical Oncology, Univ Wisconsin 1995; **Fac Appt:** Prof Med, Vanderbilt Univ

Bernard, Stephen A MD [Onc] - **Spec Exp:** Gastrointestinal Cancer; Palliative Care; Clinical Trials; **Hospital:** NC Memorial Hosp - UNC; **Address:** 170 Manning Drive Fl 3rd - rm 3105, Box 7305, Chapel Hill, NC 27599-7305; **Phone:** 919-966-0000; **Board Cert:** Internal Medicine 1987; Medical Oncology 1979; Hospice & Palliative Medicine 2008; **Med School:** Univ NC Sch Med 1973; **Resid:** Internal Medicine, Columbia-Presby Med Ctr 1976; **Fellow:** Hematology & Oncology, Wash Univ Hosps 1978; **Fac Appt:** Prof Onc, Univ NC Sch Med

Blackwell, Kimberly L MD [Onc] - **Spec Exp:** Breast Cancer; Clinical Trials; **Hospital:** Duke Univ Hosp; **Address:** Duke Univ Medical Ctr, Box 3893, Durham, NC 27710; **Phone:** 919-668-6688; **Board Cert:** Medical Oncology 2010; **Med School:** Mayo Med Sch 1994; **Resid:** Internal Medicine, Duke Univ Med Ctr 1997; **Fellow:** Medical Oncology, Duke Univ Med Ctr 2000; **Fac Appt:** Assoc Prof Med, Duke Univ

Blobe, Gerard C MD/PhD [Onc] - **Spec Exp:** Pancreatic Cancer; Colon & Rectal Cancer; Clinical Trials; **Hospital:** Duke Univ Hosp; **Address:** Duke University, Erwin Road, Box 91004, Durham, NC 27708; **Phone:** 919-668-6688; **Board Cert:** Internal Medicine 2009; Medical Oncology 2011; **Med School:** Duke Univ 1995; **Resid:** Internal Medicine, Brigham & Women's Hosp 1997; **Fellow:** Medical Oncology, Dana-Farber Cancer Inst 2000; **Fac Appt:** Assoc Prof Onc, Duke Univ

Bolger, Graeme B MD [Onc] - **Spec Exp:** Prostate Cancer; Testicular Cancer; **Hospital:** Univ of Ala Hosp at Birmingham; **Address:** 1825 University Blvd, Shel-1211, Birmingham, AL 35294; **Phone:** 205-934-2992; **Board Cert:** Internal Medicine 1984; Medical Oncology 2011; **Med School:** McGill Univ 1981; **Resid:** Internal Medicine, Johns Hopkins Hosp 1984; **Fellow:** Medical Oncology, Fred Hutchinson Cancer Rsch 1985; Oncology, Meml Sloan-Kettering Cancer Ctr 1992; **Fac Appt:** Assoc Prof Med, Univ Alabama

Boston, Barry MD [Onc] - **Spec Exp:** Gastrointestinal Cancer; Genitourinary Cancer; Prostate Cancer; **Hospital:** St. Francis Hosp - Memphis, Methodist Univ Hosp - Memphis; **Address:** 7945 Wolf River Blvd, Ste 300, BostonBaskin Cancer Foundation, Germantown, TN 38138; **Phone:** 901-752-6131; **Board Cert:** Internal Medicine 1974; Medical Oncology 1977; **Med School:** Louisiana State U, New Orleans 1971; **Resid:** Internal Medicine, Univ Tenn Hosp-VA Hosp 1973; Hematology, Univ Tenn Hosp-VA Hosp 1973; **Fellow:** Medical Oncology, Yale New Haven Hosp 1975; **Fac Appt:** Assoc Prof Med, Univ Tenn Coll Med

Brenin, Christiana M MD [Onc] - **Spec Exp:** Breast Cancer; Colon & Rectal Cancer; **Hospital:** Univ of Virginia Health Sys; **Address:** Univ Virginia Med Ctr, Division of Hematology/Oncology, Box 800716, Charlottesville, VA 22908; **Phone:** 434-924-8552; **Board Cert:** Internal Medicine 2003; Medical Oncology 2008; **Med School:** NY Med Coll 1990; **Resid:** Internal Medicine, Northwestern Meml Hosp 1993; **Fellow:** Hematology & Oncology, Northwestern Meml Hosp 1996; **Fac Appt:** Assoc Prof Med, Univ VA Sch Med

Brescia, Frank J MD [Onc] - **Spec Exp:** Palliative Care; Breast Cancer; Gastrointestinal Cancer; Ethics; **Hospital:** MUSC Med Ctr; **Address:** Low Country Hematology & Oncology, 96 Jonathan Lucas St, Charleston, SC 29425; **Phone:** 843-792-9300; **Board Cert:** Internal Medicine 1974; Medical Oncology 1975; **Med School:** UMDNJ-NJ Med Sch, Newark 1968; **Resid:** Internal Medicine, North Shore Univ Hosp 1970; **Fellow:** Medical Oncology, Meml Sloan Kettering Cancer Ctr 1974; **Fac Appt:** Prof Med, Med Univ SC

Burris III, Howard A MD [Onc] - **Spec Exp:** Drug Discovery & Development; Breast Cancer; Pancreatic Cancer; Clinical Trials; **Hospital:** Centennial Med Ctr, Baptist Hosp - Nashville; **Address:** Tennessee Oncology, 250 25th Ave N, Ste 100, Nashville, TN 37203; **Phone:** 615-986-4300; **Board Cert:** Internal Medicine 1988; Medical Oncology 2011; **Med School:** Univ S Ala Coll Med 1985; **Resid:** Internal Medicine, Brooke Army Med Ctr 1988; **Fellow:** Medical Oncology, Brooke Army Med Ctr 1991

Butler, William M MD [Onc] - **Spec Exp:** Breast Cancer; Prostate Cancer; Lung Cancer; Clinical Trials; **Hospital:** Palmetto Health Richland Mem Hosp; **Address:** South Carolina Oncology Assocs, 166 Stoneridge Drive, Columbia, SC 29210; **Phone:** 803-461-3000; **Board Cert:** Internal Medicine 1975; Medical Oncology 1979; Hematology 1980; **Med School:** Tulane Univ 1972; **Resid:** Internal Medicine, Charity Hosp 1975; **Fellow:** Hematology & Oncology, Walter Reed AMC 1980; **Fac Appt:** Clin Prof Med, Univ SC Sch Med

Carey, Lisa A MD [Onc] - **Spec Exp:** Breast Cancer; **Hospital:** NC Memorial Hosp - UNC; **Address:** Univ North Carolina-Div Hem/Onc, 170 Manning Drive, Fl 3rd, POB Campus Box 7305, Chapel Hill, NC 27599-7300; **Phone:** 919-843-6814; **Board Cert:** Internal Medicine 2003; Medical Oncology 2007; **Med School:** Johns Hopkins Univ 1990; **Resid:** Internal Medicine, Johns Hopkins Hosp 1993; **Fellow:** Oncology, Johns Hopkins Hosp 1996; **Fac Appt:** Prof Hem & Onc, Univ NC Sch Med

Carpenter Jr, John T MD [Onc] - **Spec Exp:** Breast Cancer; **Hospital:** Univ of Ala Hosp at Birmingham; **Address:** Univ Alabama Birmingham, 510 20th St S, Ste FOT-854, Birmingham, AL 35294-3412; **Phone:** 205-934-2084; **Board Cert:** Internal Medicine 1972; Hematology 1981; Medical Oncology 1975; **Med School:** Tulane Univ 1968; **Resid:** Internal Medicine, Grady Meml Hosp 1971; **Fellow:** Hematology & Oncology, Emory Univ 1973; **Fac Appt:** Prof Med, Univ Alabama

Chanan-Khan, Asher A MD [Onc] - **Spec Exp:** Multiple Myeloma; Leukemia-Chronic Lymphocytic; **Hospital:** Mayo - Jacksonville; **Address:** 4500 San Pablo Rd, Jacksonville, FL 32224; **Phone:** 716-845-3221; **Board Cert:** Medical Oncology 2001; Hematology 2004; **Med School:** Pakistan 1993; **Resid:** Internal Medicine, Harlem Hosp Ctr 1997; **Fellow:** Hematology & Oncology, NYU Med Ctr 1999; **Fac Appt:** Asst Prof Med, SUNY Buffalo

Chao, Nelson J MD [Onc] - **Spec Exp:** Bone Marrow Transplant; Lymphoma; Leukemia; **Hospital:** Duke Univ Hosp; **Address:** Duke Univ Med Ctr, Box 3961, Durham, NC 27710; **Phone:** 919-668-1002; **Board Cert:** Internal Medicine 1984; Medical Oncology 1987; **Med School:** Yale Univ 1981; **Resid:** Internal Medicine, Stanford Univ Med Ctr 1984; **Fellow:** Oncology, Stanford Univ Med Ctr 1987; **Fac Appt:** Prof Med, Duke Univ

Chung, Ki Young MD [Onc] - **Spec Exp:** Gastrointestinal Cancer; **Address:** Cancer Ctrs of the Carolinas, 120 Dillon Drive, Spartanburg, SC 29307; **Phone:** 864-699-5700; **Board Cert:** Medical Oncology 2004; **Med School:** Univ NC Sch Med 1995; **Resid:** Internal Medicine, Sinai Hosp 1999; **Fellow:** Hematology & Oncology, Meml Sloan Kettering Cancer Ctr 2003

Colon-Otero, Gerardo MD [Onc] - **Spec Exp:** Ovarian Cancer; Breast Cancer; Hematologic Malignancies; Pancreatic Cancer-Acinar Cell; **Hospital:** Mayo - Jacksonville; **Address:** Mayo Clinic, 4500 San Pablo Rd S, Jacksonville, FL 32224-1865; **Phone:** 904-953-2000; **Board Cert:** Internal Medicine 1982; Hematology 1984; Medical Oncology 1985; **Med School:** Puerto Rico 1979; **Resid:** Internal Medicine, Mayo Clinic 1982; **Fellow:** Hematology, Mayo Clinic 1984; Medical Oncology, Univ Va Med Ctr 1986; **Fac Appt:** Assoc Prof Med, Mayo Med Sch

Conry, Robert M MD [Onc] - **Spec Exp:** Melanoma; Lung Cancer; Colon & Rectal Cancer; Sarcoma; **Hospital:** Univ of Ala Hosp at Birmingham; **Address:** The Kirklin Clinic At Acton Rd, 2145 Bonner Way, Birmingham, AL 35243; **Phone:** 205-978-0250; **Board Cert:** Hematology 2011; **Med School:** Univ Alabama 1987; **Resid:** Internal Medicine, Univ Alabama Hosp 1990; **Fellow:** Medical Oncology, Univ Alabama Hosp 1993; **Fac Appt:** Assoc Prof Med, Univ Alabama

Crawford, Jeffrey MD [Onc] - **Spec Exp:** Lung Cancer; **Hospital:** Duke Univ Hosp; **Address:** Duke Univ Med Ctr, Box 3476, Durham, NC 27710; **Phone:** 919-668-6688; **Board Cert:** Internal Medicine 1977; Hematology 1980; Medical Oncology 1981; **Med School:** Ohio State Univ 1974; **Resid:** Internal Medicine, Duke Univ Med Ctr 1977; **Fellow:** Hematology & Oncology, Duke Univ Med Ctr 1981; **Fac Appt:** Prof Med, Duke Univ

Medical Oncology

De Simone, Philip MD [Onc] - **Spec Exp:** Colon Cancer; Pancreatic Cancer; **Hospital:** Univ of Kentucky Albert B. Chandler Hosp; **Address:** Markey Cancer Ctr, Dept Med Onc, 800 Rose St, rm CC-401B, Lexington, KY 40536; **Phone:** 859-323-8043; **Board Cert:** Internal Medicine 1972; Hematology 1974; **Med School:** Univ VT Coll Med 1967; **Resid:** Internal Medicine, Univ Kentucky Hosp 1972; **Fellow:** Hematology & Oncology, Univ Kentucky 1974; **Fac Appt:** Prof Med, Univ KY Coll Med

Dunphy II, Frank R MD [Onc] - **Spec Exp:** Lung Cancer; Head & Neck Cancer; **Hospital:** Duke Univ Hosp; **Address:** Duke Univ Med Ctr, Box 3198, Durham, NC 27710; **Phone:** 919-668-6688; **Board Cert:** Internal Medicine 1984; Hematology 1986; Medical Oncology 1989; **Med School:** Louisiana State U, New Orleans 1979; **Resid:** Internal Medicine, Lousiana St Univ Hosp 1983; **Fellow:** Hematology & Oncology, Louisiana St Univ Hosp 1985; **Fac Appt:** Assoc Prof Med, Duke Univ

Flinn, Ian W MD/PhD [Onc] - **Spec Exp:** Leukemia; Lymphoma; Bone Marrow Transplant; Multiple Myeloma; **Hospital:** Centennial Med Ctr; **Address:** Tennessee Oncology, 250 25th Ave N, Ste 412, Nashville, TN 37203; **Phone:** 615-986-7600; **Board Cert:** Hematology 2007; Medical Oncology 2008; **Med School:** Johns Hopkins Univ 1990; **Resid:** Internal Medicine, Univ Michigan Med Ctr 1993; **Fellow:** Hematology & Oncology, Johns Hopkins 1996

Forero, Andres MD [Onc] - **Spec Exp:** Lymphoma; **Hospital:** Univ of Ala Hosp at Birmingham; **Address:** 1530 3rd Ave S, North Pavillion, AL 35294; **Phone:** 205-934-9999; **Med School:** Colombia 1982; **Resid:** Internal Medicine, Javeriana Univ 1987; **Fellow:** Medical Oncology, Javeriana Univ 1991; **Fac Appt:** Prof Med, Univ Alabama

Fracasso, Paula M MD/PhD [Onc] - **Spec Exp:** Gynecologic Cancer; Breast Cancer; **Hospital:** Univ of Virginia Health Sys; **Address:** Univ Virginia- Dept Medicine, PO Box 800716, Charlottesville, VA 22908; **Phone:** 434-243-6143; **Board Cert:** Internal Medicine 1987; Medical Oncology 2003; **Med School:** Yale Univ 1984; **Resid:** Internal Medicine, Beth Israel Hosp 1987; **Fellow:** Cancer Research, Mass Inst Tech 1989; Hematology & Oncology, Tufts-New England Med Ctr 1991; **Fac Appt:** Prof Med, Univ VA Sch Med

Friedman, Henry S MD [Onc] - **Spec Exp:** Neuro-Oncology; Brain & Spinal Cord Tumors; Gliomas; **Hospital:** Duke Univ Hosp; **Address:** Preston R Tisch Brain Tumor Ctr, 047 Baker House, Trent Drive, DUMC, Box 3624, Durham, NC 27710; **Phone:** 919-684-5301; **Board Cert:** Pediatrics 1982; Pediatric Hematology-Oncology 1982; **Med School:** SUNY Upstate Med Univ 1977; **Resid:** Pediatrics, SUNY Upstate Med Ctr 1980; **Fellow:** Pediatric Hematology-Oncology, Duke Univ Med Ctr 1983; **Fac Appt:** Prof Neuro-Onc, Duke Univ

Garst, Jennifer L MD [Onc] - **Spec Exp:** Lung Cancer; Thoracic Cancers; Cancer Survivors-Late Effects of Therapy; **Hospital:** Duke Univ Hosp; **Address:** Duke Univ Hosp, Div Medical Oncology, 2301 Erwin Rd, Box 3198, Durham, NC 27710; **Phone:** 919-954-3050; **Board Cert:** Internal Medicine 2008; Medical Oncology 2011; **Med School:** Med Coll GA 1990; **Resid:** Internal Medicine, Univ SW Texas Hosp 1993; **Fellow:** Hematology & Oncology, Duke Univ Med Ctr 1996; **Fac Appt:** Assoc Prof Med, Duke Univ

George, Daniel J MD [Onc] - **Spec Exp:** Prostate Cancer; Kidney Cancer; **Hospital:** Duke Univ Hosp; **Address:** Duke Univ Med Ctr, Box 102002, Durham, NC 27710; **Phone:** 919-668-8108; **Board Cert:** Medical Oncology 2007; **Med School:** Duke Univ 1992; **Resid:** Internal Medicine, Johns Hopkins Hosp 1995; **Fellow:** Medical Oncology, Johns Hopkins Hosp 1998; **Fac Appt:** Assoc Prof S, Duke Univ

Gockerman, Jon Paul MD [Onc] - **Spec Exp:** Leukemia; Lymphoma; **Hospital:** Duke Univ Hosp; **Address:** Duke Univ Med Ctr, 1 Trent Drive, rm 25153, Box 3872, Morris Bldg, Durham, NC 27710; **Phone:** 919-684-8964; **Board Cert:** Internal Medicine 1972; Medical Oncology 1973; Hematology 1974; **Med School:** Univ Chicago-Pritzker Sch Med 1967; **Resid:** Internal Medicine, Duke Univ Med Ctr 1969; **Fellow:** Hematology & Oncology, Duke Univ Med Ctr 1971

Godley, Paul A MD/PhD [Onc] - **Spec Exp:** Prostate Cancer (advanced); Testicular Cancer; Penile Cancer; Bladder Cancer; **Hospital:** NC Memorial Hosp - UNC; **Address:** UNC Hematology/Oncology, POB, Campus Box 7305, 3rd Floor, 170 Manning Drive, Chapel Hill, NC 27599; **Phone:** 919-966-4431; **Board Cert:** Internal Medicine 1987; Medical Oncology 2002; **Med School:** Harvard Med Sch 1984; **Resid:** Internal Medicine, Univ Hosps 1987; **Fellow:** Epidemiology, Univ NC Sch of Public Hlth 1989; Hematology & Oncology, Univ NC Hosps 1991; **Fac Appt:** Assoc Prof Med, Univ NC Sch Med

Graham II, Mark L MD [Onc] - **Spec Exp:** Breast Cancer; Breast Cancer Genetics; **Hospital:** WakeMed Cary; **Address:** Waverly Hematology/Oncology, 300 Ashville Ave, Ste 310, Cary, NC 27518; **Phone:** 919-233-8585; **Board Cert:** Internal Medicine 1989; **Med School:** Mayo Med Sch 1982; **Resid:** Internal Medicine, Duke Univ Med Ctr 1985; **Fellow:** Medical Oncology, Univ CO Hlth Sci Ctr 1990; Medical Oncology, Mayo Clinic 1991; **Fac Appt:** Assoc Clin Prof Med, Univ NC Sch Med

Greco, F Anthony MD [Onc] - **Spec Exp:** Lung Cancer; Unknown Primary Cancer; **Hospital:** Centennial Med Ctr; **Address:** Tennessee Oncology, 250 25th Ave N, Ste 100, Nashville, TN 37203; **Phone:** 615-320-5090; **Board Cert:** Internal Medicine 1975; Medical Oncology 1977; **Med School:** W VA Univ 1972; **Resid:** Internal Medicine, Univ West Virginia Hosp 1974; **Fellow:** Medical Oncology, Natl Cancer Inst 1976

Grosh, William W MD [Onc] - **Spec Exp:** Melanoma; Sarcoma; Neuroendocrine Tumors; **Hospital:** Univ of Virginia Health Sys; **Address:** UVA Health System, Div Hem/Oncology, Box 800716, Charlottesville, VA 22908; **Phone:** 434-924-1904; **Board Cert:** Internal Medicine 1978; Medical Oncology 1985; **Med School:** Columbia P&S 1974; **Resid:** Internal Medicine, Vanderbilt Univ Med Ctr 1977; **Fellow:** Medical Oncology, Vanderbilt Univ Med Ctr 1983; **Fac Appt:** Assoc Prof Med, Univ VA Sch Med

Hande, Kenneth R MD [Onc] - **Spec Exp:** Unknown Primary Cancer; Sarcoma; Carcinoid Tumors; Drug Development; **Hospital:** Vanderbilt Univ Med Ctr (page 75), VA Tennessee Valley Healthcare System-Alvin C. Yor; **Address:** Vanderbilt Hematology/Oncology, 2220 Pierce Ave, 777 Preston Rsch Bldg, Nashville, TN 37232-6307; **Phone:** 615-936-8422; **Board Cert:** Internal Medicine 1975; Medical Oncology 1977; **Med School:** Johns Hopkins Univ 1972; **Resid:** Internal Medicine, Barnes-Jewish Hosp 1974; **Fellow:** Medical Oncology, Natl Cancer Inst 1977; **Fac Appt:** Prof Med, Vanderbilt Univ

Hurd, David MD [Onc] - **Spec Exp:** Lymphoma; Leukemia; Bone Marrow Transplant; **Hospital:** Wake Forest Baptist Med Ctr; **Address:** Medical Ctr Blvd, Winston-Salem, NC 27157-1082; **Phone:** 336-713-5440; **Board Cert:** Internal Medicine 1977; Medical Oncology 1981; **Med School:** Univ IL Coll Med 1974; **Resid:** Internal Medicine, Univ Minn Hosp 1977; **Fellow:** Medical Oncology, Univ Minn Hosp 1979; **Fac Appt:** Prof Med, Wake Forest Univ

Jahanzeb, Mohammad MD [Onc] - **Spec Exp:** Breast Cancer; Lung Cancer; Clinical Trials; **Hospital:** Boca Raton Regl Hosp, Univ of Miami Hosp & Clins/Sylvester Comp Canc Ctr; **Address:** 1192 E Newport Center Drive, Ste 200, Deerfield Beach, FL 33442; **Phone:** 954-698-3665; **Board Cert:** Medical Oncology 2003; Hematology 2005; **Med School:** Pakistan 1986; **Resid:** Internal Medicine, New Britain Genl Hosp 1990; **Fellow:** Hematology & Oncology, Washington Univ 1993; **Fac Appt:** Prof Onc, Univ Miami Sch Med

Medical Oncology

Jillella, Anand MD [Onc] - **Spec Exp:** Bone Marrow Transplant; Leukemia; Lymphoma; Multiple Myeloma; **Hospital:** Med Coll of GA Hosp and Clin (MCG Health Inc); **Address:** Med Coll Ga - BMT Program, 1120 15th St, BAA 5407, Augusta, GA 30912-3125; **Phone:** 706-721-2505; **Board Cert:** Medical Oncology 2007; **Med School:** India 1985; **Resid:** Internal Medicine, Med Coll Georgia 1992; **Fellow:** Medical Oncology, Yale-New Haven Hosp 1996; **Fac Appt:** Prof Med, Med Coll GA

Khuri, Fadlo Raja MD [Onc] - **Spec Exp:** Lung Cancer; Head & Neck Cancer; Thyroid Cancer; Mesothelioma; **Hospital:** Emory Univ Hosp, Grady Hlth Sys; **Address:** 1365 Clifton Road Rd NE, C Bldg - Ste 3000, Atlanta, GA 30322; **Phone:** 404-778-1900; **Board Cert:** Medical Oncology 2008; **Med School:** Columbia P&S 1989; **Resid:** Internal Medicine, Boston City Hosp 1992; **Fellow:** Hematology & Oncology, New England Med Ctr-Tufts 1995; **Fac Appt:** Prof Onc, Emory Univ

Kraft, Andrew S MD [Onc] - **Spec Exp:** Prostate Cancer; Sarcoma; Drug Development; Clinical Trials; **Hospital:** MUSC Med Ctr; **Address:** MUSC Hollings Cancer Ctr, 86 Jonathan Lucas St, PO Box 250955, Charleston, SC 29425; **Phone:** 843-792-8284; **Board Cert:** Internal Medicine 1980; Medical Oncology 1985; **Med School:** Univ Pennsylvania 1975; **Resid:** Internal Medicine, Mt Sinai Hosp 1979; **Fellow:** Medical Oncology, Natl Cancer Inst 1985; **Fac Appt:** Prof Med, Med Univ SC

Kucuk, Omer MD [Onc] - **Spec Exp:** Genitourinary Cancer; Nutrition in Cancer Therapy; Prostate Cancer; Nutrition & Cancer Prevention/Control; **Hospital:** Emory Univ Hosp; **Address:** Emory Winship Cancer Inst, 1365C Clifton Rd NE, Ste 2110, Atlanta, GA 30322; **Phone:** 404-778-1900; **Board Cert:** Internal Medicine 1978; Hematology 1984; Medical Oncology 1989; **Med School:** Turkey 1975; **Resid:** Internal Medicine, St Francis Hosp 1978; **Fellow:** Hematology & Oncology, Northwestern Univ 1981; **Fac Appt:** Prof Hem & Onc, Emory Univ

Kvols, Larry K MD [Onc] - **Spec Exp:** Gastrointestinal Cancer; Carcinoid Tumors; Neuroendocrine Tumors; **Hospital:** H Lee Moffitt Cancer Ctr & Research Inst (page 59); **Address:** H Lee Moffitt Cancer Ctr & Research Inst, 12902 Magnolia Drive, FOB-2, Tampa, FL 33612; **Phone:** 813-745-7257; **Board Cert:** Internal Medicine 1976; Medical Oncology 1977; **Med School:** Baylor Coll Med 1970; **Resid:** Internal Medicine, Johns Hopkins Hosp 1972; **Fellow:** Hematology & Oncology, Johns Hopkins Hosp 1973; **Fac Appt:** Prof Med, Mayo Med Sch

Lawson, David H MD [Onc] - **Spec Exp:** Melanoma; **Hospital:** Emory Univ Hosp; **Address:** Emory Winship Cancer Institute, 1365C Clifton Rd NE, Ste 2110, Atlanta, GA 30322; **Phone:** 404-778-1900; **Board Cert:** Internal Medicine 1977; Medical Oncology 1979; **Med School:** Emory Univ 1974; **Resid:** Internal Medicine, Emory Univ Hosps 1977; **Fellow:** Medical Oncology, Emory Univ 1979; **Fac Appt:** Assoc Prof Hem & Onc, Emory Univ

Lesser, Glenn J MD [Onc] - **Spec Exp:** Neuro-Oncology; Brain Tumors; **Hospital:** Wake Forest Baptist Med Ctr; **Address:** Wake Forest Univ-Div Hematolgy/Oncology, Medical Center Blvd, Winston-Salem, NC 27157-1082; **Phone:** 336-713-5440; **Board Cert:** Medical Oncology 2007; **Med School:** Penn State Coll Med 1987; **Resid:** Internal Medicine, NC Baptist Hosp/Bowman Gray Sch Med 1991; **Fellow:** Medical Oncology, Johns Hopkins Hosp 1995; **Fac Appt:** Prof Hem & Onc, Wake Forest Univ

Lilenbaum, Rogerio C MD [Onc] - **Spec Exp:** Lung Cancer; Thoracic Cancers; **Hospital:** Cleveland Clin - Weston (page 55); **Address:** 2950 Cleveland Clinic Blvd, Weston, FL 33331; **Phone:** 954-659-6391; **Board Cert:** Internal Medicine 2005; Hematology 2008; Medical Oncology 2007; **Med School:** Brazil 1986; **Resid:** Internal Medicine, Univ Hosp 1989; **Fellow:** Hematology & Oncology, Washington Univ Hosp 1992; Medical Oncology, UCSD Med Ctr 1994

Limentani, Steven A MD [Onc] - **Spec Exp:** Breast Cancer; Clinical Trials; **Hospital:** Carolinas Med Ctr; **Address:** 1100 S Tryon St, Ste 400, Charlotte, NC 28203; **Phone:** 704-446-9046; **Board Cert:** Internal Medicine 1989; Medical Oncology 2011; Hematology 2002; **Med School:** Tufts Univ 1986; **Resid:** Internal Medicine, New England Deaconess Hosp 1989; **Fellow:** Hematology & Oncology, New England Med Ctr 1992

Lippman, Marc E MD [Onc] - **Spec Exp:** Breast Cancer; **Hospital:** Univ of Miami Hosp & Clins/Sylvester Comp Canc Ctr, Univ of Miami Hosp; **Address:** Sylvester Comp Cancer Ctr, Med Oncology, 1475 NW 12th Ave, Miami, FL 33136; **Phone:** 305-243-1000; **Board Cert:** Internal Medicine 1987; Endocrinology 1975; Medical Oncology 1977; **Med School:** Yale Univ 1968; **Resid:** Internal Medicine, Johns Hopkins Hosp 1970; **Fellow:** Medical Oncology, Natl Cancer Inst 1973; Endocrinology, Yale-New Haven Hosp 1974; **Fac Appt:** Prof Med, Univ Mich Med Sch

List, Alan F MD [Onc] - **Spec Exp:** Myelodysplastic Syndromes; Leukemia; **Hospital:** H Lee Moffitt Cancer Ctr & Research Inst (page 59); **Address:** 12902 Magnolia Drive, Tampa, FL 33612-9497; **Phone:** 813-745-3980; **Board Cert:** Internal Medicine 1983; Medical Oncology 1985; Hematology 1986; **Med School:** Univ Pennsylvania 1980; **Resid:** Internal Medicine, Good Samaritan Hosp 1983; Oncology, Vanderbilt Univ Med Ctr 1985; **Fellow:** Hematology, Vanderbilt Univ Med Ctr 1986; **Fac Appt:** Prof Med, Univ S Fla Coll Med

Lossos, Izidore MD [Onc] - **Spec Exp:** Lymphoma; Hodgkin's Lymphoma; Leukemia; Lymphomas-Rare; **Hospital:** Univ of Miami Hosp & Clins/Sylvester Comp Canc Ctr, Jackson Meml Hosp; **Address:** Univ Miami - Sylvester Comp Cancer Ctr, 1475 NW 12th Ave, D8-4, Miami, FL 33136; **Phone:** 305-243-4785; **Med School:** Israel 1987; **Resid:** Internal Medicine, Hadassah Univ Hosp 1995; **Fellow:** Hematology & Oncology, Hadassah Univ Hosp 1997; Medical Oncology, Stanford Univ 2001; **Fac Appt:** Prof Hem & Onc, Univ Miami Sch Med

Lyckholm, Laurel J MD [Onc] - **Spec Exp:** Neuro-Oncology; Palliative Care; **Hospital:** Med Coll of VA Hosp; **Address:** Med Coll of VA, Div Hem/Onc, PO Box 980230, Richmond, VA 23298; **Phone:** 804-828-7999; **Board Cert:** Internal Medicine 1989; Medical Oncology 2003; Hematology 2004; Hospice & Palliative Medicine 2008; **Med School:** Creighton Univ 1985; **Resid:** Internal Medicine, Creighton Univ 1989; **Fellow:** Hematology & Oncology, Univ IA Coll Med 1992; **Fac Appt:** Assoc Prof Med, Med Coll VA

Lyman, Gary H MD [Onc] - **Spec Exp:** Breast Cancer; **Hospital:** Duke Univ Hosp; **Address:** Duke Comprehensive Cancer Center, Hock Plaza, 2424 Erwin Rd, Ste 205, Durham, NC 27705; **Phone:** 919-668-6688; **Board Cert:** Internal Medicine 1987; Medical Oncology 1977; Hematology 1978; **Med School:** SUNY Buffalo 1972; **Resid:** Internal Medicine, Univ North Carolina Hosp 1974; **Fellow:** Medical Oncology, Roswell Park Meml Inst 1976; Biostatistics, Harvard Med Sch 1982; **Fac Appt:** Prof Med, Duke Univ

Lynch Jr, James W MD [Onc] - **Spec Exp:** Lymphoma; Immunotherapy; Lung Cancer; **Hospital:** Shands at Univ of FL; **Address:** Shands Hlthcare, Div Hematology/Oncology, PO Box 100383, Gainesville, FL 32610-0383; **Phone:** 352-265-0725; **Board Cert:** Internal Medicine 1987; Medical Oncology 2012; **Med School:** Eastern VA Med Sch 1984; **Resid:** Internal Medicine, Univ Florida 1987; **Fellow:** Medical Oncology, Natl Cancer Inst 1991; **Fac Appt:** Prof Med, Univ Fla Coll Med

Marcom, Paul Kelly MD [Onc] - **Spec Exp:** Breast Cancer; Clinical Trials; Cancer Genetics; **Hospital:** Duke Univ Hosp; **Address:** Duke Univ Med Ctr, Box 3147, Durham, NC 27710; **Phone:** 919-684-3877; **Board Cert:** Internal Medicine 2003; Medical Oncology 2005; **Med School:** Baylor Coll Med 1989; **Resid:** Internal Medicine, Duke Univ Med Ctr 1992; **Fellow:** Hematology & Oncology, DukeUniv Med Ctr 1995; **Fac Appt:** Assoc Prof Med, Duke Univ

Medical Oncology

Miller, Antonius A MD [Onc] - **Spec Exp:** Lung Cancer; **Hospital:** Wake Forest Baptist Med Ctr, W.G. (Bill) Hefner VA Med Ctr; **Address:** Wake Forest University, Comprehensive Cancer Center, Medical Center Blvd, Winston-Salem, NC 27157; **Phone:** 336-713-4392; **Med School:** Germany 1977; **Resid:** Internal Medicine, Univ Essen Med Sch 1979; Internal Medicine, Univ TN Med Ctr 1987; **Fellow:** Hematology & Oncology, UT MD Anderson Cancer Ctr 1981; **Fac Appt:** Prof Med, Wake Forest Univ

Miller, Donald M MD/PhD [Onc] - **Spec Exp:** Melanoma; Lung Cancer; **Hospital:** Univ of Louisville Hosp; **Address:** James Graham Brown Cancer Center, 529 S Jackson St, Louisville, KY 40202; **Phone:** 502-562-4790; **Board Cert:** Internal Medicine 1979; **Med School:** Duke Univ 1973; **Resid:** Internal Medicine, Peter Bent Brigham Hosp 1975; **Fellow:** Internal Medicine, Peter Bent Brigham Hosp 1978; Medical Oncology, Natl Cancer Inst 1979; **Fac Appt:** Prof Med, Univ Louisville Sch Med

Moore, Joseph O MD [Onc] - **Spec Exp:** Leukemia; Hodgkin's Lymphoma; Lymphoma, Non-Hodgkin's; Neuroendocrine Tumors; **Hospital:** Duke Univ Hosp; **Address:** Duke Univ Med Ctr, Box 3872, Durham, NC 27710; **Phone:** 919-684-8964; **Board Cert:** Internal Medicine 1975; Medical Oncology 1977; **Med School:** Johns Hopkins Univ 1970; **Resid:** Internal Medicine, Johns Hopkins Hosp 1975; **Fellow:** Hematology & Oncology, Duke Univ Med Ctr 1977; **Fac Appt:** Prof Med, Duke Univ

Morgan, David S MD [Onc] - **Spec Exp:** Leukemia & Lymphoma; Hodgkin's Lymphoma; AIDS Related Lymphoma; **Hospital:** Vanderbilt Univ Med Ctr (page 75); **Address:** Vanderbilt Hematology/Oncology, 2220 Pierce Ave, 777 Preston Research Bldg, Nashville, TN 37232-6307; **Phone:** 615-936-8422; **Board Cert:** Internal Medicine 2003; Medical Oncology 2008; **Med School:** Vanderbilt Univ 1990; **Resid:** Internal Medicine, Yale-New Haven Hosp 1993; **Fellow:** Medical Oncology, Stanford Univ Med Ctr 1997; **Fac Appt:** Assoc Prof Med, Vanderbilt Univ

Muss, Hyman B MD [Onc] - **Spec Exp:** Breast Cancer; **Hospital:** NC Memorial Hosp - UNC; **Address:** Div of Hem/Onc, Physicians Office Bldg, 170 Manning Drive, Box CB#7305, Chapel Hill, NC 27599-7305; **Phone:** 919-966-4431; **Board Cert:** Internal Medicine 1973; Hematology 1974; Medical Oncology 1975; **Med School:** SUNY Downstate 1968; **Resid:** Internal Medicine, Peter Bent Brigham Hosp 1970; **Fellow:** Hematology & Oncology, Peter Bent Brigham Hosp 1974; Hematology & Oncology, Dana-Farber Cancer Ctr 1974; **Fac Appt:** Prof Onc, Univ NC Sch Med

Nabell, Lisle M MD [Onc] - **Spec Exp:** Breast Cancer; Head & Neck Cancer; **Hospital:** Univ of Ala Hosp at Birmingham; **Address:** Univ of Alabama, 1530 3rd Ave S, Ste NP2540B, Birmingham, AL 35294; **Phone:** 205-934-3061; **Board Cert:** Medical Oncology 2000; **Med School:** Univ NC Sch Med 1987; **Resid:** Internal Medicine, Univ Alabama Hosp 1990; **Fellow:** Hematology & Oncology, Univ Alabama Hosp 1992; **Fac Appt:** Assoc Prof Med, Univ Alabama

O'Regan, Ruth M MD [Onc] - **Spec Exp:** Breast Cancer; Breast Cancer Risk Assessment; Cancer Prevention; Clinical Trials; **Hospital:** Emory Univ Hosp; **Address:** Emory Winship Cancer Inst, 1365C Clifton Rd NE, Ste 2110, Atlanta, GA 30322; **Phone:** 404-778-1900; **Board Cert:** Medical Oncology 2010; **Med School:** Ireland 1988; **Resid:** Internal Medicine, Med Coll Wisconsin 1995; Internal Medicine, Northwestern Univ Hosp 1999; **Fellow:** Medical Oncology, Northwestern Univ 1998; **Fac Appt:** Assoc Prof Hem & Onc, Emory Univ

Pao, William MD/PhD [Onc] - **Spec Exp:** Thoracic Cancers; Lung Cancer; **Hospital:** Vanderbilt Univ Med Ctr (page 75); **Address:** Vanderbilt Div Hematology/Oncology, 2220 Pierce Ave, 777 Preston Rsch Bldg, Nashville, TN 37232-6307; **Phone:** 615-936-8422; **Board Cert:** Internal Medicine 2001; Medical Oncology 2003; **Med School:** Yale Univ 1998; **Resid:** Internal Medicine, New York Hosp 2000; **Fellow:** Medical Oncology, Meml Sloan Kettering Canc Ctr 2004; **Fac Appt:** Assoc Prof Med, Vanderbilt Univ

Pasche, Boris C MD/PhD [Onc] - **Spec Exp:** Colon Cancer; Gastrointestinal Cancer; **Hospital:** Univ of Ala Hosp at Birmingham; **Address:** 1802 6th Ave, Ste NP-2566, Birmingham, AL 35203; **Phone:** 205-934-9591; **Board Cert:** Medical Oncology 2008; **Med School:** Sweden 1986; **Resid:** Internal Medicine, NY Hosp/Cornell Med Ctr 1994; **Fellow:** Hematology & Oncology, Meml Sloan Kettering Cancer Ctr 1996; **Fac Appt:** Prof Med, Univ Alabama

Perez, Edith A MD [Onc] - **Spec Exp:** Breast Cancer; Breast Cancer Risk Assessment; Clinical Trials; **Hospital:** Mayo - Jacksonville; **Address:** Mayo Clinic-Jacksonville, 4500 San Pablo Rd Davis Bldg Fl 8, Jacksonville, FL 32224; **Phone:** 904-953-7283; **Board Cert:** Internal Medicine 1983; Hematology 1986; Medical Oncology 1987; **Med School:** Univ Puerto Rico 1979; **Resid:** Internal Medicine, Loma Linda Univ Med Ctr 1982; **Fellow:** Hematology & Oncology, Martinez VA Hosp/UC Davis 1987; **Fac Appt:** Prof Med, Mayo Med Sch

Posey III, James A MD [Onc] - **Spec Exp:** Gastrointestinal Cancer; Colon Cancer; Liver Cancer; Biliary Cancer; **Hospital:** Univ of Ala Hosp at Birmingham; **Address:** 1802 6th Ave S, NP-25404, Birmingham, AL 35294-3300; **Phone:** 205-934-0916; **Board Cert:** Medical Oncology 1997; **Med School:** Howard Univ 1991; **Resid:** Internal Medicine, Georgetown Univ Med Ctr 1994; **Fellow:** Hematology & Oncology, Georgetown Univ Med Ctr 1997; **Fac Appt:** Assoc Prof Med, Univ Alabama

Ready, Neal E MD/PhD [Onc] - **Spec Exp:** Lung Cancer; Head & Neck Cancer; Clinical Trials; **Hospital:** Duke Univ Hosp; **Address:** Duke Univ Medical Ctr, DUMC, Box 3198, Durham, NC 27710; **Phone:** 919-668-6688; **Board Cert:** Internal Medicine 1989; Hematology 2005; Medical Oncology 2005; **Med School:** Vanderbilt Univ 1986; **Resid:** Internal Medicine, Rhode Island Hosp 1989; **Fellow:** Hematology, Rhode Island Hosp 1992; Medical Oncology, New England Med Ctr 1994

Reed, Eddie MD [Onc] - **Spec Exp:** Ovarian Cancer; Prostate Cancer; **Hospital:** Univ of S AL Med Ctr; **Address:** USA Mitchell Cancer Institute, 1660 Springhill Ave, Mobile, AL 36604; **Phone:** 251-665-8000; **Board Cert:** Internal Medicine 1982; **Med School:** Yale Univ 1979; **Resid:** Internal Medicine, Stanford Univ Med Ctr 1982; **Fellow:** Medical Oncology, Natl Cancer Inst 1985; **Fac Appt:** Prof Med, Univ S Ala Coll Med

Robert, Nicholas J MD [Onc] - **Spec Exp:** Breast Cancer; **Hospital:** Inova Fairfax Hosp; **Address:** Virginia Cancer Specialists, 8503 Arlington Blvd, Ste 400, Fairfax, VA 22031; **Phone:** 703-280-5390; **Board Cert:** Internal Medicine 1978; Anatomic Pathology 1979; Medical Oncology 1981; Hematology 1984; **Med School:** McGill Univ 1974; **Resid:** Internal Medicine, Royal Victoria Hosp 1976; Pathology, Mass Genl Hosp 1979; **Fellow:** Hematology, Peter Bent Brigham Hosp 1980; Medical Oncology, Dana Farber Cancer Inst 1981

Robert-Vizcarrondo, Francisco MD [Onc] - **Spec Exp:** Lung Cancer; Mesothelioma; Drug Development; Clinical Trials; **Hospital:** Univ of Ala Hosp at Birmingham; **Address:** 1802 6th Ave S, rm NP-2555D, Birmingham, AL 35294-3300; **Phone:** 205-934-5077; **Board Cert:** Internal Medicine 1973; Medical Oncology 1975; Hematology 1976; **Med School:** Puerto Rico 1969; **Resid:** Internal Medicine, Univ PR Hosp 1972; Hematology, Univ PR Hosp 1974; **Fellow:** Medical Oncology, Univ AL Hosp at Birmingham 1976; **Fac Appt:** Prof Med, Univ Alabama

Romond, Edward H MD [Onc] - **Spec Exp:** Breast Cancer; Hemophilia; **Hospital:** Univ of Kentucky Albert B. Chandler Hosp; **Address:** Univ KY Med Ctr, Div Hematology/Oncology, CC413 Markey Cancer Center, 800 Rose St, Lexington, KY 40536; **Phone:** 859-323-6522; **Board Cert:** Internal Medicine 1980; Hematology 1984; Medical Oncology 1983; **Med School:** Univ KY Coll Med 1977; **Resid:** Internal Medicine, Michigan State Univ Hosps 1980; **Fellow:** Hematology & Oncology, Michigan State Univ 1983; **Fac Appt:** Prof Onc, Univ KY Coll Med

Medical Oncology

Schwartz, Michael A MD [Onc] - **Spec Exp:** Breast Cancer; Lymphoma; Prostate Cancer; **Hospital:** Mount Sinai Med Ctr - Miami; **Address:** 4306 Alton Rd, Fl 3, Miami Beach, FL 33140; **Phone:** 305-535-3310; **Board Cert:** Internal Medicine 1989; Medical Oncology 2004; Hematology 2004; **Med School:** UMDNJ-RW Johnson Med Sch 1986; **Resid:** Internal Medicine, Mt Sinai Medical Ctr 1989; **Fellow:** Hematology & Oncology, Meml Sloan Kettering Cancer Ctr 1992; **Fac Appt:** Asst Clin Prof Med, Univ Miami Sch Med

Serody, Jonathan S MD [Onc] - **Spec Exp:** Breast Cancer Vaccine Therapy; Clinical Trials; Lymphoma; **Hospital:** NC Memorial Hosp - UNC; **Address:** Lineberger Comprehensive Cancer Ctr, 450 West Drive, CB 7295, Chapel Hill, NC 27599-7295; **Phone:** 919-966-8644; **Board Cert:** Internal Medicine 1989; Hematology 2007; **Med School:** Univ VA Sch Med 1986; **Resid:** Internal Medicine, Univ NC Med Ctr 1989; **Fellow:** Hematology, Univ NC Med Ctr 1992; Bone Marrow Transplant, Fred Hutchinson Transplant Program 1993; **Fac Appt:** Prof Med, Univ NC Sch Med

Shea, Thomas MD [Onc] - **Spec Exp:** Bone Marrow Transplant; Lymphoma; Leukemia; **Hospital:** NC Memorial Hosp - UNC; **Address:** Univ N Carolina, Dept Medicine, 170 Manning Drive, CB 7305, Chapel Hill, NC 27599; **Phone:** 919-966-7746; **Board Cert:** Internal Medicine 1982; Hematology 1984; Medical Oncology 1985; **Med School:** Univ NC Sch Med 1978; **Resid:** Internal Medicine, Beth Israel Deaconess Med Ctr 1982; **Fellow:** Hematology & Oncology, Beth Israel Deaconess Med Ctr 1985; Bone Marrow Transplant, Dana Farber Cancer Inst 1988; **Fac Appt:** Prof Med, Univ NC Sch Med

Sherman, Carol A MD [Onc] - **Spec Exp:** Lung Cancer; Thoracic Cancers; **Hospital:** MUSC Med Ctr; **Address:** MUSC Hematology/Oncology, 96 Jonathan Lucas St, CSB 903, Charleston, SC 29425; **Phone:** 843-792-9621; **Board Cert:** Internal Medicine 1987; Medical Oncology 1989; **Med School:** Univ Mass Sch Med 1984; **Resid:** Internal Medicine, Univ Mass Med Ctr 1987; **Fellow:** Hematology & Oncology, Univ Mass 1989; **Fac Appt:** Assoc Prof Med, Med Univ SC

Shin, Dong Moon MD [Onc] - **Spec Exp:** Head & Neck Cancer; Mesothelioma; Thymoma; Lung Cancer; **Hospital:** Emory Univ Hosp; **Address:** Emory Winship Cancer Inst, 1365 C Clifton Rd NE, Ste 3094, Atlanta, GA 30322; **Phone:** 404-778-5990; **Board Cert:** Internal Medicine 1985; Medical Oncology 1989; **Med School:** South Korea 1975; **Resid:** Internal Medicine, Cook Co Hosp 1985; **Fellow:** Medical Oncology, UT-MD Anderson Cancer Ctr 1988; **Fac Appt:** Prof Hem & Onc, Emory Univ

Sosman, Jeffrey A MD [Onc] - **Spec Exp:** Melanoma; Skin Cancer; Immunotherapy; Drug Discovery; **Hospital:** Vanderbilt Univ Med Ctr (page 75); **Address:** Vanderbilt Hematology/Oncology, 2220 Pierce Ave, 777 Preston Rsch Bldg, Nashville, TN 37232-6307; **Phone:** 615-936-8422; **Board Cert:** Anatomic Pathology 1985; Internal Medicine 1987; Medical Oncology 1989; **Med School:** Albert Einstein Coll Med 1981; **Resid:** Anatomic Pathology, Univ Chicago Hosps 1985; Internal Medicine, Univ Wisconsin Hosp 1986; **Fellow:** Medical Oncology, Univ Wisconsin 1989; **Fac Appt:** Prof Med, Vanderbilt Univ

Sotomayor, Eduardo M MD [Onc] - **Spec Exp:** Lymphoma; Gene Therapy; Vaccine Therapy; Clinical Trials; **Hospital:** H Lee Moffitt Cancer Ctr & Research Inst (page 59); **Address:** H Lee Moffitt Cancer Inst, 12902 Magnolia Drive, FOB 3, rm 5.3125, Tampa, FL 33612; **Phone:** 813-745-3980; **Board Cert:** Medical Oncology 2009; **Med School:** Peru 1988; **Resid:** Internal Medicine, Univ Miami Sch Med 1995; **Fellow:** Immunology, Univ Miami Sch Med 1989; Oncology, Johns Hopkins Hosp 1998; **Fac Appt:** Assoc Prof Med, Univ S Fla Coll Med

Stone, Joel A MD [Onc] - **Spec Exp:** Lung Cancer; Breast Cancer; **Hospital:** St. Vincent's Med Ctr - Riverside (Jacksonville); **Address:** N Florida Hematology/Oncology Assocs, 2 Shircliff Way, Ste 800, Jacksonville, FL 32204; **Phone:** 904-388-2619; **Board Cert:** Internal Medicine 1977; Medical Oncology 1979; **Med School:** Univ VA Sch Med 1974; **Resid:** Internal Medicine, Univ KY Med Ctr 1977; **Fellow:** Hematology & Oncology, Emory Univ Hosp 1979

Sutton, Linda Marie MD [Onc] - **Spec Exp:** Breast Cancer; Palliative Care; **Hospital:** Duke Univ Hosp; **Address:** University Tower, 3100 Tower Blvd, Ste 600, Durham, NC 27707; **Phone:** 919-419-5005; **Board Cert:** Internal Medicine 2002; Medical Oncology 2003; **Med School:** Univ Mass Sch Med 1987; **Resid:** Internal Medicine, Montefiore Med Ctr 1990; **Fellow:** Hematology & Oncology, Duke Univ Med Ctr 1993

Thigpen, James T MD [Onc] - **Spec Exp:** Gynecologic Cancer; Breast Cancer; Lung Cancer; **Hospital:** Univ Mississippi Med Ctr; **Address:** Univ Mississippi Med Ctr, Div Med Onc, 2500 N State St, Jackson, MS 39216; **Phone:** 601-984-5590; **Board Cert:** Internal Medicine 1972; Hematology 1974; Medical Oncology 1975; **Med School:** Univ Miss 1969; **Resid:** Internal Medicine, Univ Miss Med Ctr 1971; **Fellow:** Hematology & Oncology, Univ Miss Med Ctr 1973; **Fac Appt:** Prof Med, Univ Miss

Torti, Frank M MD [Onc] - **Spec Exp:** Prostate Cancer; Urologic Cancer; **Hospital:** Wake Forest Baptist Med Ctr; **Address:** Wake Forest Med Ctr-Comp Cancer Ctr, Medical Center Blvd, Winston-Salem, NC 27157-1082; **Phone:** 336-716-7971; **Board Cert:** Internal Medicine 1978; Medical Oncology 1979; **Med School:** Harvard Med Sch 1974; **Resid:** Internal Medicine, Beth Israel Hosp 1976; **Fellow:** Medical Oncology, Stanford Univ Med Ctr 1979; **Fac Appt:** Prof Med, Wake Forest Univ

Troner, Michael B MD [Onc] - **Spec Exp:** Head & Neck Cancer; Urologic Cancer; **Hospital:** Baptist Hosp of Miami; **Address:** 8940 N Kendall Drive, Ste 300E, Miami, FL 33176; **Phone:** 305-595-2141; **Board Cert:** Internal Medicine 1972; Medical Oncology 1973; **Med School:** SUNY Downstate 1968; **Resid:** Internal Medicine, Univ Maryland Hosp 1971; **Fellow:** Medical Oncology, Univ Miami Med Ctr 1973

Vaughan, William P MD [Onc] - **Spec Exp:** Bone Marrow Transplant; Hematologic Malignancies; **Hospital:** Univ of Ala Hosp at Birmingham; **Address:** 1900 University Blvd, Tinsley Harrison Tower 541, Birmingham, AL 35294-0007; **Phone:** 205-975-0837; **Board Cert:** Internal Medicine 1975; Medical Oncology 1979; **Med School:** Univ Conn 1972; **Resid:** Internal Medicine, Univ Chicago Hosps 1975; **Fellow:** Oncology, Johns Hopkins Hosp 1977; **Fac Appt:** Prof Hem & Onc, Univ Alabama

Vredenburgh, James J MD [Onc] - **Spec Exp:** Brain Tumors; Gliomas; Brain Tumors-Metastatic; **Hospital:** Duke Univ Hosp; **Address:** Peter R Tisch Brain Tumor Ctr, Box 3624, Durham, NC 27710; **Phone:** 919-684-5301; **Board Cert:** Internal Medicine 1986; Hematology 1988; Medical Oncology 1989; **Med School:** Univ VT Coll Med 1983; **Resid:** Internal Medicine, St Francis Med Ctr 1986; **Fellow:** Hematology & Oncology, Dartmouth-Hitchcock Med Ctr 1989; **Fac Appt:** Prof Med, Duke Univ

Waller, Edmund K MD [Onc] - **Spec Exp:** Bone Marrow & Stem Cell Transplant; **Hospital:** Emory Univ Hosp; **Address:** 1365 Clifton Rd NE, C Bldg, Atlanta, GA 30322; **Phone:** 404-778-4342; **Board Cert:** Internal Medicine 1988; Medical Oncology 2006; **Med School:** Cornell Univ-Weill Med Coll 1985; **Resid:** Internal Medicine, Stanford Univ Med Ctr 1988; **Fellow:** Oncology, Stanford Univ Med Ctr 1992; **Fac Appt:** Prof Hem & Onc, Emory Univ

Weber, Jeffrey S MD/PhD [Onc] - **Spec Exp:** Melanoma; **Hospital:** H Lee Moffitt Cancer Ctr & Research Inst (page 59); **Address:** H Lee Moffitt Cancer Ctr, 12902 Magnolia Ave, MS SRB-2, Tampa, FL 33612; **Phone:** 813-745-2691; **Board Cert:** Internal Medicine 1983; Medical Oncology 1987; **Med School:** NYU Sch Med 1980; **Resid:** Internal Medicine, UCSD Med Ctr 1983; **Fellow:** Medical Oncology, Natl Cancer Inst 1990; **Fac Appt:** Assoc Prof Med, USC Sch Med

Medical Oncology

Weiss, Geoffrey R MD [Onc] - **Spec Exp:** Gastrointestinal Cancer; Genitourinary Cancer; Melanoma; **Hospital:** Univ of Virginia Health Sys; **Address:** Univ Virginia Hlth System, Div Hem/Onc, Box 800716, Charlottesville, VA 22908-0716; **Phone:** 434-243-0066; **Board Cert:** Internal Medicine 1977; Medical Oncology 1981; **Med School:** St Louis Univ 1974; **Resid:** Internal Medicine, Temple Univ Hosp 1978; **Fellow:** Medical Oncology, Dana Farber Cancer Inst 1982; **Fac Appt:** Prof Med, Univ VA Sch Med

Wingard, John R MD [Onc] - **Spec Exp:** Bone Marrow Transplant; Leukemia; Multiple Myeloma; Lymphoma; **Hospital:** Shands at Univ of FL; **Address:** Division of Hematology, PO Box 100278, Gainesville, FL 32610; **Phone:** 352-265-0111 x29452; **Board Cert:** Internal Medicine 1976; Medical Oncology 1983; **Med School:** Johns Hopkins Univ 1973; **Resid:** Internal Medicine, Memphis City Hosps 1976; Internal Medicine, VA Hosp 1977; **Fellow:** Medical Oncology, Johns Hopkins Hosp 1979; **Fac Appt:** Prof Med, Univ Fla Coll Med

Yunus, Furhan MD [Onc] - **Spec Exp:** Multiple Myeloma; Lymphoma; **Hospital:** Methodist Univ Hosp - Memphis, Regional Med Ctr - Memphis; **Address:** Univ TN Cancer Inst, 1331 Union Ave, Ste 800, Memphis, TN 38104; **Phone:** 901-725-1785; **Board Cert:** Medical Oncology 2008; **Med School:** Pakistan 1986; **Resid:** Internal Medicine, Methodist Hosp 1993; **Fellow:** Hematology & Oncology, Univ Ariz Coll Med Affil Hosp 1995; **Fac Appt:** Asst Prof Med, Univ Tenn Coll Med

Midwest

Adelstein, David J MD [Onc] - **Spec Exp:** Head & Neck Cancer; Esophageal Cancer; Lung Cancer; **Hospital:** Cleveland Clin (page 55); **Address:** Cleveland Clinic, Taussig Cancer Inst, 9500 Euclid Ave, R35, Cleveland, OH 44195; **Phone:** 216-444-9310; **Board Cert:** Internal Medicine 1978; Medical Oncology 1981; Hematology 1982; **Med School:** NYU Sch Med 1975; **Resid:** Internal Medicine, Univ Hosps Cleveland 1978; **Fellow:** Hematology & Oncology, Univ Hosps Cleveland 1981; **Fac Appt:** Prof Med, Cleveland Cl Coll Med/Case West Res

Albain, Kathy S MD [Onc] - **Spec Exp:** Breast Cancer; Lung Cancer; Cancer Survivors-Late Effects of Therapy; **Hospital:** Loyola Univ Med Ctr; **Address:** Loyola Univ Med Ctr, 2160 S First Ave Bldg 112 - Ste 109, Maywood, IL 60153-5590; **Phone:** 708-327-3102; **Board Cert:** Internal Medicine 1981; Medical Oncology 1983; **Med School:** Univ Mich Med Sch 1978; **Resid:** Internal Medicine, Univ Illinois Med Ctr 1981; **Fellow:** Hematology & Oncology, Univ Chicago 1984; **Fac Appt:** Prof Onc, Loyola Univ-Stritch Sch Med

Albertini, Mark R MD [Onc] - **Spec Exp:** Melanoma; Melanoma-Advanced; Immunotherapy; **Hospital:** Univ WI Hosp & Clins, Wm S Middleton Mem Vet Hosp-Madison; **Address:** 600 Highland Ave, Fl K6, rm 530 CSC, Madison, WI 53792-5669; **Phone:** 608-265-1700; **Board Cert:** Internal Medicine 1987; Medical Oncology 2002; **Med School:** Univ VT Coll Med 1984; **Resid:** Internal Medicine, Univ Wisc Hosps Clins 1987; **Fellow:** Medical Oncology, Univ Wisc Hosps Clins 1991; **Fac Appt:** Assoc Prof Onc, Univ Wisc

Benson III, Al B MD [Onc] - **Spec Exp:** Colon Cancer; Gastrointestinal Cancer; Liver Cancer; Pancreatic Cancer; **Hospital:** Northwestern Meml Hosp, Jesse Brown VA Med Ctr; **Address:** Northwestern Div Hematology/Oncology, 676 N St Clair St, Ste 850, Chicago, IL 60611; **Phone:** 312-695-0990; **Board Cert:** Internal Medicine 1979; Medical Oncology 1983; **Med School:** SUNY Buffalo 1976; **Resid:** Internal Medicine, Univ Wisc Hosps 1979; **Fellow:** Medical Oncology, Univ Wisc Hosps 1984; **Fac Appt:** Prof Onc, Northwestern Univ

Bitran, Jacob D MD [Onc] - **Spec Exp:** Breast Cancer; Bone Marrow Transplant; Lung Cancer; **Hospital:** Adv Luth Genl Hosp; **Address:** Oncology Specialists, 1700 Luther Lane, Park Ridge, IL 60068-1270; **Phone:** 866-611-1991; **Board Cert:** Internal Medicine 1974; Medical Oncology 1977; Hematology 1986; **Med School:** Univ IL Coll Med 1971; **Resid:** Pathology, Rush Presby St Lukes Hosp 1973; Internal Medicine, Michael Reese Hosp 1975; **Fellow:** Hematology & Oncology, Univ Chicago Hosps 1977; **Fac Appt:** Prof Onc, Ros Franklin Univ/Chicago Med Sch

Bolwell, Brian J MD [Onc] - **Spec Exp:** Bone Marrow Transplant; Hematologic Malignancies; **Hospital:** Cleveland Clin (page 55); **Address:** 9500 Euclid Ave, Ste R-32, Desk R32, Cleveland, OH 44195; **Phone:** 216-444-6922; **Board Cert:** Internal Medicine 1985; Medical Oncology 1987; **Med School:** Case West Res Univ 1981; **Resid:** Internal Medicine, Univ Hosp 1984; **Fellow:** Hematology & Oncology, Hosp Univ Penn 1987; **Fac Appt:** Prof Med, Cleveland Cl Coll Med/Case West Res

Bonomi, Philip D MD [Onc] - **Spec Exp:** Lung Cancer; Thymoma; Mesothelioma; **Hospital:** Rush Univ Med Ctr; **Address:** Rush University Medical Center, 1725 W Harrison St, Ste 821, Chicago, IL 60612; **Phone:** 312-942-5904; **Board Cert:** Internal Medicine 1975; Medical Oncology 1977; **Med School:** Univ IL Coll Med 1970; **Resid:** Internal Medicine, Geisinger Med Ctr 1972; Internal Medicine, Geisinger Med Ctr 1975; **Fellow:** Medical Oncology, Rush Presby-St Luke's Med Ctr 1977; **Fac Appt:** Prof Med, Rush Med Coll

Brockstein, Bruce E MD [Onc] - **Spec Exp:** Head & Neck Cancer; Sarcoma; Melanoma; **Hospital:** Evanston/North Shore Univ Hlth Sys, Highland Park/North Shore Univ Hlth Syst; **Address:** North Shore Univ Hlth Sys, Div Hematology/Oncology, 2650 Ridge Ave, rm 4816, Evanston, IL 60201; **Phone:** 847-570-2515; **Board Cert:** Internal Medicine 2003; Medical Oncology 2005; **Med School:** Univ Chicago-Pritzker Sch Med 1990; **Resid:** Internal Medicine, Hosp Univ Penn 1993; **Fellow:** Hematology & Oncology, Univ Chicago Hosps 1996; **Fac Appt:** Assoc Clin Prof Med, Northwestern Univ

Buckner, Jan Craig MD [Onc] - **Spec Exp:** Brain Tumors; Neuro-Oncology; **Hospital:** Mayo Med Ctr & Clin - Rochester; **Address:** Mayo Clinic, 200 First St SW, Rochester, MN 55905; **Phone:** 507-284-4320; **Board Cert:** Internal Medicine 1983; Medical Oncology 1985; **Med School:** Univ NC Sch Med 1980; **Resid:** Internal Medicine, Butterworth Hosp 1983; **Fellow:** Medical Oncology, Mayo Clinic 1985; **Fac Appt:** Prof Med, Mayo Med Sch

Budd, George T MD [Onc] - **Spec Exp:** Breast Cancer; **Hospital:** Cleveland Clin (page 55); **Address:** Cleveland Clinic, Taussig Cancer Ctr, 9500 Euclid Ave, Desk R35, Cleveland, OH 44195; **Phone:** 216-444-6480; **Board Cert:** Internal Medicine 1980; Medical Oncology 1983; **Med School:** Univ Kansas 1977; **Resid:** Internal Medicine, Cleveland Clinic 1980; **Fellow:** Hematology & Oncology, Cleveland Clinic 1982

Carbone, David MD/PhD [Onc] - **Spec Exp:** Lung Cancer; Mesothelioma; Thymoma; **Hospital:** Ohio St Univ Med Ctr; **Address:** 320 W 10th Ave, rm B402, Starling Loving Hall, Columbus, OH 43210; **Phone:** 614-293-6786; **Board Cert:** Internal Medicine 1988; Medical Oncology 2011; **Med School:** Johns Hopkins Univ 1985; **Resid:** Internal Medicine, Johns Hopkins Hosp 1988; **Fellow:** Medical Oncology, Natl Cancer Inst 1991; **Fac Appt:** Prof Med, Ohio State Univ

Chapman, Robert A MD [Onc] - **Spec Exp:** Lung Cancer; **Hospital:** Henry Ford Hosp; **Address:** 2799 W Grand Blvd Fl K13, Detroit, MI 48202; **Phone:** 313-916-1841; **Board Cert:** Internal Medicine 1985; Medical Oncology 1989; **Med School:** Cornell Univ-Weill Med Coll 1976; **Resid:** Internal Medicine, Henry Ford Hosp 1979; **Fellow:** Medical Oncology, Meml Sloan Kettering Cancer Ctr 1981

Medical Oncology

Chitambar, Christopher R MD [Onc] - **Spec Exp:** Lymphoma; Leukemia; Breast Cancer; **Hospital:** Froedtert and Med Ctr of WI; **Address:** Div Neoplastic Disease, 9200 W Wisconsin Ave, Milwaukee, WI 53226-3522; **Phone:** 414-805-4600; **Board Cert:** Internal Medicine 1980; Hematology 1982; Medical Oncology 1983; **Med School:** India 1977; **Resid:** Internal Medicine, Brackenridge Hosp 1980; **Fellow:** Hematology & Oncology, Univ CO Hlth Sci Ctr 1983; **Fac Appt:** Prof Med, Med Coll Wisc

Clamon, Gerald H MD [Onc] - **Spec Exp:** Lung Cancer; Palliative Care; **Hospital:** Univ Iowa Hosp & Clinics; **Address:** Holden Comprehensive Cancer Ctr, Med Onc, 200 Hawkins Drive, Ste C32GH, Iowa City, IA 52242; **Phone:** 319-384-8442; **Board Cert:** Internal Medicine 1976; Medical Oncology 1979; **Med School:** Washington Univ, St Louis 1971; **Resid:** Internal Medicine, Barnes Hosp 1976; **Fellow:** Research, Natl Cancer Inst 1974; Medical Oncology, Univ Iowa Hosp & Clinics 1977; **Fac Appt:** Prof Med, Univ Iowa Coll Med

Clark, Joseph I MD [Onc] - **Spec Exp:** Kidney Cancer; Melanoma; Head & Neck Cancer; **Hospital:** Loyola Univ Med Ctr, Edward Hines, Jr. VA Hosp; **Address:** Cardinal Bernardin Cancer Ctr, Loyola Univ Med Ctr, 2160 S 1st Ave, rm 346, Maywood, IL 60153-5500; **Phone:** 708-327-3217; **Board Cert:** Internal Medicine 2002; Medical Oncology 2006; **Med School:** Loyola Univ-Stritch Sch Med 1989; **Resid:** Internal Medicine, Loyola Univ Med Ctr/Hines VA Hosp 1992; **Fellow:** Hematology & Oncology, Fox Chase Cancer Ctr/Temple Univ Hosp 1995; **Fac Appt:** Prof Med, Loyola Univ-Stritch Sch Med

Cleary, James F MD [Onc] - **Spec Exp:** Palliative Care; Head & Neck Cancer; **Hospital:** Univ WI Hosp & Clins; **Address:** 600 Highland Ave CSC Bldg - rm k6/546, Madison, WI 53792; **Phone:** 608-262-5223; **Board Cert:** Hospice & Palliative Medicine 2011; **Med School:** Australia 1984; **Resid:** Internal Medicine, Royal Adelaide Hosp 1987; **Fellow:** Medical Oncology, Royal Adelaide Hosp 1990; **Fac Appt:** Assoc Prof Med, Univ Wisc

Clinton, Steven K MD/PhD [Onc] - **Spec Exp:** Genitourinary Cancer; Prostate Cancer; Nutrition & Cancer Prevention/Control; **Hospital:** Ohio St Univ Med Ctr; **Address:** 320 W 10th Ave, rm 456 SL, Columbus, OH 43210; **Phone:** 614-293-7560; **Board Cert:** Internal Medicine 1987; **Med School:** Univ IL Coll Med 1984; **Resid:** Internal Medicine, Univ Chicago Hosps 1987; **Fellow:** Medical Oncology, Dana Farber Cancer Inst/Harvard 1991; **Fac Appt:** Prof Med, Ohio State Univ

Cobleigh, Melody A MD [Onc] - **Spec Exp:** Breast Cancer; **Hospital:** Rush Univ Med Ctr; **Address:** Rush Univ Med Ctr, 1725 W Harrison St, Ste 821, Chicago, IL 60612-3828; **Phone:** 312-942-5904; **Board Cert:** Internal Medicine 1979; Medical Oncology 1981; **Med School:** Rush Med Coll 1976; **Resid:** Internal Medicine, Rush Presby-St Lukes Med Ctr 1979; **Fellow:** Medical Oncology, Indiana Univ 1981; **Fac Appt:** Prof Med, Rush Med Coll

Cooney, Kathleen A MD [Onc] - **Hospital:** Univ of Michigan Hosp; **Address:** U of M Internal Medicine Oncology, Cancer Center Floor B1 Reception D, 1500 E Medical Center Dr SPC 5913, Ann Arbor, MI 48109; **Phone:** 734-647-8903; **Board Cert:** Internal Medicine 1987; Medical Oncology 2001; **Med School:** Univ Pennsylvania 1984; **Resid:** Internal Medicine, U Mich Hosps 1987; Internal Medicine, U Mich Hosps 1988; **Fellow:** Hematology & Oncology, U Mich Hosps 1991; **Fac Appt:** Prof U, Univ Mich Med Sch

Dowlati, Afshin MD [Onc] - **Spec Exp:** Lung Cancer; Thoracic Cancers; **Hospital:** Univ Hosps Case Med Ctr (page 74); **Address:** UH Seidman Cancer Center, 11100 Euclid Ave, Cleveland, OH 44106; **Phone:** 216-844-1228; **Board Cert:** Internal Medicine 2010; Medical Oncology 2011; **Med School:** Belgium 1992; **Resid:** Internal Medicine, U Liege 1996; **Fellow:** Hematology & Oncology, Case Western/Univ Hosps 1998; **Fac Appt:** Assoc Prof Med, Case West Res Univ

Dreicer, Robert MD [Onc] - **Spec Exp:** Prostate Cancer; Kidney Cancer; Bladder Cancer; Testicular Cancer; **Hospital:** Cleveland Clin (page 55); **Address:** 9500 Euclid Ave, Desk R35, MS R35, 9500 Euclid Ave, Desk R35 Ave, Cleveland, OH 44195; **Phone:** 216-445-4623; **Board Cert:** Internal Medicine 1986; Medical Oncology 1989; **Med School:** Univ Tex, Houston 1983; **Resid:** Internal Medicine, Ind Univ Med Ctr 1986; **Fellow:** Medical Oncology, Univ Wisconsin Hosp 1989; **Fac Appt:** Prof Med, Cleveland Cl Coll Med/Case West Res

Einhorn, Lawrence H MD [Onc] - **Spec Exp:** Testicular Cancer; Lung Cancer; Urologic Cancer; **Hospital:** IU Health University Hosp; **Address:** IU Simon Cancer Center, 535 Barnhill Drive Fl 2, Indianapolis, IN 46202; **Phone:** 317-944-0920; **Board Cert:** Internal Medicine 1972; Medical Oncology 1975; **Med School:** UCLA 1967; **Resid:** Internal Medicine, Indiana Univ Hosp 1969; **Fellow:** Hematology & Oncology, Indiana Univ 1972; Hematology & Oncology, MD Anderson Cancer Ctr 1973; **Fac Appt:** Prof Med, Indiana Univ

Ellis, Matthew J MD/PhD [Onc] - **Spec Exp:** Breast Cancer; **Hospital:** Barnes-Jewish Hosp; **Address:** Washington University, 660 S Euclid Ave, Box 8056, St Louis, MO 63110; **Phone:** 314-747-1171; **Board Cert:** Internal Medicine 2004; Medical Oncology 2005; **Med School:** England, UK 1984; **Resid:** Internal Medicine, Hammersmith Hosp 1988; **Fellow:** Research, Georgetown Univ Med Ctr 1992; Medical Oncology, Georgetwon Univ Med Ctr 1994; **Fac Appt:** Prof Med, Washington Univ, St Louis

Ensminger, William D MD/PhD [Onc] - **Spec Exp:** Gastrointestinal Cancer; Liver Cancer; Clinical Trials; **Hospital:** Univ of Michigan Hosp; **Address:** 1050 E Med Ctr Drive Fl B1, Ann Arbor, MI 48109-5633; **Phone:** 734-647-8902; **Board Cert:** Internal Medicine 1976; Medical Oncology 1979; **Med School:** Harvard Med Sch 1973; **Resid:** Internal Medicine, Beth Israel Hosp 1975; **Fellow:** Medical Oncology, Dana Farber Cancer Inst 1977; **Fac Appt:** Prof Med, Univ Mich Med Sch

Fleming, Gini F MD [Onc] - **Spec Exp:** Breast Cancer-Novel Therapies; Gynecologic Cancer; Ovarian Cancer; **Hospital:** Univ of Chicago Med Ctr; **Address:** Univ Chicago Hosps, 5841 S Maryland MC2115, Chicago, IL 60637-1470; **Phone:** 773-702-6149; **Board Cert:** Internal Medicine 1988; Medical Oncology 2012; Hematology 2002; **Med School:** Univ IL Coll Med 1985; **Resid:** Internal Medicine, Univ Chicago Hosps 1988; **Fellow:** Hematology & Oncology, Univ Chicago Hosps 1992; **Fac Appt:** Prof Med, Univ Chicago-Pritzker Sch Med

Gaynor, Ellen MD [Onc] - **Spec Exp:** Breast Cancer; Gastrointestinal Cancer; Prostate Cancer; **Hospital:** Loyola Univ Med Ctr; **Address:** Loyola Bernardin Cancer Center, 2160 S First Ave Bldg 112 - rm 108, Maywood, IL 60153-3328; **Phone:** 708-327-3214; **Board Cert:** Internal Medicine 1982; Hematology 1986; Medical Oncology 1985; **Med School:** Univ Wisc 1978; **Resid:** Internal Medicine, Loyola Univ Med Ctr 1982; **Fellow:** Medical Oncology, Loyola Univ Med Ctr 1981; Hematology & Oncology, Univ Chicago 1984; **Fac Appt:** Prof Med, Loyola Univ-Stritch Sch Med

Gerson, Stanton L MD [Onc] - **Spec Exp:** Leukemia; Lymphoma, Non-Hodgkin's; Stem Cell Transplant; Multiple Myeloma; **Hospital:** Univ Hosps Case Med Ctr (page 74); **Address:** Seidman Cancer Ctr, 11000 Euclid Ave, Wearn Bldg, rm 151, MS 5065, Cleveland, OH 44106-5065; **Phone:** 216-844-1232; **Board Cert:** Internal Medicine 1980; Hematology 1982; Medical Oncology 1983; **Med School:** Harvard Med Sch 1977; **Resid:** Internal Medicine, Hosp Univ Penn 1980; **Fellow:** Hematology & Oncology, Hosp Univ Penn 1983; **Fac Appt:** Prof Hem & Onc, Case West Res Univ

Goldberg, Richard M MD [Onc] - **Spec Exp:** Colon & Rectal Cancer; Neuroendocrine Tumors; Gastrointestinal Cancer; Anal Cancer; **Hospital:** Ohio St Univ Med Ctr; **Address:** 300 W Tenth Ave, Ste 519, Columbus, OH 43210; **Phone:** 614-366-6355; **Board Cert:** Internal Medicine 1982; Medical Oncology 1985; **Med School:** SUNY Upstate Med Univ 1979; **Resid:** Internal Medicine, Emory Univ Med Ctr 1982; **Fellow:** Medical Oncology, Georgetown Univ Med Ctr 1984; **Fac Appt:** Prof Med, Ohio State Univ

Medical Oncology

Golomb, Harvey M MD [Onc] - **Spec Exp:** Lung Cancer; Leukemia; Lymphoma; **Hospital:** Univ of Chicago Med Ctr; **Address:** Univ Chicago Medical Ctr, 5841 S Maryland Ave, MC 2115, Chicago, IL 60637-1463; **Phone:** 773-702-3670; **Board Cert:** Internal Medicine 1975; Medical Oncology 1979; **Med School:** Univ Pittsburgh 1968; **Resid:** Internal Medicine, Johns Hopkins Hosp 1972; Clinical Genetics, Johns Hopkins Hosp 1973; **Fellow:** Hematology & Oncology, Univ Chicago Hosps 1975; **Fac Appt:** Prof Med, Univ Chicago-Pritzker Sch Med

Gradishar, William J MD [Onc] - **Spec Exp:** Breast Cancer; **Hospital:** Northwestern Meml Hosp; **Address:** 250 E Superior St, Ste 420, Chicago, IL 60611; **Phone:** 312-695-0990; **Board Cert:** Internal Medicine 1985; Medical Oncology 1989; **Med School:** Univ IL Coll Med 1982; **Resid:** Internal Medicine, Michael Reese Hosp 1985; **Fellow:** Hematology & Oncology, Univ Chicago Hosps 1990; **Fac Appt:** Prof Med, Northwestern Univ

Hayes, Daniel F MD [Onc] - **Spec Exp:** Breast Cancer; **Hospital:** Univ of Michigan Hosp; **Address:** Univ Michigan Comprehensive Cancer Ctr, 1500 E Medical Ctr Drive, Ste SPC 5916, Ann Arbor, MI 48109-5942; **Phone:** 734-936-6000; **Board Cert:** Internal Medicine 1982; Medical Oncology 1985; **Med School:** Indiana Univ 1979; **Resid:** Internal Medicine, Parkland Meml Hosp 1982; **Fellow:** Medical Oncology, Dana Farber Cancer Inst 1985; **Fac Appt:** Prof Med, Univ Mich Med Sch

Hoffman, Philip C MD [Onc] - **Spec Exp:** Lung Cancer; Breast Cancer; **Hospital:** Univ of Chicago Med Ctr, Little Company of Mary Hosp & Hlth Care Ctrs; **Address:** 5841 S Maryland Ave, MC 2115, Chicago, IL 60637-1447; **Phone:** 773-834-7424; **Board Cert:** Internal Medicine 1975; Hematology 1980; Medical Oncology 1981; **Med School:** Jefferson Med Coll 1972; **Resid:** Internal Medicine, Hosp Univ Penn 1975; **Fellow:** Hematology & Oncology, Univ Chicago Hosps 1980; **Fac Appt:** Prof Med, Univ Chicago-Pritzker Sch Med

Hussain, Maha H MD [Onc] - **Spec Exp:** Prostate Cancer; Bladder Cancer; Testicular Cancer; Genitourinary Cancer; **Hospital:** Univ of Michigan Hosp; **Address:** Univ Michigan Cancer Ctr, 1500 E Medical Ctr Drive, rm 7310, Ann Arbor, MI 48109; **Phone:** 734-936-8903; **Board Cert:** Internal Medicine 1986; Medical Oncology 1989; **Med School:** Iraq 1980; **Resid:** Internal Medicine, Wayne State Univ Affil Hosps 1986; **Fellow:** Medical Oncology, Wayne State Univ Affil Hosps 1989; **Fac Appt:** Prof Med, Univ Mich Med Sch

Ingle, James N MD [Onc] - **Spec Exp:** Breast Cancer; **Hospital:** Mayo Med Ctr & Clin - Rochester, Rochester Methodist Hosp; **Address:** Mayo Clinic, 200 First St SW, Gonda Bldg Fl 10, Rochester, MN 55905-0001; **Phone:** 507-284-4857; **Board Cert:** Internal Medicine 1974; Medical Oncology 1975; **Med School:** Johns Hopkins Univ 1971; **Resid:** Internal Medicine, Johns Hopkins Hosp 1976; Medical Oncology, Natl Cancer Inst 1975; **Fac Appt:** Prof Hem & Onc, Mayo Med Sch

Kalaycio, Matt E MD [Onc] - **Spec Exp:** Leukemia; Bone Marrow Transplant; **Hospital:** Cleveland Clin (page 55); **Address:** Taussig Cancer Ctr, 9500 Euclid Ave, Desk R35, Cleveland, OH 44195; **Phone:** 216-444-3705; **Board Cert:** Internal Medicine 2002; Hematology 2004; Medical Oncology 2005; **Med School:** W VA Univ 1988; **Resid:** Internal Medicine, Mercy Hosp 1991; **Fellow:** Hematology & Oncology, Cleveland Clinic 1994; **Fac Appt:** Prof Med, Cleveland Cl Coll Med/Case West Res

Kalemkerian, Gregory P MD [Onc] - **Spec Exp:** Lung Cancer; Mesothelioma; Thymoma; **Hospital:** Univ of Michigan Hosp; **Address:** 1500 E Medical Center Drive, C350 Med Inn - SPC 5848, Ann Arbor, MI 48109-0848; **Phone:** 734-232-6046; **Board Cert:** Internal Medicine 1988; Medical Oncology 2011; **Med School:** Northwestern Univ 1985; **Resid:** Internal Medicine, Northwestern Meml Hosp 1988; **Fellow:** Medical Oncology, Johns Hopkins Hosp 1993; **Fac Appt:** Prof Onc, Univ Mich Med Sch

Kaminski, Mark S MD [Onc] - **Spec Exp:** Lymphoma; Bone Marrow Transplant; Drug Development; Clinical Trials; **Hospital:** Univ of Michigan Hosp; **Address:** Univ Michigan Cancer Ctr, 1500 E Medical Ctr Drive, Reception B, B1-358; Ann Arbor, MI 48109; **Phone:** 734-647-8901; **Board Cert:** Internal Medicine 1981; Medical Oncology 1983; **Med School:** Stanford Univ 1978; **Resid:** Internal Medicine, Barnes Hosp 1981; **Fellow:** Medical Oncology, Stanford Univ Med Ctr 1985; **Fac Appt:** Prof Med, Univ Mich Med Sch

Kindler, Hedy Lee MD [Onc] - **Spec Exp:** Pancreatic Cancer; Mesothelioma; Gastrointestinal Cancer; **Hospital:** Univ of Chicago Med Ctr; **Address:** Univ of Chicago Medical Ctr, 5841 S Maryland Ave, Chicago, IL 60637-1470; **Phone:** 773-702-4400; **Board Cert:** Internal Medicine 2002; Medical Oncology 2005; **Med School:** SUNY Buffalo 1985; **Resid:** Internal Medicine, UCLA Med Ctr 1992; **Fellow:** Medical Oncology, Meml Sloan Kettering Cancer Ctr 1995; **Fac Appt:** Assoc Prof Onc, Univ Chicago-Pritzker Sch Med

Krishnamurthi, Smitha S MD [Onc] - **Spec Exp:** Gastrointestinal Cancer; Colon & Rectal Cancer; **Hospital:** Univ Hosps Case Med Ctr (page 74); **Address:** UH Case Medical Center, Seidman Cancer Center, 11100 Euclid Ave, Cleveland, OH 44106; **Phone:** 216-844-1006; **Board Cert:** Internal Medicine 2006; Medical Oncology 2008; **Med School:** Univ Pennsylvania 1993; **Resid:** Internal Medicine, Univ Penn Affil Hosps 1996; **Fellow:** Medical Oncology, Johns Hopkins Hosp 1996; **Fac Appt:** Asst Prof Med, Case West Res Univ

Kuzel, Timothy M MD [Onc] - **Spec Exp:** Kidney Cancer; Melanoma; Cutaneous Lymphoma; **Hospital:** Northwestern Meml Hosp; **Address:** 676 N St. Clair, Ste 850, MS 60521, Chicago, IL 60611; **Phone:** 312-695-0990; **Board Cert:** Internal Medicine 1987; Hematology 2010; Medical Oncology 1989; **Med School:** Univ Mich Med Sch 1984; **Resid:** Internal Medicine, McGraw MC-Northwestern Univ 1987; **Fellow:** Hematology & Oncology, McGraw MC-Northwestern Univ 1990; **Fac Appt:** Prof Med, Northwestern Univ

Lazarus, Hillard M MD [Onc] - **Spec Exp:** Bone Marrow & Stem Cell Transplant; Leukemia & Lymphoma; Multiple Myeloma; **Hospital:** Univ Hosps Case Med Ctr (page 74); **Address:** 11100 Euclid Ave, Wearn Bldg - Fl 3rd, rm 341, Cleveland, OH 44106-5065; **Phone:** 216-844-3629; **Board Cert:** Internal Medicine 1977; Medical Oncology 1979; Hematology 1980; **Med School:** Univ Rochester 1974; **Resid:** Internal Medicine, Univ Hosps 1977; **Fellow:** Hematology & Oncology, Univ Hosps 1979; **Fac Appt:** Prof Onc, Case West Res Univ

Loehrer, Patrick J MD [Onc] - **Spec Exp:** Thymoma; Genitourinary Cancer; Pancreatic Cancer; Esophageal Cancer; **Hospital:** IU Health University Hosp; **Address:** IU Simon Cancer Center, 535 Barnhill Drive Fl 2, Indianapolis, IN 46202; **Phone:** 317-944-0920; **Board Cert:** Internal Medicine 1981; Medical Oncology 2006; **Med School:** Rush Med Coll 1978; **Resid:** Internal Medicine, Rush-Presby-St Lukes Hosp 1981; **Fellow:** Medical Oncology, Indiana Univ 1983; **Fac Appt:** Prof Med, Indiana Univ

Loprinzi, Charles L MD [Onc] - **Spec Exp:** Breast Cancer; **Hospital:** Mayo Med Ctr & Clin - Rochester; **Address:** Mayo Clinic, Dept Med Oncology, 200 First St SW, Rochester, MN 55905-0001; **Phone:** 507-284-4849; **Board Cert:** Internal Medicine 1982; Medical Oncology 1985; **Med School:** Oregon Hlth & Sci Univ 1979; **Resid:** Internal Medicine, Maricopa Co Hosp 1982; **Fellow:** Medical Oncology, Univ Wisconsin Med Ctr 1984; **Fac Appt:** Prof Med, Mayo Med Sch

Markowitz, Sanford D MD [Onc] - **Spec Exp:** Colon & Rectal Cancer; Hereditary Cancer; **Hospital:** Univ Hosps Case Med Ctr (page 74); **Address:** Ireland Cancer Ctr, 10900 Euclid Ave, Cleveland, OH 44106-7285; **Phone:** 216-844-3951; **Board Cert:** Internal Medicine 1984; Medical Oncology 1987; **Med School:** Yale Univ 1980; **Resid:** Internal Medicine, Univ Chicago Hosp 1984; **Fellow:** Medical Oncology, Natl Cancer Inst 1986; **Fac Appt:** Prof Med, Case West Res Univ

Meropol, Neal J MD [Onc] - **Spec Exp:** Gastrointestinal Cancer; Colon Cancer; Pancreatic Cancer; **Hospital:** Univ Hosps Case Med Ctr (page 74); **Address:** 11100 Euclid Ave, Wearn Bldg, rm 145, Cleveland, OH 44106; **Phone:** 216-983-4752; **Board Cert:** Internal Medicine 1988; Medical Oncology 2011; **Med School:** Vanderbilt Univ 1985; **Resid:** Internal Medicine, Univ Hosps/Case West Res 1988; **Fellow:** Hematology & Oncology, Hosp Univ Penn 1992; **Fac Appt:** Prof Onc, Case West Res Univ

O'Brien, Timothy E MD [Onc] - **Spec Exp:** Gastrointestinal Cancer; Colon & Rectal Cancer; Multiple Myeloma; Lung Cancer; **Hospital:** MetroHealth Med Ctr; **Address:** MetroHealth Cancer Care Ctr, 2500 MetroHealth Drive, Ste C-2100, Cleveland, OH 44109-1998; **Phone:** 216-778-5802; **Board Cert:** Medical Oncology 2007; Hematology 2008; **Med School:** Univ Rochester 1989; **Resid:** Internal Medicine, Univ Hosps Cleveland 1992; **Fellow:** Hematology & Oncology, Univ Hosps Cleveland 1997; **Fac Appt:** Assoc Prof Med, Case West Res Univ

Olopade, Olufunmilayo I MD [Onc] - **Spec Exp:** Breast Cancer; Hereditary Cancer; Breast Cancer Genetics; Cancer Risk Assessment; **Hospital:** Univ of Chicago Med Ctr; **Address:** Univ Chicago Med Ctr, 5841 S Maryland Ave, MC 2115, Chicago, IL 60637-1470; **Phone:** 773-702-6149; **Board Cert:** Internal Medicine 1986; Medical Oncology 1989; **Med School:** Nigeria 1980; **Resid:** Internal Medicine, Cook Co Hosp 1986; **Fellow:** Hematology & Oncology, Univ Chicago Hosps 1991; **Fac Appt:** Prof Med, Univ Chicago-Pritzker Sch Med

Ozer, Howard MD [Onc] - **Spec Exp:** Lymphoma; **Hospital:** Univ of IL Med Ctr at Chicago; **Address:** Univ Illinois Med Ctr, Dept Onc, 1818 W Taylor St, Ste 1E, Chicago, IL 60612; **Phone:** 312-355-1625; **Board Cert:** Internal Medicine 1979; **Med School:** Yale Univ 1975; **Resid:** Internal Medicine, Mass Genl Hosp 1977; **Fellow:** Hematology & Oncology, PB Brigham/Dana Farber Cancer Inst 1979; **Fac Appt:** Prof Med, Univ IL Coll Med

Peace, David J MD [Onc] - **Spec Exp:** Prostate Cancer; Vaccine Therapy; Leukemia & Lymphoma; Immunotherapy; **Hospital:** Univ of IL Med Ctr at Chicago, MacNeal Hosp; **Address:** 840 S Wood St, CSB Bldg, Ste 820, Chicago, IL 60607; **Phone:** 312-413-1507; **Board Cert:** Internal Medicine 1983; Medical Oncology 1987; **Med School:** Univ Pittsburgh 1980; **Resid:** Internal Medicine, Univ Pittsburgh Med Ctr 1983; **Fellow:** Hematology & Oncology, Univ Washington Med Ctr 1988

Peereboom, David M MD [Onc] - **Spec Exp:** Neuro-Oncology; Brain Tumors; Drug Development; **Hospital:** Cleveland Clin (page 55); **Address:** Cleveland Clinic Taussig Cancer Ctr, 9500 Euclid Ave, Cleveland, OH 44195; **Phone:** 216-445-6068; **Board Cert:** Internal Medicine 1989; Medical Oncology 2004; **Med School:** Med Coll VA 1986; **Resid:** Internal Medicine, Univ Hosp of Cleveland 1990; **Fellow:** Medical Oncology, Johns Hopkins Hosp 1993; **Fac Appt:** Assoc Prof Onc, Cleveland Cl Coll Med/Case West Res

Peterson, Bruce MD [Onc] - **Spec Exp:** Lymphoma; Leukemia; **Hospital:** Univ Minn Med Ctr, Fairview - Riverside Campus; **Address:** Univ of Minnesota, 424 Harvard St, Minneapolis, MN 55455; **Phone:** 612-625-5411; **Board Cert:** Internal Medicine 1974; Medical Oncology 1977; **Med School:** Univ Minn 1971; **Resid:** Internal Medicine, Fletcher Allen Hlthcare 1973; Internal Medicine, Fairview-Univ Med Ctr 1974; **Fellow:** Medical Oncology, Fairview-Univ Med Ctr 1977; **Fac Appt:** Prof Med, Univ Minn

Petruska, Paul J MD [Onc] - **Spec Exp:** Leukemia & Lymphoma; Solid Tumors; **Hospital:** St. Louis Univ Hosp; **Address:** SLU, Dept Hem/Onc, 3655 Vista Ave, St Louis, MO 63110; **Phone:** 314-577-6057; **Board Cert:** Internal Medicine 1972; Hematology 1974; Medical Oncology 1979; **Med School:** St Louis Univ 1967; **Resid:** Internal Medicine, St. Louis Hosp 1969; Internal Medicine, St. Louis Hosp 1972; **Fellow:** Hematology & Oncology, St. Louis Hosp 1974; **Fac Appt:** Prof Med, St Louis Univ

Pienta, Kenneth J MD [Onc] - **Spec Exp:** Prostate Cancer; **Hospital:** Univ of Michigan Hosp; **Address:** 1500 E Med Ctr Drive, rm 7303 CCC, Ann Arbor, MI 48109-5946; **Phone:** 734-647-8903; **Board Cert:** Medical Oncology 2011; **Med School:** Johns Hopkins Univ 1986; **Resid:** Internal Medicine, Univ Chicago Hosps 1988; **Fellow:** Medical Oncology, Johns Hopkins Hosp 1991; **Fac Appt:** Prof Med, Univ Mich Med Sch

Pohlman, Brad L MD [Onc] - **Spec Exp:** Lymphoma; Lymphoma, Non-Hodgkin's; Bone Marrow Transplant; **Hospital:** Cleveland Clin (page 55); **Address:** Cleveland Clinic Fdn, 9500 Euclid Ave, Desk R35, Cleveland, OH 44195; **Phone:** 216-444-6070; **Board Cert:** Internal Medicine 1988; **Med School:** Indiana Univ 1985; **Resid:** Internal Medicine, Univ Wisconsin Hosp 1988; **Fellow:** Hematology, Univ Minnesota Hosp 1992

Ratain, Mark J MD [Onc] - **Spec Exp:** Solid Tumors; Drug Discovery & Development; **Hospital:** Univ of Chicago Med Ctr; **Address:** Univ Chicago Med Ctr, 5841 S Maryland Ave, MC 2115, Chicago, IL 60637; **Phone:** 773-702-6149; **Board Cert:** Internal Medicine 1983; Hematology 1986; Medical Oncology 1985; **Med School:** Yale Univ 1980; **Resid:** Internal Medicine, Johns Hopkins Hosp 1983; **Fellow:** Hematology & Oncology, Univ Chicago 1986; **Fac Appt:** Prof Med, Univ Chicago-Pritzker Sch Med

Richards, Jon M MD/PhD [Onc] - **Spec Exp:** Melanoma; **Hospital:** Adv Luth Genl Hosp, Skokie/North Shore Univ Htlh Syst; **Address:** Center for Advanced Care, 1700 Luther Ln Fl 2, Park Ridge, IL 60068; **Phone:** 847-268-8200; **Board Cert:** Medical Oncology 2007; **Med School:** Cornell Univ 1983; **Resid:** Internal Medicine, Univ Chicago Hosps 1985; **Fellow:** Hematology & Oncology, Univ Chicago Hosps 1988; **Fac Appt:** Assoc Prof Med, Univ IL Coll Med

Rosen, Steven T MD [Onc] - **Spec Exp:** Hematologic Malignancies; Breast Cancer; Leukemia & Lymphoma; **Hospital:** Northwestern Meml Hosp; **Address:** Northwestern Univ, 675 N St Clair St, Galter 21-100, Chicago, IL 60611; **Phone:** 312-695-0990; **Board Cert:** Internal Medicine 1979; Medical Oncology 1981; Hematology 1984; **Med School:** Northwestern Univ 1976; **Resid:** Internal Medicine, Northwestern Univ Hosp 1979; **Fellow:** Medical Oncology, Natl Cancer Inst 1981; **Fac Appt:** Prof Med, Northwestern Univ

Roth, Bruce J MD [Onc] - **Spec Exp:** Prostate Cancer; Bladder Cancer; Testicular Cancer; **Hospital:** Barnes-Jewish Hosp; **Address:** Washington University, 660 S Euclid Ave, Box 8056, St Louis, MO 63110; **Phone:** 314-747-1171; **Board Cert:** Internal Medicine 1983; Medical Oncology 1985; **Med School:** St Louis Univ 1980; **Resid:** Internal Medicine, Indiana Univ Med Ctr 1983; **Fellow:** Hematology & Oncology, Indiana Univ Med Ctr 1986; **Fac Appt:** Prof Med, Washington Univ, St Louis

Salgia, Ravi MD/PhD [Onc] - **Spec Exp:** Lung Cancer; Mesothelioma; Thoracic Cancers; **Hospital:** Univ of Chicago Med Ctr; **Address:** Univ Chicago Medical Ctr, 5841 S Maryland Ave, MC 2115, Chicago, IL 60637; **Phone:** 773-702-6149; **Board Cert:** Medical Oncology 2006; **Med School:** Loyola Univ-Stritch Sch Med 1987; **Resid:** Internal Medicine, Johns Hopkins Hosp 1990; **Fellow:** Medical Oncology, Dana-Farber Cancer Inst 1993; **Fac Appt:** Prof Med, Univ Chicago-Pritzker Sch Med

Schiffer, Charles A MD [Onc] - **Spec Exp:** Leukemia; Lymphoma; Multiple Myeloma; **Hospital:** Barbara Ann Karmanos Cancer Inst, Harper Univ Hosp; **Address:** Karmanos Cancer Inst, Cancer Research Ctr, 4100 John R St, Detroit, MI 48201; **Phone:** 800-527-6266; **Board Cert:** Internal Medicine 1972; Medical Oncology 1973; **Med School:** NYU Sch Med 1968; **Resid:** Internal Medicine, Bellevue-NY VA Hosp-NYU 1972; **Fellow:** Medical Oncology, Natl Cancer Inst 1974; **Fac Appt:** Prof Med, Wayne State Univ

Medical Oncology

Schilsky, Richard L MD [Onc] - **Spec Exp:** Gastrointestinal Cancer; Pancreatic Cancer; Drug Development; **Hospital:** Univ of Chicago Med Ctr; **Address:** Univ Chicago Med Ctr, 5841 S Maryland Ave, MC 2115, Chicago, IL 60637; **Phone:** 773-702-6149; **Board Cert:** Internal Medicine 1978; Medical Oncology 1979; **Med School:** Univ Chicago-Pritzker Sch Med 1975; **Resid:** Internal Medicine, Univ Texas 1977; **Fellow:** Medical Oncology, Natl Cancer Inst 1980; **Fac Appt:** Prof Med, Univ Chicago-Pritzker Sch Med

Schwartz, Burton S MD [Onc] - **Spec Exp:** Lymphoma; Breast Cancer; **Hospital:** Abbott - Northwestern Hosp; **Address:** 910 E 26th St, Ste 200, Minneapolis, MN 55404; **Phone:** 612-884-6300; **Board Cert:** Internal Medicine 1980; Hematology 1976; Medical Oncology 1977; **Med School:** Meharry Med Coll 1968; **Resid:** Internal Medicine, Michael Reese Hosp 1971; **Fellow:** Hematology, Univ Minn Hosp 1976; **Fac Appt:** Clin Prof Med, Univ Minn

Shapiro, Charles L MD [Onc] - **Spec Exp:** Breast Cancer; **Hospital:** Arthur G James Cancer Hosp & Research Inst; **Address:** 1145 Olentangy River Rd Fl 4, Columbus, OH 43212; **Phone:** 614-293-0066; **Board Cert:** Internal Medicine 1987; Medical Oncology 2005; **Med School:** SUNY Buffalo 1984; **Resid:** Internal Medicine, Temple Univ Hosp 1987; **Fellow:** Medical Oncology, Dana Farber Cancer Inst 1991; **Fac Appt:** Assoc Prof Med, Ohio State Univ

Shields, Peter G MD [Onc] - **Spec Exp:** Hematologic Malignancies; **Hospital:** Ohio St Univ Med Ctr; **Address:** Ohio State Univ Med Ctr, 300 W 10th Ave, Ste 519, Columbus, OH 43201; **Phone:** 614-688-6563; **Board Cert:** Medical Oncology 1989; **Med School:** Mount Sinai Sch Med 1983; **Resid:** Internal Medicine, George Washington Univ Hosp 1986; **Fellow:** Hematology & Oncology, George Washington Univ Hosp 1990; **Fac Appt:** Prof Med, Georgetown Univ

Silver, Samuel M MD/PhD [Onc] - **Spec Exp:** Hematologic Malignancies; Bleeding/Coagulation Disorders; Porphyria; Myeloproliferative Disorders; **Hospital:** Univ of Michigan Hosp; **Address:** Univ Michigan Med Ctr/Cancer Ctr, 4101 Med Sci I C- Wing, 1301 Catherine St, Ann Arbor, MI 48109-5624; **Phone:** 734-764-2204; **Board Cert:** Internal Medicine 1982; Medical Oncology 1985; Hematology 1984; **Med School:** Cornell Univ-Weill Med Coll 1979; **Resid:** Internal Medicine, UCSF-Moffit Hosp 1982; **Fellow:** Hematology & Oncology, Hosp Univ Penn 1985; **Fac Appt:** Clin Prof Onc, Univ Mich Med Sch

Silverman, Paula MD [Onc] - **Spec Exp:** Breast Cancer; **Hospital:** Univ Hosps Case Med Ctr (page 74), UH Ahuja Med Ctr (OH) (page 74); **Address:** 11100 Euclid Ave, Cleveland, OH 44106; **Phone:** 216-844-8510; **Board Cert:** Internal Medicine 1984; Medical Oncology 1989; **Med School:** Case West Res Univ 1981; **Resid:** Internal Medicine, Univ Hosps 1984; **Fellow:** Hematology & Oncology, Case Western Reserve Univ 1987; **Fac Appt:** Assoc Prof Med, Case West Res Univ

Sledge Jr, George W MD [Onc] - **Spec Exp:** Breast Cancer; **Hospital:** IU Health University Hosp, IU Health North Hosp; **Address:** IU Simon Cancer Ctr, 535 Barnhill Drive Fl 2, Indianapolis, IN 46202; **Phone:** 317-944-0920; **Board Cert:** Internal Medicine 1980; Medical Oncology 1983; **Med School:** Tulane Univ 1977; **Resid:** Internal Medicine, St Louis Univ Hosp 1980; **Fellow:** Medical Oncology, Univ Texas 1983; **Fac Appt:** Prof Med, Indiana Univ

Stadler, Walter M MD [Onc] - **Spec Exp:** Kidney Cancer; Bladder Cancer; Prostate Cancer; Testicular Cancer; **Hospital:** Univ of Chicago Med Ctr; **Address:** Univ Chicago Medical Center, 5841 S Maryland Ave, MC 2115, Chicago, IL 60637; **Phone:** 773-702-6149; **Board Cert:** Internal Medicine 2002; Medical Oncology 2003; **Med School:** Yale Univ 1988; **Resid:** Internal Medicine, Michael Reese Hosp 1991; **Fellow:** Medical Oncology, Univ Chicago Hosps 1994; **Fac Appt:** Prof Med, Univ Chicago-Pritzker Sch Med

Triozzi, Pierre L MD [Onc] - **Spec Exp:** Melanoma; Vaccine Therapy; Clinical Trials; **Hospital:** Cleveland Clin (page 55); **Address:** Cleveland Clinic Fdn, 9500 Euclid Ave, MC R40, Cleveland, OH 44195; **Phone:** 216-445-5141; **Board Cert:** Internal Medicine 1983; Medical Oncology 1987; Hematology 1988; **Med School:** Ohio State Univ 1980; **Resid:** Internal Medicine, Duke Univ Med Ctr 1983; **Fellow:** Hematology & Oncology, Duke Univ Med Ctr 1987; **Fac Appt:** Prof Med, Case West Res Univ

Urba, Susan G MD [Onc] - **Spec Exp:** Head & Neck Cancer; **Hospital:** Univ of Michigan Hosp; **Address:** 1500 E Medical Ctr Drive, Reception C, Ste B1-363, Ann Arbor, MI 48109-0922; **Phone:** 734-647-8902; **Board Cert:** Internal Medicine 1986; Medical Oncology 2002; Hospice & Palliative Medicine 2010; **Med School:** Univ Mich Med Sch 1983; **Resid:** Internal Medicine, Univ Mich Med Ctr 1986; **Fellow:** Hematology & Oncology, Univ Mich Med Ctr 1988; **Fac Appt:** Assoc Prof Med, Univ Mich Med Sch

Vokes, Everett E MD [Onc] - **Spec Exp:** Lung Cancer; Head & Neck Cancer; Esophageal Cancer; **Hospital:** Univ of Chicago Med Ctr; **Address:** Univ Chicago Hosps, 5841 S Maryland Ave, MC 2115, Chicago, IL 60637-1470; **Phone:** 773-834-3093; **Board Cert:** Internal Medicine 1983; Medical Oncology 1985; **Med School:** Germany 1980; **Resid:** Internal Medicine, Ravenswood Hosp-Univ Illinois 1982; Internal Medicine, USC Med Ctr 1983; **Fellow:** Medical Oncology, Univ Chicago 1986; **Fac Appt:** Prof Med, Univ Chicago-Pritzker Sch Med

Von Roenn, Jamie H MD [Onc] - **Spec Exp:** Palliative Care; AIDS Related Cancers; Breast Cancer; **Hospital:** Northwestern Meml Hosp; **Address:** Northwestern Medical Faculty Foundation, 676 N St Clair St, Ste 850, Chicago, IL 60611; **Phone:** 312-695-6180; **Board Cert:** Internal Medicine 1983; Medical Oncology 2009; Hospice & Palliative Medicine 2008; **Med School:** Rush Med Coll 1980; **Resid:** Internal Medicine, Rush-Presby-St Lukes Hosp 1983; **Fellow:** Medical Oncology, Rush-Presby-St Lukes Hosp 1985; **Fac Appt:** Prof Med, Northwestern Univ

Weiner, George J MD [Onc] - **Spec Exp:** Lymphoma; Leukemia; Immunotherapy; **Hospital:** Univ Iowa Hosp & Clinics; **Address:** Holden Comprehensive Cancer Ctr, Med Onc, 200 Hawkins Drive, Ste 5970HJPP, Iowa City, IA 52242; **Phone:** 319-384-8442; **Board Cert:** Internal Medicine 1985; Hematology 1988; Medical Oncology 1987; **Med School:** Ohio State Univ 1981; **Resid:** Medical Oncology, Med Coll Ohio Affil Hosp 1984; **Fellow:** Hematology & Oncology, Univ Mich Med Ctr 1987; **Fac Appt:** Prof Med, Univ Iowa Coll Med

Wicha, Max S MD [Onc] - **Spec Exp:** Breast Cancer; Stem Cell Transplant; **Hospital:** Univ of Michigan Hosp; **Address:** Comp Cancer Ctr & Geriatrics Ctr, 1500 E Med Ctr Dr, rm 6302 CC, SPC 5942, Ann Arbor, MI 48109-5942; **Phone:** 734-936-6000; **Board Cert:** Internal Medicine 1977; Medical Oncology 1983; **Med School:** Stanford Univ 1974; **Resid:** Internal Medicine, Univ Chicago Hosp 1977; **Fellow:** Medical Oncology, Natl Inst Hlth 1980; **Fac Appt:** Prof Med, Univ Mich Med Sch

Wilding, George MD [Onc] - **Spec Exp:** Prostate Cancer; Kidney Cancer; Genitourinary Cancer; Drug Discovery & Development; **Hospital:** Univ WI Hosp & Clins; **Address:** 1111 Highland Ave, Ste 7057WIMR, Madison, WI 53705; **Phone:** 608-263-8610; **Board Cert:** Internal Medicine 1983; Medical Oncology 1985; **Med School:** Univ Mass Sch Med 1980; **Resid:** Internal Medicine, Univ Mass Med Ctr 1983; **Fellow:** Medical Oncology, Natl Cancer Inst 1985; **Fac Appt:** Prof Med, Univ Wisc

Worden, Francis P MD [Onc] - **Spec Exp:** Head & Neck Cancer; Palliative Care; Clinical Trials; **Hospital:** Univ of Michigan Hosp; **Address:** Level B1363, Reception C, 1500 E Medical Ctr Drive, Ann Arbor, MI 48109; **Phone:** 734-647-8902; **Board Cert:** Medical Oncology 2010; **Med School:** Indiana Univ 1993; **Resid:** Internal Medicine & Pediatrics, Detroit Med Ctr 1997; **Fellow:** Medical Oncology, Detroit Med Ctr 2000; **Fac Appt:** Asst Clin Prof Med, Univ Mich Med Sch

Medical Oncology

Yee, Douglas MD [Onc] - **Spec Exp:** Breast Cancer; **Hospital:** Univ Minn Med Ctr, Fairview - Riverside Campus; **Address:** Masonic Cancer Ctr-Breast Ctr, 420 Delaware St SE, MMC 160, Minneapolis, MN 55455; **Phone:** 612-273-9685; **Board Cert:** Internal Medicine 1984; Medical Oncology 1987; **Med School:** Univ Chicago-Pritzker Sch Med 1981; **Resid:** Internal Medicine, Univ NC Med Ctr 1984; **Fellow:** Medical Oncology, NIH-Clin Ctr 1987; **Fac Appt:** Prof Med, Univ Minn

Great Plains and Mountains

Akerley III, Wallace L MD [Onc] - **Spec Exp:** Lung Cancer; Clinical Trials; **Hospital:** Univ Utah Hlth Care; **Address:** Huntsman Cancer Inst, 1950 Circle of Hope, Salt Lake City, UT 84112; **Phone:** 801-585-0100; **Board Cert:** Internal Medicine 1984; Medical Oncology 1987; Hematology 1988; **Med School:** Brown Univ 1981; **Resid:** Internal Medicine, USC Medical Ctr 1985; **Fellow:** Medical Oncology, USC Medical Ctr 1986; Hematology, Norris Cotton Cancer Ctr/Dartmouth 1988; **Fac Appt:** Prof Med, Univ Utah

Armitage, James MD [Onc] - **Spec Exp:** Lymphoma; Bone Marrow Transplant; Hematologic Malignancies; **Hospital:** Nebraska Med Ctr; **Address:** 987630 Nebraska Medical Center, Emile @ 42nd St, Omaha, NE 68198-7630; **Phone:** 402-559-5600; **Board Cert:** Internal Medicine 1976; Medical Oncology 1977; Hematology 1984; **Med School:** Univ Nebr Coll Med 1973; **Resid:** Internal Medicine, Univ Nebraska Med Ctr 1975; **Fellow:** Hematology & Oncology, Univ Iowa Hosp 1977; **Fac Appt:** Prof Med, Univ Nebr Coll Med

Beatty, Patrick G MD/PhD [Onc] - **Spec Exp:** Hematologic Malignancies; Lymphoma; **Hospital:** St. Patrick Hospital - Missoula; **Address:** 500 W Broadway, PO Box 7877, Missoula, MT 59807; **Phone:** 406-728-2539; **Board Cert:** Internal Medicine 1980; Medical Oncology 1985; **Med School:** Univ Chicago-Pritzker Sch Med 1976; **Resid:** Internal Medicine, Vanderbilt Univ Med Ctr 1979; **Fellow:** Oncology, Univ Washington Hosps 1982

Bierman, Philip J MD [Onc] - **Spec Exp:** Lymphoma; Bone Marrow Transplant; **Hospital:** Nebraska Med Ctr; **Address:** Nebraska Medical Ctr, Dept Hem/Oncology, 987630 Nebraska Medical Ctr, Emile @ 42nd St, Omaha, NE 68198-7630; **Phone:** 402-559-5600; **Board Cert:** Internal Medicine 1982; Medical Oncology 1985; Hematology 1986; **Med School:** Univ MO-Kansas City 1979; **Resid:** Internal Medicine, Univ Nebraska Med Ctr 1983; **Fellow:** Medical Oncology, Univ Nebraska Med Ctr 1985; Hematology, City of Hope Natl Med Ctr 1986; **Fac Appt:** Prof Med, Univ Nebr Coll Med

Bunn Jr, Paul A MD [Onc] - **Spec Exp:** Lung Cancer; Clinical Trials; Thymoma; Mesothelioma; **Hospital:** Univ of CO Hosp - Anschutz Inpatient Pav; **Address:** Univ Colorado Hosp Cancer Ctr, 12605 E 16th Ave, Aurora, CO 80045; **Phone:** 720-848-0300; **Board Cert:** Internal Medicine 1974; Medical Oncology 1975; **Med School:** Cornell Univ-Weill Med Coll 1971; **Resid:** Internal Medicine, Moffitt Hosp/ UCSF Med Ctr 1973; **Fellow:** Medical Oncology, Natl Cancer Inst 1976; **Fac Appt:** Prof Med, Univ Colorado

Buys, Saundra S MD [Onc] - **Spec Exp:** Breast Cancer; Breast Cancer Risk Assessment; Breast Cancer Genetics; **Hospital:** Univ Utah Hlth Care; **Address:** Huntsman Cancer Inst, 1950 Circle of Hope, Salt Lake City, UT 84112; **Phone:** 801-585-0100; **Board Cert:** Internal Medicine 1982; Hematology 1984; Medical Oncology 1985; **Med School:** Tufts Univ 1979; **Resid:** Internal Medicine, Univ Utah Hosps 1982; **Fellow:** Hematology & Oncology, Univ Utah Hosps 1985; **Fac Appt:** Prof Med, Univ Utah

Cowan, Kenneth H MD/PhD [Onc] - **Spec Exp:** Breast Cancer; **Hospital:** Nebraska Med Ctr; **Address:** Eppley Cancer Center, 987630 Nebraska Medical Ctr, Emile @ 42nd St, Omaha, NE 68198-7630; **Phone:** 402-559-5600; **Board Cert:** Internal Medicine 1978; Medical Oncology 1981; **Med School:** Case West Res Univ 1975; **Resid:** Internal Medicine, Parkland Meml Hosp 1977

Dakhil, Shaker MD [Onc] - **Spec Exp:** Leukemia; Mesothelioma; Lymphoma; **Hospital:** Univ of Kansas Hosp; **Address:** Cancer Ctr of Kansas, 818 N Emporia, Ste 403, Wichita, KS 67214; **Phone:** 316-262-4467; **Board Cert:** Internal Medicine 1978; Medical Oncology 1981; **Med School:** Lebanon 1976; **Resid:** Internal Medicine, Wayne State Univ Affil Hosps 1978; **Fellow:** Hematology & Oncology, Univ Michigan Med Sch 1981; **Fac Appt:** Assoc Clin Prof Med, Univ Kansas

Eckhardt, S Gail MD [Onc] - **Spec Exp:** Gastrointestinal Cancer; Drug Development; **Hospital:** Univ of CO Hosp - Anschutz Inpatient Pav; **Address:** Univ Colorado Hosp Cancer Ctr, PO Box 6510, MS F-704, 1665 Aurora Court, Aurora, CO 80045-0510; **Phone:** 720-848-0300; **Board Cert:** Internal Medicine 1988; Medical Oncology 2006; **Med School:** Univ Tex Med Br, Galveston 1985; **Resid:** Internal Medicine, Univ Virginia Med Ctr 1988; **Fellow:** Research, Scripps Clinic 1989; Medical Oncology, UCSD Med Ctr 1992; **Fac Appt:** Prof Med, Univ Colorado

Elias, Anthony D MD [Onc] - **Spec Exp:** Breast Cancer; **Hospital:** Univ of CO Hosp - Anschutz Inpatient Pav; **Address:** UCH Breast Ctr, Anschutz OPD Pavillion, 1635 Aurora Ct, MS F724, Aurora, CO 80045; **Phone:** 720-848-1030; **Board Cert:** Internal Medicine 1983; Medical Oncology 1985; **Med School:** NYU Sch Med 1980; **Resid:** Internal Medicine, Johns Hopkins Hsop 1983; **Fellow:** Medical Oncology, Dana-Farber Cancer Inst 1983; **Fac Appt:** Assoc Prof Med, Univ Colorado

Fabian, Carol J MD [Onc] - **Spec Exp:** Breast Cancer; Breast Cancer Risk Assessment; **Hospital:** Univ of Kansas Hosp; **Address:** Univ of Kansas Hosp, Dept Hem/Onc, Westwood Med Pavilion, MS 5015, 2330 Shawnee Mission Pkwy, Ste 1102, Westwood, KS 66205; **Phone:** 913-588-6029; **Board Cert:** Internal Medicine 1976; Medical Oncology 1977; **Med School:** Univ Kansas 1972; **Resid:** Internal Medicine, Wesley Med Ctr 1975; **Fellow:** Medical Oncology, Univ Kansas Med Ctr 1977; **Fac Appt:** Prof Med, Univ Kansas

Glode, L Michael MD [Onc] - **Spec Exp:** Prostate Cancer; Genitourinary Cancer; **Hospital:** Univ of CO Hosp - Anschutz Inpatient Pav; **Address:** 1665 Aurora Ct, Aurora, CO 80045; **Phone:** 720-848-0170; **Board Cert:** Internal Medicine 1975; Medical Oncology 1981; **Med School:** Washington Univ, St Louis 1972; **Resid:** Internal Medicine, Univ Texas SW Med Ctr 1973; Immunology, Natl Inst Hlth 1976; **Fellow:** Medical Oncology, Dana Farber Cancer Inst 1978; **Fac Appt:** Prof Med, Univ Colorado

Grem, Jean L MD [Onc] - **Spec Exp:** Colon & Rectal Cancer; Pancreatic Cancer; Stomach Cancer; Esophageal Cancer; **Hospital:** Nebraska Med Ctr; **Address:** 987630 Nebraska Medical Ctr, Emile @ 42nd St, Omaha, NE 68198-7630; **Phone:** 402-559-6210; **Board Cert:** Internal Medicine 1983; Medical Oncology 1985; **Med School:** Jefferson Med Coll 1980; **Resid:** Internal Medicine, Univ Iowa Hosps & Clinics 1983; **Fellow:** Medical Oncology, Univ Wisc Clin Cancer Ctr 1986; **Fac Appt:** Prof Med, Univ Nebr Coll Med

Hauke, Ralph J MD [Onc] - **Spec Exp:** Urologic Cancer; Clinical Trials; Testicular Cancer; Prostate Cancer; **Hospital:** Methodist Hosp - Omaha, Alegent Hlth - Bergan Mercy Med Ctr; **Address:** 8303 Dodge St, Ste 250, Omaha, NE 68114; **Phone:** 402-354-8124; **Board Cert:** Medical Oncology 2012; **Med School:** Panama 1990; **Resid:** Internal Medicine, Univ Nebraska Med Ctr 1996; **Fellow:** Medical Oncology, Univ Nebraska Med Ctr 2001; **Fac Appt:** Assoc Prof Onc, Univ Nebr Coll Med

Medical Oncology

Kane, Madeleine A MD/PhD [Onc] - **Spec Exp:** Head & Neck Cancer; Gastrointestinal Cancer; Neuroendocrine Tumors; **Hospital:** Univ of CO Hosp - Anschutz Inpatient Pav, VA Eastern CO Health Care Sys-Denver; **Address:** Univ Colorado Hosp Cancer Ctr, PO Box 6510, MS F-704, 1665 Aurora Court, Aurora, CO 80045; **Phone:** 720-848-0300; **Board Cert:** Internal Medicine 1981; Medical Oncology 1983; Hematology 1986; **Med School:** Univ Miami Sch Med 1978; **Resid:** Internal Medicine, Stanford Univ Med Ctr 1981; **Fellow:** Hematology & Oncology, Univ Colo Hlth Sci Ctr 1984; **Fac Appt:** Prof Med, Univ Colorado

Messersmith, Wells A MD [Onc] - **Spec Exp:** Gastrointestinal Cancer; Colon & Rectal Cancer; **Hospital:** Univ of CO Hosp - Anschutz Inpatient Pav; **Address:** Univ of CO Hosp, 12605 E 16th Ave, Aurora, CO 80045; **Phone:** 720-848-0300; **Board Cert:** Internal Medicine 2001; Medical Oncology 2003; **Med School:** Harvard Med Sch 1998; **Resid:** Medical Oncology, Mass Genl Hosp 2000; **Fellow:** Medical Oncology, Johns Hopkins Hosp 2004; **Fac Appt:** Asst Prof Med, Univ Colorado

Samuels, Brian L MD [Onc] - **Spec Exp:** Sarcoma; **Hospital:** Kootenai Med Ctr; **Address:** 1440 Mullan Ave, Post Falls, ID 83854; **Phone:** 208-619-4100; **Board Cert:** Internal Medicine 1984; Medical Oncology 1987; **Med School:** Zimbabwe 1976; **Resid:** Internal Medicine, Albert Einstein Med Ctr 1981; Internal Medicine, Albert Einstein Med Ctr 1984; **Fellow:** Hematology & Oncology, Univ Chicago Hosps 1988

Steen, Preston D MD [Onc] - **Spec Exp:** Colon & Rectal Cancer; Lung Cancer; Palliative Care; **Hospital:** Sanford Med Ctr Fargo; **Address:** 820 N Fourth St, Fargo, ND 58122; **Phone:** 701-234-6161; **Board Cert:** Internal Medicine 1987; Medical Oncology 2011; Hospice & Palliative Medicine 2010; **Med School:** Univ Minn 1984; **Resid:** Internal Medicine, Maricopa Med Ctr 1987; **Fellow:** Hematology & Oncology, Univ Utah 1990; **Fac Appt:** Clin Prof Onc, Univ ND Sch Med

Ward, John H MD [Onc] - **Spec Exp:** Breast Cancer; Gastrointestinal Cancer; Brain Tumors; Unknown Primary Cancer; **Hospital:** Univ Utah Hlth Care, St. John's Med Ctr; **Address:** Huntsman Cancer Inst, 2000 Circle of Hope, Ste 2100 - rm 2141, Salt Lake City, UT 84112-5550; **Phone:** 801-585-0255; **Board Cert:** Internal Medicine 1979; Medical Oncology 1981; Hematology 1982; **Med School:** Univ Utah 1976; **Resid:** Internal Medicine, Duke Univ Med Ctr 1979; **Fellow:** Hematology & Oncology, Univ Utah Med Ctr 1982; **Fac Appt:** Prof Med, Univ Utah

Southwest

Abbruzzese, James L MD [Onc] - **Spec Exp:** Gastrointestinal Cancer; Pancreatic Cancer; Clinical Trials; **Hospital:** UT MD Anderson Cancer Ctr; **Address:** Univ Tex MD Anderson Cancer Ctr, 1515 Holcombe Blvd, Unit 426, Houston, TX 77030; **Phone:** 713-792-2828; **Board Cert:** Internal Medicine 1981; Medical Oncology 1983; **Med School:** Univ Chicago-Pritzker Sch Med 1978; **Resid:** Internal Medicine, Johns Hopkins Hosp 1981; **Fellow:** Medical Oncology, Dana-Farber Cancer Inst 1983; **Fac Appt:** Prof Med, Univ Tex, Houston

Ahmann, Frederick R MD [Onc] - **Spec Exp:** Prostate Cancer; Testicular Cancer; Bladder Cancer; **Hospital:** Univ Arizona Med Ctr-Univ Campus; **Address:** Arizona Cancer Ctr-UMC North, 3838 N Campbell Ave, Tucson, AZ 85719; **Phone:** 520-694-2873; **Board Cert:** Internal Medicine 1977; Medical Oncology 1981; **Med School:** Univ MO-Columbia Sch Med 1974; **Resid:** Internal Medicine, Georgetown Univ Med Ctr 1977; **Fellow:** Medical Oncology, Univ Arizona 1980; **Fac Appt:** Prof Med, Univ Ariz Coll Med

Ajani, Jaffer A MD [Onc] - **Spec Exp:** Gastrointestinal Cancer; Esophageal Cancer; Stomach Cancer; Neuroendocrine Tumors; **Hospital:** UT MD Anderson Cancer Ctr; **Address:** Univ Tex MD Anderson Cancer Ctr, 1515 Holcombe Blvd, Unit 426, Houston, TX 77230; **Phone:** 713-792-2828; **Board Cert:** Internal Medicine 1979; Medical Oncology 1983; **Med School:** India 1971; **Resid:** Family Medicine, Penn State Affil Hosp 1977; Internal Medicine, Tulane Affil Hosp 1980; **Fellow:** Medical Oncology, MD Anderson Cancer Ctr 1983; **Fac Appt:** Prof Med, Univ Tex, Houston

Alberts, David S MD [Onc] - **Spec Exp:** Cancer Prevention; Ovarian Cancer; **Hospital:** Univ Arizona Med Ctr-Univ Campus; **Address:** 1515 N Campbell Ave, Tucson, AZ 85724; **Phone:** 520-626-7685; **Board Cert:** Internal Medicine 1973; Medical Oncology 1973; **Med School:** Univ VA Sch Med 1966; **Resid:** Medical Oncology, Natl Cancer Inst-NIH 1969; Internal Medicine, Univ Minn Hosps 1971; **Fellow:** Clinical Pharmacology, UCSF 1974; **Fac Appt:** Prof Med, Univ Ariz Coll Med

Argiris, Athanassios MD [Onc] - **Spec Exp:** Head & Neck Cancer; Lung Cancer; **Hospital:** Univ Hlth Syst-San Antonio; **Address:** UPMC Presbyterian Cancer Ctr, 7979 Wurzbach Rd, Fl 4th, rm Z418, San Antonio, TX 78229; **Phone:** 210-450-3838; **Board Cert:** Medical Oncology 2010; **Med School:** Greece 1990; **Resid:** Internal Medicine, Beth Israel Med Ctr 1997; **Fellow:** Medical Oncology, Yale Univ 2000; **Fac Appt:** Prof Med, Univ Tex, San Antonio

Arun, Banu K MD [Onc] - **Spec Exp:** Breast Cancer; Cancer Prevention; Clinical Trials; **Hospital:** UT MD Anderson Cancer Ctr; **Address:** 1515 Holcombe Blvd, Unit 1354, Houston, TX 77030; **Phone:** 713-792-2817; **Board Cert:** Internal Medicine 2010; Medical Oncology 2011; **Med School:** Turkey 1990; **Resid:** Internal Medicine, Univ Istanbul Affil Hosp 1994; **Fellow:** Hematology & Oncology, Lombardi Cancer Ctr-Georgetown Univ 1997; **Fac Appt:** Assoc Prof Med, Univ Tex, Houston

Benjamin, Robert S MD [Onc] - **Spec Exp:** Sarcoma; **Hospital:** UT MD Anderson Cancer Ctr; **Address:** UT MD Anderson Cancer Ctr, 1515 Holcombe Blvd, Unit 450, Houston, TX 77030; **Phone:** 713-563-9701; **Board Cert:** Internal Medicine 1973; Medical Oncology 1973; **Med School:** NYU Sch Med 1968; **Resid:** Internal Medicine, Bellevue Hosp Ctr-NYU 1970; **Fellow:** Medical Oncology, Baltimore Cancer Rsch Ctr 1972; **Fac Appt:** Prof Med, Univ Tex, Houston

Bergsagel, Peter L MD [Onc] - **Spec Exp:** Multiple Myeloma; Hematologic Malignancies; **Hospital:** Mayo Clinic - Scottsdale, Mayo Clinic - Phoenix; **Address:** Mayo Clinic-Hematology/Oncology, 13400 E Shea Blvd Fl 3, Scottsdale, AZ 85259; **Phone:** 480-301-8335; **Board Cert:** Internal Medicine 1987; Medical Oncology 1989; **Med School:** Univ Toronto 1984; **Resid:** Internal Medicine, Sunnybrook Medical Centre 1986; Internal Medicine, Stanford Univ Med Ctr 1987; **Fellow:** Medical Oncology, Natl Cancer Inst 1990; **Fac Appt:** Prof Med, Mayo Med Sch

Bruera, Eduardo MD [Onc] - **Spec Exp:** Palliative Care; **Hospital:** UT MD Anderson Cancer Ctr; **Address:** 1400 Pressler, Ste 1414, Houston, TX 77030; **Phone:** 713-792-6085; **Board Cert:** Internal Medicine 2011; **Med School:** Argentina 1979; **Resid:** Internal Medicine, Hospital Privado; **Fellow:** Medical Oncology, Cross Cancer Inst; **Fac Appt:** Prof Med, Univ Tex, Houston

Buzdar, Aman U MD [Onc] - **Spec Exp:** Breast Cancer; **Hospital:** UT MD Anderson Cancer Ctr; **Address:** UT MD Anderson Cancer Ctr, 1515 Holcome Blvd, Unit 1354, Houston, TX 77030; **Phone:** 713-792-2817; **Board Cert:** Internal Medicine 1975; Medical Oncology 1979; **Med School:** Pakistan 1967; **Resid:** Internal Medicine, Norwalk Hosp 1973; Internal Medicine, Lakewood Hosp 1971; **Fellow:** Hematology, Norwalk Hosp 1974; Oncology, MD Anderson Cancer Ctr 1975; **Fac Appt:** Prof Med, Univ Tex, Houston

Medical Oncology

Camoriano, John K MD [Onc] - **Spec Exp:** Lymphoma; Breast Cancer; Bone Marrow Transplant; Castleman's Disease; **Hospital:** Mayo Clinic - Scottsdale, Mayo Clinic - Phoenix; **Address:** Mayo Clinic-Hematology/Oncology, 13400 E Shea Blvd Fl 3, Scottsdale, AZ 85259; **Phone:** 480-301-8335; **Board Cert:** Internal Medicine 1985; Hematology 1988; Medical Oncology 1989; **Med School:** Univ Nebr Coll Med 1982; **Resid:** Internal Medicine, Univ OK Affil Hosp 1985; **Fellow:** Hematology & Oncology, Mayo Clinic 1988; Research, Mayo Clinic 1989; **Fac Appt:** Asst Prof Med, Mayo Med Sch

Chang, Jenny C N MD [Onc] - **Spec Exp:** Breast Cancer; Clinical Trials; **Hospital:** Methodist Hosp - Houston; **Address:** 6445 Main St Fl 21, Outpatient Ctr, Houston, TX 77030; **Phone:** 713-441-9948; **Board Cert:** Internal Medicine 2004; **Med School:** England, UK 1989; **Resid:** Internal Medicine 1993; **Fellow:** Medical Oncology, Royal Marsden Hosp 1997; **Fac Appt:** Assoc Prof Med, Baylor Coll Med

Fay, Joseph W MD [Onc] - **Spec Exp:** Bone Marrow Transplant; Melanoma; Leukemia & Lymphoma; **Hospital:** Baylor Univ Medical Ctr-Dallas; **Address:** 3410 Worth St, Ste 300, Sammons Cancer Ctr, Dallas, TX 75246; **Phone:** 214-370-1500; **Board Cert:** Internal Medicine 1975; Medical Oncology 1977; Hematology 1978; **Med School:** Ohio State Univ 1972; **Resid:** Internal Medicine, Duke Med Ctr 1974; Oncology, Natl Cancer Institute 1976; **Fellow:** Hematology, Duke Med Ctr 1977; **Fac Appt:** Clin Prof Med, Univ Tex SW, Dallas

Fitch, Tom R MD [Onc] - **Spec Exp:** Breast Cancer; Palliative Care; Cancer Prevention; Sarcoma; **Hospital:** Mayo Clinic - Phoenix, Mayo Clinic - Scottsdale; **Address:** Mayo Clinic-Hematology/Oncology, 5777 E Mayo Blvd, Phoenix, AZ 85054; **Phone:** 480-301-8335; **Board Cert:** Internal Medicine 1985; Medical Oncology 1987; Hematology 1988; Hospice & Palliative Medicine 2008; **Med School:** Univ Kansas 1982; **Resid:** Internal Medicine, Univ Mich Med Ctr 1985; **Fellow:** Hematology & Oncology, Mayo Clinic 1988; **Fac Appt:** Asst Prof Med, Mayo Med Sch

Fossella, Frank V MD [Onc] - **Spec Exp:** Lung Cancer; **Hospital:** UT MD Anderson Cancer Ctr; **Address:** Dept Thoracic Head/Neck Med Oncology, 1515 Holcombe Blvd, Unit 432, Houston, TX 77030; **Phone:** 713-792-6363; **Board Cert:** Internal Medicine 1985; Medical Oncology 1987; **Med School:** Baylor Coll Med 1982; **Resid:** Internal Medicine, Baylor Coll Med 1985; **Fellow:** Medical Oncology, Baylor Coll Med 1987; **Fac Appt:** Prof Med, Univ Tex, Houston

Geyer Jr, Charles E MD [Onc] - **Spec Exp:** Breast Cancer; Clinical Trials; **Hospital:** UT Southwestern Med Ctr at Dallas; **Address:** UT SW Med Ctr - Hematology/Oncology, 5323 Harry Hines Blvd, NB2.102, Dallas, TX 75390; **Phone:** 214-645-4673; **Board Cert:** Internal Medicine 1983; Medical Oncology 1987; **Med School:** Texas Tech Univ 1980; **Resid:** Internal Medicine, Baylor Affil Hosps 1983; **Fellow:** Medical Oncology, Baylor Affil Hosps 1985; **Fac Appt:** Assoc Prof Med, Univ Tex SW, Dallas

Glisson, Bonnie S MD [Onc] - **Spec Exp:** Head & Neck Cancer; Lung Cancer; **Hospital:** UT MD Anderson Cancer Ctr; **Address:** 1515 Holcombe Blvd, Unit 432, Houston, TX 77230-1402; **Phone:** 713-792-6363; **Board Cert:** Internal Medicine 1982; Medical Oncology 1985; **Med School:** Ohio State Univ 1979; **Resid:** Internal Medicine, Univ VA Med Ctr 1982; **Fellow:** Medical Oncology, Univ Fla 1985; **Fac Appt:** Prof Med, Univ Tex, Houston

Haley, Barbara MD [Onc] - **Spec Exp:** Breast Cancer; **Hospital:** UT Southwestern Med Ctr at Dallas; **Address:** 5323 Harry Hines Blvd, Ste NB2102, Dallas, TX 75390-8852; **Phone:** 214-648-4180; **Board Cert:** Internal Medicine 1979; Hematology 1984; **Med School:** Univ Tex SW, Dallas 1976; **Resid:** Internal Medicine, Parkland Meml Hosp 1979; **Fellow:** Hematology & Oncology, Parkland Meml Hosp 1981; **Fac Appt:** Prof Med, Univ Tex SW, Dallas

Hong, Waun Ki MD [Onc] - **Spec Exp:** Lung Cancer; Head & Neck Cancer; Thoracic Cancers; **Hospital:** UT MD Anderson Cancer Ctr; **Address:** Dept Thoracic Head/Neck Oncology, 1400 Holcombe Blvd, Unit 421, Houston, TX 77030; **Phone:** 713-792-6110; **Board Cert:** Internal Medicine 1976; Medical Oncology 1979; **Med School:** South Korea 1967; **Resid:** Internal Medicine, Boston VA Hosp 1973; **Fellow:** Medical Oncology, Meml Sloan-Kettering Cancer Ctr 1975; **Fac Appt:** Prof Med, Univ Tex, Houston

Hortobagyi, Gabriel N MD [Onc] - **Spec Exp:** Breast Cancer; Clinical Trials; Gene Therapy; Breast Cancer-Male; **Hospital:** UT MD Anderson Cancer Ctr; **Address:** 1155 Pressler Blvd, CPB Fl 5 - Ste 3405, MS 1354, Houston, TX 77030-1439; **Phone:** 713-792-2817; **Board Cert:** Internal Medicine 1975; Medical Oncology 1977; **Med School:** Colombia 1970; **Resid:** Internal Medicine, St Lukes Hosp 1974; **Fellow:** Medical Oncology, MD Anderson Cancer Ctr 1976; **Fac Appt:** Prof Med, Univ Tex, Houston

Hutchins, Laura F MD [Onc] - **Spec Exp:** Breast Cancer; Melanoma; **Hospital:** UAMS Med Ctr; **Address:** Univ Arkansas Med Scis, Dept Hem/Onc, 4301 W Markham St, Slot 508, Little Rock, AR 72205; **Phone:** 501-686-8511; **Board Cert:** Internal Medicine 1980; Hematology 1984; Medical Oncology 1987; **Med School:** Univ Ark 1977; **Resid:** Internal Medicine, Univ Ark Affil Hosp 1980; **Fellow:** Hematology & Oncology, Univ Arkansas 1983; **Fac Appt:** Prof Med, Univ Ark

Hwu, Patrick MD [Onc] - **Spec Exp:** Melanoma; Immunotherapy; Clinical Trials; **Hospital:** UT MD Anderson Cancer Ctr; **Address:** UT MD Anderson Cancer Center, Melanoma & Skin Center, 1515 Holcombe Blvd, Unit 347, Houston, TX 77030; **Phone:** 713-792-6800; **Board Cert:** Medical Oncology 2008; **Med School:** Med Coll PA 1987; **Resid:** Internal Medicine, Johns Hopkins Hosp 1989; **Fellow:** Medical Oncology, Natl Cancer Inst 1993

Johnson, David H MD [Onc] - **Spec Exp:** Lung Cancer; Drug Discovery & Development; **Hospital:** UT Southwestern Med Ctr at Dallas; **Address:** University of Texas Southwestern Medical, 5323 Harry Hines Blvd, rm G5.206, MS 9030, Dallas, TX 75390-9030; **Phone:** 214-648-3486; **Board Cert:** Internal Medicine 1979; Medical Oncology 2008; **Med School:** Med Coll GA 1976; **Resid:** Internal Medicine, Univ South Alabama Med Ctr 1979; Internal Medicine, Med Coll Georgia Hosp 1980; **Fellow:** Medical Oncology, Vanderbilt Univ Med Ctr 1983; **Fac Appt:** Prof Med, Univ Tex SW, Dallas

Jonasch, Eric MD [Onc] - **Spec Exp:** Kidney Cancer; Testicular Cancer; Bladder Cancer; Genitourinary Cancer; **Hospital:** UT MD Anderson Cancer Ctr; **Address:** GU Medical Oncology, 1220 Holcombe Blvd, Unit 1274, Houston, TX 77030; **Phone:** 713-792-2830; **Board Cert:** Internal Medicine 2005; Hematology 2009; Medical Oncology 2010; **Med School:** Canada 1992; **Resid:** Internal Medicine, Royal Victoria Hosp 1995; **Fellow:** Hematology & Oncology, New England Med Ctr 1997; Research, Beth Israel Deaconess Med Ctr 1999; **Fac Appt:** Assoc Prof Med, Univ Tex, Houston

Kies, Merrill S MD [Onc] - **Spec Exp:** Head & Neck Cancer; Lung Cancer; **Hospital:** UT MD Anderson Cancer Ctr; **Address:** Thoracic/Head & Neck Med Oncology, 1515 Holcombe Blvd, Unit 421, Houston, TX 77030; **Phone:** 713-792-7770; **Board Cert:** Internal Medicine 1976; Medical Oncology 1979; **Med School:** Loyola Univ-Stritch Sch Med 1973; **Resid:** Internal Medicine, Walter Reed AMC 1976; **Fellow:** Medical Oncology, Brooke AMC 1978; **Fac Appt:** Prof Med, Univ Tex, Houston

Kwak, Larry W MD/PhD [Onc] - **Spec Exp:** Lymphoma; Multiple Myeloma; Vaccine Therapy; Immunotherapy; **Hospital:** UT MD Anderson Cancer Ctr; **Address:** MD Anderson Cancer Ctr, Dept Lymphoma/Myeloma, 1515 Holcombe Blvd, Unit 429, Houston, TX 77030; **Phone:** 713-792-2860; **Board Cert:** Internal Medicine 1987; Medical Oncology 1989; **Med School:** Northwestern Univ 1982; **Resid:** Internal Medicine, Stanford Univ Hosp 1987; **Fellow:** Medical Oncology, Stanford Univ Hosp 1989

Medical Oncology

Livingston, Robert B MD [Onc] - **Spec Exp:** Breast Cancer; Breast Cancer and Pregancy; Lung Cancer; **Hospital:** Univ Arizona Med Ctr-Univ Campus; **Address:** Arizona Cancer Ctr-UMC North, 3838 N Campbell Ave, Tucson, AZ 85719; **Phone:** 520-694-2873; **Board Cert:** Internal Medicine 1972; Medical Oncology 1973; **Med School:** Univ Okla Coll Med 1965; **Resid:** Internal Medicine, Univ Oklahoma Med Ctr 1971; **Fellow:** Medical Oncology, Univ Texas Cancer Ctr 1973; **Fac Appt:** Prof Med, Univ Wash

Logothetis, Christopher J MD [Onc] - **Spec Exp:** Prostate Cancer; Bladder Cancer; **Hospital:** UT MD Anderson Cancer Ctr; **Address:** UT MD Anderson Cancer Ctr, Dept GU Onc, Unit 1274, Box 301439, Houston, TX 77230; **Phone:** 713-745-7020; **Board Cert:** Internal Medicine 1978; Medical Oncology 1981; **Med School:** Greece 1974; **Resid:** Internal Medicine, Univ Texas Affil Hosp 1979; **Fellow:** Hematology & Oncology, MD Anderson Cancer Ctr 1981; **Fac Appt:** Prof Med, Univ Tex, Houston

Makhoul, Issam MD [Onc] - **Spec Exp:** Gastrointestinal Cancer; Breast Cancer; Colon Cancer; **Hospital:** UAMS Med Ctr; **Address:** 4301 W Markham St, Slot# 721-5, Little Rock, AR 72205; **Phone:** 501-686-8530; **Board Cert:** Medical Oncology 2002; Hematology 2003; **Med School:** Syria 1980; **Resid:** Internal Medicine, Genl Hosp 1984; Internal Medicine, Penn State Affil Hosp 1999; **Fellow:** Hematology & Oncology, Hershey Med Ctr 2002; **Fac Appt:** Asst Prof Med, Univ Ark

Miller, Thomas P MD [Onc] - **Spec Exp:** Lymphoma; Lymphoma, Non-Hodgkin's; **Hospital:** Univ Arizona Med Ctr-Univ Campus; **Address:** Arizona Cancer Ctr-UMC North, 3838 N Campbell Ave, Tucson, AZ 85719; **Phone:** 520-694-2873; **Board Cert:** Internal Medicine 1977; Medical Oncology 1981; **Med School:** Univ IL Coll Med 1972; **Resid:** Internal Medicine, Univ Illinois Hosps 1977; **Fellow:** Hematology & Oncology, Arizona Univ Med Ctr 1980; **Fac Appt:** Prof Med, Univ Ariz Coll Med

Northfelt, Donald W MD [Onc] - **Spec Exp:** Breast Cancer; Colon & Rectal Cancer; Lung Cancer; **Hospital:** Mayo Clinic - Scottsdale, Mayo Clinic - Phoenix; **Address:** Mayo Clinic-Hematology/Oncology, 13400 E Shea Blvd Fl 3, Scottsdale, AZ 85259; **Phone:** 480-301-8335; **Board Cert:** Internal Medicine 1988; Medical Oncology 2011; **Med School:** Univ Minn 1985; **Resid:** Internal Medicine, UCLA Med Ctr 1988; **Fellow:** Hematology & Oncology, UCSF Med Ctr 1991; **Fac Appt:** Assoc Prof Med, Mayo Med Sch

O'Brien, Susan M MD [Onc] - **Spec Exp:** Leukemia; Lymphoma; **Hospital:** UT MD Anderson Cancer Ctr; **Address:** Dept Leukemia, Unit 428, 1515 Holcombe Blvd, Houston, TX 77230; **Phone:** 713-792-7305; **Board Cert:** Internal Medicine 1983; Medical Oncology 1987; **Med School:** UMDNJ-NJ Med Sch, Newark 1980; **Resid:** Internal Medicine, UMDNJ Med Ctr 1983; **Fellow:** Medical Oncology, Univ TX MD Anderson Med Ctr 1987; **Fac Appt:** Prof Med, Univ Tex, Houston

O'Shaughnessy, Joyce A MD [Onc] - **Spec Exp:** Breast Cancer; **Hospital:** Baylor Univ Medical Ctr-Dallas; **Address:** Texas Oncology, 3410 Worth St, Ste 400, Dallas, TX 75246; **Phone:** 214-370-1000; **Board Cert:** Internal Medicine 1985; Medical Oncology 1987; **Med School:** Yale Univ 1982; **Resid:** Internal Medicine, Mass Genl Hosp 1985; **Fellow:** Medical Oncology, National Cancer Inst 1988

Orlowski, Robert Z MD/PhD [Onc] - **Spec Exp:** Multiple Myeloma; Lymphoma, Non-Hodgkin's; Leukemia; Clinical Trials; **Hospital:** UT MD Anderson Cancer Ctr; **Address:** MD Anderson Cancer Ctr, Lymphoma & Myeloma Clinic, 1515 Holcombe Blvd, Unit 429, Houston, TX 77030; **Phone:** 713-792-3510; **Med School:** Yale Univ 1991; **Resid:** Internal Medicine, Barnes Hosp 1994; **Fellow:** Hematology & Oncology, Johns Hopkins Hosp 1998; **Fac Appt:** Assoc Prof Med, Univ Tex, Houston

Osborne, C Kent MD [Onc] - **Spec Exp:** Breast Cancer; **Hospital:** Methodist Hosp - Houston; **Address:** 1 Baylor Plaza, MS BCM600, Houston, TX 77030; **Phone:** 713-798-1641; **Board Cert:** Internal Medicine 1975; Medical Oncology 1977; **Med School:** Univ MO-Columbia Sch Med 1972; **Resid:** Internal Medicine, Johns Hopkins Hosp 1974; **Fellow:** Medical Oncology, Natl Cancer Inst 1977; **Fac Appt:** Prof Med, Baylor Coll Med

Papadopoulos, Nicholas E MD [Onc] - **Spec Exp:** Melanoma; **Hospital:** UT MD Anderson Cancer Ctr; **Address:** 1515 Holcombe Blvd, Unit 347, Houston, TX 77030; **Phone:** 713-792-6800; **Med School:** Greece 1966; **Resid:** Internal Medicine, Baylor Affil Hosp 1976; **Fellow:** Medical Oncology, MD Anderson Cancer Ctr 1978; **Fac Appt:** Assoc Prof Med, Univ Tex, Houston

Patel, Shreyaskumar MD [Onc] - **Spec Exp:** Sarcoma; **Hospital:** UT MD Anderson Cancer Ctr; **Address:** 1515 Holcombe Blvd, Box 450, Houston, TX 77030; **Phone:** 713-792-3626; **Board Cert:** Internal Medicine 1987; Medical Oncology 2011; **Med School:** India 1983; **Resid:** Internal Medicine, Wayne State Affil Hosp 1987; **Fellow:** Medical Oncology, Mayo Clinic 1990

Patt, Yehuda Z MD [Onc] - **Spec Exp:** Liver Cancer; Biliary Cancer; Colon & Rectal Cancer; Gastrointestinal Cancer; **Hospital:** Univ Hosp - New Mexico; **Address:** Univ New Mexico CRTC, Div Hem/Onc, 1201 Camino de Salud NE, Albuquerque, NM 87131; **Phone:** 505-272-4946; **Board Cert:** Internal Medicine 1982; Medical Oncology 1987; **Med School:** Israel 1967; **Resid:** Internal Medicine, Tel Aviv-Sheba Med Ctr 1974; **Fellow:** Medical Oncology, UT MD Anderson Cancer Ctr 1977; **Fac Appt:** Prof Med, Univ New Mexico

Pisters, Katherine M W MD [Onc] - **Spec Exp:** Lung Cancer; **Hospital:** UT MD Anderson Cancer Ctr; **Address:** UT MD Anderson Cancer Ctr, 1515 Holcombe Blvd, Ste 432, Houston, TX 77230-1402; **Phone:** 713-792-6110; **Board Cert:** Internal Medicine 1988; Medical Oncology 2002; **Med School:** Univ Western Ontario 1985; **Resid:** Internal Medicine, N Shore Univ Hosp 1988; **Fellow:** Medical Oncology, Meml Sloan Kettering Cancer Ctr 1991; **Fac Appt:** Prof Med, Univ Tex, Houston

Romaguera, Jorge MD [Onc] - **Spec Exp:** Lymphoma; **Hospital:** UT MD Anderson Cancer Ctr; **Address:** 1515 Holcombe Blvd, Box 429, Lymphoma & Myeloma Clinic, Houston, TX 77030; **Phone:** 713-792-3510; **Board Cert:** Internal Medicine 1988; Medical Oncology 1989; **Med School:** Univ Puerto Rico 1982; **Resid:** Internal Medicine, Univ Hosp 1985; **Fellow:** Hematology & Oncology, Univ Hosp 1987

Ross, Helen J MD [Onc] - **Spec Exp:** Lung Cancer; Mesothelioma; Esophageal Cancer; **Hospital:** Mayo Clinic - Scottsdale, Mayo Clinic - Phoenix; **Address:** Mayo Clinic-Hematology/Oncology, 13400 E Shea Blvd Fl 3, Scottsdale, AZ 85259; **Phone:** 480-301-8335; **Board Cert:** Internal Medicine 1987; Medical Oncology 1989; **Med School:** UCLA 1984; **Resid:** Internal Medicine, Cedars-Sinai Med Ctr 1987; **Fellow:** Hematology & Oncology, UCLA Med Ctr 1990; **Fac Appt:** Assoc Prof Med, Mayo Med Sch

Saiki, John H MD [Onc] - **Hospital:** Univ Hosp - New Mexico; **Address:** University of New Mexico Cancer Center, 1201 Camino de Salud NE, Albuquerque, NM 87106; **Phone:** 505-272-4946; **Board Cert:** Internal Medicine 1970; Medical Oncology 1973; **Med School:** McGill Univ 1961; **Resid:** Internal Medicine, Univ New Mexico 1968; Hematology, Univ New Mexico 1969; **Fellow:** Medical Oncology, MD Anderson Hosp 1970; **Fac Appt:** Prof Emeritus Med, Univ New Mexico

Schiller, Joan H MD [Onc] - **Spec Exp:** Lung Cancer; **Hospital:** UT Southwestern Med Ctr at Dallas; **Address:** Univ Texas Southwestern, 5323 Harry Hines Blvd, Ste NB2102, Dallas, TX 75390-8852; **Phone:** 214-648-4180; **Board Cert:** Internal Medicine 1983; Medical Oncology 1987; **Med School:** Univ IL Coll Med 1980; **Resid:** Internal Medicine, Northwestern Meml Hosp 1983; **Fellow:** Medical Oncology, Univ Wisconsin Hosp 1985; **Fac Appt:** Prof Med, Univ Wisc

Medical Oncology

Simon, George R MD [Onc] - **Spec Exp:** Mesothelioma; Lung Cancer; Thymoma; **Hospital:** UT MD Anderson Cancer Ctr; **Address:** MD Anderson Cancer Ctr, 1515 Holcombe Blvd, Unit 0432, Houston, TX 77030; **Phone:** 713-792-6363; **Board Cert:** Internal Medicine 2007; Medical Oncology 2007; **Med School:** India 1986; **Resid:** Internal Medicine, St Josephs Hosp 1995; **Fellow:** Hematology & Oncology, Univ Colorado 1997

Stopeck, Alison T MD [Onc] - **Spec Exp:** Breast Cancer; Breast Cancer Risk Assessment; **Hospital:** Univ Arizona Med Ctr-Univ Campus; **Address:** Arizona Cancer Ctr, 1515 N Campbell Ave, PO Box 245024, Tucson, AZ 85724; **Phone:** 520-626-2816; **Board Cert:** Internal Medicine 1988; Medical Oncology 2002; Hematology 2002; **Med School:** Columbia P&S 1985; **Resid:** Internal Medicine, Columbia-Presby Med Ctr 1988; **Fellow:** Hematology & Oncology, New York Hosp 1991; **Fac Appt:** Assoc Prof Med, Univ Ariz Coll Med

Taetle, Raymond MD [Onc] - **Spec Exp:** Hematologic Malignancies; Gastrointestinal Cancer; **Hospital:** St. Joseph's Hosp - Tucson; **Address:** Arizona Oncology, 6565 E Carondolet Drive, Ste 155, Tucson, AZ 85710; **Phone:** 520-886-0206; **Board Cert:** Internal Medicine 1976; Hematology 1978; Medical Oncology 1979; **Med School:** Northwestern Univ 1973; **Resid:** Internal Medicine, UCSD Med Ctr 1976; **Fellow:** Hematology & Oncology, UCSD 1979; **Fac Appt:** Clin Prof Med, Univ Ariz Coll Med

Valero, Vicente MD [Onc] - **Spec Exp:** Breast Cancer; **Hospital:** UT MD Anderson Cancer Ctr; **Address:** Univ Texas MD Anderson Cancer Ctr, 1515 Holcombe Blvd, Unit 1354, Houston, TX 77030; **Phone:** 713-792-2817; **Board Cert:** Internal Medicine 1985; Medical Oncology 1987; Hematology 1988; **Med School:** Mexico 1980; **Resid:** Internal Medicine, Univ Cincinnati Med Ctr 1985; Hematology & Oncology, Univ Cincinnati Med Ctr 1987; **Fellow:** Hematology & Oncology, Univ Texas Med Br 1988; **Fac Appt:** Prof Med, Univ Tex, Houston

Varadhachary, Gauri MD [Onc] - **Spec Exp:** Unknown Primary Cancer; Pancreatic Cancer; **Hospital:** UT MD Anderson Cancer Ctr; **Address:** 1515 Holcombe Blvd, Box 426, Houston, TX 77030; **Phone:** 713-792-2828; **Board Cert:** Internal Medicine 2004; Medical Oncology 2008; **Med School:** India 1991; **Resid:** Internal Medicine, Greater Baltimore Med Ctr 1995; **Fellow:** Hematology & Oncology, Baylor Univ Affil Hosp 1998

Von Burton, Gary MD [Onc] - **Spec Exp:** Breast Cancer; Sarcoma; Brain Tumors; **Hospital:** Louisiana State Univ Hosp; **Address:** LSU Health Shreveport, Feist-Weiller Cancer Ctr, 1501 Kings Hwy, Box 33932, Shreveport, LA 71103; **Phone:** 318-813-1200; **Board Cert:** Internal Medicine 1981; Medical Oncology 1983; **Med School:** Univ Utah 1978; **Resid:** Internal Medicine, Duke Univ Med Ctr 1981; **Fellow:** Hematology & Oncology, Duke Univ Med Ctr 1983; **Fac Appt:** Prof Med, Louisiana State U, Shrevport

Von Hoff, Daniel D MD [Onc] - **Spec Exp:** Pancreatic Cancer; Breast Cancer; Drug Discovery; **Hospital:** Scottsdale Hlthcare - Shea; **Address:** 10510 N 92nd St Ste 200, Scottsdale, AZ 85258; **Phone:** 480-323-1350; **Board Cert:** Internal Medicine 1976; Medical Oncology 1979; **Med School:** Columbia P&S 1973; **Resid:** Internal Medicine, UCSF Med Ctr 1975; **Fac Appt:** Prof Med, Univ Ariz Coll Med

Willson, James KV MD [Onc] - **Spec Exp:** Colon & Rectal Cancer; Gastrointestinal Cancer; **Hospital:** UT Southwestern Med Ctr at Dallas; **Address:** 5323 Harry Hines Blvd, MS 8590, Dallas, TX 75390-8590; **Phone:** 214-648-1677; **Board Cert:** Internal Medicine 1980; Medical Oncology 1981; **Med School:** Univ Alabama 1976; **Resid:** Internal Medicine, Johns Hopkins Hosp 1978; **Fellow:** Medical Oncology, Natl Cancer Inst-NIH 1980; **Fac Appt:** Prof Onc, Univ Tex SW, Dallas

Wolff, Robert A MD [Onc] - **Spec Exp:** Gastrointestinal Cancer; Pancreatic Cancer; Colon & Rectal Cancer; Clinical Trials; **Hospital:** UT MD Anderson Cancer Ctr; **Address:** 1515 Holcombe Blvd, Unit 421, Houston, TX 77030; **Phone:** 713-745-5476; **Board Cert:** Internal Medicine 1989; Medical Oncology 2008; **Med School:** Albany Med Coll 1986; **Resid:** Internal Medicine, Duke Univ Med Ctr 1989; **Fellow:** Hematology & Oncology, Duke Univ Med Ctr 1992

West Coast and Pacific

Aboulafia, David M MD [Onc] - **Spec Exp:** AIDS Related Cancers; Leukemia & Lymphoma; Myeloproliferative Disorders; Multiple Myeloma; **Hospital:** Virginia Mason Med Ctr; **Address:** Virginia Mason Med Ctr, Sect of Hematology/Oncology, 1100 Ninth Ave, MS C2-Hem, Seattle, WA 98101; **Phone:** 206-223-6193; **Board Cert:** Internal Medicine 1986; Medical Oncology 1989; Hematology 2003; **Med School:** Univ Mich Med Sch 1983; **Resid:** Internal Medicine, UCLA Med Ctr 1986; **Fellow:** Hematology & Oncology, UCLA Med Ctr 1989; **Fac Appt:** Clin Prof Med, Univ Wash

Abrams, Donald I MD [Onc] - **Spec Exp:** AIDS Related Cancers; Complementary Medicine; **Hospital:** San Francisco Genl Hosp; **Address:** Positive Hlth Program-SF Genl Hosp, 995 Potrero Ave, Bldg 80, Ward 84, San Francisco, CA 94110; **Phone:** 415-353-7700; **Board Cert:** Internal Medicine 1980; Medical Oncology 1983; **Med School:** Stanford Univ 1977; **Resid:** Internal Medicine, Kaiser Fdn Hosp 1980; **Fellow:** Medical Oncology, UCSF Cancer Rsch 1982; **Fac Appt:** Clin Prof Med, UCSF

Advani, Ranjana H MD [Onc] - **Spec Exp:** Lymphoma; Hematologic Malignancies; Clinical Trials; **Hospital:** Stanford Univ Hosp & Clinics; **Address:** Lymphoma Clinic, 875 Blake Wilbur Drive, Clinic C, Stanford, CA 94305; **Phone:** 650-498-6000; **Board Cert:** Internal Medicine 2001; Medical Oncology 2009; **Med School:** India 1982; **Resid:** Internal Medicine, Santa Clara Vly Med Ctr 1987; Internal Medicine, Stanford Univ 1991; **Fellow:** Hematology, Stanford Univ Med Ctr 1990; **Fac Appt:** Asst Prof Med, Stanford Univ

Appelbaum, Frederick R MD [Onc] - **Spec Exp:** Bone Marrow Transplant; Leukemia-Myeloid; Graft vs Host Disease; **Hospital:** Univ Wash Med Ctr; **Address:** 1100 Fairview Ave N, rm D5-310, PO Box 19024, Seattle, WA 98109; **Phone:** 206-288-1024; **Board Cert:** Internal Medicine 1975; Medical Oncology 1977; **Med School:** Tufts Univ 1972; **Resid:** Internal Medicine, Univ Michigan Med Ctr 1974; **Fellow:** Medical Oncology, Natl Cancer Inst 1976; **Fac Appt:** Prof Med, Univ Wash

Back, Anthony MD [Onc] - **Spec Exp:** Palliative Care; Gastrointestinal Cancer; **Hospital:** Univ Wash Med Ctr; **Address:** Seattle Cancer Care Alliance, 825 Eastlake Ave E, Box G4810, Seattle, WA 98109; **Phone:** 206-288-6797; **Board Cert:** Internal Medicine 1987; Hospice & Palliative Medicine 2008; **Med School:** Harvard Med Sch 1984; **Resid:** Internal Medicine, Univ Washington Med Ctr 1988; **Fellow:** Oncology, Univ Washington Med Ctr 1991; **Fac Appt:** Prof Med, Univ Wash

Ball, Edward D MD [Onc] - **Spec Exp:** Bone Marrow & Stem Cell Transplant; Leukemia & Lymphoma; Multiple Myeloma; Immunotherapy; **Hospital:** UCSD Med Ctr; **Address:** 3855 Health Sciences Dr, #0960, La Jolla, CA 92093-0960; **Phone:** 858-822-6600; **Board Cert:** Internal Medicine 1979; Medical Oncology 1983; Hematology 2011; **Med School:** Case West Res Univ 1976; **Resid:** Internal Medicine, Hartford Hosp 1979; **Fellow:** Hematology & Oncology, Univ Hosps Cleveland 1981; Hematology & Oncology, Dartmouth-Hitchcock Hosp 1982; **Fac Appt:** Prof Hem & Onc, UCSD

Medical Oncology

Beer, Tomasz M MD [Onc] - **Spec Exp:** Prostate Cancer; **Hospital:** OR Hlth & Sci Univ, VA Medical Center - Portland; **Address:** 3303 SW Bond Ave, CH14R, Portland, OR 97239; **Phone:** 503-494-6594; **Board Cert:** Medical Oncology 2010; **Med School:** Johns Hopkins Univ 1991; **Resid:** Internal Medicine, Oreg Hlth Scis Univ 1994; Internal Medicine, Oreg Hlth Scis Univ 1996; **Fellow:** Hematology & Oncology, Oreg Hlth Scis Univ 1999; **Fac Appt:** Prof Med, Oregon Hlth & Sci Univ

Bensinger, William I MD [Onc] - **Spec Exp:** Multiple Myeloma; Stem Cell Transplant; **Hospital:** Univ Wash Med Ctr; **Address:** Fred Hutchinson Cancer Research Ctr, 1100 Fairview Ave N, MS DS-390, Seattle, WA 98109-1024; **Phone:** 206-288-1024; **Board Cert:** Internal Medicine 1978; Medical Oncology 1979; **Med School:** Northwestern Univ 1973; **Resid:** Internal Medicine, Univ Wash Hosps 1978; **Fellow:** Medical Oncology, Univ Wash Hosps 1979; **Fac Appt:** Assoc Prof Med, Univ Wash

Berry, J Michael MD [Onc] - **Spec Exp:** Anal Cancer; HPV-Human Papilloma Virus; **Hospital:** UCSF - Mt Zion Med Ctr; **Address:** UCSF, Dysplasia Clinic, 1600 Divisadero St Fl 4th, Box 1705, San Francisco, CA 94143; **Phone:** 415-353-7100; **Board Cert:** Internal Medicine 1985; Medical Oncology 1989; **Med School:** Univ Miami Sch Med 1982; **Resid:** Internal Medicine, UCSF Med Ctr 1985; **Fellow:** Medical Oncology, Stanford Univ 1989; **Fac Appt:** Asst Clin Prof Med, UCSF

Carlson, Robert W MD [Onc] - **Spec Exp:** Breast Cancer; **Hospital:** Stanford Univ Hosp & Clinics; **Address:** Stanford Comprehensive Cancer Ctr, 900 Blake Wilbur Drive, Stanford, CA 94305; **Phone:** 650-498-6000; **Board Cert:** Internal Medicine 1981; Medical Oncology 1983; **Med School:** Stanford Univ 1978; **Resid:** Internal Medicine, Barnes Hosp 1980; Internal Medicine, Stanford Univ Hosp 1981; **Fellow:** Medical Oncology, Stanford Univ Hosp 1983; **Fac Appt:** Prof Med, Stanford Univ

Chang, Susan M MD [Onc] - **Spec Exp:** Brain Tumors; Spinal Cord Tumors; Pituitary Tumors; Acromegaly; **Hospital:** UCSF Med Ctr; **Address:** UCSF, Dept Neurological Surgery, 400 Parnassus Ave Fl 8 - rm A808, San Francisco, CA 94143; **Phone:** 415-353-2184; **Med School:** Univ British Columbia Fac Med 1985; **Resid:** Internal Medicine, Plains Hlth Ctr 1987; Internal Medicine, Toronto Genl Hosp 1989; **Fellow:** Medical Oncology, Princess Margaret Hosp 1991; Neuro-Oncology, UCSF Med Ctr 1995; **Fac Appt:** Prof Med, UCSF

Chap, Linnea MD [Onc] - **Spec Exp:** Breast Cancer; **Hospital:** St. John's Hlth Ctr, Santa Monica; **Address:** Beverly Hills Cancer Center, 8900 Wilshire Blvd Fl 2, Beverly Hills, CA 90211; **Phone:** 310-432-8900; **Board Cert:** Medical Oncology 2005; **Med School:** Univ Chicago-Pritzker Sch Med 1988; **Resid:** Internal Medicine, Northwestern Meml Hosp 1991; **Fellow:** Hematology & Oncology, UCLA Med Ctr 1992

Chew, Helen K MD [Onc] - **Spec Exp:** Breast Cancer; **Hospital:** UC Davis Med Ctr; **Address:** UC Davis Cancer Ctr, 4501 X St, Ste 3016, Sacramento, CA 95817; **Phone:** 916-734-3700; **Board Cert:** Medical Oncology 2007; **Med School:** Univ Tex, San Antonio 1991; **Resid:** Internal Medicine, UT Hlth Sci Ctr 1994; **Fellow:** Medical Oncology, UT Hlth Sci Ctr 1997

Chlebowski, Rowan T MD/PhD [Onc] - **Spec Exp:** Breast Cancer; Women's Health; **Hospital:** LAC - Harbor - UCLA Med Ctr; **Address:** 1124 W Carson St J3 Bldg, Torrance, CA 90502; **Phone:** 310-222-2218; **Board Cert:** Internal Medicine 1980; Medical Oncology 1981; **Med School:** Case West Res Univ 1974; **Resid:** Internal Medicine, MetroHealth Med Ctr 1976; Medical Oncology, LAC-USC Med Ctr 1979; **Fac Appt:** Prof Med, UCLA

Chow, Warren A MD [Onc] - **Spec Exp:** Sarcoma-Soft Tissue; Sarcoma; Melanoma; **Hospital:** City of Hope Natl Med Ctr; **Address:** 1500 E Duarte Rd, Duarte, CA 91010; **Phone:** 626-256-4673 x62961; **Board Cert:** Internal Medicine 1989; Medical Oncology 2003; Hematology 2004; **Med School:** Univ Hlth Scis, Chicago Med Sch 1986; **Resid:** Internal Medicine, Cedars-Sinai Med Ctr 1990; **Fellow:** Hematology & Oncology, City of Hope Med Ctr 1992; Molecular Genetics, City of Hope Med Ctr 1994; **Fac Appt:** Assoc Prof Onc, Ros Franklin Univ/Chicago Med Sch

Crocenzi, Todd MD [Onc] - **Spec Exp:** Gastrointestinal Cancer; **Hospital:** Providence Portland Med Ctr; **Address:** Providence Cancer Ctr, 4805 NE Glisan St, Ste 6N40, Portland, OR 97213; **Phone:** 503-215-5696; **Board Cert:** Medical Oncology 2004; **Med School:** Jefferson Med Coll 1994; **Resid:** Internal Medicine, Univ MD Med Ctr 1997; **Fellow:** Hematology & Oncology, Dartmouth Hitchcock Med Ctr 2004; Immunology, Dartmouth Hitchcock Med Ctr 2005

Daud, Adil I MD [Onc] - **Spec Exp:** Melanoma; Skin Cancer; Drug Development; **Hospital:** UCSF Med Ctr; **Address:** 1600 Divisadero St Fl 4, San Francisco, CA 94115; **Phone:** 415-353-9900; **Board Cert:** Hematology 2000; Medical Oncology 2000; **Med School:** India 1987; **Resid:** Internal Medicine, Indiana Univ Affil Hosp; **Fellow:** Hematology & Oncology, Meml Sloan Kettering Cancer Ctr

Deeg, H Joachim MD [Onc] - **Spec Exp:** Myelodysplastic Syndromes; Myeloproliferative Disorders; Bone Marrow Failure Disorders; Graft vs Host Disease; **Hospital:** Univ Wash Med Ctr; **Address:** Fred Hutchinson Cancer Research Center, 1100 Fairview Avenue N, D1-100, Box 19024, Seattle, WA 98109-1024; **Phone:** 206-667-5985; **Board Cert:** Internal Medicine 1976; Medical Oncology 1979; **Med School:** Germany 1972; **Resid:** Internal Medicine, Gennessee Hosp 1976; **Fellow:** Medical Oncology, Univ Wash Med Ctr 1978; **Fac Appt:** Prof Med, Univ Wash

Disis, Mary Lenora MD [Onc] - **Spec Exp:** Breast Cancer; Ovarian Cancer; Clinical Trials; **Hospital:** Univ Wash Med Ctr; **Address:** Univ Washington, Tumor Vaccine Group, 815 Mercer St, Box 358050, Seattle, WA 98109; **Phone:** 206-616-1823; **Board Cert:** Internal Medicine 1989; Medical Oncology 2008; **Med School:** Univ Nebr Coll Med 1986; **Resid:** Internal Medicine, Univ Illinois Med Ctr 1990; **Fellow:** Medical Oncology, Fred Hutchinson Cancer Ctr 1993; **Fac Appt:** Assoc Prof Med, Univ Wash

Druker, Brian J MD [Onc] - **Spec Exp:** Leukemia; Leukemia-Chronic Myeloid; Hematologic Malignancies; **Hospital:** OR Hlth & Sci Univ; **Address:** OHSU Ctr Hematologic Malignancies, 3181 Sam Jackson Park Rd, Multnomah Pavilion, MC UHN73A, Portland, OR 97239-3098; **Phone:** 503-494-5058; **Board Cert:** Internal Medicine 1984; Medical Oncology 1987; **Med School:** UCSD 1981; **Resid:** Internal Medicine, Barnes Jewish Hosp 1984; **Fellow:** Medical Oncology, Dana-Farber Cancer Inst 1987; **Fac Appt:** Prof Med, Oregon Hlth & Sci Univ

Ellis, Georgiana K MD [Onc] - **Spec Exp:** Breast Cancer; Clinical Trials; **Hospital:** Univ Wash Med Ctr; **Address:** Seattle Cancer Care Alliance, 825 Eastlake Ave E, Box 358081, MS G3-630, Seattle, WA 98103; **Phone:** 206-288-1000; **Board Cert:** Internal Medicine 1985; Medical Oncology 1987; **Med School:** Univ Wash 1982; **Resid:** Internal Medicine, Univ Washington Med Ctr 1985; **Fellow:** Medical Oncology, Univ Washington Med Ctr 1988; **Fac Appt:** Assoc Prof Med, Univ Wash

Estey, Elihu H MD [Onc] - **Spec Exp:** Leukemia; Leukemia-Myeloid; Clinical Trials; Myelodysplastic Syndromes; **Hospital:** Univ Wash Med Ctr; **Address:** Seattle Cancer Care Alliance, 825 Eastlake Ave E, UW Box 3587710, Seattle, WA 98109; **Phone:** 206-288-7176; **Board Cert:** Internal Medicine 1975; Medical Oncology 1981; **Med School:** Johns Hopkins Univ 1972; **Resid:** Internal Medicine, Bellevue Hosp Ctr 1975; **Fellow:** Medical Oncology, MD Anderson Cancer Ctr 1978

Medical Oncology

Figlin, Robert A MD [Onc] - **Spec Exp:** Urologic Cancer; Kidney Cancer; Immunotherapy; **Hospital:** Cedars-Sinai Med Ctr; **Address:** Cedars-Sinai Med Ctr, Division of Hematology & Oncology, 8700 Beverly Blvd, Ste 1S30, Los Angeles, CA 90048; **Phone:** 310-423-1331; **Board Cert:** Internal Medicine 1979; Medical Oncology 1983; **Med School:** Med Coll PA Hahnemann 1976; **Resid:** Internal Medicine, Cedars Sinai Med Ctr 1980; **Fellow:** Hematology & Oncology, UCLA Ctr Hlth Sci 1982; **Fac Appt:** Prof Med, UCLA

Fisher Jr, George A MD/PhD [Onc] - **Spec Exp:** Gastrointestinal Cancer; Pancreatic Cancer; **Hospital:** Stanford Univ Hosp & Clinics; **Address:** Stanford Comp Cancer Ctr, GI Onc, 875 Blake Wilbur Drive, MC 5826, Stanford, CA 94305; **Phone:** 650-498-6000; **Board Cert:** Medical Oncology 1997; **Med School:** Stanford Univ 1987; **Resid:** Internal Medicine, Stanford Univ Med Ctr 1991; **Fellow:** Medical Oncology, Stanford Univ Med Ctr 1993; **Fac Appt:** Assoc Prof Med, Stanford Univ

Ford, James M MD [Onc] - **Spec Exp:** Gastrointestinal Cancer; Colon & Rectal Cancer; Cancer Genetics; **Hospital:** Stanford Univ Hosp & Clinics; **Address:** Stanford Comp Cancer Ctr, 875 Blake Wilbur Drive, Clinic F, Stanford, CA 94305; **Phone:** 650-723-7621; **Board Cert:** Medical Oncology 2005; **Med School:** Yale Univ 1989; **Resid:** Internal Medicine, Stanford Univ Med Ctr 1991; **Fellow:** Medical Oncology, Stanford Univ Med Ctr 1994; **Fac Appt:** Assoc Prof Med, Stanford Univ

Forscher, Charles A MD [Onc] - **Spec Exp:** Bone Tumors; Sarcoma-Soft Tissue; **Hospital:** Cedars-Sinai Med Ctr, UCLA Ronald Reagan Med Ctr; **Address:** Outpatient Cancer Ctr, Lower Level, 8700 Beverly Blvd, Ste AC1042D, Los Angeles, CA 90048; **Phone:** 310-423-8045; **Board Cert:** Internal Medicine 1981; Hematology 1986; Medical Oncology 1987; **Med School:** Albert Einstein Coll Med 1978; **Resid:** Internal Medicine, Montefiore Med Ctr 1981; **Fellow:** Hematology, Montefiore Med Ctr 1983; Neoplastic Diseases, Mt Sinai Med Ctr 1985; **Fac Appt:** Clin Prof Med, UCLA

Gandara, David R MD [Onc] - **Spec Exp:** Lung Cancer; **Hospital:** UC Davis Med Ctr; **Address:** UC Davis Cancer Ctr, 4501 X St, Ste 3016, Sacramento, CA 95817; **Phone:** 916-734-3700; **Board Cert:** Internal Medicine 1976; Medical Oncology 1979; **Med School:** Univ Tex Med Br, Galveston 1973; **Resid:** Internal Medicine, Madigan Med Ctr 1976; **Fellow:** Hematology & Oncology, Letterman AMC 1978; **Fac Appt:** Prof Med, UC Davis

Ganz, Patricia A MD [Onc] - **Spec Exp:** Breast Cancer; Cancer Survivors-Late Effects of Therapy; **Hospital:** UCLA Ronald Reagan Med Ctr; **Address:** UCLA, Cancer Prev/Control Rsch, A2-125 CHS, 650 Charles Young Drive S, Box 956900, Los Angeles, CA 90095-6900; **Phone:** 310-206-6909; **Board Cert:** Internal Medicine 1976; Medical Oncology 1979; **Med School:** UCLA 1973; **Resid:** Internal Medicine, UCLA Med Ctr 1976; **Fellow:** Hematology, UCLA Med Ctr 1978; **Fac Appt:** Prof Med, UCLA

Glaspy, John A MD [Onc] - **Spec Exp:** Breast Cancer; Melanoma; Lymphoma; Gastrointestinal Cancer; **Hospital:** UCLA Ronald Reagan Med Ctr, Santa Monica - UCLA Med Ctr & Ortho Hosp; **Address:** 100 UCLA Medical Plaza, Ste 550, Los Angeles, CA 90095; **Phone:** 310-794-4955; **Board Cert:** Internal Medicine 1982; Medical Oncology 1985; Hematology 1986; **Med School:** UCLA 1979; **Resid:** Internal Medicine, UCLA Med Ctr 1982; **Fellow:** Hematology & Oncology, UCLA Med Ctr 1984; **Fac Appt:** Prof Med, UCLA

Gold, Philip J MD [Onc] - **Spec Exp:** Gastrointestinal Cancer; Clinical Trials; **Hospital:** Swedish Med Ctr-First Hill-Seattle; **Address:** Swedish Cancer Inst, 1221 Madison St, Fl 2, Ste 200, Seattle, WA 98104; **Phone:** 206-386-2121; **Board Cert:** Internal Medicine 2005; Medical Oncology 2007; **Med School:** Univ Miami Sch Med 1991; **Resid:** Internal Medicine, Univ of Washington Med Ctr 1994; **Fellow:** Medical Oncology, Fred Hutchinson Cancer Rsch Ctr 1997

Gralow, Julie MD [Onc] - **Spec Exp:** Breast Cancer; **Hospital:** Univ Wash Med Ctr; **Address:** Seattle Cancer Care Alliance, 825 Eastlake Ave E, MS G3-630, Seattle, WA 98109; **Phone:** 206-288-7222; **Board Cert:** Medical Oncology 2005; **Med School:** USC Sch Med 1988; **Resid:** Internal Medicine, Brigham & Women's Hosp 1991; **Fellow:** Oncology, Univ Wash Med Ctr 1994; **Fac Appt:** Assoc Prof Med, Univ Wash

Higano, Celestia MD [Onc] - **Spec Exp:** Genitourinary Cancer; Prostate Cancer; Testicular Cancer; **Hospital:** Univ Wash Med Ctr; **Address:** Seattle Cancer Care Alliance, 825 Eastlake Ave E, Box 19024, Seattle, WA 98109; **Phone:** 206-288-1152; **Board Cert:** Internal Medicine 1982; Medical Oncology 1985; **Med School:** Univ Mass Sch Med 1979; **Resid:** Internal Medicine, Mayo Clinic 1982; **Fellow:** Oncology, Univ Washington Med Ctr 1985; **Fac Appt:** Prof Med, Univ Wash

Jacobs, Charlotte D MD [Onc] - **Spec Exp:** Sarcoma; Unknown Primary Cancer; **Hospital:** Stanford Univ Hosp & Clinics; **Address:** 875 Blake Wilbur Drive, Clinic B, Stanford, CA 94305; **Phone:** 650-498-6000; **Board Cert:** Internal Medicine 1975; Medical Oncology 1977; **Med School:** Washington Univ, St Louis 1972; **Resid:** Internal Medicine, Barnes Hosp 1974; Internal Medicine, UCSF Med Ctr 1975; **Fellow:** Medical Oncology, Stanford Univ 1977; **Fac Appt:** Prof Med, Stanford Univ

Kaplan, Lawrence D MD [Onc] - **Spec Exp:** AIDS Related Cancers; Lymphoma; **Hospital:** UCSF Med Ctr; **Address:** UCSF Medical Center, 400 Parnassus Ave, rm 502, Box 0324, San Francisco, CA 94143-0324; **Phone:** 415-353-2421; **Board Cert:** Internal Medicine 1983; Medical Oncology 1985; **Med School:** UCLA 1980; **Resid:** Internal Medicine, Boston City Hosp 1983; **Fellow:** Hematology & Oncology, UCSF Med Ctr 1985; **Fac Appt:** Clin Prof Med, UCSF

Kelly, Karen Lee MD [Onc] - **Spec Exp:** Lung Cancer; **Hospital:** UC Davis Med Ctr; **Address:** 4501 X St, Ste 3016, Sacramento, CA 95817; **Phone:** 916-734-3735; **Board Cert:** Internal Medicine 1987; Medical Oncology 2003; **Med School:** Univ Kansas 1984; **Resid:** Internal Medicine, Univ CO Hlth Sci Ctr 1987; **Fellow:** Medical Oncology, Univ CO Hlth Sci Ctr 1990; **Fac Appt:** Prof Med, UCSD

Kesari, Santosh MD/PhD [Onc] - **Spec Exp:** Neuro-Oncology; Stem Cell Therapy; Leukoencephalopathy; **Hospital:** John M & Sally B Thornton Hosp, UCSD Med Ctr; **Address:** UCSD Moores Cancer Center, 3855 Health Sciences Drive, La Jolla, CA 92093; **Phone:** 858-822-6346; **Board Cert:** Neurology 2005; **Med School:** Univ Pennsylvania 1999; **Resid:** Neurology, Mass Genl Hosp 2003; **Fellow:** Neuro-Oncology, Dana Farber Cancer Inst 2004

Koczywas, Marianna MD [Onc] - **Spec Exp:** Lung Cancer; **Hospital:** City of Hope Natl Med Ctr; **Address:** City of Hope Med Ctr, Dept Med Onc, 1500 E Duarte Rd, Duarte, CA 91010; **Phone:** 626-471-9200; **Board Cert:** Hematology 2000; Medical Oncology 2001; **Med School:** Poland 1984; **Resid:** Internal Medicine, Troczewski City Hosp 1988; Internal Medicine, St Francis Med Ctr 1997; **Fellow:** Hematology & Oncology, City of Hope Natl Med Ctr 2000

Lim, Dean Wee MD [Onc] - **Hospital:** City of Hope Natl Med Ctr; **Address:** City of Hope Med Ctr, Dept Med Onc, 1500 E Duarte Rd, Duarte, CA 91010; **Phone:** 626-471-9200; **Board Cert:** Internal Medicine 1985; Medical Oncology 1989; **Med School:** Philippines 1980; **Resid:** Internal Medicine, Cabrini Med Ctr 1985; **Fellow:** Hematology & Oncology, St Lukes Roosevelt Hosp 1987; **Fac Appt:** Asst Clin Prof Med, USC-Keck School of Medicine

Lippman, Scott M MD [Onc] - **Spec Exp:** Cancer Prevention; Lung Cancer; Head & Neck Cancer; **Hospital:** UCSD Med Ctr; **Address:** UCSD Moore Cancer Ctr, 3855 Health Sciences Drive, La Jolla, CA 92093; **Phone:** 858-822-6168; **Board Cert:** Internal Medicine 1987; Hematology 1988; Medical Oncology 1989; **Med School:** Johns Hopkins Univ 1981; **Resid:** Internal Medicine, Harbor-UCLA Med Ctr 1983; **Fellow:** Hematology, Stanford Univ Med Ctr 1985; Hematology & Oncology, Univ Ariz Hlth Scis Ctr 1987; **Fac Appt:** Prof Med, Univ Tex, Houston

Medical Oncology

Maloney, David G MD/PhD [Onc] - **Spec Exp:** Lymphoma; Bone Marrow & Stem Cell Transplant; Vaccine Therapy; **Hospital:** Univ Wash Med Ctr; **Address:** Fred Hutchinson Cancer Rsch Ctr, 1100 Fairview Ave N, D1-100, Box 19024, Seattle, WA 98109-1024; **Phone:** 206-667-5616; **Board Cert:** Internal Medicine 1988; Medical Oncology 2005; **Med School:** Stanford Univ 1985; **Resid:** Internal Medicine, Brigham & Women's Hosp 1988; **Fellow:** Medical Oncology, Stanford Univ Med Ctr 1994; **Fac Appt:** Prof Med, Univ Wash

Margolin, Kim A MD [Onc] - **Spec Exp:** Melanoma; Kidney Cancer; Germ Cell Tumors; **Hospital:** Univ Wash Med Ctr; **Address:** Seattle Cancer Care Alliance, 825 Eastlake Ave E, MS G3-630, Seattle, WA 98109; **Phone:** 206-288-7222; **Board Cert:** Internal Medicine 1982; Medical Oncology 2006; Hematology 1986; **Med School:** Stanford Univ 1979; **Resid:** Internal Medicine, Yale-New Haven Hosp 1982; **Fellow:** Hematology & Oncology, UC San Diego Med Ctr 1983; Hematology & Oncology, City of Hope Med Ctr 1985; **Fac Appt:** Prof Med, Univ Wash

Martins, Renato G MD [Onc] - **Spec Exp:** Head & Neck Cancer; Lung Cancer; Mesothelioma; Salivary Gland Tumors; **Hospital:** Univ Wash Med Ctr; **Address:** Seattle Cancer Care Alliance, 825 Eastlake Ave E, MS G4-490, Seattle, WA 98109; **Phone:** 206-288-2048; **Board Cert:** Internal Medicine 2005; Medical Oncology 2008; **Med School:** Brazil 1992; **Resid:** Internal Medicine, Gunderson Clinic 1995; **Fellow:** Medical Oncology, Mass Genl Hosp 1998; **Fac Appt:** Assoc Prof Med, Univ Wash

McClay, Edward F MD [Onc] - **Spec Exp:** Melanoma; Brain Tumors; **Hospital:** UCSD Med Ctr; **Address:** 477 N El Camino Real, Ste D-200, Encinitas, CA 92024; **Phone:** 760-452-3340; **Board Cert:** Internal Medicine 1983; Medical Oncology 1989; **Med School:** Temple Univ 1980; **Resid:** Internal Medicine, Thomas Jefferson Univ Hosp 1983; **Fellow:** Medical Oncology, Thomas Jefferson Univ Hosp 1986

Meyskens Jr, Frank L MD [Onc] - **Spec Exp:** Melanoma; Sarcoma; **Hospital:** UC Irvine Med Ctr; **Address:** UC Irvine Cancer Ctr, 101 The City Drive, Bldg 56, rm 215, Orange, CA 92868; **Phone:** 714-456-6310; **Board Cert:** Internal Medicine 1975; Medical Oncology 1981; **Med School:** UCSF 1972; **Resid:** Internal Medicine, Moffit-Calif Hosps 1974; **Fellow:** Hematology & Oncology, Natl Cancer Inst 1977; **Fac Appt:** Prof Med, UC Irvine

Mitsuyasu, Ronald T MD [Onc] - **Spec Exp:** AIDS Related Cancers; Hematologic Malignancies; **Hospital:** UCLA Ronald Reagan Med Ctr, Santa Monica - UCLA Med Ctr & Ortho Hosp; **Address:** 1399 S Roxbury Drive, Ste 100, Los Angeles, CA 90035; **Phone:** 310-557-2273; **Board Cert:** Internal Medicine 1981; **Med School:** UCLA 1978; **Resid:** Internal Medicine, Rush Presby St Lukes Hosp 1981; **Fellow:** Hematology & Oncology, UCLA Med Ctr 1984; **Fac Appt:** Prof Hem & Onc, UCLA

Mortimer, Joanne MD [Onc] - **Spec Exp:** Breast Cancer; Clinical Trials; **Hospital:** City of Hope Natl Med Ctr; **Address:** 1500 E Duarte Rd, Duarte, CA 91010; **Phone:** 626-471-9200; **Board Cert:** Internal Medicine 1980; Medical Oncology 1983; **Med School:** Loyola Univ-Stritch Sch Med 1977; **Resid:** Internal Medicine, Cleveland Clinic 1980; **Fellow:** Medical Oncology, Cleveland Clinic 1982; **Fac Appt:** Prof Hem & Onc, Loyola Univ-Stritch Sch Med

Natale, Ronald B MD [Onc] - **Spec Exp:** Lung Cancer; **Hospital:** Cedars-Sinai Med Ctr; **Address:** Cedars-Sinai Outpatient Comp Cancer Ctr, 8700 Beverly Blvd, Ste MS-33, Los Angeles, CA 90048; **Phone:** 310-423-1101; **Board Cert:** Internal Medicine 1977; Medical Oncology 1979; **Med School:** Wayne State Univ 1974; **Resid:** Internal Medicine, Wayne State Univ 1977; **Fellow:** Hematology & Oncology, Meml Sloan Kettering 1980; **Fac Appt:** Prof Med, Univ Mich Med Sch

O'Day, Steven J MD [Onc] - **Spec Exp:** Melanoma; Melanoma-Advanced; **Hospital:** St. John's Regional Med Ctr; **Address:** Beverly Hills Cancer Ctr, 8900 Wilshire Blvd, Beverly Hills, CA 90211; **Phone:** 310-432-8900; **Med School:** Johns Hopkins Univ 1988; **Resid:** Internal Medicine, Johns Hopkins Hosp 1991; **Fellow:** Medical Oncology, Dana Farber Cancer Inst 1992; **Fac Appt:** Assoc Clin Prof Med, USC-Keck School of Medicine

Parker, Barbara A MD [Onc] - **Spec Exp:** Breast Cancer; Nutrition in Cancer Therapy; **Hospital:** UCSD Med Ctr; **Address:** Moores UCSD Cancer Ctr, Hem/Onc Dept, 3855 Health Sciences Drive, MC 0987, La Jolla, CA 92093; **Phone:** 858-822-6195; **Board Cert:** Internal Medicine 1984; Medical Oncology 1987; **Med School:** Stanford Univ 1981; **Resid:** Internal Medicine, UCSD Med Ctr 1985; **Fellow:** Medical Oncology, UCSD Med Ctr 1987; **Fac Appt:** Prof Med, UCSD

Pegram, Mark D MD [Onc] - **Spec Exp:** Breast Cancer; Breast Cancer-Novel Therapies; **Hospital:** Stanford Univ Hosp & Clinics; **Address:** Stanford Womens Cancer Ctr, 900 Blake Wilbur Drive, Stanford, CA 94305; **Phone:** 650-498-6000; **Board Cert:** Internal Medicine 1989; Medical Oncology 2003; **Med School:** Univ NC Sch Med 1986; **Resid:** Internal Medicine, Parkland Meml Hosp 1989; **Fellow:** Hematology & Oncology, UCLA Med Ctr 1993; **Fac Appt:** Prof Med, Stanford Univ

Picozzi Jr, Vincent J MD [Onc] - **Spec Exp:** Gastrointestinal Cancer; Pancreatic Cancer; Genitourinary Cancer; Hematologic Malignancies; **Hospital:** Virginia Mason Med Ctr; **Address:** Virginia Mason Med Ctr, Div Hem/Onc, 1100 Ninth Ave, MS C2-Hem, Seattle, WA 98111; **Phone:** 206-223-6193; **Board Cert:** Internal Medicine 1981; Hematology 1986; Medical Oncology 1987; **Med School:** Stanford Univ 1978; **Resid:** Internal Medicine, Peter Bent Brigham Med Ctr 1981; **Fellow:** Hematology, Stanford Univ Med Ctr 1983; Medical Oncology, Stanford Univ MEd Ctr 1983; **Fac Appt:** Clin Prof Med, Univ Wash

Pinto, Harlan A MD [Onc] - **Spec Exp:** Head & Neck Cancer; Clinical Trials; **Hospital:** Stanford Univ Hosp & Clinics, VA Hlth Care Sys - Palo Alto; **Address:** Stanford Comp Cancer Ctr, 875 Blake Wilbur Drive, Clinic C, Stanford, CA 94305; **Phone:** 650-723-7621; **Board Cert:** Internal Medicine 1986; Medical Oncology 2002; **Med School:** Yale Univ 1983; **Resid:** Internal Medicine, Mass Genl Hosp 1986; **Fellow:** Medical Oncology, Stanford Univ Med Sch 1991; **Fac Appt:** Assoc Prof Med, Stanford Univ

Prados, Michael MD [Onc] - **Spec Exp:** Neuro-Oncology; Brain Tumors; **Hospital:** UCSF Med Ctr; **Address:** UCSF Med Ctr, Div Neuro-Oncology, 400 Parnassus Ave Fl 8 - rm A-808, San Francisco, CA 94143; **Phone:** 415-353-2408; **Board Cert:** Internal Medicine 1977; **Med School:** Louisiana State U, New Orleans 1974; **Resid:** Internal Medicine, Earl K Long Hosp 1977; **Fac Appt:** Prof NS, UCSF

Press, Oliver W MD/PhD [Onc] - **Spec Exp:** Lymphoma; Bone Marrow Transplant; **Hospital:** Univ Wash Med Ctr; **Address:** Fred Hutchinson Cancer Research Center, 1100 Fairview Ave N, MS D3-190, Seattle, WA 98109; **Phone:** 206-667-1864; **Board Cert:** Internal Medicine 1982; Medical Oncology 1985; **Med School:** Univ Wash 1979; **Resid:** Internal Medicine, Mass Genl Hosp 1982; Internal Medicine, Univ Washington Med Ctr 1983; **Fellow:** Medical Oncology, Univ Washington Med Ctr 1985; **Fac Appt:** Prof Med, Univ Wash

Quinn, David I MD/PhD [Onc] - **Spec Exp:** Testicular Cancer; Bladder Cancer; Kidney Cancer; Adrenal Cancer; **Hospital:** USC Norris Cancer Hosp (page 62), Keck Med Ctr of USC (page 62); **Address:** 1441 Eastlake Ave, Ste 3440, Los Angeles, CA 90033; **Phone:** 323-865-3956; **Med School:** Australia 1987; **Resid:** Internal Medicine, St Vincents Hosp 1992; **Fellow:** Medical Oncology, St Vincents Hosp 1995; **Fac Appt:** Assoc Prof Onc, USC Sch Med

Medical Oncology

Reid, Tony R MD [Onc] - **Spec Exp:** Gastrointestinal Cancer; Pancreatic Cancer; Esophageal Cancer; Liver Cancer; **Hospital:** UCSD Med Ctr; **Address:** 3855 Health Sciences Drive, Ste 1102, MC 0987, La Jolla, CA 92093; **Phone:** 858-822-6100; **Board Cert:** Medical Oncology 1999; **Med School:** Stanford Univ 1991; **Resid:** Internal Medicine, Stanford Univ Med Ctr 1997; **Fellow:** Oncology, Stanford Univ Med Ctr 1999; Cancer Research, Stanford Univ Med Ctr 2000; **Fac Appt:** Assoc Prof Med, UCSD

Rosove, Michael H MD [Onc] - **Spec Exp:** Bleeding/Coagulation Disorders; Myeloproliferative Disorders; Myelodysplastic Syndromes; Hematologic Malignancies; **Hospital:** UCLA Ronald Reagan Med Ctr; **Address:** 100 UCLA Med Plaza, Ste 550, Los Angeles, CA 90024-6970; **Phone:** 310-794-4955; **Board Cert:** Internal Medicine 1976; Hematology 1982; Medical Oncology 1981; **Med School:** UCLA 1973; **Resid:** Internal Medicine, UCLA Med Ctr 1976; **Fellow:** Hematology & Oncology, UCLA Med Ctr 1979; Hematology & Oncology, Columbia Presby Med Ctr 1978; **Fac Appt:** Clin Prof Med, UCLA-David Geffen Sch Med

Rugo, Hope S MD [Onc] - **Spec Exp:** Breast Cancer; Complementary Medicine; Breast Cancer-Novel Therapies; **Hospital:** UCSF Med Ctr; **Address:** UCSF Comp Cancer Ctr-Breast Care Ctr, 1600 Divisadero St Fl 2, San Francisco, CA 94115; **Phone:** 415-353-7070; **Board Cert:** Internal Medicine 1987; Medical Oncology 1989; **Med School:** Univ Pennsylvania 1984; **Resid:** Internal Medicine, UCSF Med Ctr 1987; **Fellow:** Hematology & Oncology, UCSF Med Ctr 1989; **Fac Appt:** Clin Prof Med, UCSF

Russell, Christy A MD [Onc] - **Spec Exp:** Breast Cancer; **Hospital:** Keck Med Ctr of USC (page 62); **Address:** Norris Cancer Ctr, The Breast Ctr, 1441 Eastlake Ave, Ste 3448, Los Angeles, CA 90033; **Phone:** 323-865-3371; **Board Cert:** Internal Medicine 1983; Medical Oncology 1985; **Med School:** Med Coll PA Hahnemann 1980; **Resid:** Internal Medicine, Good Sam Med Ctr 1983; **Fellow:** Hematology & Oncology, LAC-USC Med Ctr 1986; **Fac Appt:** Assoc Prof Med, USC Sch Med

Samlowski, Wolfram E MD [Onc] - **Spec Exp:** Kidney Cancer; Melanoma; Sarcoma; Merkel Cell Carcinoma; **Hospital:** St. Rose Dom Hosp-San Martin, Southern Hills Hosp & Med Ctr; **Address:** 9280 W Sunset Rd W, Ste 100, One Breakthrough Way, Las Vegas, NV 89148; **Phone:** 702-952-1251; **Board Cert:** Internal Medicine 1981; Medical Oncology 1985; **Med School:** Ohio State Univ 1978; **Resid:** Internal Medicine, Wayne State Univ Affil Hosp 1981; **Fellow:** Hematology & Oncology, Univ Utah Affil Hosp 1984; **Fac Appt:** Prof Onc, Univ Nevada

Sandler, Alan B MD [Onc] - **Spec Exp:** Lung Cancer; Sarcoma; **Hospital:** OR Hlth & Sci Univ; **Address:** 3181 SW Sam Jackson Park Rd, Portland, OR 97239; **Phone:** 503-494-5586; **Board Cert:** Medical Oncology 2006; **Med School:** Rush Med Coll 1987; **Resid:** Internal Medicine, Yale-New Haven Hosp 1989; **Fellow:** Medical Oncology, Yale Univ 1993; **Fac Appt:** Prof Med, Oregon Hlth & Sci Univ

Scudder, Sidney A MD [Onc] - **Spec Exp:** Ovarian Cancer; Uterine Cancer; Cervical Cancer; **Hospital:** UC Davis Med Ctr; **Address:** 4501 X St, Ste 3016, Sacramento, CA 95817; **Phone:** 916-734-3771; **Board Cert:** Internal Medicine 1983; Medical Oncology 1985; **Med School:** Univ Fla Coll Med 1980; **Resid:** Internal Medicine, Barnes Hosp-Washington Univ 1983; **Fellow:** Medical Oncology, Stanford Univ 1987; **Fac Appt:** Prof Med, UC Davis

Sikic, Branimir I MD [Onc] - **Spec Exp:** Unknown Primary Cancer; Clinical Trials; **Hospital:** Stanford Univ Hosp & Clinics; **Address:** Stanford Comp Cancer Ctr, 875 Blake Wilbur Drive, Clinic C, Palo Alto, CA 94305; **Phone:** 650-498-6000; **Board Cert:** Internal Medicine 1975; Medical Oncology 1979; **Med School:** Ros Franklin Univ/Chicago Med Sch 1972; **Resid:** Internal Medicine, Georgetown Univ Hosp 1975; **Fellow:** Medical Oncology, Natl Cancer Inst 1978; Medical Oncology, Georgetown Univ Hosp 1979; **Fac Appt:** Prof Med, Stanford Univ

Small, Eric J MD [Onc] - **Spec Exp:** Prostate Cancer; Vaccine Therapy; Genitourinary Cancer; **Hospital:** UCSF Med Ctr; **Address:** UCSF Urologic Oncology Practice, 1600 Divisadero St Fl 3, San Francisco, CA 94115; **Phone:** 415-353-7171; **Board Cert:** Internal Medicine 1988; Medical Oncology 2001; **Med School:** Case West Res Univ 1985; **Resid:** Internal Medicine, Beth Israel Hosp 1988; **Fellow:** Hematology & Oncology, Cancer Research Inst/UCSF 1991; **Fac Appt:** Prof Med, UCSF

Stewart, Forrest M MD [Onc] - **Spec Exp:** Unknown Primary Cancer; Sarcoma; **Hospital:** Univ Wash Med Ctr; **Address:** Seattle Cancer Care Alliance, 825 Eastlake Ave E, MS G3-630, Seattle, WA 98109; **Phone:** 206-288-7222; **Board Cert:** Internal Medicine 1980; Hematology 1982; Medical Oncology 1985; **Med School:** Indiana Univ 1977; **Resid:** Internal Medicine, Indiana Univ Med Ctr 1980; Medical Oncology, Indiana Univ Med Ctr 1981; **Fellow:** Hematology, Univ Virginia Med Ctr 1983; **Fac Appt:** Prof Med, Univ Wash

Stockdale, Frank E MD/PhD [Onc] - **Spec Exp:** Breast Cancer; Tuberous Breasts; Sarcoma-Soft Tissue; **Hospital:** Stanford Univ Hosp & Clinics; **Address:** Stanford Univ Medical Ctr, 900 Blake Wilbur Drive, Stanford, CA 94305-5826; **Phone:** 650-498-6000; **Med School:** Univ Pennsylvania 1963; **Resid:** Internal Medicine, Stanford Univ Med Ctr 1967; Medical Oncology, Stanford Univ Med Ctr; **Fac Appt:** Prof Emeritus Med, Stanford Univ

Sweetenham, John W MD [Onc] - **Spec Exp:** Lymphoma; Stem Cell Transplant; Castleman's Disease; **Hospital:** UCSD Med Ctr; **Address:** UC San Diego Nevada Cancer Inst, One Breakthrough Way, Las Vegas, NV 89135-3010; **Phone:** 702-822-5433; **Med School:** England, UK 1980; **Resid:** Internal Medicine, Royal United Hosp 1984; **Fellow:** Hematology & Oncology, Univ Southampton Hosp 1989; **Fac Appt:** Prof Onc, UCSD

Tempero, Margaret A MD [Onc] - **Spec Exp:** Pancreatic Cancer; Gastrointestinal Cancer; **Hospital:** UCSF Med Ctr, VA Med Ctr - San Francisco; **Address:** 1600 Divisadero St Fl 4, San Francisco, CA 94115; **Phone:** 415-353-9888; **Board Cert:** Internal Medicine 1980; Medical Oncology 1983; Hematology 1984; **Med School:** Univ Nebr Coll Med 1977; **Resid:** Internal Medicine, Univ Nebraska Hosp 1980; **Fellow:** Medical Oncology, Univ Nebraska Hosp 1982; **Fac Appt:** Prof Med, UCSF

Thompson, John Ainslie MD [Onc] - **Spec Exp:** Melanoma; Kidney Cancer; **Hospital:** Univ Wash Med Ctr; **Address:** Seattle Cancer Care Alliance, 825 Eastlake Ave E, MS G4-200, Seattle, WA 98109-1023; **Phone:** 206-288-2015; **Board Cert:** Internal Medicine 1982; Medical Oncology 1985; **Med School:** Univ Alabama 1979; **Resid:** Internal Medicine, Univ Washington Med Ctr 1982; **Fellow:** Medical Oncology, Univ Washington Med Ctr 1985

Tripathy, Debasish MD [Onc] - **Spec Exp:** Breast Cancer; Clinical Trials; **Hospital:** USC Norris Cancer Hosp (page 62); **Address:** 1441 Eastlake Ave, Ste 3440, Los Angeles, CA 90033; **Phone:** 323-865-3900; **Board Cert:** Internal Medicine 1988; Medical Oncology 2001; **Med School:** Duke Univ 1985; **Resid:** Internal Medicine, Duke Univ Med Ctr 1988; **Fellow:** Hematology & Oncology, USCF Med Ctr 1991; **Fac Appt:** Prof Med, Univ SC Sch Med

Twardowski, Przemyslaw W MD [Onc] - **Spec Exp:** Genitourinary Cancer; **Hospital:** City of Hope Natl Med Ctr; **Address:** 1500 E Duarte Rd, Duarte, CA 91010; **Phone:** 626-256-4673; **Board Cert:** Medical Oncology 2009; **Med School:** Univ MO-Columbia Sch Med 1990; **Resid:** Internal Medicine, Northwestern Meml Hosp 1994; **Fellow:** Hematology & Oncology, Northwestern Meml Hosp 1996; **Fac Appt:** Asst Prof Med, UCLA

Medical Oncology

Urba, Walter J MD/PhD [Onc] - **Spec Exp:** Breast Cancer; **Hospital:** Providence Portland Med Ctr; **Address:** Providence Cancer Ctr, 4805 NE Glisan Rd, Portland, OR 97213; **Phone:** 503-215-5696; **Board Cert:** Internal Medicine 1985; Medical Oncology 1987; **Med School:** Univ Miami Sch Med 1981; **Resid:** Internal Medicine, Morristown Meml Hosp 1983; **Fellow:** Medical Oncology, Natl Cancer Inst 1986; **Fac Appt:** Assoc Clin Prof Med, Oregon Hlth & Sci Univ

Venook, Alan P MD [Onc] - **Spec Exp:** Gastrointestinal Cancer; Colon & Rectal Cancer; Liver Cancer; **Hospital:** UCSF Med Ctr; **Address:** UCSF Comprehensive Cancer Ctr, Multi Disciplinary Practice, 1600 Divisadero St Fl 4, San Francisco, CA 94115; **Phone:** 415-353-9888; **Board Cert:** Internal Medicine 1985; Medical Oncology 1987; Hematology 1988; **Med School:** UCSF 1980; **Resid:** Internal Medicine, UC Davis Med Ctr 1985; **Fellow:** Hematology & Oncology, UCSF Med Ctr 1987; **Fac Appt:** Prof Med

Vescio, Robert A MD [Onc] - **Spec Exp:** Multiple Myeloma; Amyloidosis; **Hospital:** Cedars-Sinai Med Ctr; **Address:** Cedars Sinai Med Ctr, Dept Hem/Oncology, 8700 Beverly Blvd, Ste AC1049, Los Angeles, CA 90048; **Phone:** 310-423-1825; **Board Cert:** Internal Medicine 1989; Hematology 2004; Medical Oncology 2003; **Med School:** UCSD 1986; **Resid:** Internal Medicine, UCSD Med Ctr 1989; **Fellow:** Hematology & Oncology, UCLA Med Ctr 1993; **Fac Appt:** Assoc Prof Med, UCLA

Vogelzang, Nicholas J MD [Onc] - **Spec Exp:** Prostate Cancer; Mesothelioma; Kidney Cancer; Genitourinary Cancer; **Hospital:** Sunrise Hosp & Med Ctr, Desert Springs Hosp Med Ctr - Las Vegas; **Address:** Comprehensive Cancer Ctr of Nevada, 3730 S Eastern Ave, Las Vegas, NV 89169; **Phone:** 702-952-3400; **Board Cert:** Internal Medicine 1977; Medical Oncology 1981; **Med School:** Univ IL Coll Med 1974; **Resid:** Internal Medicine, Rush-Presby St Luke's Med Ctr 1978; **Fellow:** Medical Oncology, Univ Minn Med Ctr 1980; **Fac Appt:** Prof Med, Univ Nevada

Volberding, Paul Arthur MD [Onc] - **Spec Exp:** AIDS Related Cancers; **Hospital:** UCSF Med Ctr, VA Med Ctr - San Francisco; **Address:** 4150 Clement St, VAMC 111, San Francisco, CA 94121; **Phone:** 415-221-4810; **Board Cert:** Internal Medicine 1978; Medical Oncology 1981; **Med School:** Univ Minn 1975; **Resid:** Internal Medicine, Univ Utah Med Ctr 1978; **Fellow:** Medical Oncology, UCSF Med Ctr 1981; **Fac Appt:** Prof Med, UCSF

Wierman, Ann MD [Onc] - **Spec Exp:** Breast Cancer; Lymphoma; Lung Cancer; **Hospital:** Mountainview Hosp - Las Vegas, Summerlin Hosp Med Ctr; **Address:** 7445 Peak Drive, Las Vegas, NV 89128; **Phone:** 702-952-2140; **Board Cert:** Internal Medicine 2002; Medical Oncology 2007; **Med School:** Baylor Coll Med 1989; **Resid:** Internal Medicine, Baylor Hosps 1992; Internal Medicine, Ben Taub Genl Hosp 1993; **Fellow:** Hematology & Oncology, Univ CO Hlth Sci Ctr 1996; **Fac Appt:** Assoc Clin Prof Med, Univ Nevada

Yen, Yun MD/PhD [Onc] - **Spec Exp:** Liver Cancer; Biliary Cancer; **Hospital:** City of Hope Natl Med Ctr; **Address:** City of Hope Comprehensive Cancer Ctr, 1500 E Duarte Rd, Duarte, CA 91010; **Phone:** 626-471-9200 x62307; **Board Cert:** Medical Oncology 2003; **Med School:** Taiwan 1982; **Resid:** Internal Medicine, St Luke's Hosp 1990; **Fellow:** Hematology & Oncology, Yale-New Haven Hosp 1993; **Fac Appt:** Prof Med, USC Sch Med

Cleveland Clinic

Every life deserves world class care.

Cleveland Clinic
Taussig Cancer Institute
9500 Euclid Avenue
Cleveland, OH 44195

Hematology and Oncology Treatment Leader

At Cleveland Clinic Taussig Cancer Institute, more than 250 top cancer specialists, researchers, nurses and technicians are dedicated to delivering the most effective medical treatments and offering access to the latest clinical trials for more than 13,000 new cancer patients every year. Our doctors are nationally and internationally known for their contributions to cancer breakthroughs and their ability to deliver superior outcomes for our patients. In recognition of these and other achievements, *U.S. News & World Report* has ranked Cleveland Clinic as one of the top cancer centers in the nation.

The Taussig Cancer Institute is a national leader in caring for and treating patients with leukemia, lymphoma, myeloma and myelodysplastic syndromes. For example, our Bone Marrow Transplant (BMT) program has unsurpassed national outcomes. We have one of the most experienced teams in the nation, having performed more than 3,600 bone marrow transplant procedures since 1977.

Our teams of nurses, social workers, pharmacists, pathologists and internationally recognized physicians work together to develop personalized treatment plans for every patient. These teams administer more than 18,000 courses of chemotherapy every year, often involving investigational drugs or drug combinations not available elsewhere.

We also have state-of-the-art, dedicated facilities with individual rooms for leukemia and BMT patients, and the most current treatments through clinical trials, many of which are developed at Cleveland Clinic. Our goal is to promote the highest quality of care for people who have hematologic cancers.

It's also important to care for the whole person. Taussig Cancer Institute provides support services that address the emotional experience for patients and their families. We have social workers, patient navigators and many other caregivers who help our patients throughout their cancer journey. We strongly believe it is important to take care of people as people. It is our goal to treat patients with the utmost dignity, empathy and compassion.

Offering Same-Day Appointments
Call 800.274.2009.

Treatment Guides

Cleveland Clinic has developed comprehensive treatment guides for many diseases and conditions. To download our free treatment guides, visit clevelandclinic.org/treatmentguides.

Online Medical Second Opinion

Call 216.444.3223 or 800.223.2273 ext. 43223 or email eclevelandclinic@ccf.org.

Out-of-State Patients Assistance

Call 800.223.2273, ext. 55580 or email medicalconcierge@ccf.org.

Visit Us At:
clevelandclinic.org

Follow Us On:
Facebook
www.facebook.com/clevelandclinic

Twitter
@ClevelandClinic

You Tube
www.youtube.com/clevelandclinic

Health Hub
health.clevelandclinic.org

Beth Israel Medical Center
Beth Israel Brooklyn
Roosevelt Hospital
St. Luke's Hospital
NY Eye and Ear Infirmary

Continuum Cancer Centers of New York

Continuum Cancer Centers of New York

212.844.6027

The hospitals of Continuum – Beth Israel Medical Center, Beth Israel Brooklyn, St. Luke's Hospital, Roosevelt Hospital and The New York Eye and Ear Infirmary – are leading providers of cancer care through Continuum Cancer Centers of New York (CCCNY).

We are dedicated to delivering care in ways that are more efficient, more attractive and more convenient for patients. Our cancer patients benefit from system-wide cancer expertise, facilities and resources. Continuum Cancer Centers feature world-renowned cancer specialists, including top-rated surgeons, medical oncologists, radiation oncologists, radiologists, pathologists, and oncology nurses.

Comprehensive diagnostic and treatment services are available for:

- Breast cancer
- Prostate cancer
- Brain cancer
- Thyroid cancer
- Skin cancer
- Lung cancer

- Colorectal cancer
- Gastrointestinal cancer
- Lymphoma/Hodgkin's Disease
- Gynecological cancer
- Head and neck cancer
- Cancer of the central nervous system

Our services also include prevention programs, expert diagnosis, outpatient treatment, inpatient services and home care. In addition, our Research Program offers patients access to investigational protocols through a wide number of clinical trials. Our physicians are leaders in both non-invasive and minimally invasive cancer treatments that focus on maximizing both the cure rate and the quality of life.

Support Services also play an important role at Continuum Cancer Centers. Our nurses, social workers, psychiatrists, chaplains, pharmacists, rehabilitation therapists and nutritionists all have specialized knowledge and expertise in the field of oncology.

In June 2011, CCCNY received a full three-year network accreditation from the American College of Surgeons Commission on Cancer (CoC), with commendation, and is the only hospital system in the metropolitan area to earn this designation.

Sponsored Page

MOFFITT CANCER CENTER

OVERVIEW

Moffitt Cancer Center is the only National Cancer Institute Comprehensive Cancer Center based in Florida. Located in Tampa, the main cancer center includes a 206-bed hospital, a 36-bed blood and marrow transplant unit, an outpatient clinic with a complete digital imaging center, state-of-the-art radiation therapy department, infusion center, 14 operating rooms and two buildings that make up the Moffitt Research Institute. Offsite locations include Moffitt Screening & Prevention; Moffitt Business Center; the Moffitt Foundation; for-profit subsidiary M2Gen®; and Moffitt at International Plaza, a 50,000-square-foot, state-of-the-art outpatient facility near Tampa International Airport.

Moffitt has also created a network of strategic partners within Florida and beyond. Moffitt is accredited by JCAHO, the American College of Surgeons Commission on Cancer, the American College of Radiology and the National Accreditation Program for Breast Centers.

ACADEMIC/CLINICAL AFFILIATIONS

Moffitt collaborates with the University of South Florida, University of Florida, Florida Agricultural and Mechanical University, Florida State University, Florida Institute for Human & Machine Cognition, Scripps Florida, University of Central Florida, University of Miami and University of Louisville.

MEDICAL STAFF

Moffitt supports a staff of more than 300 physicians, known as the Moffitt Medical Group. The clinical services are organized into disease-oriented interdisciplinary programs, along with diagnostic imaging, interventional radiology, radiation oncology, pathology, anesthesiology, internal and hospital medicine, psychosocial and palliative care, and survivorship.

PIONEERING COMPREHENSIVE MEDICAL CARE

Moffitt is at the forefront of personalized medicine with Total Cancer Care® – a system of care that encompasses prevention, genetic predisposition, the impact of lifestyle, survivorship and integrative medicine during treatment.

At the core of Total Cancer Care® is a longitudinal research study that maintains a repository of human tissue specimens and clinical data. Researchers are studying this information to discover tumor biomarkers that can be used to identify those at high risk, facilitate early detection, improve prognoses, allow drug targeting and toxicity predictions, and match individuals to the best treatment and to the right clinical trials.

Moffitt's Centers of Excellence will further its goal to be a leader in developing personalized cancer care through a unique mix of nationally recognized leadership, innovative research and multiple program collaborations. These Centers of Excellence will promote synergy across Moffitt's research and clinical programs to enhance basic, prevention and clinical discoveries in a highly focused cancer area. Centers of Excellence programs include melanoma, drug discovery, lung cancer and infection research. Additionally, the Centers of Excellence share a common mission to:

DISCOVER: Create a milieu for discovery by fostering interdisciplinary laboratory research that generates new knowledge and understanding.

TRANSLATE: Foster the translation of new scientific discoveries, made at Moffitt and elsewhere, into early phase clinical trials and ultimately into standard patient care.

DELIVER: Support the efforts of Moffitt clinicians to deliver state-of-the-art personalized cancer care and support the training and education in prevention, research and treatment.

H. LEE MOFFITT CANCER CENTER & RESEARCH INSTITUTE
AN NCI COMPREHENSIVE CANCER CENTER
TAMPA, FL | 1-888-MOFFITT | MOFFITT.ORG

MOFFITT CANCER CENTER

CLOSER TO OUR PATIENTS. CLOSER TO A CURE.®

USC Norris Cancer Hospital

Part of the Keck Medical Center of USC

1441 Eastlake Ave.
Los Angeles, CA 90033
800-700-3956
KeckMedicalCenterofUSC.org

USC NORRIS CANCER HOSPITAL

USC Norris Cancer Hospital is one of only a few facilities in Southern California built exclusively for cancer research and patient care. It is part of the USC Norris Comprehensive Cancer Center, one of the original eight comprehensive cancer centers designated by the National Cancer Institute. As such, it is home to some of the most experienced, progressive doctors and cancer treatments available.

USC Norris Cancer Hospital features two newly-renovated floors dedicated to hematology and medical oncology care. The floors are composed of 60 inpatient rooms, including 8 VIP rooms, that were recently renovated to include an updated, modern look and feel. The rooms are also outfitted with updated technology systems, including a new patient television system and a new nurse monitoring system.

STATE-OF-THE-ART PATIENT CARE

USC hospitals are equipped with cutting-edge technology, providing the most up-to-date treatment for our patients. These features include:

+ Surgical robots, including the newest da Vinci® Si™ Surgical System
+ Polestar® Intraoperative MRI Navigation System
+ Cyberknife® and Varian Trilogy Linear Accelerator for stereotactic radiosurgery, intensity modulated radiation therapy and image guided radiation therapy
+ Leksell Gamma Knife® PERFEXION™, a highly advanced radiation tool to treat brain tumors
+ Four endoscopy suites and two interventional radiology suites for endoscopic procedures for outpatients, as well as two fully equipped endoscopy suites for inpatient procedures

CLINICAL TRIALS

In the battle against devastating diseases such as cancer, a major USC effort is aimed at developing and testing new treatments — surgeries, drugs, radiation therapies, preventive therapies — that might lead to a cure. USC clinical trials contribute to finding new and better ways of treating diseases. Hundreds of clinical trials take place at USC each year, giving select patients access to therapies not available elsewhere.

SPECIALTIES & RESEARCH

USC Norris Cancer Hospital is known throughout the region for expertise and excellence in:

+ Breast cancer surgery, including clinical trials for intra-operative radiotherapy for early breast cancer

+ Prostate cancer, including nerve-sparing robotic prostatectomy

+ Head and neck oncology

+ Kidney cancer and nephron sparing surgery

+ Lung cancer

+ Neuro-oncology

+ Orthopaedic oncology

+ Radiation oncology

+ Bone marrow transplant

+ GI/GU oncology

+ Adolescents and young adults

Maimonides
Medical Center

The Maimonides Cancer Center offers a fully integrated, multimodal approach to cancer care that includes prevention, education, screening, diagnostics, treatment, palliative care and clinical research. The Lena Cymbrowitz Pavilion contains the following specialty divisions:

Radiation Oncology: equipped with state-of-the art imaging and treatment delivery technologies; offers patients the most precise treatments available, yet does so in an airy, life-affirming environment.

Medical Oncology: provides comprehensive diagnosis, oral drug therapies, intravenous chemotherapy infusions, and biological and hormonal therapies.

Pediatric Oncology: treats children with cancer and diseases of the blood in a child-friendly environment, and features special areas set aside for parent conferences.

Surgical Oncology: provides a convenient location for minor surgical procedures, as well as innovative surgical techniques such as sentinel node mapping and biopsy, skin/tissue-sparing mastectomy, and nerve-sparing prostatectomy.

Research Center: conducts basic science and genetic research, as well as clinical trials that offer appropriately screened patients, who wish to volunteer, new therapies and medications.

Resource Center: offers access to integrative (complementary) oncology services, dietary advice, as well as psychological and social services.

Located around the block from the Lena Cymbrowitz Pavilion, the newly opened Rivera Pavilion houses the **Maimonides Breast Cancer Center**. With a spa-like decor and life-affirming environment, the Center provides digital mammography, sonography, computerized interpretation, digital stereotactic biopsies, breast-specific gamma imaging, and treatment plans tailored to each patient. A genetics counselor is also on-site

Clinicians at the Maimonides Cancer Center – Brooklyn's only dedicated cancer center – are talented specialists, recruited specifically for their expertise. Our doctors emphasize multimodal care, which means that multiple methods of treatment are available to patients, sometimes simultaneously. Every week, physicians from radiology, surgery, pathology, radiation oncology, and medical oncology meet to discuss patient treatment at our case management meetings. The patient's needs, as well as the disease, are considered from many angles.

Maimonides Medical Center
Passionate about medicine.
Compassionate about people.

www.maimonidesmed.org/cancer

MOUNT SINAI
SCHOOL OF
MEDICINE

THE TISCH CANCER INSTITUTE
AT THE MOUNT SINAI MEDICAL CENTER

One Gustave L. Levy Place
Fifth Avenue and 100th Street
New York, NY 10029-6574
Physician Referral: 1-800-MD-SINAI (637-4624)
www.tischcancerinstitute.org

THE TISCH CANCER INSTITUTE is embedded within a renowned medical center that has world-class research facilities, one of the nation's top-ranked hospitals, and an outstanding medical school. Patients have access to the best possible cancer care across a variety of disciplines, including hematology and medical oncology, surgery, radiation therapy, bone marrow transplantation, radiology, palliative care, psychosocial services, and clinical trials. For fully integrated, multidisciplinary care, our patients are also treated by the best specialists in every field at Mount Sinai and can receive seamless referrals.

Services and Programs – The Tisch Cancer Institute employs a multidisciplinary treatment approach, providing access to clinical breakthroughs, innovative techniques, leading-edge technologies, and a wide range of diagnostic, therapeutic, and support services for all types of cancer. The Institute treats: breast cancer; hematological malignancies (including multiple myeloma, myelodysplastic syndrome, and myeloproliferative disorders); genitourinary cancers (including prostate, bladder, and kidney); head and neck cancers; thoracic cancer (including lung and esophagus); gynecologic cancers; brain tumors; and other diagnoses. In addition to surgical treatment, the Institute provides radiation and medical oncology therapies, as well as bone marrow transplantation. The Dubin Breast Center, consisting of 15,000 square feet, is a recently constructed facility that opened in April 2011 and significantly expands the treatment space for breast cancer patients. In 2012, the Derald H. Ruttenberg Treatment Center will double in size upon its move to the Leon and Norma Hess Center for Science and Medicine at 1470 Madison Avenue (at 101st Street).

THE RUTTENBERG TREATMENT CENTER
The Derald H. Ruttenberg Treatment Center houses the ambulatory cancer program of The Tisch Cancer Institute and is operated by the Mount Sinai Hospital.

THE DUBIN BREAST CARE CENTER
The Dubin Breast Care Center offers the latest, most innovative approaches available for breast health and the treatment of breast cancer.

The Tisch Cancer Institute encourages collaboration with colleagues across the Medical Center, drawing upon the knowledge of a vast network of specialists who are outstanding in their fields. These experts consist of award-winning physicians and surgeons specializing in cardiac care, neurology, urology, pediatrics, digestive diseases, obstetrics and gynecology, and other therapeutic areas. Oncologists, surgeons, radiation oncologists, and specialists from across the medical spectrum work together to provide the highest quality care to all cancer patients. Furthermore, Mount Sinai's nursing staff is an important part of the Medical Center's focus on delivering exceptional patient care, and it has received the prestigious Magnet Award for nursing excellence. Mount Sinai is also renowned for its palliative care program, which provides the highest level of care, focusing on the relief of pain, symptoms, and stress in cancer patients in both an inpatient and outpatient setting.

A Heritage of Breakthroughs – Teams of physicians and scientists at The Tisch Cancer Institute at Mount Sinai work together to rapidly translate laboratory research into new patient treatments. Among the advances pioneered at Mount Sinai are the first successful treatment of tumors of the bladder by transurethral electrocoagulation, the first demonstration of how asbestos can cause cancerous changes in the DNA of cells, and the first development of an ultrasound-guided technique to insert radioactive seeds into the prostate to treat prostate cancer.

THE TISCH CANCER INSTITUTE
AT THE MOUNT SINAI MEDICAL CENTER

One Gustave L. Levy Place
Fifth Avenue and 100th Street
New York, NY 10029-6574
Physician Referral: 1-800-MD-SINAI (637-4624)
www.tischcancerinstitute.org

THE TISCH CANCER INSTITUTE is embedded within a renowned medical center that has world-class research facilities, one of the nation's top-ranked hospitals, and an outstanding medical school. Patients have access to the best possible cancer care across a variety of disciplines, including hematology and medical oncology, surgery, radiation therapy, bone marrow transplantation, radiology, palliative care, psychosocial services, and clinical trials. For fully integrated, multidisciplinary care, our patients are also treated by the best specialists in every field at Mount Sinai and can receive seamless referrals.

Services and Programs – The Tisch Cancer Institute employs a multidisciplinary treatment approach, providing access to clinical breakthroughs, innovative techniques, leading-edge technologies, and a wide range of diagnostic, therapeutic, and support services for all types of cancer. The Institute treats: breast cancer; hematological malignancies (including multiple myeloma, myelodysplastic syndrome, and myeloproliferative disorders); genitourinary cancers (including prostate, bladder, and kidney); head and neck cancers; thoracic cancer (including lung and esophagus); gynecologic cancers; brain tumors; and other diagnoses. In addition to surgical treatment, the Institute provides radiation and medical oncology therapies, as well as bone marrow transplantation. The Dubin Breast Center, consisting of 15,000 square feet, is a recently constructed facility that opened in April 2011 and significantly expands the treatment space for breast cancer patients. In 2012, the Derald H. Ruttenberg Treatment Center will double in size upon its move to the Leon and Norma Hess Center for Science and Medicine at 1470 Madison Avenue (at 101st Street).

THE RUTTENBERG TREATMENT CENTER
The Derald H. Ruttenberg Treatment Center houses the ambulatory cancer program of The Tisch Cancer Institute and is operated by the Mount Sinai Hospital.

THE DUBIN BREAST CARE CENTER
The Dubin Breast Care Center offers the latest, most innovative approaches available for breast health and the treatment of breast cancer.

The Tisch Cancer Institute encourages collaboration with colleagues across the Medical Center, drawing upon the knowledge of a vast network of specialists who are outstanding in their fields. These experts consist of award-winning physicians and surgeons specializing in cardiac care, neurology, urology, pediatrics, digestive diseases, obstetrics and gynecology, and other therapeutic areas. Oncologists, surgeons, radiation oncologists, and specialists from across the medical spectrum work together to provide the highest quality care to all cancer patients. Furthermore, Mount Sinai's nursing staff is an important part of the Medical Center's focus on delivering exceptional patient care, and it has received the prestigious Magnet Award for nursing excellence. Mount Sinai is also renowned for its palliative care program, which provides the highest level of care, focusing on the relief of pain, symptoms, and stress in cancer patients in both an inpatient and outpatient setting.

A Heritage of Breakthroughs – Teams of physicians and scientists at The Tisch Cancer Institute at Mount Sinai work together to rapidly translate laboratory research into new patient treatments. Among the advances pioneered at Mount Sinai are the first successful treatment of tumors of the bladder by transurethral electrocoagulation, the first demonstration of how asbestos can cause cancerous changes in the DNA of cells, and the first development of an ultrasound-guided technique to insert radioactive seeds into the prostate to treat prostate cancer.

NewYork-Presbyterian
The University Hospital of Columbia and Cornell

Affiliated with Columbia University College of Physicians and Surgeons and Weill Cornell Medical College

Herbert Irving Comprehensive Cancer Center	Weill Cornell Cancer Center
NewYork-Presbyterian Hospital	NewYork-Presbyterian Hospital
Columbia University Medical Center	Weill Cornell Medical Center
161 Fort Washington Avenue	525 East 68th Street
New York, NY 10032	New York, NY 10065

1-877-NYP-WELL (1-877-697-9355) www.nyp.org/cancer

NewYork-Presbyterian Cancer Centers

Innovative cancer treatments. Personalized, compassionate care. Evidence-based medicine. These are the hallmarks of the cancer care available at NewYork-Presbyterian Hospital, where cutting-edge treatment goes beyond state-of-the-art. We treat more than 7,000 people who are newly diagnosed with cancer each year.

NewYork-Presbyterian features two of the country's top cancer centers: the National Cancer Institute-designated Herbert Irving Comprehensive Cancer Center (one of only three comprehensive NCI-designated cancer centers in New York State) and the Weill Cornell Cancer Center. Through a multidisciplinary team approach, we combine the expertise and talents of all of the individuals responsible for a patient's care—surgical, medical, and radiation oncologists, specialized oncology nurses, social workers, and nutritionists—to deliver seamless care in a supportive and healing environment.

Our team cares for patients with the following cancers:
- AIDS-related cancers
- Bladder cancer
- Brain and other nervous system cancers
- Breast cancer
- Colorectal, pancreatic, and other digestive cancers
- Eye cancer
- Gynecologic cancers (ovarian, cervical, endometrial)
- Head and neck cancers (oral, oropharyngeal, laryngeal)
- Kidney cancer
- Lymphomas (Hodgkin's and non-Hodgkin's)
- Leukemia and myelodysplastic syndromes
- Liver cancer
- Mesothelioma
- Myeloma
- Pediatric cancers
- Prostate cancer
- Sarcoma
- Thoracic cancers (lung, esophageal, chest wall)

Research underlies everything we do, and sets academic medical centers such as ours apart from other cancer treatment centers. Our scientists and clinical investigators are leading more than 500 clinical trials assessing new cancer management approaches in thousands of patients.

Specialized Cancer Care Includes:

- Surgical procedures for breast cancer that result in superior cosmetic outcomes, and evaluation of novel anticancer drugs for women with advanced disease
- Robotic surgery for prostate and gynecologic cancers
- Video-assisted thoracoscopy and lung-sparing surgery for some lung cancers
- Interventional endoscopy and laparoscopic surgery for colorectal and other cancers
- Targeted approaches to brain cancer treatment, including convection-enhanced chemotherapy and stereotactic radiosurgery
- Bone marrow and stem cell transplantation for hematologic cancers
- Renowned Mesothelioma Center
- Combination chemotherapy, targeted anticancer agents, novel drugs available through clinical trials, and highly targeted radiation therapy

NYU Langone Medical Center
550 First Avenue , New York, NY 10016
www.NYULMC.org

Clinical Cancer Center
160 East 34th Street, New York, NY 10016
www.NYUCI.org

**The Stephen D. Hassenfeld Children's Center
for Cancer and Blood Disorders**
160 East 32nd Street, New York, NY 10016
www.NYUMC.org/Hassenfeld

NYU CANCER INSTITUTE

The NYU Cancer Institute is an NCI-designated cancer center providing personalized patient care that is compassionate and state-of-the-art. The doctors and researchers work together to develop innovative therapies for patients. The Cancer Institute is world-renowned for excellence in cancer-focused research, personalized care, education and community outreach. Its mission is to discover the origins of human cancer and to use that knowledge to eradicate the personal and societal burden of cancer in our community, the nation and the world. For more information about our expert physicians, call 212-731-5000.

Patient-Focused Setting
The Clinical Cancer Center is the principal outpatient facility of The Cancer Institute. The Center and its multidisciplinary team of experts provide access to the latest treatment options and clinical trials, along with a variety of programs in cancer risk reduction/prevention, screening, diagnostics, genetic counseling and supportive services. In addition, the Center emphasizes the importance of a holistic approach involving integrative health, psychosocial support, survivorship and palliative care. Radiology and infusion services are available in Rego Park, NY, as well.

Renowned Expertise
The NYU Cancer Institute brings together experts from a variety of disciplines to create collaborative research endeavors and clinical care teams. It offers a continuum of personalized care, from prevention through diagnosis, treatment and post-treatment support. Additionally, we have created special programs to treat diseases such as breast cancer, brain cancer, melanoma, GI cancer, prostate cancer, hematologic malignancies and lung cancer, as well as translational programs in cancer healthcare disparities, molecularly targeted therapy, and the cell signaling pathways involved in cancer.

A Translational Approach
Our scientists and researchers excel in uncovering how cancer develops at the molecular level, and how we can harness that knowledge to reduce the risk of cancer and treat the disease.

Stephen D. Hassenfeld Children's Center for Cancer and Blood Disorders
The center is a leading pediatric outpatient facility for the treatment of childhood cancers and blood diseases. Its unique interdisciplinary and family-centered approach combines the most advanced medical treatments with psychosocial and emotional support services for young patients and their families.

Advancing Cancer Care

Penn Medicine is a national leader in developing innovative approaches to the prevention, diagnosis and treatment of cancer. Through clinical excellence, advanced research and supportive care services, patients and their families are provided with outstanding comprehensive cancer care.

Abramson Cancer Center

The Abramson Cancer Center is one of a select group of cancer centers in the country to be awarded the prestigious designation of *Comprehensive Cancer Center* by the National Cancer Institute (NCI). The Cancer Center has established a variety of interdisciplinary centers dedicated to specific cancers. Each center offers patients a complete evaluation and treatment options from a team of doctors with subspecialty, disease-specific expertise.

What Sets Abramson Apart?

- More than 400 full-time Penn faculty are actively involved in the diagnosis and treatment of patients with cancer.

- One of only 10 cancer centers in the country to offer proton therapy as part of an integrated approach to cancer treatment.

- Clinical programs offering cutting-edge treatments such as robotic surgery for prostate and gynecologic cancer, and Transoral Robotic Surgery (TORS) for head and neck cancer.

- Developing immunotherapies that use the body's own immune system to fight cancer and reduce treatment-related side effects.

- One of the first cancer risk evaluation programs in the country for women concerned about their risk for breast and ovarian cancer.

- One of the foremost cancer research centers in the country and a leader in translational research, in which scientists translate discoveries from research laboratories into new treatments that benefit cancer patients.

- Comprehensive medical care for patients with other medical conditions such as diabetes, pregnancy or heart disease.

- Utilizing personalized medicine which uses information about a person's genes, proteins, and environment to better prevent, diagnose, and treat cancer.

- Designated as a LIVESTRONG Center of Excellence™.

- Dedicated oncology nurse navigators to help patients and families access all of the treatment options and support programs the Cancer Center offers, including nutritional counseling, support groups, cancer rehabilitation, complementary and alternative therapies and pain and symptom management.

Joan Karnell Cancer Center at Pennsylvania Hospital

For patients and families facing cancer or blood-related illnesses, the Joan Karnell Cancer Center at Pennsylvania Hospital provides progressive, comprehensive and supportive cancer care through a wide range of services.

- A leader in the treatment of sarcoma and bloodless medicine.

- Committed to providing excellent cancer care in a supportive setting, offering an interdisciplinary approach to diagnosis, treatment, research and education to help patients and their families achieve the best quality of life.

The Ruth and Raymond Perelman Center for Advanced Medicine

The Perelman Center is the home of the Abramson Cancer Center, which brings together outstanding cancer specialists with state-of-the-art technology to offer the most advanced cancer treatment options available.

The Roberts Proton Therapy Center

The Roberts Proton Therapy Center is the largest, most comprehensive proton therapy center in the world, and the only one of its kind integrated with a National Cancer Institute Comprehensive Cancer Center. Proton therapy is a treatment option for several types of cancer including prostate, lung, brain, head and neck, and sarcoma.

Additional Locations

Penn cancer services are also available at:
- Abramson Cancer Center at Penn Presbyterian Medical Center
- Pennsylvania Hospital
- Penn Medicine Radnor
- Penn Medicine Cherry Hill
- Penn Medicine Valley Forge (coming early 2013)

For more information or to schedule an appointment, call 800.789.PENN (7366) or visit PennMedicine.org/cancer.

Vanderbilt-Ingram Cancer Center

2220 Pierce Ave. | Nashville, TN 37232 | Toll-free: 1 (877) 936-8422 ; Clinical Trials: 1 (800) 811-8480 | VICC.org

Overview

Vanderbilt-Ingram Cancer Center is one of only 41 in the U.S. to be named a Comprehensive Cancer Center, the National Cancer Institute's highest designation. Vanderbilt-Ingram is also a leading cancer research center, ranked in the nation's top 10 in competitive grant support from the NCI. It's also a member of the National Comprehensive Cancer Network, a nonprofit alliance working to improve care for all cancer patients.

Vanderbilt-Ingram is the only center in Tennessee ranked among the nation's Best Hospitals for cancer care by *U.S. News & World Report*.

A Specialized Approach

Cancer is not a single disease that can be treated with a generic approach. At Vanderbilt-Ingram, we provide a high level of specialization through teams of experts with the knowledge and experience to treat unique cases of all kinds.

Unlike other centers that may have a general cancer team, we have teams focused on cancers of the breast, lung, colon and other gastrointestinal organs; head and neck cancers; brain and other neurologic cancers; gynecologic cancers; bone and tissue cancers; leukemias, lymphomas and myelomas; melanoma; and pediatric cancers. We also offer expertise on rare cancers.

Personalized Cancer Medicine

We've known for some time that changes in the DNA of cancer cells can affect how they respond to treatment. Our Personalized Cancer Medicine Initiative tests patients for changes in tumor DNA known to affect treatment. The results of those tests help guide our oncologists to choose the right therapy for the patient at the right time. This approach is now used for lung, colon and breast cancers, and melanoma, with other cancers to be included soon.

Clinical Trials

Studies of promising new therapies are an important option that every cancer patient should consider. Vanderbilt-Ingram offers a wide range of clinical trials. Learn more.

Survivorship and Wellness

Living through cancer can leave lasting marks. Vanderbilt-Ingram is the only cancer center in the country to offer a dedicated program for all cancer survivors once treatment ends. It includes patients regardless of age, type of cancer or where treatment took place. Learn more.

VANDERBILT UNIVERSITY
MEDICAL CENTER

The Best in American Medicine
www.CastleConnolly.com

Hospice & Palliative Medicine

Hospice and Palliative Medicine is a subspecialty of family medicine, internal medicine, anesthesiology, emergency medicine, obstetrics and gynecology, neurology, pediatrics, physical medicine and rehabilitation, radiology and surgery.

Palliative care relieves the suffering and provides the best quality of life to people suffering from serious and severe chronic illness. Hospice care focuses on the palliation of a terminally ill patient's symptoms and also provides compassionate support to both the patient and their surrounding loved ones.

Training Required: Physicians must be board certified in one of the above ABMS specialties and complete an additional year of training in an ACGME approved Hospice and Palliative Medicine fellowship program and then pass the official examination to be board certified in this subspecialty.

HOSPICE & PALLIATIVE MEDICINE

New England

Abrahm, Janet L MD [Hospice & Palliative Med] - **Spec Exp:** Palliative Care; Pain-Cancer; **Hospital:** Dana-Farber Cancer Inst (page 57), Brigham and Women's Hosp (page 57); **Address:** Dana-Farber Cancer Institute, 450 Brookline Ave, Shields-Warren 420, Boston, MA 02215; **Phone:** 617-632-6464; **Board Cert:** Internal Medicine 1976; Medical Oncology 2010; Hematology 1978; Hospice & Palliative Medicine 2008; **Med School:** UCSF 1973; **Resid:** Internal Medicine, Mass Genl Hosp 1975; Internal Medicine, Moffitt Hosp-UCSF 1977; **Fellow:** Hematology, Mass Genl Hosp 1976; Hematology & Oncology, Hosp Univ Penn 1980; **Fac Appt:** Prof Hospice & Palliative Med, Harvard Med Sch

Block, Susan D MD [Hospice & Palliative Med] - **Spec Exp:** Psychiatry in Cancer; Palliative Care; **Hospital:** Dana-Farber Cancer Inst (page 57), Brigham and Women's Hosp (page 57); **Address:** Dana Farber Cancer Inst, 450 Brookline Ave, Shields Warren, Boston, MA 02115; **Phone:** 617-632-5788; **Board Cert:** Internal Medicine 1981; Psychiatry 1984; Hospice & Palliative Medicine 2003; **Med School:** Case West Res Univ 1977; **Resid:** Internal Medicine, Beth Israel Hosp 1980; Psychiatry, Beth Israel Hosp 1982; **Fac Appt:** Prof Psyc, Harvard Med Sch

Jackson, Vicki MD [Hospice & Palliative Med] - **Spec Exp:** Palliative Care; **Hospital:** Mass Genl Hosp; **Address:** Palliative Care Service, 55 Fruit St, FND 600, Boston, MA 02114; **Phone:** 617-724-9197; **Board Cert:** Internal Medicine 2008; Hospice & Palliative Medicine 2002; **Med School:** Univ Wisc 1995; **Resid:** Internal Medicine, Cambridge Hlth Alliance 1998

Selvaggi, Kathy J MD [Hospice & Palliative Med] - **Spec Exp:** Palliative Care; Pain-Cancer; **Hospital:** Dana-Farber Cancer Inst (page 57); **Address:** Dana Farber Cancer Inst, 450 Brookline Ave, Ste 411, Boston, MA 02215; **Phone:** 617-632-6464; **Board Cert:** Internal Medicine 1989; Medical Oncology 2005; Hospice & Palliative Medicine 2008; **Med School:** Penn State Coll Med 1985; **Resid:** Internal Medicine, UPMC Shadyside Hosp 1989; **Fellow:** Medical Oncology, UPMC Shadyside Hosp 1992; **Fac Appt:** Asst Prof Med, Harvard Med Sch

Mid Atlantic

Arnold, Robert M MD [Hospice & Palliative Med] - **Spec Exp:** Palliative Care; Ethics; Pain-HIV patients; **Hospital:** UPMC Montefiore, UPMC Presby, Pittsburgh; **Address:** UPMC Montefiore, Div Internal Medicine, Section of Palliative Care & Ethics, 3459 Fifth Ave, Ste 932W, Pittsburgh, PA 15213; **Phone:** 412-647-7228; **Board Cert:** Internal Medicine 1986; Hospice & Palliative Medicine 2008; **Med School:** Univ MO-Kansas City 1983; **Resid:** Internal Medicine, Rhode Island Hosp 1986; Internal Medicine, Hosp Univ Penn 1988; **Fellow:** Public Health, Robert Wood Johnson Univ Affil Hosp 1998; **Fac Appt:** Prof Med, Univ Pittsburgh

Portenoy, Russell MD [Hospice & Palliative Med] - **Spec Exp:** Pain Medicine; Pain-Cancer; Palliative Care; **Hospital:** Beth Israel Med Ctr - Petrie Division (page 56); **Address:** Beth Israel Med Ctr, Dept Pain Medicine/Palliative Care, First Ave at 16th St, New York, NY 10003; **Phone:** 212-844-1403; **Board Cert:** Neurology 1985; Hospice & Palliative Medicine 2008; **Med School:** Univ MD Sch Med 1980; **Resid:** Neurology, Montefiore Med Ctr 1984; **Fellow:** Pain Medicine, Meml Sloan-Kettering Cancer Ctr 1985; **Fac Appt:** Prof N, Albert Einstein Coll Med

Quill, Timothy E MD [Hospice & Palliative Med] - **Spec Exp:** Palliative Care; Chronic Illness; **Hospital:** Univ of Rochester Strong Meml Hosp; **Address:** University of Rochester Medical Ctr, 601 Elmwood Ave, Box 687, Rochester, NY 14642; **Phone:** 585-273-1154; **Board Cert:** Internal Medicine 1979; Hospice & Palliative Medicine 2008; **Med School:** Univ Rochester 1976; **Resid:** Internal Medicine, Univ Rochester/Strong Meml Hosp 1980; **Fellow:** Liaison Psychiatry, Univ Rochester Med Psych Liason Program 1981; **Fac Appt:** Prof Med, Univ Rochester

Southeast

Tulsky, James A MD [Hospice & Palliative Med] - **Spec Exp:** Palliative Care; **Hospital:** Duke Univ Hosp; **Address:** DUMC, Box 2706, Durham, NC 27710; **Phone:** 919-668-7215; **Board Cert:** Hospice & Palliative Medicine 2006; Internal Medicine 2012; **Med School:** Univ IL Coll Med 1987; **Resid:** Internal Medicine, UCSF Med Ctr 1990; **Fellow:** Research, UCSF Med Ctr 1993; **Fac Appt:** Prof Med, Duke Univ

Midwest

Bricker, Leslie J MD [Hospice & Palliative Med] - **Spec Exp:** Palliative Care; **Hospital:** Henry Ford Hosp; **Address:** Henry Ford Hospital, 2799 W Grand Blvd, CFP 5, 13th Fl, Detroit, MI 48202; **Phone:** 313-916-1859; **Board Cert:** Internal Medicine 1980; Hematology 1982; Medical Oncology 1983; Hospice & Palliative Medicine 2008; **Med School:** Wayne State Univ 1977; **Resid:** Internal Medicine, Sinai Hosp 1980; **Fellow:** Hematology & Oncology, Univ Mich Hosp 1983; **Fac Appt:** Assoc Prof Med, Wayne State Univ

Davis, Mellar P MD [Hospice & Palliative Med] - **Spec Exp:** Palliative Care; Lung Cancer (advanced); Amyloidosis; **Hospital:** Cleveland Clin (page 55); **Address:** Cleveland Clin Fdn, 9500 Euclid Ave, Desk R35, Cleveland, OH 44195; **Phone:** 216-445-4622; **Board Cert:** Internal Medicine 1980; Hematology 1982; Medical Oncology 1983; Hospice & Palliative Medicine 2004; **Med School:** Ohio State Univ 1977; **Resid:** Internal Medicine, Riverside Methodist Hosp 1979; **Fellow:** Hematology, Mayo Clinic 1981; Medical Oncology, Mayo Clinic 1982; **Fac Appt:** Prof Med, Cleveland Cl Coll Med/Case West Res

Friebert, Sarah E MD [Hospice & Palliative Med] - **Spec Exp:** Palliative Care; Cancer Survivors-Late Effects of Therapy; **Hospital:** Akron Children's Hosp; **Address:** Children's Hosp Med Ctr of Akron, One Perkins Sq Fl 5, Akron, OH 44308; **Phone:** 330-543-3343; **Board Cert:** Pediatrics 2004; Pediatric Hematology-Oncology 2008; Hospice & Palliative Medicine 2008; **Med School:** Case West Res Univ 1993; **Resid:** Pediatrics, Chldns Hosp 1996; **Fellow:** Pediatric Hematology-Oncology, Rainbow Babies-Chldns Hosp 1999; **Fac Appt:** Asst Prof Ped, NE Ohio Univ

Santa-Emma, Philip H MD [Hospice & Palliative Med] - **Spec Exp:** Palliative Care; **Hospital:** Mt Carmel W Hosp; **Address:** 1144 Dublin Rd, Columbus, OH 43215; **Phone:** 614-234-5000; **Board Cert:** Family Medicine 2010; Hospice & Palliative Medicine 2008; **Med School:** Ohio State Univ 1988; **Resid:** Family Medicine, Mt Carmel Med Ctr 1991

Great Plains and Mountains

Kutner, Jean S MD [Hospice & Palliative Med] - **Spec Exp:** Palliative Care; **Hospital:** Univ of CO Hosp - Anschutz Inpatient Pav; **Address:** 8111 E Lowry Blvd, Ste 120, Denver, CO 80230; **Phone:** 720-848-9500; **Board Cert:** Internal Medicine 2004; Geriatric Medicine 2008; Hospice & Palliative Medicine 2008; **Med School:** UCSF 1991; **Resid:** Internal Medicine, UCSF Med Ctr 1994; **Fellow:** Internal Medicine, Univ Colorado Sch Med 1996; Geriatric Medicine, Univ Colorado Sch Med 1997; **Fac Appt:** Prof Med, Univ Colorado

Hospice & Palliative Medicine

Weinstein, Sharon M MD [Hospice & Palliative Med] - **Spec Exp:** Pain-Cancer; Palliative Care; **Hospital:** Univ Utah Hlth Care; **Address:** Huntsman Cancer Institute, 2000 Circle of Hope, Salt Lake City, UT 84112; **Phone:** 801-585-0112; **Board Cert:** Neurology 1993; Pain Medicine 2010; Hospice & Palliative Medicine 2008; **Med School:** Albert Einstein Coll Med 1986; **Resid:** Neurology, Montefiore Med Ctr 1990; **Fellow:** Pain Medicine, Meml Sloan Kettering Cancer Ctr 1991; **Fac Appt:** Assoc Prof Anes, Univ Utah

Southwest

Fine, Robert L MD [Hospice & Palliative Med] - **Spec Exp:** Palliative Care; **Hospital:** Baylor Univ Medical Ctr-Dallas; **Address:** 3600 Gaston Ave, Ste 605, Dallas, TX 75204; **Phone:** 214-820-9248; **Board Cert:** Internal Medicine 1981; Hospice & Palliative Medicine 1993; **Med School:** Univ Tex SW, Dallas 1978; **Resid:** Internal Medicine, Baylor Univ Med Ctr 1981

West Coast and Pacific

Ferris, Frank D MD [Hospice & Palliative Med] - **Spec Exp:** Palliative Care; **Hospital:** San Diego Hospice; **Address:** 4311 3rd Ave, San Diego, CA 92103-1407; **Phone:** 619-688-1600; **Board Cert:** Hospice & Palliative Medicine 1998; **Med School:** Canada 1981; **Resid:** Internal Medicine, Univ Toronto; Radiation Oncology, Univ Toronto; **Fellow:** Pain Management, Toronto-Sunnybrook Reg Cancer Ctr

Pantilat, Steven MD [Hospice & Palliative Med] - **Spec Exp:** Palliative Care; **Hospital:** UCSF Med Ctr; **Address:** 521 Parnassus Ave, Box 0903, San Francisco, CA 94143-0903; **Phone:** 415-476-9019; **Board Cert:** Internal Medicine 2003; Hospice & Palliative Medicine 2001; **Med School:** UCSF 1989; **Resid:** Internal Medicine, UCSF Med Ctr 1992; **Fac Appt:** Asst Clin Prof Med, UCSF

Ritchie, Christine S MD [Hospice & Palliative Med] - **Spec Exp:** Palliative Care; **Hospital:** UCSF Med Ctr; **Address:** UCSF-Geriatrics Div, 3333 California St, Ste 340, San Francisco, CA 94118; **Phone:** 415-514-0715; **Board Cert:** Internal Medicine 2002; Geriatric Medicine 2006; Hospice & Palliative Medicine 2010; **Med School:** Univ NC Sch Med 1988; **Resid:** Internal Medicine, Univ Ala Sch Med 1992; **Fellow:** Geriatric Medicine, Univ Ala Sch Med 1994; **Fac Appt:** Assoc Prof Med, UCSF

Von Gunten, Charles MD/PhD [Hospice & Palliative Med] - **Spec Exp:** Palliative Care; **Hospital:** San Diego Hospice; **Address:** San Diego Hospice, 4311 Third Ave, San Diego, CA 92103; **Phone:** 619-688-1600; **Board Cert:** Internal Medicine 2002; Medical Oncology 2003; Hospice & Palliative Medicine 2001; **Med School:** Univ Colorado 1988; **Resid:** Internal Medicine, Northwestern Meml Hosp 1991; **Fellow:** Medical Oncology, Northwestern Meml Hosp 1993; **Fac Appt:** Assoc Clin Prof Med, UCSD

Infectious Disease

a subspecialty of Internal Medicine

An internist who deals with infectious diseases of all types and in all organs. Conditions requiring selective use of antibiotics call for this special skill. This physician often diagnoses and treats AIDS patients and patients with fevers which have not been explained. Infectious disease specialists may also have expertise in preventive medicine and conditions associated with travel.

Training Required: Three years in internal medicine *plus* additional training and examination for certification in infectious disease.

INFECTIOUS DISEASE

New England

Craven, Donald Edward MD [Inf] - **Spec Exp:** AIDS/HIV; Hepatitis C; Hospital Acquired Infections; Pneumonia; **Hospital:** Lahey Clin; **Address:** Lahey Clin Med Ctr, Infectious Diseases, 41 Mall Rd, Burlington, MA 01805; **Phone:** 781-744-8608; **Board Cert:** Internal Medicine 1973; Infectious Disease 1982; **Med School:** Albany Med Coll 1970; **Resid:** Internal Medicine, Royal Victoria Hosp-McGill 1973; Internal Medicine, Royal Victoria Hosp 1974; **Fellow:** Infectious Disease, Boston Univ Hosp 1976; NIH/Bureau of Biologics 1979; **Fac Appt:** Prof Med, Tufts Univ

Flanigan, Timothy P MD [Inf] - **Spec Exp:** AIDS/HIV; **Hospital:** Miriam Hosp, Rhode Island Hosp; **Address:** 1125 N Main St, Providence, RI 02904; **Phone:** 401-793-2928; **Board Cert:** Internal Medicine 1986; Infectious Disease 1988; **Med School:** Cornell Univ-Weill Med Coll 1983; **Resid:** Internal Medicine, Hosp Univ Penn 1986; **Fellow:** Infectious Disease, Case West Res Univ 1987; **Fac Appt:** Prof Med, Brown Univ

Quagliarello, Vincent MD [Inf] - **Spec Exp:** Meningitis; Pneumonia; Endocarditis; **Hospital:** Yale-New Haven Hosp, Yale Med Group; **Address:** Yale Univ Sch Med, TAC S169A, 300 Cedar St, New Haven, CT 06520-8022; **Phone:** 203-785-4140; **Board Cert:** Internal Medicine 1984; Infectious Disease 1988; **Med School:** Washington Univ, St Louis 1980; **Resid:** Internal Medicine, Yale-New Haven Hosp 1984; **Fellow:** Infectious Disease, Univ VA Hlth Sci Ctr 1987; **Fac Appt:** Prof Med, Yale Univ

Sax, Paul E MD [Inf] - **Spec Exp:** AIDS/HIV; **Hospital:** Brigham and Women's Hosp (page 57); **Address:** Brigham & Women's Hosp, Div Infectious Disease, 15 Francis St Fl 4, Boston, MA 02115; **Phone:** 617-732-8881; **Board Cert:** Internal Medicine 2010; Infectious Disease 2000; **Med School:** Harvard Med Sch 1987; **Resid:** Internal Medicine, Brigham & Womens Hosp 1990; **Fellow:** Infectious Disease, Mass Genl Hosp 1992

Mid Atlantic

Auwaerter, Paul MD [Inf] - **Spec Exp:** Lyme Disease; Ehrlichiosis; Tick-borne Diseases; Fevers of Unknown Origin; **Hospital:** Johns Hopkins Hosp (page 61); **Address:** 10751 Falls Rd, Ste 412, Lutherville, MD 21093; **Phone:** 410-583-2900; **Board Cert:** Internal Medicine 2002; Infectious Disease 2004; **Med School:** Columbia P&S 1988; **Resid:** Internal Medicine, Johns Hopkins Med Ctr 1992; **Fellow:** Infectious Disease, Johns Hopkins Med Ctr 1996; **Fac Appt:** Assoc Prof Med, Johns Hopkins Univ

Bartlett, John G MD [Inf] - **Spec Exp:** AIDS/HIV; Fevers of Unknown Origin; Pseudomembranous Colitis; **Hospital:** Johns Hopkins Hosp (page 61); **Address:** 1830 E Monument St, Ste 447, Baltimore, MD 21287; **Phone:** 410-955-7634; **Board Cert:** Internal Medicine 1972; **Med School:** SUNY Upstate Med Univ 1963; **Resid:** Internal Medicine, Peter Bent Brigham Hosp 1965; Internal Medicine, Univ Hosp Birmingham 1968; **Fellow:** Infectious Disease, Wadsworth VA Hosp 1970

Berkowitz, Leonard B MD [Inf] - **Spec Exp:** AIDS/HIV; **Hospital:** Brooklyn Hosp Ctr-Downtown; **Address:** 121 DeKalb Ave, Ste 5H, Brooklyn, NY 11201-5425; **Phone:** 718-250-6922; **Board Cert:** Internal Medicine 1980; Infectious Disease 1984; **Med School:** SUNY Downstate 1977; **Resid:** Internal Medicine, Kings Co Med Ctr 1981; **Fellow:** Infectious Disease, Kings Co Med Ctr 1983; **Fac Appt:** Asst Clin Prof Med, SUNY Hlth Sci Ctr

Brause, Barry MD [Inf] - **Spec Exp:** Bone/Joint Infections; Skin/Soft Tissue Infections; Infections in Prosthetic Devices; **Hospital:** Hosp For Special Surgery (page 60), NY-Presby/Weill Cornell Med Ctr, NY (page 66); **Address:** 535 E 70th St, Ste 657W, New York, NY 10021-5718; **Phone:** 212-774-7411; **Board Cert:** Internal Medicine 1973; Infectious Disease 1976; **Med School:** Univ Pittsburgh 1970; **Resid:** Internal Medicine, NY Hosp 1973; **Fellow:** Infectious Disease, NY Hosp 1975; **Fac Appt:** Clin Prof Med, Cornell Univ-Weill Med Coll

Chaisson, Richard E MD [Inf] - **Spec Exp:** AIDS/HIV; Tuberculosis; **Hospital:** Johns Hopkins Hosp (page 61); **Address:** 1550 Orleans St, 1M-08, Baltimore, MD 21231; **Phone:** 410-955-1755; **Board Cert:** Internal Medicine 1985; **Med School:** Univ Mass Sch Med 1982; **Resid:** Internal Medicine, UCSF Med Ctr 1985; **Fellow:** Infectious Disease, UCSF Med Ctr 1987; **Fac Appt:** Prof Med, Johns Hopkins Univ

Cunha, Burke A MD [Inf] - **Spec Exp:** Infections in Immunocompromised Patients; Fevers of Unknown Origin; Pneumonia; Chronic Fatigue Syndrome; **Hospital:** Winthrop Univ Hosp; **Address:** 222 Station Plz N, Ste 432, Mineola, NY 11501; **Phone:** 516-663-2507; **Board Cert:** Internal Medicine 1977; Infectious Disease 1978; **Med School:** Penn State Coll Med 1972; **Resid:** Internal Medicine, Hartford Hosp 1975; **Fellow:** Infectious Disease, Hartford Hosp 1977; **Fac Appt:** Prof Med, SUNY Stony Brook

Frank, Ian MD [Inf] - **Spec Exp:** AIDS/HIV; **Hospital:** Hosp Univ Penn - UPHS (page 72); **Address:** Hosp Univ Penn, Div Infectious Disease, 3400 Spruce St, 3 Silverstein, Ste D, Philadelphia, PA 19104; **Phone:** 215-662-6932; **Board Cert:** Internal Medicine 1983; Infectious Disease 2006; **Med School:** Dartmouth Med Sch 1980; **Resid:** Internal Medicine, Graduate Hosp 1983; **Fellow:** Infectious Disease, Hosp Univ Penn 1984; **Fac Appt:** Prof Med, Univ Pennsylvania

Gumprecht, Jeffrey P MD [Inf] - **Spec Exp:** AIDS/HIV; Travel Medicine; Infections-Surgical; **Hospital:** Mount Sinai Med Ctr (page 64); **Address:** 1100 Park Ave, Ste 1C, New York, NY 10128; **Phone:** 212-427-9550; **Board Cert:** Internal Medicine 1987; Infectious Disease 2003; **Med School:** Albany Med Coll 1983; **Resid:** Internal Medicine, Mt Sinai Hosp 1987; **Fellow:** Infectious Disease, Montefiore Med Ctr 1990; **Fac Appt:** Asst Clin Prof Med, Mount Sinai Sch Med

Hammer, Glenn S MD [Inf] - **Spec Exp:** AIDS/HIV; Hospital Acquired Infections; Infections-Surgical; **Hospital:** Mount Sinai Med Ctr (page 64); **Address:** 1100 Park Ave, Ste 1C, New York, NY 10128-1202; **Phone:** 212-427-9550; **Board Cert:** Infectious Disease 1974; Internal Medicine 1973; **Med School:** NYU Sch Med 1969; **Resid:** Internal Medicine, Mount Sinai Hosp 1972; **Fellow:** Infectious Disease, Mount Sinai Hosp 1974; **Fac Appt:** Asst Clin Prof Med, Mount Sinai Sch Med

Hammer, Scott M MD [Inf] - **Spec Exp:** AIDS/HIV; **Hospital:** NY-Presby/Columbia Univ Med Ctr, NY (page 66); **Address:** 630 W 168th St, P&S Box 82, New York, NY 10032; **Phone:** 212-305-8039; **Board Cert:** Internal Medicine 1975; Infectious Disease 1980; **Med School:** Columbia P&S 1972; **Resid:** Internal Medicine, Columbia-Presby Hosp 1975; Internal Medicine, Stanford Univ Hosp 1975; **Fellow:** Infectious Disease, Mass Genl Hosp 1981; **Fac Appt:** Prof Med, Columbia P&S

Hartman, Barry J MD [Inf] - **Spec Exp:** Endocarditis; Infections-Surgical; Parasitic Infections; **Hospital:** NY-Presby/Weill Cornell Med Ctr, NY (page 66); **Address:** 407 E 70th St, Fl 4, New York, NY 10021-5302; **Phone:** 212-744-4882; **Board Cert:** Internal Medicine 1976; Infectious Disease 1980; **Med School:** Penn State Coll Med 1973; **Resid:** Internal Medicine, NY Hosp/Cornell Med Ctr 1976; **Fellow:** Infectious Disease, NY Hosp/Cornell Med Ctr 1981; **Fac Appt:** Clin Prof Med, Cornell Univ-Weill Med Coll

Kumar, Princy N MD [Inf] - **Spec Exp:** AIDS/HIV; **Hospital:** Georgetown Univ Hosp; **Address:** Georgetown Univ Hosp, 3800 Reservoir Rd NW PHC Bldg Fl 5 - Ste 110, Washington, DC 20007; **Phone:** 202-444-0086; **Board Cert:** Internal Medicine 1988; Infectious Disease 2010; **Med School:** India 1981; **Resid:** Internal Medicine, Englewood Hosp 1988; **Fellow:** Infectious Disease, Georgetown Univ Hosp 1990; **Fac Appt:** Assoc Prof Med, Georgetown Univ

Lorber, Bennett MD [Inf] - **Spec Exp:** Foodborne illnesses; **Hospital:** Temple Univ Hosp; **Address:** Temple Univ Hosp - Inf Diseases, 3401 N Broad St, Parkinson Pavilion, Ste 501, Philadelphia, PA 19140; **Phone:** 215-707-3807; **Board Cert:** Internal Medicine 1974; Infectious Disease 1976; **Med School:** Univ Pennsylvania 1968; **Resid:** Internal Medicine, Temple Univ Hosp 1971; **Fellow:** Infectious Disease, Temple Univ Hosp 1973; **Fac Appt:** Prof Med, Temple Univ

Louie, Eddie MD [Inf] - **Spec Exp:** Lyme Disease; AIDS/HIV; Hospital Acquired Infections; **Hospital:** NYU Langone Med Ctr (page 68); **Address:** 345 E 37th St, Ste 207, New York, NY 10016; **Phone:** 212-682-9202; **Board Cert:** Internal Medicine 1982; Infectious Disease 1986; **Med School:** NYU Sch Med 1979; **Resid:** Internal Medicine, Kings County Hosp 1983; **Fellow:** Infectious Disease, NYU Med Ctr 1985; **Fac Appt:** Assoc Clin Prof Med, NYU Sch Med

Masur, Henry MD [Inf] - **Spec Exp:** Critical Care; AIDS/HIV; **Hospital:** Natl Inst of Hlth - Clin Ctr; **Address:** National Inst Hlth, 10 Center Drive, Clinical Ctr 2C145, Bethesda, MD 20892; **Phone:** 301-496-9320; **Board Cert:** Internal Medicine 1975; Infectious Disease 1978; **Med School:** Cornell Univ-Weill Med Coll 1972; **Resid:** Internal Medicine, New York Hosp 1974; Internal Medicine, Johns Hopkins Hosp 1975; **Fellow:** Infectious Disease, New York Hosp-Cornell 1977

McGowan, Joseph MD [Inf] - **Spec Exp:** AIDS/HIV; HIV in Pregnancy; HIV/Hepatitis Co-Infection; AIDS/HIV in Elderly; **Hospital:** NS-LIJ Hlth Sys (page 67); **Address:** 400 Community Drive, Manhasset, NY 11030; **Phone:** 516-562-4280; **Board Cert:** Internal Medicine 2002; Infectious Disease 2002; **Med School:** Mount Sinai Sch Med 1987; **Resid:** Internal Medicine, Montefiore Med Ctr 1990; **Fellow:** Infectious Disease, Montefiore Med Ctr 1993

Mildvan, Donna MD [Inf] - **Spec Exp:** AIDS/HIV; Clinical Trials; Infectious Disease; **Hospital:** Beth Israel Med Ctr - Petrie Division (page 56); **Address:** Beth Israel Med Ctr, Div Infectious Dis, 1st Ave at 16th St, 19BH17, New York, NY 10003; **Phone:** 212-420-4005; **Board Cert:** Internal Medicine 1972; Infectious Disease 1972; **Med School:** Johns Hopkins Univ 1967; **Resid:** Internal Medicine, Mt Sinai Hosp 1970; **Fellow:** Infectious Disease, Mt Sinai Hosp 1972; **Fac Appt:** Prof Med, Albert Einstein Coll Med

Nahass, Ronald MD [Inf] - **Spec Exp:** HIV; Hepatitis B & C; Diagnostic Problems; Bone Infections; **Hospital:** Robert Wood Johnson Univ Hosp - New Brunswick, Univ Med Ctr Princeton at Plainsboro; **Address:** 105 Raider Blvd, Ste 101, Hillsborough, NJ 08844-4254; **Phone:** 908-281-0221; **Board Cert:** Internal Medicine 1985; Infectious Disease 1988; **Med School:** UMDNJ-RW Johnson Med Sch 1982; **Resid:** Internal Medicine, RWJ Univ Hosp 1986; **Fellow:** Infectious Disease, RWJ Univ Hosp 1988

Perlman, David MD [Inf] - **Spec Exp:** AIDS/HIV; Lyme Disease; Travel Medicine; Infectious Disease; **Hospital:** Beth Israel Med Ctr - Petrie Division (page 56), Lenox Hill Hosp (page 67); **Address:** Beth Israel Med Ctr, 120 E 16th St Fl 12, New York, NY 10003; **Phone:** 212-844-8549; **Board Cert:** Internal Medicine 1986; Infectious Disease 1988; **Med School:** Albert Einstein Coll Med 1983; **Resid:** Internal Medicine, New York Hosp/Meml-Sloan Kettering 1986; **Fellow:** Infectious Disease, Montefiore Hosp 1988; **Fac Appt:** Prof Med, Albert Einstein Coll Med

Polsky, Bruce W MD [Inf] - **Spec Exp:** AIDS/HIV; Viral Infections; Infections in Cancer Patients; AIDS Related Cancers; **Hospital:** St. Luke's - Roosevelt Hosp Ctr - Roosevelt Div (page 56), St. Luke's - Roosevelt Hosp Ctr - St Luke's Hosp (page 56); **Address:** 425 W 59th St, Ste 8A, New York, NY 10019; **Phone:** 212-523-7335; **Board Cert:** Internal Medicine 1983; Infectious Disease 1986; **Med School:** Wayne State Univ 1980; **Resid:** Internal Medicine, Montefiore Hosp 1983; **Fellow:** Infectious Disease, Meml Sloan Kettering Cancer Ctr 1986; **Fac Appt:** Prof Med, Columbia P&S

Rao, Nalini G MD [Inf] - **Spec Exp:** Bone/Joint Infections; Tropical Diseases; Travel Medicine; **Hospital:** UPMC Presby, Pittsburgh, UPMC Shadyside; **Address:** Centre Commons, Suite 510, 5750 Centre Ave, Pittsburgh, PA 15206-3721; **Phone:** 412-661-1633; **Board Cert:** Internal Medicine 1975; Infectious Disease 1980; **Med School:** India 1970; **Resid:** Internal Medicine, Geo Wash Univ Hosp 1974; **Fellow:** Infectious Disease, Baylor Coll Med 1975; Infectious Disease, Univ Pittsburgh Sch Med 1977; **Fac Appt:** Clin Prof Med, Univ Pittsburgh

Romagnoli, Mario MD [Inf] - **Spec Exp:** AIDS/HIV; Bone/Joint Infections; **Hospital:** Lenox Hill Hosp (page 67); **Address:** 903 Park Ave, New York, NY 10075; **Phone:** 212-396-3390; **Board Cert:** Internal Medicine 1979; Infectious Disease 1982; **Med School:** Columbia P&S 1976; **Resid:** Internal Medicine, Columbia-Presby Med Ctr 1979; **Fellow:** Infectious Disease, Beth Israel Med Ctr 1981; **Fac Appt:** Assoc Prof Med, Columbia P&S

Segal, Brahm H MD [Inf] - **Spec Exp:** Infections in Cancer Patients; Immune Deficiencies-Primary; **Hospital:** Roswell Park Cancer Inst; **Address:** Roswell Park Cancer Inst, Elm & Carlton Streets, Buffalo, NY 14263; **Phone:** 716-845-1642; **Board Cert:** Infectious Disease 2009; **Med School:** Albert Einstein Coll Med 1992; **Resid:** Internal Medicine, New England Med Ctr 1995; **Fellow:** Infectious Disease, Natl Inst Allergy/Inf Dis 1997; **Fac Appt:** Prof Med, SUNY Buffalo

Sepkowitz, Kent A MD [Inf] - **Spec Exp:** Tuberculosis; Infections in Cancer Patients; Fungal Infections; **Hospital:** Meml Sloan-Kettering Cancer Ctr; **Address:** 1275 York Ave, New York, NY 10065; **Phone:** 800-525-2225; **Board Cert:** Internal Medicine 1983; Infectious Disease 2010; **Med School:** Univ Okla Coll Med 1980; **Resid:** Internal Medicine, Roosevelt Hosp 1984; **Fellow:** Infectious Disease, Meml Sloan Kettering Cancer Ctr 1991; **Fac Appt:** Prof Med, Cornell Univ-Weill Med Coll

Squires, Kathleen E MD [Inf] - **Spec Exp:** AIDS/HIV; AIDS/HIV in Women; **Hospital:** Thomas Jefferson Univ Hosp; **Address:** 834 Walnut St, Ste 650, Philadelphia, PA 19107; **Phone:** 215-955-7785; **Board Cert:** Internal Medicine 1984; Infectious Disease 1988; **Med School:** Med Coll PA 1981; **Resid:** Internal Medicine, Med Coll Penn 1984; **Fellow:** Infectious Disease, NY Presby Hosp/Cornell Weill Med Ctr 1988; **Fac Appt:** Prof Med, Thomas Jefferson Univ

Wallach, Frances MD [Inf] - **Spec Exp:** AIDS/HIV; Infection Control; HIV & Blood Transfusions; **Hospital:** Mount Sinai Med Ctr (page 64); **Address:** Mount Sinai Med Ctr, One Gustave L Levy Pl, New York, NY 10029; **Phone:** 212-241-7968; **Board Cert:** Internal Medicine 1989; Infectious Disease 2002; **Med School:** Albany Med Coll 1985; **Resid:** Internal Medicine, Montefiore Med Ctr 1989; **Fellow:** Nuclear Medicine, Montefiore Med Ctr 1990; Infectious Disease, NY Hosp-Cornell Med Ctr 1992; **Fac Appt:** Asst Prof Med, Mount Sinai Sch Med

Wormser, Gary P MD [Inf] - **Spec Exp:** Lyme Disease; AIDS/HIV; Diagnostic Problems; **Hospital:** Westchester Med Ctr; **Address:** New York Medical College, Munger Pavilion, rm 245, Valhalla, NY 10595; **Phone:** 914-493-8865; **Board Cert:** Internal Medicine 1978; Infectious Disease 1982; **Med School:** Johns Hopkins Univ 1972; **Resid:** Internal Medicine, Mt Sinai Hosp 1975; **Fellow:** Infectious Disease, Mt Sinai Hosp 1977; **Fac Appt:** Prof Med, NY Med Coll

Infectious Disease

Yancovitz, Stanley MD [Inf] - **Spec Exp:** Lyme Disease; AIDS/HIV; **Hospital:** Beth Israel Med Ctr - Petrie Division (page 56); **Address:** 1st Ave at 16th St, Ste 17 BH10, New York, NY 10003; **Phone:** 212-420-2600; **Board Cert:** Internal Medicine 1973; Infectious Disease 1976; **Med School:** SUNY Downstate 1967; **Resid:** Internal Medicine, Metropolitan Hosp 1969; Internal Medicine, Beth Israel Med Ctr 1972; **Fellow:** Infectious Disease, Mt Sinai Hosp 1975; **Fac Appt:** Clin Prof Med, Albert Einstein Coll Med

Southeast

Alvarez-Elcoro, Salvador MD [Inf] - **Spec Exp:** Tuberculosis; Travel Medicine; Infections-Transplant; **Hospital:** Mayo - Jacksonville; **Address:** Mayo Clinic, Div Infectious Disease, 4500 San Pablo Rd, Jacksonville, FL 32224; **Phone:** 904-953-2000; **Board Cert:** Internal Medicine 1977; Infectious Disease 1982; **Med School:** Mexico 1972; **Resid:** Internal Medicine, Charity Hosp 1977; **Fellow:** Infectious Disease, Boston City Hosp 1979; **Fac Appt:** Prof Med, Univ Fla Coll Med

Blumberg, Henry M MD [Inf] - **Spec Exp:** Tuberculosis; **Hospital:** Grady Hlth Sys, Emory Univ Hosp; **Address:** Emory Univ, Div Infectious Diseases, 49 Jesse Hill Jr Drive, Atlanta, GA 30303; **Phone:** 404-727-5096; **Board Cert:** Internal Medicine 1986; Infectious Disease 2010; **Med School:** Vanderbilt Univ 1983; **Resid:** Internal Medicine, Emory Univ Affil Hosps 1986; Internal Medicine, Crawford-Long Hosp 1988; **Fellow:** Infectious Disease, Emory Univ Affil Hosps 1992; **Fac Appt:** Prof Med, Emory Univ

Cancio, Margarita MD [Inf] - **Spec Exp:** AIDS/HIV; **Hospital:** Tampa Genl Hosp; **Address:** 4729 N Habana Ave, Tampa, FL 33614; **Phone:** 813-251-8444; **Board Cert:** Internal Medicine 1985; Infectious Disease 1988; **Med School:** Univ S Fla Coll Med 1982; **Resid:** Internal Medicine, Univ S Florida Affil Hosps 1985; **Fellow:** Infectious Disease, Univ S Florida Affil Hosps 1988; **Fac Appt:** Assoc Prof Med, Univ S Fla Coll Med

Cohen, Myron S MD [Inf] - **Spec Exp:** Infections in Immunocompromised Patients; **Hospital:** NC Memorial Hosp - UNC; **Address:** UNC-Chapel Hill, Div Infectious Diseases, 2115 Bioinformatics Bldg, 130 Mason Farm Rd, CB 7030, Chapel Hill, NC 27599-7030; **Phone:** 919-966-2536; **Board Cert:** Internal Medicine 1977; Infectious Disease 1982; **Med School:** Rush Med Coll 1974; **Resid:** Internal Medicine, Univ Michigan Hlth Ctr 1977; **Fellow:** Infectious Disease, Yale-New Haven Hosp 1979; **Fac Appt:** Prof Med, Univ NC Sch Med

Corey, G Ralph MD [Inf] - **Spec Exp:** Tropical Diseases; Travel Medicine; Endocarditis; Staphylococcal Infections; **Hospital:** Duke Univ Hosp; **Address:** 301 Trent Drive, rm 235, Trent Box 90519, Durham, NC 27708; **Phone:** 919-668-7174; **Board Cert:** Internal Medicine 1977; Infectious Disease 1980; **Med School:** Baylor Coll Med 1973; **Resid:** Internal Medicine, Duke Univ Med Ctr 1978; **Fellow:** Infectious Disease, Duke Univ Med Ctr 1980; **Fac Appt:** Prof Med, Duke Univ

Edmond, Michael B MD [Inf] - **Spec Exp:** Bone/Joint Infections; Skin/Soft Tissue Infections; Antibiotic Resistance; Hospital Acquired Infections; **Hospital:** Med Coll of VA Hosp; **Address:** VCU/Med College Virginia, Box 980019, Richmond, VA 23298-0019; **Phone:** 804-828-2121; **Board Cert:** Internal Medicine 1989; Infectious Disease 2002; **Med School:** W VA Univ 1986; **Resid:** Internal Medicine, W Virginia Univ Hosps 1989; **Fellow:** Infectious Disease, Univ Pittsburgh 1992; Epidemiology, Univ Iowa; **Fac Appt:** Prof Med, Med Coll VA

Gorensek, Margaret J MD [Inf] - **Spec Exp:** AIDS/HIV; Infections-Transplant; Chronic Fatigue Syndrome; Pediatric Infectious Disease; **Hospital:** Holy Cross Hosp - Fort Lauderdale, Broward Hlth Med Ctr; **Address:** Holy Cross Medical Group, 5601 N Dixie Hwy, Ste 107, Fort Lauderdale, FL 33334; **Phone:** 954-493-9752; **Board Cert:** Internal Medicine 1985; Pediatrics 1986; Infectious Disease 1988; Pediatric Infectious Disease 2009; **Med School:** Case West Res Univ 1981; **Resid:** Internal Medicine & Pediatrics, Cleveland Clinic 1985; **Fellow:** Infectious Disease, Cleveland Clinic 1987; Pediatric Infectious Disease, Chldns Med Ctr 1988; **Fac Appt:** Asst Clin Prof Med, Univ Miami Sch Med

Katner, Harold P MD [Inf] - **Spec Exp:** AIDS/HIV; **Hospital:** Med Ctr of Central GA; **Address:** Mercer Univ Sch Med, Dept Internal Med, 707 Pine St, Macon, GA 31201; **Phone:** 478-301-5809; **Board Cert:** Internal Medicine 1983; Infectious Disease 1986; **Med School:** Louisiana State U, New Orleans 1980; **Resid:** Internal Medicine, Univ Med Ctr 1983; **Fellow:** Infectious Disease, Ochsner Fdn Hosp 1986; **Fac Appt:** Prof Med, Mercer Univ Sch Med

Pearson, Richard D MD [Inf] - **Spec Exp:** Tropical Diseases; Travel Medicine; Infectious Disease; Parasitic Infections; **Hospital:** Univ of Virginia Health Sys; **Address:** Univ VA Sch Med, Dept Internal Med, Box 801379, Charlottesville, VA 22908-0001; **Phone:** 434-982-1700; **Board Cert:** Internal Medicine 1976; Infectious Disease 1980; **Med School:** Univ Mich Med Sch 1973; **Resid:** Internal Medicine, Strong Meml Hosp 1976; **Fellow:** Infectious Disease, Strong Meml Hosp 1979; **Fac Appt:** Prof Med, Univ VA Sch Med

Ratzan, Kenneth MD [Inf] - **Spec Exp:** AIDS/HIV; **Hospital:** Mount Sinai Med Ctr - Miami, Miami Heart Inst; **Address:** Mount Sinai Med Ctr, 4300 Alton Rd, Ste 450, Miami Beach, FL 33140-2800; **Phone:** 305-673-5490; **Board Cert:** Internal Medicine 1977; Infectious Disease 1974; **Med School:** Harvard Med Sch 1965; **Resid:** Internal Medicine, Columbia Presby Med Ctr 1967; Infectious Disease, Tufts New England Med Ctr 1972; **Fellow:** Infectious Disease, Tufts New England Med Ctr 1971; **Fac Appt:** Prof Med, Univ Miami Sch Med

Saag, Michael S MD [Inf] - **Spec Exp:** AIDS/HIV; Clinical Trials; **Hospital:** Univ of Ala Hosp at Birmingham; **Address:** UAB Div Infectious Diseases, 1530 3rd Ave S, BBRB 256, Birmingham, AL 35294; **Phone:** 205-934-7349; **Board Cert:** Internal Medicine 1985; Infectious Disease 1988; **Med School:** Univ Louisville Sch Med 1981; **Resid:** Internal Medicine, Univ Ala Hosp 1984; **Fellow:** Infectious Disease, Univ Alabama 1987; **Fac Appt:** Prof Med, Univ Alabama

Scheld, W Michael MD [Inf] - **Spec Exp:** Meningitis; Endocarditis; AIDS/HIV; Antibiotic Resistance; **Hospital:** Univ of Virginia Health Sys; **Address:** Univ VA Hlth Sci Ctr, PO Box 801342, Charlottesville, VA 22908; **Phone:** 434-924-5059; **Board Cert:** Internal Medicine 1976; Infectious Disease 1978; **Med School:** Cornell Univ-Weill Med Coll 1973; **Resid:** Internal Medicine, Univ VA Med Ctr 1976; **Fellow:** Infectious Disease, Univ VA Med Ctr 1979; **Fac Appt:** Prof Med, Univ VA Sch Med

Van Der Horst, Charles M MD [Inf] - **Spec Exp:** AIDS/HIV; Fungal Infections; Viral Infections; Immune Deficiency; **Hospital:** NC Memorial Hosp - UNC; **Address:** Univ NC-Dept Med, Box CB7030, Chapel Hill, NC 27599; **Phone:** 919-966-2536; **Board Cert:** Internal Medicine 1982; Infectious Disease 1986; **Med School:** Harvard Med Sch 1979; **Resid:** Internal Medicine, Montefiore Med Ctr 1982; **Fellow:** Infectious Disease, NC Meml Hosp 1985; **Fac Appt:** Prof Med, Univ NC Sch Med

Wallace, Mark R MD [Inf] - **Spec Exp:** Fever in Returning Travelers; Travel Medicine; Malaria; HIV; **Hospital:** Orlando Regl Med Ctr; **Address:** 77 W Underwood, Ste 4B, Orlando, FL 32806; **Phone:** 321-841-7750; **Board Cert:** Internal Medicine 1984; Infectious Disease 2010; **Med School:** St Louis Univ 1981; **Resid:** Internal Medicine, Univ Washington Hosp 1984; **Fellow:** Infectious Disease, Naval Hosp 1989; **Fac Appt:** Clin Prof Med, FSU College Medicine

Midwest

Bakken, Johan S MD/PhD [Inf] - **Spec Exp:** Human Granulocytic Anaplasmosis; Tick-borne Diseases; Diarrheal Diseases; Ehrlichiosis; **Hospital:** St. Luke's Hosp - Duluth, St. Mary's Med Ctr - Duluth; **Address:** 1001 E Superior St, Ste L201, Duluth, MN 55802; **Phone:** 218-249-7990; **Board Cert:** Internal Medicine 2009; **Med School:** Univ Wash 1972; **Resid:** Internal Medicine, Univ Wash Hosps 1978; Internal Medicine, Lillehammer Fylkessykehus 1981; **Fellow:** Infectious Disease, Ulleval Hosp 1985; Microbiology, Creighton Univ 1987; **Fac Appt:** Assoc Clin Prof FMed, Univ Minn

Campbell, J William MD [Inf] - **Spec Exp:** AIDS/HIV; **Hospital:** St. Luke's Hosp - Chesterfield, MO, Barnes-Jewish Hosp; **Address:** St Luke's Hosp, 222 S Woods Mill Rd, Ste 750 N, Chesterfield, MO 63017; **Phone:** 314-205-6600; **Board Cert:** Internal Medicine 1980; Infectious Disease 1982; **Med School:** Washington Univ, St Louis 1977; **Resid:** Internal Medicine, Barnes Hosp-Wash Univ 1980; **Fellow:** Infectious Disease, Univ Tex Hlth Sci Ctr 1981; Infectious Disease, Wash Univ 1982; **Fac Appt:** Clin Prof Med, Washington Univ, St Louis

Cohn, Susan E MD [Inf] - **Spec Exp:** AIDS/HIV; AIDS/HIV in Women; Women's Health; HIV in Pregnancy; **Hospital:** Northwestern Meml Hosp; **Address:** 645 N Michigan Ave, Ste 900, Chicago, IL 60611; **Phone:** 312-926-8358; **Board Cert:** Internal Medicine 1987; Infectious Disease 2005; **Med School:** Cornell Univ 1984; **Resid:** Internal Medicine, Boston City Hosp 1987; **Fellow:** Infectious Disease, Univ NC Affil Hosp 1992; **Fac Appt:** Prof Med, Northwestern Univ-Feinberg Sch Med

Fichtenbaum, Carl J MD [Inf] - **Spec Exp:** AIDS/HIV; **Hospital:** Univ Hosp - Cincinnati; **Address:** 231 Albert Sabin Way, ML 0560, Cincinnati, OH 45267; **Phone:** 513-584-6977; **Board Cert:** Infectious Disease 2004; Internal Medicine 2004; **Med School:** Univ MO-Kansas City 1985; **Resid:** Internal Medicine, Bridgeport Hosp 1989; Pediatrics, Bridgeport Hosp 1989; **Fellow:** Infectious Disease, Yale-New Haven Hosp 1991; Infectious Disease, Washington Univ Med Ctr 1992; **Fac Appt:** Prof Med, Univ Cincinnati

Flaherty, John P MD [Inf] - **Spec Exp:** AIDS/HIV; Travel Medicine; Orthopaedic Infectious Disease; **Hospital:** Northwestern Meml Hosp; **Address:** 676 N St Clair St, Ste 940, Chicago, IL 60611; **Phone:** 312-926-8358; **Board Cert:** Internal Medicine 1986; Infectious Disease 1988; **Med School:** Univ IL Coll Med 1983; **Resid:** Internal Medicine, Univ Iowa Hosp 1986; **Fellow:** Infectious Disease, Univ Chicago Hosps 1988; **Fac Appt:** Prof Med, Northwestern Univ

Longworth, David L MD [Inf] - **Spec Exp:** HIV; **Hospital:** Cleveland Clin (page 55); **Address:** Clevelan Clin, 9500 Euclid Ave, MC G10, Cleveland, OH 44195; **Phone:** 216-444-5665; **Board Cert:** Internal Medicine 1981; Infectious Disease 1984; **Med School:** Cornell Univ-Weill Med Coll 1978; **Resid:** Internal Medicine, UCSF-HC Moffitt Hosp 1981; **Fellow:** Infectious Disease, Brigham & Womens Hosp 1983; Research, Harvard Med School 1985; **Fac Appt:** Prof Med, Tufts Univ

Maki, Dennis G MD [Inf] - **Spec Exp:** Urinary Tract Infections; Critical Care; **Hospital:** Univ WI Hosp & Clins; **Address:** 600 Highland Ave, MC B6/242, Madison, WI 53792-2442; **Phone:** 608-263-0946; **Board Cert:** Internal Medicine 1972; Infectious Disease 1974; Critical Care Medicine 2012; **Med School:** Univ Wisc 1967; **Resid:** Infectious Disease, Mass Genl Hosp 1972; Internal Medicine, Harvard-Boston City Hosp 1973; **Fellow:** Infectious Disease, Mass Genl Hosp 1974; **Fac Appt:** Prof Med, Univ Wisc

O'Keefe, J Paul MD [Inf] - **Spec Exp:** AIDS/HIV; Fungal Infections; Infections-Surgical; Travel Medicine; **Hospital:** Loyola Univ Med Ctr; **Address:** Loyola Univ Med Ctr, 2160 S 1st Ave, Maywood, IL 60153-3304; **Phone:** 708-216-0160; **Board Cert:** Internal Medicine 1974; Infectious Disease 1978; **Med School:** Loyola Univ-Stritch Sch Med 1971; **Resid:** Internal Medicine, Loyola Univ Med Ctr 1974; **Fellow:** Infectious Disease, VA Hosp 1975; Infectious Disease, Tufts New England Med Ctr 1977; **Fac Appt:** Prof Med, Loyola Univ-Stritch Sch Med

Salata, Robert A MD [Inf] - **Spec Exp:** AIDS/HIV; **Hospital:** Univ Hosps Case Med Ctr (page 74); **Address:** UH Case Medical Center, Infectious Disease-Foley Bldg 411, 11100 Euclid Ave, Cleveland, OH 44106; **Phone:** 216-844-1709; **Board Cert:** Internal Medicine 1982; Infectious Disease 1986; **Med School:** Case West Res Univ 1979; **Resid:** Internal Medicine, Case Med Ctr 1982; **Fellow:** Infectious Disease, Univ VA Med Ctr 1985; **Fac Appt:** Prof Med, Case West Res Univ

Schmitt, Steven K MD [Inf] - **Spec Exp:** Bone/Joint Infections; **Hospital:** Cleveland Clin (page 55); **Address:** Cleveland Clinic, 9500 Euclid Ave, Desk G21, Cleveland, OH 44195; **Phone:** 216-444-5665; **Board Cert:** Internal Medicine 2002; Infectious Disease 2004; **Med School:** Univ Cincinnati 1988; **Resid:** Internal Medicine, Cleveland Clin 1991; **Fellow:** Infectious Disease, Cleveland Clin 1994

Sha, Beverly E MD [Inf] - **Spec Exp:** AIDS/HIV in Women; **Hospital:** Rush Univ Med Ctr; **Address:** 600 S Paulina St, Ste 140, Chicago, IL 60612-3806; **Phone:** 312-942-5865; **Board Cert:** Internal Medicine 1989; Infectious Disease 2002; **Med School:** Johns Hopkins Univ 1986; **Resid:** Internal Medicine, Rush-Presby St Lukes Med Ctr 1989; **Fellow:** Infectious Disease, Rush-Presby St Lukes Med Ctr 1991; **Fac Appt:** Prof Med, Rush Med Coll

Slama, Thomas G MD [Inf] - **Spec Exp:** Hematologic Infections; Bone Infections; Infective Endocarditis; Infections in Prosthetic Devices; **Hospital:** St. Vincent Indianapolis Hosp; **Address:** 8240 Naab Rd, Ste 300, Indianapolis, IN 46260; **Phone:** 317-870-1970; **Board Cert:** Internal Medicine 1976; Infectious Disease 1978; **Med School:** Indiana Univ 1973; **Resid:** Internal Medicine, Indianapolis Meth Hosp 1976; **Fellow:** Infectious Disease, Ohio State Univ Hosps 1978; **Fac Appt:** Clin Prof Med, Indiana Univ

Sobel, Jack MD [Inf] - **Spec Exp:** Vaginitis; Fungal Infections; Urinary Tract Infections; **Hospital:** Harper Univ Hosp, Detroit Receiving Hospital; **Address:** 3750 Woodward Ave, Ste 200, Detroit, MI 48201; **Phone:** 313-745-9035; **Board Cert:** Internal Medicine 1978; Infectious Disease 1982; **Med School:** South Africa 1965; **Resid:** Internal Medicine 1970; **Fellow:** Infectious Disease, Univ Penn Hosps 1977; Research, Natl Inst Hlth 1978; **Fac Appt:** Prof Med, Wayne State Univ

Tomford, J Walton MD [Inf] - **Hospital:** Cleveland Clin (page 55); **Address:** Cleveland Clinic, Dept Infectious Diseases, 9500 Euclid Ave, Desk G21, Cleveland, OH 44195; **Phone:** 216-444-5665; **Board Cert:** Internal Medicine 1978; Infectious Disease 1980; **Med School:** Johns Hopkins Univ 1975; **Resid:** Internal Medicine, Johns Hopkins Hosp 1978; Internal Medicine, Univ Hosps 1981; **Fellow:** Infectious Disease, Cleveland Univ Hosp 1980; **Fac Appt:** Assoc Prof Med, Cleveland Cl Coll Med/Case West Res

Trenholme, Gordon M MD [Inf] - **Spec Exp:** Fevers of Unknown Origin; Malaria; Tropical Diseases; **Hospital:** Rush Univ Med Ctr; **Address:** Rush Univ Med Ctr, Infectious Disease, 600 S Paulina St, Ste 143, Chicago, IL 60612-3809; **Phone:** 312-942-3665; **Board Cert:** Internal Medicine 1972; Infectious Disease 1976; **Med School:** Med Coll Wisc 1970; **Resid:** Internal Medicine, Univ Chicago Hosp 1973; **Fellow:** Infectious Disease, Rush/Presby-St Luke's Med Ctr 1975; **Fac Appt:** Prof Med, Rush Med Coll

Wilson, Walter Ray MD [Inf] - **Spec Exp:** Musculoskeletal Infections; **Hospital:** Mayo Med Ctr & Clin - Rochester; **Address:** Mayo Clin, Div Infectious Dis, 200 First St SW, Rochester, MN 55905; **Phone:** 507-255-7761; **Board Cert:** Internal Medicine 1973; Infectious Disease 1974; Medical Microbiology 1975; **Med School:** Baylor Coll Med 1967; **Resid:** Internal Medicine, Methodist Hosp 1968; Internal Medicine, Mayo Clin 1973; **Fellow:** Infectious Disease, Mayo Clin 1974; Microbiology, Mayo Clin 1975; **Fac Appt:** Prof Med, Mayo Med Sch

Infectious Disease

Great Plains and Mountains

Freifeld, Alison G MD [Inf] - **Spec Exp:** Infectious Disease during Chemotherapy; Infections in Cancer Patients; **Hospital:** Nebraska Med Ctr; **Address:** Univ Nebraska Med Ctr, 985400 Nebraska Medical Center, Omaha, NE 68198-5400; **Phone:** 402-559-8650; **Board Cert:** Internal Medicine 1985; Infectious Disease 1988; **Med School:** Johns Hopkins Univ 1982; **Resid:** Internal Medicine, Johns Hopkins Univ Med Ctr 1985

Huitt, Gwen A MD [Inf] - **Spec Exp:** Tuberculosis; Cystic Fibrosis; Mycobacterial Infections; **Hospital:** Natl Jewish Med & Rsch Ctr; **Address:** National Jewish Health, 1400 Jackson St, rm J222, Denver, CO 80206; **Phone:** 303-398-1667; **Board Cert:** Internal Medicine 2003; Infectious Disease 2004; **Med School:** Univ Colorado 1988; **Resid:** Internal Medicine, Univ Colorado Hlth Sci Ctr 1991; **Fellow:** Infectious Disease, Univ Colorado Hlth Sci Ctr 1993; **Fac Appt:** Assoc Prof Med, Univ Colorado

Johnson, Steven C MD [Inf] - **Spec Exp:** AIDS/HIV; **Hospital:** Univ of CO Hosp - Anschutz Inpatient Pav; **Address:** Univ Colorado Infectious Disease Group, 1635 Aurora Ct, MS B163, Aurora, CO 80045; **Phone:** 303-315-1540; **Board Cert:** Internal Medicine 1987; Infectious Disease 2000; **Med School:** Northwestern Univ 1984; **Resid:** Internal Medicine, Fitzsimons Army Med Ctr 1987; **Fellow:** Infectious Disease, Walter Reed Army Med Ctr 1989; **Fac Appt:** Prof Med, Univ Colorado

Southwest

DuPont, Herbert L MD [Inf] - **Spec Exp:** Tropical Diseases; Diarrheal Diseases; Travel Medicine; **Hospital:** St. Luke's Episcopal Hosp-Houston; **Address:** 6720 Bertner Ave, MC 1-164, Houston, TX 77030-1602; **Phone:** 832-355-4122; **Board Cert:** Internal Medicine 1972; **Med School:** Emory Univ 1965; **Resid:** Internal Medicine, Univ Minn Hosps 1967; **Fellow:** Infectious Disease, Univ Maryland Hosp 1969; **Fac Appt:** Prof Med, Baylor Coll Med

Galgiani, John N MD [Inf] - **Spec Exp:** Valley Fever; Infection Control; Fungal Infections; **Hospital:** Univ Ariz Med Ctr-South Campus (Kino); **Address:** Valley Fever Center for Excellence, 2800 E Ajo Way, Tuscon, AZ 85723; **Phone:** 520-626-4973; **Board Cert:** Internal Medicine 1978; **Med School:** Northwestern Univ 1972; **Resid:** Internal Medicine, Santa Clara Valley Med Ctr 1974; **Fellow:** Infectious Disease, Stanford Univ Hosp 1976; **Fac Appt:** Prof Med, Univ Ariz Coll Med

Keiser, Philip H MD [Inf] - **Spec Exp:** AIDS/HIV; International Health; **Hospital:** UT Med Br at Galveston(Joh Sealy Hosp); **Address:** 301 University Drive, MS 77555, Galveston, TX 77555; **Phone:** 409-772-2222; **Board Cert:** Internal Medicine 1989; **Med School:** Univ MD Sch Med 1986; **Resid:** Internal Medicine, Francis Scott Key Med Ctr 1989; **Fellow:** Infectious Disease, Univ Maryland 1992; **Fac Appt:** Prof Med, Univ Tex Med Br, Galveston

Luby, James P MD [Inf] - **Spec Exp:** Viral Infections; **Hospital:** Parkland Hlth & Hosp Sys, UT Southwestern Med Ctr at Dallas; **Address:** Univ Tex SW Med Ctr, Div Inf Dis, 5323 Harry Hines Blvd, Dallas, TX 75390-9113; **Phone:** 214-648-3480; **Board Cert:** Internal Medicine 1968; Infectious Disease 1972; **Med School:** Northwestern Univ 1961; **Resid:** Internal Medicine, Northwestern Univ 1964; **Fac Appt:** Prof Med, Univ Tex SW, Dallas

Patterson, Jan E MD [Inf] - **Spec Exp:** Hospital Acquired Infections; Antibiotic Resistance; **Hospital:** Audie L Murphy Meml Vets Hosp - San Antonio; **Address:** 7400 Merton Minter Blvd, San Antonio, TX 78229; **Phone:** 210-617-5300; **Board Cert:** Internal Medicine 1985; Infectious Disease 1988; **Med School:** Univ Tex, Houston 1982; **Resid:** Internal Medicine, Vanderbilt Univ Hosp 1985; **Fellow:** Infectious Disease, Yale-New Haven Hosp 1988; **Fac Appt:** Prof Med, Univ Tex, San Antonio

Patterson, Thomas F MD [Inf] - **Spec Exp:** Fungal Infections; **Hospital:** Univ Hlth Syst-San Antonio, Rio Grande State Ctr/S TX Hlthcare Sys; **Address:** Univ Texas HSC, Dept Medicine, Div Infectious Disease, 7703 Floyd Curl Drive, San Antonio, TX 78229-3900; **Phone:** 210-567-4823; **Board Cert:** Internal Medicine 1986; Infectious Disease 2009; **Med School:** Univ Tex, Houston 1983; **Resid:** Internal Medicine, Vanderbilt Univ Hosp 1985; Internal Medicine, Yale-New Haven Hosp 1986; **Fellow:** Infectious Disease, Yale-New Haven Hosp 1989; **Fac Appt:** Prof Med, Univ Tex, San Antonio

Wallace Jr, Richard James MD [Inf] - **Spec Exp:** Non Tuberculous Mycobacteria; Nocardia Infection; **Hospital:** Univ of Texas Hlth Sci Ctr at Tyler; **Address:** 11937 US Hwy 271, Tyler, TX 75708; **Phone:** 903-877-5122; **Board Cert:** Internal Medicine 1975; Infectious Disease 1976; **Med School:** Baylor Coll Med 1972; **Resid:** Internal Medicine, Boston City Hosp 1974; **Fellow:** Infectious Disease, Boston City Hosp 1975; Infectious Disease, Baylor Coll Med 1977

West Coast and Pacific

Ballon-Landa, Gonzalo MD [Inf] - **Spec Exp:** Hospital Acquired Infections; AIDS/HIV; Travel Medicine; **Hospital:** Scripps Mercy Hosp & Med Ctr; **Address:** 4136 Bachman Pl, San Diego, CA 92103; **Phone:** 619-298-1443; **Board Cert:** Internal Medicine 1980; Infectious Disease 1984; **Med School:** Northwestern Univ 1977; **Resid:** Internal Medicine, Evanston Hosp 1981; **Fellow:** Infectious Disease, UCSD Med Ctr 1983

Bayer, Arnold MD [Inf] - **Spec Exp:** Infective Endocarditis; Arthritis-Septic; Coccidioidomycosis; **Hospital:** LAC - Harbor - UCLA Med Ctr, UCLA Ronald Reagan Med Ctr; **Address:** 1124 W Carson St, RB2 Fl 2, Torrance, CA 90502; **Phone:** 310-222-3813; **Board Cert:** Internal Medicine 1973; Infectious Disease 1978; **Med School:** Temple Univ 1970; **Resid:** Internal Medicine, Thomas Jefferson Univ Hosp 1972; Internal Medicine, LAC-Harbor UCLA Med Ctr 1974; **Fellow:** Infectious Disease, VA Med Ctr 1976; Infectious Disease, LAC-Harbor UCLA Med Ctr 1977; **Fac Appt:** Prof Med, UCLA

Daar, Eric S MD [Inf] - **Spec Exp:** AIDS/HIV; **Hospital:** LAC - Harbor - UCLA Med Ctr; **Address:** 1000 W Carson St, Box 449, Torrance, CA 90502; **Phone:** 310-222-2467; **Board Cert:** Internal Medicine 1988; **Med School:** Georgetown Univ 1985; **Resid:** Internal Medicine, Cedars-Sinai Med Ctr 1988; **Fellow:** Infectious Disease, Cedars-Sinai Med Ctr 1991; **Fac Appt:** Prof Med, UCLA-David Geffen Sch Med

Edwards Jr, John Ellis MD [Inf] - **Spec Exp:** Fungal Infections; Infections in Immunocompromised Patients; **Hospital:** LAC - Harbor - UCLA Med Ctr; **Address:** 1124 W Carson St, RB2 Fl 2, Torrance, CA 90502; **Phone:** 310-222-3813; **Board Cert:** Internal Medicine 1980; Infectious Disease 1974; **Med School:** UC Irvine 1968; **Resid:** Internal Medicine, Harbor-UCLA Med Ctr 1971; **Fellow:** Infectious Disease, Harbor-UCLA Med Ctr 1973; **Fac Appt:** Prof Med, UCLA

Palefsky, Joel M MD [Inf] - **Spec Exp:** AIDS Related Cancers; **Hospital:** UCSF - Mt Zion Med Ctr; **Address:** 1600 Divisadero St, San Francisco, CA 94115; **Phone:** 415-353-7100; **Board Cert:** Internal Medicine 1984; Infectious Disease 1988; **Med School:** McGill Univ 1980; **Resid:** Internal Medicine, Royal Victoria Hosp 1984; **Fellow:** Infectious Disease, Stanford Univ 1989

Richman, Douglas D MD [Inf] - **Spec Exp:** AIDS/HIV; **Hospital:** VA San Diego Hlthcre Sys, UCSD Med Ctr; **Address:** UCSD-Stein Clin Rsch Bldg, 9500 Gilman Drive, MC 0679, La Jolla, CA 92093-0679; **Phone:** 858-552-8585 x7439; **Board Cert:** Internal Medicine 1973; Infectious Disease 1976; **Med School:** Stanford Univ 1970; **Resid:** Internal Medicine, Stanford Univ Hosp 1972; **Fellow:** Infectious Disease, NIAID/NIH 1975; Infectious Disease, Beth Israel/Chldns Hosp 1976; **Fac Appt:** Prof Med, UCSD

Infectious Disease

Schooley, Robert T MD [Inf] - **Spec Exp:** AIDS/HIV; Infectious Disease; HIV; **Hospital:** UCSD Med Ctr; **Address:** UCSD - Stein Rsch Bldg, 9500 Gilman Drive, Stein Bldg, Ste 401, La Jolla, CA 92023-0665; **Phone:** 858-822-0216; **Board Cert:** Internal Medicine 1977; **Med School:** Johns Hopkins Univ 1974; **Resid:** Internal Medicine, Johns Hopkins Hosp 1976; **Fellow:** Infectious Disease, Natl Inst Hlth 1979; Infectious Disease, Mass Genl Hosp 1981; **Fac Appt:** Prof Med, UCSD

Siegel, Martin MD [Inf] - **Spec Exp:** AIDS/HIV; Infections in Cancer Patients; Orthopaedic Infectious Disease; Travel Medicine; **Hospital:** Swedish Med Ctr-First Hill-Seattle; **Address:** 904 7th Ave Fl 8, Seattle, WA 98104; **Phone:** 206-860-4531; **Board Cert:** Internal Medicine 1976; Infectious Disease 1980; **Med School:** Case West Res Univ 1972; **Resid:** Internal Medicine, Univ N Carolina Hosp 1976; **Fellow:** Infectious Disease, Univ Washington Med Ctr 1980; **Fac Appt:** Assoc Clin Prof Med, Univ Wash

Wiviott, Lory David MD [Inf] - **Spec Exp:** AIDS/HIV; **Hospital:** CA Pacific Med Ctr-Pacific Campus, CA Pacific Med Ctr - Davies Campus; **Address:** 2100 Webster St, Ste 400, San Francisco, CA 94115; **Phone:** 415-923-3883; **Board Cert:** Internal Medicine 1986; Infectious Disease 2010; **Med School:** Albert Einstein Coll Med 1982; **Resid:** Internal Medicine, Columbia Presby Med Ctr 1985; **Fellow:** Infectious Disease, UCSF Med Ctr 1989; **Fac Appt:** Asst Clin Prof Med, UCSF

◼ Cleveland Clinic

Every life deserves world class care.

Cleveland Clinic
Infectious Disease
9500 Euclid Avenue
Cleveland, OH 44195

Infectious Disease

The Department of Infectious Disease, part of the Medicine Institute at Cleveland Clinic, provides patients with technologically advanced, compassionate medical care. We provide inpatient care, including general infectious disease consultation services and sub-specialty service lines such as solid organ transplant, bone marrow transplant, bone and joint infections, neuroinfections, cardiothoracic and medical/surgical ICU services. We also provide transition of care to outpatient for all patients discharged on parenteral antimicrobials via our Community Outpatient Parenteral Antimicrobial Therapy Program (CoPAT). Staff members participate in the CoPAT program, which has one of the highest volumes by a single center in the country and continues to grow.

Our Outpatient Sub-Specialty Clinics

Bone and Joint Infection Clinic works closely with the Orthopedic & Rheumatic Institute to treat complex infections of the musculoskeletal system.

Endocarditis Clinic evaluates and treats patients with infected heart valves, pacemakers, defibrillators and left ventricular assist devices.

Granuloma Clinic is dedicated to the care of patients with mycobacterial and fungal infections.

HIV/AIDS Clinic provides comprehensive care for HIV-infected patients.

International Travelers' Health Clinic is a full-service travel clinic that provides pre-travel health and safety advice to persons traveling abroad.

MRSA Clinic evaluates and treats patients with recurrent skin infections caused by methicillin-resistant staphylococcus aureus.

Neuroinfection Clinic is staffed with providers to treat infections of the brain, spinal cord and its linings.

Transplant Infectious Disease Clinic provides a vital role in caring for patients who are transplant candidates and recipients.

Offering Same-Day Appointments
Call 800.274.2009.

Treatment Guides
Cleveland Clinic has developed comprehensive treatment guides for many diseases and conditions. To download our free treatment guides, visit clevelandclinic.org/treatmentguides.

Online Medical Second Opinion
Call 216.444.3223 or 800.223.2273 ext. 43223 or email eclevelandclinic@ccf.org.

Out-of-State Patients Assistance
Call 800.223.2273, ext. 55580 or email medicalconcierge@ccf.org.

Visit Us At:
clevelandclinic.org

Follow Us On:
Facebook
www.facebook.com/clevelandclinic

Twitter
@ClevelandClinic

You Tube
www.youtube.com/clevelandclinic

Health Hub
health.clevelandclinic.org

INFECTIOUS DISEASES

About the Division of Infectious Diseases and Immunology
NYU Langone Medical Center has extensive expertise in the diagnosis, treatment and prevention of rare and common acute and chronic infectious diseases. Physicians and fellows within the Division of Infectious Diseases and Immunology are actively involved in the management of complicated bone and joint infections, prevention of infection in cancer and transplant patients and developing strategies for managing hepatitis B and C. They also offer the opportunity for patients with HIV to enroll in clinical trials of new drugs that are not yet widely available. We specialize in the following areas:

HIV Prevention
The Division of Infectious Diseases and Immunology has developed a unique program in HIV prevention that has gained wide recognition and has extended the hospital's expertise from New York City to West and East Africa.

AIDS Clinical Trials
The AIDS Clinical Trials Unit is one of 35 units designated and supported by the National Institute of Allergy and Infectious Diseases, and is a dedicated resource for healthcare providers, researchers and scientists working in the field of HIV/AIDS research. It is one of the most active units in the nation in enrolling adult and pediatric patients in clinical trials supported by the NIH. Data generated by the unit has supported the licensing of several drugs and plays an essential role in defining optimal therapies and preventing complications.

Population Biology of Infectious Diseases
This novel program combines laboratory and clinical studies with epidemiology and genetics to optimize patient outcomes. Researchers in the Division of Infectious Diseases and Immunology are extensively involved in local and international studies into the early diagnosis, treatment and prevention of chronic infections such as tuberculosis and Helicobacter (bacteria associated with stomach ulcers).

Medical and Molecular Parasitology
The Division of Infectious Diseases and Immunology works alongside NYU Langone Medical Center's Department of Medical Parasitology to bring malaria and other parasitic diseases under control.

Internal Medicine

A personal physician who provides long-term, comprehensive care in the office and the hospital, managing both common and complex illness of adolescents, adults and the elderly. Internists are trained in the diagnosis and treatment of cancer, infections and diseases affecting the heart, blood, kidneys, joints and digestive, respiratory and vascular systems. They are also trained in the essentials of primary care internal medicine which incorporates an understanding of disease prevention, wellness, substance abuse, mental health and effective treatment of common problems of the eyes, ears, skin, nervous system and reproductive organs.

Note: *Internal Medicine normally includes many primary care physicians. However, for purposes of this directory, no primary care physicians are included.*

Training Required: Three years

Internal Medicine

New England

Gillman, Matthew MD [IM] - **Spec Exp:** Obesity; Nutrition & Disease Prevention/Control; Diabetes in Pregnancy; Clinical Trials Only; **Hospital:** Children's Hospital - Boston, Brigham and Women's Hosp (page 57); **Address:** Harvard Pilgrim's Hlth Care, Dept of Population Medicine, 133 Brookline Ave Fl 6, Boston, MA 02215; **Phone:** 617-509-9968; **Board Cert:** Internal Medicine 1985; Pediatrics 1986; **Med School:** Duke Univ 1981; **Resid:** Internal Medicine, N Carolina Meml Hosp 1984; Pediatrics, N Carolina Meml Hosp 1985; **Fellow:** Research, Harvard Univ 1990; **Fac Appt:** Prof Med, Harvard Med Sch

Mid Atlantic

Cirigliano, Michael D MD [IM] - **Spec Exp:** Complementary Medicine; Preventive Medicine; Women's Health; **Hospital:** Hosp Univ Penn - UPHS (page 72); **Address:** 3701 Market St, Ste 370, 3701 Market St, Ste 370, Philadelphia, PA 19104; **Phone:** 215-615-3232; **Board Cert:** Internal Medicine 2005; **Med School:** Univ Pennsylvania 1990; **Resid:** Internal Medicine, Hosp Univ Penn 1993; **Fac Appt:** Assoc Prof Med, Univ Pennsylvania

Galland, Leo MD [IM] - **Spec Exp:** Nutrition; Chronic Illness; Complementary Medicine; **Address:** Foundation for Integrated Medicine, 156 Fifth Ave, Ste 519, New York, NY 10010; **Phone:** 212-989-6733; **Board Cert:** Internal Medicine 1972; **Med School:** NYU Sch Med 1968; **Resid:** Internal Medicine, Bellevue Hosp 1972; **Fellow:** Behavioral Medicine, Univ Conn Hlth Ctr 1981

Holzman, Lawrence B MD [IM] - **Spec Exp:** Glomerulonephritis; **Hospital:** Hosp Univ Penn - UPHS (page 72); **Address:** 3400 Civic Ctr Blvd, Fl 1st, Ste 300, Philadelphia, PA 19104; **Phone:** 215-662-2638; **Board Cert:** Internal Medicine 1987; **Med School:** UMDNJ-NJ Med Sch, Newark 1984; **Resid:** Internal Medicine, Med Coll Penn 1987; **Fellow:** Nephrology, Univ Michigan 1989; **Fac Appt:** Prof Med, Univ Pennsylvania

Rader, Daniel J MD [IM] - **Spec Exp:** Cholesterol/Lipid Disorders; Preventive Cardiology; Metabolic Disorders; **Hospital:** Hosp Univ Penn - UPHS (page 72), Penn Presby Med Ctr - UPHS (page 72); **Address:** Penn Heart & Vascular Ctr, Perelman Ctr for Advanced Medicine, 3400 Civic Ctr Blvd, Ste 2-150E, Philadelphia, PA 19104; **Phone:** 215-615-4949; **Board Cert:** Internal Medicine 1987; **Med School:** Med Coll PA Hahnemann 1984; **Resid:** Internal Medicine, Yale-New Haven Hosp 1987; **Fellow:** Research, Natl Inst Hlth 1992; **Fac Appt:** Prof Med, Univ Pennsylvania

Selwyn, Peter MD [IM] - **Spec Exp:** AIDS/HIV; Palliative Care; Addiction/Substance Abuse; **Hospital:** Montefiore Med Ctr-Moses Campus, NY; **Address:** Montfiore Family Hlth Ctr, 360 E 193rd St Fl 2, Bronx, NY 10458; **Phone:** 718-933-2400; **Board Cert:** Family Medicine 2005; Hospice & Palliative Medicine 2006; **Med School:** Harvard Med Sch 1981; **Resid:** Family Medicine, Montefiore Med Ctr 1984; **Fac Appt:** Prof Med, Albert Einstein Coll Med

Southeast

Braunstein, Seth N MD/PhD [IM] - **Spec Exp:** Diabetes; Preventive Medicine; **Hospital:** New Hanover Reg Med Ctr; **Address:** Wilmington Health Endocrinology Dept, 1500 Physicians Drive E Bldg, Wilmington, NC 28401; **Phone:** 910-763-6332; **Board Cert:** Internal Medicine 1975; **Med School:** NYU Sch Med 1972; **Resid:** Internal Medicine, Hosp Univ Penn 1975; **Fac Appt:** Clin Prof Med, Univ NC Sch Med

Cushman, William C MD [IM] - **Spec Exp:** Hypertension; Preventive Cardiology; Choles-terol/Lipid Disorders; **Hospital:** VA Med Ctr - Memphis; **Address:** VA Medical Ctr, 1030 Jefferson Ave, Memphis, TN 38104-2127; **Phone:** 901-523-8990 x7357; **Board Cert:** Internal Medicine 1977; **Med School:** Univ Miss 1974; **Resid:** Internal Medicine, Univ Mississippi Med Ctr 1977; **Fac Appt:** Prof Med, Univ Tenn Coll Med

Fischl, Margaret A MD [IM] - **Spec Exp:** Immunotherapy; Infectious Disease; AIDS/HIV; Clini-cal Trials; **Hospital:** Univ of Miami Hosp, Univ of Miami Hosp & Clins/Sylvester Comp Canc Ctr; **Ad-dress:** 1800 NW 10th Ave, Miami, FL 33136; **Phone:** 305-243-3838; **Board Cert:** Internal Medicine 1979; **Med School:** Univ Miami Sch Med 1976; **Resid:** Internal Medicine, Univ Miami Affil Hosps 1979; **Fellow:** Infectious Disease, Univ Miami Affil Hosps 1980; **Fac Appt:** Prof Med, Univ Miami Sch Med

Tucker, Rodney O MD [IM] - **Spec Exp:** Palliative Care; **Hospital:** Univ of Ala Hosp at Birm-ingham; **Address:** UAB Ctr for Palliative Care, Ch19, Ste 219, 1530 3rd Ave S, Birmingham, AL 35294-2041; **Phone:** 205-975-8197; **Board Cert:** Internal Medicine 2002; **Med School:** Univ Al-abama 1989; **Resid:** Internal Medicine, Carraway Methodist Med Ctr 1993; **Fac Appt:** Asst Prof Med, Univ Alabama

Midwest

Bakris, George L MD [IM] - **Spec Exp:** Hypertension; Kidney Disease; **Hospital:** Univ of Chicago Med Ctr; **Address:** ASH Comprehensive Hypertension Ctr, 5841 S Maryland St, MS 1027, Chicago, IL 60637; **Phone:** 773-702-7936; **Board Cert:** Internal Medicine 1986; **Med School:** Ros Franklin Univ/Chicago Med Sch 1981; **Resid:** Internal Medicine, Mayo Clinic 1983; Internal Medicine, Univ IL Med Ctr 1986; **Fellow:** Clinical Pharmacology, Univ Chicago Hosps 1987; Nephrology, Univ Chicago Hosps 1988; **Fac Appt:** Prof Med, Univ Chicago-Pritzker Sch Med

Burt, Richard K MD [IM] - **Spec Exp:** Stem Cell Transplant in Lupus/Crohn's; Stem Cell Trans-plant in MS; Autoimmune Disease; **Hospital:** Northwestern Meml Hosp; **Address:** Northwestern - Div Immunotherapy, 750 N Lakeshore Drive, rm 649, Chicago, IL 60611; **Phone:** 312-908-0059; **Board Cert:** Internal Medicine 1989; **Med School:** St Louis Univ 1984; **Resid:** Internal Medicine, Baylor Coll Med 1988; **Fellow:** Hematology & Oncology, NIH Clin Ctr 1993; **Fac Appt:** Assoc Prof Med, Northwestern Univ

Fischbein, Lewis C MD [IM] - **Spec Exp:** Preventive Medicine; Hypertension; **Hospital:** Barnes-Jewish Hosp; **Address:** 4921 Parkview Pl, Ste 5G, St Louis, MO 63110; **Phone:** 314-747-1970; **Board Cert:** Internal Medicine 1977; Rheumatology 1980; **Med School:** Washington Univ, St Louis 1974; **Resid:** Internal Medicine, Barnes Jewish Hosp 1977; **Fellow:** Rheumatology, Washing-ton Univ 1979; **Fac Appt:** Assoc Prof Med, Washington Univ, St Louis

Wright Jr, Jackson T MD/PhD [IM] - **Spec Exp:** Hypertension; **Hospital:** Univ Hosps Case Med Ctr (page 74); **Address:** CWRU Div Hypertension, 11100 Euclid Ave, Bolwell Bldg - rm 2200, Cleveland, OH 44106-6053; **Phone:** 216-844-5174; **Board Cert:** Internal Medicine 1980; **Med School:** Univ Pittsburgh 1976; **Resid:** Internal Medicine, Univ Michigan Hosps 1979; **Fellow:** Phar-macology, Univ Health Ctr 1980; **Fac Appt:** Prof Med, Case West Res Univ

Great Plains and Mountains

Mehler, Philip S MD [IM] - **Spec Exp:** Eating Disorders; Substance Abuse; Hypertension; Anorexia Nervosa-Severe; **Hospital:** Denver Health Med Ctr; **Address:** Denver Health Med Ctr, 777 Bannock St, MC 0278, Denver, CO 80204; **Phone:** 303-602-4971; **Board Cert:** Internal Medicine 1989; **Med School:** Univ Colorado 1983; **Resid:** Internal Medicine, Univ Colorado Affil Hosp 1987; **Fac Appt:** Prof Med, Univ Colorado

West Coast and Pacific

Bissell Jr, Dwight M MD [IM] - **Spec Exp:** Porphyria; **Hospital:** UCSF Med Ctr; **Address:** UCSF Med Ctr, Dept Gastroenterology, 350 Parnassus Ave, rm 410, San Francisco, CA 94117; **Phone:** 415-353-2318; **Board Cert:** Internal Medicine 1974; **Med School:** Harvard Med Sch 1967; **Resid:** Internal Medicine, Boston City Hosp-Harvard 1970; **Fellow:** Gastroenterology, UCSF Med Ctr 1973; **Fac Appt:** Prof Med, UCSF

Cope, Dennis W MD [IM] - **Spec Exp:** Diagnostic Problems; Complex Diagnosis; **Hospital:** Olive View-UCLA Med Ctr; **Address:** Olive View Medical Ctr, 14445 Olive View Drive, Sylmar, CA 91342; **Phone:** 818-364-3205; **Board Cert:** Internal Medicine 1973; Endocrinology 1975; **Med School:** Univ Kansas 1970; **Resid:** Internal Medicine, UCLA Med Ctr 1973; **Fellow:** Endocrinology, UCLA Med Ctr 1975

Rabow, Michael W MD [IM] - **Spec Exp:** Palliative Care; **Hospital:** UCSF - Mt Zion Med Ctr; **Address:** 1545 Divisadero St, UCSF Gen Internal Med Practice, San Francisco, CA 94115; **Phone:** 415-353-7300; **Board Cert:** Internal Medicine 2006; Hospice & Palliative Medicine 2002; **Med School:** UCSF 1993; **Resid:** Internal Medicine, UCSF Med Ctr 1996; **Fellow:** Gastroenterology, UCSF Med Ctr 1997; **Fac Appt:** Assoc Clin Prof Med, UCSF

INTERNAL MEDICINE

About the Division of General Internal Medicine, Department of Medicine
Internal medicine physicians at NYU Langone Medical Center are dedicated to treating the whole patient, and not just their disease. Bound by the highest standards of their profession, they address both the physical and psychological aspects of health and disease through clear communication and a fully integrated regimen of care. We specialize in the following areas:

Primary and Specialized Healthcare
The Division of General Internal Medicine offers a multidisciplinary medical approach to treating illnesses involving the heart, lungs, gastrointestinal tract, joints, bones, muscles, endocrine organs and kidneys. A wide range of laboratory, imaging and advanced diagnostic testing, ranging from throat cultures to the complex mapping of the electrical surface of the heart, is available on-site or by referral. Comprehensive women's healthcare, including cancer screening and osteoporosis prevention and treatment, is also available.

Geriatrics
Our geriatric specialists provide comprehensive and multidisciplinary care, consultation and follow-up for elderly patients ranging from prevention and healthy aging to the treatment and care of chronic conditions including dementia, functional impairment and degenerative disorders.

Center for Healthful Behavior Change
The Center for Healthful Behavior Change (CHBC) focuses on developing evidence-based behavioral interventions aimed at improving patient health. CHBC originates, tests and spreads innovative evidence-based behavioral interventions into everyday clinical practice and community settings for patients with high blood pressure and other conditions associated with cardiovascular risk, including obesity and high cholesterol.

The Best in American Medicine
www.CastleConnolly.com

Maternal & Fetal Medicine

a subspecialty of Obstetrics & Gynecology

An obstetrician/gynecologist possesses special knowledge, skills and professional capability in the medical and surgical care of the female reproductive system and associated disorders. This physician serves as a consultant to other physicians and as a primary physician for women.

Training Required: Four years *plus* two years in clinical practice before certification in obstetrics and gynecology is complete *plus* additional training and examination in maternal-fetal medicine.

MATERNAL & FETAL MEDICINE

New England

Acker, David B MD [MF] - **Spec Exp:** Multiple Gestation; Pregnancy-High Risk; **Hospital:** Brigham and Women's Hosp (page 57); **Address:** Brigham & Womens Hosp, Dept Ob/Gyn, 75 Francis St, ASB1-3, Boston, MA 02115; **Phone:** 617-732-5445; **Board Cert:** Obstetrics & Gynecology 2011; Maternal & Fetal Medicine 2011; **Med School:** NYU Sch Med 1968; **Resid:** Obstetrics & Gynecology, Albert Einstein Affil Hosp 1971; Obstetrics & Gynecology, Vanderbilt Univ Affil Hosp 1974; **Fellow:** Maternal & Fetal Medicine, Boston Lying-In Hosp 1979; **Fac Appt:** Assoc Prof ObG, Harvard Med Sch

Baker, Emily MD [MF] - **Spec Exp:** Ultrasound; Pregnancy-High Risk; **Hospital:** Dartmouth - Hitchcock Med Ctr; **Address:** Dartmouth-Hitchcock Med Ctr, Dept Ob/Gyn, 1 Medical Center Drive, Lebanon, NH 03756; **Phone:** 603-653-9306; **Board Cert:** Obstetrics & Gynecology 2011; Maternal & Fetal Medicine 2011; **Med School:** Stanford Univ 1986; **Resid:** Obstetrics & Gynecology, Univ Chicago Hosps 1990; Maternal & Fetal Medicine, Univ Washington Med Ctr 1991; **Fellow:** Maternal & Fetal Medicine, St Margaret's Hosp-Tufts Univ 1992; **Fac Appt:** Assoc Prof ObG, Dartmouth Med Sch

Carr, Stephen R MD [MF] - **Spec Exp:** Twin to Twin Transfusion Syndrome (TTTS); Multiple Gestation; Fetal Surgery; **Hospital:** Women & Infants Hosp of RI; **Address:** 101 Dudley St, Division of Maternal-Fetal Medicine, Providence, RI 02905; **Phone:** 401-274-1122 x7448; **Board Cert:** Obstetrics & Gynecology 2009; Maternal & Fetal Medicine 1997; **Med School:** Univ Hawaii JA Burns Sch Med 1982; **Resid:** Obstetrics & Gynecology, Univ Illinois Med Ctr 1986; **Fellow:** Maternal & Fetal Medicine, Brown Univ 1988; **Fac Appt:** Prof ObG, Brown Univ

Copel, Joshua A MD [MF] - **Spec Exp:** Prenatal Diagnosis; Fetal Echocardiography; Pregnancy-High Risk; Fetal Diagnosis & Therapy; **Hospital:** Yale-New Haven Hosp, Yale Med Group; **Address:** Yale Maternal/Fetal Medicine, 150 Sargent Drive, New Haven, CT 06511; **Phone:** 203-785-5682; **Board Cert:** Obstetrics & Gynecology 2011; Maternal & Fetal Medicine 2011; **Med School:** Tufts Univ 1979; **Resid:** Obstetrics & Gynecology, Pennsylvania Hosp 1983; **Fellow:** Maternal & Fetal Medicine, Yale-New Haven Hosp 1985; **Fac Appt:** Prof ObG, Yale Univ

Greene, Michael F MD [MF] - **Spec Exp:** Pregnancy-High Risk; Multiple Gestation; Seizure Disorders & Pregnancy; **Hospital:** Mass Genl Hosp; **Address:** Mass Genl Hosp, Dept Ob/Gyn, 55 Fruit St Yawkey Bldg - rm 4F, Boston, MA 02114; **Phone:** 617-724-2229; **Board Cert:** Obstetrics & Gynecology 2011; Maternal & Fetal Medicine 2011; **Med School:** SUNY Downstate 1976; **Resid:** Obstetrics & Gynecology, Boston Hosp Women 1980; **Fellow:** Maternal & Fetal Medicine, Brigham Hosp Women 1982; **Fac Appt:** Prof ObG, Harvard Med Sch

Heffner, Linda MD/PhD [MF] - **Spec Exp:** Pregnancy-Advanced Maternal Age; Pregnancy-High Risk; **Hospital:** Boston Med Ctr; **Address:** 85 E Concord St Fl 6, Boston, MA 02118; **Phone:** 617-414-5175; **Board Cert:** Obstetrics & Gynecology 2011; Maternal & Fetal Medicine 2011; **Med School:** Johns Hopkins Univ 1977; **Resid:** Obstetrics & Gynecology, Hosp Univ Penn 1983; **Fellow:** Maternal & Fetal Medicine, Brigham-Womens Hosp 1987; **Fac Appt:** Prof ObG, Boston Univ

Norwitz, Errol R MD/PhD [MF] - **Spec Exp:** Diabetes in Pregnancy; Critical Care; Prematurity Prevention; **Hospital:** Tufts Med Ctr; **Address:** Tufts Medical Center, 800 Washington St, Mailbox 324, Boston, MA 02111; **Phone:** 617-636-2382; **Board Cert:** Obstetrics & Gynecology 2012; Maternal & Fetal Medicine 2012; **Med School:** South Africa 1986; **Resid:** Obstetrics & Gynecology, Brigham & Women's Hosp 1996; **Fellow:** Maternal & Fetal Medicine, Brigham & Women's Hosp 1998; **Fac Appt:** Prof ObG, Tufts Univ

Paidas, Michael J MD [MF] - **Spec Exp:** Pregnancy-High Risk; Clotting Disorders in Pregnancy; Miscarriage-Recurrent; **Hospital:** Yale-New Haven Hosp, Yale Med Group; **Address:** Yale Maternal/Fetal Medicine, 150 Sargent Drive, New Haven, CT 06511; **Phone:** 203-785-5682; **Board Cert:** Obstetrics & Gynecology 2011; Maternal & Fetal Medicine 2011; **Med School:** Tufts Univ 1987; **Resid:** Obstetrics & Gynecology, Pennsylvania Hosp 1991; **Fellow:** Maternal & Fetal Medicine, Mount Sinai Med Ctr 1993; **Fac Appt:** Assoc Prof ObG, Yale Univ

Riley, Laura E MD [MF] - **Spec Exp:** AIDS/HIV in Pregnancy; Infectious Disease in Pregnancy; Pregnancy-High Risk; **Hospital:** Mass Genl Hosp; **Address:** Mass Genl Hosp, Yawkey Bldg, 32 Fruit St, Ste 4200, Boston, MA 02114; **Phone:** 617-724-2229; **Board Cert:** Obstetrics & Gynecology 2011; Maternal & Fetal Medicine 2011; **Med School:** Univ Pittsburgh 1985; **Resid:** Obstetrics & Gynecology, Univ Pittsburgh Med Ctr 1988; **Fellow:** Maternal & Fetal Medicine, Brigham & Womens Hosp 1991; Infectious Disease, Boston Univ Med Ctr 1993; **Fac Appt:** Assoc Prof ObG, Harvard Med Sch

Robinson, Julian N MD [MF] - **Spec Exp:** Prenatal Diagnosis; Fetal Echocardiography; Amniocentesis; Ultrasound; **Hospital:** Newton - Wellesley Hosp, Brigham and Women's Hosp (page 57); **Address:** Newton-Wellesley Hosp, 2014 Washington St Fl 2 West, Newton, MA 02462; **Phone:** 617-243-5909; **Board Cert:** Obstetrics & Gynecology 2011; Maternal & Fetal Medicine 2011; **Med School:** England, UK 1986; **Resid:** Obstetrics & Gynecology, Eastern VA Med Sch 1997; **Fellow:** Maternal & Fetal Medicine, Brigham & Women's Hosp 1998

Wenstrom, Katharine D MD [MF] - **Spec Exp:** Reproductive Genetics; Pregnancy-High Risk; **Hospital:** Women & Infants Hosp of RI; **Address:** Women's & Infants Hosp RI, Maternal Fetal Medicine Div, 101 Dudley St, Fl 3rd, Providence, RI 02905; **Phone:** 401-274-1122 x7452; **Board Cert:** Obstetrics & Gynecology 2006; Maternal & Fetal Medicine 2006; Clinical Genetics 1990; **Med School:** Case West Res Univ 1983; **Resid:** Obstetrics & Gynecology, Univ Illinois Hosp 1987; **Fellow:** Maternal & Fetal Medicine, Univ Illinois Hosp 1989; Clinical Genetics, Univ Iowa Med Ctr 1990; **Fac Appt:** Prof ObG, Vanderbilt Univ

Wilkins-Haug, Louise E MD/PhD [MF] - **Spec Exp:** Fetal Diagnosis & Therapy; Pregnancy-High Risk; Genetic Disorders; Fetal Surgery; **Hospital:** Brigham and Women's Hosp (page 57); **Address:** Brigham & Womens Hosp, Div Maternal Fetal Medicine, 75 Francis St, Ste 305, Boston, MA 02115; **Phone:** 617-732-4840; **Board Cert:** Obstetrics & Gynecology 2011; Maternal & Fetal Medicine 2011; **Med School:** Stanford Univ 1985; **Resid:** Obstetrics & Gynecology, Univ Colorado Med Ctr 1989; **Fellow:** Maternal & Fetal Medicine, Brigham & Women's Hosp 1992; **Fac Appt:** Assoc Prof ObG, Harvard Med Sch

Mid Atlantic

Berkowitz, Richard L MD [MF] - **Spec Exp:** Fetal Therapy; Multiple Gestation; Pregnancy & Hematologic Abnormalities; **Hospital:** NY-Presby/Columbia Univ Med Ctr, NY (page 66); **Address:** 16 E 60th St, Fl 4, New York, NY 10022; **Phone:** 212-305-0197; **Board Cert:** Obstetrics & Gynecology 2005; Maternal & Fetal Medicine 2005; **Med School:** NYU Sch Med 1965; **Resid:** Obstetrics & Gynecology, NY Hosp-Cornell Med Ctr 1972; **Fac Appt:** Prof ObG, Columbia P&S

Blakemore, Karin J MD [MF] - **Spec Exp:** Fetal Diagnosis & Therapy; Pregnancy-High Risk; Ultrasound; **Hospital:** Johns Hopkins Hosp (page 61); **Address:** Johns Hopkins Hosp, Dept Maternal/Fetal Med, 600 N Wolfe St Phipps Bldg - rm 228, Baltimore, MD 21287-1228; **Phone:** 410-955-7456; **Board Cert:** Clinical Genetics 1984; Obstetrics & Gynecology 2010; Maternal & Fetal Medicine 2010; **Med School:** Med Coll OH 1978; **Resid:** Obstetrics & Gynecology, NYU Med Ctr 1982; Clinical Genetics, Yale Univ Sch Med 1985; **Fellow:** Maternal & Fetal Medicine, Washington Univ 1987; **Fac Appt:** Assoc Prof ObG, Johns Hopkins Univ

Caritis, Steve N MD [MF] - **Spec Exp:** Pregnancy-High Risk; **Hospital:** Magee-Womens Hosp - UPMC; **Address:** Magee-Womens Hosp, Dept Maternal/Fetal Med, 300 Halket St, Ste 0610, Pittsburgh, PA 15213-3180; **Phone:** 412-641-6361; **Board Cert:** Obstetrics & Gynecology 1999; Maternal & Fetal Medicine 1999; **Med School:** W VA Univ 1969; **Resid:** Obstetrics & Gynecology, Univ Pittsburgh Med Ctr 1973; **Fellow:** Maternal & Fetal Medicine, Columbia-Presby Med Ctr 1975; **Fac Appt:** Prof ObG, Univ Pittsburgh

Cohen, Arnold N MD [MF] - **Spec Exp:** Pregnancy-High Risk; Diabetes in Pregnancy; **Hospital:** Albert Einstein Med Ctr; **Address:** AEMC 5501 Old York Rd, Lifter Bldg Fl 2, Philadelphia, PA 19141; **Phone:** 215-456-6993; **Board Cert:** Obstetrics & Gynecology 1994; Maternal & Fetal Medicine 1982; **Med School:** Cornell Univ 1971; **Resid:** Internal Medicine, Hosp Univ Penn 1973; Obstetrics & Gynecology, Hosp Univ Penn 1976; **Fellow:** Maternal & Fetal Medicine, Hosp Univ Penn 1980; **Fac Appt:** Prof ObG, Thomas Jefferson Univ

D'Alton, Mary E MD [MF] - **Spec Exp:** Pregnancy-High Risk; Multiple Gestation; Prenatal Diagnosis; **Hospital:** NY-Presby/Columbia Univ Med Ctr, NY (page 66); **Address:** 16 E 60th St, Ste 480, New York, NY 10022; **Phone:** 212-326-8951; **Board Cert:** Obstetrics & Gynecology 2010; Maternal & Fetal Medicine 2010; **Med School:** Ireland 1976; **Resid:** Obstetrics & Gynecology, Ottowa Genl Hosp 1982; **Fellow:** Maternal & Fetal Medicine, Tufts-New Eng Med Ctr 1984; **Fac Appt:** Clin Prof ObG, Columbia P&S

Dugoff, Lorraine MD [MF] - **Spec Exp:** Pregnancy-High Risk; Prenatal Diagnosis; Ultrasound; Reproductive Genetics; **Hospital:** Hosp Univ Penn - UPHS (page 72); **Address:** 579 Dulles Building, 3400 Spruce St, Philadelphia, PA 19104; **Phone:** 215-615-3739; **Board Cert:** Obstetrics & Gynecology 2011; Maternal & Fetal Medicine 2011; Clinical Genetics 2010; **Med School:** Georgetown Univ 1989; **Resid:** Obstetrics & Gynecology, Philadelphia Hosp 1990; Obstetrics & Gynecology, Univ Colorado Hlth Sci Ctr 1993; **Fellow:** Maternal & Fetal Medicine, Univ Colorado Hlth Sci Ctr 1995; Clinical Genetics, Univ Colorado Hlth Sci Ctr 1996; **Fac Appt:** Assoc Prof ObG, Univ Pennsylvania

Eddleman, Keith A MD [MF] - **Spec Exp:** Obstetric Ultrasound; Pregnancy-High Risk; Fetal Therapy; Reproductive Genetics; **Hospital:** Mount Sinai Med Ctr (page 64); **Address:** 5 E 98th St, Box 1171, New York, NY 10029; **Phone:** 212-241-5681; **Board Cert:** Obstetrics & Gynecology 2011; Maternal & Fetal Medicine 2011; Clinical Genetics 2010; **Med School:** Wake Forest Univ 1985; **Resid:** Obstetrics & Gynecology, George Washington Univ Med Ctr 1989; **Fellow:** Maternal & Fetal Medicine, Mt Sinai Med Ctr 1991; Genetics, NY-Cornell Med Ctr 1996; **Fac Appt:** Prof ObG, Mount Sinai Sch Med

Fox, Harold E MD [MF] - **Spec Exp:** Pregnancy-High Risk; Prematurity Prevention; Multiple Gestation; **Hospital:** Johns Hopkins Hosp (page 61); **Address:** Johns Hopkins Hosp, Dept Maternal/Fetal Medicine, 600 N Wolfe St Phipps Bldg - rm 264, Baltimore, MD 21287; **Phone:** 410-614-0178; **Board Cert:** Obstetrics & Gynecology 2011; Maternal & Fetal Medicine 2011; **Med School:** Univ Rochester 1972; **Resid:** Obstetrics & Gynecology, Strong Meml Hosp 1975; **Fellow:** Maternal & Fetal Medicine, Univ Rochester Hosps 1977; **Fac Appt:** Prof ObG, Johns Hopkins Univ

Genc, Mehmet R MD/PhD [MF] - **Spec Exp:** Amniocentesis; Hypertension in Pregnancy; Pregnancy-High Risk; Fetal Abnormalities; **Hospital:** NY-Presby/Weill Cornell Med Ctr, NY (page 66); **Address:** 525 E 68th St, Ste J-130, New York, NY 10065; **Phone:** 212-746-1604; **Board Cert:** Obstetrics & Gynecology 2011; Maternal & Fetal Medicine 2011; **Med School:** Turkey 1994; **Resid:** Obstetrics & Gynecology, NY-Presby/Weill Cornell Med Ctr 2000; **Fellow:** Maternal & Fetal Medicine, NY-Presby/Weill Cornell Med Ctr 2001; Maternal & Fetal Medicine, Brigham & Women's Hosp 2003; **Fac Appt:** Asst Prof ObG, Cornell Univ-Weill Med Coll

Grunebaum, Amos MD [MF] - **Spec Exp:** Pregnancy-High Risk; Amniocentesis; **Hospital:** NY-Presby/Weill Cornell Med Ctr, NY (page 66); **Address:** Dept Obstetrics & Gynecology, 525 E 68th St, Ste J-130, New York, NY 10065; **Phone:** 212-746-0714; **Board Cert:** Obstetrics & Gynecology 2011; Maternal & Fetal Medicine 2011; **Med School:** Germany 1974; **Resid:** Anesthesiology, Maimonides Med Ctr 1978; Obstetrics & Gynecology, Downstate Med Ctr 1982; **Fellow:** Maternal & Fetal Medicine, Downstate Med Ctr 1984; **Fac Appt:** Assoc Prof ObG, Columbia P&S

Landy, Helain J MD [MF] - **Spec Exp:** Pregnancy-High Risk; Miscarriage-Recurrent; Multiple Gestation; Diabetes in Pregnancy; **Hospital:** Georgetown Univ Hosp, Sibley Mem Hosp; **Address:** Georgetown Univ Dept Ob/Gyn, 3800 Reservoir Rd NW, 3PHC, Washington, DC 20007-2113; **Phone:** 202-444-8531; **Board Cert:** Obstetrics & Gynecology 2009; Maternal & Fetal Medicine 2009; **Med School:** Northwestern Univ 1982; **Resid:** Obstetrics & Gynecology, Penn Hosp 1986; **Fellow:** Maternal & Fetal Medicine, Geo Washington Univ Med Ctr 1988; **Fac Appt:** Prof ObG, Georgetown Univ

Parry, Samuel I MD [MF] - **Spec Exp:** Pregnancy-High Risk; Premature Labor; Infections in Pregnancy; Fetal Ultrasound; **Hospital:** Hosp Univ Penn - UPHS (page 72); **Address:** Univ Penn, Dept Maternal & Fetal Med, 3400 Spruce St, 2000 Courtyard, Philadelphia, PA 19104; **Phone:** 215-662-2982; **Board Cert:** Obstetrics & Gynecology 2011; Maternal & Fetal Medicine 2011; **Med School:** Columbia P&S 1990; **Resid:** Obstetrics & Gynecology, SUNY Buffalo Affil Hosp 1994; **Fellow:** Maternal & Fetal Medicine, Hosp Univ Penn 1996; **Fac Appt:** Assoc Prof ObG, Univ Pennsylvania

Pinckert, Thomas L MD [MF] - **Spec Exp:** Pregnancy-High Risk; **Hospital:** Shady Grove Adven Hosp, Holy Cross Hospital - Silver Spring; **Address:** Greater Washington Maternal-Fetal Medicine, 9707 Med Ctr Drive, Ste 230, Rockville, MD 20850; **Phone:** 301-279-6060; **Board Cert:** Obstetrics & Gynecology 2010; Clinical Genetics 1990; Maternal & Fetal Medicine 2010; **Med School:** Oregon Hlth & Sci Univ 1979; **Resid:** Obstetrics & Gynecology, David Grant Med Ctr 1983; **Fellow:** Maternal & Fetal Medicine, UCSF Med Ctr 1989; Clinical Genetics, UCSF Med Ctr 1990

Plante, Lauren A MD [MF] - **Spec Exp:** Pregnancy-High Risk; Diabetes in Pregnancy; **Hospital:** Hahnemann Univ Hosp; **Address:** Drexel Med Ctr, Women's Care, Dept Genetics & Fetal Med, 1427 Vine St Fl 7, Philadelphia, PA 19102; **Phone:** 215-762-7825; **Board Cert:** Anesthesiology 2004; Critical Care Medicine 1993; Obstetrics & Gynecology 2009; Maternal & Fetal Medicine 2008; **Med School:** Albert Einstein Coll Med 1984; **Resid:** Anesthesiology, Montefiore Med Ctr 1989; Obstetrics & Gynecology, Hahnemann Univ Hosp 1994; **Fellow:** Critical Care Medicine, Montefiore Med Ctr 1990; Maternal & Fetal Medicine, Temple Univ Med Ctr 1998; **Fac Appt:** Assoc Prof ObG, Hahnemann Univ

Repke, John T MD [MF] - **Spec Exp:** Pregnancy-High Risk; Hypertension in Pregnancy; Women's Health; **Hospital:** Penn State Milton S Hershey Med Ctr; **Address:** MS Hershey Med Ctr Maternal Fetal Med, 500 University Drive, Hershey, PA 17033; **Phone:** 717-531-3503 x4; **Board Cert:** Obstetrics & Gynecology 2011; Maternal & Fetal Medicine 2011; **Med School:** NY Med Coll 1978; **Resid:** Obstetrics & Gynecology, Johns Hopkins Hosp 1982; **Fellow:** Maternal & Fetal Medicine, Johns Hopkins Hosp 1984; **Fac Appt:** Prof ObG, Penn State Coll Med

Thomas, Ronald L MD [MF] - **Spec Exp:** Pregnancy-High Risk; **Hospital:** Western Penn Hosp; **Address:** Federal North Bldg, 1307 Federal St, Ste B100, Pittsburgh, PA 15212; **Phone:** 412-359-3437; **Board Cert:** Obstetrics & Gynecology 2011; Maternal & Fetal Medicine 2011; **Med School:** Univ Pittsburgh 1981; **Resid:** Obstetrics & Gynecology, Natl Naval Ctr 1985; **Fellow:** Maternal & Fetal Medicine, Johns Hopkins Hosp 1988; **Fac Appt:** Assoc Prof ObG, Drexel Univ Coll Med

Maternal & Fetal Medicine

Wapner, Ronald J MD [MF] - **Spec Exp:** Perinatal Medicine; Genetic Disorders; Multiple Gestation; Vomiting-Cyclic; **Hospital:** NY-Presby/Columbia Univ Med Ctr, NY (page 66); **Address:** Div Maternal/Fetal Medicine, 16 E 60th St, rm 480, New York, NY 10022; **Phone:** 212-326-8951; **Board Cert:** Obstetrics & Gynecology 2000; Maternal & Fetal Medicine 2000; Clinical Genetics 2010; **Med School:** Jefferson Med Coll 1972; **Resid:** Obstetrics & Gynecology, Jefferson Univ Hosp 1976; **Fellow:** Maternal & Fetal Medicine, Jefferson Med Coll 1978; **Fac Appt:** Prof ObG, Columbia P&S

Southeast

Abuhamad, Alfred Z MD [MF] - **Spec Exp:** Twin to Twin Transfusion Syndrome (TTTS); Prenatal Diagnosis; Prenatal Ultrasound; Multiple Gestation; **Hospital:** Sentara Norfolk Genl Hosp; **Address:** E VA Med Sch, Div Mat Fetal Med, 825 Fairfax Ave, Ste 310, Norfolk, VA 23507; **Phone:** 757-446-7900; **Board Cert:** Obstetrics & Gynecology 2009; Maternal & Fetal Medicine 2009; **Med School:** Amer Univ Beirut 1985; **Resid:** Obstetrics & Gynecology, Jackson Meml Hosp 1989; **Fellow:** Maternal & Fetal Medicine, Jackson Meml Hosp-Univ Miami 1991; Ultrasound, Yale Univ 1991; **Fac Appt:** Prof ObG, Eastern VA Med Sch

Andrews, William W MD/PhD [MF] - **Spec Exp:** Infectious Disease; Prematurity/Low Birth Weight Infants; **Hospital:** Univ of Ala Hosp at Birmingham; **Address:** UAB Dept Obstetrics & Gynecology, 619 19th St S, 176F, rm 10360, Birmingham, AL 35233; **Phone:** 205-934-7330; **Board Cert:** Obstetrics & Gynecology 2010; **Med School:** Univ Alabama 1984; **Resid:** Obstetrics & Gynecology, Univ Alabama Hosp 1988; **Fellow:** Maternal & Fetal Medicine, Univ Texas SW Med Ctr 1990

Duff, William P MD [MF] - **Spec Exp:** Pregnancy-High Risk; Infections in Pregnancy; **Hospital:** Shands at Univ of FL; **Address:** Women's Health Magnolia Parke, 3951 NW 48th Terr, Ste 101, Gainesville, FL 32606; **Phone:** 352-265-6200; **Board Cert:** Obstetrics & Gynecology 2003; Maternal & Fetal Medicine 2003; **Med School:** Georgetown Univ 1974; **Resid:** Obstetrics & Gynecology, Walter Reed Med Ctr 1978; **Fellow:** Maternal & Fetal Medicine, UT - San Antonio 1983; **Fac Appt:** Prof ObG, Univ S Fla Coll Med

Ferguson II, James E MD [MF] - **Spec Exp:** Pregnancy-High Risk; Ultrasound; Premature Labor; **Hospital:** Univ of Virginia Health Sys; **Address:** Dept Ob/Gyn, Univ Virginia Sch Med, Box 800712, Charlottesville, VA 22908-0712; **Phone:** 434-924-9937; **Board Cert:** Obstetrics & Gynecology 2009; Maternal & Fetal Medicine 2009; **Med School:** Wake Forest Univ 1977; **Resid:** Obstetrics & Gynecology, Stanford Univ Med Ctr 1980; Obstetrics & Gynecology, Wake Forest Univ Med Ctr 1981; **Fellow:** Maternal & Fetal Medicine, Stanford Univ Med Ctr 1984; **Fac Appt:** Prof ObG, Univ VA Sch Med

Grandis, Arnold MD/PhD [MF] - **Spec Exp:** Pregnancy-High Risk; **Hospital:** Wake Forest Baptist Med Ctr; **Address:** 500 Shepherd St, Ste 200, Winston-Salem, NC 27103; **Phone:** 336-716-6893; **Board Cert:** Obstetrics & Gynecology 1980; Maternal & Fetal Medicine 1982; **Med School:** Univ Pennsylvania 1974; **Resid:** Obstetrics & Gynecology, Duke Univ Med Ctr 1978; **Fellow:** Maternal & Fetal Medicine, Duke Univ Sch Med 1980; **Fac Appt:** Assoc Prof ObG, Wake Forest Univ

Heyl, Peter S MD [MF] - **Spec Exp:** Pregnancy-High Risk; **Hospital:** Univ of Louisville Hosp; **Address:** 401 E Chestnut St, Ste 410, Louisville Outpatient Ctr, Louisville, KY 40202; **Phone:** 502-271-5999; **Board Cert:** Obstetrics & Gynecology 2012; Maternal & Fetal Medicine 2012; **Med School:** Wake Forest Univ 1976; **Resid:** Obstetrics & Gynecology, Boston Hosp Women 1981; **Fellow:** Maternal & Fetal Medicine, Brigham-Womens Hosp 1983; **Fac Appt:** Prof ObG, Emory Univ

Kuller, Jeffrey MD [MF] - **Spec Exp:** Prenatal Diagnosis; **Hospital:** Duke Univ Hosp; **Address:** 2406 Blue Ridge Rd, Ste 200, Raleigh, NC 27607; **Phone:** 919-783-4299; **Board Cert:** Obstetrics & Gynecology 2012; Clinical Genetics 2010; Maternal & Fetal Medicine 2012; **Med School:** Univ Cincinnati 1984; **Resid:** Obstetrics & Gynecology, Johns Hopkins Hosp 1988; **Fellow:** Maternal & Fetal Medicine, UPMC Affil Hosp 1990; Medical Genetics, UCSF Med Ctr 1992

Mari, Giancarlo MD [MF] - **Spec Exp:** Fetal Therapy; Obstetric Ultrasound; Twin to Twin Transfusion Syndrome (TTTS); **Hospital:** Le Bonheur Chldns Med Ctr, Regional Med Ctr - Memphis; **Address:** Le Bonheur Fetal Center, 777 Washington Ave, Ste 305, Memphis, TN 38105; **Phone:** 901-287-6981; **Board Cert:** Obstetrics & Gynecology 2011; Maternal & Fetal Medicine 2011; **Med School:** Italy 1982; **Resid:** Obstetrics & Gynecology, Yale New Haven Hosp 1994; **Fellow:** Maternal & Fetal Medicine, Yale New Haven Hosp 1996; **Fac Appt:** Prof

McLaren, Rodney A MD [MF] - **Spec Exp:** Prenatal Diagnosis; Amniocentesis; Pregnancy-High Risk; **Address:** 4001 Fair Ridge Drive, Ste 304, Fairfax, VA 22033; **Phone:** 703-359-2466; **Board Cert:** Obstetrics & Gynecology 2009; Maternal & Fetal Medicine 2009; **Med School:** Tufts Univ 1983; **Resid:** Obstetrics & Gynecology, LI Coll Hosp 1987; **Fellow:** Maternal & Fetal Medicine, Georgetown Univ 1989; **Fac Appt:** Assoc Prof ObG, Georgetown Univ

Nies, Barbara MD [MF] - **Spec Exp:** Pregnancy-High Risk; Amniocentesis; **Hospital:** Inova Fairfax Hosp, Inova Fair Oaks Hosp; **Address:** 3020 Hamaker Ct, Ste 501, Fairfax, VA 22031; **Phone:** 703-698-5350; **Board Cert:** Obstetrics & Gynecology 2009; Maternal & Fetal Medicine 2009; **Med School:** Mich State Univ 1984; **Resid:** Obstetrics & Gynecology, Univ Conn Med Ctr 1988; **Fellow:** Maternal & Fetal Medicine, George Washington Univ Med Ctr 1990

Thorp Jr, John M MD [MF] - **Spec Exp:** Multiple Gestation; Premature Labor; **Hospital:** NC Memorial Hosp - UNC; **Address:** UNC School of Medicine, Obstetrics/Gynecology, 3027 Old Clinic Bldg, CB 7570, Chapel Hill, NC 27599; **Phone:** 919-966-2131; **Board Cert:** Obstetrics & Gynecology 2009; Maternal & Fetal Medicine 2008; **Med School:** E Carolina Univ 1983; **Resid:** Obstetrics & Gynecology, Univ NC Hosp 1987; **Fellow:** Maternal & Fetal Medicine, Univ NC Hosp 1989; **Fac Appt:** Prof ObG, Univ NC Sch Med

Van Dorsten, J Peter MD [MF] - **Spec Exp:** Pregnancy-High Risk; **Hospital:** MUSC Med Ctr, McLeod Reg Med Ctr; **Address:** MUSC Med Ctr, Dept Ob Gyn, 96 Jonathan Lucas St, Ste 634 MSC619, Charleston, SC 29425; **Phone:** 843-792-4509; **Board Cert:** Obstetrics & Gynecology 2008; Maternal & Fetal Medicine 2008; **Med School:** Univ NC Sch Med 1971; **Resid:** Obstetrics & Gynecology, Med Univ SC Hosp 1976; **Fellow:** Maternal & Fetal Medicine, USC-LAC Hosp 1981; **Fac Appt:** Prof ObG, Med Univ SC

Midwest

Bahado-Singh, Ray O MD [MF] - **Spec Exp:** Pregnancy-High Risk; Genetic Disorders; Obstetric Ultrasound; Twin to Twin Transfusion Syndrome (TTTS); **Hospital:** Hutzel Hosp - Detroit; **Address:** 3990 John R St, 4 Webber N, Detroit, MI 48201; **Phone:** 313-993-1379; **Board Cert:** Obstetrics & Gynecology 2007; Maternal & Fetal Medicine 2007; Clinical Genetics 2010; **Med School:** Jamaica 1979; **Resid:** Obstetrics & Gynecology, Metropolitan Hosp 1985; **Fellow:** Perinatal Medicine, UC-Irvine 1987; Clinical Genetics, Yale Univ 1993

Bartelsmeyer, James MD [MF] - **Spec Exp:** Pregnancy-High Risk; Multiple Gestation; **Hospital:** St. John's Mercy Med Ctr - St Louis; **Address:** 621 S New Ballas Rd, Ste 2007B, St Louis, MO 63141; **Phone:** 314-991-5000; **Board Cert:** Obstetrics & Gynecology 2011; Maternal & Fetal Medicine 2011; **Med School:** Univ IL Coll Med 1985; **Resid:** Obstetrics & Gynecology, Univ Illinois Affil Hosps 1989; **Fellow:** Maternal & Fetal Medicine, Barnes Hosp-Univ Wash 1991; **Fac Appt:** Assoc Prof ObG, Washington Univ, St Louis

Maternal & Fetal Medicine

Besinger, Richard MD [MF] - **Spec Exp:** Prenatal Diagnosis; Premature Labor; Critical Care; **Hospital:** Loyola Univ Med Ctr; **Address:** Loyola Univ Med Ctr, 2160 S First Ave, Outpatient Ctr, Maywood, IL 60153-5590; **Phone:** 708-216-6444; **Board Cert:** Obstetrics & Gynecology 2011; Maternal & Fetal Medicine 2011; **Med School:** Loyola Univ-Stritch Sch Med 1982; **Resid:** Obstetrics & Gynecology, Univ Mich Med Ctr 1986; **Fellow:** Maternal & Fetal Medicine, Johns Hopkins Hosp 1988; **Fac Appt:** Prof ObG, Loyola Univ-Stritch Sch Med

Dooley, Sharon L MD [MF] - **Spec Exp:** Fetal Abnormalities; Pregnancy-High Risk; Multiple Gestation; **Hospital:** Northwestern Meml Hosp; **Address:** 675 N St Clair Fl 14 - Ste 200, Chicago, IL 60611; **Phone:** 312-695-7542; **Board Cert:** Obstetrics & Gynecology 2005; Maternal & Fetal Medicine 2005; **Med School:** Univ VA Sch Med 1973; **Resid:** Obstetrics & Gynecology, Northwestern Meml Hosp 1977; **Fac Appt:** Prof ObG, Northwestern Univ

Hibbard, Judith MD [MF] - **Spec Exp:** Pregnancy-High Risk; Heart Disease in Pregnancy; Prenatal Diagnosis; Ultrasound; **Hospital:** Univ of IL Med Ctr at Chicago; **Address:** Univ Illinois at Chicago, Dept OB-GYN, 1801 W Taylor St, Ste 4C, Chicago, IL 60612; **Phone:** 312-413-7500; **Board Cert:** Obstetrics & Gynecology 2011; Maternal & Fetal Medicine 2011; **Med School:** Loyola Univ-Stritch Sch Med 1982; **Resid:** Obstetrics & Gynecology, Univ Chicago Hosps 1986; **Fellow:** Maternal & Fetal Medicine, Univ Chicago Hosps 1988; **Fac Appt:** Prof ObG, Univ IL Coll Med

Hussey, Michael J MD [MF] - **Spec Exp:** Prenatal Diagnosis; Multiple Gestation; **Hospital:** Rush Univ Med Ctr; **Address:** 1725 W Harrison St, Ste 408, Chicago, IL 60612; **Phone:** 312-997-2229; **Board Cert:** Obstetrics & Gynecology 2011; Maternal & Fetal Medicine 2011; **Med School:** Univ IL Coll Med 1986; **Resid:** Obstetrics & Gynecology, Loyola Univ Med Ctr 1993; **Fellow:** Maternal & Fetal Medicine, Rush-Presby-St Lukes Hosp 1995; Ultrasound, Univ Col Hlth Sci Ctr 1996; **Fac Appt:** Asst Prof ObG, Rush Med Coll

Ismail, Mahmoud A MD [MF] - **Spec Exp:** Pregnancy-High Risk; Perinatal Medicine; Infections-Neonatal; Infections in Pregnancy; **Hospital:** Univ of Chicago Med Ctr; **Address:** Dept Ob/Gyn, 5841 S Maryland Ave, MC 2050, Chicago, IL 60637-1463; **Phone:** 773-702-5200; **Board Cert:** Obstetrics & Gynecology 2011; Maternal & Fetal Medicine 2011; **Med School:** Egypt 1970; **Resid:** Obstetrics & Gynecology, Wayne St Univ Affil Hosps 1977; **Fellow:** Maternal & Fetal Medicine, Univ Chicago Hosps 1982; **Fac Appt:** Prof ObG, Univ Chicago-Pritzker Sch Med

Johnson, Timothy R B MD [MF] - **Spec Exp:** Prenatal Diagnosis; **Hospital:** Univ of Michigan Hosp; **Address:** Univ Mich, Dept Ob/Gyn, 1500 E Med Ctr Drive, rm L4000, Box 5276, Ann Arbor, MI 48109; **Phone:** 734-764-8123; **Board Cert:** Obstetrics & Gynecology 2001; Maternal & Fetal Medicine 2001; **Med School:** Univ VA Sch Med 1975; **Resid:** Obstetrics & Gynecology, Univ Michigan Med Ctr 1979; **Fellow:** Maternal & Fetal Medicine, Johns Hopkins Hosp 1981; **Fac Appt:** Prof ObG, Univ Mich Med Sch

Landers, Daniel V MD [MF] - **Spec Exp:** Infectious Disease; **Hospital:** Univ Minn Med Ctr, Fairview - Riverside Campus; **Address:** Univ Minn Maternal & Fetal Med Ctr, 606 24th Ave S Prof Bldg Fl 4, Minneapolis, MN 55454; **Phone:** 612-273-2223; **Board Cert:** Obstetrics & Gynecology 2011; Maternal & Fetal Medicine 2011; **Med School:** UCSF 1980; **Resid:** Obstetrics & Gynecology, UCSF Med Ctr 1984; **Fellow:** Maternal & Fetal Medicine, UCSF Med Ctr 1986; Infectious Disease, UCSF Med Ctr 1988; **Fac Appt:** Prof ObG, Univ Minn

Landon, Mark B MD [MF] - **Spec Exp:** Diabetes in Pregnancy; **Hospital:** Ohio St Univ Med Ctr; **Address:** 2050 Kenny Rd Fl 5, Columbus, OH 43221; **Phone:** 614-293-8513; **Board Cert:** Obstetrics & Gynecology 2011; Maternal & Fetal Medicine 2011; **Med School:** Cornell Univ-Weill Med Coll 1980; **Resid:** Obstetrics & Gynecology, Hosp Univ Penn 1984; **Fellow:** Maternal & Fetal Medicine, Hosp Univ Penn 1986; **Fac Appt:** Assoc Prof ObG, Ohio State Univ

Leslie, Kimberly K MD [MF] - **Spec Exp:** Uterine Cancer; **Hospital:** Univ Iowa Hosp & Clinics; **Address:** Univ Iowa Hosp & Clins, 200 Hawkins Drive, 31140-A PFP, Iowa City, IA 52242; **Phone:** 319-356-1976; **Board Cert:** Obstetrics & Gynecology 2011; Maternal & Fetal Medicine 2011; **Med School:** Univ Tex SW, Dallas 1981; **Resid:** Obstetrics & Gynecology, Georgetown Univ Med Ctr 1983; **Fellow:** Maternal & Fetal Medicine, Georgetown Univ Med Ctr 1987; **Fac Appt:** Prof ObG, Univ Iowa Coll Med

Macones, George A MD [MF] - **Spec Exp:** Pregnancy-High Risk; Premature Labor; **Hospital:** Barnes-Jewish Hosp, St. Louis Chldns Hosp; **Address:** Wash Univ, Div Maternal-Fetal Med, 660 S Euclid Ave, Box 8064, St Louis, MO 63110; **Phone:** 314-454-8181; **Board Cert:** Obstetrics & Gynecology 2012; Maternal & Fetal Medicine 2012; **Med School:** Jefferson Med Coll 1988; **Resid:** Obstetrics & Gynecology, Pennsylvania Hosp 1992; **Fellow:** Maternal & Fetal Medicine, Jefferson Univ Hosp 1994; **Fac Appt:** Prof ObG, Washington Univ, St Louis

Philipson, Elliot MD [MF] - **Spec Exp:** Pregnancy-High Risk; Amniocentesis; **Hospital:** Cleveland Clin (page 55), Hillcrest Hosp-Mayfield Hts; **Address:** Hillcrest Hosp, Dept OB/Gyn, 6770 Mayfield Rd, Ste 426, Mayfield Heights, OH 44124; **Phone:** 440-312-7774; **Board Cert:** Obstetrics & Gynecology 2011; Maternal & Fetal Medicine 2011; **Med School:** Italy 1975; **Resid:** Obstetrics & Gynecology, Albany Med Ctr 1980; **Fellow:** Maternal & Fetal Medicine, Metro Genl Hosp 1982; **Fac Appt:** Assoc Prof ObG, Cleveland Cl Coll Med/Case West Res

Samuels, Philip MD [MF] - **Spec Exp:** Epilepsy in Pregnancy; Hypertension in Pregnancy; Pregnancy & Hematologic Abnormalities; **Hospital:** Ohio St Univ Med Ctr; **Address:** 2050 Kenny Rd Fl 5, Columbus, OH 43221; **Phone:** 614-293-8513; **Board Cert:** Obstetrics & Gynecology 2011; Maternal & Fetal Medicine 2011; **Med School:** Texas Tech Univ 1980; **Resid:** Obstetrics & Gynecology, E VA Grad Sch Med 1984; **Fellow:** Maternal & Fetal Medicine, Hosp Univ Penn 1986; **Fac Appt:** Assoc Prof ObG, Ohio State Univ

Socol, Michael MD [MF] - **Spec Exp:** Diabetes in Pregnancy; Multiple Gestation; Premature Labor; **Hospital:** Northwestern Meml Hosp; **Address:** 675 N St Clair St Fl 14 - Ste 200, Chicago, IL 60611-3056; **Phone:** 312-695-7542; **Board Cert:** Obstetrics & Gynecology 1989; Maternal & Fetal Medicine 1981; **Med School:** Univ IL Coll Med 1974; **Resid:** Obstetrics & Gynecology, Univ Illinois Med Ctr 1977; **Fellow:** Maternal & Fetal Medicine, USC Med Ctr 1979; **Fac Appt:** Prof ObG, Northwestern Univ

Strassner, Howard T MD [MF] - **Spec Exp:** Pregnancy-High Risk; Amniocentesis; Obstetric Ultrasound; **Hospital:** Rush Univ Med Ctr, Resurrection Hlth Care St Joseph Hosp; **Address:** Women's Hlth Consultants, 1725 W Harrison St, Ste 408, Chicago, IL 60612; **Phone:** 312-997-2229; **Board Cert:** Obstetrics & Gynecology 2010; Maternal & Fetal Medicine 2010; **Med School:** Univ Chicago-Pritzker Sch Med 1974; **Resid:** Obstetrics & Gynecology, Columbia Presby Med Ctr 1978; **Fellow:** Maternal & Fetal Medicine, LA Co-USC Med Ctr 1980; **Fac Appt:** Prof ObG, Rush Med Coll

Treadwell, Marjorie C MD [MF] - **Spec Exp:** Ultrasound; Pregnancy-High Risk; Fetal Diagnosis & Therapy; **Hospital:** Univ of Michigan Hosp; **Address:** 1500 E Med Ctr Drive, F4806 MOTT Bldg, Ann Arbor, MI 48109-0264; **Phone:** 734-763-4264; **Board Cert:** Obstetrics & Gynecology 2011; Maternal & Fetal Medicine 2011; **Med School:** Univ Mich Med Sch 1984; **Resid:** Obstetrics & Gynecology, Wayne State Univ 1988; **Fellow:** Maternal & Fetal Medicine, Wayne State Univ 1990; **Fac Appt:** Prof ObG, Univ Mich Med Sch

Wilkins, Isabelle MD [MF] - **Spec Exp:** Multiple Gestation; Prenatal Ultrasound; Premature Labor; Prematurity/Low Birth Weight Infants; **Hospital:** Univ of IL Med Ctr at Chicago; **Address:** Center for Womens Health, 1801 W Taylor St, Ste 4C, Chicago, IL 60612; **Phone:** 312-413-7500; **Board Cert:** Obstetrics & Gynecology 2011; Maternal & Fetal Medicine 2011; **Med School:** Duke Univ 1980; **Resid:** Obstetrics & Gynecology, Mt Sinai Med Ctr 1984; **Fellow:** Maternal & Fetal Medicine, Mt Sinai Med Ctr 1986; **Fac Appt:** Prof ObG, Univ IL Coll Med

Maternal & Fetal Medicine

Winn, Hung MD [MF] - **Spec Exp:** Multiple Gestation; Pregnancy-High Risk; **Hospital:** Univ of Missouri Hosp; **Address:** 500 N Keene St, Ste 405-5, Columbia, MO 65201; **Phone:** 573-499-6041; **Board Cert:** Obstetrics & Gynecology 2000; Maternal & Fetal Medicine 2000; **Med School:** Univ IL Coll Med 1982; **Resid:** Obstetrics & Gynecology, Univ Ill Hosp 1986; **Fellow:** Maternal & Fetal Medicine, Yale-New Haven Hosp 1988; **Fac Appt:** Prof ObG, Univ MO-Columbia Sch Med

Great Plains and Mountains

Gibbs, Ronald S MD [MF] - **Spec Exp:** Infectious Disease; **Hospital:** Univ of CO Hosp - Anschutz Inpatient Pav; **Address:** Univ Colorado Womens Services, 1635 Aurora Court, MS F711, Aurora, CO 80045; **Phone:** 720-848-1060; **Board Cert:** Obstetrics & Gynecology 1989; Maternal & Fetal Medicine 1981; **Med School:** Univ Pennsylvania 1969; **Resid:** Obstetrics & Gynecology, Hosp Univ Penn 1974; **Fellow:** Maternal & Fetal Medicine, Univ Tex Hlth Sci Ctr 1978; **Fac Appt:** Prof ObG, Univ Colorado

Tomich, Paul MD [MF] - **Spec Exp:** Pregnancy-High Risk; Prenatal Ultrasound; **Hospital:** Nebraska Med Ctr; **Address:** 983255 Nebraska Med Ctr, Omaha, NE 68198-3255; **Phone:** 402-559-6150; **Board Cert:** Obstetrics & Gynecology 2011; Maternal & Fetal Medicine 2011; **Med School:** Loyola Univ-Stritch Sch Med 1973; **Resid:** Obstetrics & Gynecology, Mayo Clinic 1978; **Fellow:** Maternal & Fetal Medicine, Barnes Hosp-Wash Univ 1980; **Fac Appt:** Prof ObG, Univ Nebr Coll Med

Southwest

Adam, Karolina MD [MF] - **Spec Exp:** Pregnancy-High Risk; Heart Disease in Pregnancy; **Hospital:** Methodist Hosp - Houston, St. Luke's Episcopal Hosp-Houston; **Address:** Houston Perinatal Associates, 7900 Fannin St, Ste 2600, Houston, TX 77054; **Phone:** 713-791-9700; **Board Cert:** Obstetrics & Gynecology 2011; Maternal & Fetal Medicine 2011; **Med School:** Med Coll PA 1983; **Resid:** Obstetrics & Gynecology, Baylor Affil Hosp 1987; **Fellow:** Maternal & Fetal Medicine, Baylor Coll Med 1989

Hankins, Gary DV MD [MF] - **Spec Exp:** Pregnancy-High Risk; Hypertension in Pregnancy; **Hospital:** UT Med Br at Galveston(Joh Sealy Hosp); **Address:** 301 University Blvd, 3.400 JSA, Galveston, TX 77555-0587; **Phone:** 409-772-1957; **Board Cert:** Obstetrics & Gynecology 2000; Maternal & Fetal Medicine 2000; **Med School:** Med Coll VA 1977; **Resid:** Obstetrics & Gynecology, Wilford Hall Med Ctr 1981; **Fellow:** Critical Care Medicine, Wilford Hall Med Ctr 1982; Maternal & Fetal Medicine, Parkland Hosp 1984; **Fac Appt:** Prof ObG, Univ Tex Med Br, Galveston

Horsager, Robyn MD [MF] - **Hospital:** UT Southwestern Med Ctr at Dallas; **Address:** 5939 Harry Hines Blvd, Fl 5, Dallas, TX 75390-9102; **Phone:** 214-645-3837; **Board Cert:** Obstetrics & Gynecology 2010; Maternal & Fetal Medicine 2010; **Med School:** Univ IL Coll Med 1987; **Resid:** Obstetrics & Gynecology, Parkland Meml Hosp 1991; **Fellow:** Maternal & Fetal Medicine, Univ Texas SW Med Ctr 1993; **Fac Appt:** Assoc Prof ObG, Univ Tex SW, Dallas

Mastrobattista, Joan M MD [MF] - **Spec Exp:** Ultrasound; Prenatal Diagnosis; **Hospital:** Texas Chldns Hosp; **Address:** Dept OB/GYN-Maternal Fetal Med, 6651 Main St, Ste 1020, Houston, TX 77030; **Phone:** 713-798-5020; **Board Cert:** Obstetrics & Gynecology 2011; Maternal & Fetal Medicine 2011; **Med School:** UMDNJ-NJ Med Sch, Newark 1988; **Resid:** Obstetrics & Gynecology, New York Hosp 1992; **Fellow:** Maternal & Fetal Medicine, Univ Texas 1994

Pridjian, Gabriella C MD [MF] - **Spec Exp:** Pregnancy-High Risk; Prenatal Diagnosis; Genetic Disorders; Prenatal Ultrasound; **Hospital:** Tulane-Lakeside Hosp, Tulane Med Ctr; **Address:** Tulane Womens Health Center, 4720 S I-10 Service Road, Ste 302, Metairie, LA 70001; **Phone:** 504-988-8070; **Board Cert:** Obstetrics & Gynecology 2007; Maternal & Fetal Medicine 2007; Clinical Genetics 2010; **Med School:** Med Coll Wisc 1982; **Resid:** Obstetrics & Gynecology, Univ Chicago Affil Hosp 1986; **Fellow:** Maternal & Fetal Medicine, Univ Chicago Affil Hosp 1989; Clinical Genetics, Hayward Gentics Ctr/Tulane Univ 1994; **Fac Appt:** Prof ObG, Tulane Univ

Reed, Kathryn L MD [MF] - **Spec Exp:** Prenatal Diagnosis; Ultrasound; Fetal Echocardiography; **Hospital:** Univ Arizona Med Ctr-Univ Campus; **Address:** Univ AZ Dept Ob/Gyn-Womens Resource Ctr, 1501 N Campbell Ave Fl 8, PO Box 245078, Tucson, AZ 85724; **Phone:** 520-694-6010; **Board Cert:** Obstetrics & Gynecology 2011; Maternal & Fetal Medicine 2011; **Med School:** Univ Ariz Coll Med 1977; **Resid:** Obstetrics & Gynecology, Univ Med Ctr 1981; **Fellow:** Maternal & Fetal Medicine, Univ Arizona 1983; **Fac Appt:** Prof ObG, Univ Ariz Coll Med

Robichaux III, Alfred G MD [MF] - **Spec Exp:** Fetal Surgery; Fetal Abnormalities; Pregnancy-High Risk; **Hospital:** Ochsner Med Ctr-New Orleans; **Address:** Ochsner Clinic, 1514 Jefferson Hwy, Maternal-Fetal Medicine Fl 6, New Orleans, LA 70121; **Phone:** 504-842-4151; **Board Cert:** Obstetrics & Gynecology 2011; Maternal & Fetal Medicine 2011; **Med School:** Louisiana State U, New Orleans 1978; **Resid:** Obstetrics & Gynecology, Ochsner Clinic Fdn 1982; **Fellow:** Maternal & Fetal Medicine, George Washington Univ 1984

Saade, George R MD [MF] - **Spec Exp:** Pregnancy-High Risk; Hypertension in Pregnancy; Premature Labor; **Hospital:** UT Med Br at Galveston(Joh Sealy Hosp); **Address:** Univ of Texas Med Branch-Dept of Ob/Gyn, 301 University Blvd, Galveston, TX 77555; **Phone:** 409-772-9507; **Board Cert:** Obstetrics & Gynecology 2010; Maternal & Fetal Medicine 2010; **Med School:** Amer Univ Beirut 1985; **Resid:** Obstetrics & Gynecology, Union Meml Hosp 1991; **Fellow:** Maternal & Fetal Medicine, Baylor 1994; **Fac Appt:** Prof ObG, Univ Tex Med Br, Galveston

West Coast and Pacific

Adashek, Joseph MD [MF] - **Spec Exp:** Pregnancy-High Risk; Prematurity Prevention; Prenatal Diagnosis; **Hospital:** Southern Hills Hosp & Med Ctr, Summerlin Hosp Med Ctr; **Address:** Desert Perinatal Associates, 5761 S Fort Apache, Las Vegas, NV 89148; **Phone:** 702-341-6610; **Board Cert:** Obstetrics & Gynecology 2011; Maternal & Fetal Medicine 2011; **Med School:** Penn State Coll Med 1989; **Resid:** Obstetrics & Gynecology, Northwestern Meml Hosp 1993; **Fellow:** Maternal & Fetal Medicine, UC Irvine Med Ctr 1995

Benedetti, Thomas J MD [MF] - **Spec Exp:** Prematurity Prevention; Fetal Macrosomia; **Hospital:** Univ Wash Med Ctr, Yakima Valley Mem Hosp; **Address:** Univ Washington Dept. OB/GYN, 1959 NE Pacific St, Box 356460, Health Sci Bldg, Seattle, WA 98195-6460; **Phone:** 206-543-3729; **Board Cert:** Obstetrics & Gynecology 1980; Maternal & Fetal Medicine 1981; **Med School:** Univ Wash 1973; **Resid:** Obstetrics & Gynecology, LAC-USC Med Ctr 1977; **Fellow:** Maternal & Fetal Medicine, LAC-USC Med Ctr 1979; **Fac Appt:** Prof ObG, Univ Wash

Cheng, Edith Y MD [MF] - **Spec Exp:** Genetic Disorders; Prenatal Diagnosis; Fetal Therapy; **Hospital:** Univ Wash Med Ctr, Seattle Chldns Hosp; **Address:** Univ Washington- Dept of Ob/Gyn, 1959 NE Pacific St, Box 356460, Seattle, WA 98195; **Phone:** 206-543-3729; **Board Cert:** Clinical Genetics 2010; Obstetrics & Gynecology 2010; Maternal & Fetal Medicine 2010; **Med School:** Univ Wash 1987; **Resid:** Obstetrics & Gynecology, Univ Washington Med Ctr 1991; **Fellow:** Clinical Genetics, Univ Washington Med Ctr 1993; Maternal & Fetal Medicine, Univ Washington Med Ctr 1995; **Fac Appt:** Assoc Prof ObG, Univ Wash

Maternal & Fetal Medicine

Chmait, Ramen H MD [MF] - **Spec Exp:** Fetal Surgery; Twin to Twin Transfusion Syndrome (TTTS); **Hospital:** Hollywood Presby Med Ctr; **Address:** Hollywood Presbyterian Med Ctr, 1300 N Vermont Ave, Ste 710, Los Angles, CA 90027; **Phone:** 323-361-6074; **Board Cert:** Obstetrics & Gynecology 2007; Maternal & Fetal Medicine 2007; **Med School:** UCLA 1996; **Resid:** Obstetrics & Gynecology, LAC/USC Med Ctr 2001; **Fellow:** Maternal & Fetal Medicine, UCSD Med Ctr 2003

Druzin, Maurice L MD [MF] - **Spec Exp:** Lupus/SLE in Pregnancy; Miscarriage-Recurrent; **Hospital:** Lucile Packard Chldn's Hosp; **Address:** 770 Welch Rd, Ste 201, Palo Alto, CA 94304; **Phone:** 650-498-4069; **Board Cert:** Obstetrics & Gynecology 2011; Maternal & Fetal Medicine 2011; **Med School:** South Africa 1970; **Resid:** Obstetrics & Gynecology, Rose Med Ctr-Univ Colo 1977; **Fellow:** Maternal & Fetal Medicine, LAC-USC Med Ctr 1979; **Fac Appt:** Prof ObG, Stanford Univ

Goldberg, James D MD [MF] - **Spec Exp:** Prenatal Diagnosis; Fetal Diagnosis & Therapy; **Hospital:** CA Pacific Med Ctr-Pacific Campus; **Address:** San Francisco Perinatal Assoc, One Daniel Burnham Ct, Ste 230C, San Francisco, CA 94109; **Phone:** 415-202-1200; **Board Cert:** Obstetrics & Gynecology 2010; Clinical Genetics 1987; Maternal & Fetal Medicine 2010; **Med School:** Univ Minn 1979; **Resid:** Obstetrics & Gynecology, UCSF Med Ctr 1983; **Fellow:** Maternal & Fetal Medicine, Mt Sinai Hosp 1985; Clinical Genetics, Mt Sinai Hosp 1985

Gravett, Michael G MD [MF] - **Spec Exp:** Infectious Disease-Perinatal; Pregnancy-High Risk; Prematurity Prevention; Prematurity/Low Birth Weight Infants; **Hospital:** Univ Wash Med Ctr; **Address:** Univ Washington, Dept OB/GYN, 1959 NE Pacific St, Box 356460, Hlth Sci Bldg, Seattle, WA 98195-6460; **Phone:** 206-543-9729; **Board Cert:** Obstetrics & Gynecology 1985; Maternal & Fetal Medicine 1987; **Med School:** UCLA 1977; **Resid:** Obstetrics & Gynecology, Univ Wash Med Ctr 1981; **Fellow:** Maternal & Fetal Medicine, Univ Wash Med Ctr 1983; **Fac Appt:** Prof ObG, Univ Wash

Kelly, Thomas F MD [MF] - **Spec Exp:** Pregnancy-High Risk; **Hospital:** UCSD Med Ctr; **Address:** UCSD Med Ctr, Dept Reproductive Med, 200 W Arbor Drive, San Diego, CA 92103; **Phone:** 619-543-2384; **Board Cert:** Obstetrics & Gynecology 2011; Maternal & Fetal Medicine 2011; **Med School:** Univ Nevada 1986; **Resid:** Obstetrics & Gynecology, USCD Med Ctr 1990; **Fellow:** Maternal & Fetal Medicine, USCD Med Ctr 1992; **Fac Appt:** Clin Prof Med, UCSD

Koos, Brian J MD [MF] - **Spec Exp:** Pregnancy-High Risk; Fetal Diagnosis & Therapy; Heart Disease in Pregnancy; **Hospital:** UCLA Ronald Reagan Med Ctr; **Address:** 200 UCLA Medical Plaza, Ste 430, Los Angeles, CA 90095; **Phone:** 310-794-7852; **Board Cert:** Obstetrics & Gynecology 1999; Maternal & Fetal Medicine 1999; **Med School:** Loma Linda Univ 1975; **Resid:** Obstetrics & Gynecology, Brigham & Womens Hosp 1979; **Fellow:** Maternal & Fetal Medicine, Nuffield Inst for Med Rsch 1982; Maternal & Fetal Medicine, LAC/USC Womens Hosp 1983; **Fac Appt:** Prof ObG, UCLA

Moore, Thomas R MD [MF] - **Spec Exp:** Diabetes in Pregnancy; Fetal Diagnosis & Therapy; **Hospital:** UCSD Med Ctr, Scripps Meml Hosp - La Jolla; **Address:** 200 W Arbor Drive, MPF Bldg, Ste 170, San Diego, CA 92103; **Phone:** 619-543-7900; **Board Cert:** Obstetrics & Gynecology 2006; Maternal & Fetal Medicine 2006; **Med School:** Yale Univ 1979; **Resid:** Obstetrics & Gynecology, Naval Hosp 1983; **Fellow:** Maternal & Fetal Medicine, UCSD 1985; **Fac Appt:** Prof ObG, UCSD

Platt, Lawrence D MD [MF] - **Spec Exp:** Ultrasound; Prenatal Diagnosis; **Hospital:** Cedars-Sinai Med Ctr, St. John's Hlth Ctr, Santa Monica; **Address:** 6310 W San Vincente Blvd, Ste 520, Los Angeles, CA 90048; **Phone:** 323-857-1952; **Board Cert:** Obstetrics & Gynecology 1979; Maternal & Fetal Medicine 1981; **Med School:** Wayne State Univ 1972; **Resid:** Obstetrics & Gynecology, Sinai Hosp 1976; **Fellow:** Maternal & Fetal Medicine, USC Med Ctr 1978; **Fac Appt:** Prof ObG, UCLA

Robertson, Patricia A MD [MF] - **Spec Exp:** Pregnancy-High Risk; **Hospital:** UCSF Med Ctr; **Address:** 400 Parnassus Ave, Box 0346, San Francisco, CA 94143; **Phone:** 415-353-2566; **Board Cert:** Obstetrics & Gynecology 2011; Maternal & Fetal Medicine 2011; **Med School:** Univ Tex, San Antonio 1976; **Resid:** Obstetrics & Gynecology, UCSF Med Ctr 1980; **Fellow:** Maternal & Fetal Medicine, UCSF Med Ctr 1990; **Fac Appt:** Prof ObG, UCSF

Tabsh, Khalil M A MD [MF] - **Spec Exp:** Pregnancy-High Risk; **Hospital:** UCLA Ronald Reagan Med Ctr, Santa Monica - UCLA Med Ctr & Ortho Hosp; **Address:** 200 Med Plaza, Ste 430, Los Angeles, CA 90095; **Phone:** 310-208-4492; **Board Cert:** Obstetrics & Gynecology 1981; Maternal & Fetal Medicine 1982; **Med School:** Lebanon 1974; **Resid:** Obstetrics & Gynecology, American Univ Beirut Med Ctr 1976; Obstetrics & Gynecology, Yale-New Haven Hosp 1978; **Fellow:** Maternal & Fetal Medicine, UCLA Med Ctr 1979; **Fac Appt:** Clin Prof ObG, UCLA-David Geffen Sch Med

Zalud, Ivica MD/PhD [MF] - **Spec Exp:** Obstetric Ultrasound; Pregnancy-High Risk; **Hospital:** Kapiolani Med Ctr for Women & Chldn; **Address:** Fetal Diagnostic Center, 1319 Punahou St, Ste 540, Hololulu, HI 96826; **Phone:** 808-203-6546; **Board Cert:** Obstetrics & Gynecology 2011; Maternal & Fetal Medicine 2011; **Med School:** Croatia 1986; **Resid:** Obstetrics & Gynecology, Winthrop Univ Hosp 1997; **Fellow:** Maternal & Fetal Medicine, Georgetown Univ Med Ctr 2000; **Fac Appt:** Assoc Prof ObG, Univ Hawaii JA Burns Sch Med

Cleveland Clinic
Women's Health Institute
9500 Euclid Avenue
Cleveland, OH 44195

Maternal & Fetal Medicine

Cleveland Clinic Ob/Gyn & Women's Health Institute is designed to meet the unique and changing medical needs of women from adolescence to mature adulthood. Our team offers coordinated and supportive care. *U.S. News & World Report* has ranked our gynecology program No. 3 in the country. Our physicians are nationally and internationally known, and many serve on leadership boards for professional physician societies.

Physicians and certified nurse-midwives in the Maternal-Fetal Medicine/Obstetrics Section provide three levels of obstetrical care: Midwives offer a family-centered approach to low-risk prenatal care and delivery; general obstetricians provide care for low- and medium-risk pregnancies; and maternal/fetal medicine specialists provide diagnosis and treatment for more complicated high-risk pregnancies. Available services include genetic counseling, ultrasound, chorionic villus sampling and amniocentesis.

Cleveland Clinic Fetal Care Center, launched in 2005, is a multidisciplinary team of perinatologists, neonatologists and pediatric surgeons whose goal is to achieve the best possible outcome in pregnancies complicated by complex congenital anomalies. Through collaboration and communication, we provide accurate prenatal diagnosis using state-of-the-art techniques such as high-resolution ultrasound, fetal MRI and fetoscopy. Then we develop management and treatment plans for use during pregnancy, at delivery or immediately after birth.

The Pediatric Cardiac Catheterization Laboratory and our new Special Delivery Unit (SDU) are key components of our Fetal Care Center. The SDU offers a labor and delivery suite, operating room for C-sections and advanced newborn resuscitation and treatment room for deliveries involving complicated or maternal fetal conditions. Benefits to the patient include: access to a full range of Cleveland Clinic adult and pediatric subspecialists; pediatric OR; level III NICU; and neonatal neuro-intensive care.

Offering Same-Day Appointments
Call 800.274.2009.

Treatment Guides
Cleveland Clinic has developed comprehensive treatment guides for many diseases and conditions. To download our free treatment guides, visit clevelandclinic.org/treatmentguides.

Online Medical Second Opinion
Call 216.444.3223 or
800.223.2273 ext. 43223 or
email eclevelandclinic@ccf.org.

Out-of-State Patients Assistance
Call 800.223.2273, ext. 55580 or
email medicalconcierge@ccf.org.

Visit Us At:
clevelandclinic.org

Follow Us On:
Facebook
www.facebook.com/clevelandclinic

Twitter
@ClevelandClinic

You Tube
www.youtube.com/clevelandclinic

Health Hub
health.clevelandclinic.org

550 First Avenue *(at 31st Street)*
New York, NY 10016
www.NYULMC.org
Physician Referral: **888-7-NYU-MED** *(888-769-8633)*

MATERNAL-FETAL MEDICINE

About the Division of Maternal-Fetal Medicine

The Division of Maternal-Fetal Medicine at NYU Langone Medical Center is committed to ensuring that both mother and fetus receive the highly specialized care they need. The Division focuses on multifetal pregnancies, genetic counseling, women who have miscarried, preterm deliveries and other medical complications that can occur during pregnancy. We also specialize in helping women who have other medical conditions that may complicate a pregnancy, such as diabetes, heart problems, high blood pressure, and lupus, among others. The Division offers the latest techniques for in-utero diagnosis and treatment as well as advanced care of complex obstetrical patients. We specialize in the following areas:

Patient Care

The Division of Maternal-Fetal Medicine focuses on ensuring that each patient delivers a healthy baby. Using minimally invasive techniques, doctors at NYU Langone Medical Center are able to repair a number of life-threatening conditions in a child before it is even born, reducing the risks of preterm labor and the need for Cesarean births. Our physicians have developed numerous new treatment protocols for high-risk obstetrics that have been adopted around the world.

Research

The Division of Maternal-Fetal Medicine has generated new treatments for high-risk obstetrics patients and introduced effective new methods of diagnosis and treatment for the fetus.

The Best in American Medicine
www.CastleConnolly.com

Neonatal-Perinatal Medicine
a subspecialty of Pediatrics

A subspecialist in neonatal-perinatal medicine is a pediatrician who is the principal care provider for sick newborn infants. Clinical expertise is used for direct patient care and for consulting with obstetrical colleagues to plan for the care of mothers who have high-risk pregnancies.

Training Required: Three years in pediatrics *plus* additional training and examination.

NEONATAL-PERINATAL MEDICINE

New England

Cloherty, John MD [NP] - **Spec Exp:** Neonatology; **Hospital:** Children's Hospital - Boston, Brigham and Women's Hosp (page 57); **Address:** Longwood Pediatrics, 319 Longwood Ave Fl 4, Boston, MA 02115; **Phone:** 617-277-7320; **Board Cert:** Pediatrics 1986; Neonatal-Perinatal Medicine 1986; **Med School:** Boston Univ 1962; **Resid:** Pediatrics, Mass Genl Hosp 1969; **Fellow:** Neonatal-Perinatal Medicine, Chldns Hosp; **Fac Appt:** Assoc Clin Prof Ped, Harvard Med Sch

Davis, Jonathan M MD [NP] - **Spec Exp:** Lung Disease in Newborns; Brain Injury; Infections-Neonatal; **Hospital:** Tufts Med Ctr; **Address:** Tufts Medical Ctr, 800 Washington St, Box 44, Boston, MA 02111; **Phone:** 617-636-5322; **Board Cert:** Pediatrics 1985; Neonatal-Perinatal Medicine 1987; **Med School:** McGill Univ 1981; **Resid:** Pediatrics, Chldns Hosp 1984; **Fellow:** Neonatal-Perinatal Medicine, Chldns Hosp 1986; **Fac Appt:** Prof Ped, Tufts Univ

Ehrenkranz, Richard A MD [NP] - **Spec Exp:** Nutrition; Lung Disease in Newborns; **Hospital:** Yale-New Haven Hosp, Yale Med Group; **Address:** Yale Univ-Dept Ped, 333 Cedar Street, PO Box 208064, New Haven, CT 06520-8064; **Phone:** 203-688-2320; **Board Cert:** Pediatrics 1977; Neonatal-Perinatal Medicine 1979; **Med School:** SUNY Downstate 1972; **Resid:** Pediatrics, Yale-New Haven Hosp 1974; **Fellow:** Neonatal-Perinatal Medicine, Yale-New Haven Hosp 1978; **Fac Appt:** Prof Ped, Yale Univ

Frantz, Ivan MD [NP] - **Spec Exp:** Lung Disease in Newborns; **Address:** Children's Hospital Boston, 300 Longwood Ave, Boston, MA 02115; **Phone:** 617-919-3397; **Board Cert:** Pediatrics 1976; Neonatal-Perinatal Medicine 2009; **Med School:** Univ Minn 1971; **Resid:** Pediatrics, Univ Minn Hosp 1973; **Fellow:** Neonatal-Perinatal Medicine, McGill Royal Victoria Hosp 1974; Neonatal-Perinatal Medicine, Mass Genl Hosp 1975; **Fac Appt:** Prof Ped, Tufts Univ

Gross, Ian MD [NP] - **Spec Exp:** Breathing Disorders; Critical Care; **Hospital:** Yale-New Haven Hosp, Yale Med Group; **Address:** Yale Sch Med, Dept Pediatrics, 333 Cedar St, PO Box 208064, New Haven, CT 06520-8064; **Phone:** 203-688-2320; **Board Cert:** Pediatrics 1974; Neonatal-Perinatal Medicine 1977; **Med School:** South Africa 1967; **Resid:** Pediatrics, Univ Witwatersrand Affil Hosps 1971; Pediatrics, Chldns Hosp Med Ctr 1973; **Fellow:** Neonatal-Perinatal Medicine, Yale-New Haven Hosp 1974; **Fac Appt:** Prof Ped, Yale Univ

Van Marter, Linda J MD [NP] - **Spec Exp:** Neonatal Chronic Lung Disease (CLD); Lung Disease in Newborns; Pulmonary Hypertension of Newborn (PPHN); **Hospital:** Brigham and Women's Hosp (page 57), Children's Hospital - Boston; **Address:** Children's Hospital Boston, 300 Longwood Ave, Hunnewell 430 - Newborn Med, Boston, MA 02115; **Phone:** 617-355-6027; **Board Cert:** Pediatrics 1985; Neonatal-Perinatal Medicine 2009; **Med School:** Univ Pittsburgh 1980; **Resid:** Pediatrics, Childrens Hosp Med Ctr 1983; **Fellow:** Neonatology, Harvard Med Sch 1986; **Fac Appt:** Assoc Prof Ped, Harvard Med Sch

Mid Atlantic

Anday, Endla K MD [NP] - **Spec Exp:** Brain Injury-Neonatal; **Hospital:** St. Christopher's Hosp for Chldn; **Address:** St Christophers Hosp for Children, 3601 A St, Philadelphia, PA 19134; **Phone:** 215-427-5202; **Board Cert:** Pediatrics 1978; Neonatal-Perinatal Medicine 1981; **Med School:** Med Coll PA 1973; **Resid:** Pediatrics, Childrens Hosp 1975; **Fellow:** Neonatology, Childrens Hosp 1978; Pulmonary Disease, Univ Penn 1979; **Fac Appt:** Prof Ped, Drexel Univ Coll Med

Davidson, Dennis MD [NP] - **Spec Exp:** Lung Disease in Newborns; **Hospital:** Stony Brook Univ Med Ctr; **Address:** Stony Brook Long Island Children's Ctr, 101 Nicholls Rd, T-11060, Stony Brook, NY 11794-8111; **Phone:** 631-444-7653; **Board Cert:** Pediatrics 1980; Neonatal-Perinatal Medicine 2009; **Med School:** Loyola Univ-Stritch Sch Med 1974; **Resid:** Pediatrics, Babies Hosp-Columbia Univ 1978; **Fellow:** Neonatal-Perinatal Medicine, Babies Hosp-Columbia Univ 1981; **Fac Appt:** Clin Prof Ped, Albert Einstein Coll Med

Delivoria-Papadopoulos, Maria MD [NP] - **Spec Exp:** Neonatology; Prematurity/Low Birth Weight Infants; Breathing Disorders; Brain Injury; **Hospital:** St. Christopher's Hosp for Chldn, Hahnemann Univ Hosp; **Address:** St Christopher's Hosp for Children, 3601 A St, Ste 2212, Neonatology, Philadelphia, PA 19134; **Phone:** 215-427-5202; **Board Cert:** Pediatrics 1971; Neonatal-Perinatal Medicine 1975; **Med School:** Greece 1957; **Resid:** Pediatrics, Chldns Hosp 1959; Psychiatry, Colo State Hosp 1962; **Fellow:** Neonatology, Hosp Sick Chldn 1964; **Fac Appt:** Prof Ped

Dennery, Phyllis Armelle MD [NP] - **Spec Exp:** Lung Disease in Newborns; **Hospital:** Chldns Hosp of Philadelphia; **Address:** CHOP Bldg Div Neonatology, 34th St and Civic Ctr Blvd Fl 2, Philadelphia, PA 19104; **Phone:** 215-590-1653; **Board Cert:** Neonatal-Perinatal Medicine 2004; **Med School:** Howard Univ 1984; **Resid:** Pediatrics, Chldns Hosp Natl Med Ctr 1988; **Fellow:** Neonatal-Perinatal Medicine, Case Western Reserve Affil Hosp 1989; **Fac Appt:** Prof Ped, Univ Pennsylvania

Holzman, Ian R MD [NP] - **Spec Exp:** Neonatal Nutrition; Necrotizing Enterocolitis; Ethics; Prematurity/Low Birth Weight Infants; **Hospital:** Mount Sinai Med Ctr (page 64), Elmhurst Hosp Ctr; **Address:** Newborn Assocs, 1 Gustave L Levy Pl, Box 1508, New York, NY 10029-6500; **Phone:** 212-241-5446; **Board Cert:** Pediatrics 1974; Neonatal-Perinatal Medicine 1977; **Med School:** Univ Pittsburgh 1971; **Resid:** Pediatrics, Chldns Hosp 1975; **Fellow:** Neonatal-Perinatal Medicine, Univ Colorado Hosp 1977; **Fac Appt:** Prof Ped, Mount Sinai Sch Med

Hurt, Hallam MD [NP] - **Spec Exp:** Neonatology; **Hospital:** Chldns Hosp of Philadelphia, Hosp Univ Penn - UPHS (page 72); **Address:** Chldns Hosp of Philadelphia, 3535 Market St Fl 14, Philadelphia, PA 19104; **Phone:** 215-590-0560; **Board Cert:** Pediatrics 1976; Neonatal-Perinatal Medicine 2002; **Med School:** Univ VA Sch Med 1971; **Resid:** Pediatrics, Univ Virginia Hosp 1974; **Fellow:** Neonatal-Perinatal Medicine, Univ Virginia Hosp 1976; **Fac Appt:** Prof Ped, Univ Pennsylvania

La Gamma, Edmund F MD [NP] - **Spec Exp:** Neonatal Infections; Prematurity/Low Birth Weight Infants; Necrotizing Enterocolitis; **Hospital:** Westchester Med Ctr, Children's & Women's Phys.of Westchester; **Address:** Maria Fareri Chldns Hosp, 100 Woods Rd, rm 2215, Valhalla, NY 10595; **Phone:** 914-493-8558; **Board Cert:** Pediatrics 1981; Neonatal-Perinatal Medicine 1981; **Med School:** NY Med Coll 1976; **Resid:** Pediatrics, NY Hosp-Cornell Med Ctr 1978; **Fellow:** Neonatal-Perinatal Medicine, NY Hosp-Cornell Med Ctr 1980; Cardiovascular Disease, UCSF Med Ctr 1981; **Fac Appt:** Prof Ped, NY Med Coll

Lawson, Edward E MD [NP] - **Spec Exp:** Prematurity/Low Birth Weight Infants; Respiratory Distress Syndrome (RDS); Neonatal Critical Care; Breathing Disorders; **Hospital:** Johns Hopkins Hosp (page 61), Johns Hopkins Bayview Med Ctr (page 61); **Address:** 1800 Orleans St, Ste 8513, Baltimore, MD 21231; **Phone:** 410-955-5259; **Board Cert:** Pediatrics 1990; Neonatal-Perinatal Medicine 1997; **Med School:** Northwestern Univ 1972; **Resid:** Pediatrics, Chldns Hosp Med Ctr 1975; **Fellow:** Neonatal-Perinatal Medicine, Harvard Med Sch 1977; **Fac Appt:** Prof Ped, Johns Hopkins Univ

Neonatal-Perinatal Medicine

Nogee, Lawrence M MD [NP] - **Spec Exp:** Lung Disease in Newborns-Genetic; **Hospital:** Johns Hopkins Hosp (page 61); **Address:** Johns Hopkins Hosp, Div Neonatolgy, 600 N Wolfe St, CMSC 6-104A, Baltimore, MD 21287-3200; **Phone:** 410-614-3355; **Board Cert:** Pediatrics 1986; Neonatal-Perinatal Medicine 1987; **Med School:** Johns Hopkins Univ 1981; **Resid:** Pediatrics, Johns Hopkins Hosp 1984; **Fellow:** Neonatal-Perinatal Medicine, Chldns Hosp Med Ctr 1986; **Fac Appt:** Prof Ped, Johns Hopkins Univ

Perlman, Jeffrey M MD [NP] - **Spec Exp:** Neonatal Critical Care; Prematurity/Low Birth Weight Infants; Neonatal Neurology; Lung Disease in Newborns; **Hospital:** NY-Presby/Weill Cornell Med Ctr, NY (page 66); **Address:** 525 E 68th St, Ste N 506, New York, NY 10065; **Phone:** 212-746-3530; **Board Cert:** Pediatrics 1983; Neonatal-Perinatal Medicine 1983; **Med School:** South Africa 1974; **Resid:** Pediatrics, Johannesburg Chldns Hosp 1979; Pediatrics, St Louis Chldns Hosp 1981; **Fellow:** Neonatology, St Louis Chldns Hosp 1983; **Fac Appt:** Prof Ped, Cornell Univ-Weill Med Coll

Polin, Richard A MD [NP] - **Spec Exp:** Neonatal Infections; **Hospital:** Morgan Stanley Children's Hosp of NY-Presby, NY; **Address:** 3959 Broadway CHN 1201, New York, NY 10032; **Phone:** 212-305-5827; **Board Cert:** Pediatrics 1975; Neonatal-Perinatal Medicine 1977; **Med School:** Temple Univ 1970; **Resid:** Pediatrics, Chldns Meml Hosp 1972; Pediatrics, Babies Hosp 1973; **Fellow:** Neonatal-Perinatal Medicine, Babies Hosp-Columbia 1974; **Fac Appt:** Prof Ped, Columbia P&S

Short, Billie Lou MD [NP] - **Hospital:** Chldns Natl Med Ctr; **Address:** Div Neonatology, 111 Michigan Ave NW, Washington, DC 20010; **Phone:** 202-476-3314; **Board Cert:** Pediatrics 1979; Neonatal-Perinatal Medicine 1979; **Med School:** Univ Okla Coll Med 1974; **Resid:** Pediatrics, Chld's Hosp-Oklahoma 1977; **Fellow:** Neonatal-Perinatal Medicine, Chld's Hosp Med Ctr 1979; **Fac Appt:** Prof Ped, Geo Wash Univ

Silverman, Gary A MD/PhD [NP] - **Hospital:** Chldns Hosp of Pittsburgh - UPMC, Magee-Womens Hosp - UPMC; **Address:** Chld's Hosp Pittsburgh, 1 Chld's Hosp Drive, 4401 Penn Ave, rm 7130, Pittsburgh, PA 15224; **Phone:** 412-692-9448; **Board Cert:** Neonatal-Perinatal Medicine 2011; **Med School:** Univ Chicago-Pritzker Sch Med 1984; **Resid:** Pediatrics, Children's Hosp 1087; **Fellow:** Neonatology, St Louis Chldns Hosp 1989; Research, Washington U Sch Med 1991; **Fac Appt:** Prof Ped, Univ Pittsburgh

Watchko, Jon F MD [NP] - **Hospital:** Magee-Womens Hosp - UPMC, Chldns Hosp of Pittsburgh - UPMC; **Address:** Magee-Womens Hosp, Newborn Medicine, 300 Halket St, Pittsburgh, PA 15213; **Phone:** 412-641-1834; **Board Cert:** Pediatrics 1985; Neonatal-Perinatal Medicine 1985; **Med School:** Univ Pittsburgh 1980; **Resid:** Pediatrics, Upstate Med Ctr 1983; **Fellow:** Neonatology, Univ Washington Med Ctr 1986; **Fac Appt:** Prof Ped, Univ Pittsburgh

Zubrow, Alan B MD [NP] - **Spec Exp:** Neonatology; **Hospital:** St. Christopher's Hosp for Chldn, Hahnemann Univ Hosp; **Address:** St Christopher's Hosp for Chldn, 3601 A St, Philadelphia, PA 19134; **Phone:** 215-427-5202; **Board Cert:** Pediatrics 1980; Neonatal-Perinatal Medicine 2009; **Med School:** Univ Pennsylvania 1976; **Resid:** Pediatrics, Chldns Hosp 1979; **Fellow:** Neonatology, Columbia-Presby Med Ctr 1981; **Fac Appt:** Prof Ped, Drexel Univ Coll Med

Southeast

Bancalari, Eduardo MD [NP] - **Spec Exp:** Neonatology; **Hospital:** Jackson Meml Hosp; **Address:** Dept Pediatrics R131, 1611 NW 12 Ave, Ste 740, Miami, FL 33136; **Phone:** 305-585-2328; **Board Cert:** Neonatal-Perinatal Medicine 1993; Pediatrics 1993; **Med School:** Chile 1966; **Resid:** Pediatrics, Hosp Luis Calvo Mackenna 1969; **Fellow:** Pediatric Cardiology, Univ Miami Med Ctr; **Fac Appt:** Prof Ped, Univ Miami Sch Med

Boyle, Robert J MD [NP] - **Spec Exp:** Neonatology; Ethics; **Hospital:** Univ of Virginia Health Sys; **Address:** UVA Hlth Sci Ctr, Dept Peds, PO Box 800386, Charlottesville, VA 22908; **Phone:** 434-924-5429; **Board Cert:** Pediatrics 1978; Neonatal-Perinatal Medicine 1979; **Med School:** Johns Hopkins Univ 1973; **Resid:** Pediatrics, Rainbow Babies Chldns Hosp 1976; **Fellow:** Neonatal-Perinatal Medicine, Women & Infants Hosp 1978; **Fac Appt:** Prof Ped, Univ VA Sch Med

Bucciarelli, Richard L MD [NP] - **Spec Exp:** Neonatal Cardiology; **Hospital:** Shands at Univ of FL; **Address:** Shands Healthcare, 1600 SW Archer Rd, rm R1-118, PO Box 100296, Gainesville, FL 32610; **Phone:** 352-273-9001; **Board Cert:** Pediatrics 1977; Neonatal-Perinatal Medicine 1977; Pediatric Cardiology 1977; **Med School:** Univ Mich Med Sch 1972; **Resid:** Pediatrics, Shands Hosp-Univ Fla 1975; **Fellow:** Neonatal-Perinatal Medicine, Shands Hosp-Univ Fla 1977; Pediatric Cardiology, Shands Hosp-Univ Fla 1977; **Fac Appt:** Prof Ped, Univ Fla Coll Med

Dhanireddy, Ramasubbareddy MD [NP] - **Spec Exp:** Neonatology; Prematurity/Low Birth Weight Infants; **Hospital:** Regional Med Ctr - Memphis, Le Bonheur Chldns Med Ctr; **Address:** Univ Tennessee, Div Neonatology, 853 Jefferson Ave, rm 201, Memphis, TN 38163; **Phone:** 901-448-5950; **Board Cert:** Pediatrics 1980; Neonatal-Perinatal Medicine 2009; **Med School:** India 1974; **Resid:** Pediatrics, Lousiana State Univ Med Ctr 1978; **Fellow:** Neonatology, Georgetown Univ Med Ctr 1980; **Fac Appt:** Prof Ped, Univ Tenn Coll Med

Hendricks-Munoz, Karen MD [NP] - **Spec Exp:** Breathing Disorders; Neonatal Neurology; Retinopathy of Prematurity; **Hospital:** VCU Med Ctr; **Address:** MCU, Div of Neonatology, Critical Care Hospital, 6th Fl, P.O. Box 980276, Richmond, VA 23298; **Phone:** 804-828-9964; **Board Cert:** Pediatrics 1985; Neonatal-Perinatal Medicine 2009; **Med School:** Yale Univ 1978; **Resid:** Pediatrics, Yale-New Haven Hosp 1981; **Fellow:** Neonatology, Strong Meml Hosp 1984; **Fac Appt:** Prof Ped, Va Commonwealth Univ Sch Med

Holtzman, Ronald B MD [NP] - **Spec Exp:** Neonatology; Lung Disease in Newborns; **Hospital:** Gaston Meml Hosp; **Address:** Gaston Meml Hosp, NICU Office, 2525 Court Drive, Gastonia, NC 28056; **Phone:** 704-834-3390; **Board Cert:** Pediatrics 1987; Neonatal-Perinatal Medicine 2004; **Med School:** Rush Med Coll 1983; **Resid:** Pediatrics, Chldns Meml Hosp 1986; **Fellow:** Neonatal-Perinatal Medicine, Chldns Meml Hosp 1989

Kattwinkel, John MD [NP] - **Spec Exp:** Lung Disease in Newborns; Sudden Infant Death Syndrome (SIDS); **Hospital:** Univ of Virginia Health Sys; **Address:** Univ Va Hosp, Div Neonatology, Dept Peds, PO Box 800386, Charlottesville, VA 22908-0386; **Phone:** 434-924-5428; **Board Cert:** Pediatrics 1986; Neonatal-Perinatal Medicine 1986; **Med School:** Harvard Med Sch 1968; **Resid:** Pediatrics, Duke Univ Med Ctr 1970; **Fellow:** Neonatology, Case-West Res Univ 1974; **Fac Appt:** Prof Ped, Univ VA Sch Med

Stiles, Alan D MD [NP] - **Spec Exp:** Neonatology; **Hospital:** NC Memorial Hosp - UNC; **Address:** 260 MacNider Bldg, CB 7220, Chapel Hill, NC 27599-7220; **Phone:** 919-966-5570; **Board Cert:** Pediatrics 1984; Neonatal-Perinatal Medicine 1985; **Med School:** Univ NC Sch Med 1977; **Resid:** Pediatrics, North Carolina Meml Hosp 1982; **Fellow:** Neonatal-Perinatal Medicine, Chldns Hosp/Brigham Hosp 1985; **Fac Appt:** Prof Ped, Univ NC Sch Med

Midwest

Bell, Edward F MD [NP] - **Spec Exp:** Prematurity/Low Birth Weight Infants; Neonatal Critical Care; Neonatal Hemochromatosis; **Hospital:** Univ Iowa Hosp & Clinics; **Address:** Department of Pediatrics, University of Iowa, 200 Hawkins Drive, rm 8811 JPP, Iowa City, IA 52242; **Phone:** 319-356-4006; **Board Cert:** Pediatrics 1978; Neonatal-Perinatal Medicine 1995; **Med School:** Columbia P&S 1973; **Resid:** Pediatrics, Babies Hosp-Columbia Presby 1976; **Fellow:** Neonatology, McMaster Univ Med Ctr 1977; Neonatology, Women & Infants Hosp-Brown Univ 1979; **Fac Appt:** Prof Ped, Univ Iowa Coll Med

Cole, Francis Sessions MD [NP] - **Spec Exp:** Neonatal Chronic Lung Disease (CLD); Respiratory Distress Syndrome (RDS); Surfactant Biology; Prematurity/Low Birth Weight Infants; **Hospital:** St. Louis Chldns Hosp, Barnes-Jewish Hosp; **Address:** Wash Univ-Div Newborn Med, 660 S Euclid Ave, Box 8116, St Louis, MO 63110; **Phone:** 314-454-6148; **Board Cert:** Pediatrics 1980; Neonatal-Perinatal Medicine 1983; **Med School:** Yale Univ 1973; **Resid:** Pediatrics, Chldns Hosp Med Ctr 1978; **Fellow:** Neonatology, Brigham and Women's Hosp 1981; **Fac Appt:** Prof Ped, Washington Univ, St Louis

Donn, Steven M MD [NP] - **Spec Exp:** Breathing Disorders; Respiratory Distress Syndrome (RDS); Pulmonary Hypertension of Newborn (PPHN); Surfactant Biology; **Hospital:** Mott Chldns Hosp, Univ of Michigan Hosp; **Address:** 1540 E Hospital Drive, Mott Hosp Bldg Fl 8-621, Ann Arbor, MI 48109-5254; **Phone:** 734-763-4109; **Board Cert:** Pediatrics 1981; Neonatal-Perinatal Medicine 1981; **Med School:** Tulane Univ 1974; **Resid:** Pediatrics, Univ Vermont Med Ctr 1978; **Fellow:** Neonatology, Univ Michigan 1980; **Fac Appt:** Prof Ped, Univ Mich Med Sch

Gewolb, Ira H. MD [NP] - **Spec Exp:** Breathing Disorders; Gastroesophageal Reflux Disease (GERD); **Hospital:** Mich State Univ-Sparrow Hos; **Address:** 1215 E Michigan Ave, Fl 3, Lansing, MI 48912; **Phone:** 517-364-2670; **Board Cert:** Pediatrics 1980; Neonatal-Perinatal Medicine 1981; **Med School:** Yale Univ 1976; **Resid:** Pediatrics, Chldns Hosp Med Ctr 1979; **Fellow:** Neonatology, Yale Univ 1982; **Fac Appt:** Prof Ped, Mich State Univ

Hamvas, Aaron MD [NP] - **Spec Exp:** Lung Disease in Newborns-Genetic; **Hospital:** St. Louis Chldns Hosp, Barnes-Jewish Hosp; **Address:** Wash Univ-Div Newborn Med, 660 S Euclid Ave, Box 8116, St Louis, MO 63110; **Phone:** 314-454-6148; **Board Cert:** Neonatal-Perinatal Medicine 2006; **Med School:** Washington Univ, St Louis 1981; **Resid:** Pediatrics, St Louis Chldns Hosp 1984; **Fellow:** Neonatology, St Louis Chldns Hosp 1990; **Fac Appt:** Prof Ped, Washington Univ, St Louis

Lemons, James A MD [NP] - **Spec Exp:** Nutrition; Ethics; **Hospital:** Riley Hosp for Children, IU Health Methodist Hosp; **Address:** 699 Riley Hosp Drive, RR-208, Indianapolis, IN 46202-5119; **Phone:** 317-274-4716; **Board Cert:** Pediatrics 1993; Neonatal-Perinatal Medicine 1993; **Med School:** Northwestern Univ 1969; **Resid:** Pediatrics, Univ Mich Med Ctr 1972; **Fellow:** Neonatal-Perinatal Medicine, Univ Colo Med Ctr 1975; **Fac Appt:** Prof Ped, Indiana Univ

Martin, Richard John MD [NP] - **Spec Exp:** Breathing Disorders; **Hospital:** UH Rainbow Babies & Chldns Hosp (page 74); **Address:** 11100 Euclid Ave, Div Neonatology, Cleveland, OH 44106-6010; **Phone:** 216-844-3387; **Board Cert:** Pediatrics 1976; Neonatal-Perinatal Medicine 2005; **Med School:** Australia 1970; **Resid:** Pediatrics, Univ Missouri 1973; **Fellow:** Neonatal-Perinatal Medicine, Case West Res Univ 1975; **Fac Appt:** Prof Ped, Case West Res Univ

Meadow, William Lee MD/PhD [NP] - **Spec Exp:** Neonatal Infections; Ethics; **Hospital:** Univ of Chicago Med Ctr; **Address:** 5841 S Maryland Ave, rm 657, MC 6060, Chicago, IL 60637; **Phone:** 773-702-6210; **Board Cert:** Pediatrics 1979; Neonatal-Perinatal Medicine 1981; **Med School:** Univ Pennsylvania 1974; **Resid:** Pediatrics, Chldns Meml Hosp 1978; **Fellow:** Neonatology, Wyler Chldns Hosp 1981; Infectious Disease, Wyler Chldns Hosp 1981; **Fac Appt:** Prof Ped, Univ Chicago-Pritzker Sch Med

Muraskas, Jonathan MD [NP] - **Spec Exp:** Prematurity/Low Birth Weight Infants; Multiple Gestation; Conjoined Twins; Ethics; **Hospital:** Loyola Univ Med Ctr; **Address:** Loyola University Medical Ctr, Bldg 107, 2160 S First Ave, Russo Pavilion, Neo Unit, Rm 5811, Maywood, IL 60153-5500; **Phone:** 708-216-1067; **Board Cert:** Pediatrics 1987; Neonatal-Perinatal Medicine 1987; **Med School:** Loyola Univ-Stritch Sch Med 1982; **Resid:** Pediatrics, Loyola Univ Med Ctr 1985; **Fellow:** Neonatal-Perinatal Medicine, Loyola Univ Med Ctr 1987; **Fac Appt:** Prof Ped, Loyola Univ-Stritch Sch Med

Steinhorn, Robin H MD [NP] - **Spec Exp:** Pulmonary Hypertension; **Hospital:** Lurie Chldn's Hosp-Chicago, Northwestern Meml Hosp; **Address:** Ann & Robert H. Lurie Children's Hosp, 225 E Chicago Ave, Box 45, Chicago, IL 60611; **Phone:** 312-227-5322; **Board Cert:** Neonatal-Perinatal Medicine 2011; **Med School:** Washington Univ, St Louis 1980; **Resid:** Obstetrics & Gynecology, Barnes Hosp 1983; Pediatrics, Univ Minn Affil Hosp 1986; **Fellow:** Neonatal-Perinatal Medicine, Univ Minn Affil Hosp 1988; **Fac Appt:** Prof Ped, Northwestern Univ

Whitsett, Jeffrey A MD [NP] - **Spec Exp:** Lung Disease in Newborns-Genetic; **Hospital:** Cincinnati Chldns Hosp Med Ctr, Good Samaritan Hosp - Cincinnati; **Address:** Cincinnati Chldns Hosp, Div Neonatalogy, 3333 Burnet Ave, Cincinnati, OH 45229-3039; **Phone:** 513-636-4830; **Board Cert:** Pediatrics 1979; Neonatal-Perinatal Medicine 1979; **Med School:** Columbia P&S 1973; **Resid:** Pediatrics, Mt Sinai Hosp 1976; **Fellow:** Neonatology, Chldns Hosp Med Ctr 1977; **Fac Appt:** Prof Ped, Univ Cincinnati

Great Plains and Mountains

Milley, J Ross MD/PhD [NP] - **Spec Exp:** Nutrition; **Hospital:** Primary Children's Med Ctr, Univ Utah Hlth Care; **Address:** Univ Utah - Dept Pediatrics/Neonatology, Williams Bldg, PO Box 581289, Salt Lake City, UT 84158; **Phone:** 801-581-7085; **Board Cert:** Pediatrics 1980; Neonatal-Perinatal Medicine 1981; **Med School:** Univ Chicago-Pritzker Sch Med 1975; **Resid:** Pediatrics, Johns Hopkins Hosp 1978; **Fellow:** Neonatology, Johns Hopkins Hosp 1980; **Fac Appt:** Prof Ped, Univ Utah

Zach, Terence MD [NP] - **Spec Exp:** Neonatal Critical Care; **Hospital:** Alegent Creighton Univ Med Ctr; **Address:** Creighton Univ, Neonatal-Perinatal Med, 601 N 30th St, Omaha, NE 68198-1205; **Phone:** 402-559-6750; **Board Cert:** Pediatrics 1987; Neonatal-Perinatal Medicine 2004; **Med School:** Univ Nebr Coll Med 1983; **Resid:** Pediatrics, Univ Nebr Med Ctr 1986; **Fellow:** Neonatology, Univ Minnesota 1986; **Fac Appt:** Prof Ped, Creighton Univ

Southwest

Adams, James M MD [NP] - **Spec Exp:** Lung Disease in Newborns; **Hospital:** Texas Chldns Hosp; **Address:** 6621 Fannin St, MC WT-6104, Houston, TX 77030; **Phone:** 832-826-1380; **Board Cert:** Pediatrics 1975; Neonatal-Perinatal Medicine 1975; **Med School:** Baylor Coll Med 1970; **Resid:** Pediatrics, Baylor Affil Hosps 1973; **Fellow:** Neonatal-Perinatal Medicine, Baylor Affil Hosps 1975; **Fac Appt:** Prof Ped, Baylor Coll Med

Escobedo, Marilyn B MD [NP] - **Spec Exp:** Neonatology; Nutrition; **Hospital:** Chldns Hosp OU Med Ctr; **Address:** 1200 Everett Drive, North Pavilion Fl 7 - rm 7504, Oklahoma City, OK 73104; **Phone:** 405-271-5215; **Board Cert:** Pediatrics 1986; Neonatal-Perinatal Medicine 2004; **Med School:** Washington Univ, St Louis 1970; **Resid:** Pediatrics, Chldns Hosp 1972; Neonatal-Perinatal Medicine, Chldns Hosp 1973; **Fellow:** Neonatal-Perinatal Medicine, Vanderbilt Univ 1976; **Fac Appt:** Prof Ped, Univ Okla Coll Med

Neonatal-Perinatal Medicine

Garcia-Prats, Joseph MD [NP] - **Spec Exp:** Lung Disease in Newborns; **Hospital:** Texas Chldns Hosp, Ben Taub Genl Hosp; **Address:** 6621 Fannin St, Ste W6104, Houston, TX 77030-1608; **Phone:** 713-873-3515; **Board Cert:** Pediatrics 1977; Neonatal-Perinatal Medicine 2009; **Med School:** Tulane Univ 1972; **Resid:** Pediatrics, Baylor Affil Hosp 1975; **Fellow:** Neonatal-Perinatal Medicine, Baylor Affil Hosp 1977; **Fac Appt:** Prof Ped, Baylor Coll Med

Odom, Michael W MD [NP] - **Spec Exp:** Neonatology; **Hospital:** Univ Hlth Syst-San Antonio; **Address:** Dept Peds, 7703 Floyd Curl Drive, MC 7812, San Antonio, TX 78229-3900; **Phone:** 210-567-5225; **Board Cert:** Pediatrics 1987; Neonatal-Perinatal Medicine 2011; **Med School:** Univ Tex SW, Dallas 1983; **Resid:** Pediatrics, Vanderbilt Univ Affil Hosps 1986; **Fellow:** Neonatal-Perinatal Medicine, Mt Zion Med Ctr-UCSF 1989; **Fac Appt:** Assoc Prof Ped, Univ Tex, San Antonio

Seidner, Steven R MD [NP] - **Spec Exp:** Neonatal Chronic Lung Disease (CLD); Respiratory Distress Syndrome (RDS); Pulmonary Hypertension of Newborn (PPHN); **Hospital:** Univ Hlth Syst-San Antonio; **Address:** Dept Peds, 7703 Floyd Curl Drive, MC 7812, San Antonio, TX 78229-3901; **Phone:** 210-567-5225; **Board Cert:** Pediatrics 1987; Neonatal-Perinatal Medicine 1987; **Med School:** Univ Ariz Coll Med 1982; **Resid:** Pediatrics, Harbor-UCLA Med Ctr 1985; **Fellow:** Neonatal-Perinatal Medicine, Harbor-UCLA Med Ctr 1988; **Fac Appt:** Prof Ped, Univ Tex, San Antonio

West Coast and Pacific

Gleason, Christine A MD [NP] - **Spec Exp:** Prematurity/Low Birth Weight Infants; Neonatal Critical Care; **Hospital:** Seattle Chldns Hosp; **Address:** UW Neonatal-Perinatal Medicine, 1959 NE Pacific St, Box 356320, Seattle, WA 98195; **Phone:** 206-543-3200; **Board Cert:** Pediatrics 1994; Neonatal-Perinatal Medicine 2002; **Med School:** Univ Rochester 1979; **Resid:** Pediatrics, Univ Hosp Cleveland 1984; **Fellow:** Neonatal-Perinatal Medicine, UCSF Affil Med Ctr 1985

Simmons Jr, Charles F MD [NP] - **Hospital:** Cedars-Sinai Med Ctr; **Address:** Cedars-Sinai Medical Center, Maxine Dunitz Children's Health Center, 8700 Beverly Blvd, NT 4226, Los Angeles, CA 90048; **Phone:** 310-423-4416; **Board Cert:** Pediatrics 1986; Neonatal-Perinatal Medicine 1987; **Med School:** Harvard Med Sch 1980; **Resid:** Pediatrics, Children's Hosp 1983; **Fellow:** Neonatal-Perinatal Medicine, Children's Hosp 1986; **Fac Appt:** Prof Ped, UCLA-David Geffen Sch Med

Stevenson, David K MD [NP] - **Spec Exp:** Neonatology; **Hospital:** Lucile Packard Chldn's Hosp; **Address:** 750 Welch Rd, Ste 315, Palo Alto, CA 94304-1510; **Phone:** 650-723-5711; **Board Cert:** Pediatrics 1979; Neonatal-Perinatal Medicine 2004; **Med School:** Univ Wash 1975; **Resid:** Pediatrics, Univ Washington 1977; **Fellow:** Neonatal-Perinatal Medicine, Stanford Univ 1979; **Fac Appt:** Prof Ped, Stanford Univ

NEONATAL PERINATAL MEDICINE

Neonatal Perinatal Medicine is part of the Hassenfeld Pediatric Center, a full service specialty Children's Hospital, which supports the array of children's health services across the Medical Center where newborns, children, adolescents and young adults receive the most comprehensive and advanced care by a team of pediatricians and pediatric specialists.

The Neonatology Program at NYU Langone Medical Center addresses the unique emotional and developmental needs of infants with a program that combines family-centered care and state-of-the-art technology. We specialize in the following areas:

Neonatal Intensive Care
The Neonatal Intensive Care Unit (NICU) provides the most advanced care in New York City for neonates requiring intensive care and works closely with pediatric general and cardiac surgery, neurosurgery and craniofacial surgery. As a Regional Perinatal Center, the program additionally offers early intervention evaluation services and comprehensive family support and education.

Continuing Care
Because many premature babies may be at an increased risk for problems in growth and development, the Neonatal Comprehensive Continuing Care Program (NCCCP) follows these infants from birth through pre-school, providing evaluation and assessment of problems as soon as they arise.

Hypothermia Program
The Hypothermia Program at NYU Langone Medical Center is a full multidisciplinary service with neonatal transport and inpatient and outpatient follow-up services. The program provides rapid response treatment and assessment of infants who have birth asphyxia.

Infant Apnea and SIDS
The Infant Apnea and SIDS Program at the Bellevue Hospital Center, an affiliate of NYU Langone Medical Center, provides treatment to critically ill infants through its Neonatal Intensive Care Unit, and to other children at risk for apnea, sudden infant death syndrome (SIDS) and other life-threatening events.

Neonatal Transport
As a designated New York State Regional Perinatal Center, the Division of Neonatology cares for over one-fifth of New York City's mothers and infants. As part of that massive effort, it offers an active transport program to bring mothers and/or their newborns to NYU Langone Medical Center's Tisch Hospital for specialized intensive care.

The Best in American Medicine
www.CastleConnolly.com

Nephrology
a subspecialty of Internal Medicine

An internist who treats disorders of the kidney, high blood pressure, fluid and mineral balance and dialysis of body wastes when the kidneys do not function. This specialist consults with surgeons about kidney transplantation.

Training Required: Three years in internal medicine *plus* additional training and examination for certification in nephrology.

NEPHROLOGY

New England

Bazari, Hasan MD [Nep] - **Spec Exp:** Kidney Failure-Acute; Nephrotic Syndrome; Hypertension; **Hospital:** Mass Genl Hosp; **Address:** Renal Assocs, Mass Genl Hosp, 165 Cambridge St, Ste 302, Boston, MA 02114; **Phone:** 617-726-5050; **Board Cert:** Internal Medicine 1986; Nephrology 1988; **Med School:** Albert Einstein Coll Med 1983; **Resid:** Internal Medicine, Mass Genl Hosp 1986; **Fellow:** Nephrology, Mass Genl Hosp 1988; **Fac Appt:** Assoc Prof Med, Harvard Med Sch

Kliger, Alan MD [Nep] - **Spec Exp:** Kidney Disease; Kidney Disease-Metabolic; **Hospital:** Hosp of St Raphael; **Address:** 136 Sherman Ave, New Haven, CT 06511; **Phone:** 203-787-0117 x307; **Board Cert:** Internal Medicine 1973; Nephrology 1976; **Med School:** SUNY Upstate Med Univ 1970; **Resid:** Internal Medicine, SUNY Upstate Med Ctr 1973; **Fellow:** Nephrology, Georgetown Univ Hosp 1975; **Fac Appt:** Clin Prof Med, Yale Univ

Perrone, Ronald MD [Nep] - **Spec Exp:** Kidney Disease-Chronic; Kidney Failure-Acute; Polycystic Kidney Disease; Hypertension; **Hospital:** Tufts Med Ctr; **Address:** Tufts Med Ctr, Div Nephrology, 750 Washington St, Box 391, Boston, MA 02111; **Phone:** 617-636-5866; **Board Cert:** Internal Medicine 1979; Nephrology 1982; **Med School:** Hahnemann Univ 1975; **Resid:** Internal Medicine, Grady Meml Hosp 1978; **Fellow:** Nephrology, Boston Med Ctr 1982; **Fac Appt:** Prof Med, Tufts Univ

Salant, David MD [Nep] - **Spec Exp:** Kidney Disease-Glomerular; Kidney Disease-Autoimmune; Lupus Nephritis; Vasculitis; **Hospital:** Boston Med Ctr; **Address:** Boston Univ Med Ctr, 650 Albany St, Ste X504, Boston, MA 02118; **Phone:** 617-638-7330; **Board Cert:** Internal Medicine 1978; Nephrology 1980; **Med School:** South Africa 1969; **Resid:** Internal Medicine, Johannesburg Genl Hosp 1973; **Fellow:** Nephrology, Boston Univ Med Ctr 1978; **Fac Appt:** Prof Med, Boston Univ

Seifter, Julian L MD [Nep] - **Spec Exp:** Diabetic Kidney Disease; Kidney Failure-Chronic; Kidney Stones; **Hospital:** Brigham and Women's Hosp (page 57); **Address:** Brigham & Women's Hosp, Div Renal Med, 45 Francis St Fl 8, Boston, MA 02115; **Phone:** 617-732-6383; **Board Cert:** Internal Medicine 1978; Nephrology 1980; **Med School:** Albert Einstein Coll Med 1975; **Resid:** Internal Medicine, Bronx Muni Hosp Ctr 1981; **Fellow:** Nephrology, Yale-New Haven Hosp 1982; **Fac Appt:** Prof Med, Harvard Med Sch

Tolkoff-Rubin, Nina MD [Nep] - **Spec Exp:** Transplant Medicine-Kidney; Hypertension; Kidney Failure-Acute; Polycystic Kidney Disease; **Hospital:** Mass Genl Hosp; **Address:** Mass General Hospital, 55 Fruit St, GRB 1003J, Boston, MA 02114; **Phone:** 617-726-3706; **Board Cert:** Nephrology 1974; Internal Medicine 1972; **Med School:** Harvard Med Sch 1968; **Resid:** Internal Medicine, Mass Genl Hosp 1970; Internal Medicine, Mass Genl Hosp 1972; **Fellow:** Nephrology, Mass Genl Hosp 1971; **Fac Appt:** Assoc Prof Med, Harvard Med Sch

Mid Atlantic

Appel, Gerald B MD/PhD [Nep] - **Spec Exp:** Glomerulonephritis; Lupus Nephritis; Nephrotic Syndrome; **Hospital:** NY-Presby/Columbia Univ Med Ctr, NY (page 66); **Address:** 161 Fort Washington Ave Fl 2 - Ste 202, New York, NY 10032-3720; **Phone:** 212-305-0320 x3; **Board Cert:** Internal Medicine 1975; Nephrology 1978; **Med School:** Albert Einstein Coll Med 1972; **Resid:** Internal Medicine, Columbia Presby Hosp 1975; **Fellow:** Nephrology, Columbia Presby Hosp 1976; Nephrology, Yale-New Haven Hosp 1978; **Fac Appt:** Clin Prof Med, Columbia P&S

August, Phyllis MD [Nep] - **Spec Exp:** Hypertension; Hypertension in Pregnancy; Hypertension/Kidney Disease; **Hospital:** NY-Presby/Weill Cornell Med Ctr, NY (page 66); **Address:** 450 E 69th St, Hypertension Center, New York, NY 10021-4870; **Phone:** 212-746-2210; **Board Cert:** Internal Medicine 1980; Nephrology 1982; **Med School:** Yale Univ 1977; **Resid:** Internal Medicine, NY Hosp-Cornell Med Ctr 1980; **Fellow:** Nephrology, NY Hosp-Cornell Med Ctr 1983; **Fac Appt:** Prof Med, Cornell Univ-Weill Med Coll

Bernardo, Jose F MD [Nep] - **Spec Exp:** Kidney Disease; Dialysis Care; **Hospital:** UPMC Mercy, Pittsburgh; **Address:** UPMC Kidney Clin, 120 Lytton Ave, Ste 300, Pittsburgh, PA 15213; **Phone:** 412-802-3043; **Board Cert:** Internal Medicine 2009; Nephrology 2001; **Med School:** Peru 1984; **Resid:** Internal Medicine, Universidad Peruana 1989; Internal Medicine, UPMC 2000; **Fellow:** Nephrology, UPMC 2002; **Fac Appt:** Asst Prof Med, Univ Pittsburgh

Berns, Jeffrey S MD [Nep] - **Spec Exp:** Kidney Disease; Glomerulonephritis; Hypertension; **Hospital:** Hosp Univ Penn - UPHS (page 72); **Address:** Hosp Univ Penn, 3400 Spruce St Fl 1 - Ste 300S, 1 Founders Pavilion, Philadelphia, PA 19104; **Phone:** 215-662-7934; **Board Cert:** Internal Medicine 1984; Nephrology 2011; **Med School:** Case West Res Univ 1981; **Resid:** Internal Medicine, Univ Hosp 1984; **Fellow:** Nephrology, Yale-New Haven Hosp 1987; **Fac Appt:** Prof Med, Univ Pennsylvania

Black, Henry R MD [Nep] - **Spec Exp:** Hypertension; **Hospital:** NYU Langone Med Ctr (page 68); **Address:** NYU Medical Ctr, 530 First Ave, SKI-9U, New York, NY 10016; **Phone:** 212-263-7751; **Board Cert:** Internal Medicine 1972; Nephrology 1974; **Med School:** NYU Sch Med 1967; **Resid:** Internal Medicine, Johns Hopkins Hosp 1971; Internal Medicine, Yale-New Haven Hosp 1972; **Fellow:** Nephrology, Yale-New Haven Hosp 1974; **Fac Appt:** Clin Prof Med, NYU Sch Med

Blumenfeld, Jon D MD [Nep] - **Spec Exp:** Polycystic Kidney Disease; Hypertension; Adrenal Disorders; **Hospital:** NY-Presby/Weill Cornell Med Ctr, NY (page 66), Rockefeller Univ; **Address:** The Rogosin Institute, 505 E 70th St Fl 2, New York, NY 10021; **Phone:** 212-746-1495; **Board Cert:** Internal Medicine 1984; Nephrology 1986; **Med School:** Yale Univ 1981; **Resid:** Internal Medicine, New York Hosp 1984; **Fellow:** Nephrology, Brigham & Womens Hosp 1988; **Fac Appt:** Prof Med, Cornell Univ-Weill Med Coll

Cohen, David J MD [Nep] - **Spec Exp:** Transplant Medicine-Kidney; Glomerulonephritis; **Hospital:** NY-Presby/Columbia Univ Med Ctr, NY (page 66); **Address:** Columbia Univ Med Ctr, 622 W 168th St, rm PH 4-124, New York, NY 10032-3720; **Phone:** 212-305-0320 x4; **Board Cert:** Internal Medicine 1980; Nephrology 1984; **Med School:** Albert Einstein Coll Med 1977; **Resid:** Internal Medicine, Mount Sinai Hosp 1980; **Fellow:** Nephrology, Columbia-Presby Hosp 1981; Transplant Immunobiology, Brigham & Womens Hosp 1983; **Fac Appt:** Clin Prof Med, Columbia P&S

Dember, Laura MD [Nep] - **Spec Exp:** Kidney Failure-Chronic; Nephrotic Syndrome; Amyloidosis; **Hospital:** Hosp Univ Penn - UPHS (page 72); **Address:** Perelman Center for Advanced Medicine, South Pavilion, 1st Fl, 3400 Civic Center Blvd, Ste 1-300S, Philadelphia, PA 19104; **Phone:** 215-662-2638; **Board Cert:** Internal Medicine 2000; Nephrology 2000; **Med School:** Yale Univ 1988; **Resid:** Internal Medicine, Hosp Univ Penn 1991; **Fellow:** Nephrology, Hosp Univ Penn 1992; Nephrology, Brigham & Womens Hosp 1995; **Fac Appt:** Assoc Prof Med, Boston Univ

Johnston, James R MD [Nep] - **Spec Exp:** Diabetic Kidney Disease; Hypertension; **Hospital:** UPMC Presby, Pittsburgh; **Address:** UPMC Kidney Clinic, 120 Winton Ave, Ste 300, Pittsburgh, PA 15213; **Phone:** 412-802-3043; **Board Cert:** Internal Medicine 1982; Nephrology 1984; **Med School:** Univ Pittsburgh 1979; **Resid:** Internal Medicine, Montefiore Hosp 1982; **Fellow:** Nephrology, Univ Pittsburgh Med Ctr 1983; Nephrology, Brigham & Women's Hosp 1986; **Fac Appt:** Prof Med, Univ Pittsburgh

Kelepouris, Ellie MD [Nep] - **Spec Exp:** Kidney Stones; Hypertension; **Hospital:** Hahnemann Univ Hosp; **Address:** 219 N Broad St Fl 9, Philadelphia, PA 19107; **Phone:** 215-762-2688; **Board Cert:** Nephrology 2008; **Med School:** Greece 1976; **Resid:** Internal Medicine, Mercy Cath Med Ctr 1979; **Fellow:** Nephrology, Hosp U Penn 1982; **Fac Appt:** Prof Med, Drexel Univ Coll Med

Kobrin, Sidney M MD [Nep] - **Spec Exp:** Diabetic Kidney Disease; Kidney Failure; Hypertension; Dialysis Care; **Hospital:** Hosp Univ Penn - UPHS (page 72); **Address:** Univ Penn, Div Nephrology, Perelman Ctr for Advanced Medicine, 3400 Civic Center Blvd, Ste 1-300 S, Philadelphia, PA 19104; **Phone:** 215-662-2638; **Board Cert:** Nephrology 2002; **Med School:** South Africa 1978; **Resid:** Internal Medicine, Johannesburg Tchg Hosp 1984; **Fellow:** Nephrology, Einstein Med Ctr 1988; **Fac Appt:** Assoc Prof Med, Univ Pennsylvania

Piraino, Beth Marie MD [Nep] - **Spec Exp:** Kidney Failure; Hypertension; **Hospital:** UPMC Presby, Pittsburgh; **Address:** 3504 Fifth Ave, Ste 200, Pittsburgh, PA 15213; **Phone:** 412-383-4899; **Board Cert:** Internal Medicine 1980; Nephrology 1982; **Med School:** Med Coll PA Hahnemann 1977; **Resid:** Internal Medicine, Presby Univ Hosp 1980; **Fellow:** Nephrology, Presby Univ Hosp 1982; **Fac Appt:** Prof Med, Univ Pittsburgh

Rudnick, Michael R MD [Nep] - **Spec Exp:** Hypertension; Kidney Disease; Kidney Failure-Acute; **Hospital:** Penn Presby Med Ctr - UPHS (page 72); **Address:** Presbyterian Med Ctr, Medical Office Bldg, Penn Presbyterian - 39th and Market Sts, MOB Bldg, Ste 240, Philadelphia, PA 19104; **Phone:** 215-662-8730; **Board Cert:** Internal Medicine 1975; Nephrology 1976; **Med School:** Hahnemann Univ 1972; **Resid:** Internal Medicine, Hahnemann Univ Med Ctr 1974; **Fellow:** Nephrology, Hosp Univ Penn 1976; **Fac Appt:** Assoc Prof Med, Univ Pennsylvania

Stern, Leonard MD [Nep] - **Spec Exp:** Kidney Failure-Chronic; Transplant Medicine-Kidney; Bone Disorders-Metabolic; Dialysis Care; **Hospital:** NY-Presby/Columbia Univ Med Ctr, NY (page 66); **Address:** 622 W 168th St, rm PH4-124, New York, NY 10032-3702; **Phone:** 212-305-3273; **Board Cert:** Internal Medicine 1978; Nephrology 1980; **Med School:** NY Med Coll 1975; **Resid:** Internal Medicine, Jacobi Med Ctr 1978; **Fellow:** Nephrology, Montefiore Med Ctr 1979; Nephrology, Yale-New Haven Hosp 1981; **Fac Appt:** Assoc Clin Prof Med, Columbia P&S

Townsend, Raymond R MD [Nep] - **Spec Exp:** Hypertension-Complex; Renal Artery Stenosis; Kidney Disease-Chronic; **Hospital:** Hosp Univ Penn - UPHS (page 72); **Address:** Univ Penn, Div Nephrology, Perelman Ctr for Advanced Medicine, 3400 Civic Center Blvd, Ste 1-300 S, Philadelphia, PA 19104; **Phone:** 215-662-2638; **Board Cert:** Internal Medicine 1982; Nephrology 1984; **Med School:** Hahnemann Univ 1979; **Resid:** Internal Medicine, Allegheny Genl Hosp 1982; **Fellow:** Nephrology, Temple Univ Hosp 1984; **Fac Appt:** Prof Med, Univ Pennsylvania

Wilcox, Christopher S MD/PhD [Nep] - **Spec Exp:** Hypertension-Renovascular; Hypertension-Drug Resistent; **Hospital:** Georgetown Univ Hosp; **Address:** Georgetown Univ Med Ctr, 3800 Reservoir Rd NW, PHC, PHC Bldg Fl 6 - rm F6003, Washington, DC 20007-2113; **Phone:** 202-444-9183; **Board Cert:** Internal Medicine 1983; Nephrology 1986; **Med School:** England, UK 1968; **Resid:** Internal Medicine, Middlesex Hosp 1971; Nephrology, Middlesex Hosp 1972; **Fellow:** Nephrology, Middlesex Hosp 1975; **Fac Appt:** Prof Med, Georgetown Univ

Williams, Gail S MD [Nep] - **Spec Exp:** Kidney Failure-Chronic; Transplant Medicine-Kidney; **Hospital:** NY-Presby/Columbia Univ Med Ctr, NY (page 66); **Address:** 161 Fort Washington Ave, Ste 351, New York, NY 10032; **Phone:** 212-305-5376; **Board Cert:** Internal Medicine 1972; Nephrology 1974; **Med School:** Columbia P&S 1968; **Resid:** Internal Medicine, Columbia Presby Hosp 1973; **Fellow:** Nephrology, Columbia Presby Hosp 1974; **Fac Appt:** Assoc Clin Prof Med, Columbia P&S

Winston, Jonathan MD [Nep] - **Spec Exp:** Kidney Disease-Chronic; Kidney Failure; HIV Related Kidney Disease; Glomerulonephritis; **Hospital:** Mount Sinai Med Ctr (page 64); **Address:** 5 E 98th St Fl 11, New York, NY 10029-6501; **Phone:** 212-241-4060; **Board Cert:** Internal Medicine 1980; Nephrology 1984; **Med School:** Geo Wash Univ 1977; **Resid:** Internal Medicine, LI Jewish Med Ctr 1980; **Fellow:** Nephrology, Mt Sinai Hosp 1982; **Fac Appt:** Assoc Prof Med, Mount Sinai Sch Med

Southeast

Allon, Michael MD [Nep] - **Spec Exp:** Dialysis Care; **Hospital:** Univ of Ala Hosp at Birmingham; **Address:** UAB Nephrology, 1530 3rd Ave S, PB 226, Birmingham, AL 35294; **Phone:** 205-975-9676; **Board Cert:** Internal Medicine 1985; Nephrology 1988; **Med School:** Univ Mich Med Sch 1982; **Resid:** Internal Medicine, Emory Univ Hosp 1985; **Fellow:** Nephrology, Emory Univ 1987; **Fac Appt:** Prof Med, Univ Alabama

Bolton, W Kline MD [Nep] - **Spec Exp:** Kidney Disease-Glomerular; Kidney Disease-Chronic; Glomerulonephritis; **Hospital:** Univ of Virginia Health Sys; **Address:** Univ VA Hlth Scis Ctr, Box 800 133, Charlottesville, VA 22908-0001; **Phone:** 434-924-5125; **Board Cert:** Internal Medicine 1972; Nephrology 1974; **Med School:** Univ VA Sch Med 1969; **Resid:** Internal Medicine, Boston City Hosp 1971; **Fellow:** Nephrology, Univ Chicago 1973; **Fac Appt:** Prof Med, Univ VA Sch Med

Butterly, David W MD [Nep] - **Spec Exp:** Transplant Medicine-Kidney; Kidney Disease; **Hospital:** Duke Univ Hosp; **Address:** Duke Box 2747, 2424 Erwin Rd, Ste 605, Durham, NC 27705; **Phone:** 919-668-7630; **Board Cert:** Internal Medicine 2000; Nephrology 2000; **Med School:** Duke Univ 1987; **Resid:** Internal Medicine, Duke Univ Med Ctr 1990; **Fellow:** Nephrology, Duke Univ Med Ctr 1992

Coffman, Thomas M MD [Nep] - **Spec Exp:** Transplant Medicine-Kidney; Hypertension; **Hospital:** Duke Univ Hosp, Durham VA Med Ctr; **Address:** Duke Box 103015, Room 2018/MSRB 2, 106 Research Drive, Durham, NC 27710; **Phone:** 919-684-9708; **Board Cert:** Internal Medicine 1983; Nephrology 1988; **Med School:** Ohio State Univ 1980; **Resid:** Internal Medicine, Duke Univ Med Ctr 1983; **Fellow:** Nephrology, Duke Univ Med Ctr 1985; **Fac Appt:** Prof Med, Duke Univ

Falk, Ronald J MD [Nep] - **Spec Exp:** Glomerulonephritis; Lupus Nephritis; Wegener's Granulomatosis; Vasculitis; **Hospital:** NC Memorial Hosp - UNC; **Address:** UNC Kidney Ctr, 7024 Burnett Womack Bldg CB #7155, Chapel Hill, NC 27599-7155; **Phone:** 919-966-2561; **Board Cert:** Internal Medicine 1980; Nephrology 1982; **Med School:** Univ NC Sch Med 1977; **Resid:** Internal Medicine, Univ North Carolina Hosps 1980; Nephrology, Univ NC 1981; **Fellow:** Research, Univ Minn 1983; **Fac Appt:** Prof Med, Univ NC Sch Med

Fulop, Tibor MD [Nep] - **Hospital:** Univ Mississippi Med Ctr; **Address:** 2500 N State St, Jackson, MS 39216; **Phone:** 601-925-2292; **Board Cert:** Internal Medicine 2005; Nephrology 2007; **Med School:** Hungary 1990; **Resid:** Internal Medicine, Henry Ford Hosp 1995; **Fellow:** Nephrology, Henry Ford Hosp 1997; Nephrology, Univ of Iowa Hosp & Clin 1998

Gaston, Robert S MD [Nep] - **Spec Exp:** Transplant Medicine-Kidney; Kidney Disease; Dialysis Care; **Hospital:** Univ of Ala Hosp at Birmingham; **Address:** Univ Alabama Hosp, Div Nephrology, 1530 3rd Ave S, THT 625, Birmingham, AL 35294; **Phone:** 205-934-7220; **Board Cert:** Internal Medicine 1982; Nephrology 1986; **Med School:** St Louis Univ 1979; **Resid:** Internal Medicine, Univ Hosp Arkansas 1982; **Fellow:** Nephrology, Univ Hosp Arkansas 1986; Transplant Medicine, Univ Alabama Med Ctr 1988; **Fac Appt:** Prof Med, Univ Alabama

Nephrology

Helderman, J Harold MD [Nep] - **Spec Exp:** Transplant Medicine-Kidney; Kidney Disease-Glomerular; Kidney Disease-Autoimmune; **Hospital:** Vanderbilt Univ Med Ctr (page 75); **Address:** Vanderbilt-Div Nephrology & Hypertension, 1301 Med Ctr Drive, Ste 2501, Nashville, TN 37232; **Phone:** 615-343-7592; **Board Cert:** Internal Medicine 1974; **Med School:** SUNY Downstate 1971; **Resid:** Internal Medicine, Johns Hopkins Hosp 1973; **Fellow:** Nephrology, Harvard Univ 1976; **Fac Appt:** Prof Med, Vanderbilt Univ

Lea, Janice I MD [Nep] - **Spec Exp:** Hypertension-Complex; Kidney Disease-Chronic; Diabetic Kidney Disease; Dialysis Care; **Hospital:** Emory Univ Hosp Midtown; **Address:** Emory Midtown-Div Nephrology, 550 Peachtree St NE, Medical Office Tower, Fl 7, Atlanta, GA 30308; **Phone:** 404-686-5038; **Board Cert:** Nephrology 2005; **Med School:** Univ Tex Med Br, Galveston 1988; **Resid:** Internal Medicine, Emory Univ Affil Hosps 1991; **Fellow:** Nephrology, Emory Univ Affil Hosps 1994; **Fac Appt:** Prof Med, Emory Univ

Okusa, Mark D MD [Nep] - **Spec Exp:** Kidney Failure-Chronic; Nephrotic Syndrome; Kidney Failure-Acute; **Hospital:** Univ of Virginia Health Sys; **Address:** Univ VA Hlth Sci Ctr, Div Nephrology, Box 800133, Charlottesville, VA 22908-0001; **Phone:** 434-924-2187; **Board Cert:** Internal Medicine 1985; Nephrology 1988; **Med School:** Med Coll VA 1982; **Resid:** Internal Medicine, Med Coll Virginia 1985; **Fellow:** Nephrology, Yale Univ Sch Med 1988; **Fac Appt:** Prof Med, Univ VA Sch Med

Rakowski, Thomas A MD [Nep] - **Spec Exp:** Polycystic Kidney Disease; Kidney Disease-Glomerular; **Hospital:** Virginia Hosp Ctr - Arlington, Inova Fairfax Hosp; **Address:** Virginia Nephrology Group, 1635 N George Mason Drive, Ste 215, Arlington, VA 22205; **Phone:** 703-841-0707; **Board Cert:** Internal Medicine 1972; Nephrology 1974; **Med School:** Hahnemann Univ 1969; **Resid:** Internal Medicine, Georgetown Univ 1971; **Fellow:** Nephrology, Georgetown Univ 1973; **Fac Appt:** Assoc Prof Med, Georgetown Univ

Roth, David MD [Nep] - **Spec Exp:** Transplant Medicine-Kidney; Kidney Failure-Chronic; **Hospital:** Jackson Meml Hosp, Univ of Miami Hosp; **Address:** 1120 NW 14 th St, rm 813, PO Box 016960 (R-126), Miami, FL 33136; **Phone:** 305-243-6251; **Board Cert:** Internal Medicine 1980; Nephrology 1982; **Med School:** SUNY Downstate 1977; **Resid:** Internal Medicine, Jackson Meml Hosp 1980; **Fellow:** Nephrology, Jackson Meml Hosp 1982; **Fac Appt:** Prof Med, Univ Miami Sch Med

Warnock, David G MD [Nep] - **Spec Exp:** Liddle's Syndrome; Kidney Stones; Nephrotic Syndrome; **Hospital:** Univ of Ala Hosp at Birmingham; **Address:** UAB Nephrology, 1530 3rd Ave S, ZRB 636, Birmingham, AL 35294-0006; **Phone:** 205-934-9509; **Board Cert:** Internal Medicine 1973; Nephrology 2000; **Med School:** UCSF 1970; **Resid:** Internal Medicine, UCSF Med Ctr 1973; **Fellow:** Nephrology, Natl Inst Hlth 1975; **Fac Appt:** Prof Med, Univ Alabama

Weiner, I David MD [Nep] - **Spec Exp:** Kidney Disease; Fluid/Electrolyte Balance; Kidney Stones; Adrenal Disorders; **Hospital:** Shands at Univ of FL; **Address:** Shands at Univ Florida, Dept Nephrology, PO Box 100224, Gainesville, FL 32610-0224; **Phone:** 352-273-8821; **Board Cert:** Internal Medicine 1987; Nephrology 2011; **Med School:** Vanderbilt Univ 1984; **Resid:** Internal Medicine, UT Hlth Sci Ctr 1987; **Fellow:** Nephrology, Wash Univ 1990; **Fac Appt:** Prof Med, Univ Fla Coll Med

Midwest

Brennan, Daniel C MD [Nep] - **Spec Exp:** Transplant Medicine-Kidney; **Hospital:** Barnes-Jewish Hosp; **Address:** Wash Univ Sch Med, Div Renal Diseases, 660 S Euclid Ave, Box 8126, St Louis, MO 63110; **Phone:** 314-362-7603; **Board Cert:** Internal Medicine 1988; Nephrology 2002; **Med School:** Univ Iowa Coll Med 1985; **Resid:** Internal Medicine, Univ Iowa Hosps 1988; **Fellow:** Nephrology, Brigham and Women's Hosp 1992; **Fac Appt:** Assoc Prof Med, Washington Univ, St Louis

Coe, Fredric MD [Nep] - **Spec Exp:** Kidney Stones; Fluid/Electrolyte Balance; **Hospital:** Univ of Chicago Med Ctr; **Address:** 5841 S Maryland Ave, MC 5100, Chicago, IL 60637; **Phone:** 773-702-1475; **Board Cert:** Internal Medicine 1968; **Med School:** Univ Chicago-Pritzker Sch Med 1961; **Resid:** Internal Medicine, Michael Reese Hosp 1965; **Fellow:** Renal Disease, Univ Texas SW 1969; **Fac Appt:** Prof Med, Univ Chicago-Pritzker Sch Med

Delmez, James MD [Nep] - **Spec Exp:** Kidney Disease; **Hospital:** Barnes-Jewish Hosp, Washington Univ Physicians; **Address:** Wash Univ Sch Med, Div Renal Diseases, 660 S Euclid Ave, Box 8126, St Louis, MO 63110; **Phone:** 314-362-7603; **Board Cert:** Internal Medicine 1976; Nephrology 1982; **Med School:** Univ Rochester 1973; **Resid:** Internal Medicine, Barnes Hosp 1976; **Fellow:** Nephrology, Barnes Hosp 1978; **Fac Appt:** Prof Med, Washington Univ, St Louis

Hruska, Keith MD [Nep] - **Spec Exp:** Kidney Disease-Pediatric & Adult; Kidney Stones; Bone Disorders-Metabolic; Inherited Metabolic Disorders; **Hospital:** St. Louis Chldns Hosp, Barnes-Jewish Hosp; **Address:** St Louis Chldns Hosp, Dept Peds, 660 S Euclid Ave Fl 5MPRB, Box 8208, St Louis, MO 63110-1010; **Phone:** 314-286-2772; **Board Cert:** Internal Medicine 1972; Nephrology 1976; **Med School:** Creighton Univ 1969; **Resid:** Internal Medicine, New York Hosp-Cornell 1971; Internal Medicine, Barnes Hosp-Wash Univ 1972; **Fellow:** Nephrology, Barnes Hosp-Wash Univ 1974; **Fac Appt:** Prof Ped, Washington Univ, St Louis

Josephson, Michelle A MD [Nep] - **Spec Exp:** Transplant Medicine-Kidney; Hypertension; **Hospital:** Univ of Chicago Med Ctr; **Address:** Div Nephrology, 5841 S Maryland Ave, MC 5100, Chicago, IL 60637; **Phone:** 773-702-6134; **Board Cert:** Internal Medicine 1986; Nephrology 2010; **Med School:** Univ Pennsylvania 1983; **Resid:** Internal Medicine, Univ Chicago Hosps 1986; **Fellow:** Nephrology, Univ Chicago Hosps 1991; **Fac Appt:** Assoc Clin Prof Med, Univ Chicago-Pritzker Sch Med

Kasiske, Bertram MD [Nep] - **Spec Exp:** Transplant Medicine-Kidney; Kidney Disease-Geriatric; **Hospital:** Hennepin Cnty Med Ctr; **Address:** Hennepin Cnty Med Ctr, Div Nephrology, 701 Park Ave, Minneapolis, MN 55415; **Phone:** 612-347-6088; **Board Cert:** Internal Medicine 1980; Nephrology 1982; **Med School:** Univ Iowa Coll Med 1976; **Resid:** Internal Medicine, Hennepin Co Med Ctr 1980; **Fellow:** Nephrology, Hennepin Co Med Ctr 1983; **Fac Appt:** Prof Med, Univ Minn

Kraus, Michael A MD [Nep] - **Spec Exp:** Kidney Disease-Chronic; Kidney Failure-Acute; Dialysis Care; **Hospital:** IU Health University Hosp, IU Health North Hosp; **Address:** 8803 N Meridian St, Ste 150, Indianapolis, IN 46260; **Phone:** 317-963-6875; **Board Cert:** Internal Medicine 1988; Nephrology 2002; **Med School:** Indiana Univ 1985; **Resid:** Internal Medicine, Indiana Univ Med Ctr 1988; **Fellow:** Nephrology, Univ Iowa 1991; **Fac Appt:** Clin Prof Med, Indiana Univ

McCarthy, James T MD [Nep] - **Spec Exp:** Kidney Failure-Chronic; Dialysis Care; **Hospital:** Mayo Med Ctr & Clin - Rochester; **Address:** Mayo Clin, Div Nephrology/Hypertension, 200 First St SW, Rochester, MN 55905; **Phone:** 507-266-6711; **Board Cert:** Internal Medicine 1980; Nephrology 1982; **Med School:** Univ Kansas 1977; **Resid:** Internal Medicine, Mayo Clin 1980; **Fellow:** Nephrology, Mayo Clin 1983; **Fac Appt:** Prof Med, Mayo Med Sch

Miller, Brent W MD [Nep] - **Spec Exp:** Kidney Failure-Chronic; Transplant Medicine-Kidney; Dialysis Care; **Hospital:** Barnes-Jewish Hosp; **Address:** Wash Univ Sch Med, Div Renal Diseases, 660 S Euclid Ave, Box 8126, St Louis, MO 63110; **Phone:** 314-362-7603; **Board Cert:** Internal Medicine 2003; Nephrology 2007; **Med School:** Washington Univ, St Louis 1990; **Resid:** Internal Medicine, Washington Univ Sch Med 1994; **Fellow:** Nephrology, Washington Univ Sch Med 1998; **Fac Appt:** Assoc Prof Med, Univ Wash

Pohl, Marc MD [Nep] - **Spec Exp:** Hypertension; Kidney Disease; Diabetic Kidney Disease; **Hospital:** Cleveland Clin (page 55); **Address:** Dept Nephrology & Hypertension, 9500 Euclid Ave, Desk Q7, Cleveland, OH 44195; **Phone:** 216-444-6776; **Board Cert:** Internal Medicine 1972; Nephrology 1978; **Med School:** Case West Res Univ 1966; **Resid:** Internal Medicine, Univ Hosps 1968; Internal Medicine, Mass Genl Hosp 1971; **Fellow:** Nephrology, Boston City Hosp-Boston Univ 1972; Nephrology, Mass Genl Hosp 1973

Rodby, Roger A MD [Nep] - **Spec Exp:** Diabetic Kidney Disease; Glomerulonephritis; Lupus Nephritis; **Hospital:** Rush Univ Med Ctr; **Address:** 1426 W Washington Blvd, Chicago, IL 60607; **Phone:** 312-850-8434; **Board Cert:** Internal Medicine 1985; Nephrology 1988; **Med School:** Univ IL Coll Med 1982; **Resid:** Internal Medicine, UMDNJ-Rutgers 1985; **Fellow:** Nephrology, Rush/Presby-St Lukes 1987; **Fac Appt:** Prof Med, Rush Med Coll

Schreiber, Martin J MD [Nep] - **Spec Exp:** Dialysis Care; Diabetic Kidney Disease; Heart Failure in Kidney Disease; **Hospital:** Cleveland Clin (page 55); **Address:** Cleveland Clinic-Nephrology, 9500 Euclid Ave, Desk Q7, Cleveland, OH 44195; **Phone:** 216-444-6365; **Board Cert:** Internal Medicine 1984; Nephrology 2003; **Med School:** Wake Forest Univ 1976; **Resid:** Internal Medicine, Cleveland Clinic 1979; **Fellow:** Nephrology, Mass Genl Hosp 1980; Nephrology, Cleveland Clinic 1982

Schwartz, Gary Lee MD [Nep] - **Spec Exp:** Hypertension; Kidney Disease-Chronic; Diabetic Kidney Disease; **Hospital:** St. Mary's Hosp - Rochester MN (Mayo), Rochester Methodist Hosp; **Address:** Mayo Clinic, 200 1st St SW, Rochester, MN 55905-0002; **Phone:** 507-284-4083; **Board Cert:** Internal Medicine 1980; Nephrology 1982; **Med School:** Univ Wisc 1977; **Resid:** Internal Medicine, Mayo Clinic 1980; **Fellow:** Nephrology, Mayo Clinic 1982; **Fac Appt:** Assoc Clin Prof Med, Mayo Med Sch

Somerville, James H MD [Nep] - **Hospital:** Fairview Southdale Hosp, Fairview Ridges Hosp; **Address:** 6363 France Ave S, Ste 400, Edina, MN 55435; **Phone:** 952-920-2070; **Board Cert:** Internal Medicine 1978; Nephrology 1982; **Med School:** Univ MD Sch Med 1975; **Resid:** Internal Medicine, Hennepin Co Med Ctr 1978; **Fellow:** Nephrology, Hennepin Co Med Ctr 1980

Swartz, Richard D MD [Nep] - **Spec Exp:** Kidney Failure; Dialysis Care; **Hospital:** Univ of Michigan Hosp; **Address:** Univ Mich, Div Nephrology, 1500 E Med Ctr Drive, 3914 Taubman Ctr, Ann Arbor, MI 48109-0364; **Phone:** 734-647-9342; **Board Cert:** Internal Medicine 1975; Nephrology 1978; **Med School:** Univ Mich Med Sch 1970; **Resid:** Internal Medicine, Boston City Hosp 1975; Nephrology, Beth Israel Hosp-Harvard 1977; **Fac Appt:** Prof Med, Univ Mich Med Sch

Textor, Stephen C MD [Nep] - **Spec Exp:** Transplant Medicine-Kidney; Hypertension; Renal Artery Stenosis; **Hospital:** Mayo Med Ctr & Clin - Rochester; **Address:** Mayo Clin, Div Nephrology/Hypertension, 200 First St SW, rm MA 19-E, Rochester, MN 55905; **Phone:** 507-284-4083; **Board Cert:** Internal Medicine 1977; Nephrology 1980; **Med School:** UCLA 1973; **Resid:** Internal Medicine, Boston City Hosp 1977; **Fellow:** Nephrology, Boston Univ 1978; Hypertension, Fogarty Inst 1980; **Fac Appt:** Prof Med, Mayo Med Sch

Thomas, Christie P MD [Nep] - **Spec Exp:** Transplant Medicine-Kidney; Fabry's Disease; **Hospital:** Univ Iowa Hosp & Clinics; **Address:** UIHC Nephrology Dept, 200 Hawkins Drive, rm SE 419 GH, Iowa City, IA 52242; **Phone:** 319-356-4216; **Board Cert:** Internal Medicine 2007; Nephrology 2008; **Med School:** India 1982; **Resid:** Internal Medicine, MMM Hosp Kolenchery 1983; Internal Medicine, Genl Hosp 1986; **Fellow:** Nephrology, Univ Sheffield Hosp 1988; Nephrology, Case Western Res Univ Hosp 1991; **Fac Appt:** Prof Med, Univ Iowa Coll Med

Torres, Vicente E MD [Nep] - **Spec Exp:** Polycystic Kidney Disease; **Hospital:** Mayo Med Ctr & Clin - Rochester; **Address:** Mayo Clin, Div Nephrology/Hypertension, 200 First St SW, Mayo E-19, Rochester, MN 55905; **Phone:** 507-266-7093; **Board Cert:** Internal Medicine 1977; Nephrology 1980; **Med School:** Spain 1969; **Resid:** Internal Medicine, Mayo Med Ctr & Clin 1977; **Fellow:** Nephrology, Mayo Med Sch 1979; **Fac Appt:** Prof Med, Mayo Med Sch

Venkat, K K MD [Nep] - **Spec Exp:** Transplant Medicine-Kidney; Kidney Disease; **Hospital:** Henry Ford Hosp; **Address:** Henry Ford Hosp, Div Nephrology, 2799 W Grand Blvd, Ste K16, Detroit, MI 48202-2689; **Phone:** 313-916-2702; **Board Cert:** Internal Medicine 1977; Nephrology 1978; **Med School:** India 1970; **Resid:** Internal Medicine, Henry Ford Hosp 1976; **Fellow:** Nephrology, Henry Ford Hosp 1978

Yee, Jerry MD [Nep] - **Spec Exp:** Kidney Disease-Chronic; Hypertension; Diabetic Kidney Disease; **Hospital:** Henry Ford Hosp; **Address:** Henry Ford Hospital, 2799 W Grand Blvd, CFP-5, Detroit, MI 48202; **Phone:** 313-916-9405; **Board Cert:** Internal Medicine 1985; Nephrology 2002; **Med School:** Jefferson Med Coll 1982; **Resid:** Internal Medicine, Brooke AMC-Fort Sam 1985; **Fellow:** Nephrology, Temple Univ Hosp 1986; Hypertension, Hosp U Penn 1987; **Fac Appt:** Assoc Prof Med, Wayne State Univ

Southwest

Brennan, Stephen T MD [Nep] - **Spec Exp:** Transplant Medicine-Kidney; Kidney Stones; Kidney Failure-Chronic; **Hospital:** Methodist Hosp - Houston, St. Luke's Episcopal Hosp-Houston; **Address:** The Kidney Institute, 1415 La Concha Ln, Houston, TX 77054; **Phone:** 713-790-9080; **Board Cert:** Internal Medicine 1983; Nephrology 1988; **Med School:** Loyola Univ-Stritch Sch Med 1979; **Resid:** Internal Medicine, Loyola Univ Med Ctr 1983; **Fellow:** Nephrology, Univ Wash-Barnes Hosp 1986; **Fac Appt:** Assoc Clin Prof Med, Baylor Coll Med

Fadem, Stephen Z MD [Nep] - **Spec Exp:** Kidney Disease-Chronic; Kidney Failure; Hypertension; **Hospital:** Methodist Hosp - Houston, St. Luke's Episcopal Hosp-Houston; **Address:** 6624 Fannin St, Ste 1400, Houston, TX 77030; **Phone:** 713-795-5511; **Board Cert:** Internal Medicine 1976; Nephrology 1978; **Med School:** Univ Okla Coll Med 1973; **Resid:** Internal Medicine, UT MD Anderson Hosp 1976; **Fellow:** Renal Disease, UT San Antonio 1978; **Fac Appt:** Clin Prof Med, Baylor Coll Med

Kasinath, Balakuntalam S MD [Nep] - **Spec Exp:** Glomerulonephritis; Diabetic Kidney Disease; **Hospital:** Audie L Murphy Meml Vets Hosp - San Antonio, Univ Hlth Syst-San Antonio; **Address:** 7400 Merton Minter Blvd, San Antonio, TX 78229; **Phone:** 210-617-5300; **Board Cert:** Internal Medicine 1980; Nephrology 1982; **Med School:** India 1975; **Resid:** Internal Medicine, Ill Masonic Med Ctr 1980; **Fellow:** Nephrology, Univ Chicago Hosp 1983; **Fac Appt:** Prof Med, Univ Tex, San Antonio

Nephrology

Mitch, William MD [Nep] - **Spec Exp:** Nutrition; Hypertension; Kidney Failure; **Hospital:** St. Luke's Episcopal Hosp-Houston, Ben Taub Genl Hosp; **Address:** Baylor Internal Medicine Consultants, 6620 Main St, Ste 1375, Houston, TX 77030; **Phone:** 713-798-2500; **Board Cert:** Internal Medicine 1972; Nephrology 1978; **Med School:** Harvard Med Sch 1967; **Resid:** Internal Medicine, Brigham & Womens Hosp 1974; **Fellow:** Nephrology, Johns Hopkins Hosp 1973; **Fac Appt:** Prof Med, Baylor Coll Med

Nolan, Charles Raymond MD [Nep] - **Spec Exp:** Transplant Medicine-Kidney; Transpland Medicine-Pancreas; **Hospital:** Univ Hlth Syst-San Antonio; **Address:** University Transplant Ctr, 7703 Floyd Curl Drive, San Antonio, TX 78229; **Phone:** 210-567-5771; **Board Cert:** Internal Medicine 1983; Nephrology 1986; **Med School:** Univ Colorado 1980; **Resid:** Internal Medicine, Wilford Hall Medical Center 1983; **Fellow:** Nephrology, Univ Colorado Hosp 1985; **Fac Appt:** Prof Med, Univ Tex, San Antonio

Olivero, Juan J MD [Nep] - **Spec Exp:** Kidney Failure-Acute; Kidney Failure-Chronic; Fluid/Electrolyte Balance; Hypertension; **Hospital:** Methodist Hosp - Houston, St. Luke's Episcopal Hosp-Houston; **Address:** 6560 Fannin St, Scurlock Twr, Ste 2206, Houston, TX 77030; **Phone:** 713-790-4615; **Board Cert:** Internal Medicine 1974; Nephrology 1976; **Med School:** Guatemala 1970; **Resid:** Internal Medicine, Baylor Affil Hosps 1973; Internal Medicine, Ben Taub Genl Hosp 1974; **Fellow:** Nephrology, Baylor Affil Hosps 1975; **Fac Appt:** Clin Prof Med, Baylor Coll Med

Suki, Wadi N MD [Nep] - **Spec Exp:** Transplant Medicine-Kidney; Hypertension; Lupus Nephritis; **Hospital:** Methodist Hosp - Houston, St. Luke's Episcopal Hosp-Houston; **Address:** The Kidney Institute, 1415 La Concha Ln, Houston, TX 77054; **Phone:** 713-790-9080; **Board Cert:** Internal Medicine 1967; Nephrology 1972; **Med School:** Sudan 1959; **Resid:** Internal Medicine, Parkland Meml Hosp 1963; **Fellow:** Nephrology, Univ Tex SW Med Ctr 1961; Nephrology, Univ Tex SW Med Ctr 1965; **Fac Appt:** Clin Prof Med, Baylor Coll Med

Toto, Robert D MD [Nep] - **Spec Exp:** Hypertension/Kidney Disease; Dialysis Care; Diabetic Kidney Disease; Kidney Failure-Acute; **Hospital:** UT Southwestern Med Ctr at Dallas; **Address:** Transplant Prgm-Kidney & Liver, Professional Office Bldg 2, 5939 Harry Hines Blvd Fl 7 - Ste 700, Dallas, TX 75390; **Phone:** 214-645-1919; **Board Cert:** Internal Medicine 1980; Nephrology 1982; **Med School:** Univ IL Coll Med 1977; **Resid:** Internal Medicine, Univ Michigan Med Ctr 1979; Internal Medicine, Baylor Univ Med Ctr 1980; **Fellow:** Nephrology, US Public Hlth Svce Hosp 1981; Nephrology, UTSW Med Ctr 1983; **Fac Appt:** Prof Med, Univ Tex SW, Dallas

West Coast and Pacific

Ahmad, Suhail MD [Nep] - **Spec Exp:** Hypertension; Kidney Failure-Chronic; Kidney Stones; **Hospital:** Univ Wash Med Ctr; **Address:** Scribner Kidney Ctr, 2150 N 107th St, Ste 160, Seattle, WA 98133; **Phone:** 206-363-5090; **Med School:** India 1968; **Resid:** Internal Medicine, Univ Allahabad 1971; **Fellow:** Nephrology, Univ Washington Med Ctr 1978; **Fac Appt:** Assoc Prof Med, Univ Wash

Bennett, William M MD [Nep] - **Spec Exp:** Transplant Medicine-Kidney; **Hospital:** Legacy Good Samaritan Med Ctr; **Address:** Legacy Good Samaritan Hosp, Transplant Svcs, 1040 NW 22nd Ave, Ste 480, Portland, OR 97210; **Phone:** 503-413-6555; **Board Cert:** Internal Medicine 2002; Nephrology 2002; **Med School:** Northwestern Univ 1963; **Resid:** Internal Medicine, Chicago VA Rsch Hosp 1966; Internal Medicine, OR Hlth Sci Univ 1967; **Fellow:** Nephrology, Mass Genl Hosp 1970

Cho, Kerry C MD [Nep] - **Spec Exp:** Kidney Disease; Glomerulonephritis; **Hospital:** UCSF Med Ctr; **Address:** UCSF, Dept Nephrology, 521 Parnassus Ave, Ste C443, Box 0532, San Francisco, CA 94143-0532; **Phone:** 415-476-2173; **Board Cert:** Nephrology 2003; **Med School:** Cornell Univ-Weill Med Coll 1996; **Resid:** Internal Medicine, Univ Michigan Med Ctr 1999; **Fellow:** Nephrology, USCF Med Ctr 2002; **Fac Appt:** Asst Prof Med, UCSF

Ellison, David H MD [Nep] - **Spec Exp:** Bartter's Syndrome; Gitelman's Syndrome; Hypertension; **Hospital:** OR Hlth & Sci Univ; **Address:** OHSU-Div Nephrology, 3303 SW Bond Ave, MC CH12R, Portland, OR 97239-3098; **Phone:** 503-494-3442; **Board Cert:** Internal Medicine 1981; Nephrology 1986; **Med School:** Rush Med Coll 1978; **Resid:** Internal Medicine, Oregon Hlth Scis Univ 1981; **Fellow:** Research, Oregon Hlth Scis Univ 1982; Nephrology, Yale Univ 1985; **Fac Appt:** Prof Med, Oregon Hlth & Sci Univ

Gluck, Stephen L MD [Nep] - **Spec Exp:** Kidney Disease; Fluid/Electrolyte Balance; Hypertension; Kidney Stones; **Hospital:** UCSF Med Ctr; **Address:** UCSF, Div Nephrology, 521 Parnassus Ave, rm C443, Box 0532, San Francisco, CA 94143-0532; **Phone:** 415-476-2173; **Board Cert:** Internal Medicine 1980; Nephrology 1984; **Med School:** UCLA 1977; **Resid:** Internal Medicine, Columbia Presby Med Ctr 1980; **Fellow:** Nephrology, Columbia Presby Med Ctr 1983; **Fac Appt:** Prof Med, UCSF

Kaysen, George Alan MD/PhD [Nep] - **Spec Exp:** Kidney Disease-Metabolic; Kidney Failure-Chronic; **Hospital:** UC Davis Med Ctr, VA Northern California Health Care System; **Address:** UC Davis Med Ctr, Div Nephr, One Shields Ave, GBSF 6310, Davis, CA 95616; **Phone:** 530-752-4010; **Board Cert:** Internal Medicine 1975; Nephrology 1980; **Med School:** Albert Einstein Coll Med 1972; **Resid:** Internal Medicine, Bronx Muni Hosp 1975; **Fellow:** Renal Disease, Bronx Muni Hosp 1977; **Fac Appt:** Prof Med, UC Davis

King, Andrew J MD [Nep] - **Spec Exp:** Kidney Disease-Chronic; Hypertension; Dialysis Care; **Hospital:** Scripps Green Hosp; **Address:** Scripps Clinic Torrey Pines, 10666 N Torrey Pines Rd, Mail Drop N239, La Jolla, CA 92037-1027; **Phone:** 858-554-9765; **Board Cert:** Internal Medicine 1986; Nephrology 1988; **Med School:** Northwestern Univ 1983; **Resid:** Internal Medicine, Northwestern Meml Hosp 1986; **Fellow:** Nephrology, Brigham & Womens Hosp 1990; **Fac Appt:** Clin Prof Med, UCSD

Ott, Susan M MD [Nep] - **Spec Exp:** Bone Disorders-Metabolic; Osteoporosis; **Hospital:** Univ Wash Med Ctr; **Address:** Bone & Joint Center, UWMC- Roosevelt, 4245 Roosevelt Way NE, Box 354740, Seattle, WA 98105; **Phone:** 206-598-4288; **Board Cert:** Internal Medicine 1978; Nephrology 1982; **Med School:** Univ Wash 1974; **Resid:** Family Medicine, UC Davis Med Ctr 1978; **Fellow:** Nephrology, Univ Wash Med Ctr 1982; **Fac Appt:** Assoc Prof Med, Univ Wash

Riordan, John W MD [Nep] - **Hospital:** CA Pacific Med Ctr-Pacific Campus; **Address:** 2100 Webster St, Ste 412, San Francisco, CA 94115; **Phone:** 415-923-3815; **Board Cert:** Nephrology 2005; **Med School:** Univ Tex Med Br, Galveston 1987; **Resid:** Internal Medicine, Univ Texas Hlth Sci Ctr 1990; **Fellow:** Nephrology, UCSF Med Ctr 1995

Scandling Jr, John D MD [Nep] - **Spec Exp:** Transplant Medicine-Kidney; Transplant Medicine-Pancreas; **Hospital:** Stanford Univ Hosp & Clinics; **Address:** Stanford Nephrology/Transplant, 750 Welsh Rd, Ste 200, Palo Alto, CA 94304-1509; **Phone:** 650-725-9891; **Board Cert:** Internal Medicine 1981; Nephrology 1984; **Med School:** Med Coll VA 1978; **Resid:** Internal Medicine, West Virginia Univ Hosp 1981; **Fellow:** Nephrology, Univ Rochester 1983; **Fac Appt:** Prof Med, Stanford Univ

Nephrology

Ward, David M MD [Nep] - **Spec Exp:** Immunotherapy; Dialysis Care; Transplant Medicine-Kidney; **Hospital:** UCSD Med Ctr; **Address:** 200 W Arbor Drive, Ste 8781, San Diego, CA 92103; **Phone:** 619-543-2259; **Med School:** Scotland, UK 1971; **Resid:** Internal Medicine, Glasgow Royal Infirmary 1972; **Fellow:** Nephrology, Glasgow Royal Infirmary 1975; Immunopathology, Scripps Research Foundation 1977; **Fac Appt:** Prof Med, UCSD

◻️ Cleveland Clinic

Every life deserves world class care.

Nephrology

The Glickman Urological & Kidney Institute's Department of Nephrology & Hypertension provides comprehensive diagnostic and therapeutic services for patients with kidney disease and hypertension. The department participates in an active kidney transplant program, all modalities of dialysis care and clinical research studies of diabetic and other glomerular diseases. The nephrology program has been named #1 in the nation in *U.S. News & World Report's* Best Hospitals survey, and is renowned for expertise in renovascular hypertension, primary aldosteronism and pheochromocytoma.

Intensive Care Nephrology Services

The Department of Nephrology & Hypertension is a major participant in the intensive care setting. Our nephrologists are leaders in research into the risk factors for acute renal failure after surgeries and in evaluations and diagnosis of different techniques for treatment of acute renal failure, such as slow continuous ultrafiltration, continuous arterio-venous hemofiltration and venovenous hemofiltration.

Hypertension

We utilize the latest technology for accurate measurement of blood pressure and detailed risk assessment. Specialists tailor treatment to the individual needs of each patient. Patients with severe or uncontrolled resistant hypertension are seen in our Resistant Hypertension Clinic.

Chronic Kidney Disease (CKD)

Our CKD clinic provides health evaluation, screenings and treatment for patients. This innovative model of health management focuses on educating and involving the patient in his or her care. We focus on care of the entire patient with assessment of cardiovascular risk factors as well as care of kidney related problems.

Polycystic Kidney Disease (PKD)

Polycystic kidney disease can cause other health problems such as high blood pressure, frequent urination, low back pain and fatigue. Our nephrologists can help PKD patients create a health management plan for dealing with the disease.

Cleveland Clinic
Gickman Urological &
Kidney Institute
9500 Euclid Avenue
Cleveland, OH 44195

Offering Same-Day Appointments
Call 800.274.2009.

Treatment Guides
Cleveland Clinic has developed comprehensive treatment guides for many diseases and conditions. To download our free treatment guides, visit clevelandclinic.org/treatmentguides.

Online Medical Second Opinion
Call 216.444.3223 or
800.223.2273 ext. 43223 or
email eclevelandclinic@ccf.org.

Out-of-State Patients Assistance
Call 800.223.2273, ext. 55580 or
email medicalconcierge@ccf.org.

Visit Us At:
clevelandclinic.org

Follow Us On:
Facebook
www.facebook.com/clevelandclinic

Twitter
@ClevelandClinic

You Tube
www.youtube.com/clevelandclinic

Health Hub
health.clevelandclinic.org

MOUNT SINAI SCHOOL OF MEDICINE

THE MOUNT SINAI MEDICAL CENTER
PEDIATRIC PULMONOLOGY
One Gustave L. Levy Place
Fifth Avenue and 100th Street
New York, NY 10029-6574
Physician Referral: 1-800-MD-SINAI (637-4624)
www.kravischildrenshospital.org

PEDIATRIC PULMONOLOGY
Innovative Medicine, Family-Centered Care

At Mount Sinai's **Kravis Children's Hospital's Division of Pediatric Pulmonology**, we are dedicated to treating the full spectrum of children's respiratory illnesses, both common and complex, with a high level of skill and compassion. This dedication has led to our being **named among the top pediatric pulmonary services in America**, according to *U.S. News & World Report's* 2012-2013 ranking of "Best Children's Hospitals."

Under the direction of Alfin Vicencio, M.D., Division Chief, our team of award winning pediatric pulmonologists, nurse practitioners, nurse educators, nutritionists, social workers and respiratory therapists deliver evidence-based care to children with asthma, cystic fibrosis, chronic respiratory failure, bronchopulmonary dysplasia and other respiratory conditions.

Offering medical support and guidance, our **Children's Asthma Center** offers advanced diagnostic and treatment protocols for refractory asthma along with advanced pulmonary function testing, allergy testing, environmental assessment, nutritional evaluation, education, and family services. We teach patients and their parents or guardians to identify asthma triggers and offer a personalized asthma action plan for each patient—a process that has our patients experiencing fewer emergency department visits and hospitalizations, missing less school and enjoying more active lives. In addition, through outreach efforts and care delivered to children from East Harlem—an area with one of the highest asthma rates in the country—we have succeeded in empowering these patients to manage their disease and face the future with confidence.

To significantly enhance our pediatric flexible bronchoscopy service, we recently opened a new **Bronchoscopy Suite** that houses the most advanced technology for both diagnostic capabilities and interventional procedures.

FROM BENCH TO BEDSIDE
We have recently recruited Rosalind Wright, MD, MPH, to serve as Vice Chair for Transitional Research and as a member of the Division of Pediatric Pulmonology. Dr. Wright is recognized both nationally and internationally for her investigations into early life events in relation to the development of pediatric asthma and is a welcome addition to our team of physician-scientists.

As an accredited **Cystic Fibrosis Foundation Care Center**, we offer the latest therapies and participate in multi-center trials. With our team specially trained in caring for cystic fibrosis patients, we treat all aspects of the disease, ranging from the latest antimicrobial strategies to nutritional optimization. We offer services that include pediatric spirometry, plethysmography, and comprehensive psychosocial support and evaluation.

Our **Chronic Ventilator Program** provides the most advanced and compassionate management of children with chronic respiratory failure as well as those with muscular dystrophies and other conditions that require mechanical ventilation.

Our **Bronchopulmonary Dysplasia Program** offers the highest level of care for premature infants while they are in the hospital and, as outpatients, once they are discharged.

468

Neurological Surgery

A neurological surgeon provides the operative and non-operative management (i.e., prevention, diagnosis, evaluation, treatment, critical care and rehabilitation) of disorders of the central, peripheral and autonomic nervous systems, including their supporting structures and vascular supply; the evaluation and treatment of pathological processes which modify function or activity of the nervous system; and the operative and non-operative management of pain. A neurological surgeon treats patients with disorders of the nervous system; disorders of the brain, meninges, skull and their blood supply, including the extracranial carotid and vertebral arteries; disorders of the pituitary gland; disorders of the spinal cord, meninges and vertebral column, including those which may require treatment by spinal fusion or instrumentation; and disorders of the cranial and spinal nerves throughout their distribution.

Training Required: Seven years (including general surgery)

The American Board of Pediatric Neurological Surgery (ABPNS) is not a recognized ABMS subspecialty. However, this designation has been included because the certification process is meaningful and rigorous. It is awarded to those doctors who hold a current ABMS certification in Neurological Surgery, have completed a fully accredited one year, post-graduate fellowship in pediatric neurological surgery, and have submitted surgical logs indicating a practice of pediatric neurological surgery for one year, followed by a written examination.

NEUROLOGICAL SURGERY

New England

Al-Mefty, Ossama MD [NS] - **Spec Exp:** Skull Base Surgery; Brain Tumors; Cerebrovascular Surgery; **Hospital:** Brigham and Women's Hosp (page 57), Children's Hospital - Boston; **Address:** Brigham $ Women's Hosp, Neurosurgery, 75 Francis St, Boston, MA 02115; **Phone:** 617-525-9451; **Board Cert:** Neurological Surgery 1980; **Med School:** Syria 1972; **Resid:** Surgery, Med Coll Ohio 1974; Neurological Surgery, West Va Med Ctr 1978; **Fac Appt:** Prof NS, Harvard Med Sch

Borges, Lawrence F MD [NS] - **Spec Exp:** Spinal Surgery; Spinal Tumors; **Hospital:** Mass Genl Hosp; **Address:** Mass General Hosp, 55 Fruit St White Bldg - Ste 1205, Boston, MA 02114; **Phone:** 617-726-6156; **Board Cert:** Neurological Surgery 1986; **Med School:** Johns Hopkins Univ 1977; **Resid:** Neurological Surgery, Mass Genl Hosp 1983; **Fac Appt:** Assoc Prof S, Harvard Med Sch

Cohen, Alan R MD [NS] - **Spec Exp:** Pediatric Neurosurgery; Brain & Spinal Tumors-Pediatric; Minimally Invasive Surgery; **Hospital:** Children's Hospital - Boston; **Address:** Chldn's Hosp Boston, Dept Neurosurgery, 300 Longwood Ave Hunnewell Bldg Fl 2, Boston, MA 02115; **Phone:** 617-355-1484; **Board Cert:** Neurological Surgery 1991; Pediatric Neurological Surgery 1997; **Med School:** Cornell Univ-Weill Med Coll 1978; **Resid:** Surgery, NYU Medical Ctr 1980; Neurological Surgery, NYU Medical Ctr 1987; **Fellow:** Neurology, Natl Hosp Queen's Square 1982; **Fac Appt:** Prof NS, Harvard Med Sch

Cosgrove, Rees MD [NS] - **Spec Exp:** Epilepsy/Seizure Disorders; Brain Tumors; Spinal Disorders; Pain-Chronic; **Hospital:** Rhode Island Hosp, Miriam Hosp; **Address:** Rhode Island Hosp, Neurosurgery Dept, 593 Eddy St, APC Bldg - Fl 6, Providence, RI 02903; **Phone:** 401-793-9132; **Board Cert:** Neurological Surgery 1989; **Med School:** Queens Univ 1980; **Resid:** Neurological Surgery, Montreal Neuro Inst 1986; **Fac Appt:** Prof NS, Brown Univ

David, Carlos A MD [NS] - **Spec Exp:** Cerebrovascular Surgery; Brain Tumors; Pituitary Tumors; Carotid Artery Surgery; **Hospital:** Lahey Clin, Emerson Hosp; **Address:** Lahey Clinic, Dept Neurosurgery, 41 Mall Rd Fl 7, Burlington, MA 01805; **Phone:** 781-744-8643; **Board Cert:** Neurological Surgery 2012; **Med School:** Univ Miami Sch Med 1990; **Resid:** Neurological Surgery, Jackson Memorial Hosp 1995; **Fellow:** Cerebrovascular & Skull Base Surgery, Barrow Neuro Inst 1997; **Fac Appt:** Asst Clin Prof NS, Tufts Univ

Duhaime, Ann Christine MD [NS] - **Spec Exp:** Pediatric Neurosurgery; Brain Tumors; Epilepsy; Craniofacial Surgery; **Hospital:** Mass Genl Hosp; **Address:** Mass Genl Hosp for Children, 15 Parkman St, Ste WAC 331, Boston, MA 02114; **Phone:** 617-643-9175; **Board Cert:** Neurological Surgery 1990; Pediatric Neurological Surgery 2005; **Med School:** Univ Pennsylvania 1981; **Resid:** Neurological Surgery, Hosp Univ Penn 1987; **Fellow:** Pediatric Neurological Surgery, Chldns Hosp 1987

Goumnerova, Liliana MD [NS] - **Spec Exp:** Pediatric Neurosurgery; Brain Tumors; Endoscopic Surgery/Ventriculoscopy; **Hospital:** Children's Hospital - Boston, Dana-Farber Cancer Inst (page 57); **Address:** Children's Hospital Boston, Dept of Neurosurgery, Hunnewell 2, 300 Longwood Ave, Boston, MA 02115; **Phone:** 617-355-6364; **Board Cert:** Neurological Surgery 1992; Pediatric Neurological Surgery 2006; **Med School:** Canada 1980; **Resid:** Neurological Surgery, Univ Ottawa 1986; **Fellow:** Pediatric Neurological Surgery, Hosp for Sick Chldn 1988; Neurological Science, Univ Hosp Penn 1990; **Fac Appt:** Assoc Prof S, Harvard Med Sch

Heilman, Carl B MD [NS] - **Spec Exp:** Skull Base Surgery; Pediatric Neurosurgery; **Hospital:** Tufts Med Ctr; **Address:** Tufts Med Ctr, Dept Neurosurgery, 800 Washington St, Box 178, Bsoton, MA 02111; **Phone:** 617-636-5860; **Board Cert:** Neurological Surgery 1996; **Med School:** Univ Pennsylvania 1986; **Resid:** Neurological Surgery, Tufts New England Med Ctr 1993; **Fellow:** Skull Base Surgery, Baptist Meml Hosp 1993; **Fac Appt:** Assoc Prof NS, Tufts Univ

Madsen, Joseph R MD [NS] - **Spec Exp:** Pediatric Neurosurgery; Epilepsy/Seizure Disorders; **Hospital:** Children's Hospital - Boston; **Address:** Boston Children's Hospital, 300 Longwood Ave, Honeywell 2, Boston, MA 02115; **Phone:** 617-355-6005; **Board Cert:** Neurological Surgery 1994; Pediatric Neurological Surgery 1997; **Med School:** Harvard Med Sch 1981; **Resid:** Neurological Surgery, Mass Genl Hosp 1989; **Fellow:** Research, Beth Israel Hosp 1983; **Fac Appt:** Assoc Prof NS, Harvard Med Sch

Martuza, Robert L MD [NS] - **Spec Exp:** Brain Tumors; Acoustic Neuroma; Skull Base Surgery; **Hospital:** Mass Genl Hosp; **Address:** Mass General Hosp, Dept Neurosurgery, 55 Fruit St White Bldg - Ste 502, Boston, MA 02114; **Phone:** 617-726-8581; **Board Cert:** Neurological Surgery 1983; **Med School:** Harvard Med Sch 1973; **Resid:** Neurological Surgery, Mass Genl Hosp 1980; **Fac Appt:** Prof NS, Harvard Med Sch

Moser, Richard P MD [NS] - **Spec Exp:** Brain & Spinal Cord Tumors; Spinal Surgery; **Hospital:** UMass Memorial Med Ctr, Wing Mem Hosp-UMass; **Address:** UMass Meml Med Ctr-Univ Campus, 55 Lake Ave N, Worcester, MA 01655; **Phone:** 508-334-0605; **Board Cert:** Neurological Surgery 1985; **Med School:** Loyola Univ-Stritch Sch Med 1974; **Resid:** Surgery, Univ MN Med Coll 1977; Neurological Surgery, Univ MN Med Coll 1982; **Fellow:** Neuro-Oncology, Karolinska Inst 1982; **Fac Appt:** Prof S, Univ Mass Sch Med

Penar, Paul L MD [NS] - **Spec Exp:** Brain & Spinal Tumors; Epilepsy/Seizure Disorders; Movement Disorders; Stereotactic Radiosurgery; **Hospital:** Fletcher Allen Health Care- Med Ctr Campus; **Address:** Fletcher Allen Health Care, 111 Colchester Ave, Burlington, VT 05401; **Phone:** 802-847-4590; **Board Cert:** Neurological Surgery 1989; **Med School:** Univ Mich Med Sch 1981; **Resid:** Neurological Surgery, Yale-New Haven Hosp 1987

Piepmeier, Joseph MD [NS] - **Spec Exp:** Neuro-Oncology; Brain & Spinal Cord Tumors; **Hospital:** Yale-New Haven Hosp, Yale Med Group; **Address:** 35 Park St Fl 8, New Haven, CT 06520; **Phone:** 203-785-2791; **Board Cert:** Neurological Surgery 1984; **Med School:** Univ Tenn Coll Med 1975; **Resid:** Neurological Surgery, Yale-New Haven Hosp 1982; **Fac Appt:** Prof NS, Yale Univ

Spencer, Dennis D MD [NS] - **Spec Exp:** Epilepsy/Seizure Disorders; Brain Tumors; **Hospital:** Yale-New Haven Hosp, Yale Med Group; **Address:** Yale Univ Sch Med, Dept Neurosurgery, 333 333 Cedar St, PO Box 208082, New Haven, CT 06520; **Phone:** 203-785-4891; **Board Cert:** Neurological Surgery 1980; **Med School:** Washington Univ, St Louis 1971; **Resid:** Surgery, Barnes Hosp 1972; Neurological Surgery, Yale-New Haven Hosp 1976; **Fac Appt:** Prof NS, Yale Univ

Swearingen, Brooke MD [NS] - **Spec Exp:** Pituitary Tumors; Brain & Spinal Tumors; Neuroendocrine Tumors; Spinal Surgery; **Hospital:** Mass Genl Hosp; **Address:** 15 Parkman St, WACC 331, Boston, MA 02114-3117; **Phone:** 617-726-3910; **Board Cert:** Neurological Surgery 1993; **Med School:** Harvard Med Sch 1981; **Resid:** Neurological Surgery, Mass Genl Hosp 1987; **Fac Appt:** Assoc Prof NS, Harvard Med Sch

Neurological Surgery

Mid Atlantic

Andrews, David MD [NS] - **Spec Exp:** Brain Tumors; Stereotactic Radiosurgery; **Hospital:** Thomas Jefferson Univ Hosp; **Address:** Jefferson Neurosurgical Assocs, 909 Walnut St Fl 3, Philadelphia, PA 19107-5109; **Phone:** 215-503-7005; **Board Cert:** Neurological Surgery 1992; **Med School:** Univ Colorado 1983; **Resid:** Neurological Surgery, New York Hosp 1989; **Fellow:** Neuro-Oncology, Meml Sloan Kettering Cancer Ctr 1987; **Fac Appt:** Prof NS, Thomas Jefferson Univ

Baltuch, Gordon H MD/PhD [NS] - **Spec Exp:** Movement Disorders; Parkinson's Disease; Epilepsy/Seizure Disorders; Dystonia; **Hospital:** Hosp Univ Penn - UPHS (page 72), Pennsylvania Hosp-UPHS (page 72); **Address:** Penn Neurosurgery, 235 S 8th St, Philadelphia, PA 19106; **Phone:** 215-829-6700; **Board Cert:** Neurological Surgery 1998; **Med School:** McGill Univ 1986; **Resid:** Surgery, Montreal Genl Hosp 1988; Neurological Surgery, Montreal Neuro Inst 1994; **Fellow:** Neurological Surgery, Centre Hospitalier Univ Vaudois 1995; **Fac Appt:** Prof NS, Univ Pennsylvania

Bederson, Joshua B MD [NS] - **Spec Exp:** Brain & Spinal Cord Tumors; Aneurysm-Cerebral; Meningioma; Pituitary Tumors; **Hospital:** Mount Sinai Med Ctr (page 64); **Address:** Mount Sinai Med Ctr, 1 Gustave Levy Pl, Box 1136, New York, NY 10029; **Phone:** 212-241-2377; **Board Cert:** Neurological Surgery 1993; **Med School:** UCSF 1984; **Resid:** Neurological Surgery, UCSF Med Ctr 1990; **Fellow:** Neurovascular Surgery, Barrow Neur Inst 1990; Neurovascular Surgery, Univ Hosp Zurich 1990; **Fac Appt:** Prof NS, Mount Sinai Sch Med

Belzberg, Allan J MD [NS] - **Spec Exp:** Peripheral Nerve Disorders; Nerve Surgery & Transplantation; Nerve Tumors; Spinal Surgery; **Hospital:** Johns Hopkins Hosp (page 61); **Address:** Johns Hopkins Dept Neurosurgery, 600 N Wolfe St Meyer Bldg Fl 5 - Ste 181, Baltimore, MD 21287; **Phone:** 410-955-5810; **Board Cert:** Neurological Surgery 1997; **Med School:** Univ Calgary 1982; **Resid:** Neurological Surgery, Univ Calgary Affil Hosps 1990; **Fellow:** Neurological Surgery, Johns Hopkins Hosp 1992; **Fac Appt:** Assoc Prof NS, Johns Hopkins Univ

Bilsky, Mark H MD [NS] - **Spec Exp:** Brain & Spinal Tumors; Skull Base Tumors; Spinal Reconstructive Surgery; Spinal Cord Tumors; **Hospital:** Meml Sloan-Kettering Cancer Ctr, NY-Presby/Weill Cornell Med Ctr, NY (page 66); **Address:** 1275 York Ave MSKCC Bldg Fl c705, New York, NY 10065; **Phone:** 212-639-8526; **Board Cert:** Neurological Surgery 2010; **Med School:** Emory Univ 1988; **Resid:** Neurological Surgery, NY Hosp-Cornell Med Ctr 1994; **Fellow:** Neuro-Oncology, Louisville Univ Med Ctr 1995; **Fac Appt:** Prof NS, Cornell Univ-Weill Med Coll

Brem, Henry MD [NS] - **Spec Exp:** Brain & Spinal Cord Tumors; Skull Base Tumors; Pituitary Tumors; **Hospital:** Johns Hopkins Hosp (page 61), Johns Hopkins Bayview Med Ctr (page 61); **Address:** Johns Hopkins Div Neurosurgery, 600 N Wolfe St Meyer 7 Bldg - rm 113, Baltimore, MD 21287; **Phone:** 410-955-2248; **Board Cert:** Neurological Surgery 1986; **Med School:** Harvard Med Sch 1978; **Resid:** Neurological Surgery, Columbia-Presby Med Ctr 1984; **Fellow:** Neurological Surgery, Johns Hopkins Hosp 1980; **Fac Appt:** Prof NS, Johns Hopkins Univ

Brem, Steven MD [NS] - **Spec Exp:** Brain Tumors; Pituitary Tumors; Clinical Trials; Neuro-Oncology; **Hospital:** Hosp Univ Penn - UPHS (page 72); **Address:** Hosp of the Univ of Pennsylvania, 3 Silverstein, 3400 Spruce St, Philadelphia, PA 19104; **Phone:** 215-662-7854; **Board Cert:** Neurological Surgery 1983; **Med School:** Harvard Med Sch 1972; **Resid:** Neurological Surgery, Massachusetts Genl Hosp 1981; **Fellow:** Oncology, Natl Cancer Inst 1976; **Fac Appt:** Prof NS, Univ S Fla Coll Med

Bruce, Jeffrey MD [NS] - **Spec Exp:** Brain Tumors; Pituitary Tumors; Skull Base Surgery; Meningioma; **Hospital:** NY-Presby/Columbia Univ Med Ctr, NY (page 66); **Address:** NY Presby Hosp, Dept Neurosurgery, 710 W 168th St N1 Bldg Fl 4 - rm 434, New York, NY 10032; **Phone:** 212-305-7346; **Board Cert:** Neurological Surgery 1993; **Med School:** UMDNJ-RW Johnson Med Sch 1983; **Resid:** Neurological Surgery, Columbia-Presby Med Ctr 1990; **Fellow:** Neurological Surgery, Nat Inst Hlth 1985; **Fac Appt:** Prof NS, Columbia P&S

Caputy, Anthony J MD [NS] - **Spec Exp:** Epilepsy/Seizure Disorders; Spinal Surgery; Brain & Spinal Tumors; Minimally Invasive Surgery; **Hospital:** G Washington Univ Hosp, Suburban Hosp; **Address:** Geo Wash Univ, Dept Neurosurgery, 2150 Pennsylvania Ave NW, Ste 7-420, Washington, DC 20037; **Phone:** 202-741-2735; **Board Cert:** Neurological Surgery 1989; **Med School:** Univ VA Sch Med 1980; **Resid:** Neurological Surgery, Georgetown Univ Hosp 1986; **Fac Appt:** Prof NS, Geo Wash Univ

Carson, Benjamin S MD [NS] - **Spec Exp:** Pediatric Neurosurgery; Trigeminal Neuralgia; Brain & Spinal Cord Tumors; Brain Injury; **Hospital:** Johns Hopkins Hosp (page 61); **Address:** Johns Hopkins Div Pediatric Neurosurgery, 600 N Wolfe St, Harvey 811, Baltimore, MD 21287-8811; **Phone:** 410-955-7888; **Board Cert:** Neurological Surgery 1988; Pediatric Neurological Surgery 1997; **Med School:** Univ Mich Med Sch 1977; **Resid:** Neurological Surgery, Johns Hopkins Hosp 1983; **Fellow:** Pediatric Neurological Surgery, Queen Elizabeth II Med Ctr 1984; **Fac Appt:** Assoc Prof NS, Johns Hopkins Univ

Chen, Chun Siang MD [NS] - **Spec Exp:** Skull Base Tumors; Skull Base Surgery; Microsurgery; Brain & Spinal Tumors; **Hospital:** Mount Sinai Med Ctr (page 64); **Address:** Mount Sinai Med Ctr, Annenberg Bldg, One Gustave L Levy Pl Fl 8 - rm 10, New York, NY 10029; **Phone:** 212-241-8480; **Med School:** Brazil 1978; **Resid:** Neurological Surgery, Santa Casa de Misericordia of Sao Paulo Med Sch 1983; Neurological Surgery, Mt Sinai Med Ctr 2005; **Fellow:** Skull Base Surgery, St Lukes Roosevelt Hosp 2006; **Fac Appt:** Asst Prof NS, Mount Sinai Sch Med

Di Giacinto, George V MD [NS] - **Spec Exp:** Spinal Surgery; Pain Management; **Hospital:** St. Luke's - Roosevelt Hosp Ctr - Roosevelt Div (page 56); **Address:** 425 W 59th St, Ste 4E, New York, NY 10019; **Phone:** 212-523-8500; **Board Cert:** Neurological Surgery 1981; **Med School:** Harvard Med Sch 1970; **Resid:** Neurological Surgery, Columbia-Presby Hosp 1978

Dias, Mark S MD [NS] - **Spec Exp:** Pediatric Neurosurgery; Spina Bifida; Hydrocephalus; Craniosynostosis; **Hospital:** Penn State Milton S Hershey Med Ctr; **Address:** Penn State-Hersey Med Ctr, Dept Neurosurgery, 30 Hope Drive, MC EC110, Hersey, PA 17033; **Phone:** 717-531-8807; **Board Cert:** Neurological Surgery 1995; Pediatric Neurological Surgery 2006; **Med School:** Johns Hopkins Univ 1982; **Resid:** Neurological Surgery, Univ Pittsburgh Med Ctr 1989; **Fellow:** Pediatric Neurological Surgery, Univ Utah-Primary Chldns Hosp 1991; **Fac Appt:** Prof NS, Penn State Coll Med

Eisenberg, Howard M MD [NS] - **Spec Exp:** Acoustic Neuroma; Skull Base Surgery; Deep Brain Stimulation; Epilepsy/Seizure Disorders; **Hospital:** Univ of MD Med Ctr; **Address:** Univ MD Sch Med, Dept Neurosurg, 22 S Greene St, Ste S-12-D, Baltimore, MD 21201-1544; **Phone:** 410-328-3514; **Board Cert:** Neurological Surgery 1973; **Med School:** SUNY Downstate 1964; **Resid:** Surgery, New York Hosp 1966; Neurological Surgery, Peter Bent Brigham Hosp/Chldns Hosp 1970; **Fellow:** Harvard Univ 1970; **Fac Appt:** Prof NS, Univ MD Sch Med

Evans, James J MD [NS] - **Spec Exp:** Skull Base Surgery; Neuro-Oncology; Brain Tumors; Endoscopic Surgery; **Hospital:** Thomas Jefferson Univ Hosp; **Address:** Jefferson Neurosurgical Assocs, 909 Walnut St Fl 3, Philadelphia, PA 19107; **Phone:** 215-955-7000; **Board Cert:** Neurological Surgery 2006; **Med School:** Univ Mass Sch Med 1995; **Resid:** Neurological Surgery, Cleveland Clinic 1999; **Fellow:** Cranial Base Surgery, Fairfax Hosp 2001; **Fac Appt:** Assoc Prof NS, Thomas Jefferson Univ

Feldstein, Neil A MD [NS] - **Spec Exp:** Pediatric Neurosurgery; Chiari's Deformity; Brain Tumors-Pediatric; Spinal Cord Surgery-Pediatric; **Hospital:** Morgan Stanley Children's Hosp of NY-Presby, NY, NY-Presby/Columbia Univ Med Ctr, NY (page 66); **Address:** Neurological Inst, 710 W 168th St, Fl 2, rm 213, New York, NY 10032; **Phone:** 212-305-1396; **Board Cert:** Neurological Surgery 1995; Pediatric Neurological Surgery 2007; **Med School:** NYU Sch Med 1984; **Resid:** Neurological Surgery, Baylor Coll Med 1989; **Fellow:** Pediatric Neurological Surgery, NYU Med Ctr 1991; **Fac Appt:** Assoc Prof NS, Columbia P&S

Fenstermaker, Robert A MD [NS] - **Spec Exp:** Brain Tumors; Pituitary Tumors; Stereotactic Radiosurgery; Skull Base Surgery; **Hospital:** Roswell Park Cancer Inst; **Address:** Roswell Park Cancer Inst, Elm and Carlton Streets, Buffalo, NY 14263; **Phone:** 716-845-3154; **Board Cert:** Neurological Surgery 1991; **Med School:** NE Ohio Univ 1981; **Resid:** Neurological Surgery, Univ Hosps Cleveland 1987; **Fellow:** Pharmacology, Case Western Reserve 1989; **Fac Appt:** Prof NS, SUNY Buffalo

Gokaslan, Ziya L MD [NS] - **Spec Exp:** Spinal Tumors; Spinal Surgery-Complex; Spinal Reconstructive Surgery; **Hospital:** Johns Hopkins Hosp (page 61), Johns Hopkins Bayview Med Ctr (page 61); **Address:** Johns Hopkins Uinv, Dept Neurosurgery Spine Ctr, 600 N Wolfe St, Meyer 7-109, Baltimore, MD 21287; **Phone:** 443-287-4934; **Board Cert:** Neurological Surgery 1997; **Med School:** Turkey 1983; **Resid:** Neurological Surgery, Baylor Coll Med 1993; **Fellow:** Neurological Trauma, Baylor Coll Med 1988; Spinal Surgery, NYU Med Ctr 1994; **Fac Appt:** Prof NS, Johns Hopkins Univ

Golfinos, John G MD [NS] - **Spec Exp:** Brain Tumors; Acoustic Neuroma; Stereotactic Radiosurgery; Skull Base Surgery; **Hospital:** NYU Langone Med Ctr (page 68), Bellevue Hosp Ctr; **Address:** 530 First Ave, Ste 8R, New York, NY 10016; **Phone:** 212-263-2950; **Board Cert:** Neurological Surgery 1998; **Med School:** Columbia P&S 1988; **Resid:** Neurological Surgery, Barrow Neuro Inst 1995; **Fac Appt:** Assoc Prof NS, NYU Sch Med

Goodman, Robert R MD/PhD [NS] - **Spec Exp:** Parkinson's Disease/Movement Disorders; Epilepsy; Trigeminal Neuralgia; Hydrocephalus-Adult; **Hospital:** St. Luke's - Roosevelt Hosp Ctr - Roosevelt Div (page 56); **Address:** 1000 Tenth Ave, Ste 5G-80, New York, NY 10019; **Phone:** 212-636-3666; **Board Cert:** Neurological Surgery 1993; **Med School:** Johns Hopkins Univ 1982; **Resid:** Neurological Surgery, Columbia-Presby Med Ctr 1989; **Fac Appt:** Assoc Prof NS, Columbia P&S

Grady, M Sean MD [NS] - **Spec Exp:** Cerebrovascular Surgery; Aneurysm-Cerebral; Arteriovenous Malformations; Brain Injury-Traumatic; **Hospital:** Hosp Univ Penn - UPHS (page 72), Pennsylvania Hosp-UPHS (page 72); **Address:** Univ Penn, Dept Neurosurgery, 3400 Spruce St, Silverstein Bldg Fl 3, Philadelphia, PA 19104; **Phone:** 215-662-3483; **Board Cert:** Neurological Surgery 1990; **Med School:** Georgetown Univ 1981; **Resid:** Neurological Surgery, Univ Virginia Hosp 1987; **Fac Appt:** Prof NS, Univ Pennsylvania

Gutin, Philip H MD [NS] - **Spec Exp:** Brain Tumors; Meningioma; Acoustic Neuroma; **Hospital:** Meml Sloan-Kettering Cancer Ctr, NY-Presby/Weill Cornell Med Ctr, NY (page 66); **Address:** 1275 York Ave, New York, NY 10065; **Phone:** 212-639-8556; **Board Cert:** Neurological Surgery 1981; **Med School:** Univ Pennsylvania 1971; **Resid:** Neurological Surgery, UCSF Med Ctr 1979; **Fellow:** Neurological Surgery, Natl Cancer Inst 1976; **Fac Appt:** Prof NS, Cornell Univ-Weill Med Coll

Harbaugh, Robert E MD [NS] - **Spec Exp:** Carotid Artery Surgery; Aneurysm-Cerebral; MoyaMoya Disease; **Hospital:** Penn State Milton S Hershey Med Ctr; **Address:** Penn State Hershey Med Ctr, Dept Neurosurgery, 30 Hope Drive, Hershey, PA 17033-0850; **Phone:** 717-531-4383; **Board Cert:** Neurological Surgery 1989; **Med School:** Penn State Coll Med 1978; **Resid:** Surgery, Dartmouth-Hitchcock Med Ctr 1980; Neurological Surgery, Dartmouth-Hitchcock Med Ctr 1985; **Fac Appt:** Prof NS, Penn State Coll Med

Harrop, James S MD [NS] - **Spec Exp:** Spinal Cord Injury; Spinal Trauma; Spinal Tumors; **Hospital:** Thomas Jefferson Univ Hosp; **Address:** 909 Walnut St, Ste 200, Philadelphia, PA 19107; **Phone:** 215-955-7000; **Board Cert:** Neurological Surgery 2006; **Med School:** Jefferson Med Coll 1995; **Resid:** Neurological Surgery, Thomas Jefferson Univ Hosp 2001; **Fellow:** Neurological Surgery, Cleveland Clinic 2002; Spinal Surgery, Cleveland Clinic 2002; **Fac Appt:** Assoc Prof NS, Jefferson Med Coll

Hartl, Roger MD [NS] - **Spec Exp:** Spinal Surgery-Complex; Minimally Invasive Spinal Surgery; Spinal Disc Replacement; **Hospital:** NY-Presby/Weill Cornell Med Ctr, NY (page 66); **Address:** Cornell Neurosurgery, 525 E 68th St, Starr 651, New York, NY 10065; **Phone:** 212-746-2152; **Board Cert:** Neurological Surgery 2008; **Med School:** Germany 1993; **Resid:** Neurological Surgery, NY Presby-Cornell Med Ctr 2003; **Fellow:** Spinal Surgery, Barrow Neurological Inst

Hopkins, L Nelson MD [NS] - **Spec Exp:** Cerebrovascular Disease; Endovascular Surgery; Stroke; **Hospital:** Buffalo General Hosp; **Address:** UB Neurosurgery, 100 High St, B Wing Fl 4, Buffalo, NY 14203; **Phone:** 716-218-1000; **Board Cert:** Neurological Surgery 1977; **Med School:** Albany Med Coll 1969; **Resid:** Neurological Surgery, SUNY Buffalo Med Ctr 1975; **Fac Appt:** Prof NS, SUNY Buffalo

Huang, Judy MD [NS] - **Spec Exp:** Aneurysm-Cerebral; Cerebrovascular Surgery; Brain Tumors; Spinal Disorders; **Hospital:** Johns Hopkins Hosp (page 61), Johns Hopkins Bayview Med Ctr (page 61); **Address:** Dept of Neurosurgery, Johns Hopkins Hosp, 1800 Orleans St, Zayed Tower, Ste 6115F, Baltimore, MD 21287; **Phone:** 410-502-5767; **Board Cert:** Neurological Surgery 2006; **Med School:** Columbia P&S 1995; **Resid:** Neurological Surgery, NY Presby-Columbia Med Ctr 2002; **Fellow:** Research, NY Presby-Columbia Med Ctr 1998; Research, NY Presby-Columbia Med Ctr 2000; **Fac Appt:** Assoc Prof NS, Johns Hopkins Univ

Jallo, George I MD [NS] - **Spec Exp:** Pediatric Neurosurgery; Chiari's Deformity; Brain & Spinal Cord Tumors; Epilepsy; **Hospital:** Johns Hopkins Hosp (page 61), Johns Hopkins Bayview Med Ctr (page 61); **Address:** Johns Hopkins Hosp, Dept of Neurosurgery, 600 N Wolfe St, Ste Harvey 811, Baltimore, MD 21287; **Phone:** 410-955-7851; **Board Cert:** Neurological Surgery 2002; Pediatric Neurological Surgery 2004; **Med School:** Univ VA Sch Med 1991; **Resid:** Neurological Surgery, NYU Med Ctr 1998; **Fellow:** Pediatric Neurological Surgery, Beth Israel Med Ctr 1999; **Fac Appt:** Prof NS, Johns Hopkins Univ

Jho, Hae-Dong MD/PhD [NS] - **Spec Exp:** Minimally Invasive Surgery; Spinal Surgery; Endoscopic Surgery; **Hospital:** Allegheny General Hosp; **Address:** Jho Inst for Min Invasive Neurosurgery, 320 E North Ave, Allegheny Genl Hosp, Pittsburgh, PA 15212-4746; **Phone:** 412-359-6110; **Board Cert:** Neurological Surgery 1991; **Med School:** Korea 1971; **Resid:** Neurological Surgery, Hanyang Univ Hosp 1979; Neurological Surgery, Univ Pittsburgh 1989; **Fellow:** Microsurgery, Univ Pittsburgh 1983; **Fac Appt:** Prof NS, Drexel Univ Coll Med

Judy, Kevin MD [NS] - **Spec Exp:** Brain Tumors; Acoustic Neuroma; Skull Base Tumors; **Hospital:** Thomas Jefferson Univ Hosp; **Address:** Jefferson Neurosurgical Assocs, 909 Walnut St, 3rd Fl, Philadelphia, PA 19107; **Phone:** 215-503-7005; **Board Cert:** Neurological Surgery 1997; **Med School:** Univ Pittsburgh 1984; **Resid:** Surgery, Mercy Hosp 1986; Neurological Surgery, Johns Hopkins Hosp 1992; **Fellow:** Neurological Surgery, Johns Hopkins Hosp 1991; **Fac Appt:** Prof NS, Jefferson Med Coll

Kaiser, Michael G MD [NS] - **Spec Exp:** Spinal Surgery-Complex; Minimally Invasive Spinal Surgery; Spinal Disc Replacement; **Hospital:** NY-Presby/Columbia Univ Med Ctr, NY (page 66); **Address:** Neurological Institute, Dept Neurological Surgery, 710 W 168th St, New York, NY 10032; **Phone:** 212-305-0378; **Board Cert:** Neurological Surgery 2004; **Med School:** Yale Univ 1994; **Resid:** Neurological Surgery, Columbia Neuro Inst 2000; **Fellow:** Spinal Surgery, Emory Univ 2001; **Fac Appt:** Asst Prof NS, Columbia P&S

Kaplitt, Michael G MD/PhD [NS] - **Spec Exp:** Parkinson's Disease/Movement Disorders; Deep Brain Stimulation; Trigeminal Neuralgia; Hydrocephalus; **Hospital:** NY-Presby/Weill Cornell Med Ctr, NY (page 66); **Address:** 525 E 68th St, Box 99, New York, NY 10065; **Phone:** 212-746-4966; **Board Cert:** Neurological Surgery 2005; **Med School:** Cornell Univ-Weill Med Coll 1995; **Resid:** Neurological Surgery, New York Hosp 2000; **Fellow:** Stereo Neurological Surgery, Toronto Western Hosp 2001; **Fac Appt:** Assoc Prof NS, Cornell Univ-Weill Med Coll

Khan, Agha S MD [NS] - **Spec Exp:** Skull Base Surgery; Spinal Surgery; **Hospital:** Sinai Hosp - Baltimore, Maryland Genl Hosp; **Address:** 2411 W Belvedere Ave, Ste 402, Baltimore, MD 21215; **Phone:** 410-601-8314; **Board Cert:** Neurological Surgery 1995; **Med School:** Pakistan 1979; **Resid:** Neurological Surgery, Univ Wisconsin Hosp 1990; **Fellow:** Surgical Oncology, Roswell Park Meml Inst 1982; Neurological Surgery, Allegheny Genl Hosp 1991

Kobrine, Arthur MD/PhD [NS] - **Spec Exp:** Spinal Cord Surgery; Brain & Spinal Cord Tumors; Spinal Surgery; **Hospital:** Sibley Mem Hosp, Georgetown Univ Hosp; **Address:** 2440 M St NW, Ste 315, Washington, DC 20037-1404; **Phone:** 202-293-7136; **Board Cert:** Neurological Surgery 1976; **Med School:** Northwestern Univ 1968; **Resid:** Neurological Surgery, Northwestern Univ Hosp 1970; Neurological Surgery, Walter Reed Army Hosp 1973; **Fellow:** Physiology, Geo Wash Univ 1979; **Fac Appt:** Clin Prof NS, Georgetown Univ

Kondziolka, Douglas MD [NS] - **Spec Exp:** Brain Tumors-Adult & Pediatric; Brain Tumors-Metastatic; Stereotactic Radiosurgery; Movement Disorders; **Hospital:** UPMC Presby, Pittsburgh, Chldns Hosp of Pittsburgh - UPMC; **Address:** UPMC Presbyterian Hosp, Dept Neurological Surgery, 200 Lothrop St, Ste B400, Pittsburgh, PA 15213; **Phone:** 412-647-9990; **Board Cert:** Neurological Surgery 1994; **Med School:** Univ Toronto 1985; **Resid:** Neurological Surgery, Univ Toronto Affil Hosp 1989; **Fellow:** Stereo Neurological Surgery, Univ Pittsburgh 1991; **Fac Appt:** Prof NS, Univ Pittsburgh

Kotapka, Mark J MD [NS] - **Spec Exp:** Pituitary Tumors; Skull Base Surgery; Spinal Surgery; **Hospital:** Albert Einstein Med Ctr; **Address:** Albert Einstein Medical Ctr, Klein Bldg - Ste 400, 5401 Old York Rd, Philadelphia, PA 19141; **Phone:** 215-456-6127; **Board Cert:** Neurological Surgery 1997; **Med School:** Univ MD Sch Med 1985; **Resid:** Neurological Surgery, Hosp Univ Penn 1991; **Fellow:** Pediatric Neurological Surgery, Children's Hosp 1992; Skull Base Surgery, Univ Pittsburgh 1992; **Fac Appt:** Prof NS, Albert Einstein Coll Med

Laske, Douglas W MD [NS] - **Spec Exp:** Brain & Spinal Cord Tumors; Stereotactic Radiosurgery; Brain Tumors-Metastatic; Pituitary Tumors; **Hospital:** Temple Univ Hosp, Fox Chase Cancer Ctr (page 58); **Address:** Temple Univ Dep Neurosurgery, 3401 N Broad St, Ste C540, Phildelphia, PA 19140; **Phone:** 215-707-7200; **Board Cert:** Neurological Surgery 1996; **Med School:** Columbia P&S 1985; **Resid:** Neurological Surgery, Med Coll Virginia 1991; **Fellow:** Neurosurgical Oncology, Natl Inst Hlth 1995; **Fac Appt:** Assoc Prof NS, Temple Univ

Lavyne, Michael H MD [NS] - **Spec Exp:** Spinal Surgery; Spinal Tumors; Spinal Disorders; **Hospital:** NY-Presby/Weill Cornell Med Ctr, NY (page 66), Hosp For Special Surgery (page 60); **Address:** 110 E 55th St Fl 9, MS 10022, New York, NY 10022; **Phone:** 212-486-9100; **Board Cert:** Neurological Surgery 1982; **Med School:** Cornell Univ-Weill Med Coll 1972; **Resid:** Neurological Surgery, Mass Genl Hosp 1979; **Fellow:** Neurology, Beth Israel Hosp 1974; **Fac Appt:** Clin Prof NS, Cornell Univ-Weill Med Coll

Lunsford, L Dade MD [NS] - **Spec Exp:** Brain Tumors; Stereotactic Radiosurgery; Movement Disorders; Vascular Malformations; **Hospital:** UPMC Presby, Pittsburgh, Chldns Hosp of Pittsburgh - UPMC; **Address:** UPMC Presbyterian Hosp, 200 Lothrop St, Ste B400, Pittsburgh, PA 15213-2536; **Phone:** 412-647-0953; **Board Cert:** Neurological Surgery 1983; **Med School:** Columbia P&S 1974; **Resid:** Neurological Surgery, Univ Pittsburgh Med Ctr 1980; **Fellow:** Stereo Neurological Surgery, Karolinska Hospital 1981; **Fac Appt:** Prof NS, Univ Pittsburgh

Maroon, Joseph C MD [NS] - **Spec Exp:** Minimally Invasive Spinal Surgery; Microdiscectomy; Brain Injury-Traumatic; Pituitary Tumors; **Hospital:** UPMC Presby, Pittsburgh, UPMC Passavant-McCandless; **Address:** UPMC Presbyterian, Dept Neuro Surg, 200 Lothrop St, Ste 5-C, Pittsburgh, PA 15213; **Phone:** 412-647-3604; **Board Cert:** Neurological Surgery 1973; **Med School:** Indiana Univ 1965; **Resid:** Surgery, Georgetown Univ Hosp 1967; Neurological Surgery, Indiana Univ Med Ctr 1971; **Fellow:** Neurological Surgery, Radcliffe Infirmary 1969; Microsurgery, Univ Vermont Affil Hosp 1972; **Fac Appt:** Prof NS, Univ Pittsburgh

McCormick, Paul C MD [NS] - **Spec Exp:** Spinal Surgery; Spinal Tumors; **Hospital:** NY-Presby/Columbia Univ Med Ctr, NY (page 66); **Address:** 710 W 168th St, Ste 506, New York, NY 10032-2603; **Phone:** 212-305-7976; **Board Cert:** Neurological Surgery 1993; **Med School:** Columbia P&S 1982; **Resid:** Neurological Surgery, Columbia Presby Med Ctr 1989; **Fellow:** Neurological Surgery, Natl Inst Hlth 1984; Spinal Surgery, Med Coll Wisconsin 1990; **Fac Appt:** Prof NS, Columbia P&S

Moore, Frank M MD [NS] - **Spec Exp:** Aneurysm-Cerebral; Brain Tumors; Spinal Cord Tumors; Spinal Surgery; **Hospital:** Englewood Hosp & Med Ctr, Mount Sinai Med Ctr (page 64); **Address:** Metropolitan Neurosurgery Assocs, 309 Engle St, Ste 6, Englewood, NJ 07631; **Phone:** 201-569-7737; **Board Cert:** Neurological Surgery 1992; **Med School:** France 1983; **Resid:** Neurological Surgery, Mt Sinai Hosp 1988; **Fac Appt:** Assoc Prof NS, Mount Sinai Sch Med

Murali, Raj MD [NS] - **Spec Exp:** Trigeminal Neuralgia; Skull Base Surgery; Aneurysm-Cerebral; Pituitary Tumors; **Hospital:** Westchester Med Ctr; **Address:** Westchester Med Ctr, Dept Neurosurgery, Munger Pavilion, Ste 329, Valhalla, NY 10595; **Phone:** 914-493-8392; **Board Cert:** Neurological Surgery 1982; **Med School:** India 1968; **Resid:** Neurological Surgery, Royal Infirm-Univ Edinburgh 1974; Neurological Surgery, NYU Med Ctr 1979; **Fac Appt:** Prof NS, NY Med Coll

Naff, Neal J MD [NS] - **Spec Exp:** Brain & Spinal Cord Tumors; Stereotactic Radiosurgery; Minimally Invasive Spinal Surgery; Epilepsy/Seizure Disorders; **Hospital:** St. Joseph Med Ctr, Sinai Hosp - Baltimore; **Address:** Chesapeake Neurosurgery, 2700 Quarry Lake Drive, Ste 360, Baltimore, MD 21209; **Phone:** 410-486-0090; **Board Cert:** Neurological Surgery 2011; **Med School:** Johns Hopkins Univ 1991; **Resid:** Neurological Surgery, Johns Hopkins Hosp 1996; **Fellow:** Neurological Surgery, Johns Hopkins Hosp 2000

O'Rourke, Donald M MD [NS] - **Spec Exp:** Neuro-Oncology; Brain Tumors; Spinal Disorders; **Hospital:** Hosp Univ Penn - UPHS (page 72); **Address:** Hosp Univ Penn-Dept Neurosurgery, 3400 Spruce St, 3 Silverstein, Philadelphia, PA 19104; **Phone:** 215-662-3490; **Board Cert:** Neurological Surgery 1998; **Med School:** Univ Pennsylvania 1987; **Resid:** Neurological Surgery, Hosp Univ Penn 1994; **Fac Appt:** Assoc Prof NS, Univ Pennsylvania

Olivi, Alessandro MD [NS] - **Spec Exp:** Brain & Spinal Cord Tumors; Skull Base Tumors; Brain Tumors-Metastatic; Meningioma; **Hospital:** Johns Hopkins Hosp (page 61); **Address:** Johns Hopkins Div Neurosurgery, 600 N Wolfe St, Phipps Bldg - Ste 1-100, Baltimore, MD 21287-0001; **Phone:** 410-955-0703; **Board Cert:** Neurological Surgery 1994; **Med School:** Italy 1979; **Resid:** Neurological Surgery, Univ of Padova; Neurological Surgery, Mayfield Neur Inst 1998; **Fellow:** Neuro-Oncology, Johns Hopkins Hosp 1991; **Fac Appt:** Prof NS, Johns Hopkins Univ

Patel, Aman B MD [NS] - **Spec Exp:** Interventional Neuroradiology; Endovascular Neurosurgery; Aneurysm-Cerebral; Arteriovenous Malformations; **Hospital:** Mount Sinai Med Ctr (page 64); **Address:** One Gustave L Levy Place, Box 1136, New York, NY 10029; **Phone:** 212-241-3457; **Board Cert:** Neurological Surgery 2004; **Med School:** UCLA 1993; **Resid:** Neurological Surgery, UCLA Med Ctr 1999; **Fellow:** Interventional Neuroradiology, UCLA Med Ctr 2001; **Fac Appt:** Assoc Prof NS, Mount Sinai Sch Med

Piatt, Joseph H MD [NS] - **Spec Exp:** Brachial Plexus Palsy-Pediatric; Spasticity & Movement Disorders; Chiari's Deformity; Syringomyelia & Spinal Cord Diseases; **Hospital:** Nemours/Alfred I.duPont Hosp for Chldn; **Address:** 1600 Rockland Rd, Wilmington, DE 19803; **Phone:** 302-651-5993; **Board Cert:** Neurological Surgery 1989; Pediatric Neurological Surgery 2006; **Med School:** Univ Pennsylvania 1979; **Resid:** Neurological Surgery, Duke Univ Med Ctr 1986; **Fellow:** Pediatric Neurological Surgery, Hosp Sick Chldn 1987

Pollack, Ian F MD [NS] - **Spec Exp:** Pediatric Neurosurgery; Brain Tumors; Craniofacial Surgery; Neuro-Oncology; **Hospital:** Chldns Hosp of Pittsburgh - UPMC, UPMC Presby, Pittsburgh; **Address:** Chldns Hosp Pittsburgh, Div Neurosurgery, 4401 Penn Ave, Ste FP4129, Pittsburgh, PA 15224; **Phone:** 412-692-5881; **Board Cert:** Neurological Surgery 1996; Pediatric Neurological Surgery 2006; **Med School:** Johns Hopkins Univ 1984; **Resid:** Neurological Surgery, Univ Pittsburgh Med Ctr 1991; **Fellow:** Pediatric Neurological Surgery, Hosp Sick Chldn 1992; **Fac Appt:** Prof NS, Univ Pittsburgh

Quigley, Matthew R MD [NS] - **Spec Exp:** Brain Tumors; Spinal Cord Tumors; Neuro-Oncology; **Hospital:** Allegheny General Hosp; **Address:** Allegeny General Hosp, Neurosurgery, 420 E North Ave, Ste 302, Pittsburgh, PA 15212; **Phone:** 412-359-4764; **Board Cert:** Neurological Surgery 1991; **Med School:** Northwestern Univ-Feinberg Sch Med 1981; **Resid:** Neurological Surgery, Northwestern Meml Hosp 1987; **Fac Appt:** Assoc Prof NS, Drexel Univ Coll Med

Rigamonti, Daniele MD [NS] - **Spec Exp:** Hydrocephalus-Adult; Brain Tumors; Spinal Disorders; Vascular Neurosurgery; **Hospital:** Johns Hopkins Hosp (page 61); **Address:** Johns Hopkins Hosp, Dept Neurosurgery, 600 N Wolfe St, Phipps Bldg - Ste 126, Baltimore, MD 21287; **Phone:** 410-955-2259; **Board Cert:** Neurological Surgery 1988; **Med School:** Italy 1976; **Resid:** Neurological Surgery, Mt Sinai Hosp Med Ctr 1984; **Fellow:** Neurovascular Surgery, Barrow Neuro Inst 1987; **Fac Appt:** Prof NS, Johns Hopkins Univ

Riina, Howard A MD [NS] - **Spec Exp:** Neuroradiology; Aneurysm-Cerebral; Cerebrovascular Malformations; Stroke; **Hospital:** NYU Langone Med Ctr (page 68); **Address:** NYU Langone Med Ctr, 530 First Ave, SK1, Ste 8R, New York, NY 10016; **Phone:** 212-263-5382; **Board Cert:** Neurological Surgery 2004; **Med School:** Temple Univ 1993; **Resid:** Neurological Surgery, Hosp Univ Penn 2000; **Fellow:** Interventional Neuroradiology, Beth Israel Med Ctr 1997; Skull Base Surgery, Barrow Neuro Inst 2001; **Fac Appt:** Prof NS, NYU Sch Med

Rosenwasser, Robert H MD [NS] - **Spec Exp:** Aneurysm-Cerebral; Cerebrovascular Surgery; Arteriovenous Malformations; **Hospital:** Thomas Jefferson Univ Hosp; **Address:** Thomas Jefferson Univ Hosp, 909 Walnut St, Ste 200, Philadelphia, PA 19107; **Phone:** 215-955-7000; **Board Cert:** Neurological Surgery 1987; **Med School:** Louisiana State U, New Orleans 1979; **Resid:** Neurological Surgery, Temple Univ Hosp 1984; **Fellow:** Neurovascular Surgery, Univ West Ontarion 1985; Interventional Neuroradiology, NYU Med Ctr 1993; **Fac Appt:** Prof NS, Thomas Jefferson Univ

Schwartz, Theodore H MD [NS] - **Spec Exp:** Brain Tumors; Pituitary Tumors; Epilepsy; Minimally Invasive Surgery; **Hospital:** NY-Presby/Weill Cornell Med Ctr, NY (page 66); **Address:** Department of Neurosurgery, Box 99, 525 E 68th St, Starr Pavilion, rm 651, New York, NY 10065; **Phone:** 212-746-5620; **Board Cert:** Neurological Surgery 2002; **Med School:** Harvard Med Sch 1993; **Resid:** Neurological Surgery, Columbia-Presby Med Ctr 1999; **Fellow:** Neurological Surgery, Yale-New Haven Med Ctr 2000; **Fac Appt:** Prof NS, Cornell Univ-Weill Med Coll

Sen, Chandranath MD [NS] - **Spec Exp:** Brain Tumors; Skull Base Tumors; Trigeminal Neuralgia; Hemifacial Spasm; **Hospital:** NYU Langone Med Ctr (page 68); **Address:** NYU Langone Med Ctr, Dept Neurosurgery, 550 First Ave, Ste HCC-3F, New York, NY 10016; **Phone:** 212-263-5333; **Board Cert:** Neurological Surgery 1989; **Med School:** India 1976; **Resid:** Surgery, Univ Wisconsin Hosps 1980; Neurological Surgery, Univ Wisconsin Hosps 1985; **Fellow:** Microsurgery, Univ Pittsburgh Med Ctr 1986

Sisti, Michael B MD [NS] - **Spec Exp:** Acoustic Neuroma; Brain Tumors; Stereotactic Radiosurgery; Meningioma; **Hospital:** NY-Presby/Columbia Univ Med Ctr, NY (page 66); **Address:** 710 W 168th St, New York, NY 10032-2603; **Phone:** 212-305-1728; **Board Cert:** Neurological Surgery 1991; **Med School:** Columbia P&S 1981; **Resid:** Neurological Surgery, Neuro Inst-Columbia-Presby Med Ctr 1988; **Fellow:** Neurological Surgery, Natl Inst Hlth 1983; **Fac Appt:** Assoc Prof NS, Columbia P&S

Solomon, Robert A MD [NS] - **Spec Exp:** Aneurysm-Cerebral; Arteriovenous Malformations; **Hospital:** NY-Presby/Columbia Univ Med Ctr, NY (page 66); **Address:** 710 W 168th St, Ste 439, New York, NY 10032; **Phone:** 212-305-4118; **Board Cert:** Neurological Surgery 1988; **Med School:** Johns Hopkins Univ 1980; **Resid:** Neurological Surgery, Neuro Inst-Columbia 1986; **Fac Appt:** Prof NS, Columbia P&S

Souweidane, Mark M MD [NS] - **Spec Exp:** Pediatric Neurosurgery; Minimally Invasive Surgery; Endoscopic Surgery; Brain Tumors-Pediatric; **Hospital:** NY-Presby/Weill Cornell Med Ctr, NY (page 66), Meml Sloan-Kettering Cancer Ctr; **Address:** 525 E 68th St, Box 99, New York, NY 10065-4870; **Phone:** 212-746-2363; **Board Cert:** Neurological Surgery 2010; Pediatric Neurological Surgery 2000; **Med School:** Wayne State Univ 1988; **Resid:** Neurological Surgery, NYU Med Ctr 1994; **Fellow:** Pediatric Neurological Surgery, Hosp Sick Chldn 1995; **Fac Appt:** Prof NS, Cornell Univ-Weill Med Coll

Stieg, Philip E MD/PhD [NS] - **Spec Exp:** Cerebrovascular Surgery; Acoustic Neuroma; Skull Base Surgery; Brain Tumors; **Hospital:** NY-Presby/Weill Cornell Med Ctr, NY (page 66); **Address:** 525 E 68th St, STARR 651, New York, NY 10021-9800; **Phone:** 212-746-4684; **Board Cert:** Neurological Surgery 1992; **Med School:** Med Coll Wisc 1983; **Resid:** Neurological Surgery, Parkland Meml Hosp/Dallas Chldns Hosp 1989; **Fellow:** Neurological Biology, Karolinska Inst 1988; **Fac Appt:** Prof NS, Cornell Univ-Weill Med Coll

Sundaresan, Narayan MD [NS] - **Spec Exp:** Spinal Surgery; Brain Tumors; Neuro-Oncology; Spinal Disorders-Degenerative; **Hospital:** Mount Sinai Med Ctr (page 64), Lincoln Med & Mental Hlth Ctr; **Address:** Central Park Neurosurgery, 1148 5th Ave, New York, NY 10128; **Phone:** 212-876-7575; **Board Cert:** Neurological Surgery 1980; **Med School:** India 1969; **Resid:** Neurological Surgery, Northwestern Meml Hosp 1975; **Fellow:** Neuro-Oncology, Meml Sloan Kettering Cancer Ctr 1977; **Fac Appt:** Prof NS, Mount Sinai Sch Med

Sutton, Leslie N MD [NS] - **Spec Exp:** Brain Tumors-Pediatric; Fetal Neurosurgery; Hydrocephalus; **Hospital:** Chldns Hosp of Philadelphia; **Address:** Childrens Hosp Phila-Neurosurgery, 34th St & Civic Center Blvd, Wood Bldg Fl 6, Philadelphia, PA 19104; **Phone:** 215-590-2780; **Board Cert:** Neurological Surgery 1984; Pediatric Neurological Surgery 1996; **Med School:** Univ Pennsylvania 1975; **Resid:** Neurological Surgery, Hosp Univ Penn 1981; **Fac Appt:** Prof NS, Univ Pennsylvania

Tamargo, Rafael J MD [NS] - **Spec Exp:** Vascular Neurosurgery; Skull Base Surgery; **Hospital:** Johns Hopkins Hosp (page 61), Johns Hopkins Bayview Med Ctr (page 61); **Address:** Johns Hopkins Hospital, Neurosurgery, 1800 Orleans St, Zayed Bldg Fl 6 - Ste 6115 - rm G, Baltimore, MD 21287; **Phone:** 410-614-1533; **Board Cert:** Neurological Surgery 1995; **Med School:** Columbia P&S 1984; **Resid:** Neurological Surgery, Johns Hopkins Hosp 1992; **Fac Appt:** Prof NS, Johns Hopkins Univ

Turtz, Alan R MD [NS] - **Spec Exp:** Brain Tumors; Pituitary Tumors; Spinal Surgery; Neuro-Endoscopy; **Hospital:** Cooper Univ Hosp; **Address:** 3 Cooper Plaza, Ste 104, Camden, NJ 08103; **Phone:** 856-968-7965; **Board Cert:** Neurological Surgery 1995; **Med School:** Med Coll PA 1986; **Resid:** Neurological Surgery, Med Coll Penn 1992; **Fac Appt:** Assoc Prof NS, UMDNJ-RW Johnson Med Sch

Weiner, Howard L MD [NS] - **Spec Exp:** Pediatric Neurosurgery; Epilepsy; Tuberous Sclerosis; **Hospital:** NYU Langone Med Ctr (page 68); **Address:** NYU Med Ctr, Div Pediatric Neurosurgery, 317 E 34th St, Ste 1002, New York, NY 10016; **Phone:** 212-263-6419; **Board Cert:** Neurological Surgery 2012; **Med School:** Cornell Univ 1989; **Resid:** Neurological Surgery, NYU Med Ctr 1996; **Fellow:** Pediatric Neurological Surgery, NYU Med Ctr 1997; **Fac Appt:** Prof NS, NYU Sch Med

Weingart, Jon D MD [NS] - **Spec Exp:** Brain Tumors; Spinal Disorders; Gliomas; Chiari's Deformity; **Hospital:** Johns Hopkins Hosp (page 61); **Address:** Johns Hopkins Div Neurosurgery, 600 N Wolfe St Phipps Bldg - rm 107, Baltimore, MD 21287; **Phone:** 410-614-3052; **Board Cert:** Neurological Surgery 1998; **Med School:** Duke Univ 1987; **Resid:** Neurological Surgery, John Hopkins Hosp 1993; **Fellow:** Neurosurgical Oncology, Johns Hopkins Hosp; **Fac Appt:** Prof NS, Johns Hopkins Univ

Welch, William C MD [NS] - **Spec Exp:** Spinal Surgery; **Hospital:** Pennsylvania Hosp-UPHS (page 72); **Address:** Pennsylvania Hosp, Dept Neurosurgery, 235 S 8th St, Philadelphia, PA 19106; **Phone:** 215-829-6700; **Board Cert:** Neurological Surgery 1995; **Med School:** SUNY Downstate 1985; **Resid:** Neurological Surgery, Strong Meml Hosp 1991; **Fellow:** Neuro-Oncology, Montefiore Med Ctr 1992; Spinal Surgery, Weiler/Montefiore Med Ctr 1993; **Fac Appt:** Prof NS, Univ Pennsylvania

Whiting, Donald M MD [NS] - **Spec Exp:** Movement Disorders; Pain & Spasticity; Deep Brain Stimulation; Spinal Reconstructive Surgery; **Hospital:** Allegheny General Hosp, Washington Hosp, The; **Address:** 380 W Chestnut St, Washington, PA 15301-4657; **Phone:** 724-228-1414; **Board Cert:** Neurological Surgery 1995; **Med School:** Jefferson Med Coll 1985; **Resid:** Surgery, Geisinger Med Ctr 1986; Neurological Surgery, Cleveland Clinic 1991; **Fellow:** Neurological Trauma, Allegheny Genl Hosp 1990; **Fac Appt:** Prof NS, Drexel Univ Coll Med

Wilberger Jr, James E MD [NS] - **Spec Exp:** Epilepsy; Brain Injury; Brain Tumors-Benign; **Hospital:** Allegheny General Hosp; **Address:** Allegheny General Hosp, Neorosurgery, 420 E North Ave, Ste 302, Pittsburgh, PA 15212; **Phone:** 412-359-4764; **Board Cert:** Neurological Surgery 1986; **Med School:** Med Coll VA 1978; **Resid:** Neurological Surgery, Univ Pittsburgh Med Ctr 1984; **Fac Appt:** Prof NS, Drexel Univ Coll Med

Wisoff, Jeffrey H MD [NS] - **Spec Exp:** Pediatric Neurosurgery; Brain Tumors-Pediatric; Hydrocephalus; Chiari's Deformity; **Hospital:** NYU Langone Med Ctr (page 68), Maimonides Med Ctr (page 63); **Address:** 317 E 34th St, Ste 1002, New York, NY 10016-4974; **Phone:** 212-263-6419; **Board Cert:** Neurological Surgery 1990; Pediatric Neurological Surgery 2008; **Med School:** Geo Wash Univ 1978; **Resid:** Neurological Surgery, NYU/Bellevue Hosp 1984; **Fellow:** Pediatric Neurological Surgery, NYU Med Ctr 1985; **Fac Appt:** Assoc Prof NS, NYU Sch Med

Zager, Eric L MD [NS] - **Spec Exp:** Peripheral Nerve Disorders; Carpal Tunnel Syndrome; Pediatric Neurosurgery; Cerebrovascular Surgery; **Hospital:** Hosp Univ Penn - UPHS (page 72), Chldns Hosp of Philadelphia; **Address:** Hosp Univ Penn, Neurosurgery, 3400 Spruce St, 3 Silverstein, Philadelphia, PA 19104; **Phone:** 215-662-3497; **Board Cert:** Neurological Surgery 1992; **Med School:** Stanford Univ 1982; **Resid:** Neurological Surgery, Mass Genl Hosp 1988; **Fellow:** Peripheral Nerve Surgery, Univ Toronto 1989; Peripheral Nerve Surgery, LSU Med Ctr 1989; **Fac Appt:** Prof NS, Univ Pennsylvania

Southeast

Asher, Anthony MD [NS] - **Spec Exp:** Brain Tumors; Stereotactic Radiosurgery; Epilepsy; **Hospital:** Carolinas Med Ctr, Presby Hosp - Charlotte; **Address:** 225 Baldwin Ave, Charlotte, NC 28204; **Phone:** 704-376-1605; **Board Cert:** Neurological Surgery 1998; **Med School:** Wayne State Univ 1987; **Resid:** Neurological Surgery, Univ Mich Med Ctr 1995; **Fellow:** Surgical Oncology, Natl Cancer Inst 1991

Barrow, Daniel L MD [NS] - **Spec Exp:** Cerebrovascular Disease; Stroke; Aneurysm-Cerebral; Microsurgery; **Hospital:** Emory Univ Hosp; **Address:** Emory Univ Dept Neurosurgery, 1365B Clifton Rd NE, Ste 2200, Atlanta, GA 30322; **Phone:** 404-778-5770; **Board Cert:** Neurological Surgery 1988; **Med School:** Southern IL Univ 1979; **Resid:** Neurological Surgery, Emory Univ Affil Hosps 1985; **Fellow:** Cerebrovascular Neurosurgery, Mayo Clinic 1986; **Fac Appt:** Prof NS, Emory Univ

Boop, Frederick A MD [NS] - **Spec Exp:** Pediatric Neurosurgery; Epilepsy; Brain Tumors; **Hospital:** Le Bonheur Chldns Med Ctr, Methodist Univ Hosp - Memphis; **Address:** 6325 Humphreys Blvd, Memphis, TN 38120; **Phone:** 901-259-5340; **Board Cert:** Neurological Surgery 1993; Pediatric Neurological Surgery 2005; **Med School:** Univ Ark 1983; **Resid:** Neurological Surgery, Univ Tex Hlth Sci Ctr 1989; Neurological Surgery, Inst Neur/Hosp Sick Chldn 1987; **Fellow:** Epilepsy, Univ Minn Affil Hosp 1989; Pediatric Neurological Surgery, Ark Chldns Hosp 1990; **Fac Appt:** Assoc Prof NS, Univ Tenn Coll Med

Branch Jr, Charles L MD [NS] - **Spec Exp:** Spinal Reconstructive Surgery; Minimally Invasive Spinal Surgery; Stereotactic Radiosurgery; **Hospital:** Wake Forest Baptist Med Ctr; **Address:** Wake Forest Univ Baptist Med Ctr, Medical Center Blvd, Winston-Salem, NC 27157-1029; **Phone:** 336-716-4083; **Board Cert:** Neurological Surgery 1991; **Med School:** Univ Tex SW, Dallas 1981; **Resid:** Neurological Surgery, NC Baptist Hosp 1987; **Fellow:** Neurological Surgery, UCSF Med Ctr 1987; **Fac Appt:** Prof NS, Wake Forest Univ

Ewend, Matthew MD [NS] - **Spec Exp:** Brain Tumors; Pituitary Tumors; Pediatric Neurosurgery; Epilepsy; **Hospital:** NC Memorial Hosp - UNC, Alamance Regl Med Ctr; **Address:** Univ North Carolina Neurosurgery, 170 Manning Drive, MC 7060, Physicians Office Bldg, Chapel Hill, NC 27599; **Phone:** 919 966-1374; **Board Cert:** Neurological Surgery 2012; **Med School:** Johns Hopkins Univ 1990; **Resid:** Neurological Surgery, Johns Hopkins Hospital 1994; **Fellow:** Neuro-Oncology, National Institutes of Health 1996; **Fac Appt:** Asst Prof NS, Univ NC Sch Med

Foley, Kevin T MD [NS] - **Spec Exp:** Spinal Surgery; Minimally Invasive Spinal Surgery; **Hospital:** Methodist Univ Hosp - Memphis, Baptist Memorial Hospital-Memphis; **Address:** Semmes-Murphey Clin Neuro/Spine Inst, 6325 Humphreys Blvd, Memphis, TN 38120; **Phone:** 901-522-7700; **Board Cert:** Neurological Surgery 1987; **Med School:** UCLA 1979; **Resid:** Neurological Surgery, UCLA Med Ctr 1985; **Fac Appt:** Prof NS, Univ Tenn Coll Med

Freeman, Thomas B MD [NS] - **Spec Exp:** Parkinson's Disease; Nerve Surgery & Transplantation; Spinal Surgery; **Hospital:** Tampa Genl Hosp; **Address:** 2 Tampa Genl Cir Fl 7, Tampa, FL 33606; **Phone:** 813-259-0889; **Board Cert:** Neurological Surgery 1993; **Med School:** Johns Hopkins Univ 1981; **Resid:** Neurological Surgery, NYU Med Ctr 1988; **Fac Appt:** Prof NS, Univ S Fla Coll Med

Friedman, Allan H MD [NS] - **Spec Exp:** Brain Tumors; Skull Base Tumors; Gliomas; **Hospital:** Duke Univ Hosp; **Address:** Duke Univ Med Ctr, Box 3807, Durham, NC 27710; **Phone:** 919-681-6421; **Board Cert:** Neurological Surgery 1983; **Med School:** Univ IL Coll Med 1974; **Resid:** Neurological Surgery, Duke Univ Med Ctr 1980; **Fellow:** Vascular Surgery, Univ Western Ontario 1981; **Fac Appt:** Prof S, Duke Univ

Neurological Surgery

Green, Barth A MD [NS] - **Spec Exp:** Spinal Surgery; **Hospital:** Jackson Meml Hosp, Univ of Miami Hosp & Clins/Sylvester Comp Canc Ctr; **Address:** Univ Miami Dept Neurosurgery, 1095 NW 14th Terrace, Ste D4-6, Miami, FL 33136; **Phone:** 305-243-6946; **Board Cert:** Neurological Surgery 1978; **Med School:** Indiana Univ 1969; **Resid:** Neurological Surgery, Northwestern Univ Hosp 1975; **Fac Appt:** Prof NS, Univ Miami Sch Med

Guthrie, Barton L MD [NS] - **Spec Exp:** Brain Tumors; Stereotactic Radiosurgery; Parkinson's Disease/Movement Disorders; **Hospital:** Univ of Ala Hosp at Birmingham; **Address:** Univ Alabama, Div Neurosurg, 510 20th St S, Ste FOT 1038, Birmingham, AL 35294-3410; **Phone:** 205-934-8136; **Board Cert:** Neurological Surgery 1992; **Med School:** Univ Alabama 1980; **Resid:** Neurological Surgery, Mayo Clinic 1988; **Fellow:** Neurological Surgery, Stanford Univ Med Ctr 1988; **Fac Appt:** Assoc Prof NS, Univ Alabama

Hadley, Mark N MD [NS] - **Spec Exp:** Spinal Surgery-Complex; Spinal Disorders-Degenerative; **Hospital:** Univ of Ala Hosp at Birmingham; **Address:** UAB Div Neurosurgery, 1530 3rd Ave S, FOT 1030, Birmingham, AL 35294-3410; **Phone:** 205-934-1439; **Board Cert:** Neurological Surgery 1992; **Med School:** Albany Med Coll 1982; **Resid:** Neurological Surgery, St Josephs Hosp Med Ctr 1988; **Fac Appt:** Prof NS, Univ Alabama

Haid Jr, Regis W MD [NS] - **Spec Exp:** Spinal Surgery; Minimally Invasive Spinal Surgery; Spinal Disc Replacement; Microdiscectomy; **Hospital:** Piedmont Hosp, Shepherd Ctr - Atlanta; **Address:** Atlanta Brain & Spine Care, 2001 Peachtree Rd NE, Ste 575, Atlanta, GA 30309; **Phone:** 404-350-0106; **Board Cert:** Neurological Surgery 2011; **Med School:** W VA Univ 1982; **Resid:** Neurological Surgery, W Va Univ Hosps 1988; **Fellow:** Spinal Surgery, Univ Florida 1989; **Fac Appt:** Prof NS, Emory Univ

Heros, Roberto MD [NS] - **Spec Exp:** Cerebrovascular Surgery; Skull Base Surgery; Brain Tumors; **Hospital:** Jackson Meml Hosp, Univ of Miami Hosp & Clins/Sylvester Comp Canc Ctr; **Address:** Univ Miami, Dept Neurosurgery, 1095 NW 14th Terrace, Miami, FL 33136; **Phone:** 305-243-4572; **Board Cert:** Neurological Surgery 1979; **Med School:** Univ Tenn Coll Med 1968; **Resid:** Surgery, Mass Genl Hosp 1970; Neurological Surgery, Mass Genl Hosp 1976; **Fac Appt:** Prof NS, Univ Miami Sch Med

Hodes, Jonathan MD [NS] - **Spec Exp:** Spinal Cord Injury-Epidural Stimulation; Spinal Cord Injury; Movement Disorders; Brain Tumors; **Hospital:** Frazier Rehab Inst, Univ of Louisville Hosp; **Address:** Univ Louisville Hlth Care Outpt Ctr, Dept Neurosurgery, 3900 Kresge Way, Ste 41, Louisville, KY 40202; **Phone:** 502-899-3623; **Board Cert:** Internal Medicine 1986; Neurological Surgery 1994; **Med School:** Indiana Univ 1980; **Resid:** Internal Medicine, Indiana Univ Hosp 1983; Neurological Surgery, UCSF Med Ctr 1989; **Fellow:** Geriatric Medicine, NIH 1984; Neurological Radiology, Lariboisiere Hosp 1991

Landy, Howard J MD [NS] - **Spec Exp:** Stereotactic Radiosurgery; **Hospital:** Jackson Meml Hosp; **Address:** Univ Miami, Dept Neurosurgery, 1095 NW 14th Terrace Fl 2, Miami, FL 33136; **Phone:** 305-243-4675; **Board Cert:** Neurological Surgery 1991; **Med School:** Univ Miami Sch Med 1980; **Resid:** Neurological Surgery, Jackson Meml Hosp 1987; **Fac Appt:** Prof NS, Univ Miami Sch Med

Levi, Allan MD/PhD [NS] - **Spec Exp:** Spinal Surgery; Peripheral Nerve Disorders; Minimally Invasive Spinal Surgery; Spinal Cord Injury; **Hospital:** Jackson Meml Hosp, Univ of Miami Hosp; **Address:** 1095 NW 14th Terrace, Miami, FL 33136; **Phone:** 305-243-2088; **Board Cert:** Neurological Surgery 1999; **Med School:** Univ Ottawa 1986; **Resid:** Neurological Surgery, Univ Toronto Affil Hosp 1991; **Fellow:** Spinal Surgery, Barrow Neuro Inst 1995; **Fac Appt:** Prof NS, Univ Miami Sch Med

Markert Jr, James M MD [NS] - **Spec Exp:** Brain Tumors; Stereotactic Radiosurgery; Clinical Trials; **Hospital:** Univ of Ala Hosp at Birmingham; **Address:** Univ Alabama, Div Neurosurgery, 510 20th St S, FOT, rm 1060, Birmingham, AL 35294; **Phone:** 205-975-6985; **Board Cert:** Neurological Surgery 2010; **Med School:** Columbia P&S 1988; **Resid:** Neurological Surgery, Univ Mich Med Ctr 1995; **Fellow:** Neuro-Oncology, Mass Genl Hosp; **Fac Appt:** Prof NS, Univ Alabama

Morcos, Jacques J MD [NS] - **Spec Exp:** Cerebrovascular Surgery; Brain Tumors; Skull Base Tumors & Surgery; Arteriovenous Malformations; **Hospital:** Jackson Meml Hosp; **Address:** University of Miami, Dept Neurosurgery, 1095 NW 14th Terr Fl 2, Miami, FL 33136; **Phone:** 305-243-4675; **Board Cert:** Neurological Surgery 2010; **Med School:** Lebanon 1985; **Resid:** Neurological Surgery, Natl Hosp for Nervous Diseases 1990; Neurological Surgery, Univ Minnesota 1993; **Fellow:** Cerebrovascular Neurosurgery, Univ Florida/Shands Med Ctr 1994; Skull Base Surgery, Barrow Neurolical Inst 1995; **Fac Appt:** Assoc Prof NS, Univ Miami Sch Med

Myseros, John S MD [NS] - **Spec Exp:** Pediatric Neurosurgery; Brain Tumors; Congenital Nervous System Malformations; **Hospital:** Inova Fairfax Hosp for Chldn, Chldns Natl Med Ctr; **Address:** Children's Neurosurgery, 8501 Arlington Blvd, Ste 450, Fairfax, VA 22031; **Phone:** 571-226-8330; **Board Cert:** Neurological Surgery 2010; Pediatric Neurological Surgery 2010; **Med School:** Johns Hopkins Univ 1990; **Resid:** Neurological Surgery, Med Coll Virginia 1996; **Fellow:** Pediatric Neurological Surgery, Hosp for Sick Children 1997; **Fac Appt:** Assoc Prof NS, Geo Wash Univ

Oakes, W Jerry MD [NS] - **Spec Exp:** Pediatric Neurosurgery; Chiari's Deformity; Occult Spinal Dysraphism (OSD); **Hospital:** Children's Hospital - Birmingham; **Address:** 1600 7th Ave S Lowder Bldg - Ste 400, Birmingham, AL 35233; **Phone:** 205-638-9653; **Board Cert:** Neurological Surgery 1981; Pediatric Neurological Surgery 2005; **Med School:** Duke Univ 1972; **Resid:** Neurological Surgery, Duke Univ Hosp 1978; **Fellow:** Neurological Surgery, Hosp for Sick Chldn 1975; Neurological Surgery, Great Ormond St Hosp 1979; **Fac Appt:** Prof NS, Univ Alabama

Olson, Jeffrey J MD [NS] - **Spec Exp:** Neuro-Oncology; Brain Tumors; Skull Base Tumors; Von Hippel-Lindau Disease; **Hospital:** Emory Univ Hosp, Emory Univ Hosp Midtown; **Address:** Emory Univ, Dept Neurosurgery, 1365B Clifton Rd NE, Ste 2200, Atlanta, GA 30322; **Phone:** 404-778-5770; **Board Cert:** Neurological Surgery 1989; **Med School:** Univ Minn 1981; **Resid:** Neurological Surgery, Univ Iowa Hosps & Clinics 1987; **Fellow:** Neurological Surgery, Natl Inst Hlth 1990; **Fac Appt:** Prof NS, Emory Univ

Parent, Andrew D MD [NS] - **Spec Exp:** Pediatric Neurosurgery; Neuroendocrine Tumors; Pituitary Tumors; **Hospital:** Univ Mississippi Med Ctr; **Address:** Univ Miss Med Ctr-Dept Neurosurgery, 2500 N State St, Jackson, MS 39216-4500; **Phone:** 601-984-5702; **Board Cert:** Neurological Surgery 1981; **Med School:** Univ VT Coll Med 1970; **Resid:** Neurological Surgery, Emory Univ 1978; **Fellow:** Neurological Surgery, Univ Tex Med Br 1974; **Fac Appt:** Prof NS, Univ Miss

Patel, Sunil J MD [NS] - **Spec Exp:** Brain Tumors; Skull Base Surgery; Pain-Facial; Trigeminal Neuralgia; **Hospital:** MUSC Med Ctr, R H Johnson VA Med Ctr - Charleston; **Address:** MUSC-Adult Neurological Surgery, CSB, Ste 428, Charleston, SC 29425; **Phone:** 843-792-7700; **Board Cert:** Neurological Surgery 1996; **Med School:** Med Univ SC 1985; **Resid:** Neurological Surgery, Univ South Carolina 1991; **Fellow:** Neurological Surgery, Nagoya Univ Med School 1991; Skull Base Surgery, Univ Pittsburgh 1993; **Fac Appt:** Prof NS, Med Univ SC

Ragheb, John MD [NS] - **Spec Exp:** Pediatric Neurosurgery; Spinal Cord Tumors-Pediatric; Brain Injury-Pediatric; Epilepsy; **Hospital:** Miami Children's Hosp; **Address:** Miami Children's Hospital, Dept Neurosurgery, 3100 SW 62nd Ave, Ste 3109, Miami, FL 33155; **Phone:** 305-662-8386; **Board Cert:** Neurological Surgery 1996; Pediatric Neurological Surgery 1998; **Med School:** Univ Mich Med Sch 1985; **Resid:** Neurological Surgery, Univ Maryland Med Ctr 1991; **Fellow:** Pediatric Neurological Surgery, NYU Med Ctr 1992; **Fac Appt:** Prof NS, Univ Miami Sch Med

Reid, William S MD [NS] - **Spec Exp:** Minimally Invasive Spinal Surgery; Brain & Spinal Cord Tumors; Pituitary Tumors; Microsurgery; **Hospital:** Univ of Tennesee Med Ctr; **Address:** Univ Tenn Med Ctr, Neurological Surgery, 1932 Alcoa Hwy, Ste 280, Knoxville, TN 37920; **Phone:** 865-329-4003; **Board Cert:** Neurological Surgery 1980; **Med School:** Univ Ariz Coll Med 1971; **Resid:** Neurological Surgery, Univ Texas SW Med Ctr 1975; **Fac Appt:** Assoc Clin Prof NS, Univ Tenn Coll Med

Robertson, Jon H MD [NS] - **Spec Exp:** Brain & Spinal Cord Tumors; Skull Base Surgery; Stereotactic Radiosurgery; **Hospital:** Methodist Univ Hosp - Memphis; **Address:** Semmes-Murphey Clin Neuro/Spine Inst, 6325 Humphreys Blvd, Memphis, TN 38120; **Phone:** 901-522-7700; **Board Cert:** Neurological Surgery 1982; **Med School:** Univ Tenn Coll Med 1971; **Resid:** Surgery, City Memphis Hosp 1974; Neurological Surgery, Univ TN Med Ctr 1979; **Fac Appt:** Prof NS, Univ Tenn Coll Med

Rodts Jr, Gerald E MD [NS] - **Spec Exp:** Spinal Surgery; Spinal Trauma; Spinal Tumors; **Hospital:** Emory Univ Hosp, Emory Univ Hosp Midtown; **Address:** Emory Spine Center, 59 Executive Park South, Ste 3000, Atlanta, GA 30329; **Phone:** 404-778-7000; **Board Cert:** Neurological Surgery 1998; **Med School:** Columbia P&S 1987; **Resid:** Neurological Surgery, UCLA Med Ctr 1994; **Fellow:** Spinal Surgery, Emory Univ 1995; **Fac Appt:** Prof NS, Emory Univ

Sampson, John H MD/PhD [NS] - **Spec Exp:** Brain Tumors; Clinical Trials; **Hospital:** Duke Univ Hosp; **Address:** Duke Univ Med Ctr, Box 3050, Durham, NC 27710; **Phone:** 919-684-9041; **Board Cert:** Neurological Surgery 2002; **Med School:** Univ Manitoba 1990; **Resid:** Neurological Surgery, Duke Univ Med Ctr 1998; **Fellow:** Neurological Intensive Care, Duke Univ Med Ctr 1999; **Fac Appt:** Assoc Prof S, Duke Univ

Shaffrey, Christopher I MD [NS] - **Spec Exp:** Spinal Surgery; Spinal Surgery-Pediatric; **Hospital:** Univ of Virginia Health Sys; **Address:** Univ Virg, Dept Neurosurgery, 2 Hospital Drive, West Complex-Barringer Wing Fl 3, Charlottesville, VA 22908; **Phone:** 434-243-7026; **Board Cert:** Neurological Surgery 1997; Orthopaedic Surgery 2008; **Med School:** Univ VA Sch Med 1986; **Resid:** Neurological Surgery, Univ Virginia Med Ctr 1992; Orthopaedic Surgery, Univ Virginia Med Ctr 1995; **Fellow:** Spinal Surgery, Univ Virginia Med Ctr 1996; **Fac Appt:** Prof NS, Univ VA Sch Med

Shaffrey, Mark E MD [NS] - **Spec Exp:** Brain Tumors; Clinical Trials; Spinal Cord Tumors; Spinal Tumors; **Hospital:** Univ of Virginia Health Sys; **Address:** UVA Hlth Sys, Dept Neurosurgery, 1300 Jefferson Park Ave, Charlottesville, VA 22908; **Phone:** 434-924-1843; **Board Cert:** Neurological Surgery 2011; **Med School:** Univ VA Sch Med 1987; **Resid:** Neurological Surgery, Univ Virginia Med Ctr 1991; **Fellow:** Microvascular Physiology, NIH 1992; Neurological Pathology, Univ Virginia Med Ctr 1993; **Fac Appt:** Prof NS, Univ VA Sch Med

Sills Jr, Allen MD [NS] - **Spec Exp:** Brain & Spinal Tumors; Stereotactic Radiosurgery; Cerebrovascular Disease; **Hospital:** Vanderbilt Univ Med Ctr (page 75); **Address:** 2009 Mallory Ln, Ste 230, Franklin, TN 37067; **Phone:** 615-778-2265; **Board Cert:** Neurological Surgery 2002; **Med School:** Johns Hopkins Univ 1990; **Resid:** Neurological Surgery, Johns Hopkins Hosp 1994; **Fellow:** Neuro-Oncology, Hunterian Neurosurg Lab/Johns Hopkins 1996; **Fac Appt:** Assoc Prof NS, Vanderbilt Univ

Swaid, Swaid N MD [NS] - **Spec Exp:** Stereotactic Radiosurgery; Brain Tumors; Pituitary Tumors; Acoustic Neuroma; **Hospital:** Brookwood Med Ctr; **Address:** Neurological Surgery Assocs, 513 Brookwood Blvd, Ste 372, Birmingham, AL 35209; **Phone:** 205-949-1800; **Board Cert:** Neurological Surgery 1983; **Med School:** Univ Alabama 1976; **Resid:** Neurological Surgery, UAB Med Ctr 1981; **Fac Appt:** Assoc Prof NS, Univ Alabama

Tatter, Stephen MD/PhD [NS] - **Spec Exp:** Brain Tumors; Pituitary Tumors; Stereotactic Radio-surgery; **Hospital:** Wake Forest Baptist Med Ctr; **Address:** Wake Forest Baptist Hlth, Dept Neuro-surg, Medical Center Blvd, Winston-Salem, NC 27157-1029; **Phone:** 336-716-4047; **Board Cert:** Neurological Surgery 2004; **Med School:** Cornell Univ-Weill Med Coll 1990; **Resid:** Neurological Surgery, Mass Genl Hosp 1996; **Fellow:** Neurological Surgery, Mass Genl Hosp 1997; **Fac Appt:** Assoc Prof NS, Wake Forest Univ

Thompson, Reid C MD [NS] - **Spec Exp:** Neuro-Oncology; Brain & Spinal Cord Tumors; Neu-rovascular Surgery; Skull Base Tumors; **Hospital:** Vanderbilt Univ Med Ctr (page 75); **Address:** Van-derbilt Neurosurgery, 1500 21st Ave S, Ste 1506, Nashville, TN 37212; **Phone:** 615-322-7417; **Board Cert:** Neurological Surgery 2012; **Med School:** Johns Hopkins Univ 1989; **Resid:** Neuro-logical Surgery, Johns Hopkins Hosp 1995; **Fellow:** Neuro-Oncology, Rsch-Johns Hopkins Hosp 1996; Cerebrovascular Neurosurgery, Stanford Univ Med Ctr 1997; **Fac Appt:** Prof NS, Vanderbilt Univ

Van Loveren, Harry R MD [NS] - **Spec Exp:** Trigeminal Neuralgia; Skull Base Surgery; **Hos-pital:** Tampa Genl Hosp; **Address:** 2 Tampa General Cir, Tampa, FL 33606; **Phone:** 813-259-0965; **Board Cert:** Neurological Surgery 1988; **Med School:** Univ Cincinnati 1979; **Resid:** Neurological Surgery, Good Samaritan Hosp 1984; **Fellow:** Neurological Surgery, Universitatspital 1985; **Fac Appt:** Prof NS, Univ S Fla Coll Med

Wharen Jr, Robert E MD [NS] - **Spec Exp:** Parkinson's Disease; Brain Tumors; Epilepsy; **Hos-pital:** Mayo - Jacksonville; **Address:** Mayo Clinic, Dept Neurosurgery, 4500 San Pablo Rd, Jack-sonville, FL 32224-1865; **Phone:** 904-953-2103; **Board Cert:** Neurological Surgery 1988; **Med School:** Penn State Coll Med 1979; **Resid:** Neurological Surgery, Mayo Clinic 1985; **Fac Appt:** Prof NS, Mayo Med Sch

Wilson, John A MD [NS] - **Spec Exp:** Cerebrovascular Surgery; Skull Base Surgery; Spinal Sur-gery; MoyaMoya Disease; **Hospital:** Wake Forest Baptist Med Ctr; **Address:** Wake Forest Univ Bap-tist Medical Center, Medical Center Blvd, Winston-Salem, NC 27157-1029; **Phone:** 336-716-4020; **Board Cert:** Neurological Surgery 1996; **Med School:** Jefferson Med Coll 1982; **Resid:** Surgery, Allegheny Genl Hosp 1985; **Fellow:** Neurological Surgery, New England Med Ctr 1990; Neurologi-cal Surgery, Parcelsus Clinic 1990; **Fac Appt:** Prof NS, Wake Forest Univ

Midwest

Atkinson, John L MD [NS] - **Spec Exp:** Pituitary Surgery; Stroke; Cerebrovascular Disease; **Hospital:** Mayo Med Ctr & Clin - Rochester; **Address:** Mayo Clinic, Dept Neurosurgery, 200 First St SW, Gonda 8, Rochester, MN 55905; **Phone:** 507-284-5317; **Board Cert:** Neurological Surgery 1992; **Med School:** Univ Alabama 1984; **Resid:** Neurological Surgery, Mayo Clinic 1990; **Fac Appt:** Assoc Prof NS, Mayo Med Sch

Bailes Jr, Julian E MD [NS] - **Spec Exp:** Neuro-Oncology; Cancer Surgery; Spinal Surgery; Cerebrovascular Surgery; **Hospital:** NorthShore Univ HlthSys; **Address:** NorthShore University HealthSystem, 2650 2650 Ridge Ave, Kellogg 3rd Floor, Evaston, IL 60201; **Phone:** 847-570-4224; **Board Cert:** Neurological Surgery 1992; **Med School:** Louisiana State U, New Orleans 1982; **Resid:** Surgery, Northwestern Meml Hosp 1987; **Fellow:** Neurological Surgery, Barrow Neurological Inst 1988

Bakay, Roy AE MD [NS] - **Spec Exp:** Parkinson's Disease/Movement Disorders; Epilepsy; Stereotactic Radiosurgery; **Hospital:** Rush Univ Med Ctr; **Address:** University Neurosurgery, 1725 W Harrison St, Ste 855, Chicago, IL 60612; **Phone:** 312-942-6644; **Board Cert:** Neurological Sur-gery 1985; **Med School:** Northwestern Univ 1975; **Resid:** Neurological Surgery, Univ Washington Med Ctr 1981; **Fellow:** Neuronal Plasticity, Natl Inst Hlth 1982; **Fac Appt:** Prof NS, Rush Med Coll

Neurological Surgery

Barnett, Gene H MD [NS] - **Spec Exp:** Brain Tumors; Stereotactic Radiosurgery; Von Hippel-Lindau Disease; **Hospital:** Cleveland Clin (page 55); **Address:** Cleveland Clinic - S73, 9500 Euclid Ave, Cleveland, OH 44195; **Phone:** 216-444-5381; **Board Cert:** Neurological Surgery 1990; **Med School:** Case West Res Univ 1980; **Resid:** Neurological Surgery, Cleveland Clinic 1986; **Fellow:** Neurology, Cleveland Clinic 1982; Research, Mass Genl Hosp-Harvard 1987; **Fac Appt:** Prof NS, Cleveland Cl Coll Med/Case West Res

Bauer, Jerry MD [NS] - **Spec Exp:** Pain-Back; Minimally Invasive Surgery; Spinal Surgery; **Hospital:** Adv Luth Genl Hosp; **Address:** 1875 Dempster, Ste 410, Park Ridge, IL 60068-1168; **Phone:** 847-698-1088; **Board Cert:** Neurological Surgery 1982; **Med School:** Univ IL Coll Med 1974; **Resid:** Neurological Surgery, Univ of Illinois Med Ctr 1979; **Fac Appt:** Asst Clin Prof NS, Univ IL Coll Med

Benzel, Edward C MD [NS] - **Spec Exp:** Spinal Surgery; **Hospital:** Cleveland Clin (page 55); **Address:** 9500 Euclid Ave, Desk S80, Cleveland, OH 44195; **Phone:** 216-445-5514; **Board Cert:** Neurological Surgery 1986; **Med School:** Univ Wisc 1975; **Resid:** Neurological Surgery, Med Coll Wisc Clins 1980; **Fellow:** Spinal Cord Injury Medicine, Wood VA Med Ctr 1981; **Fac Appt:** Prof NS, Case West Res Univ

Bierbrauer, Karin S MD [NS] - **Spec Exp:** Pediatric Neurosurgery; Spina Bifida; Hydrocephalus; Hydrocephalus; **Hospital:** Cincinnati Chldns Hosp Med Ctr; **Address:** Cincinnati Childrens Hospital, 3333 Burnet Ave, MC 2016, Cincinnati, OH 45229; **Phone:** 513-636-7124; **Board Cert:** Neurological Surgery 1994; Pediatric Neurological Surgery 2007; **Med School:** Med Univ SC 1984; **Resid:** Neurological Surgery, Emory Univ Hosp 1990; **Fellow:** Pediatric Neurological Surgery, Chldns Meml Hosp 1991; **Fac Appt:** Assoc Clin Prof NS, Ohio State Univ

Bingaman, William MD [NS] - **Spec Exp:** Epilepsy; Spinal Surgery; **Hospital:** Cleveland Clin (page 55); **Address:** Cleveland Clinic, Neurological Clinic, 9500 Euclid Ave, Desk S60, Cleveland, OH 44195; **Phone:** 216-444-9058; **Board Cert:** Neurological Surgery 2011; **Med School:** Temple Univ 1990; **Resid:** Neurological Surgery, Cleveland Clinic Fdn 1996; **Fellow:** Spinal Surgery, Cleveland Clinic Fdn 1997

Brown, Frederick D MD [NS] - **Spec Exp:** Minimally Invasive Spinal Surgery; Spinal Surgery; Pain-Chronic; **Hospital:** Univ of Chicago Med Ctr; **Address:** Univ Chicago Hosp, Dept Neurosurgery, 5841 S Maryland Ave, MC 3026, Chicago, IL 60637; **Phone:** 773-702-2123; **Board Cert:** Neurological Surgery 1982; **Med School:** Ohio State Univ 1972; **Resid:** Neurological Surgery, Univ Chicago Hosps 1978; **Fac Appt:** Assoc Prof NS, Univ Chicago-Pritzker Sch Med

Bucholz, Richard D MD [NS] - **Spec Exp:** Epilepsy/Seizure Disorders; Stereotactic Radiosurgery; **Hospital:** St. Louis Univ Hosp; **Address:** 1320 S Grand Ave, O'Donnell Hall Fl 1, St Louis, MO 63104; **Phone:** 314-977-4750; **Board Cert:** Neurological Surgery 1985; **Med School:** Yale Univ 1977; **Resid:** Neurological Surgery, Yale New Haven Hosp 1983; **Fac Appt:** Prof NS, St Louis Univ

Chandler, James P MD [NS] - **Spec Exp:** Skull Base Surgery; Neuro-Oncology; Brain Tumors; Spinal Disorders; **Hospital:** Northwestern Meml Hosp; **Address:** 675 N St Clair St, Galter Pavilion, Ste 20-250, Chicago, IL 60611; **Phone:** 312-695-8143; **Board Cert:** Neurological Surgery 2002; **Med School:** Univ MD Sch Med 1990; **Resid:** Neurological Surgery, Northwestern Meml Hosp 1996; **Fellow:** Microvascular Surgery, Inst Neurologico De S√?¬£o Paulo 1996; Cranial Base Surgery, George Washington Univ Hosp 1997; **Fac Appt:** Asst Prof NS, Northwestern Univ

Chandler, William F MD [NS] - **Spec Exp:** Pituitary Surgery; Brain Tumors; **Hospital:** Univ of Michigan Hosp; **Address:** 1500 E Medical Ctr Drive, Ste 3552, Tauban Center, Ann Arbor, MI 48109; **Phone:** 734-936-5020; **Board Cert:** Neurological Surgery 1980; **Med School:** Univ Mich Med Sch 1971; **Resid:** Neurological Surgery, Michigan Hosp 1977; **Fac Appt:** Prof NS, Univ Mich Med Sch

Chiocca, E Antonio MD [NS] - **Spec Exp:** Brain Tumors; Spinal Cord Tumors; Peripheral Nerve Surgery; **Hospital:** Arthur G James Cancer Hosp & Research Inst, Ohio St Univ Med Ctr; **Address:** OSU Med Ctr, Dept Neurosurgery, 410 W 10th Ave, N1019 Doan Hall, Columbus, OH 43210; **Phone:** 614-293-9312; **Board Cert:** Neurological Surgery 2011; **Med School:** Univ Tex, Houston 1988; **Resid:** Neurological Surgery, Mass Genl Hosp 1995; **Fac Appt:** Prof NS, Ohio State Univ

Dacey Jr, Ralph G MD [NS] - **Spec Exp:** Cerebrovascular Surgery; Aneurysm-Cerebral; Brain Tumors; **Hospital:** Barnes-Jewish Hosp, Barnes-Jewish West County Hosp; **Address:** Wash Univ Dept Neurosurgery, 660 S Euclid Ave, Box 8057, St Louis, MO 63110; **Phone:** 314-362-3577; **Board Cert:** Internal Medicine 1978; Neurological Surgery 1985; **Med School:** Univ VA Sch Med 1974; **Resid:** Internal Medicine, Strong Meml Hosp 1977; Neurological Surgery, Univ Virginia Med Ctr 1983; **Fac Appt:** Prof NS, Washington Univ, St Louis

Dempsey, Robert J MD [NS] - **Spec Exp:** Vascular Neurosurgery; Aneurysm-Cerebral; Stroke; **Hospital:** Univ WI Hosp & Clins; **Address:** Dept Neurosurgery, 600 Highland Ave, rm K4-822, Madison, WI 53792; **Phone:** 608-265-5967; **Board Cert:** Neurological Surgery 1985; **Med School:** Univ Chicago-Pritzker Sch Med 1977; **Resid:** Neurological Surgery, Univ Mich Hosps 1983; **Fac Appt:** Prof NS, Univ Wisc

Diaz, Fernando G MD/PhD [NS] - **Spec Exp:** Arteriovenous Malformations; Spinal Surgery; **Hospital:** Providence Hosp - Southfield, Beaumont Hosp-Royal Oak; **Address:** Michigan Head & Spine Inst, 29275 Northwestern Hwy, Ste 100, Southfield, MI 48034; **Phone:** 877-784-3667; **Board Cert:** Neurological Surgery 1980; **Med School:** Mexico 1968; **Resid:** Surgery, Univ Kansas Med Ctr 1973; Neurological Surgery, Univ Minn Med Ctr 1978; **Fellow:** Cerebrovascular Disease, Univ Minn Med Ctr 1979; **Fac Appt:** Prof NS, Wayne State Univ

Fessler, Richard G MD/PhD [NS] - **Spec Exp:** Skull Base Surgery; Spinal Surgery; Minimally Invasive Spinal Surgery; **Hospital:** Northwestern Meml Hosp; **Address:** 676 N St Clair St, Galter Pavillion 20-250, Chicago, IL 60611; **Phone:** 312-695-8143; **Board Cert:** Neurological Surgery 1992; **Med School:** Univ Chicago-Pritzker Sch Med 1983; **Resid:** Neurological Surgery, Univ Chicago Hosp 1989; **Fac Appt:** Prof NS, Northwestern Univ

Frim, David M MD/PhD [NS] - **Spec Exp:** Pediatric Neurosurgery; Hydrocephalus; Brain & Spinal Tumors; Brain & Spinal Malformations; **Hospital:** Univ of Chicago Med Ctr; **Address:** Section of Neurosurgery, MC 3026, The University of Chicago, 5841 S Maryland Ave, Chicago, IL 60637-1463; **Phone:** 773-702-2123; **Board Cert:** Neurological Surgery 1998; Pediatric Neurological Surgery 1999; **Med School:** Harvard Med Sch 1988; **Resid:** Neurological Surgery, Mass Genl Hosp 1994; **Fellow:** Pediatric Neurological Surgery, Chldns Hosp 1996; **Fac Appt:** Prof NS, Univ Chicago-Pritzker Sch Med

Grubb Jr, Robert L MD [NS] - **Spec Exp:** Brain Tumors; Acoustic Neuroma; Trigeminal Neuralgia; Skull Base Tumors; **Hospital:** Barnes-Jewish Hosp, St. Louis Chldns Hosp; **Address:** Wash Univ Sch Med, Dept Neurosurgery, 660 S Euclid Ave, Box 8057, St Louis, MO 63110; **Phone:** 314-362-3577; **Board Cert:** Neurological Surgery 1976; **Med School:** Univ NC Sch Med 1965; **Resid:** Surgery, Barnes Jewish Hosp 1967; Neurological Surgery, Barnes Jewish Hosp 1973; **Fellow:** Neurological Surgery, National Inst Health 1969; **Fac Appt:** Prof NS, Washington Univ, St Louis

Guthikonda, Murali MD [NS] - **Spec Exp:** Skull Base Tumors; Pituitary Tumors; Aneurysm-Cerebral; Spinal Tumors; **Hospital:** Harper Univ Hosp, Beaumont Hosp-Royal Oak; **Address:** Wayne St U Physicians Grp-Neurosurgery, 4160 John R, Ste 925, Detroit, MI 48201; **Phone:** 313-831-0777; **Board Cert:** Neurological Surgery 1982; **Med School:** India 1971; **Resid:** Surgery, St Elizabeth Hosp 1976; Neurological Surgery, Med Ctr Hosp VT 1980; **Fellow:** Skull Base Surgery, Univ Cincinnati 1993; **Fac Appt:** Prof NS, Wayne State Univ

Kaufman, Bruce A MD [NS] - **Spec Exp:** Pediatric Neurosurgery; Brain & Spinal Cord Tumors; Spasticity & Movement Disorders; **Hospital:** Chldns Hosp - Wisconsin; **Address:** Chldns Corporate Ctr, Dept Neurosurg, 999 N 92nd St, Ste 310, Milwaukee, WI 53226; **Phone:** 414-266-6435; **Board Cert:** Neurological Surgery 1992; Pediatric Neurological Surgery 2006; **Med School:** Case West Res Univ 1982; **Resid:** Neurological Surgery, Univ Hosp Cleveland/Case West Res 1988; **Fellow:** Pediatric Neurological Surgery, Chldns Meml Hosp/Northwestern Univ 1989; **Fac Appt:** Prof NS, Med Coll Wisc

Kuntz IV, Charles MD [NS] - **Spec Exp:** Spinal Surgery; Peripheral Nerve Surgery; Spinal Disorders; **Hospital:** Univ Hosp - Cincinnati; **Address:** 222 Piedmont Ave, Ste 3100, Cincinnati, OH 45219; **Phone:** 513-569-5220; **Board Cert:** Neurological Surgery 2004; **Med School:** Case West Res Univ 1991; **Resid:** Surgery, Univ Wash Med Ctr 1993; Neurological Surgery, Univ Wash Med Ctr 1999; **Fellow:** Neurological Surgery, Atkinson Morley's Hosp 1996; Neurological Surgery, Univ Wash Med Ctr 2000; **Fac Appt:** Asst Prof NS, Univ Cincinnati

Link, Michael J MD [NS] - **Spec Exp:** Skull Base Tumors; Brain Tumors; Cerebrovascular Surgery; **Hospital:** Mayo Med Ctr & Clin - Rochester; **Address:** Mayo Clinic, Dept Neurosurgery, 200 First St SW, Rochester, MN 55905; **Phone:** 507-284-8008; **Board Cert:** Neurological Surgery 2011; **Med School:** Mayo Med Sch 1990; **Resid:** Neurological Surgery, Mayo Clinic 1996; **Fellow:** Cerebrovascular & Skull Base Surgery, Univ Cincinnati/Mayfield Clinic 1998; **Fac Appt:** Assoc Prof NS, Mayo Med Sch

Loftus, Christopher M MD [NS] - **Spec Exp:** Carotid Artery Surgery; Aneurysm-Cerebral; Arteriovenous Malformations; Cerebrovascular Surgery; **Hospital:** Loyola Univ Med Ctr; **Address:** Loyola Outpatient Center, 2160 S First St, Maywood, IL 60153; **Phone:** 888-584-7888; **Board Cert:** Neurological Surgery 1987; **Med School:** SUNY Downstate 1979; **Resid:** Neurological Surgery, Columbia-Presby Med Ctr 1985; **Fac Appt:** Prof NS, Temple Univ

Luken, Martin MD [NS] - **Spec Exp:** Brain Tumors; Spinal Surgery; Chiari's Deformity; **Hospital:** Ingalls Meml Hosp, Rush Univ Med Ctr; **Address:** 71 W 156th St, Ste 205, Harvey, IL 60426; **Phone:** 708-596-3344; **Board Cert:** Neurological Surgery 1983; **Med School:** Columbia P&S 1973; **Resid:** Surgery, Univ Illinois Med Ctr 1976; Neurological Surgery, Neurological Inst-Columbia Presby 1980; **Fac Appt:** Asst Prof NS, Rush Med Coll

Malik, Ghaus M MD [NS] - **Spec Exp:** Trigeminal Neuralgia; Cerebrovascular Surgery; Brain & Spinal Cord Tumors; **Hospital:** Henry Ford- W Bloomfield Hosp, Beaumont Hosp-Royal Oak; **Address:** Henry Ford Hosp, Dept Neurosurg, 6777 W Maple Rd Fl 2, West Bloomfield, MI 48322; **Phone:** 248-661-6417; **Board Cert:** Neurological Surgery 1978; **Med School:** Pakistan 1968; **Resid:** Surgery, Henry Ford Hosp 1971; Neurological Surgery, Henry Ford Hosp 1975

Menezes, Arnold MD [NS] - **Spec Exp:** Pediatric Neurosurgery; Craniocervical Disorders; Spinal Surgery-Pediatric; **Hospital:** Univ Iowa Hosp & Clinics; **Address:** Univ Iowa Hosp, Dept Neurosurgery, 200 Hawkins Drive, Iowa City, IA 52242; **Phone:** 319-356-2768; **Board Cert:** Neurological Surgery 1976; Pediatric Neurological Surgery 2009; **Med School:** India 1967; **Resid:** Surgery, Univ Iowa Hosps 1970; Neurological Surgery, Univ Iowa Hosps 1974; **Fellow:** Child Neurology, Univ Iowa Hosps; **Fac Appt:** Prof NS, Univ Iowa Coll Med

Meyer, Fredric B MD [NS] - **Spec Exp:** Cerebrovascular Disease; Brain Tumors; Epilepsy; Pituitary Tumors; **Hospital:** Mayo Med Ctr & Clin - Rochester; **Address:** Mayo Clinic, Dept Neurosurgery, 200 First St SW, Gonda 8, Rochester, MN 55905; **Phone:** 507-284-5317; **Board Cert:** Neurological Surgery 1990; **Med School:** Boston Univ 1981; **Resid:** Neurological Surgery, Mayo Clinic 1987; **Fellow:** Neurological Surgery, Mayo Clinic 1988; **Fac Appt:** Prof NS, Mayo Med Sch

Nagib, Mahmoud G MD [NS] - **Spec Exp:** Pediatric Neurosurgery; Skull Base Surgery; **Hospital:** Children's Hosps & Clinics of Minneapolis, Abbott - Northwestern Hosp; **Address:** 800 E 28th St Piper Bldg - Ste 305, Minneapolis, MN 55407; **Phone:** 612-871-7278; **Board Cert:** Neurological Surgery 1985; Pediatric Neurological Surgery 2006; **Med School:** Egypt 1973; **Resid:** Neurological Surgery, Univ Minn Hosps 1982; **Fellow:** Neurological Physiology, Univ Oslo 1976; **Fac Appt:** Clin Prof NS, Univ Minn

Park, Tae Sung MD [NS] - **Spec Exp:** Pediatric Neurosurgery; Cerebral Palsy-Select Dorsal Rhizotomy; Brachial Plexus Palsy-Pediatric; Neuro-Oncology; **Hospital:** St. Louis Chldns Hosp; **Address:** St Louis Children's Hospital, 1 Children's Place, Ste 4S20, St Louis, MO 63110; **Phone:** 314-454-2810; **Board Cert:** Neurological Surgery 1985; Pediatric Neurological Surgery 2006; **Med School:** Korea 1971; **Resid:** Neurological Surgery, Univ Virginia Hosp 1981; **Fellow:** Pediatric Neurological Surgery, Hosp for Sick Chldn 1983; **Fac Appt:** Prof NS, Washington Univ, St Louis

Raffel, Corey MD/PhD [NS] - **Spec Exp:** Pediatric Neurosurgery; Brain Tumors; Medulloblastoma; **Hospital:** Nationwide Chldn's Hosp; **Address:** Nationwide Chldn's Hosp, Dept Neurosurgery, 700 Children's Drive, Columbus, OH 43205; **Phone:** 614-722-2014; **Board Cert:** Neurological Surgery 1990; Pediatric Neurological Surgery 2006; **Med School:** UCSD 1980; **Resid:** Neurological Surgery, UCSF Med Ctr 1986; **Fellow:** Pediatric Neurological Surgery, Hosp Sick Chldn 1988

Rezai, Ali R MD [NS] - **Spec Exp:** Parkinson's Disease; Pain-Chronic; Deep Brain Stimulation; Alzheimer's Disease; **Hospital:** Ohio St Univ Med Ctr; **Address:** OSU Med Ctr, 410 W 10th Ave, rm N1043, Doan Hall, Columbus, OH 43210; **Phone:** 614-366-2420; **Board Cert:** Neurological Surgery 2003; **Med School:** USC Sch Med 1990; **Resid:** Neurological Surgery, NYU Med Ctr 1997; **Fellow:** Stereo Neurological Surgery, Univ Toronto Med Ctr 1998; Neurological Surgery, Karolinska Inst; **Fac Appt:** Prof NS, Ohio State Univ

Rich, Keith M MD [NS] - **Spec Exp:** Brain Tumors; Neurovascular Surgery; Stereotactic Radiosurgery; **Hospital:** Barnes-Jewish Hosp; **Address:** Wash Univ Dept Neurosurgery, 660 S Euclid Ave, Box 8057, St Louis, MO 63110; **Phone:** 314-362-3577; **Board Cert:** Neurological Surgery 1987; **Med School:** Indiana Univ 1977; **Resid:** Neurological Surgery, Barnes Jewish Hosp 1982; **Fellow:** Neurological Pharmacology, Barnes Jewish Hosp 1984; **Fac Appt:** Assoc Prof NS, Washington Univ, St Louis

Rock, Jack P MD [NS] - **Spec Exp:** Neuro-Oncology; Pituitary Surgery; Skull Base Surgery; Brain Tumors; **Hospital:** Henry Ford Hosp; **Address:** Henry Ford Hosp, Dept Neurosurg, 2799 W Grand Blvd Fl K11, Detroit, MI 48202; **Phone:** 313-916-2241; **Board Cert:** Neurological Surgery 1989; **Med School:** Univ Miami Sch Med 1979; **Resid:** Neurological Surgery, New York Hosp-Cornell 1985; **Fellow:** Univ Maryland 1986

Rosenblum, Mark L MD [NS] - **Spec Exp:** Brain Tumors; Spinal Surgery; Infections-Neurologic; Neuro-Oncology; **Hospital:** Henry Ford Hosp; **Address:** Henry Ford Hosp, 2799 W Grand Blvd Fl K11, Detroit, MI 48202; **Phone:** 313-916-1340; **Board Cert:** Neurological Surgery 1982; **Med School:** NY Med Coll 1969; **Resid:** Surgery, UCLA Med Ctr 1973; Neurological Surgery, UCSF Med Ctr 1979; **Fellow:** Neuro-Oncology, NIH/Natl Cancer Inst 1972

Neurological Surgery

Ruge, John R MD [NS] - **Spec Exp:** Pediatric Neurosurgery; Brain Tumors; Hydrocephalus; **Hospital:** Adv Luth Genl Hosp; **Address:** Ctr Brain & Spine Surg-Parkside Ctr, 1875 Dempster St, Ste 415, Park Ridge, IL 60068; **Phone:** 847-698-1088; **Board Cert:** Neurological Surgery 1993; **Med School:** Northwestern Univ 1983; **Resid:** Neurological Surgery, Northwestern Meml Hosp 1989; **Fellow:** Pediatric Neurological Surgery, Childrens Hosp 1990; **Fac Appt:** Asst Prof S, Rush Med Coll

Ryken, Timothy C MD [NS] - **Spec Exp:** Brain Tumors; Spinal Surgery; **Hospital:** Covenant Med Ctr; **Address:** Iowa Spine & Brain Institute, 2710 St Francis Drive, Ste 110, Waterloo, IA 50702; **Phone:** 319-272-6700; **Board Cert:** Neurological Surgery 1998; **Med School:** Univ Iowa Coll Med 1988; **Resid:** Neurological Surgery, Univ Iowa 1995; **Fellow:** Research, Cambridge Univ 1996; **Fac Appt:** Assoc Prof NS, Univ Iowa Coll Med

Selman, Warren R MD [NS] - **Spec Exp:** Stroke; Pituitary Surgery; Aneurysm-Cerebral; Microsurgery; **Hospital:** Univ Hosps Case Med Ctr (page 74); **Address:** Dept Neurosurgery, 11100 Euclid Ave, 5th Fl Hanna House, Cleveland, OH 44106; **Phone:** 216-844-5745; **Board Cert:** Neurological Surgery 1986; **Med School:** Case West Res Univ 1977; **Resid:** Neurological Surgery, Univ Hosps 1984; **Fellow:** Research, Univ Hosps 1980; Neurological Surgery, Mayo Clinic 1984; **Fac Appt:** Prof NS, Case West Res Univ

Shapiro, Scott A MD [NS] - **Spec Exp:** Brain Tumors; Aneurysm-Cerebral; Spinal Cord Injury; Pituitary Tumors; **Hospital:** IU Health Methodist Hosp, Wishard Hlth Srvs; **Address:** IU Health Methodist Hosp, 1801 N Senate Blvd, Ste 610, Indianapolis, IN 46202; **Phone:** 317-396-1300; **Board Cert:** Neurological Surgery 1990; **Med School:** Indiana Univ 1981; **Resid:** Neurological Surgery, Indiana Univ Med Ctr 1987; **Fac Appt:** Prof NS, Indiana Univ

Spinner, Robert J MD [NS] - **Spec Exp:** Peripheral Nerve Surgery; Brachial Plexus Palsy; Brain Tumors; **Hospital:** Mayo Med Ctr & Clin - Rochester; **Address:** Mayo Clinic, Dept Neurosurgery, 200 First St SW, Gonda 8, Rochester, MN 55905; **Phone:** 507-284-5317; **Board Cert:** Orthopaedic Surgery 2003; Neurological Surgery 2006; **Med School:** Mayo Med Sch 1989; **Resid:** Orthopaedic Surgery, Duke Univ Med Ctr 1996; Neurological Surgery, Mayo Clinic 2000; **Fellow:** Peripheral Nerve Surgery, LSU Med Ctr 2000; **Fac Appt:** Prof NS, Mayo Med Sch

Thompson Jr, B Gregory MD [NS] - **Spec Exp:** Acoustic Neuroma; Neurovascular Surgery; Skull Base Tumors & Surgery; Aneurysm-Cerebral; **Hospital:** Univ of Michigan Hosp; **Address:** Dept Neurosurgery, 3552 Taubman Ctr, 1500 E Medical Center Drive, Ann Arbor, MI 48109-5338; **Phone:** 734-936-7493; **Board Cert:** Neurological Surgery 1998; **Med School:** Univ Kansas 1986; **Resid:** Neurological Surgery, Univ Pittsburgh 1993; Research, Natl Inst Hlth 1992; **Fellow:** Neurological Surgery, Barrow Neuro Inst 1994; Interventional Radiology, Thomas Jefferson Univ 2005

Tomita, Tadanori MD [NS] - **Spec Exp:** Pediatric Neurosurgery; Brain Tumors-Pediatric; Hydrocephalus; **Hospital:** Lurie Chldn's Hosp-Chicago, Northwestern Meml Hosp; **Address:** Chldns Meml Hosp, Div Ped Neurosurg, 2300 Children's Plaza, Box 28, Chicago, IL 60614-3363; **Phone:** 773-880-4373; **Board Cert:** Neurological Surgery 1984; Pediatric Neurological Surgery 1996; **Med School:** Japan 1970; **Resid:** Neurological Surgery, Kobe Univ 1974; Neurological Surgery, Northwestern Meml Hosp 1980; **Fellow:** Surgery, Meml Sloan Kettering Canc Ctr 1981; **Fac Appt:** Prof NS, Northwestern Univ

Traynelis, Vincent C MD [NS] - **Spec Exp:** Spinal Surgery; **Hospital:** Rush Univ Med Ctr; **Address:** Rush Univ Med Ctr, Dept Neurosurgery, 1725 W Harrison St, Ste 1115, Chicago, IL 60612; **Phone:** 312-942-6644; **Board Cert:** Neurological Surgery 1992; **Med School:** W VA Univ 1983; **Resid:** Neurological Surgery, Univ West Virginia Med Ctr 1989; **Fac Appt:** Prof NS, Rush Med Coll

Warnick, Ronald E MD [NS] - **Spec Exp:** Neuro-Oncology; Brain Tumors; **Hospital:** Univ Hosp - Cincinnati, Good Samaritan Hosp - Cincinnati; **Address:** 222 Piedmont Ave, Ste 3100, Cincinnati, OH 45219; **Phone:** 513-569-5286; **Board Cert:** Neurological Surgery 1995; **Med School:** Univ Rochester 1982; **Resid:** Neurological Surgery, NYU Med Ctr 1989; **Fellow:** Neuro-Oncology, UCSF Med Ctr 1991; **Fac Appt:** Prof NS, Univ Cincinnati

Great Plains and Mountains

Cherny, W Bruce MD [NS] - **Spec Exp:** Pediatric Neurosurgery; Brain Tumors; Spina Bifida; **Hospital:** St. Luke's Boise Med Ctr; **Address:** Childrens Specialty Ctr, 100 E Idaho St, Ste 202, Boise, ID 83712; **Phone:** 208-381-7360; **Board Cert:** Neurological Surgery 2011; **Med School:** Univ Ariz Coll Med 1987; **Resid:** Neurological Surgery, Barrow Neuro Inst/St Joseph's Med Ctr 1994; **Fellow:** Pediatric Neurological Surgery, Primary Chldns Hosp 1995

Couldwell, William T MD/PhD [NS] - **Spec Exp:** Skull Base Surgery; Vascular Neurosurgery; Pituitary Tumors; Skull Base Tumors; **Hospital:** Univ Utah Hlth Care; **Address:** Univ Utah, Dept Neurological Surgery, 175 N Medical Drive E, Salt Lake City, UT 84132-2303; **Phone:** 801-581-6908; **Board Cert:** Neurological Surgery 1994; **Med School:** McGill Univ 1984; **Resid:** Neurological Surgery, LAC/USC Med Ctr 1989; **Fellow:** Neurological Immunology, Montreal Neur Inst/McGill Univ 1990; Neurological Surgery, CHUV 1991; **Fac Appt:** Prof Emeritus NS, Univ Utah

Johnson, Stephen D MD [NS] - **Spec Exp:** Skull Base Tumors & Surgery; **Hospital:** Presby - St Luke's Med Ctr; **Address:** Western Neurological Group, 1601 E 19th Ave, Ste 4400, Denver, CO 80218; **Phone:** 303-861-2266; **Board Cert:** Neurological Surgery 1988; **Med School:** Univ Tenn Coll Med 1974; **Resid:** Neurological Surgery, Virginia Mason Med Ctr; Neurological Surgery, New York Hosp; **Fellow:** Neurological Surgery, Univ Tennessee; **Fac Appt:** Assoc Prof NS, Univ Colorado

Kestle, John RW MD [NS] - **Spec Exp:** Pediatric Neurosurgery; Epilepsy/Seizure Disorders; **Hospital:** Primary Children's Med Ctr; **Address:** 100 N Mario Capecchi Drive, Salt Lake City, UT 84113; **Phone:** 801-662-5340; **Board Cert:** Neurological Surgery 2012; **Med School:** Canada 1984; **Resid:** Neurological Surgery, Univ Toronto 1990; **Fellow:** Pediatric Neurological Surgery, Hosp Sick Chldn 1992; **Fac Appt:** Prof NS, Univ Utah

Lillehei, Kevin O MD [NS] - **Spec Exp:** Neuro-Oncology; Pituitary Tumors; Peripheral Nerve Surgery; **Hospital:** Univ of CO Hosp - Anschutz Inpatient Pav; **Address:** Univ Colorado Hosp, Dept Neurosurgery, 12631 E 17th Ave, rm 501, MS C307, Aurora, CO 80045; **Phone:** 303-724-2280; **Board Cert:** Neurological Surgery 1989; **Med School:** Univ Minn 1979; **Resid:** Neurological Surgery, Univ Mich Med Ctr 1985; **Fac Appt:** Prof NS, Univ Colorado

Nazzaro, Jules M MD [NS] - **Spec Exp:** Parkinson's Disease; Movement Disorders; Stereotactic Radiosurgery; **Hospital:** Univ of Kansas Hosp; **Address:** Kansas University Medical Ctr, 3901 Rainbow Blvd, MS 3021, Kansas City, KS 66160; **Phone:** 913-588-6122; **Board Cert:** Neurological Surgery 1996; **Med School:** Albert Einstein Coll Med 1984; **Resid:** Neurological Surgery, NYU Med Ctr 1991; **Fellow:** Neurosurgical Oncology, Meml Sloan-Kettering Cancer Ctr 1992; **Fac Appt:** Assoc Prof NS, Univ Kansas

Origitano, Thomas C MD/PhD [NS] - **Spec Exp:** Skull Base Tumors & Surgery; Brain Tumors; Pituitary Tumors; Craniofacial Surgery; **Hospital:** Kalispell Regl Med Ctr; **Address:** Northern Rockies Neurosurgical Assocs, 350 Heritage Way, Ste 1300, Kalispell, MT 59901; **Phone:** 406-752-5170; **Board Cert:** Neurological Surgery 1995; **Med School:** Loyola Univ-Stritch Sch Med 1984; **Resid:** Neurological Surgery, Loyola Univ Med Ctr 1990

Neurological Surgery

Taylon, Charles MD [NS] - **Spec Exp:** Spinal Surgery-Cervical; Spinal Surgery-Low Back; Carpal Tunnel Syndrome; Trauma; **Hospital:** Alegent Creighton Univ Med Ctr; **Address:** Creighton Univ, Dept Surg, 601 N 30th St, Ste 3700, Omaha, NE 68131; **Phone:** 402-280-4497; **Board Cert:** Neurological Surgery 1984; **Med School:** Creighton Univ 1975; **Resid:** Neurological Surgery, Univ Wisc Hosps 1981; **Fac Appt:** Assoc Prof NS, Creighton Univ

Walker, Marion L MD [NS] - **Spec Exp:** Pediatric Neurosurgery; Spasticity & Movement Disorders; Hydrocephalus; Brain Tumors; **Hospital:** Primary Children's Med Ctr, Univ Utah Hlth Care; **Address:** Primary Chldns Med Ctr, Div Ped Neurosurgery, 100 N Mario Capecchi Drive, Ste 1475, Salt Lake City, UT 84113-1103; **Phone:** 801-662-5340; **Board Cert:** Neurological Surgery 1979; Pediatric Neurological Surgery 2006; **Med School:** Univ Tenn Coll Med 1969; **Resid:** Surgery, St Joseph's Hosp 1971; Neurological Surgery, St Joseph's Hosp-Barrow Neuro Inst 1976; **Fellow:** Pediatric Neurological Surgery, Hosp for Sick Chldn 1973; **Fac Appt:** Prof NS, Univ Utah

Zimmerman, Christian G MD [NS] - **Spec Exp:** Spinal Surgery-Complex; Head Injury; Trauma; Pain Medicine; **Hospital:** St. Alphonsus Regl Med Ctr; **Address:** 901 N Curtis Rd, Ste 503, Boise, ID 83706; **Phone:** 208-367-4000; **Board Cert:** Neurological Surgery 1996; Pain Medicine 1998; **Med School:** Univ MD Sch Med 1985; **Resid:** Surgery, Univ Md Hosp-Prince Georges Med Ctr 1987; Neurological Surgery, Oreg Hlth Sci Univ 1992; **Fellow:** Spinal Surgery, Barrow Neur Inst 1993

Southwest

Adelson, P David MD [NS] - **Spec Exp:** Pediatric Neurosurgery; Brain Injury; Epilepsy/Seizure Disorders; Spinal Cord Injury; **Hospital:** Phoenix Children's Hosp, Maricopa Med Ctr; **Address:** Phoenix Chldns Hosp, Neurosurgery, 1919 E Thomas Rd B Bldg Fl 4, Phoenix, AZ 85016; **Phone:** 602-933-0975; **Board Cert:** Neurological Surgery 1997; Pediatric Neurological Surgery 2009; **Med School:** Columbia P&S 1986; **Resid:** Neurological Surgery, UCLA Med Ctr 1992; **Fellow:** Pediatric Neurological Surgery, Children's Hosp 1994; **Fac Appt:** Prof NS, Univ Ariz Coll Med

De Monte, Franco MD [NS] - **Spec Exp:** Skull Base Tumors & Surgery; Neuro-Oncology; **Hospital:** UT MD Anderson Cancer Ctr; **Address:** UT MD Anderson Cancer Ctr, Dept Neurosurgery, 1515 Holcombe Blvd, Unit 442, Houston, TX 77030; **Phone:** 713-792-2400; **Board Cert:** Neurological Surgery 1995; **Med School:** Canada 1985; **Resid:** Neurological Surgery, Univ W Ontario Affil Hosp 1991; **Fellow:** Skull Base Surgery, Loyola Univ-Stritch 1992; **Fac Appt:** Prof NS, Baylor Coll Med

Greene Jr, Clarence S MD [NS] - **Spec Exp:** Pediatric Neurosurgery; Congenital Nervous System Malformations; Brain Tumors; **Hospital:** Children's Hospital - New Orleans; **Address:** Children's Hosp, Dept Neurosurgery, 200 Henry Clay Ave, Ste 210, New Orleans, LA 70118; **Phone:** 504-896-9458; **Board Cert:** Neurological Surgery 1984; Pediatric Neurological Surgery 2007; **Med School:** Howard Univ 1974; **Resid:** Neurological Surgery, Chldns Hosp 1981; Neurological Surgery, Peter Bent Brigham Hosp 1981; **Fellow:** Pediatric Neurology, Chldns Hosp 1984; **Fac Appt:** Assoc Clin Prof NS, UC Irvine

Hankinson, Hal L MD [NS] - **Spec Exp:** Brain Tumors; **Hospital:** Christus St Vincent Reg Med Ctr-Santa Fe; **Address:** 465 St Michael's Drive, Ste 107, Sante Fe, NM 87505; **Phone:** 505-988-3233; **Board Cert:** Neurological Surgery 1977; **Med School:** Tulane Univ 1967; **Resid:** Neurological Surgery, UCSF Med Ctr 1975; **Fac Appt:** Clin Prof NS, Univ New Mexico

Harper, Richard L MD [NS] - **Spec Exp:** Spinal Surgery; Brain Tumors & Hemifacial Spasms; **Hospital:** Methodist Hosp - Houston; **Address:** Neurosurgical Grp of Texas, 6565 Fannin St, Ste 1200, Scurlock Tower, Houston, TX 77030; **Phone:** 713-790-1211; **Board Cert:** Neurological Surgery 1983; **Med School:** Baylor Coll Med 1971; **Resid:** Neurological Surgery, Baylor Hosps 1978; **Fac Appt:** Asst Clin Prof NS, Baylor Coll Med

Jimenez, David F MD [NS] - **Spec Exp:** Pediatric Neurosurgery; Craniosynostosis; Endoscopic Strip Craniectomy; Spinal Surgery; **Hospital:** Univ Hlth Syst-San Antonio, St. Luke's Baptist Hosp; **Address:** Dept of Neurosurgery, 7703 Floyd Curl Drive, MC 7843, San Antonio, TX 78229-3900; **Phone:** 210-567-6027; **Board Cert:** Neurological Surgery 1995; **Med School:** Temple Univ 1985; **Resid:** Neurological Surgery, Temple Univ Hosp 1991; **Fellow:** Pediatric Neurological Surgery, Montefiore Med Ctr 1992; **Fac Appt:** Prof NS, Univ Tex, San Antonio

Kim, Daniel H MD [NS] - **Spec Exp:** Spinal Surgery; Peripheral Nerve Surgery; **Hospital:** St. Luke's Episcopal Hosp-Houston, Houston Hosp for Specialized Surgery; **Address:** 6620 Main St, Ste 1350, Houston, TX 77030; **Phone:** 713-798-4696; **Board Cert:** Neurological Surgery 1998; **Med School:** Tulane Univ 1989; **Resid:** Neurological Surgery, LSU Med Ctr 1995; **Fellow:** Spinal Surgery, Univ Fla 1998; **Fac Appt:** Prof NS, Baylor Coll Med

Kim, Dong H MD [NS] - **Spec Exp:** Cerebrovascular Surgery; Aneurysm-Cerebral; Brain Tumors; Arteriovenous Malformations; **Hospital:** Meml Hermann Hosp - Texas Med Ctr; **Address:** UT Neurosurgery, 6400 Fannin St, Ste 2800, Houston, TX 77030; **Phone:** 713-704-7100; **Board Cert:** Neurological Surgery 2001; **Med School:** UCSF 1990; **Resid:** Neurological Surgery, UCSF Med Ctr 1996; **Fellow:** Cerebrovascular & Skull Base Surgery, Univ Florida 1997; **Fac Appt:** Prof NS, Univ Tex, Houston

Krisht, Ali F MD [NS] - **Spec Exp:** Skull Base Surgery; Meningioma; Vascular Neurosurgery; **Hospital:** St. Vincent Health System; **Address:** Arkansas Neuroscience Inst, 5 St Vincent Circle, Ste 220, Little Rock, AR 72205; **Phone:** 501-552-6400; **Board Cert:** Neurological Surgery 2010; **Med School:** Amer Univ Beirut 1985; **Resid:** Neurological Surgery, Emory Univ Affil Hosp 1994; **Fac Appt:** Prof NS, Univ Ark

Lang Jr, Frederick F MD [NS] - **Spec Exp:** Brain & Spinal Tumors; Gliomas; Brain Tumors-Complex; Pediatric Neurosurgery; **Hospital:** UT MD Anderson Cancer Ctr; **Address:** Univ Texas MD Anderson Cancer Ctr, 1515 Holcombe Blvd, Unit 442, Houston, TX 77030; **Phone:** 713-792-6600; **Board Cert:** Neurological Surgery 2011; **Med School:** Yale Univ 1988; **Resid:** Neurological Surgery, NYU Med Ctr 1995; **Fellow:** Neurosurgical Oncology, MD Anderson Cancer Ctr 1996; **Fac Appt:** Prof NS, Univ Tex, Houston

Lemole Jr, G Michael MD [NS] - **Spec Exp:** Skull Base Surgery; Stereotactic Radiosurgery; Cerebrovascular Surgery; Minimally Invasive Surgery; **Hospital:** Univ Arizona Med Ctr-Univ Campus; **Address:** Univ Arizona Dept Neurosurgery, 1501 N Campbell Ave, 4th Fl - Ste 4303, Box 245070, Tucson, AZ 85724-5070; **Phone:** 520-694-6144; **Board Cert:** Neurological Surgery 2007; **Med School:** Univ Pennsylvania 1995; **Resid:** Neurological Surgery, St Josephs Hosp Med Ctr/Barrow Neuro Inst 2002; **Fellow:** Cerebrovascular & Skull Base Surgery, Barrow Neuro Inst 2000; Spinal Surgery, Barrow Neuro Inst 2000; **Fac Appt:** Prof NS, Univ Ariz Coll Med

Luerssen, Thomas G MD [NS] - **Spec Exp:** Pediatric Neurosurgery; Congenital Cranial Deformities; **Hospital:** Texas Chldns Hosp; **Address:** Texas Children's Hosp, Ped Neurosurgery, Clinical Care Center, Ste 1230, 6621 Fannin St, MC CC 1230.01, Houston, TX 77030-2399; **Phone:** 832-822-3950; **Board Cert:** Neurological Surgery 1985; Pediatric Neurological Surgery 2005; **Med School:** Indiana Univ 1976; **Resid:** Neurological Surgery, Indiana Univ Hosp 1981; **Fellow:** Pediatric Neurological Surgery, Chldns Hosp 1984; **Fac Appt:** Prof NS, Baylor Coll Med

Mapstone, Timothy B MD [NS] - **Spec Exp:** Brain Tumors-Adult & Pediatric; Pediatric Neurosurgery; Congenital Anomalies; **Hospital:** OU Med Ctr, Chldns Hosp OU Med Ctr; **Address:** Univ OK Hlth Sci Ctr, Dept Neurosurgery, 1000 N Lincoln Blvd, Ste 400, Oklahoma City, OK 73104; **Phone:** 405-271-4912; **Board Cert:** Neurological Surgery 1985; Pediatric Neurological Surgery 2005; **Med School:** Case West Res Univ 1977; **Resid:** Neurological Surgery, Univ Hosps 1983; **Fellow:** Research, Case West Reserve Univ; **Fac Appt:** Prof NS, Univ Okla Coll Med

Mickey, Bruce E MD [NS] - **Spec Exp:** Brain Tumors; Skull Base Surgery; Pituitary Tumors; **Hospital:** UT Southwestern Med Ctr at Dallas, Parkland Hlth & Hosp Sys; **Address:** UTSW Med Ctr, Dept Neurosurgery, 5323 Harry Hines Blvd, Dallas, TX 75390-8855; **Phone:** 214-645-2300; **Board Cert:** Neurological Surgery 1987; **Med School:** Univ Tex SW, Dallas 1978; **Resid:** Neurological Surgery, Parkland Meml Hosp 1984; **Fellow:** Research, Righospitalet 1983; **Fac Appt:** Prof NS, Univ Tex SW, Dallas

Samson, Duke S MD [NS] - **Spec Exp:** Vascular Neurosurgery; Cerebrovascular Disease; Arteriovenous Malformations; **Hospital:** UT Southwestern Med Ctr at Dallas, Parkland Hlth & Hosp Sys; **Address:** Univ Tex SW Med Ctr, Dept Neuro Surg, 5323 Harry Hines Blvd, Dallas, TX 75390-8855; **Phone:** 214-645-2300; **Board Cert:** Neurological Surgery 1978; **Med School:** Washington Univ, St Louis 1969; **Resid:** Neurological Surgery, Univ Texas SW Med Ctr 1975; **Fellow:** Neurological Surgery, Ctr Medico-Chirurgical Fech 1973; Neurological Surgery, Univ Zurich 1973; **Fac Appt:** Prof NS, Univ Tex SW, Dallas

Sandberg, David I MD [NS] - **Spec Exp:** Pediatric Neurosurgery; Brain Tumors-Pediatric; Hydrocephalus; Minimally Invasive Surgery; **Hospital:** Meml Hermann Hosp - Texas Med Ctr; **Address:** UT Physicians, Pediatric Neurological Surgery, 6410 Fannin St Fl 9 - Ste 950, Houston, TX 77030; **Phone:** 832-325-7242; **Board Cert:** Neurological Surgery 2007; Pediatric Neurological Surgery 2007; **Med School:** Johns Hopkins Univ 1997; **Resid:** Surgery, NY Presby-Cornell Med Ctr 1998; Neurological Surgery, NY Presby-Cornell Med Ctr 2002; **Fellow:** Neurosurgical Oncology, Meml Sloan Kettering Cancer Ctr 2003; Pediatric Neurological Surgery, Children's Hosp 2004; **Fac Appt:** Assoc Prof NS, Univ Tex, Houston

Sawaya, Raymond MD [NS] - **Spec Exp:** Brain Tumors; **Hospital:** UT MD Anderson Cancer Ctr; **Address:** MD Anderson Cancer Ctr, 1400 Holcombe Blvd, Houston, TX 77030; **Phone:** 713-792-2400; **Board Cert:** Neurological Surgery 1985; **Med School:** Lebanon 1974; **Resid:** Neurological Surgery, Univ Cincinnati Med Ctr 1980; Neurological Surgery, Johns Hopkins Hosp 1981; **Fellow:** Neuro-Oncology, Natl Inst Hlth 1982; **Fac Appt:** Prof NS, Baylor Coll Med

Sklar, Frederick H MD [NS] - **Spec Exp:** Pediatric Neurosurgery; Craniofacial Surgery; Hydrocephalus; **Hospital:** Chldns Med Ctr of Dallas, Texas Scottish Rite Hosp for Chldn; **Address:** Neurosurgeons for Chldn, 1935 Med District Drive, Dallas, TX 75235; **Phone:** 214-456-6660; **Board Cert:** Neurological Surgery 1978; **Med School:** Johns Hopkins Univ 1970; **Resid:** Neurological Surgery, Johns Hopkins Hosp 1976; **Fac Appt:** Assoc Clin Prof NS, Univ Tex SW, Dallas

Spetzler, Robert F MD [NS] - **Spec Exp:** Skull Base Tumors & Surgery; Cerebrovascular Surgery; **Hospital:** St. Joseph's Hosp & Med Ctr - Phoenix; **Address:** Barrow Neurosurgical Assocs, 2910 N Third Ave, Phoenix, AZ 85013; **Phone:** 602-406-3489; **Board Cert:** Neurological Surgery 1979; **Med School:** Northwestern Univ 1971; **Resid:** Neurological Surgery, UCSF Med Ctr 1977; **Fac Appt:** Prof NS, Univ Ariz Coll Med

Theodore, Nicholas MD [NS] - **Spec Exp:** Brain & Spinal Surgery; Minimally Invasive Neurosurgery; Robotic Surgery; **Hospital:** St. Joseph's Hosp & Med Ctr - Phoenix; **Address:** Barrow Neurosurgical Assocs, 2910 N Third Ave, Phoenix, AZ 85013; **Phone:** 602-406-3489; **Board Cert:** Neurological Surgery 2004; **Med School:** Georgetown Univ 1991; **Resid:** Neurological Surgery, Natl Naval Med Ctr 1997; **Fellow:** Neurological Surgery, St Josephs Hosp & Med Ctr 2001

Walsh, John W MD/PhD [NS] - **Spec Exp:** Pediatric Neurosurgery; Epilepsy; Craniofacial Surgery/Reconstruction; Vascular Malformations; **Hospital:** Tulane Med Ctr; **Address:** Pediatric Specialties, 1415 Tulane Ave Fl 5, New Orleans, LA 70112; **Phone:** 504-988-8000; **Board Cert:** Neurological Surgery 1976; **Med School:** UCLA 1969; **Resid:** Neurological Surgery, Childrens Hosp/Brigham Hosp 1974; **Fellow:** Neurological Surgery, Lahey Clin Fdn 1975; **Fac Appt:** Prof NS, Tulane Univ

Yonas, Howard MD [NS] - **Spec Exp:** Vascular Neurosurgery; Stroke; Skull Base Surgery; Trigeminal Neuralgia; **Hospital:** Univ Hosp - New Mexico; **Address:** 1 Univ of New Mexico, Dept Neurological Surgery, MSC10-5615, Albuquerque, NM 87131-0001; **Phone:** 505-272-9494; **Board Cert:** Neurological Surgery 1981; **Med School:** Ohio State Univ 1970; **Resid:** Neurological Surgery, Case West Res 1976; **Fellow:** Univ Pittsburgh 1978; **Fac Appt:** Prof NS, Univ New Mexico

West Coast and Pacific

Amar, Arun P MD/PhD [NS] - **Spec Exp:** Interventional Neuroradiology; Stroke; Stroke Prevention; **Hospital:** Keck Med Ctr of USC (page 62); **Address:** 1520 San Pablo St, Ste 3800, Los Angeles, CA 90033; **Phone:** 323-442-5720; **Board Cert:** Neurological Surgery 2005; **Med School:** UCSF 1993; **Resid:** Neurological Surgery, USC Univ Hosp 2000; **Fellow:** Interventional Neuroradiology, USC Univ Hosp 2003; **Fac Appt:** Assoc Prof NS, USC-Keck School of Medicine

Ames, Christopher P MD [NS] - **Spec Exp:** Spinal Trauma; Spinal Cord Tumors; Spinal Reconstructive Surgery; **Hospital:** UCSF Med Ctr; **Address:** Spine Center, 400 Parnassus Ave Fl 3, San Francisco, CA 94143-0332; **Phone:** 866-817-7463; **Board Cert:** Neurological Surgery 2006; **Med School:** UCLA-David Geffen Sch Med 1994; **Resid:** Neurological Surgery, UCSD Med Ctr 2000; **Fellow:** Spinal Surgery, Barrow Neurological Inst 2002; **Fac Appt:** Assoc Clin Prof NS, UCLA-David Geffen Sch Med

Apuzzo, Michael L J MD [NS] - **Spec Exp:** Brain Tumors; Epilepsy/Seizure Disorders; Stereotactic Radiosurgery; **Hospital:** LAC & USC Med Ctr, USC Norris Cancer Hosp (page 62); **Address:** 1420 San Pablo Street, PMBA106, Los Angeles, CA 90033-1029; **Phone:** 323-226-7421; **Board Cert:** Neurological Surgery 1975; **Med School:** Boston Univ 1965; **Resid:** Neurological Surgery, Hartford Hosp 1970; Neurological Surgery, Hartford Hosp 1973; **Fellow:** Neurological Physiology, Yale Univ Hosp 1972; **Fac Appt:** Prof NS, USC Sch Med

Badie, Behnam MD [NS] - **Spec Exp:** Brain Tumors; **Hospital:** City of Hope Natl Med Ctr; **Address:** City of Hope-Division of Neurosurgery, 1500 E Duarte Rd, Duarte, CA 91010; **Phone:** 626-471-7100; **Board Cert:** Neurological Surgery 1998; **Med School:** UCLA 1989; **Resid:** Neurological Surgery, UCLA Med Ctr 1996; **Fac Appt:** Assoc Prof NS, UCLA

Berger, Mitchel S MD [NS] - **Spec Exp:** Brain & Spinal Cord Tumors; Pituitary Tumors; Neuro-Oncology; Pain Management; **Hospital:** UCSF Med Ctr; **Address:** UCSF Med Ctr, Dept Neurosurgery, 505 Parnassus Avenue, M-786, San Francisco, CA 94143-0112; **Phone:** 415-353-3933; **Board Cert:** Neurological Surgery 1991; **Med School:** Univ Miami Sch Med 1979; **Resid:** Neurological Surgery, UCSF Med Ctr 1984; **Fellow:** Neuro-Oncology, UCSF Med Ctr 1985; Pediatric Neurological Surgery, Hosp Sick Chldn 1986; **Fac Appt:** Prof NS, UCSF

Black, Keith L MD [NS] - **Spec Exp:** Brain Tumors; Pineal Tumors; Spinal Tumors; Acoustic Neuroma; **Hospital:** Cedars-Sinai Med Ctr; **Address:** Cedars-Sinai Med Ctr, Dept Neurosugery, 8631 W Third St, Ste 800 East, Los Angeles, CA 90048; **Phone:** 310-423-7900; **Board Cert:** Neurological Surgery 1990; **Med School:** Univ Mich Med Sch 1981; **Resid:** Neurological Surgery, Univ Michigan Med Ctr 1987; **Fac Appt:** Prof NS

Neurological Surgery

Boggan, James E MD [NS] - **Spec Exp:** Skull Base Tumors & Surgery; Pediatric Neurosurgery; **Hospital:** UC Davis Med Ctr; **Address:** Dept Neurological Surgery, 4860 Y St, Ste 0100, Sacramento, CA 95817-2307; **Phone:** 916-734-4300; **Board Cert:** Neurological Surgery 1985; **Med School:** Univ Chicago-Pritzker Sch Med 1976; **Resid:** Neurological Surgery, UCSF Med Ctr 1982; **Fac Appt:** Prof NS, UC Davis

Bray Jr, Robert S MD [NS] - **Spec Exp:** Minimally Invasive Spinal Surgery; **Address:** DISC Sports & Spine Center, 13160 Mindanao Way, Ste 300, Marina del Rey, CA 90292; **Phone:** 310-574-0400; **Board Cert:** Neurological Surgery 1991; **Med School:** Baylor Coll Med 1980; **Resid:** Neurological Surgery, Baylor Affil Hosp 1986

Burchiel, Kim J MD [NS] - **Spec Exp:** Pain Management; Stereotactic Radiosurgery; Epilepsy; Movement Disorders; **Hospital:** OR Hlth & Sci Univ; **Address:** OHSU, Dept Neurosurgery, 3303 SW Bond Ave, MC CH8N, Portland, OR 97239; **Phone:** 503-494-4314; **Board Cert:** Neurological Surgery 1984; **Med School:** UCSD 1976; **Resid:** Neurological Surgery, Univ Wash Med Ctr 1982; **Fac Appt:** Prof NS, Oregon Hlth & Sci Univ

Chen, Thomas C MD [NS] - **Spec Exp:** Brain & Spinal Tumors; Brain Tumors-Metastatic; Gliomas; Microdiscectomy; **Hospital:** USC Norris Cancer Hosp (page 62), Keck Med Ctr of USC (page 62); **Address:** USC Health Consultation Clinic 2, 1520 San Pablo St, rm 3800, MC 9197, Los Angeles, CA 90033; **Phone:** 323-442-5720; **Board Cert:** Neurological Surgery 2000; **Med School:** UCSF 1988; **Resid:** Neurological Surgery, USC Univ Hosp 1995; **Fellow:** Spinal Surgery, Med Coll Wisconsin 1997; **Fac Appt:** Assoc Prof NS, USC-Keck School of Medicine

Danielpour, Moise MD [NS] - **Spec Exp:** Pediatric Neurosurgery; Brain Tumors; Epilepsy; Craniofacial Surgery; **Hospital:** Cedars-Sinai Med Ctr; **Address:** Cedars-Sinai Medical Center, Maxine Dunitz Neurosurgical Institute, 8631 W Third St, Ste 800 E, Los Angeles, CA 90048; **Phone:** 310-423-7900; **Board Cert:** Neurological Surgery 2004; Pediatric Neurological Surgery ; **Med School:** Albert Einstein Coll Med 1992; **Resid:** Neurological Surgery, Northwestern Univ Hosp 1999; **Fellow:** Pediatric Neurological Surgery, UCSF Med Ctr 2000

Edwards, Michael S MD [NS] - **Spec Exp:** Brain Tumors-Pediatric; Pediatric Neurosurgery; Stereotactic Radiosurgery; **Hospital:** Lucile Packard Chldn's Hosp; **Address:** Pediatric Neurosurgery, 300 Pasteur Drive, Ste R211, MC 5327, Stanford, CA 94305; **Phone:** 650-497-8775; **Board Cert:** Neurological Surgery 1980; Pediatric Neurological Surgery 2006; **Med School:** Tulane Univ 1970; **Resid:** Neurological Surgery, Oschner Fdn Hosp/Charity Hosp 1977; **Fellow:** Pediatric Neuro-Oncology, UCSF Med Ctr 1978; **Fac Appt:** Prof NS, Stanford Univ

Ellenbogen, Richard MD [NS] - **Spec Exp:** Chiari's Deformity; Brain Tumors; Minimally Invasive Surgery; Congenital Nervous System Malformations; **Hospital:** Seattle Chldns Hosp, Univ Wash Med Ctr; **Address:** 4800 Sand Point Way NE, MS W-7729, Seattle, WA 98105; **Phone:** 206-987-2544; **Board Cert:** Neurological Surgery 1992; Pediatric Neurological Surgery 2009; **Med School:** Brown Univ 1983; **Resid:** Neurological Surgery, Brigham Womens Hosp/Childrens Hosp 1989; **Fac Appt:** Prof NS, Univ Wash

Frazee, John G MD [NS] - **Spec Exp:** Vascular Neurosurgery; Spinal Surgery; Neuro-Endoscopy; Chiari's Deformity; **Hospital:** UCLA Ronald Reagan Med Ctr, VA Greater Los Angeles Hthecare Sys; **Address:** UCLA Neurosurgery, 750 Charles E Young Drive, Los Angeles, CA 90095-7039; **Phone:** 310-206-1231; **Board Cert:** Neurological Surgery 1984; **Med School:** Univ Rochester 1975; **Resid:** Neurological Surgery, UCLA Med Ctr 1982; **Fac Appt:** Clin Prof NS, UCLA

Giannotta, Steven L MD [NS] - **Spec Exp:** Aneurysm-Cerebral; Skull Base Tumors; Acoustic Neuroma; **Hospital:** Keck Med Ctr of USC (page 62), LAC & USC Med Ctr; **Address:** 1520 San Pablo St, Ste 3800, Los Angeles, CA 90033; **Phone:** 323-442-5720; **Board Cert:** Neurological Surgery 1980; **Med School:** Univ Mich Med Sch 1972; **Resid:** Neurological Surgery, Univ Michigan Med Ctr 1978; **Fac Appt:** Prof NS, USC Sch Med

Gupta, Nalin MD/PhD [NS] - **Spec Exp:** Pediatric Neurosurgery; **Hospital:** UCSF Med Ctr; **Address:** 400 Parnassus Ave, Ste A808, San Francisco, CA 94143; **Phone:** 415-353-7500; **Board Cert:** Neurological Surgery 2002; Pediatric Neurological Surgery 2003; **Med School:** Univ Toronto 1987; **Resid:** Neurological Surgery, Univ Ottawa 1989; Neurological Surgery, Univ Toronto 1997; **Fellow:** Pediatric Neurological Surgery, Hosp for Sick Chldn 1998; **Fac Appt:** Asst Prof NS, UCSF

Harsh IV, Griffith R MD [NS] - **Spec Exp:** Brain & Spinal Cord Tumors; Skull Base Tumors; Pituitary Tumors; Acoustic Neuroma; **Hospital:** Stanford Univ Hosp & Clinics; **Address:** Stanford Center for Advanced Medicine, 875 Blake Wilbur Drive, MC 5826, Stanford, CA 94305; **Phone:** 650-723-7093; **Board Cert:** Neurological Surgery 1989; **Med School:** Harvard Med Sch 1980; **Resid:** Neurological Surgery, UCSF Med Ctr 1986; **Fellow:** Neuro-Oncology, UCSF Med Ctr 1987; **Fac Appt:** Prof NS, Stanford Univ

Levy, Michael L MD/PhD [NS] - **Spec Exp:** Pediatric Neurosurgery; **Hospital:** Rady Children's Hosp - San Diego, UCSD Med Ctr; **Address:** Rady Chldn's Specialists, 8010 Frost St, Ste 502, San Diego, CA 92123; **Phone:** 858-966-8574; **Board Cert:** Neurological Surgery 1997; Pediatric Neurological Surgery 1998; **Med School:** UCSF 1986; **Resid:** Neurological Surgery, USC Med Ctr 1993; **Fellow:** Pediatric Neurological Surgery, Chldns Hosp 1995; **Fac Appt:** Prof NS, USC Sch Med

Liau, Linda M MD/PhD [NS] - **Spec Exp:** Brain Tumors; Neuro-Oncology; **Hospital:** UCLA Ronald Reagan Med Ctr; **Address:** 300 UCLA Medical Plaza, Ste B200, Los Angeles, CA 90095-6901; **Phone:** 310-267-2621; **Board Cert:** Neurological Surgery 2002; **Med School:** Stanford Univ 1991; **Resid:** Neurological Surgery, UCLA Med Ctr 1998; **Fellow:** Neuro-Oncology, UCLA Med Ctr 1998; **Fac Appt:** Prof NS, UCLA

Liker, Mark A MD [NS] - **Spec Exp:** Spinal Surgery; Deep Brain Stimulation; **Hospital:** Henry Mayo Newhall Memorial Hosp, Keck Med Ctr of USC (page 62); **Address:** 25751 McBean Pkwy, Ste 305, Valencia, CA 91355; **Phone:** 661-799-2542; **Board Cert:** Neurological Surgery 2005; **Med School:** SUNY Downstate 1995; **Resid:** Neurological Surgery, USC Med Ctr 2001; **Fellow:** Spinal Surgery, USC Med Ctr 1999; **Fac Appt:** Asst Prof NS, USC-Keck School of Medicine

Linskey, Mark E MD [NS] - **Spec Exp:** Brain Tumors; Stereotactic Radiosurgery; Skull Base Surgery; Trigeminal Neuralgia; **Hospital:** UC Irvine Med Ctr; **Address:** 101 The City Drive S Bldg 56 - Ste 400, Orange, CA 92868-3298; **Phone:** 714-456-6966; **Board Cert:** Neurological Surgery 1996; **Med School:** Columbia P&S 1986; **Resid:** Neurological Surgery, Univ Pittsburgh Hlth Ctrs 1993; **Fellow:** Neuro-Oncology, Ludwig Inst Cancer Rsch/Univ Coll London 1994; Neuro-Oncology, Pittsburgh Cancer Inst/Univ Pittsburgh 1992; **Fac Appt:** Assoc Prof NS, UC Irvine

Liu, Charles Y MD [NS] - **Spec Exp:** Epilepsy; Skull Base Tumors & Surgery; Stereotactic Radiosurgery; Meningioma; **Hospital:** Keck Med Ctr of USC (page 62); **Address:** USC Dept Neurosurgery, 1200 N State St, Ste 3300, Los Angeles, CA 90033; **Phone:** 323-442-5720; **Board Cert:** Neurological Surgery 2007; **Med School:** Yale Univ 1996; **Resid:** Neurological Surgery, LAC/USC Med Ctr 2001; **Fellow:** Spinal Surgery, LAC/USC Med Ctr 2003; **Fac Appt:** Assoc Prof NS, USC-Keck School of Medicine

Neurological Surgery

Mamelak, Adam N MD [NS] - **Spec Exp:** Brain Tumors; Epilepsy; Spinal Tumors; **Hospital:** Cedars-Sinai Med Ctr; **Address:** Maxine Dunitz Neurosurgical Institute, 8631 W Third St, Ste 800-East, Los Angeles, CA 90048; **Phone:** 310-423-7900; **Board Cert:** Neurological Surgery 2000; **Med School:** Harvard Med Sch 1990; **Resid:** Neurological Surgery, UCSF Med Ctr 1994; **Fellow:** Epilepsy, UCSF Epilepsy Research Lab 1996

Martin, Neil A MD [NS] - **Spec Exp:** Vascular Neurosurgery; Aneurysm-Cerebral; Endoscopic Surgery; Microvascular Surgery; **Hospital:** UCLA Ronald Reagan Med Ctr; **Address:** UCLA Dept Neurosurgery, Box 957039, Los Angeles, CA 90095-7039; **Phone:** 310-825-5482; **Board Cert:** Neurological Surgery 1989; **Med School:** Med Coll VA 1978; **Resid:** Neurological Surgery, UCSF Med Ctr 1984; **Fellow:** Neurovascular Surgery, Barrow Neuro Inst 1985; **Fac Appt:** Prof NS, UCLA

Mayberg, Marc R MD [NS] - **Spec Exp:** Pituitary Surgery; Skull Base Tumors; Acoustic Neuroma; **Hospital:** Swedish Med Ctr-Cherry Hill Campus, Prov Reg Med Ctr -Colby Campus; **Address:** Seattle Neuroscience Inst, 550 17th Ave, Ste 500, James Tower, Seattle, WA 98122; **Phone:** 206-320-2800; **Board Cert:** Neurological Surgery 1988; **Med School:** Mayo Med Sch 1978; **Resid:** Neurological Surgery, Mass Genl Hosp 1984; **Fellow:** Neurological Surgery, Natl Hosp for Nervous Dis 1985

McDermott, Michael W MD [NS] - **Spec Exp:** Brain Tumors; Meningioma; Stereotactic Radiosurgery; Skull Base Tumors; **Hospital:** UCSF Med Ctr; **Address:** UCSF Dept Neurosurgery, 400 Parnassus Ave, rm A808, San Francisco, CA 94143; **Phone:** 415-353-2243; **Board Cert:** Neurological Surgery 2003; **Med School:** Univ Toronto 1982; **Resid:** Neurological Surgery, Univ British Columbia 1988; **Fellow:** Neuro-Oncology, UCSF Med Ctr 1990; **Fac Appt:** Prof NS, UCSF

Neuwelt, Edward A MD [NS] - **Spec Exp:** Neuro-Oncology; Brain Tumors; **Hospital:** OR Hlth & Sci Univ; **Address:** Oregon Hlth Sci Univ, Dept Neurosurgery, 3181 SW Sam Jackson Pk Rd, MC-L603, Portland, OR 97239; **Phone:** 503-494-5626; **Board Cert:** Neurological Surgery 1980; **Med School:** Univ Colorado 1972; **Resid:** Neurological Surgery, Univ Tex SW Med Sch 1978; **Fellow:** Neuro-Oncology, Natl Canc Inst/NIH 1976; **Fac Appt:** Prof NS, Oregon Hlth & Sci Univ

Ojemann, Jeffrey G MD [NS] - **Spec Exp:** Pediatric Neurosurgery; Brain Tumors; Hydrocephalus; Epilepsy; **Hospital:** Seattle Chldns Hosp, Univ Wash Med Ctr; **Address:** 4800 Sand Point Way NE, MS W7729, Seattle, WA 98145; **Phone:** 206-987-2544; **Board Cert:** Neurological Surgery 2002; **Med School:** Washington Univ, St Louis 1992; **Resid:** Neurological Surgery, Barnes Jewish Hosp 1998; **Fellow:** Pediatric Neurological Surgery, Chldn's Hosp 2000; Neurological Surgery, Univ Wash Med Ctr 2002; **Fac Appt:** Assoc Prof NS, Univ Wash

Ott, Kenneth H MD [NS] - **Spec Exp:** Brain Tumors; Stereotactic Radiosurgery; **Hospital:** Scripps Meml Hosp - La Jolla; **Address:** Neurosurgical Med Clinic, 2100 Fifth Ave, Ste 200, San Diego, CA 92101; **Phone:** 619-297-4481 x102; **Board Cert:** Neurological Surgery 1980; **Med School:** UCSF 1970; **Resid:** Surgery, Mass Genl Hosp 1972; Neurological Surgery, Mass Genl Hosp 1976; **Fac Appt:** Assoc Clin Prof S, UCSD

Sekhar, Laligam N MD [NS] - **Spec Exp:** Aneurysm-Cerebral; Arteriovenous Malformations; Brain Tumors; Skull Base Tumors; **Hospital:** Harborview Med Ctr, Univ Wash Med Ctr; **Address:** HMC-Neurosurgery, 9th & Jeff Bldg Fl 5, 908 Jefferson St, Seattle, WA 98104-2499; **Phone:** 206-744-9300; **Board Cert:** Neurological Surgery 1986; **Med School:** India 1973; **Resid:** Neurology, Univ Cincinnati Med Ctr 1977; Neurology, Univ Pittsburgh Med Ctr 1982; **Fellow:** Skull Base Surgery, Norstadt Krankenhaus 1983; Cerebrovascular Neurosurgery, Univ Zurich Hospital; **Fac Appt:** Prof NS, Univ Wash

Sekhon, Lali MD/PhD [NS] - **Spec Exp:** Spinal Surgery; Spinal Disorders-Degenerative; Spinal Disc Replacement; Minimally Invasive Spinal Surgery; **Hospital:** Renown Reg Med Ctr, St. Mary's Reg Med Ctr; **Address:** Nevada Neurosurgery, 75 Pringle Way, Ste 1007, Reno, NV 89502; **Phone:** 775-657-8844; **Med School:** Australia 1994; **Resid:** Neurological Surgery, Univ Sidney Med Ctr 1997; **Fellow:** Neurological Surgery, Mayo Clinic 1999; Neurological Orthopaedic Surgery, Toronto Western Hosp 2000

Selden, Nathan R MD/PhD [NS] - **Spec Exp:** Pediatric Neurosurgery; Brain Tumors-Pediatric; Chiari's Deformity; Spina Bifida; **Hospital:** Doernbecher Chldns Hosp/OHSU, OR Hlth & Sci Univ; **Address:** 3303 SW Bond Ave, MC CH8N, Portland, OR 97239; **Phone:** 503-494-4314; **Board Cert:** Neurological Surgery 2004; **Med School:** Harvard Med Sch 1993; **Resid:** Neurological Surgery, Univ Michigan Med Ctr 1999; **Fellow:** Pediatric Neurological Surgery, Northwestern Meml Hosp 2000; **Fac Appt:** Prof NS, Oregon Hlth & Sci Univ

Shuer, Lawrence M MD [NS] - **Spec Exp:** Pediatric Neurosurgery; Craniosynostosis; Epilepsy; Chiari's Deformity; **Hospital:** Stanford Univ Hosp & Clinics, Lucile Packard Chldn's Hosp; **Address:** Stanford Univ Med Ctr, Dept Neurosurgery, 300 Pasteur Drive, rm R229, Stanford, CA 94305-5327; **Phone:** 650-723-5574; **Board Cert:** Neurological Surgery 1986; **Med School:** Univ Mich Med Sch 1978; **Resid:** Neurological Surgery, Stanford Univ Med Ctr 1984; **Fac Appt:** Prof NS, Stanford Univ

Silbergeld, Daniel MD [NS] - **Spec Exp:** Brain Tumors; Brain Tumors-Metastatic; Brain Mapping; **Hospital:** Univ Wash Med Ctr; **Address:** 1959 NE Pacific St, Box 356470, Seattle, WA 98195; **Phone:** 206-598-5637; **Board Cert:** Neurological Surgery 1995; **Med School:** Univ Cincinnati 1984; **Resid:** Neurological Surgery, Univ Wash Med Ctr 1990; Research, Univ Wash Med Ctr 1988; **Fellow:** Neuro-Oncology, Univ Wash Med Ctr 1991; Epilepsy, Univ Wash Med Ctr 1991; **Fac Appt:** Assoc Prof NS, Univ Wash

Steinberg, Gary K MD/PhD [NS] - **Spec Exp:** Aneurysm-Cerebral; MoyaMoya Disease; Arteriovenous Malformations; Cerebrovascular Surgery; **Hospital:** Stanford Univ Hosp & Clinics; **Address:** Stanford Univ Dept Neurosurgery, 300 Pasteur Drive, rm R281, Stanford, CA 94305-5327; **Phone:** 650-725-5562; **Board Cert:** Neurological Surgery 1989; **Med School:** Stanford Univ 1980; **Resid:** Neuropathology, Stanford Univ Med Ctr 1982; Neurological Surgery, Stanford Univ Med Ctr 1987; **Fellow:** Cerebrovascular Neurosurgery, Univ West Ontario 1985; **Fac Appt:** Prof NS, Stanford Univ

Sun, Peter P MD [NS] - **Spec Exp:** Pediatric Neurosurgery; Congenital Cranial Deformities; Brain Tumors; **Hospital:** Chldns Hosp - Oakland; **Address:** 744 52nd St, Ste 5203, Oakland, CA 94609; **Phone:** 510-428-3319; **Board Cert:** Neurological Surgery 2002; Pediatric Neurological Surgery 2006; **Med School:** Columbia P&S 1991; **Resid:** Neurological Surgery, UC Davis Med Ctr 1994; Neurological Surgery, Yale-New Haven Hosp 1996; **Fellow:** Neurological Surgery, NYU Med Ctr 1997; Pediatric Neurological Surgery, Childrens Hosp 1998; **Fac Appt:** Asst Clin Prof NS, UCSF

Yu, John S MD [NS] - **Spec Exp:** Brain Tumors; Spinal Tumors; Clinical Trials; Spinal Surgery; **Hospital:** Cedars-Sinai Med Ctr; **Address:** Maxine Dunitz Neurosurgical Institute, 8631 W 3rd St, Ste 800-East, Los Angeles, CA 90048; **Phone:** 310-423-7900; **Board Cert:** Neurological Surgery 2002; **Med School:** Harvard Med Sch 1990; **Resid:** Neurological Surgery, Mass General Hosp 1997

Cleveland Clinic

Every life deserves world class care.

Neurological Surgery

Cleveland Clinic Neurological Institute employs a multidisciplinary disease-specific focus, combining more than 300 medical, surgical and research specialists who treat children and adults with neurological and neurobehavioral disorders. Our clinical expertise, academic achievement and innovative research has earned the Neurological Institute an international reputation for excellence. *U.S. News & World Report* recently ranked our neurology, neurosurgery and pediatrics neurology/neurosurgery programs among the top 5 in the nation.

Our unique and collaborative clinical structure allows us to deliver coordinated, comprehensive and multi-disciplinary care to our patients through more efficient treatment decision-making and consultation for complex cases. Major advances in the treatment of brain tumors, epilepsy, mood disorders, stroke, movement disorders, pain and spinal disorders are improving quality of life and survival for thousands of our patients. Our innovative model of medicine will speed research and advances in treatment, resulting in better clinical care and more rapid breakthroughs in the full range of neurological and behavioral disorders.

Comprehensive Neurological Care

Cleveland Clinic offers expert diagnostic and treatment options for all neurologic conditions affecting children and adults, including Alzheimer's disease, aneurysms, arteriovenous malformations, back and neck disorders, brain and spine tumors, epilepsy, hydrocephalus, metastatic tumors, mild cognitive impairment, multiple sclerosis, movement disorders, neurofibromatosis, Parkinson's disease, pediatric and congenital neurological disorders, pituitary disorders, sleep disorders and stroke.

Cleveland Clinic
Neurological Institute
9500 Euclid Avenue
Cleveland, OH 44195

Offering Same-Day Appointments
Call 800.274.2009.

Treatment Guides
Cleveland Clinic has developed comprehensive treatment guides for many diseases and conditions. To download our free treatment guides, visit clevelandclinic.org/treatmentguides.

Online Medical Second Opinion
Call 216.444.3223 or 800.223.2273 ext. 43223 or email eclevelandclinic@ccf.org.

Out-of-State Patients Assistance
Call 800.223.2273, ext. 55580 or email medicalconcierge@ccf.org.

Visit Us At:
clevelandclinic.org

Follow Us On:
Facebook
www.facebook.com/clevelandclinic

Twitter
@ClevelandClinic

You Tube
www.youtube.com/clevelandclinic

Health Hub
health.clevelandclinic.org

MOUNT SINAI
SCHOOL OF
MEDICINE

THE MOUNT SINAI MEDICAL CENTER
NEUROSURGERY

One Gustave L. Levy Place
Fifth Avenue and 100th Street
New York, NY 10029-6574
Physician Referral: 1-800-MD-SINAI (637-4624)
www.mountsinai.org/neurosurgery

THE DEPARTMENT OF NEUROSURGERY at Mount Sinai, established in 1920, has earned a distinguished international reputation. Since assuming the position of Chair four years ago, Joshua Bederson, MD, has expanded the department by more than 50 percent through a combination of strategic recruitments, new hospital affiliations, and numerous outreach programs. Neurosurgery is the fastest growing surgical subspecialty at Mount Sinai, performing more than 2,500 procedures a year at The Mount Sinai Hospital. Areas of clinical expertise include the treatment of meningiomas and other skull base tumors, primary and metastatic brain tumors, pituitary adenomas and acoustic neuromas, deep brain stimulation for movement disorders and minimally invasive treatment of spine and spinal cord disorders. The department is a regional leader in endovascular and microsurgical treatment of aneurysms, arteriovenous malformations and stroke, microvascular decompression for trigeminal neuralgia and hemifacial spasm. We are the first medical center in the nation to use the Neurotouch virtual reality brain surgery simulator, which will be used to train our residents, assess skill level and to rehearse upcoming cases.

The Meningioma Program has pioneered endoscopic, minimally invasive surgical approaches for the treatment of meningiomas. Transnasal endoscopic tumor resections and computer-aided navigation help our surgeons achieve even greater precision during surgery. Both tactics reduce risk to the patient and help us avoid critical vascular and intracranial structures. Working with the Minimally Invasive and Endoscopic Skull Base Surgery Program, we unite specialists in neurosurgery, otolaryngology, head and neck cancer, craniofacial surgery, oral and maxillofacial surgery, and microvascular and reconstructive procedures.

The Comprehensive Brain Tumor Program collaborates with The Tisch Cancer Institute and the Departments of Neurology, Radiation Oncology, Radiology, and Pathology to provide comprehensive therapies for primary and metastatic brain tumors. We have pioneered minimally invasive approaches using imaging technology, frameless stereotaxy, awake and asleep brain mapping, and advanced microneurosurgery. Stereotactic radiosurgery, a minimally invasive treatment that does not require open surgery, gene therapy, and clinical trials are also possible options.

The Cerebrovascular Program is composed of an experienced team that provides a complete range of services for the diagnosis and treatment of patients with neurovascular disorders of the brain and spinal cord. Some current treatments include microsurgical treatment of aneurysms and AVMs with clipping and resection, endovascular treatment of aneurysms with coils and/or stents, endovascular treatment of AVMs with liquid acrylics, stereotactic radiosurgical treatment of AVMs, endovascular treatment of stenoses with stents and angioplasty and microsurgical treatment of stenoses and occlusions with bypass. We are the most experienced program in stent-assisted embolization of cerebral aneurysms and stent treatment of carotid artery disease amongst neurovascular centers in New York.

The Neurosurgery Spinal Disorders Program offers treatment for all disorders of the spinal column and spinal cord, including degenerative disorders, trauma, infections, congenital disorders (including scoliosis), and tumors. Our neurosurgeons have pioneered endoscopic, minimally invasive approaches for tumor resection and treatment of degenerative diseases. These approaches reduce pain and hospital stays, and facilitate an early return to normal activity.

The Neuroendocrine Program sees more than 200 new pituitary tumor patients each year, more than 300 follow-up patients annually, and has performed more than 2,500 transphenoidal pituitary operations.

The Center for Neuromodulation, a collaboration between the Departments of Neurology and Neurosurgery, uses the latest technology to precisely target areas of abnormal activity in the brain and spinal cord. Our physicians are focused on developing minimally invasive neurosurgical techniques that either modulate neural function, replace lost neuronal populations, or halt the neurodegenerative process altogether. Currently, deep brain stimulation dominates this field, but many technologies with great potential are on the horizon.

NEUROSURGERY

The Department of Neurosurgery at NYU Langone Medical Center offers some of the nation's most skilled and experienced surgeons in advanced, minimally invasive procedures. Patients also benefit from cutting-edge research and fully integrated approach to medical care.

Brain Tumor
The Department of Neurosurgery specializes in both malignant and benign brain tumors, including skull base tumors. Expertise includes glioblastoma, ependymoma, hemangioblastoma, other gliomas, meningiomas and vestibular schwannomas (acoustic neuromas).

Cerebrovascular Surgery
The Division of Cerebrovascular Surgery is a premier center for brain aneurysms, giant intracranial aneurysms, brain vascular malformations and cavernomas, and stroke.

Epilepsy
The Comprehensive Epilepsy Center is the largest epilepsy center in the U.S. offering patients an array of advanced surgical and medical options.

Spinal Neurosurgery
The Division of Spine Surgery provides treatment for degenerative spinal diseases, spinal tumors, spinal trauma and spinal infections.

Hyperhidrosis
The Department offers expertise in the surgical treatment of primary hyperhidrosis (excessive sweating) including Endoscopic Thoracic Sympathectomy.

Neurosurgical Technology
Our neurosurgeons remove deep-seated tumors, vascular malformations and other disease sites using a highly advanced Leksell Gamma Knife. Aided by 3-D MRI technology, the Gamma Knife bombards its target with precise doses of radiation, while preserving healthy tissue.

We also provide state-of-the-art care and research through the following divisions:
- Facial Pain: provides patients a thorough examination and, if required, nerve injections and minimally invasive surgery.
- Functional Neurosurgery: offers diagnosis and treatment of Parkinson's disease and conditions that involve involuntary muscle contractions.
- Pediatric Neurosurgery: provides treatment to children with brain and spinal cord tumors, congenital and development disorders.
- Peripheral Nerve Surgery: focuses on the diagnosis and treatment of nerve compressions, nerve tremors, Brachial Plexus (nerve fiber) and nerve injuries.

Neuro-Critical Care
Intensive care and treatment of critical neurosurgical illnesses is provided.

The Department of Neurosurgery at Penn provides comprehensive medical and surgical care for people with disorders of the brain, spinal cord and peripheral nervous system. One of the hallmarks of Penn's neurosurgery program is its integration of research and clinical practice, embracing new technologies and seeking the highest quality and best outcomes possible. More Penn neurosurgeons are listed in *The Best Doctors in America®* than are found at any other hospital or medical center in the Philadelphia region. Penn Neurology and Neurosurgery at the Hospital of the University of Pennsylvania (HUP) are ranked 21st in the nation by *U.S. News & World Report*, the only neuroscience programs in the region to be recognized.

Penn Neurosurgery is a component of the **Penn Medicine Neuroscience Center**, which facilitates and strengthens the integration of Penn's world-class neuroscience programs within the areas of clinical care, research and education. Penn's neurosurgical specialists backed by the most extensive neurodiagnostic and imaging facilities in the region, perform more than 4,500 operations each year. The neurosurgical faculty all have a particular subspecialty focus, covering the entire spectrum of surgically-treated disorders of the nervous system.

Excellence and Expertise

The Penn Gamma Knife® Center at Pennsylvania Hospital offers power, precision and hope to patients suffering from brain tumors and other serious brain disorders. Gamma Knife® Perfexion™ radiosurgery is noninvasive, effective, and safe for treating conditions including benign or malignant brain tumors, blood vessel malformations and trigeminal neuralgia.

The Center for Functional and Restorative Neurosurgery at Pennsylvania Hospital performed more deep brain stimulation procedures for the treatment of Parkinson's disease and epilepsy in the past year than any other hospital or health system in the U.S.

The Center for Cranial Base Surgery offers expert evaluation and treatment of tumors of the head, neck, face and other complex skull base disorders. With the development of innovative and endoscopic surgical procedures and state-of-the-art imaging, many of these tumors, previously inaccessible, can now be successfully treated.

The Penn Brain Tumor Center provides evaluation, diagnosis and treatment to patients with brain and spinal tumors and other cancer-related neurological central nervous system and peripheral nervous system problems. The program utilizes a patient-oriented team approach bringing together some of the nation's leading experts in the field.

The Neurosurgical Spine Center provides medical and surgical care for the most complex disorders of the spinal cord. Penn is a regional and national leader in providing quality spine care. Utilizing a multidisciplinary team approach, the Center implements the latest advances in techniques and technology.

The Neurovascular Center offers minimally invasive (endovascular) coiling and stent treatments of brain aneurysms, vascular malformations and atherosclerotic narrowing of the blood vessels of the brain, combining the skill sets of neurosurgeons and interventional neuroradiologists to obtain the best possible outcomes.

For more information or to schedule an appointment, call 800.789.PENN (7366) or visit PennMedicine.org/neurosurgery

The Next Generation in Treatment Advances

Penn neurosurgeons are advancing minimally-invasive endoscopic surgery to the next level using three-dimensional (3D) endoscopy technology. Penn Medicine is one of only a few academic medical centers in the nation, and the first in the mid-Atlantic region, to utilize this groundbreaking technology.

Penn Neurosurgery patients have access to the Roberts Proton Therapy Center, the world's largest proton therapy center associated with an academic medical center and one of only six such centers in the country. It is the world's most comprehensive proton therapy center, offering the unique ability to fully integrate conventional radiation treatment with proton radiation.

Penn Neurosurgery Programs

- Center for Brain Injury and Repair
- Center for Cranial Base Surgery
- Center for Functional and Restorative Neurosurgery
- Penn Brain Tumor Center
- Penn Gamma Knife® Center
- Neuro Intensive Care
- Neurovascular Center
- Neurosurgical Spine Center

Gamma Knife and Leksell Gamma Knife are U.S. federally registered trademarks of Elekta Instrument S.A., Geneva, Switzerland.

Locations

Hospital of the University of Pennsylvania

Pennsylvania Hospital

Penn Medicine Cherry Hill

Penn Medicine Valley Forge

Penn Medicine Bucks County

Affiliate: Doylestown Hospital

Neurology

A neurologist specializes in the diagnosis and treatment of all types of disease or impaired function of the brain, spinal cord, peripheral nerves, muscles and autonomic nervous system, as well as the blood vessels that relate to these structures. A child neurologist has special skills in the diagnosis and management of neurologic disorders of the neonatal period, infancy, early childhood and adolescence.

Training Required: Four years

NEUROLOGY

New England

Amato, Anthony A MD [N] - **Spec Exp:** Peripheral Neuropathy; Neuromuscular Disorders; Muscular Dystrophy; **Hospital:** Brigham and Women's Hosp (page 57); **Address:** Brigham & Women's Hosp, Dept Neurology, 75 Francis St, Boston, MA 02115; **Phone:** 617-732-8046; **Board Cert:** Neurology 1991; Neuromuscular Medicine 2008; **Med School:** Univ Cincinnati 1986; **Resid:** Neurology, Wilford Hall USAF Med Ctr 1990; **Fellow:** Neuromuscular Medicine, Ohio State Med Ctr 1992; **Fac Appt:** Prof N, Harvard Med Sch

Armon, Carmel MD [N] - **Spec Exp:** Amyotrophic Lateral Sclerosis (ALS); Epilepsy/Seizure Disorders; Vascular Neurology; Sleep Medicine; **Hospital:** Baystate Med Ctr; **Address:** Baystate Neurology, 3300 Main St Fl 3 - Ste 3C, Springfield, MA 01199; **Phone:** 413-794-7192; **Board Cert:** Neurology 1990; Clinical Neurophysiology 2002; Vascular Neurology 2005; Sleep Medicine 2007; **Med School:** Israel 1980; **Resid:** Neurology, Mayo Clinic 1988; **Fellow:** Neurology, Mayo Clinic 1989; Clinical Neurophysiology, Duke Univ Med Ctr 1991; **Fac Appt:** Prof N, Tufts Univ

Batchelor, Tracy T MD [N] - **Spec Exp:** Brain Tumors; Gliomas; **Hospital:** Mass Genl Hosp; **Address:** Mass Genl Hosp Cancer Ctr - Neuro-Oncology, 55 Fruit St, Ste YAW 9E, Boston, MA 02114; **Phone:** 617-724-8770; **Board Cert:** Neurology 2005; **Med School:** Emory Univ 1990; **Resid:** Neurology, Mass Genl Hosp 1994; **Fellow:** Neuro-Oncology, Meml Sloan Kettering Cancer Ctr 1995; **Fac Appt:** Prof N, Harvard Med Sch

Blum, Andrew S MD/PhD [N] - **Spec Exp:** Epilepsy; **Hospital:** Rhode Island Hosp; **Address:** Neurology Foundation Inc, 2 Dudley St, Ste 555, Providence, RI 02905; **Phone:** 401-444-3032; **Board Cert:** Neurology 2005; Clinical Neurophysiology 2006; **Med School:** Cornell Univ 1990; **Resid:** Neurology, Johns Hopkins Hosp 1994; **Fellow:** Clinical Neurophysiology, Beth Israel Deaconess Med Ctr 1995

Caplan, Louis R MD [N] - **Spec Exp:** Stroke; **Hospital:** Beth Israel Deaconess Med Ctr - Boston; **Address:** Palmer 127 West Campus BIDMC, 330 Brookline Ave, Boston, MA 02215; **Phone:** 617-632-8911; **Board Cert:** Internal Medicine 1969; Neurology 1972; Vascular Neurology 2005; **Med School:** Univ MD Sch Med 1962; **Resid:** Neurology, Boston City Hosp 1969; **Fellow:** Neurology, Harvard Univ Affil Hosp 1970; **Fac Appt:** Prof N, Harvard Med Sch

Cohen, Jeffrey Allen MD [N] - **Spec Exp:** Neuromuscular Disorders; Peripheral Neuropathy; **Hospital:** Dartmouth - Hitchcock Med Ctr; **Address:** Department of Neurology, 1 Medical Center Drive, Lebanon, NH 03756; **Phone:** 603-650-8589; **Board Cert:** Neurology 1982; Clinical Neurophysiology 2011; Neuromuscular Medicine 2008; **Med School:** Univ Okla Coll Med 1977; **Resid:** Neurology, Mt Sinai Hosp 1981; **Fellow:** Neuromuscular Disease, Mass Genl Hosp 1982; Peripheral Nerve Surgery, Mayo Clin 1986; **Fac Appt:** Prof Med, Dartmouth Med Sch

Cole, Andrew J MD [N] - **Spec Exp:** Epilepsy/Seizure Disorders; Rasmussen's Syndrome; **Hospital:** Mass Genl Hosp; **Address:** Mass Genl Hosp-Epilepsy Svc, 55 Fruit St, Wang Ambulatory Ctr, Ste 735, Boston, MA 02114; **Phone:** 617-726-3311; **Board Cert:** Neurology 1987; Clinical Neurophysiology 2009; **Med School:** Dartmouth Med Sch 1982; **Resid:** Neurology, Neuro Inst-McGill 1986; **Fellow:** Electroencephalography, Neuro Inst-McGill 1987; Neurological Surgery, Johns Hopkins Hosp 1988; **Fac Appt:** Asst Prof N, Harvard Med Sch

Cudkowicz, Merit MD [N] - **Spec Exp:** Amyotrophic Lateral Sclerosis (ALS); Neuromuscular Disorders; **Hospital:** Beth Israel Deaconess Med Ctr - Boston; **Address:** Neurology Associates, 15 Parkman St, WAC 835, Boston, MA 02114-3117; **Phone:** 617-724-3914; **Board Cert:** Neurology 2005; **Med School:** Harvard Med Sch 1990; **Resid:** Neurology, Mass Genl Hosp 1994; **Fellow:** Neurology, Mass Genl Hosp 1996; **Fac Appt:** Prof N, Harvard Med Sch

Feldmann, Edward MD [N] - **Spec Exp:** Cerebrovascular Disease; Stroke; **Hospital:** Tufts Med Ctr; **Address:** Tufts Medical Center, 800 Washington St, Box 314, Boston, MA 02111; **Phone:** 617-636-5848; **Board Cert:** Neurology 1988; Vascular Neurology 2005; **Med School:** Harvard Med Sch 1983; **Resid:** Neurology, New York Hosp 1987; **Fellow:** Cerebrovascular Disease, Tufts New Eng Med Ctr 1988; **Fac Appt:** Prof N, Brown Univ

Flaherty, Alice W MD/PhD [N] - **Spec Exp:** Parkinson's Disease; Movement Disorders; Deep Brain Stimulation; Tourette's Syndrome; **Hospital:** Mass Genl Hosp; **Address:** Neurology Assocs, 15 Parkman St, WACC 715, Boston, MA 02114; **Phone:** 617-724-9234; **Board Cert:** Neurology 2009; **Med School:** Harvard Med Sch 1994; **Resid:** Neurology, Mass Genl Hosp 1998

Furie, Karen L MD [N] - **Spec Exp:** Stroke; Cerebrovascular Disease; **Hospital:** Rhode Island Hosp; **Address:** Rhode Island Hospital, 110 Lockwood St, Ste 324, Providence, RI 02903; **Phone:** 401-444-3032; **Board Cert:** Neurology 2006; Vascular Neurology 2008; **Med School:** Brown Univ 1990; **Resid:** Neurology, Rhode Island Hosp 1994; **Fellow:** Cerebrovascular Disease, Brown Univ 1995; **Fac Appt:** Prof N, Brown Univ

Greer, David M MD [N] - **Spec Exp:** Stroke; Cerebrovascular Disease; **Hospital:** Yale-New Haven Hosp, Yale Med Group; **Address:** Yale Univ Sch Medicine, Dept Neurology, 15 York St, PO Box 208018, New Haven, CT 06520-8018; **Phone:** 203-737-1057; **Board Cert:** Neurology 2010; Vascular Neurology 2008; **Med School:** Univ Fla Coll Med 1995; **Resid:** Neurology, Mass General Hosp 1999; **Fellow:** Vascular Neurology, Mass General Hosp 2001

Gross, Paul T MD [N] - **Spec Exp:** Epilepsy; Sleep Disorders; **Hospital:** Lahey Clin; **Address:** Lahey Clinic, 41 Mall Rd, Burlington, MA 01805; **Phone:** 781-744-3263; **Board Cert:** Neurology 1981; Sleep Medicine 1992; **Med School:** Hahnemann Univ 1976; **Resid:** Neurology, Univ Wisc Hosp 1980; **Fellow:** Clinical Neurophysiology, Boston Chldn's Hosp 1981; **Fac Appt:** Clin Prof N, Tufts Univ

Jobst, Barbara C MD [N] - **Spec Exp:** Epilepsy/Seizure Disorders; Epilepsy in Women; **Hospital:** Dartmouth - Hitchcock Med Ctr; **Address:** Dartmouth-Hitchcock Medical Center, One Medical Center Drive, Lebanon, NH 03756-1000; **Phone:** 603-653-6118; **Board Cert:** Neurology 2002; **Med School:** Germany 1993; **Resid:** Neurology, Krankenhaus Barmherzigen Bruder 1996; Neurology, Dartmouth-Hitchcock Med Ctr 2000; **Fellow:** Epilepsy, Dartmouth-Hitchcock Med Ctr 2001; **Fac Appt:** Assoc Prof N, Dartmouth Med Sch

Jones Jr, H Royden MD [N] - **Spec Exp:** Neuromuscular Disorders; Amyotrophic Lateral Sclerosis (ALS); Myasthenia Gravis; Peripheral Neuropathy; **Hospital:** Lahey Clin; **Address:** Lahey Clinic, 41 Mall Rd, Burlington, MA 01805; **Phone:** 781-744-5126; **Board Cert:** Neurology 2004; Clinical Neurophysiology 2000; Neuromuscular Medicine 2006; **Med School:** Northwestern Univ 1962; **Resid:** Internal Medicine, Mayo Clinic 1965; Neurology, Mayo Clinic 1969; **Fellow:** Neurological Physiology, Mayo Clinic 1972; **Fac Appt:** Clin Prof N, Harvard Med Sch

Kase, Carlos S MD [N] - **Spec Exp:** Stroke; **Hospital:** Boston Med Ctr; **Address:** Boston Med Ctr, Shapiro Ctr, 725 Albany St Fl 7th - Ste 7B, Boston, MA 02118; **Phone:** 617-638-8456; **Board Cert:** Neurology 1980; Vascular Neurology 2005; **Med School:** Chile 1967; **Resid:** Neurology, Mass Genl Hosp 1973; Neurology, Mass Genl Hosp 1978; **Fac Appt:** Prof N, Boston Univ

Neurology

Oaklander, Anne Louise MD/PhD [N] - **Spec Exp:** Nerve Injuries; Peripheral Neuropathy; Pain-Neuropathic; Complex Regional Pain Syndromes; **Hospital:** Mass Genl Hosp; **Address:** Mass General Hosp, Dept Neurology, 55 Fruit St, Wang Bldg Fl 8 - rm 835, Boston, MA 02114; **Phone:** 617-724-3992; **Board Cert:** Neurology 1992; Pain Medicine 2000; **Med School:** Albert Einstein Coll Med 1987; **Resid:** Neurology, UMDNJ Univ Med Ctr 1991; **Fellow:** Neuromuscular Medicine, Johns Hopkins Hosp 1994; Neurological Surgery, Johns Hopkins Hosp 1995; **Fac Appt:** Assoc Prof N, Harvard Med Sch

Pennell, Page B MD [N] - **Spec Exp:** Epilepsy in Women; Epilepsy in Pregnancy; Clinical Trials; **Hospital:** Brigham and Women's Hosp (page 57); **Address:** Brigham & Womens Hosp, Div Epilepsy, EEG & Sleep Neurology, 75 Francis St, Boston, MA 02115; **Phone:** 617-732-7547; **Board Cert:** Neurology 2004; **Med School:** Univ Fla Coll Med 1989; **Resid:** Neurology, Univ Michigan Med Ctr 1993; **Fellow:** Clinical Neurophysiology, Univ Michigan 1995; **Fac Appt:** Assoc Clin Prof N, Emory Univ

Ropper, Allan MD [N] - **Spec Exp:** Guillain-Barre Syndrome; Parkinson's Disease; **Hospital:** Brigham and Women's Hosp (page 57); **Address:** Brigham & Women's Hosp, Dept Neurology, 75 Francis St, Box BB204, Boston, MA 02115; **Phone:** 617-732-8047; **Board Cert:** Internal Medicine 1977; Neurology 1980; **Med School:** Harvard Med Sch 1974; **Resid:** Internal Medicine, UCSF Med Ctr 1976; Neurology, Mass Genl Hosp 1979; **Fac Appt:** Prof N, Tufts Univ

Rutkove, Seward B MD [N] - **Spec Exp:** Neuromuscular Disorders; Amyotrophic Lateral Sclerosis (ALS); **Hospital:** Beth Israel Deaconess Med Ctr - Boston; **Address:** 330 Brookline Ave, Ste TCC-810, Boston, MA 02215; **Phone:** 617-667-8130; **Board Cert:** Neurology 2006; Clinical Neurophysiology 2007; **Med School:** Columbia P&S 1989; **Resid:** Internal Medicine, St Joseph Mercy Hosp 1991; Neurology, Harvard-Longwood Neuro Prgm 1994; **Fellow:** Clinical Neurophysiology, Brigham & Women's Hosp 1995; **Fac Appt:** Assoc Prof N, Harvard Med Sch

Samuels, Martin A MD [N] - **Spec Exp:** Neurologic Aspects of Systemic Disease; **Hospital:** Brigham and Women's Hosp (page 57), Mass Genl Hosp; **Address:** Brigham & Women's Hosp, Dept Neurology, 75 Francis St Fl 2, Boston, MA 02115; **Phone:** 617-732-7432; **Board Cert:** Internal Medicine 1974; Neurology 1978; **Med School:** Univ Cincinnati 1971; **Resid:** Internal Medicine, Boston City Hosp 1975; Neurology, Mass Genl Hosp 1977; **Fellow:** Neurological Pathology, Mass Genl Hosp 1976; **Fac Appt:** Prof N, Harvard Med Sch

Saper, Clifford MD/PhD [N] - **Spec Exp:** Sleep Disorders/Apnea; **Hospital:** Beth Israel Deaconess Med Ctr - Boston; **Address:** Beth Israel Deaconess Med Ctr, 330 Brookline Ave, Neurology, Kirstein 406, Boston, MA 02215; **Phone:** 617-667-2622; **Board Cert:** Neurology 1982; **Med School:** Washington Univ, St Louis 1977; **Resid:** Neurology, NY Hosp 1981; **Fac Appt:** Prof N, Harvard Med Sch

Taylor, Lynne P MD [N] - **Spec Exp:** Neuro-Oncology; Brain Tumors; Gliomas; Palliative Care; **Hospital:** Tufts Med Ctr; **Address:** Tufts Medical Center, 800 Washington St, South Bldg Fl 7, Box 245, Boston, MA 02111; **Phone:** 617-636-2694; **Board Cert:** Neurology 1987; Hospice & Palliative Medicine 2010; **Med School:** Washington Univ, St Louis 1982; **Resid:** Neurology, Hosp Univ Penn 1986; **Fellow:** Neuro-Oncology, Meml Sloan Kettering Cancer Ctr 1988; **Fac Appt:** Assoc Clin Prof N, Tufts Univ

Wen, Patrick Y MD [N] - **Spec Exp:** Neuro-Oncology; Brain Tumors; **Hospital:** Dana-Farber Cancer Inst (page 57), Brigham and Women's Hosp (page 57); **Address:** Dana-Farber Cancer Inst, 450 Brookline Ave, Ste SW430B, Boston, MA 02115; **Phone:** 617-632-2166; **Board Cert:** Neurology 1989; **Med School:** England, UK 1981; **Resid:** Internal Medicine, London Chest Hosp 1984; Internal Medicine, Nat'l Hosp for Nervous Disease 1984; **Fellow:** Harvard-Longwood Neurology 1988; **Fac Appt:** Prof N, Harvard Med Sch

Young, Anne MD/PhD [N] - **Spec Exp:** Huntington's Disease; Parkinson's Disease; Movement Disorders; **Hospital:** Mass Genl Hosp; **Address:** Mass Genl Hosp, Dept Neurology, 15 Parkman St Fl 7, Boston, MA 02114; **Phone:** 617-726-2385; **Board Cert:** Neurology 1981; **Med School:** Johns Hopkins Univ 1973; **Resid:** Neurology, UCSF Med Ctr 1978; **Fac Appt:** Prof N, Harvard Med Sch

Mid Atlantic

Apatoff, Brian R MD/PhD [N] - **Spec Exp:** Multiple Sclerosis; Neuro-Immunology; **Hospital:** NY-Presby/Weill Cornell Med Ctr, NY (page 66); **Address:** Multiple Sclerosis Institute, 401 E 55th St, New York, NY 10022; **Phone:** 212-593-6262; **Board Cert:** Neurology 1991; **Med School:** Univ Chicago-Pritzker Sch Med 1984; **Resid:** Neurology, Columbia Presby Med Ctr 1990; **Fellow:** Multiple Sclerosis, Neuro Inst-Columbia Univ 1992; **Fac Appt:** Assoc Prof N, Cornell Univ-Weill Med Coll

Azizi, Sayed Ausim MD/PhD [N] - **Spec Exp:** Movement Disorders; Parkinson's Disease; Stroke; **Hospital:** Temple Univ Hosp, Hahnemann Univ Hosp; **Address:** Temple Univ Sch Med, Dept of Neurology, 3401 N Broad St, Ste C525, Philadelphia, PA 19140; **Phone:** 215-707-5953; **Board Cert:** Neurology 2008; **Med School:** Univ Tex SW, Dallas 1990; **Resid:** Neurology, Yale-New Haven Hosp 1994; **Fac Appt:** Prof N, Temple Univ

Balcer, Laura J MD [N] - **Spec Exp:** Neuro-Ophthalmology; Multiple Sclerosis/Visual Disorders; Parkinson's Disease/Visual Disorders; **Hospital:** Hosp Univ Penn - UPHS (page 72); **Address:** 3400 Spruce St, Hosp University Pennsylvania, Philadelphia, PA 19104; **Phone:** 215-349-8072; **Board Cert:** Neurology 2006; **Med School:** Johns Hopkins Univ 1991; **Resid:** Neurology, Hosp Univ Penn 1995; **Fellow:** Neuro-Ophthalmology, Hosp Univ Penn/Scheie Inst 1995; **Fac Appt:** Prof N, Univ Pennsylvania

Baser, Susan M MD [N] - **Spec Exp:** Parkinson's Disease; Huntington's Disease; Dystonia; Movement Disorders; **Hospital:** Allegheny General Hosp; **Address:** Allegheny Neurology Assocs, 490 E North Ave Prof Bldg - rm 500, Pittsburgh, PA 15212; **Phone:** 412-359-8860; **Board Cert:** Neurology 1990; **Med School:** Loyola Univ-Stritch Sch Med 1983; **Resid:** Neurology, Univ Pittsburgh 1987; **Fellow:** Neuropharmacology, Natl Inst Hlth 1990; **Fac Appt:** Assoc Prof N, Thomas Jefferson Univ

Bell, Rodney D MD [N] - **Spec Exp:** Stroke; **Hospital:** Thomas Jefferson Univ Hosp; **Address:** Thomas Jefferson Univ Dept Neurology, 900 Walnut St, Ste 200, Philadelphia, PA 19107; **Phone:** 215-955-6488; **Board Cert:** Internal Medicine 1975; Neurotology 1981; Vascular Neurology 2005; **Med School:** Oregon Hlth & Sci Univ 1971; **Resid:** Internal Medicine, Parkland Meml Hosp 1975; Neurology, Parkland Meml Hosp 1978; **Fac Appt:** Prof N, Thomas Jefferson Univ

Bergey, Gregory K MD [N] - **Spec Exp:** Epilepsy/Seizure Disorders; Epilepsy in Women; Epilepsy in Pregnancy; **Hospital:** Johns Hopkins Hosp (page 61); **Address:** Johns Hopkins Epilepsy Ctr, 600 N Wolfe St, Meyer 2-147, Baltimore, MD 21287; **Phone:** 410-955-7338; **Board Cert:** Internal Medicine 1978; Neurology 1984; **Med School:** Univ Pennsylvania 1975; **Resid:** Internal Medicine, Yale-New Haven Hosp 1977; Neurology, Johns Hopkins Hosp 1981; **Fellow:** Neurological Physiology, Natl Inst Health 1983; **Fac Appt:** Prof N, Johns Hopkins Univ

Bressman, Susan MD [N] - **Spec Exp:** Parkinson's Disease; Movement Disorders; Dystonia; **Hospital:** Beth Israel Med Ctr - Petrie Division (page 56); **Address:** 10 Union Square East, Ste 5J, New York, NY 10003-3314; **Phone:** 212-844-8379; **Board Cert:** Neurology 1983; **Med School:** Columbia P&S 1977; **Resid:** Neurology, Columbia-Presby Med Ctr 1981; **Fellow:** Movement Disorders, Columbia-Presby Med Ctr 1983; **Fac Appt:** Prof N, Albert Einstein Coll Med

Neurology

Brick, John MD [N] - **Spec Exp:** Epilepsy; **Hospital:** Ruby Memorial - WVU Hosp; **Address:** 1 Stadium Drive, Morgantown, WV 26506-9180; **Phone:** 304-598-6127; **Board Cert:** Neurology 1982; Vascular Neurology 2009; **Med School:** W VA Univ 1977; **Resid:** Neurology, W Va Univ Hosp 1981; **Fellow:** Electroencephalography, Mayo Clinic 1983; **Fac Appt:** Prof N, W VA Univ

Buchholz, David W MD [N] - **Spec Exp:** Migraine; Headache; **Hospital:** Johns Hopkins Hosp (page 61); **Address:** Johns Hopkins at Green Spring Station, 10753 Falls Rd, Ste 315, Lutherville, MD 21093; **Phone:** 410-583-2830; **Board Cert:** Neurology 1984; **Med School:** Univ Pennsylvania 1979; **Resid:** Neurology, Johns Hopkins Hosp 1983; **Fac Appt:** Assoc Prof N, Johns Hopkins Univ

Busis, Neil A MD [N] - **Spec Exp:** Electromyography; Neuromuscular Disorders; Movement Disorders; Muscle Disorders; **Hospital:** UPMC Shadyside; **Address:** Pittsburgh Neurological Associates, 532 S Aiken Ave, Ste 507, Pittsburgh, PA 15232-1326; **Phone:** 412-681-2000; **Board Cert:** Neurology 1985; **Med School:** Univ Pennsylvania 1977; **Resid:** Internal Medicine, Johns Hopkins Hosp 1979; Neurology, Mass Genl Hosp 1984; **Fellow:** Electromyography, Mass Genl Hosp 1985; **Fac Appt:** Asst Clin Prof N, Univ Pittsburgh

Calabresi, Peter A MD [N] - **Spec Exp:** Multiple Sclerosis; **Hospital:** Johns Hopkins Hosp (page 61); **Address:** Johns Hopkins, dept Neuro-Immunology, 600 N Wolfe St, Pathology 627, Baltimore, MD 21287; **Phone:** 410-614-1522; **Board Cert:** Neurology 2005; **Med School:** Brown Univ 1988; **Resid:** Neurology, Strong Meml Hosp 1993; **Fellow:** Neurological Immunology, Natl Inst Hlth 1996; **Fac Appt:** Prof N, Johns Hopkins Univ

Charney, Jonathan Z MD [N] - **Spec Exp:** Headache; Stroke; **Hospital:** Mount Sinai Med Ctr (page 64); **Address:** 1111 Park Ave, Ste 1H, New York, NY 10128-1234; **Phone:** 212-831-2886; **Board Cert:** Neurology 1977; **Med School:** NY Med Coll 1969; **Resid:** Neurology, Methodist Hosp-Baylor 1971; Neurology, Columbia-Presby Med Ctr 1973; **Fac Appt:** Asst Prof N, Mount Sinai Sch Med

Cook, Stuart D MD [N] - **Spec Exp:** Multiple Sclerosis; Infectious & Demyelinating Diseases; **Hospital:** Univ Hosp-UMDNJ—Newark; **Address:** 65 Bergen St, rm 1435, Newark, NJ 07101-1709; **Phone:** 973-972-9181; **Board Cert:** Neurology 1970; **Med School:** Univ VT Coll Med 1962; **Resid:** Neurology, Albert Einstein Coll Med 1968; **Fac Appt:** Prof N, UMDNJ-NJ Med Sch, Newark

Cornblath, David R MD [N] - **Spec Exp:** Peripheral Neuropathy; **Hospital:** Johns Hopkins Hosp (page 61); **Address:** 600 N Wolfe St Meyer 6-181A, Baltimore, MD 21287-6965; **Phone:** 410-955-2229; **Board Cert:** Neurology 1982; **Med School:** Case West Res Univ 1977; **Resid:** Neurology, Hosp Univ Penn 1981; **Fellow:** Neurology, Hosp Univ Penn 1982; **Fac Appt:** Prof N, Johns Hopkins Univ

Coyle, Patricia K MD [N] - **Spec Exp:** Multiple Sclerosis; Neuro-Immunology; Lyme Disease; Infections-Neurologic; **Hospital:** Stony Brook Univ Med Ctr; **Address:** Dept Neurology, HSC T-12, rm 020, Stonybrook Univ Med Ctr, Stony Brook, NY 11794-8121; **Phone:** 631-444-2599; **Board Cert:** Neurology 2004; **Med School:** Johns Hopkins Univ 1974; **Resid:** Neurology, Johns Hopkins Hosp 1978; **Fellow:** Neurological Immunology, Johns Hopkins Hosp 1980; **Fac Appt:** Prof N, SUNY Stony Brook

DeAngelis, Lisa M MD [N] - **Spec Exp:** Neuro-Oncology; Brain Tumors; **Hospital:** Meml Sloan-Kettering Cancer Ctr; **Address:** 1275 York Avenue, New York, NY 10065; **Phone:** 212-639-7123; **Board Cert:** Neurology 1986; **Med School:** Columbia P&S 1980; **Resid:** Neurology, Neuro Inst-Presby Hosp 1984; **Fellow:** Neuro-Oncology, Neuro Inst-Presby Hosp 1985; Neuro-Oncology, Meml Sloan-Kettering Cancer Ctr 1986; **Fac Appt:** Prof N, Cornell Univ-Weill Med Coll

Devinsky, Orrin MD [N] - **Spec Exp:** Epilepsy; Tuberous Sclerosis; Behavioral Neurology; **Hospital:** NYU Langone Med Ctr (page 68), Saint Barnabas Med Ctr; **Address:** 223 E 34th St Fl Ground, New York, NY 10016-4972; **Phone:** 646-558-0803; **Board Cert:** Neurology 1987; Clinical Neurophysiology 1990; **Med School:** Harvard Med Sch 1982; **Resid:** Neurology, NY Hosp-Cornell Med Ctr 1986; **Fellow:** Epilepsy, Natl Inst Health 1988; **Fac Appt:** Prof N, NYU Sch Med

Dewberry, Robert G MD [N] - **Hospital:** Maryland Genl Hosp; **Address:** 827 Linden Ave, Armory Bldg - Fl 2 - Ste 2A, Baltimore, MD 21201; **Phone:** 410-225-8290; **Board Cert:** Neurology 1992; **Med School:** Univ MD Sch Med 1987; **Resid:** Neurology, Barnes Hosp 1991; **Fellow:** Neuromuscular Disease, Univ Virginia Hosp 1993

Fahn, Stanley MD [N] - **Spec Exp:** Movement Disorders; Parkinson's Disease; **Hospital:** NY-Presby/Columbia Univ Med Ctr, NY (page 66); **Address:** Neurological Institute, 710 W 168th St Fl 3 - rm 350, New York, NY 10032; **Phone:** 212-305-5277; **Board Cert:** Neurology 1968; **Med School:** UCSF 1958; **Resid:** Neurology, Neuro Inst-Columbia 1962; **Fellow:** Neurological Chemistry, Natl Inst Hlth 1968; **Fac Appt:** Prof N, Columbia P&S

Feinberg, Todd E MD [N] - **Spec Exp:** Alzheimer's Disease; Dementia; **Hospital:** Beth Israel Med Ctr - Petrie Division (page 56); **Address:** Beth Israel Med Ctr, Bernstein Pavilion, 10 Nathan D Perlman Pl Fl 10, New York, NY 10003; **Phone:** 212-420-4111; **Board Cert:** Psychiatry 1984; Neurology 1987; **Med School:** Mount Sinai Sch Med 1978; **Resid:** Psychiatry, Mt Sinai Med Ctr 1982; Neurology, Mt Sinai Med Ctr 1984; **Fellow:** Behavioral Neurology, Univ Florida 1986; **Fac Appt:** Clin Prof N, Albert Einstein Coll Med

Fellus, Jonathan L MD [N] - **Spec Exp:** Brain Injury; Neuro-Rehabilitation; Stroke; Dementia; **Hospital:** Meadowlands Hosp Med Ctr; **Address:** Meadowlands Hospital, 55 Meadowlands Pkwy, Secaucus, NJ 07094; **Phone:** 201-392-3524; **Board Cert:** Neurology 2009; **Med School:** UMDNJ-RW Johnson Med Sch 1992; **Resid:** Neurology, Penn Hosp 1996; **Fellow:** Neurological Rehabilitation, Kernan Hosp/Univ MD Med Ctr 1997; **Fac Appt:** Asst Clin Prof N, UMDNJ-NJ Med Sch, Newark

Fink, Matthew E MD [N] - **Spec Exp:** Cerebrovascular Disease; Stroke; **Hospital:** NY-Presby/Weill Cornell Med Ctr, NY (page 66); **Address:** NY Cornell Med Ctr Dept Neurology, 525 E 68th St, F Bldg - Fl 6 - Ste 610, New York, NY 10065; **Phone:** 212-746-4564; **Board Cert:** Internal Medicine 1980; Neurology 1983; Vascular Neurology 2005; Neurocritical Care 2010; **Med School:** Univ Pittsburgh 1976; **Resid:** Internal Medicine, Boston Med Ctr 1980; Neurology, Columbia-Presby Hosp 1982; **Fac Appt:** Prof N, Cornell Univ

Foo, Sun-Hoo MD [N] - **Spec Exp:** Stroke; Headache; Parkinson's Disease; Dementia; **Hospital:** NYU Langone Med Ctr (page 68), NY Downtown Hosp; **Address:** 650 1st Ave, Fl 4 Floor, New York, NY 10016-3240; **Phone:** 212-213-0270; **Board Cert:** Internal Medicine 1976; Neurology 1980; **Med School:** Taiwan 1972; **Resid:** Internal Medicine, St Vincent's Hosp 1976; Neurology, NYU Med Ctr 1979; **Fac Appt:** Prof N, NYU Sch Med

French, Jacqueline MD [N] - **Spec Exp:** Epilepsy/Seizure Disorders; **Hospital:** NYU Langone Med Ctr (page 68); **Address:** 223 E 34th St, New York, NY 10016; **Phone:** 646-558-0802; **Board Cert:** Neurology 1987; **Med School:** Brown Univ 1982; **Resid:** Neurology, Mount Sinai Hosp 1986; **Fellow:** Epilepsy, Mount Sinai Hosp 1988; Epilepsy, Yale-New Haven Hosp 1989; **Fac Appt:** Prof N, NYU Sch Med

Galetta, Steven MD [N] - **Spec Exp:** Neuro-Ophthalmology; Optic Nerve Disorders; Multiple Sclerosis; **Hospital:** Hosp Univ Penn - UPHS (page 72); **Address:** Hosp Univ Penn, Dept Neurology, 3W Gates Bldg, 3400 Spruce St, Philadelphia, PA 19104; **Phone:** 215-662-3381; **Board Cert:** Neurology 1988; **Med School:** Cornell Univ-Weill Med Coll 1983; **Resid:** Neurology, Hosp Univ Penn 1987; **Fellow:** Neuro-Ophthalmology, Bascom Palmer Eye Inst 1988; **Fac Appt:** Prof N, Univ Pennsylvania

Gendelman, Seymour MD [N] - **Spec Exp:** Parkinson's Disease; Dementia; Headache; **Hospital:** Mount Sinai Med Ctr (page 64); **Address:** 5 E 98th St, Fl 7, Box 1139, New York, NY 10029-6501; **Phone:** 212-241-8172; **Board Cert:** Neurology 1971; **Med School:** Geo Wash Univ 1964; **Resid:** Neurology, Mt Sinai Hosp 1968; **Fac Appt:** Clin Prof N, Mount Sinai Sch Med

Gizzi, Martin S MD/PhD [N] - **Spec Exp:** Neuro-Ophthalmology; Stroke; Progressive Supranuclear Palsy (PSP); Stroke; **Hospital:** JFK Med Ctr - Edison; **Address:** 65 James St, NJ Neuroscience Institute, Edison, NJ 08820-3947; **Phone:** 732-321-7010; **Board Cert:** Neurology 1990; Vascular Neurology 2008; **Med School:** Univ Miami Sch Med 1985; **Resid:** Neurology, Mount Sinai Hosp 1989; **Fellow:** Neuro-Ophthalmology, Mount Sinai Hosp 1991; **Fac Appt:** Prof N, Seton Hall Univ Sch Hlth & Med Scis

Glass, Jon MD [N] - **Spec Exp:** Neuro-Oncology; Brain Tumors; Spinal Tumors; **Hospital:** Thomas Jefferson Univ Hosp; **Address:** Jefferson Neurosurgical Assocs, 909 Walnut St Fl 3, Philadelphia, PA 19107; **Phone:** 215-503-7005; **Board Cert:** Neurology 1993; **Med School:** SUNY Downstate 1986; **Resid:** Neurology, Boston Univ Med Ctr 1990; **Fellow:** Neuro-Oncology, Mass Genl Hosp 1992; **Fac Appt:** Assoc Prof N, Jefferson Med Coll

Golbe, Lawrence I MD [N] - **Spec Exp:** Parkinson's Disease; Progressive Supranuclear Palsy (PSP); Movement Disorders; **Hospital:** Robert Wood Johnson Univ Hosp - New Brunswick; **Address:** 125 Paterson St Fl 6 - rm 6100, New Brunswick, NJ 08901-2160; **Phone:** 732-235-7733; **Board Cert:** Neurology 1984; **Med School:** NYU Sch Med 1978; **Resid:** Internal Medicine, Hahnemann Univ Hosp 1980; Neurology, Bellevue Hosp 1983; **Fac Appt:** Prof N, UMDNJ-RW Johnson Med Sch

Hiesiger, Emile M MD [N] - **Spec Exp:** Pain-Spine; Pain-Cancer, Spine; Pain-Back; **Hospital:** NYU Langone Med Ctr (page 68), VA NY Harbor Hlthcare Sys-Manhattan Campus; **Address:** 345 37th St, Ste 320, New York, NY 10016; **Phone:** 212-263-6123; **Board Cert:** Neurology 1983; **Med School:** NY Med Coll 1978; **Resid:** Neurology, NYU Med Ctr 1982; **Fellow:** Neurology, Meml Sloan-Kettering Cancer Ctr 1984; **Fac Appt:** Assoc Clin Prof N, NYU Sch Med

Hurtig, Howard MD [N] - **Spec Exp:** Parkinson's Disease; Movement Disorders; **Hospital:** Pennsylvania Hosp-UPHS (page 72); **Address:** Pennsylvania Hosp Neurological Inst, 330 S 9th St Fl 3, Philadelphia, PA 19107; **Phone:** 215-829-6500; **Board Cert:** Neurology 1976; **Med School:** Tulane Univ 1966; **Resid:** Internal Medicine, New York Hosp 1968; Neurology, Hosp Univ Penn 1973; **Fac Appt:** Prof N, Univ Pennsylvania

Jordan, Barry D MD [N] - **Spec Exp:** Brain Injury; Sports Neurology; Concussion; Memory Disorders; **Hospital:** Burke Rehab Hosp; **Address:** Burke Rehabilitation Hosp, 785 Mamaroneck Ave, White Plains, NY 10605; **Phone:** 914-597-2332; **Board Cert:** Neurology 1989; **Med School:** Harvard Med Sch 1981; **Resid:** Neurology, New York Hosp 1986; **Fellow:** Hosp Spec Surgery 1987; UCLA Med Ctr 1998; **Fac Appt:** Assoc Prof N, Cornell Univ-Weill Med Coll

Kasner, Scott E MD [N] - **Spec Exp:** Cerebrovascular Disease; Stroke; **Hospital:** Hosp Univ Penn - UPHS (page 72); **Address:** Univ Penn - Dept Neurology, 3400 Spruce St, 3W Gates Bldg, Philadelphia, PA 19104; **Phone:** 215-662-3564; **Board Cert:** Neurology 2007; Vascular Neurology 2006; **Med School:** Yale Univ 1992; **Resid:** Neurology, Hosp Univ Penn 1996; **Fellow:** Stroke, Univ Texas 1997; Neurocritical Care, Univ Texas 1997; **Fac Appt:** Prof N, Univ Pennsylvania

Kieburtz, Karl D MD [N] - **Spec Exp:** Huntington's Disease; Parkinson's Disease; Dementia; **Hospital:** Univ of Rochester Strong Meml Hosp; **Address:** Univ Rochester-Neurology/Mind, 265 Crittenden Blvd, CU142694, Rochester, NY 14627; **Phone:** 585-273-2153; **Board Cert:** Neurology 1990; **Med School:** Univ Rochester 1985; **Resid:** Neurology, Strong Meml Hosp/Univ Rochester 1989; **Fac Appt:** Prof N, Univ Rochester

Klein, Patricia MD [N] - **Spec Exp:** Headache; Dizziness; **Address:** 680 Kinderkamack Rd, Ste 302, Oradell, NJ 07649; **Phone:** 201-261-6222; **Board Cert:** Neurology 1980; **Med School:** UMDNJ-NJ Med Sch, Newark 1976; **Resid:** Neurology, UMDNJ 1979; **Fac Appt:** Asst Clin Prof N, UMDNJ-NJ Med Sch, Newark

Kolodny, Edwin H MD [N] - **Spec Exp:** Pediatric Neurology; Inherited Disorders of Nervous System; Gaucher Disease; Fabry's Disease; **Hospital:** NYU Langone Med Ctr (page 68), Bellevue Hosp Ctr; **Address:** 403 E 34 St Fl 2, New York, NY 10016-6402; **Phone:** 212-263-8344; **Board Cert:** Neurology 1971; Clinical Genetics 1984; Clinical Biochemical Genetics 1987; **Med School:** NYU Sch Med 1962; **Resid:** Internal Medicine, Bellevue Hosp 1964; Neurology, Mass Genl Hosp 1967; **Fellow:** Neurological Pathology, Mass Genl Hosp 1966; Neurology, Nat Inst Neurol Dis & Stroke 1970; **Fac Appt:** Prof N, NYU Sch Med

Krauss, Gregory L MD [N] - **Spec Exp:** Epilepsy/Seizure Disorders; **Hospital:** Johns Hopkins Hosp (page 61); **Address:** Johns Hopkins Hosp, Dept Neurology, 600 N Wolfe St, Meyer 2-147, Baltimore, MD 21287; **Phone:** 410-955-2822; **Board Cert:** Neurology 1990; **Med School:** Oregon Hlth & Sci Univ 1985; **Resid:** Neurology, Johns Hopkins Hosp 1989; **Fellow:** Epilepsy, Johns Hopkins Hosp 1991; **Fac Appt:** Assoc Prof N, Johns Hopkins Univ

Krumholz, Allan MD [N] - **Spec Exp:** Epilepsy/Seizure Disorders; Sleep Disorders/Apnea; **Hospital:** Univ of MD Med Ctr; **Address:** Univ Maryland Med System, Dept Neurology, 22 S Greene St, rm S12C09, Baltimore, MD 21201-1544; **Phone:** 410-328-6266; **Board Cert:** Neurology 1977; Clinical Neurophysiology 2006; **Med School:** Ros Franklin Univ/Chicago Med Sch 1970; **Resid:** Internal Medicine, Baltimore City Hosp 1972; Neurology, Johns Hopkins Hosp 1975; **Fellow:** Electroencephalography, Johns Hopkins Hosp 1980; **Fac Appt:** Prof N, Univ MD Sch Med

Kula, Roger W MD [N] - **Spec Exp:** Neuromuscular Disorders; Myasthenia Gravis; Syringomyelia & Spinal Cord Diseases; Chiari's Deformity; **Hospital:** N Shore Univ Hosp (page 67), Steven & Alexandra Cohen Chldn's Med Ctr of NY (page 67); **Address:** 611 Northern Blvd, Ste 150, Great Neck, NY 11021; **Phone:** 516-570-4425; **Board Cert:** Internal Medicine 1975; Neurology 1977; Neuromuscular Medicine 2008; **Med School:** Johns Hopkins Univ 1970; **Resid:** Internal Medicine, New York Hosp 1972; Neurology, UCSF Med Ctr 1974; **Fellow:** Neuromuscular Medicine, Natl Inst Hlth 1977; **Fac Appt:** Assoc Prof N, Hofstra N Shore-LIJ Sch Med

Kunschner, Lara MD [N] - **Spec Exp:** Neuro-Oncology; Brain Tumors; **Hospital:** Allegheny General Hosp; **Address:** Allegheny Neurological Assocs, 420 E North Ave, Ste 206, Pittsburgh, PA 15212; **Phone:** 412-359-8850; **Board Cert:** Neurology 1999; **Med School:** Univ Pittsburgh 1994; **Resid:** Neurology, Univ Michigan Hosps 1999; **Fellow:** Neuro-Oncology, MD Anderson Cancer Ctr 2000; **Fac Appt:** Assoc Prof N, Drexel Univ Coll Med

Kuzniecky, Ruben MD [N] - **Spec Exp:** Epilepsy/Seizure Disorders; MRI; Developmental Disorders; Brain Malformations; **Hospital:** NYU Langone Med Ctr (page 68); **Address:** 223 E 34th St Fl Ground, New York, NY 10016; **Phone:** 646-558-0806; **Board Cert:** Neurology 1990; **Med School:** Argentina 1980; **Resid:** Neurology, McGill Univ 1986; **Fellow:** Epilepsy, McGill Univ 1988; **Fac Appt:** Prof N, NYU Sch Med

Labar, Douglas R MD/PhD [N] - **Spec Exp:** Epilepsy/Seizure Disorders; **Hospital:** NY-Presby/Weill Cornell Med Ctr, NY (page 66); **Address:** Weill Cornell Epilepsy Center, 525 E 68th St, rm K-619, New York, NY 10065; **Phone:** 212-746-2359; **Board Cert:** Neurology 1987; **Med School:** Med Coll PA 1982; **Resid:** Neurology, Columbia Presby Med Ctr 1986; **Fellow:** Epilepsy, Columbia Presby Med Ctr 1988; **Fac Appt:** Prof N, Cornell Univ-Weill Med Coll

Lacomis, David MD [N] - **Spec Exp:** Amyotrophic Lateral Sclerosis (ALS); Muscle Disorders; Myasthenia Gravis; Neuromuscular Disorders; **Hospital:** UPMC Presby, Pittsburgh; **Address:** Dept Neurology-Kaufmann Med Bldg, 3471 Fifth Ave, Ste 810, Pittsburgh, PA 15213; **Phone:** 412-692-4917; **Board Cert:** Neurology 1992; Clinical Neurophysiology 2004; Neuromuscular Medicine 2009; **Med School:** Penn State Coll Med 1987; **Resid:** Neurology, Harvard Affil Hosp 1991; **Fellow:** Neuromuscular Disease, Univ Mass Med Ctr 1993; **Fac Appt:** Prof N, Univ Pittsburgh

Laterra, John J MD/PhD [N] - **Spec Exp:** Neuro-Oncology; Brain Tumors; **Hospital:** Johns Hopkins Hosp (page 61), Kennedy Krieger Inst; **Address:** Johns Hopkins Div Neurology, 600 N Wolfe St, Phipps 119, Baltimore, MD 21287; **Phone:** 410-614-3853; **Board Cert:** Neurology 1990; **Med School:** Case West Res Univ 1984; **Resid:** Neurology, Univ Mich Hosps 1988; **Fellow:** Research, Johns Hopkins Hosp 1989; **Fac Appt:** Prof N, Johns Hopkins Univ

Latov, Norman MD/PhD [N] - **Spec Exp:** Peripheral Neuropathy; Neuro-Immunology; **Hospital:** NY-Presby/Weill Cornell Med Ctr, NY (page 66); **Address:** 1305 York Ave Fl 2 - Ste 217, New York, NY 10021; **Phone:** 646-962-3320; **Board Cert:** Neurology 1989; **Med School:** Univ Pennsylvania 1975; **Resid:** Internal Medicine, Boston City Hosp 1976; Neurology, Columbia-Presby Med Ctr 1979; **Fellow:** Immunology, Columbia-Presby Med Ctr 1981; **Fac Appt:** Prof N, Cornell Univ-Weill Med Coll

Levine, David N MD [N] - **Spec Exp:** Dementia; Stroke; Spinal Cord Disorders; Syringomyelia & Spinal Cord Diseases; **Hospital:** NYU Langone Med Ctr (page 68); **Address:** 400 E 34th St, Ste RIRM-311, New York, NY 10016-4901; **Phone:** 212-263-7744; **Board Cert:** Neurology 1976; **Med School:** Harvard Med Sch 1968; **Resid:** Neurology, Mass Genl Hosp 1974; **Fellow:** Neurology, Mass Genl Hosp 1976; **Fac Appt:** Prof N, NYU Sch Med

Levine, Steven R MD [N] - **Spec Exp:** Stroke; Cerebrovascular Disease; **Hospital:** SUNY Downstate Med Ctr (Univ Hosp of Bklyn); **Address:** SUNY Downstate Medical Center, 470 Clarkson Ave, Box 1213, Brooklyn, NY 11203; **Phone:** 718-221-5188; **Board Cert:** Neurology 1986; Vascular Neurology 2005; **Med School:** Med Coll Wisc 1981; **Resid:** Neurology, Univ Mich Hosps 1985; **Fellow:** Cerebrovascular Disease, Henry Ford Hosp 1987; **Fac Appt:** Prof N, Mount Sinai Sch Med

Liporace, Joyce D MD [N] - **Spec Exp:** Epilepsy in Women; Women's Health; Epilepsy in Pregnancy; **Hospital:** Riddle Meml Hosp; **Address:** Center for Neuroscience, 1088 W Baltimore Pike, HCC II, Ste 2205, Media, PA 19063; **Phone:** 610-744-2960; **Board Cert:** Neurology 1993; **Med School:** Johns Hopkins Univ 1988; **Resid:** Neurology, Hosp Univ Penn 1992; **Fellow:** Clinical Neurophysiology, Graduate Hosp 1994; **Fac Appt:** Assoc Prof Med, Thomas Jefferson Univ

Lipton, Richard MD [N] - **Spec Exp:** Headache; Clinical Trials; **Hospital:** Montefiore Med Ctr-Einstein Campus, NY; **Address:** Montefiore Headache Ctr, 1575 Blondell Ave, Ste 225, Bronx, NY 10461-2662; **Phone:** 718-405-8360; **Board Cert:** Neurology 1985; **Med School:** Univ Chicago-Pritzker Sch Med 1980; **Resid:** Neurology, Montefiore Med Ctr 1984; **Fellow:** Neurological Physiology, Montefiore Med Ctr 1985; NeuroEpidemiology, Columbia Univ 1990; **Fac Appt:** Prof N, Albert Einstein Coll Med

Liu, Grant T MD [N] - **Spec Exp:** Pediatric Neuro-Ophthalmology; Neuro-Ophthalmology; **Hospital:** Hosp Univ Penn - UPHS (page 72), Chldns Hosp of Philadelphia; **Address:** Univ Penn, Dept Neurology, 3400 Spruce St, 3W Gates Bldg, Philadelphia, PA 19104; **Phone:** 215-349-8460; **Board Cert:** Neurology 1993; **Med School:** Columbia P&S 1988; **Resid:** Neurology, Harvard-Longwood Neuro Program 1992; **Fellow:** Neuro-Ophthalmology, Bascom Palmer Eye Inst 1993; **Fac Appt:** Prof N, Univ Pennsylvania

Logigian, Eric L MD [N] - **Spec Exp:** Neuromuscular Disorders; Electromyography; Lyme Disease; Peripheral Neuropathy; **Hospital:** Univ of Rochester Strong Meml Hosp, Highland Hosp of Rochester; **Address:** Univ Rochester, Dept of Neurology, 601 Elmwood Ave, Box 673, Rochester, NY 14642; **Phone:** 585-275-4568; **Board Cert:** Internal Medicine 1981; Neurology 1985; Clinical Neurophysiology 2009; **Med School:** Boston Univ 1978; **Resid:** Internal Medicine, Beth Israel Hosp 1981; Neurology, Mass Genl Hosp 1984; **Fellow:** Clinical Neurophysiology, Mass Genl Hosp 1985; **Fac Appt:** Prof N, Univ Rochester

Louis, Elan D MD [N] - **Spec Exp:** Tremor and Dystonia; Huntington's Disease; Parkinson's Disease/Movement Disorders; **Hospital:** NY-Presby/Columbia Univ Med Ctr, NY (page 66); **Address:** Neurological Inst of New York, 710 W 168th St, Ste 350, New York, NY 10032; **Phone:** 212-305-3665; **Board Cert:** Neurology 2004; **Med School:** Yale Univ 1989; **Resid:** Neurology, NY-Presby/Columbia Univ Med Ctr 1993; **Fellow:** Movement Disorders, Neurol Inst of New York 1995; Epidemiology, Neurol Inst of New York 1995; **Fac Appt:** Prof N, Columbia P&S

Lublin, Fred D MD [N] - **Spec Exp:** Multiple Sclerosis; **Hospital:** Mount Sinai Med Ctr (page 64); **Address:** Dickinson Ctr for Multiple Sclerosis, 5 E 98th St, Box 1138, New York, NY 10029-6574; **Phone:** 212-241-6854; **Board Cert:** Neurology 1977; **Med School:** Jefferson Med Coll 1972; **Resid:** Neurology, NY Hosp/Cornell Med Ctr 1976; **Fac Appt:** Prof N, Mount Sinai Sch Med

Marder, Karen S MD [N] - **Spec Exp:** Huntington's Disease; Alzheimer's Disease; Dementia; **Hospital:** NY-Presby/Columbia Univ Med Ctr, NY (page 66); **Address:** Neurological Institute, 710 W 168th St, Ste 104, New York, NY 10032-2603; **Phone:** 212-305-6939; **Board Cert:** Neurology 1989; **Med School:** Cornell Univ-Weill Med Coll 1983; **Resid:** Neurology, Columbia Presby Med Ctr 1987; **Fellow:** Behavioral Neurology, Columbia Presby Med Ctr 1989; **Fac Appt:** Assoc Prof N, Columbia P&S

Mayeux, Richard MD [N] - **Spec Exp:** Alzheimer's Disease; Dementia; **Hospital:** NY-Presby/Columbia Univ Med Ctr, NY (page 66); **Address:** 630 W 168th St, PH 19, New York, NY 10032; **Phone:** 212-305-6939; **Board Cert:** Neurology 1978; **Med School:** Univ Okla Coll Med 1972; **Resid:** Internal Medicine, Boston City Hosp 1974; Neurology, Columbia Presby Med Ctr 1977; **Fellow:** Neurology, Boston Univ 1978; **Fac Appt:** Prof N, Columbia P&S

McArthur, Justin C MD [N] - **Spec Exp:** AIDS/HIV; Multiple Sclerosis; **Hospital:** Johns Hopkins Hosp (page 61); **Address:** Johns Hopkins Hosp, Dept Neurology, 600 N Wolfe St, Meyer 6-113, Baltimore, MD 21287; **Phone:** 410-955-3730; **Board Cert:** Internal Medicine 1984; Neurology 1986; **Med School:** England, UK 1979; **Resid:** Internal Medicine, Johns Hopkins Hosp 1982; Neurology, Johns Hopkins Hosp 1985; **Fac Appt:** Prof N, Johns Hopkins Univ

McCluskey, Leo MD [N] - **Spec Exp:** Amyotrophic Lateral Sclerosis (ALS); **Hospital:** Pennsylvania Hosp-UPHS (page 72); **Address:** 330 S 9th St, Philadelphia, PA 19107; **Phone:** 215-829-3053; **Board Cert:** Neurology 1986; **Med School:** Columbia P&S 1980; **Resid:** Internal Medicine, Univ Mich 1982; Neurology, Hosp Univ Penn 1985; **Fellow:** Neuromuscular Disease, Hosp Univ Penn 1986; **Fac Appt:** Assoc Prof N, Univ Pennsylvania

Miller, Aaron E MD [N] - **Spec Exp:** Multiple Sclerosis; Autoimmune Disease; Optic Nerve Disorders; **Hospital:** Mount Sinai Med Ctr (page 64), Maimonides Med Ctr (page 63); **Address:** 5 E 98th St, Fl 1st, Box 1138, New York, NY 10029; **Phone:** 212-241-6854; **Board Cert:** Internal Medicine 1972; Neurology 1977; **Med School:** NYU Sch Med 1968; **Resid:** Internal Medicine, Jacobi Med Ctr 1970; Neurology, Montefiore Med Ctr 1975; **Fellow:** Neurovirology, Johns Hopkins Hosp 1977; **Fac Appt:** Prof N, Mount Sinai Sch Med

Mitsumoto, Hiroshi MD [N] - **Spec Exp:** Amyotrophic Lateral Sclerosis (ALS); Neuromuscular Disorders; Clinical Trials; **Hospital:** NY-Presby/Columbia Univ Med Ctr, NY (page 66); **Address:** Neurological Institute, 710 W 168th St Fl 9, New York, NY 10032; **Phone:** 212-305-1319; **Board Cert:** Neurology 1978; **Med School:** Japan 1968; **Resid:** Internal Medicine, Toho Univ Hosps 1972; Neurology, Univ Hosps 1976; **Fellow:** Neurological Pathology, Cleveland Clinic 1978; Neuromuscular Medicine, New England Med Ctr 1981; **Fac Appt:** Prof N, Columbia P&S

Mohr, JP MD [N] - **Spec Exp:** Stroke; Arteriovenous Malformations; Aphasia; MoyaMoya Disease; **Hospital:** NY-Presby/Columbia Univ Med Ctr, NY (page 66); **Address:** 710 W 168th St, Fl 6, rm 616, New York, NY 10032-2603; **Phone:** 212-305-8033; **Board Cert:** Neurology 1971; Vascular Neurology 2005; **Med School:** Univ VA Sch Med 1963; **Resid:** Neurology, Columbia Presby Med Ctr 1966; Neurology, Mass Genl Hosp 1968; **Fellow:** Neurology, Mass Genl Hosp 1969; **Fac Appt:** Prof N, Columbia P&S

Newman, Lawrence C MD [N] - **Spec Exp:** Headache; Pain-Facial; **Hospital:** St. Luke's - Roosevelt Hosp Ctr - Roosevelt Div (page 56); **Address:** St Luke's-Roosevelt Hosp-Headache Inst, 425 W 59th St Fl 4 - Ste A, New York, NY 10019; **Phone:** 212-523-5869; **Board Cert:** Neurology 2005; Headache Medicine 2006; **Med School:** Mexico 1983; **Resid:** Internal Medicine, Elmhurst Hosp 1986; Neurology, Montefiore Med Ctr 1989; **Fellow:** Headache, Montefiore Med Ctr 1990; **Fac Appt:** Prof N, Albert Einstein Coll Med

Olanow, C Warren MD [N] - **Spec Exp:** Parkinson's Disease; Movement Disorders; **Hospital:** Mount Sinai Med Ctr (page 64); **Address:** 5 E 98 St, New York, NY 10029; **Phone:** 212-241-8435; **Med School:** Univ Toronto 1965; **Resid:** Neurology, Toronto Genl Hosp 1968; Neurology, Columbia Presby Hosp 1970; **Fellow:** Neurological Anatomy, Columbia Presby Hosp 1971; **Fac Appt:** Prof N, Mount Sinai Sch Med

Pedley, Timothy A MD [N] - **Spec Exp:** Epilepsy/Seizure Disorders; **Hospital:** NY-Presby/Columbia Univ Med Ctr, NY (page 66); **Address:** The Neurological Inst of New York, 710 W 168th St, New York, NY 10032; **Phone:** 212-305-6489; **Board Cert:** Neurology 1975; **Med School:** Yale Univ 1969; **Resid:** Neurology, Stanford Univ Hosp 1973; **Fellow:** Clinical Neurophysiology, Stanford Univ Hosp 1974; Epilepsy, Stanford Univ Hosp 1975; **Fac Appt:** Prof N, Columbia P&S

Petito, Frank A MD [N] - **Spec Exp:** Multiple Sclerosis; Headache; Lyme Disease; **Hospital:** NY-Presby/Weill Cornell Med Ctr, NY (page 66); **Address:** 525 E 68th St, Ste 607, New York, NY 10065; **Phone:** 212-746-2309; **Board Cert:** Neurology 1974; **Med School:** Columbia P&S 1967; **Resid:** Neurology, New York Hosp 1971; **Fac Appt:** Prof N, Cornell Univ-Weill Med Coll

Posner, Jerome B MD [N] - **Spec Exp:** Neuro-Oncology; Brain Tumors; Paraneoplastic Syndromes; **Hospital:** Meml Sloan-Kettering Cancer Ctr; **Address:** 1275 York Ave, rm C731, New York, NY 10065; **Phone:** 212-639-7047; **Board Cert:** Neurology 1962; **Med School:** Univ Wash 1955; **Resid:** Neurology, Univ WA Affil Hosp 1959; **Fellow:** Biochemistry, Univ WA Affil Hosp 1963; **Fac Appt:** Prof N, Cornell Univ-Weill Med Coll

Pula, Thaddeus MD [N] - **Spec Exp:** Neurophysiology; Electromyography; **Hospital:** Maryland Genl Hosp; **Address:** Maryland Genl Hosp, Div Neurology, 827 Linden Ave Fl 2, Baltimore, MD 21201-4606; **Phone:** 410-225-8290; **Board Cert:** Neurology 1981; **Med School:** Univ MD Sch Med 1976; **Resid:** Internal Medicine, Mercy Hosp Med Ctr; **Fellow:** Neurology, Univ Maryland

Reich, Stephen G MD [N] - **Spec Exp:** Movement Disorders; Parkinson's Disease; Ataxia; Dystonia-Botox Therapy; **Hospital:** Univ of MD Med Ctr; **Address:** Univ Maryland Med System, Frenkil Bldg, 16 S Eutaw St Fl 3, Baltimore, MD 21201; **Phone:** 410-328-5858; **Board Cert:** Neurology 1989; **Med School:** Tulane Univ 1983; **Resid:** Neurology, Case West Res Univ Hosp 1987; **Fellow:** Movement Disorders, Johns Hopkins Hosp 1988; **Fac Appt:** Assoc Prof N, Univ MD Sch Med

Relkin, Norman R MD/PhD [N] - **Spec Exp:** Alzheimer's Disease; Dementia; Memory Disorders; **Hospital:** NY-Presby/Weill Cornell Med Ctr, NY (page 66); **Address:** Weill Cornell Memory Disorders Program, 428 E 72nd St, Ste 500, New York, NY 10021; **Phone:** 212-746-2441; **Board Cert:** Neurology 1992; **Med School:** Albert Einstein Coll Med 1987; **Resid:** Neurology, New York Hosp 1991; **Fellow:** Behavioral Neurology, New York Hosp-Cornell 1992; **Fac Appt:** Asst Prof N, Cornell Univ-Weill Med Coll

Sage, Jacob MD [N] - **Spec Exp:** Parkinson's Disease; **Hospital:** Robert Wood Johnson Univ Hosp - New Brunswick; **Address:** UMDNJ, Dept Neurology, 125 Paterson St Fl 6 - Ste 6100, New Brunswick, NJ 08901-2160; **Phone:** 732-235-7733; **Board Cert:** Neurology 1979; **Med School:** Univ Pittsburgh 1972; **Resid:** Neurology, Univ Pittsburgh Hosps 1978; **Fellow:** Neurological Chemistry, NY Hosp-Cornell 1980; **Fac Appt:** Prof N, UMDNJ-RW Johnson Med Sch

Schwartzman, Robert J MD [N] - **Spec Exp:** Reflex Sympathetic Dystrophy (RSD); Pain Management; **Hospital:** Hahnemann Univ Hosp; **Address:** Drexel Neurological Assocs, 219 N Broad St Fl 7, Philadelphia, PA 19107; **Phone:** 215-762-6915; **Board Cert:** Internal Medicine 1971; Neurology 1974; **Med School:** Univ Pennsylvania 1965; **Resid:** Internal Medicine, Duke Univ Hosp 1967; Neurology, Hosp Univ Penn 1969; **Fellow:** Neurology, NIH-Med Neur Br 1971; **Fac Appt:** Prof N, Drexel Univ Coll Med

Shefner, Jeremy M MD/PhD [N] - **Spec Exp:** Amyotrophic Lateral Sclerosis (ALS); Neuromuscular Disorders; **Hospital:** SUNY Upstate Med Univ Shos; **Address:** 90 Presidential Plaza, Syracuse, NY 13202; **Phone:** 315-464-4243; **Board Cert:** Neurology 1989; Clinical Neurophysiology 2004; **Med School:** Northwestern Univ 1983; **Resid:** Neurology, Harvard-Longwood Neur Trng 1988; **Fellow:** Neuromuscular Disease, Brigham & Womens Hosp 1990; **Fac Appt:** Prof N, SUNY Upstate Med Univ

Shulman, Lisa M MD [N] - **Spec Exp:** Movement Disorders; Movement Disorders-Botox Therapy; Parkinson's Disease; **Hospital:** Univ of MD Med Ctr; **Address:** 110 S Paca St Fl 3, Baltimore, MD 21201; **Phone:** 410-328-2164; **Board Cert:** Neurology 1994; **Med School:** Univ Miami Sch Med 1988; **Resid:** Neurology, Jackson Meml Hosp 1992; **Fellow:** Movement Disorders, Jackson Meml Hosp 1994; **Fac Appt:** Assoc Prof N, Univ MD Sch Med

Silberstein, Stephen D MD [N] - **Spec Exp:** Headache; Migraine; **Hospital:** Thomas Jefferson Univ Hosp; **Address:** Jefferson Headache Center, 111 S 11th St, Gibbon Bldg, Ste 8130, Philadelphia, PA 19107; **Phone:** 215-955-2243; **Board Cert:** Neurology 1975; Headache Medicine 2006; **Med School:** Univ Pennsylvania 1967; **Resid:** Internal Medicine, Hosp Univ Penn 1969; Neurology, Hosp Univ Penn 1975; **Fac Appt:** Clin Prof N, Temple Univ

Simpson, David M MD [N] - **Spec Exp:** Infections-CNS; AIDS-Neurologic Complications; Peripheral Neuropathy; Neuromuscular Disorders; **Hospital:** Mount Sinai Med Ctr (page 64); **Address:** Mt Sinai Med Ctr, Dept Neurology, 1 Gustave L Levy Pl, Box 1052, Annenberg, 2nd Flr, New York, NY 10029; **Phone:** 212-241-8748; **Board Cert:** Neurology 1984; Clinical Neurophysiology 2005; Neuromuscular Medicine 2008; **Med School:** SUNY Buffalo 1979; **Resid:** Neurology, NY Hosp-Cornell Med Ctr 1983; **Fellow:** Clinical Neurophysiology, Mass Genl Hosp 1984; **Fac Appt:** Prof N, Mount Sinai Sch Med

Neurology

Sirdofsky, Michael D MD [N] - **Spec Exp:** Neuromuscular Disorders; Electrodiagnosis; **Hospital:** Georgetown Univ Hosp; **Address:** Pasquerilla Health Care Bldg, Entrance 1, Fl 7, 3800 Resevoir Rd NW, Washington, DC 20007; **Phone:** 202-444-8525; **Board Cert:** Neurology 1981; **Med School:** Georgetown Univ 1976; **Resid:** Neurology, Georgetown Univ Hosp 1980; **Fac Appt:** Clin Prof N, Georgetown Univ

Sperling, Michael R MD [N] - **Spec Exp:** Epilepsy; **Hospital:** Thomas Jefferson Univ Hosp; **Address:** Thomas Jefferson Univ Hosp, Dept Neurology, 900 Walnut St, Ste 200, Philadelphia, PA 19107; **Phone:** 215-955-1222; **Board Cert:** Neurology 1984; Clinical Neurophysiology 2009; **Med School:** Temple Univ 1978; **Resid:** Neurology, Mt Sinai Hosp 1982; **Fellow:** Epilepsy, UCLA Med Ctr 1984; **Fac Appt:** Prof N, Thomas Jefferson Univ

Stern, Matthew B MD [N] - **Spec Exp:** Parkinson's Disease; Movement Disorders; Botox Therapy; **Hospital:** Pennsylvania Hosp-UPHS (page 72), Hosp Univ Penn - UPHS (page 72); **Address:** Pennsylvania Hosp, Dept Neurology, 330 S 9th St Fl 3, Philadelphia, PA 19107; **Phone:** 215-829-6500; **Board Cert:** Neurology 1983; **Med School:** Duke Univ 1978; **Resid:** Neurology, Hosp Univ Penn 1982; **Fac Appt:** Prof N, Univ Pennsylvania

Swerdlow, Michael L MD [N] - **Spec Exp:** Myasthenia Gravis; Spinal Disorders; Multiple Sclerosis; **Hospital:** Montefiore Med Ctr-Moses Campus, NY; **Address:** 3400 Bainbridge Ave, Bronx, NY 10467-2401; **Phone:** 718-920-4178; **Board Cert:** Neurology 1975; **Med School:** Univ Pennsylvania 1967; **Resid:** Internal Medicine, Mount Sinai Hosp 1969; Neurology, Montefiore Med Ctr 1972; **Fellow:** Neurology, Natl Inst Hlth 1974; **Fac Appt:** Prof N, Albert Einstein Coll Med

Tayal, Ashis H MD [N] - **Spec Exp:** Stroke; Vascular Neurology; **Hospital:** Allegheny General Hosp; **Address:** Allegheny Neurology Assocs, 490 E North Ave, Ste 500, Professional Bldg, Pittsburgh, PA 15212; **Phone:** 412-359-8870; **Board Cert:** Internal Medicine 2007; Neurology 2006; Vascular Neurology 2008; **Med School:** Tufts Univ 1994; **Resid:** Internal Medicine, Mount Sinai Med Ctr 1997; Neurology, Univ Pittsburgh Med Ctr 2001; **Fellow:** Vascular Neurology, Univ Pittsburgh Med Ctr 2006

Vas, George A MD [N] - **Spec Exp:** Stroke; Multiple Sclerosis; **Hospital:** SUNY Downstate Med Ctr (Univ Hosp of Bklyn), Kings County Hosp Ctr; **Address:** 450 Clarkson Ave N, Ste A, Brooklyn, NY 11203-2056; **Phone:** 718-270-2502; **Board Cert:** Internal Medicine 1973; Neurology 1977; Clinical Neurophysiology 2002; **Med School:** Univ Pittsburgh 1970; **Resid:** Internal Medicine, New York Hosp 1972; Neurology, New York Hosp 1975; **Fac Appt:** Prof N, SUNY Downstate

Waters, Cheryl H MD [N] - **Spec Exp:** Parkinson's Disease; Movement Disorders; **Hospital:** NY-Presby/Columbia Univ Med Ctr, NY (page 66); **Address:** 710 W 168th St Fl 3, New York, NY 10032; **Phone:** 212-305-3665; **Board Cert:** Neurology 1986; **Med School:** Univ Toronto 1980; **Resid:** Internal Medicine, Univ Toronto Med Ctr 1982; Neurology, Univ Toronto Med Ctr 1985; **Fellow:** Clinical Pharmacology, Univ Toronto Med Ctr 1987; **Fac Appt:** Prof N, Columbia P&S

Wechsler, Lawrence R MD [N] - **Spec Exp:** Cerebrovascular Disease; Stroke; **Hospital:** UPMC Presby, Pittsburgh, UPMC Shadyside; **Address:** UPMC Stroke Institute, 3471 Fifth Ave, Ste 810, Pittsburgh, PA 15213; **Phone:** 412-692-4920; **Board Cert:** Internal Medicine 1983; Neurology 1984; Vascular Neurology 2005; **Med School:** Univ Pennsylvania 1978; **Resid:** Internal Medicine, Presby-Univ Hosp 1980; Neurology, Mass Genl Hosp 1983; **Fellow:** Clinical Neurophysiology, Mass Genl Hosp 1984; Cerebrovascular Disease, Mass Genl Hosp 1985; **Fac Appt:** Prof N, Univ Pittsburgh

Weinberg, Harold J MD [N] - **Spec Exp:** Headache; Spinal Disorders; Neuromuscular Disorders; Memory Disorders; **Hospital:** NYU Langone Med Ctr (page 68); **Address:** 650 1st Ave, Fl 4, New York, NY 10016-3240; **Phone:** 212-213-9339; **Board Cert:** Neurology 1983; Electrodiagnostic Medicine 1989; **Med School:** Albert Einstein Coll Med 1978; **Resid:** Neurology, Columbia-Presby Med Ctr 1982; **Fellow:** Neuromuscular Medicine, Columbia-Presby Med Ctr 1982; **Fac Appt:** Clin Prof N, NYU Sch Med

Weiner, William J MD [N] - **Spec Exp:** Movement Disorders; Parkinson's Disease; Huntington's Disease; Progressive Supranuclear Palsy (PSP); **Hospital:** Univ of MD Med Ctr; **Address:** 110 S Paca St Fl 3 - rm 3S124, Baltimore, MD 21201; **Phone:** 410-328-2172; **Board Cert:** Neurology 1975; **Med School:** Univ IL Coll Med 1969; **Resid:** Neurology, Univ Minn 1971; Neurology, Rush-Presby Med Ctr 1973; **Fac Appt:** Prof N, Univ MD Sch Med

Wityk, Robert J MD [N] - **Spec Exp:** Stroke; Cerebrovascular Disease; **Hospital:** Johns Hopkins Hosp (page 61); **Address:** Johns Hopkins Outpatient Ctr, 601 N Caroline St, Ste 5073A, Baltimore, MD 21287; **Phone:** 410-955-2228; **Board Cert:** Internal Medicine 1988; Neurology 1992; **Med School:** Case West Res Univ 1985; **Resid:** Internal Medicine, UCSD Med Ctr 1988; Neurology, Mass Genl Hosp 1991; **Fellow:** Cardiovascular Disease, Tufts U-New Eng MC 1992; **Fac Appt:** Assoc Prof N, Johns Hopkins Univ

Zimmerman, Earl A MD [N] - **Spec Exp:** Memory Disorders; Alzheimer's Disease; Dementia; **Hospital:** Albany Med Ctr; **Address:** Albany Med Ctr-Neurology, 43 New Scotland Ave, MC 65, Albany, NY 12208; **Phone:** 518-262-0800; **Board Cert:** Neurology 1970; Internal Medicine 1970; **Med School:** Univ Pennsylvania 1963; **Resid:** Internal Medicine, Presbyterian Hosp 1965; Neurology, Neurological Inst 1968; **Fellow:** Endocrinology, Presbyterian Hosp 1972; **Fac Appt:** Prof N, Albany Med Coll

Southeast

Abou-Khalil, Bassel MD [N] - **Spec Exp:** Epilepsy; Neurophysiology; **Hospital:** Vanderbilt Univ Med Ctr (page 75); **Address:** Vanderbilt Univ-Dept Neurology, 2220 Pierce Ave, Ste B1053, Nashville, TN 37232-2551; **Phone:** 615-936-0060; **Board Cert:** Neurology 1986; Clinical Neurophysiology 2002; **Med School:** Amer Univ Beirut 1978; **Resid:** Neurology, Strong Meml Hosp/Univ Rochester 1980; Neurology, Univ Mich Hosps 1982; **Fellow:** Epilepsy, Univ Mich Hosps 1985; Electroencephalography, Univ Mich Hosps 1985; **Fac Appt:** Prof N, Vanderbilt Univ

Adams, David J MD [N] - **Spec Exp:** Diagnostic Problems; Hydrocephalus-normal pressure; Pseudotumor Cerebri; Autoimmune Disease; **Hospital:** Univ of Miami Hosp, Jackson Meml Hosp; **Address:** Univ Miami Dept Neurology, 1150 NW 14th St, Ste 609, Miami, FL 33136; **Phone:** 305-243-1691; **Board Cert:** Neurology 1977; **Med School:** Columbia P&S 1969; **Resid:** Neurology, Neurological Inst 1975; **Fac Appt:** Clin Prof N, Univ Miami Sch Med

Adams, Robert Joseph MD [N] - **Spec Exp:** Stroke; **Hospital:** MUSC Med Ctr; **Address:** MUSC Stroke Center, 19 Hagood Ave, Ste 501, Charleston, SC 29425; **Phone:** 843-792-7058; **Board Cert:** Neurology 1987; Vascular Neurology 2008; **Med School:** Univ Ark 1980; **Resid:** Neurology, Med Coll Georgia 1985; **Fac Appt:** Assoc Prof N, Med Coll GA

Alexandrov, Andrei V MD [N] - **Spec Exp:** Stroke; Cerebrovascular Disease; **Hospital:** Univ of Ala Hosp at Birmingham; **Address:** 1813 6 Ave S RWUH Bldg - Ste M226, Birmingham, AL 35249; **Phone:** 205-924-2401; **Med School:** Russia 1989; **Resid:** Neurology, Inst of Neurology, Russian Acad Med Sciences 1991; **Fellow:** Vascular Neurology, Buffalo Genl Hosp 1995; Vascular Neurology, Univ Texas Affil Hosp 2004; **Fac Appt:** Prof N, Univ Alabama

Ashizawa, Tetsuo MD [N] - **Spec Exp:** Movement Disorders; Myasthenia Gravis; Parkinson's Disease; Huntington's Disease; **Hospital:** Shands at Univ of FL; **Address:** 1600 SW Archer Rd, Box 100236, Gainesville, FL 32610; **Phone:** 352-265-8408; **Board Cert:** Neurology 1980; **Med School:** Japan 1973; **Resid:** Neurology, Baylor Coll of Med Affil Hosp 1978; **Fellow:** Neuromuscular Disease, Baylor Coll of Med Affil Hosp 1978; **Fac Appt:** Prof N, Univ Fla Coll Med

Bebin, E Martina MD [N] - **Spec Exp:** Epilepsy; Child Neurology; Tuberous Sclerosis; **Hospital:** Univ of Ala Hosp at Birmingham; **Address:** 1719 6th Ave S, Birmingham, AL 35294; **Phone:** 205-801-8986; **Board Cert:** Child Neurology 2003; **Med School:** Univ Miss 1986; **Resid:** Neurology, Mayo Clnic 1991; **Fac Appt:** Assoc Prof N, Univ Alabama

Berger, Joseph R MD [N] - **Spec Exp:** Multiple Sclerosis; AIDS/HIV; Infectious & Demyelinating Diseases; **Hospital:** Univ of Kentucky Albert B. Chandler Hosp; **Address:** Kentucky Neuroscience Clinic, 740 S Limestone St, Lexington, KY 40536; **Phone:** 859-323-5661; **Board Cert:** Internal Medicine 1977; Neurology 1983; **Med School:** Jefferson Med Coll 1974; **Resid:** Internal Medicine, Georgetown Univ Hosp 1977; Neurology, Jackson Meml Hosp 1981; **Fac Appt:** Prof N, Univ KY Coll Med

Bertorini, Tulio E MD [N] - **Spec Exp:** Clinical Neurophysiology; Neuromuscular Disorders; Electromyography; **Hospital:** Methodist Univ Hosp - Memphis; **Address:** 1211 Union Ave, Ste 400, Memphis, TN 38104; **Phone:** 901-725-8920; **Board Cert:** Neurology 1977; Clinical Neurophysiology 2011; **Med School:** Peru 1970; **Resid:** Neurology, Georgetown Univ Med Ctr 1973; Neurology, VA Hosp/Armed Forces Inst Path 1974; **Fellow:** Electrodiagnosis, Mass Genl Hosp 1975; Clinical Neurophysiology, Natl Inst Neuro Comm Dis & Stroke/NIH 1977; **Fac Appt:** Prof N, Univ Tenn Coll Med

Brooks, Benjamin R MD [N] - **Spec Exp:** Neuromuscular Disorders; Multiple Sclerosis; Neurotoxicology; **Hospital:** Carolinas Med Ctr, Levine Chldns Hosp; **Address:** CMC Dept Neurology, 1010 Edgehill Rd N, Charlotte, NC 28207-1885; **Phone:** 704-446-1900; **Board Cert:** Internal Medicine 1974; Neurology 1978; **Med School:** Harvard Med Sch 1970; **Resid:** Neurology, Mass Genl Hosp 1974; Neurology, Natl Inst Neuro Disorders & Stroke-NIH 1976; **Fellow:** Neurovirology, Johns Hopkins Hosp 1978

Corbett, James MD [N] - **Spec Exp:** Neuro-Ophthalmology; Pseudotumor Cerebri; Neurosarcoidosis; Headache; **Hospital:** Univ Mississippi Med Ctr; **Address:** Univ Mississippi Med Ctr, Dept Neurology, 2500 N State St, Jackson, MS 39216-4505; **Phone:** 601-984-5501; **Board Cert:** Neurology 2004; **Med School:** Ros Franklin Univ/Chicago Med Sch 1966; **Resid:** Internal Medicine, Rhode Island Hosp 1968; Neurology, Univ Hosp-Case Western Reserve 1971; **Fac Appt:** Prof N, Univ Miss

DeKosky, Steven T MD [N] - **Spec Exp:** Alzheimer's Disease; Dementia; Behavioral Neurology; Geriatric Neurology; **Hospital:** Univ of Virginia Health Sys; **Address:** Univ Virgina School of Med, Box 800973, Charlottesville, VA 22908; **Phone:** 434-924-5118; **Board Cert:** Neurology 2004; **Med School:** Univ Fla Coll Med 1974; **Resid:** Internal Medicine, Johns Hopkins Hosp 1975; Neurology, Univ Florida 1978; **Fellow:** Neurological Chemistry, Univ Virginia Hosp 1979; **Fac Appt:** Prof N, Univ VA Sch Med

DeLong, Mahlon R MD [N] - **Spec Exp:** Parkinson's Disease; Movement Disorders; **Hospital:** Emory Univ Hosp, Wesley Woods Ger Hosp; **Address:** Wesley Woods Health Ctr, 1841 Clifton Rd NE Fl 3, Atlanta, GA 30329; **Phone:** 404-778-3444; **Board Cert:** Neurology 1980; **Med School:** Harvard Med Sch 1966; **Resid:** Internal Medicine, Boston City Hosp 1968; Neurology, Johns Hopkins Hosp 1976; **Fellow:** Neurology, NIMH 1971; **Fac Appt:** Prof N, Emory Univ

Finkel, Alan G MD [N] - **Spec Exp:** Headache; Pain-Facial; Migraine; **Hospital:** NC Memorial Hosp - UNC; **Address:** Carolina Headache Inst, 103 Market St, Chapel Hill, NC 27516; **Phone:** 919-942-4424; **Board Cert:** Neurology 1991; Pain Medicine 2003; Headache Medicine 2006; **Med School:** SUNY Buffalo 1985; **Resid:** Neurology, NC Meml Hosp 1989; **Fellow:** Pain & Headache Medicine, Univ NC Hosp; **Fac Appt:** Prof N, Univ NC Sch Med

Finkel, Michael F MD [N] - **Spec Exp:** Movement Disorders-Lower Limb; ADD/ADHD; Headache in Women; Trauma Neurology; **Hospital:** Physicians Regl Hlthcare Med Ctr-Pine Ridge; **Address:** Physicians Regl Med Grp, 6101 Pine Ridge Rd, Naples, FL 34119; **Phone:** 239-348-4093; **Board Cert:** Neurology 1979; **Med School:** Washington Univ, St Louis 1973; **Resid:** Neurology, Strong Meml Hosp 1977

Glass, Jonathan D MD [N] - **Spec Exp:** Neuro-Pathology; Amyotrophic Lateral Sclerosis (ALS); Peripheral Neuropathy; Neuromuscular Disorders; **Hospital:** Emory Univ Hosp, Grady Hlth Sys; **Address:** The Emory Clinic, 1365B Clifton Rd NE, Ste 2200, Atlanta, GA 30322; **Phone:** 404-778-3444; **Board Cert:** Neurology 1990; Neuropathology 1997; **Med School:** Univ VT Coll Med 1985; **Resid:** Neurology, Johns Hopkins Hosp 1989; **Fellow:** Neuropathology, Johns Hopkins Univ 1991; **Fac Appt:** Prof N, Emory Univ

Goldstein, Larry B MD [N] - **Spec Exp:** Stroke; Carotid Artery Disease; **Hospital:** Duke Univ Hosp, Durham VA Med Ctr; **Address:** DUMC, Box 3651, Durham, NC 27710; **Phone:** 919-684-3801; **Board Cert:** Neurology 1987; Vascular Neurology 2005; **Med School:** Mount Sinai Sch Med 1981; **Resid:** Neurology, Mt Sinai Hosp 1985; **Fellow:** Cerebrovascular Disease, Duke Univ Med Ctr 1986; **Fac Appt:** Prof N, Duke Univ

Gress, Daryl Ray MD [N] - **Spec Exp:** Critical Care; Stroke; **Hospital:** Univ of Virginia Health Sys; **Address:** Univ of VA Health Sys, Dept Neurology, Box 800394, Charlottesville, VA 22908; **Phone:** 434-924-8371; **Board Cert:** Neurology 1989; **Med School:** Washington Univ, St Louis 1982; **Resid:** Internal Medicine, Johns Hopkins Hosp 1984; Neurology, Mass Genl Hosp 1987; **Fellow:** Stroke, Mass Genl Hosp 1988

Haley Jr, Elliott C MD [N] - **Spec Exp:** Stroke; **Hospital:** Univ of Virginia Health Sys; **Address:** Univ VA Hlth Sys, Dept Neurology, Box 800394, Charlottesville, VA 22908; **Phone:** 434-982-6952; **Board Cert:** Internal Medicine 1978; Neurology 1985; Vascular Neurology 2008; **Med School:** Tulane Univ 1974; **Resid:** Internal Medicine, Univ Va Hosp 1978; Neurology, Univ Va Hosp 1982; **Fellow:** Cerebrovascular Disease, Mass Genl Hosp 1984; **Fac Appt:** Prof N, Univ VA Sch Med

Hauser, Robert A MD [N] - **Spec Exp:** Movement Disorders; Parkinson's Disease; **Hospital:** Tampa Genl Hosp; **Address:** Parkinson's Disease/Movement Disorders Ctr, 4001 E Fletcher Ave, 6th Fl, Tampa, FL 33613; **Phone:** 813-396-0751; **Board Cert:** Neurology 1989; **Med School:** Temple Univ 1982; **Resid:** Neurological Surgery, Eastern VA Med Ctr 1985; Neurology, Eastern VA Med Ctr 1988; **Fellow:** Movement Disorders, Univ S Florida Affil Hosp 1990; **Fac Appt:** Prof N, Univ S Fla Coll Med

Heilman, Kenneth M MD [N] - **Spec Exp:** Behavioral Neurology; Memory Disorders; Aphasia; Speech Disorders; **Hospital:** Shands at Univ of FL, Malcolm Randall VA Med Ctr; **Address:** 1600 SW Archer Rd, Box 100236, Gainesville, FL 32610-0236; **Phone:** 352-273-5550; **Board Cert:** Neurology 1973; **Med School:** Univ VA Sch Med 1963; **Resid:** Internal Medicine, Bellevue Hosp Ctr 1965; Neurology, Boston City Hosp 1970; **Fac Appt:** Prof N, Univ Fla Coll Med

Hess, David C MD [N] - **Spec Exp:** Stroke; Antiphospholipid Syndrome (APS); **Hospital:** Med Coll of GA Hosp and Clin (MCG Health Inc); **Address:** Med Coll Ga Dept Neurology, 1120 15th St, rm BI-3080, Augusta, GA 30912; **Phone:** 706-721-1691; **Board Cert:** Internal Medicine 1986; Neurology 1990; Vascular Surgery 2008; **Med School:** Univ MD Sch Med 1983; **Resid:** Internal Medicine, Allegheny Genl Hosp 1985; Neurology, Med Coll Ga 1989; **Fellow:** Cerebrovascular Disease, Med Coll Ga 1990; **Fac Appt:** Prof N, Med Coll GA

Janss, Anna J MD/PhD [N] - **Spec Exp:** Brain Tumors-Pediatric; Clinical Trials; Cancer Survivors-Late Effects of Therapy; **Hospital:** Chldns Hlthcare Atlanta @ Egleston, Chldns Hlthcare Atlanta @ Scottish Rite; **Address:** Aflac Cancer & Blood Disorders Ctr, 1405 Clifton Rd NE, Outpatient Clinic, Tower 1 Fl 4, Atlanta, GA 30322; **Phone:** 404-785-1200; **Board Cert:** Neurology 1993; **Med School:** Univ Iowa Coll Med 1988; **Resid:** Neurology, Hosp Univ Penn 1992; **Fellow:** Pediatric Neuro-Oncology, Chldns Hosp 1996; **Fac Appt:** Assoc Prof N, Emory Univ

Kirshner, Howard S MD [N] - **Spec Exp:** Stroke; Aphasia; Neuro-Rehabilitation; Behavioral Neurology; **Hospital:** Vanderbilt Univ Med Ctr (page 75), Vanderbilt Stallworth Rehab Hosp (page 75); **Address:** Vanderbilt Clinic, 1301 Medical Center Drive, Ste 3930, Nashville, TN 37232-2551; **Phone:** 615-936-1354; **Board Cert:** Neurology 1980; Vascular Neurology 2005; **Med School:** Harvard Med Sch 1972; **Resid:** Neurology, Mass Genl Hosp 1978; **Fellow:** Neurological Science, Natl Inst Hlth 1975; **Fac Appt:** Prof N, Vanderbilt Univ

Kurtzke, Robert N MD [N] - **Spec Exp:** Electromyography; Neuromuscular Disorders; **Hospital:** Inova Fairfax Hosp, Reston Hosp Ctr; **Address:** Neurology Ctr of Fairfax, 3020 Hamaker Ct, Ste 400, Fairfax, VA 22031-2220; **Phone:** 703-876-0800; **Board Cert:** Neurology 1990; Clinical Neurophysiology 2004; **Med School:** Georgetown Univ 1985; **Resid:** Neurology, Neurology Inst-Columbia Presby 1989; **Fellow:** Neuromuscular Disease, Duke Univ Med Ctr 1990

Lavin, Patrick J MD [N] - **Spec Exp:** Neuro-Ophthalmology; Eye Movement Disorders; Headache; Neuro-Otology; **Hospital:** Vanderbilt Univ Med Ctr (page 75); **Address:** Vanderbilt Univ Eye Institute, 2311 Pierce Ave, Nashville, TN 37232-2551; **Phone:** 615-936-2020; **Board Cert:** Neurology 1985; **Med School:** Ireland 1970; **Resid:** Internal Medicine, St Vincent Hosp Elm Pk 1973; Internal Medicine, Genl Hosp-Royal Infirm 1976; **Fellow:** Neurology, Case Western Reserve Univ 1981; Neuro-Ophthalmology, Case Western Reserve Univ 1983; **Fac Appt:** Prof N, Vanderbilt Univ

Montgomery Jr, Erwin B MD [N] - **Spec Exp:** Parkinson's Disease; Movement Disorders; **Hospital:** Univ of Ala Hosp at Birmingham; **Address:** UAB Dept Neurology, 1720 7th Ave S, SC 350, Birmingham, AL 35233; **Phone:** 205-934-0683; **Board Cert:** Neurology 1982; **Med School:** SUNY Buffalo 1976; **Resid:** Neurology, Barnes Jewish Hosp 1980; **Fellow:** Neurological Physiology, Washington Univ 1981; **Fac Appt:** Prof N, Univ Alabama

Moots, Paul L MD [N] - **Spec Exp:** Neuro-Oncology; Brain Tumors; Neurologic Complications of Cancer; Pain-Neuropathic; **Hospital:** Vanderbilt Univ Med Ctr (page 75), TN Valley Healthcare Sys-Nashville; **Address:** Vanderbilt Dept Neurology, 1161 21st Ave S, A-0118 Med Ctr North, Nashville, TN 37232; **Phone:** 615-322-6053; **Board Cert:** Neurology 1989; **Med School:** Ohio State Univ 1980; **Resid:** Neurology, Univ Va Med Ctr 1984; **Fellow:** Neuropathology, Univ Virginia 1986; Neuro-Oncology, Meml Sloan Kettering Canc 1989; **Fac Appt:** Assoc Prof N, Vanderbilt Univ

Morgenlander, Joel C MD [N] - **Spec Exp:** Neuromuscular Disorders; Stroke; Multiple Sclerosis; **Hospital:** Duke Univ Hosp; **Address:** Duke Univ Med Ctr, 200 Trent Dr, Clinic 1-L, Durham, NC 27710; **Phone:** 919-684-6887; **Board Cert:** Neurology 1992; **Med School:** Univ Pittsburgh 1986; **Resid:** Neurology, Duke Univ Med Ctr 1990; **Fellow:** Neuromuscular Disease, Duke Univ Med Ctr 1991; **Fac Appt:** Prof N, Duke Univ

Nabors III, L Burt MD [N] - **Spec Exp:** Neuro-Oncology; Brain Tumors; **Hospital:** Univ of Ala Hosp at Birmingham; **Address:** UAB, FOT 1020, 510 20th St S, Birmingham, AL 35294-0001; **Phone:** 205-934-1432; **Board Cert:** Neurology 2009; **Med School:** Univ Tenn Coll Med 1991; **Resid:** Neurology, Univ Alabama Med Ctr; **Fellow:** Neuro-Oncology, Univ Alabama; **Fac Appt:** Prof N, Univ Alabama

Newman, Nancy J MD [N] - **Spec Exp:** Neuro-Ophthalmology; **Hospital:** Emory Univ Hosp, Chldns Hlthcare Atlanta @ Egleston; **Address:** Emory Clinic-Neuro-Ophthalmology, 1365B Clifton Rd NE, Ste 4500, Atlanta, GA 30322; **Phone:** 404-778-5360; **Board Cert:** Neurology 1989; **Med School:** Harvard Med Sch 1984; **Resid:** Neurology, Mass Genl Hosp 1988; **Fellow:** Neuro-Ophthalmology, Mass EE Infirmary 1989; **Fac Appt:** Prof N, Emory Univ

Nolan, Bruce A MD [N] - **Spec Exp:** Sleep Disorders/Apnea; **Hospital:** Jackson Meml Hosp; **Address:** Univ Miami Dept Neurology, 1501 NW 9th Ave, Miami, FL 33136; **Phone:** 305-243-5195; **Board Cert:** Neurology 1974; **Med School:** Wayne State Univ 1966; **Resid:** Neurology, Univ Miami Affil Hosp 1970; **Fac Appt:** Assoc Prof N, Univ Miami Sch Med

Oh, Shin Joong MD [N] - **Spec Exp:** Neuromuscular Disorders; Electromyography; Myasthenia Gravis; **Hospital:** Univ of Ala Hosp at Birmingham; **Address:** UAB Dept Neurology, 1530 3rd Ave S, SC 200, Birmingham, AL 35294-0017; **Phone:** 205-934-2120; **Board Cert:** Neurology 1973; Clinical Neurophysiology 2001; Neuromuscular Medicine 2009; **Med School:** Korea 1960; **Resid:** Internal Medicine, Seoul National Univ Hosp 1964; Neurology, Georgetown Univ Hosp 1967; **Fellow:** NeuroEpidemiology, Univ Minnesota Hosps 1968; **Fac Appt:** Prof N, Univ Alabama

Sacco, Ralph L MD [N] - **Spec Exp:** Stroke; Stroke Prevention; **Hospital:** Jackson Meml Hosp, Univ of Miami Hosp & Clins/Sylvester Comp Canc Ctr; **Address:** Univ of Miami-Dept of Neurology, 1120 NW 14th St Fl 13 - Ste 1352, Miami, FL 33136; **Phone:** 305-243-7519; **Board Cert:** Neurology 1989; **Med School:** Boston Univ 1983; **Resid:** Neurology, Columbia-Presby Med Ctr 1987; **Fellow:** Cerebrovascular Disease, Columbia-Presby Med Ctr 1989; **Fac Appt:** Prof N, Univ Miami Sch Med

Sadowsky, Carl H MD [N] - **Spec Exp:** Memory Disorders; Alzheimer's Disease; **Hospital:** West Palm Hosp; **Address:** Palm Beach Neurology, 4631 Congress Ave, Ste 200, West Palm Beach, FL 33407-2234; **Phone:** 561-845-0500 x129; **Board Cert:** Neurology 1977; **Med School:** Cornell Univ 1971; **Resid:** Internal Medicine, Dartmouth-Hitchcock Med Ctr 1973; Neurology, Dartmouth-Hitchcock Med Ctr 1976; **Fac Appt:** Assoc Clin Prof N, Nova SE Univ, Coll Osteo Med

Schatz, Norman J MD [N] - **Spec Exp:** Neuro-Ophthalmology; Multiple Sclerosis/Visual Disorders; Vision-Unexplained Loss; **Hospital:** Bascom Palmer Eye Inst, Univ of Miami Hosp; **Address:** 4302 Alton Rd, Ste 845, Miami Beach, FL 33140; **Phone:** 305-532-2885; **Board Cert:** Neurology 1969; **Med School:** Hahnemann Univ 1961; **Resid:** Neurology, Jefferson Hosp 1965; **Fellow:** Neuro-Ophthalmology, Bascom Palmer Eye Inst 1966; **Fac Appt:** Clin Prof N, Univ Pennsylvania

Schiff, David MD [N] - **Spec Exp:** Brain Tumors; Spinal Cord Tumors; Neurologic Complications of Cancer; Neuro-Oncology; **Hospital:** Univ of Virginia Health Sys; **Address:** Univ VA, Div of Neuro-Oncology, Box 800432, Charlottesville, VA 22908; **Phone:** 434-982-4415; **Board Cert:** Neurology 1994; **Med School:** Harvard Med Sch 1988; **Resid:** Neurology, Harvard Longwood 1992; **Fellow:** Neuro-Oncology, Meml Sloan Kettering Cancer Ctr 1993; Mayo Clinic 1994; **Fac Appt:** Assoc Prof NS, Univ VA Sch Med

Sethi, Kapil D MD [N] - **Spec Exp:** Parkinson's Disease; Restless Legs Syndrome; Movement Disorders; Botox Therapy; **Hospital:** Med Coll of GA Hosp and Clin (MCG Health Inc); **Address:** Med Coll Georgia, Dept Neurology, 1120 15th St, rm HF-1154, Augusta, GA 30912-0004; **Phone:** 706-721-2798; **Board Cert:** Neurology 1987; **Med School:** India 1976; **Resid:** Neurology, Pgimer 1981; Neurology, Med Coll Georgia 1985; **Fac Appt:** Prof N, Med Coll GA

Neurology

Singer, Carlos MD [N] - **Spec Exp:** Parkinson's Disease; Movement Disorders; Botox Therapy; **Hospital:** Jackson Meml Hosp; **Address:** Univ Miami Dept Neurology, 1150 NW 14th St, Ste 609, Miami, FL 33136; **Phone:** 305-243-3876; **Board Cert:** Internal Medicine 1976; Neurology 1981; **Med School:** Venezuela 1972; **Resid:** Internal Medicine, Montefiore Hosp 1976; Neurology, Albert Einstein Affil Hosp 1979; **Fellow:** Electromyography, Jackson Meml Hosp 1981; Movement Disorders, Univ Miami 1989; **Fac Appt:** Prof N, Univ Miami Sch Med

Watts, Ray L MD [N] - **Spec Exp:** Parkinson's Disease; Movement Disorders; **Hospital:** Univ of Ala Hosp at Birmingham; **Address:** 510 20th St S, FOT 1203, Birmingham, AL 35294; **Phone:** 205-934-0683; **Board Cert:** Neurology 1985; **Med School:** Washington Univ, St Louis 1980; **Resid:** Neurology, Mass Genl Hosp 1984; **Fellow:** Electromyography, Mass Genl Hosp 1983; **Fac Appt:** Prof N, Univ Alabama

Wooten Jr, George F MD [N] - **Spec Exp:** Movement Disorders; Parkinson's Disease; Tremor & Dystonia; **Hospital:** Univ of Virginia Health Sys; **Address:** Univ VA Hlth Sys, Box 800394, Charlottesville, VA 22908; **Phone:** 434-924-8369; **Board Cert:** Neurology 1977; **Med School:** Cornell Univ-Weill Med Coll 1970; **Resid:** Neurology, NY Hosp-Cornell 1977; **Fellow:** Pharmacology, Natl Inst Hlth-NIMH 1974; **Fac Appt:** Prof N, Univ VA Sch Med

Midwest

Adams Jr, Harold P MD [N] - **Spec Exp:** Stroke; Cerebrovascular Disease; **Hospital:** Univ Iowa Hosp & Clinics; **Address:** Univ Iowa Hosp, Dept Neurology, 200 Hawkins Drive, rm 2148-RCP, Iowa City, IA 52242; **Phone:** 319-356-4110; **Board Cert:** Neurology 2004; Vascular Neurology 2005; **Med School:** Northwestern Univ 1970; **Resid:** Neurology, Univ Iowa Hosp 1974; **Fac Appt:** Prof N, Univ Iowa Coll Med

Ahlskog, J Eric MD/PhD [N] - **Spec Exp:** Parkinson's Disease; Movement Disorders; **Hospital:** Mayo Med Ctr & Clin - Rochester, St. Mary's Hosp - Rochester MN (Mayo); **Address:** Mayo Clinic, Dept Neurology, 200 First St SW, Rochester, MN 55905; **Phone:** 507-266-5800; **Board Cert:** Neurology 1984; **Med School:** Dartmouth Med Sch 1976; **Resid:** Internal Medicine, Univ Chicago Med Ctr 1978; Neurology, Mayo Clin 1981; **Fac Appt:** Prof N, Mayo Med Sch

Alberts, Mark J MD [N] - **Spec Exp:** Stroke/Cerebrovascular Disease; **Hospital:** Northwestern Meml Hosp; **Address:** 675 N St Clair St, Galter Bldg Fl 20 - Ste 100, Chicago, IL 60611; **Phone:** 312-695-7950; **Board Cert:** Neurology 1987; Vascular Neurology 2005; **Med School:** Tufts Univ 1982; **Resid:** Neurology, Duke Univ Med Ctr 1986; **Fellow:** Cerebrovascular Disease, Duke Univ Med Ctr 1987; **Fac Appt:** Prof N, Northwestern Univ

Arnason, Barry G W MD [N] - **Spec Exp:** Multiple Sclerosis; Guillain-Barre Syndrome; Myasthenia Gravis; **Hospital:** Univ of Chicago Med Ctr; **Address:** 5841 S Maryland Ave, MC 2030, Chicago, IL 60637; **Phone:** 773-702-6222; **Board Cert:** Neurology 1971; **Med School:** Univ Manitoba 1957; **Resid:** Neurology, Mass Genl Hosp 1959; Neurology, Mass Genl Hosp 1962; **Fac Appt:** Prof N, Univ Chicago-Pritzker Sch Med

Barger, Geoffrey R MD [N] - **Spec Exp:** Neuro-Oncology; Brain Tumors; **Hospital:** Harper Univ Hosp, Barbara Ann Karmanos Cancer Inst; **Address:** Wayne State Univ Hlth Ctr, 4201 St Antoine, Ste 8A, Detroit, MI 48201; **Phone:** 313-745-4275; **Board Cert:** Neurology 1981; **Med School:** Jefferson Med Coll 1975; **Resid:** Neurology, Penn Hosp 1979; **Fellow:** Neuro-Oncology, Moffitt Hosp & Brain Tumor Ctr/UCSF 1982; **Fac Appt:** Assoc Prof N, Wayne State Univ

Barkley, Gregory L MD [N] - **Spec Exp:** Epilepsy/Seizure Disorders; **Hospital:** Henry Ford Hosp; **Address:** Henry Ford Hosp, Dept Neurology, 2799 W Grand Blvd, Detroit, MI 48202; **Phone:** 313-916-3922; **Board Cert:** Neurology 1988; Clinical Neurophysiology 2011; **Med School:** Mich State Univ 1981; **Resid:** Neurology, Henry Ford Hosp 1985; **Fellow:** Clinical Neurophysiology, Henry Ford Hosp 1986; **Fac Appt:** Assoc Prof N, Wayne State Univ

Bernstein, Richard A MD/PhD [N] - **Spec Exp:** Stroke/Cerebrovascular Disease; **Hospital:** Northwestern Meml Hosp; **Address:** 675 N St Claire St, Galter Bldg Fl 20 - Ste 100, Chicago, IL 60026; **Phone:** 312-695-7950; **Board Cert:** Neurology 2001; Vascular Neurology 2005; **Med School:** Cornell Univ-Weill Med Coll 1996; **Resid:** Neurology, Columbia-Presby Med Ctr 2000; **Fellow:** Vascular Neurology, UCSF Med Ctr 2001; Stroke, Stanford Med Ctr 2002; **Fac Appt:** Assoc Prof N, Northwestern Univ-Feinberg Sch Med

Broderick, Joseph P MD [N] - **Spec Exp:** Stroke; **Hospital:** Univ Hosp - Cincinnati; **Address:** Univ Cincinnati, Dept Neurology, 222 Piedmont Ave, Ste 3200, Cincinnati, OH 45219; **Phone:** 513-475-8730; **Board Cert:** Neurology 1988; Vascular Neurology 2005; **Med School:** Univ Cincinnati 1982; **Resid:** Neurology, Mayo Clinic 1986; **Fellow:** Cerebrovascular Disease, Mayo Clinic 1987; **Fac Appt:** Clin Prof N, Univ Cincinnati

Brown, Robert D MD [N] - **Spec Exp:** Stroke; Cerebrovascular Disease; **Hospital:** Mayo Med Ctr & Clin - Rochester; **Address:** Mayo Clinic, Dept Neurology, 200 First St SW, Rochester, MN 55905; **Phone:** 507-266-4143; **Board Cert:** Neurology 1994; Vascular Neurology 2008; **Med School:** Mayo Med Sch 1987; **Resid:** Neurology, Mayo Clin 1991; **Fellow:** Cerebrovascular Disease, Mayo Clin 1992; **Fac Appt:** Prof N, Mayo Med Sch

Burke, Allan M MD [N] - **Spec Exp:** Cerebrovascular Disease; Neurologic Imaging; **Hospital:** Northwestern Meml Hosp; **Address:** 233 E Erie St, Ste 500, Chicago, IL 60611-2912; **Phone:** 312-944-0063; **Board Cert:** Neurology 1982; Neuroimaging 2002; **Med School:** Columbia P&S 1976; **Resid:** Internal Medicine, NY Hosp 1978; Neurology, Columbia-Presby Med Ctr 1981; **Fellow:** Cerebrovascular Disease, Hosp Univ Penn 1983; **Fac Appt:** Clin Prof N, Northwestern Univ

Cascino, Terrence L MD [N] - **Spec Exp:** Neuro-Oncology; **Hospital:** Mayo Med Ctr & Clin - Rochester; **Address:** Mayo Clinic, Dept Neurology, 200 1st St SW, Rochester, MN 55905; **Phone:** 507-284-2576; **Board Cert:** Neurology 1984; **Med School:** Loyola Univ-Stritch Sch Med 1972; **Resid:** Neurology, Mayo Clinic 1980; **Fellow:** Neuro-Oncology, Meml Sloan Kettering Cancer Ctr; **Fac Appt:** Assoc Prof N, Mayo Med Sch

Chelimsky, Thomas C MD [N] - **Hospital:** Froedtert and Med Ctr of WI; **Address:** Froedtert & Medical College of WI, 9200 W Wisconsin Ave, Milwaukee, WI 53226; **Phone:** 414-805-8710; **Board Cert:** Internal Medicine 1986; Neurology 1992; **Med School:** Washington Univ, St Louis 1983; **Resid:** Internal Medicine, Mayo Clinic 1986; Neurology, Mayo Clinic 1989; **Fellow:** Physiology, Mayo Clinic 1987; **Fac Appt:** Prof N, Case West Res Univ

Cohen, Jeffrey Alan MD [N] - **Spec Exp:** Multiple Sclerosis; Neuro-Immunology; **Hospital:** Cleveland Clin (page 55); **Address:** Cleveland Clinic, 9500 Euclid Ave, Desk U10, Cleveland, OH 44195; **Phone:** 216-445-8110; **Board Cert:** Neurology 1985; **Med School:** Univ Chicago-Pritzker Sch Med 1980; **Resid:** Neurology, Hosp Univ Penn 1984; **Fellow:** Neurological Immunology, Hosp Univ Penn 1987

Corbetta, Maurizio MD [N] - **Spec Exp:** Stroke; Brain Injury Rehabilitation; Neuro-Rehabilitation; Neurologic Imaging; **Hospital:** Washington Univ Physicians, Barnes-Jewish Hosp; **Address:** 4444 Forest Park Blvd, Box 8518, St Louis, MO 63108; **Phone:** 314-362-4503; **Board Cert:** Neurology 2008; **Med School:** Italy 1985; **Resid:** Neurology, Univ Verona Affil Hosp 1990; Neurology, Barnes Jewish Hosp 1996; **Fellow:** Neuroimaging, Barnes Jewish Hosp 1992; **Fac Appt:** Prof N, Washington Univ, St Louis

Neurology

Cutrer, F Michael MD [N] - **Spec Exp:** Headache; Pain-Facial; Migraine; **Hospital:** Mayo Med Ctr & Clin - Rochester, Rochester Methodist Hosp; **Address:** Mayo Clinic, Dept Neurology, 200 First St SW, Rochester, MN 55905-0001; **Phone:** 507-266-5800; **Board Cert:** Neurology 1993; **Med School:** Univ Miss 1988; **Resid:** Neurology, UCLA Med Ctr 1992; **Fellow:** Neurology, Mass Genl Hosp-Harvard 1994; **Fac Appt:** Assoc Prof N, Mayo Med Sch

Elias, Stanton B MD [N] - **Spec Exp:** Multiple Sclerosis; Myasthenia Gravis; **Hospital:** Henry Ford Hosp; **Address:** Henry Ford Hosp, Dept Neurology, 2799 W Grand Blvd, Fl K-11, Detroit, MI 48202-2689; **Phone:** 313-916-7207; **Board Cert:** Neurology 1979; **Med School:** Univ Pittsburgh 1972; **Resid:** Neurology, Duke Univ Med Ctr 1976; **Fellow:** Neurology, Duke Univ Med Ctr 1977

Farlow, Martin R MD [N] - **Spec Exp:** Alzheimer's Disease; Neurodegenerative Disorders; Multiple Sclerosis; Prion Diseases; **Hospital:** IU Health University Hosp, Wishard Hlth Srvs; **Address:** IU Health Physicians-Dept Neurology, 355 W 16th St, Ste 3200, Indianapolis, IN 46202; **Phone:** 317-948-5450; **Board Cert:** Neurology 1988; **Med School:** Indiana Univ 1979; **Resid:** Neurology, Indiana Univ Hosp 1983; **Fac Appt:** Prof N, Indiana Univ

Feldman, Eva L MD/PhD [N] - **Spec Exp:** Neuromuscular Disorders; Amyotrophic Lateral Sclerosis (ALS); Peripheral Neuropathy; **Hospital:** Univ of Michigan Hosp; **Address:** Univ Mich, Dept Neurology, 1500 E Med Ctr Drive, Taubman 1324 SPC 5322, Ann Arbor, MI 48109; **Phone:** 734-936-9020; **Board Cert:** Neurology 1988; **Med School:** Univ Mich Med Sch 1983; **Resid:** Neurology, Johns Hopkins Hosp 1987; **Fellow:** Neuromuscular Medicine, Univ Mich Hosps 1988; **Fac Appt:** Prof N, Univ Mich Med Sch

Furlan, Anthony J MD [N] - **Spec Exp:** Stroke; Thrombolytic Therapy; **Hospital:** Univ Hosps Case Med Ctr (page 74); **Address:** Dept Neurology, 11100 Euclid Ave, Fl 5, Hanna House, Cleveland, OH 44106; **Phone:** 216-844-3193; **Board Cert:** Neurology 1979; Vascular Neurology 2005; **Med School:** Loyola Univ-Stritch Sch Med 1973; **Resid:** Neurology, Cleveland Clinic 1977; **Fellow:** Cerebrovascular Disease, Mayo Clinic 1978; **Fac Appt:** Assoc Prof N, Ohio State Univ

Gilman, Sid MD [N] - **Spec Exp:** Parkinson's Disease/Movement Disorders; Alzheimer's Disease; Multiple Sclerosis; Ataxia; **Hospital:** Univ of Michigan Hosp; **Address:** 2301 Commonwealth Blvd, 300 N Ingalls 3D15, Ann Arbor, MI 48109-0489; **Phone:** 734-936-1808; **Board Cert:** Neurology 1966; **Med School:** UCLA 1957; **Resid:** Neurology, Boston City Hosp-Harvard 1963; **Fellow:** Neurological Physiology, Boston City Hosp-Harvard 1965; **Fac Appt:** Prof N, Univ Mich Med Sch

Goetz, Christopher G MD [N] - **Spec Exp:** Movement Disorders; Parkinson's Disease; Dyskinesias; **Hospital:** Rush Univ Med Ctr; **Address:** 1725 W Harrison St, Ste 755, Chicago, IL 60612-3835; **Phone:** 312-563-2030; **Board Cert:** Neurology 1982; **Med School:** Rush Med Coll 1975; **Resid:** Neurology, Michael Reese Med Ctr 1977; Neurology, Rush-Presby-St Luke's Med Ctr 1979; **Fac Appt:** Prof N, Rush Med Coll

Goodwin, James MD [N] - **Spec Exp:** Neuro-Ophthalmology; Optic Nerve Disorders; Neuromuscular Disorder & Vision Problems; **Hospital:** Univ of IL Med Ctr at Chicago; **Address:** Univ Illinois Eye & Ear Infirm, 1855 W Taylor St, rm 3.158, MC 64, Chicago, IL 60612; **Phone:** 312-996-9120; **Board Cert:** Neurology 1975; **Med School:** Univ IL Coll Med 1969; **Resid:** Neurology, Univ Minnesota Hosps 1973; **Fellow:** Neuro-Ophthalmology, Bascom Palmer Eye Inst 1976; **Fac Appt:** Prof Oph, Univ IL Coll Med

Hain, Timothy C MD [N] - **Spec Exp:** Neuro-Otology; Balance Disorders; Motion Sickness; **Hospital:** Northwestern Meml Hosp; **Address:** 645 N Michigan Ave, Ste 410, Chicago, IL 60611; **Phone:** 312-274-0197; **Board Cert:** Neurology 1983; **Med School:** Univ IL Coll Med 1978; **Resid:** Neurology, Univ Illinois Affil Hosp 1982; **Fellow:** Neurology, Johns Hopkins Hosp 1984; Ophthalmology, Johns Hopkins Hosp 1984; **Fac Appt:** Prof N, Northwestern Univ

Hecox, Kurt E MD [N] - **Spec Exp:** Pediatric Neurology; Epilepsy/Seizure Disorders; Hearing Loss; **Hospital:** Chldns Hosp - Wisconsin; **Address:** Dept Neurology, 9000 W Wisconsin Ave, rm CCC-540, PO Box 1997, Milwaukee, WI 53226; **Phone:** 414-266-3464; **Board Cert:** Clinical Neurophysiology 1977; **Med School:** UCSD 1971; **Resid:** Neurology, Univ Texas Southwestern Med Ctr 1975; **Fellow:** Pediatric Neurology, Children's Med Ctr/Parkland Hosp 1978; **Fac Appt:** Prof N, Med Coll Wisc

Homer, Daniel MD [N] - **Spec Exp:** Stroke; **Hospital:** Evanston/North Shore Univ Hlth Sys, Highland Park/North Shore Univ Hlth Syst; **Address:** Evanston Hosp, Dept Neurology, 1000 Central St, Ste 615, Evanston, IL 60201; **Phone:** 847-570-2570; **Board Cert:** Neurology 1990; Vascular Neurology 2008; **Med School:** Northwestern Univ 1979; **Resid:** Neurology, Stanford Univ Hosp 1983; **Fellow:** Stroke, Mayo Clinic 1984; **Fac Appt:** Asst Prof N, Northwestern Univ

Josephson, David A MD [N] - **Spec Exp:** Electromyography; Epilepsy; Stroke; **Hospital:** St. Vincent Indianapolis Hosp, Gomm Hosp N - Indianapolis; **Address:** 8402 Harcourt Rd, Ste 615, Indianapolis, IN 46260; **Phone:** 317-806-6991; **Board Cert:** Neurology 2004; **Med School:** Indiana Univ 1971; **Resid:** Neurology, Univ Mich Med Ctr 1973; Neurology, Indiana Univ Med Ctr 1975; **Fac Appt:** Assoc Clin Prof N, Indiana Univ

Katirji, Bashar MD [N] - **Spec Exp:** Neuromuscular Disorders; **Hospital:** Univ Hosps Case Med Ctr (page 74); **Address:** UH Neurological Institute, 11100 Euclid Ave, Cleveland, OH 44106; **Phone:** 216-844-4854; **Board Cert:** Neurology 1985; Clinical Neurophysiology 2002; Neuromuscular Medicine 2008; **Med School:** Syria 1977; **Resid:** Internal Medicine, King Faisal Spec Hosp 1980; Neurology, Univ Pittsburgh Med Ctr 1983; **Fellow:** Electromyography, Cleveland Clinic 1984; **Fac Appt:** Prof N, Case West Res Univ

Kincaid, John C MD [N] - **Spec Exp:** Neuromuscular Disorders; Electromyography; Pain-Facial; Peripheral Neuropathy; **Hospital:** IU Health University Hosp; **Address:** IU Health Physicians-Dept Neurology, 355 W 16th St Fl 4, Indianapolis, IN 46202; **Phone:** 317-948-5450; **Board Cert:** Neurology 2010; Clinical Neurophysiology 2000; **Med School:** Indiana Univ 1975; **Resid:** Neurology, Indiana Univ Affil Hosp 1979; **Fellow:** Electromyography, Mayo Clinic 1980; **Fac Appt:** Prof N, Indiana Univ

Lewis, Richard A MD [N] - **Spec Exp:** Neuromuscular Disorders; **Hospital:** Harper Univ Hosp; **Address:** 4201 St Aintoine, Univ Health Center, Ste 8A, Detroit, MI 48201; **Phone:** 313-745-4275; **Board Cert:** Neurology 1980; **Med School:** Med Coll VA 1974; **Resid:** Neurology, Hosp Univ Penn 1978

Lisak, Robert P MD [N] - **Spec Exp:** Multiple Sclerosis; Myasthenia Gravis; Vasculitis; Demyelinating Neuropathy; **Hospital:** Harper Univ Hosp, Detroit Receiving Hospital; **Address:** 4201 St Antoine Blvd, UHC Bldg Fl 8 - Ste A, Detroit, MI 48201; **Phone:** 313-745-4240; **Board Cert:** Neurology 1975; **Med School:** Columbia P&S 1965; **Resid:** Internal Medicine, Bronx Municipal Hosp-Einstein 1969; Neurology, Hosp Univ Penn 1972; **Fac Appt:** Prof N, Wayne State Univ

Logan, William R MD [N] - **Spec Exp:** Stroke; Cerebrovascular Disease; **Hospital:** St. John's Mercy Med Ctr - St Louis; **Address:** St Johns Mercy Med Ctr, Div Neur, 621 S New Ballas Rd, Ste 5003-B, St Louis, MO 63141; **Phone:** 314-227-2020; **Board Cert:** Internal Medicine 1981; Neurology 1986; Vascular Neurology 2009; **Med School:** Univ Okla Coll Med 1978; **Resid:** Internal Medicine, Univ Missouri Hosps 1982; Neurology, Univ Texas Hlth Sci Ctr 1984

Luders, Hans MD/PhD [N] - **Spec Exp:** Epilepsy; **Hospital:** Univ Hosps Case Med Ctr (page 74); **Address:** University Hosps-Case Med Ctr, 11100 Euclid Ave, Dept Neurology, Lakeside Bldg - Ste 3200, Cleveland, OH 44106; **Phone:** 216-844-3650; **Board Cert:** Neurology 1985; **Med School:** Chile 1965; **Resid:** Neurology, Neur Inst-Kyushu Univ 1971; **Fellow:** Neurological Physiology, Mayo Grad Sch Med 1975; **Fac Appt:** Prof N, Ohio State Univ

Neurology

Maraganore, Demetrius MD [N] - **Spec Exp:** Movement Disorders; Parkinson's Disease; **Hospital:** Evanston/North Shore Univ Hlth Sys, Glenbrook Hosp-NorthShore Univ Hlth Syst; **Address:** 2150 Pfingsten Rd, Ste 3000, Glenview, IL 60026; **Phone:** 847-570-2570; **Board Cert:** Neurology 1990; **Med School:** Northwestern Univ-Feinberg Sch Med 1985; **Resid:** Neurology, Mayo Clinic 1989; **Fellow:** Movement Disorders, Natl Hosp for Nervous Disorders 1990

Mesulam, Marsel MD [N] - **Spec Exp:** Alzheimer's Disease; Tourette's Syndrome; Dementia; **Hospital:** Northwestern Meml Hosp; **Address:** 320 E Superior St Fl 11 - rm 453, Chicago, IL 60611; **Phone:** 312-908-9339; **Board Cert:** Neurology 1977; **Med School:** Harvard Med Sch 1972; **Resid:** Neurology, Boston City Hosp 1976; **Fac Appt:** Prof N, Northwestern Univ

Mikkelsen, Tom MD [N] - **Spec Exp:** Brain Tumors; Gliomas; **Hospital:** Henry Ford Hosp; **Address:** Henry Ford Hospital, 2799 W Grand Blvd Fl K11, Detroit, MI 48202; **Phone:** 313-916-2241; **Board Cert:** Neurology 2008; **Med School:** Univ Calgary 1983; **Resid:** Internal Medicine, Calgary General Hosp 1985; Neurology, Montreal Neuro Inst 1988; **Fellow:** Neuro-Oncology, Royal Victoria Hosp 1990; Neuro-Oncology, Ludwig Inst for Cancer Rsch 1992; **Fac Appt:** Assoc Prof N, Case West Res Univ

Morris, John C MD [N] - **Spec Exp:** Alzheimer's Disease; **Hospital:** Barnes-Jewish Hosp; **Address:** Memory Diagnostic Ctr, 4488 Forest Park Blvd, Ste 160, St Louis, MO 63108-2215; **Phone:** 314-286-1967; **Board Cert:** Internal Medicine 1979; Neurology 1985; **Med School:** Univ Rochester 1974; **Resid:** Internal Medicine, Akron Genl Med Ctr 1979; Neurology, Cleveland Metro Genl Hosp 1982; **Fellow:** Neuropharmacology, Washington Univ 1985; **Fac Appt:** Prof N, Washington Univ, St Louis

Newman, Daniel S MD [N] - **Spec Exp:** Amyotrophic Lateral Sclerosis (ALS); Neuromuscular Disorders; **Hospital:** Henry Ford Hosp; **Address:** Henry Ford Hospital, 2799 W Grand Blvd Fl K11, Detroit, MI 48202; **Phone:** 313-916-2594; **Board Cert:** Neurology 1992; Neuromuscular Medicine 2008; **Med School:** Univ Mich Med Sch 1983; **Resid:** Neurology, Henry Ford Hosp 1988; **Fellow:** Electromyography, Mayo Clinic 1989; **Fac Appt:** Assoc Prof N, Wayne State Univ

Newton, Herbert B MD [N] - **Spec Exp:** Neuro-Oncology; Brain & Spinal Tumors; Clinical Trials; **Hospital:** Ohio St Univ Med Ctr, Arthur G James Cancer Hosp & Research Inst; **Address:** 320 W 10th Ave, Starling Loving Bldg, rm M410, Columbus, OH 43210; **Phone:** 614-293-4448; **Board Cert:** Neurology 1989; **Med School:** SUNY Buffalo 1984; **Resid:** Neurology, Univ Michigan Med Ctr 1988; **Fellow:** Neuro-Oncology, Meml Sloan-Kettering Cancer Ctr 1990; **Fac Appt:** Prof N, Ohio State Univ

Pascuzzi, Robert M MD [N] - **Spec Exp:** Neuromuscular Disorders; Amyotrophic Lateral Sclerosis (ALS); Myasthenia Gravis; Post Polio Syndrome; **Hospital:** IU Health University Hosp, Wishard Hlth Srvs; **Address:** IU Health Physicians-Dept Neurology, 355 W 16th St, Indianapolis, IN 46202; **Phone:** 317-948-5450; **Board Cert:** Neurology 2004; **Med School:** Indiana Univ 1979; **Resid:** Neurology, Univ Va Med Ctr 1983; **Fellow:** Neuromuscular Medicine, Univ Virginia 1985; **Fac Appt:** Prof N, Indiana Univ

Perlmutter, Joel S MD [N] - **Spec Exp:** Parkinson's Disease; Movement Disorders; Huntington's Disease; **Hospital:** Barnes-Jewish Hosp; **Address:** 660 S Euclid Ave, Box 8111, St Louis, MO 63110; **Phone:** 314-362-6908; **Board Cert:** Neurology 1985; **Med School:** Univ MO-Columbia Sch Med 1979; **Resid:** Neurology, Barnes Hosp-Wash Univ 1983; **Fellow:** Movement Disorders, Barnes Hosp-Wash Univ 1984; **Fac Appt:** Prof N, Washington Univ, St Louis

Pestronk, Alan MD [N] - **Spec Exp:** Neuromuscular Disorders; Peripheral Neuropathy; **Hospital:** Barnes-Jewish Hosp; **Address:** Washington Univ Sch Med, Dept Neurology, Div Neuromuscular Disorders, 660 S Euclid Ave, Box 8111, St Louis, MO 63110; **Phone:** 314-362-6981; **Board Cert:** Neurology 1978; Neuromuscular Medicine 2008; **Med School:** Johns Hopkins Univ 1970; **Resid:** Neurology, Johns Hopkins Hosp 1974; **Fellow:** Neuromuscular Medicine, Johns Hopkins Hosp 1977; **Fac Appt:** Prof NPath, Washington Univ, St Louis

Petersen, Ronald C MD/PhD [N] - **Spec Exp:** Alzheimer's Disease; Cognitive Impairment/Mild; **Hospital:** Mayo Med Ctr & Clin - Rochester; **Address:** Mayo Clinic, Dept Neurology, 200 First St SW, Rochester, MN 55905; **Phone:** 507-266-5800; **Board Cert:** Neurology 1986; **Med School:** Mayo Med Sch 1980; **Resid:** Neurology, Mayo Clinic 1984; **Fellow:** Behavioral Neurology, Beth Israel Med Ctr 1986; **Fac Appt:** Prof N, Mayo Med Sch

Reder, Anthony T MD [N] - **Spec Exp:** Multiple Sclerosis; Tetanus; Myasthenia Gravis; Reflex Sympathetic Dystrophy (RSD); **Hospital:** Univ of Chicago Med Ctr; **Address:** Univ Chicago- Dept Neurology, 5841 S Maryland Ave, MC 2030, Chicago, IL 60637; **Phone:** 773-702-6222; **Board Cert:** Neurology 1984; **Med School:** Univ Mich Med Sch 1978; **Resid:** Neurology, Univ Minn Hosps 1982; **Fellow:** Neurological Immunology, Univ Chicago Med Ctr 1984; **Fac Appt:** Assoc Prof N, Univ Chicago-Pritzker Sch Med

Reed, Robert L MD [N] - **Spec Exp:** Multiple Sclerosis; Stroke; **Hospital:** Good Samaritan Hosp - Cincinnati; **Address:** 111 Wellington Pl, Cincinnati, OH 45219; **Phone:** 513-241-2370; **Board Cert:** Neurology 1975; **Med School:** Univ Cincinnati 1966; **Resid:** Internal Medicine, Mayo Grad Sch Med 1970; Neurology, Mayo Grad Sch Med 1973

Richerson, George B MD/PhD [N] - **Hospital:** Univ Iowa Hosp & Clinics, Iowa City VA Hlth Care Sys; **Address:** UIHC Dept Neurology, 200 Hawkins Drive, Iowa City, IA 52242; **Phone:** 319-356-4296; **Board Cert:** Neurology 1993; **Med School:** Univ Iowa Coll Med 1984; **Resid:** Neurology, Yale-New Haven Hosp 1990; **Fac Appt:** Prof N, Univ Iowa Coll Med

Rogers, Lisa R DO [N] - **Spec Exp:** Neuro-Oncology; Brain Tumors; Brain Radiation Toxicity; **Hospital:** Univ Hosps Case Med Ctr (page 74); **Address:** Univ Hosps-Case Med Ctr, Dept Neuro, MS HH 5040, 11100 Euclid Ave, Cleveland, OH 44106-5040; **Phone:** 216-844-5160; **Board Cert:** Neurology 1982; **Med School:** Kirksville Coll Osteo Med 1976; **Resid:** Neurology, Cleveland Clinic 1980; **Fellow:** Neuro-Oncology, Meml-Sloan Kettering Cancer Ctr 1982; **Fac Appt:** Prof N, Case West Res Univ

Roos, Karen L MD [N] - **Spec Exp:** Infections-Neurologic; Encephalitis; Vascular Disease; Neurofibromatosis; **Hospital:** IU Health University Hosp, Wishard Hlth Srvs; **Address:** Indiana Univ Neuroscience Ctr, 355 W 16th St, rm 4215, Indianapolis, IN 46202; **Phone:** 317-963-7441; **Board Cert:** Neurology 1986; **Med School:** Hahnemann Univ 1981; **Resid:** Neurology, Univ Virginia Med Ctr 1985; **Fac Appt:** Prof N, Indiana Univ

Roos, Raymond MD [N] - **Spec Exp:** Amyotrophic Lateral Sclerosis (ALS); Multiple Sclerosis; Neuromuscular Disorders; **Hospital:** Univ of Chicago Med Ctr; **Address:** Univ Chicago, Dept Neurology, 5841 S Maryland Ave, MS 203, Chicago, IL 60637; **Phone:** 773-702-5659; **Board Cert:** Neurology 1976; **Med School:** SUNY Downstate 1968; **Resid:** Neurology, Johns Hopkins Hosp 1974; **Fellow:** Neurology, Natl Inst Neur Dis & Stroke 1971; Neurological Viral Immunology, Johns Hopkins Hosp 1976; **Fac Appt:** Prof N, Univ Chicago-Pritzker Sch Med

Rosenfeld, Steven S MD [N] - **Spec Exp:** Brain Tumors; Gliomas; Neuro-Oncology; **Hospital:** Cleveland Clin (page 55); **Address:** Burkhardt Brain Tumor Ctr, Cleveland Clinic, 9500 Euclid Ave, Cleveland, OH 44195; **Phone:** 216-444-4461; **Board Cert:** Neurology 1994; **Med School:** Northwestern Univ 1985; **Resid:** Neurology, Duke Univ Med Ctr 1989; **Fellow:** Neuro-Oncology, Duke Univ Med Ctr 1990; **Fac Appt:** Prof N, Cleveland Cl Coll Med/Case West Res

Rubin, Susan M MD [N] - **Spec Exp:** Multiple Sclerosis in Women; Epilepsy in Pregnancy; Headache in Women; Migraine in Women; **Hospital:** Glenbrook Hosp-NorthShore Univ Hlth Syst, Evanston/North Shore Univ Hlth Sys; **Address:** Glenbrook Hosp, Dept Neurology, 2180 Pfingsten Rd, Ste 2000, Glenview, IL 60026; **Phone:** 847-503-2000; **Board Cert:** Neurology 2006; **Med School:** Univ IL Coll Med 1988; **Resid:** Neurology, Northwestern Meml Hosp 1993; **Fellow:** Neurological Physiology, Northwestern Meml Hosp 1994; **Fac Appt:** Asst Clin Prof N, Univ Chicago-Pritzker Sch Med

Saper, Joel R MD [N] - **Spec Exp:** Headache; Pain-Chronic after Head Injury; Migraine; **Hospital:** Chelsea Comm Hosp; **Address:** Michigan Head Pain & Neurological Inst, 3120 Professional Drive, Ann Arbor, MI 48104; **Phone:** 734-677-6000; **Board Cert:** Neurology 1975; Headache Medicine ; **Med School:** Univ IL Coll Med 1969; **Resid:** Neurology, Univ Mich Med Ctr 1973; **Fac Appt:** Clin Prof N, Mich State Univ

Siddique, Teepu MD [N] - **Spec Exp:** Amyotrophic Lateral Sclerosis (ALS); Muscular Dystrophy; Neurogenetics; Spasticity Management; **Hospital:** Northwestern Meml Hosp; **Address:** 675 N St Clair St, Galter Bldg Fl 20 - Ste 100, Chicago, IL 60611; **Phone:** 312-695-7950; **Board Cert:** Neurology 1980; **Med School:** Pakistan 1973; **Resid:** Neurology, UMDNJ Affil Hosp 1979; **Fellow:** Electromyography, Hosp Special Surg 1980; Neuromuscular Disease, Natl Inst Hlth 1981; **Fac Appt:** Prof N, Northwestern Univ

Sila, Cathy A MD [N] - **Spec Exp:** Cerebrovascular Disease; Stroke-Young Adults; **Hospital:** Univ Hosps Case Med Ctr (page 74); **Address:** University Hospitals - Case Me Ctr, Dept of Neurology, 11100 Euclid Ave, Cleveland, OH 44106-5040; **Phone:** 216-844-8334; **Board Cert:** Neurology 1986; Vascular Neurology 2005; **Med School:** Case West Res Univ 1981; **Resid:** Neurology, Cleveland Clin 1983; Neurology, Mayo Clin 1985; **Fellow:** Research, Cleveland Clin 1986; Vascular Neurology, Cleveland Clin 1986; **Fac Appt:** Prof N, Case West Res Univ

Swanson, Jerry W MD [N] - **Spec Exp:** Headache; Migraine; **Hospital:** Mayo Med Ctr & Clin - Rochester; **Address:** Mayo Clinic, Dept Neurology, 200 First St SW, Rochester, MN 55905-0001; **Phone:** 507-538-1036; **Board Cert:** Neurology 1984; Headache Medicine 2006; **Med School:** Northwestern Univ 1977; **Resid:** Neurology, Mayo Clinic 1982; **Fellow:** Electroencephalography, Mayo Clinic 1983; **Fac Appt:** Prof N, Mayo Med Sch

Vick, Nicholas A MD [N] - **Spec Exp:** Brain Tumors; Neuro-Oncology; **Hospital:** Evanston/North Shore Univ Hlth Sys; **Address:** Evanston Kellog Cancer Ctr, 2650 Ridge Ave, Evanston, IL 60201; **Phone:** 847-570-1808; **Board Cert:** Neurology 1971; **Med School:** Univ Chicago-Pritzker Sch Med 1965; **Resid:** Neurology, Univ Chicago Hosps 1968; **Fellow:** Neurology, Natl Inst Hlth 1970; **Fac Appt:** Prof N, Northwestern Univ

Vitek, Jerrold Lee MD/PhD [N] - **Spec Exp:** Parkinson's Disease/Movement Disorders; Tremor & Dystonia; Deep Brain Stimulation; **Hospital:** Univ Minn Med Ctr, Fairview - Riverside Campus; **Address:** Univ Minn, Dept Neurology, 516 Delaware St SE, MMC 88, Minneapolis, MN 55455; **Phone:** 612-625-9900; **Board Cert:** Neurology 1992; **Med School:** Univ Minn 1984; **Resid:** Neurology, Johns Hopkins Hosp 1988; **Fac Appt:** Prof N, Univ Minn

Windebank, Anthony J MD [N] - **Spec Exp:** Peripheral Neuropathy; Amyotrophic Lateral Sclerosis (ALS); Multiple Sclerosis; **Hospital:** Mayo Med Ctr & Clin - Rochester; **Address:** Mayo Clinic, Dept Neurology, 200 First St SW, Rochester, MN 55905; **Phone:** 507-266-5800; **Board Cert:** Neurology 1982; **Med School:** England, UK 1974; **Resid:** Internal Medicine, Radcliffe Infirm 1977; Neurology, Mayo Clin 1981; **Fellow:** Neurology, Mayo Clin 1982; **Fac Appt:** Prof N, Mayo Med Sch

Wright, Robert B MD [N] - **Spec Exp:** Myasthenia Gravis; Migraine; **Hospital:** Rush Univ Med Ctr; **Address:** 1725 W Harrison St, Ste 1118, Chicago, IL 60612-3841; **Phone:** 312-942-5936; **Board Cert:** Neurology 1988; **Med School:** Univ IL Coll Med 1982; **Resid:** Neurology, Rush Presby-St Luke's Med Ctr 1986; **Fellow:** Neuromuscular Medicine, Rush Presby-St Luke's Med Ctr 1987; **Fac Appt:** Asst Prof N, Rush Med Coll

Zimnowodzki, Simon MD [N] - **Spec Exp:** Electromyography; Amyotrophic Lateral Sclerosis (ALS); Myasthenia Gravis; Nerve Injuries; **Hospital:** Rush Univ Med Ctr, Stroger Hosp of Cook Co; **Address:** Rush Univ Medical Ctr, Dept Neurological Sciences, 1725 Harrison St, Ste 1106, Chicago, IL 60612; **Phone:** 312-942-4500; **Board Cert:** Neurology 1984; Clinical Neurophysiology 2002; Neuromuscular Medicine 2008; **Med School:** Loyola Univ-Stritch Sch Med 1978; **Resid:** Neurology, Univ Michigan Hosp 1982; **Fellow:** Neuromuscular Disease, Univ Wisconsin Med Ctr 1983; **Fac Appt:** Assoc Prof N, Rush Med Coll

Great Plains and Mountains

Barohn, Richard J MD [N] - **Spec Exp:** Peripheral Neuropathy; Myasthenia Gravis; Amyotrophic Lateral Sclerosis (ALS); Guillain-Barre Syndrome; **Hospital:** Univ of Kansas Hosp; **Address:** Univ Kansas Medical Ctr, Dept Neurology, 3599 Rainbow Blvd, MS 2012, Kansas City, KS 66160; **Phone:** 913-588-6970; **Board Cert:** Neurology 1987; Clinical Neurophysiology 2004; Neuromuscular Medicine 2008; **Med School:** Univ MO-Kansas City 1980; **Resid:** Neurology, Lackland AFB 1985

Bromberg, Mark B MD/PhD [N] - **Spec Exp:** Peripheral Neuropathy; Neuromuscular Disorders; **Hospital:** Univ Utah Hlth Care; **Address:** 175 N Medical Drive, Clinical Neurosciences Ctr, Salt Lake City, UT 84132; **Phone:** 801-585-7575; **Board Cert:** Neurology 1988; Clinical Neurophysiology 2000; **Med School:** Univ Mich Med Sch 1982; **Resid:** Neurology, Univ Mich Med Ctr 1986; **Fellow:** Electromyography, Univ Mich Med Ctr 1987; Neuromuscular Disease, Univ Mich Med Ctr 1987; **Fac Appt:** Prof N, Univ Utah

Filley, Christopher M MD [N] - **Spec Exp:** Leukoencephalopathy; Alzheimer's Disease; Brain Injury-Traumatic; Multiple Sclerosis; **Hospital:** Univ of CO Hosp - Anschutz Inpatient Pav, VA Eastern CO Health Care Sys-Denver; **Address:** Univ CO Hosp-Neurology Clinic, 1635 Aurora Ct, Ste 4200, MS F727, Aurora, CO 80045; **Phone:** 720-848-2080; **Board Cert:** Neurology 1984; Behavioral Neurology & Neuropsychiatry 2006; **Med School:** Johns Hopkins Univ 1979; **Resid:** Neurology, Univ Colorado Hosp 1983; **Fellow:** Behavioral Neurology, Boston VA Hosp 1984; **Fac Appt:** Prof N, Univ Colorado

Gilden, Donald H MD [N] - **Spec Exp:** Multiple Sclerosis; Infections-CNS; **Hospital:** Univ of CO Hosp - Anschutz Inpatient Pav; **Address:** UCH-Neurology Clinic, Anschutz Outpatient Pavilion, 1635 N Aurora Ct, Ste 4200, MS F727, Aurora, CO 80045; **Phone:** 720-848-2080; **Board Cert:** Neurology 1970; **Med School:** Univ MD Sch Med 1963; **Resid:** Neurology, Univ Chicago Med Ctr 1967; **Fellow:** Neurovirology, Johns Hopkins Hosp 1971; **Fac Appt:** Prof N, Univ Colorado

Kelly, James P MD [N] - **Spec Exp:** Brain Injury; Memory Disorders; Neurologic Rehabilitation; Brain Injury-Traumatic; **Hospital:** Univ of CO Hosp - Anschutz Inpatient Pav; **Address:** Univ Colorado, Dept Neur, Campus Box C-307, 12631 E 17th Ave, Aurora, CO 80045; **Phone:** 720-848-2080; **Board Cert:** Neurology 1991; **Med School:** Northwestern Univ 1983; **Resid:** Neurology, Univ Colorado Med Ctr 1988; **Fellow:** Behavioral Neurology, Univ Colorado Med Ctr 1989; **Fac Appt:** Prof N, Univ Colorado

Neurology

Lane, Judy C MD [N] - **Spec Exp:** Headache; Migraine; **Hospital:** Swedish Med Ctr - Denver; **Address:** CNI Head Pain Ctr, 3601 S Clarkson St, Ste 210, Englewood, CO 80113; **Phone:** 303-781-5505; **Board Cert:** Neurology 1993; Headache Medicine ; **Med School:** Univ Colorado 1987; **Resid:** Neurology, Univ N Carolina Med Ctr 1991; **Fellow:** Neurological Rehabilitation, Rocky Mountain Mult Sclerosis Ctr 1992; **Fac Appt:** Assoc Prof FMed, Univ Colorado

Pulst, Stefan M MD [N] - **Spec Exp:** Parkinson's Disease; Multiple Sclerosis; **Hospital:** Univ Utah Hlth Care; **Address:** University of Utah, Clinical Neurosciences Ctr, 175 North Medical Drive E, Salt Lake City, UT 84132; **Phone:** 801-585-6387; **Board Cert:** Neurology 1990; **Med School:** Germany 1979; **Resid:** Neurology, Hannover Med Sch 1983; Neurology, Longwood/Harvard Program; **Fellow:** Neurological Biology, UCSF Med Ctr; **Fac Appt:** Prof Med, Univ Utah

Ringel, Steven P MD [N] - **Spec Exp:** Neuromuscular Disorders; **Hospital:** Univ of CO Hosp - Anschutz Inpatient Pav; **Address:** Univ Colorado Hosp, Neuromuscular Dept, 12631 E 17th Ave, Box B185, Aurora, CO 80045; **Phone:** 303-724-2209; **Board Cert:** Neurology 1974; **Med School:** Univ Mich Med Sch 1968; **Resid:** Neurology, Rush-Presby-St Lukes Med Ctr 1972; **Fellow:** Neurology, Natl Inst Neuro Dis-NIH 1976; **Fac Appt:** Prof N, Univ Colorado

Sabo, Tonia M MD [N] - **Spec Exp:** Headache; Migraine; **Hospital:** Children's Hosp - Denver; **Address:** Migraine Headache Ctr, 340 E 1st Ave, Ste 205, Broomfield, CO 80020; **Phone:** 303-439-7777; **Board Cert:** Child Neurology 2009; Headache Medicine ; **Med School:** Bangladesh 1995; **Resid:** Child Neurology, Univ Colorado Hlth Sci Ctr 1998

Strom, Laura A MD [N] - **Spec Exp:** Epilepsy/Seizure Disorders; Sleep Disorders; **Hospital:** Univ of CO Hosp - Anschutz Inpatient Pav; **Address:** UCH-Neurology Clinic, Anschutz Outpatient Pavilion, 1635 N Aurora Ct, Ste 4200, MS F727, Aurora, CO 80045; **Phone:** 720-848-2080; **Board Cert:** Neurology 2007; **Med School:** Penn State Coll Med 1997; **Resid:** Neurology, Univ CO Hlth Sci Ctr 2002; **Fellow:** Epilepsy, Univ CO Hlth Sci Ctr 2004; **Fac Appt:** Asst Prof N, Univ Colorado

Vollmer, Timothy L MD [N] - **Spec Exp:** Multiple Sclerosis; Myasthenia Gravis; Vasculitis of the Nervous System; Stroke; **Hospital:** Univ of CO Hosp - Anschutz Inpatient Pav; **Address:** Univ Colorado Dept Neurology, MS B-185, 12631 E 17th Ave, Aurora, CO 80045; **Phone:** 720-848-2080; **Board Cert:** Neurology 1991; **Med School:** Stanford Univ 1983; **Resid:** Neurology, Stanford Univ Hosp 1987; **Fellow:** Neurological Immunology, Stanford Univ 1986; **Fac Appt:** Prof N, Univ Colorado

Southwest

Ahern, Geoffrey L MD/PhD [N] - **Spec Exp:** Behavioral Neurology; Dementia; Alzheimer's Disease; **Hospital:** Univ Arizona Med Ctr-Univ Campus; **Address:** Univ Arizona, Dept Neurology, 1501 N Campbell Ave, rm 7319, PO Box 245023, Tucson, AZ 85724; **Phone:** 520-626-6524; **Board Cert:** Neurology 1992; Behavioral Neurology & Neuropsychiatry 2006; **Med School:** Yale Univ 1984; **Resid:** Neurology, Boston Univ Affil Hosps 1988; **Fellow:** Behavioral Neurology, Beth Israel Hosp 1990; **Fac Appt:** Prof N, Univ Ariz Coll Med

Couch Jr, James R MD/PhD [N] - **Spec Exp:** Headache; Stroke; Neuro-Rehabilitation; Tourette's Syndrome; **Hospital:** OU Med Ctr, VA Med Ctr - Oklahoma City; **Address:** 711 Stanton L Young Blvd, Ste 210, Oklahoma City, OK 73104-5021; **Phone:** 405-271-3635; **Board Cert:** Neurology 1974; Clinical Neurophysiology 2002; Headache Medicine 2006; **Med School:** Baylor Coll Med 1965; **Resid:** Neurology, Washington Univ Med Ctr 1972; **Fellow:** Neuropharmacology, Natl Inst Hlth 1969; **Fac Appt:** Prof N, Univ Okla Coll Med

Coull, Bruce M MD [N] - **Spec Exp:** Stroke; **Hospital:** Univ Ariz Med Ctr-South Campus (Kino); **Address:** Univ of Arizona-Neurology, 2800 E Ajo Way UPH Clinic Bldg, Tucson, AZ 85713; **Phone:** 520-874-2700; **Board Cert:** Neurology 1979; Vascular Neurology 2005; **Med School:** Univ Pittsburgh 1972; **Resid:** Neurology, Stanford Univ Med Ctr 1976; **Fellow:** Vascular Neurology, Stanford Univ Med Ctr 1978; **Fac Appt:** Prof N, Univ Ariz Coll Med

Dodick, David W MD [N] - **Spec Exp:** Headache; Migraine; **Hospital:** Mayo Clinic - Phoenix, Mayo Clinic - Scottsdale; **Address:** Mayo Clinic-Neurology Dept, 5777 E Mayo Blvd, 5e, Phoenix, AZ 85054; **Phone:** 480-342-3078; **Board Cert:** Neurology 2006; Vascular Neurology 2005; Headache Medicine 2006; **Med School:** Dalhousie Univ 1990; **Resid:** Neurology, Mayo Clinic 1994; **Fellow:** Headache, Univ Toronto 1996; **Fac Appt:** Prof N, Mayo Med Sch

Doody, Rachelle S MD/PhD [N] - **Spec Exp:** Alzheimer's Disease; Memory Disorders; **Hospital:** Methodist Hosp - Houston; **Address:** Alzheimer's & Memory Disorder Ctr, Dept of Neurology, Medical Bldg, 1977 Butler Blvd, Ste E5.101, Houston, TX 77030; **Phone:** 713-798-4734; **Board Cert:** Neurology 1988; **Med School:** Baylor Coll Med 1983; **Resid:** Neurology, Baylor Affil Hosp 1987; **Fac Appt:** Prof N, Baylor Coll Med

Ferrendelli, James A MD [N] - **Spec Exp:** Epilepsy/Seizure Disorders; Geriatric Neurology; **Hospital:** Meml Hermann Hosp - Texas Med Ctr; **Address:** UT Neurology Physician Practice, 6410 Fannin St UTHSC Bldg - Ste 1014, Houston, TX 77030; **Phone:** 832-325-7080; **Board Cert:** Neurology 1973; **Med School:** Univ Colorado 1962; **Resid:** Neurology, Cleveland Metro Genl Hosp 1968; **Fellow:** Neuropharmacology, Washington Univ Med Sch 1971; **Fac Appt:** Prof N, Univ Tex, Houston

Frohman, Elliot M MD [N] - **Spec Exp:** Multiple Sclerosis; Neuro-Ophthalmology; **Hospital:** UT Southwestern Med Ctr at Dallas, Parkland Hlth & Hosp Sys; **Address:** UT Southwestern Med Ctr, Dept of Neurology, 5323 Harry Hines Blvd, Dallas, TX 75390-8829; **Phone:** 214-645-8800; **Board Cert:** Neurology 2005; **Med School:** UC Irvine 1990; **Resid:** Neurology, Johns Hopkins Hosp 1994; **Fellow:** Neuro-Ophthalmology, Johns Hopkins Hosp 1995; **Fac Appt:** Assoc Prof N, Univ Tex SW, Dallas

Gilbert, Mark R MD [N] - **Spec Exp:** Brain Tumors; Neuro-Oncology; **Hospital:** UT MD Anderson Cancer Ctr; **Address:** Univ Tex MD Anderson Cancer Ctr, 1515 Holcombe Blvd, Unit 431, Houston, TX 77030; **Phone:** 713-792-4008; **Board Cert:** Internal Medicine 1985; Neurology 1990; **Med School:** Johns Hopkins Univ 1982; **Resid:** Internal Medicine, Johns Hopkins Hosp 1985; Neurology, Johns Hopkins Hosp 1988; **Fellow:** Neuro-Oncology, Johns Hopkins Hosp 1988; **Fac Appt:** Assoc Prof N, Univ Tex, Houston

Grotta, James C MD [N] - **Spec Exp:** Stroke; **Hospital:** Meml Hermann Hosp - Texas Med Ctr; **Address:** UT Neurology Physician Practice, 6410 Fannin St UTHSC Bldg - Ste 1014, Houston, TX 77030; **Phone:** 832-325-7080; **Board Cert:** Neurology 1978; Vascular Neurology 2005; **Med School:** Univ VA Sch Med 1971; **Resid:** Neurology, Univ Colorado Affil Hosp 1977; **Fellow:** Diagnostic Radiology, Mass Genl Hosp 1979; **Fac Appt:** Prof N, Univ Tex, Houston

Harati, Yadollah MD [N] - **Spec Exp:** Neuromuscular Disorders; Amyotrophic Lateral Sclerosis (ALS); Myasthenia Gravis; **Hospital:** St. Luke's Episcopal Hosp-Houston; **Address:** Baylor Neurology, Smith Tower, 6550 Fannin St, Ste 1801, Houston, TX 77030; **Phone:** 713-798-7411; **Board Cert:** Neurology 1978; Neuromuscular Medicine 2011; **Med School:** Iran 1970; **Resid:** Neurology, Univ Nebraska Med Ctr 1974; Neurology, Baylor Affil Hosp 1975; **Fellow:** Neuromuscular Disease, Baylor 1976; **Fac Appt:** Prof N, Baylor Coll Med

Jankovic, Joseph MD [N] - **Spec Exp:** Movement Disorders; Parkinson's Disease; Tourette's Syndrome; **Hospital:** Methodist Hosp - Houston; **Address:** Parkinson Disease Ctr, 6550 Fannin St, Smith Tower, Ste 1801, Houston, TX 77030; **Phone:** 713-798-5998; **Board Cert:** Neurology 1979; **Med School:** Univ Ariz Coll Med 1973; **Resid:** Neurology, Columbia-Presby Med Ctr 1977; **Fac Appt:** Prof N, Baylor Coll Med

Kent, Thomas A MD [N] - **Spec Exp:** Stroke; Neuro-Psychiatry; **Hospital:** DeBakey VA Med Ctr-Houston; **Address:** 2002 Holcombe Blvd, MC 127, Houston, TX 77030; **Phone:** 713-794-7393; **Board Cert:** Psychiatry 1993; Neurology 2006; **Med School:** Univ Kansas 1979; **Resid:** Psychiatry, Univ Kansas Affil Hosp 1983; Neurology, Univ Texas Affil Hosp 1985; **Fellow:** Psychopharmacology, Univ Kansas Affil Hosp 1983; **Fac Appt:** Prof N, Baylor Coll Med

Labiner, David M MD [N] - **Spec Exp:** Epilepsy; Seizure Disorders; **Hospital:** Univ Arizona Med Ctr-Univ Campus, Yuma Regl Med Ctr; **Address:** 707 N Alvernon Way, Tucson, AZ 85711; **Phone:** 520-626-2006; **Board Cert:** Neurology 1992; **Med School:** Med Coll GA 1984; **Resid:** Neurology, Neuro Inst/Columbia 1988; **Fellow:** Epilepsy, Duke Univ Med Ctr 1989; **Fac Appt:** Prof N, Univ Ariz Coll Med

Nicholl, Jeffrey S MD [N] - **Spec Exp:** Seizure Disorders; Epilepsy; **Hospital:** Tulane Med Ctr; **Address:** Tulane Dept Neurology, 1430 Tulane Ave, Ste 8065, New Orleans, LA 70112; **Phone:** 504-988-2241; **Board Cert:** Neurology 2009; Psychiatry 2011; Clinical Neurophysiology 2011; Emergency Medicine 2004; **Med School:** Georgetown Univ 1974; **Resid:** Psychiatry, UCLA Neuro Psyc Inst 1979; Neurology, Tulane Univ 1997; **Fellow:** Clinical Neurophysiology, Tulane Univ 1998; Epilepsy, UCLA 2000; **Fac Appt:** Assoc Prof N, Tulane Univ

Oommen, Kalarickal J MD [N] - **Spec Exp:** Epilepsy; **Hospital:** Univ Med Ctr-Lubbock, Covenant Med Ctr; **Address:** 3506 21st St, Ste 400, Lubbock, TX 79410; **Phone:** 806-725-4115; **Board Cert:** Neurology 1983; **Med School:** India 1973; **Resid:** Psychiatry, Arizona Hlth Sci Ctr 1979; Neurology, Arizona Hlth Sci Ctr 1982; **Fellow:** Electroencephalography, Med Coll Georgia 1983; **Fac Appt:** Prof N, Texas Tech Univ

Patchell, Roy A MD [N] - **Spec Exp:** Neuro-Oncology; Brain Tumors; Spinal Tumors; **Hospital:** St. Joseph's Hosp & Med Ctr - Phoenix; **Address:** Barrow Neurology Clinics, 500 W Thomas Rd, Ste 300, Phoenix, AZ 85013-4409; **Phone:** 602-406-2616; **Board Cert:** Neurology 1984; **Med School:** Univ KY Coll Med 1979; **Resid:** Neurology, Johns Hopkins Hosp 1983; **Fellow:** Neuro-Oncology, Meml Sloan-Kettering Canc Ctr 1985; **Fac Appt:** Prof N, Univ KY Coll Med

Shapiro, William R MD/PhD [N] - **Spec Exp:** Neuro-Oncology; **Hospital:** St. Joseph's Hosp & Med Ctr - Phoenix; **Address:** Barrow Neurological Institute, 500 W Thomas Rd, Ste 300, Phoenix, AZ 85013; **Phone:** 602-406-6262; **Board Cert:** Neurology 1969; **Med School:** UCSF 1961; **Resid:** Neurology, NY Hosp-Cornell Med Ctr 1966; **Fellow:** Neuro-Oncology, Natl Inst Health 1969; **Fac Appt:** Prof N, Univ Ariz Coll Med

Sheikh, Kazim A MD [N] - **Spec Exp:** Amyotrophic Lateral Sclerosis (ALS); Peripheral Nerve Disorders; Neuromuscular Disorders; **Hospital:** Meml Hermann Hosp - Texas Med Ctr; **Address:** UT Physicians-Neuromuscular Program, 6410 Fannin St, Ste 1014, Houston, TX 77030; **Phone:** 713-500-7100; **Board Cert:** Neurology 1998; **Med School:** Pakistan 1987; **Resid:** Neurology, Mayo Hosp 1991; Neurology, Neuro Inst/Columbia 1996; **Fellow:** Peripheral Nerve Disorders, Johns Hopkins 1997; **Fac Appt:** Prof N, Univ Tex, Houston

Suarez, Jose MD [N] - **Spec Exp:** Stroke; Critical Care; **Hospital:** St. Luke's Episcopal Hosp-Houston; **Address:** Baylor Neurology, Smith Tower, 6550 Fannin St, Ste 1801, Houston, TX 77030; **Phone:** 713-798-7411; **Board Cert:** Neurology 2008; Vascular Neurology 2005; **Med School:** Colombia 1988; **Resid:** Neurology, Univ Hosp 1996; **Fellow:** Neurocritical Care, Johns Hopkins Univ 1998; **Fac Appt:** Assoc Prof N, Baylor Coll Med

Wolinsky, Jerry S MD [N] - **Spec Exp:** Multiple Sclerosis; Clinical Trials; **Hospital:** Meml Hermann Hosp - Texas Med Ctr; **Address:** 6410 Fannin St, Fl 10, Houston, TX 77030-1503; **Phone:** 832-325-7080; **Board Cert:** Neurology 1975; **Med School:** Univ IL Coll Med 1969; **Resid:** Neurology, UCSF Med Ctr 1973; **Fellow:** Neuropathology, VA Hosp 1975; **Fac Appt:** Prof N, Univ Tex, Houston

Yung, WK Alfred MD [N] - **Spec Exp:** Neuro-Oncology; Brain Tumors; **Hospital:** UT MD Anderson Cancer Ctr; **Address:** 1515 Holcombe Blvd, Unit 431, Houston, TX 77030-4017; **Phone:** 713-794-1285; **Board Cert:** Neurology 1980; **Med School:** Univ Chicago-Pritzker Sch Med 1975; **Resid:** Neurology, UCSD Med Ctr 1978; **Fellow:** Neuro-Oncology, Meml Sloan Kettering Cancer Ctr 1981; **Fac Appt:** Prof N, Univ Tex, Houston

West Coast and Pacific

Adornato, Bruce T MD [N] - **Spec Exp:** Stroke; Peripheral Neuropathy; Sleep Disorders/Apnea; **Hospital:** Stanford Univ Hosp & Clinics, VA Hlth Care Sys - Palo Alto; **Address:** 326 Bryant St, Palo Alto, CA 94301; **Phone:** 650-324-4300; **Board Cert:** Internal Medicine 1975; Neurology 1978; **Med School:** UCSD 1972; **Resid:** Internal Medicine, UCSF-Moffitt Hosp 1974; Neurology, UCSF-Moffitt Hosp 1976; **Fellow:** Neurology, Natl Inst Hlth 1978; **Fac Appt:** Clin Prof N, Stanford Univ

Albers, Gregory W MD [N] - **Spec Exp:** Cerebrovascular Disease; Stroke; Clinical Trials; **Hospital:** Stanford Univ Hosp & Clinics; **Address:** Stanford Univ Med Ctr, Dept Neurology, 780 Welch Rd, Ste 205, Palo Alto, CA 94304; **Phone:** 650-723-4448; **Board Cert:** Neurology 1990; Vascular Neurology 2008; **Med School:** UCSD 1984; **Resid:** Neurology, Stanford Univ Med Ctr 1988; **Fellow:** Stroke, Stanford Univ Med Ctr 1989; **Fac Appt:** Prof N, Stanford Univ

Aminoff, Michael J MD [N] - **Spec Exp:** Movement Disorders; Parkinson's Disease; **Hospital:** UCSF Med Ctr; **Address:** 505 Parnassus Ave, rm M-795, San Francisco, CA 94143-0114; **Phone:** 415-353-2273; **Board Cert:** Neurology 2004; Clinical Neurophysiology 2000; **Med School:** England, UK 1965; **Resid:** Internal Medicine, Univ London Hosps 1970; Neurology, Middlesex Hosp/Natl Hosp Queen Sq 1972; **Fac Appt:** Prof N, UCSF

Becker, Kyra J MD [N] - **Spec Exp:** Stroke/Cerebrovascular Disease; Neuro-Immunology; Stroke-Young Adults; Critical Care; **Hospital:** Harborview Med Ctr; **Address:** Harborview Medical Ctr, Dept Neurology, 325 9th Ave, Box 359859, Seattle, WA 98104; **Phone:** 206-744-6285; **Board Cert:** Neurology 2006; Vascular Neurology 2005; **Med School:** Duke Univ 1989; **Resid:** Neurology, Johns Hopkins Hosp 1993; **Fellow:** Critical Care Neurology, Johns Hopkins Hosp 1995; Research, NIH-NINDS 1996; **Fac Appt:** Assoc Prof N, Univ Wash

Bruno, Michiko K MD [N] - **Spec Exp:** Movement Disorders; Parkinson's Disease; Tourette's Syndrome; **Hospital:** Queen's Med Ctr - Honolulu; **Address:** Queens Physicians Office, 1380 Lusitana St, Ste 705, Honolulu, HI 96813; **Phone:** 808-537-9105; **Board Cert:** Neurology 2003; **Med School:** Japan 1996; **Resid:** Neurology, NY Presby-Cornell Med Ctr 2002; **Fellow:** Movement Disorders, Natl Inst Hlth 2004

Chamberlain, Marc C MD [N] - **Spec Exp:** Brain Tumors; Neuro-Oncology; Clinical Trials; **Hospital:** Univ Wash Med Ctr; **Address:** Seattle Cancer Care Alliance, 825 Eastlake Ave E, POB 10923, MS G4940, Seattle, WA 98109-1023; **Phone:** 206-288-8280; **Board Cert:** Pediatrics 1985; Child Neurology 1989; **Med School:** Columbia P&S 1977; **Resid:** Pediatrics, Montefiore Med Ctr 1981; Neurology, UCLA Med Ctr 1983; **Fellow:** Neuro-Oncology, UCSF Med Ctr 1986; **Fac Appt:** Prof N, Univ Wash

Charles, Andrew C MD [N] - **Spec Exp:** Headache; Migraine; **Hospital:** UCLA Ronald Reagan Med Ctr; **Address:** UCLA Neurological Svcs, 300 UCLA Medical Plaza, Ste B200, Los Angeles, CA 90095; **Phone:** 310-794-1195; **Board Cert:** Neurology 1992; **Med School:** UCLA 1986; **Resid:** Neurology, UCLA Med Ctr 1990; **Fellow:** Neurology, UCLA 1992; **Fac Appt:** Prof N, UCLA

Chui, Helena C MD [N] - **Spec Exp:** Stroke; Dementia; Alzheimer's Disease; **Hospital:** Keck Med Ctr of USC (page 62), Rancho Los Amigos Natl Rehab Ctr; **Address:** USC Dept Neurology, 1520 San Pablo St, Ste 3000, Los Angeles, CA 90033; **Phone:** 323-442-7591; **Board Cert:** Neurology 1984; **Med School:** Johns Hopkins Univ 1977; **Resid:** Neurology, Univ Iowa Med Ctr 1981; **Fellow:** Behavioral Neurology, Univ Iowa Med Ctr 1979; **Fac Appt:** Prof N, USC Sch Med

Cloughesy, Timothy F MD [N] - **Spec Exp:** Neuro-Oncology; Seizure Disorders; Brain Tumors; **Hospital:** UCLA Ronald Reagan Med Ctr; **Address:** 710 Westwood Plaza, Ste 1230, Los Angeles, CA 90095; **Phone:** 310-825-9113; **Board Cert:** Neurology 1993; **Med School:** Tulane Univ 1987; **Resid:** Neurology, UCLA Med Ctr 1991; **Fellow:** Neuro-Oncology, Meml Sloan-Kettering Canc Ctr; **Fac Appt:** Clin Prof N, UCLA

Corey-Bloom, Jody MD/PhD [N] - **Spec Exp:** Multiple Sclerosis; **Hospital:** UCSD Med Ctr; **Address:** 8950 Villa La Jolla Drive, Ste C129, La Jolla, CA 92037-0973; **Phone:** 858-657-8540; **Board Cert:** Neurology 1993; **Med School:** UCSD 1986; **Resid:** Neurology, UCSD Med Ctr 1990; **Fellow:** Neurology, UCSD Med Ctr 1992; **Fac Appt:** Prof N, UCSD

Cummings, Jeffrey Lee MD [N] - **Spec Exp:** Neuro-Psychiatry; Alzheimer's Disease; Clinical Trials; **Hospital:** Cleveland Clin (page 55); **Address:** Cleveland Clinic Nevada, Lou Ruvo Ctr for Brain Health, 888 W Bonneville Ave, Las Vegas, NV 89106; **Phone:** 702-483-6000; **Board Cert:** Neurology 1979; **Med School:** Univ Wash 1974; **Resid:** Neurology, Boston Univ Sch Med 1978; **Fellow:** Behavioral Neurology and Psychiatry, Boston Univ Sch Med 1979; Neurological Pathology, The Natl Hosp 1980

DeGiorgio, Christopher M MD [N] - **Spec Exp:** Epilepsy; Seizure Disorders; **Hospital:** UCLA Ronald Reagan Med Ctr; **Address:** UCLA Neurological Svcs, 300 UCLA Medical Plaza, rm B200, Los Angeles, CA 90095; **Phone:** 310-794-1195; **Board Cert:** Neurology 1987; **Med School:** Loyola Univ-Stritch Sch Med 1981; **Resid:** Neurology, Wadsworth VA Hosp 1985; **Fellow:** Epilepsy, UCLA 1987; **Fac Appt:** Prof N, UCLA

Engel, William King MD [N] - **Spec Exp:** Neuromuscular Disorders; Peripheral Neuropathy; Amyotrophic Lateral Sclerosis (ALS); Myasthenia Gravis; **Hospital:** Good Samaritan Hosp - LA, Keck Med Ctr of USC (page 62); **Address:** 637 S Lucas Ave Fl 3, Los Angeles, CA 90017; **Phone:** 213-975-9950; **Board Cert:** Neurology 1962; **Med School:** McGill Univ 1955; **Resid:** Neurology, Natl Inst Hlth 1959; Neurology, Natl Hosp 1960; **Fellow:** Neuromuscular Medicine, Natl Inst Hlth 1961; **Fac Appt:** Prof N, USC Sch Med

Engstrom, John W MD [N] - **Spec Exp:** Peripheral Neuropathy; Spinal Cord Disorders; **Hospital:** UCSF Med Ctr; **Address:** UCSF Med Ctr, Dept Neurology, 400 Parnassus Ave Fl 8, Box 0348, San Francisco, CA 94143; **Phone:** 415-353-2273; **Board Cert:** Internal Medicine 1984; Neurology 1991; Clinical Neurophysiology 2002; **Med School:** Stanford Univ 1981; **Resid:** Internal Medicine, Johns Hopkins Hosp 1984; Neurology, UCSF Med Ctr 1988; **Fellow:** Neurology, UCSF Med Ctr 1989; **Fac Appt:** Prof N, UCSF

Fisher, Mark Jay MD [N] - **Spec Exp:** Stroke; Cerebrovascular Disease; **Hospital:** UC Irvine Med Ctr, VA Long Beach Hlthcare Sys; **Address:** UC Irvine Med Ctr, Dept Neurology, 101 The City Drive S, Shanbrom Hall, rm 121, Orange, CA 92868; **Phone:** 714-456-6856; **Board Cert:** Neurology 1981; Vascular Neurology 2005; **Med School:** Univ Cincinnati 1975; **Resid:** Neurology, UCLA-Wadsworth VA Hosp 1980; **Fac Appt:** Prof N, UC Irvine

Fisher, Robert S MD [N] - **Spec Exp:** Epilepsy/Seizure Disorders; **Hospital:** Stanford Univ Hosp & Clinics; **Address:** Stanford Univ Dept Neurology, 300 Pasteur Drive, rm A-343, Stanford, CA 94305-5235; **Phone:** 650-498-3056; **Board Cert:** Neurology 1983; Clinical Neurophysiology 2002; **Med School:** Stanford Univ 1977; **Resid:** Internal Medicine, Stanford Univ 1979; **Fellow:** Neurology, Johns Hopkins Univ 1982; **Fac Appt:** Prof N, Stanford Univ

Goodin, Douglas S MD [N] - **Spec Exp:** Multiple Sclerosis; **Hospital:** UCSF Med Ctr, VA Med Ctr - San Francisco; **Address:** UCSF Multiple Sclerosis Ctr, 400 Parnassus Ave Fl 8, San Francisco, CA 94143; **Phone:** 415-353-2069; **Board Cert:** Neurology 1985; **Med School:** UC Irvine 1978; **Resid:** Neurology, UCSF Med Ctr 1981; **Fac Appt:** Clin Prof N, UCSF

Graves, Michael C MD [N] - **Spec Exp:** Amyotrophic Lateral Sclerosis (ALS); Electromyography; Guillain-Barre Syndrome; Muscular Dystrophy; **Hospital:** UCLA Ronald Reagan Med Ctr; **Address:** UCLA Neurological Svcs, 300 Medical Plaza, Ste B200, Box 956975, Los Angeles, CA 90095-6975; **Phone:** 310-794-1195; **Board Cert:** Neurology 1977; **Med School:** Stanford Univ 1970; **Resid:** Internal Medicine, UCSD Med Ctr 1972; Neurology, Johns Hopkins Hosp 1975; **Fellow:** Rockefeller Univ; **Fac Appt:** Assoc Prof N, UCLA

Guilleminault, Christian MD [N] - **Spec Exp:** Sleep Disorders/Apnea; **Hospital:** Stanford Univ Hosp & Clinics; **Address:** Stanford Sleep Medicine Center, 450 Broadway St, Pavilion B, Redwood City, CA 94063-5704; **Phone:** 650-723-6601; **Med School:** France 1962; **Resid:** Neurology, Hospital Foch 1966; Hosp de la Salpetriere 1968; **Fellow:** Univ Geneva 1967; **Fac Appt:** Prof Psyc, Stanford Univ

Hauser, Stephen L MD [N] - **Spec Exp:** Multiple Sclerosis; **Hospital:** UCSF Med Ctr; **Address:** UCSF Multiple Sclerosis Center, 400 Parnassus Ave, 8th Fl, San Francisco, CA 94143; **Phone:** 415-353-2069; **Board Cert:** Internal Medicine 1978; Neurology 1981; **Med School:** Harvard Med Sch 1975; **Resid:** Internal Medicine, NY Presby-Cornell 1977; Neurology, Mass Genl Hosp 1980; **Fellow:** Neurology, Harvard Univ 1980; **Fac Appt:** Prof N, UCSF

Heck, Christianne N MD [N] - **Spec Exp:** Epilepsy; **Hospital:** Keck Med Ctr of USC (page 62); **Address:** Neurologic Care & Research Ctr, 1520 San Pablo St, Ste 3000, Los Angeles, CA 90033; **Phone:** 323-442-5710; **Board Cert:** Neurology 2011; **Med School:** USC-Keck School of Medicine 1991; **Resid:** Neurology, LAC/USC Med Ctr 1995; **Fellow:** Epilepsy, USC Med Ctr 1996; **Fac Appt:** Assoc Prof N, USC-Keck School of Medicine

Henderson, Victor W MD [N] - **Spec Exp:** Alzheimer's Disease; Dementia; Memory Disorders; **Hospital:** Stanford Univ Hosp & Clinics; **Address:** Stanford Univ Med Ctr, Neurology, 300 Pasteur Drive, Ste A301, MC 5325, Stanford, CA 94305-5405; **Phone:** 650-723-6469; **Board Cert:** Neurology 1981; **Med School:** Johns Hopkins Univ 1976; **Resid:** Internal Medicine, Duke Univ Med Ctr 1977; Neurology, Barnes Hosp- Wash Univ 1980; **Fellow:** Behavioral Neurology, Aphasia Rsch Ctr-Boston Univ 1981; **Fac Appt:** Prof N, Stanford Univ

Langston, J William MD [N] - **Spec Exp:** Parkinson's Disease; Movement Disorders; Tremor; **Hospital:** Parkinson's Inst/Movement Disorders Trmt Ctr, The; **Address:** The Parkinsons Inst, 675 Almanor Ave, Sunnyvale, CA 94085; **Phone:** 408-542-5633; **Board Cert:** Neurology 1986; **Med School:** Univ MO-Columbia Sch Med 1967; **Resid:** Neurology, Stanford Univ 1974; **Fellow:** Electroencephalography, Stanford Univ 1974

Lew, Mark F MD [N] - **Spec Exp:** Movement Disorders; Parkinson's Disease; Dystonia; **Hospital:** Keck Med Ctr of USC (page 62); **Address:** USC Consultation Center, 1520 San Pablo St, Ste 3000, Los Angeles, CA 90033; **Phone:** 323-442-5817; **Board Cert:** Neurology 1993; **Med School:** Geo Wash Univ 1987; **Resid:** Neurology, USC-LAC Med Ctr 1991; **Fellow:** Movement Disorders, USC-LAC Med Ctr 1992; **Fac Appt:** Prof N, USC Sch Med

Longo, Frank M MD/PhD [N] - **Spec Exp:** Alzheimer's Disease; Huntington's Disease; **Hospital:** Stanford Univ Hosp & Clinics, UCSF Med Ctr; **Address:** Stanford Univ Med Ctr, Neurology, 300 Pasteur Drive, MC 5235, H3160, Stanford, CA 94305; **Phone:** 650-723-6469; **Board Cert:** Neurology 1981; **Med School:** UCSD 1981; **Resid:** Neurology, UCSF Med Ctr 1987; **Fellow:** Neurology, UCSF Med Ctr 1989; **Fac Appt:** Prof N, Stanford Univ

Lutsep, Helmi L MD [N] - **Spec Exp:** Stroke/Cerebrovascular Disease; Stroke Prevention; **Hospital:** OR Hlth & Sci Univ; **Address:** Oregon Stroke Ctr, OHSU, 3181 SW Sam Jackson Park Rd, MC CR131, Portland, OR 97239; **Phone:** 503-494-7225; **Board Cert:** Neurology 1994; Vascular Neurology 2005; **Med School:** Mayo Med Sch 1988; **Resid:** Neurology, Mayo Clinic 1992; **Fellow:** Behavioral Neurology, UC Davis Med Ctr 1995; Stroke, Stanford Univ Med Ctr 1996; **Fac Appt:** Prof N, Oregon Hlth & Sci Univ

Morrell, Martha J MD [N] - **Spec Exp:** Epilepsy; Epilepsy in Women; **Hospital:** Stanford Univ Hosp & Clinics; **Address:** Stanford Univ Dept Neurology, 300 Pasteur Drive, rm A-301, Stanford, CA 94305; **Phone:** 650-498-7551; **Board Cert:** Neurology 1989; Clinical Neurophysiology 2003; **Med School:** Stanford Univ 1984; **Resid:** Neurology, Hosp Univ Penn 1988; **Fellow:** Epilepsy, Graduate Hosp-Univ Penn 1990; **Fac Appt:** Clin Prof N, Stanford Univ

Nutt Jr, John G MD [N] - **Spec Exp:** Parkinson's Disease; Movement Disorders; **Hospital:** OR Hlth & Sci Univ; **Address:** Parkinson's Ctr of Oregon, 3181 SW Sam Jackson Park Rd, MC OP32, Portland, OR 97239; **Phone:** 503-494-7230; **Board Cert:** Neurology 1978; **Med School:** Baylor Coll Med 1970; **Resid:** Neurology, Univ Wash Med Ctr 1976; **Fellow:** Pharmacology, Natl Inst Neuro Disorders /Stroke 1978; **Fac Appt:** Prof N, Oregon Hlth & Sci Univ

Phuphanich, Surasak MD [N] - **Spec Exp:** Brain Tumors-Metastatic; Stem Cell Therapy; Spinal Tumors; Neurologic Complications of Cancer; **Hospital:** Cedars-Sinai Med Ctr; **Address:** 8631 W 3rd St, Ste 410E, Los Angeles, CA 90048; **Phone:** 310-423-4413; **Board Cert:** Neurology 1983; **Med School:** Thailand 1975; **Resid:** Neurology, Univ Illinois Med Ctr 1981; **Fellow:** Neuro-Oncology, UCSF Med Ctr 1984; **Fac Appt:** Prof Neuro-Onc

Rosenbaum, Richard B MD [N] - **Spec Exp:** Neuromuscular Disorders; Parkinson's Disease; **Hospital:** OR Hlth & Sci Univ, Providence Portland Med Ctr; **Address:** Oregon Clin, Dept Neurology, 5050 NE Hoyt St, Ste 315, Portland, OR 97213; **Phone:** 503-963-3100; **Board Cert:** Internal Medicine 1975; Neurology 1979; **Med School:** Harvard Med Sch 1971; **Resid:** Internal Medicine, Stanford Med Ctr 1973; Neurology, UCSF Med Ctr 1977; **Fac Appt:** Clin Prof N, Oregon Hlth & Sci Univ

Rothrock, John F MD [N] - **Spec Exp:** Headache; Migraine; Stroke; **Hospital:** Renown Reg Med Ctr; **Address:** 85 Kirman Ave, Ste 301, Reno, NV 89502; **Phone:** 775-982-2970; **Board Cert:** Neurology 1984; Vascular Neurology 2009; Headache Medicine 2009; **Med School:** Univ VA Sch Med 1977; **Resid:** Neurology, Univ Ariz Med Ctr 1981; **Fac Appt:** Prof N, Univ Alabama

Samii, Ali MD [N] - **Spec Exp:** Movement Disorders; Parkinson's Disease; Tremor & Dystonia; **Hospital:** Univ Wash Med Ctr; **Address:** UW Medical Center, Dept Neurology, 1959 NE Pacific St, Box 356169, Seattle, WA 98195; **Phone:** 206-598-7688; **Board Cert:** Neurology 2007; **Med School:** McGill Univ 1989; **Resid:** Neurology, UC Davis Med Ctr 1993; **Fellow:** Movement Disorders, NIH/Motor Control Sect 1996; Movement Disorders, Univ BC 1997; **Fac Appt:** Assoc Prof N, Univ Wash

Saver, Jeffrey L MD [N] - **Spec Exp:** Stroke; Stroke Prevention; **Hospital:** UCLA Ronald Reagan Med Ctr; **Address:** UCLA Stroke Ctr, 710 Westwood Plaza, rm 4126, Los Angeles, CA 90095; **Phone:** 310-794-6379; **Board Cert:** Neurology 1991; Vascular Neurology 2005; **Med School:** Harvard Med Sch 1986; **Resid:** Neurological Surgery, Brigham & Womens Hosp 1990; **Fellow:** Behavioral Neurology, Univ Iowa Hosps 1991; Cerebrovascular Disease, Rhode Island Hosp 1992; **Fac Appt:** Prof N, UCLA

Smith, Wade S MD/PhD [N] - **Spec Exp:** Stroke; Pain-Back & Shoulder; **Hospital:** UCSF Med Ctr; **Address:** UCSF Vascular Neurology, 400 Parnassus Ave Fl 8, Box 0114, San Francisco, CA 94143-0114; **Phone:** 415-353-1489; **Board Cert:** Neurology 2006; Vascular Neurology 2008; **Med School:** Univ Wash 1989; **Resid:** Neurology, UCSF-Moffitt Hosp 1993; **Fellow:** Critical Care Medicine, UCSF Med Ctr 1994; **Fac Appt:** Prof N, UCSF

Tanner, Caroline M MD/PhD [N] - **Spec Exp:** Parkinson's Disease; Movement Disorders; Dystonia; **Hospital:** Parkinson's Inst/Movement Disorders Trmt Ctr, The; **Address:** The Parkinson's Inst, 675 Almanor Ave, Sunnyvale, CA 94085; **Phone:** 408-734-2800; **Board Cert:** Neurology 1982; **Med School:** Loyola Univ-Stritch Sch Med 1976; **Resid:** Neurology, Rush-Presby-St Luke's Med Ctr 1980; **Fellow:** Neurological Pharmacology, Rush-Presby-St Luke's Med Ctr 1982

Tetrud, James W MD [N] - **Spec Exp:** Movement Disorders; Parkinson's Disease; Tremor; **Hospital:** Parkinson's Inst/Movement Disorders Trmt Ctr, The; **Address:** The Parkinson's Inst, 675 Almanor Ave, Sunnyvale, CA 94085; **Phone:** 408-734-2800; **Board Cert:** Neurology 1981; **Med School:** NYU Sch Med 1973; **Resid:** Internal Medicine, VA Med Ctr-West Los Angeles 1974; Neurology, VA Med Ctr-West Los Angeles 1978

Weiner, Leslie P MD [N] - **Spec Exp:** Multiple Sclerosis; Amyotrophic Lateral Sclerosis (ALS); **Hospital:** Keck Med Ctr of USC (page 62), LAC & USC Med Ctr; **Address:** USC Dept Neurology, 1520 San Pablo St, Ste 3000, Los Angeles, CA 90033; **Phone:** 323-442-5710; **Board Cert:** Neurology 1969; **Med School:** Univ Cincinnati 1961; **Resid:** Neurology, Baltimore City Hosp 1963; Neurology, Johns Hopkins Hosp 1965; **Fellow:** Neurology, Johns Hopkins Hosp 1969; **Fac Appt:** Prof N, USC Sch Med

Weiss, Michael D MD [N] - **Spec Exp:** Neuromuscular Disorders; Amyotrophic Lateral Sclerosis (ALS); Myasthenia Gravis; Peripheral Neuropathy; **Hospital:** Univ Wash Med Ctr; **Address:** Univ Wash Med Ctr SS 824, Box 356169, 1959 NE Pacific St, Seattle, WA 98195; **Phone:** 206-598-7688; **Board Cert:** Neurology 2006; Neuromuscular Medicine 2011; Electrodiagnostic Medicine 2011; **Med School:** Albert Einstein Coll Med 1991; **Resid:** Neurology, Georgetown Univ Hosp 1996; **Fellow:** Neurology, Univ Maryland 1997; Neuromuscular Disease, Natl Inst Hlth 1999; **Fac Appt:** Assoc Prof N, Univ Wash

Cleveland Clinic

Every life deserves world class care.

Cleveland Clinic
Neurological Institute
9500 Euclid Avenue
Cleveland, OH 44195

Neurology

Cleveland Clinic Neurological Institute employs a multidisciplinary disease-specific focus, combining more than 300 medical, surgical and research specialists who treat children and adults with neurological and neurobehavioral disorders. Our clinical expertise, academic achievement and innovative research has earned the Neurological Institute an international reputation for excellence. *U.S. News & World Report* recently ranked our neurology, neurosurgery and pediatric neurology/neurosurgery programs among the top 5 in the nation.

Our unique and collaborative clinical structure allows us to deliver coordinated, comprehensive and multidisciplinary care to our patients through more efficient treatment decision-making and consultation for complex cases. Major advances in the treatment of brain tumors, epilepsy, mood disorders, stroke, movement disorders, pain and spinal disorders are improving quality of life and survival for thousands of our patients. Our innovative model of medicine will speed research and advances in treatment, resulting in better clinical care and more rapid breakthroughs in the full range of neurological and behavioral disorders.

Comprehensive Neurological Care

Cleveland Clinic offers expert diagnostic and treatment options for all neurologic conditions affecting children and adults, including Alzheimer's disease, aneurysms, arteriovenous malformations, back and neck disorders, brain and spine tumors, epilepsy, hydrocephalus, metastatic tumors, mild cognitive impairment, multiple sclerosis, movement disorders, neurofibromatosis, Parkinson's disease, pediatric and congenital neurological disorders, pituitary disorders, sleep disorders and stroke.

Offering Same-Day Appointments
Call 800.274.2009.

Treatment Guides
Cleveland Clinic has developed comprehensive treatment guides for many diseases and conditions. To download our free treatment guides, visit clevelandclinic.org/treatmentguides.

Online Medical Second Opinion
Call 216.444.3223 or 800.223.2273 ext. 43223 or email eclevelandclinic@ccf.org.

Out-of-State Patients Assistance
Call 800.223.2273, ext. 55580 or email medicalconcierge@ccf.org.

Visit Us At:
clevelandclinic.org

Follow Us On:
Facebook
www.facebook.com/clevelandclinic

Twitter
@ClevelandClinic

You Tube
www.youtube.com/clevelandclinic

Health Hub
health.clevelandclinic.org

Neurology and Neurosurgery Expertise

800.420.4004

Continuum Health Partners, Inc.

The member hospitals of the Continuum Neurosciences consortium—St. Luke's and Roosevelt Hospitals and Beth Israel Medical Center—are home to many international leaders in neurology, neurosurgery, neuro-radiology and endovascular neurosurgery. Each of the hospitals has clinicians who are nationally and internationally recognized for their accomplishments and attract patients from throughout the United States and other countries who are looking for innovative treatment programs delivered by physicians specializing in both clinical care and research. Our expertise includes treatments for:

- Complex brain tumors, spine and spinal cord; chordomas, meningiomas, acoustic neuromas, trigeminal neuralgia and hemifacial spasms
- Headaches
- Disorders of the brain, spinal cord, peripheral nerves and muscles
- Stroke/cerebrovascular diseases
- Epilepsy and seizures
- Movement disorders (Parkinson's disease, dystonia and essential tremor)
- Neuro-ophthalmologic conditions
- Neuro-oncology-related illnesses
- Neuro-psychiatry/psychology-based conditions
- Many adult and pediatric neurologic conditions

A few of our Centers of Excellence include:

Beth Israel Medical Center

- The Alan and Barbara Mirken Department of Neurology
- Bachmann-Strauss Dystonia Center of Excellence
- National Parkinson Foundation Center of Excellence
- The Betty and Morton Yarmon Stroke Center
- Internationally respected divisions of adult and pediatric epilepsy
- ALS (Lou Gehrig's disease) Center sponsored by the ALS Association
- Adult Neurosurgery
- Pediatric Neurosurgery
- Peripheral Nerve Center

St. Luke's and Roosevelt Hospitals

- The Hyman-Newman Institute for Neurology and Neurosurgery
- Center for Endovascular Surgery
- The Vascular Birthmarks Institute
- Vascular Malformations Center of NY
- New York Brain Tumor Center
- The Headache Institute
- The Stroke Center
- Adult Neurosurgery
- Pediatric Neurosurgery

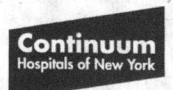

Beth Israel Medical Center
Beth Israel Brooklyn
Roosevelt Hospital
St. Luke's Hospital
NY Eye and Ear Infirmary

www.chpnyc.

MOUNT SINAI SCHOOL OF MEDICINE

THE MOUNT SINAI MEDICAL CENTER
NEUROLOGY

One Gustave L. Levy Place
Fifth Avenue and 100th Street
New York, NY 10029-6574
Physician Referral: 1-800-MD-SINAI (637-4624)
www.mountsinai.org/neurology

THE ESTELLE AND DANIEL MAGGIN DEPARTMENT OF NEUROLOGY at Mount Sinai provides compassionate, state-of-the-art, interdisciplinary care for disorders of the brain and nervous system. *US News World & Report* recently ranked Mount Sinai Neurology and Neurosurgery as a top program nationwide in recognition of our ability to care for patients with complex diseases of the nervous system.

The Robert and John M. Bendheim Parkinson and Movement Disorders Center is one of the world's leading multidisciplinary centers for clinical care and translational research aimed at Parkinson's disease, dystonia, tremor, and a variety of movement disorders. The Center incorporates a world-renowned deep-brain stimulation program, and is at the forefront in clinical trials and experimental therapeutics for movement disorders.

The Corinne Goldsmith Dickinson Center for Multiple Sclerosis is an internationally recognized comprehensive center, uniting the efforts of leading physicians and scientists from many disciplines to understand the causes and consequences of MS. The Center provides services in all aspects of diagnosis, disease management, rehabilitation, and patient support, and the opportunity for patients to participate in potentially groundbreaking clinical trials.

The Clinical Program for Cerebrovascular Disorders comprises an outstanding team of medical experts who specialize in the most advanced approaches in the evaluation, treatment, and rehabilitation of patients with cerebrovascular diseases. Services include the early diagnosis of stroke, a specialized Neurointensive Care Unit, and an advanced inpatient stroke unit. Physicians are available at all times for emergency consultation with referring physicians. The Stroke Center was the first JCAHO-certified primary stroke center in Manhattan.

The NeuroAIDS Program provides diagnosis and treatment for neurological disorders associated with HIV disease. This program is one of the few in the world to treat the various complications of the disease that affect the central and peripheral nervous systems in as many as 70 percent of patients.

The Epilepsy Center provides specific expertise in the diagnosis and treatment of epilepsy and related disorders. The Center encompasses outstanding epileptologists, a new modern inpatient epilepsy monitoring unit, and full outpatient EEG and diagnostic capabilities.

The Center for Headache and Pain Medicine is a multidisciplinary center for the diagnosis and treatment of chronic and acute headaches and other painful disorders of the skull, brain, or face in both adults and children. Specialists in neurology, pain medicine, ENT, ophthalmology, psychiatry, and rehabilitation medicine are available to evaluate and treat individuals with painful disorders.

The Division of Neuromuscular Diseases provides diagnosis, treatment, and compassionate care for patients with disorders in neuromuscular transmission, muscle diseases, peripheral nerve problems, and spasticity resulting from stroke or damage to the central nervous system.

The Center for Cognitive Health provides state-of-the-art diagnosis and treatment for memory disorders, dementias, traumatic brain injury and other cognitive disorders. Our multi-disciplinary team of neurologists, psychiatrists, neuro-psychiatrists, neuro-scientists and patient care managers bridge the brain related specialties to provide individualized comprehensive care.

Eye Movement and Vestibular Disorder Program provides outstanding diagnosis and treatment for problems, balance problems, and motion sickness. Our physicians participate in NASA programs, ...ing technology used to assess these disorders in space, and studying possible treatment applications

> **THE ESTELLE AND DANIEL MAGGIN DEPARTMENT OF NEUROLOGY** is renowned for its unique integration of outstanding patient care and cutting-edge research in neurological disease, and can bring the latest advances in treatment to our patients. Our physicians and neuroscientists have made enormous strides in basic and translational research, bringing medical breakthroughs that will change the course of neurological treatment. The department is led by some of the most prominent figures in American neurology, is #3 nationally in the number of academic neurologists trained in our residency program, and receives annual research grants of more than $20 million.

NewYork-Presbyterian
The University Hospital of Columbia and Cornell

Affiliated with Columbia University College of Physicians and Surgeons and Weill Cornell Medical College

NewYork-Presbyterian Hospital
Columbia University Medical Center
622 West 168th Street
New York, NY 10032

NewYork-Presbyterian Hospital
Weill Cornell Medical Center
525 East 68th Street
New York, NY 10065

1-877-NYP-WELL (1-877-697-9355) www.nyp.org/neuro

NewYork-Presbyterian Neuroscience

In 2012–2013, NewYork-Presbyterian's neurology and neurosurgery program was ranked 4th in the nation in the annual 'Best Hospitals' survey conducted by *U.S. News & World Report™*. Our Neuroscience Centers offer innovative treatments to improve the quality of life of patients with neurological disorders, including:

- **Stroke:** Our three comprehensive Stroke Center locations are among the few NYS designated primary stroke centers. Round-the-clock surveillance and state-of-the-art brain monitoring in our Neuro-ICU minimizes damage and maximizes the chance for a full recovery.
- **Epilepsy:** Comprehensive Epilepsy Centers use the latest monitoring and imaging tools to locate the source of a patient's seizures and tailor medical and/or surgical treatment.
- **Pediatric neurology/neurosurgery:** Specialists are sensitive to the special needs of children with epilepsy, brain tumors, stroke, craniofacial disorders, vascular anomalies, and movement disorders.
- **Spinal disorders:** Neurosurgeons, rehabilitation medicine physicians, physical therapists, pain management physicians, nurse practitioners, and neurologists personalize a plan of care for patients with neck and back pain and disorders such as scoliosis, disc disease, and compression fractures.
- **Brain and spinal tumors:** Neurosurgeons, neuro-oncologists, radiation oncologists, and others care for patients with brain and spinal tumors. Translational research programs aim to understand the biology of these diseases and develop innovative therapies.
- **Neuro-immune disorders:** Comprehensive care is delivered to patients with multiple sclerosis as well as less common diseases, such as Behcet's disease, sarcoidosis, and vasculitis.
- **Neuro-muscular disorders:** Our multidisciplinary team cares for people with neuromuscular diseases such as ALS (Lou Gehrig's Disease), Guillain-Barre syndrome, muscular dystrophy, myasthenia gravis, myopathy, and neuropathy.
- **Movement disorders:** NewYork-Presbyterian Hospital treats one of the world's largest populations of patients with movement disorders, especially Parkinson's disease. Researchers assess new drugs, imaging techniques, surgical therapies (such as deep brain stimulation), and gene therapy.
- **Memory disorders:** Our programs feature advanced care for patients with Alzheimer's disease or other memory disorders and their families, as well as clinical and laboratory research to better understand these disorders, with the goal of treating them sooner and more effectively.

Highlights:

- Researchers demonstrated that two genes associated with ALS work in tandem to support long-term survival of motor neurons.

- Neurologists, neurosurgeons, and radiologists collaborated to show that intensive medical therapy is more effective than stenting for preventing a second stroke.

- Investigators devised a computer model of the spread of dementia that can be used to predict future disease patterns years before they occur in a patient.

- NewYork-Presbyterian is participating in NeuroNEXT (Network for Excellence in Neuroscience Clinical Trials), an NIH-funded national effort to accelerate the development of therapies for people with neurological diseases.

- Neuro-oncologists are devising innovative approaches, such as the use of microcatheters, to bypass the blood-brain barrier and deliver chemotherapy directly to brain tumors.

550 First Avenue (*at 31st Street*)
New York, NY 10016
www.NYULMC.org
Physician Referral: **888-7-NYU-MED** (*888-769-8633*)

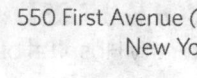

NEUROLOGY

NYU Langone Medical Center evaluates and treats adults and children with a broad spectrum of neurological diseases, including stroke, epilepsy, cerebrovascular diseases, behavioral disorders and dementia, brain tumors, genetic and degenerative diseases, nerve and muscle problems, headache and pain syndromes and movement disorders. We are home to the largest multiple sclerosis (MS) program in New York and were first primary Stroke Center in NYC.

Autonomic Diseases
Our specialized Center evaluates and treats children and adults with familial dysautonomia and other inherited or acquired autonomic nervous system diseases, including orthostatic hypotension and rare forms of hereditary sensory neuropathy.

Epilepsy
The Comprehensive Epilepsy Center offers the most advanced medical and surgical options. Complementary management approaches complete the comprehensive management plan.

Multiple Sclerosis
The Comprehensive MS Care Center provides state-of-the-art diagnostic evaluations and follow-up care as part of a comprehensive program.

Neurogenetics
We focus on inherited diseases of the nervous system. Services include diagnosis and management of inherited diseases, biochemical and molecular testing and genetic counseling.

Neuro-oncology
NYU Cancer Institute includes one of the nation's leading brain and spinal cord tumor programs, with physicians highly experienced in neuro-oncology, neurosurgery and neuroradiology.

Neuromuscular Diseases
We offer multidisciplinary programs for neuromuscular diseases, including acquired peripheral neuropathy, Charcot Marie Tooth neuropathy, myasthenia gravis, amyotrophic lateral sclerosis, spinal muscular atrophy, post-polio syndrome, muscular dystrophy and Lyme neuroborreliosis.

Parkinson's Disease and Movement Disorders
The Parkinson's disease and Movement Disorders Center helps individuals and families achieve the highest possible quality of life.

Stroke Care
The multidisciplinary Comprehensive Stroke Care Center provides rapid diagnosis, effective intervention and early rehabilitation from debilitating stroke.

The University of Pennsylvania's history of excellence in the treatment of neurological diseases dates back to the establishment of the Department of Neurology in 1874. *The Best Doctors in America®* lists more neurologists and neurosurgeons from the Hospital of the University of Pennsylvania than from any other hospital or medical center in the Philadelphia region. Penn Neurology and Neurosurgery at the Hospital of the University of Pennsylvania (HUP) are ranked 21st in the nation by *U.S. News & World Report*, the only neuroscience programs in the region to be recognized.

The Department of Neurology is a component of the **Penn Medicine Neuroscience Center**, which is dedicated to facilitating and strengthening the integration of Penn's world-class neuroscience programs within the areas of clinical care, research and education.

Excellence and Expertise

Recognized by the National Parkinson Foundation as one of its worldwide Centers of Excellence, the **Parkinson's Disease and Movement Disorders Center** is committed to providing exceptional patient care, education, and social support services. Research is an important and ongoing mission of the Center, which actively pursues the investigation of the disease as well as exploration of new medications.

The Multiple Sclerosis Center Program provides comprehensive evaluation, diagnosis and treatment for patients with MS and other demyelinating disorders of the central nervous system. In addition to maintaining the highest standards for clinical service, the Penn MS program is a leader in MS training and in clinical and laboratory-based research.

The Penn Neuro-Ophthalmology Program bridges the fields of ophthalmology and neurology through the diagnosis and management of patients with neurological disorders that affect vision and eye movements. The program is part of the Penn Medicine Neuroscience Center and the Scheie Eye Institute. With five full-time faculty members and active clinical and research components, it is one of the largest neuro-ophthalmology groups in the country. Within the areas of multiple sclerosis vision research, pediatric neuro-ophthalmology, and vision-based testing for sports-related concussion, the Penn Neuro-Ophthalmology group is a world leader.

The Penn Epilepsy Center provides the highest standard of care to patients with epilepsy and related problems. The Center offers a comprehensive, full continuum of care including state-of-the-art diagnostic techniques, cutting-edge research, medical treatments, surgery, and support services to patients with epilepsy. Both outpatient evaluation and inpatient care are available via this multidisciplinary, full-service facility.

The **Penn Stroke Center** provides emergent care to stroke patients 24 hours a day, 365 days per year. The Center employs state-of-the-art approaches to the diagnosis, treatment and prevention of stroke and critical neurologic conditions. Inpatients are cared for by physicians and nurses with specialty training in neurological diseases in different settings, depending on their needs, including the Neuroscience floor with telemetry and the **Intermediate Neurological Care Unit**. **The Neurological Intensive Care Unit** is among the most technologically advanced and sophisticated neurocritical care units in the nation, and is the only dedicated academic facility of its kind in the region.

Penn's Cognitive Neurology Program provides comprehensive, state-of-the-art assessment and treatment for patients with disorders of memory, language, attention, vision and cognition. Each patient is evaluated and treated by an experienced team of specialists and an individualized plan is developed for their ongoing care. The Center offers the latest treatment approaches available, including approved medications as well as access to numerous clinical trials of emerging treatments.

Programs

- Cognitive Neurology Program
- Center for Brain Injury and Repair
- Interventional Neuro Center
- Memory Disorders Clinic
- Multiple Sclerosis Center
- Neurological Intensive Care
- Neurogenetics Center
- Neuromuscular Disorders Program
- Neuro-Oncology Program
- Neuro-Ophthalmology Service
- Neuropsychology Service
- Parkinson's Disease and Movement Disorders Center
- Penn Epilepsy Center
- Penn Center for Sleep Disorders
- Penn Memory Center
- Stroke Center

For more information or to schedule an appointment, call 800.789.PENN (7366) or visit PennMedicine.org/neurology

The Best in American Medicine
www.CastleConnolly.com

Nuclear Medicine

A nuclear medicine specialist employs the properties of radioactive atoms and molecules in the diagnosis and treatment of disease, and in research. Radiation detection and imaging instrument systems are used to detect disease as it changes the function and metabolism of normal cells, tissues and organs. A wide variety of diseases can be found in this way, usually before the structure of the organ involved by the disease can be seen to be abnormal by any other techniques. Early detection of coronary artery disease (including acute heart attack); early cancer detection and evaluation of the effect of tumor treatment; diagnosis of infection and inflammation anywhere in the body; and early detection of blood clot in the lungs, are all possible with these techniques. Unique forms of radioactive molecules can attack and kill cancer cells (e.g., lymphoma, thyroid cancer) or can relieve the severe pain of cancer that has spread to bone.

The nuclear medicine specialist has special knowledge in the biologic effects of radiation exposure, the fundamentals of the physical sciences and the principles and operation of radiation detection and imaging instrumentation systems.

Training required: Three years

NUCLEAR MEDICINE

Mid Atlantic

Agress Jr, Harry MD [NuM] - **Spec Exp:** PET Imaging; Cancer Detection & Staging; Nuclear Oncology; CT Scan; **Hospital:** Hackensack Univ Med Ctr; **Address:** Hackensack University Medical Center, 30 Prospect Ave, Hackensack, NJ 07601; **Phone:** 201-996-2196; **Board Cert:** Nuclear Medicine 1976; Diagnostic Radiology 1978; **Med School:** Tufts Univ 1972; **Resid:** Radiology, Columbia-Presby Med Ctr 1978; **Fellow:** Nuclear Medicine, Natl Inst Hlth 1975; **Fac Appt:** Clin Prof Rad, Columbia P&S

Alavi, Abass MD [NuM] - **Spec Exp:** Brain Tumors; Neurologic Imaging; PET Imaging-Brain; Brain Infections; **Hospital:** Hosp Univ Penn - UPHS (page 72), Chldns Hosp of Philadelphia; **Address:** Hosp Univ Penn, Div Nuclear Med, 3400 Spruce St, Donner Bldg rm 117, Philadelphia, PA 19104; **Phone:** 215-662-3069; **Board Cert:** Internal Medicine 1972; Nuclear Medicine 1973; **Med School:** Iran 1964; **Resid:** Internal Medicine, Albert Einstein Med Ctr/Phila VA Hosp 1969; Hematology, Hosp Univ Penn 1970; **Fellow:** Nuclear Medicine, Hosp Univ Penn 1973; **Fac Appt:** Prof Rad, Univ Pennsylvania

Carrasquillo, Jorge A MD [NuM] - **Spec Exp:** Radioimmunotherapy of Cancer; PET Imaging; Nuclear Endocrinology; **Hospital:** Meml Sloan-Kettering Cancer Ctr; **Address:** 1275 York Ave, Nuclear Medicine Svc, Box 77, New York, NY 10065; **Phone:** 212-639-2459; **Board Cert:** Internal Medicine 1977; Nuclear Medicine 1982; **Med School:** Univ Puerto Rico 1974; **Resid:** Internal Medicine, Univ Dist Hosp 1977; Nuclear Medicine, Univ Wash Hosp 1982; **Fac Appt:** Prof NuM, SUNY Upstate Med Univ

Freeman, Leonard M MD [NuM] - **Spec Exp:** Nuclear Oncology; Gastrointestinal Disorders; PET Imaging; CT Scan; **Hospital:** Montefiore Med Ctr-Moses Campus, NY; **Address:** 111 E 210th St Foreman Bldg Fl 4, Bronx, NY 10467-2401; **Phone:** 718-920-6060; **Board Cert:** Diagnostic Radiology 1966; Nuclear Medicine 1972; Nuclear Radiology 1974; **Med School:** Ros Franklin Univ/Chicago Med Sch 1961; **Resid:** Diagnostic Radiology, Bronx Municipal Hosp 1965; **Fac Appt:** Prof NuM, Albert Einstein Coll Med

Goldsmith, Stanley J MD [NuM] - **Spec Exp:** Thyroid Cancer; PET Imaging; **Hospital:** NY-Presby/Weill Cornell Med Ctr, NY (page 66); **Address:** 525 E 68th St Starr Bldg - rm 2-21, New York, NY 10021-9800; **Phone:** 212-746-4588; **Board Cert:** Internal Medicine 1969; Nuclear Medicine 1972; Endocrinology 1972; **Med School:** SUNY Downstate 1962; **Resid:** Internal Medicine, Kings Co Hosp 1967; **Fellow:** Endocrinology, Diabetes & Metabolism, Mt Sinai Hosp 1968; Nuclear Medicine, Bronx VA Hosp 1969; **Fac Appt:** Prof Rad, Cornell Univ-Weill Med Coll

Lamonica, Dominick M MD [NuM] - **Spec Exp:** Thyroid Cancer; Lymphoma, Non-Hodgkin's; **Hospital:** Roswell Park Cancer Inst; **Address:** Dept of Nuclear Medicine, Elm & Carlton St, Buffalo, NY 14263; **Phone:** 716-845-3282; **Board Cert:** Internal Medicine 2005; Nuclear Medicine 2006; **Med School:** Mount Sinai Sch Med 1987; **Resid:** Internal Medicine, Univ Hosp-SUNY Stony Brook 1991; Diagnostic Radiology, Nassau City Med Ctr 1992; **Fellow:** Nuclear Medicine, DVAMC North Port-SUNY Stony Brook 1994; Nuclear Medicine, SUNY Buffalo-RPCI 1995; **Fac Appt:** Asst Prof, SUNY Buffalo

Majd, Massoud MD [NuM] - **Spec Exp:** Pediatric Nuclear Medicine; **Hospital:** Chldns Natl Med Ctr; **Address:** 111 Michigan Ave NW, Ste 2400, Washington, DC 20010-2978; **Phone:** 202-476-3698; **Board Cert:** Radiology 1972; Nuclear Medicine 1973; **Med School:** Iran 1960; **Resid:** Diagnostic Radiology, Georgetown Univ Hosp 1966; **Fac Appt:** Prof Rad, Geo Wash Univ

Neumann, Ronald D MD [NuM] - **Hospital:** Natl Inst of Hlth - Clin Ctr; **Address:** NIH, Bldg 10, 1C-401, 9000 Rockville Drive, MSC 1180, Bethesda, MD 20892-1180; **Phone:** 301-496-6455; **Board Cert:** Nuclear Medicine 1979; **Med School:** Yale Univ 1974; **Resid:** Pathology, Yale-New Haven Hosp 1977; Nuclear Medicine, Yale-New Haven Hosp 1979

Pandit-Taskar, Neeta MD [NuM] - **Spec Exp:** Radioimmunotherapy of Cancer; Thyroid Cancer; PET Imaging; **Hospital:** Meml Sloan-Kettering Cancer Ctr; **Address:** 1275 York Ave, Molecular Imaging and Therapy Service, Dept of Radiology, Memorial Sloan Kettering Cancer Center, New York, NY 10065; **Phone:** 212-639-3046; **Board Cert:** Nuclear Medicine 2008; **Med School:** India 1990; **Resid:** Nuclear Medicine, Mt Sinai Med Ctr 1995; **Fellow:** Nuclear Medicine, Meml Sloan Kettering Cancer Ctr 2001

Sanger, Joseph J MD [NuM] - **Spec Exp:** Nuclear Cardiology; Nuclear Oncology; **Hospital:** NYU Langone Med Ctr (page 68), Bellevue Hosp Ctr; **Address:** Old Bellevue C & D Bldg, 1st Floor, rm 7, 462 First Ave, New York, NY 10016-6402; **Phone:** 212-731-5001; **Board Cert:** Nuclear Medicine 1981; **Med School:** NYU Sch Med 1977; **Resid:** Diagnostic Radiology, NYU Med Ctr 1979; **Fellow:** Nuclear Medicine, NYU Med Ctr 1981; **Fac Appt:** Assoc Prof Rad, NYU Sch Med

Strashun, Arnold M MD [NuM] - **Spec Exp:** Neurologic Imaging; Nuclear Cardiology; Thyroid Disorders; PET Imaging-Brain; **Hospital:** SUNY Downstate Med Ctr (Univ Hosp of Bklyn), Kings County Hosp Ctr; **Address:** 450 Clarkson Ave, Box 1210, Dept Radiology, Brooklyn, NY 11203; **Phone:** 718-270-1603; **Board Cert:** Internal Medicine 1977; Nuclear Medicine 1979; **Med School:** Baylor Coll Med 1974; **Resid:** Internal Medicine, Texas Med Ctr 1977; **Fellow:** Nuclear Medicine, VA Med Ctr 1978; Nuclear Medicine, Mount Sinai Hosp 1979; **Fac Appt:** Prof NuM, SUNY Downstate

Wahl, Richard L MD [NuM] - **Spec Exp:** Radioimmunotherapy of Cancer; PET Imaging; PET Imaging-Breast; **Hospital:** Johns Hopkins Hosp (page 61); **Address:** Johns Hopkins Outpatient Ctr, 601 N Caroline St, Ste 3223-Nuclear Med, Baltimore, MD 21287; **Phone:** 410-614-3764; **Board Cert:** Diagnostic Radiology 1982; Nuclear Radiology 1983; Nuclear Medicine 1985; **Med School:** Washington Univ, St Louis 1978; **Resid:** Diagnostic Radiology, Mallinckrodt Inst 1982; **Fellow:** Nuclear Radiology, Mallinckrodt Inst 1983; **Fac Appt:** Prof Rad, Johns Hopkins Univ

Southeast

Alazraki, Naomi P MD [NuM] - **Spec Exp:** Nuclear Oncology; **Hospital:** Atlanta VA Med Ctr, Emory Univ Hosp; **Address:** VA Medical Ctr - Atlanta, 1670 Clairmont Rd, MC 115, Decatur, GA 30033; **Phone:** 404-321-6111; **Board Cert:** Nuclear Medicine 1972; Diagnostic Radiology 1972; **Med School:** Albert Einstein Coll Med 1966; **Resid:** Diagnostic Radiology, Univ Hospital 1971; **Fac Appt:** Prof Rad, Emory Univ

Sandler, Martin P MD [NuM] - **Spec Exp:** Nuclear Endocrinology; Cardiac Imaging; PET Imaging; **Hospital:** Vanderbilt Univ Med Ctr (page 75); **Address:** Vanderbilt Univ Med Ctr, CCC 1121 MCN, 1161 21st Ave S, Nashville, TN 37232-2675; **Phone:** 615-322-0860; **Board Cert:** Nuclear Medicine 1983; **Med School:** South Africa 1972; **Resid:** Internal Medicine, Groote Schur Hosp; **Fellow:** Endocrinology, Diabetes & Metabolism, Vanderbilt Univ Med Ctr 1980; Nuclear Medicine, Vanderbilt Univ Med Ctr 1982; **Fac Appt:** Prof Rad, Vanderbilt Univ

Nuclear Medicine

Ziffer, Jack A MD/PhD [NuM] - **Spec Exp:** Nuclear Cardiology; Cardiac CT Angiography; Thyroid Disease; Thyroid Cancer; **Hospital:** Baptist Hosp of Miami, Doctors' Hosp - Coral Gables (FL); **Address:** Baptist Hlth South FL/Med Group, 1500 San Remo Ave, Ste 360, Coral Gables, FL 33146; **Phone:** 786-527-9200; **Board Cert:** Diagnostic Radiology 1987; Nuclear Radiology 1988; Nuclear Medicine 1988; **Med School:** Univ Miami Sch Med 1983; **Resid:** Diagnostic Radiology, Emory Univ Affil Hosps 1987; **Fellow:** Nuclear Medicine, Emory Univ Affil Hosps 1988; **Fac Appt:** Clin Prof Rad, FIU Coll Med

Midwest

Dillehay, Gary L MD [NuM] - **Spec Exp:** Lymphoma; Bone Densitometry; PET Imaging; Thyroid Cancer; **Hospital:** Northwestern Meml Hosp; **Address:** Northwestern Meml Hosp, Dept Nuclear Medicine, 675 N St Clair St, Galter 8-110, Chicago, IL 60611; **Phone:** 312-926-5119; **Board Cert:** Nuclear Medicine 1985; Nuclear Radiology 1987; Diagnostic Radiology 2010; **Med School:** Mayo Med Sch 1979; **Resid:** Diagnostic Radiology, Northwestern Meml Hosp 1983; Nuclear Medicine, Northwestern Meml Hosp 1984; **Fac Appt:** Prof Rad, Northwestern Univ-Feinberg Sch Med

Neumann, Donald R MD [NuM] - **Spec Exp:** Nuclear Oncology; Nuclear Cardiology; Parathyroid Disease; Pheochromocytoma; **Hospital:** Cleveland Clin (page 55); **Address:** Cleveland Clinic, Dept Nuclear Medicine, 9500 Euclid Ave, MS Jb3, Cleveland, OH 44195; **Phone:** 216-444-2193; **Board Cert:** Diagnostic Radiology 1987; Nuclear Radiology 1990; **Med School:** Wright State Univ 1980; **Resid:** Diagnostic Radiology, Mount Sinai Med Ctr 1987; **Fellow:** Magnetic Resonance Imaging, Mount Sinai Med Ctr 1988

Siegel, Barry A MD [NuM] - **Spec Exp:** Cancer Detection & Staging; PET Imaging; Thyroid Disorders; **Hospital:** Barnes-Jewish Hosp, St. Louis Chldns Hosp; **Address:** 510 S Kingshighway Blvd, St Louis, MO 63110-1016; **Phone:** 314-362-2809; **Board Cert:** Nuclear Medicine 1973; Diagnostic Radiology 1977; Nuclear Radiology 1981; **Med School:** Washington Univ, St Louis 1969; **Resid:** Diagnostic Radiology, Mallinckrodt Inst Radiology 1973; **Fellow:** Nuclear Medicine, Mallinckrodt Inst Radiology 1973; **Fac Appt:** Prof Rad, Washington Univ, St Louis

Wiseman, Gregory MD [NuM] - **Spec Exp:** Lymphoma, Non-Hodgkin's; Multiple Myeloma; Radioimmunotherapy of Cancer; **Hospital:** Mayo Med Ctr & Clin - Rochester; **Address:** Mayo Clinic, Dept Nuc Med, 200 First St SW, Charlton Bldg, Rochester, MN 55905; **Phone:** 507-284-9599; **Board Cert:** Internal Medicine 1986; Hematology 1988; Nuclear Medicine 2002; **Med School:** Univ Utah 1983; **Resid:** Internal Medicine, Mayo Clinic 1986; Nuclear Medicine, Univ Washington Med Ctr 1992; **Fellow:** Hematology, Mayo Clinic 1989; Medical Oncology, Univ Washington 1991; **Fac Appt:** Asst Prof, Mayo Med Sch

Southwest

Podoloff, Donald A MD [NuM] - **Spec Exp:** Prostate Cancer; Breast Cancer; Lymphoma, Non-Hodgkin's; **Hospital:** UT MD Anderson Cancer Ctr; **Address:** UT MD Anderson Cancer Ctr, 1515 Holcombe Blvd, SCRB III Bldg, rm SCR3.3930, Box 1905, Houston, TX 77030; **Phone:** 713-745-1160; **Board Cert:** Diagnostic Radiology 1973; Nuclear Medicine 1975; Nuclear Radiology 1975; **Med School:** SUNY Downstate 1964; **Resid:** Internal Medicine, Beth Israel Med Ctr 1968; Diagnostic Radiology, Wilford Hall USAF Med Ctr 1973; **Fac Appt:** Prof NuM, Univ Tex, Houston

West Coast and Pacific

Dae, Michael W MD [NuM] - **Spec Exp:** Nuclear Cardiology; Pediatric Nuclear Medicine; **Hospital:** UCSF Med Ctr; **Address:** UCSF Med Ctr, 505 Parnassus Ave, Box 0628, San Francisco, CA 94143; **Phone:** 415-353-1905; **Board Cert:** Pediatrics 1983; Nuclear Medicine 1984; **Med School:** Duke Univ 1976; **Resid:** Pediatrics, Chldns Hosp 1978; **Fellow:** Pediatric Cardiology, UCSF Med Ctr 1982; Nuclear Cardiology, UCSF Med Ctr 1983; **Fac Appt:** Prof, UCSF

Klaas, Virginia E MD [NuM] - **Spec Exp:** Nuclear Radiology; **Hospital:** Valley Med Ctr-Renton, WA, Auburn Reg Med Ctr; **Address:** 533 S 336th St, Ste C, PO BOX 26730, Federal Way, WA 98003; **Phone:** 253-661-1700; **Board Cert:** Diagnostic Radiology 1994; Nuclear Radiology 1995; Nuclear Medicine 2004; **Med School:** UC Irvine 1989; **Resid:** Diagnostic Radiology, Stanford Univ Med Ctr 1994; **Fellow:** Nuclear Medicine, Mallinckrodt Inst of Radiology 1995

Schelbert, Heinrich R MD/PhD [NuM] - **Spec Exp:** Nuclear Cardiology; Coronary Artery Disease; **Hospital:** UCLA Ronald Reagan Med Ctr, Santa Monica - UCLA Med Ctr & Ortho Hosp; **Address:** UCLA Dept Molecular & Med Pharmacology, B2-085J CHS, Box 95648, Los Angeles, CA 90095-6948; **Phone:** 310-825-3076; **Board Cert:** Nuclear Medicine 1976; **Med School:** Germany 1964; **Resid:** Internal Medicine, Mercy Med Ctr 1968; Cardiovascular Disease, Univ Duesseldorf 1972; **Fellow:** Cardiovascular Disease, UCSD Med Ctr 1975; Nuclear Medicine, UCSD Med Ctr 1976; **Fac Appt:** Prof Pharm, UCLA-David Geffen Sch Med

Waxman, Alan D MD [NuM] - **Spec Exp:** PET Imaging-Brain; Thyroid Cancer; Cancer Detection & Staging; **Hospital:** Cedars-Sinai Med Ctr, Keck Med Ctr of USC (page 62); **Address:** Cedars-Sinai Med Ctr, Taper Imaging, 8700 Beverly Blvd, rm 1258, Los Angeles, CA 90048-1804; **Phone:** 310-423-4216; **Board Cert:** Nuclear Medicine 1972; **Med School:** USC Sch Med 1963; **Resid:** Nuclear Medicine, Wadsworth VA Hosp 1965; **Fellow:** Internal Medicine, Natl Inst Hlth 1967; **Fac Appt:** Clin Prof, USC Sch Med

Cleveland Clinic

Every life deserves world class care.

Nuclear Medicine

Cleveland Clinic Imaging Institute is one of the leading academic imaging centers in the world and one of the busiest clinical departments in the country. Each year, Cleveland Clinic imagers perform and interpret more than 1.9 million examinations, for which all images are acquired digitally.

Cleveland Clinic's Department of Nuclear Medicine's advanced imaging capabilities can identify both anatomic and physiologic changes in organ function. A Cyclotron enables on-site production of customized PET tracers for both clinical and research needs. Cleveland Clinic has 12 gamma cameras — three PET/CT scanners, three SPECT/CT scanners and six traditional gamma cameras. Our mobile PET/CT system brings main campus capabilities to Cleveland Clinic community hospitals.

Our unique expertise and unsurpassed technology are available to individualize patient diagnosis and management and treatment with the highest degree possible of accuracy and timeliness. Hybrid SPECT/CT and PET/CT fusion imaging is performed on specialized scanners that directly map the abnormal tissue depicted on the nuclear images to the affected area displayed on the high-resolution CT images.

The department possesses an abundant depth of expertise in both imaging and clinical medicine. Physicians are board-certified and clinically experienced in a broad array of specialties, including cardiology, neurology and radiology.

Patient therapy is a significant component of nuclear medicine. Treatments, and sometimes pain relief, are offered for conditions such as Graves' disease, thyroid cancer, liver cancer, cancer that has spread to the bone and refractory lymphomas. PET/CT scans also assist radiation oncologists in planning treatment with external sources of radiation.

Cleveland Clinic
Imaging Institute
9500 Euclid Avenue
Cleveland, OH 44195

Offering Same-Day Appointments
Call 800.274.2009.

Treatment Guides
Cleveland Clinic has developed comprehensive treatment guides for many diseases and conditions. To download our free treatment guides, visit clevelandclinic.org/treatmentguides.

Online Medical Second Opinion
Call 216.444.3223 or 800.223.2273 ext. 43223 or email eclevelandclinic@ccf.org.

Out-of-State Patients Assistance
Call 800.223.2273, ext. 55580 or email medicalconcierge@ccf.org.

Visit Us At:
clevelandclinic.org

Follow Us On:
Facebook
www.facebook.com/clevelandclinic

Twitter
@ClevelandClinic

You Tube
www.youtube.com/clevelandclinic

Health Hub
health.clevelandclinic.org

NUCLEAR MEDICINE

About the Division of Nuclear Medicine, Department of Radiology

Nuclear medicine at NYU Langone Medical Center spans all medical specialties to deliver safe techniques that image body physiology for the diagnosis, monitoring and prevention of disease. In addition to cutting-edge imaging, the Medical Center offers a full spectrum of radioiodine therapy protocols for the treatment of hyperthyroidism and thyroid cancer. Our nuclear medicine physicians are also experts in the field of radioimmunotherapy for lymphoma. We specialize in the following areas:

Advanced Imaging Equipment

NYU Langone Medical Center houses some of the most advanced nuclear medicine equipment in the world, including best-of-breed SPECT, SPECT and PET/CT scanners. Cameras are linked by advanced data management systems to allow rapid, accurate reading and digital report generation. Image data is available to referring physicians over a digital network that allows for timely patient management.

Nuclear Medicine

NYU Langone Medical Center's Tisch Hospital offers a wide range of nuclear medicine services, specializing in a full complement of non-invasive nuclear imaging techniques designed to diagnose and monitor disease of the neurological, cardiovascular, endocrine, gastrointestinal, pulmonary, genitourinary and hepatobiliary systems. Specialized blood volume and lymphedema evaluation protocols are also offered. Advanced dosimetry protocols are used to optimize therapy for patients with thyroid cancer and lymphoma.

PET/CT Scans

PET/CT scans allow for simultaneous imaging of metabolic processes as well as anatomic structures in the body. These advanced scanners have revolutionized the care of cancer patients and are making great strides in the diagnosis and management of neurological and cardiac diseases. NYU Langone Medical Center's nuclear medicine physicians are fellowship-trained experts in the field of PET/CT.

The Best in American Medicine
www.CastleConnolly.com

Obstetrics & Gynecology

An obstetrician/gynecologist possesses special knowledge, skills and professional capability in the medical and surgical care of the female reproductive system and associated disorders. This physician serves as a consultant to other physicians and as a primary physician for women.

Training Required: Four years *plus* two years in clinical practice before certification is complete.

OBSTETRICS & GYNECOLOGY

New England

Cramer, Daniel W MD [ObG] - **Spec Exp:** Ovarian Cancer; Ovarian Cancer-High Risk; **Hospital:** Dana-Farber Cancer Inst (page 57), Brigham and Women's Hosp (page 57); **Address:** Brigham and Women's Hosp, 221 Longwood Ave, Boston, MA 02115; **Phone:** 617-732-4895; **Board Cert:** Obstetrics & Gynecology 1979; **Med School:** Univ Colorado 1970; **Resid:** Obstetrics & Gynecology, Boston Womens Hosp 1976; **Fellow:** Public Health, Harvard Med Sch 1982; **Fac Appt:** Prof ObG, Harvard Med Sch

Eckler, Kristen MD [ObG] - **Spec Exp:** Pelvic Reconstruction; Uro-Gynecology; **Hospital:** Mass Genl Hosp; **Address:** Vincent OB/GYN Service, 55 Fruit St, YAW 4, Boston, MA 02114; **Phone:** 617-724-9019; **Board Cert:** Obstetrics & Gynecology 2011; **Med School:** Tufts Univ 1994; **Resid:** Obstetrics & Gynecology, Brigham & Women's Hosp 1998

Einarsson, Jon I MD [ObG] - **Spec Exp:** Minimally Invasive Surgery; Endometriosis; Pelvic Organ Prolapse Repair; Incontinence-Female; **Hospital:** Brigham and Women's Hosp (page 57); **Address:** Brigham & Womens Hosp, Dept Obstetrics & Gynecology, 75 Francis St, Boston, MA 02115; **Phone:** 617-525-8582; **Board Cert:** Obstetrics & Gynecology 2011; **Med School:** Iceland 1995; **Resid:** Obstetrics & Gynecology, Baylor Affil Hosp 2002; **Fellow:** Minimally Invasive Surgery, Baylor Affil Hosp 2004; **Fac Appt:** Assoc Prof ObG, Harvard Med Sch

Laufer, Marc R MD [ObG] - **Spec Exp:** Adolescent Gynecology; Endometriosis-Adolescent; Congenital Anomalies-Gynecologic; Pediatric Gynecology; **Hospital:** Children's Hospital - Boston, Brigham and Women's Hosp (page 57); **Address:** Chldns Hosp, Dept of Gynecology, 300 Longwood Ave, Boston, MA 02115; **Phone:** 617-355-5785; **Board Cert:** Obstetrics & Gynecology 2011; **Med School:** Univ Pennsylvania 1986; **Resid:** Obstetrics & Gynecology, Brigham & Womens Hosp/Mass Genl Hosp 1990; **Fellow:** Reproductive Endocrinology, Brigham & Womens Hosp/Chldns Hosp 1992; Gynecology, Chldns Hosp 1992; **Fac Appt:** Assoc Prof ObG, Harvard Med Sch

Myers, Deborah L MD [ObG] - **Spec Exp:** Uro-Gynecology; **Hospital:** Women & Infants Hosp of RI; **Address:** Women & Infants Hosp, 695 Eddy St, Providence, RI 02905; **Phone:** 401-453-7560; **Board Cert:** Obstetrics & Gynecology 2011; **Med School:** SUNY Stony Brook 1981; **Resid:** Obstetrics & Gynecology, Women & Infants Hosp 1985; **Fac Appt:** Asst Prof ObG, Brown Univ

Nour, Nawal M MD [ObG] - **Spec Exp:** Female Genital Cutting (FGC) Education; Gynecology-African women only; Pregnancy-African women only; **Hospital:** Brigham and Women's Hosp (page 57); **Address:** Brigham & Women's Hosp, Dept Ob/Gyn, 75 Francis St CWN-3 Bldg - Ste 340, Boston, MA 02115; **Phone:** 617-732-4740; **Board Cert:** Obstetrics & Gynecology 2011; **Med School:** Harvard Med Sch 1994; **Resid:** Obstetrics & Gynecology, Brgham & Women's Hosp 1998

Mid Atlantic

Bader, Thomas J MD [ObG] - **Spec Exp:** Pregnancy-High Risk; **Hospital:** Crozer - Chester Med Ctr; **Address:** 1 Medical Center Blvd, Ste 334, Upland, PA 19013; **Phone:** 610-872-7660; **Board Cert:** Obstetrics & Gynecology 2011; **Med School:** Georgetown Univ 1989; **Resid:** Obstetrics & Gynecology, Hosp Univ Penn 1993

Brodman, Michael L MD [ObG] - **Spec Exp:** Incontinence-Female; Laparoscopic Surgery; Pelvic Organ Prolapse Repair; Uro-Gynecology; **Hospital:** Mount Sinai Med Ctr (page 64); **Address:** Dept Gynecology/Urogynecology, 5 E 98th St Fl 2, New York, NY 10029; **Phone:** 212-241-7952; **Board Cert:** Obstetrics & Gynecology 2010; **Med School:** Mount Sinai Sch Med 1982; **Resid:** Obstetrics & Gynecology, Mt Sinai Hosp 1986; **Fellow:** Pelvic Surgery, Mt Sinai Hosp 1987; **Fac Appt:** Assoc Prof ObG, Mount Sinai Sch Med

Carson, Donald G MD [ObG] - **Spec Exp:** Gynecology Only; **Hospital:** Magee-Womens Hosp - UPMC; **Address:** Ob/Gyn Assocs of Pittsburgh, 3380 Boulevard of the Allies, Ste 1, Pittsburgh, PA 15213; **Phone:** 412-621-7575; **Board Cert:** Obstetrics & Gynecology 2011; **Med School:** Univ Pittsburgh 1977; **Resid:** Obstetrics & Gynecology, Magee-Womens Hosp 1981; **Fac Appt:** Assoc Clin Prof ObG, Univ Pittsburgh

De Cherney, Alan H MD [ObG] - **Spec Exp:** Infertility; Reproductive Endocrinology; Gynecologic Surgery; **Hospital:** Natl Inst of Hlth - Clin Ctr, Unif Serv Univ of the Hlth Sci; **Address:** NICHD, NIH, Bldg 10, CRC, 1 East, 10 Center Drive, rm 1-3140, MS 1109, Bethesda, MD 20892-1109; **Phone:** 301-496-5800; **Board Cert:** Obstetrics & Gynecology 1989; Reproductive Endocrinology 1979; **Med School:** Temple Univ 1967; **Resid:** Obstetrics & Gynecology, Hosp Univ Penn 1972; **Fac Appt:** Prof ObG, Uniformed Srvs Univ, Bethesda

Evans, Mark I MD [ObG] - **Spec Exp:** Reproductive Genetics; Fetal Diagnosis & Therapy; Multiple Gestation; Ultrasound; **Hospital:** Mount Sinai Med Ctr (page 64); **Address:** Comprehensive Genetics, 131 E 65th St, New York, NY 10065; **Phone:** 212-288-1422; **Board Cert:** Obstetrics & Gynecology 2011; Clinical Genetics 1984; **Med School:** SUNY Downstate 1978; **Resid:** Obstetrics & Gynecology, Lying-In Hosp 1982; **Fellow:** Clinical Genetics, Natl Inst Hlth 1984; **Fac Appt:** Prof ObG, Mount Sinai Sch Med

Goldstein, Martin S MD [ObG] - **Spec Exp:** Uterine Fibroids; Laparoscopic Surgery; Pelvic Organ Prolapse Repair; Endometriosis; **Hospital:** Mount Sinai Med Ctr (page 64); **Address:** 40 E 84th St, New York, NY 10028-1314; **Phone:** 212-472-6500; **Board Cert:** Obstetrics & Gynecology 1980; **Med School:** SUNY Hlth Sci Ctr 1966; **Resid:** Obstetrics & Gynecology, Mount Sinai Hosp 1971; **Fac Appt:** Assoc Clin Prof ObG, Mount Sinai Sch Med

Hockstein, Steven MD [ObG] - **Spec Exp:** Uterine Fibroids; **Hospital:** NY-Presby/Weill Cornell Med Ctr, NY (page 66); **Address:** 425 E 61st St Fl 11, New York, NY 10021; **Phone:** 212-821-0810; **Board Cert:** Obstetrics & Gynecology 2011; **Med School:** Univ MD Sch Med 1993; **Resid:** Obstetrics & Gynecology, McGaw Med Ctr 1997; **Fac Appt:** Asst Clin Prof ObG, Cornell Univ-Weill Med Coll

Iglesia, Cheryl MD [ObG] - **Spec Exp:** Uro-Gynecology; **Hospital:** Washington Hosp Ctr; **Address:** Washington Hosp Ctr, 106 Irving St NW, Ste 405-S, Washington, DC 20010; **Phone:** 202-877-6526; **Board Cert:** Obstetrics & Gynecology 2011; **Med School:** Univ MD Sch Med 1991; **Resid:** Obstetrics & Gynecology, Univ FL Hlth Sci Ctr 1995; **Fellow:** Uro-Gynecology, Rush Med Coll 1997

Lucente, Vincent R MD [ObG] - **Spec Exp:** Uro-Gynecology; Pelvic Floor Reconstruction; Incontinence-Female; Pelvic Organ Prolapse Repair; **Hospital:** St. Luke's Hosp - Allentown, Abington Mem Hosp; **Address:** Hamilton Court Professional Ctr, 3050 Hamilton Blvd, Ste 200, Allentown, PA 18103; **Phone:** 610-435-9575; **Board Cert:** Obstetrics & Gynecology 2011; **Med School:** SUNY Stony Brook 1985; **Resid:** Obstetrics & Gynecology, N Shore Univ Hosp 1989; **Fellow:** Uro-Gynecology, Methodist Hosp 1990; **Fac Appt:** Clin Prof ObG, Temple Univ

Maynard, Steven MD [ObG] - **Spec Exp:** Minimally Invasive Surgery; Incontinence; **Hospital:** Georgetown Univ Hosp; **Address:** 3800 Resovoir Rd NW, Pasquerilla Health Center Fl 3, Washington, DC 20007; **Phone:** 202-444-8531; **Board Cert:** Obstetrics & Gynecology 2009; **Med School:** McGill Univ 1986; **Resid:** Obstetrics & Gynecology, Women & Infants Hosp 1993; **Fac Appt:** Asst Prof ObG, Georgetown Univ

Ordorica, Steven Anthony MD [ObG] - **Spec Exp:** Pregnancy-High Risk; Miscarriage-Recurrent; Maternal & Fetal Medicine; **Hospital:** NYU Langone Med Ctr (page 68); **Address:** NYU Med Ctr, Dept OB/GYN, 530 1st Ave, Ste 10Q, New York, NY 10016-6402; **Phone:** 212-263-5982; **Board Cert:** Obstetrics & Gynecology 2011; Maternal & Fetal Medicine 2011; **Med School:** SUNY Stony Brook 1983; **Resid:** Obstetrics & Gynecology, NYU Med Ctr 1987; **Fellow:** Maternal & Fetal Medicine, NYU Med Ctr 1989; **Fac Appt:** Assoc Prof ObG, NYU Sch Med

Pfeifer, Samantha M MD [ObG] - **Spec Exp:** Infertility-Female; Endometriosis; Laparoscopic Surgery; Congenital Anomalies-Gynecologic; **Hospital:** Hosp Univ Penn - UPHS (page 72); **Address:** Penn Health for Women, 250 King of Prussia Rd, Ste 2A, Radnor, PA 19087; **Phone:** 610-902-2500; **Board Cert:** Obstetrics & Gynecology 2011; Reproductive Endocrinology 2011; **Med School:** Univ Pennsylvania 1986; **Resid:** Obstetrics & Gynecology, Hosp Univ Penn 1990; **Fellow:** Reproductive Endocrinology, Hosp Univ Penn 1993; **Fac Appt:** Assoc Prof ObG, Univ Pennsylvania

Scher, Jonathan MD [ObG] - **Spec Exp:** Miscarriage-Recurrent; Pregnancy-High Risk; Infertility-IVF Failure; **Hospital:** Mount Sinai Med Ctr (page 64); **Address:** 1126 Park Ave, New York, NY 10128-1203; **Phone:** 212-427-7400; **Board Cert:** Obstetrics & Gynecology 1981; **Med School:** South Africa 1964; **Resid:** Obstetrics & Gynecology, Groote Schuur Hosp 1970; Obstetrics & Gynecology, Kings College Hosp 1972; **Fac Appt:** Asst Clin Prof ObG, Mount Sinai Sch Med

Simon, James A MD [ObG] - **Spec Exp:** Infertility; Menopause Problems; Osteoporosis; Sexual Dysfunction; **Hospital:** G Washington Univ Hosp, Sibley Mem Hosp; **Address:** 1850 M St NW, Ste 450, Washington, DC 20036; **Phone:** 202-293-1000; **Board Cert:** Obstetrics & Gynecology 2009; Reproductive Endocrinology 2009; **Med School:** Rush Med Coll 1978; **Resid:** Obstetrics & Gynecology, George Washington Univ Hosp 1982; **Fellow:** Reproductive Endocrinology, Harbor-UCLA Medical Ctr 1984; **Fac Appt:** Clin Prof ObG, Geo Wash Univ

Wiesenfeld, Harold C MD [ObG] - **Spec Exp:** Infectious Diseases-Gynecologic; Sexually Transmitted Diseases; **Hospital:** Magee-Womens Hosp - UPMC; **Address:** Magee-Womens Hosp, Dept Ob/Gyn, 300 Halket St, Ste 0610, Pittsburgh, PA 15213; **Phone:** 412-641-6412; **Board Cert:** Obstetrics & Gynecology 2011; **Med School:** McGill Univ 1987; **Resid:** Obstetrics & Gynecology, McGill Univ 1990; **Fac Appt:** Assoc Prof ObG, Univ Pittsburgh

Witter, Frank R MD [ObG] - **Spec Exp:** Pregnancy-High Risk; Multiple Gestation; Lupus/SLE in Pregnancy; **Hospital:** Johns Hopkins Hosp (page 61), Johns Hopkins Bayview Med Ctr (page 61); **Address:** 600 N Wolfe St, Nelson 2170, Baltimore, MD 21287; **Phone:** 410-502-3200; **Board Cert:** Obstetrics & Gynecology 2011; Maternal & Fetal Medicine 2011; **Med School:** Univ Chicago-Pritzker Sch Med 1976; **Resid:** Obstetrics & Gynecology, Johns Hopkins Hosp 1980; **Fellow:** Maternal & Fetal Medicine, Johns Hopkins Hosp 1982; Clinical Pharmacology, Johns Hopkins Hosp 1984; **Fac Appt:** Prof ObG, Johns Hopkins Univ

Young, Bruce Kenneth MD [ObG] - **Spec Exp:** Infertility; Minimally Invasive Surgery; Preventive Medicine; Miscarriage-Recurrent; **Hospital:** NYU Langone Med Ctr (page 68), Bellevue Hosp Ctr; **Address:** 530 1st Ave, HCC-5th Fl, Ste 5G, New York, NY 10016; **Phone:** 212-263-6359; **Board Cert:** Obstetrics & Gynecology 1970; Maternal & Fetal Medicine 1975; **Med School:** NYU Sch Med 1963; **Resid:** Obstetrics & Gynecology, NYU Med Ctr 1968; **Fellow:** Reproductive Endocrinology, NYU Med Ctr 1968; **Fac Appt:** Prof ObG, NYU Sch Med

Southeast

Andersen, Glenna R MD [ObG] - **Hospital:** Inova Fairfax Hosp; **Address:** 8501 Arlington Blvd, Ste 300, Fairfax, VA 22031; **Phone:** 703-560-1611; **Board Cert:** Obstetrics & Gynecology 2011; **Med School:** Univ VA Sch Med 1981; **Resid:** Obstetrics & Gynecology, SUNY Buffalo Affil Hosps 1985

Berga, Sarah L MD [ObG] - **Spec Exp:** Menstrual Disorders; Hormonal Disorders; Reproductive Endocrinology; **Hospital:** Wake Forest Baptist Med Ctr; **Address:** Wake Forest Baptist Hlth, One Medical Ctr Blvd, Watlington Bldg Fl 4, Winston-Salem, NC 27157-1066; **Phone:** 336-716-6476; **Board Cert:** Obstetrics & Gynecology 2011; Reproductive Endocrinology/Infertility 2011; **Med School:** Univ VA Sch Med 1980; **Resid:** Obstetrics & Gynecology, Mass Genl Hosp 1984; **Fellow:** Reproductive Endocrinology, UCSD Med Ctr 1986; **Fac Appt:** Prof ObG, Wake Forest Univ

Filip, Stanley J MD [ObG] - **Spec Exp:** Uterine Fibroids; Menopause Problems; Hysterectomy Alternatives; Endometriosis; **Hospital:** Duke Univ Hosp, Durham Regional Hosp; **Address:** Box 3267 Med Ctr, 3116 N Duke St, Box 3267, Durham, NC 27704; **Phone:** 919-660-2370; **Board Cert:** Obstetrics & Gynecology 1985; **Med School:** Mount Sinai Sch Med 1979; **Resid:** Obstetrics & Gynecology, Univ Colo Affil Hosp 1983; **Fac Appt:** Assoc Prof ObG, Univ NC Sch Med

Hager, W David MD [ObG] - **Spec Exp:** Infectious Diseases-Gynecologic; Sexually Transmitted Diseases; HPV-Human Papilloma Virus; Laparoscopic Surgery; **Hospital:** Central Baptist Hosp, St. Joseph Hosp; **Address:** Womens Care Ctr, 1720 Nicholasville Rd, Ste 401, Lexington, KY 40503; **Phone:** 859-278-0363; **Board Cert:** Obstetrics & Gynecology 1993; **Med School:** Univ KY Coll Med 1972; **Resid:** Obstetrics & Gynecology, Univ Kentucky Med Ctr 1976; **Fac Appt:** Prof ObG, Univ KY Coll Med

Hullfish, Kathie L MD [ObG] - **Spec Exp:** Uro-Gynecology; Pelvic Reconstruction; Pelvic Organ Prolapse Repair; Incontinence; **Hospital:** Univ of Virginia Health Sys; **Address:** Univ Virginia Med Ctr, Div Urogynecology, Pelvic Reconst Med, P.O. Box 801305, Charlottesville, VA 22908-0712; **Phone:** 434-924-2103; **Board Cert:** Obstetrics & Gynecology 2009; **Med School:** Univ VA Sch Med 1992; **Resid:** Obstetrics & Gynecology, Univ Virginia Med Ctr 1996; **Fellow:** Uro-Gynecology, Rush Med Ctr 1998; **Fac Appt:** Assoc Prof ObG, Univ VA Sch Med

Jenkins, Todd MD [ObG] - **Spec Exp:** Minimally Invasive Surgery; Hysteroscopic Surgery; Endometriosis; Uterine Fibroids; **Hospital:** Univ of Ala Hosp at Birmingham; **Address:** UAB Dept Obstetrics/Gynecology, 619 19th St S, 176F 1026, Birmingham, AL 35249-7333; **Phone:** 205-996-3130; **Board Cert:** Obstetrics & Gynecology 2010; **Med School:** Univ Alabama 1994; **Resid:** Obstetrics & Gynecology, Univ Alabama Hosp 1998; **Fac Appt:** Assoc Prof ObG, Univ Alabama

Morgan, Linda S MD [ObG] - **Spec Exp:** Gynecologic Cancer; Women's Health; **Hospital:** Shands at Univ of FL; **Address:** 2000 SW Archer Rd, Ste 4101, Gainesville, FL 32608; **Phone:** 352-265-8200; **Board Cert:** Obstetrics & Gynecology 2010; Gynecologic Oncology 2010; **Med School:** Med Coll PA Hahnemann 1975; **Resid:** Obstetrics & Gynecology, Shands Hosp 1979; **Fellow:** Gynecologic Oncology, Mass Genl Hosp 1981; **Fac Appt:** Prof ObG, Univ Fla Coll Med

Sanz, Luis E MD [ObG] - **Spec Exp:** Uro-Gynecology; Robotic Surgery; Vaginal Reconstruction; Pelvic Reconstruction; **Hospital:** Virginia Hosp Ctr - Arlington; **Address:** 1625 N George Mason Drive, Ste 475, Arlington, VA 22205; **Phone:** 703-717-4000; **Board Cert:** Obstetrics & Gynecology 1982; **Med School:** Georgetown Univ 1976; **Resid:** Obstetrics & Gynecology, Georgetown Univ Hosp 1980; **Fellow:** Advanced Pelvic Surgery, Georgetown Univ 1982; **Fac Appt:** Prof ObG, Georgetown Univ

Obstetrics & Gynecology

Simpson, Joe L MD [ObG] - **Spec Exp:** Prenatal Diagnosis; Ovarian Failure; Infertility/Genetics; **Hospital:** Jackson N Med Ctr; **Address:** Florida International University, University Park AHC 693, 11200 SW 8 St, Miami, FL 33199; **Phone:** 914-997-4564; **Board Cert:** Obstetrics & Gynecology 2010; Clinical Genetics 1982; **Med School:** Duke Univ 1968; **Resid:** Obstetrics & Gynecology, NY Hosp-Cornell Med Ctr 1973; **Fac Appt:** Prof ObG, FIU Coll Med

Steege, John F MD [ObG] - **Spec Exp:** Laparoscopic Surgery; Endometriosis; Pain-Pelvic & Perineal; Gynecologic Surgery; **Hospital:** NC Memorial Hosp - UNC; **Address:** UNC-Dept OB/GYN, CB 7570, Chapel Hill, NC 27599-7570; **Phone:** 919-966-7764; **Board Cert:** Obstetrics & Gynecology 1978; **Med School:** Yale Univ 1972; **Resid:** Obstetrics & Gynecology, Yale - New Haven Hosp 1976; **Fac Appt:** Prof ObG, Univ NC Sch Med

Visco, Anthony G MD [ObG] - **Spec Exp:** Uro-Gynecology; Pelvic Organ Prolapse Repair; Robotic Hysterectomy; Minimally Invasive Surgery; **Hospital:** Duke Univ Hosp, Durham Regional Hosp; **Address:** 5324 McFarland Drive, Ste 310, Box 3192, Durham, NC 27617; **Phone:** 919-684-2471; **Board Cert:** Obstetrics & Gynecology 2008; **Med School:** SUNY Upstate Med Univ 1993; **Resid:** Obstetrics & Gynecology, Univ Rochester Med Ctr 1997; **Fellow:** Uro-Gynecology, Duke Univ Med Ctr 2000; Reconstructive Pelvic Surgery, Duke Univ Med Ctr 2000; **Fac Appt:** Assoc Prof ObG, Duke Univ

Midwest

Argenta, Peter A MD [ObG] - **Spec Exp:** Laparoscopic Surgery; Women's Health; Cervical Cancer; Ovarian Cancer; **Hospital:** Univ Minn Med Ctr, Fairview - Riverside Campus; **Address:** Womens Health Clin, 516 Delaware St SE, Clinic 1C Fl 1, Minneapolis, MN 55455; **Phone:** 612-626-3444; **Board Cert:** Obstetrics & Gynecology 2011; Gynecologic Oncology 2011; **Med School:** Duke Univ 1995; **Resid:** Obstetrics & Gynecology, Hosp U Penn 1999; **Fellow:** Gynecologic Oncology, Mt Sinai Med Ctr 2002; **Fac Appt:** Assoc Prof ObG, Univ Minn

Bartholomew, Deborah A MD [ObG] - **Spec Exp:** Gynecologic Pathology; Robotic Surgery; Minimally Invasive Surgery; **Hospital:** Ohio St Univ Med Ctr; **Address:** 4053 W Dublin Granville Rd, Dublin, OH 43017; **Phone:** 614-764-2262; **Board Cert:** Anatomic Pathology 1990; Obstetrics & Gynecology 2011; **Med School:** Med Coll VA 1983; **Resid:** Obstetrics & Gynecology, David Grant USAF Med Ctr 1987; Anatomic Pathology, UC Davis Med Ctr 1987; **Fellow:** Gynecologic Pathology, UC Davis Med Ctr 1989; **Fac Appt:** Assoc Prof ObG

Bradley, Linda D MD [ObG] - **Spec Exp:** Hysteroscopic Surgery; Menstrual Disorders; Endoscopy; Uterine Fibroids; **Hospital:** Cleveland Clin (page 55); **Address:** Cleveland Clinic Fdn, Dept Ob/Gyn, 9500 Euclid Ave, Desk A81, Cleveland, OH 44195; **Phone:** 216-444-6601; **Board Cert:** Obstetrics & Gynecology 2011; **Med School:** Univ Cincinnati 1981; **Resid:** Obstetrics & Gynecology, Cleveland Metro Genl Hosp 1985

Corteville, Jane E MD [ObG] - **Spec Exp:** Fetal Diagnosis & Therapy; Maternal & Fetal Medicine; Prenatal Genetic Diagnosis; Obstetric Ultrasound; **Hospital:** Univ Hosps Case Med Ctr (page 74); **Address:** UH MacDonald Women's Hospital, 11100 Euclid Ave, Cleveland, OH 44106; **Phone:** 216-844-8545; **Board Cert:** Obstetrics & Gynecology 2011; Clinical Genetics 2010; **Med School:** Washington Univ, St Louis 1992; **Resid:** Obstetrics & Gynecology, Barnes-Jewish Hosp 1987; **Fellow:** Ultrasound/CT, Barnes-Jewish Hosp 1989; Medical Genetics, Chldns Hosp 1992; **Fac Appt:** Asst Prof ObG, Case West Res Univ

De Lancey, John O MD [ObG] - **Spec Exp:** Uro-Gynecology; Incontinence; Pelvic Organ Prolapse Repair; **Hospital:** Univ of Michigan Hosp; **Address:** Univ Mich Med Ctr, Dept ObGyn, 1500 E Med Ctr Drive, rm L4000, Box 5276, Ann Arbor, MI 48109-0276; **Phone:** 734-764-8429; **Board Cert:** Obstetrics & Gynecology 1997; **Med School:** Univ Mich Med Sch 1977; **Resid:** Obstetrics & Gynecology, Univ Mich Med Ctr 1981; **Fac Appt:** Prof ObG, Univ Mich Med Sch

De Lia, Julian E MD [ObG] - **Spec Exp:** Fetal Surgery; Twin to Twin Transfusion Syndrome (TTTS); **Hospital:** Froedtert and Med Ctr of WI, Chldns Hosp - Wisconsin; **Address:** 9200 W Wisconsin Ave, Milwaukee, WI 53226; **Phone:** 414-805-6600; **Board Cert:** Obstetrics & Gynecology 1993; **Med School:** UMDNJ-NJ Med Sch, Newark 1972; **Resid:** Obstetrics & Gynecology, St Barnabas Med Ctr 1976; **Fac Appt:** Prof ObG, Med Coll Wisc

Famuyide, Abimbola MD [ObG] - **Spec Exp:** Minimally Invasive Surgery; Uterine Fibroids; **Hospital:** Mayo Med Ctr & Clin - Rochester; **Address:** Mayo Clinic, Dept Ob/Gyn, 200 First St SW, 4A Eisenberg, Rochester, MN 55905; **Phone:** 507-284-2511; **Board Cert:** Obstetrics & Gynecology 2011; **Med School:** Nigeria 1985; **Resid:** Obstetrics & Gynecology, Barnsley District Hosp/Central Sheffield Hosp; **Fellow:** Obstetrics & Gynecology, Mayo Grad Sch; **Fac Appt:** Asst Prof ObG, Mayo Med Sch

Gonik, Bernard MD [ObG] - **Spec Exp:** Infectious Disease in Pregnancy; Prenatal Diagnosis; Vaccinations in Pregnancy; **Hospital:** Detroit Med Ctr; **Address:** 6071 W Outer Drive, Ste M-541, Detroit, MI 48235-2624; **Phone:** 313-966-3246; **Board Cert:** Obstetrics & Gynecology 2011; Maternal & Fetal Medicine 2011; **Med School:** Mich State Univ 1978; **Resid:** Obstetrics & Gynecology, Univ Texas Med Sch 1982; **Fellow:** Maternal & Fetal Medicine, Univ Texas Med Sch 1985; **Fac Appt:** Prof ObG, Wayne State Univ

Greenfield, Marjorie L MD [ObG] - **Spec Exp:** Adolescent Gynecology; **Hospital:** Univ Hosps Case Med Ctr (page 74); **Address:** UH MacDonald Women's Hosp, Obstetrics & Gynecology, 11100 Euclid Ave, Ste 1200, Cleveland, OH 44106; **Phone:** 216-844-3941; **Board Cert:** Obstetrics & Gynecology 2011; **Med School:** Case West Res Univ 1983; **Resid:** Obstetrics & Gynecology, Univ Hosp 1987; **Fac Appt:** Assoc Prof ObG, Case West Res Univ

Hale, Douglass S MD [ObG] - **Spec Exp:** Uro-Gynecology; Pelvic Floor Reconstruction; Reconstructive Surgery; Robotic Surgery; **Hospital:** IU Health Methodist Hosp; **Address:** 1633 N Capitol Ave, Ste 436, Indianapolis, IN 46202; **Phone:** 317-962-6600; **Board Cert:** Obstetrics & Gynecology 2010; **Med School:** Med Coll OH 1989; **Resid:** Obstetrics & Gynecology, T Jefferson Univ Hosp 1993; **Fellow:** Uro-Gynecology, Methodist Hosp 1995; Reconstructive Surgery, Methodist Hosp 1995; **Fac Appt:** Assoc Clin Prof ObG, Indiana Univ

Karram, Mickey M MD [ObG] - **Spec Exp:** Uro-Gynecology; Pelvic Floor Reconstruction; Incontinence-Female; **Hospital:** Christ Hosp, The - Cincinnati; **Address:** 7759 University Drive, Ste G, Westchester, OH 45069; **Phone:** 513-463-2500; **Board Cert:** Obstetrics & Gynecology 2011; **Med School:** Egypt 1982; **Resid:** Obstetrics & Gynecology, Good Samaritan Hosp 1985; **Fellow:** Gynecologic Urology, Harbor Hosp-UCLA 1986; **Fac Appt:** Prof ObG, Univ Cincinnati

Lengyel, Ernst MD/PhD [ObG] - **Spec Exp:** Ovarian Cancer; Cervical Cancer; **Hospital:** Univ of Chicago Med Ctr; **Address:** Univ Chicago Med Ctr, Dept Gyn Onc, 5841 S Maryland Ave, rm L-264, MC 2050, Chicago, IL 60637; **Phone:** 773-702-6722; **Board Cert:** Obstetrics & Gynecology 2010; Gynecologic Oncology 2012; **Med School:** Germany 1992; **Resid:** Obstetrics & Gynecology, Univ Munich 2000; **Fellow:** Gynecologic Oncology, UCSF Med Ctr 2003; **Fac Appt:** Prof ObG, Univ Chicago-Pritzker Sch Med

Obstetrics & Gynecology

Levine, Elliot MD [ObG] - **Spec Exp:** Sexually Transmitted Diseases; Sexual Dysfunction; Vulvar & Vaginal Disorders; Vulvar Pain; **Hospital:** Adv Illinois Masonic Med Ctr-Weiss Meml Hosp; **Address:** 3000 N Halsted St, Ste 625, Chicago, IL 60657; **Phone:** 773-296-3450; **Board Cert:** Obstetrics & Gynecology 1984; **Med School:** Ros Franklin Univ/Chicago Med Sch 1978; **Resid:** Obstetrics & Gynecology, Illinois Masonic Med Ctr 1982; **Fac Appt:** Asst Prof ObG, Rush Med Coll

Merritt, Diane F MD [ObG] - **Spec Exp:** Adolescent Gynecology; Pediatric Gynecology; Endometriosis; Congenital Anomalies-Gynecologic; **Hospital:** Barnes-Jewish Hosp, St. Louis Chldns Hosp; **Address:** Washington Univ Sch Med, 660 S Euclid Ave, Box 8064, St Louis, MO 63110; **Phone:** 314-362-4211; **Board Cert:** Obstetrics & Gynecology 1984; **Med School:** NYU Sch Med 1975; **Resid:** Surgery, Barnes Hosp-Wash Univ 1977; Obstetrics & Gynecology, Barnes Hosp-Wash Univ 1980; **Fac Appt:** Prof ObG, Washington Univ, St Louis

Niebyl, Jennifer R MD [ObG] - **Spec Exp:** Premature Labor; Vomiting-Cyclic; **Hospital:** Univ Iowa Hosp & Clinics; **Address:** Univ Iowa Hosps & Clins, 200 Hawkins Drive, Dept Ob/Gyn, Iowa City, IA 52242; **Phone:** 319-384-9247; **Board Cert:** Obstetrics & Gynecology 1998; Maternal & Fetal Medicine 1998; **Med School:** Yale Univ 1967; **Resid:** Obstetrics & Gynecology, NY Hosp-Cornell Med Ctr 1970; Obstetrics & Gynecology, Johns Hopkins Hosp 1973; **Fellow:** Maternal & Fetal Medicine, Johns Hopkins Hosp 1978; **Fac Appt:** Prof ObG, Univ Iowa Coll Med

Valaitis, Sandra MD [ObG] - **Spec Exp:** Pelvic Organ Prolapse Repair; Incontinence; **Hospital:** Univ of Chicago Med Ctr; **Address:** Univ Chicago Med Ctr, Dept Ob/Gyn, 5841 S Maryland Ave, MC 2050, Chicago, IL 60637; **Phone:** 773-834-8622; **Board Cert:** Obstetrics & Gynecology 2011; **Med School:** Univ Chicago-Pritzker Sch Med 1989; **Resid:** Obstetrics & Gynecology, Univ Chicago Med Ctr 1993; **Fellow:** Uro-Gynecology, St Georges Hosp; **Fac Appt:** Assoc Prof ObG, Univ Chicago-Pritzker Sch Med

Walters, Mark D MD [ObG] - **Spec Exp:** Uro-Gynecology; Vaginal Reconstruction; Incontinence-Female; Pelvic Organ Prolapse Repair; **Hospital:** Cleveland Clin (page 55); **Address:** Cleveland Clinic, Dept Ob/Gyn, 9500 Euclid Ave, Desk A81, Cleveland, OH 44195; **Phone:** 216-444-6601; **Board Cert:** Obstetrics & Gynecology 2011; **Med School:** Ohio State Univ 1980; **Resid:** Obstetrics & Gynecology, New England Med Ctr 1984; **Fac Appt:** Prof ObG, Cleveland Cl Coll Med/Case West Res

Great Plains and Mountains

Byrne, Janice LB MD [ObG] - **Spec Exp:** Prenatal Diagnosis, Ultrasound; Reproductive Genetics; **Hospital:** Univ Utah Hlth Care; **Address:** 50 N Medical Drive, Ste 2B200, Salt Lake City, UT 84132; **Phone:** 801-581-8425; **Board Cert:** Obstetrics & Gynecology 2010; Clinical Genetics 2010; Maternal & Fetal Medicine 2010; **Med School:** Univ Tex SW, Dallas 1987; **Resid:** Obstetrics & Gynecology, Univ Utah Hosps & Clins 1991; **Fellow:** Clinical Genetics, Univ Utah Hosps & Clins 1993; Maternal & Fetal Medicine, Univ Utah Hosps & Clins 1994; **Fac Appt:** Assoc Prof ObG, Univ Utah

King, Aileen MD [ObG] - **Spec Exp:** Women's Health; **Hospital:** St. Luke's Boise Med Ctr; **Address:** Women's Health Assocs, 333 N First St, Ste 240, Boise, ID 83702; **Phone:** 208-338-8900; **Board Cert:** Obstetrics & Gynecology 2011; **Med School:** UC Irvine 1996; **Resid:** Obstetrics & Gynecology, Univ CO Hlth Sci Ctr 2000

Southwest

Bradshaw, Karen D MD [ObG] - **Spec Exp:** Women's Health; Preventive Medicine; Pediatric & Adolescent Gynecology; Menstrual Disorders; **Hospital:** UT Southwestern Med Ctr at Dallas; **Address:** Lowe Ctr for Womens Preventive Health, 5939 Harry Hines Blvd, Dallas, TX 75390-8865; **Phone:** 214-645-3888; **Board Cert:** Obstetrics & Gynecology 2010; Reproductive Endocrinology 2010; **Med School:** Univ Tex SW, Dallas 1981; **Resid:** Obstetrics & Gynecology, Parkland Hosp 1985; **Fellow:** Reproductive Endocrinology, UT-Southwestern Med Ctr 1987; **Fac Appt:** Prof ObG, Univ Tex SW, Dallas

Cornella, Jeffrey L MD [ObG] - **Spec Exp:** Pelvic Reconstruction; Robotic Surgery; Uro-Gynecology; Vaginal Reconstruction; **Hospital:** Mayo Clinic - Phoenix; **Address:** Mayo Clinic Gynecology, 5779 E Mayo Blvd, Phoenix, AZ 85054; **Phone:** 480-301-8484; **Board Cert:** Obstetrics & Gynecology 2011; **Med School:** Washington Univ, St Louis 1981; **Resid:** Obstetrics & Gynecology, Mayo Clinic 1986; **Fellow:** Uro-Gynecology, UC Irvine 1987; **Fac Appt:** Prof ObG, Mayo Med Sch

Snyder, Russell R MD [ObG] - **Spec Exp:** Gynecologic Surgery; Pap Smear Abnormalities; Vulvar & Vaginal Disorders; **Hospital:** UT Med Br at Galveston(Joh Sealy Hosp); **Address:** UTMB at Galveston,Women's Health Ctr, 301 University Blvd, Route 1386, Galveston, TX 77555-1022; **Phone:** 409-772-9507; **Board Cert:** Obstetrics & Gynecology 1994; **Med School:** Univ Tex, Houston 1978; **Resid:** Obstetrics & Gynecology, Wilford Hall USAF Med Ctr 1982; **Fellow:** Gynecologic Pathology, Armed Forces Inst Path 1984; **Fac Appt:** Assoc Prof ObG, Univ Tex Med Br, Galveston

West Coast and Pacific

Eschenbach, David A MD [ObG] - **Spec Exp:** Gynecologic Surgery-Complex; Vulvar & Vaginal Disorders; **Hospital:** Univ Wash Med Ctr; **Address:** Univ Washington Women's Health Care, 4245 Roosevelt Way NE, Box 354765, Seattle, WA 98105; **Phone:** 206-598-5500; **Board Cert:** Obstetrics & Gynecology 1975; **Med School:** Univ Wisc 1968; **Resid:** Obstetrics & Gynecology, Univ Wash Hosp 1973; **Fellow:** Infectious Disease, Univ Wash Hosp 1974; **Fac Appt:** Prof ObG, Univ Wash

Goldman, Mindy E MD [ObG] - **Spec Exp:** Breast Cancer; **Hospital:** UCSF Med Ctr; **Address:** 2356 Sutter St, San Francisco, CA 94115; **Phone:** 415-885-7788; **Board Cert:** Obstetrics & Gynecology 2007; **Med School:** Univ VT Coll Med 1989; **Resid:** Obstetrics & Gynecology, UCSF Med Ctr 1993

Parker, William H MD [ObG] - **Spec Exp:** Gynecologic Surgery; Hysteroscopic Surgery; Laparoscopic Surgery; Uterine Fibroids; **Hospital:** St. John's Hlth Ctr, Santa Monica; **Address:** 1450 10th St, Ste 404, Santa Monica, CA 90401-2804; **Phone:** 310-451-8144; **Board Cert:** Obstetrics & Gynecology 1981; **Med School:** SUNY Downstate 1974; **Resid:** Obstetrics & Gynecology, UCSD Med Ctr 1978; **Fac Appt:** Clin Prof ObG, UCLA

Sweet, Richard L MD [ObG] - **Spec Exp:** Sexually Transmitted Diseases; Infectious Diseases-Gynecologic; Women's Health; Infections in Pregnancy; **Hospital:** UC Davis Med Ctr; **Address:** UC Davis Women's Center for Health, 4860 Y St, Ste 2500, Sacramento, CA 95817; **Phone:** 916-734-6670; **Board Cert:** Obstetrics & Gynecology 1975; **Med School:** Univ Mich Med Sch 1966; **Resid:** Obstetrics & Gynecology, Univ Mich Med Ctr 1973; **Fac Appt:** Prof ObG, UC Davis

Maimonides Medical Center
STELLA AND JOSEPH PAYSON BIRTHING CENTER

Maimonides
Medical Center

4802 Tenth Avenue • Brooklyn, New York 11219
Phone: 718.283.7048 • Fax: 718.283.7167
www.maimonidesmed.org/obgyn

The Birthing Center features private suites with hardwood floors and a home-like environment. At the same time, physician coverage is provided 24/7 in our advanced Neonatal Intensive Care Unit. Our 36 obstetricians and 26 midwives have found that most families appreciate having the best of both worlds available to them.

Maimonides provides other unique services to its maternity patients. The largest doula program in the metropolitan area can be found at Maimonides. These fully-trained childbirth assistants are available to patients before, during and after delivery at no cost to families. And the maternity units utilize an electronic patient record that sets industry standards for patient safety and hospital efficiency.

This combination of family-centered services and advanced technology continues to have enormous appeal to the women served — over 7,800 of them last year alone. Our highly trained staff includes the finest nurses, physicians, midwives and specialists to ensure the safety and comfort of our patients. Several physicians specialize in high-risk pregnancy, including the Chair of Obstetrics & Gynecology, Howard Minkoff, MD.

Women who give birth at Maimonides also have a variety of other services available to them, including:

- A Perinatal Testing Center, directed by Shoshana Haberman, MD, offering amniocentesis, 3-D ultrasound, fetal echocardiograms and other diagnostic exams.

- Neonatologists on-site around-the-clock. The Norma Sutton Center for Neonatology adjoins the Payson Birthing Center and provides the most sophisticated care in a family-friendly environment.

The Stella and Joseph Payson Birthing Center is ranked among the best in the nation for maternity care by HealthGrades, the nation's leading source for independent health care quality information. In recognition of its excellence in obstetrics and pediatrics, Maimonides was designated a Regional Perinatal Center by the New York State Department of Health. More babies are delivered at Maimonides than at any other single-campus hospital in New York State.

Maimonides Medical Center
Passionate about medicine.
Compassionate about people
www.maimonidesmed.org/ob

OBSTETRICS AND GYNECOLOGY

About the Department of Obstetrics and Gynecology
NYU Langone Medical Center provides comprehensive programs and services designed specifically for women, from primary care to highly specialized programs that are supported by sophisticated research and advanced training. We specialize in the following areas:

Fertility-Related Services
NYU Langone offers state-of-the-art programs in egg donation, egg freezing and wellness (acupuncture, mind/body, psychology and yoga). Diagnosis and treatment include ovulation induction, assisted reproductive technologies and surgical options that incorporate the latest endoscopic techniques. The Center also tests for genetic abnormalities, as well as for immunity and infectious diseases.

Gynecologic Oncology
The NCI-designated NYU Cancer Institute's Women's Cancer Program specializes in the treatment of cervical cancer, endometrial cancer, ovarian cancer, uterine cancer, vaginal cancer and vulvar cancer.

Maternal Fetal Medicine
Prenatal care for high-risk pregnancies and detailed consultations before, during and after pregnancy are offered. Special attention is given to multifetal pregnancies and to women who have other medical conditions that may complicate a pregnancy, such as diabetes, heart problems, high blood pressure and lupus.

Obstetrics
We offer a broad range of obstetrical services, including prenatal care that gives equal emphasis to the well-being of the mother and the fetus; fetal monitoring through ultrasound and other techniques; childbirth preparedness and breastfeeding classes; consultation for high-risk pregnancies, including treatment for women who have experienced recurrent pregnancy loss.

Specialty Services
In addition to routine gynecological care, we offer pelvic ultrasound; aspiration of breast cysts; evaluation of infertility (including the special needs of same-sex couples); colposcopy (a diagnostic evaluation of abnormal pap smears); LEEP (a loop electrosurgical procedure used to diagnose and treat cervical cancer); cryotherapy for vaginal warts; and bone density testing.

Urogynecology and Reconstructive Pelvic Surgery
Our urogynecologists treat all forms of incontinence and pelvic disorders; malformations of the reproductive tract found at birth, during childhood or in young adults; and conditions such as overactive bladder, urinary and/or fecal incontinence and pelvic organ prolapse.

A Leader in Women's Health Care

Penn Ob/Gyn Care has a long tradition of excellence, providing women's health services for more than two centuries. The team is a pioneer in the development of new and innovative approaches to manage women's health needs and is recognized as a national leader in obstetrics, gynecology and fertility care. Penn Ob/Gyn Care specialists provide comprehensive, patient-centered care utilizing the most advanced treatment options and therapies available.

Locations

Hospital of the University of Pennsylvania

Penn Presbyterian Medical Center

Pennsylvania Hospital

Penn Medicine Radnor

Services also available at:

The Pavilions at Voorhees and satellite locations throughout New Jersey and Pennsylvania

World-Class Patient Care

- Penn offers the most comprehensive women's health program in the region, including preventive and consultative services, diagnostic imaging and testing, drug therapy and surgical treatment options. Penn specialists personalize treatment plans to match the needs of every patient.

- Penn physicians, nurses and clinical staff create a supportive environment for patients. They understand what it's like to be on the patients' side of the table. They listen and they tailor recommendations and care plans to individual needs.

- Penn's ob/gyn specialists are at the forefront of medicine. Because they teach the next generation of leaders, they are well-versed in the latest clinical practices today as well as developing promising treatment options for tomorrow.

- As a national leader in basic science, translational research and clinical trials, Penn offers patients access to the latest treatment options before they are widely available elsewhere in the region.

For more information or to schedule an appointment, call 800.789.PENN (7366) or visit PennMedicine.org/obgyn

Ophthalmology

An ophthalmologist has the knowledge and professional skills needed to provide comprehensive eye and vision care. Ophthalmologists are medically trained to diagnose, monitor and medically or surgically treat all ocular and visual disorders. This includes problems affecting the eye and its component structures, the eyelids, the orbit and the visual pathways. In so doing, an ophthalmologist prescribes vision services, including glasses and contact lenses.

Training Required: Four years

OPHTHALMOLOGY

New England

Dana, Reza MD [Oph] - **Spec Exp:** Corneal Disease & Transplant; Dry Eye Syndrome; Uveitis; **Hospital:** Mass Eye & Ear Infirmary; **Address:** Mass Eye & Ear Infirmary, 243 Charles St, Boston, MA 02114; **Phone:** 617-573-4331; **Board Cert:** Ophthalmology 2006; **Med School:** Johns Hopkins Univ 1989; **Resid:** Ophthalmology, Illinois Eye & Ear Infirm 1993; **Fellow:** Cornea & Ext Eye Disease, Wills Eye Hosp 1994; Uveitis, Mass Eye & Ear Infirm 1995; **Fac Appt:** Prof Oph, Harvard Med Sch

Duker, Jay S MD [Oph] - **Spec Exp:** Retinal Disorders; Retinal Disorders-Pediatric; Diabetic Eye Disease/Retinopathy; **Hospital:** Tufts Med Ctr; **Address:** New England Eye Center, 260 Tremont St Biewend Bldg, Boston, MA 02111; **Phone:** 617-636-4677; **Board Cert:** Ophthalmology 1989; **Med School:** Jefferson Med Coll 1984; **Resid:** Ophthalmology, Wills Eye Hosp 1988; **Fellow:** Vitreoretinal Surgery & Disease, Wills Eye Hosp 1990; **Fac Appt:** Assoc Prof Oph, Tufts Univ

Foster, C Stephen MD [Oph] - **Spec Exp:** Uveitis; Corneal Disease; Cataract Surgery; **Hospital:** Mass Eye & Ear Infirmary, Mount Auburn Hosp; **Address:** 5 Cambridge Ctr, Fl 8, Cambridge, MA 02142; **Phone:** 866-353-6377; **Board Cert:** Ophthalmology 1976; **Med School:** Duke Univ 1969; **Resid:** Ophthalmology, Barnes Hosp 1975; **Fellow:** Cornea, Mass EE Infirm-Harvard 1976; Ocular Immunology, Mass EE Infirm-Harvard 1977; **Fac Appt:** Prof Oph, Harvard Med Sch

Hedges, Thomas R MD [Oph] - **Spec Exp:** Neuro-Ophthalmology; **Hospital:** Tufts Med Ctr; **Address:** New England Eye Center, 260 Tremont St Biewend Bldg, Boston, MA 02111; **Phone:** 617-636-5488; **Board Cert:** Ophthalmology 1980; **Med School:** Tufts Univ 1975; **Resid:** Ophthalmology, Mass EE Infirm 1980; **Fellow:** Neuro-Ophthalmology, UCSF Med Ctr 1981; **Fac Appt:** Prof Oph, Tufts Univ

Hunter, David G MD/PhD [Oph] - **Spec Exp:** Pediatric Ophthalmology; Eye Muscle Disorders; Strabismus; Congenital Fibrosis-Extraocular Muscles; **Hospital:** Children's Hospital - Boston; **Address:** Children's Hospital, Fegan-4, 300 Longwood Ave, Boston, MA 02115; **Phone:** 617-355-6766; **Board Cert:** Ophthalmology 2003; Pediatric Ophthalmology ; **Med School:** Baylor Coll Med 1987; **Resid:** Ophthalmology, Mass EE Infirm 1991; **Fellow:** Pediatric Ophthalmology, Wilmer Ophthalmic Inst/Johns Hopkins 1992; **Fac Appt:** Prof Oph, Harvard Med Sch

Kornmehl, Ernest W MD [Oph] - **Spec Exp:** LASIK-Refractive Surgery; PRK-Refractive Surgery; Dry Eye Syndrome; Keratoconus; **Hospital:** Mass Eye & Ear Infirmary, Brigham and Women's Hosp (page 57); **Address:** Kornmehl Laser Eye Assoc, 54 Washington St, Brookline, MA 02445; **Phone:** 877-870-2010; **Board Cert:** Ophthalmology 1989; **Med School:** SUNY Downstate 1984; **Resid:** Ophthalmology, Yale-New Haven Hosp 1988; **Fellow:** Cornea & Ext Eye Disease, Mass E&E Infirm 1990; **Fac Appt:** Assoc Clin Prof Oph, Harvard Med Sch

Miller, Joan W MD [Oph] - **Spec Exp:** Macular Degeneration; Retinal Disorders; **Hospital:** Mass Eye & Ear Infirmary; **Address:** Mass Eye & Ear Infirm, Ophthalmology, 243 Charles St, Boston, MA 02114; **Phone:** 617-573-3915; **Board Cert:** Ophthalmology 1991; **Med School:** Harvard Med Sch 1985; **Resid:** Ophthalmology, Mass Eye & Ear Infirm 1989; **Fellow:** Retina, Mass Eye & Ear Infirm 1991; **Fac Appt:** Prof Oph, Harvard Med Sch

Mitchell, Paul R MD [Oph] - **Spec Exp:** Pediatric Ophthalmology; Nystagmus; Strabismus; **Hospital:** CT Chldns Med Ctr, Hartford Hosp; **Address:** Chldns Eye Care, 366 Colt Highway, Route 6, Bldg 2, Farmington, CT 06032; **Phone:** 860-409-0449; **Board Cert:** Ophthalmology 1977; **Med School:** Geo Wash Univ 1970; **Resid:** Ophthalmology, Wills Eye Hosp 1976; **Fellow:** Pediatric Ophthalmology, Chldns Hosp MC/Geo Wash 1977; **Fac Appt:** Asst Clin Prof Oph, Univ Conn

Rizzo III, Joseph F MD [Oph] - **Spec Exp:** Neuro-Ophthalmology; **Hospital:** Mass Eye & Ear Infirmary; **Address:** Mass Eye & Ear Infirmary, 243 Charles St Fl 9, Boston, MA 02114; **Phone:** 617-573-3412; **Board Cert:** Neurology 1984; Ophthalmology 1987; **Med School:** Louisiana State U, New Orleans 1978; **Resid:** Neurology, Tufts-New Engl Med Ctr 1982; Ophthalmology, Boston Univ 1985; **Fellow:** Neuro-Ophthalmology, Harvard Univ 1986; **Fac Appt:** Assoc Prof Oph, Harvard Med Sch

Rubin, Peter MD [Oph] - **Spec Exp:** Oculoplastic Surgery; Orbital & Eyelid Tumors/Cancer; Eyelid Cancer & Reconstruction; Eyelid Cosmetic & Reconstructive Surgery; **Hospital:** Beth Israel Deaconess Med Ctr - Boston; **Address:** Boston Eye Phys and Surgeons, 44 Washington St, Brookline, MA 02445; **Phone:** 617-232-9600; **Board Cert:** Ophthalmology 1991; **Med School:** Yale Univ 1985; **Resid:** Ophthalmology, Lenox Hill Hosp 1989; **Fellow:** Oculoplastic Surgery, Mass Eye & Ear Infirmary 1991; **Fac Appt:** Assoc Prof Oph, Univ Tenn Coll Med

Shingleton, Bradford J MD [Oph] - **Spec Exp:** Cataract Surgery; Glaucoma; **Hospital:** Mass Eye & Ear Infirmary; **Address:** Ophthalmic Consultants of Boston, 50 Stanford St, Ste 600, Boston, MA 02114; **Phone:** 617-314-2614; **Board Cert:** Ophthalmology 1982; **Med School:** Univ Mich Med Sch 1977; **Resid:** Ophthalmology, Mass E&E Infirm 1981; **Fellow:** Refractive Surgery, Mass E&E Infirm 1982; **Fac Appt:** Asst Clin Prof Oph, Harvard Med Sch

Tsai, James C MD [Oph] - **Spec Exp:** Glaucoma; **Hospital:** Yale-New Haven Hosp, Yale Med Group; **Address:** 40 Temple St, New Haven, CT 06520-8061; **Phone:** 203-785-2020; **Board Cert:** Ophthalmology 2006; **Med School:** Stanford Univ 1989; **Resid:** Ophthalmology, Doheny Eye Inst/USC 1993; **Fellow:** Glaucoma, Bascom Palmer Eye Inst 1994; Glaucoma, Moorfields Eye Hosp 1995; **Fac Appt:** Prof Oph, Yale Univ

Walton, David S MD [Oph] - **Spec Exp:** Glaucoma-Pediatric; Cataract-Pediatric; Neuro-Ophthalmology; **Hospital:** Mass Eye & Ear Infirmary, Mass Genl Hosp; **Address:** 2 Longfellow Pl, Ste 201, Boston, MA 02114; **Phone:** 617-227-3011; **Board Cert:** Ophthalmology 1969; Pediatrics 1983; **Med School:** Duke Univ 1961; **Resid:** Ophthalmology, Mass EE Infirm 1967; **Fellow:** Glaucoma, Mass EE Infirm 1968; **Fac Appt:** Prof Oph, Harvard Med Sch

Mid Atlantic

Abramson, David H MD [Oph] - **Spec Exp:** Eye Tumors/Cancer; Orbital Tumors/Cancer; Retinoblastoma; Melanoma-Choroidal (eye); **Hospital:** Meml Sloan-Kettering Cancer Ctr, NY-Presby/Weill Cornell Med Ctr, NY (page 66); **Address:** 70 E 66th St, New York, NY 10065; **Phone:** 212-744-1700; **Board Cert:** Ophthalmology 1975; **Med School:** Albert Einstein Coll Med 1969; **Resid:** Ophthalmology, Harkness Eye Inst 1974; **Fellow:** Ocular Oncology, Columbia-Presby Med Ctr 1975; **Fac Appt:** Prof Oph, Cornell Univ-Weill Med Coll

Bressler, Neil M MD [Oph] - **Spec Exp:** Retinal Disorders; **Hospital:** Johns Hopkins Hosp (page 61); **Address:** Wilmer Eye Institute, 600 N Wolfe St, Maumenee Bldg-752, Baltimore, MD 21287; **Phone:** 410-955-8342; **Board Cert:** Ophthalmology 1987; **Med School:** Johns Hopkins Univ 1982; **Resid:** Internal Medicine, Johns Hopkins Hosp 1983; Ophthalmology, Mass Eye & Ear firm 1986; **Fellow:** Retina, Wilmer Inst/Johns Hopkins Hosp 1987; **Fac Appt:** Assoc Prof Oph, J Hopkins Univ

Ophthalmology

Bressler, Susan B MD [Oph] - **Spec Exp:** Diabetic Eye Disease/Retinopathy; Retinal Disorders; Macular Degeneration; **Hospital:** Johns Hopkins Hosp (page 61); **Address:** The Johns Hopkins Hospital, Wilmer Eye Institute-Maumenee 706, 600 N Wolfe St, Baltimore, MD 21287; **Phone:** 410-955-3648; **Board Cert:** Ophthalmology 1987; **Med School:** Johns Hopkins Univ 1982; **Resid:** Ophthalmology, Mass Eye & Ear Infirmary 1986; **Fellow:** Ophthalmology, Wilmer Eye Inst 1987; Retinal Surgery, Mass Eye & Ear Infirmary 1988; **Fac Appt:** Prof Oph, Johns Hopkins Univ

Brown, Gary C MD [Oph] - **Spec Exp:** Retinal Disorders; Retinal Vascular Diseases; Macular Degeneration; **Hospital:** Wills Eye Hosp, Thomas Jefferson Univ Hosp; **Address:** Mid-Atlantic Retina, 4060 Butler Pike, Ste 200, Plymouth Meeting, PA 19462; **Phone:** 800-331-6634; **Board Cert:** Ophthalmology 2003; **Med School:** SUNY Upstate Med Univ 1975; **Resid:** Ophthalmology, Wills Eye Hosp 1979; **Fellow:** Vitreoretinal Disease, Wills Eye Hosp 1981; **Fac Appt:** Prof Oph, Jefferson Med Coll

Brucker, Alexander J MD [Oph] - **Spec Exp:** Retinal Disorders; Retina/Vitreous Surgery; Macular Degeneration; **Hospital:** Penn Presby Med Ctr - UPHS (page 72), Hosp Univ Penn - UPHS (page 72); **Address:** Penn Presby Med Ctr, Scheie Eye Inst, 51 N 39th St, Ste 517, Philadelphia, PA 19104; **Phone:** 215-662-8100; **Board Cert:** Ophthalmology 1977; **Med School:** NY Med Coll 1972; **Resid:** Ophthalmology, Friedenwald Inst 1976; **Fellow:** Retina/Vitreous, Johns Hopkins Hosp 1977; **Fac Appt:** Prof Oph, Univ Pennsylvania

Campochiaro, Peter MD [Oph] - **Spec Exp:** Retina/Vitreous Surgery; **Hospital:** Johns Hopkins Hosp (page 61); **Address:** Wilmer Ophthalmological Inst, 600 N Wolfe St, 747 Maumenee, Baltimore, MD 21287-9277; **Phone:** 410-955-5106; **Board Cert:** Ophthalmology 1983; **Med School:** Johns Hopkins Univ 1978; **Resid:** Ophthalmology, Univ Virginia 1982; **Fellow:** Retina/Vitreous, John Hopkins Univ 1984; **Fac Appt:** Prof Oph, Johns Hopkins Univ

Caputo, Anthony R MD [Oph] - **Spec Exp:** Pediatric Ophthalmology; Strabismus; **Hospital:** Clara Maass Med Ctr; **Address:** 556 Eagle Rock Ave, Ste 203, Roseland, NJ 07068-1500; **Phone:** 973-228-3111; **Board Cert:** Ophthalmology 1976; **Med School:** Italy 1969; **Resid:** Ophthalmology, UMDNJ-Univ Hosp 1974; **Fellow:** Ophthalmology, Wills Eye Hosp 1975; **Fac Appt:** Prof Oph, UMDNJ-NJ Med Sch, Newark

Chang, Stanley MD [Oph] - **Spec Exp:** Retina/Vitreous Surgery; Diabetic Eye Disease/Retinopathy; Macular Disease/Degeneration; Retinal Disorders; **Hospital:** NY Presby/Columbia Univ Med Ctr, NY (page 66); **Address:** 635 W 165th St, Box 20, New York, NY 10032; **Phone:** 212-305-9535; **Board Cert:** Ophthalmology 1979; **Med School:** Columbia P&S 1974; **Resid:** Ophthalmology, Mass Eye & Ear Infirm 1978; **Fellow:** Vitreoretinal Surgery, Bascom Palmer Eye Inst 1979; **Fac Appt:** Prof Oph, Columbia P&S

Clinch, Thomas E MD [Oph] - **Spec Exp:** Laser Vision Surgery; LASIK-Refractive Surgery; **Hospital:** Washington Hosp Ctr; **Address:** Eye Doctors of Washington, 2 Wisconsin Cir, Ste 200, Chevy Chase, MD 20815; **Phone:** 301-215-7100; **Board Cert:** Ophthalmology 1989; **Med School:** Jefferson Med Coll 1983; **Resid:** Ophthalmology, Wills Eye Hosp 1988

Cykiert, Robert MD [Oph] - **Spec Exp:** LASIK-Refractive Surgery; Cataract Surgery; Corneal Disease & Transplant; Keratoconus; **Hospital:** NYU Langone Med Ctr (page 68), New York Eye & Ear Infirm (page 65); **Address:** 345 E 37th St, Ste 210, New York, NY 10016-3217; **Phone:** 212-922-1430; **Board Cert:** Ophthalmology 1981; **Med School:** NY Med Coll 1976; **Resid:** Ophthalmology, Montefiore Med Ctr 1980; **Fellow:** Cornea, Wills Eye Hosp 1981; **Fac Appt:** Assoc Clin Prof Oph, NYU Sch Med

D'Amico, Donald J MD [Oph] - **Spec Exp:** Diabetic Eye Disease/Retinopathy; Retinal Detachment; Retinal Disorders; **Hospital:** NY-Presby/Weill Cornell Med Ctr, NY (page 66); **Address:** Weill Cornell Medical College, Dept of Ophthalmology, 1305 York Ave, Fl 11th, New York, NY 10021; **Phone:** 646-962-2020; **Board Cert:** Ophthalmology 1982; **Med School:** Univ IL Coll Med 1977; **Resid:** Ophthalmology, Mass Eye & Ear Infirm 1981; **Fellow:** Vitreoretinal Surgery, Bascom Palmer Eye Inst 1982; **Fac Appt:** Prof Oph, Cornell Univ-Weill Med Coll

Della Rocca, Robert C MD [Oph] - **Spec Exp:** Orbital Tumors/Cancer; Eyelid Tumors/Cancer; Thyroid Eye Disease; Oculoplastic Surgery; **Hospital:** New York Eye & Ear Infirm (page 65), Sound Shore Med Ctr - Westchester; **Address:** 310 E 14th St, South Bldg, rm 319, New York, NY 10003; **Phone:** 212-979-4575; **Board Cert:** Ophthalmology 1975; **Med School:** Creighton Univ 1967; **Resid:** Ophthalmology, NY Eye & Ear Infirm 1973; **Fellow:** Oculoplastic Surgery, Albany Med Ctr

Dhaliwal, Deepinder K MD [Oph] - **Spec Exp:** Refractive Surgery; Corneal & External Eye Disease; Anterior Segment Surgery; **Hospital:** UPMC Presby, Pittsburgh; **Address:** UPMC Eye Center, 203 Lothrop St, Ste 718, Pittsburgh, PA 15213; **Phone:** 412-647-2200; **Board Cert:** Ophthalmology 2007; **Med School:** Northwestern Univ-Feinberg Sch Med 1990; **Resid:** Ophthalmology, Univ Pitt Eye & Ear Inst 1994; **Fellow:** Refractive Surgery, Univ Utah 1995; **Fac Appt:** Assoc Prof Oph, Univ Pittsburgh

Dodick, Jack M MD [Oph] - **Spec Exp:** Cataract Surgery-Lens Implant; Laser Vision Surgery; **Hospital:** NYU Langone Med Ctr (page 68), Lenox Hill Hosp (Manh Eye, Ear & Throat Hosp) (page 67); **Address:** 535 Park Ave, New York, NY 10065; **Phone:** 212-288-7638; **Board Cert:** Ophthalmology 1969; **Med School:** Univ Toronto 1963; **Resid:** Ophthalmology, Manhattan EE&T Hosp 1967; **Fellow:** Anterior Segment - External Disease, Westchester Co Med Ctr 1968; **Fac Appt:** Prof Oph, NYU Sch Med

Eagle, Ralph C MD [Oph] - **Spec Exp:** Ophthalmic Pathology; **Hospital:** Wills Eye Hosp; **Address:** Wills Eye Hosp, Dept Pathology, 840 Walnut St, Ste 1410, Philadelphia, PA 19107; **Phone:** 215-928-3280; **Board Cert:** Ophthalmology 1976; **Med School:** Univ Pennsylvania 1970; **Resid:** Ophthalmology, Scheie Eye Inst 1975; **Fellow:** Ophthalmic Pathology, Armed Forces Inst Path 1978; **Fac Appt:** Prof Oph, Jefferson Med Coll

Eggers, Howard M MD [Oph] - **Spec Exp:** Pediatric Ophthalmology; Strabismus-Adult & Pediatric; **Hospital:** NY-Presby/Columbia Univ Med Ctr, NY (page 66); **Address:** Harkness Eye Institute, 635 W 165th St, New York, NY 10032-3724; **Phone:** 212-305-5409; **Board Cert:** Ophthalmology 1978; **Med School:** Columbia P&S 1971; **Resid:** Ophthalmology, Harkness Inst-Presby Hosp 1975; **Fac Appt:** Prof Oph, Columbia P&S

Feldon, Steven E MD [Oph] - **Spec Exp:** Neuro-Ophthalmology; Orbital Surgery; Strabismus; Thyroid Eye Disease; **Hospital:** Univ of Rochester Strong Meml Hosp; **Address:** 601 Elmwood Ave, Box 659, Rochester, NY 14642; **Phone:** 585-275-1126; **Board Cert:** Ophthalmology 1979; **Med School:** Albert Einstein Coll Med 1973; **Resid:** Ophthalmology, Mass Eye & Ear Infirmary 1978; **Fellow:** Neurological Surgery, Mass Genl Hosp 1975; Neuro-Ophthalmology, UCSF Med Ctr 1979; **Fac Appt:** Prof Oph, Univ Rochester

Finger, Paul T MD [Oph] - **Spec Exp:** Eye Tumors/Cancer; Melanoma-Choroidal (eye); Retinoblastoma; Orbital Tumors/Cancer; **Hospital:** New York Eye & Ear Infirm (page 65), Lenox Hill Hosp (Manh Eye, Ear & Throat Hosp) (page 67); **Address:** 115 E 61st St Fl 5 - Ste B, New York, NY 10065; **Phone:** 212-832-8170; **Board Cert:** Ophthalmology 1990; **Med School:** Tulane Univ 1982; **Resid:** Ophthalmology, Manhattan EET Hosp 1986; **Fellow:** Ocular Oncology, N Shore Univ Hosp 1987; **Fac Appt:** Clin Prof Oph, NYU Sch Med

Ophthalmology

Florakis, George J MD [Oph] - **Spec Exp:** Cornea Transplant; Corneal Disease; Keratoconus; Anterior Segment Trauma/Reconstruction; **Hospital:** NY-Presby/Columbia Univ Med Ctr, NY (page 66), White Plains Hosp; **Address:** Edward S Harkness Eye Inst, Columbia Univ Med Ctr/NY Presby Hosp, 635 W 165th St, Ste 303, New York, NY 10032; **Phone:** 212-927-2394; **Board Cert:** Ophthalmology 1989; **Med School:** Columbia P&S 1983; **Resid:** Ophthalmology, Harkness Eye Inst 1987; **Fellow:** Cornea & Ext Eye Disease, Univ Iowa Hosps & Clins 1988; **Fac Appt:** Clin Prof Oph, Columbia P&S

Friberg, Thomas R MD [Oph] - **Spec Exp:** Retinal Disorders; Diabetic Eye Disease/Retinopathy; Macular Degeneration; **Hospital:** UPMC Presby, Pittsburgh; **Address:** UPMC Eye Ctr, 203 Lothrop St, Ste 718, Pittsburgh, PA 15213-2548; **Phone:** 412-647-2200; **Board Cert:** Ophthalmology 1979; **Med School:** Univ Minn 1973; **Resid:** Ophthalmology, Stanford Univ Med Ctr 1977; **Fellow:** Retina, Mass EE Infirmary 1978; Vitreoretinal Surgery, Duke Univ Med Ctr 1979; **Fac Appt:** Prof Oph, Univ Pittsburgh

Fuchs, Wayne MD [Oph] - **Spec Exp:** Diabetic Eye Disease/Retinopathy; Macular Disease/Degeneration; Retinal Disorders; Pseudoxanthoma Elasticum; **Hospital:** Mount Sinai Med Ctr (page 64), Lenox Hill Hosp (Manh Eye, Ear & Throat Hosp) (page 67); **Address:** 121 E 60th St, Ste 5B, New York, NY 10022-1186; **Phone:** 212-319-8205; **Board Cert:** Ophthalmology 1985; **Med School:** Mount Sinai Sch Med 1979; **Resid:** Ophthalmology, Mt Sinai Hosp 1983; **Fellow:** Vitreoretinal Surgery & Disease, NY Hosp-Cornell Med Ctr 1984; **Fac Appt:** Clin Prof Oph, Mount Sinai Sch Med

Gallin, Pamela F MD [Oph] - **Spec Exp:** Pediatric Ophthalmology; Amblyopia; Strabismus; Lacrimal Gland Disorders; **Hospital:** NY-Presby/Columbia Univ Med Ctr, NY (page 66), Lenox Hill Hosp (Manh Eye, Ear & Throat Hosp) (page 67); **Address:** NY Presby/Columbia Univ, 635 W 165th St, Ste 224, New York, NY 10032-3701; **Phone:** 212-305-5407; **Board Cert:** Ophthalmology 1983; **Med School:** Washington Univ, St Louis 1978; **Resid:** Ophthalmology, Mount Sinai Med Ctr 1982; **Fellow:** Pediatric Ophthalmology, Chldns Natl Med Ctr 1983; Strabismus, Columbia-Presby Med Ctr 1983; **Fac Appt:** Clin Prof Oph, Columbia P&S

Gentile, Ronald C MD [Oph] - **Spec Exp:** Retina/Vitreous Surgery; Diabetic Eye Disease/Retinopathy; Macular Degeneration; Retinal Disorders; **Hospital:** New York Eye & Ear Infirm (page 65); **Address:** 310 E 14th St, South Bldg, Ste 319, New York, NY 10003-4201; **Phone:** 212-979-4120; **Board Cert:** Ophthalmology 2008; **Med School:** SUNY Downstate 1991; **Resid:** Ophthalmology, NY Eye & Ear Infirm 1995; **Fellow:** Vitreoretinal Surgery & Disease, Kresge Eye Inst 1998; **Fac Appt:** Prof Oph, NY Med Coll

Gibralter, Richard P MD [Oph] - **Spec Exp:** Cataract Surgery; Laser Vision Surgery; Cornea Transplant; Corneal Disease & Surgery; **Hospital:** Lenox Hill Hosp (Manh Eye, Ear & Throat Hosp) (page 67), New York Eye & Ear Infirm (page 65); **Address:** 154 E 71st St, New York, NY 10021-5123; **Phone:** 212-628-2202; **Board Cert:** Ophthalmology 1981; **Med School:** Mount Sinai Sch Med 1976; **Resid:** Ophthalmology, Manhattan EE&T Hosp 1980; **Fellow:** Cornea, Manhattan EE&T Hosp 1981; **Fac Appt:** Assoc Clin Prof Oph, NYU Sch Med

Goldberg, Daniel B MD [Oph] - **Spec Exp:** LASIK-Refractive Surgery; Cornea Transplant; Cataract Surgery; Lens Implants; **Address:** Atlantic Laser Vision Center, 180 White Rd, Ste 202, Little Silver, NJ 07739-1166; **Phone:** 732-219-9220; **Board Cert:** Ophthalmology 1979; **Med School:** SUNY Downstate 1974; **Resid:** Ophthalmology, SUNY Downstate 1978; **Fellow:** Cornea, Eye & Ear Hosp 1979; **Fac Appt:** Assoc Clin Prof Oph, Drexel Univ Coll Med

Guyton, David L MD [Oph] - **Spec Exp:** Strabismus; Pediatric Ophthalmology; **Hospital:** Johns Hopkins Hosp (page 61); **Address:** Wilmer 233, Johns Hopkins Hospital, 600 N Wolfe St, Baltimore, MD 21287; **Phone:** 410-955-5492; **Board Cert:** Ophthalmology 1977; **Med School:** Harvard Med Sch 1969; **Resid:** Ophthalmology, Johns Hopkins Hosp 1976; **Fellow:** Pediatric Ophthalmology, Baylor Coll Med 1977; **Fac Appt:** Prof Oph, Johns Hopkins Univ

Hall, Lisabeth S MD [Oph] - **Spec Exp:** Pediatric Ophthalmology; Strabismus-Adult & Pediatric; Eye Muscle Disorders; Cataract-Pediatric; **Hospital:** New York Eye & Ear Infirm (page 65); **Address:** 40 W 72nd St, New York, NY 10023; **Phone:** 212-979-4614; **Board Cert:** Ophthalmology 2009; **Med School:** SUNY Stony Brook 1992; **Resid:** Ophthalmology, Manhattan Eye & Ear Infirm 1996; **Fellow:** Pediatric Ophthalmology, Jules Stein Eye Inst 1997; **Fac Appt:** Assoc Prof Oph, NY Med Coll

Haller, Julia Allison MD [Oph] - **Spec Exp:** Retina/Vitreous Surgery; Retinal Disorders; **Hospital:** Wills Eye Hosp, Thomas Jefferson Univ Hosp; **Address:** 840 Walnut St, Ste 1510, Philadelphia, PA 19107; **Phone:** 215-928-3073; **Board Cert:** Ophthalmology 1987; **Med School:** Harvard Med Sch 1980; **Resid:** Ophthalmology, Wilmer Eye Inst/Johns Hopkins 1985; **Fellow:** Retina/Vitreous, Wilmer Eye Inst/Johns Hopkins 1986; **Fac Appt:** Prof Oph, Jefferson Med Coll

Handa, James T MD [Oph] - **Spec Exp:** Macular Degeneration; Melanoma-Choroidal (eye); Retinoblastoma; **Hospital:** Johns Hopkins Hosp (page 61); **Address:** Wilmer Eye Inst Retina Div, 600 N Wolfe St, Ste 100, Baltimore, MD 21287; **Phone:** 410-955-3518; **Board Cert:** Ophthalmology 1991; **Med School:** Univ Pennsylvania 1986; **Resid:** Ophthalmology, Wills Eye Hosp 1990; **Fellow:** Retina/Vitreous, Duke Eye Ctr 1992; Ophthalmic Oncololgy, USC Sch Med 1993; **Fac Appt:** Assoc Prof Oph, Johns Hopkins Univ

Hersh, Peter MD [Oph] - **Spec Exp:** LASIK-Refractive Surgery; Cornea Transplant; Keratoconus; **Hospital:** Univ Hosp-UMDNJ—Newark; **Address:** The Cornea & Laser Eye Institute, Glenpointe Center East, 300 Frank W Burr Blvd, Ste 71, Teaneck, NJ 07666-6704; **Phone:** 201-883-0505; **Board Cert:** Ophthalmology 1987; **Med School:** Johns Hopkins Univ 1982; **Resid:** Internal Medicine, Lenox Hill Hosp 1983; Ophthalmology, Mass Eye & Ear Infirm 1986; **Fellow:** Cornea & Ext Eye Disease, Mass Eye & Ear Infirm 1987; **Fac Appt:** Prof Oph, UMDNJ-NJ Med Sch, Newark

Ho, Allen C MD [Oph] - **Spec Exp:** Retina/Vitreous Surgery; Macular Degeneration; Diabetic Eye Disease/Retinopathy; **Hospital:** Wills Eye Hosp; **Address:** Wills Eye Institute, 840 Walnut St-Retina Service Fl 10, Plymouth Meeting, PA 19462; **Phone:** 215-928-3095; **Board Cert:** Ophthalmology 2004; **Med School:** Columbia P&S 1988; **Resid:** Ophthalmology, Wills Eye Hosp 1992; **Fellow:** Retina/Vitreous, Manhattan E&E Hosp 1994; **Fac Appt:** Prof Oph, Jefferson Med Coll

Iliff, Nicholas T MD [Oph] - **Spec Exp:** Oculoplastic Surgery; Orbital & Eyelid Tumors/Cancer; **Hospital:** Johns Hopkins Hosp (page 61); **Address:** Wilmer Eye Inst, Bayview Med Ctr, 4940 Eastern Ave, Baltimore, MD 21224; **Phone:** 410-550-2360; **Board Cert:** Ophthalmology 1978; **Med School:** Johns Hopkins Univ 1972; **Resid:** Ophthalmology, Johns Hopkins-Wilmer Inst 1977; **Fellow:** Retinal Surgery, Johns Hopkins-Wilmer Inst 1978; Oculoplastic & Reconstructive Surgery, Johns Hopkins-Wilmer Inst 1980; **Fac Appt:** Prof Oph, Johns Hopkins Univ

Jaafar, Mohamad S MD [Oph] - **Spec Exp:** Pediatric Ophthalmology; Strabismus-Adult & Pediatric; Glaucoma-Pediatric; **Hospital:** Chldns Natl Med Ctr, G Washington Univ Hosp; **Address:** Dept Ophthalmology, 111 Michigan Ave NW, Washington, DC 20010-2970; **Phone:** 202-476-3045; **Board Cert:** Ophthalmology 2008; **Med School:** Amer Univ Beirut 1978; **Resid:** Ophthalmology, Am Univ Beirut Med Ctr 1981; Ophthalmology, Washington Hosp Ctr 1994; **Fellow:** Pediatric Ophthalmology, Chldn's Hosp 1982; Pediatric Ophthalmology, Baylor Coll Med 1983; **Fac Appt:** Prof Oph, Geo Wash Univ

Jabs, Douglas MD [Oph] - **Spec Exp:** Uveitis; **Hospital:** Mount Sinai Med Ctr (page 64); **Address:** 1700 E 102 St 8W Bldg, New York, NY 10029; **Phone:** 212-241-6752; **Board Cert:** Ophthalmology 1982; Internal Medicine 1983; **Med School:** Johns Hopkins Univ 1977; **Resid:** Ophthalmology, Wilmer Eye Inst 1981; Internal Medicine, Johns Hopkins Hosp 1983; **Fellow:** Rheumatology, Johns Hopkins Hosp 1984; **Fac Appt:** Prof Oph, Mount Sinai Sch Med

Ophthalmology

Katowitz, James A MD [Oph] - **Spec Exp:** Oculoplastic & Orbital Surgery; Pediatric Ophthalmology; Corneal Disease & Surgery; **Hospital:** Chldns Hosp of Philadelphia; **Address:** Childrens Hosp, Div Ophthalmology, 3400 Civic Center Blvd, Wood Bldg Fl 1, Philadelphia, PA 19104; **Phone:** 215-590-2791; **Board Cert:** Ophthalmology 1969; **Med School:** Univ Pennsylvania 1963; **Resid:** Ophthalmology, Hosp Univ Penn 1967; **Fellow:** Oculoplastic Surgery, Queen Victoria Hosp 1968; Oculoplastic Surgery, Moorfield Eye Hosp 1968; **Fac Appt:** Prof Emeritus Oph, Univ Pennsylvania

Katz, L Jay MD [Oph] - **Spec Exp:** Glaucoma; **Hospital:** Wills Eye Hosp, Thomas Jefferson Univ Hosp; **Address:** Wills Eye Institute- Glaucoma Div, 840 Walnut St Fl 11 - Ste 1110, Philadelphia, PA 19107; **Phone:** 215-928-3197; **Board Cert:** Ophthalmology 1985; **Med School:** Yale Univ 1979; **Resid:** Ophthalmology, Yale/New Haven Hosp 1983; **Fellow:** Glaucoma, Wills Eye Hosp 1985; **Fac Appt:** Prof Oph, Thomas Jefferson Univ

Kidwell Jr, Earl MD [Oph] - **Spec Exp:** Oculoplastic Surgery; **Hospital:** Howard Univ Hosp; **Address:** Ophthalmology Associates, 2041 Georgia Ave NW, Ste 2000, Washington, DC 20060; **Phone:** 202-865-4601; **Board Cert:** Ophthalmology 1978; **Med School:** Johns Hopkins Univ 1973; **Resid:** Ophthalmology, Johns Hopkins Hosp 1977; **Fellow:** Oculoplastic Surgery, Univ Miami Hosps 1978

Koller, Harold P MD [Oph] - **Spec Exp:** Pediatric Ophthalmology; Eye Muscle Surgery; Visual Perception & Learning Disorders; Strabismus; **Hospital:** Wills Eye Hosp, Abington Mem Hosp; **Address:** Huntingdon Valley Eye Care Consultants, 1650 Huntington Pike, Ste 150, Meadowbrook, PA 19046-8001; **Phone:** 215-947-6660; **Board Cert:** Ophthalmology 1971; **Med School:** Tulane Univ 1964; **Resid:** Ophthalmology, Tulane Hosp Med Ctr 1968; **Fellow:** Pediatric Ophthalmology, Washington Chldn's Hosp 1970; **Fac Appt:** Clin Prof Oph, Thomas Jefferson Univ

Kupersmith, Mark J MD [Oph] - **Spec Exp:** Neuro-Ophthalmology; **Hospital:** St. Luke's - Roosevelt Hosp Ctr - Roosevelt Div (page 56); **Address:** Roosevelt Hosp, 1000 10th Ave, 10 INN Bldg, New York, NY 10019; **Phone:** 212-636-3200 x1; **Board Cert:** Ophthalmology 1981; Neurology 1981; **Med School:** Northwestern Univ 1974; **Resid:** Neurology, NYU Med Ctr 1978; Ophthalmology, NYU Med Ctr 1980; **Fac Appt:** Prof Oph, Albert Einstein Coll Med

Levin, Alex V MD [Oph] - **Spec Exp:** Pediatric Ophthalmology; Strabismus; Ophthalmic Genetics; Glaucoma; **Hospital:** Wills Eye Hosp; **Address:** 840 Walnut St, Ste 1210, Philadelphia, PA 19107; **Phone:** 215-928-3240; **Board Cert:** Pediatrics 1986; Ophthalmology 1991; **Med School:** Jefferson Med Coll 1982; **Resid:** Pediatrics, Chldn's Hosp 1985; Ophthalmology, Wills Eye Hosp 1989; **Fellow:** Pediatric Ophthalmology, Hosp Sick Chldn 1990

Liebmann, Jeffrey M MD [Oph] - **Spec Exp:** Glaucoma; Cataract Surgery; **Hospital:** New York Eye & Ear Infirm (page 65), Lenox Hill Hosp (Manh Eye, Ear & Throat Hosp) (page 67); **Address:** Glaucoma Associates of New York, 121 E 60th St Fl 8, New York, NY 10022; **Phone:** 212-477-7540; **Board Cert:** Ophthalmology 1989; **Med School:** Boston Univ 1983; **Resid:** Ophthalmology, SUNY Downstate Med Ctr 1987; **Fellow:** Glaucoma, New York EE Infirmary 1988; **Fac Appt:** Clin Prof Oph, NYU Sch Med

Lisman, Richard D MD [Oph] - **Spec Exp:** Oculoplastic Surgery; Eyelid/Tear Duct Reconstruction; Eyelid Cosmetic & Reconstructive Surgery; Orbital & Eyelid Tumors/Cancer; **Hospital:** NYU Langone Med Ctr (page 68), Lenox Hill Hosp (Manh Eye, Ear & Throat Hosp) (page 67); **Address:** 635 Park Ave, New York, NY 10065-6546; **Phone:** 212-585-1405; **Board Cert:** Ophthalmology 1981; **Med School:** NYU Sch Med 1976; **Resid:** Ophthalmology, Manhattan EE Hosp 1980; **Fellow:** Ophthalmic Plastic Surgery, NY Eye & Ear Infirmary 1981; Plastic Surgery, Manhattan EE&T Hosp 1982; **Fac Appt:** Clin Prof Oph, NYU Sch Med

Mackool, Richard J MD [Oph] - **Spec Exp:** Cataract Surgery; LASIK-Refractive Surgery; Lens Implants-Multifocal; Corneal Disease & Surgery; **Hospital:** New York Eye & Ear Infirm (page 65); **Address:** Mackool Eye Institute, 31-24 41st St, Astoria, NY 11103; **Phone:** 718-728-3400; **Board Cert:** Ophthalmology 2011; **Med School:** Boston Univ 1968; **Resid:** Ophthalmology, New York EE Infirm 1973; **Fac Appt:** Clin Prof Oph, NYU Sch Med

Magramm, Irene MD [Oph] - **Spec Exp:** Pediatric Ophthalmology; Strabismus; Cataract Surgery; Diplopia; **Hospital:** Lenox Hill Hosp (Manh Eye, Ear & Throat Hosp) (page 67); **Address:** 220 E 63rd St, Ste LM, New York, NY 10055; **Phone:** 212-644-5100; **Board Cert:** Ophthalmology 1987; **Med School:** Cornell Univ-Weill Med Coll 1981; **Resid:** Ophthalmology, North Shore Univ Hosp 1985; **Fellow:** Pediatric Ophthalmology, Manhattan EE&T Hosp 1986; **Fac Appt:** Asst Clin Prof Oph, Cornell Univ-Weill Med Coll

Maguire, Joseph I MD [Oph] - **Spec Exp:** Retinal Disorders; Macular Degeneration; Diabetic Eye Disease/Retinopathy; **Hospital:** Wills Eye Hosp, Lankenau Hosp; **Address:** Mid Atlantic Retina, 840 Walnut St Fl 10, Philadelphia, PA 19107; **Phone:** 800-331-6634; **Board Cert:** Ophthalmology 1989; **Med School:** Jefferson Med Coll 1983; **Resid:** Ophthalmology, Wills Eye Hosp 1987; **Fellow:** Retina/Vitreous, Wills Eye Hosp 1989; Retina, Moorfields Hosp 1990; **Fac Appt:** Assoc Prof Oph, Thomas Jefferson Univ

Mandel, Eric R MD [Oph] - **Spec Exp:** LASIK-Refractive Surgery; PRK-Refractive Surgery; Corneal Disease; **Hospital:** Lenox Hill Hosp (page 67); **Address:** 211 E 70th St, New York, NY 10021; **Phone:** 212-734-0111; **Board Cert:** Ophthalmology 1988; **Med School:** SUNY Stony Brook 1982; **Resid:** Ophthalmology, Lenox Hill Hosp 1986; **Fellow:** Cornea & Ext Eye Disease, Mass EE Infirm 1987

McDonnell, Peter J MD [Oph] - **Spec Exp:** Cornea Transplant; Corneal Disease; Refractive Surgery; **Hospital:** Johns Hopkins Hosp (page 61); **Address:** Johns Hopkins Hospital, Wilmer Eye Institute, 727 Maumenee, 600 N Wolfe St, Baltimore, MD 21287; **Phone:** 443-287-1511; **Board Cert:** Ophthalmology 1988; **Med School:** Johns Hopkins Univ 1982; **Resid:** Ophthalmology, Wilmer Eye Inst 1986; **Fellow:** Cornea & Ext Eye Disease, Doheny Eye Inst 1987; **Fac Appt:** Prof Oph, USC Sch Med

Medow, Norman MD [Oph] - **Spec Exp:** Cataract-Pediatric; Glaucoma-Pediatric; Corneal Disease-Pediatric; **Hospital:** Montefiore Med Ctr-Moses Campus, NY; **Address:** Montefiore Hosp Ctr, Dept Ophthalmology, 3400 Bainbridge Ave, Bronx, NY 10467; **Phone:** 718-920-2020; **Board Cert:** Ophthalmology 1975; **Med School:** SUNY Hlth Sci Ctr 1966; **Resid:** Ophthalmology, Manhattan EE&T Hosp 1972; **Fellow:** Cataract/Lens Implant Surgery, Charles Kelman, MD 1973; **Fac Appt:** Assoc Clin Prof Oph, Cornell Univ-Weill Med Coll

Miller, Neil MD [Oph] - **Spec Exp:** Neuro-Ophthalmology; Orbital Diseases; Thyroid Eye Disease; **Hospital:** Johns Hopkins Hosp (page 61); **Address:** Johns Hopkins - Wilmer Eye Inst, 600 N Wolfe St Wilmer Bldg - rm 233, Baltimore, MD 21287-0001; **Phone:** 410-955-8679; **Board Cert:** Ophthalmology 1976; **Med School:** Johns Hopkins Univ 1971; **Resid:** Ophthalmology, Johns Hopkins Hosp 1975; **Fellow:** Neuro-Ophthalmology, UCSF Med Ctr 1975; **Fac Appt:** Prof Oph, Johns Hopkins Univ

Mills, Monte D MD [Oph] - **Spec Exp:** Pediatric Ophthalmology; Eye Muscle Disorders; Strabismus; **Hospital:** Chldns Hosp of Philadelphia; **Address:** Chldns Hosp, Dept Ophthalmology, 34th St & Civic Ctr Blvd, Wood Bldg Fl 1, Philadelphia, PA 19104; **Phone:** 215-590-2791; **Board Cert:** Ophthalmology 2004; **Med School:** Baylor Coll Med 1988; **Resid:** Ophthalmology, Mass Eye & Ear Infirm 1992; **Fellow:** Pediatric Ophthalmology, Chldns Hosp 1993; **Fac Appt:** Assoc Clin Prof Oph, Univ Pennsylvania

Muldoon, Thomas O MD [Oph] - **Spec Exp:** Retina/Vitreous Surgery; Macular Disease/Degeneration; Diabetic Eye Disease/Retinopathy; **Hospital:** New York Eye & Ear Infirm (page 65); **Address:** 310 E 14th St, Ste 402, New York, NY 10003-4201; **Phone:** 212-979-4595; **Board Cert:** Ophthalmology 1971; **Med School:** Univ Rochester 1962; **Resid:** Surgery, St Lukes Hosp 1966; Ophthalmology, NY EE Infirm 1969; **Fellow:** Retinal Surgery, NY EE Infirm 1970; **Fac Appt:** Assoc Clin Prof Oph, NY Med Coll

Myers, Jonathan S MD [Oph] - **Spec Exp:** Glaucoma; **Hospital:** Wills Eye Hosp; **Address:** Wills Eye Institute, 840 Walnut St, Ste 1110, Philadelphia, PA 19107; **Phone:** 215-928-3197; **Board Cert:** Ophthalmology 2008; **Med School:** Univ Pennsylvania 1992; **Resid:** Ophthalmology, Wills Eye Hosp 1996; **Fellow:** Glaucoma, Duke Univ Hosp 1997; **Fac Appt:** Asst Clin Prof Oph, Thomas Jefferson Univ

Nelson, Leonard B MD [Oph] - **Spec Exp:** Pediatric Ophthalmology; Strabismus; Eye Muscle Disorders; **Hospital:** Wills Eye Hosp; **Address:** Wills Eye Hospital, 840 Walnut St, Ste 1210, Philadelphia, PA 19107; **Phone:** 215-928-3244; **Board Cert:** Ophthalmology 1981; **Med School:** Harvard Med Sch 1976; **Resid:** Ophthalmology, Bellevue Hosp Ctr-NYU 1980; **Fellow:** Pediatric Ophthalmology, Chldns Hosp Med Ctr 1981; Ocular Disease, Johns Hopkins Hosp 1982; **Fac Appt:** Assoc Prof Oph, Jefferson Med Coll

O'Brien, Joan M MD [Oph] - **Spec Exp:** Eye Tumors/Cancer; Retinoblastoma; **Hospital:** Hosp Univ Penn - UPHS (page 72); **Address:** Penn Presbyterian Med Ctr, Scheie Eye Inst, 51 N 39th St, Philadelphia, PA 19104; **Phone:** 215-662-8100; **Board Cert:** Ophthalmology 2007; **Med School:** Dartmouth Med Sch 1986; **Resid:** Internal Medicine, Beth Israel Hosp 1998; Ophthalmology, Mass Eye & Ear Infirm 1992; **Fellow:** Ophthalmic Pathology, Mass Eye & Ear Infirm 1989; Ocular Oncology, UCSF Med Ctr 1993; **Fac Appt:** Prof Oph, Univ Pennsylvania

Odel, Jeffrey G MD [Oph] - **Spec Exp:** Neuro-Ophthalmology; Retinal Disorders; Optic Nerve Disorders; **Hospital:** NY-Presby/Columbia Univ Med Ctr, NY (page 66); **Address:** Harkness Eye Institute, 635 W 165th St, rm 316, New York, NY 10032-3701; **Phone:** 212-305-5415; **Board Cert:** Ophthalmology 1981; **Med School:** Univ Rochester 1975; **Resid:** Ophthalmology, Mt Sinai Hosp 1981; **Fellow:** Ophthalmology, Bascom-Palmer Eye Inst 1977; Ophthalmology, Columbia Presby Med Ctr 1982; **Fac Appt:** Assoc Clin Prof Oph, Columbia P&S

Orlin, Stephen E MD [Oph] - **Spec Exp:** Cataract Surgery; Corneal Disease & Surgery; Refractive Surgery; **Hospital:** Penn Presby Med Ctr - UPHS (page 72), Hosp Univ Penn - UPHS (page 72); **Address:** Penn Presby Med Ctr, Scheie Eye Inst, 51 N 39th St, Ste 509, Philadelphia, PA 19104; **Phone:** 215-662-8100; **Board Cert:** Ophthalmology 1987; **Med School:** South Africa 1977; **Resid:** Ophthalmology, Scheie Eye Inst 1985; **Fellow:** Cornea & Ext Eye Disease, Scheie Eye Inst 1986; **Fac Appt:** Assoc Prof Oph, Univ Pennsylvania

Quigley, Harry A MD [Oph] - **Spec Exp:** Glaucoma; **Hospital:** Johns Hopkins Hosp (page 61); **Address:** 600 N Wolfe St, Maumenee B-110, Baltimore, MD 21287-9205; **Phone:** 410-955-6052; **Board Cert:** Ophthalmology 1976; **Med School:** Johns Hopkins Univ 1971; **Resid:** Ophthalmology, Wilmer Inst-Johns Hopkins Hosp 1975; **Fellow:** Ophthalmology, Bascom Palmer Eye Inst 1977; **Fac Appt:** Prof Oph, Johns Hopkins Univ

Quinn, Graham E MD [Oph] - **Spec Exp:** Pediatric Ophthalmology; Eye Growth/Development; **Hospital:** Chldns Hosp of Philadelphia; **Address:** Chldns Hosp, Dept Ophthalmology, 34th St & Civic Ctr Blvd, Wood Bldg Fl 1, Philadelphia, PA 19104-4399; **Phone:** 215-590-2791; **Board Cert:** Ophthalmology 1979; **Med School:** Duke Univ 1973; **Resid:** Pathology, Metro Genl Hosp 1975; Ophthalmology, Hosp Univ Penn 1978; **Fellow:** Pediatric Ophthalmology, Childrens Hosp 1979; **Fac Appt:** Prof Oph, Univ Pennsylvania

Rapuano, Christopher J MD [Oph] - **Spec Exp:** Corneal Disease; Refractive Surgery; **Hospital:** Wills Eye Hosp; **Address:** Corneal Assocs-Wills Eye Hosp, 840 Walnut St, Ste 920, Philadelphia, PA 19107; **Phone:** 215-928-3180; **Board Cert:** Ophthalmology 1991; **Med School:** Columbia P&S 1986; **Resid:** Ophthalmology, Wills Eye Hosp 1990; **Fellow:** Cornea & Ext Eye Disease, Univ Iowa Hosp & Clin 1991; **Fac Appt:** Prof Oph, Jefferson Med Coll

Regillo, Carl D MD [Oph] - **Spec Exp:** Retinal Disorders; **Hospital:** Wills Eye Hosp, Thomas Jefferson Univ Hosp; **Address:** Mid Atlantic Retina, 4060 Butler Pike, Ste 200, Wyndmoor, PA 19462; **Phone:** 800-331-6634; **Board Cert:** Ophthalmology 2004; **Med School:** Harvard Med Sch 1988; **Resid:** Ophthalmology, Wills Eye Hosp 1992; **Fellow:** Retinal Surgery, Wills Eye Hosp 1994; **Fac Appt:** Prof Oph, Jefferson Med Coll

Reynolds, James D MD [Oph] - **Spec Exp:** Pediatric Ophthalmology; Strabismus; Retinopathy of Prematurity; **Hospital:** Women & Chldn's Hosp of Buffalo, The; **Address:** 1176 Main St, Buffalo, NY 14209; **Phone:** 716-881-7900; **Board Cert:** Ophthalmology 1982; **Med School:** SUNY Buffalo 1978; **Resid:** Ophthalmology, Erie Co Med Ctr 1981; **Fellow:** Pediatric Ophthalmology, Pittsburgh EE Hospital 1982; **Fac Appt:** Prof Oph, SUNY Buffalo

Ritch, Robert MD [Oph] - **Spec Exp:** Glaucoma; Complementary Medicine; **Hospital:** New York Eye & Ear Infirm (page 65); **Address:** 310 E 14th St, South Bldg - Fl 3, New York, NY 10003-4201; **Phone:** 212-477-7540; **Board Cert:** Ophthalmology 1977; **Med School:** Albert Einstein Coll Med 1972; **Resid:** Ophthalmology, Mt Sinai Hosp 1976; **Fellow:** Glaucoma, Mt Sinai Hosp 1978; **Fac Appt:** Prof Oph, NY Med Coll

Robin, Alan L MD [Oph] - **Spec Exp:** Glaucoma; Cataract Surgery; **Hospital:** Greater Baltimore Med Ctr; **Address:** Glaucoma Specialists, 6115 Falls Rd, Ste 333, Baltimore, MD 21209; **Phone:** 410-377-2422; **Board Cert:** Ophthalmology 1979; **Med School:** Tufts Univ 1974; **Resid:** Ophthalmology, Greater Baltimore Med Ctr 1978; **Fellow:** Glaucoma, Wilmer Inst 1979; **Fac Appt:** Clin Prof Oph, Univ MD Sch Med

Schein, Oliver D MD [Oph] - **Spec Exp:** Cataract Surgery; Corneal Disease & Surgery; **Hospital:** Johns Hopkins Hosp (page 61); **Address:** Johns Hopkins Hosp, 600 N Wolfe St, Maumenee 317, Baltimore, MD 21287; **Phone:** 410-955-7677; **Board Cert:** Internal Medicine 1984; Ophthalmology 1990; **Med School:** Johns Hopkins Univ 1981; **Resid:** Internal Medicine, Johns Hopkins Hosp 1984; Ophthalmology, Mass Eye & Ear Infirm 1987; **Fellow:** Cornea & Ext Eye Disease, Mass Eye & Ear Infirm 1988; **Fac Appt:** Prof Oph, Johns Hopkins Univ

Schiff, William M MD [Oph] - **Spec Exp:** Macular Disease/Degeneration; Diabetic Eye Disease/Retinopathy; Retinal Detachment; Macular Disease/Degeneration; **Hospital:** Lenox Hill Hosp (Manh Eye, Ear & Throat Hosp) (page 67), St. Luke's - Roosevelt Hosp Ctr - Roosevelt Div (page 56); **Address:** 210 E 64th New York, NY 10065 St, Fl 7, New York, NY 10068; **Phone:** 212-702-7400; **Board Cert:** Ophthalmology 2006; **Med School:** NYU Sch Med 1988; **Resid:** Ophthalmology, New York Eye & Ear Infirm 1994; **Fellow:** Retina/Vitreous, NY Hosp-Harkness Eye Inst 1996; **Fac Appt:** Prof Oph, Columbia P&S

Schuman, Joel S MD [Oph] - **Spec Exp:** Glaucoma; Cataract Surgery; **Hospital:** UPMC Presby, Pittsburgh, UPMC Shadyside; **Address:** UPMC Eye Center, Eye & Ear Institute, Ste 816, 203 Lothrop St, Pittsburgh, PA 15213; **Phone:** 412-647-2200; **Board Cert:** Ophthalmology 1990; **Med School:** Mount Sinai Sch Med 1984; **Resid:** Ophthalmology, Med Coll Virginia Hosps 1988; **Fellow:** Glaucoma, Harvard/Mass Eye & Ear Infirmary 1990; **Fac Appt:** Prof Oph, Univ Pittsburgh

Ophthalmology

Sergott, Robert C MD [Oph] - **Spec Exp:** Neuro-Ophthalmology; Optic Nerve Disorders; Glaucoma; Thyroid Eye Disease; **Hospital:** Thomas Jefferson Univ Hosp, Wills Eye Hosp; **Address:** 840 Walnut St, Ste 930, Philadelphia, PA 19107; **Phone:** 215-928-3130; **Board Cert:** Ophthalmology 1982; **Med School:** Johns Hopkins Univ 1975; **Resid:** Ophthalmology, Wills Eye Hospital 1979; **Fellow:** Neuro-Ophthalmology, Bascom Palmer Eye Inst 1980; Neurological Immunology, Univ of Penn 1981; **Fac Appt:** Prof Oph, Thomas Jefferson Univ

Shabto, Uri MD [Oph] - **Spec Exp:** Retinopathy of Prematurity; Macular Disease/Degeneration; Diabetic Eye Disease/Retinopathy; Retinal Detachment; **Hospital:** New York Eye & Ear Infirm (page 65); **Address:** 310 E 14th St, South Bldg, Ste 419, New York, NY 10003-4201; **Phone:** 212-677-2000; **Board Cert:** Ophthalmology 1991; **Med School:** Harvard Med Sch 1986; **Resid:** Ophthalmology, NY Eye & Ear Infirm 1990; **Fellow:** Vitreoretinal Surgery, Montefiore Hosp 1991; **Fac Appt:** Asst Clin Prof Oph, NY Med Coll

Shields, Carol L MD [Oph] - **Spec Exp:** Orbital Tumors/Cancer; Melanoma-Choroidal (eye); Retinoblastoma; Pediatric Ophthalmology; **Hospital:** Wills Eye Hosp, Jefferson Reg Med Ctr - Pittsburgh; **Address:** Wills Eye Inst, Ocular Oncology Service, 840 Walnut St, Ste 1440, Phildelphia, PA 19107; **Phone:** 215-928-3105; **Board Cert:** Ophthalmology 1989; **Med School:** Univ Pittsburgh 1983; **Resid:** Ophthalmology, Willis Eye Hosp 1988; **Fellow:** Ophthalmic Pathology, Willis Eye Hosp 1988; Ophthalmic Oncololgy, Willis Eye Hosp 1989; **Fac Appt:** Prof Oph, Jefferson Med Coll

Shields, Jerry MD [Oph] - **Spec Exp:** Eye Tumors/Cancer; Pediatric Ophthalmology; Retinoblastoma; Melanoma-Choroidal (eye); **Hospital:** Wills Eye Hosp, Thomas Jefferson Univ Hosp; **Address:** Wills Eye Hosp, Ocular Oncology Svce, 840 Walnut St, Ste 1440, Philadelphia, PA 19107; **Phone:** 215-928-3105; **Board Cert:** Ophthalmology 1972; **Med School:** Univ Mich Med Sch 1964; **Resid:** Ophthalmology, Wills Eye Hosp 1970; **Fellow:** Ophthalmology, Wills Eye Hosp 1972; **Fac Appt:** Prof Oph, Thomas Jefferson Univ

Simon, John W MD [Oph] - **Spec Exp:** Pediatric Ophthalmology; Strabismus; **Hospital:** Albany Med Ctr, St. Peter's Hosp - Albany; **Address:** 1220 New Scotland Rd, Ste 202, Slingerlands, NY 12159; **Phone:** 518-533-6502; **Board Cert:** Ophthalmology 1981; **Med School:** Mount Sinai Sch Med 1976; **Resid:** Ophthalmology, Mt Sinai Hosp 1980; **Fellow:** Pediatric Ophthalmology, Wills Eye Hosp 1981; **Fac Appt:** Prof Oph, Albany Med Coll

Spaeth, George L MD [Oph] - **Spec Exp:** Glaucoma; **Hospital:** Wills Eye Hosp, Thomas Jefferson Univ Hosp; **Address:** Wills Eye Institute-Glaucoma Div, 840 Walnut St Fl 11 - Ste 1110, Philadelphia, PA 19107; **Phone:** 215-928-3197; **Board Cert:** Ophthalmology 1965; **Med School:** Harvard Med Sch 1959; **Resid:** Ophthalmology, Wills Eye Hosp 1963; **Fellow:** Glaucoma, Natl Inst Neurological Dis & Blindness 1965; **Fac Appt:** Prof Oph, Thomas Jefferson Univ

Stark, Walter J MD [Oph] - **Spec Exp:** Corneal Disease & Transplant; Cataract Surgery; Refractive Surgery; **Hospital:** Johns Hopkins Hosp (page 61); **Address:** Wilmer Eye Inst, 600 N Wolfe St Maumenee Bldg - rm 327, Baltimore, MD 21287-9238; **Phone:** 410-955-5490; **Board Cert:** Ophthalmology 1973; **Med School:** Univ Okla Coll Med 1967; **Resid:** Ophthalmology, Wilmer Inst-Johns Hopkins 1971; **Fac Appt:** Prof Oph, Johns Hopkins Univ

Stefanyszyn, Mary MD [Oph] - **Spec Exp:** Cosmetic Surgery-Eyes; Oculoplastic & Orbital Surgery; Eyelid Surgery; **Hospital:** Wills Eye Hosp; **Address:** Wills Eye Hosp, 840 Walnut St, Ste 912, Philadelphia, PA 19107; **Phone:** 215-928-3171; **Board Cert:** Ophthalmology 1983; **Med School:** Harvard Med Sch 1978; **Resid:** Ophthalmology, Wills Eye Hosp 1982; Ophthalmic Pathology, Armed Forces Inst of Pathology 1982; **Fellow:** Oculoplastic & Reconstructive Surgery, Wills Eye Hosp 1983; Orbital Surgery, Moorfields Eye Hosp 1985

Sterns, Gwen K MD [Oph] - **Spec Exp:** Geriatric Ophthalmology; Low Vision; **Hospital:** Rochester Genl Hosp, Univ of Rochester Strong Meml Hosp; **Address:** 1425 Portland Ave, Box 224, Ophthalmology Dept, Rochester, NY 14621; **Phone:** 585-922-4794; **Board Cert:** Ophthalmology 1976; **Med School:** Med Coll PA 1970; **Resid:** Ophthalmology, Nassau Co Med Ctr 1974; **Fellow:** Ophthalmology, Columbia/NY Presby Eye Inst 1975; **Fac Appt:** Clin Prof Oph, Univ Rochester

Vander, James F MD [Oph] - **Spec Exp:** Diabetic Eye Disease/Retinopathy; Retinal Disorders; Macular Degeneration; **Hospital:** Wills Eye Hosp; **Address:** Mid Atlantic Retina, 4060 Butler Pike, Ste 200, Wyndmoor, PA 19462; **Phone:** 800-331-6634; **Board Cert:** Ophthalmology 1989; **Med School:** Univ Mich Med Sch 1984; **Resid:** Ophthalmology, Univ Michigan Med Ctr 1988; **Fellow:** Retina/Vitreous, Wills Eye Hosp 1990; **Fac Appt:** Prof Oph, Thomas Jefferson Univ

Walsh, Joseph B MD [Oph] - **Spec Exp:** Diabetic Eye Disease/Retinopathy; Macular Degeneration; Retinal Disorders; **Hospital:** New York Eye & Ear Infirm (page 65); **Address:** 310 E 14th St S Bldg Fl 3 - Ste 319, New York, NY 10003-4201; **Phone:** 212-979-4282; **Board Cert:** Ophthalmology 2005; **Med School:** Georgetown Univ 1966; **Resid:** Internal Medicine, Univ Hosp 1968; Ophthalmology, NY Eye & Ear Infirm 1973; **Fellow:** Retina, Montefiore Med Ctr 1974; **Fac Appt:** Prof Oph, NY Med Coll

Wang, Frederick Mark MD [Oph] - **Spec Exp:** Pediatric Ophthalmology; Strabismus; Eye Muscle Disorders; **Hospital:** Lenox Hill Hosp (Manh Eye, Ear & Throat Hosp) (page 67), Montefiore Med Ctr-Moses Campus, NY; **Address:** 30 E 40th St, Ste 405, New York, NY 10016-1201; **Phone:** 212-684-3980; **Board Cert:** Pediatrics 1978; Ophthalmology 1980; **Med School:** Albert Einstein Coll Med 1972; **Resid:** Pediatrics, Jacobi Med Ctr 1974; Ophthalmology, Albert Einstein 1979; **Fellow:** Pediatric Ophthalmology, Children's Hosp Natl Med Ctr 1980; **Fac Appt:** Clin Prof Oph, Albert Einstein Coll Med

Yannuzzi, Lawrence MD [Oph] - **Spec Exp:** Retina/Vitreous Surgery; Macular Disease/Degeneration; Diabetic Eye Disease/Retinopathy; **Hospital:** NY-Presby/Columbia Univ Med Ctr, NY (page 66), Lenox Hill Hosp (Manh Eye, Ear & Throat Hosp) (page 67); **Address:** Vitreous-Retina-Macula Consultants of NY, 460 Park Ave Fl 5, New York, NY 10022; **Phone:** 212-861-9797; **Board Cert:** Ophthalmology 1970; **Med School:** Boston Univ 1964; **Resid:** Ophthalmology, Manhattan EE&T Hosp 1968; **Fellow:** Ophthalmology, Manhattan EE&T Hosp 1971; **Fac Appt:** Clin Prof Oph, Columbia P&S

Southeast

Afshari, Natalie A MD [Oph] - **Spec Exp:** Cataract Surgery; Cornea Transplant; LASIK-Refractive Surgery; PRK-Refractive Surgery; **Hospital:** Duke Univ Hosp; **Address:** Duke Eye Center at DUMC, 2351 Erwin Rd, Box 3802, Durham, NC 27710; **Phone:** 919-684-3799; **Board Cert:** Ophthalmology 2011; **Med School:** Stanford Univ 1995; **Resid:** Ophthalmology, Mass Eye & Ear Infirmary 1999; **Fellow:** Cornea & Refractive Surgery, Mass Eye & Ear Infirmary 2001; **Fac Appt:** Prof Oph, Duke Univ

Alfonso, Eduardo MD [Oph] - **Spec Exp:** Corneal Disease & Surgery; Cornea Transplant & Artificial Cornea; Ophthalmic Pathology; **Hospital:** Bascom Palmer Eye Inst, Jackson Meml Hosp; **Address:** Bascom Palmer Eye Institute, 900 NW 17th St, Miami, FL 33136-1119; **Phone:** 305-243-2020; **Board Cert:** Ophthalmology 1985; **Med School:** Yale Univ 1980; **Resid:** Ophthalmology, Bascom Palmer Eye Inst 1984; **Fellow:** Cornea & Ext Eye Disease, Mass Eye & Ear Hosp 1986; Ophthalmological Pathology, Mass Eye & Ear Hosp 1986; **Fac Appt:** Prof Oph, Univ Miami Sch Med

Ophthalmology

Biousse, Valerie MD [Oph] - **Spec Exp:** Neuro-Ophthalmology; Optic Nerve Disorders; **Hospital:** Emory Univ Hosp; **Address:** Emory Eye Center, 1365B Clifton Rd NE, Ste 4500, Atlanta, GA 30322; **Phone:** 404-778-2020; **Board Cert:** Ophthalmology 2004; **Med School:** France 1988; **Resid:** Neurology, Univ Paris VI Affil Hosp 1994; Ophthalmology, Emory Univ Med Ctr 2002; **Fellow:** Stroke, Univ Paris VI 1996; Neuro-Ophthalmology, Emory Univ 1996; **Fac Appt:** Prof Oph, Emory Univ

Buckley, Edward G MD [Oph] - **Spec Exp:** Pediatric Ophthalmology; Strabismus; Cataract-Pediatric; Neuro-Ophthalmology; **Hospital:** Duke Univ Hosp; **Address:** Duke Eye Center, 2351 Erwin Rd, Box 3802, Durham, NC 27710; **Phone:** 919-681-3937; **Board Cert:** Ophthalmology 2007; **Med School:** Duke Univ 1977; **Resid:** Ophthalmology, Duke Univ Eye Ctr 1981; **Fellow:** Pediatric Ophthalmology, Bascom Palmer Eye Inst 1983; Neuro-Ophthalmology, Bascom Palmer Eye Inst 1983; **Fac Appt:** Prof Oph, Duke Univ

Budenz, Donald L MD [Oph] - **Spec Exp:** Glaucoma; Cataract Surgery; **Hospital:** NC Memorial Hosp - UNC; **Address:** 5151 Bioinformatics, CB7040, Chapel Hill, NC 27599-7040; **Phone:** 919-966-5296; **Board Cert:** Ophthalmology 2003; **Med School:** Harvard Med Sch 1987; **Resid:** Ophthalmology, Scheie Eye Inst 1991; **Fellow:** Glaucoma, Bascom Palmer Eye Inst 1992; **Fac Appt:** Prof Oph, Univ NC Sch Med

Capo, Hilda MD [Oph] - **Spec Exp:** Pediatric Ophthalmology; Strabismus; Neuro-Ophthalmology; Botox Therapy; **Hospital:** Bascom Palmer Eye Inst; **Address:** Bascom Palmer Eye Institute, 900 NW 17th St, Miami, FL 33136; **Phone:** 305-243-2020; **Board Cert:** Ophthalmology 1989; **Med School:** Puerto Rico 1982; **Resid:** Ophthalmology, Univ Puerto Rico Affil Hosp 1987; **Fellow:** Neuro-Ophthalmology, NYU Med Ctr 1989; Pediatric Ophthalmology, Wilmer Institute/Hopkins 1988; **Fac Appt:** Clin Prof Oph, Univ Miami Sch Med

Carlson, Alan N MD [Oph] - **Spec Exp:** Cornea & External Eye Disease; Cornea Transplant; LASIK-Refractive Surgery; **Hospital:** Duke Univ Hosp; **Address:** Duke Univ Eye Center, 2351 Erwin Rd, Durham, NC 27710; **Phone:** 919-684-5769; **Board Cert:** Ophthalmology 1988; **Med School:** Duke Univ 1982; **Resid:** Ophthalmology, Baylor Med Ctr 1986; **Fellow:** Cornea & Ext Eye Disease, Baylor Med Ctr 1987; Cornea & Ext Eye Disease, Duke Univ Med Ctr 1988; **Fac Appt:** Prof Oph, Duke Univ

Culbertson, William MD [Oph] - **Spec Exp:** Cataract Surgery-Lens Implant; Corneal & External Eye Disease; LASIK-Refractive Surgery; **Hospital:** Bascom Palmer Eye Inst; **Address:** Bascom Palmer Eye Institute, 900 NW 17th St, Miami, FL 33136-1119; **Phone:** 305-243-2020; **Board Cert:** Ophthalmology 1976; **Med School:** Emory Univ 1970; **Resid:** Ophthalmology, Vanderbilt Univ Hosp 1974; **Fellow:** Cornea & Ext Eye Disease, Bascom Palmer Eye Inst 1979; **Fac Appt:** Prof Oph, Univ Miami Sch Med

Davis, Janet L MD [Oph] - **Spec Exp:** Uveitis; Retina/Vitreous Surgery; Macular Degeneration; Diabetic Eye Disease/Retinopathy; **Hospital:** Bascom Palmer Eye Inst; **Address:** Bascom Palmer Eye Inst, 900 NW 17th St, Miami, FL 33136-1119; **Phone:** 305-243-2020; **Board Cert:** Ophthalmology 2006; **Med School:** Baylor Coll Med 1981; **Resid:** Ophthalmology, Baylor Affil Hosp 1986; **Fellow:** Vitreoretinal Surgery, Bascom Palmer Eye Inst 1987; Ocular Immunology, NIH-Natl Eye Inst 1989; **Fac Appt:** Prof Oph, Univ Miami Sch Med

Del Priore, Lucian MD/PhD [Oph] - **Spec Exp:** Diabetic Eye Disease/Retinopathy; Macular Degeneration; Retinal Detachment; Retina-Artificial; **Hospital:** MUSC Med Ctr, Ashley River Tower; **Address:** MUSC Storm Eye Inst, 167 Ashley Ave Fl 8 - rm 825, MS 250676, Charleston, SC 29425; **Phone:** 843-792-2020; **Board Cert:** Ophthalmology 1989; **Med School:** Univ Rochester 1982; **Resid:** Ophthalmology, Wilmer Eye Inst/Johns HopkinsHosp 1987; **Fellow:** Glaucoma, Wilmer Eye Inst/Johns Hopkins Hosp 1988; Vitreoretinal Surgery, Wilmer Eye Inst/Johns Hopkins Hosp 1989; **Fac Appt:** Prof Oph, Med Univ SC

Dutton, Jonathan J MD/PhD [Oph] - **Spec Exp:** Oculoplastic Surgery; Eye Tumors/Cancer; Melanoma-Choroidal (eye); **Hospital:** NC Memorial Hosp - UNC; **Address:** Univ North Carolina - Dept Ophthalmology, 130 Mason Farm Rd, 5156 Bioinformatics, CB 7040, Chapel Hill, NC 27599; **Phone:** 919-966-5296; **Board Cert:** Ophthalmology 1983; **Med School:** Washington Univ, St Louis 1977; **Resid:** Ophthalmology, Washington Univ Med Ctr 1982; **Fellow:** Oculoplastic Surgery, Univ Iowa Med Ctr 1983; **Fac Appt:** Prof Oph, Univ NC Sch Med

Flynn Jr, Harry W MD [Oph] - **Spec Exp:** Retina/Vitreous Surgery; Diabetic Eye Disease/Retinopathy; Macular Disease/Degeneration; **Hospital:** Bascom Palmer Eye Inst; **Address:** Bascom Palmer Eye Institute, 900 NW 17th St, Miami, FL 33136-1119; **Phone:** 305-243-2020; **Board Cert:** Ophthalmology 1976; **Med School:** Univ VA Sch Med 1971; **Resid:** Ophthalmology, Univ Virginia Hosp 1975; **Fellow:** Retina, Pacific Med Ctr 1976; **Fac Appt:** Prof Oph, Univ Miami Sch Med

Forster, Richard K MD [Oph] - **Spec Exp:** Cornea Transplant; Cataract Surgery; **Hospital:** Bascom Palmer Eye Inst; **Address:** Bascom Palmer Eye Institute, 7101 Fairway Drive, Palm Beach Gardens, FL 33418; **Phone:** 561-515-1500; **Board Cert:** Ophthalmology 1971; **Med School:** Boston Univ 1963; **Resid:** Ophthalmology, Bascom Palmer Eye Inst 1969; **Fellow:** Ophthalmology, Fl Proctor Fdn/UCSF 1970; **Fac Appt:** Prof Oph, Univ Miami Sch Med

Freedman, Sharon F MD [Oph] - **Spec Exp:** Pediatric Ophthalmology; Glaucoma-Pediatric; Strabismus; Retinopathy of Prematurity; **Hospital:** Duke Univ Hosp; **Address:** Duke Eye Center, 2351 Erwin Rd, Box 3802, Durham, NC 27710; **Phone:** 919-681-3937; **Board Cert:** Ophthalmology 1991; **Med School:** Harvard Med Sch 1985; **Resid:** Ophthalmology, Mass Eye & Ear Infirm 1989; **Fellow:** Pediatric Ophthalmology, Childns Hosp 1990; Glaucoma, Duke Eye Ctr 1992; **Fac Appt:** Prof Oph, Duke Univ

Gorovoy, Mark S MD [Oph] - **Spec Exp:** Corneal Disease & Transplant; Cataract Surgery; Glaucoma; LASIK-Refractive Surgery; **Hospital:** Lee Memorial Hlth Systems; **Address:** 12381 S Cleveland Ave, Ste 300, Fort Myers, FL 33907; **Phone:** 239-939-1444; **Board Cert:** Ophthalmology 1982; **Med School:** Geo Wash Univ 1973; **Resid:** Ophthalmology, Geo Washington Univ Hosp 1980; **Fellow:** Cornea & Ext Eye Disease, Univ Florida 1982

Greenfield, David S MD [Oph] - **Spec Exp:** Glaucoma; Cataract Surgery-Lens Implant; **Hospital:** Bascom Palmer Eye Inst; **Address:** Bascom Palmer Eye Inst, 7101 Fairway Drive, Palm Beach Gardens, FL 33418; **Phone:** 561-515-1500; **Board Cert:** Ophthalmology 2007; **Med School:** NYU Sch Med 1990; **Resid:** Ophthalmology, New England Eye Center 1994; **Fellow:** Glaucoma, Bascom Palmer Eye Inst 1995; Neuro-Ophthalmology, Bascom Palmer Eye Inst 1995; **Fac Appt:** Prof Oph, Univ Miami Sch Med

Grossniklaus, Hans E MD [Oph] - **Spec Exp:** Ophthalmic Pathology; Melanoma-Choroidal (eye); Macular Disease/Degeneration; Retinal Disorders; **Hospital:** Emory Univ Hosp; **Address:** Emory Clinic - LF Montgomery Lab, 1365-B Clifton Rd NE, rm BT428, Atlanta, GA 30322; **Phone:** 404-778-4611; **Board Cert:** Ophthalmology 1985; Anatomic Pathology 1987; **Med School:** Ohio State Univ 1980; **Resid:** Ophthalmology, Case West Res Univ Hosp 1984; Pathology, Case West Res Univ Hosp 1987; **Fellow:** Ophthalmological Pathology, Johns Hopkins Hosp 1985; **Fac Appt:** Prof Oph, Emory Univ

Guy, John R MD [Oph] - **Spec Exp:** Neuro-Ophthalmology; **Hospital:** Bascom Palmer Eye Inst; **Address:** Bascom Palmer Eye Inst, 900 NW 17th St Fl 4, Miami, FL 33136; **Phone:** 305-243-2020; **Board Cert:** Ophthalmology 1983; **Med School:** Univ Miami Sch Med 1977; **Resid:** Neurology, Temple Univ Hosp 1979; Ophthalmology, Georgetown Univ Med Ctr 1988; **Fellow:** Neuro-Ophthalmology, Willis Eye Hosp 1983; **Fac Appt:** Assoc Prof Oph, Univ Miami Sch Med

Ophthalmology

Haik, Barrett MD [Oph] - **Spec Exp:** Eye Tumors/Cancer; Orbital Diseases; **Hospital:** St. Jude Children's Research Hosp; **Address:** Univ Tenn Med Group, Ophthamology, 930 Madison Ave, Ste 400, Memphis, TN 38103-3452; **Phone:** 901-448-6650; **Board Cert:** Ophthalmology 1981; **Med School:** Louisiana State U, New Orleans 1976; **Resid:** Ophthalmology, Columbia-Presby/Harkness Eye Inst 1980; **Fac Appt:** Prof Oph, Univ Tenn Coll Med

Harbour, J William MD [Oph] - **Spec Exp:** Eye Tumors/Cancer; Melanoma-Choroidal (eye); Retinoblastoma; **Hospital:** Bascom Palmer Eye Inst; **Address:** Bascom Palmer Eye Inst, 900 NW 17th St, Ste 254, Miami, FL 33136; **Phone:** 305-326-6166; **Board Cert:** Ophthalmology 2007; **Med School:** Johns Hopkins Univ 1990; **Resid:** Ophthalmology, Wills Eye Hosp 1994; **Fellow:** Retina/Vitreous, Bascom Palmer Eye Inst 1995; Ocular Oncology, UCSF Med Ctr 1996; **Fac Appt:** Prof Oph, Washington Univ, St Louis

Hess, J Bruce MD [Oph] - **Spec Exp:** Pediatric Ophthalmology; Strabismus; **Hospital:** All Children's Hosp, Bayfront Med Ctr; **Address:** 601 5th St S, Ste 601, St Petersburg, FL 33701; **Phone:** 727-767-4393; **Board Cert:** Ophthalmology 1978; **Med School:** Baylor Coll Med 1971; **Resid:** Ophthalmology, Geisinger Med Ctr 1977; **Fellow:** Ophthalmology, Wills Eye Hosp 1978; **Fac Appt:** Assoc Prof Oph, Univ S Fla Coll Med

Hodapp, Elizabeth A MD [Oph] - **Spec Exp:** Pediatric Glaucoma; **Hospital:** Bascom Palmer Eye Inst; **Address:** Bascom Palmer Eye Inst, 900 NW 17th St, Miami, FL 33136; **Phone:** 305-243-2020; **Board Cert:** Ophthalmology 1980; **Med School:** Harvard Med Sch 1975; **Resid:** Ophthalmology, Wash Univ Affil Hosp 1979; **Fellow:** Glaucoma, Washington Univ 1981

Kerr, Natalie C MD [Oph] - **Spec Exp:** Pediatric Ophthalmology; Strabismus; Cataract-Pediatric; Genetic Disorders-Eye; **Hospital:** Le Bonheur Chldns Med Ctr, St. Jude Children's Research Hosp; **Address:** Hamilton Eye Inst, 930 Madison Ave, Ste 400, Memphis, TN 38103; **Phone:** 901-448-6650; **Board Cert:** Ophthalmology 2003; **Med School:** Univ Fla Coll Med 1987; **Resid:** Ophthalmology, Shands Hosp/Univ FL 1991; **Fellow:** Pediatric Ophthalmology, Univ TN Affil Hosp 1992; **Fac Appt:** Prof Oph, Univ Tenn Coll Med

Lambert, Scott R MD [Oph] - **Spec Exp:** Pediatric Ophthalmology; Strabismus; Cataract-Pediatric; **Hospital:** Chldns Hlthcare Atlanta @ Egleston, Emory Univ Hosp; **Address:** Emory Eye Center, Pediatric Ophthalmology Clinic, 1365B Clifton Rd NE, Ste 4513, Atlanta, GA 30322; **Phone:** 404-778-3431; **Board Cert:** Ophthalmology 1989; **Med School:** Yale Univ 1983; **Resid:** Ophthalmology, UCSF Med Ctr 1987; **Fellow:** Pediatric Ophthalmology, Hosp for Sick Chldn 1988; Strabismus, Smith Kuttlewell 1988; **Fac Appt:** Prof Oph, Emory Univ

Mawn, Louise MD [Oph] - **Spec Exp:** Orbital Surgery; Reconstructive Surgery; Neuro-Ophthalmology; Eyelid/Tear Duct Reconstruction; **Hospital:** Vanderbilt Univ Med Ctr (page 75); **Address:** Vanderbilt Eye Institute, 2311 Pierce Ave, Nashville, TN 37232; **Phone:** 615-936-2020; **Board Cert:** Ophthalmology 2008; **Med School:** Wake Forest Univ 1990; **Resid:** Ophthalmology, Univ Iowa Hosps & Clin 1995; **Fellow:** Neuro-Ophthalmology, New England Med Ctr 1996; Ophthalmic Plastic & Reconstructive Surgery, Univ Ottawa Eye Inst 1997; **Fac Appt:** Assoc Prof Oph, Vanderbilt Univ

McKeown, Craig A MD [Oph] - **Spec Exp:** Pediatric Ophthalmology; Strabismus-Adult & Pediatric; Eye Muscle Disorders; **Hospital:** Bascom Palmer Eye Inst; **Address:** Bascom Palmer Eye Inst, 900 NW 17th St, Miami, FL 33136; **Phone:** 305-243-2020; **Board Cert:** Ophthalmology 1982; **Med School:** Northwestern Univ 1971; **Resid:** Ophthalmology, Walter Reed Med Ctr 1980; **Fellow:** Pediatric Ophthalmology, Chldns Hosp Natl Med Ctr 1984; Pediatric Ophthalmology, Wilmer Inst-Johns Hopkins 1985; **Fac Appt:** Clin Prof Oph, Univ Miami Sch Med

Meredith, Travis A MD [Oph] - **Spec Exp:** Retina/Vitreous Surgery; Macular Degeneration; Diabetic Eye Disease/Retinopathy; **Hospital:** NC Memorial Hosp - UNC; **Address:** 5151 Bioinformatics, CB#7040, Chapel Hill, NC 27599-7040; **Phone:** 919-966-5296; **Board Cert:** Ophthalmology 1976; **Med School:** Johns Hopkins Univ 1969; **Resid:** Ophthalmology, Wilmer Inst-Johns Hopkins 1971; Ophthalmology, Wilmer Inst-Johns Hopkins 1975; **Fellow:** Vitreoretinal Surgery, Med Coll Wisconsin 1976; **Fac Appt:** Prof Oph, Univ NC Sch Med

Murray, Timothy G MD [Oph] - **Spec Exp:** Eye Tumors/Cancer; Retinal Disorders; Macular Degeneration; Diabetic Eye Disease/Retinopathy; **Hospital:** Baptist Hosp of Miami, Miami Children's Hosp; **Address:** 6705 Red Rd, Ste 412, Murray Ocular Oncology and Retina, Coral Gables, FL 33143; **Phone:** 305-396-3830; **Board Cert:** Ophthalmology 1990; **Med School:** Johns Hopkins Univ 1985; **Resid:** Ophthalmology, UCSF Med Ctr 1989; **Fellow:** Ophthalmology, UCSF Med Ctr 1990; Vitreoretinal Disease, Med Coll Wisconsin 1991; **Fac Appt:** Prof Emeritus Oph, Univ Miami Sch Med

Nunery, William R MD [Oph] - **Spec Exp:** Orbital Surgery; Oculoplastic Surgery; Thyroid Eye Disease; **Hospital:** Univ of Louisville Hosp; **Address:** Kentucky Lions Eye Ctr, 301 E Muhammad Ali Blvd, Louisville, KY 40202; **Phone:** 502-889-1000; **Board Cert:** Ophthalmology 1980; **Med School:** Case West Res Univ 1975; **Resid:** Ophthalmology, Indiana Univ Hosp 1979; **Fellow:** Ophthalmic Plastic Surgery, Emory Univ 1980

Nussbaum, Julian MD [Oph] - **Spec Exp:** Diabetic Eye Disease/Retinopathy; Macular Degeneration; Retinopathy of Prematurity; **Hospital:** Med Coll of GA Hosp and Clin (MCG Health Inc); **Address:** 1120 15th St BA Bldg Fl 2 - rm 2331, Augusta, GA 30912; **Phone:** 706-721-1148; **Board Cert:** Ophthalmology 1981; **Med School:** Univ Miami Sch Med 1976; **Resid:** Internal Medicine, Jackson Memorial Hosp 1977; Ophthalmology, Med Coll Georgia 1980; **Fellow:** Vitreoretinal Surgery, Mass Eye & Ear Infirmary 1982; **Fac Appt:** Prof Oph, Med Coll GA

O'Brien, Terrence P MD [Oph] - **Spec Exp:** Cataract Surgery-Lens Implant; Laser Vision Surgery; Eye Infections; Corneal & External Eye Disease; **Hospital:** Bascom Palmer Eye Inst; **Address:** Bascom Palmer Eye Inst, 7101 Fairway Drive, Palm Beach Gardens, FL 33418; **Phone:** 561-515-1500; **Board Cert:** Ophthalmology 2004; **Med School:** Univ Mich Med Sch 1985; **Resid:** Ophthalmology, Wilmer Eye Inst 1991; **Fellow:** Cornea & Ext Eye Disease, Cullen Eye Inst-Baylor 1990; **Fac Appt:** Prof Oph, Univ Miami Sch Med

Olsen, Timothy W MD [Oph] - **Spec Exp:** Macular Degeneration; Diabetic Eye Disease/Retinopathy; Retinal Detachment; Retinal Disorders-Pediatric; **Hospital:** Emory Univ Hosp; **Address:** Emory Eye Center, 1365B Clifton Rd NE, Ste 3500, Atlanta, GA 30322; **Phone:** 404-778-2020; **Board Cert:** Ophthalmology 2007; **Med School:** Univ Kansas 1989; **Resid:** Ophthalmology, Univ Minn Affil Hosps 1993; **Fellow:** Vitreoretinal Surgery & Disease, Emory Univ 1996; **Fac Appt:** Prof Oph, Emory Univ

Parrish, Richard K MD [Oph] - **Spec Exp:** Glaucoma; Cataract Surgery-Lens Implant; **Hospital:** Bascom Palmer Eye Inst, Jackson Meml Hosp; **Address:** Bascom Palmer Eye Institute, 900 NW 17th St, rm 4501, Miami, FL 33136; **Phone:** 305-243-2020; **Board Cert:** Ophthalmology 1981; **Med School:** Indiana Univ 1976; **Resid:** Ophthalmology, Wills Eye Hosp 1980; **Fellow:** Glaucoma, Bascom Palmer Eye Inst 1982; **Fac Appt:** Prof Oph, Univ Miami Sch Med

Patrinely, James R MD [Oph] - **Spec Exp:** Ophthalmic Plastic Surgery; Eyelid Surgery; Orbital Surgery; **Hospital:** Methodist Hosp - Houston, St. Luke's Episcopal Hosp-Houston; **Address:** 17 E Main St, Ste 100, Pensacola, FL 32502; **Phone:** 850-473-0990; **Board Cert:** Ophthalmology 1986; **Med School:** Vanderbilt Univ 1980; **Resid:** Ophthalmology, Baylor College Med 1984; **Fellow:** Ophthalmological Pathology, Johns Hopkins Hosp 1985; Ophthalmic Plastic & Reconstructive Surgery, Univ Utah Med Ctr 1986; **Fac Appt:** Clin Prof Oph, Baylor Coll Med

Ophthalmology

Perez, Victor L MD [Oph] - **Spec Exp:** Cataract Surgery-Lens Implant; Uveitis; Cornea Transplant; Cornea & External Eye Disease; **Hospital:** Bascom Palmer Eye Inst; **Address:** 900 NW 17 St, Miami, FL 33136; **Phone:** 305-243-2020; **Board Cert:** Ophthalmology 2012; **Med School:** Univ Puerto Rico 1991; **Resid:** Ophthalmology, Mass Eye & Ear Infirmary 2000; **Fellow:** Immunology, Brigham & Womens Hosp 1996; Cornea, Mass Eye & Ear Infirmary 2002; **Fac Appt:** Assoc Prof Oph, Univ Miami Sch Med

Pollard, Zane F MD [Oph] - **Spec Exp:** Pediatric Ophthalmology; Strabismus; Tear Duct Problems; **Hospital:** Chldns Hlthcare Atlanta @ Scottish Rite, Piedmont Hosp; **Address:** Eye Consultants of Atlanta, 5445 Meridian Mark Rd, Ste 220, Atlanta, GA 30342-4722; **Phone:** 404-255-2419; **Board Cert:** Ophthalmology 1975; **Med School:** Tulane Univ 1966; **Resid:** Surgery, UCSF Med Ctr 1968; Ophthalmology, USC Med Ctr 1973; **Fellow:** Pediatric Ophthalmology, Wills Eye Hosp 1975

Rosenfeld, Philip J MD/PhD [Oph] - **Spec Exp:** Macular Disease/Degeneration; Diabetic Eye Disease/Retinopathy; Retinal Detachment; Retina/Vitreous Surgery; **Hospital:** Bascom Palmer Eye Inst; **Address:** 900 NW 17th St, rm 244, Miami, FL 33136; **Phone:** 305-326-6148; **Board Cert:** Ophthalmology 2008; **Med School:** Johns Hopkins Univ 1988; **Resid:** Ophthalmology, Mass Eye & Ear Infirm 1995; **Fellow:** Retina, Bascom Palmer Eye Inst 1996; **Fac Appt:** Prof Oph, Univ Miami Sch Med

Sherwood, Mark B MD [Oph] - **Spec Exp:** Glaucoma; **Hospital:** Shands at Univ of FL; **Address:** Shands at Univ Florida, Dept Ophthalmology, 1600 SW Archer Rd, Box 100284, Gainesville, FL 32610; **Phone:** 352-273-8708; **Med School:** England, UK 1976; **Resid:** Ophthalmology, Moorefield's Eye Hosp 1980; **Fellow:** Glaucoma, Wills Eye Hosp 1982; Glaucoma, Moorefield's Eye Hosp 1983; **Fac Appt:** Prof Oph, Univ Fla Coll Med

Solomon, Kerry D MD [Oph] - **Spec Exp:** Cataract Surgery; Corneal Disease; Refractive Surgery; Lens Implants-Multifocal; **Address:** Carolina Eyecare Physicians, 1101 Clarity Rd, Ste 100, Mt Pleasant, SC 29464; **Phone:** 843-881-3937; **Board Cert:** Ophthalmology 2004; **Med School:** Univ VT Coll Med 1987; **Resid:** Ophthalmology, Univ Kentucky Med Ctr 1992; **Fellow:** Ophthalmic Pathology, Univ Utah Hlth Sci Ctr 1988; Cornea & Ext Eye Disease, Wilmer Inst/Johns Hopkins Hosp 1993; **Fac Appt:** Clin Prof Oph, Univ SC Sch Med

Sternberg Jr, Paul MD [Oph] - **Spec Exp:** Retina/Vitreous Surgery; Macular Degeneration; Eye Tumors/Cancer; Diabetic Eye Disease/Retinopathy; **Hospital:** Vanderbilt Univ Med Ctr (page 75), Vanderbilt Monroe Carrell Jr. Chldn's Hosp (page 75); **Address:** Vanderbilt Eye Institute, 2311 Pierce Ave, Nashville, TN 37232-8808; **Phone:** 615-936-1453; **Board Cert:** Ophthalmology 1985; **Med School:** Univ Chicago-Pritzker Sch Med 1979; **Resid:** Ophthalmology, Johns Hopkins Hosp 1983; **Fellow:** Vitreoretinal Surgery, Duke Univ Med Ctr 1984; **Fac Appt:** Prof Oph, Vanderbilt Univ

Stulting, R Doyle MD/PhD [Oph] - **Spec Exp:** Corneal Disease & Transplant; Laser Vision Surgery; Cataract Surgery; Keratoconus; **Address:** Woolfson Eye Institute, 800 Mount Vernon Highway NE, Ste 125, Atlanta, GA 30328; **Phone:** 404-256-1125; **Board Cert:** Ophthalmology 1982; **Med School:** Duke Univ 1976; **Resid:** Internal Medicine, Barnes Hosp 1978; Ophthalmology, Bascom Palmer Eye Inst 1981; **Fellow:** Cornea, Emory Univ 1982

Tse, David T MD [Oph] - **Spec Exp:** Oculoplastic Surgery; Orbital Tumors/Cancer; Lacrimal Gland Disorders; Anophthalmia; **Hospital:** Bascom Palmer Eye Inst, Jackson Meml Hosp; **Address:** Bascom Palmer Eye Inst, 900 NW 17th St, Miami, FL 33136; **Phone:** 305-326-6086; **Board Cert:** Ophthalmology 2002; **Med School:** Univ Miami Sch Med 1976; **Resid:** Ophthalmology, LAC/USC Med Ctr 1981; **Fellow:** Ophthalmic Plastic Surgery, Univ Iowa 1982; Ophthalmic Oncololgy, Univ Iowa 1982; **Fac Appt:** Prof Oph, Univ Miami Sch Med

Updegraff, Stephen A MD [Oph] - **Spec Exp:** LASIK-Refractive Surgery; Corneal Disease & Surgery; Refractive Surgery; **Address:** Updegraff Vision, 1601 38th Ave N, Saint Petersburg, FL 33713; **Phone:** 727-822-4287; **Board Cert:** Ophthalmology 2008; **Med School:** Penn State Coll Med 1989; **Resid:** Ophthalmology, LSU Eye Ctr 1994; **Fellow:** Cornea, Univ Texas 1995

Wang, Ming X MD/PhD [Oph] - **Spec Exp:** Laser Vision Surgery; Corneal Disease; Cataract Surgery; **Address:** 1801 West End Ave, Ste 1150, Nashville, TN 37203; **Phone:** 615-321-8881; **Board Cert:** Ophthalmology 2009; **Med School:** Harvard Med Sch 1991; **Resid:** Ophthalmology, Wills Eye Hosp 1996; **Fellow:** Refractive Surgery, Bascom Palmer Eye Inst 1997; **Fac Appt:** Assoc Clin Prof Oph, Univ Tenn Coll Med

Waring III, George O MD [Oph] - **Spec Exp:** LASIK-Refractive Surgery; Cataract Surgery; Lens Implants; **Hospital:** Northside Hosp; **Address:** 5505 Peachtree Dunwoody Rd, Ste 220, Atlanta, GA 30342; **Phone:** 404-442-9577; **Board Cert:** Ophthalmology 1975; **Med School:** Baylor Coll Med 1967; **Resid:** Ophthalmology, Wills Eye Hosp 1973; **Fellow:** Cornea & Ext Eye Disease, Wills Eye Hosp 1974

Warman, Roberto MD [Oph] - **Spec Exp:** Pediatric Ophthalmology; Strabismus-Adult & Pediatric; Amblyopia; **Hospital:** Miami Children's Hosp; **Address:** Miami Childrens Hosp, Pediatric Ophthalmology Consultants, 3200 SW 60th Court, Ste 103, Miami, FL 33155; **Phone:** 305-662-8390; **Board Cert:** Ophthalmology 1987; **Med School:** Mexico 1981; **Resid:** Ophthalmology, Oschner Med Fndn 1985; **Fellow:** Neuro-Ophthalmology, Bascom Palmer Eye Inst 1986; Pediatric Ophthalmology, Bascom Palmer Eye Inst 1987; **Fac Appt:** Clin Prof Oph, Univ Miami Sch Med

Wilson Jr, Marion E MD [Oph] - **Spec Exp:** Cataract-Pediatric; Strabismus; Lens Implants-Pediatric; Pediatric Ophthalmology; **Hospital:** MUSC Chldns Hosp; **Address:** MUSC Storm Eye Inst, 167 Ashley Ave, Box 250676, Charleston, SC 29425; **Phone:** 843-792-7622; **Board Cert:** Ophthalmology 1987; **Med School:** Med Univ SC 1980; **Resid:** Ophthalmology, Natl Naval Med Ctr 1986; **Fellow:** Pediatric Ophthalmology, Chldns Hosp - Naval Med Ctr 1987; **Fac Appt:** Prof Oph, Med Univ SC

Wilson, Matthew W MD [Oph] - **Spec Exp:** Eye Tumors/Cancer; Retinoblastoma; Melanoma-Choroidal (eye); **Hospital:** St. Jude Children's Research Hosp, Methodist Univ Hosp - Memphis; **Address:** Univ Tenn Med Grp, Ophthalmology, 930 Madison Ave, Ste 200, Memphis, TN 38103; **Phone:** 901-448-6650; **Board Cert:** Ophthalmology 2007; **Med School:** Emory Univ 1990; **Resid:** Ophthalmology, Emory Univ Med Ctr 1994; Ophthalmic Pathology, Emory Univ Med Ctr 1995; **Fellow:** Ocular Oncology, Moorfields Eye Hosp 1996; Ophthalmic Plastic & Reconstructive Surgery, Casey Eye Inst 1998; **Fac Appt:** Assoc Prof Oph, Univ Tenn Coll Med

Yeatts, R Patrick MD [Oph] - **Spec Exp:** Oculoplastic Surgery; Orbital Tumors/Cancer; Eyelid Tumors/Cancer; Orbital Diseases; **Hospital:** Wake Forest Baptist Med Ctr; **Address:** Wake Forest Univ Eye Ctr, Janeway Clinical Sciences Bldg Fl 6, Medical Ctr Blvd, Winston-Salem, NC 27157; **Phone:** 336-716-4091; **Board Cert:** Ophthalmology 1983; **Med School:** Wake Forest Univ 1978; **Resid:** Ophthalmology, Mayo Clinic 1982; **Fellow:** Oculoplastic & Reconstructive Surgery, Mass Eye & Ear Infirmary 1983; **Fac Appt:** Prof Oph, Wake Forest Univ

Midwest

Abrams, Gary W MD [Oph] - **Spec Exp:** Retina/Vitreous Surgery; **Hospital:** Harper Univ Hosp; **Address:** Kresge Eye Inst, 4717 St Antoine St, Detroit, MI 48201; **Phone:** 313-577-8900; **Board Cert:** Ophthalmology 1977; **Med School:** Univ Okla Coll Med 1968; **Resid:** Ophthalmology, Med Coll Wisc Affil Hosps 1976; **Fellow:** Vitreoretinal Surgery, Bascom Palmer Eye Inst 1978; **Fac Appt:** Prof Oph, Wayne State Univ

Ophthalmology

Ahmad, Amjad Z MD [Oph] - **Spec Exp:** Oculoplastic & Orbital Surgery; Cosmetic & Reconstructive Surgery; Eyelid Cosmetic & Reconstructive Surgery; Tear Duct Problems; **Hospital:** Univ of IL Med Ctr at Chicago; **Address:** Univ Ill at Chicago, Dept Ophthalmology & Visual Scis, 1855 W Taylor St Fl 3 - rm 3.158, Chicago, IL 60612; **Phone:** 312-996-9120; **Board Cert:** Ophthalmology 2011; **Med School:** Univ Mich Med Sch 1994; **Resid:** Ophthalmology, Univ Michigan Affil Hosp 1998; **Fellow:** Oculoplastic & Reconstructive Surgery, Univ Michigan Affil Hosp 2000; **Fac Appt:** Asst Prof Oph, Univ IL Coll Med

Albert, Daniel M MD [Oph] - **Spec Exp:** Eye Tumors/Cancer; Ophthalmic Pathology; **Hospital:** Univ WI Hosp & Clins; **Address:** 600 Highland Ave CSC Bldg - rm K6/412, Madison, WI 53792-3284; **Phone:** 608-263-9798; **Board Cert:** Ophthalmology 1969; **Med School:** Univ Pennsylvania 1962; **Resid:** Ophthalmology, Hosp Univ Penn 1966; **Fellow:** Neuro-Ophthalmology, Natl Inst Hlth 1968; Pathology, Armed Forces Inst Path 1969; **Fac Appt:** Prof Oph, Univ Wisc

Alward, Wallace LM MD [Oph] - **Spec Exp:** Glaucoma; Anterior Segment Surgery; Cataract Surgery; Eye Tumors/Cancer; **Hospital:** Univ Iowa Hosp & Clinics; **Address:** UI Hospitals and Clinics, Department of Ophthalmology, 200 Hawkins Drive, Iowa City, IA 52242-1009; **Phone:** 319-356-3938; **Board Cert:** Ophthalmology 2006; **Med School:** Ohio State Univ 1976; **Resid:** Ophthalmology, Univ Louisville 1986; **Fellow:** Glaucoma, Univ Miami-Bascom Palmer Eye Inst 1987; **Fac Appt:** Prof Oph, Univ Iowa Coll Med

Archer, Steven M MD [Oph] - **Spec Exp:** Pediatric Ophthalmology; **Hospital:** Univ of Michigan Hosp; **Address:** Kellogg Eye Ctr, 1000 Wall St, Ann Arbor, MI 48105-1912; **Phone:** 734-764-7558; **Board Cert:** Ophthalmology 1986; **Med School:** Univ Chicago-Pritzker Sch Med 1978; **Resid:** Ophthalmology, Univ Chicago 1984; **Fellow:** Pediatric Ophthalmology, Indiana Univ 1986; **Fac Appt:** Asst Prof Oph, Univ Mich Med Sch

Augsburger, James J MD [Oph] - **Spec Exp:** Eye Tumors/Cancer; Melanoma-Choroidal (eye); Retinoblastoma; **Hospital:** Univ Hosp - Cincinnati, Cincinnati Chldns Hosp Med Ctr; **Address:** 222 Piedmont Ave, MSB Bldg Fl 1 - Ste 1500, Cincinnati, OH 45219; **Phone:** 513-475-7300; **Board Cert:** Ophthalmology 1979; **Med School:** Univ Cincinnati 1974; **Resid:** Ophthalmology, Univ Hosp-Cincinnati 1978; **Fellow:** Ocular Oncology, Wills Eye Hosp 1980; **Fac Appt:** Prof Oph, Univ Cincinnati

Azar, Dimitri T MD [Oph] - **Spec Exp:** LASIK-Refractive Surgery; **Hospital:** Univ of IL at Chicago Eye & Ear Infirm, Univ of IL Med Ctr at Chicago; **Address:** Millenium Park Eye Ctr, 30 N Michigan Ave, Ste 410, Chicago, IL 60602; **Phone:** 312-996-2020; **Board Cert:** Ophthalmology 1991; **Med School:** Lebanon 1983; **Resid:** Ophthalmology, American Univ Med Ctr 1986; Ophthalmology, Mass E&E Infirm 1991; **Fellow:** Cornea & Ext Eye Disease, Mass E&E Infirm 1988; Cornea Research, Harvard Med Sch 1991; **Fac Appt:** Prof Oph, Univ IL Coll Med

Azar, Nathalie F MD [Oph] - **Spec Exp:** Pediatric Ophthalmology; Strabismus; **Hospital:** Univ of IL at Chicago Eye & Ear Infirm; **Address:** Millenium Park Eye Ctr, 30 N Michigan Ave, Ste 410, Chicago, IL 60602; **Phone:** 312-996-2020; **Board Cert:** Ophthalmology 2007; **Med School:** Boston Univ 1990; **Resid:** Ophthalmology, George Washington U Med Ctr 1994; **Fellow:** Pediatric Ophthalmology, Wilmer Eye Inst 1995; **Fac Appt:** Assoc Clin Prof Oph, Univ IL Coll Med

Baker, John D MD [Oph] - **Spec Exp:** Pediatric Ophthalmology; **Hospital:** Chldns Hosp of Michigan; **Address:** 2355 Monroe Blvd, Ste 200, Dearborn, MI 48124-3009; **Phone:** 313-561-1777; **Board Cert:** Ophthalmology 1974; **Med School:** Wayne State Univ 1967; **Resid:** Ophthalmology, Detroit Genl Hosp 1971; **Fellow:** Pediatric Ophthalmology, Chldns Natl Med Ctr 1972; **Fac Appt:** Clin Prof Oph, Wayne State Univ

Burke, Miles J MD [Oph] - **Spec Exp:** Pediatric Ophthalmology; Eye Muscle Surgery; Amblyopia & Vision Development; Strabismus; **Hospital:** Cincinnati Chldns Hosp Med Ctr, Jewish Hosp - Kenwood - Cincinnati; **Address:** 10475 Montgomery Rd, Ste 4F, MS 45242, Cincinnati, OH 45242-5200; **Phone:** 513-984-4949; **Board Cert:** Ophthalmology 1979; **Med School:** Univ Ariz Coll Med 1974; **Resid:** Ophthalmology, Univ Michigan Med Ctr 1978; **Fellow:** Pediatric Ophthalmology, Wills Eye Hosp 1979

Cahill, Kenneth V MD [Oph] - **Spec Exp:** Eyelid Surgery; Eyelid/Tear Duct Reconstruction; Orbital Surgery; Oculoplastic Surgery; **Hospital:** Nationwide Chldn's Hosp; **Address:** The Eye Center, 262 Neil Ave, Ste 430, Columbus, OH 43215; **Phone:** 614-221-7464; **Board Cert:** Ophthalmology 1984; **Med School:** Ohio State Univ 1979; **Resid:** Ophthalmology, Univ of Pittsburgh 1983; **Fellow:** Oculoplastic Surgery, OSU Med Ctr 1984; Oculoplastic Surgery, Chldns Hosp Philadelphia 1984; **Fac Appt:** Clin Prof Oph, Ohio State Univ

Carter, Keith D MD [Oph] - **Spec Exp:** Oculoplastic & Orbital Surgery; Eyelid Surgery; Botox Therapy; **Hospital:** Univ Iowa Hosp & Clinics; **Address:** UIHC Dept Ophthalmology, 200 Hawkins Dr, PFP 11136-F, Iowa City, IA 52242; **Phone:** 319-356-2852; **Board Cert:** Ophthalmology 1988; **Med School:** Indiana Univ 1983; **Resid:** Ophthalmology, Univ Michigan Med Ctr 1987; **Fellow:** Oculoplastic Surgery, Univ Iowa 1988; **Fac Appt:** Prof Oph, Univ Iowa Coll Med

Del Monte, Monte A MD [Oph] - **Spec Exp:** Pediatric Ophthalmology; Strabismus-Adult & Pediatric; Cataract-Pediatric; Ophthalmic Genetics; **Hospital:** Univ of Michigan Hosp; **Address:** Kellogg Eye Center, 1000 Wall St, Ann Arbor, MI 48105-1912; **Phone:** 734-764-7558; **Board Cert:** Ophthalmology 1982; **Med School:** Johns Hopkins Univ 1974; **Resid:** Pediatrics, Chldns Hosp Med Ctr 1977; Ophthalmology, Wilmer Eye Inst 1981; **Fellow:** Ophthalmology, Wilmer Eye Inst 1978; Pediatric Ophthalmology, Chldns Hosp 1981; **Fac Appt:** Prof Oph, Univ Mich Med Sch

Drack, Arlene V MD [Oph] - **Spec Exp:** Eye Diseases-Hereditary; Eye Tumors/Cancer; Pediatric Ophthalmology; Strabismus; **Hospital:** Univ Iowa Hosp & Clinics; **Address:** UIHC Dept Ophthalmology, 200 Hawkins Drive, PFP 11136-F, Iowa City, IA 52242; **Phone:** 319-356-2852; **Board Cert:** Ophthalmology 1991; **Med School:** Penn State Coll Med 1986; **Resid:** Ophthalmology, Georgetown Univ Med Ctr 1990; **Fellow:** Pediatric Ophthalmology, Univ IA Hosps & Clin 1991; Molecular Genetics, Univ IA Hosps & Clin 1992; **Fac Appt:** Assoc Prof Oph, Univ Iowa Coll Med

Edwards, Paul A MD [Oph] - **Spec Exp:** Retinal Disorders; Macular Degeneration; Diabetic Eye Disease/Retinopathy; Ophthalmic Genetics; **Hospital:** Henry Ford Hosp, Henry Ford- W Bloomfield Hosp; **Address:** Henry Ford Hosp, Dept Ophthalmology, 2799 W Grand Blvd, K-10, Detroit, MI 48202; **Phone:** 313-916-3245; **Board Cert:** Ophthalmology 2005; **Med School:** West Indies 1979; **Resid:** Surgery, Washington Hosp Ctr 1984; Ophthalmology, Henry Ford Hosp 1989; **Fellow:** Research, Natl Eye Inst 1991; Retina/Vitreous, Henry Ford Hosp 1993; **Fac Appt:** Prof Oph, Wayne State Univ

Elner, Victor H MD/PhD [Oph] - **Spec Exp:** Eyelid Tumors/Cancer; Orbital Tumors/Cancer; **Hospital:** Univ of Michigan Hosp; **Address:** Kellogg Eye Ctr, 1000 Wall St, Ann Arbor, MI 48105; **Phone:** 734-763-9142; **Board Cert:** Ophthalmology 1983; Pathology 1988; **Med School:** Univ Chicago-Pritzker Sch Med 1979; **Resid:** Ophthalmology, Univ Chicago 1982; Pathology, Univ Chicago 1984; **Fellow:** Ophthalmological Pathology, Armed Forces Inst 1985; Ophthalmic Plastic & Reconstructive Surgery, Univ Wisconsin 1987; **Fac Appt:** Prof Oph, Univ Mich Med Sch

Feder, Robert S MD [Oph] - **Spec Exp:** Corneal Disease; LASIK-Refractive Surgery; Cataract Surgery; **Hospital:** Northwestern Meml Hosp; **Address:** 675 N St Clair St, Galter Bldg - Ste 15-150, Chicago, IL 60611-5975; **Phone:** 312-695-8150; **Board Cert:** Ophthalmology 1983; **Med School:** Northwestern Univ 1978; **Resid:** Ophthalmology, Barnes Hosp 1982; **Fellow:** Cornea & Eye Disease, Univ Iowa Med Ctr 1983; **Fac Appt:** Assoc Prof Oph, Northwestern Univ

Ophthalmology

Fishman, Gerald MD [Oph] - **Spec Exp:** Retinitis Pigmentosa; Retinal Disorders-Inherited; **Address:** Chicago Lighthouse, 1850 W Roosevelt Rd, Chicago, IL 60608; **Phone:** 312-997-3666; **Board Cert:** Ophthalmology 1975; **Med School:** Ohio State Univ 1969; **Resid:** Ophthalmology, Univ Illinois EE Infirmary 1973; **Fellow:** Ocular Pathology, Univ Illinois EE Infirmary 1974; **Fac Appt:** Prof Oph, Univ IL Coll Med

Greenwald, Mark MD [Oph] - **Spec Exp:** Pediatric Ophthalmology; **Hospital:** Univ of Chicago Med Ctr; **Address:** Univ Chicago Med Ctr, Dept Ophthalmology, 5758 S Maryland Ave, rm 1B, Chicago, IL 60637; **Phone:** 773-702-3937; **Board Cert:** Ophthalmology 1981; **Med School:** Harvard Med Sch 1976; **Resid:** Ophthalmology, Univ Illinois Hosp 1980; **Fellow:** Pediatric Ophthalmology, Chldns Hosp 1981; **Fac Appt:** Assoc Prof Oph, Univ Wash

Hariprasad, Seenu M MD [Oph] - **Spec Exp:** Retinal Disorders; Macular Degeneration; Diabetic Eye Disease/Retinopathy; Retinal Detachment; **Hospital:** Univ of Chicago Med Ctr, Weiss Meml Hosp; **Address:** Ctr for Advanced Medicine, 5841 S Maryland Ave, MC 2114, Chicago, IL 60637; **Phone:** 773-795-1326; **Board Cert:** Ophthalmology 2004; **Med School:** Univ Pennsylvania 1999; **Resid:** Ophthalmology, Cullen Eye Inst/Baylor Coll of Med 2003; **Fellow:** Retina/Vitreous, Barnes Retina Inst/Wash Univ 2005; **Fac Appt:** Assoc Prof Oph, Univ Chicago-Pritzker Sch Med

Heckenlively, John R MD [Oph] - **Spec Exp:** Eye Diseases-Hereditary; Retinal Disorders; Opthalmic Genetics; **Hospital:** Univ of Michigan Hosp; **Address:** Univ Michigan Kellogg Eye Ctr, 1000 Wall St, Ann Arbor, MI 48105; **Phone:** 734-763-2280; **Board Cert:** Ophthalmology 1977; **Med School:** Univ Colorado 1972; **Resid:** Ophthalmology, Univ Kentucky Affil Hosps 1976; **Fellow:** Vitreoretinal Disease, Jules Stein Eye Inst 1977; Johns Hopkins Univ 1978; **Fac Appt:** Prof Oph, Univ Mich Med Sch

Heuer, Dale K MD [Oph] - **Spec Exp:** Glaucoma; **Hospital:** Froedtert and Med Ctr of WI; **Address:** The Eye Institute, 925 N 87th St, Milwaukee, WI 53226; **Phone:** 414-955-2020; **Board Cert:** Ophthalmology 1983; **Med School:** Northwestern Univ 1978; **Resid:** Ophthalmology, Med Coll Wisc Affil Hosp 1982; **Fellow:** Glaucoma, Bascom Palmer Eye Inst 1984; **Fac Appt:** Prof Oph, Med Coll Wisc

Holland, Edward J MD [Oph] - **Spec Exp:** Corneal Disease; Refractive Surgery; Cataract Surgery; **Hospital:** St. Elizabeth Hlthcare-Edgewood; **Address:** Cincinnati Eye Institute, 1945 CEI Drive, Cincinnati, OH 45242; **Phone:** 513-984-5133; **Board Cert:** Ophthalmology 1986; **Med School:** Loyola Univ-Stritch Sch Med 1981; **Resid:** Ophthalmology, Univ Minn Med Ctr 1985; **Fellow:** Cornea & Ext Eye Disease, Univ Iowa Affil Hosp 1986; Ocular Immunology, Natl Eye Inst 1987; **Fac Appt:** Clin Prof Oph, Univ Cincinnati

John, Thomas MD [Oph] - **Spec Exp:** Cornea Transplant & Artificial Cornea; Amniotic Membrane Transplant; Cataract Surgery; Refractive Surgery; **Address:** 16532 S Oak Park Ave, Ste 201, Tinley Park, IL 60477; **Phone:** 708-429-2223; **Board Cert:** Ophthalmology 1987; **Med School:** India 1977; **Resid:** Ophthalmology, Hosp Univ Penn 1984; **Fellow:** Cornea & Ext Eye Disease, Univ Rochester Sch Med & Dentistry 1985; Cornea & Ext Eye Disease, Mass Eye & Ear Infirmary 1987; **Fac Appt:** Assoc Clin Prof Oph, Loyola Univ-Stritch Sch Med

Kaufman, Paul L MD [Oph] - **Spec Exp:** Glaucoma; **Hospital:** Univ WI Hosp & Clins; **Address:** Univ Wisconsin Hosp, Dept Ophthalmology, 2880 University Ave, MC 9030, Madison, WI 53705; **Phone:** 608-263-7171; **Board Cert:** Ophthalmology 1976; **Med School:** NYU Sch Med 1967; **Resid:** Ophthalmology, Washington Univ-Barnes Hosp 1973; **Fellow:** Ocular Pharmacology, Univ Uppsala 1975; **Fac Appt:** Prof Oph, Univ Wisc

Krueger, Ronald MD [Oph] - **Spec Exp:** Corneal Disease; Refractive Surgery; **Hospital:** Cleveland Clin (page 55); **Address:** Cleveland Clinic Fdn - Cole Eye Inst, 9500 Euclid Ave, Desk 130, Cleveland, OH 44195; **Phone:** 216-444-8158; **Board Cert:** Ophthalmology 2003; **Med School:** UMDNJ-NJ Med Sch, Newark 1987; **Resid:** Ophthalmology, Columbia Presby Med Ctr 1991; **Fellow:** Refractive Surgery, Univ Okla Hlth Sci Ctr-McGee Eye Inst 1992; Cornea, USC-Doheny Eye Inst 1993

Kushner, Burton J MD [Oph] - **Spec Exp:** Pediatric Ophthalmology; Strabismus-Adult & Pediatric; **Hospital:** Univ WI Hosp & Clins; **Address:** Pediatric Eye Clinic, 2880 University Ave, MC 9030, Madison, WI 53705; **Phone:** 608-263-7171; **Board Cert:** Ophthalmology 1975; **Med School:** Northwestern Univ 1969; **Resid:** Ophthalmology, Univ Wisc Hosp 1973; **Fellow:** Pediatric Ophthalmology, Bascom Palmer Eye Inst 1974; **Fac Appt:** Prof Oph, Univ Wisc

Kwon, Young H MD/PhD [Oph] - **Spec Exp:** Glaucoma; **Hospital:** Univ Iowa Hosp & Clinics; **Address:** UIHC Dept of Ophthalmology, 200 Hawkins Drive, PFP 11136-F, Iowa City, IA 52242; **Phone:** 319-356-2852; **Board Cert:** Ophthalmology 2008; **Med School:** Yale Univ 1991; **Resid:** Ophthalmology, Mass Eye & Ear Infirmary 1995; **Fellow:** Glaucoma, Yale Univ Affil Hosp 1996; **Fac Appt:** Prof Oph, Univ Iowa Coll Med

Lane, Stephen S MD [Oph] - **Spec Exp:** Laser Vision Surgery; Cataract Surgery; **Hospital:** United Hosp; **Address:** Associated Eye Care, 2950 Curve Crest Blvd, Stillwater, MN 55082; **Phone:** 651-275-3000; **Board Cert:** Ophthalmology 1986; **Med School:** Univ Minn 1980; **Resid:** Ophthalmology, MS Hershey Med Ctr 1984; **Fellow:** Cornea & Ext Eye Disease, Univ Minn 1984; **Fac Appt:** Clin Prof Oph, Univ Minn

Lass, Jonathan H MD [Oph] - **Spec Exp:** Cataract Surgery-Lens Implant; Corneal & External Eye Disease; **Hospital:** Univ Hosps Case Med Ctr (page 74); **Address:** UH Case Medical Center, Ophthalmology, 11100 Euclid Ave, Ste 4115, Cleveland, OH 44106; **Phone:** 216-844-8590; **Board Cert:** Ophthalmology 1978; **Med School:** Boston Univ 1973; **Resid:** Ophthalmology, Boston Univ Med Ctr 1977; **Fellow:** Ophthalmology, Mass Eye & Ear Infirmary 1979; **Fac Appt:** Prof Oph, Case West Res Univ

Lee, Paul P MD [Oph] - **Spec Exp:** Glaucoma; **Hospital:** Univ of Michigan Hosp; **Address:** Univ of Michigan Kellogg Eye Ctr, 1000 Wall St, Ann Arbor, MI 48105; **Phone:** 734-763-5874; **Board Cert:** Ophthalmology 2011; **Med School:** Univ Mich Med Sch 1986; **Resid:** Ophthalmology, Wilmer Eye Inst/Johns Hopkins 1990; **Fellow:** Glaucoma, Mass EE Infirm 1991; **Fac Appt:** Prof Oph, Univ Mich Med Sch

Lichter, Paul R MD [Oph] - **Spec Exp:** Cataract Surgery; Glaucoma; **Hospital:** Univ of Michigan Hosp; **Address:** 1000 Wall St, WK Kellogg Eye Ctr, Ann Arbor, MI 48105; **Phone:** 734-763-5874; **Board Cert:** Ophthalmology 1970; **Med School:** Univ Mich Med Sch 1964; **Resid:** Ophthalmology, Univ Mich Med Ctr 1968; **Fellow:** Ophthalmology, UCSF Med Ctr 1969; **Fac Appt:** Prof Oph, Univ Mich Med Sch

Lindstrom, Richard L MD [Oph] - **Spec Exp:** Corneal Disease; Cataract Surgery; Refractive Surgery; **Hospital:** Abbott - Northwestern Hosp, Phillips Eye Inst; **Address:** 9801 DuPont Ave S, Ste 200, Bloomington, MN 55431; **Phone:** 612-813-3600; **Board Cert:** Ophthalmology 1978; **Med School:** Univ Minn 1972; **Resid:** Ophthalmology, Univ Minn Med Ctr 1978; Ophthalmology, Univ Minn Med Ctr 1980; **Fellow:** Anterior Segment - External Disease, Mary Shields Eye Hosp; Glaucoma, Univ Hosps; **Fac Appt:** Prof Oph, Univ Minn

Lucarelli, Mark J MD [Oph] - **Spec Exp:** Ophthalmic Plastic Surgery; Reconstructive Plastic Surgery; Oculoplastic & Orbital Surgery; Thyroid Eye Disease; **Hospital:** Univ WI Hosp & Clins; **Address:** Univ Wisconsin Hosp & Clinics, 2880 University Ave, MC 9030, Madison, WI 53705; **Phone:** 608-263-7171; **Board Cert:** Ophthalmology 2008; **Med School:** Washington Univ, St Louis 1991; **Resid:** Ophthalmology, Mass Eye & Ear Infirm 1995; **Fellow:** Ophthalmic Plastic & Reconstructive Surgery, Univ Wisconsin Hosp & Clins 1997; **Fac Appt:** Prof Oph, Univ Wisc

Lueder, Gregg T MD [Oph] - **Spec Exp:** Retinoblastoma; Eye Tumors-Pediatric; Pediatric Ophthalmology; **Hospital:** St. Louis Chldns Hosp; **Address:** St Louis Children's Hospital, One Children's Pl, Ste 2 South 89, St Louis, MO 63110; **Phone:** 314-454-6026; **Board Cert:** Ophthalmology 2003; **Med School:** Univ Iowa Coll Med 1985; **Resid:** Pediatrics, St Louis Children's Hosp 1988; Ophthalmology, Univ Iowa Med Ctr 1991; **Fellow:** Pediatric Ophthalmology, Hosp for Sick Children 1993; **Fac Appt:** Assoc Prof Oph, Washington Univ, St Louis

Maguire, Leo J MD [Oph] - **Spec Exp:** Cornea Transplant; Refractive Surgery; **Hospital:** Mayo Med Ctr & Clin - Rochester; **Address:** Mayo Clinic-Ophthalmology, 200 First St SW, Rochester, MN 55905; **Phone:** 507-284-4152; **Board Cert:** Ophthalmology 1986; **Med School:** Jefferson Med Coll 1980; **Resid:** Ophthalmology, Univ Michigan Hosp 1984; **Fellow:** Cornea & Ext Eye Disease, LSU Eye Ctr 1986; **Fac Appt:** Assoc Prof Oph, Mayo Med Sch

Mets, Marilyn B MD [Oph] - **Spec Exp:** Pediatric Ophthalmology; Ophthalmic Genetics; Strabismus; Retinal Disorders; **Hospital:** Lurie Chldn's Hosp-Chicago; **Address:** Ann & Robert H. Lurie Children's Hosp, 225 E Chicago Ave, Box 70, Chicago, IL 60611; **Phone:** 312-227-6718; **Board Cert:** Ophthalmology 2005; **Med School:** Geo Wash Univ 1976; **Resid:** Ophthalmology, Cleveland Clinic Fdn 1980; **Fellow:** Pediatric Ophthalmology, Natl Chldns Hosp 1981; **Fac Appt:** Prof Oph, Northwestern Univ

Mieler, William F MD [Oph] - **Spec Exp:** Retina/Vitreous Surgery; Eye Tumors/Cancer; Macular Disease/Degeneration; Trauma; **Hospital:** Univ of IL Med Ctr at Chicago, Weiss Meml Hosp; **Address:** Univ of IL Med Ctr, Dept Ophthalmology, 1905 W Taylor St, Chicago, IL 60612; **Phone:** 312-996-6660; **Board Cert:** Ophthalmology 2009; **Med School:** Univ Wisc 1979; **Resid:** Ophthalmology, Bascom-Palmer Eye Inst 1983; **Fellow:** Vitreoretinal Surgery & Disease, Med Ctr Wisconsin Eye Inst 1984; Oculoplastic Surgery, Wills Eye Hosp 1986; **Fac Appt:** Prof Oph, Univ IL Coll Med

Mizen, Thomas R MD [Oph] - **Spec Exp:** Neuro-Ophthalmology; Optic Nerve Disorders; **Hospital:** Rush Univ Med Ctr; **Address:** 6187 S Archer Ave, Chicago, IL 60638; **Phone:** 312-942-3500; **Board Cert:** Ophthalmology 1986; **Med School:** Finch/Chicago Med Sch 1980; **Resid:** Ophthalmology, Rush-Presby-St Lukes Med Ctr 1984; **Fellow:** Neuro-Ophthalmology, Barnes Hosp/Wash Univ 1985; **Fac Appt:** Asst Prof Oph, Rush Med Coll

Nerad, Jeffrey MD [Oph] - **Spec Exp:** Orbital Tumors/Cancer; Eyelid Cancer & Reconstruction; Oculoplastic Surgery; **Address:** Cincinnati Eye Institute, 1945 CEI Drive, Cincinnati, OH 45242; **Phone:** 513-984-5133; **Board Cert:** Ophthalmology 1984; **Med School:** St Louis Univ 1979; **Resid:** Ophthalmology, St Louis Univ Med Ctr 1983; **Fellow:** Oculoplastic & Reconstructive Surgery, Univ Iowa 1984; **Fac Appt:** Prof Oph, Univ Iowa Coll Med

Olitsky, Scott E MD [Oph] - **Spec Exp:** Pediatric Ophthalmology; Strabismus; **Hospital:** Chldns Mercy Hosps & Clinics; **Address:** Chldns Mercy Hosp, Dept Oph, 2401 Gillham Rd, Kansas City, MO 64108; **Phone:** 816-234-3046; **Board Cert:** Ophthalmology 2004; **Med School:** Jefferson Med Coll 1988; **Resid:** Ophthalmology, SUNY Buffalo Med Ctr 1992; **Fellow:** Pediatric Ophthalmology, Wills Eye Inst 1993; **Fac Appt:** Prof Oph, Univ MO-Kansas City

Osher, Robert H MD [Oph] - **Spec Exp:** Cataract Surgery-Lens Implant; **Address:** 1945 CEI Drive, Cincinnati, OH 45242; **Phone:** 513-984-5133; **Board Cert:** Ophthalmology 1981; **Med School:** Univ Rochester 1976; **Resid:** Ophthalmology, Bascom Palmer Eye Inst 1980; **Fellow:** Ophthalmology, Wills Eye Hosp 1977; Ophthalmology, Bascom Palmer Eye Inst 1981; **Fac Appt:** Prof Oph, Univ Cincinnati

Page, Timothy MD [Oph] - **Spec Exp:** Cataract Surgery; Cataract Surgery-Lens Implant; Refractive Surgery; Anterior Segment Surgery; **Hospital:** Beaumont Hosp-Royal Oak; **Address:** Oakland Ophthalmic Surgery, 800 S Adams Rd, Ste 201, Birmingham, MI 48009; **Phone:** 248-644-8060; **Board Cert:** Ophthalmology 2011; **Med School:** Wayne State Univ 1994; **Resid:** Ophthalmology, William Beumont Hosp 1998

Pepose, Jay MD [Oph] - **Spec Exp:** LASIK-Refractive Surgery; Cataract Surgery; Corneal & External Eye Disease; **Hospital:** Barnes-Jewish Hosp, St. John's Mercy Med Ctr - St Louis; **Address:** 1815 Clarkson Rd, Chesterfield, MO 63017; **Phone:** 636-728-0111; **Board Cert:** Ophthalmology 1989; **Med School:** UCLA 1982; **Resid:** Ophthalmology, Johns Hopkins Hosp 1987; **Fellow:** Cornea & Ext Eye Disease, Georgetown Univ Med Ctr 1988; **Fac Appt:** Prof Oph, Washington Univ, St Louis

Petersen, Michael R MD/PhD [Oph] - **Spec Exp:** Diabetic Eye Disease/Retinopathy; Macular Degeneration; Retinal Detachment; Uveitis; **Hospital:** Bethesda North Hosp; **Address:** Cincinnati Eye Institute, 1945 CEI Drive, Cincinnati, OH 45242-5664; **Phone:** 513-984-5133; **Board Cert:** Ophthalmology 1991; **Med School:** Univ Mich Med Sch 1986; **Resid:** Ophthalmology, Kellogg Eye Ctr 1990; **Fellow:** Vitreoretinal Surgery, Univ Wash Affil Hosp 1992

Plager, David A MD [Oph] - **Spec Exp:** Pediatric Ophthalmology; Strabismus; Cataract-Pediatric; Glaucoma-Pediatric; **Hospital:** Riley Hosp for Children; **Address:** IU Pediatric Ophthalmology, 702 Rotary Circle Fl 2, Indianapolis, IN 46202; **Phone:** 317-944-8103; **Board Cert:** Ophthalmology 2006; **Med School:** Indiana Univ 1983; **Resid:** Ophthalmology, Indiana Univ Hosps 1987; **Fellow:** Pediatric Ophthalmology, Chldns Hosp Natl Med Ctr 1988; Strabismus, Chldns Hosp Natl Med Ctr 1988; **Fac Appt:** Prof Oph, Indiana Univ

Pulido, Jose S MD [Oph] - **Spec Exp:** Retina/Vitreous Surgery; Eye Tumors/Cancer; **Hospital:** Mayo Med Ctr & Clin - Rochester; **Address:** 200 1st St SW, Rochester, MN 55905; **Phone:** 507-284-3721; **Board Cert:** Ophthalmology 1986; **Med School:** Tulane Univ 1981; **Resid:** Ophthalmology, Illinois Eye & Ear Infirm 1986; **Fellow:** Vitreoretinal Surgery & Disease, Bascom-Palmer Eye Inst 1987; Ocular Oncology, Wills Eye Hosp; **Fac Appt:** Prof Oph, Mayo Med Sch

Putterman, Allen M MD [Oph] - **Spec Exp:** Oculoplastic & Orbital Surgery; Cosmetic Surgery-Face & Eyes; Thyroid Eye Disease; Eyelid Cosmetic & Reconstructive Surgery; **Hospital:** St. Joseph Hosp; **Address:** 111 N Wabash Ave, Ste 1722, Chicago, IL 60602-2002; **Phone:** 312-372-2256; **Board Cert:** Ophthalmology 1971; **Med School:** Univ Wisc 1963; **Resid:** Ophthalmology, Michael Reese Hosp 1969; **Fellow:** Oculoplastic Surgery, Manhattan Eye/Ear Infirm 1970; **Fac Appt:** Prof Oph, Univ IL Coll Med

Rogers, Gary L MD [Oph] - **Spec Exp:** Strabismus-Adult & Pediatric; **Hospital:** Nationwide Chldn's Hosp; **Address:** 555 S 18th St, Ste 4C, Columbus, OH 43205; **Phone:** 614-224-6222; **Board Cert:** Ophthalmology 1974; **Med School:** Ohio State Univ 1968; **Resid:** Ophthalmology, Mt Sinai Hosp 1972; **Fellow:** Pediatric Ophthalmology, Chldns Hosp Natl Med Ctr 1974; **Fac Appt:** Clin Prof Oph, Ohio State Univ

Ophthalmology

Rosenberg, Michael A MD [Oph] - **Spec Exp:** Refractive Surgery; Cataract Surgery; Eye Muscle Surgery; **Hospital:** Northwestern Meml Hosp; **Address:** Sorrel Rosin Eye Ctr, 675 N St Clair St, Galter Bldg - Ste 15-150, Chicago, IL 60611-5967; **Phone:** 312-695-8150; **Board Cert:** Ophthalmology 1975; **Med School:** Northwestern Univ 1967; **Resid:** Ophthalmology, Bascom Palmer Eye Inst 1973; **Fellow:** Neuro-Ophthalmology, UCSF Med Ctr 1974; Refractive Surgery, Univ Monterrey 1998; **Fac Appt:** Assoc Clin Prof Oph, Northwestern Univ

Samuelson, Thomas W MD [Oph] - **Spec Exp:** Glaucoma; Cataract Surgery; Anterior Segment Surgery; Refractive Surgery; **Hospital:** Phillips Eye Inst; **Address:** Minnesota Eye Consultants, 710 E 24th St, Ste 100, Minneapolis, MN 55404-3810; **Phone:** 612-813-3600; **Board Cert:** Ophthalmology 1991; **Med School:** Univ Minn 1985; **Resid:** Ophthalmology, Univ S Florida 1990; **Fellow:** Glaucoma, Wills Eye Hosp 1991; **Fac Appt:** Assoc Clin Prof Oph, Univ Minn

Schachat, Andrew P MD [Oph] - **Spec Exp:** Retina/Vitreous Surgery; Diabetic Eye Disease/Retinopathy; Melanoma-Choroidal (eye); **Hospital:** Cleveland Clin (page 55); **Address:** The Cleveland Clinic Fdn, Cole Eye Inst, 9500 Euclid Ave, Desk I30, Cleveland, OH 44195; **Phone:** 216-444-7963; **Board Cert:** Ophthalmology 1983; **Med School:** Johns Hopkins Univ 1979; **Resid:** Ophthalmology, Wilmer Inst-John Hopkins Hosp 1982; **Fellow:** Vitreoretinal Surgery & Disease, Wilmer Eye Inst-Johns Hopkins Hosp 1983; **Fac Appt:** Prof Oph

Stone, Edwin MD [Oph] - **Spec Exp:** Retinal Disorders; Eye Diseases-Hereditary; **Hospital:** Univ Iowa Hosp & Clinics; **Address:** UIHC Dept Ophthalmology, 200 Hawkins Dr, PFP 11136-F, Iowa City, IA 52242; **Phone:** 319-356-2852; **Board Cert:** Ophthalmology 1990; **Med School:** Baylor Coll Med 1985; **Resid:** Ophthalmology, Univ Iowa Hosps 1989; **Fellow:** Retina, Univ Iowa Hosps 1992; **Fac Appt:** Prof Oph, Univ Iowa Coll Med

Summers, C Gail MD [Oph] - **Spec Exp:** Eye Diseases-Hereditary; Albinism; **Address:** Park Plaza Bldg, 701 25th Ave S Fl 3, Minneapolis, MN 55455; **Phone:** 612-365-8350; **Board Cert:** Ophthalmology 1984; **Med School:** Univ Minn 1979; **Resid:** Ophthalmology, Univ Minnesota Med Ctr 1983; **Fellow:** Pediatric Ophthalmology, Unin Minnesota Med Ctr 1984; **Fac Appt:** Prof Oph, Univ Minn

Traboulsi, Elias Iskandar MD [Oph] - **Spec Exp:** Pediatric Ophthalmology; Glaucoma-Pediatric; **Hospital:** Cleveland Clin (page 55); **Address:** Cleveland Clinic Fdn, Cole Eye Inst, 9500 Euclid Ave, Desk I30, Cleveland, OH 44195; **Phone:** 216-444-4363; **Board Cert:** Clinical Genetics 1987; Ophthalmology 1991; **Med School:** Amer Univ Beirut 1982; **Resid:** Ophthalmology, American Univ Beirut Hosp 1985; Ophthalmology, Georgetown Hosp 1989; **Fellow:** Ophthalmology, Johns Hopkins Hosp 1986; Pediatric Ophthalmology, Chldns Hosp Natl Med Ctr 1990; **Fac Appt:** Prof Oph, Ohio State Univ

Trese, Michael T MD [Oph] - **Spec Exp:** Retina/Vitreous Surgery; Retinal Disorders-Pediatric; **Hospital:** Beaumont Hosp-Royal Oak, Chldns Hosp of Michigan; **Address:** Associated Retinal Consultants, 3535 W 13 Mile Rd, Ste 344, Royal Oak, MI 48073-6710; **Phone:** 248-288-2280; **Board Cert:** Ophthalmology 1981; **Med School:** Georgetown Univ 1976; **Resid:** Ophthalmology, Jules Stein Eye Inst-UCLA 1980; **Fellow:** Retina, Duke Univ Med Ctr 1981; **Fac Appt:** Assoc Clin Prof Oph, Wayne State Univ

Trobe, Jonathan D MD [Oph] - **Spec Exp:** Neuro-Ophthalmology; Optic Nerve Disorders; **Hospital:** Univ of Michigan Hosp; **Address:** 1500 E Medical Ctr Drive, Ann Arbor, MI 48105-1912; **Phone:** 734-763-5114; **Board Cert:** Ophthalmology 1974; Neurology 1988; **Med School:** Harvard Med Sch 1968; **Resid:** Ophthalmology, Wills Eye Hosp 1972; Neurology, Jackson Meml Hosp/U Miami 1986; **Fellow:** Neuro-Ophthalmology, Bascom Palmer Eye Inst 1977; **Fac Appt:** Prof Oph, Univ Mich Med Sch

Tychsen, Lawrence MD [Oph] - **Spec Exp:** Pediatric Ophthalmology; Strabismus; Amblyopia; **Hospital:** St. Louis Chldns Hosp, Barnes-Jewish Hosp; **Address:** Chldns Eye Ctr, 1 Children's Pl Fl 2 S-89, St Louis, MO 63110; **Phone:** 314-454-6026; **Board Cert:** Ophthalmology 1984; **Med School:** Georgetown Univ 1979; **Resid:** Ophthalmology, Univ Iowa Hosp 1983; **Fellow:** Pediatric Ophthalmology, UCSF Med Ctr 1985; **Fac Appt:** Assoc Prof Oph, Washington Univ, St Louis

Vajaranant, Thasarat S MD [Oph] - **Spec Exp:** Glaucoma; Women's Eye Health; **Hospital:** Univ of IL at Chicago Eye & Ear Infirm; **Address:** Univ Illinois Chicago Eye Ctr, Glaucoma Svc, 1855 W Taylor St, rm 3171, Chicago, IL 60612; **Phone:** 312-996-7030; **Board Cert:** Ophthalmology 2008; **Med School:** Thailand 1996; **Resid:** Ophthalmology, Univ of Illinois 2006; **Fellow:** Glaucoma, Univ of Illinois 2007; Research, Univ of Illinois 2008; **Fac Appt:** Asst Prof Oph, Univ IL Coll Med

Volpe, Nicholas J MD [Oph] - **Spec Exp:** Neuro-Ophthalmology; Strabismus; **Hospital:** Northwestern Meml Hosp; **Address:** Sorrel Rosin Eye Ctr, 675 N St Clair, Galter Pavilion, Ste 15-150, Chicago, IL 60611; **Phone:** 312-695-8150; **Board Cert:** Ophthalmology 2003; **Med School:** SUNY Downstate 1987; **Resid:** Ophthalmology, Mass E&E Infirmary 1993; **Fellow:** Neuro-Ophthalmology, Mass E&E Infirmary 1992; **Fac Appt:** Prof Oph, Northwestern Univ-Feinberg Sch Med

Williams, George A MD [Oph] - **Spec Exp:** Retinal Disorders; Macular Degeneration; **Hospital:** Beaumont Hosp-Royal Oak; **Address:** Associated Retinal Consultants, 3535 W 13 Mile Rd, Ste 344, Royal Oak, MI 48073; **Phone:** 248-288-2280; **Board Cert:** Ophthalmology 2005; **Med School:** Northwestern Univ 1978; **Resid:** Ophthalmology, Med Coll Wisconsin 1982; **Fellow:** Retina/Vitreous, Med Coll Wisconsin 1984; **Fac Appt:** Clin Prof Oph, Univ Mich Med Sch

Wilson, Steven E MD [Oph] - **Spec Exp:** LASIK-Refractive Surgery; PRK-Refractive Surgery; Corneal Disease; **Hospital:** Cleveland Clin (page 55); **Address:** Cleveland Clinic Fdn - Cole Eye Inst, 9500 Euclid Ave, Ste I32, Cleveland, OH 44195; **Phone:** 216-444-5887; **Board Cert:** Ophthalmology 1990; **Med School:** UCSD 1984; **Resid:** Ophthalmology, Mayo Clinic 1988; **Fellow:** Cornea & Ext Eye Disease, Med Ctr Louisiana-LSU 1990; **Fac Appt:** Prof Oph, Cleveland Cl Coll Med/Case West Res

Great Plains and Mountains

Anderson, Richard L MD [Oph] - **Spec Exp:** Orbital & Eyelid Tumors/Cancer; Eyelid Problems/Ptosis/Blepharospasm; Cosmetic Surgery-Face & Eyes; **Hospital:** Salt Lake Regional Med Ctr, Intermountain Shriners Hosp; **Address:** 1002 E South Temple, Ste 308, Salt Lake City, UT 84102-1525; **Phone:** 801-363-3355; **Board Cert:** Ophthalmology 1976; **Med School:** Univ Iowa Coll Med 1971; **Resid:** Ophthalmology, Univ Iowa Hosps-Clins 1975; **Fellow:** Oculoplastic & Reconstructive Surgery, Albany Med Ctr 1975; Oculoplastic & Reconstructive Surgery, UCSF Med Ctr 1976; **Fac Appt:** Prof PlS, Univ Utah

Cionni, Robert J MD [Oph] - **Spec Exp:** Cataract Surgery-Lens Implant; Refractive Surgery; **Hospital:** LDS Hosp, Univ Utah Hlth Care; **Address:** 755 E 3900 S, Salt Lake City, UT 84107; **Phone:** 801-266-2283; **Board Cert:** Ophthalmology 1991; **Med School:** Univ Cincinnati 1985; **Resid:** Ophthalmology, Univ Louisville Hosp 1987; **Fellow:** Cataract/Lens Implant Surgery, Cincinnati Eye Inst

Crandall, Alan S MD [Oph] - **Spec Exp:** Glaucoma; Cataract Surgery; **Hospital:** Univ Utah Hlth Care; **Address:** Moran Eye Ctr- Univ Utah Hosp, 65 N Mario Cappecchi Drive, Salt Lake City, UT 84132; **Phone:** 801-581-2352; **Board Cert:** Ophthalmology 1977; **Med School:** Univ Utah 1973; **Resid:** Ophthalmology, Hosp Univ Penn 1976; **Fellow:** Glaucoma, Scheie Eye Inst; **Fac Appt:** Clin Prof Oph, Univ Utah

Ophthalmology

Durrie, Daniel MD [Oph] - **Spec Exp:** LASIK-Refractive Surgery; Corneal Disease; **Hospital:** Univ of Kansas Hosp; **Address:** 5520 College Blvd, Ste 201, Overland Park, KS 66211; **Phone:** 913-491-3330; **Board Cert:** Ophthalmology 1979; **Med School:** Univ Nebr Coll Med 1975; **Resid:** Ophthalmology, Univ Nebr Med Coll Affil Hosp 1979; **Fellow:** Cornea, Filkins Eye Inst 1980; **Fac Appt:** Clin Prof Oph, Univ Kansas

Gigantelli, James W MD [Oph] - **Spec Exp:** Orbital Tumors/Cancer; Eyelid Cancer & Reconstruction; Lymphoma-Ocular (eye); **Hospital:** Nebraska Med Ctr; **Address:** 985540 Nebraska Medical Center, Omaha, NE 68198-5540; **Phone:** 402-559-4276; **Board Cert:** Ophthalmology 1991; **Med School:** Vanderbilt Univ 1985; **Resid:** Ophthalmology, Baylor Coll Med 1989; **Fellow:** Ophthalmic Plastic & Reconstructive Surgery, Duke Unv Med Ctr 1990; **Fac Appt:** Prof Oph, Univ Nebr Coll Med

McCann, John D MD/PhD [Oph] - **Spec Exp:** Cosmetic Surgery-Face & Eyes; Orbital Diseases; Botox Therapy; **Hospital:** Intermountain Med Ctr; **Address:** Center for Facial Appearances, 1002 E South Temple, Ste 308, Salt Lake City, UT 84102; **Phone:** 801-363-3355; **Board Cert:** Ophthalmology 2007; **Med School:** Univ Iowa Coll Med 1991; **Resid:** Ophthalmology, Univ CA Affil Hosp 1995; **Fellow:** Oculoplastic Surgery, Univ Utah Med Ctr 1996

Southwest

Ellis Jr, George S MD [Oph] - **Spec Exp:** Pediatric Ophthalmology; Eye Muscle Disorders; **Hospital:** Children's Hospital - New Orleans, E Jefferson Genl Hosp; **Address:** Children's Hospital, 200 Henry Clay Ave, Ste 3106, New Orleans, LA 70118; **Phone:** 504-896-9426; **Board Cert:** Ophthalmology 1982; **Med School:** Tulane Univ 1977; **Resid:** Ophthalmology, LSU-Eye Center 1979; Ophthalmology, Duke Univ-Eye Ctr 1982; **Fellow:** Pediatric Ophthalmology, Hall Eye Clinic 1982; Pediatric Ophthalmology, Chldns Hosp 1982; **Fac Appt:** Assoc Clin Prof Oph, Tulane Univ

Esmaeli-Azad, Bita MD [Oph] - **Spec Exp:** Orbital & Eyelid Tumors/Cancer; Eyelid Cancer & Reconstruction; Oculoplastic Surgery; **Hospital:** UT MD Anderson Cancer Ctr; **Address:** MD Anderson Cancer Ctr, Ophthalmology Section, 1515 Holcombe Blvd, Unit 1445, Houston, TX 77030; **Phone:** 713-792-6523; **Board Cert:** Ophthalmology 2006; **Med School:** Univ Hlth Scis, Chicago Med Sch 1990; **Resid:** Ophthalmology, Univ Mich-Kellogg Eye Ctr 1994; **Fellow:** Ophthalmic Plastic & Reconstructive Surgery, Univ Toronto 1996; **Fac Appt:** Assoc Prof Oph, Univ Tex, Houston

Eustis Jr, H Sprague MD [Oph] - **Spec Exp:** Pediatric Ophthalmology; Strabismus; **Hospital:** Ochsner Med Ctr-New Orleans, Children's Hospital - New Orleans; **Address:** Ochsner Clinic, 1514 Jefferson Hwy, Dept Ophthalmology Fl 10, New Orleans, LA 70121; **Phone:** 504-842-3995; **Board Cert:** Ophthalmology 1985; **Med School:** Louisiana State U, New Orleans 1980; **Resid:** Ophthalmology, LSU Eye Ctr 1984; **Fellow:** Pediatric Ophthalmology, Hosp Sick Chldn 1985; Pediatric Ophthalmology, Natl Chldns Med Ctr 1985; **Fac Appt:** Clin Prof Oph, Louisiana State U, New Orleans

Koch, Douglas D MD [Oph] - **Spec Exp:** Cataract Surgery; Refractive Surgery; **Hospital:** Methodist Hosp - Houston, St. Luke's Episcopal Hosp-Houston; **Address:** Baylor Eye Clinic-Alkek Eye Center, 1977 Butler Blvd Fl 2, Houston, TX 77030-2704; **Phone:** 713-798-6100; **Board Cert:** Ophthalmology 1982; **Med School:** Harvard Med Sch 1977; **Resid:** Ophthalmology, Baylor Affil Hosp 1981; **Fellow:** Cornea, Moorfields Eye Hosp 1982; Refractive Surgery, Baylor Coll Med 1982; **Fac Appt:** Prof Oph, Baylor Coll Med

Lambert, H Michael MD [Oph] - **Spec Exp:** Retina/Vitreous Surgery; Macular Degeneration; Diabetic Eye Disease/Retinopathy; **Hospital:** Methodist Hosp - Houston, St. Luke's Episcopal Hosp-Houston; **Address:** Retinia & Vitrous of Texas, 2727 Gramercy St, Ste 200, Houston, TX 77025-1633; **Phone:** 713-799-9975; **Board Cert:** Ophthalmology 1983; **Med School:** Baylor Coll Med 1977; **Resid:** Ophthalmology, Wilford Hall USAF Med Ctr 1982; **Fellow:** Vitreoretinal Surgery, Duke Univ Eye Ctr 1983; **Fac Appt:** Assoc Clin Prof Oph, Baylor Coll Med

Lee, Andrew G MD [Oph] - **Spec Exp:** Neuro-Ophthalmology; Optic Nerve Disorders; Optic Nerve Tumors; **Hospital:** Methodist Hosp - Houston; **Address:** 6560 Fannin St, Scurlock Bldg, Ste 450, Houston, TX 77030; **Phone:** 713-441-8843; **Board Cert:** Ophthalmology 2006; **Med School:** Univ VA Sch Med 1989; **Resid:** Ophthalmology, Cullen Eye Inst-Baylor 1993; **Fellow:** Neuro-Ophthalmology, Wilmer Eye Inst-Johns Hopkins 1994; **Fac Appt:** Prof Oph, Cornell Univ-Weill Med Coll

Lewis, Richard A MD [Oph] - **Spec Exp:** Eye Diseases-Hereditary; Ophthalmic Genetics; Retinal Disorders; Macular Degeneration; **Hospital:** St. Luke's Episcopal Hosp-Houston, Texas Chldns Hosp; **Address:** Cullen Eye Institute NC-206, Baylor Coll Medicine, One Baylor Plaza, Houston, TX 77030; **Phone:** 713-798-6100; **Board Cert:** Ophthalmology 1976; **Med School:** Univ Mich Med Sch 1969; **Resid:** Ophthalmology, Univ Michigan Hosp 1974; **Fellow:** Retina, Montefiore Hosp 1974; Macular Disease, Bascom Palmer Eye Inst 1975; **Fac Appt:** Prof Oph, Baylor Coll Med

McCulley, James P MD [Oph] - **Spec Exp:** Corneal & External Eye Disease; Laser Vision Surgery; Cataract Surgery; **Hospital:** UT Southwestern Med Ctr at Dallas; **Address:** Univ Tex SW Med Ctr, Dept Oph, 5323 Harry Hines Blvd, Dallas, TX 75390-9057; **Phone:** 214-645-2020; **Board Cert:** Ophthalmology 1974; **Med School:** Washington Univ, St Louis 1968; **Resid:** Ophthalmology, Mass EE Infirm 1973; **Fellow:** Cornea, Cornea Rsch-Retina Fdn 1974; Cornea, Mass EE Infirm 1974; **Fac Appt:** Prof Oph, Univ Tex SW, Dallas

Miller, Joseph M MD [Oph] - **Spec Exp:** Pediatric Ophthalmology; Strabismus; Amblyopia; **Hospital:** Univ Arizona Med Ctr-Univ Campus, Yuma Regl Med Ctr; **Address:** Univ Ariz, Dept Ophthalmology, 707 N Alvernon Way, Ste 301, Tucson, AZ 85711; **Phone:** 520-694-1460; **Board Cert:** Ophthalmology 1991; **Med School:** NE Ohio Univ 1985; **Resid:** Ophthalmology, Yale New Haven Hosp 1990; **Fellow:** Pediatric Ophthalmology, Johns Hopkins Hosp 1991; Refractive Surgery, Univ Arizona Hosp 2001; **Fac Appt:** Prof Oph, Univ Ariz Coll Med

Mims III, James Luther MD [Oph] - **Spec Exp:** Pediatric Ophthalmology; Strabismus-Adult & Pediatric; **Hospital:** Baptist Med Ctr - San Antonio, Methodist Chldns Hosp of South Texas; **Address:** 311 Camden St, Ste 511, San Antonio, TX 78215-2015; **Phone:** 210-225-0084; **Board Cert:** Ophthalmology 1977; **Med School:** Tulane Univ 1968; **Resid:** Ophthalmology, Wills Eye Hosp 1976; **Fellow:** Pediatric Ophthalmology, Wills Eye Hosp 1977; **Fac Appt:** Clin Prof Oph, Univ Tex, San Antonio

Pflugfelder, Stephen C MD [Oph] - **Spec Exp:** Corneal Disease; Refractive Surgery; Cataract Surgery; Lens Implants; **Hospital:** Methodist Hosp - Houston; **Address:** Baylor Eye Clinic-Alkek Eye Ctr, 1977 Butler Blvd Fl 2, Houston, TX 77030; **Phone:** 713-798-6100; **Board Cert:** Ophthalmology 1987; **Med School:** SUNY Upstate Med Univ 1981; **Resid:** Ophthalmology, Baylor Affil Hosp 1985; **Fellow:** Cornea & Ext Eye Disease, Bascom Palmer Eye Inst 1986; **Fac Appt:** Prof Oph, Baylor Coll Med

Richard, James M MD [Oph] - **Spec Exp:** Pediatric Ophthalmology; Eye Muscle Surgery; **Hospital:** Chldns Hosp OU Med Ctr, Integris Baptist Med Ctr - OK; **Address:** 11013 Hefner Pointe Drive, Oklahoma City, OK 73120-5050; **Phone:** 405-751-2020; **Board Cert:** Ophthalmology 1979; **Med School:** Univ Okla Coll Med 1974; **Resid:** Ophthalmology, Baylor Coll Med 1978; **Fellow:** Pediatric Ophthalmology, Chldns Hosp 1979; Ophthalmology, Johns Hopkins Hosp 1980; **Fac Appt:** Clin Prof Oph, Univ Okla Coll Med

Ophthalmology

Schiffman, Jade S MD [Oph] - **Spec Exp:** Neuro-Ophthalmology; **Hospital:** UT MD Anderson Cancer Ctr; **Address:** MD Anderson Cancer Ctr, 1515 Holcombe Blvd, Box 342, Houston, TX 77035; **Phone:** 713-792-3798; **Board Cert:** Neurology 1983; Ophthalmology 1991; **Med School:** SUNY Upstate Med Univ 1975; **Resid:** Neurology, Univ Miami Affil Hosp 1980; Ophthalmology, UCSF Med Ctr 1989; **Fellow:** Neuro-Ophthalmology, UCSF Med Ctr 1981; **Fac Appt:** Prof Oph, Univ Tex, Houston

Siatkowski, R Michael MD [Oph] - **Spec Exp:** Pediatric Ophthalmology; Neuro-Ophthalmology; Retinopathy of Prematurity; Strabismus; **Hospital:** OU Med Ctr; **Address:** 608 Stanton L. Young Blvd, rm 512, Dean McGee Eye INstitute, Oklahoma City, OK 73104; **Phone:** 405-271-1094; **Board Cert:** Ophthalmology 2009; **Med School:** Jefferson Med Coll 1987; **Resid:** Ophthalmology, St Francis Med Ctr 1991; **Fellow:** Neuro-Ophthalmology, Bascom Palmer Eye Inst 1992; Pediatric Ophthalmology, Bascom Palmer Eye Inst 1993; **Fac Appt:** Prof Oph, Univ Okla Coll Med

Soparkar, Charles MD [Oph] - **Spec Exp:** Eye Tumors/Cancer; Orbital & Eyelid Tumors/Cancer; Oculoplastic Surgery; **Hospital:** Methodist Hosp - Houston, Texas Chldns Hosp; **Address:** Plastic Eye Surg Assocs, 3730 Kirby Drive, Ste 900, Houston, TX 77098; **Phone:** 713-795-0705; **Board Cert:** Ophthalmology 2007; **Med School:** Univ Mass Sch Med 1990; **Resid:** Ophthalmology, Baylor Affil Hosps 1994; **Fellow:** Ophthalmic Oncololgy, Texas Med Ctr 1995; Ophthalmic Plastic Surgery, Texas Med Ctr 1995; **Fac Appt:** Asst Clin Prof Oph, Baylor Coll Med

Wallace III, Robert B MD [Oph] - **Spec Exp:** Refractive Surgery; Cataract Surgery; Glaucoma; **Hospital:** CHRISTUS St. Frances Cabrini Hosp; **Address:** 4110 Parliament Drive, Alexandria, LA 71303; **Phone:** 318-448-4488; **Board Cert:** Ophthalmology 1979; **Med School:** Tulane Univ 1974; **Resid:** Ophthalmology, Tulane Affil Hosp 1978; **Fac Appt:** Clin Prof Oph, Louisiana State U, New Orleans

West Coast and Pacific

Abbott, Richard L MD [Oph] - **Spec Exp:** Cornea & External Eye Disease; **Hospital:** UCSF Med Ctr; **Address:** UCSF, Dept Ophthalmology, 8 Koret Way, Ste U545, San Francisco, CA 94143-0730; **Phone:** 415-514-8200; **Board Cert:** Ophthalmology 1978; **Med School:** Geo Wash Univ 1971; **Resid:** Ophthalmology, Presby-Pacific Med Ctr 1977; **Fellow:** Cornea & Ext Eye Disease, Bascom Palmer Eye Inst 1978; **Fac Appt:** Clin Prof Oph, UCSF

Arnold, Anthony C MD [Oph] - **Spec Exp:** Neuro-Ophthalmology; **Hospital:** UCLA Ronald Reagan Med Ctr; **Address:** 100 Stein Plaza, Box 957000, Los Angeles, CA 90095-7005; **Phone:** 310-825-4344; **Board Cert:** Ophthalmology 2008; **Med School:** UCLA 1975; **Resid:** Ophthalmology, Jules Stein Eye Inst-UCLA 1979; **Fellow:** Neuro-Ophthalmology, Jules Stein Eye Inst-UCLA 1983; **Fac Appt:** Clin Prof Oph, UCLA

Baerveldt, George MD [Oph] - **Spec Exp:** Glaucoma; **Hospital:** UC Irvine Med Ctr; **Address:** 3501 Jamboree Rd, Fl 2, Ste 200 B, MS 92660, Newport Beach, CA 92660; **Phone:** 949-854-7400; **Med School:** South Africa 1967; **Resid:** Ophthalmology, Univ of Witwatersrand 1975; **Fellow:** Neuro-Ophthalmology, SUNY Downstate Med Ctr 1976; **Fac Appt:** Prof Emeritus Oph, UC Irvine

Baylis, Henry I MD [Oph] - **Spec Exp:** Oculoplastic Surgery; Eyelid Surgery; **Hospital:** UCLA Ronald Reagan Med Ctr, Hoag Meml Hosp Presby; **Address:** 1260 15th St, Ste 917, Santa Monica, CA 90404; **Phone:** 310-207-0300; **Board Cert:** Ophthalmology 1969; **Med School:** Univ Mich Med Sch 1960; **Resid:** Ophthalmology, UCLA Med Ctr 1966; **Fellow:** Oculoplastic Surgery, Manhattan EET Hosp 1967; **Fac Appt:** Clin Prof Oph, UCLA

Bernardino, Carlo R MD [Oph] - **Spec Exp:** Oculoplastic Surgery; Orbital Surgery; Thyroid Eye Disease; Anophthalmia; **Hospital:** Comm Hosp of Monterey Pen; **Address:** Vantage Eye Center, Medical Bldg B, Ste 130, 2 Upper Ragsdale Drive, Monterey, CA 93940; **Phone:** 831-647-3900; **Board Cert:** Ophthalmology 2003; **Med School:** Jefferson Med Coll 1997; **Resid:** Ophthalmology, Wills Eye Hosp 2001; **Fellow:** Oculoplastic Surgery, Mass Eye & Ear Infirm 2003; **Fac Appt:** Assoc Prof Oph, Yale Univ

Blumenkranz, Mark S MD [Oph] - **Spec Exp:** Retinal Disorders; Macular Degeneration; **Hospital:** Stanford Univ Hosp & Clinics; **Address:** Byers Eye Institute at Stanford, 2452 Watson Court, Palo Alto, CA 94303-5353; **Phone:** 650-723-6995; **Board Cert:** Ophthalmology 1980; **Med School:** Brown Univ 1975; **Resid:** Ophthalmology, Stanford Univ Hosp 1979; **Fellow:** Vitreo-retinal Surgery, Bascom Palmer Eye Inst 1980; **Fac Appt:** Prof Oph, Stanford Univ

Borchert, Mark S MD [Oph] - **Spec Exp:** Pediatric Neuro-Ophthalmology; Vision-Unexplained Loss; Optic Nerve Disorders; **Hospital:** Chldns Hosp - Los Angeles; **Address:** Chldns Hosp, Div Ophthalmology, 4650 Sunset Blvd, MS 88, Los Angeles, CA 90027-6062; **Phone:** 323-361-4510; **Board Cert:** Ophthalmology 1989; **Med School:** Baylor Coll Med 1983; **Resid:** Ophthalmology, LAC-USC Med Ctr 1987; **Fellow:** Neuro-Ophthalmology, Mass EE Infirm-Harvard 1988; **Fac Appt:** Assoc Prof Oph, USC Sch Med

Boxer Wachler, Brian S MD [Oph] - **Spec Exp:** LASIK-Refractive Surgery; Keratoconus; Corneal Disease & Surgery; Cataract Surgery; **Hospital:** Cedars-Sinai Med Ctr; **Address:** Boxer Wachler Vision Inst, 465 N Roxbury Drive, Ste 902, Beverly Hills, CA 90210; **Phone:** 310-594-5209; **Board Cert:** Ophthalmology 2010; **Med School:** Dartmouth Med Sch 1993; **Resid:** Ophthalmology, St Louis Univ Eye Inst 1997; **Fellow:** Refractive Surgery, Univ Kansas Med Ctr 1998

Boxrud, Cynthia Ann MD [Oph] - **Spec Exp:** Oculoplastic Surgery; Eye Tumors/Cancer; Orbital Diseases; **Hospital:** UCLA Ronald Reagan Med Ctr, St. John's Hlth Ctr, Santa Monica; **Address:** 2021 Santa Monica Blvd, Ste 700E, Santa Monica, CA 90404-2208; **Phone:** 310-829-9060; **Board Cert:** Ophthalmology 2008; **Med School:** Case West Res Univ 1986; **Resid:** Ophthalmology, NYU-Bellevue Hosp Ctr 1990; **Fellow:** Ophthalmic Oncololgy, New York Hosp-Cornell Med Ctr 1992; Ophthalmic Plastic Surgery, UCLA-Jules Stein Eye Inst 1993; **Fac Appt:** Asst Prof Oph, UCLA

Caprioli, Joseph MD [Oph] - **Spec Exp:** Glaucoma; Cataract Surgery; Anterior Segment Surgery; **Hospital:** UCLA Ronald Reagan Med Ctr; **Address:** UCLA-Jules Stein Eye Institute, 100 Stein Plaza Fl 2 - Ste 2-273, Los Angeles, CA 90095-7006; **Phone:** 310-794-9442; **Board Cert:** Ophthalmology 1985; **Med School:** SUNY Buffalo 1979; **Resid:** Ophthalmology, Yale-New Haven Hosp. 1983; **Fellow:** Glaucoma, Wills Eye Hosp 1984; **Fac Appt:** Prof Oph, UCLA

Caster, Andrew I MD [Oph] - **Spec Exp:** LASIK-Refractive Surgery; Laser Vision Surgery; **Hospital:** Cedars-Sinai Med Ctr; **Address:** 9100 Wilshire Blvd, Ste 265E, Beverly Hills, CA 90212; **Phone:** 310-274-1221; **Board Cert:** Ophthalmology 1986; **Med School:** Harvard Med Sch 1980; **Resid:** Ophthalmology, UCLA Jules Stein Eye Inst 1984

Char, Devron H MD [Oph] - **Spec Exp:** Eye Tumors/Cancer; Thyroid Eye Disease; Oculoplastic Surgery; **Hospital:** CA Pacific Med Ctr-Pacific Campus, UCSF Med Ctr; **Address:** 45 Castro St, Ste 309, San Francisco, CA 94114; **Phone:** 415-522-0700; **Board Cert:** Ophthalmology 1978; **Med School:** Univ Minn 1970; **Resid:** Internal Medicine, Mass Genl Hosp 1972; Ophthalmology, UCSF Med Ctr 1977; **Fellow:** Medical Oncology, Natl Cancer Inst 1974; Ophthalmology, UCSF Med Ctr 1978; **Fac Appt:** Prof Oph, Stanford Univ

Ophthalmology

Choy, Andrew MD [Oph] - **Spec Exp:** Eye Muscle Disorders; Oculoplastic & Orbital Surgery; Orbital Tumors/Cancer; **Hospital:** Long Beach Meml Med Ctr, Los Alamitos Med Ctr; **Address:** 4100 Long Beach Blvd, Ste 108, Long Beach, CA 90807-2619; **Phone:** 562-426-3925; **Board Cert:** Ophthalmology 1976; **Med School:** USC Sch Med 1969; **Resid:** Neurology, LAC-USC Med Ctr 1971; Ophthalmology, Bellevue Hosp Ctr-NYU 1974; **Fellow:** Strabismus, Columbia-Presby Med Ctr 1975; **Fac Appt:** Assoc Clin Prof Oph, UCLA

Cockerham, Kimberly P MD [Oph] - **Spec Exp:** Meningioma-Orbital (eye); Orbital Tumors/Cancer; Eyelid Cancer & Reconstruction; Neuro-Ophthalmology; **Hospital:** El Camino Hosp, Stanford Univ Hosp & Clinics; **Address:** 1801 E March Ln, Ste A160, Stockton, CA 95210; **Phone:** 209-951-1178; **Board Cert:** Ophthalmology 2004; **Med School:** Geo Wash Univ 1987; **Resid:** Ophthalmology, Walter Reed Army Med Ctr 1992; **Fellow:** Neuro-Ophthalmology, Walter Reed Army Med Ctr 1993; Neuro-Ophthalmology, Allegheny General Hosp 1995

Day, Susan H MD [Oph] - **Spec Exp:** Pediatric Ophthalmology; Strabismus-Adult & Pediatric; **Hospital:** CA Pacific Med Ctr-Pacific Campus, Chldns Hosp - Oakland; **Address:** 2340 Clay St, Ste 100, San Francisco, CA 94115; **Phone:** 415-202-1500; **Board Cert:** Ophthalmology 2009; **Med School:** Louisiana State U, New Orleans 1975; **Resid:** Ophthalmology, California Pacific Med Ctr 1979; **Fellow:** Pediatric Ophthalmology, Hosp Sick Chldn 1980

De Juan Jr, Eugene MD [Oph] - **Spec Exp:** Retina/Vitreous Surgery; **Hospital:** UCSF Med Ctr; **Address:** UCSF Dept Ophthalmology, 400 Parnassus Ave Fl 7, San Francisco, CA 94143; **Phone:** 415-353-2084; **Board Cert:** Ophthalmology 1985; **Med School:** Univ S Ala Coll Med 1979; **Resid:** Ophthalmology, Johns Hopkins Hosp 1983; **Fellow:** Vitreoretinal Surgery, Duke Univ Eye Ctr 1984; **Fac Appt:** Prof Oph, UCSF

Demer, Joseph L MD/PhD [Oph] - **Spec Exp:** Pediatric Ophthalmology; Strabismus; Nystagmus; **Hospital:** UCLA Ronald Reagan Med Ctr; **Address:** Jules Stein Eye Institute, 100 Stein Plaza, MC 7002, Los Angeles, CA 90095-7065; **Phone:** 310-825-5931; **Board Cert:** Ophthalmology 1988; **Med School:** Johns Hopkins Univ 1983; **Resid:** Ophthalmology, Baylor Coll Med 1987; **Fellow:** Pediatric Ophthalmology, Texas Chldns Hosp 1988; **Fac Appt:** Prof Oph, UCLA

Freeman, William R MD [Oph] - **Hospital:** UCSD Med Ctr; **Address:** 9415 Campus Point Drive, La Jolla, CA 92037; **Phone:** 858-534-6290; **Board Cert:** Ophthalmology 1984; **Med School:** Mount Sinai Sch Med 1979; **Resid:** Ophthalmology, Lenox Hill Hosp 1983; **Fellow:** Uveitis, Proctor Fdn-UCSF Med Ctr 1985; Retinal Surgery, Doheny Fdn-USC 1986; **Fac Appt:** Asst Prof Oph, UCSD

Gorin, Michael B MD/PhD [Oph] - **Spec Exp:** Retinal Disorders; Macular Degeneration; Eye Diseases-Hereditary; **Hospital:** UCLA Ronald Reagan Med Ctr; **Address:** Jules Stein Eye Inst, 100 Stein Plaza, Los Angeles, CA 90095-7000; **Phone:** 310-794-5400; **Board Cert:** Ophthalmology 1987; **Med School:** Univ Pennsylvania 1980; **Resid:** Ophthalmology, Jules Stein Eye Inst 1986; **Fellow:** Medical Retina, Moorfields Eye Hosp 1987; **Fac Appt:** Prof Oph, UCLA-David Geffen Sch Med

Granet, David B MD [Oph] - **Spec Exp:** Pediatric Ophthalmology; Eye Muscle Disorders; Strabismus; Nystagmus; **Hospital:** UCSD Med Ctr, Rady Children's Hosp - San Diego; **Address:** UCSD/Ratner Children's Eye Center, 9415 Campus Point Drive, La Jolla, CA 92093; **Phone:** 858-534-2020; **Board Cert:** Ophthalmology 2005; **Med School:** Yale Univ 1987; **Resid:** Ophthalmology, Bellevue Hosp-NYU 1991; **Fellow:** Pediatric Ophthalmology, Chldns Hosp & UPenn Scheie Eye Inst 1993; Strabismus, UPenn Scheie Eye Inst 1993; **Fac Appt:** Prof Oph, UCSD

Humayun, Mark S MD/PhD [Oph] - **Spec Exp:** Retina/Vitreous Surgery; Retinal Disorders; Retinal Vascular Diseases; Diabetic Eye Disease/Retinopathy; **Hospital:** Keck Med Ctr of USC (page 62); **Address:** Doheny Eye Center, 1450 San Pablo St Fl 4, Los Angeles, CA 90033; **Phone:** 323-442-6522; **Board Cert:** Ophthalmology 2006; **Med School:** Duke Univ 1989; **Resid:** Ophthalmology, Duke Univ Med Ctr 1993; **Fellow:** Vitreoretinal Surgery, Wilmer Inst-Johns Hopkins 1995; **Fac Appt:** Prof Oph, USC-Keck School of Medicine

Irvine, John A MD [Oph] - **Spec Exp:** Corneal & External Eye Disease; **Hospital:** Keck Med Ctr of USC (page 62); **Address:** USC-Doheny Eye Institute, 1450 San Pablo St, Ste 5703, Los Angeles, CA 90033; **Phone:** 323-442-6335; **Board Cert:** Ophthalmology 1989; **Med School:** USC Sch Med 1982; **Resid:** Ophthalmology, Mass Eye & Ear Infirmary 1986; **Fellow:** Cornea & Ext Eye Disease, Mass Eye & Ear Infirmary 1987; **Fac Appt:** Prof Oph, USC Sch Med

Isenberg, Sherwin Jay MD [Oph] - **Spec Exp:** Strabismus; Pediatric Ophthalmology; **Hospital:** LAC - Harbor - UCLA Med Ctr, UCLA Ronald Reagan Med Ctr; **Address:** Jules Stein Eye Inst, 100 Stein Plaza, Los Angeles, CA 90095-7000; **Phone:** 310-825-8840; **Board Cert:** Ophthalmology 1978; **Med School:** UCLA 1973; **Resid:** Ophthalmology, Illinois Ear & Eye Infirm 1977; **Fellow:** Pediatric Ophthalmology, Chldns Hosp Natl Med Ctr 1978; **Fac Appt:** Prof Oph, UCLA

Iwach, Andrew G MD [Oph] - **Spec Exp:** Glaucoma; **Hospital:** UCSF Med Ctr, CA Pacific Med Ctr-Pacific Campus; **Address:** Glaucoma Ctr of San Francisco, 55 Stevenson St, San Francisco, CA 94105; **Phone:** 415-981-2020; **Board Cert:** Ophthalmology 1991; **Med School:** UCLA 1984; **Resid:** Ophthalmology, Stanford Univ Med Ctr 1988; **Fellow:** Glaucoma, UCSF Med Ctr 1989; **Fac Appt:** Assoc Prof Oph, UCSF

Kikkawa, Don MD [Oph] - **Spec Exp:** Ophthalmic Plastic Surgery; Oculoplastic & Orbital Surgery; Thyroid Eye Disease; Lacrimal Gland Disorders; **Hospital:** UCSD Med Ctr; **Address:** Div Oph Plas& Recon Surg, UCSD-Shiley Eye Ctr, 9415 Campus Pt Drive, rm 255, MC 0946, La Jolla, CA 92093-0946; **Phone:** 858-534-7402; **Board Cert:** Ophthalmology 2003; **Med School:** St Louis Univ 1987; **Resid:** Ophthalmology, Jules Stein Eye Inst-UCLA 1991; **Fellow:** Ophthalmic Plastic & Reconstructive Surgery, Univ Wisc Med Sch 1992; **Fac Appt:** Clin Prof Oph, UCSD

Kim, Jonathan W MD [Oph] - **Spec Exp:** Oculoplastic Surgery; Orbital Tumors/Cancer; **Hospital:** USC Norris Cancer Hosp (page 62); **Address:** 1450 San Pablo St, Ste DEI4000, Los Angeles, CA 90033; **Phone:** 323-442-6335; **Board Cert:** Ophthalmology 2000; **Med School:** Univ Iowa Coll Med 1994; **Resid:** Ophthalmology, CA Pacific Med Ctr 1998; **Fellow:** Oculoplastic Surgery, Jules Stein Eye Inst/UCLA Med Ctr 2000; Orbital Surgery, Mass Eye & Ear Infirm 2004

Krauss, Howard R MD [Oph] - **Spec Exp:** Neuro-Ophthalmology; **Hospital:** UCLA Ronald Reagan Med Ctr; **Address:** Pacific Specialists, 11645 Wilshire Blvd Fl 6, Los Angeles, CA 90025; **Phone:** 310-477-5558; **Board Cert:** Ophthalmology 1982; **Med School:** NY Med Coll 1977; **Resid:** Ophthalmology, Jules Stein Eye Inst 1981; **Fellow:** Neuro-Ophthalmology, Univ Pittsburgh 1982; **Fac Appt:** Clin Prof Oph, UCLA-David Geffen Sch Med

Maloney, Robert K MD [Oph] - **Spec Exp:** Refractive Surgery; LASIK-Refractive Surgery; Cataract Surgery; **Hospital:** UCLA Ronald Reagan Med Ctr; **Address:** Maloney Vision Inst, 10921 Wilshire Blvd, Ste 900, Los Angeles, CA 90024-4002; **Phone:** 310-208-3937; **Board Cert:** Ophthalmology 1991; **Med School:** UCSF 1985; **Resid:** Ophthalmology, Johns Hopkins Hosp 1989; **Fellow:** Refractive Surgery, Emory Univ Hosp 1991; **Fac Appt:** Clin Prof Oph, UCLA

Ophthalmology

Manche, Edward E MD [Oph] - **Spec Exp:** LASIK-Refractive Surgery; Cornea Transplant; PRK-Refractive Surgery; **Hospital:** Stanford Univ Hosp & Clinics; **Address:** Byers Eye Institute at Stanford, 2452 Watson Court, Palo Alto, CA 94303-5353; **Phone:** 650-723-6995; **Board Cert:** Ophthalmology 2007; **Med School:** Albert Einstein Coll Med 1990; **Resid:** Ophthalmology, UMDNJ Affil Hosp 1994; **Fellow:** Cornea & Ext Eye Disease, Jules Stein Eye Inst-UCLA 1996; **Fac Appt:** Assoc Prof Oph, Stanford Univ

Mannis, Mark J MD [Oph] - **Spec Exp:** Cornea Transplant & Artificial Cornea; Cornea & External Eye Disease; **Hospital:** UC Davis Med Ctr; **Address:** UC Davis Med Ctr, Dept Ophthalmology, 4860 Y St, Ste 2400, Sacramento, CA 95817; **Phone:** 916-734-6602; **Board Cert:** Ophthalmology 2009; **Med School:** Univ Fla Coll Med 1975; **Resid:** Ophthalmology, Washington Univ 1979; **Fellow:** Cornea & Ext Eye Disease, Univ IA Hosps & Clins 1980; **Fac Appt:** Prof Oph, UC Davis

Marmor, Michael F MD [Oph] - **Spec Exp:** Retinal Disorders; Retinal Dystrophies; Electroretinograms (ERG); Retinal Drug Toxicity; **Hospital:** Stanford Univ Hosp & Clinics; **Address:** Byers Eye Institute at Stanford, 2452 Watson Court, Palo Alto, CA 94303-5353; **Phone:** 650-723-6995; **Board Cert:** Ophthalmology 1974; **Med School:** Harvard Med Sch 1966; **Resid:** Ophthalmology, Mass EE Infirm 1973; **Fellow:** Neurological Physiology, Natl Inst Hlth 1970; **Fac Appt:** Prof Oph, Stanford Univ

Masket, Samuel MD [Oph] - **Spec Exp:** Cataract Surgery; Cataract Surgery Revision; Congenital Eye Disorders-Rare; **Address:** 2080 Century Park E, Ste 911, Los Angeles, CA 90067; **Phone:** 310-229-1220; **Board Cert:** Ophthalmology 1974; **Med School:** NY Med Coll 1968; **Resid:** Ophthalmology, Metropolitan Hosp Ctr 1973; **Fellow:** Ophthalmology, Columbia Presby Med Ctr 1973; **Fac Appt:** Clin Prof Oph, UCLA

Mathers, William MD [Oph] - **Spec Exp:** Corneal & External Eye Disease; Refractive Surgery; Laser Surgery; **Hospital:** OR Hlth & Sci Univ; **Address:** Casey Eye Inst, 3375 SW Terwilliger Blvd Fl 4, Portland, OR 97239-4197; **Phone:** 503-494-7674; **Board Cert:** Anesthesiology 1980; Ophthalmology 1987; **Med School:** Stanford Univ 1973; **Resid:** Anesthesiology, Stanford Univ Hosp 1977; Ophthalmology, Univ Wash Med Ctr 1985; **Fellow:** Cornea, Georgetown Univ Med Ctr 1986; **Fac Appt:** Prof Oph, Oregon Hlth & Sci Univ

Miller, Kevin M MD [Oph] - **Spec Exp:** Cataract Surgery-Lens Implant; Refractive Surgery; Congenital Eye Disorders-Rare; **Hospital:** UCLA Ronald Reagan Med Ctr; **Address:** Jules Stein Eye Institute, 100 Stein Plaza, UCLA, Los Angeles, CA 90095-7000; **Phone:** 310-206-9951; **Board Cert:** Ophthalmology 2003; **Med School:** Johns Hopkins Univ 1985; **Resid:** Ophthalmology, Jules Stein Eye Inst 1991; **Fellow:** Ophthalmic Optics, Wilmer Inst/Johns Hopkins 1988; **Fac Appt:** Prof Oph, UCLA

Mondino, Bartly MD [Oph] - **Spec Exp:** Cornea & External Eye Disease; **Hospital:** UCLA Ronald Reagan Med Ctr; **Address:** UCLA Jules Stein Eye Institute, 200 Stein Plaza Fl 1, Los Angeles, CA 90095-7065; **Phone:** 310-825-5053; **Board Cert:** Ophthalmology 1976; **Med School:** Stanford Univ 1971; **Resid:** Ophthalmology, NY Hosp/Cornell Univ 1975; **Fellow:** Cornea & Ext Eye Disease, Univ Pittsburgh Eye & Ear Hosp 1976; **Fac Appt:** Prof Oph, UCLA

Murphree, A Linn MD [Oph] - **Spec Exp:** Retinoblastoma; Eye Tumors/Cancer; Ophthalmic Genetics; Pediatric Ophthalmology; **Hospital:** Chldns Hosp - Los Angeles, USC Norris Cancer Hosp (page 62); **Address:** Chldns Hosp, Dept Ophthalmology, 4650 Sunset Blvd, MS 88, Los Angeles, CA 90027-6016; **Phone:** 323-361-2347; **Board Cert:** Ophthalmology 1978; **Med School:** Baylor Coll Med 1972; **Resid:** Ophthalmology, Baylor Affil Hosp 1976; **Fellow:** Pediatric Ophthalmology, Wilmer Inst/Johns Hopkins 1977; **Fac Appt:** Prof Oph, USC Sch Med

Ng, John MD [Oph] - **Spec Exp:** Oculoplastic & Orbital Surgery; Reconstructive Surgery; Trauma; **Hospital:** OR Hlth & Sci Univ; **Address:** Casey Eye Inst, 3375 SW Terwilliger Blvd, Portland, OR 97239; **Phone:** 503-494-3004; **Board Cert:** Ophthalmology 2007; **Med School:** Geo Wash Univ 1988; **Resid:** Ophthalmology, Letterman/Madigan Army Med Ctr 1994; Ophthalmology; **Fellow:** Oculoplastic & Reconstructive Surgery, Midwest Eye Inst 1997; **Fac Appt:** Assoc Prof Oph, Oregon Hlth & Sci Univ

Paul, T Otis MD [Oph] - **Spec Exp:** Pediatric Ophthalmology; Strabismus-Adult & Pediatric; **Hospital:** Chldns Hosp - Oakland, CA Pacific Med Ctr-Pacific Campus; **Address:** 5275 Claremont Ave Fl 1, Oakland, CA 94618; **Phone:** 510-428-3050; **Board Cert:** Ophthalmology 1974; **Med School:** UCLA 1967; **Resid:** Ophthalmology, Naval Hosp 1972; **Fellow:** Pediatric Ophthalmology, Ca Pacific Med Ctr 1974

Puliafito, Carmen A MD [Oph] - **Spec Exp:** Retinal Disorders; Macular Degeneration; **Hospital:** Keck Med Ctr of USC (page 62); **Address:** USC-Doheny Eye Inst, 1450 San Pablo St, Ste 5703, Los Angeles, CA 90033; **Phone:** 323-442-6335; **Board Cert:** Ophthalmology 2012; **Med School:** Harvard Med Sch 1978; **Resid:** Ophthalmology, Mass Eye & Ear Infirm 1982; **Fellow:** Vitreoretinal Surgery, Mass Eye & Ear Infirm 1983; **Fac Appt:** Prof Oph, USC-Keck School of Medicine

Rao, Narsing A MD [Oph] - **Spec Exp:** Uveitis/AIDS; Eye Pathology; **Hospital:** Keck Med Ctr of USC (page 62); **Address:** USC Doheny Eye Center, 1450 San Pablo St, Los Angeles, CA 90033-4697; **Phone:** 323-442-6522; **Board Cert:** Pathology 1974; Ophthalmology 1977; **Med School:** India 1967; **Resid:** Pathology, Georgetown Univ Hosp 1972; Ophthalmology, Georgetown Univ Hosp 1975; **Fac Appt:** Prof Oph, USC Sch Med

Sadda, SriniVas R MD [Oph] - **Spec Exp:** Macular Degeneration; Diabetic Eye Disease/Retinopathy; Retinal Disorders-Inherited; Retinal Vascular Diseases; **Hospital:** Keck Med Ctr of USC (page 62); **Address:** USC Doheny Eye Ctr, 1450 San Pablo St Fl 4, Beverly Hills, CA 90033; **Phone:** 323-442-6522; **Board Cert:** Ophthalmology 2010; **Med School:** Johns Hopkins Univ 1994; **Resid:** Ophthalmology, Wilmer Eye Inst 1997; **Fellow:** Neuro-Ophthalmology, Wilmer Eye Inst 1998; Retina, Wilmer Eye Inst 1998; **Fac Appt:** Assoc Prof Oph, USC-Keck School of Medicine

Salz, James J MD [Oph] - **Spec Exp:** LASIK-Refractive Surgery; Cataract Surgery; **Hospital:** Cedars-Sinai Med Ctr; **Address:** 11620 Wilshire Blvd, Ste 711, Los Angeles, CA 90025; **Phone:** 310-444-1134; **Board Cert:** Ophthalmology 1971; **Med School:** Duke Univ 1965; **Resid:** Ophthalmology, LAC-USC Med Ctr 1969; **Fac Appt:** Clin Prof Oph, USC Sch Med

Savino, Peter J MD [Oph] - **Spec Exp:** Neuro-Ophthalmology; **Hospital:** UCSD Med Ctr; **Address:** Shiley Eye Ctr, 9415 Campus Point Drive, MC 0946, La Jolla, CA 92093-0946; **Phone:** 858-534-6290; **Board Cert:** Ophthalmology 1975; **Med School:** Italy 1968; **Resid:** Ophthalmology, Georgetown Med Ctr 1973; **Fellow:** Neuro-Ophthalmology, Bascom Palmer Eye Inst 1974; **Fac Appt:** Prof Oph, Thomas Jefferson Univ

Schwartz, Steven D MD [Oph] - **Spec Exp:** Diabetic Eye Disease/Retinopathy; Retinal Detachment; Retinal Disorders; Macular Degeneration; **Hospital:** UCLA Ronald Reagan Med Ctr; **Address:** Jules Stein Eye Inst, 200 Stein Plaza, Los Angeles, CA 90095; **Phone:** 310-206-7474; **Board Cert:** Ophthalmology 2005; **Med School:** USC Sch Med 1988; **Resid:** Ophthalmology, UCLA Med Ctr 1992; **Fellow:** Medical Retina, Moorfields Eye Hosp 1993; Vitreoretinal Surgery, Moorfields Eye Hosp 1994; **Fac Appt:** Prof Oph, UCLA-David Geffen Sch Med

Seibel, Barry S MD [Oph] - **Spec Exp:** Cataract Surgery; **Hospital:** Cedars-Sinai Med Ctr; **Address:** 11620 Wilshire Blvd, Ste 711, Los Angeles, CA 90025; **Phone:** 310-444-1134; **Board Cert:** Ophthalmology 1991; **Med School:** Univ Tex, Houston 1985; **Resid:** Ophthalmology, Hollywood Presby Med Ctr 1987; Ophthalmology, USC-Doheny Eye Clin 1989; **Fac Appt:** Asst Clin Prof Oph, UCLA

Seiff, Stuart R MD [Oph] - **Spec Exp:** Oculoplastic Surgery; Orbital Tumors/Cancer; **Hospital:** UCSF Med Ctr, CA Pacific Med Ctr-Pacific Campus; **Address:** 2100 Webster St, Ste 214, San Francisco, CA 94115; **Phone:** 415-923-3007; **Board Cert:** Ophthalmology 1986; **Med School:** UCSF 1980; **Resid:** Ophthalmology, UCSF Med Ctr 1984; **Fellow:** Ophthalmic Plastic & Reconstructive Surgery, UCLA Med Ctr 1985; Oculoplastic Surgery, Moorfield's Eye Hosp 1986; **Fac Appt:** Prof Oph, UCSF

Serafano, Donald N MD [Oph] - **Spec Exp:** LASIK-Refractive Surgery; Cataract Surgery; Lens Implants; **Hospital:** Los Alamitos Med Ctr, Long Beach Meml Med Ctr; **Address:** 10861 Cherry St, Ste 204, Box 250, Los Alamitos, CA 90720-5403; **Phone:** 562-598-3160; **Board Cert:** Ophthalmology 1978; **Med School:** Wayne State Univ 1971; **Resid:** Ophthalmology, Mayo Clinic 1978; **Fac Appt:** Assoc Clin Prof Oph, USC Sch Med

Shamie, Neda MD [Oph] - **Spec Exp:** Cornea Transplant; Cataract Surgery; Anterior Segment Surgery; Keratoconus; **Hospital:** Keck Med Ctr of USC (page 62); **Address:** USC Doheny Eye Ctr, 9033 Wilshire Blvd, Ste 360, Beverly Hills, CA 90210; **Phone:** 310-601-3366; **Board Cert:** Ophthalmology 2006; **Med School:** UCSF 1998; **Resid:** Ophthalmology, UC-Irvine Med Ctr 2002; **Fellow:** Cornea & Refractive Surgery, UC-Irvine Med Ctr 2993; **Fac Appt:** Assoc Clin Prof Oph, USC-Keck School of Medicine

Smith, Ronald Edward MD [Oph] - **Spec Exp:** Corneal Disease; Uveitis; **Hospital:** Keck Med Ctr of USC (page 62); **Address:** USC-Doheny Eye Center, 1450 San Pablo Rd, Ste 5703, Los Angeles, CA 90033; **Phone:** 323-442-6335; **Board Cert:** Ophthalmology 1974; **Med School:** Johns Hopkins Univ 1967; **Resid:** Ophthalmology, Wilmer Ophthal Inst 1973; **Fellow:** Research, UCSF 1972; **Fac Appt:** Prof Oph, USC Sch Med

Steinert, Roger F MD [Oph] - **Spec Exp:** Refractive Surgery; Cataract Surgery; Cornea Transplant; Corneal Disease; **Hospital:** UC Irvine Med Ctr; **Address:** 1 Medical Drive, Gottschalk Bldg - Fl 2, University of California, Irvine, Gavin Herbert Eye Institute, Irvine, CA 92697-4375; **Phone:** 949-824-2020; **Board Cert:** Ophthalmology 1982; **Med School:** Harvard Med Sch 1977; **Resid:** Ophthalmology, Mass EE Infirm 1981; **Fac Appt:** Prof Oph, UC Irvine

Stout, J Timothy MD/PhD [Oph] - **Spec Exp:** Retinal Disorders-Pediatric; Retinoblastoma; Retinopathy of Prematurity; **Hospital:** OR Hlth & Sci Univ, Providence St Vincent Med Ctr; **Address:** 3375 SW Terwilliger Blvd, Portland, OR 97239; **Phone:** 503-494-2435; **Board Cert:** Ophthalmology 2010; **Med School:** Baylor Coll Med 1989; **Resid:** Ophthalmology, Doheny Eye Inst 1993; **Fellow:** Ophthalmology, Moorfields Eye Hosp 1994; Retinal Surgery, Doheny Eye Inst 1995; **Fac Appt:** Assoc Prof Oph, Oregon Hlth & Sci Univ

Weinreb, Robert N MD [Oph] - **Spec Exp:** Glaucoma; **Hospital:** UCSD Med Ctr; **Address:** 9415 Campus Point Drive, La Jolla, CA 92093; **Phone:** 858-534-6290; **Board Cert:** Ophthalmology 1982; **Med School:** Harvard Med Sch 1975; **Resid:** Ophthalmology, UCSF Med Ctr 1981; **Fellow:** Glaucoma, UCSF Med Ctr 1982; **Fac Appt:** Prof Oph, UCSD

Weiss, Avery H MD [Oph] - **Spec Exp:** Pediatric Ophthalmology; Strabismus; Amblyopia; **Hospital:** Seattle Chldns Hosp; **Address:** 4800 Sand Point Way NE, MS W-4753, Seattle, WA 98105; **Phone:** 206-987-2177; **Board Cert:** Ophthalmology 1981; **Med School:** Univ Miami Sch Med 1974; **Resid:** Internal Medicine, Barnes-Jewish Hosp 1976; Ophthalmology, Barnes-Jewish Hosp 1980; **Fellow:** Research, Barnes-Jewish Hosp 1977; Pediatric Ophthalmology, Chldns Hosp Natl Med Ctr 1981; **Fac Appt:** Assoc Prof Oph, Univ Wash

Wilson, David Jean MD [Oph] - **Spec Exp:** Eye Tumors/Cancer; Ophthalmic Pathology; **Hospital:** OR Hlth & Sci Univ; **Address:** 3375 SW Terwilliger Blvd, Portland, OR 97239; **Phone:** 503-494-7881; **Board Cert:** Ophthalmology 2009; **Med School:** Baylor Coll Med 1981; **Resid:** Ophthalmology, Univ Oregon 1985; **Fellow:** Ophthalmic Pathology, John Hopkins Univ Hosp 1987; Retina/Vitreous, Mass Eye & Ear Infirmary 1988; **Fac Appt:** Prof Oph, Oregon Hlth & Sci Univ

Wright, Kenneth W MD [Oph] - **Spec Exp:** Cataract Surgery-Lens Implant; Strabismus-Adult & Pediatric; Pediatric Eye Surgery-Ptosis; Pediatric Ophthalmology; **Hospital:** Cedars-Sinai Med Ctr; **Address:** 520 S San Vincente Blvd, Los Angeles, CA 90048; **Phone:** 310-652-6420; **Board Cert:** Ophthalmology 1983; **Med School:** Boston Univ 1977; **Resid:** Ophthalmology, LAC-USC Med Ctr 1981; **Fellow:** Pediatric Ophthalmology, Johns Hopkins Hosp 1981; Pediatric Ophthalmology, Chldns Hosp Natl Med Ctr 1982; **Fac Appt:** Clin Prof Oph, USC Sch Med

Cleveland Clinic

Every life deserves world class care.

Orthopaedic Surgery

The Cleveland Clinic Department of Orthopaedic Surgery has a long history of excellence and innovation in treating musculoskeletal injuries and diseases. Since 1992, *U.S. News & World Report* has consistently ranked the Department of Orthopaedic Surgery among the top five orthopaedic programs in the nation.

Foot and Ankle: All specialists and surgeons have extensive training in the diagnosis and care of foot and ankle disorders.

Joint Replacement: The Center for Adult Reconstruction performs joint replacement, resurfacing and revision surgery of the hip and knee. Our experienced surgeons offer the most advanced implants and minimally invasive techniques to restore patient mobility.

Upper Extremity: This center provides a diagnosis and treatment for problems affecting the hand, wrist, elbow and shoulder.

Pediatrics: The Center for Pediatric Orthopaedics handles more than 14,000 outpatient visits each year. Our physicians offer expertise in the management of all musculoskeletal conditions in children, and sports injuries.

Center for Spine Health: The Center for Spine Health diagnoses and treats more than 13,000 patients annually. The center brings together the expertise of specialists in neurosurgery, orthopaedic surgery and non-surgical spine care.

Trauma: Cleveland Clinic is a leader in the treatment of fractures and non-union and in the development of methods to improve outcomes through advanced bone grafting techniques.

Center for Musculoskeletal Tumors: As one of the largest multidisciplinary centers of its kind, we offer expertise in treating bone and soft tissue sarcomas and performing limb salvage.

**THE MOUNT SINAI MEDICAL CENTER
OPHTHALMOLOGY**
One Gustave L. Levy Place
Fifth Avenue and 100th Street
New York, NY 10029-6574
Physician Referral: 1-800-MD-SINAI (637-4624)
www.mountsinai.org/opthalmology

Specializing in the prevention, diagnosis, and treatment of eye disorders, Mount Sinai's **DEPARTMENT OF OPHTHALMOLOGY** features faculty with wide experience in special eye problems, offers comprehensive eye care services, and houses a state-of-the-art optical shop.

Services include:

- Comprehensive ophthalmology, refractive errors, and cataract surgery
- Corneal and external diseases of the eye
- Refractive surgery
- Retinal disorders (diabetic retinopathy, macular degeneration, inherited retinal diseases, retinal detachment)
- Glaucoma
- Pediatric eye care and strabismus
- Uveitis (inflammation of the eye)
- Neuro-ophthalmic disorders
- Oculplastic surgery, including cosmetic surgery, orbital tumors, and thyroid-related eye problems

Specialized treatments and procedures include:

- LASIK and other refractive surgical procedures
- Cataract surgery, including premium intraocular lenses
- Specialists in dry eye management
- Cosmetic lid treatments, including Botox and Restalayne injections
- Laser surgery
- Management of macular degeneration, including Lucentis and Avastin injections
- Advanced management for severe uveitis, including immunosuppressive drug therapy

INTERNATIONAL LEADERS IN THE FIELD OF UVEITIS
Uveitis, a collection of 30 diseases characterized by inflammation inside the eye, is the 5th leading cause of blindness in the United States. Management of severe uveitis often requires the skilled use of systemically-administered, immunosuppressive drugs, resulting in superior outcomes. Mount Sinai ophthalmologists have been pioneers in these treatments and are internationally recognized for their leadership in the field. A team of four uveitis specialists, augmented by the only uveitis training program in New York, offer a comprehensive treatment approach to these diseases.

We offer the full range of sophisticated diagnostic tests for evaluating patient conditions, including spectral domain optical coherence tomography, fluorescein angiography, indocyanine green angiography, autofluorescence, diagnostic ultrasound, electroretinography, visually evoked potential measurements, electro-oculography, corneal topography, confocal microscopy, state-of-the-art perimetry, HRT II imaging, allowing for faster, more accurate diagnosis and help determining the best treatment plan for each patient.

We perform cataract surgery, corneal transplants, refractive, glaucoma, strabismus, laser, ophthalmic plastic and reconstructive surgery, and vitreoretinal surgery for complicated retinal problems. We also offer minimally invasive procedures to treat eye disease, including non-laser refractive surgeries, and small-incision cataract surgery.

LEADERS IN CLINICAL RESEARCH
Mount Sinai ophthalmologists helped pioneer and evaluate new treatments for eye diseases and problems, including glaucoma, uveitis, ocular infections and farsightedness.

NY Eye & Ear Infirmary

Continuum Health Partners, Inc.

THE NEW YORK EYE AND EAR INFIRMARY

310 East 14th Street
New York, New York 10003
Tel. 212.979.4000 Fax. 212.228.0664
http://www.nyee.edu

PROVIDING EXCEPTIONAL EYE CARE

The Department of Ophthalmology is the region's most comprehensive center for the delivery of primary through tertiary eye care. It is also by far the largest provider of eye care in the metropolitan area—with some 155,000 outpatient visits and 22,000 surgical cases performed each year. 365 board-certified ophthalmologists located throughout New York City and its tri-state area comprise the attending Medical Staff.

IN A HIGHLY SPECIALIZED SETTING

As a specialty hospital, The New York Eye and Ear Infirmary is uniquely qualified to handle the most complicated cases. It serves as a nationwide referral center with a commitment to teaching, research, and high-technology based patient care. Cutting edge ocular imaging instrumentation provides highest resolution to diagnose diseases of the cornea, retina and optic nerve and glaucoma. Highly experienced staff in state-of-the-art facilities have made The New York Eye and Ear Infirmary's 17 operating rooms a national benchmark in efficiency in eye surgery cases.

FOR PATIENTS OF ALL AGES

The New York Eye and Ear Infirmary's Ophthalmology staff are sensitive to the specific needs of patients of all ages. Senior citizens are the vast majority of the NYEE's 12,000 cataract patients each year, as well as individuals receiving treatment for age-related macular degeneration. Young children are now 25 percent of the patient population, with conditions such as strabismus, acquired and congenital cataracts, corneal diseases and ocular trauma. For those rare cases of children who have a disease ordinarily associated with age, the Infirmary runs New York's only Pediatric Glaucoma Service. Active adults of all ages utilize the New York Metropolitan Eye Trauma Center and Oculoplastic and Orbital Surgery Services.

Ophthalmology Clinical Services

Ambulatory Care Services
Comprehensive Eye Care
Cornea & Refractive Surgery
Eye Trauma
Glaucoma
Low Vision
Neuro-Ophthalmology
Ocular Pathology
Ocular Tumor
Oculoplastic &
Orbital Surgery
Pediatric Ophthalmology
& Strabismus
Retinal-Vitreal
Uveitis/Ocular Immunology

Facilities

Ambulatory Surgery Center
Bendheim Family Retina Center
Einhorn Clinical Trials Area
*(supporting more than 100
ophthalmology studies a year)*
Jorge N. Buxton Microsurgical
Education Center
*(for residents, fellows and
attending physicians)*

About The New York Eye and Ear Infirmary

Founded in 1820, it is the nation's first and foremost, continuously operating specialty hospital. More than 10 million people have sought treatment here since its inception.

**Physician Referral
1.800.449.HOPE (4673)**

Orthopaedic Surgery

An orthopaedic surgeon is trained in the preservation, investigation and restoration of the form and function of the extremities, spine and associated structures by medical, surgical and physical means.

An orthopaedic surgeon is involved with the care of patients whose musculoskeletal problems include congenital deformities, trauma, infections, tumors, metabolic disturbances of the musculoskeletal system, deformities, injuries and degenerative diseases of the spine, hands, feet, knee, hip, shoulder and elbow in children and adults. An orthopaedic surgeon is also concerned with primary and secondary muscular problems and the effects of central or peripheral nervous system lesions of the musculoskeletal system.

Note: *There are many Orthopaedic Surgeons who are trained in Sports Medicine and prefer to be listed under that heading; some trained in Sports Medicine prefer to be listed under Orthopaedics.*

Training Required: Five years (including general surgery training) *plus* two years in clinical practice before final certification is achieved.

ORTHOPAEDIC SURGERY

New England

Abdu, William A MD [OrS] - **Spec Exp:** Spinal Surgery; Spinal Disorders; Spinal Cord Injury; **Hospital:** Dartmouth - Hitchcock Med Ctr; **Address:** Darthmouth-Hitchcock Med Ctr, Spine Ctr, 1 Med Ctr Drive, Lebanon, NH 03756; **Phone:** 603-650-2225; **Board Cert:** Orthopaedic Surgery 2004; **Med School:** Tufts Univ 1985; **Resid:** Surgery, Darthmouth-Hitchcock Med Ctr 1990; Orthopaedic Surgery, Newington Chldns Hosp 1989; **Fellow:** Spinal Surgery, Case Western Reserve Univ Hosp 1991; **Fac Appt:** Assoc Prof OrS, Dalhousie Univ

Bono, James Vincent MD [OrS] - **Spec Exp:** Hip Surgery; Knee Surgery; **Hospital:** New England Bapt Hosp; **Address:** 125 Parker Hill Ave, Ste 573, Boston, MA 02120; **Phone:** 617-731-6337; **Board Cert:** Orthopaedic Surgery 2008; **Med School:** Albany Med Coll 1987; **Resid:** Orthopaedic Surgery, Albany Med Ctr 1993; **Fellow:** Hip & Knee Surgery, Hosp for Special Surgery 1994; **Fac Appt:** Clin Prof OrS, Tufts Univ

Brick, Gregory W MD [OrS] - **Spec Exp:** Hip Replacement; Knee Replacement; Spinal Surgery; **Hospital:** Brigham and Women's Hosp (page 57); **Address:** Brigham & Womens, Dept Orth Surg, 75 Francis St, Boston, MA 02115; **Phone:** 617-732-5386; **Med School:** New Zealand 1976; **Resid:** Surgery, Greenlane Hosp 1981; Orthopaedic Surgery, Middlemore Hosp 1984; **Fellow:** Joint Replacement Surgery, Brigham & Women's Hosp 1986; Spinal Surgery, Vanderbilt Univ Med Ctr 1987; **Fac Appt:** Assoc Clin Prof OrS, Harvard Med Sch

Browner, Bruce D MD [OrS] - **Spec Exp:** Fractures-Complex; Osteomyelitis; Bone Infections; Fractures-Non Union; **Hospital:** Univ of Conn Hlth Ctr, John Dempsey Hosp, Hartford Hosp; **Address:** Med Arts & Rsch Bldg, 263 Farmington Ave Fl 3 - Ste 2, Farmington, CT 06030-4038; **Phone:** 860-679-6650; **Board Cert:** Orthopaedic Surgery 1979; **Med School:** SUNY Downstate 1973; **Resid:** Orthopaedic Surgery, Albany Med Ctr 1978; **Fellow:** Trauma, Albany Med Ctr 1975; **Fac Appt:** Prof OrS, Univ Conn

Burke, Dennis MD [OrS] - **Spec Exp:** Knee Replacement; Hip Replacement; Reconstructive Surgery; **Hospital:** Mass Genl Hosp; **Address:** Mass General Hosp, Yawkey 3B, 55 Fruit St, Boston, MA 02114; **Phone:** 617-726-3411; **Board Cert:** Orthopaedic Surgery 2009; **Med School:** Loyola Univ-Stritch Sch Med 1978; **Resid:** Surgery, Beth Israel Deaconess Med Ctr 1980; Orthopaedic Surgery, Mass Genl Hosp 1984

DiGiovanni, Christopher W MD [OrS] - **Spec Exp:** Foot & Ankle Surgery; Sports Injuries-Foot & Ankle; **Hospital:** Rhode Island Hosp; **Address:** University Orthopedics Inc, 100 Butler Dr, Providence, RI 02906-4862; **Phone:** 401-330-1430; **Board Cert:** Orthopaedic Surgery 2001; **Med School:** Dartmouth Med Sch 1991; **Resid:** Orthopaedic Surgery, Rhode Island Hosp 1997; **Fellow:** Joint Replacement Surgery, Hosp Spec Surgery 1998; Foot & Ankle Surgery, Harborview Med Ctr 1999; **Fac Appt:** Prof OrS, Brown Univ

Einhorn, Thomas A MD [OrS] - **Spec Exp:** Hip & Knee Replacement; Bone Disorders-Metabolic; Hip & Knee Reconstruction; Osteonecrosis; **Hospital:** Boston Med Ctr; **Address:** Orthopaedic Surgical Associates, 720 Harrison Ave, Ste 808, Boston, MA 02118; **Phone:** 617-638-8435; **Board Cert:** Orthopaedic Surgery 1998; **Med School:** Cornell Univ-Weill Med Coll 1976; **Resid:** Orthopaedic Surgery, St Lukes-Roosevelt Hosp 1981; Pediatric Orthopaedic Surgery, Alfred DuPont Inst 1981; **Fellow:** Orthopaedic Surgery, Hosp Special Surgery 1982; **Fac Appt:** Prof OrS, Boston Univ

Endrizzi, Donald P MD [OrS] - **Spec Exp:** Shoulder Surgery; Rotator Cuff Surgery; Elbow Surgery; Joint Replacement; **Hospital:** Maine Med Ctr; **Address:** Maine Med Partners Orthopedics, Div Joint Replacement, 5 Bucknam Rd, Ste 1D, Falmouth, ME 04105; **Phone:** 207-781-1551; **Board Cert:** Orthopaedic Surgery 2011; **Med School:** Columbia P&S 1982; **Resid:** Surgery, Columbia-Presby Med Ctr 1984; Orthopaedic Surgery, Columbia Presby Med Ctr 1987; **Fac Appt:** Assoc Clin Prof S, Univ VT Coll Med

Friedlaender, Gary E MD [OrS] - **Spec Exp:** Bone & Soft Tissue Tumors; Limb Surgery/Reconstruction; Fractures-Complex & Non Union; Tissue Banking; **Hospital:** Yale-New Haven Hosp, Yale Med Group; **Address:** 800 Howard Ave, Yale Physicians Building YPB 133 Fl 1, New Haven, CT 06519; **Phone:** 203-737-5660; **Board Cert:** Orthopaedic Surgery 1975; **Med School:** Univ Mich Med Sch 1969; **Resid:** Surgery, Michigan Med Ctr 1971; Orthopaedic Surgery, Yale-New Haven Hosp 1974; **Fellow:** Musculoskeletal Oncology, Mass Genl Hosp 1983; **Fac Appt:** Prof OrS, Yale Univ

Fulkerson, John P MD [OrS] - **Spec Exp:** Knee-Patella Problems; Arthroscopic Surgery-Knee; Sports Medicine; Shoulder Arthroscopic Surgery; **Hospital:** Hartford Hosp, Univ of Conn Hlth Ctr, John Dempsey Hosp; **Address:** 499 Farmington Ave, Fl 3, Farmington, CT 06032; **Phone:** 860-549-8269; **Board Cert:** Orthopaedic Surgery 1980; **Med School:** Yale Univ 1972; **Resid:** Orthopaedic Surgery, Yale-New Haven Hosp 1978; **Fellow:** Knee Surgery, Berg-Sloat Traveling 1979; **Fac Appt:** Clin Prof OrS, Univ Conn

Gebhardt, Mark MD [OrS] - **Spec Exp:** Musculoskeletal Tumors; Bone Tumors; **Hospital:** Beth Israel Deaconess Med Ctr - Boston, Children's Hospital - Boston; **Address:** BIDMC-Dept of Orthopedics, 330 Brookline Ave Shapiro Bldg Fl 2, Boston, MA 02215; **Phone:** 617-667-7675; **Board Cert:** Orthopaedic Surgery 2007; **Med School:** Univ Cincinnati 1975; **Resid:** Surgery, Univ Pittsburg Med Ctr 1977; Orthopaedic Surgery, Harvard Affil Hosps 1982; **Fellow:** Pediatric Orthopaedic Surgery, Boston Chldns Hosp 1983; Orthopaedic Oncology, Mass Genl Hosp 1983; **Fac Appt:** Prof OrS, Harvard Med Sch

Green, Andrew MD [OrS] - **Spec Exp:** Shoulder Surgery; Elbow Surgery; Rotator Cuff Surgery; Arthroscopic Surgery; **Hospital:** Rhode Island Hosp, Miriam Hosp; **Address:** Univ Orthopedics Inc, 2 Dudley St, Ste 200, Providence, RI 02905-3248; **Phone:** 401-457-1533; **Board Cert:** Orthopaedic Surgery 2006; **Med School:** Columbia P&S 1987; **Resid:** Orthopaedic Surgery, Rhode Island Hosp 1992; **Fellow:** Pacific Med Ctr 1993; **Fac Appt:** Assoc Prof OrS, Brown Univ

Hornicek, Francis J MD/PhD [OrS] - **Spec Exp:** Bone Tumors; Sarcoma; Bone Tumors-Metastatic; Soft Tissue Tumors; **Hospital:** Mass Genl Hosp; **Address:** MGH Orthpaedic Oncology, 55 Fruit St, Yawkey 3B, Boston, MA 02114; **Phone:** 617-724-3700; **Board Cert:** Orthopaedic Surgery 2010; **Med School:** Univ Pittsburgh 1991; **Resid:** Orthopaedic Surgery, Jackson Meml Hosp 1996; **Fellow:** Orthopaedic Oncology, Mass Genl Hosp/Chldns Hosp 1997; **Fac Appt:** Assoc Prof OrS, Harvard Med Sch

Jokl, Peter MD [OrS] - **Spec Exp:** Knee Surgery; Sports Medicine; Shoulder Surgery; **Hospital:** Yale-New Haven Hosp, Yale Med Group; **Address:** Yale Sports Med, Dept Orthopaedics, 800 Howard Ave, New Haven, CT 06519-1369; **Phone:** 203-785-2579; **Board Cert:** Orthopaedic Surgery 1974; **Med School:** Yale Univ 1968; **Resid:** Orthopaedic Surgery, Yale-New Haven Hosp 1972; **Fac Appt:** Prof OrS, Yale Univ

Kasser, James MD [OrS] - **Spec Exp:** Pediatric Orthopaedic Surgery; **Hospital:** Children's Hospital - Boston; **Address:** Chldns Hosp, Dept Ortho Surgery, 300 Longwood Ave, Honeywell 221, Boston, MA 02115; **Phone:** 617-355-6617; **Board Cert:** Orthopaedic Surgery 2005; **Med School:** Tufts Univ 1976; **Resid:** Orthopaedic Surgery, Tufts Med Ctr 1981; **Fellow:** Pediatric Orthopaedic Surgery, Dupont Inst 1984; **Fac Appt:** Prof OrS, Harvard Med Sch

Orthopaedic Surgery

Kocher, Mininder S MD [OrS] - **Spec Exp:** Pediatric Orthopaedic Surgery; Pediatric Sports Medicine; Arthroscopic Surgery; Arthroscopic Surgery-Hip; **Hospital:** Children's Hospital - Boston, Beth Israel Deaconess Med Ctr - Boston; **Address:** Children's Hosp, Dept Orthopaedic Surg, 319 Longwood Ave Fl 6, Boston, MA 02115; **Phone:** 617-355-3501; **Board Cert:** Orthopaedic Surgery 2013; Orthopaedic Sports Medicine 2013; **Med School:** Duke Univ 1993; **Resid:** Orthopaedic Surgery, Beth Israel Deaconess Med Ctr 1999; **Fellow:** Pediatric Orthopaedic Surgery, Chldns Hosp 1999; Sports Medicine, Steadman Hawkins Clin 2000; **Fac Appt:** Asst Prof OrS, Harvard Med Sch

Laurencin, Cato T MD/PhD [OrS] - **Spec Exp:** Shoulder & Knee Surgery; Sports Medicine; **Hospital:** Univ of Conn Hlth Ctr, John Dempsey Hosp; **Address:** Univ Conn Health Ctr, 263 Farmington Ave, MC 4038, Farmington, CT 06030-3800; **Phone:** 860-679-1495; **Board Cert:** Orthopaedic Surgery 2007; **Med School:** Harvard Med Sch 1987; **Resid:** Orthopaedic Surgery, Harvard Combined Program 1993; **Fellow:** Sports Medicine & Shoulder Surgery, Hosp for Special Surg 1994; **Fac Appt:** Prof OrS, Univ Conn

Marsh, James S MD [OrS] - **Spec Exp:** Pediatric Orthopaedic Surgery; **Hospital:** Yale-New Haven Hosp, Hosp of St Raphael; **Address:** 34 York St, Ste 2, Guilford, CT 06437; **Phone:** 203-453-1088; **Med School:** Harvard Med Sch 1981; **Resid:** Orthopaedic Surgery, Stanford Univ 1986; **Fellow:** Pediatric Orthopaedic Surgery, Mass Genl Hosp 1987; **Fac Appt:** Assoc Prof OrS, Yale Univ

Minas, Tom MD [OrS] - **Spec Exp:** Arthroscopic Surgery; Cartilage Damage & Transplant; Joint Replacement; Pelvic & Acetabular Fractures; **Hospital:** Brigham and Women's Hosp (page 57); **Address:** Brigham & Wmns Hosp, Dept of Orthopedic Surg, 850 Boylston St, Ste 112, Chestnut Hill, MA 02467; **Phone:** 617-732-9967; **Board Cert:** Orthopaedic Surgery 2008; **Med School:** Univ Toronto 1982; **Resid:** Orthopaedic Surgery, University of Toronto 1988; **Fellow:** Orthopaedic Surgery, Sunnybrook Univ 1989; Joint Reconstruction, Brigham & Womens Hosp 1990; **Fac Appt:** Assoc Prof OrS, Harvard Med Sch

Ready, John E MD [OrS] - **Spec Exp:** Bone Cancer; Sarcoma-Soft Tissue; Hip & Knee Replacement in Bone Tumors; Hip & Knee Replacement; **Hospital:** Brigham and Women's Hosp (page 57), Dana-Farber Cancer Inst (page 57); **Address:** Brigham & Women's Hospital, Dept of Orthopedic Surgery, 75 Francis St, Boston, MA 02115; **Phone:** 617-732-5368; **Med School:** Dalhousie Univ 1982; **Resid:** Orthopaedic Surgery, Dalhousie Univ Hosp 1987; **Fellow:** Orthopaedic Oncology, St Michael's Hosp 1988; Orthopaedic Oncology, Mass Genl Hosp/Childns Hosp 1989

Reilly, Donald T MD [OrS] - **Spec Exp:** Knee Replacement; Hip Replacement; **Hospital:** New England Bapt Hosp; **Address:** Pro Sports Orthopaedics, 235 Cypres St, Ste 300, Brookline, MA 02445; **Phone:** 617-738-8642; **Board Cert:** Orthopaedic Surgery 1984; **Med School:** Case West Res Univ 1975; **Resid:** Orthopaedic Surgery, Harvard Combined Ortho 1981

Richmond, John C MD [OrS] - **Spec Exp:** Shoulder Injuries; Rotator Cuff Surgery; Knee Surgery; Arthroscopic Surgery; **Hospital:** New England Bapt Hosp; **Address:** Boston Sports & Shoulder Ctr, 830 Boylston St, Ste 107, Chestnut Hill, MA 02467; **Phone:** 617-264-1100; **Board Cert:** Orthopaedic Surgery 1984; Orthopaedic Sports Medicine 2011; **Med School:** Tufts Univ 1976; **Resid:** Surgery, Hosp UPenn 1978; Orthopaedic Surgery, New England Med Ctr 1981; **Fac Appt:** Prof OrS, Tufts Univ

Scott, Richard D MD [OrS] - **Spec Exp:** Knee Replacement; **Hospital:** Brigham and Women's Hosp (page 57), New England Bapt Hosp; **Address:** 125 Parker Hill Ave, Boston, MA 02120; **Phone:** 617-738-9151; **Board Cert:** Orthopaedic Surgery 1975; **Med School:** Temple Univ 1968; **Resid:** Orthopaedic Surgery, Mass Genl Hosp 1974; **Fellow:** Orthopaedic Surgery, Mass Genl Hosp 1974; Arthritis Surgery, Brigham & Women's Hosp 1975; **Fac Appt:** Prof OrS, Harvard Med Sch

Smith, Eric L MD [OrS] - **Spec Exp:** Hip & Knee Reconstruction; Hip & Knee Replacement; Trauma; **Hospital:** Tufts Med Ctr, New England Bapt Hosp; **Address:** Tufts Medical Center, 800 Washington St, Box 306, Boston, MA 02111; **Phone:** 617-636-5160; **Board Cert:** Orthopaedic Surgery 2004; **Med School:** Tulane Univ 1996; **Resid:** Orthopaedic Surgery, Tripler Army Med Ctr 2002; **Fellow:** Adult Reconstructive Surgery, New England Baptist Hosp 2007; **Fac Appt:** Asst Prof OrS, Tufts Univ

Thornhill, Thomas S MD [OrS] - **Spec Exp:** Hip & Knee Replacement; Arthritis; Shoulder & Elbow Surgery; Joint Replacement; **Hospital:** Brigham and Women's Hosp (page 57); **Address:** Brigham & Women's Hosp, Dept Orth Surg, 75 Francis St, Boston, MA 02115; **Phone:** 617-732-5383; **Board Cert:** Internal Medicine 1973; Orthopaedic Surgery 1979; **Med School:** Cornell Univ-Weill Med Coll 1970; **Resid:** Internal Medicine, Peter Brent Brigham Hosp 1972; Orthopaedic Surgery, Harvard Combined Prgm 1978; **Fellow:** Joint Replacement Surgery, Robert Breck Brigham Hosp; **Fac Appt:** Prof OrS, Harvard Med Sch

Tornetta III, Paul MD [OrS] - **Spec Exp:** Trauma; Fractures-Complex; Minimally Invasive Surgery; Fractures in the Elderly; **Hospital:** Boston Med Ctr; **Address:** Boston Medical Center, 725 Albany St, Shapiro Bldg Fl 4 - Ste 4B, Boston, MA 02118; **Phone:** 617-414-4865; **Board Cert:** Orthopaedic Surgery 2006; **Med School:** SUNY Downstate 1987; **Resid:** Orthopaedic Surgery, Downstate Med Ctr 1992; **Fellow:** Trauma, Good Samaritan Hosp 1993; **Fac Appt:** Prof OrS, Boston Univ

Weinstein, James DO [OrS] - **Spec Exp:** Pain-Back; Spinal Tumors; **Hospital:** Dartmouth - Hitchcock Med Ctr; **Address:** DHMC, Dept Orthopaedic Surgery, One Medical Ctr Drive, Lebanon, NH 03756; **Phone:** 603-650-2225; **Board Cert:** Orthopaedic Surgery 2002; **Med School:** Chicago Coll Osteo Med 1973; **Resid:** Orthopaedic Surgery, Rush Presby-St Lukes Med Ctr 1983; **Fac Appt:** Prof OrS, Dartmouth Med Sch

Zarins, Bertram MD [OrS] - **Spec Exp:** Knee Injuries/ACL; Rotator Cuff Surgery; Cartilage Damage; Shoulder Injuries; **Hospital:** Mass Genl Hosp; **Address:** MGH Sports Medicine, 175 Cambridge St, Ste 400, Boston, MA 02114; **Phone:** 617-726-3421; **Board Cert:** Orthopaedic Surgery 1994; **Med School:** SUNY Upstate Med Univ 1967; **Resid:** Surgery, Johns Hopkins Hosp 1969; Orthopaedic Surgery, Harvard Ortho Prog 1973; **Fellow:** Sports Medicine, Mass Genl Hosp 1976; **Fac Appt:** Clin Prof OrS, Harvard Med Sch

Mid Atlantic

Aboulafia, Albert J MD [OrS] - **Spec Exp:** Soft Tissue Tumors; Limb Sparing Surgery; Bone Tumors; **Hospital:** Sinai Hosp - Baltimore, Univ of MD Med Ctr; **Address:** Lapidus Cancer Inst, 2401 W Belvedere Ave, Baltimore, MD 21215; **Phone:** 410-601-9266; **Board Cert:** Orthopaedic Surgery 2004; **Med School:** Univ Mich Med Sch 1985; **Resid:** Orthopaedic Surgery, LAC/USC Sch Med 1990; **Fellow:** Orthopaedic Oncology, Chldn's Natl Med Ctr/NIH 1991; **Fac Appt:** Asst Clin Prof OrS, Univ MD Sch Med

Albert, Todd J MD [OrS] - **Spec Exp:** Spinal Surgery; Spinal Surgery-Cervical; Spinal Deformity; **Hospital:** Thomas Jefferson Univ Hosp; **Address:** Rothman Institute, 925 Chesnut St, Fl 5, Philadelphia, PA 19107; **Phone:** 800-321-9999; **Board Cert:** Orthopaedic Surgery 2006; **Med School:** Univ VA Sch Med 1987; **Resid:** Orthopaedic Surgery, Thomas Jefferson Univ Hosp 1992; **Fellow:** Spinal Surgery, Minnesota Spine Ctr 1993; **Fac Appt:** Prof OrS, Thomas Jefferson Univ

Orthopaedic Surgery

Balderston, Richard MD [OrS] - **Spec Exp:** Scoliosis; Spinal Surgery; Spinal Disc Replacement; **Hospital:** Pennsylvania Hosp-UPHS (page 72); **Address:** Pennsylvania Hosp, 800 Spruce St, Philadelphia, PA 19107; **Phone:** 215-829-2222; **Board Cert:** Orthopaedic Surgery 1985; **Med School:** Univ Pennsylvania 1977; **Resid:** Orthopaedic Surgery, Hosp Univ Penn 1982; **Fellow:** Spinal Surgery, Univ Minn Affil Hosp 1983; **Fac Appt:** Clin Prof OrS, Univ Pennsylvania

Bartolozzi, Arthur R MD [OrS] - **Spec Exp:** Sports Medicine; Arthroscopic Surgery-Knee; Knee Ligament Reconstruction; Shoulder Surgery; **Hospital:** Pennsylvania Hosp-UPHS (page 72); **Address:** Pennsylvania Hosp, 800 Spruce St, Philadelphia, PA 19107; **Phone:** 215-829-2222; **Board Cert:** Orthopaedic Surgery 2010; **Med School:** UCSD 1981; **Resid:** Orthopaedic Surgery, Hosp Univ Penn 1986; **Fellow:** Sports Medicine, UCLA Med Ctr 1987; **Fac Appt:** Assoc Clin Prof OrS, Univ Pennsylvania

Bauman, Phillip A MD [OrS] - **Spec Exp:** Foot & Ankle Surgery; Knee Surgery; Dance/Sports Medicine; Arthroscopic Surgery; **Hospital:** St. Luke's - Roosevelt Hosp Ctr - Roosevelt Div (page 56), NY-Presby/Columbia Univ Med Ctr, NY (page 66); **Address:** Orthopaedic Associates of NY, 343 W 58th St, Ste 1, New York, NY 10019; **Phone:** 212-506-0228; **Board Cert:** Orthopaedic Surgery 2011; **Med School:** Columbia P&S 1981; **Resid:** Surgery, St Lukes-Roosevelt Hosp Ctr 1983; Orthopaedic Surgery, Columbia-Presby Med Ctr 1987; **Fac Appt:** Asst Prof OrS, Columbia P&S

Benevenia, Joseph MD [OrS] - **Spec Exp:** Limb Sparing Surgery; Bone Cancer; Sarcoma-Soft Tissue; **Hospital:** Univ Hosp-UMDNJ—Newark; **Address:** 140 Bergen St, Ste ACC1610, Newark, NJ 07103; **Phone:** 973-972-2153; **Board Cert:** Orthopaedic Surgery 2012; **Med School:** UMDNJ-NJ Med Sch, Newark 1984; **Resid:** Orthopaedic Surgery, UMDNJ-NJ Med Sch Hosp 1988; **Fellow:** Orthopaedic Oncology, Case Western Reserve Univ 1991; **Fac Appt:** Prof OrS, UMDNJ-NJ Med Sch, Newark

Betz, Randal R MD [OrS] - **Spec Exp:** Spinal Cord Injury-Pediatric; Praxis Functional Electrical Stim (FES); Scoliosis; Spinal Deformity-Pediatric; **Hospital:** Philadelphia Shriners Hosp; **Address:** Shriners Hospital for Children, 3551 N Broad St, Philadelphia, PA 19140; **Phone:** 215-430-4233; **Board Cert:** Orthopaedic Surgery 1985; Spinal Cord Injury Medicine 2008; **Med School:** Temple Univ 1977; **Resid:** Orthopaedic Surgery, Shriners Hospital 1980; Orthopaedic Surgery, Temple Univ Hospital 1982; **Fellow:** Pediatric Orthopaedic Surgery, DuPont Inst 1983; **Fac Appt:** Prof OrS, Temple Univ

Bigliani, Louis U MD [OrS] - **Spec Exp:** Shoulder Surgery; Sports Medicine; Arthroscopic Surgery; Rotator Cuff Surgery; **Hospital:** NY-Presby/Columbia Univ Med Ctr, NY (page 66); **Address:** 622 W 168th St, rm 1130, New York, NY 10032-3720; **Phone:** 212-305-0998; **Board Cert:** Orthopaedic Surgery 1994; **Med School:** Loyola Univ-Stritch Sch Med 1973; **Resid:** Surgery, Roosevelt Hosp 1974; Orthopaedic Surgery, Columbia Presby Med Ctr 1977; **Fac Appt:** Prof OrS, Columbia P&S

Bitan, Fabien D MD [OrS] - **Spec Exp:** Spinal Surgery-Pediatric & Adult; Spinal Disc Replacement; Spinal Deformity; Spinal Disorders-Degenerative; **Hospital:** Lenox Hill Hosp (page 67), Beth Israel Med Ctr - Petrie Division (page 56); **Address:** 130 E 77th St, Fl 7, New York, NY 10075; **Phone:** 212-744-8114; **Med School:** France 1981; **Resid:** Orthopaedic Surgery, Hospital Beaujon 1987; Pediatric Orthopaedic Surgery, Hosp des Enfants Malades 1990; **Fellow:** Pediatric Orthopaedic Surgery, Hosp Special Surgery 1997; Spinal Surgery, Beth Israel Med Ctr 1998

Boachie-Adjei, Oheneba MD [OrS] - **Spec Exp:** Spinal Surgery; Scoliosis; **Hospital:** Hosp For Special Surgery (page 60); **Address:** Hosp for Special Surgery, 535 E 70th St, New York, NY 10021; **Phone:** 212-606-1948; **Board Cert:** Orthopaedic Surgery 2010; **Med School:** Columbia P&S 1980; **Resid:** Surgery, St Vincents Hosp 1982; Orthopaedic Surgery, Hosp Spec Surg 1986; **Fellow:** Orthopaedic Pathology, Hosp Spec Surg 1983; Spinal Surgery, Twin Cities Scoliosis r/Minn Spine Ctr 1987; **Fac Appt:** Assoc Clin Prof S, Cornell Univ-Weill Med Coll

Booth Jr, Robert E MD [OrS] - **Spec Exp:** Knee Replacement & Revision; **Hospital:** Pennsylvania Hosp-UPHS (page 72); **Address:** Pennsylvania Hosp, 800 Spruce St, Philadelphia, PA 19107; **Phone:** 215-829-2222; **Board Cert:** Orthopaedic Surgery 1978; **Med School:** Univ Pennsylvania 1971; **Resid:** Surgery, Penn Hosp 1973; Orthopaedic Surgery, Hosp Univ Penn 1977; **Fac Appt:** Clin Prof OrS, Univ Pennsylvania

Bronson, Michael J MD [OrS] - **Spec Exp:** Joint Replacement; Knee Replacement; Hip Replacement; Arthritis; **Hospital:** Mount Sinai Med Ctr (page 64); **Address:** Mt Sinai Med Ctr, Dept Orthopedic Surgery, 5 E 98th St, Box 1188, New York, NY 10029; **Phone:** 212-241-1640; **Board Cert:** Orthopaedic Surgery 1984; **Med School:** NY Med Coll 1976; **Resid:** Orthopaedic Surgery, Lenox Hill Hosp 1980; **Fellow:** Hip & Knee Surgery, Columbia-Presby Med Ctr 1981; **Fac Appt:** Assoc Prof OrS, Mount Sinai Sch Med

Bukata, Susan MD [OrS] - **Spec Exp:** Bone & Soft Tissue Tumors; Bone Cancer; Musculoskeletal Tumors; Paget's Disease of Bone; **Hospital:** Univ of Rochester Strong Meml Hosp; **Address:** Univ Rochester, Orthopaedic Surgery, 4901 Lac De Ville Blvd D Bldg, Rochester, NY 14642; **Phone:** 585-275-1725; **Board Cert:** Orthopaedic Surgery 2006; **Med School:** Columbia P&S 1995; **Resid:** Orthopaedic Surgery, Strong Meml Hosp/Univ Rochester 2002; **Fellow:** Orthopaedic Oncology, Meml Sloan Kettering Cancer Ctr 2004; Metabolic Bone Research, Hosp for Special Surgery 2004; **Fac Appt:** Assoc Prof OrS, Univ Rochester

Buly, Robert L MD [OrS] - **Spec Exp:** Hip Replacement & Revision; Arthroscopic Surgery-Hip; Knee Replacement; Arthritis; **Hospital:** Hosp For Special Surgery (page 60), NY-Presby/Weill Cornell Med Ctr, NY (page 66); **Address:** Hospital for Special Surgery, 535 E 70th St, New York, NY 10021; **Phone:** 212-606-1971; **Board Cert:** Orthopaedic Surgery 2004; **Med School:** Cornell Univ-Weill Med Coll 1985; **Resid:** Orthopaedic Surgery, Hosp for Special Surg 1990; **Fellow:** Hip Surgery, Mueller Fdn 1991; Joint Reconstruction, Case Western Res/Univ Hosp 1992; **Fac Appt:** Assoc Prof OrS, Cornell Univ-Weill Med Coll

Cammisa Jr, Frank P MD [OrS] - **Spec Exp:** Spinal Surgery; Spinal Disc Replacement; Minimally Invasive Spinal Surgery; Scoliosis; **Hospital:** Hosp For Special Surgery (page 60); **Address:** 523 E 72nd St, Fl 3, New York, NY 10021; **Phone:** 212-606-1946; **Board Cert:** Orthopaedic Surgery 2011; **Med School:** Columbia P&S 1982; **Resid:** Surgery, Columbia-Presby Hosp 1983; Orthopaedic Surgery, Hosp for Special Surgery 1987; **Fellow:** Spinal Surgery, Jackson Meml Hosp 1988; **Fac Appt:** Assoc Prof OrS, Cornell Univ-Weill Med Coll

Cappuccino, Andrew MD [OrS] - **Spec Exp:** Spinal Surgery; Spinal Disc Replacement; Minimally Invasive Spinal Surgery; **Hospital:** Kenmore Mercy Hosp, Sisters of Charity Hosp, Buffalo; **Address:** Buffalo Spine Surgery, 46 Davison Ct, Lockport, NY 14094; **Phone:** 716-438-2973; **Board Cert:** Orthopaedic Surgery 2007; Spine Surgery 2013; **Med School:** SUNY Buffalo 1988; **Resid:** Orthopaedic Surgery, Monmouth Med Ctr 1993; Pediatric Orthopaedic Surgery, Childrens Hosp 1992; **Fellow:** Spinal Surgery, Johns Hopkins/Paul McAfee, MD 1994

Chu, Constance R MD [OrS] - **Spec Exp:** Sports Medicine; Knee Injuries/ACL; Cartilage Damage; **Hospital:** UPMC Montefiore, UPMC Shadyside; **Address:** Kaufmann Bldg, 3471 5th Ave, Ste 1010, Pittsburgh, PA 15213; **Phone:** 412-687-3900; **Board Cert:** Orthopaedic Surgery 2002; **Med School:** Harvard Med Sch 1992; **Resid:** Orthopaedic Surgery, UCSD Med Ctr 1995; **Fellow:** Joint Replacement Surgery, Brigham & Women's Hosp 1999; **Fac Appt:** Assoc Prof OrS, Univ Pittsburgh

Orthopaedic Surgery

Cornell, Charles MD [OrS] - **Spec Exp:** Trauma; Joint Replacement; Hip & Knee Replacement; **Hospital:** Hosp For Special Surgery (page 60); **Address:** 535 E 70th St, Ste 306, New York, NY 10021; **Phone:** 212-606-1414; **Board Cert:** Orthopaedic Surgery 2009; **Med School:** Cornell Univ-Weill Med Coll 1980; **Resid:** Surgery, Presby Hosp 1982; Orthopaedic Surgery, Hosp For Special Surgery 1985; **Fellow:** Orthopaedic Surgery, Univ Wash Med Ctr 1986; **Fac Appt:** Clin Prof OrS, Cornell Univ-Weill Med Coll

Craig, Edward V MD [OrS] - **Spec Exp:** Shoulder Arthroscopic Surgery; Shoulder Replacement; Sports Medicine; Elbow Surgery; **Hospital:** Hosp For Special Surgery (page 60), NY-Presby/Weill Cornell Med Ctr, NY (page 66); **Address:** 535 E 70th St, New York, NY 10021; **Phone:** 212-606-1966; **Board Cert:** Orthopaedic Surgery 1984; **Med School:** Columbia P&S 1973; **Resid:** Internal Medicine, Columbia-Presby Hosp 1976; Orthopaedic Surgery, Columbia-Presby Hosp 1980; **Fellow:** Shoulder Surgery, Columbia-Presby Hosp 1981; Hand Surgery, Columbia-Presby Hosp 1982; **Fac Appt:** Clin Prof OrS, Cornell Univ-Weill Med Coll

Crossett, Lawrence MD [OrS] - **Spec Exp:** Hip Surgery; Knee Surgery; **Hospital:** UPMC Shadyside, UPMC Presby, Pittsburgh; **Address:** Shadyside Med Bldg, 5200 Centre Ave, Ste 415, Pittsburgh, PA 15232; **Phone:** 412-802-4100; **Board Cert:** Orthopaedic Surgery 2010; **Med School:** Temple Univ 1981; **Resid:** Orthopaedic Surgery, Temple Univ Hosp 1986; Orthopaedic Surgery, Shriners Children's Hosp 1984; **Fac Appt:** Assoc Prof OrS, Univ Pittsburgh

Davidson, Richard S MD [OrS] - **Spec Exp:** Limb Lengthening (Ilizarov Procedure); Limb Deformities; Foot Deformities; Clubfoot; **Hospital:** Chldns Hosp of Philadelphia; **Address:** Chldns Hosp, Dept Orthopaedics, 34th St & Civic Ctr Blvd, Wood Bldg Fl 2, Philadelphia, PA 19104; **Phone:** 215-590-1527; **Board Cert:** Orthopaedic Surgery 2007; **Med School:** NYU Sch Med 1976; **Resid:** Orthopaedic Surgery, Hosp Special Surgery 1981; **Fellow:** Pediatric Orthopaedic Surgery, Hosp for Sick Children 1982; **Fac Appt:** Assoc Prof OrS, Univ Pennsylvania

Delahay, John N MD [OrS] - **Spec Exp:** Pediatric Orthopaedic Surgery; Trauma; **Hospital:** Georgetown Univ Hosp; **Address:** 3800 Reservoir Rd NW, Washington, DC 20007; **Phone:** 202-444-1438; **Board Cert:** Orthopaedic Surgery 1975; **Med School:** Georgetown Univ 1969; **Resid:** Orthopaedic Surgery, Georgetown Univ Hosp 1974; **Fac Appt:** Prof OrS, Georgetown Univ

Deland, Jonathan T MD [OrS] - **Spec Exp:** Foot & Ankle Surgery; Sports Medicine; Arthritis; **Hospital:** Hosp For Special Surgery (page 60); **Address:** Hosp Spec Surg, Foot & Ankle Service, 535 E 70th St, New York, NY 10021-4099; **Phone:** 212-606-1665; **Board Cert:** Orthopaedic Surgery 2003; **Med School:** Columbia P&S 1980; **Resid:** Orthopaedic Surgery, St Luke's-Roosevelt Hosp Ctr 1982; Orthopaedic Surgery, Mass Genl Hosp 1987; **Fac Appt:** Asst Prof S, Cornell Univ-Weill Med Coll

Dines, David M MD [OrS] - **Spec Exp:** Shoulder Surgery; Sports Medicine; Shoulder Replacement; **Hospital:** Long Island Jewish Med Ctr (page 67), Hosp For Special Surgery (page 60); **Address:** 935 Northern Blvd, Ste 303, Great Neck, NY 11021-5309; **Phone:** 516-482-1037; **Board Cert:** Orthopaedic Surgery 1980; **Med School:** UMDNJ-NJ Med Sch, Newark 1974; **Resid:** Surgery, NY Hosp-Cornell Med Ctr 1976; Orthopaedic Surgery, Hosp Special Surg 1979; **Fac Appt:** Clin Prof OrS, Albert Einstein Coll Med

Donaldson III, William F MD [OrS] - **Spec Exp:** Spinal Surgery; **Hospital:** UPMC Presby, Pittsburgh; **Address:** Univ Pittsburgh Physicians, Orthopaedics, 3471 5th Ave, Ste 1010, Pittsburgh, PA 15213; **Phone:** 412-605-3218; **Board Cert:** Orthopaedic Surgery 2009; **Med School:** Rush Med Coll 1980; **Resid:** Surgery, Rush Presby-St Luke's Med Ctr 1981; Orthopaedic Surgery, Hosp Special Surg 1985; **Fellow:** Spinal Surgery, Hosp Special Surg 1986; **Fac Appt:** Assoc Prof OrS, Univ Pittsburgh

Dormans, John P MD [OrS] - **Spec Exp:** Bone Cancer; Spinal Surgery-Pediatric; Pediatric Orthopaedic Surgery; **Hospital:** Chldns Hosp of Philadelphia; **Address:** Childrens Hosp Phila-Orthopaedic Surg, 34th St & Civic Center Blvd, Wood Bldg Fl 2, Philadelphia, PA 19104-4399; **Phone:** 215-590-1534; **Board Cert:** Orthopaedic Surgery 2012; **Med School:** Indiana Univ 1983; **Resid:** Orthopaedic Surgery, Michigan State Univ Hosps 1988; **Fellow:** Pediatric Orthopaedic Surgery, Hosp for Sick Children 1989; **Fac Appt:** Prof OrS, Univ Pennsylvania

Errico, Thomas J MD [OrS] - **Spec Exp:** Spinal Surgery; Spinal Disc Replacement; Scoliosis; **Hospital:** NYU Langone Med Ctr (page 68), NYU Hosp For Joint Diseases (page 70); **Address:** 333 E 38th St, Fl 6, MS 10016, New York, NY 10016-6402; **Phone:** 646-501-7200; **Board Cert:** Orthopaedic Surgery 2007; **Med School:** UMDNJ-NJ Med Sch, Newark 1978; **Resid:** Orthopaedic Surgery, NYU Med Ctr 1983; **Fellow:** Spinal Surgery, Toronto Genl Hosp 1984; **Fac Appt:** Assoc Prof OrS, NYU Sch Med

Farmer, James C MD [OrS] - **Spec Exp:** Spinal Disorders-Degenerative; Trauma; Spinal Surgery; **Hospital:** Hosp For Special Surgery (page 60); **Address:** Hosp for Special Surgery, 523 E 72nd St Fl 3, New York, NY 10021; **Phone:** 212-606-1591; **Board Cert:** Orthopaedic Surgery 2007; **Med School:** Georgetown Univ 1988; **Resid:** Orthopaedic Surgery, Hosp Univ Penn 1993; **Fellow:** Orthopaedic Surgery, Jefferson Med Coll 1994; **Fac Appt:** Assoc Prof OrS, Cornell Univ-Weill Med Coll

Feldman, David S MD [OrS] - **Spec Exp:** Limb Deformities; Spinal Surgery; Pediatric Orthopaedic Surgery; Scoliosis; **Hospital:** NYU Hosp For Joint Diseases (page 70), NYU Langone Med Ctr (page 68); **Address:** 67 Irving Pl Fl 8, New York, NY 10003; **Phone:** 212-533-5310; **Board Cert:** Orthopaedic Surgery 2007; **Med School:** Albert Einstein Coll Med 1988; **Resid:** Orthopaedic Surgery, Hosp for Joint Diseases 1993; **Fellow:** Pediatric Surgery, Hosp For Sick Chldn 1994; **Fac Appt:** Asst Prof OrS, NYU Sch Med

Flatow, Evan L MD [OrS] - **Spec Exp:** Rotator Cuff Surgery; Shoulder Injuries; Shoulder Replacement; Shoulder Arthroscopic Surgery; **Hospital:** Mount Sinai Med Ctr (page 64); **Address:** 5 E 98th St, Fl 9, Box 1188, New York, NY 10029; **Phone:** 212-241-1663; **Board Cert:** Orthopaedic Surgery 2010; **Med School:** Columbia P&S 1981; **Resid:** Surgery, Roosevelt Hosp 1983; Orthopaedic Surgery, Columbia-Presby Med Ctr 1986; **Fellow:** Shoulder Surgery, Columbia-Presby Med Ctr 1987; **Fac Appt:** Prof OrS, Mount Sinai Sch Med

Frassica, Frank J MD [OrS] - **Spec Exp:** Bone Cancer; **Hospital:** Johns Hopkins Hosp (page 61), Univ of MD Med Ctr; **Address:** Johns Hopkins Outpatient Ctr, 601 N Caroline St, Ste 5215, Baltimore, MD 21287; **Phone:** 410-502-2698; **Board Cert:** Orthopaedic Surgery 2011; **Med School:** Univ SC Sch Med 1982; **Resid:** Orthopaedic Surgery, Mayo Clinic 1987; **Fellow:** Orthopaedic Oncology, Mayo Clinic 1988; **Fac Appt:** Prof OrS, Johns Hopkins Univ

Fu, Freddie H MD [OrS] - **Spec Exp:** Sports Medicine; Knee Injuries/ACL; Shoulder Injuries; **Hospital:** UPMC Presby, Pittsburgh, UPMC South Side-Out Pt Ctr; **Address:** Presbyterian Univ Hosp, Kaufmann Bldg, 3471 5th Ave, Ste 1011, Pittsburgh, PA 15213; **Phone:** 412-432-3611; **Board Cert:** Orthopaedic Surgery 1984; **Med School:** Univ Pittsburgh 1977; **Resid:** Orthopaedic Surgery, Univ Pittsburgh Med Ctr 1982; **Fellow:** Orthopaedic Research, Univ Pittsburgh Med Ctr 1979; **Fac Appt:** Prof OrS, Univ Pittsburgh

Gladstone, James N MD [OrS] - **Spec Exp:** Shoulder & Knee Surgery; Cartilage Damage; Knee-Patella Problems; Arthritis; **Hospital:** Mount Sinai Med Ctr (page 64); **Address:** Mt Sinai Med Ctr, 5 E 98th St Fl 9, Box 1188, New York, NY 10029; **Phone:** 212-241-1645; **Board Cert:** Orthopaedic Surgery 2009; Orthopaedic Sports Medicine 2007; **Med School:** Tufts Univ 1990; **Resid:** Orthopaedic Surgery, Columbia-Presby Med Ctr 1995; **Fellow:** Sports Medicine, American Sports Med Inst 1996; **Fac Appt:** Assoc Prof OrS, Mount Sinai Sch Med

Orthopaedic Surgery

Glashow, Jonathan L MD [OrS] - **Spec Exp:** Sports Medicine; Sho... ...gery; Arthroscopic Surgery; **Hospital:** Mount Sinai Med Ctr (page 64); **Addre...** 1C, New York, NY 1002); **Phone:** 212-794-5096; **Board Cert:** Orthopaedic... **School:** Cornell Univ Weill Med Coll 1984; **Resid:** Orthopaedic Surgery, Lenox... ...Arthroscopic Surgery, S Calif Ortho Inst 1990; Shoulder Surgery, Univ Texas... **App:** Assoc Clin Prof OrS, Mount Sinai Sch Med

Goldstein, Jeffrey A MD [OrS] - **Spec Exp:** Spinal Surgery; Minimally Invasive... gery; Spinal Disc Replacement; Scoliosis; **Hospital:** NYU Hosp For Joint Diseases (page... Langone Med Ctr (page 68), **Address:** NYU Hospital For Joint Diseases, 19 Benkman St, NY 10038; **Phone:** 212-718-771; **Board Cert:** Orthopaedic Surgery 2004; **Med Sc...** Downstate 1991; **Resid:** Orthopaedic Surgery, Cms West Univ Med Ctr 1995; **Fellow:** ...gery, Maryland Spine Ctr 1999; **Fac Appt:** Clin Prof OrS, NYU Sch Med

Greisberg, Justin K MD [OrS] - **Spec Exp:** Foot & Ankle Surgery; Ankle Replacem... sion; Reconstructive Surgery; Trauma; **Hospital:** NY-Presby/Columbia Univ Med Ctr, NY (page... **Address:** NY Presby/Columbia Medical Ctr, 622 W 168th St, PH-11, rm 1153, New Y... 10032; **Phone:** 212-305-5604; **Board Cert:** Orthopaedic Surgery 2004; **Med School:** Albert... stein Coll Med 1995; **Resid:** Orthopaedic Surgery, Rhode Island Hosp 2000; **Fellow:** Orthopaedic Trauma Surgery, Rhode Island Hosp 2001; Foot & Ankle Surgery, Harbor; **Fac Appt:** Assoc Prof Columbia P&S

Orelsamer, Ronald P MD [OrS] - **Spec Exp:** Knee/Patella Problems; Sports Medicine; Knee Reconstruction; Arthritis-Hip & Knee; **Hospital:** Mount Sinai Med Ctr (page 64); **Address:** Mount Sinai Medical Ctr, Dept Orthopaedics, 5 E 98th St, Box 1188, New York, NY 10029-6514; **Phone:** 212-241-2914; **Board Cert:** Orthopaedic Surgery 2006; **Med School:** Columbia P&S 1911; **Resid:** Orthopaedic Surgery, Columbia Presby Med Ctr 1984; **Fellow:** Hip & Knee Surgery, Columbia Presby Med Ctr 1985; **Fac Appt:** Assoc Prof OrS, Mount Sinai Sch Med

Haas, Steven B MD [OrS] - **Spec Exp:** Knee Surgery; Knee Replacement; Minimally Invasive Surgery; **Hospital:** Hosp For Special Surgery (page 66); **Address:** Hosp for Special Surgery, 535 E 70th St, New York, NY 10021; **Phone:** 212-606-1852; **Board Cert:** Orthopaedic Surgery 2004; **Med School:** Univ Rochester 1985; **Resid:** Orthopaedic Surgery, Hosp Special Surgery 1990; **Fellow:** Knee Surgery, Hosp Special Surgery 1991; **Fac Appt:** Clin Prof OrS, Cornell Univ-Weill Med Coll

Hannafin, Jo Anne MD/PhD [OrS] - **Spec Exp:** Sports Medicine-Women; Shoulder Arthroscopic Surgery; Knee Injuries/Ligament Surgery; Ligament Reconstruction; **Hospital:** Hosp For Special Surgery (page 66), NY-Presby/Weill Cornell Med Ctr, NY (page 66); **Address:** 535 E 70th St, New York, NY 10021-4872; **Phone:** 212-606-1469; **Board Cert:** Orthopaedic Surgery 2005; Orthopaedic Sports Medicine 2009; **Med School:** Albert Einstein Coll Med 1985; **Resid:** Orthopaedic Surgery, Montefiore Med Ctr 1990; **Fellow:** Sports Medicine, Hosp Special Surgery 1992; **Fac Appt:** Prof OrS, Cornell Univ-Weill Med Coll

Hausman, Michael R MD [OrS] - **Spec Exp:** Hand Reconstruction; Elbow Reconstruction; Reconstructive Microvascular Surgery; Arthroscopic Surgery; **Hospital:** Mount Sinai Med Ctr (page 64); **Address:** 5 E 98th St Fl 9, Box 1188, New York, NY 10029-6501; **Phone:** 212-241-1658; **Board Cert:** Orthopaedic Surgery 2010; Hand Surgery 2010; **Med School:** Yale Univ 1979; **Resid:** Surgery, Yale-New Haven Hosp 1981; Orthopaedic Surgery, Yale-New Haven Hosp 1985; **Fellow:** Hand Surgery, Roosevelt Hosp 1987; **Fac Appt:** Assoc Clin Prof OrS, Mount Sinai Sch Med

Healey, John H MD [OrS] - **Spec Exp:** Bone Tumors; Hip & Knee Replacement in Bone Tumors; Sarcoma; Sarcoma-Soft Tissue; **Hospital:** Meml Sloan-Kettering Cancer Ctr, Hosp For Special Surgery (page 60); **Address:** 1275 York Ave, New York, NY 10065; **Phone:** 212-639-7610; **Board Cert:** Orthopaedic Surgery 2007; **Med School:** Univ VT Coll Med 1978; **Resid:** Orthopaedic Surgery, Hosp Special Surg 1983; **Fellow:** Musculoskeletal Oncology, Meml Sloan Kettering Cancer Ctr 1984; Orthopaedic Surgery, Hosp Special Surgery 1984; **Fac Appt:** Prof OrS, Cornell Univ-Weill Med Coll

Hecht, Andrew MD [OrS] - **Spec Exp:** Spinal Surgery; Minimally Invasive Spinal Surgery; **Hospital:** Mount Sinai Med Ctr (page 64); **Address:** Chief Spine Surgery, Mount Sinai Med Ctr, Dept Orthopaedic Surg, 5 E 98th St, Fl 9, Box 1188, New York, NY 10029; **Phone:** 212-241-0735; **Board Cert:** Orthopaedic Surgery 2003; **Med School:** Harvard Med Sch 1994; **Resid:** Orthopaedic Surgery, Mass Genl Hosp 1999; **Fellow:** Spinal Surgery, Emory Univ Spine Ctr 2001; **Fac Appt:** Asst Prof OrS, Mount Sinai Sch Med

Helfet, David L MD [OrS] - **Spec Exp:** Fractures-Complex & Non Union; Deformity Reconstruction; Pelvic & Acetabular Fractures; Fractures-Stress; **Hospital:** Hosp For Special Surgery (page 60), NY-Presby/Weill Cornell Med Ctr, NY (page 66); **Address:** 525 E 71th St, Belaire Bldg - Fl 2, New York, NY 10021; **Phone:** 212-606-1888; **Board Cert:** Orthopedic Surgery 1984; **Med School:** South Africa 1975; **Resid:** Surgery, Edendale Hosp 1977; Orthopaedic Surgery, Johns Hopkins Hosp 1981; **Fellow:** Orthopaedic Surgery, Inselspita Hosp 1981; Orthopaedic Surgery, UCLA Med Ctr 1982; **Fac Appt:** Prof OrS, Cornell Univ-Weill Med Coll

Henshaw, Robert M MD [OrS] - **Spec Exp:** Musculoskeletal Tumors; Bone Tumors; **Hospital:** Washington Hosp Ctr, Chldns Natl Med Ctr; **Address:** 110 Irving St NW, Ste C2173, Washington, DC 20010; **Phone:** 202-877-3970; **Board Cert:** Orthopaedic Surgery 2010; **Med School:** Tufts Univ 1990; **Resid:** Orthopaedic Surgery, UCLA Med Ctr 1995; **Fellow:** Orthopaedic Surgery, Washington Hosp Ctr 1997; **Fac Appt:** Assoc Prof OrS, Georgetown Univ

Herman, Martin J MD [OrS] - **Spec Exp:** Pediatric Orthopaedic Surgery; Hip Disorders-Pediatric; Scoliosis; Musculoskeletal Disorders; **Hospital:** St. Christopher's Hosp for Chldn; **Address:** St Christophers Hosp for Children, Dept Orthopaedic Surgery, 3601 A St, Philadelphia, PA 19134; **Phone:** 215-427-3131; **Board Cert:** Orthopaedic Surgery 2009; **Med School:** Columbia P&S 1990; **Resid:** Orthopaedic Surgery, RW Johnson Univ Hosp 1995; **Fellow:** Pediatric Orthopaedic Surgery, ampbell Clinic/Univ Tenn 1996; **Fac Appt:** Assoc Prof OrS, Drexel Univ Coll Med

Herzenberg, John E MD [OrS] - **Spec Exp:** Limb Lengthening (Ilizarov Procedure); Limb Deformities; Pediatric Orthopaedic Surgery; Clubfoot; **Hospital:** Sinai Hosp - Baltimore; **Address:** International Ctr for Limb Lengthening, Sinai Hospital of Baltimore, 2401 W Belvedere Ave, Baltimore, MD 21215; **Phone:** 410-601-8700; **Board Cert:** Orthopaedic Surgery 2009; **Med School:** Boston Univ 1979; **Resid:** Orthopaedic Surgery, Duke Univ Med Ctr 1985; **Fellow:** Pediatric Orthopaedic Surgery, Hosp for Sick Children 1986; **Fac Appt:** Clin Prof OrS, Univ MD Sch Med

Hilibrand, Alan S MD [OrS] - **Spec Exp:** Spinal Surgery; Spinal Surgery-Cervical; Spinal Trauma; Minimally Invasive Spinal Surgery; **Hospital:** Bucks Specialty Inst, Thomas Jefferson Univ Hosp; **Address:** Rothman Institute, 925 Chestnut St, Fl 5, Philadelphia, PA 19107; **Phone:** 800-321-9999; **Board Cert:** Orthopaedic Surgery 2009; **Med School:** Yale Univ 1990; **Resid:** Orthopaedic Surgery, Univ Michigan Hlth System 1995; **Fellow:** Spinal Surgery, Cleveland Spine Inst 1996; **Fac Appt:** Prof OrS, Jefferson Med Coll

Orthopaedic Surgery

Hotchkiss, Robert N MD [OrS] - **Spec Exp:** Hand Surgery; Wrist Surgery; Elbow Reconstruction; Dupuytren's Contracture; **Hospital:** Hosp For Special Surgery (page 60), NY-Presby/Weill Cornell Med Ctr, NY (page 66); **Address:** 523 E 72nd St Fl 4, New York, NY 10021-4099; **Phone:** 212-606-1964; **Board Cert:** Orthopaedic Surgery 2010; Hand Surgery 2010; **Med School:** Johns Hopkins Univ 1980; **Resid:** Surgery, Johns Hopkins Hosp 1982; Orthopaedic Surgery, Johns Hopkins Hosp 1985; **Fellow:** Hand Surgery, Union Meml Hosp 1987; **Fac Appt:** Assoc Prof OrS, Cornell Univ-Weill Med Coll

Hozack, William J MD [OrS] - **Spec Exp:** Hip Surgery; Knee Surgery; Joint Replacement; **Hospital:** Thomas Jefferson Univ Hosp; **Address:** Rothman Inst, 925 Chesnut St Fl 5, Philadelphia, PA 19107; **Phone:** 800-321-9999; **Board Cert:** Orthopaedic Surgery 2010; **Med School:** McGill Univ 1981; **Resid:** Orthopaedic Surgery, Hosp Univ Penn 1986; **Fellow:** Joint Reconstruction, Penn Hosp/Thomas Jefferson Univ 1987; **Fac Appt:** Prof OrS, Jefferson Med Coll

Hume, Eric L MD [OrS] - **Spec Exp:** Hip Replacement; Knee Replacement; **Hospital:** Penn Presby Med Ctr - UPHS (page 72); **Address:** Penn Presbyterian Med Ctr, 51 N 39th St, Cupp Bldg Fl 1, Philadelphia, PA 19104; **Phone:** 215-662-3340; **Board Cert:** Orthopaedic Surgery 2007; **Med School:** SUNY Upstate Med Univ 1978; **Resid:** Orthopaedic Surgery, Jefferson Univ Hosp 1983; **Fac Appt:** Assoc Clin Prof OrS, Univ Pennsylvania

Hungerford, Marc W MD [OrS] - **Spec Exp:** Knee Replacement & Revision; Hip Replacement & Revision; Cartilage Damage; **Hospital:** Mercy Med Ctr - Baltimore; **Address:** Mercy Medical Center, Joint Replacement & Trauma Ctr, 301 Saint Paul Pl, Baltimore, MD 21202; **Phone:** 410-539-2227; **Board Cert:** Orthopaedic Surgery 2001; **Med School:** Vanderbilt Univ 1992; **Resid:** Orthopaedic Surgery, Johns Hopkins Hosp 1997; **Fac Appt:** Asst Prof OrS, Johns Hopkins Univ

Hyman, Joshua E MD [OrS] - **Spec Exp:** Pediatric Orthopaedic Surgery; Fractures-Pediatric; Scoliosis; Clubfoot/Foot Deformities in Children; **Hospital:** Morgan Stanley Children's Hosp of NY-Presby, NY, NY-Presby/Columbia Univ Med Ctr, NY (page 66); **Address:** Children's Hosp New York, 3959 Broadway, Ste 8 North, New York, NY 10032-3784; **Phone:** 212-305-5475; **Board Cert:** Orthopaedic Surgery 2002; **Med School:** Columbia P&S 1990; **Resid:** Surgery, Beth Israel Hosp 1993; Orthopaedic Surgery, Mass Genl Hosp/Beth Israel Hosp 1998; **Fellow:** Pediatric Orthopaedic Surgery, Hosp for Sick Children 1999; **Fac Appt:** Assoc Prof OrS, Columbia P&S

Johanson, Norman A MD [OrS] - **Spec Exp:** Hip Replacement & Revision; Knee Replacement & Revision; Juvenile Arthritis; **Hospital:** Hahnemann Univ Hosp; **Address:** Univ Orthopaedic Inst at Hahnenmann, 216 N Broad St, Feinstein Bldg, Fl 2, Philadelphia, PA 19102; **Phone:** 215-762-2663; **Board Cert:** Orthopaedic Surgery 2007; **Med School:** Cornell Univ 1978; **Resid:** Orthopaedic Surgery, Hosp Special Surg 1984; **Fac Appt:** Prof OrS, Drexel Univ Coll Med

Johnson, Carl A MD [OrS] - **Spec Exp:** Knee Surgery; **Hospital:** Johns Hopkins Bayview Med Ctr (page 61), Johns Hopkins Hosp (page 61); **Address:** Johns Hopkins at Whitemarsh, 4924 Campbell Blvd, Ste 130, Nottingham, MD 21236; **Phone:** 443-442-2086; **Board Cert:** Orthopaedic Surgery 1983; **Med School:** Johns Hopkins Univ 1976; **Resid:** Surgery, Johns Hopkins Hosp 1978; Orthopaedic Surgery, Johns Hopkins Hosp 1981; **Fac Appt:** Assoc Prof OrS, Johns Hopkins Univ

Kaplan, Frederick S MD [OrS] - **Spec Exp:** Bone Disorders-Metabolic; Fibrodysplasia Ossificans Progressiv FOP; Progressive Osseous Heteroplasia POH; **Hospital:** Hosp Univ Penn - UPHS (page 72); **Address:** Penn Dept Orthopaedic Surgery, 3400 Spruce St, 2 Silverstein, Philadelphia, PA 19104; **Phone:** 215-349-8727; **Med School:** Johns Hopkins Univ 1976; **Resid:** Orthopaedic Surgery, Hosp Univ Penn 1981; **Fellow:** Orthopaedic Research, Hosp Univ Penn 1982; Musculoskeletal Disorders, Dr Michael Zasloff/Univ Penn 1991; **Fac Appt:** Prof OrS, Univ Pennsylvania

Kelly, Bryan T MD [OrS] - **Spec Exp:** Hip Surgery; Arthroscopic Surgery; Sports Medicine; **Hospital:** Hosp For Special Surgery (page 60); **Address:** 535 E 70th St, New York, NY 10021; **Phone:** 212-606-1159; **Board Cert:** Orthopaedic Surgery 2006; **Med School:** Duke Univ 1996; **Resid:** Orthopaedic Surgery, Hosp Special Surg 2001; **Fellow:** Orthopaedic Sports Medicine, Hosp Special Surg 2003; Hip Sports Injuries/Arthroscopy, Univ Pittsburgh 2004; **Fac Appt:** Assoc Prof OrS, Cornell Univ-Weill Med Coll

Kenan, Samuel MD [OrS] - **Spec Exp:** Bone Tumors; **Hospital:** Lenox Hill Hosp (page 67); **Address:** 300 Old Country Rd, Ste 221, Mineola, NY 11501; **Phone:** 516-280-3733; **Med School:** Israel 1976; **Resid:** Orthopaedic Surgery, Hadassah Univ Hosp 1984; **Fellow:** Orthopaedic Pathology, Hosp for Joint Diseases 1987; **Fac Appt:** Prof OrS, NYU Sch Med

Krackow, Kenneth A MD [OrS] - **Spec Exp:** Knee Replacement; Knee Reconstruction; Hip Replacement & Revision; **Hospital:** Buffalo General Hosp; **Address:** Bufffalo Genl Hosp, Dept Orthopaedic Surgery, 100 High St, Ste B276, Buffalo, NY 14203; **Phone:** 716-859-1256; **Board Cert:** Orthopaedic Surgery 1993; **Med School:** Duke Univ 1971; **Resid:** Surgery, Johns Hopkins Hosp 1973; Orthopaedic Surgery, Johns Hopkins Hosp 1976; **Fac Appt:** Prof OrS, SUNY Buffalo

Lane, Joseph MD [OrS] - **Spec Exp:** Bone Disorders-Metabolic; Osteoporosis Spine-Kyphoplasty; Bone Cancer; **Hospital:** Hosp For Special Surgery (page 60), NY-Presby/Weill Cornell Med Ctr, NY (page 66); **Address:** Hosp for Special Surgery, 535 E 70th St, New York, NY 10021; **Phone:** 212-606-1172; **Board Cert:** Orthopaedic Surgery 1998; **Med School:** Harvard Med Sch 1965; **Resid:** Surgery, Hosp Univ Penn 1967; Orthopaedic Surgery, Hosp Univ Penn 1973; **Fac Appt:** Prof OrS, Cornell Univ-Weill Med Coll

Lauerman, William MD [OrS] - **Spec Exp:** Spinal Deformity-Pediatric & Adult; Spinal Surgery; Pain-Back; Scoliosis; **Hospital:** Georgetown Univ Hosp; **Address:** 3800 Reservoir Rd NW, Spine Surgery Clinic-1 Gorman, Washington, DC 20007; **Phone:** 202-444-8766 x2; **Board Cert:** Orthopaedic Surgery 2001; **Med School:** Georgetown Univ 1982; **Resid:** Orthopaedic Surgery, Georgetown Univ Med Ctr 1987; **Fellow:** Orthopaedic Surgery, Univ Minn-Twin Cities Scoliosis Ctr 1988; **Fac Appt:** Prof OrS, Georgetown Univ

Leadbetter, Wayne MD [OrS] - **Spec Exp:** Knee-Patella Problems; Arthritis-Knee; **Hospital:** Sinai Hosp - Baltimore; **Address:** Ctr Joint Surgery & Sports Med, 13 Western Maryland Pkwy, Ste 104, Hagerstown, MD 21740; **Phone:** 301-665-4575; **Board Cert:** Orthopaedic Surgery 1977; **Med School:** Creighton Univ 1970; **Resid:** Surgery, Johns Hopkins Hosp 1972; Orthopaedic Surgery, Johns Hopkins Hosp 1976; **Fellow:** Orthopaedic Surgery, Jonhs Hopkins Hosp 1973; **Fac Appt:** Asst Clin Prof S, Uniformed Srvs Univ, Bethesda

Lee, Francis Y MD/PhD [OrS] - **Spec Exp:** Bone & Soft Tissue Tumors; Pediatric Orthopaedic Surgery; Bone Tumors-Metastatic; Bone Tumors-Benign; **Hospital:** Morgan Stanley Children's Hosp of NY-Presby, NY, NY-Presby/Columbia Univ Med Ctr, NY (page 66); **Address:** 3959 Broadway, Ste 800N, Columbia University Medical Center, New York, NY 10032; **Phone:** 212-305-3293; **Board Cert:** Orthopaedic Surgery 2012; **Med School:** South Korea 1986; **Resid:** Orthopaedic Surgery, NJ Med Ctr 1997; **Fellow:** Orthopaedic Oncology, Harvard Med Sch 1998; Pediatric Orthopaedic Surgery, Hosp for Sick Chldn/Univ Toronto 1999; **Fac Appt:** Assoc Prof OrS, Columbia P&S

Levine, David S MD [OrS] - **Spec Exp:** Foot & Ankle Surgery; Ankle Reconstruction; **Hospital:** Hosp For Special Surgery (page 60); **Address:** Hospital for Special Surgery, 523 E 72 St Fl 5, New York, NY 10021; **Phone:** 212-606-1940; **Board Cert:** Orthopaedic Surgery 2011; **Med School:** Cornell Univ-Weill Med Coll 1992; **Resid:** Orthopaedic Surgery, Hosp for Special Surgery 1997; **Fellow:** Foot & Ankle Surgery, Harborview Med Ctr 1998

Orthopaedic Surgery

Macaulay, William B MD [OrS] - **Spec Exp:** Hip Replacement; Knee Replacement; Minimally Invasive Surgery; Reconstructive Surgery; **Hospital:** NY-Presby/Columbia Univ Med Ctr, NY (page 66); **Address:** Columbia-Orthopaedics Dept, 161 Fort Washington Ave, Irving Pavilion Fl 2, New York, NY 10032; **Phone:** 212-305-6959; **Board Cert:** Orthopaedic Surgery 2012; **Med School:** Columbia P&S 1992; **Resid:** Orthopaedic Surgery, Univ Pittsburgh Med Ctr 1997; **Fellow:** Adult Reconstructive Surgery, Hosp for Special Surgery 1999; **Fac Appt:** Prof OrS, Columbia P&S

Malawer, Martin M MD [OrS] - **Spec Exp:** Bone Tumors; Limb Sparing Surgery; Pediatric Orthopaedic Surgery; Sarcoma; **Hospital:** Georgetown Univ Hosp, G Washington Univ Hosp; **Address:** 7830 Old Georgetown Rd, Ste C15, Bethesda, MD 20814; **Phone:** 301-215-7940; **Board Cert:** Orthopaedic Surgery 1976; **Med School:** NYU Sch Med 1969; **Resid:** Surgery, Bronx Muni Hosp 1972; Orthopaedic Surgery, Bellevue Hosp Ctr 1975; **Fellow:** Orthopaedic Oncology, Shands Hosp-Univ Florida 1978; **Fac Appt:** Prof OrS, Geo Wash Univ

Marx, Robert G MD [OrS] - **Spec Exp:** Shoulder Surgery; Knee Injuries/Ligament Surgery; Knee Replacement; Sports Medicine; **Hospital:** Hosp For Special Surgery (page 60); **Address:** 535 E 70th St, New York, NY 10021; **Phone:** 212-606-1645; **Board Cert:** Orthopaedic Surgery 2003; **Med School:** McGill Univ 1991; **Resid:** Orthopaedic Surgery, Univ Toronto 1996; **Fellow:** Sports Medicine, Hosp Special Surgery 1998; **Fac Appt:** Prof OrS, Cornell Univ-Weill Med Coll

McAfee, Paul C MD [OrS] - **Spec Exp:** Spinal Reconstructive Surgery; Spinal Disc Replacement; Scoliosis; **Hospital:** St. Joseph Med Ctr; **Address:** 7505 Osler Drive, Ste 104, Towson, MD 21204; **Phone:** 410-337-8888; **Board Cert:** Orthopaedic Surgery 2007; **Med School:** SUNY Upstate Med Univ 1979; **Resid:** Orthopaedic Surgery, SUNY Upstate Med Ctr 1984; **Fellow:** Spinal Surgery, Case West Res Univ Hosps 1986; **Fac Appt:** Assoc Prof OrS, Johns Hopkins Univ

McCance, Sean E MD [OrS] - **Spec Exp:** Spinal Surgery; Scoliosis; **Hospital:** Mount Sinai Med Ctr (page 64), Lenox Hill Hosp (page 67); **Address:** 1155 Park Ave, Fl Ground, Ste E, New York, NY 10128; **Phone:** 212-360-6500; **Board Cert:** Orthopaedic Surgery 2010; Spine Surgery ; **Med School:** Columbia P&S 1991; **Resid:** Surgery, Strong Meml Hosp 1992; Orthopaedic Surgery, Strong Meml Hosp 1996; **Fellow:** Spinal Surgery, Twin Cities Spine Ctr 1998; **Fac Appt:** Asst Clin Prof OrS, Mount Sinai Sch Med

McCann, Peter D MD [OrS] - **Spec Exp:** Shoulder Surgery; Elbow Surgery; **Hospital:** Beth Israel Med Ctr - Petrie Division (page 56); **Address:** 10 Union Square E, Ste 3M, New York, NY 10003; **Phone:** 212-844-6735; **Board Cert:** Orthopaedic Surgery 2009; **Med School:** Columbia P&S 1980; **Resid:** Surgery, St Vincent's Hosp 1982; Orthopaedic Surgery, Columbia-Presby Med Ctr 1985; **Fellow:** Shoulder Surgery, Columbia-Presby Med Ctr 1986; **Fac Appt:** Assoc Prof OrS, Albert Einstein Coll Med

McFarland, Edward G MD [OrS] - **Spec Exp:** Sports Medicine; Rotator Cuff Surgery; Shoulder Surgery; **Hospital:** Johns Hopkins Hosp (page 61); **Address:** 10753 Falls Rd, Ste 215, Lutherville, MD 21093; **Phone:** 410-583-2851; **Board Cert:** Orthopaedic Surgery 2011; Orthopaedic Sports Medicine 2010; **Med School:** Univ Louisville Sch Med 1982; **Resid:** Orthopaedic Surgery, Mayo Clinic 1987; **Fellow:** Sports Medicine, Kerlan-Jobe Orthopaedic Group 1989; **Fac Appt:** Prof OrS, Johns Hopkins Univ

Myerson, Mark MD [OrS] - **Spec Exp:** Foot & Ankle Surgery; **Hospital:** Mercy Med Ctr - Baltimore; **Address:** 301 St Paul Pl, Baltimore, MD 21202; **Phone:** 410-659-2800; **Board Cert:** Orthopaedic Surgery 2008; **Med School:** South Africa 1979; **Resid:** Surgery, Sinai Hospital 1981; Orthopaedic Surgery, Johns Hopkins Hosp 1985; **Fellow:** Foot & Ankle Surgery, Hospital Joint Disease

Neuwirth, Michael MD [OrS] - **Spec Exp:** Scoliosis; Spinal Surgery; **Hospital:** Beth Israel Med Ctr - Petrie Division (page 56); **Address:** Beth Israel Med Ctr - Spine Institute, 10 Union Square E, Ste 5P, New York, NY 10003-3314; **Phone:** 212-844-8692; **Board Cert:** Orthopaedic Surgery 1980; **Med School:** SUNY Hlth Sci Ctr 1974; **Resid:** Orthopaedic Surgery, Hosp for Joint Diseases 1978; **Fellow:** Spinal Surgery, Rush-Presby Med Ctr 1979; **Fac Appt:** Assoc Clin Prof OrS, NYU Sch Med

Nicholas, Stephen J MD [OrS] - **Spec Exp:** Sports Medicine; Shoulder & Knee Surgery; Arthroscopic Surgery; **Hospital:** Lenox Hill Hosp (page 67); **Address:** 130 E 77 St Fl 5, New York, NY 10075; **Phone:** 212-737-3301; **Board Cert:** Orthopaedic Surgery 2005; **Med School:** NY Med Coll 1986; **Resid:** Orthopaedic Surgery, Hosp for Special Surgery 1991; **Fellow:** Sports Medicine, Lenox Hill Hosp 1992

O'Keefe, Regis J MD/PhD [OrS] - **Spec Exp:** Bone & Soft Tissue Tumors; Reconstructive Surgery; Bone Disorders-Metabolic; **Hospital:** Univ of Rochester Strong Meml Hosp, Highland Hosp of Rochester; **Address:** Univ Rochester, Dept Orthopaedic Surgery, 601 Elmwood Ave, Box 665, Rochester, NY 14642; **Phone:** 585-275-3100; **Board Cert:** Orthopaedic Surgery 2007; **Med School:** Harvard Med Sch 1985; **Resid:** Surgery, New Eng Deaconess Hosp/Harvard 1986; Orthopaedic Surgery, Univ Rochester 1992; **Fellow:** Orthopaedic Oncology, Mass Genl Hosp 1993; **Fac Appt:** Prof S, Univ Rochester

O'Leary, Patrick MD [OrS] - **Spec Exp:** Spinal Surgery; **Hospital:** Hosp For Special Surgery (page 60); **Address:** 1015 Madison Ave Fl 4, New York, NY 10075; **Phone:** 212-249-8100; **Board Cert:** Orthopaedic Surgery 1983; **Med School:** Ireland 1968; **Resid:** Surgery, Roosevelt Hosp 1972; Orthopaedic Surgery, Hosp Spec Surg-Cornell 1975; **Fellow:** Spinal Surgery, Univ Toronto Genl Ortho Hosp 1976; **Fac Appt:** Assoc Clin Prof OrS, Cornell Univ-Weill Med Coll

Otsuka, Norman Y MD [OrS] - **Spec Exp:** Pediatric Orthopaedic Surgery; Trauma; Neuromuscular Disorders; Cerebral Palsy; **Hospital:** NYU Hosp For Joint Diseases (page 70); **Address:** NYU Hosp for Joint Diseases, Center for Children, 301 E 17th St, Ste 303/204, New York, NY 10003; **Phone:** 212-598-6286; **Board Cert:** Orthopaedic Surgery 2009; **Med School:** Canada 1995; **Resid:** Orthopaedic Surgery, Univ of Toronto 1994; **Fellow:** Pediatric Orthopaedic Surgery, Morgan Stanley Children's Hosp of NY-Presby 1995; **Fac Appt:** Prof OrS, NYU Sch Med

Padgett, Douglas E MD [OrS] - **Spec Exp:** Hip & Knee Replacement; Arthroscopic Surgery-Hip; Arthroscopic Surgery-Knee; Dance Medicine; **Hospital:** Hosp For Special Surgery (page 60); **Address:** Hosp for Special Surgery, 535 E 70 St Fl 3, New York, NY 10021; **Phone:** 212-606-1642; **Board Cert:** Orthopaedic Surgery 2003; **Med School:** NY Med Coll 1982; **Resid:** Orthopaedic Surgery, Hosp Spec Surg 1989; **Fellow:** Orthopaedic Surgery, Rush Presby Med Ctr 1990; **Fac Appt:** Assoc Prof OrS, Cornell Univ-Weill Med Coll

Parvizi, Javad MD [OrS] - **Spec Exp:** Hip Replacement & Revision; Knee Replacement & Revision; **Hospital:** Thomas Jefferson Univ Hosp; **Address:** Rothman Institute, 925 Chestnut St, Fl 5, Philadelphia, PA 19107; **Phone:** 800-321-9999; **Board Cert:** Orthopaedic Surgery 2005; **Med School:** England, UK 1991; **Resid:** Orthopaedic Surgery, Mayo Clinic; **Fellow:** Joint Arthroplasty, Univ of Berne; **Fac Appt:** Prof OrS, Thomas Jefferson Univ

Pellicci, Paul M MD [OrS] - **Spec Exp:** Hip Replacement-Young Adults; Hip Resurfacing; Knee Replacement; Joint Replacement; **Hospital:** Hosp For Special Surgery (page 60), NY-Presby/Weill Cornell Med Ctr, NY (page 66); **Address:** 535 E 70th St, New York, NY 10021-4872; **Phone:** 212-606-1010; **Board Cert:** Orthopaedic Surgery 1982; **Med School:** Cornell Univ-Weill Med Coll 1975; **Resid:** Surgery, NY Hosp 1977; Orthopaedic Surgery, Hosp Spec Surg 1980; **Fellow:** Joint Replacement Surgery, Brigham & Womens Hosp 1981; **Fac Appt:** Prof OrS, Cornell Univ-Weill Med Coll

Pizzutillo, Peter D MD [OrS] - **Spec Exp:** Pediatric Orthopaedic Surgery; Sports Medicine; Congenital Anomalies-Orthopaedic; **Hospital:** St. Christopher's Hosp for Chldn; **Address:** St Christophers Hosp for Children, Dept Orthopaedic Surgery, 3601 A St, Philadelphia, PA 19134; **Phone:** 215-427-3131; **Board Cert:** Orthopaedic Surgery 1976; **Med School:** Jefferson Med Coll 1970; **Resid:** Orthopaedic Surgery, Thosd Jefferson Univ Hosp 1975; Pediatric Orthopaedic Surgery, Alfred I Du Pont Inst 1974; **Fac Appt:** Prof OrS, Jefferson Med Coll

Plancher, Kevin D MD [OrS] - **Spec Exp:** Shoulder Surgery; Elbow Surgery; Cartilage Damage & Transplant; Shoulder Replacement; **Hospital:** Beth Israel Med Ctr - Petrie Division (page 56), Lenox Hill Hosp (page 67); **Address:** 1160 Park Ave, New York, NY 10128; **Phone:** 212-876-5200; **Board Cert:** Orthopaedic Surgery 2007; Hand Surgery 2008; Orthopaedic Sports Medicine 2009; **Med School:** Georgetown Univ 1986; **Resid:** Orthopaedic Surgery, Mass Genl Hosp/Brigham & Womens Hosp 1991; **Fellow:** Hand Surgery, Indiana Hand Ctr 1993; Sports Medicine, Steadman-Hawkins Clinic 1994; **Fac Appt:** Assoc Clin Prof OrS, Albert Einstein Coll Med

Ramsey, Matthew L MD [OrS] - **Spec Exp:** Shoulder Surgery; Elbow Surgery; Sports Medicine; **Hospital:** Bucks Specialty Inst, Thomas Jefferson Univ Hosp; **Address:** Rothman Institute, 925 Chestnut St, Fl 5, Philadelphia, PA 19107; **Phone:** 800-321-9999; **Board Cert:** Orthopaedic Surgery 2009; **Med School:** SUNY Hlth Sci Ctr 1990; **Resid:** Orthopaedic Surgery, Thomas Jefferson Univ Hosp 1995; **Fellow:** Shoulder Surgery, Hosp Univ Penn 1996; **Fac Appt:** Assoc Prof OrS, Thomas Jefferson Univ

Rodosky, Mark W MD [OrS] - **Spec Exp:** Sports Medicine; Shoulder Surgery; Rotator Cuff Surgery; **Hospital:** UPMC South Side-Out Pt Ctr; **Address:** UPMC Center for Sports Medicine, 3200 S Water St, Pittsburgh, PA 15203; **Phone:** 412-432-3621; **Board Cert:** Orthopaedic Surgery 2008; Orthopaedic Sports Medicine 2011; **Med School:** Mount Sinai Sch Med 1987; **Resid:** Surgery, Univ Pittsburgh Med Ctr 1993; **Fellow:** Orthopaedic Surgery, NY Presby-Columbia Presby Med Ctr 1994; **Fac Appt:** Asst Prof OrS, Univ Pittsburgh

Rothman, Richard H MD/PhD [OrS] - **Spec Exp:** Hip Replacement; Knee Replacement; Joint Replacement; **Hospital:** Thomas Jefferson Univ Hosp; **Address:** Rothman Inst, 925 Chestnut St Fl 5, Philadelphia, PA 19107; **Phone:** 800-321-9999; **Board Cert:** Orthopaedic Surgery 1970; **Med School:** Univ Pennsylvania 1962; **Resid:** Orthopaedic Surgery, Jefferson Hosp 1968; **Fac Appt:** Prof OrS, Jefferson Med Coll

Roye Jr, David P MD [OrS] - **Spec Exp:** Pediatric Orthopaedic Surgery; Scoliosis; Hip Disorders-Pediatric; Neuromuscular Disorders; **Hospital:** Morgan Stanley Children's Hosp of NY-Presby, NY, NY-Presby/Columbia Univ Med Ctr, NY (page 66); **Address:** Morgan Stanley Chlds Hosp NewYork-Presby, 3959 Broadway, 8 North, New York, NY 10032-1559; **Phone:** 212-305-5475; **Board Cert:** Orthopaedic Surgery 1981; **Med School:** Columbia P&S 1975; **Resid:** Orthopaedic Surgery, Columbia-Presby Med Ctr 1979; **Fellow:** Orthopaedic Surgery, Hosp for Sick Chldn 1980; **Fac Appt:** Prof OrS, Columbia P&S

Rozbruch, S Robert MD [OrS] - **Spec Exp:** Limb Lengthening; Limb Deformities; Limb Surgery/Reconstruction; Fractures-Complex & Non Union; **Hospital:** Hosp For Special Surgery (page 60), NY-Presby/Weill Cornell Med Ctr, NY (page 66); **Address:** Hospital for Special Surgery, 535 E 70th St, River Terr Bldg - Fl 2 - Ste 204, New York, NY 10021; **Phone:** 212-606-1415; **Board Cert:** Orthopaedic Surgery 2009; **Med School:** Cornell Univ-Weill Med Coll 1990; **Resid:** Orthopaedic Surgery, Hosp Special Surgery 1995; **Fellow:** Trauma, Univ Bern Hosp 1997; Limb Lengthening, Intl Ctr Limb Length/Univ MD 1999; **Fac Appt:** Prof OrS, Cornell Univ-Weill Med Coll

Salvati, Eduardo A MD [OrS] - **Spec Exp:** Hip Replacement; Knee Replacement; **Hospital:** Hosp For Special Surgery (page 60); **Address:** Hosp for Spec Surg, 535 E 70th Street, New York, NY 10021; **Phone:** 212-606-1472; **Board Cert:** Orthopaedic Surgery 1972; **Med School:** Argentina 1963; **Resid:** Orthopaedic Surgery, Univ Florence Ortho Clinic 1965; Orthopaedic Surgery, Hosp Buenos Aires 1969; **Fellow:** Hip Surgery, Hosp For Spec Surg 1972; **Fac Appt:** Clin Prof OrS, Cornell Univ-Weill Med Coll

Sandhu, Harvinder S MD [OrS] - **Spec Exp:** Minimally Invasive Surgery; Spinal Disc Replacement; Spinal Surgery; **Hospital:** Hosp For Special Surgery (page 60); **Address:** Hosp for Special Surgery, 523 E 72nd St, New York, NY 10021; **Phone:** 212-606-1798; **Board Cert:** Orthopaedic Surgery 2007; **Med School:** Northwestern Univ 1987; **Resid:** Orthopaedic Surgery, Univ Hosp-SUNY Hlth Sci Ctr 1992; **Fellow:** Spinal Surgery, UCLA Med Ctr 1993; **Fac Appt:** Assoc Prof OrS, Cornell Univ-Weill Med Coll

Schmidt, Richard G MD [OrS] - **Spec Exp:** Bone Tumors; Sarcoma-Soft Tissue; Limb Sparing Surgery; Bone Tumors-Metastatic; **Hospital:** Lankenau Hosp, Fox Chase Cancer Ctr (page 58); **Address:** 15 N Presidential Blvd, Ste 300, Bala Cynwyd, PA 19004; **Phone:** 610-667-2663; **Board Cert:** Orthopaedic Surgery 2009; **Med School:** Penn State Coll Med 1980; **Resid:** Orthopaedic Surgery, Hosp Univ Penn 1985; **Fellow:** Orthopaedic Oncology, Shands Hosp 1986

Schwab, Frank J MD [OrS] - **Spec Exp:** Spinal Surgery; Pain-Back; Spinal Deformity; Scoliosis; **Hospital:** NYU Hosp For Joint Diseases (page 70), New York Methodist Hosp; **Address:** 306 E 15th St, Ste 1F, New York, NY 10003; **Phone:** 646-794-8646; **Board Cert:** Orthopaedic Surgery 2010; **Med School:** Columbia P&S 1990; **Resid:** Surgery, NY Presby-Columbia Med Ctr 1992; Orthopaedic Surgery, NY Presby-Columbia Med Ctr 1996; **Fellow:** Orthopaedic Surgery, Hospital Lariboisiere 1991; Spinal Surgery, Maimonides Med Ctr 1997; **Fac Appt:** Clin Prof OrS, NYU Sch Med

Scott, W Norman MD [OrS] - **Spec Exp:** Knee Injuries; Knee Replacement; Sports Medicine; **Hospital:** Lenox Hill Hosp (page 67); **Address:** 210 E 64th St Fl 4, New York, NY 10065; **Phone:** 646-293-7501; **Board Cert:** Orthopaedic Surgery 1978; **Med School:** Cornell Univ-Weill Med Coll 1972; **Resid:** Surgery, St Lukes-Roosevelt Hosp Ctr 1974; Orthopaedic Surgery, Hosp Special Surg 1977; **Fac Appt:** Clin Prof OrS, Cornell Univ-Weill Med Coll

Sharkey, Peter F MD [OrS] - **Spec Exp:** Hip Replacement; Knee Replacement; **Hospital:** Thomas Jefferson Univ Hosp, Riddle Meml Hosp; **Address:** Rothman Inst, 925 Chestnut St Fl 5, Philadelphia, PA 19107; **Phone:** 800-321-9999; **Board Cert:** Orthopaedic Surgery 2003; **Med School:** SUNY Upstate Med Univ 1984; **Resid:** Orthopaedic Surgery, Thomas Jefferson Univ Hosp 1990; **Fellow:** Hip & Knee Surgery, Rothman Inst; **Fac Appt:** Prof OrS, Thomas Jefferson Univ

Spivak, Jeffrey M MD [OrS] - **Spec Exp:** Spinal Surgery; Scoliosis; Sports Medicine Back Injuries; **Hospital:** NYU Hosp For Joint Diseases (page 70), NYU Langone Med Ctr (page 68); **Address:** Hosp for Joint Diseases, Spine Ctr, 301 E 17th St, Ste 400, New York, NY 10003-3804; **Phone:** 212-598-6696; **Board Cert:** Orthopaedic Surgery 2006; **Med School:** Cornell Univ-Weill Med Coll 1986; **Resid:** Orthopaedic Surgery, Hosp for Joint Diseases 1992; **Fellow:** Spinal Surgery, Thomas Jefferson Univ Hosp 1993; **Fac Appt:** Asst Prof OrS, NYU Sch Med

Sponseller, Paul D MD [OrS] - **Spec Exp:** Cerebral Palsy; Scoliosis; Pediatric Orthopaedic Surgery; **Hospital:** Johns Hopkins Hosp (page 61); **Address:** 601 N Caroline St, Ste 5212, Baltimore, MD 21287-0882; **Phone:** 410-955-3136; **Board Cert:** Orthopaedic Surgery 2010; **Med School:** Univ Mich Med Sch 1980; **Resid:** Orthopaedic Surgery, Univ Wisc Hosp 1985; **Fellow:** Pediatric Orthopaedic Surgery, Children's Hosp 1986; **Fac Appt:** Prof OrS, Johns Hopkins Univ

Orthopaedic Surgery

Strongwater, Allan M MD [OrS] - **Spec Exp:** Pediatric Orthopaedic Surgery; Cerebral Palsy; Deformity Reconstruction; **Hospital:** St. Joseph's Regl Med Ctr - Paterson, NYU Langone Med Ctr (page 68); **Address:** St Josephs Childrens Hospital, Dept Orthopaedic Surgery, 703 Main St - Xavier 702, Paterson, NJ 07503; **Phone:** 973-754-2414; **Board Cert:** Orthopaedic Surgery 2007; **Med School:** Rush Med Coll 1978; **Resid:** Orthopaedic Surgery, Yale-New Haven Hosp 1983; **Fellow:** Pediatric Orthopaedic Surgery, Hosp Joint Diseases 1984; **Fac Appt:** Clin Prof OrS, NYU Sch Med

Stuchin, Steven MD [OrS] - **Spec Exp:** Hand Surgery; Arthritis; Hip & Knee Replacement; Hip Resurfacing; **Hospital:** NYU Hosp For Joint Diseases (page 70), Lenox Hill Hosp (page 67); **Address:** 333 E 38th St, New York, NY 10016; **Phone:** 212-598-6708; **Board Cert:** Orthopaedic Surgery 1984; **Med School:** Columbia P&S 1976; **Resid:** Surgery, Roosevelt Hosp 1978; Orthopaedic Surgery, Hosp for Special Surg 1981; **Fellow:** Hand Surgery, Thomas Jefferson Univ Hosp 1982; **Fac Appt:** Assoc Prof OrS, NYU Sch Med

Vaccaro, Alexander R MD/PhD [OrS] - **Spec Exp:** Spinal Surgery; Spinal Trauma; Spinal Cord Injury; **Hospital:** Thomas Jefferson Univ Hosp; **Address:** 925 Chestnut St Fl 5, Philadelphia, PA 19107; **Phone:** 800-321-9999; **Board Cert:** Orthopaedic Surgery 2006; **Med School:** Georgetown Univ 1987; **Resid:** Orthopaedic Surgery, Thos Jefferson Univ Hosp 1992; **Fellow:** Spinal Surgery, UCSD Med Ctr 1993; **Fac Appt:** Prof OrS, Thomas Jefferson Univ

Wapner, Keith L MD [OrS] - **Spec Exp:** Foot & Ankle Surgery; Tendon Surgery; Arthritis; **Hospital:** Pennsylvania Hosp-UPHS (page 72); **Address:** 230 W Washington Square, The Farm Journal Bldg Fl 5, Philadelphia, PA 19106-3500; **Phone:** 215-829-3668; **Board Cert:** Orthopaedic Surgery 2009; **Med School:** Temple Univ 1980; **Resid:** Surgery, Hosp Univ Penn 1981; Orthopaedic Surgery, Hosp Univ Penn 1985; **Fellow:** Joint Reconstruction, Ohio St Univ Med Ctr 1986; Foot & Ankle Surgery, UCSF Med Ctr 1987

Warren, Russell MD [OrS] - **Spec Exp:** Knee Injuries/Ligament Surgery; Shoulder Surgery; Shoulder Replacement; Rotator Cuff Surgery; **Hospital:** Hosp For Special Surgery (page 60); **Address:** 535 E 70th St, New York, NY 10021-4892; **Phone:** 212-606-1178; **Board Cert:** Orthopaedic Surgery 1974; **Med School:** SUNY Upstate Med Univ 1966; **Resid:** Surgery, St Lukes Hosp 1968; Orthopaedic Surgery, Hosp For Special Surgery 1973; **Fellow:** Shoulder Surgery, Columbia-Presby Med Ctr 1977; **Fac Appt:** Prof OrS, Cornell Univ-Weill Med Coll

Weinfeld, Steven B MD [OrS] - **Spec Exp:** Foot & Ankle Surgery; Diabetic Leg/Foot; **Hospital:** Mount Sinai Med Ctr (page 64), Hackensack Univ Med Ctr; **Address:** 5 E 98th St Fl 9, Box 1188, New York, NY 10029; **Phone:** 212-241-1634; **Board Cert:** Orthopaedic Surgery 2009; **Med School:** Albany Med Coll 1990; **Resid:** Orthopaedic Surgery, Albany Med Ctr 1995; **Fellow:** Ankle and Foot Surgery, Union Meml Hosp 1996; **Fac Appt:** Assoc Prof OrS, Mount Sinai Sch Med

Westrich, Geoffrey H MD [OrS] - **Spec Exp:** Hip Replacement & Revision; Knee Replacement & Revision; Arthroscopic Surgery-Hip; Arthroscopic Surgery-Knee; **Hospital:** Hosp For Special Surgery (page 60), NY-Presby/Weill Cornell Med Ctr, NY (page 66); **Address:** Hospital for Special Surgery, 535 E 70th St, New York, NY 10021; **Phone:** 212-606-1510; **Board Cert:** Orthopaedic Surgery 2009; **Med School:** Tufts Univ 1990; **Resid:** Orthopaedic Surgery, Hosp for Special Surg 1995; **Fellow:** Trauma, Inselspital 1995; Adult Reconstructive Surgery, Hosp for Special Surg 1996; **Fac Appt:** Assoc Prof OrS, Cornell Univ-Weill Med Coll

Wetzel, F Todd MD [OrS] - **Spec Exp:** Spinal Surgery; Minimally Invasive Surgery; **Hospital:** Temple Univ Hosp, Jeanes Hosp; **Address:** Temple Univ Hosp Fl 5, 3509 N Broad St, Philadelphia, PA 19140; **Phone:** 215-707-2111; **Board Cert:** Orthopaedic Surgery 2011; **Med School:** Univ Pennsylvania 1981; **Resid:** Surgery, Yale-New Haven Hosp 1983; Orthopaedic Surgery, Yale Univ Affil Hosps 1986; **Fellow:** Spinal Surgery, Dr Henry LaRocca 1987; **Fac Appt:** Prof OrS, Temple Univ

Wickiewicz, Thomas L MD [OrS] - **Spec Exp:** Knee Injuries/ACL; Sports Medicine; Shoulder Surgery; Rotator Cuff Surgery; **Hospital:** Hosp For Special Surgery (page 60), NY-Presby/Weill Cornell Med Ctr, NY (page 66); **Address:** 535 E 70th St, New York, NY 10021; **Phone:** 212-606-1450; **Board Cert:** Orthopaedic Surgery 1984; **Med School:** UMDNJ-NJ Med Sch, Newark 1976; **Resid:** Orthopaedic Surgery, Hosp for Special Surg 1981; **Fellow:** Sports Medicine, UCLA Med Ctr 1982; **Fac Appt:** Clin Prof OrS, Cornell Univ-Weill Med Coll

Wiesel, Sam W MD [OrS] - **Spec Exp:** Spinal Surgery; **Hospital:** Georgetown Univ Hosp; **Address:** 3800 Reservoir Rd NW, PHC Bldg Fl Ground, Washington, DC 20007-2113; **Phone:** 202-444-8766 x2; **Board Cert:** Orthopaedic Surgery 1977; **Med School:** Univ Pennsylvania 1971; **Resid:** Orthopaedic Surgery, Hosp Univ Penn 1976; **Fellow:** Orthopaedic Surgery, Hosp Univ Penn 1973; **Fac Appt:** Prof OrS, Georgetown Univ

Williams, Gerald MD [OrS] - **Spec Exp:** Shoulder Reconstruction; Shoulder Cartilage Implant; Shoulder Replacement; Rotator Cuff Surgery; **Hospital:** Thomas Jefferson Univ Hosp, Methodist Hosp; **Address:** 925 Chestnut St Fl 5, Philadelphia, PA 19107; **Phone:** 800-321-9999; **Board Cert:** Orthopaedic Surgery 2003; **Med School:** Temple Univ 1984; **Resid:** Orthopaedic Surgery, UT San Antonio Affil Hosp 1989; **Fellow:** Shoulder Surgery, UT San Antonio Affil Hosp 1990; **Fac Appt:** Prof OrS, Thomas Jefferson Univ

Wittig, James C MD [OrS] - **Spec Exp:** Bone Tumors; Sarcoma-Soft Tissue; Hip & Knee Replacement; Shoulder Tumors; **Hospital:** Mount Sinai Med Ctr (page 64), Hackensack Univ Med Ctr; **Address:** 5 E 98th St, Fl 9, New York, NY 10029; **Phone:** 212-241-1807 x4817; **Board Cert:** Orthopaedic Surgery 2003; **Med School:** NYU Sch Med 1994; **Resid:** Orthopaedic Surgery, Columbia Presby Med Ctr 1999; **Fellow:** Orthopaedic Oncology, Washington Cancer Inst 2001; Orthopaedic Oncology, NIH 2001; **Fac Appt:** Assoc Prof OrS, Mount Sinai Sch Med

Zuckerman, Joseph D MD [OrS] - **Spec Exp:** Shoulder Surgery; Hip Replacement; Knee Replacement; Rotator Cuff Surgery; **Hospital:** NYU Hosp For Joint Diseases (page 70), NYU Langone Med Ctr (page 68); **Address:** NYU Hosp for Joint Diseases, Dept Ortho Surg, 301 E 17th St Fl 14 - Ste 1402, New York, NY 10003; **Phone:** 212-598-6674; **Board Cert:** Orthopaedic Surgery 2007; **Med School:** Med Coll Wisc 1978; **Resid:** Orthopaedic Surgery, Univ WA Med Ctr 1983; **Fellow:** Arthritis Surgery, Brigham & Womans Hosp 1984; Shoulder Surgery, Mayo Clinic 1984; **Fac Appt:** Prof OrS, NYU Sch Med

Southeast

Beaty, James H MD [OrS] - **Spec Exp:** Pediatric Orthopaedic Surgery; Clubfoot; Fractures-Pediatric; **Hospital:** Le Bonheur Chldns Med Ctr; **Address:** Campbell Clinic, 1400 S Germantown Rd, Germantown, TN 38138; **Phone:** 901-759-3125; **Board Cert:** Orthopaedic Surgery 2007; **Med School:** Univ Tenn Coll Med 1976; **Resid:** Surgery, Baptist Meml Hosp 1979; Orthopaedic Surgery, Campbell Clin Fdn 1981; **Fellow:** Pediatric Orthopaedic Surgery, Alfred I Dupont Inst 1982; **Fac Appt:** Prof OrS, Univ Tenn Coll Med

Berrey, B Hudson MD [OrS] - **Spec Exp:** Musculoskeletal Tumors; Bone Cancer; Soft Tissue Tumors; Sarcoma; **Hospital:** Shands Jacksonville Med Ctr, St. Vincent's Med Ctr - Riverside (Jacksonville); **Address:** Bone and Joint Institute, 4555 Emerson St, Ste 100, Jacksonville, FL 32207; **Phone:** 904-633-0150; **Board Cert:** Orthopaedic Surgery 1982; **Med School:** Univ Tex Med Br, Galveston 1977; **Resid:** Orthopaedic Surgery, Tripler Army Med Ctr 1981; **Fellow:** Medical Oncology, Mass Genl Hosp/Harvard 1985; **Fac Appt:** Prof OrS, Univ Fla Coll Med

Orthopaedic Surgery

Boden, Scott D MD [OrS] - **Spec Exp:** Spinal Disorders; Spinal Surgery; Spinal Disc Replacement; Microdiscectomy; **Hospital:** Emory Univ Hosp; **Address:** Emory Orthopaedics & Spine Center, 59 Executive Park South, Ste 3000, Atlanta, GA 30329; **Phone:** 404-778-7143; **Board Cert:** Orthopaedic Surgery 2005; **Med School:** Univ Pennsylvania 1986; **Resid:** Orthopaedic Surgery, Geo Washington Univ Hosp 1991; **Fellow:** Spinal Surgery, Case Western Reserve Univ 1992; **Fac Appt:** Prof OrS, Emory Univ

Curl, Walton W MD [OrS] - **Spec Exp:** Sports Medicine; Adolescent Sports Medicine; **Hospital:** Wake Forest Baptist Med Ctr; **Address:** 131 Miller St, Winston-Salem, NC 27103; **Phone:** 336-716-8091; **Board Cert:** Orthopaedic Surgery 1980; **Med School:** Duke Univ 1973; **Resid:** Orthopaedic Surgery, Letterman Army Med Ctr 1978; **Fellow:** Sports Medicine, Keller Army Hosp 1979; **Fac Appt:** Prof OrS, Wake Forest Univ

DeOrio, James K MD [OrS] - **Spec Exp:** Ankle Replacement & Revision; Foot & Ankle Surgery; Foot Deformities; **Hospital:** Duke Univ Hosp; **Address:** 4709 Creekstone Drive, Ste 200, Durham, NC 27703; **Phone:** 919-613-7797; **Board Cert:** Orthopaedic Surgery 1983; **Med School:** Geo Wash Univ 1977; **Resid:** Orthopaedic Surgery, Mayo Clinic 1982; **Fellow:** Orthopaedic Surgery, Chur Hosp 1983; **Fac Appt:** Assoc Prof OrS, Duke Univ

Diduch, David R MD [OrS] - **Spec Exp:** Sports Medicine; Knee Injuries/ACL; Shoulder Reconstruction; Rotator Cuff Surgery; **Hospital:** Univ of Virginia Health Sys; **Address:** Univ Virginia Dept Ortho Surg, Box 800159, Charlottesville, VA 22908; **Phone:** 434-243-0274; **Board Cert:** Orthopaedic Surgery 2008; Orthopaedic Sports Medicine 2009; **Med School:** Harvard Med Sch 1988; **Resid:** Orthopaedic Surgery, Univ Virginia Med Ctr 1994; **Fellow:** Sports Medicine, Insall-Scott-Kelly Inst 1995; **Fac Appt:** Prof OrS, Univ VA Sch Med

Eismont, Frank J MD [OrS] - **Spec Exp:** Spinal Surgery; Spinal Tumors; Spinal Trauma; **Hospital:** Jackson Meml Hosp, Univ of Miami Hosp; **Address:** Univ Miami Dept Orthopaedic Surg, PO Box 016960 (D-27), Miami, FL 33101-6960; **Phone:** 305-243-3000; **Board Cert:** Orthopaedic Surgery 2007; **Med School:** Univ Rochester 1973; **Resid:** Orthopaedic Surgery, Univ Hosp 1978; **Fellow:** Spinal Surgery, Case Western Res Univ 1979; Spinal Surgery, Pennsylvania Hosp 1980; **Fac Appt:** Prof OrS, Univ Miami Sch Med

Estwanik, Joseph J MD [OrS] - **Spec Exp:** Knee Surgery; **Hospital:** Carolinas Specialty Hosp; **Address:** Metrolina Ortho & Sports Med Clinic, 335 Bellingsley Rd, Ste 201, Charlotte, NC 28211; **Phone:** 704-334-4663; **Board Cert:** Orthopaedic Surgery 1979; **Med School:** Wake Forest Univ 1973; **Resid:** Orthopaedic Surgery, Cleveland Clinic 1976; Orthopaedic Surgery, North Carolina Baptist Hosp 1978; **Fac Appt:** Asst Prof OrS, Wake Forest Univ

Garrett Jr, William E MD/PhD [OrS] - **Spec Exp:** Sports Medicine; Knee Surgery; Knee Reconstruction; Arthroscopic Surgery; **Hospital:** Duke Univ Hosp; **Address:** Box 3338 Med Ctr, 305 Finch Yeager Bldg, Durham, NC 27710; **Phone:** 919-684-5678; **Board Cert:** Orthopaedic Surgery 2007; Orthopaedic Sports Medicine 2007; **Med School:** Duke Univ 1976; **Resid:** Orthopaedic Surgery, Duke Univ Med Ctr 1982; **Fac Appt:** Prof OrS, Duke Univ

Goldner, Richard D MD [OrS] - **Spec Exp:** Hand & Wrist Surgery; Hand & Wrist Reconstrction; Arthroscopic Surgery-Wrist; **Hospital:** Duke Univ Hosp; **Address:** Box 3480 Med Ctr, 5431 Hosp South, Orange Zone, Durham, NC 27710; **Phone:** 919-684-6461; **Board Cert:** Orthopaedic Surgery 1982; Hand Surgery 2000; **Med School:** Duke Univ 1974; **Resid:** Orthopaedic Surgery, Univ Virginia Med Ctr 1980; Surgery, Duke Univ Med Ctr 1976; **Fellow:** Hand Surgery, Duke Univ Med Ctr 1981; **Fac Appt:** Assoc Prof OrS, Duke Univ

Jiranek, William A MD [OrS] - **Spec Exp:** Knee Replacement; Arthritis; Minimally Invasive Surgery; Hip Replacement; **Hospital:** Med Coll of VA Hosp; **Address:** MCV Dept Orthopaedic Surgery, 9000 Stony Point Pkwy, Richmond, VA 23235; **Phone:** 804-228-4155; **Board Cert:** Orthopaedic Surgery 2005; **Med School:** Univ VA Sch Med 1985; **Resid:** Orthopaedic Surgery, Tufts Combined Program 1991; **Fellow:** Orthopaedic Surgery, Mass Genl Hosp/Harvard 1992; **Fac Appt:** Assoc Prof OrS, Med Coll VA

Johnson, Darren L MD [OrS] - **Spec Exp:** Knee Injuries; Sports Medicine; Knee Ligament Reconstruction; Arthroscopic Surgery; **Hospital:** Univ of Kentucky Albert B. Chandler Hosp; **Address:** Kentucky Clinic-Dept Orthopedic Surgery, 740 S Limestone, Ste K-401, Lexington, KY 40536-0284; **Phone:** 859-257-4969; **Board Cert:** Orthopaedic Surgery 2006; Orthopaedic Sports Medicine 2007; **Med School:** UCLA 1987; **Resid:** Orthopaedic Surgery, LAC-USC Med Ctr 1992; **Fellow:** Sports Medicine, Univ Pittsburgh 1993; **Fac Appt:** Prof OrS, Univ KY Coll Med

Karas, Spero G MD [OrS] - **Spec Exp:** Sports Medicine; Shoulder Injuries; Knee Injuries/ACL/Meniscus Tears; Cartilage Damage; **Hospital:** Emory Univ Hosp; **Address:** Emory Orthopaedics & Sports Medicine, 59 Executive Park South, Ste 1000, Atlanta, GA 30329; **Phone:** 404-778-7204; **Board Cert:** Orthopaedic Surgery 2002; Orthopaedic Sports Medicine 2008; **Med School:** Indiana Univ 1993; **Resid:** Orthopaedic Surgery, Duke Univ Med Ctr 1999; **Fellow:** Orthopaedic Surgery, Steadman Hawkins Clinic 2000; **Fac Appt:** Assoc Prof OrS, Emory Univ

Kneisl, Jeffrey S MD [OrS] - **Spec Exp:** Bone Cancer; Musculoskeletal Tumors; **Hospital:** Carolinas Med Ctr; **Address:** 1025 Morhead Medical Drive, Ste 300, Charlotte, NC 28204; **Phone:** 704-355-5982; **Board Cert:** Orthopaedic Surgery 2010; **Med School:** Northwestern Univ 1980; **Resid:** Orthopaedic Surgery, Northwestern Univ 1987; **Fellow:** Orthopaedic Oncology, Univ Chicago Med Ctr 1990

Kress, Kenneth J MD [OrS] - **Spec Exp:** Knee Replacement; Knee Reconstruction; Sports Medicine; **Hospital:** St. Joseph's Hosp - Atlanta; **Address:** Resergens Orthopaedics, 5671 Peachtree Dunwoody Rd NE, Ste 900, Atlanta, GA 30342; **Phone:** 404-847-9999; **Board Cert:** Orthopaedic Surgery 2004; **Med School:** Cornell Univ 1985; **Resid:** Orthopaedic Surgery, Hosp for Special Surg 1990; **Fellow:** Knee Reconstruction, Dr John C Garrett 1991

Lebwohl, Nathan H MD [OrS] - **Spec Exp:** Spinal Surgery; Spinal Deformity; Scoliosis; **Hospital:** Jackson Meml Hosp; **Address:** Univ Miami, Dept Orthopaedic Surgery, PO Box 016960, Miami, FL 33101-6960; **Phone:** 305-585-8225; **Board Cert:** Orthopaedic Surgery 2012; **Med School:** Harvard Med Sch 1983; **Resid:** Surgery, Mt Sinai Hosp 1985; Orthopaedic Surgery, Columbia-Presby Med Ctr 1988; **Fellow:** Spinal Surgery, Univ Louisville 1989; **Fac Appt:** Assoc Prof OrS, Univ Miami Sch Med

Miller, Mark D MD [OrS] - **Spec Exp:** Sports Medicine; Knee Ligament Reconstruction; Knee Cartilage/Meniscus Transplants; Shoulder Arthroscopic Surgery; **Hospital:** Univ of Virginia Health Sys; **Address:** Univ Virginia Dept Ortho Surg, Box 800159, Charlottesville, VA 22908; **Phone:** 434-982-4832; **Board Cert:** Orthopaedic Surgery 2006; Orthopaedic Sports Medicine 2007; **Med School:** Uniformed Srvs Univ, Bethesda 1987; **Resid:** Orthopaedic Surgery, Wilford Hall USAF Med Ctr 1992; **Fellow:** Shoulder Surgery, Univ Pittsburgh 1993; Sports Medicine, Univ Pittsburgh 1993; **Fac Appt:** Prof OrS, Univ VA Sch Med

Nunley II, James A MD [OrS] - **Spec Exp:** Foot & Ankle Surgery; Ankle Replacement & Revision; Arthritis; Sports Injuries-Foot & Ankle; **Hospital:** Duke Univ Hosp; **Address:** Duke University Med Ctr, Box 2923, Durham, NC 27710-0001; **Phone:** 919-684-4033; **Board Cert:** Orthopaedic Surgery 1981; **Med School:** Tulane Univ 1973; **Resid:** Orthopaedic Surgery, Duke Univ Med Ctr 1979; **Fellow:** Hand Surgery, Duke Univ Med Ctr 1980; **Fac Appt:** Prof OrS, Duke Univ

Orthopaedic Surgery

Paley, Dror MD [OrS] - **Spec Exp:** Limb Lengthening (Ilizarov Procedure); Limb Deformities; Pediatric Orthopaedic Surgery; **Hospital:** St. Mary's Med Ctr - W Palm Bch; **Address:** 901 45th St, Kimmel Bldg, West Palm Beach, FL 33407; **Phone:** 561-844-5255; **Board Cert:** Orthopaedic Surgery 2010; **Med School:** Univ Toronto 1979; **Resid:** Orthopaedic Surgery, Univ Toronto Hosp 1985; **Fellow:** Hand Surgery, Sunny Brook Hosp 1986; Pediatric Orthopaedic Surgery, Hosp for Sick Children 1987

Pettrone, Frank A MD [OrS] - **Spec Exp:** Sports Medicine; Shoulder & Knee Surgery; **Hospital:** Virginia Hosp Ctr - Arlington; **Address:** Commonwealth Ortho & Rehabilitation, 1635 N George Mason Drive, Ste 310, Arlington, VA 22205-3616; **Phone:** 703-525-6100; **Board Cert:** Orthopaedic Surgery 1975; **Med School:** Georgetown Univ 1969; **Resid:** Orthopaedic Surgery, Georgetown Hosp 1974; **Fac Appt:** Clin Prof OrS, Georgetown Univ

Poehling, Gary G MD [OrS] - **Spec Exp:** Hand Surgery; Arthroscopic Surgery; Sports Medicine; **Hospital:** Wake Forest Baptist Med Ctr; **Address:** Wake Forest Medical Ctr, Comp Rehab Plaza, 131 Miller St, Winston-Salem, NC 27103; **Phone:** 336-716-8091; **Board Cert:** Orthopaedic Surgery 1977; **Med School:** Marquette Sch Med 1968; **Resid:** Surgery, Duke Univ Med Ctr 1970; Orthopaedic Surgery, Duke Univ Med Ctr 1976; **Fac Appt:** Prof OrS, Wake Forest Univ

Richardson, William J MD [OrS] - **Spec Exp:** Spinal Surgery; Spinal Deformity; Spinal Disc Replacement; Spinal Trauma; **Hospital:** Duke Univ Hosp; **Address:** Box 3077 Med Ctr, 5340 Duke South, Orange Zone, Durham, NC 27710; **Phone:** 919-684-5711; **Board Cert:** Orthopaedic Surgery 2010; **Med School:** Eastern VA Med Sch 1979; **Resid:** Orthopaedic Surgery, Duke Univ Med Ctr 1986; **Fellow:** Spinal Surgery, Totonto General Hosp 1987; **Fac Appt:** Prof OrS, Duke Univ

Scarborough, Mark T MD [OrS] - **Spec Exp:** Bone Tumors; Sarcoma; **Hospital:** Shands at Univ of FL; **Address:** Shands Healthcare Univ FL, 3450 Hull Rd, Gainesville, FL 32611-2733; **Phone:** 352-273-7000; **Board Cert:** Orthopaedic Surgery 2004; **Med School:** Univ Fla Coll Med 1985; **Resid:** Orthopaedic Surgery, Univ Texas Med Ctr 1990; **Fellow:** Orthopaedic Surgery, Mass Genl Hosp 1991; **Fac Appt:** Prof OrS, Univ Fla Coll Med

Schuler, Thomas C MD [OrS] - **Spec Exp:** Spinal Surgery-Cervical; Spinal Surgery-Low Back; Sports Medicine Back Injuries; **Hospital:** Reston Hosp Ctr; **Address:** Virginia Spine Inst, 1831 Wiehle Ave, rm 200, Reston, VA 20190; **Phone:** 703-709-1114; **Board Cert:** Orthopaedic Surgery 2005; **Med School:** Indiana Univ 1986; **Resid:** Surgery, William Beaumont Hosp 1987; **Fellow:** Orthopaedic Surgery, William Beaumont Hosp 1991; Spinal Surgery, Kerlan-Jobe Orth Clinic

Schwartz, Herbert S MD [OrS] - **Spec Exp:** Bone Tumors-Metastatic; Bone Tumors; Pelvic Surgery-Complex; Musculoskeletal Tumors; **Hospital:** Vanderbilt Univ Med Ctr (page 75), Baptist Hosp - Nashville; **Address:** Vanderbilt Orthopaedic Institute, 1215 21st Ave S, Medical Ctr East, South Tower, Ste 4200, Nashville, TN 37232-8774; **Phone:** 615-343-8612; **Board Cert:** Orthopaedic Surgery 2007; **Med School:** Univ Chicago-Pritzker Sch Med 1981; **Resid:** Orthopaedic Surgery, Univ Chicago Hosps 1986; **Fellow:** Orthopaedic Oncology, Mayo Clinic 1987; **Fac Appt:** Prof OrS, Vanderbilt Univ

Siegel, Herrick J MD [OrS] - **Spec Exp:** Hip & Knee Replacement; Bone & Soft Tissue Tumors; Shoulder Replacement; Bone Tumors-Metastatic; **Hospital:** Univ of Ala Hosp at Birmingham, UAB Highlands Hosp; **Address:** 1313 13th St S, Birmingham, AL 35205; **Phone:** 205-930-8554; **Board Cert:** Orthopaedic Surgery 2005; **Med School:** NYU Sch Med 1995; **Resid:** Orthopaedic Surgery, USC Univ Hosp 2000; **Fellow:** Orthopaedic Oncology, Mayo Clinic 2002; **Fac Appt:** Assoc Prof OrS, Univ Alabama

Spengler, Dan M MD [OrS] - **Spec Exp:** Spinal Surgery; **Hospital:** Vanderbilt Univ Med Ctr (page 75); **Address:** Vanderbilt Orthopedic Inst, Medical Center E, South Tower, rm 4200, Nashville, TN 37232-8774; **Phone:** 615-343-6364; **Board Cert:** Orthopaedic Surgery 1988; **Med School:** Univ Mich Med Sch 1966; **Resid:** Orthopaedic Surgery, Univ Mich Med Ctr 1968; Orthopaedic Surgery, Univ Mich Med Ctr 1973; **Fellow:** Orthopaedic Surgery, Case West Res Hosps 1974; **Fac Appt:** Prof OrS, Vanderbilt Univ

Spindler, Kurt P MD [OrS] - **Spec Exp:** Sports Medicine; Ligament Reconstruction; Arthroscopic Surgery; Adolescent Sports Medicine; **Hospital:** Vanderbilt Univ Med Ctr (page 75); **Address:** Vanderbilt Orthopaedic Inst, Medical Center E, rm 4200, Nashville, TN 37232-8774; **Phone:** 615-343-6364; **Board Cert:** Orthopaedic Surgery 2004; Orthopaedic Sports Medicine 2007; **Med School:** Univ Pennsylvania 1985; **Resid:** Orthopaedic Surgery, Hosp Univ Penn 1990; **Fellow:** Sports Medicine, Cleveland Clinic Fdn 1991; **Fac Appt:** Prof OrS, Vanderbilt Univ

Vo, Phuc MD [OrS] - **Spec Exp:** Sports Medicine; Arthroscopic Surgery; Minimally Invasive Surgery; Joint Replacement; **Hospital:** Lakeland Regl Med Ctr; **Address:** Watson Clinic, 1600 Lakeland Hills Blvd, Lakeland, FL 33805; **Phone:** 863-680-7214; **Board Cert:** Orthopaedic Surgery 2007; Orthopaedic Sports Medicine 2007; **Med School:** Univ Fla Coll Med 1986; **Resid:** Pathology, Univ Fla/Shands Hosp 1988; Orthopaedic Surgery, Univ Fla/Shands Hosp 1993; **Fellow:** Adult Orthopedic Surgery, Univ Fla/Shands Hosp 1993; Sports Medicine, Univ Penn Sports Med Ctr 1994; **Fac Appt:** OrS, Univ Fla Coll Med

Walling, Arthur K MD [OrS] - **Spec Exp:** Bone Tumors; Soft Tissue Tumors; Foot & Ankle Surgery; **Hospital:** Tampa Genl Hosp; **Address:** Florida Orthopaedic Inst, 13020 Telecom Pkwy N, Tampa, FL 33637; **Phone:** 813-978-9700; **Board Cert:** Orthopaedic Surgery 1982; **Med School:** Creighton Univ 1976; **Resid:** Orthopaedic Surgery, Univ South Florida Affil Hosps 1980; **Fellow:** Surgical Oncology, Univ Florida 1981; **Fac Appt:** Assoc Clin Prof OrS, Univ S Fla Coll Med

Ward Sr, William G MD [OrS] - **Spec Exp:** Bone Tumors; Soft Tissue Tumors; Reconstructive Surgery, Sarcoma; **Hospital:** Wake Forest Baptist Med Ctr; **Address:** First Floor Comp Rehab, 131 Miller St, Winston-Salem, NC 27103; **Phone:** 336-716-8093; **Board Cert:** Orthopaedic Surgery 2004; **Med School:** Duke Univ 1975; **Resid:** Surgery, Duke Univ Med Ctr 1985; Orthopaedic Surgery, Duke Univ Med Ctr 1989; **Fellow:** Sports Medicine, Cleveland Clinic 1990; Orthopaedic Oncology, UCLA Med Ctr 1991; **Fac Appt:** Prof OrS, Wake Forest Univ

Webb, Lawrence X MD [OrS] - **Spec Exp:** Trauma; Pelvic & Acetabular Fractures; Fractures-Complex & Non Union; Musculoskeletal Infections; **Hospital:** Med Ctr of Central GA; **Address:** 840 Pine St, Ste 500, Macon, GA 31201; **Phone:** 478-633-8682; **Board Cert:** Orthopaedic Surgery 2007; **Med School:** Temple Univ 1978; **Resid:** Orthopaedic Surgery, Bowman Gray Affil Hosp 1983; **Fellow:** Trauma, Harborview Med Ctr 1984; **Fac Appt:** Prof OrS, Mercer Univ Sch Med

Weiner, Richard L MD [OrS] - **Spec Exp:** Trauma; Knee Replacement; Knee Reconstruction; Hip Replacement; **Hospital:** St. Mary's Med Ctr - W Palm Bch, Palm Beach Gardens Med Ctr; **Address:** Orthopaedic Care Specialists, 733 US Highway 1, North Palm Beach, FL 33408-4508; **Phone:** 561-840-1090; **Board Cert:** Orthopaedic Surgery 2004; **Med School:** Univ Pennsylvania 1986; **Resid:** Orthopaedic Surgery, UMDNJ-Univ Hosp 1991

Midwest

Albright, John P MD [OrS] - **Spec Exp:** Sports Medicine; **Hospital:** Univ Iowa Hosp & Clinics; **Address:** UI Inst Orthopaedics, Sports Med & Rehab, 2701 Prairie Meadow Drive, Iowa City, IA 52242; **Phone:** 319-384-7070; **Board Cert:** Orthopaedic Surgery 2007; **Med School:** Loyola Univ-Stritch Sch Med 1967; **Resid:** Orthopaedic Surgery, Yale-New Haven Hosp 1971; **Fellow:** Research, Yale-New Haven Hosp 1972; **Fac Appt:** Prof OrS, Univ Iowa Coll Med

An, Howard MD [OrS] - **Spec Exp:** Spinal Surgery; Scoliosis; Spinal Microdiscectomy; **Hospital:** Rush Univ Med Ctr; **Address:** 1611 W Harrison, Ste 300, Chicago, IL 60612; **Phone:** 312-243-4244; **Board Cert:** Orthopaedic Surgery 2012; **Med School:** Med Coll OH 1982; **Resid:** Orthopaedic Surgery, Med College Ohio Hosps 1988; **Fellow:** Spinal Surgery, Jefferson Med College 1989; **Fac Appt:** Prof OrS, Rush Med Coll

Anglen, Jeffrey O MD [OrS] - **Spec Exp:** Trauma; Fractures-Complex & Non Union; Bone Infections; **Hospital:** IU Health University Hosp; **Address:** Indiana Univ Dept Ortho Surgery, 541 Clinical Drive, Ste 600, Indianapolis, IN 46202; **Phone:** 317-274-7372; **Board Cert:** Orthopaedic Surgery 2011; **Med School:** Johns Hopkins Univ 1983; **Resid:** Orthopaedic Surgery, Johns Hopkins Hosp 1988; **Fellow:** Orthopaedic Trauma Surgery, Tampa Genl Hosp 1989; **Fac Appt:** Prof OrS, Indiana Univ

Archdeacon, Michael T MD [OrS] - **Spec Exp:** Trauma; Pelvic & Acetabular Fractures; **Hospital:** Univ Hosp - Cincinnati; **Address:** 222 Piedmont Ave, Ste 2200, Cincinnati, OH 45219; **Phone:** 513-475-8690; **Board Cert:** Orthopaedic Surgery 2003; **Med School:** Ohio State Univ 1993; **Resid:** Orthopaedic Surgery, Case Western Univ Hosp 2000; **Fellow:** Orthopaedic Trauma Surgery, Tampa Gen Hosp 2001; **Fac Appt:** Prof OrS, Univ Cincinnati

Bach Jr, Bernard R MD [OrS] - **Spec Exp:** Sports Medicine; Knee Surgery; Knee Injuries/ACL; Shoulder Surgery; **Hospital:** Rush Univ Med Ctr; **Address:** Midwest Orthopaedics, 1611 W Harrison St, Ste 300, Chicago, IL 60612; **Phone:** 312-243-4244; **Board Cert:** Orthopaedic Surgery 2010; Orthopaedic Sports Medicine 2010; **Med School:** Univ Cincinnati 1979; **Resid:** Surgery, New Eng Deaconess Hosp 1981; Orthopaedic Surgery, Mass Genl Hosp 1984; **Fellow:** Sports Medicine, Hosp Special Surgery 1986; **Fac Appt:** Prof OrS, Rush Med Coll

Berry, Daniel John MD [OrS] - **Spec Exp:** Hip Replacement & Revision; Knee Replacement & Revision; **Hospital:** Mayo Med Ctr & Clin - Rochester; **Address:** Mayo Clin, Dept Orth Surg, 200 1st St SW, Rochester, MN 55905; **Phone:** 507-538-3270; **Board Cert:** Orthopaedic Surgery 2004; **Med School:** Harvard Med Sch 1984; **Resid:** Orthopaedic Surgery, Harvard Univ Affil Hosps 1989; **Fellow:** Adult Reconstructive Surgery, Mauric E Muller Foundation 1990; Hip Surgery, Mayo Clinic 1991; **Fac Appt:** Prof OrS, Mayo Med Sch

Biermann, J Sybil MD [OrS] - **Spec Exp:** Sarcoma; Bone Cancer; Multiple Myeloma; Limb Sparing Surgery; **Hospital:** Univ of Michigan Hosp; **Address:** Univ Michigan Cancer Ctr, 1500 E Medical Ctr Drive, Reception C, Ste B1-363, Ann Arbor, MI 48109; **Phone:** 734-647-8902; **Board Cert:** Orthopaedic Surgery 2006; **Med School:** Stanford Univ 1987; **Resid:** Orthopaedic Surgery, Univ Iowa Hosp 1992; **Fellow:** Orthopaedic Oncology, Univ Chicago Hosps 1993; **Fac Appt:** Assoc Prof OrS, Univ Mich Med Sch

Blaha, John D MD [OrS] - **Spec Exp:** Hip & Knee Replacement; **Hospital:** Univ of Michigan Hosp; **Address:** Univ Michigan, Dept Orthopaedic Surg, 1500 E Medical Ctr Dr, Taubman 2912, Ann Arbor, MI 48109; **Phone:** 734-647-9961; **Board Cert:** Orthopaedic Surgery 1979; **Med School:** Univ Mich Med Sch 1973; **Resid:** Surgery, Univ Mich Hosp 1975; Orthopaedic Surgery, Univ Mich Hosp 1978; **Fellow:** Joint Replacement Surgery, Univ London 1980; **Fac Appt:** Prof OrS, Univ Mich Med Sch

Bridwell, Keith MD [OrS] - **Spec Exp:** Spinal Deformity; Scoliosis; Spinal Surgery; **Hospital:** Barnes-Jewish Hosp, St. Louis Chldns Hosp; **Address:** Washington Univ Sch Med, 660 S Euclid Ave, Campus Box 8233, St Louis, MO 63110; **Phone:** 314-747-2560; **Board Cert:** Orthopaedic Surgery 1985; **Med School:** Washington Univ, St Louis 1977; **Resid:** Orthopaedic Surgery, Barnes Hosp-Wash Univ 1981; **Fellow:** Spinal Surgery, Rush Presby-St Lukes Med Ctr 1982; **Fac Appt:** Prof OrS, Washington Univ, St Louis

Buckwalter IV, Joseph A MD [OrS] - **Spec Exp:** Bone Cancer; Bone Tumors-Metastatic; Fractures-Complex; **Hospital:** Univ Iowa Hosp & Clinics; **Address:** Univ Iowa Hosp & Clin, Dept Orth Surg, 200 Hawkins Drive, Iowa City, IA 52242; **Phone:** 319-356-2595; **Board Cert:** Orthopaedic Surgery 1991; **Med School:** Univ Iowa Coll Med 1974; **Resid:** Orthopaedic Surgery, Iowa Hosp 1979; **Fac Appt:** Prof OrS, Univ Iowa Coll Med

Callaghan, John J MD [OrS] - **Spec Exp:** Hip & Knee Replacement; Sports Medicine; **Hospital:** Univ Iowa Hosp & Clinics; **Address:** Univ Iowa Hosp, Dept Orthopaedics, 200 Hawkins Drive, Iowa City, IA 52242; **Phone:** 319-356-3110; **Board Cert:** Orthopaedic Surgery 2011; **Med School:** Loyola Univ-Stritch Sch Med 1978; **Resid:** Orthopaedic Surgery, Univ Iowa Hosp 1983; **Fellow:** Orthopaedic Surgery, Hosp Special Surg 1984; **Fac Appt:** Prof OrS, Univ Iowa Coll Med

Cheng, Edward Y MD [OrS] - **Spec Exp:** Bone & Soft Tissue Tumors; Reconstructive Surgery; **Hospital:** Univ Minn Med Ctr, Fairview - Riverside Campus; **Address:** Univ Minnesota, Dept Orthopaedic Surgery, 2512 S Seventh St, Ste R-200, Minneapolis, MN 55454; **Phone:** 612-273-1177; **Board Cert:** Orthopaedic Surgery 2003; **Med School:** Northwestern Univ 1983; **Resid:** Surgery, Northwestern Univ 1985; Orthopaedic Surgery, Beth Israel Hosp 1989; **Fellow:** Surgical Oncology, Mass Genl Hosp 1990; **Fac Appt:** Prof OrS, Univ Minn

Clohisy, Denis MD [OrS] - **Spec Exp:** Bone Cancer; **Hospital:** Univ Minn Med Ctr, Fairview - Riverside Campus; **Address:** Univ Minn, Dept Orthopaedic Surgery, 2512 S Seventh St, Ste R200, Minneapolis, MN 55454; **Phone:** 612-273-1177; **Board Cert:** Orthopaedic Surgery 2004; **Med School:** Northwestern Univ 1983; **Resid:** Orthopaedic Surgery, Univ Minn 1990; **Fellow:** Pathology, Wash Univ Med Ctr 1987; Musculoskeletal Oncology, Mass Genl Hosp 1991; **Fac Appt:** Prof OrS, Univ Minn

Ebraheim, Nabil A MD [OrS] - **Spec Exp:** Trauma; Fractures-Complex & Non Union; Bone Infections; Reconstructive Surgery; **Hospital:** Univ of Toledo Med Ctr; **Address:** Univ Toledo Med Ctr, Dept Orthopaedics, 3065 Arlington Ave, MS 1094, Toledo, OH 43614; **Phone:** 419-383-3761; **Board Cert:** Orthopaedic Surgery 2008; **Med School:** Egypt 1975; **Resid:** Surgery, St Clare's Hosp 1980; Orthopaedic Surgery, SUNY-Downstate Med Ctr 1983; **Fellow:** Trauma, Univ Maryland Hosps 1984; Orthopaedic Surgery, Hanover Trauma Ctr 1985; **Fac Appt:** Prof OrS, Univ Toledo, Med Univ OH

Gitelis, Steven MD [OrS] - **Spec Exp:** Bone Cancer; Soft Tissue Tumors; Limb Sparing Surgery; Hip Replacement; **Hospital:** Rush Univ Med Ctr; **Address:** 1611 W Harrison St, Ste 300, Chicago, IL 60612; **Phone:** 312-432-2397; **Board Cert:** Orthopaedic Surgery 1982; **Med School:** Rush Med Coll 1975; **Resid:** Orthopaedic Surgery, Rush Presby-St Lukes Med Ctr 1980; **Fellow:** Orthopaedic Oncology, Rizzoli Inst 1980; Orthopaedic Oncology, Mayo Clinic 1982; **Fac Appt:** Prof OrS, Rush Med Coll

Goitz, Henry MD [OrS] - **Spec Exp:** Sports Medicine; Knee Injuries/ACL/Meniscus Tears; Rotator Cuff Surgery; Elbow Surgery; **Hospital:** DMC Surgery Hosp, Harper Univ Hosp; **Address:** Detroit Med Ctr, Sports Medicine, 28800 Ryan Rd, Ste 120, Warren, MI 48092; **Phone:** 586-558-2860; **Board Cert:** Orthopaedic Surgery 2006; **Med School:** UMDNJ-Rutgers Med Sch 1985; **Resid:** Orthopaedic Surgery, Univ Virginia Affil Hosp 1991; **Fellow:** Sports Medicine & Hand Surgery, Univ Virginia Affil Hosp 1991; Sports Medicine, American Sports Med Inst 1992

Goldstein, Wayne MD [OrS] - **Spec Exp:** Hip Replacement; Knee Replacement; **Hospital:** Adv Luth Genl Hosp; **Address:** Illinois Bone & Joint Institute, 9000 Waukegan Rd, Ste 200, Morton Grove, IL 60053; **Phone:** 847-375-3000; **Board Cert:** Orthopaedic Surgery 2007; **Med School:** Univ IL Coll Med 1978; **Resid:** Orthopaedic Surgery, Univ Ilinois Med Ctr 1983; **Fellow:** Arthritis Surgery, Brigham & Women's Hosp 1984; **Fac Appt:** Assoc Clin Prof OrS, Univ Chicago-Pritzker Sch Med

Orthopaedic Surgery

Graf, Ben K MD [OrS] - **Spec Exp:** Sports Medicine; **Hospital:** Univ WI Hosp & Clins; **Address:** 621 Science Drive, Madison, WI 53711; **Phone:** 608-263-8850; **Board Cert:** Orthopaedic Surgery 2008; Orthopaedic Sports Medicine 2007; **Med School:** Univ Wisc 1979; **Resid:** Orthopaedic Surgery, Univ Wisc Hosps 1984; **Fellow:** Sports Medicine, Long Beach Meml Hosp 1985; **Fac Appt:** Assoc Prof S, Univ Wisc

Hanssen, Arlen D MD [OrS] - **Spec Exp:** Hip Surgery; Knee Surgery; **Hospital:** Mayo Med Ctr & Clin - Rochester; **Address:** Mayo Clin, Dept Orth Surg, 200 First St SW, Rochester, MN 55905; **Phone:** 507-284-2884; **Board Cert:** Orthopaedic Surgery 2011; **Med School:** St Louis Univ 1983; **Resid:** Orthopaedic Surgery, Mayo Clin 1988; **Fac Appt:** Prof OrS, Mayo Med Sch

Iannotti, Joseph MD/PhD [OrS] - **Spec Exp:** Shoulder Surgery; Rotator Cuff Surgery; **Hospital:** Cleveland Clin (page 55); **Address:** Cleveland Clinic, Dept Orthopaedic Surg, 9500 Euclid Ave, Desk A40, Cleveland, OH 44195-5027; **Phone:** 216-445-5151; **Board Cert:** Orthopaedic Surgery 2007; **Med School:** Northwestern Univ 1979; **Resid:** Orthopaedic Surgery, Hosp Univ Penn 1984; **Fellow:** Orthopaedic Research, Hosp Univ Penn 1985; **Fac Appt:** Prof OrS, Cleveland Cl Coll Med/Case West Res

Irwin, Ronald B MD [OrS] - **Spec Exp:** Bone Cancer; Limb Sparing Surgery; Sarcoma-Soft Tissue; **Hospital:** Mount Clemens Regional Med Ctr; **Address:** 1080 Harrington Blvd, Ste 201, Mount Clemens, MI 48043; **Phone:** 586-493-7575; **Board Cert:** Orthopaedic Surgery 1979; **Med School:** Univ Mich Med Sch 1971; **Resid:** Orthopaedic Surgery, William Beaumont Hosp 1978; **Fellow:** Orthopaedic Oncology, Mayo Clinic 1978

Jacobs, Joshua J MD [OrS] - **Spec Exp:** Hip Replacement & Revision; Knee Replacement & Revision; **Hospital:** Rush Univ Med Ctr; **Address:** 1611 W Harrison St, Ste 300, Chicago, IL 60612; **Phone:** 312-243-4344; **Board Cert:** Orthopaedic Surgery 2011; **Med School:** Univ IL Coll Med 1981; **Resid:** Orthopaedic Surgery, Harvard Univ Affil Hosp 1987; **Fellow:** Joint Replacement Surgery, Rush Univ Med Ctr 1988; **Fac Appt:** Prof OrS, Rush Med Coll

Joyce, Michael J MD [OrS] - **Spec Exp:** Bone & Soft Tissue Tumors; Fractures-Complex & Non Union; Musculoskeletal Tissue Banking; Pelvic & Acetabular Fractures; **Hospital:** Cleveland Clin (page 55); **Address:** 9500 Euclid Ave, Desk A41, Cleveland Clinic Dept Orthopaedic Surgery, Cleveland, OH 44195; **Phone:** 216-444-4282; **Board Cert:** Orthopaedic Surgery 1985; **Med School:** Univ Louisville Sch Med 1976; **Resid:** Surgery, Johns Hopkins Hosp 1978; Orthopaedic Surgery, Harvard Combined Program 1981; **Fellow:** Orthopaedic Oncology, Mass General Hosp 1982; Trauma, Univ Toronto-Sunnybrook Hosp 1983; **Fac Appt:** Assoc Clin Prof OrS, Case West Res Univ

Kaeding, Christopher C MD [OrS] - **Spec Exp:** Sports Medicine; Knee Injuries/ACL; Shoulder Injuries; Rotator Cuff Surgery; **Hospital:** Ohio St Univ Med Ctr; **Address:** OSU Sports Med Ctr, 2050 Kenny Rd, Ste 3100, Columbus, OH 43221; **Phone:** 614-293-8813; **Board Cert:** Orthopaedic Surgery 2012; Orthopaedic Sports Medicine 2012; **Med School:** Northwestern Univ 1983; **Resid:** Orthopaedic Surgery, Northwestern Univ 1988; **Fellow:** Sports Medicine, Cleveland Clinic 1989; **Fac Appt:** Clin Prof OrS, Ohio State Univ

Kenter, Keith MD [OrS] - **Spec Exp:** Sports Medicine; Shoulder Reconstruction; Knee Surgery; **Hospital:** Univ Hosp - Cincinnati; **Address:** University of Cincinnati Physicians, 222 Piedmont Ave, Ste 2200, Cincinnati, OH 45219; **Phone:** 513-475-8690; **Board Cert:** Orthopaedic Surgery 2010; Orthopaedic Sports Medicine 2007; **Med School:** Univ MO-Columbia Sch Med 1990; **Resid:** Surgery, Duke Univ Med Ctr 1992; Orthopaedic Surgery, Duke Univ Med Ctr 1996; **Fellow:** Sports Medicine & Shoulder Surgery, Hosp for Special Surgery 1997; **Fac Appt:** Asst Prof OrS, Univ Cincinnati

Kraay, Matthew J MD [OrS] - **Spec Exp:** Arthritis; Reconstructive Surgery; Joint Replacement; **Hospital:** Univ Hosps Case Med Ctr (page 74); **Address:** UH Case Medical Center, Dept of Orthopaedic Surgery, 11100 Euclid Ave, Cleveland, OH 44106; **Phone:** 216-844-8372; **Board Cert:** Orthopaedic Surgery 2004; **Med School:** Wayne State Univ 1983; **Resid:** Orthopaedic Surgery, Univ Hosps 1989; **Fellow:** Adult Reconstructive Surgery, Univ Hosps 1990; Orthopaedic Surgery, Hosp Special Surgery 1991; **Fac Appt:** Prof OrS, Case West Res Univ

Lenke, Lawrence G MD [OrS] - **Spec Exp:** Spinal Surgery; Spinal Deformity; Scoliosis; Spinal Reconstructive Surgery; **Hospital:** Barnes-Jewish Hosp, St. Louis Chldns Hosp; **Address:** Washington Univ Sch Med, 660 S Euclid Ave, Campus Box 8233, St Louis, MO 63110; **Phone:** 314-747-2509; **Board Cert:** Orthopaedic Surgery 2005; **Med School:** Northwestern Univ 1986; **Resid:** Orthopaedic Surgery, Barnes-Jewish Hosp 1989; **Fellow:** Spinal Surgery, Barnes-Jewish Hosp 1992; **Fac Appt:** Prof OrS, Washington Univ, St Louis

Les, Kimberly A MD [OrS] - **Spec Exp:** Bone Cancer; **Hospital:** Beaumont Hosp-Royal Oak; **Address:** Rose Cancer Treatment Ctr, 3577 W 13 Mile Rd, Ste 402, Royal Oak, MI 48073; **Phone:** 248-551-9910; **Board Cert:** Orthopaedic Surgery 2011; **Med School:** Geo Wash Univ 1992; **Resid:** Orthopaedic Surgery, Henry Ford Hosp 1997; **Fellow:** Orthopaedic Oncology, Univ Chicago Hosps 1978

Lock, Terrence Ralph MD [OrS] - **Spec Exp:** Sports Medicine; Arthroscopic Surgery; Shoulder & Knee Reconstruction; **Hospital:** Henry Ford Hosp, Henry Ford Med Ctr-Cottage; **Address:** Henry Ford Hosp, Ctr for Athletic Med, 6525 Second Ave, Detroit, MI 48202; **Phone:** 313-972-4060; **Board Cert:** Orthopaedic Surgery 2012; Orthopaedic Sports Medicine 2007; **Med School:** Wayne State Univ 1983; **Resid:** Orthopaedic Surgery, Wayne St Univ Sch Med 1988; **Fellow:** Sports Medicine, Mass Genl Hosp 1989

Manoli II, Arthur MD [OrS] - **Spec Exp:** Foot & Ankle Surgery; Reconstructive Surgery; **Hospital:** St. Joseph Mercy Oakland Hosp; **Address:** 44555 Woodward Ave, Ste 503, Pontiac, MI 48341; **Phone:** 248-858-6773; **Board Cert:** Orthopaedic Surgery 2007; **Med School:** Univ Mich Med Sch 1970; **Resid:** Surgery, Oakwood Hosp 1972; Orthopaedic Surgery, Wayne St Univ Affil Hosps 1975; **Fellow:** Ankle and Foot Surgery, Univ Wash/Vanderbilt Univ 1990

Mayerson, Joel L MD [OrS] - **Spec Exp:** Bone Tumors; Sarcoma-Soft Tissue; Limb Surgery/Reconstruction; Musculoskeletal Tumors; **Hospital:** Ohio St Univ Med Ctr; **Address:** Ohio State, Div of Musculoskeletal Onc, 410 W 10 Ave N Doan Hall Bldg - rm 1049, Columbus, OH 43210; **Phone:** 614-293-4420; **Board Cert:** Orthopaedic Surgery 2003; **Med School:** Johns Hopkins Univ 1994; **Resid:** Orthopaedic Surgery, Cleveland Clinic 1999; **Fellow:** Orthopaedic Oncology, Univ Wash Med Ctr 2000; **Fac Appt:** Assoc Prof OrS, Ohio State Univ

McCarthy, James J MD [OrS] - **Spec Exp:** Lower Limb Surgery in Children; Arthroscopic Surgery-Hip; Pediatric Orthopaedic Surgery; Hip Disorders-Pediatric; **Hospital:** Cincinnati Chldns Hosp Med Ctr; **Address:** Cincinnati Chldn's, Dept Ped Ortho Surg, 3333 Burnet Ave, ML 2017, Cincinnati, OH 45229; **Phone:** 513-636-4454; **Board Cert:** Orthopaedic Surgery 2010; **Med School:** Univ NC Sch Med 1991; **Resid:** Orthopaedic Surgery, Cleveland Clinic 1996; **Fellow:** Arthroscopic Surgery, Children's Hosp 1997; **Fac Appt:** Prof OrS, Univ Wisc

McDonald, Douglas J MD [OrS] - **Spec Exp:** Bone & Soft Tissue Tumors; Ewing's Sarcoma; Sarcoma; Hip & Knee Reconstruction; **Hospital:** Barnes-Jewish Hosp, St. Louis Chldns Hosp; **Address:** Ctr Advanced Med, Orthopaedic Surg Ctr, 4921 Parkview Pl Fl 6 - Ste A, Box 8605, St Louis, MO 63110; **Phone:** 314-747-2500; **Board Cert:** Orthopaedic Surgery 2011; **Med School:** Univ Minn 1982; **Resid:** Orthopaedic Surgery, Mayo Clinic 1987; **Fellow:** Orthopaedic Oncology, Mayo Clinic 1988; Orthopaedic Surgery, Rizzoli Inst 1989; **Fac Appt:** Prof OrS, Washington Univ, St Louis

Morcuende, Jose A MD/PhD [OrS] - **Spec Exp:** Clubfoot; Pediatric Orthopaedic Surgery; **Hospital:** Univ Iowa Hosp & Clinics; **Address:** UIHC Dept Orthopaedics & Rehab, 200 Hawkins Drive, Iowa City, IA 52242; **Phone:** 319-356-2223; **Board Cert:** Orthopaedic Surgery 2004; **Med School:** Spain 1981; **Resid:** Orthopaedic Surgery, Univ IA Hosp & Clin 2001; **Fellow:** Pediatric Orthopaedic Surgery, Univ IA Hosp & Clin 2002; **Fac Appt:** Assoc Prof OrS, Univ Iowa Coll Med

Mott, Michael P MD [OrS] - **Spec Exp:** Soft Tissue Tumors; Musculoskeletal Tumors; Bone Cancer; **Hospital:** Henry Ford Hosp, Henry Ford- W Bloomfield Hosp; **Address:** Henry Ford Hosp, Dept Ortho Surg, 2799 W Grand Blvd Fl 12, Detroit, MI 48202; **Phone:** 313-916-1961; **Board Cert:** Orthopaedic Surgery 2007; **Med School:** Univ Mich Med Sch 1989; **Resid:** Orthopaedic Surgery, Wayne State Univ Affil Hosp 1994; **Fellow:** Musculoskeletal Oncology, Mass Genl Hosp 1995; Orthopaedic Oncology, Wayne State Univ 1996; **Fac Appt:** Assoc Prof OrS, Wayne State Univ

Muschler, George F MD [OrS] - **Spec Exp:** Hip Replacement; Knee Replacement; Fractures-Complex & Non Union; **Hospital:** Cleveland Clin (page 55); **Address:** Cleveland Clinic, Dept Orthopaedic Surg, 9500 Euclid Ave, Desk A40, Cleveland, OH 44195-0001; **Phone:** 216-444-2601; **Board Cert:** Orthopaedic Surgery 2011; **Med School:** Northwestern Univ 1981; **Resid:** Orthopaedic Surgery, Univ Texas SW Med Ctr 1986; **Fellow:** Metabolic Bone Research, Hosp Special Surgery 1988; Musculoskeletal Oncology, Meml Sloan Kettering Cancer Ctr 1988; **Fac Appt:** Prof OrS, Cleveland Cl Coll Med/Case West Res

Nepola, James V MD [OrS] - **Spec Exp:** Trauma; Shoulder Reconstruction; **Hospital:** Univ Iowa Hosp & Clinics; **Address:** UIHC Dept Orthopaedics & Rehab, 200 Hawkins Drive, Iowa City, IA 52242; **Phone:** 319-356-2223; **Board Cert:** Orthopaedic Surgery 2009; **Med School:** Columbia P&S 1978; **Resid:** Surgery, Roosevelt Hosp 1980; Orthopaedic Surgery, NY-Presby Hosp/Columbia 1983; **Fellow:** Orthopaedic Trauma Surgery, NY-Presby Hosp/Columbia 1984; **Fac Appt:** Prof OrS, Univ Iowa Coll Med

Nuber, Gordon W MD [OrS] - **Spec Exp:** Shoulder Reconstruction; Rotator Cuff Surgery; Cartilage Damage; Arthroscopic Surgery-Knee; **Hospital:** Northwestern Meml Hosp; **Address:** Northwestern Orthopaedic Inst, 680 N Lake Shore, Ste 924, Chicago, IL 60611-4451; **Phone:** 312-664-6848; **Board Cert:** Orthopaedic Surgery 2007; **Med School:** Wayne State Univ 1978; **Resid:** Orthopaedic Surgery, Northwestern Meml Hosp 1983; **Fellow:** Sports Medicine, Natl Athletic Hlth Inst 1984; **Fac Appt:** Clin Prof OrS, Northwestern Univ

O'Driscoll, Shawn MD/PhD [OrS] - **Spec Exp:** Sports Medicine; Shoulder Surgery; Elbow Surgery; Cartilage Damage; **Hospital:** Mayo Med Ctr & Clin - Rochester; **Address:** Mayo Clin, Dept Orth Surg, 200 1st St SW, Rochester, MN 55905; **Phone:** 507-538-1953; **Board Cert:** Orthopaedic Surgery 2003; Orthopaedic Sports Medicine 2007; **Med School:** Univ Toronto 1980; **Resid:** Orthopaedic Surgery, Univ Toronto 1987; **Fellow:** Arthroscopic Surgery, Toronto Western Hosp; Elbow & Shoulder Surgery, Mayo Clinic 1988; **Fac Appt:** Prof OrS, Mayo Med Sch

Parsons III, Theodore W MD [OrS] - **Spec Exp:** Bone & Soft Tissue Tumors; Reconstructive Surgery; **Hospital:** Henry Ford Hosp; **Address:** Henry Ford Hosp, Dept Orthopaedics, 2799 West Grand Blvd Fl 12, Detroit, MI 48202; **Phone:** 313-916-1964; **Board Cert:** Orthopaedic Surgery 2005; **Med School:** Uniformed Srvs Univ, Bethesda 1986; **Resid:** Orthopaedic Surgery, Wilford Hall USAF Med Ctr 1991; **Fellow:** Pediatric Oncology, Boston Chldns Hosp 1992; Orthopaedic Oncology, Mass Genl Hosp 1992; **Fac Appt:** Prof OrS, Wayne State Univ

Peabody, Terrance D MD [OrS] - **Spec Exp:** Soft Tissue Tumors; Bone Tumors; Pediatric Orthopaedic Cancers; Limb Sparing Surgery; **Hospital:** Northwestern Meml Hosp; **Address:** Northwestern Meml Hosp, Galter Pavilion, 675 N St Clair, rm 17-100, Chicago, IL 60611; **Phone:** 312-695-6800; **Board Cert:** Orthopaedic Surgery 2004; **Med School:** UC Irvine 1985; **Resid:** Orthopaedic Surgery, UC Irvine Med Ctr 1990; **Fellow:** Orthopaedic Oncology, Univ Chicago Med Ctr 1991; **Fac Appt:** Prof OrS, Univ Chicago-Pritzker Sch Med

Pinzur, Michael S MD [OrS] - **Spec Exp:** Diabetes-Amputation; Foot & Ankle Surgery; Amputation Surgery; Charcot Foot; **Hospital:** Loyola Univ Med Ctr; **Address:** Loyola University Medical Center, 2160 S 1st Ave, Maywood, IL 60153-3304; **Phone:** 708-216-4993; **Board Cert:** Orthopaedic Surgery 1980; **Med School:** Rush Med Coll 1974; **Resid:** Orthopaedic Surgery, Northwestern Meml Hosp 1979; **Fac Appt:** Prof OrS, Loyola Univ-Stritch Sch Med

Polly, David W MD [OrS] - **Spec Exp:** Spinal Surgery; Scoliosis; Aging; **Address:** Univ Minn Orthopaedic Clin, 2512 S 7th St, rm R-102, Minneapolis, MN 55454; **Phone:** 612-273-9400; **Board Cert:** Orthopaedic Surgery 2005; **Med School:** Uniformed Srvs Univ, Bethesda 1985; **Resid:** Orthopaedic Surgery, Walter Reed Army Med Ctr 1991; **Fellow:** Spinal Surgery, Univ Minn Affil Hosp 1992

Riew, K Daniel MD [OrS] - **Spec Exp:** Spinal Surgery-Cervical; Minimally Invasive Spinal Surgery; Spinal Microdiscectomy; **Hospital:** Barnes-Jewish Hosp; **Address:** Ctr for Advanced Med-Spine Ctr, 4921 Parkview Pl, CAM Bldg Fl 12 - Ste A, St Louis, MO 63110; **Phone:** 314-514-3500; **Board Cert:** Internal Medicine 1987; Orthopaedic Surgery 2008; **Med School:** Case West Res Univ 1984; **Resid:** Internal Medicine, NY Hosp-Cornell Med Ctr 1987; Orthopaedic Surgery, G Washington Univ Hosp 1994; **Fellow:** Spinal Surgery, Case West Res Univ 1995; **Fac Appt:** Prof OrS, Washington Univ, St Louis

Romeo, Anthony A MD [OrS] - **Spec Exp:** Shoulder Reconstruction; Shoulder Problems-Complex; Sports Medicine; Elbow Surgery; **Hospital:** Rush Univ Med Ctr, Rush Oak Park Hosp; **Address:** 1611 W Harrison St, Ste 300, Chicago, IL 60612; **Phone:** 312-432-2342; **Board Cert:** Orthopaedic Surgery 2008; Orthopaedic Sports Medicine 2010; **Med School:** St Louis Univ 1987; **Resid:** Orthopaedic Surgery, Cleveland Clinic 1992; **Fellow:** Shoulder Surgery, Univ Washington 1993; **Fac Appt:** Assoc Prof OrS, Rush Med Coll

Schafer, Michael F MD [OrS] - **Spec Exp:** Sports Medicine; Spinal Surgery; Scoliosis; **Hospital:** Northwestern Meml Hosp; **Address:** 675 N St Clair St, Galter Bldg Fl 17 - Ste 100, Chicago, IL 60611-5968; **Phone:** 312-695-6800; **Board Cert:** Orthopaedic Surgery 1983; **Med School:** Univ Iowa Coll Med 1967; **Resid:** Orthopaedic Surgery, Northwestern Univ Hosp 1972; **Fellow:** Spinal Surgery, Natl Fdn Traveling Fellowship 1973; **Fac Appt:** Prof OrS, Northwestern Univ

Shelbourne, K Donald MD [OrS] - **Spec Exp:** Knee Surgery; Arthroscopic Surgery; Knee Rehabilitation (Non-Surgical); Knee Ligament Reconstruction; **Hospital:** IU Health Methodist Hosp; **Address:** 1815 N Capitol Ave, Ste 600, Indianapolis, IN 46202; **Phone:** 317-924-8636; **Board Cert:** Orthopaedic Surgery 1984; **Med School:** Indiana Univ 1976; **Resid:** Orthopaedic Surgery, Indiana Univ Hosp 1981; **Fellow:** Sports Medicine, Univ Wisconsin 1982; **Fac Appt:** Assoc Clin Prof OrS, Indiana Univ

Sim, Franklin H MD [OrS] - **Spec Exp:** Sarcoma; Bone Cancer; **Hospital:** Mayo Med Ctr & Clin - Rochester; **Address:** Mayo Clinic, Orthopaedic Surg, Gonda 14, 200 1st St SW, Rochester, MN 55905; **Phone:** 507-284-3661; **Board Cert:** Orthopaedic Surgery 1971; **Med School:** Dalhousie Univ 1965; **Resid:** Orthopaedic Surgery, Mayo Clinic 1970; **Fac Appt:** Prof OrS, Mayo Med Sch

Stulberg, S David MD [OrS] - **Spec Exp:** Hip & Knee Replacement; **Hospital:** Northwestern Meml Hosp; **Address:** 680 N Lake Shore Drive, Ste 924, Chicago, IL 60611; **Phone:** 312-664-6848; **Board Cert:** Orthopaedic Surgery 1977; **Med School:** Univ Mich Med Sch 1969; **Resid:** Orthopaedic Surgery, Mass Genl Hosp 1974; **Fellow:** Research, Toronto Hosp Sick Chldn 1976; **Fac Appt:** Prof OrS, Northwestern Univ

Orthopaedic Surgery

Swiontkowski, Marc F MD [OrS] - **Spec Exp:** Osteomyelitis; Fractures-Non Union; Trauma; Bone Infections; **Address:** Tria Orthopedic Ctr, 8100 Northland Drive, Bloomington, MN 55431; **Phone:** 952-831-8742; **Board Cert:** Orthopaedic Surgery 2008; **Med School:** USC Sch Med 1979; **Resid:** Orthopaedic Surgery, Univ Washington Med Ctr 1984; **Fac Appt:** Prof OrS, Univ Minn

Thompson, George H MD [OrS] - **Spec Exp:** Pediatric Orthopaedic Surgery; Scoliosis; Spinal Deformity-Pediatric; **Hospital:** UH Rainbow Babies & Chldns Hosp (page 74); **Address:** UH Rainbow Babies & Children's Hospital, Ped Ortho Surg, 11100 Euclid Ave, MS RBC6081, Cleveland, OH 44106; **Phone:** 216-844-5416; **Board Cert:** Orthopaedic Surgery 1994; **Med School:** Univ Okla Coll Med 1970; **Resid:** Surgery, UCLA Med Ctr 1972; Orthopaedic Surgery, UCLA Med Ctr 1977; **Fellow:** Pediatric Orthopaedic Surgery, Hosp for Sick Chldn; **Fac Appt:** Prof OrS, Case West Res Univ

Weinstein, Stuart L MD [OrS] - **Spec Exp:** Scoliosis; Hip Disorders & Dysplasia; Hip Disorders-Pediatric; Spinal Deformity; **Hospital:** Univ Iowa Hosp & Clinics; **Address:** 01026 JPP 200 Hawkins Drive, Iowa City, IA 52242-1009; **Phone:** 319-356-1872; **Board Cert:** Orthopaedic Surgery 2007; **Med School:** Univ Iowa Coll Med 1972; **Resid:** Orthopaedic Surgery, Univ Iowa Hosps 1976; **Fac Appt:** Prof OrS, Univ Iowa Coll Med

Wixson, Richard L MD [OrS] - **Spec Exp:** Hip & Knee Replacement; **Hospital:** Northwestern Meml Hosp; **Address:** 680 N Lake Shore Drive, rm 924, Chicago, IL 60611; **Phone:** 312-664-6848; **Board Cert:** Orthopaedic Surgery 1979; **Med School:** Univ Wisc 1972; **Resid:** Orthopaedic Surgery, Henry Ford Hosp 1977; Orthopaedic Surgery, New Eng Baptist Hosp 1979; **Fellow:** Orthopaedic Surgery, Mass Genl Hosp 1978; **Fac Appt:** Clin Prof OrS, Northwestern Univ

Wurtz, L Daniel MD [OrS] - **Spec Exp:** Bone & Soft Tissue Tumors; Limb Sparing Surgery; Sarcoma; Pediatric Orthopaedic Cancers; **Hospital:** IU Health University Hosp, Riley Hosp for Children; **Address:** University Orthopaedic Assocs, 541 Clinical Drive, Ste 600, Indianapolis, IN 46202; **Phone:** 317-274-3227; **Board Cert:** Orthopaedic Surgery 2004; **Med School:** Univ S Ala Coll Med 1985; **Resid:** Orthopaedic Surgery, Wilford Hall USAF Med Ctr 1990; **Fellow:** Musculoskeletal Oncology, Univ Chicago; **Fac Appt:** Assoc Prof OrS, Indiana Univ

Yamaguchi, Ken MD [OrS] - **Spec Exp:** Shoulder Surgery; Elbow Surgery; Rotator Cuff Surgery; **Hospital:** Barnes-Jewish Hosp; **Address:** Washington Univ Sch Med, 660 S Euclid Ave, Campus Box 8233, St Louis, MO 63110; **Phone:** 314-747-2534; **Board Cert:** Orthopaedic Surgery 2008; **Med School:** Geo Wash Univ 1989; **Resid:** Orthopaedic Surgery, G Washington Univ Hosp 1994; **Fellow:** Shoulder Surgery, NY-Presby/Columbia Univ Med Ctr 1995; **Fac Appt:** Prof OrS, Washington Univ, St Louis

Zdeblick, Thomas MD [OrS] - **Spec Exp:** Spinal Surgery; **Hospital:** Univ WI Hosp & Clins; **Address:** 621 Science Drive, Madison, WI 53711; **Phone:** 608-265-3207; **Board Cert:** Orthopaedic Surgery 2012; **Med School:** Tufts Univ 1982; **Resid:** Orthopaedic Surgery, Case West Res Univ 1988; **Fellow:** Spinal Surgery, Johns Hopkins Hosp 1989; **Fac Appt:** Prof OrS, Univ Wisc

Great Plains and Mountains

Coughlin, Michael J MD [OrS] - **Spec Exp:** Foot & Ankle Surgery; **Hospital:** St. Alphonsus Regl Med Ctr; **Address:** 1075 N Curtis Rd, Ste 300, Boise, ID 83706; **Phone:** 208-367-3330; **Board Cert:** Orthopaedic Surgery 1980; **Med School:** Oregon Hlth & Sci Univ 1974; **Resid:** Orthopaedic Surgery, UCSF Med Ctr 1978; **Fellow:** Foot & Ankle Surgery, Samuel Merrit Hosp 1979; **Fac Appt:** Clin Prof OrS, Oregon Hlth & Sci Univ

Garvin, Kevin L MD [OrS] - **Spec Exp:** Hip Surgery; Knee Surgery; Joint Replacement; **Hospital:** Nebraska Med Ctr; **Address:** UNMC Orthopaedic Clinic, 44th & Emily, Omaha, NE 68198-9265; **Phone:** 402-559-8000; **Board Cert:** Orthopaedic Surgery 2011; **Med School:** Med Coll Wisc 1982; **Resid:** Orthopaedic Surgery, Univ Arkansas Hosp 1987; **Fellow:** Hip Surgery, Hosp for Special Surgery 1988; **Fac Appt:** Prof OrS, Univ Nebr Coll Med

Heiden, Eric A MD [OrS] - **Spec Exp:** Sports Medicine; Knee Surgery; **Hospital:** Ortho Spec Hosp, The (TOSH); **Address:** 2200 Park Ave D Bldg - Ste 100, Park City, UT 84060; **Phone:** 801-703-8397; **Board Cert:** Orthopaedic Surgery 2011; **Med School:** Stanford Univ 1991; **Resid:** Orthopaedic Surgery, UC Davis Med Ctr 1996; **Fellow:** Sports Medicine, Amer Sports Med Inst 1997

Kelly, Cynthia M MD [OrS] - **Spec Exp:** Osteonecrosis; Bone Tumors; Soft Tissue Tumors; Bone Cancer; **Hospital:** Presby - St Luke's Med Ctr; **Address:** 1601 E 19th Ave, Ste 3300, Denver, CO 80218; **Phone:** 303-837-0072; **Board Cert:** Orthopaedic Surgery 2011; **Med School:** UCLA 1989; **Resid:** Orthopaedic Surgery, Harbor-UCLA Med Ctr 1994; **Fellow:** Orthopaedic Oncology, UCLA Med Ctr 1995

Millett, Peter J MD [OrS] - **Spec Exp:** Shoulder Surgery; Sports Medicine; Arthroscopic Surgery; **Hospital:** Vail Valley Med Ctr; **Address:** The Steadman Clinic, 181 W Meadow Drive, Ste 400, Vail, CO 81657; **Phone:** 970-476-1100; **Board Cert:** Orthopaedic Surgery 2003; **Med School:** Dartmouth Med Sch 1995; **Resid:** Orthopaedic Surgery, Hosp Special Surgery 2000; **Fellow:** Sports Medicine, Steadman Hawkins Clinic 2001

Philippon, Marc J MD [OrS] - **Spec Exp:** Arthroscopic Surgery-Hip; Sports Medicine; **Hospital:** Vail Valley Med Ctr; **Address:** Steadman Clinic, 181 W Meadow Drive, Ste 400, Vail, CO 81657; **Phone:** 970-476-1100; **Board Cert:** Orthopaedic Surgery 2010; **Med School:** Canada 1990; **Resid:** Orthopaedic Surgery, Jackson Meml Hosp 1995; **Fac Appt:** , Univ Pittsburgh

Randall, R Lor L MD [OrS] - **Spec Exp:** Bone Tumors; Sarcoma-Soft Tissue; Pediatric Orthopaedic Surgery; **Hospital:** Univ Utah Hlth Care, Primary Children's Med Ctr; **Address:** 2000 Circle of Hope, Ste 4260, Salt Lake City, UT 84113; **Phone:** 801-585-0300; **Board Cert:** Orthopaedic Surgery 2012; **Med School:** Yale Univ 1992; **Resid:** Orthopaedic Surgery, UCSF Med Ctr 1997; **Fellow:** Musculoskeletal Oncology, Univ WA Med Ctr 1998; **Fac Appt:** Assoc Prof OrS, Univ Utah

Rosenberg, Thomas D MD [OrS] - **Spec Exp:** Knee Surgery; Sports Medicine; **Hospital:** Ortho Spec Hosp, The (TOSH); **Address:** 900 Round Valley Drive, Ste 100, Park City, UT 84060; **Phone:** 435-655-6600; **Board Cert:** Orthopaedic Surgery 1979; **Med School:** Univ Utah 1973; **Resid:** Orthopaedic Surgery, Univ Utah Affil Hosps 1977; **Fellow:** Sports Medicine, Univ Wisconsin Hosp 1978

Saltzman, Charles L MD [OrS] - **Spec Exp:** Foot & Ankle Surgery; **Hospital:** Univ Utah Hlth Care; **Address:** Dept Orthopaedic Surgery, 590 Wakara Way, Salt Lake City, UT 84108; **Phone:** 801-587-7100; **Board Cert:** Orthopaedic Surgery 2004; **Med School:** Univ NC Sch Med 1985; **Resid:** Orthopaedic Surgery, Univ Michigan Med Ctr; **Fellow:** Orthopaedic Surgery, Mayo Clinic; **Fac Appt:** Prof OrS, Univ Utah

Steadman, J Richard MD [OrS] - **Spec Exp:** Knee-Microfracture Surgery; Sports Medicine; **Hospital:** Vail Valley Med Ctr; **Address:** The Steadman Clinic, 181 W Meadow Drive, Ste 400, Vail, CO 81657; **Phone:** 970-476-1100; **Board Cert:** Orthopaedic Surgery 1972; **Med School:** Univ Tex SW, Dallas 1963; **Resid:** Orthopaedic Surgery, Charity Hosp 1966; Orthopaedic Surgery, Louisiana St Univ Hosp 1967

Orthopaedic Surgery

Wilkins, Ross M MD [OrS] - **Spec Exp:** Bone Cancer; Bone Infections; Fractures-Non Union; **Hospital:** Presby - St Luke's Med Ctr; **Address:** 1601 E 19th Ave, Ste 3300, Denver, CO 80218; **Phone:** 303-837-0072; **Board Cert:** Orthopaedic Surgery 2007; **Med School:** Wayne State Univ 1978; **Resid:** Orthopaedic Surgery, Univ Colorado Med Ctr 1983; **Fellow:** Orthopaedic Oncology, Mayo Clinic 1984

Southwest

Agarwal, Animesh MD [OrS] - **Spec Exp:** Trauma; Reconstructive Surgery; **Hospital:** Univ Hlth Syst-San Antonio; **Address:** UTHSCSA Div Orthopaedic Trauma, 7703 Floyd Curl Drive, MC 7774, San Antonio, TX 78229-3900; **Phone:** 210-567-5154; **Board Cert:** Orthopaedic Surgery 2011; **Med School:** Univ Tex, San Antonio 1992; **Resid:** Orthopaedic Surgery, Unix TX Med Ctr 1997; **Fellow:** Trauma, Grant Med Ctr 1998; **Fac Appt:** Prof OrS, Univ Tex, San Antonio

Aronson, James MD [OrS] - **Spec Exp:** Limb Lengthening (Ilizarov Procedure); Hip Disorders & Dysplasia; Clubfoot; Limb Deformities; **Hospital:** Arkansas Chldns Hosp; **Address:** Arkansas Chldns Hosp, Dept Orthopaedics, 1 Children's Way, Slot 839, Little Rock, AR 72202; **Phone:** 501-364-1468; **Board Cert:** Orthopaedic Surgery 2007; **Med School:** Univ Pittsburgh 1975; **Resid:** Surgery, Maine Med Ctr 1977; Orthopaedic Surgery, Duke Univ Med Ctr 1982; **Fellow:** Pediatric Orthopaedic Surgery, Alfred I DuPont Inst 1983; **Fac Appt:** Prof OrS, Univ Ark

Brodsky, James W MD [OrS] - **Spec Exp:** Foot & Ankle Surgery; **Hospital:** Baylor Univ Medical Ctr-Dallas; **Address:** 3900 Junius St, Ste 500, Dallas, TX 75246; **Phone:** 214-823-7090; **Board Cert:** Orthopaedic Surgery 2008; **Med School:** Case West Res Univ 1979; **Resid:** Orthopaedic Surgery, Bellevue Hosp Ctr/NYU 1981; Orthopaedic Surgery, Baylor Coll Med 1984; **Fellow:** Foot & Ankle Surgery, Rancho Los Amigos/USC/LAC Hosp 1985; **Fac Appt:** Clin Prof OrS, Univ Tex SW, Dallas

Bucholz, Robert W MD [OrS] - **Spec Exp:** Hip & Knee Replacement; **Hospital:** UT Southwestern Med Ctr at Dallas, Parkland Hlth & Hosp Sys; **Address:** Dept Ortho Surg, 1801 Inwood Rd, Dallas, TX 75390-8882; **Phone:** 214-645-3300; **Board Cert:** Orthopaedic Surgery 2005; **Med School:** Yale Univ 1973; **Resid:** Orthopaedic Surgery, Yale-New Haven Hosp 1977; **Fac Appt:** Prof OrS, Univ Tex SW, Dallas

Cooper, Daniel E MD [OrS] - **Spec Exp:** Sports Medicine; Knee Injuries/ACL; Arthroscopic Surgery; Reconstructive Surgery; **Hospital:** Baylor Univ Medical Ctr-Dallas, Mary Shiels Hosp; **Address:** WB Carrell Clin, 9301 N Central Expwy, Ste 400, Tower 1, Dallas, TX 75231; **Phone:** 214-220-2468; **Board Cert:** Orthopaedic Surgery 2003; **Med School:** Univ Tex SW, Dallas 1984; **Resid:** Orthopaedic Surgery, Univ Texas Health Scis Ctr 1989; **Fellow:** Sports Medicine, Hosp for Special Surgery 1990

Gugenheim Jr, Joseph J MD [OrS] - **Spec Exp:** Limb Lengthening (Ilizarov Procedure); Limb Deformities; **Hospital:** Texas Ortho Hosp; **Address:** Fondren Orthopaedic Group, 7401 S Main St, Houston, TX 77030; **Phone:** 713-799-2300; **Board Cert:** Orthopaedic Surgery 1978; **Med School:** Northwestern Univ 1972; **Resid:** Orthopaedic Surgery, Baylor Affil Hosp 1976; **Fellow:** Pediatric Orthopaedic Surgery, Boston Chldns Hosp 1977; **Fac Appt:** Assoc Prof S, Baylor Coll Med

Hochschuler, Stephen H MD [OrS] - **Spec Exp:** Spinal Surgery; **Hospital:** TX Hlth Presby Hosp Plano; **Address:** Texas Back Institute, 6020 W Parker Rd, Ste 200, Plano, TX 75093-7916; **Phone:** 972-608-5000; **Board Cert:** Orthopaedic Surgery 1978; **Med School:** Harvard Med Sch 1968; **Resid:** Surgery, Boston City Hosp 1971; Orthopaedic Surgery, Univ Texas SW Med Ctr 1976

Lewis, Valerae O MD [OrS] - **Spec Exp:** Bone Tumors; Soft Tissue Tumors; **Hospital:** UT MD Anderson Cancer Ctr; **Address:** 1400 Pressler St, Houston, TX 77030; **Phone:** 713-792-5073; **Board Cert:** Orthopaedic Surgery 2002; **Med School:** Harvard Med Sch 1993; **Resid:** Orthopaedic Surgery, Harvard Comb Ortho Program 1999

Mabrey, Jay D MD [OrS] - **Spec Exp:** Knee Replacement & Revision; Hip Replacement & Revision; Arthroscopic Surgery-Hip; **Hospital:** Baylor Univ Medical Ctr-Dallas, Mary Shiels Hosp; **Address:** 3600 Gaston Ave, Ste 1101, Dallas, TX 75246; **Phone:** 214-820-7010; **Board Cert:** Orthopaedic Surgery 2009; **Med School:** Cornell Univ-Weill Med Coll 1981; **Resid:** Surgery, Duke Univ Med Ctr 1983; Orthopaedic Surgery, Duke Univ Med Ctr 1987; **Fellow:** Joint Replacement Surgery, Hosp Special Surg 1991; **Fac Appt:** Clin Prof OrS, Univ Tex SW, Dallas

Seltzer, Dana G MD [OrS] - **Spec Exp:** Sports Medicine; Trauma; Arthroscopic Surgery; Shoulder Surgery-Complex; **Hospital:** St. Joseph's Hosp & Med Ctr - Phoenix; **Address:** 500 W Thomas Rd, Ste 850, Phoenix, AZ 85013; **Phone:** 602-406-2663; **Board Cert:** Orthopaedic Surgery 2007; **Med School:** USC-Keck School of Medicine 1986; **Resid:** Orthopaedic Surgery, Univ Miami-Jackson Meml Hosp 1991; **Fellow:** Sports Medicine, Kerlan-Jobe Orthopedic Clin 1992; Shoulder Surgery, UTSA 1993

Souryal, Tarek O MD [OrS] - **Spec Exp:** Sports Medicine; Knee Injuries/ACL; **Hospital:** TX Hlth Presby Hosp Dallas; **Address:** 6901 Snider Plaza, Ste 200, Dallas, TX 75205; **Phone:** 214-369-7733; **Board Cert:** Orthopaedic Surgery 2011; **Med School:** Univ Tex, San Antonio 1982; **Resid:** Orthopaedic Surgery, UTSW Med Ctr 1987; **Fellow:** Sports Medicine, Sports Med Clin N Tex 1987; Sports Medicine, Hughston Ortho Clinic 1988; **Fac Appt:** Clin Prof OrS, Univ Tex SW, Dallas

Williams, Ronald P MD [OrS] - **Spec Exp:** Bone Tumors; **Address:** 901 W 38th St, Ste 200, Austin, TX 78705; **Phone:** 512-421-4100; **Board Cert:** Orthopaedic Surgery 2003; **Med School:** Univ Tex, San Antonio 1984; **Resid:** Orthopaedic Surgery, Univ Kans Sch Med 1989; **Fellow:** Orthopaedic Oncology, Case West Res Univ 1990

Wirth, Michael A MD [OrS] - **Spec Exp:** Shoulder Surgery; Shoulder Replacement; **Hospital:** Univ Hlth Syst-San Antonio, Methodist Hosp-San Antonio; **Address:** 8300 Floyd Curl Drive Fl 3, San Antonio, TX 78229; **Phone:** 210-450-9300; **Board Cert:** Orthopaedic Surgery 2004; **Med School:** Oregon Hlth & Sci Univ 1985; **Resid:** Orthopaedic Surgery, Univ Texas Hlth Sci Ctr 1990; **Fellow:** Shoulder Surgery, Charles Rockwood Jr MD 1991; **Fac Appt:** Prof OrS, Univ Tex, San Antonio

West Coast and Pacific

Anderson, Lesley J MD [OrS] - **Spec Exp:** Knee Injuries/ACL; Knee Cartilage/Meniscus Transplants; Cartilage Damage; Stem Cells in Orthopedics; **Hospital:** CA Pacific Med Ctr-Pacific Campus, St. Francis Memorial Hosp; **Address:** 2100 Webster St, Ste 309, San Francisco, CA 94115; **Phone:** 415-923-3029; **Board Cert:** Orthopaedic Surgery 2007; **Med School:** Penn State Coll Med 1976; **Resid:** Orthopaedic Surgery, UCLA Med Ctr 1983; **Fellow:** Sports Medicine/Knee Surgery, Blazina Ortho Clinic 1984; **Fac Appt:** Asst Clin Prof OrS, UCSF

Bos, Gary D MD [OrS] - **Spec Exp:** Musculoskeletal Tumors; Sarcoma; Reconstructive Surgery; **Hospital:** Kittitas Valley Community Hosp, Kaiser Sunnyside Med Ctr; **Address:** 611 S Chestnut St, Ste D, Ellensburg, WA 98926; **Phone:** 509-933-8700; **Board Cert:** Orthopaedic Surgery 2008; **Med School:** Univ Chicago-Pritzker Sch Med 1978; **Resid:** Orthopaedic Surgery, Case West Reserve Univ 1984; **Fellow:** Orthopaedic Surgery, Case West Reserve Univ 1980; Orthopaedic Oncology, Mayo Clinic 1985; **Fac Appt:** Asst Clin Prof OrS

Orthopaedic Surgery

Brage, Michael E MD [OrS] - **Spec Exp:** Foot & Ankle Surgery-Complex; Ankle Replacement & Revision; Cartilage Damage; Fractures; **Hospital:** Harborview Med Ctr, Univ Wash Med Ctr; **Address:** 325 Ninth Ave, Box 359798, Seattle, WA 98104; **Phone:** 206-744-4631; **Board Cert:** Orthopaedic Surgery 2005; **Med School:** Univ IL Coll Med 1986; **Resid:** Orthopaedic Surgery, Univ Chicago Hosps 1991; **Fellow:** Foot & Ankle Surgery, Univ Washington Med Ctr 1992; **Fac Appt:** Assoc Prof OrS

Brien, Earl Warren MD [OrS] - **Spec Exp:** Bone & Soft Tissue Tumors; **Hospital:** Cedars-Sinai Med Ctr; **Address:** 8700 Beverly Blvd, rm AC1058, Los Angeles, CA 90048; **Phone:** 310-423-9887; **Board Cert:** Orthopaedic Surgery 2006; **Med School:** Howard Univ 1986; **Resid:** Orthopaedic Surgery, LAC-King Drew Med Ctr 1992; **Fellow:** Musculoskeletal Disorders, Memorial Sloan Kettering 1993; Metabolic Bone Research, Hosp for Special Surgery 1994

Caillouette, James Thompson MD [OrS] - **Spec Exp:** Joint Replacement; Hip & Knee Reconstruction; **Hospital:** Hoag Meml Hosp Presby; **Address:** 22 Corporate Plaza, Newport Beach, CA 92660; **Phone:** 949-722-5000; **Board Cert:** Orthopaedic Surgery 2011; **Med School:** USC Sch Med 1983; **Resid:** Orthopaedic Surgery, Univ CA Affil Hosp 1988; **Fac Appt:** Assoc Clin Prof OrS, UC Irvine

Carragee, Eugene J MD [OrS] - **Spec Exp:** Spinal Surgery; Spinal Disc Replacement; **Hospital:** Stanford Univ Hosp & Clinics; **Address:** Orthopaedic Spine Center, 450 Broadway St, Pavilion A, 1st Fl, Redwood City, CA 94063-6110; **Phone:** 650-725-5905; **Board Cert:** Orthopaedic Surgery 2005; **Med School:** Stanford Univ 1982; **Resid:** Internal Medicine, Stanford Univ Hosp 1984; Orthopaedic Surgery, Stanford Univ Hosp 1988; **Fac Appt:** Prof OrS, Stanford Univ

Chapman, Jens Robert MD [OrS] - **Spec Exp:** Spinal Disorders; Spinal Cord Injury; Spinal Surgery-Neck; **Hospital:** Univ Wash Med Ctr, Harborview Med Ctr; **Address:** Roosevelt Bone & Joint Surgery Ctr, 4245 Roosevelt Way NE Fl 2, Box 354740, Seattle, WA 98105; **Phone:** 206-598-4288; **Board Cert:** Orthopaedic Surgery 2004; **Med School:** Germany 1983; **Resid:** Surgery, Klinkum F.D. Isar 1985; Orthopaedic Surgery, Univ Texas Southern Med Ctr 1990; **Fellow:** Trauma, Harborview Med Ctr 1990; Spinal Surgery, Univ Washington Med School 1991; **Fac Appt:** Prof OrS, Univ Wash

Conrad, E Chappie MD [OrS] - **Spec Exp:** Pediatric Orthopaedic Surgery; Bone Tumors; **Hospital:** Seattle Chldns Hosp, Univ Wash Med Ctr; **Address:** 4800 Sand Point Way NE, #W7706, Box 359300, Seattle, WA 98105; **Phone:** 206-987-5678; **Board Cert:** Orthopaedic Surgery 2009; **Med School:** Univ VA Sch Med 1979; **Resid:** Orthopaedic Surgery, Hosp for Special Surgery 1984; **Fellow:** Orthopaedic Oncology, Univ Fla Coll Med 1985; Pediatric Orthopaedic Surgery, Hosp for Sick Chldn 1986; **Fac Appt:** Prof OrS, Univ Wash

Copp, Steven N MD [OrS] - **Spec Exp:** Hip & Knee Replacement; Reconstructive Surgery-Complex; **Hospital:** Scripps Green Hosp; **Address:** Scripps Clinic Torrey Pines, 10666 N Torrey Pines Rd, MS 116, La Jolla, CA 92037; **Phone:** 858-554-8519; **Board Cert:** Orthopaedic Surgery 2012; **Med School:** UCSD 1983; **Resid:** Orthopaedic Surgery, UCSD Med Ctr 1988

Delamarter, Rick B MD [OrS] - **Spec Exp:** Spinal Surgery; Minimally Invasive Spinal Surgery; Spinal Disc Replacement; Spinal Reconstructive Surgery; **Hospital:** Cedars-Sinai Med Ctr; **Address:** Spine Institute of Santa Monica, 444 S San Vincente Blvd, Ste 900, Los Angeles, CA 90048; **Phone:** 310-248-7300; **Board Cert:** Orthopaedic Surgery 2010; **Med School:** Oregon Hlth & Sci Univ 1981; **Resid:** Orthopaedic Surgery, UCLA Med Ctr 1986; **Fac Appt:** Assoc Prof S, UCLA

Dillingham, Michael F MD [OrS] - **Spec Exp:** Sports Medicine; **Hospital:** Sequoia Hosp; **Address:** 500 Arguello St, Ste 100, Redwood City, CA 94063; **Phone:** 650-851-4900; **Board Cert:** Orthopaedic Surgery 1977; Physical Medicine & Rehabilitation 1979; **Med School:** Stanford Univ 1971; **Resid:** Orthopaedic Surgery, Standford Univ Med Ctr 1975; Physical Medicine & Rehabilitation, Santa Clara Valley Med Ctr 1977; **Fellow:** Spinal Surgery, Santa Clara Valley Med Ctr 1976; **Fac Appt:** Clin Prof OrS, Stanford Univ

Dorr, Lawrence D MD [OrS] - **Spec Exp:** Hip & Knee Replacement; **Hospital:** Good Samaritan Hosp - LA; **Address:** Dorr Arthritis Institute, 637 S Lucas Ave, Ste 101, Los Angeles, CA 90017; **Phone:** 213-977-2280; **Board Cert:** Orthopaedic Surgery 1978; **Med School:** Univ Iowa Coll Med 1967; **Resid:** Orthopaedic Surgery, LAC-USC Med Ctr 1976; **Fellow:** Joint Replacement Surgery, Hosp Special Surgery 1977

Eckardt, Jeffrey J MD [OrS] - **Spec Exp:** Bone Tumors; Soft Tissue Tumors; Limb Sparing Surgery; **Hospital:** Santa Monica - UCLA Med Ctr & Ortho Hosp, UCLA Ronald Reagan Med Ctr; **Address:** UCLA Med Ctr, Dept Ortho Surg/Oncology, 1250 16th St Tower # 713, Santa Monica, CA 90404; **Phone:** 310-319-1234; **Board Cert:** Orthopaedic Surgery 1981; **Med School:** Cornell Univ-Weill Med Coll 1971; **Resid:** Orthopaedic Surgery, UCLA Med Ctr 1979; **Fellow:** Orthopaedic Oncology, Mayo Clinic 1980; **Fac Appt:** Prof OrS, UCLA

Elattrache, Neal S MD [OrS] - **Spec Exp:** Shoulder & Elbow Surgery; Knee Surgery; Sports Medicine; **Hospital:** Keck Med Ctr of USC (page 62); **Address:** Kerlan-Jobe Orthopaedic Clin, 6801 Park Terrace Drive, Los Angeles, CA 90045; **Phone:** 310-665-7257; **Board Cert:** Orthopaedic Surgery 2004; Orthopaedic Sports Medicine 2007; **Med School:** Univ Pittsburgh 1985; **Resid:** Orthopaedic Surgery, Univ Pittsburgh Med Ctr 1990; **Fellow:** Sports Medicine, Kerlan-Jobe Orthpaedic Clin 1991; **Fac Appt:** Assoc Clin Prof OrS, USC-Keck School of Medicine

Finerman, Gerald MD [OrS] - **Spec Exp:** Sports Medicine; Hip & Knee Replacement; **Hospital:** UCLA Ronald Reagan Med Ctr, Santa Monica - UCLA Med Ctr & Ortho Hosp; **Address:** 1245 16 St, Ste 202, Santa Monica, CA 90404; **Phone:** 310-825-6019; **Board Cert:** Orthopaedic Surgery 1971; **Med School:** Johns Hopkins Univ 1962; **Resid:** Surgery, Johns Hopkins Hosp 1964; Orthopaedic Surgery, Johns Hopkins Hosp 1969; **Fac Appt:** Prof Emeritus OrS, UCLA

Garfin, Steven R MD [OrS] - **Spec Exp:** Spinal Surgery; Minimally Invasive Spinal Surgery; **Hospital:** UCSD Med Ctr; **Address:** UCSD, Dept Orthopedic Surgery, 9350 Campus Pointe Drive, Ste 1B, La Jolla, CA 92037; **Phone:** 858-657-8200; **Board Cert:** Orthopaedic Surgery 1982; **Med School:** Univ Minn 1972; **Resid:** Orthopaedic Surgery, UCSD Med Ctr 1980; **Fellow:** Spinal Surgery, Pennsylvania Hosp 1981; **Fac Appt:** Prof OrS, UCSD

Goodman, Stuart B MD/PhD [OrS] - **Spec Exp:** Arthritis; Joint Replacement; Reconstructive Surgery; **Hospital:** Stanford Univ Hosp & Clinics, Lucile Packard Chldn's Hosp; **Address:** Joint Replacement Center, 450 Broadway St, Redwood City, CA 94063-6110; **Phone:** 650-723-5643; **Board Cert:** Orthopaedic Surgery 2008; **Med School:** Univ Toronto 1978; **Resid:** Orthopaedic Surgery, Univ Toronto Affil Hosp 1984; **Fellow:** Trauma, Univ Toronto 1985; **Fac Appt:** Prof OrS, Stanford Univ

Gorab II, Robert S MD [OrS] - **Spec Exp:** Knee Replacement; Hip Replacement; Arthritis; **Hospital:** Hoag Hosp Irvine, St. Joseph's Hosp - Orange; **Address:** Orthopaedic Specialty Inst, 280 S Main St, Ste 200, Orange, CA 92868; **Phone:** 714-937-2136; **Board Cert:** Orthopaedic Surgery 2006; **Med School:** Univ Pittsburgh 1989; **Resid:** Orthopaedic Surgery, UC-Irvine Med Ctr 1995; **Fellow:** Joint Reconstruction, Cleveland Clinic 1996; **Fac Appt:** Assoc Prof OrS, UC Irvine

Orthopaedic Surgery

Howe, Kevin MD [OrS] - **Spec Exp:** Arthritis-Hip & Knee; Hip Replacement; **Hospital:** Santa Rosa Meml Hosp, Healdsburg Dist Hosp; **Address:** Redwood Orthopaedic Surgery Assocs, 208 Concourse Blvd, Ste 1, Santa Rosa, CA 95403; **Phone:** 707-544-3400; **Board Cert:** Orthopaedic Surgery 2012; **Med School:** UCLA 1994; **Resid:** Orthopaedic Surgery, UC Davis Med Ctr 1998; **Fellow:** Joint Replacement Surgery, New England Bapt Hosp 2001

Johnson, Eric E MD [OrS] - **Spec Exp:** Pelvic & Acetabular Fractures; Trauma; Limb Lengthening; Hip Replacement; **Hospital:** UCLA Ronald Reagan Med Ctr; **Address:** UCLA Med Ctr-Dept Orthopedic Surgery, 10833 Le Conte Ave, rm 76-143 CHF, Los Angeles, CA 90095-6902; **Phone:** 310-206-1169; **Board Cert:** Orthopaedic Surgery 1985; **Med School:** Univ Utah 1976; **Resid:** Surgery, Univ Utah Med Ctr 1978; Orthopaedic Surgery, UCLA Med Ctr 1981; **Fellow:** Orthopaedic Trauma Surgery, Univ Hanover 1982; Hip Surgery, Univ Paris 1984; **Fac Appt:** Prof OrS, UCLA

Kim, Choll W MD/PhD [OrS] - **Spec Exp:** Minimally Invasive Spinal Surgery; Spinal Surgery; Scoliosis; Spinal Surgery-Cervical; **Hospital:** UCSD Med Ctr, Alvarado Hosp & Med Ctr; **Address:** Spine Institute of San Diego, Ctr for Minimally Invasive Spine Surgery, 6719 Alvarado Rd, Ste 308, San Diego, CA 92120; **Phone:** 619-265-7912; **Board Cert:** Orthopaedic Surgery 2005; **Med School:** Harvard Med Sch 1996; **Resid:** Orthopaedic Surgery, UCSD Affil Hosp 2001; **Fellow:** Spinal Surgery, Mayo Clin 2002; **Fac Appt:** Assoc Clin Prof OrS, UCSD

Lowenberg, David W MD [OrS] - **Spec Exp:** Osteomyelitis; Limb Lengthening (Ilizarov Procedure); Fractures-Complex & Non Union; Limb Deformities; **Hospital:** Stanford Univ Hosp & Clinics; **Address:** 450 Broadway, Pavilion A, Redwood City, CA 94063; **Phone:** 650-723-5643; **Board Cert:** Orthopaedic Surgery 2003; **Med School:** UCLA 1985; **Resid:** Orthopaedic Surgery, UCSF Med Ctr 1990; **Fac Appt:** Prof OrS, Stanford Univ

Luck Jr, James V MD [OrS] - **Spec Exp:** Hemophilia Related Disease; Hip & Knee Replacement; Musculoskeletal Tumors; **Hospital:** Santa Monica - UCLA Med Ctr & Ortho Hosp; **Address:** 2400 S Flower St,, Los Angeles, CA 90007; **Phone:** 213-749-8255; **Board Cert:** Orthopaedic Surgery 2000; **Med School:** USC Sch Med 1967; **Resid:** Orthopaedic Surgery, Orthopaedic Hosp 1973; **Fellow:** Orthopaedic Oncology, Orthopaedic Hosp 1974; Reconstructive Surgery, Rancho Los Amigos 1974; **Fac Appt:** Prof OrS, UCLA

Mandelbaum, Bert R MD [OrS] - **Spec Exp:** Sports Medicine; Knee Injuries/ACL; Cartilage Damage; **Hospital:** St. John's Hlth Ctr, Santa Monica; **Address:** Santa Monica Orthopaedic Group, 2020 Santa Monica Blvd Fl 4, Santa Monica, CA 90404; **Phone:** 310-829-2663; **Board Cert:** Orthopaedic Surgery 2009; Orthopaedic Sports Medicine 2010; **Med School:** Washington Univ, St Louis 1980; **Resid:** Orthopaedic Surgery, Johns Hopkins Hosp 1985

Matsen III, Frederick A MD [OrS] - **Spec Exp:** Shoulder Replacement; Rotator Cuff Surgery; **Hospital:** Univ Wash Med Ctr; **Address:** Bone & Joint Ctr, 4245 Roosevelt Way NE, Box 354740, Seattle, WA 98105; **Phone:** 206-598-4288; **Board Cert:** Orthopaedic Surgery 1978; **Med School:** Baylor Coll Med 1968; **Resid:** Orthopaedic Surgery, Univ Washington Med Ctr 1974; **Fac Appt:** Prof OrS, Univ Wash

Menendez, Lawrence R MD [OrS] - **Spec Exp:** Musculoskeletal Tumors; Bone Tumors; Reconstructive Surgery; Musculoskeletal Infections; **Hospital:** Keck Med Ctr of USC (page 62), USC Norris Cancer Hosp (page 62); **Address:** USC Orthopaedic Surgery Assocs, 1520 San Pablo St, Ste 2000, Los Angeles, CA 90033; **Phone:** 800-872-2273; **Board Cert:** Orthopaedic Surgery 2008; **Med School:** NYU Sch Med 1979; **Resid:** Orthopaedic Surgery, NYU Med Ctr 1984; **Fellow:** Orthopaedic Oncology, Univ Fla 1985; **Fac Appt:** Clin Prof OrS, USC-Keck School of Medicine

O'Donnell, Richard John MD [OrS] - **Spec Exp:** Bone Cancer; Sarcoma-Soft Tissue; Pediatric Orthopaedic Cancers; **Hospital:** UCSF Med Ctr; **Address:** UCSF Helen Diller Cancer Ctr, 1600 Divisadero St Fl 4, San Francisco, CA 94115; **Phone:** 415-885-3800; **Board Cert:** Orthopaedic Surgery 2010; **Med School:** Harvard Med Sch 1989; **Resid:** Orthopaedic Surgery, Mass Genl Hosp 1995; **Fellow:** Musculoskeletal Oncology, Univ WA Med Ctr 1996; **Fac Appt:** Assoc Prof OrS, UCSF

Oakes, Daniel A MD [OrS] - **Spec Exp:** Hip & Knee Replacement; Hip & Knee Reconstruction; Hip Resurfacing; Osteonecrosis; **Hospital:** Keck Med Ctr of USC (page 62); **Address:** USC Univ Hospital, Dept Orthopaedics, 1520 San Pablo St, Ste 2000, Los Angeles, CA 90033; **Phone:** 323-442-5860; **Board Cert:** Orthopaedic Surgery 2006; **Med School:** Harvard Med Sch 1997; **Resid:** Orthopaedic Surgery, UCLA Med Ctr 2003; **Fellow:** Joint Reconstruction, Mayo Clinic 2004; **Fac Appt:** Assoc Prof OrS, UCLA

Oppenheim, William L MD [OrS] - **Spec Exp:** Limb Lengthening; Clubfoot/Foot Deformities in Children; Pediatric Orthopaedic Surgery; Cerebral Palsy; **Hospital:** UCLA Ronald Reagan Med Ctr, Santa Monica - UCLA Med Ctr & Ortho Hosp; **Address:** Luskin Childrens Clinic, 1250 16th St, Ste 2100B, Santa Monica, CA 90404; **Phone:** 310-206-6345; **Board Cert:** Orthopaedic Surgery 1992; **Med School:** Georgetown Univ 1970; **Resid:** Orthopaedic Surgery, Univ Washington Hosp 1976; **Fellow:** Pediatric Orthopaedic Surgery, Orthopaedic Hosp UCLA 1979; **Fac Appt:** Prof OrS, UCLA

Peterson, Davis C MD [OrS] - **Spec Exp:** Spinal Surgery; Scoliosis; Trauma; **Hospital:** Providence Alaska Med Ctr, Alaska Regl Hosp; **Address:** Anchorage Fracture & Orthopaedics, 3831 Piper St, Ste 220, Anchorage, AK 99508; **Phone:** 907-563-3145; **Board Cert:** Orthopaedic Surgery 2009; **Med School:** Baylor Coll Med 1980; **Resid:** Orthopaedic Surgery, Madigan Army Med Ctr 1986; **Fellow:** Spinal Surgery, St Luke's Med Ctr 1990

Rajacich, Nicholas MD [OrS] - **Spec Exp:** Pediatric Orthopaedic Surgery; **Hospital:** Mary Bridge Chldns Hosp & Hlth Ctr, Tacoma Genl Hosp; **Address:** Mary Bridge Orthopaedic Clin, 311 S L St, Tacoma, WA 98405; **Phone:** 253-403-1507; **Board Cert:** Orthopaedic Surgery 2012; **Med School:** Johns Hopkins Univ 1982; **Resid:** Surgery, Rhode Island Hosp 1985; Orthopaedic Surgery, St Mary's Hosp 1989; **Fellow:** Pediatric Orthopaedic Surgery, Hosp for Sick Chldn 1990

Sangeorzan, Bruce J MD [OrS] - **Spec Exp:** Foot & Ankle Surgery; Trauma; Ankle Replacement & Revision; **Hospital:** Harborview Med Ctr, Univ Wash Med Ctr; **Address:** 908 Jefferson St, MS 359799, Seattle, WA 98104; **Phone:** 206-744-4830; **Board Cert:** Orthopaedic Surgery 2010; **Med School:** Wayne State Univ 1981; **Resid:** Orthopaedic Surgery, Wayne State Univ 1986; **Fellow:** Trauma, Univ Washington Med Ctr 1986; Foot & Ankle Reconstruction, Univ Washington Med Ctr 1987; **Fac Appt:** Prof OrS, Univ Wash

Schmalzried, Thomas P MD [OrS] - **Spec Exp:** Hip & Knee Replacement; **Hospital:** St. Vincent's Med Ctr - Los Angeles; **Address:** The Joint Replacement Inst, 2200 W 3rd St, Ste 400, Los Angeles, CA 90057; **Phone:** 213-484-7600; **Board Cert:** Orthopaedic Surgery 2004; **Med School:** UCLA 1984; **Resid:** Orthopaedic Surgery, UCLA Med Ctr 1990; **Fellow:** Joint Replacement Surgery, UCLA Med Ctr 1987; Hip Surgery, Mass Genl Hosp/Harvard 1991; **Fac Appt:** Asst Prof OrS, UCLA

Singer, Daniel I MD [OrS] - **Spec Exp:** Hand Surgery; Bone Cancer; Hand & Upper Extremity Tumors; **Hospital:** Queen's Med Ctr - Honolulu; **Address:** Queen's Physicians' Office Blg 1, 1380 Lusitana St, Ste 615, Honolulu, HI 96813-2442; **Phone:** 808-521-8109; **Board Cert:** Orthopaedic Surgery 2010; Hand Surgery 2010; **Med School:** Boston Univ 1979; **Resid:** Surgery, Univ Conn Hlth Ctr 1981; Orthopaedic Surgery, Univ Hawaii Affil Hosp 1984; **Fellow:** Hand Surgery, Thomas Jefferson Univ Hosp 1985; Microvascular Surgery, St Vincent's Hosp 1986; **Fac Appt:** Assoc Prof OrS, Univ Hawaii JA Burns Sch Med

Smith, Douglas George MD [OrS] - **Spec Exp:** Amputation Surgery; Foot & Ankle Surgery; Limb Sparing Surgery; **Hospital:** Harborview Med Ctr; **Address:** Harborview Medical Center, 325 9th Ave, Box 359798, Seattle, WA 98104; **Phone:** 206-744-3462; **Board Cert:** Orthopaedic Surgery 2003; **Med School:** Univ Chicago-Pritzker Sch Med 1984; **Resid:** Orthopaedic Surgery, Loyola Univ Hosp 1989; **Fellow:** Foot & Ankle Surgery, Harborview Med Ctr 1990; **Fac Appt:** Prof OrS, Univ Wash

Thomas, Bert J MD [OrS] - **Spec Exp:** Hip Replacement & Revision; Hip Resurfacing; Knee Replacement & Revision; Arthroscopic Surgery; **Hospital:** UCLA Ronald Reagan Med Ctr, Santa Monica - UCLA Med Ctr & Ortho Hosp; **Address:** 1250 16th St, Santa Monica, CA 90404; **Phone:** 310-319-3828; **Board Cert:** Orthopaedic Surgery 2008; **Med School:** Univ Pennsylvania 1979; **Resid:** Orthopaedic Surgery, UCLA Med Ctr 1984; **Fellow:** Hip Replacement Surgery, Hosp Special Surg 1985; **Fac Appt:** Clin Prof OrS, UCLA-David Geffen Sch Med

Tolo, Vernon T MD [OrS] - **Spec Exp:** Pediatric Orthopaedic Surgery; Spinal Surgery-Pediatric; Spinal Deformity-Pediatric; Scoliosis; **Hospital:** Chldns Hosp - Los Angeles, Keck Med Ctr of USC (page 62); **Address:** Chldns Hosp LA, Orthopaedic Surgery, 4650 W Sunset Blvd, MS 69, Los Angeles, CA 90027-6062; **Phone:** 323-361-4658; **Board Cert:** Orthopaedic Surgery 1977; **Med School:** Johns Hopkins Univ 1968; **Resid:** Orthopaedic Surgery, Johns Hopkins Hosp 1975; **Fellow:** Pediatric Orthopaedic Surgery, Hosp Sick Chldn 1976; **Fac Appt:** Prof OrS, USC Sch Med

Vail, Thomas P MD [OrS] - **Spec Exp:** Hip & Knee Replacement; Hip Resurfacing; Arthritis; Osteonecrosis; **Hospital:** UCSF Med Ctr; **Address:** 1500 Owens St Fl 2, 500 Parnassus Ave, Box MU320W, San Francisco, CA 94143-0728; **Phone:** 415-502-5183; **Board Cert:** Orthopaedic Surgery 2005; **Med School:** Loyola Univ-Stritch Sch Med 1985; **Resid:** Thoracic Surgery, Duke Univ Med Ctr 1987; Orthopaedic Surgery, Duke Univ Med Ctr 1991; **Fellow:** Reconstructive Surgery, Duke Univ Med Ctr 1992; **Fac Appt:** Prof OrS, UCSF

Wang, Jeffrey C MD [OrS] - **Spec Exp:** Spinal Surgery; Spinal Cord Injury; Spinal Tumors; Spinal Trauma; **Hospital:** UCLA Ronald Reagan Med Ctr, Santa Monica - UCLA Med Ctr & Ortho Hosp; **Address:** UCLA Spine Center, 1250 16th St, Ste 3145, Santa Monica, CA 90404; **Phone:** 424-259-9875; **Board Cert:** Orthopaedic Surgery 2010; **Med School:** Univ Pittsburgh 1991; **Resid:** Orthopaedic Surgery, Orthopaedic Hosp UCLA 1996; **Fellow:** Spinal Surgery, Case Western Reserve Univ 1997; **Fac Appt:** Prof OrS, UCLA-David Geffen Sch Med

Watkins III, Robert G MD [OrS] - **Spec Exp:** Spinal Surgery; Spinal Disc Replacement; **Hospital:** Marina Del Rey Hosp; **Address:** 4640 Admiralty Way, Ste 600, Marina Del Rey, CA 90292; **Phone:** 310-448-7890; **Board Cert:** Orthopaedic Surgery 1982; **Med School:** Univ Tenn Coll Med 1969; **Resid:** Orthopaedic Surgery, LAC-USC Med Ctr 1978; **Fellow:** Spinal Surgery, Jones-Hunt Orth Hosp 1979; **Fac Appt:** Assoc Prof OrS, USC Sch Med

Yoo, Jung MD [OrS] - **Spec Exp:** Spinal Surgery; **Hospital:** OR Hlth & Sci Univ; **Address:** 3181 SW Sam Jackson Park Rd, MC OP31, Portland, OR 97239; **Phone:** 503-494-6400; **Board Cert:** Orthopaedic Surgery 2004; **Med School:** Univ Chicago-Pritzker Sch Med 1984; **Resid:** Orthopaedic Surgery, Case Western Reserve Univ 1990; **Fellow:** Orthopaedic Surgery, SUNY Hlth Sci Ctr 1991; **Fac Appt:** Prof OrS, Oregon Hlth & Sci Univ

Cleveland Clinic

Every life deserves world class care.

Orthopaedic Surgery

The Cleveland Clinic Department of Orthopaedic Surgery has a long history of excellence and innovation in treating musculoskeletal injuries and diseases. Since 1992, *U.S. News & World Report* has consistently ranked the Department of Orthopaedic Surgery among the top five orthopaedic programs in the nation.

Foot and Ankle: All specialists and surgeons have extensive training in the diagnosis and care of foot and ankle disorders.

Joint Replacement: The Center for Adult Reconstruction performs joint replacement, resurfacing and revision surgery of the hip and knee. Our experienced surgeons offer the most advanced implants and minimally invasive techniques to restore patient mobility.

Upper Extremity: This center provides a diagnosis and treatment for problems affecting the hand, wrist, elbow and shoulder.

Pediatrics: The Center for Pediatric Orthopaedics handles more than 14,000 outpatient visits each year. Our physicians offer expertise in the management of all musculoskeletal conditions in children, and sports injuries.

Center for Spine Health: The Center for Spine Health diagnoses and treats more than 13,000 patients annually. The center brings together the expertise of specialists in neurosurgery, orthopaedic surgery and non-surgical spine care.

Trauma: Cleveland Clinic is a leader in the treatment of fractures and non-union and in the development of methods to improve outcomes through advanced bone grafting techniques.

Center for Musculoskeletal Tumors: As one of the largest multidisciplinary centers of its kind, we offer expertise in treating bone and soft tissue sarcomas and performing limb salvage.

THE MOUNT SINAI MEDICAL CENTER ORTHOPAEDICS

One Gustave L. Levy Place
Fifth Avenue and 100th Street
New York, NY 10029-6574
Physician Referral: 1-800-MD-SINAI (637-4624)
www.mountsinai.org/orthopaedics

Beyond its reputation for depth and breadth of expertise, **THE LENI AND PETER W. MAY DEPARTMENT OF ORTHOPAEDICS** at The Mount Sinai Medical Center is known for personalized care. The faculty and staff invest the time to get to know their patients as individuals, ensuring that they receive direct care from superb subspecialty-trained orthopedists. The faculty share expertise in surgery of the foot and ankle, knee, hip, hand, elbow, shoulder, and spine; total joint replacement; microvascular surgery; cancer surgery; and minimally invasive surgery. Taking a whole-patient approach to care, they work in close collaboration with specialists in geriatrics, neurology, oncology, pathology, and rehabilitation medicine.

Investigation and Innovation – Recent years have seen successive refinements in the techniques of orthopedic surgery at Mount Sinai, including joint replacement, minimally invasive fracture repair, and microvascular surgery. Faculty members have been instrumental in the design and perfection of hip and shoulder prostheses. Additionally, Mount Sinai has broadened the applications of arthroscopic surgery—the fiber optic technology that first heralded the arrival of minimally invasive surgery.

Mount Sinai orthopedic bone, spine and tendon scientists are known for their studies of diseases of the skeletal system. Researchers are currently investigating disc degeneration in the spine; rotator cuff degeneration; and the fundamental molecular mechanisms of tendon failure and regeneration.

Use of Cutting-Edge Techniques – Mount Sinai uses innovative, minimally invasive approaches for joint replacement and fracture repair. The Department's Oncology Service is renowned for saving limbs with both bone and joint malignancies.

The Sports Service provides patients with the full spectrum of non-operative and operative treatment including arthroscopic surgery of the hip, shoulder, knee, and elbow. Patients have the ability to return to activities faster and with less pain with this minimally invasive procedure. Our arthroscopists also specialize in cartilage preservation techniques, including cartilage transplantation, allowing patients to preserve their own joints and delaying the need for joint replacement surgery.

GROUNDBREAKING PROCEDURES ENHANCE QUALITY OF LIFE

Today at Mount Sinai, arthroscopy is used to repair not only the knee but virtually every joint. Converting what used to be major open surgery to outpatient procedures has dramatically shortened rehabilitation and return to work times. More significantly, it has allowed many more patients to get help for painful, function-limiting conditions. That is the case for many elderly or frail patients who are physically unable to undergo major surgery. The fact that such procedures are now more widely accessible is enhancing the quality of life for many patients and allowing them to lead more active lives.

HOSPITAL FOR JOINT DISEASES

About the Hospital for Joint Diseases

The Hospital for Joint Diseases at NYU Langone Medical Center (HJD) is one of the nation's leading inpatient orthopaedic and rheumatologic specialty hospitals, and is ranked among the nation's top 10 for both orthopaedics and rheumatology in the 2012-2013 *U.S. News & World Report* annual survey of "Best Hospitals" in America. HJD is dedicated to the prevention and treatment of musculoskeletal diseases, providing some of the most advanced programs in the region for musculoskeletal disorders and the largest pediatric orthopaedic program in New York City. HJD also offers a number of unique and highly specialized services to provide tailored, world-class care to patients with specific musculoskeletal conditions and needs. We specialize in the following areas:

Orthopaedic Surgery

The clinical expertise of our internationally-renowned surgeons represents the full range of subspecialty areas of orthopaedic surgery, including Adult Reconstructive, Sports Medicine, Spine, Shoulder & Elbow, Foot & Ankle, Hand Surgery, Trauma & Fracture, Orthopaedic Oncology, and Pediatric Orthopaedics; additional areas of focus include minimally-invasive hip surgery and robotic-assisted joint replacement.

Rheumatology

HJD houses the Division of Rheumatology's Osteoporosis Center, offering a multidisciplinary approach to the evaluation and treatment of osteoporosis, including a range of advanced drug therapies.

Rehabilitation

Rehabilitation care at HJD is provided by the world-renowned Rusk Rehabilitation. Rusk's CARF-Accredited Brain Injury Rehabilitation Program is a center of innovation and excellence for the treatment of disabling neurological and neurocognitive disorders. HJD also houses Rusk's Orthopaedic Rehabilitation Unit, where an expert multidisciplinary rehabilitation team aids patients in their recovery after orthopaedic surgery or injury.

Neurology – Spine & Nerve

HJD provides a broad range of diagnostic and therapeutic services to patients with neurological disorders. Its outstanding clinical staff includes specialists in pain management, spine and nerve pain, and cerebral palsy.

Radiology

HJD provides complete diagnostic orthopaedic radiology services, including MRI, computed tomography, ultrasonography and conventional radiography, as well as a multitude of musculoskeletal interventional procedures. The medical team includes several internationally-known musculoskeletal radiologists with expertise in all aspects of osteoradiology.

550 First Avenue *(at 31st Street)*
New York, NY 10016

www.NYULMC.org

Physician Referral: **888-7-NYU-MED** *(888-769-8633)*

ORTHOPAEDIC PROGRAMS

The **Department of Orthopaedic Surgery** at NYU Langone Medical Center continues to be recognized as a national leader, ranked #6 nationwide in *U.S. News & World Report's* 2012-2013 "Best Hospitals" survey. Expert physicians combine extensive experience with cutting-edge research and technology to address bone and joint problems that affect a patient's ability to function. The department provides care at NYU Langone's premier outpatient facility, The Center for Musculoskeletal Care, as well as at the Hospital for Joint Diseases, our internationally-renowned inpatient musculoskeletal hospital. The clinical expertise of our world-class orthopaedic surgeons represents the full range of subspecialty areas including Adult Reconstructive, Sports Medicine, Spine, Shoulder & Elbow, Foot & Ankle, Hand Surgery, Trauma & Fracture, Orthopaedic Oncology, and Pediatric Orthopaedics; additional areas of focus include minimally-invasive surgery and robotic-assisted joint replacement.

The department also features a number of specialized orthopaedic patient care centers:
The Bone Healing Center evaluates and treats problem fractures and are leaders in technologies and procedures to help patients facing a long and difficult recovery from complex fracture reconstruction or fracture healing problems.
Harkness Center for Dance Injuries offers many subsidized and free services for dancers, including clinics staffed by orthopaedists and dance physical therapists. The Center also offers state-of-the-art rehabilitation technology and free injury prevention screenings and lectures.
The Diabetes Foot and Ankle Center focuses on the prevention and recurrence of foot and ankle problems associated with complications of diabetes.
The Hip Center evaluates and treats developmental, traumatic, and degenerative hip disorders and specializes in the cutting-edge, minimally invasive anterior total hip replacement technique.
The Orthopaedic Immediate Care Center ("i-Care"), New York City's only walk-in orthopaedic clinic, uses state-of-the-art diagnostic equipment to evaluate and treat hand and foot injuries, hip, arm or leg fractures, dislocation or joint injury, sprains, and bone or joint infection.
The Joint Preservation Center (JPC) is dedicated to operative and non-operative treatment of joint problems, aiming to reduce symptoms, restore function and delay the onset of degenerative arthritis and potential need for an eventual joint replacement.
Joint Replacement Center physicians are experts in knee, hip and shoulder replacements, complex joint revisions, and minimally invasive surgeries, conducting 3,000+ procedures annually.
The Occupational and Industrial Orthopaedic Center (OIOC) provides clinical, educational, research and consulting services in the prevention and treatment of musculoskeletal injuries and disorders that arise from work or the work environment.
The Spine Center specializes in spine disorders, including lower back and neck pain, scoliosis, osteoporosis and complex spine problems. The Center performs minimally invasive spinal fusions and was one of the first in the country to successfully perform artificial disc implantation.

Penn Orthopaedics, a leader in treating patients with musculoskeletal injuries and disorders from the most common to the most complex, provides comprehensive, quality care that ranks among the very best in the nation. Our multidisciplinary team of surgeons and staff use the latest technology and techniques to get people – grandparents and professional athletes alike – back in motion.

Programs

Penn Orthopaedics offers specialized services and programs to treat a wide range of orthopaedic problems, including:

- Foot and ankle
- General orthopaedics
- Hand and wrist
- Hip and knee replacement
- Neuro-orthopaedics

- Orthopaedic oncology
- Shoulder and elbow
- Spine
- Sports medicine
- Trauma and fracture

Leadership

As recognized clinical leaders, our doctors offer state-of-the-art treatment options, including:

- Advanced minimally invasive joint replacement procedures.
- Upper extremity services dedicated to the treatment of shoulder, elbow, wrist and hand disorders.
- Treatment for malignant and benign tumors of the bone and soft tissue.

Our physicians serve on the boards of the nation's premiere orthopaedic organizations and publish articles in many of the leading orthopaedic journals in the world.

Also a noted research group, Penn Orthopaedics is helping to create the next generation of orthopaedic care, in areas including tissue engineering, tendon healing and biomechanics of the shoulder and spine. Penn Orthopaedics is the 3rd ranked orthopaedic department in the country for orthopaedic grants from the National Institutes of Health.

Expertise

Penn Orthopaedics is consistently recognized as a national leader in outstanding care. *U.S. News & World Report* ranked the Hospital of the University of Pennsylvania among the best in Philadelphia region for outstanding orthopaedic care. Many of our surgeons are listed among the *Best Doctors in America*®, and a number of our physicians are listed annually in *Philadelphia* magazine's " *Top Docs* " issue.

Locations

Hospital of the University of Pennsylvania

Penn Presbyterian Medical Center

Pennsylvania Hospital

Penn Sports Medicine Center— Weightman Hall

Penn Medicine Cherry Hill

Penn Medicine Radnor

Penn Medicine Valley Forge

For more information or to schedule an appointment, call 800.789.PENN (7366) or visit PennMedicine.org/ortho

Otolaryngology

An otolaryngologist-head and neck surgeon provides comprehensive medical and surgical care for patients with diseases and disorders that affect the ears, nose, throat, the respiratory and upper alimentary systems and related structures of the head and neck.

An otolaryngologist diagnoses and provides medical and/or surgical therapy or prevention of diseases, allergies, neoplasms, deformities, disorders and/or injuries of the ears, nose, sinuses, throat, respiratory and upper alimentary systems, face, jaws and the other head and neck systems. Head and neck oncology, facial plastic and reconstructive surgery and the treatment of disorders of hearing and voice are fundamental areas of expertise.

Training Required: Five years

Certification in the following subspecialty requires additional training and examination.

Plastic Surgery within the Head and Neck: An otolaryngologist with additional training in plastic and reconstructive procedures within the head, face, neck and associated structures, including cutaneous head and neck oncology and reconstruction, management of maxillofacial trauma, soft tissue repair and neural surgery.

Facial Plastic and Reconstructive Surgery is not a recognized ABMS subspecialty. However this designation has been included because the certification process is meaningful and rigorous. It is awarded to those doctors who hold a current ABMS certification in Otolaryngology, but those board certified in Plastic Surgery, Ophthalmology, or Dermatology are also eligible. Certification requires a post-graduate fellowship in Facial Plastic and Reconstructive Surgery followed by a written examination.

This field is diverse and involves a wide age range of patients, from the newborn to the aged. While both cosmetic and reconstructive surgeries are practiced, there are many additional procedures which interface with them.

OTOLARYNGOLOGY

New England

Bhattacharyya, Neil MD [Oto] - **Spec Exp:** Sinus Disorders; Endoscopic Sinus Surgery; Sleep Apnea; **Hospital:** Brigham and Women's Hosp (page 57), Dana-Farber Cancer Inst (page 57); **Address:** Brigham & Women's Hospital, Div of Otolaryngology, 45 Francis St Fl 2, Boston, MA 02115; **Phone:** 617-525-6540; **Board Cert:** Otolaryngology 1998; **Med School:** Univ IL Coll Med 1992; **Resid:** Otolaryngology, Mass Eye & Ear Infirm 1997; **Fac Appt:** Prof Oto, Harvard Med Sch

Burns, James A MD [Oto] - **Spec Exp:** Laryngeal & Vocal Cord Surgery; Laryngeal & Tracheal Disorders; Voice Disorders; **Hospital:** Mass Genl Hosp; **Address:** Ctr for Laryngeal Surgery, One Bowdoin Square Fl 11, BS01-11, Boston, MA 02114; **Phone:** 617-726-1444; **Board Cert:** Otolaryngology 1997; **Med School:** Univ VA Sch Med 1991; **Resid:** Otolaryngology, Univ Virginia Affil Hosp 1996; **Fellow:** Laryngology, Mass Eye & Ear Infirmary 2003

Couch, Marion E MD [Oto] - **Spec Exp:** Head & Neck Cancer; Thyroid & Parathyroid Cancer & Surgery; Microvascular Surgery; Airway Reconstruction; **Hospital:** Fletcher Allen Health Care- Med Ctr Campus; **Address:** 111 Colchester Ave, Div Otolaryngology, Burlington, VT 05401; **Phone:** 802-847-4537; **Board Cert:** Otolaryngology 1997; **Med School:** Rush Med Coll 1990; **Resid:** Surgery, Johns Hopkins Hosp 1991; Otolaryngology, Johns Hopkins Hosp 1995; **Fac Appt:** Assoc Prof Oto, Univ VT Coll Med

Deschler, Daniel G MD [Oto] - **Spec Exp:** Head & Neck Cancer; Head & Neck Reconstruction; Salivary Gland Tumors & Surgery; Voice after Laryngeal Cancer Surgery; **Hospital:** Mass Eye & Ear Infirmary, Mass Genl Hosp; **Address:** Mass Eye & Ear Infirmary, Head & Neck Surgery Dept, 243 Charles St Fl 11 - Ste 1199, Boston, MA 02114; **Phone:** 617-573-4100; **Board Cert:** Otolaryngology 1996; **Med School:** Harvard Med Sch 1990; **Resid:** Otolaryngology, UCSF Med Ctr 1995; **Fellow:** Head & Neck Surgical Oncology, Hahneman Univ Med Ctr 1996; **Fac Appt:** Assoc Prof Oto, Harvard Med Sch

Gliklich, Richard E MD [Oto] - **Spec Exp:** Cosmetic Surgery-Face & Neck; Rhinoplasty; Skin Laser Surgery-Resurfacing; **Hospital:** Mass Eye & Ear Infirmary; **Address:** Mass Eye & Ear Infirmary, 243 Charles St Fl 9, Boston, MA 02114; **Phone:** 617-573-4105; **Board Cert:** Otolaryngology 1994; Facial Plastic & Reconstr Surgery 1996; **Med School:** Harvard Med Sch 1988; **Resid:** Otolaryngology, Mass E&E Infirm 1993; **Fellow:** Facial Plastic Surgery, Harvard Univ 1994; **Fac Appt:** Prof Oto, Harvard Med Sch

Gosselin, Benoit J MD [Oto] - **Spec Exp:** Head & Neck Cancer; Facial Plastic & Reconstructive Surgery; Head & Neck Reconstruction; **Hospital:** Dartmouth - Hitchcock Med Ctr; **Address:** Dartmouth-Hitchcock Med Ctr, Dept Oto, 1 Med Ctr Drive, Lebanon, NH 03756; **Phone:** 603-650-8123; **Board Cert:** Otolaryngology 1994; **Med School:** Univ Ottawa 1988; **Resid:** Head and Neck Surgery, Univ Ottawa 1993; **Fellow:** Head and Neck Surgery, Univ Toronto 1994; Facial Plastic Surgery, Mercy Hosp 1995; **Fac Appt:** Assoc Clin Prof Oto, Dartmouth Med Sch

Grillone, Gregory A MD [Oto] - **Spec Exp:** Laryngeal Disorders; Laryngeal Cancer; Head & Neck Cancer; Voice Disorders; **Hospital:** Boston Med Ctr; **Address:** BMC-Dept Otolaryngology, 830 Harrison Ave, Moakley Bldg - Ste 1400, Boston, MA 02118; **Phone:** 617-638-8124; **Board Cert:** Otolaryngology 1988; **Med School:** Mount Sinai Sch Med 1983; **Resid:** Otolaryngology, Boston Univ Med Ctr 1988; **Fac Appt:** Assoc Prof Oto, Boston Univ

Otolaryngology

Grundfast, Kenneth M MD [Oto] - **Spec Exp:** Hearing Loss; Pediatric Otolaryngology; **Hospital:** Boston Med Ctr, VA Boston Hlthcare Sys-Jamaica Plain Div; **Address:** Boston Med Ctr, 830 Harrison Ave, Moakley Bldg - Ste 1400, Boston, MA 02118; **Phone:** 617-638-8124; **Board Cert:** Otolaryngology 1977; **Med School:** SUNY Upstate Med Univ 1969; **Resid:** Surgery, Sibley Meml Hosp 1974; Otolaryngology, Boston-Affil Hosps 1977; **Fellow:** Pediatric Otolaryngology, Chldns Hosp 1978; **Fac Appt:** Prof Oto, Boston Univ

Hadlock, Theresa MD [Oto] - **Spec Exp:** Facial Paralysis; **Hospital:** Mass Eye & Ear Infirmary; **Address:** Mass Eye & Ear Infirm, Facial Plastic Surgey, 243 Charles St, Boston, MA 02114; **Phone:** 617-573-3641; **Board Cert:** Otolaryngology 2012; **Med School:** Harvard Med Sch 1994; **Resid:** Otolaryngology, Mass Eye & Ear Infirm 1998; **Fellow:** Facial Plastic Surgery, Mass Eye & Ear Infirm 1999; **Fac Appt:** Asst Prof Oto, Harvard Med Sch

Kim, Daniel Y MD [Oto] - **Spec Exp:** Head & Neck Surgery; Head & Neck Tumors; Skull Base Tumors & Surgery; Thyroid & Parathyroid Surgery; **Hospital:** UMass Memorial Med Ctr, UMass Mem Med Ctr-Memorial Campus; **Address:** UMass Meml Med Ctr-Univ Campus, 55 Lake Ave N, Worcester, MA 01655; **Phone:** 508-856-4161; **Board Cert:** Otolaryngology 1986; **Med School:** UMDNJ-RW Johnson Med Sch 1980; **Resid:** Surgery, Boston Univ Med Ctr 1982; Otolaryngology, NYU Med Ctr 1985; **Fellow:** Head & Neck Surgical Oncology, Montefiore Med Ctr 1986; **Fac Appt:** Assoc Clin Prof Oto, Univ Mass Sch Med

Kveton, John F MD [Oto] - **Spec Exp:** Ear Disorders/Surgery; Cochlear Implants; Acoustic Neuroma; Hearing Loss; **Hospital:** Yale-New Haven Hosp; **Address:** ENT Med & Surgical Grp, 46 Prince St, Ste 601, New Haven, CT 06519-1634; **Phone:** 203-752-1726; **Board Cert:** Otolaryngology 1982; Neurotology 2004; **Med School:** St Louis Univ 1978; **Resid:** Otolaryngology, Yale-New Haven Hosp 1982; **Fellow:** Neurotology, The Otology Group 1983; **Fac Appt:** Clin Prof Oto, Yale Univ

McKenna, Michael J MD [Oto] - **Spec Exp:** Skull Base Surgery; Otology; Neuro-Otology; **Hospital:** Mass Eye & Ear Infirmary; **Address:** Massachusetts Eye & Ear Infirm, 243 Charles St Fl 2, Boston, MA 02114-3002; **Phone:** 617-573-3672; **Board Cert:** Otolaryngology 1988; Neurotology 2004; **Med School:** USC Sch Med 1982; **Resid:** Otolaryngology, Mass Eye & Ear Infirm 1988; **Fellow:** Neurotology, Otologic Med Grp 1989; **Fac Appt:** Prof Oto, Harvard Med Sch

Metson, Ralph MD [Oto] - **Spec Exp:** Sinus Disorders/Surgery; **Hospital:** Mass Eye & Ear Infirmary; **Address:** Zero Emerson Pl, Ste 2D, Boston, MA 02114; **Phone:** 617-227-4366; **Board Cert:** Otolaryngology 1985; **Med School:** UCSD 1979; **Resid:** Otolaryngology, UCLA Med Ctr 1985; **Fac Appt:** Assoc Clin Prof Oto, Harvard Med Sch

Randolph, Gregory W MD [Oto] - **Spec Exp:** Thyroid Disorders; Thyroid Cancer; Parathyroid Disease; **Hospital:** Mass Eye & Ear Infirmary; **Address:** Mass Eye & Ear Infirmary, 243 Charles St, Ste 271, Boston, MA 02114; **Phone:** 617-573-4115; **Board Cert:** Otolaryngology 1993; **Med School:** Cornell Univ-Weill Med Coll 1987; **Resid:** Otolaryngology, Mass Eye & Ear Infirmary 1992; **Fellow:** Thyroid Oncology, Mass Eye & Ear Infirmary 1993; **Fac Appt:** Asst Prof Oto, Harvard Med Sch

Rauch, Steven D MD [Oto] - **Spec Exp:** Hearing & Balance Disorders; Meniere's Disease; Neuro-Otology; **Hospital:** Mass Eye & Ear Infirmary; **Address:** Mass Eye & Ear Infirm Dept Otolary, 243 Charles St, Boston, MA 02114; **Phone:** 617-573-3644; **Board Cert:** Otolaryngology 1984; **Med School:** Univ Cincinnati 1979; **Resid:** Surgery, U Mass Med Ctr 1981; Otolaryngology, Mass Eye & Ear Infirm 1984; **Fac Appt:** Assoc Prof Oto, Harvard Med Sch

Rebeiz, Elie E MD [Oto] - **Spec Exp:** Head & Neck Surgery; Sinus Disorders/Surgery; Skull Base Surgery; **Hospital:** Tufts Med Ctr; **Address:** Tufts Med Ctr, Dept Otolaryngology, 800 Washington St, Boston, MA 02111; **Phone:** 617-636-1664; **Board Cert:** Otolaryngology 2000; **Med School:** Lebanon 1984; **Resid:** Otolaryngology, Amer Univ Med Ctr 1988; **Fellow:** Otolaryngology, Mass E&E Infirm 1990; **Fac Appt:** Prof Oto, Tufts Univ

Sasaki, Clarence T MD [Oto] - **Spec Exp:** Head & Neck Cancer; Swallowing Disorders; Zenker Diverticulum; Voice Disorders; **Hospital:** Yale-New Haven Hosp, Yale Med Group; **Address:** Yale Sch Med, Dept Otolaryngology, 333 Cedar St, Box 208041, New Haven, CT 06520-8041; **Phone:** 203-785-2592; **Board Cert:** Otolaryngology 1973; **Med School:** Yale Univ 1966; **Resid:** Surgery, Mary Hitchcock Hosp 1968; Otolaryngology, Yale-New Haven Hosp 1973; **Fellow:** Head and Neck Surgery, Univ of Milan 1978; Skull Base Surgery, Univ Zurich 1982; **Fac Appt:** Prof Oto, Yale Univ

Silverman, Damon A MD [Oto] - **Spec Exp:** Head & Neck Cancer & Surgery; Voice Disorders; Throat Disorders; **Hospital:** Fletcher Allen Health Care- Med Ctr Campus; **Address:** Fletcher Allen Otolaryngology, West Pavilion, Level 4, Med Ctr Campus, 111 Colchester Ave, MS 210WP4, Burlington, VT 05401; **Phone:** 802-847-4041; **Board Cert:** Otolaryngology 2004; **Med School:** UC Davis 1997; **Resid:** Otolaryngology, Cleveland Clinic 2003; **Fellow:** Laryngology, Vanderbilt Univ 2004; **Fac Appt:** Asst Prof Oto, Univ VT Coll Med

Spiegel, Jeffrey H MD [Oto] - **Spec Exp:** Head & Neck Cancer & Surgery; Reconstructive Surgery; Cosmetic Surgery-Face; **Hospital:** Boston Med Ctr; **Address:** Advanced Facial Aesthetics, 1200 Boylston St, Chestnut Hill, MA 02467; **Phone:** 617-566-3223; **Board Cert:** Otolaryngology 2000; Facial Plastic & Reconstr Surgery 2001; **Med School:** Univ Mich Med Sch 1994; **Resid:** Otolaryngology, UCSF Med Ctr 1999; **Fellow:** Facial Plastic & Reconstr Surgery, Mass Eye & Ear Infirmary 2000; **Fac Appt:** Assoc Prof Oto, Boston Univ

Vining, Eugenia M MD [Oto] - **Spec Exp:** Sinus Disorders/Surgery; Skull Base Tumors; Sinus Tumors; **Hospital:** Yale-New Haven Hosp; **Address:** ENT Medical & Surgical Grp, 46 Prince St, Ste 601, New Haven, CT 06519; **Phone:** 203-752-1726; **Board Cert:** Otolaryngology 1993; **Med School:** Yale Univ 1987; **Resid:** Otolaryngology, Yale-New Haven Hosp 1991; Otolaryngology, Yale-New Haven Hosp 1992; **Fellow:** Sinus Surgery, Univ Penn 1993

Yarbrough, Wendell G MD [Oto] - **Spec Exp:** Head & Neck Cancer; **Hospital:** Yale-New Haven Hosp; **Address:** 800 Howard Ave Fl 4, New Haven, CT 06519; **Phone:** 203-785-4862; **Board Cert:** Otolaryngology 1995; **Med School:** Univ NC Sch Med 1989; **Resid:** Otolaryngology, Univ NC Hosps 1994; **Fellow:** Surgical Oncology, Univ NC Med Sch 1996

Zeitels, Steven MD [Oto] - **Spec Exp:** Laryngeal Cancer; Voice Disorders; Head & Neck Cancer & Surgery; **Hospital:** Mass Genl Hosp; **Address:** MGH Center for Laryngeal Surgery, 1 Bowdoin Square Fl 11, Boston, MA 02114; **Phone:** 617-726-0218; **Board Cert:** Otolaryngology 1988; **Med School:** Boston Univ 1982; **Resid:** Surgery, Univ Hosp-Boston City Hosp 1983; Otolaryngology, Boston Univ-Tufts Univ Affil Hosps 1987; **Fellow:** Head and Neck Surgery, Boston VA Med Ctr 1988; **Fac Appt:** Prof Oto, Harvard Med Sch

Mid Atlantic

Aviv, Jonathan MD [Oto] - **Spec Exp:** Voice Disorders; Swallowing Disorders; Cough; Endoscopy; **Hospital:** Mount Sinai Med Ctr (page 64); **Address:** 210 E 86th St, Fl 9, New York, NY 10028; **Phone:** 212-722-5570; **Board Cert:** Otolaryngology 1990; **Med School:** Columbia P&S 1985; **Resid:** Surgery, Mt Sinai Med Ctr 1987; Otolaryngology, Mt Sinai Med Ctr 1990; **Fellow:** Otolaryngology, Mt Sinai Med Ctr 1991; **Fac Appt:** Prof Oto, Mount Sinai Sch Med

Blitzer, Andrew MD/DDS [Oto] - **Spec Exp:** Voice Disorders; Swallowing Disorders; Nasal & Sinus Surgery; Botox Therapy; **Hospital:** St. Luke's - Roosevelt Hosp Ctr - Roosevelt Div (page 56); **Address:** 425 W 59th St Fl 10, New York, NY 10019-1104; **Phone:** 212-262-9500; **Board Cert:** Otolaryngology 1977; **Med School:** Mount Sinai Sch Med 1973; **Resid:** Surgery, Beth Israel Med Ctr 1974; Otolaryngology, Mt Sinai Hosp 1977; **Fac Appt:** Clin Prof Oto, Columbia P&S

Califano III, Joseph A MD [Oto] - **Spec Exp:** Head & Neck Cancer; Thyroid Cancer; Skull Base Tumors; Melanoma; **Hospital:** Johns Hopkins Hosp (page 61), Greater Baltimore Med Ctr; **Address:** Johns Hopkins Outpatient Clin, 601 N Caroline St Fl 6th, Baltimore, MD 21287; **Phone:** 443-849-8940; **Board Cert:** Otolaryngology 2000; **Med School:** Harvard Med Sch 1993; **Resid:** Otolaryngology, Johns Hopkins Hosp 1999; **Fellow:** Otolaryngology, Meml Sloan Kettering Cancer Ctr 2000; **Fac Appt:** Prof Oto, Johns Hopkins Univ

Carey, John P MD [Oto] - **Spec Exp:** Skull Base Surgery; Hearing Disorders; Neuro-Otology; **Hospital:** Johns Hopkins Hosp (page 61); **Address:** John Hopkins Outpt Ctr, 601 N Caroline St, rm 6255, Baltimore, MD 21287; **Phone:** 443-997-6467; **Board Cert:** Otolaryngology 1999; Neurotology 2008; **Med School:** Univ Wash 1991; **Resid:** Internal Medicine, Univ Washington 1998; **Fellow:** Otolaryngology, John Hopkins Med Inst 1999; **Fac Appt:** Prof Oto, Johns Hopkins Univ

Caruana, Salvatore M MD [Oto] - **Spec Exp:** Head & Neck Cancer; Thyroid & Parathyroid Cancer & Surgery; Nasal & Sinus Disorders; Laser Surgery; **Hospital:** NY-Presby/Columbia Univ Med Ctr, NY (page 66); **Address:** 180 Fort Washington Ave, Harkness Bldg Fl 7, New York, NY 10032; **Phone:** 212-305-5335; **Board Cert:** Otolaryngology 1996; **Med School:** Mount Sinai Sch Med 1989; **Resid:** Otolaryngology, NY EE Infirm 1995; **Fellow:** Head & Neck Surgical Oncology, Meml Sloan-Kettering Canc Ctr 1997; **Fac Appt:** Asst Prof Oto, Columbia P&S

Chalian, Ara A MD [Oto] - **Spec Exp:** Head & Neck Cancer; Head & Neck Reconstruction; Thyroid Cancer; Reconstructive Surgery; **Hospital:** Hosp Univ Penn - UPHS (page 72); **Address:** Hosp Univ Penn, Dept Otolaryngology, 3400 Spruce St, 5 Silverstein, Philadelphia, PA 19104; **Phone:** 215-349-5559; **Board Cert:** Otolaryngology 1994; **Med School:** Indiana Univ 1988; **Resid:** Surgery, Indiana Univ Hosp 1990; Otolaryngology, Indiana Univ Hosp 1993; **Fellow:** Molecular Biology, Hosp Univ Penn 1994; Head and Neck Surgery, Hosp Univ Penn 1995; **Fac Appt:** Assoc Prof Oto, Univ Pennsylvania

Close, Lanny G MD [Oto] - **Spec Exp:** Skull Base Surgery; Head & Neck Cancer; Sinus Disorders/Surgery; Endoscopic Sinus Surgery; **Hospital:** NY-Presby/Columbia Univ Med Ctr, NY (page 66); **Address:** 16 E 60th St, Ste 470, New York, NY 10022; **Phone:** 212-326-8475; **Board Cert:** Otolaryngology 1977; **Med School:** Baylor Coll Med 1972; **Resid:** Surgery, Johns Hopkins Hosp 1974; Otolaryngology, Baylor Affil Hosps 1977; **Fellow:** Head and Neck Surgery, MD Anderson Cancer Ctr 1979; **Fac Appt:** Prof Oto, Columbia P&S

Costantino, Peter D MD [Oto] - **Spec Exp:** Skull Base Tumors; Head & Neck Cancer; Craniofacial Surgery/Reconstruction; **Hospital:** Lenox Hill Hosp (page 67); **Address:** 130 E 77th St Fl 10, New York, NY 10075; **Phone:** 212-434-4500; **Board Cert:** Otolaryngology 1990; Facial Plastic & Reconstr Surgery 2000; **Med School:** Northwestern Univ 1984; **Resid:** Surgery, Northwestern Meml Hosp 1986; Otolaryngology, Northwestern Meml Hosp 1989; **Fellow:** Head and Neck Surgery, Northwestern Meml Hosp 1990; Skull Base Surgery, Univ Pittsburgh 1991; **Fac Appt:** Prof Oto, Columbia P&S

Davidson, Bruce J MD [Oto] - **Spec Exp:** Head & Neck Cancer; Thyroid Disorders; **Hospital:** Georgetown Univ Hosp; **Address:** Georgetown Univ Med Ctr, Dept Otolaryngology-Head & Neck Surgery, 3800 Reservoir Rd NW, Gorman Bldg - Fl 1, Washington, DC 20007; **Phone:** 202-444-1351; **Board Cert:** Otolaryngology 1993; **Med School:** W VA Univ 1987; **Resid:** Otolaryngology, Georgetown Univ Med Ctr 1992; **Fellow:** Head and Neck Surgery, Memorial Sloan-Kettering Cancer Ctr 1994; **Fac Appt:** Asst Prof Oto, Georgetown Univ

Edelstein, David R MD [Oto] - **Spec Exp:** Endoscopic Sinus Surgery; Nasal Reconstruction; Rhinoplasty; Sleep Disorders/Apnea; **Hospital:** Lenox Hill Hosp (Manh Eye, Ear & Throat Hosp) (page 67); **Address:** 1421 3rd Ave, Fl 4, New York, NY 10028; **Phone:** 212-452-1500; **Board Cert:** Otolaryngology 1985; **Med School:** Boston Univ 1980; **Resid:** Otolaryngology, Mount Sinai Hosp 1984; **Fac Appt:** Clin Prof Oto, Cornell Univ-Weill Med Coll

Eisele, David W MD [Oto] - **Spec Exp:** Salivary Gland Tumors & Surgery; Head & Neck Cancer; Thyroid Cancer; Neck Masses; **Hospital:** Johns Hopkins Hosp (page 61); **Address:** 601 N Caroline St, Baltimore, MD 21287; **Phone:** 443-287-2658; **Board Cert:** Otolaryngology 1988; **Med School:** Cornell Univ-Weill Med Coll 1982; **Resid:** Surgery, Univ Wash Med Ctr 1984; Otolaryngology, Univ Wash Med Ctr 1988; **Fac Appt:** Prof Oto, Johns Hopkins Univ

Feghali, Joseph G MD [Oto] - **Spec Exp:** Ear Disorders/Surgery; Acoustic Neuroma; Hearing Disorders; Neuro-Otology; **Hospital:** Montefiore Med Ctr-Moses Campus, NY; **Address:** 182 E 210th St, Bronx, NY 10467; **Phone:** 718-881-3277; **Board Cert:** Otolaryngology 1990; **Med School:** Lebanon 1978; **Resid:** Otolaryngology, American Univ Beirut 1982; Otolaryngology, Montefiore Med Ctr 1990; **Fellow:** Otology & Neurotology, House Ear Inst 1983; Neurological Surgery, Meml Sloan Kettering Cancer Ctr 1984; **Fac Appt:** Clin Prof Oto, Albert Einstein Coll Med

Ferris, Robert L MD/PhD [Oto] - **Spec Exp:** Head & Neck Cancer; Thyroid & Parathyroid Cancer & Surgery; Salivary Gland Tumors; Laryngeal Cancer; **Hospital:** UPMC Presby, Pittsburgh; **Address:** University ENT Specialists, Eye & Ear Institute, 203 Lothrop St, Ste 500, Pittsburgh, PA 15213; **Phone:** 412-647-2100; **Board Cert:** Otolaryngology 2002; **Med School:** Johns Hopkins Univ 1995; **Resid:** Otolaryngology, Johns Hopkins Hosp 2001; **Fac Appt:** Assoc Prof Oto, Univ Pittsburgh

Fried, Marvin P MD [Oto] - **Spec Exp:** Endoscopic Sinus Surgery; Head & Neck Tumors; Laryngeal & Voice Disorders; Sinus Disorders/Surgery; **Hospital:** Montefiore Med Ctr-Moses Campus, NY, Montefiore Med Ctr-Einstein Campus, NY; **Address:** 3400 Bainbridge Ave, Fl 3, Bronx, NY 10467; **Phone:** 718-920-4646; **Board Cert:** Otolaryngology 1975; **Med School:** Tufts Univ 1969; **Resid:** Surgery, Jewish Hosp 1971; Otolaryngology, Barnes Hosp 1975; **Fellow:** Stroke, Washington Univ 1976; **Fac Appt:** Prof Oto, Albert Einstein Coll Med

Genden, Eric M MD [Oto] - **Spec Exp:** Head & Neck Cancer & Surgery; Head & Neck Cancer Reconstruction; Airway Reconstruction; Thyroid & Parathyroid Cancer & Surgery; **Hospital:** Mount Sinai Med Ctr (page 64); **Address:** Mt Sinai Dept Otolaryngology, 1 Gustave L Levy Pl, Box 1191, New York, NY 10029; **Phone:** 212-241-9410; **Board Cert:** Otolaryngology 1999; Facial Plastic & Reconstr Surgery 2000; **Med School:** Mount Sinai Sch Med 1992; **Resid:** Otolaryngology, Barnes Jewish Hosp 1998; **Fellow:** Head and Neck Surgery, Mt Sinai Med Ctr 1999; **Fac Appt:** Assoc Prof Oto, Mount Sinai Sch Med

Gold, Scott D MD [Oto] - **Spec Exp:** Endoscopic Sinus Surgery; Sinus Disorders/Surgery; **Hospital:** Beth Israel Med Ctr - Petrie Division (page 56), Mount Sinai Med Ctr (page 64); **Address:** 36A E 36th St, Ste 200, New York, NY 10016-3401; **Phone:** 212-889-8575; **Board Cert:** Otolaryngology 1983; **Med School:** Mount Sinai Sch Med 1979; **Resid:** Otolaryngology, Mt Sinai Med Ctr 1983; **Fac Appt:** Asst Clin Prof Oto, Mount Sinai Sch Med

Goldenberg, David MD [Oto] - **Spec Exp:** Head & Neck Cancer & Surgery; Thyroid & Parathyroid Cancer & Surgery; Salivary Gland Tumors & Surgery; **Hospital:** Penn State Milton S Hershey Med Ctr; **Address:** Otolaryngology-Head and Neck Surgery, 500 University Drive, Hershey, PA 17033-0850; **Phone:** 717-531-8945; **Med School:** Israel 1995; **Resid:** Otolaryngology, Rambam Med Ctr; **Fellow:** Head & Neck Surgical Oncology, Johns Hopkins Med Ctr; **Fac Appt:** Prof S, Penn State Coll Med

Otolaryngology

Grandis, Jennifer R MD [Oto] - **Spec Exp:** Head & Neck Cancer; **Hospital:** UPMC Presby, Pittsburgh, Magee-Womens Hosp - UPMC; **Address:** University ENT Specialists, Eye & Ear Institute, 203 Lothrop St, Ste 300, Pittsburgh, PA 15213; **Phone:** 412-647-2100; **Board Cert:** Otolaryngology 1994; **Med School:** Univ Pittsburgh 1987; **Resid:** Otolaryngology, Univ Pittsburgh Med Ctr 1993; **Fellow:** Univ Pittsburgh 1992; **Fac Appt:** Prof Oto, Univ Pittsburgh

Hammerschlag, Paul E MD [Oto] - **Spec Exp:** Cochlear Implants; Hearing Loss; Meniere's Disease; Balance Disorders; **Hospital:** NYU Langone Med Ctr (page 68), New York Eye & Ear Infirm (page 65); **Address:** 650 First Ave, New York, NY 10016-3240; **Phone:** 212-889-2600; **Board Cert:** Otolaryngology 1978; **Med School:** Albert Einstein Coll Med 1972; **Resid:** Surgery, Virginia Mason Hosp 1974; Otolaryngology, Mass Eye & Ear Infirm 1978; **Fellow:** Otolaryngology, Mass Eye & Ear Infirm 1978; **Fac Appt:** Assoc Clin Prof Oto, NYU Sch Med

Har-El, Gady MD [Oto] - **Spec Exp:** Head & Neck Cancer; Thyroid & Parathyroid Surgery; Sinus Tumors; Skull Base Tumors; **Hospital:** Lenox Hill Hosp (page 67), Lenox Hill Hosp (Manh Eye, Ear & Throat Hosp) (page 67); **Address:** 186 E 76th St E Fl 2, MS 10021, New York, NY 10021; **Phone:** 212-744-4368; **Board Cert:** Otolaryngology 1992; **Med School:** Israel 1982; **Resid:** Otolaryngology, SUNY Downstate Med Ctr 1991; **Fellow:** Head and Neck Surgery, Long Island Coll Hosp 1987; **Fac Appt:** Prof Oto, SUNY Hlth Sci Ctr

Hicks Jr, Wesley L MD/DDS [Oto] - **Spec Exp:** Head & Neck Cancer & Surgery; Reconstructive Surgery; **Hospital:** Roswell Park Cancer Inst; **Address:** Roswell Park Cancer Inst, Dept Head & Neck Surgery, Elm & Carlton Sts, Buffalo, NY 14263; **Phone:** 716-845-3158; **Board Cert:** Otolaryngology 1993; **Med School:** SUNY Buffalo 1984; **Resid:** Otolaryngology, Manhattan Eye Ear & Throat Hosp 1988; Otolaryngology, New York Hosp/Meml Sloan Kettering Cancer Ctr 1989; **Fellow:** Head and Neck Surgery, Stanford Univ Med Ctr 1990; **Fac Appt:** Prof Oto, SUNY Buffalo

Hirsch, Barry E MD [Oto] - **Spec Exp:** Neuro-Otology; Skull Base Tumors; Facial Nerve Disorders; Cochlear Implants; **Hospital:** UPMC Presby, Pittsburgh, UPMC St Margaret; **Address:** University ENT Specialists, Eye & Ear Institute, 203 Lothrop St, Ste 300, Pittsburgh, PA 15213; **Phone:** 412-647-2100; **Board Cert:** Otolaryngology 1982; Neurotology 2005; **Med School:** Univ Pennsylvania 1977; **Resid:** Otolaryngology, Univ Pittsburgh Med Ctr 1982; **Fellow:** Neurotology, Univ Pittsburgh 1985; Neurotology, Univ Zurich 1986; **Fac Appt:** Prof Oto, Univ Pittsburgh

Hoffman, Ronald A MD [Oto] - **Spec Exp:** Cochlear Implants; Balance Disorders; Ear Disorders/Surgery; **Hospital:** New York Eye & Ear Infirm (page 65); **Address:** 380 2nd Ave Fl 9, New York, NY 10010; **Phone:** 212-614-8388; **Board Cert:** Otolaryngology 1976; **Med School:** Jefferson Med Coll 1971; **Resid:** Otolaryngology, NYU Med Ctr 1976; **Fellow:** Otology & Neurotology, Lenox Hill Hosp 1977; **Fac Appt:** Prof Oto, Albert Einstein Coll Med

Holliday, Michael J MD [Oto] - **Spec Exp:** Neuro-Otology; Skull Base Surgery; Otology; **Hospital:** Johns Hopkins Hosp (page 61), Johns Hopkins Bayview Med Ctr (page 61); **Address:** Johns Hopkins Outpatient Clin, 601 N Caroline St Fl 6, Baltimore, MD 21287; **Phone:** 410-955-1686; **Board Cert:** Otolaryngology 1976; **Med School:** Marquette Sch Med 1969; **Resid:** Otolaryngology, Johns Hopkins Hosp 1976; **Fellow:** Neurotology, Univ Zurich 1979; **Fac Appt:** Assoc Prof Oto, Johns Hopkins Univ

Hopping, Steven B MD [Oto] - **Spec Exp:** Cosmetic Surgery-Face; Hair Restoration/Transplant; **Hospital:** G Washington Univ Hosp; **Address:** The Center for Cosmetic Surgery, 2311 M St NW, Ste 503, Washington, DC 20037; **Phone:** 202-785-3175; **Board Cert:** Otolaryngology 1980; Facial Plastic & Reconstr Surgery 1986; Hair Restoration Surgery 1990; **Med School:** Univ Cincinnati 1975; **Resid:** Surgery, George Washington Hosp 1977; Otolaryngology, Maa E&E Infirmary 1980; **Fellow:** Plastic Surgery, Mass E&E Infirmary 1981; **Fac Appt:** Clin Prof S, Geo Wash Univ

Hurst, Michael K MD/DDS [Oto] - **Spec Exp:** Nasal Allergy; Sleep Disorders/Apnea; Thyroid Surgery; **Hospital:** Ruby Memorial - WVU Hosp, Monongalia Genl Hosp; **Address:** 1188 Pineview Drive, Morgantown, WV 26505; **Phone:** 304-599-3959; **Board Cert:** Otolaryngology 1994; **Med School:** Marshall Univ 1988; **Resid:** Otolaryngology, Univ West Virginia Hosps 1993; Head and Neck Surgery, Univ West Virginia Hosps 1993; **Fac Appt:** Assoc Prof Oto, W VA Univ

Jacobs, Joseph B MD [Oto] - **Spec Exp:** Endoscopic Sinus Surgery; Sinus Disorders/Surgery; Sinus Surgery-Revision; **Hospital:** NYU Langone Med Ctr (page 68); **Address:** 345 E 37 St, Ste 306, MS 10016, Ave, New York, NY 10016-6402; **Phone:** 646-754-1203; **Board Cert:** Otolaryngology 1978; **Med School:** Albert Einstein Coll Med 1974; **Resid:** Otolaryngology, NYU Med Ctr 1978; **Fellow:** Plastic/Reconstructive Surgery, UCLA Med Ctr 1979; **Fac Appt:** Prof Oto, NYU Sch Med

Johnson, Jonas T MD [Oto] - **Spec Exp:** Head & Neck Surgery; Head & Neck Cancer; Sleep Disorders/Apnea/Snoring; Parotid Gland Tumors; **Hospital:** UPMC Presby, Pittsburgh, Magee-Womens Hosp - UPMC; **Address:** University ENT Specialists, 203 Lothrop St, Ste 300, Pittsburgh, PA 15213; **Phone:** 412-647-2100; **Board Cert:** Otolaryngology 1977; **Med School:** SUNY Upstate Med Univ 1972; **Resid:** Surgery, Med Coll Virginia Hosps 1974; Otolaryngology, SUNY-Univ Hosp 1977; **Fac Appt:** Prof Oto, Univ Pittsburgh

Josephson, Jordan S MD [Oto] - **Spec Exp:** Rhinoplasty Revision; Endoscopic Sinus Surgery; Nasal & Sinus Disorders; Sleep Apnea; **Hospital:** Lenox Hill Hosp (Manh Eye, Ear & Throat Hosp) (page 67); **Address:** 205 E 76th St, Ste M1, New York, NY 10021; **Phone:** 212-717-1773; **Board Cert:** Otolaryngology 1988; **Med School:** SUNY Downstate 1983; **Resid:** Otolaryngology, LI Jewish Med Ctr 1988; **Fellow:** Sinus Surgery, Johns Hopkins Hosp 1989

Keane, William M MD [Oto] - **Spec Exp:** Head & Neck Cancer & Surgery; Thyroid Cancer; Parathyroid Surgery; **Hospital:** Thomas Jefferson Univ Hosp; **Address:** Jefferson Univ Physicians, Dept Otolaryngology, 925 Chestnut St Fl 6, Philadelphia, PA 19107; **Phone:** 215-955-6760; **Board Cert:** Otolaryngology 1978; **Med School:** Harvard Med Sch 1970; **Resid:** Surgery, Strong Meml Hosp 1972; Otolaryngology, Hosp Univ Penn 1977; **Fac Appt:** Prof Oto, Thomas Jefferson Univ

Kennedy, David W MD [Oto] - **Spec Exp:** Sinus Disorders/Surgery; Skull Base Tumors & Surgery; Minimally Invasive Surgery; Esthesioneuroblastoma; **Hospital:** Hosp Univ Penn - UPHS (page 72), Pennsylvania Hosp-UPHS (page 72); **Address:** Univ of Penn Hosp, 3400 Spruce St, Ravdin Bldg - Fl 5, Philadelphia, PA 19104-4229; **Phone:** 215-662-6971; **Board Cert:** Otolaryngology 1978; **Med School:** Ireland 1972; **Resid:** Surgery, Johns Hopkins Hosp 1974; Otolaryngology, Johns Hopkins Hosp 1978; **Fac Appt:** Prof Oto, Univ Pennsylvania

Koch, Wayne M MD [Oto] - **Spec Exp:** Head & Neck Cancer; Sinus Tumors; **Hospital:** Johns Hopkins Hosp (page 61); **Address:** Johns Hopkins Outpatient Clin, 601 N Caroline St Fl 6, Baltimore, MD 21287; **Phone:** 410-955-1686; **Board Cert:** Otolaryngology 1987; **Med School:** Univ Pittsburgh 1982; **Resid:** Otolaryngology, Tufts-Boston Univ Hosps 1987; **Fellow:** Surgical Oncology, Johns Hopkins Hosp 1989; **Fac Appt:** Assoc Prof Oto, Johns Hopkins Univ

Koufman, Jamie A MD [Oto] - **Spec Exp:** Voice Disorders; Laryngeal Disorders; **Hospital:** New York Eye & Ear Infirm (page 65); **Address:** 200 W 57th St, Ste 1203, New York, NY 10019; **Phone:** 212-463-8014; **Board Cert:** Otolaryngology 1978; **Med School:** Boston Univ 1973; **Resid:** Surgery, Hartford Hosp 1975; Otolaryngology, Boston Univ Med Ctr 1978

Kraus, Dennis H MD [Oto] - **Spec Exp:** Head & Neck Cancer; Skull Base Tumors; Thyroid & Parathyroid Surgery; Sarcoma; **Hospital:** Lenox Hill Hosp (page 67); **Address:** 130 E 77th St, Fl 10, New York, NY 10075-1851; **Phone:** 212-434-4500; **Board Cert:** Otolaryngology 1990; **Med School:** Univ Rochester 1985; **Resid:** Surgery, Cleveland Clinic 1987; Otolaryngology, Cleveland Clinic 1990; **Fellow:** Head and Neck Surgery, Meml Sloan Kettering Cancer Ctr 1991; **Fac Appt:** Prof Oto, Cornell Univ-Weill Med Coll

Krespi, Yosef P MD [Oto] - **Spec Exp:** Nasal & Sinus Cancer & Surgery; Sleep Disorders/Apnea; Head & Neck Cancer & Surgery; Snoring/Sleep Apnea; **Hospital:** Lenox Hill Hosp (Manh Eye, Ear & Throat Hosp) (page 67); **Address:** 110 E 59th St, Ste 10A, New York, NY 10019-1128; **Phone:** 212-434-4500; **Board Cert:** Otolaryngology 1981; **Med School:** Israel 1973; **Resid:** Surgery, Mt Sinai Hosp 1976; Otolaryngology, Mt Sinai Hosp 1980; **Fellow:** Surgery, Northwestern Meml Hosp 1981; **Fac Appt:** Clin Prof Oto, Columbia P&S

Kuhel, William I MD [Oto] - **Spec Exp:** Head & Neck Cancer & Surgery; Thyroid Cancer; Parathyroid Cancer; **Hospital:** NY-Presby/Weill Cornell Med Ctr, NY (page 66); **Address:** 1305 York Ave Fl 5, New York, NY 10021; **Phone:** 646-962-6325; **Board Cert:** Otolaryngology 1988; **Med School:** Univ Mich Med Sch 1983; **Resid:** Surgery, St Vincent's Hosp 1985; Otolaryngology, Indiana Univ 1988; **Fellow:** Head and Neck Surgery, MD Anderson Cancer Ctr 1989; **Fac Appt:** Assoc Clin Prof Oto, Cornell Univ-Weill Med Coll

Lalwani, Anil K MD [Oto] - **Spec Exp:** Ear Disorders/Surgery; Facial Nerve Disorders; Pediatric Otolaryngology; Skull Base Surgery; **Hospital:** NY-Presby/Columbia Univ Med Ctr, NY (page 66); **Address:** 180 Fort Washington Ave, Harkness Pavilion Fl 7, New York, NY 10032; **Phone:** 212-305-1696; **Board Cert:** Otolaryngology 1992; Neurotology 2010; **Med School:** Univ Mich Med Sch 1985; **Resid:** Surgery, Duke Univ Med Ctr 1987; Otolaryngology, UCSF Med Ctr 1991; **Fellow:** Skull Base Surgery, UCSF Med Ctr 1992; **Fac Appt:** Prof Oto, Columbia P&S

Lawson, William MD [Oto] - **Spec Exp:** Sinus Disorders/Surgery; Endoscopic Sinus Surgery; **Hospital:** Mount Sinai Med Ctr (page 64); **Address:** 5 E 98th St Fl 8, Box 1191, New York, NY 10029-6501; **Phone:** 212-241-9410; **Board Cert:** Otolaryngology 1974; **Med School:** NYU Sch Med 1965; **Resid:** Surgery, Bronx VA Hosp 1967; Otolaryngology, Mt Sinai Hosp 1973; **Fellow:** Otolaryngology, Mt Sinai Hosp 1970; **Fac Appt:** Prof Oto, Mount Sinai Sch Med

Lebovics, Robert S MD [Oto] - **Spec Exp:** Head & Neck Inflammatory Disorders; Head & Neck Autoimmune Disease; Head & Neck Infectious Disease; Relapsing Polychondritis; **Hospital:** St. Luke's - Roosevelt Hosp Ctr - Roosevelt Div (page 56); **Address:** 425 W 59th St Fl 10, New York, NY 10019; **Phone:** 212-262-2002; **Board Cert:** Otolaryngology 1988; **Med School:** SUNY Downstate 1982; **Resid:** Surgery, Montefiore-Weiler Einstein Div 1983; Otolaryngology, Montefiore-Weiler Einstein Div 1987

Linstrom, Christopher J MD [Oto] - **Spec Exp:** Cochlear Implants; Acoustic Neuroma; Encephalocele; Cholesteatoma; **Hospital:** New York Eye & Ear Infirm (page 65); **Address:** NY Eye & Ear Infirmary, Dept Otolaryngology, 310 E 14th St, New York, NY 10003-4201; **Phone:** 212-979-4200; **Board Cert:** Otolaryngology 1987; Neurotology 2004; **Med School:** McGill Univ 1982; **Resid:** Surgery, Geo Wash Med Ctr 1984; Otolaryngology, NY Hosp 1987; **Fellow:** Otology & Neurotology, Michigan Ear Inst 1989; **Fac Appt:** Assoc Prof Oto, NY Med Coll

Mirza, Natasha MD [Oto] - **Spec Exp:** Vocal Cord Disorders; Voice Disorders; Laryngeal Disorders; Swallowing Disorders; **Hospital:** Hosp Univ Penn - UPHS (page 72); **Address:** Hosp Univ Penn, Dept Otolaryngology, 3400 Spruce St, Silverstein Bldg Fl 5, Philadelphia, PA 19104; **Phone:** 215-662-2777; **Board Cert:** Otolaryngology 1993; **Med School:** India 1983; **Resid:** Surgery, Ohio State Univ Hosp 1987; Otolaryngology, UC Irvine Med Ctr 1992; **Fac Appt:** Prof Oto, Univ Pennsylvania

Newkirk, Kenneth Allen MD [Oto] - **Spec Exp:** Head & Neck Cancer; Sinus Disorders; **Hospital:** Georgetown Univ Hosp; **Address:** 3800 Reservoir Rd NW, Gorman Bldg, 1st Fl, rm G-104, Washington, DC 20007; **Phone:** 202-444-8186; **Board Cert:** Otolaryngology 2002; **Med School:** Mount Sinai Sch Med 1993; **Resid:** Otolaryngology, Lombardi Cancer Center 2000; **Fellow:** Otolaryngology, Lombardi Cancer Center 2003; Otolaryngology, MD Anderson Cancer Ctr 2005; **Fac Appt:** Asst Prof Oto, Georgetown Univ

Niparko, John MD [Oto] - **Spec Exp:** Ear Disorders/Surgery; Neuro-Otology; **Hospital:** Johns Hopkins Hosp (page 61); **Address:** Johns Hopkins Hosp, Dept Otolaryngology, 601 N Caroline St, rm 6223, Baltimore, MD 21287-0910; **Phone:** 410-955-2689; **Board Cert:** Otolaryngology 1986; Neurotology 2004; **Med School:** Univ Mich Med Sch 1980; **Resid:** Surgery, William Beaumont Hosp 1982; Otolaryngology, Univ Michigan Hosp 1986; **Fellow:** Otolaryngology, Univ Michigan Hosp; **Fac Appt:** Prof Oto, Johns Hopkins Univ

O'Malley Jr, Bert W MD [Oto] - **Spec Exp:** Head & Neck Cancer; Sinus Tumors; Skull Base Tumors; **Hospital:** Hosp Univ Penn - UPHS (page 72); **Address:** Hosp Univ Penn, Dept Otolaryngology, 3400 Spruce St, 5 Ravdin, Philadelphia, PA 19104; **Phone:** 215-615-4325; **Board Cert:** Otolaryngology 1995; **Med School:** Univ Tex SW, Dallas 1988; **Resid:** Surgery, Parkland Meml Hosp 1989; Otolaryngology, Baylor Affil Hosp 1993; **Fellow:** Head & Neck Oncology, Univ Pittsburgh 1994; Skull Base Surgery, Univ Pittsburgh 1995; **Fac Appt:** Prof Oto, Univ Pennsylvania

Papel, Ira D MD [Oto] - **Spec Exp:** Rhinoplasty; Cosmetic Surgery-Face; Reconstructive Surgery-Face; Skin Cancer/Facial Reconstruction; **Hospital:** Greater Baltimore Med Ctr, Johns Hopkins Hosp (page 61); **Address:** 1838 Greene Tree Rd, Ste 370, Baltimore, MD 21208; **Phone:** 410-486-3400; **Board Cert:** Otolaryngology 1986; Facial Plastic & Reconstr Surgery 1991; **Med School:** Boston Univ 1981; **Resid:** Otolaryngology, Johns Hopkins Hosp 1986; **Fellow:** Facial Plastic Surgery, UCSF Med Ctr 1987; **Fac Appt:** Assoc Prof Oto, Johns Hopkins Univ

Parisier, Simon C MD [Oto] - **Spec Exp:** Cochlear Implants; Hearing Loss; Ear Disorders/Surgery; Cholesteatoma; **Hospital:** New York Eye & Ear Infirm (page 65); **Address:** NY Eye & Ear Infirmary - Otolaryngology, 380 2nd Ave Fl 9, New York, NY 10010; **Phone:** 212-979-4542; **Board Cert:** Otolaryngology 1967; **Med School:** Boston Univ 1961; **Resid:** Otolaryngology, Mount Sinai Hosp 1966; **Fac Appt:** Prof Oto, NY Med Coll

Persky, Mark S MD [Oto] - **Spec Exp:** Head & Neck Cancer; Skull Base Tumors; Thyroid Cancer; Vascular Lesions-Head & Neck; **Hospital:** Beth Israel Med Ctr - Petrie Division (page 56), New York Eye & Ear Infirm (page 65); **Address:** 10 Union Square East, Ste 4J, New York, NY 10003; **Phone:** 212-844-8648; **Board Cert:** Otolaryngology 1976; **Med School:** SUNY Upstate Med Univ 1972; **Resid:** Otolaryngology, Bellevue Hosp 1976; **Fellow:** Head and Neck Surgery, Beth Israel Med Ctr 1977; **Fac Appt:** Clin Prof Oto, Albert Einstein Coll Med

Picken, Catherine A MD [Oto] - **Spec Exp:** Head & Neck Reconstruction; Thyroid Disorders; Sinus Disorders/Surgery; **Hospital:** Georgetown Univ Hosp, Sibley Mem Hosp; **Address:** 2440 M St NW, Ste 620, Washington, DC 20037; **Phone:** 202-785-5000; **Board Cert:** Otolaryngology 1989; **Med School:** Northwestern Univ 1979; **Resid:** Surgery, Natl Heart Lung Blood Inst 1983; Otolaryngology, Georgetown Univ Hosp 1989; **Fac Appt:** Assoc Prof Oto, Georgetown Univ

Pribitkin, Edmund A MD [Oto] - **Spec Exp:** Rhinoplasty; Thyroid Disorders; Facial Plastic Surgery; **Hospital:** Thomas Jefferson Univ Hosp; **Address:** 925 Chestnut St Fl 6, Philadelphia, PA 19107; **Phone:** 215-955-6760; **Board Cert:** Otolaryngology 1992; **Med School:** Univ Pennsylvania 1986; **Resid:** Otolaryngology, Univ Penn Hosp 1991; **Fellow:** Facial Plastic & Reconstr Surgery, Stanford Univ Hosp 1992; **Fac Appt:** Assoc Prof Oto, Thomas Jefferson Univ

Quatela, Vito C MD [Oto] - **Spec Exp:** Facial Plastic Surgery; Rhinoplasty; Reconstructive Surgery; **Hospital:** Univ of Rochester Strong Meml Hosp, Rochester Genl Hosp; **Address:** 973 East Ave, Ste 100, Rochester, NY 14607; **Phone:** 585-244-1000; **Board Cert:** Otolaryngology 1985; Facial Plastic & Reconstr Surgery 1991; **Med School:** Northwestern Univ 1979; **Resid:** Surgery, Med Ctr Hosp Vermont 1981; Otolaryngology, Northwestern Univ Hosp 1985; **Fellow:** Facial Plastic Surgery, Tulane Univ 1986; Facial Plastic Surgery, Oregon Hlth Science Univ 1987; **Fac Appt:** Assoc Clin Prof Oto, Univ Rochester

Rassekh, Christopher H. MD [Oto] - **Spec Exp:** Laryngeal Cancer-Organ Preservation; Skull Base Tumors; Salivary Gland Tumors & Surgery; **Hospital:** Hosp Univ Penn - UPHS (page 72); **Address:** 3400 Spruce St, Sliverstei Bldg - Fl 5th, Philadelphia, PA 19104; **Phone:** 215-662-2777; **Board Cert:** Otolaryngology 1993; **Med School:** Univ Iowa Coll Med 1986; **Resid:** Otolaryngology, Univ Iowa Med Ctr 1992; **Fellow:** Head and Neck Surgery, Univ Pittsburgh Med Ctr 1993; **Fac Appt:** Assoc Prof Oto, Univ Pennsylvania

Roland Sr, J Thomas MD [Oto] - **Spec Exp:** Acoustic Neuroma; Cochlear Implants; Neuro-Otology; Facial Nerve Disorders; **Hospital:** NYU Langone Med Ctr (page 68), Bellevue Hosp Ctr; **Address:** 550 First Avenue, Ste 7Q, New York, NY 10016; **Phone:** 212-263-5565; **Board Cert:** Otolaryngology 1993; Neurotology 2004; **Med School:** Temple Univ 1983; **Resid:** Otolaryngology, NYU Med Ctr 1992; **Fellow:** Neurotology, NYU Med Ctr 1993; **Fac Appt:** Assoc Prof Oto, NYU Sch Med

Rosen, Clark A MD [Oto] - **Spec Exp:** Voice Disorders; **Hospital:** UPMC Mercy, Pittsburgh, UPMC Presby, Pittsburgh; **Address:** UPMC The Voice Ctr, 1400 Locust St, D Bldg Fl 2 - Ste 2100, Pittsburgh, PA 15219; **Phone:** 412-232-7464; **Board Cert:** Otolaryngology 1995; **Med School:** Rush Med Coll 1989; **Resid:** Otolaryngology, Oregon Hlth Sci Univ 1994; **Fellow:** Otolaryngology, Univ Tenn Med Ctr 1995; **Fac Appt:** Prof Oto, Univ Pittsburgh

Sataloff, Robert T MD [Oto] - **Spec Exp:** Neuro-Otology; Voice Disorders; Laryngeal Disorders; Throat Disorders; **Hospital:** Hahnemann Univ Hosp, St. Christopher's Hosp for Chldn; **Address:** 1721 Pine Street, Philadelphia, PA 19103-6701; **Phone:** 215-545-3322; **Board Cert:** Otolaryngology 1980; **Med School:** Jefferson Med Coll 1975; **Resid:** Otolaryngology, Univ Mich Hosp 1980; **Fellow:** Neurotology, Univ Mich Hosp 1981; **Fac Appt:** Prof Oto, Drexel Univ Coll Med

Schaefer, Steven D MD [Oto] - **Spec Exp:** Sinus Disorders/Surgery; Head & Neck Surgery; Endoscopic Sinus Surgery; **Hospital:** Lenox Hill Hosp (Manh Eye, Ear & Throat Hosp) (page 67), Beth Israel Med Ctr - Petrie Division (page 56); **Address:** 110 E 59th St, Fl 10, Ste 10A, New York, NY 10022; **Phone:** 212-434-4500; **Board Cert:** Otolaryngology 1978; **Med School:** UC Irvine 1972; **Resid:** Surgery, UCLA Med Ctr 1974; Otolaryngology, Stanford Med Ctr 1977; **Fac Appt:** Prof Oto, NY Med Coll

Schaitkin, Barry M MD [Oto] - **Spec Exp:** Sinus Disorders/Surgery; Endoscopic Sinus Surgery; Rhinosinusitis; **Hospital:** UPMC Shadyside; **Address:** Shadyside Medical Bldg, 5200 Centre Ave, Ste 211, Pittsburgh, PA 15232; **Phone:** 412-621-0123; **Board Cert:** Otolaryngology 1990; **Med School:** Penn State Coll Med 1984; **Resid:** Otolaryngology, Hershey Med Ctr 1990; **Fac Appt:** Assoc Prof Oto, Univ Pittsburgh

Schantz, Stimson P MD [Oto] - **Spec Exp:** Head & Neck Surgery; Head & Neck Cancer; Thyroid Cancer; **Hospital:** New York Eye & Ear Infirm (page 65), Beth Israel Med Ctr - Petrie Division (page 56); **Address:** 310 E 14th St Fl 6N, New York, NY 10003; **Phone:** 212-979-4535; **Board Cert:** Surgery 2005; **Med School:** Univ Cincinnati 1975; **Resid:** Surgery, Georgetown Univ Med CtrGeorgetown Univ Med Ctr 1982; Otolaryngology, Univ Illinois Eye & Ear Infirm 1980; **Fellow:** Surgical Oncology, MD Anderson Cancer Ctr 1984; **Fac Appt:** Prof Oto, NY Med Coll

Schley, W Shain MD [Oto] - **Spec Exp:** Nasal & Sinus Disorders; Throat Disorders; Voice Disorders; Sleep Disorders; **Hospital:** NY-Presby/Weill Cornell Med Ctr, NY (page 66); **Address:** 449 E 68th St, Fl 2, Ste DS 10, New York, NY 10065-6310; **Phone:** 212-746-2223; **Board Cert:** Otolaryngology 1973; **Med School:** Emory Univ 1966; **Resid:** Surgery, Roosevelt Hosp 1968; Otolaryngology, New York Hosp 1973; **Fac Appt:** Assoc Clin Prof Oto, Cornell Univ-Weill Med Coll

Setzen, Michael MD [Oto] - **Spec Exp:** Nasal & Sinus Surgery; Rhinoplasty; Sleep Disorders/Apnea; Snoring/Sleep Apnea; **Hospital:** N Shore Univ Hosp (page 67), St. Francis Hosp - The Heart Ctr (page 73); **Address:** 600 Northern Blvd, Ste 312, Great Neck, NY 11021-5200; **Phone:** 516-829-0045; **Board Cert:** Otolaryngology 1982; **Med School:** South Africa 1974; **Resid:** Surgery, Cleveland Clinic Fdn 1978; Otolaryngology, Barnes Jewish Hosp 1982; **Fac Appt:** Assoc Clin Prof Oto, NYU Sch Med

Shapshay, Stanley M MD [Oto] - **Spec Exp:** Laryngeal Cancer; Vocal Cord Disorders; Sleep Apnea; **Hospital:** Albany Med Ctr; **Address:** University Ear, Nose & Throat Ctr, 35 Hackett Blvd, Albany, NY 12208-3420; **Phone:** 518-262-5575; **Board Cert:** Otolaryngology 1975; **Med School:** Med Coll VA 1968; **Resid:** Surgery, New England Med Ctr 1971; Otolaryngology, Boston Med Ctr 1975; **Fellow:** Surgery, Serafimer Hosp/Karolinska Med Sch 1972; **Fac Appt:** Prof Oto, Albany Med Coll

Singh, Bhuvanesh MD/PhD [Oto] - **Spec Exp:** Head & Neck Cancer & Surgery; Thyroid Cancer; **Hospital:** Meml Sloan-Kettering Cancer Ctr; **Address:** 1275 York Ave, MC C1073, New York, NY 10065; **Phone:** 212-639-2024; **Board Cert:** Otolaryngology 1998; **Med School:** SUNY Downstate 1991; **Resid:** Otolaryngology, SUNY Downstate Med Ctr 1997; **Fellow:** Head and Neck Surgery, Meml Sloan-Kettering Canc Ctr 1999; **Fac Appt:** Assoc Prof Oto, Cornell Univ-Weill Med Coll

Snyderman, Carl H MD [Oto] - **Spec Exp:** Skull Base Tumors & Surgery; Sinus Tumors; Head & Neck Cancer; Endoscopic Surgery; **Hospital:** UPMC Presby, Pittsburgh, Chldns Hosp of Pittsburgh - UPMC; **Address:** 200 Lothrop St, EEI Bldg - Fl 3 - Ste 300, Pittsburgh, PA 15213; **Phone:** 412-647-2100; **Board Cert:** Otolaryngology 1987; **Med School:** Univ Chicago-Pritzker Sch Med 1982; **Resid:** Otolaryngology, Eye-Ear Hosp/Univ Pittsburgh 1987; **Fellow:** Skull Base Surgery, Eye-Ear Hosp/Univ Pittsburgh 1988; **Fac Appt:** Prof Oto, Univ Pittsburgh

Stewart, Michael G MD [Oto] - **Spec Exp:** Nasal & Sinus Disorders; Sleep Disorders/Apnea; Head & Neck Surgery; **Address:** Weill Greenberg Center, 1305 York Ave Fl 5, New York, NY 10021; **Phone:** 646-962-6673; **Board Cert:** Otolaryngology 1995; **Med School:** Johns Hopkins Univ 1988; **Resid:** Otolaryngology, Baylor Coll Med 1994; **Fac Appt:** Prof Oto, Cornell Univ-Weill Med Coll

Strome, Marshall MD [Oto] - **Spec Exp:** Voice Disorders; Swallowing Disorders; Head & Neck Cancer Reconstruction; Head & Neck Cancer & Surgery; **Hospital:** St. Luke's - Roosevelt Hosp Ctr - St Luke's Hosp (page 56), Mount Sinai Med Ctr (page 64); **Address:** 425 W 59th St, Fl 10, New York, NY 10019; **Phone:** 212-262-4444; **Board Cert:** Otolaryngology 1970; **Med School:** Univ Mich Med Sch 1964; **Resid:** Surgery, Harper Hosp 1966; Otolaryngology, Univ Michigan Hosp 1970; **Fac Appt:** Prof Oto

Strome, Scott E MD [Oto] - **Spec Exp:** Microsurgery; Head & Neck Cancer; Head & Neck Reconstruction; Laryngeal Cancer; **Hospital:** Univ of MD Med Ctr; **Address:** UMMC Dept Otorhinolaryngology, 16 S Eutaw St, Ste 500, Baltimore, MD 21201; **Phone:** 410-328-6467; **Board Cert:** Otolaryngology 1998; **Med School:** Harvard Med Sch 1991; **Resid:** Otolaryngology, Univ Michigan 1997; **Fellow:** Head and Neck Surgery, Allegheny Genl Hosp 1998; Microvascular Surgery, Allegheny Genl Hosp 1998; **Fac Appt:** Prof Oto, Univ MD Sch Med

Otolaryngology

Sulica, Radu Lucian MD [Oto] - **Spec Exp:** Laryngeal & Vocal Cord Surgery; Voice Disorders; Vocal Cord Disorders; Botox Therapy; **Hospital:** NY-Presby/Weill Cornell Med Ctr, NY (page 66); **Address:** 1305 York Ave, Fl 5th Floor, New York, NY 10021; **Phone:** 646-962-4734; **Board Cert:** Otolaryngology 2000; **Med School:** Georgetown Univ 1993; **Resid:** Surgery, Georgetown Univ Hosp 1995; Otolaryngology, Georgetown Univ Hosp 1999; **Fellow:** Laryngology, St Lukes Roosevelt Hosp 2000; **Fac Appt:** Assoc Prof Oto, Cornell Univ-Weill Med Coll

Thaler, Erica R MD [Oto] - **Spec Exp:** Apnea/Robotic Surgery; Thyroid Surgery; Sinus Disorders/Surgery; **Hospital:** Hosp Univ Penn - UPHS (page 72); **Address:** Hosp Univ Penn, Dept Otolaryngology, 3400 Spruce St, 5 Silverstein, Philadelphia, PA 19104; **Phone:** 215-662-2777; **Board Cert:** Otolaryngology 1996; **Med School:** Harvard Med Sch 1990; **Resid:** Otolaryngology, Hosp Univ Penn 1995; **Fac Appt:** Prof Oto, Univ Pennsylvania

Tufano, Ralph P MD [Oto] - **Spec Exp:** Thyroid Disorders; Parathyroid Surgery; Head & Neck Cancer; **Hospital:** Johns Hopkins Hosp (page 61); **Address:** Johns Hopkins Outpatient Clin, 601 N Caroline St, Ste 6242, Baltimore, MD 21287; **Phone:** 410-955-3628; **Board Cert:** Otolaryngology 2001; **Med School:** SUNY Buffalo 1995; **Resid:** Otolaryngology, Univ Penn Affil Hosps 2000; **Fellow:** Head and Neck Surgery, Johns Hopkins Hosp 2001; **Fac Appt:** Assoc Prof Oto, Johns Hopkins Univ

Urken, Mark MD [Oto] - **Spec Exp:** Head & Neck Cancer & Surgery; Head & Neck Cancer Reconstruction; Thyroid & Parathyroid Cancer & Surgery; Salivary Gland Tumors; **Hospital:** Beth Israel Med Ctr - Petrie Division (page 56); **Address:** Inst for Head, Neck & Thyroid Cancer, 10 Union Square E, Ste 5B, New York, NY 10003-3314; **Phone:** 212-844-8775; **Board Cert:** Otolaryngology 1986; **Med School:** Univ VA Sch Med 1981; **Resid:** Otolaryngology, Mt Sinai Hosp 1986; **Fellow:** Microvascular Surgery, Mercy Hosp 1987; **Fac Appt:** Prof Oto, Albert Einstein Coll Med

Waner, Milton MD [Oto] - **Spec Exp:** Pediatric Facial Plastic Surgery; Birthmarks/Hemangiomas; Vascular Malformations; **Hospital:** St. Luke's - Roosevelt Hosp Ctr - St Luke's Hosp (page 56), Beth Israel Med Ctr - Petrie Division (page 56); **Address:** Vascular Birthmark Institute, 126 W 60th St, New York, NY 10023; **Phone:** 212-636-3970; **Med School:** South Africa 1977; **Resid:** Surgery, Univ of Witwatersrand 1980; Otolaryngology, Univ of Witwatersrand 1984; **Fellow:** Otolaryngology, Univ Cincinnatti Med Ctr 1985

Weinstein, Gregory MD [Oto] - **Spec Exp:** Head & Neck Cancer; Laryngeal Cancer; **Hospital:** Hosp Univ Penn - UPHS (page 72); **Address:** Hosp Univ Penn, Dept Otolaryngology, 3400 Spruce St, 5 Ravdin, Philadelphia, PA 19104; **Phone:** 215-349-5390; **Board Cert:** Otolaryngology 1990; **Med School:** NY Med Coll 1985; **Resid:** Otolaryngology, Univ Iowa Hosp 1990; **Fellow:** Head & Neck Oncology, UC Davis 1991; **Fac Appt:** Prof Oto, Univ Pennsylvania

Wong, Richard J MD [Oto] - **Spec Exp:** Head & Neck Cancer; Thyroid Cancer; **Hospital:** Meml Sloan-Kettering Cancer Ctr; **Address:** 1275 York Ave, C-1069, New York, NY 10065; **Phone:** 212-639-7638; **Board Cert:** Otolaryngology 2000; **Med School:** Harvard Med Sch 1994; **Resid:** Otolaryngology, Mass General Hosp 1999; **Fellow:** Head & Neck Surgical Oncology, Meml Sloan Kettering Cancer Ctr 2000

Woo, Peak MD [Oto] - **Spec Exp:** Voice Disorders; Laryngeal Disorders; Laryngeal Cancer; **Hospital:** Mount Sinai Med Ctr (page 64); **Address:** 300 Central Park West, Ste 1-H, New York, NY 10024; **Phone:** 212-580-1004; **Board Cert:** Otolaryngology 1983; **Med School:** Boston Univ 1978; **Resid:** Otolaryngology, Boston Univ Med Ctr 1983; **Fac Appt:** Clin Prof Oto, Mount Sinai Sch Med

Zalzal, George MD [Oto] - **Spec Exp:** Airway Disorders; Laryngeal & Tracheal Disorders; Ear Disorders/Surgery; **Hospital:** Chldns Natl Med Ctr; **Address:** Childrens Natl Med Ctr, Dept Otolaryngology, 111 Michigan Ave NW Fl 1 - Ste 1000, Washington, DC 20010; **Phone:** 202-476-2159; **Board Cert:** Otolaryngology 1996; **Med School:** Lebanon 1979; **Resid:** Otolaryngology, American Univ Hosp 1983; **Fellow:** Pediatric Otolaryngology, Univ Cincinnati 1985; **Fac Appt:** Prof Ped, Geo Wash Univ

Zwillenberg, Seth MD [Oto] - **Spec Exp:** Pediatric Otolaryngology; **Hospital:** Albert Einstein Med Ctr, St. Christopher's Hosp for Chldn; **Address:** 10 Presidential Blvd, Ste 100, Bala Cynwyd, PA 19004; **Phone:** 610-660-8071; **Board Cert:** Otolaryngology 1987; **Med School:** SUNY Downstate 1981; **Resid:** Surgical Pathology, St. Vincent's Hosp 1983; Otolaryngology, Hosp Univ Penn 1986; **Fellow:** Pediatric Otolaryngology, Med Coll Penn 1987; **Fac Appt:** Assoc Prof Oto, Drexel Univ Coll Med

Southeast

Balkany, Thomas J MD [Oto] - **Spec Exp:** Ear Disorders/Surgery; Neuro-Otology; Cochlear Implants; Hearing Loss; **Hospital:** Jackson Meml Hosp; **Address:** Univ Miami Dept Otolaryngology, PO Box 016960, Miami, FL 33101; **Phone:** 305-243-2000; **Board Cert:** Otolaryngology 1977; Neurotology 2004; **Med School:** Univ Miami Sch Med 1972; **Resid:** Surgery, St Joseph Hosp 1974; Otolaryngology, Colorado Med Ctr 1977; **Fellow:** Otology & Neurotology, House Ear Inst 1978; **Fac Appt:** Clin Prof Oto, Univ Miami Sch Med

Becker, Ferdinand F MD [Oto] - **Spec Exp:** Cosmetic Surgery-Face; **Hospital:** Indian River Med Ctr; **Address:** 5070 N A1A, Ste A, Vero Beach, FL 32963-1229; **Phone:** 772-234-3700; **Board Cert:** Otolaryngology 1972; **Med School:** Tulane Univ 1965; **Resid:** Surgery, Charity Hosp 1969; Otolaryngology, Charity Hosp 1972; **Fac Appt:** Asst Clin Prof Oto, Univ Fla Coll Med

Bolger, William E MD [Oto] - **Spec Exp:** Sinus Disorders/Surgery; Nasal Surgery; Sinus Tumors; **Hospital:** Mayo - Jacksonville; **Address:** Mayo Clinic, Otolaryngology Dept, 4500 San Pablo Rd, Davis E-3B, Jacksonville, FL 32224; **Phone:** 904-953-2217; **Board Cert:** Otolaryngology 1992; **Med School:** Uniformed Srvs Univ, Bethesda 1986; **Resid:** Otolaryngology, Willford Hall USAF Med Ctr 1991; **Fellow:** Rhinology, Hosp Univ Penn 1992; **Fac Appt:** Prof S, Mayo Med Sch

Browne, J Dale MD [Oto] - **Spec Exp:** Head & Neck Cancer; Thyroid Cancer; Skull Base Surgery; Head & Neck Reconstruction; **Hospital:** Wake Forest Baptist Med Ctr; **Address:** Medical Ctr Blvd, Winston Salem, NC 27103; **Phone:** 336-716-3854; **Board Cert:** Otolaryngology 1987; **Med School:** Med Coll GA 1982; **Resid:** Otolaryngology, NC Baptist Hosp 1987; **Fellow:** Otolaryngology, Univ Hosp 1991; **Fac Appt:** Prof Oto, Wake Forest Univ

Bumpous, Jeffrey MD [Oto] - **Spec Exp:** Head & Neck Cancer; Head & Neck Reconstruction; Thyroid & Parathyroid Cancer & Surgery; **Hospital:** Univ of Louisville Hosp, Norton Hosp; **Address:** Univ Surgical Assocs, 401 E Chestnut St, Ste 710, Louisville, KY 40202-1845; **Phone:** 502-583-8303; **Board Cert:** Otolaryngology 1994; **Med School:** Univ Louisville Sch Med 1988; **Resid:** Otolaryngology, Univ Louisville Hosp 1993; **Fellow:** Head and Neck Surgery, Univ Pittsburgh 1994; **Fac Appt:** Prof Oto, Univ Louisville Sch Med

Civantos, Francisco J MD [Oto] - **Spec Exp:** Head & Neck Cancer; Skull Base Surgery; **Hospital:** Univ of Miami Hosp & Clins/Sylvester Comp Canc Ctr; **Address:** Sylvester Cancer Ctr, Otolaryngology, 1475 NW 12th Ave, Ste 3550, Miami, FL 33136; **Phone:** 305-243-5276; **Board Cert:** Otolaryngology 1992; **Med School:** Columbia P&S 1986; **Resid:** Otolaryngology, Univ Illinois Coll Med 1991; **Fellow:** Head & Neck Oncology, Vanderbilt Univ 1992; **Fac Appt:** Assoc Prof Oto, Univ Miami Sch Med

Otolaryngology

Day, Terry A MD [Oto] - **Spec Exp:** Head & Neck Cancer; Reconstructive Microvascular Surgery; Skull Base Surgery; **Hospital:** MUSC Med Ctr; **Address:** 135 Rutledge Ave, MSC Bldg, Box 550, Charleston, SC 29425; **Phone:** 843-792-0719; **Board Cert:** Otolaryngology 1996; **Med School:** Univ Okla Coll Med 1989; **Resid:** Otolaryngology, LSU Med Ctr 1995; **Fellow:** Head & Neck Surgical Oncology, UC Davis Med Ctr 1996; Maxillofacial Surgery, Univ Hosp 1994; **Fac Appt:** Prof Oto, Med Univ SC

DiNardo, Laurence J MD [Oto] - **Spec Exp:** Head & Neck Cancer; Endoscopic Sinus Surgery; Skull Base Surgery; Sinus Disorders/Surgery; **Hospital:** Med Coll of VA Hosp; **Address:** VCU Dept Otolaryngology, 401 N 11th St Nelson Bldg, Richmond, VA 23298-0146; **Phone:** 804-628-4368; **Board Cert:** Otolaryngology 1992; **Med School:** Stanford Univ 1986; **Resid:** Otolaryngology, Hosp Univ Penn 1991; **Fac Appt:** Prof Oto, Va Commonwealth Univ Sch Med

Epstein, Jeffrey S MD [Oto] - **Spec Exp:** Hair Restoration/Transplant; Facial Plastic Surgery; **Hospital:** South Miami Hosp; **Address:** 6280 Sunset Drive, Ste 504, Miami, FL 33143; **Phone:** 305-666-1774; **Board Cert:** Otolaryngology 1994; Facial Plastic & Reconstr Surgery 1995; Hair Restoration Surgery 1998; **Med School:** Univ VT Coll Med 1988; **Resid:** Otolaryngology, Jackson Meml Hosp 1993; **Fellow:** Facial Plastic Surgery, Sheldon S Kabaker MD 1994; **Fac Appt:** Clin Prof Oto, Univ Miami Sch Med

Farrior, Edward H MD [Oto] - **Spec Exp:** Rhinoplasty; Ear Reshaping (Otoplasty); Facial Plastic Surgery; **Hospital:** Tampa Genl Hosp, St. Joseph's Hosp - Tampa; **Address:** 2908 W Azeele St, Tampa, FL 33609-3109; **Phone:** 813-875-3223; **Board Cert:** Otolaryngology 1987; Facial Plastic & Reconstr Surgery 1992; **Med School:** Univ VA Sch Med 1982; **Resid:** Otolaryngology, Univ Mich Hosps 1987; **Fellow:** Facial Plastic & Reconstr Surgery, Tampa Genl Hosp 1988; **Fac Appt:** Assoc Clin Prof S, Univ S Fla Coll Med

Farrior III, Joseph Brown MD [Oto] - **Spec Exp:** Otosclerosis/Stapedectomy; Hearing Loss; Meniere's Disease; Otology; **Hospital:** St. Joseph's Hosp - Tampa, Tampa Genl Hosp; **Address:** Farrior Ear Clinic, 2727 W Martin Luther King Jr Blvd, Ste 520, Tampa, FL 33607; **Phone:** 813-879-0810; **Board Cert:** Otolaryngology 1981; **Med School:** Emory Univ 1975; **Resid:** Surgery, Johns Hopkins Hosp 1977; Otolaryngology, Johns Hopkins Hosp 1981; **Fellow:** Otolaryngology, Farrior Clin/St Josephs Hosp 1980; **Fac Appt:** Assoc Clin Prof Oto, Univ S Fla Coll Med

Goodwin, W Jarrard MD [Oto] - **Spec Exp:** Head & Neck Cancer; **Hospital:** Univ of Miami Hosp & Clins/Sylvester Comp Canc Ctr, Jackson Meml Hosp; **Address:** Sylvester Comp Cancer Ctr, Dept Otolaryngology, 1475 NW 12th Ave, rm 4037, Miami, FL 33136-1015; **Phone:** 305-243-6520; **Board Cert:** Otolaryngology 1978; **Med School:** Albany Med Coll 1972; **Resid:** Surgery, Jackson Meml Hosp 1974; Otolaryngology, Jackson Meml Hosp 1977; **Fellow:** Head & Neck Surgical Oncology, MD Anderson Hosp 1980; **Fac Appt:** Prof Oto, Univ Miami Sch Med

Haynes, David S MD [Oto] - **Spec Exp:** Otology; Neuro-Otology; Hearing Disorders; Cochlear Implants; **Hospital:** Vanderbilt Univ Med Ctr (page 75), Saint Thomas Hosp - Nashville; **Address:** Otology Group of Vanderbilt, 1215 21st Ave S, Medical Center East, Ste 7209, Nashville, TN 37232; **Phone:** 615-322-6180; **Board Cert:** Otolaryngology 1994; Neurotology 2004; **Med School:** Univ Tenn Coll Med 1987; **Resid:** Surgery, Vanderbilt Univ Med Ctr 1989; Otolaryngology, Vanderbilt Univ Med Ctr 1993; **Fellow:** Otology & Neurotology, Otology Grp/ Ear Fdn 1995; **Fac Appt:** Assoc Prof Oto, Vanderbilt Univ

Kesser, Bradley W MD [Oto] - **Spec Exp:** Aural Atresia Repair; Neuro-Otology; **Hospital:** Univ of Virginia Health Sys; **Address:** Dept. Oto-HNS, Unviersity of Virginia Health System, Box 800713, Charlottesville, VA 22908-0713; **Phone:** 434-924-2040; **Board Cert:** Otolaryngology 1999; Neurotology 2008; **Med School:** Univ VA Sch Med 1993; **Resid:** Otolaryngology, Univ Va Med Ctr 1998; **Fellow:** Otology & Neurotology, House Ear Clinic 2000; **Fac Appt:** Assoc Prof Oto, Univ VA Sch Med

Kuhn, Frederick MD [Oto] - **Spec Exp:** Endoscopic Sinus Surgery; Allergic Fungal Sinusitis; Rhinoplasty Revision; **Hospital:** Meml Hlth Univ Med Ctr - Savannah, St. Joseph's-Candler Hosp; **Address:** Georgia Nasal & Sinus Inst, 4750 Waters Ave, Ste 112, Savannah, GA 31404; **Phone:** 912-355-1070; **Board Cert:** Otolaryngology 1972; **Med School:** Univ Okla Coll Med 1966; **Resid:** Surgery, St Lukes Hosp 1968; **Fellow:** Otolaryngology, Barnes Hosp/Wash Univ 1972

Lambert, Paul R MD [Oto] - **Spec Exp:** Neuro-Otology; Acoustic Neuroma; Meniere's Disease; Cholesteatoma; **Hospital:** MUSC Med Ctr; **Address:** MUSC, Dept Otolaryngology, 135 Rutledge Ave, Box 550, Charleston, SC 29425; **Phone:** 843-792-3531; **Board Cert:** Otolaryngology 1981; Neurotology 2004; **Med School:** Duke Univ 1976; **Resid:** Surgery, UCLA Med Ctr 1978; Otolaryngology, UCLA Med Ctr 1981; **Fellow:** Neurotology, Otologic Med Group 1982; **Fac Appt:** Prof Oto, Med Univ SC

Lanza, Donald C MD [Oto] - **Spec Exp:** Skull Base Tumors; Sinus Disorders/Surgery; Rhinitis; Graves' Disease-Eye; **Hospital:** St. Anthony's Hosp - St Petersburg, All Children's Hosp; **Address:** 550 94th Ave N, St Petersburg, FL 33702; **Phone:** 727-573-0074; **Board Cert:** Otolaryngology 1990; **Med School:** SUNY Hlth Sci Ctr 1985; **Resid:** Surgery, Albany Med Ctr 1987; Otolaryngology, Albany Med Ctr 1990; **Fellow:** Rhinology, Johns Hopkins Univ 1990; Rhinology, Univ Penn 1991

Levine, Paul A MD [Oto] - **Spec Exp:** Head & Neck Cancer; Head & Neck Reconstruction; Skull Base Tumors; **Hospital:** Univ of Virginia Health Sys; **Address:** UVA Health System, PO Box 800713, Charlottesville, VA 22908; **Phone:** 434-924-5593; **Board Cert:** Otolaryngology 1978; **Med School:** Albany Med Coll 1973; **Resid:** Otolaryngology, Yale-New Haven Hosp 1977; **Fellow:** Head and Neck Surgery, Stanford Med Ctr 1978; **Fac Appt:** Prof Oto, Univ VA Sch Med

Mangat, Devinder S MD [Oto] - **Spec Exp:** Cosmetic & Reconstructive Surgery-Face; **Hospital:** St. Elizabeth Hlthcare-Edgewood; **Address:** 133 Barnwood Drive, Edgewood, KY 41017; **Phone:** 513-984-3223; **Board Cert:** Otolaryngology 1978; Facial Plastic & Reconstr Surgery 2007; **Med School:** Univ KY Coll Med 1973; **Resid:** Surgery, Univ KY Med Ctr 1975; Otolaryngology, Univ Okla Hlth Scis Ctr 1978; **Fellow:** Facial Plastic Surgery, McCullough Clinic 1979; **Fac Appt:** Assoc Prof Oto, Univ Cincinnati

Mattox, Douglas E MD [Oto] - **Spec Exp:** Neuro-Otology; Meniere's Disease; Hearing Loss; Cochlear Implants; **Hospital:** Emory Univ Hosp, Chldns Hlthcare Atlanta @ Egleston; **Address:** Emory Univ Dept Otolaryngology, 550 Peachtree St, Ste 4400, Atlanta, GA 30322; **Phone:** 404-778-3381; **Board Cert:** Otolaryngology 1977; Neurotology 2004; **Med School:** Yale Univ 1973; **Resid:** Otolaryngology, Stanford Univ Hosp 1977; **Fellow:** Neurotology, Ugo Fisch, MD 1985; **Fac Appt:** Prof Oto, Emory Univ

Netterville, James L MD [Oto] - **Spec Exp:** Head & Neck Surgery; Head & Neck Cancer; Vocal Cord Disorders; Skull Base Tumors; **Hospital:** Vanderbilt Univ Med Ctr (page 75), Vanderbilt Monroe Carrell Jr. Chldn's Hosp (page 75); **Address:** Vanderbilt Univ Med Ctr, Dept Oto, 7209 Med Ctr East, South Twr, 1215 21st Ave S, Nashville, TN 37232-8605; **Phone:** 615-322-6180; **Board Cert:** Otolaryngology 1985; **Med School:** Univ Tenn Coll Med 1980; **Resid:** Surgery, Methodist Hosp 1982; Otolaryngology, Univ Tenn Med Ctr 1985; **Fellow:** Surgical Oncology, Univ Iowa 1986; **Fac Appt:** Prof Oto, Vanderbilt Univ

Ossoff, Robert H MD/DMD [Oto] - **Spec Exp:** Voice Disorders; Laryngeal Disorders; Vocal Cord Disorders; Endoscopic Surgery; **Hospital:** Vanderbilt Univ Med Ctr (page 75); **Address:** 1500 21st Ave S, Ste 3100, Nashville, TN 37212-8200; **Phone:** 615-343-0429; **Board Cert:** Otolaryngology 1982; **Med School:** Tufts Univ 1975; **Resid:** Otolaryngology, Northwestern Meml Hosp 1980; **Fellow:** Head and Neck Surgery, Northwestern Meml Hosp 1981; **Fac Appt:** Prof Oto, Vanderbilt Univ

Peters, Glenn E MD [Oto] - **Spec Exp:** Thyroid & Parathyroid Cancer & Surgery; **Hospital:** Univ of Ala Hosp at Birmingham; **Address:** UAB Med Ctr, Div of Head & Neck Surgery, 1530 3rd Ave S, Ste BDB 563, Birmingham, AL 35294-0012; **Phone:** 205-934-9767; **Board Cert:** Otolaryngology 1985; **Med School:** Louisiana State U, New Orleans 1980; **Resid:** Surgery, Baptist Med Ctr 1982; Otolaryngology, Univ Alabama Hosp 1984; **Fellow:** Head & Neck Surgical Oncology, Johns Hopkins Hosp 1987; **Fac Appt:** Prof S, Univ Alabama

Petruzzelli, Guy MD/PhD [Oto] - **Spec Exp:** Head & Neck Cancer & Surgery; Skull Base Tumors; Thyroid Cancer; Pituitary Tumors; **Hospital:** Meml Hlth Univ Med Ctr - Savannah; **Address:** 4700 Waters Ave ACI Bldg, Savannah, GA 31404; **Phone:** 912-350-0688; **Board Cert:** Otolaryngology 1993; **Med School:** Rush Med Coll 1987; **Resid:** Otolaryngology, Univ Pittsburgh Med Ctr 1992; **Fellow:** Head & Neck Oncology, Univ Pittsburgh Med Ctr 1993; Skull Base Surgery, Univ Pittsburgh Ctr Cranial Base Surg 1993; **Fac Appt:** Prof S, Mercer Univ Sch Med

Pillsbury, Harold C MD [Oto] - **Spec Exp:** Cochlear Implants; Neuro-Otology; Ear Disorders/Surgery; **Hospital:** NC Memorial Hosp - UNC; **Address:** UNC Dept of Otolaryngology/HSN Drive, G125 Physicians Office Bldg, 170 Manning Drive, CB 7070, Chapel Hill, NC 27599-7070; **Phone:** 919-966-6483; **Board Cert:** Otolaryngology 1978; Neurotology 2004; **Med School:** Geo Wash Univ 1972; **Resid:** Surgery, Univ NC Hosp 1973; Otolaryngology, NC Meml Hosp 1976; **Fac Appt:** Prof Oto, Univ NC Sch Med

Pitman, Karen MD [Oto] - **Spec Exp:** Head & Neck Cancer & Surgery; Thyroid & Parathyroid Cancer & Surgery; Sentinel Node Surgery; **Hospital:** Univ Mississippi Med Ctr; **Address:** Univ Miss Med Ctr, Dept Otolaryngology, 2500 N State St, Jackson, MS 39216; **Phone:** 601-984-5160; **Board Cert:** Otolaryngology 1995; **Med School:** Uniformed Srvs Univ, Bethesda 1987; **Resid:** Otolaryngology, Naval Med Ctr 1994; **Fellow:** Head & Neck Oncology, Univ Pittsburgh 1996; **Fac Appt:** Prof Oto, Univ Miss

Poole, Michael D MD/PhD [Oto] - **Spec Exp:** Pediatric Otolaryngology; Ear Infections; Sleep Disorders/Apnea; Sinus Disorders; **Hospital:** Meml Hlth Univ Med Ctr - Savannah, St. Joseph's-Candler Hosp; **Address:** Georgia Ear Institute, 4700 Waters Ave, Savannah, GA 31404; **Phone:** 912-356-1515; **Board Cert:** Otolaryngology 1986; **Med School:** Univ NC Sch Med 1981; **Resid:** Otolaryngology, NC Meml Hosp 1986; **Fac Appt:** Prof Oto, Mercer Univ Sch Med

Postma, Gregory N MD [Oto] - **Spec Exp:** Voice Disorders; **Hospital:** Med Coll of GA Hosp and Clin (MCG Health Inc); **Address:** Med Coll Georgia, Voice & Swallowing Center, 1447 Harper St, Augusta, GA 30912; **Phone:** 706-721-4400; **Board Cert:** Otolaryngology 1994; **Med School:** Hahnemann Univ 1984; **Resid:** Otolaryngology, Oakland Naval Hosp 1992; Otolaryngology, Univ N Carolina Hosps 1993; **Fellow:** Otolaryngology, Vanderbilt Univ 1996; **Fac Appt:** Prof Oto, Med Coll GA

Ries, W Russell MD [Oto] - **Spec Exp:** Facial Plastic & Reconstructive Surgery; Cosmetic Surgery-Face; Skin Laser Surgery; **Hospital:** Vanderbilt Univ Med Ctr (page 75); **Address:** Otology Group of Vanderbilt, 1215 21st Ave S, Medical Center East, Ste 7209, Nashville, TN 37232; **Phone:** 615-322-6180; **Board Cert:** Otolaryngology 1985; Facial Plastic & Reconstr Surgery 1992; **Med School:** Univ Tenn Coll Med 1978; **Resid:** Surgery, Baptist Meml Hosp 1981; Otolaryngology, Northwestern Meml Hosp 1984; **Fellow:** Facial Plastic Surgery, Tulane Med Ctr 1985; **Fac Appt:** Prof Oto, Vanderbilt Univ

Rosenthal, Eben MD [Oto] - **Spec Exp:** Head & Neck Cancer; Microvascular Surgery; Reconstructive Surgery; Minimally Invasive Surgery; **Hospital:** Univ of Ala Hosp at Birmingham; **Address:** 2000 6th Ave S, Birmingham, AL 35233; **Phone:** 205-934-9766; **Board Cert:** Otolaryngology 2001; **Med School:** Univ Mich Med Sch 1994; **Resid:** Otolaryngology, Univ MI Med Ctr 2000; **Fellow:** Head and Neck Surgery, OR Hlth Sci Univ 2001; **Fac Appt:** Prof S, Univ Alabama

Samant, Sandeep MD [Oto] - **Spec Exp:** Head & Neck Cancer & Surgery; Skull Base Surgery; Endoscopic Surgery; Thyroid & Parathyroid Cancer & Surgery; **Hospital:** Methodist Univ Hosp - Memphis; **Address:** UT Med Grp-Oto-Head & Neck Surgery, 7945 Wolf River Blvd, Ste 220, Germantown, TN 38138; **Phone:** 901-347-8220; **Board Cert:** Otolaryngology 2009; **Med School:** India 1986; **Resid:** Otolaryngology, ALL-Indian Inst 1989; Otolaryngology, Royal Coll Surgeons 1994; **Fellow:** Head and Neck Surgery, Univ Miami/Sylvester Comprehensive Cancer Ctr 1995; Head & Neck Oncology, Univ TN Med Ctr 1996

Senior, Brent A MD [Oto] - **Spec Exp:** Sinus Disorders/Surgery; Nasal Allergy; Sleep Disorders; **Hospital:** NC Memorial Hosp - UNC; **Address:** UNC, Otolaryngology Dept, Physicians Office Building, G-120, 170 Manning Drive, CB 7070, Chapel Hill, NC 27599-7070; **Phone:** 919-966-6483; **Board Cert:** Otolaryngology 1996; **Med School:** Univ Mich Med Sch 1990; **Resid:** Otolaryngology, Boston Univ/Tufts Univ Affil Hosp 1995; **Fellow:** Sinus Surgery, HOsp Univ Penn 1996; **Fac Appt:** Prof Oto, Univ NC Sch Med

Shockley, William W MD [Oto] - **Spec Exp:** Facial Plastic & Reconstructive Surgery; Rhinoplasty; Skin Cancer; Salivary Gland Tumors & Surgery; **Hospital:** NC Memorial Hosp - UNC; **Address:** 170 Manning Drive, Physicians Office Bldg, CB 7070, Chapel Hill, NC 27599-7070; **Phone:** 919-966-3342; **Board Cert:** Otolaryngology 1981; Facial Plastic & Reconstr Surgery ; **Med School:** Indiana Univ 1976; **Resid:** Otolaryngology, Univ Cincinnati Hosps 1981; **Fellow:** Head and Neck Surgery, H&N Surg Assoc 1982; **Fac Appt:** Prof Oto, Univ NC Sch Med

Sillers, Michael J MD [Oto] - **Spec Exp:** Nasal & Sinus Disorders; Sinus Disorders/Surgery; **Hospital:** St. Vincent's Hosp - Birmingham; **Address:** Alabama Nasal & Sinus Ctr, 7191 Cahaba Valley Rd, Ste 301, Birmingham, AL 35242; **Phone:** 205-980-2091; **Board Cert:** Otolaryngology 1994; **Med School:** Univ Alabama 1988; **Resid:** Otolaryngology, Univ Alabama Hosp 1993; **Fellow:** Sinus Surgery, Med Coll Georgia 1994; **Fac Appt:** Asst Prof S, Univ Alabama

Silverstein, Herbert MD [Oto] - **Spec Exp:** Ear Disorders/Surgery; Meniere's Disease; **Hospital:** Sarasota Meml Hosp; **Address:** Silverstein Institute, 1901 Floyd St, Sarasota, FL 34239; **Phone:** 941-366-9222; **Board Cert:** Otolaryngology 1967; **Med School:** Temple Univ 1961; **Resid:** Surgery, Hosp Univ Penn 1963; Otolaryngology, Mass EE Infirm 1966; **Fac Appt:** Clin Prof S, Univ S Fla Coll Med

Stringer, Scott P MD [Oto] - **Spec Exp:** Rhinitis; Skull Base Surgery; **Hospital:** Univ Mississippi Med Ctr, G.V. (Sonny) Montgomery VA Med Ctr - Jackson; **Address:** Univ Miss Med Ctr, Dept Otolaryngology, 2500 N State St, Jackson, MS 39216-4505; **Phone:** 601-984-5160; **Board Cert:** Otolaryngology 1987; **Med School:** Univ Tex SW, Dallas 1982; **Resid:** Surgery, Univ Tex SW Med Ctr 1984; Otolaryngology, Univ Tex SW Med Ctr 1987; **Fac Appt:** Prof Oto, Univ Miss

Telischi, Fred F MD [Oto] - **Spec Exp:** Ear Disorders/Surgery; Hearing Loss; Cochlear Implants; Neuro-Otology; **Hospital:** Jackson Meml Hosp; **Address:** Univ Miami Sch Med, Dept Otolaryngology, 1120 NW 14th St Fl 5, Box 016960, Miami, FL 33101; **Phone:** 305-243-2000; **Board Cert:** Otolaryngology 1990; Neurotology 2010; **Med School:** Univ Miami Sch Med 1985; **Resid:** Otolaryngology, Jackson Meml Hosp 1990; **Fellow:** Neurotology, House Ear Clinic 1992; **Fac Appt:** Prof Oto, Univ Miami Sch Med

Terris, David J MD [Oto] - **Spec Exp:** Thyroid Surgery; Thyroid Cancer; Parathyroid Disease; **Hospital:** Med Coll of GA Hosp and Clin (MCG Health Inc), Doctors Hosp; **Address:** MCG Health - Dept Otolaryngology, 1120 15th St, rm BP-4109, Augusta, GA 30912; **Phone:** 706-721-4400; **Board Cert:** Otolaryngology 1994; **Med School:** Duke Univ 1988; **Resid:** Surgery, Stanford Univ Med Ctr 1989; Otolaryngology, Stanford Univ Med Ctr 1993; **Fellow:** Head and Neck Surgery, Stanford Univ Med Ctr 1994; **Fac Appt:** Prof Oto, Med Coll GA

Otolaryngology

Tucci, Debara L MD [Oto] - **Spec Exp:** Skull Base Surgery; Otology; Cochlear Implants; Hearing & Balance Disorders; **Hospital:** Duke Univ Hosp; **Address:** Box 3805 Med Ctr, 3556 Hosp South, Blue Zone, Durham, NC 27710; **Phone:** 919-684-6968; **Board Cert:** Otolaryngology 1990; Neurotology 2004; **Med School:** Univ VA Sch Med 1985; **Resid:** Otolaryngology, Univ Va Med ctr 1990; **Fellow:** Otology & Neurotology, Univ Mich Med Ctr 1992; **Fac Appt:** Prof S, Duke Univ

Valentino, Joseph MD [Oto] - **Spec Exp:** Head & Neck Cancer; Reconstructive Microvascular Surgery; Thyroid Cancer; **Hospital:** Univ of Kentucky Albert B. Chandler Hosp; **Address:** UKMC ENT Dept, 740 S Limestone, Fl 3/Wing C, Lexington, KY 40536; **Phone:** 859-257-5405; **Board Cert:** Otolaryngology 1993; **Med School:** UMDNJ-RW Johnson Med Sch 1987; **Resid:** Otolaryngology, Univ Minn 1992; **Fellow:** Otolaryngology, Univ Iowa Coll Med 1993; **Fac Appt:** Assoc Prof Oto, Univ KY Coll Med

Wazen, Jack J MD [Oto] - **Spec Exp:** Skull Base Surgery; Meniere's Disease; Acoustic Neuroma; Hearing & Balance Disorders; **Hospital:** Sarasota Meml Hosp; **Address:** Silverstein Institute, 1901 Floyd St, Sarasota, FL 34239; **Phone:** 941-366-9222; **Board Cert:** Otolaryngology 1983; Neurotology 2012; **Med School:** Lebanon 1978; **Resid:** Surgery, St Lukes Hosp 1980; Otolaryngology, Columbia Presby Hosp 1983; **Fellow:** Neurotology, Ear Rsch Fdn 1984

Weissler, Mark C MD [Oto] - **Spec Exp:** Head & Neck Cancer; Laryngeal & Tracheal Disorders; Voice Disorders; Salivary Gland Tumors; **Hospital:** NC Memorial Hosp - UNC; **Address:** 170 Manning Drive, G106 Physician's Office Bldg, Campus Box 7070, Chapel Hill, NC 27599-7070; **Phone:** 919-843-4820; **Board Cert:** Otolaryngology 1985; **Med School:** Boston Univ 1980; **Resid:** Surgery, Mass Genl Hosp 1982; Otolaryngology, Mass Eye & Ear Infirm 1985; **Fellow:** Head & Neck Oncology, Univ Cincinnati 1986; **Fac Appt:** Prof Oto, Univ NC Sch Med

Midwest

Akervall, Jan A MD/PhD [Oto] - **Spec Exp:** Head & Neck Cancer; Head & Neck Reconstruction; Minimally Invasive Surgery; **Hospital:** Beaumont Hosp-Royal Oak, St. Joseph Mercy Hosp - Ann Arbor; **Address:** 28300 Orchard Lake Rd, Ste 100, Farmington Hills, MI 48334; **Phone:** 248-737-4030; **Med School:** Sweden 1990; **Resid:** Otolaryngology, Lund Univ Fac Med 1998; **Fellow:** Head & Neck Oncology, Univ MI Hosps 2002; **Fac Appt:** Clin Prof Oto, Oakland Univ-William Beaumont Med Sch

Alam, Daniel Syed MD [Oto] - **Spec Exp:** Nasal Reconstruction; Head & Neck Reconstruction; Parotid Gland Tumors; Cancer Reconstruction; **Hospital:** Cleveland Clin (page 55); **Address:** Cleveland Clin Main Campus, 9500 Euclid Ave, MC A71, Cleveland, OH 44195; **Phone:** 216-445-6594; **Board Cert:** Otolaryngology 2002; **Med School:** Johns Hopkins Univ 1996; **Resid:** Otolaryngology, Mass Genl Hosp 2001; **Fellow:** Facial Plastic & Reconstr Surgery, UCLA Med Ctr 2002

Arts, H Alexander MD [Oto] - **Spec Exp:** Skull Base Tumors & Surgery; Neuro-Otology; Hearing Loss; Cochlear Implants; **Hospital:** Univ of Michigan Hosp; **Address:** CS Mott Chldns Hosp, Dept Otolaryngology, 1500 E Medical Ctr Drive, Ste 1904, Ann Arbor, MI 48109; **Phone:** 734-936-8006; **Board Cert:** Otolaryngology 1992; Neurotology 2004; **Med School:** Baylor Coll Med 1983; **Resid:** Surgery, Univ Washington Med Ctr 1985; Otolaryngology, Univ Washington Med Ctr 1990; **Fellow:** Neurotology, Univ Virginia 1991; **Fac Appt:** Prof Oto, Univ Mich Med Sch

Baim, Howard M MD [Oto] - **Spec Exp:** Head & Neck Surgery; Sleep Disorders/Apnea; Sinus Disorders; **Hospital:** Adv Illinois Masonic Med Ctr, Highland Park/North Shore Univ Hlth Syst; **Address:** 2532 N Lincoln Ave, Chicago, IL 60614-2468; **Phone:** 773-883-1177; **Board Cert:** Otolaryngology 1978; **Med School:** Univ IL Coll Med 1973; **Resid:** Surgery, Illinois Met Grp Hosps 1975; Otolaryngology, Illinois EE Infirmary 1978; **Fac Appt:** Asst Clin Prof Oto, Univ IL Coll Med

Baker, Shan R MD [Oto] - **Spec Exp:** Cosmetic Surgery-Face & Neck; Reconstructive Surgery; **Hospital:** Univ of Michigan Hosp; **Address:** Ctr Facial & Cosmetic Surgery, 19900 Haggerty Rd, Ste 103, Livonia, MI 48152-1054; **Phone:** 734-432-7634; **Board Cert:** Otolaryngology 1977; Facial Plastic & Reconstr Surgery 1990; **Med School:** Univ Iowa Coll Med 1971; **Resid:** Surgery, UCSD Med Ctr 1973; Otolaryngology, Univ Iowa Hosps 1977; **Fac Appt:** Prof Oto, Univ Mich Med Sch

Bastian, Robert W MD [Oto] - **Spec Exp:** Voice Disorders; Swallowing Disorders; Laryngeal Disorders; **Hospital:** Adv Good Samaritan Hosp; **Address:** Bastian Voice Inst, 3010 Highland Parkway, Ste 550, Downers Grove, IL 60515-5500; **Phone:** 630-724-1100; **Board Cert:** Otolaryngology 1983; **Med School:** Washington Univ, St Louis 1978; **Resid:** Surgery, Barnes Hosp 1979; Otolaryngology, Barnes Hosp 1983; **Fellow:** Otolaryngology, Hosp Foch 1983

Beatty, Charles W MD [Oto] - **Spec Exp:** Otology & Neuro-Otology; Acoustic Neuroma; Meniere's Disease; Cochlear Implants; **Hospital:** Mayo Med Ctr & Clin - Rochester; **Address:** Mayo Clin-Dept Ear, Nose and Throat, 200 First St SW, Gonda-12, Rochester, MN 55905; **Phone:** 507-284-8532; **Board Cert:** Otolaryngology 1982; **Med School:** Univ Iowa Coll Med 1977; **Resid:** Otolaryngology, Mayo Clinic 1982; **Fac Appt:** Prof Oto, Mayo Med Sch

Benninger, Michael S MD [Oto] - **Spec Exp:** Voice Disorders; Nasal & Sinus Disorders; Sinus Disorders/Surgery; Laryngeal Disorders; **Hospital:** Cleveland Clin (page 55); **Address:** Cleveland Clinic, 9500 Euclid Ave, Cleveland, OH 44195; **Phone:** 216-444-6686; **Board Cert:** Otolaryngology 1988; **Med School:** Case West Res Univ 1983; **Resid:** Surgery, Cleveland Clin Fdn 1985; Otolaryngology, Cleveland Clin Fdn 1988; **Fac Appt:** Prof S, Cleveland Cl Coll Med/Case West Res

Blair, Elizabeth MD [Oto] - **Spec Exp:** Head & Neck Cancer & Surgery; Thyroid & Parathyroid Surgery; Salivary Gland Tumors; Skull Base Tumors; **Hospital:** Univ of Chicago Med Ctr; **Address:** Univ Chicago Med Ctr, Otol/ENT Clin, 5841 S Maryland Ave, MC 1035, Chicago, IL 60637; **Phone:** 773-702-1865; **Board Cert:** Otolaryngology 1994; **Med School:** Creighton Univ 1988; **Resid:** Otolaryngology, Univ Pittsburgh Med Ctr 1993; **Fellow:** Head & Neck Surgical Oncology, MD Anderson Cancer Ctr 1994; **Fac Appt:** Assoc Prof Oto, Univ Chicago-Pritzker Sch Med

Bojrab, Dennis I MD [Oto] - **Spec Exp:** Otology & Neuro-Otology; Facial Nerve Disorders; Skull Base Tumors; **Hospital:** Beaumont Hosp-Royal Oak; **Address:** Michigan Ear Inst, 30055 Northwestern Hwy, Ste 101, Farmington Hills, MI 48334; **Phone:** 248-865-4444; **Board Cert:** Otolaryngology 1985; Neurotology 2005; **Med School:** Indiana Univ 1979; **Resid:** Surgery, Butterworth Hosp 1981; Otolaryngology, Univ Indiana Sch Med 1984; **Fellow:** Skull Base Surgery, Vanderbilt Univ Med Ctr 1985; **Fac Appt:** Prof Oto, Oakland Univ-William Beaumont Med Sch

Bradford, Carol MD [Oto] - **Spec Exp:** Head & Neck Cancer; Melanoma-Head & Neck; Skin Cancer-Head & Neck; **Hospital:** Univ of Michigan Hosp; **Address:** Univ of Michigan Hlth Sys, 1500 E Medical Ctr Drive, rm 1904-TC, Ann Arbor, MI 48109-0312; **Phone:** 734-936-8029; **Board Cert:** Otolaryngology 1993; **Med School:** Univ Mich Med Sch 1986; **Resid:** Otolaryngology, Univ Michigan Med Ctr 1992; **Fellow:** Head and Neck Surgery, Univ Michigan Med Ctr 1988; **Fac Appt:** Prof Oto, Univ Mich Med Sch

Branham, Gregory H MD [Oto] - **Spec Exp:** Cosmetic & Reconstructive Surgery-Face; Nasal Surgery; Botox Therapy; Skin Laser Surgery-Resurfacing; **Hospital:** Barnes-Jewish West County Hosp, Barnes-Jewish Hosp; **Address:** 605 Old Ballas Rd, Ste 100, St Louis, MO 63141; **Phone:** 314-432-7760; **Board Cert:** Otolaryngology 1989; Facial Plastic & Reconstr Surgery 1993; **Med School:** Univ SC Sch Med 1983; **Resid:** Otolaryngology, St Louis Univ Hosp 1989; **Fellow:** Facial Plastic & Reconstr Surgery, Washington Univ Affil Hosp 1990; **Fac Appt:** Prof Oto, St Louis Univ

Burkey, Brian MD [Oto] - **Spec Exp:** Parotid Gland Tumors; Head & Neck Cancer; Reconstructive Surgery; **Hospital:** Cleveland Clin (page 55); **Address:** Head & Neck Inst, Desk A71, The Cleveland Clinic, 9500 Euclid Ave, Cleveland, OH 44195; **Phone:** 216-445-8837; **Board Cert:** Otolaryngology 1992; **Med School:** Univ VA Sch Med 1986; **Resid:** Otolaryngology, Univ Mich Med Ctr 1991; **Fellow:** Microsurgery, Ohio State Univ 1991; **Fac Appt:** Prof Oto, Vanderbilt Univ

Caldarelli, David D MD [Oto] - **Spec Exp:** Laryngeal & Vocal Cord Surgery; Sinus Disorders/Surgery; Ear Disorders/Surgery; Meniere's Disease; **Hospital:** Rush Univ Med Ctr; **Address:** Rush Otolaryngology, 1611 W Harrison St, Ste 550, Chicago, IL 60612; **Phone:** 312-733-4341; **Board Cert:** Otolaryngology 1970; **Med School:** Univ IL Coll Med 1965; **Resid:** Surgery, Presby-St Lukes Hosp 1967; Otolaryngology, Univ Illinois Eye/Ear Infirm 1970; **Fac Appt:** Prof Oto, Rush Med Coll

Campbell, Bruce H MD [Oto] - **Spec Exp:** Head & Neck Cancer; Thyroid Surgery; **Hospital:** Froedtert and Med Ctr of WI, Chldns Hosp - Wisconsin; **Address:** Med Coll Wisc-Dept Oto, 9200 W Wisconsin Ave, Milwaukee, WI 53226; **Phone:** 414-805-5583; **Board Cert:** Otolaryngology 1986; **Med School:** Rush Med Coll 1980; **Resid:** Otolaryngology, Med Coll Wisconsin 1985; **Fellow:** Head and Neck Surgery, MD Anderson Cancer Ctr 1987; **Fac Appt:** Prof Oto, Med Coll Wisc

Corey, Jacquelynne P MD [Oto] - **Spec Exp:** Nasal & Sinus Disorders; Allergy; Voice Disorders; **Hospital:** Univ of Chicago Med Ctr; **Address:** 5841 S Maryland Ave, MC 1035, Chicago, IL 60637; **Phone:** 773-702-1865; **Board Cert:** Otolaryngology 1985; **Med School:** Univ IL Coll Med 1979; **Resid:** Otolaryngology, Rush Presby-St Lukes Med Ctr 1984; **Fac Appt:** Assoc Prof Oto, Univ Chicago-Pritzker Sch Med

Driscoll, Colin L W MD [Oto] - **Spec Exp:** Acoustic Neuroma; Cochlear Implants; Skull Base Tumors; **Hospital:** Mayo Med Ctr & Clin - Rochester; **Address:** Mayo Clinic, Dept of Ear, Nose and Throat, 200 First St SW, Rochester, MN 55905; **Phone:** 507-284-4065; **Board Cert:** Otolaryngology 1998; Neurology 2006; **Med School:** Univ New Mexico 1992; **Resid:** Otolaryngology, Mayo Clinic 1997; **Fellow:** Neurotology, UCSF Med Ctr 1998; Skull Base Surgery, UCSF Med Ctr 1999; **Fac Appt:** Assoc Prof Oto, Mayo Med Sch

Ford, Charles N MD [Oto] - **Spec Exp:** Voice Disorders; Laryngeal Disorders; **Hospital:** Univ WI Hosp & Clins; **Address:** Univ of WI Hosp & Clinics, 600 Highland Ave, G3/225 Otolaryngology, MC 2400, Madison, WI 53792-3284; **Phone:** 608-263-6190; **Board Cert:** Otolaryngology 1971; **Med School:** Univ Louisville Sch Med 1965; **Resid:** Otolaryngology, Henry Ford Hosp 1970; **Fac Appt:** Prof Oto, Univ Wisc

Friedman, Michael MD [Oto] - **Spec Exp:** Sleep Disorders/Apnea/Snoring; Thyroid & Parathyroid Surgery; Sinus Disorders/Surgery; **Hospital:** Adv Illinois Masonic Med Ctr, Rush Univ Med Ctr; **Address:** 3000 N Halsted St, Ste 400, Chicago, IL 60657; **Phone:** 312-236-3642; **Board Cert:** Otolaryngology 1977; **Med School:** Univ IL Coll Med 1972; **Resid:** Surgery, Illinois Masonic Hosp 1974; Otolaryngology, Univ Illinois Med Ctr 1977; **Fac Appt:** Prof Oto, Rush Med Coll

Funk, Gerry F MD [Oto] - **Spec Exp:** Head & Neck Cancer; Head & Neck Reconstruction; Head & Neck Trauma; **Hospital:** Univ Iowa Hosp & Clinics; **Address:** Univ Iowa Hosp & Clinics, 200 Hawkins Drive, PFP-Otolaryngology, Iowa City, IA 52242; **Phone:** 319-356-2201; **Board Cert:** Otolaryngology 1992; **Med School:** Univ Chicago-Pritzker Sch Med 1986; **Resid:** Surgery, LAC-USC Med Ctr 1987; Otolaryngology, LAC-USC Med Ctr 1991; **Fellow:** Head and Neck Surgery, Univ Iowa Hosp 1992; **Fac Appt:** Prof Oto, Univ Iowa Coll Med

Gantz, Bruce J MD [Oto] - **Spec Exp:** Cochlear Implants; Neuro-Otology; Skull Base Surgery; **Hospital:** Univ Iowa Hosp & Clinics; **Address:** Univ Hosp & Clins, Dept Otolaryngology, 200 Hawkins Drive, rm 21201 PFP, Iowa City, IA 52242-1078; **Phone:** 319-356-2173; **Board Cert:** Otolaryngology 1980; Neurotology 2004; **Med School:** Univ Iowa Coll Med 1974; **Resid:** Otolaryngology, Univ Iowa Hosps 1980; **Fellow:** Neurotology, Univ Zurich 1982; **Fac Appt:** Prof Oto, Univ Iowa Coll Med

Goebel, Joel Alan MD [Oto] - **Spec Exp:** Dizziness; Hearing Disorders; Otology & Neuro-Otology; **Hospital:** Barnes-Jewish Hosp, St. Louis Chldns Hosp; **Address:** Barnes Jewish Hosp South, Campus Box 8115, St Louis, MO 63110; **Phone:** 314-362-7509; **Board Cert:** Otolaryngology 1985; **Med School:** Washington Univ, St Louis 1980; **Resid:** Otolaryngology, Barnes Hosp/Wash Univ 1985; **Fac Appt:** Prof Oto, Washington Univ, St Louis

Hartig, Gregory K MD [Oto] - **Spec Exp:** Head & Neck Cancer; Skull Base Tumors; **Hospital:** Univ WI Hosp & Clins; **Address:** 600 Highland Ave, rm K4/720, Madison, WI 53792-7375; **Phone:** 608-263-6190; **Board Cert:** Otolaryngology 1994; **Med School:** Univ Mich Med Sch 1988; **Resid:** Otolaryngology, Univ Mich Med Ctr 1993; **Fellow:** Otolaryngology, Univ Penn Med Ctr 1994; **Fac Appt:** Prof Oto, Univ Mich Med Sch

Haughey, Bruce H MD [Oto] - **Spec Exp:** Reconstructive Surgery-Face; Head & Neck Cancer; Head & Neck Reconstruction; **Hospital:** Barnes-Jewish Hosp, St. Louis Chldns Hosp; **Address:** Barnes Jewish Hosp South, 660 S Euclid Ave, Box 8115, St Louis, MO 63110; **Phone:** 314-362-7509; **Board Cert:** Otolaryngology 1984; **Med School:** New Zealand 1976; **Resid:** Surgery, Univ Auckland 1981; Otolaryngology, Univ Iowa Med Ctr 1984; **Fellow:** Otolaryngology, Univ Iowa Med Ctr 1985; **Fac Appt:** Prof Oto, Washington Univ, St Louis

Hilger, Peter A MD [Oto] - **Spec Exp:** Head & Neck Surgery; Facial Plastic Surgery; **Hospital:** Regions Hosp - St Paul, Fairview Southdale Hosp; **Address:** Centennial Lakes Med Bldg, 7373 France Ave S, Ste 410, Edina, MN 55435; **Phone:** 952-844-0404; **Board Cert:** Otolaryngology 1979; **Med School:** Univ Minn 1974; **Resid:** Surgery, Univ Minn Hosp 1975; Otolaryngology, Univ Minn Hosp 1979; **Fellow:** Plastic Surgery, Mass Eye & Ear Infirm 1980; **Fac Appt:** Asst Prof Oto, Univ Minn

Hoffman, Henry T MD [Oto] - **Spec Exp:** Voice Disorders; Head & Neck Cancer; Salivary Gland Tumors & Surgery; **Hospital:** Univ Iowa Hosp & Clinics; **Address:** Univ Iowa Hosp & Clins, 200 Hawkins Drive, PFP-Otolaryngology, Iowa City, IA 52242; **Phone:** 319-356-2201; **Board Cert:** Otolaryngology 1985; **Med School:** UCSD 1980; **Resid:** Otolaryngology, Univ Iowa Hosp & Clinics 1985; **Fellow:** Head & Neck Oncology, Univ Michigan Hosp 1989; **Fac Appt:** Clin Prof Oto, Univ Iowa Coll Med

Hogikyan, Norman D MD [Oto] - **Spec Exp:** Voice Disorders; Vocal Cord Disorders; Swallowing Disorders; Airway Disorders; **Hospital:** Univ of Michigan Hosp; **Address:** 1500 E Medical Center Drive, 1904 Taubman Center/5312, Ann Arbor, MI 48109-5312; **Phone:** 734-936-7633; **Board Cert:** Otolaryngology 1995; **Med School:** Univ Mich Med Sch 1988; **Resid:** Otolaryngology, Barnes Jewish Med Ctr 1994; **Fellow:** Otolaryngology, Loyola Univ Med Ctr 1995; **Fac Appt:** Prof Oto, Univ Mich Med Sch

Hotaling, Andrew J MD [Oto] - **Spec Exp:** Pediatric Otolaryngology; Sleep Disorders/Apnea; Neck Masses; Ear Infections; **Hospital:** Loyola Univ Med Ctr; **Address:** Loyola Univ Med Ctr, 2160 S First Ave Bldg 105 - rm 1870, Maywood, IL 60153-5590; **Phone:** 708-216-9183; **Board Cert:** Otolaryngology 1985; **Med School:** Case West Res Univ 1979; **Resid:** Surgery, Case Western 1981; Otolaryngology, Northwestern Meml Hosp 1984; **Fellow:** Pediatric Otolaryngology, Univ Pittsburgh Med Ctr 1985; **Fac Appt:** Prof Oto, Loyola Univ-Stritch Sch Med

Jones, Paul J MD [Oto] - **Spec Exp:** Pediatric Otolaryngology; **Hospital:** Rush Univ Med Ctr; **Address:** 1611 W Harrison St, Ste 550, Chicago, IL 60612; **Phone:** 312-942-6100; **Board Cert:** Otolaryngology 1989; **Med School:** Rush Med Coll 1983; **Resid:** Otolaryngology, Rush Presby-St Lukes Med Ctr 1988; **Fac Appt:** Asst Prof Oto, Rush Med Coll

Kartush, Jack MD [Oto] - **Spec Exp:** Ear Disorders/Surgery; Balance Disorders; **Hospital:** Providence Hosp - Southfield; **Address:** Michigan Ear Inst, 30055 Northwestern Hwy, Ste 101, Farmington Hills, MI 48334; **Phone:** 248-865-4444; **Board Cert:** Otolaryngology 1984; **Med School:** Univ Mich Med Sch 1978; **Resid:** Otolaryngology, Univ Mich Med Ctr 1984; **Fellow:** Neurotology, Univ Mich Med Ctr 1985; **Fac Appt:** Assoc Clin Prof Oto, Wayne State Univ

Kern, Robert C MD [Oto] - **Spec Exp:** Sinus Disorders/Surgery; Nasal & Sinus Disorders; Snoring/Sleep Apnea; Taste & Smell Disorders; **Hospital:** Northwestern Meml Hosp; **Address:** Northwestern Medical Faculty Fdn, 675 N St Clair St Fl 15, Chicago, IL 60611; **Phone:** 312-695-8182; **Board Cert:** Otolaryngology 1990; **Med School:** Jefferson Med Coll 1985; **Resid:** Otolaryngology, Wayne State Affil Hosp 1990; **Fellow:** Research, Natl Inst Hlth 1991; **Fac Appt:** Prof Oto, Northwestern Univ

Lavertu, Pierre MD [Oto] - **Spec Exp:** Thyroid Cancer; Head & Neck Cancer; Skull Base Tumors; **Hospital:** Univ Hosps Case Med Ctr (page 74); **Address:** 11100 Euclid Ave, Cleveland, OH 44106-5045; **Phone:** 216-844-4773; **Board Cert:** Otolaryngology 1981; **Med School:** Univ Montreal 1976; **Resid:** Otolaryngology, Univ Montreal Med Ctr 1981; **Fellow:** Head and Neck Surgery, Univ Montreal Med Ctr 1982; Head and Neck Surgery, Cleveland Clinic 1983; **Fac Appt:** Prof Oto, Case West Res Univ

Leonetti, John P MD [Oto] - **Spec Exp:** Skull Base Tumors & Surgery; Neuro-Otology; Head & Neck Cancer; Facial Paralysis; **Hospital:** Loyola Univ Med Ctr; **Address:** Loyola University Medical Ctr, Dept Otolaryngology, 2160 S First Ave Bldg 105 - rm 1870, Maywood, IL 60153; **Phone:** 708-216-4804; **Board Cert:** Otolaryngology 1987; **Med School:** Loyola Univ-Stritch Sch Med 1982; **Resid:** Otolaryngology, Loyola Univ Med Ctr 1987; Research, House Ear Inst 1987; **Fellow:** Neurotology, Barnes Jewish Hosp 1988; **Fac Appt:** Prof Oto, Loyola Univ-Stritch Sch Med

Marentette, Lawrence J MD [Oto] - **Spec Exp:** Skull Base Tumors & Surgery; Facial Plastic & Reconstructive Surgery; **Hospital:** Univ of Michigan Hosp; **Address:** 1500 E Med Ctr Drive, 1904 Taubman Ctr, Ann Arbor, MI 48109-5312; **Phone:** 734-936-8051; **Board Cert:** Otolaryngology 1981; Facial Plastic & Reconstr Surgery 1995; **Med School:** Wayne State Univ 1976; **Resid:** Otolaryngology, Wayne State Univ 1980; **Fellow:** Maxillofacial Surgery, Univ of Zurich 1985; **Fac Appt:** Prof Oto, Univ Mich Med Sch

Miyamoto, Richard T MD [Oto] - **Spec Exp:** Neuro-Otology; Acoustic Neuroma; Ear Disorders/Surgery; Cochlear Implants; **Hospital:** IU Health University Hosp, Riley Hosp for Children; **Address:** 705 Riley Hosp Drive, Ste 0860, Indianapolis, IN 46202; **Phone:** 317-274-3556; **Board Cert:** Otolaryngology 1975; Neurotology 2004; **Med School:** Univ Mich Med Sch 1970; **Resid:** Surgery, Butterworth Hosp 1972; Otolaryngology, Indiana Univ Hosps 1975; **Fellow:** Otology & Neurotology, Otologic Med Grp 1978; **Fac Appt:** Prof Oto, Indiana Univ

Naclerio, Robert M MD [Oto] - **Spec Exp:** Sinus Disorders/Surgery; Pediatric Otolaryngology; Rhinitis; **Hospital:** Univ of Chicago Med Ctr; **Address:** Univ Chicago Med Ctr, 5841 S Maryland Ave, MC1035, Chicago, IL 60637; **Phone:** 773-702-0080; **Board Cert:** Otolaryngology 1983; **Med School:** Baylor Coll Med 1976; **Resid:** Surgery, Johns Hopkins Hosp 1978; Otolaryngology, Baylor Coll Med 1983; **Fellow:** Clinical Immunology, Johns Hopkins Hosp 1982; **Fac Appt:** Prof Oto, Univ Chicago-Pritzker Sch Med

Olsen, Kerry D MD [Oto] - **Spec Exp:** Head & Neck Cancer & Surgery; Esthesioneuroblastoma; Salivary Gland Tumors & Surgery; Skull Base Tumors; **Hospital:** Mayo Med Ctr & Clin - Rochester; **Address:** Mayo Clinic, Dept Otolaryngology, 200 1st St SW, Rochester, MN 55905-0001; **Phone:** 507-284-3542; **Board Cert:** Otolaryngology 1981; **Med School:** Mayo Med Sch 1976; **Resid:** Otolaryngology, Mayo Clinic 1981; **Fac Appt:** Prof Oto, Mayo Med Sch

Ozer, Enver MD [Oto] - **Spec Exp:** Head & Neck Cancer; Head & Neck Surgery; **Hospital:** Ohio St Univ Med Ctr; **Address:** 456 W 10th Ave, Ste 4A, Columbus, OH 43210; **Phone:** 614-293-8074; **Med School:** Turkey 1994; **Resid:** Otolaryngology, Marmara Univ Med Sch 1996; Head and Neck Surgery, Marmara Univ Med Sch 2000; **Fellow:** Head & Neck Oncology, Ohio St Univ Med Ctr 2005; **Fac Appt:** Asst Prof Oto, Ohio State Univ

Paparella, Michael M MD [Oto] - **Spec Exp:** Hearing Disorders; Neuro-Otology; Meniere's Disease; Ear Infections; **Hospital:** Univ Minn Med Ctr, Fairview - Riverside Campus, Maple Grove Hosp; **Address:** 701 25th Ave S, Ste 200, 9825 Hospital Drive, Fl LL, Ste 10, Minneapolis, MN 55454-1443; **Phone:** 612-339-2836; **Board Cert:** Otolaryngology 1963; **Med School:** Univ Mich Med Sch 1957; **Resid:** Otolaryngology, Henry Ford Hosp 1961; **Fac Appt:** Clin Prof Oto, Univ Minn

Patil, Yash J MD [Oto] - **Spec Exp:** Thyroid & Parathyroid Cancer & Surgery; Head & Neck Cancer & Surgery; Airway Disorders; **Hospital:** Univ Hosp - Cincinnati; **Address:** 222 Piedmont Ave, Cincinnati, OH 45219; **Phone:** 513-475-8400; **Board Cert:** Otolaryngology 2002; **Med School:** Vanderbilt Univ 1996; **Resid:** Otolaryngology, Chicago Medical Center 2000; **Fellow:** Microvascular Surgery, Washington Univ School of Med 2002; **Fac Appt:** Asst Prof Oto, Univ Cincinnati

Pelzer, Harold J MD/DDS [Oto] - **Spec Exp:** Head & Neck Cancer; Swallowing Disorders; **Hospital:** Northwestern Meml Hosp; **Address:** Northwestern Dept Otolaryngology, 675 N St Clair St Fl 15, Chicago, IL 60611; **Phone:** 312-695-8182; **Board Cert:** Otolaryngology 1985; **Med School:** Northwestern Univ 1979; **Resid:** Surgery, Northwestern Meml Hosp 1983; **Fellow:** Head and Neck Surgery, Northwestern Meml Hosp 1985; **Fac Appt:** Assoc Prof Oto, Northwestern Univ

Pensak, Myles L MD [Oto] - **Spec Exp:** Skull Base Tumors; Facial Paralysis; Hearing & Balance Disorders; **Hospital:** Univ Hosp - Cincinnati, Good Samaritan Hosp - Cincinnati; **Address:** Univ Medical Arts Building, 222 Piedmont Ave, Ste 5200, Cincinnati, OH 45219; **Phone:** 513-475-8400; **Board Cert:** Otolaryngology 1983; Neurotology 2004; **Med School:** NY Med Coll 1978; **Resid:** Surgery, Upstate Med Ctr 1980; Otolaryngology, Yale Univ 1983; **Fellow:** Otology & Neurotology, The Otology Group 1984; **Fac Appt:** Prof Oto, Univ Cincinnati

Piccirillo, Jay MD [Oto] - **Spec Exp:** Sleep Disorders/Apnea; Sinus Disorders/Surgery; **Hospital:** Barnes-Jewish Hosp; **Address:** Barnes Jewish Hosp South, Campus Box 8115, St Louis, MO 63110; **Phone:** 314-362-7509; **Board Cert:** Otolaryngology 1990; **Med School:** Univ VT Coll Med 1985; **Resid:** Otolaryngology, Albany Med Ctr 1990; **Fellow:** Yale Univ 1992; **Fac Appt:** Asst Prof Oto, Washington Univ, St Louis

Siegel, Gordon J MD [Oto] - **Spec Exp:** Head & Neck Cancer; Nasal & Sinus Disorders; **Hospital:** Northwestern Meml Hosp, Lurie Chldn's Hosp-Chicago; **Address:** 3 E Huron St Fl 1, Chicago, IL 60611-2705; **Phone:** 312-988-7777; **Board Cert:** Otolaryngology 1984; **Med School:** Ros Franklin Univ/Chicago Med Sch 1978; **Resid:** Otolaryngology, Northwestern Univ Affil Hosp 1982; **Fac Appt:** Asst Clin Prof Oto, Northwestern Univ

Stankiewicz, James MD [Oto] - **Spec Exp:** Endoscopic Sinus Surgery; Rhinosinusitis; Nasal & Sinus Disorders; **Hospital:** Loyola Univ Med Ctr; **Address:** Loyola Univ Med Ctr, Dept Oto, 2160 S First Ave, Maywood, IL 60153-5590; **Phone:** 708-216-9183; **Board Cert:** Otolaryngology 1978; **Med School:** Univ Chicago-Pritzker Sch Med 1974; **Resid:** Otolaryngology, Univ Chicago Hosp 1978; **Fac Appt:** Prof Oto, Loyola Univ-Stritch Sch Med

Otolaryngology

Stenson, Kerstin M MD [Oto] - **Spec Exp:** Head & Neck Cancer & Surgery; Head & Neck Cancer Reconstruction; Trauma; Vocal Cord Disorders; **Hospital:** Univ of Chicago Med Ctr; **Address:** Univ Chicago Med Ctr, Otol/ENT Clin, 5841 S Maryland Ave, MC 1035, Chicago, IL 60637-1463; **Phone:** 773-702-1865; **Board Cert:** Otolaryngology 1994; **Med School:** Ros Franklin Univ/Chicago Med Sch 1988; **Resid:** Otolaryngology, Univ Illinois Affil Hosps 1993; **Fellow:** Head & Neck Oncology, Univ Michigan Hosp 1994; Microvascular Surgery, Univ Michigan Hosp 1994; **Fac Appt:** Prof S, Univ Chicago-Pritzker Sch Med

Szachowicz II, Edward H MD [Oto] - **Spec Exp:** Cosmetic Surgery-Face; Rhinoplasty; **Hospital:** Abbott - Northwestern Hosp; **Address:** Centennial Lakes Med Bldg, 7373 France Ave S, Ste 508, Edina, MN 55435-4538; **Phone:** 952-835-5665; **Board Cert:** Otolaryngology 1984; **Med School:** Univ IL Coll Med 1979; **Resid:** Surgery, Fairview Univ Med Ctr 1980; Otolaryngology, Fairview Univ Med Ctr 1984; **Fellow:** Facial Plastic Surgery, Fairview Univ Med Ctr 1986; **Fac Appt:** Asst Clin Prof Oto, Univ Minn

Teknos, Theodoros N MD [Oto] - **Spec Exp:** Head & Neck Cancer; Thyroid Cancer; Facial Plastic & Reconstructive Surgery; Reconstructive Microvascular Surgery; **Hospital:** Ohio St Univ Med Ctr; **Address:** 456 W 10th Ave, Ste 4A, Columbus, OH 43210; **Phone:** 614-293-8074; **Board Cert:** Otolaryngology 1997; **Med School:** Harvard Med Sch 1991; **Resid:** Otolaryngology, Mass Eye & Ear Hosp 1996; **Fellow:** Head and Neck Surgery, Vanderbilt Univ Med Ctr 1997; Microvascular Surgery, Vanderbilt Univ Med Ctr 1997; **Fac Appt:** Prof Oto, Ohio State Univ

Telian, Steven A MD [Oto] - **Spec Exp:** Cochlear Implants; Ear Disorders/Surgery; Acoustic Neuroma; **Hospital:** Univ of Michigan Hosp; **Address:** Univ Mich Med Ctr, Dept Otolaryngology-Head & Neck Surgery, 1500 E Med Ctr Drive, 1904 Taubman Ctr, Ann Arbor, MI 48109-0312; **Phone:** 734-936-8006; **Board Cert:** Otolaryngology 1985; Neurotology 2004; **Med School:** Univ Pennsylvania 1980; **Resid:** Otolaryngology, Hosp Univ Penn 1985; **Fellow:** Neurotology, Univ Mich Med Ctr 1986; **Fac Appt:** Prof Oto, Univ Mich Med Sch

Toriumi, Dean MD [Oto] - **Spec Exp:** Rhinoplasty; Cosmetic Surgery-Face; Reconstructive Plastic Surgery; **Hospital:** Univ of IL Med Ctr at Chicago; **Address:** 60 E Delaware Pl, Ste 1460, Chicago, IL 60611; **Phone:** 312-255-8812; **Board Cert:** Otolaryngology 1988; **Med School:** Rush Med Coll 1981; **Resid:** Surgery, Univ Illinois Med Ctr 1985; Otolaryngology, Northwestern Univ Med Sch 1987; **Fellow:** Facial Plastic Surgery, Tulane Med Sch 1988; Facial Plastic Surgery, Virginia Mason Med Ctr 1989; **Fac Appt:** Assoc Prof Oto, Univ IL Coll Med

Wiet, Richard J MD [Oto] - **Spec Exp:** Acoustic Neuroma; Hearing Loss; Otosclerosis/Stapedectomy; Cochlear Implants; **Hospital:** Adventist Hinsdale Hosp, Northwestern Meml Hosp; **Address:** Ear Institute of Chicago, 11 Salt Creek Ln, Ste 101, Hinsdale, IL 60521; **Phone:** 630-789-3110; **Board Cert:** Otolaryngology 1976; Neurotology 2004; **Med School:** Loyola Univ-Stritch Sch Med 1971; **Resid:** Otolaryngology, Cincinnati Med Ctr 1976; **Fellow:** Neurotology, Univ Zurich/Ear Fdn 1979; **Fac Appt:** Clin Prof Oto, Northwestern Univ

Wilson, Keith M MD [Oto] - **Spec Exp:** Head & Neck Cancer & Surgery; Voice Disorders; **Hospital:** Univ Hosp - Cincinnati; **Address:** 7700 University Ct, Ste 3900, Westchester, OH 45069; **Phone:** 513-475-8400; **Board Cert:** Otolaryngology 1992; **Med School:** Cornell Univ-Weill Med Coll 1986; **Resid:** Otolaryngology, St Louis Univ Med Ctr 1991; **Fellow:** Head & Neck Surgical Oncology, Ohio State Med Ctr 1992; **Fac Appt:** Assoc Prof Oto, Univ Cincinnati

Wolf, Gregory T MD [Oto] - **Spec Exp:** Head & Neck Cancer; Laryngeal Cancer; **Hospital:** Univ of Michigan Hosp; **Address:** Univ Mich Med Ctr, Dept Oto-HNS, 1500 E Med Ctr, Taubman Ctr, rm 1903, Ann Arbor, MI 48109-0312; **Phone:** 734-936-9178; **Board Cert:** Otolaryngology 1978; Facial Plastic & Reconstr Surgery 1994; **Med School:** Univ Mich Med Sch 1973; **Resid:** Surgery, Georgetown Univ Hosp 1975; Otolaryngology, SUNY Upstate Med Ctr 1978; **Fellow:** Immunology, NIH 1980; **Fac Appt:** Prof Oto, Univ Mich Med Sch

Woodson, B Tucker MD [Oto] - **Spec Exp:** Sleep Disorders/Apnea; **Hospital:** Froedtert and Med Ctr of WI, Chldns Hosp - Wisconsin; **Address:** Froedtert West ENT Clinic, 9200 W Wisconsin Ave, Milwaukee, WI 53226-3522; **Phone:** 414-805-7667; **Board Cert:** Otolaryngology 1988; **Med School:** Univ MO-Columbia Sch Med 1983; **Resid:** Surgery, Henry Ford Hosp 1984; Otolaryngology, Henry Ford Hosp 1988; **Fac Appt:** Assoc Prof Oto, Med Coll Wisc

Woodson, Gayle Ellen MD [Oto] - **Spec Exp:** Voice Disorders; Swallowing Disorders; **Hospital:** St. John's Hosp - Springfield, Memorial Med Ctr-Springfield; **Address:** Div Otolaryngology, 301 N 8 St Fl 5, Box 19662, Springfield, IL 62701; **Phone:** 217-545-6099; **Board Cert:** Otolaryngology 1981; **Med School:** Baylor Coll Med 1975; **Resid:** Surgery, Johns Hopkins Hosp 1978; Otolaryngology, Baylor Coll Med 1981; **Fellow:** Laryngology, Inst Laryngology and Otology 1982; **Fac Appt:** Prof Oto, Southern IL Univ

Yoo, George H MD [Oto] - **Spec Exp:** Laryngeal Cancer; Oral Cancer; Thyroid Cancer; Sinus Tumors; **Hospital:** Barbara Ann Karmanos Cancer Inst; **Address:** Barbara Ann Karmanos Cancer Inst, 4100 John R, Detroit, MI 48201; **Phone:** 313-576-9782; **Board Cert:** Otolaryngology 1996; **Med School:** Univ Kansas 1990; **Resid:** Otolaryngology, Johns Hopkins Hosp 1994; **Fellow:** Head and Neck Surgery, Johns Hopkins Hosp 1997; **Fac Appt:** Prof Oto, Wayne State Univ

Young, Nancy MD [Oto] - **Spec Exp:** Cochlear Implants; Cholesteatoma; Hearing Loss; Baha Implant; **Hospital:** Lurie Chldn's Hosp-Chicago, Glenbrook Hosp-NorthShore Univ Hlth Syst; **Address:** Children's Memorial, Div Otolaryngology, 2300 Children's Plaza, Box 265, Chicago, IL 60614; **Phone:** 773-880-3020; **Board Cert:** Otolaryngology 1987; **Med School:** NYU Sch Med 1982; **Resid:** Surgery, Montefiore Med Ctr 1984; Otolaryngology, Northwestern Univ Hosp 1987; **Fellow:** Neurotology, Hinsdale Hosp 1988; **Fac Appt:** Assoc Prof Oto, Northwestern Univ

Yueh, Bevan MD [Oto] - **Spec Exp:** Head & Neck Cancer; Hearing Loss; **Address:** Univ Minnesota Med Ctr PWB Bldg Fl 8, MMC 396, 516 Delaware St SE, Ste 8A, Minneapolis, MN 55455-0932; **Phone:** 612-625-2410; **Board Cert:** Otolaryngology 1995; **Med School:** Stanford Univ 1989; **Resid:** Otolaryngology, Johns Hopkins Hosp 1994; **Fellow:** Otolaryngology, Johns Hopkins Hosp 1995; **Fac Appt:** Assoc Prof Oto, Univ Minn

Great Plains and Mountains

Abaza, Mona M MD [Oto] - **Spec Exp:** Voice Disorders; Swallowing Disorders; **Hospital:** Univ of CO Hosp - Anschutz Inpatient Pav; **Address:** Univ Colorado Dept ENT, 1635 Aurora Court Fl 6, Aurora, CO 80045; **Phone:** 720-848-2820; **Board Cert:** Otolaryngology 1999; **Med School:** Med Coll PA Hahnemann 1991; **Resid:** Otolaryngology, Univ Texas Affil Hosps 1998; **Fellow:** Research, Natl Insts of Deafness & Communicative Disorders 1994; Laryngology, Jefferson Univ Hosp 1999; **Fac Appt:** Assoc Prof Oto, Univ Colorado

Chowdhury, Khalid MD [Oto] - **Spec Exp:** Skull Base Tumors & Surgery; Craniofacial Surgery; Maxillofacial Surgery; Head & Neck Cancer; **Hospital:** Porter Adventist Hosp, Rocky Mountain Hosp for Children; **Address:** 1601 E 19th Ave, Ste 3000, MS 80218, Denver, CO 80218; **Phone:** 303-839-5155; **Board Cert:** Otolaryngology 1990; Facial Plastic & Reconstr Surgery 1995; **Med School:** Univ Saskatchewan 1982; **Resid:** Surgery, Univ Saskatchewan Hosp 1985; Otolaryngology, McGill Univ Hosps 1989; **Fellow:** Craniofacial Surgery, Univ Bern Hosp 1990; Facial Plastic & Reconstr Surgery, Univ Bern Hosp 1990; **Fac Appt:** Assoc Prof Oto, Univ Colorado

Otolaryngology

Denenberg, Steven M MD [Oto] - **Spec Exp:** Cosmetic Surgery-Face; Rhinoplasty; **Hospital:** Nebraska Meth Hosp, Alegent Hlth - Bergan Mercy Med Ctr; **Address:** 7640 Pacific St, Omaha, NE 68114-5421; **Phone:** 402-391-7640; **Board Cert:** Otolaryngology 1984; Facial Plastic & Reconstr Surgery 1992; **Med School:** Univ Nebr Coll Med 1980; **Resid:** Otolaryngology, Stanford Univ Med Ctr 1984; **Fellow:** Facial Plastic Surgery, McCollough Ctr 1985; **Fac Appt:** Asst Clin Prof Oto, Univ Nebr Coll Med

Jenkins, Herman A MD [Oto] - **Spec Exp:** Ear Disorders/Surgery; Neuro-Otology; Acoustic Neuroma; Cochlear Implants; **Hospital:** Univ of CO Hosp - Anschutz Inpatient Pav, Chldn's Hosp - Aurora (CO); **Address:** Univ Colorado Hosp, Dept Otolaryngology, 1635 Aurora Ct Fl 6, Aurora, CO 80045; **Phone:** 720-848-2820; **Board Cert:** Otolaryngology 1977; Neurotology 2004; **Med School:** Vanderbilt Univ 1970; **Resid:** Surgery, UCLA Med Ctr 1972; Otolaryngology, UCLA Med Ctr 1977; **Fellow:** Neurotology, Univ Hosp 1980; **Fac Appt:** Prof Oto, Univ Colorado

Kang, Dong-Kyoo Richard MD [Oto] - **Spec Exp:** Cochlear Implants; Ear Disorders/Surgery; **Hospital:** Boys Town Natl Rsch Hosp; **Address:** Boystown Medical Campus-Downtown Clinic, 555 N 30th St, Omaha, NE 68131; **Phone:** 402-498-6540; **Board Cert:** Otolaryngology 1986; **Med School:** Boston Univ 1980; **Resid:** Otolaryngology, Naval Med Ctr 1986; **Fellow:** Pediatric Otolaryngology, St. Louis Chldn's Hosp 1991; Pediatric Otolaryngology, San Diego Chldn's Hosp 1993; **Fac Appt:** Assoc Clin Prof Oto, Ohio State Univ

Kingdom, Todd T MD [Oto] - **Spec Exp:** Nasal & Sinus Disorders; Endoscopic Sinus Surgery; Skull Base Surgery; **Hospital:** Univ of CO Hosp - Anschutz Inpatient Pav, Natl Jewish Med & Rsch Ctr; **Address:** Univ Colorado Hospital, 1635 Aurora Court, MS F737, Aurora, CO 80045; **Phone:** 720-848-2820; **Board Cert:** Otolaryngology 1997; **Med School:** Emory Univ 1991; **Resid:** Otolaryngology, UCSF Med Ctr 1996; **Fac Appt:** Assoc Prof Oto, Univ Colorado

Lydiatt, Daniel D MD/DDS [Oto] - **Spec Exp:** Head & Neck Cancer; **Hospital:** Nebraska Med Ctr, Methodist Hosp - Omaha; **Address:** Nebraska Med Ctr, Dept Otolaryngology, 981225 Nebraska Medical Ctr, Omaha, NE 68198-1225; **Phone:** 402-559-6500; **Board Cert:** Otolaryngology 1992; **Med School:** Univ Nebr Coll Med 1983; **Resid:** Otolaryngology, Univ Nebraska Med Ctr 1990; **Fellow:** Head and Neck Surgery, MD Anderson Med Ctr 1991; **Fac Appt:** Assoc Prof Oto, Univ Nebr Coll Med

Lydiatt, William M MD [Oto] - **Spec Exp:** Head & Neck Cancer; Thyroid Cancer; Salivary Gland Tumors & Surgery; **Hospital:** Nebraska Med Ctr, Nebraska Meth Hosp; **Address:** 981225 Nebraska Medical Ctr, Omaha, NE 68198-7630; **Phone:** 402-559-6500; **Board Cert:** Otolaryngology 1994; **Med School:** Univ Nebr Coll Med 1988; **Resid:** Otolaryngology, Univ Nebraska Med Ctr 1993; **Fellow:** Head and Neck Surgery, Meml Sloan Kettering Cancer Ctr 1995; **Fac Appt:** Prof Oto, Univ Nebr Coll Med

Shelton, Clough MD [Oto] - **Spec Exp:** Facial Nerve Disorders; Acoustic Neuroma; Hearing & Balance Disorders; Cochlear Implants; **Hospital:** Univ Utah Hlth Care; **Address:** Univi Utah Sch Med, 50 N Med Drive, 1900 East, Ste 3C120, Salt Lake City, UT 84132; **Phone:** 801-585-5450; **Board Cert:** Otolaryngology 1986; Neurotology 2004; **Med School:** Univ Tex SW, Dallas 1981; **Resid:** Otolaryngology, Stanford Univ Med Ctr 1986; **Fellow:** Neurotology, Otologic Med Group 1987; **Fac Appt:** Prof Oto, Univ Utah

Smith, Russell B MD [Oto] - **Spec Exp:** Head & Neck Cancer; Thyroid Cancer; Skull Base Tumors; **Hospital:** Nebraska Med Ctr, Nebraska Meth Hosp; **Address:** 981225 Nebraska Medical Center, Omaha, NE 68198-1225; **Phone:** 402-559-6500; **Board Cert:** Otolaryngology 2001; **Med School:** Univ MO-Columbia Sch Med 1995; **Resid:** Otolaryngology, Univ Missouri Med Ctr 2000; **Fellow:** Head & Neck Surgical Oncology, Univ Iowa Hosps & Clins 2001; **Fac Appt:** Assoc Prof Oto, Univ Nebr Coll Med

Song, John I MD [Oto] - **Spec Exp:** Head & Neck Cancer; Skull Base Tumors; Swallowing Disorders; **Hospital:** Univ of CO Hosp - Anschutz Inpatient Pav; **Address:** Univ Colorado Hosp, Otolaryngology, 1635 Aurora Ct, MS F737, Aurora, CO 80045; **Phone:** 720-848-2820; **Board Cert:** Otolaryngology 1998; **Med School:** NYU Sch Med 1991; **Resid:** Otolaryngology, UCLA Med Ctr 1997; **Fellow:** Head and Neck Surgery, Univ Pittsburgh Med Ctr 1998; **Fac Appt:** Asst Prof Oto, Univ Colorado

Southwest

Amedee, Ronald G MD [Oto] - **Spec Exp:** Otology & Neuro-Otology; Skull Base Surgery; Sinus Disorders/Surgery; Hearing & Balance Disorders; **Hospital:** Ochsner Med Ctr-New Orleans, Tulane Med Ctr; **Address:** 1514 Jefferson Hwy Fl 4 - Ste ENT Clinic, New Orleans, LA 70121; **Phone:** 504-842-3640; **Board Cert:** Otolaryngology 1987; **Med School:** Louisiana State U, New Orleans 1981; **Resid:** Surgery, Charity Hosp 1983; Otolaryngology, Charity Hosp 1986; **Fellow:** Skull Base Surgery, Klinikum der Albert Ludwigs 1988; **Fac Appt:** Prof Oto, Tulane Univ

Arriaga, Moises A MD [Oto] - **Spec Exp:** Meniere's Disease; Skull Base Surgery; Acoustic Neuroma; Cochlear Implants; **Hospital:** Our Lady of the Lake Regl Med Ctr, Children's Hospital - New Orleans; **Address:** Hearing & Balance Ctr, 7777 Hennessy Blvd, Ste 709, Baton Rouge, LA 70808; **Phone:** 225-765-7735; **Board Cert:** Otolaryngology 1990; Neurotology 2004; **Med School:** Brown Univ 1985; **Resid:** Otolaryngology, Univ Pittsburgh Med Ctr 1990; **Fellow:** Neurotology, House Ear Clinic 1991; **Fac Appt:** Prof Oto, Louisiana State U, New Orleans

Clark, Keith F MD/PhD [Oto] - **Spec Exp:** Pediatric Otolaryngology; Airway Reconstruction; Voice Disorders; Vocal Cord Disorders-Botox Therapy; **Hospital:** St. Anthony Hosp -Oklahoma City; **Address:** 535 NW 9th St, Ste 300, Oklahoma City, OK 73102; **Phone:** 405-272-6027; **Board Cert:** Otolaryngology 1983; **Med School:** Univ Mich Med Sch 1978; **Resid:** Otolaryngology, Univ Iowa Med Ctr 1983

Clayman, Gary Lee MD/DMD [Oto] - **Spec Exp:** Thyroid Cancer & Surgery; Salivary Gland Tumors & Surgery; Head & Neck Cancer; Thyroid & Parathyroid Surgery; **Hospital:** UT MD Anderson Cancer Ctr; **Address:** Univ TX/MD Anderson Cancer Center, 1515 Holcombe Blvd, Unit 1445, Houston, TX 77030-4009; **Phone:** 713-792-8837; **Board Cert:** Otolaryngology 1992; **Med School:** NE Ohio Univ 1986; **Resid:** Surgery, Hennepin Co Med Ctr 1987; Otolaryngology, Univ Minn Med Ctr 1991; **Fellow:** Head and Neck Surgery, MD Anderson Cancer Ctr 1993; **Fac Appt:** Prof Oto, Univ Tex, Houston

Diaz, Eduardo M MD [Oto] - **Spec Exp:** Head & Neck Cancer; Laryngeal Cancer; Laryngeal Cancer-Organ Preservation; Tongue Cancer; **Hospital:** UT MD Anderson Cancer Ctr; **Address:** UT MD Anderson Cancer Center, Head & Neck Center, 1515 Holcombe Blvd, Unit 460, Houston, TX 77030; **Phone:** 713-792-6920; **Board Cert:** Otolaryngology 1995; **Med School:** Baylor Coll Med 1989; **Resid:** Surgery, Univ Tex Affil Hosp 1991; Ophthalmology, Univ Tex Affil Hosp 1994; **Fellow:** Head & Neck Surgical Oncology, UT MD Anderson Cancer Ctr 1995; **Fac Appt:** Prof Oto, Univ Tex, Houston

Donovan, Donald T MD [Oto] - **Spec Exp:** Head & Neck Cancer; Voice Disorders; Vocal Cord Disorders; Thyroid Disorders; **Hospital:** Methodist Hosp - Houston, St. Luke's Episcopal Hosp-Houston; **Address:** Baylor-Dept of Otolaryngology, Smith Tower, 6550 Fannin St, Ste 1701, Houston, TX 77030; **Phone:** 713-798-5900; **Board Cert:** Otolaryngology 1981; **Med School:** Baylor Coll Med 1976; **Resid:** Surgery, Baylor Affil Hosps 1978; Otolaryngology, Baylor Affil Hosps 1981; **Fellow:** Head and Neck Surgery, Columbia-Presby Med Ctr 1982; **Fac Appt:** Prof Oto, Baylor Coll Med

Otolaryngology

Dornhoffer, John L MD [Oto] - **Spec Exp:** Hearing & Balance Disorders; Neuro-Otology; Hearing Loss; **Hospital:** UAMS Med Ctr; **Address:** UAMS, Dept Otolaryngology, Head & Neck Surgery, 4301 W Markham St, Slot 547-05, Little Rock, AR 72205; **Phone:** 501-686-5878; **Board Cert:** Otolaryngology 1994; **Med School:** Univ Kansas 1988; **Resid:** Otolaryngology, UAMS Med Ctr 1992; **Fellow:** Otology, Univ of Zurich Affil Hosp 1994; Otology, Univ of Wuzburg Affil Hosp 1994; **Fac Appt:** Prof Oto, Univ Ark

Gianoli, Gerard Joseph MD [Oto] - **Spec Exp:** Dizziness; Hearing Loss; Ear Disorders/Surgery; Balance Disorders; **Hospital:** North Oaks Med Ctr; **Address:** The Ear and Balance Institute, 1401 Ochsner Blvd, Ste A, Covington, LA 70433; **Phone:** 985-809-1111; **Board Cert:** Otolaryngology 1993; Neurotology 2004; **Med School:** Tulane Univ 1986; **Resid:** Pediatrics, Tulane Univ 1988; Otolaryngology, Tulane Univ 1992; **Fellow:** Otology & Neurotology, Michigan Ear Inst; **Fac Appt:** Assoc Clin Prof Oto, Tulane Univ

Graham III, H Devon MD [Oto] - **Spec Exp:** Cosmetic & Reconstructive Surgery-Face; Snoring/Sleep Apnea; Nasal Reconstruction; Facial Rejuvenation; **Hospital:** Ochsner Med Ctr-New Orleans; **Address:** 1514 Jefferson Hwy Fl 4, New Orleans, LA 70121; **Phone:** 504-842-4080; **Board Cert:** Otolaryngology 1989; Facial Plastic & Reconstr Surgery 1993; **Med School:** Louisiana State U, New Orleans 1984; **Resid:** Surgery, Ochsner Fdn Hosp 1986; Otolaryngology, Tulane Univ Med Ctr 1989; **Fellow:** Facial Plastic Surgery, Baptist Hosp 1990; Facial Plastic Surgery, St Joseph Hosp 1990; **Fac Appt:** Asst Clin Prof Oto, Tulane Univ

Hanna, Ehab YN MD [Oto] - **Spec Exp:** Skull Base Tumors & Surgery; Head & Neck Cancer & Surgery; **Hospital:** UT MD Anderson Cancer Ctr; **Address:** Univ Tex MD Anderson Cancer Ctr, 1515 Holcolmbe Blvd, Unit 1445, Houston, TX 77030; **Phone:** 713-745-1815; **Board Cert:** Otolaryngology 1994; **Med School:** Egypt 1982; **Resid:** Otolaryngology, Cleveland Clinic 1989; Otolaryngology, Cleveland Clinic 1993; **Fellow:** Otolaryngology, Univ Pittsburgh Med Ctr 1994; **Fac Appt:** Prof Oto, Univ Tex, Houston

Hayden, Richard E MD [Oto] - **Spec Exp:** Head & Neck Surgery; Thyroid & Parathyroid Surgery; Facial Plastic & Reconstructive Surgery; Microvascular Surgery; **Hospital:** Mayo Clinic - Phoenix; **Address:** Mayo Clinic, Dept Otolaryngology, 5777 E Mayo Blvd, Phoenix, AZ 85054; **Phone:** 480-342-2912; **Board Cert:** Otolaryngology 1978; **Med School:** McGill Univ 1974; **Resid:** Otolaryngology, Univ Toronto Affil Hosp 1978; **Fellow:** Head & Neck Oncology, MD Anderson Hosp 1979; Radiation Oncology, Princess Margaret Hosp 1980; **Fac Appt:** Prof Oto, Mayo Med Sch

Johnson Jr, Calvin M MD [Oto] - **Spec Exp:** Ear Disorders/Surgery; Nasal Surgery; Cosmetic Surgery-Face; **Address:** Hedgewood Surgical Ctr, 2427 St Charles Ave, New Orleans, LA 70130; **Phone:** 504-895-7642; **Board Cert:** Otolaryngology 1974; Facial Plastic & Reconstr Surgery 1991; **Med School:** Tulane Univ 1967; **Resid:** Surgery, Tulane Univ Sch Med 1971; Otolaryngology, Tulane Univ Sch Med 1974; **Fellow:** Facial Plastic Surgery, Amer Academy Facial Plastic & Recon Surg 1975

Macias, John D MD [Oto] - **Spec Exp:** Otology; Neuro-Otology; Cochlear Implants; Hearing Loss; **Hospital:** Banner Good Samaritan Regl Med Ctr - Phoenix, Phoenix Children's Hosp; **Address:** 1515 N 9th St, Ste B, Phoenix, AZ 85006-2523; **Phone:** 602-257-4228; **Board Cert:** Otolaryngology 1994; Neurotology 2005; **Med School:** Stanford Univ 1988; **Resid:** Otolaryngology, Univ Iowa Hosps & Clins 1993; **Fellow:** Otology & Neurotology, Ear Fdn/Otology Grp 1994

Medina, Jesus E MD [Oto] - **Spec Exp:** Head & Neck Cancer & Surgery; **Hospital:** OU Med Ctr; **Address:** 825 NE 10th St, Fl 4, Ste 4200, Oklahoma City, OK 73104; **Phone:** 405-271-7559; **Board Cert:** Otolaryngology 1980; **Med School:** Peru 1974; **Resid:** Surgery, Wayne St Univ Affil Hosp 1977; Otolaryngology, Wayne St Univ Affil Hosp 1980; **Fellow:** Head and Neck Surgery, MD Anderson Hosp 1981; **Fac Appt:** Prof Oto, Univ Okla Coll Med

Miller, Frank R MD [Oto] - **Spec Exp:** Head & Neck Cancer & Surgery; **Hospital:** Univ Hlth Syst-San Antonio; **Address:** 8300 Floyd Curl Drive, MARC Bldg - Fl 6th - Ste 6-B, MS 8300, San Antonio, TX 78229; **Phone:** 210-450-0719; **Board Cert:** Otolaryngology 1995; **Med School:** Brown Univ 1989; **Resid:** Otolaryngology, Cleveland Clinic 1994; **Fellow:** Head & Neck Oncology, Vancerbilt Univ Hosp 1998; **Fac Appt:** Prof Oto, Univ Tex, San Antonio

Myers, Jeffrey N MD/PhD [Oto] - **Spec Exp:** Head & Neck Cancer; Melanoma-Head & Neck; Tongue Cancer; **Hospital:** UT MD Anderson Cancer Ctr; **Address:** Univ Texas MD Anderson Cancer Ctr, 1515 Holcombe Blvd, Unit 1445, Houston, TX 77030; **Phone:** 713-745-2667; **Board Cert:** Otolaryngology 1997; **Med School:** Univ Pennsylvania 1991; **Resid:** Otolaryngology, Univ Pittsburgh Med Ctr 1996; **Fellow:** Head & Neck Surgical Oncology, MD Anderson Cancer Ctr 1997; **Fac Appt:** Assoc Prof Oto, Univ Tex, Houston

Nuss, Daniel W MD [Oto] - **Spec Exp:** Head & Neck Cancer; Skull Base Tumors & Surgery; **Hospital:** Our Lady of the Lake Regl Med Ctr; **Address:** Our Lady of the Lake Regl Med Ctr, 4950 Essen Ln, Ste 400, Baton Rouge, LA 70809; **Phone:** 225-765-1765; **Board Cert:** Otolaryngology 1987; **Med School:** Louisiana State U, New Orleans 1981; **Resid:** Surgery, Charity Hosp 1983; Otolaryngology, LSU Med Ctr 1987; **Fellow:** Surgical Oncology, MD Anderson Hosp & Tumor Inst 1984; Head and Neck Surgery, Ctr Cranial Base Surg-Univ Pittsburgh 1991; **Fac Appt:** Prof Oto, Louisiana State U, New Orleans

Otto, Randal A MD [Oto] - **Spec Exp:** Head & Neck Cancer; Thyroid & Parathyroid Cancer & Surgery; Sinus Disorders/Surgery; **Hospital:** Univ Hlth Syst-San Antonio; **Address:** 8300 Floyd Curl Drive, MSC 7777, San Antonio, TX 78229-3900; **Phone:** 210-450-0700; **Board Cert:** Otolaryngology 1987; **Med School:** Univ MO-Columbia Sch Med 1981; **Resid:** Pathology, Queens Med Ctr 1982; Otolaryngology, Univ of Missouri 1987; **Fac Appt:** Prof Emeritus Oto, Univ Tex, San Antonio

Stasney, C Richard MD [Oto] - **Spec Exp:** Voice Disorders; Vocal Cord Disorders; Laryngeal Disorders; **Hospital:** Methodist Hosp - Houston; **Address:** Texas Voice Center, 6550 Fannin St, Ste 2025, Houston, TX 77030; **Phone:** 713-796-2181; **Board Cert:** Otolaryngology 1974; **Med School:** Baylor Coll Med 1969; **Resid:** Surgery, Baylor Affil Hosps 1971; Otolaryngology, Baylor Affil Hosps 1974; **Fac Appt:** Assoc Clin Prof Oto, Cornell Univ-Weill Med Coll

Suen, James Y MD [Oto] - **Spec Exp:** Head & Neck Cancer; Vascular Lesions-Head & Neck; Laryngeal Disorders; Thyroid Cancer; **Hospital:** UAMS Med Ctr, Arkansas Chldns Hosp; **Address:** Univ Hosp Arkansas Med Scis, 4301 W Markham St, Slot 543, Little Rock, AR 72205; **Phone:** 501-686-7009; **Board Cert:** Otolaryngology 1973; **Med School:** Univ Ark 1966; **Resid:** Surgery, Univ Arkansas Med Ctr 1970; Otolaryngology, Univ Arkansas Med Ctr 1973; **Fellow:** Head and Neck Surgery, MD Anderson Cancer Ctr 1974; **Fac Appt:** Prof Oto, Univ Ark

Weber, Randal S MD [Oto] - **Spec Exp:** Skin Cancer; Thyroid & Parathyroid Cancer & Surgery; Salivary Gland Tumors & Surgery; Head & Neck Cancer; **Hospital:** UT MD Anderson Cancer Ctr; **Address:** 1400 Pressler St, Unit 1445, Houston, TX 77030-4009; **Phone:** 713-745-0497; **Board Cert:** Otolaryngology 1985; **Med School:** Univ Tenn Coll Med 1976; **Resid:** Surgery, Baylor Affil Hosp 1982; Otolaryngology, Baylor Affil Hosp 1985; **Fellow:** Head and Neck Surgery, MD Anderson Cancer Ctr 1986; **Fac Appt:** Prof Oto, Univ Tex, Houston

Weber, Samuel C MD [Oto] - **Spec Exp:** Thyroid Cancer; Parathyroid Cancer; Nasal & Sinus Surgery; Head & Neck Surgery; **Hospital:** St. Luke's Episcopal Hosp-Houston, Methodist Hosp - Houston; **Address:** 6624 Fannin St, Ste 1480, Houston, TX 77030-2385; **Phone:** 713-795-5343; **Board Cert:** Otolaryngology 1972; **Med School:** Univ Tenn Coll Med 1965; **Resid:** Surgery, Baylor Affil Hosp 1971; Otolaryngology, Baylor Affil Hosp 1972; **Fac Appt:** Clin Prof Oto, Baylor Coll Med

Otolaryngology

West Coast and Pacific

Andersen, Peter MD [Oto] - **Spec Exp:** Laryngeal Cancer; Nasal & Sinus Cancer & Surgery; Head & Neck Cancer & Surgery; Neck Masses; **Hospital:** OR Hlth & Sci Univ; **Address:** Dept of Otolaryngology, 3181 SW Sam Jackson Park Rd, MC PV-01, Portland, OR 97239; **Phone:** 503-494-5355; **Board Cert:** Otolaryngology 1994; **Med School:** Washington Univ, St Louis 1988; **Resid:** Otolaryngology, Oregon Hlth & Science Univ 1993; **Fellow:** Head & Neck Surgical Oncology, Meml Sloan Kettering Cancer Ctr 1995; **Fac Appt:** Prof Oto, Oregon Hlth & Sci Univ

Berke, Gerald S MD [Oto] - **Spec Exp:** Head & Neck Surgery; Head & Neck Cancer; Voice Disorders; Laryngeal Disorders; **Hospital:** UCLA Ronald Reagan Med Ctr; **Address:** 200 UCLA Med Plaza, Ste 550, Los Angeles, CA 90095; **Phone:** 310-794-8634; **Board Cert:** Otolaryngology 1984; **Med School:** USC Sch Med 1978; **Resid:** Otolaryngology, LAC-USC Med Ctr 1979; **Fellow:** Head and Neck Surgery, UCLA Med Ctr 1984; **Fac Appt:** Prof Oto, UCLA

Blackwell, Keith Edward MD [Oto] - **Spec Exp:** Head & Neck Reconstruction; Head & Neck Cancer & Surgery; Microvascular Surgery; **Hospital:** UCLA Ronald Reagan Med Ctr; **Address:** 200 UCLA Med Plaza, Ste 550, Los Angeles, CA 90095; **Phone:** 310-206-6688; **Board Cert:** Otolaryngology 1995; **Med School:** Northwestern Univ 1988; **Resid:** Otolaryngology, UCLA Med Ctr1 1994; **Fellow:** Otolaryngology, Mount Sinai Med Ctr 1995; **Fac Appt:** Prof Oto, UCLA

Brackmann, Derald E MD [Oto] - **Spec Exp:** Ear Disorders/Surgery; Facial Nerve Disorders; Acoustic Neuroma; Otosclerosis/Stapedectomy; **Hospital:** St. Vincent's Med Ctr - Los Angeles, Good Samaritan Hosp - LA; **Address:** House Clinic, 2100 W 3rd St, Fl 1st, Los Angeles, CA 90057-1902; **Phone:** 213-483-9930; **Board Cert:** Otolaryngology 1971; Neurotology 2005; **Med School:** Univ IL Coll Med 1962; **Resid:** Otolaryngology, LAC/USC Med Ctr 1970; **Fellow:** Otology & Neurotology, House Ear Clinic 1971; **Fac Appt:** Clin Prof Oto, USC-Keck School of Medicine

Courey, Mark S MD [Oto] - **Spec Exp:** Laryngeal Disorders; Swallowing Disorders; Laryngeal Cancer; **Hospital:** UCSF - Mt Zion Med Ctr, UCSF Med Ctr; **Address:** UCSF Voice & Swallowing Ctr, 2330 Post St Fl 5 - Ste 526, San Francisco, CA 94115; **Phone:** 415-885-7700; **Board Cert:** Otolaryngology 1993; **Med School:** SUNY Buffalo 1987; **Resid:** Otolaryngology, SUNY-Buffalo Med Ctr 1992; **Fellow:** Laryngology, Vanderbilt Univ 1993; **Fac Appt:** Prof Oto, UCSF

Donald, Paul J MD [Oto] - **Spec Exp:** Skull Base Tumors & Surgery; Head & Neck Cancer; **Hospital:** UC Davis Med Ctr; **Address:** 2521 Stockton Blvd, Ste 5200, Sacramento, CA 95817; **Phone:** 916-734-5400; **Board Cert:** Otolaryngology 1973; **Med School:** Univ British Columbia Fac Med 1964; **Resid:** Surgery, St Pauls Hosp 1969; Otolaryngology, Univ Iowa Hosp 1973; **Fac Appt:** Prof Oto, UC Davis

Duckert, Larry G MD/PhD [Oto] - **Spec Exp:** Otology & Neuro-Otology; Otosclerosis/Stapedectomy; Acoustic Neuroma; Skull Base Surgery; **Hospital:** Univ Wash Med Ctr; **Address:** 1959 NE Pacific St, Box 356161, Seattle, WA 98195; **Phone:** 206-598-4022; **Board Cert:** Otolaryngology 1978; **Med School:** Univ Minn 1972; **Resid:** Otolaryngology, Univ Minnesota Hosp 1978; **Fellow:** Research, Ohio State Univ Coll of Med 1972; Otology & Neurotology, Univ Wuzburg Affil Hosp 1990; **Fac Appt:** Prof Oto, Univ Wash

Fee Jr, Willard E MD [Oto] - **Spec Exp:** Head & Neck Cancer; Parotid Gland Tumors; Thyroid Cancer; **Hospital:** Stanford Univ Hosp & Clinics; **Address:** Stanford Cancer Ctr, 875 Blake Lake Wilbur Dr, CC-2227, Stanford, CA 94305-5826; **Phone:** 650-725-6500; **Board Cert:** Otolaryngology 1974; **Med School:** Univ Colorado 1969; **Resid:** Surgery, Wadsworth VA Hosp 1971; Otolaryngology, UCLA Med Ctr 1974; **Fac Appt:** Prof Emeritus Oto, Stanford Univ

Flint, Paul W MD [Oto] - **Spec Exp:** Voice Disorders; Laryngeal Disorders; **Hospital:** OR Hlth & Sci Univ; **Address:** Oregon Health & Science Univ, 3181 SW Sam Jackson Park Rd, MC PV01, Portland, OR 97239; **Phone:** 503-494-5947; **Board Cert:** Otolaryngology 1989; **Med School:** Baylor Coll Med 1983; **Resid:** Surgery, Univ Washington 1985; Otolaryngology, Univ Washington 1989; **Fellow:** Otolaryngology, Guys Hosp 1989; **Fac Appt:** Prof Oto, Oregon Hlth & Sci Univ

Futran, Neal D MD/DMD [Oto] - **Spec Exp:** Head & Neck Cancer & Surgery; Head & Neck Cancer Reconstruction; Skull Base Tumors & Surgery; **Hospital:** Univ Wash Med Ctr, Harborview Med Ctr; **Address:** UWMC, Otolaryngology, 1959 NE Pacific St, Box 356515, Seattle, WA 98195-6515; **Phone:** 206-543-3060; **Board Cert:** Otolaryngology 1993; **Med School:** SUNY Downstate 1987; **Resid:** Surgery, Kings Co-SUNY Downstate 1985; Otolaryngology, Univ Rochester Med Ctr 1992; **Fellow:** Microvascular Surgery, Mt Sinai Hosp 1993; **Fac Appt:** Prof Oto, Univ Wash

Harris, Jeffrey P MD/PhD [Oto] - **Spec Exp:** Neuro-Otology; Hearing & Balance Disorders; Skull Base Surgery; Meniere's Disease; **Hospital:** UCSD Med Ctr, VA San Diego Hlthcre Sys; **Address:** UCSD Med Ctr, 9350 Campus Point Drive, La Jolla, CA 92037; **Phone:** 858-657-8590; **Board Cert:** Otolaryngology 1979; Neurotology 2004; **Med School:** Univ Pennsylvania 1974; **Resid:** Otolaryngology, Mass EE Infirmary 1979; **Fellow:** Neurological Surgery, Univ Zurich Med Ctr 1983; **Fac Appt:** Prof S, UCSD

Jackler, Robert K MD [Oto] - **Spec Exp:** Neuro-Otology; Skull Base Surgery; Ear Tumors; **Hospital:** Stanford Univ Hosp & Clinics; **Address:** Stanford Univ Med Ctr, Dept Head & Neck Surg, 801 Welch Rd Fl 2, Stanford, CA 94305-5739; **Phone:** 650-723-5281; **Board Cert:** Otolaryngology 1984; Neurotology 2004; **Med School:** Boston Univ 1979; **Resid:** Otolaryngology, UCSF Med Ctr 1984; **Fellow:** Otolaryngology, Oto Med Grp 1985; **Fac Appt:** Prof Oto, Stanford Univ

Kaplan, Michael J MD [Oto] - **Spec Exp:** Head & Neck Surgery; Skull Base Surgery; Head & Neck Cancer; **Hospital:** Stanford Univ Hosp & Clinics; **Address:** 875 Blake Wilbur Drive, Clinic B, Stanford, CA 94305-5739; **Phone:** 650-498-6000; **Board Cert:** Otolaryngology 1982; **Med School:** Harvard Med Sch 1977; **Resid:** Surgery, Beth Israel-Chldns Hosps 1979; Otolaryngology, Mass EE Infirm 1982; **Fellow:** Head and Neck Surgery, Univ Virginia 1984; **Fac Appt:** Prof Oto, Stanford Univ

Keller, Gregory S MD [Oto] - **Spec Exp:** Cosmetic Surgery-Face; **Hospital:** Santa Barbara Cottage Hosp, UCLA Ronald Reagan Med Ctr; **Address:** 221 W Pueblo St, Ste A, Santa Barbara, CA 93105; **Phone:** 805-687-6408; **Board Cert:** Otolaryngology 1976; **Med School:** Univ IL Coll Med 1971; **Resid:** Surgery, Cottage Hosp 1973; Otolaryngology, Univ Illinois Affil Hosp 1976; **Fac Appt:** Assoc Clin Prof S, UCLA

Larrabee Jr, Wayne F MD [Oto] - **Spec Exp:** Cosmetic Surgery-Face; Eyelid Surgery; Rhinoplasty; Nasal Surgery; **Hospital:** Swedish Med Ctr-First Hill-Seattle; **Address:** Facial Plastic Surgery Ctr, 600 Broadway Ste 280, Seattle, WA 98122-5371; **Phone:** 206-386-3550; **Board Cert:** Otolaryngology 1979; Facial Plastic & Reconstr Surgery 1999; **Med School:** Tulane Univ 1971; **Resid:** Surgery, Charity Hosp 1976; Otolaryngology, Tulane Univ Med Ctr 1979; **Fac Appt:** Clin Prof Oto, Univ Wash

Lustig, Lawrence R MD [Oto] - **Spec Exp:** Cochlear Implants; Hearing Loss; **Hospital:** UCSF Med Ctr; **Address:** Cochlear Implant Center, 2380 Sutter St Fl 1, San Francisco, CA 94115; **Phone:** 415-353-2464; **Board Cert:** Otolaryngology 1998; Neurotology 2006; **Med School:** UCSF 1992; **Resid:** Otolaryngology, UCSF Med Ctr 1997; **Fellow:** Neurotology, John Hopkins Hosp 1999

Otolaryngology

McMenomey, Sean O MD [Oto] - **Spec Exp:** Otology & Neuro-Otology; Skull Base Tumors & Surgery; Head & Neck Surgery; Stereotactic Radiosurgery; **Hospital:** OR Hlth & Sci Univ, Providence St Vincent Med Ctr; **Address:** Oregon Hlth & Sci Univ, Dept Otolaryngology, 3181 SW Sam Jackson Park Rd, MC PV-01, Portland, OR 97239; **Phone:** 503-494-8135; **Board Cert:** Otolaryngology 1993; Neurotology 2004; **Med School:** St Louis Univ 1987; **Resid:** Otolaryngology, Oregon Hlth Sci Ctr 1992; **Fellow:** Otology & Neurotology, Baptist Hosp 1993; **Fac Appt:** Prof Oto, Oregon Hlth & Sci Univ

Moe, Kristen MD [Oto] - **Spec Exp:** Facial Plastic & Reconstructive Surgery; Skull Base Surgery; Cosmetic Surgery-Face; **Hospital:** Harborview Med Ctr, Univ Wash Med Ctr; **Address:** Head & Neck Surgery-4 West Clinic, 325 Ninth Ave, Seattle, WA 98104; **Phone:** 206-744-4132; **Board Cert:** Otolaryngology 1996; **Med School:** Univ Wash 1989; **Resid:** Surgery, Univ Washington Med Ctr 1991; Otolaryngology, Univ Michigan Med Ctr 1994; **Fellow:** Skull Base Surgery, Univ Bern Hosp; Facial Plastic & Reconstr Surgery, Univ Zurich Hosp; **Fac Appt:** Prof Oto, Univ Wash

O'Leary, Michael J MD [Oto] - **Spec Exp:** Skull-Base Tumors & Surgery; Pituitary Tumors; Neuro-Otology; Cochlear Implants; **Hospital:** Alvarado Hosp & Med Ctr, Scripps Hlth; **Address:** Senta Clinic, 6645 Alvarado Rd, Ste 4000, San Diego, CA 92120-5208; **Phone:** 619-229-4903; **Board Cert:** Otolaryngology 1987; Neurotology 2012; **Med School:** Georgetown Univ 1980; **Resid:** Otolaryngology, Naval Medical Ctr 1986; **Fellow:** Skull Base Surgery, House Ear Clinic 1990; Microvascular Surgery, Washington Univ 1991

Oghalai, John S MD [Oto] - **Spec Exp:** Neuro-Otology; **Hospital:** Stanford Univ Hosp & Clinics, Lucile Packard Chldn's Hosp; **Address:** Stanford Univ, 801 Welch Rd, Stanford, CA 94305; **Phone:** 650-723-5281; **Board Cert:** Otolaryngology 2002; Neurotology 2010; **Med School:** Univ Wisc 1994; **Resid:** Otolaryngology, Baylor Coll Med Ctr 2001; **Fellow:** Otolaryngology, UCSF Med Ctr 2003; Neurological Surgery, UCSF Med Ctr 2003; **Fac Appt:** Assoc Prof Oto, Baylor Coll Med

Orloff, Lisa MD [Oto] - **Spec Exp:** Thyroid & Parathyroid Cancer & Surgery; Minimally Invasive Surgery; Head & Neck Surgery; **Hospital:** UCSF Med Ctr; **Address:** Head & Neck Surg Canc Clin, 2380 Sutter St Fl 2, San Francisco, CA 94115; **Phone:** 415-885-7528; **Board Cert:** Otolaryngology 1993; **Med School:** UCLA 1986; **Resid:** Surgery, Univ Washington 1988; Otolaryngology, Univ Washington 1992; **Fellow:** Microvascular Surgery, Mt Sinai Med Ctr; **Fac Appt:** Assoc Prof S, UCSD

Rice, Dale H MD [Oto] - **Spec Exp:** Head & Neck Cancer; Sinus Disorders/Surgery; **Hospital:** Keck Med Ctr of USC (page 62), USC Norris Cancer Hosp (page 62); **Address:** 1520 San Pablo St, Ste 4600, Los Angeles, CA 90033-1029; **Phone:** 323-442-5790; **Board Cert:** Otolaryngology 1976; **Med School:** Univ Mich Med Sch 1968; **Resid:** Surgery, Univ of Michigan Hosp 1970; Otolaryngology, Univ of Michigan Hosp 1976; **Fac Appt:** Prof Oto, USC Sch Med

Rubinstein, Jay T MD/PhD [Oto] - **Spec Exp:** Cochlear Implants; Acoustic Neuroma; Hearing Loss; Neuro-Otology; **Hospital:** Univ Wash Med Ctr, Seattle Chldns Hosp; **Address:** Univeristy of Washington Medical Center, 1959 NE Pacific St, Box 356161, Seattle, WA 98195; **Phone:** 206-598-4022; **Board Cert:** Otolaryngology 1995; Neurotology 2005; **Med School:** Univ Wash 1987; **Resid:** Otolaryngology, Mass Eye & Ear Infirmary 1994; **Fellow:** Research, Mass Eye & Ear Infirmary 1990; Otology & Neurotology, Univ Iowa Affil Hosp 1995; **Fac Appt:** Prof Oto, Univ Wash

Senders, Craig W MD [Oto] - **Spec Exp:** Pediatric Otolaryngology; Cleft Palate/Lip; Endoscopic Sinus Surgery; Sleep Disorders/Apnea; **Hospital:** UC Davis Med Ctr; **Address:** UC Davis, Dept Otolaryngology, 2521 Stockton Blvd, Ste 7200, Sacramento, CA 95817; **Phone:** 916-734-5400; **Board Cert:** Otolaryngology 1984; **Med School:** Oregon Hlth & Sci Univ 1979; **Resid:** Otolaryngology, Univ Iowa Hosps & Clins 1983; **Fellow:** Maxillofacial Surgery, Univ Iowa Hosps & Clins 1984; **Fac Appt:** Prof Oto, UC Davis

Shindo, Maisie L MD [Oto] - **Spec Exp:** Thyroid Cancer & Surgery; Parathyroid Surgery; Parathyroid Cancer; Head & Neck Surgery; **Hospital:** OR Hlth & Sci Univ, Providence St Vincent Med Ctr; **Address:** Thyroid & Parathyroid Clinic, 3181 SW Sam Jackson Park Rd, MC PV-01, Portland, OR 97239-3098; **Phone:** 503-494-2544; **Board Cert:** Otolaryngology 1989; **Med School:** USC-Keck School of Medicine 1984; **Resid:** Otolaryngology, LAC-USC Med Ctr 1989; **Fellow:** Head and Neck Surgery, Northwestern Meml Hosp 1991; **Fac Appt:** Prof Oto, Oregon Hlth & Sci Univ

Singer, Mark I MD [Oto] - **Spec Exp:** Head & Neck Surgery; Head & Neck Cancer; Melanoma; **Hospital:** CA Pacific Med Ctr-Pacific Campus; **Address:** 2340 Clay St Fl 2, San Francisco, CA 94115; **Phone:** 415-600-3800; **Board Cert:** Otolaryngology 1976; **Med School:** Columbia P&S 1970; **Resid:** Surgery, Northwestern Meml Hosp 1973; Otolaryngology, Northwestern Meml Hosp 1976; **Fellow:** Oncology, Northwestern Meml Hosp 1976

Sinha, Uttam K MD [Oto] - **Spec Exp:** Head & Neck Cancer; Voice Disorders; Thyroid Cancer; Swallowing Disorders; **Hospital:** Keck Med Ctr of USC (page 62), House Ear Inst; **Address:** 1520 San Pablo St, Ste 4600, Los Angeles, CA 90033; **Phone:** 323-442-5790; **Board Cert:** Otolaryngology 1998; **Med School:** India 1985; **Resid:** Otolaryngology, LAC-USC Med Ctr 1995; **Fellow:** Microvascular Surgery, Mount Sinai Med Ctr 1996; Laryngology 1997; **Fac Appt:** Assoc Prof Oto, USC Sch Med

Wackym, P Ashley MD [Oto] - **Spec Exp:** Cochlear Implants; Acoustic Neuroma; Head & Neck Surgery; **Hospital:** Legacy Good Samaritan Med Ctr, Randall Chldns Hosp at Legacy; **Address:** Ear and Skull Base Center, 1225 NE 2nd Ave, Ste 305, Portland, OR 97232; **Phone:** 503-233-6068; **Board Cert:** Otolaryngology 1992; Neurotology 2004; **Med School:** Vanderbilt Univ 1985; **Resid:** Neurological Surgery, UCLA Med Ctr 1987; Head and Neck Surgery, UCLA Med Ctr 1991; **Fellow:** Otology & Neurotology, Univ Iowa 1992; Neurological Science, UCLA Med Ctr 1989; **Fac Appt:** Prof Oto

Wang, Steven J MD [Oto] - **Spec Exp:** Head & Neck Cancer; Head & Neck Surgery; **Hospital:** UCSF Med Ctr; **Address:** 2380 Sutter St Fl 2, San Francisco, CA 94115; **Phone:** 415-885-7528; **Board Cert:** Otolaryngology 2002; **Med School:** Harvard Med Sch 1995; **Resid:** Otolaryngology, UCLA Med Ctr 2001; Head and Neck Surgery, UCLA Med Ctr 2001; **Fellow:** Head & Neck Surgical Oncology, Univ Michigan 2003; **Fac Appt:** Assoc Prof Oto, UCSF

Wax, Mark K MD [Oto] - **Spec Exp:** Facial Nerve Disorders; Skull Base Tumors & Surgery; Facial Plastic & Reconstructive Surgery; Microvascular Surgery; **Hospital:** OR Hlth & Sci Univ; **Address:** Oregon Hlth Scis Univ, Dept Ototlaryngology, 3181 SW Sam Jackson Park Rd, MC PV-01, Portland, OR 97201; **Phone:** 503-494-5355; **Board Cert:** Otolaryngology 1985; Facial Plastic & Reconstr Surgery 2000; **Med School:** Univ Toronto 1980; **Resid:** Otolaryngology, Univ Toronto 1985; Surgery, Cedars-Sinai Med Ctr 1983; **Fellow:** Head and Neck Surgery, St Michaels Hosp 1991; **Fac Appt:** Prof Oto, Oregon Hlth & Sci Univ

Weisman, Robert A MD [Oto] - **Spec Exp:** Head & Neck Cancer; Clinical Trials; Thyroid & Parathyroid Cancer & Surgery; Head & Neck Cancer Reconstruction; **Hospital:** UCSD Med Ctr; **Address:** Moores-UCSD Cancer Center, 3855 Hlth Sci Drive, MC 0987, La Jolla, CA 92093-0987; **Phone:** 858-822-6197; **Board Cert:** Otolaryngology 1978; **Med School:** Washington Univ, St Louis 1973; **Resid:** Head and Neck Surgery, UCLA Med Ctr 1978; **Fac Appt:** Prof S, UCSD

Weymuller Jr, Ernest MD [Oto] - **Spec Exp:** Head & Neck Cancer; Sinus Disorders/Surgery; **Hospital:** Univ Wash Med Ctr; **Address:** 1959 NE Pacific St, Box 356161, Seattle, WA 98195; **Phone:** 206-598-4022; **Board Cert:** Otolaryngology 1973; **Med School:** Harvard Med Sch 1966; **Resid:** Surgery, Vanderbilt Univ Hosp 1968; Otolaryngology, Mass Eye and Ear Infirm 1973; **Fac Appt:** Prof Oto, Univ Wash

Otolaryngology

Wong, Brian JF MD [Oto] - **Spec Exp:** Facial Plastic & Reconstructive Surgery; Head & Neck Surgery; Vascular Malformations; **Hospital:** UC Irvine Med Ctr; **Address:** UC Irvine, Dept Head & Neck Surgery, 101 The City Drive, Pavillion II, 1st Fl, Orange, CA 92868; **Phone:** 714-456-7017; **Board Cert:** Otolaryngology 1998; Facial Plastic & Reconstr Surgery 2007; **Med School:** Johns Hopkins Univ 1990; **Resid:** Otolaryngology, UC Irvine Med Ctr 1996; **Fellow:** Facial Plastic & Reconstr Surgery, UC Irvine Med Ctr 1998; **Fac Appt:** Prof Oto, UC Irvine

Cleveland Clinic

Every life deserves world class care.

Otolaryngology

Cleveland Clinic's Head & Neck Institute is recognized nationally and internationally in this multidisciplinary field and is ranked #2 in the nation by *U.S. News & World Report*. The Institute is composed of extensively trained specialists in these areas:

Audiology: Comprehensive evaluation and treatment through assistive listening devices, hearing aids, bone anchored auditory implants and cochlear implants.

Facial Plastic and Reconstructive Surgery: Treatments range from office-based injectables to rhinoplasty, face-lifts and major facial reconstructive surgery, including the world's first near-total face transplant.

Head and Neck Surgery: Evaluation and treatment of benign and malignant tumors.

Laryngotracheal Reconstruction: Laryngeal airway obstruction, esophageal reflux, tracheal aspiration, voice preservation/rehabilitation and removal of respiratory foreign bodies.

Nasal and Sinus Disorders: Sinusitis, polyps, septal deviation, nasal obstruction and allergies. Minimally invasive, computer-aided techniques for sinus and skull base surgery.

Otology-Neurotology: Middle and posterior cranial fossa surgery for cerebellopontine and skull base tumors, immune-mediated inner ear disease (deafness), Meniere's disease and cochlear implantation are handled here.

Pediatric Otolaryngology: Treatment of all forms of pediatric disorders.

Speech-Language Pathology: Evaluation and treatment for pediatric through geriatric patients with speech, language, voice, cognitive and swallowing disorders.

Vestibular and Balance Disorders: Diagnosis and vestibular rehabilitation for dizziness and disequilibrium.

Voice Center: Voice therapies and effective management options for all conditions related to the voice.

Mount Sinai

M S S M

MOUNT SINAI
SCHOOL OF
MEDICINE

THE MOUNT SINAI MEDICAL CENTER
OTOLARYNGOLOGY – EAR, NOSE, AND THROAT

One Gustave L. Levy Place
Fifth Avenue and 100th Street
New York, NY 10029-6574
Physician Referral: 1-800-MD-SINAI (637-4624)
www.mountsinai.org/ENT

Mount Sinai's **DEPARTMENT OF OTOLARYNGOLOGY – HEAD AND NECK SURGERY** – ranks as one of the finest in the nation. In 2012, *U.S. News & World Report* again placed us among the top 15 in the United States, continuing our impressive history of achievement. Since the early nineteenth century, we have pioneered surgical advances in endoscopy, otology, skull-base surgery, laryngology, rhinology, facial plastic surgery, and head and neck oncology and reconstruction. More recently, we have incorporated advanced technology in robotic and endoscopic surgery, basic science research, and translational science programs.

Robotic Head and Neck Surgery – We are a world leader in robotic head and neck surgery. Our surgeons and researchers have published techniques that have changed the paradigm for management of head and neck cancer, allowing for endoscopic surgery without external incisions, shortening hospital stays, and improving outcomes.

Endoscopic Laser Surgery of the Larynx and Trachea – Our surgeons and scientists have introduced techniques in laryngeal and tracheal surgery, including endoscopic laser surgery, tracheal transplantation, and reconstructive surgery, allowing removal of malignant disease while preserving voice and swallowing functions.

The Grabscheid Voice Center – Our multidisciplinary group provides professional singers and patients in need with cutting-edge treatments, using endoscopic laser and minimally invasive surgery. We pioneered office-based procedures that offer patients the opportunity to undergo therapy without the need for general anesthesia.

Cranial Base Surgery – Techniques in endoscopic trans-nasal surgery have revolutionized the management of skull base tumors and cerebrospinal leaks. We have developed procedures for accessing the cranial base and frontal lobes of the brain through the nose, delivering excellent outcomes with lower complications rates.

Thyroid and Parathyroid Surgery – We are nationally recognized for excellence in clinical care and clinical outcomes research. Our minimally invasive and robotic surgical techniques offer patients surgery through tiny incisions. Cure rates for thyroid cancer using these techniques are higher than 95 percent. Parathyroid surgery is performed using similar techniques and intraoperative parathyroid hormone monitoring.

Otology and Neurotology – Long recognized among the best in the nation, our otologic surgeons have pioneered surgical techniques to manage chronic ear disease and cochlear implantation that have resulted in excellent outcomes.

THE MULTIDISCIPLINARY HEAD AND NECK ONCOLOGY TEAM—Acclaimed as one of the finest in the country, our multidisciplinary team includes 35 physicians, surgeons, and ancillary staff from 12 departments. We offer top-rated courses, training and research fellowships and enjoy national recognition for expertise in head, neck, and skull-base cancer. Our minimally invasive and endoscopic team includes surgeons and oncologists focused on treating tumors of the oral cavity, jaw, and larynx, while preserving each patient's quality of life. Speech and swallowing rehabilitation therapists work with patients to help them recover, all of which keeps Mount Sinai on the cutting edge of head and neck cancer therapy, reconstruction, and rehabilitation.

The Center for Comprehensive Management of Nasal and Sinus Disease – We deliver the most advanced care for patients suffering from allergic and invasive fungal sinusitis, acute and chronic sinusitis, benign and malignant tumors of the sinonasal cavity, cerebrospinal fluid leaks and encephalocele treatment and inflammatory polyp disease.

The Sleep Surgery Center – We offer comprehensive management and treatment of obstructive sleep apnea (OSA) and snoring. Collaboration with the divisions of pulmonary medicine, sleep medicine and endocrinology, provides the collective expertise of a multidisciplinary approach, which is necessary to address all conditions in sleep disordered breathing.

Center for Facial Plastic and Reconstructive Surgery – Our plastic surgeons provide expertise in the areas of facial plastic surgery and complex reconstructive surgery. Our team is expert in the areas of congenital and traumatic deformities, skin cancer, and facial nerve paralysis with reanimation. With expertise, they reverse the signs of aging, remove contour irregularities or deformities, and make the overall appearance of the face more natural and youthful.

NY Eye & Ear Infirmary

Continuum Health Partners, Inc.

THE NEW YORK EYE AND EAR INFIRMARY

310 East 14th Street
New York, New York 10003
Tel. 212.979.4000 Fax. 212.228.0664
http://www.nyee.edu

PROVIDING EXCEPTIONAL CARE OF THE EAR, NOSE, THROAT, AND HEAD & NECK

Established in 1820 the Department of Otolaryngology/Head & Neck Surgery is the first training program in this specialty in the Western Hemisphere. Over nearly two centuries the department has evolved to be an international referral center for the medical and surgical treatment of diseases of the ear, nose, throat and face.

OUTSTANDING SERVICES:

Ear Institute (Otology – Neuro-otology): Specializing in the care of acute and chronic ear disease including hearing loss, cochlear implantation, dizziness, tinnitus, intra cranial tumors and facial nerve disorders. Our advanced otologic and vestibular diagnostic labs assist physicians in treatment.

Facial Plastic Surgery: Highly specialized and renowned surgeons perform in-office or ambulatory procedures utilizing state-of-the-art technology and techniques to produce outstanding results with minimal incisions, rapid recovery and a natural, youthful appearance.

Facial Paralysis: Comprehensive center treating all causes and offering reconstruction of the paralyzed face.

Head & Neck Oncology: A multi-disciplinary team including board-certified surgeons, medical & radiation oncologists, nutritionists and rehabilitation specialists insure rapid recovery from complex, life-saving surgical procedures and return to daily activities.

Pediatric Otolaryngology: Treating children has long been a priority at the Infirmary. Pediatric care ranges from middle ear infection, tonsil and adenoid disease, and neck masses to complex sinus and airway diseases.

Rhinology and Sinus Surgery: Internationally known specialists utilize minimally invasive techniques to treat disorders from sinusitis to intra cranial tumors.

Thyroid Center: A comprehensive program to streamline the diagnosis and treatment of thyroid diseases and cancers. A highly skilled team of surgeons, endocrinologists and radiologists manage the patient's care.

Voice & Swallowing Institute: Combining the expertise of physicians, speech pathologists and a voice physiologist to diagnose and treat voice problems – not only for performing artists but also for teachers, stockbrokers, receptionists, salespeople – anyone for whom voice is an important part of life.

Otolaryngology Clinical Services

General Otolaryngology *plus*
Facial Plastic & Reconstructive Surgery
Cochlear Implantation
Voice & Vocal Dynamics
Head & Neck Oncology
Laryngology
Otology & Neuro-otology
Pediatric Otolaryngology
Rhinology & Sinus Surgery
Swallowing Disorders
Thyroid Center

Facilities

Academic Faculty Practice,
including multiple locations throughout metropolitan NY
Hearing Aid Dispensary
Vestibular Rehabilitation
Ambulatory Care Services

About The New York Eye and Ear Infirmary

The New York Eye and Ear Infirmary is the nation's first specialty hospital and one of the most experienced in terms of the number of patients it treats and complexity of its cases. Each year the otolaryngology department performs more than 6,000 surgeries and sees more than 70,000 visits from outpatients.

**Physician Referral
1.800.449.HOPE (4673)**

OTOLARYNGOLOGY

About the Department of Otolaryngology
The Department of Otolaryngology at NYU Langone Medical Center provides the highest quality treatment for ear, nose, throat, head and neck disorders, including one of the premier head and neck surgery programs in the country. We specialize in the following areas:

Cochlear Implants
Patients are provided with extensive evaluation, device programming and speech rehabilitation both pre- and post-operatively.

Facial Plastic and Reconstructive Surgery
Care is provided to patients requiring facial reconstructive surgery for a wide variety of facial deformities, and to those seeking facial cosmetic surgery. Specialties include functional and aesthetic rhinoplasty, facial rejuvenation surgery, injectable fillers, Botulinum Toxin (Botox) for facial spasm or wrinkles, and chemical peels and microdermabrasion.

General Otolaryngology and Sleep Surgery
Care is provided to adult patients with voice, sleep, allergy and nasal breathing disorders. Additionally, services for children are provided through our pediatric otolaryngologists.

Head and Neck Surgery and Oncology
Care is provided to patients with cancer of the head and neck, including cancer of the larynx, oral cavity, throat, nasal cavity and sinuses, salivary glands and lymph nodes in the neck.

Neutology/Skull Base Program
The Otolaryngology team provides expert care to patients with hearing loss, facial nerve palsy, vertigo and tinnitus, and treats lesions such as acoustic neuromas and skull base meningiomas. Featured services include facial palsy rehabilitation, auditory brainstem implants, cochlear implants, laser surgery and endoscopic anterior and lateral skull base surgery.

Voice and Swallowing Disorders
We treat voice and swallowing disorders, including sore throat, chronic cough, hoarseness, voice loss, swallowing dysfunction, benign growths and cancerous tumors, vocal cord paralysis, the aging voice, recurrent or chronic laryngitis, gastroesophageal reflux, and injuries from overuse and misuse of the voice.

Audiology treats patients suffering with hearing or balance disorders; Head and Neck Speech Pathology treats voice, speech or swallowing problems; Rhinology treats all diseases of the paranasal sinuses, nose and related structures; Skull Base Surgery offers a minimally invasive and advanced surgical approach to tumors of the anterior and posterior skull base.

The Best in American Medicine
www.CastleConnolly.com

Pain Medicine

subspecialty of Anesthesiology, Neurology, and in Physical Medicine and Rehabilitation or Psychiatry

Some physicians who have their primary board certification in anesthesiology, neurology, physical medicine and rehabilitation, or psychiatry have completed additional training and passed an examination in the subspecialty called pain management. These doctors provide a high level of care, either as a primary physician or consultant, for patients experiencing problems with acute, chronic and/or cancer pain in both hospital and ambulatory settings.

For more information about the main specialties of these physicians, see **Anesthesiology, Neurology, Physical Medicine** and **Rehabilitation** or **Psychiatry** section(s).

Training Required: Number of years required for primary specialty *plus* additional training and examination

PAIN MEDICINE

New England

Berde, Charles Benjamin MD/PhD [PM] - **Spec Exp:** Pain Management-Pediatric; Critical Care; Reflex Sympathetic Dystrophy (RSD); **Hospital:** Children's Hospital - Boston, Spaulding Rehab Hosp; **Address:** Chldns Hosp, PTS, 333 Longwood Ave Fl 5, Boston, MA 02115; **Phone:** 617-355-7040; **Board Cert:** Pediatrics 1988; Anesthesiology 2009; Pain Medicine 2004; **Med School:** Stanford Univ 1980; **Resid:** Pediatrics, Chldns Hosp 1983; Anesthesiology, Mass Genl Hosp 1985; **Fellow:** Pediatric Anesthesiology, Chldns Hosp 1985; **Fac Appt:** Prof Ped, Harvard Med Sch

Loder, Elizabeth W MD [PM] - **Spec Exp:** Headache; Migraine; **Hospital:** Brigham and Women's Hosp (page 57), Brigham and Women's Faulkner Hosp; **Address:** 1153 Centre St, Ste 4970, Boston, MA 02130; **Phone:** 617-983-7580; **Board Cert:** Internal Medicine 2010; **Med School:** Univ ND Sch Med 1985; **Resid:** Internal Medicine, Faulkner Hosp 1989; **Fellow:** Headache, Graham Headache Ctr 1990; **Fac Appt:** Asst Prof Med, Harvard Med Sch

Peeters-Asdourian, Christine MD [PM] - **Hospital:** Beth Israel Deaconess Med Ctr - Boston; **Address:** Arnold Pain Management Ctr, One Brookline Pl, Ste 105, Brookline, MA 02445; **Phone:** 617-278-8000; **Board Cert:** Anesthesiology 1987; Pain Medicine 2004; **Med School:** Belgium 1978; **Resid:** Anesthesiology, U Mass Med Ctr 1982; **Fac Appt:** Asst Prof Anes, Univ Mass Sch Med

Ross, Edgar L MD [PM] - **Hospital:** Brigham and Women's Hosp (page 57); **Address:** Brigham & Women's Dept of Pain Medicine, 850 Boylston St Fl 3 - Ste 320, Chestnut Hill, MA 02467; **Phone:** 617-732-9056; **Board Cert:** Anesthesiology 1984; Pain Medicine 2004; **Med School:** Wayne State Univ 1980; **Resid:** Anesthesiology, Case West Univ Hosps 1983; **Fellow:** Pain Medicine, Case West Univ Hosps 1984; **Fac Appt:** Asst Prof Anes, Harvard Med Sch

Mid Atlantic

Argoff, Charles E MD [PM] - **Spec Exp:** Pain Management; Headache; Botox for Pain; Pain-Inverventional Techniques; **Hospital:** Albany Med Ctr, St. Catherine's of Siena Med Ctr; **Address:** AMC Neurology Group, 47 New Scotland Ave, MC 70, Physicians Pavilion, 1st Fl, Albany, NY 12208; **Phone:** 518-262-5226; **Board Cert:** Neurology 1990; Pain Medicine 2009; **Med School:** Northwestern Univ-Feinberg Sch Med 1984; **Resid:** Neurology, Stony Brook Univ Affil Hosp 1988; **Fellow:** Neurology, Natl Inst of Hlth 1990; **Fac Appt:** Prof N, Albany Med Coll

Christo, Paul J MD [PM] - **Spec Exp:** Reflex Sympathetic Dystrophy (RSD); Spinal Cord Stimulation; Pain-Spine; Pain-Low Back; **Hospital:** Johns Hopkins Hosp (page 61); **Address:** Pain Treatment Ctr, 601 N Caroline St, Ste 3062, Baltimore, MD 21287; **Phone:** 410-955-7246; **Board Cert:** Anesthesiology 2001; Pain Medicine 2002; **Med School:** Univ Louisville Sch Med 1995; **Resid:** Anesthesiology, Mass General Hosp 2000; **Fellow:** Pain Medicine, Johns Hopkins Hosp 2001; **Fac Appt:** Assoc Prof Anes, Johns Hopkins Univ

Cope, Doris K MD [PM] - ; **Address:** KURE Pain, 116 Defense Hwy, Ste 403, Annapolis, MD 21401; **Phone:** 410-571-2946; **Board Cert:** Anesthesiology 1989; Pain Medicine 2007; **Med School:** Med Coll GA 1982; **Resid:** Anesthesiology, Univ S Alabama 1986; **Fac Appt:** Prof Anes, Univ Pittsburgh

DeLeon, Oscar A MD [PM] - **Spec Exp:** Pain-Acute; Pain-Chronic; Pain-Cancer; **Hospital:** Roswell Park Cancer Inst; **Address:** Roswell Park Cancer Inst, Dept Anesthesia/Pain Medicine, Elm & Carlton Sts, Buffalo, NY 14263; **Phone:** 716-845-4595; **Board Cert:** Anesthesiology 1991; Critical Care Medicine 1993; Pain Medicine 2005; **Med School:** Guatemala 1982; **Resid:** Surgery, SUNY-Downstate Med Ctr 1986; Anesthesiology, Univ Buffalo 1989; **Fac Appt:** Prof Anes, SUNY Buffalo

Diwan, Sudhir MD [PM] - **Spec Exp:** Pain-after Spinal Intervention; Pain-Musculoskeletal; Pain-Neuropathic; Pain-Cancer; **Hospital:** Staten Island Univ Hosp - North (page 67); **Address:** Spine & Pain Inst of New York, 1534 Victory Blvd, Staten Island, NY 10314; **Phone:** 718-667-3577; **Board Cert:** Anesthesiology 2012; Pain Medicine 2002; **Med School:** India 1983; **Resid:** Surgery, St Luke's-Roosevelt Hosp Ctr 1994; Anesthesiology, St Luke's-Roosevelt Hosp Ctr 1997; **Fellow:** Pain Medicine, NY Presby Hosp 1998

Falco, Frank J.E. MD [PM] - **Spec Exp:** Spinal Disorders; Pain-Musculoskeletal-Spine; Pain-Chronic; **Hospital:** Christiana Hospital; **Address:** Mid Atlantic Spine & Pain Ctr, 100 Biddle Ave, Ste 101, Newark, DE 19702; **Phone:** 302-392-6501; **Board Cert:** Pain Medicine 2011; Physical Medicine & Rehabilitation 2003; Sports Medicine 2007; Electrodiagnostic Medicine 2004; **Med School:** Temple Univ 1988; **Resid:** Physical Medicine & Rehabilitation, Temple Univ Hosp 1992; **Fellow:** Pain Management, Georgia Spine & Sports Ctr 1994; **Fac Appt:** Asst Clin Prof PMR, Temple Univ

Gharibo, Christopher G MD [PM] - **Spec Exp:** Pain-Back & Neck; Pain-Neuropathic; Pain-Chronic; Complex Regional Pain Syndromes; **Hospital:** NYU Langone Med Ctr (page 68), NYU Hosp For Joint Diseases (page 70); **Address:** 333 E 38th St N, Fl 6, New York, NY 10016; **Phone:** 646-501-7246; **Board Cert:** Anesthesiology 1997; Pain Medicine 2009; **Med School:** UMDNJ-NJ Med Sch, Newark 1992; **Resid:** Anesthesiology, NYU Med Ctr 1997; **Fellow:** Pain Medicine, Jefferson Univ Hosp 1997; **Fac Appt:** Assoc Prof Anes, NYU Sch Med

Jain, Subhash MD [PM] - **Spec Exp:** Pain-Cancer; Pain-Pelvic; Reflex Sympathetic Dystrophy (RSD); Complex Regional Pain Syndromes; **Hospital:** Beth Israel Med Ctr - Petrie Division (page 56); **Address:** 360 E 72nd St, Ste C, New York, NY 10021; **Phone:** 212-439-6100; **Board Cert:** Anesthesiology 1994; Pain Medicine 1998; **Med School:** India 1968; **Resid:** Surgery, St Vincent Med Ctr 1977; Anesthesiology, New York Hosp 1979; **Fellow:** Pain Medicine, New York Hosp/Meml Sloan Kettering Cancer Ctr 1980; **Fac Appt:** Assoc Prof Anes, Cornell Univ-Weill Med Coll

Kreitzer, Joel M MD [PM] - **Spec Exp:** Pain-Back; Pain-Cancer; Pain-Neuropathic; **Hospital:** Mount Sinai Med Ctr (page 64), Mount Sinai Hosp of Queens (page 64); **Address:** Upper East Side Pain Medicine, 1540 York Ave, New York, NY 10028; **Phone:** 212-288-2180; **Board Cert:** Anesthesiology 1990; Pain Medicine 2004; **Med School:** Albert Einstein Coll Med 1985; **Resid:** Anesthesiology, Mt Sinai Hosp 1989; **Fellow:** Pain Medicine, Mt Sinai Hosp 1989; **Fac Appt:** Assoc Clin Prof Anes, Mount Sinai Sch Med

Ngeow, Jeffrey MD [PM] - **Spec Exp:** Pain-Musculoskeletal-Spine & Neck; Reflex Sympathetic Dystrophy (RSD); Acupuncture; Pain-Neuropathic; **Hospital:** Hosp For Special Surgery (page 60); **Address:** 635 Madison Ave Fl 5, New York, NY 10022; **Phone:** 212-224-7918; **Board Cert:** Anesthesiology 1980; Pain Medicine 2005; **Med School:** England, UK 1971; **Resid:** Anesthesiology, Peter Bent Brigham Hosp 1977; **Fellow:** Pain Medicine, Tufts New England Med Ctr 1978; **Fac Appt:** Assoc Clin Prof Anes, Cornell Univ-Weill Med Coll

Raja, Srinivasa MD [PM] - **Spec Exp:** Pain-Neuropathic; Herpetic Neuralgia (Shingles); Reflex Sympathetic Dystrophy (RSD); **Hospital:** Johns Hopkins Hosp (page 61); **Address:** 601 N Caroline St, Ste 3062, Baltimore, MD 21287; **Phone:** 410-955-7246; **Board Cert:** Anesthesiology 1982; Pain Medicine 2004; **Med School:** India 1974; **Resid:** Anesthesiology, Univ Washington Med Ctr 1979; **Fellow:** Pain Medicine, Univ Virginia Hosp 1981; **Fac Appt:** Prof Anes, Johns Hopkins Univ

Pain Medicine

Richman, Daniel MD [PM] - **Spec Exp:** Pain-Back & Neck; Complex Regional Pain Syndromes; Reflex Sympathetic Dystrophy (RSD); **Hospital:** Hosp For Special Surgery (page 60); **Address:** 535 E 70th St, New York, NY 10021-4872; **Phone:** 212-606-1768; **Board Cert:** Anesthesiology 1999; Pain Medicine 2005; **Med School:** UMDNJ-NJ Med Sch, Newark 1986; **Resid:** Anesthesiology, Hartford Hosp 1990; **Fellow:** Pain Medicine, Hosp Special Surgery 1991; **Fac Appt:** Assoc Clin Prof Anes, Cornell Univ-Weill Med Coll

Staats, Peter MD [PM] - **Spec Exp:** Pain-Cancer; Pain-Back; **Hospital:** Riverview Med Ctr, CentraState Med Ctr; **Address:** Premier Pain Centers, 160 Avenue at the Commons, Ste 1, Shrewsbury, NJ 07702; **Phone:** 732-380-0200; **Board Cert:** Anesthesiology 1994; Pain Medicine 2005; **Med School:** Univ Mich Med Sch 1989; **Resid:** Anesthesiology, Johns Hopkins Hosp 1993; **Fellow:** Pain Medicine, Johns Hopkins Hosp 1994

Weinberger, Michael L MD [PM] - **Spec Exp:** Pain-Cancer; Pain-Back; Palliative Care; **Hospital:** NY-Presby/Columbia Univ Med Ctr, NY (page 66); **Address:** 630 W 168th St, PH5, rm 500, New York, NY 10032-3720; **Phone:** 212-305-7114; **Board Cert:** Internal Medicine 1986; Anesthesiology 1990; Pain Medicine 2004; Hospice & Palliative Medicine 2006; **Med School:** Columbia P&S 1983; **Resid:** Internal Medicine, St Vincent's Hosp 1986; Anesthesiology, Columbia-Presby Med Ctr 1989; **Fellow:** Pain Medicine, Meml Sloan Kettering Cancer Ctr 1990; **Fac Appt:** Assoc Prof Anes, Columbia P&S

Southeast

Anghelescu, Doralina L MD [PM] - **Spec Exp:** Pain Management-Pediatric; Pain-Cancer; **Hospital:** St. Jude Children's Research Hosp; **Address:** St Jude Chldn's Rsch Hosp, Dept Anesthesiology/Pain Management, 262 Danny Thomas Pl, MS 130, Memphis, TN 38105; **Phone:** 901-595-4034; **Board Cert:** Anesthesiology 1998; **Med School:** Romania 1985; **Resid:** Anesthesiology, Univ N Mex Hosp 1997; **Fellow:** Pain Medicine, Chldns Natl Med Ctr 1998; Pain Medicine, Univ N Mex Hosp 1999

Baumann, Patricia L MD [PM] - **Spec Exp:** Pain-Back; Pain-Neuropathic; Spinal Disorders; Complex Regional Pain Syndromes; **Hospital:** Emory Univ Hosp Midtown, Emory Univ Hosp; **Address:** Emory Center for Pain Management, 550 Peachtree St NE, Ste 7085, Atlanta, GA 30308; **Phone:** 404-686-2410; **Board Cert:** Anesthesiology 1993; Pain Medicine 2005; **Med School:** Emory Univ 1988; **Resid:** Anesthesiology, Emory Univ Med Ctr 1992; **Fac Appt:** Asst Prof Anes, Emory Univ

Gobrial, Wagih W MD [PM] - **Hospital:** Cleveland Clin - Weston (page 55); **Address:** Cleveland Clinic Florida, 2950 Cleveland Clinic Blvd, Weston, FL 33331; **Phone:** 954-659-5045; **Board Cert:** Anesthesiology 1997; Pain Medicine 2009; **Med School:** Egypt 1976; **Resid:** Anesthesiology, Cleveland Clinic 1996; **Fellow:** Pain Management, Cleveland Clinic 1997; **Fac Appt:** Asst Prof Anes, FAU/Schmidt Coll Med

Huntoon, Marc MD [PM] - **Spec Exp:** Pain-Cancer; Pain-after Spinal Intervention; Palliative Care; **Hospital:** Vanderbilt Univ Med Ctr (page 75); **Address:** 719 Thompson Ln, Nashville, TN 37204; **Phone:** 615-322-4311; **Board Cert:** Anesthesiology 2003; Pain Medicine 2004; Hospice & Palliative Medicine 2004; **Med School:** Wayne State Univ 1985; **Resid:** Anesthesiology, Naval Hosp Med Ctr 1991; **Fellow:** Pain Medicine, Naval Hosp Med Ctr 1992; **Fac Appt:** Prof Anes, Vanderbilt Univ

Rauck, Richard L MD [PM] - **Spec Exp:** Pain-Cancer; Spinal Cord Stimulation; Complex Regional Pain Syndromes; **Hospital:** Forsyth Med Ctr, Wake Forest Baptist Med Ctr; **Address:** Carolinas Pain Institute, 145 Kimel Park Drive, Ste 330, Winston-Salem, NC 27103; **Phone:** 336-765-6181; **Board Cert:** Anesthesiology 1987; Pain Medicine 2005; **Med School:** Bowman Gray 1982; **Resid:** Anesthesiology, Univ Cincinnati Hosp 1985; **Fellow:** Pain Medicine, Univ Cincinnati Hosp 1986; **Fac Appt:** Assoc Prof Anes, Wake Forest Univ

Vetter, Thomas R MD [PM] - **Spec Exp:** Pain Management-Pediatric; Pain-Chronic; **Hospital:** Children's Hospital - Birmingham, Univ of Ala Hosp at Birmingham; **Address:** UAB Anesthesiology/Pain Medicine, 619 19th St S, JT 865, Birmingham, AL 35249-6810; **Phone:** 205-934-6501; **Board Cert:** Anesthesiology 2009; Pain Medicine 2009; **Med School:** Ohio State Univ 1984; **Resid:** Anesthesiology, Univ Pittsburgh Med Ctr 1988; **Fellow:** Pain Management, Childrens Hosp 1989; **Fac Appt:** Prof Anes, Univ Alabama

Midwest

Abram, Stephen E MD [PM] - **Hospital:** Froedtert and Med Ctr of WI; **Address:** Pain Management Clinic/Med College WI, 1155 N Mayfair Rd, Wauwatosa, WI 53226; **Phone:** 414-456-7600; **Board Cert:** Anesthesiology 2001; Pain Medicine 2004; **Med School:** Jefferson Med Coll 1970; **Resid:** Anesthesiology, Mary Hitchcock Meml Hosp 1973; **Fac Appt:** Prof Anes, Med Coll Wisc

Benzon, Honorio T MD [PM] - **Spec Exp:** Pain-Back; Complex Regional Pain Syndromes; Pain-Neuropathic; Pain-Cancer; **Hospital:** Northwestern Meml Hosp; **Address:** 675 N Saint Clair St, Fl 17 - Ste 200, Chicago, IL 60611-3015; **Phone:** 312-695-2500; **Board Cert:** Anesthesiology 2009; Pain Medicine 2004; **Med School:** Philippines 1971; **Resid:** Anesthesiology, Univ Cincinnati Med Ctr 1975; Anesthesiology, Northwestern Meml Hosp 1976; **Fellow:** Research, Brigham & Womens Hosp 1986; **Fac Appt:** Prof Anes, Northwestern Univ

Covington, Edward C MD [PM] - **Spec Exp:** Pain-Chronic; **Hospital:** Cleveland Clin (page 55); **Address:** Cleveland Clinic, 9500 Euclid Ave, Desk C21, Cleveland, OH 44195; **Phone:** 216-444-5964; **Board Cert:** Psychiatry 1978; **Med School:** Univ Tenn Coll Med 1970; **Resid:** Psychiatry, Mayo Clinic 1975

Green, Carmen R MD [PM] - **Spec Exp:** Pain Care-Racial/Ethnic Disparities; **Hospital:** Univ of Michigan Hosp; **Address:** Univ Mich Hlth Sys, Dept Anesthesiology, rm 1H247, 1500 E Med Ctr Drive, SPC5048, Ann Arbor, MI 48109-5048; **Phone:** 734-936-4240; **Board Cert:** Anesthesiology 1996; Pain Medicine 2009; **Med School:** Mich State Univ 1987; **Resid:** Anesthesiology, Univ Mich Med Ctr 1989; **Fellow:** Pain Medicine, Univ Mich Med Ctr 1992; **Fac Appt:** Asst Prof Anes, Univ Mich Med Sch

Hooten, William Michael MD [PM] - **Spec Exp:** Pain-Interventional Techniques; **Hospital:** Mayo Med Ctr & Clin - Rochester, St. Mary's Hosp - Rochester MN (Mayo); **Address:** Mayo Clinic, Dept Anesthesia/Pain, 200 First St SW, Rochester, MN 55905; **Phone:** 507-266-9240; **Board Cert:** Anesthesiology 2004; Pain Medicine 2005; Psychiatry 2010; **Med School:** St Louis Univ 1993; **Resid:** Internal Medicine, Mayo Clinic 1985; Psychiatry, Johns Hopkins Hosp 1998; **Fellow:** Pain Medicine, Barnes Jewish Hosp 2005; **Fac Appt:** Assoc Prof Anes, Mayo Med Sch

Macadaeg, Kevin E MD [PM] - **Spec Exp:** Spinal Disorders; Pain-Spine; Pain-Interventional Techniques; **Hospital:** St. Vincent Indianapolis Hosp; **Address:** Indiana Spine Group, 8402 Harcourt Rd, Ste 400, Indianapolis, IN 46260; **Phone:** 317-228-7000; **Board Cert:** Anesthesiology 1992; Pain Medicine 2004; **Med School:** Wayne State Univ 1988; **Resid:** Anesthesiology, SUNY Upstate Med Ctr 1992; **Fac Appt:** Asst Clin Prof Anes, Indiana Univ

Mekhail, Nagy A MD/PhD [PM] - **Spec Exp:** Pain-Back & Neck; Pain-Chronic; Pain-Neuropathic; Pain-Cancer; **Hospital:** Cleveland Clin (page 55); **Address:** Cleveland Clinic, 10524 Euclid Ave, Cleveland, OH 44106; **Phone:** 216-445-7370; **Board Cert:** Anesthesiology 1993; Pain Medicine 2004; **Med School:** Egypt 1975; **Resid:** Anesthesiology, Cleveland Clinic 1991; **Fellow:** Pain Medicine, Cleveland Clinic 1992; **Fac Appt:** Prof Anes, Cleveland Cl Coll Med/Case West Res

Robbins, Larry D MD [PM] - **Spec Exp:** Headache; Migraine; Psychopharmacology; Pain Management; **Address:** 60 Revere Drive, Ste 330, Northbrook, IL 60062; **Phone:** 847-480-9399; **Board Cert:** Anesthesiology 2005; **Med School:** Univ IL Coll Med 1981; **Resid:** Neurology, Univ Illinois Med Ctr 1985; **Fellow:** Pain Medicine, Diamond Headache Clinic 1986

Rosenquist, Richard W MD [PM] - **Spec Exp:** Complex Regional Pain Syndromes; Pain-Back; Pain-Facial; Headache; **Hospital:** Cleveland Clin (page 55); **Address:** Cleveland Clinic-Pain Management, 10524 Euclid Ave, MC C25, Cleveland, OH 44106; **Phone:** 216-445-7370; **Board Cert:** Anesthesiology 1988; Pain Medicine 2004; **Med School:** Northwestern Univ 1984; **Resid:** Anesthesiology, Northwestern Univ Med Ctr 1987; **Fellow:** Anesthesiology & Pain Management, Emory Univ Hosp 1988

Suresh, Santhanam MD [PM] - **Hospital:** Lurie Chldn's Hosp-Chicago; **Address:** Chldns Meml Hosp, 225 E Chicago Ave, Chicago, IL 60611; **Phone:** 312-227-5157; **Board Cert:** Pediatrics 2011; Anesthesiology 2012; Pain Medicine 2009; **Med School:** India 1983; **Resid:** Pediatrics, Cook Co Hosp 1988; Anesthesiology, Loyola Univ Med Ctr 1990; **Fellow:** Pediatric Anesthesiology, Northwestern Meml Hosp 1991; **Fac Appt:** Prof Anes, Northwestern Univ-Feinberg Sch Med

Swarm, Robert A MD [PM] - **Spec Exp:** Pain-Acute; Pain-Chronic; Pain-Cancer; **Hospital:** Barnes-Jewish Hosp; **Address:** Ctr for Advanced Med-Pain Mngmt Ctr, 4921 Parkview Pl, Ste 10A, St Louis, MO 63110; **Phone:** 314-362-8820; **Board Cert:** Anesthesiology 1990; Pain Medicine 2004; **Med School:** Washington Univ, St Louis 1983; **Resid:** Surgery, Barnes Hosp 1986; Anesthesiology, Barnes Hosp 1989; **Fellow:** Pain Medicine, Univ Sydney 1991; **Fac Appt:** Assoc Prof Anes, Washington Univ, St Louis

Weisman, Steven J MD [PM] - **Spec Exp:** Pain Management-Pediatric; Palliative Care-Pediatric; Complex Regional Pain Syndromes; Pain-Cancer; **Hospital:** Chldns Hosp - Wisconsin; **Address:** Children's Hospital of Wisconsin, 9000 W Wisconsin Ave, Box 1997, Milwaukee, WI 53201-1997; **Phone:** 414-266-2775; **Board Cert:** Pediatrics 1982; Pediatric Hematology-Oncology 1984; Anesthesiology 2009; **Med School:** Albert Einstein Coll Med 1978; **Resid:** Pediatrics, Chldns Hosp 1981; Anesthesiology, Univ Conn Hlth Ctr 1994; **Fellow:** Pediatric Hematology-Oncology, Indiana Univ Sch Med 1984; **Fac Appt:** Prof Anes, Med Coll Wisc

Wellington, Joshua R MD [PM] - **Spec Exp:** Pain-Spine; Pain-Cancer; Pain-Neuropathic; Pain-Pediatric; **Hospital:** IU Health University Hosp; **Address:** IU Dept Anesthesiology, Fesler Hall, 1120 South Drive, rm 204, Indianapolis, IN 46202; **Phone:** 317-944-2891; **Board Cert:** Physical Medicine & Rehabilitation 2004; Pain Medicine 2005; **Med School:** Med Coll OH 1999; **Resid:** Physical Medicine & Rehabilitation, Spaulding Rehab Hosp 2003; **Fellow:** Pain Management, Chldns Hosp/Brigham & Womens Hosp/Beth Israel 2004; **Fac Appt:** Asst Clin Prof PMR, Indiana Univ

Great Plains and Mountains

Fine, Perry G MD [PM] - **Spec Exp:** Pain-Cancer; Palliative Care; Pain-Chronic; **Hospital:** Univ Utah Hlth Care; **Address:** 546 S Chipeta Way, Ste 220, Salt Lake City, UT 84108; **Phone:** 801-581-7246; **Board Cert:** Anesthesiology 1985; Pain Medicine 2004; **Med School:** Med Coll VA 1981; **Resid:** Anesthesiology, Univ Utah Hlth Sci Ctr 1984; **Fellow:** Pain Medicine, Univ Toronto Affil Hosp 1985; **Fac Appt:** Prof Anes, Univ Utah

Southwest

Burton, Allen W MD [PM] - **Spec Exp:** Pain-Cancer; Palliative Care; **Hospital:** St. Luke's Episcopal Hosp-Houston; **Address:** 7700 Main St, Ste 400, Houston, TX 77030; **Phone:** 832-553-1336; **Board Cert:** Anesthesiology 1996; Pain Medicine 2009; **Med School:** Baylor Coll Med 1991; **Resid:** Anesthesiology, Brigham & Women's Hosp 1995; **Fellow:** Pain Medicine, Univ Texas Med Branch 1998; **Fac Appt:** Assoc Prof Anes, Univ Tex Med Br, Galveston

Driver, Larry C MD [PM] - **Spec Exp:** Pain-Cancer; Palliative Care; **Hospital:** UT MD Anderson Cancer Ctr; **Address:** UT MD Anderson Cancer Ctr, Dept Pain Medicine, 1400 Holcombe Blvd, Unit 409, Houston, TX 77030; **Phone:** 713-745-7246; **Board Cert:** Anesthesiology 1992; Pain Medicine 2002; **Med School:** Univ Tex, San Antonio 1980; **Resid:** Anesthesiology, Univ CO Affil Hosp 1984; **Fellow:** Pain Medicine, UT MD Anderson Cancer Ctr 1999; **Fac Appt:** Assoc Prof Anes, Univ Tex, Houston

Freitag, Frederick G DO [PM] - **Spec Exp:** Headache; Migraine-Chronic; Botox Therapy; **Hospital:** Baylor Univ Medical Ctr-Dallas; **Address:** 9101 N Central Expressway, Ste 400, Dallas, TX 75231; **Phone:** 214-820-9272; **Board Cert:** Family Medicine 1982; Pain Medicine 2001; **Med School:** Chicago Coll Osteo Med 1979; **Resid:** Family Medicine, Brentwood Hosp 1981; **Fellow:** Headache, Cleveland Clinic 1982; **Fac Appt:** Assoc Clin Prof FMed, Baylor Coll Med

Noe, Carl E MD [PM] - **Spec Exp:** Pain-Back & Neck; **Hospital:** UT Southwestern Med Ctr at Dallas; **Address:** 1801 Inwood Rd, Dallas, TX 75390-9189; **Phone:** 214-645-8450; **Board Cert:** Anesthesiology 1989; Pain Medicine 2004; Critical Care Medicine 1989; **Med School:** Univ Tex, San Antonio 1984; **Resid:** Anesthesiology, TX Tech Univ Hlth Sci Ctr 1987; Anesthesiology, Stanford Univ Med Ctr 1988; **Fellow:** Critical Care Medicine, Stanford Univ Med Ctr 1988; Pain Management, TX Tech Univ Hlth Sci Ctr 1989; **Fac Appt:** Assoc Prof Anes, Univ Tex SW, Dallas

Racz, Gabor MD [PM] - **Spec Exp:** Pain-after Spinal Intervention; Reflex Sympathetic Dystrophy (RSD); Pain-Back, Head & Neck; Headache/Facial Pain; **Hospital:** Univ Med Ctr-Lubbock; **Address:** 3601 4th St, MS 8182, Lubbock, TX 79430-0002; **Phone:** 806-743-3112; **Board Cert:** Anesthesiology 1993; Pain Medicine 2004; **Med School:** England, UK 1962; **Resid:** Anesthesiology, SUNY Upstate Med Ctr 1969; **Fac Appt:** Prof Anes, Texas Tech Univ

Ramamurthy, Somayaji MD [PM] - **Spec Exp:** Pain-Back; Pain-Chronic; **Hospital:** Univ Hlth Syst-San Antonio; **Address:** UT Medicine Pain Consultants, 5282 Medical Drive, Ste 614, San Antonio, TX 78229; **Phone:** 210-450-9857; **Board Cert:** Anesthesiology 1972; Pain Medicine 2004; **Med School:** India 1965; **Resid:** Anesthesiology, Cook Co Hosp 1970; **Fac Appt:** Prof Anes, Univ Tex, San Antonio

Walsh, Nicolas E MD [PM] - **Spec Exp:** Pain-Back; Trauma Rehabilitation; Post Polio Syndrome; **Hospital:** Univ Hlth Syst-San Antonio, Audie L Murphy Meml Vets Hosp - San Antonio; **Address:** Univ Tex Hlth Sci Ctr, Rehab Med, 7703 Floyd Curl Drive, MC 7798, San Antonio, TX 78229-3901; **Phone:** 210-358-0770; **Board Cert:** Physical Medicine & Rehabilitation 2009; Pain Medicine 2000; **Med School:** Univ Colorado 1979; **Resid:** Physical Medicine & Rehabilitation, Univ Tex Hlth Sci Ctr 1982; **Fac Appt:** Prof PMR, Univ Tex, San Antonio

West Coast and Pacific

Audell, Laura G MD [PM] - **Spec Exp:** Complex Regional Pain Syndromes; Reflex Sympathetic Dystrophy (RSD); Herpetic Neuralgia (Shingles); Spinal Cord Disorders; **Hospital:** Cedars-Sinai Med Ctr; **Address:** 444 S San Vincente, Ste 1101, Los Angeles, CA 90048; **Phone:** 310-423-9600; **Board Cert:** Internal Medicine 1986; Anesthesiology 1988; Pain Medicine 2007; **Med School:** Univ Wash 1982; **Resid:** Internal Medicine, UCLA-Hosps 1985; Anesthesiology, UCLA-Hosps 1987; **Fellow:** Pain Medicine, UCLA-Hosps 1988

Ballantyne, Jane C MD [PM] - **Spec Exp:** Pain-Chronic; Pain-Cancer; **Hospital:** Harborview Med Ctr; **Address:** Univ Wash Pain Ctr, 4225 Roosevelt Way NE Fl 4 - Ste 401, Seattle, WA 98105; **Phone:** 206-598-4282; **Board Cert:** Anesthesiology 2007; **Med School:** England, UK 1978; **Resid:** Surgery, London & Oxford 1985; Anesthesiology, John Radcliffe Hosp 1990; **Fellow:** Anesthesiology, Mass Genl Hosp 1992; Pain Medicine, Mass Genl Hosp 1994; **Fac Appt:** Prof Anes, Univ Wash

Ferrante, F Michael MD [PM] - **Spec Exp:** Pain-Back & Neck; Reflex Sympathetic Dystrophy (RSD); Botox for Pain; Pain-Neuropathic; **Hospital:** Santa Monica - UCLA Med Ctr & Ortho Hosp, UCLA Ronald Reagan Med Ctr; **Address:** UCLA Pain Program, 1245 16th St, Ste 225, Santa Monica, CA 90404; **Phone:** 310-319-2241; **Board Cert:** Internal Medicine 1985; Anesthesiology 1987; Pain Medicine 2004; **Med School:** NY Med Coll 1980; **Resid:** Internal Medicine, Emroy Univ Affil Hosp 1983; Anesthesiology, Emroy Univ Affil Hosp 1986; **Fellow:** Infectious Disease, Barnes Hosp-Wash Univ 1984; Pain Medicine, Brigham & Womens Hosp 1987; **Fac Appt:** Prof Anes, UCLA

Fishman, Scott M MD [PM] - **Spec Exp:** Pain-Cancer; Pain-Chronic; **Hospital:** UC Davis Med Ctr; **Address:** UC Davis Med Ctr, Pain Management Clinic, 4860 Y St, Ste 2700, Sacramento, CA 95817; **Phone:** 916-734-7246; **Board Cert:** Psychiatry 1998; Pain Medicine 1995; **Med School:** Univ Mass Sch Med 1990; **Resid:** Internal Medicine, Greenwich Hosp 1993; Psychiatry, Mass Genl Hosp 1996; **Fellow:** Pain Medicine, Mass Genl Hosp 1995; **Fac Appt:** Prof Anes, UC Davis

Fitzgibbon, Dermot R MD [PM] - **Spec Exp:** Pain-Cancer; **Hospital:** Univ Wash Med Ctr; **Address:** Univ Wash Med Ctr, Dept Anesthesiology, 1959 NE Pacific St, Box 356043, Seattle, WA 98195; **Phone:** 206-598-4100; **Board Cert:** Anesthesiology 1996; Pain Medicine 2009; **Med School:** Ireland 1983; **Resid:** Anesthesiology, St Vincent's Hosp 1992; Anesthesiology, Univ Washington Med Ctr 1995; **Fellow:** Pain Medicine, Univ Wash-Pain Mngmt Clinic 1994; **Fac Appt:** Assoc Prof Anes, Univ Wash

Fuller, Nicholas S MD [PM] - **Hospital:** Cedars-Sinai Med Ctr; **Address:** 120 S Spalding Drive, Ste 301, Beverly Hills, CA 90212; **Phone:** 310-883-3388; **Board Cert:** Anesthesiology 1996; **Med School:** SUNY Buffalo 1991; **Resid:** Anesthesiology, Brigham & Women's Hosp 1995; **Fellow:** Pain Medicine, Univ Washington Med Ctr 1997

Jasmin, Luc MD/PhD [PM] - **Spec Exp:** Spinal Cord Stimulation; Spasticity & Movement Disorders; Stereotactic Radiosurgery; Pain-Cancer; **Hospital:** Cedars-Sinai Med Ctr; **Address:** 8635 W Third St, Ste 1080-W, Los Angeles, CA 90048; **Phone:** 310-779-6636; **Med School:** Canada 1981; **Resid:** Neurological Surgery, Notre-Dame Hospital; **Fellow:** Research, UCSF Med Ctr; Neurosurgical Oncology, UCSF Med Ctr

Koh, Jeffrey MD [PM] - **Spec Exp:** Pain Management-Pediatric; **Hospital:** Doernbecher Chldns Hosp/OHSU, OR Hlth & Sci Univ; **Address:** 3181 SW Sam Jackson Park Rd, MC UHS-2, Portland, OR 97239; **Phone:** 503-418-5188; **Board Cert:** Pediatrics 2011; Anesthesiology 1993; Pain Medicine 2007; **Med School:** Wayne State Univ 1985; **Resid:** Pediatrics, Emory Univ Hosp 1988; Anesthesiology, Brigham & Women's Hosp 1991; **Fellow:** Pediatric Anesthesiology, Chldn's Hosp 1992; Pediatric Pain Management, UCLA Med Ctr 1993; **Fac Appt:** Prof Ped, Oregon Hlth & Sci Univ

Mackey, Sean C MD/PhD [PM] - **Spec Exp:** Pain-Cancer; Pain-Chronic; **Hospital:** Stanford Univ Hosp & Clinics; **Address:** 780 Welch Rd, Ste 208, Palo Alto, CA 94304-5340; **Phone:** 650-725-9636; **Board Cert:** Anesthesiology 2009; Pain Medicine 2011; **Med School:** Univ Ariz Coll Med 1994; **Resid:** Anesthesiology, Stanford Univ Med Ctr 1998; **Fellow:** Pain Medicine, Stanford Univ Med Ctr 1999; **Fac Appt:** Assoc Prof Anes, Stanford Univ

Prager, Joshua P MD [PM] - **Spec Exp:** Complex Regional Pain Syndromes; **Hospital:** UCLA Ronald Reagan Med Ctr; **Address:** California Pain Medicine Ctr, 100 UCLA Medical Plaza, Ste 760, Los Angeles, CA 90095; **Phone:** 310-794-7246 x100; **Board Cert:** Internal Medicine 1984; Anesthesiology 1987; Pain Medicine 2004; **Med School:** Stanford Univ 1981; **Resid:** Internal Medicine, UCLA Med Ctr 1984; Anesthesiology, Mass Genl Hosp 1986

Rosner, Howard L MD [PM] - **Spec Exp:** Pain-after Spinal Intervention; Pain-Back; Reflex Sympathetic Dystrophy (RSD); **Hospital:** Cedars-Sinai Med Ctr; **Address:** 444 S San Vincente Blvd, Ste 1101, Los Angeles, CA 90048; **Phone:** 310-423-9600; **Board Cert:** Anesthesiology 1989; Pain Medicine 2004; **Med School:** Univ Miami Sch Med 1980; **Resid:** Anesthesiology, Mass Genl Hosp 1983; **Fellow:** Pain Medicine, Columbia-Presby Med Ctr 1984

Slatkin, Neal E MD [PM] - **Spec Exp:** Pain-Cancer; Palliative Care; **Hospital:** El Camino Hosp, Good Samaritan Hosp - San Jose; **Address:** 4850 Union Ave, San Jose, CA 95124-5156; **Phone:** 408-559-5600; **Board Cert:** Neurology 1982; Pain Medicine 2000; **Med School:** SUNY Stony Brook 1976; **Resid:** Neurology, Bellevue Hosp Ctr-NYU 1978; Neurology, Med Coll Va Hosps 1981; **Fellow:** Neurology, Med Coll Va 1982; Neuro-Oncology, Meml Sloan-Kettering Cancer Ctr 1984

Wallace, Mark Steven MD [PM] - **Spec Exp:** Pain-Chronic; Pain-Cancer; Palliative Care; **Hospital:** UCSD Med Ctr; **Address:** 9350 Campus Point Drive, Ste 2C, La Jolla, CA 92037; **Phone:** 858-657-6035; **Board Cert:** Anesthesiology 1992; Pain Medicine 2005; **Med School:** Creighton Univ 1987; **Resid:** Anesthesiology, Univ Maryland Hosp 1991; **Fellow:** Pain Medicine, UCSD Med Ctr 1994

Cleveland Clinic

Every life deserves world class care.

Cleveland Clinic
Anesthesiology Institute
9500 Euclid Avenue
Cleveland, OH 44195

Pain Management

At Cleveland Clinic's Department of Pain Management, 28 board-certified pain management physicians and researchers are dedicated to the goal of helping every patient with chronic pain return to a normal, productive lifestyle. Our committed staff uses the latest in diagnostic technology, paired with medical and interventional therapeutics, to work with patients to identify the source of the pain, eliminate or reduce the pain and teach them to manage it.

Cleveland Clinic Pain Management specialists treat chronic pain related to any type of disease, injury or accident, including:

- Back and neck pain, including herniated discs, spinal stenosis, tumors and arthritis
- Chronic abdominal pain and pelvic pain
- Complex regional pain syndrome (also known as reflex sympathetic dystrophy or RSD)
- Muscle and joint pain and arthritis
- Headache
- Sports injuries
- Disorders of the nervous system, including shingles and trigeminal and occipital neuralgia (facial pain)
- Pain associated with AIDS
- Sickle cell anemia
- Cancer pain
- Intractable spasticity associated with multiple sclerosis or spinal cord injuries
- Pain associated with osteoporosis and vertebral compression fractures

The mission of Cleveland Clinic's Department of Pain Management is to be the leader in patient care, education and outcomes-oriented clinical and basic research in pain medicine. The department is home to one of the largest and most sought-after pain medicine fellowship programs in the world.

Offering Same-Day Appointments
Call 800.274.2009.

Treatment Guides
Cleveland Clinic has developed comprehensive treatment guides for many diseases and conditions. To download our free treatment guides, visit clevelandclinic.org/treatmentguides.

Online Medical Second Opinion
Call 216.444.3223 or 800.223.2273 ext. 43223 or email eclevelandclinic@ccf.org.

Out-of-State Patients Assistance
Call 800.223.2273, ext. 55580 or email medicalconcierge@ccf.org.

Visit Us At:
clevelandclinic.org

Follow Us On:
Facebook
www.facebook.com/clevelandclinic

Twitter
@ClevelandClinic

You Tube
www.youtube.com/clevelandclinic

Health Hub
health.clevelandclinic.org

Pathology

A pathologist deals with the causes and nature of disease and contributes to diagnosis, prognosis and treatment through knowledge gained by the laboratory application of the biologic, chemical and physical sciences.

A pathologist uses information gathered from the microscopic examination of tissue specimens, cells and body fluids, and from clinical laboratory tests on body fluids and secretions for the diagnosis, exclusion and monitoring of disease.

Training Required: Five to seven years

Certification in the following subspecialty requires additional training and examination.

Dermatopathology: A dermatopathologist has the expertise to diagnose and monitor diseases of the skin including infectious, immunologic, degenerative and neoplastic diseases. This entails the examination and interpretation of specially prepared tissue sections, cellular scrapings and smears of skin lesions by means of routine and special (electron and flourescent) microscopes.

PATHOLOGY

New England

Bhan, Atul K MD [Path] - **Spec Exp:** Immunopathology; Liver Pathology; Liver Cancer; **Hospital:** Mass Genl Hosp; **Address:** Mass Genl Hosp, Dept Pathology, 55 Fruit St, Warren 501, Boston, MA 02114-2620; **Phone:** 617-726-2588; **Board Cert:** Anatomic Pathology 1976; Immunopathology 1985; **Med School:** India 1965; **Resid:** Pathology, Boston Univ Hosp 1971; Pathology, Chldns Univ Hosp 1974; **Fac Appt:** Prof Path, Harvard Med Sch

Connolly, James L MD [Path] - **Spec Exp:** Breast Pathology; Breast Cancer; **Hospital:** Beth Israel Deaconess Med Ctr - Boston, Brigham and Women's Hosp (page 57); **Address:** BIDMC-Dept of Anatomic Pathology, 330 Brookline Ave, Ste E106, Boston, MA 02215; **Phone:** 617-667-5754; **Board Cert:** Anatomic Pathology 1980; **Med School:** Vanderbilt Univ 1974; **Resid:** Anatomic Pathology, Beth Israel Deaconess Med Ctr 1978; **Fac Appt:** Prof Path, Harvard Med Sch

De Las Morenas, Antonio MD [Path] - **Spec Exp:** Thyroid Disorders; Gynecologic Pathology; Breast Pathology; **Hospital:** Boston Med Ctr; **Address:** Boston Med Ctr, 670 Albany St Fl 3rd - Ste 307, Boston, MA 02118; **Phone:** 617-414-5059; **Board Cert:** Pathology 1989; Cytopathology 1990; **Med School:** Spain 1978; **Resid:** Anatomic Pathology, Mallory Inst 1987; **Fellow:** Cytopathology, Hosp UPenn 1988; **Fac Appt:** Prof Path, Boston Univ

Fletcher, Christopher DM MD [Path] - **Spec Exp:** Soft Tissue Tumors; Sarcoma; Surgical Pathology; **Hospital:** Brigham and Women's Hosp (page 57), Dana-Farber Cancer Inst (page 57); **Address:** Brigham & Women's Hosp, Dept Pathology, 75 Francis St, Boston, MA 02115-6110; **Phone:** 617-732-8558; **Med School:** England, UK 1981; **Resid:** Pathology, St Thomas Hosp 1985; **Fellow:** Pathology, St Thomas Hosp 1986; **Fac Appt:** Prof Path, Harvard Med Sch

Gottlieb, Geoffrey J MD [Path] - **Spec Exp:** Dermatopathology; Melanoma; **Address:** StrataDx & Strata Pathology Services, One Cranberry Hill, Ste 303, Lexington, MA 02421; **Phone:** 617-252-6880; **Board Cert:** Anatomic Pathology 1979; Dermatopathology 1982; **Med School:** Cornell Univ-Weill Med Coll 1976; **Resid:** Pathology, NY Hosp-Cornell Med Ctr 1979; **Fellow:** Dermatopathology, NYU Med Ctr 1982

Harris, Nancy L MD [Path] - **Spec Exp:** Lymphoma; Hematopathology; **Hospital:** Mass Genl Hosp; **Address:** Mass Genl Hosp, Dept Pathology, 55 Fruit St, Warren-2, Boston, MA 02114; **Phone:** 617-726-5155; **Board Cert:** Anatomic & Clinical Pathology 1978; **Med School:** Stanford Univ 1970; **Resid:** Pathology, Beth Israel Hosp 1978; **Fellow:** Immunopathology, Mass Genl Hosp 1980; **Fac Appt:** Prof Path, Harvard Med Sch

Kaufman, Richard Max MD [Path] - **Spec Exp:** Transfusion Medicine; **Hospital:** Brigham and Women's Hosp (page 57), Dana-Farber Cancer Inst (page 57); **Address:** Brigham & Women's Hosp, 75 Francis St, Boston, MA 02115; **Phone:** 617-732-4749; **Board Cert:** Clinical Pathology 2000; Blood Banking Transfusion Medicine 2002; **Med School:** Washington Univ, St Louis 1992; **Resid:** Pathology, Washington Univ 2000; **Fellow:** Blood Banking Transfusion Medicine, Washington Univ 2001; **Fac Appt:** Asst Prof Path, Harvard Med Sch

Mark, Eugene J MD [Path] - **Spec Exp:** Pulmonary Pathology; Forensic Pathology; Occupational Lung Disease; Lung Pathology-Rare Tumors; **Hospital:** Mass Genl Hosp; **Address:** Mass Genl Hosp, Dept Path, 55 Fruit St, Warren 246, Boston, MA 02114; **Phone:** 617-726-8891; **Board Cert:** Anatomic & Clinical Pathology 1973; Dermatopathology 1975; **Med School:** Harvard Med Sch 1967; **Resid:** Pathology, Mass Genl Hosp 1972; **Fellow:** Pathology, Kantonspital 1966; **Fac Appt:** Prof Path, Harvard Med Sch

Morrow, Jon S MD/PhD [Path] - **Spec Exp:** Kidney Cancer; Colon Cancer; Breast Cancer; Hematopathology; **Hospital:** Yale-New Haven Hosp; **Address:** Yale Pathology, Bady Memorial Laboratory, 310 Cedar St, BML 140, New Haven, CT 06510; **Phone:** 203-785-3624; **Board Cert:** Pathology 1980; **Med School:** Yale Univ 1976; **Resid:** Pathology, Yale-New Haven Hosp 1978; **Fellow:** Pathology, Yale-New Haven Hosp 1980; **Fac Appt:** Prof Path, Yale Univ

O'Brien, Michael J MD [Path] - **Hospital:** Boston Med Ctr; **Address:** 670 Albany St Biosquare3 Bldg - rm 672, Boston, MA 02118; **Phone:** 617-414-5314; **Board Cert:** Anatomic Pathology 1983; Cytopathology 1997; Cytopathology ; **Med School:** Ireland 1971; **Resid:** Pathology, Univ Hosp 1976; Pathology, Boston City Hosp/Mallory Inst Path 1978; **Fellow:** Gastrointestinal Pathology, Boston City Hosp/Mallory Inst Path Inst Path 1979; **Fac Appt:** Prof Path, Boston Univ

Odze, Robert D MD [Path] - **Spec Exp:** Gastrointestinal Pathology; Liver Pathology; Esophageal Cancer; **Hospital:** Brigham and Women's Hosp (page 57); **Address:** Brigham & Women's Hosp, Dept Pathology, 75 Francis St, Boston, MA 02115; **Phone:** 617-732-7549; **Board Cert:** Anatomic Pathology 1990; **Med School:** McGill Univ 1984; **Resid:** Surgery, McGill Univ 1987; Pathology, McGill Univ 1990; **Fellow:** Gastrointestinal Pathology, New England Deaconess Med Ctr 1991; **Fac Appt:** Prof Path, Harvard Med Sch

Rennke, Helmut G MD [Path] - **Spec Exp:** Kidney Pathology; **Hospital:** Brigham and Women's Hosp (page 57); **Address:** Brigham & Womens Hosp, Dept Pathology, 75 Francis St Emory Bldg - rm AL 380, Boston, MA 02115; **Phone:** 617-732-6518; **Board Cert:** Anatomic Pathology 1980; **Med School:** Chile 1971; **Resid:** Pathology, Boston City Hosp 1974; Pathology, Peter Bent Brigham Hosp 1977; **Fac Appt:** Prof Path, Harvard Med Sch

Schnitt, Stuart J MD [Path] - **Spec Exp:** Breast Pathology; Breast Cancer; **Hospital:** Beth Israel Deaconess Med Ctr - Boston; **Address:** BIDMC-Dept of Anatomic Pathology, 330 Brookline Ave, Ste E106, Boston, MA 02215-5400; **Phone:** 617-667-4344; **Board Cert:** Anatomic & Clinical Pathology 1983; **Med School:** Albany Med Coll 1979; **Resid:** Anatomic Pathology, Beth Israel Deaconess Med Ctr 1983; **Fellow:** Surgical Pathology, Beth Israel Deaconess Med Ctr 1984; **Fac Appt:** Assoc Prof Path, Harvard Med Sch

Smith, Thomas W MD [Path] - **Spec Exp:** Neuropathology; **Hospital:** UMass Meml Med Ctr - Univ Campus; **Address:** Univ Mass Dept Pathology, Div Neuropathology, 55 Lake Ave N, Worcester, MA 01655; **Phone:** 508-856-2331; **Board Cert:** Neuropathology 1976; **Med School:** Cornell Univ 1972; **Resid:** Neuropathology, Peter Bent Brigham Hosp 1976; Radiology, Mass General Hosp 1977; **Fellow:** Anatomic Pathology, Peter Bent Brigham Hosp 1978; **Fac Appt:** Prof Path, Univ Mass Sch Med

Young, Robert H MD [Path] - **Spec Exp:** Ovarian Cancer; Gynecologic Cancer; **Hospital:** Mass Genl Hosp; **Address:** Mass General Hosp, Dept Pathology, 55 Fruit St Warren Bldg - Ste 215, Boston, MA 02114; **Phone:** 617-726-8892; **Board Cert:** Anatomic Pathology 1980; **Med School:** Ireland 1974; **Resid:** Pathology, Mass Genl Hosp 1979; Pathology, Dublin Univ 1977; **Fac Appt:** Prof Path, Harvard Med Sch

Mid Atlantic

Antonescu, Cristina R MD [Path] - **Spec Exp:** Bone Pathology; Sarcoma-Soft Tissue; Ewing's Sarcoma; **Hospital:** Meml Sloan-Kettering Cancer Ctr; **Address:** Meml Sloan Kettering Cancer Ctr, Dept Pathology, 1275 York Ave, New York, NY 10021; **Phone:** 212-639-5905; **Board Cert:** Anatomic Pathology 1998; **Med School:** Romania 1992; **Resid:** Anatomic Pathology, Lenox Hill Hosp 1996; **Fellow:** Pathology-Oncology, Meml Sloan-Kettering Canc Ctr 1997; **Fac Appt:** Assoc Prof Path, Cornell Univ-Weill Med Coll

Bagg, Adam MD [Path] - **Spec Exp:** Hematopathology; Leukemia & Lymphoma; Myelodysplastic Syndromes; **Hospital:** Hosp Univ Penn - UPHS (page 72); **Address:** Hosp Univ Penn, Dept Pathology & Lab Med, 3400 Spruce St, 7 Founders, Phildelphia, PA 19104; **Phone:** 215-662-6550; **Board Cert:** Clinical Pathology 1992; Hematology 1999; **Med School:** South Africa 1981; **Resid:** Internal Medicine, Univ Witwatersrand 1992; Clinical Pathology, Georgetown Univ 1992; **Fellow:** Hematopathology, Georgetown Univ 1993; **Fac Appt:** Prof Path, Univ Pennsylvania

Bleiweiss, Ira J MD [Path] - **Spec Exp:** Breast Pathology; Breast Cancer; **Hospital:** Mount Sinai Med Ctr (page 64); **Address:** Mt Sinai Med Ctr, Dept Pathology, 1 Gustave Levy Pl, Box 1194, New York, NY 10029-6504; **Phone:** 212-241-9159; **Board Cert:** Anatomic & Clinical Pathology 1988; **Med School:** West Indies 1984; **Resid:** Pathology, Mt Sinai Med Ctr 1988; **Fellow:** Surgical Pathology, Mt Sinai Med Ctr 1989; Surgical Pathology, Meml-Sloan Kettering Cancer Ctr 1990; **Fac Appt:** Prof Path, Mount Sinai Sch Med

Brooks, John S MD [Path] - **Spec Exp:** Bone & Soft Tissue Pathology; Sarcoma; **Hospital:** Pennsylvania Hosp-UPHS (page 72); **Address:** Pennsylvania Hospital, Preston 6 FL, 800 Spruce St, Philadelphia, PA 19107; **Phone:** 215-829-3541; **Board Cert:** Anatomic Pathology 1978; Immunopathology 1983; **Med School:** Thomas Jefferson Univ 1974; **Resid:** Pathology, Hosp Univ Penn 1978; **Fellow:** Immunopathology, Hosp Univ Penn 1978; **Fac Appt:** Prof Path, Univ Pennsylvania

Burger, Peter MD [Path] - **Spec Exp:** Brain Tumors; Neuro-Pathology; **Hospital:** Johns Hopkins Hosp (page 61); **Address:** Johns Hopkins Hosp, Div Pathology, 600 N Wolfe St, Baltimore, MD 21287; **Phone:** 410-955-8378; **Board Cert:** Anatomic Pathology 1976; Neuropathology 1976; **Med School:** Northwestern Univ 1966; **Resid:** Anatomic Pathology, Duke Univ Med Ctr 1973; **Fellow:** Neuropathology, Duke Univ Med Ctr 1973

Crawford, James M MD/PhD [Path] - **Spec Exp:** Liver Pathology; Gastrointestinal Pathology; Gastrointestinal Cancer; **Hospital:** N Shore Univ Hosp (page 67), Long Island Jewish Med Ctr (page 67); **Address:** N Shore-LIJ Laboratories, 10 Nevada Drive, Lake Success, NY 11042-1114; **Phone:** 516-719-1060; **Board Cert:** Anatomic Pathology 1987; **Med School:** Duke Univ 1982; **Resid:** Pathology, Brigham & Women's Hosp 1984; **Fellow:** Gastrointestinal Pathology, Brigham & Women's Hosp 1987; Pathology, Royal Free hosp 1989

Demetris, Anthony J MD [Path] - **Spec Exp:** Transplant Pathology; Liver Pathology; **Hospital:** UPMC Montefiore; **Address:** UPMC - Montefiore, 3459 5th Ave, rm E741, Pittsburgh, PA 15213; **Phone:** 412-647-2067; **Board Cert:** Anatomic & Clinical Pathology 1987; **Med School:** Univ Pittsburgh 1982; **Resid:** Anatomic & Clinical Pathology, Univ Pittsburgh Med Ctr 1986; **Fac Appt:** Prof Path, Univ Pittsburgh

Ehya, Hormoz MD [Path] - **Spec Exp:** Cytopathology; Breast Pathology; Lung Pathology; Fine Needle Aspiration Biopsy; **Hospital:** Fox Chase Cancer Ctr (page 58); **Address:** Fox Chase Cancer Center, 333 Cottman Ave, rm C427, Philadelphia, PA 19111-2497; **Phone:** 215-728-5389; **Board Cert:** Anatomic Pathology 1979; Cytopathology 1989; **Med School:** Iran 1974; **Resid:** Pathology, Univ Miss Med Ctr 1979; **Fellow:** Cytopathology, Meml Sloan-Kettering Cancer Ctr 1980; **Fac Appt:** Prof Path

Epstein, Jonathan MD [Path] - **Spec Exp:** Bladder Cancer; Prostate Cancer; Urologic Pathology; **Hospital:** Johns Hopkins Hosp (page 61); **Address:** 401 N Broadway, Weinberg 2242, Baltimore, MD 21231; **Phone:** 410-955-5043; **Board Cert:** Anatomic Pathology 1986; **Med School:** Boston Univ 1981; **Resid:** Pathology, Johns Hopkins Hosp 1985; **Fellow:** Pathology, Meml Sloan Kettering Cancer Ctr 1984; **Fac Appt:** Prof Path, Johns Hopkins Univ

Fogt, Franz MD/PhD [Path] - **Spec Exp:** Gastrointestinal Pathology; Ophthalmic Pathology; **Hospital:** Penn Presby Med Ctr - UPHS (page 72); **Address:** Penn Presbyterian-Dept Pathology, 51 N 39th St, W542 Wright Saunders Bldg, Philadelphia, PA 19104; **Phone:** 215-662-8077; **Board Cert:** Anatomic & Clinical Pathology 1995; **Med School:** Germany 1988; **Resid:** Anatomic & Clinical Pathology, New England Deaconess Hosp 1995; **Fellow:** Gastrointestinal Pathology, New England Deaconess Hosp 1996; **Fac Appt:** Prof Path, Univ Pennsylvania

Gupta, Prabodh K MD [Path] - **Spec Exp:** Lung Pathology; Cervical Cancer; Fine Needle Aspiration Biopsy; **Hospital:** Hosp Univ Penn - UPHS (page 72); **Address:** 3400 Spruce St, Philadelphia, PA 19104; **Phone:** 215-662-3238; **Board Cert:** Anatomic Pathology 1975; Cytopathology 1989; **Med School:** India 1960; **Resid:** Pathology, All India Inst Med Scis 1967; **Fellow:** Pathology, Mass Genl Hosp 1968; Cytopathology, Johns Hopkins Hosp 1969; **Fac Appt:** Prof Path, Univ Pennsylvania

Heller, Debra S MD [Path] - **Spec Exp:** Gynecologic Pathology; Pediatric Pathology; Perinatal Pathology; **Hospital:** Univ Hosp-UMDNJ—Newark; **Address:** UMDNJ-NJ Med Sch Dept Pathology, 185 S Orange Ave, UH/E158, Newark, NJ 07101; **Phone:** 973-972-0751; **Board Cert:** Anatomic Pathology 1988; Obstetrics & Gynecology 2011; Pediatric Pathology 1999; **Med School:** NY Med Coll 1977; **Resid:** Obstetrics & Gynecology, Beth Israel Med Ctr 1981; Anatomic Pathology, Mt Sinai Med Ctr 1988; **Fellow:** Pediatric Pathology, Mt Sinai Med Ctr 1987; Gynecologic Pathology, Mt Sinai Med Ctr 1989; **Fac Appt:** Prof Path, UMDNJ-NJ Med Sch, Newark

Hoda, Syed A MD [Path] - **Spec Exp:** Breast Cancer; Surgical Pathology; **Hospital:** NY-Presby/Weill Cornell Med Ctr, NY (page 66); **Address:** 525 E 68th St, 1028 Starr, New York, NY 10021-4870; **Phone:** 212-746-2700; **Board Cert:** Anatomic & Clinical Pathology 1990; Cytopathology 1991; Pathology 2001; **Med School:** Pakistan 1984; **Resid:** Anatomic & Clinical Pathology, Tulane Univ Affil Hosps 1990; **Fellow:** Cytopathology, Meml Sloan Kettering Cancer Ctr 1991; Pathology, Meml Sloan Kettering Cancer Ctr 1992; **Fac Appt:** Clin Prof Path, Cornell Univ-Weill Med Coll

Hruban, Ralph H MD [Path] - **Spec Exp:** Gastrointestinal Pathology; Pancreatic Cancer; **Hospital:** Johns Hopkins Hosp (page 61); **Address:** Johns Hopkins Hosp, Dept Pathology, 401 N Broadway, Weinberg Bldg - rm 2242, Baltimore, MD 21231; **Phone:** 410-955-2163; **Board Cert:** Anatomic Pathology 1990; **Med School:** Johns Hopkins Univ 1985; **Resid:** Pathology, Johns Hopkins Hosp 1990; **Fellow:** Anatomic Pathology, Meml Sloan-Kettering Cancer Ctr 1989; **Fac Appt:** Prof Path, Johns Hopkins Univ

Jones, Robert V MD [Path] - **Spec Exp:** Neuro-Pathology; Brain Tumors; **Hospital:** G Washington Univ Hosp; **Address:** GWUMC, Dept Path, 2300 I (Eye) St NW, Ross Hall, Ste 502, Washington, DC 20037; **Phone:** 202-994-3391; **Board Cert:** Anatomic & Clinical Pathology 1981; Neuropathology 1994; **Med School:** Univ VA Sch Med 1977; **Resid:** Anatomic & Clinical Pathology, Walter Reed AMC 1981; **Fellow:** Neurological Pathology, ARmed Forces Inst Path 1990; **Fac Appt:** Assoc Prof Path, Geo Wash Univ

Kahn, Leonard B MD [Path] - **Spec Exp:** Bone Pathology; Head & Neck Pathology; Soft Tissue Tumors; Jaw Tumors; **Hospital:** Long Island Jewish Med Ctr (page 67), N Shore Univ Hosp (page 67); **Address:** 6 Ohio Drive, Ste 202, rm 621, Lake Success, NY 10042; **Phone:** 516-304-7264; **Board Cert:** Anatomic Pathology 1980; **Med School:** South Africa 1960; **Resid:** Pathology, Univ Cape Town 1966; **Fellow:** Pathology, Washington Univ 1969; **Fac Appt:** Prof Path, Albert Einstein Coll Med

Pathology

Katzenstein, Anna-Luise A MD [Path] - **Spec Exp:** Lung Cancer; Pulmonary Pathology; Interstitial Lung Disease; **Hospital:** SUNY Upstate Med Univ Shos; **Address:** SUNY Upstate Medical Univ, 750 E Adams St, UH Bldg, rm 6709, Syracuse, NY 13210; **Phone:** 315-464-7125; **Board Cert:** Anatomic Pathology 1976; **Med School:** Johns Hopkins Univ 1971; **Resid:** Pathology, Univ Hosp 1975; **Fellow:** Surgical Pathology, Barnes Hosp-Wash Univ 1976; **Fac Appt:** Prof Path, SUNY Upstate Med Univ

Klimstra, David MD [Path] - **Spec Exp:** Gastrointestinal Pathology; Pulmonary Pathology; **Hospital:** Meml Sloan-Kettering Cancer Ctr; **Address:** Meml Sloan Kettering Canc Ctr, Dept Pathology, 1275 York Ave, New York, NY 10065; **Phone:** 212-639-2410; **Board Cert:** Anatomic Pathology 1992; **Med School:** Yale Univ 1988; **Resid:** Pathology, Yale New Haven Hosp 1991; **Fellow:** Pathology, Meml Sloan Kettering Canc Ctr 1992; **Fac Appt:** Asst Prof Path, Cornell Univ

Kurman, Robert J MD [Path] - **Spec Exp:** Gynecologic Pathology; Ovarian Cancer; Uterine Cancer; **Hospital:** Johns Hopkins Hosp (page 61); **Address:** Johns Hopkins Hosp, Div Gyn Pathology, 401 N Broadway, Weinberg 2242, Baltimore, MD 21231; **Phone:** 443-287-4996; **Board Cert:** Anatomic Pathology 1972; Obstetrics & Gynecology 1980; **Med School:** SUNY Upstate Med Univ 1968; **Resid:** Pathology, Peter Bent Brigham Hosp/Mass Genl Hosp 1977; Obstetrics & Gynecology, LAC Hosp/USC 1978; **Fellow:** Obstetrics & Gynecology, Harvard Univ 1973; **Fac Appt:** Prof Path, Johns Hopkins Univ

Li Volsi, Virginia A MD [Path] - **Spec Exp:** Endocrine Cancers; Thyroid Cancer; Gynecologic Cancer; **Hospital:** Hosp Univ Penn - UPHS (page 72); **Address:** Hosp Univ Penn - Pathology, 3400 Spruce St, Founders Bldg Fl 6 - rm 6009, Philadelphia, PA 19104; **Phone:** 215-662-6545; **Board Cert:** Anatomic Pathology 1974; **Med School:** Columbia P&S 1969; **Resid:** Anatomic Pathology, Presbyterian Hosp 1974; **Fac Appt:** Prof Path, Univ Pennsylvania

Melamed, Jonathan MD [Path] - **Spec Exp:** Prostate Cancer; Tumor Banking-Prostate; **Hospital:** NYU Langone Med Ctr (page 68); **Address:** NYU Medical Ctr, Dept Pathology, TH-461, 560 First Ave, New York, NY 10016; **Phone:** 212-263-8927; **Board Cert:** Anatomic & Clinical Pathology 1992; **Med School:** South Africa 1985; **Resid:** Pathology, Lenox Hill Hosp 1991; **Fellow:** Pathology, Meml Sloan Kettering Cancer Ctr 1992; Urologic Pathology, Meml Sloan Kettering Cancer Ctr 1993; **Fac Appt:** Assoc Prof Path, NYU Sch Med

Mies, Carolyn MD [Path] - **Spec Exp:** Breast Cancer; Breast Pathology; **Hospital:** Hosp Univ Penn - UPHS (page 72); **Address:** Hosp Univ Penn-Surgical Pathology, 3400 Spruce St, 6 Founders, Philadelphia, PA 19104; **Phone:** 215-662-6503; **Board Cert:** Anatomic Pathology 1984; **Med School:** Rush Med Coll 1980; **Resid:** Pathology, Tufts-New England Med Ctr 1982; Pathology, New England Deaconess Hosp 1984; **Fellow:** Surgical Pathology, Meml Sloan Kettering Cancer Ctr 1986; **Fac Appt:** Assoc Prof Path, Univ Pennsylvania

Montgomery, Elizabeth A MD [Path] - **Spec Exp:** Barrett's Esophagus; Gastrointestinal Pathology; Soft Tissue Pathology; **Hospital:** Johns Hopkins Hosp (page 61); **Address:** Johns Hopkins Univ, Dept Pathology, 401 N Broadway Weinberg Bldg - rm 2242, Baltimore, MD 21231; **Phone:** 410-614-2308; **Board Cert:** Anatomic Pathology 1988; Cytopathology 1994; **Med School:** Geo Wash Univ 1984; **Resid:** Pathology, Walter Reed AMC 1988; **Fac Appt:** Prof Path, Johns Hopkins Univ

Orazi, Attilio MD [Path] - **Spec Exp:** Hematopathology; Bone Marrow Pathology; Lymph Node Pathology; Spleen Pathology; **Hospital:** NY-Presby/Weill Cornell Med Ctr, NY (page 66); **Address:** NY Presby-Cornell Medical Ctr, 525 E 68th St, Starr Pavilion, rm 707, New York, NY 10065; **Phone:** 212-746-2050; **Board Cert:** Anatomic Pathology 1997; Hematology 1998; **Med School:** Italy 1979; **Resid:** Internal Medicine, Leicester Royal Infirmary 1982; Histopathology, Northampton Genl Hosp 1983; **Fellow:** Anatomic Pathology, Natl Cancer Inst 1985; **Fac Appt:** Prof Path, Cornell Univ-Weill Med Coll

Patchefsky, Arthur S MD [Path] - **Spec Exp:** Breast Cancer; Pulmonary Pathology; Sarcoma; **Hospital:** Fox Chase Cancer Ctr (page 58); **Address:** Fox Chase Cancer Center, 333 Cottman Ave, rm C433, Philadelphia, PA 19111; **Phone:** 215-728-5390; **Board Cert:** Anatomic Pathology 1969; **Med School:** Hahnemann Univ 1963; **Resid:** Pathology, John Hopkins Hosp 1966; Pathology, Hosp Univ Penn 1967; **Fellow:** Pathology, Meml Sloan Kettering Cancer Ctr 1968; **Fac Appt:** Prof Path, Thomas Jefferson Univ

Reuter, Victor E MD [Path] - **Spec Exp:** Prostate Cancer; Genitourinary Pathology; Bladder Cancer; Testicular Cancer; **Hospital:** Meml Sloan-Kettering Cancer Ctr; **Address:** Memorial Sloan Kettering Cancer Ctr, Dept Pathology, 1275 York Ave, New York, NY 10021; **Phone:** 212-639-8225; **Board Cert:** Anatomic & Clinical Pathology 1983; **Med School:** Dominican Republic 1978; **Resid:** Anatomic Pathology, Thos Jefferson Univ Hosp 1981; Clinical Pathology, Thos Jefferson Univ Hosp 1983; **Fellow:** Surgical Pathology, Meml Sloan Kettering Cancer Ctr 1985; **Fac Appt:** Prof Path, Cornell Univ-Weill Med Coll

Rosenblum, Marc K MD [Path] - **Spec Exp:** Neuropathology; Brain Tumors; **Hospital:** Meml Sloan-Kettering Cancer Ctr; **Address:** 1275 York Ave, Meml Sloan-Kettering Cancer Ctr, New York, NY 10065; **Phone:** 212-639-3844; **Board Cert:** Anatomic Pathology 1984; Neuropathology 1988; **Med School:** Univ Miami Sch Med 1979; **Resid:** Anatomic Pathology, Mt Sinai Med Ctr 1984; **Fellow:** Pathology, Meml Sloan-Kettering Cancer Ctr 1985; Neurological Pathology, Bellevue-NYU Med Ctr 1987; **Fac Appt:** Prof Path, Cornell Univ-Weill Med Coll

Ross, Jeffrey S MD [Path] - **Spec Exp:** Urologic Cancer; Prostate Cancer; Breast Cancer; **Hospital:** Albany Med Ctr; **Address:** Albany Med Coll, Dept Path, 47 New Scotland Ave, MC 81, Albany, NY 12208; **Phone:** 518-262-5471; **Board Cert:** Anatomic & Clinical Pathology 1974; **Med School:** SUNY Buffalo 1970; **Resid:** Pathology, Mass Genl Hosp 1974; **Fellow:** Pathology, Harvard Med Sch 1974; **Fac Appt:** Prof Path, Albany Med Coll

Sanchez, Miguel A MD [Path] - **Spec Exp:** Breast Cancer; Thyroid Cancer; **Hospital:** Englewood Hosp & Med Ctr; **Address:** 350 Engle St, Dean Bldg - Fl LL1, Englewood, NJ 07631-1898; **Phone:** 201-894-3423; **Board Cert:** Anatomic Pathology 1975; Clinical Pathology 1979; Cytopathology 1991; **Med School:** Spain 1969; **Resid:** Pathology, Englewood Hosp 1972; Pathology, Temple Univ 1973; **Fellow:** Pathology, Meml Sloan Kettering Cancer Ctr 1974; Clinical Pathology, St Vincents Hosp 1975; **Fac Appt:** Assoc Prof Path, Mount Sinai Sch Med

Schiller, Alan L MD [Path] - **Spec Exp:** Bone & Joint Pathology; Soft Tissue Pathology; Bone Tumors; **Hospital:** Mount Sinai Med Ctr (page 64); **Address:** Mt Sinai Sch Med, Dept Pathology, 1 Gustave Levy Pl, Box 1194, New York, NY 10029-6500; **Phone:** 212-241-8014; **Board Cert:** Anatomic Pathology 1973; **Med School:** Ros Franklin Univ/Chicago Med Sch 1967; **Resid:** Pathology, Mass Genl Hosp 1972; **Fac Appt:** Prof Emeritus Path, Mount Sinai Sch Med

Silverman, Jan F MD [Path] - **Spec Exp:** Fine Needle Aspiration Biopsy; Surgical Pathology; Gastrointestinal Pathology; Cytopathology; **Hospital:** Allegheny General Hosp, West Penn Hosp-Forbes Campus; **Address:** Allegheny Gen Hosp-Dept Lab Medicine, 320 E North Ave, Pittsburgh, PA 15212; **Phone:** 412-359-6886; **Board Cert:** Anatomic & Clinical Pathology 1975; Cytopathology 1989; **Med School:** Med Coll VA 1970; **Resid:** Pathology, Med Coll Virginia Hosps 1975; **Fellow:** Surgical Pathology, Med Coll Virginia 1975; **Fac Appt:** Prof Path, Drexel Univ Coll Med

Soslow, Robert A MD [Path] - **Spec Exp:** Gynecologic Pathology; **Hospital:** Meml Sloan-Kettering Cancer Ctr; **Address:** 1275 York Avenue, Pathology Department, New York, NY 10065; **Phone:** 800-525-2225; **Board Cert:** Anatomic Pathology 1995; **Med School:** Univ Pennsylvania 1991; **Resid:** Anatomic Pathology, Stanford Univ Med Ctr 1994; **Fellow:** Immunopathology, Stanford Univ Med Ctr 1995; **Fac Appt:** Assoc Prof Path, Cornell Univ

Pathology

Swerdlow, Steven H MD [Path] - **Spec Exp:** Lymphoma; Hematopathology; Transplant Pathology; **Hospital:** UPMC Presby, Pittsburgh; **Address:** Div Hematopathology, 200 Lothrop St, Ste G-300, Pittsburgh, PA 15213-2536; **Phone:** 412-647-5191; **Board Cert:** Anatomic & Clinical Pathology 2005; **Med School:** Harvard Med Sch 1975; **Resid:** Pathology, Beth Israel Hosp 1979; **Fellow:** Hematopathology, Vanderbilt Univ 1981; Hematopathology, St Bartholmew's Hosp 1983; **Fac Appt:** Prof Path, Univ Pittsburgh

Tomaszewski, John E MD [Path] - **Spec Exp:** Kidney Pathology; Genitourinary Pathology; Immunopathology; **Hospital:** Buffalo General Hosp; **Address:** Pathology and Anatomical Sciences, 206 Farber Hall, 3435 Main St, Buffalo, NY 14214; **Phone:** 716-352-7370; **Board Cert:** Anatomic Pathology 1982; Immunopathology 1983; **Med School:** Univ Pennsylvania 1977; **Resid:** Pathology, Hosp Univ Penn 1982; **Fellow:** Surgical Pathology, Univ Penn 1983; Renal Pathology, Columbia Univ 1984; **Fac Appt:** Prof Path, SUNY Buffalo

Tornos, Carmen MD [Path] - **Spec Exp:** Gynecologic Cancer; Breast Cancer; Ovarian Cancer; **Hospital:** Stony Brook Univ Med Ctr; **Address:** Stony Brook Univ Hosp, Dept Pathology, Level 2, rm 766, Stony Brook, NY 11794; **Phone:** 631-444-2222; **Board Cert:** Anatomic & Clinical Pathology 1989; **Med School:** Spain 1977; **Resid:** Hematology, Ciudad Sanitaria Valle de Hebron 1982; Anatomic & Clinical Pathology, Univ Texas HSC 1989; **Fellow:** Surgical Pathology, MD Anderson Cancer Ctr 1990; **Fac Appt:** Prof Path, SUNY Stony Brook

Travis, William D MD [Path] - **Spec Exp:** Pulmonary Pathology; Lung Cancer; Interstitial Lung Disease; **Hospital:** Meml Sloan-Kettering Cancer Ctr; **Address:** 1275 York Ave, MSKCC Bldg, Pathology Dept, New York, NY 10065; **Phone:** 212-639-6364; **Board Cert:** Anatomic & Clinical Pathology 1985; **Med School:** Univ Fla Coll Med 1981; **Resid:** Anatomic Pathology, New England Deaconess Hosp 1983; Clinical Pathology, Mayo Clinic 1985; **Fellow:** Surgical Pathology, Mayo Clinic 1986

Wang, Beverly Y MD [Path] - **Spec Exp:** Head & Neck Pathology; **Hospital:** Beth Israel Med Ctr - Petrie Division (page 56); **Address:** Beth Israel Medical Ctr, Dept Pathology, First Avenue at 16th St, Silver Bldg Fl 11, New York, NY 10003; **Phone:** 212-844-1959; **Board Cert:** Anatomic Pathology 1998; Cytopathology 1999; **Med School:** China 1982; **Resid:** Pathology, Mount Sinai Med Ctr 1998; **Fellow:** Cytopathology, Mount Sinai Med Ctr 1999; **Fac Appt:** Prof Path, Albert Einstein Coll Med

Yousem, Samuel A MD [Path] - **Spec Exp:** Pulmonary Pathology; Transplant-Lung (Pathology); Lung Cancer; **Hospital:** UPMC Presby, Pittsburgh; **Address:** UPMC Presbyterian Hosp, Dept Pathology, 200 Lothrop St, A-610, Pittsburgh, PA 15213; **Phone:** 412-647-6193; **Board Cert:** Anatomic Pathology 1985; Cytopathology 1997; **Med School:** Univ MD Sch Med 1981; **Resid:** Pathology, Stanford Univ Med Ctr 1983; **Fellow:** Surgical Pathology, Stanford Univ 1984; **Fac Appt:** Prof Path, Univ Pittsburgh

Zagzag, David MD/PhD [Path] - **Spec Exp:** Neuropathology; Brain Tumors; Tumor Banking-Brain; **Hospital:** NYU Langone Med Ctr (page 68), Bellevue Hosp Ctr; **Address:** NYU Med Ctr, Dept Pathology, 550 First Ave, Div Neuropathology, NB-4N30, New York, NY 10016; **Phone:** 212-263-6449; **Board Cert:** Anatomic Pathology 1993; Neuropathology 1993; **Med School:** France 1984; **Resid:** Surgical Pathology, NYU Med Ctr 1990; **Fellow:** Neurological Pathology, NYU Med Ctr 1992; **Fac Appt:** Assoc Prof Path, NYU Sch Med

Southeast

Banks, Peter MD [Path] - **Spec Exp:** Hematopathology; Lymphoma; **Hospital:** Carolinas Med Ctr; **Address:** Dept Pathology, 1000 Blythe Blvd Fl 4, Charlotte, NC 28203; **Phone:** 704-355-2251; **Board Cert:** Anatomic Pathology 2008; **Med School:** Harvard Med Sch 1971; **Resid:** Pathology, National Cancer Inst 1974; Pathology, Duke Univ Med Ctr 1975; **Fellow:** Surgical Pathology, Univ Minn Med Ctr 1976; **Fac Appt:** Prof Path, Univ NC Sch Med

Bostwick, David MD [Path] - **Spec Exp:** Urologic Pathology; Prostate Cancer; Bladder Cancer; Gastrointestinal Pathology; **Address:** 4355 Innslake Drive, Glen Allen, VA 23060; **Phone:** 804-967-9225; **Board Cert:** Anatomic Pathology 2003; **Med School:** Univ MD Sch Med 1979; **Resid:** Pathology, Stanford Univ Med Ctr 1981; **Fellow:** Surgical Pathology, Stanford Univ Med Ctr 1984

Chesney, Carolyn M MD [Path] - **Spec Exp:** Hematopathology; Bleeding/Coagulation Disorders; **Hospital:** Baptist Memorial Hospital-Memphis; **Address:** Pathology Group of the MidSouth, 7550 Wolf River Blvd, Ste 200, Germantown, TN 38138; **Phone:** 901-542-6800; **Board Cert:** Internal Medicine 1972; Hematology 1999; **Med School:** Vanderbilt Univ 1968; **Resid:** Internal Medicine, Vanderbilt Univ Hosp 1970; **Fellow:** Hematology, Mass Genl Hosp 1972; **Fac Appt:** Prof Med, Univ Tenn Coll Med

Cote, Richard J MD [Path] - **Spec Exp:** Lymph Node Pathology; Bladder Cancer; Breast Cancer; **Hospital:** Univ of Miami Hosp; **Address:** 1120 NW 14th St, CRB Bldg - Ste 1416, Miami, FL 33136; **Phone:** 305-243-2683; **Board Cert:** Anatomic Pathology 1987; **Med School:** Univ Chicago-Pritzker Sch Med 1980; **Resid:** Pathology, New York Hosp 1987; **Fellow:** Pathology, Meml Sloan-Kettering Cancer Ctr 1990; **Fac Appt:** Prof Path, USC-Keck School of Medicine

Faye-Petersen, Ona MD [Path] - **Spec Exp:** Perinatal Pathology; Fetal Pathology; Neonatal Pathology; Pediatric Pathology; **Hospital:** Univ of Ala Hosp at Birmingham, UAB Highlands Hosp; **Address:** UAB Dept Pathology, 619 19th St S, NP 3547, Birmingham, AL 35249; **Phone:** 205-975-8880; **Board Cert:** Anatomic & Clinical Pathology 1987; Pediatric Pathology 1991; **Med School:** Univ Colorado 1980; **Resid:** Pathology, Presby-Denver Hosp 1985; **Fellow:** Surgical Pathology, Meml Sloan Ketter Cancer Ctr 1986; Pediatric Pathology, Mt Sinai Hosp 1987; **Fac Appt:** Prof Path, Univ Alabama

Lage, Janice M MD [Path] - **Spec Exp:** Obstetric Pathology; Gynecologic Pathology; Breast Pathology; **Hospital:** MUSC Med Ctr; **Address:** MUSC Med Ctr, Pathology Dept, 171 Ashley Ave, MS 908, Charleston, SC 29425; **Phone:** 843-792-3121; **Board Cert:** Anatomic Pathology 1985; **Med School:** Washington Univ, St Louis 1980; **Resid:** Pathology, Barnes Hosp/Wash Univ 1982; Obstetrics & Gynecology, Barnes Hosp/Wash Univ 1983; **Fellow:** Surgical Pathology, Barnes Hosp/Wash Univ 1984; **Fac Appt:** Prof Path, Med Univ SC

Masood, Shahla MD [Path] - **Spec Exp:** Breast Cancer; Breast Pathology; **Hospital:** Shands Jacksonville Med Ctr; **Address:** Univ of Florida, Dept Pathology, 655 W 8th St, Jacksonville, FL 32209-6511; **Phone:** 904-244-4387; **Board Cert:** Anatomic & Clinical Pathology 1977; Cytopathology 1990; **Med School:** Iran 1973; **Resid:** Anatomic Pathology, Univ Hosp 1977; **Fac Appt:** Prof Path, Univ Fla Coll Med

Mills, Stacey E MD [Path] - **Spec Exp:** Breast Pathology; Ear, Nose & Throat Pathology; Surgical Pathology; Bone Pathology; **Hospital:** Univ of Virginia Health Sys; **Address:** 1215 Lee St, rm 3022, PO Box 800214, Charlottesville, VA 22908-0214; **Phone:** 434-982-4406; **Board Cert:** Anatomic Pathology 2009; **Med School:** Univ VA Sch Med 1977; **Resid:** Pathology, Univ Virginia Med Ctr 1980; **Fellow:** Pathology, Univ Virginia Med Ctr 1981; **Fac Appt:** Prof Path, Univ VA Sch Med

Pathology

Nicosia, Santo MD [Path] - **Spec Exp:** Ovarian Cancer; Cytopathology; **Hospital:** H Lee Moffitt Cancer Ctr & Research Inst (page 59); **Address:** 12901 Bruce B Downs Blvd, MDC Box 11, Tampa, FL 33612-4742; **Phone:** 813-974-3133; **Board Cert:** Anatomic Pathology 1978; Cytopathology 1990; **Med School:** Italy 1967; **Resid:** Anatomic Pathology, Michael Reese Hosp 1972; **Fellow:** Hosp Univ Penn 1973; **Fac Appt:** Prof Path, Univ S Fla Coll Med

Norenberg, Michael D MD [Path] - **Spec Exp:** Liver Pathology; Parkinson's Disease; **Hospital:** Jackson Meml Hosp; **Address:** Jackson Meml Hosp, Dept Pathology, 1611 NW 12th Ave Holtz Ctr, rm 2142, Miami, FL 33136; **Phone:** 305-585-7017; **Board Cert:** Anatomic Pathology 1972; Neuropathology 1974; **Med School:** Univ Rochester 1965; **Resid:** Pathology, Strong Meml Hosp 1970; **Fellow:** Neuropathology, Strong Meml Hosp 1972; **Fac Appt:** Prof Path, Univ Miami Sch Med

Petito, Carol K MD [Path] - **Spec Exp:** Neuro-Pathology; **Hospital:** Jackson Meml Hosp; **Address:** Univ Miami Dept Pathology (R-5), 1550 NW 10th Ave, PAP Bldg, rm 417, Miami, FL 33136; **Phone:** 305-585-8970; **Board Cert:** Anatomic Pathology 1973; Neuropathology 1973; **Med School:** Columbia P&S 1967; **Resid:** Pathology, NY Hosp-Cornell Med Ctr 1970; Neuropathology, Armed Forces Inst; **Fac Appt:** Prof Path, Univ Miami Sch Med

Rosenberg, Andrew E MD [Path] - **Spec Exp:** Bone & Joint Pathology; **Hospital:** Univ of Miami Hosp; **Address:** University of Miami Hosp, 1400 NW 12th Ave, rm 4076, Miami, FL 33136; **Phone:** 305-243-8730; **Board Cert:** Anatomic Pathology 1985; **Med School:** Temple Univ 1981; **Resid:** Anatomic Pathology, Mass Genl Hosp 1984; **Fellow:** Immunopathology, Mass Genl Hosp 1985

Sewell, C Whitaker MD [Path] - **Spec Exp:** Breast Pathology; Surgical Pathology; **Hospital:** Emory Univ Hosp; **Address:** Emory Univ Hosp, Dept Pathology, 1364 Clifton Rd NE, rm H185C, Atlanta, GA 30322; **Phone:** 404-712-7003; **Board Cert:** Anatomic & Clinical Pathology 1974; **Med School:** Emory Univ 1969; **Resid:** Pathology, Emory Univ Hosp 1974; **Fac Appt:** Prof Path, Emory Univ

Weiss, Sharon A W MD [Path] - **Spec Exp:** Soft Tissue Pathology; Surgical Pathology; Sarcoma; **Hospital:** Emory Univ Hosp; **Address:** Emory Univ Hosp, Dept Pathology, 1364 Clifton Rd NE, rm H176, Atlanta, GA 30322; **Phone:** 404-712-0708; **Board Cert:** Anatomic Pathology 1974; **Med School:** Johns Hopkins Univ 1971; **Resid:** Pathology, Johns Hopkins Hosp 1975; **Fac Appt:** Prof Path, Emory Univ

Midwest

Allred, D Craig MD [Path] - **Spec Exp:** Breast Cancer; Breast Pathology; Breast Cancer Risk Assessment; **Hospital:** Barnes-Jewish Hosp; **Address:** Washington Univ Sch Med, Path & Immunology, 660 S Euclid Ave, Box 8118, St Louis, MO 63110; **Phone:** 314-362-6313; **Board Cert:** Anatomic Pathology 1984; **Med School:** Univ Utah 1979; **Resid:** Anatomic Pathology, Univ Conn Hlth Ctr 1983; **Fellow:** Immunopathology, Univ Conn Hlth Ctr 1982; **Fac Appt:** Prof Path, Baylor Coll Med

Appelman, Henry MD [Path] - **Spec Exp:** Gastrointestinal Pathology; Liver Pathology; **Hospital:** Univ of Michigan Hosp; **Address:** 1301 Catherine St, rm M5220, Box 5602, Ann Arbor, MI 48109-5602; **Phone:** 734-936-6770; **Board Cert:** Anatomic & Clinical Pathology 1966; **Med School:** Univ Mich Med Sch 1961; **Resid:** Pathology, Univ Mich Med Ctr 1966; **Fac Appt:** Prof Path, Univ Mich Med Sch

Balla, Andre K MD/PhD [Path] - **Spec Exp:** Prostate Cancer; Gynecologic Pathology; Tumor Banking; **Hospital:** Univ of IL Med Ctr at Chicago; **Address:** Univ Illinois Chicago, Dept Pathology, 840 S Wood St, 130 CSN Bldg, MC 847, Chicago, IL 60612; **Phone:** 312-996-3879; **Board Cert:** Anatomic & Clinical Pathology 1988; **Med School:** Brazil 1972; **Resid:** Pathology, Hahnemann Univ Hosp 1988; **Fellow:** Clinical Immunology, Scripps Clin Rsch Fdn 1981; **Fac Appt:** Prof Path, Univ IL Coll Med

Behm, Frederick G MD [Path] - **Spec Exp:** Hematopathology; **Hospital:** Univ of IL Med Ctr at Chicago; **Address:** Univ Illinois Chicago, Dept Pathology, 840 S Wood St, 130 CSN Bldg, MC 847, Chicago, IL 60612-7335; **Phone:** 312-996-3150; **Board Cert:** Anatomic & Clinical Pathology 1980; Hematology 1983; **Med School:** Med Coll Wisc 1974; **Resid:** Pathology, Med Coll of VA Hosp 1979; **Fac Appt:** Prof Path, Univ IL Coll Med

Bell, Debra A MD [Path] - **Spec Exp:** Gynecologic Pathology; Ovarian Cancer; **Hospital:** Mayo Med Ctr & Clin - Rochester; **Address:** Mayo Clinic-Pathology Dept, 200 First St SW, Rochester, MN 55905; **Phone:** 507-284-1800; **Board Cert:** Anatomic Pathology 1980; Cytopathology 1989; **Med School:** Albany Med Coll 1976; **Resid:** Pathology, NYU Med Ctr 1981; **Fellow:** Cytopathology, Meml Sloan Kettering Cancer Ctr 1982; **Fac Appt:** Assoc Prof Path, Mayo Med Sch

Cho, Kathleen R MD [Path] - **Spec Exp:** Gynecologic Pathology; Ovarian Cancer; Cervical Cancer; **Hospital:** Univ of Michigan Hosp; **Address:** Univ Michigan Med Sch, 109 Zina Pitcher Pl, rm 1506, Ann Arbor, MI 48109-2200; **Phone:** 734-764-1549; **Board Cert:** Anatomic Pathology 1990; **Med School:** Vanderbilt Univ 1984; **Resid:** Pathology, Johns Hopkins Hosp 1988; **Fellow:** Gynecologic Pathology, Johns Hopkins Hosp 1990; **Fac Appt:** Prof Path, Univ Mich Med Sch

Dahmoush, Laila MD [Path] - **Spec Exp:** Breast Pathology; Gynecologic Pathology; Urologic Pathology; **Hospital:** Univ Iowa Hosp & Clinics; **Address:** UIHC Dept of Pathology, 200 Hawkins Dr 5216D RCP, Iowa City, IA 52242; **Phone:** 319-356-4440; **Board Cert:** Anatomic & Clinical Pathology 1999; Cytopathology 2001; **Med School:** Egypt 1983; **Resid:** Anatomic & Clinical Pathology, G Washington Univ Hosp 1997; Anatomic & Clinical Pathology, Univ MD Med Sys 1999; **Fellow:** Surgical Pathology, Univ MD Med Sys 2000; Cytopathology, Natl Inst Hlth/Natl Canc Inst 2001; **Fac Appt:** Assoc Clin Prof Path, Univ Iowa Coll Med

Gambetti, Pierluigi MD [Path] - **Spec Exp:** Neuro-Pathology; Neurodegenerative Disorders; Creutzfeldt-Jakob Disease (CJD); Huntington's Disease; **Hospital:** Univ Hosps Case Med Ctr (page 74); **Address:** Case Western Reserve Univ, Inst Path, 2085 Adelbert Rd, rm 419, Cleveland, OH 44106; **Phone:** 216-368-0587; **Board Cert:** Neuropathology 1981; **Med School:** Italy 1960; **Resid:** Neurology, Univ Bologna Med Ctr 1963; **Fellow:** Neurological Pathology, Institut Bunge 1965; Neurological Pathology, Hosp Univ Penn 1968; **Fac Appt:** Prof Path, Case West Res Univ

Goldblum, John R MD [Path] - **Spec Exp:** Soft Tissue Pathology; Esophageal Cancer; Gastrointestinal Pathology; Sarcoma; **Hospital:** Cleveland Clin (page 55); **Address:** Cleveland Clinic, Anatomic Pathology L25, 9500 Euclid Ave, Cleveland, OH 44195; **Phone:** 216-444-8238; **Board Cert:** Anatomic Pathology 1993; **Med School:** Univ Mich Med Sch 1989; **Resid:** Anatomic Pathology, Univ Michigan Hosps 1993; **Fac Appt:** Prof Path, Cleveland Cl Coll Med/Case West Res

Greenson, Joel K MD [Path] - **Spec Exp:** Liver Cancer; Gastrointestinal Pathology; Liver Pathology; **Hospital:** Univ of Michigan Hosp; **Address:** Univ Michigan Hospitals, Dept Pathology, 1301 Catherine St, Med Sci 1 Bldg, rm 5218, Ann Arbor, MI 48109-5602; **Phone:** 734-936-6770; **Board Cert:** Anatomic & Clinical Pathology 1988; **Med School:** Univ Mich Med Sch 1984; **Resid:** Pathology, Cedars-Sinai Med Ctr 1988; **Fellow:** Gastrointestinal Pathology, Johns Hopkins Hosp 1990; **Fac Appt:** Prof Path, Univ Mich Med Sch

Pathology

Kurtin, Paul J MD [Path] - **Spec Exp:** Lymph Node Pathology; Bone Marrow Pathology; Lymphoma; **Hospital:** Mayo Med Ctr & Clin - Rochester; **Address:** Mayo Clinic - Div Hematopathology, 200 First St SW, Hilton 1160A, Rochester, MN 55905; **Phone:** 507-284-4939; **Board Cert:** Anatomic & Clinical Pathology 1983; Hematology 1988; **Med School:** Med Coll Wisc 1979; **Resid:** Anatomic & Clinical Pathology, Vanderbilt Univ Med Ctr 1983; **Fellow:** Hematopathology, Brigham & Women's Hosp 1984; Surgical Pathology, Brigham & Women's Hosp 1986; **Fac Appt:** Prof Path, Mayo Med Sch

Lucas, David R MD [Path] - **Spec Exp:** Bone Tumors; Soft Tissue Tumors; Surgical Pathology; **Hospital:** Univ of Michigan Hosp; **Address:** 1500 E Med Ctr Drive, Ste 2G332 UH, Ann Arbor, MI 48109; **Phone:** 734-232-0022; **Board Cert:** Anatomic Pathology 1993; **Med School:** Wayne State Univ 1988; **Resid:** Pathology, Wayne State Univ Med Ctr 1991; **Fellow:** Surgical Pathology, Mayo Clinic 1993; **Fac Appt:** Prof Path, Univ Mich Med Sch

Moore, Steven A MD/PhD [Path] - **Spec Exp:** Muscular Dystrophy; Neuropathology; **Hospital:** Univ Iowa Hosp & Clinics; **Address:** UIHC Dept of Pathology, 200 Hawkins Dr 5239B RCP, Iowa City, IA 52242; **Phone:** 319-384-9084; **Board Cert:** Anatomic Pathology 1986; Neuropathology 1986; **Med School:** Indiana Univ 1982; **Resid:** Pathology, Univ IA Hosp & Clin 1984; **Fellow:** Neurological Pathology, Univ IA Hosp & Clin 1986; **Fac Appt:** Prof NPath, Univ Iowa Coll Med

Myers, Jeffrey L MD [Path] - **Spec Exp:** Lung Cancer; Lung Pathology; **Hospital:** Univ of Michigan Hosp; **Address:** 1500 E Med Ctr Drive, Ste 2G332 UH, Ann Arbor, MI 48109-5912; **Phone:** 734-936-1888; **Board Cert:** Anatomic Pathology 1986; **Med School:** Washington Univ, St Louis 1981; **Resid:** Anatomic Pathology, Barnes Jewish Hosp 1984; **Fellow:** Surgical Pathology, Univ Alabama Med Ctr 1985; **Fac Appt:** Prof Path, Univ Mich Med Sch

Petras, Robert E MD [Path] - **Spec Exp:** Gastrointestinal Pathology; **Address:** Ameripath Cleveland, 7730 First Pl, Ste A, Oakwood Village, OH 44146; **Phone:** 440-703-2100; **Board Cert:** Anatomic & Clinical Pathology 2004; **Med School:** Ohio State Univ 1978; **Resid:** Anatomic & Clinical Pathology, Cleveland Clinic 1982; **Fellow:** Gastrointestinal Pathology, St Marks Hosp; **Fac Appt:** Assoc Clin Prof Path, NE Ohio Univ

Rubin, Brian P MD [Path] - **Spec Exp:** Bone & Soft Tissue Pathology; Sarcoma; **Hospital:** Cleveland Clin (page 55); **Address:** Cleveland Clinic, Dept Anatomic Pathology, L25, 9500 Euclid Ave, Cleveland, OH 44195; **Phone:** 216-445-5551; **Board Cert:** Anatomic Pathology 1999; **Med School:** Cornell Univ-Weill Med Coll 1995; **Resid:** Pathology, Brigham & Womens Hosp 2000; **Fac Appt:** Asst Prof Path, Univ Wash

Suster, Saul M MD [Path] - **Spec Exp:** Surgical Pathology; Mediastinal Tumors; Thyroid Cancer; Thyroid Disorders; **Hospital:** Froedtert and Med Ctr of WI; **Address:** Med College of Wisconsin, Dept Pathology, Dynacare Lab Bldg, rm 226, 9200 W Wisconsin Ave, Milwaukee, WI 53226; **Phone:** 414-805-6968; **Board Cert:** Anatomic & Clinical Pathology 1988; **Med School:** Ecuador 1976; **Resid:** Anatomic Pathology, Tel Aviv Univ Med Ctr 1984; Anatomic & Clinical Pathology, Mt Sinai Med Ctr 1988; **Fellow:** Surgical Pathology, Yale-New Haven Hosp 1990; **Fac Appt:** Prof Path, Med Coll Wisc

Ulbright, Thomas M MD [Path] - **Spec Exp:** Testicular Cancer; Gynecologic Pathology; **Hospital:** IU Health University Hosp; **Address:** IU Health Pathology Laboratory, 350 W 11th St, rm 4078, Indianapolis, IN 46202; **Phone:** 317-491-6498; **Board Cert:** Anatomic Pathology 1980; **Med School:** Washington Univ, St Louis 1975; **Resid:** Pathology, Barnes Jewish Hosp 1978; Surgical Pathology, Barnes Jewish Hosp 1979; **Fellow:** Gynecologic Pathology, St Johns Mercy Med Ctr 1980; **Fac Appt:** Prof Path, Indiana Univ

Great Plains and Mountains

Cohen, Michael B MD [Path] - **Spec Exp:** Urologic Cancer; Cytopathology; **Hospital:** Univ Utah Hlth Care, Huntsman Cancer Hosp; **Address:** Univ of Utah - Dept Pathology, 1950 Circle of Hope, Ste N3100, Salt Lake City, UT 84112; **Phone:** 801-213-4341; **Board Cert:** Anatomic Pathology 2008; Cytopathology 1996; **Med School:** Albany Med Coll 1982; **Resid:** Pathology, UCSF Hosps & Clinics 1986; **Fellow:** Cytopathology, UCSF Hosps & Clinics 1987; **Fac Appt:** Prof Path, Univ Utah

De Masters, Bette K MD [Path] - **Spec Exp:** Neuro-Pathology; Brain Tumors; **Hospital:** Univ of CO Hosp - Anschutz Inpatient Pav, Chldn's Hosp - Aurora (CO); **Address:** Univ CO Hlth Sci Ctr, Dept Pathology, 12605 E 16th Ave, rm 3026, MS F-768, Aurora, CO 80045; **Phone:** 720-848-4421; **Board Cert:** Anatomic & Clinical Pathology 1982; Neuropathology 1985; **Med School:** Univ Wisc 1977; **Resid:** Pathology, Univ Colo Med Sch 1982; **Fellow:** Neurological Pathology, Univ Colo/Univ Kansas 1984; **Fac Appt:** Prof Path, Univ Colorado

Thor, Ann D MD [Path] - **Spec Exp:** Breast Cancer; Gynecologic Cancer; **Hospital:** Univ of CO Hosp - Anschutz Inpatient Pav; **Address:** 12631 E 17th Ave, rm L15-2215, MS B216, Aurora, CO 80045-0508; **Phone:** 303-724-3704; **Board Cert:** Anatomic Pathology 1987; Cytopathology 1989; **Med School:** Vanderbilt Univ 1981; **Resid:** Pathology, Vanderbilt Univ 1983; **Fellow:** Immunopathology, Natl Cancer Inst 1986; Gynecologic Pathology, Mass Genl Hosp 1990; **Fac Appt:** Prof Path, Univ Colorado

Weisenburger, Dennis D MD [Path] - **Spec Exp:** Hematopathology; Lymphoma; **Hospital:** Nebraska Med Ctr; **Address:** Dept Pathology and Microbiology, 983135 Nebraska Medical Center, Omaha, NE 68198-3135; **Phone:** 402-559-7688; **Board Cert:** Anatomic & Clinical Pathology 1979; **Med School:** Univ Minn 1974; **Resid:** Anatomic Pathology, Univ Iowa Hosps 1978; **Fellow:** Hematopathology, City of Hope Natl Med Ctr 1980; **Fac Appt:** Prof Path, Univ Nebr Coll Med

Southwest

Bruner, Janet M MD [Path] - **Spec Exp:** Brain Tumors; Neuro-Pathology; **Hospital:** UT MD Anderson Cancer Ctr; **Address:** MD Anderson Cancer Ctr, 1515 Holcombe Blvd, Ste 85, Houston, TX 77030; **Phone:** 713-792-6127; **Board Cert:** Anatomic Pathology 1982; Neuropathology 1984; **Med School:** Med Coll OH 1979; **Resid:** Anatomic & Clinical Pathology, Med Coll Ohio Hosp 1982; **Fellow:** Neurological Pathology, Baylor Coll Med 1984; **Fac Appt:** Prof Path, Univ Tex, Houston

Cagle, Philip MD [Path] - **Spec Exp:** Pulmonary Pathology; Lung Cancer; Mesothelioma; **Hospital:** Methodist Hosp - Houston; **Address:** Methodist Hospital, Dept Pathology, 6565 Fannin St, Ste 227, Houston, TX 77030; **Phone:** 713-441-6478; **Board Cert:** Anatomic & Clinical Pathology 1985; **Med School:** Univ Tenn Coll Med 1981; **Resid:** Pathology, Baylor Affil Hosp 1985; **Fellow:** Pulmonary Pathology, Univ British Columbia 1987; **Fac Appt:** Prof Path, Baylor Coll Med

Foucar, M Kathryn MD [Path] - **Spec Exp:** Leukemia; Lymph Node Pathology; Bone Marrow Pathology; **Hospital:** Univ Hosp - New Mexico; **Address:** TriCore Reference Lab, Hematopathology, 1001 Woodward Pl NE, Albuquerque, NM 87102; **Phone:** 505-938-8122; **Board Cert:** Anatomic & Clinical Pathology 1978; **Med School:** Ohio State Univ 1974; **Resid:** Anatomic Pathology, Univ NM Health & Sci Ctr 1976; Anatomic Pathology, Univ Minn Med Ctr 1978; **Fellow:** Surgical Pathology, Univ Minn Med Ctr 1979; **Fac Appt:** Prof Path, Univ New Mexico

Pathology

Hamilton, Stanley R MD [Path] - **Spec Exp:** Gastrointestinal Pathology; Liver Pathology; **Hospital:** UT MD Anderson Cancer Ctr; **Address:** Univ Texas MD Anderson Cancer Ctr, 1515 Holcombe Blvd, Unit 085, Houston, TX 77030-4009; **Phone:** 713-792-2040; **Board Cert:** Anatomic & Clinical Pathology 1978; **Med School:** Indiana Univ 1973; **Resid:** Pathology, Johns Hopkins Hosp 1979; **Fellow:** St Marks Hosp 1980; **Fac Appt:** Prof Path, Univ Tex, Houston

Kinney, Marsha C MD [Path] - **Spec Exp:** Hematopathology; Lymphoma; Leukemia; **Hospital:** Univ Hlth Syst-San Antonio; **Address:** Univ Texas Hlth & Sci Ctr, Dept Path, 7703 Floyd Curl Drive, MC 7750, San Antonio, TX 78229-3900; **Phone:** 210-567-4072; **Board Cert:** Anatomic & Clinical Pathology 1985; Hematology 1998; **Med School:** Univ Tex SW, Dallas 1981; **Resid:** Pathology, Vanderbilt Univ Med Ctr 1985; **Fellow:** Hematopathology, Vanderbilt Univ Med Ctr 1988; **Fac Appt:** Prof Path, Univ Tex, San Antonio

Leslie, Kevin O MD [Path] - **Spec Exp:** Pulmonary Pathology; Lung Cancer; Surgical Pathology; **Hospital:** Mayo Clinic - Scottsdale, Mayo Clinic - Phoenix; **Address:** Mayo Clinic-Pathology Div, 13400 E Shea Blvd, Scottsdale, AZ 85259; **Phone:** 480-301-8021; **Board Cert:** Anatomic & Clinical Pathology 1982; **Med School:** Albert Einstein Coll Med 1978; **Resid:** Anatomic & Clinical Pathology, Univ Colorado Hlth Sci Ctr 1982; **Fellow:** Surgical Pathology, Stanford Univ Med Ctr 1983; **Fac Appt:** Prof Path, Mayo Med Sch

Moran, Cesar A MD [Path] - **Spec Exp:** Lung Cancer; Mediastinal Tumors; Mesothelioma; **Hospital:** UT MD Anderson Cancer Ctr; **Address:** MD Anderson Cancer Ctr, Dept Pathology, 1515 Holcombe Blvd, rm G1-3738, Houston, TX 77030; **Phone:** 713-792-8134; **Board Cert:** Anatomic Pathology 1992; **Med School:** Guatemala 1981; **Resid:** Anatomic Pathology, Mt Sinai Med Ctr 1988; **Fellow:** Surgical Pathology, Yale-New Haven Med Ctr 1989; **Fac Appt:** Prof Path, Univ Tex, Houston

Prieto, Victor G MD/PhD [Path] - **Spec Exp:** Dermatopathology; Melanoma; Skin Cancer; **Hospital:** UT MD Anderson Cancer Ctr; **Address:** MD Anderson Cancer Ctr, Dept Pathology, 1515 Holcombe Blvd, Box 85, Houston, TX 77030-4000; **Phone:** 713-792-0918; **Board Cert:** Anatomic Pathology 1995; Dermatopathology 1997; **Med School:** Spain 1986; **Resid:** Pathology, New York Hosp 1993; **Fellow:** Pathology, Meml Sloan Kettering Cancer Ctr 1995; Dermatopathology, New York Hosp-Cornell Med Ctr 1996; **Fac Appt:** Prof Path, Univ Tex, Houston

Rashid, Asif MD/PhD [Path] - **Spec Exp:** Gastrointestinal Pathology; Liver Pathology; **Hospital:** UT MD Anderson Cancer Ctr; **Address:** MD Anderson Cancer Ctr, Dept Pathology, 1515 Holcombe Blvd, Box 85, Houston, TX 77030; **Phone:** 713-745-1101; **Board Cert:** Anatomic Pathology 1994; **Med School:** Pakistan 1984; **Resid:** Anatomic Pathology, Mass Genl Hosp 1993; **Fellow:** Anatomic Pathology, Mass Genl Hosp 1994; Anatomic Pathology, Johns Hopkins 1996

Roberts, William C MD [Path] - **Spec Exp:** Cardiac Pathology; **Hospital:** Baylor Univ Medical Ctr-Dallas; **Address:** Baylor Univ Med Ctr, Heart & Vascular Inst, 3500 Gaston Ave, Ste H-030, Dallas, TX 75246-2017; **Phone:** 214-820-7911; **Board Cert:** Anatomic Pathology 1965; **Med School:** Emory Univ 1958; **Resid:** Anatomic Pathology, Natl Heart Inst-NIH 1962; Internal Medicine, Johns Hopkins Hosp 1963; **Fellow:** Cardiovascular Disease, Natl Heart Inst-NIH 1964

Sahin, Aysegul MD [Path] - **Spec Exp:** Breast Cancer; **Hospital:** UT MD Anderson Cancer Ctr; **Address:** 1515 Holcombe Blvd, Box 0085, Houston, TX 77030; **Phone:** 713-794-1500; **Board Cert:** Pathology 1987; **Med School:** Turkey 1980; **Resid:** Pathology, Oregon HSU Affil Hosp 1986; **Fellow:** Surgical Pathology, Univ Iowa Hosps & Clins 1987; **Fac Appt:** Prof Path, Univ Tex, Houston

Silva, Elvio G MD [Path] - **Spec Exp:** Gynecologic Pathology; Gynecologic Cancer; **Hospital:** UT MD Anderson Cancer Ctr, Cedars-Sinai Med Ctr; **Address:** MD Anderson Cancer Ctr, Dept Pathology, 1515 Holcombe Blvd, Unit 85, rm G1-3563B, Houston, TX 77030; **Phone:** 713-792-3154; **Board Cert:** Anatomic Pathology 2007; **Med School:** Argentina 1969; **Resid:** Pathology, National Univ Med Ctr 1975; Anatomic Pathology, Univ Toronto Affil Hosp 1978; **Fellow:** Surgical Pathology, MD Anderson Cancer Ctr 1979

Walker, David H MD [Path] - **Spec Exp:** Infections-Emerging; Tropical Diseases; Bioterrorism Preparedness; **Hospital:** UT Med Br at Galveston(Joh Sealy Hosp); **Address:** UT Med Br Galveston, Dept Path, 301 University Blvd, Galveston, TX 77555-0609; **Phone:** 409-772-2856; **Board Cert:** Anatomic & Clinical Pathology 1974; **Med School:** Vanderbilt Univ 1969; **Resid:** Anatomic & Clinical Pathology, Peter Bent Brigham Hosp 1973; **Fellow:** Pathology, Harvard Univ 1974; **Fac Appt:** Prof Path, Univ Tex Med Br, Galveston

Wheeler, Thomas M MD [Path] - **Spec Exp:** Thyroid Disorders; Thyroid Cancer; Genitourinary Cancer; **Hospital:** Ben Taub Genl Hosp; **Address:** Baylor Coll Med, Dept Pathology, One Baylor Plaza, rm T203, MS 315, Houston, TX 77030; **Phone:** 713-798-4664; **Board Cert:** Anatomic & Clinical Pathology 1981; Cytopathology 1990; **Med School:** Baylor Coll Med 1977; **Resid:** Pathology, Baylor Affil Hosps 1981; **Fac Appt:** Prof Path, Baylor Coll Med

West Coast and Pacific

Amin, Mahul MD [Path] - **Spec Exp:** Genitourinary Pathology; Bladder Cancer; **Hospital:** Cedars-Sinai Med Ctr; **Address:** Cedars Sinai Med Ctr, 8700 Beverly Blvd, Ste 8709, Los Angeles, CA 90048; **Phone:** 310-423-6631; **Board Cert:** Anatomic & Clinical Pathology 1996; **Med School:** India 1983; **Resid:** Pathology, Henry Ford Hosp 1992; **Fellow:** Surgical Pathology, MD Anderson Cancer Ctr 1993; **Fac Appt:** Prof Path, UCLA-David Geffen Sch Med

Arber, Daniel A MD [Path] - **Spec Exp:** Bone Marrow Pathology; Lymph Node Pathology; Spleen Pathology; **Hospital:** Stanford Univ Hosp & Clinics, Lucile Packard Chldn's Hosp; **Address:** Clinic Laboratories, Stanford Univ Med Ctr, 300 Pasteur Drive, rm H1507, Stanford, CA 94305; **Phone:** 650-725-5604; **Board Cert:** Anatomic & Clinical Pathology 1991; Hematology 1993; **Med School:** Univ Tex, San Antonio 1986; **Resid:** Anatomic & Clinical Pathology, Scott & White Meml Hosp 1991; **Fellow:** Hematopathology, City of Hope Natl Med Ctr 1993; **Fac Appt:** Prof Path, Stanford Univ

Bastian, Boris C MD/PhD [Path] - **Spec Exp:** Melanoma; Skin Cancer; Dermatopathology; **Hospital:** UCSF Med Ctr; **Address:** 1701 Divisadero St, Fl 2, UCSF Dermatopathology Service, San Francisco, CA 94115; **Phone:** 415-502-0267; **Med School:** Germany 1988; **Resid:** Dermatology, University of Wurzburg 1994; **Fellow:** Hematology, Ludwig-Maximilian-University 1989; Genetics, UCSF Helen Diller Comprehensive Cancer Ctr 1999; **Fac Appt:** Prof D, UCSF

Bollen, Andrew W MD [Path] - **Spec Exp:** Neuro-Pathology; Brain Tumors; Brain Infections; **Hospital:** UCSF Med Ctr, San Francisco Genl Hosp; **Address:** UCSF School of Medicine, Dept Pathology/Neuropathology, 505 Parnassus Ave, rm M553, Box 0102, San Francisco, CA 94143-0511; **Phone:** 415-476-5236; **Board Cert:** Neuropathology 1992; Anatomic Pathology 1992; Clinical Pathology 1993; **Med School:** UCSD 1985; **Resid:** Anatomic Pathology, UCSF Med Ctr 1991; **Fellow:** Neuropathology, UCSF Med Ctr 1989; **Fac Appt:** Prof Path, UCSF

Pathology

Chandrasoma, Parakrama T MD [Path] - **Spec Exp:** Gastrointestinal Pathology; Gastrointestinal Cancer; Neuro-Pathology; **Hospital:** LAC & USC Med Ctr; **Address:** LAC-USC Med Ctr, Dept Path, Clinic Tower Fl 7 - rm A7A127, 1100 N State St, Los Angeles, CA 90033; **Phone:** 323-226-2622; **Board Cert:** Anatomic Pathology 1982; **Med School:** Sri Lanka 1971; **Resid:** Anatomic Pathology, Univ Sri Lanka 1978; Anatomic Pathology, LAC-USC Med Ctr 1982; **Fac Appt:** Prof Path, USC Sch Med

Chang, Karen L MD [Path] - **Spec Exp:** Leukemia; Lymphoma; **Hospital:** Kaiser Permanente LA Med Ctr; **Address:** SCPMG Regional Reference Laboratories, 11668 Sherman Way, North Hollywood, CA 91605; **Phone:** 818-503-6769; **Board Cert:** Anatomic & Clinical Pathology 1992; **Med School:** Mount Sinai Sch Med 1985; **Resid:** Anatomic Pathology, Stanford Univ Med Ctr 1988; Clinical Pathology, Stanford Univ Med Ctr 1991; **Fellow:** Surgical Pathology, Stanford Univ Med Ctr 1989

Chen, Yunn-Yi MD/PhD [Path] - **Spec Exp:** Breast Pathology; Breast Cancer; **Hospital:** UCSF Med Ctr; **Address:** 505 Parnassus Ave, rm M545, San Francisco, CA 94143; **Phone:** 415-353-1613; **Board Cert:** Anatomic & Clinical Pathology 1998; **Med School:** China 1985; **Resid:** Pathology, Beth Israel Deaconess Med Ctr 1998; **Fellow:** Surgical Pathology, UCSF Med Ctr 1999; **Fac Appt:** Assoc Prof Path, UCSF

Cochran, Alistair J MD [Path] - **Spec Exp:** Melanoma; Dermatopathology; **Hospital:** UCLA Ronald Reagan Med Ctr; **Address:** UCLA Med Ctr, Dept Path & Med, 10833 Le Conte Ave, rm A4-215CHS, MC 173216, Los Angeles, CA 90095-1732; **Phone:** 310-825-8182; **Med School:** Scotland, UK 1959; **Resid:** Dermatopathology, Western Infirmary 1968; Pathology, Western Infirmary 1968; **Fellow:** Immunology, Karolinska Inst 1970; **Fac Appt:** Prof Path, UCLA

Dubeau, Louis MD/PhD [Path] - **Spec Exp:** Ovarian Cancer; **Hospital:** USC Norris Cancer Hosp (page 62); **Address:** 1441 Eastlake Ave, Ezralow To Bldg, Ste 6338, Los Angeles, CA 90033-1048; **Phone:** 323-865-0720; **Board Cert:** Anatomic Pathology 1984; **Med School:** McGill Univ 1979; **Resid:** Anatomic Pathology, McGill Univ Med Ctr 1984; **Fellow:** Molecular Biology, USC/Norris Comprehensive Cancer Ctr 1987; **Fac Appt:** Prof Path, USC Sch Med

Ferrell, Linda MD [Path] - **Spec Exp:** Liver Pathology; **Hospital:** UCSF Med Ctr; **Address:** UCSF Med Ctr, Dept Pathology, 505 Parnassus Ave, rm M590, Box 0102, San Francisco, CA 94143-0102; **Phone:** 415-353-1090; **Board Cert:** Anatomic Pathology 1982; **Med School:** Univ Kansas 1977; **Resid:** Anatomic Pathology, Univ Kansas Med Ctr 1979; Anatomic Pathology, UCSF Med Ctr 1981; **Fac Appt:** Prof Path, UCSF

Fishbein, Michael C MD [Path] - **Spec Exp:** Cardiovascular Pathology; Pulmonary Pathology; **Hospital:** UCLA Ronald Reagan Med Ctr; **Address:** UCLA Pathology & Lab Medicine, 10833 Le Conte Ave, Los Angeles, CA 90095-1732; **Phone:** 310-825-8940; **Board Cert:** Anatomic & Clinical Pathology 1975; **Med School:** Univ IL Coll Med 1971; **Resid:** Anatomic & Clinical Pathology, UCLA-Harbor General Hosp 1975; **Fellow:** Pathology, Heart Lung Inst-NIH 1975; **Fac Appt:** Prof Path, UCLA

Govindarajan, Sugantha MD [Path] - **Spec Exp:** Liver Pathology; **Hospital:** Rancho Los Amigos Natl Rehab Ctr; **Address:** Rancho Los Amigos Natl Rehab Ctr, 7601 E Imperial Hwy, Bldg JPI - rm B170, Dept Pathology, Downey, CA 90242; **Phone:** 562-401-8996; **Board Cert:** Anatomic Pathology 1976; **Med School:** India 1969; **Resid:** Pathology, St Lukes Hosp 1976; **Fellow:** Pathology, Cleveland Clinic 1977; **Fac Appt:** Prof Path, USC Sch Med

Hammar, Samuel P MD [Path] - **Spec Exp:** Lung Cancer; Pulmonary Pathology; **Hospital:** Harrison Med Ctr; **Address:** Diagnostic Specialties Laboratory, 700 Lebo Blvd, Bremerton, WA 98310; **Phone:** 360-479-7707; **Board Cert:** Anatomic & Clinical Pathology 1975; **Med School:** Univ Wash 1970

Kanel, Gary MD [Path] - **Spec Exp:** Liver Pathology; **Hospital:** Keck Med Ctr of USC (page 62); **Address:** USC Univ Hosp, Dept Pathology, 1500 San Pablo St Fl 2, Los Angeles, CA 90033; **Phone:** 323-442-8591; **Board Cert:** Anatomic & Clinical Pathology 1979; **Med School:** Tufts Univ 1974; **Resid:** Pathology, Tufts-New England Med Ctr 1976; Pathology, Univ Chicago Hosp 1977; **Fellow:** Pathology, Tufts-New England Med Ctr 1979; **Fac Appt:** Prof Path, USC Sch Med

Koss, Michael N MD [Path] - **Spec Exp:** Pulmonary Pathology; Lung Cancer; Kidney Pathology; **Hospital:** USC Norris Cancer Hosp (page 62), Keck Med Ctr of USC (page 62); **Address:** 2222 Ocean View Ave, Ste 212, Los Angeles, CA 90057; **Phone:** 213-381-2260; **Board Cert:** Anatomic Pathology 1979; **Med School:** Stanford Univ 1970; **Resid:** Pathology, Columbia Presby Med Ctr 1974; **Fellow:** Renal Pathology, Columbia Presby Med Ctr 1975; Pulmonary Pathology, Armed Forces Inst Path 1978; **Fac Appt:** Prof Path, USC Sch Med

Le Boit, Philip E MD [Path] - **Spec Exp:** Cutaneous Lymphoma; Skin Cancer; Dermatopathology; **Hospital:** UCSF Med Ctr; **Address:** UCSF - Dermatopathology Section, 1701 Divisadero St, rm 280, San Francisco, CA 94115; **Phone:** 415-353-7546; **Board Cert:** Anatomic Pathology 1983; Dermatopathology 1983; Clinical Pathology 1986; **Med School:** Albany Med Coll 1979; **Resid:** Anatomic Pathology, UCSF Med Ctr 1981; Clinical Pathology, Mt Sinai Hosp 1982; **Fellow:** Dermatopathology, New York Hosp-Cornell Med Ctr 1983; **Fac Appt:** Prof Path, UCSF

Ljung, Britt-Marie E MD [Path] - **Spec Exp:** Breast Cancer; Fine Needle Aspiration Biopsy; **Hospital:** UCSF - Mt Zion Med Ctr; **Address:** UCSF - Dept Pathology, 1600 Divisadero St, Box 1785, R-200, San Francisco, CA 94143-1785; **Phone:** 415-353-7320; **Board Cert:** Anatomic Pathology 1985; Cytopathology 1989; **Med School:** Sweden 1975; **Resid:** Pathology, Karolinska Hosp 1979; Anatomic Pathology, UCLA Med Ctr 1983; **Fac Appt:** Prof Path, UCSF

Mischel, Paul S MD [Path] - **Spec Exp:** Neuro-Pathology; Brain Tumors; **Hospital:** UCLA Ronald Reagan Med Ctr; **Address:** UCLA Med Ctr, Div Neuropathology, 10833 Le Conte Ave, rm 13-188 CHS, Los Angeles, CA 90095-1732; **Phone:** 310-825-2783; **Board Cert:** Anatomic Pathology 1997; Neuropathology 1997; **Med School:** Cornell Univ-Weill Med Coll 1991; **Resid:** Anatomic & Clinical Pathology, UCLA Med Center 1996; **Fellow:** Neurological Pathology, UCLA 1995; Research, Howard Hughes Med Inst/UCSF 1998; **Fac Appt:** Prof Path, UCLA

Nathwani, Bharat N MD [Path] - **Spec Exp:** Hematopathology; Leukemia; Lymphoma; **Hospital:** Cedars-Sinai Med Ctr; **Address:** Cedars-Sinai Dept Pathology, 8700 Beverly Blvd, South Tower, rm 7706, Los Angeles, CA 90048; **Phone:** 310-248-6659; **Board Cert:** Anatomic Pathology 1977; **Med School:** India 1969; **Resid:** Pathology, JJ Group-Grant Med Ctr 1972; Pathology, Rush-Presby-St Lukes Med Ctr 1974; **Fellow:** Hematopathology, City Hope Natl Med Ctr 1975; **Fac Appt:** Prof Path, USC Sch Med

Perry, Arie MD [Path] - **Spec Exp:** Neuro-Pathology; Brain Tumors; **Hospital:** UCSF Med Ctr; **Address:** UCSF-Dept of Neuropathology, 505 Parnassus Ave, rm M-551, San Francisco, CA 94143; **Phone:** 415-476-5236; **Board Cert:** Anatomic & Clinical Pathology 1995; Neuropathology 1997; **Med School:** Univ Tex SW, Dallas 1990; **Resid:** Pathology, Univ Tex SW 1994; **Fellow:** Surgical Pathology, Mayo Clin 1995; Neurological Pathology, Mayo Clin 1998; **Fac Appt:** Assoc Prof Path, Washington Univ, St Louis

Rutgers, Joanne MD [Path] - **Spec Exp:** Gynecologic Cancer; Gastrointestinal Pathology; **Hospital:** Long Beach Meml Med Ctr; **Address:** 2801 Atlantic Ave, Dept of Pathology, Long Beach, CA 90806; **Phone:** 562-933-0717; **Board Cert:** Clinical Pathology 1992; Anatomic Pathology 1985; Cytopathology 1997; **Med School:** UCSD 1981; **Resid:** Pathology, Montefiore Med Ctr 1983; Pathology, NYU Med Ctr 1985; **Fellow:** Gynecologic Pathology, Mass Genl Hosp 1989; **Fac Appt:** Clin Prof Path, UC Irvine

Pathology

Sibley, Richard K MD [Path] - **Spec Exp:** Kidney Pathology; Breast Pathology; Liver Pathology; **Hospital:** Stanford Univ Hosp & Clinics; **Address:** Stanford Univ Med Ctr, Surg Path Lab, 300 Pasteur Drive, rm H2110, MC 5324, Stanford, CA 94305; **Phone:** 650-723-7211; **Board Cert:** Anatomic Pathology 1975; **Med School:** Univ Tex SW, Dallas 1971; **Resid:** Anatomic Pathology, Univ Chicago Hosps 1974; **Fellow:** Stanford Univ Med Ctr 1975; **Fac Appt:** Prof Path, Stanford Univ

Triche, Timothy J MD/PhD [Path] - **Spec Exp:** Pediatric Pathology; Pediatric Cancers; Sarcoma; **Hospital:** Chldns Hosp - Los Angeles; **Address:** 4650 Sunset Blvd, MS 133, Los Angeles, CA 90027; **Phone:** 323-361-8898; **Board Cert:** Anatomic Pathology 1975; **Med School:** Tulane Univ 1971; **Resid:** Anatomic Pathology, Barnes Hosp-Wash Univ 1973; Surgical Pathology, Barnes Hosp 1974; **Fellow:** Pathology, Natl Cancer Inst 1975; **Fac Appt:** Prof Path, USC Sch Med

True, Lawrence D MD [Path] - **Spec Exp:** Urologic Pathology; Prostate Cancer; Bladder Cancer; **Hospital:** Univ Wash Med Ctr; **Address:** Univ Wash Med Ctr, Dept Anatomic Path, Campus Box 356100, rm NE110, 1959 NE Pacific St, Seattle, WA 98195-6100; **Phone:** 206-598-6400; **Board Cert:** Anatomic Pathology 1981; **Med School:** Tulane Univ 1971; **Resid:** Pathology, Univ Colo Hlth Sci Ctr 1980; **Fac Appt:** Prof Path, Univ Wash

Warnke, Roger A MD [Path] - **Spec Exp:** Lymphoma; Hematopathology; **Hospital:** Stanford Univ Hosp & Clinics; **Address:** Stanford Hosp, 1291 Welch Rd, Pathology, rm L235, Stanford, CA 94305-5324; **Phone:** 650-498-6458; **Board Cert:** Anatomic Pathology 1975; **Med School:** Washington Univ, St Louis 1971; **Resid:** Pathology, Stanford Univ Med Ctr 1974; **Fellow:** Surgical Pathology, Stanford Univ Med Ctr 1975; Immunology, Stanford Univ Med Ctr 1976; **Fac Appt:** Prof Path, Stanford Univ

Weiss, Lawrence M MD [Path] - **Spec Exp:** Lymphoma; Hematopathology; Adrenal Pathology; **Address:** Clarient, 31 Columbia, Aliso Viejo, CA 92656; **Phone:** 888-443-3311; **Board Cert:** Anatomic Pathology 1985; **Med School:** Univ MD Sch Med 1981; **Resid:** Pathology, Brigham & Women's Hosp 1983; **Fellow:** Surgical Pathology, Stanford Univ Hosp 1984

Wilczynski, Sharon P MD/PhD [Path] - **Spec Exp:** Gynecologic Cancer; Breast Cancer; Ovarian Cancer; Clinical Trials; **Hospital:** City of Hope Natl Med Ctr; **Address:** City Hope Natl Med Ctr-Dept of Pathology, 1500 E Duarte Rd, Duarte, CA 91010; **Phone:** 626-256-4673 x62456; **Board Cert:** Anatomic & Clinical Pathology 1985; Cytopathology 1991; **Med School:** Med Coll PA Hahnemann 1981; **Resid:** Pathology, Hosp Univ Penn 1983; Anatomic & Clinical Pathology, Long Beach Meml Hosp 1985; **Fac Appt:** Prof Path, USC-Keck School of Medicine

Pediatrics

A pediatrician is concerned with the physical, emotional and social health of children from birth to young adulthood. Care encompasses a broad spectrum of health services ranging from preventive health-care to the diagnosis and treatment of acute and chronic diseases.

A pediatrician deals with biological, social and environmental influences on the developing child, and with the impact of disease and dysfunction on development.

Training Required: Three years

Pediatric Allergy and Immunology: An allergist-immunologist is trained in evaluation, physical and laboratory diagnosis and management of disorders involving the immune system. Selected examples of such conditions include asthma, anaphylaxis, rhinitis, eczema and adverse reactions to drugs, foods and insect stings as well as immune deficiency diseases (both acquired and congenital), defects in host defense and problems related to autoimmune disease, organ transplantation or malignancies of the immune system. As our understanding of the immune system develops, the scope of this specialty is widening.

Training Required: Prior certification in pediatrics *plus* two years in allergy/immunology. (Training programs are available at some medical centers to provide individuals with expertise in both allergy/immunology and pediatric pulmonology. Such individuals are candidates for dual certification.)

(continued on next page)

Certification in one of the following subspecialties requires additional training and examination.

Pediatric Cardiology: A pediatric cardiologist provides comprehensive care to patients with cardiovascular problems. This specialist is skilled in selecting, performing and evaluating the structural and functional assessment of the heart and blood vessels and the clinical evaluation of cardiovascular disease.

Pediatric Critical Care Medicine: A pediatrician who cares for children who are victims of life threatening disorders such as severe accidents, shock and diabetic acidosis.

Pediatric Endocrinology: A pediatrician who provides expert care to infants, children and adolescents who have diseases that result from an abnormality in the endocrine glands (glands which secrete hormones). These diseases include diabetes mellitus, growth failure, unusual size for age, early or late pubertal development, birth defects, the genital anomalies and disorders of the thyroid, the adrenal and pituitary glands.

Pediatric Gastroenterology: A pediatrician who specializes in the diagnosis and treatment of diseases of the digestive systems of infants, children and adolescents. This specialist treats conditions such as abdominal pain, ulcers, diarrhea, cancer and jaundice and performs complex diagnostic and therapeutic procedures using lighted scopes to see internal organs.

Pediatric Hematology-Oncology: A pediatrician trained in the combination of pediatrics, hematology and oncology to recognize and manage pediatric blood disorders and cancerous diseases.

Pediatric Infectious Diseases: A pediatrician trained to care for children in the diagnosis, treatment and prevention of infectious diseases. This specialist can apply specific knowledge to effect a better outcome for pediatric infections with complicated courses, underly-

ing diseases that predispose to unusual or severe infections, unclear diagnoses, uncommon diseases and complex or investigational treatments.

Pediatric Nephrology: A pediatrician who deals with the normal and abnormal development and maturation of the kidney and urinary tract, the mechanisms by which the kidney can be damaged, the evaluation and treatment of renal diseases, fluid and electrolyte abnormalities, hypertension and renal replacement therapy.

Pediatric Otolaryngology: A pediatric otolaryngologist has special expertise in the management of infants and children with disorders that include congenital and acquired conditions involving the aerodigestive tract, nose and paranasal sinuses, the ear and other areas of the head and neck. The pediatric otolaryngologist has special skills in the diagnosis, treatment and management of childhood disorders of voice, speech, language and hearing.

Pediatric Pulmonology: A pediatrician dedicated to the prevention and treatment of all respiratory diseases affecting infants, children and young adults. This specialist is knowledgeable about the growth and development of the lung, assessment of respiratory function in infants and children and experienced in a variety of invasive and noninvasive diagnostic techniques.

Pediatric Rheumatology: A pediatrician who treats diseases of joints, muscle, bones and tendons. A pediatric rheumatologist diagnoses and treats arthritis, back pain, muscle strains, common athletic injuries and "collagen" diseases.

Pediatric Surgery: A surgeon with expertise in the management of surgical conditions in premature and newborn infants, children and adolescents.

PEDIATRICS

New England

Miller, Karen J MD [Ped] - **Spec Exp:** Developmental & Behavioral Disorders; **Hospital:** Tufts Med Ctr; **Address:** Tufts Med Ctr, 800 Washington St, rm 334, Boston, MA 02111; **Phone:** 617-636-7242; **Board Cert:** Internal Medicine 1982; Developmental-Behavioral Pediatrics 2002; **Med School:** Tulane Univ 1977; **Resid:** Pediatrics, Georgetown Univ Hosp 1980; **Fellow:** Developmental-Behavioral Pediatrics, Schneider's Chldns Hosp 1996; **Fac Appt:** Assoc Prof Ped, Tufts Univ

Palfrey, Judith S MD [Ped] - **Spec Exp:** Special Health Care Needs (CSHCN); Developmental Disorders; **Hospital:** Children's Hospital - Boston; **Address:** Chldns Hosp, 300 Longwood Ave, Honeywell 201.3, Boston, MA 02115; **Phone:** 617-355-4662; **Board Cert:** Pediatrics 1976; Developmental-Behavioral Pediatrics 2002; **Med School:** Columbia P&S 1971; **Resid:** Pediatrics, Montefiore Med Ctr 1974; **Fac Appt:** Prof Ped, Harvard Med Sch

Rappaport, Leonard MD [Ped] - **Spec Exp:** Developmental & Behavioral Disorders; **Hospital:** Children's Hospital - Boston; **Address:** Chldns Hosp, Fegan 10, 300 Longwood Ave, Boston, MA 02115; **Phone:** 617-355-4683; **Board Cert:** Pediatrics 1983; Developmental-Behavioral Pediatrics 2002; **Med School:** Yale Univ 1977; **Resid:** Pediatrics, Chldns Hosp 1980; **Fellow:** Developmental-Behavioral Pediatrics, Chldns Hosp 1982; **Fac Appt:** Prof Ped, Harvard Med Sch

Mid Atlantic

Berlin Jr, Cheston M MD [Ped] - **Spec Exp:** Phenylketonuria (PKU); Tourette's Syndrome; **Hospital:** Penn State Milton S Hershey Med Ctr; **Address:** PennState Hershey Children's Hospital, MS HS83, 35 Hope Drive, MS HS83, Hershey, PA 17033-0850; **Phone:** 717-531-8006; **Board Cert:** Pediatrics 1982; **Med School:** Harvard Med Sch 1962; **Resid:** Pediatrics, Chldns Hosp 1967; **Fac Appt:** Prof Ped, Penn State Coll Med

Burgess, David B MD [Ped] - **Spec Exp:** Developmental & Behavioral Disorders; ADD/ADHD; Autism; **Hospital:** Chldns Hosp of Philadelphia; **Address:** 4009 Black Horse Pike, Mays Landing, NJ 08330; **Phone:** 609-677-7895; **Board Cert:** Pediatrics 1978; Developmental-Behavioral Pediatrics 2004; **Med School:** Univ Wisc 1973; **Resid:** Pediatrics, Charity Hosp 1977; **Fellow:** Child Development, JFK Child Dev Ctr, Univ Colorado 1980; **Fac Appt:** Assoc Clin Prof Ped, Univ Pennsylvania

Gartner Jr, J Carlton MD [Ped] - **Spec Exp:** Diagnostic Problems; Multisystem Disorders; **Hospital:** Nemours/Alfred I. duPont Hosp for Chldn; **Address:** Alfred I duPont Hosp for Children, 1600 Rockland Rd, rm 3B367, Wilmington, DE 19803; **Phone:** 302-651-5946; **Board Cert:** Pediatrics 2007; **Med School:** Johns Hopkins Univ 1971; **Resid:** Pediatrics, Childrens Hosp 1974; **Fac Appt:** Prof Ped, Thomas Jefferson Univ

Hofkosh, Dena MD [Ped] - **Spec Exp:** Developmental & Behavioral Disorders; Developmental Disorders; **Hospital:** Chldns Hosp of Pittsburgh - UPMC; **Address:** Chldns Hosp, Child Development Unit, Chldn's Oakland Med Bldg, 3420 5th Ave Fl 2, Pittsburgh, PA 15213; **Phone:** 412-692-5560; **Board Cert:** Pediatrics 2009; Neurodevelopmental Disabilities 2012; **Med School:** NYU Sch Med 1979; **Resid:** Pediatrics, Univ Pittsburgh Med Ctr 1982; **Fellow:** Ambulatory Pediatrics, Univ Pittsburgh Med Ctr 1984; **Fac Appt:** Prof Ped, Univ Pittsburgh

Morton, D Holmes MD [Ped] - **Spec Exp:** Genetic Disorders; Rare Disorders; **Hospital:** Lancaster Genl Hosp; **Address:** Clinic For Special Children, 535 Bunker Hill Rd, PO Box 128, Strasburg, PA 17579; **Phone:** 717-687-9407; **Board Cert:** Pediatrics 1987; **Med School:** Harvard Med Sch 1983; **Resid:** Pediatrics, Childrens Hosp 1986; **Fellow:** Research, Childrens Hosp 1988

Oeffinger, Kevin MD [Ped] - **Spec Exp:** Cancer Survivors-Late Effects of Therapy; **Hospital:** Meml Sloan-Kettering Cancer Ctr; **Address:** 300 E 66th St, New York, NY 10065; **Phone:** 646-888-4730; **Board Cert:** Family Medicine 2006; **Med School:** Univ Tex, San Antonio 1984; **Resid:** Family Medicine, Baylor Coll Med 1985; **Fellow:** Family Medicine, Fam Practice Faculty Dev Ctr 1999; Natl Cancer Inst 2000

Vining, Eileen P MD [Ped] - **Spec Exp:** Pediatric Neurology; Epilepsy; Rasmussen's Syndrome; **Hospital:** Johns Hopkins Hosp (page 61); **Address:** 600 N Wolfe St Meyer Bldg Fl 2 - rm 147, Baltimore, MD 21227; **Phone:** 410-502-0964; **Board Cert:** Pediatrics 1977; **Med School:** Johns Hopkins Univ 1972; **Resid:** Pediatrics, Chldns Hosp 1974; **Fellow:** Developmental-Behavioral Pediatrics, JFK Inst/Johns Hopkins Hosp 1976; **Fac Appt:** Assoc Prof Ped, Johns Hopkins Univ

Zitelli, Basil MD [Ped] - **Spec Exp:** Complex Diagnosis; **Hospital:** Chldns Hosp of Pittsburgh - UPMC; **Address:** Childrens Hospital Drive, 4401 Penn Ave, Faculty Pavilion Fl 3, Pittsburgh, PA 15201; **Phone:** 412-692-5135; **Board Cert:** Pediatrics 1976; **Med School:** Univ Pittsburgh 1971; **Resid:** Pediatrics, Johns Hopkins Hosp 1974; **Fellow:** Pediatrics, Johns Hopkins Hosp 1978; **Fac Appt:** Prof Ped, Univ Pittsburgh

Southeast

Hershorin, Eugene R MD [Ped] - **Spec Exp:** ADD/ADHD; Developmental & Mood Disorders; Learning Disorders; **Hospital:** Jackson Meml Hosp, Baptist Hosp of Miami; **Address:** 8932 SW 97th Ave, Ste D, Miami, FL 33176; **Phone:** 305-270-5050; **Board Cert:** Pediatrics 1980; Developmental-Behavioral Pediatrics 2004; **Med School:** Penn State Coll Med 1976; **Resid:** Pediatrics, Chldn's Hosp 1979; **Fac Appt:** Assoc Prof Ped, Univ Miami Sch Med

Midwest

Berman, Brian W MD [Ped] - **Spec Exp:** Sickle Cell Disease; Thrombotic Disorders; Thalassemia; Fanconi Aplastic Anemia; **Hospital:** Beaumont Hosp-Royal Oak; **Address:** 3601 W 13 Mile Road, Med Office Bldg - Ste 709, Royal Oak, MI 48073; **Phone:** 248-551-1644; **Board Cert:** Pediatrics 2009; Pediatric Hematology-Oncology 1989; **Med School:** Temple Univ 1975; **Resid:** Pediatrics, St Chris Hosp for Chldn 1978; **Fellow:** Pediatric Hematology-Oncology, Yale-New Haven Hosp 1980; **Fac Appt:** Prof Ped, Oakland Univ-William Beaumont Med Sch

Bull, Marilyn J MD [Ped] - **Spec Exp:** Developmental Disorders; Down Syndrome; Birth Defects; **Hospital:** Riley Hosp for Children; **Address:** 705 Riley Hospital Drive, rm 1601, Indianapolis, IN 46202; **Phone:** 317-944-4846; **Board Cert:** Pediatrics 1973; Clinical Genetics 1982; Neurodevelopmental Disabilities 2012; **Med School:** Univ Mich Med Sch 1968; **Resid:** Pediatrics, Childrens Meml Hosp 1972; **Fellow:** Genetics, Boston Floating Hosp 1973; **Fac Appt:** Prof Ped, Indiana Univ

Fost, Norman C MD [Ped] - **Spec Exp:** Ethics; **Hospital:** Univ WI Hosp & Clins; **Address:** Dept Pediatrics 4108, 600 Highland Ave, Madison, WI 53792-4108; **Phone:** 608-265-6050; **Board Cert:** Pediatrics 1970; **Med School:** Yale Univ 1964; **Resid:** Pediatrics, Johns Hopkins Hosp 1971; **Fellow:** Pediatrics, Harvard Sch Public Hlth 1973; **Fac Appt:** Prof Ped, Univ Wisc

Pediatrics

Jacob, Molly MD [Ped] - **Spec Exp:** Asthma; ADD/ADHD; Nutrition; **Hospital:** Lurie Chldn's Hosp-Chicago, Adv Illinois Masonic Med Ctr; **Address:** 2742 W Montrose Ave, Chicago, IL 60610; **Phone:** 773-463-0136; **Board Cert:** Pediatrics 1980; **Med School:** India 1968; **Resid:** Pediatrics, Ill Masonic Med Ctr 1979; **Fellow:** Ambulatory Pediatrics, Ill Masonic Med Ctr 1979; **Fac Appt:** Asst Clin Prof Ped, Univ IL Coll Med

Lantos, John D MD [Ped] - **Spec Exp:** Ethics; Palliative Care; Ethics Issues in Neonatalogy; **Hospital:** Chldns Mercy Hosps & Clinics; **Address:** Children's Mercy Bioethics Ctr, 2401 Gilham Rd, Kansas City, MO 64108; **Phone:** 816-701-5284; **Board Cert:** Pediatrics 2009; **Med School:** Univ Pittsburgh 1981; **Resid:** Pediatrics, Chldns Natl Med Ctr 1984; **Fellow:** Clinical Ethics, Univ Chicago Hosps 1987; **Fac Appt:** Prof Ped, Univ MO-Kansas City

Roizen, Nancy Jean M MD [Ped] - **Spec Exp:** Down Syndrome; Autism; ADD/ADHD; **Hospital:** UH Rainbow Babies & Chldns Hosp (page 74), Univ Hosps Case Med Ctr (page 74); **Address:** UH Rainbow Specialty Center - Westlake, 10524 Euclid Ave, rm 3150, Cleveland, OH 44106; **Phone:** 216-844-3230; **Board Cert:** Pediatrics 1987; Neurodevelopmental Disabilities 2011; Developmental-Behavioral Pediatrics 2012; **Med School:** Tufts Univ 1972; **Resid:** Pediatrics, Johns Hopkins Hosp 1974; **Fellow:** Neurodevelopmental Disabilities, Johns Hopkins Hosp 1975; Behavioral Pediatrics, UCSF 1976; **Fac Appt:** Prof Psyc, Case West Res Univ

Southwest

Infante, Anthony J MD/PhD [Ped] - **Spec Exp:** Immune Deficiencies-Primary; Autoimmune Disease; Fevers-Periodic; **Hospital:** Christus Santa Rosa Children's Hosp; **Address:** 333 Santa Rosa St Fl 8th, San Antonio, TX 78207; **Phone:** 210-704-2187; **Board Cert:** Pediatrics 2004; **Med School:** Indiana Univ 1978; **Resid:** Pediatrics, Mayo Clinic 1980; **Fellow:** Pediatric Immunology, Mayo Clinic 1981; Immunology, Stanford Univ Hosp 1983; **Fac Appt:** Prof Ped, Univ Tex, San Antonio

Kleinerman, Eugenie S MD [Ped] - **Spec Exp:** Ewing's Sarcoma; Cancer Survivors-Late Effects of Therapy; **Hospital:** UT MD Anderson Cancer Ctr; **Address:** MD Anderson Cancer Ctr, Dept Pediatrics, 1515 Holcombe Blvd, Unit 87, Houston, TX 77030; **Phone:** 713-792-8110; **Board Cert:** Pediatrics 1980; **Med School:** Duke Univ 1975; **Resid:** Pediatrics, Chldns Hosp-Natl Med Ctr 1978; **Fellow:** Immunology, Natl Cancer Inst 1981; **Fac Appt:** Prof Ped, Univ Tex, Houston

West Coast and Pacific

Berkowitz, Carol D MD [Ped] - **Spec Exp:** Child Abuse; **Hospital:** LAC - Harbor - UCLA Med Ctr; **Address:** LAC-Harbor-UCLA Med Ctr, 1000 W Carson St, Box 437, Torrance, CA 90509-2910; **Phone:** 310-222-3091; **Board Cert:** Pediatrics 2000; Pediatric Emergency Medicine 2006; Child Abuse Pediatrics 2009; **Med School:** Columbia P&S 1969; **Resid:** Pediatrics, Roosevelt Hosp 1972; **Fac Appt:** Clin Prof Ped, UCLA

Feldman, Kenneth W MD [Ped] - **Spec Exp:** Child Abuse; **Hospital:** Seattle Chldns Hosp; **Address:** Odessa Brown Chldns Clin, 2101 E Yesler Way, Ste 100, Seattle, WA 98122; **Phone:** 206-987-7225; **Board Cert:** Pediatrics 1975; Child Abuse Pediatrics 2009; **Med School:** Univ Wisc 1970; **Resid:** Pediatrics, Chldns Regl Med Ctr 1974; **Fac Appt:** Clin Prof Ped, Univ Wash

Jones Jr, Kenneth Lyons MD [Ped] - **Spec Exp:** Genetic Disorders; Dysmorphology; **Hospital:** Rady Children's Hosp - San Diego, UCSD Med Ctr; **Address:** 9500 Gilman Drive, MC 0828, Dept Pediatrics, La Jolla, CA 92093-0828; **Phone:** 858-246-0047; **Board Cert:** Pediatrics 1971; **Med School:** Hahnemann Univ 1966; **Resid:** Pediatrics, Chldns Ortho Hosp 1969; **Fac Appt:** Prof Ped, UCSD

Walker, William O MD [Ped] - **Spec Exp:** Developmental & Behavioral Disorders; Autism; Cerebral Palsy; Hydrocephalus; **Hospital:** Seattle Chldns Hosp; **Address:** 4800 Sand Point Way NE, MS A-7938, Seattle, WA 98145-5005; **Phone:** 206-987-2210; **Board Cert:** Pediatrics 1984; Developmental-Behavioral Pediatrics 2010; **Med School:** Tulane Univ 1979; **Resid:** Pediatrics, W Beaumont Army Med Ctr 1982; **Fellow:** Behavioral Pediatrics, W Beaumont Army Med Ctr 1987; **Fac Appt:** Prof Ped, Univ Wash

Zeltzer, Lonnie K MD [Ped] - **Spec Exp:** Pain Management; Complementary Medicine; **Hospital:** Mattel Chldns Hosp at UCLA; **Address:** UCLA Pediatric Pain Program, 200 Medial Plaza, Ste 265, Los Angeles, CA 90024; **Phone:** 310-825-0731; **Board Cert:** Pediatrics 1976; **Med School:** Univ Cincinnati 1970; **Resid:** Pediatrics, Univ Ariz Hosp 1973; **Fellow:** Adolescent Medicine, Chldns Hosp 1976; **Fac Appt:** Prof Ped, UCLA

PEDIATRIC ALLERGY & IMMUNOLOGY

New England

Klein, Robert B MD [PA&I] - **Spec Exp:** Asthma; **Hospital:** Rhode Island Hosp; **Address:** Rhode Island Hosp, Dept of Pediatrics, 593 Eddy St, Providence, RI 02903; **Phone:** 401-444-5648; **Board Cert:** Pediatrics 1976; Allergy & Immunology 1977; **Med School:** Switzerland 1971; **Resid:** Pediatrics, Dartmouth/Hitchcock Med Ctr 1974; **Fellow:** Allergy & Immunology, UCLA Med Ctr 1976; **Fac Appt:** Prof Ped, Brown Univ

Mid Atlantic

Ehrlich, Paul M MD [PA&I] - **Spec Exp:** Asthma; Food Allergy; **Hospital:** New York Eye & Ear Infirm (page 65), NYU Langone Med Ctr (page 68); **Address:** 35 E 35th St, Ste 202, New York, NY 10016-3823; **Phone:** 212-685-4225; **Board Cert:** Pediatrics 1975; Allergy & Immunology 1977; **Med School:** NYU Sch Med 1970; **Resid:** Pediatrics, Bellevue Hosp Ctr 1973; **Fellow:** Allergy & Immunology, Walter Reed Army Med Ctr 1976; **Fac Appt:** Assoc Clin Prof Ped, NYU Sch Med

Josephs, Shelby H MD [PA&I] - **Spec Exp:** Food Allergy; **Hospital:** Georgetown Univ Hosp; **Address:** 6000 Executive Blvd, Ste 615, North Bethesda, MD 20852; **Phone:** 240-747-5750; **Board Cert:** Pediatrics 1979; Allergy & Immunology 1985; **Med School:** Duke Univ 1975; **Resid:** Pediatrics, Chldns Hosp 1977; Allergy & Immunology, Duke Univ Med Ctr 1979; **Fac Appt:** Assoc Clin Prof Ped, Georgetown Univ

Kamani, Naynesh R MD [PA&I] - **Spec Exp:** Stem Cell Transplant; Immunotherapy; Bone Marrow Transplant; **Hospital:** Chldns Natl Med Ctr; **Address:** Chldns Natl Med Ctr, Div Hematology, 111 Michigan Ave NW, Washington, DC 20010; **Phone:** 202-476-2140; **Board Cert:** Pediatrics 1983; Allergy & Immunology 1983; Diagnostic Lab Immunology 1986; **Med School:** Ethiopia 1975; **Resid:** Pediatrics, Downstate Med Ctr-Kings Co Hosp 1981; **Fellow:** Pediatric Allergy & Immunology, Chldns Hosp 1983; **Fac Appt:** Prof Ped, Geo Wash Univ

Sampson Jr, Hugh A MD [PA&I] - **Spec Exp:** Food Allergy; Eczema; Atopic Dermatitis; **Hospital:** Mount Sinai Med Ctr (page 64); **Address:** Mt Sinai Sch Med, Dept Peds, 1 Gustave Levy Pl, Box 1198, New York, NY 10029; **Phone:** 212-241-5548; **Board Cert:** Pediatrics 1980; Allergy & Immunology 1981; **Med School:** SUNY Buffalo 1975; **Resid:** Pediatrics, Chldns Meml Hosp 1979; **Fellow:** Allergy & Immunology, Duke Univ Med Ctr 1980; **Fac Appt:** Prof Ped, Mount Sinai Sch Med

Pediatric Allergy & Immunology

Schuberth, Kenneth Charles MD [PA&I] - **Spec Exp:** Allergy; Asthma; **Hospital:** Johns Hopkins Hosp (page 61), Greater Baltimore Med Ctr; **Address:** 10807 Falls Rd, Ste 200, Lutherville, MD 21093; **Phone:** 410-321-9393; **Board Cert:** Pediatrics 1979; Allergy & Immunology 1983; **Med School:** Johns Hopkins Univ 1973; **Resid:** Pediatrics, Johns Hopkins Hosp 1978; **Fellow:** Allergy & Immunology, Johns Hopkins Hosp 1980; **Fac Appt:** Assoc Prof Ped, Johns Hopkins Univ

Sicherer, Scott H MD [PA&I] - **Spec Exp:** Food Allergy; Drug Allergy; Eczema; **Hospital:** Mount Sinai Med Ctr (page 64); **Address:** 5 E 98th St Fl 10, New York, NY 10029-6500; **Phone:** 212-241-5548; **Board Cert:** Pediatrics 2008; Allergy & Immunology 2007; **Med School:** Johns Hopkins Univ 1990; **Resid:** Pediatrics, Mt Sinai Hosp 1994; **Fellow:** Allergy & Immunology, Johns Hopkins Hosp 1997; **Fac Appt:** Prof Ped, Mount Sinai Sch Med

Skoner, David Peter MD [PA&I] - **Spec Exp:** Asthma & Allergy; Rhinitis; **Hospital:** Allegheny General Hosp; **Address:** Allegheny Genl Hosp, Div Asthma, Allergy & Immunology, 320 E North Ave, Fl 7-South Tower, Pittsburgh, PA 15212; **Phone:** 412-359-6640; **Board Cert:** Pediatrics 1985; Allergy & Immunology 1985; **Med School:** Temple Univ 1980; **Resid:** Pediatrics, Chldns Hosp Med Ctr 1983; **Fellow:** Allergy & Immunology, Chldns Hosp 1985; **Fac Appt:** Prof Ped, Drexel Univ Coll Med

Sly, R Michael MD [PA&I] - **Spec Exp:** Asthma; Allergy; Atopic Dermatitis; **Hospital:** Chldns Natl Med Ctr; **Address:** 9850 Key West Ave Fl 4, Rockville, MD 20850; **Phone:** 301-765-5400; **Board Cert:** Pediatric Allergy & Immunology 1967; Pediatrics 1980; Allergy & Immunology 1987; **Med School:** Washington Univ, St Louis 1960; **Resid:** Pediatrics, St Louis Chldns Hosp 1962; Pediatrics, Univ Kentucky Med Ctr 1963; **Fellow:** Pediatric Allergy & Immunology, UCLA Med Ctr 1967; **Fac Appt:** Prof Ped, Geo Wash Univ

Spergel, Jonathan Michael MD/PhD [PA&I] - **Spec Exp:** Atopic Dermatitis; Food Allergy; Asthma; Eosinophilic Esophagitis; **Hospital:** Chldns Hosp of Philadelphia; **Address:** 3550 Market St, Fl 3, Philadelphia, PA 19104; **Phone:** 215-590-2549; **Board Cert:** Allergy & Immunology 2006; **Med School:** Mount Sinai Sch Med 1992; **Resid:** Pediatrics, Yale New Haven Hosp 1994; **Fellow:** Allergy & Immunology, Chldn's Hosp 1995; **Fac Appt:** Assoc Prof Ped, Univ Pennsylvania

Sullivan, Kathleen E MD/PhD [PA&I] - **Spec Exp:** Immune Deficiency; **Hospital:** Chldns Hosp of Philadelphia; **Address:** Chldn's Hosp, Dept Immunology, 3550 Market St Fl 3, Philadelphia, PA 19104; **Phone:** 215-590-2549; **Board Cert:** Pediatrics 2008; Pediatric Rheumatology 2009; **Med School:** UCSF 1988; **Resid:** Pediatrics, UCSF 1990; **Fellow:** Pediatric Rheumatology, Jonhs Hopkins Hosp 1993; **Fac Appt:** Prof Ped, Univ Pennsylvania

Wood, Robert A MD [PA&I] - **Spec Exp:** Food Allergy; Asthma; **Hospital:** Johns Hopkins Hosp (page 61); **Address:** Johns Hopkins Children's Ctr, 600 N Wolfe St, CMSC-1102, Baltimore, MD 21287; **Phone:** 410-955-5883; **Board Cert:** Pediatrics 1987; Allergy & Immunology 2010; **Med School:** Univ Rochester 1982; **Resid:** Pediatrics, Johns Hopkins Hosp 1986; **Fellow:** Allergy & Immunology, Johns Hopkins Hosp 1988; **Fac Appt:** Prof Ped, Johns Hopkins Univ

Southeast

Burks Jr, A Wesley MD [PA&I] - **Spec Exp:** Asthma; Allergic Rhinitis; Food Allergy; Anaphylaxis; **Hospital:** NC Memorial Hosp - UNC; **Address:** Department of Pediatrics, Box 7220, University of North Carolina at Chapel Hill, Chapel Hill, NC 27599; **Phone:** 919-966-1505; **Board Cert:** Pediatrics 1985; Allergy & Immunology 1985; **Med School:** Univ Ark 1980; **Resid:** Pediatrics, Ark Chldns Hosp 1983; **Fellow:** Allergy & Immunology, Duke Univ Med Ctr 1985; **Fac Appt:** Prof Ped, Duke Univ

Kelly, Cynthia S MD [PA&I] - **Spec Exp:** Asthma; Rhinitis; Sinusitis; **Hospital:** Chldns Hosp of King's Daughters; **Address:** Chlds Hosp of The Kings Daughters, 601 Childrens Lane, Fl 4th, Norfolk, VA 23507; **Phone:** 757-668-8255; **Board Cert:** Pediatrics 2004; Allergy & Immunology 2007; **Med School:** Wayne State Univ 1985; **Resid:** Pediatrics, Univ Mich 1987; **Fellow:** Allergy & Immunology, UCLA Med Ctr 1988; Pediatric Infectious Disease, Vanderbilt Univ 1989; **Fac Appt:** Assoc Prof Ped, Eastern VA Med Sch

Ownby, Dennis R MD [PA&I] - **Spec Exp:** Food Allergy; Anaphylaxis; Latex Allergy; Asthma; **Hospital:** Med Coll of GA Hosp and Clin (MCG Health Inc); **Address:** Allergy & Immunology, 1446 Harper St, Augusta, GA 30912-0004; **Phone:** 706-721-2390; **Board Cert:** Pediatrics 1977; Allergy & Immunology 2006; Clinical & Laboratory Immunology 1986; **Med School:** Med Coll OH 1972; **Resid:** Pediatrics, Duke Univ Med Ctr 1974; **Fellow:** Pediatric Allergy & Immunology, Duke Univ Med Ctr 1977; **Fac Appt:** Prof Ped, Med Coll GA

Sleasman, John W MD [PA&I] - **Spec Exp:** Infectious Disease; Immunodeficiency Disorders; Hypogammaglobulinemia; **Hospital:** All Children's Hosp; **Address:** All Childrens Hosp, Div Ped Immun/Rheumatology, 601 5th St S, Ste 304, St Petersburg, FL 33701; **Phone:** 727-767-4150; **Board Cert:** Pediatrics 1988; Diagnostic Lab Immunology 1990; **Med School:** Univ Tenn Coll Med 1981; **Resid:** Pediatrics, Shands Hosp 1984; **Fellow:** Pediatric Infectious Disease, Shands Hosp 1987; Immunology, Dana Farber Cancer Inst 1988

Midwest

Lemanske Jr, Robert F MD [PA&I] - **Spec Exp:** Asthma; Allergy; Immune Deficiency; **Hospital:** Univ WI Hosp & Clins; **Address:** 451 Junction Rd, Madison, WI 53717; **Phone:** 608-263-6180; **Board Cert:** Pediatrics 1980; Allergy & Immunology 1981; **Med School:** Univ Wisc 1975; **Resid:** Pediatrics, Univ Wisc Hosp 1978; **Fellow:** Allergy & Immunology, Univ Wisc Hosp 1980; Allergy & Immunology, Natl Inst Hlth 1983; **Fac Appt:** Prof Ped, Univ Wisc

Pongracic, Jacqueline MD [PA&I] - **Spec Exp:** Latex Allergy; Asthma; Food Allergy; **Hospital:** Lurie Chldn's Hosp-Chicago; **Address:** 225 E Chicago Ave, Box 60, Chicago, IL 60611; **Phone:** 312-227-6010; **Board Cert:** Internal Medicine 1988; Allergy & Immunology 2012; **Med School:** Northwestern Univ 1985; **Resid:** Internal Medicine, North Shore Univ Hosp 1988; **Fellow:** Allergy & Immunology, Johns Hopkins Hosp 1991; **Fac Appt:** Prof Ped, Northwestern Univ-Feinberg Sch Med

Strunk, Robert C MD [PA&I] - **Spec Exp:** Asthma; **Hospital:** St. Louis Chldns Hosp; **Address:** 660 S Euclid Ave, Box 8116, St Louis, MO 63110; **Phone:** 314-454-2694; **Board Cert:** Pediatrics 1974; Allergy & Immunology 1987; **Med School:** Northwestern Univ 1968; **Resid:** Pediatrics, Cincinnati Chldns Hosp 1970; **Fellow:** Pediatric Allergy & Immunology, Boston Chldns Hosp 1974; **Fac Appt:** Prof Ped, Washington Univ, St Louis

Wolf, Raoul MD [PA&I] - **Spec Exp:** Asthma; Allergy; Immune Deficiency; **Hospital:** Univ of Chicago Med Ctr, La Rabida Chlds Hosp; **Address:** 5841 S Maryland St, Wyler Bldg - Ste C101, MS 5044, Chicago, IL 60637; **Phone:** 773-834-4010; **Board Cert:** Pediatrics 1980; Allergy & Immunology 1983; **Med School:** South Africa 1969; **Resid:** Pediatrics, Baragwanath Hosp 1973; Pediatrics, Transvaal Meml Hosp Chldn 1976; **Fellow:** Allergy & Immunology, Chldns Hosp Med Ctr 1979; **Fac Appt:** Prof Ped, Univ Chicago-Pritzker Sch Med

Pediatric Allergy & Immunology

Great Plains and Mountains

Bock, Samuel A MD [PA&I] - **Spec Exp:** Asthma up to age 50; Allergy up to age 50; Food Allergy; **Hospital:** Boulder Community Hospital, Natl Jewish Med & Rsch Ctr; **Address:** Boulder Valley Asthma And Allergy, 3950 Broadway, Boulder, CO 80304; **Phone:** 303-444-5995; **Board Cert:** Pediatrics 1977; Allergy & Immunology 1977; **Med School:** Univ MD Sch Med 1972; **Resid:** Pediatrics, Colo Med Ctr/Natl Jewish Med Ctr 1974; **Fellow:** Allergy & Immunology, Colo Med Ctr/Natl Jewish Med Ctr 1976; **Fac Appt:** Clin Prof Ped, Univ Colorado

Gelfand, Erwin W MD [PA&I] - **Spec Exp:** Immune Deficiency; Asthma; Allergy; **Hospital:** Natl Jewish Med & Rsch Ctr, Chldn's Hosp - Aurora (CO); **Address:** National Jewish Health, 1400 Jackson St, Denver, CO 80206; **Phone:** 303-398-1196; **Board Cert:** Pediatrics 1972; **Med School:** McGill Univ 1966; **Resid:** Pediatrics, Montreal Childrens Hosp 1968; Pediatrics, Childrens Hosp Med Ctr 1969; **Fellow:** Immunology, Childrens Hosp Med Ctr 1971; **Fac Appt:** Prof Ped, Univ Colorado

Leung, Donald YM MD/PhD [PA&I] - **Spec Exp:** Atopic Dermatitis; Asthma; Food Allergy; **Hospital:** Natl Jewish Med & Rsch Ctr, Chldn's Hosp - Aurora (CO); **Address:** National Jewish Health, 1400 Jackson St, Goodman Bldg, K926i, Denver, CO 80206; **Phone:** 303-398-1379; **Board Cert:** Pediatrics 1982; Allergy & Immunology 1983; Diagnostic Lab Immunology 1990; **Med School:** Univ Chicago-Pritzker Sch Med 1977; **Resid:** Pediatrics, Chldn's Hosp 1979; **Fellow:** Allergy & Immunology, Chldn's Hosp 1981; **Fac Appt:** Prof Ped, Univ Colorado

Southwest

Bahna, Sami L MD [PA&I] - **Spec Exp:** Food Allergy; Asthma; Eczema; **Hospital:** Louisiana State Univ Hosp; **Address:** LSU Hlth Scis Ctr, 1501 Kings Hwy, rm 5-323, Department Peds, Sect A&I, Shreveport, LA 71103; **Phone:** 318-675-7625; **Board Cert:** Pediatrics 1980; Allergy & Immunology 1981; **Med School:** Egypt 1964; **Resid:** Pediatrics, Univ Maryland Hosp 1975; **Fellow:** Allergy & Immunology, Harbor-UCLA Med Ctr 1978; **Fac Appt:** Prof Ped, Louisiana State U, New Orleans

Orange, Jordan MD/PhD [PA&I] - **Spec Exp:** Immunodeficiency Disorders; **Hospital:** Texas Chldns Hosp; **Address:** Texas Children's Hospital, Dept Allergy & Immunology, 6621 Fannin St, Houston, TX 77030; **Phone:** 832-824-2030; **Board Cert:** Pediatrics 2008; Allergy & Immunology 2003; **Med School:** Brown Univ 1997; **Resid:** Pediatrics, Chldn's Hosp 2000; **Fellow:** Allergy & Immunology, Chldn's Hosp 2003; **Fac Appt:** Assoc Prof Ped, Univ Tex, Houston

Shearer, William T MD/PhD [PA&I] - **Spec Exp:** AIDS/HIV; Immune Deficiency; **Hospital:** Texas Chldns Hosp; **Address:** 1102 Bates Ave, Feigin Ctr, Ste 330, Houston, TX 77030-2399; **Phone:** 832-824-1319; **Board Cert:** Pediatrics 1986; Allergy & Immunology 1989; Clinical & Laboratory Immunology 1986; **Med School:** Washington Univ, St Louis 1970; **Resid:** Pediatrics, Chldns Hosp-Wash Univ 1972; **Fellow:** Allergy & Immunology, Barnes Hosp-Wash Univ 1974; **Fac Appt:** Prof Ped, Baylor Coll Med

Wasserman, Richard L MD/PhD [PA&I] - **Spec Exp:** Immunodeficiency Disorders; Food Allergy; Asthma; Allergy; **Hospital:** Med City Dallas Hosp, Chldns Med Ctr of Dallas; **Address:** 7777 Forest Ln B Bldg - Ste 332, Dallas, TX 75230; **Phone:** 972-566-7788; **Board Cert:** Pediatrics 1982; Allergy & Immunology 1987; **Med School:** Univ Tex SW, Dallas 1977; **Resid:** Pediatrics, Chldns Hosp of Philadelphia 1979; **Fellow:** Immunology, Chldns Hosp of Philadelphia 1980; Rheumatology, Rockefeller Univ 1982; **Fac Appt:** Clin Prof A&I, Univ Tex SW, Dallas

West Coast and Pacific

Church, Joseph A MD [PA&I] - **Spec Exp:** Immunodeficiency Disorders; AIDS/HIV; **Hospital:** Chldns Hosp - Los Angeles; **Address:** 4650 Sunset Blvd, Los Angeles, CA 90027; **Phone:** 323-361-2501; **Board Cert:** Pediatrics 1977; Allergy & Immunology 1977; **Med School:** UMDNJ-NJ Med Sch, Newark 1972; **Resid:** Pediatrics, Chldns Hosp/Natl Med Ctr 1974; **Fellow:** Allergy & Immunology, Georgetown Med Ctr 1976; **Fac Appt:** Prof Ped, USC-Keck School of Medicine

Cowan, Morton J MD [PA&I] - **Spec Exp:** Immunodeficiency Disorders; Stem Cell Transplant-Fetal; Bone Marrow Transplant; **Hospital:** UCSF Med Ctr; **Address:** UCSF Med Ctr, Peds BMT Program, 505 Parnassus Ave, rm M659, San Francisco, CA 94143-1278; **Phone:** 415-476-2188; **Board Cert:** Pediatrics 1981; Allergy & Immunology 1983; **Med School:** Univ Pennsylvania 1970; **Resid:** Surgery, Duke Univ Med Ctr 1972; Pediatrics, UCSF Med Ctr 1977; **Fellow:** Research, Natl Inst Hlth 1975; Immunology, UCSF Med Ctr 1979; **Fac Appt:** Prof Ped, UCSF

Epstein, Stuart MD [PA&I] - **Spec Exp:** Asthma & Allergy; Food Allergy; **Hospital:** Cedars-Sinai Med Ctr, UCLA Ronald Reagan Med Ctr; **Address:** 9735 Wilshire Blvd, Ste 121, Beverly Hills, CA 90212-2101; **Phone:** 310-274-6853; **Board Cert:** Allergy & Immunology 1999; **Med School:** Univ IL Coll Med 1978; **Resid:** Pediatrics, Cedars Sinai Med Ctr 1980; **Fellow:** Pediatrics, UC Irvine 1981; Pediatrics, USC Med Ctr 1982; **Fac Appt:** Assoc Clin Prof Ped, UCLA

Fanous, Yvonne F MD [PA&I] - **Spec Exp:** Asthma & Allergy; Cystic Fibrosis; Immune Deficiency; **Hospital:** Loma Linda Univ Med Ctr; **Address:** Loma Linda Hlth Care Pediatrics, 250 E Caroline St, Ste J, San Bernardino, CA 92408; **Phone:** 909-651-1900; **Board Cert:** Pediatrics 1983; Allergy & Immunology 1985; **Med School:** Egypt 1973; **Resid:** Pediatrics, Texas Tech Univ Hosp 1980; Pediatrics, Loma Linda Univ 1981; **Fellow:** Allergy & Immunology, UC Irvine 1984; **Fac Appt:** Assoc Prof A&I, Loma Linda Univ

PEDIATRIC CARDIOLOGY

New England

De Moor, Michael MD [PCd] - **Spec Exp:** Interventional Cardiology; **Hospital:** Floating Hosp for Children at Tufts Med Ce; **Address:** Floating Hosp for Chldn at Tufts Med Ctr, 800 Washington St, Box 313, Boston, MA 02111; **Phone:** 617-636-7435; **Med School:** South Africa 1976; **Resid:** Internal Medicine, Red Cross Chldns Hosp 1983; **Fellow:** Pediatric Cardiology, Red Cross Chldns Hosp 1985; **Fac Appt:** Assoc Prof Ped, Tufts Univ

Hellenbrand, William E MD [PCd] - **Spec Exp:** Interventional Cardiology; **Hospital:** Yale-New Haven Hosp; **Address:** 333 cedar St, Box 208064, LLCI Bldg, rm 301, New Haven, CT 06520-8064; **Phone:** 203-785-2022; **Board Cert:** Pediatrics 1975; Pediatric Cardiology 1977; **Med School:** SUNY Downstate 1970; **Resid:** Pediatrics, Yale-New Haven Hosp 1972; **Fellow:** Pediatric Cardiology, Yale-New Haven Hosp 1976; **Fac Appt:** Prof Ped, Columbia P&S

Lang, Peter MD [PCd] - **Spec Exp:** Interventional Cardiology; Cardiac Catheterization; **Hospital:** Children's Hospital - Boston; **Address:** Chldns Hosp, Dept Cardiology, 300 Longwood Ave, Boston, MA 02114; **Phone:** 617-355-8539; **Board Cert:** Pediatrics 1977; Pediatric Cardiology 1979; **Med School:** Mount Sinai Sch Med 1972; **Resid:** Pediatrics, Babies Hosp-Presby Med Ctr 1975; **Fellow:** Pediatric Cardiology, Chldns Hosp Med Ctr 1978; **Fac Appt:** Assoc Prof Ped, Harvard Med Sch

Pediatric Cardiology

Lock, James E MD [PCd] - **Spec Exp:** Interventional Cardiology; Angioplasty-Pulmonary Artery; Cardiac Catheterization; Fetal Surgery; **Hospital:** Children's Hospital - Boston; **Address:** Chldns Hosp, Dept Cardiology, 300 Longwood Ave, Boston, MA 02115-5724; **Phone:** 617-355-7313; **Board Cert:** Pediatrics 1978; Pediatric Cardiology 1981; **Med School:** Stanford Univ 1973; **Resid:** Pediatrics, Univ Minn Hosp 1975; Pediatric Cardiology, Univ Minn Hosp 1977; **Fellow:** Cardiovascular Disease, Hosp Sick Chldn 1979; **Fac Appt:** Prof Ped, Harvard Med Sch

Newburger, Jane MD [PCd] - **Spec Exp:** Kawasaki Disease; Congenital Heart Disease; **Hospital:** Children's Hospital - Boston, Brigham and Women's Hosp (page 57); **Address:** Chldns Hosp, Dept Ped Cardiology, 300 Longwood Ave, Farley Bldg Fl 2, Boston, MA 02115; **Phone:** 617-355-5427; **Board Cert:** Pediatrics 1979; Pediatric Cardiology 1983; **Med School:** Harvard Med Sch 1974; **Resid:** Pediatrics, Chldns Hosp Med Ctr 1976; **Fellow:** Pediatric Cardiology, Chldns Hosp Med Ctr 1979; **Fac Appt:** Prof Ped, Harvard Med Sch

Walsh, Edward P MD [PCd] - **Spec Exp:** Arrhythmias; **Hospital:** Children's Hospital - Boston; **Address:** Chldns Hosp, Dept Cardiology, 300 Longwood Ave Bader Bldg Fl 2, Boston, MA 02115; **Phone:** 617-355-6328; **Board Cert:** Pediatrics 1985; Pediatric Cardiology 1985; **Med School:** Univ Pennsylvania 1979; **Resid:** Pediatrics, Chldns Hosp 1982; **Fellow:** Pediatric Cardiology, Chldns Hosp 1985; **Fac Appt:** Assoc Prof Ped, Harvard Med Sch

Mid Atlantic

Beerman, Lee B MD [PCd] - **Spec Exp:** Congenital Heart Disease-Adult & Child; Arrhythmias; **Hospital:** Chldns Hosp of Pittsburgh - UPMC; **Address:** Chldns Hosp-Heart Ctr, 4401 Penn Ave Fl 5, Faculty Pavilion, Pittsburgh, PA 15224; **Phone:** 412-692-5540; **Board Cert:** Pediatrics 1979; Pediatric Cardiology 1979; **Med School:** Univ Pittsburgh 1974; **Resid:** Pediatrics, Chldns Hosp 1977; **Fellow:** Pediatric Cardiology, Chldns Hosp 1979; **Fac Appt:** Prof Ped, Univ Pittsburgh

Biancaniello, Thomas MD [PCd] - **Spec Exp:** Congenital Heart Disease; Fetal Echocardiography; Interventional Cardiology; Cardiac Catheterization; **Hospital:** Morgan Stanley Children's Hosp of NY-Presby, NY; **Address:** 226 N Belle Mead Rd, East Setauket, NY 11733; **Phone:** 631-265-3300; **Board Cert:** Pediatrics 1979; Pediatric Cardiology 1981; **Med School:** NY Med Coll 1975; **Resid:** Pediatrics, North Shore Univ Hosp 1977; **Fellow:** Pediatric Cardiology, Cincinnati Chldns Hosp 1980; **Fac Appt:** Prof Ped, Columbia P&S

Bierman, Fredrick MD [PCd] - **Spec Exp:** Fetal Echocardiography; Kawasaki Disease; Congenital Heart Disease; Echocardiography; **Hospital:** Westchester Med Ctr; **Address:** Munger Bldg, Ste 618, Ave, rm 139, Valhalla, NY 10595; **Phone:** 914-594-4370; **Board Cert:** Pediatrics 1978; Pediatric Cardiology 1981; **Med School:** SUNY Downstate 1973; **Resid:** Pediatrics, Mount Sinai Med Ctr 1976; **Fellow:** Pediatric Cardiology, Harvard Chldns Hosp 1979; **Fac Appt:** Prof Ped, Albert Einstein Coll Med

Brenner, Joel I MD [PCd] - **Spec Exp:** Congenital Heart Disease; **Hospital:** Johns Hopkins Hosp (page 61); **Address:** Johns Hopkins Hosp, Pediatric Cardiology, 1800 Orleans St, Baltimore, MD 21287; **Phone:** 410-955-5987; **Board Cert:** Pediatrics 1975; Pediatric Cardiology 1977; **Med School:** NY Med Coll 1970; **Resid:** Pediatrics, NY Hosp 1972; **Fellow:** Pediatric Cardiology, Yale-New Haven Hosp 1974; **Fac Appt:** Assoc Prof Ped, Johns Hopkins Univ

Cooper, Rubin MD [PCd] - **Spec Exp:** Congenital Heart Disease; Rheumatic Heart Disease; Kawasaki Disease; **Hospital:** Steven & Alexandra Cohen Chldn's Med Ctr of NY (page 67); **Address:** Steven & Alexandra Cohen Chldns Med Ctr, 269-01 76th Ave, Ste 139, New Hyde Park, NY 11040; **Phone:** 718-470-3661; **Board Cert:** Pediatrics 1976; Pediatric Cardiology 1979; **Med School:** NY Med Coll 1971; **Resid:** Pediatrics, Strong Meml Hosp 1973; **Fellow:** Pediatric Cardiology, Strong Meml Hosp 1975; **Fac Appt:** Prof Ped, Cornell Univ-Weill Med Coll

Crosson, Jane MD [PCd] - **Spec Exp:** Congenital Heart Disease-Adult & Child; Pacemakers; Syncope; Fetal Echocardiography; **Hospital:** Johns Hopkins Hosp (page 61); **Address:** 1800 Orleans St, Baltimore, MD 21287; **Phone:** 410-955-5987; **Board Cert:** Pediatrics 1987; Pediatric Cardiology 2010; **Med School:** Med Coll GA 1982; **Resid:** Pediatrics, Univ MD Hosp 1986; **Fellow:** Pediatric Cardiology, Univ Minn Hosp 1990

Gelb, Bruce D MD [PCd] - **Spec Exp:** Noonan Syndrome; Marfan's Syndrome; **Hospital:** Mount Sinai Med Ctr (page 64); **Address:** 1 Gustave Levy Pl, Box 1201, New York, NY 10029; **Phone:** 212-241-8592; **Board Cert:** Pediatric Cardiology 2006; **Med School:** Univ Rochester 1984; **Resid:** Pediatrics, NYPresby-Columbia Univ Med Ctr 1987; **Fellow:** Pediatric Cardiology, Baylor College Med 1991; **Fac Appt:** Prof Ped, Mount Sinai Sch Med

Gewitz, Michael MD [PCd] - **Spec Exp:** Neonatal Cardiology; Kawasaki Disease; Echocardiography; Heart Failure; **Hospital:** Westchester Med Ctr, Children's & Women's Phys.of Westchester; **Address:** Maria Fareri Children's Hospital, Munger Pavillion, Ste 618, Valhalla, NY 10595; **Phone:** 914-594-4370; **Board Cert:** Pediatrics 1979; Pediatric Cardiology 1981; **Med School:** Hahnemann Univ 1974; **Resid:** Pediatrics, Chldns Hosp 1976; Pediatrics, Hosp Sick Chldn 1977; **Fellow:** Pediatric Cardiology, Yale-New Haven Hosp 1979; **Fac Appt:** Prof Ped, NY Med Coll

Hanna, Brian D MD/PhD [PCd] - **Spec Exp:** Pulmonary Hypertension; Cardiac Catheterization; Autonomic Disorders; Congenital Heart Disease; **Hospital:** Chldns Hosp of Philadelphia; **Address:** Childrens Hosp Phila, Pulmonary Hypertension Program, 34th St & Civic Center Blvd, Philadelphia, PA 19104; **Phone:** 215-590-5248; **Board Cert:** Pediatric Cardiology 2009; **Med School:** Canada 1983; **Resid:** Pediatrics, Montreal Chldns Hosp 1986; **Fellow:** Pediatric Cardiology, Montreal Chldns Hosp 1987; Pediatric Cardiology, Childrens Hosp 1989; **Fac Appt:** Clin Prof Ped, Univ Pennsylvania

Hsu, Daphne MD [PCd] - **Spec Exp:** Interventional Cardiology; Heart Failure; Transplant Medicine-Heart; **Hospital:** Montefiore Med Ctr-Moses Campus, NY; **Address:** Chldn's Hosp at Montefiore, 3415 Bainbridge Ave, Bronx, NY 10467; **Phone:** 718-741-2315; **Board Cert:** Pediatrics 1988; Pediatric Cardiology 2010; **Med School:** Yale Univ 1982; **Resid:** Pediatrics, Columbia Babies & Chldn's Hosp 1985; **Fellow:** Pediatric Cardiology, Columbia Babies & Chldn's Hosp 1988; **Fac Appt:** Prof Ped, Albert Einstein Coll Med

Murphy, John D MD [PCd] - **Spec Exp:** Cardiac Catheterization; Interventional Cardiology; **Hospital:** St. Christopher's Hosp for Chldn; **Address:** St Christophers Hosp for Children, The Heart Center, 3601 A St, Philadelphia, PA 19134; **Phone:** 215-427-4820; **Board Cert:** Pediatrics 1980; Pediatric Cardiology 1981; **Med School:** Univ VT Coll Med 1975; **Resid:** Pediatrics, Chldns Hosp 1977; **Fellow:** Pediatric Cardiology, Chldns Hosp Med Ctr 1980; **Fac Appt:** Prof Ped, Drexel Univ Coll Med

Parness, Ira A MD [PCd] - **Spec Exp:** Echocardiography; Congenital Heart Disease; Fetal Echocardiography; **Hospital:** Mount Sinai Med Ctr (page 64), Englewood Hosp & Med Ctr; **Address:** 1 Gustave L Levy Pl, Anbg Bldg - rm 3-40, Box 1201, New York, NY 10029-6500; **Phone:** 212-241-6640; **Board Cert:** Pediatrics 1984; Pediatric Cardiology 1985; **Med School:** SUNY Downstate 1979; **Resid:** Pediatrics, Brookdale Hosp 1982; **Fellow:** Pediatric Cardiology, Chldns Hosp 1985; **Fac Appt:** Prof Ped, Mount Sinai Sch Med

Radtke, Wolfgang MD [PCd] - **Spec Exp:** Interventional Cardiology; Cardiac Catheterization; Congenital Heart Disease-Adult & Child; **Hospital:** Nemours/Alfred I. duPont Hosp for Chldn; **Address:** Nemours Cardiac Ctr, 1600 Rockland Rd, Wilmington, DE 19803; **Phone:** 302-651-6600; **Board Cert:** Pediatrics 2011; Pediatric Cardiology 2012; **Med School:** Germany 1980; **Resid:** Pediatrics, Kiel Univ Chldns Hosp 1985; **Fellow:** Pediatric Cardiology, Chldns Hosp 1988; **Fac Appt:** Prof Ped, Jefferson Med Coll

Pediatric Cardiology

Rome, Jonathan J MD [PCd] - **Spec Exp:** Interventional Cardiology; Percutaneous ASD/PFO Closure; Congenital Heart Disease; **Hospital:** Chldns Hosp of Philadelphia; **Address:** Childrens Hosp Philadelphia, Cardiac Center, 34th St & Civic Center Blvd, Philadelphia, PA 19104; **Phone:** 215-590-4040 x1; **Board Cert:** Pediatrics 1987; Pediatric Cardiology 2010; **Med School:** Stanford Univ 1982; **Resid:** Pediatrics, Children's Hosp 1986; **Fellow:** Pediatric Cardiology, Children's Hosp 1989; **Fac Appt:** Assoc Prof Ped, Univ Pennsylvania

Rychik, Jack MD [PCd] - **Spec Exp:** Echocardiography; Fetal Cardiology; Congenital Heart Disease; **Hospital:** Chldns Hosp of Philadelphia; **Address:** Childrens Hosp Phila, Fetal Heart Program, 34th St & Civic Center Blvd, Philadelphia, PA 19104; **Phone:** 215-590-4040 x1; **Board Cert:** Pediatric Cardiology 2006; **Med School:** SUNY Downstate 1985; **Resid:** Pediatrics, Albert Einstein Affil Hosp 1988; **Fellow:** Pediatric Cardiology, Children's Hosp 1991; **Fac Appt:** Prof Ped, Univ Pennsylvania

Shaddy, Robert E MD [PCd] - **Spec Exp:** Transplant Medicine-Heart; Heart Failure; **Hospital:** Chldns Hosp of Philadelphia; **Address:** CHOP - Division Cardiology, 34th St & Civic Center Blvd, Philadelphia, PA 19104; **Phone:** 215-590-4040 x1; **Board Cert:** Pediatrics 1984; Pediatric Cardiology 2000; **Med School:** Creighton Univ 1980; **Resid:** Pediatrics, Univ Iowa Hosp & Clinics 1983; **Fellow:** Pediatric Cardiology, UCSF 1986; **Fac Appt:** Prof Ped, Univ Pennsylvania

Sherman, Frederick S MD [PCd] - **Hospital:** Chldns Hosp of Pittsburgh - UPMC, Magee-Womens Hosp - UPMC; **Address:** Children's Hosp Heart Ctr, 4401 Penn Ave Fl 5, Pittsburgh, PA 15224; **Phone:** 412-692-5540; **Board Cert:** Pediatrics 1980; Pediatric Cardiology 1985; **Med School:** Yale Univ 1975; **Resid:** Internal Medicine, Univ Virginia Hosp 1978; **Fellow:** Pediatric Cardiology, Boston Children's Hosp 1984; **Fac Appt:** Prof Ped, Univ Pittsburgh

Sommer, Robert J MD [PCd] - **Spec Exp:** Congenital Heart Disease; Atrial Septal Defect; Cardiac Catheterization; **Hospital:** NY-Presby/Columbia Univ Med Ctr, NY (page 66), St. Joseph's Regl Med Ctr - Paterson; **Address:** 161 Fort Washington Ave Fl 6, New York, NY 10032; **Phone:** 212-342-0886; **Board Cert:** Pediatric Cardiology 2006; **Med School:** NYU Sch Med 1985; **Resid:** Pediatrics, Mt Sinai Med Ctr 1988; **Fellow:** Pediatric Cardiology, Mt Sinai Med Ctr 1991; Interventional Cardiology, Childrens Hosp 1991; **Fac Appt:** Assoc Prof Ped, Columbia P&S

Steinherz, Laurel J MD [PCd] - **Spec Exp:** Cardiac Effects of Cancer/Cancer Therapy; **Hospital:** Meml Sloan-Kettering Cancer Ctr, NY-Presby/Weill Cornell Med Ctr, NY (page 66); **Address:** 1275 York Ave, New York, NY 10021; **Phone:** 212-639-8103; **Board Cert:** Pediatrics 1976; Pediatric Cardiology 1978; **Med School:** Albert Einstein Coll Med 1970; **Resid:** Pediatrics, NY Hosp-Cornell Med Ctr 1971; Pediatrics, Chldns Hosp 1972; **Fellow:** Pediatric Cardiology, NY Hosp-Cornell Med Ctr 1975; **Fac Appt:** Prof Ped, Cornell Univ-Weill Med Coll

Velvis, Harmannus MD [PCd] - **Spec Exp:** Cardiac Catheterization; Congenital Heart Disease; Heart Disease in Down Syndrome; Interventional Cardiology; **Hospital:** Albany Med Ctr, St. Peter's Hosp - Albany; **Address:** Capital Dist Ped Cardio Assoc, 319 S Manning Blvd, Ste 203, Albany, NY 12208-1743; **Phone:** 518-489-3292; **Board Cert:** Pediatric Cardiology 2009; **Med School:** Netherlands 1980; **Resid:** Pediatrics, Albany Med Ctr 1987; **Fellow:** Pediatric Cardiology, UCSF Med Ctr 1990; **Fac Appt:** Assoc Clin Prof Ped, Albany Med Coll

Walsh, Christine A MD [PCd] - **Spec Exp:** Arrhythmias; Congenital Heart Disease; Sudden Infant Death Syndrome (SIDS); **Hospital:** Montefiore Med Ctr-Moses Campus, NY; **Address:** 3415 Bainbridge Ave Fl 5, Bronx, NY 10467-2401; **Phone:** 718-741-2343; **Board Cert:** Pediatrics 1978; Pediatric Cardiology 1983; Pediatric Critical Care Medicine 2003; **Med School:** Yale Univ 1973; **Resid:** Pediatrics, Columbia-Presby Med Ctr 1976; **Fellow:** Pediatric Cardiology, Columbia-Presby Med Ctr 1978; Cardiac Electrophysiology, Columbia P&S 1980; **Fac Appt:** Prof Ped, Albert Einstein Coll Med

Weinberg, Paul M MD [PCd] - **Spec Exp:** Cardiac MRI; **Hospital:** Chldns Hosp of Philadelphia; **Address:** Chldns Hosp, Div Cardiology, 34th St & Civic Ctr Blvd, Ste 8NW90, Philadelphia, PA 19104; **Phone:** 215-590-3274; **Board Cert:** Pediatrics 1974; Pediatric Cardiology 1975; **Med School:** Jefferson Med Coll 1969; **Resid:** Pediatrics, Chldns Hosp 1971; Cardiology & Pathology, Chldns Hosp 1977; **Fellow:** Pediatric Cardiology, Chldns Hosp 1973; **Fac Appt:** Prof Ped, Univ Pennsylvania

Southeast

Colvin, Edward V MD [PCd] - **Spec Exp:** Congenital Heart Disease-Adult & Child; Fetal Echocardiography; Transplant Medicine-Heart; **Hospital:** Children's Hospital - Birmingham, Univ of Ala Hosp at Birmingham; **Address:** UAB Pediatric Cardiology, 1700 6th Ave S, 176F, Ste 9100, Birmingham, AL 35249; **Phone:** 205-934-3460; **Board Cert:** Pediatrics 1982; Pediatric Cardiology 1985; **Med School:** Univ Alabama 1977; **Resid:** Pediatrics, Chldns Hosp 1980; **Fellow:** Pediatric Cardiology, Baylor Coll Med 1983; **Fac Appt:** Prof Ped, Univ Alabama

Epstein, Michael L MD [PCd] - **Spec Exp:** Congenital Heart Disease; **Hospital:** All Children's Hosp; **Address:** All Children's Hosp, 601 5th St S, St Petersburg, FL 33701; **Phone:** 727-767-3333; **Board Cert:** Pediatrics 1976; Pediatric Cardiology 1981; **Med School:** Univ Tex Med Br, Galveston 1971; **Resid:** Pediatrics, Univ Ariz Hlth Sci Ctr 1974; **Fellow:** Pediatric Cardiology, Univ Minn Hosp 1979; **Fac Appt:** Prof Ped, Univ S Fla Coll Med

Fish, Frank A MD [PCd] - **Spec Exp:** Arrhythmias-Pediatric & Adult; Congenital Heart Disease-Adult; Pacemakers; Cardiac Electrophysiology; **Hospital:** Vanderbilt Monroe Carrell Jr. Chldn's Hosp (page 75), Vanderbilt Univ Med Ctr (page 75); **Address:** Vanderbilt Chldns Hosp, Div Pediatric Cardiology, 2200 Children's Way, 5230 DOT, Nashville, TN 37232-9119; **Phone:** 615-322-7447; **Board Cert:** Pediatrics 1987; Pediatric Cardiology 2006; **Med School:** Indiana Univ 1983; **Resid:** Pediatrics, Indiana Univ Hosp 1986; **Fellow:** Pediatric Cardiology, Vanderbilt Univ Med Ctr 1989; Cardiac Electrophysiology, Chldns Meml Hosp 1990; **Fac Appt:** Assoc Prof Ped, Vanderbilt Univ

Fricker, Frederick Jay MD [PCd] - **Spec Exp:** Transplant Medicine-Heart; **Hospital:** Shands at Univ of FL; **Address:** Shands Hlthcre, Div Pediatric Cardiology, 1600 SW Archer Rd, Box 100296, Gainesville, FL 32610-0296; **Phone:** 352-273-7770; **Board Cert:** Pediatrics 1975; Pediatric Cardiology 1981; **Med School:** Loyola Univ-Stritch Sch Med 1970; **Resid:** Pediatrics, Chldns Hosp 1973; **Fellow:** Pediatric Cardiology, Chldns Hosp 1977; **Fac Appt:** Prof Ped, Univ Fla Coll Med

Gullquist, Scott D MD [PCd] - **Hospital:** VCU Med Ctr; **Address:** VCU Medical Ctr, Pediatric Cardiology, Box 980301, Richmond, VA 23298; **Phone:** 804-828-5745; **Board Cert:** Pediatric Cardiology 2009; **Med School:** Georgetown Univ 1987; **Resid:** Pediatrics, Chldns Hosp 1990; **Fellow:** Pediatric Cardiology, Chldns Hosp 1993; **Fac Appt:** Assoc Prof Ped, Med Coll VA

Latson, Larry A MD [PCd] - **Spec Exp:** Congenital Heart Disease-Adult & Child; Interventional Cardiology; Cardiac Catheterization; **Hospital:** Joe DiMaggio Chldns Hosp, Meml Regl Hosp; **Address:** 1150 N 35th Ave, Ste 575, Hollywood, FL 33021; **Phone:** 954-265-3437; **Board Cert:** Pediatrics 1981; Pediatric Cardiology 1983; Pediatric Critical Care Medicine 2010; **Med School:** Baylor Coll Med 1976; **Resid:** Pediatrics, Baylor Affil Hosp 1978; **Fellow:** Pediatric Cardiology, Baylor Coll Med 1981

Moskowitz, William B MD [PCd] - **Spec Exp:** Patent Foramen Ovale; Cardiac Catheterization; Coarctation of the Aorta; Congenital Heart Disease-Adult & Child; **Hospital:** Med Coll of VA Hosp; **Address:** Childrens Heart Ctr, Med Coll Virginia, 1200 E Broad St, PO Box 980543, Richmond, VA 23298; **Phone:** 804-828-9143; **Board Cert:** Pediatrics 1983; Pediatric Cardiology 1985; **Med School:** Univ S Fla Coll Med 1978; **Resid:** Pediatrics, Chldns Hosp 1981; **Fellow:** Pediatric Cardiology, Chldns Hosp 1984; **Fac Appt:** Prof Ped, Med Coll VA

Pediatric Cardiology

Young, Ming-Lon MD [PCd] - **Spec Exp:** Arrhythmias; Syncope; **Hospital:** Joe DiMaggio Chldns Hosp, Jackson Meml Hosp; **Address:** Joe DiMaggio Childrens Hosp, 1150 N 35th Ave, Ste 575, Hollywood, FL 33021; **Phone:** 954-265-3437; **Board Cert:** Pediatrics 1985; Pediatric Cardiology 2009; **Med School:** Taiwan 1976; **Resid:** Preventive Medicine, Johns Hopkins Hosp 1979; Pediatrics, St Agnes Hosp 1981; **Fellow:** Pediatric Cardiology, Univ Miami 1985; Pediatric Cardiac Electrophysiology, Univ Miami 1985; **Fac Appt:** Prof Ped, Univ Miami Sch Med

Midwest

Ackerman, Michael J MD/PhD [PCd] - **Spec Exp:** Long QT Interval Syndrome; Sudden Infant Death Syndrome (SIDS); Hypertrophic Cardiomyopathy; Sudden Unexplained Death Syndrome (SUDS); **Hospital:** Mayo Med Ctr & Clin - Rochester; **Address:** Mayo Clin, Dept Ped Cardiology, 200 First St SW, Rochester, MN 55905; **Phone:** 507-284-0101; **Board Cert:** Pediatric Cardiology 2010; **Med School:** Mayo Med Sch 1995; **Resid:** Pediatric & Adolescent Medicine, Mayo Clin 1998; **Fellow:** Pediatric Cardiology, Mayo Clin 2000; **Fac Appt:** Prof Ped, Mayo Med Sch

Agarwala, Brojendra MD [PCd] - **Spec Exp:** Congenital Heart Disease; **Hospital:** Univ of Chicago Med Ctr; **Address:** 5841 S Maryland Ave, rm C-104, MC 4051, Chicago, IL 60637; **Phone:** 773-702-6172; **Board Cert:** Pediatrics 1970; Pediatric Cardiology 1978; **Med School:** India 1965; **Resid:** Pediatrics, St Vincent Hosp Med Ctr 1969; **Fellow:** Pediatric Cardiology, NYU Med Ctr 1972; **Fac Appt:** Prof Ped, Univ Chicago-Pritzker Sch Med

Beekman III, Robert H MD [PCd] - **Spec Exp:** Interventional Cardiology; Cardiac Catheterization; **Hospital:** Cincinnati Chldns Hosp Med Ctr; **Address:** Cincinnati Chldns Hosp Med Ctr, Heart Institute, 3333 Burnet Ave, Cincinnati, OH 45229-3026; **Phone:** 513-636-7072; **Board Cert:** Pediatrics 1981; Pediatric Cardiology 1983; **Med School:** Duke Univ 1976; **Resid:** Pediatrics, UCLA Med Ctr 1979; **Fellow:** Pediatric Cardiology, Univ Mich Hosp 1981; **Fac Appt:** Prof Ped, Univ Cincinnati

Caldwell, Randall L MD [PCd] - **Spec Exp:** Transplant Medicine-Heart; Echocardiography; Congenital Heart Disease; **Hospital:** Riley Hosp for Children; **Address:** Riley Hosp for Chldn-Ped Cardiology, 705 Riley Hosp Drive, RR-127, Indianapolis, IN 46202-5128; **Phone:** 317-274-8906; **Board Cert:** Pediatrics 1976; Pediatric Cardiology 1978; **Med School:** Indiana Univ 1971; **Resid:** Pediatrics, Indiana Univ Med Ctr 1974; **Fellow:** Pediatric Cardiology, Indiana Univ Med Ctr 1978; **Fac Appt:** Prof Ped, Indiana Univ

Cetta Jr, Frank MD [PCd] - **Spec Exp:** Congenital Heart Disease-Adult; Congenital Heart Disease; **Hospital:** Mayo Med Ctr & Clin - Rochester; **Address:** Mayo Clinic, 200 1st St SW, Gonda 6-138 SW, Rochester, MN 55905; **Phone:** 507-266-0676; **Board Cert:** Pediatric Cardiology 2011; **Med School:** Loyola Univ-Stritch Sch Med 1987; **Resid:** Internal Medicine & Pediatrics, Loyola Med Ctr 1991; **Fac Appt:** Assoc Prof Ped, Mayo Med Sch

Cheatham, John P MD [PCd] - **Spec Exp:** Congenital Heart Disease-Adult & Child; Cardiac Catheterization; **Hospital:** Nationwide Chldn's Hosp; **Address:** The Heart Center, 700 Children's Drive, Columbus, OH 43205; **Phone:** 614-722-2459; **Board Cert:** Pediatrics 1981; Pediatric Cardiology 1983; **Med School:** Univ Okla Coll Med 1976; **Resid:** Pediatrics, Children's Hosp 1978; **Fellow:** Pediatric Cardiology, Texas Children's Hosp 1981; **Fac Appt:** Prof Ped, Ohio State Univ

Dick, Macdonald MD [PCd] - **Spec Exp:** Congenital Heart Disease; **Hospital:** Mott Chldns Hosp; **Address:** Motts Chldns Hosp, Dept Ped Cardio, 1500 E Med Ctr Drive, rm L1242, Box 0204, Ann Arbor, MI 48109; **Phone:** 734-936-7418; **Board Cert:** Pediatrics 1989; Pediatric Cardiology 2007; **Med School:** Univ VA Sch Med 1967; **Resid:** Pediatrics, Univ Va Hosp 1971; **Fellow:** Pediatric Cardiology, Chldns Hosp Med Ctr 1974; **Fac Appt:** Prof Ped, Univ Mich Med Sch

Driscoll, David J MD [PCd] - **Spec Exp:** Exercise Physiology; Klippel-Trenaunay Syndrome; Cardiomyopathy; **Hospital:** Mayo Med Ctr & Clin - Rochester; **Address:** Mayo Clin, Div Ped Cardiology, 200 First St SW, Rochester, MN 55905; **Phone:** 507-284-3682; **Board Cert:** Pediatrics 1976; Pediatric Cardiology 2006; **Med School:** Marquette Sch Med 1970; **Resid:** Pediatrics, Milwaukee Chldns Hosp 1972; Pediatrics, Milwaukee Chldns Hosp 1975; **Fellow:** Pediatric Cardiology, Baylor Coll Med 1978; **Fac Appt:** Prof Ped, Mayo Med Sch

Feltes, Timothy F MD [PCd] - **Spec Exp:** Congenital Heart Disease; **Hospital:** Nationwide Chldn's Hosp; **Address:** 700 Children's Drive, rm ED619, Nationwide Chldn's Hosp, Columbus, OH 43205; **Phone:** 614-722-2565; **Board Cert:** Pediatrics 1985; Pediatric Cardiology 2010; **Med School:** Univ Toledo, Med Univ OH 1980; **Resid:** Pediatrics, Emory Univ Med Ctr 1983; **Fellow:** Pediatric Cardiology, Texas Children's Hosp 1986; **Fac Appt:** Clin Prof Ped, Ohio State Univ

Hardin, Joel T MD [PCd] - **Spec Exp:** Congenital Heart Disease-Adult & Child; Cardiac Intensive Care; Marfan's Syndrome; **Hospital:** Loyola Univ Med Ctr; **Address:** Loyola University Medical Center, 2160 S 1st Ave Maguire Bldg - rm 3312, Maywood, IL 60153-3328; **Phone:** 708-327-9103; **Board Cert:** Pediatrics 2005; Pediatric Cardiology 2009; **Med School:** Univ Tenn Coll Med 1987; **Resid:** Pediatrics, St Louis Children's Hosp 1990; **Fellow:** Pediatric Cardiology, St Louis Children's Hosp 1993; **Fac Appt:** Assoc Prof Ped, Loyola Univ-Stritch Sch Med

Hijazi, Ziyad M MD [PCd] - **Spec Exp:** Interventional Cardiology; Congenital Heart Disease; Coarctation of the Aorta; **Hospital:** Rush Univ Med Ctr; **Address:** 1653 W Congress Pkwy, Ste 770 Jones, Chicago, IL 60612; **Phone:** 312-942-8941; **Board Cert:** Pediatric Cardiology 2007; **Med School:** Jordan 1982; **Resid:** Pediatrics, Yale-New Haven Hosp 1988; **Fellow:** Pediatric Cardiology, Yale-New Haven Hosp 1991; **Fac Appt:** Prof Ped, Rush Med Coll

Hoyer, Mark H MD [PCd] - **Spec Exp:** Cardiac Catheterization; Congenital Heart Disease-Adult; **Hospital:** Riley Hosp for Children; **Address:** Riley Hosp Div Cardiology, 702 Barnhill Drive, RR 104, Indianapolis, IN 46202; **Phone:** 317-274-8906; **Board Cert:** Pediatric Cardiology 2006; **Med School:** Ohio State Univ 1985; **Resid:** Pediatrics, Wright-Patterson AFB Med Ctr 1988; **Fellow:** Pediatric Cardiac Surgery, Chldns Hosp 1991; **Fac Appt:** Clin Prof Ped, Indiana Univ

Pahl, Elfriede MD [PCd] - **Spec Exp:** Transplant Medicine-Heart; Heart Failure; Congenital Heart Disease; Kawasaki Disease; **Hospital:** Lurie Chldn's Hosp-Chicago; **Address:** Lurie Chldn's Hosp, Ped Cardiology, 225 E Chicago Ave, Box 21, Chicago, IL 60611; **Phone:** 773-880-4553; **Board Cert:** Pediatrics 1987; Pediatric Cardiology 2010; **Med School:** Northwestern Univ 1983; **Resid:** Pediatrics, Chldns Meml Hosp 1986; **Fellow:** Pediatric Cardiology, Chldns Hosp of Pittsburgh 1988; **Fac Appt:** Prof Ped, Northwestern Univ

Rocchini, Albert P MD [PCd] - **Spec Exp:** Congenital Heart Disease; Interventional Cardiology; Hypertension in Obesity; **Hospital:** Univ of Michigan Hosp; **Address:** Mott Chldns Hosp, Dept Ped Cardiology, 1500 E Med Ctr Drive, rm L1242, Box 0204, Ann Arbor, MI 48109-0204; **Phone:** 734-936-8993; **Board Cert:** Pediatrics 1989; Pediatric Cardiology 1989; **Med School:** Univ Pittsburgh 1972; **Resid:** Pediatrics, Univ Minn 1974; **Fellow:** Pediatric Cardiology, Chldns Hosp 1977; **Fac Appt:** Prof Ped, Univ Mich Med Sch

Great Plains and Mountains

Minich, Lois LuAnn MD [PCd] - **Spec Exp:** Echocardiography; **Hospital:** Primary Children's Med Ctr; **Address:** Dept Ped Cardiology, 100 N Mario Capecchi Drive, Ste 1500, Salt Lake City, UT 84113; **Phone:** 801-662-5400; **Board Cert:** Pediatric Cardiology 2007; **Med School:** W VA Univ 1986; **Resid:** Pediatrics, Fletcher Allen Health Care 1989; **Fellow:** Pediatric Cardiology, Univ Michigan Hosps 1992

Pediatric Cardiology

Southwest

Bricker, John T MD [PCd] - **Spec Exp:** Transplant Medicine-Heart; Congenital Heart Disease-Adult & Child; **Hospital:** Meml Hermann Hosp - Texas Med Ctr; **Address:** UT Physicians- Pediatric Cardiology, 6410 Fannin St, Ste 425, Houston, TX 77030; **Phone:** 832-325-7200; **Board Cert:** Pediatrics 1981; Pediatric Cardiology 1997; **Med School:** Ohio State Univ 1976; **Resid:** Pediatrics, Tex Chldns Hosp 1980; **Fellow:** Pediatric Cardiology, Tex Chldns Hosp 1983; **Fac Appt:** Prof Ped, Univ Tex, Houston

Dreyer, William J MD [PCd] - **Spec Exp:** Congenital Heart Disease; Transplant Medicine-Heart; **Hospital:** Texas Chldns Hosp; **Address:** 6621 Fannin St, West Tower Fl 20, MC 19345-C, Houston, TX 77030; **Phone:** 832-826-5659; **Board Cert:** Pediatrics 1987; Pediatric Cardiology 2006; **Med School:** Univ Fla Coll Med 1981; **Resid:** Pediatrics, UCSF Med Ctr 1984; **Fellow:** Pediatric Cardiology, Baylor Coll Med 1988; **Fac Appt:** Assoc Prof Ped, Baylor Coll Med

Gillette, Paul C MD [PCd] - **Spec Exp:** Arrhythmias; **Hospital:** Cook Chldns Med Ctr, Harris Methodist Hosp - Fort Worth; **Address:** 209 N Bonnie Brae, Bldg 3 - Fl 1 - Ste 100, MS 76201, Denton, TX 76201; **Phone:** 940-243-0104; **Board Cert:** Pediatrics 1974; Pediatric Cardiology 1975; **Med School:** Med Univ SC 1969; **Resid:** Pediatrics, Baylor Coll Med 1972; **Fellow:** Pediatric Cardiology, Baylor Coll Med 1974

Mahony, Lynn MD [PCd] - **Spec Exp:** Congenital Heart Disease; Marfan's Syndrome; Congestive Heart Failure; Complex Diagnosis; **Hospital:** Chldns Med Ctr of Dallas; **Address:** 1935 Medical District Drive, Ste C3210, Dept Cardiology, Dallas, TX 75235; **Phone:** 214-456-2333; **Board Cert:** Pediatrics 1979; Pediatric Cardiology 1997; **Med School:** Stanford Univ 1975; **Resid:** Pediatrics, Stanford Univ 1978; **Fellow:** Pediatric Cardiology, UCSF Med Ctr 1981; **Fac Appt:** Prof Ped, Univ Tex SW, Dallas

Moodie, Douglas S MD [PCd] - **Spec Exp:** Marfan's Syndrome; Congenital Heart Disease-Adult & Child; **Hospital:** Texas Chldns Hosp; **Address:** 6621 Fannin St Fl 20, MC 19345-C, Houston, TX 77030; **Phone:** 832-826-5659; **Board Cert:** Pediatrics 1977; Pediatric Cardiology 1977; **Med School:** Med Coll Wisc 1972; **Resid:** Pediatrics, Mayo Clinic 1974; **Fellow:** Pediatric Cardiology, Mayo Clinic 1977; **Fac Appt:** Assoc Prof Ped, Baylor Coll Med

Rogers Jr, James H MD [PCd] - **Spec Exp:** Congenital Heart Disease; **Hospital:** Christus Santa Rosa Children's Hosp, Univ Hlth Syst-San Antonio; **Address:** Chldns Heart Network, 1901 Babcock Rd, Ste 301, San Antonio, TX 78229; **Phone:** 210-341-7722; **Board Cert:** Pediatrics 1976; Pediatric Cardiology 2009; **Med School:** Med Coll GA 1971; **Resid:** Pediatrics, Wilford Hall USAF Med Ctr 1974; **Fellow:** Pediatric Cardiology, Med Coll Georgia 1976; **Fac Appt:** Assoc Clin Prof Ped, Univ Tex, San Antonio

West Coast and Pacific

Bernstein, Daniel MD [PCd] - **Spec Exp:** Transplant Medicine-Heart; Congenital Heart Disease; Heart Failure; **Hospital:** Lucile Packard Chldn's Hosp, Stanford Univ Hosp & Clinics; **Address:** Lucile Packard Chldns Hosp, Div Ped Card, 750 Welch Rd, Ste 305, Palo Alto, CA 94304-5731; **Phone:** 650-721-2121; **Board Cert:** Pediatrics 1984; Pediatric Cardiology 1985; **Med School:** NYU Sch Med 1978; **Resid:** Pediatrics, Montefiore Hosp-Einstein 1982; **Fellow:** Pediatric Cardiology, UCSF Med Ctr 1986; **Fac Appt:** Prof Ped, Stanford Univ

Lewin, Mark MD [PCd] - **Spec Exp:** Echocardiography; Fetal Cardiology; **Hospital:** Seattle Chldns Hosp, Univ Wash Med Ctr; **Address:** Seattle Chldn's Hosp, 4800 Sand Point Way NE, G-0035-Cardiology Admin, Seattle, WA 98105; **Phone:** 206-987-2015; **Board Cert:** Pediatric Cardiology 2006; **Med School:** USC-Keck School of Medicine 1991; **Resid:** Pediatrics, Chldns Hosp 1994; **Fellow:** Pediatric Cardiology, Texas Chldns Hosp 1998; **Fac Appt:** Assoc Prof Ped, Univ Wash

Perry, Stanton Bruce MD [PCd] - **Spec Exp:** Interventional Cardiology; **Hospital:** Lucile Packard Chldn's Hosp; **Address:** Lucile Packard Chldns Hosp, Dept Ped Cardiology, 750 Welch Rd, Ste 305, Palo Alto, CA 94304; **Phone:** 650-721-2121; **Board Cert:** Pediatrics 1986; **Med School:** Iceland 1978; **Resid:** Pediatrics, St Louis Chldn's Hosp 1983; **Fellow:** Pediatric Cardiology, Chldns Hosp 1984; **Fac Appt:** Assoc Prof Ped, Stanford Univ

Teitel, David F MD [PCd] - **Spec Exp:** Cardiac Catheterization; Congenital Heart Disease; **Hospital:** UCSF Med Ctr; **Address:** UCSF, Pediatric Heart Center, 400 Parnassus Ave, 2nd Fl, San Francisco, CA 94143-0544; **Phone:** 415-353-2008; **Board Cert:** Pediatrics 1980; Pediatric Cardiology 2004; **Med School:** Univ Toronto 1975; **Resid:** Pediatrics, Chldns Hosp 1980; **Fellow:** Pediatric Cardiology, UCSF Med Ctr 1982; **Fac Appt:** Prof Ped, UCSF

Zahn, Evan M MD [PCd] - **Spec Exp:** Interventional Cardiology; Ventricular Septal Defect (Amplatzer R); Congenital Heart Disease; **Hospital:** Cedars-Sinai Med Ctr; **Address:** Cedar-Sinai Med Ctr, 8700 Beverly Blvd, Los Angeles, CA 90048; **Phone:** 310-423-1153; **Board Cert:** Pediatric Cardiology 2007; **Med School:** NY Med Coll 1986; **Resid:** Pediatrics, Univ Colorado Hosp 1989; **Fellow:** Pediatric Cardiology, Hosp for Sick Children 1991; Interventional Cardiology, Hosp for Sick Children 1992

PEDIATRIC CRITICAL CARE MEDICINE

Mid Atlantic

Thompson, Ann Ellen MD [PCCM] - **Spec Exp:** Mechanical Ventilation; Critical Care; Respiratory Failure; **Hospital:** Chldns Hosp of Pittsburgh - UPMC; **Address:** Chldns Hosp, Dept Ped Crit Care, 4401 Penn Ave Fl 2, Pittsburgh, PA 15224; **Phone:** 412-692-5164; **Board Cert:** Pediatrics 1992; Anesthesiology 1980; Pediatric Critical Care Medicine 2010; **Med School:** Tufts Univ 1974; **Resid:** Pediatrics, Chldns Hosp 1977; Anesthesiology, Hosp Univ Penn 1980; **Fellow:** Pediatric Critical Care Medicine, Chldns Hosp 1979; **Fac Appt:** Prof Ped, Univ Pittsburgh

Southeast

Anand, Kanwaljeet Singh MD/PhD [PCCM] - **Spec Exp:** Pain Management; Critical Care; **Hospital:** Le Bonheur Chldns Med Ctr, St. Jude Children's Research Hosp; **Address:** 50 N Dunlap St, rm 351R, Memphis, TN 38103-2893; **Phone:** 901-287-6303; **Board Cert:** Pediatric Critical Care Medicine 2011; **Med School:** India 1981; **Resid:** Pediatrics, Chldns Hosp 1991; Neonatal-Perinatal Medicine, John Radcliffe Hosp 1985; **Fellow:** Pediatric Critical Care Medicine, Mass Genl Hosp 1993; **Fac Appt:** Prof Ped, Univ Tenn Coll Med

Pediatric Critical Care Medicine

Midwest

Sarnaik, Ashok P MD [PCCM] - **Spec Exp:** Critical Care; Perinatal Medicine; **Hospital:** Chldns Hosp of Michigan; **Address:** Chldns Hosp, Div Crit Care Med, 3901 Beaubien St, Carl's Bldg - Ste 4134, Detroit, MI 48201-2119; **Phone:** 313-745-5629; **Board Cert:** Pediatrics 1975; Neonatal-Perinatal Medicine 1979; Pediatric Critical Care Medicine 2003; **Med School:** India 1969; **Resid:** Pediatrics, JJ Hosp-Bombay Univ 1971; Pediatrics, Chldns Hosp Mich 1974; **Fellow:** Neonatal-Perinatal Medicine, Chldns Hosp Mich 1975; **Fac Appt:** Prof Ped, Wayne State Univ

Sichting, Kay A MD [PCCM] - **Hospital:** Peyton Manning Children's Hosp at St. Vincent; **Address:** Peyton Manning Chldns Hosp-PICU, 2001 W 86th St, Indianapolis, IN 46260; **Phone:** 317-338-5230; **Board Cert:** Pediatric Critical Care Medicine 2006; **Med School:** Indiana Univ 1990; **Resid:** Pediatrics, Riley Hosp for Chldn 1993; **Fellow:** Pediatric Critical Care Medicine, Riley Hosp for Chldn 1994; Pediatric Critical Care Medicine, Chldns Hosp of WI 1997

Great Plains and Mountains

Dean, J. Michael MD [PCCM] - **Hospital:** Primary Children's Med Ctr; **Address:** Pediatric Critical Care, Univ Utah, 100 N Mario Capecchi Drive, Salt Lake City, UT 84158; **Phone:** 801-662-2400; **Board Cert:** Pediatrics 1981; Pediatric Critical Care Medicine 2010; **Med School:** Northwestern Univ 1977; **Resid:** Pediatrics, Children's Hosp 1981; **Fellow:** Pediatric Critical Care Medicine, Johns Hopkins Hosp 1983; **Fac Appt:** Prof Ped, Univ Utah

Southwest

Easley, Ronald B MD [PCCM] - **Spec Exp:** Congenital Heart Disease; **Hospital:** Texas Chldns Hosp; **Address:** 6621 Fannin St, Houston, TX 77030; **Phone:** 832-824-5800; **Board Cert:** Pediatric Critical Care Medicine 2012; Pediatrics 2006; Anesthesiology 2003; **Med School:** Univ MO-Columbia Sch Med 1995; **Resid:** Pediatrics, Univ MO Hosp 1999; Anesthesiology, Johns Hopkins Hosp 2002; **Fellow:** Pediatric Critical Care Medicine, Johns Hopkins Hosp 2004; **Fac Appt:** Asst Prof Ped, Baylor Coll Med

Fuhrman, Bradley P MD [PCCM] - **Spec Exp:** Disaster Preparedness; **Hospital:** El Paso Chldns Hosp; **Address:** Professor and Chair Department of Pediatrics, Paul L. Foster School of Medicine, 4800 Alberta Ave, El Paso, TX 79905-2799; **Phone:** 915-545-6921; **Board Cert:** Pediatrics 1992; Pediatric Critical Care Medicine 2010; Neonatal-Perinatal Medicine 1979; Pediatric Cardiology 1979; **Med School:** NYU Sch Med 1971; **Resid:** Pediatrics, Univ Minnesota Med Ctr 1973; **Fellow:** Pediatric Cardiology, Univ Minnesota 1979; Neonatal-Perinatal Medicine, Univ Minnesota 1979; **Fac Appt:** Prof Ped, Texas Tech Univ

Perez Fontan, J Julio MD [PCCM] - **Spec Exp:** Respiratory Failure; **Hospital:** UT Southwestern Med Ctr at Dallas, Chldns Med Ctr of Dallas; **Address:** UT SW Med Ctr, Dept Peds, 5323 Harry Hines Blvd, Ste K4.500, Dallas, TX 75390-9063; **Phone:** 214-648-9618; **Board Cert:** Pediatrics 1987; Pediatric Critical Care Medicine 2003; **Med School:** Spain 1977; **Resid:** Pediatrics, Chldns Hosp/Univ Barcelona 1981; **Fellow:** Critical Care Medicine, UCSF Med Ctr 1984; **Fac Appt:** Prof Ped, Univ Tex SW, Dallas

Taylor, Richard P MD [PCCM] - **Hospital:** Christus Santa Rosa Children's Hosp, Univ Hlth Syst-San Antonio; **Address:** Dept Ped Critical Care, 7703 Floyd Curl Drive, San Antonio, TX 78229; **Phone:** 210-562-5816; **Board Cert:** Internal Medicine 1988; Pediatric Critical Care Medicine 2004; **Med School:** Univ Tex Med Br, Galveston 1984; **Resid:** Internal Medicine, St Joseph Mercy Hosp 1988; Pediatrics, UNiv Michigan Med Ctr 1988; **Fellow:** Pediatric Critical Care Medicine, Univ Michigan Med Ctr 1995; **Fac Appt:** Prof Ped, Univ Tex, San Antonio

West Coast and Pacific

Schwarz, Adam J MD [PCCM] - **Hospital:** Chldns Hosp Orange Co; **Address:** Chldns Hosp of Orange, 455 S Main St, Orange, CA 92868; **Phone:** 714-532-8620; **Board Cert:** Pediatric Critical Care Medicine 2011; Pediatrics 2009; **Med School:** Stanford Univ 1990; **Resid:** Pediatrics, Stanford Med Ctr 1993; **Fellow:** Pediatric Critical Care Medicine, Harbor-UCLA Med Ctr 1996; **Fac Appt:** Assoc Clin Prof Ped

Zimmerman, Jerry John MD [PCCM] - **Spec Exp:** Inflammation in Critical Illness; Sepsis; Septic Shock; **Hospital:** Seattle Chldns Hosp, Harborview Med Ctr; **Address:** Seattle Chldn's Hosp, 4800 Sand Point Way NE, MS W8866, Seattle, WA 98145-5440; **Phone:** 206-987-3862; **Board Cert:** Pediatrics 1992; Pediatric Critical Care Medicine 2010; **Med School:** Univ Wisc 1979; **Resid:** Pediatrics, Univ Wisconsin Hosp 1982; **Fellow:** Pediatric Critical Care Medicine, Chldns Natl Med Ctr 1984; **Fac Appt:** Prof Ped, Univ Wash

PEDIATRIC ENDOCRINOLOGY

New England

Casella, Samuel Joseph MD [PEn] - **Spec Exp:** Thyroid Disorders; Growth/Development Disorders; **Hospital:** Dartmouth - Hitchcock Med Ctr; **Address:** Dartmouth-Hitchcock Med Ctr, Dept Ped Endo, 1 Med Ctr Drive Fl 6M, Lebanon, NH 03756; **Phone:** 603-653-9877; **Board Cert:** Pediatrics 1985; Pediatric Endocrinology 1986; **Med School:** SUNY Upstate Med Univ 1981; **Resid:** Pediatrics, Upstate Med Ctr 1984; **Fellow:** Pediatric Endocrinology, NC Meml Hosp-Univ NC 1986; **Fac Appt:** Assoc Prof Ped, Johns Hopkins Univ

Gordon, Catherine M MD [PEn] - **Spec Exp:** Bone Disorders-Metabolic; **Hospital:** Rhode Island Hosp; **Address:** Hasbro Children's Hospital, 593 Eddy St, Providence, RI 02903; **Phone:** 401-444-4712; **Board Cert:** Pediatric Endocrinology 2007; Adolescent Medicine 2009; **Med School:** Univ NC Sch Med 1991; **Resid:** Pediatrics, Chldns Hosp 1994; **Fellow:** Pediatric Endocrinology, Chldns Hosp 1996

Levitsky, Lynne Li MD [PEn] - **Spec Exp:** Diabetes; Growth/Development Disorders; Cushing's Syndrome; **Hospital:** Mass Genl Hosp; **Address:** MGH Pediatric Endocrine Assocs, 55 Fruit St Yawkey Bldg Fl 6 - rm 6C, Boston, MA 02114; **Phone:** 617-726-2909; **Board Cert:** Pediatrics 1971; Pediatric Endocrinology 1978; **Med School:** Yale Univ 1966; **Resid:** Pediatrics, Albert Einstein Coll of Med 1967; Pediatrics, Chldns Hosp 1968; **Fellow:** Pediatric Endocrinology, Univ Maryland Hosp 1970; **Fac Appt:** Assoc Prof Ped, Harvard Med Sch

Ludwig, David S MD/PhD [PEn] - **Spec Exp:** Obesity; Nutrition; **Hospital:** Children's Hospital - Boston; **Address:** Chldns Hosp, Div Endocrinology, 333 Longwood Ave Fl 6 - rm 624, Boston, MA 02115; **Phone:** 617-355-7476; **Board Cert:** Pediatric Endocrinology 2003; **Med School:** Stanford Univ 1990; **Resid:** Pediatrics, Chldns Hosp 1993; **Fellow:** Pediatric Endocrinology, Chldns Hosp 1995; **Fac Appt:** Asst Prof Ped, Harvard Med Sch

Spack, Norman P MD [PEn] - **Spec Exp:** Transgender Issues; **Hospital:** Children's Hospital - Boston; **Address:** Chldns Hosp, Div Endocrinology, 300 Longwood Ave, Boston, MA 02115; **Phone:** 617-355-7476; **Board Cert:** Pediatrics 1975; Pediatric Endocrinology 2003; **Med School:** Univ Rochester 1969; **Resid:** Pediatrics, Boston City Hosp/Chldns Hosp 1972; **Fellow:** Adolescent Medicine, Chldns Hosp 1975; Pediatric Endocrinology, Chldns Hosp 1978; **Fac Appt:** Assoc Prof Ped, Harvard Med Sch

Pediatric Endocrinology

Tamborlane, William V MD [PEn] - **Spec Exp:** Diabetes; **Hospital:** Yale-New Haven Hosp, Yale Med Group; **Address:** Yale Pediatric Endocrinology, 333 Cedar St, rm 3091-LMP, New Haven, CT 06519; **Phone:** 203-764-6747; **Board Cert:** Pediatrics 1978; Pediatric Endocrinology 1986; **Med School:** Georgetown Univ 1972; **Resid:** Pediatrics, Georgetown Univ Hosp 1975; **Fellow:** Pediatric Endocrinology, Yale-New Haven Hosp 1977; **Fac Appt:** Prof Ped, Yale Univ

Mid Atlantic

Alter, Craig A MD [PEn] - **Spec Exp:** Diabetes; Growth Disorders; Thyroid Disorders; Pubertal Disorders; **Hospital:** Chldns Hosp of Philadelphia; **Address:** Children's Hosp of Philadelphia, Dept Pediatric Endocrinology, 34th & Civic Ctr Blvd, Philadelphia, PA 19104; **Phone:** 215-590-3174; **Board Cert:** Pediatrics 2012; Pediatric Endocrinology 2010; **Med School:** Harvard Med Sch 1987; **Resid:** Pediatrics, Boston Childrens Hosp 1990; **Fellow:** Pediatric Endocrinology, Childrens Hosp 1993; **Fac Appt:** Clin Prof Ped, Univ Pennsylvania

Arslanian, Silva A MD [PEn] - **Spec Exp:** Obesity; Diabetes; **Hospital:** Chldns Hosp of Pittsburgh - UPMC; **Address:** Childrens Hosp Pittsburgh-Endocrinology, 4401 Penn Ave Fl 3, Pittsburgh, PA 15224; **Phone:** 412-692-6935; **Board Cert:** Pediatrics 1983; Pediatric Endocrinology 1983; **Med School:** Lebanon 1978; **Resid:** Pediatrics, American Univ Hosp 1980; **Fellow:** Pediatric Endocrinology, Chldns Hosp 1983; **Fac Appt:** Prof Ped, Univ Pittsburgh

Becker, Dorothy J MD [PEn] - **Spec Exp:** Diabetes; **Hospital:** Chldns Hosp of Pittsburgh - UPMC; **Address:** Childrens Hosp Pittsburgh-Endocrinology, 4401 Penn Ave, Faculty Pavilion Fl 8, Pittsburgh, PA 15224; **Phone:** 412-692-5172; **Board Cert:** Pediatrics 1978; Pediatric Endocrinology 1978; **Med School:** South Africa 1964; **Resid:** Pediatrics, Univ Capetown 1972; **Fellow:** Endocrinology, Diabetes & Metabolism, Univ Capetown 1974; Pediatric Endocrinology, Univ Pittsburgh Hosp 1976; **Fac Appt:** Prof Ped, Univ Pittsburgh

DeLuca, Francesco MD [PEn] - **Spec Exp:** Growth Disorders; Metabolic Syndrome; Osteoporosis; **Hospital:** St. Christopher's Hosp for Chldn; **Address:** St Christophers Hosp for Children, Endocrinology Section, Ste 3303, 3601 A St, Philadelphia, PA 19134; **Phone:** 215-427-8100; **Board Cert:** Pediatric Endocrinology 2010; **Med School:** Italy 1983; **Resid:** Pediatrics, Cath Univ Sacred Heart Affil Hosp; Pediatrics, Albert Einstein Med Ctr; **Fellow:** Pediatric Endocrinology, St Christophers Hosp; Pediatric Endocrinology, Natl Inst Hlth; **Fac Appt:** Prof Ped, Drexel Univ Coll Med

Garibaldi, Luigi R MD [PEn] - **Spec Exp:** Pubertal Disorders; Growth Disorders; **Hospital:** Chldns Hosp of Pittsburgh - UPMC; **Address:** Chldns Hosp Pittsburgh-Div Endocrinology, 4401 Penn Ave, Faculty Pavilion Fl 8, Pittsburgh, PA 15224; **Phone:** 412-692-5170; **Board Cert:** Pediatrics 1986; Pediatric Endocrinology 1986; **Med School:** Italy 1973; **Resid:** Pediatrics, Gaslini Inst-Chldn's Hosp 1978; Pediatrics, Univ Michigan Affil Hosp 1985; **Fellow:** Pediatric Endocrinology, Temple Univ Hosp 1981; Pediatric Endocrinology, Univ Chicago 1986; **Fac Appt:** Prof Ped, Univ Pittsburgh

Levine, Michael A MD [PEn] - **Spec Exp:** Bone Disorders-Metabolic; Osteoporosis; **Hospital:** Chldns Hosp of Philadelphia; **Address:** Childrens Hosp Philadelphia, Div Endocrinology, 34th St & Civic Center Blvd, Philadelphia, PA 19104; **Phone:** 215-590-3174; **Board Cert:** Internal Medicine 1979; Endocrinology, Diabetes & Metabolism 1981; **Med School:** Hahnemann Univ 1976; **Resid:** Internal Medicine, Johns Hopkins Hosp 1979; **Fellow:** Endocrinology, Natl Inst Hlth 1981; Genetics, Natl Inst Hlth 1981; **Fac Appt:** Prof Med, Univ Pennsylvania

Maclaren, Noel K MD [PEn] - **Spec Exp:** Diabetes; Obesity; Metabolic Syndrome; **Hospital:** Lenox Hill Hosp (page 67); **Address:** Bioseek Endocrine Clinic, 200 W 57th St, Ste 610, New York, NY 10019; **Phone:** 212-371-0658; **Board Cert:** Pediatrics 1977; Pediatric Endocrinology 1978; **Med School:** New Zealand 1963; **Resid:** Pediatrics, Wellington Public Hosp 1967; **Fellow:** Pediatric Endocrinology, Johns Hopkins Hosp 1973; **Fac Appt:** Prof Ped, Cornell Univ-Weill Med Coll

New, Maria I MD [PEn] - **Spec Exp:** Adrenal Disorders; Growth/Development Disorders; **Hospital:** Mount Sinai Med Ctr (page 64); **Address:** Mount Sinai Medical Ctr, 5 E 98th St Fl 10, New York, NY 10029; **Phone:** 212-241-8210; **Board Cert:** Pediatrics 1960; **Med School:** Univ Pennsylvania 1954; **Resid:** Pediatrics, New York Hosp 1957; **Fellow:** Pediatric Endocrinology, New York Hosp 1958; Endocrinology, Diabetes & Metabolism, New York Hosp 1964; **Fac Appt:** Prof Ped, Cornell Univ-Weill Med Coll

Oberfield, Sharon E MD [PEn] - **Spec Exp:** Adrenal Disorders; Neuroendocrine Growth Disorders; Growth Disorders; **Hospital:** Morgan Stanley Children's Hosp of NY-Presby, NY; **Address:** 630 W 168th St, PH East Bldg Fl 5 East - Ste 522, New York, NY 10032; **Phone:** 212-305-6559; **Board Cert:** Pediatrics 1979; Pediatric Endocrinology 2000; **Med School:** Cornell Univ-Weill Med Coll 1974; **Resid:** Pediatrics, NY Hosp-Cornell 1976; **Fellow:** Pediatric Endocrinology, NY Hosp-Cornell 1979; **Fac Appt:** Prof Ped, Columbia P&S

Plotnick, Leslie P MD [PEn] - **Spec Exp:** Diabetes; Growth Disorders; Thyroid Disorders; Pubertal Disorders; **Hospital:** Johns Hopkins Hosp (page 61); **Address:** Rubenstein Child Health Building, 200 N Wolfe St, Pediatric Endocrinology #3120, Baltimore, MD 21287; **Phone:** 410-955-6463; **Board Cert:** Pediatrics 1975; Pediatric Endocrinology 2009; **Med School:** Univ MD Sch Med 1970; **Resid:** Pediatrics, Johns Hopkins Hosp 1972; **Fellow:** Pediatric Endocrinology, Johns Hopkins Hosp 1974; **Fac Appt:** Prof Ped, Univ MD Sch Med

Sklar, Charles A MD [PEn] - **Spec Exp:** Cancer Survivors-Late Effects of Therapy; Growth Disorders in Childhood Cancer; Pituitary Disorders; **Hospital:** Meml Sloan-Kettering Cancer Ctr; **Address:** 1275 York Avenue, New York, NY 10065; **Phone:** 212-639-8138; **Board Cert:** Pediatrics 1979; Pediatric Endocrinology 1980; **Med School:** USC Sch Med 1974; **Resid:** Pediatrics, Childrens Hosp 1976; **Fellow:** Pediatric Endocrinology, UCSF Med Ctr 1979; **Fac Appt:** Assoc Prof Ped, Cornell Univ-Weill Med Coll

Sperling, Mark A MD [PEn] - **Spec Exp:** Diabetes; Growth/Development Disorders; Hypoglycemia; Neonatal Diabetes; **Hospital:** Chldns Hosp of Pittsburgh - UPMC, UPMC Presby, Pittsburgh; **Address:** 4401 Penn Ave, Faculty Pavillion, rm 8139, Pittsburgh, PA 15224-1334; **Phone:** 412-692-5172; **Board Cert:** Pediatrics 1986; Pediatric Endocrinology 1986; **Med School:** Australia 1962; **Resid:** Pediatrics, Royal Chldns Hosp 1968; **Fellow:** Endocrinology, Chldns Hosp 1970; **Fac Appt:** Prof Ped, Univ Pittsburgh

Stanley, Charles A MD [PEn] - **Spec Exp:** Hyperinsulinism-Congenital; Hypoglycemia; **Hospital:** Chldns Hosp of Philadelphia; **Address:** Chldns Hosp, Div Endocrinology, 34th St & Civic Ctr Blvd, Philadelphia, PA 19104; **Phone:** 215-590-3174; **Board Cert:** Pediatrics 1976; Pediatric Endocrinology 1978; **Med School:** Univ VA Sch Med 1970; **Resid:** Pediatrics, Children's Hosp 1972; **Fellow:** Pediatric Endocrinology, Children's Hosp 1976; **Fac Appt:** Prof Emeritus Ped, Univ Pennsylvania

Southeast

Diamond, Frank B MD [PEn] - **Spec Exp:** Growth Disorders; Obesity; Calcium Disorders in Newborn; **Hospital:** All Children's Hosp, Tampa Genl Hosp; **Address:** 501 6th Ave S, MS 33701, ACH Box 6900, St Petersburg, FL 33701; **Phone:** 727-767-3636; **Board Cert:** Pediatrics 1979; Pediatric Endocrinology 1980; **Med School:** Penn State Coll Med 1974; **Resid:** Pediatrics, Chldns Hosp-Univ Alabama 1976; **Fellow:** Pediatric Endocrinology, Chldns Hosp-Univ Penn 1978; **Fac Appt:** Prof Ped, Univ S Fla Coll Med

Pediatric Endocrinology

Freemark, Michael S MD [PEn] - **Spec Exp:** Prader-Willi Syndrome; Growth Disorders; Pubertal Disorders; Diabetes; **Hospital:** Duke Univ Hosp, Durham Regional Hosp; **Address:** DUMC, Box 102820, 3000 Erwin Rd, Lenox Baker Bldg, Ste 200, Durham, NC 27710; **Phone:** 919-684-8350; **Board Cert:** Pediatrics 1980; Pediatric Endocrinology 2010; **Med School:** Duke Univ 1976; **Resid:** Pediatrics, Duke Univ Med Ctr 1979; **Fellow:** Pediatric Endocrinology, Duke Univ Med Ctr 1983; Pediatric Endocrinology, Hospital Necker Enfants Malades 1993; **Fac Appt:** Prof Ped, Duke Univ

Meacham, Lillian R MD [PEn] - **Spec Exp:** Growth Disorders in Childhood Cancer; Cancer Survivors-Late Effects of Therapy; **Hospital:** Chldns Hlthcare Atlanta @ Scottish Rite, Chldns Hlthcare Atlanta @ Egleston; **Address:** Aflac Outpatient Center, 5455 Meridian Mark Rd NE, Ste 400, Atlanta, GA 30342; **Phone:** 404-785-3240; **Board Cert:** Pediatrics 2006; Pediatric Endocrinology 2006; **Med School:** Emory Univ 1984; **Resid:** Pediatrics, Emory Univ Hosp 1987; **Fellow:** Pediatric Endocrinology, Emory Univ Hosp 1990; **Fac Appt:** Prof Ped, Emory Univ

Rivkees, Scott A MD [PEn] - **Spec Exp:** Thyroid Disorders; Adrenal Disorders; Neuroendocrinology; Growth Disorders; **Hospital:** Children's Hosp at Shands/University of Florid; **Address:** UF Coll Medicine, Dept Pediatrics, 1600 SW Archer Rd, rm R1-118, Gainesville, FL 32610-0296; **Phone:** 352-273-5625; **Board Cert:** Pediatrics 1987; Pediatric Endocrinology 2012; **Med School:** UMDNJ-NJ Med Sch, Newark 1982; **Resid:** Pediatrics, Mass Genl Hosp 1985; **Fellow:** Pediatric Endocrinology, Mass Genl Hosp 1986; **Fac Appt:** Prof Ped, Univ Fla Coll Med

Silverstein, Janet H MD [PEn] - **Spec Exp:** Diabetes; Growth/Development Disorders; Obesity; **Hospital:** Shands at Univ of FL; **Address:** Univ Florida - Shands Hlthcare, 1701 SW Archer Rd, Gainesville, FL 32610-3003; **Phone:** 352-334-1390; **Board Cert:** Pediatrics 1975; Pediatric Endocrinology 2004; **Med School:** Univ Pennsylvania 1970; **Resid:** Pediatrics, Chldns Hosp 1972; Pediatrics, Chldns Hosp 1975; **Fellow:** Pediatric Endocrinology, Duke Univ Med Ctr 1977; **Fac Appt:** Prof Ped, Univ Fla Coll Med

Midwest

Allen, David B MD [PEn] - **Spec Exp:** Growth Disorders; Pubertal Disorders; Diabetes; **Hospital:** Univ WI Hosp & Clins; **Address:** UW American Family Chldn's Hosp, H4/448 CSC-Pediatrics, 600 Highland Ave, Madison, WI 53792-4108; **Phone:** 608-263-9059; **Board Cert:** Pediatrics 1986; Pediatric Endocrinology 2011; **Med School:** Duke Univ 1980; **Resid:** Pediatrics, Univ Wisconsin Hosp 1985; **Fellow:** Pediatric Endocrinology, Univ Wisconsin 1988; **Fac Appt:** Prof Ped, Univ Wisc

Cuttler, Leona MD [PEn] - **Hospital:** UH Rainbow Babies & Chldns Hosp (page 74); **Address:** Rainbow Babies & Children's Hosp, Div Pediatric Endocrinology, 11100 Euclid Ave, Ste 737, Cleveland, OH 44106; **Phone:** 216-844-3661; **Board Cert:** Pediatrics 1980; Pediatric Endocrinology 1983; **Med School:** McGill Univ 1975; **Resid:** Pediatrics, Hosp for Sick Chldn 1980; **Fellow:** Pediatric Endocrinology, Hosp for Sick Chldn 1982; Pediatric Endocrinology, UCSF Med Ctr 1984; **Fac Appt:** Prof Ped, Case West Res Univ

DiMeglio, Linda A MD [PEn] - **Spec Exp:** Diabetes; Bone Disorders-Metabolic; Clinical Trials; **Hospital:** Riley Hosp for Children; **Address:** Riley Hosp for Children, Div Endocrinology, 705 Riley Hospital Drive, rm 5960, Indianapolis, IN 46202; **Phone:** 317-944-3889; **Board Cert:** Pediatrics 2011; Pediatric Endocrinology 2007; **Med School:** Univ Pennsylvania 1993; **Resid:** Pediatrics, Chldns Meml Hosp 1996; **Fellow:** Pediatric Endocrinology, Indiana Univ Med Ctr 1999; **Fac Appt:** Assoc Prof Ped, Indiana Univ

Eugster, Erica A MD [PEn] - **Spec Exp:** Pubertal Disorders; Turner Syndrome; Growth/Development Disorders; Sex Development Disorders; **Hospital:** Riley Hosp for Children, Franciscan St. Francis Hlth-Indianapolis; **Address:** Riley Childrens Hosp, Pediatric Endocrinology, 705 Riley Hospital Drive, rm 5960, Indianapolis, IN 46202; **Phone:** 317-944-3889; **Board Cert:** Pediatric Endocrinology 2012; **Med School:** Med Coll PA 1990; **Resid:** Pediatrics, Marshfield Clin-St Josephs Hosp 1994; **Fellow:** Pediatric Endocrinology, Univ Minn 1997; **Fac Appt:** Prof Ped, Indiana Univ

Gutai, James P MD [PEn] - **Hospital:** Chldns Hosp of Michigan, Marquette Genl Hosp; **Address:** Comprehensive Diabetes Ctr, 4201 St Antoine St, Univ Hlth Ctr, Ste 6G14, Detroit, MI 48201; **Phone:** 313-577-0133; **Board Cert:** Pediatrics 1977; Pediatric Endocrinology 1980; **Med School:** Temple Univ 1970; **Resid:** Pediatrics, Johns Hopkins Hosp 1977; **Fellow:** Pediatric Endocrinology, Johns Hopkins Hosp 1980; **Fac Appt:** Prof Ped, Wayne State Univ

Levy, Richard A MD [PEn] - **Spec Exp:** Growth Disorders; Pituitary Disorders; Thyroid Disorders; **Hospital:** Rush Univ Med Ctr; **Address:** 1725 W Harrison St, Ste 328, Chicago, IL 60612-3863; **Phone:** 312-942-8989; **Board Cert:** Internal Medicine 1976; Pediatrics 1983; Endocrinology 1985; Pediatric Endocrinology 1986; **Med School:** Louisiana State U, New Orleans 1971; **Resid:** Internal Medicine, Univ Mass Med Ctr 1978; Pediatrics, Beth Israel Hosp 1979; **Fellow:** Endocrinology, Diabetes & Metabolism, Barnes Jewish Hosp 1982; **Fac Appt:** Asst Prof Ped, Rush Med Coll

Menon, Ram K MD [PEn] - **Spec Exp:** Growth/Development Disorders; Diabetes; **Hospital:** Univ of Michigan Hosp, Mott Chldns Hosp; **Address:** Mott Chldns Hosp-Pediatric Endocrinology, 1500 E Med Ctr Drive, D1205 MPB-SPC5718, Ann Arbor, MI 48109; **Phone:** 734-764-5175; **Board Cert:** Pediatrics 2009; Pediatric Endocrinology 2010; **Med School:** India 1979; **Resid:** Pediatrics, India Inst Med Sci 1984; **Fellow:** Endocrinology & Metabolism, Royal Free Hosp & Med Coll 1986; Pediatric Endocrinology, Chldn's Hosp Med Ctr 1989; **Fac Appt:** Assoc Prof Ped, Univ Mich Med Sch

Mirmira, Raghu G MD/PhD [PEn] - **Spec Exp:** Diabetes; **Hospital:** Riley Hosp for Children; **Address:** Riley Hosp Chldn-Endocrinology, 705 Riley Hospital Drive, rm 5960, Indianapolis, IN 46202; **Phone:** 317-944-3889; **Board Cert:** Endocrinology, Diabetes & Metabolism 2008; **Med School:** Univ Chicago-Pritzker Sch Med 1993; **Resid:** Internal Medicine, UCSF Med Ctr 1995; **Fellow:** Endocrinology, Diabetes & Metabolism, UCSF 1998; **Fac Appt:** Assoc Prof Ped, Indiana Univ

Norris, Andrew W MD/PhD [PEn] - **Spec Exp:** Diabetes; **Hospital:** Univ Iowa Hosp & Clinics; **Address:** UIHC Pediatric Endocrinology, 200 Hawkins Dr 2857 JPP, Iowa City, IA 52242; **Phone:** 319-356-2229; **Board Cert:** Pediatric Endocrinology 2011; **Med School:** Washington Univ, St Louis 1997; **Resid:** Pediatrics, Univ IA Hosp & Clin 2000; **Fellow:** Pediatric Endocrinology, Chldns Hosp 2003; **Fac Appt:** Asst Prof Ped, Univ Wash

Rogers, Douglas G MD [PEn] - **Spec Exp:** Diabetes; Growth/Development Disorders; Thyroid Disorders; **Hospital:** Cleveland Clin (page 55); **Address:** Cleveland Clinic Foundation, Center for Pediatric Endocrinology, 9500 Euclid Ave, MS A-120, Cleveland, OH 44195-0001; **Phone:** 216-444-5515; **Board Cert:** Pediatrics 1984; Pediatric Endocrinology 1986; **Med School:** Ros Franklin Univ/Chicago Med Sch 1978; **Resid:** Pediatrics, Cardinal Glennon Chldns Hosp 1981; **Fellow:** Pediatric Endocrinology, St Louis Chldns Hosp 1985

White, Neil H MD [PEn] - **Spec Exp:** Diabetes; **Hospital:** St. Louis Chldns Hosp; **Address:** St Louis Chldns Hosp, One Children's Pl, CB 8116, St Louis, MO 63110-1010; **Phone:** 314-454-6051; **Board Cert:** Pediatrics 1981; Pediatric Endocrinology 1983; **Med School:** Albert Einstein Coll Med 1975; **Resid:** Pediatrics, St Louis Chldns Hosp 1980; **Fellow:** Endocrinology, Diabetes & Metabolism, Washington Univ 1983; **Fac Appt:** Prof Ped, Washington Univ, St Louis

Pediatric Endocrinology

Zimmerman, Donald MD [PEn] - **Spec Exp:** Growth Disorders in Childhood Cancer; Thyroid Cancer; Thyroid Disorders; Growth/Development Disorders; **Hospital:** Lurie Chldn's Hosp-Chicago; **Address:** Children's Memorial Hosp, 2300 Children's Plaza, Div Endocrinology, Box 54, Chicago, IL 60614; **Phone:** 312-227-6090; **Board Cert:** Internal Medicine 1977; Endocrinology 1979; Pediatrics 1983; Pediatric Endocrinology 2001; **Med School:** Univ IL Coll Med 1974; **Resid:** Internal Medicine, Johns Hopkins Hosp 1977; Pediatrics, Mayo Clinic 1981; **Fellow:** Endocrinology, Diabetes & Metabolism, Mayo Clinic 1980; **Fac Appt:** Prof Ped, Northwestern Univ

Great Plains and Mountains

Foster, Carol M MD [PEn] - **Spec Exp:** Diabetes; Growth/Development Disorders; Pubertal Disorders; **Hospital:** Primary Children's Med Ctr, Univ Utah Hlth Care; **Address:** Utah Diabetes Ctr, 615 Arapeen Drive, Ste 100, Salt Lake City, UT 84108; **Phone:** 801-581-7761; **Board Cert:** Pediatrics 1983; Pediatric Endocrinology 1983; **Med School:** Washington Univ, St Louis 1978; **Resid:** Pediatrics, Univ Utah Hlth Scis Ctr 1981; **Fellow:** Pediatric Endocrinology, Natl Inst Hlth 1984; **Fac Appt:** Prof Med, Univ Utah

Kappy, Michael S MD/PhD [PEn] - **Spec Exp:** Growth/Development Disorders; Thyroid Disorders; Pubertal Disorders; **Hospital:** Chldn's Hosp - Aurora (CO); **Address:** Chldns Hosp-Dept Endocrinology, 13123 E 16th Ave, Box B265, Aurora, CO 80045; **Phone:** 720-777-6128; **Board Cert:** Pediatrics 1972; Pediatric Endocrinology 1980; **Med School:** Univ Wisc 1967; **Resid:** Pediatrics, Univ Colorado Med Ctr 1972; **Fellow:** Pediatric Endocrinology, Johns Hopkins Hosp 1980; **Fac Appt:** Prof Ped, Univ Colorado

Klingensmith, Georgeanna J MD [PEn] - **Spec Exp:** Diabetes; **Hospital:** Chldn's Hosp - Aurora (CO), Univ of CO Hosp - Anschutz Inpatient Pav; **Address:** Barbara Davis Center, 1775 Aurora Court, MS A140, Aurora, CO 80045; **Phone:** 303-724-2323; **Board Cert:** Pediatrics 1976; Pediatric Endocrinology 2000; **Med School:** Duke Univ 1971; **Resid:** Pediatrics, Childrens Hosp 1974; **Fellow:** Pediatric Endocrinology, Johns Hopkins Univ 1976; **Fac Appt:** Prof Ped, Univ Colorado

Rewers, Marian J MD/PhD [PEn] - **Spec Exp:** Diabetes; **Hospital:** Chldn's Hosp - Aurora (CO), Univ of CO Hosp - Anschutz Inpatient Pav; **Address:** CO Chldns Hosp-Barbara Davis Ctr, 1775 N Ursula St, MS A140 PO Box 6511, Aurora, CO 80045; **Phone:** 303-315-3828; **Board Cert:** Pediatrics 2011; Pediatric Endocrinology 2012; **Med School:** Poland 1981; **Resid:** Pediatrics, Inst Pediatrics 1984; **Fellow:** Pediatric Endocrinology, U Pittsburgh/Chldns Hosp 1988; **Fac Appt:** Prof Ped, Univ Colorado

West Coast and Pacific

Geffner, Mitchell E MD [PEn] - **Spec Exp:** Growth Disorders; Pubertal Disorders; Thyroid Disorders; Pituitary Disorders; **Hospital:** Chldns Hosp - Los Angeles; **Address:** Chlds Hosp LA, Div Endocrinology, 4650 Sunset Blvd, MS 61, Los Angeles, CA 90027; **Phone:** 323-361-2185; **Board Cert:** Pediatrics 1980; Pediatric Endocrinology 2006; **Med School:** Albert Einstein Coll Med 1975; **Resid:** Pediatrics, LAC-USC Med Ctr 1979; **Fellow:** Pediatric Endocrinology, UCLA Med Ctr 1982; **Fac Appt:** Prof Ped, USC Sch Med

Gitelman, Stephen E MD [PEn] - **Spec Exp:** Diabetes; **Hospital:** UCSF Med Ctr; **Address:** UCSF Madison Clinic-Pediatric Diabetes, 400 Parnassus Ave Fl 4, San Francisco, CA 94143; **Phone:** 415-514-8500; **Board Cert:** Pediatric Endocrinology 2006; **Med School:** Univ NC Sch Med 1984; **Resid:** Pediatrics, UCSF Med Ctr 1987; **Fellow:** Pediatric Endocrinology, UCSF Med Ctr 1990; **Fac Appt:** Clin Prof Ped, UCSF

Lustig, Robert H MD [PEn] - **Spec Exp:** Obesity; Metabolic Syndrome; Neuroendocrinology; Hyperinsulinism; **Hospital:** UCSF Med Ctr; **Address:** UCSF Medical Ctr, Div Pediatric Endocrinology, 513 Parnassus Ave, San Francisco, CA 94143; **Phone:** 415-353-2813; **Board Cert:** Pediatrics 1984; Pediatric Endocrinology 1986; **Med School:** Cornell Univ-Weill Med Coll 1980; **Resid:** Pediatrics, St Louis Children's Hosp 1983; **Fellow:** Pediatric Endocrinology, UCSF Medical Ctr 1984; **Fac Appt:** Prof Ped, UCSF

Rosenthal, Stephen M MD [PEn] - **Spec Exp:** Diabetes; **Hospital:** UCSF Med Ctr; **Address:** UCSF Pediatric Specialty Clinic, 400 Parnassus Ave Fl 2, San Fransisco, CA 94143; **Phone:** 415-353-7337; **Board Cert:** Pediatrics 1982; Pediatric Endocrinology 1983; **Med School:** Columbia P&S 1976; **Resid:** Pediatrics, NY Presby-Columbia Med Ctr 1979; **Fellow:** Pediatric Endocrinology, UCSF Med Ctr 1982; **Fac Appt:** Prof Ped, UCSF

Wilson, Darrell M MD [PEn] - **Spec Exp:** Diabetes; Growth Disorders; Weight Management; **Hospital:** Lucile Packard Chldn's Hosp, Stanford Univ Hosp & Clinics; **Address:** Pediatric Diabetes & Endocrinology Clin, 730 Welch Rd Fl 2, Stanford, CA 94305-5208; **Phone:** 650-723-5791 x3; **Board Cert:** Pediatrics 1982; Pediatric Endocrinology 2010; **Med School:** UCSD 1977; **Resid:** Pediatrics, Stanford Univ Med Ctr 1980; **Fellow:** Endocrinology, Diabetes & Metabolism, Stanford Univ Med Ctr 1984; **Fac Appt:** Asst Prof Ped, Stanford Univ

PEDIATRIC GASTROENTEROLOGY

New England

Jonas, Maureen M MD [PGe] - **Spec Exp:** Liver Disease; Transplant Medicine-Liver; Hepatitis; **Hospital:** Children's Hospital - Boston, Brigham and Women's Hosp (page 57); **Address:** Chldns Hosp, Dept Ped Gastroenterology, 300 Longwood Ave, Boston, MA 02115; **Phone:** 617-355-5837; **Board Cert:** Pediatrics 1982; Pediatric Gastroenterology 2005; Pediatric Transplant Hepatology 2006; **Med School:** Univ Miami Sch Med 1977; **Resid:** Pediatrics, Chldns Hosp 1980; **Fellow:** Pediatric Gastroenterology, Chldns Hosp 1982; **Fac Appt:** Assoc Prof Ped, Harvard Med Sch

Kleinman, Ronald E MD [PGe] - **Spec Exp:** Transplant Medicine-Liver; Nutrition; **Hospital:** Mass Genl Hosp, N Shore Children's Hosp; **Address:** Mass Genl Hosp, Div Ped GI/Nutrition, 55 Fruit St, VBK 107, Boston, MA 02114; **Phone:** 617-726-8705; **Board Cert:** Pediatrics 1992; Pediatric Gastroenterology 2005; **Med School:** NY Med Coll 1972; **Resid:** Pediatrics, Montefiore Med Ctr 1977; **Fellow:** Pediatric Gastroenterology, Mass Genl Hosp 1980; **Fac Appt:** Prof Ped, Harvard Med Sch

Leichtner, Alan M MD [PGe] - **Spec Exp:** Inflammatory Bowel Disease; Celiac Disease; Nutrition; **Hospital:** Children's Hospital - Boston; **Address:** Chldns Hosp, Div Gastroenterology, 300 Longwood Ave, Hunnewell-Ground, Boston, MA 02115; **Phone:** 617-355-2946; **Board Cert:** Pediatrics 1982; Pediatric Gastroenterology 2005; **Med School:** Harvard Med Sch 1977; **Resid:** Pediatrics, Chldn's Hosp 1980; **Fellow:** Pediatric Gastroenterology, Chldn's Hosp 1983; **Fac Appt:** Assoc Prof Ped, Harvard Med Sch

Pediatric Gastroenterology

Mid Atlantic

Baker Jr, Robert D MD/PhD [PGe] - **Spec Exp:** Gastroesophageal Reflux Disease (GERD); Cystic Fibrosis; Nutrition; Malabsorption Syndrome; **Hospital:** Women & Chldn's Hosp of Buffalo, The; **Address:** Digestive Disease & Nutrition Ctr, Women & Children's Hosp Buffalo, 239 Bryant St Fl 2, Buffalo, NY 14222-2006; **Phone:** 716-878-7793; **Board Cert:** Pediatrics 1978; Pediatric Gastroenterology 2010; **Med School:** Temple Univ 1972; **Resid:** Pediatrics, Buffalo Chldns Hosp 1975; **Fellow:** Gastroenterology, Mass Genl Hosp/Chldns Hosp Med Ctr 1983; Nutritional Biochemistry, MIT 1984; **Fac Appt:** Prof Ped, SUNY Buffalo

Baker, Susan S MD/PhD [PGe] - **Spec Exp:** Nutrition; Obesity; Liver Disease; Gastroesophageal Reflux Disease (GERD); **Hospital:** Women & Chldn's Hosp of Buffalo, The; **Address:** Digestive Disease & Nutrition Ctr, Women & Chldns Hosp Buffalo, 239 Bryant St Fl 2, Buffalo, NY 14201-2099; **Phone:** 716-878-7793; **Board Cert:** Pediatrics 1978; Pediatric Gastroenterology 2010; **Med School:** Temple Univ 1972; **Resid:** Pediatrics, Buffalo Chldns Hosp 1975; **Fellow:** Nutrition, MIT 1981; Gastroenterology, Mass Genl Hosp/Harvard 1984; **Fac Appt:** Prof Ped, SUNY Buffalo

Baldassano, Robert N MD [PGe] - **Spec Exp:** Inflammatory Bowel Disease; Ulcerative Colitis; Crohn's Disease; **Hospital:** Chldns Hosp of Philadelphia; **Address:** Children's Hospital of Philadelphia Blvd, MS 19104, 324 S 34th St, Philadelphia, PA 19104-4399; **Phone:** 215-426-5123; **Board Cert:** Pediatric Gastroenterology 2007; **Med School:** SUNY Downstate 1984; **Resid:** Pediatrics, Childrens Hosp 1988; **Fellow:** Pediatric Gastroenterology, Childrens Hosp 1991; **Fac Appt:** Prof Ped, Univ Pennsylvania

Baldridge, Alan D MD [PGe] - **Spec Exp:** Inflammatory Bowel Disease; Celiac Disease; **Hospital:** Cooper Univ Hosp; **Address:** 3 Cooper Plaza, Ste 309, Div Pediatric Gastroenterology, Camden, NJ 08034; **Phone:** 856-342-2001; **Board Cert:** Pediatrics 2008; Pediatric Gastroenterology 2005; **Med School:** Med Coll VA 1988; **Resid:** Pediatrics, Boston City Hosp 1991; **Fellow:** Pediatric Gastroenterology, Mass Genl Hosp 1994; **Fac Appt:** Asst Prof Med, Drexel Univ Coll Med

Benkov, Keith J MD [PGe] - **Spec Exp:** Inflammatory Bowel Disease/Crohn's; Liver Disease; Celiac Disease; **Hospital:** Mount Sinai Med Ctr (page 64), Englewood Hosp & Med Ctr; **Address:** Mt Sinai Div Ped Gastroenterology, 5 E 98th St Fl 10, New York, NY 10029; **Phone:** 212-241-5415; **Board Cert:** Pediatrics 1984; Pediatric Gastroenterology 2005; **Med School:** Mount Sinai Sch Med 1979; **Resid:** Pediatrics, Mt Sinai Hosp 1982; **Fellow:** Pediatric Gastroenterology, Mt Sinai Hosp 1984; **Fac Appt:** Assoc Prof Ped, Mount Sinai Sch Med

Fasano, Alessio MD [PGe] - **Spec Exp:** Celiac Disease; Diarrheal Diseases; Nutrition; **Hospital:** Univ of MD Med Ctr; **Address:** 22 S Greene St, rm N5W40, Baltimore, MD 21201; **Phone:** 410-328-6749; **Med School:** Italy 1981; **Resid:** Pediatrics, Univ Naples 1985; **Fac Appt:** Prof Med, Univ MD Sch Med

Levy, Joseph MD [PGe] - **Spec Exp:** Celiac Disease; Irritable Bowel Syndrome; Gastroesophageal Reflux Disease (GERD); Nutrition in Autism; **Hospital:** NYU Langone Med Ctr (page 68); **Address:** 160 E 32nd St Fl L3 Medical, New York, NY 10016; **Phone:** 212-263-5407; **Board Cert:** Pediatrics 1981; Pediatric Gastroenterology 2005; **Med School:** Israel 1973; **Resid:** Pediatrics, Beth Israel Med Ctr 1977; **Fellow:** Research, Columbia-Presby Med Ctr 1975; Pediatric Gastroenterology, Columbia-Presby Med Ctr 1979; **Fac Appt:** Prof Ped, NYU Sch Med

Oliva-Hemker, Maria M MD [PGe] - **Spec Exp:** Inflammatory Bowel Disease/Crohn's; Ulcerative Colitis; Malabsorption Syndrome; **Hospital:** Johns Hopkins Hosp (page 61), Greater Baltimore Med Ctr; **Address:** Johns Hopkins Hosp, Ped GI & Nutrition, 600 N Wolfe St, Brady 320, Baltimore, MD 21287-2631; **Phone:** 410-955-8769; **Board Cert:** Pediatrics 2007; Pediatric Gastroenterology 2007; **Med School:** Johns Hopkins Univ 1986; **Resid:** Pediatrics, Johns Hopkins Hosp 1989; **Fellow:** Gastroenterology, Johns Hopkins Hosp 1992; **Fac Appt:** Assoc Prof Ped, Johns Hopkins Univ

Piccoli, David A MD [PGe] - **Spec Exp:** Liver Disease; **Hospital:** Chldns Hosp of Philadelphia; **Address:** Chlds Hosp of Philadelphia, Div Gastroenterology/Nutrition, 324 S 34th St, Philadelphia, PA 19104; **Phone:** 215-590-3630; **Board Cert:** Pediatrics 1984; Pediatric Gastroenterology 2005; **Med School:** Harvard Med Sch 1979; **Resid:** Pediatrics, Chldns Hosp Med Ctr 1983; **Fellow:** Gastroenterology, Chldns Hosp 1986; **Fac Appt:** Prof Ped, Univ Pennsylvania

Schwarz, Kathleen B MD [PGe] - **Spec Exp:** Hepatitis B & C; Transplant Medicine-Liver; Liver Disease; **Hospital:** Johns Hopkins Hosp (page 61); **Address:** Johns Hopkins Pediatric GI, 600 N Wolfe St, Brady 320, Baltimore, MD 21287-0005; **Phone:** 410-955-8769; **Board Cert:** Pediatrics 1977; Pediatric Gastroenterology 2005; Pediatric Transplant Hepatology 2006; **Med School:** Washington Univ, St Louis 1972; **Resid:** Pediatrics, St Louis Chldns Hosp 1974; **Fellow:** Pediatric Gastroenterology, St Louis Chldns Hosp 1976; **Fac Appt:** Prof Ped, Johns Hopkins Univ

Schwarz, Steven M MD [PGe] - **Spec Exp:** Gastroesophageal Reflux Disease (GERD); Nutrition; Endoscopy; Inflammatory Bowel Disease; **Hospital:** SUNY Downstate Med Ctr (Univ Hosp of Bklyn), Beth Israel Med Ctr - Petrie Division (page 56); **Address:** Children's Hosp at SUNY Downstate, 445 Lenox Rd, Box 49, Brooklyn, NY 11203; **Phone:** 718-270-4714; **Board Cert:** Pediatrics 1979; Pediatric Gastroenterology 2005; **Med School:** Columbia P&S 1974; **Resid:** Pediatrics, Columbia-Presby Med Ctr 1977; **Fellow:** Pediatric Gastroenterology, Stanford Univ Med Ctr 1978; Pediatric Gastroenterology, Columbia-Presby Med Ctr 1980; **Fac Appt:** Prof Ped, SUNY Downstate

Snyder, John David MD [PGe] - **Spec Exp:** Celiac Disease; Gastroesophageal Reflux Disease (GERD); **Hospital:** Chldns Natl Med Ctr; **Address:** Children's National Med Ctr, 111 Michigan Ave NW, Ste 300, Washington, DC 20010; **Phone:** 202-476-3032; **Board Cert:** Pediatrics 1982; Pediatric Gastroenterology 2005; **Med School:** UCLA 1975; **Resid:** Pediatrics, Duke Univ Med Ctr 1978; **Fellow:** Pediatric Gastroenterology, Mass Genl Hosp 1984

Spivak, William MD [PGe] - **Spec Exp:** Ulcerative Colitis; Crohn's Disease; Nutrition; Intestinal Disorders; **Hospital:** NY-Presby/Weill Cornell Med Ctr, NY (page 66), Lenox Hill Hosp (page 67); **Address:** 177 E 87th St, Ste 305, New York, NY 10128; **Phone:** 212-369-7700; **Board Cert:** Pediatrics 1981; Pediatric Gastroenterology 2005; **Med School:** Albert Einstein Coll Med 1976; **Resid:** Pediatrics, Jacobi Med Ctr/Albert Einstein Med Sch 1979; **Fellow:** Gastroenterology, Childrens Hosp 1982; Research, Brigham & Womens Hosp 1982; **Fac Appt:** Clin Prof Ped, Cornell Univ-Weill Med Coll

Squires Jr, Robert H MD [PGe] - **Spec Exp:** Liver Disease; Intestinal Disorders; **Hospital:** Chldns Hosp of Pittsburgh - UPMC; **Address:** Children's Hosp Pittsburgh, Pediatric Gastroenterology, 4401 Penn Ave Fl 3, Pittsburgh, PA 15201; **Phone:** 412-692-5180; **Board Cert:** Pediatrics 1981; Pediatric Gastroenterology 2005; Pediatric Transplant Hepatology 2006; **Med School:** Univ Tex Med Br, Galveston 1977; **Resid:** Pediatrics, Children's Hosp 1979; **Fellow:** Pediatric Gastroenterology, Children's Hosp 1982; **Fac Appt:** Prof Ped, Univ Pittsburgh

Pediatric Gastroenterology

Southeast

Black, Dennis D MD [PGe] - **Spec Exp:** Nutrition; Obesity; **Hospital:** Le Bonheur Chldns Med Ctr; **Address:** 7945 Wolf River Rd, Ste 250, Germantown, TN 38138; **Phone:** 901-866-8821; **Board Cert:** Pediatrics 1983; Pediatric Gastroenterology 2012; **Med School:** Univ Tenn Coll Med 1978; **Resid:** Pediatrics, Le Bonheur Chldns Med Ctr 1981; **Fellow:** Pediatric Gastroenterology, Univ Tenn Hlth Sci Ctr 1984; **Fac Appt:** Prof Ped, Univ Tenn Coll Med

Hill, Ivor D MD [PGe] - **Spec Exp:** Celiac Disease; Inflammatory Bowel Disease; Malabsorption Syndrome; Diarrheal Diseases; **Hospital:** Brenner Chldrn's Hosp, Wake Forest Baptist Med Ctr; **Address:** Wake Forest Univ Sch Med, Div Ped Gastro, Medical Center Blvd, Winston-Salem, NC 27157; **Phone:** 336-716-3009; **Board Cert:** Pediatrics 2007; Pediatric Gastroenterology 2012; **Med School:** South Africa 1972; **Resid:** Pediatrics, Addington Hosp 1976; Pediatrics, Red Cross Chldns Hosp 1977; **Fellow:** Pediatric Gastroenterology, Red Cross Chlds Hosp 1980; **Fac Appt:** Prof Ped, Wake Forest Univ

Novak, Donald A MD [PGe] - **Spec Exp:** Liver Disease; Nutrition; Obesity; **Hospital:** Shands at Univ of FL; **Address:** UF Pediatrics, 1600 SW Archer Rd, rm RG120, Gainesville, FL 32610; **Phone:** 352-273-9350; **Board Cert:** Pediatrics 1988; Pediatric Gastroenterology 2010; **Med School:** Univ S Fla Coll Med 1981; **Resid:** Pediatrics, Univ South Fla Affil Hosp 1984; **Fellow:** Pediatric Gastroenterology, Chldn's Hosp 1987; **Fac Appt:** Prof Ped, Univ Fla Coll Med

Ulshen, Martin H MD [PGe] - **Spec Exp:** Liver Disease; Inflammatory Bowel Disease; Irritable Bowel Syndrome; **Hospital:** Duke Univ Hosp; **Address:** Duke Univ Med Ctr, Box 102375, Durham, NC 27710; **Phone:** 919-684-5068; **Board Cert:** Pediatrics 1993; Pediatric Gastroenterology 2005; **Med School:** Univ Rochester 1969; **Resid:** Pediatrics, Univ Colorado Med Ctr 1974; **Fellow:** Pediatric Gastroenterology, Univ Colorado Med Ctr 1975; Pediatric Gastroenterology, Chldns Hosp 1977; **Fac Appt:** Prof Ped, Duke Univ

Midwest

Berman, James MD [PGe] - **Spec Exp:** Inflammatory Bowel Disease/Crohn's; Nutrition; Ulcerative Colitis; **Hospital:** Loyola Univ Med Ctr, Adv Luth Genl Hosp; **Address:** Loyola Univ Med Ctr, Dept Ped Gastro, 2160 S 1st Ave Bldg 105 Fl 3, Outpatient Ctr, Maywood, IL 60153-3304; **Phone:** 708-327-9073; **Board Cert:** Pediatrics 1986; Pediatric Gastroenterology 2005; **Med School:** Univ Pittsburgh 1981; **Resid:** Pediatrics, Chldns Hosp 1984; **Fellow:** Pediatric Gastroenterology, Mass Genl Hosp/Chldns Hosp 1987; **Fac Appt:** Assoc Clin Prof Ped, Loyola Univ-Stritch Sch Med

Bishop, Warren P MD [PGe] - **Spec Exp:** Liver Disease; Constipation; Diarrheal Diseases; Inflammatory Bowel Disease; **Hospital:** Univ Iowa Hosp & Clinics; **Address:** Univ Iowa Chldns Hosp, 200 Hawkins Drive, 2869 JPP, Iowa City, IA 52242; **Phone:** 319-356-2229; **Board Cert:** Pediatrics 1984; Pediatric Gastroenterology 2012; **Med School:** Univ Wisc 1979; **Resid:** Pediatrics, Univ Michigan Hlth Sys 1982; **Fellow:** Pediatric Gastroenterology, Univ NC Affil Hosp 1989; **Fac Appt:** Prof Ped, Univ Iowa Coll Med

Cohen, Mitchell B MD [PGe] - **Spec Exp:** Inflammatory Bowel Disease; Diarrheal Diseases; Celiac Disease; **Hospital:** Cincinnati Chldns Hosp Med Ctr; **Address:** Chldns Hosp Med Ctr, 3333 Burnet Ave, MLC 2010, Cincinnati, OH 45229; **Phone:** 513-636-4415; **Board Cert:** Pediatrics 1981; Pediatric Gastroenterology 2005; **Med School:** Mount Sinai Sch Med 1977; **Resid:** Pediatrics, Johns Hopkins Hosp 1980; **Fellow:** Pediatric Gastroenterology, Chldns Hosp Med Ctr 1986; **Fac Appt:** Prof Ped, Univ Cincinnati

Di Lorenzo, Carlo MD [PGe] - **Spec Exp:** Gastrointestinal Motility Disorders; Gastrointestinal Functional Disorders; **Hospital:** Nationwide Chldn's Hosp; **Address:** Nationwide Children's Hospital, Div Gastroenterology & Nutrition, 700 Children's Drive, Columbus, OH 43205; **Phone:** 614-722-3450; **Board Cert:** Pediatric Gastroenterology 2012; **Med School:** Italy 1984; **Resid:** Pediatrics, Univ Naples Medical Ctr 1988; **Fellow:** Pediatric Gastroenterology, Harbor-UCLA Medical Ctr 1989; **Fac Appt:** Prof Ped, Ohio State Univ

El-Youssef, Mounif MD [PGe] - **Spec Exp:** Liver Disease; **Hospital:** Mayo Med Ctr & Clin - Rochester; **Address:** Mayo Clin, Div Ped Gastroenterology, 200 First St SW, Rochester, MN 55905; **Phone:** 507-266-4950; **Board Cert:** Pediatric Gastroenterology 2012; Pediatric Transplant Hepatology 2012; **Med School:** Belgium 1982; **Resid:** Pediatrics, Cleveland Clin 1987; **Fellow:** Pediatric Gastroenterology, Harvard Med Sch 1990

Guandalini, Stefano MD [PGe] - **Spec Exp:** Celiac Disease; Digestive Disorders; Diarrheal Diseases; **Hospital:** Univ Chicago-Comer Chldn's Hosp; **Address:** Univ Chicago Med Ctr, 5841 S Maryland Ave, MC 4065, Chicago, IL 60637; **Phone:** 773-702-6418; **Med School:** Italy 1971; **Resid:** Pediatrics, Univ Messina Affil Hosp 1974; **Fellow:** Pediatric Gastroenterology, Univ Naples Affil Hosp; **Fac Appt:** Prof Ped, Univ Chicago-Pritzker Sch Med

Gunasekaran, T S MD [PGe] - **Spec Exp:** Gastroesophageal Reflux Disease (GERD); Esophageal Disorders; Inflammatory Bowel Disease; Pain-Abdominal Recurrent; **Hospital:** Adv Luth Genl Hosp, Loyola Univ Med Ctr; **Address:** Lutheran Genl Chldns Hosp, Dept Ped GI, Dept Ped GI, 1675 Dempster St, Park Ridge, IL 60068; **Phone:** 847-723-7700; **Board Cert:** Pediatric Gastroenterology 2007; **Med School:** India 1977; **Resid:** Pediatrics, Univ Madras 1982; Pediatrics, Chldn's Hosp 1987; **Fellow:** Pediatric Gastroenterology, Chldn's Hosp 1992; **Fac Appt:** Assoc Clin Prof Ped, Loyola Univ-Stritch Sch Med

Gupta, Sandeep K MD [PGe] - **Spec Exp:** Eosinophilic Esophagitis; Gastroesophageal Reflux Disease (GERD); Nutrition; Obesity; **Hospital:** Riley Hosp for Children; **Address:** Riley Hosp for Chldn, Div Ped Gastroenterology, 705 Riley Hosp Drive, ROC 4210, Indianapolis, IN 46202; **Phone:** 317-944-3774; **Board Cert:** Pediatric Gastroenterology 2012; **Med School:** Nigeria 1986; **Resid:** Pediatrics, Univ Conn Hlth Ctr; **Fellow:** Pediatric Gastroenterology, Indiana Univ; **Fac Appt:** Clin Prof Ped, Indiana Univ

Kirschner, Barbara S MD [PGe] - **Spec Exp:** Ulcerative Colitis; Pain-Abdominal Recurrent; Inflammatory Bowel Disease/Crohn's; **Hospital:** Univ Chicago-Comer Chldn's Hosp; **Address:** Univ Chicago Med Ctr, 5839 S Maryland Ave, MC 4065, Chicago, IL 60637; **Phone:** 773-702-6418; **Board Cert:** Pediatrics 1972; Pediatric Gastroenterology 2005; **Med School:** Med Coll PA 1967; **Resid:** Pediatrics, Univ Chicago Hosps 1970; **Fellow:** Pediatric Gastroenterology, Univ Chicago Hosps 1977; **Fac Appt:** Prof Ped, Univ Chicago-Pritzker Sch Med

Molleston, Jean P MD [PGe] - **Spec Exp:** Liver Disease; Hepatitis; Transplant Medicine-Liver; Graft vs Host Disease; **Hospital:** Riley Hosp for Children, IU Health North Hosp; **Address:** Riley Hosp for Chldn, Div Ped Gastroenterology, 705 Riley Hosp Drive, ROC 4210, Indianapolis, IN 46202-5225; **Phone:** 317-944-3774; **Board Cert:** Pediatrics 2009; Pediatric Gastroenterology 2010; Pediatric Transplant Hepatology 2006; **Med School:** Washington Univ, St Louis 1986; **Resid:** Pediatrics, Chldns Hosp 1988; **Fellow:** Pediatric Gastroenterology, Washington Univ 1991; **Fac Appt:** Clin Prof Ped, Indiana Univ

Mousa, Hayat M MD [PGe] - **Spec Exp:** Gastroesophageal Reflux Disease (GERD); Gastrointestinal Motility Disorders; Gastrointestinal Functional Disorders; **Hospital:** Nationwide Chldn's Hosp; **Address:** Nationwide Children's Hospital, Div Gastroenterology & Nutrition, 700 Children's Drive, Columbus, OH 43205; **Phone:** 614-722-3450; **Board Cert:** Pediatric Gastroenterology 2007; **Med School:** Syria 1982; **Resid:** Pediatrics, Henry Ford Hosp 1993; **Fellow:** Pediatric Gastroenterology, Chldns Hosp 1998; **Fac Appt:** Assoc Clin Prof Ped, Ohio State Univ

Pediatric Gastroenterology

Rothbaum, Robert J MD [PGe] - **Spec Exp:** Inflammatory Bowel Disease; **Hospital:** St. Louis Chldns Hosp, Barnes-Jewish Hosp; **Address:** St Louis Chldns Hosp, 1 Chldns Pl, NW Tower, Fl 9, Box 8116, St Louis, MO 63110; **Phone:** 314-454-6173; **Board Cert:** Pediatrics 1981; Pediatric Gastroenterology 2012; **Med School:** Univ Chicago-Pritzker Sch Med 1976; **Resid:** Pediatrics, St Louis Chldns Hosp 1978; **Fellow:** Ambulatory Pediatrics, St Louis Chldns Hosp 1979; Pediatric Gastroenterology, Chldns Hosp Med Ctr 1982; **Fac Appt:** Prof Ped, Washington Univ, St Louis

Whitington, Peter F MD [PGe] - **Spec Exp:** Transplant Medicine-Liver; Liver Disease; **Hospital:** Lurie Chldn's Hosp-Chicago; **Address:** Lurie Chldn's Hosp, Div Ped Gastro, 225 E Chicago Ave, Box 57, Chicago, IL 60611; **Phone:** 312-227-4599; **Board Cert:** Pediatrics 1977; Pediatric Gastroenterology 2005; Pediatric Transplant Hepatology 2006; **Med School:** Univ Tenn Coll Med 1971; **Resid:** Pediatrics, Univ Tenn Hosp 1975; **Fellow:** Gastroenterology, Johns Hopkins Hosp 1977; Gastroenterology, Univ Wisconsin Affil Hosp 1978; **Fac Appt:** Prof Ped, Northwestern Univ

Wyllie, Robert MD [PGe] - **Spec Exp:** Inflammatory Bowel Disease/Crohn's; Ulcerative Colitis; **Hospital:** Cleveland Clin (page 55); **Address:** 9500 Euclid Ave, Crile Bldg - Fl 11, Cleveland, OH 44195; **Phone:** 216-444-2237; **Board Cert:** Pediatrics 1982; Pediatric Gastroenterology 2005; **Med School:** Indiana Univ 1976; **Resid:** Pediatrics, Indiana Univ Med Ctr 1978; **Fellow:** Pediatric Gastroenterology, Indiana Univ Med Ctr 1981; **Fac Appt:** Prof Ped, Cleveland Cl Coll Med/Case West Res

Great Plains and Mountains

Hoffenberg, Edward J MD [PGe] - **Spec Exp:** Inflammatory Bowel Disease; Celiac Disease; Liver Disease; Pancreatic Disease; **Hospital:** Chldn's Hosp - Aurora (CO); **Address:** Chldns Hosp-Div Gastroenterology, 13123 E 16th Ave, Box B290, Aurora, CO 80045; **Phone:** 720-777-6669; **Board Cert:** Pediatric Gastroenterology 2007; **Med School:** Case West Res Univ 1986; **Resid:** Pediatrics, Rainbow Babies & Chldns Hosp 1989; **Fellow:** Pediatric Gastroenterology, Chldns Hosp 1992; **Fac Appt:** Assoc Prof Ped, Univ Colorado

Krebs, Nancy F MD [PGe] - **Spec Exp:** Obesity; Nutrition; Weight Management; **Hospital:** Chldn's Hosp - Aurora (CO); **Address:** 12700 E 19th Ave, Box C225, Aurora, CO 80045; **Phone:** 303-724-3260; **Board Cert:** Pediatrics 2009; Pediatric Gastroenterology 2010; **Med School:** Univ Colorado 1987; **Resid:** Pediatrics, Univ Colorado Affil Hosp 1990; **Fellow:** Pediatric Gastroenterology, Univ Colorado 1992; Nutrition, Univ Colorado 1993; **Fac Appt:** Prof Ped, Univ Colorado

Narkewicz, Michael R MD [PGe] - **Spec Exp:** Transplant Medicine-Liver; Liver Disease; **Hospital:** Chldn's Hosp - Aurora (CO); **Address:** Children's Hospital, Dept Liver Disease and Nutrition, 13123 E 16th Ave, Aurora, CO 80045; **Phone:** 720-777-6669; **Board Cert:** Pediatrics 1988; Pediatric Gastroenterology 2005; Pediatric Transplant Hepatolgy 2006; **Med School:** Univ VT Coll Med 1983; **Resid:** Pediatrics, Univ Colorado Med Ctr 1986; **Fellow:** Pediatric Gastroenterology, Univ Colorado Med Ctr 1989; **Fac Appt:** Prof Ped, Univ Colorado

Sokol, Ronald Jay MD [PGe] - **Spec Exp:** Liver Disease; Transplant Medicine - Liver; Nutrition; Cystic Fibrosis; **Hospital:** Chldn's Hosp - Aurora (CO); **Address:** Children's Hospital Colorado, 13123 E 16th Ave, Box B290, Aurora, CO 80045; **Phone:** 720-777-6669; **Board Cert:** Pediatrics 1981; Pediatric Gastroenterology 2005; Pediatric Transplant Hepatology 2010; **Med School:** Univ Chicago-Pritzker Sch Med 1976; **Resid:** Pediatrics, Univ Colo Med Ctr 1980; **Fellow:** Pediatric Gastroenterology, Chldns Hosp 1983; **Fac Appt:** Prof Ped, Univ Colorado

Suchy, Frederick J MD [PGe] - **Spec Exp:** Hepatitis; Liver Disease; Neonatal Cholestasis; **Hospital:** Chldn's Hosp - Aurora (CO); **Address:** Children's Hosp Colorado, 13123 E 16th Ave, Box B290, Aurora, CO 80045; **Phone:** 720-777-6669; **Board Cert:** Pediatrics 1982; Pediatric Gastroenterology 2005; Pediatric Transplant Hepatology 2006; **Med School:** Univ Cincinnati 1974; **Resid:** Pediatrics, Chldns Hosp Med Ctr 1978; **Fellow:** Pediatric Gastroenterology, Chldns Hosp Med Ctr 1981; **Fac Appt:** Prof Ped, Univ Colorado

Vanderhoof, Jon A MD [PGe] - **Spec Exp:** Nutrition; Short Bowel Syndrome; **Hospital:** Boys Town Natl Rsch Hosp, Children's Hosp - Omaha; **Address:** Boystown Hosp & Clin, 14080 Hosp Rd, Boystown, NE 68010; **Phone:** 402-778-6820; **Board Cert:** Pediatrics 1993; Pediatric Gastroenterology 2005; **Med School:** Univ Nebr Coll Med 1972; **Resid:** Pediatrics, Univ Nebr Coll Med 1974; **Fellow:** Pediatric Gastroenterology, UCLA Med Ctr 1976; **Fac Appt:** Prof Ped, Univ Nebr Coll Med

Southwest

Mittal, Naveen K MD [PGe] - **Spec Exp:** Transplant Medicine-Liver; Liver Disease; Short Bowel Syndrome; **Hospital:** Christus Santa Rosa Children's Hosp, Univ Hlth Syst-San Antonio; **Address:** 333 N Santa Rosa St, Ste 2658, San Antonio, TX 78207; **Phone:** 210-562-5844; **Board Cert:** Pediatrics 2009; Pediatric Gastroenterology 2007; Pediatric Transplant Hepatology 2006; **Med School:** India 1988; **Resid:** Pediatrics, S Cleveland Hosp 1990; Pediatrics, Hahnemann Univ Hosp 1993; **Fellow:** Pediatric Gastroenterology, Bristol Royal Hosp 1991; Pediatric Gastroenterology, Univ Chicago Hosp 1993; **Fac Appt:** Prof Ped, Univ Tex, San Antonio

Rhoads, J Marc MD [PGe] - **Spec Exp:** Diarrheal Diseases; Inflammatory Bowel Disease; Intestinal Disorders; **Hospital:** Meml Hermann Hosp - Texas Med Ctr; **Address:** UT Physicians-Pediatric Gastroenterology, 6410 Fannin St, Ste 500, Houston, TX 77030; **Phone:** 832-325-6516; **Board Cert:** Pediatrics 1986; Pediatric Gastroenterology 2012; **Med School:** Johns Hopkins Univ 1980; **Resid:** Pediatrics, UCLA Med Ctr 1983; **Fellow:** Pediatric Gastroenterology, Hosp for Sick Chldn 1986; **Fac Appt:** Prof Ped, Univ Tex, Houston

West Coast and Pacific

Christie, Dennis L MD [PGe] - **Spec Exp:** Inflammatory Bowel Disease; **Hospital:** Seattle Chldns Hosp; **Address:** Chldns Hosp Med Ctr, Div Gastroenterology, 4800 Sand Point Way NE, MS A-5950, Seattle, WA 98105-3901; **Phone:** 206-987-2521; **Board Cert:** Pediatrics 1992; Pediatric Gastroenterology 2005; **Med School:** Northwestern Univ 1968; **Resid:** Pediatrics, Univ Wash Med Ctr 1971; **Fellow:** Pediatric Gastroenterology, UCLA Ctr Hlth Sci 1976; **Fac Appt:** Prof Ped, Univ Wash

Dubinsky, Marla C MD [PGe] - **Spec Exp:** Inflammatory Bowel Disease; Crohn's Disease; Ulcerative Colitis; Clinical Trials; **Hospital:** Cedars-Sinai Med Ctr; **Address:** 8635 W 3rd St, Ste 1165W, Los Angeles, CA 90048; **Phone:** 310-423-7100; **Board Cert:** Pediatric Gastroenterology 2009; **Med School:** Canada 1993; **Fac Appt:** Asst Prof Ped, UCLA

Heyman, Melvin B MD [PGe] - **Spec Exp:** Inflammatory Bowel Disease/Crohn's; Short Bowel Syndrome; Gastroesophageal Reflux Disease (GERD); Nutrition; **Hospital:** UCSF Med Ctr; **Address:** UCSF, Dept Ped Gastroenterology, 500 Parnassus Ave, Ste MU 4E, Box 0136, San Francisco, CA 94143-0136; **Phone:** 415-476-5892; **Board Cert:** Pediatrics 1981; Pediatric Gastroenterology 2005; **Med School:** UCLA 1976; **Resid:** Pediatrics, LAC-USC Med Ctr 1979; **Fellow:** Gastroenterology, UCLA Med Ctr 1981; Nutrition, Human Nutrition Res Ctr 1990; **Fac Appt:** Prof Ped, UCSF

Pediatric Gastroenterology

McDiarmid, Suzanne V MD [PGe] - **Spec Exp:** Transplant Medicine-Liver; Transplant Medicine-Bowel; Transplant Immunology; Liver Disease; **Hospital:** UCLA Ronald Reagan Med Ctr; **Address:** UCLA Pediatric Gastroenterology, 18033 Le Conte Ave, Room 12-383 MDCC, Los Angeles, CA 90095; **Phone:** 310-206-6136; **Board Cert:** Pediatrics 1984; Pediatric Gastroenterology 2007; **Med School:** New Zealand 1976; **Resid:** Pediatrics, Chldns Hosp Kings Daughters 1982; Pediatrics, Valley Med Ctr 1983; **Fellow:** Pediatric Gastroenterology, UCLA 1988; **Fac Appt:** Prof Ped, UCLA

Murray, Karen MD [PGe] - **Spec Exp:** Liver Disease; Hepatitis B & C; **Hospital:** Seattle Chldns Hosp; **Address:** Dept of Gastroenterology, 4800 Sand Point Way NE, MS A-5950, Seattle, WA 98105; **Phone:** 206-987-2521; **Board Cert:** Pediatrics 2008; Pediatric Gastroenterology 2005; Transplant Hepatology 2006; **Med School:** Johns Hopkins Univ 1990; **Resid:** Pediatrics, Chldn's Hosp & Med Ctr 1993; **Fellow:** Gastroenterology, Chldn's Hosp 1996; **Fac Appt:** Prof Med, Univ Wash

Thomas, Dan W MD [PGe] - **Spec Exp:** Gastrointestinal Disorders-Neonatal; Transplant Medicine-Liver; Inflammatory Bowel Disease; Nutrition in Bowel Disorders; **Hospital:** Chldns Hosp - Los Angeles; **Address:** Childrens Hosp LA-Peds Gastroenterology, 4650 Sunset Blvd, MS 78, Los Angeles, CA 90027; **Phone:** 323-361-2181; **Board Cert:** Pediatrics 1979; Pediatric Gastroenterology 2012; Pediatric Transplant Hepatology 2006; **Med School:** Univ Cincinnati 1974; **Resid:** Pediatrics, Chldns Hosp 1977; **Fellow:** Pediatric Gastroenterology, Chldns Hosp 1979; **Fac Appt:** Clin Prof Ped, USC Sch Med

PEDIATRIC HEMATOLOGY-ONCOLOGY

New England

Altman, Arnold MD [PHO] - **Spec Exp:** Leukemia; **Hospital:** CT Chldns Med Ctr; **Address:** CT Childrens Med Ctr, Hematology/Oncology, 282 Washington St, Ste 5A, Hartford, CT 06106; **Phone:** 860-545-9630; **Board Cert:** Pediatrics 1971; Pediatric Hematology-Oncology 1974; **Med School:** Johns Hopkins Univ 1965; **Resid:** Pediatrics, Chldns Hosp Med Ctr 1970; **Fellow:** Pediatric Hematology-Oncology, Chldns Hosp Med Ctr 1972; **Fac Appt:** Prof Ped, Univ Conn

Billett, Amy L MD [PHO] - **Spec Exp:** Hodgkin's Lymphoma; Lymphoma, Non-Hodgkin's; **Hospital:** Dana-Farber Cancer Inst (page 57), Children's Hospital - Boston; **Address:** Div Hematology/Onc, 44 Binney St, Ste 312A, Boston, MA 02215; **Phone:** 617-632-5640; **Board Cert:** Pediatric Hematology-Oncology 2009; **Med School:** Harvard Med Sch 1984; **Resid:** Pediatrics, Univ Wash Affil Hosps 1987; **Fellow:** Pediatric Hematology-Oncology, Children's Hosp 1990; **Fac Appt:** Assoc Prof Ped, Harvard Med Sch

Diller, Lisa R MD [PHO] - **Spec Exp:** Neuroblastoma; Cancer Survivors-Late Effects of Therapy; **Hospital:** Children's Hospital - Boston, Dana-Farber Cancer Inst (page 57); **Address:** Dana-Farber Cancer Inst, Dept Pediatric Onc, 450 Brookline Ave, Ste SW-312, Boston, MA 02215; **Phone:** 617-632-5642; **Board Cert:** Pediatric Hematology-Oncology 2007; **Med School:** UCSD 1985; **Resid:** Pediatrics, Chldns Hosp 1988; **Fellow:** Pediatric Hematology-Oncology, Chldns Hosp-Dana Farber Cancer Inst 1991; **Fac Appt:** Assoc Prof Ped, Harvard Med Sch

Guinan, Eva C MD [PHO] - **Spec Exp:** Bone Marrow Transplant; Anemia-Aplastic; **Hospital:** Dana-Farber Cancer Inst (page 57), Children's Hospital - Boston; **Address:** Dana Faber Cancer Inst, 450 Brookline Ave, Boston, MA 02215; **Phone:** 617-632-4932; **Board Cert:** Pediatrics 1986; Pediatric Hematology-Oncology 2005; **Med School:** Harvard Med Sch 1980; **Resid:** Internal Medicine, Children's Hosp 1982; **Fellow:** Pediatric Hematology-Oncology, Dana Farber Cancer Inst 1985; **Fac Appt:** Assoc Prof Ped, Harvard Med Sch

Homans, Alan C MD [PHO] - **Spec Exp:** Leukemia; **Hospital:** Fletcher Allen Health Care-Med Ctr Campus; **Address:** Fletcher Allen Healthcare, 111 Colchester Ave Smith Bldg - Ste 559A, Burlington, VT 05401; **Phone:** 802-847-2850; **Board Cert:** Pediatrics 1985; Pediatric Hematology-Oncology 1987; **Med School:** Ohio State Univ 1979; **Resid:** Pediatrics, Med Ctr Hosp 1981; Pediatrics, Univ Mass Med Ctr 1982; **Fellow:** Pediatric Hematology-Oncology, Rhode Island Hosp 1985; **Fac Appt:** Prof Ped, Univ VT Coll Med

Kieran, Mark W MD/PhD [PHO] - **Spec Exp:** Brain Tumors; Neuro-Oncology; **Hospital:** Dana-Farber Cancer Inst (page 57), Children's Hospital - Boston; **Address:** Dana Farber Cancer Inst, 450 Brookline Ave, Ste SW-331, Boston, MA 02115; **Phone:** 617-632-4386; **Board Cert:** Pediatric Hematology-Oncology 2011; **Med School:** Univ Calgary 1986; **Resid:** Pediatrics, Montreal Chldns Hosp 1992; **Fellow:** Pediatric Hematology-Oncology, Chldns Hosp 1995; **Fac Appt:** Assoc Prof Ped, Harvard Med Sch

Sallan, Stephen E MD [PHO] - **Spec Exp:** Pediatric Cancers; Leukemia; **Hospital:** Children's Hospital - Boston, Dana-Farber Cancer Inst (page 57); **Address:** Dana Farber Cancer Inst, Dept Pediatric Onc, 450 Brookline Ave Dana Bldg - Ste 1642, Boston, MA 02215; **Phone:** 617-632-3316; **Board Cert:** Pediatrics 1972; **Med School:** Wayne State Univ 1967; **Resid:** Pediatrics, Chldns Hosp 1969; Pediatrics, Hosp Sick Chldn 1970; **Fellow:** Pediatric Oncology, Chldns Hosp Med Ctr 1975; **Fac Appt:** Prof Ped, Harvard Med Sch

Schwartz, Cindy Lee MD [PHO] - **Spec Exp:** Hodgkin's Lymphoma; Bone Cancer; Cancer Survivors-Late Effects of Therapy; **Hospital:** Rhode Island Hosp; **Address:** Rhode Island Hospital, Div Pediatric Hematology/Oncology, 593 Eddy St, MPS rm 117, Providence, RI 02903-4923; **Phone:** 401-444-5171; **Board Cert:** Pediatrics 1985; Pediatric Hematology-Oncology 2009; **Med School:** Brown Univ 1979; **Resid:** Pediatrics, Johns Hopkins Hosp 1982; **Fellow:** Pediatric Hematology-Oncology, Johns Hopkins Hosp 1985; **Fac Appt:** Prof Ped, Brown Univ

van Hoff, Jack MD [PHO] - **Spec Exp:** Brain Tumors; Clinical Trials; **Hospital:** Dartmouth - Hitchcock Med Ctr; **Address:** DHMC, Dept Pediatric Hem/Onc, One Medical Center Drive, Lebanon, NH 03756; **Phone:** 603-650-5541; **Board Cert:** Pediatrics 1985; Pediatric Hematology-Oncology 1987; **Med School:** UMDNJ-NJ Med Sch, Newark 1981; **Resid:** Pediatrics, Yale New Haven Hosp 1984; **Fellow:** Pediatric Hematology-Oncology, Yale New Haven Hosp 1986

Weinstein, Howard J MD [PHO] - **Spec Exp:** Bone Marrow Transplant; Leukemia; Lymphoma; **Hospital:** Mass Genl Hosp, Dana-Farber Cancer Inst (page 57); **Address:** Mass General Hosptial, 55 Fruit St, Yawkey 8B, Boston, MA 02114-2622; **Phone:** 617-726-2737; **Board Cert:** Pediatrics 1977; **Med School:** Univ MD Sch Med 1972; **Resid:** Pediatrics, Mass Genl Hosp 1974; **Fellow:** Pediatric Hematology-Oncology, Dana Farber Cancer Inst/Chldns Hosp 1977; **Fac Appt:** Prof Ped, Harvard Med Sch

Wolff, Johannes MD [PHO] - **Spec Exp:** Brain Tumors; Neuro-Oncology; **Hospital:** Floating Hosp for Children at Tufts Med Ce; **Address:** Floating Hosp for Chldn at Tufts Med Ctr, Div Ped Hem/Onc, 800 Washington St, Box 14, Boston, MA 02111; **Phone:** 617-636-5535; **Med School:** Germany 1986; **Resid:** Pediatrics, Univ Hosp of Muenster 1989; **Fellow:** Pediatric Hematology-Oncology, Johns Hopkins Hosp 1991; **Fac Appt:** Prof Ped, Tufts Univ

Pediatric Hematology-Oncology

Mid Atlantic

Adamson, Peter C MD [PHO] - **Spec Exp:** Drug Development; Clinical Trials; Rhabdomyosarcoma; Pediatric Cancers; **Hospital:** Chldns Hosp of Philadelphia; **Address:** Chldns Hosp of Philadelphia, Div Onc, 34th St & Civic Ctr Blvd Abramson Bldg, Philadelphia, PA 19104; **Phone:** 215-590-3025; **Board Cert:** Pediatric Hematology-Oncology 2005; **Med School:** Cornell Univ-Weill Med Coll 1984; **Resid:** Pediatrics, Chldns Hosp 1987; **Fellow:** Pediatric Hematology-Oncology, Natl Cancer Inst 1990; **Fac Appt:** Clin Prof Ped, Univ Pennsylvania

Aledo, Alexander MD [PHO] - **Spec Exp:** Leukemia; Lymphoma; Bone Tumors; **Hospital:** NY-Presby/Weill Cornell Med Ctr, NY (page 66), NY Hosp Queens; **Address:** 525 E 68th St, rm P695, New York, NY 10021-4870; **Phone:** 212-746-3494; **Board Cert:** Pediatric Hematology-Oncology 2004; **Med School:** NYU Sch Med 1984; **Resid:** Pediatrics, NYPresby/Weill Cornell Med Ctr 1987; **Fellow:** Pediatric Hematology-Oncology, Meml Sloan Kettering Cancer Ctr 1990; **Fac Appt:** Assoc Clin Prof Ped, Cornell Univ-Weill Med Coll

Angiolillo, Anne L MD [PHO] - **Spec Exp:** Leukemia; Lymphoma; **Hospital:** Chldns Natl Med Ctr; **Address:** Chldns Natl Med Ctr-Hem/Onc, 111 Michigan Ave NW, Washington, DC 20010; **Phone:** 202-476-2140; **Board Cert:** Pediatric Hematology-Oncology 2011; **Med School:** NY Med Coll 1989; **Resid:** Pediatrics, Chldns Natl Med Ctr 1992; **Fellow:** Pediatric Hematology-Oncology, Chldns Natl Med Ctr 1995

Arceci, Robert J MD/PhD [PHO] - **Spec Exp:** Leukemia; Histiocytoma; Bone Marrow Transplant; **Hospital:** Johns Hopkins Hosp (page 61); **Address:** Sidney Kimmel Comprehensive Cancer Ctr, Bunting Blaustein Rsch Bldg, 1650 Orleans St, rm I-207, Baltimore, MD 21231; **Phone:** 410-502-7519; **Board Cert:** Pediatrics 1987; Pediatric Hematology-Oncology 2005; **Med School:** Univ Rochester 1981; **Resid:** Pediatrics, Chldns Hosp 1983; **Fellow:** Pediatric Hematology-Oncology, Chldns Hosp/Dana Farber Cancer Ctr 1986; **Fac Appt:** Prof Ped, Johns Hopkins Univ

Brecher, Martin L MD [PHO] - **Spec Exp:** Brain Tumors; Lymphoma; Hodgkin's Lymphoma; Leukemia; **Hospital:** Roswell Park Cancer Inst, Women & Chldn's Hosp of Buffalo, The; **Address:** Roswell Park Cancer Inst, Dept Pediatrics, Elm & Carlton Sts, Buffalo, NY 14263; **Phone:** 716-845-2333; **Board Cert:** Pediatrics 1977; Pediatric Hematology-Oncology 1978; **Med School:** SUNY Buffalo 1972; **Resid:** Pediatrics, Buffalo Chldns Hosp 1975; **Fellow:** Hematology & Oncology, Buffalo Chldns Hosp/Roswell Park Cancer Inst 1977; **Fac Appt:** Assoc Prof Ped, SUNY Buffalo

Bussel, James MD [PHO] - **Spec Exp:** Bleeding/Coagulation Disorders; Platelet Disorders; Wiskott-Aldrich Syndrome; **Hospital:** NY-Presby/Weill Cornell Med Ctr, NY (page 66), Lenox Hill Hosp (page 67); **Address:** 525 E 68th St, rm P-695, New York, NY 10065; **Phone:** 212-746-3400; **Board Cert:** Pediatrics 1979; Pediatric Hematology-Oncology 1980; **Med School:** Columbia P&S 1975; **Resid:** Pediatrics, Chldns Hosp 1978; **Fellow:** Pediatric Hematology-Oncology, NY Presby Hosp/Cornell 1981; **Fac Appt:** Prof Ped, Cornell Univ-Weill Med Coll

Cairo, Mitchell S MD [PHO] - **Spec Exp:** Bone Marrow Transplant; Stem Cell Transplant; Leukemia; Lymphoma; **Hospital:** Westchester Med Ctr, Children's & Women's Phys.of Westchester; **Address:** New York Medical College, Munger Pavilion, rm 110, Valhalla, NY 10595; **Phone:** 914-594-3650; **Board Cert:** Pediatrics 1980; Pediatric Hematology-Oncology 1982; **Med School:** UCSF 1976; **Resid:** Pediatrics, UCLA Med Ctr 1979; **Fellow:** Pediatric Hematology-Oncology, Indiana Univ Med Ctr 1981; **Fac Appt:** Prof Ped, NY Med Coll

Carroll, William L MD [PHO] - **Spec Exp:** Leukemia; **Hospital:** NYU Langone Med Ctr (page 68); **Address:** NYU Med Ctr, Div Ped Hem/Onc, 160 E 32nd Level L3 St, New York, NY 10016; **Phone:** 212-263-8400; **Board Cert:** Pediatrics 1984; Pediatric Hematology-Oncology 1987; **Med School:** UC Irvine 1978; **Resid:** Pediatrics, Chldns Hosp Med Ctr 1981; **Fellow:** Pediatric Hematology-Oncology, Stanford Univ 1987; **Fac Appt:** Prof Ped, NYU Sch Med

Chen, Allen R MD/PhD [PHO] - **Spec Exp:** Bone Marrow Transplant; Hodgkin's Lymphoma; Immunotherapy; Graft vs Host Disease; **Hospital:** Johns Hopkins Hosp (page 61); **Address:** Johns Hopkins Hosp, Div Peds Oncology, 1650 Orleans St CRB Bldg Fl 2M - rm 53, Baltimore, MD 21287; **Phone:** 410-955-8751; **Board Cert:** Pediatric Hematology-Oncology 2006; **Med School:** Duke Univ 1986; **Resid:** Pediatrics, Chldns Hosp Med Ctr 1989; **Fellow:** Pediatric Hematology-Oncology, Fred Hutchinson Canc Ctr 1993; Bone Marrow Transplant, Fred Hutchinson Canc Ctr 1994; **Fac Appt:** Assoc Prof Ped, Johns Hopkins Univ

Cheung, Nai-Kong V MD/PhD [PHO] - **Spec Exp:** Neuroblastoma; **Hospital:** Meml Sloan-Kettering Cancer Ctr; **Address:** 1275 York Ave, New York, NY 10065; **Phone:** 646-888-2313; **Board Cert:** Pediatrics 1987; Pediatric Hematology-Oncology 2012; **Med School:** Harvard Med Sch 1978; **Resid:** Pediatrics, Stanford Univ Hosp 1980; **Fellow:** Pediatric Hematology-Oncology, Stanford Univ Hosp 1982; **Fac Appt:** Assoc Prof Ped, Cornell Univ-Weill Med Coll

Cohen, Kenneth J MD [PHO] - **Spec Exp:** Brain Tumors; Spinal Tumors; **Hospital:** Johns Hopkins Hosp (page 61); **Address:** Johns Hopkins Hosp, 600 N Wolfe St, rm CMSC-800, Baltimore, MD 21287; **Phone:** 410-614-5055; **Board Cert:** Pediatric Hematology-Oncology 2009; **Med School:** SUNY Upstate Med Univ 1987; **Resid:** Pediatrics, Univ Colo Hlth Sci Ctr 1990; **Fellow:** Pediatric Hematology-Oncology, Johns Hopkins Hospital 1994; **Fac Appt:** Assoc Prof Ped, Johns Hopkins Univ

Dome, Jeffrey S MD [PHO] - **Spec Exp:** Solid Tumors; Wilms' Tumor; Bone Cancer; **Hospital:** Chldns Natl Med Ctr; **Address:** Sheikh Zayed Campus, 111 Michigan Ave NW, Washington, DC 20010; **Phone:** 202-476-2800; **Board Cert:** Pediatric Hematology-Oncology 2006; **Med School:** Univ Pennsylvania 1991; **Resid:** Pediatrics, Yale-New Haven Hosp 1994; **Fellow:** Hematology & Oncology, Johns Hopkins Hosp 1997

Drachtman, Richard A MD [PHO] - **Spec Exp:** Pediatric Cancers; Sickle Cell Disease; **Hospital:** Robert Wood Johnson Univ Hosp - New Brunswick, Jersey Shore Univ Med Ctr; **Address:** Cancer Inst of New Jersey, 195 Little Albany St, rm 3507, New Brunswick, NJ 08903; **Phone:** 732-235-5437; **Board Cert:** Pediatric Hematology-Oncology 2007; **Med School:** Ros Franklin Univ/Chicago Med Sch 1984; **Resid:** Pediatrics, N Shore Univ Hosp 1988; **Fellow:** Pediatric Hematology-Oncology, Mount Sinai Hosp 1991; **Fac Appt:** Prof Ped, UMDNJ-RW Johnson Med Sch

Dunkel, Ira J MD [PHO] - **Spec Exp:** Retinoblastoma; Brain & Spinal Cord Tumors; Brain Tumors; Pediatric Cancers; **Hospital:** Meml Sloan-Kettering Cancer Ctr; **Address:** 1275 York Ave, Box 185, New York, NY 10065; **Phone:** 212-639-2153; **Board Cert:** Pediatric Hematology-Oncology 2007; **Med School:** Duke Univ 1985; **Resid:** Pediatrics, Duke Univ Med Ctr 1988; **Fellow:** Pediatric Hematology-Oncology, Memorial-Sloan Kettering 1992; **Fac Appt:** Assoc Prof Ped, Cornell Univ-Weill Med Coll

Felix, Carolyn A MD [PHO] - **Spec Exp:** Leukemia; Leukemia in Infants; **Hospital:** Chldns Hosp of Philadelphia; **Address:** Colket Translational Research Bldg, 3501 Civic Ctr Blvd, Fl 4 - rm 4006, Philadelphia, PA 19104; **Phone:** 215-590-2831; **Board Cert:** Pediatrics 1987; Pediatric Hematology-Oncology 1987; **Med School:** Boston Univ 1981; **Resid:** Pediatrics, Chldns Hosp 1984; **Fellow:** Pediatric Hematology-Oncology, Natl Cancer Inst 1987; **Fac Appt:** Prof Ped, Univ Pennsylvania

Frantz, Christopher N MD [PHO] - **Spec Exp:** Solid Tumors; Neuroblastoma; Leukemia; **Hospital:** Nemours/Alfred I. duPont Hosp for Chldn, Wilmington Hosp; **Address:** Alfred I duPont Hosp for Chldn, 1600 Rockland Rd, Box 269, Wilmington, DE 19803; **Phone:** 302-651-5500; **Board Cert:** Pediatrics 1977; Pediatric Hematology-Oncology 2012; **Med School:** Albert Einstein Coll Med 1971; **Resid:** Pediatrics, Chldns Hosp 1976; **Fellow:** Pediatric Hematology-Oncology, Chldns Hosp/Dana Farber Cancer Inst 1979

Pediatric Hematology-Oncology

Friedman, Alan D MD [PHO] - **Spec Exp:** Leukemia; **Hospital:** Johns Hopkins Hosp (page 61); **Address:** Bunting Blaustein Cancer Rsch Bldg 1, 1650 Orleans St, rm 253, Baltimore, MD 21287; **Phone:** 410-955-8751; **Board Cert:** Pediatrics 1987; Pediatric Hematology-Oncology 2005; **Med School:** Harvard Med Sch 1983; **Resid:** Pediatrics, Chldns Hosp 1986; **Fellow:** Pediatric Hematology-Oncology, Johns Hopkins Hosp 1987; **Fac Appt:** Prof Ped, Johns Hopkins Univ

Garvin Jr, James H MD/PhD [PHO] - **Spec Exp:** Brain Tumors; Pediatric Cancers; Bone Marrow Transplant; **Hospital:** Morgan Stanley Children's Hosp of NY-Presby, NY; **Address:** 161 Fort Washington Ave, Fl 7, rm 708, New York, NY 10032-3729; **Phone:** 212-305-5808; **Board Cert:** Pediatrics 1982; Pediatric Hematology-Oncology 1984; **Med School:** Jefferson Med Coll 1976; **Resid:** Pediatrics, Chldns Hosp 1978; Pediatrics, Middlesex Hosp 1979; **Fellow:** Pediatric Hematology-Oncology, Dana Farber Cancer Inst/Childrens Hosp 1982; **Fac Appt:** Clin Prof Ped, Columbia P&S

Giardina, Patricia J V MD [PHO] - **Spec Exp:** Thalassemia; **Hospital:** NY-Presby/Weill Cornell Med Ctr, NY (page 66); **Address:** 525 E 68th St, Payson Pavilion 695, New York, NY 10065; **Phone:** 212-746-3400; **Board Cert:** Pediatrics 1973; Pediatric Hematology-Oncology 1974; **Med School:** NY Med Coll 1968; **Resid:** Pediatrics, New York Hosp 1971; **Fellow:** Pediatric Hematology-Oncology, New York Hosp-Cornell 1974; **Fac Appt:** Clin Prof Ped, Cornell Univ-Weill Med Coll

Greenberg, Jay N MD [PHO] - **Hospital:** Chldns Natl Med Ctr, Inova Fairfax Hosp; **Address:** Pediatric Hematology/Oncology, 111 Michigan Ave NW Fl 4 W Wing, Washington, DC 20010; **Phone:** 202-476-2140; **Board Cert:** Pediatrics 1981; Pediatric Hematology-Oncology 1982; **Med School:** Univ Pennsylvania 1976; **Resid:** Pediatrics, Univ MI Hosp 1978; Pediatrics, Chldns Hosp 1979; **Fellow:** Pediatric Hematology-Oncology, Chldns Hosp 1982

Grupp, Stephan A MD/PhD [PHO] - **Spec Exp:** Stem Cell Transplant; Neuroblastoma; Bone Marrow Transplant; **Hospital:** Chldns Hosp of Philadelphia; **Address:** Childrens Hosp - Oncology, 34th St & Civic Ctr Blvd, Abramson Bldg, Philadelphia, PA 19104; **Phone:** 215-590-2821; **Board Cert:** Pediatric Hematology-Oncology 2009; **Med School:** Univ Cincinnati 1987; **Resid:** Pediatrics, Chldns Hosp 1990; **Fellow:** Pediatric Hematology-Oncology, Dana Farber Cancer Inst/Chldns Hosp 1992; **Fac Appt:** Asst Prof Ped, Univ Pennsylvania

Guarini, Ludovico MD [PHO] - **Spec Exp:** Leukemia; Solid Tumors; Sickle Cell Disease; **Hospital:** Maimonides Med Ctr (page 63); **Address:** MMC Dept of Pediatrics, 6300 Eighth Ave Fl 2, Brooklyn, NY 11220; **Phone:** 718-765-2671; **Board Cert:** Pediatrics 1984; Pediatric Hematology-Oncology 2007; **Med School:** Italy 1974; **Resid:** Pediatrics, Beth Israel Hosp 1981; **Fellow:** Pediatric Hematology-Oncology, Columbia-Presby Med Ctr 1984; **Fac Appt:** Assoc Prof Ped, SUNY Hlth Sci Ctr

Halligan, Gregory E MD [PHO] - **Spec Exp:** Clinical Trials; Solid Tumors; **Hospital:** St. Christopher's Hosp for Chldn; **Address:** St Christophers Hosp for Children, Dept Oncology, 3601 A St, Philadelphia, PA 19134; **Phone:** 215-427-4447; **Board Cert:** Pediatrics 1982; Pediatric Hematology-Oncology 1984; **Med School:** Belgium 1977; **Resid:** Pediatrics, St Christophers Hosp for Chldn 1981; **Fellow:** Pediatric Hematology-Oncology, St Christophers Hosp for Chldn 1984; **Fac Appt:** Assoc Prof Ped, Drexel Univ Coll Med

Halpern, Steven L MD [PHO] - **Spec Exp:** Leukemia & Lymphoma; Brain Tumors; Hodgkin's Lymphoma; Hemophilia; **Hospital:** Morristown Med Ctr, Overlook Med Ctr; **Address:** 100 Madison Ave, Morristown, NJ 07960; **Phone:** 973-971-6720; **Board Cert:** Pediatrics 1981; Pediatric Hematology-Oncology 1982; **Med School:** Ros Franklin Univ/Chicago Med Sch 1976; **Resid:** Pediatrics, St Christophers Hosp for Children 1979; **Fellow:** Pediatric Hematology-Oncology, Childrens Hosp 1982; **Fac Appt:** Asst Prof Ped, UMDNJ-NJ Med Sch, Newark

Harris, Michael B MD [PHO] - **Spec Exp:** Leukemia & Lymphoma; Bone Tumors; Cancer Survivors-Late Effects of Therapy; **Hospital:** Hackensack Univ Med Ctr; **Address:** Tomorrows Chldns Inst, JM Sanzari Chldns Hosp, 30 Prospect Ave, Imus 1-TCI, rm PC116, Hackensack, NJ 07601; **Phone:** 201-996-5437; **Board Cert:** Pediatrics 1974; Pediatric Hematology-Oncology 1974; **Med School:** Albert Einstein Coll Med 1969; **Resid:** Pediatrics, Chldns Hosp 1971; **Fellow:** Pediatric Hematology-Oncology, Chldns Hosp 1974; **Fac Appt:** Prof Ped, UMDNJ-NJ Med Sch, Newark

Helman, Lee Jay MD [PHO] - **Spec Exp:** Solid Tumors; **Hospital:** Natl Inst of Hlth - Clin Ctr; **Address:** National Cancer Inst, 31 Center Drive, rm 3A11, Bethesda, MD 20892; **Phone:** 301-496-4257; **Board Cert:** Internal Medicine 1983; Medical Oncology 1985; **Med School:** Univ MD Sch Med 1980; **Resid:** Internal Medicine, Barnes Hosp 1983; **Fellow:** Oncology, Natl Inst Hlth 1986

Hoots, William K MD [PHO] - **Spec Exp:** Hemophilia; **Hospital:** Natl Inst of Hlth - Clin Ctr; **Address:** Nat Inst Hlth-Clin Ctr, 6701 Rockledge Drive, Ste 9030 - rm 9136, Bethesda, MD 20892; **Phone:** 301-435-0080; **Board Cert:** Pediatrics 1980; Pediatric Hematology-Oncology 1980; **Med School:** Univ NC Sch Med 1975; **Resid:** Pediatrics, Chldns Med Ctr 1978; **Fellow:** Pediatric Hematology-Oncology, Univ NC Med Ctr 1980; **Fac Appt:** Prof Ped, Univ Tex, Houston

Jakacki, Regina I MD [PHO] - **Spec Exp:** Neuro-Oncology; Clinical Trials; Palliative Care; **Hospital:** Chldns Hosp of Pittsburgh - UPMC; **Address:** Childrens Hosp-Div Hematology/Oncology, One Childrens Hosp Drive, 4401 Penn Ave Fl 8, Pittsburgh, PA 15224; **Phone:** 412-692-5055; **Board Cert:** Pediatric Hematology-Oncology 2007; **Med School:** Univ Pennsylvania 1985; **Resid:** Pediatrics, Childrens Hosp 1988; **Fellow:** Pediatric Hematology-Oncology, Childrens Hosp 1991; **Fac Appt:** Assoc Prof Ped, Univ Pittsburgh

Kamen, Barton A MD/PhD [PHO] - **Spec Exp:** Drug Development; Leukemia; **Hospital:** Robert Wood Johnson Univ Hosp - New Brunswick; **Address:** Cancer Inst of New Jersey, 195 Little Albany St, rm 3549, New Brunswick, NJ 08903; **Phone:** 732-235-5437; **Board Cert:** Pediatrics 1981; Pediatric Hematology-Oncology 1987; **Med School:** Case West Res Univ 1976; **Resid:** Pediatrics, Yale-New Haven Hosp 1978; **Fellow:** Pediatric Hematology-Oncology, Yale-New Haven Hosp 1980; **Fac Appt:** Prof Ped, UMDNJ-RW Johnson Med Sch

Korones, David N MD [PHO] - **Spec Exp:** Brain Tumors; Palliative Care; Pediatric Cancers; **Hospital:** Univ of Rochester Strong Meml Hosp; **Address:** Golisano Childrens Hosp at Strong, 601 Elmwood Ave, Box 777, Rochester, NY 14642-8777; **Phone:** 585-275-2981; **Board Cert:** Pediatrics 1987; Pediatric Hematology-Oncology 2006; Hospice & Palliative Medicine 2002; **Med School:** Vanderbilt Univ 1983; **Resid:** Pediatrics, Strong Meml Hosp 1986; **Fellow:** Pediatrics, Yale Univ 1988; Pediatric Hematology-Oncology, Strong Meml Hosp 1991; **Fac Appt:** Prof Ped, Univ Rochester

Kramer, Kim MD [PHO] - **Spec Exp:** Neuroblastoma; Brain & Spinal Cord Tumors; **Hospital:** Meml Sloan-Kettering Cancer Ctr; **Address:** 1275 York, Box 429, New York, NY 10021; **Phone:** 212-639-6410; **Board Cert:** Pediatric Hematology-Oncology 2011; **Med School:** SUNY Upstate Med Univ 1989; **Resid:** Pediatrics, Strong Meml Hosp 1992; **Fellow:** Pediatric Hematology-Oncology, Meml Sloan Kettering Cancer Ctr 1994

Kushner, Brian H MD [PHO] - **Spec Exp:** Neuroblastoma; Bone Marrow Transplant; Immunotherapy; **Hospital:** Meml Sloan-Kettering Cancer Ctr; **Address:** 1275 York Avenue, New York, NY 10065; **Phone:** 212-639-6793; **Board Cert:** Pediatrics 1983; Pediatric Hematology-Oncology 1987; **Med School:** Johns Hopkins Univ 1976; **Resid:** Pediatrics, Columbia-Presby Med Ctr 1978; Pediatrics, NY Hosp 1979; **Fellow:** Pediatric Hematology-Oncology, Boston Chldns Hosp 1980; Pediatric Hematology-Oncology, Meml Sloan Kettering Cancer Ctr 1986; **Fac Appt:** Prof Ped, Cornell Univ-Weill Med Coll

Pediatric Hematology-Oncology

Kuttesch, John F MD/PhD [PHO] - **Spec Exp:** Brain Tumors; Brain Tumors-Recurrent; Solid Tumors; **Hospital:** Penn State Chldns Hosp; **Address:** Penn State Hershey Div Pediatric Hem/Onc, 500 University Drive, MC HO85, Hershey, PA 17033-0850; **Phone:** 717-531-6012; **Board Cert:** Pediatrics 2008; Pediatric Hematology-Oncology 2007; **Med School:** Univ Tex, Houston 1985; **Resid:** Pediatrics, Vanderbilt Univ Med Ctr 1988; **Fellow:** Pediatric Hematology-Oncology, St Judes Chldns Hosp 1990; **Fac Appt:** Prof Ped, Penn State Coll Med

Lange, Beverly J MD [PHO] - **Spec Exp:** Leukemia; Brain & Spinal Cord Tumors; Cognitive Rehabilitation; **Hospital:** Chldns Hosp of Philadelphia; **Address:** Chldns Hosp Phila, Medical Oncology, 34th St & Civic Ctr Blvd, Wood Center Fl 4, Philadelphia, PA 19104; **Phone:** 215-590-3025; **Board Cert:** Pediatrics 1976; Pediatric Hematology-Oncology 1997; **Med School:** Temple Univ 1971; **Resid:** Pediatrics, Philadelphia Genl Hosp 1973; **Fellow:** Pediatric Oncology, Chldns Hosp; **Fac Appt:** Prof Ped, Univ Pennsylvania

Lipton, Jeffrey M MD/PhD [PHO] - **Spec Exp:** Bone Marrow Failure Disorders; Stem Cell Transplant; Bone Marrow Transplant; Bone Marrow Failure Disorders; **Hospital:** Steven & Alexandra Cohen Chldn's Med Ctr of NY (page 67); **Address:** Cohen Children's Medical Center of NY, 269-01 76th Ave, New Hyde Park, NY 11040-1433; **Phone:** 718-470-3460; **Board Cert:** Pediatrics 1981; **Med School:** St Louis Univ 1975; **Resid:** Pediatrics, Boston Chldns Hosp 1977; **Fellow:** Pediatric Hematology-Oncology, Boston Chldns Hosp/Dana Farber Cancer Inst 1979; **Fac Appt:** Prof Ped, Hofstra N Shore-LIJ Sch Med

Loeb, David M MD/PhD [PHO] - **Spec Exp:** Bone Marrow Transplant; Bone Cancer; **Hospital:** Johns Hopkins Hosp (page 61); **Address:** Charlotte R Bloomberg Chldns Ctr, Pediatric Onc Clin, Bloomberg 11-N, 1800 Orleans St, Baltimore, MD 21287; **Phone:** 410-502-4997; **Board Cert:** Pediatric Hematology-Oncology 2008; **Med School:** Columbia P&S 1994; **Resid:** Pediatrics, John Hopkins Hosp 1997; **Fellow:** Pediatric Oncology, John Hopkins Hosp 1997; **Fac Appt:** Asst Prof Ped, Johns Hopkins Univ

Luchtman-Jones, Lori MD [PHO] - **Spec Exp:** Leukemia; Bleeding/Coagulation Disorders; **Hospital:** Chldns Natl Med Ctr; **Address:** Chldn's Natl Med Ctr, 111 Michigan Ave NW Fl 4 - Ste 4043, Washington, DC 20010; **Phone:** 202-476-2140; **Board Cert:** Pediatric Hematology-Oncology 2011; **Med School:** UCSD 1987; **Resid:** Pediatrics, UCSD School Med 1990; **Fellow:** Pediatric Hematology-Oncology, Washington Univ 1995; **Fac Appt:** Asst Prof Ped, Washington Univ, St Louis

Marcus, Judith R MD [PHO] - **Spec Exp:** Leukemia; Lymphoma; Bleeding/Coagulation Disorders; Solid Tumors; **Hospital:** Morgan Stanley Children's Hosp of NY-Presby, NY, White Plains Hosp; **Address:** 161 Ft Washington Ave, Ste 7I, New York, NY 10032; **Phone:** 212-305-5808; **Board Cert:** Pediatrics 1997; Pediatric Hematology-Oncology 1997; **Med School:** NYU Sch Med 1971; **Resid:** Pediatrics, Bronx Muni Hosp-Albert Einstein 1974; **Fellow:** Pediatric Hematology-Oncology, Meml Sloan Kettering Cancer Ctr 1979; **Fac Appt:** Clin Prof Ped, Columbia P&S

Maris, John M MD [PHO] - **Spec Exp:** Neuroblastoma; Clinical Trials; **Hospital:** Chldns Hosp of Philadelphia; **Address:** Chldns Hosp Philadelphia - Oncology, 3501 Civic Ctr Blvd CTRB Bldg - rm 3060, Philadelphia, PA 19104-4318; **Phone:** 215-590-5244; **Board Cert:** Pediatric Hematology-Oncology 2004; **Med School:** Univ Pennsylvania 1989; **Resid:** Pediatrics, Chldns Hosp 1992; **Fellow:** Pediatric Hematology-Oncology, Chldns Hosp 1996

Meyers, Paul A MD [PHO] - **Spec Exp:** Pediatric Cancers; Bone Tumors; Sarcoma; **Hospital:** Meml Sloan-Kettering Cancer Ctr, NY-Presby/Weill Cornell Med Ctr, NY (page 66); **Address:** 1275 York Ave, New York, NY 10065; **Phone:** 212-639-5952; **Board Cert:** Pediatrics 1978; Pediatric Hematology-Oncology 1978; **Med School:** Mount Sinai Sch Med 1973; **Resid:** Pediatrics, Mt Sinai Hosp 1976; **Fellow:** Pediatric Hematology-Oncology, NY Hosp-Cornell Med Ctr 1979; **Fac Appt:** Prof Ped, Cornell Univ-Weill Med Coll

O'Reilly, Richard MD [PHO] - **Spec Exp:** Bone Marrow Transplant; **Hospital:** Meml Sloan-Kettering Cancer Ctr, NY-Presby/Weill Cornell Med Ctr, NY (page 66); **Address:** 1275 York Avenue, New York, NY 10065; **Phone:** 212-639-5957; **Board Cert:** Pediatrics 1974; **Med School:** Univ Rochester 1968; **Resid:** Pediatrics, Chldrns Hosp 1972; **Fellow:** Infectious Disease, Chldrns Hosp 1973; **Fac Appt:** Prof Ped, Cornell Univ-Weill Med Coll

Parker, Robert MD [PHO] - **Spec Exp:** Pediatric Cancers; Bleeding/Coagulation Disorders; Platelet Disorders; Lymphoma; **Hospital:** Stony Brook Univ Med Ctr; **Address:** Stony Brook Univ Hosp, Dept Peds, HSC T-11, Rm 029, Stony Brook, NY 11794-8111; **Phone:** 631-444-7720; **Board Cert:** Pediatrics 1983; Pediatric Hematology-Oncology 1984; **Med School:** Brown Univ 1976; **Resid:** Internal Medicine, Roger Williams Med Ctr 1977; Pediatrics, Rhode Island Hosp 1979; **Fellow:** Pediatric Hematology-Oncology, Natl Cancer Inst 1981; Hematology, Natl Cancer Inst 1984; **Fac Appt:** Prof Ped, SUNY Stony Brook

Reaman, Gregory H MD [PHO] - **Spec Exp:** Leukemia; Lymphoma; Cancer Survivors-Late Effects of Therapy; **Hospital:** Chldns Natl Med Ctr; **Address:** 111 Michigan Ave NW, West Bldg Fl 4 - Ste 600, Washington, DC 20010-2916; **Phone:** 202-476-2800; **Board Cert:** Pediatrics 1978; Pediatric Hematology-Oncology 1978; **Med School:** Loyola Univ-Stritch Sch Med 1973; **Resid:** Hematology, Montreal Chldns Hosp 1975; Pediatrics, Montreal Chldns Hosp 1976; **Fellow:** Pediatric Oncology, Natl Cancer Inst 1979; **Fac Appt:** Prof Ped, Geo Wash Univ

Rheingold, Susan R MD [PHO] - **Spec Exp:** Leukemia; Complementary Medicine; Clinical Trials; **Hospital:** Chldns Hosp of Philadelphia; **Address:** Chldns Hosp Phila - Div Oncology, 3501 Civic Ctr Blvd, CTRB Fl 10 - rm 10052, Philadelphia, PA 19104; **Phone:** 215-590-3079; **Board Cert:** Pediatrics 2010; Pediatric Hematology-Oncology 2008; **Med School:** Univ Pennsylvania 1992; **Resid:** Pediatrics, Johns Hopkins Hosp 1995; **Fellow:** Pediatric Hematology-Oncology, Chldns Hosp 1999; **Fac Appt:** Assoc Clin Prof Ped, Univ Pennsylvania

Ritchey, A Kim MD [PHO] - **Spec Exp:** Leukemia; Bleeding/Coagulation Disorders; Hematologic Malignancies; Clinical Trials; **Hospital:** Chldns Hosp of Pittsburgh - UPMC; **Address:** Chldns Hosp, Div Hematology/Oncology, One Children's Hosp Drive, 4401 Penn Ave, Faculty Pavilion Fl 8, Pittsburgh, PA 15224; **Phone:** 412-692-5055; **Board Cert:** Pediatrics 1977; Pediatric Hematology-Oncology 2007; **Med School:** Univ Cincinnati 1972; **Resid:** Pediatrics, Johns Hopkins Hosp 1975; **Fellow:** Pediatric Hematology-Oncology, Yale-New Haven Hosp 1980; **Fac Appt:** Prof Ped, Univ Pittsburgh

Rood, Brian R MD [PHO] - **Spec Exp:** Brain Tumors; **Hospital:** Chldns Natl Med Ctr; **Address:** CNMC Div Ped Onc, 111 Michigan Ave NW, Washington, DC 20010; **Phone:** 202-476-2140; **Board Cert:** Pediatrics 2006; Pediatric Hematology-Oncology 2010; **Med School:** Jefferson Med Coll 1995; **Resid:** Pediatrics, Univ VT Hosp 1998; **Fellow:** Pediatric Hematology-Oncology, Chldns Natl Med Ctr 1998; Research, Chldns Natl Med Ctr 2001

Shearer, Patricia C MD [PHO] - **Spec Exp:** Cancer Survivors-Late Effects of Therapy; **Hospital:** Univ of MD Med Ctr; **Address:** Univ Maryland Medical Center, 22 S Greene St, Baltimore, MD 21201; **Phone:** 410-328-2808; **Board Cert:** Pediatric Hematology-Oncology 2007; **Med School:** Louisiana State U, New Orleans 1986; **Resid:** Pediatrics, Johns Hopkins Hosp 1989; **Fellow:** Pediatric Hematology-Oncology, St Jude Chldns Rsch Hosp 1992; **Fac Appt:** Assoc Clin Prof Ped, Univ Fla Coll Med

Small, Donald MD [PHO] - **Spec Exp:** Leukemia; Lymphoma; **Hospital:** Johns Hopkins Hosp (page 61); **Address:** Bunting Blaustein Cancer Rsch Bldg, 1650 Orleans St, rm 251, Baltimore, MD 21231; **Phone:** 410-955-8817; **Board Cert:** Pediatric Hematology-Oncology 2002; **Med School:** Johns Hopkins Univ 1985; **Resid:** Pediatrics, Johns Hopkins Hosp 1987; **Fellow:** Pediatric Hematology-Oncology, Johns Hopkins Hosp 1990; **Fac Appt:** Prof Ped, Johns Hopkins Univ

Pediatric Hematology-Oncology

Steinherz, Peter G MD [PHO] - **Spec Exp:** Leukemia & Lymphoma; Pediatric Cancers; Wilms' Tumor; **Hospital:** Meml Sloan-Kettering Cancer Ctr, NY-Presby/Weill Cornell Med Ctr, NY (page 66); **Address:** 1275 York Avenue, New York, NY 10065; **Phone:** 212-639-7951; **Board Cert:** Pediatrics 1973; Pediatric Hematology-Oncology 1978; **Med School:** Albert Einstein Coll Med 1968; **Resid:** Pediatrics, NYPresby/Weill Cornell Med Ctr 1971; **Fellow:** Pediatric Hematology-Oncology, NYPresby/Weill Cornell Med Ctr 1975; **Fac Appt:** Prof Ped, Cornell Univ-Weill Med Coll

Weinblatt, Mark E MD [PHO] - **Spec Exp:** Leukemia & Lymphoma; Sickle Cell Disease; Bleeding/Coagulation Disorders; Thalassemia; **Hospital:** Winthrop Univ Hosp; **Address:** 120 Mineola Blvd, Ste 460, Mineola, NY 11501; **Phone:** 516-663-9400; **Board Cert:** Pediatrics 1980; Pediatric Hematology-Oncology 1982; **Med School:** Albert Einstein Coll Med 1976; **Resid:** Pediatrics, Jacobi Med Ctr 1979; **Fellow:** Pediatric Hematology-Oncology, Children's Hosp 1981; **Fac Appt:** Prof Ped, SUNY Stony Brook

Weiner, Michael A MD [PHO] - **Spec Exp:** Hodgkin's Lymphoma; Lymphoma; Leukemia; **Hospital:** Morgan Stanley Children's Hosp of NY-Presby, NY; **Address:** 161 Fort Washington Ave, Irving Pavilion-FL 7, New York, NY 10032-3710; **Phone:** 212-305-9770; **Board Cert:** Pediatrics 1980; Pediatric Hematology-Oncology 1980; **Med School:** SUNY Hlth Sci Ctr 1972; **Resid:** Pediatrics, Montefiore Med Ctr 1974; **Fellow:** Pediatric Hematology-Oncology, NYU Med Ctr 1976; Pediatric Hematology-Oncology, Johns Hopkins Hosp 1977; **Fac Appt:** Prof Ped, Columbia P&S

Wexler, Leonard MD [PHO] - **Spec Exp:** Rhabdomyosarcoma; Bone Cancer; Gastrointestinal Stromal Tumors; Sarcoma-Soft Tissue; **Hospital:** Meml Sloan-Kettering Cancer Ctr; **Address:** 1275 York Avenue, New York, NY 10065; **Phone:** 212-639-7990; **Board Cert:** Pediatrics 2007; Pediatric Hematology-Oncology 2007; **Med School:** Boston Univ 1985; **Resid:** Pediatrics, Montefiore Med Ctr 1988; **Fellow:** Pediatric Hematology-Oncology, National Cancer Inst 1991; **Fac Appt:** Assoc Prof Ped, Columbia P&S

Wiley, Joseph M MD [PHO] - **Hospital:** Sinai Hosp - Baltimore; **Address:** Sinai Hosp, Div Pediatric Hem/Onc, 2401 W Belvedere Ave, Baltimore, MD 21215; **Phone:** 410-601-5864; **Board Cert:** Pediatrics 1986; Pediatric Hematology-Oncology 2005; **Med School:** Univ MD Sch Med 1982; **Resid:** Pediatrics, Johns Hopkins Hosp 1995; **Fellow:** Pediatric Hematology-Oncology, Johns Hopkins Hosp 1998; **Fac Appt:** Assoc Prof Ped, Johns Hopkins Univ

Wolfe, Lawrence C MD [PHO] - **Spec Exp:** Palliative Care; Adrenal Cancer; Congenital Hemolytic Anemia; Hemochromatosis; **Hospital:** Steven & Alexandra Cohen Chldn's Med Ctr of NY (page 67); **Address:** Steven & Alexandra Cohen Chldn's Med Ctr, Div Pediatric Hematology/Oncology, 269-01 76th Ave, New Hyde Park, NY 11040; **Phone:** 718-470-3460; **Board Cert:** Pediatrics 1981; Pediatric Hematology-Oncology 1987; Hospice & Palliative Medicine 2011; **Med School:** Harvard Med Sch 1976; **Resid:** Pediatrics, Chldns Hosp 1978; **Fellow:** Pediatric Hematology-Oncology, Chldns Hosp 1991; **Fac Appt:** Prof Ped

York, Teresa A MD [PHO] - **Spec Exp:** Leukemia; **Hospital:** Univ of MD Med Ctr; **Address:** Greenebaum Cancer Center, 22 S Greene St, rm N5E16, Baltimore, MD 21201; **Phone:** 410-328-2808; **Board Cert:** Pediatric Hematology-Oncology 2004; **Med School:** W VA Univ 1997; **Resid:** Pediatrics, W VA Univ Chldns Hosp 2000; **Fellow:** Pediatric Hematology-Oncology, Med Univ SC Hosp 2000; **Fac Appt:** Asst Prof Ped, Univ MD Sch Med

Southeast

Barredo, Julio C MD [PHO] - **Spec Exp:** Leukemia; Bone Marrow Transplant; Cancer Survivors-Late Effects of Therapy; Stem Cell Transplant; **Hospital:** Univ of Miami Hosp & Clins/Sylvester Comp Canc Ctr; **Address:** Univ Miami Dept Pediatrics (R-131), PO Box 016960, Miami, FL 33101; **Phone:** 305-585-5635; **Board Cert:** Pediatric Hematology-Oncology 2007; **Med School:** Peru 1982; **Resid:** Pediatrics, Kings Co Hosp 1987; **Fellow:** Pediatric Hematology-Oncology, Chldns Hosp/USC 1988; **Fac Appt:** Prof Ped, Univ Miami Sch Med

Bertolone, Salvatore MD [PHO] - **Spec Exp:** Bone Marrow Transplant; Kasabach-Merritt Syndrome (KMS); Sickle Cell Disease; **Hospital:** Kosair Chldn's Hosp, Norton Hosp; **Address:** Pediatric Hem/Onc Specs, 601 S Floyd St, Ste 403, Louisville, KY 40202; **Phone:** 502-629-7750; **Board Cert:** Pediatrics 1975; Pediatric Hematology-Oncology 1976; **Med School:** Univ Louisville Sch Med 1970; **Resid:** Pediatrics, Univ Louisville Affil Hosps 1972; **Fellow:** Pediatric Hematology-Oncology, Univ Colorado 1974; **Fac Appt:** Prof Ped, Univ Louisville Sch Med

Blatt, Julie MD [PHO] - **Spec Exp:** Neuroblastoma; Cancer Survivors-Late Effects of Therapy; **Hospital:** NC Memorial Hosp - UNC; **Address:** UNC, Dept Ped Hematology Oncology, 170 Manning Drive, Campus Box 7236, Chapel Hill, NC 27599-7236; **Phone:** 919-966-1178; **Board Cert:** Pediatrics 1981; Pediatric Hematology-Oncology 1982; **Med School:** Johns Hopkins Univ 1976; **Resid:** Pediatrics, Columbia-Presby Hosp 1978; **Fellow:** Pediatric Oncology, Natl Cancer Inst 1982; **Fac Appt:** Prof Ped, Univ NC Sch Med

Castellino, Sharon M MD [PHO] - **Spec Exp:** Cancer Survivors-Late Effects of Therapy; Leukemia; Lymphoma; **Hospital:** Brenner Chldrn's Hosp; **Address:** Wake Forest Univ Baptist Med Ctr, Div Pediatric Hematology/Oncology, Medical Center Blvd, Winston-Salem, NC 27157; **Phone:** 336-716-4324; **Board Cert:** Pediatrics 2003; Pediatric Hematology-Oncology 2006; **Med School:** Duke Univ 1992; **Resid:** Pediatrics, Childrens Hosp 1994; Pediatrics, Duke Univ Med Ctr 1995; **Fellow:** Pediatric Hematology-Oncology, Duke Univ Med Ctr 1997; **Fac Appt:** Asst Prof Ped, Wake Forest Univ

Frangoul, Haydar A MD [PHO] - **Spec Exp:** Stem Cell Transplant; Pediatric Cancers; **Hospital:** Vanderbilt Monroe Carrell Jr. Chldn's Hosp (page 75); **Address:** VUMC-Ped Hematology/Oncology, 1215 21st Ave S, 397 Preston Research Bldg, Nashville, TN 37232-6310; **Phone:** 615-936-1762; **Board Cert:** Pediatric Hematology-Oncology 2008; **Med School:** Amer Univ Beirut 1990; **Resid:** Pediatrics, Duke Univ Med Ctr 1993; **Fellow:** Pediatric Hematology-Oncology, Duke Univ Med Ctr 1994; Pediatric Hematology-Oncology, Seattle Chldns/Fred Hutchinson Cancer Ctr 1996; **Fac Appt:** Prof Ped, Vanderbilt Univ

Friedman, Debra L MD [PHO] - **Spec Exp:** Cancer Survivors-Late Effects of Therapy; Hodgkin's Lymphoma; Retinoblastoma; Pediatric Cancers; **Hospital:** Vanderbilt Monroe Carrell Jr. Chldn's Hosp (page 75), Vanderbilt Univ Med Ctr (page 75); **Address:** 2220 Children's Way, 6th Floor Doctor's Office Tower, Nashville, TN 37232-6310; **Phone:** 615-936-1762; **Board Cert:** Pediatric Hematology-Oncology 2006; **Med School:** UMDNJ-RW Johnson Med Sch 1991; **Resid:** Pediatrics, Chldns Hosp 1994; **Fellow:** Pediatric Hematology-Oncology, Chldns Hosp 1997; Cancer Epidemiology, Univ Penn; **Fac Appt:** Assoc Prof Ped, Vanderbilt Univ

Furman, Wayne L MD [PHO] - **Spec Exp:** Neuroblastoma; Liver Cancer; Drug Development; **Hospital:** St. Jude Children's Research Hosp; **Address:** St Jude Children's Research Hospital, 262 Danny Thomas Pl, MS 260, Memphis, TN 38105; **Phone:** 901-595-2800; **Board Cert:** Pediatrics 1985; Pediatric Hematology-Oncology 1987; **Med School:** Ohio State Univ 1979; **Resid:** Pediatrics, Children's Hosp 1983; **Fellow:** Pediatric Hematology-Oncology, St Jude Chldn's Rsch Hosp 1985; **Fac Appt:** Prof Ped, Univ Tenn Coll Med

Pediatric Hematology-Oncology

Gajjar, Amar J MD [PHO] - **Spec Exp:** Brain Tumors; Medulloblastoma; Neuro-Oncology; Drug Development; **Hospital:** St. Jude Children's Research Hosp; **Address:** St Judes Childrens Research Hosp, Neuro-Oncology, 262 Danny Thomas Pl, MS 260, Memphis, TN 38105-2794; **Phone:** 901-595-4599; **Board Cert:** Pediatric Hematology-Oncology 2007; **Med School:** India 1984; **Resid:** Pediatrics, All Chldns Hosp 1989; **Fellow:** Hematology & Oncology, St Jude Chldns Hosp 1992; **Fac Appt:** Prof Ped, Univ Tenn Coll Med

Godder, Kamar MD/PhD [PHO] - **Spec Exp:** Stem Cell Transplant; Leukemia; Palliative Care; **Hospital:** Med Coll of VA Hosp; **Address:** 401-09 N 11th St Fl 2, Richmond, VA 23298; **Phone:** 804-828-9300; **Med School:** Israel 1980; **Resid:** Pediatrics, Hadassah-Mt Scopus 1984; **Fellow:** Pediatric Hematology-Oncology, Meml Sloan Kettering Cancer Ctr 1988; **Fac Appt:** Prof Ped, Va Commonwealth Univ Sch Med

Gold, Stuart H MD [PHO] - **Spec Exp:** Leukemia; Brain Tumors; Cancer Survivors-Late Effects of Therapy; **Hospital:** NC Memorial Hosp - UNC; **Address:** UNC, Dept Ped Hem-Onc, 1185A Physicians Office Bldg, 170 Manning Drive, Campus Box 7236, Chapel Hill, NC 27599-7236; **Phone:** 919-966-1178; **Board Cert:** Pediatrics 1986; Pediatric Hematology-Oncology 1987; **Med School:** Vanderbilt Univ 1981; **Resid:** Pediatrics, Univ Colorado Hlth Sci Ctr 1984; **Fellow:** Pediatric Hematology-Oncology, Univ Colorado Hlth Sci Ctr 1989; **Fac Appt:** Prof Ped, Univ NC Sch Med

Green, Daniel M MD [PHO] - **Spec Exp:** Wilms' Tumor; Fertility in Cancer Survivors; Cancer Survivors-Late Effects of Therapy; **Hospital:** St. Jude Children's Research Hosp; **Address:** Department of Epidemiology and Cancer Control, St Jude Children's Research Hospital, 262 Danny Thomas Pl, MS 735, Memphis, TN 38105-2794; **Phone:** 901-595-5915; **Board Cert:** Pediatrics 1986; Pediatric Hematology-Oncology 1997; **Med School:** St Louis Univ 1973; **Resid:** Pediatrics, Boston City Hosp 1975; **Fellow:** Pediatric Hematology-Oncology, Chldns Hosp Med Ctr 1978

Gururangan, Sridharan MD [PHO] - **Spec Exp:** Brain Tumors; Spinal Cord Tumors; Neuro-Oncology; **Hospital:** Duke Univ Hosp; **Address:** Robert Tisch Brain Tumor Ctr at Duke, Hanes House, rm 307, Box 102382, 315 Trent Drive, Durham, NC 27710; **Phone:** 919-668-6288; **Med School:** India 1958; **Resid:** Pediatrics, Le Bonheur Children's Med Ctr 1992; **Fellow:** Pediatric Hematology-Oncology, St Jude Children's Hosp 1993; Pediatric Hematology-Oncology, Meml Sloan Kettering Cancer Ctr 1996; **Fac Appt:** Prof Ped, Duke Univ

Hudson, Melissa M MD [PHO] - **Spec Exp:** Cancer Survivors-Late Effects of Therapy; Hodgkin's Lymphoma; **Hospital:** St. Jude Children's Research Hosp; **Address:** St Jude Children's Research Hosp, 262 Danny Thomas Pl, Memphis, TN 38105; **Phone:** 901-595-3445; **Board Cert:** Pediatrics 1988; Pediatric Hematology-Oncology 2006; **Med School:** Univ Tex SW, Dallas 1983; **Resid:** Pediatrics, Univ Texas Affil Hosps 1986; **Fellow:** Pediatric Hematology-Oncology, MD Anderson Cancer Ctr 1989

Johnston, J Martin MD [PHO] - **Spec Exp:** Leukemia; Lymphoma; Hemophilia; **Hospital:** Meml Hlth Univ Med Ctr - Savannah; **Address:** Backus Children's Hosp Outpatient Ctr, 4700 Waters Ave, PO Box 23089, Savannah, GA 31403-3089; **Phone:** 912-350-8194; **Board Cert:** Pediatric Hematology-Oncology 2009; **Med School:** Duke Univ 1984; **Resid:** Pediatrics, Univ Utah Med Ctr 1988; **Fellow:** Pediatric Hematology-Oncology, Barnes Jewish Hosp 1991; **Fac Appt:** Assoc Prof Ped, Mercer Univ Sch Med

Keller Jr, Frank G MD [PHO] - **Spec Exp:** Leukemia; Hodgkin's Lymphoma; **Hospital:** Chldns Hlthcare Atlanta @ Egleston; **Address:** Aflac Cancer Ctr at Egleston, 1405 Clifton Rd NE, Tower 1, 4th Fl, Atlanta, GA 30322; **Phone:** 404-785-1200; **Board Cert:** Pediatric Hematology-Oncology 2009; **Med School:** Univ NC Sch Med 1986; **Resid:** Pediatrics, Vanderbilt Univ Med Ctr 1990; **Fellow:** Pediatric Hematology-Oncology, Duke Univ Med Ctr 1993; **Fac Appt:** Assoc Prof Ped, Emory Univ

Kreissman, Susan G MD [PHO] - **Spec Exp:** Neuroblastoma; Clinical Trials; **Hospital:** Duke Univ Hosp; **Address:** Duke Univ Med Ctr, Box 102382, Durham, NC 27710; **Phone:** 919-684-3401; **Board Cert:** Pediatric Hematology-Oncology 2004; **Med School:** Mount Sinai Sch Med 1985; **Resid:** Pediatrics, Chldns Hosp 1988; **Fellow:** Pediatric Hematology-Oncology, Chldns Hosp/Dana Farber Cancer Inst 1991; **Fac Appt:** Clin Prof Ped, Duke Univ

Kurtzberg, Joanne MD [PHO] - **Spec Exp:** Stem Cell Transplant; Bone Marrow Transplant; **Hospital:** Duke Univ Hosp; **Address:** Duke Univ Med Ctr, Box 3350, Durham, NC 27705; **Phone:** 919-668-1102; **Board Cert:** Pediatrics 1982; Pediatric Hematology-Oncology 1982; **Med School:** NY Med Coll 1976; **Resid:** Pediatrics, Dartmouth Med Ctr 1977; Pediatrics, Upstate Med Ctr 1979; **Fellow:** Pediatric Hematology-Oncology, Upstate Med Ctr 1980; Pediatric Hematology-Oncology, Duke Med Ctr 1983; **Fac Appt:** Prof Ped, Duke Univ

Laver, Joseph H MD [PHO] - **Spec Exp:** Stem Cell Transplant; Lymphoma, Non-Hodgkin's; **Hospital:** St. Jude Children's Research Hosp; **Address:** St Jude's Chldns Rsch Hosp, rm C-7045E, 262 Danny Thomas Pl, Memphis, TN 38105-3678; **Phone:** 901-595-3532; **Board Cert:** Pediatrics 1985; Pediatric Hematology-Oncology 1987; **Med School:** Israel 1979; **Resid:** Pediatrics, Assaf Harofeh Med Ctr 1982; **Fellow:** Pediatric Hematology-Oncology, Meml Sloan Kettering 1985

Leung, Wing H MD/PhD [PHO] - **Spec Exp:** Bone Marrow & Stem Cell Transplant; **Hospital:** St. Jude Children's Research Hosp; **Address:** 262 Danny Thomas Pl, Memphis, TN 38105-3678; **Phone:** 901-495-3300; **Board Cert:** Pediatrics 2008; Pediatric Hematology-Oncology 2006; **Med School:** Hong Kong 1988; **Resid:** Pediatrics, Univ Hosp Downstate Med Ctr 1994; **Fellow:** Pediatric Hematology-Oncology, Johns Hopkins Hosp 1997; **Fac Appt:** Prof Hem & Onc, Univ Tenn Coll Med

McLean, Thomas W MD [PHO] - **Hospital:** Brenner Chldrn's Hosp, Wake Forest Baptist Med Ctr; **Address:** Medical Ctr Blvd, Winston-Salem, NC 27157; **Phone:** 336-716-4085; **Board Cert:** Pediatrics 2009; Pediatric Hematology-Oncology 2006; **Med School:** Med Univ SC 1990; **Resid:** Pediatrics, Chldns Hosp 1993; **Fellow:** Pediatric Hematology-Oncology, Great Ormons St Hosp for Sick Chldn 1994; Pediatric Hematology-Oncology, Dana Farber Chldns Hosp 1997; **Fac Appt:** Assoc Prof Ped, Wake Forest Univ

Moscow, Jeffrey A MD [PHO] - **Spec Exp:** Pediatric Cancers; **Hospital:** Univ of Kentucky Albert B. Chandler Hosp; **Address:** 725 Rose St, MDS Bldg, Ste 401, MS 0284, Lexington, KY 40536; **Phone:** 859-257-4554; **Board Cert:** Pediatrics 1988; Pediatric Hematology-Oncology 2007; **Med School:** Dartmouth Med Sch 1982; **Resid:** Pediatrics, Univ Texas SW Med Ctr 1985; **Fellow:** Pediatric Hematology-Oncology, Natl Cancer Inst 1989; **Fac Appt:** Prof Ped, Univ KY Coll Med

Neuberg, Ronnie W MD [PHO] - **Spec Exp:** Pediatric Cancers; Brain Tumors; Gene Therapy; Clinical Trials; **Hospital:** Palmetto Health Richland Mem Hosp, MUSC Chldns Hosp; **Address:** Childrens Ctr-Cancer & Blood Disorders, 7 Richland Medical Park Drive, Ste 7215, Columbia, SC 29203; **Phone:** 803-434-3533; **Board Cert:** Pediatrics 1982; Pediatric Hematology-Oncology 1982; **Med School:** SUNY Buffalo 1977; **Resid:** Pediatrics, Chldns Hosp 1980; **Fellow:** Pediatric Hematology-Oncology, SUNY Upstate Med Ctr 1982; **Fac Appt:** Assoc Clin Prof Ped, Univ SC Sch Med

Olson, Thomas A MD [PHO] - **Spec Exp:** Platelet Disorders; Germ Cell Tumors; Retinoblastoma; Sarcoma; **Hospital:** Chldns Hlthcare Atlanta @ Egleston; **Address:** Childrens at Egleston Aflac Cancer Ctr, 1405 Clifton Rd NE, Tower 1, 4th Fl, Atlanta, GA 30322; **Phone:** 404-785-1200; **Board Cert:** Pediatrics 1982; Pediatric Hematology-Oncology 1984; **Med School:** Loyola Univ-Stritch Sch Med 1978; **Resid:** Pediatrics, Walter Reed AMC 1981; **Fellow:** Pediatric Hematology-Oncology, Walter Reed AMC 1983; **Fac Appt:** Assoc Prof Ped, Emory Univ

Pediatric Hematology-Oncology

Pui, Ching-Hon MD [PHO] - **Spec Exp:** Leukemia; Lymphoma; **Hospital:** St. Jude Children's Research Hosp; **Address:** St Jude Chldns Rsch Hosp, 262 Danny Thomas Pl, Memphis, TN 38105; **Phone:** 901-595-3606; **Board Cert:** Pediatrics 1980; Pediatric Hematology-Oncology 1982; **Med School:** Taiwan 1976; **Resid:** Pediatrics, St Jude Chldns Rsch Hosp 1979; **Fellow:** Hematology & Oncology, St Jude Chldns Rsch Hosp 1981; **Fac Appt:** Prof Ped, Univ Tenn Coll Med

Ribeiro, Raul C MD [PHO] - **Spec Exp:** Leukemia & Lymphoma; **Hospital:** St. Jude Children's Research Hosp; **Address:** St Jude's Chldns Rsch Hosp, 262 Danny Thomas Pl, rm S-2012, MS 721, Memphis, TN 38105-3678; **Phone:** 901-595-3694; **Board Cert:** Pediatric Hematology-Oncology 2009; **Med School:** Brazil 1975; **Resid:** Pediatrics, Univ Parana Sch Med 1978; **Fellow:** Hematology & Oncology, St Jude's Chldns Rsch Hosp 1987; **Fac Appt:** Prof Ped, Univ Tenn Coll Med

Rosoff, Philip M MD [PHO] - **Spec Exp:** Cancer Survivors-Late Effects of Therapy; Down Syndrome; Leukemia; **Hospital:** Duke Univ Hosp; **Address:** Duke Univ Med Ctr, Box 102382, 330 Trent Drive, Durham, NC 27710-0001; **Phone:** 919-684-3401; **Board Cert:** Pediatrics 1984; Pediatric Hematology-Oncology 2009; **Med School:** Case West Res Univ 1978; **Resid:** Pediatrics, Chldns Hosp 1980; **Fellow:** Pediatric Hematology-Oncology, Chldns Hosp/Dana Farber Cancer Inst 1984; **Fac Appt:** Assoc Prof Ped, Duke Univ

Russo, Carolyn MD [PHO] - **Spec Exp:** Brain Tumors; Cancer Survivors-Late Effects of Therapy; Palliative Care; **Hospital:** Huntsville Hosp, The; **Address:** 910 Adams St, Ste 310, huntsville, AL 35801; **Phone:** 256-265-5833; **Board Cert:** Pediatric Hematology-Oncology 2005; **Med School:** UCLA 1984; **Resid:** Pediatrics, Harbor-UCLA Med Ctr 1987; **Fellow:** Pediatric Hematology-Oncology, Stanford Med Ctr 1990

Sandler, Eric MD [PHO] - **Spec Exp:** Bone Marrow Transplant; Leukemia; Bone Tumors; Sickle Cell Disease; **Hospital:** Wolfson Chldns Hosp; **Address:** 807 Childrens Way, Jacksonville, FL 32207; **Phone:** 904-697-3793; **Board Cert:** Pediatrics 2008; Pediatric Hematology-Oncology 2007; **Med School:** Univ VT Coll Med 1985; **Resid:** Pediatrics, UCSF Med Ctr 1988; **Fellow:** Pediatric Hematology-Oncology, Univ Fla Med Sch 1991; **Fac Appt:** Assoc Prof Ped, Mayo Med Sch

Sandlund Jr, John T MD [PHO] - **Spec Exp:** Lymphoma, Non-Hodgkin's; Leukemia & Lymphoma; Ataxia Telangiectasia; **Hospital:** St. Jude Children's Research Hosp, Le Bonheur Chldns Med Ctr; **Address:** St Jude Children's Research Hosp, 262 Danny Thomas Pl, MS 260, Memphis, TN 38105; **Phone:** 901-595-2153; **Board Cert:** Pediatrics 1986; Pediatric Hematology-Oncology 1987; **Med School:** Ohio State Univ 1980; **Resid:** Pediatrics, Columbus Chldns Hosp 1983; **Fellow:** Hematology, Natl Cancer Inst 1986; Research, Natl Cancer Inst 1987; **Fac Appt:** Prof Ped, Univ Tenn Coll Med

Santana, Victor M MD [PHO] - **Spec Exp:** Solid Tumors; Clinical Trials; Ethics; **Hospital:** St. Jude Children's Research Hosp; **Address:** St Jude Chldns Rsch Hosp, Dept Oncology, 262 Danny Thomas Pl, MS 274, Memphis, TN 38105-2794; **Phone:** 901-595-2801; **Board Cert:** Pediatrics 1982; Pediatric Hematology-Oncology 1984; **Med School:** Puerto Rico 1978; **Resid:** Pediatrics, Johns Hopkins Hosp 1981; **Fellow:** Pediatric Hematology-Oncology, Johns Hopkins Hosp 1984; **Fac Appt:** Prof Ped, Univ Tenn Coll Med

Tebbi, Cameron MD [PHO] - **Spec Exp:** Hemophilia; Hodgkin's Lymphoma; Leukemia; Sickle Cell Disease; **Hospital:** St. Josephs Chldns Hosp, Tampa Genl Hosp; **Address:** University of South Florida, 2 Tampa General Drive Fl 5, Tampa, FL 33607; **Phone:** 813-601-4400; **Board Cert:** Pediatrics 1974; Pediatric Hematology-Oncology 1980; **Med School:** Iran 1968; **Resid:** Pediatrics, Cincinnati Chldns Hosp 1972; Pediatric Hematology-Oncology, MD Anderson Cancer Inst 1972; **Fellow:** Pediatric Hematology-Oncology, St Louis Chldns Hosp 1973; Medical Oncology, Ontario Cancer Inst 1974

Wang, Winfred C MD [PHO] - **Spec Exp:** Sickle Cell Disease; Bone Marrow Failure Disorders; Anemia-Aplastic; **Hospital:** St. Jude Children's Research Hosp, Le Bonheur Chldns Med Ctr; **Address:** St Jude Chldn Rsch Hosp, 262 Danny Thomas Pl, MS 800, Memphis, TN 38105-2729; **Phone:** 901-595-2051; **Board Cert:** Pediatrics 1972; Pediatric Hematology-Oncology 1974; **Med School:** Univ Chicago-Pritzker Sch Med 1967; **Resid:** Pediatrics, Montefiore Med Ctr 1969; Pediatrics, Kauikeolani Chldns Hosp 1970; **Fellow:** Pediatric Hematology-Oncology, UCSF Med Ctr 1975; **Fac Appt:** Prof Ped, Univ Tenn Coll Med

Wechsler, Daniel S MD/PhD [PHO] - **Spec Exp:** Leukemia & Lymphoma; Neuroblastoma; **Hospital:** Duke Univ Hosp; **Address:** Duke Univ Med Ctr-Ped Hem/Onc, Box 102382, Durham, NC 27710; **Phone:** 919-684-3401; **Board Cert:** Pediatric Hematology-Oncology 2009; **Med School:** Canada 1987; **Resid:** Pediatrics, Johns Hopkins Hosp 1990; **Fellow:** Pediatric Hematology-Oncology, Johns Hopkins Hosp 1994; **Fac Appt:** Assoc Prof Ped, Duke Univ

Midwest

Arndt, Carola A MD [PHO] - **Spec Exp:** Sarcoma; Brain Tumors; Stem Cell Transplant; **Hospital:** Mayo Med Ctr & Clin - Rochester; **Address:** Mayo Clinic, Dept Pediatrics, 200 1st St SW, Rochester, MN 55905; **Phone:** 507-284-2652; **Board Cert:** Pediatrics 1982; Pediatric Hematology-Oncology 1987; **Med School:** Boston Univ 1978; **Resid:** Pediatrics, Naval Reg Med Ctr 1981; **Fellow:** Pediatric Hematology-Oncology, Natl Inst Hlth 1984

Beyer, Eric C MD/PhD [PHO] - **Spec Exp:** Pediatric Cancers; Bleeding/Coagulation Disorders; Anemia; **Hospital:** Univ of Chicago Med Ctr; **Address:** Univ Chicago Med Ctr, Dept Ped Hem/Onc, 900 E 57th St, MC KCBD-5, Chicago, IL 60637; **Phone:** 773-702-6808; **Board Cert:** Pediatrics 1987; **Med School:** UCSD 1982; **Resid:** Pediatrics, Chldns Hosp 1984; **Fellow:** Hematology & Oncology, Dana Farber Cancer Inst 1987; **Fac Appt:** Prof Ped, Univ Chicago-Pritzker Sch Med

Blum, Kristie MD [PHO] - **Spec Exp:** Lymphoma; Lymphoma, Non-Hodgkin's; Lymphomas-Rare; **Hospital:** Ohio St Univ Med Ctr; **Address:** B315 Starling-Loving Hall, 320 W 10th Ave, Columbus, OH 43210; **Phone:** 614-293-8508; **Board Cert:** Medical Oncology 2004; Hematology 2004; **Med School:** Univ Miami Sch Med 1997; **Resid:** Internal Medicine, Univ VA Hlth Sci Ctr 2000; **Fellow:** Hematology & Oncology, Vanderbilt Univ Med Ctr 2001; Hematology & Oncology, Wash Univ Affil Hosp 2003; **Fac Appt:** Asst Prof Med, Ohio State Univ

Boxer, Laurence Alan MD [PHO] - **Spec Exp:** Congenital Neutropenia-Severe; Anemias & Red Cell Disorders; Bone Marrow Failure Disorders; Anemia-Aplastic; **Hospital:** Univ of Michigan Hosp; **Address:** MPB Bldg, rm D3251, Box 5718, 1500 E Medical Center Drive, Ann Arbor, MI 48109-5718; **Phone:** 734-764-7126; **Board Cert:** Pediatrics 1971; Pediatric Hematology-Oncology 1974; **Med School:** Stanford Univ 1966; **Resid:** Pediatrics, Yale-New Haven Hosp 1968; Pediatrics, Stanford Univ Hosp 1969; **Fellow:** Hematology & Oncology, Chldns Hosp-Harvard 1974; **Fac Appt:** Prof Ped, Univ Mich Med Sch

Camitta, Bruce M MD [PHO] - **Spec Exp:** Leukemia; Anemia-Aplastic; Bone Marrow Transplant; **Hospital:** Chldns Hosp - Wisconsin; **Address:** MACC Fund Ctr for Cancer/Blood Disorders, 8701 Watertown Plank Rd, Ste 3018, Milwaukee, WI 53226; **Phone:** 414-266-2421; **Board Cert:** Pediatrics 1971; Pediatric Hematology-Oncology 1976; **Med School:** Johns Hopkins Univ 1966; **Resid:** Pediatrics, Chldns Hosp 1968; Pediatrics, Johns Hopkins Hosp 1969; **Fellow:** Pediatric Hematology-Oncology, Chldns Hosp 1973; **Fac Appt:** Prof Ped, Med Coll Wisc

Pediatric Hematology-Oncology

Castle, Valerie P MD [PHO] - **Spec Exp:** Neuroblastoma; Bleeding/Coagulation Disorders; Cancer Survivors-Late Effects of Therapy; **Hospital:** Univ of Michigan Hosp; **Address:** Univ Mich Comp Cancer Ctr, 1540 E Hospital Drive, Ste SPC 4259, Ann Arbor, MI 48109-0911; **Phone:** 734-936-9814; **Board Cert:** Pediatric Hematology-Oncology 2006; **Med School:** McMaster Univ 1983; **Resid:** Pediatrics, McMaster Univ Med Ctr 1986; **Fellow:** Pediatric Hematology-Oncology, Univ Mich Hosps 1989; **Fac Appt:** Prof Ped, Univ Mich Med Sch

Cohn, Susan L MD [PHO] - **Spec Exp:** Pediatric Cancers; Neuroblastoma; **Hospital:** Univ of Chicago Med Ctr; **Address:** 900 E 57th St, KCBM Bldg, rm 5100, Chicago, IL 60637; **Phone:** 773-702-6808; **Board Cert:** Pediatrics 1985; Pediatric Hematology-Oncology 1987; **Med School:** Univ IL Coll Med 1980; **Resid:** Pediatrics, Michael Reese Hosp 1984; **Fellow:** Hematology & Oncology, Chldns Meml Hosp 1987; **Fac Appt:** Prof Ped, Univ Chicago-Pritzker Sch Med

Corey, Seth J MD [PHO] - **Spec Exp:** Bone Marrow Failure Disorders; Leukemia; Myelodysplastic Syndromes; Ataxia Telangiectasia; **Hospital:** Lurie Chldn's Hosp-Chicago; **Address:** Robert Lurie Comp Cancer Ctr, 303 E Superior St, Chicago, IL 60611; **Phone:** 312-503-6694; **Board Cert:** Pediatrics 1986; Pediatric Hematology-Oncology 2004; **Med School:** Tulane Univ 1982; **Resid:** Pediatrics, St Louis Chldns Hosp 1985; **Fellow:** Hematology & Oncology, Tufts Univ 1992; Renal Pathology, Boston Chldns-Dana Farber Ctr 1989; **Fac Appt:** Prof Ped, Northwestern Univ-Feinberg Sch Med

Croop, James M MD/PhD [PHO] - **Spec Exp:** Solid Tumors; Clinical Trials; **Hospital:** Riley Hosp for Children; **Address:** Riley Hospital for Children, Pediatric Hematology/Oncology RI 4340, 705 Riley Hospital Drive, Indianapolis, IN 46202; **Phone:** 317-944-2143; **Board Cert:** Pediatrics 1985; Pediatric Hematology-Oncology 2010; **Med School:** Univ Pennsylvania 1980; **Resid:** Pediatrics, Chldns Hosp of Philadelphia 1983; **Fellow:** Pediatric Hematology-Oncology, Boston Chldns Hosp 1985; **Fac Appt:** Prof Ped, Indiana Univ

Cunningham, John M MD [PHO] - **Spec Exp:** Stem Cell Transplant; Sickle Cell Disease; Thalassemia; Clinical Trials; **Hospital:** Univ of Chicago Med Ctr; **Address:** Univ of Chicago Med Ctr, 5841 S Maryland Ave, MC 4060, Chicago, IL 60637; **Phone:** 773-702-2616; **Med School:** Ireland 1982; **Resid:** Pediatrics, St Laurence's Hosp 1985; Pediatrics, Mater Misericordiae Hosp 1987; **Fellow:** Pediatric Hematology-Oncology, Royal Free Hosp 1991; Transplant Surgery, Natl Heart, Lung, & Blood Inst/NIH 1993; **Fac Appt:** Prof Ped, Univ Chicago-Pritzker Sch Med

Davies, Stella M MD/PhD [PHO] - **Spec Exp:** Leukemia; Bone Marrow Transplant; Stem Cell Transplant; **Hospital:** Cincinnati Chldns Hosp Med Ctr; **Address:** Cincinnati Chldns Hosp Med Ctr, 3333 Burnet Ave, MLC 7015, Cincinnati, OH 45229-3039; **Phone:** 513-636-2469; **Med School:** England, UK 1981; **Resid:** Pediatrics, Univ Newcastle Med Ctr 1985; **Fellow:** Pediatric Hematology-Oncology, Univ Minn Med Ctr 1993; **Fac Appt:** Prof Ped, Univ Cincinnati

Fallon, Robert J MD/PhD [PHO] - **Spec Exp:** Lymphoma; Hodgkin's Lymphoma; Stem Cell Transplant; **Hospital:** Riley Hosp for Children; **Address:** Riley Hosp for Children, Hem/Onc, 705 Riley Hospital Drive, rm 4340, Indianapolis, IN 46202; **Phone:** 317-944-2143; **Board Cert:** Internal Medicine 1983; Medical Oncology 1985; **Med School:** NYU Sch Med 1980; **Resid:** Internal Medicine, Brigham & Womens Hosp 1983; **Fellow:** Hematology & Oncology, Brigham & Womens Hosp/Dana Farber Cancer Inst 1985; **Fac Appt:** Prof Ped, Indiana Univ

Ferrara, James MD [PHO] - **Spec Exp:** Bone Marrow Transplant; Graft vs Host Disease; Inflammatory Cytokines; **Hospital:** Univ of Michigan Hosp; **Address:** Univ Michigan Comprehensive Cancer Ctr, 1500 E Medical Center Drive, Ste 6308, Ann Arbor, MI 48109-5942; **Phone:** 734-615-1340; **Board Cert:** Pediatrics 2005; Pediatric Hematology-Oncology 2006; **Med School:** Georgetown Univ 1980; **Resid:** Pediatrics, Children's Hosp 1982; **Fellow:** Pediatric Hematology-Oncology, Children's Hosp 1985; **Fac Appt:** Prof Ped, Univ Mich Med Sch

Goldman, Stewart MD [PHO] - **Spec Exp:** Neuro-Oncology; Brain Tumors; Clinical Trials; **Hospital:** Lurie Chldn's Hosp-Chicago; **Address:** Childrens Meml Hosp, Div Hem/Onc, 2300 Childrens Plaza, Box 30, Chicago, IL 60614; **Phone:** 773-880-3004; **Board Cert:** Pediatric Hematology-Oncology 2011; **Med School:** Loyola Univ-Stritch Sch Med 1985; **Resid:** Pediatrics, Univ Chicago Hosps 1988; **Fellow:** Pediatric Hematology-Oncology, Univ Chicago Hosps 1991

Haut, Paul R MD [PHO] - **Spec Exp:** Stem Cell Transplant; Bone Marrow Transplant; Leukemia; **Hospital:** Riley Hosp for Children, IU Health North Hosp; **Address:** Riley Hospital for Children, 705 Riley Hospital Drive, RI Bldg, rm 1960, Indianapolis, IN 46202; **Phone:** 317-944-4093; **Board Cert:** Pediatric Hematology-Oncology 2008; **Med School:** Univ Ark 1990; **Resid:** Pediatrics, Arkansas Childrens Hosp 1994; **Fellow:** Pediatric Hematology-Oncology, Children's Meml Hosp 1997; **Fac Appt:** Assoc Prof Ped, Indiana Univ

Hayani, Ammar MD [PHO] - **Spec Exp:** Leukemia; Solid Tumors; Lymphoma; **Hospital:** Adv Christ Med Ctr, Adv Good Samaritan Hosp; **Address:** Hope Childrens Hosp, 4440 W 95th St, Oak Lawn, IL 60453-2600; **Phone:** 708-684-4094; **Board Cert:** Pediatric Hematology-Oncology 2011; **Med School:** Syria 1982; **Resid:** Pediatrics, LSU Hosp 1987; **Fellow:** Pediatric Hematology-Oncology, Baylor Affil Hosp 1991

Hayashi, Robert J MD [PHO] - **Spec Exp:** Bone Marrow Transplant; Cancer Survivors-Late Effects of Therapy; Leukemia; **Hospital:** St. Louis Chldns Hosp; **Address:** St Louis Chldns Hosp, Div Ped Hem Onc, One Children's Pl, Ste 9 South, Box 8116, St Louis, MO 63110; **Phone:** 314-454-6018; **Board Cert:** Pediatrics 2007; Pediatric Hematology-Oncology 2007; **Med School:** Washington Univ, St Louis 1986; **Resid:** Pediatrics, St Louis Childrens Hosp 1989; **Fellow:** Pediatric Hematology-Oncology, Johns Hopkins Hosp 1992; **Fac Appt:** Assoc Prof Ped, Washington Univ, St Louis

Hetherington, Maxine MD [PHO] - **Spec Exp:** Brain Tumors; **Hospital:** Chldns Mercy Hosps & Clinics; **Address:** Childrens Mercy Hosptial, 2401 Gillham Rd, Kansas City, MO 64108; **Phone:** 816-234-3265; **Board Cert:** Pediatrics 1983; Pediatric Hematology-Oncology 1987; **Med School:** Univ Tenn Coll Med 1978; **Resid:** Pediatrics, Childrens Med Ctr 1981; **Fellow:** Pediatric Hematology-Oncology, Univ Texas Hlth Sci Ctr 1987; **Fac Appt:** Assoc Prof Ped, Univ MO-Kansas City

Hord, Jeffrey D MD [PHO] - **Spec Exp:** Hematologic Malignancies; Bone Marrow Failure Disorders; Sickle Cell Disease; Pediatric Cancers; **Hospital:** Akron Children's Hosp; **Address:** Akron Childrens Hosp, Hematology/Oncology, One Perkins Square, Akron, OH 44308; **Phone:** 330-543-8580; **Board Cert:** Pediatric Hematology-Oncology 2004; **Med School:** Univ KY Coll Med 1989; **Resid:** Pediatrics, Childrens Hosp 1992; **Fellow:** Pediatric Hematology-Oncology, Vanderbilt Univ Med Ctr 1995; **Fac Appt:** Prof Ped, NE Ohio Univ

Hutchinson, Raymond MD [PHO] - **Spec Exp:** Leukemia; Hodgkin's Lymphoma; **Hospital:** Univ of Michigan Hosp; **Address:** CS Mott Chldns Hosp, Dept Hematology/Onc, 1540 E Hospital Drive, Ann Arbor, MI 48109-4259; **Phone:** 734-936-9814; **Board Cert:** Pediatrics 1979; Pediatric Hematology-Oncology 1980; **Med School:** Harvard Med Sch 1973; **Resid:** Pediatrics, New England Med Ctr 1975; **Fellow:** Pediatric Hematology-Oncology, Childrens Hosp 1978; **Fac Appt:** Prof Ped, Univ Mich Med Sch

Lusher, Jeanne M MD [PHO] - **Hospital:** Chldns Hosp of Michigan; **Address:** Children's Hospital Michigan, Div Hem/Onc, 3901 Beaubien Blvd Carls Bldg Fl 2, Detroit, MI 48201; **Phone:** 313-745-5515; **Board Cert:** Pediatrics 1986; Pediatric Hematology-Oncology 1986; **Med School:** Univ Cincinnati 1960; **Resid:** Pediatrics, Charity Hosp/Tulane Univ 1963; **Fellow:** Hematology & Oncology, Charity Hosp/Tulane Univ 1965; Hematology & Oncology, Saint Louis Children's Hosp 1966; **Fac Appt:** Prof Ped, Wayne State Univ

Pediatric Hematology-Oncology

Manera, Ricarchito B MD [PHO] - **Spec Exp:** Leukemia & Lymphoma; Brain Tumors; **Hospital:** Loyola Univ Med Ctr; **Address:** Loyola University Med Ctr, Div Pediatric Hematology/Oncology, 2160 S First Ave, Maywood, IL 60611; **Phone:** 708-327-9136; **Board Cert:** Pediatrics 2010; Pediatric Hematology-Oncology 2011; **Med School:** Philippines 1984; **Resid:** Pediatrics, Bronx-Lebanon Hosp Ctr 1995; **Fellow:** Pediatric Hematology-Oncology, MD Anderson Cancer Ctr 1994; Pediatric Hematology-Oncology, Columbia-Presby Med Ctr 1996; **Fac Appt:** Assoc Prof Ped, Loyola Univ-Stritch Sch Med

Morgan, Elaine MD [PHO] - **Spec Exp:** Leukemia; Palliative Care; Ethics; Hemophagocytic Syndrome; **Hospital:** Lurie Chldn's Hosp-Chicago; **Address:** Ann & Robert H. Lurie Chldn's Hosp, 225 E Chicago Ave, Box 30, Chicago, IL 60611; **Phone:** 312-227-4090; **Board Cert:** Pediatrics 1976; Pediatric Hematology-Oncology 2009; Hospice & Palliative Medicine 2008; **Med School:** Univ Pennsylvania 1971; **Resid:** Pediatrics, Chldns Hosp 1974; **Fellow:** Pediatric Hematology-Oncology, Chldns Hosp Med Ctr 1975; Pediatric Hematology-Oncology, Chldns Meml Med Ctr 1976; **Fac Appt:** Prof Ped, Northwestern Univ-Feinberg Sch Med

Neglia, Joseph MD [PHO] - **Spec Exp:** Cancer Survivors-Late Effects of Therapy; **Hospital:** Univ Minn Med Ctr, Fairview - Riverside Campus; **Address:** Univ Minnesota-Div Ped Hem/Oncology, 2450 Riverside Ave, Minneapolis, MN 55455; **Phone:** 612-624-3113; **Board Cert:** Pediatrics 1986; Pediatric Hematology-Oncology 1987; **Med School:** Loma Linda Univ 1981; **Resid:** Pediatrics, Baylor Coll Med 1984; **Fellow:** Pediatric Hematology-Oncology, Univ Minn Hosp 1987; **Fac Appt:** Prof Ped, Univ Minn

O'Dorisio, M Sue MD/PhD [PHO] - **Spec Exp:** Neuroblastoma; Medulloblastoma; Neuroendocrine Tumors; **Hospital:** Univ Iowa Hosp & Clinics; **Address:** Univ Iowa Hosp & Clin, Dept Ped Hem/Onc, 200 Hawkins Drive JCP Bldg - rm 2520, Iowa City, IA 52242; **Phone:** 319-356-7873; **Board Cert:** Pediatrics 2007; Pediatric Hematology-Oncology 2009; **Med School:** Ohio State Univ 1985; **Resid:** Pediatrics, Chldns Hosp 1988; **Fellow:** Pediatric Hematology-Oncology, Chldns Hosp 1992; **Fac Appt:** Prof Ped, Univ Iowa Coll Med

Olshefski, Randal S MD [PHO] - **Spec Exp:** Brain Tumors; **Hospital:** Nationwide Chldn's Hosp; **Address:** Nationwide Chldn's Hosp: Hemology/Onc, 700 Children's Drive, Columbus, OH 43205; **Phone:** 614-722-3552; **Board Cert:** Pediatric Hematology-Oncology 2004; **Med School:** Univ Pittsburgh 1988; **Resid:** Pediatrics, Nationwide Chldn's Hosp 1991; **Fellow:** Hematology & Oncology, Children's Natl Med Ctr 1995; **Fac Appt:** Clin Prof Ped, Ohio State Univ

Plautz, Gregory E MD [PHO] - **Spec Exp:** Brain Tumors; Leukemia & Lymphoma; Wilms' Tumor; Cancer Survivors-Late Effects of Therapy; **Hospital:** Cleveland Clin (page 55); **Address:** 9500 Euclid Ave, S Bldg - Fl 2, MS S20, Cleveland, OH 44195; **Phone:** 216-445-4044; **Board Cert:** Pediatric Hematology-Oncology 2005; **Med School:** Indiana Univ 1984; **Resid:** Pediatrics, Johns Hopkins Hosp 1987; **Fellow:** Pediatric Hematology-Oncology, Univ Michigan Affil Hosp 1990; **Fac Appt:** Prof Ped, Case West Res Univ

Puccetti, Diane M MD [PHO] - **Spec Exp:** Brain Tumors; Neuro-Oncology; Cancer Survivors-Late Effects of Therapy; **Hospital:** Univ WI Hosp & Clins; **Address:** Univ Wisconsin Childrens Hosp, 1675 Highland Ave Fl 2, Madison, WI 53792; **Phone:** 608-263-6420; **Board Cert:** Pediatric Hematology-Oncology 2007; **Med School:** Med Coll OH 1985; **Resid:** Pediatrics, UC-Irvine Med Ctr 1986; Pediatrics, Med Coll Ohio 1988; **Fellow:** Pediatric Hematology-Oncology, Riley Hosp Chldn 1991; **Fac Appt:** Assoc Clin Prof Ped, Univ Wisc

Razzouk, Bassem I MD [PHO] - **Spec Exp:** Leukemia; Clinical Trials; Lymphoma; Langerhans Cell Histiocytosis (LCH); **Hospital:** Peyton Manning Children's Hosp at St. Vincent; **Address:** Peyton Manning Chldns Hosp, Center for Cancer & Blood Diseases, 2001 W 86th St, Indianapolis, IN 46260; **Phone:** 317-338-4673; **Board Cert:** Pediatrics 2008; Pediatric Hematology-Oncology 2011; **Med School:** Lebanon 1987; **Resid:** Pediatrics, American Univ Med Ctr 1990; Pediatrics, SUNY Hlth Sci Ctr 1992; **Fellow:** Hematology & Oncology, St Jude Chldns Rsch Hosp 1995

Rubin, Charles M MD [PHO] - **Spec Exp:** Brain Tumors; Retinoblastoma; Bone Marrow Transplant; **Hospital:** Univ Chicago-Comer Chldn's Hosp; **Address:** Univ Chicago Med Ctr, 5841 S Maryland Ave, MC 4060, Chicago, IL 60637; **Phone:** 773-702-6808; **Board Cert:** Pediatrics 1984; Clinical Cytogenetics 1987; Pediatric Hematology-Oncology 1984; **Med School:** Tufts Univ 1979; **Resid:** Pediatrics, Chldn's Hosp 1982; Pediatric Hematology-Oncology, Univ Minnesota Hosp 1985; **Fellow:** Cytogenetics, Univ Chicago-Pritzker School of Med 1987; **Fac Appt:** Assoc Prof Ped, Univ Chicago-Pritzker Sch Med

Salvi, Sharad MD [PHO] - **Spec Exp:** Leukemia & Lymphoma; Bleeding/Coagulation Disorders; Anemia; Solid Tumors; **Hospital:** Adv Christ Med Ctr, Central DuPage Hosp; **Address:** Hope Chldns Hosp, 4440 W 95th St, Oak Lawn, IL 60453; **Phone:** 708-684-4094; **Board Cert:** Pediatrics 1982; Pediatric Hematology-Oncology 1982; **Med School:** India 1974; **Resid:** Pediatrics, Lincoln Meml Hosp 1979; **Fellow:** Pediatric Hematology-Oncology, Chldns Hosp/Roswell Park Meml Cancer Inst 1981

Sencer, Susan F MD [PHO] - **Spec Exp:** Pediatric Cancers; Complementary Medicine; **Hospital:** Children's Hosps & Clinics of Minneapolis; **Address:** Chldns Specialty Clinic, Hem/Onc Clin, 2525 Chicago Ave S, Ste CSC-175, Minneapolis, MN 55404; **Phone:** 612-813-5940; **Board Cert:** Pediatric Hematology-Oncology 2007; **Med School:** Univ Minn 1984; **Resid:** Pediatrics, Univ Minnesota Affil Hosp 1988; **Fellow:** Pediatric Hematology-Oncology, Univ Minnesota Affil Hosp 1991

Shapiro, Amy D MD [PHO] - **Spec Exp:** Hemophilia; Bleeding/Coagulation Disorders; **Hospital:** Peyton Manning Children's Hosp at St. Vincent; **Address:** Indiana Hemophilia & Thrombosis Ctr, 8402 Harcourt Rd, Ste 500, Indianapolis, IN 46260; **Phone:** 317-871-0000; **Board Cert:** Pediatrics 1986; Pediatric Hematology-Oncology 1987; **Med School:** NYU Sch Med 1980; **Resid:** Pediatrics, Univ Colo Affil Hosp 1982; **Fellow:** Pediatric Hematology-Oncology, Univ Colo Hlth Sci Ctr 1983

Sondel, Paul M MD/PhD [PHO] - **Spec Exp:** Immunotherapy; Stem Cell Transplant; Pediatric Cancers; Neuroblastoma; **Hospital:** Univ WI Hosp & Clins; **Address:** 4159 WIMR, 1111 Highland Ave, Madison, WI 53705; **Phone:** 608-263-6200; **Board Cert:** Pediatrics 1981; **Med School:** Harvard Med Sch 1977; **Resid:** Pediatrics, Univ MN Hosp 1978; Pediatrics, Univ Wisconsin Hosp 1980; **Fellow:** Research, Sidney Farber Cancer Inst/Harvard 1977; **Fac Appt:** Prof Ped, Univ Wisc

Valentino, Leonard Anthony MD [PHO] - **Spec Exp:** Bleeding/Coagulation Disorders; Thrombotic Disorders; Hemophilia; Hereditary Hemorrhagic Telangiectasia; **Hospital:** Rush Univ Med Ctr, Rush Copley Med Ctr; **Address:** 1725 W Harrison St, Ste 710, Chicago, IL 60612-3828; **Phone:** 312-942-5983; **Board Cert:** Pediatrics 2007; Pediatric Hematology-Oncology 2005; **Med School:** Creighton Univ 1984; **Resid:** Pediatrics, Univ Illinios Med Ctr 1987; **Fellow:** Pediatric Hematology-Oncology, UCLA Med Ctr 1990; **Fac Appt:** Prof Ped, Rush Med Coll

Vik, Terry A MD [PHO] - **Spec Exp:** Neuroblastoma; Cancer Survivors-Late Effects of Therapy; Leukemia; Drug Development; **Hospital:** Riley Hosp for Children; **Address:** Riley Hospital for Children, 705 Riley Hospital Drive, rm 4340, Indianapolis, IN 46202; **Phone:** 317-944-2143; **Board Cert:** Pediatrics 1987; Pediatric Hematology-Oncology 2004; **Med School:** Johns Hopkins Univ 1983; **Resid:** Pediatrics, UCLA Med Ctr 1986; **Fellow:** Pediatric Hematology-Oncology, Chldns Hosp/Dana Farber 1989; **Fac Appt:** Assoc Prof Ped, Indiana Univ

Pediatric Hematology-Oncology

Yaddanapudi, Ravindranath MD [PHO] - **Spec Exp:** Leukemia; **Hospital:** Chldns Hosp of Michigan; **Address:** Children's Hospital Michigan, Div Hem/Onc, 3901 Beaubien Blvd Carls Bldg Fl 2, Detroit, MI 48201; **Phone:** 313-745-5515; **Board Cert:** Pediatrics 1970; Pediatric Hematology-Oncology 1974; **Med School:** India 1964; **Resid:** Pathology, Western Penn Hosp 1967; Pediatrics, Children's Hosp 1969; **Fellow:** Pediatric Hematology-Oncology, Children's Hosp Michigan 1971; **Fac Appt:** Prof Ped, Wayne State Univ

Great Plains and Mountains

Abromowitch, Minnie MD [PHO] - **Hospital:** Children's Hosp - Omaha; **Address:** Children's Hosp & Med Ctr, Dept Pediatric Hem Onc, 8200 Dodge St, Omaha, NE 68114; **Phone:** 402-955-3950; **Board Cert:** Pediatrics 1980; Pediatric Hematology-Oncology 1982; **Med School:** Univ Manitoba 1973; **Resid:** Pediatrics, Hospital for Sick Children 1976; Pediatric Hematology-Oncology, Univ Manitoba 1978; **Fellow:** Pediatric Hematology-Oncology, St Jude Chldns Research Hosp 1980; **Fac Appt:** Assoc Prof Ped, Univ Nebr Coll Med

Bruggers, Carol S MD [PHO] - **Spec Exp:** Brain Tumors; Clinical Trials; **Hospital:** Primary Children's Med Ctr, Univ Utah Hlth Care; **Address:** Primary Children's Medical Ctr, 100 Mario Capecchi Drive, Salt Lake City, UT 84113; **Phone:** 801-662-4700; **Board Cert:** Pediatrics 2008; Pediatric Hematology-Oncology 2008; **Med School:** Mich State Univ 1984; **Resid:** Pediatrics, Univ Colorado Health Sci Ctr 1987; **Fellow:** Pediatric Hematology-Oncology, Duke Univ Med Ctr 1991; **Fac Appt:** Prof Ped, Univ Utah

Coccia, Peter F MD [PHO] - **Spec Exp:** Bone Marrow Transplant; Leukemia & Lymphoma; Bone Marrow Failure Disorders; Osteopetrosis; **Hospital:** Nebraska Med Ctr, Children's Hosp - Omaha; **Address:** Univ Nebr Med Ctr, Dept Pediatrics, 982168 Nebraska Med Ctr, Omaha, NE 68198-2168; **Phone:** 402-559-7257; **Board Cert:** Clinical Pathology 1972; Hematology 1975; Pediatrics 1976; Pediatric Hematology-Oncology 1976; **Med School:** SUNY Upstate Med Univ 1968; **Resid:** Pathology, Upstate Med Ctr 1970; Pediatrics, Univ Minn 1973; **Fellow:** Pediatric Hematology-Oncology, Univ Minn 1974; **Fac Appt:** Prof Ped, Univ Nebr Coll Med

Hilden, Joanne M MD [PHO] - **Spec Exp:** Leukemia in Infants; Brain Tumors; Leukemia & Lymphoma; Leukemia in Down Syndrome; **Hospital:** Chldn's Hosp - Aurora (CO); **Address:** 13123 E 16th St, MS B115, Aurora, CO 80045; **Phone:** 720-777-2843; **Board Cert:** Pediatrics 2006; Pediatric Hematology-Oncology 2009; Hospice & Palliative Medicine 2008; **Med School:** Univ Minn 1988; **Resid:** Pediatrics, Univ Minn Med Ctr 1991; **Fellow:** Pediatric Hematology-Oncology, Univ Minnesota 1994; **Fac Appt:** Assoc Prof Ped, Univ Colorado

Kobrinsky, Nathan L MD [PHO] - **Spec Exp:** Pediatric Cancers; Immunotherapy; Hemophilia; Bleeding/Coagulation Disorders; **Hospital:** Sanford Med Ctr Fargo; **Address:** Sanford Roger Maris Cancer Ctr, 820 4th St N, Fargo, ND 58122; **Phone:** 701-234-7544; **Board Cert:** Pediatrics 1981; Pediatric Hematology-Oncology 1982; **Med School:** Univ Manitoba 1976; **Resid:** Pediatrics, Chldns Hlth Sci Ctr 1978; **Fellow:** Pediatric Hematology-Oncology, Chldns Hlth Sci Ctr 1979; Pediatric Hematology-Oncology, Univ Minn 1981; **Fac Appt:** Prof Ped, Univ ND Sch Med

Manco-Johnson, Marilyn MD [PHO] - **Spec Exp:** Hemophilia; Thrombotic Disorders; **Hospital:** Chldn's Hosp - Aurora (CO), Univ of CO Hosp - Anschutz Inpatient Pav; **Address:** Univ Colorado Hemophilia Ctr, 13199 E Montview Blvd, Ste 100, MS F416, Aurora, CO 80045; **Phone:** 303-724-0365; **Board Cert:** Pediatrics 1979; Pediatric Hematology-Oncology 1980; **Med School:** Jefferson Med Coll 1974; **Resid:** Pediatrics, Univ Colorado Affil Hosps 1977; **Fellow:** Pediatric Hematology-Oncology, Chldns Hosp 1981; **Fac Appt:** Prof Ped, Univ Colorado

Southwest

Albritton, Karen H MD [PHO] - **Spec Exp:** Sarcoma; **Hospital:** Cook Chldns Med Ctr, Harris Methodist Hosp - Fort Worth; **Address:** 1500 Cooper St Fl 5, Fort Worth, TX 76104; **Phone:** 682-885-4007; **Board Cert:** Pediatric Hematology-Oncology 2002; **Med School:** Univ Tex, San Antonio 1992; **Resid:** Internal Medicine & Pediatrics, Univ NC Hosps 1996; **Fellow:** Hematology & Oncology, Univ NC Hosps 2000; Pediatric Hematology-Oncology, Univ NC Hosps 2000; **Fac Appt:** Assoc Prof Ped, Univ N Tex Hlth Sci Ctr, Coll Osteo Med

Berg, Stacey MD [PHO] - **Spec Exp:** Drug Discovery & Development; Brain Tumors; Solid Tumors; **Hospital:** Texas Chldns Hosp; **Address:** Texas Chldns Cancer Ctr, Dept Ped Hem-Onc, 6701 Fannin St, Ste CC 1400, Houston, TX 77030; **Phone:** 832-822-4242; **Board Cert:** Pediatrics 2007; Pediatric Hematology-Oncology 2007; **Med School:** Univ Pittsburgh 1985; **Resid:** Pediatrics, Chldns Hosp 1988; **Fellow:** Pediatric Hematology-Oncology, Natl Inst Hlth 1991; **Fac Appt:** Prof Ped, Baylor Coll Med

Blaney, Susan MD [PHO] - **Spec Exp:** Brain Tumors; Neuro-Oncology; Drug Development; Clinical Trials; **Hospital:** Texas Chldns Hosp; **Address:** 6701 Fannin St, Ste 1410.00, Houston, TX 77030; **Phone:** 832-822-1482; **Board Cert:** Pediatric Hematology-Oncology 2005; **Med School:** Med Coll OH 1984; **Resid:** Pediatrics, Letterman AMC 1987; **Fellow:** Pediatric Oncology, Walter Reed AMC 1990; **Fac Appt:** Prof Ped, Baylor Coll Med

Buchanan, George R MD [PHO] - **Spec Exp:** Sickle Cell Disease; Thrombotic Disorders; Hemophilia; Leukemia; **Hospital:** Chldns Med Ctr of Dallas; **Address:** Univ Texas SW Med Ctr, Peds Hem Onc, 5323 Harry Hines Blvd, MC 9063, Dallas, TX 75390-9063; **Phone:** 214-456-2382; **Board Cert:** Pediatrics 1975; Pediatric Hematology-Oncology 2000; **Med School:** Univ Chicago-Pritzker Sch Med 1970; **Resid:** Pediatrics, Chldns Meml Hosp 1973; **Fellow:** Hematology & Oncology, Chldns Meml Hosp 1975; **Fac Appt:** Prof Ped, Univ Tex SW, Dallas

Cooper, Laurence J N MD/PhD [PHO] - **Spec Exp:** Bone Marrow Transplant; **Hospital:** UT MD Anderson Cancer Ctr; **Address:** 1515 Holcombe Blvd, SCR 1.2028, Houston, TX 77030; **Phone:** 713-792-5410; **Med School:** Case West Res Univ 1994; **Resid:** Pediatrics, Seattle Chldn's Hosp 1996; **Fellow:** Pediatric Hematology-Oncology, Fred Hutchinson Cancer Rsch Ctr 1999; **Fac Appt:** Prof Ped, Univ Tex, Houston

Dreyer, ZoAnn E MD [PHO] - **Spec Exp:** Cancer Survivors-Late Effects of Therapy; Leukemia in Infants; **Hospital:** Texas Chldns Hosp; **Address:** Texas Childrens Hosp, Clinical Care Ctr, 6701 Fannin St Fl 14, MC CC1400, Houston, TX 77030; **Phone:** 832-822-4242; **Board Cert:** Pediatrics 1988; Pediatric Hematology-Oncology 2005; **Med School:** UC Davis 1982; **Resid:** Pediatrics, Baylor Affil Hosps 1985; **Fellow:** Pediatric Hematology-Oncology, Baylor Coll Med 1988; **Fac Appt:** Assoc Prof Ped, Baylor Coll Med

Goldman, Stanton C MD [PHO] - **Spec Exp:** Leukemia; Lymphoma; Stem Cell Transplant; **Hospital:** Med City Dallas Hosp; **Address:** 7777 Forest Ln D Bldg - Ste 400, Dallas, TX 75230; **Phone:** 972-566-6647; **Board Cert:** Pediatric Hematology-Oncology 2004; Pediatrics 2008; **Med School:** Boston Univ 1990; **Resid:** Pediatrics, Chldns Natl Med Ctr 1996; **Fellow:** Pediatric Hematology-Oncology, Johns Hopkins Hosp

Graham, Michael L MD [PHO] - **Spec Exp:** Bone Marrow Transplant; Leukemia; Stem Cell Transplant; **Hospital:** Cardon Children's Med Ctr; **Address:** Banner Hlth Clin-Heme/Onc Dept, 1432 S Dobson Rd, Ste 107, Mesa, AZ 85202; **Phone:** 480-412-4100; **Board Cert:** Pediatrics 1980; Pediatric Hematology-Oncology 1984; **Med School:** Brown Univ 1975; **Resid:** Pediatrics, Johns Hopkins Hosp 1978; Pediatric Hematology-Oncology, Johns Hopkins Hosp 1980; **Fellow:** Medical Oncology, Yale-New Haven Hosp 1982; **Fac Appt:** Assoc Prof Ped, Univ Ariz Coll Med

Pediatric Hematology-Oncology

Kane, Javier R MD [PHO] - **Spec Exp:** Palliative Care; Pediatric Cancers; **Hospital:** Scott & White Mem Hosp; **Address:** Temple Clinic, Pediatric Hematology/Oncology, 2401 S 31st St, Temple, TX 76508; **Phone:** 254-724-2006; **Board Cert:** Pediatrics 2007; Pediatric Hematology-Oncology 2012; Hospice & Palliative Medicine 2008; **Med School:** Mexico 1986; **Resid:** Pediatrics, Chldns Hosp 1992; **Fellow:** Pediatric Hematology-Oncology, St Judes Chldns Rsch Hosp 1995; **Fac Appt:** Prof Ped, Texas A&M Univ

Meyer, William H MD [PHO] - **Spec Exp:** Sarcoma; Pediatric Cancers; **Hospital:** Chldns Hosp OU Med Ctr; **Address:** 1200 Children's Ave, Fl 10, Ste 10000, Jimmy Everest Center for Cancer and Blood Disorders, Oklahoma City, OK 73104; **Phone:** 405-271-4412; **Board Cert:** Pediatrics 1980; Pediatric Hematology-Oncology 1980; **Med School:** Jefferson Med Coll 1974; **Resid:** Pediatrics, Wilmington Med Ctr 1977; **Fellow:** Pediatric Hematology-Oncology, Johns Hopkins Hosp 1980; **Fac Appt:** Prof Ped, Univ Okla Coll Med

Tomlinson, Gail E MD [PHO] - **Spec Exp:** Cancer Survivors-Late Effects of Therapy; Cancer Genetics; Liver Cancer; Kidney Cancer; **Hospital:** Christus Santa Rosa Children's Hosp, Univ Hlth Syst-San Antonio; **Address:** UT HSC at San Antonio, 7703 Floyd Curl Drive, MC 7810, San Antonio, TX 78229; **Phone:** 210-704-3405; **Board Cert:** Pediatrics 2008; Pediatric Hematology-Oncology 2009; **Med School:** Geo Wash Univ 1984; **Resid:** Pediatrics, Chldns Hosp Natl Med Ctr 1987; **Fellow:** Pediatric Hematology-Oncology, MD Anderson Cancer Ctr 1989; Pediatric Hematology-Oncology, Univ Texas SW Med Ctr 1992; **Fac Appt:** Prof Ped, Univ Tex, San Antonio

Williams, James A MD [PHO] - **Spec Exp:** Solid Tumors; **Hospital:** Phoenix Children's Hosp; **Address:** Phoenix Childrens Hosp, 5131 E Southern Ave, Mesa, AZ 85206; **Phone:** 602-546-0920; **Board Cert:** Pediatric Hematology-Oncology 2008; **Med School:** Wayne State Univ 1993; **Resid:** Pediatrics, Wayne St Univ Med Ctr 1996; **Fellow:** Pediatric Hematology-Oncology, Wayne St Univ Med Ctr 1999

Winick, Naomi J MD [PHO] - **Spec Exp:** Leukemia; **Hospital:** Chldns Med Ctr of Dallas; **Address:** Ctr for Cancer & Blood Disorders, 1935 Medical District Drive Fl 3, Dallas, TX 75235-7794; **Phone:** 214-456-2382; **Board Cert:** Pediatrics 1984; Pediatric Hematology-Oncology 1987; **Med School:** Northwestern Univ 1978; **Resid:** Pediatrics, Babies Hosp-Columbia Presbyterian Med Ctr 1981; **Fellow:** Pediatric Hematology-Oncology, Sloan-Kettering Cancer Ctr 1983; **Fac Appt:** Prof Ped, Univ Tex SW, Dallas

West Coast and Pacific

Andrews, Robert G MD [PHO] - **Spec Exp:** Bone Marrow Transplant; Leukemia; Lymphoma; **Hospital:** Seattle Chldns Hosp; **Address:** 1100 Fairview Ave N, MS D2-373, Seattle, WA 98109; **Phone:** 206-667-5000; **Board Cert:** Pediatrics 1984; Pediatric Hematology-Oncology 1984; **Med School:** Univ Minn 1976; **Resid:** Pediatrics, New England Med Ctr 1979; **Fellow:** Pediatric Hematology-Oncology, Children's Hosp Med Ctr 1983; **Fac Appt:** Assoc Prof Ped, Univ Wash

Banerjee, Anuradha MD [PHO] - **Spec Exp:** Brain Tumors; **Hospital:** UCSF Med Ctr; **Address:** UC San Francisco, Div Ped Oncology/Neuro Oncology, 400 Parnassus Ave, rm A101, San Francisco, CA 94107; **Phone:** 415-353-2986; **Board Cert:** Pediatrics 2011; Pediatric Hematology-Oncology 2012; **Med School:** Tulane Univ 1992; **Resid:** Pediatrics, UCSF Med Ctr 1996; **Fellow:** Pediatric Hematology-Oncology, UCSF Med Ctr 1997; **Fac Appt:** Assoc Clin Prof Ped, UCSF

Carpenter, Paul MD [PHO] - **Spec Exp:** Graft vs Host Disease; Bone Marrow Transplant; **Hospital:** Seattle Chldns Hosp; **Address:** Fred Hutchinson Cancer Rsch Ctr, FHCRC, Box 358080, MS D5-290, PO Box 19024, Seattle, WA 98109; **Phone:** 206-667-3786; **Med School:** Australia 1988; **Resid:** Pediatrics, Chldns Hosp 1992; **Fellow:** Pediatric Hematology-Oncology, Chldns Hosp 1994; Pediatric Hematology-Oncology, Univ Washington Med Ctr 1998

Ducore, Jonathan M MD [PHO] - **Spec Exp:** Brain Tumors; Bone & Soft Tissue Tumors; Bleeding/Coagulation Disorders; **Hospital:** UC Davis Med Ctr; **Address:** UC Davis Med Ctr, Dept Pediatrics, Div Pediatric Hematology/Oncology, 2521 Stockton Blvd, Ste 3200, Sacramento, CA 95817; **Phone:** 916-734-8336; **Board Cert:** Pediatrics 1978; Pediatric Hematology-Oncology 1978; **Med School:** Duke Univ 1973; **Resid:** Pediatrics, Chldns Med Ctr 1975; **Fellow:** Pediatric Hematology-Oncology, Univ Colorado Med Ctr 1977; Cancer Research, Natl Cancer Inst 1980; **Fac Appt:** Assoc Prof Ped, UC Davis

Finklestein, Jerry Z MD [PHO] - **Spec Exp:** Cancer Survivors-Late Effects of Therapy; Anemias & Red Cell Disorders; **Hospital:** Long Beach Meml Med Ctr, LAC - Harbor - UCLA Med Ctr; **Address:** 2653 Elm Ave, Ste 200, Long Beach, CA 90806-1652; **Phone:** 562-728-5000; **Board Cert:** Pediatrics 1980; Pediatric Hematology-Oncology 1974; **Med School:** McGill Univ 1963; **Resid:** Pediatrics, Montreal Chldns Hosp 1966; **Fellow:** Pediatric Hematology-Oncology, LA Chldns Hosp 1968; **Fac Appt:** Clin Prof Ped, UCLA

Finlay, Jonathan MD [PHO] - **Spec Exp:** Brain Tumors; **Hospital:** Chldns Hosp - Los Angeles, Chldns Hosp - Oakland; **Address:** 4650 Sunset Blvd, MS 54, Los Angeles, CA 90027-6016; **Phone:** 323-361-8147; **Board Cert:** Pediatrics 1984; Pediatric Hematology-Oncology 1987; **Med School:** England, UK 1973; **Resid:** Pediatrics, Univ Birmingham 1975; Pediatrics, Christie Hosp 1976; **Fellow:** Pediatric Allergy & Immunology, Univ Wisconsin Hosp 1978; Pediatric Hematology-Oncology, Univ Wisconsin Hosp 1980; **Fac Appt:** Prof Ped, USC-Keck School of Medicine

Geyer, J Russell MD [PHO] - **Spec Exp:** Pediatric Cancers; Neuro-Oncology; Brain Tumors; **Hospital:** Seattle Chldns Hosp, Univ Wash Med Ctr; **Address:** Seattle Chldns Hosp - Div Hem/Onc, 4800 Sand Point Way NE, MS B-6553, Seattle, WA 98105; **Phone:** 206-987-2106; **Board Cert:** Pediatrics 1983; Pediatric Hematology-Oncology 1987; **Med School:** Wayne State Univ 1977; **Resid:** Pediatrics, Chldns Hosp Michigan 1980; **Fellow:** Pediatric Hematology-Oncology, Univ Michigan Med Ctr 1981; **Fac Appt:** Prof Ped, Univ Wash

Glader, Bertil MD/PhD [PHO] - **Spec Exp:** Genetic Disorders-Blood; Hemophilia; **Hospital:** Lucile Packard Chldn's Hosp; **Address:** Pediatric Hematology/Oncology, 1000 Welch Rd, Ste 300, Box 5798, Palo Alto, CA 94304; **Phone:** 650-497-8953; **Board Cert:** Pediatrics 1982; Pediatric Hematology-Oncology 2005; Hematology 1983; **Med School:** Northwestern Univ 1968; **Resid:** Pediatrics, Chldns Hosp Med Ctr 1973; **Fellow:** Hematology, Chldns Hosp Med Ctr 1975; **Fac Appt:** Prof Ped, Stanford Univ

Hawkins, Douglas MD [PHO] - **Spec Exp:** Bone Tumors; Ewing's Sarcoma; Leukemia; Rhabdomyosarcoma; **Hospital:** Seattle Chldns Hosp; **Address:** 4800 Sand Point Way NE, MS B6553, Seattle, WA 98105; **Phone:** 206-987-2106; **Board Cert:** Pediatric Hematology-Oncology 2004; **Med School:** Harvard Med Sch 1990; **Resid:** Pediatrics, Univ Washington Med Ctr 1993; **Fellow:** Pediatric Hematology-Oncology, Fred Hutchinson Cancer Research Ctr 1996; **Fac Appt:** Assoc Prof Ped, Univ Wash

Horn, Biljana N MD [PHO] - **Spec Exp:** Bone Marrow Transplant; Brain Tumors; Stem Cell Transplant; Immunotherapy; **Hospital:** UCSF Med Ctr; **Address:** UCSF Med Ctr, Pediatric BMT Prgm, 505 Parnassus Ave, rm M-659, San Francisco, CA 94143; **Phone:** 415-476-2188; **Board Cert:** Pediatrics 2006; Pediatric Hematology-Oncology 2004; **Med School:** Croatia 1983; **Resid:** Pediatrics, Rainbow Babies & Chldns Hosp 1991; **Fellow:** Pediatric Hematology-Oncology, Natl Cancer Inst 1994; Pediatric Neuro-Oncology, UCSF Med Ctr 1998; **Fac Appt:** Assoc Prof Ped, UCSF

Kapoor, Neena MD [PHO] - **Spec Exp:** Bone Marrow Transplant; Immune Deficiency; **Hospital:** Chldns Hosp - Los Angeles; **Address:** Chlds Hosp LA-Rsch Immunology/BMT, 4650 Sunset Blvd, MS 62, Los Angeles, CA 90027; **Phone:** 323-361-2546; **Board Cert:** Pediatrics 1978; **Med School:** India 1972; **Resid:** Pediatrics, Rhode Island Hosp 1976; **Fellow:** Pediatric Hematology-Oncology, Meml Sloan-Kettering Cancer Ctr 1978; **Fac Appt:** Prof Ped, USC Sch Med

Pediatric Hematology-Oncology

Kung, Faith H MD [PHO] - **Spec Exp:** Leukemia & Lymphoma; Bleeding/Coagulation Disorders; Sickle Cell Disease; Hemophilia; **Hospital:** Rady Children's Hosp - San Diego; **Address:** UCSD Med Ctr, Div Ped Hem/Oncology, 200 W Arbor Drive, San Diego, CA 92103-8447; **Phone:** 858-246-0027; **Board Cert:** Pediatrics 1967; Pediatric Hematology-Oncology 1974; **Med School:** Univ VA Sch Med 1957; **Resid:** Pediatrics, NC Meml Hosp 1960; **Fellow:** Pediatric Hematology-Oncology, Chldns Hosp/Babies Hosp 1962; **Fac Appt:** Prof Ped, UCSD

Link, Michael P MD [PHO] - **Spec Exp:** Stem Cell Transplant; Pediatric Cancers; **Hospital:** Lucile Packard Chldn's Hosp, Stanford Univ Hosp & Clinics; **Address:** 1000 Welch Rd, Ste 300, Palo Alto, CA 94304; **Phone:** 650-723-5535; **Board Cert:** Pediatrics 1979; Pediatric Hematology-Oncology 1980; **Med School:** Stanford Univ 1974; **Resid:** Pediatrics, Chldns Hosp Med Ctr 1976; **Fellow:** Hematology & Oncology, Dana Farber Cancer Inst 1979; **Fac Appt:** Prof Ped, Stanford Univ

Marina, Neyssa MD [PHO] - **Spec Exp:** Sarcoma; Cancer Survivors-Late Effects of Therapy; Germ Cell Tumors; **Hospital:** Lucile Packard Chldn's Hosp; **Address:** Pediatric Hematology & Oncology, 725 Walsh Rd, Bass Ctr, rm 160, Palo Alto, CA 94304; **Phone:** 650-497-8953; **Board Cert:** Pediatrics 1987; Pediatric Hematology-Oncology 2005; **Med School:** Puerto Rico 1983; **Resid:** Pediatrics, Univ Pediatric Hosp 1986; **Fellow:** Pediatric Hematology-Oncology, St Jude Children's Hosp 1989; **Fac Appt:** Prof Ped, Stanford Univ

Matthay, Katherine K MD [PHO] - **Spec Exp:** Neuroblastoma; Bone Marrow & Stem Cell Transplant; **Hospital:** UCSF Med Ctr; **Address:** UCSF, Dept Ped Onc, 505 Parnassus Ave, Box 0106, San Francisco, CA 94143; **Phone:** 415-476-3831; **Board Cert:** Pediatrics 1979; Pediatric Hematology-Oncology 1980; **Med School:** Univ Pennsylvania 1973; **Resid:** Pediatrics, Univ Colorado 1976; **Fellow:** Pediatric Hematology-Oncology, UCSF 1979; **Fac Appt:** Prof Ped, UCSF

Nicholson, H Stacy MD [PHO] - **Spec Exp:** Brain Tumors; Cancer Survivors-Late Effects of Therapy; Histiocytoma; **Hospital:** Doernbecher Chldns Hosp/OHSU, OR Hlth & Sci Univ; **Address:** OR Hlth Scis Univ, 707 SW Gaines Rd, CDRCP, Portland, OR 97239; **Phone:** 503-494-4265; **Board Cert:** Pediatrics 2008; Pediatric Hematology-Oncology 2007; **Med School:** Med Coll GA 1985; **Resid:** Pediatrics, Chldns National Med Ctr 1988; **Fellow:** Pediatric Hematology-Oncology, Chldns National Med Ctr 1991; **Fac Appt:** Prof Ped, Oregon Hlth & Sci Univ

Olson, Janice MD [PHO] - **Spec Exp:** Hodgkin's Lymphoma; Neuro-Oncology; Bone Marrow Transplant; **Hospital:** Randall Chldns Hosp at Legacy; **Address:** Chldn's Cancer & Blood Disorders Program, Randall Chldns Hosp, 2801 N Ganenbein Ave Fl 3, Portland, OR 97227; **Phone:** 503-276-9300; **Board Cert:** Pediatrics 2005; Pediatric Hematology-Oncology 2009; **Med School:** Univ Utah 1985; **Resid:** Pediatrics, Baylor/TX Chldn's Hosp 1988; **Fellow:** Hematology & Oncology, Duke Univ Med Ctr 1992

Park, Julie MD [PHO] - **Spec Exp:** Pediatric Cancers; Neuroblastoma; Lymphoma, Non-Hodgkin's; **Hospital:** Seattle Chldns Hosp; **Address:** Seattle Chldn's-Hem/Onc Dept, 4800 Sandpoint Way NE, Box B6553, Seattle, WA 98105; **Phone:** 206-987-2106; **Board Cert:** Pediatric Hematology-Oncology 2004; **Med School:** Univ VT Coll Med 1988; **Resid:** Pediatrics, Univ Wash Affil Hosp 1991; **Fellow:** Pediatric Hematology-Oncology, Univ Wash/Fred Hutchinson Cancer Rsch Ctr 1994; Pediatric Hematology-Oncology, Leukemia Soc/Fred Hutchinson Cancer Rsch Ctr 1996; **Fac Appt:** Assoc Prof Ped, Univ Wash

Pendergrass, Thomas W MD [PHO] - **Spec Exp:** Pediatric Cancers; Hematologic Disorders; Retinoblastoma; **Hospital:** Seattle Chldns Hosp, Univ Wash Med Ctr; **Address:** Seattle Chldn's Hosp, 4800 Sandpoint Way NE, Box 5371, MS B6553, Seattle, WA 98105; **Phone:** 206-987-2106; **Board Cert:** Pediatrics 1978; **Med School:** Univ Tenn Coll Med 1971; **Resid:** Pediatrics, Children's Memorial Hosp 1973; **Fellow:** Pediatric Hematology-Oncology, Children's Hosp Med Ctr 1977; **Fac Appt:** Prof Ped, Univ Wash

Recht, Michael MD/PhD [PHO] - **Spec Exp:** Hemophilia; Bleeding/Coagulation Disorders; Hematologic Disorders; **Hospital:** Doernbecher Chldns Hosp/OHSU; **Address:** Peds Hem/Onc 10C, 3181 SW Sam Jackson Park Rd, MC CDRC, Portland, OR 97239; **Phone:** 503-494-8716; **Board Cert:** Pediatric Hematology-Oncology 2006; **Med School:** Univ Wisc 1992; **Resid:** Pediatrics, Yale/New Haven Hosp 1995; **Fellow:** Pediatric Hematology-Oncology, Yale/New Haven Hosp 1998

Rosenthal, Joseph MD [PHO] - **Spec Exp:** Bone Marrow Transplant; Clinical Trials; **Hospital:** Chldns Hosp Central CA; **Address:** City Of Hope National Medical Center, 1500 Duarte Rd, Duarte, CA 91010; **Phone:** 626-359-8111; **Board Cert:** Pediatrics 2003; Pediatric Hematology-Oncology 2004; **Med School:** Israel 1984; **Resid:** Pediatrics, Soroka Med Ctr 1988; Pediatrics, Chldn Hosp 1995; **Fellow:** Pediatric Hematology-Oncology, Univ Colorado Affil Hosp 1991; Pediatric Hematology-Oncology, Chldn Hosp 1994; **Fac Appt:** Assoc Prof Ped, USC-Keck School of Medicine

Sakamoto, Kathleen M MD/PhD [PHO] - **Spec Exp:** Leukemia; Pediatric Cancers; Bone Marrow Transplant; **Hospital:** Lucile Packard Chldn's Hosp; **Address:** 269 Campus Drive, 1215C CSSR Bldg, Stanford, CA 94305-5162; **Phone:** 650-725-7126; **Board Cert:** Pediatrics 2007; Pediatric Hematology-Oncology 2007; **Med School:** Univ Cincinnati 1985; **Resid:** Pediatrics, Chldn's Hosp 1988; **Fellow:** Pediatric Hematology-Oncology, Chldn's Hosp 1991; **Fac Appt:** Prof Hem & Onc, Stanford Univ

Siegel, Stuart E MD [PHO] - **Spec Exp:** Leukemia & Lymphoma; Infections in Cancer Patients; Psychosocial Support in Childhood Cancer; Solid Tumors; **Hospital:** Chldns Hosp - Los Angeles, Ventura Cnty Med Ctr; **Address:** Chldns Hosp, 4650 Sunset Blvd, MS 54, Los Angeles, CA 90027-6062; **Phone:** 323-361-2205; **Board Cert:** Pediatrics 1973; Pediatric Hematology-Oncology 1976; **Med School:** Boston Univ 1967; **Resid:** Pediatrics, Univ Minnesota Hosps 1969; **Fellow:** Pediatric Hematology-Oncology, Natl Cancer Inst 1972; **Fac Appt:** Prof Ped, USC-Keck School of Medicine

Thomas, Gregory A MD [PHO] - **Spec Exp:** Palliative Care; Anemias & Red Cell Disorders; Bleeding/Coagulation Disorders; **Hospital:** Doernbecher Chldns Hosp/OHSU; **Address:** 707 SW Gaines Rd, MC 1104-CDRCP, Portland, OR 97239; **Phone:** 503-346-0644; **Board Cert:** Pediatrics 1986; Pediatric Hematology-Oncology 2005; **Med School:** Oregon Hlth & Sci Univ 1981; **Resid:** Pediatrics, Univ Utah Med Ctr 1984; **Fellow:** Pediatric Hematology-Oncology, Univ Utah Med Ctr 1987; **Fac Appt:** Assoc Prof Ped, Oregon Hlth & Sci Univ

PEDIATRIC INFECTIOUS DISEASE

New England

Andiman, Warren A MD [PInf] - **Spec Exp:** AIDS/HIV; Viral Infections; Lyme Disease; Infectious Mononucleosis; **Hospital:** Yale-New Haven Hosp, Yale Med Group; **Address:** Yale Univ Sch Med, Dept Pediatrics, 333 Cedar St, Box 208064, New Haven, CT 06520-8064; **Phone:** 203-785-4730; **Board Cert:** Pediatrics 1975; **Med School:** Albert Einstein Coll Med 1969; **Resid:** Pediatrics, Babies Hosp-Columbia Presby 1971; **Fellow:** Pediatric Infectious Disease, Yale Un 1973; **Fac Appt:** Prof Ped, Yale Univ

Baltimore, Robert MD [PInf] - **Spec Exp:** Neonatal Infections; Hospital Acquired Infections; Tuberculosis; **Hospital:** Yale-New Haven Hosp, Yale Med Group; **Address:** Yale Univ Sch Med, Dept Pediatrics, 333 Cedar St, Box 208064, New Haven, CT 06520-8064; **Phone:** 203-785-4750; **Board Cert:** Pediatrics 1975; Pediatric Infectious Disease 2009; **Med School:** SUNY Buffalo 1968; **Resid:** Pediatrics, Univ Chicago Hosps 1971; **Fellow:** Infectious Disease, Boston City Hosp-Harvard 1976; **Fac Appt:** Prof Ped, Yale Univ

Pediatric Infectious Disease

Durbin Jr, William Applebee MD [PInf] - **Spec Exp:** AIDS/HIV; Lyme Disease; **Hospital:** UMass Memorial Med Ctr; **Address:** UMass Meml Med Ctr-Univ Campus, 55 Lake Ave N, Worcester, MA 01655; **Phone:** 774-442-3947; **Board Cert:** Pediatrics 1978; Pediatric Infectious Disease 2009; **Med School:** Columbia P&S 1972; **Resid:** Pediatrics, Boston Chldns Hosp 1977; **Fellow:** Infectious Disease, Boston Chldns Hosp/Beth Israel 1979; **Fac Appt:** Prof Ped, Univ Mass Sch Med

Meissner, H Cody MD [PInf] - **Spec Exp:** Infections-Respiratory; Kawasaki Disease; **Hospital:** Tufts Med Ctr; **Address:** Tufts Medical Center, 800 Washington St, Ste 321, Boston, MA 02111; **Phone:** 617-636-8100; **Board Cert:** Pediatrics 1981; Pediatric Infectious Disease 2009; **Med School:** Tufts Univ 1973; **Resid:** Pediatrics, New England Med Ctr 1975; Pediatrics, Natl Inst of Health 1977; **Fellow:** Infectious Disease, Chldns Hosp Med Ctr 1998; **Fac Appt:** Assoc Prof Ped, Tufts Univ

Raszka Jr, William V MD [PInf] - **Hospital:** Fletcher Allen Health Care- Med Ctr Campus; **Address:** Chldns Specialty Clin, Dept Ped Infect Disease, 111 Colchester Avenue, Burlington, VT 05401; **Phone:** 802-847-8200; **Board Cert:** Pediatrics 2008; Pediatric Infectious Disease 2009; **Med School:** Boston Univ 1985; **Resid:** Pediatrics, Tripler Army Med Ctr 1988; **Fellow:** Pediatric Infectious Disease, Uniformed Servs Hlth Ctr 1993; **Fac Appt:** Prof Ped, Univ VT Coll Med

Shapiro, Eugene D MD [PInf] - **Spec Exp:** Lyme Disease; Vaccines; **Hospital:** Yale-New Haven Hosp, Yale Med Group; **Address:** Yale Univ Sch Med, Dept Pediatrics, 333 Cedar St, Box 208064, New Haven, CT 06520-8064; **Phone:** 203-688-4518; **Board Cert:** Pediatrics 1980; Pediatric Infectious Disease 2009; **Med School:** UCSF 1976; **Resid:** Pediatrics, Chldns Hosp 1979; **Fellow:** Pediatric Infectious Disease, Chldns Hosp 1981; Research, Yale Univ 1983; **Fac Appt:** Prof Ped, Yale Univ

Mid Atlantic

Bell, Louis MD [PInf] - **Hospital:** Chldns Hosp of Philadelphia; **Address:** Children's Hospital of Philadelphia, 34th and Civic Center Blvd, Philadelphia, PA 19104; **Phone:** 215-590-2195; **Board Cert:** Pediatrics 1985; Pediatric Infectious Disease 2007; **Med School:** Univ MD Sch Med 1980; **Resid:** Pediatrics, Hahnemann Univ Med Ctr 1983; **Fellow:** Pediatric Infectious Disease, Chldns Hosp 1985; **Fac Appt:** Prof Ped, Univ Pennsylvania

Green, Michael D MD [PInf] - **Spec Exp:** Infections-Transplant; **Hospital:** Chldns Hosp of Pittsburgh - UPMC; **Address:** Chldns Hosp Pittsburgh, 4401 Penn Ave Fl 3, Pittsburgh, PA 15224; **Phone:** 412-692-7885; **Board Cert:** Pediatrics 1987; Pediatric Infectious Disease 2009; **Med School:** Univ IL Coll Med 1983; **Resid:** Pediatrics, Children's Hosp 1986; **Fellow:** Pediatric Infectious Disease, Children's Hosp 1989; **Fac Appt:** Assoc Prof Ped, Univ Pittsburgh

Kotloff, Karen MD [PInf] - **Spec Exp:** Diarrheal Diseases; Infectious Disease; Sexually Transmitted Diseases; **Hospital:** Univ of MD Med Ctr; **Address:** Ctr for Vaccine Development, 685 W Baltimore St HSF Bldg - Ste 480, Baltimore, MD 21201; **Phone:** 410-706-5328; **Board Cert:** Pediatrics 1985; Pediatric Infectious Disease 2002; **Med School:** Temple Univ 1979; **Resid:** Pediatrics, Chldn's Hosp 1983; **Fellow:** Pediatric Infectious Disease, Univ Maryland Med Ctr 1986; **Fac Appt:** Prof Ped, Univ MD Sch Med

Krilov, Leonard MD [PInf] - **Spec Exp:** Infections-Respiratory; Infections in Int'l Adopted Children; Chronic Fatigue Syndrome; Lyme Disease; **Hospital:** Winthrop Univ Hosp; **Address:** 120 Mineola Blvd, Ste 210, Mineola, NY 11501; **Phone:** 516-663-4600; **Board Cert:** Pediatrics 1983; Pediatric Infectious Disease 2009; **Med School:** Columbia P&S 1978; **Resid:** Pediatrics, Johns Hopkins Hosp 1981; **Fellow:** Pediatric Infectious Disease, Children's Hosp 1984; **Fac Appt:** Prof Ped, SUNY Stony Brook

Long, Sarah S MD [PInf] - **Spec Exp:** Whooping Cough; Vaccines; Antibiotic Resistance; **Hospital:** St. Christopher's Hosp for Chldn; **Address:** St Christopher's Hosp for Children, 3601 A St, Ste 1112, Philadelphia, PA 19134; **Phone:** 215-427-5201; **Board Cert:** Pediatrics 2002; Pediatric Infectious Disease 2009; **Med School:** Jefferson Med Coll 1970; **Resid:** Pediatrics, St Christophers Hosp Chldn 1973; **Fellow:** Pediatric Infectious Disease, Temple Univ Sch Med 1975; **Fac Appt:** Prof Ped, Drexel Univ Coll Med

Michaels, Marian G MD [PInf] - **Spec Exp:** Infections in Immunocompromised Patients; Infectious Disease-Perinatal; AIDS/HIV; **Hospital:** Chldns Hosp of Pittsburgh - UPMC, Magee-Womens Hosp - UPMC; **Address:** Children's Hosp Pittsburgh, 4401 Penn Ave, AOB Bldg, Ste 3300, Pittsburgh, PA 15224; **Phone:** 412-864-8977; **Board Cert:** Pediatric Infectious Disease 2009; **Med School:** Univ Pennsylvania 1985; **Resid:** Pediatrics, Children's Hosp 1988; Pediatrics, Hosp for Sick Children 1989; **Fellow:** Pediatric Infectious Disease, Univ Pittsburgh 1992; **Fac Appt:** Prof Ped, Univ Pittsburgh

Offit, Paul A MD [PInf] - **Spec Exp:** Vaccines; **Hospital:** Chldns Hosp of Philadelphia; **Address:** Children's Hospital of Philadelphia, Abramson Bldg, 34th St & Civic Center Blvd, Ste 1202D, Philadelphia, PA 19104; **Phone:** 215-590-2017; **Board Cert:** Pediatrics 1982; **Med School:** Univ MD Sch Med 1977; **Resid:** Pediatrics, Children's Hosp 1980; **Fac Appt:** Prof Ped, Univ Pennsylvania

Saiman, Lisa MD [PInf] - **Spec Exp:** Cystic Fibrosis Infection; Fungal Infections; Tick-borne Diseases; Tuberculosis; **Hospital:** Morgan Stanley Children's Hosp of NY-Presby, NY; **Address:** 3959 Broadway, rm 106, New York, NY 10032; **Phone:** 212-305-4558; **Board Cert:** Pediatrics 1987; Pediatric Infectious Disease 2009; **Med School:** Albert Einstein Coll Med 1983; **Resid:** Pediatrics, Babies Hosp/NY Presby 1986; **Fellow:** Infectious Disease, Babies Hosp/NY Presby 1989; **Fac Appt:** Assoc Clin Prof Ped, Columbia P&S

Singh, Nalini MD [PInf] - **Hospital:** Chldns Natl Med Ctr; **Address:** Div Infectious Disease, 111 Michigan Ave NW, Ste 3100, Washington, DC 20010; **Phone:** 202-476-5051; **Board Cert:** Pediatrics 1982; Pediatric Infectious Disease 2005; **Med School:** India 1973; **Resid:** Pediatrics, Univ Mass Med Ctr 1979; **Fellow:** Infectious Disease, Natl Inst Hlth 1981; **Fac Appt:** Assoc Prof Ped, Geo Wash Univ

Southeast

Edwards, Kathryn M MD [PInf] - **Spec Exp:** Vaccines; Clinical Trials; **Hospital:** Vanderbilt Univ Med Ctr (page 75); **Address:** Vanderbilt Div Infectious Diseases, 1161 21st Ave S, CCC-5311, Med Ctr North, Nashville, TN 37232; **Phone:** 615-322-2250; **Board Cert:** Pediatrics 1978; Pediatric Infectious Disease 2005; **Med School:** Univ Iowa Coll Med 1973; **Resid:** Pediatrics, Chldns Meml Hosp 1976; **Fellow:** Pediatric Infectious Disease, Chldns Meml Hosp 1980; **Fac Appt:** Prof Ped, Vanderbilt Univ

Emmanuel, Patricia MD [PInf] - **Spec Exp:** Infections in Immunocompromised Patients; AIDS/HIV; Congenital Infections; **Hospital:** Tampa Genl Hosp, All Children's Hosp; **Address:** 17 Davis Blvd, Ste 200, Tampa, FL 33604; **Phone:** 813-259-8800; **Board Cert:** Pediatrics 2005; Pediatric Infectious Disease 2009; **Med School:** Univ Fla Coll Med 1986; **Resid:** Pediatrics, Univ S Florida Affil Hosp 1989; **Fellow:** Infectious Disease, Univ S Florida Affil Hosp 1993; **Fac Appt:** Assoc Prof Ped, Univ S Fla Coll Med

Pediatric Infectious Disease

Flynn, Patricia M MD [PInf] - **Spec Exp:** AIDS/HIV; Infections in Immunocompromised Patients; Clinical Trials; **Hospital:** St. Jude Children's Research Hosp, Le Bonheur Chldns Med Ctr; **Address:** 262 Danny Thomas Pl, MS 600, Memphis, TN 38105; **Phone:** 901-595-2338; **Board Cert:** Pediatrics 1986; Pediatric Infectious Disease 2009; **Med School:** Louisiana State U, New Orleans 1981; **Resid:** Pediatrics, LeBonheur Chldns Med Ctr 1984; **Fellow:** Pediatric Infectious Disease, St Jude Chldns Rsch Hosp 1987; **Fac Appt:** Prof Ped, Univ Tenn Coll Med

Givner, Laurence B MD [PInf] - **Spec Exp:** Streptococcal Infections; Rocky Mountain Spotted Fever; **Hospital:** Brenner Chldrn's Hosp, Wake Forest Baptist Med Ctr; **Address:** Medical Ctr Blvd, Winston-Salem, NC 27157-0001; **Phone:** 336-716-6568; **Board Cert:** Pediatrics 1984; Pediatric Infectious Disease 2009; **Med School:** Univ MD Sch Med 1978; **Resid:** Pediatrics, Univ Maryland Affil Hosp 1982; **Fellow:** Infectious Disease, Baylor Coll Med 1984; **Fac Appt:** Prof Ped, Wake Forest Univ

Ingram, David L MD [PInf] - **Hospital:** WakeMed-Raleigh Campus; **Address:** WakeMed Faculty Physicians, Pediatrics, 3024 New Bern Ave, Ste 307, Raleigh, NC 27610; **Phone:** 919-350-8009; **Board Cert:** Pediatrics 1980; Pediatric Infectious Disease 2009; **Med School:** Yale Univ 1967; **Resid:** Pediatrics, Yale-New Haven Hosp 1971; **Fellow:** Pediatric Infectious Disease, Chldns Hosp Med Ctr 1973; **Fac Appt:** Prof Ped, Univ NC Sch Med

McKinney Jr, Ross E MD [PInf] - **Spec Exp:** Infections in Immunocompromised Patients; Fevers of Unknown Origin; AIDS/HIV; **Hospital:** Duke Univ Hosp; **Address:** Duke Univ Med Ctr, Box 3461, Durham, NC 27710; **Phone:** 919-668-9000; **Board Cert:** Pediatrics 1983; Pediatric Infectious Disease 2009; **Med School:** Univ Rochester 1979; **Resid:** Pediatrics, Duke Univ Med Ctr 1982; **Fellow:** Pediatric Infectious Disease, Duke Univ Med Ctr 1985; **Fac Appt:** Prof Ped, Duke Univ

Mitchell, Charles D MD [PInf] - **Spec Exp:** AIDS/HIV; Viral Infections; **Hospital:** Jackson Meml Hosp; **Address:** Univ Miami Div Ped Inf Disease, PO Box 016960 (D4-4), Miami, FL 33101; **Phone:** 305-243-2700; **Board Cert:** Pediatrics 1986; Pediatric Infectious Disease 2009; **Med School:** Univ Tex Med Br, Galveston 1977; **Resid:** Pediatrics, Univ Minn Hosp 1981; **Fellow:** Pediatric Infectious Disease, Univ Minn Hosp 1984; **Fac Appt:** Clin Prof Ped, Univ Miami Sch Med

Scott, Gwendolyn B MD [PInf] - **Spec Exp:** AIDS/HIV; **Hospital:** Jackson Meml Hosp, Univ of Miami Hosp & Clins/Sylvester Comp Canc Ctr; **Address:** Univ Miami Div Ped Inf Disease, 1580 NW 10th Ave, rm BCRI 286 (D4-4), Miami, FL 33136; **Phone:** 305-243-6522; **Board Cert:** Pediatrics 1978; Pediatric Infectious Disease 2009; **Med School:** UCSF 1972; **Resid:** Pediatrics, San Francisco Genl Hosp 1973; Pediatrics, Univ Maryland Hosp 1975; **Fellow:** Pediatric Infectious Disease, Univ Miami Hosp 1978; **Fac Appt:** Prof Ped, Univ Miami Sch Med

Midwest

Alexander, Kenneth MD/PhD [PInf] - **Spec Exp:** HPV-Human Papilloma Virus; Infections in Immunocompromised Patients; Fevers of Unknown Origin; Antibiotic Resistance; **Hospital:** Univ of Chicago Med Ctr; **Address:** The Univ of Chicago Medicine, 5841 S Maryland Ave, MC 3055, Chicago, IL 60637; **Phone:** 773-702-6169; **Board Cert:** Pediatric Infectious Disease 2005; **Med School:** Univ Wash 1989; **Resid:** Pediatrics, Chldn's Hosp 1992; **Fellow:** Pediatric Infectious Disease, Duke Univ Hosp 1995; **Fac Appt:** Assoc Prof Ped, Univ Chicago-Pritzker Sch Med

Belcher, Christopher E MD [PInf] - **Spec Exp:** Travel Medicine; Drug-Resistant Infections; Histoplasmosis; Fungal Infections; **Hospital:** Peyton Manning Children's Hosp at St. Vincent, St. Vincent Carmel Hosp; **Address:** Infectious Disease of Indiana, 11455 N Meridian St, Ste 200, Carmel, IN 46032; **Phone:** 317-582-8180; **Board Cert:** Pediatrics 2006; Pediatric Infectious Disease 2009; **Med School:** UCSD 1994; **Resid:** Pediatrics, Stanford Univ Hosp 1997; **Fellow:** Pediatric Infectious Disease, Barnes Jewish Hosp 1998; Pediatric Infectious Disease, Stanford Univ Med Ctr 2000

Bernstein, David I MD [PInf] - **Spec Exp:** Vaccines; Viral Infections; **Hospital:** Cincinnati Chldns Hosp Med Ctr; **Address:** Cincinnatti Children's Hosp, Dept Infectious Diseases, 3333 Burnet Ave, Cincinnati, OH 45229-3039; **Phone:** 513-636-7625; **Board Cert:** Pediatrics 1982; **Med School:** SUNY Buffalo 1977; **Resid:** Pediatrics, Tufts-New Englan Med Ctr 1981; **Fellow:** Infectious Disease, UCLA Med Ctr 1981; **Fac Appt:** Prof Ped, Univ Cincinnati

Christenson, John C MD [PInf] - **Spec Exp:** Travel Medicine; Lyme Disease; Viral Infections; Histoplasmosis; **Hospital:** Riley Hosp for Children; **Address:** Riley Hosp for Chldn, Div Infectious Disease, 705 Riley Hosp Drive, ROC 4380, Indianapolis, IN 46202; **Phone:** 317-944-7260; **Board Cert:** Pediatrics 1986; Pediatric Infectious Disease 2009; **Med School:** Univ Puerto Rico 1981; **Resid:** Pediatrics, Univ Pediatric Hosp 1984; **Fellow:** Pediatric Infectious Disease, Okla Chldns Meml Hosp 1987; **Fac Appt:** Clin Prof Ped, Indiana Univ

Kleiman, Martin B MD [PInf] - **Spec Exp:** Histoplasmosis; Blastomycosis; Meningitis; AIDS/HIV; **Hospital:** Riley Hosp for Children; **Address:** Riley Hosp for Chldn, 705 Riley Hosp Drive, ROC 4380, Indianapolis, IN 46202; **Phone:** 317-944-7260; **Board Cert:** Pediatrics 1973; Pediatric Infectious Disease 2009; **Med School:** SUNY Upstate Med Univ 1968; **Resid:** Pediatrics, Upstate Med Ctr 1971; **Fellow:** Infectious Disease, Johns Hopkins Hosp 1976; **Fac Appt:** Prof Emeritus Ped, Indiana Univ

Leonard, Ethan G MD [PInf] - **Hospital:** UH Rainbow Babies & Chldns Hosp (page 74); **Address:** UH Rainbow Babies & Children's Hospital, Pediatric Infectious Disease, 11100 Euclid Ave, MS 6008B, Cleveland, OH 44106; **Phone:** 216-844-3645; **Board Cert:** Pediatrics 2007; Pediatric Infectious Disease 2011; **Med School:** Case West Res Univ 1996; **Resid:** Pediatrics, Univ Hosps 2000; **Fellow:** Pediatric Infectious Disease, Univ Hosps 2003; **Fac Appt:** Assoc Prof Ped, Case West Res Univ

McComsey, Grace A MD [PInf] - **Spec Exp:** AIDS/HIV; Infections in Immunocompromised Patients; **Hospital:** UH Rainbow Babies & Chldns Hosp (page 74); **Address:** 11100 Euclid Ave, Pediatric Infectious Disease, Cleveland, OH 44106; **Phone:** 216-844-3607; **Board Cert:** Internal Medicine 2005; Pediatric Infectious Disease 2005; Infectious Disease 2007; **Med School:** Lebanon 1989; **Resid:** Internal Medicine & Pediatrics, Metrohealth Med Ctr 1994; **Fellow:** Infectious Disease, Univ Hosps 1997; **Fac Appt:** Prof Med, Case West Res Univ

Shulman, Stanford MD [PInf] - **Spec Exp:** Kawasaki Disease; Streptococcal Infections; **Hospital:** Lurie Chldn's Hosp-Chicago, Northwestern Meml Hosp; **Address:** 225 E Chicago Ave, Box 20, Chicago, IL 60614-3318; **Phone:** 773-880-4187; **Board Cert:** Pediatrics 1972; Pediatric Infectious Disease 2010; **Med School:** Univ Chicago-Pritzker Sch Med 1967; **Resid:** Pediatrics, Univ Chicago Hosps 1970; **Fellow:** Infectious Disease, Shands Hosp 1973; **Fac Appt:** Prof Ped, Northwestern Univ

Wald, Ellen Rashkow MD [PInf] - **Spec Exp:** Urinary Tract Infections; Infections-Respiratory; Meningitis; Ear Infections; **Hospital:** Univ WI Hosp & Clins; **Address:** American Family Childrens Hosp, Dept Pediatrics, Box 4108, 600 Highland Ave, Madison, WI 57392; **Phone:** 608-263-8558; **Board Cert:** Pediatrics 1973; Pediatric Infectious Disease 2009; **Med School:** SUNY Downstate 1968; **Resid:** Pediatrics, Kings Co Hosp 1971; **Fellow:** Infectious Disease, Univ Maryland Hosp 1973; **Fac Appt:** Prof Ped, Univ Wisc

Pediatric Infectious Disease

Southwest

Baker, Carol J MD [PInf] - **Spec Exp:** Streptococcal Infections; Neonatal Infections; Vaccines; **Hospital:** Texas Chldns Hosp; **Address:** 1102 Bates St, Feigin Ctr Fl 11 - Ste 1120, Houston, TX 77030; **Phone:** 832-824-1780; **Board Cert:** Pediatrics 1973; Pediatric Infectious Disease 2009; **Med School:** Baylor Coll Med 1968; **Resid:** Pediatrics, Baylor Affil Hosp 1971; **Fellow:** Pediatric Infectious Disease, Baylor Coll Med 1973; Infectious Disease, Boston City Hosp/Harvard 1974; **Fac Appt:** Prof Ped, Baylor Coll Med

Demmler-Harrison, Gail J MD [PInf] - **Spec Exp:** Viral Infections; Vaccines; **Hospital:** Texas Chldns Hosp; **Address:** 6701 Fannin St Fl 16, MC 3-2371, Houston, TX 77030; **Phone:** 832-824-4330; **Board Cert:** Pediatrics 1981; Pediatric Infectious Disease 2009; **Med School:** Texas Tech Univ 1977; **Resid:** Pediatrics, Baylor Univ Med Ctr 1980; **Fellow:** Pediatric Infectious Disease, Baylor Univ Med Ctr 1984; Virology, NY-Presby/Columbia Univ Med Ctr 1987; **Fac Appt:** Prof Ped, Baylor Coll Med

Jacobs, Richard F MD [PInf] - **Spec Exp:** Viral Infections; Drug Discovery & Development; Neonatal Infections; **Hospital:** Arkansas Chldns Hosp, UAMS Med Ctr; **Address:** 1 Childrens Way, Slot 512-11, Little Rock, AR 72202-3591; **Phone:** 501-364-1416; **Board Cert:** Pediatrics 1982; Pediatric Infectious Disease 2009; **Med School:** Univ Ark 1977; **Resid:** Pediatrics, Ark Chldns Hosp 1980; **Fellow:** Infectious Disease, Univ Washington 1982; **Fac Appt:** Prof Ped, Univ Ark

Kaplan, Sheldon MD [PInf] - **Spec Exp:** Pneumococcal Infections; Meningitis; **Hospital:** Texas Chldns Hosp; **Address:** Div Infectious Disease, 1102 Bates St, Ste 1150, Houston, TX 77030; **Phone:** 832-824-4330; **Board Cert:** Pediatrics 1978; Pediatric Infectious Disease 2009; **Med School:** Univ MO-Columbia Sch Med 1973; **Resid:** Pediatrics, St Louis Chldns Hosp 1975; **Fellow:** Pediatric Infectious Disease, St Louis Chldns Hosp 1977; **Fac Appt:** Prof Ped, Baylor Coll Med

Kline, Mark W. MD [PInf] - **Spec Exp:** AIDS/HIV; **Hospital:** Texas Chldns Hosp; **Address:** Texas Children's Hosp, 6621 Fannin St, Houston, TX 77030; **Phone:** 832-824-2233; **Board Cert:** Pediatrics 1987; Pediatric Infectious Disease 2009; **Med School:** Baylor Coll Med 1981; **Resid:** Pediatrics, Baylor Affil Hosp 1985; **Fellow:** Pediatric Infectious Disease, Baylor Coll Med 1987; **Fac Appt:** Prof Ped, Baylor Coll Med

McCracken Jr, George H MD [PInf] - **Spec Exp:** Meningitis; Antibiotic Resistance; **Hospital:** UT Southwestern Med Ctr at Dallas; **Address:** Dept Pediatric Infectious Disease, 1935 Med District Drive, Dallas, TX 75235; **Phone:** 214-648-3720; **Board Cert:** Pediatrics 1966; **Med School:** Cornell Univ-Weill Med Coll 1962; **Resid:** Pediatrics, NY-Cornell Med Ctr 1965; Pediatrics, Univ Texas SW Med Ctr 1966; **Fac Appt:** Prof Ped, Univ Tex SW, Dallas

West Coast and Pacific

Bradley, John S MD [PInf] - **Spec Exp:** Meningitis; Brain Infections; **Hospital:** Rady Children's Hosp - San Diego, UCSD Med Ctr; **Address:** 3020 Chldns Way, MC 5041, San Diego, CA 92123; **Phone:** 858-966-7785; **Board Cert:** Pediatrics 1981; Pediatric Infectious Disease 2009; **Med School:** UC Davis 1976; **Resid:** Pediatrics, UC Davis Med Ctr 1980; **Fellow:** Pediatric Infectious Disease, Stanford Univ Hosp 1981; **Fac Appt:** Assoc Clin Prof Ped, UCSD

Bryson, Yvonne J MD [PInf] - **Spec Exp:** AIDS/HIV; Herpes Simplex; Clinical Trials; Toxoplasmosis; **Hospital:** UCLA Ronald Reagan Med Ctr; **Address:** UCLA Pediatric Infectious Disease, 10833 Le Conte Ave, rm 22-442 MDCC, Los Angeles, CA 90095-1752; **Phone:** 310-825-5235; **Board Cert:** Pediatrics 1976; **Med School:** Univ Tex SW, Dallas 1970; **Resid:** Pediatrics, UCSD Med Ctr 1974; **Fellow:** Pediatric Infectious Disease, UCSD Med Ctr 1976; **Fac Appt:** Prof Ped, UCLA

Mason, Wilbert H MD [PInf] - **Spec Exp:** Kawasaki Disease; **Hospital:** Chldns Hosp - Los Angeles, Keck Med Ctr of USC (page 62); **Address:** Chldns Hosp, Div Inf Dis, 4650 West Sunset Blvd, MS 51, Los Angeles, CA 90027-6062; **Phone:** 323-361-2509; **Board Cert:** Pediatrics 1975; Pediatric Infectious Disease 2009; **Med School:** UC Irvine 1970; **Resid:** Pediatrics, Chldns Hosp 1973; **Fellow:** Infectious Disease, Chldns Hosp 1974; **Fac Appt:** Assoc Clin Prof Ped, USC Sch Med

Petru, Ann MD [PInf] - **Spec Exp:** AIDS/HIV; **Hospital:** Chldns Hosp - Oakland; **Address:** Chldns Hosp, Div Infectious Disease, 744 52nd St, Oakland, CA 94609; **Phone:** 510-428-3336; **Board Cert:** Pediatrics 1983; Pediatric Infectious Disease 2002; **Med School:** UCSF 1978; **Resid:** Pediatrics, Chldns Hosp Med Ctr 1982; **Fellow:** Pediatric Infectious Disease, Chldns Hosp Med Ctr 1983; **Fac Appt:** Asst Clin Prof Med, UCSF

PEDIATRIC NEPHROLOGY

New England

Harmon, William E MD [PNep] - **Spec Exp:** Nephrotic Syndrome; **Hospital:** Children's Hospital - Boston; **Address:** Chldns Hosp, Div Nephrology, 300 Longwood Ave, Hunnewell 319, Boston, MA 02115; **Phone:** 617-355-6129; **Board Cert:** Pediatrics 1976; **Med School:** Case West Res Univ 1971; **Resid:** Pediatrics, Chldns Hosp Med Ctr 1976; **Fellow:** Pediatric Nephrology, Chldns Hosp Med Ctr 1979; **Fac Appt:** Prof Ped, Harvard Med Sch

Mid Atlantic

Conley, Susan B MD [PNep] - **Spec Exp:** Transplant Medicine-Kidney; Dialysis Care; **Hospital:** St. Christopher's Hosp for Chldn; **Address:** St Christophers Hosp for Children, Kidney Center for Children, Fl 3, 3601 A St, Philadelphia, PA 19134; **Phone:** 215-427-5190; **Board Cert:** Pediatrics 1978; Pediatric Nephrology 1979; **Med School:** Univ Mich Med Sch 1973; **Resid:** Pediatrics, Children's Hosp 1975; **Fellow:** Pediatric Nephrology, Children's Hosp 1977; **Fac Appt:** Prof Ped, Drexel Univ Coll Med

Ellis, Demetrius MD [PNep] - **Spec Exp:** Transplant Medicine-Kidney; Hypertension; **Hospital:** Chldns Hosp of Pittsburgh - UPMC; **Address:** Children's Hospital, Dept Nephrology, 4401 Penn Ave, Pittsburgh, PA 15224; **Phone:** 412-692-5182; **Board Cert:** Pediatrics 1978; Pediatric Nephrology 1979; **Med School:** SUNY Buffalo 1973; **Resid:** Pediatrics, Chldns Hosp 1975; **Fellow:** Pediatric Nephrology, Chldns Hosp-Natl Med Ctr 1977; **Fac Appt:** Prof Ped, Univ Pittsburgh

Fivush, Barbara A MD [PNep] - **Spec Exp:** Transplant Medicine-Kidney; **Hospital:** Johns Hopkins Hosp (page 61); **Address:** Johns Hopkins Hosp-Div Nephrology, 200 N Wolfe St, rm 3055, Baltimore, MD 21287; **Phone:** 410-955-2467; **Board Cert:** Pediatrics 1984; Pediatric Nephrology 2010; **Med School:** Boston Univ 1978; **Resid:** Pediatrics, Johns Hopkins Hosp 1981; **Fellow:** Pediatric Nephrology, Johns Hopkins Hosp 1983; Pediatric Nephrology, Chldns Hosp Natl Med Ctr 1984; **Fac Appt:** Assoc Prof Ped, Johns Hopkins Univ

Kaplan, Bernard S MD [PNep] - **Spec Exp:** Hemolytic Uremic Syndrome; Polycystic Kidney Disease; **Hospital:** Chldns Hosp of Philadelphia; **Address:** Chldns Hosp of Philadelphia, Div Nephrology, 34 St & Civic Ctr Blvd, rm 1E15, Philadelphia, PA 19104; **Phone:** 215-590-2449; **Board Cert:** Pediatrics 1972; Pediatric Nephrology 1974; **Med School:** South Africa 1964; **Resid:** Pediatrics, Baragwanath Hosp, Transvaal Meml Hosp 1970; Nephrology, Royal Victoria Hosp 1973; **Fellow:** Nephrology, Montreal Chldns Hosp 1972; **Fac Appt:** Prof Ped, Univ Pennsylvania

Pediatric Nephrology

Mendley, Susan MD [PNep] - **Spec Exp:** Transplant Medicine-Kidney; Hypertension; Dialysis Care; Glomerulonephritis; **Hospital:** Univ of MD Med Ctr; **Address:** Univ Maryland Med Ctr, 22 S Greene St, Pediatric Nephrol N5W67, Baltimore, MD 21201; **Phone:** 410-328-5303; **Board Cert:** Internal Medicine 1988; Nephrology 2012; **Med School:** Boston Univ 1984; **Resid:** Internal Medicine, Univ Chicago Hosps 1987; **Fellow:** Nephrology, Univ Chicago 1990; Pediatric Nephrology, Chldns Meml Hosp/Northwestern Univ 1991; **Fac Appt:** Assoc Prof Ped, Univ MD Sch Med

Roskes, Saul David MD [PNep] - **Hospital:** Johns Hopkins Hosp (page 61); **Address:** 10807 Falls Rd, Ste 200, Lutherville, MD 21093; **Phone:** 410-321-9393; **Board Cert:** Pediatrics 1970; Pediatric Nephrology 1976; **Med School:** Johns Hopkins Univ 1963; **Resid:** Pediatrics, Bronx Muni Hosp Ctr 1965; Pediatrics, Johns Hopkins Hosp 1968; **Fac Appt:** Assoc Prof Ped, Johns Hopkins Univ

Southeast

Ault, Bettina H MD [PNep] - **Spec Exp:** Hemolytic Uremic Syndrome; Kidney Failure; Anemia; **Hospital:** Le Bonheur Chldns Med Ctr; **Address:** 777 Washington Ave, Ste 400, Memphis, TN 38105; **Phone:** 901-866-8821; **Board Cert:** Pediatrics 2006; Pediatric Nephrology 2006; **Med School:** Univ Tenn Coll Med 1984; **Resid:** Pediatrics, Johns Hopkins Hosp 1987; **Fellow:** Pediatric Nephrology, Univ Tn Med Ctr 1990; **Fac Appt:** Assoc Prof

Benfield, Mark R MD [PNep] - **Spec Exp:** Hypertension; Glomerulonephritis; Nephrotic Syndrome; Transplant Medicine-Kidney; **Hospital:** Children's Hospital - Birmingham; **Address:** 1425 Richard Arriington Jr Blvd S, Ste 206, Birmingham, AL 35205; **Phone:** 205-558-3200; **Board Cert:** Pediatric Nephrology 2006; **Med School:** Tulane Univ 1984; **Resid:** Pediatrics, Chldn's Hosp 1987; **Fellow:** Pediatric Nephrology, Univ Minnesota 1990; **Fac Appt:** Prof Ped, Univ Alabama

Chandar, Jayanthi J MD [PNep] - **Spec Exp:** Kidney Disease; Transplant Medicine-Kidney; Renal Replacement Therapy; **Hospital:** Jackson Meml Hosp; **Address:** Univ Miami Div Ped Nephrology, PO Box 016960 (M-714), Miami, FL 33101; **Phone:** 305-585-6726; **Board Cert:** Pediatrics 2012; Pediatric Nephrology 2010; **Med School:** India 1983; **Resid:** Pediatrics, Jackson Memorial Hosp 1987; **Fellow:** Pediatric Nephrology, Jackson Memorial Hosp 1993; **Fac Appt:** Assoc Prof Ped, Univ Miami Sch Med

Jabs, Kathy MD [PNep] - **Spec Exp:** Transplant Medicine-Kidney; Kidney Failure-Chronic; Dialysis Care; Hypertension; **Hospital:** Vanderbilt Monroe Carrell Jr. Chldn's Hosp (page 75); **Address:** Vanderbilt Chldns Hosp, Div Ped Nephrology, 10111 Doctor's Office Tower, Nashville, TN 37232-9560; **Phone:** 615-322-7416; **Board Cert:** Pediatrics 1987; Pediatric Nephrology 2010; **Med School:** Columbia P&S 1982; **Resid:** Pediatrics, Columbia-Presby Hosp 1985; **Fellow:** Pediatric Nephrology, Chldns Hosp 1988; **Fac Appt:** Assoc Prof Ped, Vanderbilt Univ

Neiberger, Richard E MD/PhD [PNep] - **Spec Exp:** Kidney Disease-Genetic; Hypertension; Kidney Failure; **Hospital:** Shands at Univ of FL; **Address:** UF Pediatrics, Div Pediatric Nephrology, 1600 SW Archer Rd, HD Bldg - Fl 2, rm 216, Gainesville, FL 32610; **Phone:** 352-273-9180; **Board Cert:** Pediatrics 2006; Nephrology 2006; **Med School:** Univ Louisville Sch Med 1982; **Resid:** Pediatrics, Montefiore Med Ctr 1985; **Fellow:** Pediatric Nephrology, Montefiore Med Ctr 1988; **Fac Appt:** Assoc Prof Ped, Univ Fla Coll Med

Wyatt, Robert J MD [PNep] - **Spec Exp:** Kidney Disease-Autoimmune; Berger's Disease (IgA Nephropathy); **Hospital:** Le Bonheur Chldns Med Ctr; **Address:** Univ Tennessee, Dept Peds, 777 Washington Ave, Ste 400, Memphis, TN 38105; **Phone:** 901-866-8821; **Board Cert:** Pediatrics 1978; Pediatric Nephrology 1979; **Med School:** Med Coll GA 1973; **Resid:** Pediatrics, Kentucky Med Ctr 1975; Pediatric Nephrology, Kentucky Med Ctr 1976; **Fellow:** Pediatric Nephrology, Cincinnati Chldns Hosp 1979; **Fac Appt:** Prof Ped, Univ Tenn Coll Med

Zilleruelo, Gaston E MD [PNep] - **Spec Exp:** Transplant Medicine-Kidney; Nephrotic Syndrome; Congenital Anomalies-Genitourinary; **Hospital:** Jackson Meml Hosp, Broward Hlth Med Ctr; **Address:** PO Box 016960 (M-714), Miami, FL 33136; **Phone:** 305-585-6726; **Board Cert:** Pediatrics 1979; Pediatric Nephrology 1991; **Med School:** Chile 1969; **Resid:** Pediatrics, L Calvo-Mackenna Chldns Hosp 1972; Pediatrics, Jackson Meml Hosp 1977; **Fellow:** Pediatric Nephrology, Jackson Meml Hosp 1978; **Fac Appt:** Prof Ped, Univ Miami Sch Med

Midwest

Andreoli, Sharon P MD [PNep] - **Spec Exp:** Kidney Failure; Kidney Failure-Chronic; Osteodystrophy; Glomerulonephritis; **Hospital:** Riley Hosp for Children, IU Health Methodist Hosp; **Address:** Riley Hosp for Chldn-Ped Nephrology, 699 Riley Hosp Drive, rm RR230, Indianapolis, IN 46202; **Phone:** 317-274-2563; **Board Cert:** Pediatrics 1983; Pediatric Nephrology 1985; **Med School:** Indiana Univ 1978; **Resid:** Pediatrics, Riley Hosp Chldn 1981; **Fellow:** Pediatric Nephrology, Univ Minnesota 1981; Pediatric Nephrology, Indiana Univ 1984; **Fac Appt:** Prof Ped, Indiana Univ

Brophy, Patrick D MD [PNep] - **Spec Exp:** Polycystic Kidney Disease; Transplant Medicine-Kidney; Dialysis Care; **Hospital:** Univ Iowa Hosp & Clinics; **Address:** Univ Iowa Chldns Hosp, Ped Nephrology, 200 Hawkins Drive, Iowa City, IA 52242; **Phone:** 319-356-7249; **Board Cert:** Pediatrics 2012; Pediatric Nephrology 2009; **Med School:** Canada 1994; **Resid:** Pediatrics, Univ Manitoba Affil Hosp 1998; **Fellow:** Pediatric Nephrology, Univ Michigan Hosps 2001; **Fac Appt:** Assoc Prof Ped, Univ Iowa Coll Med

Cohn, Richard Allan MD [PNep] - **Spec Exp:** Transplant Medicine-Kidney; Nephrotic Syndrome; Kidney Disease-Chronic; **Hospital:** Lurie Chldn's Hosp-Chicago; **Address:** Ann & Robert H Lurie Chldn's Hosp, 225 E Chicago Ave, MS 37, Chicago, IL 60611; **Phone:** 312-227-6160; **Board Cert:** Pediatrics 1978; Pediatric Nephrology 1979; **Med School:** Albert Einstein Coll Med 1972; **Resid:** Pediatrics, Johns Hopkins Hosp 1975; **Fellow:** Pediatric Nephrology, Univ Minnesota Hosp 1978; **Fac Appt:** Prof Ped, Northwestern Univ

Friedman, Aaron L MD [PNep] - **Spec Exp:** Hypertension; Transplant Medicine-Kidney; Growth Disorders; Fanconi Syndrome; **Address:** Discovery Clin-Ped Specialty Care, 2512 S 7th St Fl 3, Minneapolis, MN 55454; **Phone:** 612-365-6777; **Board Cert:** Pediatrics 1979; Pediatric Nephrology 2003; **Med School:** SUNY Upstate Med Univ 1974; **Resid:** Pediatrics, Univ Wisconsin Med Ctr 1976; **Fellow:** Pediatric Nephrology, Univ Wisconsin 1980; **Fac Appt:** Prof Ped, Univ Minn

Kashtan, Clifford E MD [PNep] - **Spec Exp:** Transplant Medicine-Kidney; Kidney Disease-Genetic; **Hospital:** Univ Minn Med Ctr, Fairview - Riverside Campus; **Address:** Univ Minn Amplatz Chldns Hosp, Div Ped Nephrology, 2450 Riverside Ave Fl 6, Minneapolis, MN 55454; **Phone:** 612-626-2922; **Board Cert:** Pediatrics 1983; Pediatric Nephrology 2010; **Med School:** Wayne State Univ 1978; **Resid:** Pediatrics, Boston City Hosp 1981; **Fellow:** Pediatric Nephrology, Mass Genl Hosp 1984; Pediatric Nephrology, Univ Minnesota Hosp 1987; **Fac Appt:** Prof Ped, Univ Minn

Langman, Craig MD [PNep] - **Spec Exp:** Kidney Stones; Osteoporosis-Juvenile; Oxalosis; **Hospital:** Lurie Chldn's Hosp-Chicago, Evanston/North Shore Univ Hlth Sys; **Address:** Lurie Chldn's Hosp of Chicago, 225 E Chicago Ave, Box 37, Chicago, IL 60611; **Phone:** 312-227-6555; **Board Cert:** Pediatrics 1982; Pediatric Nephrology 1992; **Med School:** Hahnemann Univ 1977; **Resid:** Pediatrics, Chldns Hosp 1979; **Fellow:** Pediatric Nephrology, Chldns Hosp 1981; **Fac Appt:** Prof Ped, Northwestern Univ

Pediatric Nephrology

Warady, Bradley A MD [PNep] - **Spec Exp:** Dialysis Care; Transplant Medicine-Kidney; Kidney Disease-Chronic; Birth Defects; **Hospital:** Chldns Mercy Hosps & Clinics; **Address:** Chldns Mercy Hosps & Clins, 2401 Gillham Rd, Kansas City, MO 64108; **Phone:** 816-234-3010; **Board Cert:** Pediatrics 1984; Pediatric Nephrology 1985; **Med School:** Univ IL Coll Med 1979; **Resid:** Pediatrics, Chldns Mercy Hosp 1982; **Fellow:** Pediatric Nephrology, Colorado Univ Med Ctr 1984; **Fac Appt:** Prof Ped, Univ MO-Kansas City

West Coast and Pacific

Ettenger, Robert B MD [PNep] - **Spec Exp:** Transplant Medicine-Kidney; Hypertension in Children; Urinary Tract Infections; Kidney Disease; **Hospital:** UCLA Ronald Reagan Med Ctr, Mattel Chldns Hosp at UCLA; **Address:** UCLA Pediatric Nephrology, 10833 Le Conte Ave, Box 951752, A2-383 MDCC, Los Angeles, CA 90095; **Phone:** 310-206-6987; **Board Cert:** Pediatrics 1986; Pediatric Nephrology 1986; **Med School:** Univ Pennsylvania 1968; **Resid:** Pediatrics, St Christophers Hosp Chldn 1971; **Fellow:** Pediatric Nephrology, Chldns Hosp 1975; **Fac Appt:** Prof Ped, UCLA

Flynn, Joseph T MD [PNep] - **Spec Exp:** Hypertension; Dialysis Care; Kidney Disease; Obesity; **Hospital:** Seattle Chldns Hosp; **Address:** Children's Hospital, Ped Nephrology, 4800 Sand Point Way NE, MS A-7931, Seattle, WA 98105; **Phone:** 206-987-2524; **Board Cert:** Pediatric Nephrology 2008; **Med School:** SUNY Upstate Med Univ 1987; **Resid:** Pediatrics, St Christophers Hosp 1990; **Fellow:** Pediatric Nephrology, St Christophers Hosp 1993; **Fac Appt:** Prof Ped, Univ Wash

Fouser, Laurie S MD [PNep] - **Spec Exp:** Congenital Kidney Disease; Glomerulonephritis; Hypertension in Children; Kidney Failure; **Hospital:** Swedish Med Ctr-First Hill-Seattle; **Address:** Swedish Ped Spec Care, 1101 Madison St, Ste 800, Seattle, WA 98104; **Phone:** 206-215-2700; **Board Cert:** Pediatrics 1985; Pediatric Nephrology 2003; **Med School:** Univ Nebr Coll Med 1979; **Resid:** Pediatrics, Chldns Ortho Hosp-Univ WA 1982; **Fellow:** Pediatric Nephrology, Univ Minnesota Hosp 1987; Research, Univ Washington Med Ctr 1989; **Fac Appt:** Asst Prof Ped, Univ Wash

Jordan, Stanley C MD [PNep] - **Spec Exp:** Transplant Medicine-Kidney; **Hospital:** Cedars-Sinai Med Ctr; **Address:** Cedars Sinai Med Ctr, Div Ped Nephrology, 8635 W 3rd St, Ste 590W, Los Angeles, CA 90048; **Phone:** 310-423-2641; **Board Cert:** Pediatrics 1978; Pediatric Nephrology 1979; Clinical & Laboratory Immunology 1988; **Med School:** Univ NC Sch Med 1973; **Resid:** Pediatrics, UCLA Med Ctr 1976; Pediatric Nephrology, UCLA Med Ctr 1977; **Fellow:** Renal Immunology, Scripps Clinic 1978; Dialysis & Tranplantation, Chldns Hosp 1980; **Fac Appt:** Prof Ped, UCLA

McDonald, Ruth A MD [PNep] - **Spec Exp:** Transplant Medicine-Kidney; Kidney Disease; **Hospital:** Seattle Chldns Hosp; **Address:** 4800 Sand Point Way NE, MS A-7931, Seattle, WA 98105; **Phone:** 206-987-2524; **Board Cert:** Pediatric Nephrology 2005; **Med School:** Univ Minn 1987; **Resid:** Pediatrics, Chldns Hosp & Med Ctr 1990; **Fellow:** Pediatric Nephrology, Chldns Hosp & Med Ctr 1993; **Fac Appt:** Assoc Prof Ped, Univ Wash

PEDIATRIC OTOLARYNGOLOGY

New England

Cunningham, Michael J MD [PO] - **Spec Exp:** Head & Neck Tumors; Sinus Disorders; Hemangiomas; Vascular Malformations; **Hospital:** Children's Hospital - Boston; **Address:** Chldns Hosp Boston, Dept Otolaryngology, 300 Longwood Ave, Ste Lo-367, Boston, MA 02115; **Phone:** 617-355-6460; **Board Cert:** Otolaryngology 1988; **Med School:** Univ Rochester 1981; **Resid:** Pediatrics, Mass Genl Hosp 1983; Otolaryngology, Univ Pittsburgh Eye & Ear Hosp 1988; **Fellow:** Pediatric Otolaryngology, Mass Eye & Ear Infirm 1989; **Fac Appt:** Prof Oto, Harvard Med Sch

McGill, Trevor J MD [PO] - **Spec Exp:** Head & Neck Tumors; Cholesteatoma; Lymphatic Malformations-Head & Neck; Hemangiomas; **Hospital:** Children's Hospital - Boston; **Address:** Childrens Hosp, Dept Otolaryngology, 300 Longwood Ave, Boston, MA 02115; **Phone:** 617-355-6460; **Board Cert:** Otolaryngology 1988; **Med School:** Ireland 1967; **Resid:** Otolaryngology, Royal Natl Throat Nose & Ear Hosp 1974; **Fellow:** Otolaryngology, Mass Eye & Ear Infirm 1976; **Fac Appt:** Prof Oto, Harvard Med Sch

Poe, Dennis MD [PO] - **Spec Exp:** Cochlear Implants; Neuro-Otology; Ear Disorders/Surgery; **Hospital:** Children's Hospital - Boston; **Address:** Chldns Hosp, Dept Otolaryngology, 300 Longwood Ave, Box 00367, Boston, MA 02115-5724; **Phone:** 617-355-3794; **Board Cert:** Otolaryngology 1987; Neurotology 2004; **Med School:** SUNY Upstate Med Univ 1982; **Resid:** Surgery, Univ Mass Med Ctr 1983; Otolaryngology, Univ Chicago Hosps 1987; **Fellow:** Otology & Neurotology, Otology Group 1988; **Fac Appt:** Assoc Prof Oto, Harvard Med Sch

Mid Atlantic

April, Max M MD [PO] - **Spec Exp:** Sinus Disorders; Neck Masses; Laryngeal Disorders; Sleep Apnea; **Hospital:** NY-Presby/Weill Cornell Med Ctr, NY (page 66), Long Island Jewish Med Ctr (page 67); **Address:** 428 E 72nd St, Ste 100, New York, NY 10021; **Phone:** 646-962-2224; **Board Cert:** Otolaryngology 1990; **Med School:** Boston Univ 1985; **Resid:** Otolaryngology, Boston Univ Med Ctr 1990; **Fellow:** Pediatric Otolaryngology, Johns Hopkins Hosp 1991; **Fac Appt:** Clin Prof Oto, Cornell Univ-Weill Med Coll

Casselbrant, Margaretha L MD/PhD [PO] - **Spec Exp:** Ear Infections; **Hospital:** Chldns Hosp of Pittsburgh - UPMC; **Address:** Chldn's Hosp, Dept Otolaryngology, 4401 Penn Ave Fl 3, Pittsburgh, PA 15224; **Phone:** 412-692-5460; **Board Cert:** Otolaryngology 1992; **Med School:** Sweden 1973; **Resid:** Otolaryngology, Malmo Genl Hosp-Univ Lund 1978; **Fellow:** Otolaryngology, Univ Pittsburgh Med Ctr 1982; **Fac Appt:** Prof Oto, Univ Pittsburgh

Dolitsky, Jay MD [PO] - **Spec Exp:** Ear Infections; Neck Masses; Tonsil/Adenoid Disorders; Sleep Disorders; **Hospital:** New York Eye & Ear Infirm (page 65); **Address:** 261 Fifth Ave, Fl 9, Ste 901, MS 10016, New York, NY 10016; **Phone:** 212-679-3499; **Board Cert:** Otolaryngology 1990; **Med School:** SUNY Downstate 1981; **Resid:** Surgery, NYU/Bellevue Hosp 1986; Otolaryngology, Manhattan EET Hosp 1990; **Fellow:** Pediatric Otolaryngology, Children's Hosp 1992

Goldsmith, Ari J MD [PO] - **Spec Exp:** Voice Disorders; Airway Disorders; Hearing Loss; Sleep Apnea; **Hospital:** SUNY Downstate Med Ctr (Univ Hosp of Bklyn) - LICH; **Address:** 921 49th St, Brooklyn, NY 11209; **Phone:** 718-283-6260; **Board Cert:** Otolaryngology 1994; **Med School:** Albert Einstein Coll Med 1988; **Resid:** Otolaryngology, LI Jewish Hosp 1993; **Fellow:** Pediatric Otolaryngology, Chldns Hosp 1994; **Fac Appt:** Assoc Prof Oto, SUNY Hlth Sci Ctr

Pediatric Otolaryngology

Haddad Jr, Joseph MD [PO] - **Spec Exp:** Ear Infections; Sinus Disorders; Cleft Palate/Lip; **Hospital:** Morgan Stanley Children's Hosp of NY-Presby, NY; **Address:** Morgan Stanley Chldns Hosp of NY-Presby, 3959 Broadway, Ste 501N, New York, NY 10032-1559; **Phone:** 212-305-8933; **Board Cert:** Otolaryngology 1988; **Med School:** NYU Sch Med 1983; **Resid:** Surgery, Columbia-Presby Hosp 1985; Otolaryngology, Columbia-Presby Hosp 1988; **Fellow:** Pediatric Otolaryngology, Chldns Hosp 1990; **Fac Appt:** Clin Prof Oto, Columbia P&S

Harley, Earl H MD [PO] - **Spec Exp:** Infectious Disease; **Hospital:** Georgetown Univ Hosp; **Address:** Georgetown Univ Hosp, 3800 Reservoir Rd NW, Gorman Bldg Fl 1, Washington, DC 20007; **Phone:** 202-444-8186; **Board Cert:** Otolaryngology 1984; **Med School:** Howard Univ 1971; **Resid:** Pediatrics, San Diego Naval Hosp 1973; Otolaryngology, Oakland Naval Hosp 1984; **Fellow:** Pediatric Otolaryngology, Chldn's Hosp Natl Med Ctr 1988; Pediatric Otolaryngology, Mass EE Infirm/Harvard Med Sch 1989; **Fac Appt:** Asst Prof Oto, Georgetown Univ

Jones, Jacqueline MD [PO] - **Spec Exp:** Sinus Disorders/Surgery; Ear Infections; **Hospital:** NY-Presby/Weill Cornell Med Ctr, NY (page 66), Lenox Hill Hosp (page 67); **Address:** 1175 Park Ave, Ste 1A, New York, NY 10128; **Phone:** 212-996-2559; **Board Cert:** Otolaryngology 1989; **Med School:** Cornell Univ-Weill Med Coll 1984; **Resid:** Otolaryngology, Hosp Univ Penn 1989; **Fellow:** Pediatric Otolaryngology, Chldns Hosp 1990; **Fac Appt:** Assoc Prof Oto, Cornell Univ-Weill Med Coll

Kazahaya, Ken MD [PO] - **Spec Exp:** Cochlear Implants; Skull Base Surgery; Otology; Thyroid Surgery; **Hospital:** Chldns Hosp of Philadelphia; **Address:** Children's Hosp of Philadelphia, Div Pediatric Otolaryngology, 34th St & Civic Ctr Blvd Wood Bldg Fl 1, Philadelphia, PA 19104; **Phone:** 215-590-3440; **Board Cert:** Otolaryngology 1999; **Med School:** Univ Pennsylvania 1993; **Resid:** Otolaryngology, Hosp U Penn 1998; **Fellow:** Pediatric Otolaryngology, Children's Hosp 2000; **Fac Appt:** Assoc Clin Prof Oto, Univ Pennsylvania

Rosenfeld, Richard M MD [PO] - **Spec Exp:** Sinus Disorders/Surgery; Head & Neck Surgery; Ear Disorders/Surgery; **Hospital:** SUNY Downstate Med Ctr (Univ Hosp of Bklyn), SUNY Downstate Med Ctr (Univ Hosp of Bklyn) - LICH; **Address:** Univ Otolaryngologists, 134 Atlantic Ave, Brooklyn, NY 11201; **Phone:** 718-780-1498; **Board Cert:** Otolaryngology 1989; **Med School:** SUNY Buffalo 1984; **Resid:** Surgery, Mount Sinai Med Ctr 1986; Otolaryngology, Mount Sinai Med Ctr 1989; **Fellow:** Pediatric Otolaryngology, Chldn's Hosp 1991; **Fac Appt:** Prof Oto, SUNY Downstate

Tunkel, David E MD [PO] - **Spec Exp:** Laryngeal Disorders; Otology; Head & Neck Surgery; **Hospital:** Johns Hopkins Hosp (page 61), Greater Baltimore Med Ctr; **Address:** 601 N Caroline St, rm 6161, Baltimore, MD 21287; **Phone:** 410-955-1559; **Board Cert:** Otolaryngology 1990; **Med School:** Johns Hopkins Univ 1984; **Resid:** Surgery, Johns Hopkins Hosp 1986; Otolaryngology, Johns Hopkins Hosp 1990; **Fellow:** Pediatric Otolaryngology, Chldns Natl Med Ctr 1991; **Fac Appt:** Assoc Prof Oto, Johns Hopkins Univ

Ward, Robert MD [PO] - **Spec Exp:** Airway Disorders; Sinus Disorders/Surgery; Choanal Atresia; **Hospital:** NY-Presby/Weill Cornell Med Ctr, NY (page 66), Lenox Hill Hosp (Manh Eye, Ear & Throat Hosp) (page 67); **Address:** Weill Cornell Med Ctr, Otolaryngology, 428 E 72nd St, Ste 100, New York, NY 10021; **Phone:** 646-962-2224; **Board Cert:** Otolaryngology 1986; **Med School:** Cornell Univ-Weill Med Coll 1981; **Resid:** Surgery, NY Hosp 1983; Otolaryngology, NY Hosp 1986; **Fellow:** Pediatric Otolaryngology, Chldns Hosp 1986; **Fac Appt:** Assoc Clin Prof Oto, Cornell Univ-Weill Med Coll

Southeast

Darrow, David H MD/DDS [PO] - **Spec Exp:** Airway Disorders; Sinus Disorders; Otology; Neck Masses; **Hospital:** Chldns Hosp of King's Daughters; **Address:** Chldns Hosp of Kings Daughters, Div Otolaryngology, 601 Childrens Lane, Norfolk, VA 23507; **Phone:** 757-668-9327; **Board Cert:** Otolaryngology 1994; **Med School:** Duke Univ 1987; **Resid:** Otolaryngology, UCSD Med Ctr 1993; **Fellow:** Pediatric Otolaryngology, Chldns Meml Hosp 1994; **Fac Appt:** Assoc Prof Oto, Eastern VA Med Sch

Drake, Amelia F MD [PO] - **Spec Exp:** Head & Neck Surgery; **Hospital:** NC Memorial Hosp - UNC; **Address:** 170 Manning Drive, Box 7070, Physicians Office Bldg, Rm G116, Chapel Hill, NC 27599-7070; **Phone:** 919-966-3342; **Board Cert:** Otolaryngology 1987; **Med School:** Univ NC Sch Med 1981; **Resid:** Otolaryngology, Univ Michigan Hosps 1986; **Fac Appt:** Prof Oto, Univ NC Sch Med

Eavey, Roland D MD [PO] - **Spec Exp:** Ear Reconstruction/Microtia; Ear Disorders/Surgery; Otology; Hearing Loss; **Hospital:** Vanderbilt Monroe Carrell Jr. Chldn's Hosp (page 75); **Address:** Vanderbilt Pediatric Otolaryngology, 2200 Childrens Way, Doctors Office Tower Fl 7, Nashville, TN 37232; **Phone:** 615-936-8176; **Board Cert:** Otolaryngology 1981; Pediatrics 1982; **Med School:** Univ Pennsylvania 1975; **Resid:** Pediatrics, Chldns Hosp 1977; Surgery, Kaiser Fdn Hosp 1978; **Fellow:** Otolaryngology, Mass EE Infirm 1981; **Fac Appt:** Prof Oto, Vanderbilt Univ

Midwest

Arjmand, Ellis M MD/PhD [PO] - **Spec Exp:** Hearing Loss; Cochlear Implants; Sinus Disorders; **Hospital:** Cincinnati Chldns Hosp Med Ctr; **Address:** Cinncinatti Chldns Hosp-Otolaryngology, 3333 Burnet Ave, Fl C3, ML 2018, Cincinnati, OH 45229; **Phone:** 513-636-4355; **Board Cert:** Otolaryngology 1994; **Med School:** Northwestern Univ 1986; **Resid:** Otolaryngology, Barnes Jewish Hosp 1993; **Fellow:** Pediatric Otolaryngology, St Louis Chldns Hosp 1994; **Fac Appt:** Prof Oto, Univ Cincinnati

Arnold, James E MD [PO] - **Spec Exp:** Airway Disorders; Otology; Ear Tumors; **Hospital:** UH Rainbow Babies & Chldns Hosp (page 74), Univ Hosps Case Med Ctr (page 74); **Address:** 11100 Euclid Ave, Lakeside Bldg Fl 4, Cleveland, OH 44106-5045; **Phone:** 216-844-5031; **Board Cert:** Otolaryngology 1982; **Med School:** Univ Tex, San Antonio 1977; **Resid:** Otolaryngology, Fitzsimons Army Med Ctr 1982; **Fellow:** Pediatric Otolaryngology, Childrens Hosp 1987; **Fac Appt:** Prof Oto, Case West Res Univ

Cotton, Robin MD [PO] - **Spec Exp:** Tracheal Surgery; Head & Neck Surgery; Airway Reconstruction; **Hospital:** Cincinnati Chldns Hosp Med Ctr; **Address:** Cincinnati Chldns Hosp-Otolaryngology, 3333 Burnet Ave Fl C3, ML 2018, Cincinnati, OH 45229; **Phone:** 513-636-4355; **Board Cert:** Otolaryngology 1972; **Med School:** England, UK 1965; **Resid:** Otolaryngology, Univ Birmingham 1968; Otolaryngology, Univ Toronto Med Ctr 1972; **Fellow:** Head and Neck Surgery, Univ Cincinnati Med Ctr 1973; **Fac Appt:** Prof Oto, Univ Cincinnati

Holinger, Lauren D MD [PO] - **Spec Exp:** Airway Disorders; Swallowing Disorders; Cough-Chronic; Voice Disorders; **Hospital:** Lurie Chldn's Hosp-Chicago; **Address:** Lurie Chldn's Hosp, Dept Otolaryngology, 225 E Chicago Ave, Box 25, Chicago, IL 60611; **Phone:** 312-227-6805; **Board Cert:** Otolaryngology 1975; **Med School:** Ros Franklin Univ/Chicago Med Sch 1971; **Resid:** Surgery, Univ Colorado Affil Hosp 1972; Otolaryngology, Univ Colorado Affil Hosp 1975; **Fellow:** Pediatric Otolaryngology, Chldns Meml Hosp 1976; **Fac Appt:** Prof Oto, Northwestern Univ

Pediatric Otolaryngology

Katz, Robert L MD [PO] - **Spec Exp:** Ear Infections; Sinus Disorders/Surgery; Hearing Loss; **Hospital:** Cleveland Clin (page 55); **Address:** 8701 Darrow Rd, CCF Bldg - Fl 2nd, Twinsburg, OH 44087; **Phone:** 330-888-4000; **Board Cert:** Otolaryngology 1968; **Med School:** Case West Res Univ 1963; **Resid:** Surgery, Mount Sinai Hosp 1965; Otolaryngology, Mass EE Infirm/Chldns Hosp 1968; **Fac Appt:** Clin Prof Oto, Cleveland Cl Coll Med/Case West Res

Miller, Robert Paul MD [PO] - **Spec Exp:** Ear Disorders/Surgery; Airway Disorders; Sinus Disorders; Tonsil/Adenoid Disorders; **Hospital:** Adv Luth Genl Hosp, Lurie Chldn's Hosp-Chicago; **Address:** 8780 W Golf Rd, Ste 200, Niles, IL 60714; **Phone:** 847-674-5585; **Board Cert:** Otolaryngology 1978; **Med School:** Loyola Univ-Stritch Sch Med 1974; **Resid:** Otolaryngology, Univ Illinois Hosps 1978; **Fellow:** Pediatric Otolaryngology, Chldns Hosp Med Ctr 1987; **Fac Appt:** Asst Clin Prof Oto, Univ IL Coll Med

Myer III, Charles M MD [PO] - **Spec Exp:** Airway Disorders; Head & Neck Tumors; Neck Masses; **Hospital:** Cincinnati Chldns Hosp Med Ctr, Univ Hosp - Cincinnati; **Address:** Cincinnati Chldn's Hosp-Otolaryngology, 3333 Burnet Ave Fl C3, ML 2018, Cincinnati, OH 45229; **Phone:** 513-636-4355; **Board Cert:** Otolaryngology 1984; **Med School:** Univ Alabama 1978; **Resid:** Otolaryngology, Univ Cincinnati Med Ctr 1984; **Fellow:** Pediatric Otolaryngology, Chldns Hosp 1985; **Fac Appt:** Prof Oto, Univ Cincinnati

Great Plains and Mountains

Chan, Kenny H MD [PO] - **Spec Exp:** Ear Infections; Sinusitis; Hearing Disorders; **Hospital:** Chldn's Hosp - Aurora (CO), Parker Adventist Hosp; **Address:** Chldns Hosp, Dept Otolaryngology, 13123 E 16th Ave, Box B455, Aurora, CO 80045; **Phone:** 720-777-8501; **Board Cert:** Otolaryngology 1984; **Med School:** Loma Linda Univ 1977; **Resid:** Otolaryngology, Loma Linda Univ Hosp 1983; **Fellow:** Pediatric Otolaryngology, Chldns Hosp 1987; **Fac Appt:** Prof Oto, Univ Colorado

Lusk, Rodney P MD [PO] - **Spec Exp:** Cochlear Implants; Sinus Disorders/Surgery; Sleep Disorders/Apnea; **Hospital:** Boys Town Natl Rsch Hosp, Children's Hosp - Omaha; **Address:** Boystown National Research Hosp, 555 N 30th St, Omaha, NE 68131; **Phone:** 402-498-6502; **Board Cert:** Otolaryngology 1982; **Med School:** Univ MO-Columbia Sch Med 1977; **Resid:** Head and Neck Surgery, Univ Iowa Hosp & Clinics 1982; **Fellow:** Pediatric Otolaryngology, Chldn's Hosp 1983

Southwest

Bower, Charles MD [PO] - **Spec Exp:** Airway Disorders; Sleep Disorders/Apnea; Sinus Disorders/Surgery; **Hospital:** Arkansas Chldns Hosp; **Address:** Arkansas Chldns Hosp, Dept Ped Oto, 1 Children's Way, Slot 836, Little Rock, AR 72202-3510; **Phone:** 501-364-1047; **Board Cert:** Otolaryngology 1990; **Med School:** Univ Ark 1985; **Resid:** Otolaryngology, Univ Ark Med Ctr 1991; **Fellow:** Pediatric Otolaryngology, Chldns Hosp 1992; **Fac Appt:** Assoc Prof Oto, Univ Ark

Duncan III, Newton O MD [PO] - **Spec Exp:** Sinus Disorders; Airway Disorders; Head & Neck Surgery; **Hospital:** Texas Chldns Hosp, Methodist Hosp - Houston; **Address:** 6550 Fannin St, Ste 2001, Houston, TX 77030-2709; **Phone:** 713-796-2001; **Board Cert:** Otolaryngology 1986; **Med School:** Baylor Coll Med 1978; **Resid:** Surgery, Baylor Affil Hosp 1983; Otolaryngology, Baylor Affil Hosp 1986; **Fellow:** Pediatric Otolaryngology, Univ Wash 1991; Pediatric Otolaryngology, Royal Alexandra Hosp Chld 1992; **Fac Appt:** Asst Clin Prof Oto, Baylor Coll Med

Friedman, Ellen M MD [PO] - **Spec Exp:** Airway Disorders; Lymphatic Malformations-Head & Neck; **Hospital:** Texas Chldns Hosp, Methodist Hosp - Houston; **Address:** 6701 Fannin, Ste 540, MC CC6102, Houston, TX 77030; **Phone:** 832-822-3250; **Board Cert:** Otolaryngology 1981; **Med School:** Albert Einstein Coll Med 1975; **Resid:** Surgery, Montefiore Hosp 1976; Otolaryngology, Washington Hosp Ctr 1979; **Fellow:** Pediatric Otolaryngology, Boston Chldns Hosp; **Fac Appt:** Prof Oto, Baylor Coll Med

West Coast and Pacific

Crockett, Dennis M MD [PO] - **Spec Exp:** Head & Neck Cancer; Airway Disorders; **Hospital:** Mission Hosp-Mission Viejo, Saddleback Meml Med Ctr-San Clemente; **Address:** 26726 Crown Valley Pkwy, Ste 200, Mission Viejo, CA 92691; **Phone:** 949-364-4361; **Board Cert:** Otolaryngology 1985; **Med School:** USC Sch Med 1979; **Resid:** Otolaryngology, LAC & USC Med Ctr 1984; **Fellow:** Pediatrics, Boston Chldns Hosp 1985; **Fac Appt:** Assoc Prof Oto, USC Sch Med

Geller, Kenneth Allen MD [PO] - **Spec Exp:** Airway Disorders; Sinus Disorders/Surgery; Head & Neck Cancer; **Hospital:** Chldns Hosp - Los Angeles, Huntington Memorial Hosp; **Address:** Chldns Hosp, Div Otolaryngology, 4650 Sunset Blvd, MS 58, Los Angeles, CA 90027; **Phone:** 323-361-2145; **Board Cert:** Otolaryngology 1978; **Med School:** USC Sch Med 1972; **Resid:** Surgery, Wadsworth VA Hosp 1975; Otolaryngology, UCLA Hlth Scis Ctr 1978; **Fellow:** Pediatric Otolaryngology, Chldns Hosp 1979; **Fac Appt:** Assoc Clin Prof Oto, USC Sch Med

Inglis, Andrew MD [PO] - **Spec Exp:** Airway Disorders; Voice Disorders; **Hospital:** Seattle Chldns Hosp; **Address:** Children's Hospital & Medical Ctr, 4800 Sand Point Way NE, MS W6640, Seattle, WA 98105-0371; **Phone:** 206-987-2105; **Board Cert:** Otolaryngology 1987; **Med School:** Med Coll PA Hahnemann 1981; **Resid:** Surgery, Virginia Mason Hosp 1983; Otolaryngology, Univ Washington Hosps 1987; **Fellow:** Pediatric Otolaryngology, Royal Alexandria Hosp Chldn 1987; **Fac Appt:** Assoc Prof Oto, Univ Wash

Parikh, Sanjay R MD [PO] - **Spec Exp:** Airway Reconstruction; Sinus Disorders/Surgery; Vocal Cord Disorders; Hearing Disorders; **Hospital:** Seattle Chldns Hosp; **Address:** Seattle Children's Hosp, Div Pediatric Otolaryngology, 4800 Sand Point Way, NE, W-7729, Seattle, WA 98105; **Phone:** 206-987-2105; **Board Cert:** Otolaryngology 2000; **Med School:** Rush Med Coll 1994; **Resid:** Surgery, Harbor UCLA Med Ctr 1996; Otolaryngology, Univ Toronto 1999; **Fellow:** Pediatric Otolaryngology, Chldns Hosp 2001; **Fac Appt:** Assoc Prof Oto, Univ Wash

Richardson, Mark A MD [PO] - **Spec Exp:** Sinus Disorders; Airway Disorders; Lymphatic Malformations-Head & Neck; **Hospital:** Doernbecher Chldns Hosp/OHSU; **Address:** 3181 SW Sam Jackson Park Rd, MC PV01, Portland, OR 97239; **Phone:** 503-494-5350; **Board Cert:** Otolaryngology 1979; **Med School:** Med Univ SC 1975; **Resid:** Otolaryngology, Med Univ Hosp 1979; **Fellow:** Pediatric Otolaryngology, Chldns Hosp Med Ctr 1980; **Fac Appt:** Prof Oto, Oregon Hlth & Sci Univ

Rosbe, Kristina W MD [PO] - **Spec Exp:** Airway Disorders; Sinus Disorders/Surgery; Cochlear Implants; Neck Masses; **Hospital:** UCSF Med Ctr; **Address:** UCSF Med Ctr, Dept Otolaryngology, 2380 Sutter St, San Francisco, CA 94115; **Phone:** 415-353-2757; **Board Cert:** Otolaryngology 1999; **Med School:** Dartmouth Med Sch 1993; **Resid:** Surgery, Univ N Carolina Hosps 1994; Otolaryngology, Univ N Carolina Hosps 1998; **Fellow:** Pediatric Otolaryngology, Chldns Hosp 2000; **Fac Appt:** Assoc Prof Ped, UCSF

PEDIATRIC PULMONOLOGY

New England

Dorkin, Henry L MD [PPul] - **Spec Exp:** Cystic Fibrosis; **Hospital:** Children's Hospital - Boston; **Address:** Chldn's Hosp Boston, Div Respiratory Diseases, 300 Longwood Ave, Box 343, Boston, MA 02111-1854; **Phone:** 617-355-1900; **Board Cert:** Pediatrics 1993; Pediatric Pulmonology 2003; **Med School:** Johns Hopkins Univ 1974; **Resid:** Pediatrics, Johns Hopkins Hosp 1977; **Fellow:** Pulmonary Disease, Chldn's Hosp Med Ctr 1980; **Fac Appt:** Assoc Prof Ped, Harvard Med Sch

Lapey, Allen MD [PPul] - **Spec Exp:** Cystic Fibrosis; Asthma; Food Allergy; **Hospital:** Mass Genl Hosp; **Address:** 275 Cambridge St, Ste 530, Professional Office Bldg, Boston, MA 02114; **Phone:** 617-726-8707; **Board Cert:** Pediatrics 1972; Allergy & Immunology 1979; **Med School:** Univ Rochester 1966; **Resid:** Pediatrics, Chldns Hosp 1968; **Fellow:** Pediatric Pulmonology, Mass Genl Hosp 1972; Allergy & Immunology, Mass Genl Hosp 1972; **Fac Appt:** Asst Clin Prof Ped, Harvard Med Sch

Mid Atlantic

Borowitz, Drucy S MD [PPul] - **Spec Exp:** Cystic Fibrosis; Clinical Trials; Nutrition; **Hospital:** Women & Chldn's Hosp of Buffalo, The; **Address:** Women & Childrens Hospital, The Lung Center, 219 Bryant St, Buffalo, NY 14222; **Phone:** 716-878-7561; **Board Cert:** Pediatrics 1984; Pediatric Gastroenterology 2007; **Med School:** Cornell Univ-Weill Med Coll 1979; **Resid:** Pediatrics, UCSF Med Ctr 1982; **Fellow:** Nutrition, UCSF 1983; **Fac Appt:** Clin Prof Ped, SUNY Buffalo

Dovey, Mark E MD [PPul] - **Spec Exp:** Cystic Fibrosis; **Hospital:** St. Christopher's Hosp for Chldn; **Address:** St Christopher's Hosp for Children, Div Pediatric Pulmonology, 3601 A St, Ste 2215, Philadelphia, PA 19134; **Phone:** 215-427-5183; **Board Cert:** Pediatric Pulmonology 2006; **Med School:** Duke Univ 1989; **Resid:** Pediatrics, Johns Hopkins Hosp 1992; **Fellow:** Pediatric Pulmonology, Childrens Hosp 1995; **Fac Appt:** Assoc Prof Ped, Temple Univ

Dozor, Allen J MD [PPul] - **Spec Exp:** Asthma; Cystic Fibrosis; **Hospital:** Westchester Med Ctr, Children's & Women's Phys.of Westchester; **Address:** NY Med College, Munger Pavilion, Pediatric Pulmonology, Ste 106, Valhalla, NY 10595-1600; **Phone:** 914-493-7585; **Board Cert:** Pediatrics 1981; Pediatric Pulmonology 2003; **Med School:** Penn State Coll Med 1977; **Resid:** Pediatrics, St Vincent's Hosp & Med Ctr 1980; **Fellow:** Pediatric Pulmonology, Chldns Hosp 1982; **Fac Appt:** Prof Ped, NY Med Coll

Kattan, Meyer MD [PPul] - **Spec Exp:** Asthma; Cystic Fibrosis; Chronic Lung Disease; **Hospital:** NY-Presby/Columbia Univ Med Ctr, NY (page 66), Englewood Hosp & Med Ctr; **Address:** 3959 Broadway, CHC 7-701, New York, NY 10032; **Phone:** 212-305-5122; **Board Cert:** Pediatrics 1980; Pediatric Pulmonology 2010; **Med School:** McGill Univ 1973; **Resid:** Pediatrics, Chldns Hosp 1975; Pediatrics, Hosp for Sick Chldn 1976; **Fellow:** Pulmonary Disease, Hosp for Sick Chldn 1978; **Fac Appt:** Prof Ped, Columbia P&S

Kurland, Geoffrey MD [PPul] - **Spec Exp:** Transplant Medicine-Lung; **Hospital:** Chldns Hosp of Pittsburgh - UPMC; **Address:** Chldns Hosp, Dept Ped Pulmonology, 4401 Penn Ave AOB Bldg - Ste 3300, Pittsburgh, PA 15224; **Phone:** 412-692-5630; **Board Cert:** Pediatrics 1978; Allergy & Immunology 1979; Pediatric Pulmonology 2010; **Med School:** Stanford Univ 1973; **Resid:** Pediatrics, Stanford Affil Hosps 1976; **Fellow:** Allergy & Immunology, Stanford Affil Hosps 1978; **Fac Appt:** Prof Ped, Univ Pittsburgh

Loughlin, Gerald M MD [PPul] - **Spec Exp:** Sleep Disorders/Apnea; Swallowing Disorders; Asthma & Chronic Lung Disease; Breathing Disorders; **Hospital:** NY-Presby/Weill Cornell Med Ctr, NY (page 66); **Address:** Cornell Med Coll, Dept Peds, 525 E 68th St, rm M-622, New York, NY 10021-4870; **Phone:** 646-962-3410; **Board Cert:** Pediatrics 1993; Pediatric Pulmonology 2012; **Med School:** Univ Rochester 1973; **Resid:** Pediatrics, Univ Ariz Med Ctr 1973; **Fellow:** Pediatric Pulmonology, Univ Ariz Med Ctr 1977; **Fac Appt:** Prof Ped, Cornell Univ-Weill Med Coll

Marcus, Carole L MD [PPul] - **Spec Exp:** Sleep Disorders/Apnea; **Hospital:** Chldns Hosp of Philadelphia; **Address:** Div of Pulmonology, 34th & Civic Ctr Blvd Wood Bldg Fl 5, Philadelphia, PA 19104; **Phone:** 215-590-3749; **Board Cert:** Pediatric Pulmonology 2007; Sleep Medicine 2007; **Med School:** South Africa 1982; **Resid:** Pediatrics, LIJ/SUNY Brooklyn Med Ctr 1986; **Fellow:** Pediatric Pulmonology, Chldns Hosp 1991; **Fac Appt:** Prof Ped, Univ Pennsylvania

Mcgrath-Morrow, Sharon A MD [PPul] - **Spec Exp:** Lung Injury-Neonatal; Bronchopulmonary Dysplasia; Ataxia Telangiectasia; Swallowing Disorders; **Hospital:** Johns Hopkins Hosp (page 61); **Address:** Johns Hopkins Ped Pulmonology, Rubenstein Chldns Hlth Bldg, 200 N Wolfe St, Ste 3029, Baltimore, MD 21287; **Phone:** 410-955-2035; **Board Cert:** Pediatrics 2007; Pediatric Pulmonology 2007; **Med School:** Univ VA Sch Med 1985; **Resid:** Pediatrics, Johns Hopkins Hosp 1988; **Fellow:** Pulmonary Critical Care Medicine, Johns Hopkins 1992; **Fac Appt:** Assoc Prof Ped, Johns Hopkins Univ

Orenstein, David M MD [PPul] - **Spec Exp:** Cystic Fibrosis; **Hospital:** Chldns Hosp of Pittsburgh - UPMC; **Address:** Chldns Hosp, Dept Ped Pulmonology, 4401 Penn Ave AOB Bldg - Ste 3300, Pittsburgh, PA 15224; **Phone:** 412-692-5630; **Board Cert:** Pediatrics 1979; Pediatric Pulmonology 2004; **Med School:** Case West Res Univ 1973; **Resid:** Pediatrics, Rainbow Babies & Chldn's Hosp 1975; **Fellow:** Pediatric Pulmonology, Rainbow Babies & Chldn's Hosp 1977; **Fac Appt:** Prof Ped, Univ Pittsburgh

Panitch, Howard B MD [PPul] - **Spec Exp:** Chronic Obstructive Lung Disease (COPD); Cystic Fibrosis; **Hospital:** Chldns Hosp of Philadelphia; **Address:** Div Pulmonology, 34th & Civic Ctr Blvd Wood Bldg Fl 5, Philadelphia, PA 19104; **Phone:** 215-590-3749; **Board Cert:** Pediatrics 1987; Pediatric Pulmonology 2011; **Med School:** Univ Pittsburgh 1982; **Resid:** Pediatrics, Children's Hosp 1985; **Fellow:** Pediatric Pulmonology, St Christopher's Hosp 1988; **Fac Appt:** Prof Ped, Univ Pennsylvania

Quittell, Lynne M MD [PPul] - **Spec Exp:** Cystic Fibrosis; Asthma; **Hospital:** Morgan Stanley Children's Hosp of NY-Presby, NY, NY-Presby/Columbia Univ Med Ctr, NY (page 66); **Address:** Morgan Stanley Children's Hosp of NY, 3959 Broadway, CHONY Bldg - Fl 7, New York, NY 10032; **Phone:** 212-305-5122; **Board Cert:** Pediatrics 1986; Pediatric Pulmonology 2011; **Med School:** Israel 1981; **Resid:** Pediatrics, Schneider Chldns Hosp 1984; **Fellow:** Pediatric Pulmonology, St Christopher's Hosp 1988; **Fac Appt:** Assoc Prof Ped, Columbia P&S

Tauber, Danna MD [PPul] - **Spec Exp:** Sleep Disorders; Cystic Fibrosis; **Hospital:** St. Christopher's Hosp for Chldn; **Address:** St. Christopher's Hosp for Chldn, 3601 A St, Phildelphia, PA 19134; **Phone:** 215-427-5000; **Board Cert:** Pediatric Pulmonology 2012; Sleep Medicine 2009; **Med School:** Tulane Univ 1997; **Resid:** Pediatrics, Montefiore Med Ctr 2000; **Fellow:** Pediatric Pulmonology, Chldn's Hosp Phildelphia 2003; **Fac Appt:** Asst Prof Ped, Drexel Univ Coll Med

Zeitlin, Pamela L MD [PPul] - **Spec Exp:** Cystic Fibrosis; **Hospital:** Johns Hopkins Hosp (page 61), Mt Washington Ped Hosp; **Address:** Johns Hopkins Ped Pulmonology, 200 N Wolfe St, rm 3075, Baltimore, MD 21287; **Phone:** 410-955-2035; **Board Cert:** Pediatrics 1988; Pediatric Pulmonology 2007; **Med School:** Yale Univ 1983; **Resid:** Pediatrics, Johns Hopkins Hosp 1986; **Fellow:** Pediatric Pulmonology, Johns Hopkins Hosp 1989; **Fac Appt:** Prof Ped, Johns Hopkins Univ

Pediatric Pulmonology

Southeast

Murphy, Thomas M MD [PPul] - **Spec Exp:** Cystic Fibrosis; Asthma; Chronic Lung Disease of Infancy; Pneumonia-Recurrent; **Hospital:** Duke Univ Hosp; **Address:** DUMC Pediatric Pulmonology, 2301 Erwin Rd, Box 102360, Durham, NC 27710; **Phone:** 919-684-3364; **Board Cert:** Internal Medicine 1976; Pediatrics 2003; Pediatric Pulmonology 2004; **Med School:** Univ Rochester 1973; **Resid:** Internal Medicine, Georgetown Univ Hosp 1976; **Fellow:** Pediatric Pulmonology, Georgetown Univ Hosp 1978; **Fac Appt:** Assoc Prof Ped, Duke Univ

Rubin, Bruce Kalman MD [PPul] - **Spec Exp:** Asthma; Cystic Fibrosis; Cough-Chronic; Plastic Bronchitis; **Hospital:** Children's Hosp, Med Coll of VA Hosp; **Address:** Children's Hospital of Richmond at VCU, 1001 E Marshall St, Fl 2, Richmond, VA 23298; **Phone:** 804-828-2980; **Board Cert:** Pediatrics 1984; Pediatric Pulmonology 2005; **Med School:** Tulane Univ 1979; **Resid:** Pediatrics, Tulane Univ 1981; Pediatric Pulmonology, Hosp for Sick Children 1983; **Fellow:** Pediatric Pulmonary & Critical Care, Hosp for Sick Children 1983; **Fac Appt:** Prof Ped, Va Commonwealth Univ Sch Med

Sallent, Jorge A MD [PPul] - **Spec Exp:** Chronic Lung Disease of Infancy; Asthma & Chronic Lung Disease; Lung Injuries-RSV related; **Hospital:** St. Mary's Med Ctr - W Palm Bch, Palms - West Hosp; **Address:** Pediatric Respiratory Ctr, 500 Federal Highway (US 1), Lake Park, FL 33403-3598; **Phone:** 561-863-0105; **Board Cert:** Pediatrics 1984; Pediatric Pulmonology 2010; **Med School:** Dominican Republic 1978; **Resid:** Pediatrics, Orlando Regional Med Ctr 1983; **Fellow:** Pediatric Pulmonology, Univ Florida 1986; **Fac Appt:** Asst Clin Prof Ped, Univ Fla Coll Med

Sherman, James MD [PPul] - **Spec Exp:** Asthma; Airway Disorders; Cough-Chronic; **Hospital:** Carilion Roanoke Meml Hosp; **Address:** 1906 Bellview Ave, 12 South, Roanoke, VA 24013; **Phone:** 540-266-6013; **Board Cert:** Pediatrics 1981; Pediatric Pulmonology 2003; **Med School:** Univ S Fla Coll Med 1975; **Resid:** Pediatrics, SUNY Upstate Med Ctr 1977; Pediatrics, Tampa Genl Hosp- Univ So Florida 1978; **Fellow:** Pediatric Pulmonology, Rainbow Babies & Children's Hosp 1981; **Fac Appt:** Prof Ped, Univ Fla Coll Med

Midwest

Givan, Deborah C MD [PPul] - **Spec Exp:** Sleep Disorders/Apnea; Apnea in Infants; Asthma; Pulmonary Complications-Neurodisability; **Hospital:** Riley Hosp for Children; **Address:** Riley Hosp for Chldn, Pulmonary Medicine, 705 Riley Hosp Drive, Ste 4270, Indianapolis, IN 46202; **Phone:** 317-274-7208; **Board Cert:** Pediatrics 1982; Pediatric Pulmonology 2010; Sleep Medicine 2011; **Med School:** Indiana Univ 1977; **Resid:** Pediatrics, Meethodist Hosp 1980; **Fellow:** Pediatric Pulmonology, Riley Chldns Hosp 1981; Pediatric Pulmonology, Texas Chldns Hosp 1982; **Fac Appt:** Clin Prof Ped, Indiana Univ

Green, Thomas P MD [PPul] - **Spec Exp:** Respiratory Failure; Breathing Disorders; **Hospital:** Lurie Chldn's Hosp-Chicago, Northwestern Meml Hosp; **Address:** Lurie Chldn's Hosp, Dept Pulm/Crit Care, 225 E Chicago Ave, Box 86, Chicago, IL 60611; **Phone:** 312-227-6260; **Board Cert:** Pediatrics 1992; Pediatric Pulmonology 2009; Pediatric Critical Care Medicine 2010; **Med School:** Stanford Univ 1974; **Resid:** Pediatrics, Univ Minn Med Ctr 1977; **Fellow:** Pharmacology, Univ Minn Med Ctr 1979; Pediatric Pulmonology, Univ Minn Med Ctr 1994; **Fac Appt:** Prof Ped, Northwestern Univ

Kemp, James S MD [PPul] - **Spec Exp:** Sudden Infant Death Syndrome (SIDS); Breathing Disorders; Sleep Disorders; **Hospital:** St. Louis Chldns Hosp; **Address:** Wash Univ, Div Pulm Med, 660 S Euclid Ave, Box 8116, St Louis, MO 63110; **Phone:** 314-454-2694; **Board Cert:** Pediatrics 1981; Sleep Medicine 2007; **Med School:** Creighton Univ 1976; **Resid:** Pediatrics, Cardinal Glennon Chldns Hosp 1978; Pediatrics, Baylor Univ 1979; **Fellow:** Pediatric Pulmonology, Texas Chldns Hosp 1988; **Fac Appt:** Assoc Prof Ped, Washington Univ, St Louis

Kim, Young-Jee MD [PPul] - **Spec Exp:** Asthma; Rare Lung Disease-Pediatric; Pulmonary Complications-Sickle Cell Dis; Pulmonary Complications-Cancer Therapy; **Hospital:** Riley Hosp for Children; **Address:** 705 Riley Hospital Drive, rm ROC4270, Indianapolis, IN 46202-5128; **Phone:** 317-274-7208; **Board Cert:** Pediatric Pulmonology 2006; **Med School:** South Korea 1982; **Resid:** Pediatrics, Duke Univ Med Ctr 1995; **Fellow:** Pediatric Pulmonology, Yale Univ Med Sch 1991; Pediatric Pulmonology, Riley Hosp Chldn 1998; **Fac Appt:** Assoc Clin Prof Ped, Indiana Univ

Konstan, Michael W MD [PPul] - **Spec Exp:** Cystic Fibrosis; Asthma; **Hospital:** UH Rainbow Babies & Chldns Hosp (page 74); **Address:** Div Ped Pulmonology, 11100 Euclid Ave, MS RBC6040, Cleveland, OH 44106; **Phone:** 216-844-1997; **Board Cert:** Pediatrics 1986; Pediatric Pulmonology 2011; **Med School:** Case West Res Univ 1982; **Resid:** Pediatrics, Chldn's Hosp 1985; **Fellow:** Pediatric Pulmonology, Rainbow Babies & Chldns Hosp 1988; **Fac Appt:** Prof Ped, Case West Res Univ

Kurachek, Stephen MD [PPul] - **Spec Exp:** Critical Care; Asthma; **Hospital:** Children's Hosps & Clinics of Minneapolis; **Address:** 2530 Chicago Ave S, Ste 400, Minneapolis, MN 55404; **Phone:** 612-813-3300; **Board Cert:** Pediatrics 1985; Pediatric Critical Care Medicine 2010; Pediatric Pulmonology 2011; **Med School:** Univ Miami Sch Med 1978; **Resid:** Pediatrics, Univ Hosp 1981; **Fellow:** Pulmonary Disease, Boston Chldns Hosp 1984; **Fac Appt:** Asst Clin Prof Ped, Univ Minn

McCoy, Karen S MD [PPul] - **Spec Exp:** Cystic Fibrosis; Asthma; **Hospital:** Nationwide Chldn's Hosp; **Address:** Nationwide Children's Hosp, Section of Pulmonary Medicine, 555 S 18th St, Columbus, OH 43205; **Phone:** 614-722-4766; **Board Cert:** Pediatrics 1991; Pediatric Pulmonology 2010; **Med School:** Univ NC Sch Med 1975; **Resid:** Pediatrics, NC Meml Hosp 1979; **Fellow:** Pulmonary Disease, Arizona Hlth Scis Ctr 1982; **Fac Appt:** Assoc Prof Ped, Ohio State Univ

Great Plains and Mountains

Fan, Leland Lane MD [PPul] - **Spec Exp:** Interstitial Lung Disease; **Hospital:** Chldn's Hosp - Aurora (CO); **Address:** The Chldn's Hosp Pulmonary Med, 13123 E 16th Ave, Ste B395, Aurora, CO 80045; **Phone:** 720-777-6181; **Board Cert:** Pediatrics 1978; Pediatric Pulmonology 2003; Pediatric Critical Care Medicine 2003; **Med School:** Baylor Coll Med 1973; **Resid:** Pediatrics, UCSF Med Ctr 1975; Pediatrics, Univ Colo Hlth Sci Ctr 1976; **Fellow:** Pediatric Pulmonary & Critical Care, Univ Colo Hlth Sci Ctr 1978; **Fac Appt:** Prof Ped, Univ Colorado

Southwest

Morgan, Wayne J MD [PPul] - **Spec Exp:** Cystic Fibrosis; Asthma; **Hospital:** Univ Arizona Med Ctr-Univ Campus, Tucson Med Ctr; **Address:** Univ Arizona Hlth Sci Ctr, Div Pediatric Pulmonology, 1501 N Campbell Ave, Box 245073, Tucson, AZ 85724; **Phone:** 520-626-7780; **Board Cert:** Pediatrics 1982; Pediatric Pulmonology 2010; **Med School:** McGill Univ 1976; **Resid:** Pediatrics, Montreal Chldns Hosp 1980; **Fellow:** Pediatric Pulmonology, Univ Ariz 1982; **Fac Appt:** Prof Ped, Univ Ariz Coll Med

Warren, Robert H MD [PPul] - **Spec Exp:** Pulmonary Complications-Neurodisability; Pulmonary Rehabilitation; Ventilation Management-Long Term; **Hospital:** Arkansas Chldns Hosp; **Address:** Arkansas Chldns Hosp, Pulmonary Med, 1 Children's Way, Slot 512-17, Little Rock, AR 72202; **Phone:** 501-364-1006; **Board Cert:** Pediatrics 1973; Pediatric Pulmonology 2010; **Med School:** Univ Ark 1967; **Resid:** Pediatrics, LSU Med Ctr 1971; **Fellow:** Pediatric Pulmonology, Tulane Univ Sch Med 1974; Pediatric Pulmonary & Critical Care, Children's Meml Hosp 1974; **Fac Appt:** Assoc Prof Ped, Univ Ark

Pediatric Pulmonology

West Coast and Pacific

Cooper, Dan M MD [PPul] - **Hospital:** Chldns Hosp Orange Co; **Address:** Chldns Hosp Orange Co, Dept Ped Pulmology, 455 S Main St, Orange, CA 92868; **Phone:** 714-532-7983; **Board Cert:** Pediatrics 1980; Pediatric Pulmonology 2009; **Med School:** UCSF 1974; **Resid:** Internal Medicine, Hadassah Hosp; Pediatrics, Chldns Hosp Med Ctr 1980; **Fellow:** Pediatric Pulmonology, Babies Hosp-Columbia Univ 1994; **Fac Appt:** Prof Ped, UC Irvine

Gibson, Ronald MD/PhD [PPul] - **Spec Exp:** Pulmonary Infections; Sleep Disorders; Cystic Fibrosis; Asthma; **Hospital:** Seattle Chldns Hosp; **Address:** Seattle Children's, 4800 Sand Point Way NE, Ste A-5937, Seattle, WA 98105; **Phone:** 206-987-2174; **Board Cert:** Pediatrics 1988; Pediatric Pulmonology 2007; **Med School:** Washington Univ, St Louis 1982; **Resid:** Pediatrics, Univ Washington Med Ctr 1985; **Fellow:** Pediatric Pulmonology, Univ Washington Med Ctr 1988; **Fac Appt:** Prof Ped, Univ Wash

Keens, Thomas G MD [PPul] - **Spec Exp:** Sudden Infant Death Syndrome (SIDS); Breathing Disorders; **Hospital:** Chldns Hosp - Los Angeles; **Address:** Chldns Hosp, Div Pulmonology, 4650 W Sunset Blvd, MS 83, Los Angeles, CA 90027-6062; **Phone:** 323-361-2101; **Board Cert:** Pediatrics 1978; Neonatal-Perinatal Medicine 1983; Pediatric Pulmonology 2010; **Med School:** UCSD 1972; **Resid:** Pediatrics, Chldns Hosp 1975; **Fellow:** Pediatric Pulmonology, Hosp Sick Chldn 1977; **Fac Appt:** Prof Ped, USC Sch Med

Nielson, Dennis W MD/PhD [PPul] - **Spec Exp:** Cystic Fibrosis; Bronchopulmonary Dysplasia; **Hospital:** UCSF Med Ctr; **Address:** UCSF Dept Padiatric Pulmonology, 521 Parnassus Ave, rm C344, San Francisco, CA 94143; **Phone:** 415-476-2072; **Board Cert:** Pediatrics 1986; Pediatric Pulmonology 2003; **Med School:** Univ Utah 1976; **Resid:** Pediatrics, UCSF Med Ctr 1978; **Fellow:** Pediatric Pulmonology, UCSF Med Ctr 1981; **Fac Appt:** Prof Ped, UCSF

Platzker, Arnold CG MD [PPul] - **Spec Exp:** Asthma; Chronic Lung Disease; Cystic Fibrosis; HIV and Lung Disease; **Hospital:** Chldns Hosp - Los Angeles, Mattel Chldns Hosp at UCLA; **Address:** Chldns Hosp, Div Ped Pulmonology, 4650 W Sunset Blvd, MS 83, Los Angeles, CA 90027-6062; **Phone:** 323-361-2101; **Board Cert:** Pediatrics 1967; Neonatal-Perinatal Medicine 1975; Pediatric Pulmonology 2010; **Med School:** Tufts Univ 1962; **Resid:** Pediatrics, City Hosp 1964; Pediatrics, Stanford Univ Med Ctr 1966; **Fellow:** Pediatric Pulmonology, UCSF Med Ctr 1971; Neonatal-Perinatal Medicine, UCSF Med Ctr 1971; **Fac Appt:** Prof Ped, USC Sch Med

Ramsey, Bonnie W MD [PPul] - **Spec Exp:** Cystic Fibrosis; **Hospital:** Seattle Chldns Hosp; **Address:** 4800 Sand Point Way NE, Ste A-5937, Seattle, WA 98105; **Phone:** 206-987-2174; **Board Cert:** Pediatrics 1981; Pediatric Pulmonology 2007; **Med School:** Harvard Med Sch 1976; **Resid:** Pediatrics, Chldns Hosp 1978; Pediatrics, Chldns Hosp 1979; **Fellow:** Pediatric Critical Care Medicine, Chldns Hosp 1981; **Fac Appt:** Prof Ped, Univ Wash

Redding, Gregory MD [PPul] - **Spec Exp:** Chest Wall Deformities; Interstitial Lung Disease; Sleep Disorders; Thoracic Insufficiency Syndrome; **Hospital:** Seattle Chldns Hosp; **Address:** Seattle Children's Hospital, 4800 Sand Point Way NE, rm A-5937, Seattle, WA 98105; **Phone:** 206-987-2174; **Board Cert:** Pediatrics 1992; Pediatric Pulmonology 2003; **Med School:** Stanford Univ 1974; **Resid:** Pediatrics, Harbor-UCLA Affil Hosps 1977; **Fellow:** Pediatric Pulmonology, Univ Colo Affil Hosps 1979; **Fac Appt:** Prof Ped, Univ Wash

Wall, Michael A MD [PPul] - **Spec Exp:** Cystic Fibrosis; Asthma; Pneumonia; **Hospital:** Doernbecher Chldns Hosp/OHSU, OR Hlth & Sci Univ; **Address:** OHSU, MC CDRC-P, 707 SW Gaines St, Portland, OR 97239; **Phone:** 503-494-8023; **Board Cert:** Pediatrics 1992; Pediatric Pulmonology 2010; **Med School:** Univ NC Sch Med 1973; **Resid:** Pediatrics, Mass Genl Hosp 1976; **Fellow:** Pulmonary Disease, Chldns Hosp 1978; **Fac Appt:** Prof Ped, Oregon Hlth & Sci Univ

Pediatric Rheumatology

New England

McCarthy, Paul L MD [PRhu] - **Spec Exp:** Lupus/SLE; Juvenile Arthritis; Dermatomyositis; Vasculitis; **Hospital:** Yale-New Haven Hosp, Yale Med Group; **Address:** Yale Sch Med, 333 Cedar St, Box 208064, New Haven, CT 06520-3206; **Phone:** 203-688-2475; **Board Cert:** Pediatrics 1974; Pediatric Rheumatology 2007; **Med School:** Georgetown Univ 1969; **Resid:** Pediatrics, Chldns Hosp 1972; **Fellow:** Pediatrics, Chldns Hosp 1974; **Fac Appt:** Prof Ped, Yale Univ

Mid Atlantic

Goldsmith, Donald P MD [PRhu] - **Spec Exp:** Arthritis; Juvenile Arthritis; Vasculitis; **Hospital:** St. Christopher's Hosp for Chldn; **Address:** St Christophers Hosp for Children, Rheumatology Section, 3601 A St, Philadelphia, PA 19134; **Phone:** 215-427-5051; **Board Cert:** Pediatrics 1974; Allergy & Immunology 1975; Pediatric Rheumatology 2007; **Med School:** Univ VT Coll Med 1967; **Resid:** Pediatrics, St Christophers Hosp for Chldn 1973; **Fellow:** Allergy Immunology & Rheumatology, St Christophers Hosp for Chldn 1975; **Fac Appt:** Prof Ped, Drexel Univ Coll Med

Haines, Kathleen A MD [PRhu] - **Spec Exp:** Juvenile Arthritis; Lupus/SLE; Immune Deficiency; Scleroderma; **Hospital:** Hackensack Univ Med Ctr, NYU Langone Med Ctr (page 68); **Address:** 30 Prospect Ave Fl 3, Pediatric Ctr, Hackensack, NJ 07601; **Phone:** 551-996-5306; **Board Cert:** Pediatrics 1980; Allergy & Immunology 1981; Pediatric Rheumatology 2007; **Med School:** Albert Einstein Coll Med 1975; **Resid:** Pediatrics, New York Hosp 1977; **Fellow:** Allergy & Immunology, New York Hosp 1980; Rheumatology, NYU Med Sch 1982; **Fac Appt:** Assoc Prof Ped, UMDNJ-NJ Med Sch, Newark

Ilowite, Norman T MD [PRhu] - **Spec Exp:** Juvenile Arthritis; Lyme Disease; Lupus/SLE; Dermatomyositis; **Hospital:** Montefiore Med Ctr Moses Campus, NY, Jacobi Med Ctr; **Address:** Chldns Hosp-Montefiore, Rheumatology, 3415 Bainbridge Ave Fl Rosenthal3, Bronx, NY 10467; **Phone:** 718-741-2456; **Board Cert:** Pediatrics 1985; Clinical & Laboratory Immunology 1990; Pediatric Rheumatology 2007; **Med School:** SUNY Downstate 1979; **Resid:** Pediatrics, Chldns Hosp Natl Med Ctr 1982; **Fellow:** Pediatric Rheumatology, Univ WA Med Ctr 1984; **Fac Appt:** Prof Ped, Albert Einstein Coll Med

Lehman, Thomas MD [PRhu] - **Spec Exp:** Arthritis; Scleroderma; Lupus/SLE; Rheumatoid Arthritis; **Hospital:** Hosp For Special Surgery (page 60), NY-Presby/Weill Cornell Med Ctr, NY (page 66); **Address:** Hospital for Special Surgery, 535 E 70 St, New York, NY 10021-4872; **Phone:** 212-606-1151; **Board Cert:** Pediatrics 1979; Pediatric Rheumatology 2007; **Med School:** Jefferson Med Coll 1974; **Resid:** Pediatrics, Chldns Hosp 1976; Pediatrics, UCSF Med Ctr 1977; **Fellow:** Pediatric Rheumatology, Chldns Hosp 1979; Rheumatology, Natl Inst Hlth 1983; **Fac Appt:** Prof Ped, Cornell Univ-Weill Med Coll

Sherry, David D MD [PRhu] - **Spec Exp:** Pain-Musculoskeletal; Reflex Sympathetic Dystrophy (RSD); Juvenile Arthritis; Lupus/SLE; **Hospital:** Chldns Hosp of Philadelphia; **Address:** Chldns Hosp of Phildelphia, Div Rheum, 3405 Civic Ctr Blvd, Philadelphia, PA 19104; **Phone:** 215-590-2547; **Board Cert:** Pediatrics 1981; Pediatric Rheumatology 2007; **Med School:** Texas Tech Univ 1977; **Resid:** Pediatrics, Duke Univ Med Ctr 1980; **Fellow:** Pediatric Rheumatology, Univ British Columbia 1982; **Fac Appt:** Prof Ped, Univ Pennsylvania

Pediatric Rheumatology

Sills, Edward M MD [PRhu] - **Spec Exp:** Juvenile Arthritis; Lupus/SLE; Dermatomyositis; Vasculitis; **Hospital:** Johns Hopkins Hosp (page 61); **Address:** Johns Hopkins Hosp, 200 N Wolfe St, Ste 2-127, Baltimore, MD 21205; **Phone:** 410-955-6145; **Board Cert:** Pediatrics 1968; **Med School:** NYU Sch Med 1963; **Resid:** Pediatrics, Bronx Muni Hosp 1967; **Fac Appt:** Assoc Prof Ped, Johns Hopkins Univ

Southeast

Finkel, Terri H MD [PRhu] - **Spec Exp:** Juvenile Arthritis; Lupus/SLE; Vasculitis; **Hospital:** Nemours Chldns Hosp - Orlando; **Address:** Nemours Children's Clinic, Div Pediatric Rheumatology, 13535 Nemours Pkwy, Orlando, FL 32827; **Phone:** 407-650-7280; **Board Cert:** Pediatrics 1988; Pediatric Rheumatology 2009; **Med School:** Stanford Univ 1982; **Resid:** Pediatrics, Univ Colorado Med Ctr 1985; **Fellow:** Pediatric Rheumatology, Natl Jewish Med Ctr 1990; **Fac Appt:** Prof Ped, Univ Fla Coll Med

Passo, Murray H MD [PRhu] - **Hospital:** MUSC Med Ctr; **Address:** MUSC, Dept Pediatrics, Div Pediatric Rheumatology, 135 Rutledge Ave, MSC 561, Charleston, SC 29425-5610; **Phone:** 843-792-5696; **Board Cert:** Pediatrics 1979; Pediatric Rheumatology 2007; **Med School:** Indiana Univ 1974; **Resid:** Pediatrics, Riley Chldns Hosp 1977; **Fellow:** Rheumatology, Indiana Univ Hosps 1979

Schanberg, Laura E MD [PRhu] - **Spec Exp:** Lupus/SLE; Juvenile Arthritis; Dermatomyositis; Spondyloarthropathies; **Hospital:** Duke Univ Hosp; **Address:** Duke Univ Med Ctr, 2301 Erwin Rd, Durham, NC 27710; **Phone:** 919-684-6627; **Board Cert:** Pediatric Rheumatology 2007; **Med School:** Duke Univ 1984; **Resid:** Pediatrics, Duke Univ Med Ctr 1987; **Fellow:** Pediatric Rheumatology, Duke Univ Med Ctr 1991; **Fac Appt:** Asst Prof Ped, Duke Univ

Warren, Robert W MD/PhD [PRhu] - **Spec Exp:** Juvenile Arthritis; Lupus/SLE; **Hospital:** MUSC Med Ctr; **Address:** 261 Calhoun St, rm 316 MSC186, Charleston, SC 29425; **Phone:** 843-876-1985; **Board Cert:** Pediatrics 1983; Allergy & Immunology 1983; Pediatric Rheumatology 2007; **Med School:** Washington Univ, St Louis 1978; **Resid:** Pediatrics, Duke Univ Med Ctr 1980; **Fellow:** Rheumatology, Duke Univ Med Ctr 1983; **Fac Appt:** Assoc Prof Ped, Baylor Coll Med

Midwest

Klein-Gitelman, Marisa MD [PRhu] - **Spec Exp:** Lupus/SLE; Juvenile Arthritis; **Hospital:** Lurie Chldn's Hosp-Chicago; **Address:** Lurie Chldns Hosp, 225 E Chicago Ave, Box 50, Chicago, IL 60611; **Phone:** 312-227-6270; **Board Cert:** Pediatrics 2006; Pediatric Rheumatology 2009; **Med School:** Washington Univ, St Louis 1985; **Resid:** Pediatrics, Columbia-Presby Med Ctr 1989; **Fellow:** Pediatric Rheumatology, New England Med Ctr 1993; **Fac Appt:** Assoc Prof Ped, Northwestern Univ

Wagner-Weiner, Linda MD [PRhu] - **Spec Exp:** Lupus/SLE; Juvenile Arthritis; Vasculitis; Dermatomyositis; **Hospital:** Univ Chicago-Comer Chldn's Hosp, La Rabida Chlds Hosp; **Address:** 5841 S Maryland, rm C101, Chicago, IL 60637; **Phone:** 773-702-2406; **Board Cert:** Pediatrics 1984; Pediatric Rheumatology 2007; **Med School:** Rush Med Coll 1979; **Resid:** Pediatrics, Univ Chicago Hosps 1982; **Fellow:** Pediatric Rheumatology, Univ Chicago/La Rabida Chldns Hosp 1984; **Fac Appt:** Assoc Prof Ped, Univ Chicago-Pritzker Sch Med

Southwest

Myones, Barry Lee MD [PRhu] - **Spec Exp:** Vasculitis; Kawasaki Disease; Dermatomyositis; Scleroderma; **Hospital:** Texas Chldns Hosp; **Address:** Pediatric Rheumatology Ctr, 6701 Fannin St Fl 11, Houston, TX 77030; **Phone:** 832-824-3830; **Board Cert:** Pediatrics 1983; Pediatric Rheumatology 2007; **Med School:** Albany Med Coll 1977; **Resid:** Pediatrics, Duke Univ Med Ctr 1980; **Fellow:** Pediatric Rheumatology, Chldns Hosp-Stanford 1983; Rheumatology, Univ N Carolina 1988; **Fac Appt:** Assoc Clin Prof Ped, Baylor Coll Med

Wilking, Andrew P MD [PRhu] - **Spec Exp:** Arthritis; Lupus/SLE; Dermatomyositis; **Hospital:** Texas Chldns Hosp, Driscoll Chldn's Hosp; **Address:** Pediatric Rheumatology Ctr, 6701 Fannin St Fl 11, Houston, TX 77030; **Phone:** 832-824-3830; **Board Cert:** Pediatrics 1985; **Med School:** Columbia P&S 1978; **Resid:** Pediatrics, Babies Hosp 1981; **Fellow:** Pediatric Rheumatology, Tex Chldns Hosp 1983; **Fac Appt:** Prof Ped, Baylor Coll Med

PEDIATRIC SURGERY

New England

Caty, Michael G MD [PS] - **Spec Exp:** Neonatal Surgery; Thoracic Surgery; Gastrointestinal Motility Disorders; Laparoscopic Surgery; **Hospital:** Yale-New Haven Hosp; **Address:** Yale Pediatric Surgery, 330 Cedar St, FMB-131, PO Box 208062, New Haven, CT 06520-8062; **Phone:** 203-785-2701; **Board Cert:** Surgery 2001; Pediatric Surgery 2003; **Med School:** Univ Mass Sch Med 1985; **Resid:** Surgery, Univ Michigan Hosps 1991; Pediatric Surgery, Boston Chldns Hosp 1993; **Fac Appt:** Prof S, Yale Univ

Chwals, Walter J MD [PS] - **Spec Exp:** Necrotizing Enterocolitis; Cancer Surgery; Endocrine Surgery; Congenital Anomalies; **Hospital:** Tufts Med Ctr; **Address:** Tufts Med Ctr, Floating Hosp, 800 Washington St, Ste 207, Box 344, Boston, MA 02111; **Phone:** 617-636-5025; **Board Cert:** Pediatric Surgery 2007; **Med School:** Poland 1980; **Resid:** Surgery, Univ Mass Med Ctr 1985; **Fellow:** Nutrition, New England Deaconess Hosp 1986; Pediatric Surgery, Chldns Hosp 1988; **Fac Appt:** Prof S, Case West Res Univ

Doody, Daniel P MD [PS] - **Spec Exp:** Neonatal Surgery; Inflammatory Bowel Disease; Hirschsprung's Disease; Minimally Invasive Surgery; **Hospital:** Mass Genl Hosp, Newton - Wellesley Hosp; **Address:** MGH, Dept Pediatric Surgery, 55 Fruit St, Warren Bldg Fl 11, Boston, MA 02114-2621; **Phone:** 617-726-2913; **Board Cert:** Surgery 2006; Pediatric Surgery 2007; **Med School:** Univ IL Coll Med 1977; **Resid:** Surgery, Univ Illinois Hosps 1984; Pediatric Surgery, Chldn's Hosp 1987; **Fellow:** Transplant Research, Mass Genl Hosp 1985; **Fac Appt:** Assoc Prof S, Harvard Med Sch

Jennings, Russell W MD [PS] - **Spec Exp:** Fetal Surgery; Pediatric Cardiac Surgery; Robotic Surgery; Esophageal Surgery; **Hospital:** Children's Hospital - Boston, Brigham and Women's Hosp (page 57); **Address:** Children's Hospital, Fegan 3, 300 Longwood Ave, Boston, MA 02115; **Phone:** 617-355-3038; **Board Cert:** Surgery 2005; Pediatric Surgery 2007; **Med School:** UCSF 1986; **Resid:** Surgery, UCSF Med Ctr 1991; **Fellow:** Fetal Surgery, Fetal Trmt Ctr/UCSF Med Ctr 1994; Pediatric Surgery, Chldns Hosp 1996; **Fac Appt:** Asst Prof S, Harvard Med Sch

Pediatric Surgery

Latchaw, Laurie A MD [PS] - **Spec Exp:** Pediatric Thoracic Surgery; Cancer Surgery; Neonatal Surgery; Lung Disease in Newborns; **Hospital:** Dartmouth - Hitchcock Med Ctr; **Address:** DHMC, Clinic 6M, One Medical Center Drive, Lebanon, NH 03756; **Phone:** 603-653-9883; **Board Cert:** Surgery 2001; Pediatric Surgery 2011; **Med School:** Rush Med Coll 1976; **Resid:** Surgery, Univ Texas 1981; **Fellow:** Pediatric Surgery, Montreal Chldns Hosp 1983; **Fac Appt:** Assoc Prof S, Dartmouth Med Sch

Lillehei, Craig W MD [PS] - **Spec Exp:** Pediatric Thoracic Surgery; **Hospital:** Children's Hospital - Boston; **Address:** Chldns Hosp, Dept Surgery-Fagen Bldg, 300 Longwood Ave Fl 3, Boston, MA 02115; **Phone:** 617-355-3039; **Board Cert:** Surgery 2006; Pediatric Surgery 2007; Surgical Critical Care 2011; **Med School:** Harvard Med Sch 1976; **Resid:** Surgery, Mass Genl Hosp 1984; **Fellow:** Pediatric Surgery, Mass Genl Hosp 1986

Shamberger, Robert C MD [PS] - **Spec Exp:** Wilms' Tumor; Neuroblastoma; Inflammatory Bowel Disease; **Hospital:** Children's Hospital - Boston; **Address:** Boston Children's Hosptial, 300 Longwood Ave, Fegan Bldg Fl 3 - Ste 304, Boston, MA 02115; **Phone:** 617-355-8326; **Board Cert:** Surgery 2002; Pediatric Surgery 2003; **Med School:** Harvard Med Sch 1975; **Resid:** Surgery, Massachusetts Genl Hosp 1978; Pediatric Surgery, Children's Hosp 1985; **Fellow:** Surgical Oncology, NCI-Surgical Branch 1980; **Fac Appt:** Prof S, Harvard Med Sch

Tracy Jr, Thomas F MD [PS] - **Spec Exp:** Hepatobiliary Surgery; Endoscopic Surgery; Fetal Surgery; Hirschsprung's Disease; **Hospital:** Rhode Island Hosp, Women & Infants Hosp of RI; **Address:** 2 Dudley St, Ste 190, Providence, RI 02905; **Phone:** 401-421-1939; **Board Cert:** Surgery 2006; Pediatric Surgery 2006; **Med School:** Israel 1981; **Resid:** Surgery, Med Coll Virginia 1986; **Fellow:** Pediatric Surgery, Columbia Presby Med Ctr 1988; **Fac Appt:** Prof S, Brown Univ

Mid Atlantic

Adzick, N Scott MD [PS] - **Spec Exp:** Fetal Surgery; Congenital Hyperinsulinism; Neonatal Surgery; Twin to Twin Transfusion Syndrome (TTTS); **Hospital:** Chldns Hosp of Philadelphia; **Address:** 34th St & Civic Center Blvd, Wood Bldg Fl 5 - Ste 5113, Philadelphia, PA 19104-4399; **Phone:** 215-590-2727; **Board Cert:** Surgery 2006; Pediatric Surgery 2007; **Med School:** Harvard Med Sch 1979; **Resid:** Surgery, Mass Genl Hosp 1986; Pediatric Surgery, Chldns Hosp 1988; **Fellow:** Research, UCSF Med Ctr 1985; **Fac Appt:** Prof S, Univ Pennsylvania

Alexander, Frederick MD [PS] - **Spec Exp:** Inflammatory Bowel Disease; Solid Tumors; Congenital Anomalies-Gastrointestinal; **Hospital:** Hackensack Univ Med Ctr; **Address:** 30 W Century Rd Fl 2 - Ste 235, Paramas, NJ 07652; **Phone:** 201-225-9440; **Board Cert:** Pediatric Surgery 1999; **Med School:** Columbia P&S 1977; **Resid:** Surgery, Brigham-Womens Hosp 1984; **Fellow:** Pediatric Surgery, Chldns Hosp 1986; **Fac Appt:** Clin Prof S

Colombani, Paul M MD [PS] - **Spec Exp:** Pediatric Cardiothoracic Surgery; Transplant-Kidney; Transplant-Liver; Cancer Surgery; **Hospital:** Johns Hopkins Hosp (page 61); **Address:** Johns Hopkins Hosp, Ped Surgery, 600 N Wolfe St, Harvey Bldg - rm 319, Baltimore, MD 21287; **Phone:** 410-955-5210; **Board Cert:** Surgery 2003; Pediatric Surgery 2003; **Med School:** Univ KY Coll Med 1976; **Resid:** Surgery, Geo Wash Univ Hosp 1981; **Fellow:** Pediatric Surgery, Johns Hopkins Hosp 1983; **Fac Appt:** Prof S, Johns Hopkins Univ

Dolgin, Stephen MD [PS] - **Spec Exp:** Neonatal Surgery; Ulcerative Colitis; Inflammatory Bowel Disease/Crohn's; Ovarian Masses in Children/Adolescents; **Hospital:** Steven & Alexandra Cohen Chldn's Med Ctr of NY (page 67), N Shore Univ Hosp (page 67); **Address:** Cohen Chldn's Med Ctr, Pediatric Surgery, 269-01 76th Ave, Ste 158, New Hyde Park, NY 11040; **Phone:** 718-470-3636; **Board Cert:** Surgery 2011; Pediatric Surgery 2003; Surgical Critical Care 2000; **Med School:** NYU Sch Med 1977; **Resid:** Surgery, Peter Bent Brigham Hosp/Harvard Univ 1982; **Fellow:** Pediatric Surgery, Chldns Meml Hosp/Northwestern Univ 1984; **Fac Appt:** Prof S, Hofstra N Shore-LIJ Sch Med

Flake, Alan W MD [PS] - **Spec Exp:** Fetal Surgery; Stem Cell Transplant-Fetal; Neonatal Surgery; **Hospital:** Chldns Hosp of Philadelphia; **Address:** Dept Pediatric Surgery, 34th St & Civic Center Blvd, Wood Bldg - Ste 5113, Philadelphia, PA 19104; **Phone:** 215-590-2744; **Board Cert:** Surgery 2010; Pediatric Surgery 2011; **Med School:** Univ Ark 1981; **Resid:** Surgery, UCSF Med Ctr 1988; **Fellow:** Pediatric Surgery, Chldns Hosp Med Ctr 1990; **Fac Appt:** Prof S, Univ Pennsylvania

Gaines, Barbara A MD [PS] - **Spec Exp:** Trauma; Critical Care; Minimally Invasive Surgery; **Hospital:** Chldns Hosp of Pittsburgh - UPMC; **Address:** Chldn's Hosp Pittsburgh, One Chldn's Hosp Drive, 4401 Penn Ave, Faculty Pavilion Fl 7, Pittsburgh, PA 15224; **Phone:** 412-692-8288; **Board Cert:** Surgery 2007; Surgical Critical Care 2007; Pediatric Surgery 2009; **Med School:** Univ VA Sch Med 1990; **Resid:** Surgery, Vanderbilt Univ Hosp 1995; **Fellow:** Pediatric Surgery, Children's Hosp 1998; **Fac Appt:** Asst Prof S, Univ Pittsburgh

Ginsburg, Howard B MD [PS] - **Spec Exp:** Neonatal Surgery; Tumor Surgery; Pediatric Urology; Gastrointestinal Surgery; **Hospital:** NYU Langone Med Ctr (page 68), Bellevue Hosp Ctr; **Address:** 530 First Ave, Ste 10W, New York, NY 10016-6402; **Phone:** 212-263-7391; **Board Cert:** Pediatric Surgery 2001; **Med School:** Univ Cincinnati 1972; **Resid:** Surgery, NYU-Bellvue Hosp 1977; Pediatric Surgery, Columbia-Presby Med Ctr 1979; **Fellow:** Pediatric Surgery, Mass Genl Hosp 1980; **Fac Appt:** Assoc Prof PS, NYU Sch Med

Gittes, George K MD [PS] - **Spec Exp:** Gastrointestinal Surgery; **Hospital:** Chldns Hosp of Pittsburgh - UPMC; **Address:** Childrens Hosp Pittsburgh, Dept Surgery, 4401 Penn Ave, Pittsburgh, PA 15224; **Phone:** 412-692-7291; **Board Cert:** Surgery 2003; Pediatric Surgery 2007; **Med School:** Harvard Med Sch 1987; **Resid:** Surgery, UCSF Med Ctr 1994; **Fellow:** Pediatric Surgery, Childrens Mercy Hosp 1995; **Fac Appt:** Prof S, Univ Pittsburgh

Glick, Philip L MD [PS] - **Spec Exp:** Robotic Surgery; Neonatal Surgery; Fetal Surgery; Chest Wall Deformities; **Hospital:** Women & Chldn's Hosp of Buffalo, The, Roswell Park Cancer Inst; **Address:** Womens & Childrens Hosp, Dept Pediatric Surgery, 219 Bryant St, Buffalo, NY 14222-2006; **Phone:** 716-878-7449; **Board Cert:** Surgery 2006; Pediatric Surgery 2009; Surgical Critical Care 1999; **Med School:** UCSF 1979; **Resid:** Surgery, UCSF Med Ctr 1985; **Fellow:** Fetal Surgery, UCSF Med Ctr 1984; Pediatric Surgery, Chldns Hosp Med Ctr 1988; **Fac Appt:** Prof S, SUNY Buffalo

Kane, Timothy D MD [PS] - **Spec Exp:** Minimally Invasive Surgery; Neonatal Surgery; **Hospital:** Chldns Natl Med Ctr; **Address:** Children's National Medical Ctr, Dept Surgery, 111 Michigan Ave NW Fl 4, Washington, DC 20010; **Phone:** 202-476-2151; **Board Cert:** Surgery 2001; Pediatric Surgery 2004; **Med School:** SUNY Upstate Med Univ 1992; **Resid:** Surgery, Univ Cincinnati Hosp 1999; **Fellow:** Pediatric Surgery, UAB Chldns Hosp 2001; **Fac Appt:** Assoc Prof S, Univ Wash

La Quaglia, Michael MD [PS] - **Spec Exp:** Cancer Surgery; Neuroblastoma; Liver Cancer; Colon & Rectal Cancer; **Hospital:** Meml Sloan-Kettering Cancer Ctr, NY-Presby/Weill Cornell Med Ctr, NY (page 66); **Address:** 1275 York Ave, Ste H1315, New York, NY 10065; **Phone:** 212-639-7002; **Board Cert:** Surgery 2003; Pediatric Surgery 2007; **Med School:** UMDNJ-NJ Med Sch, Newark 1976; **Resid:** Surgery, Mass Genl Hosp 1983; **Fellow:** Cardiothoracic Surgery, Broadgreen Ctr 1984; Pediatric Surgery, Chldns Hosp 1985; **Fac Appt:** Prof S, Cornell Univ-Weill Med Coll

Nance, Michael L MD [PS] - **Spec Exp:** Trauma; Neonatal Surgery; Brain Injury; Congenital Anomalies; **Hospital:** Chldns Hosp of Philadelphia; **Address:** Chldns Hosp of Philadelphia, Dept Surgery, 34th & Civic Ctr Blvd Wood Bldg Fl 5, Philadelphia, PA 19104; **Phone:** 215-590-5932; **Board Cert:** Surgery 2005; Surgical Critical Care 2008; Pediatric Surgery 2007; **Med School:** Louisiana State U, New Orleans 1988; **Resid:** Surgery, Hosp Univ Penn 1995; **Fellow:** Surgical Critical Care, Hosp Univ Penn 1996; Pediatric Surgery, Chldns Hosp 1997; **Fac Appt:** Prof S, Univ Pennsylvania

Quaegebeur, Jan M MD [PS] - **Spec Exp:** Arterial Switch; Heart Valve Surgery; Pediatric Cardiac Surgery; **Hospital:** Morgan Stanley Children's Hosp of NY-Presby, NY; **Address:** Morgan Stanley Chlds Hosp of NY-Presby, 3959 Broadway, Ste BN276, New York, NY 10032; **Phone:** 212-305-5975; **Med School:** Belgium 1969; **Resid:** Surgery, St Michel Clinic 1973; **Fellow:** Thoracic Surgery, Baylor Coll Med 1974; Thoracic Surgery, Univ Hosp 1978; **Fac Appt:** Prof S, Columbia P&S

Schwartz, Marshall Z MD [PS] - **Spec Exp:** Gastrointestinal Surgery; Neonatal Surgery; Transplant-Kidney; Inflammatory Bowel Disease; **Hospital:** St. Christopher's Hosp for Chldn, St. Luke's Hosp - Bethlehem; **Address:** St Christopher's Hosp for Chldn, Dept of Surgery, 3601 A St, Ste 2204, Philadelphia, PA 19134; **Phone:** 215-427-5292; **Board Cert:** Surgery 2009; Pediatric Surgery 1999; **Med School:** Univ Minn 1970; **Resid:** Surgery, Univ Minnesota Hosp 1972; Pediatric Surgery, Chldns Hosp Med Ctr - Harvard Med Sch 1974; **Fellow:** Surgery, Univ Minnesota Hosp 1975; **Fac Appt:** Prof S, Jefferson Med Coll

Spigland, Nitsana A MD [PS] - **Spec Exp:** Congenital Anomalies; Pediatric Thoracic Surgery; Cancer Surgery; Minimally Invasive Surgery; **Hospital:** NY-Presby/Weill Cornell Med Ctr, NY (page 66); **Address:** NY Hosp-Cornell Med Ctr, 505 E 70th St, New York, NY 10021; **Phone:** 212-746-5648; **Board Cert:** Pediatric Surgery 2003; **Med School:** NY Med Coll 1982; **Resid:** Surgery, Lenox Hill Hosp 1987; **Fellow:** Pediatric Surgery, St Justine Chldn's Hosp 1989; **Fac Appt:** Assoc Prof S, Cornell Univ-Weill Med Coll

Strauch, Eric D MD [PS] - **Spec Exp:** Pediatric Cancers; Neonatal Surgery; Conjoined Twins; **Hospital:** Univ of MD Med Ctr; **Address:** 419 W Redwood St, Ste 300, Baltimore, MD 21201; **Phone:** 410-328-5730; **Board Cert:** Surgery 2003; Pediatric Surgery 2005; **Med School:** Univ MD Sch Med 1988; **Resid:** Surgery, Univ of MD Med Ctr 1994; **Fellow:** Pediatric Surgery, John Hopkins Hosp 1996; **Fac Appt:** Assoc Prof S, Univ MD Sch Med

Stylianos, Steven MD [PS] - **Spec Exp:** Trauma; Neonatal Surgery; Chest Wall Deformities; Congenital Anomalies; **Hospital:** Steven & Alexandra Cohen Chldn's Med Ctr of NY (page 67); **Address:** 269-01 76th Ave, New Hyde Park, NY 11040; **Phone:** 718-470-3636; **Board Cert:** Surgery 2002; Pediatric Surgery 2003; **Med School:** NYU Sch Med 1983; **Resid:** Surgery, Columbia-Presby Med Ctr 1988; Pediatric Surgery, Chldns Hosp 1992; **Fellow:** Pediatric Trauma, New England Med Ctr 1990; **Fac Appt:** Prof S, FIU Coll Med

Velcek, Francisca T MD [PS] - **Spec Exp:** Anorectal Malformations; Pediatric Gynecology; Neonatal Surgery; Hernia; **Hospital:** Lenox Hill Hosp (page 67), SUNY Downstate Med Ctr (Univ Hosp of Bklyn) - LICH; **Address:** 965 5th Ave, New York, NY 10075; **Phone:** 212-744-9396; **Board Cert:** Surgery 1974; Pediatric Surgery 2007; **Med School:** Philippines 1966; **Resid:** Surgery, St Clares Hosp 1971; Pediatric Surgery, SUNY Downstate Med Ctr 1975; **Fellow:** Pediatric Surgery, SUNY Downstate Med Ctr 1973; **Fac Appt:** Prof S, SUNY Hlth Sci Ctr

Voigt, Roger W MD [PS] - **Spec Exp:** Minimally Invasive Surgery; Neonatal Surgery; Pediatric Urology; **Hospital:** Univ of MD Med Ctr; **Address:** UMMC, Dept Pediatric Surgery, 22 S Greene St, N4E37, Baltimore, MD 21201; **Phone:** 410-328-5730; **Med School:** New Zealand 1980; **Resid:** Surgery, Univ Aukland 1984; **Fellow:** Pediatric Surgery, Royal Children's Hosp; Pediatric Urology, Univ Maryland Med Ctr; **Fac Appt:** Asst Prof S, Univ MD Sch Med

Southeast

Bond, Sheldon J MD [PS] - **Spec Exp:** Pediatric Cancers; Fetal Surgery; Trauma; **Hospital:** Univ of Louisville Hosp, Kosair Chldn's Hosp; **Address:** University Pediatric Surgery Assocs, 234 E Gray St, Medical Tower South, Ste 766, Louisville, KY 40202; **Phone:** 502-583-7337; **Board Cert:** Surgery 2008; Pediatric Surgery 2009; Surgical Critical Care 2001; **Med School:** Med Coll Wisc 1983; **Resid:** Surgery, Univ Louisville Med Ctr 1989; **Fellow:** Fetal Surgery, UCSF Med Ctr; Pediatric Surgery, Chldns Natl Med Ctr 1991; **Fac Appt:** Prof S, Univ Louisville Sch Med

Chen, Mike K MD [PS] - **Spec Exp:** Gastrointestinal Surgery; Transplant Surgery-Pediatric; **Hospital:** Children's Hospital - Birmingham; **Address:** UAB Pediatric Surgery, 1600 7th Ave S, ACC 300, Birmingham, AL 35233; **Phone:** 205-939-9688; **Board Cert:** Surgery 2003; Pediatric Surgery 2007; **Med School:** Univ Tex, Houston 1987; **Resid:** Surgery, Univ Fla/Shands Med Ctr 1993; **Fellow:** Transplant Surgery, Univ Fla/Shands Med Ctr 1994; Pediatric Surgery, Univ Tennessee Med Ctr 1996

Davidoff, Andrew M MD [PS] - **Spec Exp:** Neuroblastoma; Cancer Surgery; **Hospital:** St. Jude Children's Research Hosp, Le Bonheur Chldns Med Ctr; **Address:** St Jude Chldns Rsch Hosp, Dept Surg, 262 Danny Thomas Pl, MS 133, Memphis, TN 38105; **Phone:** 901-595-4060; **Board Cert:** Surgery 2005; Pediatric Surgery 2007; **Med School:** Univ Pennsylvania 1987; **Resid:** Surgery, Duke Med Ctr 1994; **Fellow:** Pediatric Surgery, Chldns Hosp 1996; **Fac Appt:** Assoc Prof S, Univ Tenn Coll Med

Fallat, Mary E MD [PS] - **Spec Exp:** Trauma; Burn Care; **Hospital:** Kosair Chldn's Hosp, Univ of Louisville Hosp; **Address:** 234 E Gray St, Ste 766, MS 40202, University Pediatric Surgery Associates, Louisville, KY 40202; **Phone:** 502-583-7337; **Board Cert:** Surgery 2005; **Med School:** SUNY Upstate Med Univ 1979; **Resid:** Surgery, Univ Louisville Med Ctr 1985; **Fellow:** Research, Mass Genl Hosp 1983; Pediatric Surgery, Chldns Natl Med Ctr 1987; **Fac Appt:** Prof S, Univ Louisville Sch Med

Morgan III, Walter M MD [PS] - **Spec Exp:** Germ Cell Tumors; Neuroblastoma; Bone Cancer; Congenital Anomalies; **Hospital:** Vanderbilt Monroe Carrell Jr. Chldn's Hosp (page 75), Vanderbilt Univ Med Ctr (page 75); **Address:** Vanderbilt Dept Pediatric Surgery, 2200 Children's Way, 7100 Doctors Office Tower, Nashville, TN 37232-9780; **Phone:** 615-936-1050; **Board Cert:** Pediatric Surgery 2001; **Med School:** Vanderbilt Univ 1982; **Resid:** Surgery, Johns Hopkins Hosp 1988; **Fellow:** Pediatric Surgery, Johns Hopkins Hosp 1990; **Fac Appt:** Asst Prof S, Vanderbilt Univ

Nakayama, Don K MD [PS] - **Spec Exp:** Neonatal Surgery; Minimally Invasive Surgery; **Hospital:** Med Ctr of Central GA; **Address:** 777 Hemlock St, MSC 140, Macon, GA 31201; **Phone:** 478-633-1367; **Board Cert:** Surgery 2003; Pediatric Surgery 2005; **Med School:** UCSF 1978; **Resid:** Surgery, UCSF Hosps 1984; **Fellow:** Pediatric Surgery, Childrens Hosp 1986; **Fac Appt:** Prof S, Mercer Univ Sch Med

Paidas, Charles N MD [PS] - **Spec Exp:** Pediatric Cancers; Chest Wall Deformities; Transplant Surgery-Pediatric; Hernia; **Hospital:** Tampa Genl Hosp; **Address:** USF Dept Surgery, 2 Tampa Cir, Tampa, FL 33606; **Phone:** 813-259-0929; **Board Cert:** Surgery 2010; Pediatric Surgery 2011; Surgical Critical Care 2002; **Med School:** NY Med Coll 1981; **Resid:** Surgery, NY Med Coll Affil Hosps 1987; **Fellow:** Pediatric Surgery, Johns Hopkins Hosp 1991; **Fac Appt:** Prof S, Univ S Fla Coll Med

Rice, Henry MD [PS] - **Spec Exp:** Neonatal Surgery; Cancer Surgery; **Hospital:** Duke Univ Hosp; **Address:** Duke Univ Med Ctr, Dept Ped Surg, DUMC, Box 3815, Durham, NC 27710; **Phone:** 919-681-5077; **Board Cert:** Surgery 2006; Pediatric Surgery 2009; **Med School:** Yale Univ 1988; **Resid:** Surgery, Univ Wash Affil Hosps 1996; **Fellow:** Pediatric Surgery, Chldns Hosp of Buffalo 1998; **Fac Appt:** Assoc Prof S, Duke Univ

Pediatric Surgery

Ricketts, Richard R MD [PS] - **Spec Exp:** Neonatal Surgery; Cancer Surgery; Gastrointestinal Surgery; Hirschsprung's Disease; **Hospital:** Chldns Hlthcare Atlanta @ Egleston, Chldns Hlthcare Atlanta @ Scottish Rite; **Address:** Emory Univ-CHOA Div Pediatric Surgery, 1975 Century Blvd, Ste 6, Atlanta, GA 30345; **Phone:** 404-982-9938; **Board Cert:** Surgery 2004; Pediatric Surgery 2001; **Med School:** Northwestern Univ 1973; **Resid:** Surgery, LAC-USC Med Ctr 1978; **Fellow:** Pediatric Surgery, Chldns Meml Hosp 1980; **Fac Appt:** Prof S, Emory Univ

Rodgers, Bradley M MD [PS] - **Spec Exp:** Pediatric Thoracic Surgery; Neonatal Surgery; Minimally Invasive Surgery; **Hospital:** Univ of Virginia Health Sys; **Address:** Box 800709, Charlottesville, VA 22908; **Phone:** 434-924-2673; **Board Cert:** Surgery 1997; Pediatric Surgery 2005; Thoracic Surgery 1975; **Med School:** Johns Hopkins Univ 1966; **Resid:** Surgery, Duke Univ Med Ctr 1968; Cardiothoracic Surgery, Duke Univ Med Ctr 1973; **Fellow:** Pediatric Surgery, Chldns Hosp 1974; **Fac Appt:** Prof S, Univ VA Sch Med

Shochat, Stephen J MD [PS] - **Spec Exp:** Cancer Surgery; Chest Wall Deformities; Pediatric Cancers; **Hospital:** St. Jude Children's Research Hosp; **Address:** St Jude Childrens Research Hosp, Dept Surgery, 262 Danny Thomas Pl, MS 133, Memphis, TN 38105; **Phone:** 901-595-2911; **Board Cert:** Surgery 1969; Thoracic & Cardiac Surgery 1975; Pediatric Surgery 2005; **Med School:** Med Coll VA 1963; **Resid:** Surgery, Barnes Hosp 1968; Pediatric Surgery, Boston Chldns Hosp 1970; **Fellow:** Thoracic Surgery, George Washington Univ 1974; **Fac Appt:** Prof S, Univ Tenn Coll Med

Midwest

Aiken, John J MD [PS] - **Spec Exp:** Tumor Surgery; Chest Wall Deformities; Hernia; Solid Tumors; **Hospital:** Chldns Hosp - Wisconsin; **Address:** 999 N 92nd St, Ste C-320, Milwaukee, WI 53226; **Phone:** 414-266-6550; **Board Cert:** Surgery 2004; Pediatric Surgery 2010; **Med School:** Univ Cincinnati 1984; **Resid:** Surgery, Mass Genl Hosp 1991; **Fellow:** Pediatric Surgery, Chldns Hosp 1993; **Fac Appt:** Assoc Prof S, Med Coll Wisc

Andrews, Walter S MD [PS] - **Spec Exp:** Transplant-Liver; Transplant-Kidney; **Hospital:** Chldns Mercy Hosps & Clinics; **Address:** Chldns Mercy Hosp, Surg Clin, 2401 Gillham Rd, Kansas City, MO 64108; **Phone:** 816-234-3199; **Board Cert:** Surgery 2002; Pediatric Surgery 2003; **Med School:** Boston Univ 1975; **Resid:** Surgery, Univ CO Hlth Science Ctr 1981; Pediatric Surgery, Univ Pittsburgh Med Ctr 1983; **Fellow:** Transplant Surgery, Univ Pittsburgh Med Ctr 1984; **Fac Appt:** Prof S, Univ MO-Kansas City

Arensman, Robert MD [PS] - **Spec Exp:** Congenital Anomalies; **Hospital:** Alexian Brothers Med Ctr; **Address:** Alexian Brothers Pediatric Surgery, 1555 Barrington Rd Bldg 1 - Ste 415, Hoffman Estates, IL 60169; **Phone:** 847-490-4222; **Board Cert:** Pediatric Surgery 2010; **Med School:** Univ IL Coll Med 1969; **Resid:** Surgery, Univ Illinois Med Ctr 1972; Surgery, Univ Illinois Med Ctr 1976; **Fellow:** Pediatric Surgery, Chldns Natl Med Ctr 1978; Surgical Research, Boston Chldn's Hosp

Barksdale Jr, Edward M MD [PS] - **Spec Exp:** Gastrointestinal Surgery; Nutrition in Bowel Disorders; Neuroblastoma; Minimally Invasive Surgery; **Hospital:** UH Rainbow Babies & Chldns Hosp (page 74); **Address:** Rainbow Babies & Children's Hosp, 11100 Euclid Ave, rm 122, Cleveland, OH 44106; **Phone:** 216-844-8623; **Board Cert:** Surgery 2002; Pediatric Surgery 2003; **Med School:** Harvard Med Sch 1984; **Resid:** Surgery, Mass Genl Hosp 1992; Pediatric Surgery, Chldns Hosp 1994; **Fellow:** Surgical Research, Mass Genl Hosp 1989; **Fac Appt:** Prof S, Ohio State Univ

Bove, Edward L MD [PS] - **Spec Exp:** Pediatric Cardiothoracic Surgery; Hypoplastic Left Heart Syndrome; Congenital Heart Surgery; **Hospital:** Univ of Michigan Hosp; **Address:** 1500 E Med Ctr Drive, 5144 CVC, Ann Arbor, MI 48109-5864; **Phone:** 734-936-4980; **Board Cert:** Thoracic Surgery 2009; Congenital Cardiac Surgery 2009; **Med School:** Albany Med Coll 1972; **Resid:** Surgery, Univ Mich Med Ctr 1976; Thoracic Surgery, Univ Mich Med Ctr 1979; **Fellow:** Pediatric Cardiac Surgery, Hosp Sick Chldn 1980; **Fac Appt:** Prof S, Univ Mich Med Sch

Dillon, Patrick A MD [PS] - **Spec Exp:** Pediatric Cancers; Trauma; Gastrointestinal Disorders; Congenital Anomalies; **Hospital:** St. Louis Chldns Hosp, Barnes-Jewish Hosp; **Address:** St Louis Chldns Hosp, 1 Chldns Pl, Ste 5 South 40, St Louis, MO 63110; **Phone:** 314-454-6022; **Board Cert:** Surgery 2004; Pediatric Surgery 2007; **Med School:** Georgetown Univ 1988; **Resid:** Surgery, Barnes Hosp 1995; **Fellow:** Pediatric Surgery, Johns Hopkins Hosp 1997; **Fac Appt:** Assoc Prof S, Washington Univ, St Louis

Ehrlich, Peter F MD [PS] - **Spec Exp:** Pediatric Cancers; Wilms' Tumor; Thyroid Cancer; **Hospital:** Mott Chldns Hosp; **Address:** Mott Children's Hospital, 1540 E Hospital Drive, rm SPC 4217, Ann Arbor, MI 48109; **Phone:** 734-764-4151; **Board Cert:** Surgery 2007; Pediatric Surgery 2009; **Med School:** Canada 1989; **Resid:** Surgery, Univ Toronto Med Ctr 1996; **Fellow:** Pediatric Surgery, Children's Natl Med Ctr 1998; **Fac Appt:** Assoc Prof S, Univ Mich Med Sch

Holterman, Mark J MD [PS] - **Spec Exp:** Minimally Invasive Surgery; Neonatal Surgery; Head & Neck Surgery; Congenital Anomalies; **Hospital:** OSF Saint Francis Med Ctr; **Address:** Chdn's Hosp Illinois, 420 NE Glen Oak Ave, Hillcrest Bldg - Ste 201, Peoria, IL 61637; **Phone:** 309-655-2343; **Board Cert:** Surgery 2001; Pediatric Surgery 2007; **Med School:** Univ VA Sch Med 1988; **Resid:** Surgery, Univ Virginia Hosp 1993; **Fellow:** Pediatric Surgery, Chldns Hosp & Med Ctr 1993; **Fac Appt:** Assoc Prof S, Univ IL Coll Med

Moss, R Lawrence MD [PS] - **Spec Exp:** Congenital Anomalies; Cancer Surgery; Minimally Invasive Surgery; **Hospital:** Nationwide Chldn's Hosp; **Address:** 700 Children's Drive, OCC Bldg - Fl 7th, rm FMB132, Columbus, OH 43205; **Phone:** 614-722-5163; **Board Cert:** Surgery 2010; Pediatric Surgery 2003; Surgical Critical Care 2011; **Med School:** UCSD 1986; **Resid:** Surgery, Virginia Mason Med Ctr 1991; Surgical Critical Care, Chldns Meml Hosp 1992; **Fellow:** Pediatric Surgery, Chldns Meml Hosp 1994; **Fac Appt:** Prof S, Yale Univ

Oldham, Keith T MD [PS] - **Spec Exp:** Neonatal Surgery; Pediatric Thoracic Surgery; Gastrointestinal Surgery; **Hospital:** Chldns Hosp - Wisconsin; **Address:** 9000 W Wisconsin Ave, Milwaukee, WI 53201; **Phone:** 414-266-6550; **Board Cert:** Surgery 2000; Pediatric Surgery 2009; **Med School:** Med Coll VA 1976; **Resid:** Surgery, Univ Wash Med Ctr 1981; **Fellow:** Pediatric Surgery, Univ Cincinnati Chldns Hosp 1983; **Fac Appt:** Prof S, Med Coll Wisc

Pena, Alberto MD [PS] - **Spec Exp:** Imperforate Anus; Anorectal Malformations; Colon & Rectal Surgery; **Hospital:** Cincinnati Chldns Hosp Med Ctr; **Address:** Cincinnati Chlds Hosp Med Ctr, 3333 Burnet Ave, ML 2023, Cincinnati, OH 45229; **Phone:** 513-636-3240; **Med School:** Mexico 1962; **Resid:** Surgery, Military Hosp 1966; **Fellow:** Pediatric Surgery, Childrens Hosp 1971; Cardiovascular Surgery, Childrens Hosp 1969

Rescorla, Frederick J MD [PS] - **Spec Exp:** Neonatal Surgery; Cancer Surgery; Head & Neck Surgery; Gastrointestinal Surgery; **Hospital:** Riley Hosp for Children; **Address:** Riley Hospital for Children, 705 Riley Hospital Drive, rm 2500, Indianapolis, IN 46202; **Phone:** 317-274-4681; **Board Cert:** Surgery 2004; Surgical Critical Care 2009; Pediatric Surgery 2007; **Med School:** Univ Wisc 1981; **Resid:** Surgery, Indiana Univ Med Ctr 1986; Pediatric Surgery, Indiana Univ Med Ctr 1988; **Fac Appt:** Prof S, Indiana Univ

Pediatric Surgery

Reynolds, Marleta MD [PS] - **Spec Exp:** Critical Care; Trauma; Congenital Anomalies; Pediatric Cancers; **Hospital:** Lurie Chldn's Hosp-Chicago; **Address:** Lurie Chldns Hosp, Dept Ped Surg, 225 E Chicago Ave, Box 63, Chicago, IL 60611; **Phone:** 312-227-4210; **Board Cert:** Surgery 2001; Pediatric Surgery 2003; Thoracic & Cardiac Surgery 2006; **Med School:** Tulane Univ 1976; **Resid:** Surgery, Tulane Univ Affil Hosp 1981; Pediatric Surgery, Chldns Meml Hosp 1983; **Fellow:** Cardiothoracic Surgery, Northwestern Univ 1985; **Fac Appt:** Prof S, Northwestern Univ

Sato, Thomas T MD [PS] - **Spec Exp:** Neonatal Surgery; Congenital Anomalies; **Hospital:** Chldns Hosp - Wisconsin; **Address:** 999 N 92nd St, Ste C320, Milwaukee, WI 53226; **Phone:** 414-607-5280; **Board Cert:** Surgery 2006; Pediatric Surgery 2007; **Med School:** USC Sch Med 1988; **Resid:** Surgery, Univ Wash Med Ctr 1995; Pediatric Surgery, Chldns Natl Med Ctr 1997; **Fellow:** Trauma, Harborview Med Ctr 1993; **Fac Appt:** Prof S, Med Coll Wisc

Warner, Brad MD [PS] - **Spec Exp:** Gastrointestinal Surgery; Neonatal Surgery; Pediatric Cancers; Short Bowel Syndrome; **Hospital:** St. Louis Chldns Hosp; **Address:** 1 Children's Pl, Ste 5S40, St Louis, MO 63110; **Phone:** 314-454-6022; **Board Cert:** Surgery 2009; Pediatric Surgery 2011; **Med School:** Univ MO-Kansas City 1982; **Resid:** Surgery, Univ Cincinnati Med Ctr 1989; **Fellow:** Pediatric Surgery, Chldns Hosp Med Ctr 1991; **Fac Appt:** Prof S, Univ Cincinnati

Weber, Thomas R MD [PS] - **Spec Exp:** Neonatal Surgery; Short Bowel Syndrome; Chest Wall Deformities; **Hospital:** Rush Univ Med Ctr, Rush Children's Hosp; **Address:** 1725 W Harrison St, Professional Bldg, Ste 710, Chicago, IL 60612; **Phone:** 708-684-2016; **Board Cert:** Surgery 2001; Pediatric Surgery 2011; Surgical Critical Care 2002; **Med School:** Ohio State Univ 1971; **Resid:** Surgery, Univ MI Hosp & Hlth Ctr 1976; **Fellow:** Pediatric Surgery, Chldns Natl Med Ctr 1979; **Fac Appt:** Prof S, Rush Med Coll

Great Plains and Mountains

Crombleholme, Timothy M MD [PS] - **Spec Exp:** Fetal Surgery; Twin to Twin Transfusion Syndrome (TTTS); **Hospital:** Chldn's Hosp - Aurora (CO); **Address:** Chldn's Hosp of CO, Pediatric Surgery, 13123 E 16th Ave, Box 323, Cincinnati, CO 80045-7106; **Phone:** 720-777-6571; **Board Cert:** Surgery 2003; Pediatric Surgery 2007; **Med School:** Tufts Univ 1984; **Resid:** Surgery, UCSF Med Ctr 1991; **Fellow:** Pediatric Surgery, Tufts-New England Med Ctr 1993; **Fac Appt:** Prof S, Univ Cincinnati

Karrer, Frederick M MD [PS] - **Spec Exp:** Liver Surgery; Transplant-Liver; Critical Care; Neonatal Surgery; **Hospital:** Chldn's Hosp - Aurora (CO), Denver Health Med Ctr; **Address:** Chldn's Hosp, Dept Surgery, 13123 E 16th Ave, Box B323, Aurora, CO 80045; **Phone:** 720-777-6571; **Board Cert:** Surgery 2007; Pediatric Surgery 2009; **Med School:** Univ Nebr Coll Med 1979; **Resid:** Surgery, Univ Ariz Med Ctr 1984; Pediatric Surgery, Chldns Meml Hosp 1986; **Fellow:** Transplant Surgery, Univ Pittsburgh Affil Hosp 1988; **Fac Appt:** Prof S, Univ Colorado

Meyers, Rebecka L MD [PS] - **Spec Exp:** Transplant-Liver; Tumor Surgery; Biliary Surgery; Pancreatic Surgery; **Hospital:** Primary Children's Med Ctr, Univ Utah Hlth Care; **Address:** Primary Chlds Med Ctr, Dept Ped Surg, 100 N Mario Capecchi Drive, Ste 2600, Salt Lake City, UT 84113-1103; **Phone:** 801-662-2950; **Board Cert:** Surgery 2003; Pediatric Surgery 2005; **Med School:** Oregon Hlth & Sci Univ 1985; **Resid:** Surgery, UCSF Med Ctr 1990; **Fellow:** Research, Cardio Rsch Inst-UCSF 1992; Pediatric Surgery, St Christophers Hosp for Chldn 1994; **Fac Appt:** Assoc Prof S, Univ Utah

Southwest

Black, C Thomas MD [PS] - **Spec Exp:** Neonatal Surgery; Minimally Invasive Surgery; Chest Wall Deformities; **Hospital:** Cook Chldns Med Ctr; **Address:** 7000 W Plano Pkwy, Ste 200, Plano, TX 75093; **Phone:** 214-483-9300; **Board Cert:** Pediatric Surgery 2007; Surgery 2005; **Med School:** Baylor Coll Med 1979; **Resid:** Surgery, Baylor College Affil Hosp 1984; **Fellow:** Pediatric Surgery, Riley Childrens Hospital 1985; Pediatric Surgery-ECMO, Chldn's Meml Hosp 1987

Cass, Darrell L MD [PS] - **Spec Exp:** Fetal Surgery; Neonatal Surgery; Chest Wall Deformities; **Hospital:** Texas Chldns Hosp, St. Luke's Episcopal Hosp-Houston; **Address:** Clinical Care Ctr, 6701 Fannin St, Ste 1210, Houston, TX 77030-2303; **Phone:** 832-822-3135; **Board Cert:** Surgery 2010; Pediatric Surgery 2011; **Med School:** UCLA-David Geffen Sch Med 1991; **Resid:** Surgery, UCSF Med Ctr 1999; **Fellow:** Pediatric Surgery, Baylor Coll Med 2001; **Fac Appt:** Assoc Prof PS, Baylor Coll Med

Foglia, Robert P MD [PS] - **Spec Exp:** Congenital Anomalies; Burn Care; Gastroesophageal Reflux Disease (GERD); **Hospital:** Chldns Med Ctr of Dallas; **Address:** 1935 Medical District Drive, Ste B3250, Dallas, TX 75235; **Phone:** 214-456-6040; **Board Cert:** Surgery 2002; Pediatric Surgery 2005; Surgical Critical Care 1993; **Med School:** Georgetown Univ 1974; **Resid:** Surgery, UCLA Med Ctr 1981; **Fellow:** Pediatric Surgery, Chldns Hosp Natl Med Ctr 1983; **Fac Appt:** Prof S, Univ Tex SW, Dallas

Graziano, Kathleen D MD [PS] - **Spec Exp:** Congenital Reproductive Anomalies; Sexual Anomalies; **Hospital:** Phoenix Children's Hosp; **Address:** Pediatric Surgeons of Phoenix, 1920 E Cambridge Ave, Ste 201, Phoenix, AZ 85006; **Phone:** 602-254-5561; **Board Cert:** Surgery 2004; Pediatric Surgery 2006; **Med School:** Columbia P&S 1996; **Resid:** Surgery, Univ Michigan Med Ctr 2003; **Fellow:** Pediatric Surgery, Univ MI/CS Mott Chldns Hosp 2005

Jackson, Richard J MD [PS] - **Spec Exp:** Pediatric Cancers; Neonatal Surgery; Robotic Surgery; **Hospital:** Arkansas Chldns Hosp; **Address:** Arkansas Children's Hospital, 1 Children's Way, Slot 837, Little Rock, AR 72202-3591; **Phone:** 501-364-1446; **Board Cert:** Surgery 2008; Pediatric Surgery 2001; Surgical Critical Care 1998; **Med School:** W VA Univ 1983; **Resid:** Surgery, W Va Univ Hosps 1988; Pediatric Surgery, Chldns Hosp 1989; **Fellow:** Surgical Critical Care, Chldns Hosp-Univ Pittsburgh 1990; Pediatric Surgery, Chldns Hosp-Univ Pittsburgh 1992

McGill, Leigh C MD [PS] - **Spec Exp:** Congenital Anomalies; **Hospital:** Phoenix Children's Hosp, St. Joseph's Hosp & Med Ctr - Phoenix; **Address:** 1920 E Cambridge Ave, Ste 201, Phoenix, AZ 85006; **Phone:** 602-254-5561; **Board Cert:** Pediatric Surgery 2011; **Med School:** Univ Colorado 1976; **Resid:** Surgery, Maricopa Co General Hosp 1981; **Fellow:** Pediatric Surgery, Denver Childrens Hosp 1983; Pediatric Urology, Royal Children's Hosp; **Fac Appt:** Asst Clin Prof S, Univ Ariz Coll Med

Notrica, David MD [PS] - **Spec Exp:** Biliary Surgery; Inflammatory Bowel Disease; Laparoscopic Surgery-Complex; Hirschsprung's Disease; **Hospital:** Phoenix Children's Hosp, St. Joseph's Hosp & Med Ctr - Phoenix; **Address:** Pediatric Surgeons of Phoenix, 1920 E Cambridge Ave, Ste 201, Phoenix, AZ 85006; **Phone:** 602-254-5561; **Board Cert:** Surgery 2005; Pediatric Surgery 2000; **Med School:** Emory Univ 1992; **Resid:** Surgery, Emory Univ Hosps 1997; **Fellow:** Pediatric Surgery, Texas Chldns Hosp 1999; **Fac Appt:** Asst Clin Prof S, Univ Ariz Coll Med

Nuchtern, Jed G MD [PS] - **Spec Exp:** Pediatric Thoracic Surgery; Cancer Surgery; Laparoscopic Surgery; **Hospital:** Texas Chldns Hosp, Ben Taub Genl Hosp; **Address:** Texas Children's Hosp, 6701 Fannin St, MC CCC1210, Houston, TX 77030; **Phone:** 832-822-3135; **Board Cert:** Surgery 2003; Surgical Critical Care 2002; Pediatric Surgery 2007; **Med School:** Harvard Med Sch 1985; **Resid:** Surgery, Univ Washington Med ctr 1992; Pediatric Surgery, Baylor Affil Hosp 1995; **Fellow:** Cellular Molecular Biology, Natl Inst Hlth 1990; **Fac Appt:** Prof S, Baylor Coll Med

Pediatric Surgery

Skinner, Michael A MD [PS] - **Spec Exp:** Endocrine Cancers; Thyroid Cancer; **Hospital:** UT Southwestern Med Ctr at Dallas; **Address:** UT Southwestern Med Ctr at Dallas, 1935 Medical District Drive, MC B3.01, Dallas, TX 75235; **Phone:** 214-456-6040; **Board Cert:** Surgery 2010; Pediatric Surgery 2003; **Med School:** Rush Med Coll 1984; **Resid:** Surgery, Duke Univ Med Ctr 1991; **Fellow:** Pediatric Surgery, Indiana Univ 1993; **Fac Appt:** Assoc Prof S, Univ Tex SW, Dallas

Tuggle, David W MD [PS] - **Spec Exp:** Trauma; Critical Care; Reconstructive Surgery; **Hospital:** Chldns Hosp OU Med Ctr; **Address:** OU Div Pediatric Surgery, 1200 N Phillips Ave, Ste 2700, Oklahoma City, OK 73104; **Phone:** 405-271-4357; **Board Cert:** Surgery 2004; Pediatric Surgery 2005; Surgical Critical Care 2007; **Med School:** Univ Tex SW, Dallas 1979; **Resid:** Surgery, Parkland Meml Hosp 1985; Pediatric Surgery, Chldns Meml Hosp 1987; **Fac Appt:** Prof S, Univ Okla Coll Med

West Coast and Pacific

Albanese, Craig T MD [PS] - **Spec Exp:** Fetal Surgery; Laparoscopic Surgery; Twin to Twin Transfusion Syndrome (TTTS); **Hospital:** Lucile Packard Chldn's Hosp; **Address:** 780 Welch Rd, Ste 206, MC 5733, Palo Alto, CA 94304; **Phone:** 650-724-3664; **Board Cert:** Surgery 2000; Pediatric Surgery 2003; **Med School:** SUNY Hlth Sci Ctr 1986; **Resid:** Surgery, Mt Sinai Med Ctr 1991; **Fellow:** Pediatric Surgery, Chldns Hosp 1994; **Fac Appt:** Prof S, Stanford Univ

Farmer, Diana MD [PS] - **Spec Exp:** Pediatric Cancers; Fetal Surgery; Spina Bifida; Twin to Twin Transfusion Syndrome (TTTS); **Hospital:** UC Davis Med Ctr; **Address:** 2315 Stockton Blvd, Sacramento, CA 95817; **Phone:** 916-734-2011; **Board Cert:** Surgery 2001; Pediatric Surgery 2005; **Med School:** Univ Wash 1983; **Resid:** Surgery, UCSF Med Ctr 1993; **Fellow:** Pediatric Surgery, Childrens Hosp 1995; **Fac Appt:** Assoc Prof S, UCSF

Ford, Henri R MD [PS] - **Spec Exp:** Minimally Invasive Surgery; Trauma; **Hospital:** Chldns Hosp - Los Angeles, Long Beach Meml Med Ctr; **Address:** 4650 Sunset Blvd, MS 72, Los Angeles, CA 90027; **Phone:** 323-361-2104; **Board Cert:** Surgery 2002; Pediatric Surgery 2005; **Med School:** Harvard Med Sch 1984; **Resid:** Surgery, New York Hosp 1991; **Fellow:** Pediatric Surgery, Chldns Hosp Pittsburgh 1995

Grikscheit, Tracy C MD [PS] - **Spec Exp:** Congenital Anomalies; Short Bowel Syndrome; Necrotizing Enterocolitis; Neonatal Surgery; **Hospital:** Chldns Hosp - Los Angeles; **Address:** 4650 Sunset Blvd, Pediatric Surgery, MS 100, Los Angeles, CA 90027; **Phone:** 323-361-5901; **Board Cert:** Surgery 2005; Pediatric Surgery 2008; **Med School:** Columbia P&S 1997; **Resid:** Surgery, Mass General Hosp 2002; **Fellow:** Pediatric Surgery, Seattle Children's Hosp 2004; **Fac Appt:** Asst Prof S, UCLA

Healey, Patrick J MD [PS] - **Spec Exp:** Transplant Surgery-Pediatric; Transplant-Kidney; Transplant-Liver; Congenital Anomalies; **Hospital:** Seattle Chldns Hosp; **Address:** 4800 Sand Point Way, Dept Surgery, Box 359300, MS W7729, Seattle, WA 98105; **Phone:** 206-987-1800; **Board Cert:** Surgery 2002; Pediatric Surgery 2009; **Med School:** Boston Univ 1987; **Resid:** Surgery, Hartford Hosp 1992; **Fellow:** Transplant Surgery, Univ WA Med Ctr 1995; Pediatric Surgery, Chldns Hosp 1997; **Fac Appt:** Asst Prof S, Univ Wash

Hilfiker, Mary L MD/PhD [PS] - **Hospital:** Rady Children's Hosp - San Diego; **Address:** 8010 Frost St, Ste 414, San Diego, CA 92123; **Phone:** 858-966-7711; **Board Cert:** Surgery 2004; Pediatric Surgery 2007; **Med School:** Wright State Univ 1988; **Resid:** Surgery, Univ New Mexico Med Ctr 1993; **Fellow:** Pediatric Surgery, SUNY-Children's Hosp 1995; **Fac Appt:** Assoc Clin Prof S, UCSD

Krummel, Thomas M MD [PS] - **Spec Exp:** Minimally Invasive Surgery; Robotic Surgery; Fetal Surgery; **Hospital:** Lucile Packard Chldn's Hosp, Stanford Univ Hosp & Clinics; **Address:** Neurosciences & Pediatric Surgery, 750 Welch Rd Fl 2, Palo Alto, CA 94304; **Phone:** 650-724-4270; **Board Cert:** Surgery 2004; Pediatric Surgery 2007; **Med School:** Univ Wisc 1977; **Resid:** Surgery, Med Coll Va Hosp 1983; Pediatric Surgery, Chldns Hosp 1985; **Fellow:** Fetal Surgery, UCSF Med Ctr 1985; **Fac Appt:** Prof S, Stanford Univ

Lobe, Thom E MD [PS] - **Spec Exp:** Minimally Invasive Surgery; Robotic Surgery; Pediatric Urology; **Address:** 50 N La Cienega, Ste 215, Beverly Hills, CA 90211; **Phone:** 310-935-4320; **Board Cert:** Surgery 2000; Pediatric Surgery 2001; **Med School:** Univ MD Sch Med 1975; **Resid:** Surgery, Ohio State Univ Med Ctr 1979; Pediatric Surgery, Childrens Hosp 1981

Proctor, Monja L MD [PS] - **Spec Exp:** Fetal Surgery; Neonatal Surgery; Hirschsprung's Disease; **Hospital:** Swedish Med Ctr-First Hill-Seattle; **Address:** Swedish Med Ctr-Ped Spec Care, 1101 Madison St, Ste 800, Seattle, WA 98104; **Phone:** 206-215-2700; **Board Cert:** Pediatrics 2003; Pediatric Surgery 2004; **Med School:** Univ Tex SW, Dallas 1993; **Resid:** Pediatrics, Univ TX SW Meml Med Ctr 2000; **Fellow:** Pediatric Surgery, Hosp For Sick Chldn 2002

Sawin, Robert S MD [PS] - **Spec Exp:** Pediatric Cancers; Pediatric Thoracic Surgery; Neonatal Surgery-Gastrointestinal; Transplant-Liver; **Hospital:** Seattle Chldns Hosp; **Address:** Seattle Chldn's Hosp, 4800 Sand Point Way NE, MS W7729, Seattle, WA 98145-5005; **Phone:** 206-987-2039; **Board Cert:** Surgical Critical Care 2001; Pediatric Surgery 2009; **Med School:** Univ Pittsburgh 1982; **Resid:** Surgery, Brigham Women's Hosp 1987; **Fellow:** Pediatric Surgery, Chldns Hosp 1989; **Fac Appt:** Prof S, Univ Wash

Stein, James E MD [PS] - **Hospital:** Chldns Hosp - Los Angeles; **Address:** Chdns Hosp-LA, Dept Pediatric Surgery, 4650 Sunset Blvd, MS 100, Los Angeles, CA 90027; **Phone:** 323-361-2491; **Board Cert:** Surgery 2004; Pediatric Surgery 2005; **Med School:** Tufts Univ 1986; **Resid:** Surgery, Tufts New England Med Ctr 1993; **Fellow:** Pediatric Surgery, Royal Chldns Hosp 1994; Pediatric Surgery, Babies Hosp/Columbia Presby 1996; **Fac Appt:** Assoc Prof S, USC Sch Med

Waldhausen, John HT MD [PS] - **Spec Exp:** Minimally Invasive Surgery; Laparoscopic Surgery; Neonatal Surgery; Congenital Anomalies; **Hospital:** Seattle Chldns Hosp; **Address:** 4800 Sand Point Way, Dept Surgery, MS W-7729, Seattle, WA 98105; **Phone:** 206-987-2794; **Board Cert:** Surgery 2010; Pediatric Surgery 2005; **Med School:** Penn State Coll Med 1986; **Resid:** Surgery, Univ Virginia Med Ctr 1992; **Fellow:** Pediatric Surgery, Chldns Hosp Med Ctr - Washington Univ 1994; **Fac Appt:** Prof S, Univ Wash

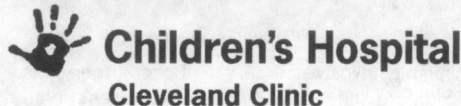
Children's Hospital
Cleveland Clinic

Pediatrics

Cleveland Clinic Children's Hospital is ranked among the best pediatric hospitals in the nation by *U.S. News & World Report*, and more than 80 pediatricians and pediatric specialists are recognized as "Best Doctors in America." Our specialists are nationally recognized for sophisticated diagnosis and innovative care for complex or chronic medical conditions. Their nationally funded research initiatives are leading to advanced treatments for young patients.

Our Center for Pediatric and Congenital Heart Diseases, the largest and most experienced in Northern Ohio, is known for groundbreaking catheter and surgical treatments. Our Department of Pediatric Gastroenterology offers breakthrough technology to diagnose and treat gastrointestinal problems. Our pediatric epilepsy specialists offer specialized diagnosis and surgery for different seizure disorders.

Children's Hospital oncologists are national leaders in the treatment of childhood cancers. Our Fetal Care Center is staffed by pediatric specialists and maternal-fetal medicine specialists who diagnose fetal problems and can treat them immediately after birth or in the womb. Our Special Delivery Unit and adjoining Pediatric Cardiac Catheterization Laboratory are key components of the Fetal Care Center.

Cleveland Clinic Children's Hospital has the only comprehensive pediatric transplant center in Northern Ohio, offering heart, lung, liver, kidney, pancreas, bone marrow and intestinal transplantation and follow-up.

Our Pediatric ICU offers outstanding outcomes, saving many more young lives than the national standard, largely due to the 24-hour presence of seasoned critical care specialists.

Our expertise in specialty pediatrics extends into the realm of long-term care for developmental, behavioral and rehabilitation needs.

Cleveland Clinic
Children's Hospital
9500 Euclid Avenue
Cleveland, OH 44195

Offering Same-Day Appointments
Call 800.274.2009.

Treatment Guides
Cleveland Clinic has developed comprehensive treatment guides for many diseases and conditions. To download our free treatment guides, visit clevelandclinic.org/treatmentguides.

Online Medical Second Opinion
Call 216.444.3223 or
800.223.2273 ext. 43223 or
email eclevelandclinic@ccf.org.

Out-of-State Patients Assistance
Call 800.223.2273, ext. 55580 or
email medicalconcierge@ccf.org.

Visit Us At:
clevelandclinicchildrens.org

Follow Us On:
Facebook
www.facebook.com/clevelandclinic

Twitter
@ClevelandClinic

You Tube
www.youtube.com/clevelandclinic

Health Hub
health.clevelandclinic.org

MOUNT SINAI
SCHOOL OF
MEDICINE

THE MOUNT SINAI MEDICAL CENTER
PEDIATRIC DIABETES AND ENDOCRINOLOGY

One Gustave L. Levy Place
Fifth Avenue and 100th Street
New York, NY 10029-6574
Physician Referral: 1-800-MD-SINAI (637-4624)
www.kravischildrenshospital.org

PEDIATRIC DIABETES AND ENDOCRINOLOGY
INNOVATIVE MEDICINE, FAMILY-CENTERED CARE

The Hall Family Center for Pediatric Endocrinology and Diabetes at Kravis Children's Hospital at Mount Sinai is dedicated to excellence in clinical care, education and research – a fact that has led to our being **named among the top 25 pediatric diabetes and endocrinology services in America,** according to *The U.S. News & World Report's* 2012-2013 ranking of "Best Children's Hospitals."

Under the direction of Robert Rapaport, M.D., Division Chief, we use a team approach, which is patient and family centered, to manage:

- Diabetes (type 1 and type 2, medication-related, monogenic and pre-diabetes)

- Short stature

- Growth disorders, including growth hormone deficiency, growth in children born small for gestational age, and early and late puberty

- Genetic disorders, including Turner Syndrome and Noonan Syndrome

- Congenital and acquired hypothyroidism and hyperthyroidism

- Hyperparathyroidism

- Congenital adrenal hyperplasia/hypoplasia

- Obesity and other nutritional disorders, including Vitamin D deficiency.

Diabetes – We offer the complete spectrum of high level diagnostic and treatment services, including simulation testing, for children and adolescents and bring families into their circle of care. Since education and support are vital to managing diabetes, we offer a variety of programs for patients and their families, including "Toddlers and Grandparents," "College Prep," for teens entering college, and a free one-week day camp in Central Park in conjunction with the Barton Center for Diabetes Education.

We are currently collaborating with four other medical centers on the **R.O.A.D. (Reduce Obesity and Diabetes)** project, to study and educate middle school children in Harlem. By identifying the metabolic factors that lead from obesity to diabetes, we will develop a protocol for detecting which children will most likely develop diabetes, allowing us to streamline interventions and identify where best to allocate resources.

Endocrine Disorders and Growth - With our faculty leading investigations into both international and multi-center trials, we enjoy a stellar reputation for identifying and treating a host of common and complex endocrine disorders, including growth hormone deficiency, growth in children born small for gestational age, and other disorders caused by Turner or Noonan Syndrome, and congenital hypothyroidism. In addition to offering expert consultations, we employ early screening methods and breakthrough growth hormone therapy that enables children to grow and develop normally.

ANNUAL SYMPOSIUM

Our physician-scientists conduct investigations into the causes and treatments of childhood endocrine conditions, and we are committed to translating research into better methods of clinical care. To that end, we hold an annual symposium each November to update pediatricians practicing within the community on the latest advances in pediatric endocrinology and diabetes.

We also excel at diagnosing and treating children with **precocious or delayed puberty** and have developed methods to identify and manage these conditions before they appear clinically obvious.

814

THE MOUNT SINAI MEDICAL CENTER
PEDIATRIC GASTROENTEROLOGY
One Gustave L. Levy Place
Fifth Avenue and 100th Street
New York, NY 10029-6574
Physician Referral: 1-800-MD-SINAI (637-4624)
www.mountsinai.org/kravis

PEDIATRIC GASTROENTEROLOGY
Innovative Medicine, Family-Centered Care

In recognition of our tradition of excellence in patient care, research and education, **Mount Sinai's Kravis Children's Hospital was named among the country's best in Pediatric Gastroenterology**, according to *U.S. News and World Report's* 2012-2013 edition of "America's Best Children's Hospitals."

Under the direction of Keith Benkov, M.D., Chief of Pediatric Gastroenterology, we deliver expert consultation and compassionate, evidence-based care to pediatric patients with common and complex digestive disorders, including inflammatory bowel disease, celiac disease, gastroesophageal reflux disease and irritable bowel syndrome.

With a reputation for providing the highest level of innovative and comprehensive care to patients with Crohn's disease and ulcerative colitis, our nationally recognized **Children's IBD Center** receives referrals from across the country. We are currently following over 500 children and have seen over 1700 patients with IBD in the last 10 years. The combination of this extensive experience, our focus on basic science and clinical research, and our collaboration with Mount Sinai's internationally renowned adult IBD program, enables us to deliver a unique approach to IBD care in children.

To optimize outcomes, our entire team of healthcare professionals participates in every patient's circle of care. We address each patient's specific needs, including management, nutrition, growth, body image and coping methods for a chronic illness. The center fosters family participation and encourages patients to gather to share ideas. Lectures, discussions and support groups are open to all families.

In addition, we continually strive to advance our knowledge of IBD and its treatments through research. In conjunction with Department of Pediatric Allergy and Immunology, we are currently investigating the benefits of an herbal medicine developed as a complementary therapy for children with Crohn's disease.

IBD runs the spectrum from mild to severe disease. No matter how seriously a child is affected, our ultimate goal is to help every child who comes to us with IBD lead a normal, productive life and achieve all his or her personal aspirations.

Mount Sinai

MOUNT SINAI
SCHOOL OF
MEDICINE

THE MOUNT SINAI MEDICAL CENTER
PEDIATRIC NEPHROLOGY AND HYPERTENSION
One Gustave L. Levy Place
Fifth Avenue and 100th Street
New York, NY 10029-6574
Physician Referral: 1-800-MD-SINAI (637-4624)
www.mountsinai.org/kravis

Pediatric Nephrology and Hypertension
Innovative Medicine, Family-Centered Care

Mount Sinai's Kravis Children's Hospital's Division of Pediatric Nephrology and Hypertension recognized as one of America's best by *U.S.News & World Report's* 2012-2013 ranking of "Best Children Hospitals."

We are recognized as one of the country's largest and most respected centers for pediatric kidney car and a pioneer in research and education. Under the direction of Jeffrey Saland, M.D., Division Chief, w deliver specialized, evidence-based care to children with kidney disease, high blood pressure, urinar tract infections and a wide variety of related conditions, both common and complex.

Our patients benefit from our multidisciplinary team of pediatric nephrologists, urologists, transplantatio specialists, psychiatrists, registered nurses, social workers, nutritionists and child life specialists workin together to deliver the most effective care. Understanding that children require a special level of suppo and service, we bring families into their circle of care, and, as our patients become young adults, we hel transition them into our excellent adult kidney program.

Our teaching and research programs in pediatric kidney disease serve to drive and maintain our expertis at the highest level. Working closely with our colleagues in diagnostic radiology and pediatric urology, w offer advanced diagnostic services and confident and experienced care for all kidney-related condition including:

• Kidney failure

• Dialysis (hemodialysis or peritoneal dialysis)

• Hypertension (high blood pressure)

• Kidney transplant, multiple organ transplant

We are a major referral center for children with high blood pressure, offering state-of-the art diagnostic such as ambulatory blood pressure monitoring (ABPM), a home-based measure that allows us to be sur hypertension is present, and we provide comprehensive treatment plans that include a focus on die physical activity, and stress factors.

As a **Center of Excellence in Transplantation**, we are one of the most sought after pediatric kidne transplant centers in the country. During the past five years, we provided kidney transplants to twic as many children as any other New York hospital, and, even more significant, the outcomes of thos transplants were superior, as verified by the Organ Procurement and Transplantation Network (OPTN and the Scientific Registry of Transplantation Recipients (SRTR), under contract from the US Departmer of Health and Human Services.

We offer fast appointments and a streamlined admitting process for admitting physicians.

**MOUNT SINAI
SCHOOL OF
MEDICINE**

THE MOUNT SINAI MEDICAL CENTER
PEDIATRIC PULMONOLOGY

One Gustave L. Levy Place
Fifth Avenue and 100th Street
New York, NY 10029-6574
Physician Referral: 1-800-MD-SINAI (637-4624)
www.kravischildrenshospital.org

PEDIATRIC PULMONOLOGY
Innovative Medicine, Family-Centered Care

At Mount Sinai's **Kravis Children's Hospital's Division of Pediatric Pulmonology**, we are dedicated to treating the full spectrum of children's respiratory illnesses, both common and complex, with a high level of skill and compassion. This dedication has led to our being **named among the top pediatric pulmonary services in America**, according to *U.S. News & World Report's* 2012-2013 ranking of "Best Children's Hospitals."

Under the direction of Alfin Vicencio, M.D., Division Chief, our team of award winning pediatric pulmonologists, nurse practitioners, nurse educators, nutritionists, social workers and respiratory therapists deliver evidence-based care to children with asthma, cystic fibrosis, chronic respiratory failure, bronchopulmonary dysplasia and other respiratory conditions.

Offering medical support and guidance, our **Children's Asthma Center** offers advanced diagnostic and treatment protocols for refractory asthma along with advanced pulmonary function testing, allergy testing, environmental assessment, nutritional evaluation, education, and family services. We teach patients and their parents or guardians to identify asthma triggers and offer a personalized asthma action plan for each patient—a process that has our patients experiencing fewer emergency department visits and hospitalizations, missing less school and enjoying more active lives. In addition, through outreach efforts and care delivered to children from East Harlem—an area with one of the highest asthma rates in the country—we have succeeded in empowering these patients to manage their disease and face the future with confidence.

To significantly enhance our pediatric flexible bronchoscopy service, we recently opened a new **Bronchoscopy Suite** that houses the most advanced technology for both diagnostic capabilities and interventional procedures.

FROM BENCH TO BEDSIDE
We have recently recruited Rosalind Wright, MD, MPH, to serve as Vice Chair for Transitional Research and as a member of the Division of Pediatric Pulmonology. Dr. Wright is recognized both nationally and internationally for her investigations into early life events in relation to the development of pediatric asthma and is a welcome addition to our team of physician-scientists.

As an accredited **Cystic Fibrosis Foundation Care Center**, we offer the latest therapies and participate in multi-center trials. With our team specially trained in caring for cystic fibrosis patients, we treat all aspects of the disease, ranging from the latest antimicrobial strategies to nutritional optimization. We offer services that include pediatric spirometry, plethysmography, and comprehensive psychosocial support and evaluation.

Our **Chronic Ventilator Program** provides the most advanced and compassionate management of children with chronic respiratory failure as well as those with muscular dystrophies and other conditions that require mechanical ventilation.

Our **Bronchopulmonary Dysplasia Program** offers the highest level of care for premature infants while they are in the hospital and, as outpatients, once they are discharged.

MOUNT SINAI
SCHOOL OF
MEDICINE

THE KRAVIS CHILDREN'S HOSPITAL AT THE MOUNT SINAI MEDICAL CENTER

One Gustave L. Levy Place
Fifth Avenue and 100th Street
New York, NY 10029-6574
Physician Referral: 1-800-MD-SINAI (637-4624)
www.mountsinai.org/kravis

THE KRAVIS CHILDREN'S HOSPITAL AT THE MOUNT SINAI MEDICAL CENTER

At the Kravis Children's Hospital at The Mount Sinai Medical Center, we offer the most advanced treatments and technologies available, supported by groundbreaking research, because the health and care of your child is our first priority.

This year the Kravis Children's Hospital saw significant gains in the *U.S. News & World Report* pediatric rankings, which **placed it among the country's best children's hospitals in six of the ten pediatric specialties**, as noted in the 2012-13 edition of the annual "Best Children's Hospitals" report. The six specialties are: gastroenterology (ranked #21 nationally), diabetes and endocrinology (#23), urology (#23), nephrology (#29), cancer (#32), and pulmonology (#34).

The rankings reflect not only double-digit gains within specialties, but also **first-time rankings in two new areas – cancer and urology** – placing these specialties among the best pediatric programs in the United States.

In all of our services, including 31 subspecialty areas of care, we offer advanced treatments, supported by research, community outreach, and advocacy programs. Our ongoing efforts to recruit the finest physicians and scientists have resulted in our ability to provide fundamental insights into the causes of childhood diseases and to deliver breakthrough treatments.

We will soon be opening a new Pediatric Intensive Care Unit (PICU), a 15-bed unit that will wed state-of-the-art medical technology with a family-friendly facility for our most critically ill children. Upon completion of the PICU in the fall of 2012, construction will immediately begin on a new 46-bed Neonatal Intensive Care Unit (NICU).

THE ZONE SPACE AT KRAVIS

An especially unique feature of the Kravis Children's Hospital at Mount Sinai is the Zone - a 3,000 square foot state-of-the-art therapeutic and educational play environment for pediatric patients and their families. **The Zone space at Kravis is the only one of its kind in the northeast region of the United States.**

The area is staffed by the Child Life and Creative Arts Therapy Department, a full-time pediatric medical librarian, and numerous consultants and volunteers who share their talents in art, music, cooking, knitting and more. The facility includes a lounge, theatre, family resource center, teen area, full kitchen and performing space. **The Zone features KidsZone TV (KZTV), the first live, interactive broadcast studio in a children's hospital.** The space is also used as a pediatric television programming training site for hospitals across the country and abroad.

NewYork-Presbyterian
The University Hospital of Columbia and Cornell

Affiliated with Columbia University College of Physicians and Surgeons and Weill Cornell Medical College

NewYork-Presbyterian
Morgan Stanley Children's Hospital
Columbia University Medical Center
3959 Broadway
New York, NY 10032

NewYork-Presbyterian
Phyllis and David Komansky
Center for Children's Health
Weill Cornell Medical Center
525 East 68th Street
New York, NY 10065

1-800-245-KIDS (1-800-245-5437) www.childrensnyp.org

Accreditation: The Joint Commission

Overview

The pediatric services of NewYork-Presbyterian Hospital are comprised of NewYork-Presbyterian Morgan Stanley Children's Hospital, which is affiliated with Columbia University College of Physicians and Surgeons, and the NewYork-Presbyterian Phyllis and David Komansky Center for Children's Health, which is affiliated with Weill Cornell Medical College. Together, they serve as one of the nation's premier centers for comprehensive pediatric care. Skilled and experienced physicians, surgeons, nurses and other pediatric healthcare professionals manage some of the most complex medical conditions of children at every stage of development. Their expertise includes general pediatric care and the full range of medical and surgical subspecialties:

- Adolescent Medicine
- Allergy and Immunology
- Anesthesiology
- Blood Disorders
- Blood and Marrow Transplantation
- Cancer
- Cardiology and Cardiac Surgery
- Craniofacial and Plastic Surgery
- Critical Care
- Dermatology
- Digestive Disease
- Ear, Nose and Throat
- Emergency Department, including specialized units for burns and trauma injuries
- Endocrinology, Diabetes and Metabolism
- Epilepsy
- Genetics
- Infectious Diseases

- Kidney Disease
- Liver Disease
- Lung Disease
- Maternal Fetal Medicine (high-risk pregnancy)
- Neonatal Medicine
- Neurology and Neurological Surgery
- Nutrition
- Obesity and Bariatric Surgery
- Ophthalmology
- Oral and Maxillofacial Surgery and Pediatric Dentistry
- Organ Transplantation
- Orthopaedic Surgery
- Pain Medicine
- Pediatric Surgery
- Pregnancy and Newborn Services
- Primary Care/General Pediatrics
- Psychiatry
- Radiology
- Rheumatology
- Urology

Highlights at a Glance:

- A national leader in pediatric heart surgery with one of the largest heart transplant programs in the nation.
- A pediatric kidney and liver transplant program, which includes a Living Donor Program and leading edge therapies to help reduce the side effects of anti-rejection drugs.
- Pediatric cardiac surgeons at the forefront of ventricular assist devices for infants and small children as a bridge to recovery or transplantation.
- One of three Level 1-designated Regional Pediatric Trauma Centers in New York State and the only one in New York City.
- Maternal-Fetal Medicine Divison designated a Regional Perinatal Center, the highest hospital classification, able to care for the most complex, highest-risk cases.
- One of the largest Type 1 diabetes programs in New York State.
- Outstanding neonatal intensive care programs setting standards of care nationwide for extremely ill newborns.
- The only program in the New York tri-state area that has active programs in both liver and small bowel transplantation.

550 First Avenue *(at 31st Street)*
New York, NY 10016
www.NYULMC.org
Physician Referral: **888-7-NYU-MED** *(888-769-8633)*

PEDIATRIC CRITICAL CARE

Pediatric Critical Care is part of the Hassenfeld Pediatric Center, a full service specialty Children's Hospital, which supports the array of children's health services across the Medical Center where newborns, children, adolescents and young adults receive the most comprehensive and advanced care by a team of pediatricians and pediatric specialists.

About the Pediatric Critical Care Team
Pediatric critical care specialists at NYU Langone Medical Center are highly trained and experienced in the treatment of seriously ill children, providing a supportive environment for patients and their families. In addition to these dedicated pediatric intensivists, the Medical Center's 12-bed Laurence D. and Lori Weider Fink Pediatric Intensive Care Unit (PICU) is staffed by a team of specially trained pediatric nurses who care for children from babies through young adults. In addition to managing children who require days or weeks of intense therapy, the Pediatric Critical Care team's responsibilities include caring for children recovering from postsurgical anesthesia, as well as overnight monitoring of patients after surgery or other procedures in the PICU. The Pediatric Critical Care team collaborates with all of the pediatric surgical specialties at NYU Langone, as well as with medical specialties and pediatric anesthesia. Social workers dedicated to the PICU are also an integral part of the team. We specialize in the following areas:

Ventilator Support
Children who require ventilator support benefit from the knowledge and experience of physicians who assess and carefully negotiate the proper timing of extubation. They are also skilled in the management of pain for each young patient.

Parent Education
Educating parents of critical ill children is a very important part of our services. The Pediatric Critical Care team is committed to fostering a supportive environment by continually engaging parents in dialogue. This includes "demystifying" the PICU, which can be an intimidating environment for children given its elaborate equipment and unfamiliar sounds. Parents are also encouraged to participate in daily rounds, and to listen and contribute to medical updates regarding their child's condition. Particularly comforting to the parents of critically ill children is the availability of round-the-clock, unlimited visitation.

Children with Complex Conditions
Because of their expertise with various congenital and acquired conditions, pediatric critical care specialists at NYU Langone are highly experienced in caring for children with complex conditions, including severely handicapped youngsters with special needs. Primary care pediatricians are encouraged to visit their patients at the PICU, and our team of caregivers communicates frequently with these physicians in-person and by telephone.

PEDIATRIC EMERGENCY MEDICINE

Pediatric Emergency Medicine is part of the Hassenfeld Pediatric Center, a full service specialty Children's Hospital, which supports the array of children's health services across the Medical Center where newborns, children, adolescents and young adults receive the most comprehensive and advanced care by a team of pediatricians and pediatric specialists.

About the Division of Pediatric Emergency Medicine, Department of Pediatrics
The Division of Pediatric Emergency Medicine at NYU Langone Medical Center offers patients compassionate, state-of-the-art emergency medical care. Our physicians are specially trained in pediatric emergency medicine and are expert in managing emergencies specific to infants, children, adolescents and young adults. They are recognized as national leaders for the training of Pediatric Emergency Medicine physicians, as well as for their research and advocacy. We specialize in the following areas:

Pediatric Emergency Medicine
The Tisch Hospital Pediatric Emergency Medicine Program at NYU Langone Medical Center provides the highest level of care to all pediatric patients. Ill and injured children receive treatment in an atmosphere that is child-friendly and family-focused. Pediatric sub-specialty physicians and pediatric surgeons are available for consultation in the Emergency Department 24 hours a day, 365 days a year.

Pediatric Emergency Services
Pediatric Emergency Services (PES) at Bellevue Hospital Center, an affiliate of NYU Langone Medical Center, is dedicated to the care of acutely ill and injured children. Each year approximately 25,000 children and young adults are evaluated by PES, which is staffed around the clock by board-certified pediatric emergency medicine physicians and nurses who specialize in the emergency care of children. PES manages patients with a wide range of medical, surgical and psychiatric problems, including asthma, appendicitis, child abuse, orthopaedic injuries, major trauma, poisoning and suicide.

Pediatric Transport
The Pediatric Transport Program at NYU Langone Medical Center transfers critically ill pediatric patients from outlying facilities to the Medical Center. In-house teams are available 24 hours a day, 7 days a week to allow a rapid response to medical transports from more than 50 hospitals. The transport team includes a physician as well as a respiratory therapist and pediatric critical care nurse. Patients are provided with the most advanced care possible from the beginning of the transport at the referring facility to their final destination.

PEDIATRIC GASTROENTEROLOGY

Pediatric Gastroenterology is part of the Hassenfeld Pediatric Center, a full service specialty Children's Hospital, which supports the array of children's health services across the Medical Center where newborns, children, adolescents and young adults receive the most comprehensive and advanced care by a team of pediatricians and pediatric specialists.

About the Division of Pediatric Gastroenterology, Department of Pediatrics

Pediatric gastroenterologists at NYU Langone Medical Center are committed to the highest quality medical care and state-of-the-art techniques in the evaluation and management of gastrointestinal, liver and nutritional disorders from infancy to young adulthood. With access to the latest in endoscopic procedures performed at one of the country's leading academic medical centers, patients receive comprehensive and multidisciplinary treatments for a wide range of conditions. Our pediatric gastroenterologists are particularly adept at providing family-centered, integrated care with a focus on the physical and psychological well-being of the child. We specialize in the following areas:

Clinical Care

Most children will occasionally experience one or more gastrointestinal symptoms during their childhood years. Some children, however, develop recurrent symptoms, which interrupt their normal lives and are the presenting features of serious but treatable diseases. The gastrointestinal and nutritional concerns impacting on the health and quality of life of children on the autism spectrum is an area of particular interest at NYU Langone. We are in the forefront of the evaluation and management of celiac disease and food allergies, including allergic involvement of the esophagus (eosinophilic esophagitis), and our experts use the latest techniques to pinpoint problems and determine the most effective therapy. We offer a vast range of therapeutic services, as well as access to clinical nutrition services, pediatric rehabilitation and some of the country's best surgeons.

Specialty Care

Pediatric gastroenterologists at NYU Langone Medical Center evaluate and treat a variety of disorders including abdominal pain, celiac spruce, congenital bowel dysfunction, congenital liver disorders and chronic liver disease, chronic constipation, feeding problems in infants, failure to thrive, food allergies, lactose intolerance, gastrointestinal bleeding, gastroesophageal reflux, hepatitis, malabsorption syndromes, pancreatitis, peptic ulcer disease, ulcerative colitis and Crohn's disease.

HASSENFELD PEDIATRIC CENTER

The new Hassenfeld Pediatric Center (HPC) is a full-service specialty children's hospital that works as a cohesive team across all children's health services provided at NYU Langone Medical Center. At HPC, newborns, children, adolescents and young adults receive the most comprehensive and advanced care possible from a team of pediatricians and pediatric specialists across more than 30 medical and surgical disciplines. With more than 150 full-time pediatric specialists, as well as pediatric nurses, child life specialists and social workers, the Hassenfeld Pediatric Center is uniquely equipped to provide innovative pediatric subspecialty care in a highly personalized manner.

About Children's Services at NYU Langone

NYU Langone Medical Center is nationally recognized in many pediatric specialty fields, including craniofacial anomalies, cardiac surgery, orthopaedic surgery, rehabilitation medicine, brain tumors, leukemia, sarcoma, and epilepsy. Our specialists work collaboratively to optimize care for each child, from the operating room and pediatric intensive care unit to the Emergency Department and pediatric inpatient unit.

A Family-Centered Approach

Integral to the care we provide is a myriad of support services for children and their families. We recognize that the best outcomes are achieved when the child's family is actively involved in every step of care. For that reason, our trained specialists address the needs of not just the patient, but of parents and siblings through ongoing education and communication.

The Future Shape of Pediatric Care at HPC

In 2017, a 160,000 square foot pediatric hospital, on the Medical Center's main campus, will become the inpatient centerpiece of the Hassenfeld Pediatric Center. This state-of-the-art facility will enhance the Center's ability to deliver world-class care through all private rooms, a feature that increases patient safety by decreasing exposure to infections, while providing a private, supportive environment for the patients and their families. HPC will be the only pediatric inpatient facility in Manhattan with this amenity, which will also include a "family zone" offering a sleep-in couch, storage, and Web access for each room.

The new pediatric hospital will also include a child-friendly pre-operative unit along with recovery bays where parents can be by the child's bedside during post-operation. Rounding out the new hospital will be a Family Center for orientation activities geared to patients, space for child-life activities and performances, as well as support, education and respite services for families.

PEDIATRIC HEMATOLOGY/ONCOLOGY

Pediatric Hemaology/Oncology is part of the Hassenfeld Pediatric Center, a full service specialty Children's Hospital, which supports the array of children's health services across the Medical Center where newborns, children, adolescents and young adults receive the most comprehensive and advanced care by a team of pediatricians and pediatric specialists.

We are committed to providing modern, family-centered and highly personalized care to children with cancer and blood disorders. Teams of specialists deliver personalized care in a healing environment promoting physical, emotional and spiritual well-being of children and their families.

Hematologic Malignancies
We offer new treatments for childhood acute lymphoblastic leukemia (ALL) and are a national leader in clinical trials for children with newly diagnosed leukemia and recurrent diseases.

Hematology
We provide treatment for children and adolescents with all types of blood disorders including Sickle Cell Disease, other hemoglobinopathies, bleeding disorders and aplastic anemia.

Pediatric Neuro-Oncology
We provide multidisciplinary comprehensive care for children from infants to young adults with primary central nervous system, slow-growing and malignant tumors assuring the safest and most effective treatments for newly diagnosed or recurrent tumors.

Pediatric Special Hematology Laboratory
NYU Langone offers comprehensive homeostasis and red cell testing incorporating the latest developments in the field.

Psychosocial Services
Our holistic approach to care includes art therapy, relaxation training, play therapy, psychiatric evaluation, neuropsychological assessment, individual/group counseling and patient education.

Sarcoma and Solid Tumor Program
We offer cutting-edge medical, surgical and radiotherapy treatments for bone and soft tissue sarcomas, and all pediatric solid tumors including Wilms' Tumor and neuroblastoma and are developing national trials for the treatment of sarcomas and offer a number of clinical trials.

Stephen D. Hassenfeld Children's Center for Cancer and Blood Disorders
As a member of the NCI-designated NYU Cancer Institute, we are constantly developing new ways to treat childhood cancer. Our unique interdisciplinary and family-centered approach combines the most advanced medical treatments with psychosocial and emotional support.

PEDIATRIC PULMONOLOGY

Pediatric Pulmonology is part of the Hassenfeld Pediatric Center, a full service specialty Children's Hospital, which supports the array of children's health services across the Medical Center where newborns, children, adolescents and young adults receive the most comprehensive and advanced care by a team of pediatricians and pediatric specialists.

About Pediatric Pulmonology, Department of Pediatrics

The Division of Pediatric Pulmonology provides comprehensive care to children -- from infancy to adolescence to young adulthood -- with a variety of conditions affecting the respiratory system. Physicians in the Division are committed to providing both family-centered and multidisciplinary care, collaborating with specialists in other divisions throughout NYU Langone Medical Center. For example, physicians in the Division work closely with the Infant Apnea/SIDS Program to follow children discharged from the Neonatal Intensive Care Unit; with the Division of Pediatric Gastroenterology and the Swallowing Center to follow children with feeding difficulties and swallowing dysfunction; with the Division of Pediatric Surgery to follow children with congenital lung lesions through minimally invasive surgery; and with the Division of Orthopaedics to optimize the care of children with neuromuscular disease undergoing spine surgery. We specialize in the following areas:

Pulmonologists in the Division care for children with a wide range of problems, including asthma, bronchopulmonary dysplasia (chronic lung disease of prematurity), cystic fibrosis, chronic respiratory failure and pulmonary complications of neuromuscular disease, congenital lung malformations, chest wall deformities, interstitial lung disease, and obstructive sleep apnea. Consultation for chronic cough, noisy breathing, and exercise intolerance is also provided.

Flexible bronchoscopy

Using specialized pediatric equipment, the airways of even the tiniest infants can be examined in the state-of-the-art endoscopy suite at NYU Langone Medical Center, with multiple specialists often involved in the procedure. Because the equipment is mobile, procedures can also be performed at bedside in the Pediatric Intensive Care Unit.

550 First Avenue *(at 31st Street)*
New York, NY 10016

www.NYULMC.org

Physician Referral: **888-7-NYU-MED** *(888-769-8633)*

PEDIATRIC RHEUMATOLOGY

Pediatric Rheumatology is part of the Hassenfeld Pediatric Center, a full service specialty Children's Hospital, which supports the array of children's health services across the Medical Center where newborns, children, adolescents and young adults receive the most comprehensive and advanced care by a team of pediatricians and pediatric specialists.

About the Division of Pediatric Rheumatology, Department of Pediatrics

Pediatric rheumatology specialists at the NYU Langone Medical Center are dedicated to the complete care of children with rheumatic disease. In conjunction with our multidisciplinary team of specialists, we treat children with a variety of rheumatologic conditions, including Juvenile Idiopathic Arthritis (JIA), systemic lupus erythematosus, juvenile dermatomyositis, Kawasaki's disease, and others. Through early diagnosis and appropriately intensive treatment we aim to achieve disease quiescence as quickly and safely as possible, with the ultimate goal of returning children to full physical functionality.

In addition to our clinical services, we are committed to the continued formal education of residents, rheumatology fellows and medical students, as well as the general public through our community outreach programs and in collaboration with the adult Rheumatology Division, we have initiated an annual pediatric rheumatology CME course which is well-attended by general physicians and rheumatologists. Our emphasis on providing high-level clinical services and teaching is complemented by the Division's collaboration with national pediatric rheumatology research organizations in several clinical research projects pertaining to drug exposure in children with rheumatic disease. We specialize in the following areas:

Juvenile Idiopathic Arthritis

An umbrella term for several different patterns of arthritis in children, juvenile idiopathic arthritis (JIA) refers to arthritic disorders caused by an autoimmune reaction. Our Pediatric rheumatologists diagnose and treat different types of JIA. The use of methotrexate in combination with newly discovered biologic agents, such as Etanercept and Infliximab, gives even greater reason for optimism. Juvenile arthritis, once a crippler of children, is fast becoming a highly manageable disease.

Pediatric Arthritis

A bacterial joint infection in children, known as septic arthritis, is a painful condition requiring urgent care to prevent the spread of infection and the possibility of permanent damage to the joint. At the first sign of septic arthritis, NYU Langone's Pediatric staff takes quick action to fight the infection at its source.

PEDIATRIC ORTHOPAEDICS

Pediatric Orthopaedics is part of the Hassenfeld Pediatric Center, a full service specialty Children's Hospital, which supports the array of children's health services across the Medical Center where newborns, children, adolescents and young adults receive the most comprehensive and advanced care by a team of pediatricians and pediatric specialists.

From common injuries to the most complex congenital disorders, NYU Langone's pediatric orthopaedic service, based at the Hospital for Joint Diseases (HJD), is one of the most extensive orthopaedic programs for children in the country and is a renowned multidisciplinary center featuring a strong collaborative approach to care. Areas of specialization include scoliosis, limb deformities, hip dysplasia, cerebral palsy, congenital insensitivity to pain, arthrogryposis, sports injuries, anterior cruciate ligament injuries, bone tumors, juvenile idiopathic arthritis, Charcot-Marie-Tooth disease, and brachial plexus injuries.

Specialized Orthopaedic Services
The Center for Children at HJD is a full-service pediatric outpatient facility that offers multidisciplinary management of pediatric musculoskeletal and neuromuscular disorders and brings together outstanding board-certified pediatric specialists in orthopaedic surgery, rheumatology, genetics, neurology, rehabilitation and pediatrics.

The Orthopaedic Immediate Care Center (i-Care), New York City's only walk-in orthopaedic clinic, uses state-of-the-art diagnostic equipment to evaluate and treat urgent orthopaedic injuries, such as fractures, dislocation or joint injury, sprains, and bone or joint infection.

The Ambulatory Care Clinic is available for convenient, streamlined treatment of both children and adults. A team of pediatric hospitalists evaluates patients with multiple medical problems prior to surgery, and helps to manage their postoperative care.

Nationally Recognized Surgical Care
The Wallace B. Lehman, MD, Center for Pediatric Orthopaedic Surgery at HJD is at the forefront of specialized surgery and personalized care for children. The Center is proud to be the largest teaching program in the country to offer a pediatric orthopaedic surgical residency, as well as fellowship training. It is also a recognized leader in surgical innovation and advanced technology, which helps ensure that patients receive the best possible care.

Convenient Satellite Sites
Satellite locations in the outlying areas of Westchester, Long Island, Rockland and New Jersey provide added convenience for parents seeking top orthopaedic care for their children within their own communities.

550 First Avenue *(at 31st Street)*
New York, NY 10016
www.NYULMC.org
Physician Referral: **888-7-NYU-MED** *(888-769-8633)*

PEDIATRIC SURGERY

Pediatric Surgery is part of the Hassenfeld Pediatric Center, a full service specialty Children's Hospital, which supports the array of children's health services across the Medical Center where newborns, children, adolescents and young adults receive the most comprehensive and advanced care by a team of pediatricians and pediatric specialists.

The Division of Pediatric Surgery at NYU Langone Medical Center provides comprehensive pediatric surgical care for the smallest preterm infant to the adolescent. Our surgeons are experts at minimally invasive procedures (resulting in shorter hospitals stays and faster recoveries), as well as in conventional surgical techniques. In addition to highly-skilled surgeons and surgical nurses, we offer a wide array of Child Life Services to help children and their families become familiar with the hospital environment and lessen fears.

Surgical Expertise
NYU Langone Medical Center is renowned for its achievements in the full spectrum of pediatric surgical specialties, including abdominal and thoracic surgery, neonatal surgery, surgery for all congenital anomalies, cancer surgery, urology, cardiac surgery, neurosurgery, orthopaedics, plastic and reconstructive surgery, repair of cleft lips and palates, ophthalmology, and ENT, among others.

Pediatric Anesthesia
We are proud of our expert team of fellowship-trained pediatric anesthesiologists who serve the pediatric population. These anesthesiologists are involved in preoperative and postoperative care as well as in administering anesthesia, and they have close working relationships with our pediatric surgeons.

Child Life Services
The pediatric unit is home to The Child Life Program which is focused on creating a supportive environment for children undergoing surgery and their families through a total care approach. Child Life personnel meet with parents and their child prior to surgery and provide a continuum of care to the entire family throughout the hospital experience.

Pre-Admission Orientation and Information
Informational packets about what to expect are given to families during the pre-admission testing process. Parents and their children are also encouraged to attend an orientation session.

Facilities
Day surgery facilities include an expansive playroom with computers, games and Child Life personnel to care for the family. A separate recovery room area provides a calming environment for children during their emergence from anesthesia.

550 First Avenue (*at 31st Street*)
New York, NY 10016
www.NYULMC.org
Children's Services Access Line: **855-NYU-KIDS**

HASSENFELD PEDIATRIC CENTER

The new Hassenfeld Pediatric Center (HPC) is a full-service specialty children's hospital that works as a cohesive team across all children's health services at NYU Langone Medical Center. At HPC, newborns, children, adolescents and young adults receive the most comprehensive and advanced care possible from a team of pediatricians and pediatric specialists across more than 30 medical and surgical disciplines. With more than 150 full-time pediatric specialists, as well as pediatric nurses, child life specialists and social workers, the Hassenfeld Pediatric Center is uniquely equipped to provide innovative pediatric subspecialty care in a highly personalized manner.

About Children's Services at NYU Langone

NYU Langone Medical Center is nationally recognized in many pediatric specialty fields, including craniofacial anomalies, cardiac surgery, orthopaedic surgery, rehabilitation medicine, brain tumors, leukemia, sarcoma, and epilepsy. Our specialists work collaboratively to optimize care for each child, from the operating room and pediatric intensive care unit to the Emergency Department and pediatric inpatient unit.

A Family-Centered Approach

Integral to the care we provide is a myriad of support services for children and their families. We recognize that the best outcomes are achieved when the child's family is actively involved in every step of care. For that reason, our trained specialists address the needs of not just the patient, but of parents and siblings through ongoing education and communication.

The Future Shape of Pediatric Care at HPC

In 2017, a 160,000 square foot pediatric hospital, on the Medical Center's main campus, will become the inpatient centerpiece of the Hassenfeld Pediatric Center. This state-of-the-art facility will enhance the Center's ability to deliver world-class care through all private rooms, a feature that increases patient safety by decreasing exposure to infections, while providing a private, supportive environment for the patients and their families. HPC will be the only pediatric inpatient facility in Manhattan with this amenity, which will also include a "family zone" offering a sleep-in couch, storage, and Web access for each room.

The new pediatric hospital will also include a child-friendly pre-operative unit along with recovery bays where parents can be by the child's bedside during post-operation. Rounding out the new hospital will be a Family Center for orientation activities geared to patients, space for child-life activities and performances, as well as support, education and respite services for families.

Rusk Rehabilitation
400 East 34th Street *(between 1st Avenue and FDR Drive)*
New York, NY 10016
HJD: 301 East 17th Street *(at 2nd Avenue)*
New York, NY 10003
www.NYULMC.org/RUSK
Children's Services Access Line: **855-NYU-KIDS**

PEDIATRIC REHABILITATION MEDICINE

Pediatric Rehabilitation is part of the Hassenfeld Pediatric Center, a full service specialty Children's Hospital, which supports the array of children's health services across the Medical Center where newborns, children, adolescents and young adults receive the most comprehensive and advanced care by a team of pediatricians and pediatric specialists.

About the Pediatric Rehabilitation Program
The Pediatric Rehabilitation Medicine Division is a key component Rusk Rehabilitation at NYU Langone (Rusk), providing world-class inpatient and outpatient rehabilitation services for children, from birth through early adulthood. Rusk has been ranked the best rehabilitation hospital in New York and among the top ten in the country by *U.S. News & World Report* for 23 consecutive years. At Rusk, the focus is on early intervention and a family-centered approach that includes sibling and family support groups and counseling.

Areas of Expertise
The pediatric rehabilitation team is particularly skilled in treating the multiple challenges of children with developmental disorders such as cerebral palsy, spina bifida, muscular dystrophy, reflex sympathetic dystrophy, limb deficiencies, arthrogryposis, and spinal cord injuries. Children with traumatic brain injuries, brain tumors, and oncologic diagnoses (such as bone tumors or musculoskeletal disease) also benefit from our specialized services, as do youngsters affected by stroke or cerebrovascular accidents, viral infections or inflammatory diseases, and rheumatic disease.

Spanning the Continuum of Care
In addition to inpatient services, we offer extensive outpatient programs for young patients, including physical therapy, occupational therapy, speech therapy, feeding and swallowing, vocational services, psychological services, and other specialized therapies.

Rusk's pediatric services are delivered at Rusk's 34th Street location as well as at the world-renowned Hospital for Joint Diseases. Moreover, specialized rehabilitation care for premature infants is provided by the Medical Center's neonatal intensive care unit.

Monroe Carell Jr. Children's Hospital at Vanderbilt

Vanderbilt University Medical Center
2200 Children's Way
Nashville, TN 37232
(800) 288-5000

Monroe Carell Jr.
children's Hospital
at Vanderbilt

Overview

Monroe Carell Jr. Children's Hospital at Vanderbilt is a nationally recognized leader in pediatric health care. Children's Hospital offers an extremely high level of care within an elite teaching and research facility. A recent 33-bed expansion to our 243-bed facility will help meet the growing demands for pediatric care in our region.

While Children's Hospital primarily serves children in Middle Tennessee, southern Kentucky and northern Alabama, patients from across the country seek treatment here. Every child who needs our services is given care, regardless of ability to pay.

Among the Nation's Best

Children's Hospital is ranked as one of the top children's hospitals in the nation by *U.S. News & World Report* in 10 out of 10 possible specialties:

Cancer

Cardiology and heart surgery

Diabetes and endocrinology

Gastroenterology

Neurology and neurosurgery

Neonatology

Orthopaedics

Pulmonology

Urology

Junior League Fetal Center at Vanderbilt

The Junior League Fetal Center at Vanderbilt gives babies and their families the best care possible. Patients from across the country turn to us for care of complications during pregnancy. Our internationally recognized experts offer superior care that leads to very high patient satisfaction.

Fetal Repair of Spina Bifida

A landmark study co-led by experts at Vanderbilt has proven that babies who have surgery to repair spina bifida while still in the womb have better outcomes than babies who have surgery after birth. Members of the fetal surgery team at Vanderbilt pioneered the surgery to repair myelomeningocele, the most serious form of spina bifida. Noel Tulipan, M.D., internationally renowned neurosurgeon and director of pediatric neurosurgery, has performed more than 200 prenatal surgeries to repair the spina bifida defect. Learn more.

Family-centered Care

At Children's Hospital, your family is our family. Children heal faster with their loved ones nearby, and staying at a place that doesn't feel like a hospital helps families focus on rest and recuperation. We offer a robust Family Resource Center, serenity gardens, quiet rooms for families, a beautiful chapel and other features to promote healing and reduce stress. Learn more.

ChildrensHospital.Vanderbilt.org

Physical Medicine & Rehabilitation

Physical medicine and rehabilitation, also referred to as rehabilitation medicine, is the medical specialty concerned with diagnosing, evaluating and treating patients with physical disabilities. These disabilities may arise from conditions affecting the musculoskeletal system such as neck and back pain, sports injuries, or other painful conditions affecting the limbs, for example carpal tunnel syndrome. Alternatively, the disabilities may result from neurological trauma or disease such as spinal cord injury, head injury or stroke.

A physician certified in physical medicine and rehabilitation is often called a physiatrist. The primary goal of the physiatrist is to achieve maximal restoration of physical, psychological, social and vocational function through comprehensive rehabilitation. Pain management is often an important part of the role of the physiatrist. For diagnosis and evaluation, a physiatrist may include the techniques of electromyography to supplement the standard history, physical, X-ray and laboratory examinations. The physiatrist has expertise in the appropriate use of therapeutic exercise, prosthetics (artificial limbs), orthotics and mechanical and electrical devices.

Training Required: Four years *plus* one year clinical practice.

Certification in the following subspecialty requires additional training and examination.

Spinal Cord Injury Medicine: A physician who addresses the prevention, diagnosis, treatment and management of traumatic spinal cord injury and non-traumatic etiologies of spinal cord dysfunction by working in an interdisciplinary manner. Care is provided to patients of all ages on a lifelong basis and covers related medical, physical, psychological and vocational disabilities and complications.

PHYSICAL MEDICINE & REHABILITATION

New England

Bloch, Rina M MD [PMR] - **Spec Exp:** Spinal Cord Injury; Brain Injury Rehabilitation; Geriatric Rehabilitation; Musculoskeletal Disorders; **Hospital:** Tufts Med Ctr; **Address:** Tufts Medical Ctr, Rehab Medicine, 800 Washington St, Box 400, Boston, MA 02111; **Phone:** 617-636-3003; **Board Cert:** Physical Medicine & Rehabilitation 1989; Spinal Cord Injury Medicine 2008; Electrodiagnostic Medicine 1997; **Med School:** Univ Louisville Sch Med 1983; **Resid:** Physical Medicine & Rehabilitation, Rehab Inst of Chicago 1987

Borg-Stein, Joanne MD [PMR] - **Spec Exp:** Pain Management; Sports Medicine; Acupuncture; Spinal Rehabilitation; **Hospital:** Spaulding Rehab Hosp, Newton - Wellesley Hosp; **Address:** Spaulding-Wellesley Outpatient Center, 65 Walnut St, Wellesley, MA 02481; **Phone:** 781-431-9144; **Board Cert:** Physical Medicine & Rehabilitation 1990; Pain Medicine 2011; Sports Medicine 2008; **Med School:** Albert Einstein Coll Med 1984; **Resid:** Physical Medicine & Rehabilitation, Columbia-Presby Med Ctr 1988; **Fac Appt:** Asst Prof PMR, Harvard Med Sch

Glenn, Mel B MD [PMR] - **Spec Exp:** Brain Injury Rehabilitation; Spasticity Management; **Hospital:** Spaulding Rehab Hosp, Mass Genl Hosp; **Address:** Spaulding Rehab Hosp, 125 Nashua St, rm 707, Boston, MA 02114; **Phone:** 617-573-2200; **Board Cert:** Physical Medicine & Rehabilitation 1982; **Med School:** NYU Sch Med 1978; **Resid:** Physical Medicine & Rehabilitation, NYU Med Ctr 1981; **Fellow:** Spinal Cord Injury Medicine, NYU Med Ctr 1982; **Fac Appt:** Assoc Prof PMR, Harvard Med Sch

Richter, Edwin MD [PMR] - **Spec Exp:** Neuro-Rehabilitation; Brain Injury Rehabilitation; Amputee Rehabilitation; Lymphedema; **Hospital:** Stamford Hosp; **Address:** 166 W Broad St, Ste 305, Stamford, CT 06902; **Phone:** 203-316-0610; **Board Cert:** Physical Medicine & Rehabilitation 1992; **Med School:** NYU Sch Med 1987; **Resid:** Physical Medicine & Rehabilitation, NYU Med Ctr 1991; **Fac Appt:** Asst Clin Prof PMR, NYU Sch Med

Webster, Harry C MD [PMR] - **Spec Exp:** Pediatric Rehabilitation; Cerebral Palsy; Muscular Dystrophy; Spasticity Management; **Hospital:** Tufts Med Ctr; **Address:** Tufts Med Ctr, 800 Washington St, Box 387, Boston, MA 02111; **Phone:** 617-636-5626; **Board Cert:** Pediatrics 1983; Physical Medicine & Rehabilitation 1988; **Med School:** UCSF 1977; **Resid:** Pediatrics, Chldns Hosp 1980; Physical Medicine & Rehabilitation, Tufts Med Ctr 1987; **Fac Appt:** Asst Prof PMR, Tufts Univ

Zafonte, Ross D DO [PMR] - **Spec Exp:** Brain Injury Rehabilitation; Spinal Cord Injury; **Hospital:** Spaulding Rehab Hosp; **Address:** Spaulding Rehab Hosp, 125 Nashua St, rm 707, Boston, MA 02114; **Phone:** 617-573-2200; **Board Cert:** Physical Medicine & Rehabilitation 1990; **Med School:** Nova SE Univ, Coll Osteo Med 1985; **Resid:** Physical Medicine & Rehabilitation, Mt Sinai Med Ctr 1989; **Fac Appt:** Clin Prof PMR, Boston Univ

Mid Atlantic

Ahn, Jung Hwan MD [PMR] - **Spec Exp:** Spinal Cord Injury; Stroke Rehabilitation; Neurologic Rehabilitation; **Hospital:** NYU Langone Med Ctr (page 68); **Address:** Ambulatory Care Ctr, 240 E 38th St Fl 15, New York, NY 10016; **Phone:** 212-263-6122; **Board Cert:** Physical Medicine & Rehabilitation 1980; Spinal Cord Injury Medicine 2008; **Med School:** South Korea 1970; **Resid:** Obstetrics & Gynecology, Elmhurst City Hosp - Mt Sinai 1976; Physical Medicine & Rehabilitation, NYU Med Ctr 1979; **Fellow:** Spinal Cord Injury Medicine, NYU Med Ctr 1980; **Fac Appt:** Clin Prof PMR, NYU Sch Med

Aseff, John N MD [PMR] - **Spec Exp:** Electrodiagnosis; Pain-Soft Tissue; **Hospital:** Natl Rehab Hosp, Washington Hosp Ctr; **Address:** National Rehabilitation Hosp, 102 Irving St NW, Washington, DC 20010; **Phone:** 202-877-1916; **Board Cert:** Physical Medicine & Rehabilitation 1978; **Med School:** Ohio State Univ 1973; **Resid:** Surgery, Univ Hosps Cleveland 1975; Physical Medicine & Rehabilitation, Ohio State Univ Hosp 1977; **Fac Appt:** Assoc Clin Prof PMR, Georgetown Univ

Bach, John MD [PMR] - **Spec Exp:** Neuromuscular Disorders; Amyotrophic Lateral Sclerosis (ALS); Post Polio Syndrome/Rehabilitation; **Hospital:** Univ Hosp-UMDNJ—Newark; **Address:** 90 Bergen St Fl 3 - Ste 3100, Newark, NJ 07103; **Phone:** 973-972-7195; **Board Cert:** Physical Medicine & Rehabilitation 1986; **Med School:** UMDNJ-NJ Med Sch, Newark 1976; **Resid:** Physical Medicine & Rehabilitation, NYU Med Ctr 1980; **Fellow:** Neuromuscular Disease, Univ Hosp 1983; **Fac Appt:** Prof PMR, UMDNJ-NJ Med Sch, Newark

Ballard, Pamela H MD [PMR] - **Spec Exp:** Spinal Cord Injury; Spasticity Management; Neuromuscular Disorders; **Hospital:** Natl Rehab Hosp; **Address:** MedStar Natl Rehab Hosp, 102 Irving St NW, Washington, DC 20010; **Phone:** 202-877-1621; **Board Cert:** Physical Medicine & Rehabilitation 1991; Spinal Cord Injury Medicine 2009; **Med School:** Howard Univ 1986; **Resid:** Physical Medicine & Rehabilitation, Sinai Hosp 1990

Braddom, Randall L MD [PMR] - **Spec Exp:** Electromyography; Pain-Neck; Pain-Low Back; Musculoskeletal Disorders; **Hospital:** Riverview Med Ctr; **Address:** 1801 Market St, Ste 200, Philadelphia, PA 19103; **Phone:** 215-569-9500; **Board Cert:** Physical Medicine & Rehabilitation 1974; **Med School:** Ohio State Univ 1968; **Resid:** Physical Medicine & Rehabilitation, Ohio State Univ Hosp 1973; **Fac Appt:** Clin Prof PMR, UMDNJ-NJ Med Sch, Newark

De Lateur, Barbara J MD [PMR] - **Spec Exp:** Frailty Syndrome; **Hospital:** Johns Hopkins Bayview Med Ctr (page 61), Good Samaritan Hosp; **Address:** Johns Hopkins Bayview Med Ctr, Rehab, 4940 Eastern Ave, Baltimore, MD 21224; **Phone:** 410-550-5299; **Board Cert:** Physical Medicine & Rehabilitation 1970; **Med School:** Univ Wash 1963; **Resid:** Physical Medicine & Rehabilitation, Univ Wash Hosp 1968; **Fac Appt:** Prof PMR, Johns Hopkins Univ

Dillard, James N MD [PMR] - **Spec Exp:** Pain Management; Acupuncture; Complementary Medicine; Nutrition; **Hospital:** Southampton Hosp; **Address:** 110 E 59th St, Ste 10A, New York, NY 10022; **Phone:** 212-265-4038; **Board Cert:** Physical Medicine & Rehabilitation 2005; **Med School:** Rush Med Coll 1990; **Resid:** Physical Medicine & Rehabilitation, Columbia-Presby Med Ctr 1994; **Fac Appt:** Asst Clin Prof PMR, Columbia P&S

Esquenazi, Alberto M MD [PMR] - **Spec Exp:** Amputee Rehabilitation; Mobility Evaluation & Treatment; Post Polio Syndrome/Rehabilitation; Spasticity Management; **Hospital:** Moss Rehab Hosp; **Address:** Moss Rehab Hosp, 60 Township Line Rd, Elkins Park, PA 19027; **Phone:** 215-663-6676; **Board Cert:** Physical Medicine & Rehabilitation 1986; **Med School:** Mexico 1981; **Resid:** Physical Medicine & Rehabilitation, Temple Univ Hosp 1985; **Fellow:** Gait and Prosthetics, Moss Rehab Hosp 1986; **Fac Appt:** Prof PMR, Jefferson Med Coll

Evans, Sarah H MD [PMR] - **Spec Exp:** Pediatric Rehabilitation; White Matter Disorders; Encephalitis; **Hospital:** Chldns Natl Med Ctr, Natl Rehab Hosp; **Address:** Children's National Medical Ctr, Pediatric Rehabilitation, 111 Michigan Ave NW, Ste 1090, Washington, DC 20010; **Phone:** 202-476-3080; **Board Cert:** Physical Medicine & Rehabilitation 1992; Pediatrics 2002; Pediatric Rehabilitation Medicine 2003; **Med School:** Univ MD Sch Med 1984; **Resid:** Pediatrics, Univ Colorado Hlth Sci Ctr 1987; **Fellow:** Physical Medicine & Rehabilitation, Univ Colorado Hlth Sci Ctr 1988; Pediatric Rehabilitation Medicine, Chldns Hosp 1989; **Fac Appt:** Assoc Prof PMR, Univ Colorado

Feinberg, Joseph H MD [PMR] - **Spec Exp:** Peripheral Neuropathy; Spinal Rehabilitation; Electrodiagnosis; Sports Medicine; **Hospital:** Hosp For Special Surgery (page 60), Kessler Inst for Rehab - W Orange; **Address:** 535 E 70th St, Hospital for Special Surgery, New York, NY 10021-4872; **Phone:** 212-606-1568; **Board Cert:** Physical Medicine & Rehabilitation 1991; Sports Medicine 2009; **Med School:** Albany Med Coll 1983; **Resid:** Surgery, Mt Sinai Hosp 1985; Physical Medicine & Rehabilitation, Rusk Inst Rehab 1990; **Fellow:** Orthopaedic Pathology, Hosp Spec Surg 1986; Orthopaedic Biomechanics, Univ Iowa Hosp & Clins 1987; **Fac Appt:** Assoc Prof PMR, Cornell Univ-Weill Med Coll

Flanagan, Steven R MD [PMR] - **Spec Exp:** Brain Injury Rehabilitation; Stroke Rehabilitation; **Hospital:** NYU Langone Med Ctr (page 68), NYU Rusk Inst (page 71); **Address:** Ambulatory Care Ctr, 240 E 38th St Fl 15, New York, NY 10016; **Phone:** 212-263-6037; **Board Cert:** Physical Medicine & Rehabilitation 2003; **Med School:** UMDNJ-NJ Med Sch, Newark 1988; **Resid:** Physical Medicine & Rehabilitation, Mt Sinai Hosp 1992; **Fac Appt:** Prof PMR, NYU Sch Med

Francis, Kathleen D MD [PMR] - **Spec Exp:** Lymphedema; **Address:** Lymphedema Physician Services, 200 S Orange Ave, Ste 111, Livingston, NJ 07039; **Phone:** 973-322-7366; **Board Cert:** Physical Medicine & Rehabilitation 2004; **Med School:** UMDNJ-NJ Med Sch, Newark 1989; **Resid:** Physical Medicine & Rehabilitation, UMDNJ-Kessler Inst Rehab 1993; **Fac Appt:** Asst Clin Prof PMR, UMDNJ-NJ Med Sch, Newark

Fried, Guy W MD [PMR] - **Spec Exp:** Brain Injury Rehabilitation; Spinal Cord Injury; Neurogenic Bladder; **Hospital:** Magee Rehab Hosp; **Address:** Magee Rehab Hosp, 1513 Race St, Philadelphia, PA 19102-1177; **Phone:** 215-587-3394; **Board Cert:** Physical Medicine & Rehabilitation 1990; Spinal Cord Injury Medicine 2009; Pain Medicine 2011; **Med School:** Yale Univ 1985; **Resid:** Physical Medicine & Rehabilitation, Thomas Jefferson Univ Hosp 1988; Preventive Medicine, Thomas Jefferson Univ Hosp 1989; **Fac Appt:** Asst Prof PMR, Thomas Jefferson Univ

Kirshblum, Steven C MD [PMR] - **Spec Exp:** Spinal Cord Injury; Spasticity Management; **Hospital:** Kessler Inst for Rehab - W Orange, Saint Barnabas Med Ctr; **Address:** Kessler Institute, 1199 Pleasant Valley Way, West Orange, NJ 07052-1424; **Phone:** 973-731-3600 x2258; **Board Cert:** Physical Medicine & Rehabilitation 1991; Spinal Cord Injury Medicine 2008; **Med School:** Univ Hlth Scis, Chicago Med Sch 1986; **Resid:** Physical Medicine & Rehabilitation, Mount Sinai Med Ctr 1990; **Fac Appt:** Prof PMR, UMDNJ-NJ Med Sch, Newark

Lutz, Christopher MD [PMR] - **Spec Exp:** Pain-Low Back; Pain-Spine; Pain-Lower Back (IDET Procedure); Electromyography; **Hospital:** Hosp For Special Surgery (page 60); **Address:** Hosp for Special Surgery, 75th Street Campus, 429 E 75th St Fl 3, New York, NY 10021; **Phone:** 212-606-1494; **Board Cert:** Physical Medicine & Rehabilitation 2012; **Med School:** Georgetown Univ 1996; **Resid:** Physical Medicine & Rehabilitation, UMDNJ-Kessler Inst for Rehab 2000; **Fellow:** Sports Medicine, Hosp for Special Surgery 2001

Lutz, Gregory MD [PMR] - **Spec Exp:** Spinal Rehabilitation; Sports Medicine; Pain-Low Back; **Hospital:** Hosp For Special Surgery (page 60), Univ Med Ctr Princeton at Plainsboro; **Address:** 429 E 75 St Fl 3, New York, NY 10021; **Phone:** 212-606-1648; **Board Cert:** Physical Medicine & Rehabilitation 2003; **Med School:** Georgetown Univ 1988; **Resid:** Physical Medicine & Rehabilitation, Mayo Clinic 1992; **Fellow:** Sports Medicine, Hosp For Spec Surg 1993; **Fac Appt:** Assoc Prof PMR, Cornell Univ-Weill Med Coll

Ma, Dong M MD [PMR] - **Spec Exp:** Electromyography; Musculoskeletal Disorders; **Hospital:** NYU Rusk Inst (page 71), NYU Langone Med Ctr (page 68); **Address:** NYU Ctr for Musculoskeletal Care, 2333 E 38th St Fl 5, New York, NY 10016; **Phone:** 646-501-7277; **Board Cert:** Physical Medicine & Rehabilitation 1979; **Med School:** South Korea 1968; **Resid:** Physical Medicine & Rehabilitation, NYU Med Ctr 1975; **Fellow:** Physical Medicine & Rehabilitation, NYU Med Ctr 1977; **Fac Appt:** Clin Prof PMR, NYU Sch Med

Marino, Ralph J MD [PMR] - **Spec Exp:** Spinal Cord Injury; Spasticity Management; **Hospital:** Thomas Jefferson Univ Hosp; **Address:** 25 S 9th St, Philadelphia, PA 19107; **Phone:** 215-955-1200; **Board Cert:** Physical Medicine & Rehabilitation 1988; Spinal Cord Injury Medicine 2010; **Med School:** Jefferson Med Coll 1982; **Resid:** Physical Medicine & Rehabilitation, Thos Jefferson Univ Hosp 1987; **Fac Appt:** Assoc Prof PMR, Jefferson Med Coll

Mayer, Nathaniel H MD [PMR] - **Spec Exp:** Motor Control Analysis; Spasticity Management; Brain Injury Rehabilitation; **Hospital:** Moss Rehab Hosp; **Address:** Drucker Brain Injury Ctr/Moss Rehab, 60 Township Line Rd, Elkins Park, PA 19027; **Phone:** 215-663-6677; **Board Cert:** Physical Medicine & Rehabilitation 1976; **Med School:** Albert Einstein Coll Med 1968; **Resid:** Physical Medicine & Rehabilitation, Temple Univ Hosp 1973; **Fac Appt:** Prof PMR, Temple Univ

Miknevich, Mary Ann MD [PMR] - **Spec Exp:** Amputee Rehabilitation; Electrodiagnosis; Spasticity Management; Geriatric Rehabilitation; **Hospital:** UPMC Mercy, Pittsburgh, UPMC McKeesport; **Address:** Mercy Professional Bldg., Building C, 1350 Locust St, Ste 409, Pittsburgh, PA 15219; **Phone:** 412-232-7608; **Board Cert:** Physical Medicine & Rehabilitation 1985; **Med School:** Univ Pittsburgh 1980; **Resid:** Physical Medicine & Rehabilitation, St Francis Med Ctr 1983; **Fac Appt:** Asst Clin Prof PMR, Univ Pittsburgh

Munin, Michael C MD [PMR] - **Spec Exp:** Spasticity Management; Amputee Rehabilitation; Electrodiagnosis; Electrodiagnosis; **Hospital:** UPMC Presby, Pittsburgh, UPMC Mercy, Pittsburgh; **Address:** 3471 Fifth Avenue, Pittsuburgh PA Ave, Ste 1103, MS 15213, Pittsburgh, PA 15213; **Phone:** 412-692-4400; **Board Cert:** Physical Medicine & Rehabilitation 2003; **Med School:** Jefferson Med Coll 1988; **Resid:** Physical Medicine & Rehabilitation, Thomas Jefferson Univ Hosp 1992; **Fac Appt:** Prof PMR, Univ Pittsburgh

Palmer, Jeffrey B MD [PMR] - **Spec Exp:** Swallowing Disorders; Neuro-Rehabilitation; Stroke Rehabilitation; **Hospital:** Johns Hopkins Hosp (page 61), Good Samaritan Hosp; **Address:** The Johns Hopkins Hospital, 600 N Wolfe St Phipps Bldg - Ste 160, Baltimore, MD 21287; **Phone:** 410-502-2446; **Board Cert:** Physical Medicine & Rehabilitation 1984; Electrodiagnostic Medicine 1998; **Med School:** NYU Sch Med 1980; **Resid:** Physical Medicine & Rehabilitation, Univ Wash Med Ctr 1983; **Fac Appt:** Prof PMR, Johns Hopkins Univ

Ragnarsson, Kristjan T MD [PMR] - **Spec Exp:** Spinal Cord Injury; Brain Injury Rehabilitation; Pain-Back & Neck; **Hospital:** Mount Sinai Med Ctr (page 64); **Address:** 5 E 98th St, Fl 6, New York, NY 10029-6501; **Phone:** 212-659-9370; **Board Cert:** Physical Medicine & Rehabilitation 1976; **Med School:** Iceland 1969; **Resid:** Physical Medicine & Rehabilitation, NYU Med Ctr 1974; **Fellow:** Spinal Cord & Brain Injury Rehab, NYU Med Ctr 1975; **Fac Appt:** Prof PMR, Mount Sinai Sch Med

Schwartz, L Matthew MD [PMR] - **Spec Exp:** Pain-Musculoskeletal; Cancer Rehabilitation; Lymphedema; Head & Neck Cancer; **Hospital:** Chestnut Hill Hosp; **Address:** Montgomery Rehab Assocs, 8601 Stenton Ave, Wyndmoor, PA 19038; **Phone:** 215-233-6226; **Board Cert:** Physical Medicine & Rehabilitation 1992; Pain Medicine 2003; **Med School:** UMDNJ-NJ Med Sch, Newark 1987; **Resid:** Physical Medicine & Rehabilitation, Hosp Univ Penn 1989; Physical Medicine & Rehabilitation, Thos Jefferson Univ Hosp 1991; **Fac Appt:** Asst Clin Prof PMR, Univ Pennsylvania

Stubblefield, Michael Dean MD [PMR] - **Spec Exp:** Cancer Rehabilitation; Pain-Cancer; Pain-Neuropathic; Pain-Musculoskeletal; **Hospital:** Meml Sloan-Kettering Cancer Ctr; **Address:** Sillerman Center for Rehabilitation, Meml Sloan-Kettering Cancer Ctr, 515 Madison Ave Fl 5, New York, NY 10022; **Phone:** 646-888-1936; **Board Cert:** Internal Medicine 2011; Physical Medicine & Rehabilitation 2012; Electrodiagnostic Medicine 2003; **Med School:** Columbia P&S 1996; **Resid:** Internal Medicine, Columbia Presby Med Ctr 2001; Physical Medicine & Rehabilitation, Columbia Presby Med Ctr 2001; **Fac Appt:** Assoc Prof PMR, Cornell Univ-Weill Med Coll

Southeast

Alexander, Joshua MD [PMR] - **Spec Exp:** Pediatric Rehabilitation; Cerebral Palsy; Spina Bifida; **Hospital:** NC Memorial Hosp - UNC; **Address:** UNC- Physical Med & Rehab, 101 Manning Drive, Campus Box 7200, Chapel Hill, NC 27599-7200; **Phone:** 919-966-5165; **Board Cert:** Pediatrics 2010; Physical Medicine & Rehabilitation 2006; Pediatric Rehabilitation Medicine 2005; **Med School:** Temple Univ 1990; **Resid:** Pediatrics, Baylor Coll of Med 1995; Physical Medicine & Rehabilitation, Baylor Coll of Med 1995; **Fac Appt:** Assoc Prof PMR, Univ NC Sch Med

Cardenas, Diana D MD [PMR] - **Spec Exp:** Spinal Cord Injury; Spina Bifida; Neurogenic Bladder; Urinary Tract Infections; **Hospital:** Univ of Miami Hosp & Clins/Sylvester Comp Canc Ctr, Jackson Meml Hosp; **Address:** 1475 NW 12th Ave, Miami, FL 33136; **Phone:** 305-243-4000; **Board Cert:** Physical Medicine & Rehabilitation 1977; Electrodiagnostic Medicine 1989; **Med School:** Univ Tex SW, Dallas 1973; **Resid:** Physical Medicine & Rehabilitation, Univ Wash Affil Hosps 1976; **Fac Appt:** Prof PMR, Univ Miami Sch Med

Creamer, Michael J DO [PMR] - **Spec Exp:** Spinal Cord Injury; Pain Management; Electrodiagnosis; **Hospital:** Florida Hosp - Orlando, Orlando Regl Med Ctr; **Address:** Rehab Medical Group, 100 W Gore St, Ste 500, Orlando, FL 32806; **Phone:** 407-649-8707; **Board Cert:** Physical Medicine & Rehabilitation 1992; Spinal Cord Injury Medicine 2008; Pain Medicine 2011; **Med School:** Chicago Coll Osteo Med 1987; **Resid:** Physical Medicine & Rehabilitation, Rehab Inst Chicago 1991; **Fac Appt:** Asst Clin Prof Med, Univ Fla Coll Med

Diamond, Paul T MD [PMR] - **Spec Exp:** Neuro-Rehabilitation; Geriatric Rehabilitation; **Hospital:** Univ of Virginia Health Sys; **Address:** Univ of Virginia Hlth Sci Ctr, Dept Rehabilitation, Box 801004, Charlottesville, VA 22908-1004; **Phone:** 434-243-5622; **Board Cert:** Internal Medicine 1989; Physical Medicine & Rehabilitation 2003; **Med School:** Univ VA Sch Med 1986; **Resid:** Internal Medicine, Johns Hospkins Bayview Hosp 1989; Physical Medicine & Rehabilitation, Sinai/Johns Hopkins Hosp 1992; **Fac Appt:** Assoc Prof PMR, Univ VA Sch Med

Gater Jr, David R MD/PhD [PMR] - **Spec Exp:** Spinal Cord Injury; Exercise Physiology; Electrodiagnosis; **Hospital:** Hunter Holmes McGuire VA Med Ctr - Richmond, VCU Med Ctr; **Address:** 1201 Broadrock Blvd, MS 652/128, Richmond, VA 23249; **Phone:** 804-675-5000 x6583; **Board Cert:** Physical Medicine & Rehabilitation 2007; Spinal Cord Injury Medicine 2009; Electrodiagnostic Medicine 1998; **Med School:** Univ Ariz Coll Med 1992; **Resid:** Physical Medicine & Rehabilitation, UC Davis Med Ctr 1996; **Fac Appt:** Prof PMR, Va Commonwealth Univ Sch Med

Jackson, Amie B MD [PMR] - **Spec Exp:** Spinal Cord Injury; **Hospital:** UAB Spain Rehab Ctr, Univ of Ala Hosp at Birmingham; **Address:** Univ Alabama at Birmingham, Spain Rehab Center, 1717 6th Ave S, rm 190, Birmingham, AL 35249-7330; **Phone:** 205-934-3330; **Board Cert:** Physical Medicine & Rehabilitation 1990; **Med School:** Univ Alabama 1984; **Resid:** Physical Medicine & Rehabilitation, Univ Alabama Med Ctr 1987; **Fac Appt:** Prof PMR, Univ Alabama

Kezar, Laura B MD [PMR] - **Spec Exp:** Pain-Back; Pain-Spine; **Hospital:** UAB Spain Rehab Ctr; **Address:** Spain Rehabilitation Ctr, 1717 6th Ave S, Birmingham, AL 35233; **Phone:** 205-934-4179; **Board Cert:** Physical Medicine & Rehabilitation 2006; **Med School:** Emory Univ 1985; **Resid:** Physical Medicine & Rehabilitation, Univ Alabama Hosp 1994; **Fac Appt:** Assoc Prof PMR, Univ Alabama

King Jr, Richard W MD [PMR] - **Spec Exp:** Cancer Rehabilitation; Lymphedema; Soft Tissue Radiation Necrosis; Soft Tissue Radiation Necrosis-Breast; **Hospital:** WellStar Windy Hill Hosp, WellStar Cobb Hosp; **Address:** HyOx Medical Treatment Ctr, 2550 Windy Hill Rd, Ste 110, Marietta, GA 30067; **Phone:** 678-303-3200; **Board Cert:** Physical Medicine & Rehabilitation 1988; Undersea & Hyperbaric Medicine 2012; **Med School:** Emory Univ 1979; **Resid:** Physical Medicine & Rehabilitation, Emory Univ Hosp 1987; **Fac Appt:** Asst Clin Prof PMR, Emory Univ

Leslie, Donald P MD [PMR] - **Spec Exp:** Brain/Spinal Cord Injury; **Hospital:** Shepherd Ctr - Atlanta; **Address:** Shepherd Center, 2020 Peachtree Rd NW, Atlanta, GA 30309; **Phone:** 404-352-2020; **Board Cert:** Physical Medicine & Rehabilitation 1989; **Med School:** Univ Tenn Coll Med 1972; **Resid:** Internal Medicine, Mayo Clinic 1975; Physical Medicine & Rehabilitation, Emory Univ Hosp 1986

McKinley, William O MD [PMR] - **Spec Exp:** Spinal Cord Injury; **Hospital:** VCU Med Ctr; **Address:** Ambulatory Care Ctr, 417 N 11th St, Richmond, VA 23298; **Phone:** 804-828-4097; **Board Cert:** Physical Medicine & Rehabilitation 1990; Spinal Cord Injury Medicine 2008; **Med School:** Albany Med Coll 1985; **Resid:** Physical Medicine & Rehabilitation, Med Coll Va 1989; **Fac Appt:** Prof PMR, Va Commonwealth Univ Sch Med

Stewart, Paula JB MD [PMR] - **Spec Exp:** Lymphedema; Brain Tumors; Spinal Cord Tumors; Cancer Rehabilitation; **Hospital:** Healthsouth Lakeshore Rehab Hosp; **Address:** Healthsouth Lakeshore Rehab Hosp, 3800 Ridgeway Drive, Birmingham, AL 35209; **Phone:** 205-868-2347; **Board Cert:** Physical Medicine & Rehabilitation 2006; Spinal Cord Injury Medicine 2010; **Med School:** Univ Minn 1987; **Resid:** Physical Medicine & Rehabilitation, Mayo Clinic 1991

Midwest

Brown, Allen W MD [PMR] - **Spec Exp:** Brain Injury; Stroke; **Hospital:** St. Mary's Hosp - Rochester MN (Mayo), Rochester Methodist Hosp; **Address:** Mayo Clinic PM&R, 200 1st St SW, Rochester, MN 55905; **Phone:** 507-255-3116; **Board Cert:** Physical Medicine & Rehabilitation 1994; **Med School:** Univ Minn 1998; **Resid:** Physical Medicine & Rehabilitation, Mayo Med Ctr & Clin 1992; **Fac Appt:** Asst Prof PMR, Mayo Med Sch

Chen, David MD [PMR] - **Spec Exp:** Spinal Cord Injury; **Hospital:** Rehab Inst of Chicago; **Address:** 345 E Superior St, Ste 1146, Chicago, IL 60611; **Phone:** 312-238-1000; **Board Cert:** Physical Medicine & Rehabilitation 1992; Spinal Cord Injury Medicine 2008; **Med School:** Univ IL Coll Med 1987; **Resid:** Physical Medicine & Rehabilitation, Northwestern Med Sch 1991; **Fac Appt:** Asst Prof PMR, Northwestern Univ

Cheville, Andrea L MD [PMR] - **Spec Exp:** Lymphedema; Cancer Rehabilitation; Pain-Cancer; **Hospital:** Mayo Med Ctr & Clin - Rochester; **Address:** Mayo Clinic, Dept Physical Med & Rehab, 200 1st St SW, Rochester, MN 55905; **Phone:** 507-284-2747; **Board Cert:** Physical Medicine & Rehabilitation 2008; Pain Medicine 2004; Hospice & Palliative Medicine 2008; **Med School:** Harvard Med Sch 1993; **Resid:** Physical Medicine & Rehabilitation, UMDNJ Med Ctr 1997; **Fellow:** Pain & Palliative Care, Meml Sloan Kettering Cancer Ctr 1999; **Fac Appt:** Assoc Prof PMR, Mayo Med Sch

Clairmont, Albert C MD [PMR] - **Spec Exp:** Spasticity Management; Electrodiagnosis; **Hospital:** Ohio St Univ Med Ctr; **Address:** 480 Medical Center Drive, Columbus, OH 43210; **Phone:** 614-293-7604; **Board Cert:** Physical Medicine & Rehabilitation 1985; Pediatrics 1985; **Med School:** Jamaica 1974; **Resid:** Pediatrics, Columbus Chldns Hosp 1981; Physical Medicine & Rehabilitation, Ohio St Univ Hosps 1983; **Fac Appt:** Assoc Clin Prof PMR, Ohio State Univ

Colachis III, Samuel C MD [PMR] - **Spec Exp:** Spinal Cord Injury; Electrodiagnosis; **Hospital:** Ohio St Univ Med Ctr; **Address:** 480 Medical Center Drive, Columbus, OH 43210; **Phone:** 614-293-7604; **Board Cert:** Physical Medicine & Rehabilitation 1988; Spinal Cord Injury Medicine 2003; **Med School:** USC Sch Med 1984; **Resid:** Physical Medicine & Rehabilitation, Ohio State Univ Hosps 1987; **Fellow:** Electrodiagnosis, Ohio State Univ Hosps 1988; **Fac Appt:** Assoc Prof PMR, Ohio State Univ

DePompolo, Robert W MD [PMR] - **Spec Exp:** Cancer Rehabilitation; Lymphedema; **Hospital:** St. Mary's Hosp - Rochester MN (Mayo), Mayo Med Ctr & Clin - Rochester; **Address:** Mayo Clinic, Dept Phys Med & Rehab, 200 1st St SW, Rochester, MN 55905; **Phone:** 507-255-3116; **Board Cert:** Physical Medicine & Rehabilitation 1981; **Med School:** Wayne State Univ 1977; **Resid:** Physical Medicine & Rehabilitation, Univ Minnesota Affil Hosp 1980

Feldman, Joseph L MD [PMR] - **Spec Exp:** Lymphedema; **Hospital:** Evanston/North Shore Univ Hlth Sys; **Address:** 1000 Central St, Ste 800, Evanston, IL 60201; **Phone:** 847-570-2066; **Board Cert:** Physical Medicine & Rehabilitation 1971; **Med School:** Univ IL Coll Med 1965; **Resid:** Physical Medicine & Rehabilitation, Univ Ilinois Med Ctr 1969; **Fac Appt:** Asst Prof PMR, Northwestern Univ

Frost, Frederick S MD [PMR] - **Spec Exp:** Spinal Cord Injury; Stroke Rehabilitation; Geriatric Rehabilitation; **Hospital:** Cleveland Clin (page 55); **Address:** Cleveland Clinic Fdn, 9500 Euclid Ave, Desk S-31, Cleveland, OH 44195; **Phone:** 216-445-2006; **Board Cert:** Physical Medicine & Rehabilitation 1988; Spinal Cord Injury Medicine 2008; **Med School:** Northwestern Univ 1983; **Resid:** Physical Medicine & Rehabilitation, Northwestern Meml Hosp 1987; **Fellow:** Spinal Cord Injury Medicine, Rehab Inst Chicago; **Fac Appt:** Asst Prof PMR, Cleveland Cl Coll Med/Case West Res

Gamble, Gail L MD [PMR] - **Spec Exp:** Lymphedema; Cancer Rehabilitation; **Hospital:** Rehab Inst of Chicago; **Address:** Rehab Inst of Chicago, 345 E Superior St, Ste 1136, Chicago, IL 60611; **Phone:** 312-238-7670; **Board Cert:** Physical Medicine & Rehabilitation 1985; **Med School:** Mayo Med Sch 1979; **Resid:** Physical Medicine & Rehabilitation, Mayo Clinic 1983

Gittler, Michelle S MD [PMR] - **Spec Exp:** Spinal Cord Injury; Amputee Rehabilitation; **Hospital:** Schwab Rehab Hosp, Univ of Chicago Med Ctr; **Address:** 1401 S California Blvd, Chicago, IL 60608; **Phone:** 773-522-6617; **Board Cert:** Physical Medicine & Rehabilitation 2003; Spinal Cord Injury Medicine 2008; **Med School:** Univ IL Coll Med 1988; **Resid:** Physical Medicine & Rehabilitation, Rehab Inst Chicago 1992; **Fac Appt:** Assoc Clin Prof S, Univ Chicago-Pritzker Sch Med

Haig, Andrew John MD [PMR] - **Spec Exp:** International Health; Pain-Back & Neck; Electrodiagnosis; **Hospital:** Univ of Michigan Hosp; **Address:** 325 E Eisenhower, Burlington Bldg - Ste 100, Ann Arbor, MI 48108-3346; **Phone:** 734-763-4200; **Board Cert:** Physical Medicine & Rehabilitation 1987; Pain Medicine 2002; **Med School:** Med Coll Wisc 1983; **Resid:** Physical Medicine & Rehabilitation, Northwestern Univ 1986; **Fac Appt:** Prof PMR, Univ Mich Med Sch

Keen, Mary MD [PMR] - **Spec Exp:** Pediatric Rehabilitation; Spasticity Management; Neurodevelopmental Disabilities; Autism; **Hospital:** Marianjoy Rehab Hosp, Central DuPage Hosp; **Address:** Marianjoy Rehab Medical Clinic, 26 W 171 Roosevelt Rd, Wheaton, IL 60187; **Phone:** 630-909-7000 x2; **Board Cert:** Physical Medicine & Rehabilitation 1984; Pediatrics 2012; Neurodevelopmental Disabilities 2012; Pediatric Rehabilitation Medicine 2003; **Med School:** Northwestern Univ 1979; **Resid:** Physical Medicine & Rehabilitation, Univ Wash Med Ctr 1983; Pediatrics, Loyola Univ Med Ctr 1990; **Fac Appt:** Assoc Clin Prof Ped, Loyola Univ-Stritch Sch Med

Kirschner, Kristi MD [PMR] - **Spec Exp:** Spina Bifida-Adult; Neuromuscular Disorders; Women's Health/Disabilities; **Hospital:** Schwab Rehab Hosp, Northwestern Meml Hosp; **Address:** Schwab Rehab Hosp, 1401 S California Ave, Chicago, IL 60608; **Phone:** 773-522-6617; **Board Cert:** Physical Medicine & Rehabilitation 1991; **Med School:** Northwestern Univ-Feinberg Sch Med 1986; **Resid:** Physical Medicine & Rehabilitation, Rehab Inst of Chicago/Northwestern Univ 1990; **Fellow:** Clinical Ethics, Maclean Ctr/Univ Chicago 1995; **Fac Appt:** Prof PMR, Northwestern Univ-Feinberg Sch Med

Kuiken, Todd A MD/PhD [PMR] - **Spec Exp:** Amputee Rehabilitation; Prosthesis Control; Gait Disorders; **Hospital:** Rehab Inst of Chicago; **Address:** Rehabilitation Institute of Chicago, 345 E Superior St, rm 1309, Chicago, IL 60611; **Phone:** 312-238-8072; **Board Cert:** Physical Medicine & Rehabilitation 2006; **Med School:** Northwestern Univ 1990; **Resid:** Physical Medicine & Rehabilitation, Rehab Inst Chicago 1995; **Fac Appt:** Prof PMR, Northwestern Univ

La Ban, Myron M MD [PMR] - **Spec Exp:** Pain-Back; Electromyography; Neuromuscular Disorders; **Hospital:** Beaumont Hosp-Royal Oak; **Address:** 3535 W 13 Mile Rd, Ste 437, Royal Oak, MI 48073; **Phone:** 248-288-2237; **Board Cert:** Physical Medicine & Rehabilitation 1967; **Med School:** Univ Mich Med Sch 1961; **Resid:** Physical Medicine & Rehabilitation, Univ Ohio Hosps 1965; **Fac Appt:** Clin Prof PMR, Ohio State Univ

Leonard Jr, James A MD [PMR] - **Spec Exp:** Amputee Rehabilitation; Electrodiagnosis; **Hospital:** Univ of Michigan Hosp; **Address:** Eisenhower Corporate Park, 2850 S Industrial Hwy, Ste 400, Ann Arbor, MI 48104; **Phone:** 734-973-2400; **Board Cert:** Physical Medicine & Rehabilitation 1977; **Med School:** Univ Mich Med Sch 1972; **Resid:** Physical Medicine & Rehabilitation, Univ Mich Med Ctr 1975; **Fac Appt:** Clin Prof PMR, Univ Mich Med Sch

Mysiw, W Jerry MD [PMR] - **Spec Exp:** Brain Injury Rehabilitation; **Hospital:** Ohio St Univ Med Ctr; **Address:** 480 Medical Center Drive, Columbus, OH 43210-1245; **Phone:** 614-293-7604; **Board Cert:** Physical Medicine & Rehabilitation 1985; **Med School:** Ohio State Univ 1981; **Resid:** Physical Medicine & Rehabilitation, Ohio State Univ Med Ctr 1984; **Fac Appt:** Assoc Prof PMR, Ohio State Univ

Nobunaga, Austin MD [PMR] - **Spec Exp:** Spinal Cord Injury; Electrodiagnosis; **Hospital:** Univ Hosp - Cincinnati; **Address:** Drake Center, 151 W Galbraith Rd, South Pavillion, Cincinnati, OH 45216; **Phone:** 513-418-2707; **Board Cert:** Physical Medicine & Rehabilitation 1990; Spinal Cord Injury Medicine 2009; **Med School:** Univ Mich Med Sch 1985; **Resid:** Physical Medicine & Rehabilitation, Rehab Inst Chicago 1989

Press, Joel MD [PMR] - **Spec Exp:** Sports Medicine; Pain-Back; Musculoskeletal Injuries; **Hospital:** Rehab Inst of Chicago; **Address:** Ctr for Spine, Sports & Occup Rehab, 1030 N Clark St, Ste 500, Chicago, IL 60610; **Phone:** 312-238-7767; **Board Cert:** Physical Medicine & Rehabilitation 1989; Sports Medicine 2009; **Med School:** Univ IL Coll Med 1984; **Resid:** Physical Medicine & Rehabilitation, Northwestern Meml Hosp 1988; **Fac Appt:** Assoc Clin Prof PMR, Northwestern Univ

Roth, Elliot MD [PMR] - **Spec Exp:** Stroke Rehabilitation; Neurologic Rehabilitation; Geriatric Rehabilitation; **Hospital:** Rehab Inst of Chicago, Northwestern Meml Hosp; **Address:** Rehab Inst Chicago, 345 E Superior St, Ste 1146, Chicago, IL 60611-2654; **Phone:** 312-238-1000; **Board Cert:** Physical Medicine & Rehabilitation 1987; **Med School:** Northwestern Univ 1982; **Resid:** Physical Medicine & Rehabilitation, Northwestern Univ 1985; **Fellow:** Physical Medicine & Rehabilitation, Rehab Inst Chicago 1986; **Fac Appt:** Prof PMR, Northwestern Univ

Sisung, Charles MD [PMR] - **Spec Exp:** Rheumatic Diseases of Childhood; Trauma Rehabilitation; Burn Care; **Hospital:** Rehab Inst of Chicago; **Address:** 345 E Superior St, rm 1158, Chicago, IL 60611; **Phone:** 312-238-1246; **Board Cert:** Pediatrics 2011; Physical Medicine & Rehabilitation 1991; Pediatric Rehabilitation Medicine 2003; **Med School:** Univ Mich Med Sch 1981; **Resid:** Pediatrics, Mott Chldns Hosp/Univ Mich 1984; Physical Medicine & Rehabilitation, Schwab Rehab Hosp 1989; **Fellow:** Pediatric Rheumatology, Univ Chicago Hosps 1991; **Fac Appt:** Asst Prof PMR, Northwestern Univ

Physical Medicine & Rehabilitation

Sliwa, James A DO [PMR] - **Spec Exp:** Post Polio Syndrome/Rehabilitation; Multiple Sclerosis; Pain-Back; **Hospital:** Rehab Inst of Chicago; **Address:** Rehab Inst Chicago, 345 E Superior St, rm 1509, Chicago, IL 60611-3015; **Phone:** 312-238-4093; **Board Cert:** Physical Medicine & Rehabilitation 2005; **Med School:** Chicago Coll Osteo Med 1980; **Resid:** Physical Medicine & Rehabilitation, Rehab Institute Chicago 1984; **Fac Appt:** Prof PMR, Northwestern Univ

Volshteyn, Oksana MD [PMR] - **Spec Exp:** Spinal Cord Injury; Amputee Rehabilitation; **Hospital:** Rehab Inst St. Louis, Barnes-Jewish Hosp; **Address:** 4444 Forest Park Blvd, Ste 8518, St Louis, MO 63108; **Phone:** 314-362-4503; **Board Cert:** Physical Medicine & Rehabilitation 1986; Spinal Cord Injury Medicine 2009; **Med School:** Russia 1976; **Resid:** Physical Medicine & Rehabilitation, Barnes-Jewish Hosp 1985; **Fac Appt:** Assoc Prof N, Washington Univ, St Louis

Great Plains and Mountains

Mason, Kristin D MD [PMR] - **Spec Exp:** Neurologic Rehabilitation; Electrodiagnosis; Musculoskeletal Injuries; **Hospital:** Swedish Med Ctr - Denver; **Address:** Rehab Assocs Colorado, 9025 Grant St, Ste 103, Thornton, CO 80229; **Phone:** 303-286-2888; **Board Cert:** Physical Medicine & Rehabilitation 2003; **Med School:** Baylor Coll Med 1988; **Resid:** Physical Medicine & Rehabilitation, Rehab Inst Chicago 1992

Matthews, Dennis J MD [PMR] - **Spec Exp:** Pediatric Rehabilitation; Brain Injury Rehabilitation; Neuromuscular Disorders; Cerebral Palsy; **Hospital:** Chldn's Hosp - Aurora (CO); **Address:** Chldns Hosp, Dept Rehabilitation, 13123 E 16th Ave, Box 285, Aurora, CO 80045; **Phone:** 720-777-3907; **Board Cert:** Physical Medicine & Rehabilitation 1979; Pediatric Rehabilitation Medicine 2003; Neuromuscular Medicine 2008; **Med School:** Univ Colorado 1975; **Resid:** Physical Medicine & Rehabilitation, Univ Minnesota Hosps 1978; **Fellow:** Research, Univ Minnesota Hosps 1978; **Fac Appt:** Prof PMR, Univ Colorado

Southwest

Currie, Donald M MD [PMR] - **Spec Exp:** Pediatric Rehabilitation; Neuro-Rehabilitation; **Hospital:** Univ Hlth Syst-San Antonio, Christus Santa Rosa Med Ctr Hosp; **Address:** Univ Hospital, 4502 Medical Drive, MS 64-1, San Antonio, TX 78229; **Phone:** 210-358-0500; **Board Cert:** Physical Medicine & Rehabilitation 1978; **Med School:** Univ Tex SW, Dallas 1972; **Resid:** Physical Medicine & Rehabilitation, Baylor Univ Med Ctr 1975; Physical Medicine & Rehabilitation, Univ Washington Affil Hosp 1977; **Fac Appt:** Prof PMR, Univ Tex, San Antonio

Dumitru, Daniel MD/PhD [PMR] - **Spec Exp:** Electrodiagnosis; **Hospital:** Univ Hlth Syst-San Antonio; **Address:** 4502 Med Drive, MS 33-1, San Antonio, TX 78229-3900; **Phone:** 210-358-0770; **Board Cert:** Physical Medicine & Rehabilitation 1984; **Med School:** Univ Cincinnati 1980; **Resid:** Physical Medicine & Rehabilitation, VA Hosp 1983; **Fac Appt:** Prof PMR, Univ Tex, San Antonio

Francisco, Gerard E MD [PMR] - **Spec Exp:** Spasticity Management; Brain Injury Rehabilitation; Stroke Rehabilitation; **Hospital:** TIRR-Inst for Rehab and Research, Meml Hermann Hosp - Texas Med Ctr; **Address:** 1333 Moursund Ave, Houston, TX 77030; **Phone:** 713-797-5246; **Board Cert:** Physical Medicine & Rehabilitation 2005; **Med School:** Philippines 1989; **Resid:** Physical Medicine & Rehabilitation, UMDNJ-Univ Hosp 1994; **Fellow:** Physical Medicine & Rehabilitation, Baylor Coll Med 1995; **Fac Appt:** Clin Prof PMR, Univ Tex, Houston

Harris, David K MD [PMR] - **Spec Exp:** Spinal Rehabilitation; Spinal Cord Injury; Pain-Back; Pain-Spine; **Address:** Ctr for Healing & Regenerative Med, 7307 Creekbluff Drive, Austin, TX 78750; **Phone:** 512-614-3300; **Board Cert:** Physical Medicine & Rehabilitation 2004; Pain Medicine 2004; **Med School:** Univ Tex SW, Dallas 1988; **Resid:** Physical Medicine & Rehabilitation, Univ Colorado Hlth Sci Ctr 1992

Ivanhoe, Cindy MD [PMR] - **Spec Exp:** Brain Injury Rehabilitation; Spasticity Management; Movement Disorders; **Hospital:** TIRR-Inst for Rehab and Research, Meml Hermann Hosp - Texas Med Ctr; **Address:** 1312 Hermann Drive, Park Plaza Bldg - Ste 740, Houston, TX 77098; **Phone:** 713-942-7300; **Board Cert:** Physical Medicine & Rehabilitation 2003; **Med School:** Mexico 1984; **Resid:** Physical Medicine & Rehabilitation, Univ Illinois Affil Hosp 1992; **Fellow:** Brain Injury, Baylor Coll Med 1993; **Fac Appt:** Assoc Prof PMR, Baylor Coll Med

Kevorkian, Charles G MD [PMR] - **Spec Exp:** Stroke Rehabilitation; Neuromuscular Disorders; Electrodiagnosis; **Hospital:** St. Luke's Episcopal Hosp-Houston; **Address:** Dept Physical Med & Rehab, 6624 Fannin St, Ste 2330, Houston, TX 77030-2335; **Phone:** 713-798-4061; **Board Cert:** Physical Medicine & Rehabilitation 1980; **Med School:** Australia 1972; **Resid:** Physical Medicine & Rehabilitation, Prince Henry Hosp 1976; Physical Medicine & Rehabilitation, Mayo Clinic 1979; **Fac Appt:** Assoc Prof PMR, Baylor Coll Med

King, John C MD [PMR] - **Spec Exp:** Stroke Rehabilitation; Pain-Chronic; Spinal Cord Injury; Electrodiagnosis; **Hospital:** Univ Hlth Syst-San Antonio; **Address:** 4502 Medical Drive, San Antonio, TX 78229; **Phone:** 210-358-0770; **Board Cert:** Physical Medicine & Rehabilitation 1987; Spinal Cord Injury Medicine 2000; Pain Medicine 2002; **Med School:** Oral Roberts Sch Med 1983; **Resid:** Physical Medicine & Rehabilitation, Baylor Coll Med 1986; **Fac Appt:** Prof PMR, Univ Tex, San Antonio

Nelson, Maureen R MD [PMR] - **Spec Exp:** Pediatric Rehabilitation; Brachial Plexus Palsy; Electrodiagnosis; **Hospital:** Dell Children's Med Ctr of Central Texas; **Address:** 1301 Barbara Jordan Blvd, Ste 200, Austin, TX 78723; **Phone:** 512-628-1896; **Board Cert:** Physical Medicine & Rehabilitation 1990; Pediatric Rehabilitation Medicine 2003; **Med School:** Univ IL Coll Med 1985; **Resid:** Physical Medicine & Rehabilitation, Univ Tex Hlth Scis Ctr 1989; **Fellow:** Pediatric Rehabilitation Medicine, Alfred I Dupont Inst 1990

Wilson, Amy J MD [PMR] - **Spec Exp:** Amputee Rehabilitation; Stroke Rehabilitation; **Hospital:** Baylor Inst for Rehabilitation; **Address:** Baylor Institute for Rehabilitation, 909 N Washington Ave, Dallas, TX 75246; **Phone:** 214-820-9300; **Board Cert:** Physical Medicine & Rehabilitation 2007; **Med School:** Univ Tex, Houston 1992; **Resid:** Physical Medicine & Rehabilitation, Baylor Univ Med Ctr 1996

West Coast and Pacific

Herring, Stanley A MD [PMR] - **Spec Exp:** Muskuloskeletal Disorders; Spinal Rehabilitation; Concussion; Sports Medicine; **Hospital:** Harborview Med Ctr; **Address:** 908 Jefferson St, Box 359721, Seattle, WA 98104; **Phone:** 206-744-0401; **Board Cert:** Physical Medicine & Rehabilitation 1983; **Med School:** Univ Tex SW, Dallas 1979; **Resid:** Physical Medicine & Rehabilitation, Univ Washington Med Ctr 1982; **Fac Appt:** Clin Prof PMR, Univ Wash

Massagli, Teresa L MD [PMR] - **Spec Exp:** Spinal Cord Injury-Pediatric; Brain Injury Rehabilitation-Pediatric; Neuromuscular Disorders; Pediatric Rehabilitation; **Hospital:** Seattle Chldns Hosp, Harborview Med Ctr; **Address:** Seattle Children's Hosp, 4800 Sand Point Way NE, PO Box 50010, MS W6847, Seattle, WA 98145; **Phone:** 206-987-2180; **Board Cert:** Pediatrics 1987; Physical Medicine & Rehabilitation 2009; Spinal Cord Injury Medicine 2008; Pediatric Rehabilitation Medicine 2009; **Med School:** Yale Univ 1982; **Resid:** Pediatrics, Yale-New Haven Hosp 1985; **Fellow:** Physical Medicine & Rehabilitation, Univ Washington Med Ctr 1988; **Fac Appt:** Prof PMR, Univ Wash

Robinson, Lawrence R MD [PMR] - **Spec Exp:** Electrodiagnosis; Electromyography; Botox Therapy; **Hospital:** Harborview Med Ctr, Univ Wash Med Ctr; **Address:** Harborview Medical Ctr, 325 Ninth Ave, Box 356490, Seattle, WA 98104; **Phone:** 206-744-5862; **Board Cert:** Physical Medicine & Rehabilitation 1987; **Med School:** Baylor Coll Med 1982; **Resid:** Physical Medicine & Rehabilitation, Northwestern Meml Hosp 1985; **Fac Appt:** Prof PMR, Univ Wash

Saal, Jeffrey A MD [PMR] - **Spec Exp:** Pain-Lower Back (IDET procedure); Spinal Rehabilitation; Sports Medicine; **Address:** 500 Arguello St, Ste 100, Redwood City, CA 94063; **Phone:** 650-851-4900; **Board Cert:** Internal Medicine 1978; Physical Medicine & Rehabilitation 1982; **Med School:** Tulane Univ 1975; **Resid:** Internal Medicine, VA Med Ctr 1978; Physical Medicine & Rehabilitation, Stanford Univ Affil Hosps 1981; **Fac Appt:** Assoc Clin Prof PMR, UC Irvine

 Cleveland Clinic

Every life deserves world class care.

Physical Medicine & Rehabilitation

Comprehensive rehabilitation programs can help patients regain lost skills, improve function, relearn tasks and maximize independence. The Cleveland Clinic Department of Physical Medicine & Rehabilitation, part of the Cleveland Clinic Neurological Institute, engages innovative treatments through disease-specific physician evaluations combined with physical, occupational and speech therapy programs.

Our physician faculty members serve as medical directors to nearly 100 acute inpatient rehabilitation beds throughout Greater Cleveland. Consulting services are provided to inpatient, outpatient and sub-acute settings. Patients benefit from rapid access to Cleveland Clinic medical and surgical specialists.

Our senior therapists have achieved certifications and qualifications in more than a dozen subspecialties. Members of our staff hold neuroclinical specialized certification and have training in Neuro-Developmental Treatment, offering special benefits for our patients with disorders such as stroke.

Primary conditions we see:

- Stroke, brain tumors and aneurysms
- Brain injury
- Orthopaedic conditions
- Back and neck pain
- Spinal cord injury
- Cancer
- Parkinson's disease
- Organ transplant
- Cardiac disorders
- MS and transverse myelitis
- Vestibular rehabilitation
- Osteoporosis rehabilitation
- Falls and injury prevention

PEDIATRIC REHABILITATION MEDICINE

Pediatric Rehabilitation is part of the Hassenfeld Pediatric Center, a full service specialty Children's Hospital, which supports the array of children's health services across the Medical Center where newborns, children, adolescents and young adults receive the most comprehensive and advanced care by a team of pediatricians and pediatric specialists.

About the Pediatric Rehabilitation Program
The Pediatric Rehabilitation Medicine Division is a key component Rusk Rehabilitation at NYU Langone (Rusk), providing world-class inpatient and outpatient rehabilitation services for children, from birth through early adulthood. Rusk has been ranked the best rehabilitation hospital in New York and among the top ten in the country by *U.S. News & World Report* for 23 consecutive years. At Rusk, the focus is on early intervention and a family-centered approach that includes sibling and family support groups and counseling.

Areas of Expertise
The pediatric rehabilitation team is particularly skilled in treating the multiple challenges of children with developmental disorders such as cerebral palsy, spina bifida, muscular dystrophy, reflex sympathetic dystrophy, limb deficiencies, arthrogryposis, and spinal cord injuries. Children with traumatic brain injuries, brain tumors, and oncologic diagnoses (such as bone tumors or musculoskeletal disease) also benefit from our specialized services, as do youngsters affected by stroke or cerebrovascular accidents, viral infections or inflammatory diseases, and rheumatic disease.

Spanning the Continuum of Care
In addition to inpatient services, we offer extensive outpatient programs for young patients, including physical therapy, occupational therapy, speech therapy, feeding and swallowing, vocational services, psychological services, and other specialized therapies.

Rusk's pediatric services are delivered at Rusk's 34th Street location as well as at the world-renowned Hospital for Joint Diseases. Moreover, specialized rehabilitation care for premature infants is provided by the Medical Center's neonatal intensive care unit.

The Best in American Medicine
www.CastleConnolly.com

Plastic Surgery

A plastic surgeon deals with the repair, reconstruction or replacement of physical defects of form or function involving the skin, musculoskeletal system, craniomaxillofacial structures, hand, extremities, breast and trunk and external genitalia. He/she uses aesthetic surgical principles not only to improve undesirable qualities of normal structures (commonly called "cosmetic surgery") but in all reconstructive procedures as well.

A plastic surgeon possesses special knowledge and skill in the design and surgery of grafts, flaps, free tissue transfer and replantation. Competence in the management of complex wounds, the use of implantable materials, and in tumor surgery is required.

Training Required: Five to seven years

Certification in one of the following subspecialties requires additional training and examination.

Plastic Surgery within the Head and Neck: A plastic surgeon with additional training in plastic and reconstructive procedures within the head, face, neck and associated structures, including cutaneous head and neck oncology and reconstruction, management of maxillofacial trauma, soft tissue repair and neural surgery.

The field is diverse and involves a wide age range of patients, from the newborn to the aged. While both cosmetic and reconstructive surgery are practiced, there are many additional procedures which interface with them.

Surgery of the Hand (see Hand Surgery)

PLASTIC SURGERY

New England

Ariyan, Stephan MD [PlS] - **Spec Exp:** Melanoma; **Hospital:** Yale-New Haven Hosp; **Address:** New Haven Hosp, 60 Temple St, Ste 4B, New Haven, CT 06510-2716; **Phone:** 203-786-3000; **Board Cert:** Plastic Surgery 1978; **Med School:** NY Med Coll 1966; **Resid:** Surgery, Yale-New Haven Hosp 1975; Plastic Surgery, Yale-New Haven Hosp 1976; **Fellow:** Surgical Oncology, Yale-New Haven Hosp 1971; **Fac Appt:** Clin Prof S, Yale Univ

Collins, Dale C MD [PlS] - **Spec Exp:** Breast Cancer; Breast Reconstruction; **Hospital:** Dartmouth - Hitchcock Med Ctr; **Address:** Div Plastic Surgery, 1 Medical Center Drive, Lebanon, NH 03756; **Phone:** 603-650-5148; **Board Cert:** Plastic Surgery 2007; **Med School:** Emory Univ 1989; **Resid:** Plastic Surgery, Washington Univ Med Ctr 1994; **Fellow:** Microsurgery, Washington Univ Med Ctr 1995; **Fac Appt:** Prof S, Dartmouth Med Sch

Constantian, Mark B MD [PlS] - **Spec Exp:** Rhinoplasty; Rhinoplasty Revision; Cosmetic Surgery-Face; Breast Surgery; **Hospital:** St. Joseph Hosp & Trauma Ctr, Southern NH Med Ctr; **Address:** 19 Tyler St, Ste 302, Nashua, NH 03060-2951; **Phone:** 603-880-7700; **Board Cert:** Plastic Surgery 2009; **Med School:** Univ VA Sch Med 1972; **Resid:** Surgery, Boston Univ Med Ctr 1976; **Fellow:** Plastic/Reconstructive Surgery, Medical Coll VA 1978

Eriksson, Elof K MD [PlS] - **Spec Exp:** Abdominoplasty; Cosmetic Surgery-Breast; Facial Plastic & Reconstructive Surgery; **Hospital:** Brigham and Women's Hosp (page 57), Children's Hospital - Boston; **Address:** Brigham & Women's Hosp, Div Plas Surg, 75 Francis St, Boston, MA 02115; **Phone:** 617-732-5093; **Board Cert:** Plastic Surgery 2007; **Med School:** Sweden 1969; **Resid:** Surgery, Chicago Affil Hosps 1977; **Fellow:** Plastic Surgery, Med Coll Va 1979; **Fac Appt:** Prof PlS, Harvard Med Sch

Feldman, Joel J MD [PlS] - **Spec Exp:** Cosmetic Surgery-Face & Neck; Burns-Reconstructive Plastic Surgery; Reconstructive Surgery; **Hospital:** Mount Auburn Hosp; **Address:** Doctors Office Bldg, 300 Mt Auburn St, Ste 304, Cambridge, MA 02138; **Phone:** 617-661-5998; **Board Cert:** Surgery 1975; Plastic Surgery 1977; **Med School:** Harvard Med Sch 1969; **Resid:** Surgery, Mass Genl Hosp 1974; Plastic Surgery, Johns Hopkins Hosp 1976; **Fac Appt:** Assoc Clin Prof PlS, Harvard Med Sch

Gallico III, G Gregory MD [PlS] - **Spec Exp:** Liposuction & Body Contouring; Rhinoplasty; Abdominoplasty; Breast Surgery; **Hospital:** Mass Genl Hosp, Mass Eye & Ear Infirmary; **Address:** Boston Ctr for Ambulatory Surgery, 170 Commonwealth Ave, Boston, MA 02116; **Phone:** 617-267-5553; **Board Cert:** Plastic Surgery 1982; **Med School:** Harvard Med Sch 1973; **Resid:** Surgery, Mass Genl Hosp 1980; Plastic Surgery, Mass Genl Hosp 1981; **Fellow:** Immunology, Oxford Univ Med Sch 1977; **Fac Appt:** Assoc Clin Prof S, Harvard Med Sch

Meara, John MD/DMD [PlS] - **Spec Exp:** Cleft Palate/Lip; Craniofacial Surgery-Pediatric; **Hospital:** Children's Hospital - Boston; **Address:** Dept Plastic Surgery, 300 Longwood Ave, Enders 1, Boston, MA 02115; **Phone:** 617-355-4401; **Board Cert:** Plastic Surgery 2011; Otolaryngology 1998; **Med School:** Univ Mich Med Sch 1990; **Resid:** Plastic Surgery, Brigham & Womens & The Chldns Hosps 1999; Otolaryngology, Mass Eye & Ear Infirmary 1997; **Fellow:** Craniofacial Surgery, Royal Chldns Hosp 2000; **Fac Appt:** Assoc Prof PlS, Harvard Med Sch

Mulliken, John B MD [PlS] - **Spec Exp:** Pediatric Plastic Surgery; Cleft Palate/Lip; Vascular Malformations; **Hospital:** Children's Hospital - Boston; **Address:** Chldns Hosp, Div Plastic Surgery, 300 Longwood Ave, Hunnewell-1, Boston, MA 02115-5724; **Phone:** 617-355-7686; **Board Cert:** Surgery 1972; Plastic Surgery 1975; **Med School:** Columbia P&S 1964; **Resid:** Surgery, Mass Genl Hosp 1970; Plastic Surgery, Johns Hopkins Hosp 1974; **Fac Appt:** Prof S, Harvard Med Sch

Orgill, Dennis MD [PlS] - **Spec Exp:** Wound Healing/Care; Burns-Reconstructive Plastic Surgery; **Hospital:** Brigham and Women's Hosp (page 57); **Address:** Brigham & Women's Hosp, Dept Plas Surg, 75 Francis St, Boston, MA 02115; **Phone:** 617-732-5456; **Board Cert:** Surgery 2011; Plastic Surgery 2007; **Med School:** Harvard Med Sch 1985; **Resid:** Surgery, Brigham & Women's Hosp 1990; **Fellow:** Plastic Surgery, Brigham & Women's Hosp 1992; **Fac Appt:** Prof S, Harvard Med Sch

Persing, John A MD [PlS] - **Spec Exp:** Craniofacial Surgery; Vascular Malformations; Cosmetic Surgery; **Hospital:** Yale-New Haven Hosp, Yale Med Group; **Address:** Yale Plastic Surgery, 330 Cedar St Boardroom Bldg Fl 3, New Haven, CT 06519-3218; **Phone:** 203-785-2570; **Board Cert:** Plastic Surgery 1985; Neurological Surgery 1986; **Med School:** Univ VT Coll Med 1974; **Resid:** Surgery, Univ Arizona Med Ctr 1976; Neurological Surgery, Univ Virginia Med Ctr 1982; **Fellow:** Plastic Surgery, Univ Virginia Med Ctr 1984; **Fac Appt:** Prof PlS, Yale Univ

Slavin, Sumner MD [PlS] - **Spec Exp:** Breast Reconstruction; Cosmetic Surgery-Face; Liposuction & Body Contouring; **Hospital:** Beth Israel Deaconess Med Ctr - Boston; **Address:** 1101 Beacon St, Ste 7E, Brookline, MA 02446; **Phone:** 617-277-7010; **Board Cert:** Plastic Surgery 1983; **Med School:** Univ VT Coll Med 1973; **Resid:** Surgery, Beth Israel Hosp 1978; Plastic Surgery, NYU Med Ctr 1980; **Fellow:** Hand & Microvascular Surgery, Bellevue Hosp-NYU Med Ctr 1981; **Fac Appt:** Assoc Clin Prof S, Harvard Med Sch

Stadelmann, Wayne K MD [PlS] - **Spec Exp:** Melanoma-Head & Neck; Breast Reconstruction; Breast Augmentation; **Hospital:** Concord Hospital, New London Hosp; **Address:** 246 Pleasant St, Ste 210, MS 03301, Concord, NH 03301; **Phone:** 603-224-5200; **Board Cert:** Plastic Surgery 2009; **Med School:** Univ Chicago-Pritzker Sch Med 1990; **Resid:** Surgery, Univ Chicago Hosps 1994; Plastic Surgery, Univ S Florida/H Lee Moffit Cancer Ctr 1997

Stahl, Richard S MD [PlS] - **Spec Exp:** Abdominal Wall Reconstruction; Chest Wall Reconstruction; Breast Reconstruction; Chest Wall Deformities; **Hospital:** Yale-New Haven Hosp, Hosp of St Raphael; **Address:** 5 Durham Rd, Guilford, CT 06437; **Phone:** 203-458-4440; **Board Cert:** Surgery 2001; Plastic Surgery 1984; **Med School:** Vanderbilt Univ 1976; **Resid:** Surgery, Yale New Haven Hosp 1981; **Fellow:** Plastic Surgery, Emory Univ Med Ctr 1983; **Fac Appt:** Clin Prof S, Yale Univ

Stotland, Mitchell A MD [PlS] - **Spec Exp:** Cleft Palate/Lip; Craniofacial Surgery-Pediatric; Pediatric Plastic Surgery; **Hospital:** Dartmouth - Hitchcock Med Ctr; **Address:** DHMC, Dept Plastic Surgery, 1 Medical Center Drive, Lebanon, NH 03756-1000; **Phone:** 603-650-8068; **Board Cert:** Plastic Surgery 2010; **Med School:** McGill Univ 1989; **Resid:** Surgery, McGill Univ Med Ctr 1994; Plastic Surgery, UCLA Med Ctr 1997; **Fac Appt:** Assoc Prof S, Dartmouth Med Sch

Sullivan, Patrick K MD [PlS] - **Spec Exp:** Cosmetic Surgery-Face; Cosmetic Surgery-Breast; Rhinoplasty; Eyelid Surgery; **Hospital:** Rhode Island Hosp; **Address:** 235 Plain St, Ste 502, Providence, RI 02905; **Phone:** 401-831-8300; **Board Cert:** Otolaryngology 1985; Plastic Surgery 1989; **Med School:** Mayo Med Sch 1979; **Resid:** Otolaryngology, Univ Colo Hlth Scis Ctr 1984; Plastic Surgery, Rhode Island Hosp 1986; **Fellow:** Craniofacial Surgery, Dr Paul Tessier & Dr Hugo Obwegeser 1987; **Fac Appt:** Assoc Prof PlS, Brown Univ

Mid Atlantic

Ascherman, Jeffrey MD [PlS] - **Spec Exp:** Breast Cosmetic & Reconstructive Surgery; Craniofacial Surgery; Cleft Palate/Lip; Cosmetic Surgery; **Hospital:** NY-Presby/Columbia Univ Med Ctr, NY (page 66), New York Eye & Ear Infirm (page 65); **Address:** 161 Ft Washington Ave, Ste 509, New York, NY 10032-3713; **Phone:** 212-305-9612; **Board Cert:** Plastic Surgery 2007; **Med School:** Columbia P&S 1988; **Resid:** Surgery, Columbia-Presby Med Ctr 1991; Plastic Surgery, Columbia-Presby Med Ctr 1994; **Fellow:** Craniofacial Surgery, Hosp Necke-Enfants Malades 1995; **Fac Appt:** Prof S, Columbia P&S

Aston, Sherrell MD [PlS] - **Spec Exp:** Cosmetic Surgery-Face & Body; Rhinoplasty; Cosmetic Surgery-Breast; Liposuction & Body Contouring; **Hospital:** Lenox Hill Hosp (page 67), NYU Langone Med Ctr (page 68); **Address:** 728 Park Ave, New York, NY 10021; **Phone:** 212-249-6000; **Board Cert:** Surgery 1974; Plastic Surgery 1978; **Med School:** Univ VA Sch Med 1968; **Resid:** Surgery, UCLA Med Ctr 1973; Plastic Surgery, NY Univ 1975; **Fellow:** Surgery, Johns Hopkins Hosp 1970; **Fac Appt:** Prof PlS, NYU Sch Med

Attinger, Christopher E MD [PlS] - **Spec Exp:** Limb Surgery/Reconstruction; Diabetic Leg/Foot; Wound Healing/Care; Lower Limb Reconstruction; **Hospital:** Georgetown Univ Hosp; **Address:** Georgetown Univ Hosp-Wound Healing Ctr, 3800 Reservoir Rd NW 1 Bles Bldg, Washington, DC 20007; **Phone:** 202-444-6161; **Board Cert:** Plastic Surgery 1992; **Med School:** Yale Univ 1981; **Resid:** Surgery, Brigham & Women's Hosp 1986; Plastic Surgery, NYU Med Ctr 1989; **Fellow:** Vascular Surgery, Brigham & Women's Hosp 1987; Hand Surgery, NYU Med Ctr 1990; **Fac Appt:** Prof PlS, Georgetown Univ

Baker III, Daniel MD [PlS] - **Spec Exp:** Cosmetic Surgery-Face; Reconstructive Surgery-Face; Rhinoplasty; **Address:** 65 E 66th St, New York, NY 10065; **Phone:** 212-734-9695; **Board Cert:** Plastic Surgery 1978; **Med School:** Columbia P&S 1968; **Resid:** Surgery, UCSF Med Ctr 1975; Plastic Surgery, NYU Med Ctr 1977; **Fellow:** Head and Neck Surgery, NYU Med Ctr/St Vincents Hosp 1978; **Fac Appt:** Assoc Prof PlS, NYU Sch Med

Baker, Stephen B MD/DDS [PlS] - **Spec Exp:** Craniofacial Surgery/Reconstruction; Facial Trauma/Fractures; Cosmetic Surgery-Face; Cleft Palate/Lip; **Hospital:** Georgetown Univ Hosp, Inova Fairfax Hosp; **Address:** 3800 Reservoir Rd NW, PHC Bldg - Fl 1ST, MS 20007, Washington, DC 20007; **Phone:** 202-444-9302; **Board Cert:** Plastic Surgery 2002; **Med School:** Univ Pennsylvania 1993; **Resid:** Oral & Maxillofacial Surgery, Hosp Univ Penn 1996; Plastic Surgery, Hosp Univ Penn 2000; **Fellow:** Craniofacial Surgery, Childrens Hosp 2001; **Fac Appt:** Prof PlS, Georgetown Univ

Bartlett, Scott P MD [PlS] - **Spec Exp:** Craniofacial Surgery/Reconstruction; Cosmetic Surgery-Face; Reconstructive Surgery-Face; Pediatric Plastic Surgery; **Hospital:** Hosp Univ Penn - UPHS (page 72), Chldns Hosp of Philadelphia; **Address:** Childrens Hospital Phila, 34th St and Civic Center Blvd, Wood Bldg, 1st Fl, Philadelphia, PA 19104-4227; **Phone:** 215-662-2096; **Board Cert:** Plastic Surgery 2007; **Med School:** Washington Univ, St Louis 1975; **Resid:** Surgery, Mass Genl Hosp 1983; Plastic Surgery, Mass Genl Hosp 1985; **Fellow:** Craniofacial Surgery, Hosp Univ Penn 1986; **Fac Appt:** Prof PlS, Univ Pennsylvania

Boyajian, Michael J MD [PlS] - **Spec Exp:** Pediatric Plastic Surgery; Craniofacial Surgery; Cleft Palate/Lip; Vascular Malformations; **Hospital:** Chldns Natl Med Ctr; **Address:** 111 Michigan Ave NW, Ste 4W-100, Washington, DC 20010-2978; **Phone:** 202-476-2157; **Board Cert:** Plastic Surgery 1984; **Med School:** NYU Sch Med 1976; **Resid:** Surgery, Univ Colo Med Ctr 1979; Surgery, Univ Cincinnati Hosp 1981; **Fellow:** Plastic Surgery, Brigham & Women's Hosp 1983; Craniofacial Surgery, Chldns Hosp 1983; **Fac Appt:** Asst Prof S, Geo Wash Univ

Bucky, Louis P MD [PlS] - **Spec Exp:** Cosmetic Surgery-Face; Cosmetic Surgery-Breast; Liposuction & Body Contouring; Breast Reconstruction; **Hospital:** Pennsylvania Hosp-UPHS (page 72), Hosp Univ Penn - UPHS (page 72); **Address:** 230 W Washington Square, Ste 101, Philadelphia, PA 19106; **Phone:** 215-829-6320; **Board Cert:** Plastic Surgery 2006; **Med School:** Harvard Med Sch 1986; **Resid:** Surgery, Mass Genl Hosp 1992; Plastic Surgery, Mass Genl Hosp 1994; **Fellow:** Microsurgery, Meml Sloan Kettering Cancer Ctr 1995; Craniofacial Surgery, Miami Chldns Hosp 1996; **Fac Appt:** Clin Prof S, Univ Pennsylvania

Chang, Benjamin MD [PlS] - **Spec Exp:** Hand Surgery; Melanoma; Microsurgery; Pediatric Plastic Surgery; **Hospital:** Hosp Univ Penn - UPHS (page 72), Chldns Hosp of Philadelphia; **Address:** Univ Penn, Div Plastic Surgery, 3400 Spruce St, 10 Penn Tower, Philadelphia, PA 19104-4306; **Phone:** 215-662-4283; **Board Cert:** Plastic Surgery 2006; Hand Surgery 2006; **Med School:** Harvard Med Sch 1986; **Resid:** Surgery, NYU Med Ctr 1992; Plastic Surgery, NYU Med Ctr 1994; **Fellow:** Hand Surgery, NYU Med Ctr 1995; **Fac Appt:** Assoc Clin Prof S, Univ Pennsylvania

Chiu, David T W MD [PlS] - **Spec Exp:** Hand & Microvascular Surgery; Cosmetic Surgery-Face; Peripheral Nerve Surgery; **Hospital:** NYU Langone Med Ctr (page 68), Lenox Hill Hosp (page 67); **Address:** 900 Park Ave, New York, NY 10075; **Phone:** 212-879-8880; **Board Cert:** Plastic Surgery 1982; Hand Surgery 2010; **Med School:** Columbia P&S 1973; **Resid:** Surgery, Barnes Jewish Hosp 1977; Plastic Surgery, Columbia-Presby Med Ctr 1979; **Fellow:** Hand Surgery, NYU Med Ctr 1980; **Fac Appt:** Prof PlS, NYU Sch Med

Cordeiro, Peter G MD [PlS] - **Spec Exp:** Reconstructive Surgery; Breast Reconstruction; Facial Plastic & Reconstructive Surgery; **Hospital:** Meml Sloan-Kettering Cancer Ctr, Lenox Hill Hosp (Manh Eye, Ear & Throat Hosp) (page 67); **Address:** 1275 York Ave, New York, NY 10065; **Phone:** 212-639-2521; **Board Cert:** Surgery 2008; Plastic Surgery 2007; **Med School:** Harvard Med Sch 1983; **Resid:** Surgery, New Engl Deaconess Hosp-Harvard 1989; Plastic Surgery, NYU Med Ctr 1991; **Fellow:** Microsurgery, Meml Sloan-Kettering Cancer Ctr. 1992; Craniofacial Surgery, Univ Miami 1992; **Fac Appt:** Prof S, Cornell Univ-Weill Med Coll

Dagum, Alexander B MD [PlS] - **Spec Exp:** Reconstructive Plastic Surgery; Cleft Palate/Lip; Hand Surgery; Microsurgery; **Hospital:** Stony Brook Univ Med Ctr; **Address:** 24 Research Way, Ste 100, East Setauket, NY 11733; **Phone:** 631-444-4666; **Board Cert:** Plastic Surgery 2003; Hand Surgery 2004; **Med School:** Canada 1987; **Resid:** Surgery, Univ Ottawa Civic Hosp 1988; Plastic Surgery, Univ Toronto Med Ctr 1993; **Fellow:** Microsurgery, Univ Toronto Med Ctr 1984; Hand Surgery, Stony Brook Univ Hosp 1995; **Fac Appt:** Prof S, SUNY Stony Brook

Dick, Gregory O MD [PlS] - **Spec Exp:** Cosmetic Surgery-Face; Facial Rejuvenation; Cosmetic Surgery-Breast; Liposuction & Body Contouring; **Hospital:** Shady Grove Adven Hosp; **Address:** 9711 Medical Ctr Drive, Ste 100, Rockville, MD 20850; **Phone:** 301-251-2600; **Board Cert:** Plastic Surgery 1989; **Med School:** NY Med Coll 1980; **Resid:** Surgery, New Britain Genl Hosp 1985; Plastic Surgery, Univ Pittsbugh Med Ctr 1987; **Fac Appt:** Clin Prof S, Uniformed Srvs Univ, Bethesda

Disa, Joseph MD [PlS] - **Spec Exp:** Cancer Reconstruction; Breast Reconstruction; Head & Neck Reconstruction; Microsurgery; **Hospital:** Meml Sloan-Kettering Cancer Ctr; **Address:** 1275 York Ave, New York, NY 10065; **Phone:** 212-639-5022; **Board Cert:** Surgery 2005; Plastic Surgery 2009; **Med School:** Univ Mass Sch Med 1988; **Resid:** Surgery, Univ Md Med Ctr 1994; Plastic Surgery, Johns Hopkins Univ 1996; **Fellow:** Reconstructive Microsurgery, Meml Sloan-Kettering Cancer Ctr.; **Fac Appt:** Prof PlS, Cornell Univ-Weill Med Coll

Ducic, Ivica MD/PhD [PlS] - **Spec Exp:** Reconstructive Surgery; Peripheral Nerve Surgery; **Hospital:** Georgetown Univ Hosp; **Address:** Dept of Plastic Surgery, 3800 Reservoir Rd NW, Washington, DC 20007; **Phone:** 202-444-8929; **Board Cert:** Plastic Surgery 2004; **Med School:** Croatia 1991; **Resid:** Plastic Surgery, Georgetown Univ Hosp 2002; **Fellow:** Peripheral Nerve Surgery, Inst Peripheral Nerve Surg 2003; **Fac Appt:** Prof PlS, Georgetown Univ

Dufresne, Craig R MD [PlS] - **Spec Exp:** Craniofacial Surgery; Reconstructive Surgery; Cosmetic Surgery-Face; Liposuction & Body Contouring; **Hospital:** Inova Fairfax Hosp, Sibley Mem Hosp; **Address:** Aesthetic, Plastic & Reconstructive Surg, 5530 Wisconsin Ave, Ste 1208, Chevy Chase, MD 20815; **Phone:** 301-654-9151; **Board Cert:** Plastic Surgery 1986; **Med School:** Columbia P&S 1977; **Resid:** Surgery, Johns Hopkins Hosp 1982; Plastic Surgery, NYU Med Ctr 1984; **Fellow:** Craniofacial Surgery, NYU Med Ctr 1985; **Fac Appt:** Clin Prof PlS, Georgetown Univ

Fox IV, James W MD [PlS] - **Spec Exp:** Breast Cancer & Surgery; Breast Cosmetic & Reconstructive Surgery; Cosmetic Surgery-Face; Facial Rejuvenation; **Hospital:** Thomas Jefferson Univ Hosp; **Address:** 840 Walnut St Fl 15, Philadelphia, PA 19107; **Phone:** 215-625-6630; **Board Cert:** Plastic Surgery 1978; **Med School:** Jefferson Med Coll 1970; **Resid:** Surgery, Jefferson Hosp 1974; **Fellow:** Plastic Surgery, Univ Virginia Med Ctr 1976; **Fac Appt:** Prof S, Jefferson Med Coll

Glat, Paul M MD [PlS] - **Spec Exp:** Pediatric & Adult Plastic Surgery; Burns-Reconstructive Plastic Surgery; Craniofacial Surgery; Cleft Palate/Lip; **Hospital:** St. Christopher's Hosp for Chldn, Bryn Mawr Hosp; **Address:** 191 Presidential Blvd, Ste 101, Bala Cynwyd, PA 19004; **Phone:** 610-980-4000; **Board Cert:** Plastic Surgery 2009; **Med School:** NYU Sch Med 1988; **Resid:** Surgery, NYU Med Ctr 1994; Plastic Surgery, NYU Med Ctr 1996; **Fellow:** Craniofacial Surgery, Univ Penn 1997; **Fac Appt:** Assoc Prof PlS, Drexel Univ Coll Med

Herman, Charles K MD [PlS] - **Spec Exp:** Cosmetic Surgery-Breast; Cosmetic Surgery-Face; Rhinoplasty; **Hospital:** Pocono Med Ctr; **Address:** 100 Plaza Ct, Ste C, E. Stroudsburg, PA 18301; **Phone:** 570-420-6220; **Board Cert:** Plastic Surgery 2006; **Med School:** Albany Med Coll 2000; **Resid:** Surgery, Montefiore Med Ctr 2003; Plastic/Reconstructive Surgery, Montefiore Med Ctr 2005; **Fac Appt:** Asst Clin Prof PlS, Albert Einstein Coll Med

Hidalgo, David A MD [PlS] - **Spec Exp:** Cosmetic Surgery-Face; Cosmetic Surgery-Breast; Rhinoplasty; Reconstructive Surgery; **Hospital:** NY-Presby/Weill Cornell Med Ctr, NY (page 66), Lenox Hill Hosp (page 67); **Address:** 655 Park Ave, New York, NY 10065; **Phone:** 212-517-9777; **Board Cert:** Plastic Surgery 1987; **Med School:** Georgetown Univ 1978; **Resid:** Surgery, NYU Med Ctr 1983; Plastic Surgery, NYU Med Ctr 1985; **Fellow:** Microsurgery, NYU Med Ctr 1986; **Fac Appt:** Clin Prof S, Cornell Univ-Weill Med Coll

Hoffman, Lloyd A MD [PlS] - **Spec Exp:** Cosmetic Surgery-Face; Liposuction & Body Contouring; Breast Reconstruction; Facial Rejuvenation; **Hospital:** NY-Presby/Weill Cornell Med Ctr, NY (page 66), Lenox Hill Hosp (page 67); **Address:** 12A E 68th St, New York, NY 10021; **Phone:** 212-861-1640; **Board Cert:** Plastic Surgery 1989; **Med School:** Northwestern Univ 1978; **Resid:** Surgery, New York Hosp 1983; Plastic Surgery, NYU Med Ctr 1986; **Fellow:** Hand Surgery, NYU Med Ctr 1987; **Fac Appt:** Assoc Prof PlS, Cornell Univ-Weill Med Coll

Hurwitz, Dennis J MD [PlS] - **Spec Exp:** Body Contouring; Cosmetic Surgery-Face; Rhinoplasty; Breast Cosmetic & Reconstructive Surgery; **Hospital:** Magee-Womens Hosp - UPMC; **Address:** 3109 Forbes Ave, Ste 500, Pittsburgh, PA 15213; **Phone:** 412-802-6100; **Board Cert:** Plastic Surgery 2005; **Med School:** Univ MD Sch Med 1970; **Resid:** Surgery, Dartmouth Med Ctr 1975; Plastic Surgery, Univ Pittsburgh Med Ctr 1977; **Fac Appt:** Prof S, Univ Pittsburgh

Imber, Gerald MD [PlS] - **Spec Exp:** Cosmetic Surgery-Face; Eyelid Surgery; **Hospital:** NY-Presby/Weill Cornell Med Ctr, NY (page 66); **Address:** 121A E 83rd St, New York, NY 10028; **Phone:** 212-472-1800; **Board Cert:** Plastic Surgery 1976; **Med School:** SUNY Downstate 1966; **Resid:** Surgery, LI Jewish Med Ctr 1972; Plastic Surgery, NY Hosp 1974; **Fac Appt:** Asst Clin Prof S, Cornell Univ-Weill Med Coll

Leipziger, Lyle S MD [PIS] - **Spec Exp:** Cosmetic Surgery-Face & Eyes; Cosmetic Surgery-Breast; Breast Reconstruction; Liposuction & Body Contouring; **Hospital:** N Shore Univ Hosp (page 67), Long Island Jewish Med Ctr (page 67); **Address:** 825 Northern Blvd Fl 3, Great Neck, NY 11021; **Phone:** 516-465-8787; **Board Cert:** Plastic Surgery 1994; **Med School:** Cornell Univ-Weill Med Coll 1985; **Resid:** Plastic Surgery, New York Hosp 1990; **Fellow:** Craniofacial Surgery, Johns Hopkins Hosp 1991; **Fac Appt:** Asst Prof S, Albert Einstein Coll Med

Levin, Lawrence Scott MD [PIS] - **Spec Exp:** Toe-to-Hand Transfer; Reconstructive Microvascular Surgery; Microsurgery; **Hospital:** Penn Presby Med Ctr - UPHS (page 72), Pennsylvania Hosp-UPHS (page 72); **Address:** Hosp Univ Penn, Dept Orth Surg, 2 Silverstein, 3400 Spruce St, Philadelphia, PA 19104; **Phone:** 215-349-5803; **Board Cert:** Plastic Surgery 2010; Orthopaedic Surgery 2004; Hand Surgery 2004; **Med School:** Temple Univ 1982; **Resid:** Orthopaedic Surgery, Duke Univ Med Ctr 1988; Plastic Surgery, Duke Univ Med Ctr 1989; **Fac Appt:** Prof S, Univ Pennsylvania

Levine, Joshua L MD [PIS] - **Spec Exp:** Breast Reconstruction; Microsurgery; **Hospital:** New York Eye & Ear Infirm (page 65), Montefiore Med Ctr-Einstein Campus, NY; **Address:** 1776 Broadway at 57th St, Ste 1200, New York, NY 10019; **Phone:** 212-245-8140; **Board Cert:** Plastic Surgery 2005; **Med School:** Med Coll GA 1994; **Resid:** Plastic Surgery, Montefiore Med Ctr 2000; Plastic Surgery, Montefiore Med Ctr 2001; **Fellow:** Cosmetic Plastic Surgery, NY Eye & Ear Infirm 2003; Reconstructive Microsurgery, Louisiana State Univ 2004

Little, John W MD [PIS] - **Spec Exp:** Cosmetic Surgery-Face; **Hospital:** Georgetown Univ Hosp, G Washington Univ Hosp; **Address:** 1145 19th St NW, Ste 802, Washington, DC 20036; **Phone:** 202-467-6700; **Board Cert:** Surgery 1975; Plastic Surgery 1977; **Med School:** Harvard Med Sch 1969; **Resid:** Surgery, Case Western Reserve Affil Hosps 1974; Plastic Surgery, Case Western Reserve Affil Hosps 1975; **Fellow:** Plastic Surgery, Jackson Meml Hosp 1977; **Fac Appt:** Clin Prof PIS, Georgetown Univ

Loree, Thom R MD [PIS] - **Spec Exp:** Head & Neck Cancer; Thyroid Cancer; Reconstructive Surgery; Breast Reconstruction; **Hospital:** Erie County Med Ctr; **Address:** Erie County Med Ctr, Dept Head & Neck/Plastic & Recon Surg, 462 Grider St, Main Bldg-Ground Fl, Buffalo, NY 14215; **Phone:** 716-898-3698; **Board Cert:** Surgery 2010; Plastic Surgery 2004; **Med School:** Geo Wash Univ 1982; **Resid:** Surgery, St Lukes-Roosevelt Hosp 1987; Plastic Surgery, St Lukes-Roosevelt Hosp 1989; **Fellow:** Head & Neck Surgical Oncology, Meml Sloan-Kettering Cancer Ctr 1990; **Fac Appt:** Assoc Prof S, SUNY Buffalo

Losee, Joseph E MD [PIS] - **Spec Exp:** Pediatric Plastic Surgery; Cleft Palate/Lip; Craniofacial Surgery/Reconstruction; **Hospital:** Chldns Hosp of Pittsburgh - UPMC; **Address:** Dept of Pediatric Surgery, 1 Chldn's Hosp Drive, 4401 Penn Ave Fl 3, Pittsburgh, PA 15224; **Phone:** 412-692-7949; **Board Cert:** Plastic Surgery 2011; **Med School:** Univ Rochester 1994; **Resid:** Plastic Surgery, Strong Meml Hosp 1999; **Fellow:** Pediatric Plastic Surgery, Childrens Hosp 2000; Craniofacial Surgery, Hosp Univ Penn 2000; **Fac Appt:** Assoc Prof S, Univ Pittsburgh

Low, David W MD [PIS] - **Spec Exp:** Microsurgery; Cosmetic & Reconstructive Surgery; Vascular Malformations; Cleft Palate/Lip; **Hospital:** Hosp Univ Penn - UPHS (page 72), Chldns Hosp of Philadelphia; **Address:** Univ Penn Div Plastic Surgery, 3400 Spruce St, 10 Penn Tower, Philadelphia, PA 19104; **Phone:** 215-662-4283; **Board Cert:** Plastic Surgery 1991; **Med School:** Harvard Med Sch 1980; **Resid:** Surgery, Hosp Univ Penn 1986; **Fellow:** Plastic/Reconstructive Surgery, Hosp Univ Penn 1989; **Fac Appt:** Prof S, Univ Pennsylvania

Plastic Surgery

Mackay, Donald R MD/DDS [PlS] - **Spec Exp:** Pediatric Plastic Surgery; Craniofacial Surgery; Cleft Palate/Lip; Cosmetic Surgery-Face; **Hospital:** Penn State Milton S Hershey Med Ctr; **Address:** Hershey Med Ctr, Div Plastic Surg, 500 University Drive, MC HU71, Hershey, PA 17033-0850; **Phone:** 717-531-8952; **Board Cert:** Plastic Surgery 2006; **Med School:** South Africa 1980; **Resid:** Plastic Surgery, Univ Teaching Hosps 1984; Plastic Surgery, MS Hershey Med Ctr 1995; **Fac Appt:** Prof PlS, Penn State Coll Med

Manders, Ernest K MD [PlS] - **Spec Exp:** Facial Nerve Disorders; **Hospital:** UPMC Presby, Pittsburgh, Magee-Womens Hosp - UPMC; **Address:** UPMC Presbyterian, 3601 Fifth Ave Falk Med Bldg - Ste 6B, Pittsburgh, PA 15213; **Phone:** 412-648-9670; **Board Cert:** Surgery 2009; Plastic Surgery 1982; **Med School:** Harvard Med Sch 1972; **Resid:** Surgery, Univ Michigan Med Ctr 1979; Plastic Surgery, Univ Michigan Med Ctr 1981; **Fellow:** Viral Oncology, Natl Insts of Allergy-Infectious Disease 1975; **Fac Appt:** Prof S, Univ Pittsburgh

Manson, Paul MD [PlS] - **Spec Exp:** Facial Trauma/Fractures; Skin Cancer; Reconstructive Surgery; Cosmetic Surgery-Face; **Hospital:** Johns Hopkins Hosp (page 61), Univ of MD Med Ctr; **Address:** 601 N Caroline St, McElderry-8152F, Baltimore, MD 21287; **Phone:** 410-955-9470; **Board Cert:** Plastic Surgery 1979; **Med School:** Northwestern Univ 1968; **Resid:** Surgery, New Eng Deaconess Hosp 1971; Plastic Surgery, Johns Hopkins Hosp 1978; **Fellow:** Surgery, Lahey Clinic 1974; **Fac Appt:** Prof PlS, Johns Hopkins Univ

Matarasso, Alan MD [PlS] - **Spec Exp:** Cosmetic Surgery-Face & Eyes; Rhinoplasty; Liposuction; Abdominoplasty; **Hospital:** Lenox Hill Hosp (Manh Eye, Ear & Throat Hosp) (page 67); **Address:** 1009 Park Ave, New York, NY 10028-0936; **Phone:** 212-249-7500; **Board Cert:** Plastic Surgery 1986; **Med School:** Univ Miami Sch Med 1979; **Resid:** Surgery, Montefiore Med Ctr 1983; Plastic Surgery, Montefiore Med Ctr 1985; **Fellow:** Plastic Surgery, Manhattan EET Hosp/NYU 1985; **Fac Appt:** Clin Prof PlS, Albert Einstein Coll Med

McCarthy, Joseph G MD [PlS] - **Spec Exp:** Craniofacial Surgery-Pediatric; Reconstructive Surgery-Face; Cosmetic Surgery-Face; **Hospital:** NYU Langone Med Ctr (page 68), Lenox Hill Hosp (Manh Eye, Ear & Throat Hosp) (page 67); **Address:** 722 Park Ave, New York, NY 10021-4954; **Phone:** 212-628-4420; **Board Cert:** Surgery 1972; Plastic Surgery 1978; **Med School:** Columbia P&S 1964; **Resid:** Surgery, Columbia-Presby Med Ctr 1971; Plastic Surgery, NYU Med Ctr 1973; **Fac Appt:** Prof PlS, NYU Sch Med

Mehrara, Babak J MD [PlS] - **Spec Exp:** Breast Reconstruction; Cancer Reconstruction; Microsurgery; Reconstructive Surgery-Face; **Hospital:** Meml Sloan-Kettering Cancer Ctr; **Address:** 1275 York Ave, New York, NY 10065; **Phone:** 212-639-8639; **Board Cert:** Plastic Surgery 2003; **Med School:** Columbia P&S 1993; **Resid:** Surgery, NYU Med Ctr 1996; Plastic Surgery, NYU Med Ctr 2001; **Fellow:** Microsurgery, UCLA Med Ctr 2002; **Fac Appt:** Assoc Prof S, Cornell Univ-Weill Med Coll

Nahabedian, Maurice Y MD [PlS] - **Spec Exp:** Breast Reconstruction & Augmentation; Cosmetic Surgery-Face; Abdominoplasty; **Hospital:** Georgetown Univ Hosp; **Address:** Georgetown Univ Hosp, Dept Plastic Surgery, 3800 Reservoir Rd NW, Fl 1PHC, Washington, DC 20007; **Phone:** 202-444-6576; **Board Cert:** Plastic Surgery 2005; **Med School:** UC Irvine 1987; **Resid:** Surgery, UC Irvine Med Ctr 1992; Plastic Surgery, Johns Hopkins Univ Hosp 1995; **Fac Appt:** Prof PlS, Geo Wash Univ

Napoli, Joseph A MD/DDS [PlS] - **Spec Exp:** Cleft Palate/Lip; Maxillofacial Surgery; Cranio-facial Surgery-Pediatric; Beckwith-Wiedemann Syndrome; **Hospital:** Nemours/Alfred I. duPont Hosp for Chldn, Wilmington Hosp; **Address:** Al duPont Hosp for Children, Div Plastic Surgery, 1600 Rockland Rd, Wilmington, DE 19803; **Phone:** 302-651-6301; **Board Cert:** Plastic Surgery 2004; **Med School:** Columbia P&S 1987; **Resid:** Oral & Maxillofacial Surgery, Columbia-Presby Med Ctr 1985; Plastic/Reconstructive Surgery, Dartmouth-Hitchcock Med Ctr 2001; **Fellow:** Craniofacial Surgery, Royal Chldns Hosp 2002; Pediatric Plastic Surgery, Royal Chldns Hosp 2002; **Fac Appt:** Asst Prof S, Jefferson Med Coll

Noone, R Barrett MD [PlS] - **Spec Exp:** Breast Cosmetic & Reconstructive Surgery; Cosmetic Surgery-Face; Liposuction & Body Contouring; **Hospital:** Bryn Mawr Hosp; **Address:** 888 Glenbrook Ave, Bryn Mawr, PA 19010-2506; **Phone:** 610-527-4833; **Board Cert:** Surgery 1972; Plastic Surgery 2007; **Med School:** Univ Pennsylvania 1965; **Resid:** Surgery, Hosp Univ Penn 1971; Plastic Surgery, Hosp Univ Penn 1973; **Fac Appt:** Clin Prof S, Univ Pennsylvania

Olding, Michael Joseph MD [PlS] - **Spec Exp:** Breast Reconstruction; Liposuction & Body Contouring; Cosmetic Surgery-Face & Breast; **Hospital:** G Washington Univ Hosp; **Address:** GWU Med Faculty Assocs, 2150 Pennslyvania Ave NW Fl 9, Washington, DC 20037; **Phone:** 202-741-3241; **Board Cert:** Plastic Surgery 1986; **Med School:** Univ KY Coll Med 1980; **Resid:** Surgery, NY Presy Hosp/Weill Cornell 1982; Plastic Surgery, Mcgill Univ Hosps 1985; **Fac Appt:** Prof PlS, Geo Wash Univ

Pitman, Gerald H MD [PlS] - **Spec Exp:** Cosmetic Surgery-Face; Liposuction; Abdominoplasty; **Hospital:** Lenox Hill Hosp (Manh Eye, Ear & Throat Hosp) (page 67), NYU Langone Med Ctr (page 68); **Address:** 170 E 73rd St, New York, NY 10021; **Phone:** 212-517-2600; **Board Cert:** Plastic Surgery 1978; **Med School:** Univ Pennsylvania 1968; **Resid:** Surgery, Columbia-Presby Hosp 1975; Plastic Surgery, NYU Med Ctr 1977; **Fellow:** Microsurgery, NYU Med Ctr 1981; **Fac Appt:** Clin Prof PlS, NYU Sch Med

Posnick, Jeffrey C MD/DMD [PlS] - **Spec Exp:** Cosmetic Surgery-Face; Craniofacial Surgery/Reconstruction; Maxillofacial Surgery; **Hospital:** Georgetown Univ Hosp; **Address:** 5530 Wisconsin Ave, Ste 1250, Chevy Chase, MD 20815; **Phone:** 301-986-9475; **Board Cert:** Plastic Surgery 1988; **Med School:** Vanderbilt Univ 1979; **Resid:** Surgery, Mass Genl Hosp 1983; Plastic Surgery, Eastern Va Affil HOsp 1986; **Fellow:** Craniofacial Surgery, Hosp Univ Penn/Chldns Hosp 1983; **Fac Appt:** Clin Prof PlS, Georgetown Univ

Price, G Wesley MD [PlS] - **Spec Exp:** Cosmetic Surgery-Face & Breast; Liposuction & Body Contouring; **Hospital:** Sibley Mem Hosp; **Address:** Center for Plastic Surgery, 5550 Friendshop Blvd, Ste 130, Chevy Chase, MD 20815; **Phone:** 301-652-7700; **Board Cert:** Plastic Surgery 1987; **Med School:** Bowman Gray 1977; **Resid:** Surgery, Geo Wash Univ Hosp 1982; Plastic Surgery, NYU Med Ctr 1984; **Fellow:** Facial Plastic & Reconstr Surgery, Univ Miami 1985

Rodriguez, Eduardo De Jesus MD/DDS [PlS] - **Spec Exp:** Facial Plastic & Reconstructive Surgery; Transplant-Face; Cranofacial Surgery/Reconstruction; Microsurgery; **Hospital:** Univ of MD Med Ctr; **Address:** Univ MD Med Ctr, 22 S Greene St, Baltimore, MD 21201; **Phone:** 410-328-2999; **Board Cert:** Plastic Surgery 2005; **Med School:** Va Commonwealth Univ Sch Med 1999; **Resid:** Surgery, Johns Hopkins Hosp 2003; Plastic Surgery, Johns Hopkins Hosp 2005; **Fellow:** Reconstructive Microsurgery, Chang Gung Meml Hosp; **Fac Appt:** Assoc Prof PlS, Univ MD Sch Med

Plastic Surgery

Rose, Elliott H MD [PlS] - **Spec Exp:** Facial Plastic & Reconstructive Surgery; Cosmetic Surgery-Face & Body; Facial Paralysis Reconstruction; Burns-Reconstructive Plastic Surgery; **Hospital:** Mount Sinai Med Ctr (page 64); **Address:** The Aesthetic Surgery Center, 895 Park Ave, New York, NY 10021-0327; **Phone:** 212-639-1346; **Board Cert:** Plastic Surgery 1979; **Med School:** Univ Tex Med Br, Galveston 1970; **Resid:** Surgery, Johns Hopkins Hosp 1973; Plastic Surgery, Stanford Univ Med Ctr 1977; **Fellow:** Hand & Microvascular Surgery, UCSF Med Ctr 1978; **Fac Appt:** Assoc Clin Prof PlS, Mount Sinai Sch Med

Serletti, Joseph M MD [PlS] - **Spec Exp:** Breast Reconstruction; Head & Neck Reconstruction; Cosmetic Surgery; Reconstructive Surgery; **Hospital:** Hosp Univ Penn - UPHS (page 72); **Address:** Hosp Univ Penn, Dept Plastic Surgery, 10 Penn Tower, 3400 Spruce St, Philadelphia, PA 19104; **Phone:** 215-662-3743; **Board Cert:** Plastic Surgery 2003; **Med School:** Univ Rochester 1982; **Resid:** Surgery, Strong Meml Hosp 1986; Plastic Surgery, Strong Meml Hosp 1988; **Fellow:** Reconstructive Surgery, Johns Hopkins Hosp 1990; **Fac Appt:** Prof PlS, Univ Pennsylvania

Seyfer, Alan MD [PlS] - **Spec Exp:** Chest Wall Reconstruction; Cleft Palate/Lip; Reconstructive Surgery; Abdominal Wall Reconstruction; **Hospital:** Walter Reed Natl Military Med Ctr; **Address:** USUHS-School of Medicine, 4301 Jones Bridge Rd, Bethesda, MD 20814; **Phone:** 301-295-0441; **Board Cert:** Hand Surgery 1999; Plastic Surgery 1982; **Med School:** Louisiana State U, New Orleans 1973; **Resid:** Surgery, Fitzsimons AMC 1978; Plastic Surgery, Walter Reed AMC 1981; **Fellow:** Hand Surgery, Duke Univ Med Ctr 1980; **Fac Appt:** Prof S, Uniformed Srvs Univ, Bethesda

Singh, Navin MD [PlS] - **Spec Exp:** Cosmetic Surgery-Face & Breast; Liposuction & Body Contouring; Abdominoplasty; Facial Rejuvenation; **Hospital:** Sibley Mem Hosp; **Address:** 5454 Wisconsin Ave, Ste 1710, Chevy Chase, MD 20815; **Phone:** 301-244-0277; **Board Cert:** Plastic Surgery 2011; **Med School:** Brown Univ 1993; **Resid:** Surgery, Johns Hopkins Hosp 1997; Plastic/Reconstructive Surgery, Johns Hopkins Hosp 1999; **Fellow:** Craniofacial Surgery, Johns Hopkins Hosp 2000; **Fac Appt:** Asst Prof PlS, Johns Hopkins Univ

Slezak, Sheri MD [PlS] - **Spec Exp:** Breast Reconstruction; Cosmetic Surgery-Breast; **Hospital:** Univ of MD Med Ctr; **Address:** Univ Maryland, Dept Plastic Surgery, 22 S Greene St, rm S8D18, Baltimore, MD 21201; **Phone:** 410-328-2360; **Board Cert:** Plastic Surgery 2008; **Med School:** Harvard Med Sch 1980; **Resid:** Surgery, NY-Presby/Columbia Univ Med Ctr 1986; Plastic Surgery, Johns Hopkins Hosp 1989; **Fellow:** Immunology, Johns Hopkins Hosp 1986; **Fac Appt:** Prof PlS, Univ MD Sch Med

Spence, Robert J MD [PlS] - **Spec Exp:** Burns-Reconstructive Plastic Surgery; Burn Care; Tissue Banking; **Hospital:** Good Samaritan Hosp; **Address:** 5601 Loch Raven Blvd, Baltimore, MD 21239; **Phone:** 443-444-2876; **Board Cert:** Plastic Surgery 1981; **Med School:** Johns Hopkins Univ 1972; **Resid:** Surgery, Johns Hopkins Hosp 1974; Surgery, Hershey Med Ctr 1978; **Fellow:** Plastic Surgery, Johns Hopkins Hosp 1980; **Fac Appt:** Assoc Prof S, Johns Hopkins Univ

Spinelli, Henry M MD [PlS] - **Spec Exp:** Cosmetic Surgery-Face; Craniofacial Surgery/Reconstruction; Oculoplastic & Orbital Surgery; Eyelid Surgery/Blepharoplasty; **Hospital:** NY-Presby/Weill Cornell Med Ctr, NY (page 66), Lenox Hill Hosp (Manh Eye, Ear & Throat Hosp) (page 67); **Address:** 875 Fifth Ave, New York, NY 10021-4952; **Phone:** 212-570-6235; **Board Cert:** Ophthalmology 1987; Plastic Surgery 1993; **Med School:** NYU Sch Med 1981; **Resid:** Ophthalmology, Manhattan EET Hosp 1985; Plastic/Reconstructive Surgery, NYU-Bellevue Hosp 1990; **Fellow:** Craniofacial Surgery, NYU Med Ctr 1991; **Fac Appt:** Clin Prof S, Cornell Univ-Weill Med Coll

Staffenberg, David A MD [PlS] - **Spec Exp:** Craniofacial Surgery/Reconstruction; Pediatric Plastic Surgery; Ear Reconstruction/Microtia; Cosmetic Surgery-Face; **Hospital:** NYU Langone Med Ctr (page 68); **Address:** NYU Med Ctr, 305 E 33rd St, New York, NY 10016; **Phone:** 212-263-8065; **Board Cert:** Plastic Surgery 2009; **Med School:** NY Med Coll 1989; **Resid:** Surgery, Maimonides Med Ctr 1995; Plastic Surgery, Emory Univ Med Ctr 1997; **Fellow:** Craniofacial Surgery, UCLA Med Ctr 1998; **Fac Appt:** Assoc Prof PlS, Albert Einstein Coll Med

Sultan, Mark R MD [PlS] - **Spec Exp:** Breast Reconstruction; Cosmetic Surgery-Breast; Cosmetic Surgery-Face; Liposuction & Body Contouring; **Hospital:** St. Luke's - Roosevelt Hosp Ctr - Roosevelt Div (page 56); **Address:** 1100 Park Ave, New York, NY 10128; **Phone:** 212-360-0700; **Board Cert:** Plastic Surgery 1992; **Med School:** Columbia P&S 1982; **Resid:** Surgery, Columbia-Presby Hosp 1987; Plastic Surgery, Columbia-Presby Hosp 1990; **Fellow:** Head and Neck Surgery, Emory Univ Hosp 1989; **Fac Appt:** Assoc Prof S, Columbia P&S

Tabbal, Nicolas MD [PlS] - **Spec Exp:** Rhinoplasty; Cosmetic Surgery-Face; Eyelid Surgery; **Hospital:** Lenox Hill Hosp (Manh Eye, Ear & Throat Hosp) (page 67), NYU Langone Med Ctr (page 68); **Address:** 521 Park Ave, rm 1, New York, NY 10021-8140; **Phone:** 212-644-5800; **Board Cert:** Plastic Surgery 1980; **Med School:** Lebanon 1972; **Resid:** Surgery, Am Univ Med Ctr 1976; Plastic Surgery, Akron City Hosp 1979; **Fellow:** Surgery, Upstate Med Ctr 1977; Reconstructive Microsurgery, NYU Med Ctr 1980

Taub, Peter J MD [PlS] - **Spec Exp:** Pediatric Plastic Surgery; Craniofacial Surgery; Cosmetic Surgery; Maxillofacial Surgery; **Hospital:** Mount Sinai Med Ctr (page 64), Westchester Med Ctr; **Address:** 5 E 98th St, Fl 14th, Ste B, New York, NY 10029-6574; **Phone:** 212-241-4178; **Board Cert:** Surgery 2009; Plastic Surgery 2003; **Med School:** Albert Einstein Coll Med 1993; **Resid:** Surgery, Mt Sinai Med Ctr 1999; Plastic Surgery, UCLA Med Ctr 2001; **Fellow:** Craniofacial Surgery, UCLA Med Ctr 2002; **Fac Appt:** Prof S, Mount Sinai Sch Med

Thorne, Charles H MD [PlS] - **Spec Exp:** Cosmetic Surgery-Face; Ear Reconstruction/Microtia; Craniofacial Surgery; Rhinoplasty; **Hospital:** NYU Langone Med Ctr (page 68), Lenox Hill Hosp (Manh Eye, Ear & Throat Hosp) (page 67); **Address:** 812 Park Ave, New York, NY 10021-2759; **Phone:** 212-794-0044; **Board Cert:** Plastic Surgery 2007; **Med School:** UCLA 1981; **Resid:** Surgery, Mass Genl Hosp 1986; Plastic Surgery, NYU Med Ctr 1988; **Fellow:** Craniofacial Surgery, NYU Med Ctr 1989; **Fac Appt:** Assoc Prof PlS, NYU Sch Med

Ting, Jess MD [PlS] - **Spec Exp:** Breast Reconstruction; Cosmetic Surgery; **Hospital:** Mount Sinai Med Ctr (page 64), Mount Sinai Hosp of Queens (page 64); **Address:** 5 E 98th St, Fl 14, Ste B, Box 1259, New York, NY 10029; **Phone:** 212-241-4410; **Board Cert:** Plastic Surgery 2002; Hand Surgery 2003; **Med School:** Columbia P&S 1995; **Resid:** Surgery, Columbia Presby Med Ctr 1998; Plastic Surgery, Univ Pittsburgh Med Ctr 2000; **Fellow:** Hand Surgery, Hosp Special Surgery 2001; **Fac Appt:** Asst Prof S, Mount Sinai Sch Med

Topham, Neal MD [PlS] - **Spec Exp:** Breast Reconstruction; Head & Neck Reconstruction; Microsurgery; **Hospital:** Fox Chase Cancer Ctr (page 58); **Address:** Fox Chase Cancer Center, Dept Surgical Oncology, 333 Cottman Ave, C308, Philadelphia, PA 19111; **Phone:** 215-728-2662; **Board Cert:** Plastic Surgery 2005; **Med School:** Case West Res Univ 1994; **Resid:** Surgery, Akron Med Ctr 1998; Plastic Surgery, Case Western Reserve Univ 2000; **Fellow:** Microvascular Surgery, MD Anderson Cancer Ctr 2003; **Fac Appt:** Asst Clin Prof S, Univ Pennsylvania

Plastic Surgery

Tufaro, Anthony P MD/DDS [PlS] - **Spec Exp:** Head & Neck Cancer; Skin Cancer-Head & Neck; Merkel Cell Carcinoma; Craniofacial Surgery/Reconstruction; **Hospital:** Johns Hopkins Hosp (page 61); **Address:** 601 N caroline St, McElderry Bldg - Fl 8th, MS 21287, Baltimore, MD 21287; **Phone:** 410-955-9846; **Board Cert:** Plastic Surgery 2000; **Med School:** Hahnemann Univ 1993; **Resid:** Surgery, Johns Hopkins Hosp 1995; **Fellow:** Plastic Surgery, Johns Hopkins Hosp 1997; Head and Neck Surgery, Meml Sloan Kettering Cancer Ctr 1998; **Fac Appt:** Assoc Prof S, Johns Hopkins Univ

Vander Kolk, Craig A MD [PlS] - **Spec Exp:** Cosmetic Surgery-Face; Cleft Palate/Lip; Craniofacial Surgery/Reconstruction; Cosmetic Surgery-Breast; **Hospital:** Mercy Med Ctr - Baltimore; **Address:** Cosmetic Medicine at Mercy, 227 St Paul Place Fl 6, Baltimore, MD 21202; **Phone:** 410-332-9700; **Board Cert:** Plastic Surgery 1989; **Med School:** Univ Mich Med Sch 1980; **Resid:** Surgery, Univ Mich Med Ctr 1983; Plastic Surgery, Univ Mich Med Ctr 1986; **Fellow:** Hand Surgery, St Vincents Hosp 1985; Craniofacial Surgery, Chldns Hosp 1987; **Fac Appt:** Prof PlS, Johns Hopkins Univ

Zide, Barry M MD/DMD [PlS] - **Spec Exp:** Facial Surgery-Chin & Lip; Birthmarks/Hemangiomas; Reconstructive Plastic Surgery; Melanoma; **Hospital:** NYU Langone Med Ctr (page 68), Lenox Hill Hosp (page 67); **Address:** 420 E 55th St, Ste 1D, New York, NY 10022-5140; **Phone:** 212-421-2424; **Board Cert:** Plastic Surgery 1981; **Med School:** Tufts Univ 1973; **Resid:** Surgery, Stanford Med Ctr 1976; Plastic Surgery, Univ NC Hosp 1978; **Fellow:** Head & Neck Oncology, Roswell Park Cancer Inst 1979; Craniofacial Surgery, NYU Med Ctr 1980; **Fac Appt:** Prof PlS, NYU Sch Med

Southeast

Allen, Robert J MD [PlS] - **Spec Exp:** Breast Reconstruction; Microsurgery; **Hospital:** Roper Hosp; **Address:** 125 Doughty St, Ste 590, Charleston, SC 29403; **Phone:** 888-890-3437; **Board Cert:** Plastic Surgery 1985; **Med School:** Med Univ SC 1976; **Resid:** Surgery, LSU Med Ctr 1982; Plastic Surgery, LSU Med Ctr 1981; **Fellow:** Microsurgery, NYU Med Ctr 1983; **Fac Appt:** Assoc Clin Prof PlS, Louisiana State U, New Orleans

Beasley, Michael E MD [PlS] - **Spec Exp:** Breast Reconstruction & Augmentation; Liposuction & Body Contouring; Facial Rejuvenation; **Address:** Charlotte Plastic Surgery, 2215 Randolph Rd, Charlotte, NC 28207-1523; **Phone:** 704-372-6846; **Board Cert:** Plastic Surgery 1989; **Med School:** Univ NC Sch Med 1980; **Resid:** Surgery, NC Meml Hosp 1985; Plastic Surgery, Emory Univ Hosp 1987; **Fellow:** Plastic Surgery, St Joseph's Hosp 1987; **Fac Appt:** Clin Prof PlS, Univ NC Sch Med

Burstein, Fernando D MD [PlS] - **Spec Exp:** Craniofacial Surgery-Pediatric; Cosmetic Surgery-Face; Maxillofacial Surgery; Rhinoplasty; **Hospital:** Chldns Hlthcare Atlanta @ Scottish Rite, Northside Hosp; **Address:** Ped Plastic Surg. & Craniofacial Assocs, 975 Johnson Ferry Rd NE, Ste 100, Atlanta, GA 30342; **Phone:** 404-256-1311; **Board Cert:** Otolaryngology 1986; Plastic Surgery 1991; **Med School:** Univ Kansas 1980; **Resid:** Otolaryngology, UCLA Med Ctr 1986; Plastic Surgery, Yale Univ 1988; **Fellow:** Craniofacial Surgery, UCLA Med Ctr 1989; **Fac Appt:** Clin Prof PlS, Emory Univ

Carraway, James Howard MD [PlS] - **Spec Exp:** Oculoplastic Surgery; Cosmetic Surgery-Face; Eyelid Surgery; Breast Surgery; **Hospital:** Sentara Leigh Hosp; **Address:** 5589 Greenwich Rd, Ste 100, Virginia Beach, VA 23462; **Phone:** 757-557-0300; **Board Cert:** Surgery 1972; Plastic Surgery 1974; **Med School:** Univ VA Sch Med 1962; **Resid:** Surgery, Norfolk Med Ctr 1970; Plastic Surgery, Eastern VA Med Ctr 1973; **Fellow:** Plastic Surgery, Glasgow Royal Infirmary 1970; **Fac Appt:** Prof PlS, Eastern VA Med Sch

Colen, Lawrence B MD [PlS] - **Spec Exp:** Cosmetic Surgery-Face; Cosmetic Surgery-Breast; Breast Reconstruction; **Hospital:** Sentara Norfolk Genl Hosp; **Address:** Norfolk Plastic Surgery, 6261 E Virginia Beach Blvd, Ste 100, Norfolk, VA 23502; **Phone:** 757-466-1000; **Board Cert:** Plastic Surgery 2007; **Med School:** Dartmouth Med Sch 1975; **Resid:** Surgery, UCSF Med Ctr 1979; **Fellow:** Plastic Surgery, UCSF Med Ctr 1983; **Fac Appt:** Assoc Prof PlS, Eastern VA Med Sch

Cruse, C Wayne MD [PlS] - **Spec Exp:** Burns-Reconstructive Plastic Surgery; Cancer Reconstruction; **Hospital:** Tampa Genl Hosp, H Lee Moffitt Cancer Ctr & Research Inst (page 59); **Address:** 12902 Magnolia Dr, Ste 4035, Tampa, FL 33612; **Phone:** 813-844-8546; **Board Cert:** Plastic Surgery 1981; **Med School:** Univ Louisville Sch Med 1972; **Resid:** Surgery, Univ S Fla Hosp 1977; Plastic Surgery, Univ KY Hosp-Chandler Med Ctr 1979; **Fac Appt:** Prof S, Univ S Fla Coll Med

Davis, Glenn M MD [PlS] - **Spec Exp:** Cosmetic Surgery-Breast; Abdominoplasty; Liposuction & Body Contouring; Facial Rejuvenation; **Hospital:** Rex HlthCare, WakeMed-Raleigh Campus; **Address:** 2304 Wesvill Ct, Ste 360, Raleigh, NC 27607-2981; **Phone:** 919-785-1220; **Board Cert:** Plastic Surgery 1986; **Med School:** Med Univ SC 1974; **Resid:** Surgery, National Naval Med Ctr 1982; Plastic Surgery, Eastern Va Affil Hosp 1985; **Fac Appt:** Assoc Clin Prof PlS, Univ NC Sch Med

Erdmann, Detlev MD/PhD [PlS] - **Spec Exp:** Body Contouring after Weight Loss; Abdominoplasty; Cosmetic Surgery-Breast; Hand Surgery; **Hospital:** Duke Univ Hosp; **Address:** Box 3181 Med Ctr, 131 Baker House, Brown Zone, Durham, NC 27710; **Phone:** 919-684-3320; **Board Cert:** Plastic Surgery 2000; Hand Surgery 2003; **Med School:** Germany 1990; **Resid:** Surgery, Univ Heidelberg Affil Hosp 1998; **Fellow:** Plastic Surgery, Univ Heidelberg 2000; Hand Surgery, Univ Heidelberg 2003; **Fac Appt:** Assoc Prof S, Duke Univ

Fix, R Jobe MD [PlS] - **Spec Exp:** Breast Reconstruction; Hand Surgery; Microsurgery; **Hospital:** Univ of Ala Hosp at Birmingham, Children's Hospital - Birmingham; **Address:** Univ of Alabama Hosp, Div Plastic Surg, 1530 3rd Ave S, Ste FOT-1102, Birmingham, AL 35294-3411; **Phone:** 205-801-8500; **Board Cert:** Surgery 2009; Plastic Surgery 1991; Hand Surgery 2001; **Med School:** Univ Nebr Coll Med 1982; **Resid:** Surgery, Valley Med Ctr 1987; Plastic Surgery, Univ Ala Hosp 1989; **Fac Appt:** Prof PlS, Univ Alabama

Georgiade, Gregory S MD [PlS] - **Spec Exp:** Breast Reconstruction; Cleft Palate/Lip; **Hospital:** Duke Univ Hosp; **Address:** Duke Univ Med Ctr, Box 3960, Durham, NC 27710; **Phone:** 919-684-3039; **Board Cert:** Surgery 2011; Plastic Surgery 1981; **Med School:** Duke Univ 1973; **Resid:** Surgery, Duke Univ Med Ctr 1978; Plastic Surgery, Duke Univ Med Ctr 1980; **Fac Appt:** Prof S, Duke Univ

Gregory, Richard O MD [PlS] - **Spec Exp:** Skin Laser Surgery; Cosmetic Surgery-Face; Facial Rejuvenation; Liposuction & Body Contouring; **Hospital:** Florida Hosp Celebration Hlth, Florida Hosp - Orlando; **Address:** Inst of Aesthetic Surgery, 400 Celebration Pl, Ste A320, Kissimmee, FL 34747; **Phone:** 407-303-4250; **Board Cert:** Plastic Surgery 1981; **Med School:** Indiana Univ 1971; **Resid:** Surgery, Duke Univ Med Ctr 1977; Plastic Surgery, Duke Univ Med Ctr 1979; **Fellow:** Hand Surgery, Univ Louisville 1979; **Fac Appt:** Assoc Clin Prof PlS, Univ S Fla Coll Med

Grotting, James C MD [PlS] - **Spec Exp:** Cosmetic Surgery-Face & Body; Cosmetic Surgery-Breast; Breast Reconstruction; Liposuction & Body Contouring; **Hospital:** UAB Highlands Hosp, St. Vincent's Hosp - Birmingham; **Address:** One Inverness Ctr Pkwy, Ste 100, Birmingham, AL 35242-4865; **Phone:** 205-930-1600; **Board Cert:** Plastic Surgery 1986; **Med School:** Univ Minn 1978; **Resid:** Surgery, Univ Wash Affil Hosps 1983; Plastic Surgery, UCSF Med Ctr 1985; **Fac Appt:** Clin Prof PlS, Univ Alabama

Hagan, Kevin F MD [PlS] - **Spec Exp:** Reconstructive Surgery; Cosmetic Surgery-Breast; Cosmetic Surgery; **Hospital:** Vanderbilt Univ Med Ctr (page 75); **Address:** Vanderbilt Univ Med Ctr, Dept Plastic Surgery, D-4207 Medical Center N, Nashville, TN 37232-2345; **Phone:** 615-936-3574; **Board Cert:** Plastic Surgery 1983; **Med School:** Johns Hopkins Univ 1974; **Resid:** Surgery, Med Coll VA Hosps 1979; Plastic Surgery, UCSF Med Ctr 1982; **Fellow:** Microsurgery, Dr Harry Buncke Med Clinic 1980; **Fac Appt:** Assoc Prof PlS, Vanderbilt Univ

Hester Jr, T Roderick MD [PlS] - **Spec Exp:** Cosmetic Surgery-Face; **Hospital:** Emory Univ Hosp, Northside Hosp; **Address:** Paces Plastic Surgery, 3200 Downwood Cir NW, Ste 640, Atlanta, GA 30327-1610; **Phone:** 404-351-0051; **Board Cert:** Surgery 1973; Plastic Surgery 2007; **Med School:** Emory Univ 1967; **Resid:** Surgery, Emory Affil Hosps 1972; Plastic/Reconstructive Surgery, Emory Affil Hosps 1978; **Fac Appt:** Assoc Prof S, Emory Univ

Hultman, C Scott MD [PlS] - **Spec Exp:** Breast Reconstruction; Burns-Reconstructive Plastic Surgery; Reconstructive Plastic Surgery; Cosmetic Surgery; **Hospital:** NC Memorial Hosp - UNC; **Address:** UNC Div Plastic & Reconstructive Surgery, CB 7195, Chapel Hill, NC 27599-7195; **Phone:** 919-966-2300; **Board Cert:** Surgery 1999; Plastic Surgery 2001; Surgical Critical Care 2002; **Med School:** Univ Pittsburgh 1990; **Resid:** Surgery, Univ NC Hosps 1996; Plastic Surgery, Emory Univ Med Ctr 2000; **Fellow:** Surgical Critical Care, Univ N Carolina 1998; **Fac Appt:** Assoc Prof S, Univ NC Sch Med

Hunstad, Joseph P MD [PlS] - **Spec Exp:** Facial Plastic & Reconstructive Surgery; Body Contouring after Weight Loss; Abdominoplasty; **Hospital:** Carolinas Med Ctr-Univ, Presby Hosp - Charlotte; **Address:** The Hunstad Center, 11208 Statesville Rd, Ste 300, Huntersville, NC 28078; **Phone:** 704-659-9000; **Board Cert:** Plastic Surgery 1989; **Med School:** Mich State Univ 1981; **Resid:** Surgery, Butterworth Hosp 1984; Plastic Surgery, Grand Rapids Area Med Ed Ct 1986; **Fellow:** Reconstructive Microsurgery, MECOM MicSurg Inst 1987

Kelly, Kevin J MD/DDS [PlS] - **Spec Exp:** Craniofacial Surgery; Pediatric Plastic Surgery; Cleft Palate/Lip; Ear Reshaping (Otoplasty); **Hospital:** Vanderbilt Univ Med Ctr (page 75), Vanderbilt Monroe Carrell Jr. Chldn's Hosp (page 75); **Address:** Vanderbilt Univ Med Ctr, Dept Plastic Surgery, D-4207 Med Ctr North, Nashville, TN 37232-2345; **Phone:** 615-936-3574; **Board Cert:** Plastic Surgery 1991; **Med School:** SUNY Downstate 1982; **Resid:** Surgery, Albany Med Ctr 1986; Plastic Surgery, Albany Med Ctr 1988; **Fellow:** Craniofacial Surgery, Johns Hopkins Med Ctr 1989; **Fac Appt:** Assoc Prof PlS, Vanderbilt Univ

Magee Jr, William P MD/DDS [PlS] - **Spec Exp:** Cleft Palate/Lip; Craniofacial Surgery; **Hospital:** Chldns Hosp of King's Daughters; **Address:** Institute for Craniofacial/Plastic Surg, 400 W Brambleton Ave, Ste 301, Norfolk, VA 23510; **Phone:** 757-627-6700; **Board Cert:** Plastic Surgery 1979; **Med School:** Geo Wash Univ 1972; **Resid:** Surgery, Univ Va Med Ctr 1974; Plastic Surgery, Univ Va Med Ctr 1974; **Fellow:** Craniofacial Surgery, Hosp Foch 1978

Mast, Bruce A MD [PlS] - **Spec Exp:** Breast Cosmetic & Reconstructive Surgery; Body Contouring; Cosmetic Surgery-Face; Skin Cancer Reconstruction; **Hospital:** Shands at Univ of FL, Children's Hosp at Shands/University of Florid; **Address:** 4340 Newberry Rd, Ste 203, Gainesville, FL 32607; **Phone:** 352-271-5367; **Board Cert:** Plastic Surgery 2008; **Med School:** UMDNJ-RW Johnson Med Sch 1987; **Resid:** Surgery, Med Coll Virginia Hosp 1993; **Fellow:** Plastic Surgery, Univ Pittsburgh Med Ctr 1995; **Fac Appt:** Assoc Prof PlS, Univ Fla Coll Med

Matthews, David C MD [PlS] - **Spec Exp:** Craniofacial Surgery/Reconstruction; Facial Trauma/Fractures; Cosmetic Surgery-Face; Cleft Palate/Lip; **Hospital:** Carolinas Med Ctr; **Address:** 1719 South Blvd, Ste B, Charlotte, NC 28203-2747; **Phone:** 704-375-2955; **Board Cert:** Plastic Surgery 1983; **Med School:** Univ Cincinnati 1974; **Resid:** Surgery, Hosp Univ Penn 1980; Plastic Surgery, Hosp Univ Penn 1982; **Fellow:** Craniofacial Surgery, Royal Melbourne Hosp 1982; **Fac Appt:** Clin Prof PlS, Univ NC Sch Med

Maxwell, G Patrick MD [PlS] - **Spec Exp:** Cosmetic Surgery-Breast; Cosmetic Surgery-Face; Breast Reconstruction; Liposuction & Body Contouring; **Hospital:** Baptist Hosp - Nashville, Centennial Med Ctr; **Address:** 2020 21st Ave S, Nashville, TN 37212; **Phone:** 615-932-7700; **Board Cert:** Plastic Surgery 1981; **Med School:** Vanderbilt Univ 1972; **Resid:** Surgery, Johns Hopkins Hosp 1976; Plastic Surgery, Johns Hopkins Hosp 1979; **Fellow:** Microsurgery, Davies Med Ctr 1975; **Fac Appt:** Asst Clin Prof PlS, Vanderbilt Univ

Molnar, Joseph MD/PhD [PlS] - **Spec Exp:** Burns-Reconstructive Plastic Surgery; Reconstructive Microvascular Surgery; Hand Surgery; Wound Healing/Care; **Hospital:** Wake Forest Baptist Med Ctr, Moses H Cone Mem Hosp; **Address:** Wake Forest Univ Sch Med, Dept Plastic Surgery, Medical Center Blvd, Winston-Salem, NC 27157-1075; **Phone:** 336-716-4171; **Board Cert:** Plastic Surgery 2005; Hand Surgery 2000; **Med School:** Ohio State Univ 1977; **Resid:** Surgery, Univ Wash Med Ctr 1989; Plastic Surgery, Med Coll VA 1992; **Fellow:** Microsurgery, Med Coll Wisc 1199; Hand Surgery, Med Coll Wisc 1994; **Fac Appt:** Assoc Prof PlS, Wake Forest Univ

Morgan, Raymond F MD [PlS] - **Spec Exp:** Hand Surgery; Cosmetic Surgery; **Hospital:** Univ of Virginia Health Sys; **Address:** UVA Hand Center, Fontaine Research Park, 415 Ray C. Hunt Drive Fl 3, Charlottesville, VA 22908; **Phone:** 434-924-2413; **Board Cert:** Plastic Surgery 2007; Hand Surgery 2005; **Med School:** W VA Univ 1976; **Resid:** Surgery, Johns Hopkins Hosp 1980; Plastic Surgery, Johns Hopkins Hosp 1982; **Fellow:** Hand Surgery, Raymond M. Curtis Natl Hand Ctr; **Fac Appt:** Prof OrS, Univ VA Sch Med

Smith Jr, David J MD [PlS] - **Spec Exp:** Breast Reconstruction; Burns-Reconstructive Plastic Surgery; Reconstructive Surgery; Body Contouring after Weight Loss; **Hospital:** Tampa Genl Hosp; **Address:** USF Dept Plastic Surgery, 2 Tampa General Circle Fl 7, Tampa, FL 33606; **Phone:** 813-844-8783; **Board Cert:** Plastic Surgery 2006; **Med School:** Indiana Univ 1973; **Resid:** Surgery, Grady Hosp 1988; Plastic Surgery, Indiana Univ Med Ctr 1980; **Fellow:** Hand Surgery, Univ Louisville 1979; **Fac Appt:** Prof S, Univ S Fla Coll Med

Smith, Paul D MD [PlS] - **Spec Exp:** Facial Plastic Surgery; Reconstructive Surgery-Face; Breast Reconstruction; **Hospital:** H Lee Moffitt Cancer Ctr & Research Inst (page 59); **Address:** 2 Tampa Genl Cir Fl 7, Tampa, FL 33606-3589; **Phone:** 813-844-8783; **Board Cert:** Plastic Surgery 2012; **Med School:** Univ IL Coll Med 1994; **Resid:** Surgery, Univ IL Med Ctr 1999; **Fellow:** Plastic Surgery, Univ Texas SW Med Ctr 2001; **Fac Appt:** Prof PlS, Univ S Fla Coll Med

Stuzin, James M MD [PlS] - **Spec Exp:** Facial Rejuvenation; Skin Laser Surgery-Resurfacing; Cosmetic Surgery-Face & Neck; Rhinoplasty; **Hospital:** Mercy Hosp; **Address:** 3225 Aviation Ave, Ste 100, Coconut Grove, FL 33133; **Phone:** 305-854-8828; **Board Cert:** Plastic Surgery 1989; **Med School:** Univ Fla Coll Med 1978; **Resid:** Surgery, Univ Wash Affil Hosp 1983; Plastic Surgery, NYU Med Ctr 1986; **Fellow:** Craniofacial Surgery, UCLA Med Ctr 1987

Thaller, Seth R MD/DMD [PlS] - **Spec Exp:** Cosmetic Surgery-Face; Rhinoplasty; Pediatric Plastic Surgery; Reconstructive Plastic Surgery; **Hospital:** Jackson Meml Hosp, Univ of Miami Hosp; **Address:** Univ Miami Dept Plastic Surgery, 1120 NW 14th St Fl 4, Miami, FL 33136; **Phone:** 305-243-4500; **Board Cert:** Otolaryngology 1985; Plastic Surgery 2007; **Med School:** Univ Louisville Sch Med 1975; **Resid:** Otolaryngology, Mass Eye & Ear Infirmary 1983; Plastic Surgery, Montefiore Med Ctr 1985; **Fellow:** Craniofacial Surgery, UCLA Med Ctr 1986; **Fac Appt:** Prof PlS, Univ Miami Sch Med

Tobin, Gordon R MD [PlS] - **Spec Exp:** Reconstructive Plastic Surgery; Transplant-Hand; Cosmetic Surgery; Pelvic Reconstruction After Cancer; **Hospital:** Univ of Louisville Hosp, Jewish Hosp Med Ctr (KY); **Address:** 401 E Chestnut St, Ste 710, Louisville, KY 40202; **Phone:** 502-583-8303; **Board Cert:** Plastic Surgery 1978; **Med School:** UCSF 1969; **Resid:** Surgery, Univ Ariz Affil Hosps 1975; Plastic Surgery, Univ Ariz Affil Hosps 1976; **Fellow:** Pediatric Plastic Surgery, Univ Miami 1973; Cosmetic Plastic Surgery, Univ Miami 1973; **Fac Appt:** Prof PlS, Univ Louisville Sch Med

Plastic Surgery

Vasconez, Henry C MD [PlS] - **Spec Exp:** Craniofacial Surgery/Reconstruction; Pediatric Plastic Surgery; Breast Reconstruction; Cosmetic Surgery; **Hospital:** Univ of Kentucky Albert B. Chandler Hosp; **Address:** 740 S Limestone St, Ste K454, Lexington, KY 40536; **Phone:** 859-257-7171; **Board Cert:** Plastic Surgery 2007; **Med School:** Ecuador 1978; **Resid:** Surgery, Cook Co Hosp 1984; Plastic Surgery, Emory Univ Med Ctr 1986; **Fellow:** Craniofacial Surgery, Baylor Med Ctr/International Craniofacial Inst 1987; **Fac Appt:** Prof S, Univ KY Coll Med

Wilhelmi, Bradon J MD [PlS] - **Spec Exp:** Cosmetic Surgery; Hand Surgery; Reconstructive Plastic Surgery; **Hospital:** Norton Hosp, Univ of Louisville Hosp; **Address:** University Surgical Assocs, 401 E Chestnut St, Ste 710, Louisville, KY 40202; **Phone:** 502-583-8303; **Board Cert:** Plastic Surgery 2011; Hand Surgery 2011; **Med School:** Rush Med Coll 1992; **Resid:** Surgery, Northwestern Univ 1996; Plastic Surgery, Univ Texas Med Ctr 1998; **Fellow:** Hand & Microvascular Surgery, Mass General Hosp 1999; **Fac Appt:** Prof PlS, Univ Louisville Sch Med

Wolfe, S Anthony MD [PlS] - **Spec Exp:** Craniofacial Surgery/Reconstruction; Maxillofacial Surgery; Cosmetic Surgery; **Hospital:** Miami Children's Hosp; **Address:** 3100 SW 62 Ave, Ste 2230, Miami, FL 33155; **Phone:** 305-662-4111; **Board Cert:** Surgery 2003; Plastic Surgery 1973; **Med School:** Harvard Med Sch 1965; **Resid:** Surgery, Peter Bent Brigham Hosp 1972; Plastic Surgery, Jackson Meml Hosp 1974; **Fac Appt:** Assoc Clin Prof PlS, Univ Miami Sch Med

Yu, Jack C MD/DMD [PlS] - **Spec Exp:** Facial Plastic & Reconstructive Surgery; Facial Tumors; Craniofacial Surgery; Cleft Palate/Lip; **Hospital:** Med Coll of GA Hosp and Clin (MCG Health Inc); **Address:** Med College of Georgia Health, 1447 Harper St Fl 3, Augusta, GA 30912; **Phone:** 706-721-4147; **Board Cert:** Surgery 2003; Plastic Surgery 2004; **Med School:** Univ Pennsylvania 1985; **Resid:** Surgery, Hosp Univ Penn 1991; Plastic Surgery, Hosp Univ Penn 1993; **Fellow:** Craniofacial Surgery, Chldn's Hosp 1994; **Fac Appt:** Prof PlS, Med Coll GA

Midwest

Bauer, Bruce S MD [PlS] - **Spec Exp:** Cleft Palate/Lip; Vascular Birthmarks; Ear Reconstruction/Microtia; Pigmented Lesions; **Hospital:** Highland Park/North Shore Univ Hlth Syst, Lurie Chldn's Hosp-Chicago; **Address:** 501 Skokie Blvd, Northbrook, IL 60062; **Phone:** 847-504-2300; **Board Cert:** Plastic Surgery 1980; **Med School:** Northwestern Univ 1974; **Resid:** Surgery, Northwestern Meml Hosp 1977; Plastic Surgery, Northwestern Meml Hosp 1979; **Fac Appt:** Clin Prof S, Northwestern Univ

Bentz, Michael L MD [PlS] - **Spec Exp:** Pediatric Plastic Surgery; Facial Deformities/Reconstruction; Pediatric Hand Surgery; Reconstructive Surgery; **Hospital:** Univ WI Hosp & Clins, Meriter Hosp; **Address:** Univ Wisconsin Hosp, 600 Highland Ave, CSC, rm G5-361, Madison, WI 53792-3236; **Phone:** 608-263-1367; **Board Cert:** Surgery 2009; Plastic Surgery 1994; **Med School:** Temple Univ 1984; **Resid:** Surgery, Temple Univ Hosp 1989; Plastic Surgery, Univ Pittsburgh Med Ctr 1992; **Fellow:** Research, Univ Pittsburgh 1990; **Fac Appt:** Prof S, Univ Wisc

Billmire, David A MD [PlS] - **Spec Exp:** Cleft Palate/Lip; Reconstructive Plastic Surgery; **Hospital:** Cincinnati Chldns Hosp Med Ctr, Univ Hosp - Cincinnati; **Address:** 3333 Burnet Ave, MC 2020, Cincinnati, OH 45229; **Phone:** 513-636-7181; **Board Cert:** Plastic Surgery 1985; **Med School:** Ohio State Univ 1975; **Resid:** Surgery, Univ Hosp 1982; Plastic Surgery, Univ Hosp 1984; **Fellow:** Craniofacial Surgery, Texas Craniofacial Fdn 1985; **Fac Appt:** Assoc Clin Prof S, Univ Cincinnati

Brandt, Keith E MD [PlS] - **Spec Exp:** Breast Reconstruction; Cancer Reconstruction; Micro-surgery; Reconstructive Surgery-Complex; **Hospital:** Barnes-Jewish Hosp, Barnes-Jewish West County Hosp; **Address:** 4921 Parkview Pl, Ste 6G, St Louis, MO 63110-1010; **Phone:** 314-362-7388; **Board Cert:** Hand Surgery 2005; Plastic Surgery 2003; **Med School:** Univ Tex, Houston 1983; **Resid:** Surgery, Univ Nebraska Med Ctr 1989; Plastic Surgery, Univ Tennessee 1991; **Fellow:** Hand Surgery, Wash Univ 1992; Microsurgery, Wash Univ 1993; **Fac Appt:** Prof S, Washington Univ, St Louis

Buchman, Steven R MD [PlS] - **Spec Exp:** Pediatric Plastic Surgery; Craniofacial Surgery-Pedi-atric; Craniofacial Surgery; **Hospital:** Mott Chldns Hosp, Univ of Michigan Hosp; **Address:** Mott Chldns Hosp, 1500 E Med Ctr Drive, rm 7859, Ann Arbor, MI 48109-5219; **Phone:** 734-763-8063; **Board Cert:** Plastic Surgery 2005; **Med School:** Univ VA Sch Med 1985; **Resid:** Surgery, Hosp Univ Penn 1990; Plastic Surgery, Hosp Univ Penn 1992; **Fellow:** Craniofacial Surgery, UCLA Med Ctr 1993; **Fac Appt:** Prof PlS, Univ Mich Med Sch

Cederna, Paul S MD [PlS] - **Spec Exp:** Burns-Reconstructive Plastic Surgery; Cosmetic Surgery-Face; Facial Rejuvenation; Body Contouring; **Hospital:** Univ of Michigan Hosp; **Address:** 2130 Taubman Center, 1500 E Medical Center Drive, Ann Arbor, MI 48109-0340; **Phone:** 734-998-6022; **Board Cert:** Plastic Surgery 2009; **Med School:** Univ Mich Med Sch 1989; **Resid:** Surgery, Univ Iowa Hosp & Clin 1994; **Fellow:** Microsurgery, Univ Iowa Hosp & Clin 1995; Plastic Surgery, Univ Michigan Hosps 1997; **Fac Appt:** Prof PlS, Univ Mich Med Sch

Coleman III, John J MD [PlS] - **Spec Exp:** Cancer Reconstruction; Breast Reconstruction; Head & Neck Surgery; Pediatric Plastic Surgery; **Hospital:** IU Health University Hosp, Riley Hosp for Chil-dren; **Address:** IU Plastic Surgery Assocs, 545 Barnhill Dr, Emerson Hall, Ste 232, Indianapolis, IN 46202-5120; **Phone:** 317-274-8106; **Board Cert:** Plastic Surgery 1981; **Med School:** Harvard Med Sch 1973; **Resid:** Surgery, Emory Univ Affil Hosp 1978; Plastic Surgery, Emory Univ Affil Hosp 1979; **Fellow:** Surgical Oncology, Univ Maryland Med Ctr 1981; **Fac Appt:** Prof S, Indiana Univ

Gottlieb, Lawrence Jay MD [PlS] - **Spec Exp:** Burn Care; Reconstructive Plastic Surgery; **Hospital:** Univ of Chicago Med Ctr; **Address:** Univ Chicago Med Ctr, 5841 S Maryland Ave, MC 6035, Chicago, IL 60637-1447; **Phone:** 773-702-6302; **Board Cert:** Plastic Surgery 2007; **Med School:** Penn State Coll Med 1977; **Resid:** Surgery, Yale-New Haven Hosp 1982; Plastic Surgery, LAC-USC Med Ctr 1984; **Fac Appt:** Prof S, Univ Chicago-Pritzker Sch Med

Hammond, Dennis C MD [PlS] - **Spec Exp:** Cosmetic Surgery-Breast; Breast Reconstruction; Body Contouring after Weight Loss; **Hospital:** Spectrum Hlth Blodgett Campus; **Address:** 4070 Lake Drive SE, Ste 202, Grand Rapids, MI 49546; **Phone:** 616-464-4420; **Board Cert:** Plastic Surgery 1994; **Med School:** Univ Mich Med Sch 1985; **Resid:** Surgery, Blodgett Meml Med Ctr 1988; Plas-tic/Reconstructive Surgery, Grand Rapids Area Med Educ Ctr 1990; **Fellow:** Plastic Surgery, Baptist Hosp 1991; Hand & Microvascular Surgery, Med Coll Wisconsin 1992; **Fac Appt:** Prof PlS, Univ Mich Med Sch

Kirschner, Richard Eugene MD [PlS] - **Spec Exp:** Cleft Palate/Lip; Craniofacial Surgery; **Hospital:** Nationwide Chldn's Hosp; **Address:** Nationwide Chldn's Hosp: Education Bldg, 700 Chil-dren's Drive, Fl 2nd, Ste 260, Columbus, OH 43205; **Phone:** 614-722-6692; **Board Cert:** Plastic Surgery 2009; Surgery 2006; **Med School:** Univ Miami Sch Med 1989; **Resid:** Surgery, NY-Presby Hosp/Cornell 1995; Plastic Surgery, Univ Penn 1997; **Fellow:** Plastic Surgery, Chldn's Hosp Philadel-phia 1997

Kuzon Jr, William M MD/PhD [PlS] - **Spec Exp:** Facial Paralysis Reconstruction; Abdominal Wall Reconstruction; Gender Reassignment Surgery; **Hospital:** Univ of Michigan Hosp, John D. Dingell VA Med Ctr, Detroit; **Address:** 1500 E Med Ctr Drive, 2130 Taubman Ctr, Ann Arbor, MI 48109-0340; **Phone:** 734-998-6022; **Board Cert:** Plastic Surgery 2006; **Med School:** Univ Rochester 1981; **Resid:** Plastic Surgery, Univ Toronto Med Ctr 1990; **Fellow:** Microvascular Surgery, Univ Toronto Med Ctr 1991; Hand & Microvascular Surgery, Univ Pittsburgh Med Ctr 1992; **Fac Appt:** Prof PlS, Univ Mich Med Sch

Lee, Raphael MD [PlS] - **Spec Exp:** Reconstructive Surgery; Trauma-Reconstructive Plastic Surgery; Burns-Reconstructive Plastic Surgery; Nerve Injuries/Surgery; **Hospital:** Univ of Chicago Med Ctr; **Address:** 5841 S Maryland Ave, MC 6035, Chicago, IL 60637; **Phone:** 773-702-6302; **Board Cert:** Plastic Surgery 1989; **Med School:** Temple Univ 1975; **Resid:** Surgery, Univ Chicago Hosp 1981; Plastic Surgery, Mass Genl Hosp 1983; **Fellow:** Research, Harvard Med School 1979; **Fac Appt:** Prof PlS, Univ Chicago-Pritzker Sch Med

MacKinnon, Susan E MD [PlS] - **Spec Exp:** Nerve Surgery & Transplantation; Hand Surgery; Reconstructive Surgery; Peripheral Nerve Surgery; **Hospital:** Barnes-Jewish Hosp; **Address:** Washington Univ Sch Med, 660 S Euclid Ave, Box 8238, St Louis, MO 63110; **Phone:** 314-362-4586; **Med School:** Canada 1975; **Resid:** Surgery, Queens Univ-Kingston 1978; Plastic Surgery, Univ Toronto Med Ctr 1980; **Fellow:** Neurological Surgery, Univ Toronto Med Ctr 1981; Hand Surgery, Union Meml Hosp 1982; **Fac Appt:** Prof S, Washington Univ, St Louis

Marsh, Jeffrey L MD [PlS] - **Spec Exp:** Cleft Palate/Lip; Craniofacial Surgery/Reconstruction; Pediatric Plastic Surgery; **Hospital:** St. John's Mercy Med Ctr - St Louis; **Address:** 621 S New Ballas Rd, Ste 260A, St Louis, MO 63141; **Phone:** 314-251-4772; **Board Cert:** Plastic Surgery 1979; **Med School:** Johns Hopkins Univ 1970; **Resid:** Surgery, UCLA Med Ctr 1975; Plastic Surgery, Univ Virginia Hosp 1977; **Fellow:** Craniofacial Surgery, Cannisburn Hosp; Craniofacial Surgery, Clinic Belvedere; **Fac Appt:** Clin Prof PlS, St Louis Univ

Medalie, Daniel A MD [PlS] - **Spec Exp:** Cosmetic Surgery-Breast; Liposuction & Body Contouring; Genital Enhancement; Gender Reassignment Surgery; **Hospital:** MetroHealth Med Ctr; **Address:** MetroHealth Medical Ctr, 2500 MetroHealth Drive, Ste H953, Cleveland, OH 44109; **Phone:** 216-778-4450; **Board Cert:** Plastic Surgery 2010; **Med School:** Cornell Univ 1991; **Resid:** Surgery, Univ Pittsburgh Med Ctr 1995; Plastic Surgery, Univ Pittsburgh Med Ctr 1997; **Fellow:** Research, Mass Genl Hosp 1999; **Fac Appt:** Asst Prof PlS, Case West Res Univ

Miller, Michael John MD [PlS] - **Spec Exp:** Cancer Reconstruction; Breast Reconstruction; Head & Neck Reconstruction; **Hospital:** Ohio St Univ Med Ctr; **Address:** OSU Div of Plastic Surgery, 915 Olentangy River Rd, Ste 2100, Columbus, OH 43212; **Phone:** 614-293-8566; **Board Cert:** Plastic Surgery 2003; **Med School:** Univ Mass Sch Med 1983; **Resid:** Surgery, Berkshire Med Ctr 1987; **Fellow:** Plastic Surgery, Ohio State Univ Med Ctr 1989; **Fac Appt:** Prof S, Ohio State Univ

Mustoe, Thomas A MD [PlS] - **Spec Exp:** Cosmetic Surgery-Face; Cosmetic Surgery-Breast; Rhinoplasty; Body Contouring; **Hospital:** Northwestern Meml Hosp; **Address:** NW Med Faculty Fdn-Plastic Surgery, 675 N St Clair St Fl 19 - Ste 250, Chicago, IL 60611-5975; **Phone:** 312-695-6022; **Board Cert:** Otolaryngology 1983; Plastic Surgery 2007; **Med School:** Harvard Med Sch 1978; **Resid:** Surgery, Brigham & Womens Hosp 1980; Otolaryngology, Mass Eye & Ear Infirm 1983; **Fellow:** Plastic Surgery, Brigham & Womens Hosp 1985; **Fac Appt:** Prof S, Northwestern Univ

Ness, John A MD [PlS] - **Spec Exp:** Cosmetic Surgery-Breast; Facial Plastic Surgery; Abdomino-plasty; Cosmetic Surgery-Face; **Hospital:** Maple Grove Hosp; **Address:** 2805 Campus Drive, Ste 485, Plymouth, MN 55441; **Phone:** 763-559-4500; **Board Cert:** Otolaryngology 1992; Plastic Surgery 2009; Facial Plastic & Reconstr Surgery 1996; **Med School:** Univ Minn 1986; **Resid:** Otolaryngology, Loyola Univ Med Ctr 1991; Plastic Surgery, UC Davis Med Ctr 1998; **Fellow:** Facial Plastic & Reconstr Surgery, UC Davis 1993; Craniofacial Surgery, Australian Craniofacial Inst 1996; **Fac Appt:** Asst Clin Prof PlS, Univ Minn

Neumeister, Michael W MD [PlS] - **Spec Exp:** Hand Surgery; Microsurgery; Breast Reconstruction & Augmentation; Cleft Palate/Lip; **Hospital:** Memorial Med Ctr-Springfield; **Address:** SIU Div Plastic Surgery, Baylis Med Bldg, 747 N Rutledge St Fl 3, Springfield, IL 62702; **Phone:** 217-545-6314; **Board Cert:** Plastic Surgery 2005; Hand Surgery 2006; **Med School:** Univ Toronto 1988; **Resid:** Surgery, Dalhousie Univ Affil Hosp 1991; Plastic Surgery, Univ Manitoba Affil Hosp 1994; **Fellow:** Microsurgery, Brigham & Womens Hosp 1996; Hand & Microvascular Surgery, Southern Illinois Univ 2007; **Fac Appt:** Prof S, Southern IL Univ

Papay, Francis A MD [PlS] - **Spec Exp:** Craniofacial Surgery/Reconstruction; Maxillofacial Surgery; Cosmetic Surgery-Face; Pediatric Plastic Surgery; **Hospital:** Cleveland Clin (page 55); **Address:** Cleveland Clinic, 9500 Euclid Ave, Desk A60, Cleveland, OH 44195; **Phone:** 216-444-6906; **Board Cert:** Otolaryngology 1989; Plastic Surgery 2007; **Med School:** NE Ohio Univ 1983; **Resid:** Otolaryngology, Cleveland Clinic 1989; Plastic/Reconstructive Surgery, Cleveland Clinic 1991; **Fellow:** Craniofacial & Maxillofacial Surgery, Primary Chldns Med Ctr 1992; **Fac Appt:** Assoc Prof S, Cleveland Cl Coll Med/Case West Res

Patel, Pravin K MD [PlS] - **Spec Exp:** Pediatric Plastic Surgery; Craniofacial Surgery; Cleft Palate/Lip; Reconstructive Surgery-Complex; **Hospital:** Lurie Chldn's Hosp-Chicago, Shriners Hosp for Children-Chicago; **Address:** Lurie Chldn's Hosp, Div Plastic Surgery, 225 E Chicago Ave, Box 93, Chicago, IL 60611; **Phone:** 312-227-6250; **Board Cert:** Plastic Surgery 2009; **Med School:** Hahnemann Univ 1985; **Resid:** Surgery, Mayo Clinic 1989; Plastic Surgery, Northwestern Univ 1993; **Fellow:** Craniofacial Surgery, UCLA Med Ctr 1994; **Fac Appt:** Assoc Prof S, Northwestern Univ-Feinberg Sch Med

Polley, John W MD [PlS] - **Spec Exp:** Craniofacial Surgery; Pediatric Plastic Surgery; Maxillofacial Surgery; **Hospital:** Rush Univ Med Ctr; **Address:** Rush Cranio Facial Ctr, 1725 W Harrison St, Ste 425, Chicago, IL 60612; **Phone:** 312-563-3000; **Board Cert:** Plastic Surgery 1992; **Med School:** Northwestern Univ 1983; **Resid:** Surgery, Mich State Univ Med Ctr 1986; Plastic Surgery, Mich State Univ Med Ctr 1988; **Fellow:** Craniofacial & Maxillofacial Surgery, Chang Gung Meml Hosp 1989; Pediatric Craniofacial Surgery, Hosp for Sick Chldn 1990; **Fac Appt:** Prof PlS, Rush Med Coll

Puckett, Charles L MD [PlS] - **Spec Exp:** Cosmetic & Reconstructive Surgery; Breast Surgery; **Hospital:** Univ of Missouri Hosp, Columbia Regional Hosp; **Address:** 1 Hospital Drive, Ste M349, Columbia, MO 65212; **Phone:** 573-882-2275; **Board Cert:** Surgery 1972; Plastic Surgery 2006; **Med School:** Wake Forest Univ 1966; **Resid:** Surgery, Duke Univ Med Ctr 1971; Plastic Surgery, Duke Univ Med Ctr 1976; **Fellow:** Hand Surgery, Kleinert Hand Fellowship; **Fac Appt:** Prof S, Univ MO-Columbia Sch Med

Sanger, James R MD [PlS] - **Spec Exp:** Reconstructive Surgery; Hand Surgery; Microsurgery; **Hospital:** Froedtert and Med Ctr of WI, Chldns Hosp - Wisconsin; **Address:** 8700 Watertown Plank Rd, Dept Plastic Surg, Milwaukee, WI 53226; **Phone:** 414-805-5451; **Board Cert:** Plastic Surgery 2008; Hand Surgery 2009; **Med School:** Univ Wisc 1974; **Resid:** Surgery, LAC-Harbor UCLA Med Ctr 1979; Plastic Surgery, Med Coll Wisc Affil Hosps 1981; **Fellow:** Hand Surgery, Med Coll Wisc Affil Hosps 1982; **Fac Appt:** Prof PlS, Med Coll Wisc

Plastic Surgery

Siebert, John W MD [PlS] - **Spec Exp:** Facial Plastic & Reconstructive Surgery; Microsurgery; Cosmetic Surgery-Face; **Hospital:** Univ WI Hosp & Clins, New York Eye & Ear Infirm (page 65); **Address:** UW Hospital and Clinics, Div of Plastic & Reconstructive Surgery, 600 Highland Ave, Madison, WI 53792; **Phone:** 212-737-8300; **Board Cert:** Plastic Surgery 1991; **Med School:** Univ Wisc 1981; **Resid:** Surgery, Mass Genl Hosp 1986; Plastic Surgery, NYU Med Ctr 1988; **Fellow:** Microsurgery, NYU Med Ctr 1989; **Fac Appt:** Assoc Prof S, Univ Wisc

Siemionow, Maria MD/PhD [PlS] - **Spec Exp:** Microsurgery; Peripheral Nerve Surgery; Reconstructive Plastic Surgery; Transplant-Face; **Hospital:** Cleveland Clin (page 55); **Address:** Cleveland Clin Fdn, 9500 Euclid Ave, Desk A60, Cleveland, OH 44195; **Phone:** 216-445-2405; **Med School:** Poland 1974; **Resid:** Surgery, Inst Orth & Rehab Med; **Fellow:** Plastic Surgery, Univ Hosp; Microsurgery, Univ Louisville Hosp

Sood, Rajiv MD [PlS] - **Spec Exp:** Burns-Reconstructive Plastic Surgery; Pediatric Hand Surgery; Breast Cosmetic & Reconstructive Surgery; Body Contouring after Weight Loss; **Hospital:** IU Health University Hosp, Riley Hosp for Children; **Address:** Richard Fairbanks Burn Ctr, 1001 W 10th St, Dunlap Bldg Fl 4, Indianapolis, IN 46202; **Phone:** 317-278-1022; **Board Cert:** Plastic Surgery 2007; Hand Surgery 2006; **Med School:** Albany Med Coll 1984; **Resid:** Surgery, Temple Univ Hosp 1989; **Fellow:** Plastic Surgery, Cleveland Clinic Fdn 1991; Hand Surgery, Union Meml Hosp 1992; **Fac Appt:** Prof S, Indiana Univ

Vogt, Peter MD [PlS] - **Spec Exp:** Cosmetic Surgery; **Hospital:** Mercy Hosp - Coon Rapids, Unity Hosp - Fridley; **Address:** 319 Barry Ave S, Ste 300, Wayzata, MN 55391; **Phone:** 952-473-1111; **Board Cert:** Plastic Surgery 1974; **Med School:** Univ Manitoba 1965; **Resid:** Surgery, Montreal Genl Hosp 1970; Plastic Surgery, Winnipeg Hlth Scis Ctr 1973

Walton Jr, Robert L MD [PlS] - **Spec Exp:** Nasal Reconstruction; Breast Reconstruction; Ear Reconstruction/Microtia; Cosmetic Surgery-Face; **Hospital:** Resurrection Hlth Care St Joseph Hosp, Lurie Chldn's Hosp-Chicago; **Address:** 60 E Delaware Pl, Ste 1430, Chicago, IL 60611-1495; **Phone:** 312-337-7795; **Board Cert:** Plastic Surgery 1980; **Med School:** Univ Kansas 1972; **Resid:** Surgery, Johns Hopkins Hosp 1974; Plastic Surgery, Yale-New Haven Hosp 1978; **Fellow:** Hand Surgery, Hartford Hosp 1978; **Fac Appt:** Prof PlS, Northwestern Univ-Feinberg Sch Med

Wilkins, Edwin G MD [PlS] - **Spec Exp:** Breast Reconstruction; Lower Limb Reconstruction; Microsurgery; **Hospital:** Univ of Michigan Hosp; **Address:** Univ Mich, Div Plastic Surg, 1500 E Med Ctr Drive, rm 2130 Taubman Ctr, Ann Arbor, MI 48109-5340; **Phone:** 734-998-6022; **Board Cert:** Plastic Surgery 1991; **Med School:** Wake Forest Univ 1981; **Resid:** Surgery, Charlotte Meml Hosp 1986; Plastic Surgery, Vanderbilt Univ Med Ctr 1988; **Fellow:** Reconstructive Microsurgery, Univ Louisville Sch Med 1989; **Fac Appt:** Assoc Prof PlS, Univ Mich Med Sch

Yetman, Randall MD [PlS] - **Spec Exp:** Breast Reconstruction; Melanoma; Microsurgery; **Hospital:** Cleveland Clin (page 55); **Address:** 9500 Euclid Ave, Desk A60, Cleveland, OH 44195; **Phone:** 216-444-6908; **Board Cert:** Plastic Surgery 1984; **Med School:** Univ Miami Sch Med 1975; **Resid:** Surgery, Montefiore Med Ctr 1979; Plastic Surgery, NY Cornell Med Ctr 1981; **Fellow:** Plastic Surgery, Cleveland Clin Fdn 1982

Young, V Leroy MD [PlS] - **Spec Exp:** Breast Augmentation; Skin Laser Surgery-Resurfacing; Body Contouring after Weight Loss; **Hospital:** Barnes-Jewish West County Hosp; **Address:** 969 N Mason Rd, Ste 170, St Louis, MO 63141; **Phone:** 314-628-8200; **Board Cert:** Plastic Surgery 1981; **Med School:** Univ KY Coll Med 1970; **Resid:** Surgery, Univ KY Med Ctr 1977; Plastic Surgery, Barnes Hosp-Wash Univ 1979; **Fac Appt:** Prof S, Washington Univ, St Louis

Zins, James E MD [PIS] - **Spec Exp:** Cosmetic Surgery-Face; Rhinoplasty; Facial Rejuvenation; Maxillofacial Surgery; **Hospital:** Cleveland Clin (page 55); **Address:** Department of Plastic Surgery, 9500 Euclid Ave, Desk A-60, Cleveland, OH 44195; **Phone:** 216-444-6901; **Board Cert:** Plastic Surgery 2007; **Med School:** Univ Pennsylvania 1974; **Resid:** Surgery, Hosp Univ Penn 1980; Plastic Surgery, Hosp Univ Penn 1982; **Fellow:** Craniofacial Surgery, Hosp Univ Penn 1978; Maxillofacial Surgery, Hosp Sick Chldn 1983

Great Plains and Mountains

Deleyiannis, Frederic W B MD [PIS] - **Spec Exp:** Head & Neck Reconstruction; Maxillofacial Surgery; Craniofacial Surgery; Pediatric Plastic Surgery; **Hospital:** Univ of CO Hosp - Anschutz Inpatient Pav, Chldn's Hosp - Aurora (CO); **Address:** 13123 E 16th Ave, Box B467, Aurora, CO 80045; **Phone:** 720-777-3880; **Board Cert:** Otolaryngology 2000; Plastic Surgery 2003; **Med School:** Yale Univ 1992; **Resid:** Otolaryngology, Univ Washington Med Ctr 1999; Plastic Surgery, Univ Pittsburgh Med Ctr 2002; **Fellow:** Head and Neck Surgery, Univ Oviedo Med Ctr 2000; **Fac Appt:** Assoc Prof PIS, Univ Colorado

Grossman, John A MD [PIS] - **Spec Exp:** Cosmetic Surgery; **Hospital:** Rose Med Ctr, Cedars-Sinai Med Ctr; **Address:** Grossman Plastic Surgery, 4600 E Hale Pkwy, Denver, CO 80220; **Phone:** 303-320-5566; **Board Cert:** Surgery 1974; Plastic Surgery 1976; **Med School:** Cornell Univ-Weill Med Coll 1967; **Resid:** Surgery, Boston City Hosp 1973; Plastic Surgery, Univ Colo Hlth Scis Ctr 1975; **Fellow:** Surgery, Harvard Med Sch 1973

Rockwell, William MD [PIS] - **Spec Exp:** Microsurgery; Sarcoma; Breast Reconstruction; Hand Surgery; **Hospital:** Univ Utah Hlth Care; **Address:** 30 N 1900 E, Ste 3B400, Salt Lake City, UT 84132; **Phone:** 801-585-3253; **Board Cert:** Plastic Surgery 2007; Hand Surgery 2006; **Med School:** Washington Univ, St Louis 1984; **Resid:** Surgery, Univ Washington/Barnes Hosp 1987; Plastic Surgery, Univ Rochester Affil Hosp 1991; **Fellow:** Hand Surgery, Univ Rochester Affil Hosp 1992; **Fac Appt:** Assoc Prof PIS, Univ Utah

Southwest

Barone, Constance M MD [PIS] - **Spec Exp:** Cosmetic Surgery; Cosmetic Surgery-Breast; Rhinoplasty; Craniofacial Surgery; **Hospital:** Christus Santa Rosa Med Ctr Hosp, Univ Hlth Syst-San Antonio; **Address:** 2829 Babcock Rd, Tower 1 Bldg - Fl 6 - Ste 615, MS 78229, Ste 615, San Antonio, TX 78229; **Phone:** 210-614-0400; **Board Cert:** Plastic Surgery 1991; **Med School:** Mount Sinai Sch Med 1982; **Resid:** Surgery, Temple Univ Hosp 1987; Plastic Surgery, NYU Med Ctr 1989; **Fellow:** Craniofacial Surgery, Montefiore-Weiler Einstein Div 1992; **Fac Appt:** Prof NS, Univ Tex, San Antonio

Barton Jr, Fritz E MD [PIS] - **Spec Exp:** Cosmetic Surgery-Face; Liposuction & Body Contouring; Cosmetic Surgery-Breast; Facial Rejuvenation; **Hospital:** Baylor Univ Medical Ctr-Dallas; **Address:** 4311 Oak Lawn Ave, Ste 380, Dallas, TX 75219; **Phone:** 214-821-9355; **Board Cert:** Surgery 1975; Plastic Surgery 1977; **Med School:** Univ Tex SW, Dallas 1967; **Resid:** Surgery, Parkland Meml Hosp 1974; Plastic/Reconstructive Surgery, NYU Med Ctr 1976; **Fac Appt:** Clin Prof PIS, Univ Tex SW, Dallas

Beals, Stephen P MD [PlS] - **Spec Exp:** Craniofacial Surgery; Pediatric Plastic Surgery; Cosmetic Surgery-Face & Breast; Liposuction & Body Contouring; **Hospital:** St. Joseph's Hosp & Med Ctr - Phoenix, Phoenix Children's Hosp; **Address:** 500 W Thomas Rd, Ste 960, Phoenix, AZ 85013-4223; **Phone:** 602-266-9066; **Board Cert:** Plastic Surgery 1986; **Med School:** Wayne State Univ 1978; **Resid:** Surgery, William Beaumont Hosp 1983; Plastic Surgery, Phoenix Plastic Surgery Inst 1985; **Fellow:** Craniofacial Surgery, Hospital for Sick Chldn 1985; **Fac Appt:** Assoc Prof PlS, Mayo Med Sch

Burns, A Jay MD [PlS] - **Spec Exp:** Cosmetic Surgery-Face; Cosmetic Surgery-Breast; Facial Rejuvenation; Vascular Birthmarks; **Hospital:** Baylor Univ Medical Ctr-Dallas, Chldns Med Ctr of Dallas; **Address:** 9101 N Central Expresswy St, Ste 600, Dallas, TX 75231; **Phone:** 214-823-1978; **Board Cert:** Plastic Surgery 1990; **Med School:** Univ Tex SW, Dallas 1981; **Resid:** Surgery, Univ Utah Hosp 1986; Plastic Surgery, Univ Tex SW Med Ctr 1988; **Fellow:** Vascular Anomalies, Chldns Hosp 1988; **Fac Appt:** Asst Prof PlS, Univ Tex SW, Dallas

Butler, Charles E MD [PlS] - **Spec Exp:** Breast Reconstruction; **Hospital:** UT MD Anderson Cancer Ctr; **Address:** UT MD Anderson Cancer Ctr, 1515 Holcombe Blvd, Ste 1488, PO Box 301402, Houston, TX 77030; **Phone:** 713-794-1247; **Board Cert:** Plastic Surgery 2010; Surgery 2008; **Med School:** Univ Pennsylvania 1990; **Resid:** Surgery, Mass Genl Hosp 1993; Plastic Surgery, Brigham & Women's Hosp 1995; **Fellow:** Research, Brigham & Women's Hosp 1998; **Fac Appt:** Prof PlS, Case West Res Univ

Byrd, H Stephenson MD [PlS] - **Spec Exp:** Rhinoplasty; Cosmetic Surgery-Face; Cosmetic Surgery-Breast; Liposuction & Body Contouring; **Hospital:** Baylor Univ Medical Ctr-Dallas; **Address:** 9101 N Central Expressway, Ste 600, Dallas, TX 75231; **Phone:** 214-821-9662; **Board Cert:** Plastic Surgery 1980; **Med School:** Univ Tex Med Br, Galveston 1972; **Resid:** Surgery, Univ Utah Med Ctr 1977; Plastic Surgery, Dallas Co Hosp-Parkland Meml 1979; **Fac Appt:** Clin Prof PlS, Univ Tex SW, Dallas

Hamra, Sameer T MD [PlS] - **Spec Exp:** Cosmetic Surgery-Face; Rhinoplasty; **Hospital:** Mary Shiels Hosp; **Address:** 9301 N Central Expressway, Tower II, Ste 551, Dallas, TX 75231; **Phone:** 214-754-9001; **Board Cert:** Surgery 1970; Plastic Surgery 1977; **Med School:** Univ Okla Coll Med 1963; **Resid:** Surgery, Univ Okla 1968; Plastic Surgery, NYU Med Ctr 1973; **Fellow:** Surgery, Univ Lausanne 1966; **Fac Appt:** Clin Prof S, Univ Tex SW, Dallas

Kane, Alex A MD [PlS] - **Spec Exp:** Pediatric Plastic Surgery; Craniofacial Surgery; Cleft Palate/Lip; Hemangiomas/Birthmarks; **Hospital:** Chldns Med Ctr of Dallas; **Address:** 2350 N Stemmons Freeway, Ambulatory Care Pavilion Fl 4, Dallas, TX 75207; **Phone:** 214-456-2240; **Board Cert:** Plastic Surgery 2001; **Med School:** Dartmouth Med Sch 1991; **Resid:** Surgery, Barnes Jewish Hosp 1994; Plastic Surgery, Barnes Jewish Hosp 1998; **Fellow:** Craniofacial Surgery, Chang-Gung Meml Hosp 1999; Craniofacial Imaging, Nat'l Lab for Diagnostic Rsch 1999; **Fac Appt:** Prof S, Univ Tex SW, Dallas

Kenkel, Jeffrey M MD [PlS] - **Spec Exp:** Cosmetic Surgery-Face; Laser Surgery; Cosmetic Surgery-Breast; Body Contouring after Weight Loss; **Hospital:** UT Southwestern Med Ctr at Dallas; **Address:** UTSW Plastic Surgery, 1801 Inwood Rd Fl 5, Dallas, TX 75390; **Phone:** 214-645-2353; **Board Cert:** Plastic Surgery 2008; **Med School:** Georgetown Univ 1990; **Resid:** Surgery, Georgetown Univ Med Ctr 1994; Plastic Surgery, UT Southwestern Med Ctr 1996; **Fac Appt:** Prof PlS, Univ Tex SW, Dallas

Kronowitz, Steven J MD [PlS] - **Spec Exp:** Reconstructive Surgery; **Hospital:** UT MD Anderson Cancer Ctr; **Address:** 1400 Pressler Unit 1488, Houston, TX 77030; **Phone:** 713-794-1247; **Board Cert:** Surgery 2007; Plastic Surgery 2002; **Med School:** Univ Miami Sch Med 1992; **Resid:** Surgery, Mt Sinai Hosp 1997; Plastic Surgery, Mt Sinai Hosp 2000; **Fellow:** Microsurgery, MD Anderson Cancer Center 2001; **Fac Appt:** Prof S, Univ Tex, Houston

Leighton, William D MD [PlS] - **Spec Exp:** Burns-Reconstructive Plastic Surgery; Facial Plastic & Reconstructive Surgery; Breast Cosmetic & Reconstructive Surgery; Conjoined Twins; **Hospital:** Scottsdale Hlthcare - Shea, Scottsdale Hlthcare - Osborn; **Address:** 7425 E Shea Blvd, Ste 103, Scottsdale, AZ 85260; **Phone:** 480-948-3250; **Board Cert:** Plastic Surgery 2008; **Med School:** Univ IL Coll Med 1978; **Resid:** Surgery, Mayo Clinic 1983; Plastic Surgery, Mayo Clinic 1985; **Fellow:** Microsurgery, S Illinois Univ Med Ctr 1986; **Fac Appt:** Assoc Prof S, Mayo Med Sch

Meltzer, Toby R MD [PlS] - **Spec Exp:** Gender Reassignment Surgery; Penile Inversion Technique; Breast Augmentation; Cosmetic Surgery-Face & Breast; **Hospital:** Scottsdale Hlthcare - Osborn; **Address:** 7025 N Scottsdale Rd, Ste 302, Scottsdale, AZ 85253; **Phone:** 480-657-7006; **Board Cert:** Plastic Surgery 1992; **Med School:** Louisiana State U, New Orleans 1983; **Resid:** Surgery, Charity Hosp Louisiana 1988; Plastic Surgery, Univ Michigan Med Ctr 1990; **Fellow:** Burn Surgery, Wayne State Univ 1987; **Fac Appt:** Asst Clin Prof S, Univ Ariz Coll Med

Menick, Frederick J MD [PlS] - **Spec Exp:** Reconstructive Surgery-Face; Nasal Reconstruction; Cancer Reconstruction; Rhinoplasty; **Hospital:** St. Joseph's Hosp - Tucson; **Address:** 1102 N Eldorado Pl, Tucson, AZ 85715; **Phone:** 520-881-4525; **Board Cert:** Plastic Surgery 1983; **Med School:** Yale Univ 1970; **Resid:** Surgery, Stanford Med Ctr 1974; Surgery, Univ Ariz Med Ctr 1979; **Fellow:** Plastic Surgery, UC Irvine 1981; Plastic Surgery, Univ Miami 1982; **Fac Appt:** Assoc Clin Prof S, Univ Ariz Coll Med

Metzinger, Stephen E MD [PlS] - **Spec Exp:** Rhinoplasty; Eyelid Surgery/Blepharoplasty; Cosmetic Surgery-Face; Cosmetic Surgery-Breast; **Hospital:** E Jefferson Genl Hosp; **Address:** Aesthetic Surgery Assocs, 3223 8th St, Ste 200, Metairie, LA 70002; **Phone:** 504-309-7061; **Board Cert:** Otolaryngology 1994; Plastic Surgery 2008; Facial Plastic & Reconstr Surgery; **Med School:** Louisiana State U, New Orleans 1987; **Resid:** Otolaryngology, LSU Med Ctr 1993; Plastic Surgery, Johns Hopkins Affil Hosp 1996; **Fellow:** Facial Plastic & Reconstr Surgery, McCollough Aesthetic Med Ctr 1994; Craniofacial Surgery, Univ Maryland Trauma Ctr 1996; **Fac Appt:** Assoc Prof PlS, Louisiana State U, New Orleans

Moses, Michael H MD [PlS] - **Spec Exp:** Cosmetic Surgery-Face; Cosmetic Surgery-Breast; Liposuction & Body Contouring; Rhinoplasty; **Hospital:** Touro Infirmary, Children's Hospital - New Orleans; **Address:** 1603 2nd St, New Orleans, LA 70130; **Phone:** 504-895-7200; **Board Cert:** Plastic Surgery 1985; **Med School:** Tulane Univ 1977; **Resid:** Surgery, Yale-New Haven Hosp 1982; Plastic Surgery, Mass Genl Hosp 1984; **Fellow:** Craniofacial Surgery, Childrens Hosp 1985; **Fac Appt:** Assoc Clin Prof PlS, Tulane Univ

Rappaport, Norman H MD/DDS [PlS] - **Spec Exp:** Cosmetic Surgery-Face; Breast Cosmetic & Reconstructive Surgery; Body Contouring after Weight Loss; Facial Rejuvenation; **Hospital:** Methodist Hosp - Houston, St. Luke's Episcopal Hosp-Houston; **Address:** Houston Center for Plastic Surgery, 6560 Fannin St, Ste 1812 Scurlock Tower, Houston, TX 77030-2775; **Phone:** 713-790-4500; **Board Cert:** Plastic Surgery 2007; **Med School:** Hahnemann Univ 1975; **Resid:** Surgery, Abingdon Meml Hosp 1978; Plastic Surgery, Baylor Coll Med 1980; **Fellow:** Plastic Surgery, Hosp Univ Penn 1978; **Fac Appt:** Assoc Clin Prof S, Baylor Coll Med

Robb, Geoffrey L MD [PlS] - **Spec Exp:** Breast Reconstruction; Head & Neck Cancer Reconstruction; Facial Plastic & Reconstructive Surgery; **Hospital:** UT MD Anderson Cancer Ctr, St. Luke's Episcopal Hosp-Houston; **Address:** UT MD Anderson Cancer Ctr, 1515 Holcombe Blvd, Ste 1418, PO Box 301402, Houston, TX 77030; **Phone:** 713-794-1247; **Board Cert:** Otolaryngology 1979; Plastic Surgery 1986; **Med School:** Univ Miami Sch Med 1974; **Resid:** Otolaryngology, Naval Reg Med Ctr 1979; Plastic Surgery, Univ Pittsburgh Med Ctr 1985; **Fellow:** Microvascular Surgery, Univ Pittsburgh 1986; **Fac Appt:** Prof PlS, Univ Tex, Houston

Plastic Surgery

Rohrich, Rod J MD [PlS] - **Spec Exp:** Rhinoplasty; Cosmetic Surgery-Face; Facial Rejuvenation; Liposuction & Body Contouring; **Hospital:** UT Southwestern Med Ctr at Dallas, Baylor Univ Medical Ctr-Dallas; **Address:** Univ Tex SW Med Ctr, Plastic Surgery, 1801 Inwood Rd, MS 9132, Dallas, TX 75390-9132; **Phone:** 214-645-2353; **Board Cert:** Plastic Surgery 1987; Hand Surgery 1990; **Med School:** Baylor Coll Med 1979; **Resid:** Plastic Surgery, Univ Mich Hosp 1985; Plastic Surgery, Radcliffe Infirm/Oxford 1983; **Fellow:** Hand Surgery, Mass Genl Hosp 1987; **Fac Appt:** Prof PlS, Univ Tex SW, Dallas

Schusterman, Mark A MD [PlS] - **Spec Exp:** Breast Reconstruction; Cancer Reconstruction; Cosmetic Surgery-Face & Breast; Liposuction & Body Contouring; **Hospital:** Methodist Hosp - Houston, St. Luke's Episcopal Hosp-Houston; **Address:** 1200 Binz St, Ste 1200, Houston, TX 77004; **Phone:** 713-794-0368; **Board Cert:** Plastic Surgery 1989; **Med School:** Univ Louisville Sch Med 1980; **Resid:** Surgery, Univ Hosp 1985; Plastic Surgery, Univ Pittsburgh Med Ctr 1987; **Fellow:** Micro-surgery, Univ Pittsburgh 1988; **Fac Appt:** Clin Prof PlS, Baylor Coll Med

Tebbetts, John B MD [PlS] - **Spec Exp:** Cosmetic Surgery-Breast; Rhinoplasty; Liposuction; **Hospital:** Mary Shiels Hosp, Baylor Univ Medical Ctr-Dallas; **Address:** 2801 Lemmon Ave W, Ste 300, Dallas, TX 75204; **Phone:** 214-220-2712; **Board Cert:** Plastic Surgery 1980; **Med School:** Univ Tex Med Br, Galveston 1972; **Resid:** Surgery, Univ Utah Med Ctr 1977; Plastic Surgery, Dallas Co Hosp-Parkland Meml Hosp 1979; **Fac Appt:** Asst Clin Prof PlS, Univ Tex SW, Dallas

Wilcox, Robert D MD [PlS] - **Spec Exp:** Cosmetic Surgery-Face; Cosmetic Surgery-Breast; Lipo-suction & Body Contouring; **Hospital:** Columbia Med Ctr - Plano; **Address:** Plastic & Cosmetic Surgery Ctr of Texas, 5316 W Plano Pkwy, Plano, TX 75093; **Phone:** 972-620-1700; **Board Cert:** Plastic Surgery 1994; Hand Surgery 2003; **Med School:** Univ Tex SW, Dallas 1984; **Resid:** Surgery, Univ Florida Hlth Sci Ctr 1989; Plastic/Reconstructive Surgery, Univ Texas-SW Med Sch 1991; **Fellow:** Hand Surgery, Univ Texas-SW Med Sch 1992

Yuen, James C MD [PlS] - **Spec Exp:** Hand Reconstruction; Breast Reconstruction; Head & Neck Cancer Reconstruction; Chest Wall Reconstruction; **Hospital:** UAMS Med Ctr; **Address:** 4301 W Markham, Ste 720, Little Rock, AR 72205; **Phone:** 501-686-8711; **Board Cert:** Surgery 2001; Plastic Surgery 2004; **Med School:** Med Coll VA 1985; **Resid:** Surgery, West Va Med Ctr 1990; Plastic/Reconstructive Surgery, Duke Univ Med Ctr 1993; **Fellow:** Hand & Microvascular Surgery, Kleinert Inst of Hand & Microsurgery 1991; **Fac Appt:** Assoc Prof S, Univ Ark

West Coast and Pacific

Alter, Gary J MD [PlS] - **Spec Exp:** Genitourinary Reconstruction; Gender Reassignment Surgery; Genital Enhancement; **Hospital:** Cedars-Sinai Med Ctr, UCLA Ronald Reagan Med Ctr; **Address:** 416 N Bedford Drive, Ste 400, Beverly Hills, CA 90210-4318; **Phone:** 310-275-5566; **Board Cert:** Urology 1981; Plastic Surgery 2007; **Med School:** UCLA 1973; **Resid:** Urology, Baylor Med Ctr 1979; Plastic Surgery, Mayo Clin 1992; **Fellow:** Genitourinary Surgery, Eastern Va Med Sch 1992; **Fac Appt:** Clin Prof PlS, UCLA

Aly, Al Said MD [PlS] - **Spec Exp:** Abdominoplasty; Body Contouring after Weight Loss; Breast Augmentation; **Hospital:** UC Irvine Med Ctr; **Address:** 200 S Manchester Ave, Ste 650, Orange, CA 92868; **Phone:** 714-456-5471; **Board Cert:** Otolaryngology 1993; Plastic Surgery 2009; **Med School:** Georgetown Univ 1983; **Resid:** Otolaryngology, Vanderbilt Univ Med Ctr 1992; Plastic Surgery, Jackson Meml Med Ctr 1997; **Fellow:** Facial Plastic & Reconstr Surgery, UC Irvine Med Ctr 1993; **Fac Appt:** Prof PlS, UC Irvine

Andersen, James S MD [PIS] - **Spec Exp:** Breast Reconstruction; Head & Neck Reconstruction; Microsurgery; **Hospital:** City of Hope Natl Med Ctr, Huntington Memorial Hosp; **Address:** 1500 E Duarte Rd, Duarte, CA 91010; **Phone:** 626-471-7100; **Board Cert:** Plastic Surgery 1994; **Med School:** Jefferson Med Coll 1983; **Resid:** Surgery, Hosp Univ Penn 1989; Plastic Surgery, Hosp Univ Penn 1991; **Fellow:** Microsurgery, USC Med Ctr 1992; **Fac Appt:** Assoc Clin Prof S, USC Sch Med

Bradley, James P MD [PIS] - **Spec Exp:** Facial Plastic & Reconstructive Surgery; Cosmetic Surgery-Face; Pediatric Plastic Surgery; Cleft Palate/Lip; **Hospital:** UCLA Ronald Reagan Med Ctr; **Address:** Div Plastic & Reconstructive Surgery, 200 UCLA Medical Plaza, Ste 465, Los Angeles, CA 90095; **Phone:** 310-825-5510; **Board Cert:** Plastic Surgery 2011; Surgery 2011; **Med School:** Thomas Jefferson Univ 1991; **Resid:** Surgery, Pennsylvania Hosp 1996; Plastic Surgery, NYU Med Ctr 1998; **Fellow:** Craniofacial Surgery, UCLA Med Ctr 1999; **Fac Appt:** Prof PIS, UCLA-David Geffen Sch Med

Cohen, Steven R MD [PIS] - **Spec Exp:** Craniofacial Surgery-Pediatric; Craniofacial Surgery/Reconstruction; Cosmetic Surgery-Face; Rhinoplasty; **Hospital:** Rady Children's Hosp - San Diego, UCSD Med Ctr; **Address:** 4510 Executive Drive, Ste 200, San Diego, CA 92121; **Phone:** 858-453-7224; **Board Cert:** Plastic Surgery 1992; **Med School:** Geo Wash Univ 1980; **Resid:** Surgery, Dartmouth-Hitchcock Med Ctr 1987; Plastic Surgery, Hosp Univ Penn/Chldns Hosp 1989; **Fellow:** Craniofacial Surgery, UCLA Med Ctr 1990; **Fac Appt:** Clin Prof PIS, UCSD

Da Lio, Andrew L MD [PIS] - **Spec Exp:** Cosmetic Surgery-Face; Cosmetic Surgery-Breast; Breast Reconstruction; Liposuction & Body Contouring; **Hospital:** UCLA Ronald Reagan Med Ctr; **Address:** Div of Plastic & Reconstructive Surgery, 200 UCLA Medical Plaza, Ste 465, Los Angeles, CA 90095; **Phone:** 310-825-5510; **Board Cert:** Plastic Surgery 2010; **Med School:** Univ Mich Med Sch 1989; **Resid:** Surgery, Dartmouth-Hitchcock Med Ctr 1994; Plastic Surgery, USC Med Ctr 1995; **Fellow:** Microsurgery, UCLA Med Ctr 1996; **Fac Appt:** Clin Prof PIS, UCLA-David Geffen Sch Med

Daniel, Rollin K MD [PIS] - **Spec Exp:** Rhinoplasty; **Hospital:** Hoag Meml Hosp Presby; **Address:** 1441 Avocado Ave, Ste 308, Newport Beach, CA 92660; **Phone:** 949-721-0494; **Board Cert:** Plastic Surgery 1977; **Med School:** Columbia P&S 1972; **Resid:** Plastic Surgery, McGill Univ Affil Hosps 1975; Hand Surgery, Univ Louisville Hosp 1976; **Fellow:** Craniofacial Surgery, Univ Toronto 1984

Edwards, Michael C MD [PIS] - **Spec Exp:** Breast Cosmetic & Reconstructive Surgery; Liposuction & Body Contouring; Body Contouring after Weight Loss; **Hospital:** Summerlin Hosp Med Ctr, Mountainview Hosp - Las Vegas; **Address:** 653 N Town Center Drive, Ste 214, Las Vegas, NV 89144; **Phone:** 702-248-8989; **Board Cert:** Surgery 2006; Plastic Surgery 2008; **Med School:** Uniformed Srvs Univ, Bethesda 1988; **Resid:** Surgery, David Grant Med Ctr 1993; **Fellow:** Plastic Surgery, Wilford Hall Med Ctr 1996

Evans, Gregory R MD [PIS] - **Spec Exp:** Cosmetic Surgery-Face; Cosmetic Surgery-Breast; Body Contouring; Cancer Reconstruction; **Hospital:** UC Irvine Med Ctr; **Address:** Aesthetic & Plastic Surgery Inst, 200 S Manchester Ave, Ste 650, Orange, CA 92868; **Phone:** 714-456-3077; **Board Cert:** Surgery 2001; Plastic Surgery 2008; **Med School:** USC Sch Med 1985; **Resid:** Surgery, LAC/USC Med Ctr 1990; Plastic Surgery, Johns Hopkins Hosp 1993; **Fac Appt:** Prof S, UC Irvine

Fisher, Garth MD [PIS] - **Spec Exp:** Cosmetic Surgery-Face; Cosmetic Surgery-Breast; Rhinoplasty; Body Contouring; **Address:** 120 S Spalding Drive, Ste 222, Beverly Hills, CA 90212; **Phone:** 310-273-5995; **Board Cert:** Plastic Surgery 1993; **Med School:** Univ Miss 1984; **Resid:** Surgery, UC Irvine Med Ctr 1989; Plastic Surgery, UC Irvine Med Ctr 1991; **Fellow:** Plastic Surgery, Bruce Connelly 1992

Plastic Surgery

Fodor, Peter B MD [PlS] - **Spec Exp:** Facial Rejuvenation; Liposuction & Body Contouring; Cosmetic Surgery-Breast; **Hospital:** Olympia Med Ctr; **Address:** 2080 Century Park East, Ste 710, Los Angeles, CA 90067; **Phone:** 310-203-9818; **Board Cert:** Plastic Surgery 1977; **Med School:** Univ Wisc 1966; **Resid:** Surgery, Columbia-Presby Med Ctr 1968; Plastic Surgery, St Luke's Hosp 1976; **Fac Appt:** Assoc Clin Prof S, UCLA

Garner, Warren L MD [PlS] - **Spec Exp:** Burns-Reconstructive Plastic Surgery; Wound Healing/Care; Skin Healing; **Hospital:** LAC & USC Med Ctr, Keck Med Ctr of USC (page 62); **Address:** 1510 San Pablo St, Ste 415, Los Angeles, CA 90033; **Phone:** 323-442-7920; **Board Cert:** Plastic Surgery 2008; Surgical Critical Care 2010; **Resid:** Surgery, Ohio State Univ Hosp 1985; Plastic Surgery, Wash Univ Hosp 1989; **Fellow:** Critical Care Medicine, Ohio State Univ Hosp 1986; **Fac Appt:** Assoc Prof PlS, USC Sch Med

Gruss, Joseph MD [PlS] - **Spec Exp:** Maxillofacial & Craniofacial Surgery; Facial Trauma/Fractures; Cleft Palate/Lip; Pediatric Plastic Surgery; **Hospital:** Seattle Chldns Hosp, Harborview Med Ctr; **Address:** Seattle Children's, 4800 Sand Point Way NE, MS W7847, Seattle, WA 98105; **Phone:** 206-987-2759; **Board Cert:** Plastic Surgery 1977; **Med School:** South Africa 1969; **Resid:** Plastic Surgery, Toronto Western Hosp 1976; Plastic Surgery, Hosp for Sick Children 1976; **Fellow:** Surgical Oncology, Princess Margaret Hosp 1977; Head and Neck Surgery, Princess Margaret Hosp 1977; **Fac Appt:** Prof PlS, Univ Wash

Hansen, Juliana MD [PlS] - **Spec Exp:** Breast Reconstruction; Cancer Reconstruction; **Hospital:** OR Hlth & Sci Univ; **Address:** 3303 SW Bond Ave, MC CH5P, Portland, OR 97239; **Phone:** 503-494-6687; **Board Cert:** Plastic Surgery 2008; **Med School:** Univ Wash 1988; **Resid:** Surgery, UCSF Med Ctr 1994; Plastic Surgery, UCSF Med Ctr 1996

Hardesty, Robert MD [PlS] - **Spec Exp:** Cosmetic Surgery-Face & Body; Reconstructive Surgery; Body Contouring; Cosmetic Surgery-Breast; **Hospital:** Riverside Comm Hosp, Loma Linda Univ Med Ctr; **Address:** Riverside Plastic Surgery, 4646 Brockton Ave, Ste 302, Riverside, CA 92506; **Phone:** 951-686-7600; **Board Cert:** Plastic Surgery 1989; **Med School:** Loma Linda Univ 1978; **Resid:** Surgery, Loma Linda Univ Med Ctr 1983; Plastic Surgery, Univ Pittsburgh Med Ctr 1986; **Fellow:** Pediatric Plastic Surgery, Washington Univ 1987; **Fac Appt:** Clin Prof PlS, Loma Linda Univ

Hoffman, William Y MD [PlS] - **Spec Exp:** Pediatric Plastic Surgery; Cleft Palate/Lip; Craniofacial Surgery; Reconstructive Surgery; **Hospital:** UCSF Med Ctr, UCSF - Mt Zion Med Ctr; **Address:** UCSF Plastic Surgery, 350 Parnassus Ave, Ste 509, Box 0932, San Francisco, CA 94143-0932; **Phone:** 415-353-4287; **Board Cert:** Plastic Surgery 1987; **Med School:** Univ Rochester 1977; **Resid:** Surgery, UCSF Med Ctr 1983; Plastic Surgery, UCSF Med Ctr 1985; **Fellow:** Craniofacial Surgery, NYU Med Ctr 1986; **Fac Appt:** Prof PlS, UCSF

Horowitz, Jed H MD [PlS] - **Spec Exp:** Cosmetic Surgery-Breast; Cosmetic Surgery-Face; Transumbilical Breast Augmentation(TUBA); **Hospital:** Hoag Meml Hosp Presby, Orange Coast Memorial Med Ctr; **Address:** 7677 Center Ave, Ste 401, Huntington Beach, CA 92647-3098; **Phone:** 714-902-1100; **Board Cert:** Plastic Surgery 1986; **Med School:** SUNY Buffalo 1977; **Resid:** Surgery, Grady Meml Hosp 1983; **Fellow:** Plastic Surgery, Univ Virginia 1985; **Fac Appt:** Asst Clin Prof PlS, USC Sch Med

Isik, F. Frank MD [PlS] - **Spec Exp:** Cosmetic Surgery; Breast Reconstruction; Cosmetic Surgery-Breast; Liposuction & Body Contouring; **Hospital:** Swedish Med Ctr-First Hill-Seattle; **Address:** The Polyclinic, 1145 Broadway, Ste 1T, Seattle, WA 98122; **Phone:** 206-860-4566; **Board Cert:** Surgery 2001; Plastic Surgery 2007; **Med School:** Mount Sinai Sch Med 1985; **Resid:** Surgery, Boston Univ Hosps 1990; Plastic Surgery, Univ Wash Affil Hosp 1995; **Fellow:** Research, NIH / Univ Washington 1992

Jewell, Mark L MD [PlS] - **Spec Exp:** Liposuction & Body Contouring; Cosmetic Surgery-Face; Breast Reconstruction; Cosmetic Surgery-Breast; **Hospital:** Sacred Heart Med Ctr; **Address:** 10 Coburg Rd, Ste 300, Eugene, OR 97401; **Phone:** 541-683-3234; **Board Cert:** Plastic Surgery 1981; **Med School:** Univ Kansas 1973; **Resid:** Surgery, LAC-Harbor Med Ctr 1976; Plastic Surgery, Erlanger Hosp 1979; **Fellow:** Burn Surgery, LAC-USC Med Ctr 1977; **Fac Appt:** Asst Clin Prof PlS, Oregon Hlth & Sci Univ

Koplin, Lawrence M MD [PlS] - **Spec Exp:** Cosmetic Surgery-Face; Breast Cosmetic & Reconstructive Surgery; Facial Rejuvenation; Liposuction & Body Contouring; **Hospital:** Cedars-Sinai Med Ctr; **Address:** 465 N Roxbury Drive, Ste 800, Beverly Hills, CA 90210; **Phone:** 310-277-3223; **Board Cert:** Plastic Surgery 1985; **Med School:** Baylor Coll Med 1976; **Resid:** Surgery, Kaiser Fdn Hosp 1981; Plastic Surgery, St Joseph Hosp 1983

Leaf, Norman MD [PlS] - **Spec Exp:** Cosmetic Surgery-Face & Neck; Cosmetic Surgery-Breast; Eyelid Surgery/Blepharoplasty; **Hospital:** Cedars-Sinai Med Ctr, UCLA Ronald Reagan Med Ctr; **Address:** 436 N Bedford Drive, Ste 104, Beverly Hills, CA 90210-4310; **Phone:** 310-274-8001; **Board Cert:** Surgery 1973; Plastic Surgery 1974; **Med School:** Univ Chicago-Pritzker Sch Med 1966; **Resid:** Surgery, Univ Chicago Hosps 1972; Plastic Surgery, Univ Chicago Hosps 1973; **Fellow:** Research, Univ Chicago Hosps 1969; **Fac Appt:** Assoc Clin Prof PlS, UCLA

Lesavoy, Malcolm A MD [PlS] - **Spec Exp:** Cosmetic Surgery-Face & Neck; Cosmetic Surgery-Breast; Abdominoplasty; Reconstructive Surgery; **Hospital:** UCLA Ronald Reagan Med Ctr; **Address:** 16311 Ventura Blvd, Ste 555, Encino, CA 91436-4314; **Phone:** 818-986-8270; **Board Cert:** Plastic Surgery 1977; **Med School:** Ros Franklin Univ/Chicago Med Sch 1969; **Resid:** Surgery, Univ Chicago Hosps 1974; Plastic Surgery, Univ Miami Hosp/Clinics 1976; **Fac Appt:** Clin Prof PlS, UCLA

Markowitz, Bernard L MD [PlS] - **Spec Exp:** Cosmetic Surgery-Face & Body; Abdominoplasty; Facial Rejuvenation; Craniofacial Surgery/Reconstruction; **Hospital:** UCLA Ronald Reagan Med Ctr, Cedars-Sinai Med Ctr; **Address:** 9675 Brighton Way, Ste 350, Beverly Hills, CA 90210; **Phone:** 310-205-5557; **Board Cert:** Plastic Surgery 1989; **Med School:** NYU Sch Med 1979; **Resid:** Surgery, NYU Med Ctr 1984; Plastic Surgery, NYU Med Ctr 1986; **Fellow:** Maxillofacial Surgery, Johns Hopkins Hosp 1987; Microvascular Surgery, Johns Hopkins Hosp 1987; **Fac Appt:** Clin Prof PlS, UCLA

Marten, Timothy J MD [PlS] - **Spec Exp:** Cosmetic Surgery-Face & Neck; Facial Rejuvenation; **Hospital:** CA Pacific Med Ctr-Pacific Campus, St. Mary's Med Ctr - San Fran; **Address:** 450 Sutter St, Ste 2222, San Francisco, CA 94108-4207; **Phone:** 415-677-9937; **Board Cert:** Plastic Surgery 1993; **Med School:** UC Davis 1982; **Resid:** Surgery, Kaiser Fdn Hosp 1987; Plastic Surgery, Univ Illinois Chicago Hosp 1989; **Fellow:** Cosmetic Plastic Surgery, Connell Aesthetic Network 1990; Cosmetic Plastic Surgery, Baker, Gordon, & Stuzin 1990

Miller, Timothy A MD [PlS] - **Spec Exp:** Cosmetic Surgery-Face; Eyelid Surgery; Nasal Reconstruction; Burns-Reconstructive Plastic Surgery; **Hospital:** UCLA Ronald Reagan Med Ctr; **Address:** 200 UCLA Medical Plaza, Ste 463, Los Angeles, CA 90095-8344; **Phone:** 310-825-5644; **Board Cert:** Surgery 1971; Plastic Surgery 1973; **Med School:** UCLA 1963; **Resid:** Surgery, Johns Hopkins Hosp 1967; Thoracic Surgery, UCLA Med Ctr 1969; **Fellow:** Plastic Surgery, Univ Pittsburgh 1971; **Fac Appt:** Prof S, UCLA

Nichter, Larry S MD [PlS] - **Spec Exp:** Cosmetic Surgery-Face & Body; Cosmetic Surgery-Breast; Liposuction & Body Contouring; Congenital Breast Anomalies; **Hospital:** Hoag Meml Hosp Presby, Orange Coast Memorial Med Ctr; **Address:** 7677 Center Ave, Ste 401, Huntington Beach, CA 92647-3098; **Phone:** 714-902-1100; **Board Cert:** Plastic Surgery 1986; **Med School:** Boston Univ 1978; **Resid:** Surgery, UCLA Medical Ctr 1982; Plastic Surgery, Univ Virginia Med Ctr 1985; **Fellow:** Hand & Microvascular Surgery, Univ Virginia 1983; Craniofacial Surgery, Univ Virginia 1985; **Fac Appt:** Clin Prof PlS, USC-Keck School of Medicine

Ousterhout, Douglas K MD/DDS [PIS] - **Spec Exp:** Cosmetic Surgery-Face; Gender Reassignment Surgery; Craniofacial Surgery; Facial Feminization Surgery (FFS); **Hospital:** CA Pacific Med Ctr - Davies Campus; **Address:** 45 Castro St, Ste 150, San Francisco, CA 94114; **Phone:** 415-626-2888; **Board Cert:** Plastic Surgery 1974; **Med School:** Univ Mich Med Sch 1965; **Resid:** Surgery, Univ Mich Hosps 1969; Plastic Surgery, Stanford Univ 1972; **Fellow:** Craniofacial Surgery, Clinic Belvedere 1973; **Fac Appt:** Clin Prof PIS, UCSF

Paul, Malcolm D MD [PIS] - **Spec Exp:** Cosmetic Surgery-Face & Neck; Cosmetic Surgery-Breast; Liposuction & Body Contouring; **Hospital:** Hoag Meml Hosp Presby; **Address:** 1401 Avocado Ave, Ste 810, Newport Beach, CA 92660-8708; **Phone:** 949-760-5047; **Board Cert:** Plastic Surgery 1976; **Med School:** Univ MD Sch Med 1969; **Resid:** Surgery, Geo Wash Med Ctr 1973; Plastic Surgery, Geo Wash Med Ctr 1975; **Fac Appt:** Clin Prof S, UC Irvine

Rand, Richard P MD [PIS] - **Spec Exp:** Cosmetic Surgery-Face; Cosmetic Surgery-Breast; Liposuction & Body Contouring; Facial Rejuvenation; **Hospital:** Overlake Hosp Med Ctr; **Address:** 1135 116th Ave NE, Ste 630, Bellevue, WA 98004; **Phone:** 425-688-8828; **Board Cert:** Plastic Surgery 1991; **Med School:** Univ Mich Med Sch 1981; **Resid:** Surgery, Tufts-New England Med Ctr 1986; Plastic Surgery, Emory Univ Hosp 1989; **Fellow:** Craniofacial Surgery, Univ Miami Hosp 1989; **Fac Appt:** Assoc Prof S, Univ Wash

Reinisch, John F MD [PIS] - **Spec Exp:** Birthmarks/Hemangiomas; Ear Reconstruction/Microtia; Pediatric Plastic Surgery; **Hospital:** Cedars-Sinai Med Ctr; **Address:** 250 N Robertson Blvd, Ste 506, Beverly Hills, CA 90211; **Phone:** 310-385-6090; **Board Cert:** Plastic Surgery 1980; **Med School:** Harvard Med Sch 1970; **Resid:** Surgery, Univ Mich Med Ctr 1975; Plastic Surgery, Univ Virginia Hosp 1978; **Fac Appt:** Prof S, USC Sch Med

Ristow, Brunno MD [PIS] - **Spec Exp:** Cosmetic Surgery-Face; Facial Plastic & Reconstructive Surgery; Rhinoplasty; Nasal Reconstruction; **Hospital:** CA Pacific Med Ctr-Pacific Campus; **Address:** 2100 Webster St, Ste 501, San Francisco, CA 94115-2381; **Phone:** 415-202-1507; **Board Cert:** Plastic Surgery 1975; **Med School:** Brazil 1966; **Resid:** Surgery, New York Hosp 1971; Plastic Surgery, NYU Med Ctr 1973; **Fellow:** Plastic Surgery, NYU Med Ctr 1968

Romano, James John MD [PIS] - **Spec Exp:** Body Contouring; Cosmetic Surgery-Breast; Tuberous Breasts; Facial Rejuvenation; **Hospital:** CA Pacific Med Ctr - CA Campus, Seton Med Ctr; **Address:** 1650 Jackson St, Ste 101, San Francisco, CA 94109; **Phone:** 415-981-3911; **Board Cert:** Plastic Surgery 1990; **Med School:** Eastern VA Med Sch 1980; **Resid:** Surgery, Georgetown Univ Hosp 1985; Plastic Surgery, Johns Hopkins Hosp 1988; **Fac Appt:** Asst Prof PIS, USC Sch Med

Rosenberg, Howard L MD [PIS] - **Spec Exp:** Cosmetic Surgery-Face; Cosmetic Surgery-Breast; Liposuction & Body Contouring; Facial Rejuvenation; **Hospital:** El Camino Hosp; **Address:** 2204 Grant Rd, Ste 201, Mountain View, CA 94040; **Phone:** 650-961-2652; **Board Cert:** Surgery 1975; Plastic Surgery 1977; **Med School:** Johns Hopkins Univ 1969; **Resid:** Surgery, UCLA Med Ctr 1974; Plastic Surgery, Stanford Univ Med Ctr 1976; **Fac Appt:** Asst Clin Prof PIS, Stanford Univ

Sanders, George H MD [PIS] - **Spec Exp:** Eyelid Surgery; Liposuction; **Address:** 16633 Ventura Blvd, Ste 110, Encino, CA 91436-1834; **Phone:** 818-981-3333; **Board Cert:** Plastic Surgery 1986; **Med School:** Harvard Med Sch 1978; **Resid:** Surgery, UCLA Med Ctr 1980; Surgery, Cedars-Sinai Hosp 1983; **Fellow:** Plastic Surgery, UCLA Med Ctr 1985

Sherman, Randolph MD [PIS] - **Spec Exp:** Facial Paralysis; Breast Reconstruction; Limb Surgery/Reconstruction; **Hospital:** Cedars-Sinai Med Ctr; **Address:** 8635 W 3rd St, Ste 777-W, Los Angeles, CA 90048; **Phone:** 310-423-2129; **Board Cert:** Surgery 2004; Plastic Surgery 1986; Hand Surgery 2000; **Med School:** Univ MO-Columbia Sch Med 1977; **Resid:** Surgery, UCSF Hosps 1981; Surgery, State Univ of New York 1983; **Fellow:** Plastic Surgery, USC Med Ctr 1985; **Fac Appt:** Prof S, USC Sch Med

Singer, Robert MD [PlS] - **Spec Exp:** Cosmetic Surgery-Face; Cosmetic Surgery-Breast; Liposuction & Body Contouring; **Hospital:** Scripps Meml Hosp - La Jolla; **Address:** 9834 Genesee Ave, Ste 100, La Jolla, CA 92037-1214; **Phone:** 858-455-0290; **Board Cert:** Plastic Surgery 1977; **Med School:** SUNY Buffalo 1967; **Resid:** Surgery, Stanford Univ Med Ctr 1969; Plastic Surgery, Vanderbilt Univ Hosp 1976; **Fellow:** Neurological Surgery, Rigs Hosp-Kommunes Hosp 1976

Stevens, W Grant MD [PlS] - **Spec Exp:** Cosmetic Surgery-Breast; Liposuction & Body Contouring; Cosmetic Surgery-Face; **Hospital:** St. John's Hlth Ctr, Santa Monica, Marina Del Rey Hosp; **Address:** 4644 Lincoln Blvd, Ste 552, Marina Del Rey, CA 90292-6391; **Phone:** 310-827-2653; **Board Cert:** Plastic Surgery 1989; **Med School:** Washington Univ, St Louis 1980; **Resid:** Surgery, Harbor/UCLA Med Ctr 1983; **Fellow:** Hand Surgery, Washington Univ Sch Med 1984; Plastic Surgery, Washington Univ Sch Med 1986; **Fac Appt:** Assoc Clin Prof PlS, USC Sch Med

Urata, Mark M MD/DDS [PlS] - **Spec Exp:** Craniofacial Surgery-Pediatric; Maxillofacial Surgery; Cosmetic Surgery-Head & Neck; **Hospital:** Chldns Hosp - Los Angeles, Keck Med Ctr of USC (page 62); **Address:** Chldns Hosp LA, Dept Plastic Surgery, 4650 W Sunset Blvd, MS 96, Los Angeles, CA 90027; **Phone:** 323-361-2154; **Board Cert:** Plastic Surgery 2005; **Med School:** USC Sch Med 1996; **Resid:** Oral & Maxillofacial Surgery, USC Med Ctr 1993; Plastic Surgery, USC Med Ctr 2002; **Fellow:** Craniofacial Surgery, UCLA Med Ctr 2003; **Fac Appt:** Prof PlS, USC-Keck School of Medicine

Wells, James H MD [PlS] - **Spec Exp:** Cleft Palate/Lip; Breast Surgery; **Hospital:** Long Beach Meml Med Ctr; **Address:** 2880 Atlantic Ave, Ste 290, Long Beach, CA 90806; **Phone:** 562-595-6543; **Board Cert:** Plastic Surgery 2009; **Med School:** Univ Tex Med Br, Galveston 1966; **Resid:** Surgery, Ochsner Fdn Hosp 1971; Plastic Surgery, Univ Virginia Hosp 1975

Plastic Surgery

Cleveland Clinic's Department of Plastic Surgery, part of the Cleveland Clinic Dermatology & Plastic Surgery Institute, offers a full array of subspecialized care for adult and pediatric patients. The department includes a team of surgeons extremely adept at handling all types of traumatic, congenital and work-related hand, peripheral nerve and upper extremity problems. Pediatric surgery and craniofacial surgery are strong specialties in the department. Among the department's major advancements is the successful completion of the first near-total face transplant in the United States. This achievement has progressed into our Reconstructive Transplant Center which provides an alternative for patients seeking new avenues in reconstruction of difficult facial, abdominal, laryngeal and hand deformities and dysfunction.

Cleveland Clinic plastic surgeons offer numerous methods of breast reconstruction that can be performed either at the time of mastectomy or as a secondary procedure. These techniques include breast implants and expanders; pedicled transverse rectus abdominis myocutaneous flaps (using abdominal skin and muscle); and free-tissue transfers such as deep inferior epigastric perforator (or DIEP) flap.

The Department of Plastic Surgery focuses on minimally invasive techniques in facial cosmetic surgery. This includes alternatives to face lift and neck lift surgery, short-scar face lifts and minimally invasive face lift techniques. In addition to standard body contouring procedures including abdominoplasty and a wide variety of liposuction techniques, the department is particularly interested in plastic surgery after significant weight loss.

THE NEW YORK EYE AND EAR INFIRMARY

310 East 14th Street
New York, New York 10003
Tel. 212.979.4000 Fax. 212.228.0664
http://www.nyee.edu

PROVIDING EXCEPTIONAL CARE

The Department of Plastic & Reconstructive Surgery is one of the region's most comprehensive centers for surgery which restores the body and spirit. More than 1,500 procedures a year are performed here, and 50 of the most noted board-certified plastic surgeons located throughout New York City and tri-state area comprise the attending medical staff.

IN A HIGHLY SPECIALIZED SETTING

As a specialty hospital, the Infirmary is uniquely qualified to handle the most complicated cases. It serves as a nationwide referral center with a commitment to teaching, research, and high-technology based patient care. Highly experienced staff using state-of-the-art instrumentation have made the Infirmary's 17 operating rooms a national benchmark in efficiency. In addition, private premium patient accommodations are available to assure that the hospital experience is as comfortable and convenient as possible.

FOR PATIENTS OF ALL AGES

The Department treats more than 1,500 patients a year who seek reconstructive surgery of the body as well as facial area as a result of accident, birth defect or cancer, and those who elect cosmetic surgery. It is one of the few hospitals in the region to perform breast reconstruction after mastectomy with microvascular surgery to harvest tissue from patients' lower body to create living, natural, and normal looking breasts, often preferred to artificial implants. State-of-the-art lymph node transfer to cure post-mastectomy lymphedema is also available.

Childhood problems, such as cleft lip and palate and ear deformities also fall under the care of our surgeons.

Innovative cosmetic surgery procedures such as endoscopic and other minimally invasive operations are offered. The Center for Nasal Plastic specializes in closed (no scar) nasal plastic techniques as well as repair of previous nasal surgeries, the secondary nasal plasty. Liposuction using the latest instrumentation and fat grafting by the latest technology is also available as are the latest variants of the abdominoplasty (tummy tuck) operation.

The latest version of a skin tightening Fraxel Re:pair laser enables many patients to avoid a surgical face and eyelid plastic operation.

The hospital has a Post Graduate Cosmetic Surgery Program which offers a year of intensive cosmetic surgery training to surgeons who have completed a formal plastic surgery residency. The program is the largest and most sought-after in the US and also provides a source for affordable cosmetic surgery for the community.

Plastic Surgery Clinical Services

Facial plasty

Eyelid plastic operations

Nasal plastic operations

Breast augmentation
Breast reduction procedures and suspension

Breast reconstruction using patient's own tissue (DIEP, S-GAP, I-GAP and SIEA flap procedures)

Liposuction

Abdominoplasty

Facial resurfacing and dermabrasion

Fraxel laser

Botox

About The New York Eye and Ear Infirmary

Founded in 1820, it is the nation's oldest, continuously operating specialty hospital. Throughout its history, the Infirmary has led clinical advances and research in vision, hearing, speech and restoration of the physical appearance.

**Physician Referral
1.800.449.HOPE (4673)**

The Best in American Medicine
www.CastleConnolly.com

Preventive & Occupational Medicine

A preventive medicine specialist focuses on the health of individuals and defined populations in order to protect, promote and maintain health and well-being, and to prevent disease, disability and premature death. A preventive medicine physician may be a specialist in general preventive medicine, public health, occupational medicine, or aerospace medicine. This specialist works with large population groups as well as with individual patients to promote health and understand the risks of disease, injury, disability, and death, seeking to modify and eliminate these risks.

Training Required: Three years

OCCUPATIONAL MEDICINE

Mid Atlantic

Gochfeld, Michael MD/PhD [OM] - **Spec Exp:** Environmental Medicine; Mercury Toxic Exposure; Chemical Exposure; **Hospital:** Robert Wood Johnson Univ Hosp - New Brunswick; **Address:** Enviro & Occupational Health-EOHSI, 170 Frelinghuysen Rd, Ste 200, Piscataway, NJ 08854; **Phone:** 848-445-0123; **Board Cert:** Occupational Medicine 1983; **Med School:** Albert Einstein Coll Med 1965; **Resid:** Behavioral Medicine, Rockefeller Univ 1977; **Fac Appt:** Prof OM, UMDNJ-RW Johnson Med Sch

Kipen, Howard M MD [OM] - **Spec Exp:** Environmental Medicine; Occupational Lung Disease; **Hospital:** Robert Wood Johnson Univ Hosp - New Brunswick; **Address:** UMDNJ-RWJ Med Sch, EOHSI, 170 Frelinghuysen Rd, Ste 200, Piscataway, NJ 08854; **Phone:** 848-445-0123; **Board Cert:** Internal Medicine 1982; Occupational Medicine 1986; **Med School:** UCSF 1979; **Resid:** Internal Medicine, Columbia Presby Med Ctr 1982; Occupational Medicine, Mt Sinai Hosp 1984; **Fac Appt:** Prof Med, UMDNJ-RW Johnson Med Sch

Landrigan, Philip MD [OM] - **Spec Exp:** Environmental Health in Children; **Hospital:** Mount Sinai Med Ctr (page 64); **Address:** Dept Preventive Med, One Gustave L Levy Pl, Box 1057, New York, NY 10029-6500; **Phone:** 212-824-7018; **Board Cert:** Pediatrics 1973; Public Health & Genl Preventive Med 1979; Occupational Medicine 1983; **Med School:** Harvard Med Sch 1967; **Resid:** Internal Medicine, Metro Genl Hosp 1968; Pediatrics, Chldns Hosp 1970; **Fellow:** Epidemiology, Ctrs for Disease Control 1973; Occupational Medicine, Univ London 1977; **Fac Appt:** Prof Ped, Mount Sinai Sch Med

Southwest

Harber, Philip I MD [OM] - **Spec Exp:** Occupational Lung Disease; Occupational Asthma; Beryllium-induced Lung Disease; Asbestos-related Lung Disease; **Address:** College of Public Health, Univ Arizona, Community, Environment & Policy Div, 1656 E Mabel St, MRB rm 112, Tucson, AZ 85724; **Phone:** 310-433-5342; **Board Cert:** Internal Medicine 1979; Pulmonary Disease 1980; Occupational Medicine 1982; **Med School:** Univ Pennsylvania 1972; **Resid:** Internal Medicine, Georgetown Univ Med Ctr 1978; Occupational Medicine, Johns Hopkins Hosp 1980; **Fellow:** Pulmonary Disease, Johns Hopkins Hosp 1980; **Fac Appt:** Prof PrM, Univ Ariz Coll Med

PREVENTIVE MEDICINE

Mid Atlantic

Cahill, John MD [PrM] - **Spec Exp:** Tropical Diseases; Travel Medicine; Parasitic Infections; International Health; **Hospital:** St. Luke's - Roosevelt Hosp Ctr - Roosevelt Div (page 56); **Address:** 425 W 59th St, Ste 8A, New York, NY 10019; **Phone:** 212-492-5500; **Board Cert:** Emergency Medicine 2011; **Med School:** Mount Sinai Sch Med 1996; **Resid:** Emergency Medicine, Rhode Island Hosp 1997; Emergency Medicine, Rhode Island Hosp 2000; **Fellow:** Tropical Medicine, Royal Coll Surgeons 1998; **Fac Appt:** Asst Clin Prof Med, Columbia P&S

Cahill, Kevin M MD [PrM] - **Spec Exp:** Tropical Diseases; International Health; Parasitic Infections; Tropical Diseases; **Hospital:** Lenox Hill Hosp (page 67); **Address:** 850 5th Ave, New York, NY 10065; **Phone:** 212-434-2477; **Board Cert:** Public Health & Genl Preventive Med 1970; **Med School:** Cornell Univ-Weill Med Coll 1961; **Resid:** Internal Medicine, US Navy Med Res Unit 1965; Public Health & Genl Preventive Med, US Navy Med Res Unit 1965; **Fac Appt:** Clin Prof Med, NYU Sch Med

Hoffman, Robert S MD [PrM] - **Spec Exp:** Poison Control; Disaster Preparedness; **Hospital:** NYU Langone Med Ctr (page 68), Bellevue Hosp Ctr; **Address:** NY Poison Control Ctr, 455 1st Ave, rm 123, New York, NY 10016; **Phone:** 212-340-4494; **Board Cert:** Internal Medicine 1987; Emergency Medicine 2005; Medical Toxicology 2008; **Med School:** NYU Sch Med 1984; **Resid:** Internal Medicine, NYU Med Ctr 1987; **Fellow:** Medical Toxicology, NYU Med Ctr 1989; **Fac Appt:** Assoc Prof Med, NYU Sch Med

Pearson, Thomas A MD/PhD [PrM] - **Spec Exp:** Preventive Cardiology; Cholesterol/Lipid Disorders; **Hospital:** Univ of Rochester Strong Meml Hosp; **Address:** Dept Community & Preventive Medicine, 2400 S Clinton Ave G Bldg, Rochester, NY 14618; **Phone:** 585-341-7759; **Board Cert:** Internal Medicine 1983; Public Health & Genl Preventive Med 1986; **Med School:** Johns Hopkins Univ 1976; **Resid:** Preventive Medicine, Johns Hopkins Hosp 1979; Internal Medicine, Johns Hopkins Hosp 1980; **Fellow:** Cardiovascular Disease, Johns Hopkins Hosp 1983; **Fac Appt:** Prof PrM, Univ Rochester

THE JOAN H. TISCH CENTER FOR WOMEN'S HEALTH

About the Joan H. Tisch Center for Women's Health

Because many diseases and conditions impact women differently than men, NYU Langone Medical Center has created the Joan H. Tisch Center for Women's Health. Offering a comprehensive array of primary and specialty care, the Joan H. Tisch Center for Women's Health is New York City's premier destination for healthcare services tailored to the special needs of women. Conveniently located in the heart of Manhattan's Upper East Side, the Center combines NYU Langone's tradition of excellence with a multidisciplinary approach to providing individuals with the best possible medical care. At the Joan H. Tisch Center for Women's Health, the goal is maintaining excellent health and the vehicle is a caring, nurturing environment which understands that women are more than a collection of symptoms and medical conditions.

Expert Staff

Primary and specialty care physicians at the Joan H. Tisch Center for Women's Health have been carefully chosen for their ability to render quality, compassionate care to women. These healthcare professionals are focused on the holistic needs of patients in a state-of-the-art setting that relies heavily on teamwork. As part of a major academic medical institution, the Center is able to draw on additional healthcare resources and innovative research, when the need arises.

Comprehensive Range of Services

The Joan H. Tisch Center for Women's Health offers a wide range of primary and specialty medical care geared to women at a single location. Specialty services include breast health, cardiology, dermatology, endocrinology, ear/nose/throat, gastroenterology, gynecology, internal medicine, mental health, neurology, orthopaedics, plastic surgery, podiatry, pulmonary medicine, rehabilitation medicine, rheumatology, urology, vascular and women's imaging.

Technology Edge

The Joan H. Tisch Center for Women's Health has incorporated sophisticated technology into all levels of the patient experience. This ranges from the Center's informative website to its use of Epic, the Medical Center's up-to-the-minute electronic medical records system. In addition, patients can confidentially view their medical records and test results, as well as make appointment, request prescriptions and communicate with their physicians, through myNYULMC, a secure online service.

Joan H. Tisch Center for Women's Health
207 East 84th Street *(at 3rd Avenue)*
New York, NY

www.NYULMC.org

646-754-3300

Physician Referral: **888-7-NYU-MED** *(888-769-8633)*

THE JOAN H. TISCH CENTER FOR WOMEN'S HEALTH

About the Joan H. Tisch Center for Women's Health

Because many diseases and conditions impact women differently than men, NYU Langone Medical Center has created the Joan H. Tisch Center for Women's Health. Offering a comprehensive array of primary and specialty care, the Joan H. Tisch Center for Women's Health is New York City's premier destination for healthcare services tailored to the special needs of women. Conveniently located in the heart of Manhattan's Upper East Side, the Center combines NYU Langone's tradition of excellence with a multidisciplinary approach to providing individuals with the best possible medical care. At the Joan H. Tisch Center for Women's Health, the goal is maintaining excellent health and the vehicle is a caring, nurturing environment which understands that women are more than a collection of symptoms and medical conditions.

Expert Staff

Primary and specialty care physicians at the Joan H. Tisch Center for Women's Health have been carefully chosen for their ability to render quality, compassionate care to women. These healthcare professionals are focused on the holistic needs of patients in a state-of-the-art setting that relies heavily on teamwork. As part of a major academic medical institution, the Center is able to draw on additional healthcare resources and innovative research, when the need arises.

Comprehensive Range of Services

The Joan H. Tisch Center for Women's Health offers a wide range of primary and specialty medical care geared to women at a single location. Specialty services include breast health, cardiology, dermatology, endocrinology, ear/nose/throat, gastroenterology, gynecology, internal medicine, mental health, neurology, orthopaedics, plastic surgery, podiatry, pulmonary medicine, rehabilitation medicine, rheumatology, urology, vascular and women's imaging.

Technology Edge

The Joan H. Tisch Center for Women's Health has incorporated sophisticated technology into all levels of the patient experience. This ranges from the Center's informative website to its use of Epic, the Medical Center's up-to-the-minute electronic medical records system. In addition, patients can confidentially view their medical records and test results, as well as make appointment, request prescriptions and communicate with their physicians, through myNYULMC, a secure online service.

The Best in American Medicine
www.CastleConnolly.com

Psychiatry

A psychiatrist specializes in the prevention, diagnosis and treatment of mental, addictive and emotional disorders such as schizophrenia and other psychotic disorders, mood disorders, anxiety disorders, substance-related disorders, sexual and gender identity disorders and adjustment disorders. The psychiatrist is able to understand the biologic, psychologic and social components of illness, and therefore is uniquely prepared to treat the whole person. A psychiatrist is qualified to order diagnostic laboratory tests and to prescribe medications, evaluate and treat psychologic and interpersonal problems and to intervene with families who are coping with stress, crises and other problems in living.

Training Required: Four years

Certification in one of the following subspecialties requires additional training and examination.

Addiction Psychiatry: A psychiatrist who focuses on the evaluation and treatment of individuals with alcohol, drug, or other substance-related disorders and of individuals with the dual diagnosis of substance-related and other psychiatric disorders.

Child and Adolescent Psychiatry: A psychiatrist with additional training in the diagnosis and treatment of developmental, behavioral, emotional and mental disorders of childhood and adolescence.

Geriatric Psychiatry: A psychiatrist with expertise in the prevention, evaluation, diagnosis and treatment of mental and emotional disorders in the elderly. The geriatric psychiatrist seeks to improve the psychiatric care of the elderly both in health and in disease.

PSYCHIATRY

New England

Adler, David A MD [Psyc] - **Spec Exp:** Depression; Personality Disorders; Schizophrenia; **Hospital:** Tufts Med Ctr; **Address:** Tufts Med Ctr, Dept Psyc, 800 Washington St, Ste 1007, Boston, MA 02111; **Phone:** 617-636-8755; **Board Cert:** Psychiatry 1977; **Med School:** Yale Univ 1973; **Resid:** Psychiatry, Mass Mental Hlth Ctr 1976; **Fac Appt:** Prof Psyc, Tufts Univ

Benes, Francine M MD/PhD [Psyc] - **Spec Exp:** Schizophrenia; Bipolar/Mood Disorders; Neuro-Pathology; **Hospital:** McLean Hosp; **Address:** McLean Hosp, Harvard Brain Tissue Resource Ctr, 115 Mill St, Mailman Rsch Bldg, Belmont, MA 02478-1064; **Phone:** 617-855-2401; **Board Cert:** Psychiatry 1987; **Med School:** Yale Univ 1978; **Resid:** Psychiatry, McLean Hosp 1982; **Fac Appt:** Prof Psyc, Harvard Med Sch

Ellison, James M MD [Psyc] - **Spec Exp:** Geriatric Psychiatry; **Hospital:** McLean Hosp; **Address:** McLean Hospital, 115 Mill St, Belmont, MA 02478; **Phone:** 617-855-2532; **Board Cert:** Psychiatry 1984; Geriatric Psychiatry 2007; **Med School:** UCSF 1978; **Resid:** Psychiatry, Mass Genl Hosp 1982; **Fac Appt:** Assoc Prof Psyc, Harvard Med Sch

Friedman, Matthew J MD/PhD [Psyc] - **Spec Exp:** Post Traumatic Stress Disorder; Psychopharmacology; Anxiety & Mood Disorders; **Hospital:** White River Junction VA Med Ctr, Dartmouth - Hitchcock Med Ctr; **Address:** National Ctr for PTSD, VA Med Ctr, 215 N Main St, White River Junction, VT 05009; **Phone:** 802-296-5132; **Board Cert:** Psychiatry 1976; **Med School:** Univ KY Coll Med 1976; **Resid:** Psychiatry, Mass Genl Hosp 1972; Psychiatry, Dartmouth Hitchcock Med Ctr 1973; **Fac Appt:** Prof Psyc, Dartmouth Med Sch

Greenberg, Benjamin D MD/PhD [Psyc] - **Spec Exp:** Obsessive-Compulsive Disorder; **Hospital:** Butler Hosp; **Address:** 345 Blackstone Blvd, Providence, RI 02906; **Phone:** 401-455-6602; **Board Cert:** Psychiatry 1994; **Med School:** Univ Miami Sch Med 1987; **Resid:** Neurology, Columbian Univ/Presbyterian Hosp 1989; Psychiatry, Johns Hopkins Hosp 1992; **Fac Appt:** Psyc, Johns Hopkins Univ

Greenberg, Donna B MD [Psyc] - **Spec Exp:** Psychiatry in Cancer; **Hospital:** Mass Genl Hosp; **Address:** Mass Genl Hosp, Psychiatry Assocs, 55 Fruit St Warren Bldg Fl 6, Boston, MA 02114-2696; **Phone:** 617-726-2984; **Board Cert:** Internal Medicine 1978; Psychiatry 1990; **Med School:** Univ Rochester 1975; **Resid:** Internal Medicine, Boston City Hosp 1978; Psychiatry, Mass Genl Hosp 1989; **Fellow:** Psychiatry, Mass Genl Hosp 1979; **Fac Appt:** Assoc Prof Psyc, Harvard Med Sch

Greenberg, William E MD [Psyc] - **Hospital:** Beth Israel Deaconess Med Ctr - Boston; **Address:** Beth Israel Deaconess Med Ctr, Dept Psychiatry, 330 Brookline Ave, Boston, MA 02215-5400; **Phone:** 617-667-4766; **Board Cert:** Psychiatry 1981; **Med School:** Univ Pennsylvania 1976; **Resid:** Psychiatry, Beth Israel Deaconess Med Ctr 1981; **Fac Appt:** Asst Prof Psyc, Harvard Med Sch

Gunderson, John G MD [Psyc] - **Spec Exp:** Personality Disorders; Personality Disorders-Borderline; Psychotherapy; **Hospital:** McLean Hosp; **Address:** McLean Hospital, 115 Mill St, Belmont, MA 02478; **Phone:** 617-855-2293; **Board Cert:** Psychiatry 1974; **Med School:** Harvard Med Sch 1967; **Resid:** Psychiatry, Mass Mental Hlth Ctr 1971; **Fac Appt:** Prof Psyc, Harvard Med Sch

Jenike, Michael A MD [Psyc] - **Spec Exp:** Obsessive-Compulsive Disorder; Geriatric Psychiatry; **Hospital:** Mass Genl Hosp; **Address:** Obsessive Compulsive Disorders Unit, 185 Cambridge St, Ste 2000, Boston, MA 02114; **Phone:** 617-726-6766; **Board Cert:** Psychiatry 1984; **Med School:** Univ Okla Coll Med 1978; **Resid:** Psychiatry, Mass Genl Hosp 1982; **Fellow:** Psychiatry, Harvard Med Sch; Psychiatry, Mass Genl Hosp; **Fac Appt:** Prof Psyc, Harvard Med Sch

Jimerson, David C MD [Psyc] - **Spec Exp:** Eating Disorders; **Hospital:** Beth Israel Deaconess Med Ctr - Boston; **Address:** Beth Israel Deaconess Med Ctr, Dept Psyc, 330 Brookline Ave, Boston, MA 02215-5400; **Phone:** 617-667-4667; **Board Cert:** Psychiatry 1977; **Med School:** Cornell Univ-Weill Med Coll 1972; **Resid:** Psychiatry, UC-San Diego 1974; Psychiatry, NIMH 1975; **Fac Appt:** Prof Psyc, Harvard Med Sch

McGlashan, Thomas H MD [Psyc] - **Spec Exp:** Schizophrenia-Early Detection/Treatment; Personality Disorders; Schizophrenia-Clinical Trials; Personality Disorders-Clinical Trials; **Hospital:** Connecticut Mental Hlth Ctr, Yale-New Haven Hosp; **Address:** Univ CT Hlth Ctr, 263 Farmington Ave, Farmington, CT 06030; **Phone:** 203-974-7346; **Board Cert:** Psychiatry 1973; **Med School:** Univ Pennsylvania 1967; **Resid:** Psychiatry, Mass Mental Hlth Ctr 1971; **Fac Appt:** Prof Psyc, Yale Univ

Phillips, Katharine A MD [Psyc] - **Spec Exp:** Body Dysmorphic Disorder (BDD); Obsessive-Compulsive Disorder; **Hospital:** Rhode Island Hosp; **Address:** BDD Program, Coro Center West, 1 Hoppin St, Ste 2.030, Providence, RI 02903; **Phone:** 401-444-1646; **Board Cert:** Psychiatry 1992; **Med School:** Dartmouth Med Sch 1987; **Resid:** Psychiatry, McLean Hosp 1991; **Fellow:** Research, McLean Hosp 1994; **Fac Appt:** Prof Psyc, Brown Univ

Price, Lawrence H MD [Psyc] - **Spec Exp:** Anxiety & Mood Disorders; Depression; Bipolar/Mood Disorders; Obsessive-Compulsive Disorder; **Hospital:** Butler Hosp, Kent Hosp; **Address:** Butler Hospital, Dept Psychiatry, 345 Blackstone Blvd, Providence, RI 02906; **Phone:** 401-455-6533; **Board Cert:** Psychiatry 1983; **Med School:** Univ Mich Med Sch 1978; **Resid:** Psychiatry, Yale-New Haven Hosp 1982; **Fellow:** Psychiatry, Yale-New Haven Hosp 1983; **Fac Appt:** Prof Psyc, Brown Univ

Rasmussen, Steven A MD [Psyc] - **Spec Exp:** Obsessive-Compulsive Disorder; **Hospital:** Butler Hosp; **Address:** Butler Hosp, 345 Blackstone Blvd, Providence, RI 02906; **Phone:** 401-455-6209; **Board Cert:** Psychiatry 1983; **Med School:** Brown Univ 1977; **Resid:** Psychiatry, Yale Univ 1981; **Fac Appt:** Assoc Prof Psyc, Brown Univ

Rauch, Paula K MD [Psyc] - **Spec Exp:** Parent Guidance in Parental Cancer; Psychiatry in Physical Illness; **Hospital:** Mass Genl Hosp; **Address:** Mass General Hosp, Dept Child Psychiatry, 55 Fruit St, Yawkey 6A, Boston, MA 02114; **Phone:** 617-724-3923; **Board Cert:** Psychiatry 1990; Child & Adolescent Psychiatry 1991; **Med School:** Univ Cincinnati 1981; **Resid:** Psychiatry, Mass Genl Hosp 1984; **Fellow:** Child Psychiatry, Cambridge Hosp 1986; **Fac Appt:** Assoc Prof Psyc, Harvard Med Sch

Salzman, Carl MD [Psyc] - **Spec Exp:** Psychopharmacology; Psychotherapy; **Hospital:** MA Mental Hlth Ctr, Beth Israel Deaconess Med Ctr - Boston; **Address:** 1330 Beacon St, Brookline, MA 02446; **Phone:** 617-754-1264; **Board Cert:** Psychiatry 1970; **Med School:** SUNY Upstate Med Univ 1963; **Resid:** Psychiatry, Mass Mental Hlth Ctr 1967; Psychiatry, Natl Inst Mental Hlth 1969; **Fac Appt:** Prof Psyc, Harvard Med Sch

Shapiro, Edward R MD [Psyc] - **Spec Exp:** Psychoanalysis; **Hospital:** Austen Riggs Ctr; **Address:** Austen Riggs Ctr, 25 Main St, PO Box 962, Stockbridge, MA 01262; **Phone:** 413-298-5511; **Board Cert:** Psychiatry 1974; **Med School:** Harvard Med Sch 1968; **Resid:** Psychiatry, Mass Mental Hlth Ctr 1972; **Fellow:** Psychiatry, Natl Inst Mental Hlth 1974; **Fac Appt:** Assoc Clin Prof Psyc, Harvard Med Sch

Psychiatry

Summergrad, Paul MD [Psyc] - **Hospital:** Tufts Med Ctr; **Address:** Tufts Med Ctr, 800 Washington St, Ste 1007, Boston, MA 02111; **Phone:** 617-636-5773; **Board Cert:** Internal Medicine 1981; Psychiatry 1986; Geriatric Psychiatry 2007; Psychosomatic Medicine 2005; **Med School:** SUNY Buffalo 1978; **Resid:** Internal Medicine, Boston City Hosp 1981; **Fellow:** Psychiatry, Mass Genl Hosp 1985; **Fac Appt:** Prof Psyc, Tufts Univ

Vanderkolk, Bessel MD [Psyc] - **Spec Exp:** Post Traumatic Stress Disorder; Child Abuse; **Hospital:** Boston Med Ctr; **Address:** 16 Braddock Park, Boston, MA 02116-5804; **Phone:** 617-247-1720; **Board Cert:** Psychiatry 1976; **Med School:** Univ Chicago-Pritzker Sch Med 1970; **Resid:** Psychiatry, Harvard Med Sch 1974; **Fac Appt:** Prof Psyc, Boston Univ

Mid Atlantic

Akhtar, Salman MD [Psyc] - **Spec Exp:** Psychoanalysis; **Hospital:** Thomas Jefferson Univ Hosp; **Address:** Jefferson Med College, Dept Psychiatry, 833 Chestnut St, Ste 210, Philadelphia, PA 19107; **Phone:** 215-955-2547; **Board Cert:** Psychiatry 1977; **Med School:** India 1968; **Resid:** Psychiatry, UMDNJ Med Ctr 1974; Psychiatry, Univ Virginia Med Ctr 1976; **Fellow:** Psychoanalysis, Philadelphia Psych Inst 1986; **Fac Appt:** Prof Psyc, Thomas Jefferson Univ

Appelbaum, Paul S MD [Psyc] - **Spec Exp:** Forensic Psychiatry; Depression; Anxiety & Mood Disorders; **Hospital:** NY-Presby/Columbia Univ Med Ctr, NY (page 66); **Address:** NY State Psychiatric Inst, 1051 Riverside Drive, rm 6714, Box 122, New York, NY 10032; **Phone:** 212-543-4184; **Board Cert:** Psychiatry 1981; Forensic Psychiatry 2004; **Med School:** Harvard Med Sch 1976; **Resid:** Psychiatry, Mass Mental Health Ctr 1980; **Fac Appt:** Prof Psyc, Columbia P&S

Arnold, Steven E MD [Psyc] - **Spec Exp:** Alzheimer's Disease; Memory Disorders; Dementia; Cognitive Impairment-Mild; **Hospital:** Hosp Univ Penn - UPHS (page 72); **Address:** Ralston House, 3615 Chestnut St, Philadelphia, PA 19104; **Phone:** 215-662-7810; **Board Cert:** Psychiatry 1988; Neurology 1991; **Med School:** Boston Univ 1983; **Resid:** Psychiatry, NYS Psychiatric Inst 1987; Neurology, Univ IA Hosps & Clins 1990; **Fellow:** Behavioral Neurology, Univ IA Hosps & Clins 1990; **Fac Appt:** Prof Psyc, Univ Pennsylvania

Basch, Samuel MD [Psyc] - **Spec Exp:** Psychopharmacology; Psychiatry in Physical Illness; Psychiatry in Cancer; Psychoanalysis; **Hospital:** Mount Sinai Med Ctr (page 64); **Address:** 10 E 85th St, Ste 1B, New York, NY 10028; **Phone:** 212-427-0344; **Board Cert:** Psychiatry 1970; **Med School:** Hahnemann Univ 1961; **Resid:** Psychiatry, Mount Sinai Hosp 1965; **Fellow:** Psychoanalysis, Columbia Presby Hosp 1976; **Fac Appt:** Prof Psyc, Mount Sinai Sch Med

Boronow, John Joseph MD [Psyc] - **Spec Exp:** Psychotic Disorders; Schizophrenia; **Hospital:** Sheppard Pratt Hlth Sys; **Address:** 6501 N Charles St, rm TJ-113, Towson, MD 21284; **Phone:** 410-938-4306; **Board Cert:** Psychiatry 1983; **Med School:** Yale Univ 1977; **Resid:** Psychiatry, New York Hosp 1981; **Fellow:** Psychopharmacology, Natl Inst Mntl Hlth 1983; **Fac Appt:** Assoc Clin Prof Psyc, Univ MD Sch Med

Brandt, Harry A MD [Psyc] - **Spec Exp:** Eating Disorders; **Hospital:** St. Joseph Med Ctr, Sheppard Pratt Hlth Sys; **Address:** Ctr for Eating Disorders, 6535 N Charles St, Ste 300, Towson, MD 21204; **Phone:** 410-938-5252; **Board Cert:** Psychiatry 1989; **Med School:** Univ MD Sch Med 1983; **Resid:** Psychiatry, Univ Maryland Hosp 1986; **Fellow:** Biological Psychiatry, Natl Inst Mental Hlth 1988; **Fac Appt:** Assoc Clin Prof Psyc, Univ MD Sch Med

Breitbart, William MD [Psyc] - **Spec Exp:** Psychiatry in Cancer; AIDS Related Cancers; Pain-Cancer; Palliative Care; **Hospital:** Meml Sloan-Kettering Cancer Ctr; **Address:** 1275 York Ave, New York, NY 10065; **Phone:** 646-888-0100; **Board Cert:** Internal Medicine 1982; Psychiatry 1986; Psychosomatic Medicine 2005; **Med School:** Albert Einstein Coll Med 1978; **Resid:** Internal Medicine, Bronx Muni Hosp Ctr 1982; Psychiatry, Bronx Muni Hosp Ctr 1984; **Fellow:** Psychiatric Oncology, Meml Sloan Kettering Cancer Ctr 1986; **Fac Appt:** Prof Psyc, Cornell Univ-Weill Med Coll

Brodkin, Edward S MD [Psyc] - **Spec Exp:** Autism; Asperger's Syndrome; **Hospital:** Hosp Univ Penn - UPHS (page 72), Pennsylvania Hosp-UPHS (page 72); **Address:** Univ Penn Sch Med, Translational Rsch Lab, 125 S 31st St, rm 2220, Philadelphia, PA 19104-3403; **Phone:** 215-746-0118; **Board Cert:** Psychiatry 2006; **Med School:** Harvard Med Sch 1992; **Resid:** Psychiatry, Yale-New Haven Hosp 1996; **Fellow:** Neurological Science, Yale Univ Sch Med 1998; Genetics, Princeton Univ 2002; **Fac Appt:** Asst Prof Psyc, Univ Pennsylvania

Bronheim, Harold E MD [Psyc] - **Spec Exp:** Psychiatry in Body Image Awareness; Relationship Problems; Psychiatry in Physical Illness; Anxiety & Depression; **Hospital:** Mount Sinai Med Ctr (page 64); **Address:** 1155 Park Ave, New York, NY 10028; **Phone:** 212-996-5777; **Board Cert:** Psychiatry 1985; Internal Medicine 1986; Psychosomatic Medicine 2005; Geriatric Psychiatry 2011; **Med School:** SUNY Downstate 1980; **Resid:** Psychiatry, Mount Sinai Hosp 1984; **Fellow:** Internal Medicine, Beth Israel Hosp 1985; **Fac Appt:** Clin Prof Psyc, Mount Sinai Sch Med

Buysse, Daniel J MD [Psyc] - **Spec Exp:** Sleep Disorders; **Hospital:** UPMC Presby, Pittsburgh; **Address:** 3811 O'Hara St, rm E-1127, Pittsburgh, PA 15213; **Phone:** 412-246-6413; **Board Cert:** Psychiatry 1988; Sleep Medicine 2007; **Med School:** Univ Mich Med Sch 1983; **Resid:** Psychiatry, Western Psych Inst 1987; **Fellow:** Sleep Medicine, Univ of Pittsburgh; **Fac Appt:** Asst Prof Psyc, Univ Pittsburgh

Cohen, Mitchell Joseph MD [Psyc] - **Spec Exp:** Pain-Chronic; Psychiatry in Physical Illness; Anxiety Disorders; **Hospital:** Thomas Jefferson Univ Hosp; **Address:** 833 Chestnut St E, Ste 210B, Philadelphia, PA 19107; **Phone:** 215-955-6592; **Board Cert:** Psychiatry 1989; Pain Medicine 2002; **Med School:** Med Coll PA 1984; **Resid:** Psychiatry, Johns Hopkins Hosp 1988; **Fac Appt:** Assoc Prof Psyc, Thomas Jefferson Univ

DePaulo Jr, J Raymond MD [Psyc] - **Spec Exp:** Bipolar/Mood Disorders; Depression; **Hospital:** Johns Hopkins Hosp (page 61); **Address:** Johns Hopkins Hosp, Dept Psychiatry, 600 N Wolfe St, Meyer 4-113, Baltimore, MD 21287-7413; **Phone:** 410-955-3130; **Board Cert:** Psychiatry 1977; **Med School:** Johns Hopkins Univ 1972; **Resid:** Psychiatry, Johns Hopkins Hosp 1977; **Fac Appt:** Prof Psyc, Johns Hopkins Univ

Doghramji, Karl MD [Psyc] - **Spec Exp:** Sleep Disorders/Apnea; Narcolepsy; Restless Legs Syndrome; **Hospital:** Thomas Jefferson Univ Hosp; **Address:** 211 S Ninth St, Ste 500, Philadelphia, PA 19107; **Phone:** 215-955-6175; **Board Cert:** Psychiatry 1986; Sleep Medicine 1985; **Med School:** Thomas Jefferson Univ 1980; **Resid:** Psychiatry, Thomas Jefferson Univ Hosp 1984; **Fellow:** Sleep Medicine, Montefiore Med Ctr; **Fac Appt:** Prof Psyc, Thomas Jefferson Univ

Eaton Jr, James S MD [Psyc] - **Spec Exp:** Anxiety Disorders; Sexual Identity Issues; Depression; Diagnostic Second Opinions; **Hospital:** Georgetown Univ Hosp; **Address:** 4214 50th St NW, Washington, DC 20016; **Phone:** 202-333-5796; **Board Cert:** Psychiatry 1976; **Med School:** Tulane Univ 1962; **Resid:** Internal Medicine, Tulane Univ Med Ctr 1966; Psychiatry, Tulane Univ Med Ctr 1968; **Fellow:** Psychoanalysis, Tulane Univ Med Ctr 1973; **Fac Appt:** Clin Prof Psyc, Georgetown Univ

Fallon, Brian A MD [Psyc] - **Spec Exp:** Lyme Disease-Neuro Complications; Psychosomatic Disorders; Obsessive-Compulsive Disorder; Psychiatry in Physical Illness; **Hospital:** NY-Presby/Columbia Univ Med Ctr, NY (page 66); **Address:** NYS Psychiatric Institute, 1051 Riverside Drive, Room 3724, Unit/Box 69, New York, NY 10032; **Phone:** 212-543-5487; **Board Cert:** Psychiatry 1991; **Med School:** Columbia P&S 1985; **Resid:** Psychiatry, NYS Psychiatric Inst 1989; **Fellow:** Psychiatric Research, NYS Psychiatric Inst 1992; Psychodynamic Psychotherapy, Columbia Univ Psychoanalytic Inst 1990; **Fac Appt:** Prof Psyc, Columbia P&S

First, Michael B MD [Psyc] - **Spec Exp:** Psychotherapy; Psychopharmacology; Forensic Psychiatry; Sexual Addiction; **Hospital:** NY-Presby/Columbia Univ Med Ctr, NY (page 66); **Address:** NY State Psychiatric Inst, Unit 60, 1051 Riverside Drive, New York, NY 10032; **Phone:** 212-543-5531; **Board Cert:** Psychiatry 1989; **Med School:** Univ Pittsburgh 1983; **Resid:** Psychiatry, NY State Psych Inst 1987; **Fellow:** Psychiatric Research, NY State Psych Inst 1988; **Fac Appt:** Clin Prof Psyc, Columbia P&S

Fyer, Abby J MD [Psyc] - **Spec Exp:** Anxiety Disorders; Panic Disorder; **Hospital:** NY State Psychiatric Inst; **Address:** 1051 Riverside Dr, Box 82, New York, NY 10032; **Phone:** 212-543-5372; **Board Cert:** Psychiatry 1980; **Med School:** NYU Sch Med 1973; **Resid:** Psychiatry, Montefiore Med Ctr 1978; **Fac Appt:** Prof Psyc, Columbia P&S

Goff, Donald C MD [Psyc] - **Spec Exp:** Schizophrenia; Psychopharmacology; **Hospital:** NYU Langone Med Ctr (page 68); **Address:** 1 Park Ave Fl 8 - rm 8-212, New York, NY 10016; **Phone:** 646-754-4843; **Board Cert:** Psychiatry 1986; **Med School:** UCLA 1980; **Resid:** Psychiatry, Mass Genl Hosp 1984; **Fellow:** Psychopharmacology, Tufts-New England Med Ctr 1985; **Fac Appt:** Assoc Clin Prof Psyc, NYU Sch Med

Guarda, Angela S MD [Psyc] - **Spec Exp:** Eating Disorders; **Hospital:** Johns Hopkins Hosp (page 61); **Address:** Johns Hopkins Hosp, Eating Disorder Program, 600 N Wolfe St Meyer Bldg - Ste 101, Baltimore, MD 21287; **Phone:** 410-614-4624; **Board Cert:** Psychiatry 2006; **Med School:** Univ MD Sch Med 1991; **Resid:** Psychiatry, Johns Hopkins Hosp 1995; **Fac Appt:** Assoc Prof Psyc, Johns Hopkins Univ

Hollander, Eric MD [Psyc] - **Spec Exp:** Obsessive-Compulsive Disorder; Anxiety Disorders; Autism; Body Dysmorphic Disorder (BDD); **Hospital:** Montefiore Med Ctr-Moses Campus, NY, Lenox Hill Hosp (page 67); **Address:** 901 Fifth Ave, New York, NY 10021; **Phone:** 212-873-4051; **Board Cert:** Psychiatry 1987; **Med School:** SUNY Hlth Sci Ctr 1982; **Resid:** Internal Medicine, Mount Sinai Hosp 1983; Psychiatry, Mount Sinai Hosp 1986; **Fellow:** Psychiatry, Columbia-Presby Med Ctr 1988; **Fac Appt:** Prof Psyc, Albert Einstein Coll Med

Karasu, T Byram MD [Psyc] - **Spec Exp:** Depression; Personality Disorders; Psychotherapy; **Hospital:** Montefiore Med Ctr-Moses Campus, NY; **Address:** 2 E 88th St, New York, NY 10128-0555; **Phone:** 212-426-5208; **Board Cert:** Psychiatry 1972; **Med School:** Turkey 1959; **Resid:** Psychiatry, Yale-New Haven Hosp 1969; **Fac Appt:** Prof Psyc, Albert Einstein Coll Med

Kavey, Neil B MD [Psyc] - **Spec Exp:** Sleep Medicine; Narcolepsy; Sleep Disorders/Apnea; **Hospital:** NY-Presby/Columbia Univ Med Ctr, NY (page 66), Rockefeller Univ; **Address:** The Sleep Disorders Center, Columbia University Medical Center, 161 Fort Washington Ave, Irving Pav Bldg, New York, NY 10032; **Phone:** 212-305-1860; **Board Cert:** Psychiatry 1976; Sleep Medicine 2003; **Med School:** Columbia P&S 1969; **Resid:** Psychiatry, Columbia Presby Med Ctr 1973; **Fac Appt:** Clin Prof Psyc, Columbia P&S

Klagsbrun, Samuel C MD [Psyc] - **Spec Exp:** Psychiatry in Cancer; Psychiatry in Terminal Illness; **Hospital:** Four Winds Hosp; **Address:** 800 Cross River Rd, Katonah, NY 10536; **Phone:** 914-763-8151 x2222; **Board Cert:** Psychiatry 1977; **Med School:** Ros Franklin Univ/Chicago Med Sch 1962; **Resid:** Psychiatry, Yale-New Haven Hosp 1966; **Fac Appt:** Clin Prof Psyc, Albert Einstein Coll Med

Krueger, Richard B MD [Psyc] - **Spec Exp:** Sexual Behavior-Compulsive; **Hospital:** NY-Presby/Columbia Univ Med Ctr, NY (page 66); **Address:** 210 E 68th St, Ste 1H, New York, NY 10021-6047; **Phone:** 212-517-6624; **Board Cert:** Psychiatry 1984; Internal Medicine 1980; Addiction Psychiatry 2007; Forensic Psychiatry 2006; **Med School:** Harvard Med Sch 1977; **Resid:** Internal Medicine, Boston VA Hosp 1980; **Fellow:** Psychiatry, Boston Univ Hosp 1983; **Fac Appt:** Assoc Prof Psyc, Columbia P&S

Kunkel, Elisabeth J MD [Psyc] - **Spec Exp:** Psychiatry in Cancer; Psychiatry in Physical Illness; **Hospital:** Thomas Jefferson Univ Hosp, Methodist Hosp; **Address:** Thomas Jefferson Univ, Dept Psychiatry, 1020 Samson St, Thompson Bldg, Ste 1652, Philadelphia, PA 19107; **Phone:** 215-955-9545; **Board Cert:** Psychiatry 1989; Psychosomatic Medicine 2005; **Med School:** McGill Univ 1983; **Resid:** Psychiatry, NYU Med Ctr 1987; **Fellow:** Liaison Psychiatry, Meml Sloan Kettering Cancer Ctr 1989; Consultation Psychiatry, Meml Sloan Kettering Cancer Ctr 1989; **Fac Appt:** Prof Psyc, Jefferson Med Coll

Kupfer, David J MD [Psyc] - **Spec Exp:** Bipolar/Mood Disorders; **Hospital:** Western Psych Inst & Clin-UPMC; **Address:** Univ of Pittsburgh School of Med, Psychiatry Dept, 3811 O'Hara St, Pittsburgh, PA 15213-2593; **Phone:** 412-246-6777; **Board Cert:** Psychiatry 1978; **Med School:** Yale Univ 1965; **Resid:** Psychiatry, Yale-New Haven Hosp 1970; Psychiatry, Natl Inst Mental Hlth 1969; **Fellow:** Psychiatry, Yale-New Haven Hosp 1967; **Fac Appt:** Prof Psyc, Univ Pittsburgh

Lawson, William B MD/PhD [Psyc] - **Spec Exp:** Bipolar/Mood Disorders; Addiction/Substance Abuse; Dual Diagnosis; **Hospital:** Howard Univ Hosp; **Address:** Dept of Psychiatry, Howard Univ Hlth Sciences, 2041 Georgia Ave NW, Fl 5th, Ste 5B02, Washington, DC 20060; **Phone:** 202-865-6611; **Board Cert:** Psychiatry 1984; Addiction Psychiatry 2006; **Med School:** Univ Chicago-Pritzker Sch Med 1978; **Resid:** Psychiatry, Stanford Univ Med Ctr 1981; Psychiatry, Natl Inst Mental Hlth 1982; **Fellow:** Neuropsychiatry, Natl Inst Mental Hlth 1984; **Fac Appt:** Prof Psyc, Howard Univ

Loewenstein, Richard J. MD [Psyc] - **Spec Exp:** Trauma Psychiatry; Dissociative Disorders; Post Traumatic Stress Disorder; Psychopharmacology; **Hospital:** Sheppard Pratt Hlth Sys; **Address:** 6501 N Charles St, Ste PJ106, Baltimore, MD 21204; **Phone:** 410-938-5075; **Board Cert:** Psychiatry 1980; **Med School:** Yale Univ 1975; **Resid:** Psychiatry, Yale Affil Hosps 1979; **Fellow:** Psychiatry, NIH,NIMH-Biol Psych Br 1982; **Fac Appt:** Assoc Clin Prof Psyc, Univ MD Sch Med

Manevitz, Alan MD [Psyc] - **Spec Exp:** Marital/Family/Sex Therapy; Depression-TMS Therapy; ADD/PTSD; Frbromyalgia Syndrome (FMS); **Hospital:** NY-Presby/Weill Cornell Med Ctr, NY (page 66), Lenox Hill Hosp (page 67); **Address:** 60 Sutton Place South, Ste 1CN, New York, NY 10022; **Phone:** 212-751-5072; **Board Cert:** Psychiatry 1987; **Med School:** Columbia P&S 1980; **Resid:** Psychiatry, NY Hosp 1984; **Fellow:** Psychopharmacology, NY Hosp 1985; **Fac Appt:** Assoc Clin Prof Psyc, Cornell Univ-Weill Med Coll

Mann, J John MD/PhD [Psyc] - **Spec Exp:** Mood Disorders; Clinical Trials; Suicide; **Hospital:** NY-Presby/Columbia Univ Med Ctr, NY (page 66); **Address:** NYS Psychiatric Institute, 1051 Riverside Drive, Box 42, New York, NY 10032; **Phone:** 212-543-5571; **Board Cert:** Psychiatry 1980; **Med School:** Australia 1978; **Resid:** Psychiatry, Royal Melbourne Hosp 1976; **Fac Appt:** Prof Psyc, Columbia P&S

Marin, Deborah B MD [Psyc] - **Spec Exp:** Memory Disorders; Depression; Depression in the Elderly; Geriatric Psychiatry; **Hospital:** Mount Sinai Med Ctr (page 64); **Address:** 1 Gustave Levy Pl, Box 1068, MS 10029, New York, NY 10029; **Phone:** 212-659-8092; **Board Cert:** Psychiatry 1990; **Med School:** Mount Sinai Sch Med 1984; **Resid:** Psychiatry, Mount Sinai Hosp 1988; **Fellow:** Psychiatry, NY Hosp-Cornell Med Ctr 1991; **Fac Appt:** Prof Psyc, Mount Sinai Sch Med

McCann, Merle C MD [Psyc] - **Hospital:** Sheppard Pratt Hlth Sys; **Address:** Sheppard & Enoch Pratt Hosp, 6501 N Charles St,, rm PJ-111, Baltimore, MD 21204; **Phone:** 410-938-3000; **Board Cert:** Psychiatry 1986; **Med School:** Med Coll VA 1981; **Resid:** Psychiatry, Geo Wash Univ Hosp 1985; **Fac Appt:** Asst Clin Prof Psyc, Univ MD Sch Med

Roose, Steven MD [Psyc] - **Spec Exp:** Depression in the Elderly; **Hospital:** NY-Presby/Columbia Univ Med Ctr, NY (page 66); **Address:** NY State Psychiatric Institute, 1051 Riverside Drive, New York, NY 10032; **Phone:** 212-831-8644; **Board Cert:** Psychiatry 1979; **Med School:** Mount Sinai Sch Med 1974; **Resid:** Psychiatry, NY Psychiatric Inst 1978; **Fellow:** Research, Columbia-Presby Med Ctr 1981; **Fac Appt:** Clin Prof Psyc, Columbia P&S

Rosenthal, Norman E MD [Psyc] - ; **Address:** 11110 Stephalee Ln, Rockville, MD 20852; **Phone:** 301-770-3843; **Board Cert:** Psychiatry 1980; **Med School:** South Africa 1973; **Resid:** Psychiatry, NY State Psych Inst 1979; **Fellow:** Psychiatry, Natl Inst Mental Health 1981; **Fac Appt:** Clin Prof Psyc, Georgetown Univ

Rosenthal, Richard N MD [Psyc] - **Spec Exp:** Anxiety & Mood Disorders; Addiction/Substance Abuse; **Hospital:** St. Luke's - Roosevelt Hosp Ctr - Roosevelt Div (page 56), Beth Israel Med Ctr - Petrie Division (page 56); **Address:** 1090 Amerstdam Ave, Fl 16, Ste G, New York, NY 10025; **Phone:** 212-523-5366; **Board Cert:** Psychiatry 1985; Addiction Psychiatry 2012; **Med School:** SUNY Hlth Sci Ctr 1980; **Resid:** Psychiatry, Mount Sinai Hosp 1984; **Fac Appt:** Prof Psyc, Columbia P&S

Rosse, Richard B MD [Psyc] - **Hospital:** VA Med Ctr - Washington; **Address:** VA Med Ctr, 50 Irving St NW, Washington, DC 20422-0001; **Phone:** 202-745-8156; **Board Cert:** Psychiatry 1986; **Med School:** Univ MD Sch Med 1980; **Resid:** Psychiatry, Georgetown Univ Med Ctr 1984; **Fac Appt:** Prof Psyc, Howard Univ

Roth, Andrew J MD [Psyc] - **Spec Exp:** Psychiatry of Prostate Cancer; Geriatric Psychiatry; **Hospital:** Meml Sloan-Kettering Cancer Ctr; **Address:** 641 Lexington Ave Fl 7, New York, NY 10022; **Phone:** 646-888-0024; **Board Cert:** Psychiatry 1993; Geriatric Psychiatry 2007; Psychosomatic Medicine 2005; **Med School:** NY Med Coll 1988; **Resid:** Psychiatry, Mt Sinai Med Ctr 1992; **Fellow:** Liaison Psychiatry, Meml Sloan-Kettering Canc Ctr 1994; **Fac Appt:** Clin Prof Psyc, Cornell Univ-Weill Med Coll

Sadock, Virginia MD [Psyc] - **Spec Exp:** Psychotherapy; Sexual Dysfunction; Anxiety & Depression; Marital/Family/Sex Therapy; **Hospital:** NYU Langone Med Ctr (page 68); **Address:** 4 E 89th St, Ste 1E, New York, NY 10128; **Phone:** 212-427-0885; **Board Cert:** Psychiatry 1975; **Med School:** NY Med Coll 1970; **Resid:** Psychiatry, Metropolitan Hosp 1973; **Fac Appt:** Clin Prof Psyc, NYU Sch Med

Samberg, Eslee MD [Psyc] - **Spec Exp:** Psychoanalysis; **Hospital:** NY-Presby/Weill Cornell Med Ctr, NY (page 66); **Address:** 165 W End Ave, Ste 1M, New York, NY 10024; **Phone:** 212-874-7725; **Board Cert:** Psychiatry 1983; **Med School:** Cornell Univ-Weill Med Coll 1978; **Resid:** Psychiatry, NY Hosp-Cornell Med Ctr 1982; **Fac Appt:** Assoc Clin Prof Psyc, Cornell Univ-Weill Med Coll

Scott, C Paul MD [Psyc] - **Spec Exp:** Anxiety & Mood Disorders; Psychoanalysis; **Hospital:** UPMC Presby, Pittsburgh; **Address:** 401 Shady Ave, Ste C202, Pittsburgh, PA 15206; **Phone:** 412-661-2354; **Board Cert:** Psychiatry 1976; **Med School:** Case West Res Univ 1968; **Resid:** Internal Medicine, Univ Cleveland Hosps 1970; Psychiatry, Western Psych Inst 1975; **Fellow:** Psychoanalysis, Western Psych Inst 1982; **Fac Appt:** Clin Prof Psyc, Univ Pittsburgh

Sussman, Norman MD [Psyc] - **Spec Exp:** Psychopharmacology; Anxiety & Mood Disorders; Bipolar/Mood Disorders; **Hospital:** NYU Langone Med Ctr (page 68); **Address:** 150 E 58th St, Fl 27, New York, NY 10155; **Phone:** 212-588-9722; **Board Cert:** Psychiatry 1980; **Med School:** NY Med Coll 1975; **Resid:** Psychiatry, Metropolitan Hosp Ctr 1977; Psychiatry, Westchester Co Med Ctr 1978; **Fac Appt:** Prof Psyc, NYU Sch Med

Thase, Michael E MD [Psyc] - **Spec Exp:** Anxiety & Mood Disorders; Psychopharmacology; Depression; **Hospital:** Hosp Univ Penn - UPHS (page 72); **Address:** Univ Penn, Dept Psychiatry, 3535 Market St, Ste 670, Philadelphia, PA 19104; **Phone:** 215-746-6680; **Board Cert:** Psychiatry 1984; **Med School:** Ohio State Univ 1979; **Resid:** Psychiatry, Western Psych Inst 1983; **Fellow:** Research, Univ Pittsburgh 1984; **Fac Appt:** Prof Psyc, Univ Pennsylvania

Wait, Susan B MD [Psyc] - **Spec Exp:** Post Traumatic Stress Disorder; Dissociative Disorders; Anxiety & Mood Disorders; Dialectical Behavioral Therapy; **Hospital:** Sheppard Pratt Hlth Sys; **Address:** Sheppard Pratt Hlth Sys, 6501 N Charles St, Baltimore, MD 21285; **Phone:** 410-938-5076; **Board Cert:** Psychiatry 1993; **Med School:** Med Coll PA Hahnemann 1987; **Resid:** Psychiatry, Sheppard Pratt Hosp 1991; **Fac Appt:** Assoc Clin Prof Psyc, Univ MD Sch Med

Walsh, B Timothy MD [Psyc] - **Spec Exp:** Eating Disorders; **Hospital:** NY State Psychiatric Inst, NY-Presby/Columbia Univ Med Ctr, NY (page 66); **Address:** NY State Psychiatric Inst-Unit 98, 1051 Riverside Dr, New York, NY 10032-2695; **Phone:** 212-543-5739; **Board Cert:** Psychiatry 1978; **Med School:** Harvard Med Sch 1972; **Resid:** Internal Medicine, Dartmouth Affil Hosps 1973; Psychiatry, Bronx Muni Hosp Ctr 1977; **Fac Appt:** Prof Psyc, Columbia P&S

Southeast

Blazer II, Dan G MD/PhD [Psyc] - **Spec Exp:** Geriatric Psychiatry; Mood Disorders; **Hospital:** Duke Univ Hosp; **Address:** Duke Univ Med Ctr, Dept Psychiatary, 3521 Hospital South, Box 3003, Durham, NC 27710-3003; **Phone:** 919-684-4128; **Board Cert:** Psychiatry 1977; **Med School:** Univ Tenn Coll Med 1969; **Resid:** Psychiatry, Duke Univ Med Ctr 1975; **Fellow:** Liaison Psychiatry, Montefiore Hosp 1976; **Fac Appt:** Prof Psyc, Duke Univ

Canterbury II, Randolph J MD [Psyc] - **Spec Exp:** Panic Disorder; Depression; Substance Abuse; **Hospital:** Univ of Virginia Health Sys; **Address:** Univ Virginia Dept Psychiatry, Div Outpatient Psychiatry, Box 800623, Charlottesville, VA 22908-0623; **Phone:** 434-924-2241; **Board Cert:** Internal Medicine 1983; Psychiatry 1985; Psychosomatic Medicine 2005; **Med School:** W VA Univ 1979; **Resid:** Internal Medicine, Univ Va Hosp 1983; Psychiatry, Univ Va Hosp 1985; **Fac Appt:** Prof Psyc, Univ VA Sch Med

Eth, Spencer MD [Psyc] - **Spec Exp:** Forensic Psychiatry; Post Traumatic Stress Disorder; **Hospital:** VA Med Ctr - Miami, Univ of Miami Hosp; **Address:** VA Medical Center, 1201 NW 16th St, Miami, FL 33125; **Phone:** 305-575-3301; **Board Cert:** Child & Adolescent Psychiatry 1982; Geriatric Psychiatry 2010; Forensic Psychiatry 2005; Addiction Psychiatry 2009; **Med School:** UCLA 1976; **Resid:** Psychiatry, NY Cornell Med Ctr 1979; **Fellow:** Child & Adolescent Psychiatry, Cedars-Sinai Med Ctr 1981; **Fac Appt:** Prof Psyc, Univ Miami Sch Med

Psychiatry

Giustra Jr, Lawrence J MD [Psyc] - **Spec Exp:** Psychotherapy; Marital/Family/Sex Therapy; Depression; **Hospital:** Emory Univ Hosp; **Address:** 1945 Cliff Valley Way NE, Ste 202, Atlanta, GA 30329; **Phone:** 404-325-2139; **Board Cert:** Psychiatry 1982; **Med School:** Johns Hopkins Univ 1976; **Resid:** Psychiatry, Mass Genl Hosp 1980; **Fac Appt:** Asst Prof Psyc, Emory Univ

Klapheke, Martin M MD [Psyc] - **Spec Exp:** Transplantation Psychiatry; Psychoanalysis; **Address:** College of Medicine Rm427, 6850 Lake Nona Blvd, Orlando, FL 32827; **Phone:** 407-266-1100; **Board Cert:** Psychiatry 1985; **Med School:** Univ KY Coll Med 1979; **Resid:** Psychiatry, Mayo Grad Sch Med 1982; **Fellow:** Child & Adolescent Psychiatry, Mayo Grad Sch Med 1984; Psychoanalysis, Topeka Inst Psychoanalysis 1994; **Fac Appt:** Prof Psyc, Univ C Fla Coll Med

Levy, Steven T MD [Psyc] - **Spec Exp:** Depression; Anxiety & Mood Disorders; Bipolar/Mood Disorders; **Hospital:** Emory Univ Hosp, Grady Hlth Sys; **Address:** Emory Univ Psychoanalytic Inst, 2004 Ridgewood Drive, Ste 300, Atlanta, GA 30322; **Phone:** 404-727-5886; **Board Cert:** Psychiatry 1976; **Med School:** Duke Univ 1969; **Resid:** Psychiatry, Yale-New Haven Hosp 1973; **Fac Appt:** Prof Psyc, Emory Univ

Powers, Pauline MD [Psyc] - **Spec Exp:** Eating Disorders; **Hospital:** Tampa Genl Hosp; **Address:** 3515 E Fletcher Ave, Tampa, FL 33613; **Phone:** 813-974-1074; **Board Cert:** Psychiatry 1977; **Med School:** Univ Iowa Coll Med 1971; **Resid:** Psychiatry, Univ Iowa Med Ctr 1974; Psychiatry, UC Davis Med Ctr 1975; **Fac Appt:** Prof Psyc, Univ S Fla Coll Med

Salloum, Ihsan M MD [Psyc] - **Spec Exp:** Bipolar/Mood Disorders; Addiction/Substance Abuse; **Hospital:** Univ of Miami Hosp; **Address:** 1120 NW 14th St, Ste 1450, Miami, FL 33136; **Phone:** 305-243-7931; **Board Cert:** Psychiatry 1994; Addiction Psychiatry 2007; **Med School:** Italy 1980; **Resid:** Psychiatry, Univ Hlth Sci Ctr 1988; **Fellow:** Research, Univ Pittsburgh Med Ctr 1989; **Fac Appt:** Prof Psyc, Univ Miami Sch Med

Weiner, Richard D MD/PhD [Psyc] - **Spec Exp:** Bipolar/Mood Disorders; Electroconvulsive Therapy (ECT); Depression; Schizophrenia; **Hospital:** Duke Univ Hosp, Durham VA Med Ctr; **Address:** Duke Univ Medical Ctr, Box 3309, Durham, NC 27710; **Phone:** 919-681-8742; **Board Cert:** Psychiatry 1979; Clinical Neurophysiology 2003; **Med School:** Duke Univ 1973; **Resid:** Psychiatry, Duke Univ Med Ctr 1976; **Fellow:** Electroencephalography, Duke Univ Med Ctr 1977; **Fac Appt:** Prof Psyc, Duke Univ

Weisler, Richard H MD [Psyc] - **Spec Exp:** Depression; Bipolar/Mood Disorders; Clinical Trials; **Hospital:** NC Memorial Hosp - UNC; **Address:** 700 Spring Forest Rd, Ste 125, Raleigh, NC 27609; **Phone:** 919-872-5900; **Board Cert:** Psychiatry 1982; **Med School:** Univ NC Sch Med 1977; **Resid:** Psychiatry, Duke Univ Med Ctr 1982; **Fac Appt:** Assoc Prof Psyc, Duke Univ

Wilson, Daniel R MD/PhD [Psyc] - **Spec Exp:** Psychopharmacology; Neuro-Psychiatry; Forensic Psychiatry; **Hospital:** Shands Jacksonville Med Ctr; **Address:** University of Florida HSC, 653 W 8th St, Jacksonville, FL 32209; **Phone:** 904-244-3131; **Board Cert:** Psychiatry 1989; Forensic Psychiatry 2009; **Med School:** Univ Iowa Coll Med 1983; **Resid:** Psychiatry, McLean Hosp 1986; **Fellow:** Geriatric Psychiatry, McLean Hosp 1987; Genetics, Cambridge Univ 1993; **Fac Appt:** Prof Psyc, Univ Fla Coll Med

Midwest

Black, Donald W MD [Psyc] - **Spec Exp:** Obsessive-Compulsive Disorder; Personality Disorders; Bipolar/Mood Disorders; Psychotic Disorders; **Hospital:** Univ Iowa Hosp & Clinics; **Address:** Univ Iowa Hosp & Clinics, 500 Newton Rd, MEB Bldg - rm 2-126B, Iowa City, IA 52242; **Phone:** 319-353-4431; **Board Cert:** Psychiatry 1988; **Med School:** Univ Utah 1982; **Resid:** Psychiatry, Univ Iowa Hosp & Clincs 1988; **Fellow:** Epidemiology, Univ Iowa Hosp & Clincs 1989; **Fac Appt:** Prof Psyc, Univ Iowa Coll Med

Black, Kevin J MD [Psyc] - **Spec Exp:** Neuro-Psychiatry; **Hospital:** Barnes-Jewish Hosp; **Address:** Washington Univ Sch Med, Dept Neurology, 660 S Euclid Ave, Box 8111, St Louis, MO 63110; **Phone:** 314-362-6908; **Board Cert:** Psychiatry 2005; **Med School:** Duke Univ 1990; **Resid:** Psychiatry, Barnes Hosp-Washington Univ 1994; **Fellow:** Movement Disorders, Barnes Hosp-Washington Univ 1996; **Fac Appt:** Assoc Prof Psyc, Washington Univ, St Louis

Calabrese, Joseph R MD [Psyc] - **Spec Exp:** Bipolar/Mood Disorders; **Hospital:** Univ Hosps Case Med Ctr (page 74); **Address:** Case Western Reserve Univ, 10524 Euclid Ave, Ste 12-135, Cleveland, OH 44106; **Phone:** 216-844-2865; **Board Cert:** Psychiatry 1989; **Med School:** Ohio State Univ 1980; **Resid:** Psychiatry, Cleveland Clinic 1984; **Fellow:** Biological Psychiatry, Natl Inst Mental Hlth 1986; **Fac Appt:** Prof Psyc, Case West Res Univ

Cloninger, C Robert MD [Psyc] - **Spec Exp:** Personality Disorders; **Hospital:** Barnes-Jewish Hosp; **Address:** Wash Univ Sch Med, Dept Psyc, 660 S Euclid Ave, Box 8134, St Louis, MO 63110; **Phone:** 314-362-7005; **Board Cert:** Psychiatry 1975; **Med School:** Washington Univ, St Louis 1970; **Resid:** Psychiatry, Barnes Hosp 1973; Psychiatry, Renard Hosp-Wash Univ 1973; **Fac Appt:** Prof Psyc, Washington Univ, St Louis

Crow, Scott J MD [Psyc] - **Spec Exp:** Eating Disorders; Obesity; **Address:** The Emily Program, 2265 Como Ave, St Paul, MN 55108; **Phone:** 651-645-5323; **Board Cert:** Psychiatry 1994; **Med School:** Univ Minn 1988; **Resid:** Psychiatry, Univ Minn Med Ctr 1991; **Fellow:** Psychiatry, Univ Minn 1992; **Fac Appt:** Prof Psyc, Univ Minn

Greden, John F MD [Psyc] - **Spec Exp:** Depression; **Hospital:** Univ of Michigan Hosp; **Address:** Univ Michigan Comp Depression Ctr, Rachel Upjohn Bldg, 4250 Plymouth Rd, Ann Arbor, MI 48109-2700; **Phone:** 734-763-9629; **Board Cert:** Psychiatry 1975; **Med School:** Univ Minn 1967; **Resid:** Psychiatry, Univ Minn Med Ctr 1969; Psychiatry, Walter Reed AMC 1972; **Fac Appt:** Prof Psyc, Univ Mich Med Sch

Janicak, Philip G MD [Psyc] - **Spec Exp:** Psychopharmacology; Mood Disorders; Psychotic Disorders; **Hospital:** Rush Univ Med Ctr; **Address:** Rush Univ Med Ctr, Dept Psych, 2150 W Harrison St, rm 253, Chicago, IL 60612; **Phone:** 312-942-7287; **Board Cert:** Psychiatry 1978; **Med School:** Loyola Univ-Stritch Sch Med 1973; **Resid:** Psychiatry, McGaw Hosp/Loyola Med Ctr 1976; **Fac Appt:** Prof Psyc, Rush Med Coll

Levine, Stephen B MD [Psyc] - **Spec Exp:** Sexual Dysfunction; Relationship Problems; Sexual Identity Issues; **Hospital:** Univ Hosps Case Med Ctr (page 74); **Address:** 23425 Commerce Park Rd, Ste 104, Beachwood, OH 44122-5446; **Phone:** 216-831-2900; **Board Cert:** Psychiatry 1976; **Med School:** Case West Res Univ 1967; **Resid:** Psychiatry, Univ Hosps Cleveland 1973; **Fac Appt:** Clin Prof Psyc, Case West Res Univ

Locala, Joseph MD [Psyc] - **Spec Exp:** Psychiatry in Transplant Patients; Psychiatry in Physical Illness; Anxiety & Mood Disorders; Neuro-Psychiatry; **Hospital:** Univ Hosps Case Med Ctr (page 74); **Address:** WO Walker Ctr, 10524 Euclid Ave Fl 13, Cleveland, OH 44106; **Phone:** 216-844-2400; **Board Cert:** Psychiatry 2006; Psychosomatic Medicine 2006; **Med School:** Temple Univ 1990; **Resid:** Psychiatry, Medical Ctr Hosp 1994; **Fellow:** Psychosomatic Medicine, Cleveland Clinic 1995; **Fac Appt:** Assoc Prof Psyc, Case West Res Univ

McCallum, Kimberli E MD [Psyc] - **Spec Exp:** Eating Disorders; **Hospital:** St. Louis Univ Hosp; **Address:** McCallum Place, 231 W Lockwood Ave, Ste 201, Webster Groves, MO 63119; **Phone:** 314-968-1900; **Board Cert:** Psychiatry 1993; Child & Adolescent Psychiatry 1994; **Med School:** Yale Univ 1986; **Resid:** Psychiatry, UCLA Neuropsyc Inst 1991; **Fellow:** Child Psychiatry, Washington Univ 1993; **Fac Appt:** Assoc Clin Prof Psyc, Washington Univ, St Louis

Nurnberger Jr, John I MD/PhD [Psyc] - **Spec Exp:** Bipolar/Mood Disorders; Depression; Psychiatric Genetics; **Hospital:** IU Health University Hosp, Wishard Hlth Srvs; **Address:** Inst Psychiatric Rsch-IUMC, 791 Union Drive, Indianapolis, IN 46202-4887; **Phone:** 317-944-7422; **Board Cert:** Psychiatry 1981; **Med School:** Indiana Univ 1975; **Resid:** Psychiatry, Columbia-Presby Med Ctr 1978; **Fellow:** Psychiatry & Genetics, NIMH Clinical Ctr 1983; **Fac Appt:** Prof Psyc, Indiana Univ

Riba, Michelle B MD [Psyc] - **Spec Exp:** Psychiatry in Cancer; **Hospital:** Univ of Michigan Hosp; **Address:** Mott Chldns Hosp, MCHC F6236, 1500 E Medical Ctr Drive, Ste SPC 5295, Ann Arbor, MI 48109-0295; **Phone:** 734-764-6879; **Board Cert:** Psychiatry 1991; Psychosomatic Medicine 2005; **Med School:** Univ Conn 1985; **Resid:** Psychiatry, Univ Connecticut 1988; **Fac Appt:** Clin Prof Psyc, Univ Mich Med Sch

Strakowski, Stephen M MD [Psyc] - **Spec Exp:** Bipolar/Mood Disorders; Psychotic Disorders; Dual Diagnosis; Addiction/Substance Abuse; **Hospital:** Univ Hosp - Cincinnati, Cincinnati Chldns Hosp Med Ctr; **Address:** Univ Cincinnati Coll Med, Dept Psychiatry, 231 Albert Sabin Way, Cincinnati, OH 45267-0559; **Phone:** 513-558-4274; **Board Cert:** Psychiatry 1993; **Med School:** Vanderbilt Univ 1988; **Resid:** Psychiatry, McLean Hosp-Harvard Med Sch 1992; **Fac Appt:** Prof Psyc, Univ Cincinnati

Wooten, Virgil D MD [Psyc] - **Spec Exp:** Sleep Disorders; **Hospital:** Univ Hosp - Cincinnati, University Pointe Surgical Hosp; **Address:** UC Health Univ Hosp Sleep Medicine Ctr, 200 Albert Sabin Way Holmes Bldg Fl 3, Cincinnati, OH 45219; **Phone:** 513-475-7500; **Board Cert:** Psychiatry 1985; Sleep Medicine 2007; **Med School:** Univ Ark 1980; **Resid:** Psychiatry, Univ Hosp-VA Hosp 1984; **Fellow:** Sleep Medicine, Univ Hosp 1984; **Fac Appt:** Prof Psyc, Univ Cincinnati

Great Plains and Mountains

Freedman, Robert MD [Psyc] - **Spec Exp:** Schizophrenia; **Hospital:** Univ of CO Hosp - Anschutz Inpatient Pav; **Address:** Univ Colorado Hosp, Dept Psychiatry, 13001 E 17th Place, Campus Box F546, Aurora, CO 80045; **Phone:** 303-724-4940; **Board Cert:** Psychiatry 1980; **Med School:** Harvard Med Sch 1972; **Resid:** Psychiatry, Univ Chicago Hosps 1978; **Fellow:** Neuropharmacology, NIMH/St Elizabeth's Hosp 1975; **Fac Appt:** Prof Psyc, Univ Colorado

Greiner, Carl B MD [Psyc] - **Spec Exp:** Psychiatry in Cancer; Psychiatry in Physical Illness; Forensic Psychiatry; Post Traumatic Stress Disorder; **Hospital:** Nebraska Med Ctr; **Address:** UNMC, Dept Psychiatry, 985575 Nebraska Medical Ctr, Omaha, NE 68198-5575; **Phone:** 402-552-6002; **Board Cert:** Psychiatry 1984; Forensic Psychiatry 2008; **Med School:** Univ Cincinnati 1978; **Resid:** Psychiatry, Univ Cincinnati Med Ctr 1982; **Fac Appt:** Prof Psyc, Univ Nebr Coll Med

Hoffman, Daniel A MD [Psyc] - **Spec Exp:** ADD/ADHD; Mood Disorders; **Hospital:** Rose Med Ctr; **Address:** Neuro-Therapy Clinic, 7800 E Orchard Rd, Ste 340, Greenwood Village, CO 80111; **Phone:** 303-741-4800; **Board Cert:** Psychiatry 1981; **Med School:** Wayne State Univ 1974; **Resid:** Psychiatry, Univ Colo Affil Hosp 1977

McIntosh, J Michael MD [Psyc] - **Spec Exp:** Depression; Schizophrenia; Anxiety Disorders; Bipolar/Mood Disorders; **Hospital:** Univ Utah Hlth Care; **Address:** 30 N 1900 East, rm 5R110, Salt Lake City, UT 84108; **Phone:** 801-581-7951; **Board Cert:** Psychiatry 1994; **Med School:** UCLA 1987; **Resid:** Psychiatry, Univ Colo Hlth Sci Ctr 1991; Psychiatry, Univ Utah Hosps 1992; **Fac Appt:** Clin Prof Psyc, Univ Utah

Mitchell III, James E MD [Psyc] - **Spec Exp:** Eating Disorders; **Hospital:** Sanford Med Ctr Fargo; **Address:** NeuroPsychiatric Research Inst, 120 8th St S, Fargo, ND 58103; **Phone:** 701-293-1335; **Board Cert:** Psychiatry 1979; **Med School:** Northwestern Univ 1972; **Resid:** Psychiatry, Fairview-Univ Med Ctr 1976; **Fac Appt:** Prof Psyc, Univ ND Sch Med

Moench, Louis A MD [Psyc] - **Hospital:** LDS Hosp; **Address:** 324 Kent Ave, Ste 178, Salt Lake City, UT 84103; **Phone:** 801-408-8500; **Board Cert:** Psychiatry 1978; Forensic Psychiatry 2004; **Med School:** Univ Utah 1970; **Resid:** Psychiatry, Hosp Univ Penn 1976; **Fellow:** Forensic Psychiatry, Hosp Univ Penn 1976; **Fac Appt:** Clin Prof Psyc, Univ Utah

Weiner, Kenneth L MD [Psyc] - **Spec Exp:** Eating Disorders; **Hospital:** Univ of CO Hosp - Anschutz Inpatient Pav; **Address:** Eating Recovery Center, 1830 Franklin St, Ste 500, Denver, CO 80218; **Phone:** 303-825-8584; **Board Cert:** Psychiatry 1983; **Med School:** Tufts Univ 1977; **Resid:** Psychiatry, Univ Colorado Hlth Sci Ctr 1981; **Fac Appt:** Asst Clin Prof Psyc, Univ Colorado

Southwest

Avery, Eric N MD [Psyc] - **Spec Exp:** Depression; Dementia; Arts in the Healing Process; AIDS/HIV Liaison Psychiatry; **Hospital:** UT Med Br at Galveston(Joh Sealy Hosp); **Address:** Dept Psychiatry, 301 University Blvd, Galveston, TX 77555-0193; **Phone:** 409-747-9789; **Board Cert:** Psychiatry 2003; **Med School:** Univ Tex Med Br, Galveston 1974; **Resid:** Psychiatry, NY State Psych Inst 1978; **Fellow:** Liaison Psychiatry for AIDS/HIV, NY State Psych Inst 1994; **Fac Appt:** Assoc Clin Prof Psyc, Univ Tex Med Br, Galveston

Baile, Walter F MD [Psyc] - **Spec Exp:** Psychiatry in Cancer; **Hospital:** UT MD Anderson Cancer Ctr; **Address:** PO Box 301402, Unit 1426, Texas, TX 77230; **Phone:** 713-563-1484; **Board Cert:** Psychiatry 1980; **Med School:** Italy 1973; **Resid:** Psychiatry, Johns Hopkins Hosp 1976; **Fellow:** Behavioral Medicine, Natl Inst Aging 1978; **Fac Appt:** Prof Psyc, Univ Tex, Houston

Bowden, Charles L MD [Psyc] - **Spec Exp:** Bipolar/Mood Disorders; **Hospital:** Univ Hlth Syst-San Antonio; **Address:** Univ Tex Hlth Sci Ctr, Dept Psychiatry, 7526 Louis Pasteur Drive, Ste 318, San Antonio, TX 78229-3900; **Phone:** 210-567-5555; **Board Cert:** Psychiatry 1970; **Med School:** Baylor Coll Med 1964; **Resid:** Psychiatry, NY State Psyc Inst/Columbia-Presby Med Ctr 1968; **Fac Appt:** Prof Psyc, Univ Tex, San Antonio

Davidson, Joyce E MD [Psyc] - **Spec Exp:** Obsessive-Compulsive Disorder; Bipolar/Mood Disorders; Schizophrenia; **Hospital:** Menninger Clinic; **Address:** The Menninger Clinic, 2801 Gessner Drive, Houston, TX 77080; **Phone:** 713-275-5000; **Board Cert:** Psychiatry 1988; **Med School:** Univ MO-Kansas City 1979; **Resid:** Psychiatry, Menninger Clinic 1982; **Fellow:** Child & Adolescent Psychiatry, Karl Menninger Sch Psyc 1984; **Fac Appt:** Asst Prof Psyc, Baylor Coll Med

Psychiatry

Gabbard, Glen O MD [Psyc] - **Spec Exp:** Personality Disorders-Borderline; Cognitive Psychotherapy; Psychoanalysis; **Address:** 6750 W Loop S, Ste 460, Bellaire, TX 77401; **Phone:** 713-665-1607; **Board Cert:** Psychiatry 1979; **Med School:** Rush Med Coll 1975; **Resid:** Psychiatry, Menninger Clinic 1978; **Fellow:** Psychoanalysis, Topeka Inst Psychoanalysis 1984; **Fac Appt:** Clin Prof Psyc, Univ Kansas

Haque, Waheedul MD [Psyc] - **Spec Exp:** Depression; Panic Disorder; **Hospital:** UT Med Br at Galveston(Joh Sealy Hosp); **Address:** Dept Psychiatry, 301 University Blvd, Route 0190, Galveston, TX 77555; **Phone:** 409-747-9722; **Board Cert:** Psychiatry 1970; **Med School:** Pakistan 1962; **Resid:** Psychiatry, Barnes Jewish Med Ctr 1969; **Fac Appt:** Prof Psyc, Univ Tex Med Br, Galveston

Hirschfeld, Robert M A MD [Psyc] - **Spec Exp:** Bipolar/Mood Disorders; Schizophrenia; Depression; Suicide; **Hospital:** UT Med Br at Galveston(Joh Sealy Hosp); **Address:** Dept Psychiatry, 301 University Blvd, Route 0188, Galveston, TX 77555-0188; **Phone:** 409-747-9791; **Board Cert:** Psychiatry 1975; **Med School:** Univ Mich Med Sch 1968; **Resid:** Psychiatry, Stanford Univ Med Ctr 1972; **Fac Appt:** Prof Psyc, Univ Tex Med Br, Galveston

Mohl, Paul C MD [Psyc] - **Spec Exp:** Psychopharmacology; Psychotherapy; **Hospital:** UT Southwestern Med Ctr at Dallas; **Address:** 5323 Harry Hines Blvd, Dallas, TX 75390-9070; **Phone:** 214-645-8500; **Board Cert:** Psychiatry 1977; **Med School:** Duke Univ 1971; **Resid:** Psychiatry, Duke Univ Hosp 1974; **Fac Appt:** Prof Psyc, Univ Tex SW, Dallas

Valentine, Alan D MD [Psyc] - **Spec Exp:** Psychiatry in Cancer; Palliative Care; **Hospital:** UT MD Anderson Cancer Ctr; **Address:** MD Anderson Cancer Center, Dept Psychiatry Unit 1454, PO Box 301402, Houston, TX 77230-1402; **Phone:** 713-745-3344; **Board Cert:** Psychiatry 1992; Geriatric Psychiatry 2006; Psychosomatic Medicine 2005; **Med School:** Univ Tex, Houston 1986; **Resid:** Psychiatry, Univ Texas Affil Hosps 2000; **Fac Appt:** Assoc Prof Psyc, Univ Tex, Houston

Weiner, Myron MD [Psyc] - **Spec Exp:** Geriatric Psychiatry; Alzheimer's Disease; Dementia; Memory Disorders; **Hospital:** UT Southwestern Med Ctr at Dallas; **Address:** Univ Texas SW Med Ctr, 5323 Harry Hines Blvd, Dallas, TX 75390-9129; **Phone:** 214-648-9394; **Board Cert:** Psychiatry 1966; Geriatric Psychiatry 2001; **Med School:** Tulane Univ 1957; **Resid:** Psychiatry, Parkland Hosp 1963; **Fellow:** Geriatric Psychiatry, Mt Sinai Med Ctr 1985; **Fac Appt:** Prof Psyc, Univ Tex SW, Dallas

West Coast and Pacific

Blumenfield, Michael MD [Psyc] - **Spec Exp:** Psychotherapy; Psychopharmacology; Psychosomatic Disorders; Disaster Psychiatry; **Address:** 5901 Nita Ave, Woodland Hills, CA 91367; **Phone:** 818-564-4207; **Board Cert:** Psychiatry 1970; Psychosomatic Medicine 2005; **Med School:** SUNY Downstate 1964; **Resid:** Psychiatry, Kings County Hosp 1968; **Fellow:** Psychosomatic Medicine, Kings County Hosp 1971; **Fac Appt:** Prof Emeritus Psyc, NY Med Coll

Burt, Vivien K MD/PhD [Psyc] - **Spec Exp:** Women's Health-Mental Health; Impulse-Control Disorders; Psychiatry in Pregnancy; Postpartum Depression; **Hospital:** Resnick Neuropsychiatric Hosp at UCLA; **Address:** 300 UCLA Med Plaza, Ste 2337, Los Angeles, CA 90095; **Phone:** 310-562-4942; **Board Cert:** Psychiatry 1990; **Med School:** McGill Univ 1984; **Resid:** Psychiatry, UCLA-Neurpsyc Inst 1988; **Fac Appt:** Assoc Prof Psyc, UCLA

Bystritsky, Alexander MD/PhD [Psyc] - **Spec Exp:** Obsessive-Compulsive Disorder; Anxiety Disorders; Psychopharmacology; Body Dysmorphic Disorder (BDD); **Hospital:** Resnick Neuropsychiatric Hosp at UCLA; **Address:** UCLA Anxiety Disorders Clin, 300 UCLA Med Plaza, Ste 2200, Box 956968, Los Angeles, CA 90095-6968; **Phone:** 310-206-5133; **Board Cert:** Psychiatry 1988; **Med School:** Russia 1977; **Resid:** Psychiatry, NYU Med Ctr 1985; **Fellow:** Psychiatry, UCLA 1987; **Fac Appt:** Prof Psyc, UCLA

Eisendrath, Stuart J MD [Psyc] - **Spec Exp:** Depression; Munchausen Syndrome; Cognitive Psychotherapy; **Hospital:** UCSF Med Ctr; **Address:** UCSF Med Ctr, 401 Parnassus Ave, Ste 278, MS 0984, San Francisco, CA 94143-0984; **Phone:** 415-476-7868; **Board Cert:** Psychiatry 1980; Psychosomatic Medicine 2008; **Med School:** Med Coll Wisc 1974; **Resid:** Psychiatry, Langley Porter Neuropsych Inst 1978; **Fellow:** Liaison Psychiatry, Langley Porter Neuropsych Inst 1979; **Fac Appt:** Prof Psyc, UCSF

Fann, Jesse R MD [Psyc] - **Spec Exp:** Psychiatry in Physical Illness; Psychiatry in Cancer; Neuro-Psychiatry; **Hospital:** Univ Wash Med Ctr, Harborview Med Ctr; **Address:** 1959 NE Pacific St, Box 356560, Seattle, WA 98195-6560; **Phone:** 206-685-4280; **Board Cert:** Psychiatry 2005; **Med School:** Northwestern Univ 1989; **Resid:** Psychiatry, Univ Washington Med Ctr 1993; **Fellow:** Liaison Psychiatry, Univ Washington Med Ctr 1995; Epidemiology, Univ Washington Med Ctr 1996; **Fac Appt:** Prof Psyc, Univ Wash

Friedman, Barry MD [Psyc] - **Spec Exp:** Psychopharmacology; Psychoanalysis; **Address:** 9171 Wilshire Blvd, Ste 310, Beverly Hills, CA 90210; **Phone:** 310-274-4372; **Board Cert:** Psychiatry 1974; **Med School:** UCSF 1965; **Resid:** Psychiatry, UCLA Med Ctr 1971; **Fellow:** Psychoanalysis, Los Angeles Psychoanalytic Inst 1992; **Fac Appt:** Assoc Clin Prof Psyc, UCLA

Gitlin, Michael Jay MD [Psyc] - **Spec Exp:** Mood Disorders; **Hospital:** Resnick Neuropsychiatric Hosp at UCLA; **Address:** UCLA NPI-Mood Disorders Clin, 300 Med Plaza, Ste 2200, Los Angeles, CA 90095-6968; **Phone:** 310-206-3654; **Board Cert:** Psychiatry 1981; **Med School:** Univ Pennsylvania 1975; **Resid:** Psychiatry, UCLA Med Ctr 1979; **Fac Appt:** Prof Psyc, UCLA

Keepers, George MD [Psyc] - **Spec Exp:** Neuro-Psychiatry; ADD/ADHD; **Hospital:** OR Hlth & Sci Univ; **Address:** Dept of Psychiatry, 3181 SW Sam Jackson Park Rd, MC UHN80, Portland, OR 97239; **Phone:** 503-494-8144; **Board Cert:** Psychiatry 1984; **Med School:** Baylor Coll Med 1977; **Resid:** Psychiatry, Oregon Hlth Sci Univ 1981; **Fac Appt:** Prof Psyc, Oregon Hlth & Sci Univ

Leuchter, Andrew F MD [Psyc] - **Spec Exp:** Depression; **Hospital:** Resnick Neuropsychiatric Hosp at UCLA; **Address:** UCLA Neuropsychiatric Inst, 760 Westwood Pl, rm 57-456, Los Angeles, CA 90024; **Phone:** 310-825-0207; **Board Cert:** Psychiatry 1986; Geriatric Psychiatry 2001; **Med School:** Baylor Coll Med 1980; **Resid:** Psychiatry, UCLA-Neuro Psyc Inst & Hosp 1984; **Fellow:** Geriatric Psychiatry, UCLA Med Ctr 1986; **Fac Appt:** Prof Psyc, UCLA

Liberman, Robert Paul MD [Psyc] - **Spec Exp:** Schizophrenia; Psychotic Disorders; Psychiatric Rehabilitation; Family Therapy; **Hospital:** Resnick Neuropsychiatric Hosp at UCLA; **Address:** UCLA Neuropsychiatric Inst, 760 Westwood Plaza, Ste C9-400, Los Angeles, CA 90024; **Phone:** 310-206-1616; **Board Cert:** Psychiatry 1969; **Med School:** Johns Hopkins Univ 1963; **Resid:** Psychiatry, Mass Mntl Hlth Ctr 1968; **Fellow:** Pharmacology, UCSF Med Ctr 1961; Research, Harvard Med Sch 1968; **Fac Appt:** Prof Psyc, UCLA

Marder, Stephen R MD [Psyc] - **Spec Exp:** Schizophrenia; Psychopharmacology; **Hospital:** VA Greater Los Angeles Hthcare Sys, UCLA Ronald Reagan Med Ctr; **Address:** West Los Angeles VA - Gr LA Hlth Svcs, 11301 Wilshire Blvd, Bldg MIRECC 210A, Los Angeles, CA 90073; **Phone:** 310-268-3647; **Board Cert:** Psychiatry 1977; **Med School:** SUNY Buffalo 1971; **Resid:** Psychiatry, LAC-USC Med Ctr 1975; **Fac Appt:** Prof Psyc, UCLA

Nelson, J Craig MD [Psyc] - **Spec Exp:** Geriatric Psychiatry; Dementia; Depression; Psychopharmacology; **Hospital:** UCSF Med Ctr; **Address:** UCSF-Langley Porter Psychiatric Inst, 401 Parnassus Ave, Box 0984, San Francisco, CA 94143-0984; **Phone:** 415-476-7405; **Board Cert:** Psychiatry 1974; Geriatric Psychiatry 2002; **Med School:** Univ Wisc 1968; **Resid:** Psychiatry, Yale-New Haven Hosp 1970; Psychiatry, Yale-New Haven Hosp 1974; **Fac Appt:** Prof Psyc, UCSF

Neppe, Vernon M MD/PhD [Psyc] - **Spec Exp:** Behavioral Neurology; Neuro-Psychiatry; Psychopharmacology; Forensic Psychiatry; **Hospital:** Overlake Hosp Med Ctr, Northwest Hosp - Seattle; **Address:** Pacific Neuropsychiatric Institute, 6300 Ninth Ave NE, Ste 353, Seattle, WA 98115; **Phone:** 206-527-6289; **Board Cert:** Psychiatry 1988; Behavioral Neurology & Neuropsychiatry 2006; **Med School:** South Africa 1973; **Resid:** Neurology, Univ Witwatersrand 1979; Psychiatry, Univ Witwatersrand 1980; **Fellow:** Psychopharmacology, Cornell Med Ctr 1983; Neuropsychiatry, Cornell Med Ctr 1983

Norman, Kim P MD [Psyc] - **Spec Exp:** Eating Disorders/Obesity; Personality Disorders; Dual Diagnosis; **Hospital:** UCSF Med Ctr; **Address:** UCSF-Langley Porter Psychiatric Inst, 401 Parnassus Ave, Box CAF-0984, San Francisco, CA 94143-0984; **Phone:** 415-476-7402; **Board Cert:** Psychiatry 1983; **Med School:** Albert Einstein Coll Med 1977; **Resid:** Psychiatry, Langley Porter Psych Inst 1981; **Fac Appt:** Clin Prof Psyc, UCSF

Pi, Edmond H MD [Psyc] - **Spec Exp:** Psychopharmacology; Cross Cultural Psychiatry; Anxiety Disorders; Mood Disorders; **Hospital:** LAC & USC Med Ctr; **Address:** LAC & USC Med Ctr, Dept Psyc, 1200 N State St, Los Angeles, CA 90033-1029; **Phone:** 323-226-7975; **Board Cert:** Psychiatry 1980; Psychosomatic Medicine 2008; **Med School:** South Korea 1972; **Resid:** Psychiatry, SUNY Affil Hosps 1977; Psychiatry, Univ Kentucky Hosp-Chandler Med Ctr 1978; **Fac Appt:** Clin Prof Psyc, USC Sch Med

Pynoos, Robert S MD [Psyc] - **Spec Exp:** Post Traumatic Stress Disorder; Disaster Psychiatry; **Hospital:** Resnick Neuropsychiatric Hosp at UCLA; **Address:** Natl Ctr for Chld Traumatic Stress-UCLA, 11150 W Olympic Blvd, Ste 650, Los Angeles, CA 90064; **Phone:** 310-235-2633; **Board Cert:** Psychiatry 1980; **Med School:** Columbia P&S 1972; **Resid:** Pediatrics, Mt Sinai Hosp; Psychiatry, NY Presby-Cornell Med Ctr; **Fac Appt:** Prof Psyc, UCLA

Raskind, Murray MD [Psyc] - **Spec Exp:** Geriatric Psychiatry; Alzheimer's Disease; Post Traumatic Stress Disorder; **Hospital:** VA Puget Sound Hlth Care Sys, Univ Wash Med Ctr; **Address:** VA Puget Sound Health Care System, 1660 S Columbian Way, Box 358280, Seattle, WA 98108; **Phone:** 206-764-2702; **Board Cert:** Psychiatry 1976; Geriatric Psychiatry 2001; **Med School:** Columbia P&S 1968; **Resid:** Internal Medicine, Harlem Hosp Ctr 1970; Psychiatry, Univ Wash Affil Hosps 1973; **Fac Appt:** Prof Psyc, Univ Wash

Reus, Victor I MD [Psyc] - **Spec Exp:** Psychopharmacology; Bipolar/Mood Disorders; Behavioral Disorders; Depression; **Hospital:** UCSF Med Ctr; **Address:** Langley Porter Institute, 401 Parnassus Ave, San Francisco, CA 94143-0984; **Phone:** 415-476-7478; **Board Cert:** Psychiatry 1977; Geriatric Psychiatry 2010; **Med School:** Univ MD Sch Med 1973; **Resid:** Psychiatry, Univ Wisc Med Ctr 1976; **Fellow:** Biological Psychiatry, Natl Inst Mntl Hlth 1978; **Fac Appt:** Prof Psyc, UCSF

Roy-Byrne, Peter P MD [Psyc] - **Spec Exp:** Anxiety & Mood Disorders; Panic Disorder; Bipolar/Mood Disorders; Post Traumatic Stress Disorder; **Address:** Psychiatric Medicine Assoc, 1505 Westlake Ave N, Ste 920, Seattle, WA 98109; **Phone:** 206-386-3103; **Board Cert:** Psychiatry 1983; **Med School:** Tufts Univ 1978; **Resid:** Psychiatry, UCLA Neuropsych Inst 1982; **Fellow:** Biological Psychiatry, Natl Inst Hlth-NIMH 1984; **Fac Appt:** Prof Psyc, Univ Wash

Saxena, Sanjaya MD [Psyc] - **Spec Exp:** Obsessive-Compulsive Disorder; Anxiety Disorders; Body Dysmorphic Disorder (BDD); Tourette's Syndrome; **Hospital:** UCSD Med Ctr; **Address:** UCSD Outpatient Psychiatric Services, 140 Arbor Drive, MS 0851, San Diego, CA 92103; **Phone:** 619-543-6883; **Board Cert:** Psychiatry 2006; **Med School:** Univ Minn 1990; **Resid:** Psychiatry, UCLA Neuropsychiatric Hosp 1994; **Fellow:** Neuroimaging, UCLA Ctr for Hlth Scis 1996; **Fac Appt:** Prof Psyc, UCSD

Schatzberg, Alan F MD [Psyc] - **Spec Exp:** Psychopharmacology; Anxiety & Mood Disorders; Depression; **Hospital:** Stanford Univ Hosp & Clinics; **Address:** Stanford Univ Dept Psychiatry, 401 Quarry Rd, Stanford, CA 94305-5797; **Phone:** 650-723-6811; **Board Cert:** Psychiatry 1975; **Med School:** NYU Sch Med 1968; **Resid:** Psychiatry, Mass Mental Hlth Ctr 1972; **Fellow:** Psychiatry, Mass Mental Hlth Ctr/Harvard 1972; **Fac Appt:** Prof Psyc, Stanford Univ

Spiegel, David MD [Psyc] - **Spec Exp:** Hypnosis; Psychiatry in Cancer; Post Traumatic Stress Disorder; **Hospital:** Stanford Univ Hosp & Clinics; **Address:** 401 Quarry Rd, Ste 2325, MC 5718, Stanford, CA 94305-5718; **Phone:** 650-723-2423; **Board Cert:** Psychiatry 1976; **Med School:** Harvard Med Sch 1971; **Resid:** Psychiatry, Harvard Univ/Mass Mental Hlth Ctr 1974; Psychiatry, Cambridge Hosp-Harvard Med Sch 1974; **Fellow:** Community Psychiatry, Harvard Univ Med School 1974; **Fac Appt:** Prof Psyc, Stanford Univ

Stein, Murray B MD [Psyc] - **Spec Exp:** Anxiety Disorders; Panic Disorder; Post Traumatic Stress Disorder; **Hospital:** UCSD Med Ctr, VA San Diego Hlthcre Sys; **Address:** UCSD Dept Psychiatry, 8939 Villa La Jolla Drive, Ste 200, MS 0855, La Jolla, CA 92037; **Phone:** 858-534-6400; **Board Cert:** Psychiatry 1989; **Med School:** Univ Manitoba 1983; **Resid:** Psychiatry, Univ Toronto Hosp 1986; Psychiatry, Natl Inst Mental Hlth-NIH 1987; **Fellow:** Anxiety Disorder, Natl Inst Mental Hlth-NIH 1990; **Fac Appt:** Prof Psyc, UCSD

Strouse, Thomas B MD [Psyc] - **Spec Exp:** Psychiatry in Cancer; Pain-Cancer; Psychiatry in Physical Illness; Palliative Care; **Hospital:** UCLA Ronald Reagan Med Ctr, Cedars-Sinai Med Ctr; **Address:** UCLA Resnick Neuropsychiatric Hosp, 757 Westwood Plaza, Ste 4230B, Los Angeles, CA 90095; **Phone:** 310-267-9159; **Board Cert:** Psychiatry 1993; Hospice & Palliative Medicine 2008; Psychosomatic Medicine 2009; **Med School:** Case West Res Univ 1987; **Resid:** Psychiatry, UCLA Med Ctr 1991; **Fac Appt:** Clin Prof Psyc, UCLA

Weinstock, Robert MD [Psyc] - **Spec Exp:** Adolescent Psychiatry; Addiction/Substance Abuse; **Hospital:** Cedars-Sinai Med Ctr; **Address:** 1823 Sawtelle Blvd, Los Angeles, CA 90025; **Phone:** 310-477-9933; **Board Cert:** Psychiatry 1975; Forensic Psychiatry 2004; **Med School:** NYU Sch Med 1966; **Resid:** Psychiatry, McLean Hosp 1970; McLean Hosp 1972; **Fellow:** Psychiatric Research, Boston Univ 1974; **Fac Appt:** Clin Prof Psyc, UCLA

Zerbe, Kathryn J MD [Psyc] - **Spec Exp:** Eating Disorders; Women's Health-Mental Health; Psychoanalysis; **Address:** 4800 SW Macadam Ave, Ste 340, Portland, OR 97239; **Phone:** 503-295-9909; **Board Cert:** Psychiatry 1984; **Med School:** Temple Univ 1978; **Resid:** Psychiatry, Menninger Clin 1982; Psychoanalysis, Topeka Inst for Psychoanalysis 1992; **Fac Appt:** Prof Psyc, Oregon Hlth & Sci Univ

ADDICTION PSYCHIATRY

New England

Ciraulo, Domenic A MD [AdP] - **Spec Exp:** Alcohol Abuse; Psychopharmacology; Anxiety & Depression; **Hospital:** Boston Med Ctr; **Address:** Boston Univ, Div Psychiatry, 720 Harrison Ave, Ste 914, Boston, MA 02118; **Phone:** 617-414-1995; **Board Cert:** Psychiatry 1980; Addiction Psychiatry 2003; **Med School:** Georgetown Univ 1975; **Resid:** Psychiatry, Inst Living 1977; **Fellow:** Psychopharmacology, Mass Mental Hlth Ctr 1978; **Fac Appt:** Prof Psyc, Boston Univ

Greenfield, Shelly F MD [AdP] - **Spec Exp:** Addiction/Substance Abuse; Alcohol Abuse; Women & Addiction; **Hospital:** McLean Hosp; **Address:** McLean Hospital, 115 Mill St, Belmont, MA 02478; **Phone:** 617-855-2241; **Board Cert:** Psychiatry 1992; Addiction Psychiatry 2006; **Med School:** Harvard Med Sch 1986; **Resid:** Psychiatry, McLean Hosp 1990; **Fellow:** Epidemiology, Univ North Carolina 1992; Research, NIH-Natl Inst Drug Abuse 1993; **Fac Appt:** Assoc Prof Psyc, Harvard Med Sch

Nitenson, Nancy C MD [AdP] - **Spec Exp:** Alcohol Abuse; Addiction/Substance Abuse; **Address:** Ten Post Office Square Fl 8, Boston, MA 02109; **Phone:** 617-850-9005; **Board Cert:** Psychiatry 1992; Addiction Psychiatry 2006; **Med School:** Univ Mass Sch Med 1986; **Resid:** Psychiatry, U Mass Med Ctr 1990; **Fellow:** Psychopharmacology, McLean Hosp 1991

Mid Atlantic

Collins, Eric D MD [AdP] - **Spec Exp:** Addiction/Substance Abuse; Alcohol Abuse; **Hospital:** NY-Presby/Columbia Univ Med Ctr, NY (page 66); **Address:** 180 Ft Washington Ave, Box HP-260, New York, NY 10032; **Phone:** 212-305-8732; **Board Cert:** Psychiatry 2005; Addiction Psychiatry 2007; Psychosomatic Medicine 2008; **Med School:** Columbia P&S 1990; **Resid:** Psychiatry, NY State Psyc Inst 1994; **Fellow:** Psychosomatic Medicine, NY-Presby/Columbia Univ Med Ctr 1995; Substance Abuse, NY State Psyc Inst 1996; **Fac Appt:** Asst Prof Psyc, Columbia P&S

Frances, Richard J MD [AdP] - **Spec Exp:** Addiction/Substance Abuse; Anxiety & Mood Disorders; Forensic Psychiatry; **Hospital:** Silver Hill Hosp, NYU Langone Med Ctr (page 68); **Address:** 510 E 86th St, Ste 1D, New York, NY 10028; **Phone:** 212-861-0570; **Board Cert:** Psychiatry 1976; Addiction Psychiatry 2002; **Med School:** NYU Sch Med 1971; **Resid:** Psychiatry, Bronx Meml Hosp 1974; **Fellow:** Psychoanalysis, NY Psychoanalitic Inst 1984; **Fac Appt:** Clin Prof Psyc, NYU Sch Med

Galanter, I Marc MD [AdP] - **Spec Exp:** Alcohol Abuse; Drug Abuse; **Hospital:** NYU Langone Med Ctr (page 68), Bellevue Hosp Ctr; **Address:** 285 Central Park West, New York, NY 10024-3006; **Phone:** 212-877-4093; **Board Cert:** Psychiatry 1974; Addiction Psychiatry 2011; **Med School:** Albert Einstein Coll Med 1967; **Resid:** Psychiatry, Bronx Muni Hosp-Einstein 1971; **Fac Appt:** Prof Psyc, NYU Sch Med

Kampman, Kyle M MD [AdP] - **Spec Exp:** Addiction/Substance Abuse; Cocaine Addiction; Opiate Addiction; Alcohol Abuse; **Hospital:** Hosp Univ Penn - UPHS (page 72); **Address:** Charles O'Brien Treatment Ctr, 3900 Chesnut St, Philadelphia, PA 19104; **Phone:** 215-222-3200; **Board Cert:** Psychiatry 2004; Addiction Psychiatry 2006; **Med School:** Tulane Univ 1985; **Resid:** Psychiatry, Hosp Univ Penn 1993; **Fellow:** Substance Abuse, Hosp Univ Penn 1994; **Fac Appt:** Assoc Prof Psyc, Univ Pennsylvania

Kleber, Herbert MD [AdP] - **Spec Exp:** Opiate Addiction; Cocaine Addiction; Drug Abuse; **Hospital:** NY-Presby/Columbia Univ Med Ctr, NY (page 66), NY State Psychiatric Inst; **Address:** 1051 Riverside Drive, Room 3713, Unit 66, New York, NY 10032-1007; **Phone:** 212-543-5570; **Med School:** Jefferson Med Coll 1960; **Resid:** Psychiatry, Yale-New Haven Hosp 1964; **Fac Appt:** Prof Psyc, Columbia P&S

Serota, Ronald D MD [AdP] - **Spec Exp:** Addiction/Substance Abuse; **Hospital:** Thomas Jefferson Univ Hosp; **Address:** 833 Chestnut St, Ste 210, Philadelphia, PA 19107; **Phone:** 215-955-4834; **Board Cert:** Internal Medicine 1974; Psychiatry 1990; **Med School:** Thomas Jefferson Univ 1968; **Resid:** Internal Medicine, Mt Zion Hosp 1972; Psychiatry, Thomas Jefferson Univ Hosp 1981; **Fac Appt:** Asst Prof Psyc, Thomas Jefferson Univ

Strain, Eric C MD [AdP] - **Spec Exp:** Addiction/Substance Abuse; Dual Diagnosis; Opiate Addiction; **Hospital:** Johns Hopkins Bayview Med Ctr (page 61); **Address:** 5510 Mathen Shock Drive Fl 3 - Ste 3046, Baltimore, MD 21224; **Phone:** 410-550-1191; **Board Cert:** Psychiatry 1989; Addiction Psychiatry 2002; **Med School:** Ohio State Univ 1984; **Resid:** Psychiatry, Johns Hopkins Hosp 1988; **Fellow:** Addiction Psychiatry, Johns Hopkins Hosp 1990; **Fac Appt:** Prof Psyc, Johns Hopkins Univ

Southeast

Anton, Raymond F MD [AdP] - **Spec Exp:** Alcohol Abuse; Clinical Trials; **Hospital:** MUSC Med Ctr; **Address:** MUSC Dept Psychiatry, 67 President St, Box 250861, Charleston, SC 29425; **Phone:** 843-792-1226; **Board Cert:** Psychiatry 1982; **Med School:** UMDNJ-Rutgers Med Sch 1976; **Resid:** Psychiatry, Yale-New Haven Hosp/CT Mental Health Ctr 1980; **Fac Appt:** Prof Psyc, Med Univ SC

Midwest

Stine, Susan M MD/PhD [AdP] - **Spec Exp:** Addiction/Substance Abuse; Opiate Addiction; **Hospital:** John D. Dingell VA Med Ctr, Detroit; **Address:** Wayne State Univ Sch Med, Dept Psychiatry, 2761 E Jefferson Ave, Detroit, MI 48207; **Phone:** 313-993-9879; **Board Cert:** Psychiatry 1993; Addiction Psychiatry 2002; **Med School:** Univ Miami Sch Med 1983; **Resid:** Psychiatry, Yale-New Haven Hosp 1987; **Fac Appt:** Assoc Prof Psyc, Wayne State Univ

Great Plains and Mountains

Howell, Elizabeth F MD [AdP] - **Spec Exp:** Opiate Addiction; Alcohol Abuse; Addiction/Substance Abuse; Pain Management; **Hospital:** Univ Utah Hlth Care, Lakeview Hosp; **Address:** Univ Utah Neuropsychiatric Inst, 501 Chipeta Way, Salt Lake City, UT 84108; **Phone:** 801-583-2500; **Board Cert:** Psychiatry 1985; Addiction Psychiatry 2003; Addiction Medicine 1986; **Med School:** Med Univ SC 1980; **Resid:** Pediatrics, MUSC Med Ctr 1981; Psychiatry, MUSC Med Ctr 1984; **Fellow:** Psychiatric Research, MUSC Med Ctr 1985; **Fac Appt:** Assoc Clin Prof Psyc, Univ Utah

Addiction Psychiatry

Southwest

Kosten, Thomas MD [AdP] - **Spec Exp:** Cocaine Addiction; Alcohol Abuse; Psychopharmacology; Opiate Addiction; **Hospital:** DeBakey VA Med Ctr-Houston, UT MD Anderson Cancer Ctr; **Address:** Michael DeBakey VA Medical Ctr, 2002 Holcombe Blvd, Research - Building 110, Houston, TX 77030; **Phone:** 713-794-7032; **Board Cert:** Psychiatry 1984; Addiction Psychiatry 2002; **Med School:** Cornell Univ-Weill Med Coll 1977; **Resid:** Psychiatry, Yale-New Haven Hosp 1981; **Fellow:** Epidemiology, Yale-New Haven Hosp 1983; **Fac Appt:** Prof Psyc, Baylor Coll Med

West Coast and Pacific

Schuckit, Marc A MD [AdP] - **Spec Exp:** Alcohol Abuse; Substance Abuse; Psychopharmacology; **Hospital:** UCSD Med Ctr; **Address:** UCSD Dept Psychiatry, 8950 Villa La Jolla Drive, Ste B-218, La Jolla, CA 92037; **Phone:** 858-822-0880; **Board Cert:** Psychiatry 1974; **Med School:** Washington Univ, St Louis 1968; **Resid:** Psychiatry, Wash Univ Affil Hosp 1971; Psychiatry, UCSD Med Ctr 1972; **Fac Appt:** Prof Psyc, UCSD

Walker, R Dale MD [AdP] - **Spec Exp:** Alcohol Abuse-Consultation; Drug Abuse-Consultation; Substance Abuse-Consultation; **Hospital:** OR Hlth & Sci Univ; **Address:** OHSU/One Sky Ctr, 3181 SW Sam Jackson Pk Rd, GH 151, Portland, OR 97239; **Phone:** 503-494-3703; **Board Cert:** Psychiatry 1982; **Med School:** Univ Okla Coll Med 1972; **Resid:** Psychiatry, Univ Oklahoma Med Ctr 1973; Psychiatry, UCSD Med Ctr 1977; **Fellow:** Public Health & Genl Preventive Med, Andriga Stampur; **Fac Appt:** Prof Psyc, Oregon Hlth & Sci Univ

CHILD & ADOLESCENT PSYCHIATRY

New England

Biederman, Joseph MD [ChAP] - **Spec Exp:** ADD/ADHD; Anxiety & Mood Disorders; Psychopharmacology; **Hospital:** Mass Genl Hosp; **Address:** 55 Fruit St Yawkey Bldg - rm 6900, Boston, MA 02114; **Phone:** 617-726-1743; **Board Cert:** Psychiatry 1983; Child & Adolescent Psychiatry 1984; **Med School:** Argentina 1971; **Resid:** Psychiatry, Hadassah Univ Hosp 1977; Psychiatry, Mass Genl Hosp 1981; **Fellow:** Child Psychiatry, Childrens Hosp 1979; **Fac Appt:** Prof Psyc, Harvard Med Sch

Herzog, David B MD [ChAP] - **Spec Exp:** Eating Disorders; Psychiatry in Physical Illness; **Hospital:** Mass Genl Hosp; **Address:** 2 Longfellow Place, Ste 200, Boston, MA 02114; **Phone:** 617-726-8470; **Board Cert:** Pediatrics 1980; Psychiatry 1982; Child & Adolescent Psychiatry 1986; **Med School:** Mexico 1973; **Resid:** Pediatrics, Univ Wisc 1975; Pediatrics, Boston City Hosp 1976; **Fellow:** Child & Adolescent Psychiatry, Chldns Hosp 1978; Psychiatry, Mass Genl Hosp 1980; **Fac Appt:** Prof Psyc, Harvard Med Sch

Hudziak, James MD [ChAP] - **Spec Exp:** ADD/ADHD; Obsessive-Compulsive Disorder; Psychopharmacology; **Hospital:** Fletcher Allen Health Care- Med Ctr Campus; **Address:** Univ Hlth Ctr, Dept Psychiatry, St Joseph's, rm 3213, Box 364SJ3, 1 S Prospect Drive, Burlington, VT 05401; **Phone:** 802-656-1084; **Board Cert:** Psychiatry 2005; Child & Adolescent Psychiatry 2005; **Med School:** Univ Minn 1988; **Resid:** Psychiatry, St Louis Chldns Hosp 1991; **Fac Appt:** Assoc Prof Psyc, Univ VT Coll Med

Leckman, James F MD [ChAP] - **Spec Exp:** Tourette's Syndrome; Obsessive-Compulsive Disorder; Autism; **Hospital:** Yale-New Haven Hosp, Yale Med Group; **Address:** Yale Child Study Ctr, 230 S Frontage Rd, Box 207900, New Haven, CT 06520-7900; **Phone:** 203-785-7971; **Board Cert:** Psychiatry 1980; Child & Adolescent Psychiatry 1982; **Med School:** Univ New Mexico 1973; **Resid:** Psychiatry, Yale Univ 1979; Child Psychiatry, Yale Chld Stdy Ctr 1980; **Fellow:** Psychiatry, Natl Inst Mental Hlth 1976; **Fac Appt:** Prof Psyc, Yale Univ

McDougle, Christopher J MD [ChAP] - **Spec Exp:** Autism & Developmental Disorders; Obsessive-Compulsive Disorder; Mental Retardation; **Hospital:** Mass Genl Hosp; **Address:** Lurie Center for Autism, 1 Maguire Rd, Lexington, MA 02421; **Phone:** 781-860-1700; **Board Cert:** Psychiatry 1992; Child & Adolescent Psychiatry 2006; **Med School:** Indiana Univ 1986; **Resid:** Psychiatry, Yale Univ Affil Hosp 1990; **Fellow:** Child & Adolescent Psychiatry, Yale Child Study Ctr 1995; **Fac Appt:** Prof Psyc, Harvard Med Sch

Sargent II, Albert J MD [ChAP] - **Spec Exp:** Eating Disorders; Suicide; Family Therapy; Trauma Psychiatry; **Hospital:** Tufts Med Ctr; **Address:** Tufts Medical Center, 800 Washington St, Box 1007, Boston, MA 02111; **Phone:** 617-636-8768; **Board Cert:** Pediatrics 1979; Psychiatry 1988; Child & Adolescent Psychiatry 1989; **Med School:** Univ Rochester 1973; **Resid:** Pediatrics, Univ Wisc Hosp 1977; Psychiatry, Hosp Univ Penn 1987; **Fellow:** Ambulatory Pediatrics, Univ Wisconsin Hosp 1976; Child Psychiatry, Philadelphia Child Guidance Ctr 1980; **Fac Appt:** Prof Psyc, Tufts Univ

Spencer, Thomas MD [ChAP] - **Spec Exp:** ADD/ADHD; **Hospital:** Mass Gen Hosp; **Address:** Mass Gen Hosp, 55 Fruit St, Ste YAW 6A, Boston, MA 02114; **Phone:** 617-724-5600; **Board Cert:** Psychiatry 1983; Child & Adolescent Psychiatry 1992; **Med School:** Univ Wisc 1978; **Resid:** Psychiatry, New England Med Ctr 1984; **Fellow:** Child & Adolescent Psychiatry, Mass Genl Hosp 1992; **Fac Appt:** Assoc Prof Psyc, Harvard Med Sch

Wilens, Timothy MD [ChAP] - **Spec Exp:** ADD/ADHD; Bipolar/Mood Disorders; Addiction/Substance Abuse; **Hospital:** Mass Genl Hosp; **Address:** Mass Genl Hosp, Dept Psyc, 55 Fruit St Yawkey Bldg - Ste 6A, Boston, MA 02114; **Phone:** 617-724-5600; **Board Cert:** Psychiatry 1990; Child & Adolescent Psychiatry 1991; Addiction Psychiatry 2004; **Med School:** Univ Mich Med Sch 1985; **Resid:** Internal Medicine, Henry Ford Hosp 1986; Psychiatry, Mass Genl Hosp 1988; **Fellow:** Child & Adolescent Psychiatry, Mass Genl Hosp 1990; **Fac Appt:** Assoc Prof Psyc, Harvard Med Sch

Mid Atlantic

Abright, A Reese MD [ChAP] - **Spec Exp:** Mood Disorders; ADD/ADHD; Anxiety Disorders; **Hospital:** Elmhurst Hosp Ctr; **Address:** 140 E 40th St, Ste 1B, New York, NY 10016; **Phone:** 212-867-3131; **Board Cert:** Psychiatry 1978; Child & Adolescent Psychiatry 1981; **Med School:** Univ Tex SW, Dallas 1973; **Resid:** Psychiatry, St Vincent's Hosp 1974; Psychiatry, NY Hosp-Cornell Med Ctr 1977; **Fellow:** Child & Adolescent Psychiatry, NY Hosp-Cornell Med Ctr 1979; **Fac Appt:** Clin Prof Psyc, NY Med Coll

Bird, Hector MD [ChAP] - **Spec Exp:** ADD/ADHD; Anxiety & Depression; Personality Disorders; **Address:** 300 W 72nd St, Ste 1F, New York, NY 10023-2004; **Phone:** 212-874-5311; **Board Cert:** Psychiatry 1975; Child & Adolescent Psychiatry 1977; **Med School:** Yale Univ 1965; **Resid:** Psychiatry, NY State Psych Inst 1971; NY State Psych Inst 1972; **Fellow:** Psychoanalysis, WA White Institute 1977; **Fac Appt:** Prof Emeritus Psyc, Columbia P&S

Child & Adolescent Psychiatry

Birmaher, Boris MD [ChAP] - **Spec Exp:** Bipolar/Mood Disorders; Anxiety Disorders; **Hospital:** Western Psych Inst & Clin-UPMC; **Address:** Western Psych Inst & Clinic-UPMC, 3811 O'Hara St, Pittsburgh, PA 15213; **Phone:** 412-246-5788; **Board Cert:** Psychiatry 1989; Child & Adolescent Psychiatry 1990; **Med School:** Colombia 1975; **Resid:** Psychiatry, Haddassah Med Coll-Hebrew U 1983; Psychiatry, Montefiore Med Ctr 1984; **Fellow:** Child Psychiatry, NY Presby-Columbia Med Ctr 1986; Child Psychiatry, NY Psych Inst-Columbia U 1987; **Fac Appt:** Prof Psyc, Univ Pittsburgh

Bogrov, Michael MD [ChAP] - **Spec Exp:** ADD/ADHD; Mood Disorders; **Hospital:** Sheppard Pratt Hlth Sys, Johns Hopkins Hosp (page 61); **Address:** 6501 N Charles St, P.O. Box 6815, Towson, MD 21204-6815; **Phone:** 410-938-4913; **Board Cert:** Psychiatry 1993; Child & Adolescent Psychiatry 1994; **Med School:** Emory Univ 1987; **Resid:** Psychiatry, Univ Maryland 1990; Critical Care Obstetrics, Johns Hopkins Hosp 1992; **Fac Appt:** Asst Prof Psyc, Johns Hopkins Univ

Brent, David A MD [ChAP] - **Spec Exp:** Suicide; **Hospital:** Western Psych Inst & Clin-UPMC; **Address:** Western Psych Inst & Clin, 3811 O'Hara St, Ste 315 BFT, Pittsburgh, PA 15213-2593; **Phone:** 412-246-5619; **Board Cert:** Pediatrics 1981; Psychiatry 1982; Child & Adolescent Psychiatry 1983; **Med School:** Jefferson Med Coll 1974; **Resid:** Psychiatry, Western Psych Inst 1982; **Fellow:** Psychiatry, Univ Colorado Med Ctr 1976; **Fac Appt:** Prof Psyc, Univ Pittsburgh

Coffey, Barbara J MD [ChAP] - **Spec Exp:** Tourette's Syndrome; ADD/ADHD; Obsessive-Compulsive Disorder; Psychopharmacology; **Hospital:** Mount Sinai Med Ctr (page 64); **Address:** Tics & Tourette's Clin & Rsch Program, 1240 Park Ave, New York, NY 10029; **Phone:** 212-659-1663; **Board Cert:** Psychiatry 1981; Child & Adolescent Psychiatry 1986; **Med School:** Tufts Univ 1975; **Resid:** Psychiatry, Boston Univ Med Ctr 1978; **Fellow:** Child & Adolescent Psychiatry, Tufts Univ 1980; **Fac Appt:** Prof Psyc, Mount Sinai Sch Med

Foley, Carmel A MD [ChAP] - **Spec Exp:** Mood Disorders; **Hospital:** Steven & Alexandra Cohen Chldn's Med Ctr of NY (page 67); **Address:** 420 Lakeville Rd, 1st Floor, New Hyde Park, NY 11040; **Phone:** 718-470-3550; **Board Cert:** Psychiatry 1979; Child & Adolescent Psychiatry 1981; Psychosomatic Medicine 2009; **Med School:** Ireland 1972; **Resid:** Psychiatry, St Patrick's Hosp 1976; Psychiatry, Lafayette Clinic 1977; **Fellow:** Child & Adolescent Psychiatry, Lafayette Clinic 1979; **Fac Appt:** Assoc Prof Psyc, Albert Einstein Coll Med

Fornari, Victor MD [ChAP] - **Spec Exp:** Eating Disorders; Trauma Psychiatry; Post Traumatic Stress Disorder; **Hospital:** Zucker Hillside Hosp (page 67); **Address:** Zucker Hillside Hospital, Ambulatory Care Pavilion Lower Level, 75-59 263rd St, Glen Oaks, NY 11004; **Phone:** 718-470-3510; **Board Cert:** Psychiatry 1984; Child & Adolescent Psychiatry 1985; **Med School:** SUNY Downstate 1979; **Resid:** Psychiatry, Hosp Univ Penn 1982; **Fellow:** Child & Adolescent Psychiatry, LIJ Med Ctr 1984; **Fac Appt:** Prof Psyc, NYU Sch Med

Hertzig, Margaret MD [ChAP] - **Spec Exp:** Developmental Disorders; ADD/ADHD; **Hospital:** NY-Presby/Weill Cornell Med Ctr, NY (page 66); **Address:** 525 E 68th St, Box 140, New York, NY 10021-4870; **Phone:** 212-746-5712; **Board Cert:** Psychiatry 1968; Child & Adolescent Psychiatry 1975; **Med School:** NYU Sch Med 1960; **Resid:** Pediatrics, Jewish Hosp 1962; Psychiatry, Bellevue Psych Hosp 1964; **Fellow:** Psychiatric Research, NYU Sch Med 1966; **Fac Appt:** Prof Psyc, Cornell Univ-Weill Med Coll

Hirsch, Glenn S MD [ChAP] - **Spec Exp:** Anxiety & Mood Disorders; Tourette's Syndrome; Bipolar/Mood Disorders; ADD/ADHD; **Hospital:** NYU Langone Med Ctr (page 68), Bellevue Hosp Ctr; **Address:** NYU Child Study Center, 1 Park Ave Fl 7, New York, NY 10016; **Phone:** 212-263-8704; **Board Cert:** Psychiatry 1984; Child & Adolescent Psychiatry 1985; **Med School:** Albert Einstein Coll Med 1979; **Resid:** Psychiatry, New York Hosp-Cornell 1982; **Fellow:** Child & Adolescent Psychiatry, Columbia-Presby Med Ctr 1984; **Fac Appt:** Asst Prof ChAP, NYU Sch Med

Koplewicz, Harold S MD [ChAP] - **Spec Exp:** Anxiety & Mood Disorders; Psychopharmacology; ADD/ADHD; **Address:** Child Mind Inst, 445 Park Ave at 56th St, New York, NY 10022; **Phone:** 212-308-3118; **Board Cert:** Psychiatry 1983; Child & Adolescent Psychiatry 1984; **Med School:** Albert Einstein Coll Med 1978; **Resid:** Psychiatry, NY Hosp-Westchester Div 1981; Psychiatry, NY State Psych Inst 1983; **Fellow:** Psychiatric Research, NY State Psych Inst 1985

Leventhal, Bennett MD [ChAP] - **Spec Exp:** Autism; ADD/ADHD; Psychopharmacology; **Hospital:** NYU Langone Med Ctr (page 68); **Address:** 577 First Ave, New York, NY 10016; **Phone:** 212-263-8696; **Board Cert:** Psychiatry 1979; Child & Adolescent Psychiatry 1980; **Med School:** Louisiana State U, New Orleans 1974; **Resid:** Psychiatry, Duke Univ Med Ctr 1978; **Fellow:** Child & Adolescent Psychiatry, Duke Univ Med Ctr 1977; **Fac Appt:** Prof Psyc, NYU Sch Med

Pomeroy, John C MD [ChAP] - **Spec Exp:** Autism; Mental Retardation; Developmental Disorders; **Hospital:** Stony Brook Univ Med Ctr; **Address:** The Cody Center for Autism, 37 Research Way, East Setauket, NY 11733; **Phone:** 631-444-4660; **Board Cert:** Psychiatry 1984; Child & Adolescent Psychiatry 1988; **Med School:** England, UK 1973; **Resid:** Psychiatry, St Mary's Hosp 1979; **Fellow:** Child & Adolescent Psychiatry, Univ Iowa Hosps 1981; **Fac Appt:** Assoc Prof Psyc, SUNY Stony Brook

Rapoport, Judith MD [ChAP] - **Spec Exp:** Schizophrenia; Obsessive-Compulsive Disorder; **Hospital:** Natl Inst of Hlth - Clin Ctr; **Address:** 3010 44th Place NW, Washington, DC 20016; **Phone:** 202-966-7355; **Board Cert:** Psychiatry 1969; Child & Adolescent Psychiatry 1969; **Med School:** Harvard Med Sch 1959; **Resid:** Psychiatry, Mass Mental Hlth Ctr 1961; Psychiatry, St Elizabeth Hosp 1962; **Fellow:** Psychiatry, Karolinska Inst 1964; Child & Adolescent Psychiatry, Childns Hosp 1966

Riddle, Mark A MD [ChAP] - **Spec Exp:** Psychopharmacology; Anxiety Disorders; Mood Disorders; **Hospital:** Johns Hopkins Hosp (page 61); **Address:** 600 N Wolfe St, CMSC-346, Baltimore, MD 21287-3325; **Phone:** 410-955-2320; **Board Cert:** Psychiatry 1982; Child & Adolescent Psychiatry 1986; **Med School:** Indiana Univ 1977; **Resid:** Psychiatry, Yale-New Haven Hosp 1981; **Fellow:** Child & Adolescent Psychiatry, Yale Child Study Ctr 1983; **Fac Appt:** Prof Psyc, Johns Hopkins Univ

Rostain, Anthony L MD [ChAP] - **Spec Exp:** ADD/ADHD; Autism; Tourette's Syndrome; Asperger's Syndrome; **Hospital:** Penn Presby Med Ctr - UPHS (page 72); **Address:** Hosp Univ Penn, Dept Psychiatry, 3535 Market St Fl 2, Philadelphia, PA 19104; **Phone:** 215-746-7210; **Board Cert:** Pediatrics 1985; Psychiatry 1988; Child & Adolescent Psychiatry 1989; **Med School:** NYU Sch Med 1980; **Resid:** Pediatrics, Chldn's Hosp 1983; Psychiatry, Hosp Univ Penn 1987; **Fellow:** Child Psychiatry, Philadelphia Child Guidance Clin 1985; **Fac Appt:** Prof Psyc, Univ Pennsylvania

Turecki, Stanley K MD [ChAP] - **Spec Exp:** Temperamentally Difficult Child; ADD/ADHD; Parenting Issues; **Hospital:** Lenox Hill Hosp (page 67); **Address:** 136 E 64th St, Ste 1B, New York, NY 10065; **Phone:** 212-355-2535; **Board Cert:** Psychiatry 1978; Child & Adolescent Psychiatry 1981; **Med School:** South Africa 1961; **Resid:** Psychiatry, Tara Hospital 1969; Psychiatry, Mt Sinai Hosp 1971

Walkup, John MD [ChAP] - **Spec Exp:** Anxiety Disorders; **Hospital:** NY-Presby/Weill Cornell Med Ctr, NY (page 66); **Address:** NY Presby Hosp-Weill Cornell, Dept Psych, 525 E 68th St, Box 140, New York, NY 10065; **Phone:** 212-746-1891; **Board Cert:** Psychiatry 1987; Child & Adolescent Psychiatry 1992; **Med School:** Univ Minn 1982; **Resid:** Psychiatry, Yale Univ Med Sch 1985; **Fellow:** Child Psychiatry, Yale Chld Study Ctr 1988; **Fac Appt:** Asst Prof Psyc, Johns Hopkins Univ

Child & Adolescent Psychiatry

Southeast

Deas, Deborah V MD [ChAP] - **Spec Exp:** Addiction/Substance Abuse; Dual Diagnosis; Substance Abuse in ADHD Patients; **Hospital:** MUSC Med Ctr; **Address:** MUSC, Ctr for Drug & Alcohol Programs, 67 President St, Charleston, SC 29425; **Phone:** 843-792-5214; **Board Cert:** Psychiatry 2005; Child & Adolescent Psychiatry 2007; **Med School:** Med Univ SC 1989; **Resid:** Psychiatry, MUSC Med Ctr 1992; **Fellow:** Child & Adolescent Psychiatry, MUSC Med Ctr 1994; Addiction Psychiatry, MUSC/Natl Inst Alcohol Abuse & Alcoholism 1994; **Fac Appt:** Prof Psyc, Med Univ SC

Heston, Jerry D MD [ChAP] - **Spec Exp:** ADD/ADHD; Depression; Asperger's Syndrome; **Hospital:** Le Bonheur Chldns Med Ctr, St. Jude Children's Research Hosp; **Address:** Child & Adolescent Psychiatric Assocs, 1135 Cully Rd, Ste 100, Cordova, TN 38016; **Phone:** 901-752-1980; **Board Cert:** Psychiatry 1988; Child & Adolescent Psychiatry 1989; **Med School:** Univ S Fla Coll Med 1981; **Resid:** Pediatrics, LeBonheur Chldns Hosp 1984; Psychiatry, Univ Tennessee Affil Hosp 1986; **Fellow:** Child & Adolescent Psychiatry, Univ Tennessee Affil Hosp 1988; **Fac Appt:** Clin Prof Psyc, Univ Tenn Coll Med

Sexson, Sandra G B MD [ChAP] - **Spec Exp:** Psychiatry in Transplant Patients; Death & Dying; **Hospital:** Med Coll of GA Hosp and Clin (MCG Health Inc); **Address:** Medical College Georgia, Dept Psych & Health Behavior, 997 St Sebastian Way, Augusta, GA 30912; **Phone:** 706-721-6699; **Board Cert:** Psychiatry 1980; Child & Adolescent Psychiatry 2004; **Med School:** Univ Miss 1971; **Resid:** Psychiatry, Tex Hlth Sci Ctr 1974; Child Psychiatry, Washington Univ Affil Hosp 1978; **Fac Appt:** Prof Psyc, Med Coll GA

Midwest

Alessi, Norman E MD [ChAP] - **Spec Exp:** Mood Disorders; Autism; Cognitive Psychotherapy; ADD/ADHD; **Hospital:** Univ of Michigan Hosp; **Address:** 325 E Eisenhower Pkwy, Ste 6, Ann Arbor, MI 48108; **Phone:** 734-222-6222; **Board Cert:** Psychiatry 1982; Child & Adolescent Psychiatry 1985; **Med School:** Emory Univ 1976; **Resid:** Psychiatry, Univ Mich Med Ctr 1980; Child Psychiatry, Univ Mich Med Ctr 1981; **Fellow:** Child & Adolescent Psychiatry, Univ Mich Med Ctr 1983; **Fac Appt:** Prof Emeritus Psyc, Univ Mich Med Sch

Boxer, Gary H MD [ChAP] - **Spec Exp:** ADD/ADHD; Parenting Issues; Mood Disorders; Behavioral Disorders; **Hospital:** St. Louis Chldns Hosp, Barnes-Jewish Hosp; **Address:** St Louis Chldns Hosp, Dept Psychiatry, 24 S Kingshighway Blvd, St Louis, MO 63108; **Phone:** 314-286-1700; **Board Cert:** Psychiatry 1986; Child & Adolescent Psychiatry 1988; **Med School:** Univ Colorado 1980; **Resid:** Psychiatry, Univ Michigan Med Ctr 1983; **Fellow:** Child Psychiatry, Univ Colorado 1985; **Fac Appt:** Assoc Prof Psyc, Washington Univ, St Louis

Campo, John V MD [ChAP] - **Spec Exp:** Psychosomatic Disorders; Psychiatry in Physical Illness; **Hospital:** Nationwide Chldn's Hosp, Ohio St Univ Med Ctr; **Address:** Columbus Chldn's Hosp, 700 Childrens Drive, Dept Psychiatry, Columbus, OH 43205; **Phone:** 614-722-2291; **Board Cert:** Pediatrics 1986; Psychiatry 1989; Child & Adolescent Psychiatry 1993; **Med School:** Univ Pennsylvania 1982; **Resid:** Pediatrics, Childrens Hosp 1985; Psychiatry, West Psych Inst Clin 1989; **Fac Appt:** Prof Psyc, Ohio State Univ

Dulcan, Mina K MD [ChAP] - **Spec Exp:** ADD/ADHD; **Hospital:** Lurie Chldn's Hosp-Chicago, Northwestern Meml Hosp; **Address:** Lurie Chldn's Hosp, Dept Psych, 225 E Chicago Ave, Box 10, Chicago, IL 60611; **Phone:** 312-227-3413; **Board Cert:** Psychiatry 1978; Child & Adolescent Psychiatry 1979; **Med School:** Penn State Coll Med 1974; **Resid:** Psychiatry, Western Psych Inst/Clinic 1977; **Fellow:** Child Psychiatry, Western Psych Inst 1978; **Fac Appt:** Prof Psyc, Northwestern Univ

Luby, Joan L MD [ChAP] - **Spec Exp:** Mood Disorders; **Hospital:** Barnes-Jewish Hosp; **Address:** Wash Univ Sch Med, Dept Psyc, 660 S Euclid Ave, Box 8134, St Louis, MO 63110; **Phone:** 314-286-1700; **Board Cert:** Psychiatry 1993; Child & Adolescent Psychiatry 1993; **Med School:** Wayne State Univ 1985; **Resid:** Psychiatry, Stanford Univ Sch Med 1988; **Fellow:** Child & Adolescent Psychiatry, Stanford Univ Sch Med 1990; **Fac Appt:** Assoc Prof Psyc, Washington Univ, St Louis

Slomowitz, Marcia MD [ChAP] - **Spec Exp:** ADD/ADHD; Bipolar/Mood Disorders; Anxiety & Depression; **Hospital:** Northwestern Meml Hosp; **Address:** 333 N Michigan Ave, Ste 1125, Chicago, IL 60601; **Phone:** 312-726-1083; **Board Cert:** Psychiatry 1982; Child & Adolescent Psychiatry 1983; **Med School:** Univ Wisc 1977; **Resid:** Psychiatry, Univ Cincinnati Affil Hosp 1980; **Fellow:** Child & Adolescent Psychiatry, Univ Cincinnati Affil Hosp 1982; **Fac Appt:** Asst Prof Psyc, Northwestern Univ

Great Plains and Mountains

Hagman, Jennifer O MD [ChAP] - **Spec Exp:** Eating Disorders; Depression; Anxiety Disorders; **Hospital:** Chldn's Hosp - Aurora (CO); **Address:** Chldns Hosp, Dept Psychiatry, 13123 E 16th Ave, B130, Aurora, CO 80045; **Phone:** 720-777-2539; **Board Cert:** Psychiatry 1992; Child & Adolescent Psychiatry 1992; **Med School:** Univ Kansas 1986; **Resid:** Psychiatry, UC Irvine Med Ctr 1990; **Fellow:** Child & Adolescent Psychiatry, UC Irvine Med Ctr 1991; **Fac Appt:** Assoc Prof Psyc, Univ Colorado

Martini, D Richard MD [ChAP] - **Spec Exp:** Psychiatry in Physical Illness; Post Traumatic Stress Disorder; ADD/ADHD; Brain Injury; **Hospital:** Primary Children's Med Ctr; **Address:** Primary Chldns Med Ctr, 100 N Mario Capecchi Drive, Salt Lake City, UT 84113; **Phone:** 801-662-6755; **Board Cert:** Psychiatry 1987; Child & Adolescent Psychiatry 1990; **Med School:** Univ Nebr Coll Med 1982; **Resid:** Psychiatry, Univ Pittsburgh Med Ctr 1985; Child Psychiatry, Univ Pittsburgh Med Ctr 1987; **Fac Appt:** Prof Psyc, Univ Utah

Wamboldt, Marianne Z MD [ChAP] - **Hospital:** Chldn's Hosp - Aurora (CO); **Address:** Children's Hosp, Dept Psychiatry, 13123 E 16th Ave, B130, Aurora, CO 80045; **Phone:** 720-777-6096; **Board Cert:** Psychiatry 1986; Child & Adolescent Psychiatry 1991; **Med School:** Univ Wisc 1982; **Resid:** Psychiatry, Univ Wisconsin Hosp 1986

Southwest

Bleiberg, Efrain MD [ChAP] - **Spec Exp:** Trauma Psychiatry; Personality Disorders; **Hospital:** Menninger Clinic; **Address:** Menninger Hosp & Clinic, 2801 Gessner Drive, Box 809045, Houston, TX 77280-9045; **Phone:** 713-275-5213; **Board Cert:** Psychiatry 1985; Child & Adolescent Psychiatry 1986; **Med School:** Mexico 1976; **Resid:** Psychiatry, Menninger Fdn 1980; **Fellow:** Child & Adolescent Psychiatry, Menninger Fdn 1981

Emslie, Graham J MD [ChAP] - **Spec Exp:** Depression; **Hospital:** Chldns Med Ctr of Dallas; **Address:** UT SW Med Ctr at Dallas, 5323 Harry Hines Blvd, Dallas, TX 75235; **Phone:** 214-456-5900; **Board Cert:** Psychiatry 1981; **Med School:** Scotland, UK 1974; **Resid:** Psychiatry, Univ Rochester 1978; Child Psychiatry, Stanford Med Ctr 1981; **Fac Appt:** Prof Psyc, Univ Tex SW, Dallas

Zeanah Jr, Charles H MD [ChAP] - **Spec Exp:** Attachment Disorders; Abuse/Neglect; Post Traumatic Stress Disorder; Infant-Toddler Psychiatry; **Hospital:** Tulane Med Ctr; **Address:** Tulane University School of Med, 1430 Tulane Ave, Box 8055, New Orleans, LA 70112; **Phone:** 504-988-5402; **Board Cert:** Psychiatry 1983; Child & Adolescent Psychiatry 1983; **Med School:** Tulane Univ 1977; **Resid:** Psychiatry, Duke Univ Med Ctr 1980; Child Psychiatry, Stanford Univ Med Ctr 1982; **Fellow:** Research, Stanford Univ 1984; **Fac Appt:** Prof Psyc, Tulane Univ

Child & Adolescent Psychiatry

West Coast and Pacific

King, Bryan H MD [ChAP] - **Spec Exp:** Autism; Developmental Disorders; Behavioral Disorders; **Hospital:** Seattle Chldns Hosp; **Address:** Seattle Children's Hospital, PO Box 5371, Seattle, WA 98145; **Phone:** 206-987-4080; **Board Cert:** Psychiatry 1991; Child & Adolescent Psychiatry 2004; **Med School:** Med Coll Wisc 1983; **Resid:** Psychiatry, UCLA Neuropsych Inst 1987; **Fellow:** Child & Adolescent Psychiatry, UCLA Neuropsych Inst 1990; **Fac Appt:** Prof Psyc, Univ Wash

Kwon, Hower MD [ChAP] - **Spec Exp:** Anxiety & Mood Disorders; ADD/ADHD; Developmental Disorders; **Hospital:** Univ Wash Med Ctr; **Address:** Bellevue Child Behavior Ctr, 365 118th Ave SE, Ste 118, Bellevue, WA 98005; **Phone:** 425-454-2911; **Board Cert:** Psychiatry 2009; Child & Adolescent Psychiatry 2009; **Med School:** NYU Sch Med 1993; **Resid:** Psychiatry, UCLA Neuropsychiatric Ins 1996; **Fellow:** Child & Adolescent Psychiatry, UCLA Neuropsychiatric Inst 1999; **Fac Appt:** Asst Clin Prof Psyc, Univ Wash

McCracken, James T MD [ChAP] - **Spec Exp:** Obsessive-Compulsive Disorder; Tourette's Syndrome; **Hospital:** Resnick Neuropsychiatric Hosp at UCLA; **Address:** UCLA Neuropsychiatric Inst, 760 Westwood Plaza, Ste 48-270, Los Angeles, CA 90024; **Phone:** 310-825-0470; **Board Cert:** Psychiatry 1986; Child & Adolescent Psychiatry 1988; **Med School:** Baylor Coll Med 1980; **Resid:** Psychiatry, Duke Univ Med Ctr 1984; **Fellow:** Child & Adolescent Psychiatry, UCLA Neuropsych Inst 1985; **Fac Appt:** Prof Psyc, UCLA

McKelvey, Robert S MD [ChAP] - **Spec Exp:** Suicide; Depression; Cross Cultural Psychiatry; Anxiety Disorders; **Hospital:** Doernbecher Chldns Hosp/OHSU; **Address:** 5520 SW Macadam Ave, Ste 265, Portland, OR 97239; **Phone:** 971-219-8363; **Board Cert:** Psychiatry 1980; Child & Adolescent Psychiatry 1982; **Med School:** Dartmouth Med Sch 1974; **Resid:** Psychiatry, Cambridge Hosp 1977; **Fellow:** Child Psychiatry, McLean Hosp 1979; **Fac Appt:** Prof Psyc, Oregon Hlth & Sci Univ

Ponton, Lynn Elisabeth MD [ChAP] - **Spec Exp:** Behavioral Disorders; Eating Disorders; **Hospital:** UCSF Med Ctr; **Address:** 201 Edgewood Ave, San Francisco, CA 94117; **Phone:** 415-664-3039; **Board Cert:** Psychiatry 1985; Child & Adolescent Psychiatry 1985; **Med School:** Univ Wisc 1978; **Resid:** Psychiatry, Hosp Univ Penn 1980; Psychiatry, UCSF Med Ctr 1981; **Fellow:** Child & Adolescent Psychiatry, UCSF Med Ctr 1983; **Fac Appt:** Prof Psyc, UCSF

Russell, Andrew T MD [ChAP] - **Spec Exp:** ADD/ADHD; Schizophrenia; Developmental Disorders; **Hospital:** Resnick Neuropsychiatric Hosp at UCLA; **Address:** Semel Inst, 760 Westwood Plaza, Ste 48-240B, Los Angeles, CA 90095; **Phone:** 310-825-0389; **Board Cert:** Psychiatry 1980; Child & Adolescent Psychiatry 2004; **Med School:** Univ Colorado 1970; **Resid:** Psychiatry, UCLA Med Ctr 1973; **Fellow:** Child & Adolescent Psychiatry, UCLA Med Ctr 1977; **Fac Appt:** Clin Prof Psyc, UCLA

Steiner, Hans MD [ChAP] - **Spec Exp:** Aggression Disorders; Eating Disorders; Trauma Psychiatry; Psychosomatic Disorders; **Hospital:** Stanford Univ Hosp & Clinics, Lucile Packard Chldn's Hosp; **Address:** 401 Quarry Rd, rm 3324, Stanford, CA 94305-5719; **Phone:** 650-723-5511; **Board Cert:** Psychiatry 1979; Child & Adolescent Psychiatry 1981; **Med School:** Austria 1972; **Resid:** Psychiatry, SUNY Syracuse Med Ctr 1976; **Fellow:** Child & Adolescent Psychiatry, Univ Mich Hosps 1978; **Fac Appt:** Prof Emeritus Psyc, Stanford Univ

Terr, Lenore MD [ChAP] - **Spec Exp:** Trauma Psychiatry; **Hospital:** UCSF Med Ctr; **Address:** Dept Psychiatry, 505 Parnassus Ave, San Francisco, CA 94143; **Phone:** 415-433-7800; **Board Cert:** Psychiatry 1968; Child & Adolescent Psychiatry 1969; **Med School:** Univ Mich Med Sch 1961; **Resid:** Psychiatry, Univ Mich Med Ctr 1964; **Fellow:** Child & Adolescent Psychiatry, Univ Mich 1966; **Fac Appt:** Clin Prof Psyc, UCSF

GERIATRIC PSYCHIATRY

Mid Atlantic

Greenwald, Blaine MD [GerPsy] - **Spec Exp:** Depression; Dementia; **Hospital:** Zucker Hillside Hosp (page 67), N Shore Univ Hosp (page 67); **Address:** Zucker Hillside Hospital - ACP 2102, North Shore-Long Island Jewish Health System, 75-59 263rd St, Glen Oaks, NY 11004; **Phone:** 718-470-8159; **Board Cert:** Psychiatry 1983; Geriatric Psychiatry 2000; **Med School:** NY Med Coll 1978; **Resid:** Psychiatry, Mt Sinai Hosp 1982; **Fellow:** Geriatric Psychiatry, Mt Sinai Hosp/Bronx VA Hosp 1983; **Fac Appt:** Assoc Prof Psyc, Hofstra N Shore-LIJ Sch Med

Kennedy, Gary MD [GerPsy] - **Spec Exp:** Alzheimer's Disease; Dementia; Depression; **Hospital:** Montefiore Med Ctr-Moses Campus, NY; **Address:** Dept of Psychiatry & Behavioral Sciences, Montefiore Medical Center, 111 E 210th St, Bronx, NY 10467-2490; **Phone:** 718-920-6270; **Board Cert:** Psychiatry 1980; Geriatric Psychiatry 2010; Psychosomatic Medicine 2005; **Med School:** Univ Tex, San Antonio 1975; **Resid:** Psychiatry, VA Hosp-Univ Texas 1979; **Fellow:** Geriatric Psychiatry, Montefiore Med Ctr 1981; Psychosomatic Medicine, Montefiore Med Ctr 1983; **Fac Appt:** Prof Psyc, Albert Einstein Coll Med

Lyketsos, Constantine G MD [GerPsy] - **Spec Exp:** Alzheimer's Disease; Neuro-Psychiatry; Depression; Dementia; **Hospital:** Johns Hopkins Bayview Med Ctr (page 61), Johns Hopkins Hosp (page 61); **Address:** Johns Hopkins Bayview Med Ctr, 5300 Alpha Commons Drive Fl 4, Baltimore, MD 21224; **Phone:** 410-550-0062; **Board Cert:** Psychiatry 1994; Psychosomatic Medicine 2005; **Med School:** Washington Univ, St Louis 1988; **Resid:** Psychiatry, Johns Hopkins Hosp 1992; **Fellow:** Neuropsychiatry, Johns Hopkins Hosp 1994; **Fac Appt:** Prof Psyc, Johns Hopkins Univ

Reisberg, Barry MD [GerPsy] - **Spec Exp:** Alzheimer's Disease; Dementia; Cognitive Loss in Aging; Depression; **Hospital:** NYU Langone Med Ctr (page 68); **Address:** 145 E 32 St, Fl 5, Ste 508, rm 508, New York, NY 10016-6055; **Phone:** 212-263-8550; **Board Cert:** Psychiatry 1976; Geriatric Psychiatry 2012; **Med School:** NY Med Coll 1972; **Resid:** Psychiatry, Metropolitan Hosp 1975; **Fellow:** Psychiatric Research, Univ London 1975; **Fac Appt:** Prof Psyc, NYU Sch Med

Rovner, Barry W MD [GerPsy] - **Spec Exp:** Alzheimer's Disease; Behavioral Problems & Dementia; **Hospital:** Thomas Jefferson Univ Hosp; **Address:** Jefferson Hosp Neuroscience, 900 Walnut St, Ste 200, Philadelphia, PA 19107; **Phone:** 215-503-1254; **Board Cert:** Psychiatry 1985; Geriatric Psychiatry 2011; **Med School:** Jefferson Med Coll 1980; **Resid:** Psychiatry, Johns Hopkins Hosp 1984; **Fac Appt:** Assoc Prof Psyc, Jefferson Med Coll

Streim, Joel E MD [GerPsy] - **Spec Exp:** Psychiatry in Physical Illness; Psychiatric Barriers to Physical Rehab; Alzheimer's Disease; **Hospital:** Hosp Univ Penn - UPHS (page 72), VA Med Ctr - Philadelphia; **Address:** Univ Penn Geriatric Psychiatry, 3535 Market St, rm 3053, Philadelphia, PA 19104; **Phone:** 215-615-3086; **Board Cert:** Psychiatry 1988; Geriatric Psychiatry 2009; **Med School:** Univ Rochester 1978; **Resid:** Internal Medicine, Rochester Genl Hosp 1981; Psychiatry, Univ Wisconsin Hosp 1985; **Fellow:** Liaison Psychiatry, Univ Rochester/Strong Mem 1981; Geriatric Psychiatry, VA Med Ctr 1988; **Fac Appt:** Prof Psyc, Univ Pennsylvania

Geriatric Psychiatry

Southeast

Holroyd, Suzanne MD [GerPsy] - **Spec Exp:** Dementia; Psychoses-Late Onset; Mood Disorders; **Hospital:** Univ of Virginia Health Sys; **Address:** Univ of Virginia Health Sys, Dept Psych, Box 800623, Charlottesville, VA 22908; **Phone:** 434-924-2241; **Board Cert:** Psychiatry 1992; Geriatric Psychiatry 2004; **Med School:** Univ VA Sch Med 1986; **Resid:** Psychiatry, Johns Hopkins Hosp 1990; **Fellow:** Geriatric Psychiatry, Johns Hopkins Hosp 1991; **Fac Appt:** Prof Psyc, Univ VA Sch Med

Tune, Larry E MD [GerPsy] - **Spec Exp:** Alzheimer's Disease; Dementia; Psychopharmacology; Psychoses-Late Onset; **Hospital:** Wesley Woods Ger Hosp, Emory Univ Hosp; **Address:** Wesley Woods Ctr, Dept Psychiatry, 1841 Clifton Rd NE, Atlanta, GA 30329; **Phone:** 404-728-6690; **Board Cert:** Psychiatry 1991; Geriatric Psychiatry 2004; **Med School:** Univ VA Sch Med 1975; **Resid:** Psychiatry, Johns Hopkins Hosp 1979; Neurology, Johns Hopkins Hosp 1983; **Fellow:** Psychopharmacology, Johns Hopkins Univ 1981; **Fac Appt:** Prof Psyc, Emory Univ

Midwest

Grossberg, George MD [GerPsy] - **Spec Exp:** Alzheimer's Disease; Depression; Behavioral Problems & Dementia; **Hospital:** St. Louis Univ Hosp; **Address:** St Louis Univ Sch Med, Dept Neurology and Psychiatry, 1438 S Grand Blvd, St Louis, MO 63104; **Phone:** 314-977-4850; **Board Cert:** Psychiatry 1982; Geriatric Psychiatry 2011; **Med School:** St Louis Univ 1975; **Resid:** Psychiatry, St Louis Univ Med Ctr 1979; **Fac Appt:** Prof N, St Louis Univ

Manepalli, Jothika M MD [GerPsy] - **Spec Exp:** Mood Disorders; Dementia; Depression; Palliative Care; **Hospital:** St. Louis Univ Hosp; **Address:** St Louis Univ Sch Med, Dept Neurology and Psychiatry, 1438 S Grand Blvd, St Louis, MO 63104; **Phone:** 314-977-4850; **Board Cert:** Psychiatry 1994; Geriatric Psychiatry 2007; **Med School:** India 1977; **Resid:** Psychiatry, Duke Univ Med Ctr 1987; Psychiatry, Barnes Hosp 1989; **Fellow:** Geriatric Psychiatry, St Louis Univ Hosp 1990; **Fac Appt:** Prof Psyc, St Louis Univ

Mellow, Alan M MD/PhD [GerPsy] - **Spec Exp:** Dementia; Depression; **Hospital:** VA Ann Arbor Healthcare Sys, Univ of Michigan Hosp; **Address:** Dept VA Affairs, (10N11), VISN Office, PO Box 134002, Ann Arbor, MI 48113-4002; **Phone:** 734-222-4350; **Board Cert:** Psychiatry 1988; Geriatric Psychiatry 2002; **Med School:** Northwestern Univ 1981; **Resid:** Internal Medicine, Univ Chicago Hosp 1982; Psychiatry, McLean Hosp-Harvard 1985; **Fellow:** Psychiatry, Natl Inst Mental Hlth 1988; **Fac Appt:** Prof Psyc, Univ Mich Med Sch

Great Plains and Mountains

Burke, William J MD [GerPsy] - **Spec Exp:** Alzheimer's Disease; Dementia; Depression; Panic Disorder; **Hospital:** Nebraska Med Ctr; **Address:** 986150 Nebraska Medical Center, Omaha, NE 68198-6150; **Phone:** 402-552-6062; **Board Cert:** Psychiatry 1986; Geriatric Psychiatry 2001; **Med School:** Univ Nebr Coll Med 1980; **Resid:** Internal Medicine, Univ Nebraska Med Ctr 1981; Psychiatry, Wash Univ Barnes Hosp 1984; **Fac Appt:** Prof Psyc, Univ Nebr Coll Med

West Coast and Pacific

Borson, Soo MD [GerPsy] - **Spec Exp:** Alzheimer's Disease; Psychiatry in Physical Illness; Dementia; Memory Disorders; **Hospital:** Univ Wash Med Ctr; **Address:** Univ Washington Med Ctr, 4225 Roosevelt Way NE, Ste 306, Seattle, WA 98105-6099; **Phone:** 206-598-7792; **Board Cert:** Psychiatry 1985; **Med School:** Stanford Univ 1969; **Resid:** Psychiatry, Univ Washington Med Ctr 1979; **Fellow:** Geriatric Psychiatry, Univ Washington Med Ctr 1981; **Fac Appt:** Prof Psyc, Univ Wash

Kramer, Barry A MD [GerPsy] - **Spec Exp:** Electroconvulsive Therapy (ECT); Depression; **Hospital:** Olympia Med Ctr, Kaiser Permanente LA Med Ctr; **Address:** PO Box 5792, Beverly Hills, CA 90209-5792; **Phone:** 323-932-5475; **Board Cert:** Psychiatry 1978; Geriatric Psychiatry 2001; **Med School:** Hahnemann Univ 1974; **Resid:** Psychiatry, Montefiore Hosp Med Ctr 1977; **Fellow:** Geriatric Psychiatry, UCLA-USC Long Term Gero Ctr 1986

Small, Gary W MD [GerPsy] - **Spec Exp:** Dementia; Alzheimer's Disease; Memory Loss; **Hospital:** UCLA Ronald Reagan Med Ctr; **Address:** 760 Westwood Plaza, 38-251 Semel Inst, Los Angeles, CA 90095-1759; **Phone:** 310-825-0291; **Board Cert:** Psychiatry 1983; **Med School:** USC Sch Med 1977; **Resid:** Psychiatry, Mass Genl Hosp 1981; **Fellow:** Psychiatry, UCLA Med Ctr 1983; **Fac Appt:** Prof Psyc, UCLA

Stein, Elliott M MD [GerPsy] - **Spec Exp:** Anxiety & Depression; Memory Disorders; Dementia; Stress Management; **Address:** Jewish Home of San Francisco, 302 Silver Ave, San Francisco, CA 94112; **Phone:** 415-406-1516; **Board Cert:** Psychiatry 1979; Geriatric Psychiatry 2001; **Med School:** Univ Miami Sch Med 1973; **Resid:** Psychiatry, Herrick Meml Hosp 1976; **Fac Appt:** Assoc Clin Prof Psyc, Univ Miami Sch Med

Veith, Richard C MD [GerPsy] - **Spec Exp:** Depression in Cardiovascular Disease; **Hospital:** Univ Wash Med Ctr; **Address:** Univ Washington Med Ctr, 1959 NE Pacific St, BB 1644, Box 356560, Seattle, WA 98195; **Phone:** 206-543-3752; **Board Cert:** Psychiatry 1979; Geriatric Psychiatry 2000; **Med School:** Univ Wash 1973; **Resid:** Psychiatry, Univ Wash Med Ctr 1977; **Fac Appt:** Prof Psyc, Univ Wash

Cleveland Clinic

Every life deserves world class care.

Cleveland Clinic
Center for Behavioral Health
9500 Euclid Avenue
Cleveland, OH 44195

Psychiatry and Psychology

Cleveland Clinic Center for Behavioral Health offers the full range of mental health and behavioral services for children, adolescents and adults. Our staff, who offer expert clinical evaluation and treatment, includes psychiatrists, psychologists, clinical nurse specialists, social workers, counselors and therapists. In addition to evaluating and treating patients, our proven staff educates trainees, professionals and the public on the latest developments in psychiatry and the behavioral sciences.

The Center for Behavioral Health includes:

- Adult psychiatry
- Child and adolescent psychiatry
- Chemical dependency
- General psychology
- Habit management
- Neuropsychology
- Psychosomatic medicine
- Psychiatric occupational therapy

The center is part of Cleveland Clinic Neurological Institute, a fully integrated entity with a disease-specific focus, combining medical, surgical and research specialists who treat children and adults with neurological and neurobehavioral disorders. Our staff of more than 300 specialists works with one of the largest and most diverse patient populations in the country. Our clinical expertise, academic achievement and innovative research have earned Cleveland Clinic Neurological Institute an international reputation for excellence and advanced patient care.

Our staff also serves as consultants for patients admitted to Cleveland Clinic medical and surgical units, and as key team members in the treatment of many conditions including epilepsy, movement disorders, organ transplantation, morbid obesity, chronic pain, headaches and cancer.

Offering Same-Day Appointments
Call 800.274.2009.

Treatment Guides
Cleveland Clinic has developed comprehensive treatment guides for many diseases and conditions. To download our free treatment guides, visit clevelandclinic.org/treatmentguides.

Online Medical Second Opinion
Call 216.444.3223 or 800.223.2273 ext. 43223 or email eclevelandclinic@ccf.org.

Out-of-State Patients Assistance
Call 800.223.2273, ext. 55580 or email medicalconcierge@ccf.org.

Visit Us At:
clevelandclinic.org

Follow Us On:
Facebook
www.facebook.com/clevelandclinic

Twitter
@ClevelandClinic

You Tube
www.youtube.com/clevelandclinic

Health Hub
health.clevelandclinic.org

MOUNT SINAI
SCHOOL OF
MEDICINE

THE MOUNT SINAI MEDICAL CENTER PSYCHIATRY
One Gustave L. Levy Place
Fifth Avenue and 100th Street
New York, NY 10029-6574
Physician Referral: 1-800-MD-SINAI (637-4624)
www.mountsinai.org/psychiatry
www.mssm.edu/psychiatry

THE DEPARTMENT OF PSYCHIATRY at Mount Sinai strives to bring breakthrough discoveries from neuroscience research to clinical care today. We provide services for children, adolescents, adults, and seniors, offering mental health evaluation and treatment for autism, attention-deficit hyperactivity disorder (ADHD), behavioral disorders, schizophrenia, Alzheimer's disease, mood and anxiety disorders, obsessive-compulsive disorder (OCD), tics and Tourette's Disorder (TD), substance abuse, post-traumatic stress disorder (PTSD), eating disorders, and personality disorders.

Clinical Services – The Department of Psychiatry is organized around key Centers of Excellence that link academic thought leaders to clinicians throughout the department. We offer a full range of diagnostic and treatment services, including psychotherapy, psychopharmacology, emergency services, electroconvulsive therapy, neuropsychological testing, and management of difficult clinical cases. We also provide mental health services in the Mount Sinai's World Trade Center Medical Monitoring and Treatment Program.

Specialty Programs – The Seaver Autism Center of Excellence offers a comprehensive assessment and treatment program that provides the finest patient care informed by the latest research. Our expert clinical staff is experienced in autism spectrum disorders, specializing in personalized and evidence-based treatment for very young children and high-functioning adults, as well as those individuals considered most difficult to assess and treat. The ADHD Center serves children and adults providing state-of-the-art psychiatric evaluation, psychological testing, behavioral and cognitive-behavioral treatments, and medication management. Our Center for Eating and Weight Disorders serves adults and children, offering innovative and evidence-based treatment for anorexia nervosa, bulimia nervosa, binge eating disorder, and obesity.

The Mood and Anxiety Disorders Program (MAP) is devoted to understanding the causes of mood and anxiety disorders and aims to advance the latest integrative treatment strategies for patients who suffer from major depression, bipolar disorder, PTSD, panic attacks, generalized anxiety disorder, and social phobia. MAP at Mount Sinai uses state-of-the-art brain imaging, and genetic, and clinical trials methods to enhance our understanding of brain processes associated with these disorders.

TRANSLATING KNOWLEDGE INTO NEW SOLUTIONS
Mount Sinai is at the forefront of unlocking the interactions between biological processes and the myriad states of the human mind. Among our major research programs in psychiatry are the Alzheimer's Disease Research Center, which conducts both basic science and clinical research, and The Seaver Autism Center for Research and Treatment, which is dedicated to unraveling the biological causes of this disorder and to developing innovative treatment strategies. In shedding important new light on mental illness, psychiatrists at Mount Sinai are frequently able to offer experimental interventions for treatment-resistant cases of depression, OCD, and other disorders.

The OCD Center of Excellence provides state-of-the-art diagnostic evaluation and specializes in treating severe or treatment-resistant OCD. The Center offers comprehensive evaluations, expert consultations, outpatient services, novel and evidence-based treatments, and research studies. We specialize in biological interventions for patients who have not responded to conventional therapies. In addition, the **Tics and TD Clinical and Research Program** is dedicated to enhancing the understanding, evaluation, and treatment of children, adolescents, and adults with tics, TD, and related problems such as OCD and ADHD.

BEHAVIORAL HEALTH

About the Behavioral Health Program
The Behavioral Health Program at NYU Langone Medical Center offers the most up-to-date treatments available for a wide range of disorders, including stress/anxiety, schizophrenia, depression (including medicine resistant depression), shyness, insomnia, low self-esteem, women's issues, sexual difficulties, panic attacks and phobias, manic-depression, obsession and compulsions and attention-deficit/hyperactivity disorder. The program serves its patients through a variety of approaches, including career counseling, assertiveness training, marital/couples counseling, and individual, group or family therapy. We specialize in the following areas:

Inpatient Services
An inpatient unit serves an adult population and includes a special Young Adult Program. The service combines comprehensive diagnostic assessment and treatment, including psychopharmacology, neuropsychology, psychotherapies and electroconvulsive therapy (a treatment in which seizures are electronically induced in anesthetized patients for therapeutic effect). A multidisciplinary team approach provides a continuum of behavioral and therapeutic modalities.

Outpatient Psychiatry
The Outpatient Psychiatry Program at Tisch Hospital provides expert treatment to individuals suffering from a broad range of mental disorders and emotional problems, including anxiety, depression (including medicine resistant depression), insomnia, manic-depression, reproductive psychiatry, attention-deficit hyperactivity disorder and schizophrenia. Our multidisciplinary team of licensed psychiatrists, psychologists and social workers offers the most up-to-date and scientifically validated treatments, such as psychotherapy, medication, or a combination of the two. Direct treatment with a member of faculty is also available as an option.

Scientific Innovation
At NYU Langone Medical Center, scientific innovation goes hand-in-hand with patient care. Our physician-scientists continue to lead the way in psychopharmacology and test new treatments for depression and bipolar disorder, with potentially life-altering results for the millions who suffer from these debilitating illnesses.

Sleep Disorders
The Sleep Disorders Consultation and Treatment Service provides thorough evaluation for a full range of sleep problems, including insomnia, nightmares, narcolepsy, sleepwalking and restless leg syndrome. Both behavioral and medication treatments are available to treat sleep disorders.

CHILD STUDY CENTER

The Child Study Center is the world's leading institution for transformative science and innovation in the diagnosis and treatment of children with mental illness and learning disabilities. Since 1997, The Child Study Center has treated thousands of children from around the world at its Faculty Group Practices in Manhattan and satellite clinical campuses in New Jersey and Long Island. Through its website, www.AboutOurKids.org, and through professional education programs, parents and practitioners are provided with the tools and knowledge needed to promote children's mental health. The Child Study Center, part of the Hassenfeld Pediatric Center, as well as NYU Langone's Department of Child and Adolescent Psychiatry, provides the following services:

Anxiety and Mood Disorders
The Anita Saltz Institute for Anxiety and Mood Disorders offers the most advanced treatment and evaluation of children, adolescents and young adults. Our psychopharmacologists are experts in understanding the issues of treating children with bipolar disorder and our researchers explore treatments for children with severe temper outbursts and adolescent depression.

Attention Deficit Hyperactivity and Behavior Disorders
The Institute for Attention Deficit Hyperactivity and Behavior Disorders focuses on the treatment of ADHD. Our Parent-Child Interaction Therapy Program (PCIT) offers state-of-the-art treatment for behavioral problems in young children and is the largest program of its kind in the Northeast.

Autism, Asperger's Syndrome and Communication Disorders
The Autism Spectrum programs at the Child Study Center provide extensive evaluations for toddlers and preschoolers with social and communication difficulties. Our Early Social Interaction treatment is a home-based intervention for children identified with symptoms of autism. Center specialists are also experienced at supporting the needs of teens and young adults who have been diagnosed with Asperger's.

Learning Disorders
The Institute for Learning and Academic Achievement evaluates children with suspected learning weaknesses or poor academic achievement using a multidisciplinary team-based approach.

Tics and Tourette Disorder
The Center's Tics and Tourette Clinical and Research programs are dedicated to the evaluation and treatment of individuals with tics, Tourette disorder and related problems. Treatment includes Habit Reversal Therapy (HRT).

PSYCHIATRY

About the Department of Psychiatry
The Department of Psychiatry is dedicated to improving the health and well-being of patients by delivering peerless psychiatric services and care. The Department is home to some of the nation's most respected clinical psychiatrists and psychologists, with specialties in psychoanalysis, psychopharmacology, behavioral therapy, child psychiatry, geriatric psychiatry and neuropsychiatry. We specialize in the following areas:

Inpatient Services
The Inpatient Services Unit combines comprehensive diagnostic assessment and treatment, including psychopharmacology, neuropsychology, psychotherapies and electroconvulsive therapy.

Outpatient Psychiatry
The Outpatient Psychiatry Program provides expert treatment to individuals suffering from a broad range of mental disorders and emotional problems, including anxiety, depression (including medicine resistant depression), insomnia, manic-depression, reproductive psychiatry, attention-deficit hyperactivity disorder and schizophrenia. Multidisciplinary teams of licensed psychiatrists, psychologists and social workers offer the most up-to-date, scientifically validated treatments, such as psychotherapy, medication, or a combination of both.

Post-Traumatic Stress Disorder
The Department of Psychiatry offers assessment and treatment of PTSD for victims of sexual and physical assault, natural disasters, terrorism and combat trauma. Treatment includes end-based cognitive behavioral therapy and evaluation of strategies for the prevention of insomnia, stress, anxiety and depression.

Memory Impairment
The Pearl Barlow Center for Memory Evaluation and Treatment specializes in treating patients with memory impairments caused by neurological, psychological and physical ailments, as well as memory issues resulting from medication side effects, anxiety, depression and the effects of normal aging from illnesses like Alzheimer's disease. The Center's multidisciplinary medical approach, integrated with advanced research, represents a first-of-its-kind in New York City for the treatment of memory disorders.

Human Sexuality
The Human Sexuality Treatment Program provides comprehensive evaluation of a full range of sexual dysfunction, including erectile disorder, premature ejaculation, male orgasmic disorder, female orgasmic and arousal disorders, vaginismus, dyspareunia, lack of desire, and unconsummated marriage and sexual incompatibility between partners.

Pulmonary Disease

a subspecialty of Internal Medicine

An internist who treats diseases of the lungs and airways. The pulmonologist diagnoses and treats cancer, pneumonia, pleurisy, asthma, occupational diseases, bronchitis, sleep disorders, emphysema and other complex disorders of the lungs.

Training Required: Three years in internal medicine *plus* additional training and examination for certification in pulmonary disease.

PULMONARY DISEASE

New England

Berk, John L MD [Pul] - **Spec Exp:** Amyloidosis; Interstitial Lung Disease; Pulmonary Fibrosis; **Hospital:** Boston Med Ctr; **Address:** Amyloid Treatment & Research Program, 72 E Concord St, Boston, MA 02118; **Phone:** 617-638-4317; **Board Cert:** Critical Care Medicine 2002; Internal Medicine 1986; Pulmonary Disease 2000; **Med School:** Case West Res Univ 1983; **Resid:** Internal Medicine, Univ Hosp/VAMC 1986; **Fellow:** Pulmonary Critical Care Medicine, Boston Univ Med Ctr 1991; **Fac Appt:** Assoc Prof Med, Boston Univ

Celli, Bartolome MD [Pul] - **Spec Exp:** Chronic Obstructive Lung Disease (COPD); Mechanical Ventilation; Respiratory Failure; **Hospital:** Brigham and Women's Hosp (page 57); **Address:** Brigham & Women's Hosp, Pulmonary Div, 75 Francis St, PBB Clin 3, Boston, MA 02115; **Phone:** 617-132-6770; **Board Cert:** Internal Medicine 1975; Pulmonary Disease 1978; **Med School:** Venezuela 1971; **Resid:** Internal Medicine, St Vincent Hosp 1973; Internal Medicine, Boston City Hosp 1976; **Fellow:** Pulmonary Disease, Boston Univ Med Ctr 1977; **Fac Appt:** Prof Med, Tufts Univ

Christiani, David MD [Pul] - **Spec Exp:** Occupational Lung Disease; **Hospital:** Mass Genl Hosp; **Address:** Mass Genl Hosp, Pulmonary Assocs, 55 Fruit St Cox 201B, Boston, MA 02114; **Phone:** 617-726-1721; **Board Cert:** Internal Medicine 1979; Occupational Medicine 1984; Pulmonary Disease 1988; **Med School:** Tufts Univ 1976; **Resid:** Internal Medicine, Boston City Hosp 1979; Occupational Medicine, Harvard Sch Public Hlth 1981; **Fellow:** Pulmonary Disease, Mass Genl Hosp 1987; **Fac Appt:** Prof Med, Harvard Med Sch

Enelow, Richard Ian MD [Pul] - **Spec Exp:** Interstitial Lung Disease; Lung Disease; **Hospital:** Dartmouth - Hitchcock Med Ctr; **Address:** Dartmouth-Hitchcock Medical Ctr, Dept Pulmonary & Critical Care Med, 1 Medical Center Drive, Lebanon, NH 03756; **Phone:** 603-650-5533; **Board Cert:** Internal Medicine 1986; Pulmonary Disease 2002; **Med School:** Boston Univ 1983; **Resid:** Internal Medicine, New Engl Deaconess Med Ctr 1986; **Fellow:** Pulmonary Disease, Univ VA Hlth Scis Ctr 1992; **Fac Appt:** Prof Med, Dartmouth Med Sch

Ernst, Armin MD [Pul] - **Spec Exp:** Interventional Pulmonology; Tracheal Stenosis; Airway Disorders; Lung Cancer; **Hospital:** Steward St Elizabeth's Med Ctr-Boston; **Address:** St. Elizabeth's Pulm $ Sleep Med Clin, 77 Warren St Fl 2, Brighton, MA 02135; **Phone:** 617-789-2936; **Board Cert:** Internal Medicine 2003; Pulmonary Disease 2006; Critical Care Medicine 2007; **Med School:** Germany 1988; **Resid:** Internal Medicine, Thoraxklinik-Univ Heidelberg; Internal Medicine, Univ Tex Hlth Sci Ctr 1993; **Fellow:** Pulmonary Critical Care Medicine, Deaconess Med Ctr/Brigham & Women's 1996; Interventional Pulmonology, Thoraxklinik-Univ Heidelberg; **Fac Appt:** Assoc Prof Med, Harvard Med Sch

Fanta, Christopher MD [Pul] - **Spec Exp:** Asthma; Chronic Obstructive Lung Disease (COPD); Bronchiectasis; **Hospital:** Brigham and Women's Hosp (page 57), Brigham and Women's Faulkner Hosp; **Address:** Brigham & Women's Hosp, 15 Francis St, Boston, MA 02115; **Phone:** 617-732-6770; **Board Cert:** Internal Medicine 1978; Pulmonary Disease 1980; **Med School:** Harvard Med Sch 1975; **Resid:** Internal Medicine, Peter Bent Brigham Hosp 1978; **Fellow:** Pulmonary Disease, Peter Bent Brigham Hosp 1980; **Fac Appt:** Assoc Prof Med, Harvard Med Sch

Friedman, Lloyd Neal MD [Pul] - **Spec Exp:** Tuberculosis; **Hospital:** Milford Hosp, Yale-New Haven Hosp; **Address:** Milford Hospital, 300 Seaside Ave, Milford, CT 06460; **Phone:** 203-876-4070; **Board Cert:** Internal Medicine 1983; Pulmonary Disease 1988; Critical Care Medicine 2009; **Med School:** Yale Univ 1979; **Resid:** Internal Medicine, Beth Israel Med Ctr 1980; Internal Medicine, Oregon Hlth Scis Univ 1983; **Fellow:** Pulmonary Intensive Care, Yale-New Haven Hosp 1988; **Fac Appt:** Clin Prof Med, Yale Univ

Hill, Nicholas S MD [Pul] - **Spec Exp:** Pulmonary Hypertension; **Hospital:** Tufts Med Ctr; **Address:** Tufts Med Ctr, 800 Washington St, #257, Boston, MA 02111; **Phone:** 617-636-4288; **Board Cert:** Internal Medicine 1978; Pulmonary Disease 1982; Critical Care Medicine 2009; **Med School:** Dartmouth Med Sch 1975; **Resid:** Internal Medicine, New England Med Ctr 1977; Cardiovascular Disease, Boston VA Med Ctr 1978; **Fellow:** Pulmonary Disease, Univ Mass Med Ctr 1979; Critical Care Medicine, Boston Univ Med Ctr 1982; **Fac Appt:** Prof Med, Tufts Univ

Irwin, Richard S MD [Pul] - **Spec Exp:** Cough; Asthma; Critical Care; **Hospital:** UMass Memorial Med Ctr; **Address:** UMass Meml Med Ctr-Univ Campus, 55 Lake Ave N, Worcester, MA 01655-0002; **Phone:** 508-856-1919; **Board Cert:** Internal Medicine 1972; Pulmonary Disease 1974; Critical Care Medicine 2007; **Med School:** Tufts Univ 1968; **Resid:** Internal Medicine, Tufts-New England Med Ctr 1970; **Fellow:** Pulmonary Disease, Columbia-Presby Hosp 1972; **Fac Appt:** Prof Med, Univ Mass Sch Med

Mahler, Donald A MD [Pul] - **Spec Exp:** Chronic Obstructive Lung Disease (COPD); Asthma; Breathing Disorders; **Hospital:** Dartmouth - Hitchcock Med Ctr; **Address:** Dartmouth-Hitchcock Med Ctr, Div Pulmonary Med, 1 Medical Center Drive, Lebanon, NH 03756-0001; **Phone:** 603-650-5533; **Board Cert:** Internal Medicine 1978; Pulmonary Disease 1980; **Med School:** Loyola Univ-Stritch Sch Med 1972; **Resid:** Internal Medicine, Dartmouth-Hitchcock Med Ctr 1977; **Fellow:** Pulmonary Disease, Yale-New Haven Hosp 1980; **Fac Appt:** Prof Med, Dartmouth Med Sch

Metersky, Mark L MD [Pul] - **Spec Exp:** Pulmonary Infections; Asthma; Bronchiectasis; **Hospital:** Univ of Conn Hlth Ctr, John Dempsey Hosp; **Address:** Univ Conn Hlth Ctr, 263 Farmington Ave, Farmington, CT 06030-2204; **Phone:** 860-679-8300; **Board Cert:** Internal Medicine 1988; Pulmonary Disease 2003; Critical Care Medicine 2003; Sleep Medicine 2009; **Med School:** NYU Sch Med 1985; **Resid:** Internal Medicine, Boston City Hosp 1988; **Fellow:** Pulmonary Critical Care Medicine, UCSD Med Ctr 1992; **Fac Appt:** Prof Med, Univ Conn

Millman, Richard P MD [Pul] - **Spec Exp:** Sleep Disorders/Apnea; **Hospital:** Rhode Island Hosp, Miriam Hosp; **Address:** 1 James P Murphy Hwy, West Warwick, RI 02893; **Phone:** 401-615-5878; **Board Cert:** Internal Medicine 1979; Pulmonary Disease 1982; Sleep Medicine 2009; **Med School:** Univ Pennsylvania 1976; **Resid:** Internal Medicine, Univ Mich Hosp 1979; **Fellow:** Pulmonary Disease, Univ Penn Hosp 1981; **Fac Appt:** Prof Med, Brown Univ

Nardell, Edward MD [Pul] - **Spec Exp:** Tuberculosis; Mycobacterial Infections; **Hospital:** Brigham and Women's Hosp (page 57); **Address:** Brigham & Women's Hosp, 15 Francis St, Boston, MA 02115; **Phone:** 617-732-6770; **Board Cert:** Internal Medicine 1975; Pulmonary Disease 1982; **Med School:** Hahnemann Univ 1972; **Resid:** Internal Medicine, Hahnemann Univ Hosp 1975; **Fellow:** Pulmonary Disease, Mass Genl Hosp 1977; **Fac Appt:** Assoc Prof Med, Harvard Med Sch

Redlich, Carrie MD [Pul] - **Spec Exp:** Occupational Lung Disease; **Hospital:** Yale-New Haven Hosp, Yale Med Group; **Address:** Yale Occupational & Environmental Med, 135 College St Fl 3 - Ste 392, New Haven, CT 06510; **Phone:** 203-785-4197; **Board Cert:** Internal Medicine 1986; Occupational Medicine 1990; Pulmonary Disease 2002; **Med School:** Yale Univ 1982; **Resid:** Internal Medicine, Yale-New Haven Hosp 1986; Occupational Medicine, Yale-New Haven Hosp 1987; **Fellow:** Pulmonary Disease, Univ Washington 1989; **Fac Appt:** Assoc Prof Med, Yale Univ

Pulmonary Disease

Rochester, Carolyn L MD [Pul] - **Spec Exp:** Chronic Obstructive Lung Disease (COPD); **Hospital:** VA Conn Hlthcre Sys-W Haven Campus, Yale-New Haven Hosp; **Address:** Yale Univ Sch Med, Pulm & Crit Care Sect, 300 Cedar St, Box 208057, New Haven, CT 06520-8057; **Phone:** 203-785-3207; **Board Cert:** Internal Medicine 1986; Pulmonary Disease 2002; Critical Care Medicine 2006; **Med School:** Columbia P&S 1983; **Resid:** Internal Medicine, Columbia Presby Med Ctr 1986; **Fellow:** Pulmonary Disease, Columbia Presby Med Ctr 1988; **Fac Appt:** Asst Prof Med, Yale Univ

Villanueva, Andrew G MD [Pul] - **Spec Exp:** Asthma; Chronic Obstructive Lung Disease (COPD); Pleural Disease; **Hospital:** Lahey Clin; **Address:** Lahey Clinic, Dept Pulmonary & Critical Care Med, 41 Mall Rd, Burlington, MA 01805; **Phone:** 781-744-8480; **Board Cert:** Internal Medicine 1983; Pulmonary Disease 1986; Critical Care Medicine 2007; **Med School:** UCSD 1980; **Resid:** Internal Medicine, Boston Univ Med Ctr 1984; **Fellow:** Pulmonary Disease, Boston Univ Med Ctr 1988; **Fac Appt:** Asst Clin Prof Med, Tufts Univ

White, David P MD [Pul] - **Spec Exp:** Sleep Disorders/Apnea; **Hospital:** Brigham and Women's Hosp (page 57); **Address:** 1505 Commonwealth Ave Fl 5, Boston, MA 02135; **Phone:** 617-783-1441; **Board Cert:** Internal Medicine 1978; Pulmonary Disease 1982; Sleep Medicine 2007; **Med School:** Emory Univ 1975; **Resid:** Internal Medicine, Univ Colo Med Ctr 1978; **Fellow:** Pulmonary Disease, Univ Colo Med Ctr 1982; **Fac Appt:** Prof Med, Harvard Med Sch

Mid Atlantic

Ahya, Vivek N MD [Pul] - **Spec Exp:** Transplant Medicine-Lung; Lymphangioleiomyomatosis(LAM); **Hospital:** Hosp Univ Penn - UPHS (page 72); **Address:** Penn Lung Center, Perelman Ctr for Advanced Medicine, 3400 Civic Center Blvd, 1st Fl W, Philadelphia, PA 19104; **Phone:** 215-662-3202; **Board Cert:** Pulmonary Disease 2010; Critical Care Medicine 2011; **Med School:** Boston Univ 1994; **Resid:** Internal Medicine, Barnes Jewish Hosp 1997; **Fellow:** Pulmonary Critical Care Medicine, Univ Penn 1998; **Fac Appt:** Assoc Prof Med, Univ Pennsylvania

Arcasoy, Selim M MD [Pul] - **Spec Exp:** Transplant Medicine-Lung; Chronic Obstructive Lung Disease (COPD); Interstitial Lung Disease; Pulmonary Embolism; **Hospital:** NY-Presby/Columbia Univ Med Ctr, NY (page 66); **Address:** Ctr for Advanced Lung Dis/Transp, 622 W 168th St PH Bldg Fl 14E - rm 104, New York, NY 10032-3720; **Phone:** 212-305-6589; **Board Cert:** Internal Medicine 2003; Pulmonary Disease 2006; Critical Care Medicine 2007; **Med School:** Turkey 1990; **Resid:** Internal Medicine, SUNY Downstate Med Ctr 1994; **Fellow:** Pulmonary Critical Care Medicine, Univ Pittsburgh Med Ctr 1998; **Fac Appt:** Prof Med, Columbia P&S

Bascom, Rebecca MD [Pul] - **Spec Exp:** Environmental Medicine; Chemical Exposure; Occupational Medicine; Pulmonary Fibrosis; **Hospital:** Penn State Milton S Hershey Med Ctr; **Address:** Hershey Med Ctr, Pulmonary Div, 500 University Drive, MC HO41, Hershey, PA 17033-0850; **Phone:** 717-531-6525 x7; **Board Cert:** Internal Medicine 1982; Occupational Medicine 1987; Pulmonary Disease 1988; **Med School:** Oregon Hlth & Sci Univ 1979; **Resid:** Internal Medicine, Johns Hopkins Hosp 1982; **Fellow:** Pulmonary Disease, Johns Hopkins 1986; Occupational Medicine, Johns Hopkins 1985; **Fac Appt:** Prof Med, Penn State Coll Med

Burschtin, Omar E MD [Pul] - **Spec Exp:** Sleep Disorders/Apnea; Airway Disorders; Asthma; **Hospital:** NYU Langone Med Ctr (page 68); **Address:** Sleep Medicine Assocs NYC, 11 E 26th St Fl 13, New York, NY 10010; **Phone:** 212-481-1818; **Board Cert:** Pulmonary Disease 2008; Sleep Medicine 2009; **Med School:** Uruguay 1988; **Resid:** Internal Medicine, NYU Downtown Hosp 1994; **Fellow:** Pulmonary Critical Care Medicine, NYU 1998; **Fac Appt:** Asst Prof Med, NYU Sch Med

Christie, Jason D MD [Pul] - **Spec Exp:** Transplant Medicine-Lung; **Hospital:** Penn Presby Med Ctr - UPHS (page 72); **Address:** Penn Lung Ctr, Pearlman Ctr, West Pavilion Fl 1, 3400 Civic Ctr Blvd, Philadelphia, PA 19104; **Phone:** 215-615-5864; **Board Cert:** Internal Medicine 2006; Pulmonary Disease 2009; Critical Care Medicine 2010; **Med School:** Columbia P&S 1993; **Resid:** Internal Medicine, Hosp Univ Penn 1996; **Fellow:** Pulmonary Disease, Hosp Univ Penn 1998; **Fac Appt:** Assoc Prof Med, Univ Pennsylvania

Cooke, Joseph T MD [Pul] - **Spec Exp:** Asthma; Lung Cancer; Critical Care; Emphysema; **Hospital:** NY-Presby/Weill Cornell Med Ctr, NY (page 66); **Address:** Weill Greenberg Center, Pulmonary/Critical Care Medicine, 1305 York Ave Fl 4, New York, NY 10021; **Phone:** 646-962-2333; **Board Cert:** Internal Medicine 1989; Pulmonary Disease 2002; Critical Care Medicine 2003; **Med School:** SUNY Downstate 1985; **Resid:** Internal Medicine, New York Hosp 1988; **Fellow:** Pulmonary Intensive Care, New York Hosp 1991; **Fac Appt:** Assoc Clin Prof Med, Cornell Univ-Weill Med Coll

Criner, Gerard J MD [Pul] - **Spec Exp:** Chronic Obstructive Lung Disease (COPD); Pulmonary Fibrosis; Pulmonary Hypertension; Critical Care; **Hospital:** Temple Univ Hosp; **Address:** Temple Univ Hosp, Pulmonary Med, 3401 N Broad St Fl 5, Philadelphia, PA 19140; **Phone:** 215-707-5555; **Board Cert:** Internal Medicine 1982; Pulmonary Disease 1986; Critical Care Medicine 2007; **Med School:** Temple Univ 1979; **Resid:** Internal Medicine, Temple Univ Hosp 1983; **Fellow:** Pulmonary Disease, Boston Univ 1986; **Fac Appt:** Prof Med, Temple Univ

Deitz, Joel L MD [Pul] - **Spec Exp:** Respiratory Failure; Chronic Obstructive Lung Disease (COPD); Cough; **Hospital:** Penn Presby Med Ctr - UPHS (page 72), Hosp Univ Penn - UPHS (page 72); **Address:** Penn-Presby Med Ctr, Pulmonology, 51 N 39th St, Philadelphia Heart Inst, Fl 1 Rear, Philadelphia, PA 19104; **Phone:** 215-662-8585; **Board Cert:** Internal Medicine 1980; Pulmonary Disease 1984; Critical Care Medicine 2007; **Med School:** Tufts Univ 1977; **Resid:** Internal Medicine, Med Coll Va Med Ctr 1980; **Fellow:** Pulmonary Disease, Duke Univ Med Ctr 1984; **Fac Appt:** Assoc Clin Prof Med, Univ Pennsylvania

Donahoe, Michael MD [Pul] - **Spec Exp:** Critical Care; Respiratory Distress Syndrome (ARDS); Chronic Obstructive Lung Disease (COPD); **Hospital:** UPMC Montefiore; **Address:** UPMC Montefiore Hosp, NW628, 3601 Fifth Ave Fl 4, Pittsburgh, PA 15213; **Phone:** 412-648-6161; **Board Cert:** Internal Medicine 1986; Pulmonary Disease 1988; Critical Care Medicine 2010; **Med School:** Hahnemann Univ 1983; **Resid:** Internal Medicine, UPMC Presbyterian 1086; **Fellow:** Pulmonary Critical Care Medicine, UPMC Presbyterian 1989; **Fac Appt:** Assoc Prof Med, Univ Pittsburgh

Greenberg, Harly MD [Pul] - **Spec Exp:** Sleep Disorders/Apnea; Lung Disease; Critical Care; **Hospital:** Long Island Jewish Med Ctr (page 67), N Shore Univ Hosp (page 67); **Address:** North Shore LIJ Sleep Disorders Ctr, 410 Lakeville Rd, Ste 107, New Hyde Park, NY 11040; **Phone:** 516-465-3899; **Board Cert:** Internal Medicine 1985; Pulmonary Disease 1988; Sleep Medicine 2011; **Med School:** NYU Sch Med 1982; **Resid:** Internal Medicine, North Shore Univ Hosp 1985; **Fellow:** Pulmonary Disease, NYU-Bellevue Hosp Ctr 1987; **Fac Appt:** Assoc Prof Med, Albert Einstein Coll Med

Hansen-Flaschen, John MD [Pul] - **Spec Exp:** Diagnostic Problems; Interstitial Lung Disease; Chronic Obstructive Lung Disease (COPD); **Hospital:** Hosp Univ Penn - UPHS (page 72); **Address:** Penn Lung Center, Perelman Center for Advanced Medicine, 3400 Civic Center Blvd, 1st Fl W, Philadelphia, PA 19104; **Phone:** 215-662-3202; **Board Cert:** Internal Medicine 1979; Pulmonary Disease 1982; **Med School:** NYU Sch Med 1976; **Resid:** Internal Medicine, Hosp Univ Penn 1981; **Fellow:** Pulmonary Critical Care Medicine, Hosp Univ Penn 1982; **Fac Appt:** Prof Med, Univ Pennsylvania

Pulmonary Disease

King, Earl D MD [Pul] - **Spec Exp:** Lung Cancer; Critical Care; Sleep Disorders; **Hospital:** Fox Chase Cancer Ctr (page 58); **Address:** Fox Chase Cancer Center, 333 Cottman Ave, Philadelphia, PA 19111; **Phone:** 215-728-5703; **Board Cert:** Internal Medicine 1989; Pulmonary Disease 2002; Critical Care Medicine 2003; Sleep Medicine 1995; **Med School:** Penn State Coll Med 1986; **Resid:** Internal Medicine, Temple Univ Med Ctr 1989; **Fellow:** Pulmonary Critical Care Medicine, Johns Hopkins Hosp 1993; Sleep Medicine, Johns Hopkins Hosp 1993

Kotloff, Robert M MD [Pul] - **Spec Exp:** Transplant Medicine-Lung; Lung Disease-Complex; Interstitial Lung Disease; Lymphangioleiomyomatosis(LAM); **Hospital:** Hosp Univ Penn - UPHS (page 72); **Address:** Perelman Ctr for Advanced Medicine, 3400 Civic Center Blvd, West Pavilion, 1st Fl, Philadelphia, PA 19104; **Phone:** 215-662-3202; **Board Cert:** Internal Medicine 1986; Pulmonary Disease 2005; Critical Care Medicine 2005; **Med School:** Yale Univ 1983; **Resid:** Internal Medicine, Temple Univ Hosp 1986; **Fellow:** Pulmonary Disease, Hosp Univ Penn 1990; **Fac Appt:** Prof Med, Univ Pennsylvania

Libby, Daniel M MD [Pul] - **Spec Exp:** Asthma; Lung Cancer; Interstitial Lung Disease; Chronic Obstructive Lung Disease (COPD); **Hospital:** NY-Presby/Weill Cornell Med Ctr, NY (page 66); **Address:** 635 Madison Ave, Ste 1101, New York, NY 10022; **Phone:** 212-628-6611; **Board Cert:** Internal Medicine 1977; Pulmonary Disease 1980; **Med School:** Baylor Coll Med 1974; **Resid:** Internal Medicine, NY Hosp 1977; **Fellow:** Pulmonary Disease, NY Hosp 1979; **Fac Appt:** Clin Prof Med, Cornell Univ-Weill Med Coll

Maxfield, Roger A MD [Pul] - **Spec Exp:** Emphysema & Asthma; Occupational Lung Disease; Lung Cancer; Bronchoscopy; **Hospital:** NY-Presby/Columbia Univ Med Ctr, NY (page 66); **Address:** Columbia Presbyterian Eastside, 16 E 60th St, Ste 320, New York, NY 10022-1002; **Phone:** 212-326-8415; **Board Cert:** Internal Medicine 1980; Pulmonary Disease 1986; **Med School:** Brown Univ 1977; **Resid:** Internal Medicine, Georgetown Univ Hosp 1980; **Fellow:** Pulmonary Disease, Bellevue-NYU Med Ctr 1985; **Fac Appt:** Clin Prof Med, Columbia P&S

Nash, Thomas MD [Pul] - **Spec Exp:** Asthma; Cough; Pneumonia; **Hospital:** NY-Presby/Weill Cornell Med Ctr, NY (page 66), Hosp For Special Surgery (page 60); **Address:** 310 E 72nd St, New York, NY 10021-4726; **Phone:** 212-734-6612; **Board Cert:** Internal Medicine 1981; Infectious Disease 1984; Pulmonary Disease 1988; **Med School:** NYU Sch Med 1978; **Resid:** Internal Medicine, New York Hosp-Cornell 1981; **Fellow:** Infectious Disease, New York Hosp-Cornell 1983; Pulmonary Disease, Meml Sloan Kettering Cancer Ctr 1985; **Fac Appt:** Assoc Clin Prof Med, NYU Sch Med

Nelson, Judith E MD [Pul] - **Spec Exp:** Palliative Care; Critical Care; **Hospital:** Mount Sinai Med Ctr (page 64); **Address:** Mt Sinai Medical Ctr, One Gustave Levy Pl, Box 1232, New York, NY 10029; **Phone:** 212-241-2587; **Board Cert:** Internal Medicine 1989; Pulmonary Disease 2002; Critical Care Medicine 2003; Hospice & Palliative Medicine 2005; **Med School:** NYU Sch Med 1986; **Resid:** Internal Medicine, Mt Sinai Med Ctr 1989; **Fellow:** Pulmonary Critical Care Medicine, Mt Sinai Med Ctr 1992; **Fac Appt:** Assoc Prof Med, Mount Sinai Sch Med

Niederman, Michael S MD [Pul] - **Spec Exp:** Infections-Respiratory; Emphysema; Respiratory Failure; Pneumonia; **Hospital:** Winthrop Univ Hosp; **Address:** 222 Station Plaza N, Ste 400, Mineola, NY 11501-3893; **Phone:** 516-663-2834; **Board Cert:** Internal Medicine 1980; Pulmonary Disease 1982; Critical Care Medicine 2007; **Med School:** Boston Univ 1977; **Resid:** Internal Medicine, Northwestern Univ Med Ctr 1980; **Fellow:** Pulmonary Disease, Yale-New Haven Hosp 1983; **Fac Appt:** Prof Med, SUNY Stony Brook

O'Donnell, Anne E MD [Pul] - **Spec Exp:** Bronchiectasis; Critical Care; Sleep Medicine; **Hospital:** Georgetown Univ Hosp; **Address:** Georgetown Univ Hosp-Pulm CCM, 3800 Reservoir Rd NW PHC Bldg Fl 5, Washington, DC 20007; **Phone:** 202-444-8830; **Board Cert:** Internal Medicine 1985; Pulmonary Disease 1988; Sleep Medicine 2007; Critical Care Medicine 2009; **Med School:** Georgetown Univ 1982; **Resid:** Internal Medicine, Georgetown Univ Hosp 1985; **Fellow:** Pulmonary Disease, Georgetown Univ Hosp 1988; **Fac Appt:** Assoc Prof Med, Georgetown Univ

Pack, Allan I MD/PhD [Pul] - **Spec Exp:** Sleep Disorders/Apnea; **Hospital:** Hosp Univ Penn - UPHS (page 72); **Address:** Penn Sleep Ctr, 3624 Market St, Ste 201, Philadelphia, PA 19104; **Phone:** 215-662-7772; **Med School:** Scotland, UK 1967; **Resid:** Internal Medicine, Univ Glasgow Med Ctr 1972; **Fellow:** Pulmonary Disease, Univ Glasgow 1975; **Fac Appt:** Prof Med, Univ Pennsylvania

Padilla, Maria L MD [Pul] - **Spec Exp:** Pulmonary Fibrosis; Transplant Medicine-Lung; Sarcoidosis; Pulmonary Hypertension; **Hospital:** Mount Sinai Med Ctr (page 64); **Address:** Mt Sinai Med Ctr, Div Pulmonology, One Gustave L Levy Pl, Box 1232, New York, NY 10029-6574; **Phone:** 212-241-5656; **Board Cert:** Internal Medicine 1978; Pulmonary Disease 1980; **Med School:** Mount Sinai Sch Med 1975; **Resid:** Internal Medicine, Mt Sinai Hosp 1978; **Fellow:** Pulmonary Disease, Mt Sinai Hosp 1980; Critical Care Medicine, Mt Sinai Hosp 1991; **Fac Appt:** Prof Med, Mount Sinai Sch Med

Palevsky, Harold I MD [Pul] - **Spec Exp:** Pulmonary Hypertension; Pulmonary Vascular Disease; Thromboembolic Disorders; Pulmonary Embolism; **Hospital:** Penn Presby Med Ctr - UPHS (page 72), Hosp Univ Penn - UPHS (page 72); **Address:** Penn Lung Ctr at Penn Presby Med Ctr, 51 N 39th St PHI Bldg Fl 1 Rear, Philadelphia, PA 19104; **Phone:** 215-662-8766; **Board Cert:** Internal Medicine 2007; Pulmonary Disease 2007; Critical Care Medicine 2007; **Med School:** Med Coll VA 1978; **Resid:** Internal Medicine, Hosp Univ Penn 1981; **Fellow:** Pulmonary Critical Care Medicine, Hosp Univ Penn 1984; **Fac Appt:** Prof Med, Univ Pennsylvania

Rossman, Milton D MD [Pul] - **Spec Exp:** Beryllium-induced Lung Disease; Sarcoidosis; Interstitial Lung Disease; Pulmonary Fibrosis; **Hospital:** Hosp Univ Penn - UPHS (page 72); **Address:** Penn Lung Center, Perelman Ctr for Advanced Medicine, 3400 Civic Center Blvd, 1st Fl W, Philadelphia, PA 19104-4283; **Phone:** 215-662-3202; **Board Cert:** Internal Medicine 1975; Pulmonary Disease 1978; **Med School:** Jefferson Med Coll 1970; **Resid:** Internal Medicine, Univ Hosps 1975; **Fellow:** Pulmonary Disease, Univ Penn 1977; **Fac Appt:** Prof Med, Univ Pennsylvania

Schluger, Neil MD [Pul] - **Spec Exp:** Tuberculosis; **Hospital:** NY-Presby/Columbia Univ Med Ctr, NY (page 66); **Address:** Div Pulm, Allergy & Crit Care Med, 630 W 168th St, PH-8 East, Rm 101, New York, NY 10032; **Phone:** 212-305-1544; **Board Cert:** Internal Medicine 1988; Pulmonary Disease 2003; **Med School:** Univ Pennsylvania 1985; **Resid:** Internal Medicine, St Lukes Hosp 1989; **Fellow:** Pulmonary Critical Care Medicine, NY Hosp-Cornell 1992; **Fac Appt:** Prof Med, Columbia P&S

Schwab, Richard MD [Pul] - **Spec Exp:** Sleep Disorders/Apnea; **Hospital:** Hosp Univ Penn - UPHS (page 72); **Address:** Penn Sleep Ctr, 3624 Market St, Fl 2, Ste 201, Philadelphia, PA 19104; **Phone:** 215-662-7772; **Board Cert:** Internal Medicine 1986; Sleep Medicine 2009; **Med School:** Univ Pennsylvania 1983; **Resid:** Internal Medicine, Hosp Univ Penn 1986; **Fellow:** Pulmonary Critical Care Medicine, Hosp Univ Penn 1991; **Fac Appt:** Prof Med, Univ Pennsylvania

Steiger, David MD [Pul] - **Spec Exp:** Rheumatologic Diseases of the Lung; Thromboembolic Disorders; Pulmonary Hypertension; Critical Care; **Hospital:** NYU Hosp For Joint Diseases (page 70), NYU Langone Med Ctr (page 68); **Address:** 305 2nd Ave, Ste 16, New York, NY 10003; **Phone:** 212-598-6422; **Board Cert:** Internal Medicine 1987; Pulmonary Disease 2002; Critical Care Medicine 2005; **Med School:** England, UK 1981; **Resid:** Internal Medicine, St Thomas's Hosp 1984; Internal Medicine, St Lukes Hosp 1989; **Fellow:** Pulmonary Disease, UCSF Med Ctr 1994; **Fac Appt:** Asst Prof Med, NYU Sch Med

Steinberg, Harry MD [Pul] - **Spec Exp:** Asthma; Emphysema; Lung Cancer; Pulmonary Hypertension; **Hospital:** Long Island Jewish Med Ctr (page 67), N Shore Univ Hosp (page 67); **Address:** 410 Lakeville Rd, Ste 107, 270-05 76th Ave, New Hyde Park, NY 11040; **Phone:** 516-465-5400; **Med School:** Temple Univ 1966; **Resid:** Internal Medicine, LI Jewish Med Ctr 1969; Pulmonary Critical Care Medicine, LI Jewish Med Ctr 1970; **Fellow:** Pulmonary Disease, Hosp Univ Penn 1974; **Fac Appt:** Prof Med, Hofstra N Shore-LIJ Sch Med

Sterman, Daniel H MD [Pul] - **Spec Exp:** Interventional Pulmonology; Lung Cancer; Mesothelioma; Gene Therapy; **Hospital:** Hosp Univ Penn - UPHS (page 72); **Address:** Penn Lung Center, Perelman Ctr for Advanced Medicine, 3400 Civic Ctr Blvd, 1st Fl W, Philadelphia, PA 19104-4283; **Phone:** 215-662-3202; **Board Cert:** Internal Medicine 2007; Pulmonary Disease 2007; Critical Care Medicine 2007; **Med School:** Cornell Univ-Weill Med Coll 1989; **Resid:** Internal Medicine, Hosp Univ Penn 1992; **Fellow:** Pulmonary Critical Care Medicine, Hosp Univ Penn 1997; **Fac Appt:** Assoc Prof Med, Univ Pennsylvania

Stover-Pepe, Diane E MD [Pul] - **Spec Exp:** Interstitial Lung Disease; Pulmonary Infections; Pulmonary Disease/Immunocompromised; Bronchiolitis Obliterans; **Hospital:** Meml Sloan-Kettering Cancer Ctr; **Address:** 1275 York Ave, New York, NY 10065; **Phone:** 212-639-8380; **Board Cert:** Internal Medicine 1975; Pulmonary Disease 1978; **Med School:** Albert Einstein Coll Med 1970; **Resid:** Internal Medicine, Harlem Hosp Ctr 1972; Internal Medicine, NY Hosp-Cornell Med Ctr 1975; **Fellow:** Pulmonary Disease, Montefiore Med Ctr 1977; **Fac Appt:** Prof Med, Cornell Univ-Weill Med Coll

Strollo, Patrick J MD [Pul] - **Spec Exp:** Sleep Disorders/Apnea; Respiratory Failure; **Hospital:** UPMC Montefiore, UPMC Presby, Pittsburgh; **Address:** Montefiore Univ Hosp, 3459 5th Ave, Ste S639.11, Pittsburgh, PA 15213; **Phone:** 412-692-2880; **Board Cert:** Internal Medicine 1984; Pulmonary Disease 1988; Sleep Medicine 2007; **Med School:** Uniformed Srvs Univ, Bethesda 1981; **Resid:** Internal Medicine, Wilford Hall Med Ctr 1984; **Fellow:** Pulmonary Disease, Wilford Hall Med Ctr 1987; **Fac Appt:** Prof Med, Univ Pittsburgh

Thomashow, Byron MD [Pul] - **Spec Exp:** Emphysema; Asthma; Respiratory Failure; Chronic Obstructive Lung Disease (COPD); **Hospital:** NY-Presby/Columbia Univ Med Ctr, NY (page 66); **Address:** 161 Fort Washington Ave, rm 311, New York, NY 10032; **Phone:** 212-305-5261; **Board Cert:** Internal Medicine 1977; Pulmonary Disease 1980; **Med School:** Columbia P&S 1974; **Resid:** Internal Medicine, Roosevelt Hosp 1977; Pulmonary Disease, Roosevelt Hosp 1978; **Fellow:** Pulmonary Disease, Harlem Hosp Ctr 1979; **Fac Appt:** Clin Prof Med, Columbia P&S

Tino, Gregory MD [Pul] - **Spec Exp:** Interstitial Lung Disease; Bronchiectasis; Chronic Obstructive Lung Disease (COPD); Pulmonary Fibrosis; **Hospital:** Hosp Univ Penn - UPHS (page 72); **Address:** Dvi Pulmonary & Critical Care, Perelman Ctr for Advanced Medicine, 3400 Civic Ctr Blvd, Fl 1 West, Philadelphia, PA 19104; **Phone:** 215-662-3202; **Board Cert:** Internal Medicine 1989; Pulmonary Disease 2009; Critical Care Medicine 2009; **Med School:** Mount Sinai Sch Med 1986; **Resid:** Internal Medicine, Hosp Univ Penn 1989; **Fellow:** Pulmonary Disease, Hosp Univ Penn 1992; **Fac Appt:** Assoc Prof Med, Univ Pennsylvania

Unger, Michael MD [Pul] - **Spec Exp:** Lung Cancer; Lung Cancer in Women; Cancer Prevention; Interventional Pulmonology; **Hospital:** Fox Chase Cancer Ctr (page 58); **Address:** Fox Chase Cancer Center, 333 Cottman Ave, Philadelphia, PA 19111; **Phone:** 215-728-5703; **Board Cert:** Internal Medicine 1977; Pulmonary Disease 1978; **Med School:** France 1971; **Resid:** Internal Medicine, Mt Sinai Hosp 1974; **Fellow:** Pulmonary Disease, NY Hosp-Cornell 1976; **Fac Appt:** Clin Prof Med, Thomas Jefferson Univ

Wenzel, Sally E MD [Pul] - **Spec Exp:** Asthma & Allergy; Bronchiectasis; Autoimmune Lung Disease; Inflammatory Pulmonary Diseases; **Hospital:** UPMC Montefiore; **Address:** UPMC Montefiore, 3459 5th Ave Montefiore Bldg - Ste NW931, Falk Medical Bldg, Fl 4, Pittsburgh, PA 15213; **Phone:** 412-802-6859; **Board Cert:** Internal Medicine 1984; Pulmonary Disease 1986; **Med School:** Univ Fla Coll Med 1981; **Resid:** Internal Medicine, NC Baptist Hosp 1984; **Fellow:** Pulmonary Disease, Med Coll VA Hosp 1986; **Fac Appt:** Prof Med, Univ Pittsburgh

Young Jr, K Randall MD [Pul] - **Spec Exp:** Transplant Medicine-Lung; Cystic Fibrosis; **Hospital:** Albert Einstein Med Ctr; **Address:** Albert Einstein Med Ctr, 5401 Old York Rd, Ste 363, Philadelphia, PA 19141; **Phone:** 215-456-6950; **Board Cert:** Internal Medicine 1982; Pulmonary Disease 2009; Allergy & Immunology 1987; **Med School:** Jefferson Med Coll 1978; **Resid:** Internal Medicine, Yale-New Haven Hosp 1982; Pulmonary Critical Care Medicine, Yale-New Haven Hosp 1985; **Fellow:** Allergy & Immunology, Nat Inst Hlth 1988

Southeast

Alberts, W Michael MD [Pul] - **Spec Exp:** Lung Cancer; **Hospital:** H Lee Moffitt Cancer Ctr & Research Inst (page 59); **Address:** H Lee Moffitt Cancer Ctr, Thoracic Onc, 12902 Magnolia Drive, MCC VP Suite, Tampa, FL 33612; **Phone:** 813-979-3067; **Board Cert:** Internal Medicine 1980; Pulmonary Disease 1982; **Med School:** Univ IL Coll Med 1977; **Resid:** Internal Medicine, Ohio State Univ Hosp 1980; **Fellow:** Pulmonary Critical Care Medicine, UCSD Med Ctr 1983; **Fac Appt:** Prof Med, Univ S Fla Coll Med

Antony, Veena B MD [Pul] - **Hospital:** UAB Med West; **Address:** Univ of Alabama at Birmingham, The Kirklin Clinic, 2000 6th Ave S, Birmingham, AL 35233; **Phone:** 205-975-3258; **Board Cert:** Internal Medicine 1979; Pulmonary Disease 1982; **Med School:** India 1974; **Resid:** Internal Medicine, Kingsbrook Jewish Med Ctr 1978; **Fellow:** Pulmonary Disease, Univ Co Hlth Sci Ctr 1981; Pulmonary Disease, Natl Jewish Hosp-Asthma Ctr; **Fac Appt:** Prof Med, Univ Alabama

Brooks, Stuart M MD [Pul] - **Spec Exp:** Occupational Lung Disease; Asthma; Lung Injuries-Inhalation Induced; **Hospital:** Tampa Genl Hosp, H Lee Moffitt Cancer Ctr & Research Inst (page 59); **Address:** 4572 Bardsdale Drive, Palm Harbor, FL 34685; **Phone:** 813-389-6000; **Board Cert:** Internal Medicine 1977; Pulmonary Disease 1969; Occupational Medicine 1987; **Med School:** Univ Cincinnati 1962; **Resid:** Internal Medicine, Boston City Hosp 1967; **Fellow:** Pulmonary Disease, Boston City Hosp 1969; **Fac Appt:** Prof Med, Univ S Fla Coll Med

Campbell Jr, G Douglas MD [Pul] - **Spec Exp:** Infectious Disease-Lung; **Hospital:** Univ Mississippi Med Ctr, G.V. (Sonny) Montgomery VA Med Ctr - Jackson; **Address:** Univ Mississippi Med Ctr, Div Pulmonology, 2500 N State St, Jackson, MS 39216; **Phone:** 601-362-4471; **Board Cert:** Internal Medicine 1979; Pulmonary Disease 1986; **Med School:** Univ Miss 1976; **Resid:** Internal Medicine, Univ Miss Hosp 1979; **Fellow:** Pulmonary Disease, Univ Tex Hlth Sci Ctr 1983; Infectious Disease, Univ Calgary HSC 1985; **Fac Appt:** Prof Med, Univ Miss

Pulmonary Disease

Christman, Brian W MD [Pul] - **Spec Exp:** Chronic Obstructive Lung Disease (COPD); Sepsis; Critical Care; Respiratory Distress Syndrome (ARDS); **Hospital:** TN Valley Healthcare Sys-Nashville; **Address:** VA Tennessee Valley Hlth Care Sys, 1310 24th Ave So (111), Nashville, TN 37212; **Phone:** 615-873-6979; **Board Cert:** Internal Medicine 1984; Pulmonary Disease 1986; Critical Care Medicine 2010; **Med School:** Univ Okla Coll Med 1981; **Resid:** Internal Medicine, Vanderbilt Univ Med Ctr 1984; **Fellow:** Pulmonary Disease, Vanderbilt Univ Med Ctr 1987; **Fac Appt:** Prof Med, Vanderbilt Univ

Cooper, J Allen D MD [Pul] - **Spec Exp:** Drug Induced Lung Disease; Chronic Obstructive Lung Disease (COPD); **Hospital:** Univ of Ala Hosp at Birmingham, Birmingham, Alabama VA Med Ctr; **Address:** UAB Pulmonary Medicine, 1530 3rd Ave S, TNT 422, Birmingham, AL 35294; **Phone:** 205-934-5400; **Board Cert:** Internal Medicine 1981; Pulmonary Disease 1984; **Med School:** Duke Univ 1978; **Resid:** Internal Medicine, Univ Virginia Hosp 1981; **Fellow:** Pulmonary Disease, Yale Univ 1985; **Fac Appt:** Prof Med, Univ Alabama

Cooper, William R MD [Pul] - **Spec Exp:** Lung Cancer; Asthma; Chronic Obstructive Lung Disease (COPD); **Hospital:** Sentara VA Beach Genl Hosp; **Address:** 1008 First Colonial Rd, Virginia Beach, VA 23454-3071; **Phone:** 757-481-2515; **Board Cert:** Internal Medicine 1972; Pulmonary Disease 1974; Critical Care Medicine 2009; **Med School:** Univ VA Sch Med 1969; **Resid:** Internal Medicine, Cleveland Metro Genl Hosp 1971; Pulmonary Disease, Univ Va Hosp 1973; **Fellow:** Pulmonary Disease, Mt Sinai Med Ctr 1974

Doherty, Dennis E MD [Pul] - **Spec Exp:** Asthma; Chronic Obstructive Lung Disease (COPD); Interstitial Lung Disease; **Hospital:** Univ of Kentucky Albert B. Chandler Hosp, Lexington VA Med Ctr-Leestown Div; **Address:** Univ Kentucky Med Ctr, Div Pulm & Crit Care, Div Pulm & Crit Care, 740 S Limestone St, rm L-543, Lexington, KY 40536; **Phone:** 859-323-5045; **Board Cert:** Internal Medicine 1985; Pulmonary Disease 1988; **Med School:** Ohio State Univ 1980; **Resid:** Internal Medicine, Ohio State Univ Hosp 1983; **Fellow:** Pulmonary Disease, Univ Colorado Hlth Sci Ctr 1986; **Fac Appt:** Prof Med, Univ KY Coll Med

Donohue, James F MD [Pul] - **Spec Exp:** Asthma; Chronic Obstructive Lung Disease (COPD); Sarcoidosis; Pulmonary Fibrosis; **Hospital:** NC Memorial Hosp - UNC; **Address:** UNC, Div Pulmonary Disease, 102 Mason Farm Rd, CB 7020, Chapel Hill, NC 27599-7020; **Phone:** 919-966-2531; **Board Cert:** Internal Medicine 1975; Pulmonary Disease 1976; **Med School:** UMDNJ-NJ Med Sch, Newark 1969; **Resid:** Internal Medicine, UMDNJ-Newark 1971; Internal Medicine, NC Meml Hosp 1974; **Fellow:** Pulmonary Disease, Univ North Carolina 1976; **Fac Appt:** Prof Med, Univ NC Sch Med

Fulkerson Jr, William J MD [Pul] - **Spec Exp:** Asthma; Chronic Obstructive Lung Disease (COPD); Pulmonary Fibrosis; **Hospital:** Duke Univ Hosp; **Address:** Duke Univ Med Ctr, Box 3708, Durham, NC 27710; **Phone:** 919-684-1860; **Board Cert:** Internal Medicine 1981; Pulmonary Disease 1984; **Med School:** Univ NC Sch Med 1977; **Resid:** Internal Medicine, Vanderbilt Univ Med Ctr 1980; **Fellow:** Pulmonary Disease, Vanderbilt Univ Med Ctr 1983; **Fac Appt:** Prof Med, Duke Univ

Garver Jr, Robert MD [Pul] - **Spec Exp:** Lung Cancer; Lung Disease; **Hospital:** Mobile Infirmary Med Ctr; **Address:** 109 Med Park Drive, Ste C, Andalusia, AL 36420; **Phone:** 888-681-5864; **Board Cert:** Internal Medicine 1984; Pulmonary Disease 1986; Critical Care Medicine 2008; **Med School:** Johns Hopkins Univ 1981; **Resid:** Internal Medicine, Johns Hopkins Hosp 1984; **Fellow:** Pulmonary Disease, NHLBI 1985; **Fac Appt:** Prof Med, Univ Alabama

Goldman, Allan L MD [Pul] - **Spec Exp:** Occupational Lung Disease; Airway Disorders; Lung Cancer; **Hospital:** Tampa Genl Hosp, James A Haley VA Hosp; **Address:** USF Coll Med, Dept Internal Medicine, 12901 Bruce B Downs Blvd, Box MDC19, Tampa, FL 33612-4742; **Phone:** 813-974-2271; **Board Cert:** Internal Medicine 1972; Pulmonary Disease 1972; **Med School:** Univ Minn 1968; **Resid:** Internal Medicine, Brooke Army Hosp 1970; **Fellow:** Pulmonary Disease, Walter Reed Army Hosp 1972; **Fac Appt:** Prof Med, Univ S Fla Coll Med

Harman, Eloise M MD [Pul] - **Spec Exp:** Critical Care; Diagnostic Problems; Mechanical Ventilation; **Hospital:** Malcolm Randall VA Med Ctr; **Address:** 1601 SW Archer Rd, Gainesville, FL 32608; **Phone:** 352-376-1611; **Board Cert:** Internal Medicine 1973; Pulmonary Disease 1976; Critical Care Medicine 2007; **Med School:** Johns Hopkins Univ 1970; **Resid:** Internal Medicine, Johns Hopkins Hosp 1972; **Fellow:** Pulmonary Disease, NY Hosp-Cornell Med Ctr 1974; **Fac Appt:** Prof Med, Univ Fla Coll Med

Haynes Jr, Johnson MD [Pul] - **Spec Exp:** Sickle Cell Disease-Lung; Chronic Obstructive Lung Disease (COPD); **Hospital:** Univ of S AL Med Ctr; **Address:** 2451 Fillingim St, Moore Clin Bldg - rm 1505, MS 36617, Mobile, AL 36617; **Phone:** 251-470-5893; **Board Cert:** Internal Medicine 1983; Pulmonary Disease 1986; **Med School:** Univ S Ala Coll Med 1980; **Resid:** Internal Medicine, Univ S Alabama Med Ctr 1983; **Fellow:** Pulmonary Disease, Univ S Alabama 1986; Univ Colorado 1988; **Fac Appt:** Prof Med, Univ S Ala Coll Med

Henke, David C MD [Pul] - **Spec Exp:** Asthma; Chronic Obstructive Lung Disease (COPD); Vasculitis; **Hospital:** NC Memorial Hosp - UNC; **Address:** UNC SOM Div of Pulmonary Medicine, 4136 Bioinformatics Bldg, CB 7020, 130 Mason Farm Rd, Chapel Hill, NC 27599-7020; **Phone:** 919-966-2531; **Board Cert:** Internal Medicine 1980; Dermatology 1983; Pulmonary Disease 1988; **Med School:** Univ NC Sch Med 1977; **Resid:** Internal Medicine, NC Memorial Hosp 1980; Dermatology, NC Meml NIEHS 1984; **Fellow:** Pulmonary Disease, NC Memorial Hosp 1987; **Fac Appt:** Assoc Prof Med, Univ NC Sch Med

Johnson, Bruce Ellsworth MD [Pul] - **Spec Exp:** Sleep Disorders/Apnea; **Hospital:** Sentara VA Beach Genl Hosp; **Address:** 1008 First Colonial Rd, Virginia Beach, VA 23454-3002; **Phone:** 757-481-2515; **Board Cert:** Internal Medicine 1981; Pulmonary Disease 1986; Critical Care Medicine 2001; Sleep Medicine 2009; **Med School:** Med Coll GA 1978; **Resid:** Internal Medicine, Univ VA Med Ctr 1981; **Fellow:** Pulmonary Disease, Univ VA Med Ctr 1983

Light, Richard W MD [Pul] - **Spec Exp:** Pleural Disease; **Hospital:** Vanderbilt Univ Med Ctr (page 75); **Address:** Vanderbilt Univ Med Ctr-Pulmonary Medicine, 1161 21st Ave S, T1218 MCN, Nashville, TN 37232-2650; **Phone:** 615-322-3412; **Board Cert:** Internal Medicine 1972; Pulmonary Disease 1974; **Med School:** Johns Hopkins Univ 1968; **Resid:** Internal Medicine, Johns Hopkins Hosp 1970; **Fellow:** Pulmonary Disease, Johns Hopkins Hosp 1972; **Fac Appt:** Prof Med, Vanderbilt Univ

LoRusso, Thomas J MD [Pul] - **Spec Exp:** Critical Care; Sleep Disorders/Apnea; **Hospital:** Inova Fairfax Hosp; **Address:** 1800 Town Ctr Drive, Ste 419, Reston, VA 20190; **Phone:** 703-620-3926; **Board Cert:** Internal Medicine 2001; Pulmonary Disease 2002; Critical Care Medicine 2003; Sleep Medicine 2009; **Med School:** SUNY Upstate Med Univ 1987; **Resid:** Internal Medicine, Univ Hosp-SUNY 1990; **Fellow:** Pulmonary Disease, Cedars Sinai Med Ctr 1993

Loyd, James E MD [Pul] - **Spec Exp:** Pulmonary Fibrosis; Interstitial Lung Disease; Transplant Medicine-Lung; Pulmonary Hypertension; **Hospital:** Vanderbilt Univ Med Ctr (page 75); **Address:** Vanderbilt Univ Div Pulmonary Medicine, 1161 21st Ave S, T-1218 Medical Center N, Nashville, TN 37232-2650; **Phone:** 615-322-3412; **Board Cert:** Internal Medicine 1978; Pulmonary Disease 1984; **Med School:** W VA Univ 1973; **Resid:** Internal Medicine, Vanderbilt Univ Hosp 1976; **Fellow:** Pulmonary Disease, Vanderbilt Univ Hosp 1978; **Fac Appt:** Prof Med, Vanderbilt Univ

Sahn, Steven A MD [Pul] - **Spec Exp:** Pleural Disease; Interstitial Lung Disease; Chronic Obstructive Lung Disease (COPD); Pulmonary Fibrosis; **Hospital:** MUSC Med Ctr, R H Johnson VA Med Ctr - Charleston; **Address:** MUSC, Div Pulm & Crit Care Med, 96 Jonathan Lucas St, Box 250630, Charleston, SC 29425-8900; **Phone:** 843-792-3167; **Board Cert:** Internal Medicine 1974; Pulmonary Disease 1974; **Med School:** Univ Louisville Sch Med 1968; **Resid:** Internal Medicine, Univ Iowa Hosp 1971; **Fellow:** Pulmonary Disease, Univ CO Hlth Sci Ctr 1973; **Fac Appt:** Prof Med, Med Univ SC

Staton Jr, Gerald W MD [Pul] - **Spec Exp:** Interstitial Lung Disease; Chronic Obstructive Lung Disease (COPD); Pulmonary Fibrosis; Sarcoidosis; **Hospital:** Emory Univ Hosp Midtown, Wesley Woods Ger Hosp; **Address:** Emory Midtown-Pulmonary Medicine, 550 Peachtree St NE Fl 6, Atlanta, GA 30308; **Phone:** 404-686-2505; **Board Cert:** Internal Medicine 1979; Pulmonary Disease 1982; Critical Care Medicine 2007; **Med School:** Med Coll GA 1976; **Resid:** Internal Medicine, Stanford Univ Med Ctr 1979; **Fellow:** Pulmonary Disease, Mass Genl Hosp 1981; **Fac Appt:** Prof Med, Emory Univ

Tapson, Victor F MD [Pul] - **Spec Exp:** Pulmonary Hypertension; Thromboembolic Disorders; Chronic Obstructive Lung Disease (COPD); Emphysema; **Hospital:** Duke Univ Hosp; **Address:** DUMC 102351, Durham, NC 27710; **Phone:** 919-684-6237; **Board Cert:** Internal Medicine 1986; Pulmonary Disease 2000; **Med School:** Hahnemann Univ 1982; **Resid:** Internal Medicine, Duke Univ Med Ctr 1986; **Fellow:** Pulmonary Disease, Boston Univ 1989; **Fac Appt:** Prof Med, Duke Univ

Vaughey, Ellen MD [Pul] - **Spec Exp:** Critical Care; Sleep Disorders/Apnea; Asthma; **Hospital:** Inova Fairfax Hosp, Virginia Hosp Ctr - Arlington; **Address:** 3289 Woodburn Rd, Ste 350, Annandale, VA 22003; **Phone:** 703-641-8616; **Board Cert:** Internal Medicine 2001; Pulmonary Disease 2002; Critical Care Medicine 2003; **Med School:** Georgetown Univ 1987; **Resid:** Internal Medicine, Thomas Jefferson Univ Hosp 1990; **Fellow:** Pulmonary Disease, Roger Williams Hosp-Brown Univ 1993

Voelkel, Norbert F MD [Pul] - **Spec Exp:** Pulmonary Hypertension; Asthma; Emphysema; **Hospital:** Med Coll of VA Hosp; **Address:** 417 N 11th St, Richmond, VA 23298; **Phone:** 804-828-7929; **Med School:** Germany 1972; **Resid:** Internal Medicine, Univ Hamburg 1977; **Fellow:** Research, Univ Colorado 1978; Pulmonary Disease, Univ Colorado 1981; **Fac Appt:** Prof Med, Univ Colorado

Wanner, Adam MD [Pul] - **Spec Exp:** Asthma; **Hospital:** Jackson Meml Hosp, Univ of Miami Hosp; **Address:** Univ Miami Sch Med, Div Pulm & Crit Care, 1600 NW 10th Ave, rm 7056, Miami, FL 33136; **Phone:** 305-243-3045; **Board Cert:** Internal Medicine 1973; Pulmonary Disease 1974; **Med School:** Switzerland 1966; **Resid:** Internal Medicine, Kantonsspital Aarau 1970; **Fellow:** Pulmonary Disease, Mt Sinai Med Ctr 1972; **Fac Appt:** Prof Med, Univ Miami Sch Med

Wheeler, Arthur P MD [Pul] - **Spec Exp:** Critical Care; Sepsis; Respiratory Distress Syndrome (ARDS); **Hospital:** Vanderbilt Univ Med Ctr (page 75); **Address:** Vanderbilt Univ Medical Ctr, 1161 21st Ave S, rm T-1218 MCN, Nashville, TN 37232-2650; **Phone:** 615-322-3412; **Board Cert:** Internal Medicine 1985; Pulmonary Disease 1988; **Med School:** Univ MD Sch Med 1982; **Resid:** Internal Medicine, Vanderbilt Univ Med Ctr 1985; **Fellow:** Pulmonary Disease, Vanderbilt Univ Med Ctr 1986; **Fac Appt:** Assoc Prof Med, Vanderbilt Univ

Midwest

Balk, Robert A MD [Pul] - **Spec Exp:** Asthma; Cystic Fibrosis; Respiratory Failure; Lung Injury/ARDS; **Hospital:** Rush Univ Med Ctr; **Address:** 1725 W Harrison St, Ste 054, Chicago, IL 60612; **Phone:** 312-942-6744; **Board Cert:** Internal Medicine 1981; Pulmonary Disease 1986; Critical Care Medicine 2008; **Med School:** Univ MO-Kansas City 1978; **Resid:** Internal Medicine, Univ MO-Kansas City Affil Hosps 1981; **Fellow:** Pulmonary Critical Care Medicine, Univ Ark Hosp 1983; **Fac Appt:** Prof Med, Rush Med Coll

Bijwadia, Jagdeep S MD [Pul] - **Spec Exp:** Sleep Medicine; **Address:** HealthPartners Spec Ctr, Lung & Sleep Hlth, 401 Phalen Blvd, St Paul, MN 55130; **Phone:** 651-254-7670 x3; **Board Cert:** Internal Medicine 2001; Pulmonary Disease 2004; Sleep Medicine 2007; **Med School:** India 1986; **Resid:** Internal Medicine, Nassau Co MC 1992; **Fellow:** Pulmonary Critical Care Medicine, USC Univ Hosp 1992; **Fac Appt:** Asst Prof Med, Univ Minn

Fahey, Patrick J MD [Pul] - **Hospital:** Loyola Univ Med Ctr, Edward Hines, Jr. VA Hosp; **Address:** Loyola Univ Med Ctr-Pulmonary Disease, 2160 S 1st Ave, Maywood, IL 60153-3304; **Phone:** 708-216-8563; **Board Cert:** Internal Medicine 1976; Pulmonary Disease 1978; **Med School:** Univ Wisc 1973; **Resid:** Internal Medicine, St Elizabeth's Hosp 1976; **Fellow:** Pulmonary Disease, Strong Meml Hosp 1980; **Fac Appt:** Prof Med, Loyola Univ-Stritch Sch Med

Fletcher, Eugene MD [Pul] - **Spec Exp:** Chronic Obstructive Lung Disease (COPD); Sleep Disorders/Apnea; **Hospital:** Reid Hosp & Hlth Care Servs; **Address:** 428 Vincennes St, New Albany, IN 47150; **Phone:** 812-948-5841; **Board Cert:** Internal Medicine 1974; Pulmonary Disease 1980; Critical Care Medicine 2010; **Med School:** Temple Univ 1971; **Resid:** Internal Medicine, Univ Colo Affil Hosps 1973; Internal Medicine, Fitzsimons Army Med Ctr 1974; **Fellow:** Pulmonary Disease, Univ Okla Hlth Scis Ctr 1974; **Fac Appt:** Clin Prof Med, Univ Louisville Sch Med

Garrity Jr, Edward R MD [Pul] - **Spec Exp:** Transplant Medicine-Lung; Pulmonary Vascular Disease; Asthma; Cystic Fibrosis; **Hospital:** Univ of Chicago Med Ctr; **Address:** Lung Transplant Prgrm, 5841 S Maryland Ave, MS 0999, Chicago, IL 60637; **Phone:** 773-834-7235 x1655; **Board Cert:** Internal Medicine 2003; Pulmonary Disease 1998; **Med School:** Loyola Univ-Stritch Sch Med 1976; **Resid:** Internal Medicine, Loyola Univ Med Ctr 1979; **Fellow:** Pulmonary Disease, Univ Chicago Hosps 1983; **Fac Appt:** Prof Med, Univ Chicago-Pritzker Sch Med

Grum, Cyril M MD [Pul] - **Spec Exp:** Asthma; Cystic Fibrosis; **Hospital:** Univ of Michigan Hosp; **Address:** Univ Michigan Hosp-Div Pulm Med, 1500 E Med Ctr Drive, 3916 TC, Ann Arbor, MI 48109; **Phone:** 734-647-9342; **Board Cert:** Internal Medicine 1980; Pulmonary Disease 1982; **Med School:** Med Coll Wisc 1977; **Resid:** Internal Medicine, Cleveland Clin; **Fellow:** Pulmonary Disease, Univ Mich; **Fac Appt:** Asst Prof Med, Univ Mich Med Sch

Hall, Jesse MD [Pul] - **Spec Exp:** Respiratory Failure; Critical Care; **Hospital:** Univ of Chicago Med Ctr; **Address:** 5841 S Maryland Ave, rm W656, MC 6076, Chicago, IL 60637; **Phone:** 773-702-1454; **Board Cert:** Internal Medicine 1980; Critical Care Medicine 2011; **Med School:** Univ Chicago-Pritzker Sch Med 1977; **Resid:** Internal Medicine, Univ Chicago Hosps 1982; **Fac Appt:** Prof Med, Univ Chicago-Pritzker Sch Med

Hertz, Marshall I MD [Pul] - **Spec Exp:** Transplant Medicine-Lung; Transplant Medicine-Heart & Lung; Pulmonary Hypertension; **Hospital:** Univ Minn Med Ctr, Fairview - Riverside Campus; **Address:** Pulmonary, Allergy & Critical Care Med, 420 Delaware St SE, MMC 276, Minneapolis, MN 55455; **Phone:** 612-624-0999; **Board Cert:** Internal Medicine 1981; Pulmonary Disease 1984; **Med School:** Univ Mich Med Sch 1978; **Resid:** Internal Medicine, Univ Minn Med Ctr 1982; **Fellow:** Pulmonary Critical Care Medicine, Univ Minn Med Ctr 1984; **Fac Appt:** Prof Med, Univ Minn

Pulmonary Disease

Hyers, Thomas M MD [Pul] - **Spec Exp:** Thromboembolic Disorders; Chronic Obstructive Lung Disease (COPD); Occupational Medicine; **Hospital:** SSM St. Clare Hlth Ctr, St. John's Mercy Med Ctr - St Louis; **Address:** CARE Clin Research, 522 N New Ballas Rd, Ste 350, St Louis, MO 63141; **Phone:** 314-699-9383; **Board Cert:** Internal Medicine 1974; Pulmonary Disease 1980; **Med School:** Duke Univ 1968; **Resid:** Internal Medicine, Univ Wash Med Ctr 1975; Pulmonary Disease, Univ Colorado Hosp 1977; **Fellow:** Pulmonary Disease, Natl Inst Hlth 1972; **Fac Appt:** Clin Prof Med, St Louis Univ

Ingbar, David H MD [Pul] - **Spec Exp:** Critical Care; Pulmonary Infections; Respiratory Failure; **Hospital:** Univ Minn Med Ctr, Fairview - Riverside Campus, Fairview Southdale Hosp; **Address:** Univ Minn Med Ctr, Div Pulm & Crit Care, 420 Delaware St SE, MMC 276, Minneapolis, MN 55455; **Phone:** 612-626-6100; **Board Cert:** Internal Medicine 1981; Critical Care Medicine 2007; Pulmonary Disease 1984; **Med School:** Harvard Med Sch 1978; **Resid:** Internal Medicine, Univ Wash Med Ctr 1981; **Fellow:** Pulmonary Disease, Yale Univ-New Haven Hosp 1985; **Fac Appt:** Prof Med, Univ Minn

Kaye, Mitchell MD [Pul] - **Spec Exp:** Chronic Obstructive Lung Disease (COPD); Asthma; **Hospital:** Abbott - Northwestern Hosp; **Address:** Minnesota Lung Ctr, 920 E 28th St, Ste 700, Minneapolis, MN 55407; **Phone:** 952-567-7400; **Board Cert:** Internal Medicine 1987; Pulmonary Disease 2010; Critical Care Medicine 2001; **Med School:** Univ Minn 1984; **Resid:** Internal Medicine, Univ IL Med Ctr 1987; **Fellow:** Pulmonary Disease, Northwestern Univ 1989

Kovitz, Kevin L MD [Pul] - **Spec Exp:** Interventional Pulmonology; **Hospital:** Central DuPage Hosp, Alexian Brothers Med Ctr; **Address:** Chicago Chest Ctr/Suburban Lung Assocs, 800 Biesterfield Rd, Ste 510, Elk Grove Village, IL 60007; **Phone:** 847-498-5864; **Board Cert:** Internal Medicine 1988; Pulmonary Disease 2002; Critical Care Medicine 2005; **Med School:** Israel 1985; **Resid:** Internal Medicine, Univ Maryland Hosps 1988; **Fellow:** Pulmonary Intensive Care, Johns Hopkins Hosp 1992; Interventional Pulmonology, Sainte Marguerite Hosp 1993

Krowka, Michael J MD [Pul] - **Spec Exp:** Hepatopulmonary Syndrome; Pulmonary Hypertension; Chronic Obstructive Lung Disease (COPD); **Hospital:** Mayo Med Ctr & Clin - Rochester; **Address:** Mayo Clin, Div Pulm & Crit Care Med, 200 First St SW, Gonda-18 S, Rochester, MN 55905; **Phone:** 507-284-2158; **Board Cert:** Internal Medicine 1983; Pulmonary Disease 1986; **Med School:** Univ Nevada 1980; **Resid:** Internal Medicine, Evanston Hosp 1983; **Fellow:** Pulmonary Disease, Mayo Clinic 1986; **Fac Appt:** Prof Med, Mayo Med Sch

Lem, Vincent M MD [Pul] - **Spec Exp:** Asthma; **Hospital:** St. Luke's Hosp of Kansas City; **Address:** 4321 Washington St, Ste 6000, Kansas City, MO 64111; **Phone:** 816-756-2255; **Board Cert:** Internal Medicine 1982; Pulmonary Disease 1984; Critical Care Medicine 2004; **Med School:** Univ Kansas 1978; **Resid:** Internal Medicine, St Luke's Hosp 1982; **Fellow:** Pulmonary Disease, Univ Texas Hlth Sci Ctr 1984; **Fac Appt:** Assoc Clin Prof Med, Univ MO-Kansas City

Marini, John Joseph MD [Pul] - **Spec Exp:** Critical Care; Mechanical Ventilation; Chronic Obstructive Lung Disease (COPD); **Hospital:** Regions Hosp - St Paul; **Address:** 401 Phelon Blvd, St Paul, MN 55130; **Phone:** 651-254-7670; **Board Cert:** Internal Medicine 2003; Pulmonary Disease 2003; Critical Care Medicine 2002; **Med School:** Johns Hopkins Univ 1973; **Resid:** Internal Medicine, Univ Wash Med Ctr 1976; **Fellow:** Pulmonary Disease, Univ Wash Med Ctr 1978; **Fac Appt:** Prof Med, Univ Minn

Martinez, Fernando J MD [Pul] - **Spec Exp:** Lung Disease; Critical Care; **Hospital:** Univ of Michigan Hosp; **Address:** Univ Michigan Hosp-Div Pulm Med, 1500 E Med Ctr Drive, 3916 TC, Ann Arbor, MI 48109; **Phone:** 734-647-9342; **Board Cert:** Internal Medicine 1986; Pulmonary Disease 1988; Critical Care Medicine 2010; **Med School:** Univ Fla Coll Med 1983; **Resid:** Internal Medicine, Beth Israel Hosp 1986; **Fellow:** Pulmonary Disease, Boston Univ 1989; **Fac Appt:** Prof Med, Univ Mich Med Sch

Matuschak, George M MD [Pul] - **Spec Exp:** Chronic Obstructive Lung Disease (COPD); Asthma; **Hospital:** St. John's Mercy Med Ctr - St Louis; **Address:** 621 S New Ballas Rd, Ste 228A, St Louis, MO 63141; **Phone:** 314-251-4966; **Board Cert:** Internal Medicine 1980; Critical Care Medicine 2008; Pulmonary Disease 2008; **Med School:** Temple Univ 1977; **Resid:** Internal Medicine, Strong Meml Hosp 1980; **Fellow:** Critical Care Medicine, Univ Htlh Ctr 1981; Pulmonary Disease, Univ Hlth Ctr 1984; **Fac Appt:** Prof Med, St Louis Univ

Popovich Jr, John MD [Pul] - **Spec Exp:** Lung Disease; Pulmonary Embolism; Interstitial Lung Disease; Critical Care; **Hospital:** Henry Ford Hosp; **Address:** Henry Ford Hosp, Dept Int Med, 2799 W Grand Blvd, Detroit, MI 48202; **Phone:** 313-916-8058; **Board Cert:** Internal Medicine 1978; Pulmonary Disease 1980; **Med School:** Univ Mich Med Sch 1975; **Resid:** Internal Medicine, Henry Ford Hosp 1978; **Fellow:** Pulmonary Disease, Henry Ford Hosp 1980; **Fac Appt:** Prof Med, Wayne State Univ

Prakash, Udaya MD [Pul] - **Spec Exp:** Bronchoscopy; **Hospital:** Mayo Med Ctr & Clin - Rochester; **Address:** Mayo Clin, Div Pulm & Crit Care Med, 200 First St SW, Gonda-18 S, Rochester, MN 55905; **Phone:** 507-284-2158; **Board Cert:** Internal Medicine 1987; Pulmonary Disease 1976; **Med School:** India 1970; **Resid:** Internal Medicine, Mayo Clin 1973; **Fellow:** Pulmonary Disease, Mayo Clin 1976; **Fac Appt:** Prof Med, Mayo Med Sch

Rosenbluth, Daniel B MD [Pul] - **Spec Exp:** Cystic Fibrosis; **Hospital:** Barnes-Jewish Hosp; **Address:** Washington Univ Sch Med, 660 S Euclid Ave, Box 8052, St Louis, MO 63110; **Phone:** 314-454-8762; **Board Cert:** Internal Medicine 2002; Pulmonary Disease 2004; Critical Care Medicine 2005; **Med School:** Mount Sinai Sch Med 1989; **Resid:** Internal Medicine, Northwestern Meml Hosp 1992; **Fellow:** Pulmonary Critical Care Medicine, Barnes Hosp 1995; **Fac Appt:** Prof Med, Washington Univ, St Louis

Shore, Bernard L MD [Pul] - **Spec Exp:** Lung Disease; Palliative Care; Pain Management; **Hospital:** Barnes-Jewish Hosp; **Address:** 1110 Highlands Plaza E, Ste 375, St Louis, MO 63110; **Phone:** 314-367-3113; **Board Cert:** Internal Medicine 1980; Pulmonary Disease 1982; **Med School:** Washington Univ, St Louis 1977; **Resid:** Internal Medicine, Barnes Hosp 1980; **Fellow:** Pulmonary Disease, Wash Univ Sch Med 1982; **Fac Appt:** Assoc Clin Prof Med, Washington Univ, St Louis

Silver, Michael R MD [Pul] - **Spec Exp:** Chronic Obstructive Lung Disease (COPD); Lung Cancer; Asthma; **Hospital:** Rush Univ Med Ctr, Rush Oak Park Hosp; **Address:** Rush Univ Med Ctr, Professional Office Bldg 3, 1725 W Harrison St, Ste 054, Chicago, IL 60612; **Phone:** 312-942-6744; **Board Cert:** Internal Medicine 1984; Pulmonary Disease 1988; Critical Care Medicine 2009; **Med School:** Albany Med Coll 1981; **Resid:** Internal Medicine, Rush-Presby-St Lukes Med Ctr 1985; **Fellow:** Pulmonary Critical Care Medicine, Rush-Presby-St Lukes Med Ctr 1987; **Fac Appt:** Assoc Prof Med, Rush Med Coll

Simon, Richard H MD [Pul] - **Spec Exp:** Cystic Fibrosis; **Hospital:** Univ of Michigan Hosp; **Address:** Univ Michigan Hosp-Div Pulm Med, 1500 E Med Ctr Drive, 3916 TC, Ann Arbor, MI 48109; **Phone:** 734-647-9342; **Board Cert:** Internal Medicine 1976; Pulmonary Disease 1980; **Med School:** Duke Univ 1972; **Resid:** Internal Medicine, UCSF Med Ctr 1975; Internal Medicine, Univ Colorado Affil Hosps 1976; **Fellow:** Pulmonary Disease, Univ Colorado 1981; **Fac Appt:** Prof Med, Univ Mich Med Sch

Pulmonary Disease

Stoller, James MD [Pul] - **Spec Exp:** Emphysema/Alpha-1 Antitrypsin Deficiency; **Hospital:** Cleveland Clin (page 55); **Address:** Cleveland Clinic, Dept Education, 9500 Euclid Ave, Desk NA22, Cleveland, OH 44195; **Phone:** 216-444-1960; **Board Cert:** Internal Medicine 1982; Pulmonary Disease 1984; Critical Care Medicine 2007; **Med School:** Yale Univ 1979; **Resid:** Internal Medicine, Peter Bent Brigham Hosp 1982; **Fellow:** Pulmonary Disease, Brigham & Women's Hosp 1983; Critical Care Medicine, Mass Genl Hosp 1985; **Fac Appt:** Prof Med, Cleveland Cl Coll Med/Case West Res

Tobin, Martin MD [Pul] - **Spec Exp:** Mechanical Ventilation; Chronic Obstructive Lung Disease (COPD); **Hospital:** Edward Hines, Jr. VA Hosp, Loyola Univ Med Ctr; **Address:** Hines VA Hosp (111N), Fifth Ave and Roosevelt Rd, Bldg 1 - rm E438, Hines, IL 60141; **Phone:** 708-202-2705; **Board Cert:** Internal Medicine 1983; Pulmonary Disease 1984; **Med School:** Ireland 1975; **Resid:** Internal Medicine, Trinity Coll Hosps 1979; Pulmonary Disease, Kings Coll Hosp 1980; **Fellow:** Pulmonary Critical Care Medicine, Mt Sinai Hosp 1983; Pulmonary Critical Care Medicine, Univ Pittsburgh 1983; **Fac Appt:** Prof Med, Loyola Univ-Stritch Sch Med

Trulock, Elbert MD [Pul] - **Spec Exp:** Transplant Medicine-Lung; Emphysema-Lung Volume Reduction; Pulmonary Hypertension; Cystic Fibrosis; **Hospital:** Barnes-Jewish Hosp; **Address:** 216 S Kings Hwy, MS 90-32-680, St Louis, MO 63110; **Phone:** 314-362-5378; **Board Cert:** Internal Medicine 1981; Pulmonary Disease 1984; **Med School:** Emory Univ 1978; **Resid:** Internal Medicine, Barnes Hosp 1981; **Fellow:** Pulmonary Disease, Wash Univ Med Ctr 1983; **Fac Appt:** Prof Med, Washington Univ, St Louis

Wiedemann, Herbert P MD [Pul] - **Spec Exp:** Respiratory Distress Syndrome (ARDS); Asthma; Emphysema; **Hospital:** Cleveland Clin (page 55); **Address:** Cleveland Clinic-Pulmonary & Allergy, 9500 Euclid Ave, Desk A90, Cleveland, OH 44195; **Phone:** 216-444-8335; **Board Cert:** Internal Medicine 1980; Pulmonary Disease 1984; **Med School:** Cornell Univ 1977; **Resid:** Internal Medicine, Univ Wash Hosps 1980; Internal Medicine, Harborview Hosp 1981; **Fellow:** Pulmonary Disease, Yale Univ 1984

Great Plains and Mountains

Brown, Kevin K MD [Pul] - **Spec Exp:** Pulmonary Fibrosis; Interstitial Lung Disease; Autoimmune Lung Disease; Clinical Trials; **Hospital:** Natl Jewish Med & Rsch Ctr, Univ of CO Hosp - Anschutz Inpatient Pav; **Address:** Natl Jewish Health, 1400 Jackson St, Denver, CO 80206-2762; **Phone:** 303-398-1621; **Board Cert:** Internal Medicine 1989; Pulmonary Disease 2005; **Med School:** Univ Minn 1984; **Resid:** Internal Medicine, Providence Med Ctr 1989; **Fellow:** Pulmonary Disease, Maine Med Ctr 1992; Pulmonary Disease, Univ Colo Hlth Scis Ctr 1994; **Fac Appt:** Prof Med, Univ Colorado

Elliott, C. Gregory MD [Pul] - **Spec Exp:** Pulmonary Hypertension; Thromboembolic Disorders; **Hospital:** Intermountain Med Ctr, LDS Hosp; **Address:** Intermountain Med Ctr, Dept Medicine, 5121 S Cottonwood St, Ste 307, Murray, UT 84107; **Phone:** 801-507-3373; **Board Cert:** Internal Medicine 1976; Pulmonary Disease 1978; **Med School:** Univ MD Sch Med 1973; **Resid:** Internal Medicine, Univ Maryland Hosp 1976; **Fellow:** Pulmonary Disease, Univ Utah 1978; **Fac Appt:** Prof Med, Univ Utah

Iseman, Michael MD [Pul] - **Spec Exp:** Tuberculosis; Mycobacterial Infections; **Hospital:** Natl Jewish Med & Rsch Ctr; **Address:** Natl Jewish Med & Rsch Ctr, 1400 Jackson St, rm J223, Denver, CO 80206; **Phone:** 303-398-1667; **Board Cert:** Internal Medicine 1972; Pulmonary Disease 1976; **Med School:** Columbia P&S 1965; **Resid:** Internal Medicine, Bellevue Hosp 1967; Internal Medicine, Harlem Hosp 1970; **Fellow:** Pulmonary Disease, Harlem Hosp 1972; **Fac Appt:** Prof Med, Univ Colorado

Kaplan, James D MD [Pul] - **Spec Exp:** Critical Care; Sleep Disorders/Apnea; **Hospital:** Overland Pk Regl Med Ctr; **Address:** 10550 Quivira, Ste 335, Overland Park, KS 66215-2304; **Phone:** 913-599-3800; **Board Cert:** Internal Medicine 1987; Pulmonary Disease 2010; Critical Care Medicine 2003; **Med School:** Univ MO-Kansas City 1984; **Resid:** Internal Medicine, Barnes Hosp 1987; **Fellow:** Pulmonary Disease, Barnes Hosp-Wash Univ 1987

Kern, Jeffrey A MD [Pul] - **Spec Exp:** Lung Cancer; **Hospital:** Natl Jewish Med & Rsch Ctr; **Address:** National Jewish Health, 1400 Jackson St, Denver, CO 80206; **Phone:** 877-225-5654; **Board Cert:** Internal Medicine 1982; Pulmonary Disease 1986; **Med School:** Univ Wisc 1979; **Resid:** Internal Medicine, Parkland Meml Hosp 1982; **Fellow:** Pulmonary Critical Care Medicine, Hosp Univ of Penn 1984

Martin, Richard J MD [Pul] - **Spec Exp:** Asthma; Vocal Cord Disorders; Chronic Obstructive Lung Disease (COPD); **Hospital:** Natl Jewish Med & Rsch Ctr, Univ of CO Hosp - Anschutz Inpatient Pav; **Address:** 1400 Jackson St, Denver, CO 80206-2762; **Phone:** 303-398-1847; **Board Cert:** Internal Medicine 1976; Pulmonary Disease 1978; **Med School:** Univ Mich Med Sch 1971; **Resid:** Internal Medicine, Tulane Univ Affil Hosp 1976; **Fellow:** Pulmonary Disease, Univ Oklahoma 1978; **Fac Appt:** Prof Med, Univ Colorado

Rennard, Stephen I MD [Pul] - **Spec Exp:** Chronic Obstructive Lung Disease (COPD); Emphysema; **Hospital:** Nebraska Med Ctr; **Address:** Univ Nebraska Med Ctr, 985910 Nebraska Med Ctr, Omaha, NE 68198-5910; **Phone:** 402-559-7313; **Board Cert:** Internal Medicine 1978; Pulmonary Disease 1982; **Med School:** Baylor Coll Med 1975; **Resid:** Internal Medicine, Barnes Hosp-Washington Univ 1977; **Fac Appt:** Prof Med, Univ Nebr Coll Med

Rose, Cecile MD [Pul] - **Spec Exp:** Occupational Lung Disease; Sarcoidosis; Pneumoconiosis; Asbestos-related Lung Disease; **Hospital:** Natl Jewish Med & Rsch Ctr, Univ of CO Hosp - Anschutz Inpatient Pav; **Address:** 1400 Jackson St, rm G-211, Denver, CO 80206-2761; **Phone:** 303-398-1867; **Board Cert:** Internal Medicine 1983; Pulmonary Disease 1986; Occupational Medicine 1987; **Med School:** Univ IL Coll Med 1980; **Resid:** Internal Medicine, Med Coll Virginia Hosp 1983; **Fellow:** Pulmonary Disease, Med Coll Virginia Hosp 1985; **Fac Appt:** Assoc Prof Med, Univ Colorado

Schwartz, David A MD [Pul] - **Spec Exp:** Pulmonary Fibrosis; Asthma; Occupational Lung Disease; **Hospital:** Univ of CO Hosp - Anschutz Inpatient Pav, Natl Jewish Med & Rsch Ctr; **Address:** 12631 E 17th Ave, MS B178, Aurora, CO 80045; **Phone:** 303-724-1783; **Board Cert:** Internal Medicine 1984; Occupational Medicine 1987; Pulmonary Disease 1988; **Med School:** UCSD 1979; **Resid:** Internal Medicine, Boston City Hosp 1986; Preventive Medicine, Harvard Sch Public Health 1986; **Fellow:** Pulmonary Disease, Univ Seattle Medical Ctr 1988

Schwarz, Marvin I MD [Pul] - **Spec Exp:** Interstitial Lung Disease; Pulmonary Vascular Disease; Pulmonary Fibrosis; **Hospital:** Univ of CO Hosp - Anschutz Inpatient Pav, Natl Jewish Med & Rsch Ctr; **Address:** Div of Pulmonary Science & Critical Care, 12700 E 19th Ave, C-272 Ave, Aurora, CO 80045; **Phone:** 303-724-4075; **Board Cert:** Internal Medicine 1970; Pulmonary Disease 1971; **Med School:** Tulane Univ 1964; **Resid:** Internal Medicine, Charity Hosp 1967; **Fellow:** Pulmonary Disease, Charity Hosp/Tulane Univ 1969; **Fac Appt:** Prof Med, Univ Colorado

Sutherland, Everett Rand MD [Pul] - **Spec Exp:** Allergy; Occupational Asthma; Chronic Obstructive Lung Disease (COPD); **Hospital:** Natl Jewish Med & Rsch Ctr; **Address:** 1400 Jackson St, rm J-201, Denver, CO 80206; **Phone:** 303-398-1081; **Board Cert:** Internal Medicine 2007; Pulmonary Disease 2010; **Med School:** Univ Chicago-Pritzker Sch Med 1994; **Resid:** Internal Medicine, UCSF 1997; **Fellow:** Pulmonary Critical Care Medicine, Univ Colorado Denver 2001; **Fac Appt:** Assoc Prof Med, Univ Colorado

Pulmonary Disease

Southwest

Arroliga, Alejandro C MD [Pul] - **Spec Exp:** Pulmonary Hypertension; Respiratory Distress Syndrome (ARDS); Critical Care; **Hospital:** Scott & White Mem Hosp; **Address:** 2401 S 31st St, Temple, TX 76508; **Phone:** 254-724-9887; **Board Cert:** Internal Medicine 2010; Pulmonary Disease 2000; Critical Care Medicine 2003; **Med School:** Mexico 1984; **Resid:** Internal Medicine, Coney Island Hosp 1990; **Fellow:** Pulmonary Critical Care Medicine, Yale-New Haven Hosp 1993; **Fac Appt:** Prof Med, Cleveland Cl Coll Med/Case West Res

Guidry, George G MD [Pul] - **Spec Exp:** Chronic Obstructive Lung Disease (COPD); Asthma; Pneumonia; Lung Cancer; **Hospital:** Lafayette Genl Med Ctr; **Address:** 155 Hospital Drive, Ste 206, Lafayette, LA 70503-2852; **Phone:** 337-234-3204; **Board Cert:** Internal Medicine 1988; Pulmonary Disease 2010; **Med School:** Louisiana State U, New Orleans 1985; **Resid:** Internal Medicine, LSU Med Ctr 1988; **Fellow:** Pulmonary Disease, LSU Med Ctr 1991; **Fac Appt:** Assoc Clin Prof Med, Louisiana State U, New Orleans

Levin, David C MD [Pul] - **Spec Exp:** Asthma; Chronic Obstructive Lung Disease (COPD); **Hospital:** OU Med Ctr, VA Med Ctr - Oklahoma City; **Address:** OU Physicians Building, 825 NE 10th St, Ste 2500, Oklahoma City, OK 73104; **Phone:** 405-271-7001; **Board Cert:** Internal Medicine 1973; Pulmonary Disease 1976; **Med School:** Case West Res Univ 1970; **Resid:** Internal Medicine, Univ Colorado Affil Hosp 1974; **Fellow:** Pulmonary Disease, Univ Colorado 1975; **Fac Appt:** Prof Med, Univ Okla Coll Med

Perret, Philip S MD [Pul] - **Spec Exp:** Chronic Obstructive Lung Disease (COPD); **Hospital:** Our Lady of Lourdes Reg Med Ctr - Lafayette, Lafayette Genl Med Ctr; **Address:** 614 W St Mary Blvd, Lafayette, LA 70506; **Phone:** 337-232-6435; **Board Cert:** Internal Medicine 1978; Pulmonary Disease 1980; **Med School:** Emory Univ 1974; **Resid:** Internal Medicine, Emory Univ Hosp 1977; **Fellow:** Pulmonary Disease, Emory Univ 1979

Shellito, Judd E MD [Pul] - **Spec Exp:** Pulmonary Infections; Occupational Lung Disease; **Hospital:** Ochsner Med Ctr-Kenner; **Address:** LSU Pulmonary Medicine, 1901 Perdido St, Ste 3205, New Orleans, LA 70112; **Phone:** 504-568-4634; **Board Cert:** Internal Medicine 1977; Pulmonary Disease 1980; **Med School:** Tulane Univ 1974; **Resid:** Internal Medicine, Evanston Hosp 1978; **Fellow:** Pulmonary Critical Care Medicine, Univ New Mexico Hosp 1980; **Fac Appt:** Prof Med, Louisiana State U, New Orleans

Weissler, Jonathan C MD [Pul] - **Spec Exp:** Interstitial Lung Disease; Asthma; **Hospital:** UT Southwestern Med Ctr at Dallas, Parkland Hlth & Hosp Sys; **Address:** 5909 Harry Hines Blvd, Dallas, TX 75390-8225; **Phone:** 214-645-1825; **Board Cert:** Internal Medicine 1982; Pulmonary Disease 1984; Critical Care Medicine 2007; **Med School:** NYU Sch Med 1979; **Resid:** Internal Medicine, UT Hlth Sci Ctr 1982; **Fellow:** Pulmonary Disease, UT Hlth Sci Ctr 1985; **Fac Appt:** Prof Med, Univ Tex SW, Dallas

West Coast and Pacific

Albertson, Timothy MD/PhD [Pul] - **Spec Exp:** Critical Care; Toxicology; **Hospital:** UC Davis Med Ctr; **Address:** UC Davis Medical Group- Pulmonology Dept, 2825 J St, Ste 400, Sacramento, CA 95816; **Phone:** 916-734-2737 x2; **Board Cert:** Pulmonary Disease 1984; Critical Care Medicine 2007; Emergency Medicine 2007; Medical Toxicology 2005; **Med School:** UC Davis 1977; **Resid:** Internal Medicine, Univ Arizona 1980; Internal Medicine, UC Davis Med Ctr 1981; **Fellow:** Pulmonary Critical Care Medicine, UC Davis Med Ctr 1983; **Fac Appt:** Prof Med, UC Davis

Auger, William R MD [Pul] - **Spec Exp:** Thromboembolic Disorders; Pulmonary Hypertension; **Hospital:** UCSD Med Ctr; **Address:** Thornton Hosp, UCSD, 9300 Campus Point Drive, La Jolla, CA 92037; **Phone:** 858-657-7140; **Board Cert:** Internal Medicine 1986; Pulmonary Disease 1988; **Med School:** Univ Rochester 1982; **Resid:** Internal Medicine, Strong Meml Hosp 1985; **Fellow:** Critical Care Medicine, Ellis Hosp 1986; Pulmonary Disease, UCSD Med Ctr 1989; **Fac Appt:** Clin Prof Med, UCSD

Balmes, John Randolph MD [Pul] - **Spec Exp:** Beryllium-induced Lung Disease; **Hospital:** San Francisco Genl Hosp, UCSF Med Ctr; **Address:** UCSF, Div Occup & Envr Med, Campus Box 0843, 1001 Potrero Ave, rm 5K1, San Francisco, CA 94110; **Phone:** 415-206-8314; **Board Cert:** Internal Medicine 1979; Pulmonary Disease 1984; **Med School:** Mount Sinai Sch Med 1976; **Resid:** Internal Medicine, Mount Sinai Hosp 1979; **Fellow:** Pulmonary Disease, Yale-New Haven Hosp 1981; **Fac Appt:** Prof Med, UCSF

Bellamy, Paul E MD [Pul] - **Spec Exp:** Critical Care; **Hospital:** Kaiser Permanente Woodland Hills Med Ctr; **Address:** Kaiser Woodland Hills Med Ctr, Pulm Div, 5601 De Soto Ave, Med Office Twr, Fl 4, Woodland Hills, CA 91367; **Phone:** 818-719-3530; **Board Cert:** Internal Medicine 1978; Pulmonary Disease 1980; Critical Care Medicine 2007; **Med School:** SUNY Buffalo 1975; **Resid:** Internal Medicine, Univ Hosps-Case West Res 1978; **Fellow:** Pulmonary Disease, UCLA Med Ctr 1980; **Fac Appt:** Clin Prof Med, UCLA

Boushey Jr, Homer A MD [Pul] - **Spec Exp:** Asthma; Lung Injuries-Inhalation Induced; **Hospital:** UCSF Med Ctr; **Address:** UCSF Med Ctr, Pulmonary Medicine, 505 Parnassus Ave, Box 0130, Room M1292, San Francisco, CA 94143; **Phone:** 415-476-8019; **Board Cert:** Internal Medicine 1972; Pulmonary Disease 1974; **Med School:** UCSF 1968; **Resid:** Internal Medicine, UCSF Med Ctr 1970; Internal Medicine, Beth Israel Hosp 1971; **Fellow:** Pulmonary Disease, Oxford Univ 1972; Pulmonary Disease, UCSF Hosp 1974; **Fac Appt:** Prof Med, UCSF

Catanzaro, Antonino MD [Pul] - **Spec Exp:** Tuberculosis; Coccidioidomycosis; Mycobacterial Infections; **Hospital:** UCSD Med Ctr; **Address:** 9500 Gilman Drive Stein Bldg - rm 105, La Jolla, CA 92093; **Phone:** 619-543-5550; **Board Cert:** Internal Medicine 1972; Pulmonary Disease 1976; **Med School:** SUNY Buffalo 1965; **Resid:** Internal Medicine, Georgetown Univ Hosp 1970; **Fellow:** Pulmonary Critical Care Medicine, UCSD Med Ctr 1972; Research, Scripps Clin Rsch Fdn 1972; **Fac Appt:** Prof Med, UCSD

Gerboth, Gregory D MD [Pul] - **Spec Exp:** Asthma; Critical Care; **Hospital:** Providence Alaska Med Ctr; **Address:** Internal Medicine Assocs, 2841 De Barre Rd, Ste 50, Anchorage, AK 99508; **Phone:** 907-276-2811; **Board Cert:** Internal Medicine 2000; Pulmonary Disease 2000; Critical Care Medicine 2000; **Med School:** Med Coll Wisc 1987; **Resid:** Internal Medicine, Med Coll Wisc Med Ctr 1990; **Fellow:** Pulmonary Critical Care Medicine, Med Coll Wisc Med Ctr 1991

Heffner, John E MD [Pul] - **Spec Exp:** Critical Care; Respiratory Failure; **Hospital:** Providence Portland Med Ctr; **Address:** 5050 NE Hoyt St, Ste 540, Portland, OR 97213; **Phone:** 503-215-6258; **Board Cert:** Internal Medicine 1977; Pulmonary Disease 1982; Critical Care Medicine 2005; **Med School:** UCLA 1974; **Resid:** Internal Medicine, Univ Colo Med Ctr 1978; **Fac Appt:** Prof Med, Med Univ SC

Hopewell, Philip C MD [Pul] - **Spec Exp:** AIDS/HIV; Tuberculosis; Infectious Disease-Lung; **Hospital:** San Francisco Genl Hosp; **Address:** San Francisco Genl Hosp, 1001 Potrero Ave, 5K1, San Francisco, CA 94110; **Phone:** 415-206-8314; **Board Cert:** Internal Medicine 1973; Pulmonary Disease 1974; **Med School:** W VA Univ 1965; **Resid:** Internal Medicine, UCSF Med Ctr 1971; **Fellow:** Pulmonary Disease, UCSF Med Ctr 1973; **Fac Appt:** Prof Med, UCSF

Pulmonary Disease

Huang, Laurence MD [Pul] - **Spec Exp:** AIDS/HIV; Pneumocystis Carinii Pneumonia (PCP); **Hospital:** San Francisco Genl Hosp; **Address:** UCSF Positive Health Program-SFGH, 995 Potrero Ave, Bldg 80-Ward 84, San Francisco, CA 94110; **Phone:** 415-206-2484; **Board Cert:** Internal Medicine 2003; Pulmonary Disease 2006; Critical Care Medicine 2007; **Med School:** Columbia P&S 1989; **Resid:** Internal Medicine, Columbia-Presby Hosp 1992; Pulmonary Critical Care Medicine, UCSF Med Ctr 1995; **Fac Appt:** Assoc Clin Prof Med, UCSF

Jacoby, David B MD [Pul] - **Spec Exp:** Viral Infections; Infections-Respiratory; Asthma; **Hospital:** OR Hlth & Sci Univ; **Address:** 3181 SW Sam Jackson Park Rd, MC UHN67, Dept Pulmonary/Crit Care, Portland, OR 97239; **Phone:** 503-494-6158; **Board Cert:** Internal Medicine 1983; Pulmonary Disease 1986; **Med School:** NY Med Coll 1980; **Resid:** Internal Medicine, Temple Univ Hosp 1984; **Fellow:** Pulmonary Critical Care Medicine, UCSF Hosp 1987; **Fac Appt:** Prof Med, Oregon Hlth & Sci Univ

King Jr, Talmadge E MD [Pul] - **Spec Exp:** Interstitial Lung Disease; Sarcoidosis; Asthma; Pulmonary Fibrosis; **Hospital:** UCSF Med Ctr; **Address:** UCSF Dept Medicine, 505 Parnassus Ave, M994, Box 0120, San Francisco, CA 94143-0120; **Phone:** 415-476-0909; **Board Cert:** Internal Medicine 1977; Pulmonary Disease 2009; **Med School:** Harvard Med Sch 1974; **Resid:** Internal Medicine, Emory Univ Affil Hosps 1977; **Fellow:** Pulmonary Critical Care Medicine, Univ Colorado 1979; **Fac Appt:** Prof Med, UCSF

Lynch, Joseph P MD [Pul] - **Spec Exp:** Transplant Medicine-Lung; Interstitial Lung Disease; Pulmonary Fibrosis; Lymphangioleiomyomatosis(LAM); **Hospital:** UCLA Ronald Reagan Med Ctr; **Address:** UCLA - Div Pulmonary Medicine, 200 Medical Plaza Ave, Ste 365B, Los Angeles, CA 90095; **Phone:** 310-825-7921; **Board Cert:** Internal Medicine 1976; Pulmonary Disease 1980; **Med School:** Harvard Med Sch 1973; **Resid:** Internal Medicine, Univ Mich Med Ctr 1976; **Fellow:** Pulmonary Disease, Univ Mich 1978; **Fac Appt:** Prof Med, UCLA

Mosenifar, Zab MD [Pul] - **Spec Exp:** Chronic Obstructive Lung Disease (COPD); Interstitial Lung Disease; Asthma; Pulmonary Hypertension; **Hospital:** Cedars-Sinai Med Ctr; **Address:** Cedars-Sinai Med Ctr, Div Pulmonary Med, 8700 Beverly Blvd, rm 6732 South Twr, Los Angeles, CA 90048-1804; **Phone:** 310-423-1835; **Board Cert:** Internal Medicine 1978; Pulmonary Disease 1980; **Med School:** Iran 1973; **Resid:** Internal Medicine, Thomas Jefferson Univ Hosp; Internal Medicine, UCLA Med Ctr; **Fellow:** Pulmonary Disease, UCLA Med Ctr; **Fac Appt:** Prof Med, UCLA

Patterson, James R MD [Pul] - **Spec Exp:** Sleep Disorders/Apnea; **Hospital:** Providence Portland Med Ctr; **Address:** 1111 NE 99th Ave, Ste 200, Portland, OR 97220; **Phone:** 503-963-3030; **Board Cert:** Internal Medicine 1972; Pulmonary Disease 1974; **Med School:** Columbia P&S 1968; **Resid:** Internal Medicine, Columbia-Presby Med Ctr 1970; **Fellow:** Pulmonary Disease, Fitzsimons Army Med Ctr 1973; **Fac Appt:** Clin Prof Med, Oregon Hlth & Sci Univ

Raghu, Ganesh MD [Pul] - **Spec Exp:** Interstitial Lung Disease; Pulmonary Fibrosis; Sarcoidosis; Transplant-Lung; **Hospital:** Univ Wash Med Ctr; **Address:** 1959 NE Pacific St, Box 356166, Seattle, WA 98195-6166; **Phone:** 206-598-4615; **Board Cert:** Internal Medicine 1982; **Med School:** India 1974; **Resid:** Internal Medicine, Univ Rochester-Strong Meml Hosp 1978; Internal Medicine, SUNY Buffalo Med Ctr 1981; **Fellow:** Pulmonary Critical Care Medicine, Univ Washington Med Ctr 1984; **Fac Appt:** Prof Med, Univ Wash

Rizk, Norman W MD [Pul] - **Spec Exp:** Critical Care; Asthma; Pulmonary Infections; **Hospital:** Stanford Univ Hosp & Clinics; **Address:** 300 Pasteur Drive, rm A175, Stanford, CA 94305; **Phone:** 650-725-7061; **Board Cert:** Internal Medicine 1979; Pulmonary Disease 1984; Critical Care Medicine 2007; **Med School:** Yale Univ 1976; **Resid:** Internal Medicine, San Fran Genl Hosp 1980; **Fellow:** Pulmonary Disease, Moffitt Hosp-UCSF 1983; **Fac Appt:** Prof Med, Stanford Univ

Rubin, Lewis J MD [Pul] - **Spec Exp:** Pulmonary Hypertension; Pulmonary Vascular Disease; **Hospital:** UCSD Med Ctr; **Address:** UCSD Med Ctr, Pulmonary & Crit Care, 9300 Campus Point Drive, La Jolla, CA 92037-7381; **Phone:** 858-657-8700; **Board Cert:** Internal Medicine 1978; Pulmonary Disease 1980; **Med School:** Albert Einstein Coll Med 1975; **Resid:** Internal Medicine, Duke Univ Med Ctr 1978; **Fellow:** Pulmonary Disease, Duke Univ Med Ctr 1979; **Fac Appt:** Prof Med, UCSD

Sharma, Om Prakash MD [Pul] - **Spec Exp:** Sarcoidosis; Interstitial Lung Disease; Hypersensitivity Pneumonitis; **Hospital:** LAC & USC Med Ctr, Keck Med Ctr of USC (page 62); **Address:** 2020 Zonal Ave, IRD/178, Los Angeles, CA 90033; **Phone:** 323-226-7923; **Board Cert:** Internal Medicine 1987; **Med School:** India 1959; **Resid:** Internal Medicine, Norwalk Hosp 1963; Internal Medicine, Montefiore Med Ctr 1965; **Fellow:** Pulmonary Disease, Montefiore Med Ctr 1966; Research, Royal Coll Physicians 1969; **Fac Appt:** Prof Med, USC Sch Med

Tharratt, Robert S MD [Pul] - **Spec Exp:** Disaster Preparedness; Critical Care; Toxicology; **Hospital:** UC Davis Med Ctr; **Address:** UC Davis Medical Center- Pulmonology, Patient Support Services Bldg, 4150 V St, Ste 3100, Sacramento, CA 95817-2214; **Phone:** 916-734-0779 x2; **Board Cert:** Pulmonary Disease 1988; Critical Care Medicine 2009; Medical Toxicology 2004; Emergency Medicine 2007; **Med School:** UCLA 1983; **Resid:** Internal Medicine, UC Davis Med Ctr 1986; **Fellow:** Pulmonary Critical Care Medicine, UC Davis Med Ctr 1989; **Fac Appt:** Prof Med, UC Davis

Wallace, Jeanne M MD [Pul] - **Spec Exp:** Pulmonary Infections; Sleep Disorders/Apnea; Asthma; **Hospital:** Olive View-UCLA Med Ctr; **Address:** Olive View UCLA Med Ctr, 14445 Olive View, Dept Medicine 2B 182, Sylmar, CA 91342-1437; **Phone:** 818-364-3205; **Board Cert:** Internal Medicine 1977; Pulmonary Disease 1980; Sleep Medicine 2007; **Med School:** UCLA 1974; **Resid:** Internal Medicine, UCSF Med Ctr 1977; **Fellow:** Pulmonary Disease, UCSD Med Ctr 1980; **Fac Appt:** Clin Prof Med, UCLA

Wolfe, Robert N MD [Pul] - **Hospital:** Cedars-Sinai Med Ctr; **Address:** 8635 W 3rd St, Ste 965, Los Angeles, CA 90048-6101; **Phone:** 310-657-3792; **Board Cert:** Internal Medicine 1978; Pulmonary Disease 1980; **Med School:** UCLA 1975; **Resid:** Internal Medicine, UCLA Med Ctr 1978; **Fellow:** Pulmonary Disease, Wadsworth VA Med Ctr 1979; **Fac Appt:** Assoc Clin Prof Med, UCLA

Cleveland Clinic

Every life deserves world class care.

Pulmonary Disease

Individuals with all types of acute or chronic lung diseases, as well as sleep disordered breathing (sleep apnea) can access specialty care at Cleveland Clinic. In 2010, physicians in the Department of Pulmonary, Allergy and Critical Care Medicine provided more than 95,000 outpatient visits.

Lung Transplantation

Cleveland Clinic's Lung Transplant Program is the largest in Ohio and among the largest in the United States. In 2010 our program performed 122 lung transplants. The average wait time for a lung transplantation at Cleveland Clinic is significantly lower than the national average.

Sarcoidosis Center of Excellence

Cleveland Clinic established a Sarcoidosis Center of Excellence in 2003. The only such center in Northeastern Ohio, the center aims to raise awareness of pulmonary sarcoidosis, improve the quality of sarcoidosis care and minimize the degree to which it can affect quality of life.

Areas of Expertise

Cleveland Clinic specializes in diagnosing and curing acute respiratory distress syndrome, allergic rhinitis and allergies (drug and food; latex) We have doctors and specialists in the field of aspirin desensitization, asthma and Beryllium-induced lung disease.

In collaboration with Cleveland Clinic thoracic surgeons, patients are evaluated for:

- Lung transplantation
- Lung volume reduction surgery (LVRS) for emphysema
- Pulmonary thromboendarterectomy (for chronic pulmonary hypertension secondary to thromboemboli)

Cleveland Clinic
Pulmonology, Allergy and
Critical Care Medicine
9500 Euclid Avenue
Cleveland, OH 44195

Offering Same-Day Appointments
Call 800.274.2009.

Treatment Guides
Cleveland Clinic has developed comprehensive treatment guides for many diseases and conditions. To download our free treatment guides, visit clevelandclinic.org/treatmentguides.

Online Medical Second Opinion
Call 216.444.3223 or
800.223.2273 ext. 43223 or
email eclevelandclinic@ccf.org.

Out-of-State Patients Assistance
Call 800.223.2273, ext. 55580 or
email medicalconcierge@ccf.org.

Visit Us At:
clevelandclinic.org

Follow Us On:
Facebook
www.facebook.com/clevelandclinic

Twitter
@ClevelandClinic

You Tube
www.youtube.com/clevelandclinic

Health Hub
health.clevelandclinic.org

MOUNT SINAI SCHOOL OF MEDICINE

THE MOUNT SINAI MEDICAL CENTER
PULMONARY MEDICINE
One Gustave L. Levy Place
Fifth Avenue and 100th Street
New York, NY 10029-6574
Physician Referral: 1-800-MD-SINAI (637-4624)
www.mountsinai.org/pulmonary

The mission of Mount Sinai's **DIVISION OF PULMONARY, CRITICAL CARE, AND SLEEP MEDICINE** is to offer state-of-the-art clinical care to patients with all forms of lung disease and critical illness, cutting-edge research that will translate into improved patient care and outcomes, and hands-on training of future leaders in the field.

To achieve this goal, every faculty member is charged with the success of a specific program. Mount Sinai's Pulmonary Division has a long history of providing specialized care and key research in several disease areas that include sarcoidosis and occupational lung diseases. Mount Sinai's Sarcoidosis Service, the largest of its kind in the world, is a Center of Excellence for sarcoidosis research. It is the only site in the United States that performs the diagnostic Kveim- Siltzbach skin test for sarcoidosis, which eliminates the need for more invasive, uncomfortable, and expensive procedures. Through its Pulmonary Physiology Laboratory, Mount Sinai has been instrumental in establishing normal values for various pulmonary function tests and is currently conducting clinical studies of new tests for obesity, sarcoidosis, asthma, and lung cancer.

Pulmonary specialists at Mount Sinai are investigating asthma and emphysema, lung cancer, collagen vascular diseases, pulmonary infections, and occupational lung diseases. Mount Sinai has the largest screening program for workers and anyone in the general population exposed to polluted air at the World Trade Center catastrophe site. Our critical care physicians are experts in treating liver disease and acute and chronic respiratory failure, using the most modern forms of delivery of intensive care and providing compassionate end-of-life care.

The Asthma Program uses a multidisciplinary team approach, focusing on patient education and skill-building to foster self-management.

The Chronic Obstructive Pulmonary Disease Program offers a screening and a coordinated approach of exercise, treatment, and education that improves symptoms and quality of life, for one of the nation's most underdiagnosed conditions.

The Critical Care Medicine Program features state-of-the-art medical intensive care and respiratory care units.

The Interventional Pulmonary Service performs cutting-edge diagnostic and therapeutic procedures for patients with advanced pulmonary diseases.

The Lung Cancer/Thoracic Oncology Service provides specialized care for lung cancer diagnosis and staging and for coordinating multidisciplinary medical care for lung cancer.

The Occupational Lung Disorders Program specializes in the diagnosis and management of occupational lung disorders, such as occupational asthma and bronchitis, asbestosis, silicosis, and heavy metal lung injury.

The Pulmonary Fibrosis/Interstitial Lung Disease Program treats patients with chronic inflammatory and scarring disorders of the lungs, including idiopathic pulmonary fibrosis and collagen vascular-associated pulmonary diseases.

The Pulmonary Physiology Laboratory, performs the full range of physiological lung function and cardiopulmonary exercise testing for lung disease.

The Pulmonary Rehabilitation Program provides occupational, physical, and cardiopulmonary rehabilitation programs for patients with disabling lung disorders, as well as pre- and post-operative consultation and therapy.

The Thoracic Oncology Service provides multidisciplinary medical care for lung cancer, as a joint effort with the Department of Cardiothoracic Surgery.

The Sarcoidosis Service, which has passed its 20,000 enrollee count, offers standard care as well as the opportunity to participate in new clinical trials to 60 new enrollees per week.

PULMONOLOGY

About the Division of Pulmonary, Critical Care and Sleep Medicine
NYU Langone's Pulmonary, Critical Care and Sleep Medicine Division offers a full range of services for the diagnosis and treatment of inpatient and ambulatory patients. Services include pulmonary function laboratories; specialized medical critical care units at Tisch Hospital and the Hospital for Joint Diseases; and a multidisciplinary interventional bronchoscopy program integrated with thoracic radiology at Tisch Hospital. Research grant support includes the National Institutes of Health and the Centers for Disease Control and Prevention. We specialize in the following areas:

Asthma
The Division of Pulmonary Medicine is experienced in treating all aspects of asthma and airway disorders. The Bellevue Asthma Clinic at Bellevue Hospital Center, an affiliate of NYU Langone Medical Center, offers an active research program dealing exclusively with particulate matter pollution and asthma.

Pulmonary Services
The Division of Pulmonary Medicine provides clinical chest services at Tisch Hospital which care for patients with tuberculosis, lung cancer, asthma and interstitial fibrosis. Hospital consultation services are available for interstitial lung diseases, sarcoidosis, pulmonary hypertension, COPD, lung cancer, occupational lung diseases, bronchiectasis, and myobacterial other than TB.

Interventional Bronchoscopy
The Interventional Bronchoscopy Program at Tisch Hospital employs leading-edge techniques to diagnose and treat tumors and inflammatory conditions of the lung.

Lung Cancer Screening Program
Individuals at high risk for lung cancer may schedule a CT-scan as part of our lung cancer screening program. Eligible patients are also choose to contribute to our research efforts by participating in our lung cancer biomarker screening study.

Sleep Disorders
The Sleep Disorders Center at NYU Langone Medical Center offers clinical and research services for physicians and patients in the diagnosis and treatment of severe or prolonged sleeping difficulties. The Center is also equipped for limited home or in-hospital patient monitoring.

Radiation Oncology

a subspecialty of Radiology

A radiation oncologist deals with the therapeutic applications of radiant energy and its modifiers and the study and management of disease, especially malignant tumors.

Training Required: Four years in radiology *plus* additional training and examination.

RADIATION ONCOLOGY

New England

Choi, Noah C MD [RadRO] - **Spec Exp:** Lung Cancer; Esophageal Cancer; Mesothelioma; **Hospital:** Mass Genl Hosp; **Address:** Mass Genl Hosp, Dept Rad Oncology, 100 Blossom St, Cox 3, Boston, MA 02114; **Phone:** 617-726-6050; **Board Cert:** Therapeutic Radiology 1970; **Med School:** South Korea 1963; **Resid:** Radiation Oncology, Princess Margaret Hosp 1970; **Fac Appt:** Prof RadRO, Harvard Med Sch

D'Amico, Anthony V MD/PhD [RadRO] - **Spec Exp:** Prostate Cancer; Brachytherapy; Urologic Cancer; **Hospital:** Dana-Farber Cancer Inst (page 57), Brigham and Women's Hosp (page 57); **Address:** Brigham & Women's Hosp, Radiation Oncology, 75 Francis St, Ste ASB1-L2, Boston, MA 02115; **Phone:** 617-732-8821; **Board Cert:** Radiation Oncology 2010; **Med School:** Univ Pennsylvania 1990; **Resid:** Radiation Oncology, Hosp Univ Penn 1994; **Fac Appt:** Prof RadRO, Harvard Med Sch

DeLaney, Thomas F MD [RadRO] - **Spec Exp:** Sarcoma; Proton Beam Therapy; **Hospital:** Mass Genl Hosp; **Address:** Francis H. Burr Proton Therapy Ctr, MGH Radiation Oncology, 30 Fruit St, Boston, MA 02114; **Phone:** 617-726-6876; **Board Cert:** Therapeutic Radiology 1986; **Med School:** Harvard Med Sch 1982; **Resid:** Therapeutic Radiology, Mass Genl Hosp 1986; **Fac Appt:** Assoc Prof RadRO, Harvard Med Sch

Harris, Jay R MD [RadRO] - **Spec Exp:** Breast Cancer; **Hospital:** Brigham and Women's Hosp (page 57), Dana-Farber Cancer Inst (page 57); **Address:** Dana-Farber Cancer Institute, 450 Brookline Ave, Boston, MA 02215; **Phone:** 617-632-2291; **Board Cert:** Therapeutic Radiology 1976; **Med School:** Stanford Univ 1970; **Resid:** Radiation Therapy, Joint Ctr Rad Ther 1976; **Fellow:** Radiation Therapy, Harvard Med Sch 1977; **Fac Appt:** Prof RadRO, Harvard Med Sch

Hartford, Alan C MD/PhD [RadRO] - **Spec Exp:** Prostate Cancer; Brain & Spinal Tumors; **Hospital:** Dartmouth - Hitchcock Med Ctr; **Address:** Darthmouth-Hitchcock Med Ctr, 1 Med Ctr Drive, Lebanon, NH 03756; **Phone:** 603-650-6602; **Board Cert:** Radiation Oncology 2010; **Med School:** Harvard Med Sch 1992; **Resid:** Radiation Oncology, Mass Genl Hosp 1998; **Fellow:** Radiation Oncology, Mass Genl Hosp 1999; **Fac Appt:** Assoc Prof RadRO, Dartmouth Med Sch

Heimann, Ruth MD [RadRO] - **Spec Exp:** Breast Cancer; Gastrointestinal Cancer; Lung Cancer; **Hospital:** Fletcher Allen Health Care- Med Ctr Campus; **Address:** Fletcher Allen Radiation Medicine, 111 Colchester Ave, Burlington, VT 05401; **Phone:** 802-847-3506; **Board Cert:** Radiation Oncology 1995; **Med School:** UMDNJ-NJ Med Sch, Newark 1989; **Resid:** Radiation Oncology, Meml Sloan-Kettering Cancer Ctr 1993; **Fac Appt:** Prof Med, Univ VT Coll Med

Kachnic, Lisa A MD [RadRO] - **Spec Exp:** Breast Cancer; Gastrointestinal Cancer; Thoracic Cancers; **Hospital:** Boston Med Ctr; **Address:** BMC-Dept Rad Onc, 830 Harrison Ave, Ste LL-100, Boston, MA 02118; **Phone:** 617-638-7070; **Board Cert:** Radiation Oncology 2006; **Med School:** Tufts Univ 1991; **Resid:** Radiation Oncology, Mass Genl Hosp 1996; **Fac Appt:** Prof RadRO, Boston Univ

Kaplan, Irving D MD [RadRO] - **Spec Exp:** Prostate Cancer; Brachytherapy; **Hospital:** Beth Israel Deaconess Med Ctr - Boston; **Address:** BIDMC-Dept of Rad Onc, 330 Brookline Ave, Finard Basment, Boston, MA 02215; **Phone:** 617-667-2345; **Board Cert:** Radiation Oncology 1989; **Med School:** Stanford Univ 1985; **Resid:** Radiation Oncology, Stanford Univ Med Ctr 1989; **Fac Appt:** Asst Prof RadRO, Harvard Med Sch

Loeffler, Jay S MD [RadRO] - **Spec Exp:** Stereotactic Radiosurgery; Brain Tumors-Benign; Meningioma; Acoustic Neuroma; **Hospital:** Mass Genl Hosp; **Address:** Mass Genl Hosp, Radiation Oncology, 100 Blossom St, Boston, MA 02114; **Phone:** 617-724-1548; **Board Cert:** Therapeutic Radiology 1986; **Med School:** Brown Univ 1982; **Resid:** Radiation Oncology, Harvard Joint Ctr for Rad Ther 1986; **Fellow:** Cancer Biology, Harvard Sch Pub Hlth 1985; **Fac Appt:** Prof RadRO, Harvard Med Sch

Peschel, Richard E MD [RadRO] - **Spec Exp:** Prostate Cancer; Testicular Cancer; **Hospital:** Yale-New Haven Hosp, Yale Med Group; **Address:** 35 Park St, rm LL-510, MS 06510, New Haven, CT 06510; **Phone:** 203-785-2958; **Board Cert:** Therapeutic Radiology 1982; **Med School:** Yale Univ 1977; **Resid:** Radiation Oncology, Yale-New Haven Hosp 1981; **Fac Appt:** Prof RadRO, Yale Univ

Recht, Abram MD [RadRO] - **Spec Exp:** Breast Cancer; Gynecologic Cancer; **Hospital:** Beth Israel Deaconess Med Ctr - Boston; **Address:** Beth Israel Deaconess Med Ctr, 330 Brookline Ave Finard Bldg - rm B25, Boston, MA 02215; **Phone:** 617-667-2345; **Board Cert:** Therapeutic Radiology 1984; **Med School:** Johns Hopkins Univ 1980; **Resid:** Radiation Oncology, Joint Ctr Radiation Therapy 1984; **Fac Appt:** Prof RadRO, Harvard Med Sch

Roberts, Kenneth MD [RadRO] - **Spec Exp:** Pediatric Cancers; Lymphoma; Hodgkin's Lymphoma; **Hospital:** Yale-New Haven Hosp, Yale Med Group; **Address:** Yale Univ Sch Med, Dept Radiation Therapy, 15 York St, New Haven, CT 06520-8040; **Phone:** 203-785-2957; **Board Cert:** Internal Medicine 1987; Medical Oncology 1989; Radiation Oncology 1995; **Med School:** Duke Univ 1984; **Resid:** Internal Medicine, Ohio State Univ Hosps 1987; Radiation Oncology, Duke Univ Med Ctr 1992; **Fellow:** Hematology & Oncology, Duke Univ Med Ctr 1989; **Fac Appt:** Assoc Prof Rad, Yale Univ

Russell, Anthony Henryk MD [RadRO] - **Spec Exp:** Gynecologic Cancer; Intensity Modulated Radiotherapy (IMRT); Proton Beam Therapy; **Hospital:** Mass Genl Hosp; **Address:** Clark Ctr for Radiology Oncology, 100 Blossom St, COX LL, Boston, MA 02114; **Phone:** 617-726-7559; **Board Cert:** Therapeutic Radiology 1978; **Med School:** Harvard Med Sch 1974; **Resid:** Radiation Oncology, Mass Genl Hosp 1978

Taghian, Alphonse G MD/PhD [RadRO] - **Spec Exp:** Breast Cancer; **Hospital:** Mass Genl Hosp; **Address:** MGH Dept Radiation Oncology, 100 Blossom St, COX LL, Boston, MA 02114; **Phone:** 617-726-7559; **Board Cert:** Radiation Oncology 2006; **Med School:** Egypt 1980; **Resid:** Radiation Oncology, Vautrin Cancer Ctr 1987; Radiation Oncology, Inst Gustave Roussy 1989; **Fellow:** Radiation Oncology, Mass Genl Hosp 1993; **Fac Appt:** Assoc Prof RadRO, Harvard Med Sch

Tarbell, Nancy MD [RadRO] - **Spec Exp:** Brain Tumors-Pediatric; Proton Beam Therapy; **Hospital:** Mass Genl Hosp; **Address:** Mass Genl Hosp, Proton Therapy Ctr, 55 Fruit St, Ste 107, Boston, MA 02114; **Phone:** 617-724-1836; **Board Cert:** Therapeutic Radiology 1983; **Med School:** SUNY Upstate Med Univ 1979; **Resid:** Therapeutic Radiology, Harvard Med School 1983; **Fac Appt:** Prof RadRO, Harvard Med Sch

Wazer, David E MD [RadRO] - **Spec Exp:** Breast Cancer; Melanoma; Gastrointestinal Cancer; **Hospital:** Rhode Island Hosp, Tufts Med Ctr; **Address:** Rhode Island Hospital, Dept Radiation Oncology, 593 Eddy St, Providence, RI 02903; **Phone:** 401-444-8311; **Board Cert:** Radiation Oncology 1988; **Med School:** NYU Sch Med 1982; **Resid:** Radiation Oncology, Tufts New Eng Med Ctr 1988; **Fellow:** Neurological Chemistry, NYU Med Ctr 1984; **Fac Appt:** Prof RadRO, Tufts Univ

Radiation Oncology

Wilson, Lynn D MD [RadRO] - **Spec Exp:** Cutaneous Lymphoma; Lung Cancer; Head & Neck Cancer; **Hospital:** Yale-New Haven Hosp, Yale Med Group; **Address:** Yale Univ Sch Med, Dept Therapeutic Rad, PO Box 208040, New Haven, CT 06520-8040; **Phone:** 203-737-1202; **Board Cert:** Radiation Oncology 2004; **Med School:** Geo Wash Univ 1990; **Resid:** Therapeutic Radiology, Yale-New Haven Hosp 1994; **Fac Appt:** Prof RadRO, Yale Univ

Zietman, Anthony L MD [RadRO] - **Spec Exp:** Prostate Cancer; Urologic Cancer; Proton Beam Therapy; **Hospital:** Mass Genl Hosp; **Address:** Mass General Hosp, 55 Fruit St, Ste YAW 7E, Boston, MA 02114; **Phone:** 617-724-1158; **Board Cert:** Radiation Oncology 1994; **Med School:** England, UK 1983; **Resid:** Internal Medicine, St Stephens & Westminster Hosp 1986; Radiation Oncology, Mass Genl Hosp 1989; **Fellow:** Radiation Oncology, Middlesex Hosp 1991; Radiation Oncology, Mass Genl Hosp 1994; **Fac Appt:** Prof RadRO, Harvard Med Sch

Mid Atlantic

Berg, Christine D MD [RadRO] - **Spec Exp:** Breast Cancer-Early Detection; Breast Cancer-High Risk Women; **Hospital:** Natl Inst of Hlth - Clin Ctr; **Address:** National Cancer Inst, Executive Plaza North, 6130 Executive Blvd, rm 3100, Bethesda, MD 20892-7346; **Phone:** 301-496-1071; **Board Cert:** Internal Medicine 1980; Medical Oncology 1983; Therapeutic Radiology 1986; **Med School:** Northwestern Univ 1977; **Resid:** Internal Medicine, Northwestern Meml Hosp 1981; Radiation Oncology, Georgetown Univ Hosp 1986; **Fellow:** Medical Oncology, Natl Cancer Inst-NIH 1984

Bogart, Jeffrey A MD [RadRO] - **Spec Exp:** Lung Cancer; Thoracic Cancers; Prostate Cancer; Clinical Trials; **Hospital:** SUNY Upstate Med Univ Shos, Crouse Hosp; **Address:** SUNY Upstate Medical Ctr, Dept Radiation Oncology, 750 E Adams St, rm 222, Syracuse, NY 13210; **Phone:** 315-464-5276; **Board Cert:** Radiation Oncology 1994; **Med School:** SUNY Upstate Med Univ 1989; **Resid:** Radiation Oncology, SUNY Hlth Sci Ctr 1993; **Fac Appt:** Prof RadRO, SUNY Upstate Med Univ

Chao, KS Clifford MD [RadRO] - **Spec Exp:** Intensity Modulated Radiotherapy (IMRT); **Hospital:** NY-Presby/Weill Cornell Med Ctr, NY (page 66); **Address:** 622 W 168th St, New York, NY 10032; **Phone:** 212-305-9987; **Board Cert:** Radiation Oncology 2010; **Med School:** Taiwan 1982; **Resid:** Radiation Oncology, Mallinckrodt Inst Rad-Wash Med Ctr 1993; **Fellow:** Radiation Oncology, Mallinckrodt Inst Rad-Wash Med Ctr 1994; **Fac Appt:** Prof RadRO, Cornell Univ-Weill Med Coll

Constine III, Louis Sanders MD [RadRO] - **Spec Exp:** Pediatric Cancers; Lymphoma; Cancer Survivors-Late Effects of Therapy; Sarcoma; **Hospital:** Univ of Rochester Strong Meml Hosp; **Address:** 601 Elmwood Ave, Box 647, Rochester, NY 14642; **Phone:** 585-275-5622; **Board Cert:** Pediatrics 1978; Pediatric Hematology-Oncology 1978; Therapeutic Radiology 1981; **Med School:** Johns Hopkins Univ 1973; **Resid:** Pediatrics, Moffitt Hosp-UCSF Med Ctr 1975; Pediatrics, Stanford Hosp Med Ctr 1976; **Fellow:** Pediatric Hematology-Oncology, Univ Wash/Chldns Ortho Hosp 1978; Therapeutic Radiology, Stanford Hosp Med Ctr 1978; **Fac Appt:** Prof RadRO, Univ Rochester

Cooper, Jay MD [RadRO] - **Spec Exp:** Head & Neck Cancer; Skin Cancer; Chemo-Radiation Combined Therapy; Intensity Modulated Radiotherapy (IMRT); **Hospital:** Maimonides Med Ctr (page 63); **Address:** 6300 8th Ave, Brooklyn, NY 11220; **Phone:** 718-765-2700; **Board Cert:** Therapeutic Radiology 1977; **Med School:** NYU Sch Med 1973; **Resid:** Radiation Oncology, NYU Med Ctr 1977; **Fac Appt:** Prof RadRO, Albert Einstein Coll Med

DeWeese, Theodore L MD [RadRO] - **Spec Exp:** Urologic Cancer; Prostate Cancer; Testicular Cancer; **Hospital:** Johns Hopkins Hosp (page 61); **Address:** Sidney Kimmel Cancer Ctr, 401 N Broadway, Weinberg Bldg - rm 1343, Baltimore, MD 21231; **Phone:** 410-955-8964; **Board Cert:** Radiation Oncology 2005; **Med School:** Univ Colorado 1990; **Resid:** Radiation Oncology, Johns Hopkins Hosp 1994; **Fellow:** Urologic Oncology, Johns Hopkins Hosp 1995; **Fac Appt:** Prof RadRO, Johns Hopkins Univ

Dicker, Adam P MD/PhD [RadRO] - **Spec Exp:** Prostate Cancer; Urologic Cancer; **Hospital:** Thomas Jefferson Univ Hosp; **Address:** Jefferson Radiation Oncology, 111 South 11th St, Ste G-301, Philadelphia, PA 19107-5097; **Phone:** 215-955-6702; **Board Cert:** Radiation Oncology 2000; **Med School:** Cornell Univ 1992; **Resid:** Radiation Oncology, Meml Sloan Kettering Cancer Ctr 1997; **Fellow:** Radiation Oncology, Meml Sloan Kettering Cancer Ctr 1998; **Fac Appt:** Prof RadRO, Thomas Jefferson Univ

Donahue, Bernadine R MD [RadRO] - **Spec Exp:** Brain Tumors; Gastrointestinal Cancer; Pediatric Cancers; Solid Tumors; **Hospital:** Maimonides Med Ctr (page 63); **Address:** Maimonides Med Ctr, Dept Radiation Oncology, 6300 8th Ave, Lower Level, Brooklyn, NY 11220; **Phone:** 718-765-2700; **Board Cert:** Internal Medicine 1987; Radiation Oncology 1991; **Med School:** Boston Univ 1984; **Resid:** Internal Medicine, Boston Univ Med Ctr 1987; **Fellow:** Radiation Oncology, NYU Med Ctr 1990

Dritschilo, Anatoly MD [RadRO] - **Spec Exp:** Prostate Cancer; Breast Cancer; Pediatric Cancers; **Hospital:** Georgetown Univ Hosp; **Address:** Georgetown Univ Hosp, Dept Radiation Medicine, LL-Bles, 3800 Reservoir Rd NW, Washington, DC 20007; **Phone:** 202-444-3320; **Board Cert:** Therapeutic Radiology 1977; **Med School:** UMDNJ-NJ Med Sch, Newark 1973; **Resid:** Radiation Therapy, Harvard Joint Rad Ther Ctr 1977; **Fac Appt:** Prof Med, Georgetown Univ

Ennis, Ronald D MD [RadRO] - **Spec Exp:** Prostate Cancer; Brachytherapy; Breast Cancer; Stereotactic Radiosurgery; **Hospital:** St. Luke's - Roosevelt Hosp Ctr - Roosevelt Div (page 56), Beth Israel Med Ctr - Petrie Division (page 56); **Address:** 1000 10th Ave, Lower Level, Dept Radiation Oncology, Roosevelt Hospital, New York, NY 10019; **Phone:** 212-523-7165; **Board Cert:** Radiation Oncology 2004; **Med School:** Yale Univ 1990; **Resid:** Therapeutic Radiology, Yale-New Haven Hosp 1994; **Fac Appt:** Assoc Prof RadRO, Albert Einstein Coll Med

Flickinger, John C MD [RadRO] - **Spec Exp:** Neuro-Oncology; Brain & Spinal Tumors; **Hospital:** UPMC Shadyside, UPMC Presby, Pittsburgh; **Address:** UPMC Shadyside, Dept Radiation Oncology, 5230 Centre Ave, Pittsburgh, PA 15213; **Phone:** 412-623-6720; **Board Cert:** Therapeutic Radiology 1985; **Med School:** Univ Chicago-Pritzker Sch Med 1981; **Resid:** Radiation Therapy, Mass Genl Hosp 1985; **Fac Appt:** Prof RadRO, Univ Pittsburgh

Formenti, Silvia C MD [RadRO] - **Spec Exp:** Breast Cancer; Chemo-Radiation Combined Therapy; **Hospital:** NYU Langone Med Ctr (page 68); **Address:** NYU Med Ctr, Dept Radiation Oncology, 160 E 34th St, New York, NY 10016; **Phone:** 212-263-2601; **Board Cert:** Radiation Oncology 1991; **Med School:** Italy 1980; **Resid:** Internal Medicine, San Carlo Borromeo Hosp 1983; Medical Oncology, Univ of Pavia Med Ctr 1985; **Fellow:** Radiation Oncology, USC Med Ctr 1990; **Fac Appt:** Prof RadRO, NYU Sch Med

Freedman, Gary M MD [RadRO] - **Spec Exp:** Breast Cancer; **Hospital:** Hosp Univ Penn - UPHS (page 72); **Address:** Radiation Oncology, PCAM / TRC 4 West, 3400 Civic Ctr Blvd, Philadelphia, PA 19104; **Phone:** 215-662-2428; **Board Cert:** Radiation Oncology 2011; **Med School:** Temple Univ 1993; **Resid:** Radiation Oncology, Fox Chase Cancer Ctr 1997; **Fac Appt:** Assoc Prof RadRO, Univ Pennsylvania

Radiation Oncology

Gejerman, Glen MD [RadRO] - **Spec Exp:** Prostate Cancer; Intensity Modulated Radiotherapy (IMRT); Brachytherapy; Urologic Cancer; **Hospital:** Hackensack Univ Med Ctr; **Address:** Hackensack University Medical Center, 92 Second St, Hackensack, NJ 07601; **Phone:** 201-996-2464; **Board Cert:** Radiation Oncology 2006; **Med School:** UMDNJ-NJ Med Sch, Newark 1990; **Resid:** Radiation Oncology, Montefiore Med Ctr 1995; **Fac Appt:** Asst Clin Prof RadRO, Albert Einstein Coll Med

Goodman, Robert L MD [RadRO] - **Spec Exp:** Breast Cancer; Lymphoma; Prostate Cancer; Brain Tumors; **Hospital:** Saint Barnabas Med Ctr; **Address:** 631 Grand St, Jersey City, NJ 07304; **Phone:** 201-942-3999; **Board Cert:** Internal Medicine 1971; Therapeutic Radiology 1974; Medical Oncology 1975; **Med School:** Columbia P&S 1966; **Resid:** Internal Medicine, Beth Israel Hosp 1970; Radiation Therapy, Harvard Joint Ctr Rad Therapy 1974; **Fellow:** Hematology, NY-Presby Hosp 1969; **Fac Appt:** Prof RadRO, Univ Pennsylvania

Greenberger, Joel S MD [RadRO] - **Spec Exp:** Lung Cancer; Esophageal Cancer; **Hospital:** UPMC Shadyside, UPMC Presby, Pittsburgh; **Address:** UPMC Shadyside, Dept Radiation Oncology, 5230 Centre Ave, Pittsburgh, PA 15232; **Phone:** 412-623-6720; **Board Cert:** Therapeutic Radiology 1977; **Med School:** Harvard Med Sch 1971; **Resid:** Radiation Therapy, Jointa Ctr Radiation Therapy 1977; **Fac Appt:** Prof RadRO, Univ Pittsburgh

Haffty, Bruce MD [RadRO] - **Spec Exp:** Breast Cancer; Head & Neck Cancer; **Hospital:** Robert Wood Johnson Univ Hosp - New Brunswick; **Address:** The Cancer Institute of New Jersey, 195 Little Albany St, rm 2038, New Brunswick, NJ 08903; **Phone:** 732-253-3939; **Board Cert:** Radiation Oncology 1988; **Med School:** Yale Univ 1984; **Resid:** Radiation Oncology, Yale-New Haven Hosp 1988; **Fac Appt:** Prof RadRO, UMDNJ-RW Johnson Med Sch

Hahn, Stephen M MD [RadRO] - **Spec Exp:** Lung Cancer; Prostate Cancer; Sarcoma; Photodynamic Therapy; **Hospital:** Hosp Univ Penn - UPHS (page 72), Penn Presby Med Ctr - UPHS (page 72); **Address:** Hosp of the Univ of Penn, 3400 Spruce St Donner Bldg Fl 2, Philadelphia, PA 19104; **Phone:** 215-662-7296; **Board Cert:** Internal Medicine 1987; Medical Oncology 2001; Radiation Oncology 2004; **Med School:** Temple Univ 1984; **Resid:** Internal Medicine, UCSF Med Ctr 1988; Medical Oncology, Natl Inst Hlth 1991; **Fellow:** Radiation Oncology, Natl Inst Hlth 1994; **Fac Appt:** Prof RadRO, Univ Pennsylvania

Harrison, Louis B MD [RadRO] - **Spec Exp:** Brachytherapy; Head & Neck Cancer; Radiation Therapy-Intraoperative; **Hospital:** Beth Israel Med Ctr - Petrie Division (page 56), St. Luke's - Roosevelt Hosp Ctr - Roosevelt Div (page 56); **Address:** Beth Israel Med Ctr, Dept Rad Onc, 10 Union Square East, Ste 4G, New York, NY 10003-3314; **Phone:** 212-844-8087; **Board Cert:** Therapeutic Radiology 1986; **Med School:** SUNY Downstate 1982; **Resid:** Therapeutic Radiology, Yale-New Haven Hosp 1986; **Fac Appt:** Prof RadRO, Albert Einstein Coll Med

Horwitz, Eric MD [RadRO] - **Spec Exp:** Prostate Cancer; Intensity Modulated Radiotherapy (IMRT); Brachytherapy; **Hospital:** Fox Chase Cancer Ctr (page 58); **Address:** Fox Chase Cancer Ctr, Dept Radiation Oncology, 333 Cottman Ave, Philadelphia, PA 19111; **Phone:** 215-728-5641; **Board Cert:** Radiation Oncology 2010; **Med School:** Albany Med Coll 1992; **Resid:** Radiation Oncology, William Beaumont Hosp 1997

Isaacson, Steven R MD [RadRO] - **Spec Exp:** Brain Tumors; Neuro-Oncology; Stereotactic Radiosurgery; Gliomas; **Hospital:** NY-Presby/Columbia Univ Med Ctr, NY (page 66); **Address:** NY Presbyterian-Columbia Med Ctr, Dept Radiation Oncology, 622 W 168th St BHN Bldg - rm B-11, New York, NY 10032-3720; **Phone:** 212-305-2611; **Board Cert:** Radiation Oncology 1988; Otolaryngology 1978; **Med School:** Jefferson Med Coll 1973; **Resid:** Otolaryngology, Hosp Univ Penn 1978; Radiation Oncology, SUNY Hlth Sci Ctr 1988; **Fac Appt:** Clin Prof RadRO, Columbia P&S

Kalnicki, Shalom MD [RadRO] - **Spec Exp:** Lung Cancer; Head & Neck Cancer; Gynecologic Cancer; Prostate Cancer; **Hospital:** Montefiore Med Ctr-Moses Campus, NY, Montefiore Med Ctr-Einstein Campus, NY; **Address:** Montefiore Medical Group, 1625 Poplar St Fl 2, Bronx, NY 10461; **Phone:** 718-920-5280; **Board Cert:** Therapeutic Radiology 1979; **Med School:** Israel 1974; **Resid:** Radiation Therapy, Montefiore Med Ctr 1978; **Fac Appt:** Clin Prof Rad, Albert Einstein Coll Med

Kleinberg, Lawrence MD [RadRO] - **Spec Exp:** Brain & Spinal Cord Tumors; Brain Tumors-Metastatic; Stereotactic Radiosurgery; Esophageal Cancer; **Hospital:** Johns Hopkins Hosp (page 61); **Address:** Johns Hopkins Oncology Ctr, 401 N Broadway, Weinberg Bldg - Ste 1440, Baltimore, MD 21231; **Phone:** 410-614-2597; **Board Cert:** Radiation Oncology 1994; **Med School:** Yale Univ 1989; **Resid:** Radiation Oncology, Meml Sloan-Kettering Canc Ctr 1993; **Fac Appt:** Assoc Prof RadRO, Johns Hopkins Univ

Knisely, Jonathan P S MD [RadRO] - **Spec Exp:** Brain Tumors; Stereotactic Radiosurgery; **Hospital:** NS-LIJ Hlth Sys (page 67); **Address:** North Shore University Hospital, 300 Community Drive, Manhasset, NY 11030; **Phone:** 516-470-7190; **Board Cert:** Internal Medicine 1989; Radiation Oncology 1993; **Med School:** Univ Pennsylvania 1986; **Resid:** Internal Medicine, Michael Reese Hosp 1989; Radiation Oncology, Univ Toronto Med Ctr 1992; **Fac Appt:** Assoc Prof RadRO, Hofstra N Shore-LIJ Sch Med

Kuettel, Michael R MD/PhD [RadRO] - **Spec Exp:** Prostate Cancer; **Hospital:** Roswell Park Cancer Inst; **Address:** Roswell Park Cancer Inst, Radiation Med, Elm and Carlton Streets, Buffalo, NY 14263; **Phone:** 716-845-1562; **Board Cert:** Radiation Oncology 1992; **Med School:** Northwestern Univ 1985; **Resid:** Internal Medicine, Northwestern Hosp 1986; Radiation Oncology, Johns Hopkins Hosp 1990; **Fac Appt:** Prof RadRO, SUNY Buffalo

Lepanto, Philip B MD [RadRO] - **Hospital:** St. Mary's Med Ctr - Huntington, Cabell Huntington Hosp; **Address:** St Mary's Med Ctr, Dept Rad/Onc, 2900 First Ave, Huntington, WV 25702; **Phone:** 304-526-1143; **Board Cert:** Therapeutic Radiology 1975; **Med School:** Univ Louisville Sch Med 1970; **Resid:** Diagnostic Radiology, Graduate Hosp 1972; Radiation Therapy, Hosp Univ Penn 1975; **Fac Appt:** Clin Prof Rad, Marshall Univ

McCormick, Beryl MD [RadRO] - **Spec Exp:** Breast Cancer; Eye Tumors/Cancer; **Hospital:** Meml Sloan-Kettering Cancer Ctr; **Address:** 1275 York Avenue, New York, NY 10065; **Phone:** 212-639-6828; **Board Cert:** Therapeutic Radiology 1977; **Med School:** UMDNJ-NJ Med Sch, Newark 1973; **Resid:** Therapeutic Radiology, Meml Sloan Kettering Cancer Ctr 1977; **Fac Appt:** Prof RadRO, Cornell Univ-Weill Med Coll

Nicolaou, Nicos MD [RadRO] - **Spec Exp:** Lymphoma; Hodgkin's Lymphoma; Urologic Cancer; Breast Cancer; **Address:** Phila Cancer Treatment, 1 Presidential Blvd, Ste 100, Bala Cynwyd, PA 19004; **Phone:** 610-632-4100; **Board Cert:** Radiation Oncology 2010; **Med School:** South Africa 1984; **Resid:** Radiation Oncology, Univ British Columbia Cancer Ctr 1994; **Fellow:** Radiation Oncology, Fox Chase Cancer Ctr 1995

Nori, Dattatreyudu MD [RadRO] - **Spec Exp:** Prostate Cancer; Brachytherapy; Lung Cancer; Breast Cancer; **Hospital:** NY-Presby/Weill Cornell Med Ctr, NY (page 66), NY Hosp Queens; **Address:** 525 E 68th St, Box 575, New York, NY 10065; **Phone:** 212-746-3679; **Board Cert:** Therapeutic Radiology 1979; **Med School:** India 1970; **Resid:** Radiation Oncology, Meml Sloan Kettering Cancer Ctr 1975; **Fellow:** Radiation Oncology, Meml Sloan Kettering Cancer Ctr 1978; **Fac Appt:** Prof RadRO, Cornell Univ-Weill Med Coll

Porrazzo, Michael S MD [RadRO] - **Spec Exp:** Prostate Cancer; Central Nervous System Cancer; Breast Cancer; Stereotactic Radiosurgery; **Hospital:** Washington Hosp Ctr; **Address:** Wash Hosp Ctr-Dept Radiation Onc, 110 Irving St NW, Ste CG-116, Washington, DC 20010; **Phone:** 202-877-3925; **Board Cert:** Radiation Oncology 1990; **Med School:** Meharry Med Coll 1985; **Resid:** Radiation Oncology, SUNY Hlth Sci Ctr 1989

Randolph-Jackson, Pamela D MD [RadRO] - **Spec Exp:** Breast Cancer; Lung Cancer; Gastrointestinal Cancer; **Hospital:** Washington Hosp Ctr; **Address:** 110 Irving St NW, Ste CG-116, Washington, DC 20010; **Phone:** 202-877-3925; **Board Cert:** Radiation Oncology 2004; **Med School:** E Tenn State Univ 1988; **Resid:** Radiology, Howard Univ Hosp 1992; **Fellow:** Radiation Oncology, Jefferson Med Coll 1993

Regine, William F MD [RadRO] - **Spec Exp:** Stereotactic Radiosurgery; Brain & Spinal Tumors; Gastrointestinal Cancer; **Hospital:** Univ of MD Med Ctr; **Address:** Univ MD Med System-Greenbaum Cancer Ctr, 22 S Green St, Baltimore, MD 21201; **Phone:** 410-328-6080; **Board Cert:** Radiation Oncology 1992; **Med School:** SUNY Upstate Med Univ 1987; **Resid:** Radiation Oncology, Thomas Jefferson Univ Hosp 1991; **Fellow:** Radiation Oncology, Thomas Jefferson Univ Hosp 1992; **Fac Appt:** Prof RadRO, Univ MD Sch Med

Rotman, Marvin Z MD [RadRO] - **Spec Exp:** Bladder Cancer; Gynecologic Cancer; Eye Tumors/Cancer; Prostate Cancer; **Hospital:** SUNY Downstate Med Ctr (Univ Hosp of Bklyn), SUNY Downstate Med Ctr (Univ Hosp of Bklyn) - LICH; **Address:** 450 Clarkson Ave, Box 1211, Brooklyn, NY 11203-2056; **Phone:** 718-270-2181; **Board Cert:** Diagnostic Radiology 1966; Radiation Oncology 1999; **Med School:** Jefferson Med Coll 1958; **Resid:** Internal Medicine, Albert Einstein Med Ctr 1960; Radiation Oncology, Montefiore Hosp Med Ctr 1965; **Fac Appt:** Prof RadRO, SUNY Downstate

Schiff, Peter B MD/PhD [RadRO] - **Spec Exp:** Prostate Cancer; Gynecologic Cancer; Lung Cancer; **Hospital:** NYU Langone Med Ctr (page 68); **Address:** NYU Clinical Cancer Ctr, 160 E 34th St Fl 1, New York, NY 10016; **Phone:** 212-731-5003; **Board Cert:** Radiation Oncology 1990; **Med School:** Albert Einstein Coll Med 1984; **Resid:** Radiation Oncology, Meml Sloan Kettering Cancer Ctr 1988; **Fac Appt:** Prof RadRO, NYU Sch Med

Solin, Lawrence J MD [RadRO] - **Spec Exp:** Breast Cancer; **Hospital:** Albert Einstein Med Ctr; **Address:** 5501 Old York Rd, Radiation Oncology Dept, Philadelphia, PA 19141; **Phone:** 215-456-6280; **Board Cert:** Therapeutic Radiology 1984; **Med School:** Brown Univ 1978; **Resid:** Surgery, Thos Jefferson Univ Hosp 1981; Radiation Oncology, Thos Jefferson Univ Hosp 1982; **Fellow:** Radiation Oncology, Hosp Univ Penn 1984; **Fac Appt:** Prof Emeritus RadRO, Univ Pennsylvania

Stock, Richard MD [RadRO] - **Spec Exp:** Prostate Cancer; Urologic Cancer; **Hospital:** Mount Sinai Med Ctr (page 64); **Address:** Dept Radiation Oncology, 1184 5th Ave, Box 1236, New York, NY 10029; **Phone:** 212-241-7502; **Board Cert:** Radiation Oncology 1993; **Med School:** Mount Sinai Sch Med 1988; **Resid:** Radiation Oncology, Meml Sloan Kettering Cancer Ctr 1992; **Fac Appt:** Prof RadRO, Mount Sinai Sch Med

Streeter Jr, Oscar E MD [RadRO] - **Spec Exp:** Lung Cancer; Head & Neck Cancer; **Hospital:** Howard Univ Hosp; **Address:** Howard Univ Hosp, Dept Radiation Onc, 2041 Georgia Ave NW, Washington, DC 20060; **Phone:** 202-865-6100; **Board Cert:** Radiation Oncology 1989; **Med School:** Howard Univ 1982; **Resid:** Radiation Oncology, Howard Univ 1986; Radiation Oncology, USC Sch Med 1994; **Fac Appt:** Assoc Prof RadRO, USC Sch Med

Suntharalingam, Mohan MD [RadRO] - **Spec Exp:** Head & Neck Cancer; Lung Cancer; Esophageal Cancer; **Hospital:** Univ of MD Med Ctr; **Address:** 22 S Greene St, Ste GGK-0101, Baltimore, MD 21201; **Phone:** 410-328-6236; **Board Cert:** Radiation Oncology 2005; **Med School:** Thomas Jefferson Univ 1990; **Resid:** Radiation Oncology, Univ of MD Med Ctr 1993; **Fellow:** Radiation Oncology, Univ of MD Med Ctr 1994; **Fac Appt:** Prof RadRO, Univ MD Sch Med

Weiss, Marisa C MD [RadRO] - **Spec Exp:** Breast Cancer; **Hospital:** Lankenau Hosp; **Address:** Lankenau Hospital, Dept Rad Oncology, 100 E Lancaster Ave, Wynnewood, PA 19096; **Phone:** 484-476-2433; **Board Cert:** Radiation Oncology 1988; **Med School:** Univ Pennsylvania 1984; **Resid:** Radiation Oncology, Hosp Univ Penn 1988; **Fellow:** Radiological Biology, Hosp Univ Penn 1990

Werner-Wasik, Maria MD [RadRO] - **Spec Exp:** Brain Tumors; Lung Cancer; Melanoma; Breast Cancer; **Hospital:** Thomas Jefferson Univ Hosp; **Address:** Jefferson Radiation Oncology, 111 S 11th St, Ste G-301, Philadelphia, PA 19107; **Phone:** 215-955-6702; **Board Cert:** Radiation Oncology 1994; **Med School:** Poland 1979; **Resid:** Internal Medicine, Framingham Union Hosp 1990; Radiation Oncology, Tufts/New England Med Ctr 1993; **Fellow:** Radiation Oncology, Hosp Univ Penn 1994; **Fac Appt:** Prof RadRO, Thomas Jefferson Univ

Yahalom, Joachim MD [RadRO] - **Spec Exp:** Lymphoma; Hodgkin's Lymphoma; Multiple Myeloma; **Hospital:** Meml Sloan-Kettering Cancer Ctr; **Address:** 1275 York Ave, SM03, Dept Radiation Onc, New York, NY 10065; **Phone:** 212-639-5999; **Board Cert:** Radiation Oncology 1988; **Med School:** Israel 1976; **Resid:** Internal Medicine, Hadassah Hosp 1979; Radiation Oncology, Hadassah Hosp 1984; **Fellow:** Radiation Oncology, Meml Sloan Kettering Canc Ctr 1986; **Fac Appt:** Prof RadRO, Cornell Univ-Weill Med Coll

Zelefsky, Michael J MD [RadRO] - **Spec Exp:** Prostate Cancer; Brachytherapy; Head & Neck Cancer; **Hospital:** Meml Sloan-Kettering Cancer Ctr; **Address:** 1275 York Ave, New York, NY 10065; **Phone:** 212-639-6802; **Board Cert:** Radiation Oncology 1991; **Med School:** Albert Einstein Coll Med 1986; **Resid:** Radiation Oncology, Meml Sloan Kettering Cancer Ctr 1990; **Fac Appt:** Prof RadRO, Cornell Univ-Weill Med Coll

Southeast

Anscher, Mitchell S MD [RadRO] - **Spec Exp:** Prostate Cancer; Brachytherapy; Penile Cancer; Testicular Cancer; **Hospital:** Med Coll of VA Hosp, Hunter Holmes McGuire VA Med Ctr - Richmond; **Address:** 401 College St, Box 980058, Department of Radiation Oncology, Richmond, VA 23298-0058; **Phone:** 804-828-7238; **Board Cert:** Internal Medicine 1984; Radiation Oncology 1987; **Med School:** Med Coll VA 1981; **Resid:** Internal Medicine, St Marys Hosp 1984; Radiation Oncology, Duke Univ Med Ctr 1987; **Fac Appt:** Prof RadRO, Va Commonwealth Univ Sch Med

Beitler, Jonathan J MD [RadRO] - **Spec Exp:** Head & Neck Cancer; Breast Cancer; Lung Cancer; Brachytherapy; **Hospital:** Emory Univ Hosp, Emory Univ Hosp Midtown; **Address:** Winship Cancer Institute, Dept Radiation Oncology, 1365C Clifton Rd NE, Atlanta, GA 30322; **Phone:** 404-778-3473; **Board Cert:** Radiation Oncology 1990; **Med School:** Med Coll PA Hahnemann 1982; **Resid:** Surgery, Downstate Med Ctr 1985; Radiation Oncology, Meml Sloan Kettering Cancer Ctr 1988; **Fac Appt:** Prof RadRO, Emory Univ

Blackstock Jr, A William MD [RadRO] - **Spec Exp:** Lung Cancer; Gastrointestinal Cancer; Clinical Trials; **Hospital:** Wake Forest Baptist Med Ctr; **Address:** Wake Forest, Comprehensive Cancer Ctr, Dept Radiation Oncology, Medical Center Blvd, Winston-Salem, NC 27157; **Phone:** 336-713-3600; **Board Cert:** Radiation Oncology 2006; **Med School:** E Carolina Univ 1989; **Resid:** Radiation Oncology, Univ NC Hosps 1994; **Fac Appt:** Prof RadRO, Wake Forest Univ

Brizel, David M MD [RadRO] - **Spec Exp:** Head & Neck Cancer; Sarcoma; **Hospital:** Duke Univ Hosp; **Address:** Duke Univ Med Ctr, Dept Rad Onc, Box 3085, Durham, NC 27710-0001; **Phone:** 919-668-5637; **Board Cert:** Radiation Oncology 1987; **Med School:** Northwestern Univ 1983; **Resid:** Radiation Oncology, Harvard Joint Ctr Radiation Ther 1987; **Fac Appt:** Prof RadRO, Duke Univ

Chakravarthy, Anuradha (Bapsi) MD [RadRO] - **Spec Exp:** Breast Cancer; Gastrointestinal Cancer; **Hospital:** Vanderbilt Univ Med Ctr (page 75); **Address:** Vanderbilt Radiation Oncology, 22nd St at Pierce Ave, B-1003 TVC Bldg, Nashville, TN 37232; **Phone:** 615-322-2555; **Board Cert:** Radiation Oncology 1994; Internal Medicine 1986; Medical Oncology 1989; **Med School:** Geo Wash Univ 1983; **Resid:** Internal Medicine, Mayo Clinic 1986; Hematology & Oncology, Univ Maryland Cancer Ctr 1990; **Fellow:** Radiation Oncology, Johns Hopkins Univ 1993; **Fac Appt:** Assoc Prof RadRO, Vanderbilt Univ

Cmelak, Anthony J MD [RadRO] - **Spec Exp:** Brain Tumors; Stereotactic Radiosurgery; **Hospital:** Vanderbilt Univ Med Ctr (page 75); **Address:** 2220 Pierce Ave, PRB Bldg, rm B-1003, Nashville, TN 37232-5671; **Phone:** 615-322-2555; **Board Cert:** Radiation Oncology 2008; **Med School:** Northwestern Univ 1992; **Resid:** Radiation Oncology, Stanford Univ Med Ctr 1996; **Fac Appt:** Prof RadRO, Vanderbilt Univ

Crocker, Ian R MD [RadRO] - **Spec Exp:** Brain Tumors; Eye Tumors/Cancer; Melanoma-Choroidal (eye); **Hospital:** Emory Univ Hosp, Emory Univ Hosp Midtown; **Address:** The Emory Clinic, Dept Radiation Onc, 1365C Clifton Rd NE, CT-104, Atlanta, GA 30322; **Phone:** 404-778-3473; **Board Cert:** Therapeutic Radiology 1983; Internal Medicine 1980; **Med School:** Univ Saskatchewan 1976; **Resid:** Internal Medicine, Univ Hosp 1980; Radiation Oncology, Princess Margaret Hosp 1983; **Fac Appt:** Prof RadRO, Emory Univ

Fiveash, John MD [RadRO] - **Spec Exp:** Brain Tumors; Pediatric Cancers; **Hospital:** Univ of Ala Hosp at Birmingham; **Address:** Hazelrig-Salter Radiation-Oncology Ctr, 1700 6th Ave, Birmingham, AL 35249; **Phone:** 205-975-0224; **Board Cert:** Radiation Oncology 2009; **Med School:** Med Coll GA 1993; **Resid:** Radiation Oncology, GA Hlth Sci Univ 1997

Henderson, Randal H MD [RadRO] - **Spec Exp:** Gynecologic Cancer; Prostate Cancer; Brachytherapy; Proton Beam Therapy; **Hospital:** Shands at Univ of FL; **Address:** Univ Florida Proton Therapy Inst, 2015 N Jefferson St, Jacksonville, FL 32206; **Phone:** 904-588-1800; **Board Cert:** Therapeutic Radiology 1984; **Med School:** Texas Tech Univ 1979; **Resid:** Radiation Oncology, Univ Florida/Shands Hosp 1983; **Fac Appt:** Prof RadRO, Univ Fla Coll Med

Kudrimoti, Mahesh R MD [RadRO] - **Spec Exp:** Lung Cancer; Head & Neck Cancer; Brachytherapy; **Hospital:** Univ of Kentucky Albert B. Chandler Hosp; **Address:** Chandler Medical Center, 800 Rose St UKMC Bldg, Lexington, KY 40536; **Phone:** 859-323-0283; **Board Cert:** Radiation Oncology 2003; **Med School:** India 1992; **Resid:** Radiation Oncology, Univ KY Chandler Med Ctr 2001; **Fac Appt:** Assoc Prof RadRO, Univ KY Coll Med

Kun, Larry E MD [RadRO] - **Spec Exp:** Brain Tumors; Pediatric Cancers; **Hospital:** St. Jude Children's Research Hosp, Le Bonheur Chldns Med Ctr; **Address:** St Jude Chldns Research Hosp, 262 Danny Thomas Pl, MS 220, Memphis, TN 38105; **Phone:** 901-595-3565; **Board Cert:** Therapeutic Radiology 1973; **Med School:** Jefferson Med Coll 1968; **Resid:** Therapeutic Radiology, Penrose Cancer Hosp 1972; **Fellow:** Radiation Oncology, Natl Cancer Inst 1974; Radiation Oncology, Rotterdam Radiotherapy Inst 1975; **Fac Appt:** Prof, Univ Tenn Coll Med

Landry, Jerome C MD [RadRO] - **Spec Exp:** Gastrointestinal Cancer; Sarcoma-Soft Tissue; **Hospital:** Emory Univ Hosp, Grady Hlth Sys; **Address:** Emory Dept Radiation Oncology, 1365C Clifton Rd NE, Atlanta, GA 30322; **Phone:** 404-778-3473; **Board Cert:** Radiation Oncology 1988; **Med School:** Harvard Med Sch 1983; **Resid:** Radiation Oncology, Mass Genl Hosp 1987; **Fac Appt:** Prof RadRO, Emory Univ

Larner, James M MD [RadRO] - **Spec Exp:** Neuro-Oncology; Brain Tumors; **Hospital:** Univ of Virginia Health Sys; **Address:** Univ Virginia Medical Ctr, Dept Radiation Oncology, 1240 Lee St, Charlottesville, VA 22908; **Phone:** 434-924-5191; **Board Cert:** Internal Medicine 1983; Medical Oncology 1987; Hematology 1988; Radiation Oncology 1989; **Med School:** Univ VA Sch Med 1980; **Resid:** Internal Medicine, Thos Jefferson Univ Hosp 1983; Radiation Oncology, Montefiore-Einstein Med Ctr 1989; **Fellow:** Hematology & Oncology, Thos Jefferson Univ Hosp 1986; **Fac Appt:** Assoc Prof Med, Univ VA Sch Med

Lee, W Robert MD [RadRO] - **Spec Exp:** Prostate Cancer; Brachytherapy; Intensity Modulated Radiotherapy (IMRT); **Hospital:** Duke Univ Hosp; **Address:** Duke Univ Med Ctr, Div Radiation Oncology, Box 3085, Durham, NC 27710; **Phone:** 919-668-5640; **Board Cert:** Radiation Oncology 1994; **Med School:** Univ VA Sch Med 1989; **Resid:** Radiation Oncology, Univ Fl Affil Hosp 1993; **Fac Appt:** Prof RadRO, Duke Univ

Lewin, Alan A MD [RadRO] - **Spec Exp:** Breast Cancer; Lung Cancer; Brain & Spinal Cord Tumors; **Hospital:** Baptist Hosp of Miami; **Address:** Baptist Hosp Miami, Dept Radiation Oncology, 8900 N Kendall Drive, Miami, FL 33176-2118; **Phone:** 786-596-6566; **Board Cert:** Internal Medicine 1976; Hematology 1978; Medical Oncology 1981; Therapeutic Radiology 1982; **Med School:** Geo Wash Univ 1973; **Resid:** Internal Medicine, Mt Sinai Hosp 1976; **Fellow:** Hematology & Oncology, Beth Israel Med Ctr 1978; Radiation Oncology, Joint Ctr Radiation Therapy 1980; **Fac Appt:** Clin Prof RadRO, Univ Miami Sch Med

Malcolm, Arnold W MD [RadRO] - **Spec Exp:** Prostate Cancer; Breast Cancer; Brachytherapy; **Hospital:** Vanderbilt Univ Med Ctr (page 75); **Address:** Vanderbilt Radiation Oncology, 2220 Pierce Ave, B-1003 Preston Research Bldg, Nashville, TN 37232; **Phone:** 615-322-2555; **Board Cert:** Radiation Oncology 1977; **Med School:** Meharry Med Coll 1973; **Resid:** Radiation Oncology, Joint Ctr Radiation Therapy 1977; **Fac Appt:** Assoc Prof RadRO, Vanderbilt Univ

Marcus Jr, Robert B MD [RadRO] - **Spec Exp:** Pediatric Cancers; Proton Beam Therapy; Bone Cancer; Brain & Spinal Cord Tumors; **Hospital:** Shands Jacksonville Med Ctr; **Address:** 2015 N Jefferson St, Jacksonville, FL 32206; **Phone:** 904-588-1800; **Board Cert:** Therapeutic Radiology 1980; **Med School:** Univ Fla Coll Med 1975; **Resid:** Radiation Oncology, Shands Hosp 1979; **Fac Appt:** Prof RadRO, Univ Fla Coll Med

Markoe, Arnold M MD [RadRO] - **Spec Exp:** Eye Tumors/Cancer; Orbital Tumors/Cancer; Central Nervous System Cancer; Lymphoma; **Hospital:** Univ of Miami Hosp & Clins/Sylvester Comp Canc Ctr, Jackson Meml Hosp; **Address:** Univ of Miami Sylvester Comp Cancer Ctr, 1475 NW 12th Ave Ave NW, rm 1508, Miami, FL 33136; **Phone:** 305-243-4319; **Board Cert:** Therapeutic Radiology 1983; **Med School:** Hahnemann Univ 1977; **Resid:** Radiation Oncology, Hahnemann Hosp 1981; **Fac Appt:** Prof RadRO, Univ Miami Sch Med

Marks, Lawrence B MD [RadRO] - **Spec Exp:** Breast Cancer; Lung Cancer; **Hospital:** NC Memorial Hosp - UNC, Rex HlthCare; **Address:** NC Cancer Hosp, Dept Rad Onc, 101 Manning Drive, rm CB 295, Level B, Campus Box 7512, Chapel Hill, NC 27599-7512; **Phone:** 919-966-0400; **Board Cert:** Radiation Oncology 1989; **Med School:** Univ Rochester 1985; **Resid:** Radiation Oncology, Mass Genl Hosp 1989; **Fac Appt:** Prof RadRO, Univ NC Sch Med

McGarry, Ronald C MD/PhD [RadRO] - **Spec Exp:** Lung Cancer; Lymphoma; Clinical Trials; Stereotactic Radiosurgery; **Hospital:** Univ of Kentucky Albert B. Chandler Hosp; **Address:** Chandler Medical Ctr, Radiation Medicine, 800 Rose St, rm C114C, Lexington, KY 40536; **Phone:** 859-323-6486; **Board Cert:** Radiation Oncology 2010; **Med School:** Canada 1992; **Resid:** Radiation Oncology, Univ W Ontario Regl Cancer Ctr 1997; **Fac Appt:** Prof RadRO, Univ KY Coll Med

Mendenhall, Nancy P MD [RadRO] - **Spec Exp:** Breast Cancer; Lymphoma; Hodgkin's Lymphoma; Prostate Cancer; **Hospital:** Shands at Univ of FL; **Address:** Univ Florida, Proton Therapy Inst, 2015 N Jefferson St, Jacksonville, FL 32206; **Phone:** 904-588-1800; **Board Cert:** Therapeutic Radiology 1985; **Med School:** Univ Fla Coll Med 1980; **Resid:** Diagnostic Radiology, Shands-Univ of Florida 1984; **Fac Appt:** Prof RadRO, Univ Fla Coll Med

Mendenhall, William M MD [RadRO] - **Spec Exp:** Head & Neck Cancer; Stereotactic Radiosurgery; Gastrointestinal Cancer; Gynecologic Cancer; **Hospital:** Shands at Univ of FL; **Address:** Univ Florida, Dept Radiation Oncology, Box 100385, Gainesville, FL 32610-0385; **Phone:** 352-265-0287; **Board Cert:** Therapeutic Radiology 1983; **Med School:** Univ S Fla Coll Med 1978; **Resid:** Radiation Oncology, Univ Fla Affil Hosp 1983; **Fac Appt:** Prof RadRO, Univ Fla Coll Med

Merchant, Thomas E DO [RadRO] - **Spec Exp:** Brain Tumors-Pediatric; **Hospital:** St. Jude Children's Research Hosp; **Address:** St Jude Chldns Rsch Hosp, 262 Danny Thomas Pl, MS 220, Memphis, TN 38105; **Phone:** 901-595-3604; **Board Cert:** Radiation Oncology 2004; **Med School:** Chicago Coll Osteo Med 1989; **Resid:** Radiation Oncology, Meml Sloan Kettering Cancer Ctr 1994

Meredith, Ruby F MD [RadRO] - **Spec Exp:** Multiple Myeloma; Breast Cancer; Radionuclide Therapy; Bone Tumors-Metastatic; **Hospital:** Univ of Ala Hosp at Birmingham; **Address:** 1700 S 6th Ave S, 176 F Bldg, rm 2232Q, MS 35249, 619 19th St S, MS 35233, Birmingham, AL 35249; **Phone:** 205-934-2763; **Board Cert:** Radiation Oncology 1987; **Med School:** Ohio State Univ 1983; **Resid:** Radiation Oncology, Med College Va Hosps 1987; **Fac Appt:** Prof RadRO, Univ Alabama

Morris, Monica M MD [RadRO] - **Spec Exp:** Breast Cancer; Lung Cancer; **Hospital:** Univ of Virginia Health Sys; **Address:** Univ VA Hlth Sciences-Radiation Onc, PO Box 800383, Charlottesville, VA 22908; **Phone:** 434-924-5192; **Board Cert:** Radiation Oncology 2009; **Med School:** Baylor Coll Med 1993; **Resid:** Radiation Oncology, Mass Genl Hosp 1998; **Fac Appt:** Assoc Prof RadRO, Univ VA Sch Med

Pollack, Alan MD/PhD [RadRO] - **Spec Exp:** Prostate Cancer; Genitourinary Cancer; Sarcoma; **Hospital:** Univ of Miami Hosp & Clins/Sylvester Comp Canc Ctr; **Address:** 1475 NW 12th Ave, Ste 1501, Miami, FL 33136; **Phone:** 305-243-4916; **Board Cert:** Radiation Oncology 1993; **Med School:** Univ Miami Sch Med 1987; **Resid:** Radiation Oncology, MD Anderson Cancer Ctr 1992; **Fac Appt:** Prof RadRO, Univ Miami Sch Med

Prosnitz, Leonard MD [RadRO] - **Spec Exp:** Lymphoma; Breast Cancer; Hyperthermia Treatment of Cancer; Sarcoma; **Hospital:** Duke Univ Hosp; **Address:** Duke Univ Med Ctr, Dept Rad Onc, Box 3085, Durham, NC 27710; **Phone:** 919-668-5637; **Board Cert:** Therapeutic Radiology 1970; **Med School:** SUNY Downstate 1961; **Resid:** Internal Medicine, Dartmouth Affil Hosps 1963; Radiation Oncology, Yale-New Haven Hosp 1969; **Fellow:** Hematology & Oncology, Yale-New Haven Hosp 1967; **Fac Appt:** Prof RadRO, Duke Univ

Randall, Marcus E MD [RadRO] - **Spec Exp:** Gynecologic Cancer; Stereotactic Radiosurgery; **Hospital:** Univ of Kentucky Albert B. Chandler Hosp; **Address:** Univ Kentucky Medical Ctr, 800 Rose St, rm C 114D, Office of Radiation Medicine, Lexington, KY 40536-0001; **Phone:** 859-257-7618; **Board Cert:** Therapeutic Radiology 1986; **Med School:** Univ NC Sch Med 1982; **Resid:** Radiation Oncology, Univ Va Med Ctr 1986; **Fellow:** Radiation Oncology, Univ Va Med Ctr 1986; **Fac Appt:** Prof RadRO, Univ KY Coll Med

Rich, Tyvin A MD [RadRO] - **Spec Exp:** Colon & Rectal Cancer; Chemo-Radiation Combined Therapy; Gastrointestinal Cancer; Gallbladder & Biliary Cancer; **Hospital:** Univ of Virginia Health Sys; **Address:** Univ Va Hlth Sys, Dept Rad Onc, 1240 Lee St, PO Box 800383, Charlottesville, VA 22908-0383; **Phone:** 434-924-5191; **Board Cert:** Radiation Oncology 1978; **Med School:** Univ VA Sch Med 1973; **Resid:** Radiation Oncology, Mass Genl Hosp 1978; **Fellow:** Radiation Oncology, Mt Vernon Hosp/Gray Lab 1978; **Fac Appt:** Prof RadRO, Univ VA Sch Med

Rosenman, Julian MD/PhD [RadRO] - **Spec Exp:** Lung Cancer; Breast Cancer; Prostate Cancer; **Hospital:** NC Memorial Hosp - UNC; **Address:** UNC Cancer Hosp, Dept Rad Onc, 101 Manning Drive, Level B, Campus Box 7512, Chapel Hill, NC 27514; **Phone:** 919-966-0400; **Board Cert:** Therapeutic Radiology 1981; **Med School:** Univ Tex SW, Dallas 1977; **Resid:** Therapeutic Radiology, Mass Genl Hosp 1981; **Fac Appt:** Prof RadRO, Univ NC Sch Med

Sailer, Scott MD [RadRO] - **Spec Exp:** Breast Cancer; Genitourinary Cancer; Head & Neck Cancer; **Hospital:** WakeMed Cary, WakeMed-Raleigh Campus; **Address:** Cancer Centers of North Carollina, 300 Ashville Ave, Ste 110, Cary, NC 27518; **Phone:** 919-854-4588; **Board Cert:** Radiation Oncology 1988; **Med School:** Harvard Med Sch 1984; **Resid:** Radiation Therapy, Mass Genl Hosp 1988

Shaw, Edward G MD [RadRO] - **Spec Exp:** Stereotactic Radiosurgery; Brain Tumors; **Hospital:** Wake Forest Baptist Med Ctr; **Address:** Wake Forest Baptist Health, Dept of Radiation Oncology, Medical Ctr Blvd, Winston-Salem, NC 27157; **Phone:** 336-713-6506; **Board Cert:** Radiation Oncology 1987; **Med School:** Rush Med Coll 1983; **Resid:** Radiation Oncology, Mayo Grad Sch Med 1987; **Fac Appt:** Prof RadRO, Wake Forest Univ

Song, Shiyu MD/PhD [RadRO] - **Spec Exp:** Head & Neck Cancer; Lymphoma; **Hospital:** VCU Med Ctr; **Address:** 401 College St, Box 980058, Richmond, VA 23298-0037; **Phone:** 804-828-7232; **Board Cert:** Radiation Oncology 2006; **Med School:** China 1983; **Resid:** Radiation Oncology, Univ Wisc Hosp & Clins; **Fellow:** Radiation Oncology, Johns Hopkins Hosp; **Fac Appt:** Assoc Prof RadRO, Va Commonwealth Univ Sch Med

St Clair, William H MD/PhD [RadRO] - **Spec Exp:** Brain Tumors; Urologic Cancer; Intensity Modulated Radiotherapy (IMRT); **Hospital:** Univ of Kentucky Albert B. Chandler Hosp; **Address:** UKMC Radiation Med Clin, 800 Rose St, rm CC-112A, Lexington, KY 40536; **Phone:** 859-323-6486; **Board Cert:** Radiation Oncology 2000; **Med School:** Univ KY Coll Med 1995; **Resid:** Radiation Oncology, Mass Genl Hosp 2000; **Fellow:** Radiation Oncology, Mass Genl Hosp 2000; **Fac Appt:** Assoc Prof RadRO, Univ KY Coll Med

Tepper, Joel E MD [RadRO] - **Spec Exp:** Gastrointestinal Cancer; Sarcoma; Rectal Cancer; **Hospital:** NC Memorial Hosp - UNC; **Address:** UNC Cancer Hosp, Dept Rad Onc, 101 Manning Drive, Level B, Campus Box 7512, Chapel Hill, NC 27599-7512; **Phone:** 919-445-5216; **Board Cert:** Therapeutic Radiology 1976; **Med School:** Washington Univ, St Louis 1972; **Resid:** Therapeutic Radiology, Mass Genl Hosp 1976; **Fellow:** Therapeutic Radiology, Mass Genl Hosp 1977; **Fac Appt:** Prof RadRO, Univ NC Sch Med

Radiation Oncology

Toonkel, Leonard M MD [RadRO] - **Spec Exp:** Prostate Cancer; Breast Cancer; Brachytherapy; **Hospital:** Mount Sinai Med Ctr - Miami; **Address:** 4300 Alton Rd, BLUM Bldg - Fl 1st, Miami Beach, FL 33140; **Phone:** 305-535-3400; **Board Cert:** Therapeutic Radiology 1979; **Med School:** Univ Miami Sch Med 1975; **Resid:** Radiation Therapy, Jackson Meml Hosp 1977; Diagnostic Radiology, MD Anderson Hosp 1978; **Fellow:** Radiation Oncology, MD Anderson Hosp 1979; **Fac Appt:** Assoc Clin Prof Rad, Univ Miami Sch Med

Vijayakumar, Srinivasan MD [RadRO] - **Spec Exp:** Brachytherapy; Prostate Cancer; **Hospital:** Univ Mississippi Med Ctr; **Address:** 350 Woodrow Wilson Drive, Jackson, MS 39213; **Phone:** 601-984-2550; **Board Cert:** Therapeutic Radiology 1986; **Med School:** India 1978; **Resid:** Radiation Oncology, Madras Univ Med Ctr 1981; Radiation Oncology, Michael Reese Hosp 1984; **Fellow:** Brachytherapy, Univ Chicago Hosps 1985; **Fac Appt:** Prof RadRO, Univ Miss

Willett, Christopher MD [RadRO] - **Spec Exp:** Gastrointestinal Cancer; Clinical Trials; **Hospital:** Duke Univ Hosp; **Address:** Duke Univ Med Ctr, PO Box 3085, Durham, NC 27710; **Phone:** 919-668-5640; **Board Cert:** Therapeutic Radiology 1985; **Med School:** Tufts Univ 1981; **Resid:** Radiation Oncology, Mass Genl Hosp 1986; **Fac Appt:** Prof RadRO, Duke Univ

Wolfson, Aaron H MD [RadRO] - **Spec Exp:** Gynecologic Cancer; Sarcoma; Gastrointestinal Cancer; **Hospital:** Univ of Miami Hosp & Clins/Sylvester Comp Canc Ctr; **Address:** UMHC Sylvester Comp Cancer Ctr, 1475 NW 12th Ave, Ste D31, Miami, FL 33136; **Phone:** 305-243-4210; **Board Cert:** Radiation Oncology 1999; **Med School:** Univ Fla Coll Med 1982; **Resid:** Radiation Oncology, Med Coll of Virginia 1989; **Fac Appt:** Prof RadRO, Univ Miami Sch Med

Woo, Shiao Y MD [RadRO] - **Spec Exp:** Brain Tumors-Adult & Pediatric; Proton Beam Therapy; Stereotactic Radiosurgery; Pediatric Cancers; **Hospital:** Univ of Louisville Hosp; **Address:** James Graham Brown Cancer Ctr, 529 S Jackson St, Lower Level, Louisville, KY 40202; **Phone:** 502-562-4759; **Board Cert:** Radiation Oncology 1988; Pediatrics 1980; **Med School:** Malaysia 1972; **Resid:** Pediatrics, Georgetown Univ Hosp 1978; **Fellow:** Pediatric Hematology-Oncology, Georgetown Univ Hosp 1980; Radiation Oncology, Georgetown Univ Hosp 1988; **Fac Appt:** Prof RadRO, Univ Louisville Sch Med

Midwest

Abrams, Ross A MD [RadRO] - **Spec Exp:** Gastrointestinal Cancer; Lymphoma; **Hospital:** Rush Univ Med Ctr; **Address:** Women's Board Ctr for Radiation Therapy, 500 S Paulina, Ground Floor Atrium, Chicago, IL 60612; **Phone:** 312-942-5751; **Board Cert:** Internal Medicine 1976; Medical Oncology 1979; Hematology 1982; Radiation Oncology 1987; **Med School:** Univ Pennsylvania 1973; **Resid:** Internal Medicine, Pennsylvania Hosp 1975; Hematology & Oncology, Hosp Univ Penn 1976; **Fellow:** Hematology & Oncology, Natl Cancer Inst 1978; Radiation Oncology, Med Coll Wisconsin 1987; **Fac Appt:** Prof RadRO, Rush Med Coll

Awan, Azhar M MD [RadRO] - **Spec Exp:** Brain Tumors; Prostate Cancer; Breast Cancer; **Hospital:** Sherman Hosp, Univ of Chicago Med Ctr; **Address:** Sherman Hosp Cancer Care Ctr, 1425 N Randall Rd, Elgin, IL 60123; **Phone:** 224-783-8746; **Board Cert:** Therapeutic Radiology 1985; **Med School:** Loyola Univ-Stritch Sch Med 1981; **Resid:** Therapeutic Radiology, Rush Med Ctr 1985; **Fac Appt:** Assoc Prof RadRO, Univ Chicago-Pritzker Sch Med

Bradley, Jeffrey D MD [RadRO] - **Spec Exp:** Lung Cancer; Esophageal Cancer; Thoracic Cancers; Clinical Trials; **Hospital:** Barnes-Jewish Hosp; **Address:** Ctr for Advanced Medicine, Rad Oncology, 4921 Parkview Pl Fl LL, St Louis, MO 63110; **Phone:** 314-747-7236; **Board Cert:** Radiation Oncology 2009; **Med School:** Univ Ark 1993; **Resid:** Radiation Oncology, Univ Chicago 1998; **Fac Appt:** Assoc Prof RadRO, Washington Univ, St Louis

Buatti, John M MD [RadRO] - **Spec Exp:** Central Nervous System Cancer; **Hospital:** Univ Iowa Hosp & Clinics; **Address:** Univ Iowa Hosp & Clin, Dept Rad Onc, 200 Hawkins Drive PFP Bldg - rm 01626, Iowa City, IA 52242; **Phone:** 319-356-2699; **Board Cert:** Radiation Oncology 1994; **Med School:** Georgetown Univ 1986; **Resid:** Internal Medicine, Georgetown Univ 1989; **Fellow:** Radiation Oncology, Univ Arizona 1993; **Fac Appt:** Prof RadRO, Univ Iowa Coll Med

Chakravarti, Arnab MD [RadRO] - **Spec Exp:** Brain Tumors; **Hospital:** Ohio St Univ Med Ctr; **Address:** Arthur G James Comp Cancer Ctr, Ohio State Univ Medical School, 300 W 10th Ave, rm 080B, Columbus, OH 43210; **Phone:** 614-293-8415; **Board Cert:** Radiation Oncology 2010; **Med School:** Univ VA Sch Med 1995; **Resid:** Radiation Oncology, Mass General Hosp 2000; **Fac Appt:** Prof RadRO, Ohio State Univ

Ciezki, Jay P MD [RadRO] - **Spec Exp:** Brachytherapy; Prostate Cancer; Genitourinary Cancer; **Hospital:** Cleveland Clin (page 55); **Address:** Cleveland Clinic, 9500 Euclid Ave, MC T28, Cleveland, OH 44195; **Phone:** 216-445-9465; **Board Cert:** Radiation Oncology 2005; **Med School:** Med Coll Wisc 1991; **Resid:** Radiation Oncology, Cleveland Clinic 1995; **Fellow:** Brachytherapy, Cleveland Clinic 1996

Eisbruch, Avraham MD [RadRO] - **Spec Exp:** Head & Neck Cancer; **Hospital:** Univ of Michigan Hosp; **Address:** Univ MI Hlth Sys, 1500 E Med Ctr Drive, Fl B2 - rm C490, Ann Arbor, MI 48109; **Phone:** 734-936-4319; **Board Cert:** Radiation Oncology 1992; **Med School:** Israel 1979; **Resid:** Radiology, Washington Univ 1992; **Fellow:** Medical Oncology, Univ TX MD Anderson Cancer Ctr 1996; **Fac Appt:** Assoc Clin Prof RadRO, Univ Mich Med Sch

Emami, Bahman MD [RadRO] - **Spec Exp:** Head & Neck Cancer; Lung Cancer; **Hospital:** Loyola Univ Med Ctr, Edward Hines, Jr. VA Hosp; **Address:** Loyola Univ Med Ctr, Dept Rad Onc, 2160 S First Ave Bldg 150 - rm 0300, Maywood, IL 60153-3328; **Phone:** 708-216-2729; **Board Cert:** Therapeutic Radiology 1976; **Med School:** Iran 1968; **Resid:** Radiation Therapy, St Vincents Hosp 1973; Radiation Therapy, New England Med Ctr 1977; **Fac Appt:** Prof RadRO, Loyola Univ-Stritch Sch Med

Forman, Jeffrey D MD [RadRO] - **Spec Exp:** Neutron Therapy for Advanced Cancer; Genitourinary Cancer; Prostate Cancer; **Hospital:** Botsford Hosp; **Address:** 70 Fulton St, Pontiac, MI 48341; **Phone:** 248-338-0300; **Board Cert:** Radiation Oncology 1986; **Med School:** NYU Sch Med 1982; **Resid:** Radiation Oncology, Johns Hopkins Hosp 1986; **Fellow:** Therapeutic Radiology, Johns Hopkins Hosp 1987; **Fac Appt:** Prof RadRO, Wayne State Univ

Grigsby, Perry W MD [RadRO] - **Spec Exp:** Gynecologic Cancer; Thyroid Cancer; **Hospital:** Barnes-Jewish Hosp, St. Louis Chldns Hosp; **Address:** Ctr for Advanced Medicine, Rad Oncology, 4921 Parkview Pl Fl LL, St Louis, MO 63110; **Phone:** 314-747-7236; **Board Cert:** Radiation Oncology 1987; **Med School:** Univ KY Coll Med 1982; **Resid:** Radiation Oncology, Barnes Jewish Hosp 1985; **Fac Appt:** Prof RadRO, Washington Univ, St Louis

Halpern, Howard J MD/PhD [RadRO] - **Spec Exp:** Breast Cancer; Esophageal Cancer; Gynecologic Cancer; **Hospital:** Univ of Chicago Med Ctr, Univ of IL Med Ctr at Chicago; **Address:** Univ Chicago Med Ctr, Dept Radiation Onc, 5758 S Maryland Ave, MC 9006, Chicago, IL 60637; **Phone:** 773-702-6870; **Board Cert:** Therapeutic Radiology 1984; **Med School:** Univ Miami Sch Med 1980; **Resid:** Therapeutic Radiology, Harvard Jnt Ctr Rad Ther 1984; **Fellow:** Therapeutic Radiology, Harvard Jnt Ctr Rad Ther 1985; **Fac Appt:** Prof RadRO, Univ Chicago-Pritzker Sch Med

Radiation Oncology

Haraf, Daniel J MD [RadRO] - **Spec Exp:** Head & Neck Cancer; Lung Cancer; Prostate Cancer; **Hospital:** Univ of Chicago Med Ctr; **Address:** Univ Chicago Med Ctr, Dept Radiation Onc, 5841 S Maryland Ave, rm 1D, MC 9006, Chicago, IL 60637; **Phone:** 773-702-6870; **Board Cert:** Internal Medicine 1985; Radiation Oncology 1990; **Med School:** Ros Franklin Univ/Chicago Med Sch 1982; **Resid:** Internal Medicine, Michael Reese Hosp 1985; **Fellow:** Radiation Oncology, Michael Reese Hosp 1988; **Fac Appt:** Prof RadRO, Univ Chicago-Pritzker Sch Med

Harari, Paul M MD [RadRO] - **Spec Exp:** Head & Neck Cancer; **Hospital:** Univ WI Hosp & Clins; **Address:** Dept of Human Oncology, 600 Highland Ave, Ste K4/B100, Madison, WI 53792; **Phone:** 608-263-8500; **Board Cert:** Radiation Oncology 1990; **Med School:** Univ VA Sch Med 1984; **Resid:** Radiation Oncology, Univ Arizona Med Ctr 1990; **Fac Appt:** Prof RadRO, Univ Wisc

Hayman, James A MD [RadRO] - **Spec Exp:** Breast Cancer; Stomach Cancer; Lung Cancer; Brain Tumors; **Hospital:** Univ of Michigan Hosp; **Address:** Univ Michigan Hosp, 1500 E Medical Ctr Drive, rm UH B2C490, Ann Arbor, MI 48109-0010; **Phone:** 734-647-9956; **Board Cert:** Radiation Oncology 2004; **Med School:** Univ Chicago-Pritzker Sch Med 1991; **Resid:** Radiation Therapy, Joint Ctr for Radiation Therapy 1996; **Fac Appt:** Assoc Prof RadRO, Univ Mich Med Sch

Johnstone, Peter A S MD [RadRO] - **Spec Exp:** Prostate Cancer; Proton Beam Therapy; Head & Neck Cancer; **Hospital:** IU Health University Hosp; **Address:** 535 Barnhill Drive, Ste 041, Indianapolis, IN 46202; **Phone:** 317-944-2524; **Board Cert:** Radiation Oncology 2010; **Med School:** Uniformed Srvs Univ, Bethesda 1989; **Resid:** Radiation Oncology, Natl Cancer Inst 1993; **Fac Appt:** Prof RadRO, Indiana Univ

Jose, Baby Oliapuram MD [RadRO] - **Spec Exp:** Head & Neck Cancer; Lung Cancer; Gynecologic Cancer; Prostate Cancer; **Hospital:** Floyd Meml Hosp & Hlth Svcs; **Address:** Univ Radiotherapy Assocs, Cancer Ctr of Indiana, 2210 Green Valley Rd, New Albany, IN 47150; **Phone:** 812-945-4000; **Board Cert:** Therapeutic Radiology 1978; **Med School:** India 1971; **Resid:** Surgery, Christian Med Coll Hosp 1974; Radiation Oncology, Christian Med Coll Hosp 1976; **Fellow:** Radiation Oncology, Brown Univ-RI Hosp 1979; **Fac Appt:** Prof RadRO, Univ Louisville Sch Med

Konski, Andre MD [RadRO] - **Spec Exp:** Esophageal Cancer; Rectal Cancer; Pancreatic Cancer; Gastrointestinal Cancer; **Hospital:** Barbara Ann Karmanos Cancer Inst; **Address:** Dept Radiation Oncology, 4100 John R St, Detroit, MI 48201; **Phone:** 313-576-9620; **Board Cert:** Radiation Oncology 2000; **Med School:** NY Med Coll 1984; **Resid:** Radiation Oncology, Stong Meml/Genesee Hosp 1988; **Fac Appt:** Prof RadRO, Wayne State Univ

Lawrence, Theodore S MD/PhD [RadRO] - **Spec Exp:** Gastrointestinal Cancer; Liver Cancer; Pancreatic Cancer; **Hospital:** Univ of Michigan Hosp; **Address:** Univ of Mich Hosp, Dept Rad Onc, 1500 E Med Ctr Dr, SPC5010, Box 5010, UH-B2-C502, Ann Arbor, MI 48109-5010; **Phone:** 734-936-4300; **Board Cert:** Internal Medicine 1983; Medical Oncology 1985; Radiation Oncology 1987; **Med School:** Cornell Univ-Weill Med Coll 1980; **Resid:** Internal Medicine, Stanford Univ Hosp 1983; Radiation Oncology, Natl Cancer Inst 1987; **Fellow:** Medical Oncology, Natl Cancer Inst 1986; **Fac Appt:** Prof RadRO, Univ Mich Med Sch

Lee, Chung K MD [RadRO] - **Spec Exp:** Head & Neck Cancer; Breast Cancer; Lymphoma; Gastrointestinal Cancer; **Hospital:** Univ Minn Med Ctr, Fairview - Riverside Campus; **Address:** Univ Minn, Dept Radiation Oncology, 420 Delaware St SE, MMC 400, Minneapolis, MN 55455; **Phone:** 612-273-6700; **Board Cert:** Therapeutic Radiology 1976; **Med School:** Korea 1965; **Resid:** Radiation Oncology, Yonsei Univ Hosp 1971; Therapeutic Radiology, Univ of Minn Hosp 1976; **Fellow:** Yonsei Univ Hosp; **Fac Appt:** Prof RadRO, Univ Minn

Machtay, Mitchell MD [RadRO] - **Spec Exp:** Head & Neck Cancer; Skin Cancer; Skull Base Tumors; **Hospital:** Univ Hosps Case Med Ctr (page 74); **Address:** UH Case Medical Center/Seidman Cancer Center, Dept Rad Onc, 11100 Euclid Ave, Cleveland, OH 44106; **Phone:** 216-844-2530; **Board Cert:** Radiation Oncology 1994; **Med School:** NYU Sch Med 1989; **Resid:** Radiation Oncology, Hosp Univ Penn 1993; **Fac Appt:** Assoc Prof RadRO, Jefferson Med Coll

Macklis, Roger M MD [RadRO] - **Spec Exp:** Radioimmunotherapy of Cancer; Breast Cancer; Lymphoma; **Hospital:** Cleveland Clin (page 55); **Address:** Cleveland Cin Fdn, Dept Rad Onc, 9500 Euclid Ave, Desk T28, Cleveland, OH 44195; **Phone:** 216-444-5576; **Board Cert:** Radiation Oncology 1989; **Med School:** Harvard Med Sch 1983; **Resid:** Radiation Oncology, Joint Ctr Radiotherapy Inst 1987; **Fellow:** Research, Dana Farber Cancer Inst 1987; **Fac Appt:** Prof RadRO, Case West Res Univ

Martenson Jr, James A MD [RadRO] - **Spec Exp:** Mucositis; Esophageal Cancer; Gastrointestinal Cancer; **Hospital:** Mayo Med Ctr & Clin - Rochester; **Address:** Mayo Clinic, Dept Rad/Onc, 200 First St SW, Rochester, MN 55905; **Phone:** 507-284-4561; **Board Cert:** Therapeutic Radiology 1985; **Med School:** Univ Wash 1981; **Resid:** Radiation Oncology, Mayo Clinic 1985; **Fac Appt:** Prof RadRO, Mayo Med Sch

Michalski, Jeff M MD [RadRO] - **Spec Exp:** Prostate Cancer; Sarcoma; Pediatric Cancers; **Hospital:** Barnes-Jewish Hosp, St. Louis Chldns Hosp; **Address:** Ctr for Advanced Medicine, Rad Oncology, 4921 Parkview Pl Fl LL, St Louis, MO 63110; **Phone:** 314-747-7236; **Board Cert:** Radiation Oncology 1991; **Med School:** Med Coll Wisc 1986; **Resid:** Radiation Oncology, Columbia Presby Med Ctr 1988; Radiation Oncology, Mallinckrodt Inst of Radiology 1990; **Fellow:** Radiation Oncology, Mallinckrodt Inst of Radiology 1991; **Fac Appt:** Prof RadRO, Washington Univ, St Louis

Mittal, Bharat B MD [RadRO] - **Spec Exp:** Head & Neck Cancer; Lymphoma; Skin Cancer; **Hospital:** Northwestern Meml Hosp; **Address:** 251 E Huron St, Galter LC-178, Chicago, IL 60611; **Phone:** 312-926-2520; **Board Cert:** Therapeutic Radiology 1981; **Med School:** India 1975; **Resid:** Internal Medicine, Christian Med Coll 1976; Radiation Oncology, Northwestern Meml Hosp 1980; **Fellow:** Radiation Oncology, Mallinckrodt Inst 1981; **Fac Appt:** Prof RadRO, Northwestern Univ

Movsas, Benjamin MD [RadRO] - **Spec Exp:** Lung Cancer; Brain Tumors; Prostate Cancer; Stereotactic Radiosurgery; **Hospital:** Henry Ford Hosp; **Address:** Henry Ford Health Sys, Dept Rad Oncology, 2799 W Grand Blvd, Detroit, MI 48202-2608; **Phone:** 313-916-1021; **Board Cert:** Radiation Oncology 2010; **Med School:** Washington Univ, St Louis 1990; **Resid:** Radiation Oncology, National Cancer Inst 1995

Myerson, Robert J MD [RadRO] - **Spec Exp:** Gastrointestinal Cancer; Breast Cancer; Hyperthermia Treatment of Cancer; **Hospital:** Barnes-Jewish Hosp; **Address:** Ctr for Advanced Med, Rad Oncology, 4921 Parkview Pl Fl LL, St Louis, MO 63110; **Phone:** 314-747-7236; **Board Cert:** Therapeutic Radiology 1985; **Med School:** Univ Miami Sch Med 1980; **Resid:** Radiation Therapy, Hosp Univ Penn 1984; **Fac Appt:** Prof RadRO, Washington Univ, St Louis

Pierce, Lori J MD [RadRO] - **Spec Exp:** Breast Cancer; **Hospital:** Univ of Michigan Hosp; **Address:** Univ of Michigan Hosp, Dept Rad Onc, 1500 E Medical Ctr Drive, rm B2C440, Ann Arbor, MI 48109-5099; **Phone:** 734-936-4300; **Board Cert:** Radiation Oncology 1989; **Med School:** Duke Univ 1985; **Resid:** Radiation Oncology, Hosp Univ Penn 1989; **Fac Appt:** Prof RadRO, Univ Mich Med Sch

Radiation Oncology

Schomberg, Paula J MD [RadRO] - **Spec Exp:** Brain Tumors; Pediatric Cancers; **Hospital:** Mayo Med Ctr & Clin - Rochester; **Address:** Mayo Clinic - Charlton Bldg, Desk R, 200 1st St SW, Rochester, MN 55905; **Phone:** 507-284-4561; **Board Cert:** Therapeutic Radiology 1984; **Med School:** Med Coll Wisc 1979; **Resid:** Radiation Therapy, Mayo Clinic 1983; **Fac Appt:** Prof RadRO, Mayo Med Sch

Small Jr, William MD [RadRO] - **Spec Exp:** Gynecologic Cancer; Gastrointestinal Cancer; Breast Cancer; Pancreatic Cancer; **Hospital:** Northwestern Meml Hosp; **Address:** 251 E Huron St, Galter Bldg, Ste 178, Chicago, IL 60611; **Phone:** 312-472-3650; **Board Cert:** Radiation Oncology 2004; **Med School:** Northwestern Univ 1990; **Resid:** Radiation Oncology, Northwestern Univ 1994; **Fac Appt:** Prof RadRO, Northwestern Univ

Suh, John H MD [RadRO] - **Spec Exp:** Brain Tumors-Adult & Pediatric; Stereotactic Radio-surgery; Stereotactic Body Radiation Therapy; **Hospital:** Cleveland Clin (page 55); **Address:** Cleveland Clinic, Dept Rad/Onc, 9500 Euclid Ave, Desk T28, Cleveland, OH 44195-0001; **Phone:** 216-444-5574; **Board Cert:** Radiation Oncology 2011; **Med School:** Univ Miami Sch Med 1990; **Resid:** Radiation Oncology, Cleveland Clinic 1994; **Fellow:** Radiation Oncology, Cleveland Clinic 1995

Vicini, Frank A MD [RadRO] - **Spec Exp:** Breast Cancer; Prostate Cancer; Brachytherapy; **Hospital:** Botsford Hosp; **Address:** Botsford Radiation Oncology Ctr, 28595 Orchard Lake Rd, Ste 110, Farmington Hills, MI 48334; **Phone:** 248-553-0606; **Board Cert:** Radiation Oncology 1999; **Med School:** Wayne State Univ 1985; **Resid:** Radiation Oncology, Beaumont Hosp 1989; **Fellow:** Radiation Oncology, Harvard Med Sch/Joint Ctr for Rad Ther 1990; **Fac Appt:** Clin Prof RadRO, Oakland Univ-William Beaumont Med Sch

Videtic, Gregory M MD [RadRO] - **Spec Exp:** Lung Cancer; Mesothelioma; Esophageal Cancer; Thymoma; **Hospital:** Cleveland Clin (page 55); **Address:** Cleveland Clinic, Radiation Oncology, 9500 Euclid Ave, MC T28, Cleveland, OH 44195; **Phone:** 216-444-9797; **Board Cert:** Radiation Oncology 2009; **Med School:** McGill Univ 1986; **Resid:** Radiation Oncology, Dalhousie Univ 1988; Radiation Oncology, London Regl Cancer Ctr 1997; **Fellow:** Radiation Oncology, Wayne State Univ 1998; **Fac Appt:** Assoc Prof Rad, Cleveland Cl Coll Med/Case West Res

Weichselbaum, Ralph R MD [RadRO] - **Spec Exp:** Gene Targeted Radiotherapy; Pancreatic Cancer; Rectal Cancer; **Hospital:** Univ of Chicago Med Ctr; **Address:** Univ Chicago Med Ctr, Dept Radiation Onc, 5841 S Maryland Ave, rm 1D, MC 9006, Chicago, IL 60637; **Phone:** 773-702-6870; **Board Cert:** Therapeutic Radiology 1975; **Med School:** Univ IL Coll Med 1971; **Resid:** Therapeutic Radiology, Harvard Jt Ctr Rad Therapy 1975; **Fellow:** Harvard Univ 1976; **Fac Appt:** Prof RadRO, Univ Chicago-Pritzker Sch Med

Wilson, J Frank MD [RadRO] - **Spec Exp:** Breast Cancer; Skin Cancer; **Hospital:** Froedtert and Med Ctr of WI; **Address:** Dept Radiation Oncology, 9200 W Wisconsin Ave, Milwaukee, WI 53226; **Phone:** 414-805-4400; **Board Cert:** Therapeutic Radiology 1971; **Med School:** Univ MO-Columbia Sch Med 1965; **Resid:** Radiation Therapy, Penrose Cancer Hosp 1969; **Fellow:** Radiation Therapy, Natl Cancer Inst/NIH 1971; **Fac Appt:** Prof RadRO, Med Coll Wisc

Great Plains and Mountains

Gaffney, David K MD/PhD [RadRO] - **Spec Exp:** Breast Cancer; Gynecologic Cancer; **Hospital:** Univ Utah Hlth Care; **Address:** Huntsman Cancer Hosp, Dept Rad Oncology, 1950 Circle of Hope, rm 1440, Salt Lake City, UT 84112-5560; **Phone:** 801-581-2396; **Board Cert:** Radiation Oncology 2007; **Med School:** Med Coll Wisc 1992; **Resid:** Radiation Oncology, Univ Utah Hosps 1996; **Fac Appt:** Assoc Prof, Univ Utah

Rabinovitch, Rachel A MD [RadRO] - **Spec Exp:** Breast Cancer; Lymphoma; **Hospital:** Univ of CO Hosp - Anschutz Inpatient Pav; **Address:** Anschutz Cancer Pavilion, Dept Rad Oncology, 1665 Aurora Court, Ste 1032, MS F-706, Aurora, CO 80045; **Phone:** 720-848-0156; **Board Cert:** Radiation Oncology 1994; **Med School:** Albert Einstein Coll Med 1989; **Resid:** Radiation Oncology, Meml Sloan Kettering Cancer Ctr 1993; **Fac Appt:** Assoc Prof RadRO, Univ Colorado

Shrieve, Dennis C MD/PhD [RadRO] - **Spec Exp:** Brain Tumors-Adult & Pediatric; Genitourinary Cancer; Gastrointestinal Cancer; **Hospital:** Univ Utah Hlth Care, Primary Children's Med Ctr; **Address:** Huntsman Cancer Inst, Dept Rad Oncology, 1950 Circle of Hope, rm 1440, Salt Lake City, UT 84112; **Phone:** 801-581-2396; **Board Cert:** Radiation Oncology 1993; **Med School:** Univ Miami Sch Med 1989; **Resid:** Radiation Oncology, UCSF Med Ctr 1993; **Fac Appt:** Prof RadRO, Univ Utah

Smalley, Stephen R MD [RadRO] - **Spec Exp:** Colon Cancer; Gastrointestinal Cancer; **Hospital:** Olathe Med Ctr; **Address:** Olathe Medical Center, 20375 W 151st St, Doctors Bldg, Ste 180, Olathe, KS 66061-4575; **Phone:** 913-768-7200; **Board Cert:** Internal Medicine 1982; Radiation Oncology 1987; Medical Oncology 1985; **Med School:** Univ MO-Kansas City 1979; **Resid:** Internal Medicine, Mayo Clinic 1982; Radiation Oncology, Mayo Clinic 1986; **Fellow:** Medical Oncology, Mayo Clinic 1984; **Fac Appt:** Prof RadRO, Univ Kansas

Southwest

Ang, Kie-Kian MD/PhD [RadRO] - **Spec Exp:** Head & Neck Cancer; **Hospital:** UT MD Anderson Cancer Ctr; **Address:** UT MD Anderson Cancer Ctr, 1515 Holcombe Blvd, Unit 97, Houston, TX 77030; **Phone:** 713-563-2323; **Board Cert:** Radiation Oncology 1987; **Med School:** Belgium 1975; **Resid:** Radiation Oncology, Univ Hosp 1980; **Fac Appt:** Prof, Univ Tex, Houston

Buchholz, Thomas A MD [RadRO] - **Spec Exp:** Breast Cancer; **Hospital:** UT MD Anderson Cancer Ctr; **Address:** Univ Texas MD Anderson Cancer Ctr, 1515 Holcombe Blvd, Unit 97, Houston, TX 77030; **Phone:** 713-794-4892; **Board Cert:** Radiation Oncology 1993; **Med School:** Tufts Univ 1988; **Resid:** Radiation Oncology, Univ Washington Med Ctr 1993; **Fellow:** Research, Univ Washington 1994; **Fac Appt:** Prof RadRO, Univ Tex, Houston

Choy, Hak MD [RadRO] - **Spec Exp:** Lung Cancer; **Hospital:** UT Southwestern Med Ctr at Dallas; **Address:** UT SW Med Ctr - Dallas, Dept Rad-Onc, 5801 Forest Park Rd, Dallas, TX 75390-9183; **Phone:** 214-645-7600; **Board Cert:** Radiation Oncology 1993; **Med School:** Univ Tex Med Br, Galveston 1987; **Resid:** Radiation Oncology, Ohio State Univ Hosp 1989; Radiation Oncology, Univ Texas Hlth Sci Ctr 1991; **Fac Appt:** Prof RadRO, Univ Tex SW, Dallas

Cox, James D MD [RadRO] - **Spec Exp:** Lung Cancer; Esophageal Cancer; Thymoma; Thoracic Cancers; **Hospital:** UT MD Anderson Cancer Ctr; **Address:** Univ Tex MD Anderson Cancer Ctr, 1515 Holcombe Blvd, Unit 97, Houston, TX 77030; **Phone:** 713-563-2316; **Board Cert:** Therapeutic Radiology 1971; **Med School:** Univ Rochester 1965; **Resid:** Diagnostic Radiology, Penrose Cancer Hosp 1969; **Fellow:** Therapeutic Radiology, Inst Gustave-Roussy 1970; **Fac Appt:** Prof RadRO, Univ Tex, Houston

Crane, Christopher H MD [RadRO] - **Spec Exp:** Gastrointestinal Cancer; **Hospital:** UT MD Anderson Cancer Ctr; **Address:** UT MD Anderson Cancer Ctr, Dept Rad Onc, 1515 Holcombe Blvd, Unit 1202, Houston, TX 77030; **Phone:** 713-563-6830; **Board Cert:** Radiation Oncology 2009; **Med School:** Univ VA Sch Med 1993; **Resid:** Radiation Oncology, Univ Virginia 1998; **Fac Appt:** Prof RadRO, Univ Tex, Houston

Radiation Oncology

Eifel, Patricia J MD [RadRO] - **Spec Exp:** Cervical Cancer; Uterine Cancer; Vulvar Disease/Cancer; Vaginal Cancer; **Hospital:** UT MD Anderson Cancer Ctr; **Address:** MD Anderson Cancer Ctr, Dept Rad Onc, 1515 Holcombe Blvd, Unit 1202, Houston, TX 77030-4009; **Phone:** 713-563-6830; **Board Cert:** Therapeutic Radiology 1983; **Med School:** Stanford Univ 1977; **Resid:** Radiation Oncology, Stanford Univ Med Ctr 1981; **Fellow:** Therapeutic Radiology, Stanford Univ Med Ctr 1982

Grado, Gordon L MD [RadRO] - **Spec Exp:** Prostate Cancer; Brachytherapy; **Hospital:** Scottsdale Hlthcare - Shea; **Address:** Southwest Oncology Centers, 2926 N Civic Center Plaza, Scottsdale, AZ 85251; **Phone:** 480-614-6300; **Board Cert:** Therapeutic Radiology 1981; **Med School:** Southern IL Univ 1977; **Resid:** Therapeutic Radiology, Mayo Clinic 1981; **Fac Appt:** Assoc Prof RadRO, Univ Minn

Halyard, Michele MD [RadRO] - **Spec Exp:** Breast Cancer; Head & Neck Cancer; **Hospital:** Mayo Clinic - Scottsdale; **Address:** Mayo Clinic-Radiation Oncology, 13400 E Shea Blvd, Scottsdale, AZ 85259-5404; **Phone:** 480-342-1262; **Board Cert:** Radiation Oncology 1989; **Med School:** Howard Univ 1984; **Resid:** Radiation Therapy, Howard Univ Hosp 1987; **Fellow:** Radiation Oncology, Mayo Clinic 1989; **Fac Appt:** Assoc Prof RadRO, Mayo Med Sch

Herman, Terence S MD [RadRO] - **Spec Exp:** Breast Cancer; Sarcoma; Brain Tumors; **Hospital:** OU Med Ctr; **Address:** Oklahoma Univ Health Sci Ctr, 800 NE 10th St, Level L, Oklahoma City, OK 73104-5417; **Phone:** 405-271-5641; **Board Cert:** Internal Medicine 1975; Medical Oncology 1977; Therapeutic Radiology 1985; **Med School:** Univ Conn 1972; **Resid:** Internal Medicine, Univ Arizona Med Ctr 1975; Radiation Oncology, Stanford Univ Med Ctr 1985; **Fellow:** Medical Oncology, Univ Arizona 1977; **Fac Appt:** Prof RadRO, Univ Okla Coll Med

Jhingran, Anuja MD [RadRO] - **Spec Exp:** Gynecologic Cancer; Brachytherapy; **Hospital:** UT MD Anderson Cancer Ctr; **Address:** MD Anderson Cancer Ctr, Dept Rad Onc, 1515 Holcombe Blvd, Unit 1202, Houston, TX 77030; **Phone:** 713-563-6830; **Board Cert:** Radiation Oncology 1993; **Med School:** Texas Tech Univ 1988; **Resid:** Radiation Oncology, Baylor Affil Hosp 1993; **Fac Appt:** Assoc Prof RadRO, Univ Tex, Houston

Komaki, Ritsuko U MD [RadRO] - **Spec Exp:** Lung Cancer; Thymoma; Esophageal Cancer; **Hospital:** UT MD Anderson Cancer Ctr; **Address:** UT MD Anderson Cancer Ctr, Dept Rad Onc, 1515 Holcombe Blvd, Unit 97, Houston, TX 77030; **Phone:** 713-563-2300; **Board Cert:** Therapeutic Radiology 1977; **Med School:** Japan 1969; **Resid:** Radiation Oncology, Med Coll Wisconsin Hosp 1978; **Fac Appt:** Prof RadRO, Univ Tex, Houston

Kuban, Deborah MD [RadRO] - **Spec Exp:** Genitourinary Cancer; **Hospital:** UT MD Anderson Cancer Ctr; **Address:** 1515 Holcombe Blvd Unit 1202, Houston, TX 77030-9904; **Phone:** 713-563-2329; **Board Cert:** Therapeutic Radiology 1986; **Med School:** Med Coll GA 1981; **Resid:** Radiation Oncology, EVMS Affil Hosp 1985; **Fac Appt:** Prof RadRO, Univ Tex, Houston

Kuske, Robert R MD [RadRO] - **Spec Exp:** Breast Cancer; **Hospital:** Scottsdale Hlthcare - Shea; **Address:** Arizona Breast Cancer Specialists, 9055 E Del Camino Drive, Scottsdale, AZ 85258; **Phone:** 480-922-4600; **Board Cert:** Therapeutic Radiology 1985; **Med School:** Univ Cincinnati 1980; **Resid:** Radiation Oncology, Univ Cincinnati Med Ctr 1984

Lee, Andrew K MD [RadRO] - **Spec Exp:** Prostate Cancer; Proton Beam Therapy; Genitourinary Cancer; **Hospital:** UT MD Anderson Cancer Ctr; **Address:** MD Anderson Cancer Ctr, 1515 Holcombe Blvd, Unit 97, Houston, TX 77030; **Phone:** 713-563-2300; **Board Cert:** Radiation Oncology 2011; **Med School:** Univ Minn 1996; **Resid:** Radiation Oncology, Joint Ctr for Radiation Therapy/Harvard 2001; **Fac Appt:** Assoc Prof RadRO, Univ Tex, Houston

Medbery, Clinton A MD [RadRO] - **Spec Exp:** Breast Cancer; Prostate Cancer; Brachytherapy; Stereotactic Radiosurgery; **Hospital:** St. Anthony Hosp -Oklahoma City; **Address:** Southwest Radiation Oncology, 1011 N Dewey Ave, Ste 101, Oklahoma City, OK 73101; **Phone:** 405-272-7311; **Board Cert:** Internal Medicine 1980; Medical Oncology 1983; Radiation Oncology 1987; **Med School:** Med Univ SC 1976; **Resid:** Internal Medicine, Naval Hosp 1980; Radiation Oncology, Natl Cancer Inst 1987; **Fellow:** Medical Oncology, Naval Hosp 1982

Minsky, Bruce D MD [RadRO] - **Spec Exp:** Gastrointestinal Cancer; Esophageal Cancer; Colon & Rectal Cancer; Pancreatic Cancer; **Hospital:** UT MD Anderson Cancer Ctr; **Address:** MD Anderson Cancer Center, 1515 Holcombe Blvd, Box 97, Houston, TX 77030; **Phone:** 713-563-2304; **Board Cert:** Radiation Oncology 1987; **Med School:** Univ Mass Sch Med 1982; **Resid:** Radiation Oncology, Harvard Jt Ctr Rad Ther 1986; **Fac Appt:** Prof RadRO, Univ Tex, Houston

Morrison, William H MD [RadRO] - **Spec Exp:** Head & Neck Cancer; Skin Cancer; Merkel Cell Carcinoma; **Hospital:** UT MD Anderson Cancer Ctr; **Address:** 1515 Holcombe Blvd, #97, Houston, TX 77030-4000; **Phone:** 713-794-1974; **Board Cert:** Internal Medicine 1981; Therapeutic Radiology 1985; **Med School:** Johns Hopkins Univ 1978; **Resid:** Internal Medicine, Rush Presby/St Lukes Med Ctr 1981; Therapeutic Radiology, Stanford Univ Hosp 1985; **Fac Appt:** Prof RadRO, Univ Tex, Houston

Schild, Steven E MD [RadRO] - **Spec Exp:** Lung Cancer; Prostate Cancer; Genitourinary Cancer; **Hospital:** Mayo Clinic - Scottsdale; **Address:** Mayo Clinic-Radiation Oncology, 13400 E Shea Blvd, Scottsdale, AZ 85259; **Phone:** 480-342-1262; **Board Cert:** Radiation Oncology 1989; **Med School:** Creighton Univ 1985; **Resid:** Radiation Oncology, Mayo Clinic 1989; **Fac Appt:** Prof RadRO, Mayo Med Sch

Senzer, Neil N MD [RadRO] - **Spec Exp:** Clinical Trials; Gene Therapy; **Hospital:** Med City Dallas Hosp, Baylor Univ Medical Ctr-Dallas; **Address:** Mary Crowley Cancer Research Ctr, 7777 Forest Ln C Bldg - Ste 707, Dallas, TX 75230; **Phone:** 972-566-3000; **Board Cert:** Pediatrics 1976; Pediatric Hematology-Oncology 1978; Therapeutic Radiology 1985; **Med School:** SUNY Buffalo 1971; **Resid:** Pediatrics, Johns Hopkins Hosp 1974; Radiation Oncology, St Barnabas Med Ctr 1985; **Fellow:** Pediatric Hematology-Oncology, St Jude Chldns Rsch Hosp 1978

Shina, Donald C MD [RadRO] - **Spec Exp:** Breast Cancer; **Hospital:** Christus St Vincent Reg Med Ctr-Santa Fe; **Address:** Santa Fe Cancer Ctr at St Vincent Hosp, 455 Saint Michael's Drive, Santa Fe, NM 87505; **Phone:** 505-820-5233; **Board Cert:** Internal Medicine 1977; Medical Oncology 1979; Therapeutic Radiology 1981; **Med School:** Case West Res Univ 1974; **Resid:** Internal Medicine, Univ Hosps 1977; **Fellow:** Radiation Oncology, Univ Hosps 1980; Medical Oncology, Univ Hosps 1980

Stea, Baldassarre MD/PhD [RadRO] - **Spec Exp:** Brain Tumors; Stereotactic Radiosurgery; Pediatric Cancers; Lymphoma; **Hospital:** Univ Arizona Med Ctr-Univ Campus, St. Joseph's Hosp - Tucson; **Address:** 1501 N Campbell Ave, Tucson, AZ 85724-0001; **Phone:** 520-626-6724; **Board Cert:** Radiation Oncology 1987; **Med School:** Geo Wash Univ 1983; **Resid:** Radiation Oncology, Natl Cancer Inst 1987; **Fac Appt:** Prof RadRO, Univ Ariz Coll Med

West Coast and Pacific

Donaldson, Sarah S MD [RadRO] - **Spec Exp:** Pediatric Cancers; Hodgkin's Lymphoma; Sarcoma; Breast Cancer; **Hospital:** Stanford Univ Hosp & Clinics; **Address:** 875 Blake Wilbur Drive, CC Bldg Fl G - rm 226, MC 5847, Stanford, CA 94305-5847; **Phone:** 650-723-6195; **Board Cert:** Therapeutic Radiology 1974; **Med School:** Harvard Med Sch 1968; **Resid:** Radiation Oncology, Stanford Univ Med Ctr 1972; **Fellow:** Pediatric Hematology-Oncology, Inst Gustave-Roussy 1973; Pediatric Hematology-Oncology, MD Anderson Cancer Ctr 1971; **Fac Appt:** Prof RadRO, Stanford Univ

Fowble, Barbara MD [RadRO] - **Spec Exp:** Breast Cancer; **Hospital:** UCSF Med Ctr; **Address:** 1600 Divisadero St, Ste H1031, San Francisco, CA 94115; **Phone:** 415-353-7175; **Board Cert:** Therapeutic Radiology 1976; **Med School:** Jefferson Med Coll 1972; **Resid:** Therapeutic Radiology, Bellevue Hosp Ctr-NYU 1975; Therapeutic Radiology, Hahnemann 1976; **Fellow:** Radiation Therapy, Jefferson Hosp 1977; **Fac Appt:** Prof RadRO, UCSF

Fuss, Martin MD/PhD [RadRO] - **Spec Exp:** Intensity Modulated Radiotherapy (IMRT); Stereotactic Body Radiation Therapy; Stereotactic Radiosurgery; Bladder Cancer; **Hospital:** OR Hlth & Sci Univ; **Address:** Dept of Radiation Medicine, 3181 SW Sam Jackson Park Rd, MC KPV4, Portland, OR 97239; **Phone:** 503-494-8756; **Med School:** Germany 1994; **Resid:** Radiation Oncology, Univ of Heidelberg; **Fellow:** Radiation Therapy, Loma Linda Univ; **Fac Appt:** Prof RadRO, Oregon Hlth & Sci Univ

Halberg, Francine MD [RadRO] - **Spec Exp:** Breast Cancer; **Hospital:** Marin Genl Hosp, UCSF Med Ctr; **Address:** Marin Cancer Inst-Dept of Rad.Oncology, 1350 S Eliseo Drive, Ste 100, Greenbrae, CA 94904; **Phone:** 415-925-7326; **Board Cert:** Internal Medicine 1981; Therapeutic Radiology 1984; **Med School:** Cornell Univ-Weill Med Coll 1978; **Resid:** Internal Medicine, USPHS Hosp 1981; **Fellow:** Radiation Oncology, Stanford Univ Med Ctr 1984; **Fac Appt:** Assoc Prof RadRO, UCSF

Hancock, Steven MD [RadRO] - **Spec Exp:** Prostate Cancer; Breast Cancer; Cancer Survivors-Late Effects of Therapy; **Hospital:** Stanford Univ Hosp & Clinics; **Address:** Stanford Cancer Center-Dept Rad Onc, 875 Blake Wilbur Drive, MC 5847, Stanford, CA 94305; **Phone:** 650-723-6440; **Board Cert:** Internal Medicine 1980; Therapeutic Radiology 1982; **Med School:** Stanford Univ 1976; **Resid:** Radiation Therapy, Stanford Univ Med Ctr 1981; Internal Medicine, Stanford Univ Med Ctr 1979; **Fac Appt:** Prof RadRO, Stanford Univ

Hoppe, Richard T MD [RadRO] - **Spec Exp:** Lymphoma; Hodgkin's Lymphoma; Cutaneous Lymphoma; **Hospital:** Stanford Univ Hosp & Clinics; **Address:** 875 Blake Wilbur Drive, Clinic D, Stanford, CA 94305-5847; **Phone:** 650-723-5510; **Board Cert:** Therapeutic Radiology 1976; **Med School:** Cornell Univ-Weill Med Coll 1971; **Resid:** Radiation Therapy, Stanford Univ Med Ctr 1976; **Fac Appt:** Prof, Stanford Univ

Koh, Wui-Jin MD [RadRO] - **Spec Exp:** Gynecologic Cancer; Brachytherapy; Gastrointestinal Cancer; **Hospital:** Univ Wash Med Ctr; **Address:** Seattle Cancer Care Alliance, 825 Eastlake Ave E, Box 19023, MS G1-101, Seattle, WA 98109; **Phone:** 206-288-7318; **Board Cert:** Radiation Oncology 1988; **Med School:** Loma Linda Univ 1984; **Resid:** Radiation Oncology, Univ Washington Med Ctr 1988; **Fellow:** Tumor Imaging, Univ Washington Med Ctr 1988; **Fac Appt:** Prof RadRO, Univ Wash

Kupelian, Patrick A MD [RadRO] - **Spec Exp:** Genitourinary Cancer; Clinical Trials; Stereotactic Body Radiation Therapy; Stereotactic Radiosurgery; **Hospital:** UCLA Ronald Reagan Med Ctr; **Address:** UCLA Jonsson Comprehensive Cancer Center, 200 UCLA Medical Plaza, Ste B265, Los Angeles, CA 90095-6951; **Phone:** 310-825-9775; **Board Cert:** Radiation Oncology 2004; **Med School:** Lebanon 1989; **Resid:** Radiation Oncology, MD Anderson Cancer Ctr 1994; **Fellow:** Radiation Oncology, Cleveland Clinic 1995; **Fac Appt:** Prof RadRO, UCLA

Laramore, George E MD/PhD [RadRO] - **Spec Exp:** Neutron Therapy for Advanced Cancer; Salivary Gland Tumors; Head & Neck Cancer; Skin Cancer; **Hospital:** Univ Wash Med Ctr, Harborview Med Ctr; **Address:** Univ Washington Med Ctr, Dept Rad Onc Box 356043, Seattle, WA 98195; **Phone:** 206-598-4121; **Board Cert:** Therapeutic Radiology 1980; Radiation Oncology 2010; **Med School:** Univ Miami Sch Med 1976; **Resid:** Radiation Oncology, Univ Washington Med Ctr 1980; **Fac Appt:** Prof RadRO, Univ Wash

Larson, David A MD/PhD [RadRO] - **Spec Exp:** Neuro-Oncology; Brain Tumors; Stereotactic Radiosurgery; **Hospital:** UCSF Med Ctr, Washington Hosp; **Address:** UCSF Med Ctr, Dept Rad Onc, 505 Parnassus Ave, rm L-75, San Francisco, CA 94143-0226; **Phone:** 415-353-8900; **Board Cert:** Therapeutic Radiology 1986; **Med School:** Univ Miami Sch Med 1981; **Resid:** Radiation Therapy, Joint Ctr for Radiation Therapy 1985; **Fac Appt:** Prof RadRO, UCSF

Le, Quynh-Thu Xuan MD [RadRO] - **Spec Exp:** Head & Neck Cancer; Lung Cancer; Thoracic Cancers; Clinical Trials; **Hospital:** Stanford Univ Hosp & Clinics; **Address:** Stanford Univ, Dept Rad Oncology, 875 Blake Wilbur Drive, MC 5847, Clinic D, Stanford, CA 94305; **Phone:** 650-723-6171; **Board Cert:** Radiation Oncology 2008; **Med School:** UCSF 1993; **Resid:** Radiation Oncology, UCSF Med Ctr 1997; **Fac Appt:** Prof RadRO, Stanford Univ

Mundt, Arno J MD [RadRO] - **Spec Exp:** Gynecologic Cancer; Intensity Modulated Radiotherapy (IMRT); **Hospital:** UCSD Med Ctr; **Address:** 3855 Hlth Sciences Drive, MC 0843, La Jolla, CA 92093-0843; **Phone:** 858-822-6046; **Board Cert:** Radiation Oncology 1994; **Med School:** Univ Mich Med Sch 1987; **Resid:** Physical Medicine & Rehabilitation, George Washington Univ Hosp 1990; Radiation Oncology, Univ Chicago Hosps 1993; **Fellow:** Physical Medicine & Rehabilitation, Univ Chicago Hosps 1994; **Fac Appt:** Prof RadRO, UCSD

Park, Catherine C MD [RadRO] - **Spec Exp:** Breast Cancer; Lymphoma; **Hospital:** UCSF Med Ctr; **Address:** UCSF Radiation Oncology, 1600 Divisadero St, Ste H1031, San Francisco, CA 94115; **Phone:** 415-353-9807; **Board Cert:** Radiation Oncology 2000; **Med School:** UCLA 1995; **Resid:** Radiation Oncology, Mass Genl Hosp 2000; **Fac Appt:** Assoc Prof RadRO, UCSF

Pezner, Richard D MD [RadRO] - **Spec Exp:** Sarcoma-Soft Tissue; Breast Cancer; Stereotactic Radiosurgery; **Hospital:** City of Hope Natl Med Ctr; **Address:** City of Hope Med Ctr-Div Radiation Onc, 1500 E Duarte Rd, Duarte, CA 91010-3000; **Phone:** 626-301-8247; **Board Cert:** Therapeutic Radiology 1979; **Med School:** Northwestern Univ 1975; **Resid:** Radiation Oncology, Oregon Health Sci Ctr 1979; **Fac Appt:** Clin Prof RadRO, UC Irvine

Quivey, Jeanne M MD [RadRO] - **Spec Exp:** Head & Neck Cancer; Breast Cancer; Eye Tumors/Cancer; Intensity Modulated Radiotherapy (IMRT); **Hospital:** UCSF Med Ctr; **Address:** UCSF Med Ctr @ Mt Zion, Radiation Onc Dept, 1600 Divisadero St, Ste H1031, Box 1708, San Francisco, CA 94143-1708; **Phone:** 415-353-7175; **Board Cert:** Therapeutic Radiology 1974; **Med School:** UCSF 1970; **Resid:** Radiation Therapy, UCSF Med Ctr 1974; **Fac Appt:** Prof RadRO, UCSF

Roach III, Mack MD [RadRO] - **Spec Exp:** Prostate Cancer; Genitourinary Cancer; Lung Cancer; **Hospital:** UCSF - Mt Zion Med Ctr, UCSF Med Ctr; **Address:** UCSF Radiation Oncology, 1600 Divisadero St Fl 3, San Francisco, CA 94143-1708; **Phone:** 415-353-9807; **Board Cert:** Internal Medicine 1984; Medical Oncology 1985; Radiation Oncology 1987; **Med School:** Stanford Univ 1979; **Resid:** Internal Medicine, ML King Genl Hosp 1981; Radiation Oncology, Stanford Univ Med Ctr 1987; **Fellow:** Medical Oncology, UCSF Med Ctr 1983; **Fac Appt:** Prof RadRO, UCSF

Rose, Christopher M MD [RadRO] - **Spec Exp:** Prostate Cancer; Breast Cancer; Intensity Modulated Radiotherapy (IMRT); **Hospital:** Providence St Joseph Med Ctr, Providence Tarzana Med Ctr; **Address:** 9292 Wilshire Blvd, Beverly Hills, CA 90210; **Phone:** 310-651-9292; **Board Cert:** Radiation Oncology 1999; Therapeutic Radiology 1979; **Med School:** Harvard Med Sch 1974; **Resid:** Internal Medicine, Beth Israel Deaconess 1976; Radiation Oncology, Joint Ctr Rad Therapy 1979; **Fellow:** Cancer Research, British Inst Cancer Rsch 1979; **Fac Appt:** Clin Prof RadRO, USC Sch Med

Radiation Oncology

Rossi, Carl John MD [RadRO] - **Spec Exp:** Prostate Cancer; Proton Beam Therapy; **Hospital:** Scripps Green Hosp; **Address:** 10666 N Torrey Pines Rd MS B1, La Jolla, CA 92037; **Phone:** 858-678-6866; **Board Cert:** Radiation Oncology 1994; **Med School:** Loyola Univ-Stritch Sch Med 1988; **Resid:** Radiation Oncology, Loma Linda Univ Med Ctr 1992; **Fac Appt:** Asst Prof RadRO, Loma Linda Univ

Russell, Kenneth J MD [RadRO] - **Spec Exp:** Genitourinary Cancer; Prostate Cancer; Lymphoma; **Hospital:** Univ Wash Med Ctr; **Address:** Seattle Cancer Care Alliance, 825 Eastlake Ave E, Box 19023, MS G1-101, Seattle, WA 98109; **Phone:** 206-288-7318; **Board Cert:** Therapeutic Radiology 1984; **Med School:** Harvard Med Sch 1979; **Resid:** Radiation Therapy, Stanford Univ Med Ctr 1983; **Fellow:** Radiological Biology, Stanford Univ Med Ctr 1985; **Fac Appt:** Prof Rad, Univ Wash

Sandler, Howard M MD [RadRO] - **Spec Exp:** Prostate Cancer; Genitourinary Cancer; Brain Tumors; **Hospital:** Cedars-Sinai Med Ctr; **Address:** S Oschin Comprehensive Cancer Inst, Cedars-Sinai Med Ctr, 8700 Beverly Blvd, Los Angeles, CA 90048; **Phone:** 310-423-4234; **Board Cert:** Radiation Oncology 1989; **Med School:** Univ Conn 1985; **Resid:** Radiation Oncology, Hosp Univ Penn 1989

Seung, Steven K MD/PhD [RadRO] - **Spec Exp:** Stereotactic Radiosurgery; Brain Tumors; Esophageal Cancer; Lung Cancer; **Hospital:** Providence Portland Med Ctr; **Address:** 4805 NE Glisan St, Garden Level, Portland, OR 97213; **Phone:** 503-215-6029; **Board Cert:** Radiation Oncology 2010; **Med School:** Univ Chicago-Pritzker Sch Med 1994; **Resid:** Radiation Oncology, UCSF Med Ctr 1998

Thomas Jr, Charles R MD [RadRO] - **Spec Exp:** Gastrointestinal Cancer; Esophageal Cancer; Colon & Rectal Cancer; **Hospital:** OR Hlth & Sci Univ; **Address:** 3181 SW Sam Jackson Park Rd, MC KPV4, Portland, OR 97239; **Phone:** 503-494-8756; **Board Cert:** Internal Medicine 1989; Radiation Oncology 2010; **Med School:** Univ IL Coll Med 1985; **Resid:** Internal Medicine, Baylor Coll Med 1988; Radiation Oncology, Univ Wash Med Ctr 1997; **Fellow:** Medical Oncology, Rush Univ Med Ctr 1999; **Fac Appt:** Prof RadRO, Oregon Hlth & Sci Univ

Tripuraneni, Prabhakar MD [RadRO] - **Spec Exp:** Prostate Cancer; Head & Neck Cancer; Lymphoma; **Hospital:** Scripps Green Hosp, Scripps Meml Hosp - La Jolla; **Address:** Scripps Clinic, Div Radiation Oncology, 10666 N Torrey Pines Rd, MSB 1, La Jolla, CA 92037; **Phone:** 858-554-2000; **Board Cert:** Therapeutic Radiology 1983; **Med School:** India 1976; **Resid:** Radiation Oncology, Univ Alberta 1981; Radiation Oncology, UCSF Med Ctr 1983; **Fac Appt:** Clin Prof RadRO, UCSD

Wara, William M MD [RadRO] - **Spec Exp:** Brain & Spinal Tumors; Sarcoma; Pediatric Cancers; **Hospital:** Kaiser Permanente S San Francisco Med Ctr; **Address:** Cancer Treatment Ctr, 220 Oyster Pt Blvd, South San Francisco, CA 94080; **Phone:** 650-827-6500; **Board Cert:** Therapeutic Radiology 1974; **Med School:** UC Irvine 1969; **Resid:** Therapeutic Radiology, UCSF Medical Ctr 1973; **Fac Appt:** Prof RadRO, UCSF

Wong, Jeffrey Y C MD [RadRO] - **Spec Exp:** Radioimmunotherapy of Cancer; Prostate Cancer; Intensity Modulated Radiotherapy (IMRT); Multiple Myeloma; **Hospital:** City of Hope Natl Med Ctr; **Address:** City of Hope Med Ctr-Dept Radiation Onc, 1500 E Duarte Rd, Duarte, CA 91768-3012; **Phone:** 626-359-8111 x62969; **Board Cert:** Therapeutic Radiology 1985; **Med School:** Johns Hopkins Univ 1981; **Resid:** Radiation Oncology, UCSF Med Ctr 1985; **Fac Appt:** Prof RadRO, UC Irvine

Cleveland Clinic

Every life deserves world class care.

Radiation Oncology

At Cleveland Clinic Taussig Cancer Institute, more than 250 top cancer specialists, researchers, nurses and technicians are dedicated to delivering the most effective medical treatments and offering access to the latest clinical trials for more than 13,000 new cancer patients every year. Our doctors are known nationally and internationally for their contributions to cancer breakthroughs and their ability to deliver superior outcomes for our patients. *U.S. News & World Report* has ranked Cleveland Clinic one of the top cancer centers in the nation.

The Taussig Cancer Institute offers a full range of advanced technology equipment, including 16 linear accelerators, fully integrated CT simulators and various image-guided treatment technologies. Using multiple imaging modalities including PET/CT, SPECT/CT and MRI, we offer patients accurately targeted treatment, and our state-of-the-art computer technologies provide precise external beam radiation. The department is equipped with a combined X-ray and optical imaging tracking system; kilovoltage and mega-voltage cone-beam computerized tomography; electromagnetic emission detectors and ultrasound imaging to provide optimal cancer treatment.

Our program was one of the first to implement intensity-modulated radiation therapy, image-guided radiation therapy and radioimmunotherapy. In addition to intra-cavitary, intraoperative and intraluminal treatments, we have developed many novel approaches to brachytherapy, especially with prostate cancer.

Cleveland Clinic is active in a number of in-house pharmaceutical and cooperative group trials. We are one of the leading enrollers in national studies and in combining novel agents such as radiation sensitizers with radiation therapy. In addition, the Department of Radiation Oncology houses one of the largest prostate cancer databases in the nation.

Cleveland Clinic
Taussig Cancer Institute
9500 Euclid Avenue
Cleveland, OH 44195

Offering Same-Day Appointments
Call 800.274.2009.

Treatment Guides
Cleveland Clinic has developed comprehensive treatment guides for many diseases and conditions. To download our free treatment guides, visit clevelandclinic.org/treatmentguides.

Online Medical Second Opinion
Call 216.444.3223 or 800.223.2273 ext. 43223 or email eclevelandclinic@ccf.org.

Out-of-State Patients Assistance
Call 800.223.2273, ext. 55580 or email medicalconcierge@ccf.org.

Visit Us At:
clevelandclinic.org

Follow Us On:
Facebook
www.facebook.com/clevelandclinic

Twitter
@ClevelandClinic

You Tube
www.youtube.com/clevelandclinic

Health Hub
health.clevelandclinic.org

The Best in American Medicine
www.CastleConnolly.com

Radiology

A radiologist utilizes radiologic methodologies to diagnose and treat disease. Physicians practicing in the field of radiology most often specialize in radiology, diagnostic radiology, radiation oncology or radiological physics.

Diagnostic Radiology: A radiologist who utilizes X-ray, radionuclides, ultrasound and electromagnetic radiation to diagnose and treat disease.

Training Required: Four years

Radiation Oncology: A radiologist who deals with the therapeutic applications of radiant energy and its modifiers and the study and management of disease, especially malignant tumors.

Certification in one of the following subspecialties requires additional training and examination.

Neuroradiology: A radiologist who diagnoses and treats diseases utilizing imaging procedures as they relate to the brain, spine and spinal cord, head, neck and organs of special sense in adults and children.

Pediatric Radiology: A radiologist who is proficient in all forms of diagnostic imaging as it pertains to the treatment of diseases in the newborn, infant, child and adolescent. This specialist has knowledge of both imaging and interventional procedures related to the care and management of diseases of children. A pediatric radiologist must be highly knowledgeable of all organ systems as they relate to growth and development, congenital malformations, diseases peculiar to infants and children and diseases that begin in childhood but cause substantial residual impairment in adulthood.

Vascular and Interventional Radiology: A radiologist who diagnoses and treats diseases by various radiologic imaging modalities. These include fluoroscopy, digital radiography, computed tomography, sonography and magnetic resonance imaging.

DIAGNOSTIC RADIOLOGY

New England

Benson, Carol B MD [DR] - **Spec Exp:** Obstetric Ultrasound; Thyroid Ultrasound; Fetal Surgical Imaging; Gynecologic Imaging; **Hospital:** Brigham and Women's Hosp (page 57); **Address:** Brigham & Women's Hospital, Dept Radiology, 75 Francis St, Boston, MA 02115; **Phone:** 617-732-6280; **Board Cert:** Diagnostic Radiology 1984; **Med School:** Univ Pennsylvania 1980; **Resid:** Diagnostic Radiology, New York Hosp-Cornell 1984; **Fellow:** Ultrasound, Brigham & Womens Hosp 1985; **Fac Appt:** Prof Rad, Harvard Med Sch

Black, William C MD [DR] - **Spec Exp:** Chest Radiology; Lung Cancer; CT Chest Scan; **Hospital:** Dartmouth - Hitchcock Med Ctr; **Address:** Dartmouth Hitchcock Med Ctr, Dept Radiology, 1 Medical Center Drive, Lebanon, NH 03756; **Phone:** 603-650-7443; **Board Cert:** Diagnostic Radiology 1983; **Med School:** Med Coll VA 1979; **Resid:** Diagnostic Radiology, Univ Virginia Hosp 1983; **Fellow:** Ultrasound/CT, Univ Virginia Hosp 1984; **Fac Appt:** Prof Rad, Dartmouth Med Sch

Doubilet, Peter MD [DR] - **Spec Exp:** Ultrasound; Obstetric Ultrasound; **Hospital:** Brigham and Women's Hosp (page 57); **Address:** Brigham & Women's Hosp, Dept Radiology, 75 Francis St, Boston, MA 02115; **Phone:** 617-732-6757; **Board Cert:** Diagnostic Radiology 1981; **Med School:** Columbia P&S 1977; **Resid:** Diagnostic Radiology, Brigham & Women's Hosp 1981; **Fac Appt:** Prof Rad, Harvard Med Sch

McCarthy, Shirley M MD/PhD [DR] - **Spec Exp:** Gynecologic Cancer; Pelvic Imaging; **Hospital:** Yale-New Haven Hosp, Yale Med Group; **Address:** Yale-New Haven Hosp, 333 Cedar St, Ste TE2, PO Box 208042, New Haven, CT 06520-3206; **Phone:** 203-785-2384; **Board Cert:** Diagnostic Radiology 1983; **Med School:** Yale Univ 1979; **Resid:** Diagnostic Radiology, Yale-New Haven Hosp 1983; **Fellow:** Cross Sectional Imaging, UCSF Med Ctr 1984; **Fac Appt:** Prof Rad, Yale Univ

Newman, Joel S MD [DR] - **Spec Exp:** Musculoskeletal Imaging; **Hospital:** New England Bapt Hosp; **Address:** New England Baptist Hosp, Dept Radiology, 125 Parker Hill Ave, Converse 2, Boston, MA 02120; **Phone:** 617-754-6687; **Board Cert:** Diagnostic Radiology 1992; **Med School:** Northwestern Univ-Feinberg Sch Med 1987; **Resid:** Diagnostic Radiology, Tufts Med Ctr 1992; **Fellow:** Cross Sectional Imaging, Michigan Hosp & Med Ctr 1993; Musculoskeletal Imaging, Michigan Hosp & Med Ctr 1994; **Fac Appt:** Clin Prof Rad, Tufts Univ

Palmer, William E MD [DR] - **Spec Exp:** Musculoskeletal Imaging; Sports Medicine Radiology; Pain Management; Musculoskeletal Imaging; **Hospital:** Mass Genl Hosp; **Address:** Mass General Hospital, Yawkey 6 Radiology, 55 Fruit St YAW Bldg - rm 6033, Boston, MA 02114; **Phone:** 617-726-7717; **Board Cert:** Internal Medicine 1987; Diagnostic Radiology 1991; **Med School:** Yale Univ 1984; **Resid:** Internal Medicine, Hosp Univ Penn 1987; Diagnostic Radiology, Mass Genl Hosp 1991; **Fac Appt:** Asst Prof Rad, Harvard Med Sch

Weinreb, Jeffrey C MD [DR] - **Spec Exp:** MRI; Breast Cancer; Abdominal Imaging; CT Body Scan; **Hospital:** Yale-New Haven Hosp, Yale Med Group; **Address:** Yale Univ Sch Medicine, Dept Radiology, 333 Cedar St, rm MRC165, Box 208042, New Haven, CT 06520-8042; **Phone:** 203-785-5913; **Board Cert:** Diagnostic Radiology 1983; **Med School:** Mount Sinai Sch Med 1978; **Resid:** Diagnostic Radiology, LI Jewish Med Ctr 1982; **Fellow:** Ultrasound/CT, Hosp Univ Penn 1983; **Fac Appt:** Prof Rad, Yale Univ

Diagnostic Radiology

Mid Atlantic

Adler, Ronald S MD/PhD [DR] - **Spec Exp:** Musculoskeletal Imaging; Ultrasound; Power Doppler Imaging; **Hospital:** NYU Langone Med Ctr (page 68), NYU Hosp For Joint Diseases (page 70); **Address:** Ctr for Musculoskeletal Care-Radiology Dept, 333 E 38th St Fl 6, New York, NY 10016; **Phone:** 646-501-7289; **Board Cert:** Diagnostic Radiology 1988; **Med School:** Wayne State Univ 1984; **Resid:** Diagnostic Radiology, Univ Mich Med Ctr 1988; **Fellow:** Ultrasound/CT/MRI, Univ Mich Med Ctr 1989; **Fac Appt:** Prof Rad, Cornell Univ-Weill Med Coll

Austin, John H M MD [DR] - **Spec Exp:** Lung Cancer; Thoracic Radiology; **Hospital:** NY-Presby/Columbia Univ Med Ctr, NY (page 66); **Address:** 177 Fort Washington Ave, Milstein Hosp Bldg 3-202C, New York, NY 10032-3784; **Phone:** 212-305-2639; **Board Cert:** Diagnostic Radiology 1970; **Med School:** Yale Univ 1965; **Resid:** Diagnostic Radiology, UCSF Med Ctr 1968; **Fellow:** Diagnostic Radiology, UCSF Med Ctr 1970; **Fac Appt:** Prof Emeritus Rad, Columbia P&S

Bluemke, David A MD/PhD [DR] - **Spec Exp:** Cardiac Imaging; MRI; **Hospital:** Natl Inst of Hlth - Clin Ctr; **Address:** 9000 Rockville Pike, Bldg 10 - Ste 1C351, Bethesda, MD 20892; **Phone:** 301-402-1854; **Board Cert:** Diagnostic Radiology 1993; **Med School:** Univ Chicago-Pritzker Sch Med 1989; **Resid:** Diagnostic Radiology, Johns Hopkins Hosp 1993; **Fellow:** Diagnostic Imaging, Johns Hopkins Hosp 1994; **Fac Appt:** Prof Rad, Johns Hopkins Univ

Brem, Rachel F MD [DR] - **Spec Exp:** Breast Imaging; Breast Cancer; **Hospital:** G Washington Univ Hosp; **Address:** GWU Med Faculty Assocs, Mammography Clin, 2150 Pennsylvania Ave NW, DC Level, Washington, DC 20037; **Phone:** 202-741-3036; **Board Cert:** Diagnostic Radiology 1990; **Med School:** Columbia P&S 1984; **Resid:** Diagnostic Radiology, Johns Hopkins Hosp 1989; **Fellow:** Mammography, Johns Hopkins Hosp 1990; **Fac Appt:** Prof Rad, Geo Wash Univ

Cohen, Burton A MD [DR] - **Spec Exp:** CT Scan; MRI; PET Imaging; **Hospital:** Mount Sinai Med Ctr (page 64); **Address:** 165 E 84th St, New York, NY 10028; **Phone:** 212-535-9770; **Board Cert:** Diagnostic Radiology 1979; **Med School:** NY Med Coll 1975; **Resid:** Diagnostic Radiology, Mt Sinai Hosp 1979; **Fac Appt:** Assoc Clin Prof Rad, Mount Sinai Sch Med

Coleman, Beverly G MD [DR] - **Spec Exp:** Ultrasound; **Hospital:** Hosp Univ Penn - UPHS (page 72); **Address:** Univ Penn Radiology, Ground Dulles, 3400 Spruce St, Philadelphia, PA 19104; **Phone:** 215-662-3046; **Board Cert:** Diagnostic Radiology 1978; **Med School:** Harvard Med Sch 1974; **Resid:** Diagnostic Radiology, Univ Penn Hosp 1975; Diagnostic Radiology, Univ Mich Hosp 1977; **Fellow:** Ultrasound, Univ Penn Hosp 1979; **Fac Appt:** Prof Rad, Univ Pennsylvania

Conant, Emily F MD [DR] - **Spec Exp:** Breast Cancer; Breast Imaging; **Hospital:** Hosp Univ Penn - UPHS (page 72); **Address:** Penn Radiology (Breast Imaging), 3400 Spruce St, 1 Silverstein, Philadelphia, PA 19104; **Phone:** 215-662-4032; **Board Cert:** Diagnostic Radiology 1989; **Med School:** Univ Pennsylvania 1984; **Resid:** Diagnostic Radiology, Hosp Univ Penn 1986; **Fellow:** Breast Imaging, Hosp Univ Penn 1989; **Fac Appt:** Prof Rad, Univ Pennsylvania

Dalinka, Murray MD [DR] - **Spec Exp:** Bone Disorders-Metabolic; Musculoskeletal Imaging; MRI; **Hospital:** Hosp Univ Penn - UPHS (page 72); **Address:** Univ Penn Radiology, Ground Dulles, 3400 Spruce St, Philadelphia, PA 19104; **Phone:** 215-662-3019; **Board Cert:** Diagnostic Radiology 1969; **Med School:** Univ Mich Med Sch 1964; **Resid:** Diagnostic Radiology, Montefiore Med Ctr 1968; **Fac Appt:** Prof Emeritus Rad, Univ Pennsylvania

Dershaw, D David MD [DR] - **Spec Exp:** Breast Imaging; Breast Cancer; Mammography; **Hospital:** Meml Sloan-Kettering Cancer Ctr; **Address:** 300 E 66th St, rm 727, New York, NY 10065; **Phone:** 646-888-4505; **Board Cert:** Diagnostic Radiology 1978; **Med School:** Jefferson Med Coll 1974; **Resid:** Diagnostic Radiology, New York Hosp 1978; **Fellow:** Ultrasound, Thos Jefferson Univ Hosp 1979; **Fac Appt:** Prof Rad, Cornell Univ-Weill Med Coll

Edelstein, Barbara A MD [DR] - **Spec Exp:** Breast Cancer; Women's Imaging; **Address:** 1045 Park Ave, New York, NY 10028; **Phone:** 212-860-7700; **Board Cert:** Diagnostic Radiology 1983; **Med School:** NY Med Coll 1977; **Resid:** Diagnostic Radiology, Montefiore Hosp 1982

Evers, Kathryn A MD [DR] - **Spec Exp:** Breast Cancer; Mammography; MRI-Breast; **Hospital:** Fox Chase Cancer Ctr (page 58); **Address:** Fox Chase Cancer Ctr, Diagnostic Imaging, 333 Cottman Ave, Philadelphia, PA 19111; **Phone:** 215-728-2646; **Board Cert:** Diagnostic Radiology 1980; **Med School:** NYU Sch Med 1975; **Resid:** Diagnostic Radiology, Hosp Univ Penn 1980; **Fellow:** Diagnostic Radiology, Hosp Univ Penn 1981; **Fac Appt:** Asst Clin Prof Rad, Temple Univ

Fishman, Elliot Keith MD [DR] - **Spec Exp:** CT Body Scan; Abdominal Imaging; Cardiac Imaging; Cancer Imaging; **Hospital:** Johns Hopkins Hosp (page 61); **Address:** Johns Hopkins Hosp, Dept Radiology, 601 N Caroline St, JHOC 3254, Baltimore, MD 21287-0006; **Phone:** 410-955-5173; **Board Cert:** Diagnostic Radiology 1981; **Med School:** Univ MD Sch Med 1977; **Resid:** Diagnostic Radiology, Sinai Hosp 1980; **Fellow:** Computerized Tomography, Johns Hopkins Hosp 1981; **Fac Appt:** Prof Rad, Johns Hopkins Univ

Fuhrman, Carl R MD [DR] - **Spec Exp:** Thoracic Imaging; **Hospital:** UPMC Presby, Pittsburgh; **Address:** UPMC-Dept Radiology, 200 Lothrop St, rm E177-PUH, Pittsburgh, PA 15213; **Phone:** 412-647-7288; **Board Cert:** Diagnostic Radiology 1983; **Med School:** Univ Pittsburgh 1979; **Resid:** Diagnostic Radiology, Presby Univ Hosp 1983; **Fac Appt:** Prof Rad, Univ Pittsburgh

Gefter, Warren B MD [DR] - **Spec Exp:** Thoracic Imaging; **Hospital:** Hosp Univ Penn - UPHS (page 72); **Address:** Univ Penn Radiology, Ground Dulles, 3400 Spruce St, Philadelphia, PA 19104; **Phone:** 215-662-6724; **Board Cert:** Diagnostic Radiology 1978; **Med School:** Univ Pennsylvania 1974; **Resid:** Diagnostic Radiology, Hosp Univ Penn 1978; **Fac Appt:** Prof Rad, Univ Pennsylvania

Henschke, Claudia L MD/PhD [DR] - **Spec Exp:** Lung Cancer; Lung Disease; Thoracic Radiology; **Hospital:** Mount Sinai Med Ctr (page 64); **Address:** Mt Sinai Med Ctr, Radiology Dept, 1 Gustave Levy Pl, Box 1234, New York, NY 10029; **Phone:** 212-241-2420; **Board Cert:** Diagnostic Radiology 1981; **Med School:** Howard Univ 1977; **Resid:** Diagnostic Radiology, Brigham & Womens Hosp 1983; **Fac Appt:** Prof Rad, Cornell Univ-Weill Med Coll

Holliday, Roy MD [DR] - **Spec Exp:** Head & Neck Radiology; **Hospital:** New York Eye & Ear Infirm (page 65), Beth Israel Med Ctr - Petrie Division (page 56); **Address:** 310 E 14th St, New York, NY 10003; **Phone:** 212-979-4397; **Board Cert:** Diagnostic Radiology 1986; **Med School:** NYU Sch Med 1982; **Resid:** Diagnostic Radiology, NYU Med Ctr 1986; **Fellow:** Neurological Radiology, NYU Med Ctr 1987; **Fac Appt:** Clin Prof Rad, NYU Sch Med

Hricak, Hedvig MD/PhD [DR] - **Spec Exp:** Prostate Cancer-MR Spectroscopy (MRSI); Breast Imaging; Breast Cancer; **Hospital:** Meml Sloan-Kettering Cancer Ctr; **Address:** 1275 York Ave, Ste C278, New York, NY 10065; **Phone:** 800-525-2225; **Board Cert:** Diagnostic Radiology 1978; **Med School:** Yugoslavia 1970; **Resid:** Diagnostic Radiology, St Joseph Mercy Hosp 1977; **Fellow:** Ultrasound/CT, Henry Ford Hosp 1978; **Fac Appt:** Prof Rad, Cornell Univ-Weill Med Coll

Jaramillo, Diego MD [DR] - **Spec Exp:** Pediatric Radiology; **Hospital:** Chldns Hosp of Philadelphia; **Address:** CHOP, Dept Radiology, 34th & Civic Center Blvd, rm 3NW-17, Philadelphia, PA 19104; **Phone:** 267-425-7110; **Board Cert:** Diagnostic Radiology 1987; Pediatric Radiology 2005; **Med School:** Colombia 1981; **Resid:** Diagnostic Radiology, Univ Texas 1987; **Fellow:** Pediatric Radiology, Children's Hosp 1989; **Fac Appt:** Prof Rad, Univ Pennsylvania

Kanal, Emanuel MD [DR] - **Spec Exp:** Neuroradiology; MRI; **Hospital:** UPMC Presby, Pittsburgh; **Address:** Univ Pittsburgh Med Ctr, Dept Radiology, 200 Lothrop St, rm D132, Pittsburgh, PA 15213-2582; **Phone:** 412-647-3540; **Board Cert:** Diagnostic Radiology 1985; **Med School:** Univ Pittsburgh 1981; **Resid:** Diagnostic Radiology, Univ Pittsburgh Med Ctr 1985; **Fellow:** Magnetic Resonance Imaging, Pittsburgh NMR Inst 1986; Neurological Radiology, Univ Pittsburgh Med Ctr 1993; **Fac Appt:** Prof Rad, Univ Pittsburgh

Kurtz, Alfred B MD [DR] - **Spec Exp:** Obstetric Ultrasound; **Hospital:** Thomas Jefferson Univ Hosp; **Address:** Thomas Jefferson Univ Hosp, Radiology, 111 S 11th St, Ste 3350A-B, Philadelphia, PA 19107; **Phone:** 215-955-6226; **Board Cert:** Diagnostic Radiology 1977; **Med School:** Stanford Univ 1972; **Resid:** Internal Medicine, Montefiore Med Ctr 1974; Diagnostic Radiology, Montefiore Med Ctr 1977; **Fellow:** Ultrasound, Thomas Jefferson Univ Hosp 1978; **Fac Appt:** Prof Rad, Jefferson Med Coll

Levy, Angela D MD [DR] - **Spec Exp:** Abdominal Imaging; **Hospital:** Georgetown Univ Hosp, Armed Forces Inst of Path; **Address:** Georgetown University Hospital, 3800 Reservoir Rd NW, CCC Bldg Fl Ground, Washington, DC 20007; **Phone:** 202-444-3380; **Board Cert:** Diagnostic Radiology 1993; **Med School:** Uniformed Srvs Univ, Bethesda 1988; **Resid:** Diagnostic Radiology, Walter Reed Army Hosp 1992; **Fac Appt:** Assoc Prof Rad, Uniformed Srvs Univ, Bethesda

Logan-Young, Wende MD [DR] - **Spec Exp:** Breast Cancer; **Address:** Elizabeth Wende Breast Care, 170 Sawgrass Drive, Rochester, NY 14620; **Phone:** 585-442-2190; **Board Cert:** Diagnostic Radiology 1970; **Med School:** SUNY Buffalo 1961; **Resid:** Internal Medicine, Highland Hospital 1964; **Fellow:** Radiology, Univ Rochester 1969

Megibow, Alec J MD [DR] - **Spec Exp:** Abdominal Imaging; Gastrointestinal Imaging; CT Body Scan; **Hospital:** NYU Langone Med Ctr (page 68), Bellevue Hosp Ctr; **Address:** 550 1st Ave, HHC 232, New York, NY 10016; **Phone:** 212-263-5222; **Board Cert:** Diagnostic Radiology 1978; **Med School:** SUNY Upstate Med Univ 1974; **Resid:** Diagnostic Radiology, Bellevue/NYU Med Ctr 1978; **Fellow:** Abdominal Imaging, NYU Med Ctr 1978; **Fac Appt:** Prof Rad, NYU Sch Med

Mirvis, Stuart E MD [DR] - **Spec Exp:** Trauma Radiology; **Hospital:** Univ of MD Med Ctr, Good Samaritan Hosp; **Address:** Univ Maryland Med Ctr, Dept Radiology, 22 S Greene St, Baltimore, MD 21201; **Phone:** 410-328-8845; **Board Cert:** Diagnostic Radiology 1984; **Med School:** Johns Hopkins Univ 1979; **Resid:** Diagnostic Radiology, Univ Maryland Med Ctr 1984; **Fellow:** Trauma Radiology, Univ Maryland Med Ctr 1985; **Fac Appt:** Prof Rad, Univ MD Sch Med

Mitnick, Julie MD [DR] - **Spec Exp:** Mammography; Breast Cancer; **Address:** 650 1st Ave, New York, NY 10016; **Phone:** 212-686-4440; **Board Cert:** Diagnostic Radiology 1977; **Med School:** NYU Sch Med 1972; **Resid:** Diagnostic Radiology, NYU Med Ctr 1977; **Fellow:** Pediatric Radiology, NYU Med Ctr 1978; **Fac Appt:** Assoc Clin Prof Rad, NYU Sch Med

Mountz, James M MD/PhD [DR] - **Spec Exp:** Neurologic Imaging; Brain Imaging; **Hospital:** UPMC Presby, Pittsburgh; **Address:** UPMC Hlth Sys, Presby Univ Hosp, 200 Lothrop St, PET Facility, rm B932, Pittsburgh, PA 15213; **Phone:** 412-647-0104; **Board Cert:** Diagnostic Radiology 1985; Nuclear Medicine 1986; **Med School:** Case West Res Univ 1981; **Resid:** Diagnostic Radiology, Univ Michigan Hosps 1985; **Fellow:** Nuclear Medicine, Univ Michigan Hosps 1986; **Fac Appt:** Prof Rad, Univ Pittsburgh

Panicek, David M MD [DR] - **Spec Exp:** Bone Cancer; Soft Tissue Tumors; Musculoskeletal Tumor Imaging; **Hospital:** Meml Sloan-Kettering Cancer Ctr; **Address:** 1275 York Ave, Ste C276G, Meml Sloan Kettering Cancer Ctr, New York, NY 10065; **Phone:** 800-525-2225; **Board Cert:** Diagnostic Radiology 1984; **Med School:** Cornell Univ-Weill Med Coll 1980; **Resid:** Diagnostic Radiology, NY Hosp-Cornell Med Ctr 1984; **Fac Appt:** Prof Rad, Cornell Univ-Weill Med Coll

Parsons, Rosaleen B MD [DR] - **Spec Exp:** CT Body Scan; Genitourinary Cancer; Genitourinary Radiology; **Hospital:** Fox Chase Cancer Ctr (page 58); **Address:** Fox Chase Cancer Ctr, Dept of Diagnostic Imaging, 333 Cottman Ave, Philadelphia, PA 19111; **Phone:** 215-728-3024; **Board Cert:** Diagnostic Radiology 1991; **Med School:** Med Coll PA Hahnemann 1986; **Resid:** Diagnostic Radiology, Med Coll Penn Affil Hosp 1991; **Fac Appt:** Prof Rad, Med Coll PA

Pavlov, Helene MD [DR] - **Spec Exp:** Sports Medicine Radiology; Musculoskeletal Imaging; Orthopaedic Imaging; **Hospital:** Hosp For Special Surgery (page 60), NY-Presby/Weill Cornell Med Ctr, NY (page 66); **Address:** Hosp for Special Surgery, 535 E 70th St, New York, NY 10021-4892; **Phone:** 212-606-1132; **Board Cert:** Diagnostic Radiology 1976; **Med School:** Temple Univ 1972; **Resid:** Diagnostic Radiology, Germantown Hosp 1976; **Fellow:** Musculoskeletal Imaging, Hosp For Special Surg 1977; **Fac Appt:** Prof Rad, Cornell Univ-Weill Med Coll

Potter, Hollis G MD [DR] - **Spec Exp:** Musculoskeletal Imaging; Cartilage Damage; Arthroplasty Imaging; **Hospital:** Hosp For Special Surgery (page 60); **Address:** Hosp for Special Surgery, MRI-basement, 535 E 70th St, Ste MRI, New York, NY 10021-4892; **Phone:** 212-606-1023; **Board Cert:** Diagnostic Radiology 1990; **Med School:** NY Med Coll 1985; **Resid:** Diagnostic Radiology, North Shore Univ Hosp 1990; **Fellow:** Diagnostic Radiology, Hosp Special Surgery 1991; **Fac Appt:** Prof Rad, Cornell Univ-Weill Med Coll

Prince, Martin R MD/PhD [DR] - **Spec Exp:** MRI Angiography; Abdominal Imaging; **Hospital:** NY-Presby/Weill Cornell Med Ctr, NY (page 66), NY-Presby/Columbia Univ Med Ctr, NY (page 66); **Address:** 416 E 55th St, New York, NY 10022; **Phone:** 212-746-6880; **Board Cert:** Diagnostic Radiology 1993; **Med School:** Harvard Med Sch 1985; **Resid:** Radiology, Mass Genl Hosp 1993; **Fellow:** Magnetic Resonance Imaging, Mass Genl Hosp 1993; Angiography, Mass Genl Hosp 1989; **Fac Appt:** Prof Rad, Cornell Univ-Weill Med Coll

Rao, Vijay M MD [DR] - **Spec Exp:** Head & Neck Tumors Imaging; TMJ Imaging; Ear Nose & Throat Imaging; **Hospital:** Thomas Jefferson Univ Hosp; **Address:** Jefferson Dept Radiology, 132 S 10th St, 1087 Main Bldg, Philadelphia, PA 19107-4824; **Phone:** 215-955-4804; **Board Cert:** Diagnostic Radiology 1978; **Med School:** India 1973; **Resid:** Diagnostic Radiology, Thomas Jefferson Univ Hosp 1978; **Fac Appt:** Prof Rad, Thomas Jefferson Univ

Reinus, William R MD [DR] - **Spec Exp:** Musculoskeletal Imaging; MRI; **Hospital:** Temple Univ Hosp; **Address:** Radiology Dept, 3401 N Broad St, Philadelphia, PA 19140; **Phone:** 215-707-9745; **Board Cert:** Diagnostic Radiology 1983; **Med School:** NYU Sch Med 1979; **Resid:** Radiology, Mallinkradt Inst Rad 1983; **Fellow:** Musculoskeletal Imaging, Mallinkradt Inst Rad 1984; **Fac Appt:** Prof Rad, Temple Univ

Roth, Susan Orel MD [DR] - **Spec Exp:** Breast Imaging; Breast Cancer; **Hospital:** Hosp Univ Penn - UPHS (page 72); **Address:** Penn Radiology, 3400 Spruce St, 1 Silverstein, Philadelphia, PA 19104; **Phone:** 215-614-0124; **Board Cert:** Diagnostic Radiology 1989; **Med School:** Univ Pennsylvania 1984; **Resid:** Diagnostic Radiology, Johns Hopkins Hosp 1989; **Fac Appt:** Prof Rad, Univ Pennsylvania

Teal, James S MD [DR] - **Spec Exp:** Interventional Radiology; Neuroradiology; **Hospital:** Howard Univ Hosp; **Address:** 2041 Georgia Ave NW, Washington, DC 20060; **Phone:** 202-865-1571; **Board Cert:** Diagnostic Radiology 1970; **Med School:** Univ Tex Med Br, Galveston 1964; **Resid:** Diagnostic Radiology, Mt Zion Hosp 1969; **Fellow:** Neuroradiology, LAC-USC Med Ctr 1970; **Fac Appt:** Prof Rad, Howard Univ

Diagnostic Radiology

White, Charles S MD [DR] - **Spec Exp:** Thoracic Imaging; **Hospital:** Univ of MD Med Ctr; **Address:** Univ Maryland Med Ctr, Dept Radiology, 22 S Greene St, Baltimore, MD 21201; **Phone:** 410-328-3477; **Board Cert:** Diagnostic Radiology 1991; Internal Medicine 1987; **Med School:** SUNY Buffalo 1984; **Resid:** Internal Medicine, Columbia-Presby Hosp 1987; Diagnostic Radiology, Columbia-Presby Hosp 1991; **Fellow:** Thoracic Radiology, Columbia-Presby Med Ctr; **Fac Appt:** Prof, Univ MD Sch Med

Yankelevitz, David MD [DR] - **Spec Exp:** Lung Cancer; Thoracic Radiology; **Hospital:** Mount Sinai Med Ctr (page 64); **Address:** Mt Sinai Med Ctr, Radiology Dept, 1 Gustave Levy Pl, Box 1234, New York, NY 10029; **Phone:** 212-241-2420; **Board Cert:** Diagnostic Radiology 1987; Nuclear Medicine 1987; **Med School:** SUNY Hlth Sci Ctr 1981; **Resid:** Diagnostic Radiology, Long Island Coll Hosp 1984; Nuclear Medicine, NY-Cornell Med Ctr 1987; **Fellow:** Diagnostic Radiology, NY-Cornell Med Ctr 1987; **Fac Appt:** Prof Rad, Cornell Univ-Weill Med Coll

Yoon, Sydney S MD [DR] - **Spec Exp:** MRI; CT Scan; Neuroradiology; Interventional Radiology; **Hospital:** South Nassau Comm Hosp; **Address:** 1 Healthy Way, Dept of Radiology, Oceanside, NY 11572; **Phone:** 516-632-4660; **Board Cert:** Internal Medicine 1989; Diagnostic Radiology 1993; Vascular & Interventional Radiology 2011; Neuroradiology 2006; **Med School:** Univ Chicago-Pritzker Sch Med 1986; **Resid:** Internal Medicine, Johns Hopkins Hosp 1989; Diagnostic Radiology, UCLA Med Ctr 1993; **Fellow:** Neuroradiology, Columbia Presby Med Ctr 1995; Vascular & Interventional Radiology, UCLA Med Ctr 1997

Zeman, Robert K MD [DR] - **Spec Exp:** Cardiovascular Imaging; Cardiac CT Angiography; **Hospital:** G Washington Univ Hosp; **Address:** GM Medical Faculty Associates, Diagnostic Radiology, 900 23rd St NW, Washington, DC 20037; **Phone:** 202-715-5154; **Board Cert:** Diagnostic Radiology 1980; **Med School:** Northwestern Univ 1976; **Resid:** Diagnostic Radiology, Yale-New Haven Hosp 1980; **Fellow:** Nuclear Medicine, Yale-New Haven Hosp 1980; **Fac Appt:** Prof Rad, Geo Wash Univ

Southeast

Abbitt, Patricia L MD [DR] - **Spec Exp:** Ultrasound; Interventional Radiology; Breast Imaging; Breast Cancer; **Hospital:** Shands at Univ of FL; **Address:** Shands Healthcare, Dept Radiology, 1600 SW Archer Rd, PO Box 100374, Gainesville, FL 32610; **Phone:** 352-265-0291; **Board Cert:** Diagnostic Radiology 1986; **Med School:** Tufts Univ 1981; **Resid:** Diagnostic Radiology, Univ VA Med Ctr 1986; **Fellow:** Breast Imaging, Univ VA Med Ctr 1987; **Fac Appt:** Prof Rad, Univ Fla Coll Med

Berland, Lincoln L MD [DR] - **Spec Exp:** Abdominal Imaging; Gastrointestinal Imaging; **Hospital:** Univ of Ala Hosp at Birmingham; **Address:** UAB Diagnostic Radiology, N348 Jefferson Tower Bldg, 619 19th St S, Birmingham, AL 35249-6830; **Phone:** 205-934-7978; **Board Cert:** Diagnostic Radiology 1980; **Med School:** Washington Univ, St Louis 1975; **Resid:** Diagnostic Radiology, Med Coll Wisconsin Hosps 1979; **Fellow:** Ultrasound/CT, Med Coll Wisconsin Hosps 1980; **Fac Appt:** Prof Rad, Univ Alabama

Cardenosa, Gilda MD [DR] - **Spec Exp:** Breast Imaging; **Hospital:** Med Coll of VA Hosp; **Address:** VCU Med Ctr at Stony Point, Dept Radiology, 9000 Stony Point Pkwy, Richmond, VA 23235; **Phone:** 804-560-8906 x7862; **Board Cert:** Diagnostic Radiology 1989; **Med School:** Columbia P&S 1984; **Resid:** Diagnostic Radiology, Mass Genl Hosp 1989; **Fac Appt:** Prof Rad, Med Coll VA

Chiles, Caroline MD [DR] - **Spec Exp:** Thoracic Radiology; Lung Cancer; **Hospital:** Wake Forest Baptist Med Ctr; **Address:** Wake Forest Baptist Med Ctr, Medical Ctr Blvd, Winston-Salem, NC 27157; **Phone:** 336-716-4316; **Board Cert:** Diagnostic Radiology 1984; **Med School:** Duke Univ 1979; **Resid:** Diagnostic Radiology, Stanford Univ Hosp 1984; **Fellow:** Thoracic Radiology, Duke Univ Med Ctr 1985; **Fac Appt:** Assoc Prof Rad, Bowman Gray

Cohen, Harris L MD [DR] - **Spec Exp:** Pediatric Radiology; Fetal Ultrasound/Obstetrical Imaging; Ultrasound; **Hospital:** Le Bonheur Chldns Med Ctr; **Address:** Le Bonheur Children's Hosp, Dept Radiology Fl Ground, 50 N Dunlap St, Memphis, TN 38103-2807; **Phone:** 901-287-7041; **Board Cert:** Diagnostic Radiology 1980; Pediatric Radiology 2005; **Med School:** SUNY Downstate 1976; **Resid:** Diagnostic Radiology, Univ Hosp 1980; **Fellow:** Pediatric Radiology, Chldns Hosp 1981; **Fac Appt:** Prof Rad, Univ Tenn Coll Med

Elster, Allen D MD [DR] - **Spec Exp:** MRI; Neurologic Imaging; Brain Tumors; Spinal Tumor Imaging; **Hospital:** Wake Forest Baptist Med Ctr; **Address:** Wake Forest Baptist Med Ctr, Medical Center Blvd, Winston Salem, NC 27157-1088; **Phone:** 336-716-7095; **Board Cert:** Diagnostic Radiology 1987; Neuroradiology 2005; **Med School:** Baylor Coll Med 1980; **Resid:** Surgery, Mass Genl Hosp 1983; Diagnostic Radiology, Univ Texas Hlth Sci Ctr 1986; **Fellow:** Neuroradiology, Bowman Gray Sch Med 1987; **Fac Appt:** Prof Rad, Wake Forest Univ

Freimanis, Rita I MD [DR] - **Spec Exp:** Breast Cancer; Breast Imaging; **Hospital:** Wake Forest Baptist Med Ctr; **Address:** Wake Forest Baptist Med Ctr, One Medical Center Blvd, Winston-Salem, NC 27157; **Phone:** 336-713-4019; **Board Cert:** Diagnostic Radiology 1990; **Med School:** Bowman Gray 1985; **Resid:** Diagnostic Radiology, NC Bapt Hosp 1990; **Fac Appt:** Assoc Prof Rad, Wake Forest Univ

Mancuso, Anthony A MD [DR] - **Spec Exp:** Head & Neck Radiology; Neuroradiology; **Hospital:** Shands at Univ of FL; **Address:** Shands Hosp, Univ Florida, Dept Radiology, 1600 SW Archer Rd, Ste G393, Gainesville, FL 32610; **Phone:** 352-265-0296; **Board Cert:** Diagnostic Radiology 1978; **Med School:** Univ Miami Sch Med 1973; **Resid:** Diagnostic Radiology, UCLA Med Ctr 1977; **Fellow:** Neuroradiology, UCLA Med Ctr 1978; **Fac Appt:** Prof Rad, Univ Fla Coll Med

Partain, Clarence L MD/PhD [DR] - **Spec Exp:** MRI; Nuclear Radiology; Chest Radiology; **Hospital:** Vanderbilt Univ Med Ctr (page 75); **Address:** Vanderbilt Univ Med Ctr, Dept Radiology, 1161 21st Ave S, rm RR1223 MCN, Nashville, TN 37232-2675; **Phone:** 615-343-3588; **Board Cert:** Nuclear Medicine 1979; Diagnostic Radiology 1980; Nuclear Radiology 1981; **Med School:** Washington Univ, St Louis 1975; **Resid:** Diagnostic Radiology, Univ North Carolina 1979; Nuclear Medicine, Univ North Carolina 1979; **Fac Appt:** Prof, Vanderbilt Univ

Patz Jr, Edward F MD [DR] - **Spec Exp:** Thoracic Radiology; PET Imaging; Lung Cancer; **Hospital:** Duke Univ Hosp; **Address:** Duke Univ Med Ctr, Dept Radiology, Box 3808, Durham, NC 27710; **Phone:** 919-684-7999; **Board Cert:** Diagnostic Radiology 1990; **Med School:** Univ MD Sch Med 1985; **Resid:** Diagnostic Radiology, Brigham & Womens Hosp 1990; **Fellow:** Thoracic Radiology, Brigham & Womens Hosp 1990; **Fac Appt:** Prof, Duke Univ

Rubin, Geoffrey D MD [DR] - **Spec Exp:** Cardiovascular Imaging; Cardiac Imaging; Thoracic Radiology; **Hospital:** Duke Univ Hosp; **Address:** Duke Univ Med Ctr, 2301 Erwin Rd, rm 1529, DUMC 3808, Durham, NC 27710-3808; **Phone:** 919-684-7289; **Board Cert:** Diagnostic Radiology 1992; **Med School:** UCSD 1987; **Resid:** Diagnostic Radiology, Stanford Univ Med Ctr 1992; **Fellow:** Body Imaging, Stanford Univ Med Ctr 1993; **Fac Appt:** Prof Rad, Duke Univ

Diagnostic Radiology

Zagoria, Ronald J MD [DR] - **Spec Exp:** Abdominal Imaging; Genitourinary Radiology; Interventional Radiology; MRI; **Hospital:** Wake Forest Baptist Med Ctr; **Address:** Wake Forest Univ Bapt Med Ctr, Medical Center Blvd, MRI Bldg - Fl 3, Winston-Salem, NC 27157; **Phone:** 336-716-2471; **Board Cert:** Diagnostic Radiology 1987; Vascular & Interventional Radiology 2004; **Med School:** Univ MD Sch Med 1983; **Resid:** Radiology, Bowman Gray Med Ctr 1987; **Fellow:** Abdominal Imaging, Bowman Gray Med Ctr 1987; **Fac Appt:** Prof Rad, Wake Forest Univ

Midwest

Charboneau, J William MD [DR] - **Spec Exp:** Radiofrequency Tumor Ablation; Liver Cancer; Thyroid Cancer; **Hospital:** Mayo Med Ctr & Clin - Rochester; **Address:** Mayo Clinic Dept of Radiology, 200 First St SW, Rochester, MN 55905-0002; **Phone:** 507-284-2097; **Board Cert:** Diagnostic Radiology 1980; **Med School:** Univ Wisc 1976; **Resid:** Diagnostic Radiology, Mayo Clin 1980; **Fac Appt:** Prof, Mayo Med Sch

Edelman, Robert R MD [DR] - **Spec Exp:** MRI; Cardiac CT Angiography; Cardiac MRI; **Hospital:** Evanston/North Shore Univ Hlth Sys; **Address:** Evanston Hosp, Dept Radiology, 2650 Ridge Ave Walgreen Bldg - rm G534, Evanston, IL 60201; **Phone:** 847-570-2553; **Board Cert:** Diagnostic Radiology 1984; **Med School:** Boston Univ 1980; **Resid:** Diagnostic Radiology, Beth Israel Deaconess Med Ctr 1984; **Fac Appt:** Prof Rad, Northwestern Univ

Fidler, Jeff L MD [DR] - **Spec Exp:** Gastrointestinal Imaging; CT Colonography; MRI; **Hospital:** Mayo Med Ctr & Clin - Rochester; **Address:** Mayo Clinic, Div Radiology, 200 First St SW, Rochester, MN 55905-0002; **Phone:** 507-284-2311; **Board Cert:** Diagnostic Radiology 1993; **Med School:** Univ Nebr Coll Med 1988; **Resid:** Radiology, Duke Univ Hosp 1993; **Fellow:** Abdominal Imaging, Duke Univ 1994; **Fac Appt:** Assoc Prof Rad, Mayo Med Sch

Flamm, Scott D MD [DR] - **Spec Exp:** Cardiac MRI; Cardiovascular Imaging; Congenital Heart Disease; **Hospital:** Cleveland Clin (page 55); **Address:** 9500 Euclid Ave, MS J1-4, Cleveland, OH 44195; **Phone:** 216-444-2740; **Board Cert:** Diagnostic Radiology 1993; **Med School:** Geo Wash Univ 1988; **Resid:** Diagnostic Radiology, UCLA Med Ctr 1993; **Fellow:** Cardiovascular Disease, UCSF Med Ctr 1994; **Fac Appt:** Assoc Prof Rad, Case West Res Univ

Goodman, Lawrence R MD [DR] - **Spec Exp:** Thoracic Imaging; Pulmonary Embolism; Lung Disease; **Hospital:** Froedtert and Med Ctr of WI; **Address:** Dept Radiology, 9200 W Wisconsin Ave, Milwaukee, WI 53226; **Phone:** 414-805-2060; **Board Cert:** Diagnostic Radiology 1973; **Med School:** SUNY Downstate 1968; **Resid:** Diagnostic Radiology, Boston Univ/City Hosp 1972; **Fellow:** Thoracic Radiology, UCSF Med Ctr 1973; **Fac Appt:** Prof Rad, Med Coll Wisc

Helvie, Mark A MD [DR] - **Spec Exp:** Breast Imaging; Breast Cancer; Mammography; **Hospital:** Univ of Michigan Hosp; **Address:** Univ Of Michigan Hospital, Taubman Center, 1500 E Medical Center Drive, rm 2910N, Ann Arbor, MI 48109-0326; **Phone:** 734-936-4367; **Board Cert:** Internal Medicine 1983; Diagnostic Radiology 1986; **Med School:** Univ NC Sch Med 1980; **Resid:** Internal Medicine, Univ Michigan Hosps 1983; Diagnostic Radiology, Univ Michigan Hosps 1986; **Fellow:** Breast Imaging, Univ Michigan Hosps 1987; **Fac Appt:** Prof Rad, Univ Mich Med Sch

Jackson, Valerie P MD [DR] - **Spec Exp:** Breast Imaging; **Hospital:** IU Health University Hosp, Wishard Hlth Srvs; **Address:** Indiana Univ Dept Radiology, 550 N University Blvd, rm 0663, Indianapolis, IN 46202; **Phone:** 317-944-1866; **Board Cert:** Diagnostic Radiology 1982; **Med School:** Indiana Univ 1978; **Resid:** Diagnostic Radiology, Indiana Univ Med Ctr 1982; **Fac Appt:** Prof Rad, Indiana Univ

Monsees, Barbara MD [DR] - **Spec Exp:** Mammography; Breast Cancer; **Hospital:** Barnes-Jewish Hosp; **Address:** 510 S Kingshighway Blvd, Campus Box 8131, St Louis, MO 63110; **Phone:** 314-454-7500; **Board Cert:** Diagnostic Radiology 1980; **Med School:** Washington Univ, St Louis 1975; **Resid:** Pediatrics, St Louis Chldns Hosp 1977; Diagnostic Radiology, Mallinckrodt Inst Radiology 1980; **Fac Appt:** Prof, Washington Univ, St Louis

Sivit, Carlos J MD [DR] - **Spec Exp:** Pediatric Radiology; Abdominal Imaging; Trauma Radiology; **Hospital:** UH Rainbow Babies & Chldns Hosp (page 74); **Address:** Dept Radiology, 11100 Euclid Ave, Cleveland, OH 44106-1736; **Phone:** 216-844-1172; **Board Cert:** Pediatrics 1987; Diagnostic Radiology 1987; **Med School:** Univ VA Sch Med 1981; **Resid:** Pediatrics, Vanderbilt Univ Hosp 1984; Diagnostic Radiology, George Washington Univ Hosp 1987; **Fellow:** Pediatric Radiology, Chldns Natl Med Ctr 1989; **Fac Appt:** Prof Rad, Case West Res Univ

Swensen, Stephen J MD [DR] - **Spec Exp:** Lung Cancer; Lung Disease; **Hospital:** Mayo Med Ctr & Clin - Rochester; **Address:** Mayo Clinic - Diagnostic Radiology, 200 1st St SW, Rochester, MN 55905; **Phone:** 507-284-8550; **Board Cert:** Diagnostic Radiology 1986; **Med School:** Univ Wisc 1981; **Resid:** Diagnostic Radiology, Mayo Clinic 1986; **Fellow:** Pulmonary Radiology, Brigham & Womens Hosp 1987; **Fac Appt:** Prof Rad, Mayo Med Sch

Thompson, Brad H MD [DR] - **Spec Exp:** Cardiovascular Imaging; **Hospital:** Univ Iowa Hosp & Clinics; **Address:** UIHC, Dept Radiology, 200 Hawkins Drive, rm 3895 JPP, Iowa City, IA 52242; **Phone:** 319-356-3444; **Board Cert:** Diagnostic Radiology 1990; **Med School:** Univ Iowa Coll Med 1986; **Resid:** Diagnostic Radiology, Univ Iowa Hosp & Clins 1990; **Fac Appt:** Assoc Prof Rad, Univ Iowa Coll Med

Wells, Robert G MD [DR] - **Spec Exp:** Pediatric Radiology; **Hospital:** Chldns Hosp - Wisconsin; **Address:** Pediatric Diagnostic Imaging, 10500 W Loomis Rd, Ste 120, Franklin, WI 53132; **Phone:** 414-529-3100; **Board Cert:** Diagnostic Radiology 1984; Pediatric Radiology 2004; Vascular & Interventional Radiology 2004; **Med School:** Med Coll Wisc 1980; **Resid:** Diagnostic Radiology, St Lukes Hosp 1984; **Fellow:** Pediatric Radiology, Milwaukee Chldns Hosp 1985; **Fac Appt:** Assoc Clin Prof Rad, Med Coll Wisc

White, Richard D MD [DR] - **Spec Exp:** Cardiovascular Imaging; Congenital Heart Disease-Adult & Child; **Hospital:** Ohio St Univ Med Ctr; **Address:** 395 W 12th Ave, Ste 452A, Columbus, OH 43210; **Phone:** 614-293-4456; **Board Cert:** Diagnostic Radiology 1986; **Med School:** Duke Univ 1981; **Resid:** Diagnostic Radiology, UCSF Med Ctr 1985; **Fellow:** Cardiovascular Radiology, UCSF Med Ctr 1987; **Fac Appt:** Prof, Univ Fla Coll Med

Great Plains and Mountains

Dodd III, Gerald Dewey MD [DR] - **Spec Exp:** Abdominal Imaging; Liver Cancer; **Hospital:** Univ of CO Hosp - Anschutz Inpatient Pav; **Address:** Univ Co Hosp, Dept Radiology, 12605 E 16th Ave, Leprino Bldg, MS L954, Aurora, CO 80045; **Phone:** 720-848-6608; **Board Cert:** Diagnostic Radiology 1987; **Med School:** Univ Tex, Houston 1983; **Resid:** Diagnostic Radiology, Univ Hosp 1987; **Fellow:** Abdominal Imaging & Angio-Interventional, Univ Hosp 1988; **Fac Appt:** Prof, Univ Tex, San Antonio

Hubbard, Anne M MD [DR] - **Spec Exp:** Pediatric Radiology; Fetal MRI; Fetal Imaging; **Hospital:** Nebraska Med Ctr; **Address:** 981045 Nebraska Medical Ctr, Omaha, NE 68198-1045; **Phone:** 402-559-1010; **Board Cert:** Diagnostic Radiology 1983; Pediatric Radiology 2005; **Med School:** Univ Nebr Coll Med 1977; **Resid:** Internal Medicine, Mayo Clinic 1980; Diagnostic Radiology, Med Coll Wisc Affil Hosp 1983; **Fellow:** Pediatric Radiology, Milwaukee Chldns Hosp 1984; **Fac Appt:** Prof Rad, Univ Nebr Coll Med

Diagnostic Radiology

Southwest

Erasmus, Jeremy J MD [DR] - **Spec Exp:** Lung Cancer; CT Body Scan; PET Imaging; **Hospital:** UT MD Anderson Cancer Ctr; **Address:** MD Anderson Cancer Ctr, Dept of Rad, 1515 Holcombe Blvd, Unit 1478, Houston, TX 77030; **Phone:** 713-792-5878; **Board Cert:** Diagnostic Radiology 1993; **Med School:** South Africa 1982; **Resid:** Diagnostic Radiology, Queens Univ Affil Hosp 1993; **Fac Appt:** Prof Rad, Univ Tex, Houston

Huynh, Phan T MD [DR] - **Spec Exp:** Mammography; Breast Cancer; **Hospital:** St. Luke's Episcopal Hosp-Houston; **Address:** 6624 Fannin St, St Luke's Medical Towers, Women's Center, Fl 10, Houston, TX 77030; **Phone:** 832-355-8130; **Board Cert:** Diagnostic Radiology 1994; **Med School:** Univ VA Sch Med 1989; **Resid:** Diagnostic Radiology, Univ Virginia Med Ctr 1994; **Fellow:** Mammography, Univ Virginia 1995; **Fac Appt:** Assoc Clin Prof Rad, Baylor Coll Med

Otto, Pamela MD [DR] - **Spec Exp:** Breast Imaging; Breast Cancer; **Hospital:** Univ Hlth Syst-San Antonio, Audie L Murphy Meml Vets Hosp - San Antonio; **Address:** UTHSC-Dept Radiology, 7703 Floyd Curl Drive, MC 7800, San Antonio, TX 78229-7800; **Phone:** 210-567-3448; **Board Cert:** Diagnostic Radiology 1993; **Med School:** Univ MO-Columbia Sch Med 1988; **Resid:** Diagnostic Radiology, Univ Texas Hlth Sci Ctr 1993; **Fellow:** Breast Imaging, Univ Texas Hlth Sci Ctr 1993; **Fac Appt:** Assoc Prof Rad, Univ Tex, San Antonio

Stough, Rebecca G MD [DR] - **Spec Exp:** MRI-Breast; Breast Cancer; **Hospital:** Mercy Hlth Ctr - Oklahoma City; **Address:** Mercy Womens Center, Breast MRI of Oklahoma, 4625 Southwestern, Oklahoma City, OK 73109; **Phone:** 405-632-2323; **Board Cert:** Diagnostic Radiology 1981; **Med School:** Univ Okla Coll Med 1975; **Resid:** Diagnostic Radiology, Univ Oklahoma Affil Hosp 1980

Ulissey, Michael J MD [DR] - **Spec Exp:** Breast Imaging; Breast Cancer; Mammography; **Hospital:** UT Southwestern Med Ctr at Dallas; **Address:** Univ SW Med Ctr, Parkland Comprehensive Breast Ctr, 5701 Maple Ave, Ste 300, Dallas, TX 75235; **Phone:** 214-266-3300; **Board Cert:** Diagnostic Radiology 1998; **Med School:** Texas A&M Univ 1991; **Resid:** Diagnostic Radiology, Univ Oklahoma Hlth Ctr 1998; **Fellow:** Radiology, Univ TX SW Clin Breast Radiology 1999; Magnetic Resonance Imaging, UT Southwestern Med Ctr 2004; **Fac Appt:** Assoc Prof Rad, Univ Tex SW, Dallas

West Coast and Pacific

Bahn, Duke K MD [DR] - **Spec Exp:** Prostate Cancer-Cryosurgery; Ultrasound; Immunotherapy; **Hospital:** Comm Meml Hosp - Ventura; **Address:** 168 N Brent St, Ste 402, Ventura, CA 93003; **Phone:** 805-585-3082; **Board Cert:** Diagnostic Radiology 1978; **Med School:** Korea 1970; **Resid:** Diagnostic Radiology, Wayne State Univ Med Ctr 1978; **Fac Appt:** Clin Prof Rad, Korea

Bassett, Lawrence W MD [DR] - **Spec Exp:** Breast Imaging; **Hospital:** UCLA Ronald Reagan Med Ctr; **Address:** 200 UCLA Med Plaza, rm 165-47, Los Angeles, CA 90095; **Phone:** 310-206-9608; **Board Cert:** Diagnostic Radiology 1975; **Med School:** UC Irvine 1968; **Resid:** Diagnostic Radiology, UCLA Med Ctr 1972; **Fac Appt:** Prof Rad, UCLA

Coakley, Fergus V MD [DR] - **Spec Exp:** Abdominal Imaging; Anal Cancer; Liver Cancer; Esophageal Cancer; **Hospital:** OHSU Hlthcare; **Address:** Oregon Health & Science University, 3181 SW Sam Jackson Park Road, Mail Code: L340, Portland, OR 97239; **Phone:** 503-494-4511; **Board Cert:** Diagnostic Radiology 2001; **Med School:** Ireland 1988; **Resid:** Internal Medicine, Mater & St. Vincents Hosp 1991; Radiology, Leicester Univ Hosp 1996; **Fellow:** Body Imaging, Meml Sloan-Kettering Cancer Ctr 1997; **Fac Appt:** Prof Rad, UCSF

Federle, Michael P MD [DR] - **Spec Exp:** Abdominal Imaging; Gastrointestinal Imaging; **Hospital:** Stanford Univ Hosp & Clinics; **Address:** Stanford Diagnostic Radiology, 300 Pasteur Drive, SO92, MC 5105, Stanford, CA 94305; **Phone:** 650-721-6411; **Board Cert:** Diagnostic Radiology 1978; **Med School:** Georgetown Univ 1974; **Resid:** Diagnostic Radiology, Univ Cincinnati Hosp 1978; **Fellow:** Body Imaging, UCSF Med Ctr 1979; **Fac Appt:** Prof Rad, Stanford Univ

Feig, Stephen A MD [DR] - **Spec Exp:** Breast Imaging; Breast Cancer; **Hospital:** UC Irvine Med Ctr; **Address:** UCI Medical Ctr, 101 City Drive South Route 140, Orange, CA 92868-3298; **Phone:** 714-456-6905; **Board Cert:** Diagnostic Radiology 1972; **Med School:** NYU Sch Med 1967; **Resid:** Radiology, Bronx Muni Hosp-Einstein 1971; **Fac Appt:** Prof Rad, UC Irvine

Filly, Roy A MD [DR] - **Spec Exp:** Obstetric Ultrasound; **Hospital:** UCSF Med Ctr; **Address:** UCSF Med Ctr, Dept Diagnostic Radiology, 505 Parnassus Ave, Box 0628, San Francisco, CA 94143-0628; **Phone:** 415-353-1628; **Board Cert:** Diagnostic Radiology 1974; **Med School:** Ohio State Univ 1970; **Resid:** Diagnostic Radiology, Stanford Univ Med Ctr 1974; **Fac Appt:** Prof Rad, UCSF

Gilsanz, Vicente MD [DR] - **Spec Exp:** Pediatric Radiology; Bone Disorders-Metabolic; **Hospital:** Chldns Hosp - Los Angeles; **Address:** Chdns Hosp LA, 4650 Sunset Blvd, MS 81, Los Angeles, CA 90027; **Phone:** 323-361-4571; **Board Cert:** Internal Medicine 1973; Diagnostic Radiology 1976; Pediatric Radiology 2004; **Med School:** Spain 1969; **Resid:** Internal Medicine, Mayo Clin 1973; Diagnostic Radiology, Mt Sinai Hosp 1976; **Fellow:** Pediatric Radiology, Chldns Hosp 1978; **Fac Appt:** Prof Rad, USC Sch Med

Grant, Edward G MD [DR] - **Spec Exp:** Ultrasound; Thyroid Ultrasound; Liver & Biliary Imaging; Abdominal Imaging; **Hospital:** Keck Med Ctr of USC (page 62), USC Norris Cancer Hosp (page 62); **Address:** UCLA Med Ctr Dept Rad, Los Angeles, CA 90024-1301; **Phone:** 323-442-7450; **Board Cert:** Diagnostic Radiology 1978; **Med School:** Temple Univ 1974; **Resid:** Diagnostic Radiology, Georgetown Univ Med Ctr 1978; **Fellow:** Ultrasound, Herlev Hosp 1979; **Fac Appt:** Prof Rad, USC-Keck School of Medicine

Lehman, Constance D MD/PhD [DR] - **Spec Exp:** Breast Imaging; Breast Cancer; MRI-Breast; Mammography; **Hospital:** Univ Wash Med Ctr; **Address:** Seattle Cancer Care Alliance, 825 Eastlake Ave E, MS G2600, Seattle, WA 98109-1023; **Phone:** 206-288-2046; **Board Cert:** Diagnostic Radiology 1995; **Med School:** Yale Univ 1990; **Resid:** Diagnostic Radiology, Univ Washington Med Ctr 1995; **Fellow:** Breast Imaging, Univ Washington Med Ctr 1996; **Fac Appt:** Prof Rad, Univ Wash

Parikh, Jay Rajendra MD [DR] - **Spec Exp:** Breast Imaging; Breast Cancer; Mammography; **Hospital:** Swedish Med Ctr-First Hill-Seattle; **Address:** The Swedish Breast Imaging Ctr, 1101 Madison St, Ste 310, MS 98104, Seattle, WA 98104; **Phone:** 206-215-3939; **Board Cert:** Diagnostic Radiology 1996; **Med School:** Univ Ottawa 1990; **Resid:** Diagnostic Radiology, Queens Univ Faculty Hlth Scics 1996; **Fellow:** Breast Imaging, Univ of IL Med Ctr 1997; **Fac Appt:** Asst Clin Prof Rad, Univ Wash

Pathria, Mini N MD [DR] - **Spec Exp:** Musculoskeletal Imaging; **Hospital:** UCSD Med Ctr; **Address:** UCSD Med Ctr, Dept Radiology, 200 W Arbor Drive, MC 8756, San Diego, CA 92103-8756; **Phone:** 619-543-6222; **Board Cert:** Diagnostic Radiology 1986; **Med School:** McMaster Univ 1982; **Resid:** Diagnostic Radiology, Mcmaster Univ 1983; **Fellow:** Skeletal Radiology, UCSD Med Ctr 1987; **Fac Appt:** Clin Prof Rad, UCSD

Diagnostic Radiology

Shaw, Dennis MD [DR] - **Spec Exp:** Pediatric Neuroradiology; Interventional Radiology; **Hospital:** Seattle Chldns Hosp; **Address:** 4800 Sand Point Way NE, R-5417 Radiology, Seattle, WA 98105; **Phone:** 206-987-2133; **Board Cert:** Diagnostic Radiology 1990; Pediatric Radiology 2006; **Med School:** Univ Wash 1983; **Resid:** Neurological Surgery, Univ Washington Med Ctr 1985; Diagnostic Radiology, Univ Washington Med Ctr 1990; **Fellow:** Pediatric Radiology, Chldn's Hosp & Med Ctr 1991; **Fac Appt:** Prof Rad, Univ Wash

Thurmond, Amy S MD [DR] - **Spec Exp:** Women's Imaging; Gynecologic Imaging; **Hospital:** OR Hlth & Sci Univ; **Address:** Siker Medical Imaging, 1800 NE 2nd Ave, Portland, OR 97212; **Phone:** 503-595-3967; **Board Cert:** Diagnostic Radiology 1987; **Med School:** UCLA 1982; **Resid:** Cardiovascular Disease, St Vincent Hosp Med Ctr 1984; Diagnostic Radiology, Oreg Hlth Scis Univ 1987; **Fellow:** Interventional Radiology, Oreg Hlth Scis Univ 1988; **Fac Appt:** Assoc Prof Rad, Oregon Hlth & Sci Univ

Wood, Beverly MD/PhD [DR] - **Spec Exp:** Pediatric Radiology; **Hospital:** LAC & USC Med Ctr, Loma Linda Chldns Hosp; **Address:** Loma Linda Univ Chldns Hosp, Div Pediatric Radiology, 11234 Anderson St, rm 2835, Loma Linda, CA 92354; **Phone:** 909-558-8205; **Board Cert:** Diagnostic Radiology 1972; Pediatric Radiology 2003; **Med School:** Univ Rochester 1965; **Resid:** Diagnostic Radiology, Strong Meml Hosp 1971; **Fellow:** Pediatric Radiology, Strong Meml Hosp 1972; **Fac Appt:** Prof Rad, USC Sch Med

NEURORADIOLOGY

New England

Curtin, Hugh D MD [NRad] - **Spec Exp:** Head & Neck Radiology; **Hospital:** Mass Eye & Ear Infirmary; **Address:** Mass Eye & Ear Infirmary, Dept Radiology, 243 Charles St, Boston, MA 02114; **Phone:** 617-573-3563 x4; **Board Cert:** Diagnostic Radiology 1976; Neuroradiology 2011; **Med School:** SUNY Upstate Med Univ 1972; **Resid:** Diagnostic Radiology, Presby Univ Hosp 1976; **Fellow:** Neuroradiology, Foundation Rothschild; **Fac Appt:** Prof Rad, Harvard Med Sch

Hackney, David B MD [NRad] - **Hospital:** Beth Israel Deaconess Med Ctr - Boston; **Address:** BIDMC, Dept Radiology, 330 Brookline Ave, Boston, MA 02215; **Phone:** 617-754-2009; **Board Cert:** Diagnostic Radiology 1984; Neuroradiology 2005; **Med School:** Cornell Univ 1980; **Resid:** Diagnostic Radiology, UCSD Med Ctr 1983; **Fellow:** Neurological Radiology, Mass Genl Hosp 1985; **Fac Appt:** Prof Rad, Harvard Med Sch

Hirsch, Joshua A MD [NRad] - **Spec Exp:** Interventional Neuroradiology; Endovascular Surgery; Minimally Invasive Spinal Surgery; Osteoporosis Spine-Vertebroplasty; **Hospital:** Mass Genl Hosp; **Address:** Mass General Hosp, Interventional Neuroradiology GRB-241, 55 Fruit St, Boston, MA 02114; **Phone:** 617-726-1767; **Board Cert:** Diagnostic Radiology 1996; **Med School:** Univ Pennsylvania 1991; **Resid:** Diagnostic Radiology, Hosp Univ Penn 1996; **Fellow:** Neuroradiology, Hosp Univ Penn 1995; Interventional Neuroradiology, Lahey Clinic 1998; **Fac Appt:** Asst Prof Rad, Harvard Med Sch

Norbash, Alexander M MD [NRad] - **Spec Exp:** Interventional Neuroradiology; Aneurysm-Cerebral; Osteoporosis Spine-Kyphoplasty; Arteriovenous Malformations; **Hospital:** Boston Med Ctr; **Address:** BMC, Dept Radiology, 820 Harrison Ave, Boston, MA 02118; **Phone:** 617-638-6610; **Board Cert:** Diagnostic Radiology 1991; Neuroradiology 2004; **Med School:** Univ MO-Kansas City 1986; **Resid:** Diagnostic Radiology, St Francis Hosp 1990; Diagnostic Radiology, Presby Univ Hosp 1991; **Fellow:** Neurological Radiology, Stanford Univ Hosp 1993; Interventional Radiology, Stanford Univ Hosp 1994; **Fac Appt:** Prof Rad, Boston Univ

Orbach, Darren MD/PhD [NRad] - **Spec Exp:** Stroke in Children; Vascular Malformations; Interventional Neuroradiology; **Hospital:** Children's Hospital - Boston; **Address:** Boston Children's Hospital, Interventional Radiology Dept, 300 Longwood Ave, Boston, MA 02115; **Phone:** 617-355-6579; **Board Cert:** Diagnostic Radiology 2004; Neurology 2004; Neuroradiology 2005; **Med School:** Cornell Univ 1998; **Resid:** Diagnostic Radiology, NYU Med Ctr 2002; Neurology, NYU Med Ctr 2004; **Fellow:** Neuroradiology, NYU Med Ctr 2005; **Fac Appt:** Asst Prof Rad, Harvard Med Sch

Sze, Gordon K MD [NRad] - **Spec Exp:** Brain Tumors; Spinal Cord Tumors; Head & Neck Cancer; MRI; **Hospital:** Yale-New Haven Hosp, Yale Med Group; **Address:** Yale-New Haven Hospital, Yale Diagnostic Radiology, 20 York St, New Haven, CT 06510; **Phone:** 203-785-3667; **Board Cert:** Diagnostic Radiology 1985; Neuroradiology 2008; **Med School:** Harvard Med Sch 1981; **Resid:** Diagnostic Radiology, UCSF Med Ctr 1985; **Fellow:** Neuroradiology, UCSF Med Ctr 1986; **Fac Appt:** Prof Rad, Yale Univ

Mid Atlantic

Berenstein, Alejandro MD [NRad] - **Spec Exp:** Interventional Neuroradiology; Aneurysm-Cerebral; Endovascular Surgery; Vascular Malformations; **Hospital:** St. Luke's - Roosevelt Hosp Ctr - Roosevelt Div (page 56); **Address:** Center for Endovascular Surgery, 1000 10th Ave, 10th Fl, Ste 10G - INN, New York, NY 10019; **Phone:** 212-636-3400; **Board Cert:** Diagnostic Radiology 1976; **Med School:** Mexico 1970; **Resid:** Diagnostic Radiology, Mt Sinai Med Ctr 1976; **Fellow:** Neuroradiology, NYU Med Ctr 1978; **Fac Appt:** Prof Rad, Albert Einstein Coll Med

Drayer, Burton P MD [NRad] - **Spec Exp:** Parkinson's Disease/Aging Brain; Alzheimer's Disease; Vascular Neurology; MRI & CT of Brain & Spine; **Hospital:** Mount Sinai Med Ctr (page 64); **Address:** 1 Gustave Levy Pl, Box 1234, New York, NY 10029; **Phone:** 212-241-6403; **Board Cert:** Neurology 1976; Diagnostic Radiology 1978; Neuroradiology 2006; **Med School:** Ros Franklin Univ/Chicago Med Sch 1971; **Resid:** Neurology, Univ Vt Med Ctr 1975; Diagnostic Radiology, Univ Pitt Hlth Ctr 1978; **Fellow:** Neuroradiology, Univ Pitt Hlth Ctr 1978; **Fac Appt:** Prof Rad, Mount Sinai Sch Med

Faro, Scott H MD [NRad] - **Spec Exp:** Brain Mapping; Brain Tumors; Epilepsy; Spinal Cord Injury; **Hospital:** Temple Univ Hosp; **Address:** Temple Univ Div Neuroradiology, 3401 N Broad St, Philadelphia, PA 19140; **Phone:** 215-707-5003; **Board Cert:** Diagnostic Radiology 1993; Neuroradiology 2006; **Med School:** UMDNJ-Rutgers Med Sch 1986; **Resid:** Diagnostic Radiology, Med Ctr Delaware 1991; **Fellow:** Neuroradiology, Jefferson Med Ctr 1992; Pediatric Neuroradiology, Childrens Hosp 1993; **Fac Appt:** Prof Rad, Temple Univ

Hurst, Robert W MD [NRad] - **Spec Exp:** Interventional Neuroradiology; Aneurysm; Carotid Artery Stent Placement; Intracranial Angioplasty & Stent; **Hospital:** Hosp Univ Penn - UPHS (page 72); **Address:** HUP Radiology/Neuroradiology, 3400 Spruce St, 2 Dulles, Philadelphia, PA 19104; **Phone:** 215-662-3064; **Board Cert:** Neurology 1986; Diagnostic Radiology 1989; Neuroradiology 2005; Vascular Neurology 2009; **Med School:** Univ Tex, Houston 1981; **Resid:** Neurology, Univ Virginia Hosp 1985; Diagnostic Radiology, Univ Virginia Hosp 1989; **Fellow:** Neurological Radiology, Hosp Univ Penn 1990; Interventional Radiology, NYU Med Ctr 1991; **Fac Appt:** Prof Rad, Univ Pennsylvania

Khandji, Alexander G MD [NRad] - **Spec Exp:** Pituitary Disorders; Spine Imaging & Intervention; MRI; Headache; **Hospital:** NY-Presby/Columbia Univ Med Ctr, NY (page 66); **Address:** 177 Ft Washington Ave, Ste 4-156, New York, NY 10032-3173; **Phone:** 212-305-7669; **Board Cert:** Diagnostic Radiology 1985; Neuroradiology 2006; **Med School:** SUNY Downstate 1980; **Resid:** Surgery, MS Hershey Med Ctr 1982; Diagnostic Radiology, Columbia-Presby Med Ctr 1985; **Fellow:** Neuroradiology, Columbia-Presby Med Ctr 1987; **Fac Appt:** Prof Rad, Columbia P&S

Neuroradiology

Lis, Eric MD [NRad] - **Spec Exp:** Spinal Cord Tumors; Brain Tumors; **Hospital:** Meml Sloan-Kettering Cancer Ctr; **Address:** 1275 York Ave, Ste MRI1158, New York, NY 10065; **Phone:** 212-639-8330; **Board Cert:** Diagnostic Radiology 1995; Neuroradiology 2008; **Med School:** UMDNJ-NJ Med Sch, Newark 1990; **Resid:** Internal Medicine, Mountainside Hosp 1991; Diagnostic Radiology, UMDNJ-RW Johnson Med Sch 1995; **Fellow:** Neuroradiology, NY-Presby-Weill Cornell Med Ctr 1997

Loevner, Laurie A MD [NRad] - **Spec Exp:** Head & Neck Cancer; Thyroid Cancer; Brain Tumor Imaging; Spinal Tumor Imaging; **Hospital:** Hosp Univ Penn - UPHS (page 72); **Address:** Penn Radiology, 3400 Spruce St, Fl 2 Dulles, Philadelphia, PA 19104; **Phone:** 215-662-3020; **Board Cert:** Diagnostic Radiology 1993; Neuroradiology 2006; **Med School:** Univ Pennsylvania 1988; **Resid:** Diagnostic Radiology, Univ Michigan Med Ctr 1993; **Fellow:** Neuroradiology, Hosp Univ Penn 1995; **Fac Appt:** Prof Rad, Univ Pennsylvania

Pile-Spellman, John MD [NRad] - **Spec Exp:** Interventional Neuroradiology; Cerebrovascular Disease; Aneurysm; Arteriovenous Malformations; **Hospital:** Winthrop Univ Hosp; **Address:** Neurological Surgery, 1991 Marcus Ave, Ste 108, Lake Success, NY 11042; **Phone:** 516-442-2250; **Board Cert:** Diagnostic Radiology 1984; **Med School:** Tufts Univ 1978; **Resid:** Neurological Surgery, New England Med Ctr 1981; Neurological Radiology, Mass Genl Hosp 1984; **Fellow:** Interventional Neuroradiology, NYU Med Ctr 1986; **Fac Appt:** Prof Rad, Columbia P&S

Tenner, Michael MD [NRad] - **Spec Exp:** Stroke; Brain & Spinal Tumors; Carotid Artery Stent Placement; **Hospital:** Westchester Med Ctr; **Address:** NY Med Coll, Dept Radiology, 100 Woods Rd, Valhalla, NY 10595; **Phone:** 914-493-6692; **Board Cert:** Diagnostic Radiology 1967; Neuroradiology 2007; **Med School:** Univ MD Sch Med 1960; **Resid:** Diagnostic Radiology, Univ Maryland Hosp 1962; Diagnostic Radiology, Univ Maryland Hosp 1966; **Fellow:** Neuroradiology, Neurological Inst-Columbia Presby 1968; **Fac Appt:** Prof Rad, NY Med Coll

Vezina, L Gilbert MD [NRad] - **Spec Exp:** Pediatric Neuroradiology; Brain Tumors; Neurofibromatosis; **Hospital:** Chldns Natl Med Ctr; **Address:** Chldns Natl Med Ctr, Dept Radiology, 111 Michigan Ave NW, Washington, DC 20010-2970; **Phone:** 202-476-3651; **Board Cert:** Diagnostic Radiology 1987; Neuroradiology 2008; **Med School:** McGill Univ 1983; **Resid:** Diagnostic Radiology, Mass Genl Hosp 1987; **Fellow:** Neurological Radiology, Mass Genl Hosp 1989; Pediatric Neuroradiology, Chldns Natl Med Ctr 1991; **Fac Appt:** Prof, Geo Wash Univ

Yousem, David M MD [NRad] - **Hospital:** Johns Hopkins Hosp (page 61); **Address:** Johns Hopkins Hosp, Div Neuroradiology, 600 N Wolfe St Phipps Bldg - rm B-100, Baltimore, MD 21287; **Phone:** 410-955-2353; **Board Cert:** Diagnostic Radiology 1987; Neuroradiology 2005; **Med School:** Univ Mich Med Sch 1983; **Resid:** Diagnostic Radiology, Johns Hopkins Hosp 1987; **Fellow:** Neuroradiology, Hosp Univ Penn 1990; **Fac Appt:** Prof Rad, Johns Hopkins Univ

Zimmerman, Robert A MD [NRad] - **Spec Exp:** Pediatric Neuroradiology; **Hospital:** Chldns Hosp of Philadelphia; **Address:** Childrens Hosp Philadelphia, Radiology, 324 S 34th St Wood Bldg - rm 2115, Philadelphia, PA 19104; **Phone:** 215-590-2569; **Board Cert:** Diagnostic Radiology 1970; Neuroradiology 2005; **Med School:** Georgetown Univ 1964; **Resid:** Diagnostic Radiology, Hosp Univ Penn 1969; **Fac Appt:** Prof Rad, Univ Pennsylvania

Zinreich, S James MD [NRad] - **Spec Exp:** Head & Neck Radiology; **Hospital:** Johns Hopkins Hosp (page 61); **Address:** Johns Hopkins Hosp, 600 N Wolfe St Phipps Bldg - rm B-100, Baltimore, MD 21287; **Phone:** 410-614-3020; **Board Cert:** Diagnostic Radiology 1982; Neuroradiology 2006; **Med School:** Belgium 1976; **Resid:** Diagnostic Radiology, Sinai Hosp; **Fac Appt:** Prof Oto, Johns Hopkins Univ

Southeast

Burdette, Jonathan Hill MD [NRad] - **Spec Exp:** Brain Injury; MRI; **Hospital:** Wake Forest Baptist Med Ctr; **Address:** Medical Center Blvd, Winston-Salem, NC 27157; **Phone:** 336-716-1286; **Board Cert:** Diagnostic Radiology 1997; Neuroradiology 2011; **Med School:** Univ Tenn Coll Med 1993; **Resid:** Diagnostic Radiology, Univ Mich Affil Hosps 1997; **Fellow:** Neurological Radiology, Wake Forest Baptist Med Ctr 1999; **Fac Appt:** Prof Rad

Dion, Jacques E MD [NRad] - **Spec Exp:** Interventional Neuroradiology; Aneurysm-Cerebral; Intracranial Angioplasty & Stent; **Hospital:** Emory Univ Hosp; **Address:** Emory Univ-Interventional Radiology, 1364 Clifton Rd NE, rm AG21, Atlanta, GA 30322; **Phone:** 404-712-4991; **Board Cert:** Diagnostic Radiology 1982; Neuroradiology 2009; **Med School:** Univ Ottawa 1978; **Resid:** Diagnostic Radiology, Harbor-UCLA Med Ctr 1981; Diagnostic Radiology, Notre Dame Hosp 1983; **Fellow:** Neuroradiology, Univ Hosp 1985; **Fac Appt:** Prof Rad, Emory Univ

Jensen, Mary E MD [NRad] - **Spec Exp:** Interventional Neuroradiology; Osteoporosis Spine-Vertebroplasty; Aneurysm-Cerebral; **Hospital:** Univ of Virginia Health Sys; **Address:** Univ of Virginia Med Ctr, Dept Radiology, Box 800170, Charlottsville, VA 22908; **Phone:** 434-924-9719; **Board Cert:** Diagnostic Radiology 1987; **Med School:** Med Coll VA 1982; **Resid:** Diagnostic Radiology, Univ Virginia Med Ctr 1991; **Fellow:** Interventional Neuroradiology, UCLA Med Ctr 1992; **Fac Appt:** Prof Rad, Univ VA Sch Med

Johnson, Annette MD [NRad] - **Spec Exp:** Brain Tumors; MRI; **Hospital:** Wake Forest Baptist Med Ctr; **Address:** Wake Forest Baptist Hlth, Dept Radiology, One Medical Ctr Blvd, Winston-Salem, NC 27157; **Phone:** 336-716-2872; **Board Cert:** Diagnostic Radiology 1996; Neuroradiology 2009; **Med School:** Med Coll VA 1992; **Resid:** Diagnostic Radiology, Geisinger Med Ctr 1996; **Fellow:** Diagnostic Radiology, Mallinckrodt Inst Radiology/Washingtno Univ 1998; **Fac Appt:** Assoc Prof Rad, Wake Forest Univ

Joseph, Gregory J MD [NRad] - **Spec Exp:** Stroke; Aneurysm-Cerebral; Intracranial Angioplasty & Stent; **Hospital:** Presby Hosp - Charlotte; **Address:** Presbyterian Hosp, Dept Radiology, 200 Hawthorne Ln, Charlotte, NC 28204; **Phone:** 704-384-9654; **Board Cert:** Diagnostic Radiology 1989; Neuroradiology 2010; **Med School:** Georgetown Univ 1984; **Resid:** Diagnostic Radiology, Georgetown Univ Hosp 1989; Vascular & Interventional Radiology, Emory Univ Hosp 1990; **Fellow:** Neuroradiology, Emory Univ Hosp 1991

Maldjian, Joseph MD [NRad] - **Spec Exp:** Brain Tumors; Stroke; **Hospital:** Wake Forest Baptist Med Ctr; **Address:** Wake Forest Univ Med Ctr, Dept Radiology, Medical Center Blvd MRI Bldg Fl 3, Winston-Salem, NC 27157; **Phone:** 336-716-7849; **Board Cert:** Diagnostic Radiology 1993; Neuroradiology 2005; **Med School:** UMDNJ-NJ Med Sch, Newark 1988; **Resid:** Diagnostic Radiology, Mount Sinai Med Ctr 1993; **Fellow:** Neuroradiology, Hosp U Penn 1995

Morris, P Pearse MD [NRad] - **Spec Exp:** Interventional Neuroradiology; Endovascular Neurosurgery; Aneurysm-Cerebral; Arteriovenous Malformations; **Hospital:** Wake Forest Baptist Med Ctr; **Address:** Medical Ctr Blvd, MRI Bldg Fl 3, Winston-Salem, NC 27157; **Phone:** 336-716-7849; **Board Cert:** Psychiatry 1989; Diagnostic Radiology 1994; Neuroradiology 2008; **Med School:** Ireland 1983; **Resid:** Psychiatry, Johns Hopkins Hosp 1987; Diagnostic Radiology, Mass Genl Hosp 1994; **Fellow:** Geriatric Psychiatry, Cornell Univ 1988; Neuroradiology, Mass Genl Hosp 1995; **Fac Appt:** Prof Rad, Wake Forest Univ

Neuroradiology

Murtagh, F Reed MD [NRad] - **Spec Exp:** Neuro-Oncology; Brain Tumor Imaging; Spinal Tumor Imaging; Memory Disorders; **Hospital:** H Lee Moffitt Cancer Ctr & Research Inst (page 59); **Address:** Univ Diagnostic Institute-USF, 3301 Alumni Drive, Tampa, FL 33612; **Phone:** 813-972-3351; **Board Cert:** Diagnostic Radiology 1978; Neuroradiology 2004; **Med School:** Temple Univ 1971; **Resid:** Diagnostic Radiology, Jackson Meml Hosp 1978; **Fellow:** Neurological Radiology, Univ Miami 1979; **Fac Appt:** Prof Rad, Univ S Fla Coll Med

Provenzale, James M MD [NRad] - **Spec Exp:** Brain Tumor Imaging; Multiple Sclerosis Imaging; Brain Imaging-Pediatric; **Hospital:** Duke Univ Hosp, Durham VA Med Ctr; **Address:** Duke University Medical Ctr, Dept Radiology, Box 3808, Durham, NC 27710; **Phone:** 919-684-7218; **Board Cert:** Neurology 1988; Diagnostic Radiology 1991; **Med School:** Albany Med Coll 1983; **Resid:** Neurology, NC Memorial Hosp 1987; Diagnostic Radiology, Mass Genl Hosp 1991; **Fellow:** Neuroradiology, Mass Genl Hosp 1992; **Fac Appt:** Prof Rad, Duke Univ

Quencer, Robert MD [NRad] - **Spec Exp:** Spinal Cord Injury; **Hospital:** Univ of Miami Hosp & Clins/Sylvester Comp Canc Ctr; **Address:** Univ Miami, Dept Radiology, 1150 NW 14th St, Ste 511, MC M828, Miami, FL 33136-2116; **Phone:** 305-243-4701; **Board Cert:** Diagnostic Radiology 1972; Neuroradiology 2006; **Med School:** SUNY Upstate Med Univ 1967; **Resid:** Diagnostic Radiology, Columbia-Presbyterian Med Ctr 1971; **Fellow:** Neuroradiology, Neurological Inst 1972; **Fac Appt:** Prof, Univ Miami Sch Med

Midwest

Ball Jr, William S MD [NRad] - **Spec Exp:** Pediatric Neuroradiology; **Hospital:** Cincinnati Chldns Hosp Med Ctr; **Address:** Cincinnati Chldns Hosp, Dept Neuroradiology, 3333 Burnet Ave, ML 5031, Cincinnati, OH 45229-3039; **Phone:** 513-636-4251; **Board Cert:** Diagnostic Radiology 1982; Pediatrics 1982; Neuroradiology 2011; **Med School:** Tulane Univ 1974; **Resid:** Pediatrics, Oschner Fdn Hosp 1977; Diagnostic Radiology, Univ New Mexico 1978; **Fellow:** Pediatric Radiology, Chldns Hosp Med Ctr 1981; Neuroradiology, Univ New Mexico Med Ctr 1979; **Fac Appt:** Prof, Univ Cincinnati

Cross III, DeWitte T MD [NRad] - **Spec Exp:** Interventional Neuroradiology; Aneurysm-Cerebral; Stroke; **Hospital:** Barnes-Jewish Hosp, St. Louis Chldns Hosp; **Address:** Wash Univ, Dept Radiology, 510 S Kingshighway Blvd, Box 8131, St Louis, MO 63110-1016; **Phone:** 314-362-5949; **Board Cert:** Diagnostic Radiology 1985; Neuroradiology 2006; **Med School:** Univ Alabama 1980; **Resid:** Diagnostic Radiology, Naval Hosp 1985; **Fellow:** Neuroradiology, NY Med Coll 1988; Neuroradiology, Columbia Univ 1989; **Fac Appt:** Prof Rad, Washington Univ, St Louis

Grobelny, Thomas MD [NRad] - **Spec Exp:** Interventional Neuroradiology; Aneurysm-Cerebral; Stroke; Arteriovenous Malformations; **Hospital:** Evanston/North Shore Univ Hlth Sys, Adv Christ Med Ctr; **Address:** 9669 Kenton Ave, Ste 500, Skokie, IL 60076; **Phone:** 847-933-3700; **Board Cert:** Diagnostic Radiology 1996; Neuroradiology 2010; **Med School:** Poland 1986; **Resid:** Diagnostic Radiology, Harlem Hospital 1995; **Fellow:** Neurocritical Care, Thos Jefferson Univ Hosp 1998; Interventional Neuroradiology, UCLA Med Ctr 1989

Haughton III, Victor M MD [NRad] - **Spec Exp:** Spinal Imaging; **Hospital:** Univ WI Hosp & Clins; **Address:** Univ WI Hosps & Clins, Dept Radiology, 600 Highland Ave, MC 3252, Madison, WI 53792; **Phone:** 608-263-9179; **Board Cert:** Diagnostic Radiology 1974; **Med School:** Yale Univ 1967; **Resid:** Diagnostic Radiology, Peter Bent Brigham Hosp 1973; **Fellow:** Neurological Radiology, Peter Bent Brigham Hosp 1974; **Fac Appt:** Prof Rad, Univ Wisc

Kallmes, David F MD [NRad] - **Spec Exp:** Aneurysm-Cerebral; Stroke; Osteoporosis Spine-Vertebroplasty; **Hospital:** Mayo Med Ctr & Clin - Rochester; **Address:** Mayo Clinic, 200 First St SW, OL 1-115, Rochester, MN 55905; **Phone:** 507-266-3350; **Board Cert:** Diagnostic Radiology 1994; Neuroradiology 2009; **Med School:** Univ Mass Sch Med 1989; **Resid:** Diagnostic Radiology, Duke Univ Med Ctr 1993; **Fellow:** Neuroradiology, Univ Virginia Med Ctr 1995; **Fac Appt:** Assoc Prof Rad, Mayo Med Sch

Koeller, Kelly K MD [NRad] - **Spec Exp:** Brain Tumor Imaging; Head & Neck Tumors Imaging; Spinal Tumor Imaging; **Hospital:** Mayo Med Ctr & Clin - Rochester, St. Mary's Hosp - Rochester MN (Mayo); **Address:** Mayo Clinic, 200 First St SW Charlton Bldg - rm 2-290, Rochester, MN 55905; **Phone:** 507-266-3412; **Board Cert:** Diagnostic Radiology 1990; Neuroradiology 2004; **Med School:** Univ Tenn Coll Med 1982; **Resid:** Diagnostic Radiology, Naval Hosp 1990; **Fellow:** Neuro-radiology, UCSF Med Ctr 1992; **Fac Appt:** Assoc Prof Rad, Mayo Med Sch

Masaryk, Thomas MD [NRad] - **Spec Exp:** Cerebrovascular Disease; Aneurysm-Cerebral; Vascular Lesions of the CNS; Carotid Artery Stent Placement; **Hospital:** Cleveland Clin (page 55); **Address:** Cleveland Clinic, Dept Radiology, 9500 Euclid Ave, MC P34, Cleveland, OH 44195; **Phone:** 216-444-6653; **Board Cert:** Diagnostic Radiology 1985; Neuroradiology 2005; **Med School:** Med Coll OH 1981; **Resid:** Diagnostic Radiology, Cleveland Clinic 1984; **Fellow:** Neuro-logical Radiology, Cleveland Clinic 1985

Modic, Michael MD [NRad] - **Spec Exp:** MRI; Spinal Imaging; **Hospital:** Cleveland Clin (page 55); **Address:** Cleveland Clinic, Dept Radiology, 9500 Euclid Ave, MC T13, Cleveland, OH 44195; **Phone:** 216-444-9308; **Board Cert:** Diagnostic Radiology 1979; Neuroradiology 2003; **Med School:** Case West Res Univ 1975; **Resid:** Diagnostic Radiology, Cleveland Clin Fdn 1978; **Fellow:** Neuroradiology, Cleveland Clin Fdn 1979; **Fac Appt:** Prof Rad, Cleveland Cl Coll Med/Case West Res

Moran, Christopher J MD [NRad] - **Spec Exp:** Aneurysm-Cerebral; Cerebrovascular Dis-ease/Stroke; Carotid Artery Stent Placement; Interventional Neuroradiology; **Hospital:** Barnes-Jewish Hosp; **Address:** Mallinckrodt Inst Radiology, Wash Univ Sch Med, Campus Box 8131, 510 S King-shighway Blvd, St Louis, MO 63110; **Phone:** 314-362-5949; **Board Cert:** Diagnostic Radiology 1978; Neuroradiology 2004; **Med School:** St Louis Univ 1974; **Resid:** Diagnostic Radiology, Mallinckrodt Inst Rad/Wash U 1978; **Fellow:** Neuroradiology, Mallinckrodt Inst Rad/Wash U 1979; **Fac Appt:** Prof Rad, Washington Univ, St Louis

Mukherji, Suresh K MD [NRad] - **Spec Exp:** Head & Neck Radiology; Head & Neck Tumors Imaging; **Hospital:** Univ of Michigan Hosp; **Address:** Univ of Michigan-Dept Radiology, 1500 E Med Ctr Drive Fl UH-B2 - rm A209B, Ann Arbor, MI 48109-0030; **Phone:** 734-936-8865; **Board Cert:** Diagnostic Radiology 1992; Neuroradiology 2006; **Med School:** Georgetown Univ 1987; **Resid:** Diagnostic Radiology, Brigham & Women's Hosp 1992; **Fellow:** Neuroradiology, Univ Florida 1994; **Fac Appt:** Prof Rad, Univ Mich Med Sch

Rowley, Howard A MD [NRad] - **Spec Exp:** Epilepsy; Cerebrovascular Disease/Stroke; **Hospital:** Univ WI Hosp & Clins; **Address:** Dept Neuroradiology, 600 Highland Ave, MC 3252, Madison, WI 53792; **Phone:** 608-263-9179; **Board Cert:** Neurology 1991; Diagnostic Radiology 1993; Neuroradiology 2008; **Med School:** Washington Univ, St Louis 1985; **Resid:** Neurology, UCSF Med Ctr 1989; Diagnostic Radiology, UCSF Med Ctr 1991; **Fellow:** Neurological Radiology, UCSF Med Ctr 1991; **Fac Appt:** Prof Rad, Univ Wisc

Thulborn, Keith R MD/PhD [NRad] - **Spec Exp:** MRI; **Hospital:** Univ of IL Med Ctr at Chicago; **Address:** Univ Illinois Med Ctr, 1801 W Taylor St, Ste 1A, Chicago, IL 60612; **Phone:** 312-413-4900; **Board Cert:** Diagnostic Radiology 1989; **Med School:** Washington Univ, St Louis 1984; **Resid:** Diagnostic Radiology, Mass Genl Hosp 1989; **Fellow:** Neuroradiology, Mass Genl Hosp 1991; **Fac Appt:** Prof Rad, Univ IL Coll Med

Neuroradiology

Great Plains and Mountains

Frei, Donald MD [NRad] - **Spec Exp:** Interventional Neuroradiology; Aneurysm-Cerebral; Cerebrovascular Disease/Stroke; **Hospital:** Swedish Med Ctr - Denver, Exempla Lutheran Med Ctr; **Address:** 8200 E Belleview Ave, Ste 600E, Englewood, CO 80112; **Phone:** 720-493-3406; **Board Cert:** Diagnostic Radiology 1994; Neuroradiology 2008; **Med School:** Univ Cincinnati 1989; **Resid:** Diagnostic Radiology, Tulane Univ Med Ctr 1994; **Fellow:** Neurological Radiology, Mallinckrodt Inst Rad-Barnes Hosp 1996; Interventional Neuroradiology, Mallinckrodt Inst Rad-Barnes Hosp 1996

Osborn, Anne G MD [NRad] - **Spec Exp:** Spinal Imaging; Brain Imaging; Head & Neck Radiology; **Hospital:** Univ Utah Hlth Care; **Address:** Dept Radiology, 30 N 1900 E, rm 1A71, Salt Lake City, UT 84132-2140; **Phone:** 801-581-7553; **Board Cert:** Diagnostic Radiology 1974; Neuroradiology 2004; **Med School:** Stanford Univ 1970; **Resid:** Diagnostic Radiology, Stanford Univ Hosp 1974; **Fellow:** Diagnostic Radiology, Univ Utah Hosp 1977; **Fac Appt:** Prof, Univ Utah

Southwest

Hunter, Jill V MD [NRad] - **Spec Exp:** Pediatric Neuroradiology; Brain Injury-Pediatric; Autism; **Hospital:** Texas Chldns Hosp, St. Luke's Episcopal Hosp-Houston; **Address:** 6621 Fannin St, MC W-1120, Houston, TX 77030; **Phone:** 832-822-5324; **Board Cert:** Diagnostic Radiology 1997; Neuroradiology 2009; **Med School:** England, UK 1975; **Resid:** Diagnostic Radiology, Baylor Affil Hosp 1978; **Fellow:** Neuroradiology, Queen Square Hosp 1992; **Fac Appt:** Assoc Prof Rad, Baylor Coll Med

Mawad, Michel E MD [NRad] - **Spec Exp:** Interventional Neuroradiology; **Hospital:** St. Luke's Episcopal Hosp-Houston; **Address:** 6720 Bertner Ave, Box 4-267, Houston, TX 77030; **Phone:** 713-798-2200; **Board Cert:** Diagnostic Radiology 1980; Neuroradiology 2006; **Med School:** Lebanon 1976; **Resid:** Diagnostic Radiology, St Luke's-Roosevelt Hosp 1979; **Fellow:** Neurological Radiology, Columbia-Presby Med Ctr 1980; **Fac Appt:** Prof N, Baylor Coll Med

West Coast and Pacific

Atlas, Scott W MD [NRad] - **Spec Exp:** MRI-Brain & Spine; Brain Tumors; **Hospital:** Stanford Univ Hosp & Clinics; **Address:** Stanford Univ Med Ctr, Dept Rad, Stanford, CA 94305-5105; **Phone:** 650-723-0340; **Board Cert:** Diagnostic Radiology 1985; Neuroradiology 2005; **Med School:** Univ Chicago-Pritzker Sch Med 1981; **Resid:** Diagnostic Radiology, Northwestern Univ Med Ctr 1985; **Fellow:** Neuroradiology, Hosp Univ Penn 1987; **Fac Appt:** Prof Rad, Stanford Univ

Barkovich, A James MD [NRad] - **Spec Exp:** Pediatric Neuroradiology; MRI; Brain Development Abnormalities; Stroke-Neonatal; **Hospital:** UCSF Med Ctr; **Address:** UCSF Med Ctr, Div Neuroradiology, 505 Parnassus Ave, rm L371, Box 0628, San Francisco, CA 94143-0628; **Phone:** 415-352-2000; **Board Cert:** Diagnostic Radiology 1984; Neuroradiology 2006; **Med School:** Geo Wash Univ 1980; **Resid:** Diagnostic Radiology, Letterman AMC 1984; **Fellow:** Neuroradiology, Walter Reed AMC 1986; **Fac Appt:** Prof Rad, UCSF

Barnes, Patrick D MD [NRad] - **Spec Exp:** Pediatric Neuroradiology; Brain Injury-Pediatric; Brain Development Abnormalities; Fetal Neuroradiology; **Hospital:** Lucile Packard Chldn's Hosp; **Address:** Lucile Packard Chldns Hosp, Pediatric Radiology, 725 Welch Rd, Palo Alto, CA 94304; **Phone:** 650-497-8376; **Board Cert:** Diagnostic Radiology 1977; Neuroradiology 2008; **Med School:** Univ Okla Coll Med 1973; **Resid:** Diagnostic Radiology, Univ Okla Coll Med 1976; **Fellow:** Pediatric Neuroradiology, Chldns Hosp/Harvard Med Sch 1977; **Fac Appt:** Prof, Stanford Univ

Cha, Soonmee MD [NRad] - **Spec Exp:** Brain Tumors; **Hospital:** UCSF Med Ctr; **Address:** 505 Parnassus Ave, rm L-358, San Francisco, CA 94143; **Phone:** 415-353-8913; **Board Cert:** Diagnostic Radiology 1996; Neuroradiology 2008; **Med School:** Georgetown Univ 1991; **Resid:** Diagnostic Radiology, North Shore Univ Hosp 1996; **Fellow:** Neuroradiology, NYU Med Ctr 1998; **Fac Appt:** Assoc Prof Rad, UCSF

Dillon, William P MD [NRad] - **Spec Exp:** Brain Tumors; **Hospital:** UCSF Med Ctr; **Address:** 505 Parnassus Ave, rm L 371, San Francisco, CA 94143-0628; **Phone:** 415-353-1668; **Board Cert:** Diagnostic Radiology 1982; Neuroradiology 2006; **Med School:** UCLA 1978; **Resid:** Diagnostic Radiology, Univ Utah Hosp 1982; **Fellow:** Neuroradiology, UCSF Med Ctr 1983; **Fac Appt:** Prof Rad, UCSF

Hesselink, John R MD [NRad] - **Spec Exp:** MRI & CT of Brain & Spine; Stroke; Brain Tumor Imaging; **Hospital:** UCSD Med Ctr; **Address:** UCSD Med Ctr, Div Neuroradiology, 200 W Arbor Drive, MC 8749, San Diego, CA 92013; **Phone:** 619-543-3856; **Board Cert:** Diagnostic Radiology 1975; Neuroradiology 2005; **Med School:** Univ Wisc 1971; **Resid:** Diagnostic Radiology, Univ Wisconsin-Madison 1975; **Fellow:** Neuroradiology, Mass Genl Hosp- Harvard Univ 1979; **Fac Appt:** Prof Rad, UCSD

Higashida, Randall T MD [NRad] - **Spec Exp:** Aneurysm-Cerebral; Stroke; Intracranial Angioplasty & Stent; **Hospital:** UCSF Med Ctr; **Address:** UCSF Med Ctr, Dept Interven Neurorad, 505 Parnassus Ave, rm L352, San Francisco, CA 94143-0628; **Phone:** 415-353-1863; **Board Cert:** Diagnostic Radiology 1984; **Med School:** Tulane Univ 1980; **Resid:** Diagnostic Radiology, UCLA Med Ctr 1984; **Fellow:** Neuroradiology, UCLA Med Ctr 1985; **Fac Appt:** Clin Prof Rad, UCSF

Jarvik, Jeffrey G MD [NRad] - **Spec Exp:** Spinal Imaging; Brain Imaging; **Hospital:** Harborview Med Ctr, Univ Wash Med Ctr; **Address:** Dept. of Radiology, Box 359728, 325 Ninth Ave, Box 359728, Seattle, WA 98104; **Phone:** 206-744-3561; **Board Cert:** Diagnostic Radiology 1992; Neuroradiology 2005; **Med School:** UCSD 1987; **Resid:** Diagnostic Radiology, Hosp Univ Penn 1992; **Fellow:** Neuroradiology, Hosp Univ Penn 1993; **Fac Appt:** Prof Rad, Univ Wash

Larsen, Donald W MD [NRad] - **Spec Exp:** Interventional Neuroradiology; Stroke; Stroke Prevention; Aneurysm-Cerebral; **Hospital:** Keck Med Ctr of USC (page 62); **Address:** 1500 San Pablo St, Keck Hosp Bldg - Fl 1st - Ste Admin, Los Angeles, CA 90033; **Phone:** 323-442-9906; **Board Cert:** Diagnostic Radiology 1990; **Med School:** Ros Franklin Univ/Chicago Med Sch 1985; **Resid:** Diagnostic Radiology, USC Med Ctr 1990; **Fellow:** Vascular & Interventional Radiology, USC Med Ctr 1991; Neuroradiology, USF Med Ctr 1995; **Fac Appt:** Assoc Prof Rad, USC-Keck School of Medicine

Teitelbaum, George P MD [NRad] - **Spec Exp:** Interventional Neuroradiology; Aneurysm-Cerebral; Carotid Artery Stent Placement; Vascular Lesions of the CNS; **Hospital:** Providence St Joseph Med Ctr; **Address:** 501 S Buena Vista St, Burbank, CA 91505; **Phone:** 818-847-4835; **Board Cert:** Diagnostic Radiology 1984; Neuroradiology 2008; **Med School:** UCSD 1980; **Resid:** Diagnostic Radiology, UC Irvine Med Ctr 1984; Interventional Radiology, George Washington 1985; **Fellow:** Magnetic Resonance Imaging, Huntington Med Research Inst 1988; Interventional Radiology, UCSF Med Ctr 1994; **Fac Appt:** Prof NS, USC-Keck School of Medicine

Vinuela, Fernando MD [NRad] - **Spec Exp:** Stroke; Intracranial Angioplasty & Stent; Aneurysm-Cerebral; **Hospital:** UCLA Ronald Reagan Med Ctr; **Address:** 757 Westwood Plaza, Ste 2129, Los Angeles, CA 90095-7437; **Phone:** 310-267-8765; **Board Cert:** Diagnostic Radiology 1979; **Med School:** Uruguay 1970; **Resid:** Diagnostic Radiology, Westminster Hosp 1975; Diagnostic Radiology, Victoria Hosp 1977; **Fellow:** Neuroradiology, Univ Hosp 1979; **Fac Appt:** Prof Rad, UCLA

VASCULAR & INTERVENTIONAL RADIOLOGY

New England

Aruny, John E MD [VIR] - **Spec Exp:** Thrombolytic Therapy; Dialysis Access; Vascular Disease; Vein Disorders; **Hospital:** Yale-New Haven Hosp, Yale Med Group; **Address:** Yale Univ School of Medicine, 333 Cedar St, New Haven, CT 06520; **Phone:** 203-785-7026; **Board Cert:** Diag Rad with Spec Comp in Nuc Rad 1989; Vascular & Interventional Radiology 2009; **Med School:** Mexico 1983; **Resid:** Diagnostic Radiology, Westch Co Med Ctr 1989; **Fellow:** Interventional Radiology, Brigham & Women's Hosp 1992; **Fac Appt:** Assoc Prof Rad, Yale Univ

Hallisey, Michael J MD [VIR] - **Spec Exp:** Uterine Fibroid Embolization; Liver Cancer/Chemoembolization; Peripheral Vascular Disease; **Hospital:** Hartford Hosp; **Address:** 399 Farmington Ave, Farmington, CT 06032; **Phone:** 860-676-0110; **Board Cert:** Diagnostic Radiology 1991; Vascular & Interventional Radiology 2009; **Med School:** Univ Conn 1986; **Resid:** Diagnostic Radiology, Hospital of St Raphael 1991; **Fac Appt:** Assoc Clin Prof Rad, Univ Conn

Murphy, Timothy P MD [VIR] - **Spec Exp:** Uterine Fibroid Embolization; Aneurysm-Aortic; Hypertension-Renovascular; **Hospital:** Rhode Island Hosp; **Address:** RI Hosp, Diagnostic Imaging, 593 Eddy St Fl 3, Providence, RI 02903-4970; **Phone:** 401-444-5194; **Board Cert:** Diagnostic Radiology 1992; Vascular & Interventional Radiology 2005; **Med School:** Boston Univ 1987; **Resid:** Diagnostic Radiology, Rhode Island Hosp 1992; **Fellow:** Vascular & Interventional Radiology, Rhode Island Hosp 1993; **Fac Appt:** Prof Rad, Brown Univ

White Jr, Robert I MD [VIR] - **Spec Exp:** Uterine Fibroid Embolization; Pelvic Congestion Syndrome; Varicocele Embolization; Hereditary Hemorrhagic Telangiectasia; **Hospital:** Yale-New Haven Hosp, Yale Med Group; **Address:** Yale Univ Sch Med, Vasc & Interventional Rad, PO Box 208042, New Haven, CT 06520-8042; **Phone:** 203-737-5395; **Board Cert:** Diagnostic Radiology 1970; **Med School:** Baylor Coll Med 1963; **Resid:** Internal Medicine, Johns Hopkins Hosp 1967; Diagnostic Radiology, Johns Hopkins Hosp 1969; **Fellow:** Cardiovascular Disease, Johns Hopkins Hosp 1958; Cardiovascular Radiology, Univ Minn Med Ctr 1971; **Fac Appt:** Prof Rad, Yale Univ

Mid Atlantic

Brown, Daniel B MD [VIR] - **Spec Exp:** Liver Cancer/Radioembolization; Radiofrequency Tumor Ablation; **Hospital:** Thomas Jefferson Univ Hosp; **Address:** 132 S 10th St, Main Bldg - Fl 7 - Ste 766, Dept Radiology, Philadelphia, PA 19107; **Phone:** 215-955-6440; **Board Cert:** Diagnostic Radiology 2012; Vascular & Interventional Radiology 2012; **Med School:** Hahnemann Univ 1993; **Resid:** Diagnostic Radiology, Bryn Mawr Hosp 1997; **Fellow:** Vascular & Interventional Radiology, Penn State 1999; **Fac Appt:** Prof Rad, Thomas Jefferson Univ

Brown, Karen T MD [VIR] - **Spec Exp:** Liver Cancer; Radiofrequency Tumor Ablation; **Hospital:** Meml Sloan-Kettering Cancer Ctr; **Address:** 1275 York Ave, New York, NY 10065; **Phone:** 212-639-5882; **Board Cert:** Diagnostic Radiology 1984; Vascular & Interventional Radiology 2004; **Med School:** Boston Univ 1979; **Resid:** Diagnostic Radiology, Mass Genl Hosp 1984; **Fellow:** Vascular & Interventional Radiology, Mass Genl Hosp 1985; **Fac Appt:** Prof Rad, Cornell Univ-Weill Med Coll

Cohen, Gary S MD [VIR] - **Spec Exp:** Uterine Fibroid Embolization; Cancer Chemoembolization; Liver Cancer/Chemoembolization; Portal Hypertension; **Hospital:** Temple Univ Hosp, Jeanes Hosp; **Address:** 3401 N Broad St, MS 19140, Parkinson Bldg Fl 1 - Ste C, Philadelphia, PA 19140; **Phone:** 215-707-7002; **Board Cert:** Diagnostic Radiology 1992; Vascular & Interventional Radiology 2006; **Med School:** Mount Sinai Sch Med 1988; **Resid:** Diagnostic Radiology, Temple Univ Hosp 1992; **Fellow:** Vascular & Interventional Radiology, Temple Univ Hosp 1993; **Fac Appt:** Prof Rad, Temple Univ

Denny, Donald F MD [VIR] - **Spec Exp:** Dialysis Access; Uterine Fibroids; **Hospital:** Univ Med Ctr Princeton at Plainsboro; **Address:** Princeton Radiology Assocs, 1 Plainsboro Rd, Plainsboro, NJ 08536; **Phone:** 609-497-4310; **Board Cert:** Diagnostic Radiology 1982; Vascular & Interventional Radiology 2005; **Med School:** Hahnemann Univ 1978; **Resid:** Diagnostic Radiology, Yale-New Haven Hosp 1982; **Fellow:** Diagnostic Radiology, Brigham & Womens Hosp 1983; **Fac Appt:** Assoc Clin Prof Rad, Yale Univ

Geschwind, Jean-Francois H MD [VIR] - **Spec Exp:** Liver Cancer/Chemoembolization; Cancer Chemoembolization; Cancer Radiotherapy; **Hospital:** Johns Hopkins Hosp (page 61); **Address:** Johns Hopkins Hosp, Int Radiology, 1800 Orleans St, Ste 3287, Baltimore, MD 21287; **Phone:** 410-614-2227; **Board Cert:** Diagnostic Radiology 1998; **Med School:** Boston Univ 1991; **Resid:** Diagnostic Radiology, UCSF Med Ctr 1995; **Fellow:** Interventional Radiology, Johns Hopkins Hosp 1998; **Fac Appt:** Assoc Prof Rad, Johns Hopkins Univ

Haskal, Ziv MD [VIR] - **Spec Exp:** Uterine Fibroid Embolization; Vascular Malformations; Liver Cancer/Chemoembolization; **Hospital:** Univ of MD Med Ctr; **Address:** 22 S Greene St, Ste 110, Baltimore, MD 21201; **Phone:** 410-328-0000; **Board Cert:** Diagnostic Radiology 1991; Vascular & Interventional Radiology 2010; **Med School:** Boston Univ 1986; **Resid:** Diagnostic Radiology, UCSF Med Ctr 1991; **Fellow:** Vascular & Interventional Radiology, UCSF Med Ctr 1992; **Fac Appt:** Prof Rad, Univ MD Sch Med

McLean, Gordon K MD [VIR] - **Spec Exp:** Uterine Fibroid Embolization; Angioplasty & Stent Placement; **Hospital:** Western Penn Hosp; **Address:** Western Pennsylvania Hosp, Dept Radiology, 4800 Friendship Ave, Pittsburgh, PA 15224-1722; **Phone:** 412-578-7412; **Board Cert:** Diagnostic Radiology 1979; Vascular & Interventional Radiology 2005; **Med School:** Dartmouth Med Sch 1975; **Resid:** Diagnostic Radiology, Hosp Univ Penn 1979; **Fellow:** Angiography, Hosp Univ Penn 1980; **Fac Appt:** Prof Rad, Univ Pennsylvania

Shlansky-Goldberg, Richard MD [VIR] - **Spec Exp:** Uterine Fibroid Embolization; Varicocele Embolization; Pelvic Congestion Syndrome; **Hospital:** Hosp Univ Penn - UPHS (page 72); **Address:** Hosp Univ Penn, Dept Radiology, 3400 Spruce St, 1 Silverstein, Philadelphia, PA 19104; **Phone:** 215-662-6839; **Board Cert:** Diagnostic Radiology 1989; Vascular & Interventional Radiology 2008; **Med School:** Univ Rochester 1984; **Resid:** Diagnostic Radiology, Thomas Jefferson Univ Hosp 1989; **Fellow:** Interventional Radiology, Hosp Univ Penn 1991; **Fac Appt:** Assoc Prof Rad, Univ Pennsylvania

Solomon, Stephen B MD [VIR] - **Spec Exp:** Radiofrequency Tumor Ablation; Kidney Cancer; Liver Cancer; Lung Cancer; **Hospital:** Meml Sloan-Kettering Cancer Ctr; **Address:** Meml Sloan-Kettering Cancer Ctr, Ctr for Image Guided Intervention, 1275 York Ave, New York, NY 10021; **Phone:** 212-639-5012; **Board Cert:** Diagnostic Radiology 1998; **Med School:** Yale Univ 1993; **Resid:** Diagnostic Radiology, Johns Hopkins Hosp 1998

Soulen, Michael C MD [VIR] - **Spec Exp:** Liver Cancer/Chemoembolization; Kidney Cancer; Radiofrequency Tumor Ablation; **Hospital:** Hosp Univ Penn - UPHS (page 72); **Address:** Hosp Univ Penn, Interventional Radiology, 3400 Spruce St, Philadelphia, PA 19104; **Phone:** 215-615-4135; **Board Cert:** Diagnostic Radiology 1989; Vascular & Interventional Radiology 2006; **Med School:** Univ Pennsylvania 1984; **Resid:** Diagnostic Radiology, Johns Hopkins Med Inst 1989; **Fellow:** Vascular & Interventional Radiology, Thomas Jefferson Univ Hosp 1991; **Fac Appt:** Prof Rad, Univ Pennsylvania

Trerotola, Scott O MD [VIR] - **Spec Exp:** Uterine Fibroid Embolization; Hereditary Hemorrhagic Telangiectasia; Varicocele Embolization; **Hospital:** Hosp Univ Penn - UPHS (page 72), Penn Presby Med Ctr - UPHS (page 72); **Address:** Hosp Univ Penn, Dept Radiology, 3400 Spruce St, 1 Silverstein, Philadelphia, PA 19104; **Phone:** 215-615-3540; **Board Cert:** Diagnostic Radiology 1991; Vascular & Interventional Radiology 2005; **Med School:** Univ Pennsylvania 1986; **Resid:** Diagnostic Radiology, Johns Hopkins Hosp 1991; **Fellow:** Vascular & Interventional Radiology, Johns Hopkins Hosp 1992; **Fac Appt:** Prof Rad, Univ Pennsylvania

Weintraub, Joshua L MD [VIR] - **Spec Exp:** Gastrointestinal Cancer; Chemoembolization & Tumor Ablation; Uterine Fibroid Embolization; Vascular Malformations; **Hospital:** NY-Presby/Columbia Univ Med Ctr, NY (page 66); **Address:** NY Presbyterian-Columbia Med Ctr, Dept Radiology, 622 W 168th St, New York, NY 10032; **Phone:** 212-305-7094; **Board Cert:** Diagnostic Radiology 1996; Vascular & Interventional Radiology 1998; **Med School:** Wayne State Univ 1991; **Resid:** Diagnostic Radiology, Beth Israel Hosp 1996; **Fellow:** Vascular & Interventional Radiology, Hosp Univ Penn 1997; **Fac Appt:** Assoc Prof Rad, Columbia P&S

Wood, Bradford J MD [VIR] - **Spec Exp:** Radiofrequency Tumor Ablation; Cancer Radiotherapy; Adrenal Cancer; Liver Cancer; **Hospital:** Natl Inst of Hlth - Clin Ctr; **Address:** National Institutes of Health, 10 Center Drive, MS 1182, Bethesda, MD 20892; **Phone:** 301-443-8191; **Board Cert:** Diagnostic Radiology 1996; Vascular & Interventional Radiology 2011; **Med School:** Univ VA Sch Med 1991; **Resid:** Diagnostic Radiology, Georgetown Univ Med Ctr 1996; **Fellow:** Abdominal/Interventional Radiology, Mass Genl Hosp-Harvard Med Sch 1997; Interventional Radiology, Mass Genl Hosp-Harvard Med Sch 1998; **Fac Appt:** Rad

Southeast

Benenati, James F MD [VIR] - **Spec Exp:** Uterine Fibroid Embolization; Aneurysm-Abdominal Aortic; Peripheral Vascular Disease; **Hospital:** Baptist Hosp of Miami; **Address:** 8900 N Kendall Drive, Miami, FL 33176; **Phone:** 786-596-5990; **Board Cert:** Diagnostic Radiology 1988; Vascular & Interventional Radiology 2005; **Med School:** Univ S Fla Coll Med 1984; **Resid:** Diagnostic Radiology, Indiana Univ Hosp 1988; **Fellow:** Vascular & Interventional Radiology, Johns Hopkins Hosp 1989; **Fac Appt:** Prof Rad, Univ S Fla Coll Med

Coldwell, Douglas M MD [VIR] - **Spec Exp:** Palliative Care; Brachytherapy & Theraspheres; Radiofrequency Tumor Ablation; **Hospital:** Univ of Louisville Hosp; **Address:** 530 S Jackson St, Louisville, KY 40202; **Phone:** 502-852-5875; **Board Cert:** Diagnostic Radiology 1986; Vascular & Interventional Radiology 1995; **Med School:** Univ Tex Med Br, Galveston 1980; **Resid:** Diagnostic Radiology, Hershey Med Ctr-Penn St Univ 1983; **Fellow:** Vascular & Interventional Radiology, MD Anderson Hosp-Tumor Inst 1984; **Fac Appt:** Prof Rad, Univ Louisville Sch Med

Katzen, Barry T MD [VIR] - **Spec Exp:** Peripheral Vascular Disease; Aneurysm-Aortic; Carotid Artery Disease; **Hospital:** Baptist Hosp of Miami; **Address:** 8900 N Kendall Drive, Miami, FL 33176; **Phone:** 786-596-5990; **Board Cert:** Diagnostic Radiology 1974; Vascular & Interventional Radiology 2004; **Med School:** Univ Miami Sch Med 1970; **Resid:** Diagnostic Radiology, NY-Presby/Weill Cornell Med Ctr 1974

Lewis, Curtis A MD [VIR] - **Spec Exp:** Interventional Radiology; Vein Disorders; **Hospital:** Grady Hlth Sys, Emory Univ Hosp; **Address:** Grady Meml Hosp, Dept Radiology, 80 Jesse Hill Jr Drive, 1B Admin Suite, Box 26298, Atlanta, GA 30303; **Phone:** 404-616-4261; **Board Cert:** Diagnostic Radiology 1991; Vascular & Interventional Radiology 2007; **Med School:** Emory Univ 1986; **Resid:** Diagnostic Radiology, Emory Univ Affil Hosps 1991; **Fellow:** Interventional Radiology, Emory Univ 1992; **Fac Appt:** Asst Prof Rad, Emory Univ

Matsumoto, Alan H MD [VIR] - **Spec Exp:** Aneurysm-Abdominal Aortic; Carotid Artery Disease; Vascular Disease; Endovascular Stent Grafts; **Hospital:** Univ of Virginia Health Sys; **Address:** Univ VA Hlth Systems Radiology, Box 800170, Charlottesville, VA 22908; **Phone:** 434-982-0211; **Board Cert:** Internal Medicine 1983; Diagnostic Radiology 1987; Vascular & Interventional Radiology 2005; **Med School:** Wake Forest Univ 1980; **Resid:** Internal Medicine, U Mass Med Ctr 1983; Diagnostic Radiology, Univ NC Med Ctr 1987; **Fellow:** Interventional Radiology, Georgetown Univ Hosp 1988; **Fac Appt:** Prof Med, Univ VA Sch Med

Mauro, Matthew A MD [VIR] - **Spec Exp:** Cancer Chemoembolization; Cancer Radiotherapy; Gastrointestinal Cancer; **Hospital:** NC Memorial Hosp - UNC; **Address:** University NC Hosps, Dept Radiology, CB 7510, 2006 Old Clinic Bldg, 101 Manning Drive, Chapel Hill, NC 27599; **Phone:** 919-966-4238; **Board Cert:** Diagnostic Radiology 1981; Vascular & Interventional Radiology 2003; **Med School:** Cornell Univ-Weill Med Coll 1977; **Resid:** Diagnostic Radiology, Univ NC Hosps 1980; **Fellow:** Interventional Radiology, Univ NC Hosp 1981; Abdominal/Interventional Radiology, Mallinckrodt Inst 1982; **Fac Appt:** Prof Rad, Univ NC Sch Med

Midwest

Cho, Kyung J MD [VIR] - **Spec Exp:** Chemoembolization & Tumor Ablation; Vascular Malformations; Peripheral Vascular Disease; **Hospital:** Univ of Michigan Hosp; **Address:** Univ Michigan Med Ctr, Dept Radiology, 1500 E Med Ctr Drive, CVC 5582, Ann Arbor, MI 48109-5868; **Phone:** 734-936-4466; **Board Cert:** Diagnostic Radiology 1974; Vascular & Interventional Radiology 2005; **Med School:** Korea 1966; **Resid:** Diagnostic Radiology, Wayne Med Ctr 1973; **Fellow:** Cardiovascular Radiology, Univ Michigan 1975; **Fac Appt:** Prof Rad, Univ Mich Med Sch

Darcy, Michael MD [VIR] - **Spec Exp:** Portal Hypertension; Chemoembolization & Tumor Ablation; **Hospital:** Barnes-Jewish Hosp; **Address:** Washington Univ, Mallinckrodt Inst Radiology, 510 S Kingshighway Blvd, St Louis, MO 63110; **Phone:** 314-362-2900; **Board Cert:** Diagnostic Radiology 1985; Vascular & Interventional Radiology 2004; **Med School:** Ohio State Univ 1979; **Resid:** Surgery, Univ Minn Hosps 1982; Diagnostic Radiology, Univ Minn Hosps 1985; **Fellow:** Interventional Radiology, Univ Minn 1987; **Fac Appt:** Prof Rad, Washington Univ, St Louis

Johnson, Matthew S MD [VIR] - **Spec Exp:** Liver Tumors; Uterine Fibroid Embolization; Portal Hypertension; Varicocele Embolization; **Hospital:** IU Health University Hosp, IU Health Methodist Hosp; **Address:** Indiana Univ Hospital, Interventional Radiology, 550 N University Blvd, rm 0290, Indianapolis, IN 46202-5253; **Phone:** 317-944-0849; **Board Cert:** Diagnostic Radiology 1992; Vascular & Interventional Radiology 2006; **Med School:** Univ Mich Med Sch 1986; **Resid:** Surgery, Loyola Univ Med Ctr 1988; Diagnostic Radiology, Loyola Univ Med Ctr 1992; **Fellow:** Interventional Radiology, Johns Hopkins Univ 1994; **Fac Appt:** Prof Rad, Indiana Univ

Ketcham, Douglas B MD [VIR] - **Spec Exp:** Uterine Fibroid Embolization; Varicocele Embolization; Osteoporosis Spine-Vertebroplasty; **Hospital:** United Hosp, Regions Hosp - St Paul; **Address:** St Paul Radiology, 166 4th St E, St Paul, MN 55101; **Phone:** 651-632-5700; **Board Cert:** Diagnostic Radiology 1972; Vascular & Interventional Radiology 2005; **Med School:** Univ Wisc 1965; **Resid:** Diagnostic Radiology, Univ Minn Hosp 1971; **Fellow:** Neuroradiology, Univ Minn Hosp 1972

Vascular & Interventional Radiology

Nemcek Jr, Albert A MD [VIR] - **Spec Exp:** Radiofrequency Tumor Ablation; Vascular Disease; Liver Tumors; **Hospital:** Northwestern Meml Hosp; **Address:** Northwestern Meml Hosp, Dept Radiology, Feinberg Pavillion, rm 4-710T, 251 E Huron St, Chicago, IL 60611; **Phone:** 312-926-5302; **Board Cert:** Diagnostic Radiology 1986; Vascular & Interventional Radiology 2005; **Med School:** UCSD 1982; **Resid:** Diagnostic Radiology, UCSD Med Ctr 1986; **Fellow:** Interventional Radiology, Northwestern Meml Hosp 1987; **Fac Appt:** Assoc Prof Rad, Northwestern Univ

Rilling, William S MD [VIR] - **Spec Exp:** Liver Cancer/Chemoembolization; Arteriovenous Malformations; Uterine Fibroid Embolization; **Hospital:** Froedtert and Med Ctr of WI; **Address:** Froedtert Hosp, Dept Radiology, 9200 W Wisconsin Ave, Milwaukee, WI 53226; **Phone:** 414-805-3028; **Board Cert:** Diagnostic Radiology 1995; Vascular & Interventional Radiology 2007; **Med School:** Univ Wisc 1990; **Resid:** Diagnostic Radiology, Univ Wisc Affil Hosps 1995; **Fellow:** Vascular & Interventional Radiology, Northwestern Meml Hosp 1996; **Fac Appt:** Assoc Prof Rad, Univ Wisc

Salem, Riad MD [VIR] - **Spec Exp:** Cancer Radiotherapy; Cancer Chemoembolization; Liver Cancer/Chemoembolization; **Hospital:** Northwestern Meml Hosp; **Address:** Northwestern Univ Dept Radiology, 676 N St Clair St, Ste 800, Chicago, IL 60611; **Phone:** 312-695-1791; **Board Cert:** Diagnostic Radiology 1997; Vascular & Interventional Radiology 2010; **Med School:** McGill Univ 1993; **Resid:** Diagnostic Radiology, Geo Washington Univ Hosp 1997; **Fellow:** Interventional Radiology, Chldns Hosp 1998; Interventional Radiology, Hosp Univ Penn 1998; **Fac Appt:** Assoc Prof Rad, Northwestern Univ

Smith, Steven J MD [VIR] - **Spec Exp:** Angioplasty-Peripheral; Uterine Fibroid Embolization; Varicocele Embolization; Arteriovenous Malformations; **Hospital:** La Grange Meml Hosp, Adventist Hinsdale Hosp; **Address:** 911 N Elm St, Ste 327, Hinsdale, IL 60521; **Phone:** 630-856-7460; **Board Cert:** Diagnostic Radiology 1983; Vascular & Interventional Radiology 2006; **Med School:** Wayne State Univ 1979; **Resid:** Diagnostic Radiology, Henry Ford Hosp 1983; **Fellow:** Vascular & Interventional Radiology, Northwestern Meml Hosp 1984; **Fac Appt:** Assoc Clin Prof Rad, Northwestern Univ

Vogelzang, Robert MD [VIR] - **Spec Exp:** Uterine Fibroid Embolization; Varicocele Embolization; Vascular Malformations; **Hospital:** Northwestern Meml Hosp; **Address:** Northwestern Meml Hosp, Dept Radiology, 251 E Huron St, Feinberg Bldg - Ste 4-710, Chicago, IL 60611; **Phone:** 312-926-5112; **Board Cert:** Diagnostic Radiology 1981; Vascular & Interventional Radiology 2005; **Med School:** Ros Franklin Univ/Chicago Med Sch 1977; **Resid:** Diagnostic Radiology, Northwestern Meml Hosp 1982; **Fellow:** Interventional Radiology, Northwestern Meml Hosp; **Fac Appt:** Prof Rad, Northwestern Univ

Great Plains and Mountains

Durham, Janette D MD [VIR] - **Spec Exp:** Uterine Fibroid Embolization; Peripheral Vascular Disease; Liver Cancer; **Hospital:** Univ of CO Hosp - Anschutz Inpatient Pav; **Address:** Univ Colorado Dept Radiology, 12401 E 17th Ave, MS L954, Aurora, CO 80045; **Phone:** 303-724-3796; **Board Cert:** Diagnostic Radiology 1987; Vascular & Interventional Radiology 2006; **Med School:** Indiana Univ 1983; **Resid:** Diagnostic Radiology, Indiana Univ Hosp 1987; **Fellow:** Vascular & Interventional Radiology, Mass General Hosp 1988; **Fac Appt:** Prof Rad, Univ Colorado

Kumpe, David A MD [VIR] - **Spec Exp:** Aneurysm-Cerebral; Stroke; Arterial & Venous Stents; Interventional Neuroradiology; **Hospital:** Univ of CO Hosp - Anschutz Inpatient Pav, Chldn's Hosp - Aurora (CO); **Address:** Univ Hosp, Dept Radiology, 12605 E 16th Ave, Aurora, CO 80045; **Phone:** 720-848-7620; **Board Cert:** Diagnostic Radiology 1972; Vascular & Interventional Radiology 2005; **Med School:** Harvard Med Sch 1967; **Resid:** Diagnostic Radiology, Mass Genl Hosp 1971; **Fellow:** Neurological Radiology, Kantonsspital 1976; Angiography, Kantonsspital 1976; **Fac Appt:** Prof Rad, Univ Colorado

Yakes, Wayne F MD [VIR] - **Spec Exp:** Vascular Malformations; Interventional Neuroradiology; **Hospital:** Swedish Med Ctr - Denver; **Address:** Vasacular Malformation Ctr, 501 E Hampden Ave, Ste 4600, Englewood, CO 80113; **Phone:** 303-788-4280; **Board Cert:** Diagnostic Radiology 1983; **Med School:** Creighton Univ 1979; **Resid:** Diagnostic Radiology, Fitzsimons Med Ctr 1983; **Fellow:** Angiography, Walter Reed Med Ctr 1984; Interventional Neuroradiology, Baptist Hosp 1992; **Fac Appt:** Clin Prof, Univ Colorado

Southwest

Hicks, Marshall E MD [VIR] - **Spec Exp:** Liver Cancer; Lung Cancer; **Hospital:** UT MD Anderson Cancer Ctr; **Address:** UT MD Anderson Cancer Ctr, Diagnostic Imaging, 1515 Holcombe Blvd, Houston, TX 77030; **Phone:** 713-563-7900; **Board Cert:** Diagnostic Radiology 1987; Vascular & Interventional Radiology 2004; **Med School:** Univ KY Coll Med 1982; **Resid:** Diagnostic Radiology, Indiana Univ Med Ctr 1987; **Fellow:** Interventional Radiology, Univ Colorado 1988; **Fac Appt:** Prof Rad, Univ Tex, Houston

Kay, Dennis MD [VIR] - **Spec Exp:** Radiofrequency Tumor Ablation; **Hospital:** Ochsner Med Ctr-New Orleans; **Address:** Ochsner Clin, Dept Interven Radiology, 1514 Jefferson Hwy, New Orleans, LA 70121-2429; **Phone:** 504-842-3470; **Board Cert:** Diagnostic Radiology 1986; Vascular & Interventional Radiology 2004; **Med School:** Tulane Univ 1981; **Resid:** Diagnostic Radiology, Ochsner Fdn Hosp 1985; **Fellow:** Vascular & Interventional Radiology, Beth Israel Hosp 1986; **Fac Appt:** Assoc Clin Prof Rad, Tulane Univ

West Coast and Pacific

Dake, Michael D MD [VIR] - **Spec Exp:** Aortic Stent Grafts; Endovascular Stent Grafts; Vascular Disease; Aneurysm; **Hospital:** Stanford Univ Hosp & Clinics; **Address:** Stanford Dept Cardiothoracic Surgery, 300 Pasteur Drive, Falk Research Bldg, 2nd Fl, Stanford, CA 94305-5407; **Phone:** 650-724-0831; **Board Cert:** Internal Medicine 1981; Pulmonary Disease 1986; Diagnostic Radiology 1986; Vascular & Interventional Radiology 2006; **Med School:** Baylor Coll Med 1978; **Resid:** Internal Medicine, Baylor Affil Hosp 1982; Diagnostic Radiology, UCSF Med Ctr 1986; **Fellow:** Pulmonary Disease, UCSF Med Ctr 1983; Interventional Radiology, UCSF Med Ctr 1987; **Fac Appt:** Prof TS, Stanford Univ

Gomes, Antoinette S MD [VIR] - **Spec Exp:** Cardiovascular Interventional Radiology; Vascular Malformations; Chemoembolization & Tumor Ablation; **Hospital:** UCLA Ronald Reagan Med Ctr, Santa Monica - UCLA Med Ctr & Ortho Hosp; **Address:** Dept Radiological Sciences, Ronald Reagan UCLA Med Ctr, 757 Westwood Plaza, Ste 2125, Los Angeles, CA 90095; **Phone:** 310-267-8769; **Board Cert:** Diagnostic Radiology 1975; Vascular & Interventional Radiology 2004; **Med School:** Med Coll PA Hahnemann 1969; **Resid:** Internal Medicine, LAC-USC Med Ctr 1972; Diagnostic Radiology, Stanford Univ Med Ctr 1975; **Fellow:** Cardiovascular Radiology, UCLA Med Ctr 1976; Cardiovascular Radiology, Univ Minn 1978; **Fac Appt:** Prof Rad, UCLA

Goodwin, Scott C MD [VIR] - **Spec Exp:** Uterine Fibroids; Liver Cancer; **Hospital:** UC Irvine Med Ctr; **Address:** 101 City Drive S, MS 104, Orange, CA 92868; **Phone:** 714-456-7517; **Board Cert:** Diagnostic Radiology 1989; Vascular & Interventional Radiology 2007; **Med School:** Harvard Med Sch 1984; **Resid:** Diagnostic Radiology, UCLA Medical Ctr 1988; **Fellow:** Vascular & Interventional Radiology, UCLA Medical Ctr 1989; **Fac Appt:** Prof Rad, UCLA

Hovsepian, David M MD [VIR] - **Spec Exp:** Uterine Fibroid Embolization; Aneurysm-Aortic; Vascular Malformations; **Hospital:** Stanford Univ Hosp & Clinics; **Address:** Dept Interventional Radiology, 300 Pasteur Drive, rm H3630, MC 5642, Stanford, CA 94305-5642; **Phone:** 650-724-7362; **Board Cert:** Diagnostic Radiology 1991; Vascular & Interventional Radiology 2006; **Med School:** Columbia P&S 1986; **Resid:** Diagnostic Radiology, Columbia Presby Hosp 1991; **Fellow:** Interventional Radiology, Thomas Jefferson Univ Hosp 1993; **Fac Appt:** Prof Rad, Stanford Univ

Kaufman, John A MD [VIR] - **Spec Exp:** Uterine Fibroid Embolization; Angioplasty & Stent Placement; **Hospital:** OR Hlth & Sci Univ; **Address:** Dotter Interven Inst-OHSU Hosps & Clins, 3181 SW Sam Jackson Park Rd, Portland, OR 97239; **Phone:** 503-494-7660; **Board Cert:** Diagnostic Radiology 1990; Vascular & Interventional Radiology 2005; **Med School:** Boston Univ 1982; **Resid:** Diagnostic Radiology, Boston Univ Med Ctr 1990; **Fellow:** Vascular & Interventional Radiology, Boston Univ Med Ctr 1991; **Fac Appt:** Prof Rad, Oregon Hlth & Sci Univ

Keller, Frederick S MD [VIR] - **Spec Exp:** Uterine Fibroid Embolization; Arterial & Venous Stents; Urinary Tract Interventions; **Hospital:** OR Hlth & Sci Univ; **Address:** Dotter Interventional Inst, 3181 SW Sam Jackson Park Rd, rm L605, Portland, OR 97239; **Phone:** 503-494-7660; **Board Cert:** Diagnostic Radiology 1977; Vascular & Interventional Radiology 2003; **Med School:** Univ Pennsylvania 1968; **Resid:** Diagnostic Radiology, Univ Oreg Hlth Scis Ctr 1977; **Fac Appt:** Prof, Oregon Hlth & Sci Univ

McGahan, John P MD [VIR] - **Spec Exp:** Radiofrequency Tumor Ablation; Liver Cancer; Kidney Cancer; **Hospital:** UC Davis Med Ctr; **Address:** UC Davis Medical Ctr, Dept Radiology, 4860 Y St ACC3100, Sacramento, CA 95817; **Phone:** 916-734-0655; **Board Cert:** Diagnostic Radiology 1979; **Med School:** Oregon Hlth & Sci Univ 1974; **Resid:** Surgery, UC Davis Med Ctr 1976; Diagnostic Radiology, UC Davis Med Ctr 1979; **Fac Appt:** Prof Rad, UC Davis

Roberts, Anne C MD [VIR] - **Spec Exp:** Uterine Fibroids; Pelvic Congestion Syndrome; Vascular Disease; **Hospital:** UCSD Med Ctr; **Address:** UCSD Medical Ctr-Thornton Hosp, 9300 Campus Point Drive, La Jolla, CA 92037; **Phone:** 619-543-3405; **Board Cert:** Diagnostic Radiology 1986; Vascular & Interventional Radiology 2004; **Med School:** UCSD 1982; **Resid:** Diagnostic Radiology, Mass Genl Hospital 1986; **Fellow:** Vascular & Interventional Radiology, Mass Genl Hospital 1987; **Fac Appt:** Prof Rad, UCSD

Valji, Karim MD [VIR] - **Spec Exp:** Thrombolytic Therapy; **Hospital:** Univ Wash Med Ctr; **Address:** Univ of WA Med Ctr-Dept Rad, 1959 NE Pacific St, Box 357115, Seattle, WA 98195-7115; **Phone:** 206-598-7200; **Board Cert:** Diagnostic Radiology 1989; Vascular & Interventional Radiology 2009; **Med School:** Harvard Med Sch 1982; **Resid:** Internal Medicine, UCSF Med Ctr 1984; Diagnostic Radiology, UCSD Med Ctr 1988; **Fellow:** Angiography, UCSD Med Ctr 1989

Cleveland Clinic

Every life deserves world class care.

Cleveland Clinic
Imaging Institute
9500 Euclid Avenue
Cleveland, OH 44195

Diagnostic Radiology, Neuroradiology

Cleveland Clinic Imaging Institute is one of the leading academic imaging centers in the world and one of the busiest clinical departments in the country. Each year, more than 1.9 million examinations are performed and interpreted by Cleveland Clinic radiologists.

Imaging Institute radiologists are leaders in their specialties. They are responsible for the publication of numerous peer-reviewed manuscripts each year, serve on committees of the most prestigious radiologic societies and are involved in cutting-edge research. This research encompasses treatment of acute stroke, magnetic resonance angiography, 3-D imaging, digital radiography, digital mammography, cardiac magnetic resonance, cartilage imaging, electronic image distribution and intravascular ultrasound.

Neuroradiology specializes in imaging and diagnosing neurological disorders such as epilepsy, brain tumors, multiple sclerosis and problems of the ear-nose-throat system. Patients are referred from around the United States and the world to seek insights, treatments and opinions from our dedicated team of professionals.

Interventional Radiology supports some of the most cutting-edge therapies offered at Cleveland Clinic. Organ transplantation, thoracic surgery and hepato-biliary surgery have been developed in unison with image-guided techniques for the management of issues that arise during surgery. Interventional radiology performs more than 9,500 procedures annually.

Cardiovascular Imaging is equipped with state-of-the-art CT and MRI equipment. The staff is expert in the diagnosis and planning of treatment for conditions that include acquired cardiac disease in adults and congenital heart disease in children and adults. The advanced technology used includes two MRI scanners for cardiac analysis and two CT scanners.

Offering Same-Day Appointments
Call 800.274.2009.

Treatment Guides
Cleveland Clinic has developed comprehensive treatment guides for many diseases and conditions. To download our free treatment guides, visit clevelandclinic.org/treatmentguides.

Online Medical Second Opinion
Call 216.444.3223 or 800.223.2273 ext. 43223 or email eclevelandclinic@ccf.org.

Out-of-State Patients Assistance
Call 800.223.2273, ext. 55580 or email medicalconcierge@ccf.org.

Visit Us At:
clevelandclinic.org

Follow Us On:
Facebook
www.facebook.com/clevelandclinic

Twitter
@ClevelandClinic

You Tube
www.youtube.com/clevelandclinic

Health Hub
health.clevelandclinic.org

Sponsored Page

MOUNT SINAI
SCHOOL OF
MEDICINE

THE MOUNT SINAI MEDICAL CENTER
RADIOLOGY
One Gustave L. Levy Place
Fifth Avenue and 100th Street
New York, NY 10029-6574
Physician Referral: 1-800-MD-SINAI (637-4624)
www.mountsinai.org/imaging

THE DEPARTMENT OF RADIOLOGY at Mount Sinai offers patients one of the world's most comprehensive and sophisticated arrays of diagnostic and interventional radiology services. The department uses filmless digital technology that spans magnetic resonance imaging (MRI), multi-slice computed tomography (CT), positron emission tomography CT (PET-CT), single photon emission computed tomography CT (SPECT-CT), advanced ultrasound, conventional radiography, angiography, digital mammography, and state-of-the-art Picture Archiving Communication System (PACS) technology.

Comprehensive Diagnostic Services – Mount Sinai provides the entire range of diagnostic radiology services in a patient-friendly environment. Its nationally renowned radiologic physicians specialize in every area of disease diagnosis, as well as disease prevention and innovative therapeutic approaches. The combination of state-of-the-art imaging equipment with the finest imaging physicians makes Mount Sinai Radiology the place to go for all your imaging needs.

Early Detection Programs – We are committed to special screening approaches for early disease detection. We provide radiological screenings for colon, breast, and lung cancer and atherosclerosis. The early detection programs use a variety of imaging techniques, such as CT and MRI for atherosclerosis, CT for lung and colon cancer, PET for oncology, digital and 3D mammography, MRI, ultrasound, and computer-aided diagnosis for breast cancer.

Minimally Invasive Procedures – Radiology at Mount Sinai has moved beyond diagnosis to the most sophisticated therapeutic interventions. Interventional radiologists at Mount Sinai perform biopsies, vascular therapies, and uterine artery embolization for fibroids—an alternative to hysterectomy—as well as treatments for aneurysms, atherosclerosis, and many types of cancer. In addition, advanced CT and MR angiography techniques are widely utilized to diagnose vascular diseases in a minimally invasive yet highly accurate manner.

Oncology Imaging – Radiologists work closely with surgeons, oncologists, and other caregivers to optimize the diagnosis and treatment of patients with head and neck, liver, lung, breast, and gastrointestinal cancers. State of the art CT, MRI, ultrasound, SPECT and PET CT are utilized to make the most accurate, least invasive and lowest dose diagnosis.

DEVELOPING NEW DIAGNOSTIC TOOLS
Radiology at Mount Sinai is an active center of imaging research and development. Mount Sinai physicians and scientists developed a special form of MRI to diagnose heart disease and atherosclerosis noninvasively and thereby identify patients at greatest risk for stroke and heart attack. We actively collaborate with other disciplines to develop and refine imaging tools that will make prevention and diagnosis increasingly effective. That is the case, for example, in neuroscience, where the imaging innovations impact our understanding of neurodegenerative conditions, such as Parkinson's disease, multiple sclerosis, stroke, brain tumors, and various psychiatric disorders; cardiovascular disease, where studies are under way to predict the risk associated with atherosclerotic plaques and assess new therapies for aortic and cerebral artery aneurysms; and liver disease, where radiologists, transplant surgeons, and hepatologists collaborate closely to develop optimal therapeutic strategies.

550 First Avenue *(at 31st Street)*
New York, NY 10016

www.NYULMC.org

Physician Referral: **888-7-NYU-MED** *(888-769-8633)*

RADIOLOGY

The Department of Radiology at NYU Langone Medical Center is committed to capturing the best images possible with the lowest dose of radiation. As an academic medical center, our radiologists are in a unique position to take the lead in helping to define and advance radiology in today's rapidly advancing technological environment.

Expertise

NYU Langone Medical Center's board certified radiologists and licensed technologists specialize in imaging and are involved in a variety of innovative collaborations and research initiatives. The Department consists of over 100 sub-specialized academic radiologists, many of them acknowledged leaders and innovators in their fields.

Advanced Technology

NYU Langone uses some of the most advanced imaging equipment in the world, including high and ultra high-field MRI imaging systems (known as 1.5T and 3T magnets). Its MRI scanners are shorter and wider than ever, making for a more patient-friendly experience. The Center for Biomedical Imaging, an advanced research facility, features a powerful 7T magnet.

Recognition for Safety and Quality

We continually follow a rigorous set of quality standards and maintain accreditation by the American College of Radiology (ACR). We are designated by the ACR as a "Breast Imaging Center of Excellence" and maintaining high practice standards in image quality, personnel qualifications, facility equipment, quality control procedures and quality assurance programs.

Patient Focused Approach

We are conveniently located and participate in many insurance plans. We ensure timely delivery of reports and images and allow physicians to view patient exam status, reports and images online from their office. In addition to our convenient hours, weekend, evening and often same-day appointments are available. Language interpretation services are available as needed.

Our Areas of Specialization

We offer an extensive range of diagnostic services around MRI, CT, ultrasound, PET/CT, X-ray, interventional radiology and nuclear medicine. Sub-specialized radiologists provide diagnostic interpretation in abdominal, biomedical, breast, cardiac, chest, emergency, general, musculoskeletal, neuroradiology, neuro interventional, nuclear medicine, pediatric, vascular interventional and women's imaging. Specialty procedures include coronary artery disease and virtual colonoscopy screening, stereotactic biopsy capability, minimally invasive techniques including radiofrequency ablation, chemoembolization, radioimmunotherapy and bone densitometry.

The Best in American Medicine
www.CastleConnolly.com

Reproductive Endocrinology

a subspecialty of Obstetrics & Gynecology

An obstetrician/gynecologist who is capable of managing complex problems relating to reproductive endocrinology and infertility.

Training Required: Four years *plus* two years in clinical practice before certification in obstetrics and gynecology is complete *plus* additional training and examination in reproductive endocrinology.

REPRODUCTIVE ENDOCRINOLOGY

New England

Buster, John E MD [RE] - **Spec Exp:** Infertility-IVF; Reproductive Surgery; **Hospital:** Tufts Med Ctr; **Address:** Tufts Med Ctr, 800 Washington St, Boston, MA 02111; **Phone:** 617-636-0053; **Board Cert:** Obstetrics & Gynecology 2011; Reproductive Endocrinology 2011; **Med School:** UCLA 1966; **Resid:** Obstetrics & Gynecology, Harbor-UCLA Med Ctr 1971; **Fellow:** Reproductive Endocrinology, Harbor-UCLA Med Ctr 1973; **Fac Appt:** Prof ObG, Tufts Univ

Carson, Sandra A MD [RE] - **Spec Exp:** Infertility-IVF; Laparoscopic Surgery; Endometriosis; Sexual Dysfunction; **Hospital:** Women & Infants Hosp of RI; **Address:** Women & Infants Hosp of RI, 90 Plain St Fl 3, Providence, RI 02903; **Phone:** 401-453-7500; **Board Cert:** Obstetrics & Gynecology 2012; Reproductive Endocrinology 2012; **Med School:** Northwestern Univ 1977; **Resid:** Obstetrics & Gynecology, Prentice Womens Hosp 1981; **Fellow:** Reproductive Endocrinology, Michael Reese Hosp 1983; **Fac Appt:** Prof ObG, Brown Univ

Crowley Jr, William F MD [RE] - **Spec Exp:** Pituitary Disorders; Kallmann's Syndrome; Fertility Preservation in Cancer; **Hospital:** Mass Genl Hosp; **Address:** Mass Genl Hosp, Reproductive Endocrine Unit, 55 Fruit St, Ste BHX 511, Boston, MA 02114; **Phone:** 617-726-8433; **Board Cert:** Internal Medicine 1974; Endocrinology 1977; **Med School:** Tufts Univ 1969; **Resid:** Internal Medicine, Mass Genl Hosp 1971; Internal Medicine, Mass Genl Hosp 1974; **Fellow:** Endocrinology, Mass Genl Hosp 1976; **Fac Appt:** Prof Med, Harvard Med Sch

Ginsburg, Elizabeth S MD [RE] - **Spec Exp:** Infertility-IVF; Fertility Preservation in Cancer; **Hospital:** Brigham and Women's Hosp (page 57); **Address:** Brigham & Womens Hosp, Reproductive Med, 75 Francis St ASB1 Bldg - Ste 3300, Boston, MA 02115; **Phone:** 617-732-4222; **Board Cert:** Obstetrics & Gynecology 2011; Reproductive Endocrinology 2011; **Med School:** Mount Sinai Sch Med 1985; **Resid:** Obstetrics & Gynecology, Brigham & Womens Hosp 1989; **Fellow:** Reproductive Endocrinology, Brigham & Womens Hosp 1991; **Fac Appt:** Assoc Prof ObG, Harvard Med Sch

Hill III, Joseph A MD [RE] - **Spec Exp:** Miscarriage-Recurrent; Infertility-Female; Infertility-IVF; **Hospital:** Portsmouth Regl Hosp, Winchester Hosp; **Address:** Fertility Ctr of New England, 875 Greenland Rd, Orchard Park C Bldg, Portsmouth, NH 03801; **Phone:** 781-942-7000 x601; **Board Cert:** Obstetrics & Gynecology 2008; Reproductive Endocrinology 2008; **Med School:** Med Coll GA 1981; **Resid:** Obstetrics & Gynecology, Med Coll Ga 1985; **Fellow:** Reproductive Endocrinology, Brigham-Womens Hosp/Harvard 1987; Reproductive Immunology, Brigham-Womens Hosp/Harvard 1988; **Fac Appt:** Prof ObG, Harvard Med Sch

Hornstein, Mark D MD [RE] - **Spec Exp:** Infertility-IVF; Endometriosis; Laparoscopic Surgery; Hysteroscopic Surgery; **Hospital:** Brigham and Women's Hosp (page 57), Newton - Wellesley Hosp; **Address:** Brigham & Women's Hosp, 75 Francis St, Boston, MA 02115; **Phone:** 617-732-4648; **Board Cert:** Obstetrics & Gynecology 2011; Reproductive Endocrinology 2011; **Med School:** Univ Cincinnati 1982; **Resid:** Obstetrics & Gynecology, Brigham & Women's Hosp 1986; **Fellow:** Reproductive Endocrinology, Brigham & Women's Hosp 1988; **Fac Appt:** Assoc Prof ObG, Harvard Med Sch

Isaacson, Keith B MD [RE] - **Spec Exp:** Infertility; Endometriosis; Minimally Invasive Surgery; **Hospital:** Newton - Wellesley Hosp, Mass Genl Hosp; **Address:** 2014 Washington St Fl 2 West, Newton, MA 02462; **Phone:** 617-243-5205; **Board Cert:** Obstetrics & Gynecology 2011; Reproductive Endocrinology 2011; **Med School:** Med Coll GA 1983; **Resid:** Obstetrics & Gynecology, Ochsner Fdn Hosp 1987; **Fellow:** Reproductive Endocrinology, Hosp Univ Penn 1989; **Fac Appt:** Assoc Prof ObG, Harvard Med Sch

Johnson, Julia V MD [RE] - **Spec Exp:** Infertility-IVF; Endometriosis; Menopause Problems; **Hospital:** UMass Memorial Med Ctr; **Address:** U Mass Medical Ctr-Memorial Campus, 33 Belmont St, Worcester, MA 01605; **Phone:** 508-334-1345; **Board Cert:** Obstetrics & Gynecology 2011; Reproductive Endocrinology/Infertility 2011; **Med School:** Med Coll GA 1984; **Resid:** Obstetrics & Gynecology, Med Coll of Georgia 1988; **Fellow:** Reproductive Endocrinology, Univ Texas Hlth Sci Ctr 1990; **Fac Appt:** Prof ObG, Univ Mass Sch Med

Luciano, Anthony A MD [RE] - **Spec Exp:** Infertility; Endometriosis; Menopause Problems; Osteoporosis; **Hospital:** Hosp of Central CT at New Britain, Hartford Hosp; **Address:** Center for Fertility & Womens Health, 100 Grand St, Ste E3, New Britain, CT 06050; **Phone:** 860-224-5467; **Board Cert:** Obstetrics & Gynecology 1980; Reproductive Endocrinology 1981; **Med School:** Univ Conn 1973; **Resid:** Obstetrics & Gynecology, Univ Conn Hosp 1977; **Fellow:** Reproductive Endocrinology, Univ Conn Hosp 1979; **Fac Appt:** Prof ObG, Univ Conn

Oskowitz, Selwyn P MD [RE] - **Spec Exp:** Infertility-IVF; **Hospital:** Beth Israel Deaconess Med Ctr - Boston; **Address:** Boston IVF, 1 Brookline Pl, Ste 302, Brookline, MA 02445; **Phone:** 617-735-9000; **Board Cert:** Obstetrics & Gynecology 1981; **Med School:** South Africa 1970; **Resid:** Obstetrics & Gynecology, Univ Colorado Med Ctr 1977; **Fellow:** Reproductive Endocrinology, Beth Israel Deaconess Med Ctr 1984; **Fac Appt:** Asst Prof ObG, Harvard Med Sch

Patrizio, Pasquale MD [RE] - **Spec Exp:** Infertility-IVF; Fertility Preservation in Cancer; **Hospital:** Yale-New Haven Hosp, Yale Med Group; **Address:** Yale Fertility Ctr, Dept OB/GYN, 150 Sargent Drive, New Haven, CT 06511; **Phone:** 203-785-4708; **Board Cert:** Obstetrics & Gynecology 2007; Reproductive Endocrinology 2010; **Med School:** Italy 1983; **Resid:** Obstetrics & Gynecology, Univ Naples 1987; Reproductive Endocrinology, Univ Pisa 1990; **Fellow:** Infertility, UC Irvine 1995; **Fac Appt:** Prof ObG, Yale Univ

Petrozza, John C MD [RE] - **Spec Exp:** Pain-Chronic Pelvic; Endometriosis; Minimally Invasive Surgery; Infertility-IVF; **Hospital:** Mass Genl Hosp; **Address:** Mass Genl Hosp, Fetility Ctr, 55 Fruit St Yawkey Bldg - Ste 10A, Boston, MA 02114; **Phone:** 617-726-8868; **Board Cert:** Obstetrics & Gynecology 2011; Reproductive Endocrinology/Infertility 2011; **Med School:** Univ Tex Med Br, Galveston 1990; **Resid:** Obstetrics & Gynecology, Univ Texas Affil Hosp 1994; **Fellow:** Reproductive Endocrinology, Tufts New England Med Ctr 1996; **Fac Appt:** Asst Prof ObG, Harvard Med Sch

Toth, Thomas L MD [RE] - **Spec Exp:** Infertility-IVF; **Hospital:** Mass Genl Hosp, Newton - Wellesley Hosp; **Address:** Mass Genl Hosp, Fertility Ctr, 55 Fruit St Yawkey Bldg - Ste 10A, Boston, MA 02114-2621; **Phone:** 617-726-8868; **Board Cert:** Obstetrics & Gynecology 2011; Reproductive Endocrinology/Infertility 2011; **Med School:** Univ MO-Kansas City 1986; **Resid:** Obstetrics & Gynecology, Mass Genl Hosp/Brigham & Womens Hosp 1990; **Fellow:** Reproductive Endocrinology, E Virginia Med Sch Hosps 1992; **Fac Appt:** Assoc Prof ObG, Harvard Med Sch

Zinaman, Michael J MD [RE] - **Spec Exp:** Endometriosis; Infertility; Uterine Fibroids; **Hospital:** Steward St Elizabeth's Med Ctr-Boston; **Address:** Caritas St Elizabeth's Med Ctr SMC5, 736 Cambridge St, Boston, MA 02135; **Phone:** 617-562-7018; **Board Cert:** Obstetrics & Gynecology 2011; Reproductive Endocrinology 2011; **Med School:** SUNY Downstate 1981; **Resid:** Obstetrics & Gynecology, Univ Chicago Hosps 1985; **Fellow:** Reproductive Endocrinology, Georgetown Univ 1987

Reproductive Endocrinology

Mid Atlantic

Copperman, Alan B MD [RE] - **Spec Exp:** Infertility-IVF; Fertility Preservation in Cancer; Hysteroscopic Surgery; **Hospital:** Mount Sinai Med Ctr (page 64); **Address:** 635 Madison Ave, Fl 10, New York, NY 10022; **Phone:** 212-756-5777; **Board Cert:** Obstetrics & Gynecology 2011; Reproductive Endocrinology 2011; **Med School:** NY Med Coll 1989; **Resid:** Obstetrics & Gynecology, Yale-New Haven Hosp 1993; **Fellow:** Reproductive Endocrinology, Mt Sinai Med Ctr 1995; **Fac Appt:** Clin Prof ObG, Mount Sinai Sch Med

Coutifaris, Christos MD/PhD [RE] - **Spec Exp:** Infertility-IVF; Fertility Preservation in Cancer; Polycystic Ovarian Syndrome; **Hospital:** Hosp Univ Penn - UPHS (page 72); **Address:** Penn Fertility Care, 3701 Market St Fl 8 - Ste 800, Philadelphia, PA 19104; **Phone:** 215-662-6100; **Board Cert:** Obstetrics & Gynecology 2011; Reproductive Endocrinology 2011; **Med School:** Univ Pennsylvania 1982; **Resid:** Obstetrics & Gynecology, Hosp Univ Penn 1986; **Fellow:** Reproductive Endocrinology, Hosp Univ Penn 1987; **Fac Appt:** Prof ObG, Univ Pennsylvania

Gracia, Clarisa R MD [RE] - **Spec Exp:** Gynecology in Cancer Patients; Infertility in Cancer Patients; Fertility Preservation in Cancer; **Hospital:** Hosp Univ Penn - UPHS (page 72); **Address:** Penn Fertility Care, 3701 Market St, Ste 800, Philadelphia, PA 19104; **Phone:** 215-662-6100; **Board Cert:** Obstetrics & Gynecology 2007; Reproductive Endocrinology 2007; **Med School:** SUNY Buffalo 1997; **Resid:** Obstetrics & Gynecology, Hosp Univ Penn 2000; **Fellow:** Reproductive Endocrinology, Hosp Univ Penn; **Fac Appt:** Asst Prof ObG, Univ Pennsylvania

Grazi, Richard MD [RE] - **Spec Exp:** Infertility-IVF; Preimplantation Genetic Diagnosis; Fertility Preservation in Cancer; **Hospital:** Maimonides Med Ctr (page 63), Richmond Univ Med Ctr; **Address:** 1355 84th St, Brooklyn, NY 11228-3030; **Phone:** 718-283-8600; **Board Cert:** Obstetrics & Gynecology 2006; Reproductive Endocrinology/Infertility 2006; **Med School:** SUNY Buffalo 1981; **Resid:** Obstetrics & Gynecology, NYU Med Ctr 1985; **Fellow:** Reproductive Endocrinology, UMDNJ Med Ctr 1987; **Fac Appt:** Assoc Clin Prof ObG, Mount Sinai Sch Med

Grifo, James A MD/PhD [RE] - **Spec Exp:** Preimplantation Genetic Diagnosis; Fertility Preservation in Cancer; Hysteroscopic Surgery; Laparoscopic Surgery; **Hospital:** NYU Langone Med Ctr (page 68); **Address:** 660 1st Ave, Fl 5, New York, NY 10016; **Phone:** 212-263-7978; **Board Cert:** Obstetrics & Gynecology 2011; Reproductive Endocrinology 2011; **Med School:** Case West Res Univ 1984; **Resid:** Obstetrics & Gynecology, NY Hosp-Cornell Med Ctr 1988; **Fellow:** Reproductive Endocrinology, Yale-New Haven Hosp 1990; **Fac Appt:** Prof ObG, NYU Sch Med

Grunfeld, Lawrence MD [RE] - **Spec Exp:** Infertility-IVF; Hysteroscopic Surgery; Laparoscopic Surgery; **Hospital:** Mount Sinai Med Ctr (page 64), Lenox Hill Hosp (page 67); **Address:** 635 Madison Ave, Fl 10, New York, NY 10022-1009; **Phone:** 212-756-5777; **Board Cert:** Obstetrics & Gynecology 2011; Reproductive Endocrinology 2011; **Med School:** Mount Sinai Sch Med 1979; **Resid:** Obstetrics & Gynecology, Montefiore Med Ctr 1984; **Fellow:** Reproductive Endocrinology, Montefiore Med Ctr 1987; **Fac Appt:** Assoc Clin Prof ObG, Mount Sinai Sch Med

Keltz, Martin D MD [RE] - **Spec Exp:** Infertility-IVF; Pregnancy Loss-Recurrent; **Hospital:** St. Luke's - Roosevelt Hosp Ctr - Roosevelt Div (page 56); **Address:** 425 W 59th St, Ste 5A, New York, NY 10019; **Phone:** 212-523-7751; **Board Cert:** Obstetrics & Gynecology 2010; Reproductive Endocrinology 2010; **Med School:** NYU Sch Med 1989; **Resid:** Obstetrics & Gynecology, NYU/Bellevue Hosp 1993; **Fellow:** Reproductive Endocrinology, Yale-New Haven Hosp 1996; **Fac Appt:** Assoc Clin Prof ObG, Columbia P&S

Legro, Richard S MD [RE] - **Spec Exp:** Polycystic Ovarian Syndrome; Menstrual Disorders; Ovarian Failure; Infertility-IVF; **Hospital:** Penn State Milton S Hershey Med Ctr; **Address:** Hershey Med Ctr, 500 University Drive, Box 850, MC H103, Hershey, PA 17033-0850; **Phone:** 717-531-8478; **Board Cert:** Obstetrics & Gynecology 2011; Reproductive Endocrinology 2011; **Med School:** Mount Sinai Sch Med 1987; **Resid:** Obstetrics & Gynecology, Magee-Womens Hosp 1991; **Fellow:** Reproductive Endocrinology, USC Women's Hosp 1993; **Fac Appt:** Prof ObG, Penn State Coll Med

Licciardi, Frederick L MD [RE] - **Spec Exp:** Infertility-IVF; Infertility; Fertility Preservation in Cancer; **Hospital:** NYU Langone Med Ctr (page 68); **Address:** NYU Medical Ctr, 660 First Ave, 5th Fl, New York, NY 10016; **Phone:** 212-263-7754; **Board Cert:** Obstetrics & Gynecology 2007; Reproductive Endocrinology 2007; **Med School:** UMDNJ-Rutgers Med Sch 1986; **Resid:** Obstetrics & Gynecology, St Barnabas Med Ctr 1990; **Fellow:** Reproductive Endocrinology, NY Hosp-Cornell Med Ctr 1992; **Fac Appt:** Assoc Prof ObG, NYU Sch Med

McClamrock, Howard D MD [RE] - **Spec Exp:** Infertility-IVF; Prenatal Genetic Diagnosis; **Hospital:** Univ of MD Med Ctr, St. Joseph Med Ctr; **Address:** 720 Aliceanna St, Ste 300, Baltimore, MD 21201; **Phone:** 443-825-3340; **Board Cert:** Obstetrics & Gynecology 2009; Reproductive Endocrinology 2009; **Med School:** Univ NC Sch Med 1981; **Resid:** Obstetrics & Gynecology, Univ Maryland Affil Hosp 1986; **Fellow:** Reproductive Endocrinology, Univ Maryland 1988; **Fac Appt:** Assoc Prof ObG, Univ MD Sch Med

McGovern, Peter G MD [RE] - **Spec Exp:** Infertility-IVF; Fertility Preservation in Cancer; **Hospital:** Univ Hosp-UMDNJ—Newark, Hackensack Univ Med Ctr; **Address:** University Reproductive Assocs, 214 Terrace Ave, Hasbrouck Heights, NJ 07604; **Phone:** 201-288-6330; **Board Cert:** Obstetrics & Gynecology 2011; Reproductive Endocrinology/Infertility 2011; **Med School:** NYU Sch Med 1986; **Resid:** Obstetrics & Gynecology, NYU-Bellevue Hosp Ctr 1990; **Fellow:** Reproductive Endocrinology, UMDNJ-Newark 1992; **Fac Appt:** Assoc Prof ObG, UMDNJ-NJ Med Sch, Newark

Mukherjee, Tanmoy MD [RE] - **Spec Exp:** Infertility-IVF; Endometriosis; Uterine Fibroids; **Hospital:** Mount Sinai Med Ctr (page 64); **Address:** 635 Madison Ave, Fl 10, New York, NY 10022; **Phone:** 212-756-5777; **Board Cert:** Obstetrics & Gynecology 2011; Reproductive Endocrinology 2011; **Med School:** Albert Einstein Coll Med 1990; **Resid:** Obstetrics & Gynecology, Montefiore Med Ctr 1994; **Fellow:** Reproductive Endocrinology, Mt Sinai Hosp 1996; **Fac Appt:** Asst Clin Prof ObG, Mount Sinai Sch Med

Noyes, Nicole MD [RE] - **Spec Exp:** Infertility-IVF; Fertility Preservation in Cancer; Reproductive Surgery; **Hospital:** NYU Langone Med Ctr (page 68); **Address:** NYU Fertility Clinic, 660 First Ave, 5th FL, New York, NY 10016; **Phone:** 212-263-7981; **Board Cert:** Obstetrics & Gynecology 2011; Reproductive Endocrinology 2011; **Med School:** Univ VT Coll Med 1986; **Resid:** Obstetrics & Gynecology, NY Hosp-Cornell Med Ctr 1990; **Fellow:** Reproductive Endocrinology, NY Hosp-Cornell Med Ctr 1992; **Fac Appt:** Assoc Prof ObG, NYU Sch Med

Rosenwaks, Zev MD [RE] - **Spec Exp:** Infertility-IVF; Genetic Disorders; Fertility Preservation in Cancer; **Hospital:** NY-Presby/Weill Cornell Med Ctr, NY (page 66); **Address:** Ctr For Reproductive Medicine & Infertility, 1305 York Ave Fl 6, New York, NY 10021-4872; **Phone:** 646-962-3743; **Board Cert:** Obstetrics & Gynecology 1978; Reproductive Endocrinology 1981; **Med School:** SUNY Downstate 1972; **Resid:** Obstetrics & Gynecology, LI Jewish Med Ctr 1976; **Fellow:** Reproductive Endocrinology, Johns Hopkins Hosp 1978; **Fac Appt:** Prof ObG, Cornell Univ-Weill Med Coll

Reproductive Endocrinology

Sanfilippo, Joseph S MD [RE] - **Spec Exp:** Adolescent Gynecology; Pediatric Gynecology; Minimally Invasive Surgery; Infertility; **Hospital:** Magee-Womens Hosp - UPMC, Chldns Hosp of Pittsburgh - UPMC; **Address:** Ctr for Fertility & Repro Endocrinology, Magee-Womens Hosp, 300 Halket St, rm 2309, Pittsburgh, PA 15213; **Phone:** 412-641-1204; **Board Cert:** Obstetrics & Gynecology 2007; Reproductive Endocrinology 2007; **Med School:** Univ Hlth Scis, Chicago Med Sch 1973; **Resid:** Obstetrics & Gynecology, SUNY Upstate Med Ctr 1977; **Fellow:** Reproductive Endocrinology, Univ Louisville 1979; **Fac Appt:** Prof ObG, Univ Pittsburgh

Sauer, Mark V MD [RE] - **Spec Exp:** Infertility-IVF; **Hospital:** NY-Presby/Columbia Univ Med Ctr, NY (page 66); **Address:** 1790 Broadway, Fl 2, New York, NY 10019; **Phone:** 646-756-8282; **Board Cert:** Obstetrics & Gynecology 2011; Reproductive Endocrinology 2011; **Med School:** Univ IL Coll Med 1980; **Resid:** Obstetrics & Gynecology, Univ Illinois Med Ctr 1984; **Fellow:** Reproductive Endocrinology, Harbor-UCLA Med Ctr 1986; **Fac Appt:** Prof ObG, Columbia P&S

Schlaff, William D MD [RE] - **Spec Exp:** Infertility; Endometriosis; Vaginal/Uterine Abnormalities; **Hospital:** Thomas Jefferson Univ Hosp; **Address:** Jefferson Univ Hosp, Dept OB&Gyn, 834 Chestnut St, Ste 300, Philadelphia, PA 19107; **Phone:** 215-955-5000; **Board Cert:** Obstetrics & Gynecology 2011; Reproductive Endocrinology 2011; **Med School:** Univ Mich Med Sch 1977; **Resid:** Obstetrics & Gynecology, Univ Mich Hosps 1981; **Fellow:** Reproductive Endocrinology, Johns Hopkins Med Ctr 1985; **Fac Appt:** Prof ObG, Jefferson Med Coll

Seifer, David B MD [RE] - **Spec Exp:** Infertility-IVF; Infertility-Advanced Maternal Age; Fertility Preservation in Cancer; **Hospital:** Maimonides Med Ctr (page 63), Richmond Univ Med Ctr; **Address:** 1355 84th St, Brooklyn, NY 11228; **Phone:** 718-283-8600; **Board Cert:** Obstetrics & Gynecology 2011; Reproductive Endocrinology/Infertility 2011; **Med School:** Univ IL Coll Med 1981; **Resid:** Obstetrics & Gynecology, Stanford Univ Hosp 1985; **Fellow:** Reproductive Endocrinology, Yale-New Haven Hosp 1991; **Fac Appt:** Prof ObG, Mount Sinai Sch Med

Sondheimer, Steven J MD [RE] - **Spec Exp:** Infertility-Female; Infertility-IVF; Endometriosis; **Hospital:** Hosp Univ Penn - UPHS (page 72); **Address:** Penn Fertility Care, 3701 Market St Fl 8, Philadelphia, PA 19104; **Phone:** 215-662-6100; **Board Cert:** Obstetrics & Gynecology 2005; Reproductive Endocrinology 2005; **Med School:** Univ Pennsylvania 1974; **Resid:** Obstetrics & Gynecology, Hosp Univ Penn 1978; **Fellow:** Endocrinology, Hosp Univ Penn 1980; **Fac Appt:** Prof ObG, Univ Pennsylvania

Wallach, Edward E MD [RE] - **Spec Exp:** Uterine Fibroids; Infertility-IVF; **Hospital:** Johns Hopkins Hosp (page 61), Johns Hopkins Bayview Med Ctr (page 61); **Address:** Johns Hopkins at Greenspring Station, 2330 W Joppa Rd, Ste 301, Lutherville, MD 21093; **Phone:** 410-583-2751; **Board Cert:** Obstetrics & Gynecology 1979; Reproductive Endocrinology 1975; **Med School:** Cornell Univ-Weill Med Coll 1958; **Resid:** Obstetrics & Gynecology, Kings Co Hosp 1963; **Fellow:** Reproductive Endocrinology, Worcester Fdn Exper Biol 1962; **Fac Appt:** Prof ObG, Johns Hopkins Univ

Weiss, Gerson MD [RE] - **Spec Exp:** Infertility; Menopause Problems; **Hospital:** Hackensack Univ Med Ctr, Univ Hosp-UMDNJ—Newark; **Address:** 214 Terrace Ave, Hasbrouck Heights, NJ 07604-1815; **Phone:** 201-288-6330; **Board Cert:** Obstetrics & Gynecology 2011; Reproductive Endocrinology 2011; **Med School:** NYU Sch Med 1964; **Resid:** Obstetrics & Gynecology, Bellevue Hosp Ctr 1969; **Fellow:** Reproductive Endocrinology, Univ Pittsburgh 1973; **Fac Appt:** Prof ObG, UMDNJ-NJ Med Sch, Newark

Widra, Eric A MD [RE] - **Spec Exp:** Infertility-IVF; **Hospital:** Georgetown Univ Hosp; **Address:** Shady Grove Fertility, 2021 K St NW, Ste 701, Washington, DC 20006; **Phone:** 202-296-2595; **Board Cert:** Obstetrics & Gynecology 2009; Reproductive Endocrinology/Infertility 2009; **Med School:** UMDNJ-RW Johnson Med Sch 1990; **Resid:** Obstetrics & Gynecology, Thomas Jefferson Univ Hosp 1994; **Fellow:** Reproductive Endocrinology, George Washington Univ Hosp 1996; **Fac Appt:** Assoc Prof ObG, Georgetown Univ

Zacur, Howard A MD/PhD [RE] - **Spec Exp:** Prolactin Disorders; Uterine Fibroids; Hormonal Disorders; Infertility-IVF; **Hospital:** Johns Hopkins Hosp (page 61); **Address:** Johns Hopkins at Green Spring Station, 2330 W Joppa Rd, Ste 301, Lutherville, MD 21093; **Phone:** 410-583-2751; **Board Cert:** Obstetrics & Gynecology 1994; Reproductive Endocrinology 1984; **Med School:** Univ Miami Sch Med 1973; **Resid:** Obstetrics & Gynecology, Johns Hopkins Hosp 1980; **Fellow:** Reproductive Endocrinology, Johns Hopkins Hosp 1982; **Fac Appt:** Prof ObG, Johns Hopkins Univ

Southeast

Azziz, Ricardo MD [RE] - **Spec Exp:** Infertility-Female; Reproductive Surgery; Polycystic Ovarian Syndrome; **Hospital:** Med Coll of GA Hosp and Clin (MCG Health Inc); **Address:** Med Coll GA, Kelly Admin Bldg, rm 311, 1120 15th St, Augusta, GA 30912; **Phone:** 706-721-2301; **Board Cert:** Obstetrics & Gynecology 2007; Reproductive Endocrinology 2007; **Med School:** Penn State Coll Med 1981; **Resid:** Obstetrics & Gynecology, Georgetown Univ Hosp 1985; **Fellow:** Reproductive Endocrinology, Johns Hopkins Hosp 1987; **Fac Appt:** Prof ObG, UCLA

Bateman, Bruce MD [RE] - **Spec Exp:** Infertility-IVF; **Hospital:** Univ of Virginia Health Sys; **Address:** 595 Martha Jefferson Drive, Ste 390, Charlottesville, VA 22911; **Phone:** 434-654-8520; **Board Cert:** Obstetrics & Gynecology 1977; Reproductive Endocrinology/Infertility 1985; **Med School:** Med Coll GA 1970; **Resid:** Obstetrics & Gynecology, Univ Va Med Ctr 1975; **Fellow:** Reproductive Endocrinology, Univ Va Med Ctr 1975

Blackwell, Richard E MD/PhD [RE] - **Spec Exp:** Infertility-Female; Women's Health; Menopause Problems; **Hospital:** Univ of Ala Hosp at Birmingham; **Address:** Women & Infants Ctr, 1700 6 Ave S, rm 10390, Birmingham, AL 35249; **Phone:** 205-996-3160; **Board Cert:** Obstetrics & Gynecology 1982; Reproductive Endocrinology 1987; **Med School:** Baylor Coll Med 1975; **Resid:** Obstetrics & Gynecology, Univ Alabama Hosp 1979; **Fellow:** Reproductive Endocrinology, Univ Alabama 1981; **Fac Appt:** Prof Emeritus ObG, Univ Alabama

DeVane, Gary W MD [RE] - **Spec Exp:** Infertility-IVF; Miscarriage-Recurrent; Endometriosis; Vaginal/Uterine Abnormalities; **Hospital:** Florida Hosp - Orlando, Winnie Palmer Hosp for Women & Babies; **Address:** Center for Reproductive Medicine, 3435 Pinehurst Ave, Orlando, FL 32804-4049; **Phone:** 407-740-0909; **Board Cert:** Obstetrics & Gynecology 1977; Reproductive Endocrinology 1982; **Med School:** Baylor Coll Med 1971; **Resid:** Obstetrics & Gynecology, UCSD Hosp 1975; **Fellow:** Reproductive Endocrinology, Univ Texas SW Hosp 1980; **Fac Appt:** Assoc Clin Prof ObG, Univ Fla Coll Med

Durso, Nancy MD [RE] - **Spec Exp:** Infertility-IVF; Uterine Fibroids; Endometriosis; **Hospital:** Inova Fairfax Hosp; **Address:** 8501 Arlington Blvd, Ste 500, Fairfax, VA 22031; **Phone:** 703-876-6311; **Board Cert:** Obstetrics & Gynecology 2009; Reproductive Endocrinology/Infertility 2009; **Med School:** Univ VA Sch Med 1983; **Resid:** Obstetrics & Gynecology, St Louis/Washington Univ 1987; **Fellow:** Reproductive Endocrinology, Washington Univ Sch Med 1989

Fritz, Marc A MD [RE] - **Spec Exp:** Infertility-IVF; Menopause Problems; **Hospital:** NC Memorial Hosp - UNC; **Address:** UNC School Medicine, Dept Ob/Gyn, 4001 Old Clinic Bldg, CB 7570, Chapel Hill, NC 27599-7570; **Phone:** 919-966-5283; **Board Cert:** Obstetrics & Gynecology 1996; Reproductive Endocrinology 1996; **Med School:** Tulane Univ 1977; **Resid:** Obstetrics & Gynecology, Wright-Patterson USAF Med Ctr 1981; **Fellow:** Reproductive Endocrinology, Oregon Hlth Sci Univ 1983; **Fac Appt:** Prof ObG, Univ NC Sch Med

Reproductive Endocrinology

Kutteh, William H MD/PhD [RE] - **Spec Exp:** Miscarriage-Recurrent; Infertility; **Hospital:** Baptist Memorial Hospital-Memphis, Methodist LeBonheur Germantown Hosp; **Address:** Fertility Assocs of Memphis, 80 Humphrey's Center, Ste 307, Memphis, TN 38120-2363; **Phone:** 901-747-2229; **Board Cert:** Obstetrics & Gynecology 2011; Reproductive Endocrinology/Infertility 2011; **Med School:** Wake Forest Univ 1985; **Resid:** Obstetrics & Gynecology, UAB Med Ctr 1989; **Fellow:** Reproductive Endocrinology, Univ Tennessee Affil Hosp 1991; **Fac Appt:** Prof Med, Univ Tenn Coll Med

Ory, Steven J MD [RE] - **Spec Exp:** Infertility-IVF; Hormonal Disorders; Endometriosis; Uterine Fibroids; **Hospital:** Northwest Med Ctr, Meml Regl Hosp; **Address:** 2960 N State Road 7, Ste 300, Margate, FL 33063-5737; **Phone:** 954-247-6200; **Board Cert:** Obstetrics & Gynecology 2011; Reproductive Endocrinology 2011; **Med School:** Baylor Coll Med 1976; **Resid:** Obstetrics & Gynecology, Mayo Clinic 1980; **Fellow:** Reproductive Endocrinology, Duke Univ 1982; **Fac Appt:** Prof ObG, FIU Coll Med

Session, Donna R MD [RE] - **Spec Exp:** Infertility-IVF; Reproductive Surgery; Polycystic Ovarian Syndrome; Ultrasound; **Hospital:** Emory Univ Hosp, Emory Univ Hosp Midtown; **Address:** Emory Reproductive Center, 550 Peachtree St NE, 18th Fl MOT, Atlanta, GA 30308; **Phone:** 404-778-3401; **Board Cert:** Obstetrics & Gynecology 2004; Reproductive Endocrinology 2004; **Med School:** Eastern VA Med Sch 1986; **Resid:** Obstetrics & Gynecology, Winthrop Hosp 1990; **Fellow:** Reproductive Endocrinology, Columbia-Presby Med Ctr 1993; **Fac Appt:** Assoc Prof ObG, Emory Univ

Steinkampf, Michael P MD [RE] - **Spec Exp:** Infertility-IVF; **Hospital:** Brookwood Med Ctr, St. Vincent's Hosp - Birmingham; **Address:** Alabama Fertility Specialists, 2700 Highway 280 South, Ste 370 East, Birmingham, AL 35223; **Phone:** 205-874-0000; **Board Cert:** Obstetrics & Gynecology 2010; Reproductive Endocrinology 2010; **Med School:** Louisiana State U, New Orleans 1981; **Resid:** Obstetrics & Gynecology, Parkland Meml Hosp 1985; **Fellow:** Reproductive Endocrinology, Univ Texas SW Med Ctr 1987; **Fac Appt:** Prof ObG, Univ Alabama

Walmer, David K MD/PhD [RE] - **Spec Exp:** Infertility-IVF; Miscarriage-Recurrent; Polycystic Ovarian Syndrome; Asherman's Syndrome; **Hospital:** Duke Univ Hosp; **Address:** 5704 Fayetteville Rd, Durham, NC 27713; **Phone:** 919-572-4673; **Board Cert:** Obstetrics & Gynecology 2009; Reproductive Endocrinology 2009; **Med School:** Univ NC Sch Med 1983; **Resid:** Obstetrics & Gynecology, Univ Texas Affil Hosp 1987; **Fellow:** Reproductive Endocrinology, Duke Univ 1989; **Fac Appt:** Assoc Prof ObG, Duke Univ

Midwest

Barnes, Randall B MD [RE] - **Spec Exp:** Infertility-IVF; Polycystic Ovarian Syndrome; Miscarriage-Recurrent; **Hospital:** Northwestern Meml Hosp; **Address:** 675 N St Clair St Fl 14 - Ste 200, Chicago, IL 60611; **Phone:** 312-695-7269; **Board Cert:** Obstetrics & Gynecology 2011; Reproductive Endocrinology 2011; **Med School:** Johns Hopkins Univ 1979; **Resid:** Obstetrics & Gynecology, LAC-USC Med Ctr 1983; **Fellow:** Reproductive Endocrinology, LAC-USC Med Ctr 1985; **Fac Appt:** Assoc Prof ObG, Northwestern Univ

Christman, Gregory MD [RE] - **Spec Exp:** Infertility-IVF; Uterine Fibroids; Endometriosis; Microsurgery; **Hospital:** Univ of Michigan Hosp; **Address:** UofM Ctr for Reproductive Med, 475 Market Pl, Ste B, Ann Arbor, MI 48108; **Phone:** 734-763-4323; **Board Cert:** Obstetrics & Gynecology 2011; Reproductive Endocrinology 2011; **Med School:** Univ Wisc 1983; **Resid:** Obstetrics & Gynecology, Univ Wisconsin Hosps 1987; **Fellow:** Reproductive Endocrinology, Univ North Carolina 1992; **Fac Appt:** Assoc Prof ObG, Univ Mich Med Sch

Coddington III, Charles C MD [RE] - **Spec Exp:** Reproductive Surgery; Endometriosis; Infertility-IVF; **Hospital:** Mayo Med Ctr & Clin - Rochester; **Address:** Mayo Clin, Dept Reproductive Med, 200 First St SW, rm 3127, Rochester, MN 55905; **Phone:** 507-284-9792; **Board Cert:** Obstetrics & Gynecology 2006; Reproductive Endocrinology 2006; **Med School:** Med Univ SC 1977; **Resid:** Obstetrics & Gynecology, Natl Naval Med Ctr 1981; **Fellow:** Reproductive Endocrinology, Natl Inst Hlth 1985; **Fac Appt:** Prof ObG, Mayo Med Sch

Diamond, Michael P MD [RE] - **Spec Exp:** Infertility-IVF; Endometriosis; Polycystic Ovarian Syndrome; Hysteroscopic Surgery; **Hospital:** Hutzel Hosp - Detroit, Harper Univ Hosp; **Address:** Univ Physicians, 26400 W 12 Mile Rd, Southfield, MI 48034; **Phone:** 248-352-8200; **Board Cert:** Obstetrics & Gynecology 2011; Reproductive Endocrinology 2011; **Med School:** Vanderbilt Univ 1981; **Resid:** Obstetrics & Gynecology, Vanderbilt Univ Med Ctr 1985; **Fellow:** Reproductive Endocrinology, Yale-New Haven Hosp 1987; **Fac Appt:** Prof ObG, Wayne State Univ

Dodds, William G MD [RE] - **Spec Exp:** Infertility; Endometriosis; **Hospital:** Spectrum Hlth Butterworth Campus; **Address:** The Fertility Center, 3230 Eagle Park Drive NE, Ste 100, Grand Rapids, MI 49525; **Phone:** 616-988-2229; **Board Cert:** Obstetrics & Gynecology 2011; Reproductive Endocrinology 2011; **Med School:** Ohio State Univ 1982; **Resid:** Obstetrics & Gynecology, Ohio State Univ Med Ctr 1986; **Fellow:** Reproductive Endocrinology, Ohio State Univ 1988; **Fac Appt:** Assoc Prof ObG, Univ Mich Med Sch

Falcone, Tommaso MD [RE] - **Spec Exp:** Minimally Invasive Surgery; Infertility-IVF; Endometriosis; Hysteroscopic Surgery; **Hospital:** Cleveland Clin (page 55); **Address:** Cleveland Clin, Dept Ob/Gyn, 9500 Euclid Ave, Desk A81, Cleveland, OH 44195-0001; **Phone:** 216-444-1758; **Board Cert:** Obstetrics & Gynecology 2011; Reproductive Endocrinology 2011; **Med School:** McGill Univ 1981; **Resid:** Obstetrics & Gynecology, McGill Univ Hlth Ctr 1986; **Fellow:** Reproductive Endocrinology, McGill Univ 1989; **Fac Appt:** Prof ObG, Cleveland Cl Coll Med/Case West Res

Friedman, Chad MD [RE] - **Spec Exp:** Infertility-IVF; Polycystic Ovarian Syndrome; **Hospital:** Ohio St Univ Med Ctr; **Address:** 4830 Knightsbridge Blvd, Ste E, Columbus, OH 43214; **Phone:** 614-451-2280; **Board Cert:** Obstetrics & Gynecology 1982; Reproductive Endocrinology/Infertility 1983; **Med School:** Univ Chicago-Pritzker Sch Med 1975; **Resid:** Obstetrics & Gynecology, Ohio State Univ Hosp 1979; **Fellow:** Reproductive Endocrinology, Ohio State Univ Hosp 1981; **Fac Appt:** Assoc Prof ObG, Ohio State Univ

Goldberg, Jeffrey M MD [RE] - **Spec Exp:** Infertility-IVF; Endoscopic Surgery; Microsurgery; **Hospital:** Cleveland Clin (page 55); **Address:** Beachwood Family Health Ctr, 26900 Cedar Rd, MC BD20, Beechwood, OH 44122; **Phone:** 216-839-3150; **Board Cert:** Obstetrics & Gynecology 2011; Reproductive Endocrinology 2011; **Med School:** UMDNJ-NJ Med Sch, Newark 1983; **Resid:** Obstetrics & Gynecology, Emory Univ Med Ctr 1987; **Fellow:** Reproductive Endocrinology, Ohio State Univ 1989; **Fac Appt:** Prof ObG, Cleveland Cl Coll Med/Case West Res

Haney, Arthur F MD [RE] - **Spec Exp:** Infertility-Female; DES-Exposed Females; Minimally Invasive Gynecologic Surgery; **Hospital:** Univ of Chicago Med Ctr; **Address:** 5841 S Maryland Ave, MC 2050, Chicago, IL 60637; **Phone:** 773-702-6127; **Board Cert:** Obstetrics & Gynecology 2010; Reproductive Endocrinology 2010; **Med School:** Univ Ariz Coll Med 1972; **Resid:** Obstetrics & Gynecology, Duke Univ Med Ctr 1976; **Fellow:** Reproductive Endocrinology, Duke Univ Med Ctr 1978; **Fac Appt:** Prof ObG, Univ Chicago-Pritzker Sch Med

Jacobs, Laurence A MD [RE] - **Spec Exp:** Infertility-IVF; Polycystic Ovarian Syndrome; Endometriosis; Obesity; **Hospital:** Adv Luth Genl Hosp, Northwest Comm Hosp; **Address:** 135 N Arlington Hts Rd, Ste 195, Buffalo Grove, IL 60089; **Phone:** 847-215-8899; **Board Cert:** Obstetrics & Gynecology 1981; **Med School:** Northwestern Univ 1975; **Resid:** Obstetrics & Gynecology, Northwestern Meml Hosp 1979; **Fellow:** Reproductive Endocrinology, Mayo Clinic 1988; **Fac Appt:** Assoc Prof ObG, Northwestern Univ-Feinberg Sch Med

Reproductive Endocrinology

Kazer, Ralph R MD [RE] - **Spec Exp:** Polycystic Ovarian Syndrome; Infertility-IVF; **Hospital:** Northwestern Meml Hosp; **Address:** Northwestern Meml Hosp, 675 N St Clair St Fl 14 - Ste 200, Galter Pavillion, Chicago, IL 60611; **Phone:** 312-695-7269; **Board Cert:** Obstetrics & Gynecology 2011; Reproductive Endocrinology 2011; **Med School:** Tufts Univ 1979; **Resid:** Obstetrics & Gynecology, Tufts Univ Med Ctr 1983; **Fellow:** Reproductive Endocrinology, UC San Diego Med Ctr 1986; **Fac Appt:** Prof ObG, Northwestern Univ

Milad, Magdy P MD [RE] - **Spec Exp:** Reproductive Surgery; Infertility; Uterine Fibroids; **Hospital:** Northwestern Meml Hosp; **Address:** Northwestern Med Fac Fdn, 675 N St Clair St, Galter Pavilion Fl 14 - Ste 200, Chicago, IL 60611-5975; **Phone:** 312-695-7269; **Board Cert:** Obstetrics & Gynecology 2011; Reproductive Endocrinology 2011; **Med School:** Wayne State Univ 1987; **Resid:** Obstetrics & Gynecology, William Beaumont Hosp 1991; **Fellow:** Reproductive Endocrinology, Mayo Clinic 1993; **Fac Appt:** Prof ObG, Northwestern Univ

Miller, Charles E MD [RE] - **Spec Exp:** Infertility-IVF; Minimally Invasive Surgery; Endometriosis; Uterine Fibroids; **Hospital:** Edward Hosp, Adv Luth Genl Hosp; **Address:** 120 Osler Drive, Ste 100, Naperville, IL 60540; **Phone:** 630-428-2229; **Board Cert:** Obstetrics & Gynecology 1984; **Med School:** Northwestern Univ 1977; **Resid:** Obstetrics & Gynecology, Univ Texas SW Med Ctr 1980; **Fellow:** Reproductive Endocrinology, Hosp Univ Penn 1983; **Fac Appt:** Assoc Clin Prof ObG, Univ Chicago-Pritzker Sch Med

Molo, Mary W MD [RE] - **Spec Exp:** Infertility-IVF; Uterine Fibroids; Fertility Preservation in Cancer; **Hospital:** Rush Univ Med Ctr; **Address:** 1725 W Harrison St, Ste 408 East, Chicago, IL 60612; **Phone:** 312-997-2229; **Board Cert:** Obstetrics & Gynecology 2011; Reproductive Endocrinology 2011; **Med School:** Southern IL Univ 1982; **Resid:** Obstetrics & Gynecology, Southern Illinois Affil Hosps 1984; Obstetrics & Gynecology, Rush Presby St Lukes Hosp 1987; **Fellow:** Reproductive Endocrinology, Rush Presby St Lukes Hosp 1989; **Fac Appt:** Asst Prof ObG, Rush Med Coll

Odem, Randall R MD [RE] - **Spec Exp:** Infertility; Reproductive Surgery; Miscarriage-Recurrent; Asherman's Syndrome; **Hospital:** Barnes-Jewish Hosp; **Address:** Ctr for Reproductive Med, 4444 Forest Park Ave, Ste 3100, St Louis, MO 63108-2212; **Phone:** 314-286-2400; **Board Cert:** Obstetrics & Gynecology 2011; Reproductive Endocrinology 2011; **Med School:** Univ Iowa Coll Med 1981; **Resid:** Obstetrics & Gynecology, Univ Illinois Affil Hosps 1985; **Fellow:** Reproductive Endocrinology, Washington Univ 1987; **Fac Appt:** Prof ObG, Washington Univ, St Louis

Ratts, Valerie S MD [RE] - **Spec Exp:** Infertility-IVF; Miscarriage-Recurrent; Endometriosis; Adolescent Gynecology; **Hospital:** Barnes-Jewish Hosp; **Address:** Ctr for Reproductive Med, 4444 Forest Park Ave, Ste 3100, St Louis, MO 63108-2212; **Phone:** 314-286-2400; **Board Cert:** Obstetrics & Gynecology 2011; Reproductive Endocrinology 2011; **Med School:** Johns Hopkins Univ 1987; **Resid:** Obstetrics & Gynecology, Johns Hopkins Hosp 1991; **Fellow:** Reproductive Endocrinology, Johns Hopkins Hosp 1993; **Fac Appt:** Assoc Prof ObG, Washington Univ, St Louis

Smith, Yolanda R MD [RE] - **Spec Exp:** Infertility-IVF; Pediatric & Adolescent Gynecology; Polycystic Ovarian Syndrome; Menopause Problems; **Hospital:** Univ of Michigan Hosp; **Address:** UofM Ctr for Reproductive Med, 475 Market Pl, Ste B, Ann Arbor, MI 48108; **Phone:** 734-763-4323; **Board Cert:** Obstetrics & Gynecology 2011; Reproductive Endocrinology 2011; **Med School:** Wake Forest Univ 1989; **Resid:** Obstetrics & Gynecology, Univ Mich Hosp 1993; **Fellow:** Reproductive Endocrinology, Johns Hopkins Univ 1995; **Fac Appt:** Assoc Prof ObG, Univ Mich Med Sch

Stewart, Elizabeth A MD [RE] - **Spec Exp:** Uterine Fibroids; Hysteroscopic Surgery; Infertility-IVF; **Hospital:** Mayo Med Ctr & Clin - Rochester; **Address:** Mayo Clin, Dept Reproductive Med, 200 First St SW, rm 3127, Rochester, MN 55905; **Phone:** 507-284-9792; **Board Cert:** Obstetrics & Gynecology 2011; Reproductive Endocrinology 2011; **Med School:** Harvard Med Sch 1985; **Resid:** Obstetrics & Gynecology, Brigham & Womens Hosp 1989; **Fellow:** Reproductive Endocrinology, Brigham & Womens Hosp 1992; **Fac Appt:** Prof ObG, Mayo Med Sch

Van Voorhis, Bradley MD [RE] - **Spec Exp:** Infertility; Endometriosis; Uterine Fibroids; **Hospital:** Univ Iowa Hosp & Clinics; **Address:** Univ Iowa Hosps & Clinics, 200 Hawkins Drive, Dept Reproductive Endocrinology 3PFP, Iowa City, IA 52242; **Phone:** 319-356-1767; **Board Cert:** Obstetrics & Gynecology 2011; Reproductive Endocrinology 2011; **Med School:** Univ Iowa Coll Med 1984; **Resid:** Obstetrics & Gynecology, Med Coll Va 1988; **Fellow:** Reproductive Endocrinology, Brigham & Women's Hosp 1991; **Fac Appt:** Prof ObG, Univ Iowa Coll Med

Great Plains and Mountains

Richardson, Marilyn MD [RE] - **Spec Exp:** Menopause Problems; Hormonal Disorders; **Address:** 12616 W 62nd Terr, Ste 112, Shawnee, KS 66216; **Phone:** 913-631-0277; **Board Cert:** Obstetrics & Gynecology 2011; **Med School:** Univ Kansas 1979; **Resid:** Obstetrics & Gynecology, Truman Med Ctr 1983; **Fellow:** Reproductive Endocrinology, Univ Texas Hlth Scis Ctr 1985; **Fac Appt:** Asst Clin Prof ObG, Univ Kansas

Surrey, Eric S MD [RE] - **Spec Exp:** Infertility-IVF; Endometriosis; **Hospital:** Sky Ridge Med Ctr, Swedish Med Ctr - Denver; **Address:** CO Center for Reproductive Medicine, 10290 RidgeGate Cir, Lone Tree, CO 80124; **Phone:** 303-788-8300; **Board Cert:** Obstetrics & Gynecology 2011; Reproductive Endocrinology 2011; **Med School:** Univ Pennsylvania 1981; **Resid:** Obstetrics & Gynecology, UCLA Med Ctr 1986; **Fellow:** Reproductive Endocrinology, UCLA Med Ctr 1988

Southwest

Brzyski, Robert MD/PhD [RE] - **Spec Exp:** Infertility-IVF; Polycystic Ovarian Syndrome; **Hospital:** Univ Hlth Syst-San Antonio; **Address:** 8300 Floyd Curl Drive, San Antonio, TX 78229; **Phone:** 210-450-9500; **Board Cert:** Obstetrics & Gynecology 2011; Reproductive Endocrinology 2011; **Med School:** St Louis Univ 1983; **Resid:** Obstetrics & Gynecology, Yale-New Haven Hosp 1987; **Fellow:** Reproductive Endocrinology, E VA Med School/Jones Inst for Reproductive Med 1989; **Fac Appt:** Prof ObG, Univ Tex, San Antonio

Carr, Bruce R MD [RE] - **Spec Exp:** Infertility-Female; **Hospital:** UT Southwestern Med Ctr at Dallas, Parkland Hlth & Hosp Sys; **Address:** 1801 Inwood Rd Fl 6 - Ste 616, Dallas, TX 75390; **Phone:** 214-645-3858; **Board Cert:** Obstetrics & Gynecology 2000; Reproductive Endocrinology 2000; **Med School:** Univ Mich Med Sch 1971; **Resid:** Obstetrics & Gynecology, Parkland Meml Hosp 1975; **Fellow:** Reproductive Endocrinology, Univ Texas SW Med Ctr 1980; **Fac Appt:** Prof ObG, Univ Tex SW, Dallas

Clisham, P Ronald MD [RE] - **Spec Exp:** Infertility-IVF; Endometriosis; Uterine Fibroids; Laparoscopic Surgery; **Hospital:** Tulane Med Ctr; **Address:** Audubon Fertility & Reproductive Med, 4321 Magnolia St, New Orleans, LA 70115; **Phone:** 504-891-1390; **Board Cert:** Obstetrics & Gynecology 2011; Reproductive Endocrinology 2011; **Med School:** Louisiana State U, New Orleans 1982; **Resid:** Obstetrics & Gynecology, Charity Hosp 1986; **Fellow:** Reproductive Endocrinology, UCLA Med Ctr 1988; **Fac Appt:** Prof ObG, Tulane Univ

Dickey, Richard P MD/PhD [RE] - **Spec Exp:** Infertility-IVF; **Hospital:** Tulane-Lakeside Hosp; **Address:** 800 N Causeway Blvd, Ste 2C, Mandeville, LA 70448; **Phone:** 985-892-7621; **Board Cert:** Obstetrics & Gynecology 1967; Reproductive Endocrinology/Infertility 1976; **Med School:** Case West Res Univ 1960; **Resid:** Obstetrics & Gynecology, Ohio State Univ Hosp 1965; **Fellow:** Reproductive Endocrinology, Ohio State Univ Hosp 1966; **Fac Appt:** Clin Prof ObG, Louisiana State U, New Orleans

Reproductive Endocrinology

Huang, Jaou-Chen MD [RE] - **Spec Exp:** Infertility-IVF; Endometriosis; Hysteroscopic Surgery; Uterine Fibroids; **Hospital:** Meml Hermann Hosp - Texas Med Ctr; **Address:** UT Physicians Womens Center, 6410 Fannin St, Ste 250, Houston, TX 77030; **Phone:** 832-325-7131; **Board Cert:** Obstetrics & Gynecology 2011; Reproductive Endocrinology/Infertility 2011; **Med School:** Taiwan 1980; **Resid:** Obstetrics & Gynecology, Natl Taiwan Univ Hosp 1985; Obstetrics & Gynecology, Harlem Hosp 1992; **Fellow:** Reproductive Endocrinology, Brigham & Women's Hosp 1993; **Fac Appt:** Asst Clin Prof ObG, Univ Tex, Houston

Moffitt, Drew MD [RE] - **Spec Exp:** Infertility-IVF; Reproductive Surgery; **Hospital:** Banner Good Samaritan Regl Med Ctr - Phoenix; **Address:** Arizona Reproductive Medicine, 1701 E Thomas Rd Bldg 1 - Ste 101, Phoenix, AZ 85016; **Phone:** 602-343-2767; **Board Cert:** Obstetrics & Gynecology 2011; Reproductive Endocrinology/Infertility 2011; **Med School:** UCLA 1988; **Resid:** Obstetrics & Gynecology, UCLA Med Ctr 1992; **Fellow:** Reproductive Endocrinology, Jones Inst/Eastern Va Med Sch 1994; **Fac Appt:** Assoc Prof ObG, Univ Ariz Coll Med

Putman, John M MD [RE] - **Spec Exp:** Infertility-IVF; Uterine Fibroids; Endometriosis; Minimally Invasive Surgery; **Hospital:** Baylor Univ Medical Ctr-Dallas; **Address:** Fertility Center of Dallas, 3900 Junius St, Ste 610, Dallas, TX 75246; **Phone:** 214-823-2692; **Board Cert:** Obstetrics & Gynecology 1980; **Med School:** Med Coll GA 1979; **Resid:** Obstetrics & Gynecology, Baylor Univ Med Ctr 1977; **Fac Appt:** Assoc Clin Prof ObG, Univ Tex SW, Dallas

Schenken, Robert S MD [RE] - **Spec Exp:** Infertility; Endometriosis; **Hospital:** Univ Hlth Syst-San Antonio, Baptist Hlth Sys; **Address:** Dept OB/GYN, 7703 Floyd Curl Dr, MSC 7836, San Antonio, TX 78229-3900; **Phone:** 210-567-4950; **Board Cert:** Obstetrics & Gynecology 1995; Reproductive Endocrinology 1995; **Med School:** Baylor Coll Med 1977; **Resid:** Obstetrics & Gynecology, Bexar Co Hosp 1981; **Fellow:** Reproductive Endocrinology, Natl Inst Hlth 1982; Reproductive Endocrinology, Univ Tex Hlth Sci Ctr 1983; **Fac Appt:** Prof ObG, Univ Tex, San Antonio

Wilson, Ellen E MD [RE] - **Spec Exp:** Infertility; Uterine Fibroids; Polycystic Ovarian Syndrome; Pediatric & Adolescent Gynecology; **Hospital:** UT Southwestern Med Ctr at Dallas; **Address:** UTSW Fertility & Reproductive Medicine, 1801 Inwood Rd Fl 6 - Ste 616, Dallas, TX 75390-8539; **Phone:** 214-645-3858; **Board Cert:** Obstetrics & Gynecology 2009; Reproductive Endocrinology/Infertility 2009; **Med School:** Baylor Coll Med 1984; **Resid:** Obstetrics & Gynecology, George Washington Univ Hosp 1989; **Fellow:** Reproductive Endocrinology, UTSW Southwestern 1991; Laparoscopic Surgery, Womens Hosp 1992; **Fac Appt:** Assoc Prof ObG, Univ Tex SW, Dallas

West Coast and Pacific

Adamson, G David MD [RE] - **Spec Exp:** Infertility; Endometriosis; Laparoscopic Surgery; **Hospital:** Stanford Univ Hosp & Clinics, Good Samaritan Hosp - San Jose; **Address:** Fertility Phsyicians of N California, 2581 Samaritan Drive, Ste 302, San Jose, CA 95124; **Phone:** 408-356-5000; **Board Cert:** Obstetrics & Gynecology 1980; Reproductive Endocrinology 1982; **Med School:** Univ Toronto 1973; **Resid:** Obstetrics & Gynecology, Toronto Genl Hosp 1977; **Fellow:** Obstetrics & Gynecology, Toronto Genl Hosp 1978; Reproductive Endocrinology, Stanford Univ 1980; **Fac Appt:** Clin Prof ObG, Stanford Univ

Agarwal, Sanjay K MD [RE] - **Spec Exp:** Infertility-IVF; Endometriosis; **Hospital:** UCSD Med Ctr; **Address:** Univ California-San Diego Medical Ctr, 9350 Campus Point Drive, Ste LL-C, La Jolla, CA 92037-1300; **Phone:** 858-657-8745; **Board Cert:** Obstetrics & Gynecology 2011; Reproductive Endocrinology/Infertility 2011; **Med School:** England, UK 1986; **Resid:** Obstetrics & Gynecology, Duke Univ Med Ctr 1993; **Fellow:** Reproductive Endocrinology, UCLA Med Ctr 1995; **Fac Appt:** Clin Prof ObG, UCSD

Cedars, Marcelle I MD [RE] - **Spec Exp:** Infertility-IVF; Polycystic Ovarian Syndrome; **Hospital:** UCSF Med Ctr; **Address:** UCSF Ctr for Reproductive Hlth, 2356 Sutter St Fl 7, San Francisco, CA 94115; **Phone:** 415-353-7475; **Board Cert:** Obstetrics & Gynecology 2011; Reproductive Endocrinology 2011; **Med School:** Univ Tex SW, Dallas 1981; **Resid:** Obstetrics & Gynecology, Parkland Meml Hosp 1985; **Fellow:** Reproductive Endocrinology, UCLA Med Ctr 1987; **Fac Appt:** Prof ObG, UCSF

Chang, R Jeffrey MD [RE] - **Spec Exp:** Polycystic Ovarian Syndrome; Hormonal Disorders; Menstrual Disorders; Pituitary Tumors; **Hospital:** UCSD Med Ctr; **Address:** UCSD Reproductive Medicine, 9350 Campus Point Drive, Ste LL-C, La Jolla, CA 92037; **Phone:** 858-657-8745; **Board Cert:** Obstetrics & Gynecology 2002; Reproductive Endocrinology/Infertility 2002; **Med School:** Oregon Hlth & Sci Univ 1969; **Resid:** Obstetrics & Gynecology, Harbor Genl Hosp-UCLA 1974; **Fellow:** Reproductive Endocrinology, Harbor Genl Hosp-UCLA 1975; Reproductive Endocrinology, UCSF Med Ctr 1977; **Fac Appt:** Prof ObG, UCSD

Dumesic, Daniel A MD [RE] - **Spec Exp:** Infertility-Female; Hormonal Disorders; Polycystic Ovarian Syndrome; Hysteroscopic Surgery; **Hospital:** UCLA Ronald Reagan Med Ctr; **Address:** 200 UCLA Medical Plaza, Ste 430, Los Angeles, CA 90095; **Phone:** 310-794-7274; **Board Cert:** Obstetrics & Gynecology 2011; Reproductive Endocrinology 2011; **Med School:** Univ Wisc 1978; **Resid:** Obstetrics & Gynecology, UCSF Med Ctr 1982; **Fellow:** Reproductive Endocrinology, UCSF 1987

Giudice, Linda C MD/PhD [RE] - **Spec Exp:** Infertility-IVF; Endometriosis; **Hospital:** UCSF Med Ctr; **Address:** Center for Reproductive Health, 2356 Sutter St Fl 7, San Francisco, CA 94115; **Phone:** 415-353-7475; **Board Cert:** Obstetrics & Gynecology 2011; Reproductive Endocrinology 2011; **Med School:** Stanford Univ 1982; **Resid:** Obstetrics & Gynecology, Stanford Univ Med Ctr 1984; Obstetrics & Gynecology, Barnes Hosp-Wash Univ Med Ctr 1986; **Fellow:** Reproductive Endocrinology, Stanford Univ Med Ctr 1987; **Fac Appt:** Prof ObG, UCSF

Houmard, Brenda MD/PhD [RE] - **Spec Exp:** Infertility; Menstrual Disorders; Miscarriage-Recurrent; **Hospital:** Univ Wash Med Ctr; **Address:** University Reproductive Care, 4245 Roosevelt Way NE, Box 354765, Seattle, WA 98105; **Phone:** 206-598-4225; **Board Cert:** Obstetrics & Gynecology 2011; **Med School:** Ohio State Univ 1994; **Resid:** Obstetrics & Gynecology, OSU Med Ctr 1998; **Fellow:** Reproductive Endocrinology, Univ Wash Med Ctr 2001; **Fac Appt:** Asst Prof ObG, Univ Wash

Marrs, Richard P MD [RE] - **Spec Exp:** Infertility-Female; Endometriosis; Uterine Fibroids; **Address:** 11818 Wilshire Blvd, Ste 300, Los Angeles, CA 90025; **Phone:** 310-828-4008; **Board Cert:** Obstetrics & Gynecology 1980; Reproductive Endocrinology 1983; **Med School:** Univ Tex Med Br, Galveston 1974; **Resid:** Obstetrics & Gynecology, Univ Tex Hosps 1977; **Fellow:** Reproductive Endocrinology, USC Med Ctr 1979

Paulson, Richard J MD [RE] - **Spec Exp:** Infertility-IVF; Infertility-Advanced Maternal Age; **Hospital:** LAC & USC Med Ctr, Good Samaritan Hosp - LA; **Address:** USC Fertility, 1127 Wilshire Blvd, Ste 1400, Los Angeles, CA 90017; **Phone:** 213-975-9990; **Board Cert:** Obstetrics & Gynecology 2011; Reproductive Endocrinology 2011; **Med School:** UCLA 1980; **Resid:** Obstetrics & Gynecology, Harbor-UCLA Med Ctr 1984; **Fellow:** Reproductive Endocrinology, LAC-USC Med Ctr 1986; **Fac Appt:** Prof ObG, USC Sch Med

Smikle, Collin B MD [RE] - **Spec Exp:** Infertility-IVF; Laparoscopic Surgery; Fertility Preservation in Cancer; **Hospital:** CA Pacific Med Ctr-Pacific Campus; **Address:** Laurel Fertility Care, 1700 California St, Ste 570, San Francisco, CA 94109; **Phone:** 415-673-9199; **Board Cert:** Obstetrics & Gynecology 2010; Reproductive Endocrinology/Infertility 2010; **Med School:** Yale Univ 1985; **Resid:** Obstetrics & Gynecology, Brigham & Women's Hosp 1989; **Fellow:** Reproductive Endocrinology, UCSF Med Ctr 1991

Reproductive Endocrinology

Soules, Michael R MD [RE] - **Spec Exp:** Infertility-IVF; Polycystic Ovarian Syndrome; Endometriosis; **Hospital:** Northwest Hosp - Seattle; **Address:** 1505 Westlake Ave N, Ste 400, Seattle, WA 98109; **Phone:** 206-301-5000; **Board Cert:** Obstetrics & Gynecology 2002; Reproductive Endocrinology 2002; **Med School:** UCLA 1972; **Resid:** Obstetrics & Gynecology, Univ Colorado Med Ctr 1976; **Fellow:** Reproductive Endocrinology, Duke Univ Hosp 1978; **Fac Appt:** Prof ObG, Univ Wash

Winer, Sharon A MD [RE] - **Spec Exp:** Hormonal Disorders; Infertility-IVF; Vaginitis; **Hospital:** Cedars-Sinai Med Ctr, Keck Med Ctr of USC (page 62); **Address:** 9400 Brighton Way, Ste 206, Beverly Hills, CA 90210-4709; **Phone:** 310-274-9100; **Board Cert:** Obstetrics & Gynecology 2010; Reproductive Endocrinology 2010; **Med School:** USC Sch Med 1978; **Resid:** Obstetrics & Gynecology, LAC-USC Med Ctr 1982; **Fellow:** Microsurgery, Hammersmith Hosp 1983; Reproductive Endocrinology, LAC-USC Med Ctr 1985; **Fac Appt:** Clin Prof ObG, USC Sch Med

Yee, Billy MD [RE] - **Spec Exp:** Infertility-IVF; Microsurgery; Laparoscopic Surgery; Hysteroscopic Surgery; **Hospital:** Long Beach Meml Med Ctr; **Address:** 13950 Milton Ave, Ste 100, Westminster, CA 92683; **Phone:** 714-702-3001; **Board Cert:** Obstetrics & Gynecology 2011; Reproductive Endocrinology 2011; **Med School:** UC Davis 1978; **Resid:** Obstetrics & Gynecology, LAC-USC Med Ctr 1982; **Fellow:** Reproductive Endocrinology, USC Med Ctr 1985; **Fac Appt:** Assoc Clin Prof ObG, UC Irvine

Cleveland Clinic

Every life deserves world class care.

Reproductive Endocrinology

Cleveland Clinic Ob/Gyn & Women's Health Institute is designed to meet the unique and changing medical needs of women from adolescence to mature adulthood. Our team offers coordinated and supportive care. *U.S. News & World Report* has ranked our gynecology program No. 3 in the country. Our physicians are nationally and internationally known, and many serve on leadership boards for professional physician societies.

Reproductive Endocrinology and Infertility Section physicians provide comprehensive evaluation for infertile couples. Treatments encompass all assisted reproductive technologies, including artificial insemination, ovulation induction, intracytoplasmic sperm injection, in vitro fertilization and reproductive surgery, including microsurgery (sterilization reversal) – both robotic and conventional – and advanced endoscopic techniques for problems such as stage IV endometriosis.

For maximum patient convenience, Cleveland Clinic's Fertility Center has several locations throughout the area. In vitro fertilization retrievals and transfers are performed at the Fertility Center at Beachwood, while initial fertility consultations and testing are available at Main Campus, the Beachwood Fertility Center, the Richard E. Jacobs Health Center in Avon, and the Solon, Strongsville and Twinsburg Family Health Centers. Telemed consults are also offered at Youngstown and night appointments offered at the Richard E. Jacobs Health Center in Avon.

Offering Same-Day Appointments
Call 800.274.2009.

Treatment Guides
Cleveland Clinic has developed comprehensive treatment guides for many diseases and conditions. To download our free treatment guides, visit clevelandclinic.org/treatmentguides.

Online Medical Second Opinion
Call 216.444.3223 or 800.223.2273 ext. 43223 or email eclevelandclinic@ccf.org.

Out-of-State Patients Assistance
Call 800.223.2273, ext. 55580 or email medicalconcierge@ccf.org.

Visit Us At:
clevelandclinic.org

Follow Us On:
Facebook
www.facebook.com/clevelandclinic

Twitter
@ClevelandClinic

You Tube
www.youtube.com/clevelandclinic

Health Hub
health.clevelandclinic.org

PROGRAM FOR IVF REPRODUCTIVE SURGERY AND INFERTILITY

About the Division of Reproductive Endocrinology and Infertility, Department of Obstetrics and Gynecology

The Division of Reproductive Endocrinology and Infertility offers the most advanced technology available to help infertile women and men realize their dreams of parenthood. The Division is highly experienced in all aspects of reproductive endocrinology, including the diagnosis and treatment of endometriosis, fibroids, problems with ovulation or sperm function, and recurring pregnancy loss. Its clinical staff includes seasoned technicians and physicians who have pioneered new innovations and been honored for their contributions to the field.

Patient-Centered Care

From the initial diagnosis through all stages of treatment, couples at NYU Langone Medical Center receive state-of-the-art, compassionate care tailored to their specific needs. After a comprehensive evaluation to determine the cause of infertility, couples are counseled on whether assisted reproduction is necessary.

In Vitro Fertilization (IVF)

When medical conditions prevent the sperm from reaching the egg, skilled physicians and laboratory staff at the Fertility Center assist patients with retrieving their eggs, insemination in the lab, and insertion back into the patient's uterus as embryos. Preimplantation Genetic Screening (PGS) at the Fertility Center offers tests for aneuploidy (an abnormal number of chromosomes). Some of the genetic disorders identified with PGS include cystic fibrosis, Down syndrome, hemophilia, Huntington's disease, Marfan's disease, muscular dystrophy and sickle cell anemia. State-of-the-art technology is also used to increase chances of delivery in some women with a history of recurrent miscarriage or previous IVF failures.

Complex Cases

The Center offers the most advanced care available for complex cases of infertility including those which may not have been successful in other centers and may even have been told there is no hope.

IVF for Male Factor Infertility

The Fertility Center provides male patients with experienced urologists who can provide expert fertility treatment. Men receive a complete evaluation, including a fertility history, physical exam, blood testing and semen analysis. Surgical treatment of male infertility is performed on-site at the Center's surgical suites on an outpatient basis and may include testicular biopsy, vasectomy reversal, epididymal tissue repair and varicose vein repair.

OBSTETRICS AND GYNECOLOGY

About the Department of Obstetrics and Gynecology
NYU Langone Medical Center provides comprehensive programs and services designed specifically for women, from primary care to highly specialized programs that are supported by sophisticated research and advanced training. We specialize in the following areas:

Fertility-Related Services
NYU Langone offers state-of-the-art programs in egg donation, egg freezing and wellness (acupuncture, mind/body, psychology and yoga). Diagnosis and treatment include ovulation induction, assisted reproductive technologies and surgical options that incorporate the latest endoscopic techniques. The Center also tests for genetic abnormalities, as well as for immunity and infectious diseases.

Gynecologic Oncology
The NCI-designated NYU Cancer Institute's Women's Cancer Program specializes in the treatment of cervical cancer, endometrial cancer, ovarian cancer, uterine cancer, vaginal cancer and vulvar cancer.

Maternal Fetal Medicine
Prenatal care for high-risk pregnancies and detailed consultations before, during and after pregnancy are offered. Special attention is given to multifetal pregnancies and to women who have other medical conditions that may complicate a pregnancy, such as diabetes, heart problems, high blood pressure and lupus.

Obstetrics
We offer a broad range of obstetrical services, including prenatal care that gives equal emphasis to the well-being of the mother and the fetus; fetal monitoring through ultrasound and other techniques; childbirth preparedness and breastfeeding classes; consultation for high-risk pregnancies, including treatment for women who have experienced recurrent pregnancy loss.

Specialty Services
In addition to routine gynecological care, we offer pelvic ultrasound; aspiration of breast cysts; evaluation of infertility (including the special needs of same-sex couples); colposcopy (a diagnostic evaluation of abnormal pap smears); LEEP (a loop electrosurgical procedure used to diagnose and treat cervical cancer); cryotherapy for vaginal warts; and bone density testing.

Urogynecology and Reconstructive Pelvic Surgery
Our urogynecologists treat all forms of incontinence and pelvic disorders; malformations of the reproductive tract found at birth, during childhood or in young adults; and conditions such as overactive bladder, urinary and/or fecal incontinence and pelvic organ prolapse.

The Best in American Medicine
www.CastleConnolly.com

Rheumatology

a subspecialty of Internal Medicine

An internist who treats diseases of joints, muscle, bones and tendons. This specialist diagnoses and treats arthritis, back pain, muscle strains, common athletic injuries and "collagen" diseases.

Training Required: Three years in internal medicine *plus* additional training and examination for certification in rheumatology.

RHEUMATOLOGY

New England

Albert, Daniel A MD [Rhu] - **Spec Exp:** Juvenile Arthritis; **Hospital:** Dartmouth - Hitchcock Med Ctr; **Address:** Dartmouth-Hitchcock Med Ctr, Dept Rheumatology, One Medical Center Drive, Lebanon, NH 03756; **Phone:** 603-650-8622; **Board Cert:** Internal Medicine 1977; Rheumatology 1980; **Med School:** NYU Sch Med 1974; **Resid:** Internal Medicine, NC Meml Hosp 1977; **Fellow:** Rheumatology, UCSD Med Ctr 1981; **Fac Appt:** Prof Med, Univ Pennsylvania

Coblyn, Jonathan S MD [Rhu] - **Spec Exp:** Rheumatoid Arthritis; Lupus/SLE; Vasculitis; Musculoskeletal Disorders; **Hospital:** Brigham and Women's Hosp (page 57), New England Bapt Hosp; **Address:** Brigham & Women's Hosp, Div Rheumatology, 75 Francis St, PBB-B3, Boston, MA 02115; **Phone:** 617-732-5347; **Board Cert:** Internal Medicine 1977; Rheumatology 1980; **Med School:** Johns Hopkins Univ 1974; **Resid:** Internal Medicine, Peter Bent Brigham Hosp 1976; Internal Medicine, Stanford Univ Hosps 1977; **Fellow:** Rheumatology, Peter Bent Brigham Hosp 1979; **Fac Appt:** Assoc Prof Med, Harvard Med Sch

Kay, Jonathan MD [Rhu] - **Spec Exp:** Rheumatoid Arthritis; Psoriatic Arthritis; Ankylosing Spondylitis; Nephrogenic Systemic Fibrosis; **Hospital:** UMass Memorial Med Ctr; **Address:** Rheumatology Ctr, UMass Meml Med Ctr-Meml Campus, 119 Belmont St, Worcester, MA 01605; **Phone:** 508-334-6273; **Board Cert:** Internal Medicine 1986; Rheumatology 1988; **Med School:** UCSF 1983; **Resid:** Internal Medicine, Hosp Univ Penn 1986; **Fellow:** Rheumatology/Immunology, Brigham & Womens Hosp 1989; **Fac Appt:** Prof Med, Univ Mass Sch Med

Massarotti, Elena M MD [Rhu] - **Spec Exp:** Lupus/SLE; Rheumatoid Arthritis; Psoriatic Arthritis; Gout; **Hospital:** Brigham and Women's Hosp (page 57); **Address:** Brigham & Women's Hosp, Div Rheumatology, PBB-B3, 75 Francis St, Boston, MA 02115; **Phone:** 617-732-6523; **Board Cert:** Internal Medicine 1989; Rheumatology 2000; **Med School:** Tufts Univ 1984; **Resid:** Internal Medicine, Tufts-New England Med Ctr 1987; **Fellow:** Rheumatology, Tufts-New England Med Ctr 1989; **Fac Appt:** Assoc Prof Med, Tufts Univ

McAlindon, Timothy E MD [Rhu] - **Spec Exp:** Arthritis; Autoimmune Rheumatic Disorders; **Hospital:** Tufts Med Ctr; **Address:** Tufts Med Ctr, Div Rheumatology, 800 Washington St, Box 599, Boston, MA 02111; **Phone:** 617-636-5990; **Board Cert:** Internal Medicine 2003; **Med School:** England, UK 1982; **Resid:** Internal Medicine, Torbay Hosp 1985; Internal Medicine, Southmead Hosp 1988; **Fellow:** Rheumatology, Bristol Royal Infirmary 1990; Rheumatology, St Thomas Hosp 1995; **Fac Appt:** Prof Med, Tufts Univ

Polisson, Richard P MD [Rhu] - **Spec Exp:** Rheumatoid Arthritis; Lupus/SLE; **Hospital:** Mass Genl Hosp; **Address:** Mass General Hospital, 55 Fruit St Yawkey Bldg - Ste 2C, Boston, MA 02114; **Phone:** 617-726-7938; **Board Cert:** Internal Medicine 1979; Rheumatology 1984; **Med School:** Duke Univ 1976; **Resid:** Internal Medicine, Duke Univ Med Ctr 1978; Internal Medicine, Natl Inst Hlth/NCI 1980; **Fellow:** Rheumatology, Mass Genl Hosp 1982; **Fac Appt:** Assoc Prof Med, Harvard Med Sch

Schoen, Robert T MD [Rhu] - **Spec Exp:** Rheumatoid Arthritis; Lyme Disease; Osteoporosis; **Hospital:** Yale-New Haven Hosp; **Address:** 60 Temple St, Ste 6A, New Haven, CT 06510-2716; **Phone:** 203-789-2255; **Board Cert:** Internal Medicine 1979; Rheumatology 1982; **Med School:** Columbia P&S 1976; **Resid:** Internal Medicine, Yale New Haven Hosp 1979; **Fellow:** Rheumatology, Brigham & Womens Hosp 1981; **Fac Appt:** Clin Prof Med, Yale Univ

Seton, Margaret P MD [Rhu] - **Spec Exp:** Paget's Disease of Bone; **Hospital:** Mass Genl Hosp; **Address:** Rheumatology Assocs, 55 Fruit St Yawkey Bldg - Ste 2C, Boston, MA 02114; **Phone:** 617-726-7938; **Board Cert:** Internal Medicine 1986; Rheumatology 2002; **Med School:** Med Coll VA 1980; **Resid:** Internal Medicine, Univ Hosp 1984; **Fellow:** Immunology, Mass Genl Hosp 1986; Rheumatology, Mass Genl Hosp 1991; **Fac Appt:** Asst Prof Med, Harvard Med Sch

Shadick, Nancy A MD [Rhu] - **Spec Exp:** Lyme Disease; Rheumatoid Arthritis; Osteoarthritis; **Hospital:** Brigham and Women's Hosp (page 57); **Address:** Brigham & Womens Hosp, Arthritis Ctr, Dept Rheumatology, 75 Francis St, Boston, MA 02115-6105; **Phone:** 617-732-5325; **Board Cert:** Internal Medicine 1989; Rheumatology 2002; **Med School:** NYU Sch Med 1986; **Resid:** Internal Medicine, Columbia-Presby Hosp 1989; **Fellow:** Rheumatology, Brigham & Womens Hosp 1992; **Fac Appt:** Asst Prof Med, Harvard Med Sch

Simms, Robert W MD [Rhu] - **Spec Exp:** Scleroderma; Rheumatoid Arthritis; Lyme Disease; **Hospital:** Boston Med Ctr; **Address:** Boston Univ Medical Center, 725 Albany St, Shapiro Center, Ste 7B, Boston, MA 02118; **Phone:** 617-638-4312; **Board Cert:** Internal Medicine 1985; Rheumatology 1988; **Med School:** Univ Rochester 1980; **Resid:** Internal Medicine, N Shore Hosp 1982; Internal Medicine, Brigham & Women's Hosp 1985; **Fellow:** Rheumatology, Boston Univ Med Ctr 1987; **Fac Appt:** Prof Med, Boston Univ

Tsokos, George MD [Rhu] - **Spec Exp:** Lupus/SLE; **Hospital:** Beth Israel Deaconess Med Ctr - Boston; **Address:** Beth Israel Deaconess Med Ctr, Dept Rheumatology, 110 Francis St, Ste 4B, Boston, MA 02215; **Phone:** 617-632-8658; **Board Cert:** Internal Medicine 1983; Diagnostic Lab Immunology 1986; Rheumatology 1984; **Med School:** Greece 1975; **Resid:** Internal Medicine, Natl Univ 1979; Immunology, Natl Inst of Hlth 1981; **Fellow:** Rheumatology, Natl Inst of Hlth 1983

Weinblatt, Michael E MD [Rhu] - **Spec Exp:** Rheumatoid Arthritis; **Hospital:** Brigham and Women's Hosp (page 57); **Address:** Brigham & Womens Hosp, Arthritis Ctr, 75 Francis St, Boston, MA 02115; **Phone:** 617-732-5331; **Board Cert:** Internal Medicine 1978; Rheumatology 1980; **Med School:** Univ MD Sch Med 1975; **Resid:** Internal Medicine, Univ Maryland Hosp 1978; **Fellow:** Rheumatology, Peter Bent Brigham Hosp 1980; **Fac Appt:** Prof Med, Harvard Med Sch

Mid Atlantic

Allman, Richard L MD [Rhu] - **Spec Exp:** Arthritis; **Hospital:** Albert Einstein Med Ctr; **Address:** 5401 Old York Rd Klein Bldg Fl 3 - Ste 331, Philadelphia, PA 19141; **Phone:** 215-456-8220; **Board Cert:** Internal Medicine 1987; Rheumatology 1974; **Med School:** Jefferson Med Coll 1969; **Resid:** Internal Medicine, Allentown State Hosp 1972; **Fellow:** Rheumatology, Tufts Med Ctr 1974; **Fac Appt:** Assoc Prof Med, Jefferson Med Coll

Belmont, H Michael MD [Rhu] - **Spec Exp:** Lupus/SLE; Antiphospholipid Syndrome (APS); Wegener's Granulomatosis; Rheumatoid Arthritis; **Hospital:** NYU Hosp For Joint Diseases (page 70), NYU Langone Med Ctr (page 68); **Address:** 333 E 30th St, Fl 4, MS 10016, New York, NY 10016; **Phone:** 646-501-7400 x7213; **Board Cert:** Internal Medicine 1983; Rheumatology 1986; **Med School:** Univ Pittsburgh 1980; **Resid:** Internal Medicine, Mt Sinai Hosp 1983; **Fellow:** Rheumatology, NYU/Bellevue Hosp 1985; **Fac Appt:** Assoc Prof Med, NYU Sch Med

Blume, Ralph S MD [Rhu] - **Spec Exp:** Vasculitis; Lupus/SLE; Rheumatoid Arthritis; **Hospital:** NY-Presby/Columbia Univ Med Ctr, NY (page 66); **Address:** 161 Fort Washington Ave, Ste 537, New York, NY 10032-3713; **Phone:** 212-305-5512; **Board Cert:** Internal Medicine 1972; Rheumatology 1974; **Med School:** Columbia P&S 1964; **Resid:** Internal Medicine, NY-Presby/Columbia Univ Med Ctr 1968; **Fellow:** Rheumatology, NY-Presby/Columbia Univ Med Ctr 1970; **Fac Appt:** Clin Prof Med, Columbia P&S

Rheumatology

Bunning, Robert D MD [Rhu] - **Spec Exp:** Exercise Physiology; Rheumatoid Arthritis; Musculoskeletal Disorders; **Hospital:** Natl Rehab Hosp; **Address:** MedStar Natl Rehab Hosp, 102 Irving St NW, Washington, DC 20010; **Phone:** 202-877-1660; **Board Cert:** Internal Medicine 1984; Rheumatology 1986; **Med School:** Univ Cincinnati 1979; **Resid:** Internal Medicine, Wash Hosp Ctr 1984; **Fellow:** Rheumatology, Wash Hosp Ctr 1983; **Fac Appt:** Asst Clin Prof Med, Geo Wash Univ

Buyon, Jill P MD [Rhu] - **Spec Exp:** Lupus/SLE in Pregnancy; Lupus/SLE in Menopause; **Hospital:** NYU Hosp For Joint Diseases (page 70), NYU Langone Med Ctr (page 68); **Address:** Ctr for Musculoskeletal Care, 333 E 38th St, New York, NY 10016; **Phone:** 646-501-7400; **Board Cert:** Internal Medicine 1981; Rheumatology 1984; **Med School:** Albert Einstein Coll Med 1978; **Resid:** Internal Medicine, Montefiore Med Ctr 1981; **Fellow:** Rheumatology, NYU Med Ctr 1983; **Fac Appt:** Prof Med, NYU Sch Med

Cupps, Thomas R MD [Rhu] - **Spec Exp:** Vasculitis; Hepatitis B-Immune Response; **Hospital:** Georgetown Univ Hosp; **Address:** 3800 Resevoir Rd NW, George Univ Hosp, Dept of Med, Pasquerilla Bldg, Ste 3004, Washington, DC 20007; **Phone:** 202-444-6200; **Board Cert:** Internal Medicine 1978; Allergy & Immunology 1981; **Med School:** Stanford Univ 1975; **Resid:** Internal Medicine, Strong Meml Hosp 1978; **Fellow:** Allergy & Immunology, Natl Inst Allergy & Inf Dis 1980; **Fac Appt:** Assoc Prof Med, Georgetown Univ

Farber, Martin S MD/PhD [Rhu] - **Hospital:** Sunnyview Hosp & Rehab Ctr, Ellis Hosp; **Address:** 124 Rosa Rd, Ste 381, Schenectady, NY 12308-2198; **Phone:** 518-386-3644; **Board Cert:** Internal Medicine 1982; Rheumatology 1984; **Med School:** Albert Einstein Coll Med 1979; **Resid:** Internal Medicine, Boston City Hosp 1982; **Fellow:** Rheumatology, Boston Univ Sch Med 1984; **Fac Appt:** Asst Clin Prof Med, Albany Med Coll

Fields, Theodore R MD [Rhu] - **Spec Exp:** Gout; Rheumatoid Arthritis; Osteoarthritis; **Hospital:** Hosp For Special Surgery (page 60), NY-Presby/Weill Cornell Med Ctr, NY (page 66); **Address:** 535 E 70th St, Fl 8, Ste 848F, New York, NY 10021-4872; **Phone:** 212-606-1286; **Board Cert:** Internal Medicine 1979; Rheumatology 1982; **Med School:** SUNY Downstate 1976; **Resid:** Internal Medicine, Nassau Co Med Ctr 1979; **Fellow:** Rheumatology, Univ Hosp 1982; **Fac Appt:** Clin Prof Med, Cornell Univ-Weill Med Coll

Gorevic, Peter D MD [Rhu] - **Spec Exp:** Autoimmune Disease; Amyloidosis/Joint Disease; Cryoglobulinemia; **Hospital:** Mount Sinai Med Ctr (page 64), Huntington Hosp (page 67); **Address:** 5 E 98th St Fl 11, New York, NY 10029; **Phone:** 212-241-1671; **Board Cert:** Internal Medicine 1973; Rheumatology 1976; Allergy & Immunology 1977; Diagnostic Lab Immunology 1986; **Med School:** NYU Sch Med 1970; **Resid:** Internal Medicine, NYU Med Ctr 1973; **Fellow:** Rheumatology, NYU Med Ctr 1975; Allergy & Immunology, NYU Med Ctr 1977; **Fac Appt:** Prof Med, Mount Sinai Sch Med

Gourley, Mark F MD [Rhu] - **Spec Exp:** Autoimmune Disease; Lupus/SLE; **Hospital:** Natl Inst of Hlth - Clin Ctr; **Address:** Natl Inst Hlth, 10 Center Drive Bldg 10 - rm 6N216F, Bethesda, MD 20892-1616; **Phone:** 301-451-6807; **Board Cert:** Internal Medicine 1988; Rheumatology 2002; **Med School:** Tulane Univ 1985; **Resid:** Internal Medicine, Univ Wisconsin Hosps 1988; **Fellow:** Rheumatology, Natl Inst Hlth 1996

Hochberg, Marc C MD [Rhu] - **Spec Exp:** Osteoporosis; Osteoarthritis; Rheumatoid Arthritis; **Hospital:** Univ of MD Med Ctr, Kernan Hosp; **Address:** Univ MD Sch Med, Div Rheum, 10 S Pine St, MSTF 8-34, Baltimore, MD 21201; **Phone:** 410-706-6474; **Board Cert:** Internal Medicine 1976; Rheumatology 1978; **Med School:** Johns Hopkins Univ 1973; **Resid:** Internal Medicine, Johns Hopkins Hosp 1975; **Fellow:** Rheumatology, Johns Hopkins Hosp 1977; **Fac Appt:** Prof Med, Univ MD Sch Med

Lahita, Robert G MD/PhD [Rhu] - **Spec Exp:** Lupus/SLE; Endocrinology & Joint Disorders; Immunodeficiency Disorders; Vasculitis; **Hospital:** Newark Beth Israel Med Ctr; **Address:** 201 Lyons Ave Fl 4, Newark, NJ 07112; **Phone:** 973-926-7472; **Board Cert:** Internal Medicine 2004; Rheumatology 2007; **Med School:** Jefferson Med Coll 1973; **Resid:** Internal Medicine, New York Hosp-Cornell 1976; **Fellow:** Rheumatology, Rockefeller Hosp 1978; **Fac Appt:** Prof Med, Mount Sinai Sch Med

Magid, Steven K MD [Rhu] - **Spec Exp:** Rheumatoid Arthritis; Osteoarthritis; Lyme Disease; Polymyalgia Rheumatica; **Hospital:** Hosp For Special Surgery (page 60); **Address:** 535 E 70th St, Fl 7, New York, NY 10021; **Phone:** 212-606-1060; **Board Cert:** Internal Medicine 1979; Rheumatology 1984; **Med School:** Cornell Univ-Weill Med Coll 1976; **Resid:** Internal Medicine, New York Hosp 1979; **Fellow:** Rheumatology, Hosp For Special Surgery 1981; **Fac Appt:** Clin Prof Med, Cornell Univ-Weill Med Coll

Manzi, Susan MD [Rhu] - **Spec Exp:** Lupus/SLE; Lupus/SLE in Women; **Hospital:** Western Penn Hosp, Allegheny General Hosp; **Address:** WPAHS-Lupus Ctr Excellence, 4815 Liberty Ave, Ste 222, Pittsburgh, PA 15224; **Phone:** 412-578-1152; **Board Cert:** Internal Medicine 1988; Rheumatology 2000; **Med School:** Univ Pittsburgh 1985; **Resid:** Internal Medicine, Duke Univ Med Ctr 1988; **Fellow:** Rheumatology, Univ Pittsburgh 1991; **Fac Appt:** Assoc Prof Med, Drexel Univ Coll Med

Medsger Jr, Thomas A MD [Rhu] - **Spec Exp:** Scleroderma; Raynaud's Disease; Polymyositis; Dermatomyositis; **Hospital:** UPMC Presby, Pittsburgh; **Address:** Arthritis & Autoimmunity Ctr, 3601 Fifth Ave Falk Med Bldg - Ste 2B, Pittsburgh, PA 15213; **Phone:** 412-647-6700; **Board Cert:** Internal Medicine 1972; Rheumatology 1972; **Med School:** Univ Pennsylvania 1962; **Resid:** Internal Medicine, Univ Pittsburgh 1968; **Fellow:** Rheumatology, Univ Pittsburgh 1966; Rheumatology, Univ Tenn Coll Med 1969; **Fac Appt:** Prof Med, Univ Pittsburgh

Mitnick, Hal J MD [Rhu] - **Spec Exp:** Rheumatoid Arthritis; Psoriatic Arthritis; Osteoporosis; Dermatomyositis; **Hospital:** NYU Langone Med Ctr (page 68); **Address:** 333 E 34th St, Ste 1C, New York, NY 10016-4977; **Phone:** 212-889-7217; **Board Cert:** Internal Medicine 1976; Rheumatology 1978; **Med School:** NYU Sch Med 1972; **Resid:** Internal Medicine, Bellevue Hosp 1976; **Fellow:** Rheumatology, NYU Med Ctr 1978; **Fac Appt:** Clin Prof Med, NYU Sch Med

Oddis, Chester V MD [Rhu] - **Spec Exp:** Polymyositis; Dermatomyositis; Connective Tissue Disorders; **Hospital:** UPMC Presby, Pittsburgh; **Address:** UPMC-Div Rheumatology, 3601 Fifth Ave Falk Med Bldg - Ste 2B, Pittsburgh, PA 15213; **Phone:** 412-647-6700; **Board Cert:** Internal Medicine 1983; Rheumatology 1986; **Med School:** Penn State Coll Med 1980; **Resid:** Internal Medicine, Hershey Med Ctr 1984; **Fellow:** Rheumatology, Univ Pittsburgh 1986; **Fac Appt:** Prof Med, Univ Pittsburgh

Paget, Stephen MD [Rhu] - **Spec Exp:** Rheumatoid Arthritis; Lupus/SLE; Vasculitis; Connective Tissue Disorders; **Hospital:** Hosp For Special Surgery (page 60); **Address:** 535 E 70th St Fl 7, New York, NY 10021; **Phone:** 212-606-1845; **Board Cert:** Internal Medicine 1974; Rheumatology 2009; **Med School:** SUNY Downstate 1971; **Resid:** Internal Medicine, Johns Hopkins Hosp 1973; **Fellow:** Rheumatology, Hosp Special Surg 1975; **Fac Appt:** Prof Med, Cornell Univ-Weill Med Coll

Petri, Michelle A MD [Rhu] - **Spec Exp:** Lupus/SLE; Antiphospholipid Syndrome (APS); Autoimmune Disease; **Hospital:** Johns Hopkins Hosp (page 61); **Address:** Jonhs Hopkins Lupus Ctr, Div Rheumatology, 1830 E Monument St, Ste 7500, Baltimore, MD 21205-2100; **Phone:** 410-955-9114; **Board Cert:** Internal Medicine 1983; Allergy & Immunology 1985; Rheumatology 1986; **Med School:** Harvard Med Sch 1980; **Resid:** Internal Medicine, Mass Genl Hosp 1983; **Fellow:** Allergy & Immunology, UCSF Med Ctr 1985; Rheumatology, UCSF Med Ctr 1986; **Fac Appt:** Prof Med, Johns Hopkins Univ

Rheumatology

Plotz, Paul MD [Rhu] - **Hospital:** Natl Inst of Hlth - Clin Ctr; **Address:** 50 S Drive Bldg 50 - rm 1503, Bethesda, MD 20814; **Phone:** 301-496-9904; **Board Cert:** Internal Medicine 1970; **Med School:** Harvard Med Sch 1963; **Resid:** Internal Medicine, Beth Israel Hosp 1965; **Fellow:** Rheumatology, Clin Ctr- NIH 1968

Rothenberg, Russell R MD [Rhu] - **Spec Exp:** Fibromyalgia; Lupus/SLE; Rheumatoid Arthritis; Preventive Medicine; **Hospital:** G Washington Univ Hosp; **Address:** 10215 Fernwood Rd, Ste 401, Bethesda, MD 20817; **Phone:** 301-571-2273; **Board Cert:** Internal Medicine 1980; Rheumatology 1982; **Med School:** Albany Med Coll 1977; **Resid:** Internal Medicine, LIJ Med Ctr 1980; **Fellow:** Rheumatology, Mt Sinai Med Ctr 1982; **Fac Appt:** Assoc Prof Med, Geo Wash Univ

Salmon, Jane E MD [Rhu] - **Spec Exp:** Lupus/SLE; Antiphospholipid Syndrome (APS); Rheumatoid Arthritis; **Hospital:** Hosp For Special Surgery (page 60); **Address:** 535 E 70th St, New York, NY 10021-4872; **Phone:** 212-606-1728; **Board Cert:** Internal Medicine 1981; Rheumatology 1984; **Med School:** Columbia P&S 1978; **Resid:** Internal Medicine, New York Hosp 1981; **Fellow:** Rheumatology, Hosp Special Surgery 1983; **Fac Appt:** Prof Med, Cornell Univ-Weill Med Coll

Schubert, Richard D MD [Rhu] - **Spec Exp:** Arthritis; **Hospital:** Sibley Mem Hosp, Georgetown Univ Hosp; **Address:** 3301 New Mexico Ave NW, Ste 348, Washington, DC 20016; **Phone:** 202-362-4467; **Board Cert:** Rheumatology 1978; Internal Medicine 1975; **Med School:** SUNY Downstate 1972; **Resid:** Internal Medicine, Peter Bent Brigham Hosp 1975; **Fellow:** Rheumatology, Peter Bent Brigham Hosp 1978; **Fac Appt:** Assoc Clin Prof Med, Georgetown Univ

Solitar, Bruce M MD [Rhu] - **Spec Exp:** Arthritis; Fibromyalgia; Reiter's Syndrome; Retroperitoneal Fibrosis; **Hospital:** NYU Langone Med Ctr (page 68), NYU Hosp For Joint Diseases (page 70); **Address:** 333 E 34th St, New York, NY 10016; **Phone:** 212-889-7217; **Board Cert:** Internal Medicine 2012; Rheumatology 2004; **Med School:** NYU Sch Med 1988; **Resid:** Internal Medicine, NYU/Bellevue Med Ctr 1992; **Fellow:** Rheumatology, NYU/Bellevue Med Ctr 1994; **Fac Appt:** Assoc Clin Prof Med, NYU Sch Med

Solomon, Gary MD [Rhu] - **Spec Exp:** Psoriatic Arthritis; Rheumatoid Arthritis; Autoimmune Disease; **Hospital:** NYU Hosp For Joint Diseases (page 70), NYU Langone Med Ctr (page 68); **Address:** Ctr for Musculoskeletal Care, 333 E 38th St, New York, NY 10016; **Phone:** 646-501-7400; **Board Cert:** Internal Medicine 1980; Rheumatology 1982; **Med School:** Mount Sinai Sch Med 1977; **Resid:** Internal Medicine, Mt Sinai Med Ctr 1980; **Fellow:** Rheumatology, Montefiore Med Ctr 1982; **Fac Appt:** Assoc Clin Prof Med, NYU Sch Med

Spiera, Harry MD [Rhu] - **Spec Exp:** Lupus/SLE; Scleroderma; Vasculitis; Behcet's Syndrome; **Hospital:** Mount Sinai Med Ctr (page 64), NY-Presby/Weill Cornell Med Ctr, NY (page 66); **Address:** Rheumatology Assocs, 1088 Park Ave, New York, NY 10128-1132; **Phone:** 212-860-4000 x2; **Board Cert:** Internal Medicine 1965; Rheumatology 1972; **Med School:** NYU Sch Med 1958; **Resid:** Internal Medicine, VA Med Ctr 1960; Internal Medicine, Mt Sinai Hosp 1961; **Fellow:** Rheumatology, Columbia-Presby Med Ctr 1963; **Fac Appt:** Clin Prof Med, Mount Sinai Sch Med

Starz, Terence W MD [Rhu] - **Spec Exp:** Arthritis; **Hospital:** UPMC Shadyside, UPMC St Margaret; **Address:** Arthritis & Int Medicine Assocs-UPMC, 3500 Fifth Ave Hieber Bldg Fl 4, Pittsburgh, PA 15213; **Phone:** 412-682-2434; **Board Cert:** Internal Medicine 1975; Rheumatology 1978; **Med School:** Jefferson Med Coll 1971; **Resid:** Internal Medicine, Presby-Univ Hosp 1975; **Fellow:** Rheumatology, Presby-Univ Hosp 1977; **Fac Appt:** Clin Prof Med, Univ Pittsburgh

Steen, Virginia MD [Rhu] - **Spec Exp:** Scleroderma; Lupus/SLE; Polymyositis; **Hospital:** Georgetown Univ Hosp; **Address:** 3800 Reservoir Rd NW, Pasquerilla Bldg, Ste 3004, Washington, DC 20007; **Phone:** 202-444-6200; **Board Cert:** Internal Medicine 1978; Rheumatology 1980; **Med School:** Univ Pittsburgh 1975; **Resid:** Internal Medicine, Hosp Univ Penn 1978; **Fellow:** Rheumatology, Presby Hosp 1980; **Fac Appt:** Prof Med, Georgetown Univ

Vivino, Frederick B MD [Rhu] - **Spec Exp:** Sjogren's Syndrome; **Hospital:** Penn Presby Med Ctr - UPHS (page 72); **Address:** Penn Rheumatology Assocs & Sjogren's Ctr, 3910 Powelton Ave Fl 2, Philadelphia, PA 19104; **Phone:** 215-662-4333; **Board Cert:** Internal Medicine 1986; Rheumatology 1988; **Med School:** Temple Univ 1983; **Resid:** Internal Medicine, Hosp Univ Penn 1986; **Fellow:** Rheumatology, Hosp Univ Penn 1989; **Fac Appt:** Assoc Clin Prof Med, Univ Pennsylvania

Weinstein, Arthur MD [Rhu] - **Spec Exp:** Lupus/SLE; Lyme Disease; Rheumatoid Arthritis; Gout; **Hospital:** Washington Hosp Ctr; **Address:** Washington Hospital Center, 110 Irving St NW, rm 2A-66, Washington, DC 20010; **Phone:** 202-877-0333; **Board Cert:** Rheumatology 1976; Diagnostic Lab Immunology 1986; **Med School:** Univ Toronto 1967; **Resid:** Internal Medicine, Toronto Genl Hosp 1972; Rheumatology, Hammersmith Hosp 1971; **Fellow:** Rheumatology, Toronto Wellesley Hosp 1973; **Fac Appt:** Prof Med, Georgetown Univ

Wigley, Frederick M MD [Rhu] - **Spec Exp:** Scleroderma; Raynaud's Disease; **Hospital:** Johns Hopkins Bayview Med Ctr (page 61), Johns Hopkins Hosp (page 61); **Address:** 5501 Hopkins Bayview Cir, Ste 1B32, Baltimore, MD 21224; **Phone:** 410-550-7715; **Board Cert:** Internal Medicine 1975; Rheumatology 1980; **Med School:** Univ Fla Coll Med 1972; **Resid:** Internal Medicine, Johns Hopkins Hosp 1975; **Fellow:** Rheumatology, Johns Hopkins Hosp 1979; **Fac Appt:** Prof Med, Johns Hopkins Univ

Southeast

Allen, Nancy B MD [Rhu] - **Spec Exp:** Vasculitis; Wegener's Granulomatosis; Lupus/SLE; Temporal Arteritis; **Hospital:** Duke Univ Hosp; **Address:** Duke Box 3440, 4140 Purple Zone Hosp South, 201 Trent Drive, Durham, NC 27710; **Phone:** 919-684-2965; **Board Cert:** Internal Medicine 1981; Rheumatology 1984; **Med School:** Tufts Univ 1978; **Resid:** Internal Medicine, Duke Univ Med Ctr 1981; **Fellow:** Rheumatology, Duke Univ Med Ctr 1983; **Fac Appt:** Prof Med, Duke Univ

Chatham, W Winn MD [Rhu] - **Spec Exp:** Lupus/SLE; Connective Tissue Disorders; Rheumatoid Arthritis; **Hospital:** Univ of Ala Hosp at Birmingham; **Address:** UAB Med Ctr, FOT Bldg, Ste 802, 1530 3rd Ave S, Birmingham, AL 35294-3408; **Phone:** 205-801-8191; **Board Cert:** Internal Medicine 1983; Rheumatology 1988; **Med School:** Vanderbilt Univ 1980; **Resid:** Internal Medicine, North Carolina Meml Hosp 1983; **Fellow:** Rheumatology, Univ Alabama Birmingham 1988; **Fac Appt:** Prof Med, Univ Alabama

Crofford, Leslie J MD [Rhu] - **Spec Exp:** Fibromyalgia; Rheumatoid Arthritis; Lupus/SLE; **Hospital:** Univ of Kentucky Albert B. Chandler Hosp; **Address:** 740 S Limestone St, rm J509, Lexington, KY 40536-0284; **Phone:** 859-323-6700; **Board Cert:** Internal Medicine 1987; Rheumatology 2003; **Med School:** Univ Tenn Coll Med 1984; **Resid:** Internal Medicine, Barnes/Wash Univ 1987; **Fellow:** Rheumatology, Natl Inst Hlth Clin Ctr 1992; **Fac Appt:** Prof Med, Univ KY Coll Med

Hadler, Nortin M MD [Rhu] - **Spec Exp:** Musculoskeletal Disorders; Occupational Musculoskeletal Disorders; Spondylitis; Pain-Back; **Hospital:** NC Memorial Hosp - UNC; **Address:** UNC,Div Rheumatology, 3330 Thurston Building, Box 7280, Chapel Hill, NC 27599-7280; **Phone:** 919-966-0566; **Board Cert:** Rheumatology 1974; Allergy & Immunology 1975; Internal Medicine 1987; **Med School:** Harvard Med Sch 1968; **Resid:** Internal Medicine, Mass Genl Hosp 1973; **Fellow:** Rheumatology, Natl Inst Hlth 1972; Allergy & Immunology, Clin Res Ctr 1974; **Fac Appt:** Prof Med, Univ NC Sch Med

Rheumatology

Kimberly, Robert P MD [Rhu] - **Spec Exp:** Lupus/SLE; Rheumatoid Arthritis; Vasculitis; Autoimmune Disease; **Hospital:** Univ of Ala Hosp at Birmingham; **Address:** University of Alabama at Birmingham, 1825 University Blvd, Shelby Bldg - Ste 172B, Birmingham, AL 35294; **Phone:** 205-934-0245; **Board Cert:** Internal Medicine 1976; Rheumatology 1978; **Med School:** Harvard Med Sch 1973; **Resid:** Internal Medicine, Hosp Univ Penn 1975; **Fellow:** Rheumatology, NIAMS, NIH 1977; Rheumatology, Hosp Special Surgery 1979; **Fac Appt:** Prof Med, Univ Alabama

Moore, Walter J MD [Rhu] - **Spec Exp:** Rheumatoid Arthritis; Lupus/SLE; **Hospital:** Med Coll of GA Hosp and Clin (MCG Health Inc); **Address:** Medical College of Georgia, 1120 15th St, rm BI 5083, Augusta, GA 30912; **Phone:** 706-721-2981; **Board Cert:** Internal Medicine 1980; Rheumatology 1984; **Med School:** Georgetown Univ 1977; **Resid:** Internal Medicine, Walter Reed AMC 1980; **Fellow:** Rheumatology, Walter Reed AMC 1983; **Fac Appt:** Assoc Prof Med, Med Coll GA

Sergent, John S MD [Rhu] - **Spec Exp:** Vasculitis; **Hospital:** Vanderbilt Univ Med Ctr (page 75); **Address:** Vanderbilt Rheumatology, 1301 Medical Center Drive, Ste 2501, Nashville, TN 27232; **Phone:** 615-322-1900; **Board Cert:** Internal Medicine 1972; Rheumatology 1974; **Med School:** Vanderbilt Univ 1966; **Resid:** Internal Medicine, Johns Hopkins Hosp 1968; Internal Medicine, Vanderbilt Univ Hosp 1972; **Fellow:** Rheumatology, Hosp Special Surgery 1974; **Fac Appt:** Prof Med, Vanderbilt Univ

Silver, Richard M MD [Rhu] - **Spec Exp:** Scleroderma & Lung Disease; Pediatric Rheumatology; Connective Tissue Disorders; **Hospital:** MUSC Med Ctr; **Address:** MUSC Med Ctr, 96 Jonathan Lucas St, Ste 912, Charleston, SC 29425; **Phone:** 843-876-0500; **Board Cert:** Internal Medicine 1978; Rheumatology 1982; **Med School:** Vanderbilt Univ 1975; **Resid:** Internal Medicine, Univ NC Hosps 1978; **Fellow:** Rheumatology, UCSD Med Ctr 1981; **Fac Appt:** Prof Med, Med Univ SC

Wise, Christopher M MD [Rhu] - **Spec Exp:** Gout; Sjogren's Syndrome; Rheumatoid Arthritis; **Hospital:** Med Coll of VA Hosp; **Address:** Virginia Commonwealth Univ/MCV Campus, Box 980647, Richmond, VA 23219; **Phone:** 804-828-9341; **Board Cert:** Internal Medicine 1980; Rheumatology 1982; **Med School:** Univ NC Sch Med 1977; **Resid:** Internal Medicine, Med Coll Virginia Hosp 1980; **Fellow:** Rheumatology, Med Coll Virginia Hosp 1982; **Fac Appt:** Prof Med, Va Commonwealth Univ Sch Med

Midwest

Adams, Elaine MD [Rhu] - **Spec Exp:** Rheumatoid Arthritis; Lupus/SLE; Spondyloarthropathies; **Hospital:** Loyola Univ Med Ctr, Edward Hines, Jr. VA Hosp; **Address:** Loyola Univ Med Ctr, Dept Rheumatology, 2160 S 1st Ave, Bldg 54 - rm 121, Maywood, IL 60153-5590; **Phone:** 708-216-8563; **Board Cert:** Internal Medicine 1981; Rheumatology 1984; **Med School:** Loyola Univ-Stritch Sch Med 1978; **Resid:** Internal Medicine, Loyola Univ Med Ctr 1981; **Fellow:** Rheumatology, Univ Wisconsin Med Ctr 1983; **Fac Appt:** Prof Med, Loyola Univ-Stritch Sch Med

Brasington, Richard MD [Rhu] - **Hospital:** Barnes-Jewish Hosp; **Address:** 660 S Euclid Ave, Box 8602, St Louis, MO 63110; **Phone:** 314-286-2635; **Board Cert:** Internal Medicine 1985; Rheumatology 1986; **Med School:** Duke Univ 1980; **Resid:** Internal Medicine, Univ Iowa Med Ctr 1982; Internal Medicine, Univ Iowa Med Ctr 1985; **Fellow:** Rheumatology, Univ Iowa 1986; **Fac Appt:** Assoc Prof Med, Washington Univ, St Louis

Chang, Rowland W MD [Rhu] - **Spec Exp:** Rheumatoid Arthritis; Arthritis; Ankylosing Spondylitis; **Hospital:** Rehab Inst of Chicago, Northwestern Meml Hosp; **Address:** Rehab Inst of Chicago Arthritis Ctr, 345 E Superior St Fl 3, Chicago, IL 60611-2654; **Phone:** 312-238-2784; **Board Cert:** Internal Medicine 1979; Rheumatology 1982; **Med School:** Tufts Univ 1976; **Resid:** Internal Medicine, Mt Auburn Hosp 1979; **Fellow:** Rheumatology, Hammersmith Hosp 1980; Rheumatology, Brigham & Womens Hosp 1982; **Fac Appt:** Prof Med, Northwestern Univ

Curran, James J MD [Rhu] - **Spec Exp:** Rheumatoid Arthritis; Polymyositis; Sjogren's Syndrome; Lupus/SLE; **Hospital:** Univ of Chicago Med Ctr; **Address:** 5841 S Maryland Ave, MS 093, Chicago, IL 60637-1463; **Phone:** 773-702-1232; **Board Cert:** Internal Medicine 1980; Rheumatology 1982; **Med School:** Univ IL Coll Med 1976; **Resid:** Internal Medicine, Bethesda Naval Hosp 1980; **Fellow:** Rheumatology, Univ Chicago Hosps 1982; **Fac Appt:** Prof Med, Univ Chicago-Pritzker Sch Med

Fife, Rose S MD [Rhu] - **Spec Exp:** Women's Health; Arthritis; **Hospital:** IU Health University Hosp; **Address:** IU Health Physicians Rheumatology, 550 N University Blvd, Ste 2180, Indianapolis, IN 46202; **Phone:** 317-944-7718; **Board Cert:** Internal Medicine 1978; Rheumatology 1982; **Med School:** Johns Hopkins Univ 1975; **Resid:** Internal Medicine, Johns Hopkins Hosp 1978; **Fellow:** Rheumatology, Univ Washington Med Ctr 1981; **Fac Appt:** Prof Med, Indiana Univ

Hugenberg, Steven T MD [Rhu] - **Spec Exp:** Rheumatoid Arthritis; Osteoarthritis; Psoriatic Arthritis; Ankylosing Spondylitis; **Hospital:** IU Health University Hosp; **Address:** IU Health Physicians Rheumatology, 550 N University Blvd, Ste 2180, Indianapolis, IN 46202; **Phone:** 317-944-7718; **Board Cert:** Internal Medicine 1985; Rheumatology 1988; **Med School:** Ohio State Univ 1982; **Resid:** Internal Medicine, Indiana Univ Med Ctr 1985; **Fellow:** Rheumatology, Indiana Univ Med Ctr 1987; **Fac Appt:** Assoc Prof Med, Indiana Univ

Katz, Robert S MD [Rhu] - **Spec Exp:** Rheumatoid Arthritis; Lupus/SLE; Fibromyalgia; Vasculitis; **Hospital:** Rush Univ Med Ctr, Northwestern Meml Hosp; **Address:** 1725 W Harrison St, Ste 365, Chicago, IL 60612-3841; **Phone:** 312-942-2159; **Board Cert:** Internal Medicine 1975; Rheumatology 1976; **Med School:** Univ MD Sch Med 1970; **Resid:** Internal Medicine, Washington Univ Med Ctr 1972; **Fellow:** Rheumatology, Johns Hopkins Hosp 1976; **Fac Appt:** Prof Med, Rush Med Coll

Langford, Carol MD [Rhu] - **Spec Exp:** Vasculitis; **Hospital:** Cleveland Clin (page 55); **Address:** Cleveland Clinic, 9500 Euclid Ave, Ste A50, Cleveland, OH 44195; **Phone:** 216-445-6056; **Board Cert:** Rheumatology 2000; **Med School:** UCLA 1987; **Resid:** Internal Medicine, Univ Mich Hosps & Med Ctr 1990; **Fellow:** Rheumatology, Duke Univ Med Ctr 1991

Luggen, Michael MD [Rhu] - **Hospital:** Univ Hosp - Cincinnati, Deaconess Hosp - Cincinnati; **Address:** 2123 Auburn Ave, Ste 630, Cincinnati, OH 45219; **Phone:** 513-585-1970; **Board Cert:** Internal Medicine 1978; Rheumatology 1982; **Med School:** Columbia P&S 1974; **Resid:** Internal Medicine, Cinn Genl Hosp 1977; **Fellow:** Rheumatology, Univ Cincinnati 1982; **Fac Appt:** Prof Med, Univ Cincinnati

Luthra, Harvinder Singh MD [Rhu] - **Spec Exp:** Rheumatoid Arthritis; Ankylosing Spondylitis; Relapsing Polychondritis; **Hospital:** St. Mary's Hosp - Rochester MN (Mayo), Rochester Methodist Hosp; **Address:** Mayo Clin, 200 First St SW, Rochester, MN 55905-0002; **Phone:** 507-266-4439; **Board Cert:** Internal Medicine 1973; Rheumatology 2002; **Med School:** India 1967; **Resid:** Ophthalmology, Christian Med Coll; Internal Medicine, Mount Sinai Hosp 1972; **Fellow:** Rheumatology, Mayo Grad Sch Affil Hosp 1974; **Fac Appt:** Prof Med, Mayo Med Sch

McCune, W Joseph MD [Rhu] - **Spec Exp:** Lupus/SLE; Rheumatoid Arthritis; **Hospital:** Univ of Michigan Hosp; **Address:** Univ Mich, Dept Rheumatology, 300 N Ingalls St, Ste 7C27, SPC 5422, Ann Arbor, MI 48109-0358; **Phone:** 734-647-5900; **Board Cert:** Internal Medicine 1978; Rheumatology 2011; **Med School:** Univ Cincinnati 1975; **Resid:** Internal Medicine, Univ Mich Hosps 1978; **Fellow:** Rheumatology, Brigham Womens Hosp 1981; **Fac Appt:** Prof Med, Univ Mich Med Sch

Rheumatology

Moder, Kevin G MD [Rhu] - **Spec Exp:** Rheumatoid Arthritis; Lupus/SLE; **Hospital:** Mayo Med Ctr & Clin - Rochester; **Address:** Mayo Clin, Div Rheumatology, 200 First St SW, Rochester, MN 55905-0002; **Phone:** 507-284-4550; **Board Cert:** Rheumatology 2000; **Med School:** Univ MO-Columbia Sch Med 1987; **Resid:** Internal Medicine, Mayo Clinic 1990; **Fellow:** Rheumatology, Mayo Clinic 1993; **Fac Appt:** Asst Prof Med, Mayo Med Sch

Pope, Richard M MD [Rhu] - **Spec Exp:** Rheumatoid Arthritis; Sjogren's Syndrome; Psoriatic Arthritis; **Hospital:** Northwestern Meml Hosp; **Address:** 675 N St Clair Fl 14 - Ste 100, Chicago, IL 60611-5966; **Phone:** 312-695-8628; **Board Cert:** Internal Medicine 1973; Rheumatology 1976; Clinical & Laboratory Immunology 1986; **Med School:** Loyola Univ-Stritch Sch Med 1970; **Resid:** Internal Medicine, Michael Reese Hosp 1972; **Fellow:** Rheumatology, Univ Wash Med Ctr 1974; **Fac Appt:** Prof Med, Northwestern Univ

Warner, Ann E MD [Rhu] - **Hospital:** St. Luke's Hosp of Kansas City; **Address:** 4330 Wornall St, Ste 40, Kansas City, MO 64111-3210; **Phone:** 816-531-0930; **Board Cert:** Internal Medicine 1986; Rheumatology 1988; **Med School:** Univ Kansas 1983; **Resid:** Internal Medicine, St Luke's Hosp 1986; **Fellow:** Rheumatology, Univ Kansas Med Ctr 1989; **Fac Appt:** Asst Clin Prof Med, Univ MO-Kansas City

Great Plains and Mountains

O'Dell, James R MD [Rhu] - **Spec Exp:** Osteoarthritis; Rheumatoid Arthritis; **Hospital:** Nebraska Med Ctr; **Address:** Durham Outpatient Center, 42nd & Emile St, Omaha, NE 68198-9500; **Phone:** 402-559-4015; **Board Cert:** Internal Medicine 1980; Rheumatology 1984; **Med School:** Univ Nebr Coll Med 1977; **Resid:** Internal Medicine, Univ Nebraska Med Ctr 1981; **Fellow:** Rheumatology, Univ Colorado 1984; **Fac Appt:** Prof Med, Univ Nebr Coll Med

West, Sterling G MD [Rhu] - **Spec Exp:** Lupus/SLE; Vasculitis; Osteoporosis; **Hospital:** Univ of CO Hosp - Anschutz Inpatient Pav; **Address:** Univ Colorado Rheumatology Practice, 1635 Aurora Court, MS F721, Box 6510, Aurora, CO 80045; **Phone:** 720-848-1940; **Board Cert:** Internal Medicine 1979; Rheumatology 2005; **Med School:** Emory Univ 1976; **Resid:** Internal Medicine, Fitzsimons Army Med Ctr 1979; **Fellow:** Rheumatology, Walter Reed Army Med Ctr 1981; **Fac Appt:** Prof Med, Univ Colorado

Southwest

Chang-Miller, April MD [Rhu] - **Spec Exp:** Spondyloarthritis-Consult; Inflammatory Arthritis-Consult; **Hospital:** Mayo Clinic - Scottsdale; **Address:** 13400 E Shea Blvd, Scottsdale, AZ 85259; **Phone:** 480-301-4342; **Board Cert:** Internal Medicine 1986; Rheumatology 2000; **Med School:** Yale Univ 1983; **Resid:** Internal Medicine, Mayo Clinic 1985; **Fellow:** Rheumatology, Mayo Clinic 1989; Biochemical and Molecular Biology, Mayo Clinic 1990; **Fac Appt:** Asst Prof Med, Mayo Med Sch

Davis, William Eugene MD [Rhu] - **Spec Exp:** Lupus/SLE; Rheumatoid Arthritis; Gout; **Hospital:** Ochsner Med Ctr-New Orleans; **Address:** Ochsner Clinic, 1514 Jefferson Hwy, Rheumatology Fl 5, New Orleans, LA 70121-2483; **Phone:** 504-842-3920; **Board Cert:** Internal Medicine 1987; Rheumatology 1988; **Med School:** Louisiana State U, New Orleans 1983; **Resid:** Internal Medicine, Ochsner Fdn Hosp 1986; **Fellow:** Rheumatology, Univ Michigan 1988

Lindsey, Stephen M MD [Rhu] - **Spec Exp:** Osteoporosis; Rheumatoid Arthritis; **Hospital:** Ochsner Med Ctr-Baton Rouge; **Address:** Ochsner Hlth Ctr, 9001 Summa Ave, Baton Rouge, LA 70809; **Phone:** 225-761-5481; **Board Cert:** Internal Medicine 1975; Rheumatology 1980; **Med School:** Louisiana State U, New Orleans 1972; **Resid:** Internal Medicine, Letterman AMC 1975; **Fellow:** Rheumatology, Walter Reed AMC 1979; **Fac Appt:** Clin Prof Med, Louisiana State U, New Orleans

Lipstate, James M MD [Rhu] - **Spec Exp:** Arthritis; Osteoporosis; **Hospital:** Our Lady of Lourdes Reg Med Ctr - Lafayette, Lafayette Genl Med Ctr; **Address:** Lafayette Arthritis & Endocrine Clinic, 401 Audubon Blvd, Ste 102B, Lafayette, LA 70503; **Phone:** 337-237-7801; **Board Cert:** Internal Medicine 1983; Rheumatology 1986; **Med School:** Tulane Univ 1980; **Resid:** Internal Medicine, Univ Alabama Hosp 1983; **Fellow:** Rheumatology, Univ Alabama 1986; **Fac Appt:** Asst Clin Prof Med, Louisiana State U, New Orleans

Mayes, Maureen D MD [Rhu] - **Spec Exp:** Scleroderma; **Hospital:** Meml Hermann Hosp - Texas Med Ctr, LBJ General Hosp; **Address:** UT Physicians, Rheumatology, 6410 Fannin St, Ste 450, Houston, TX 77030-1501; **Phone:** 713-486-3100; **Board Cert:** Internal Medicine 1980; Rheumatology 1982; **Med School:** Eastern VA Med Sch 1976; **Resid:** Internal Medicine, Cleveland Clinic 1979; **Fellow:** Rheumatology, Cleveland Clinic 1981; **Fac Appt:** Prof Med, Univ Tex, Houston

Sessoms, Sandra L MD [Rhu] - **Spec Exp:** Arthritis; Lupus/SLE; Autoimmune Disease; **Hospital:** Methodist Hosp - Houston; **Address:** 7501 Fannin St, Univ General Hosp Bldg, Ste 730, Houston, TX 77054; **Phone:** 713-790-0102; **Board Cert:** Internal Medicine 1981; Rheumatology 1984; **Med School:** Baylor Coll Med 1978; **Resid:** Internal Medicine, Baylor Affil Hosp 1979; **Fellow:** Rheumatology, Baylor Coll Med 1983; **Fac Appt:** Assoc Prof Med, Baylor Coll Med

West Coast and Pacific

Bobrove, Arthur M MD [Rhu] - **Spec Exp:** Psoriatic Arthritis; Ankylosing Spondylitis; Rheumatoid Arthritis; Lupus/SLE; **Hospital:** Stanford Univ Hosp & Clinics; **Address:** 795 El Camino Real, Palo Alto, CA 94301; **Phone:** 650-853-2083; **Board Cert:** Internal Medicine 1972; Rheumatology 1976; **Med School:** Temple Univ 1967; **Resid:** Internal Medicine, Univ Mich Hosp 1969; Internal Medicine, Univ Mich Hosp 1972; **Fellow:** Immunology, Stanford Univ Hosp 1974; **Fac Appt:** Clin Prof Med, Stanford Univ

Clements, Philip J MD [Rhu] - **Spec Exp:** Scleroderma; Raynaud's Disease; **Hospital:** UCLA Ronald Reagan Med Ctr; **Address:** UCLA Sch Med, Rehab 32-59, 1000 Veteran Ave, Los Angeles, CA 90095-1670; **Phone:** 310-825-8414; **Board Cert:** Internal Medicine 1972; Rheumatology 1974; **Med School:** Indiana Univ 1965; **Resid:** Internal Medicine, Cedars-Sinai Med Ctr 1971; **Fellow:** Rheumatology, UCLA Med Ctr 1974; **Fac Appt:** Prof Med, UCLA

Ehresmann, Glenn R MD [Rhu] - **Spec Exp:** Rheumatoid Arthritis; Scleroderma; Rehabilitation for Rheumatic Diseases; Lupus/SLE; **Hospital:** Keck Med Ctr of USC (page 62); **Address:** 1520 San Pablo St, Ste 1000, Los Angeles, CA 90033; **Phone:** 323-442-5100; **Board Cert:** Internal Medicine 1977; Rheumatology 1978; **Med School:** UC Irvine 1973; **Resid:** Internal Medicine, LAC-USC Med Ctr 1976; **Fellow:** Rheumatology, LAC-USC Med Ctr 1978; **Fac Appt:** Assoc Prof Med, USC-Keck School of Medicine

Rheumatology

Gershwin, Merrill E MD [Rhu] - **Spec Exp:** Allergy; Rheumatoid Arthritis; **Hospital:** UC Davis Med Ctr; **Address:** UC Davis Sch Med, Div Rheum, 451 Health Sciences Drive, Ste 6510, Davis, CA 95616; **Phone:** 530-752-2884; **Board Cert:** Internal Medicine 1974; Rheumatology 1976; Allergy & Immunology 1979; **Med School:** Stanford Univ 1971; **Resid:** Internal Medicine, Tufts-New Eng Med Ctr 1972; Allergy & Immunology, Tufts-New Eng Med Ctr 1973; **Fellow:** Rheumatology, Natl Inst Hlth 1975; Allergy & Immunology, Natl Inst Hlth 1977; **Fac Appt:** Prof Med, UC Davis

Lawry II, George Vance MD [Rhu] - **Spec Exp:** Gout; Rheumatoid Arthritis; Vasculitis; **Hospital:** UC Irvine Med Ctr; **Address:** UC Irvine Med Ctr, 101 The City Drive S Fl 4, South Orange, CA 92868; **Phone:** 714-456-7662; **Board Cert:** Internal Medicine 1978; Rheumatology 1982; **Med School:** Johns Hopkins Univ 1975; **Resid:** Internal Medicine, Mass Genl Hosp 1977; Internal Medicine, Stanford Hosp 1978; **Fellow:** Rheumatology, Wadsworth VA-UCLA Med Ctr 1981; **Fac Appt:** Clin Prof Med, Univ Iowa Coll Med

Mease, Philip J MD [Rhu] - **Spec Exp:** Arthritis; Autoimmune Disease; Osteoporosis; **Hospital:** Swedish Med Ctr-First Hill-Seattle, Swedish Med Ctr-Cherry Hill Campus; **Address:** 1101 Madison St, Ste 1000, Seattle, WA 98104; **Phone:** 206-386-2000; **Board Cert:** Internal Medicine 1980; Rheumatology 1982; **Med School:** Stanford Univ 1977; **Resid:** Internal Medicine, Univ Wash Med Ctr 1981; **Fellow:** Rheumatology, Univ Wash Med Ctr 1982; **Fac Appt:** Clin Prof Med, Univ Wash

Peng, Stanford L MD [Rhu] - **Spec Exp:** Lupus/SLE; Inflammatory Arthritis; Scleroderma; Vasculitis; **Hospital:** Virginia Mason Med Ctr; **Address:** Virginia Mason, 1100 9th Ave, Ste X6-RHE, Seattle, WA 98101; **Phone:** 206-223-6824; **Board Cert:** Rheumatology 2002; **Med School:** Yale Univ 1997; **Resid:** Internal Medicine, Univ Penn Hosp 1999; **Fellow:** Rheumatology, Brigham & Women's Hosp 2002

Wallace, Daniel J MD [Rhu] - **Spec Exp:** Lupus/SLE; Rheumatoid Arthritis; Scleroderma; **Hospital:** Cedars-Sinai Med Ctr, UCLA Ronald Reagan Med Ctr; **Address:** 8737 Beverly Blvd, Ste 302, Los Angeles, CA 90048-1828; **Phone:** 310-652-0920; **Board Cert:** Internal Medicine 1978; Rheumatology 1982; **Med School:** USC Sch Med 1974; **Resid:** Internal Medicine, Cedars-Sinai Med Ctr 1977; **Fellow:** Rheumatology, UCLA Med Ctr 1979; **Fac Appt:** Clin Prof Med, UCLA

Wener, Mark MD [Rhu] - **Spec Exp:** Lupus/SLE; Vasculitis; Scleroderma; Autoimmune Disease; **Hospital:** Univ Wash Med Ctr, Harborview Med Ctr; **Address:** Univ Washington Med Ctr, Medical Specialties, 1959 NE Pacific St, Box 356166, Seattle, WA 98195; **Phone:** 206-598-4615; **Board Cert:** Internal Medicine 1978; Rheumatology 1980; Clinical & Laboratory Immunology 1986; **Med School:** Washington Univ, St Louis 1974; **Resid:** Internal Medicine, Univ Iowa Hosps 1978; **Fellow:** Rheumatology, Univ Iowa Hosp 1980; Immunology, Univ Washington Med Ctr 1981; **Fac Appt:** Prof Med, Univ Wash

Wofsy, David MD [Rhu] - **Spec Exp:** Rheumatoid Arthritis; Lupus/SLE; Autoimmune Disease; Clinical Trials; **Hospital:** VA Med Ctr - San Francisco, UCSF Med Ctr; **Address:** 533 Parnassus Ave, Box 0633, San Francisco, CA 94143-0633; **Phone:** 415-750-2104; **Board Cert:** Internal Medicine 1977; Rheumatology 1980; **Med School:** UCSD 1974; **Resid:** Internal Medicine, UCSF Hosps 1977; **Fellow:** Rheumatology, UCSF 1979; **Fac Appt:** Prof Med, UCSF

Cleveland Clinic

Every life deserves world class care.

Rheumatology

Cleveland Clinic's Department of Rheumatic and Immunologic Diseases has a long-standing commitment to excellence and innovation in the research and care of patients with illnesses such as arthritis, osteoporosis and vasculitis. Since 1993, *U.S. News & World Report* has consistently ranked it among the nation's top 10 rheumatology programs.

Arthritis: Our department's Arthritis & Musculoskeletal Center is a multidisciplinary clinic combining the expertise of non-operative orthopaedists and rheumatologists in one location for patients with joint pain. Our doctors have a specific interest in joint pain problems, including rheumatoid arthritis and osteoarthritis, and work together to provide patients with the highest level of care so that they can return to their usual level of activity.

Osteoporosis: Our Center for Osteoporosis and Metabolic Bone Diseases is devoted to the evaluation and treatment of patients with osteoporosis and other diseases that affect bones. The Center's goal is to evaluate patients at an early stage to prevent the complications and additional disease manifestations of osteoporosis and other treatable diseases.

Vasculitis: Cleveland Clinic's Center for Vasculitis Care and Research aims to ensure the best possible care for patients with vasculitis, discover the causes of these diseases, identify improved therapies and alleviate discomfort. The department has established extensive collaborations with other Cleveland Clinic departments to bring complementary skills to both patient care and research.

Autoimmune Disease: Our Department of Rheumatic and Immunologic Diseases also provides expert care for autoimmune diseases, such as systemic lupus, scleroderma, myositis, polychondritis and vasculitis.

Cleveland Clinic
Rheumatic and Immunologic Diseases
9500 Euclid Avenue
Cleveland, OH 44195

Offering Same-Day Appointments
Call 800.274.2009.

Treatment Guides
Cleveland Clinic has developed comprehensive treatment guides for many diseases and conditions. To download our free treatment guides, visit clevelandclinic.org/treatmentguides.

Online Medical Second Opinion
Call 216.444.3223 or 800.223.2273 ext. 43223 or email eclevelandclinic@ccf.org.

Out-of-State Patients Assistance
Call 800.223.2273, ext. 55580 or email medicalconcierge@ccf.org.

Visit Us At:
clevelandclinic.org

Follow Us On:
Facebook
www.facebook.com/clevelandclinic

Twitter
@ClevelandClinic

You Tube
www.youtube.com/clevelandclinic

Health Hub
health.clevelandclinic.org

HOSPITAL FOR JOINT DISEASES

About the Hospital for Joint Diseases
The Hospital for Joint Diseases at NYU Langone Medical Center (HJD) is one of the nation's leading inpatient orthopaedic and rheumatologic specialty hospitals, and is ranked among the nation's top 10 for both orthopaedics and rheumatology in the 2012-2013 *U.S. News & World Report* annual survey of "Best Hospitals" in America. HJD is dedicated to the prevention and treatment of musculoskeletal diseases, providing some of the most advanced programs in the region for musculoskeletal disorders and the largest pediatric orthopaedic program in New York City. HJD also offers a number of unique and highly specialized services to provide tailored, world-class care to patients with specific musculoskeletal conditions and needs. We specialize in the following areas:

Orthopaedic Surgery
The clinical expertise of our internationally-renowned surgeons represents the full range of subspecialty areas of orthopaedic surgery, including Adult Reconstructive, Sports Medicine, Spine, Shoulder & Elbow, Foot & Ankle, Hand Surgery, Trauma & Fracture, Orthopaedic Oncology, and Pediatric Orthopaedics; additional areas of focus include minimally-invasive hip surgery and robotic-assisted joint replacement.

Rheumatology
HJD houses the Division of Rheumatology's Osteoporosis Center, offering a multidisciplinary approach to the evaluation and treatment of osteoporosis, including a range of advanced drug therapies.

Rehabilitation
Rehabilitation care at HJD is provided by the world-renowned Rusk Rehabilitation. Rusk's CARF-Accredited Brain Injury Rehabilitation Program is a center of innovation and excellence for the treatment of disabling neurological and neurocognitive disorders. HJD also houses Rusk's Orthopaedic Rehabilitation Unit, where an expert multidisciplinary rehabilitation team aids patients in their recovery after orthopaedic surgery or injury.

Neurology – Spine & Nerve
HJD provides a broad range of diagnostic and therapeutic services to patients with neurological disorders. Its outstanding clinical staff includes specialists in pain management, spine and nerve pain, and cerebral palsy.

Radiology
HJD provides complete diagnostic orthopaedic radiology services, including MRI, computed tomography, ultrasonography and conventional radiography, as well as a multitude of musculoskeletal interventional procedures. The medical team includes several internationally-known musculoskeletal radiologists with expertise in all aspects of osteoradiology.

RHEUMATOLOGY

Rheumatologists at NYU Langone Medical Center are dedicated to the diagnosis and treatment of patients with rheumatic illnesses, particularly autoimmune diseases. *U.S. News and World Report* has repeatedly recognized the Division of Rheumatology as one of the best in the country, ranking #7 nationwide in the 2012-2013 "Best Hospitals" survey. The division provides care at NYU Langone's premier outpatient facility, The Center for Musculoskeletal Care; the internationally-renowned, inpatient Hospital for Joint Diseases; and at the medical center's Tisch Hospital.

Arthritis and Autoimmunity: We offer a comprehensive program for the prevention, diagnosis and treatment of all rheumatologic conditions. Patients also have access to complete rheumatologic evaluations, orthopaedic and neurological consultative services, and participation in clinical trials using the most advanced interventional therapies, highly sophisticated diagnostic testing, and complementary medicine.

Behçet's Syndrome: We have the largest North American Behçet's Center for research and the evaluation and treatment of patients with Behçet's Syndrome, a disease that involves inflammation of the blood vessels.

Biological Treatment: Biological treatments for inflammatory arthritis, rheumatoid arthritis, lupus, psoriatic arthritis, vasculitis, and osteoporosis are administered by the Medical Center's infusion centers.

Lupus: The Center for Lupus Care and Research is devoted to the treatment and research of patients with this autoimmune disease. Patients have access to world renowned specialists in lupus, lupus and pregnancy, and related sub-specialties.

Osteoporosis: We offer comprehensive care for the prevention, evaluation and treatment of osteoporosis, including state-of-the art bone densitometers, a range of advanced drug therapies, and programs in balance training and exercise.

Psoriatic Arthritis: Patients at the Psoriatic Arthritis Center, a collaborative effort with the Department of Dermatology, are seen by both a rheumatologist and dermatologist who specialize in psoriasis and psoriatic arthritis.

We are also leaders in rheumatology research, focusing on the study of drugs, drug delivery systems and protocols, and the roles genes play in the development and treatment of rheumatic diseases, positioning us at the forefront of basic science and translational research, personalized medicine and the genetics of rheumatic diseases. The Peter D. Seligman Center for Advanced Therapeutics, renowned for breakthrough research in arthritis and Systematic Lupus Erythematosus, conducts clinical studies using a wide variety of newly developed therapies.

The Best in American Medicine
www.CastleConnolly.com

Sports Medicine

a subspecialty of Internal Medicine, Family Practice, Pediatrics, Physical Medicine & Rehabilitation, or Orthopaedics

A specialist trained to be responsible for continuous care in the field of sports medicine, not only for the enhancement of health and fitness, but also for the prevention of injury and illness. A sports medicine physician must have knowledge and experience in the promotion of wellness and the prevention of injury. Knowledge about special areas of medicine such as exercise physiology, biomechanics, nutrition, psychology, physical rehabilitation, epidemiology, physical evaluation, injuries (treatment and prevention and referral practice) and the role of exercise in promoting a healthy life style are essential to the practice of sports medicine. The sports medicine physician requires special education to provide the knowledge to improve the healthcare of the individual engaged in physical exercise (sports) whether as an individual or in team participation.

Training Required: Three years in internal medicine, family practice, or pediatrics or seven years in orthopaedics *plus* additional training and examination for certification in sports medicine.

For more information about the main specialties of these physicians, see **Internal Medicine, Family Practice, Pediatrics, Physical Medicine & Rehabilitation, Orthopaedics** section(s).

SPORTS MEDICINE

New England

Asnis, Peter MD [SM] - **Spec Exp:** Arthroscopic Surgery-Hip; Shoulder Injuries; Rotator Cuff Surgery; Ligament Reconstruction; **Hospital:** Mass Genl Hosp; **Address:** Massachusetts General Hospital, 175 Cambridge St Fl 4, Yawkey 3200, Boston, MA 02114; **Phone:** 617-643-0803; **Board Cert:** Orthopaedic Surgery 2008; **Med School:** Cornell Univ-Weill Med Coll 1999; **Resid:** Orthopaedic Surgery, Hosp Special Surg 2005; **Fellow:** Orthopaedic Sports Medicine, Mass Genl Hosp 2006

Gill IV, Thomas J MD [SM] - **Spec Exp:** Knee Injuries; Shoulder Injuries; Arthroscopic Surgery; **Hospital:** Mass Genl Hosp; **Address:** MGH Sports Medicine Ctr, 175 Cambridge St Fl 4, CPZS 4, Boston, MA 02114-2723; **Phone:** 617-726-7797; **Board Cert:** Orthopaedic Surgery 2011; **Med School:** Harvard Med Sch 1990; **Resid:** Orthopaedic Surgery, Hosp Special Surgery 1992; Orthopaedic Surgery, Brigham & Women's Hosp 1996; **Fellow:** Sports Medicine, Steadman Hawkins Clinic 1998; **Fac Appt:** Assoc Prof OrS, Harvard Med Sch

Micheli, Lyle J MD [SM] - **Spec Exp:** Pediatric Sports Medicine; Dance/Ballet Injuries; Ostechondritis Dissecans (OCD); Knee Injuries/ACL; **Hospital:** Children's Hospital - Boston, Beth Israel Deaconess Med Ctr - Boston; **Address:** Chldns Hosp, Div Sports Medicine, 319 Longwood Ave, Boston, MA 02115; **Phone:** 617-355-3501; **Board Cert:** Orthopaedic Surgery 1973; **Med School:** Harvard Med Sch 1966; **Resid:** Surgery, Univ Hosps 1968; Orthopaedic Surgery, Mass Genl Hosp/Chldns Hosp 1972; **Fellow:** Pediatric Orthopaedic Surgery, Orth Rsch Soc-Traveling 1973; **Fac Appt:** Assoc Clin Prof OrS, Harvard Med Sch

Scheller, Arnold D MD [SM] - **Spec Exp:** Sports Injuries; Ankle Surgery; Shoulder Surgery; Knee Surgery; **Hospital:** New England Bapt Hosp; **Address:** Pro Sports Orthopaedics, 840 Winter St, Waltham, MA 02451; **Phone:** 781-487-9444; **Board Cert:** Orthopaedic Surgery 1980; **Med School:** Rush Med Coll 1973; **Resid:** Orthopaedic Surgery, New England Hosp 1983; **Fac Appt:** Asst Clin Prof OrS, Tufts Univ

Steiner, Mark E MD [SM] - **Spec Exp:** Shoulder Injuries; Knee Injuries; Arthroscopic Surgery; **Hospital:** New England Bapt Hosp; **Address:** 830 Boylston St, Ste 205, Chestnut Hill, MA 02467; **Phone:** 617-739-2003; **Board Cert:** Orthopaedic Surgery 2008; Orthopaedic Sports Medicine 2011; **Med School:** Columbia P&S 1978; **Resid:** Surgery, Mass General Hosp 1980; Orthopaedic Surgery, Mass General Hosp 1984; **Fellow:** Sports Medicine, U Oklahoma Med Ctr 1985

Mid Atlantic

Altchek, David MD [SM] - **Spec Exp:** Shoulder Surgery; Elbow Surgery; Knee Surgery; Arthroscopic Surgery; **Hospital:** Hosp For Special Surgery (page 60), NY-Presby/Weill Cornell Med Ctr, NY (page 66); **Address:** Hospital for Special Surgery, 535 E 70th St, New York, NY 10021; **Phone:** 212-606-1909; **Board Cert:** Orthopaedic Surgery 2011; **Med School:** Cornell Univ-Weill Med Coll 1982; **Resid:** Orthopaedic Surgery, Hosp for Special Surg 1987; **Fellow:** Sports Medicine, Hosp for Special Surg 1988; **Fac Appt:** Assoc Prof OrS, Cornell Univ-Weill Med Coll

Bradley, James Philip\p MD [SM] - **Spec Exp:** Reconstructive Surgery; Shoulder Surgery; Knee Surgery; **Hospital:** UPMC St Margaret, UPMC Shadyside; **Address:** 200 Delafield Rd, Ste 4010, Pittsburgh, PA 15215; **Phone:** 412-784-5770; **Board Cert:** Orthopaedic Surgery 2011; **Med School:** Georgetown Univ 1982; **Resid:** Surgery, Univ Tennessee Affil Hosp 1984; Orthopaedic Surgery, Univ Hlth Ctr 1987; **Fellow:** Sports Medicine, Kerlan-Jobe Ortho Clinic 1988; **Fac Appt:** Clin Prof OrS, Univ Pittsburgh

Burke, Charles J MD [SM] - **Spec Exp:** Knee Injuries; Shoulder Injuries; **Hospital:** UPMC St Margaret, UPMC Shadyside; **Address:** 200 Delafield Rd, Ste 4010, Pittsburgh, PA 15215; **Phone:** 412-784-5779; **Board Cert:** Orthopaedic Surgery 2009; **Med School:** Univ Cincinnati 1981; **Resid:** Therapeutic Radiology, Univ Mass Med Ctr 1983; Orthopaedic Surgery, Univ Pittsburgh Med Ctr 1986; **Fac Appt:** Asst Prof OrS, Univ Pittsburgh

Ciccotti, Michael G MD [SM] - **Spec Exp:** Knee Reconstruction; Elbow Reconstruction; Shoulder Reconstruction; Arthroscopic Surgery; **Hospital:** Thomas Jefferson Univ Hosp, Bryn Mawr Hosp; **Address:** Rothman Inst, 925 Chestnut St Fl 5, Philadelphia, PA 19107; **Phone:** 800-321-9999; **Board Cert:** Orthopaedic Surgery 2005; **Med School:** Georgetown Univ 1986; **Resid:** Orthopaedic Surgery, Thos Jefferson Univ Med Ctr 1991; **Fellow:** Sports Medicine, Kerlan-Jobe Clinic/USC 1992; **Fac Appt:** Assoc Prof OrS, Jefferson Med Coll

Harner, Christopher D MD [SM] - **Spec Exp:** Knee Injuries; **Hospital:** UPMC South Side-Out Pt Ctr; **Address:** UPMC Ctr for Sports Med, 3200 S Water St, Pittsburgh, PA 15203; **Phone:** 412-432-3661; **Board Cert:** Orthopaedic Surgery 2010; Orthopaedic Sports Medicine 2007; **Med School:** Univ Mich Med Sch 1981; **Resid:** Orthopaedic Surgery, Univ Pittsburgh 1986; **Fellow:** Sports Medicine/Knee Surgery, Salt Lake City Knee & Sport 1987; **Fac Appt:** Prof OrS, Univ Pittsburgh

Hershman, Elliott MD [SM] - **Spec Exp:** Knee Injuries; Knee Surgery; Arthroscopic Surgery; Ligament Reconstruction; **Hospital:** Lenox Hill Hosp (page 67); **Address:** 130 E 77th St Fl 7, New York, NY 10075; **Phone:** 212-744-8114; **Board Cert:** Orthopaedic Surgery 2008; **Med School:** Univ Rochester 1979; **Resid:** Orthopaedic Surgery, Lenox Hill Hosp 1984; **Fellow:** Sports Medicine, Cleveland Clin 1985; **Fac Appt:** Asst Clin Prof OrS, Mount Sinai Sch Med

Levine, William N MD [SM] - **Spec Exp:** Arthroscopic Surgery; Shoulder & Elbow Surgery; Knee Injuries; **Hospital:** NY-Presby/Columbia Univ Med Ctr, NY (page 66); **Address:** 622 W 168th St, Fl PH-11, rm 1117, New York, NY 10032; **Phone:** 212-305-0762; **Board Cert:** Orthopaedic Surgery 2010; Orthopaedic Sports Medicine 2008; **Med School:** Case West Res Univ 1990; **Resid:** Surgery, Beth Israel Hosp 1991; Orthopaedic Surgery, New Eng Med Ctr Hosps 1995; **Fellow:** Shoulder Surgery, Columbia-Presby Med Ctr 1996; Sports Medicine, Univ MD Med Ctr 1998; **Fac Appt:** Clin Prof OrS, Columbia P&S

Metzl, Jordan D MD [SM] - **Spec Exp:** Adolescent Sports Medicine; Running Injuries; Dance/Ballet Injuries; **Hospital:** Hosp For Special Surgery (page 60); **Address:** 519 E 72nd St, Ste 206, New York, NY 10021; **Phone:** 212-606-1678; **Board Cert:** Sports Medicine 2011; **Med School:** Univ MO-Columbia Sch Med 1993; **Resid:** Pediatrics, Tufts-New Engl Med Ctr 1996; **Fellow:** Sports Medicine, Vanderbilt Univ Med Ctr 1997; Sports Medicine, Harvard Med Sch 1998; **Fac Appt:** Assoc Prof Ped, Cornell Univ-Weill Med Coll

Nisonson, Barton MD [SM] - **Spec Exp:** Shoulder & Knee Surgery; Arthroscopic Surgery; Knee Replacement; **Hospital:** Lenox Hill Hosp (page 67); **Address:** 130 E 77th St Fl 8, New York, NY 10021-1851; **Phone:** 212-570-9120; **Board Cert:** Orthopaedic Surgery 1974; **Med School:** Columbia P&S 1966; **Resid:** Surgery, Columbia-Presby Med Ctr 1968; Orthopaedic Surgery, Columbia-Presby Med Ctr 1973

Sports Medicine

Rodeo, Scott A MD [SM] - **Spec Exp:** Knee Injuries; Cartilage Damage; **Hospital:** Hosp For Special Surgery (page 60); **Address:** Hosp for Special Surgery, 535 E 70th St, New York, NY 10021; **Phone:** 212-606-1513; **Board Cert:** Orthopaedic Surgery 2009; Orthopaedic Sports Medicine 2007; **Med School:** Cornell Univ-Weill Med Coll 1989; **Resid:** Orthopaedic Surgery, Hosp Special Surgery 1994; **Fellow:** Sports Medicine, Hosp Special Surgery 1996; **Fac Appt:** Assoc Clin Prof OrS, Cornell Univ-Weill Med Coll

Sennett, Brian J MD [SM] - **Spec Exp:** Arthroscopic Surgery; Cartilage Damage; Sports Injuries; Upper Extremity Trauma; **Hospital:** Hosp Univ Penn - UPHS (page 72); **Address:** Penn Sports Medicine Center, Weightman Hall, Fl 1, 235 S 33rd St, Philadelphia, PA 19104; **Phone:** 215-662-3340; **Board Cert:** Orthopaedic Surgery 2009; Orthopaedic Sports Medicine 2008; **Med School:** Univ Pennsylvania 1988; **Resid:** Orthopaedic Surgery, Hosp Univ Penn 1993; **Fellow:** Sports Medicine, Univ Penn Sports Med Ctr 1994; Hand Surgery, Hosp Univ Penn 1994; **Fac Appt:** Assoc Prof OrS, Univ Pennsylvania

Williams, Riley J MD [SM] - **Spec Exp:** Cartilage Damage & Transplant; Shoulder Arthroscopic Surgery; Knee Injuries/ACL; Knee Surgery; **Hospital:** Hosp For Special Surgery (page 60), NY-Presby/Weill Cornell Med Ctr, NY (page 66); **Address:** Hosp Special Surgery, 535 E 70th St Fl Blair 1, New York, NY 10021; **Phone:** 212-606-1855; **Board Cert:** Orthopaedic Sports Medicine 2009; **Med School:** Stanford Univ 1992; **Resid:** Orthopaedic Surgery, Hosp Special Surgery 1997; **Fellow:** Sports Medicine & Shoulder Surgery, Hosp Special Surgery 1998; **Fac Appt:** Assoc Prof OrS, Cornell Univ-Weill Med Coll

Southeast

Andrews, James R MD [SM] - **Spec Exp:** Shoulder Surgery; Elbow Surgery; Knee Surgery; **Hospital:** Baptist Hosp - Pensacola, St. Vincent's Hosp - Birmingham; **Address:** Inst Orthopaedics & Sports Medicine, 1040 Gulf Breeze Pkwy, Gulf Breeze, FL 32561; **Phone:** 850-916-8700; **Board Cert:** Orthopaedic Surgery 1974; **Med School:** Louisiana State U, New Orleans 1967; **Resid:** Orthopaedic Surgery, USPHS Hosp 1969; Orthopaedic Surgery, Touro Infirm-Tulane 1970; **Fellow:** Orthopaedic Sports Medicine, Univ Va Med Ctr 1972; **Fac Appt:** Clin Prof OrS, Univ Alabama

Byrd, J.W. Thomas MD [SM] - **Spec Exp:** Arthroscopic Surgery; Hip Surgery; **Hospital:** Baptist Hosp - Nashville; **Address:** Nashville Sports Med & Ortho Ctr, 2011 Church St, Ste 100, Nashville, TN 37203; **Phone:** 615-284-5800; **Board Cert:** Orthopaedic Surgery 2011; Orthopaedic Sports Medicine 2007; **Med School:** Vanderbilt Univ 1982; **Resid:** Orthopaedic Surgery, Univ Louisville Hosp 1987; **Fellow:** Sports Medicine, Amer Sprts Inst 1988; Joint Replacement Surgery, New England Baptist Hosp 1989

Garth Jr, William P MD [SM] - **Spec Exp:** Knee Ligament Reconstruction; Shoulder Reconstruction; **Hospital:** Univ of Ala Hosp at Birmingham, Children's Hospital - Birmingham; **Address:** UAB Sports Medicine, 1600 7th Ave S, Ste 402, Birmingham, AL 35233-1711; **Phone:** 205-934-1041; **Board Cert:** Orthopaedic Surgery 1980; Orthopaedic Sports Medicine 2007; **Med School:** Tulane Univ 1973; **Resid:** Surgery, Duke Univ Hosp 1975; Orthopaedic Surgery, Campbell Clinic 1979; **Fellow:** Sports Medicine, Sports Med Clinic 1984; **Fac Appt:** Prof OrS, Univ Alabama

Taft, Timothy N MD [SM] - **Spec Exp:** Sports Medicine; Knee Injuries/ACL; Shoulder Surgery; **Hospital:** NC Memorial Hosp - UNC; **Address:** 3154 Bioinformatics Bldg, 130 Mason Farm Rd, Chapel Hill, NC 27599; **Phone:** 919-962-6637; **Board Cert:** Orthopaedic Surgery 1976; **Med School:** Univ MO-Columbia Sch Med 1969; **Resid:** Orthopaedic Surgery, UNC Hosps 1974; Orthopaedic Surgery, N Carolina Ortho Hosp 1972; **Fac Appt:** Prof OrS, Univ NC Sch Med

Xerogeanes, John W MD [SM] - **Spec Exp:** Knee Surgery; Shoulder Surgery; Knee Injuries/ACL; Arthroscopic Surgery; **Hospital:** Emory Univ Hosp; **Address:** Emory Sports Medicine Ctr, 59 Executive Park S, Ste 1000, Atlanta, GA 30329; **Phone:** 404-778-3350; **Board Cert:** Orthopaedic Surgery 2012; Orthopaedic Sports Medicine 2008; **Med School:** Emory Univ 1992; **Resid:** Orthopaedic Surgery, Univ Pittsburgh Med Ctr 1997; **Fellow:** Sports Medicine, Steadman-Hawkins Clinic 1998; **Fac Appt:** Assoc Prof OrS, Emory Univ

Midwest

Arendt, Elizabeth A MD [SM] - **Spec Exp:** Sports Medicine; Knee Ligament Reconstruction; Knee Injuries; **Hospital:** Univ Minn Med Ctr, Fairview - Riverside Campus; **Address:** Univ Minn Med Ctr-Fairview, 2450 Riverside Ave S, R102, MMC 88, Minneapolis, MN 55454; **Phone:** 612-273-9400; **Board Cert:** Orthopaedic Surgery 2008; Orthopaedic Sports Medicine 2007; **Med School:** Univ Rochester 1979; **Resid:** Surgery, Univ Rochester Med Ctr 1981; Orthopaedic Surgery, Univ Rochester Med Ctr 1984; **Fellow:** Sports Medicine, Univ Minn Med Ctr 1985; **Fac Appt:** Prof OrS, Univ Miss

Bush-Joseph, Charles MD [SM] - **Spec Exp:** Knee Reconstruction; Cartilage Damage; Sports Medicine; Rotator Cuff Surgery; **Hospital:** Rush Univ Med Ctr, Rush Oak Park Hosp; **Address:** Midwest Orthopaedics at Rush, 1611 W Harrison St, Ste 400, Chicago, IL 60612; **Phone:** 312-243-4244; **Board Cert:** Orthopaedic Surgery 2003; Orthopaedic Sports Medicine 2007; **Med School:** Univ Mich Med Sch 1983; **Resid:** Orthopaedic Surgery, Rush Med Ctr 1988; **Fellow:** Sports Medicine, Cincinnati Sports Med Ctr 1989; **Fac Appt:** Prof OrS, Rush Med Coll

Ho, Sherwin S W MD [SM] - **Spec Exp:** Shoulder & Knee Surgery; Arthroscopic Surgery; Cartilage Damage; **Hospital:** Univ of Chicago Med Ctr; **Address:** Univ Chicago Dept Surgery, 5841 S Maryland Ave, MC 3079, Chicago, IL 60637-3079; **Phone:** 773-702-5978; **Board Cert:** Orthopaedic Surgery 2005; Orthopaedic Sports Medicine 2008; **Med School:** Univ Hawaii JA Burns Sch Med 1985; **Resid:** Orthopaedic Surgery, Univ Hawaii Med Ctr 1991; **Fellow:** Sports Medicine, Univ Chicago 1992; **Fac Appt:** Assoc Prof S, Univ Chicago-Pritzker Sch Med

Miniaci, Anthony MD [SM] - **Spec Exp:** Shoulder Reconstruction; Shoulder Arthroscopic Surgery; Knee Reconstruction; Cartilage Damage; **Hospital:** Cleveland Clin (page 55); **Address:** Cleveland Clinic, Sports Hlth Ctr, 5555 Transportation Blvd, Garfield Heights, OH 44125; **Phone:** 216-518-3444; **Med School:** Univ Western Ontario 1982; **Resid:** Orthopaedic Surgery, Univ Western Ontario 1987; **Fellow:** Sports Medicine, Kerlan-Jobe Orthopaedic Clin 1989; Orthopaedic Research, Univ Calgary 1990; **Fac Appt:** Prof S, Case West Res Univ

Paletta, George A MD [SM] - **Spec Exp:** Ankle Surgery; Knee Surgery; Shoulder & Elbow Surgery; **Address:** The Orthopedic Ctr of St Louis, 14825 N Outer Forty Rd, Ste 200, Chesterfield, MO 63017; **Phone:** 314-336-2555; **Board Cert:** Orthopaedic Surgery 2009; **Med School:** Johns Hopkins Univ 1988; **Resid:** Orthopaedic Surgery, Cornell Univ Med Ctr 1994; **Fellow:** Sports Medicine, Cleveland Clin Fnd 1995; Pediatric Sports Medicine, Chldns Hosp Michigan; **Fac Appt:** Assoc Prof OrS, Washington Univ, St Louis

Great Plains and Mountains

Saint-Phard, Deborah MD [SM] - **Spec Exp:** Sports Medicine-Women; Spinal Rehabilitation; **Hospital:** Univ of CO Hosp - Anschutz Inpatient Pav; **Address:** Univ Sports Med, 2000 S Colorado Blvd, Ste 4500, Denver, CO 80222; **Phone:** 720-848-8200; **Board Cert:** Physical Medicine & Rehabilitation 2007; Pain Medicine 2004; Sports Medicine 2008; **Med School:** Temple Univ 1992; **Resid:** Physical Medicine & Rehabilitation, Univ Colorado Med Ctr 1996; **Fellow:** Sports Medicine, Mayo Clin 1997; **Fac Appt:** Assoc Prof PMR, Univ Colorado

Sports Medicine

Southwest

Jones, Deryk G MD [SM] - **Spec Exp:** Arthroscopic Surgery; Cartilage Damage & Transplant; **Hospital:** Ochsner Med Ctr-Kenner; **Address:** Ochsner Sports Medicine, 1201 S Clearview Pkwy, Ste 104, Jefferson, LA 70121; **Phone:** 504-736-4800; **Board Cert:** Orthopaedic Surgery 2011; Orthopaedic Sports Medicine 2009; **Med School:** Stanford Univ 1991; **Resid:** Orthopaedic Surgery, Harvard Combined Prog 1997; **Fellow:** Sports Medicine, Univ Pittsburgh Med Ctr 1998; **Fac Appt:** Asst Clin Prof OrS, Tulane Univ

West Coast and Pacific

Fronek, Jan MD [SM] - **Spec Exp:** Knee Injuries; Shoulder Injuries; Arthroscopic Surgery; Rotator Cuff Surgery; **Hospital:** Scripps Green Hosp; **Address:** Scripps Clinic, 10666 N Torrey Pines Rd, La Jolla, CA 92037; **Phone:** 858-554-9753; **Board Cert:** Orthopaedic Surgery 2009; Orthopaedic Sports Medicine 2011; **Med School:** Univ Rochester 1978; **Resid:** Orthopaedic Surgery, UCSD Med Ctr 1984; **Fellow:** Sports Medicine, Hosp Special Surgery 1985

Gambardella, Ralph A MD [SM] - **Spec Exp:** Cartilage Damage; Shoulder & Elbow Surgery; Knee Surgery; **Hospital:** Marina Del Rey Hosp, White Memorial Med Ctr; **Address:** Kerlan-Jobe Clinic, 6801 Park Terr, Ste 400, Los Angeles, CA 90045; **Phone:** 310-665-7200; **Board Cert:** Orthopaedic Surgery 1985; **Med School:** USC Sch Med 1977; **Resid:** Orthopaedic Surgery, USC Med Ctr 1982; **Fellow:** Sports Medicine, Southwestern Ortho Grp 1983; **Fac Appt:** Assoc Clin Prof S, USC Sch Med

Ma, C Benjamin MD [SM] - **Spec Exp:** Shoulder Surgery; Knee Surgery; Arthroscopic Surgery; **Hospital:** UCSF Med Ctr; **Address:** Sports Medicine Center, 1500 Owens St, San Francisco, CA 94158; **Phone:** 415-353-2808; **Board Cert:** Orthopaedic Surgery 2005; Orthopaedic Sports Medicine 2008; **Med School:** Johns Hopkins Univ 1996; **Resid:** Orthopaedic Surgery, Univ Pittsburgh Med Ctr 2002; **Fellow:** Shoulder Surgery, Hosp for Special Surg 2003; Macular Disease, Hosp for Special Surg 2003

Mirzayan, Raffy MD [SM] - **Spec Exp:** Arthroscopic Surgery; Shoulder & Elbow Surgery; Ligament Reconstruction; Knee Injuries; **Hospital:** Kaiser Permanente Baldwin Pk Med Ctr; **Address:** Kaiser Permanente Med Ctr, Orthopaedics, 1011 Baldwin Park Blvd, Baldwin Park, CA 91706; **Phone:** 626-851-5256; **Board Cert:** Orthopaedic Surgery 2003; Sports Medicine 2007; **Med School:** USC Sch Med 1995; **Resid:** Orthopaedic Surgery, LAC/USC Med Ctr 2000; **Fellow:** Sports Medicine, Kerlan Jobe Ortho Clin 2001; **Fac Appt:** Clin Prof OrS, USC-Keck School of Medicine

Schechter, David L MD [SM] - **Spec Exp:** Pain-Back; Sports Injuries; Muscle Pain-Stress Related; **Hospital:** Cedars-Sinai Med Ctr; **Address:** 8500 Wilshire Blvd, Ste 705, Beverly Hills, CA 90211; **Phone:** 310-657-1022; **Board Cert:** Family Medicine 2008; Sports Medicine 2003; **Med School:** NYU Sch Med 1984; **Resid:** Family Medicine, UCLA/Santa Monica Hosp 1987; **Fac Appt:** Assoc Clin Prof FMed, USC Sch Med

Teitz, Carol C MD [SM] - **Spec Exp:** Sports Injuries; Musculoskeletal Injuries in Dancers; Foot & Ankle Surgery; Knee Surgery; **Hospital:** Univ Wash Med Ctr; **Address:** University of Washington, Box 354060, Seattle, WA 98195; **Phone:** 206-543-1552; **Board Cert:** Orthopaedic Surgery 1981; Orthopaedic Sports Medicine 2007; **Med School:** Yale Univ 1974; **Resid:** Orthopaedic Surgery, Univ Wash Affil Hosps 1980; **Fellow:** Arthroscopic Surgery, J McGinty MD, Newton-Wellesley Hosp 1983; **Fac Appt:** Prof OrS, Univ Wash

Cleveland Clinic

Every life deserves world class care.

Sports Health

Cleveland Clinic Sports Health brings together top orthopaedic surgeons, primary care sports medicine physicians, physical therapists, athletic trainers, nutritionists, radiologists and exercise physiologists to keep athletes in the game and get injured players back on the field sooner.

All athletes deserve the best sports-related care and treatment that is focused, one-on-one and state-of-the art.

At Cleveland Clinic Sports Health, our experts treat athletes in all sports and at all ages and skill levels.

Our comprehensive services include rehabilitation and injury prevention, athletic training, imaging, nutrition, evaluation and management for sports-related concussions, injury treatment and help in improving performance. Our staff is involved in research every day to discover new treatments to improve the patient care of tomorrow.

Our world-renowned team of physicians is trained in diagnosing and treating the unique problems of amateur to high-performance athletes. We've provided the physicians for Cleveland's professional sports teams for more than 25 years.

Athletic Performance
Sports Rehabilitation and Injury Prevention Programs offer services such as motion analysis, injury prevention, sport-specific evaluations and rehabilitation programs — all tailored to particular sports.

Cleveland Clinic Sports Health is dedicated to building performance and strives to provide athletes with advanced understanding of body mechanics and capabilities that are as unique as each athlete. Performance Training Services are strength-building and functional fitness training programs designed to meet the goals of each athlete.

The Best in American Medicine
www.CastleConnolly.com

Surgery

A surgeon manages a broad spectrum of surgical conditions affecting almost any area of the body. The surgeon establishes the diagnosis and provides the preoperative, operative and postoperative care to surgical patients and is usually responsible for the comprehensive management of the trauma victim and the critically ill surgical patient.

The surgeon uses a variety of diagnostic techniques, including endoscopy, for observing internal structures and may use specialized instruments during operative procedures. A general surgeon is expected to be familiar with the salient features of other surgical specialties in order to recognize problems in those areas and to know when to refer a patient to another specialist.

Training Required: Five years

For a description of the subspecialty **Hand Surgery**, **Pediatric Surgery** and **Vascular Surgery** see the corresponding section(s).

SURGERY

New England

Ashley, Stanley W MD [S] - **Spec Exp:** Gastrointestinal Cancer & Surgery; **Hospital:** Brigham and Women's Hosp (page 57), Dana-Farber Cancer Inst (page 57); **Address:** Brigham & Womens Hosp, Dept Surgery, 75 Francis St ASBII Bldg Fl 3, Boston, MA 02115; **Phone:** 617-732-6730; **Board Cert:** Surgery 2004; Surgical Critical Care 1999; **Med School:** Cornell Univ-Weill Med Coll 1981; **Resid:** Surgery, Barnes Jewish Med Ctr 1989; **Fac Appt:** Prof S, Harvard Med Sch

Becker, James M MD [S] - **Spec Exp:** Inflammatory Bowel Disease; Gastrointestinal Cancer; Gastrointestinal Surgery; **Hospital:** Newton - Wellesley Hosp, Mass Genl Hosp; **Address:** 2014 Washington St Green Bldg - Ste 563, Newton, MA 02462; **Phone:** 617-219-1285; **Board Cert:** Surgery 2010; **Med School:** Case West Res Univ 1975; **Resid:** Surgery, Univ Utah Med Ctr 1980; **Fellow:** Research, Mayo Clinic 1982; **Fac Appt:** Prof S, Boston Univ

Brooks, David C MD [S] - **Spec Exp:** Gastrointestinal Surgery; **Hospital:** Brigham and Women's Hosp (page 57); **Address:** Brigham & Women's Hospital, Dept Surgery, 75 Francis St, ASB II Fl 3, Boston, MA 02115; **Phone:** 617-732-6337; **Board Cert:** Surgery 2003; **Med School:** Brown Univ 1976; **Resid:** Surgery, Brigham & Women's Hosp 1983; **Fac Appt:** Assoc Prof S, Harvard Med Sch

Burke, Peter A MD [S] - **Spec Exp:** Trauma; Critical Care; **Hospital:** Boston Med Ctr; **Address:** Carl & Ruth Shapiro Ambulatory Care Ctr, 725 Albany St Fl 3, Boston, MA 02118; **Phone:** 617-414-8056; **Board Cert:** Surgery 2011; Surgical Critical Care 2001; **Med School:** Tufts Univ 1983; **Resid:** Surgery, New England Deaconess Med Ctr 1990; **Fac Appt:** Prof S, Boston Univ

Callery, Mark P MD [S] - **Spec Exp:** Pancreatic Cancer; Liver Cancer; Laparoscopic Surgery; **Hospital:** Beth Israel Deaconess Med Ctr - Boston; **Address:** Beth Israel Deaconess Med Ctr, 330 Brookline Ave Shapiro Bldg Fl 3, Boston, MA 02215; **Phone:** 617-667-3798; **Board Cert:** Surgery 2004; **Med School:** Albany Med Coll 1985; **Resid:** Surgery, Albany Med Coll Hosp 1987; Surgery, Barnes Jewish Med Ctr 1992; **Fellow:** Research, Wash Univ Sch Med 1990; **Fac Appt:** Assoc Prof S, Harvard Med Sch

Cioffi, William G MD [S] - **Spec Exp:** Liver & Biliary Cancer; Trauma; Critical Care; Esophageal Cancer; **Hospital:** Rhode Island Hosp, Miriam Hosp; **Address:** Rhode Island Hosp, Dept Surg, 2 Dudley St, Ste 470, Providence, RI 02905; **Phone:** 401-553-8348; **Board Cert:** Surgery 2007; Surgical Critical Care 2008; **Med School:** Univ VT Coll Med 1981; **Resid:** Surgery, Medical Ctr Hosp 1986; **Fac Appt:** Prof S, Brown Univ

Cusack Jr, James C MD [S] - **Spec Exp:** Gastrointestinal Cancer; Colon & Rectal Cancer; Melanoma; Merkel Cell Carcinoma; **Hospital:** Mass Genl Hosp; **Address:** Mass Genl Hosp, Div Surgical Oncology, 55 Fruit St, Yawkey Bldg - Fl 7, Boston, MA 02114-2621; **Phone:** 617-724-4093; **Board Cert:** Surgery 2011; **Med School:** Emory Univ 1986; **Resid:** Surgery, Tufts-New England Med Ctr 1991; **Fellow:** Surgery, Brigham & Women's Hosp 1992; Surgical Oncology, MD Anderson Cancer Ctr 1992; **Fac Appt:** Assoc Prof S, Harvard Med Sch

Cushing, Brad M MD [S] - **Spec Exp:** Trauma; Critical Care; **Hospital:** Maine Med Ctr; **Address:** Maine Medical Partners Surgical Assocs, 22 Bram Hall, Portland, ME 04102-3113; **Phone:** 207-774-2381; **Board Cert:** Surgery 2005; Surgical Critical Care 2003; **Med School:** Univ Rochester 1980; **Resid:** Surgery, St Francis Hosp 1985; **Fellow:** Trauma/Critical Care, Univ Maryland 1987; **Fac Appt:** Clin Prof S, Univ VT Coll Med

Doherty, Gerard M MD [S] - **Spec Exp:** Endocrine Surgery; Adrenal Surgery; Laparoscopic Surgery; Thyroid Surgery; **Hospital:** Boston Med Ctr; **Address:** Boston Med Ctr, 88 E Newton St, Boston, MA 02118; **Phone:** 617-638-8609; **Board Cert:** Surgery 2003; **Med School:** Yale Univ 1986; **Resid:** Surgery, UCSF Med Ctr 1993; **Fellow:** Surgical Oncology, Natl Cancer Inst 1991; **Fac Appt:** Prof Med, Boston Univ

Eisenberg, Burton L MD [S] - **Spec Exp:** Breast Cancer; Melanoma; Sarcoma; **Hospital:** Dartmouth - Hitchcock Med Ctr; **Address:** DHMC, Dept General Surgery, One Medical Center Drive, Lebanon, NH 03756; **Phone:** 603-650-9479; **Board Cert:** Surgery 2010; **Med School:** Univ Tenn Coll Med 1974; **Resid:** Surgery, Wilford Hall USAF Med Ctr 1979; **Fellow:** Surgical Oncology, Meml Sloan-Kettering Cancer Ctr 1981; **Fac Appt:** Prof S, Dartmouth Med Sch

Emre, Sukru MD [S] - **Spec Exp:** Transplant-Liver-Adult & Pediatric; Hepatobiliary Surgery; Liver Cancer; Portal Hypertension; **Hospital:** Yale-New Haven Hosp, Yale Med Group; **Address:** 330 Cedar St, FMB121 Bldg - Fl 1, FMB 121, New Haven, CT 07520-8062; **Phone:** 203-737-2804; **Med School:** Turkey 1977; **Resid:** Surgery, Univ Istanbul 1982; **Fellow:** Hepatobiliary Surgery, Univ Istanbul 1988; Transplant Surgery, Mount Sinai Med Ctr 1994; **Fac Appt:** Prof S, Yale Univ

Gawande, Atul A MD [S] - **Spec Exp:** Endocrine Surgery; Cancer Surgery; Gastrointestinal Surgery; **Hospital:** Brigham and Women's Hosp (page 57), Dana-Farber Cancer Inst (page 57); **Address:** Brigham & Womens Hosp, 75 Francis St ASB2 Bldg Fl 3, Boston, MA 02115; **Phone:** 617-732-6830; **Board Cert:** Surgery 2004; **Med School:** Harvard Med Sch 1995; **Resid:** Surgery, Brigham & Womens Hosp 2003; **Fac Appt:** Assoc Prof S, Harvard Med Sch

Goodman, Martin D MD [S] - **Spec Exp:** Gastrointestinal Cancer; Peritoneal Carcinomatosis; **Hospital:** Tufts Med Ctr; **Address:** Tufts Med Ctr, Surgical Oncology, 800 Washington St, Box 9248, Boston, MA 02111; **Phone:** 617-636-9248; **Board Cert:** Surgery 2010; **Med School:** UMDNJ-RW Johnson Med Sch 1994; **Resid:** Surgery, Cooper Hosp 2000; **Fellow:** Surgical Oncology, UPMC 2002; **Fac Appt:** Asst Prof S, Tufts Univ

Graham, Roger A MD [S] - **Spec Exp:** Thyroid Cancer; Breast Cancer & Surgery; Gastrointestinal Cancer; Melanoma; **Hospital:** Tufts Med Ctr; **Address:** Tufts Med Ctr, Div Surg Onc, 800 Washington St, Box 1043, Boston, MA 02111; **Phone:** 617-636-8270; **Board Cert:** Surgery 2006; **Med School:** Johns Hopkins Univ 1982; **Resid:** Surgery, Tufts Med Ctr 1987; **Fellow:** Surgical Oncology, MD Anderson Cancer Ctr 1989; **Fac Appt:** Assoc Prof S, Tufts Univ

Gupta, Rajan MD [S] - **Spec Exp:** Trauma; Critical Care; **Hospital:** Dartmouth - Hitchcock Med Ctr; **Address:** Dartmouth Hitchcock Med Ctr, Dept Surgery, One Medical Center Drive, Lebanon, NH 03756; **Phone:** 603-650-8022; **Board Cert:** Surgery 2010; Surgical Critical Care 2002; **Med School:** Boston Univ 1991; **Resid:** Surgery, Dartmouth-Hitchcock Med Ctr 1997; **Fellow:** Trauma/Critical Care, Hosp Univ Penn 1999; **Fac Appt:** Asst Prof S, Dartmouth Med Sch

Hebert, James C MD [S] - **Spec Exp:** Biliary Surgery; Colon & Rectal Surgery; **Hospital:** Fletcher Allen Health Care- Med Ctr Campus; **Address:** Fletcher Allen Hlth Care, 111 Colchester Ave, Burlington, VT 05401; **Phone:** 802-847-3344; **Board Cert:** Surgery 2000; **Med School:** Univ VT Coll Med 1977; **Resid:** Surgery, Med Ctr Hosp 1982; **Fac Appt:** Prof S, Univ VT Coll Med

Hodin, Richard A MD [S] - **Spec Exp:** Thyroid Cancer; Inflammatory Bowel Disease; Adrenal Tumors; Endocrine Surgery; **Hospital:** Mass Genl Hosp; **Address:** Mass General Hospital, 15 Parkman St Wang Bldg Fl 3 - Ste 360, Boston, MA 02114; **Phone:** 617-724-2570; **Board Cert:** Surgery 2010; **Med School:** Tulane Univ 1984; **Resid:** Surgery, Beth Israel Deaconess Med Ctr 1990; **Fellow:** Research, Brigham & Women's Hosp 1989; **Fac Appt:** Prof S, Harvard Med Sch

Hughes, Kevin S MD [S] - **Spec Exp:** Breast Cancer; Ovarian Cancer; Breast Cancer-High Risk Women; Hereditary Cancer; **Hospital:** Mass Genl Hosp, Newton - Wellesley Hosp; **Address:** Mass Genl Hosp, Dept Surgery, 55 Fruit St YAW Bldg Fl 9A, Boston, MA 02114; **Phone:** 617-724-4800; **Board Cert:** Surgery 2006; **Med School:** Dartmouth Med Sch 1979; **Resid:** Surgery, Mercy Hosp 1984; **Fellow:** Surgical Oncology, National Cancer Inst 1986; **Fac Appt:** Assoc Prof S, Harvard Med Sch

Iglehart, James Dirk MD [S] - **Spec Exp:** Breast Cancer; **Hospital:** Dana-Farber Cancer Inst (page 57); **Address:** Dana-Farber Cancer Institute, 450 Brookline Ave, Smith 958, Boston, MA 02215; **Phone:** 617-632-5178 x1; **Board Cert:** Surgery 2005; **Med School:** Harvard Med Sch 1975; **Resid:** Surgery, Duke Univ Med Ctr 1981; Thoracic Surgery, Duke Univ Med Ctr 1984; **Fac Appt:** Prof S, Harvard Med Sch

Jabbour, Nicolas MD [S] - **Spec Exp:** Hepatobiliary Surgery; Transplant Surgery; Transplant-Liver; **Hospital:** UMass Memorial Med Ctr; **Address:** UMass Meml Med Ctr-Univ Campus, 55 Lake Ave N, Worcester, MA 01655; **Phone:** 508-334-2023; **Board Cert:** Surgery 2001; Surgical Critical Care 2003; **Med School:** Belgium 1984; **Resid:** Surgery, Lincoln Hosp 1991; **Fellow:** Transplant Surgery, UPMC/Chldn's Hosp 1993; **Fac Appt:** Prof S, Univ Mass Sch Med

Jenkins, Roger L MD [S] - **Spec Exp:** Transplant-Liver; Liver & Biliary Cancer; Pancreatic Cancer; **Hospital:** Lahey Clin, Children's Hospital - Boston; **Address:** Lahey Clinic, 41 Mall Rd Fl 4, Burlington, MA 01805; **Phone:** 781-744-2500; **Board Cert:** Surgery 2005; **Med School:** Univ VT Coll Med 1977; **Resid:** Surgery, New Eng Deaconess Hosp 1982; **Fellow:** Cardiac Surgery, New Eng Deaconess Hosp 1983; Transplant Surgery, Univ Pittsburgh Hosp 1983; **Fac Appt:** Prof S, Tufts Univ

Kavanah, Maureen MD [S] - **Spec Exp:** Breast Cancer; Gynecologic Cancer; Melanoma; **Hospital:** Boston Med Ctr; **Address:** BMC-Dept Surgical Onc & Endocrinology, 820 Harrison Ave, Ste 1200, Boston, MA 02118; **Phone:** 617-638-2778; **Board Cert:** Surgery 2009; **Med School:** Tufts Univ 1975; **Resid:** Surgery, Steward St Elizabeth's Med Ctr 1979; **Fellow:** Surgical Oncology, Boston Med Ctr 1981; **Fac Appt:** Assoc Prof S, Boston Univ

Krag, David N MD [S] - **Spec Exp:** Sentinel Node Surgery; Breast Cancer; Cancer Surgery; Melanoma; **Hospital:** Fletcher Allen Health Care- Med Ctr Campus; **Address:** Univ Vermont Coll Med, Dept Surgery, 89 Beaumont Ave, Given Bldg - E309C, Burlington, VT 05405; **Phone:** 802-656-5830; **Board Cert:** Surgery 2006; **Med School:** Loyola Univ-Stritch Sch Med 1980; **Resid:** Surgery, UC Davis Med Ctr 1983; **Fellow:** Surgical Oncology, UCLA Med Ctr 1984; **Fac Appt:** Assoc Prof S, Univ VT Coll Med

Lannin, Donald R MD [S] - **Spec Exp:** Breast Cancer; Breast Surgery; **Hospital:** Yale-New Haven Hosp, Yale Med Group; **Address:** Yale-New Haven Breast Ctr, 20 York St, New Haven, CT 06510; **Phone:** 203-785-2328; **Board Cert:** Surgery 2002; **Med School:** Univ Minn 1974; **Resid:** Surgery, Univ Minnesota Med Ctr 1982; **Fac Appt:** Prof S, Yale Univ

Lillemoe, Keith D MD [S] - **Spec Exp:** Pancreatic Cancer; Colon Cancer; Pancreatic & Biliary Surgery; Gastrointestinal Cancer; **Hospital:** Mass Genl Hosp; **Address:** Mass General Hospital, 55 Fruit St WHT Bldg - rm 506, Boston, MA 02114; **Phone:** 617-643-1010; **Board Cert:** Surgery 2007; **Med School:** Johns Hopkins Univ 1978; **Resid:** Surgery, Johns Hopkins Hosp 1985; **Fac Appt:** Prof S, Harvard Med Sch

Lipkowitz, George S MD [S] - **Spec Exp:** Transplant-Kidney; Dialysis Access; **Hospital:** Baystate Med Ctr, Mercy Med Ctr - Springfield, MA; **Address:** 208 Ashley Ave, West Springfield, MA 01089; **Phone:** 413-747-4170 x151; **Board Cert:** Surgery 2006; **Med School:** SUNY Downstate 1980; **Resid:** Surgery, SUNY Kings Co Hosp 1985; **Fellow:** Transplant Surgery, SUNY Hlth Scis Ctr 1986; **Fac Appt:** Assoc Prof S, Tufts Univ

Markmann, James F MD/PhD [S] - **Spec Exp:** Transplant-Liver; Transplant-Kidney; Transplant-Pancreas; Pancreatic Islet Cell Transplant; **Hospital:** Mass Genl Hosp; **Address:** MGH Transplantation Ctr, WHT 517, 55 Fruit St, Boston, MA 02114; **Phone:** 617-643-4533; **Board Cert:** Surgery 2006; **Med School:** Univ Pennsylvania 1986; **Resid:** Surgery, Hosp UPenn 1992; **Fellow:** Transplant Surgery, UCLA Med Ctr 1994; **Fac Appt:** Prof S, Harvard Med Sch

McAneny, David B MD [S] - **Spec Exp:** Gastrointestinal Cancer & Surgery; Endocrine Tumors; Pancreatic Cancer; Biliary Surgery; **Hospital:** Boston Med Ctr; **Address:** Boston Medical Center, 830 Harrison Ave, Ste 3400, Boston, MA 02118; **Phone:** 617-638-8446; **Board Cert:** Surgery 2008; **Med School:** Georgetown Univ 1983; **Resid:** Surgery, Boston Med Ctr 1988; **Fellow:** Gastrointestinal Surgery, Lahey Clinic 1989; **Fac Appt:** Assoc Prof S, Boston Univ

McFadden, David W MD [S] - **Spec Exp:** Pancreatic Cancer; **Hospital:** Univ of Conn Hlth Ctr, John Dempsey Hosp; **Address:** UConn Health Center, Dept Surgery, 263 Farmington Ave, Farmington, CT 06030; **Phone:** 860-679-4801; **Board Cert:** Surgery 2007; Surgical Critical Care 2003; **Med School:** Univ VA Sch Med 1980; **Resid:** Surgery, Johns Hopkins Hosp 1986; **Fellow:** Surgery, Johns Hopkins Hosp 1988; **Fac Appt:** Prof S, Univ VT Coll Med

Moore Jr, Francis D MD [S] - **Spec Exp:** Endocrine Surgery; Thyroid Cancer; **Hospital:** Brigham and Women's Hosp (page 57); **Address:** Brigham & Womens Hosp-Dept Surgery, 75 Francis St ASB2 Bldg Fl 3, Boston, MA 02115; **Phone:** 617-732-6830; **Board Cert:** Surgery 2004; **Med School:** Harvard Med Sch 1976; **Resid:** Surgery, Brigham & Womens Hosp 1984; **Fellow:** Immunology, Brigham & Womens Hosp 1981; **Fac Appt:** Prof S, Harvard Med Sch

Ponn, Teresa MD [S] - **Spec Exp:** Breast Cancer; **Hospital:** Elliot Hosp; **Address:** Elliot Breast Health Center, 185 Queen city Ave, Ste 1, MS 03109, Manchester, NH 03109; **Phone:** 603-668-3067; **Board Cert:** Surgery 2000; **Med School:** Univ Fla Coll Med 1976; **Resid:** Surgery, Stanford Univ Med Ctr 1982

Rattner, David W MD [S] - **Spec Exp:** Gastrointestinal Cancer & Surgery; Minimally Invasive Surgery; Gastroesophageal Reflux Disease (GERD); Natural Orifice Surgery (NOTES); **Hospital:** Mass Genl Hosp; **Address:** Mass General Hosp, Dept Surgery, 15 Parkman St, WACC 460, Boston, MA 02114-3117; **Phone:** 617-726-1893; **Board Cert:** Surgery 2004; **Med School:** Johns Hopkins Univ 1978; **Resid:** Surgery, Mass General Hosp 1985; **Fac Appt:** Prof S, Harvard Med Sch

Ryan, Colleen M MD [S] - **Spec Exp:** Burn Care; Toxic Epidermal Neurolysis; Wound Healing/Care; **Hospital:** Mass Genl Hosp, Shriners Hosp for Chldn-Boston; **Address:** MGH Burn Assocs, 55 Fruit St GRB Bldg - Ste 1303, Boston, MA 02114-2621; **Phone:** 617-726-3712; **Board Cert:** Surgery 2009; Surgical Critical Care 2003; **Med School:** Georgetown Univ 1982; **Resid:** Surgery, NE Deaconess Hosp 1988; **Fellow:** Hepatology, Hammersmith Hosp 1986; Burn Surgery, Mass Genl Hosp 1989; **Fac Appt:** Assoc Prof S, Harvard Med Sch

Salem, Ronald R MD [S] - **Spec Exp:** Cancer Surgery; Liver & Biliary Surgery; Gastrointestinal Cancer; Liver Cancer; **Hospital:** Yale-New Haven Hosp, Yale Med Group; **Address:** Dept Surgery, 333 Cedar St, FMB 130, New Haven, CT 06520-8062; **Phone:** 203-785-3577; **Board Cert:** Surgery 2011; **Med School:** Zimbabwe 1978; **Resid:** Surgery, Hammersmith Hosp 1985; Surgery, New England Deaconess Hosp 1989; **Fac Appt:** Prof S, Yale Univ

Shikora, Scott A MD [S] - **Spec Exp:** Obesity/Bariatric Surgery; Laparoscopic Abdominal Surgery; **Hospital:** Brigham and Women's Hosp (page 57); **Address:** Brigham & Women's Hosp, Dept Surgery, ASBII- 3rd Fl, 75 Francis St, Boston, MA 02115; **Phone:** 617-525-8570; **Board Cert:** Surgery 2011; **Med School:** Columbia P&S 1985; **Resid:** Surgery, New England Deaconess Hosp 1991; **Fellow:** Nutrition & Metabolism, New England Deaconess Hos 1989; **Fac Appt:** Prof S, Tufts Univ

Smith, Barbara L MD/PhD [S] - **Spec Exp:** Breast Cancer; Breast Cancer-High Risk Women; **Hospital:** Mass Genl Hosp; **Address:** MGH Cancer Center, 55 Fruit St, Ste YAW 9A, Boston, MA 02114; **Phone:** 617-724-1074; **Board Cert:** Surgery 2009; **Med School:** Harvard Med Sch 1983; **Resid:** Surgery, Brigham & Women's Hosp 1989; **Fac Appt:** Asst Prof S, Harvard Med Sch

Sosa, Julie A MD [S] - **Spec Exp:** Thyroid Cancer; Parathyroid Cancer; Endocrine Cancers; **Hospital:** Yale-New Haven Hosp; **Address:** 800 Howard Ave, New Haven, CT 06520; **Phone:** 203-785-2314; **Board Cert:** Surgery 2004; **Med School:** Johns Hopkins Univ 1994; **Resid:** Surgery, Johns Hopkins Hosp 2001; **Fellow:** Surgical Oncology, Johns Hoplins Hosp 2002; **Fac Appt:** Assoc Prof S, Yale Univ

Sutton Jr, John E MD [S] - **Spec Exp:** Esophageal Cancer; Liver & Biliary Surgery; Pancreatic Cancer; **Hospital:** White River Junction VA Med Ctr; **Address:** 215 N Main St, White River Junction, VT 05009; **Phone:** 802-295-9363 x6194; **Board Cert:** Surgery 2011; Surgical Critical Care 2007; **Med School:** Georgetown Univ 1974; **Resid:** Surgery, Dartmouth-Hitchcock Med Ctr 1981; **Fellow:** Surgical Critical Care, Dartmouth-Hitchcock Med Ctr 1983; **Fac Appt:** Prof S, Dartmouth Med Sch

Tanabe, Kenneth K MD [S] - **Spec Exp:** Liver Cancer; Colon & Rectal Cancer; Melanoma; **Hospital:** Mass Genl Hosp; **Address:** Mass General Hosp, Div Surgical Oncology, 55 Fruit St, YAW 7B, Boston, MA 02114; **Phone:** 617-724-3868; **Board Cert:** Surgery 2010; **Med School:** UCSD 1985; **Resid:** Surgery, New York Hosp-Cornell 1990; **Fellow:** Surgical Oncology, MD Anderson Cancer Ctr 1993; **Fac Appt:** Prof S, Harvard Med Sch

Thayer, Sarah P MD/PhD [S] - **Spec Exp:** Pancreatic Cancer; Gastrointestinal Cancer & Surgery; Hepatobiliary Surgery; Breast Cancer & Surgery; **Hospital:** Mass Genl Hosp; **Address:** Mass Genl Hosp, 15 Parkman St, WAC 460, Boston, MA 02114; **Phone:** 617-726-0624; **Board Cert:** Surgery 2010; **Med School:** Univ VA Sch Med 1991; **Resid:** Surgery, Mass Genl Hosp 1994; Surgery, Mass Genl Hosp 2001; **Fellow:** Research, Meml Sloan Kettering Cancer Ctr 1998; **Fac Appt:** Assoc Prof Surg & Onc, Harvard Med Sch

Udelsman, Robert MD [S] - **Spec Exp:** Parathyroid Cancer; Adrenal Tumors; Thyroid Cancer; Endocrine Surgery; **Hospital:** Yale-New Haven Hosp, Yale Med Group; **Address:** Yale-New Haven Hosp, Dept Surgery, 330 Cedar St, Box 208062, New Haven, CT 06520-8062; **Phone:** 203-785-2697; **Board Cert:** Surgery 2009; **Med School:** Geo Wash Univ 1981; **Resid:** Surgery, Natl Inst Hlth 1986; Surgery, Johns Hopkins Hosp 1989; **Fellow:** Gastrointestinal Surgery, Johns Hopkins Hosp 1990; Surgical Oncology, Natl Cancer Inst 1985; **Fac Appt:** Prof S, Yale Univ

Ward, Barbara A MD [S] - **Spec Exp:** Breast Cancer; Breast Surgery; Breast Disease; **Hospital:** Greenwich Hosp; **Address:** 77 Lafayette Pl, Ste 302, Greenwich, CT 06830-5426; **Phone:** 203-863-4250; **Board Cert:** Surgery 2002; **Med School:** Temple Univ 1983; **Resid:** Surgery, Yale-New Haven Hosp 1990; **Fellow:** Surgical Oncology, Natl Cancer Inst 1987; **Fac Appt:** Assoc Clin Prof S, Yale Univ

Winchell, Robert J MD [S] - **Spec Exp:** Critical Care; Trauma; Burn Care; **Hospital:** Maine Med Ctr; **Address:** Maine Medical Partners Surgical Assocs, 22 Bram Hall, Portland, ME 04102-3113; **Phone:** 207-774-2381; **Board Cert:** Surgery 2010; Surgical Critical Care 2001; **Med School:** Yale Univ 1984; **Resid:** Surgery, UCSD Med Ctr 1990; **Fellow:** Trauma/Critical Care, UCSD Med Ctr 1991; **Fac Appt:** Assoc Clin Prof S, Univ VT Coll Med

Zinner, Michael MD [S] - **Spec Exp:** Colon & Rectal Cancer & Surgery; Pancreatic Cancer; Stomach Cancer; Gastrointestinal Stromal Tumors; **Hospital:** Brigham and Women's Hosp (page 57), Dana-Farber Cancer Inst (page 57); **Address:** Brigham & Women's Hosp, Dept Surgery, 75 Francis St, Boston, MA 02115; **Phone:** 617-732-8973; **Board Cert:** Surgery 2010; **Med School:** Univ Fla Coll Med 1971; **Resid:** Surgery, Johns Hopkins Hosp 1974; Surgery, Johns Hopkins Hosp 1980; **Fac Appt:** Prof S, Harvard Med Sch

Mid Atlantic

Alexander Jr, H Richard MD [S] - **Spec Exp:** Gastrointestinal Cancer & Surgery; Liver Cancer-Metastatic; Pancreatic Cancer; **Hospital:** Univ of MD Med Ctr; **Address:** UMMC, Dept Surgerical Oncology, 22 S Greene St, rm S4B12, Baltimore, MD 21201; **Phone:** 410-328-7321; **Board Cert:** Surgery 2004; **Med School:** Georgetown Univ 1979; **Resid:** Surgery, Bethesda Naval Hosp 1985; **Fellow:** Surgical Oncology, Meml Sloan Kettering Cancer Ctr 1989; **Fac Appt:** Prof S, Univ MD Sch Med

Alfonso II, Antonio E MD [S] - **Spec Exp:** Thyroid Cancer; Head & Neck Surgery; Breast Cancer; **Hospital:** SUNY Downstate Med Ctr (Univ Hosp of Bklyn) - LICH, SUNY Downstate Med Ctr (Univ Hosp of Bklyn); **Address:** Long Island Coll Hosp, 339 Hicks St, Brooklyn, NY 11201; **Phone:** 718-875-3244; **Board Cert:** Surgery 1973; **Med School:** Philippines 1968; **Resid:** Surgery, Temple Univ Hosp 1972; **Fellow:** Surgical Oncology, Meml Sloan Kettering Cancer Ctr 1974; **Fac Appt:** Prof Emeritus S, SUNY Downstate

August, David MD [S] - **Spec Exp:** Pancreatic Cancer; Esophageal Cancer; Stomach Cancer; Sarcoma-Soft Tissue; **Hospital:** Robert Wood Johnson Univ Hosp - New Brunswick; **Address:** CINJ-195 Little Albany St, New Brunswick, NJ 08903; **Phone:** 732-235-7701; **Board Cert:** Surgery 2005; **Med School:** Yale Univ 1980; **Resid:** Surgery, Yale-New Haven Hosp 1986; **Fellow:** Surgical Oncology, Natl Cancer Inst 1984; **Fac Appt:** Prof S, UMDNJ-RW Johnson Med Sch

Axelrod, Deborah MD [S] - **Spec Exp:** Breast Cancer; Breast Disease; **Hospital:** NYU Langone Med Ctr (page 68); **Address:** NYU Clinical Cancer Ctr, 160 E 34th St Fl 3, New York, NY 10016; **Phone:** 212-731-5366; **Board Cert:** Surgery 2008; **Med School:** Israel 1982; **Resid:** Surgery, Beth Israel Med Ctr 1988; **Fellow:** Surgical Oncology, Meml Sloan Kettering Cancer Ctr 1986; **Fac Appt:** Assoc Prof S, NYU Sch Med

Barie, Philip MD [S] - **Spec Exp:** Trauma; Critical Care; Hernia; Gastrointestinal Surgery; **Hospital:** NY-Presby/Weill Cornell Med Ctr, NY (page 66), Hosp For Special Surgery (page 60); **Address:** Weill Med College-Cornell Univ, 525 E 68th St, Box 206, New York, NY 10065; **Phone:** 212-746-5401; **Board Cert:** Surgery 2004; Surgical Critical Care 2005; **Med School:** Boston Univ 1977; **Resid:** Surgery, NY Hosp-Cornell Med Ctr 1984; **Fellow:** Trauma, Albany Med Coll 1981; **Fac Appt:** Prof S, Cornell Univ-Weill Med Coll

Bartlett, David L MD [S] - **Spec Exp:** Peritoneal Carcinomatosis; Pancreatic Cancer; Liver Cancer; Appendix Cancer; **Hospital:** UPMC Shadyside; **Address:** UPMC Cancer Pavilion-Surgical Oncology, 5150 Centre Ave Fl 4 - rm 415, Pittsburgh, PA 15232; **Phone:** 412-692-2852; **Board Cert:** Surgery 2004; **Med School:** Univ Tex, Houston 1987; **Resid:** Surgery, Hosp Univ Penn 1993; **Fellow:** Surgical Oncology, Meml Sloan-Kettering Cancer Ctr 1995; **Fac Appt:** Prof S, Univ Pittsburgh

Bartlett, Stephen T MD [S] - **Spec Exp:** Transplant-Pancreas; Transplant-Kidney; **Hospital:** Univ of MD Med Ctr; **Address:** 22 S Greene St, Ste N4E40, Baltimore, MD 21201; **Phone:** 410-328-8407; **Board Cert:** Surgery 2004; Vascular Surgery 2007; **Med School:** Univ Chicago-Pritzker Sch Med 1979; **Resid:** Surgery, Hosp Univ Penn 1985; **Fellow:** Vascular Surgery, Northwestern Univ Affil Hosp 1986; **Fac Appt:** Prof S, Univ MD Sch Med

Bessey, Palmer Q MD [S] - **Spec Exp:** Burn Care; Wound Healing/Care; Nutrition; **Hospital:** NY-Presby/Weill Cornell Med Ctr, NY (page 66); **Address:** 525 E 68th St, Box 137, New York, NY 10065; **Phone:** 212-746-0242; **Board Cert:** Surgery 2011; Surgical Critical Care 2005; **Med School:** Univ VT Coll Med 1975; **Resid:** Surgery, Univ Alabama Hosp 1981; **Fellow:** Metabolism, Brigham & Women's Hosp 1983; **Fac Appt:** Prof S, Cornell Univ-Weill Med Coll

Bessler, Marc MD [S] - **Spec Exp:** Obesity/Bariatric Surgery; Laparoscopic Surgery; Gastrointestinal Metabolic Surgery; Natural Orifice Surgery (NOTES); **Hospital:** NY-Presby/Columbia Univ Med Ctr, NY (page 66); **Address:** NY Presby Med Ctr, Dept of Surgery, 161 Fort Washington Ave Fl 5 - rm 524, New York, NY 10032; **Phone:** 212-305-9506; **Board Cert:** Surgery 2007; **Med School:** NYU Sch Med 1989; **Resid:** Surgery, Columbia Presby Med Ctr 1995; **Fac Appt:** Clin Prof S, Columbia P&S

Boraas, Marcia MD [S] - **Spec Exp:** Breast Cancer; Breast Disease; **Hospital:** Fox Chase Cancer Ctr (page 58); **Address:** Fox Chase Cancer Center, 333 Cottman Ave, rm P2131, Philadelphia, PA 19111; **Phone:** 215-728-2982; **Board Cert:** Surgery 2005; **Med School:** Univ Pennsylvania 1977; **Resid:** Surgery, Hosp U Penn 1983

Borgen, Patrick I MD [S] - **Spec Exp:** Breast Cancer; Breast Cancer & Surgery; **Hospital:** Maimonides Med Ctr (page 63); **Address:** Maimonides Breast Ctr, 6300 8th Ave, Brooklyn, NY 11220; **Phone:** 718-765-2570; **Board Cert:** Surgery 2002; **Med School:** Louisiana State U, New Orleans 1984; **Resid:** Surgery, Ochsner Fdn Hosp 1989; **Fellow:** Surgical Oncology, Meml Sloan Kettering Canc Ctr 1990; **Fac Appt:** Prof S, Cornell Univ-Weill Med Coll

Brady, Mary Sue MD [S] - **Spec Exp:** Melanoma; Merkel Cell Carcinoma; Sarcoma-Soft Tissue; **Hospital:** Meml Sloan-Kettering Cancer Ctr; **Address:** 1275 York Ave, rm H1211, New York, NY 10065; **Phone:** 212-639-8347; **Board Cert:** Surgery 2009; **Med School:** Univ Miami Sch Med 1983; **Resid:** Surgery, NY Hosp-Cornell Med Ctr 1988; **Fellow:** Surgical Oncology, Meml Sloan-Kettering Cancer Ctr 1990; Immunology, Meml Sloan-Kettering Cancer Ctr 1992; **Fac Appt:** Assoc Prof S, Cornell Univ-Weill Med Coll

Brodsky, Jeffrey T MD [S] - **Spec Exp:** Esophageal Cancer; Gastrointestinal Cancer; Pancreatic Cancer; Minimally Invasive Surgery; **Hospital:** Aria Health- Torresdale; **Address:** 3398 Red Lion Rd, Med Office Bldg, Ste 235, Philadelphia, PA 19114; **Phone:** 215-612-5630; **Board Cert:** Surgery 2009; **Med School:** Univ Pennsylvania 1984; **Resid:** Surgery, NYU Med Ctr 1989; **Fellow:** Surgical Oncology, Meml Sloan-Kettering Cancer Ctr 1991

Brody, Fred J MD [S] - **Spec Exp:** Gastrointestinal Surgery; Laparoscopic Surgery; Hernia; **Hospital:** G Washington Univ Hosp; **Address:** George Washington Univ Dept Surgery, 2150 Pennsylvania Ave NW, Ste 6B, Washington, DC 20037; **Phone:** 202-741-2587; **Board Cert:** Surgery 2008; **Med School:** Univ NC Sch Med 1991; **Resid:** Surgery, George Washington Univ Med Ctr 1997; **Fellow:** Laparoscopic Surgery, Duke Univ Med Ctr 1998; **Fac Appt:** Assoc Prof S, Geo Wash Univ

Bromberg, Jonathan S MD/PhD [S] - **Spec Exp:** Transplant-Kidney; Transplant-Pancreas; **Hospital:** Univ of MD Med Ctr; **Address:** Univ Maryland Med Ctr, 29 S Greene St, Ste 200, Baltimore, MD 21201; **Phone:** 410-328-5408; **Board Cert:** Surgery 2009; **Med School:** Harvard Med Sch 1983; **Resid:** Surgery, Univ Washington Med Ctr 1988; **Fellow:** Transplant Surgery, Hosp U Penn 1990; **Fac Appt:** Prof S, Univ MD Sch Med

Brooks, Ari D MD [S] - **Spec Exp:** Breast Cancer; Minimally Invasive Surgery; **Hospital:** Hahnemann Univ Hosp; **Address:** Drexel Surgical Assocs, 219 N Broad St Fl 8, Philadelphia, PA 19107; **Phone:** 215-762-2295; **Board Cert:** Surgery 2010; **Med School:** Hahnemann Univ 1992; **Resid:** Surgery, NYU Med Ctr 1999; **Fellow:** Surgical Oncology, Meml Sloan-Kettering Cancer Ctr 2001; **Fac Appt:** Assoc Prof S, Drexel Univ Coll Med

Cameron, John L MD [S] - **Spec Exp:** Pancreatic Cancer; Pancreatic Surgery; Biliary Cancer; Liver Cancer; **Hospital:** Johns Hopkins Hosp (page 61); **Address:** Johns Hopkins Hosp, 600 N Wolfe St Blalock Bldg - Ste 679, Baltimore, MD 21287; **Phone:** 410-955-5166; **Board Cert:** Surgery 1970; Thoracic Surgery 1971; **Med School:** Johns Hopkins Univ 1962; **Resid:** Surgery, Johns Hopkins Hosp 1970; **Fellow:** Thoracic Surgery, Johns Hopkins Hosp 1971; **Fac Appt:** Prof S, Johns Hopkins Univ

Cance, William G MD [S] - **Spec Exp:** Pancreatic Cancer; Endocrine Cancers; Colon & Rectal Cancer; **Hospital:** Roswell Park Cancer Inst; **Address:** Roswell Park Cancer Inst, Elm and Carlton Streets, Buffalo, NY 14263; **Phone:** 716-845-4010; **Board Cert:** Surgery 2009; **Med School:** Duke Univ 1982; **Resid:** Surgery, Barnes Jewish Hosp 1988; **Fellow:** Surgical Oncology, Meml Sloan Kettering Canc Ctr 1990; **Fac Appt:** Prof S, SUNY Buffalo

Carty, Sally E MD [S] - **Spec Exp:** Endocrine Surgery; Endocrine Tumors; Parathyroid Surgery; Von Hippel-Lindau Disease; **Hospital:** UPMC Montefiore, UPMC Presby, Pittsburgh; **Address:** 3471 Fifth Ave, Kaufmann Bldg, Ste 101, Pittsburgh, PA 15213; **Phone:** 412-647-0467; **Board Cert:** Surgery 2010; **Med School:** Penn State Coll Med 1984; **Resid:** Surgery, Penn State Hershey Med Ctr 1989; **Fellow:** Surgical Oncology, Natl Cancer Inst 1991; **Fac Appt:** Prof S, Univ Pittsburgh

Chabot, John A MD [S] - **Spec Exp:** Liver & Biliary Surgery; Pancreatic Cancer; Pancreatic Surgery; Thyroid & Parathyroid Surgery; **Hospital:** NY-Presby/Columbia Univ Med Ctr, NY (page 66); **Address:** NY Presby-Columbia Medical Ctr, 161 Ft Washington Ave Fl 8 - Ste 819, New York, NY 10032; **Phone:** 212-305-9468; **Board Cert:** Surgery 2010; **Med School:** Dartmouth Med Sch 1983; **Resid:** Surgery, Columbia-Presby Med Ctr 1990; **Fac Appt:** Prof S, Columbia P&S

Cherqui, Daniel MD [S] - **Spec Exp:** Liver Cancer; Transplant-Liver; Hepatobiliary Surgery; Minimally Invasive Surgery; **Hospital:** NY-Presby/Weill Cornell Med Ctr, NY (page 66); **Address:** 525 E 68th St, Box 287, New York, NY 10065; **Phone:** 212-746-2127; **Med School:** France 1980; **Resid:** Surgery, Hospitaux de Paris 1986; **Fellow:** Hepatobiliary Surgery, Paul Brousse Hosp 1987; Transplant Surgery, Univ Chicago Med Ctr; **Fac Appt:** Prof S, Cornell Univ-Weill Med Coll

Choti, Michael A MD [S] - **Spec Exp:** Pancreatic Cancer; Liver Cancer-Metastatic; Carcinoid Tumors; **Hospital:** Johns Hopkins Hosp (page 61); **Address:** Johns Hopkins Hosp, 600 N Wolfe St Blalock Bldg - rm 665, Baltimore, MD 21287; **Phone:** 410-955-7113; **Board Cert:** Surgery 2002; **Med School:** Yale Univ 1983; **Resid:** Surgery, Hosp Univ Penn 1990; **Fellow:** Surgical Oncology, Meml Sloan-Kettering Cancer Ctr 1992; **Fac Appt:** Prof S, Johns Hopkins Univ

Cohen, Murray J MD [S] - **Spec Exp:** Trauma; Critical Care; **Hospital:** Thomas Jefferson Univ Hosp, Paoli Hosp; **Address:** 1100 Walnut St, Ste 702, Philadelphia, PA 19107; **Phone:** 215-955-2600; **Board Cert:** Surgery 2006; Surgical Critical Care 2008; **Med School:** Temple Univ 1981; **Resid:** Surgery, Albert Einstein Med Ctr 1986; **Fellow:** Trauma, Hartford Hosp 1987; **Fac Appt:** Assoc Prof S, Thomas Jefferson Univ

Coit, Daniel G MD [S] - **Spec Exp:** Melanoma; Pancreatic Cancer; Stomach Cancer; **Hospital:** Meml Sloan-Kettering Cancer Ctr; **Address:** 1275 York Avenue, New York, NY 10065; **Phone:** 646-497-9072; **Board Cert:** Surgery 2004; **Med School:** Univ Cincinnati 1976; **Resid:** Internal Medicine, New Eng Deaconess Hosp 1978; Surgery, New Eng Deaconess Hosp 1983; **Fellow:** Surgical Oncology, Meml Sloan Kettering Canc Ctr 1985; **Fac Appt:** Prof S, Cornell Univ-Weill Med Coll

Conti, David J MD [S] - **Spec Exp:** Transplant-Kidney; **Hospital:** Albany Med Ctr; **Address:** Albany Medical Center, 47 New Scotland Ave, f Bldg, Ste 212, Albany, NY 12208; **Phone:** 518-262-5614; **Board Cert:** Surgery 2008; **Med School:** Northwestern Univ 1981; **Resid:** Surgery, Northwestern Meml Hosp 1987; **Fellow:** Transplant Surgery, Mass Genl Hosp 1989; **Fac Appt:** Prof S, Albany Med Coll

Cornwell III, Edward E MD [S] - **Spec Exp:** Trauma; **Hospital:** Howard Univ Hosp; **Address:** Howard Univ Hospital, 2041 Georgia Ave NW, Ste 4B02, Washington, DC 20060; **Phone:** 202-865-1441; **Board Cert:** Surgery 2006; **Med School:** Howard Univ 1982; **Resid:** Surgery, LAC-USC Med Ctr 1987; **Fellow:** Trauma, Emer/Med Svcs System 1989; **Fac Appt:** Assoc Prof S, Johns Hopkins Univ

Courcoulas, Anita P MD [S] - **Spec Exp:** Obesity/Bariatric Surgery; Minimally Invasive Surgery; **Hospital:** Magee-Womens Hosp - UPMC, UPMC Shadyside; **Address:** Magee-Womens Hosp, 3380 Boulevard of the Allies, Ste 390, Pittsburgh, PA 15213; **Phone:** 412-641-3632; **Board Cert:** Surgery 2005; **Med School:** Boston Univ 1988; **Resid:** Surgery, Univ Pitts Med Ctr 1996; **Fac Appt:** Assoc Prof S, Univ Pittsburgh

Curcillo, Paul G MD [S] - **Spec Exp:** Minimally Invasive Surgery; Gastrointestinal Cancer & Surgery; Natural Orifice Surgery (NOTES); **Hospital:** Fox Chase Cancer Ctr (page 58); **Address:** Fox Chase Cancer Ctr-Surgical Oncology, 333 Cottman Ave, Philadelphia, PA 19111; **Phone:** 215-728-5363; **Board Cert:** Surgery 2007; **Med School:** Univ Pennsylvania 1989; **Resid:** Surgery, T Jefferson Univ Hosp 1996; **Fellow:** Clinical Nutrition, Hosp Univ Penn 1991; **Fac Appt:** Assoc Prof S, Drexel Univ Coll Med

Czerniecki, Brian J MD/PhD [S] - **Spec Exp:** Breast Cancer & Surgery; Sentinel Node Surgery; Melanoma; **Hospital:** Hosp Univ Penn - UPHS (page 72); **Address:** Rena Rowan Breast Ctr, 3rd Fl West, 3400 Civic Ctr Blvd, Philadelphia, PA 19104; **Phone:** 215-615-5858; **Board Cert:** Surgery 2004; **Med School:** Univ Pennsylvania 1988; **Resid:** Surgery, Ohio State Univ Hosp 1993; **Fellow:** Surgical Oncology, Natl Inst Hlth 1995; **Fac Appt:** Assoc Prof S, Univ Pennsylvania

Dayton, Merril T MD [S] - **Spec Exp:** Gastrointestinal Surgery; Inflammatory Bowel Disease; Pancreatic & Biliary Surgery; **Hospital:** Buffalo General Hosp; **Address:** Buffalo Genl Hosp, Dept Surgery, 100 High St, Ste C3, Buffalo, NY 14203; **Phone:** 716-859-3911; **Board Cert:** Surgery 2004; **Med School:** Univ Utah 1976; **Resid:** Surgery, UCLA Med Ctr 1982; **Fellow:** Gastrointestinal Surgery, Wadsworth VA Hosp 1980; **Fac Appt:** Prof S, SUNY Buffalo

Deitch, Edwin A MD [S] - **Spec Exp:** Burn Care; Abdominal Wall Reconstruction; Critical Care; **Hospital:** Univ Hosp-UMDNJ—Newark; **Address:** 185 S Orange Ave, MSB, rm G506, Newark, NJ 07103; **Phone:** 973-972-6639; **Board Cert:** Surgery 2009; Surgical Critical Care 2006; **Med School:** Univ MD Sch Med 1973; **Resid:** Surgery, US Public Hlth Svc Hosp 1976; Surgery, US Public Hlth Svc Hosp 1978; **Fac Appt:** Prof S, UMDNJ-NJ Med Sch, Newark

Dempsey, Daniel T MD [S] - **Spec Exp:** Gastrointestinal Surgery; Laparoscopic Surgery; Gastroesophageal Reflux Disease (GERD); Esophageal Surgery; **Hospital:** Hosp Univ Penn - UPHS (page 72); **Address:** University of Pennsylvania - Dept Surgery, 3400 Spruce Street, 4 Silverstein Pvln., Philadelphia, PA 19104; **Phone:** 215-614-0092; **Board Cert:** Surgery 2006; **Med School:** Univ Rochester 1979; **Resid:** Surgery, Hosp Univ Penn 1986; **Fac Appt:** Prof S, Univ Pennsylvania

Drebin, Jeffrey A MD/PhD [S] - **Spec Exp:** Pancreatic Cancer; Liver Cancer; Biliary Cancer; Gastrointestinal Cancer; **Hospital:** Hosp Univ Penn - UPHS (page 72); **Address:** Hosp Univ Penn, Dept Surgery, 3400 Spruce St, 4 Silverstein Pavilion, Philadelphia, PA 19104; **Phone:** 215-662-7539; **Board Cert:** Surgery 2004; **Med School:** Harvard Med Sch 1987; **Resid:** Surgery, Johns Hopkins Hosp 1994; **Fellow:** Surgical Oncology, Johns Hopkins Hosp 1991; Surgical Oncology, Johns Hopkins Hosp 1995; **Fac Appt:** Prof S, Univ Pennsylvania

Duncan, Mark D MD [S] - **Spec Exp:** Gastrointestinal Cancer & Surgery; Minimally Invasive Surgery; **Hospital:** Johns Hopkins Bayview Med Ctr (page 61); **Address:** Johns Hopkins Bayview Med Ctr, Genl Surgery Clinic, 4940 Eastern Ave, Bldg A Fl 5, Baltimore, MD 21224; **Phone:** 410-550-1226; **Board Cert:** Surgery 2006; **Med School:** Mayo Med Sch 1987; **Resid:** Surgery, Georgetown Univ Hosp 1994; **Fellow:** Surgery, VA Medical Ctr 1991

Edge, Stephen B MD [S] - **Spec Exp:** Breast Cancer; Cancer Surgery; **Hospital:** Roswell Park Cancer Inst; **Address:** Roswell Park Cancer Inst, Elm & Carlton Streets, Buffalo, NY 14263; **Phone:** 716-845-2918; **Board Cert:** Surgery 2006; **Med School:** Case West Res Univ 1979; **Resid:** Surgery, Univ Hosp 1986; **Fellow:** Surgical Oncology, Natl Cancer Inst 1984; **Fac Appt:** Prof S, SUNY Buffalo

Edington, Howard D MD [S] - Spec Exp: Melanoma; Breast Reconstruction; Reconstructive Surgery; Wound Healing/Care; **Hospital:** Magee-Womens Hosp - UPMC; **Address:** Magee-Womens Surgical Assocs, 300 Halket St, Ste 2502, Pittsburgh, PA 15213; **Phone:** 412-641-1342; **Board Cert:** Surgery 2008; Plastic Surgery 1993; **Med School:** Temple Univ 1983; **Resid:** Surgery, Univ Pittsburgh Med Ctr 1989; Plastic Surgery, Univ Pittsburgh Med Ctr 1990; **Fellow:** Hand Surgery, Univ Pittsburgh 1991; Surgical Oncology, National Cancer Inst 1993; **Fac Appt:** Assoc Prof S, Univ Pittsburgh

Edye, Michael MD [S] - Spec Exp: Laparoscopic Abdominal Surgery; Colon Cancer; Diverticulitis; Obesity/Bariatric Surgery; **Hospital:** Mount Sinai Med Ctr (page 64); **Address:** 17 E 102nd St Fl 5, Ctr for Advanced Medicine Bldg, New York, NY 10029; **Phone:** 212-241-0872; **Med School:** Australia 1977; **Resid:** Surgery, St Vincents Hosp 1980; Surgery, Royal N Shore Hosp 1984; **Fellow:** Laparoscopic Surgery, Univ Bordeaux 1992; **Fac Appt:** Assoc Clin Prof S, Mount Sinai Sch Med

Emond, Jean C MD [S] - Spec Exp: Transplant-Liver; Liver Cancer; Liver & Biliary Cancer; Hepatobiliary Surgery; **Hospital:** NY-Presby/Columbia Univ Med Ctr, NY (page 66), Holy Name Med Ctr; **Address:** 622 W 168th St, PH - Fl 14, New York, NY 10032; **Phone:** 212-305-9691; **Board Cert:** Surgery 2006; **Med School:** Univ Chicago-Pritzker Sch Med 1979; **Resid:** Surgery, Cook Cty Hosp 1984; **Fellow:** Surgery, Hopital P Brousse/Univ de Paris Sud 1985; Transplant Surgery, Univ Chicago Hosps 1987; **Fac Appt:** Prof S, Columbia P&S

Estabrook, Alison MD [S] - Spec Exp: Breast Cancer; Breast Disease; Breast Cancer-High Risk Women; **Hospital:** St. Luke's - Roosevelt Hosp Ctr - Roosevelt Div (page 56); **Address:** Comprehensive Breast Center, 425 W 59th St Fl 7 - Ste 7A, New York, NY 10019-1104; **Phone:** 212-523-7500; **Board Cert:** Surgery 2004; **Med School:** NYU Sch Med 1978; **Resid:** Surgery, Columbia Presby Med Ctr 1984; **Fellow:** Surgical Oncology, Columbia Presby Med Ctr 1982; **Fac Appt:** Prof S, Columbia P&S

Fahey III, Thomas J MD [S] - Spec Exp: Endocrine Surgery; Pheochromocytoma; Pancreatic Cancer; Minimally Invasive Surgery; **Hospital:** NY-Presby/Weill Cornell Med Ctr, NY (page 66); **Address:** NY Presby Cornell Med Ctr, Dept Surgery, 525 E 68 St, rm Starr 8, Box 249, New York, NY 10065; **Phone:** 212-746 5130; **Board Cert:** Surgery 2002; **Med School:** Cornell Univ-Weill Med Coll 1986; **Resid:** Surgery, New York Hosp 1992; **Fellow:** Endocrine Surgery, Royal North Shore Hosp 1993; **Fac Appt:** Prof S, Cornell Univ-Weill Med Coll

Fong, Yuman MD [S] - Spec Exp: Pancreatic Cancer; Liver & Biliary Cancer; Stomach Cancer; **Hospital:** Meml Sloan-Kettering Cancer Ctr, NY-Presby/Weill Cornell Med Ctr, NY (page 66); **Address:** 1275 York Ave, rm C887, New York, NY 10065; **Phone:** 212-639-2016; **Board Cert:** Surgery 2002; **Med School:** Cornell Univ-Weill Med Coll 1984; **Resid:** Surgery, NY Hosp-Cornell Med Ctr 1992; **Fellow:** Surgical Oncology, Meml Sloan-Kettering Cancer Ctr 1994; **Fac Appt:** Prof S, Cornell Univ-Weill Med Coll

Fraker, Douglas L MD [S] - Spec Exp: Melanoma; Endocrine Surgery; Liver Cancer; Sarcoma; **Hospital:** Hosp Univ Penn - UPHS (page 72); **Address:** Hosp Univ Penn, Dept Surgery, 3400 Spruce St, 4 Silverstein, Philadelphia, PA 19104; **Phone:** 215-662-7866; **Board Cert:** Surgery 2002; **Med School:** Harvard Med Sch 1983; **Resid:** Surgery, UCSF Med Ctr 1986; Surgery, UCSF Med Ctr 1991; **Fellow:** Surgical Oncology, National Cancer Inst 1989; **Fac Appt:** Prof S, Univ Pennsylvania

Frazier, Thomas G MD [S] - Spec Exp: Breast Cancer; Breast Disease; **Hospital:** Bryn Mawr Hosp; **Address:** 101 S Bryn Mawr Ave, Ste 201, Bryn Mawr, PA 19010; **Phone:** 610-520-0700; **Board Cert:** Surgery 2004; **Med School:** Univ Pennsylvania 1968; **Resid:** Surgery, Hosp Univ Penn 1975; **Fellow:** Surgical Oncology, MD Anderson Cancer Ctr 1976; **Fac Appt:** Clin Prof S, Drexel Univ Coll Med

Surgery

Geller, David A MD [S] - **Spec Exp:** Liver Cancer; Laparoscopic Surgery; Clinical Trials; **Hospital:** UPMC Presby, Pittsburgh, UPMC Passavant-McCandless; **Address:** UPMC Liver Cancer Center, 3459 5th Ave, Pittsburgh, PA 15213-2582; **Phone:** 412-692-2001; **Board Cert:** Surgery 2005; **Med School:** Northwestern Univ 1988; **Resid:** Surgery, UPMC-Presbyterian Hosp 1993; **Fellow:** Hepatobiliary Surgery, Univ Pittsburgh 1998; Transplant Surgery, Univ Pittsburgh 1998; **Fac Appt:** Prof S, Univ Pittsburgh

Gibbs, John F MD [S] - **Spec Exp:** Gastrointestinal Cancer; Stomach Cancer; Pancreatic Cancer; Liver Cancer; **Hospital:** Buffalo General Hosp; **Address:** University Surgeons, 100 High St, C319, Buffalo, NY 14203; **Phone:** 716-859-2268; **Board Cert:** Surgery 2009; **Med School:** UCSD 1985; **Resid:** Surgery, Rush Presby-St Lukes Med Ctr 1990; **Fellow:** Transplant Surgery, Baylor Univ Med Ctr 1992; Surgical Oncology, Roswell Park Cancer Inst 1996; **Fac Appt:** Prof S, SUNY Buffalo

Haith Jr, Linwood R MD [S] - **Spec Exp:** Burn Care; **Hospital:** Crozer - Chester Med Ctr; **Address:** One Medical Ctr Blvd, Ste 241, Upland, PA 19013; **Phone:** 610-619-7400; **Board Cert:** Surgery 2002; Surgical Critical Care 2007; **Med School:** Harvard Med Sch 1976; **Resid:** Surgery, Yale-New Haven Hosp 1982; **Fellow:** Surgical Critical Care, Thomas Jefferson Univ Hosp 1987; **Fac Appt:** Assoc Clin Prof S, Temple Univ

Hanna, Nader N MD [S] - **Spec Exp:** Pancreatic Cancer; Adrenal Tumors; Peritoneal Carcinomatosis; Sarcoma-Soft Tissue; **Hospital:** Univ of MD Med Ctr; **Address:** 22 S Greene St, Ste S4B12, Baltimore, MD 21201; **Phone:** 410-328-7320; **Board Cert:** Surgery 2005; **Med School:** Egypt 1985; **Resid:** Surgery, St. Elizabeth's Med Ctr-Tuft's Univ 1994; **Fellow:** Surgical Oncology, Univ of Chicago Med Ctr 1997; **Fac Appt:** Assoc Prof S, Univ MD Sch Med

Hiotis, Spiros P MD/PhD [S] - **Spec Exp:** Liver Cancer; Gallbladder & Biliary Cancer; Pancreatic Cancer; Stomach Cancer; **Hospital:** Mount Sinai Med Ctr (page 64); **Address:** Surgical Oncology Assocs, 5 E 98th St Fl 12, Box 1259, New York, NY 100 129; **Phone:** 212-241-2891; **Board Cert:** Surgery 2010; **Med School:** Univ MD Sch Med 1992; **Resid:** Surgery, USF Med Ctr 1998; **Fellow:** Surgical Oncology, Meml Sloan Kettering Cancer Ctr 2000; **Fac Appt:** Asst Prof S, Mount Sinai Sch Med

Hoffman, John P MD [S] - **Spec Exp:** Pancreatic Cancer; Gastrointestinal Cancer; Hepatobiliary Surgery; Liver Cancer; **Hospital:** Fox Chase Cancer Ctr (page 58); **Address:** Fox Chase Cancer Ctr, 333 Cottman Ave, Philadelphia, PA 19111-2497; **Phone:** 215-728-3518; **Board Cert:** Surgery 2010; **Med School:** Case West Res Univ 1970; **Resid:** Surgery, Virginia Mason Hosp 1977; **Fellow:** Surgical Oncology, Meml Sloan Kettering Cancer Ctr 1980; **Fac Appt:** Prof S, Temple Univ

Jarnagin, William MD [S] - **Spec Exp:** Hepatobiliary Surgery; Liver Cancer; Pancreatic Cancer; Gallbladder & Biliary Cancer; **Hospital:** Meml Sloan-Kettering Cancer Ctr; **Address:** 1275 York Ave, New York, NY 10065; **Phone:** 212-639-7601; **Board Cert:** Surgery 2006; **Med School:** Rush Med Coll 1988; **Resid:** Surgery, Univ Calif San Francisco 1996; **Fellow:** Hepatopancreatobiliary Surgery, Meml Sloan-Kettering Cancer Ctr 1997; **Fac Appt:** Prof S, Cornell Univ

Johnson, Lynt B MD [S] - **Spec Exp:** Transplant Surgery; Liver Surgery; Pancreatic Surgery; **Hospital:** Georgetown Univ Hosp; **Address:** 3800 Reservoir Rd NW PHC Bldg Fl 4, Washington, DC 20007; **Phone:** 202-444-4557; **Board Cert:** Surgery 1992; **Med School:** Harvard Med Sch 1985; **Resid:** Surgery, Mass Genl Hosp 1991; **Fellow:** Transplant Surgery, Beth Israel Deaconess Med Ctr 1993; **Fac Appt:** Prof S, Georgetown Univ

Johnson, Ronald R MD [S] - **Spec Exp:** Breast Cancer; Breast Disease; **Hospital:** Magee-Womens Hosp - UPMC, UPMC Presby, Pittsburgh; **Address:** Magee-Womens Surgical Assocs, 300 Halket St, Ste 2601, Pittsburgh, PA 15213; **Phone:** 412-641-1225; **Board Cert:** Surgery 2010; **Med School:** Univ Pittsburgh 1983; **Resid:** Surgery, Univ Pittsburgh Med Ctr 1989; **Fac Appt:** Assoc Prof S, Univ Pittsburgh

Julian, Thomas B MD [S] - **Spec Exp:** Breast Cancer & Surgery; Clinical Trials; **Hospital:** Allegheny General Hosp; **Address:** Allegheny Cancer Ctr, 320 E North Ave, Fl 5, Pittsburgh, PA 15212; **Phone:** 412-359-8229; **Board Cert:** Surgery 2001; **Med School:** Univ Pittsburgh 1976; **Resid:** Surgery, Univ Pittsburgh Med Ctr 1982; **Fac Appt:** Prof S, Temple Univ

Kapur, Sandip MD [S] - **Spec Exp:** Transplant-Kidney; Pancreatic Islet Cell Transplant; Transplant-Pancreas; **Hospital:** NY-Presby/Weill Cornell Med Ctr, NY (page 66), NY-Presby/Columbia Univ Med Ctr, NY (page 66); **Address:** 525 E 68th St, Baker Bldg Fl 19 - Ste F1919, Box 98, New York, NY 10065; **Phone:** 212-746-5330; **Board Cert:** Surgery 2007; **Med School:** Cornell Univ-Weill Med Coll 1990; **Resid:** Surgery, Cornell Univ Med Ctr 1996; **Fellow:** Research, The Rogosin Inst 1994; Transplant Surgery, Thomas E Starzl Transplant Inst 1998; **Fac Appt:** Assoc Prof S, Cornell Univ-Weill Med Coll

Karpeh Jr, Martin S MD [S] - **Spec Exp:** Gastrointestinal Cancer; Esophageal Cancer; Pancreatic Cancer; Liver Cancer; **Hospital:** Beth Israel Med Ctr - Petrie Division (page 56); **Address:** Beth Israel Medical Center, Philips Ambulatory Care Center, 10 Union Square E, Ste 4D, New York, NY 10003; **Phone:** 212-420-4041; **Board Cert:** Surgery 2006; **Med School:** Penn State Coll Med 1983; **Resid:** Surgery, Hosp Univ Penn 1989; **Fellow:** Surgical Oncology, Meml Sloan Kettering Cancer Ctr 1991; **Fac Appt:** Prof S, Mount Sinai Sch Med

Kato, Tomoaki MD [S] - **Spec Exp:** Transplant-Liver; Transplant Surgery-Pediatric; Transplant-Multi Organ; Transplant-Auto Transplantation; **Hospital:** NY-Presby/Columbia Univ Med Ctr, NY (page 66); **Address:** Columbia Univ Med Ctr, 622 W 168th St PH 14 Bldg - rm 105, New York, NY 10032; **Phone:** 212-305-5101; **Med School:** Japan 1991; **Resid:** Surgery, Itami City Hospital 1995; **Fellow:** Transplant Surgery, Jackson Meml Hosp 1997; **Fac Appt:** Prof S, Columbia P&S

Kinkhabwala, Milan M MD [S] - **Spec Exp:** Transplant-Liver; Hepatobiliary Surgery; Liver & Biliary Surgery; Liver & Biliary Cancer; **Hospital:** Montefiore Med Ctr-Moses Campus, NY, Montefiore Med Ctr-Einstein Campus, NY; **Address:** 111 E 210th St, Bronx, NY 10467; **Phone:** 718-920-6659; **Board Cert:** Surgery 2004; **Med School:** Cornell Univ-Weill Med Coll 1989; **Resid:** Surgery, NY Presby/Weil Cornell 1994; **Fellow:** Hepatobiliary Surgery, UCLA Med Ctr; **Fac Appt:** Prof S, Albert Einstein Coll Med

Leach, Steven D MD [S] - **Spec Exp:** Pancreatic Cancer; **Hospital:** Johns Hopkins Hosp (page 61); **Address:** Johns Hopkins Med Outpatient Ctr, 601 N Caroline St, Baltimore, MD 21287; **Phone:** 410-933-1233; **Board Cert:** Surgery 2004; **Med School:** Emory Univ 1986; **Resid:** Surgery, Yale-New Haven Hosp 1993; **Fellow:** Surgical Oncology, MD Anderson Cancer Ctr 1995; **Fac Appt:** Prof S, Johns Hopkins Univ

Lee, Kenneth Kwock MD [S] - **Spec Exp:** Pancreatic Cancer; Gastrointestinal Cancer & Surgery; Minimally Invasive Surgery; **Hospital:** UPMC Presby, Pittsburgh, UPMC Shadyside; **Address:** 3550 Terrace St, Ste 497, Scaife Hall, Pittsburgh, PA 15261; **Phone:** 412-647-0457; **Board Cert:** Surgery 2008; **Med School:** Univ Chicago-Pritzker Sch Med 1981; **Resid:** Surgery, Univ Chicago Hosps 1988; **Fellow:** Univ Chicago; **Fac Appt:** Assoc Prof S, Univ Pittsburgh

Libutti, Steven K MD [S] - **Spec Exp:** Liver Cancer; Neuroendocrine Tumors; Gastrointestinal Cancer; **Hospital:** Montefiore Med Ctr-Einstein Campus, NY, Montefiore Med Ctr-Moses Campus, NY; **Address:** Montefiore-Einstein Ctr for Cancer Care, 1521 Jarret Pl, Bronx, NY 10461; **Phone:** 718-862-8840; **Board Cert:** Surgery 2004; **Med School:** Columbia P&S 1990; **Resid:** Surgery, Columbia Presby Med Ctr 1995; **Fellow:** Surgical Oncology, Natl Cancer Inst 1996; **Fac Appt:** Prof S, Albert Einstein Coll Med

Lieberman, Michael D MD [S] - **Spec Exp:** Gastrointestinal Cancer; Colon & Rectal Cancer & Surgery; Hepatobiliary Surgery; Pancreatic Cancer; **Hospital:** NY-Presby/Weill Cornell Med Ctr, NY (page 66); **Address:** 1315 York Ave, Box 216, New York, NY 10021; **Phone:** 212-746-5434; **Board Cert:** Surgery 2003; **Med School:** UMDNJ-NJ Med Sch, Newark 1985; **Resid:** Surgery, Hosp Univ Penn 1992; **Fellow:** Surgical Oncology, Hosp Univ Penn 1990; Surgical Oncology, Meml Sloan-Kettering Cancer Ctr 1994; **Fac Appt:** Assoc Prof S, Cornell Univ-Weill Med Coll

Mannella Jr, William J MD [S] - **Spec Exp:** Vascular Surgery; Peripheral Vascular Disease; Wound Healing/Care; **Hospital:** Crozer - Chester Med Ctr; **Address:** One Medical Ctr Blvd, ACP Bldg - Ste 233, Upland, PA 19013; **Phone:** 610-499-0400; **Board Cert:** Surgery 2009; **Med School:** Hahnemann Univ 1973; **Resid:** Surgery, Hahnemann Univ Hosp 1978; **Fac Appt:** Clin Prof S, Drexel Univ Coll Med

Marsh Jr, James W MD [S] - **Spec Exp:** Transplant-Liver; Liver Cancer; Pancreatic Cancer; **Hospital:** UPMC Presby, Pittsburgh, Monongahela Valley Hosp; **Address:** Starzl Transplantation Inst, UPMC Montefiore 7 South, 3459 Fifth Ave, Pittsburgh, PA 15213-2582; **Phone:** 412-647-5800; **Board Cert:** Surgery 2003; **Med School:** Univ Ark 1979; **Resid:** Surgery, St Paul Hosp 1984; **Fellow:** Transplant Surgery, Mayo Clinic 1985; Transplant Surgery, Univ Pittsburgh 1986; **Fac Appt:** Prof S, Univ Pittsburgh

Meyers, William C MD [S] - **Spec Exp:** Hernia; Liver & Biliary Surgery; **Address:** 4623 S Broad St, Philadelphia, PA 19112; **Phone:** 215-334-1274; **Board Cert:** Surgery 2004; **Med School:** Columbia P&S 1975; **Resid:** Surgery, Duke Univ Med Ctr 1982; Surgery, Duke Univ Med Ctr 1983; **Fellow:** Gastroenterology, Duke Univ Med Ctr 1983; **Fac Appt:** Prof S, Drexel Univ Coll Med

Michelassi, Fabrizio MD [S] - **Spec Exp:** Gastrointestinal Cancer; Crohn's Disease; Ulcerative Colitis; Colon Cancer; **Hospital:** NY-Presby/Weill Cornell Med Ctr, NY (page 66); **Address:** 525 E 68th St Fl 7 - rm F-739, Box 129, New York, NY 10065; **Phone:** 212-746-6006; **Board Cert:** Surgery 2002; **Med School:** Italy 1975; **Resid:** Surgery, NYU Med Ctr 1981; **Fellow:** Research, Mass Genl Hosp 1983; **Fac Appt:** Prof S, Cornell Univ-Weill Med Coll

Montgomery, Robert A MD/PhD [S] - **Spec Exp:** Transplant-Kidney; **Hospital:** Johns Hopkins Hosp (page 61); **Address:** Johns Hopkins Hosp, Transplant Surgery, 720 Rutland Ave Ross Bldg - Ste 765, Baltimore, MD 21205; **Phone:** 410-614-8297; **Board Cert:** Surgery 2006; **Med School:** Univ Rochester 1987; **Resid:** Surgery, Johns Hopkins Hosp 1995; **Fellow:** Transplant Surgery, Johns Hopkins Hosp 1997; **Fac Appt:** Prof S, Johns Hopkins Univ

Morrow, Monica MD [S] - **Spec Exp:** Breast Cancer; **Hospital:** Meml Sloan-Kettering Cancer Ctr; **Address:** 300 E 66th St Fl 4, New York, NY 10065; **Phone:** 646-888-5354; **Board Cert:** Surgery 2011; **Med School:** Jefferson Med Coll 1976; **Resid:** Surgery, Med Ctr Hosp Vermont 1981; **Fellow:** Surgical Oncology, Meml Sloan Kettering Cancer Ctr 1983; **Fac Appt:** Prof S, Cornell Univ-Weill Med Coll

Newman, Elliot MD [S] - **Spec Exp:** Gastrointestinal Cancer; Robotic Surgery; Liver & Biliary Cancer; Colon & Rectal Cancer; **Hospital:** NYU Langone Med Ctr (page 68); **Address:** NYU Clinical Cancer Ctr, 160 E 34th St, New York, NY 10016; **Phone:** 212-731-5466; **Board Cert:** Surgery 2004; **Med School:** NYU Sch Med 1986; **Resid:** Surgery, NYU Med Ctr 1989; Surgery, NYU Med Ctr 1993; **Fellow:** Research, Meml Sloan Kettering Cancer Ctr 1991; Surgical Oncology, Meml Sloan Kettering Cancer Ctr 1995; **Fac Appt:** Assoc Prof S, NYU Sch Med

Nowak, Eugene J MD [S] - **Spec Exp:** Breast Cancer; Hernia; Sentinel Node Surgery; Gastrointestinal Surgery; **Hospital:** NY-Presby/Weill Cornell Med Ctr, NY (page 66); **Address:** 325 E 79th St, Ground Fl, New York, NY 10075-0954; **Phone:** 212-517-6693; **Board Cert:** Surgery 2002; **Med School:** UMDNJ-NJ Med Sch, Newark 1975; **Resid:** Surgery, New York Hosp 1980; **Fac Appt:** Asst Clin Prof S, Cornell Univ-Weill Med Coll

O'Hea, Brian J MD [S] - **Spec Exp:** Breast Cancer; Sentinel Node Surgery; **Hospital:** Stony Brook Univ Med Ctr; **Address:** HSC T-18, Rm 060, Dept of Surgery, Stony Brook, NY 11794-8191; **Phone:** 631-444-1795; **Board Cert:** Surgery 2002; **Med School:** Georgetown Univ 1986; **Resid:** Surgery, St Vincent's Hosp 1991; **Fellow:** Breast Disease, Meml Sloan-Kettering Cancer Ctr 1996; **Fac Appt:** Asst Prof S, SUNY Stony Brook

Olson Jr, John A MD/PhD [S] - **Spec Exp:** Endocrine Cancers; Breast Cancer; Melanoma; Clinical Trials; **Hospital:** Univ of MD Med Ctr; **Address:** 22 Greene St, S4B18, Baltimore, MD 21201; **Phone:** 410-328-6187; **Board Cert:** Surgery 2009; **Med School:** Univ Fla Coll Med 1992; **Resid:** Surgery, Barnes Hospital/Wash Univ 1998; Surgery, Royal Infirm of Edingurgh 1997; **Fellow:** Surgical Oncology, Meml Sloan-Kettering Cancer Ctr 2000; **Fac Appt:** Prof S, Univ MD Sch Med

Olthoff, Kim M MD [S] - **Spec Exp:** Transplant-Liver-Adult & Pediatric; Liver & Biliary Surgery; Liver Cancer; Transplant-Pancreas; **Hospital:** Hosp Univ Penn - UPHS (page 72), Chldns Hosp of Philadelphia; **Address:** Univ Penn - Dept Surgery, 3400 Spruce St, 2 Dulles, Philadelphia, PA 19104; **Phone:** 215-662-6136; **Board Cert:** Surgery 2003; **Med School:** Univ Chicago-Pritzker Sch Med 1986; **Resid:** Surgery, UCLA Med Ctr 1988; **Fellow:** Surgery, UCLA 1990; Transgender Surgery, UCLA 1995; **Fac Appt:** Prof S, Univ Pennsylvania

Osborne, Michael P MD [S] - **Spec Exp:** Breast Cancer & Surgery; Breast Disease; Breast Reconstruction; **Hospital:** Beth Israel Med Ctr - Petrie Division (page 56); **Address:** 325 W 15 St, Beth Israel Comprehensive Cancer Center, New York, NY 10011; **Phone:** 212-367-0133; **Med School:** England, UK 1970; **Resid:** Surgery, Charing Cross Hosp 1977; Surgery, Royal Marsden Hosp 1980; **Fellow:** Surgical Oncology, Meml Sloan-Kettering Canc Ctr 1981; **Fac Appt:** Prof S, Cornell Univ-Weill Med Coll

Pachter, H Leon MD [S] - **Spec Exp:** Adrenal Surgery; Gastrointestinal Surgery; Pancreatic Cancer; Hernia; **Hospital:** NYU Langone Med Ctr (page 68), Bellevue Hosp Ctr; **Address:** 530 1st Ave, Ste 6C, New York, NY 10016; **Phone:** 212-263-7302; **Board Cert:** Surgery 2009; **Med School:** NYU Sch Med 1971; **Resid:** Surgery, NYU Med Ctr 1976; **Fac Appt:** Prof S, NYU Sch Med

Patel, Sameer A MD [S] - **Spec Exp:** Breast Reconstruction; Head & Neck Reconstruction; **Hospital:** Fox Chase Cancer Ctr (page 58), Virtua West Jersey Hosp - Voorhees; **Address:** Fox Chase Cancer Ctr, 333 Cottman Ave, Philadelphia, PA 19111; **Phone:** 215-728-3559; **Board Cert:** Surgery 2005; Plastic Surgery 2008; **Med School:** UMDNJ-NJ Med Sch, Newark 1998; **Resid:** Surgery, Montefiore Med Ctr 2003; Plastic/Reconstructive Surgery, Montefiore Med Ctr 2004; **Fellow:** Microsurgery, MD Anderson Cancer Ctr 2005

Paty, Philip B MD [S] - **Spec Exp:** Colon & Rectal Cancer; Gastrointestinal Cancer; Pelvic Tumors; **Hospital:** Meml Sloan-Kettering Cancer Ctr; **Address:** 1275 York Avenue, New York, NY 10065; **Phone:** 646-497-9065; **Board Cert:** Surgery 2001; **Med School:** Stanford Univ 1983; **Resid:** Surgery, UCSF Med Ctr 1990; **Fellow:** Surgical Oncology, Meml Sloan Kettering Cancer Ctr 1992; **Fac Appt:** Prof S, Cornell Univ-Weill Med Coll

Pawlik, Timothy M MD [S] - **Spec Exp:** Liver Cancer; Pancreatic Cancer; Gastrointestinal Cancer; Gallbladder & Biliary Cancer; **Hospital:** Johns Hopkins Hosp (page 61); **Address:** Johns Hopkins Hosp, 600 N Wolfe St, Harvey Bldg - rm 611, Baltimore, MD 21287; **Phone:** 410-933-1233; **Board Cert:** Surgery 2004; **Med School:** Tufts Univ 1995; **Resid:** Surgery, Univ Michigan Hosp 2002; **Fellow:** Research, Mass Genl Hosp 2004; Surgical Oncology, UT MD Anderson Cancer Ctr 2006; **Fac Appt:** Assoc Prof S, Johns Hopkins Univ

Peitzman, Andrew B MD [S] - **Spec Exp:** Trauma; **Hospital:** UPMC Presby, Pittsburgh; **Address:** UPMC, Dept Surg, 200 Lothrop St, Ste F1281, Pittsburgh, PA 15213; **Phone:** 412-647-0635; **Board Cert:** Surgery 2003; **Med School:** Univ Pittsburgh 1976; **Resid:** Surgery, Univ Pittsburgh Med Ctr 1979; Surgery, Univ Pittsburgh Med Ctr 1984; **Fellow:** Surgery, NY Hosp-Cornell Med Ctr 1981; **Fac Appt:** Prof S, Univ Pittsburgh

Peters, Jeffrey H MD [S] - **Spec Exp:** Esophageal Surgery; Gastroesophageal Reflux Disease (GERD); **Hospital:** Univ of Rochester Strong Meml Hosp; **Address:** 601 Elmwood Ave, Box SURG, Rochester, NY 14642-8410; **Phone:** 585-275-2725; **Board Cert:** Surgery 2007; **Med School:** Ohio State Univ 1981; **Resid:** Surgery, Johns Hopkins Hosp 1988; **Fellow:** Allergy & Immunology, Johns Hopkins Hosp 1985; Esophageal Surgery, Creighton Univ; **Fac Appt:** Prof S, Univ Rochester

Philosophe, Benjamin MD [S] - **Spec Exp:** Transplant-Liver; Transplant-Pancreas; Hepatobiliary Surgery; Liver Cancer; **Hospital:** Univ of MD Med Ctr; **Address:** UMMC Transplant Ctr, 29 S Greene St, Ste 200, Baltimore, MD 21201; **Phone:** 410-328-1145; **Board Cert:** Surgery 2001; **Med School:** Boston Univ 1990; **Resid:** Surgery, Barnes Jewish Hosp 1995; **Fellow:** Hepatopancreatobiliary Surgery, Toronto Hosp 1996; Transplant Surgery, Toronto Hosp 1997; **Fac Appt:** Assoc Prof S, Univ MD Sch Med

Pomp, Alfons MD [S] - **Spec Exp:** Obesity/Bariatric Surgery; Laparoscopic Abdominal Surgery; Hernia; **Hospital:** NY-Presby/Weill Cornell Med Ctr, NY (page 66); **Address:** Weill Cornell College of Medicine, 525 E 68th St, Box 294, New York, NY 10065; **Phone:** 212-746-5294; **Board Cert:** Surgery 2010; **Med School:** Univ Sherbrooke 1980; **Resid:** Surgery, Univ Montreal Med Ctr 1985; **Fellow:** Nutrition, Rhode Island Hosp 1988; **Fac Appt:** Prof S, Cornell Univ-Weill Med Coll

Ramanathan, Ramesh Chandran MD [S] - **Spec Exp:** Obesity/Bariatric Surgery; Minimally Invasive Surgery; Colon Cancer; Clinical Trials; **Hospital:** Magee-Womens Hosp - UPMC; **Address:** Magee-Womens Hosp, 3380 Boulevard of the Allies, Ste 390, Pittsburgh, PA 15213; **Phone:** 412-641-3632; **Board Cert:** Surgery 2004; **Med School:** India 1988; **Resid:** Surgery, Univ Pitts Med Ctr 2003; **Fellow:** Surgical Oncology, Univ Pitts Med Ctr 1999; Minimally Invasive Surgery, Univ Pitts Med Ctr 2000; **Fac Appt:** Asst Prof S, Univ Pittsburgh

Reich, David J MD [S] - **Spec Exp:** Transplant-Liver; Hepatobiliary Surgery; Liver Cancer; Transplant-Kidney; **Hospital:** Hahnemann Univ Hosp, Abington Mem Hosp; **Address:** Transplant Center, 216 N Broad St, Feinstein Bldg Fl 5, Philadelphia, PA 19102; **Phone:** 215-762-8153; **Board Cert:** Surgery 2003; **Med School:** McGill Univ 1989; **Resid:** Surgery, Beth Israel Med Ctr 1994; **Fellow:** Transplant Surgery, Mt Sinai Med Ctr 1996; **Fac Appt:** Prof S, Drexel Univ Coll Med

Reiner, Mark A MD [S] - **Spec Exp:** Laparoscopic Surgery; Hernia; Esophageal Surgery; Pancreatic Surgery; **Hospital:** Mount Sinai Med Ctr (page 64); **Address:** 1010 5th Ave, Ste 82 & 83, New York, NY 10028-0130; **Phone:** 212-879-6677; **Board Cert:** Surgery 2011; **Med School:** SUNY Downstate 1974; **Resid:** Surgery, Mt Sinai Hosp 1979; **Fac Appt:** Clin Prof S, Mount Sinai Sch Med

Ridge, John Andrew MD/PhD [S] - **Spec Exp:** Head & Neck Cancer & Surgery; Thyroid Cancer & Surgery; Laryngeal Cancer; Robotic Surgery; **Hospital:** Fox Chase Cancer Ctr (page 58); **Address:** 333 Cottman Ave, Philadelphia, PA 19111; **Phone:** 215-728-3517; **Board Cert:** Surgery 2006; **Med School:** Stanford Univ 1981; **Resid:** Surgery, Univ Colorado Med Ctr 1987; **Fellow:** Cancer Research, Meml Sloan-Kettering Cancer Ctr 1985; Surgical Oncology, Meml Sloan-Kettering Cancer Ctr 1989; **Fac Appt:** Prof S, Temple Univ

Rosenberg, Steven A MD/PhD [S] - **Spec Exp:** Melanoma; Kidney Cancer; **Hospital:** Natl Inst of Hlth - Clin Ctr; **Address:** National Cancer Inst, Surgery Branch, 9000 Rockville Pike, Bldg 10 - rm 3-3940, Bethesda, MD 20892; **Phone:** 301-496-4164; **Board Cert:** Surgery 1975; **Med School:** Johns Hopkins Univ 1964; **Resid:** Surgery, Peter Bent Brigham Hosp 1974; **Fac Appt:** Prof S, Uniformed Srvs Univ, Bethesda

Roses, Daniel F MD [S] - **Spec Exp:** Breast Cancer; Melanoma; Thyroid Cancer; Parathyroid Cancer; **Hospital:** NYU Langone Med Ctr (page 68); **Address:** 530 First Ave, Ste 6B, New York, NY 10016-6402; **Phone:** 212-263-7329; **Board Cert:** Surgery 1975; **Med School:** NYU Sch Med 1969; **Resid:** Surgery, NYU-Bellevue Hosp 1974; **Fellow:** Surgical Oncology, NYU-Bellevue Hosp 1978; **Fac Appt:** Prof Surg & Onc, NYU Sch Med

Rubino, Francesco MD [S] - **Spec Exp:** Gastrointestinal Metabolic Surgery; Diabetes Surgery-Rubino's Procedure; Obesity/Bariatric Surgery; **Hospital:** NY-Presby/Weill Cornell Med Ctr, NY (page 66); **Address:** NY Presbyterian Hosp/Weill Cornell, 525 E 68th St, rm P714, New York, NY 10021; **Phone:** 212-746-5925; **Med School:** Italy 1994; **Resid:** Surgery, Catholic Univ/Policlinico Gemelli; **Fellow:** Laparoscopic Surgery, European Inst of Telesurgery; Research, Catholic Univ; **Fac Appt:** Asst Prof S, Cornell Univ-Weill Med Coll

Salky, Barry A MD [S] - **Spec Exp:** Laparoscopic Abdominal Surgery; Gastroesophageal Reflux Disease (GERD); Colon Cancer; Ulcerative Colitis; **Hospital:** Mount Sinai Med Ctr (page 64); **Address:** Mt Sinai Medical Center, Div of Laparoscopic Surgery, 5 E 98th St Fl 14 - Ste C, Box 1259, New York, NY 10029; **Phone:** 212-241-6156; **Board Cert:** Surgery 2010; **Med School:** Univ Tenn Coll Med 1970; **Resid:** Surgery, Mount Sinai Hosp 1973; Surgery, Mount Sinai Hosp 1978; **Fac Appt:** Prof S, Mount Sinai Sch Med

Sataloff, Dahlia M MD [S] - **Spec Exp:** Breast Cancer; Breast Disease; **Hospital:** Pennsylvania Hosp-UPHS (page 72); **Address:** 700 Spruce St, Ste B03, Philadelphia, PA 19106; **Phone:** 215-829-8461; **Board Cert:** Surgery 2005; **Med School:** Univ Mich Med Sch 1978; **Resid:** Surgery, St Joseph Mercy Hosp 1980; Surgery, Pennsylvania Hosp 1985; **Fac Appt:** Clin Prof S, Univ Pennsylvania

Scantlebury, Velma P MD [S] - **Spec Exp:** Transplant-Kidney; **Hospital:** Wilmington Hosp, Christiana Hospital; **Address:** 4735 Ogletown-Stanton Rd, Med Arts Pavilion II, Ste 2224, Newark, DE 19713; **Phone:** 302-623-3866; **Board Cert:** Surgery 2001; **Med School:** Columbia P&S 1981; **Resid:** Surgery, Harlem Hosp 1986; **Fellow:** Transplant Surgery, Univ Pittsburgh Med Ctr 1988

Schnabel, Freya MD [S] - **Spec Exp:** Breast Cancer; Breast Cancer-High Risk Women; **Hospital:** NYU Langone Med Ctr (page 68); **Address:** 160 E 34th St Fl 3, New York, NY 10016; **Phone:** 212-731-5367; **Board Cert:** Surgery 2008; **Med School:** NYU Sch Med 1982; **Resid:** Surgery, NYU Med Ctr 1987; **Fellow:** Research, SUNY Hlth Sci Ctr 1988; **Fac Appt:** Prof S, NYU Sch Med

Schraut, Wolfgang H MD [S] - **Spec Exp:** Inflammatory Bowel Disease; Gastrointestinal Surgery; Colon & Rectal Cancer & Surgery; Minimally Invasive Surgery; **Hospital:** UPMC Presby, Pittsburgh, UPMC Shadyside; **Address:** 3550 Terrace St, Ste 497, Scaife Hall, Pittsburgh, PA 15261; **Phone:** 412-647-0457; **Board Cert:** Surgery 2009; **Med School:** Germany 1970; **Resid:** Surgery, Univ Chicago Hosps 1978; **Fellow:** Surgery, Univ Chicago; **Fac Appt:** Prof S, Univ Pittsburgh

Shah, Jatin P MD/PhD [S] - **Spec Exp:** Head & Neck Cancer & Surgery; Thyroid Cancer; Skull Base Tumors; Salivary Gland Tumors & Surgery; **Hospital:** Meml Sloan-Kettering Cancer Ctr; **Address:** 1275 York Ave, New York, NY 10065; **Phone:** 646-497-9161; **Board Cert:** Surgery 1975; **Med School:** India 1964; **Resid:** Surgery, SSG Hosp 1967; Surgery, NY Eye & Ear Infirm 1974; **Fellow:** Head & Neck Surgical Oncology, Meml Sloan-Kettering Hosp 1972; **Fac Appt:** Prof S, Cornell Univ-Weill Med Coll

Shaked, Abraham MD/PhD [S] - **Spec Exp:** Transplant Surgery; Transplant-Liver; Hepatobiliary Surgery; **Hospital:** Hosp Univ Penn - UPHS (page 72); **Address:** Hosp Univ Penn, Liver Transplant Unit, 2 Dulles, 3400 Spruce St, Philadelphia, PA 19104; **Phone:** 215-662-6723; **Board Cert:** Surgery 2010; **Med School:** Israel 1982; **Resid:** Surgery, Mt Sinai Hosp 1989; **Fellow:** Transplant Surgery, UCLA Med Ctr 1990; **Fac Appt:** Prof S, Univ Pennsylvania

Shapiro, Richard L MD [S] - **Spec Exp:** Breast Cancer; Melanoma; Thyroid & Parathyroid Surgery; Cancer Surgery; **Hospital:** NYU Langone Med Ctr (page 68); **Address:** NYU Medical Clinical Cancer Center, 160 E 34th St Fl 4, New York, NY 10016; **Phone:** 212-731-5347; **Board Cert:** Surgery 2004; **Med School:** NYU Sch Med 1988; **Resid:** Surgery, NYU Langone Med Ctr 1993; **Fellow:** Surgical Oncology, NYU Langone Med Ctr 1995; **Fac Appt:** Assoc Prof S, NYU Sch Med

Shapiro, Ron MD [S] - **Spec Exp:** Transplant-Kidney; Transplant-Pancreas; Pancreatic Islet Cell Transplant; **Hospital:** UPMC Presby, Pittsburgh, Chldns Hosp of Pittsburgh - UPMC; **Address:** Starzl Transplantation Inst, UPMC Montefiore - 7 South, 3459 Fifth Ave, Pittsburgh, PA 15213-2582; **Phone:** 412-647-5800; **Board Cert:** Surgery 2005; **Med School:** Stanford Univ 1980; **Resid:** Surgery, Mt Sinai Hosp 1986; **Fellow:** Transplant Surgery, Univ Pittsburgh 1988; **Fac Appt:** Prof S, Univ Pittsburgh

Sigurdson, Elin R MD [S] - **Spec Exp:** Breast Cancer; Colon & Rectal Cancer; Melanoma; Liver Cancer; **Hospital:** Fox Chase Cancer Ctr (page 58); **Address:** 333 Cottman Ave, Philadelphia, PA 19111-2412; **Phone:** 215-728-3519; **Board Cert:** Surgery 2006; **Med School:** Univ Toronto 1980; **Resid:** Surgery, Univ Toronto Affil Hosp 1984; **Fellow:** Surgical Oncology, Meml Sloan-Kettering Cancer Ctr 1987

Simmons, Rache M MD [S] - **Spec Exp:** Breast Cancer & Surgery; Minimally Invasive Surgery; **Hospital:** NY-Presby/Weill Cornell Med Ctr, NY (page 66); **Address:** Weill Cornell Breast Ctr, 425 E 61st St Fl 10, New York, NY 10065; **Phone:** 212-821-0853; **Board Cert:** Surgery 2005; **Med School:** Duke Univ 1988; **Resid:** Surgery, Univ NC Hosp 1993; **Fellow:** Surgical Oncology, NY Hosp-Cornell Hosp 1994; **Fac Appt:** Assoc Prof S, Cornell Univ-Weill Med Coll

Singer, Samuel MD [S] - **Spec Exp:** Sarcoma-Soft Tissue; **Hospital:** Meml Sloan-Kettering Cancer Ctr; **Address:** 1275 York Ave, Ste H1210, New York, NY 10065; **Phone:** 646-497-9072; **Board Cert:** Surgery 2010; **Med School:** Harvard Med Sch 1982; **Resid:** Surgery, Brigham & Women's Hosp 1988; **Fellow:** Surgical Oncology, Dana Farber Cancer Inst 1990; **Fac Appt:** Assoc Prof S, Cornell Univ-Weill Med Coll

Skinner, Kristin A MD [S] - **Spec Exp:** Breast Cancer; **Hospital:** Univ of Rochester Strong Meml Hosp; **Address:** URMC Comprehensive Breast Care Ctr, 601 Elmwood Ave, Box SURG, Rochester, NY 14642; **Phone:** 585-276-4504; **Board Cert:** Surgery 2005; **Med School:** Johns Hopkins Univ 1988; **Resid:** Surgery, UCLA Med Ctr 1995; **Fellow:** Surgical Oncology, UCLA Med Ctr 1994; **Fac Appt:** Assoc Prof S, Univ Rochester

Sugarbaker, Paul H MD [S] - **Spec Exp:** Appendix Cancer; Peritoneal Carcinomatosis; Cystadenocarcinoma; Ovarian Cancer; **Hospital:** Washington Hosp Ctr; **Address:** Washington Hosp Ctr, 106 Irving St NW, Ste 3900N, Washington, DC 20010; **Phone:** 202-877-3908; **Board Cert:** Surgery 1973; **Med School:** Cornell Univ-Weill Med Coll 1967; **Resid:** Surgery, Peter Bent Brigham Hosp 1973; **Fellow:** Surgical Oncology, Mass Genl Hosp 1976; **Fac Appt:** Prof S, Univ Wash

Swistel, Alexander J MD [S] - **Spec Exp:** Breast Cancer & Surgery; Cancer Reconstruction; Nipple Sparing Mastectomy; **Hospital:** NY-Presby/Weill Cornell Med Ctr, NY (page 66), St. Luke's - Roosevelt Hosp Ctr - Roosevelt Div (page 56); **Address:** 425 E 61st St, Fl 10, New York, NY 10065; **Phone:** 212-821-0602; **Board Cert:** Surgery 2005; **Med School:** Brown Univ 1975; **Resid:** Surgery, St Luke's Roosevelt Hosp Ctr 1981; **Fellow:** Surgical Oncology, Meml Sloan Kettering Canc Ctr 1983; **Fac Appt:** Assoc Clin Prof S, Cornell Univ-Weill Med Coll

Tafra, Lorraine MD [S] - **Spec Exp:** Breast Cancer; **Hospital:** Anne Arundel Med Ctr; **Address:** AAMC Breast Ctr, 2000 Medical Pkwy, Ste 200, Annapolis, MD 21401; **Phone:** 443-481-5300; **Board Cert:** Surgery 2005; **Med School:** Case West Res Univ 1986; **Resid:** Surgery, Rhode Island Hosp 1988; Surgery, Hosp Univ Penn 1992; **Fellow:** Surgical Oncology, John Wayne Cancer Inst 1994

Tartter, Paul MD [S] - **Spec Exp:** Breast Cancer; Breast Cancer in Elderly; Sentinel Node Surgery; **Hospital:** St. Luke's - Roosevelt Hosp Ctr - Roosevelt Div (page 56); **Address:** 425 W 59th St, Ste 7A, New York, NY 10019-1104; **Phone:** 212-523-7500; **Board Cert:** Surgery 2011; **Med School:** Brown Univ 1977; **Resid:** Surgery, Mt Sinai Hosp 1982; **Fac Appt:** Assoc Prof S, Columbia P&S

Tchou, Julia Chok-Moua MD/PhD [S] - **Spec Exp:** Breast Cancer; Breast Disease; Breast Cancer Risk Assessment; **Hospital:** Hosp Univ Penn - UPHS (page 72); **Address:** Abramson Cancer Ctr, Rena Rowan Breast Ctr Fl 3 West, 3400 Civic Ctr Blvd, Philadelphia, PA 19104; **Phone:** 215-615-7575; **Board Cert:** Surgery 2002; **Med School:** SUNY Stony Brook 1995; **Resid:** Surgery, Johns Hopkins Hosp 2001; **Fellow:** Gastrointestinal Surgery, Johns Hopkins Hosp 2002; Breast Surgery, Northwestern Meml Hosp 2003; **Fac Appt:** Asst Prof S, Univ Pennsylvania

Teperman, Lewis W MD [S] - **Spec Exp:** Transplant-Liver; Transplant-Kidney; Liver Cancer; Hepatobiliary Surgery; **Hospital:** NYU Langone Med Ctr (page 68); **Address:** NYU Transplant Associates, 403 E 34th St Fl 3, New York, NY 10016; **Phone:** 212-263-8134; **Board Cert:** Surgery 2007; **Med School:** Mount Sinai Sch Med 1981; **Resid:** Surgery, Columbia Presby Med Ctr 1984; Surgery, LI Jewish Med Ctr 1986; **Fellow:** Transplant Surgery, Univ Pittsburgh 1988; **Fac Appt:** Assoc Prof S, NYU Sch Med

Tsangaris, Theodore N MD [S] - **Spec Exp:** Nipple Sparing Mastectomy; **Hospital:** Johns Hopkins Hosp (page 61); **Address:** Johns Hopkins Hospital, 600 N Wolfe St, Carnegie 686, Baltimore, MD 21287; **Phone:** 443-287-2778; **Board Cert:** Surgery 2005; **Med School:** Geo Wash Univ 1983; **Resid:** Surgery, Geo Washington Univ Med Ctr 1989; **Fellow:** Surgical Oncology, Baylor Univ Med Ctr 1990; **Fac Appt:** Assoc Prof S, Johns Hopkins Univ

Van Zee, Kimberly J MD [S] - **Spec Exp:** Breast Cancer; **Hospital:** Meml Sloan-Kettering Cancer Ctr; **Address:** Meml Sloan Kettering Cancer Ctr, Evelyn H Lauder Breast Center, 300 E 66th St, New York, NY 10065; **Phone:** 800-525-2225; **Board Cert:** Surgery 2003; **Med School:** Harvard Med Sch 1987; **Resid:** Surgery, NY Hosp-Cornell Univ Med Ctr 1990; Surgery, NY Hosp-Cornell Univ Med Ctr 1994; **Fellow:** Research, NY Hosp-Cornell Univ Med Ctr 1993; **Fac Appt:** Prof S, Cornell Univ-Weill Med Coll

Surgery

Willey, Shawna C MD [S] - **Spec Exp:** Breast Cancer; Clinical Trials; **Hospital:** Georgetown Univ Hosp; **Address:** 3800 Reservoir Rd NW, PHC Bldg Fl 4, Washington, DC 20007; **Phone:** 202-444-0241; **Board Cert:** Surgery 2009; **Med School:** Univ Iowa Coll Med 1982; **Resid:** Surgery, George Washington Univ Med Ctr 1988; **Fac Appt:** Asst Prof S, Georgetown Univ

Yang, James C MD [S] - **Spec Exp:** Kidney Cancer; Clinical Trials; Immunotherapy; **Hospital:** Natl Inst of Hlth - Clin Ctr; **Address:** National Cancer Inst, Surgery Branch, 9000 Rockville Pike, Bldg 10 - rm 2B37, Bethesda, MD 20892; **Phone:** 301-496-1574; **Board Cert:** Surgery 2005; **Med School:** UCSD 1978; **Resid:** Surgery, UCSD Med Ctr 1984; **Fellow:** Surgical Oncology, Natl Cancer Inst 1986

Yeo, Charles J MD [S] - **Spec Exp:** Pancreatic Cancer; Biliary Cancer; Gastrointestinal Surgery; Pancreatic Endocrine Tumors; **Hospital:** Thomas Jefferson Univ Hosp; **Address:** 1015 Walnut St, Ste 620, Philadelphia, PA 19107; **Phone:** 215-955-9402; **Board Cert:** Surgery 2005; **Med School:** Johns Hopkins Univ 1979; **Resid:** Surgery, Johns Hopkins Hosp 1985; **Fellow:** Research, SUNY Downstate 1982; **Fac Appt:** Prof S, Thomas Jefferson Univ

Yurt, Roger W MD [S] - **Spec Exp:** Burn Care; Wound Healing/Care; Hyperbaric Medicine; Critical Care; **Hospital:** NY-Presby/Weill Cornell Med Ctr, NY (page 66); **Address:** 525 E 68th St, rm L706, New York, NY 10021-4885; **Phone:** 212-746-5410; **Board Cert:** Surgery 2008; **Med School:** Univ Miami Sch Med 1972; **Resid:** Surgery, Parkland Meml Hosp 1974; Surgery, New York Hosp-Cornell Med Ctr 1980; **Fellow:** Internal Medicine, Brigham & Womens Hosp 1978; **Fac Appt:** Prof S, Cornell Univ-Weill Med Coll

Southeast

Adams, Reid B MD [S] - **Spec Exp:** Hepatobiliary Surgery; Liver Cancer; Pancreatic & Biliary Surgery; **Hospital:** Univ of Virginia Health Sys; **Address:** UVA Health System, Dept Surgery, PO Box 800709, Charlottesville, VA 22908; **Phone:** 434-924-2839; **Board Cert:** Surgery 2003; **Med School:** Univ VA Sch Med 1987; **Resid:** Surgery, Univ Va Hlth Sci Ctr 1994; **Fellow:** Hepatopancreatobiliary Surgery, Univ Toronto Med Ctr 1995; **Fac Appt:** Assoc Prof S, Univ VA Sch Med

Andreoni, Kenneth A MD [S] - **Spec Exp:** Transplant-Kidney-Adult & Pediatric; Transplant-Liver-Adult & Pediatric; Transplant-Pancreas; **Hospital:** Shands at Univ of FL; **Address:** Shands Transplant Center at UF, 1600 SW Archer Rd, Gainsville, FL 32608; **Phone:** 352-265-0111 x44082; **Board Cert:** Surgery 2004; **Med School:** Yale Univ 1988; **Resid:** Surgery, Johns Hopkins Hosp; **Fellow:** Transplant Surgery, OSU Med Ctr 1998; **Fac Appt:** Assoc Prof S, Ohio State Univ

Baker, Christopher C MD [S] - **Spec Exp:** Trauma/Critical Care; Colon & Rectal Surgery; Hernia; Incontinence-Fecal; **Hospital:** Carilion Roanoke Meml Hosp; **Address:** Carillion Clinic, General Surgery, 3 Riverside Cir, Roanoke, VA 24016; **Phone:** 540-224-5170; **Board Cert:** Surgery 2002; Surgical Critical Care 2007; **Med School:** Harvard Med Sch 1974; **Resid:** Surgery, UCSF Med Ctr 1981; **Fellow:** Trauma, San Francisco Genl Hosp 1979; **Fac Appt:** Prof S, Louisiana State U, New Orleans

Ballantyne, Garth H MD [S] - **Spec Exp:** Laparoscopic Surgery; Gastroesophageal Reflux Disease (GERD); Colon Cancer; Obesity/Bariatric Surgery; **Hospital:** Charlie Norwood VA Med Ctr - Augusta; **Address:** 1 Freedom Way, Augusta, GA 30904; **Phone:** 706-733-0188; **Board Cert:** Surgery 2006; Colon & Rectal Surgery 1985; **Med School:** Columbia P&S 1977; **Resid:** Surgery, UCLA Med Ctr 1980; Surgery, Northwestern Meml Hosp 1982; **Fellow:** Colon & Rectal Surgery, Mayo Clinic 1984

Bear, Harry D MD/PhD [S] - **Spec Exp:** Breast Cancer; Melanoma; Gastrointestinal Cancer; **Hospital:** Med Coll of VA Hosp; **Address:** Med Coll Virginia - VCU, PO Box 980011, Richmond, VA 23298; **Phone:** 804-828-9325; **Board Cert:** Surgery 2003; **Med School:** Med Coll VA 1975; **Resid:** Surgery, Brigham & Women's Hosp 1983; **Fellow:** Surgical Oncology, Med Coll Virgina 1984; **Fac Appt:** Prof Surg & Onc, Med Coll VA

Beauchamp, Robert D MD [S] - **Spec Exp:** Esophageal Cancer; Colon & Rectal Cancer; Gastrointestinal Cancer; Breast Cancer; **Hospital:** Vanderbilt Univ Med Ctr (page 75), TN Valley Healthcare Sys-Nashville; **Address:** Vanderbilt Dept Surgery, Medical Center North D-4316, 1161 21st Ave S, Nashville, TN 37232-2730; **Phone:** 615-322-2363; **Board Cert:** Surgery 2007; **Med School:** Univ Tex Med Br, Galveston 1982; **Resid:** Surgery, Univ Tex Med Br 1987; **Fellow:** Cellular Molecular Biology, Vanderbilt Univ 1989; **Fac Appt:** Prof S, Vanderbilt Univ

Behrns, Kevin E MD [S] - **Spec Exp:** Pancreatic Cancer; Gastrointestinal Cancer & Surgery; **Hospital:** Shands at Univ of FL; **Address:** Shands Healthcare at Univ Florida, 1600 SW Archer Rd, Gainesville, FL 32610; **Phone:** 352-265-0604; **Board Cert:** Surgery 2011; **Med School:** Mayo Med Sch 1988; **Resid:** Surgery, Mayo Clinic 1995; **Fac Appt:** Prof S, Univ Fla Coll Med

Bland, Kirby MD [S] - **Spec Exp:** Breast Cancer; Colon Cancer; Thyroid & Parathyroid Cancer & Surgery; **Hospital:** Univ of Ala Hosp at Birmingham; **Address:** UAB, Dept Surgery, 1530 3rd Ave S, BDB 502, Birmingham, AL 35294-0002; **Phone:** 205-975-2193; **Board Cert:** Surgery 2011; **Med School:** Univ Alabama 1968; **Resid:** Surgery, Univ Fla Hosp 1970; Surgery, Univ Fla Hosp 1976; **Fellow:** Surgical Oncology, MD Anderson Cancer Ctr 1977; **Fac Appt:** Prof S, Univ Alabama

Britt, L D MD [S] - **Spec Exp:** Trauma; Head Injury; Thyroid Surgery; **Hospital:** Sentara Norfolk Genl Hosp; **Address:** Eastern Virginia Med Sch, Dept Surgery, 825 Fairfax Ave, Ste 610, Norfolk, VA 23507; **Phone:** 757-446-8950; **Board Cert:** Surgery 2003; Surgical Critical Care 2006; **Med School:** Harvard Med Sch 1977; **Resid:** Surgery, Barnes Hosp-Wash Univ 1979; Surgery, Univ Illinois Chicago Med Ctr 1984; **Fellow:** Trauma, Md Inst Emer Med Serv Sys 1986; **Fac Appt:** Prof S, Eastern VA Med Sch

Buchman, Timothy G MD/PhD [S] - **Spec Exp:** Critical Care; Pilonidal Disease; Wound Healing/Care; Sepsis; **Hospital:** Emory Univ Hosp, Emory Univ Hosp Midtown; **Address:** The Emory Clinic, 1440 Clifton Rd NE, Ste 313A, Atlanta, GA 30322; **Phone:** 404-712-2602; **Board Cert:** Surgery 2004; Surgical Critical Care 2005; **Med School:** Univ Chicago-Pritzker Sch Med 1980; **Resid:** Surgery, Johns Hopkins Hosp 1985; **Fellow:** Trauma, Maryland Inst for Emergency Med 1987; **Fac Appt:** Prof S, Emory Univ

Cairns, Bruce A MD [S] - **Spec Exp:** Burn Care; Wound Healing/Care; Electrical Injury; **Hospital:** NC Memorial Hosp - UNC; **Address:** Univ N Carolina Dept Surgery, N Carolina Jaycee Burn Ctr, Box 7600, 101 Manning Drive, Chapel Hill, NC 27599-7212; **Phone:** 919-966-3693; **Board Cert:** Surgery 2005; Surgical Critical Care 2000; **Med School:** Univ Pennsylvania 1989; **Resid:** Surgery, Univ NC Hosps 1994; **Fellow:** Surgical Critical Care, Univ NC Hosps 1996; **Fac Appt:** Assoc Prof S, Univ NC Sch Med

Calvo, Benjamin MD [S] - **Spec Exp:** Colon Cancer; Endocrine Cancers; Breast Cancer; **Hospital:** NC Memorial Hosp - UNC; **Address:** UNC, Dept of Surgery, 170 Manning Drive, 1150 POB, CB #7213, Chapel Hill, NC 27599; **Phone:** 919-966-5221; **Board Cert:** Surgery 2010; **Med School:** Univ MD Sch Med 1981; **Resid:** Surgery, George Washington Univ Hosp 1988; Surgery, Natl Inst Hlth 1991; **Fellow:** Surgery, Meml Sloan Kettering Cancer Ctr 1993; **Fac Appt:** Assoc Prof S, Univ NC Sch Med

Cole, David J MD [S] - **Spec Exp:** Breast Cancer; Gastrointestinal Cancer; Vaccine Therapy; **Hospital:** MUSC Med Ctr; **Address:** MUSC Surgery Dept, 96 Jonathan Lucas St, MSC 613 /CSB 420, Charleston, SC 29425; **Phone:** 843-792-4638; **Board Cert:** Surgery 2010; **Med School:** Cornell Univ 1986; **Resid:** Surgery, Emory Univ Affil Hosp 1991; **Fellow:** Surgical Oncology, Natl Cancer Inst 1994; **Fac Appt:** Prof S, Med Univ SC

Daneker Jr, George W MD [S] - **Spec Exp:** Gastrointestinal Surgery; Cancer Surgery; Laparoscopic Surgery; Pancreatic Surgery; **Hospital:** CTCA at Southeastern Regl Med Ctr; **Address:** CTCA at Southeastern Regional Med Ctr, 600 Parkway North, Newnan, GA 30265; **Phone:** 770-400-7000; **Board Cert:** Surgery 2002; **Med School:** Univ MD Sch Med 1983; **Resid:** Surgery, Univ Cincinnati Med Ctr 1990; **Fellow:** Cancer Research, New Engl Deaconess Med Ctr 1988; Surgical Oncology, UT MD Anderson Cancer Ctr 1992

Eason, James D MD [S] - **Spec Exp:** Transplant-Kidney; Transplant-Pancreas & Liver; Liver Cancer; **Hospital:** Methodist Univ Hosp - Memphis; **Address:** Transplant Inst, 1265 Union Ave, Memphis, TN 38104; **Phone:** 901-516-7469; **Board Cert:** Surgery 2002; **Med School:** Univ Tenn Coll Med 1987; **Resid:** Surgery, Wilford Hall USAF Med Ctr 1992; **Fellow:** Transplant Surgery, Mass Genl Hosp 1994; **Fac Appt:** Prof S, Univ Tenn Coll Med

Eckhoff, Devin E MD [S] - **Spec Exp:** Transplant-Liver; Hepatobiliary Surgery; Transplant-Kidney; Pancreatic Islet Cell Transplant; **Hospital:** Univ of Ala Hosp at Birmingham; **Address:** UAB Transplant Surgery, 1530 3rd Ave S, LHRB 710, Birmingham, AL 35294-0007; **Phone:** 205-975-7622; **Board Cert:** Surgery 2010; Surgical Critical Care 2001; **Med School:** Univ Minn 1986; **Resid:** Surgery, Univ Wisconsin Med Ctr 1992; **Fellow:** Transplant Surgery, Univ Wisconsin 1994; **Fac Appt:** Prof S, Univ Alabama

Feliciano, David V MD [S] - **Spec Exp:** Trauma; **Hospital:** Atlanta Med Ctr, Med Ctr of Central GA; **Address:** 315 Boulevard NE, Ste 500, Atlanta, GA 30312; **Phone:** 404-265-3635; **Board Cert:** Surgery 2008; **Med School:** Georgetown Univ 1970; **Resid:** Surgery, Mayo Clinic 1978; **Fellow:** Cardiovascular Surgery, Texas Med Ctr/Baylor 1978; **Fac Appt:** Prof S, Mercer Univ Sch Med

Flynn, Michael B MD [S] - **Spec Exp:** Head & Neck Cancer; Head & Neck Surgery; Thyroid & Parathyroid Surgery; **Hospital:** Univ of Louisville Hosp, Norton Hosp; **Address:** Univ Surgical Associates, 410 E Chestnut St, Ste 710, Louisville, KY 40202; **Phone:** 502-583-8303; **Board Cert:** Surgery 1972; **Med School:** Ireland 1962; **Resid:** Surgery, Univ Maryland Hosp 1969; **Fellow:** Surgical Oncology, MD Anderson Hosp 1970; Head and Neck Surgery, MD Anderson Hosp 1971; **Fac Appt:** Prof S, Univ Louisville Sch Med

Gabram, Sheryl G A MD [S] - **Spec Exp:** Breast Cancer; Breast Cancer-High Risk Women; Breast Disease; **Hospital:** Emory Univ Hosp, Grady Hlth Sys; **Address:** Winship Cancer Institute, 1365C Clifton Rd NE Fl 2, Atlanta, GA 30322; **Phone:** 404-778-1230; **Board Cert:** Surgery 2006; **Med School:** Georgetown Univ 1982; **Resid:** Surgery, Washington Hosp Ctr 1987; **Fellow:** Trauma, Hartford Hosp 1988; **Fac Appt:** Prof S, Emory Univ

Galloway, John R MD [S] - **Spec Exp:** Gastrointestinal Surgery; Pancreatic Surgery; Pancreatic Islet Cell Transplant; Hepatobiliary Surgery; **Hospital:** Emory Univ Hosp; **Address:** Emory Univ Hosp, Dept Surgery, 1365A Clifton Rd NE, Ste A 3300, Atlanta, GA 30322; **Phone:** 404-778-3712; **Board Cert:** Surgery 2008; **Med School:** Emory Univ 1981; **Resid:** Surgery, Emory Affil Hosps 1986; **Fellow:** Emory Univ Hosp 1987; **Fac Appt:** Prof S, Emory Univ

Greene, Frederick L MD [S] - **Spec Exp:** Gastrointestinal Surgery; Gastrointestinal Cancer; Hernia; **Hospital:** Carolinas Med Ctr; **Address:** Carolinas Medical Ctr, 1025 Morehead Medical Drive, Ste 300, Charlotte, NC 28204; **Phone:** 704-355-1813; **Board Cert:** Surgery 2009; **Med School:** Univ VA Sch Med 1970; **Resid:** Surgery, Yale-New Haven Hosp 1976; **Fellow:** Surgical Oncology, Yale-New Haven Hosp 1973; **Fac Appt:** Prof S, Univ NC Sch Med

Hanks, John B MD [S] - **Spec Exp:** Endocrine Cancers; Breast Cancer; Thyroid Cancer & Surgery; Endocrine Surgery; **Hospital:** Univ of Virginia Health Sys; **Address:** Univ VA Hlth Sys, Dept Surgery, PO Box 800709, Charlottesville, VA 22908-0709; **Phone:** 434-924-0376; **Board Cert:** Surgery 2001; **Med School:** Univ Rochester 1973; **Resid:** Surgery, Duke Univ Med Ctr 1982; **Fac Appt:** Prof S, Univ VA Sch Med

Herrmann, Virginia M MD [S] - **Spec Exp:** Breast Cancer; Breast Cancer Genetics; Breast Surgery; Nutrition & Cancer Prevention/Control; **Hospital:** Hilton Head Reg Med Ctr, MUSC Med Ctr; **Address:** Hilton Head Regional Med Ctr, 25 Hospital Center Blvd, Breast Health Ctr, Ste 300, Hilton Head, SC 29926; **Phone:** 843-682-7377; **Board Cert:** Surgery 2009; **Med School:** St Louis Univ 1974; **Resid:** Surgery, St Louis Univ Hosps 1979; **Fellow:** Surgery, Brigham & Women's Hosp 1980; **Fac Appt:** Prof S, Med Univ SC

Heslin, Martin J MD [S] - **Spec Exp:** Gastrointestinal Cancer; Pancreatic Cancer; Biliary Cancer; Sarcoma-Soft Tissue; **Hospital:** Univ of Ala Hosp at Birmingham; **Address:** Univ Alabama, 1922 7th Ave S, Ste 321, Birmingham, AL 35294-0016; **Phone:** 205-934-3064; **Board Cert:** Surgery 2006; **Med School:** SUNY Upstate Med Univ 1987; **Resid:** Surgery, NYU Med Ctr 1994; Surgery, Meml Sloan-Kettering Canc Ctr 1991; **Fellow:** Surgical Oncology, Meml Sloan-Kettering Cancer Ctr 1996; **Fac Appt:** Prof S, Univ Alabama

Howerton, Russell M MD [S] - **Spec Exp:** Hepatobiliary Surgery; Pancreatic Surgery; Colon & Rectal Surgery; Laparoscopic Surgery; **Hospital:** Wake Forest Baptist Med Ctr; **Address:** Medical Ctr Blvd, Winston-Salem, NC 27157; **Phone:** 336-716-0664; **Board Cert:** Surgery 2008; **Med School:** Vanderbilt Univ 1983; **Resid:** Surgery, Tufts/New England Med Ctr 1989; **Fellow:** Hepatobiliary Surgery, Hammersmith Hosp 1992; **Fac Appt:** Assoc Prof S, Wake Forest Univ

Kelley, Mark C MD [S] - **Spec Exp:** Breast Cancer; Melanoma; **Hospital:** Vanderbilt Univ Med Ctr (page 75), TN Valley Healthcare Sys-Nashville; **Address:** Vanderbilt Div Surgical Oncology, 2220 Pierce Ave, 597 Preston Rsch Bldg, Nashville, TN 37232-6860; **Phone:** 615-322-2391; **Board Cert:** Surgery 2005; **Med School:** Univ Fla Coll Med 1989; **Resid:** Surgery, Shands Hosp 1995; **Fellow:** Surgical Oncology, John Wayne Cancer Inst 1997; **Fac Appt:** Assoc Prof S, Vanderbilt Univ

Knechtle, Stuart J MD [S] - **Spec Exp:** Transplant-Liver; Transplant-Kidney; Transplant Immunology; Hepatobiliary Surgery; **Hospital:** Emory Univ Hosp; **Address:** Emory Transplant Surgery Program, 1365B Clifton Rd NE, Ste 6400, Atlanta, GA 30322; **Phone:** 404-712-5676; **Board Cert:** Surgery 2009; **Med School:** Cornell Univ 1982; **Resid:** Surgery, Duke Univ Med Ctr 1989; **Fellow:** Transplant Surgery, Univ Wisconsin Hosp 1991; **Fac Appt:** Prof S, Emory Univ

Koruda, Mark J MD [S] - **Spec Exp:** Gastrointestinal Surgery; Minimally Invasive Surgery; Inflammatory Bowel Disease; **Hospital:** NC Memorial Hosp - UNC; **Address:** Div Gastrointestinal Surgery, 4035 Burnett-Womack Bldg, Campus Box 7081, Chapel Hill, NC 27599-7081; **Phone:** 919-966-8436; **Board Cert:** Surgery 1999; **Med School:** Yale Univ 1981; **Resid:** Surgery, Hosp Univ Penn 1988; **Fac Appt:** Prof S, Univ NC Sch Med

Krontiras, Helen MD [S] - **Spec Exp:** Breast Cancer; **Hospital:** Univ of Ala Hosp at Birmingham; **Address:** The Kirklin Clinic, 2000 6th Ave S, Birmingham, AL 35233; **Phone:** 205-801-8266; **Board Cert:** Surgery 2010; **Med School:** Univ Alabama 1991; **Resid:** Surgery, Univ AL Hosp 2000; **Fellow:** Surgical Oncology, Northwestern Univ Med Ctr 2001; **Fac Appt:** Assoc Prof S, Univ Alabama

Larsen, Christian P MD/PhD [S] - **Spec Exp:** Pancreatic Islet Cell Transplant; Transplant-Pancreas; Transplant-Kidney; Transplant Immunology; **Hospital:** Emory Univ Hosp; **Address:** Emory Kidney/Pancreas Transplant Prgm, 1365B Clifton Rd NE, Ste 6400, Atlanta, GA 30322; **Phone:** 404-727-0717; **Board Cert:** Surgery 2011; **Med School:** Emory Univ 1984; **Resid:** Surgery, Emory Univ Hosp 1988; **Fellow:** Surgical Research, Oxford Univ 1990; Transplant Surgery, Emory Univ Hosp 1993; **Fac Appt:** Prof S, Emory Univ

Levi, Joe U MD [S] - **Spec Exp:** Pancreatic Cancer; Liver Disease; Liver Cancer; Biliary Surgery; **Hospital:** Jackson Meml Hosp, Univ of Miami Hosp & Clins/Sylvester Comp Canc Ctr; **Address:** 1120 NW 14th St, M875, Clinical Research Bldg, Miami, FL 33136; **Phone:** 305-243-4211; **Board Cert:** Surgery 1975; **Med School:** Univ Fla Coll Med 1967; **Resid:** Surgery, Johns Hopkins Hosp 1969; Surgery, Jackson Meml Hosp 1974; **Fac Appt:** Prof S, Univ Miami Sch Med

Levine, Edward A MD [S] - **Spec Exp:** Breast Cancer; Esophageal Cancer; Peritoneal Carcinomatosis; Sarcoma; **Hospital:** Wake Forest Baptist Med Ctr; **Address:** Wake Forest Univ Baptist Med Ctr, Dept Surgery, Med Ctr Blvd Fl 5, Winston-Salem, NC 27157; **Phone:** 336-716-4276; **Board Cert:** Surgery 2010; **Med School:** Ros Franklin Univ/Chicago Med Sch 1985; **Resid:** Surgery, Michael Reese Hosp 1990; **Fellow:** Surgical Oncology, Univ Illinois 1992; **Fac Appt:** Prof S, Wake Forest Univ

Livingstone, Alan S MD [S] - **Spec Exp:** Liver & Biliary Cancer; Stomach Cancer; Esophageal Cancer; Pancreatic Cancer; **Hospital:** Jackson Meml Hosp, Univ of Miami Hosp & Clins/Sylvester Comp Canc Ctr; **Address:** 1150 NW 14th St Fl 4, Miami, FL 33136; **Phone:** 305-243-4902; **Board Cert:** Surgery 2007; **Med School:** McGill Univ 1971; **Resid:** Surgery, Montreal Genl Hosp 1976; Surgery, Jackson Meml Hosp 1975; **Fac Appt:** Prof S, Univ Miami Sch Med

Luterman, Arnold MD [S] - **Spec Exp:** Burn Care; Wound Healing/Care; Critical Care; **Hospital:** Univ of S AL Med Ctr; **Address:** Univ of S Alabama Med Ctr, Mastin Bldg, 2451 Fillingim St, Ste 101, Mobile, AL 36617; **Phone:** 251-445-8282; **Board Cert:** Surgery 2006; **Med School:** McGill Univ 1970; **Resid:** Surgery, Jewish Gen Hosp 1976; Surgery, Sinai Hospital 1973; **Fellow:** Burn Surgery, Univ Washington 1976; **Fac Appt:** Prof S, Univ S Ala Coll Med

MacDonald Jr, Kenneth G MD [S] - **Spec Exp:** Gastrointestinal Surgery; Obesity/Bariatric Surgery; Pancreatic Surgery; **Hospital:** Univ Hlth Sys-Vidant Med Ctr, Nash Genl Hosp; **Address:** Physicians East, 1850 W Arlington Blvd, Greenville, NC 27834; **Phone:** 252-413-6735; **Board Cert:** Surgery 2009; **Med School:** W VA Univ 1981; **Resid:** Surgery, NC Baptist Hosp 1984; Surgery, Univ Med Ctr E Carolina 1987; **Fac Appt:** Prof S, E Carolina Univ

McGrath, Patrick C MD [S] - **Spec Exp:** Breast Cancer; Cancer Surgery; **Hospital:** Univ of Kentucky Albert B. Chandler Hosp; **Address:** 800 Rose St UKMC Bldg - rm C-224, Dept General Surgery, Lexington, KY 40536-0293; **Phone:** 859-323-6346 x240; **Board Cert:** Surgery 2008; **Med School:** Univ IL Coll Med 1980; **Resid:** Surgery, Med Coll Virginia Hosp 1986; **Fellow:** Surgical Oncology, Med Coll Virginia Hosp 1988; **Fac Appt:** Prof S, Univ KY Coll Med

McMasters, Kelly M MD [S] - **Spec Exp:** Melanoma; Breast Cancer; Liver Cancer; **Hospital:** Univ of Louisville Hosp; **Address:** Univ Surgical Assocs, 401 E Chestnut St, Ste 710, Louisville, KY 40202; **Phone:** 502-583-8303; **Board Cert:** Surgery 2005; **Med School:** UMDNJ-RW Johnson Med Sch 1989; **Resid:** Surgery, Univ Louisville Hosp 1994; **Fellow:** Surgical Oncology, Univ Texas-M D Anderson Cancer Ctr 1996; **Fac Appt:** Prof S, Univ Louisville Sch Med

Meyer, Anthony A MD [S] - **Spec Exp:** Trauma; Burn Care; **Hospital:** NC Memorial Hosp - UNC; **Address:** UNC-Sch Med, Dept Surgery, 4041 Burnett-Womack Bldg, CB 7050, Chapel Hill, NC 27599-7050; **Phone:** 919-966-3284; **Board Cert:** Surgery 2001; Surgical Critical Care 2005; **Med School:** Univ Chicago-Pritzker Sch Med 1977; **Resid:** Surgery, UCSF Med Ctr 1982; **Fac Appt:** Prof S, Univ NC Sch Med

Neifeld, James P MD [S] - **Spec Exp:** Melanoma; Head & Neck Cancer; Gastrointestinal Cancer; Cancers-Rare & Unusual; **Hospital:** Med Coll of VA Hosp; **Address:** Medical College Virginia Hosp, Box 980645, Richmond, VA 23298-0645; **Phone:** 804-828-9324; **Board Cert:** Surgery 2008; **Med School:** Med Coll VA 1972; **Resid:** Surgery, Med Coll Va Hosps 1978; **Fac Appt:** Prof S, Va Commonwealth Univ Sch Med

Newell, Kenneth A MD/PhD [S] - **Spec Exp:** Transplant-Kidney; Transplant-Pancreas; **Hospital:** Emory Univ Hosp; **Address:** Emory Kidney/Pancreas Transplant Prgm, 1365B Clifton Rd NE, Ste 6400, Atlanta, GA 30322; **Phone:** 404-727-0717; **Board Cert:** Surgery 2008; **Med School:** Univ Mich Med Sch 1984; **Resid:** Surgery, Loyola Univ Med Ctr 1989; **Fellow:** Transplant Surgery, Univ Chicago 1994; **Fac Appt:** Prof S, Emory Univ

Norman Jr, James G MD [S] - **Spec Exp:** Parathyroid Surgery; **Hospital:** Tampa Genl Hosp; **Address:** 2400 Cypress Glen Drive, Wesley Chapel, FL 33544; **Phone:** 813-972-0000; **Board Cert:** Surgery 2002; **Med School:** Oral Roberts Sch Med 1986; **Resid:** Surgery, Univ S Fla 1991; **Fellow:** Univ S Fla 1992

Pappas, Theodore N MD [S] - **Spec Exp:** Pancreatic Surgery; Laparoscopic Surgery; **Hospital:** Duke Univ Hosp; **Address:** Duke Univ Med Ctr, Dept Surgery, DUMC Box 3479, Durham, NC 27710; **Phone:** 919-681-3442; **Board Cert:** Surgery 2009; **Med School:** Ohio State Univ 1981; **Resid:** Surgery, Brigham & Womens Hosp 1988; **Fellow:** Research, Wadworth VA Med Ctr 1985; **Fac Appt:** Prof S, Duke Univ

Pinson, C Wright MD [S] - **Spec Exp:** Transplant-Liver; Liver & Biliary Cancer; Pancreatic Cancer; Liver & Biliary Surgery; **Hospital:** Vanderbilt Univ Med Ctr (page 75); **Address:** 1161 21st Ave S, Ste D3300MCN, Nashville, TN 37232-5545; **Phone:** 615-343-9324; **Board Cert:** Surgery 2007; Surgical Critical Care 2007; **Med School:** Vanderbilt Univ 1980; **Resid:** Surgery, Oregon Health Sci Ctr 1986; **Fellow:** Gastrointestinal Surgery, Lahey Clinic 1987; Transplant Surgery, Deaconess Hosp 1988; **Fac Appt:** Prof S, Vanderbilt Univ

Richards, William O MD [S] - **Spec Exp:** Laparoscopic Surgery; Obesity/Bariatric Surgery; Esophageal Disorders; Gastrointestinal Surgery; **Hospital:** Univ of S AL Med Ctr; **Address:** Univ S Alabama Dept Surgery, 2451 Fillingim St, Ste 101, Mobile, AL 36617; **Phone:** 251-445-8282; **Board Cert:** Surgery 2004; **Med School:** Univ MD Sch Med 1979; **Resid:** Surgery, Univ Maryland Med Ctr 1984; **Fellow:** Gastrointestinal Surgery, Emory Univ 1985; Vanderbilt Univ 1987; **Fac Appt:** Prof S, Univ S Ala Coll Med

Roh, Mark S MD [S] - **Spec Exp:** Liver Cancer; Cancer Surgery; **Hospital:** MD Anderson Cancer Ctr-Orlando; **Address:** 1400 S Orange Ave, MP 760, Orlando, FL 32806; **Phone:** 321-841-5134; **Board Cert:** Surgery 2006; **Med School:** Ohio State Univ 1979; **Resid:** Surgery, Univ Pittsburgh Med Ctr 1982; Surgery, Univ Pittsburgh Med Ctr 1986; **Fellow:** Surgical Oncology, Meml Sloan-Kettering Cancer Ctr 1984; Surgical Oncology, Meml Sloan-Kettering Cancer Ctr 1987; **Fac Appt:** Prof S, Drexel Univ Coll Med

Rosemurgy, Alexander S MD [S] - **Spec Exp:** Pancreatic Cancer; Gastrointestinal Surgery; Minimally Invasive Surgery; Portal Hypertension; **Hospital:** Florida Hosp-Tampa; **Address:** 3000 Medical Park Drive, Ste 310, Lifehope Bldg, Tampa, FL 33613; **Phone:** 813-615-7030; **Board Cert:** Surgery 2005; **Med School:** Univ Mich Med Sch 1979; **Resid:** Surgery, Univ Chicago Hosps 1984

Salo, Jonathan C MD [S] - **Spec Exp:** Gastrointestinal Cancer; Esophageal Cancer; **Hospital:** Carolinas Med Ctr; **Address:** Carolinas Med Ctr, 1025 Medical Ctr Drive, Charlotte, NC 28203; **Phone:** 704-355-2884; **Board Cert:** Surgery 2005; **Med School:** UCSF 1981; **Resid:** Surgery, UCSF Med Ctr 1993; **Fellow:** Surgical Oncology, Natl Cancer Inst 1991; Surgical Oncology, Meml Sloan-Kettering Cancer Ctr 1998; **Fac Appt:** Asst Prof S, Univ NC Sch Med

Surgery

Schirmer, Bruce D MD [S] - **Spec Exp:** Laparoscopic Surgery; Gastrointestinal Surgery; Pancreatic Surgery; Liver Surgery; **Hospital:** Univ of Virginia Health Sys; **Address:** Univ VA Hlth Sys, Dept Surgery, PO Box 800709, Charlottesville, VA 22908; **Phone:** 434-924-2104; **Board Cert:** Surgery 2005; **Med School:** Duke Univ 1978; **Resid:** Surgery, Duke Univ Med Ctr 1985; **Fac Appt:** Prof S, Univ VA Sch Med

Sharp, Kenneth MD [S] - **Spec Exp:** Gastrointestinal Surgery; Esophageal Disorders; Laparoscopic Surgery; Pancreatic Surgery; **Hospital:** Vanderbilt Univ Med Ctr (page 75); **Address:** Vanderbilt Univ Med Ctr, Div Gen Surgery, 1161 21st Ave, D-4303 MCN, Nashville, TN 37232; **Phone:** 615-322-0259; **Board Cert:** Surgery 2003; **Med School:** Johns Hopkins Univ 1977; **Resid:** Surgery, Johns Hopkins Univ Med Ctr 1984; **Fellow:** Hepatobiliary Surgery, Loch Raven VA Hosp 1981; Surgery, John Radcliffe Hosp 1982; **Fac Appt:** Prof S, Vanderbilt Univ

Shen, Perry MD [S] - **Spec Exp:** Liver & Biliary Cancer; Pancreatic Cancer; Gastrointestinal Cancer; Melanoma; **Hospital:** Wake Forest Baptist Med Ctr; **Address:** Wake Forest Univ Baptist Med Ctr, Dept Surgery, Medical Center Blvd Fl 5, Winston-Salem, NC 27157; **Phone:** 336-716-0545; **Board Cert:** Surgery 2008; **Med School:** USC Sch Med 1992; **Resid:** Surgery, LAC-USC Med Ctr 1998; **Fellow:** Surgical Oncology, John Wayne Cancer Inst 2000; **Fac Appt:** Assoc Prof S, Wake Forest Univ

Shibata, David MD [S] - **Spec Exp:** Colon & Rectal Cancer; Minimally Invasive Surgery; Laparoscopic Surgery; **Hospital:** H Lee Moffitt Cancer Ctr & Research Inst (page 59); **Address:** 12902 Magnolia Drive, FOB Bldg - Fl 2, Tampa, FL 33612; **Phone:** 813-745-6898; **Board Cert:** Surgery 2008; **Med School:** McGill Univ 1991; **Resid:** Surgery, Deaconess Hosp 1994; Surgery, Beth Israel Med Ctr 1998; **Fellow:** Research, Harvard Univ Med Sch 1996; Surgical Oncology, Meml Sloan-Kettering Cancer Ctr 2000; **Fac Appt:** Assoc Prof S, Univ S Fla Coll Med

Slingluff Jr, Craig L MD [S] - **Spec Exp:** Melanoma; Immunotherapy; **Hospital:** Univ of Virginia Health Sys; **Address:** UVA Health System, Dept Surgery, PO Box 800709, Charlottesville, VA 22908; **Phone:** 434-924-1730; **Board Cert:** Surgery 2011; **Med School:** Univ VA Sch Med 1984; **Resid:** Surgery, Duke Univ Med Ctr 1991; **Fellow:** Surgical Research, Duke Univ Med Ctr 1992; **Fac Appt:** Prof S, Univ VA Sch Med

Solorzano, Carmen C MD [S] - **Spec Exp:** Endocrine Cancers; Neuroendocrine Tumors; Thyroid & Parathyroid Cancer & Surgery; Adrenal Cancer; **Hospital:** Vanderbilt Univ Med Ctr (page 75), VA Tennessee Valley Healthcare System-Alvin C. Yor; **Address:** 2220 Pierce Ave, PRB Bldg Fl 5 - Ste 97, MS 37232, Nashville, TN 37232; **Phone:** 615-322-2391; **Board Cert:** Surgery 2009; **Med School:** Univ Fla Coll Med 1993; **Resid:** Surgery, Univ Florida Affil Hosp 1999; **Fellow:** Surgical Oncology, UT MD Anderson Cancer Ctr 2002; **Fac Appt:** Assoc Prof S, Vanderbilt Univ

Sondak, Vernon K MD [S] - **Spec Exp:** Cancer Surgery; Melanoma; Sarcoma; **Hospital:** H Lee Moffitt Cancer Ctr & Research Inst (page 59); **Address:** H Lee Moffitt Cancer Ctr, Cutaneous Program, 12902 Magnolia Drive, Tampa, FL 33612; **Phone:** 813-745-8482; **Board Cert:** Surgery 2008; **Med School:** Boston Univ 1980; **Resid:** Surgery, UCLA Med Ctr 1987; **Fellow:** Surgical Oncology, UCLA Med Ctr 1984; **Fac Appt:** Prof S, Univ S Fla Coll Med

Staley, Charles A MD [S] - **Spec Exp:** Gastrointestinal Cancer & Rare Tumors; Pancreatic Cancer; Liver & Biliary Cancer; **Hospital:** Emory Univ Hosp; **Address:** Emory - Winship Cancer Inst, 1365C Clifton Rd NE Fl 2, Atlanta, GA 30322; **Phone:** 404-778-3307; **Board Cert:** Surgery 2010; **Med School:** Dartmouth Med Sch 1987; **Resid:** Surgery, Univ Pittsburgh Med Ctr 1992; **Fellow:** Surgical Oncology, MD Anderson Cancer Ctr 1995; **Fac Appt:** Prof S, Emory Univ

Stratta, Robert J MD [S] - **Spec Exp:** Transplant-Pancreas; Transplant-Kidney; Dialysis Access; **Hospital:** Wake Forest Baptist Med Ctr; **Address:** Medical Ctr Blvd, Winston-Salem, NC 27157-1095; **Phone:** 336-716-6371; **Board Cert:** Surgery 2006; **Med School:** Univ Chicago-Pritzker Sch Med 1980; **Resid:** Surgery, Univ Utah Med Ctr 1986; **Fellow:** Transplant Surgery, Univ Wisc Hosps & Clins 1988; **Fac Appt:** Prof S, Wake Forest Univ

Sweeney, John F MD [S] - **Spec Exp:** Obesity/Bariatric Surgery; Laparoscopic Surgery; Gastroesophageal Reflux Disease (GERD); Minimally Invasive Surgery; **Hospital:** Emory Univ Hosp; **Address:** Emory Univ Dept Surgery, 1365A Clifton Rd NE, Ste A 3300, Atlanta, GA 30322; **Phone:** 404-778-3712; **Board Cert:** Surgery 2004; **Med School:** Rush Med Coll 1988; **Resid:** Surgery, Univ S Florida Affil Hosps 1995; **Fellow:** Surgical Research, Univ S Florida 1993; **Fac Appt:** Prof S, Emory Univ

Tyler, Douglas S MD [S] - **Spec Exp:** Melanoma; Pancreatic Cancer; Gastrointestinal Cancer; Melanoma; **Hospital:** Duke Univ Hosp, Durham VA Med Ctr; **Address:** Duke University Med Ctr, Box 3118, Durham, NC 27710; **Phone:** 919-684-6858; **Board Cert:** Surgery 2010; **Med School:** Dartmouth Med Sch 1985; **Resid:** Surgery, Duke Univ Med Ctr 1992; **Fellow:** Surgical Oncology, MD Anderson Cancer Ctr 1994; **Fac Appt:** Prof S, Duke Univ

Unger, Stephen W MD [S] - **Spec Exp:** Laparoscopic Surgery; **Hospital:** Mount Sinai Med Ctr - Miami; **Address:** 4302 Alton Rd, Ste 720, Miami Beach, FL 33140-2893; **Phone:** 305-532-4835; **Board Cert:** Surgery 2000; **Med School:** Duke Univ 1975; **Resid:** Surgery, Univ VA Sch Med 1982; **Fellow:** Surgical Oncology, Univ VA Sch Med 1979

Urist, Marshall M MD [S] - **Spec Exp:** Cancer Surgery; Breast Cancer; Melanoma; **Hospital:** Univ of Ala Hosp at Birmingham; **Address:** Univ Alabama Sch Med, Dept Surgery, 1922 7th Ave S, Kracke Bldg, Ste 321, Birmingham, AL 35294; **Phone:** 205-934-3065; **Board Cert:** Surgery 2010; **Med School:** Univ Chicago-Pritzker Sch Med 1971; **Resid:** Surgery, Johns Hopkins Hosp 1978; **Fellow:** Surgical Oncology, UCLA Med Ctr 1976; **Fac Appt:** Prof S, Univ Alabama

Weber, Collin J MD [S] - **Spec Exp:** Endocrine Surgery; Thyroid & Parathyroid Surgery; Adrenal Surgery; Pancreatic Islet Cell Transplant; **Hospital:** Emory Univ Hosp; **Address:** Emory Clinic, Dept Surgery, 1365A Clifton Rd NE, Atlanta, GA 30322; **Phone:** 404-778-3322; **Board Cert:** Surgery 2008; **Med School:** Columbia P&S 1971; **Resid:** Surgery, Columbia Presby Med Ctr 1978; **Fellow:** Research, Natl Inst Hlth 1975; **Fac Appt:** Prof S, Emory Univ

White Jr, Richard L MD [S] - **Spec Exp:** Breast Cancer; Melanoma; Sarcoma; Immunotherapy; **Hospital:** Carolinas Med Ctr; **Address:** Carolinas Medical Center, 1025 Morehead Medical Drive, Charlotte, NC 28204; **Phone:** 704-355-2884; **Board Cert:** Surgery 2002; **Med School:** Columbia P&S 1986; **Resid:** Surgery, Georgetown Univ Hosp 1992; **Fellow:** Surgical Oncology, NIH-Natl Cancer Inst 1995; **Fac Appt:** Clin Prof S, Univ NC Sch Med

Whitworth, Pat W MD [S] - **Spec Exp:** Breast Cancer; **Hospital:** Baptist Hosp - Nashville, Centennial Med Ctr; **Address:** Nashville Breast Center, 300 20th Ave N, Ste 401, Nashville, TN 37203; **Phone:** 615-620-5535; **Board Cert:** Surgery 2009; **Med School:** Univ Tenn Coll Med 1983; **Resid:** Surgery, Univ Louisville Med Ctr 1988; **Fellow:** Surgical Oncology, MD Anderson Cancer Ctr 1991; **Fac Appt:** Assoc Clin Prof S, Vanderbilt Univ

Yeatman, Timothy J MD [S] - **Spec Exp:** Liver Cancer; **Hospital:** H Lee Moffitt Cancer Ctr & Research Inst (page 59); **Address:** H Lee Moffitt Cancer Ctr, 12902 Magnolia Drive, Tampa, FL 33612-9497; **Phone:** 813-979-7292; **Board Cert:** Surgery 2010; **Med School:** Emory Univ 1984; **Resid:** Surgery, Univ Florida 1990; **Fellow:** Surgical Oncology, MD Anderson Cancer Ctr 1992; **Fac Appt:** Prof S, Univ S Fla Coll Med

Surgery

Midwest

Abecassis, Michael MD [S] - **Spec Exp:** Transplant-Liver; Transplant-Kidney; Pancreatic & Biliary Surgery; Liver Cancer; **Hospital:** Northwestern Meml Hosp; **Address:** Northwestern Med Faculty Fdn, 676 N St Clair St, Galter Pavilion Fl 19 - Ste 100, Chicago, IL 60611; **Phone:** 312-695-8900; **Board Cert:** Surgery 2009; **Med School:** Univ Toronto 1983; **Resid:** Surgery, Toronto Genl Hosp 1989; **Fellow:** Hepatopancreatobiliary Surgery, Toronto Genl Hosp 1990; Transplant Surgery, Univ Iowa Hosp 1991; **Fac Appt:** Prof S, Northwestern Univ-Feinberg Sch Med

Abouljoud, Marwan S MD [S] - **Spec Exp:** Transplant-Liver; Liver Cancer; Liver Surgery; **Hospital:** Henry Ford Hosp; **Address:** Henry Ford Hospital, 2799 W Grand Blvd Fl K16, Detroit, MI 48202; **Phone:** 313-916-2941; **Board Cert:** Surgery 2002; **Med School:** Lebanon 1985; **Resid:** Surgery, Univ of Mich igan Med Ctr 1988; Surgery, Henry Ford Hosp 1992; **Fellow:** Transplant Surgery, Univ Alabama 1994; Transplant Surgery, Baylor Univ Med Ctr 1996; **Fac Appt:** Prof S, Wayne State Univ

Angelos, Peter MD/PhD [S] - **Spec Exp:** Thyroid & Parathyroid Cancer & Surgery; Pheochromocytoma; Adrenal Tumors; Ethics; **Hospital:** Univ of Chicago Med Ctr; **Address:** Univ Chicago Med Ctr, Dept Surg, 5841 S Maryland Ave, MC 4052, Chicago, IL 60637; **Phone:** 773-702-4429; **Board Cert:** Surgery 2004; **Med School:** Boston Univ 1989; **Resid:** Surgery, Northwestern Univ 1995; **Fellow:** Medical Ethics, Univ of Chicago Hosps 1992; Endocrine Surgery, Univ of Michigan Med Sch 1996; **Fac Appt:** Prof S, Univ Chicago-Pritzker Sch Med

Aranha, Gerard V MD [S] - **Spec Exp:** Pancreatic & Biliary Surgery; Stomach Cancer; Esophageal Cancer; **Hospital:** Loyola Univ Med Ctr, Edward Hines, Jr. VA Hosp; **Address:** 2160 S first Ave Bldg 110 - rm 3236, Maywood, IL 60153-3328; **Phone:** 708-327-2391; **Board Cert:** Surgery 2006; **Med School:** India 1969; **Resid:** Surgery, Loyola Univ Med Ctr 1975; **Fellow:** Surgical Oncology, Univ Minn Hosp 1977; **Fac Appt:** Prof S, Loyola Univ-Stritch Sch Med

Averbook, Bruce J MD [S] - **Spec Exp:** Melanoma; Cancer Surgery; Clinical Trials; **Hospital:** MetroHealth Med Ctr; **Address:** MetroHealth Medical Center, Cancer Care Pavilion, 2500 MetroHealth Drive, rm C2110, Cleveland, OH 44109; **Phone:** 216-778-4795; **Board Cert:** Surgery 2010; **Med School:** Geo Wash Univ 1983; **Resid:** Surgery, UC Irvine Med Ctr 1990; **Fellow:** Surgical Oncology, Natl Cancer Inst 1993; **Fac Appt:** Assoc Prof S, Case West Res Univ

Becker, Yolanda T MD [S] - **Spec Exp:** Transplant Surgery; Transplant-Kidney; Transplant-Pancreas; Dialysis Access; **Hospital:** Univ of Chicago Med Ctr; **Address:** Univ Chicago Med Ctr-Surgery Dept, 5841 S Maryland Ave, MC 5026, Chicago, IL 60637; **Phone:** 773-702-6319; **Board Cert:** Surgery 2006; **Med School:** Johns Hopkins Univ 1990; **Resid:** Surgery, Vanderbilt Univ Med Ctr 1997; **Fellow:** Transplant Surgery, Univ Wisconsin Hosp 1999; **Fac Appt:** Prof S, Univ Chicago-Pritzker Sch Med

Benedetti, Enrico MD [S] - **Spec Exp:** Transplant-Liver; Transplant-Pancreas; Transplant-Kidney; Transplant-Bowel; **Hospital:** Univ of IL Med Ctr at Chicago; **Address:** Univ Illinois, Dept Surg/Transplant, 840 S Wood St, rm 402, Chicago, IL 60612; **Phone:** 312-996-6771; **Board Cert:** Surgery 2003; **Med School:** Italy 1985; **Resid:** Surgery, Univ IL at Chicago Med Ctr 1993; **Fellow:** Transplant Surgery, Univ Minn Med Ctr 1994; **Fac Appt:** Prof S, Univ IL Coll Med

Brems, John J MD [S] - **Spec Exp:** Pancreatic Cancer; Liver Cancer; Transplant-Liver; Liver Disease; **Hospital:** Sherman Hosp; **Address:** 1435 N Randall Rd, Ste 107, Elgin, IL 60123; **Phone:** 224-359-0100; **Board Cert:** Surgery 2004; Surgical Critical Care 2000; **Med School:** St Louis Univ 1981; **Resid:** Surgery, St Louis Univ 1986; **Fellow:** Transplant Surgery, UCLA Med Ctr 1987; **Fac Appt:** Prof S, Loyola Univ-Stritch Sch Med

Brown, Charles K MD [S] - **Spec Exp:** Melanoma; Sarcoma; **Hospital:** CTCA at Midwestern Reg Med Ctr; **Address:** Cancer Treatments Ctrs America, 2520 Elishe Ave, Zion, IL 60099; **Phone:** 800-955-2822; **Board Cert:** Surgery 2010; **Med School:** Univ Fla Coll Med 1992; **Resid:** Surgery, Univ Arizona Med Ctr 1998; **Fellow:** Surgical Oncology, UPMC Med Ctr 1999; Surgical Oncology, Univ Chicago Med Ctr 2000

Brown, Eric A MD [S] - **Spec Exp:** Breast Cancer & Surgery; **Hospital:** Beaumont Hosp-Troy; **Address:** Beaumont Comprehensive Breast Care Ctr, 44199 Dequindre, Ste 612, Troy, MI 48085; **Phone:** 248-687-7300; **Board Cert:** Surgery 2004; **Med School:** Univ Hlth Scis, Chicago Med Sch 1989; **Resid:** Surgery, St John Hosp & Med Ctr 1994

Brunt, L Michael MD [S] - **Spec Exp:** Minimally Invasive Surgery; Adrenal Tumors; Hernia; Hernia-Sports; **Hospital:** Barnes-Jewish Hosp; **Address:** Washington Univ Sch Med, Dept Surgery, 660 S Euclid Ave, Box 8109, St Louis, MO 63110; **Phone:** 314-454-7194 x2; **Board Cert:** Surgery 2006; **Med School:** Johns Hopkins Univ 1980; **Resid:** Surgery, Barnes Jewish Hosp 1987; **Fellow:** Surgery, Barnes Jewish Hosp 1984; **Fac Appt:** Prof S, Washington Univ, St Louis

Chand, Bipan MD [S] - **Spec Exp:** Obesity/Bariatric Surgery; Gastrointestinal Metabolic Surgery; Gastroesophageal Reflux Disease (GERD); Barrett's Esophagus; **Hospital:** Loyola Univ Med Ctr; **Address:** Loyola Univ Med Ctr, 2160 S First Ave Bldg 110 - rm 3224, Maywood, IL 60153; **Phone:** 708-327-2845; **Board Cert:** Surgery 2003; **Med School:** Univ MO-Kansas City 1996; **Resid:** Surgery, Cleveland Clinic 2002; **Fellow:** Laparoscopic Surgery, Cleveland Clinic 2003; **Fac Appt:** Assoc Prof S, Loyola Univ-Stritch Sch Med

Chang, Alfred E MD [S] - **Spec Exp:** Cancer Surgery; Breast Cancer; Gastrointestinal Cancer; Melanoma; **Hospital:** Univ of Michigan Hosp; **Address:** 1500 E Medical Center Drive, 3302 Cancer Geriatric Ctr SPC 5932, Ann Arbor, MI 48109-5932; **Phone:** 734-936-4392; **Board Cert:** Surgery 2011; **Med School:** Harvard Med Sch 1974; **Resid:** Surgery, Duke Univ Med Ctr 1976; Surgery, Hosp Univ Penn 1982; **Fellow:** Surgical Oncology, Natl Cancer Inst 1979; **Fac Appt:** Prof S, Univ Mich Med Sch

Chapman, William C MD [S] - **Spec Exp:** Transplant-Liver-Adult & Pediatric; Liver Cancer; Liver & Biliary Surgery; **Hospital:** Barnes-Jewish Hosp, St. Louis Chldns Hosp; **Address:** Washington Univ Sch Med, 660 S Euclid Ave, Box 8109, St Louis, MO 63110; **Phone:** 314-362-7792; **Board Cert:** Surgery 2011; Surgical Critical Care 2001; **Med School:** Med Univ SC 1984; **Resid:** Surgery, Vanderbilt Univ Med Ctr 1991; **Fellow:** Hepatobiliary Surgery, Kings College Hosp 1992; **Fac Appt:** Prof S, Washington Univ, St Louis

Cronin II, David C MD/PhD [S] - **Spec Exp:** Transplant-Liver; Transplant Surgery-Pediatric; Liver & Biliary Surgery; Pancreatic Surgery; **Hospital:** Froedtert and Med Ctr of WI; **Address:** Div Transplant Surgery, 9200 W Wisconsin Ave, Ste E5700, Milwaukee, WI 53226; **Phone:** 414-955-6920; **Board Cert:** Surgery 2005; **Med School:** Mount Sinai Sch Med 1987; **Resid:** Surgery, Univ Chicago Hosp 1995; **Fellow:** Transplant Surgery, Univ Chicago Hosp 1997; Medical Ethics, Univ Chicago Hosp 2002; **Fac Appt:** Assoc Prof S, Univ Wisc

Crowe Jr, Joseph P MD [S] - **Spec Exp:** Breast Cancer; Tumor Surgery; **Hospital:** Cleveland Clin (page 55); **Address:** Cleveland Clinic Fdn, Dept Surg, 9500 Euclid Ave, Desk A80, Cleveland, OH 44195; **Phone:** 216-444-3024; **Board Cert:** Surgery 2004; **Med School:** Case West Res Univ 1978; **Resid:** Surgery, Univ Hosp-Case West Reserve 1983; **Fellow:** Surgical Oncology, Meml Sloan Kettering Cancer Ctr 1985

Deziel, Daniel J MD [S] - **Spec Exp:** Hepatobiliary Surgery; Pancreatic Surgery; Laparoscopic Surgery; **Hospital:** Rush Univ Med Ctr; **Address:** 1725 W Harrison St, Ste 810/818, Chicago, IL 60612; **Phone:** 312-942-6500; **Board Cert:** Surgery 2003; **Med School:** Univ Minn 1979; **Resid:** Surgery, Rush-Presby-St Luke's Med Ctr 1984; **Fellow:** Gastrointestinal Surgery, Lahey Clinic 1985; **Fac Appt:** Prof S, Rush Med Coll

Donohue, John H MD [S] - **Spec Exp:** Gastrointestinal Cancer; Breast Cancer; Stomach Cancer; **Hospital:** Mayo Med Ctr & Clin - Rochester; **Address:** Mayo Clinic, Dept General Surgery, 200 First St SW, Rochester, MN 55905; **Phone:** 507-284-0362; **Board Cert:** Surgery 2005; **Med School:** Harvard Med Sch 1978; **Resid:** Surgery, UCSF Med Ctr 1981; Surgery, UCSF Med Ctr 1985; **Fellow:** Surgery, Natl Inst Hlth 1983; Surgical Oncology, Meml Sloan-Kettering Canc Ctr 1987; **Fac Appt:** Prof S, Mayo Med Sch

Dulchavsky, Scott A MD/PhD [S] - **Spec Exp:** Trauma; **Hospital:** Henry Ford Hosp; **Address:** Henry Ford Hospital, 2799 W Grand Blvd, CFP1, Detroit, MI 48202; **Phone:** 313-916-3152; **Board Cert:** Surgery 2007; **Med School:** Wayne State Univ 1983; **Resid:** Surgery, Wayne State 1989; **Fac Appt:** Prof S, Wayne State Univ

Eberlein, Timothy J MD [S] - **Spec Exp:** Breast Cancer; Melanoma; Immunotherapy; **Hospital:** Barnes-Jewish Hosp, St. Louis Chldns Hosp; **Address:** Wash Univ School Med, Dept Surgery, 660 S Euclid Ave, Box 8109, St Louis, MO 63110-1093; **Phone:** 314-362-8020; **Board Cert:** Surgery 2006; **Med School:** Univ Pittsburgh 1977; **Resid:** Surgery, Peter Bent Brigham Hosp 1979; Surgery, Brigham-Womens Hosp 1985; **Fellow:** Immunology, Natl Inst Hlth 1982; **Fac Appt:** Prof S, Washington Univ, St Louis

Edwards, Michael J MD [S] - **Spec Exp:** Breast Cancer; Melanoma; **Hospital:** Univ Hosp - Cincinnati; **Address:** 234 Goodman St, ML 0772, Cincinnati, OH 45219; **Phone:** 513-584-8900; **Board Cert:** Surgery 2005; **Med School:** Emory Univ 1981; **Resid:** Surgery, Univ Louisville Hosp 1986; **Fellow:** Surgical Oncology, MD Anderson Cancer Ctr 1987; **Fac Appt:** Prof S, Univ Cincinnati

Ellison, E Christopher MD [S] - **Spec Exp:** Biliary Surgery; Biliary Cancer; Pancreatic Cancer; **Hospital:** Ohio St Univ Med Ctr; **Address:** 1654 Upham Drive, Ste 327 Means Hall, Columbus, OH 43210-1236; **Phone:** 614-293-4499; **Board Cert:** Surgery 2011; **Med School:** Univ Wisc 1976; **Resid:** Surgery, Ohio State Univ 1981; **Fac Appt:** Prof S, Ohio State Univ

Evans, Douglas B MD [S] - **Spec Exp:** Pancreatic Cancer; Thyroid Cancer; Endocrine Cancers; **Hospital:** Froedtert and Med Ctr of WI; **Address:** Medical Coll Wisconsin, Dept Surgery, 9200 W Wisconsin Ave, Ste 3510, Milwaukee, WI 53226-6533; **Phone:** 414-805-5706; **Board Cert:** Surgery 2008; **Med School:** Boston Univ 1983; **Resid:** Surgery, Dartmouth-Hitchcock Med Ctr 1988; **Fellow:** Surgical Oncology, MD Anderson Cancer Ctr 1990; **Fac Appt:** Prof S, Med Coll Wisc

Farley, David R MD [S] - **Spec Exp:** Endocrine Surgery; Hepatobiliary Surgery; Laparoscopic Surgery; Hernia; **Hospital:** Mayo Med Ctr & Clin - Rochester; **Address:** Mayo Clin, Dept Surg, 200 1st St SW, Mayo West, Fl 12, Rochester, MN 55905; **Phone:** 507-284-2644; **Board Cert:** Surgery 2002; **Med School:** Univ Wisc 1988; **Resid:** Surgery, Mayo Clin 1994; **Fellow:** Endocrinology, Mayo Clin 1995; **Fac Appt:** Assoc Prof S, Mayo Med Sch

Farrar, William B MD [S] - **Spec Exp:** Breast Cancer; Thyroid Cancer; **Hospital:** Arthur G James Cancer Hosp & Research Inst, Ohio St Univ Med Ctr; **Address:** 410 W 10th Ave, N924 Doan Hall, Columbus, OH 43210; **Phone:** 614-293-8890; **Board Cert:** Surgery 2010; **Med School:** Univ VA Sch Med 1975; **Resid:** Surgery, Ohio State Univ Hosps 1980; **Fellow:** Surgical Oncology, Meml Sloan-Kettering Cancer Ctr 1982; **Fac Appt:** Prof S, Ohio State Univ

Frantzides, Constantine T MD/PhD [S] - **Spec Exp:** Minimally Invasive Surgery; Laparoscopic Surgery; Obesity/Bariatric Surgery; Laparoscopic Abdominal Surgery; **Hospital:** St. Francis Hosp - Evanston, Evanston/North Shore Univ Hlth Sys; **Address:** Chicago Inst of Minimally Invasive Surg, 4905 Old Orchard Ctr, Ste 409, Skokie, IL 60077; **Phone:** 847-676-2200; **Med School:** Greece 1976; **Resid:** Surgery, Athens Univ Affil Hosp 1982; **Fellow:** Surgery, Queen Mary's Hosp 1978; Surgery, Med Coll Wisc 1985; **Fac Appt:** Prof S, Univ IL Coll Med

Fung, John J MD/PhD [S] - **Spec Exp:** Transplant-Liver; Transplant-Kidney; Liver & Biliary Cancer; Laparoscopic Surgery; **Hospital:** Cleveland Clin (page 55), Hillcrest Hosp-Mayfield Hts; **Address:** 9500 Euclid Ave, MS A100, Cleveland, OH 44195; **Phone:** 216-444-3776; **Board Cert:** Surgery 2008; **Med School:** Univ Chicago-Pritzker Sch Med 1982; **Resid:** Surgery, Strong Meml Hosp 1988; **Fellow:** Transplant Surgery, Univ Pittsburgh Med Ctr 1986; **Fac Appt:** Prof S, Cleveland Cl Coll Med/Case West Res

Gamelli, Richard L MD [S] - **Spec Exp:** Burn Care; Trauma/Critical Care; **Hospital:** Loyola Univ Med Ctr; **Address:** 2160 S First Ave Bldg 103 - rm 1175, Maywood, IL 60153; **Phone:** 708-216-4444; **Board Cert:** Surgery 2009; **Med School:** Univ VT Coll Med 1974; **Resid:** Surgery, Vermont Med Ctr Hosp 1979; **Fac Appt:** Prof S, Loyola Univ-Stritch Sch Med

Goulet Jr, Robert J MD [S] - **Spec Exp:** Breast Cancer; Breast Surgery; **Hospital:** Commun Hosp E - Indianapolis; **Address:** Community Hospital Breast Care, 1400 N Ritter Ave, Ste 485, Indianapolis, IN 46219; **Phone:** 317-355-2727; **Board Cert:** Surgery 2006; **Med School:** SUNY Downstate 1979; **Resid:** Surgery, SUNY-Downstate Med Ctr 1986; **Fellow:** Surgical Research, SUNY-Downstate Med Ctr 1983

Grant, Clive S MD [S] - **Spec Exp:** Thyroid & Parathyroid Cancer & Surgery; Adrenal Tumors; Breast Cancer; **Hospital:** Mayo Med Ctr & Clin - Rochester; **Address:** Mayo Clinic, Dept Surgery, 200 First St SW, Rochester, MN 55905-0001; **Phone:** 507-284-2644; **Board Cert:** Surgery 2010; **Med School:** Univ Colorado 1975; **Resid:** Surgery, Mayo Clinic 1980; **Fac Appt:** Prof S, Mayo Med Sch

Gruber, Scott A MD/PhD [S] - **Spec Exp:** Transplant-Kidney; Transplant-Pancreas; **Hospital:** John D. Dingell VA Med Ctr, Detroit, Harper Univ Hosp; **Address:** 4646 John R St, Detroit, MI 48201; **Phone:** 313-576-3327; **Board Cert:** Surgery 2011; **Med School:** SUNY Downstate 1983; **Resid:** Surgery, Univ Minnesota Med Ctr 1986; **Fellow:** Surgery, Univ Minnesota Med Ctr 1989; Transplant Surgery, Univ Minnesota Med Ctr 1993; **Fac Appt:** Prof S, Wayne State Univ

Hansen, Nora M MD [S] - **Spec Exp:** Sentinel Node Surgery; Breast Cancer-High Risk Women; Breast Cancer Risk Assessment; **Hospital:** Northwestern Meml Hosp, Prentice Women's Hosp; **Address:** Lynn Sage Breast Surgery Ctr, 250 E Superior St Fl 4 - Ste 420, Chicago, IL 60611; **Phone:** 312-695-1156; **Board Cert:** Surgery 2006; **Med School:** NY Med Coll 1988; **Resid:** Surgery, Univ Chicago Hosps 1995; **Fellow:** Surgical Oncology, Univ Chicago Hosps 1996; **Fac Appt:** Assoc Prof S, Northwestern Univ

Hering, Bernhard J MD [S] - **Spec Exp:** Pancreatic Islet Cell Transplant; Diabetes; **Hospital:** Univ Minn Med Ctr, Fairview - Riverside Campus; **Address:** Schulze Diabetes Inst, MMC 280 Mayo, 8280A, 420 Delaware St SE, Minneapolis, MN 55455; **Phone:** 612-626-5697; **Med School:** Germany 1983; **Resid:** Research, Islet Transplant Lab, Justus Liebig Univ 1986; Internal Medicine, Justus Liebig Univ 1995; **Fellow:** Endocrinology, Justus Liebig Univ 1996; **Fac Appt:** Prof S, Univ Minn

Hinshaw, Daniel B MD [S] - **Spec Exp:** Palliative Care; **Hospital:** VA Ann Arbor Healthcare Sys, Univ of Michigan Hosp; **Address:** VA Medical Ctr, 2215 Fuller Rd, rm 530, MS 112, Ann Arbor, MI 48105; **Phone:** 734-769-7100 x5939; **Board Cert:** Surgery 2003; Hospice & Palliative Medicine 2008; **Med School:** Loma Linda Univ 1978; **Resid:** Surgery, Loma Linda U Med Ctr 1983; **Fellow:** Immunology, Scripps Clinic Rsch Fdn 1985; Cleveland Clin 2001; **Fac Appt:** Clin Prof S, Univ Mich Med Sch

Howe, James R MD [S] - **Spec Exp:** Endocrine Surgery; Gastrointestinal Cancer; Colon & Rectal Cancer; **Hospital:** Univ Iowa Hosp & Clinics; **Address:** Univ Iowa Hosp & Clinics, Dept Surg, 200 Hawkins Drive JCP Bldg - rm 4644, Iowa City, IA 52242-1086; **Phone:** 319-356-1727; **Board Cert:** Surgery 2006; **Med School:** Univ VT Coll Med 1987; **Resid:** Surgery, Barnes Hosp-Wash Univ 1994; **Fellow:** Research, Wash Univ-NCI 1991; Surgical Oncology, Meml Sloan-Kettering Cancer Ctr 1996; **Fac Appt:** Prof S, Univ Iowa Coll Med

Ikramuddin, Sayeed MD [S] - **Spec Exp:** Minimally Invasive Surgery; Obesity/Bariatric Surgery; **Hospital:** Univ Minn Med Ctr, Fairview - Riverside Campus; **Address:** Univ Minn Med Ctr, Fairview, P Wagenstein Bldg, Fl 1, Clin 1E-MMC88, 516 Delaware St SE, Minneapolis, MN 55454; **Phone:** 612-625-8446; **Board Cert:** Surgery 2007; **Med School:** Albany Med Coll 1990; **Resid:** Surgery, SUNY Hlth Sci Ctr 1992; Surgery, SUNY Hlth Sci Ctr 1996; **Fellow:** Research, SUNY Hlth Sci Ctr 1993; Laparoscopic Surgery, Ohio State Univ Affil Hosp 1997; **Fac Appt:** Assoc Prof S, Univ Minn

Johnson Miller, Denise L MD [S] - **Spec Exp:** Breast Cancer; Breast Cancer-High Risk Women; Melanoma; Neuroendocrine Tumors; **Hospital:** Franciscan St. Francis Hlth-Indianapolis; **Address:** 8111 S Emerson Ave, Ste 104, Indianapolis, IN 46237; **Phone:** 317-781-7391; **Board Cert:** Surgery 2001; **Med School:** Washington Univ, St Louis 1978; **Resid:** Immunology, Univ Texas SW Med Ctr 1982; Surgery, Univ Illinois Med Ctr 1986; **Fellow:** Surgical Oncology, City of Hope Med Ctr 1988

Kagan, Richard J MD [S] - **Spec Exp:** Burn Care; **Hospital:** Cincinnati Shriners Hosp, Univ Hosp - Cincinnati; **Address:** Cincinnati Shriners Hosp, 3229 Burnet Ave, Cincinnati, OH 45229; **Phone:** 513-872-6210; **Board Cert:** Surgery 2007; **Med School:** St Louis Univ 1974; **Resid:** Surgery, Univ IL Hosp 1980; **Fac Appt:** Prof S, Univ Cincinnati

Kaufman, Howard L MD [S] - **Spec Exp:** Cancer Surgery; Vaccine Therapy; Melanoma; Immunotherapy; **Hospital:** Rush Univ Med Ctr; **Address:** 1725 W Harrison St, Ste 845, Chicago, IL 60612-3244; **Phone:** 312-942-0600; **Board Cert:** Surgery 2007; **Med School:** Loyola Univ-Stritch Sch Med 1986; **Resid:** Surgery, Boston Univ Hosp 1995; **Fellow:** Surgical Oncology, Natl Cancer Inst 1996; **Fac Appt:** Prof S, Loyola Univ-Stritch Sch Med

Kendrick, Michael L MD [S] - **Spec Exp:** Pancreatic Cancer; Liver Cancer; Hepatobiliary Surgery; Laparoscopic Surgery; **Hospital:** Mayo Med Ctr & Clin - Rochester; **Address:** Mayo Clinic Atten: Dept of Surgery, 200 First St SW, Rochester, MN 55905; **Phone:** 507-284-2511; **Board Cert:** Surgery 2004; **Med School:** Geo Wash Univ 1997; **Resid:** Surgery, Mayo Clinic 2003; **Fellow:** Hepatopancreatobiliary Surgery, Mayo Clinic 2004; Laparoscopic Surgery, Mt Sinai Med Ctr 2005; **Fac Appt:** Assoc Prof S, Mayo Med Sch

Kim, Julian A MD [S] - **Spec Exp:** Melanoma; Breast Cancer; Gastrointestinal Cancer; Immunotherapy; **Hospital:** Univ Hosps Case Med Ctr (page 74); **Address:** 11100 Euclid Ave, LKS 5047, Cleveland, OH 44106-1716; **Phone:** 216-844-8247; **Board Cert:** Surgery 2002; **Med School:** Med Univ Ohio at Toledo 1986; **Resid:** Surgery, Univ Maryland Hosps 1991; **Fellow:** Surgical Oncology, Arthur James Cancer Hosp & Rsch Inst 1993; Immunotherapy, Ohio State Univ Comp Cancer Ctr 1994; **Fac Appt:** Prof S, Case West Res Univ

Leeming, Rosemary A MD [S] - **Spec Exp:** Breast Cancer & Surgery; Breast Disease; Clinical Trials; **Hospital:** Univ Hosps Case Med Ctr (page 74); **Address:** 3909 Orange Pl, Ste 4400, Orange Village, OH 44122; **Phone:** 216-591-1909; **Board Cert:** Surgery 2009; **Med School:** Hahnemann Univ 1983; **Resid:** Surgery, Mt Sinai Med Ctr 1989; **Fellow:** Breast Disease, Univ Pitts-Shadyside Hosp 1989; **Fac Appt:** Asst Prof S, Case West Res Univ

Mahvi, David M MD [S] - **Spec Exp:** Gastrointestinal Cancer & Surgery; Liver Cancer; Pancreatic Cancer; **Hospital:** Northwestern Meml Hosp; **Address:** Northwestern Memorial Hospital, 675 N St Clair, Galter 21-700, Chicago, IL 60611; **Phone:** 312-695-0990; **Board Cert:** Surgery 2007; **Med School:** Med Univ SC 1981; **Resid:** Surgery, Duke Univ Med Ctr 1989; **Fac Appt:** Prof S, Northwestern Univ

Mamounas, Eleftherios P MD [S] - **Spec Exp:** Breast Cancer; **Hospital:** Aultman Hosp; **Address:** Aultman Cancer Ctr, 2600 6th St SW, Canton, OH 44710; **Phone:** 330-363-6281; **Board Cert:** Surgery 2009; **Med School:** Greece 1983; **Resid:** Surgery, McKeesport Hosp 1989; **Fellow:** Clinical Oncology, Univ Pittsburgh 1991; Surgical Oncology, Roswell Park Cancer Inst 1992; **Fac Appt:** Prof S, NE Ohio Univ

Marks, Jeffrey M MD [S] - **Spec Exp:** Gastrointestinal Surgery; Endoscopy; Laparoscopic Surgery; Natural Orifice Surgery (NOTES); **Hospital:** Univ Hosps Case Med Ctr (page 74); **Address:** Univ Hospitals Case Medical Ctr, Dept Surgery, 11100 Euclid Ave, Cleveland, OH 44106; **Phone:** 216-844-7874; **Board Cert:** Surgery 2001; **Med School:** Tufts Univ 1987; **Resid:** Surgery, Mt Sinai Hosp 1992; **Fellow:** Endoscopy, Mt Sinai Hosp 1992; **Fac Appt:** Assoc Prof S, Case West Res Univ

Matas, Arthur J MD [S] - **Spec Exp:** Transplant-Kidney; **Hospital:** Univ Minn Med Ctr, Fairview - Riverside Campus; **Address:** Univ Minn Med Ctr, Dept Surg, 420 Delaware St SE, MMC 328, Minneapolis, MN 55455; **Phone:** 612-624-1927; **Board Cert:** Surgery 2010; **Med School:** Univ Manitoba 1972; **Resid:** Surgery, Univ Minn Hosps 1979; **Fellow:** Transplant Surgery, Univ Minn Hosps 1980; **Fac Appt:** Prof S, Univ Minn

Matthews, Jeffrey MD [S] - **Spec Exp:** Gastrointestinal Surgery; Pancreatic Surgery; Liver & Biliary Surgery; **Hospital:** Univ of Chicago Med Ctr; **Address:** 5841 S Maryland Ave, Ste 0220, MC 5029, Chicago, IL 60637; **Phone:** 773-702-0881; **Board Cert:** Surgery 2001; **Med School:** Harvard Med Sch 1985; **Resid:** Surgery, Beth Israel Hosp 1990; **Fellow:** Hepatobiliary Surgery, Univ Bern 1989; **Fac Appt:** Prof S, Univ Chicago-Pritzker Sch Med

McHenry, Christopher R MD [S] - **Spec Exp:** Adrenal Surgery; Thyroid Surgery; Parathyroid Surgery; **Hospital:** MetroHealth Med Ctr; **Address:** MetroHealth Medical Ctr, Dept Surgery, 2500 Metro Health Drive, Cleveland, OH 44109; **Phone:** 216-778-4753; **Board Cert:** Surgery 2009; **Med School:** NE Ohio Univ 1984; **Resid:** Surgery, Loyola Univ Med Ctr 1989; **Fellow:** Endocrinology, Univ Toronto Med Ctr 1990; Head and Neck Surgery, Univ Toronto Med Ctr 1990; **Fac Appt:** Prof S, Case West Res Univ

Melvin, W Scott MD [S] - **Spec Exp:** Liver & Biliary Surgery; Pancreatic Cancer; Laparoscopic Surgery; **Hospital:** Ohio St Univ Med Ctr; **Address:** 410 W 10th Ave, rm N729, North Doan Hall, Columbus, OH 43210; **Phone:** 614-293-4499; **Board Cert:** Surgery 2002; **Med School:** Med Coll OH 1987; **Resid:** Surgery, Univ Maryland 1992; **Fellow:** Gastrointestinal Surgery, Grant Med Ctr 1993; **Fac Appt:** Prof S, Ohio State Univ

Millis, J Michael MD [S] - **Spec Exp:** Transplant-Liver-Adult & Pediatric; Liver Cancer; Transplant-Pancreas; Liver Disease; **Hospital:** Univ of Chicago Med Ctr; **Address:** Univ Chicago Med Ctr, Dept Surg, 5841 S Maryland Ave, MC 5027, Chicago, IL 60637; **Phone:** 773-702-6319; **Board Cert:** Surgery 2001; Surgical Critical Care 2001; **Med School:** Univ Tenn Coll Med 1985; **Resid:** Surgery, UCLA Med Ctr 1991; **Fellow:** Transplant Surgery, UCLA Med Ctr 1994; **Fac Appt:** Prof S, Univ Chicago-Pritzker Sch Med

Moley, Jeffrey F MD [S] - **Spec Exp:** Thyroid Cancer & Surgery; Endocrine Cancers; Melanoma; **Hospital:** Barnes-Jewish Hosp; **Address:** Washington Univ School Med, Dept Surgery, 660 S Euclid Ave, Box 8109, St Louis, MO 63110; **Phone:** 314-362-2280; **Board Cert:** Surgery 2005; **Med School:** Columbia P&S 1980; **Resid:** Surgery, Yale-New Haven Hosp 1985; **Fellow:** Surgical Oncology, National Cancer Inst 1987; **Fac Appt:** Prof S, Washington Univ, St Louis

Nagorney, David M MD [S] - **Spec Exp:** Pancreatic Cancer; Hepatobiliary Surgery; Gastrointestinal Cancer; **Hospital:** Mayo Med Ctr & Clin - Rochester; **Address:** Mayo Clin, Dept Surgery, 200 1st St SW, Mayo E12, Rochester, MN 55905; **Phone:** 507-284-0362; **Board Cert:** Surgery 2011; **Med School:** Univ Kansas 1975; **Resid:** Surgery, Mayo Clin 1982; **Fellow:** Hepatobiliary Surgery, Hammersmith Hosp 1985; **Fac Appt:** Prof S, Mayo Med Sch

Nathanson, S David MD [S] - **Spec Exp:** Breast Cancer; Breast Cancer Risk Assessment; Melanoma; Sarcoma; **Hospital:** Henry Ford- W Bloomfield Hosp, Henry Ford Hosp; **Address:** 6777 W Maple Rd, West Bloomfield, MI 48322; **Phone:** 248-661-6592; **Board Cert:** Surgery 2002; **Med School:** South Africa 1966; **Resid:** Surgery, Univ Witwaterstrand 1974; Surgical Oncology, UCLA Med Ctr 1980; **Fellow:** Surgery, UC Davis Med Ctr 1982; **Fac Appt:** Prof S, Wayne State Univ

Newman, Lisa A MD [S] - **Spec Exp:** Breast Cancer; **Hospital:** Univ of Michigan Hosp; **Address:** Univ Michigan Cancer Center, 1500 E Medical Center Drive, rm 3308-CGC, Ann Arbor, MI 48109-5932; **Phone:** 734-936-8771; **Board Cert:** Surgery 2001; **Med School:** SUNY Downstate 1985; **Resid:** Surgery, Downstate Med Ctr 1990; **Fac Appt:** Assoc Prof S, Univ Mich Med Sch

Oberholzer, Jose MD [S] - **Spec Exp:** Diabetes; Transplant-Pancreas; Pancreatic Islet Cell Transplant; Hepatobiliary Surgery; **Hospital:** Univ of IL Med Ctr at Chicago, Adv Luth Genl Hosp; **Address:** University of Illinois at Chicago, Div Transplant Surgery, 840 S Wood St CSB Bldg - Ste 405, MS 958, Chicago, IL 60612; **Phone:** 312-996-6771; **Med School:** Switzerland 1992; **Resid:** Surgery, Triemli Hosp 1996; Surgery, Univ Geneva Hosp 1998; **Fellow:** Transplant Surgery, Univ Geneva Hosp 2002; Hepatopancreatobiliary Surgery, Univ Alberta Hosp 2003; **Fac Appt:** Prof S, Univ IL Coll Med

Onders, Raymond P MD [S] - **Spec Exp:** Laparoscopic Surgery; Diaphragm Pacing via Laparoscopy; Gastrointestinal Cancer; **Hospital:** Univ Hosps Case Med Ctr (page 74); **Address:** 11100 Euclid Ave, MS LKS 5047, Cleveland, OH 44106-5047; **Phone:** 216-844-5797; **Board Cert:** Surgery 2001; **Med School:** NE Ohio Univ 1988; **Resid:** Surgery, Case Western Reserve Univ 1993; **Fac Appt:** Assoc Prof S, NE Ohio Univ

Ponsky, Jeffrey L MD [S] - **Spec Exp:** Minimally Invasive Surgery; Gastrointestinal Surgery; Endoscopy; **Hospital:** Univ Hosps Case Med Ctr (page 74); **Address:** Univ Hosps Cleveland, Dept Surgery, 11100 Euclid Ave, Cleveland, OH 44106; **Phone:** 216-844-3209; **Board Cert:** Surgery 2007; **Med School:** Case West Res Univ 1971; **Resid:** Surgery, Univ Hosps 1976; **Fac Appt:** Prof S, Case West Res Univ

Posner, Mitchell C MD [S] - **Spec Exp:** Pancreatic Cancer; Gastrointestinal Cancer; Esophageal Cancer; **Hospital:** Univ of Chicago Med Ctr; **Address:** Univ Chicago Med Ctr, Dept Surg, 5841 S Maryland Ave, Ste G209, MC 5094, Chicago, IL 60637-1447; **Phone:** 773-834-4007; **Board Cert:** Surgery 2006; **Med School:** SUNY Buffalo 1981; **Resid:** Surgery, Univ Colorado Med Ctr 1986; **Fellow:** Surgical Oncology, Meml Sloan-Kettering Cancer Ctr 1988; **Fac Appt:** Prof S, Univ Chicago-Pritzker Sch Med

Prinz, Richard A MD [S] - **Spec Exp:** Adrenal Surgery; Thyroid & Parathyroid Surgery; Pancreatic & Biliary Surgery; Laparoscopic Surgery; **Hospital:** Evanston/North Shore Univ Hlth Sys, Highland Park/North Shore Univ Hlth Syst; **Address:** 2650 N Ridge Ave, Evanston, IL 60201; **Phone:** 847-570-1700; **Board Cert:** Surgery 2007; **Med School:** Loyola Univ-Stritch Sch Med 1972; **Resid:** Surgery, Barnes Hosp 1974; Surgery, Loyola Univ Hosp 1977; **Fellow:** Endocrine Surgery, Hammersmith Hosp 1980; **Fac Appt:** Prof S, Univ Chicago-Pritzker Sch Med

Reed, Alan I MD [S] - **Spec Exp:** Hepatobiliary Surgery; Transplant-Liver; Transplant-Kidney; Transplant-Pancreas; **Hospital:** Univ Iowa Hosp & Clinics; **Address:** 200 Hawkins Drive, Ste SE427 GH, Organ Transplant Ctr, Iowa City, IA 52242-1009; **Phone:** 319-356-4778; **Board Cert:** Surgery 2010; **Med School:** Cornell Univ-Weill Med Coll 1984; **Resid:** Surgery, NY Hosp/Cornell 1989; **Fellow:** Transplant Surgery, Univ Wisc Hosp 1984; **Fac Appt:** Prof S, Univ Iowa Coll Med

Renz, John MD/PhD [S] - **Spec Exp:** Transplant-Liver; Transplant-Liver-Adult & Pediatric; Transplant Surgery; **Hospital:** Univ of Chicago Med Ctr; **Address:** Univ Chicago Med Ctr-Surgery Dept, 5841 S Maryland Ave, MC 5027, Chicago, IL 60637; **Phone:** 773-702-4500; **Board Cert:** Surgery 2003; **Med School:** Jefferson Med Coll 1992; **Resid:** Surgery, UCSF Med Ctr 1999; **Fellow:** Transplant Surgery, UCLA Med Ctr 2002; **Fac Appt:** Prof S, Univ Chicago-Pritzker Sch Med

Rosen, Charles B MD [S] - **Spec Exp:** Transplant-Liver; Transplant-Bile Duct; **Hospital:** Mayo Med Ctr & Clin - Rochester; **Address:** Mayo Clin, Dept Surg-Div Transplantation, 200 First St SW, Charlton 10A, Rochester, MN 55905-0001; **Phone:** 507-266-6640; **Board Cert:** Surgery 2009; **Med School:** Mayo Med Sch 1984; **Resid:** Surgery, Mayo Clin 1989; **Fellow:** Transplant Surgery, Mayo Clin 1991; **Fac Appt:** Prof S, Mayo Med Sch

Rosen, Michael J MD [S] - **Spec Exp:** Hernia; Gastrointestinal Surgery; Minimally Invasive Surgery; **Hospital:** Univ Hosps Case Med Ctr (page 74); **Address:** Univ Hosp Case Med Ctr, 11100 Euclid Ave, LKS5047, Cleveland, OH 44106; **Phone:** 216-844-2763; **Board Cert:** Surgery 2005; **Med School:** USC-Keck School of Medicine 1997; **Resid:** Surgery, Mass Gen Hosp 2004; **Fellow:** Minimally Invasive Surgery, Cleveland Clinic 2002; Laparoscopic Surgery, Carolinas Med Ctr 2005; **Fac Appt:** Asst Prof S, Case West Res Univ

Saha, Sukamal MD [S] - **Spec Exp:** Sentinel Node Surgery; Colon Cancer; Head & Neck Cancer & Surgery; **Hospital:** McLaren Reg Med Ctr, Genesys Reg Med Ctr - St Joseph Campus; **Address:** 3500 Calkins Rd, Ste A, Flint, MI 48532; **Phone:** 810-230-9600 x500; **Board Cert:** Surgery 2010; **Med School:** India 1977; **Resid:** Surgery, Hahnemann Univ Hosp 1985; Surgery, Easton Hosp 1987; **Fellow:** Surgical Oncology, Tulane Univ Med Ctr 1989; Head and Neck Surgery, Roswell Park Meml Hosp 1990; **Fac Appt:** Asst Prof S, Mich State Univ

Sarr, Michael G MD [S] - **Spec Exp:** Pancreatic Cancer; Gastrointestinal Cancer; Obesity/Bariatric Surgery; Gastrointestinal Motility Disorders; **Hospital:** Mayo Med Ctr & Clin - Rochester; **Address:** Mayo Clinic, 200 First St SW, Dept Surg, Desk West 12A, Rochester, MN 55905; **Phone:** 507-284-0362; **Board Cert:** Surgery 2001; **Med School:** Johns Hopkins Univ 1976; **Resid:** Surgery, Johns Hopkins Hosp 1982; **Fellow:** Surgery, Mayo Clinic 1984; Surgery, Johns Hopkins Hosp 1985; **Fac Appt:** Prof S, Mayo Med Sch

Schauer, Philip MD [S] - **Spec Exp:** Obesity/Bariatric Surgery; Minimally Invasive Surgery; **Hospital:** Cleveland Clin (page 55); **Address:** Cleveland Clinic, 9500 Euclid Ave, MC M61, Cleveland, OH 44195; **Phone:** 216-444-4794; **Board Cert:** Surgery 2004; **Med School:** Baylor Coll Med 1986; **Resid:** Surgery, Univ Texas Med Ctr 1991; **Fellow:** Laparoscopic Surgery, Duke Univ Med Ctr 1992; **Fac Appt:** Prof S, Cleveland Cl Coll Med/Case West Res

Schulak, James A MD [S] - **Spec Exp:** Transplant-Kidney-Adult & Pediatric; Transplant-Pancreas & Liver; Pancreatic Surgery; **Hospital:** Univ Hosps Case Med Ctr (page 74); **Address:** Univ Hosps of Cleveland, Dept Surgery, 11100 Euclid Ave, MS 5047, Cleveland, OH 44106-5407; **Phone:** 216-844-0307; **Board Cert:** Surgery 2010; **Med School:** Univ Chicago-Pritzker Sch Med 1974; **Resid:** Surgery, Univ Chicago Hosp 1980; **Fellow:** Transplant Surgery, Univ Chicago Hosp 1981; **Fac Appt:** Prof S, Case West Res Univ

Schwartzentruber, Douglas J MD [S] - **Spec Exp:** Cancer Surgery; Melanoma; Kidney Cancer; **Hospital:** IU Health Methodist Hosp, IU Health University Hosp; **Address:** Indiana Univ Hlth Cancer Services, 550 N University Blvd, AOC Bldg Fl 6 - Ste 6237, Indianapolis, IN 46202; **Phone:** 317-948-7449; **Board Cert:** Surgery 2008; **Med School:** Indiana Univ 1982; **Resid:** Surgery, Indiana Univ Med Ctr 1987; **Fellow:** Surgical Oncology, Natl Cancer Inst 1990; **Fac Appt:** Assoc Clin Prof S, Indiana Univ

Scott-Conner, Carol E H MD/PhD [S] - **Spec Exp:** Breast Cancer; Cancer Surgery; Laparoscopic Surgery; **Hospital:** Univ Iowa Hosp & Clinics, Iowa City VA Hlth Care Sys; **Address:** Univ Iowa Hosp & Clinics, Dept Surg, 200 Hawkins Drive JCP Bldg - rm 4622, Iowa City, IA 52242-1086; **Phone:** 319-356-0330; **Board Cert:** Surgery 2010; **Med School:** NYU Sch Med 1976; **Resid:** Surgery, NYU Med Ctr 1981; **Fac Appt:** Prof S, Univ Iowa Coll Med

Shenk, Robert R MD [S] - **Spec Exp:** Breast Cancer; Melanoma; Pancreatic Cancer; Stomach Cancer; **Hospital:** Univ Hosps Case Med Ctr (page 74); **Address:** Univ Hosp Case Med Ctr, 11100 Euclid Ave, Dept General Surgery, Cleveland, OH 44106; **Phone:** 216-844-3026; **Board Cert:** Surgery 2004; **Med School:** Case West Res Univ 1978; **Resid:** Surgery, Univ Hosp 1985; Immunology, Natl Cancer Inst 1982; **Fellow:** Surgical Oncology, MD Anderson Cancer Ctr 1987; **Fac Appt:** Assoc Prof S, Case West Res Univ

Sielaff, Timothy D MD/PhD [S] - **Spec Exp:** Liver Cancer; Pancreatic Cancer; Gallbladder & Biliary Cancer; **Hospital:** Abbott - Northwestern Hosp; **Address:** Virginia Piper Cancer Inst, Liver and Pancreas Clinic, 800 E 28th St, Minneapolis, MN 55407; **Phone:** 612-863-7553; **Board Cert:** Surgery 2008; **Med School:** Med Coll VA 1989; **Resid:** Surgery, Univ Minn Hosps 1997; **Fellow:** Transplant Surgery, Univ Toronto Affil Hosp 1998; **Fac Appt:** Assoc Prof S, Univ Minn

Simeone, Diane M MD [S] - **Spec Exp:** Pancreatic Cancer; Cancer Surgery; **Hospital:** Univ of Michigan Hosp; **Address:** Univ Michigan Hlth Sys, 1500 E Med Ctr Drive, 2210B Taubman Center SPC 5343, Ann Arbor, MI 48109-5343; **Phone:** 734-615-1600; **Board Cert:** Surgery 2005; **Med School:** Duke Univ 1988; **Resid:** Surgery, Univ Mich Med Ctr 1995; **Fac Appt:** Prof S, Univ Mich Med Sch

Siperstein, Allan E MD [S] - **Spec Exp:** Laparoscopic Surgery; Endocrine Tumors; Thyroid & Parathyroid Cancer & Surgery; **Hospital:** Cleveland Clin (page 55); **Address:** Cleveland Clinic, Dept Endocrine Surg, 9500 Euclid Ave, MC F20, Cleveland, OH 44195; **Phone:** 216-444-5664; **Board Cert:** Surgery 2007; **Med School:** Univ Tex SW, Dallas 1983; **Resid:** Surgery, UCSF Med Ctr 1990; **Fellow:** Research, UCSF Med Ctr 1988

Soper, Nathaniel MD [S] - **Spec Exp:** Laparoscopic Surgery; Gastroesophageal Reflux Disease (GERD); Biliary Surgery; **Hospital:** Northwestern Meml Hosp; **Address:** Northwestern Med Faculty Fdn, 675 N St Clair St, Galter Bldg Fl 17 - Ste 250, Chicago, IL 60611; **Phone:** 312-695-8918; **Board Cert:** Surgery 2005; **Med School:** Univ Iowa Coll Med 1980; **Resid:** Surgery, Univ Utah Hosps 1986; **Fellow:** Digestive Dis, Mayo Clinic 1988; **Fac Appt:** Prof S, Northwestern Univ

Stahl, Donna L MD [S] - **Spec Exp:** Breast Cancer; Breast Surgery; **Hospital:** Jewish Hosp - Kenwood - Cincinnati; **Address:** 4750 E Galbraith Rd, Ste 112, Cincinnati, OH 45236; **Phone:** 513-686-3109; **Med School:** Univ Iowa Coll Med 1971; **Resid:** Surgery, Univ Cincinnati Hosps 1978

Sundaram, Magesh MD [S] - **Spec Exp:** Gastrointestinal Cancer & Surgery; Pancreatic Cancer; Stomach Cancer; Liver & Biliary Cancer; **Hospital:** Carle Foundation Hosp; **Address:** Carle Cancer Ctr, 611 W Park St, Urbana, IL 61801; **Phone:** 217-383-5701; **Board Cert:** Surgery 2006; **Med School:** Univ MD Sch Med 1990; **Resid:** Surgery, Delaware Med Ctr 1995; **Fellow:** Surgical Oncology, Jackson Meml Hosp 1997; **Fac Appt:** Assoc Prof S, Univ IL Coll Med

Talamonti, Mark S MD [S] - **Spec Exp:** Pancreatic Cancer; Liver Cancer; Gastrointestinal Cancer & Surgery; Melanoma; **Hospital:** Evanston/North Shore Univ Hlth Sys, Highland Park/North Shore Univ Hlth Syst; **Address:** North Shore Dept Surgery, 2560 Ridge Ave Walgreen Bldg - rm 2555, Evanston, IL 60201; **Phone:** 847-570-1700; **Board Cert:** Surgery 2009; **Med School:** Northwestern Univ 1983; **Resid:** Surgery, Northwestern Meml Hosp 1989; **Fellow:** Surgical Oncology, MD Anderson Cancer Ctr 1991; **Fac Appt:** Clin Prof S, Univ Chicago-Pritzker Sch Med

Thistlethwaite, J Richard MD/PhD [S] - **Spec Exp:** Transplant-Kidney; Transplant-Pancreas; Transplant-Liver; Transplant Surgery-Pediatric; **Hospital:** Univ of Chicago Med Ctr; **Address:** 5841 S Maryland Ave, rm J-517, MC 5026, Chicago, IL 60637; **Phone:** 773-702-6319; **Board Cert:** Surgery 2008; **Med School:** Duke Univ 1977; **Resid:** Surgery, Mass Genl Hosp 1983; **Fellow:** Surgical Oncology, Natl Inst Hlth 1981; Transplant Surgery, Mass Genl Hosp 1984; **Fac Appt:** Prof S, Univ Chicago-Pritzker Sch Med

Tuttle, Todd M MD [S] - **Spec Exp:** Breast Cancer; Minimally Invasive Surgery; Cancer Surgery; **Hospital:** Univ Minn Med Ctr, Fairview - Riverside Campus; **Address:** Univ Minn, Dept Surgery, 420 Delaware St SE, MMC 195, Minneapolis, MN 55455; **Phone:** 612-625-2991; **Board Cert:** Surgery 2004; **Med School:** Johns Hopkins Univ 1988; **Resid:** Surgery, Med Coll Virginia Hosps 1994; **Fellow:** Surgical Oncology, MD Anderson Cancer Ctr 1996; **Fac Appt:** Assoc Prof S

Tzakis, Andreas G MD [S] - **Spec Exp:** Transplant-Liver; Transplant-Bowel; **Hospital:** Cleveland Clin (page 55); **Address:** Cleveland Clinic-Transplant Center, 9500 Euclid Ave, Bldg A, Fl 10, Cleveland, OH 44195; **Phone:** 216-444-5914; **Board Cert:** Surgery 2003; **Med School:** Greece 1974; **Resid:** Surgery, Mt Sinai Hosp 1979; Surgery, SUNY Stony Brook 1983; **Fellow:** Transplant Surgery, Univ Pittsburgh 1985; **Fac Appt:** Prof S, Univ Miami Sch Med

Vickers, Selwyn M MD [S] - **Spec Exp:** Pancreatic Cancer; Liver Cancer; Gastrointestinal Surgery; **Hospital:** Univ Minn Med Ctr, Fairview - Riverside Campus; **Address:** University of Minnesota, 420 Delaware St SE, Phillips Wangensteen Bldg, MMC 195, Minneapolis, MN 55455; **Phone:** 612-626-1999; **Board Cert:** Surgery 2003; **Med School:** Johns Hopkins Univ 1986; **Resid:** Surgery, Johns Hopkins Hosp 1992; **Fellow:** NIH-Dept Aging 1987; **Fac Appt:** Prof S, Johns Hopkins Univ

Wakefield, Thomas MD [S] - **Spec Exp:** Thrombotic Disorders; Bleeding/Coagulation Disorders; Pulmonary Embolism; **Hospital:** Univ of Michigan Hosp, VA Ann Arbor Healthcare Sys; **Address:** Univ Mich, Dept Surg, Div Vasc Surg, 1500 E Med Ctr Drive, CVC5463 SPC5867, Ann Arbor, MI 48109; **Phone:** 734-936-5820; **Board Cert:** Surgery 2002; Vascular Surgery 2005; Surgical Critical Care 2000; **Med School:** Med Coll OH 1978; **Resid:** Surgery, Univ Mich Med Ctr 1984; **Fellow:** Peripheral Vascular Surgery, Univ Mich Med Ctr 1986; **Fac Appt:** Prof S, Univ Mich Med Sch

Walker, Alonzo P MD [S] - **Spec Exp:** Breast Cancer; **Hospital:** Froedtert and Med Ctr of WI; **Address:** Cinical Cancer Ctr-Surgery Dept, 9200 W Wisconsin Ave, Milwaukee, WI 53226-3522; **Phone:** 414-805-5737; **Board Cert:** Surgery 2004; **Med School:** Univ Fla Coll Med 1976; **Resid:** Surgery, Univ Maryland Hosps 1983; **Fac Appt:** Prof S, Med Coll Wisc

Walsh, R Matthew MD [S] - **Spec Exp:** Pancreatic Cancer; Gastrointestinal Surgery; Hepatobiliary Surgery; **Hospital:** Cleveland Clin (page 55); **Address:** Cleveland Clin, Dept Surgery, 9500 Euclid Ave, Desk A100, Cleveland, OH 44195; **Phone:** 216-445-7576; **Board Cert:** Surgery 2009; **Med School:** Med Coll Wisc 1985; **Resid:** Surgery, Loyola Univ Hosp 1990; **Fellow:** Endoscopy, Mass General Hosp 1991; Hepatopancreatobiliary Surgery, Cleveland Clinic 1991; **Fac Appt:** Assoc Prof S, Cleveland Cl Coll Med/Case West Res

Weber, Sharon M MD [S] - **Spec Exp:** Liver Cancer; Pancreatic & Biliary Surgery; Colon & Rectal Cancer; Sarcoma; **Hospital:** Univ WI Hosp & Clins, Wm S Middleton Mem Vet Hosp-Madison; **Address:** 600 Highland Ave, Madison, WI 53792; **Phone:** 608-265-0500; **Board Cert:** Surgery 2009; **Med School:** Med Coll Wisc 1993; **Resid:** Surgery, Univ Wisc Med Ctr 1999; **Fellow:** Tumor Immunology, Univ Wisc Med Ctr 1997; Hepatobiliary Surgery, Meml Sloan Kettering Cancer Ctr 2001; **Fac Appt:** Assoc Prof S, Univ Wisc

Weigel, Ronald J MD/PhD [S] - **Spec Exp:** Breast Cancer; Endocrine Surgery; **Hospital:** Univ Iowa Hosp & Clinics; **Address:** University of IA, Carver College of Med, 200 Hawkins Drive, JCP Bldg, rm 1509, Iowa City, IA 52242; **Phone:** 319-353-7474; **Board Cert:** Surgery 2001; **Med School:** Yale Univ 1986; **Resid:** Surgery, Duke Univ Med Ctr 1992; **Fellow:** Immunology, Duke Univ Med Ctr; **Fac Appt:** Prof S, Univ Iowa Coll Med

Weigelt, John A MD [S] - **Spec Exp:** Trauma; Critical Care; **Hospital:** Froedtert and Med Ctr of WI; **Address:** Froedtert Hospital, Dept Surgery, 9200 W Wisconsin Ave, rm 295B, Milwaukee, WI 53226; **Phone:** 414-805-8636; **Board Cert:** Surgery 2010; Surgical Critical Care 2006; **Med School:** Med Coll Wisc 1974; **Resid:** Surgery, UT SW Hosps 1979; **Fac Appt:** Prof S, Med Coll Wisc

Winchester, David J MD [S] - **Spec Exp:** Breast Cancer; **Hospital:** Evanston/North Shore Univ Hlth Sys; **Address:** Evanston Hospital, Dept Surgery, 2650 Ridge Ave, Walgreen-Ste 2507, Evanston, IL 60201; **Phone:** 847-570-1700; **Board Cert:** Surgery 2001; **Med School:** Northwestern Univ 1986; **Resid:** Surgery, Northwestern Meml Hosp 1992; **Fellow:** Surgical Oncology, MD Anderson Cancer Ctr 1994; **Fac Appt:** Clin Prof S, Northwestern Univ

Witt, Thomas R MD [S] - **Spec Exp:** Breast Cancer; Breast Disease; **Hospital:** Rush Univ Med Ctr; **Address:** Surgical Oncology Group, 1725 W Harrison St, Ste 409, Chicago, IL 60612-3828; **Phone:** 312-942-2302; **Board Cert:** Surgery 2010; **Med School:** Northwestern Univ 1975; **Resid:** Surgery, Rush Presby-St Lukes Med Ctr 1980; **Fellow:** Surgical Oncology, Meml Sloan Kettering Cancer Ctr 1982; **Fac Appt:** Assoc Prof S, Rush Med Coll

Great Plains and Mountains

Edney, James A MD [S] - **Spec Exp:** Breast Cancer; Thyroid & Parathyroid Cancer & Surgery; Cancer Surgery; Melanoma; **Hospital:** Nebraska Med Ctr; **Address:** Univ Nebraska Med Ctr, Dept Surgery, 984030 Nebraska Medical Ctr, Omaha, NE 68198-4030; **Phone:** 402-559-7272; **Board Cert:** Surgery 2010; **Med School:** Univ Nebr Coll Med 1975; **Resid:** Surgery, Univ Nebraska Med Ctr 1980; **Fellow:** Surgical Oncology, Univ Colorado Med Ctr 1981; **Fac Appt:** Prof S, Univ Nebr Coll Med

Finlayson, Christina A MD [S] - **Spec Exp:** Breast Cancer; Breast Disease; **Hospital:** Univ of CO Hosp - Anschutz Inpatient Pav; **Address:** 12631 E 17th Ave, Box C313, Auora, CO 80045; **Phone:** 303-724-2728; **Board Cert:** Surgery 2004; **Med School:** Univ Utah 1989; **Resid:** Surgery, Univ CO Hlth Sci Ctr 1994; **Fellow:** Surgical Oncology, Fox Chase Cancer Ctr 1996; **Fac Appt:** Prof S, Univ Colorado

Fitzgibbons Jr, Robert J MD [S] - **Spec Exp:** Abdominal Wall Reconstruction; Minimally Invasive Surgery; Gastrointestinal Surgery; Hernia; **Hospital:** Alegent Creighton Univ Med Ctr, Bergan Mercy Med Ctr-Alegant Hlth; **Address:** Creighton Univ, Dept Surgery, 601 N 30th St, Ste 3700, Omaha, NE 68131-2100; **Phone:** 402-280-4503; **Board Cert:** Surgery 2011; **Med School:** Creighton Univ 1974; **Resid:** Surgery, Charity Hosp/LA State Univ 1979; **Fellow:** Surgical Oncology, Lahey Clinic 1980; **Fac Appt:** Prof S, Creighton Univ

Loggie, Brian W MD [S] - **Spec Exp:** Mesothelioma; Solid Tumors; Melanoma; Pseudomyxoma Peritonei; **Hospital:** Alegent Creighton Univ Med Ctr; **Address:** 601 N 30th St, Ste 2803, Omaha, NE 68131; **Phone:** 402-280-5200; **Board Cert:** Surgery 2010; **Med School:** McGill Univ 1979; **Resid:** Surgery, Montreal Genl Hosp 1986; **Fellow:** Surgical Oncology, Univ Illinois 1988; **Fac Appt:** Prof S, Creighton Univ

McIntyre Jr, Robert C MD [S] - **Spec Exp:** Endocrine Surgery; Trauma; Critical Care; **Hospital:** Univ of CO Hosp - Anschutz Inpatient Pav, Chldn's Hosp - Aurora (CO); **Address:** Univ Colorado at Denver & Hlth Sci Ctr, 12631 E 17th Ave, MS C313, Aurora, CO 80045; **Phone:** 303-724-2724; **Board Cert:** Surgery 2002; Surgical Critical Care 2003; **Med School:** Tulane Univ 1987; **Resid:** Surgery, Univ Colorado 1992; **Fac Appt:** Prof S, Univ Colorado

Mistry, Bhargav M MD [S] - **Spec Exp:** Transplant-Kidney; Transplant-Liver; Transplant-Pancreas; Trauma/Critical Care; **Hospital:** Sanford Med Ctr Fargo; **Address:** MeritCare Broadway Hlth Ctr, Transplantation Surgery, 736 Broadway N, Fargo, ND 58122; **Phone:** 701-234-3400; **Board Cert:** Surgery 2009; Surgical Critical Care 2009; **Med School:** India 1984; **Resid:** Surgery, St Louis Univ Med Ctr 2000; **Fellow:** Surgical Critical Care, St Louis Univ 1995; Transplant Surgery, St Louis Univ 1998; **Fac Appt:** Assoc Clin Prof S, Univ ND Sch Med

Moore Jr, Ernest E MD [S] - **Spec Exp:** Liver Trauma; Aortic Injuries; Thoracic Aortic Surgery; Pelvic Surgery; **Hospital:** Denver Health Med Ctr, Yampa Valley Med Ctr; **Address:** Denver Hlth Med Ctr, 655 Broadway St, Ste 365, Denver, CO 80204-4597; **Phone:** 303-436-6558; **Board Cert:** Surgery 2006; Surgical Critical Care 2006; **Med School:** Univ Pittsburgh 1972; **Resid:** Surgery, Univ VT Med Ctr 1976; **Fac Appt:** Prof S, Univ Colorado

Mulvihill, Sean J MD [S] - **Spec Exp:** Gastrointestinal Surgery; Liver & Biliary Cancer; Pancreatic Cancer; **Hospital:** Univ Utah Hlth Care; **Address:** Univ Utah, Dept Surgery, 30 N 1900 E, rm 3B110, Salt Lake City, UT 84132; **Phone:** 801-581-7304; **Board Cert:** Surgery 2008; **Med School:** USC Sch Med 1981; **Resid:** Surgery, UCLA Med Ctr 1987; **Fac Appt:** Prof S, Univ Utah

Nelson, Edward W MD [S] - **Spec Exp:** Breast Cancer; **Hospital:** Univ Utah Hlth Care; **Address:** Univ Utah Med Ctr, Div Genl Surgery, 30 N 1900 E, rm 3B322, Salt Lake City, UT 84132; **Phone:** 801-581-7738; **Board Cert:** Surgery 2008; **Med School:** Univ Utah 1974; **Resid:** Surgery, Univ Utah Med Ctr 1979; **Fac Appt:** Prof S, Univ Utah

Petelin, Joseph B MD [S] - **Spec Exp:** Laparoscopic Abdominal Surgery; **Hospital:** Shawnee Mission Med Ctr; **Address:** 9119 W 74th St, Ste 255, Shawnee Mission, KS 66204; **Phone:** 913-432-5420; **Board Cert:** Surgery 2010; **Med School:** Univ Kansas 1976; **Resid:** Surgery, Univ Kansas 1981; **Fac Appt:** Assoc Clin Prof S, Univ Kansas

Saffle, Jeffrey R MD [S] - **Spec Exp:** Burn Care; Wound Healing/Care; **Hospital:** Univ Utah Hlth Care; **Address:** Dept Surgery, 50 N 1900 E, rm 3B306, Salt Lake City, UT 84132; **Phone:** 801-581-3595; **Board Cert:** Surgery 2002; Surgical Critical Care 2007; **Med School:** Univ Chicago-Pritzker Sch Med 1976; **Resid:** Surgery, Univ Utah Med Ctr 1982; **Fellow:** Burn Surgery, Univ Utah Med Ctr 1980; **Fac Appt:** Prof S, Univ Utah

Sasson, Aaron R MD [S] - **Spec Exp:** Gastrointestinal Cancer; Pancreatic Cancer; Liver Cancer; Neuroendocrine Tumors; **Hospital:** Nebraska Med Ctr; **Address:** 984030 Univ Nebraska Med Ctr, Omaha, NE 68198-4030; **Phone:** 402-559-8941; **Board Cert:** Surgery 2010; **Med School:** UMDNJ-NJ Med Sch, Newark 1993; **Resid:** Surgery, UCSD Med Ctr 1999; **Fellow:** Surgical Oncology, Fox Chase Cancer Ctr 2001; **Fac Appt:** Assoc Prof S, Univ Nebr Coll Med

Sauter, Edward R MD/PhD [S] - **Spec Exp:** Breast Cancer; Breast Cancer Risk Assessment; Clinical Trials; **Hospital:** Fargo VA Med Ctr, Sanford Med Ctr Fargo; **Address:** Univ North Dakota Dept Surgery, 501 N Columbia Rd, MS 9037, Grand Forks, ND 58202; **Phone:** 701-777-4862; **Board Cert:** Surgery 2010; **Med School:** Louisiana State U, New Orleans 1986; **Resid:** Surgery, Ochsner Fdn Hosp 1991; **Fellow:** Surgical Oncology, Fox Chase Cancer Ctr 1993; **Fac Appt:** Prof S, Univ ND Sch Med

Schulick, Richard D MD [S] - **Spec Exp:** Liver Cancer; Biliary Cancer; Pancreatic Cancer; Adrenal Tumors; **Hospital:** Univ of CO Hosp - Anschutz Inpatient Pav; **Address:** Univ Colorado Hosp, 12361 E 17th Ave, MS C305, Aurora, CO 80045; **Phone:** 720-848-3532; **Board Cert:** Surgery 2007; **Med School:** Johns Hopkins Univ 1989; **Resid:** Surgery, Johns Hopkins Hosp 1994; **Fellow:** Clinical Pharmacology, NIH 1995; Thyroid Oncology, Meml Sloan-Kettering Cancer Ctr 1996; **Fac Appt:** Prof Surg & Onc, Univ Colorado

Traynor, Michael D MD [S] - **Spec Exp:** Endocrine Surgery; Thyroid & Parathyroid Surgery; Vascular Surgery; **Hospital:** Sanford Med Ctr Fargo; **Address:** MeritCare Broadway Health Ctr, 737 Broadway, Fargo, ND 58122; **Phone:** 701-234-2251; **Board Cert:** Surgery 2009; **Med School:** Univ ND Sch Med 1986; **Resid:** Surgery, Mayo Clinic 1991; **Fac Appt:** Clin Prof S, Univ ND Sch Med

Southwest

Ames, Frederick C MD [S] - **Spec Exp:** Breast Cancer; **Hospital:** UT MD Anderson Cancer Ctr; **Address:** MD Anderson Cancer Ctr, Dept Surgery, 1400 Pressler St Unit 1484, Houston, TX 77030-4009; **Phone:** 713-792-6929; **Board Cert:** Surgery 1975; **Med School:** Univ Tex Med Br, Galveston 1969; **Resid:** Surgery, Univ Texas Med Branch Hosp 1971; Surgery, St Joseph Hosp 1974; **Fellow:** Surgical Oncology, MD Anderson Cancer Ctr 1975; **Fac Appt:** Prof S, Univ Tex, Houston

Babiera, Gildy V MD [S] - **Spec Exp:** Breast Cancer; **Hospital:** UT MD Anderson Cancer Ctr; **Address:** MD Anderson Cancer Ctr, Dept Surgical Oncology, Unit 444, 1515 Holcombe Blvd, Houston, TX 77030-1402; **Phone:** 713-792-2121; **Board Cert:** Surgery 2007; **Med School:** NY Med Coll 1991; **Resid:** Surgery, NYU Med Ctr 1995; Surgery, NYU Med Ctr 1997; **Fellow:** Surgical Oncology, MD Anderson Cancer Ctr 1996; **Fac Appt:** Assoc Prof Surg & Onc, Univ Tex, Houston

Beitsch, Peter D MD [S] - **Spec Exp:** Breast Cancer; **Hospital:** Med City Dallas Hosp; **Address:** 7777 Forrest Ln, C Bldg, Ste 760, Dallas, TX 75230; **Phone:** 972-566-8039; **Board Cert:** Surgery 2002; **Med School:** Univ Tex SW, Dallas 1986; **Resid:** Surgery, Univ TX SW Med Ctr 1993; **Fellow:** Surgical Oncology, MD Anderson Cancer Ctr 1990; Surgical Oncology, John Wayne Cancer Inst 1994

Bellows, Charles F MD [S] - **Spec Exp:** Gastrointestinal Surgery; Minimally Invasive Surgery; Hernia-Complex; Abdominal Wall Reconstruction; **Hospital:** Tulane Med Ctr; **Address:** Tulane Univ Dept Surgery, 1430 Tulane Ave, New Orleans, LA 70112; **Phone:** 504-988-2307; **Board Cert:** Surgery 2002; **Med School:** Med Coll PA 1995; **Resid:** Surgery, Tulane Univ Hosp 2001; **Fellow:** Surgical Research, Tulane 1998; **Fac Appt:** Assoc Prof S, Tulane Univ

Bentley, Frederick R MD [S] - **Spec Exp:** Transplant-Kidney; Colon Cancer; **Hospital:** UAMS Med Ctr; **Address:** 4301 W Markham St, Slot 520, Little Rock, AR 72205; **Phone:** 501-526-7053; **Board Cert:** Surgery 2006; **Med School:** Louisiana State U, New Orleans 1977; **Resid:** Surgery, LSU Med Ctr 1983; **Fellow:** Research, Univ Minnesota Affil Hosp 1982; Transplant Surgery, Univ Minnesota Affil Hosp 1984; **Fac Appt:** Assoc Prof S, Univ Louisville Sch Med

Blackstone, Robin S MD [S] - **Spec Exp:** Obesity/Bariatric Surgery; Laparoscopic Surgery; **Hospital:** Scottsdale Hlthcare - Shea; **Address:** Scottsdale Healthcare Bariatric Ctr, 10200 N 92nd St, Ste 101, Scottsdale, AZ 85258; **Phone:** 480-391-3885; **Board Cert:** Surgery 2005; **Med School:** Univ Tex, San Antonio 1988; **Resid:** Surgery, Univ Colorado Med Ctr 1993

Bolton, John S MD [S] - **Spec Exp:** Cancer Surgery; Esophageal Cancer; Pancreatic Cancer; Liver Cancer; **Hospital:** Ochsner Med Ctr-New Orleans; **Address:** Ochsner Clin, Dept Surg, 1514 Jefferson Hwy Fl 8, New Orleans, LA 70121; **Phone:** 504-842-4072; **Board Cert:** Surgery 2002; **Med School:** Louisiana State U, New Orleans 1976; **Resid:** Surgery, Charity Hosp 1981; **Fellow:** Hepatopancreatobiliary Surgery, Lahey Clinic 1980; Surgical Oncology, Meml Sloan Kettering Cancer Ctr 1982; **Fac Appt:** Asst Clin Prof S, Louisiana State U, New Orleans

Curley, Steven A MD [S] - **Spec Exp:** Colon & Rectal Cancer; Liver Cancer; Hepatobiliary Surgery; **Hospital:** UT MD Anderson Cancer Ctr; **Address:** MD Anderson Cancer Ctr, Dept Surg Oncology, 1515 Holcome Blvd, Unit 1484, Houston, TX 77230-1402; **Phone:** 713-792-2022; **Board Cert:** Surgery 2008; **Med School:** Univ Tex, Houston 1982; **Resid:** Surgery, Univ New Mexico Hosps 1988; **Fellow:** Surgical Oncology, MD Anderson Cancer Ctr 1990; **Fac Appt:** Prof S, Univ Tex, Houston

Demarest III, Gerald B MD [S] - **Spec Exp:** Trauma; Burn Care; **Hospital:** Univ Hosp - New Mexico; **Address:** Univ New Mexico Surgical Clin, 2211 Lomas Blvd NE, Albuquerque, NM 87106; **Phone:** 505-272-2336; **Board Cert:** Surgery 2008; Surgical Critical Care 2005; **Med School:** Columbia P&S 1973; **Resid:** Surgery, Univ Washington Med Ctr 1978; **Fellow:** Burn Surgery, Harborview Med Ctr 1979; Harborview Med Ctr 1980; **Fac Appt:** Assoc Prof S, Univ New Mexico

Dooley, William C MD [S] - **Spec Exp:** Breast Cancer; Tumors-Rare & Multiple; Sarcoma; Melanoma; **Hospital:** OU Med Ctr, St. Anthony Hosp -Oklahoma City; **Address:** 825 NE 10th St, Ste 4500, Oklahoma City, OK 73104; **Phone:** 405-271-7867; **Board Cert:** Surgery 2010; **Med School:** Vanderbilt Univ 1982; **Resid:** Surgery, Johns Hopkins Hosp 1987; Surgical Oncology, Oxford Univ 1986; **Fellow:** Surgical Oncology, Johns Hopkins 1988; **Fac Appt:** Prof S, Univ Okla Coll Med

Surgery

Ellis, Lee M MD [S] - **Spec Exp:** Colon & Rectal Cancer; Metastatic Cancer; Peritoneal Carcinomatosis; **Hospital:** UT MD Anderson Cancer Ctr; **Address:** MD Anderson Cancer Ctr, Dept Surgery & Cancer Biology, 1515 Holcombe Blvd, Box 173, Houston, TX 77030; **Phone:** 713-792-6926; **Board Cert:** Surgery 2009; **Med School:** Univ VA Sch Med 1983; **Resid:** Surgery, Univ Fla-Shands Hosp 1990; **Fellow:** Surgical Oncology, MD Anderson Cancer Ctr 1992; **Fac Appt:** Prof S, Univ Tex, Houston

Euhus, David M MD [S] - **Spec Exp:** Breast Cancer; **Hospital:** UT Southwestern Med Ctr at Dallas; **Address:** 2201 Inwood Rd Fl 3, Dallas, TX 75390-9155; **Phone:** 214-645-4673; **Board Cert:** Surgery 2010; **Med School:** St Louis Univ 1984; **Resid:** Surgery, UCLA Med Ctr 1991; **Fellow:** Surgical Oncology, UCLA Med Ctr 1988; Breast Disease, Queens Med Ctr 1990; **Fac Appt:** Prof S, Univ Tex SW, Dallas

Feig, Barry W MD [S] - **Spec Exp:** Gastrointestinal Cancer; Sarcoma; Breast Cancer; **Hospital:** UT MD Anderson Cancer Ctr; **Address:** UT MD Anderson Cancer Ctr, Dept Surg Onc, 1400 Pressler St, Unit 1484, Houston, TX 77030; **Phone:** 713-792-2022; **Board Cert:** Surgery 2008; **Med School:** SUNY Upstate Med Univ 1984; **Resid:** Surgery, Northwestern Meml Hosp 1990; **Fellow:** Trauma, Univ Minn Affil Hosp 1991; Surgical Oncology, UT MD Anderson Cancer Ctr 1994; **Fac Appt:** Prof S, Univ Tex, Houston

Fisher, William E MD [S] - **Spec Exp:** Pancreatic Cancer; **Hospital:** St. Luke's Episcopal Hosp-Houston; **Address:** 6620 Main St, Ste 1475, Houston, TX 77030; **Phone:** 713-798-8070; **Board Cert:** Surgery 2006; **Med School:** Univ Cincinnati 1990; **Resid:** Surgery, Ohio State Univ Hosps 1996; **Fellow:** Cancer Research, Ohio State Univ Hosps 1998; **Fac Appt:** Prof S, Baylor Coll Med

Franklin, Morris E MD [S] - **Spec Exp:** Laparoscopic Surgery; Colon & Rectal Surgery; **Hospital:** Baptist Hlth Sys, Baptist Med Ctr - San Antonio; **Address:** 4242 E Southcross Blvd, Ste 1, San Antonio, TX 78222; **Phone:** 210-333-7510; **Board Cert:** Surgery 1973; **Med School:** Univ Tex SW, Dallas 1967; **Resid:** Surgery, Univ Hlth Syst 1972; **Fac Appt:** Clin Prof S, Univ Tex, San Antonio

Friese, Randall S MD [S] - **Spec Exp:** Trauma; Critical Care; **Hospital:** Univ Arizona Med Ctr-Univ Campus; **Address:** University Med Ctr - Trauma, 1501 N Campbell Ave, rm 5411, PO Box 245063, Tucson, AZ 85724; **Phone:** 520-694-6144; **Board Cert:** Surgery 2005; Surgical Critical Care 2002; **Med School:** Univ MD Sch Med 1990; **Resid:** Surgery, Univ Colorado Affil Hosp 1997; **Fellow:** Trauma/Critical Care, Univ Texas SW Med Ctr 2002; **Fac Appt:** Assoc Prof S, Univ Ariz Coll Med

Grant, Michael D MD [S] - **Spec Exp:** Breast Cancer; Breast Surgery; **Hospital:** Baylor Univ Medical Ctr-Dallas; **Address:** 3900 Junius St, Ste 220, Baylor Med Pavillion, Dallas, TX 75246; **Phone:** 214-826-7300; **Board Cert:** Surgery 2001; **Med School:** Univ Tex, Houston 1987; **Resid:** Surgery, Baylor Univ Med Ctr 1992; **Fellow:** Breast Cancer, Baylor Univ Med Ctr 1993

Gray, Richard J MD [S] - **Spec Exp:** Cancer Surgery; Breast Cancer; Melanoma; **Hospital:** Mayo Clinic - Phoenix, Mayo Clinic - Scottsdale; **Address:** Mayo Clinic-Surgical Oncology, 5777 E Mayo Blvd, Phoenix, AZ 85054; **Phone:** 480-342-2849; **Board Cert:** Surgery 2001; **Med School:** Mich State Univ 1995; **Resid:** Surgery, Mayo Clinic 2000; **Fellow:** Surgical Oncology, H Lee Moffitt Cancer Ctr 2002; **Fac Appt:** Assoc Prof S, Mayo Med Sch

Griswold, John A MD [S] - **Spec Exp:** Burn Care; **Hospital:** Univ Med Ctr-Lubbock; **Address:** Dept Surgery, 3601 4th St, MS 9905, Lubbock, TX 79430; **Phone:** 806-743-2373; **Board Cert:** Surgery 2009; Surgical Critical Care 2000; **Med School:** Creighton Univ 1981; **Resid:** Surgery, Texas Tech Univ Hlth Scis Ctr 1986; **Fellow:** Burn Surgery, Univ Washington 1988

Halff, Glenn A MD [S] - **Spec Exp:** Transplant-Liver; Liver Surgery; **Hospital:** Univ Hlth Syst-San Antonio, Christus Santa Rosa Children's Hosp; **Address:** Univ Transplant Center, 7703 Floyd Curl Drive, MC 785, San Antonio, TX 78229; **Phone:** 210-567-5771; **Board Cert:** Surgery 2007; Surgical Critical Care 2000; **Med School:** Univ Tex, Houston 1983; **Resid:** Surgery, NYU Med Ctr 1987; **Fellow:** Transplant Surgery, Univ Pittsburgh 1989; **Fac Appt:** Assoc Prof S, Univ Tex, San Antonio

Holcomb, John B MD [S] - **Spec Exp:** Trauma; **Hospital:** Meml Hermann Hosp - Texas Med Ctr; **Address:** Univ Texas Dept Surgery, 6431 Fannin St, MSB 4.170, Houston, TX 77030; **Phone:** 713-500-5493; **Board Cert:** Surgery 2002; Surgical Critical Care 2004; **Med School:** Univ Ark 1985; **Resid:** Surgery, Wm Beaumont AMC 1991; **Fellow:** Surgical Critical Care, Univ Texas 2002; **Fac Appt:** Prof S, Univ Tex, Houston

Hollingsworth, Alan B MD [S] - **Spec Exp:** Breast Cancer; **Hospital:** Mercy Hlth Ctr - Oklahoma City; **Address:** 4300 McAuley Blvd, Oklahoma City, OK 73120; **Phone:** 405-936-5455; **Board Cert:** Surgery 2009; **Med School:** Univ Okla Coll Med 1975; **Resid:** Surgery, Univ Oklahoma Hlth Sci Ctr 1980; **Fellow:** Anatomic Pathology, UCLA Med Ctr 1978; **Fac Appt:** Prof S, Univ Okla Coll Med

Hunt, John L MD [S] - **Spec Exp:** Trauma; Burn Care; **Hospital:** UT Southwestern Med Ctr at Dallas; **Address:** Dept Surgery, 5323 Harry Hines Blvd, MC 9158, Dallas, TX 75390-9158; **Phone:** 214-648-2152; **Board Cert:** Surgery 1972; Surgical Critical Care 1996; **Med School:** Univ Cincinnati 1964; **Resid:** Surgery, Cincinnati Genl Hosp 1971; **Fac Appt:** Prof S, Univ Tex SW, Dallas

Hunt, Kelly K MD [S] - **Spec Exp:** Breast Cancer; Sarcoma-Soft Tissue; Gene Therapy; **Hospital:** UT MD Anderson Cancer Ctr; **Address:** MD Anderson Cancer Ctr, 1400 Pressler St, Unit 1484, Houston, TX 77030-4000; **Phone:** 713-792-7216; **Board Cert:** Surgery 2001; **Med School:** Univ Tenn Coll Med 1986; **Resid:** Surgery, UCLA Med Ctr 1993; **Fellow:** Surgical Oncology, MD Anderson Cancer Ctr 1996; **Fac Appt:** Prof S, Univ Tex, Houston

Huth, James F MD [S] - **Spec Exp:** Melanoma; Skin Cancer; Vaccine Therapy; Sarcoma-Soft Tissue; **Hospital:** UT Southwestern Med Ctr at Dallas; **Address:** UTSW Med Ctr, Dept Surgery, 5323 Harry Hines Blvd, Box 9155, Dallas, TX 75390-9155; **Phone:** 214-645-4673; **Board Cert:** Surgery 2010; **Med School:** Univ Rochester 1975; **Resid:** Surgery, Univ Wash Med Ctr 1980; **Fellow:** Surgical Oncology, UCLA Med Ctr 1981; **Fac Appt:** Prof S, Univ Tex SW, Dallas

Jackson, Gilchrist MD [S] - **Spec Exp:** Thyroid & Parathyroid Surgery; Head & Neck Cancer & Surgery; Laparoscopic Surgery; Gastrointestinal Cancer; **Hospital:** St. Luke's Episcopal Hosp-Houston, Woman's Hosp TX; **Address:** 2727 W Holcombe Blvd Fl 3-A, Houston, TX 77025; **Phone:** 713-442-1132; **Board Cert:** Surgery 2008; **Med School:** Univ Louisville Sch Med 1974; **Resid:** Surgery, Parkland Hosp 1979; **Fellow:** Surgical Oncology, MD Anderson Hosp 1980; **Fac Appt:** Assoc Clin Prof S, Baylor Coll Med

Jayaseelan, Nirmal S MD [S] - **Spec Exp:** Obesity/Bariatric Surgery; **Hospital:** Med City Dallas Hosp; **Address:** 11970 N Central Expressway, Ste 670, Dallas, TX 75243; **Phone:** 972-331-1111; **Board Cert:** Surgery 2002; **Med School:** Texas Tech Univ 1994; **Resid:** Surgery, Emanuel Hosp 1999

Kim, Lawrence Thomas MD [S] - **Spec Exp:** Endocrine Surgery; Thyroid Cancer; Parathyroid Parathyroid Surgery; **Hospital:** UAMS Med Ctr; **Address:** 4301 W Markham, Slot 725, Little Rock, AR 72205; **Phone:** 501-686-8211; **Board Cert:** Surgery 2005; **Med School:** Univ Tex SW, Dallas 1987; **Resid:** Surgery, South Western Med Ctr 1994; **Fellow:** Research, South Western Med Ctr 1991; Research, Natl Inst Health 1996; **Fac Appt:** Prof S, Univ Ark

Klimberg, Vicki S MD [S] - **Spec Exp:** Breast Cancer; Radiofrequency Tumor Ablation; Sentinel Node Surgery; **Hospital:** UAMS Med Ctr; **Address:** Univ Arkansas Medical Sciences, 4301 W Markham, MS 725, Little Rock, AR 72205-7199; **Phone:** 501-686-5669; **Board Cert:** Surgery 1999; **Med School:** Univ Fla Coll Med 1984; **Resid:** Surgery, Univ Fla Med Ctr 1989; **Fellow:** Clinical Oncology, Univ Fla 1990; Breast Disease, Univ Arkansas for Med Scis 1991; **Fac Appt:** Prof S, Univ Ark

Krouse, Robert S MD [S] - **Spec Exp:** Cancer Surgery; Gastrointestinal Cancer; Palliative Care; **Hospital:** Southern AZ VA Health Care Sys - Tucson; **Address:** Southern AZ VA Health Care System, Surg Care Line, 2-112, 3601 S 6th Ave, Tucson, AZ 85723-0001; **Phone:** 520-792-1450 x6145; **Board Cert:** Surgery 2007; **Med School:** Hahnemann Univ 1991; **Resid:** Surgery, Univ Hawaii Integrated Surg Prog 1993; Immunotherapy, Natl Cancer Inst 1994; **Fellow:** Surgery, W Virginia Univ Sch Med 1997; Surgical Oncology, City of Hope Natl Med Ctr 2000; **Fac Appt:** Prof S, Univ Ariz Coll Med

Kuhn, Joseph A MD [S] - **Spec Exp:** Liver Cancer; Peritoneal Carcinomatosis; Melanoma; Thyroid Cancer; **Hospital:** Baylor Univ Medical Ctr-Dallas; **Address:** 7777 Forest Ln, Ste C-400, Dallas, TX 75230; **Phone:** 214-823-5000; **Board Cert:** Surgery 2009; Surgical Critical Care 2003; **Med School:** Univ Tex Med Br, Galveston 1984; **Resid:** Surgery, Baylor Univ Med Ctr 1989; **Fellow:** Surgical Oncology, City Hosp Natl Med Ctr 1992

Lee, Jeffrey E MD [S] - **Spec Exp:** Melanoma; Pancreatic Cancer; Endocrine Tumors; Adrenal Cancer; **Hospital:** UT MD Anderson Cancer Ctr; **Address:** UT MD Anderson Cancer Ctr, 1400 Pressler St, FCT Bldg - rm 17.6000, Unit 1484, Houston, TX 77030-4009; **Phone:** 713-792-7218; **Board Cert:** Surgery 2010; **Med School:** Stanford Univ 1984; **Resid:** Surgery, Stanford Univ Hosp 1987; Surgery, Stanford Univ Hosp 1991; **Fellow:** Immunology, Stanford Univ 1989; Surgical Oncology, UT-MD Anderson Cancer Ctr 1993; **Fac Appt:** Prof S, Univ Tex, Houston

Leitch, A Marilyn MD [S] - **Spec Exp:** Breast Cancer & Surgery; Melanoma; Sarcoma; **Hospital:** UT Southwestern Med Ctr at Dallas; **Address:** UT Southwestern Med Ctr - Dept Surgery, 5323 Harry Hines Blvd, Dallas, TX 75390-9155; **Phone:** 214-648-3039; **Board Cert:** Surgery 2003; **Med School:** Univ Tex SW, Dallas 1978; **Resid:** Surgery, UCLA Med Ctr 1984; **Fellow:** Surgical Oncology, MD Anderson Cancer Ctr 1985; **Fac Appt:** Prof S, Univ Tex SW, Dallas

Lentz, Christopher W MD [S] - **Spec Exp:** Burn Care; Trauma; Critical Care; Wound Healing/Care; **Hospital:** Univ Hosp - New Mexico; **Address:** Univ New Mexico Surgical Clin, 2211 Lomas Blvd NE, Albuquerque, NM 87131-0001; **Phone:** 505-272-2336; **Board Cert:** Surgery 2005; Surgical Critical Care 2006; **Med School:** Wayne State Univ 1988; **Resid:** Surgery, Med Coll Wisc 1994; **Fellow:** Surgical Critical Care, Shriners Burns Inst 1991; Burn Surgery, Univ N Carolina Med Ctr 1996; **Fac Appt:** Assoc Prof S, Univ Rochester

Li, Benjamin D L MD [S] - **Spec Exp:** Gastrointestinal Cancer; Sarcoma; Breast Cancer; **Hospital:** Willis-Knighton Med Ctr; **Address:** LSU Hlth Scis Ctr, Dept Surgery, 1501 Kings Hwy, rm 3203, Shreveport, LA 71103; **Phone:** 318-675-6100; **Board Cert:** Surgery 2002; **Med School:** Yale Univ 1986; **Resid:** Surgery, Northwestern Univ-McGraw Med Ctr 1992; **Fellow:** Surgical Oncology, Roswell Park Cancer Inst 1995; **Fac Appt:** Prof S, Louisiana State U, New Orleans

Livingston, Edward H MD [S] - **Spec Exp:** Gastrointestinal Surgery; Endocrine Surgery; Obesity/Bariatric Surgery; Hernia-Complex; **Hospital:** UT Southwestern Med Ctr at Dallas; **Address:** 1801 Inwood Rd Fl 7 - Ste 100, Dallas, TX 75390-9156; **Phone:** 214-648-7956; **Board Cert:** Surgery 2003; **Med School:** UCLA 1985; **Resid:** Surgery, UCLA Med Ctr 1992; **Fac Appt:** Prof S, Univ Tex SW, Dallas

Mansfield, Paul F MD [S] - **Spec Exp:** Appendix Cancer; Stomach Cancer; Colon Cancer; Melanoma; **Hospital:** UT MD Anderson Cancer Ctr; **Address:** UT MD Anderson Cancer Ctr, 1515 Holcombe Blvd, Unit 1485, Houston, TX 77030; **Phone:** 713-794-5499; **Board Cert:** Surgery 2006; **Med School:** Jefferson Med Coll 1983; **Resid:** Surgery, Pennsylvania Hosp 1988; **Fellow:** Surgical Oncology, MD Anderson Cancer Ctr 1991; **Fac Appt:** Prof Surg & Onc, Univ Tex, Houston

McCabe, Daniel P MD [S] - **Spec Exp:** Cancer Surgery; Melanoma; Gastrointestinal Cancer; **Hospital:** Tucson Med Ctr; **Address:** Southwestern Surgical Assocs, 1951 N Wilmot Rd Bldg 2, Tucson, AZ 85712; **Phone:** 520-795-5845; **Board Cert:** Surgery 2002; **Med School:** Creighton Univ 1979; **Resid:** Surgery, St Joseph Hosp 1982; Surgery, Baystate Med Ctr 1984; **Fellow:** Surgical Oncology, James Cancer Ctr/Ohio State 1986; **Fac Appt:** Asst Clin Prof S, Univ Ariz Coll Med

Meric-Bernstam, Funda MD [S] - **Spec Exp:** Breast Cancer & Surgery; Clinical Trials; **Hospital:** UT MD Anderson Cancer Ctr; **Address:** UT MD Anderson Cancer Center, 1400 Pressler St, Unit 1484, Houston, TX 77030; **Phone:** 713-745-4453; **Board Cert:** Surgery 2007; **Med School:** Yale Univ 1991; **Resid:** Surgery, Univ Mich Med Ctr 1998; **Fellow:** Surgical Oncology, UT MD Anderson Cancer Ctr 2001; **Fac Appt:** Prof Surg & Onc, Univ Tex, Houston

Pisters, Peter MD [S] - **Spec Exp:** Pancreatic Cancer; Sarcoma-Soft Tissue; Gastrointestinal Cancer; **Hospital:** UT MD Anderson Cancer Ctr; **Address:** MD Anderson Cancer Ctr, 1515 Holcombe Blvd, Unit 1484, Houston, TX 77230-1402; **Phone:** 713-792-2022; **Board Cert:** Surgery 2001; **Med School:** Univ Western Ontario 1985; **Resid:** Surgery, NYU/Bellevue Hosp 1992; **Fellow:** Surgical Research, Meml Sloan-Kettering Cancer Ctr 1989; Surgical Oncology, Meml Sloan-Kettering Cancer Ctr 1994; **Fac Appt:** Prof S, Univ Tex, Houston

Pockaj, Barbara A MD [S] - **Spec Exp:** Cancer Surgery; Breast Cancer; Melanoma; Stomach Cancer; **Hospital:** Mayo Clinic - Phoenix, Mayo Clinic - Scottsdale; **Address:** Mayo Clinic-Surgery, 5777 E Mayo Blvd, Phoenix, AZ 85054; **Phone:** 480-342-2849; **Board Cert:** Surgery 2005; **Med School:** Vanderbilt Univ 1987; **Resid:** Surgery, Univ Hosps 1995; **Fellow:** Surgical Oncology, Natl Inst Hlth 1992; Immunotherapy, Natl Cancer Inst-Natl Inst Hlth 1993; **Fac Appt:** Assoc Prof S, Mayo Med Sch

Pollock, Raphael E MD/PhD [S] - **Spec Exp:** Sarcoma; **Hospital:** UT MD Anderson Cancer Ctr; **Address:** UT MD Anderson Cancer Ctr, Dept Surg Oncology, 1400 Pressler, Unit 1447, Houston, TX 77030; **Phone:** 713-792-6928; **Board Cert:** Surgery 2003; **Med School:** St Louis Univ 1977; **Resid:** Surgery, Univ Chicago Hosps 1979; Surgery, Rush Presby-St Lukes Hosp 1982; **Fellow:** Surgical Oncology, MD Anderson Cancer Ctr 1984; **Fac Appt:** Prof S, Univ Tex, Houston

Postier, Russell G MD [S] - **Spec Exp:** Cancer Surgery; Pancreatic Cancer; Biliary Surgery; Gastrointestinal Surgery; **Hospital:** OU Med Ctr; **Address:** OU Physicians, Dept Surgery, 825 NE 10th St, Ste 4500, Oklahoma City, OK 73104; **Phone:** 405-271-1400; **Board Cert:** Surgery 2000; **Med School:** Univ Okla Coll Med 1975; **Resid:** Surgery, Johns Hopkins Hosp 1981; **Fac Appt:** Prof S, Univ Okla Coll Med

Rege, Robert V MD [S] - **Spec Exp:** Gastrointestinal Surgery; Laparoscopic Surgery; Hernia; **Hospital:** UT Southwestern Med Ctr at Dallas; **Address:** GI Endocrine Surgery, Dept Surgery, 1801 Inwood Rd Fl 7 - Ste 100, Dallas, TX 75390; **Phone:** 214-645-2900; **Board Cert:** Surgery 2000; **Med School:** Penn State Coll Med 1975; **Resid:** Surgery, Milton S. Hershey Med Ctr 1976; Surgery, Milton S. Hershey Med Ctr 1982; **Fellow:** Research, Gastrointestinal Research Fel 1983; **Fac Appt:** Prof S, Univ Tex SW, Dallas

Surgery

Rhee, Peter M MD [S] - **Spec Exp:** Trauma; Critical Care; **Hospital:** Univ Arizona Med Ctr-Univ Campus; **Address:** 1501 N Campbell Ave, Box 245063, Tucson, AZ 85274; **Phone:** 520-626-5056; **Board Cert:** Surgery 2002; Surgical Critical Care 2006; **Med School:** Uniformed Srvs Univ, Bethesda 1987; **Resid:** Surgery, UC Irvine Med Ctr 1992; **Fellow:** Trauma, Harborview Med Ctr 1995; **Fac Appt:** Prof S, Univ Ariz Coll Med

Ross, Merrick I MD [S] - **Spec Exp:** Sentinel Node Surgery; Breast Cancer; Melanoma; **Hospital:** UT MD Anderson Cancer Ctr; **Address:** 1515 Holcombe Blvd, Ste 1484, Houston, TX 77030; **Phone:** 713-792-2022; **Board Cert:** Surgery 2007; **Med School:** Univ IL Coll Med 1980; **Resid:** Surgery, Univ IL Hosp & Clin 1982; Surgery, Univ IL Hosp & Clin 1987; **Fellow:** Research, Scripps Clin & Rsch 1984; Surgical Oncology, UT-MD Anderson Cancer Ctr 1989; **Fac Appt:** Prof S, Univ Tex, Houston

Schlinkert, Richard T MD [S] - **Spec Exp:** Endocrine Surgery; Laparoscopic Surgery; Gastrointestinal Surgery; Adrenal Surgery; **Hospital:** Mayo Clinic - Phoenix; **Address:** Mayo Clin, Dept Surgery, 5779 E Mayo Blvd, Phoenix, AZ 85054; **Phone:** 480-342-1051; **Board Cert:** Surgery 2006; **Med School:** Med Coll OH 1981; **Resid:** Surgery, Mayo Clinic 1986; **Fellow:** Hepatobiliary Surgery, Royal Infirmary 1987; **Fac Appt:** Prof S, Mayo Med Sch

Skibber, John M MD [S] - **Spec Exp:** Rectal Cancer/Sphincter Preservation; Colon & Rectal Cancer-Familial Polyposis; **Hospital:** UT MD Anderson Cancer Ctr; **Address:** UT MD Anderson Cancer Ctr, Dept Surgical Oncology, Unit 1484, PO Box 301402, Houston, TX 77230-1402; **Phone:** 713-792-5165; **Board Cert:** Surgery 2009; **Med School:** Jefferson Med Coll 1981; **Resid:** Surgery, NYU Med Ctr 1989; **Fellow:** Surgical Oncology, UT MD Anderson Cancer Ctr 1991; **Fac Appt:** Prof S, Univ Tex, Houston

Staren, Edgar D MD/PhD [S] - **Spec Exp:** Breast Cancer; Endocrine Cancers; Liver Cancer; **Hospital:** CTCA at Western Regl Med Ctr; **Address:** Cancer Treatment Ctrs America, 14200 W Fillmore St, MS 85338, Goodyear, AZ 85338; **Phone:** 623-207-3000; **Board Cert:** Surgery 2006; **Med School:** Loyola Univ-Stritch Sch Med 1982; **Resid:** Surgery, Rush-Presby-St Lukes Med Ctr 1987; **Fellow:** Surgical Oncology, Rush-Presby-St Lukes Med Ctr 1988

Stewart, Ronald M MD [S] - **Spec Exp:** Trauma; **Hospital:** Univ Hlth Syst-San Antonio; **Address:** Univ Tex Hlth Sci Ctr, Dept Surg-Trauma, 7703 Floyd Curl Drive, MC 7740, San Antonio, TX 78229-3900; **Phone:** 210-567-3623; **Board Cert:** Surgery 2009; Surgical Critical Care 2002; **Med School:** Univ Tex, San Antonio 1985; **Resid:** Surgery, Univ Tex Hlth Sci Ctr 1991; **Fellow:** Trauma, Univ Tenn Coll Med 1993; **Fac Appt:** Assoc Prof S, Univ Tex, San Antonio

Stolier, Alan J MD [S] - **Spec Exp:** Breast Cancer; **Hospital:** St. Charles Surgical Hosp; **Address:** St Charles Surgical Hosp, 1717 St Charles Ave, New Orleans, LA 70130; **Phone:** 504-529-6600; **Board Cert:** Surgery 2006; **Med School:** Louisiana State U, New Orleans 1970; **Resid:** Surgery, Charity Hosp 1974; **Fellow:** Surgical Oncology, MD Anderson Hosp 1976; **Fac Appt:** Clin Prof S, Tulane Univ

Vauthey, Jean-Nicholas MD [S] - **Spec Exp:** Hepatobiliary Surgery; Liver Cancer; Gallbladder & Biliary Cancer; **Hospital:** UT MD Anderson Cancer Ctr; **Address:** UT MD Anderson Cancer Ctr -Surg Oncology, 1515 Holcombe Blvd, Unit 1484, Houston, TX 77030; **Phone:** 713-792-2022; **Board Cert:** Surgery 2008; **Med School:** Switzerland 1979; **Resid:** Surgery, Ochsner Med Fdn 1989; **Fellow:** Hepatobiliary Surgery, Med Fac Univ Bern 1991; Surgical Oncology, Meml Sloan-Kettering Cancer Ctr 1993; **Fac Appt:** Prof S, Univ Tex, Houston

Woltering, Eugene MD [S] - **Spec Exp:** Neuroendocrine Tumors; **Hospital:** Ochsner Med Ctr-New Orleans; **Address:** Ochsner Med Ctr, 200 W Esplanade, Ste 200, Kenner, LA 70065; **Phone:** 504-464-8500; **Board Cert:** Surgery 2002; **Med School:** Ohio State Univ 1975; **Resid:** Surgery, Vanderbilt Med Ctr 1982; Surgical Oncology, Natl Inst Hlth 1979; **Fellow:** Surgical Oncology, Ohio State Univ 1984; **Fac Appt:** Prof S, Louisiana State U, New Orleans

Wood, R Patrick MD [S] - **Spec Exp:** Liver Cancer; Transplant-Liver; Biliary Surgery; Laparoscopic Surgery; **Hospital:** St. Luke's Episcopal Hosp-Houston; **Address:** Transplantation/Genl Surgery Assocs, 6624 Fannin St, Ste 1200, Houston, TX 77030; **Phone:** 713-795-8994; **Board Cert:** Surgery 2004; **Med School:** Univ Rochester 1979; **Resid:** Surgery, NYU/Bellevue Hosp Ctr 1984; **Fellow:** Transplant Surgery, Univ Pittsburgh 1985; **Fac Appt:** Clin Prof S, Univ Tex, Houston

Zannis, Victor J MD [S] - **Spec Exp:** Breast Cancer; Breast Surgery; **Hospital:** Phoenix Baptist Hosp & Med Ctr, J C Lincoln Hosp - North Mountain; **Address:** Breast Care Ctr, 2525 W Greenway Rd, Ste 130, Phoenix, AZ 85023; **Phone:** 602-942-8000; **Board Cert:** Surgery 2010; **Med School:** UCLA 1976; **Resid:** Surgery, Maricopa Med Ctr 1982

West Coast and Pacific

Anderson, Benjamin O MD [S] - **Spec Exp:** Breast Cancer & Surgery; **Hospital:** Univ Wash Med Ctr; **Address:** Univ Washington Dept Surgery, 1959 NE Pacific St, Box 356410, Seattle, WA 98195-6410; **Phone:** 206-288-6806; **Board Cert:** Surgery 2002; **Med School:** Albert Einstein Coll Med 1985; **Resid:** Surgery, Univ Colorado Affil Hosp 1992; **Fellow:** Surgical Oncology, Meml Sloan Kettering Cancer Ctr 1994; **Fac Appt:** Prof S, Univ Wash

Ascher, Nancy L MD/PhD [S] - **Spec Exp:** Transplant-Liver; Transplant-Kidney; **Hospital:** UCSF Med Ctr; **Address:** 513 Parnassus Ave, Box 0104, San Francisco, CA 94143-0104; **Phone:** 415-476-1236; **Board Cert:** Surgery 2002; **Med School:** Univ Mich Med Sch 1974; **Resid:** Surgery, Univ Minn Hosp 1981; **Fellow:** Transplant Surgery, Univ Minn Hosp 1982; **Fac Appt:** Prof S, UCSF

Bilchik, Anton J MD/PhD [S] - **Spec Exp:** Gastrointestinal Cancer; Laparoscopic Surgery; **Hospital:** St. John's Hlth Ctr, Santa Monica, Cedars-Sinai Med Ctr; **Address:** 2200 Santa Monica Blvd, Ste 113, Santa Monica, CA 90404; **Phone:** 310-696-0716; **Board Cert:** Surgery 2004; **Med School:** South Africa 1985; **Resid:** Surgery, UCLA Med Ctr 1996; **Fellow:** John Wayne Cancer Inst. 1998; **Fac Appt:** Asst Clin Prof S, UCLA

Billingsley, Kevin MD [S] - **Spec Exp:** Cancer Surgery; Liver Tumors; Hepatobiliary Surgery; Pancreatic Surgery; **Hospital:** OR Hlth & Sci Univ; **Address:** Surgical Oncology Div, 3181 SW Sam Jackson Park Rd, MC L619, Portland, OR 97239; **Phone:** 503-494-5501; **Board Cert:** Surgery 2007; **Med School:** Johns Hopkins Univ 1989; **Resid:** Surgery, Oregon Hlth Science Univ 1996; **Fellow:** Surgical Oncology, Natl Cancer Inst 1994; Surgical Oncology, Meml Sloan Kettering Cancer Ctr 1998; **Fac Appt:** Assoc Prof S, Oregon Hlth & Sci Univ

Bouvet, Michael MD [S] - **Spec Exp:** Endocrine Surgery; Pancreatic Cancer; Biliary Cancer; **Hospital:** UCSD Med Ctr; **Address:** UCSD Moores Cancer Ctr, 3855 Health Science Drive, La Jolla, CA 92093-0987; **Phone:** 858-822-6191; **Board Cert:** Surgery 2004; **Med School:** Univ Wash 1989; **Resid:** Surgery, UCSD Med Ctr 1995; **Fellow:** Surgical Oncology, MD Anderson Cancer Ctr 1998; **Fac Appt:** Assoc Prof S, UCSD

Surgery

Brunicardi, F Charles MD [S] - **Spec Exp:** Pancreatic Islet Cell Transplant; Pancreatic Cancer; Gastroesophageal Reflux Disease (GERD); **Hospital:** Santa Monica - UCLA Med Ctr & Ortho Hosp; **Address:** 1304 15 St, Ste 213, Santa Monica, CA 90404; **Phone:** 310-394-7069; **Board Cert:** Surgery 2009; **Med School:** UMDNJ-Rutgers Med Sch 1980; **Resid:** Surgery, SUNY Brooklyn Hlth Sci Ctr 1989; **Fellow:** Pancreatic Physiology, SUNY Brooklyn Hlth Sci Ctr 1986; **Fac Appt:** Prof S, UCLA-David Geffen Sch Med

Busuttil, Ronald W MD/PhD [S] - **Spec Exp:** Transplant-Liver; Liver Cancer; **Hospital:** UCLA Ronald Reagan Med Ctr; **Address:** 200 UCLA Medical Plaza, Ste 214, Los Angeles, CA 90095-7430; **Phone:** 310-825-5318; **Board Cert:** Surgery 2007; **Med School:** Tulane Univ 1971; **Resid:** Surgery, UCLA Med Ctr 1976; **Fellow:** Surgery, UCLA Med Ctr 1975; **Fac Appt:** Prof S, UCLA

Butler, John A MD [S] - **Spec Exp:** Breast Cancer; Thyroid Cancer; Adrenal Tumors; Small Bowel Cancer; **Hospital:** UC Irvine Med Ctr; **Address:** UC-Irvine Medical Ctr-Zot 5376, 101 City Drive S, Rte 81 Bldg 56 - Ste 256, Orange, CA 92868-3298; **Phone:** 714-456-8030; **Board Cert:** Surgery 2003; **Med School:** Loyola Univ-Stritch Sch Med 1976; **Resid:** Surgery, LAC-USC Med Ctr 1982; Surgery, Harbor-UCLA Med Ctr 1982; **Fellow:** Surgical Oncology, Meml Sloan-Kettering Cancer Ctr 1984; **Fac Appt:** Prof S, UC Irvine

Byrd, David MD [S] - **Spec Exp:** Cancer Surgery; Thyroid Cancer; Melanoma; Breast Cancer & Surgery; **Hospital:** Univ Wash Med Ctr; **Address:** Univ Washington Med Ctr, Dept Surgical Specialites Center, 1959 NE Pacific St, Box 356165, Seattle, WA 98195; **Phone:** 206-598-4477; **Board Cert:** Surgery 2008; **Med School:** Tulane Univ 1982; **Resid:** Surgery, Univ Wash Med Ctr 1987; **Fellow:** Surgical Oncology, Univ Tex-MD Anderson Cancer Ctr 1992; **Fac Appt:** Assoc Prof S, Univ Wash

Chang, Helena MD [S] - **Spec Exp:** Breast Cancer; Cancer Surgery; **Hospital:** UCLA Ronald Reagan Med Ctr; **Address:** 200 UCLA Medical Plaza Drive, Ste B265-1, Revlon Breast Clinic, Los Angeles, CA 90024; **Phone:** 310-825-2144; **Board Cert:** Surgery 1997; **Med School:** Temple Univ 1981; **Resid:** Surgery, Episcopal Hosp 1986; **Fellow:** Cellular Molecular Biology, Temple Univ 1977; Surgical Oncology, Meml Sloan-Kettering Cancer Ctr 1988; **Fac Appt:** Prof S, UCLA

Clark, Orlo H MD [S] - **Spec Exp:** Thyroid Cancer & Surgery; Neuroendocrine Tumors; Parathyroid Cancer; **Hospital:** UCSF - Mt Zion Med Ctr, UCSF Med Ctr; **Address:** UCSF Mt Zion Med Ctr, 1600 Divisadero St, Fl 3, Box 1926, San Francisco, CA 94115-1926; **Phone:** 415-353-7687; **Board Cert:** Surgery 1974; **Med School:** Cornell Univ-Weill Med Coll 1967; **Resid:** Surgery, UCSF Med Ctr 1970; Surgery, UCSF Med Ctr 1973; **Fellow:** Surgery, Royal Med Sch London 1971; **Fac Appt:** Prof S, UCSF

Colquhoun, Steven D MD [S] - **Spec Exp:** Liver Cancer; Transplant-Liver; Pancreatic Cancer; Hepatobiliary Surgery; **Hospital:** Cedars-Sinai Med Ctr; **Address:** Cedars-Sinai Med Center, 8635 W 3rd St, Ste 590-W, Los Angeles, CA 90048; **Phone:** 310-423-2641; **Board Cert:** Surgery 2003; Surgical Critical Care 2008; **Med School:** Loyola Univ-Stritch Sch Med 1984; **Resid:** Surgery, UCLA Med Ctr 1990; **Fellow:** Surgical Oncology, UCLA Med Ctr 1993; Transplant Surgery, UCLA Med Ctr 1994; **Fac Appt:** Assoc Clin Prof S, UCLA

Crookes, Peter F MD [S] - **Spec Exp:** Obesity/Bariatric Surgery; Laparoscopic Surgery; Gastroesophageal Reflux Disease (GERD); Esophageal Surgery; **Hospital:** Keck Med Ctr of USC (page 62); **Address:** USC Healthcare Consultation Ctr, Ste 514, 1510 San Pablo St, Los Angeles, CA 90033-4612; **Phone:** 323-442-6236; **Med School:** Ireland 1978; **Resid:** Surgery, Royal Victoria Hosp 1989; Surgery, St Vincent's Hosp 1990; **Fellow:** Research, Creighton Univ 1992; Research, Univ SC 1994; **Fac Appt:** Assoc Prof S, Univ SC Sch Med

Dixon, Sherwood M MD [S] - **Spec Exp:** Wound Healing/Care; **Hospital:** Northern Nevada Med Ctr; **Address:** 1500 E 2nd St, Ste 206, Reno, NV 89502; **Phone:** 775-789-7000; **Board Cert:** Surgery 2009; **Med School:** Univ Alabama 1976; **Resid:** Surgery, UC Davis Med Ctr 1981; **Fellow:** Vascular Surgery, UCLA Ctr Hlth Scis 1982

Duh, Quan-Yang MD [S] - **Spec Exp:** Endocrine Surgery; Thyroid & Parathyroid Cancer & Surgery; Adrenal Tumors; Minimally Invasive Surgery; **Hospital:** UCSF Med Ctr, VA Med Ctr - San Francisco; **Address:** UCSF Medical Ctr, 1600 Divisadero St Fl 3, San Francisco, CA 94115; **Phone:** 415-353-7687; **Board Cert:** Surgery 2007; **Med School:** UCSF 1981; **Resid:** Surgery, UCSF Med Ctr 1988; **Fellow:** Endocrine Surgery, UCSF Med Ctr 1987; **Fac Appt:** Prof S, UCSF

Easter, David W MD [S] - **Spec Exp:** Breast Cancer; Gastrointestinal Cancer; **Hospital:** VA San Diego Hlthcre Sys; **Address:** VA San Diego Healthcare Sys, 3350 La Jolla Village Drive, San Diego, CA 92161; **Phone:** 858-552-8585; **Board Cert:** Surgery 2010; **Med School:** Yale Univ 1983; **Resid:** Surgery, UCSD Med Ctr 1989; **Fellow:** Surgical Oncology, Ninewells, Dundee 1990; **Fac Appt:** Clin Prof S, UCSD

Eilber, Frederick R MD [S] - **Spec Exp:** Sarcoma; **Hospital:** UCLA Ronald Reagan Med Ctr; **Address:** 200 UCLA Medical Plaza, Ste 120, Los Angeles, CA 90095; **Phone:** 310-825-7086; **Board Cert:** Surgery 1973; **Med School:** Univ Mich Med Sch 1965; **Resid:** Surgery, Univ Maryland Hosp 1972; **Fellow:** Surgery, Univ Tex-MD Anderson Hosp 1973; **Fac Appt:** Prof S, UCLA

Ellenhorn, Joshua D MD [S] - **Spec Exp:** Gastrointestinal Cancer; Breast Cancer; Cancer Surgery; **Hospital:** Cedars-Sinai Med Ctr, St. John's Hlth Ctr, Santa Monica; **Address:** 8635 W THIRD St, Ste 1090W, Los Angeles, CA 90048; **Phone:** 310-659-9011; **Board Cert:** Surgery 2010; **Med School:** Boston Univ 1984; **Resid:** Surgery, Univ Cincinnati Hosp 1991; **Fellow:** Surgical Oncology, Meml Sloan-Kettering Cancer Ctr 1993; **Fac Appt:** Prof S

Esquivel, Carlos O MD [S] - **Spec Exp:** Transplant-Liver-Adult & Pediatric; **Hospital:** Stanford Univ Hosp & Clinics, Lucile Packard Chldn's Hosp; **Address:** 750 Welch Rd, Ste 319, Palo Alto, CA 94304; **Phone:** 650-498-5689; **Board Cert:** Surgery 2003; **Med School:** Costa Rica 1975; **Resid:** Surgery, UC- Davis Med Ctr 1984; **Fellow:** Transplant Surgery, Univ Pittsburgh 1985; **Fac Appt:** Prof S, Stanford Univ

Esserman, Laura J MD [S] - **Spec Exp:** Breast Cancer; **Hospital:** UCSF - Mt Zion Med Ctr, UCSF Med Ctr; **Address:** UCSF-Helen Diller Family Comp Cancer Ctr, 1600 Divisadero St Fl 2, San Francisco, CA 94115; **Phone:** 415-353-7070; **Board Cert:** Surgery 2001; **Med School:** Stanford Univ 1983; **Resid:** Surgery, Stanford Univ Med Ctr 1991; **Fellow:** Oncology, Stanford Univ Med Ctr 1988; **Fac Appt:** Assoc Prof S, UCSF

Essner, Richard MD [S] - **Spec Exp:** Sentinel Node Surgery; Melanoma; Gastrointestinal Surgery; **Hospital:** St. John's Hlth Ctr, Santa Monica; **Address:** 2336 Santa Monica Blvd, Ste 206, Santa Monica, CA 90404-2302; **Phone:** 310-295-2522; **Board Cert:** Surgery 2002; **Med School:** Emory Univ 1985; **Resid:** Surgery, Univ NC Hosps 1992; **Fac Appt:** Asst Clin Prof S, USC Sch Med

Fisher, Jonathan S MD [S] - **Spec Exp:** Transplant-Kidney; Transplant-Liver; Transplant-Pancreas; Pancreatic Islet Cell Transplant; **Hospital:** Scripps Green Hosp; **Address:** Scripps Clinic Torrey Pines, 10666 N Torrey Pines Rd, MC 200N, La Jolla, CA 92037; **Phone:** 858-554-4310; **Board Cert:** Surgery 2002; **Med School:** Columbia P&S 1994; **Resid:** Surgery, Univ Chicago Hosps 2001; **Fellow:** Transplant Surgery, Univ Tennessee 2003

Giuliano, Armando E MD [S] - **Spec Exp:** Breast Cancer; Sentinel Node Surgery; Thyroid Cancer; **Hospital:** Cedars-Sinai Med Ctr; **Address:** Saul & Joyce Brandman Breast Ctr, 310 N San Vincente Blvd Fl 3, Los Angeles, CA 90048; **Phone:** 310-423-9331 x0; **Board Cert:** Surgery 2009; **Med School:** Univ Chicago-Pritzker Sch Med 1973; **Resid:** Surgery, UCSF Med Ctr 1980; **Fellow:** Surgical Oncology, UCLA Med Ctr 1978; **Fac Appt:** Prof S, UCLA

Goodson III, William H MD [S] - **Spec Exp:** Breast Cancer; **Hospital:** CA Pacific Med Ctr-Pacific Campus, UCSF - Mt Zion Med Ctr; **Address:** 2100 Webster St, Ste 401, San Francisco, CA 94115-2378; **Phone:** 415-923-3925; **Board Cert:** Surgery 2006; **Med School:** Harvard Med Sch 1971; **Resid:** Surgery, Univ Hosps 1976; Surgery, Childrens Hosp 1977

Gosnell, Jessica E MD [S] - **Spec Exp:** Thyroid Cancer & Surgery; Parathyroid Surgery; **Hospital:** UCSF - Mt Zion Med Ctr; **Address:** 1600 Divisardero St Fl 3, San Francisco, CA 94115; **Phone:** 415-353-7687; **Board Cert:** Surgery 2004; **Med School:** UCSF 1995; **Resid:** Surgery, UCSF Med Ctr 2002; **Fellow:** Research, San Francisco Genl Hosp 2000; Endocrine Surgery, Univ Sydney 2003; **Fac Appt:** Asst Prof S, UCSF

Gower, Roland E MD [S] - **Spec Exp:** Breast Surgery; Biliary Surgery; Thyroid Surgery; **Hospital:** Providence Alaska Med Ctr, Alaska Regl Hosp; **Address:** 2841 De Barr Rd, Ste 41, Anchorage, AK 99508-2973; **Phone:** 907-279-3564; **Board Cert:** Surgery 2008; **Med School:** Vanderbilt Univ 1971; **Resid:** Surgery, Kansas Med Ctr 1975

Greenhalgh, David G MD [S] - **Spec Exp:** Burn Care; Nutrition; Wound Healing/Care; **Hospital:** Northern CA Shriners Hosp, UC Davis Med Ctr; **Address:** Shriners Hosp Chldn, 2425 Stockton Blvd, Sacramento, CA 95817; **Phone:** 916-453-2050; **Board Cert:** Surgery 2005; Surgical Critical Care 2008; **Med School:** SUNY Upstate Med Univ 1981; **Resid:** Surgery, MC Hosp of VT 1986; **Fellow:** Burn Surgery, Univ Wash Hosp 1989; **Fac Appt:** Prof S, UC Davis

Hemming, Alan W MD [S] - **Spec Exp:** Liver Cancer; Transplant-Liver; Hepatobiliary Surgery; Pancreatic Cancer; **Hospital:** UCSD Med Ctr, Rady Children's Hosp - San Diego; **Address:** UC San Diego Center for Hepatobiliary Disease and Transplantation, 200 W Arbor Drive, MS 8401, San Diego, CA 92103-8401; **Phone:** 619-543-5870; **Board Cert:** Surgery 2004; **Med School:** Univ British Columbia Fac Med 1987; **Resid:** Surgery, Univ British Columbia Med Ctr 1994; **Fellow:** Transplant Surgery, Univ of Toronto Hosp 1995; Hepatobiliary Surgery, Univ of Toronto Hosp 1996; **Fac Appt:** Prof S, UCSD

Horvath, Karen MD [S] - **Spec Exp:** Colon & Rectal Surgery; Gastrointestinal Surgery; Minimally Invasive Surgery; Pancreatic Surgery; **Hospital:** Univ Wash Med Ctr; **Address:** 1959 NE Pacific St, Box 356165, Seattle, WA 98195; **Phone:** 206-598-4477; **Board Cert:** Surgery 2007; **Med School:** NY Med Coll 1990; **Resid:** Surgery, NY Presby Hosp/Columbia 1997; **Fellow:** Surgical Critical Care, Mt Sinai Hosp 1994; Laparoscopic Surgery, Oregon Hlth Sci Ctr 1998; **Fac Appt:** Assoc Prof S, Univ Wash

Hunter, John G MD [S] - **Spec Exp:** Gastrointestinal Surgery; Laparoscopic Abdominal Surgery; Gastroesophageal Reflux Disease (GERD); Esophageal Surgery; **Hospital:** OR Hlth & Sci Univ; **Address:** Digestive Hlth Ctr, 3303 SW Bond Ave Fl 6, MC CH6D, Portland, OR 97239; **Phone:** 503-494-4373; **Board Cert:** Surgery 2006; **Med School:** Univ Pennsylvania 1981; **Resid:** Surgery, Univ Utah Med Ctr 1987; **Fellow:** Gastrointestinal Surgery, Mass Genl Hosp 1988; Endoscopy, Univ West Ontario 1989; **Fac Appt:** Assoc Prof S, Oregon Hlth & Sci Univ

Karlan, Scott R MD [S] - **Spec Exp:** Breast Cancer & Surgery; **Hospital:** Cedars-Sinai Med Ctr; **Address:** 310 N San Vicente Blvd Fl 3, Los Angeles, CA 90048; **Phone:** 310-423-9331; **Board Cert:** Surgery 2005; **Med School:** Harvard Med Sch 1982; **Resid:** Surgery, Yale-New Haven Hosp 1987; **Fac Appt:** Clin Prof S, UCLA

Kaufman, Cary S MD [S] - **Spec Exp:** Breast Cancer & Surgery; Breast Disease; **Hospital:** St. Joseph Hosp - Bellingham; **Address:** 2940 Squalicum Pkwy, Ste 101, Bellingham, WA 98225; **Phone:** 360-671-9877; **Board Cert:** Surgery 2011; **Med School:** UCLA 1973; **Resid:** Surgery, Univ Wash Med Ctr 1975; Surgery, Harbor-UCLA Med Ctr 1979; **Fac Appt:** Assoc Clin Prof S, Univ Wash

Kirgan, Daniel MD [S] - **Spec Exp:** Cancer Surgery; Breast Cancer & Surgery; **Hospital:** Univ Med Ctr - Las Vegas; **Address:** 1707 W Charleston Blvd, Ste 160, Las Vegas, NV 89102; **Phone:** 702-671-5150; **Board Cert:** Surgery 2004; **Med School:** Geo Wash Univ 1986; **Resid:** Surgery, Univ Med Ctr 1992; **Fellow:** Surgical Oncology, John Wayne Cancer Inst 1994; **Fac Appt:** Assoc Prof S, Univ Nevada

Klein, Andrew S MD [S] - **Spec Exp:** Transplant-Liver; Liver Cancer; Liver Failure; **Hospital:** Cedars-Sinai Med Ctr; **Address:** Liver & Transplant Ctr at Cedars-Sinai, 8635 W Third St, Ste 590W, Los Angeles, CA 90048; **Phone:** 310-423-2641; **Board Cert:** Surgery 2007; **Med School:** Johns Hopkins Univ 1979; **Resid:** Surgery, Johns Hopkins Hosp 1982; Surgery, Johns Hopkins Hosp 1986; **Fellow:** Transplant Surgery, UCLA-CHS 1988; **Fac Appt:** Clin Prof S, UCLA

Knudson, Mary Margaret MD [S] - **Spec Exp:** Breast Cancer; Trauma; **Hospital:** San Francisco Genl Hosp; **Address:** 1001 Potrero Ave, Ste 3A, San Francisco, CA 94110; **Phone:** 415-206-4623; **Board Cert:** Surgery 2011; Surgical Critical Care 2008; **Med School:** Univ Mich Med Sch 1976; **Resid:** Surgery, Beth Israel Hosp 1979; Surgery, Univ Mich Med Ctr 1982; **Fellow:** Pediatric Surgery, Stanford Univ Hosps 1983; **Fac Appt:** Assoc Prof S, UCSF

Lowy, Andrew M MD [S] - **Spec Exp:** Pancreatic Cancer; Gastrointestinal Cancer; Peritoneal Carcinomatosis; Clinical Trials; **Hospital:** UCSD Med Ctr; **Address:** 3855 Health Sciences Drive, Fl 2, La Jolla, CA 92093-0987; **Phone:** 858-822-2124; **Board Cert:** Surgery 2003; **Med School:** Cornell Univ-Weill Med Coll 1988; **Resid:** Surgery, NY-Cornell Med Ctr 1996; **Fellow:** Surgical Oncology, MD Anderson Cancer Ctr 1996; **Fac Appt:** Prof S, UCSD

Moossa, AR MD [S] - **Spec Exp:** Pancreatic Cancer; Gastrointestinal Cancer; Hepatobiliary Surgery; **Hospital:** UCSD Med Ctr; **Address:** 9300 Campus Point Drive, La Jolla, CA 92037; **Phone:** 858-657-6113; **Med School:** England, UK 1965; **Resid:** Surgery, Liverpool Univ Hosps 1970; **Fellow:** Surgical Oncology, Johns Hopkins Hosp 1972; **Fac Appt:** Prof S, UCSD

Morton, John M MD [S] - **Spec Exp:** Obesity/Bariatric Surgery; Minimally Invasive Surgery; **Hospital:** Stanford Univ Hosp & Clinics; **Address:** Surgical Specialties, 300 Pasteur Drive, rm H3680, Stanford, CA 94305-5655; **Phone:** 650-725-9777; **Board Cert:** Surgery 2002; **Med School:** Tulane Univ 1993; **Resid:** Surgery, Tulane Univ Hosp 1999; Surgery, Swedish Med Ctr 2001; **Fellow:** Laparoscopic Surgery, Univ N Carolina Affil Hosp 2003; **Fac Appt:** Assoc Prof S, Stanford Univ

Nakakura, Eric MD/PhD [S] - **Spec Exp:** Pancreatic Cancer; Liver Cancer; Gastrointestinal Cancer; Sarcoma; **Hospital:** UCSF Med Ctr; **Address:** 1600 Divisadero St Fl 4, Box 1705, San Francisco, CA 94115; **Phone:** 415-353-9888; **Board Cert:** Surgery 2004; **Med School:** Stanford Univ 1995; **Resid:** Surgery, Johns Hopkins Hosp 2000; **Fellow:** Surgical Oncology, Johns Hopkins Hosp 2004; **Fac Appt:** Asst Prof S, UCSF

Nguyen, Ninh T MD [S] - **Spec Exp:** Laparoscopic Surgery; Obesity/Bariatric Surgery; Gastrointestinal Cancer & Surgery; **Hospital:** UC Irvine Med Ctr; **Address:** Div Gastrointestinal Surgery, 333 City Blvd W, Ste 850, Orange, CA 92868; **Phone:** 714-456-8598; **Board Cert:** Surgery 2006; **Med School:** Univ Tex, San Antonio 1990; **Resid:** Surgery, Mt Sinai Med Ctr 1995; **Fellow:** Surgical Oncology, Univ Pittsburgh Med Ctr 1997; Laparoscopic Surgery, Univ Pittsburgh Med Ctr 1998; **Fac Appt:** Assoc Prof S, UC Irvine

Nissen, Nicholas N MD [S] - **Spec Exp:** Liver Cancer; Transplant-Liver; Pancreatic Cancer; Minimally Invasive Surgery; **Hospital:** Cedars-Sinai Med Ctr; **Address:** Cedars-Sinai Medical Center, 8635 W 3rd St, Ste 590-W, Los Angeles, CA 90048; **Phone:** 310-423-2641; **Board Cert:** Surgery 1999; Surgical Critical Care 1999; **Med School:** Univ Minn 1991; **Resid:** Surgery, Loyola Univ Med Ctr 1998; **Fellow:** Surgical Critical Care, Univ Pittsburgh Med Ctr 1999; Hepatobiliary Surgery, UCLA Med Ctr 2001

Norton, Jeffrey A MD [S] - **Spec Exp:** Pancreatic Cancer; Gastrointestinal Cancer & Surgery; Endocrine Surgery; **Hospital:** Stanford Univ Hosp & Clinics; **Address:** 875 Blake Wilbur Drive, Clin F, Stanford, CA 94305; **Phone:** 650-723-5461; **Board Cert:** Surgery 2001; **Med School:** SUNY Upstate Med Univ 1973; **Resid:** Surgery, Duke Univ Med Ctr 1982; **Fellow:** Research, Natl Cancer Inst 1989; **Fac Appt:** Prof S, Stanford Univ

Paz, Isaac Benjamin MD [S] - **Spec Exp:** Breast Cancer; Esophageal Cancer; **Hospital:** City of Hope Natl Med Ctr; **Address:** 1500 E Duarte Rd, Duarte, CA 91010; **Phone:** 626-256-4673 x67100; **Board Cert:** Surgery 2000; **Med School:** Chile 1981; **Resid:** Surgery, Univ Catolica de Chile 1985; Surgery, Univ Arizona 1990; **Fellow:** Surgical Oncology, City of Hope Med Ctr 1993

Pellegrini, Carlos MD [S] - **Spec Exp:** Esophageal Cancer; Esophageal Surgery; Barrett's Esophagus; Gastrointestinal Cancer & Surgery; **Hospital:** Univ Wash Med Ctr; **Address:** Univ Washington Medical Ctr, Dept Surgery, 1959 NE Pacific St, Box 356165, Seattle, WA 98195; **Phone:** 206-598-4547; **Board Cert:** Surgery 2010; **Med School:** Argentina 1971; **Resid:** Surgery, Granadero Hosp 1975; Surgery, Univ Chicago Hosps 1979; **Fac Appt:** Prof S, Univ Wash

Perkins, James D MD [S] - **Spec Exp:** Transplant-Pancreas; Transplant-Liver; Transplant-Kidney; **Hospital:** Univ Wash Med Ctr, Seattle Chldns Hosp; **Address:** Univ Wash Med Ctr, Dept Surg, 1959 NE Pacific St, Box 356410, Seattle, WA 98195; **Phone:** 206-543-3825; **Board Cert:** Surgery 2004; **Med School:** Univ Ark 1979; **Resid:** Surgery, St Francis Regl Med Ctr 1984; **Fellow:** Transplant Surgery, Mayo Grad Sch 1985; **Fac Appt:** Prof S, Univ Wash

Peterson, Laura D MD [S] - **Spec Exp:** Breast Cancer; Breast Surgery; **Hospital:** Kapiolani Med Ctr for Women & Chldn, Straub Clinic & Hosp; **Address:** Kapi'olani Womens Ctr, 1907 S Beretania St, Ste 501, Honolulu, HI 96826; **Phone:** 808-949-3444; **Board Cert:** Surgery 2004; **Med School:** UCSD 1998; **Resid:** Surgery, Univ Hawaii Affil Hosp 2004; **Fellow:** Minimally Invasive Surgery, Kaiser Permanente 2005; Surgical Oncology, Kaiser Permanente 2005

Phillips, Edward H MD [S] - **Spec Exp:** Laparoscopic Surgery; Obesity/Bariatric Surgery; **Hospital:** Cedars-Sinai Med Ctr; **Address:** 8635 W 3rd St, Ste 795 West, Los Angeles, CA 90048-6101; **Phone:** 310-423-8350; **Board Cert:** Surgery 2008; **Med School:** USC Sch Med 1973; **Resid:** Surgery, USC Medical Ctr 1978; Vascular Surgery, Los Angeles Co-USC Medical Ctr 1979; **Fac Appt:** Assoc Clin Prof S, USC Sch Med

Posselt, Andrew M MD/PhD [S] - **Spec Exp:** Obesity/Bariatric Surgery; Pancreatic Islet Cell Transplant; Transplant-Liver; Transplant-Pancreas; **Hospital:** UCSF Med Ctr; **Address:** UCSF Medical Ctr, Dept Surgery, 505 Parnassus Ave, M884, San Francisco, CA 94143; **Phone:** 415-353-2161; **Board Cert:** Surgery 2011; **Med School:** Univ Pennsylvania 1993; **Resid:** Internal Medicine, UCSF Med Ctr 1996; Surgery, UCSF Med Ctr 2001; **Fellow:** Transplant Surgery, UCSF Med Ctr 2002; **Fac Appt:** Asst Prof S, UCSF

Potenza, Bruce M MD [S] - **Spec Exp:** Burn Care; Critical Care; **Hospital:** UCSD Med Ctr; **Address:** UCSD Med Ctr, 200 W Arbor Drive, MC 8896, San Diego, CA 92103-8896; **Phone:** 619-543-6001; **Board Cert:** Surgery 2004; Internal Medicine 1988; Surgical Critical Care 2007; Critical Care Medicine 2006; **Med School:** Loyola Univ-Stritch Sch Med 1983; **Resid:** Internal Medicine, Good Samaritan Med Ctr 1987; Surgery, SUNY Syracuse Med Ctr 1993; **Fac Appt:** Clin Prof S, UCSD

Rassman, William R MD [S] - **Spec Exp:** Hair Restoration/Transplant; **Address:** 5757 Wilshire Blvd, Ste 607, Promenade 2, Los Angeles, CA 90036; **Phone:** 310-553-9113; **Board Cert:** Surgery 1975; **Med School:** Med Coll VA 1966; **Resid:** Surgery, New York Hos -Cornell 1969; Surgery, Dartmouth Med Ctr 1973

Reber, Howard A MD [S] - **Spec Exp:** Pancreatic Cancer; Pancreatic Surgery; Gastrointestinal Cancer; **Hospital:** UCLA Ronald Reagan Med Ctr; **Address:** UCLA General Surgery, 200 UCLA Medical Plaza, Ste 214, Los Angeles, CA 90095; **Phone:** 310-794-7788; **Board Cert:** Surgery 1971; **Med School:** Univ Pennsylvania 1964; **Resid:** Surgery, Hosp Univ Penn 1970; **Fac Appt:** Prof S, UCLA

Reyes, Jorge D MD [S] - **Spec Exp:** Transplant Surgery; Transplant Surgery-Pediatric; Transplant-Liver; Hepatobiliary Surgery; **Hospital:** Univ Wash Med Ctr, Seattle Chldns Hosp; **Address:** UWMC, Liver & Kidney Care, 1959 NE Pacific St, Box 356175, Seattle, WA 98195; **Phone:** 206-598-4973; **Board Cert:** Surgery 2011; **Med School:** Brazil 1979; **Resid:** Surgical Pathology, New Eng Deaconess Hosp 1983; Surgery, Lincoln Hosp/NY Med Coll 1988; **Fellow:** Transplant Surgery, Presby Univ Hosp 1989; **Fac Appt:** Prof S, Univ Wash

Roberts, John Paul MD [S] - **Spec Exp:** Transplant-Liver; **Hospital:** UCSF Med Ctr; **Address:** UCSF Medical Ctr, Div Transplant Surgery, 505 Parnassus Ave, rm M896, Box 0780, San Francisco, CA 94143-0780; **Phone:** 415-353-1888; **Board Cert:** Surgery 2006; **Med School:** UCSD 1980; **Resid:** Surgery, Univ Wash 1983; Surgery, Univ Wash 1987; **Fellow:** Surgery, Cornell-New York Hosp 1986; Transplant Surgery, Univ Minn Med Ctr 1988; **Fac Appt:** Prof S, UCSF

Rogers, Stanley J MD [S] - **Spec Exp:** Minimally Invasive Surgery; Gastrointestinal Surgery; Obesity/Bariatric Surgery; **Hospital:** UCSF Med Ctr, San Francisco Genl Hosp; **Address:** UCSF Med Ctr, Dept Surgery, 400 Parnassus Ave, Ste 665, Campus Box 0338, San Francisco, CA 94143; **Phone:** 415-353-2161; **Board Cert:** Surgery 2006; **Med School:** Univ Utah 1991; **Resid:** Surgery, UCSF Med Ctr 1997; **Fac Appt:** Assoc Prof S, UCSF

Satava, Richard M MD [S] - **Spec Exp:** Laparoscopic Abdominal Surgery; Gastrointestinal Surgery; **Hospital:** Univ Wash Med Ctr; **Address:** Univ Washington Med Ctr, Dept Surgery, 1959 NE Pacific St, Box 356410, Seattle, WA 98195; **Phone:** 206-598-4477; **Board Cert:** Surgery 2000; **Med School:** Hahnemann Univ 1968; **Resid:** Surgery, Mayo Clinic 1974; **Fellow:** Research, Mayo Clinic 1972

Schaffer, Randolph L MD [S] - **Spec Exp:** Transplant-Liver; Transplant-Kidney; Transplant-Pancreas; **Hospital:** Scripps Green Hosp; **Address:** Scripps Clinic Torrey Pines, 10666 N Torrey Pines Rd, MC 200N, La Jolla, CA 92037; **Phone:** 858-544-4310; **Board Cert:** Surgery 2011; **Med School:** Baylor Coll Med 1995; **Resid:** Surgery, Baylor Affil Hosp 2001; **Fellow:** Transplant Surgery, Univ Chicago 2003

Selby, Robert R MD [S] - **Spec Exp:** Liver & Biliary Surgery; Liver Cancer; **Hospital:** Keck Med Ctr of USC (page 62); **Address:** 1510 San Pablo St, Ste 514, Los Angeles, CA 90033-4612; **Phone:** 323-442-7172; **Board Cert:** Surgery 2008; Surgical Critical Care 2011; **Med School:** Univ MO-Columbia Sch Med 1979; **Resid:** Internal Medicine, Good Samaritan Hosp 1981; Surgery, Good Samaritan Hosp 1986; **Fellow:** Transplant Surgery, Presby Univ Hosp 1988; **Fac Appt:** Prof S, USC Sch Med

Sener, Stephen F MD [S] - **Spec Exp:** Breast Cancer; Lymphedema; Thyroid Cancer; Melanoma; **Hospital:** Keck Med Ctr of USC (page 62); **Address:** USC Norris Comprehensive Cancer Ctr, 1510 San Pablo, Ste 412, Los Angeles, CA 90033; **Phone:** 323-865-3535; **Board Cert:** Surgery 2001; **Med School:** Northwestern Univ 1977; **Resid:** Surgery, Northwestern Univ 1982; **Fellow:** Surgery, Meml Sloan Kettering Cancer Ctr 1984; **Fac Appt:** Prof S, USC-Keck School of Medicine

Surgery

Silverstein, Melvin J MD [S] - **Spec Exp:** Breast Cancer; **Hospital:** Hoag Meml Hosp Presby; **Address:** 1 Hoag Drive, MS 6100, Breast Care Ctr, Newport Beach, CA 92658; **Phone:** 949-764-8281; **Board Cert:** Surgery 1971; **Med School:** Albany Med Coll 1965; **Resid:** Surgery, Boston City Hosp-Tufts Univ 1970; **Fellow:** Surgical Oncology, UCLA Med Ctr 1975

Sinanan, Mika N MD [S] - **Spec Exp:** Gastrointestinal Surgery; Gastrointestinal Cancer; Liver & Biliary Cancer; Colon & Rectal Cancer; **Hospital:** Univ Wash Med Ctr; **Address:** Univ Washington, Dept Surgery, 1959 NE Pacific St, Box 356165, Seattle, WA 98195-6410; **Phone:** 206-598-4477; **Board Cert:** Surgery 2008; **Med School:** Johns Hopkins Univ 1980; **Resid:** Surgery, Univ Washington Hosp 1988; **Fellow:** Gastrointestinal Surgery, Univ Brit Columbia Med Ctr 1986; **Fac Appt:** Prof S, Univ Wash

Swanstrom, Lee L MD [S] - **Spec Exp:** Esophageal Surgery; Esophageal Disorders; Minimally Invasive Surgery; Gastrointestinal Motility Disorders; **Hospital:** Providence Portland Med Ctr; **Address:** 4805 NE Glisan St, Ste 6N60, Portland, OR 97213; **Phone:** 503-281-0561; **Board Cert:** Surgery 2009; **Med School:** Creighton Univ 1983; **Resid:** Surgery, Emanuel Hosp 1988; **Fac Appt:** Clin Prof S, Oregon Hlth & Sci Univ

Trisal, Vijay MD [S] - **Spec Exp:** Skin Cancer; **Hospital:** City of Hope Natl Med Ctr; **Address:** City of Hope Med Ctr, Dept Surgery, 1500 E Duarte Rd, Duarte, CA 91010; **Phone:** 626-256-4673 x67100; **Board Cert:** Surgery 2003; **Med School:** India 1993; **Resid:** Surgery, Providence Hosp & Med Ctrs 2002; **Fellow:** Surgical Oncology, City of Hope Natl Med Ctr 2004

Vetto, John MD [S] - **Spec Exp:** Cancer Surgery; **Hospital:** OR Hlth & Sci Univ; **Address:** 3181 SW Sam Jackson Park Rd, MC L619, Portland, OR 97239; **Phone:** 503-494-5501; **Board Cert:** Surgery 2009; **Med School:** Oregon Hlth & Sci Univ 1982; **Resid:** Surgery, Brigham & Women's Hosp 1984; Surgery, UCLA Med Ctr 1989; **Fellow:** Surgical Oncology, Natl Cancer Inst 1986; Surgical Oncology, Meml Sloan Kettering Cancer Ctr 1991; **Fac Appt:** Assoc Prof S, Oregon Hlth & Sci Univ

Wagman, Lawrence D MD [S] - **Spec Exp:** Liver Cancer; Gastrointestinal Cancer; Carcinoid Tumors; **Hospital:** St. Joseph's Hosp - Orange, City of Hope Natl Med Ctr; **Address:** 1010 W La Veta Ave, Ste 470, Orange, CA 92868; **Phone:** 714-835-8300; **Board Cert:** Surgery 2004; **Med School:** Columbia P&S 1978; **Resid:** Surgery, Med Coll Virginia Hosp 1985; **Fellow:** Surgical Oncology, Natl Inst of Hlth - Clin Ctr 1982; **Fac Appt:** Assoc Clin Prof S, UCSD

Wallace, Anne Marie MD [S] - **Spec Exp:** Breast Cancer; Breast Reconstruction; Melanoma; **Hospital:** UCSD Med Ctr; **Address:** UCSD Moores Cancer Ctr, 3855 Health Sciences Drive #0987, La Jolla, CA 92093; **Phone:** 858-822-6193; **Board Cert:** Surgery 2011; Plastic Surgery 2005; **Med School:** Creighton Univ 1987; **Resid:** Surgery, Washington Hosp Ctr 1992; Plastic Surgery, UCSD Med Ctr 1994; **Fellow:** Surgical Breast Oncology, MD Anderson Cancer Ctr 1995; **Fac Appt:** Clin Prof S, UCSD

Wapnir, Irene L MD [S] - **Spec Exp:** Breast Surgery; Breast Cancer; **Hospital:** Stanford Univ Hosp & Clinics; **Address:** Stanford Univ Medical Ctr, 900 Blake Wilbur Drive, Stanford, CA 94305; **Phone:** 650-498-6000; **Board Cert:** Surgery 2008; **Med School:** Mexico 1980; **Resid:** Surgery, Lincoln Hosp 1985; **Fellow:** Breast Disease, RW Johnson Univ Med Ctr 1986; **Fac Appt:** Assoc Prof S, Stanford Univ

Warren, Robert S MD [S] - **Spec Exp:** Gastrointestinal Cancer; Liver Cancer; Biliary Cancer; **Hospital:** UCSF Med Ctr; **Address:** UCSF Comprehensive Cancer Center, GI Surgery & Oncology Clinic, 1600 Divisadero St, San Francisco, CA 94115; **Phone:** 415-353-9888; **Med School:** Univ Minn 1980; **Resid:** Surgery, Univ Minn Hosps 1988; **Fellow:** Surgical Oncology, Meml Sloan-Kettering Cancer Ctr 1986; **Fac Appt:** Prof S, UCSF

Yeung, Raymond S W MD [S] - **Spec Exp:** Liver & Biliary Cancer; Liver Cancer; Melanoma; Breast Cancer; **Hospital:** Univ Wash Med Ctr; **Address:** Univ of Washington, Dept Surgery, 1959 NE Pacific St, Box 356165, Seattle, WA 98195; **Phone:** 206-598-4477; **Board Cert:** Surgery 2009; **Med School:** Univ Toronto 1982; **Resid:** Surgery, University of Toronto 1987; **Fellow:** Surgical Oncology, Fox Chase Cancer Ctr 1992; **Fac Appt:** Prof S, Univ Wash

Cleveland Clinic

Every life deserves world class care.

General Surgery

Cleveland Clinic's Digestive Disease Institute (DDI) is one of the largest digestive programs in the country and is ranked No. 2 in the nation by *U.S. News & World Report*. DDI was the first to fully integrate its departments of Colorectal Surgery, Gastroenterology & Hepatology, General Surgery and Nutrition. Combining these disciplines in one location facilitates unprecedented patient care, multidisciplinary education and collaborative research. In 2011, DDI physicians performed more than 16,000 surgical cases and close to 51,000 endoscopic cases. Transplant surgeons completed more than 150 digestive disease-related organ transplants, including liver, pancreas and intestinal transplantation, achieving outstanding outcomes.

Highlights of the Department of General Surgery:

- Our general surgeons performed the nation's first robotic single-port gallbladder removal surgery.
- Cleveland Clinic is one of only a few programs in the country to offer Hyperthermic (or Heated) Intraoperative Peritoneal Chemotherapy to treat cancers that have spread to the lining of the abdominal cavity.
- Our Hernia Center performs more than 2,100 hernia repairs annually at 16 locations, from the routine to the most complex cases.
- The Acute Care Surgery program has a dedicated operating room 24/7 for emergent cases.
- Our Liver Tumor Clinic cares for patients with benign and cancerous liver tumors with treatment aimed at preserving liver function and quality of life.
- Our Pancreas Clinic is one of the few centers in the nation specializing in multidisciplinary, patient-centered treatments and frontline research for complicated acute pancreatitis, chronic pancreatitis, pancreatic cancer and pancreatic-biliary disorders.

SURGICAL ONCOLOGY

Studies show that experienced surgeons provide better surgical outcomes. At Fox Chase, our surgeons are fellowship-trained, meaning they have up to four years of additional training in the highly complex techniques of cancer surgery. They have extensive experience, focused entirely on cancer care and treat nearly all types of cancers with minimally invasive techniques. In addition, our plastic and reconstructive surgeons specialize in restoring form and function with excellent results for patients needing reconstructive surgery after cancer treatment.

Breast Cancer: Through our Women's Cancer Center—the first of its kind in the Philadelphia region—we offer the most advanced diagnostic techniques, including digital mammography, stereotactic breast biopsy and sentinel lymph-node surgery. Treatment options include breast-preserving surgery with radiation therapy as well as skin-sparing mastectomy with cosmetic reconstructive surgery. In addition, Fox Chase's inflammatory breast cancer clinic offers specialized care for women with this aggressive form of breast cancer.

Gastrointestinal Cancers: Our gastrointestinal surgeons have extensive expertise with colorectal, pancreatic, stomach, liver and other bowel cancers and are the most experienced laparoscopic and robotic experts in the region. We also offer the most advanced endoscopic and minimally invasive techniques to avoid major surgery. In addition, Fox Chase offers personalized care for patients with Barrett's esophagus—a condition that increases the risk of gastrointestinal cancer—to prevent the need for surgery and the development of cancer.

Genitourinary Cancers: Our urologic surgical oncologists have extensive expertise in the treatment of prostate, bladder, kidney, ureteral, adrenal, testicular and penile cancers. Our urologists emphasize organ preservation, quality of life and minimally invasive/robotic approaches to cancer surgery.

Gynecologic Cancers: Gynecologic surgeons in our Women's Cancer Center offer the most advanced laparoscopic and robotic techniques as well as complex open surgery for women with cancers of the uterus, ovary and cervix.

Head and Neck Cancers: Fox Chase provides patients with one-stop consultations with surgical, radiation and medical oncologists. Expertise includes otolaryngology, transoral laser surgery, plastic and microvascular reconstruction as well as robotic surgery.

Lung and Esophageal Cancers: Our thoracic surgeons offer a variety of minimally invasive techniques for patients with lung and esophageal cancers, including video-assisted thoracic surgery (VATS) and laparoscopic esophageal surgery. Fox Chase was one of the first centers in the country to offer these options.

Minimally Invasive Surgery

At Fox Chase, we offer the broadest range of minimally invasive treatment options for your cancer. Minimally invasive procedures allow the surgeon to reach the tumor through tiny incisions with pinpoint accuracy. This benefits patients because it means less scarring, reduced pain, less bleeding, fewer complications, and a faster recovery.

Fox Chase was one of the first institutions worldwide to use robot-assisted surgery to treat nearly all types of cancers, including prostate, gynecologic, kidney, bladder, colon, lung, and head and neck cancers. In addition, Fox Chase's highly skilled surgeons have extensive experience performing laparoscopic surgery for cancers of the liver, pancreas, bile ducts, and gallbladder; video-assisted thoracic surgery (VATS) for lung and other thoracic cancers; and transoral laser surgery for cancers of the head and neck.

For more about Fox Chase physicians and services, visit our website, www.foxchase.org, or call 1-888-FOX CHASE.

MOUNT SINAI
SCHOOL OF
MEDICINE

**THE MOUNT SINAI MEDICAL CENTER
TRANSPLANTATION**
One Gustave L. Levy Place
Fifth Avenue and 100th Street
New York, NY 10029-6574
Physician Referral: 1-800-MD-SINAI (637-4624)
212-731-RMTI (7684)
www.mountsinai.org/rmti

Scientific breakthroughs, technological advances, and improved clinical therapies make it possible to save more lives through organ transplantation than ever before. The Mount Sinai Medical Center's **RECANATI MILLER/TRANSPLANTATION INSTITUTE (RMTI)** has been a world leader in these advances. The RMTI brings together clinical programs in adult and pediatric liver, kidney, pancreas, and intestinal transplantation. It is one of the largest transplant centers in the United States and performs more than 350 transplant procedures annually. In addition, RMTI surgeons also perform complex hepatobiliary surgical procedures.

History of Achievement – The kidney transplant program was instituted at Mount Sinai in 1967 and is now one of the largest adult and pediatric programs in the nation, having performed more than 2,500 transplants. The first liver transplant to be performed in New York State was in 1988 at Mount Sinai. There have been many other firsts in the program's 22-year history, including the first pediatric liver transplant and the first adult-to-adult living-donor liver transplant in New York State. Our surgeons have successfully performed more than 3,000 liver transplants and over 250 living donor liver transplants.

Tradition of Excellence – Mount Sinai is one of the few hospitals in the country that offers comprehensive, multi-organ transplant services for both children and adults. Our physicians are able to accept and care for the sickest and most complex patients.

Innovative Programs

- **HIV/Protocol Study** – Since 2001, the RMTI has been one of the only transplant centers to participate in a National Institutes of Health study on transplantation for carefully selected patients with HIV.

- **Living Donor Program** – Mount Sinai has an active living-donor program. The newly endowed **Zweig Family Center for Living Donation** is the first multi-organ living donor center where dedicated resources ensure the well-being of these heroes who give one, or a part, of their own organs to save another person's life. We also participate in local and national paired-exchange and donor-chain initiatives.

- **Multi-organ Transplantation and Intestinal Rehabilitation Program** – We have performed many combined transplant procedures. Our rehabilitation program offers patients with intestinal failure the opportunity, when possible, to avoid transplantation through medical and/or surgical interventions.

- **Translational Research** – Our scientists are actively investigating new and innovative ways to detect, prevent and treat rejection. We have nationally-recognized and well-funded transplant, genomic, and proteomic projects.

MOUNT SINAI SCHOOL OF MEDICINE

THE MOUNT SINAI MEDICAL CENTER
DEPARTMENT OF SURGERY

One Gustave L. Levy Place
Fifth Avenue and 100th Street
New York, NY 10029-6574
Physician Referral: 1-800-MD-SINAI (637-4624)
www.mountsinai.org/surgery

THE DEPARTMENT OF SURGERY continues to build upon the legacy of those who have gone before, caring for the very sickest of patients while developing new therapies and training tomorrow's physicians to save and enhance lives. Patients today are experiencing less pain, shorter hospital stays, and faster recovery times than was ever imaginable just 20 years ago.

Bariatric Surgery – The latest minimally invasive techniques are used to perform laparoscopic gastric bypass, lap band placement, duodenal switch, and sleeve gastrectomy.

Colon and Rectal Surgery – Leaders in the treatment of gastrointestinal disorders, our surgeons care for a wide range of diseases, including: inflammatory bowel disease (Crohn's disease and ulcerative colitis), diverticulitis, colon and rectal cancer, and fecal incontinence. We offer many important procedures not commonly available.

General Surgery – The Division of General Surgery specializes in the treatment of abdominal surgical conditions. These include benign and malignant diseases of the gallbladder and gastrointestinal track (stomach, intestine, and colon). Our Comprehensive Hernia Center offers state-of-the-art repair of inguinal, ventral and hiatal hernias. We use minimally invasive and evidence-based surgery to deliver the highest standard of care to our patients.

Laparoscopic and Minimally Invasive Surgery – Mount Sinai surgeons rank as some of the world's most respected and innovative surgeons, performing more laparoscopic procedures than surgeons at any other hospital in New York.

Metabolic, Endocrine and Minimally Invasive Surgery – This division was formed to serve as the backbone for several disease-specific multidisciplinary programs. Ours is a truly novel metabolic surgery program that brings together traditional endocrine, bariatric and laparoscopic techniques to treat diseases of metabolism and the endocrine system.

Pediatric Surgery – Surgeries involving children can be met with even more apprehension than those for adults. Fortunately, Mount Sinai surgeons offer a full range of pediatric surgical procedures in a family-focused, child-sensitive environment.

Plastic and Reconstructive Surgery – Surgical care from aesthetic to complex reconstruction is offered for benign and malignant disease, as well as for deformities that are either congenital or acquired. The aim is to restore function and correct deformities caused by birth defects, aging, accident, or illness.

Surgical Oncology – Our surgeons provide expert care for both minimally invasive and open complex malignancies. Patients are seen promptly and are cared for by a multidisciplinary team of medical and surgical experts, enabling them to benefit from the opinions of dozens of nationally renowned doctors.

Vascular Surgery – Mount Sinai is a recognized world leader in the development of new minimally invasive techniques for the treatment of aortic aneurysms, carotid stenosis for the prevention of stroke and lower extremity ischemia. Mount Sinai performs research in areas ranging from stem cell therapy to specialized vascular devices. Our research serves to advance the field of vascular surgery. A wide array of advanced patient services is available, ensuring that conditions are managed successfully.

TOP-RANKING MINIMALLY INVASIVE SURGEONS
In surveys of leading minimally invasive surgeons in a variety of specialties, Mount Sinai's physicians are consistently at the top of the list in surgery of the colon and rectum, liver and bile ducts, thyroid, hernia, chest, and blood vessels.

MINIMALLY INVASIVE SURGERY

NYU Langone Medical Center has been at the forefront of minimally invasive surgery for more than 20 years, treating conditions from heart disease and prostate cancer to obesity and fetal abnormalities in utero.

Robotic Surgery
NYU Langone Medical Center was the first hospital in New York City to use the minimally invasive da Vinci Si HD robotic surgical system which allows a 40 percent higher definition view of the surgical field. The Robotic Surgery Center combines world-class experience with the latest technology to treat a number of cardiac, gynecologic, thoracic, and urologic conditions.

Laparoscopic Surgery
Surgeons at NYU Langone Medical Center use laparoscopic techniques to manage kidney cancers, remove adrenal glands, perform renal biopsies, remove renal cysts and perform innovative urinary reconstruction. Kidney donations can also be performed laparoscopically.

Cardiac Surgery
Since 1996, over 6,000 minimally invasive heart surgery procedures have been performed by our cardiac surgeons. Most patients are candidates for minimally invasive procedures.

Thoracic Surgery
We offer a minimally invasive thoracic surgery program, incorporating video-assisted techniques along with the newest methods for post-operative pain relief.

Neurosurgical Technology
NYU Langone Medical Center was the first hospital in the Northeast with the highly advanced Leksell Gamma Knife, allowing neurosurgeons to remove deep-seated tumors, vascular malformations and other disease sites with outstanding results. Assisted by three-dimensional MRI technology, the Leksell Gamma Knife bombards its target with precise doses of radiation, while preserving healthy tissue.

Gynecologic Surgery
Minimally invasive gynecological surgery, including surgery for endometriosis and laparoscopic hysterectomy, are routinely performed at NYU Langone Medical Center.

Varicose Veins
Our physicians pioneered two minimally invasive procedures that do not require surgical incisions to treat varicose veins. They are endovascular closure, which uses radio heat waves to close down inadequate valves, and scope-based varicose vein treatment which allows veins to be removed without an open incision.

For more than 200 years, Penn has expanded the frontiers of medicine. Today, surgeons at Penn Medicine are leading the way in robotic-assisted surgery.

A Leading Program in the United States

Penn is home to eight daVinci® Surgical Systems making it one of the largest robotic-assisted surgical programs in the United States. The equipment has been used for some time in urologic/prostate procedures, cardiac surgery, gastrointestinal and gynecological operations.

In addition, Penn surgeons have pioneered new procedures in head and neck surgery using robotic-assisted technology. Penn was the first medical center in the world with an approved study to perform this surgery and many patients have benefited from transoral robotic surgery (TORS).

Benefits of Robotic Surgery

The advantages of robotic-assisted surgery include a tremendous enhancement in the surgeon's control of the instruments and the ability to perform more intricate procedures. For patients, the benefits of robotic-assisted surgery may include:

- Less post-operative pain
- Less risk of infection
- Less anesthesia
- Less blood loss
- Shorter hospital stay
- Faster and more complete recovery
- Quicker return to normal daily activities

Experience Makes the Difference

Because of its many benefits, robotic-assisted surgery has gained increased popularity among the medical community in recent years. But technology is only as good as the hands that control it. Robotic technology is meant to be operated by skilled and experienced surgeons. The robotic surgery program at Penn is staffed by surgeons who far exceed the recommended level of experience required for its use. In addition, Penn is one of the largest, state-of-the-art surgical training centers in the country.

As the medical community embraces robotic-assisted surgery, our researchers, nurses, and surgeons remain at the forefront of this field by relentlessly advancing the application of this technology as well as educating the next generation of surgeons who will use it. The result is that Penn is the first place surgeons turn to learn the technology of tomorrow and the first place you should turn for answers.

Robotic Surgery
Available at Penn:

- **Cancer:** Head and Neck, Throat, Mouth and Tongue, Prostate, Bladder, Kidney, Heart, Uterus, Cervix

- **Colon & Rectal Surgery:** Abdominal Perineal Resection; Proctocolectomy with IPAA and Temporary Loop Ileostomy; Right Colectomy; Sigmoid Resection with Rectoplexy

- **Gastrointestinal:** Bariatric LAP-BAND® and Sleeve Gastrectomy

- **Gynecology:** Pelvic Floor Reconstruction, Hysterectomy, Fibroid Removal, Myomectomy, Tubal Anastomosis

- **Heart:** Mitral Valve Repair, MIDCAB/CABG – Coronary Revascularization, Atrial Septal Defect Closure, Atrial Tumor Excision, Atrial Fibrillation

- **Otorhinolaryngology—Head and Neck Surgery:** TORS; Thyroidectomy; Tongue, Palate and Tonsil Surgery; Sleep Apnea

- **Thoracic:** Lobectomy; Thymectomy; Resection of Esophageal and Mediastinal Masses, Tumors and Cysts

- **Urology:** Prostatectomy, Nephrectomy, Cystectomy, Pelvic Reconstruction, Retroperitoneal Lymph Node Dissection, Retroperitoneal Mass Removal, Adrenalectomy, Ureteropelvic Junction Repair

For more information or to schedule an appointment, call 800.789.PENN (7366) or visit PennMedicine.org

Thoracic & Cardiac Surgery

A thoracic and cardiac surgeon provides the operative, perioperative care and critical care of patients with pathologic conditions within the chest. Included is the surgical care of coronary artery disease, cancers of the lung, esophagus and chest wall, abnormalities of the trachea, abnormalities of the great vessels and heart valves, congenital anomalies, tumors of the mediastinum and diseases of the diaphragm. The management of the airway and injuries of the chest is within the scope of the specialty.

Thoracic and cardiac surgeons have the knowledge, experience and technical skills to accurately diagnose, operate upon safely and effectively manage patients with thoracic diseases of the chest. This requires substantial knowledge of cardiorespiratory physiology and oncology, as well as capability in the use of heart assist devices, management of abnormal heart rhythms and drainage of the chest cavity, respiratory support systems, endoscopy and invasive and noninvasive diagnostic techniques.

Training Required: Seven to eight years

THORACIC & CARDIAC SURGERY

New England

Akins, Cary W MD [T&CS] - **Spec Exp:** Heart Valve Surgery; Coronary Artery Surgery; Aneurysm-Thoracic Aortic; **Hospital:** Mass Genl Hosp; **Address:** Mass Genl Hosp, Dept Surgery, 55 Fruit St Cox Bldg - rm 648, Boston, MA 02114; **Phone:** 617-726-8218; **Board Cert:** Thoracic Surgery 2005; **Med School:** Harvard Med Sch 1970; **Resid:** Cardiovascular Surgery, Mass Genl Hosp 1975; **Fac Appt:** Clin Prof S, Harvard Med Sch

Bolman III, Ralph Morton MD [T&CS] - **Spec Exp:** Heart Failure & Ventricular Containment; Ventricular Assist Device (LVAD); Mitral Valve Surgery; Aneurysm; **Hospital:** Brigham and Women's Hosp (page 57); **Address:** Brigham & Womens Hosp, Dept Cardiac Surg, 75 Francis St, rm CA211, Boston, MA 02115; **Phone:** 617-732-7678; **Board Cert:** Thoracic Surgery 2004; **Med School:** St Louis Univ 1973; **Resid:** Surgery, Duke Univ Med Ctr 1980; **Fellow:** Thoracic Surgery, Univ Minn Hosp 1982; **Fac Appt:** Prof S, Harvard Med Sch

Brinckerhoff, Laurence H MD [T&CS] - **Spec Exp:** Lung Cancer; Esophageal Cancer; Minimally Invasive Thoracic Surgery; **Hospital:** Tufts Med Ctr; **Address:** Tufts Medical Center, 750 Washington St, Boston, MA 02111; **Phone:** 617-636-5589; **Board Cert:** Surgery 2002; Thoracic Surgery 2006; **Med School:** Dartmouth Med Sch 1994; **Resid:** Surgery, Univ Virginia Med Ctr 2001; **Fellow:** Cardiothoracic Surgery, Univ Colorado Hlth Sci Ctr 2004

Bueno, Raphael MD [T&CS] - **Spec Exp:** Lung Cancer; Minimally Invasive Thoracic Surgery; Minimally Invasive Esophageal Surgery; Mesothelioma; **Hospital:** Brigham and Women's Hosp (page 57), Dana-Farber Cancer Inst (page 57); **Address:** Brigham and Women's Hospital, Div of Thoracic Surgery, 75 Francis St, Boston, MA 02115; **Phone:** 617-732-6824; **Board Cert:** Thoracic Surgery 2006; Surgery 2002; Surgical Critical Care 2003; **Med School:** Harvard Med Sch 1985; **Resid:** Surgery, Brigham & Women's Hosp 1992; **Fellow:** Surgical Critical Care, Brigham & Women's Hosp 1993; Thoracic Surgery, Mass Genl Hosp 1995; **Fac Appt:** Assoc Prof S, Harvard Med Sch

Colson, Yolonda L MD/PhD [T&CS] - **Spec Exp:** Lung Cancer; Mesothelioma; Thoracic Cancers; **Hospital:** Brigham and Women's Hosp (page 57), Dana-Farber Cancer Inst (page 57); **Address:** Brigham & Women's Hosp, Dept Surgery, 75 Francis St, Boston, MA 02115; **Phone:** 617-732-6824; **Board Cert:** Surgery 2010; Thoracic Surgery 2010; **Med School:** Mayo Med Sch 1989; **Resid:** Surgery, Univ Pittsburg Med Ctr 1995; **Fellow:** Research, Univ Pittsburg Med Ctr 1996; Cardiothoracic Surgery, Brigham & Women's Hosp 2001; **Fac Appt:** Assoc Prof S, Harvard Med Sch

Del-Nido, Pedro J MD [T&CS] - **Spec Exp:** Heart Valve Surgery-Pediatric; Congenital Heart Disease; Minimally Invasive Surgery; Robotic Surgery; **Hospital:** Children's Hospital - Boston; **Address:** Children's Hospital Boston, Dept Cardiac Surgery, 300 Longwood Ave, Bader 273, Boston, MA 02115; **Phone:** 617-355-8290; **Board Cert:** Surgery 2006; Thoracic Surgery 2004; Congenital Cardiac Surgery 2011; **Med School:** Univ Wisc 1977; **Resid:** Surgery, Boston Univ Med Ctr 1982; Thoracic Surgery, Toronto Genl Hosp 1985; **Fellow:** Pediatric Cardiothoracic Surgery, Hosp Sick Children 1986; **Fac Appt:** Prof S, Harvard Med Sch

Elefteriades, John MD [T&CS] - **Spec Exp:** Aneurysm-Thoracic Aortic; Transplant-Heart; Ventricular Assist Device (LVAD); **Hospital:** Yale-New Haven Hosp, Yale Med Group; **Address:** 333 Cedar St, Boardman 2, Dept Cardiothoracic Surgery, PO Box 208039, New Haven, CT 06520; **Phone:** 203-785-2705; **Board Cert:** Thoracic Surgery 2004; **Med School:** Yale Univ 1976; **Resid:** Surgery, Yale-New Haven Hosp 1981; Cardiothoracic Surgery, Yale-New Haven Hosp 1983; **Fellow:** Cardiothoracic Surgery, Yale-New Haven Hosp 1983; **Fac Appt:** Prof S, Yale Univ

Fernando, Hiran C MD [T&CS] - **Spec Exp:** Esophageal Cancer; Lung Cancer; Esophageal Disorders; Minimally Invasive Thoracic Surgery; **Hospital:** Boston Med Ctr; **Address:** 88 E Newton St, Robinson B402, Boston, MA 02118; **Phone:** 617-638-5600; **Board Cert:** Surgery 2005; Thoracic Surgery 2009; **Med School:** England, UK 1986; **Resid:** Surgery, LAC - Harbor - UCLA Med Ctr 1993; Thoracic Surgery, UC Davis Med Ctr 1998; **Fellow:** Minimally Invasive Surgery, UPMC 2001; **Fac Appt:** Assoc Prof TS, Boston Univ

Gaissert, Henning A MD [T&CS] - **Spec Exp:** Esophageal Cancer; Tracheal Surgery; Lung Cancer; Thymoma; **Hospital:** Mass Genl Hosp, Newton - Wellesley Hosp; **Address:** Mass Genl Hosp, 55 Fruit St, BLK 1570, Boston, MA 02114; **Phone:** 617-726-5341; **Board Cert:** Surgery 2010; Thoracic & Cardiac Surgery 2004; **Med School:** Germany 1984; **Resid:** Surgery, Mass Genl Hosp 1989; Surgery, Barnes Jewish Hosp 1991; **Fellow:** Research, Harvard Med Sch 1993; Cardiothoracic Surgery, Barnes Jewish Hosp 1996; **Fac Appt:** Assoc Prof S, Harvard Med Sch

Hashim, Sabet W MD [T&CS] - **Spec Exp:** Mitral Valve Surgery; Heart Valve Surgery; Maze Procedure for Atrial Fibrillation; **Hospital:** Yale-New Haven Hosp, Yale Med Group; **Address:** Yale Univ Cardiothoracic Surgery, 330 Cedar St, Ste BB204, PO Box 208039, New Haven, CT 06520-8039; **Phone:** 203-785-6214; **Board Cert:** Thoracic Surgery 2001; **Med School:** Lebanon 1975; **Resid:** Surgery, St Lukes Roosevely Hosp 1979; Cardiothoracic Surgery, Yale-New Haven Hosp 1981; **Fac Appt:** Assoc Prof S, Yale Univ

Kopf, Gary S MD [T&CS] - **Spec Exp:** Cardiac Surgery; Pediatric Cardiothoracic Surgery; Congenital Heart Disease; **Hospital:** Yale-New Haven Hosp, Yale Med Group; **Address:** Yale Univ Sch Med, Dept of Surgery, Box 208039, New Haven, CT 06520-8039; **Phone:** 203-785-2702; **Board Cert:** Thoracic Surgery 2011; **Med School:** Harvard Med Sch 1970; **Resid:** Surgery, Peter Bent Brigham Hosp 1977; Cardiothoracic Surgery, Chldns Hosp Med Ctr 1980; **Fellow:** Cardiothoracic Surgery, Peter Bent Brigham Hosp 1980; **Fac Appt:** Prof S, Yale Univ

Lazar, Harold L MD [T&CS] - **Spec Exp:** Aortic Surgery; Coronary Artery Surgery; Heart Valve Surgery; Esophageal Surgery; **Hospital:** Boston Med Ctr; **Address:** Boston Med Ctr, 88 E Newton St Robinson Bldg - Ste B-402, Boston, MA 02118; **Phone:** 617-638-7350; **Board Cert:** Thoracic Surgery 2003; Surgery 2001; **Med School:** Boston Univ 1974; **Resid:** Surgery, Univ Michigan Med Ctr 1981; Cardiothoracic Surgery, Columbia-Presbyterian Med Ctr 1983; **Fellow:** Cardiovascular Research, UCLA Med Ctr 1979; **Fac Appt:** Prof TS, Boston Univ

Mathisen, Douglas MD [T&CS] - **Spec Exp:** Tracheal Surgery; Lung Cancer; Esophageal Cancer; **Hospital:** Mass Genl Hosp, Newton - Wellesley Hosp; **Address:** Mass Genl Hosp, Thoracic Surgery, 55 Fruit St, Blake 1570, Boston, MA 02114; **Phone:** 617-726-6826; **Board Cert:** Thoracic Surgery 2002; **Med School:** Univ IL Coll Med 1974; **Resid:** Surgery, Mass Genl Hosp 1981; Thoracic Surgery, Mass Genl Hosp 1982; **Fellow:** Surgical Oncology, Natl Cancer Inst 1979; **Fac Appt:** Prof S, Harvard Med Sch

Mayer Jr, John E MD [T&CS] - **Spec Exp:** Pediatric Cardic Surgery; Cardiovascular Surgery; Transplant-Heart; **Hospital:** Children's Hospital - Boston; **Address:** Chldns Hosp, Dept Cardiac Surg, 300 Longwood Ave, Bader 273, Boston, MA 02115; **Phone:** 617-355-8258; **Board Cert:** Thoracic & Cardiac Surgery 2010; Congenital Cardiac Surgery 2009; **Med School:** Yale Univ 1972; **Resid:** Surgery, Univ Minn Med Ctr 1979; **Fellow:** Cardiothoracic Surgery, Univ Minn Med Ctr 1981; **Fac Appt:** Prof S, Harvard Med Sch

Nugent, William C MD [T&CS] - **Spec Exp:** Thoracic Cancers; Hyperhidrosis-Palmar; **Hospital:** Dartmouth - Hitchcock Med Ctr; **Address:** Dartmouth-Hitchcock Med Ctr, Dept Cardiothoracic Surgery, 1 Medical Center Drive, Lebanon, NH 03756; **Phone:** 603-650-8572; **Board Cert:** Thoracic Surgery 2002; **Med School:** Albany Med Coll 1975; **Resid:** Surgery, Beth Israel Hosp 1980; Thoracic Surgery, Univ Michigan Med Ctr 1983; **Fellow:** Cardiothoracic Surgery, Mass Genl Hosp 1981; **Fac Appt:** Prof S, Dartmouth Med Sch

Thoracic & Cardiac Surgery

Rastegar, Hassan MD [T&CS] - **Spec Exp:** Cardiac Surgery-Adult; Heart Valve Surgery; Minimally Invasive Cardiac Surgery; **Hospital:** Tufts Med Ctr; **Address:** Tufts Medical Center, 800 Washington St, Box 266, Boston, MA 02111; **Phone:** 617-636-5528; **Board Cert:** Thoracic Surgery 2003; **Med School:** Iran 1974; **Resid:** Surgery, Hosp Univ Penn 1980; Cardiothoracic Surgery, Northwestern Univ 1982; **Fac Appt:** Prof S, Tufts Univ

Sellke, Frank W MD [T&CS] - **Spec Exp:** Heart Valve Surgery; Aortic Surgery; Coronary Artery Surgery; Cardiac Tumors/Cancer; **Hospital:** Rhode Island Hosp, Miriam Hosp; **Address:** 2 Dudley St, MOC Bldg - Fl 3 - Ste 360, Providence, RI 02905; **Phone:** 401-274-7546; **Board Cert:** Surgery 2005; Thoracic Surgery 2009; **Med School:** Indiana Univ 1981; **Resid:** Surgery, Akron City Hosp 1987; Cardiothoracic Surgery, Univ Iowa Hosps & Clinics 1990; **Fac Appt:** Prof S, Brown Univ

Singh, Arun K MD [T&CS] - **Spec Exp:** Cardiac Surgery; **Hospital:** Rhode Island Hosp; **Address:** University Cardiovascular Surgical, 2 Dudley St, Ste 360, Providence, RI 02905-3248; **Phone:** 401-274-7546; **Board Cert:** Surgery 1973; Thoracic Surgery 1975; **Med School:** India 1967; **Resid:** Surgery, Columbia Presby Med Ctr 1972; Cardiothoracic Surgery, Rhode Island Hosp 1974; **Fellow:** Cardiac Surgery, Hosp Sick Chldn 1975; **Fac Appt:** Clin Prof S, Brown Univ

Sugarbaker, David J MD [T&CS] - **Spec Exp:** Mesothelioma; Transplant-Lung; Esophageal Cancer; **Hospital:** Brigham and Women's Hosp (page 57), Dana-Farber Cancer Inst (page 57); **Address:** Brigham & Women's Hosp, Div Thoracic Surgery, 75 Francis St Fl 2, Boston, MA 02115-6110; **Phone:** 617-732-6824; **Board Cert:** Thoracic Surgery 2009; **Med School:** Cornell Univ-Weill Med Coll 1979; **Resid:** Surgery, Brigham & Women's Hosp 1982; Surgery, Brigham & Women's Hosp 1986; **Fellow:** Thoracic Surgery, Toronto Genl Hosp 1988; **Fac Appt:** Assoc Prof S, Harvard Med Sch

Swanson, Scott J MD [T&CS] - **Spec Exp:** Lung Cancer; Video Assisted Thoracic Surgery (VATS); Esophageal Cancer; **Hospital:** Brigham and Women's Hosp (page 57), Dana-Farber Cancer Inst (page 57); **Address:** Brigham & Women's Hosp, Div Thoracic Surgery, 75 Francis St Fl 2, Boston, MA 02115; **Phone:** 617-732-6824; **Board Cert:** Surgery 2003; Thoracic Surgery 2006; **Med School:** Harvard Med Sch 1985; **Resid:** Surgery, Brigham & Womens Hosp 1990; **Fellow:** Cardiothoracic Surgery, Brigham & Womens Hosp 1994; **Fac Appt:** Prof S, Harvard Med Sch

Vander Salm, Thomas MD [T&CS] - **Spec Exp:** Heart Valve Surgery-Mitral; Cardiovascular Surgery; **Hospital:** N Shore Med Ctr - Salem Hosp; **Address:** Salem Hosp, Div Cardiac Surgery, 81 Highland Ave, Axelrod Fl 5th, Salem, MA 01970; **Phone:** 978-354-2500; **Board Cert:** Surgery 1974; Thoracic Surgery 2006; **Med School:** Johns Hopkins Univ 1966; **Resid:** Surgery, Mass Genl Hosp 1968; Thoracic Surgery, Johns Hopkins Hosp 1969; **Fac Appt:** Prof S, Univ Mass Sch Med

Vlahakes, Gus J MD [T&CS] - **Spec Exp:** Cardiac Surgery; Transplant-Heart; Maze Procedure for Atrial Fibrillation; **Hospital:** Mass Genl Hosp; **Address:** Mass Genl Hosp, 55 Fruit St, Ste COX 652, Boston, MA 02114; **Phone:** 617-726-1861; **Board Cert:** Surgery 2002; Surgical Critical Care 2000; Thoracic Surgery 2005; **Med School:** Harvard Med Sch 1975; **Resid:** Surgery, Mass Genl Hosp 1983; Cardiothoracic Surgery, Mass Genl Hosp 1985; **Fellow:** Pediatric Cardiac Surgery, Chldns Hosp 1985; **Fac Appt:** Prof S, Harvard Med Sch

Wain, John MD [T&CS] - **Spec Exp:** Transplant-Lung; Lung Cancer; Esophageal Cancer; **Hospital:** Mass Genl Hosp; **Address:** Mass Genl Hosp, Div Thoracic Surgery, 55 Fruit St, Blake 1570B, Boston, MA 02114; **Phone:** 617-726-5200; **Board Cert:** Thoracic Surgery 2010; **Med School:** Jefferson Med Coll 1980; **Resid:** Surgery, Mass Genl Hosp 1985; **Fellow:** Cardiothoracic Surgery, Mass Genl Hosp 1988; **Fac Appt:** Asst Prof TS, Harvard Med Sch

Warner, Kenneth G MD [T&CS] - **Spec Exp:** Cardiac Surgery-Adult & Pediatric; Congenital Heart Surgery; Heart Valve Surgery; Aortic Surgery; **Hospital:** Tufts Med Ctr; **Address:** Tufts Medical Center, 800 Washington St, Box 266, Boston, MA 02111-1526; **Phone:** 617-636-0033; **Board Cert:** Surgery 2007; Thoracic Surgery 2009; Surgical Critical Care 2001; **Med School:** Univ Mich Med Sch 1982; **Resid:** Surgery, Brigham & Women's Hosp 1984; Cardiothoracic Surgery, Brigham & Women's Hosp 1990; **Fellow:** Research, West Roxbury VA Hosp 1986; **Fac Appt:** Assoc Prof S, Tufts Univ

Whyte, Richard MD [T&CS] - **Spec Exp:** Lung Cancer; Esophageal Cancer; Chest Wall Tumors; **Hospital:** Beth Israel Deaconess Med Ctr - Boston; **Address:** Beth Israel Deaconess Med Ctr, 330 Brookline Ave Shapiro Bldg Fl 9, Boston, MA 02215; **Phone:** 617-632-8252; **Board Cert:** Surgery 2011; Thoracic Surgery 2003; **Med School:** Univ Pittsburgh 1983; **Resid:** Surgery, Mass Genl Hosp 1990; Thoracic Surgery, Univ Michigan Hosp 1992

Wright, Cameron D MD [T&CS] - **Spec Exp:** Lung Cancer; Esophageal Cancer; Tracheal Surgery; **Hospital:** Mass Genl Hosp; **Address:** Mass Genl Hosp, Div Thoracic Surg, 55 Fruit St, Blake 1570, Boston, MA 02114; **Phone:** 617-726-5801; **Board Cert:** Surgery 2006; Thoracic Surgery 2007; **Med School:** Univ Mich Med Sch 1980; **Resid:** Surgery, Mass Genl Hosp 1986; Thoracic Surgery, Mass Genl Hosp 1988; **Fac Appt:** Assoc Prof S, Harvard Med Sch

Mid Atlantic

Acker, Michael A MD [T&CS] - **Spec Exp:** Transplant-Heart; Ventricular Assist Device (LVAD); Coronary Artery Surgery; Heart Valve Surgery; **Hospital:** Hosp Univ Penn - UPHS (page 72); **Address:** Univ Penn Dept Surgery, 3400 Spruce St, 6 Silverstein, Philadelphia, PA 19104-4227; **Phone:** 215-349-8305; **Board Cert:** Surgery 2001; Thoracic & Cardiac Surgery 2001; **Med School:** Brown Univ 1981; **Resid:** Surgery, Hosp Univ Penn 1988; Cardiothoracic Surgery, Johns Hopkins Hosp 1991; **Fac Appt:** Prof S, Univ Pennsylvania

Adams, David H MD [T&CS] - **Spec Exp:** Mitral Valve Surgery; Heart Valve Surgery; Minimally Invasive Cardiac Surgery; Aortic Surgery; **Hospital:** Mount Sinai Med Ctr (page 64); **Address:** The Mount Sinai Medical Center, Department of Cardiothoracic Surgery, 1190 Fifth Ave, MS 1028, New York, NY 10029; **Phone:** 212-659-6820; **Board Cert:** Thoracic Surgery 2003; **Med School:** Duke Univ 1983; **Resid:** Surgery, Brigham & Women's Hosp 1990; Thoracic & Cardiac Surgery, Brigham & Women's Hosp/Chldn's Hosp 1992; **Fellow:** Research, Harvard Med Sch 1988; Surgery, Harvard Med Sch 1992; **Fac Appt:** Prof T&CS, Mount Sinai Sch Med

Altorki, Nasser K MD [T&CS] - **Spec Exp:** Esophageal Cancer; Lung Cancer; Thoracic Cancers; Vaccine Therapy; **Hospital:** NY-Presby/Weill Cornell Med Ctr, NY (page 66); **Address:** 525 E 68th St, M-404, New York, NY 10065; **Phone:** 212-746-5156; **Board Cert:** Surgery 2006; Thoracic Surgery 2007; **Med School:** Egypt 1978; **Resid:** Surgery, Univ Chicago Hosps 1985; **Fellow:** Cardiothoracic Surgery, Univ Chicago Hosps 1987; **Fac Appt:** Prof S, Cornell Univ-Weill Med Coll

Argenziano, Michael MD [T&CS] - **Spec Exp:** Robotic Cardiac Surgery; Coronary Artery Surgery; Maze Procedure for Atrial Fibrillation; **Hospital:** NY-Presby/Columbia Univ Med Ctr, NY (page 66); **Address:** NY Presby Med Ctr, Milstein Bldg, 177 Fort Washington Ave, rm 7-435, New York, NY 10032; **Phone:** 212-305-5888; **Board Cert:** Thoracic Surgery 2002; **Med School:** Columbia P&S 1992; **Resid:** Surgery, Columbia Presby Med Ctr 1998; **Fellow:** Cardiothoracic Surgery, Columbia Presby Med Ctr 1999; **Fac Appt:** Asst Prof S, Columbia P&S

Thoracic & Cardiac Surgery

Bacha, Emile A MD [T&CS] - **Spec Exp:** Pediatric Cardiac Surgery; Congenital Heart Surgery; Neonatal & Infant Cardiac Surgery; Minimally Invasive Cardiac Surgery; **Hospital:** NY-Presby/Columbia Univ Med Ctr, NY (page 66), Morgan Stanley Children's Hosp of NY-Presby, NY; **Address:** Morgan Stanley Chldns Hosp North, Columbia Univ Medical Ctr, 3959 Broadway, rm 274, New York, NY 10032; **Phone:** 212-305-2688; **Board Cert:** Thoracic & Cardiac Surgery 2009; Congenital Cardiac Surgery 2009; **Med School:** Germany 1989; **Resid:** Thoracic Surgery, Mass Genl Hosp 1993; Surgery, Emory Univ Med Ctr 1995; **Fellow:** Pediatric Cardiac Surgery, Hosp Marie Lanne Longe 1996; Pediatric Cardiac Surgery, Mass Genl Hosp 1998; **Fac Appt:** Prof S, Columbia P&S

Bains, Manjit MD [T&CS] - **Spec Exp:** Cardiothoracic Surgery; Esophageal Cancer; Lung Cancer; **Hospital:** Meml Sloan-Kettering Cancer Ctr; **Address:** 1275 York Ave, rm C861, New York, NY 10065; **Phone:** 212-639-7450; **Board Cert:** Surgery 1971; Thoracic Surgery 1972; **Med School:** India 1963; **Resid:** Surgery, Rochester Genl Hosp 1970; **Fellow:** Thoracic Surgery, Sloan Kettering Cancer Ctr 1972; **Fac Appt:** Clin Prof S, Cornell Univ-Weill Med Coll

Battafarano, Richard J MD [T&CS] - **Spec Exp:** Lung Cancer; Barrett's Esophagus; Esophageal Surgery; Mesothelioma; **Hospital:** Univ of MD Med Ctr; **Address:** Greenebaum Cancer Ctr-Dept Thoracic Surgery, 29 S Greene St, Ste 504, Baltimore, MD 21201; **Phone:** 410-328-6366; **Board Cert:** Surgery 2008; Thoracic Surgery 2000; **Med School:** Hahnemann Univ 1988; **Resid:** Surgery, Univ Minn Hosp & Clin 1997; **Fellow:** Thoracic Surgery, Meml Sloan Kettering Cancer Ctr 1999; **Fac Appt:** Assoc Prof S, Univ MD Sch Med

Bavaria, Joseph E MD [T&CS] - **Spec Exp:** Aortic Surgery; Transplant-Heart & Lung; Heart Valve Surgery; **Hospital:** Hosp Univ Penn - UPHS (page 72); **Address:** Univ Penn Dept Surgery, 3400 Spruce St, 6 Silverstein, Philadelphia, PA 19104; **Phone:** 215-662-2017; **Board Cert:** Thoracic Surgery 2001; **Med School:** Tulane Univ 1983; **Resid:** Surgery, Hosp Univ Penn 1990; Cardiothoracic Surgery, Hosp Univ Penn/Children's Hosp 1992; **Fac Appt:** Prof S, Univ Pennsylvania

Chen, Jonathan M MD [T&CS] - **Spec Exp:** Pediatric Cardiothoracic Surgery; Arrhythmias; Congenital Heart Disease; **Hospital:** Morgan Stanley Children's Hosp of NY-Presby, NY, NY-Presby/Columbia Univ Med Ctr, NY (page 66); **Address:** NY Presbyterian-Weill Cornell Med Ctr, 525 E 68th St, Ste M404, New York, NY 10065; **Phone:** 212-746-5014; **Board Cert:** Surgery 2001; Thoracic Surgery 2003; **Med School:** Columbia P&S 1994; **Resid:** Surgery, NY Columbia Presby Hosp 2000; **Fellow:** Cardiothoracic Surgery, NY Columbia Presby Hosp 2001; **Fac Appt:** Asst Prof S, Columbia P&S

Cohen, Neri M MD/PhD [T&CS] - **Spec Exp:** Hyperhidrosis-Palmar; Minimally Invasive Surgery; Radiofrequency Tumor Ablation; **Hospital:** Greater Baltimore Med Ctr; **Address:** Greater Baltimore Thoracic Surgery, 6569 N Charles St, Ste 701, Baltimore, MD 21204; **Phone:** 443-849-3470; **Board Cert:** Surgery 2009; Thoracic Surgery 2008; **Med School:** Univ MD Sch Med 1989; **Resid:** Surgery, Med Coll Virginia Hosp 1996; **Fellow:** Cardiothoracic Surgery, Med Coll Virginia Hosp 1997; Thoracic Surgery, Cleveland Clinic 1998

Conte Jr, John V MD [T&CS] - **Spec Exp:** Transplant-Heart; Transplant-Lung; Cardiac Surgery-Adult; Coronary Artery Surgery; **Hospital:** Johns Hopkins Hosp (page 61); **Address:** 1800 Orleans St, Ste 7107, Baltimore, MD 21287-4618; **Phone:** 410-955-1753; **Board Cert:** Thoracic Surgery 2007; **Med School:** Georgetown Univ 1986; **Resid:** Surgery, Georgetown Univ Med Ctr 1992; Thoracic Surgery, Stanford Univ Med Ctr 1995; **Fac Appt:** Prof S, Johns Hopkins Univ

Cooper, Joel D MD [T&CS] - **Spec Exp:** Transplant-Lung; Emphysema-Lung Volume Reduction; Lung Surgery; **Hospital:** Hosp Univ Penn - UPHS (page 72); **Address:** Univ Penn Dept Surgery, 3400 Spruce St, 4 Silverstein, Philadelphia, PA 19104; **Phone:** 215-662-2022; **Board Cert:** Surgery 1971; Thoracic & Cardiac Surgery 1972; **Med School:** Harvard Med Sch 1964; **Resid:** Surgery, Mass Genl Hosp 1968; Thoracic Surgery, Frenchay Hosp; **Fellow:** Research, Hammersmith Hosp; Thoracic Surgery, Mass Genl Hosp; **Fac Appt:** Prof S, Univ Pennsylvania

Demmy, Todd L MD [T&CS] - **Spec Exp:** Lung Cancer; Thoracic Cancers; Esophageal Cancer; Minimally Invasive Thoracic Surgery; **Hospital:** Roswell Park Cancer Inst, Buffalo General Hosp; **Address:** Roswell Park Cancer Inst, Thoracic Surgery Dept, Elm & Carlton Sts, Buffalo, NY 14263; **Phone:** 716-845-1229; **Board Cert:** Surgery 2008; Thoracic Surgery 2010; Surgical Critical Care 2010; **Med School:** Jefferson Med Coll 1983; **Resid:** Surgery, Baylor Affil Hosp 1988; Thoracic Surgery, Allegheny Genl Hosp 1991; **Fac Appt:** Assoc Prof S, SUNY Buffalo

DeRose Jr, Joseph J MD [T&CS] - **Spec Exp:** Robotic Cardiac Surgery; Minimally Invasive Cardiac Surgery; Aortic Surgery; Mitral Valve Surgery; **Hospital:** Montefiore Med Ctr-Einstein Campus, NY, Montefiore Med Ctr-Moses Campus, NY; **Address:** Montefiore-Weiler Medical Ctr, Dept Cardiothoracic Surgery, 1575 Blondell Ave, Ste 125, Bronx, NY 10461; **Phone:** 718-405-8371; **Board Cert:** Thoracic Surgery 2002; **Med School:** Columbia P&S 1993; **Resid:** Surgery, Columbia Presby Med Ctr 1999; **Fellow:** Cardiothoracic Surgery, Columbia Presby Med Ctr 2001; **Fac Appt:** Assoc Prof TS, Albert Einstein Coll Med

Diehl, James T MD [T&CS] - **Spec Exp:** Cardiac Surgery-Adult; Aortic Surgery; Heart Valve Surgery-Aortic; Heart Valve Surgery-Mitral; **Hospital:** Thomas Jefferson Univ Hosp; **Address:** 1025 Walnut St, Ste 607, Philadelphia, PA 19107; **Phone:** 215-955-6996; **Board Cert:** Thoracic Surgery 2004; **Med School:** Albert Einstein Coll Med 1978; **Resid:** Surgery, Cleveland Clinic 1984; Cardiothoracic Surgery, Univ Toronto Med Ctr 1986; **Fac Appt:** Prof S, Thomas Jefferson Univ

Downey, Robert J MD [T&CS] - **Spec Exp:** Lung Cancer; Thoracic Cancers; **Hospital:** Meml Sloan-Kettering Cancer Ctr; **Address:** 1275 York Avenue, New York, NY 10065; **Phone:** 212-639-8124; **Board Cert:** Surgery 2002; Surgical Critical Care 2006; Thoracic & Cardiac Surgery 2005; **Med School:** Columbia P&S 1985; **Resid:** Surgery, Columbia-Presby Med Ctr 1991; **Fellow:** Thoracic Surgery, Mayo Clinic 1992; Thoracic Surgery, Columbia-Presby Med Ctr 1994

Edwards, Niloo M MD [T&CS] - **Spec Exp:** Transplant-Heart; Cardiac Surgery-Geriatric; **Hospital:** St. Peter's Hosp - Albany; **Address:** 319 S Manning Blvd, Ste 110, Albany, NY 12208; **Phone:** 518-525-2525; **Board Cert:** Surgery 2004; Thoracic Surgery 2006; **Med School:** Columbia P&S 1986; **Resid:** Surgery, Strong Meml Hosp 1992; **Fellow:** Cardiothoracic Surgery, Columbia-Presby Med Ctr 1996; **Fac Appt:** Assoc Prof TS, Univ Wisc

Filsoufi, Farzan MD [T&CS] - **Spec Exp:** Mitral Valve Surgery; Minimally Invasive Heart Valve Surgery; Heart Valve Surgery; Robotic Cardiac Surgery; **Hospital:** Mount Sinai Med Ctr (page 64), Elmhurst Hosp Ctr; **Address:** Mt Sinai Med Ctr, Dept Cardiothoracic Surg, 1190 5th Ave, Box 1028, New York, NY 10029; **Phone:** 212-659-6813; **Med School:** France 1991; **Resid:** Surgery, Univ Paris Hosps 1994; Thoracic Surgery, Hospital Broussais/U of Paris 1995; **Fellow:** Cardiothoracic Surgery, Hospital Broussais/U of Paris 1996; Heart Valve Surgery, Brigham & Women's Hosp 2000; **Fac Appt:** Prof TS, Mount Sinai Sch Med

Flores, Raja M MD [T&CS] - **Spec Exp:** Mesothelioma; Lung Cancer; Video Assisted Thoracic Surgery (VATS); Esophageal Cancer; **Hospital:** Mount Sinai Med Ctr (page 64); **Address:** Mt. Sinai Medical Ctr, 1440 Madison Ave, New York, NY 10029; **Phone:** 212-241-9466; **Board Cert:** Surgery 2009; Thoracic & Cardiac Surgery 2010; **Med School:** Albert Einstein Coll Med 1992; **Resid:** Surgery, Columbia Presby Med Ctr 1997; **Fellow:** Thoracic Surgery, Brigham & Womens Hosp/Dana Faber Cancer Inst 2000; **Fac Appt:** Assoc Prof TS, Cornell Univ-Weill Med Coll

Fontana, Gregory MD [T&CS] - **Spec Exp:** Minimally Invasive Surgery; Cardiac Surgery-Pediatric; Mitral Valve Surgery; Coronary Artery Surgery; **Hospital:** Lenox Hill Hosp (page 67); **Address:** Lenox Hill Hosp, Cardiothoracic Dept, 130 E 77th St Fl 4, New York, NY 10075; **Phone:** 212-434-3792; **Board Cert:** Thoracic Surgery 2004; **Med School:** UCLA 1984; **Resid:** Surgery, Duke Univ Med Ctr 1990; Thoracic Surgery, Duke Univ Med Ctr 1993; **Fellow:** Pediatric Cardiac Surgery, UCLA Med Ctr; Pediatric Cardiac Surgery, Chldns Hosp; **Fac Appt:** Clin Prof S, UCLA

Friedberg, Joseph MD [T&CS] - **Spec Exp:** Mesothelioma; Pleural Disease; Lung Cancer; Thoracic Cancers; **Hospital:** Penn Presby Med Ctr - UPHS (page 72), Hosp Univ Penn - UPHS (page 72); **Address:** Penn-Presbyterian Medical Ctr, 51 N 39th St, rm W250, Philadelphia, PA 19104; **Phone:** 215-662-9194; **Board Cert:** Surgery 2006; Thoracic Surgery 2006; **Med School:** Harvard Med Sch 1986; **Resid:** Surgery, Mass General Hosp 1994; **Fellow:** Cardiothoracic Surgery, Brigham & Womens Hosp 1996; **Fac Appt:** Assoc Prof TS, Univ Pennsylvania

Furukawa, Satoshi MD [T&CS] - **Spec Exp:** Transplant-Heart & Lung; Cardiac Surgery-High Risk; Heart Valve Surgery; Minimally Invasive Cardiac Surgery; **Hospital:** Temple Univ Hosp; **Address:** 7500 Central Ave, Ste 208, Jeanes Physician Office Bldg, Philadelphia, PA 19111; **Phone:** 215-728-4866; **Board Cert:** Surgery 2003; Thoracic Surgery 2005; **Med School:** Univ Pennsylvania 1984; **Resid:** Surgery, Hosp Univ Penn 1991; Thoracic & Cardiac Surgery, Hosp Univ Penn 1993; **Fac Appt:** Prof TS, Temple Univ

Galloway, Aubrey MD [T&CS] - **Spec Exp:** Minimally Invasive Heart Valve Surgery; Mitral Valve Surgery; Coronary Artery Surgery; Robotic Surgery; **Hospital:** NYU Langone Med Ctr (page 68); **Address:** 530 1st Ave, Ste 9V, New York, NY 10016-6402; **Phone:** 212-263-7185; **Board Cert:** Thoracic Surgery 2006; **Med School:** Tulane Univ 1978; **Resid:** Surgery, Univ Colo Hlth Sci Ctr 1983; Cardiovascular Surgery, NYU Med Ctr 1985; **Fellow:** Research, Boston Chldns Hosp 1981; Cardiothoracic Surgery, NYU Med Ctr 1985; **Fac Appt:** Prof TS, NYU Sch Med

Gaynor, J William MD [T&CS] - **Spec Exp:** Pediatric Cardiothoracic Surgery; Congenital Heart Surgery; Transplant-Heart; **Hospital:** Chldns Hosp of Philadelphia; **Address:** CHOP, Div of Cardiothoracic Surgery, Main Bldg - rm 2NW10, 34th St & Civic Ctr Blvd, Philadelphia, PA 19104; **Phone:** 215-590-2708; **Board Cert:** Thoracic Surgery 2004; Congenital Cardiac Surgery 2009; **Med School:** Med Univ SC 1982; **Resid:** Surgery, Parkland Meml Hosp; Thoracic Surgery, Duke Univ Med Ctr; **Fellow:** Congenital Heart Surgery, Hosp for Sick Childn; **Fac Appt:** Assoc Prof TS, Univ Pennsylvania

Gharagozloo, Farid MD [T&CS] - **Spec Exp:** Video Assisted Thoracic Surgery (VATS); Lung Cancer; **Hospital:** G Washington Univ Hosp, Harbor Hosp; **Address:** 2175 K St NW, Ste 300, Washington, DC 20037; **Phone:** 202-775-8600; **Board Cert:** Thoracic Surgery 2001; **Med School:** Johns Hopkins Univ 1983; **Resid:** Surgery, Mayo Clinic 1989; Research, Harvard Med Sch 1986; **Fellow:** Cardiothoracic Surgery, Mayo Clinic 1992; **Fac Appt:** Prof S, Geo Wash Univ

Ginsburg, Mark E MD [T&CS] - **Spec Exp:** Lung Cancer; Transplant-Lung; Emphysema-Lung Volume Reduction; **Hospital:** NY-Presby/Columbia Univ Med Ctr, NY (page 66), Good Samaritan Hosp - Suffern; **Address:** 161 Ft Washington Ave Fl 3 - Ste 301, New York, NY 10032; **Phone:** 212-305-3408; **Board Cert:** Surgery 2005; Thoracic Surgery 2006; **Med School:** Tufts Univ 1980; **Resid:** Surgery, Strong Meml Hosp 1985; **Fellow:** Thoracic Surgery, Strong Meml Hosp 1987; **Fac Appt:** Asst Clin Prof S, Columbia P&S

Girardi, Leonard N MD [T&CS] - **Spec Exp:** Aneurysm-Aortic; Cardiac Surgery; Marfan's Syndrome; Cardiothoracic Surgery; **Hospital:** NY-Presby/Weill Cornell Med Ctr, NY (page 66); **Address:** Cardiothoracic Surgery Dept, 525 E 68th St, Ste M404, New York, NY 10065; **Phone:** 212-746-5194; **Board Cert:** Surgery 2005; Thoracic Surgery 2007; **Med School:** Cornell Univ-Weill Med Coll 1989; **Resid:** Surgery, NY Presby/Cornell Univ Med Ctr 1994; **Fellow:** Cardiothoracic Surgery, NY Presby Hosp/Cornell Univ Med Ctr 1996; Cardiothoracic Surgery, Baylor Coll Med 1997; **Fac Appt:** Assoc Prof TS, Cornell Univ-Weill Med Coll

Graver, L Michael MD [T&CS] - **Spec Exp:** Minimally Invasive Heart Valve Surgery; Coronary Artery Surgery; Aortic Surgery; Heart Valve Surgery; **Hospital:** Long Island Jewish Med Ctr (page 67); **Address:** 270-05 76th Ave, Ste O-4000, Long Island Jewish Med Ctr, New Hyde Park, NY 11040-1433; **Phone:** 718-470-7460; **Board Cert:** Surgery 2003; Thoracic Surgery 2004; **Med School:** Albany Med Coll 1977; **Resid:** Surgery, St Luke's-Roosevelt Hosp Ctr 1982; Cardiovascular Surgery, Deaconness Hosp 1983; **Fellow:** Cardiovascular Pathology, NY Hosp-Cornell Med Ctr 1985; **Fac Appt:** Prof TS, Hofstra N Shore-LIJ Sch Med

Griffith, Bartley MD [T&CS] - **Spec Exp:** Transplant-Heart & Lung; Aneurysm-Aortic; Heart Valve Surgery; **Hospital:** Univ of MD Med Ctr; **Address:** Univ Maryland, Div Cardiac Surg, 110 S Paca St Fl 7, Baltimore, MD 21201; **Phone:** 410-328-3822; **Board Cert:** Thoracic Surgery 2001; **Med School:** Jefferson Med Coll 1974; **Resid:** Surgery, Univ Hlth Ctr Hosps 1979; Thoracic Surgery, Univ Hlth Ctr Hosps 1981; **Fellow:** Research, Univ Hlth Ctr Hosps 1978; **Fac Appt:** Prof S, Univ MD Sch Med

Grossi, Eugene A MD [T&CS] - **Spec Exp:** Minimally Invasive Cardiac Surgery; Mitral Valve Surgery; Cardiac Tumors, Myxomas; **Hospital:** NYU Langone Med Ctr (page 68); **Address:** NYU Langone Med Ctr, 530 1st Ave, Ste 9V, New York, NY 10016-6402; **Phone:** 212-263-7452; **Board Cert:** Thoracic Surgery 2011; **Med School:** Columbia P&S 1981; **Resid:** Surgery, NYU Med Ctr 1987; Thoracic Surgery, NYU Med Ctr 1991; **Fac Appt:** Prof S, NYU Sch Med

Guy, T Sloane MD [T&CS] - **Spec Exp:** Robotic Cardiac Surgery; Minimally Invasive Heart Valve Surgery; **Hospital:** Temple Univ Hosp; **Address:** Parkinson Pavillion, Fl 9, 3401 Broad St, Philadelphia, PA 19140; **Phone:** 215-707-3601 x1; **Board Cert:** Surgery 2011; Thoracic & Cardiac Surgery 2005; **Med School:** Univ Pennsylvania 1994; **Resid:** Surgery, Hosp Univ Penn 2002; **Fellow:** Thoracic & Cardiac Surgery, Hosp Univ Penn 2004; **Fac Appt:** Assoc Prof S, Temple Univ

Hargrove III, W Clark MD [T&CS] - **Spec Exp:** Mitral Valve Robotic Surgery; Heart Valve Surgery; Minimally Invasive Cardiac Surgery; **Hospital:** Penn Presby Med Ctr - UPHS (page 72); **Address:** Philadelphia Heart Inst, 51 N 39th St, Ste 2A, Philadelphia, PA 19104; **Phone:** 215-662-9595; **Board Cert:** Thoracic Surgery 2004; **Med School:** Wake Forest Univ 1973; **Resid:** Surgery, Hosp Univ Penn 1979; Cardiothoracic Surgery, Hosp Univ Penn 1984; **Fellow:** Vascular Surgery, Hosp Univ Penn 1981; **Fac Appt:** Clin Prof S, Univ Pennsylvania

Heitmiller, Richard F MD [T&CS] - **Spec Exp:** Esophageal Cancer; Lung Cancer; **Hospital:** Union Meml Hosp-Baltimore; **Address:** Union Memorial Hosp, 3333 N Calvert St, Ste 610, Baltimore, MD 21218-2867; **Phone:** 410-554-2063; **Board Cert:** Thoracic & Cardiac Surgery 2008; **Med School:** Johns Hopkins Univ 1979; **Resid:** Surgery, Mass Genl Hosp 1985; **Fellow:** Thoracic Surgery, Mass Genl Hosp 1987; **Fac Appt:** Assoc Prof Surg & Onc, Johns Hopkins Univ

Horvath, Keith MD [T&CS] - **Spec Exp:** Minimally Invasive Cardiac Surgery; Heart Valve Surgery; Heart Laser Revascularization; **Hospital:** Suburban Hosp, Johns Hopkins Hosp (page 61); **Address:** Suburban Hospital, 8600 Old Georgetown Rd, Bethesda, MD 20814; **Phone:** 301-896-7610; **Board Cert:** Thoracic Surgery 2005; **Med School:** Univ Chicago-Pritzker Sch Med 1987; **Resid:** Surgery, Brigham & Women's Hosp 1994; Brigham & Women's Hosp 1996; **Fellow:** Research, Mass Genl Hosp 1991; **Fac Appt:** Assoc Prof S, Northwestern Univ

Isom, O Wayne MD [T&CS] - **Spec Exp:** Cardiac Surgery; Coronary Artery Surgery; Heart Valve Surgery; **Hospital:** NY-Presby/Weill Cornell Med Ctr, NY (page 66), NY Hosp Queens; **Address:** 525 E 68th St, rm M-404, New York, NY 10065; **Phone:** 212-746-5151; **Board Cert:** Surgery 1971; Thoracic Surgery 1972; **Med School:** Univ Tex, Houston 1965; **Resid:** Surgery, Parkland Meml Hosp 1970; **Fellow:** Thoracic Surgery, NYU Med Ctr 1972; **Fac Appt:** Prof TS, Cornell Univ-Weill Med Coll

Thoracic & Cardiac Surgery

Jonas, Richard A MD [T&CS] - **Spec Exp:** Pediatric Cardiothoracic Surgery; Congenital Heart Disease; **Hospital:** Chldns Natl Med Ctr, Georgetown Univ Hosp; **Address:** 111 Michigan Ave NW, Washington, DC 20010; **Phone:** 202-476-2811; **Med School:** Australia 1974; **Resid:** Surgery, Royal Melbourne Hosp 1979; Thoracic Surgery, Green Lane Hosp 1982; **Fellow:** Thoracic Surgery, Brigham & Women's Hosp 1984; **Fac Appt:** Prof S, Geo Wash Univ

Kaiser, Larry R MD [T&CS] - **Spec Exp:** Lung Cancer; Esophageal Cancer; Mediastinal Tumors; Myasthenia Gravis; **Hospital:** Temple Univ Hosp; **Address:** Temple Univ Sch Medicine, 3500 N Broad St, MERB-11th Fl, Philadelphia, PA 19140; **Phone:** 215-707-8773; **Board Cert:** Surgery 2005; Thoracic Surgery 2006; **Med School:** Tulane Univ 1977; **Resid:** Surgery, UCLA Med Ctr 1983; Cardiothoracic Surgery, Univ Toronto Hosps 1985; **Fellow:** Surgical Oncology, UCLA 1981; **Fac Appt:** Prof TS, Temple Univ

Kanda, Louis T MD [T&CS] - **Spec Exp:** Heart Valve Surgery; **Hospital:** Washington Hosp Ctr; **Address:** 110 Irving St NW, Ste 1041, Washington, DC 20010; **Phone:** 202-877-5039; **Board Cert:** Thoracic Surgery 2002; **Med School:** Geo Wash Univ 1970; **Resid:** Surgery, Washington Hosp Ctr 1975; **Fellow:** Cardiothoracic Surgery, Cleveland Clin Fdn 1980; **Fac Appt:** Asst Prof S, Howard Univ

Keenan, Robert J MD [T&CS] - **Spec Exp:** Lung Cancer; Esophageal Cancer; Mediastinal Tumors; Emphysema-Lung Volume Reduction; **Hospital:** Allegheny General Hosp, West Penn Hosp-Forbes Campus; **Address:** Center for Thoracic Surgery, Allegheny Cancer Ctr, Ste 363, 320 E North Ave, Pittsburgh, PA 15212; **Phone:** 412-359-6137; **Board Cert:** Surgery 2009; **Med School:** Univ Alberta 1984; **Resid:** Surgery, Univ Toronto Affil Hosp 1989; **Fellow:** Thoracic Surgery, Univ Pittsburgh 1990; Thoracic Surgery, Univ Toronto 1992; **Fac Appt:** Prof TS, Drexel Univ Coll Med

Keller, Steven M MD [T&CS] - **Spec Exp:** Lung Cancer; Esophageal Cancer; Mediastinal Tumors; Hyperhidrosis-Palmar; **Hospital:** Montefiore Med Ctr-Moses Campus, NY, Montefiore Med Ctr-Einstein Campus, NY; **Address:** Montefiore-Einstein Medical Ctr, 1575 Blondell Ave, Ste 125, Bronx, NY 10461; **Phone:** 718-405-8378; **Board Cert:** Thoracic Surgery 2007; **Med School:** Albany Med Coll 1977; **Resid:** Surgery, Mount Sinai Hosp 1985; Thoracic Surgery, Mem Sloan Kettering Cancer Ctr 1987; **Fellow:** Surgical Oncology, NIH/National Cancer Inst 1983; **Fac Appt:** Prof TS, Albert Einstein Coll Med

Kiev, Jonathan MD [T&CS] - **Spec Exp:** Chest Wall Tumors; Esophageal Cancer; Lung Cancer; **Hospital:** Cabell Huntington Hosp; **Address:** Cabell Huntington Hosp, Thoracic Surg, 1600 Medical Ctr Drive, Ste 2500, Huntington, WV 25701; **Phone:** 304-691-1200; **Board Cert:** Surgery 2005; Thoracic Surgery 2010; **Med School:** Tulane Univ 1989; **Resid:** Surgery, Hahnemann Univ Hosp 1996; Cardiothoracic Surgery, Loma Linda Univ 2000; **Fellow:** Thoracic Surgery, Univ Pittsburgh 2001; Thoracic Surgery, Mayo Clinic 2001

Kormos, Robert MD [T&CS] - **Spec Exp:** Transplant-Heart; Artificial Heart Devices; **Hospital:** UPMC Presby, Pittsburgh; **Address:** UPMC Presby Hosp, 200 Lothrop, Ste C714, Pittsburgh, PA 15213; **Phone:** 412-648-6259; **Med School:** Univ Western Ontario 1976; **Resid:** Surgery, Toronto Western Hosp 1980; Cardiothoracic Surgery, Toronto Genl Hosp/Hosp for Sick Chldn 1983; **Fellow:** Transplant Surgery, Univ Pittsburgh Med Ctr 1987; **Fac Appt:** Prof S, Univ Pittsburgh

Krellenstein, Daniel J MD/PhD [T&CS] - **Spec Exp:** Lung Cancer; Minimally Invasive Thoracic Surgery; Asbestos-related Lung Disease; **Hospital:** Mount Sinai Med Ctr (page 64), Lenox Hill Hosp (page 67); **Address:** 16 E 98th St, Ste 1F, New York, NY 10029-6545; **Phone:** 212-423-9311; **Board Cert:** Surgery 1974; Thoracic & Cardiac Surgery 2006; **Med School:** SUNY Buffalo 1964; **Resid:** Surgery, SUNY Downstate Med Ctr 1971; **Fellow:** Thoracic & Cardiac Surgery, Kings County Hosp Ctr 1972; **Fac Appt:** Assoc Clin Prof TS, Mount Sinai Sch Med

Krieger, Karl H MD [T&CS] - **Spec Exp:** Heart Valve Surgery; Coronary Artery Surgery; Cardiac Surgery-Adult; **Hospital:** NY-Presby/Weill Cornell Med Ctr, NY (page 66), NY Hosp Queens; **Address:** Cardiothoracic Surgery Dept, 525 E 68th St, Ste M404, New York, NY 10065; **Phone:** 212-746-5152; **Board Cert:** Thoracic Surgery 2004; **Med School:** Johns Hopkins Univ 1975; **Resid:** Surgery, Johns Hopkins 1976; Bellevue Hosp 1979; **Fellow:** Thoracic Surgery, NYU Med Ctr 1981; **Fac Appt:** Prof S, Cornell Univ-Weill Med Coll

Kucharczuk, John C MD [T&CS] - **Spec Exp:** Lung Cancer; Esophageal Cancer; Chest Wall Tumors; Mediastinal Tumors; **Hospital:** Hosp Univ Penn - UPHS (page 72); **Address:** 3400 Spruce St, 6 White Bldg, Philadelphia, PA 19104; **Phone:** 215-662-4988; **Board Cert:** Surgery 2008; Thoracic Surgery 2010; **Med School:** Univ Pennsylvania 1992; **Resid:** Surgery, Hosp Univ Penn 1999; **Fellow:** Cardiothoracic Surgery, Hosp Univ Penn 2001; **Fac Appt:** Assoc Prof S, Univ Pennsylvania

Landreneau, Rodney J MD [T&CS] - **Spec Exp:** Lung Cancer; Esophageal Cancer; Mesothelioma; Video Assisted Thoracic Surgery (VATS); **Hospital:** UPMC Shadyside; **Address:** Lung Center at UPMC Shadyside, 5200 Centre Ave, Ste 715, Pittsburgh, PA 15232; **Phone:** 412-623-3859; **Board Cert:** Thoracic & Cardiac Surgery 2005; **Med School:** Louisiana State U, New Orleans 1978; **Resid:** Surgery, Parkland Meml Hosp 1983; **Fellow:** Cardiothoracic Surgery, Univ Mich 1985; **Fac Appt:** Prof S, Univ Pittsburgh

Lang, Samuel J MD [T&CS] - **Spec Exp:** Minimally Invasive Cardiac Surgery; Heart Valve Surgery; Cardiothoracic Surgery; **Hospital:** NY Hosp Queens; **Address:** 56-45 Main St, rm 387, Flushing, NY 11355; **Phone:** 718-670-1137; **Board Cert:** Thoracic Surgery 2006; **Med School:** Univ Alabama 1978; **Resid:** Surgery, UCLA Med Ctr 1982; Thoracic Surgery, NYU Med Ctr 1983; **Fellow:** Cardiothoracic Surgery, UCLA Med Ctr 1985; Pediatric Cardiac Surgery, Hosp for Sick Chldn 1986

Lansman, Steven L MD/PhD [T&CS] - **Spec Exp:** Coronary Artery Surgery; Heart Valve Surgery; Ventricular Assist Device (LVAD); Transplant-Heart; **Hospital:** Westchester Med Ctr; **Address:** Westchester Medical Ctr, 100 Woods Rd, Macy Pavilion, rm 114W, Valhalla, NY 10595; **Phone:** 914-493-8793; **Board Cert:** Thoracic Surgery 2004; **Med School:** SUNY Hlth Sci Ctr 1977; **Resid:** Surgery, Montefiore Med Ctr 1982; **Fellow:** Thoracic Surgery, Univ Hosp 1984; **Fac Appt:** Prof S, NY Med Coll

Lazzaro, Richard S MD [T&CS] - **Spec Exp:** Robotic Surgery; Minimally Invasive Surgery; Thoracic Surgery; **Hospital:** Lenox Hill Hosp (page 67), N Shore Univ Hosp (page 67); **Address:** Lenox Hill Hospital, Dept Cardiothoracic Surgery, 130 E 77th St, Black Hall-4th Fl, New York, NY 10075; **Phone:** 212-434-3000; **Board Cert:** Surgery 2006; Thoracic & Cardiac Surgery 2007; **Med School:** Albany Med Coll 1988; **Resid:** Surgery, North Shore Univ Hosp 1994; **Fellow:** Cardiothoracic Surgery, SUNY Downstate Med Ctr 1997; Thoracic Surgery, Univ Pittsburgh 1998

Loulmet, Didier F MD [T&CS] - **Spec Exp:** Heart Valve Surgery; Robotic Cardiac Surgery; Minimally Invasive Cardiac Surgery; Aneurysm-Aortic; **Hospital:** NYU Langone Med Ctr (page 68); **Address:** NYU Medical Ctr, Cardiothoracic Surgery, 530 1st Ave, Ste 9V, New York, NY 10016; **Phone:** 212-263-2329; **Med School:** France 1984; **Resid:** Cardiothoracic Surgery, Paris Univ Hosp 1990; Cardiothoracic Surgery, Brigham & Women's Hosp 1991; **Fellow:** Pediatric Cardiac Surgery, Children's Hosp 1992; **Fac Appt:** Assoc Prof TS, NYU Sch Med

Magovern Jr, George J MD [T&CS] - **Spec Exp:** Cardiac Surgery; Ventricular Assist Device (LVAD); **Hospital:** Allegheny General Hosp; **Address:** Cardiovascular Surgery Ctr, CVI-1, 320 E North Ave, NW Wing-Snyder Pavilion, Allegheny Genl Hosp, Pittsburgh, PA 15212; **Phone:** 412-359-8820; **Board Cert:** Thoracic Surgery 2005; **Med School:** Univ Pittsburgh 1978; **Resid:** Surgery, Johns Hopkins Hosp 1981; Cardiovascular Surgery, Johns Hopkins Hosp 1985; **Fac Appt:** Prof S, Drexel Univ Coll Med

Marshall, M Blair MD [T&CS] - **Spec Exp:** Lung Cancer; Esophageal Cancer; Thymoma; Chest Wall Tumors; **Hospital:** Georgetown Univ Hosp, Sibley Mem Hosp; **Address:** Georgetown Univ Hosp, Dept Thoracic Surg, 3800 Reservoir Rd NW, 4PHC, Washington, DC 20007; **Phone:** 202-444-5045; **Board Cert:** Surgery 2009; Thoracic Surgery 2010; **Med School:** Georgetown Univ 1991; **Resid:** Surgery, Georgetown Univ Med Ctr 1995; Cardiothoracic Surgery, Hosp Univ Penn 2001; **Fellow:** Research, Chldn's Hosp 1998; **Fac Appt:** Assoc Prof S, Georgetown Univ

Morris, Rohinton J MD [T&CS] - **Spec Exp:** Transplant-Heart; Ventricular Assist Device (LVAD); Coronary Artery Surgery; **Hospital:** Abington Mem Hosp; **Address:** Abington Memorial Hospital, Toll Bldg Fl 5, 1200 Old York Rd, Abington, PA 19001; **Phone:** 215-481-4200; **Board Cert:** Thoracic Surgery 2003; **Med School:** Hahnemann Univ 1984; **Resid:** Surgery, Hahnemann Univ Hosp 1989; Thoracic Surgery, Hahnemann Univ Hosp 1992; **Fac Appt:** Assoc Clin Prof S, Univ Pennsylvania

Naka, Yoshifumi MD/PhD [T&CS] - **Spec Exp:** Transplant-Heart & Lung; Ventricular Assist Device (LVAD); Heart Failure & Ventricular Containment; Mitral Valve Surgery; **Hospital:** NY-Presby/Columbia Univ Med Ctr, NY (page 66); **Address:** 177 Fort Washington Ave, MHB Bldg Fl 7 - rm 435, New York, NY 10032; **Phone:** 212-305-0828; **Med School:** Japan 1984; **Resid:** Surgery, Osaka Police Hosp 1991; **Fellow:** Cardiovascular Surgery, Osaka Police Hosp 1993; Cardiothoracic Surgery, Columbia Univ Med Ctr 1998; **Fac Appt:** Asst Prof S, Columbia P&S

Oz, Mehmet C MD [T&CS] - **Spec Exp:** Transplant-Heart; Heart Valve Surgery; Minimally Invasive Cardiac Surgery; **Hospital:** NY-Presby/Columbia Univ Med Ctr, NY (page 66); **Address:** NY Presby Hosp, Dept Cardiothoracic Surg, 177 Ft Washington Ave, MHB- Rm 7, GN435, New York, NY 10032; **Phone:** 212-305-4434; **Board Cert:** Thoracic Surgery 2003; **Med School:** Univ Pennsylvania 1986; **Resid:** Surgery, Columbia Presby Med Ctr 1991; **Fellow:** Cardiothoracic Surgery, Columbia Presby Med Ctr 1993; **Fac Appt:** Prof S, Columbia P&S

Park, Bernard J MD [T&CS] - **Spec Exp:** Lung Cancer; Esophageal Cancer; Mediastinal Tumors; Robotic Surgery; **Hospital:** Hackensack Univ Med Ctr; **Address:** 30 Prospect Ave, Ste 5640, Hackensack, NJ 07601; **Phone:** 551-996-4218; **Board Cert:** Surgery 2011; Thoracic Surgery 2003; **Med School:** Univ Pennsylvania 1993; **Resid:** Surgery, New York Hosp 1996; Surgery, New York Hosp 2000; **Fellow:** Cardiothoracic Surgery, NY Presby/Cornell 2002; Thoracic Surgery, Meml Sloan Kettering Cancer Ctr 2002; **Fac Appt:** Asst Clin Prof TS, UMDNJ-NJ Med Sch, Newark

Pass, Harvey I MD [T&CS] - **Spec Exp:** Lung Cancer; Mesothelioma; Clinical Trials; Robotic Surgery; **Hospital:** NYU Langone Med Ctr (page 68); **Address:** NYU Cancer Ctr, 160 E 34th St, Fl 8, New York, NY 10016; **Phone:** 212-731-5414; **Board Cert:** Thoracic & Cardiac Surgery 2001; **Med School:** Duke Univ 1973; **Resid:** Surgery, Duke Univ Med Ctr 1975; Surgery, Univ Miss Med Ctr 1980; **Fellow:** Cardiothoracic Surgery, MUSC Med Ctr 1982; Thoracic Oncology, Natl Cancer Inst 1985; **Fac Appt:** Prof T&CS, NYU Sch Med

Pechet, Taine MD [T&CS] - **Spec Exp:** Lung Cancer; Lung Surgery; Video Assisted Thoracic Surgery (VATS); Palliative Care; **Hospital:** Penn Presby Med Ctr - UPHS (page 72); **Address:** Penn Presby Med Ctr, Wright-Saunders, Ste 266, 51 N 39th St, Philadelphia, PA 19104; **Phone:** 215-662-9195; **Board Cert:** Surgery 2009; Thoracic Surgery 2002; **Med School:** Harvard Med Sch 1992; **Resid:** Surgery, Brigham & Women's Hosp 2000; **Fellow:** Thoracic Surgery, Barnes-Jewish Hosp 2002; **Fac Appt:** Assoc Clin Prof S, Univ Pennsylvania

Pierson III, Richard N MD [T&CS] - **Spec Exp:** Transplant-Lung; Lung Cancer; Transplant-Heart; **Hospital:** Univ of MD Med Ctr, VA Med Ctr - Washington; **Address:** UMMC-Dept Cardiothoracic Surg, 419 W Redwood St, Ste 300, Baltimore, MD 21201; **Phone:** 410-328-5842; **Board Cert:** Surgery 2011; Thoracic Surgery 2002; **Med School:** Columbia P&S 1983; **Resid:** Surgery, Univ Mich Med Ctr 1990; **Fellow:** Cardiothoracic Surgery, Mass Genl Hosp 1992; **Fac Appt:** Assoc Prof TS, Univ MD Sch Med

Rosengart, Todd MD [T&CS] - **Spec Exp:** Transfusion Free Surgery; Gene Therapy-Cardiac Angiogenesis; Minimally Invasive Surgery; Cardiac Surgery; **Hospital:** Stony Brook Univ Med Ctr; **Address:** Stonybrook Univ Hosp, Health Sci Ctr, Cardiothoracic Surgery, HSC-T19, rm 020, Stonybrook, NY 11794-0001; **Phone:** 631-444-7875; **Board Cert:** Surgery 2010; Thoracic Surgery 2001; **Med School:** Northwestern Univ 1983; **Resid:** Surgery, NYU Med Ctr 1985; Surgery, NYU Med Ctr 1989; **Fellow:** Thoracic Surgery, Natl Inst Hlth 1987; Cardiothoracic Surgery, NY-Cornell Med Ctr 1991; **Fac Appt:** Prof S, SUNY Stony Brook

Rusch, Valerie MD [T&CS] - **Spec Exp:** Mesothelioma; Lung Cancer; Esophageal Cancer; **Hospital:** Meml Sloan-Kettering Cancer Ctr; **Address:** 1275 York Ave, New York, NY 10021-6094; **Phone:** 212-639-5873; **Board Cert:** Surgery 2011; Thoracic Surgery 2003; **Med School:** Columbia P&S 1975; **Resid:** Surgery, Univ Wash Med Ctr 1980; Cardiothoracic Surgery, Univ Wash Med Ctr 1982; **Fac Appt:** Prof TS, Cornell Univ-Weill Med Coll

Samuels, Louis E MD [T&CS] - **Spec Exp:** Transplant-Heart; Artificial Heart Devices; Ventricular Assist Device (LVAD); **Hospital:** Paoli Hosp, Bryn Mawr Hosp; **Address:** Main Line Cardiothoracic Surgery, 830 Old Lancaster Rd, MOB North, Ste 210, Bryn Mawr, PA 19010; **Phone:** 610-527-1600; **Board Cert:** Thoracic & Cardiac Surgery 2005; **Med School:** Hahnemann Univ 1987; **Resid:** Surgery, Hahnemann Hosp 1992; Thoracic Surgery, Hahnemann Hosp 1995; **Fac Appt:** Prof S, Hahnemann Univ

Scott, Walter J MD [T&CS] - **Spec Exp:** Lung Cancer; Esophageal Cancer; Mediastinal Tumors; Video Assisted Thoracic Surgery (VATS); **Hospital:** Fox Chase Cancer Ctr (page 58); **Address:** Fox Chase Cancer Ctr, 333 Cottman Ave, rm C308, Philadelphia, PA 19111; **Phone:** 215-214-1427; **Board Cert:** Thoracic & Cardiac Surgery 2010; **Med School:** Univ Chicago-Pritzker Sch Med 1981; **Resid:** Surgery, Univ Chicago Med Ctr 1987; **Fellow:** Cardiothoracic Surgery, Univ Chicago 1989

Smith, Craig R MD [T&CS] - **Spec Exp:** Mitral Valve Surgery; Transplant-Heart; Minimally Invasive Cardiac Surgery; Robotic Cardiac Surgery; **Hospital:** NY-Presby/Columbia Univ Med Ctr, NY (page 66); **Address:** Columbia Presbyterian Med Ctr, 177 Fort Washington Ave Fl 7 - Ste 435, New York, NY 10032; **Phone:** 212-305-8312; **Board Cert:** Thoracic Surgery 2004; **Med School:** Case West Res Univ 1977; **Resid:** Surgery, Strong Meml Hosp 1982; **Fellow:** Cardiothoracic Surgery, Columbia Presby Med Ctr 1984; **Fac Appt:** Prof S, Columbia P&S

Soberman, Mark S MD [T&CS] - **Spec Exp:** Thoracic Cancers; Lung Cancer; Esophageal Cancer; Esophageal Surgery; **Hospital:** Frederick Mem Hospital; **Address:** 501 W 7th St, Ste D, Frederick, MD 21701; **Phone:** 301-694-5861; **Board Cert:** Thoracic & Cardiac Surgery 2003; **Med School:** Emory Univ 1983; **Resid:** Surgery, Emory Univ Hosp 1990; Cardiothoracic Surgery, George Wash Univ Hosp 1992; **Fellow:** Thoracic & Cardiac Surgery, Cleveland Clinic 1992; 1993; **Fac Appt:** Assoc Clin Prof T&CS, Georgetown Univ

Sonett, Joshua R MD [T&CS] - **Spec Exp:** Minimally Invasive Thoracic Surgery; Transplant-Lung; Thoracic Cancers; Emphysema-Lung Volume Reduction; **Hospital:** NY-Presby/Columbia Univ Med Ctr, NY (page 66); **Address:** 161 Fort Washington Ave, Ste 301, New York, NY 10032; **Phone:** 212-305-8086; **Board Cert:** Surgery 2004; Thoracic Surgery 2007; **Med School:** E Carolina Univ 1988; **Resid:** Surgery, Univ Mass Med Ctr 1993; **Fellow:** Cardiothoracic Surgery, Univ Pittsburgh Med Ctr 1994; Thoracic Surgery, Meml Sloan Kettering Cancer Ctr; **Fac Appt:** Prof S, Columbia P&S

Thoracic & Cardiac Surgery

Spray, Thomas L MD [T&CS] - **Spec Exp:** Cardiac Surgery-Adult & Pediatric; Transplant-Heart & Lung; Neonatal & Infant Cardiac Surgery; Congenital Heart Disease-Adult; **Hospital:** Chldns Hosp of Philadelphia, Hosp Univ Penn - UPHS (page 72); **Address:** Childrens Hosp, Div Cardiothoracic Surg, 34th St & Civic Ctr Blvd, Ste 12NW10, Philadelphia, PA 19104; **Phone:** 215-590-2708; **Board Cert:** Thoracic Surgery 2004; Congenital Cardiac Surgery 2009; **Med School:** Duke Univ 1973; **Resid:** Surgery, Duke Univ Med Ctr 1975; Cardiothoracic Surgery, Duke Univ Med Ctr 1983; **Fac Appt:** Prof S, Univ Pennsylvania

Stewart, Allan MD [T&CS] - **Spec Exp:** Heart Valve Surgery-Aortic; Aneurysm-Aortic; Aortic Surgery; **Hospital:** NY-Presby/Columbia Univ Med Ctr, NY (page 66); **Address:** 177 Fort Washington Ave, Milstein Hosp Bldg Fl 7 - rm 435, New York, NY 10030; **Phone:** 212-305-4980; **Board Cert:** Surgery 2003; Thoracic Surgery 2006; **Med School:** UMDNJ-NJ Med Sch, Newark 1995; **Resid:** Surgery, Univ PA Hlth Sys 2002; **Fellow:** Thoracic Surgery, NY Presby Hosp 2004; **Fac Appt:** Asst Prof TS, Columbia P&S

Swistel, Daniel MD [T&CS] - **Spec Exp:** Coronary Artery Surgery; Minimally Invasive Surgery; Heart Valve Surgery; Hypertrophic Cardiomyopathy; **Hospital:** St. Luke's - Roosevelt Hosp Ctr - St Luke's Hosp (page 56); **Address:** 1111 Amsterdam Ave, MU 2 Section A, New York, NY 10025; **Phone:** 212-523-4088; **Board Cert:** Thoracic Surgery 2006; **Med School:** UMDNJ-RW Johnson Med Sch 1979; **Resid:** Surgery, St Lukes-Roosevelt Hosp 1984; Cardiothoracic Surgery, Montefiore Med Ctr 1986; **Fac Appt:** Assoc Clin Prof TS, Columbia P&S

Szeto, Wilson Y MD [T&CS] - **Spec Exp:** Thoracic Aortic Surgery; Heart Valve Disease; Ventricular Assist Device (VAD); Endovascular Stent Grafts; **Hospital:** Penn Presby Med Ctr - UPHS (page 72), Hosp Univ Penn - UPHS (page 72); **Address:** Hosp Univ Pennsylvania, 3400 Spruce St, 6 Silverstein Pavilion, Philadelphia, PA 19104; **Phone:** 215-615-1642; **Board Cert:** Surgery 2004; Thoracic Surgery 2006; **Med School:** Med Coll VA 1996; **Resid:** Surgery, Hosp U Penn 2002; **Fellow:** Thoracic & Cardiac Surgery, Hosp U Penn 2004; **Fac Appt:** Assoc Prof S, Univ Pennsylvania

Toyoda, Yoshiya MD/PhD [T&CS] - **Spec Exp:** Cardiothoracic Surgery; Transplant-Heart; Heart Valve Surgery; Coronary Artery Surgery; **Hospital:** Temple University Hosp-Episcopal Campus; **Address:** Parkinson Pavilion, Zone C, 3401 N Broad St, Ste 301, Philadelphia, PA 19140; **Phone:** 215-707-3601; **Med School:** Japan 1990; **Resid:** Surgery, Kobe Univ Hosp 1994; Cardiothoracic Surgery, Kove Univ Hosp 1997; **Fellow:** Cardiothoracic Research, Harvard Med School 2001; Cardiovascular Surgery, Havard Univ Affil Hosp 2004; **Fac Appt:** Assoc Prof S, Univ Pittsburgh

Tranbaugh, Robert MD [T&CS] - **Spec Exp:** Coronary Artery Surgery; Heart Valve Surgery; Aneurysm-Thoracic Aortic; **Hospital:** Beth Israel Med Ctr - Petrie Division (page 56), St. Luke's - Roosevelt Hosp Ctr - Roosevelt Div (page 56); **Address:** 317 E 17th St, Fl 11, Division of Cardiac Surgery, Beth Israel Medical Center, New York, NY 10003; **Phone:** 212-420-2584; **Board Cert:** Thoracic Surgery 2004; **Med School:** Univ Pennsylvania 1976; **Resid:** Surgery, UCSF Med Ctr 1983; Cardiothoracic Surgery, UCSF Med Ctr 1985; **Fac Appt:** Assoc Prof T&CS, Albert Einstein Coll Med

Watson, Thomas J MD [T&CS] - **Spec Exp:** Esophageal Cancer; Gastroesophageal Reflux Disease (GERD); Lung Cancer; **Hospital:** Univ of Rochester Strong Meml Hosp, Highland Hosp of Rochester; **Address:** 601 Elmwood Ave, Box SURG, Rochester, NY 14642; **Phone:** 585-275-1509; **Board Cert:** Surgery 2003; Thoracic Surgery 2007; **Med School:** USC-Keck School of Medicine 1988; **Resid:** Surgery, LAC-USC Med Ctr 1993; Cardiothoracic Surgery, LAC-USC Med Ctr 1996; **Fellow:** Esophageal Surgery, LAC-USC Med Ctr 1994; **Fac Appt:** Assoc Prof S, Univ Rochester

Weksler, Benny MD [T&CS] - **Spec Exp:** Minimally Invasive Thoracic Surgery; Lung Cancer; Esophageal Cancer; Thymoma; **Hospital:** UPMC Presby, Pittsburgh, VA Pittsburgh Hlth Care Sys-Univ Dr; **Address:** 200 Lothrop St, PUH Bldg - Fl C800, Pittsburgh, PA 15213; **Phone:** 412-648-6271; **Board Cert:** Surgery 2007; Thoracic & Cardiac Surgery 2007; **Med School:** Brazil 1987; **Resid:** Surgery, Lincoln Med Ctr 1995; Research, Meml Sloan Kettering Cancer Ctr 1993; **Fellow:** Cardiothoracic Surgery, New York Hosp/MSK Cancer Ctr 1997; Minimally Invasive Surgery, Univ Pittsburgh 2008; **Fac Appt:** Assoc Prof TS, Univ Pittsburgh

Williams, Mathew R MD [T&CS] - **Spec Exp:** Interventional Cardiology; Heart Valve Surgery; **Hospital:** NY-Presby/Columbia Univ Med Ctr, NY (page 66); **Address:** Milstein Hospital Bldg Fl 7 - rm 435, 177 Fort Washington Ave, New York, NY 10032; **Phone:** 212-305-9320; **Board Cert:** Thoracic Surgery 2007; **Med School:** Columbia P&S 1996; **Resid:** Surgery, UCLA Med Ctr 1998; Surgery, NY Presby Hosp/Columbia 2003; **Fellow:** Cardiothoracic Surgery, NY Presby Hosp/Columbia 2005; Interventional Cardiology, NY Presby Hosp/Columbia 2006; **Fac Appt:** Asst Prof S, Columbia P&S

Woo, Y Joseph MD [T&CS] - **Spec Exp:** Minimally Invasive Cardiac Surgery; Robotic Cardiac Surgery; Aneurysm-Abdominal & Thoracic Aortic; Mitral Valve Robotic Surgery; **Hospital:** Hosp Univ Penn - UPHS (page 72); **Address:** Univ Penn Dept Surgery, 3400 Spruce St, 6 Silverstein, Philadelphia, PA 19104; **Phone:** 215-662-2956; **Board Cert:** Surgery 2009; Thoracic & Cardiac Surgery 2010; **Med School:** Univ Pennsylvania 1992; **Resid:** Surgery, Hosp Univ Penn 1998; Thoracic Surgery, Hosp Univ Penn 2001; **Fac Appt:** Assoc Prof S, Univ Pennsylvania

Yang, Stephen C MD [T&CS] - **Spec Exp:** Mesothelioma; Lung Cancer; Esophageal Cancer; Robotic Surgery; **Hospital:** Johns Hopkins Hosp (page 61), Johns Hopkins Bayview Med Ctr (page 61); **Address:** Johns Hopkins Hosp, 600 N Wolfe St Blalock Bldg - rm 240, Baltimore, MD 21287; **Phone:** 410-933-1233; **Board Cert:** Surgery 2003; Thoracic Surgery 2005; **Med School:** Med Coll VA 1984; **Resid:** Surgery, Univ Tex Hlth Sci Ctr 1990; **Fellow:** Thoracic Surgery, MD Anderson Cancer Ctr 1992; Cardiothoracic Surgery, Med Coll Virginia 1994; **Fac Appt:** Assoc Prof TS, Johns Hopkins Univ

Southeast

Athanasuleas, Constantine MD [T&CS] - **Spec Exp:** Cardiac Surgery; Heart Failure; **Hospital:** Univ of Ala Hosp at Birmingham; **Address:** 1900 University Blvd, Tinsley Harrison Tower 720, Birmingham, AL 35294; **Phone:** 205-934-2536; **Board Cert:** Thoracic & Cardiac Surgery 2006; **Med School:** Univ Chicago-Pritzker Sch Med 1975; **Resid:** Surgery, Stanford Univ Med Ctr 1980; Thoracic & Cardiac Surgery, Stanford Univ Med Ctr 1982; **Fac Appt:** Prof S, Univ Alabama

Bichell, David P MD [T&CS] - **Spec Exp:** Cardiac Surgery-Neonatal; Cardiac Surgery-Pediatric; Congenital Heart Surgery; Minimally Invasive Cardiac Surgery; **Hospital:** Vanderbilt Monroe Carrell Jr. Chldn's Hosp (page 75), Vanderbilt Univ Med Ctr (page 75); **Address:** Vanderbilt Childrens Hosp, Div Pediatric Cardiac Surgery, 2200 Childrens Way, 5247 DOT, Nashville, TN 37232-9292; **Phone:** 615-343-6525; **Board Cert:** Thoracic Surgery 2006; **Med School:** Columbia P&S 1987; **Resid:** Surgery, Barnes Jewish Hosp 1994; Cardiothoracic Surgery, Brigham & Womens Hosp/Chldns Hosp 1996; **Fellow:** Cardiac Surgery, Brigham & Womens Hosp 1997; **Fac Appt:** Prof TS, Vanderbilt Univ

Bridges, Charles R MD [T&CS] - **Spec Exp:** Minimally Invasive Cardiac Surgery; Maze Procedure for Atrial Fibrillation; Aneurysm-Aortic; Heart Valve Surgery; **Hospital:** Carolinas Med Ctr-Univ, Carolinas Med Ctr-Pineville; **Address:** Sanger Heart & Vascular Inst, 1001 Blythe Blvd Fl 3 - Ste 300, Charlotte, NC 28203; **Phone:** 704-373-0212; **Board Cert:** Surgery 2003; Thoracic Surgery 2004; **Med School:** Harvard Med Sch 1981; **Resid:** Internal Medicine, Brigham & Women's Hosp 1984; Surgery, Hosp Univ Penn 1991; **Fellow:** Cardiothoracic Surgery, Hosp Univ Penn 1993; **Fac Appt:** Clin Prof T&CS, Univ NC Sch Med

Brunsting III, Louis A MD [T&CS] - **Spec Exp:** Robotic Cardiac Surgery; **Hospital:** Univ of Ala Hosp at Birmingham; **Address:** UAB, The Kirklin Clinic, 2000 6th Ave S, Birmingham, AL 35233; **Phone:** 205-934-3853; **Board Cert:** Thoracic Surgery 2011; **Med School:** UCSD 1983; **Resid:** Surgery, Univ Rochester 1985; Surgery, Univ Rochester 1989; **Fellow:** Surgery, Duke Univ 1987; Thoracic Surgery, Duke Univ 1991; **Fac Appt:** Assoc Prof T&CS, Univ Alabama

Burke, Redmond P MD [T&CS] - **Spec Exp:** Pediatric Cardiac Surgery; Congenital Heart Surgery; **Hospital:** Miami Children's Hosp; **Address:** 3200 SW 60th Ct, Ste 102, Miami Children's Hosp, Miami, FL 33155; **Phone:** 305-663-8401; **Board Cert:** Thoracic Surgery 2001; Surgery 2002; **Med School:** Harvard Med Sch 1984; **Resid:** Surgery, Brigham & Women's Hosp 1989; **Fellow:** Research, Brigham & Women's Hosp 1990; Cardiothoracic Surgery, Brigham & Women's Hosp 1992

Byrne, John G MD [T&CS] - **Spec Exp:** Cardiothoracic Surgery; Heart Failure; Heart Valve Surgery; Transplant-Heart; **Hospital:** Vanderbilt Univ Med Ctr (page 75); **Address:** Vanderbilt Heart Inst, 1215 21 Ave S, Ste 5025, MCE-North Tower, Nashville, TN 37232-8802; **Phone:** 615-343-9195; **Board Cert:** Thoracic Surgery 2008; **Med School:** Boston Univ 1987; **Resid:** Surgery, Univ Illinois Affil Hosp 1995; Thoracic Surgery, Brigham & Women's Hosp 1997; **Fellow:** Cardiothoracic Research, Harvard Med School 1992; **Fac Appt:** Prof S, Vanderbilt Univ

Cerfolio, Robert J MD [T&CS] - **Spec Exp:** Lung Cancer; Tracheal Surgery; Chest Wall Tumors; Esophageal Cancer; **Hospital:** Univ of Ala Hosp at Birmingham; **Address:** 703 19th St S, 739 Zeigler Bldg, Birmingham, AL 35294-0007; **Phone:** 205-934-5937; **Board Cert:** Surgery 2003; Thoracic Surgery 2006; **Med School:** Univ Rochester 1988; **Resid:** Surgery, Cornell-NY Hosp 1990; Surgery, Mayo Clinic 1993; **Fellow:** Cardiothoracic Surgery, Mayo Clinic 1996; **Fac Appt:** Prof TS, Univ Alabama

Chitwood Jr, W Randolph MD [T&CS] - **Spec Exp:** Robotic Cardiac Surgery; Minimally Invasive Cardiac Surgery; Heart Valve Surgery; Mitral Valve Surgery; **Hospital:** Univ Hlth Sys-Vidant Med Ctr; **Address:** East Carolina Heart Inst, 115 Heart Drive, rm 3107, Greenville, NC 27834; **Phone:** 252-744-4536; **Board Cert:** Thoracic & Cardiac Surgery 2005; **Med School:** Univ VA Sch Med 1974; **Resid:** Surgery, Duke Univ Med Ctr 1983; **Fellow:** Cardiovascular Surgery, Duke Univ Med Ctr 1984; **Fac Appt:** Prof S, E Carolina Univ

Christian, Karla G MD [T&CS] - **Spec Exp:** Congenital Heart Surgery; Transplant-Heart-Pediatric; Cardiac Surgery-Adult & Pediatric; **Hospital:** Vanderbilt Monroe Carrell Jr. Chldn's Hosp (page 75), Vanderbilt Univ Med Ctr (page 75); **Address:** Vanderbilt Chldns Hosp, Cardiac Surgery, 2200 Childrens Way, 5247 Doctors Office Tower, Nashville, TN 37232-9292; **Phone:** 615-343-6525; **Board Cert:** Surgery 2001; Thoracic Surgery 2003; **Med School:** Univ Wash 1985; **Resid:** Surgery, Univ Washington Med Ctr 1987; Surgery, Vanderbilt Univ Med Ctr 1991; **Fellow:** Cardiothoracic Surgery, Vanderbilt Univ Med Ctr 1994; **Fac Appt:** Assoc Prof S, Vanderbilt Univ

D'Amico, Thomas MD [T&CS] - **Spec Exp:** Lung Cancer; Esophageal Cancer; **Hospital:** Duke Univ Hosp; **Address:** Duke Univ Med Ctr, Dept Thoracic Surg, Box 3496, Durham, NC 27710; **Phone:** 919-684-4891; **Board Cert:** Surgery 2004; Thoracic Surgery 2006; **Med School:** Columbia P&S 1987; **Resid:** Surgery, Duke Univ Med Ctr 1989; Cardiothoracic Surgery, Duke Univ Med Ctr 1996; **Fellow:** Thoracic Oncology, Meml Sloan Kettering Cancer Ctr; **Fac Appt:** Assoc Prof S, Duke Univ

Dabal, Robert Joseph MD [T&CS] - **Spec Exp:** Pediatric Cardiac Surgery; Neonatal & Infant Cardiac Surgery; **Hospital:** Univ of Ala Hosp at Birmingham, Children's Hospital - Birmingham; **Address:** 1900 University Blvd, THT 712, Birmingham, AL 35294; **Phone:** 205-934-3368; **Board Cert:** Surgery 2002; Thoracic Surgery 2004; **Med School:** Duke Univ 1995; **Resid:** Surgery, NY Presby Hosp/Columbia 2000; Thoracic Surgery, Univ Washington Med Ctr 2003; **Fellow:** Pediatric Cardiothoracic Surgery, Chldn's Hosp 2004; Pediatric Cardiothoracic Surgery, Chldn's Hosp 2005; **Fac Appt:** Asst Prof S, Univ Alabama

Drinkwater Jr, Davis C MD [T&CS] - **Spec Exp:** Cardiac Surgery-Adult & Pediatric; Heart Valve Surgery; Congenital Heart Surgery; **Hospital:** Centennial Med Ctr, Vanderbilt Monroe Carrell Jr. Chldn's Hosp (page 75); **Address:** 2400 Patterson St, Ste 307, Nashville, TN 37203; **Phone:** 615-342-6900; **Board Cert:** Thoracic Surgery 2005; **Med School:** Univ VT Coll Med 1976; **Resid:** Surgery, McGill Univ 1981; Cardiothoracic Surgery, McGill Univ 1983; **Fellow:** Cardiothoracic Surgery, Childrens Hosp 1984; **Fac Appt:** Clin Prof TS, Vanderbilt Univ

Feins, Richard H MD [T&CS] - **Spec Exp:** Thoracic Cancers; Lung Cancer; Robotic Surgery; Esophageal Surgery; **Hospital:** NC Memorial Hosp - UNC; **Address:** UNC Dept Surgery, Div Cardiothoracic Surgery, 3040 Burnett-Womack Bldg, CB#7065, Chapel Hill, NC 27599-7065; **Phone:** 919-966-3383; **Board Cert:** Thoracic Surgery 2003; **Med School:** Univ VT Coll Med 1973; **Resid:** Surgery, Strong Meml Hosp 1980; Cardiothoracic Surgery, Univ Rochester Affil Hosp 1982; **Fac Appt:** Prof S, Univ NC Sch Med

Glassford Jr, David M MD [T&CS] - **Spec Exp:** Cardiothoracic Surgery; **Hospital:** Saint Thomas Hosp - Nashville; **Address:** Cardiovascular Surgery Assocs, 4230 Harding Rd, Ste 430, Nashville, TN 37205; **Phone:** 615-385-4781; **Board Cert:** Thoracic Surgery 2007; **Med School:** Univ Tex Med Br, Galveston 1970; **Resid:** Surgery, Univ Texas Med Br 1975; Thoracic Surgery, Ochsner Clinic 1977; **Fac Appt:** Asst Clin Prof TS, Vanderbilt Univ

Guyton, Robert A MD [T&CS] - **Spec Exp:** Coronary Artery Surgery; Minimally Invasive Cardiac Surgery; Heart Valve Surgery-Percutaneous; **Hospital:** Emory Univ Hosp Midtown, Emory Univ Hosp; **Address:** Emory Dept Cardiothoracic Surgery, 550 Peachtree St NE Fl 6 MOT, Atlanta, GA 30308; **Phone:** 404-686-2513; **Board Cert:** Thoracic & Cardiac Surgery 2010; **Med School:** Harvard Med Sch 1971; **Resid:** Surgery, Mass Genl Hosp 1978; **Fellow:** Thoracic Surgery, National Heart Lung Inst 1975; Cardiothoracic Surgery, Mass Genl/Childrens Hosp 1979; **Fac Appt:** Prof S, Emory Univ

Harpole Jr, David H MD [T&CS] - **Spec Exp:** Lung Cancer; Mesothelioma; Esophageal Cancer; **Hospital:** Duke Univ Hosp; **Address:** 3627 DUMC, Hock Plaza-2424 Erwin Rd, Ste 403 - rm 4017, Durham, NC 27705; **Phone:** 919-668-8413; **Board Cert:** Surgery 2011; Thoracic Surgery 2003; **Med School:** Univ VA Sch Med 1984; **Resid:** Surgery, Duke Univ Med Ctr 1991; **Fellow:** Thoracic Surgery, Duke Univ Med Ctr 1993; **Fac Appt:** Prof S, Duke Univ

Jones, David R MD [T&CS] - **Spec Exp:** Lung Cancer; Esophageal Cancer; Minimally Invasive Thoracic Surgery; **Hospital:** Univ of Virginia Health Sys; **Address:** Univ Virginnia Hlth Sys, Dept Surgery, 1215 Lee St, rm 4065, Charlottesville, VA 22908; **Phone:** 434-243-6443; **Board Cert:** Surgery 2005; Thoracic Surgery 2007; **Med School:** W VA Univ 1989; **Resid:** Surgery, West Va Univ 1995; **Fellow:** Thoracic Surgery, Univ North Carolina 1998; **Fac Appt:** Assoc Prof S, Univ VA Sch Med

Kanter, Kirk R MD [T&CS] - **Spec Exp:** Pediatric Cardiac Surgery; Transplant-Heart-Pediatric; Transplant-Lung-Pediatric; **Hospital:** Chldns Hlthcare Atlanta @ Egleston, Emory Univ Hosp; **Address:** Childrens Hlthcare Atlanta at Egleston, Pediatric Cardiothoracic Surgery, 1405 Clifton Rd NE Fl 2, Atlanta, GA 30322; **Phone:** 404-785-6330; **Board Cert:** Thoracic & Cardiac Surgery 2008; Congenital Cardiac Surgery 2009; **Med School:** Albany Med Coll 1976; **Resid:** Surgery, Johns Hopkins Hosp 1982; Thoracic Surgery, Johns Hopkins Hosp 1984; **Fellow:** Pediatric Cardiac Surgery, Brompton/Harefield Hosps 1985; **Fac Appt:** Prof S, Emory Univ

Kiernan, Paul D MD [T&CS] - **Spec Exp:** Lung Cancer; Esophageal Cancer; Mediastinal Tumors; **Hospital:** Inova Fairfax Hosp, Inova Alexandria Hosp; **Address:** Cardiac/Vascular/Thoracic Surgery Assocs, 2921 Telestar Ct Fl 2, Falls Church, VA 22042; **Phone:** 703-280-5858; **Board Cert:** Thoracic Surgery 2002; **Med School:** Georgetown Univ 1974; **Resid:** Surgery, Mayo Clinic 1979; Cardiothoracic Surgery, Mayo Clinic 1981; **Fellow:** Vascular Surgery, Mayo Clinic 1982; **Fac Appt:** Assoc Clin Prof S, Georgetown Univ

Kirklin, James K MD [T&CS] - **Spec Exp:** Transplant-Heart-Adult & Pediatric; Cardiac Surgery-Adult & Pediatric; Transplant-Heart & Lung; **Hospital:** Univ of Ala Hosp at Birmingham; **Address:** UAB CardioThoracic Surgery, 1900 University Blvd, THT 760, Birmingham, AL 35294; **Phone:** 205-934-3368; **Board Cert:** Thoracic Surgery 2000; **Med School:** Harvard Med Sch 1973; **Resid:** Surgery, Mass Genl Hosp 1977; Cardiothoracic Surgery, Mass Genl Hosp 1979; **Fellow:** Cardiothoracic Surgery, Chidren's Hosp Med Ctr 1979; **Fac Appt:** Prof S, Univ Alabama

Kron, Irving L MD [T&CS] - **Spec Exp:** Coronary Artery Surgery; Transplant-Heart; **Hospital:** Univ of Virginia Health Sys; **Address:** Univ VA Hlth Sys, Div Cardiovascular Surg, PO Box 800679, Charlottesville, VA 22908; **Phone:** 434-924-2158; **Board Cert:** Surgery 1999; Thoracic Surgery 2011; Vascular Surgery 2006; **Med School:** Med Coll Wisc 1975; **Resid:** Surgery, Maine Med Ctr 1980; **Fellow:** Cardiothoracic Surgery, Univ Virginia Med Ctr 1982; **Fac Appt:** Prof S, Univ VA Sch Med

Lau, Christine L MD [T&CS] - **Spec Exp:** Lung Cancer; Transplant-Lung; Esophageal Cancer; **Hospital:** Univ of Virginia Health Sys; **Address:** Univ VA Hlth System, Div Thoracic & Cardiovascular Surg, 1215 Lee St, Box 800679, Charlottesville, VA 22908; **Phone:** 434-924-8016; **Board Cert:** Surgery 2003; Thoracic Surgery 2007; **Med School:** Dartmouth Med Sch 1995; **Resid:** Surgery, Duke Affil Hosp 2003; **Fellow:** Cardiothoracic Surgery, Washington Univ Affil Hosps 2005; **Fac Appt:** Assoc Prof S, Univ VA Sch Med

Martin, Tomas D MD [T&CS] - **Spec Exp:** Cardiothoracic Surgery; Aortic Surgery; Aneurysm-Abdominal Aortic; **Hospital:** Shands at Univ of FL; **Address:** 1600 SW Archer Rd, Box 100129, Gainesville, FL 32608; **Phone:** 352-273-5505; **Board Cert:** Thoracic Surgery 2008; **Med School:** Univ Tex, Houston 1981; **Resid:** Surgery, Baylor Coll Med 1986; Vascular Surgery, Baylor Coll Med 1987; **Fellow:** Cardiothoracic Surgery, Shands/Univ Florida 1989; **Fac Appt:** Assoc Prof S, Univ Fla Coll Med

Mavroudis, Constantine MD [T&CS] - **Spec Exp:** Pediatric Cardiac Surgery; Congenital Heart Disease; Transplant-Heart & Lung; **Hospital:** Florida Hosp - Orlando; **Address:** Florida Hospital for Children, 2501 N Orange Ave, Ste 540, Orlando, FL 32804; **Phone:** 407-303-3697; **Board Cert:** Thoracic & Cardiac Surgery 2010; Congenital Cardiac Surgery 2009; **Med School:** Univ VA Sch Med 1973; **Resid:** Surgery, UCSF Med Ctr 1979; **Fellow:** Thoracic Surgery, UCSF Med Ctr 1977; **Fac Appt:** Prof S, Northwestern Univ

McGiffin, David C MD [T&CS] - **Spec Exp:** Coronary Artery Surgery; Heart Valve Surgery; Transplant-Lung; **Hospital:** Univ of Ala Hosp at Birmingham; **Address:** 1900 University Blvd, Tinsley Harrison Tower 760, Birmingham, AL 35294; **Phone:** 205-934-6580; **Med School:** Australia 1975; **Resid:** Surgery, Princess Alexandra Hosp 1979; Cardiovascular Surgery, Prince Charles Hosp 1982; **Fellow:** Cardiothoracic Surgery, Univ of Alabama Hosp 1983; **Fac Appt:** Prof S, Univ Alabama

Mill, Michael R MD [T&CS] - **Spec Exp:** Pediatric Cardiac Surgery; Transplant-Heart-Adult & Pediatric; Transplant-Heart & Lung; Heart Valve Surgery; **Hospital:** NC Memorial Hosp - UNC; **Address:** UNC Sch Med, Cardiothoracic Surgery, 3040 Burnett Womack Bldg, CB.7065, Chapel Hill, NC 27599-7965; **Phone:** 919-966-3381; **Board Cert:** Thoracic Surgery 2009; Congenital Cardiac Surgery 2009; **Med School:** Univ Colorado 1980; **Resid:** Surgery, Univ Colorado Hlth Sci Ctr 1985; **Fellow:** Cardiothoracic Surgery, Stanford Univ Med Ctr 1987; Transplant Surgery, Stanford Univ Med Ctr 1988; **Fac Appt:** Prof S, Univ NC Sch Med

Miller, Daniel L MD [T&CS] - **Spec Exp:** Esophageal Cancer; Lung Cancer; Mesothelioma; Emphysema-Lung Volume Reduction; **Hospital:** Emory Univ Hosp, Emory Univ Hosp Midtown; **Address:** The Emory Clinic, 1365A Clifton Rd NE, Ste 2219, Atlanta, GA 30322; **Phone:** 404-778-3755; **Board Cert:** Thoracic & Cardiac Surgery 2005; Surgery 2001; **Med School:** Univ KY Coll Med 1985; **Resid:** Surgery, Georgetown Univ Hosp 1991; **Fellow:** Cardiothoracic Surgery, Mayo Clinic 1994; **Fac Appt:** Prof TS, Emory Univ

Moore, John E MD [T&CS] - **Spec Exp:** Lung Cancer; Esophageal Cancer; Thoracic Cancers; **Hospital:** Northside Hosp, St. Joseph's Hosp - Atlanta; **Address:** Atlanta Cardiac & Thoracic Surg Assocs, 960 Johnson Ferry Rd, Ste 100, Atlanta, GA 30342; **Phone:** 404-252-9063; **Board Cert:** Thoracic & Cardiac Surgery 2005; **Med School:** Univ Louisville Sch Med 1975; **Resid:** Surgery, Emory Univ Affil Hosps 1980; Cardiovascular Surgery, Emory Univ Affil Hosps 1983

Mullett, Timothy W MD [T&CS] - **Spec Exp:** Lung Cancer; Transplant-Heart & Lung; Cardiac Surgery-Adult & Pediatric; Esophageal Surgery; **Hospital:** Univ of Kentucky Albert B. Chandler Hosp; **Address:** Univ Kentucky Hlth Care-Cardio Thor Clin, 740 S Limestone St, Ste A-301, Lexington, KY 40536; **Phone:** 859-323-6494; **Board Cert:** Surgery 2005; Thoracic Surgery 2007; **Med School:** Univ Fla Coll Med 1987; **Resid:** Surgery, Shands/Univ of FL 1990; **Fellow:** Pediatric Surgery, Shands/Univ of FL 1994; Cardiothoracic Surgery, Shands/Univ of FL 1995; **Fac Appt:** Assoc Prof S, Univ KY Coll Med

Murphy, Douglas A MD [T&CS] - **Spec Exp:** Robotic Surgery; Minimally Invasive Cardiac Surgery; Heart Valve Surgery; Mitral Valve Robotic Surgery; **Hospital:** St. Joseph's Hosp - Atlanta; **Address:** Peachtree Cardiovascular Surgeons, 5665 Peachtree Dunwoody Rd NE, Ste 200, Atlanta, GA 30342; **Phone:** 404-252-6104; **Board Cert:** Internal Medicine 1978; Thoracic & Cardiac Surgery 2004; **Med School:** Univ Pennsylvania 1975; **Resid:** Internal Medicine, Mass Genl Hosp 1977; Surgery, Mass Genl Hosp 1981; **Fellow:** Thoracic Surgery, Emory Univ Affil Hosp 1983; **Fac Appt:** Prof TS, Emory Univ

Nesbitt, Jonathan C MD [T&CS] - **Spec Exp:** Lung Cancer; Esophageal Cancer; Chest Diseases-Benign; Minimally Invasive Thoracic Surgery; **Hospital:** Vanderbilt Univ Med Ctr (page 75), Williamson Med Ctr; **Address:** 1313 21st Ave S, Oxford Hse Bldg - Fl 6th - Ste 609, Nashville, TN 37232; **Phone:** 615-322-0064; **Board Cert:** Thoracic Surgery 2009; **Med School:** Georgetown Univ 1981; **Resid:** Surgery, Vanderbilt Univ Med Ctr 1987; Cardiothoracic Surgery, Albany Med Ctr 1989; **Fac Appt:** Assoc Prof TS, Vanderbilt Univ

Nguyen, Dao M MD [T&CS] - **Spec Exp:** Thoracic Cancers; Lung Cancer; Minimally Invasive Thoracic Surgery; **Hospital:** Univ of Miami Hosp, Jackson Meml Hosp; **Address:** 1611 NW 12th Ave Fl 3, East Tower 3072, Miami, FL 33136; **Phone:** 305-585-5271; **Board Cert:** Thoracic Surgery 2005; **Med School:** McGill Univ 1986; **Resid:** Surgery, McGill Univ Affil Hosp 1992; Thoracic Surgery, McGill Univ Affil Hosp 1994; **Fellow:** Thoracic Oncology, MD Anderson Cancer Ctr 1996; **Fac Appt:** Prof S, Univ Miami Sch Med

Thoracic & Cardiac Surgery

Ninan, Mathew MD [T&CS] - **Spec Exp:** Lung Cancer; Robotic Surgery; Esophageal Cancer; Transplant-Lung; **Hospital:** Centennial Med Ctr; **Address:** TriStar-Sarah Cannon Cancer Ctr, 2410 Patterson St, Ste 212, Nashville, TN 37203; **Phone:** 615-342-7345; **Med School:** India 1988; **Resid:** Surgery, Univ London Affil Hosp 1994; **Fellow:** Cardiothoracic Surgery, Univ Pittsburgh 1998; **Fac Appt:** Assoc Prof TS, Vanderbilt Univ

Oaks, Timothy E MD [T&CS] - **Spec Exp:** Cardiothoracic Surgery; Lung Cancer; Lung Surgery; **Hospital:** Alamance Regl Med Ctr; **Address:** 3940 Arrowhead Blvd, Ste 230, Mebane, NC 27302; **Phone:** 919-304-1081; **Board Cert:** Thoracic Surgery 2011; **Med School:** Penn State Coll Med 1984; **Resid:** Surgery, Penn State-Hershey Med Ctr 1990; **Fellow:** Cardiothoracic Surgery, Penn State-Hershey Med Ctr 1992; Cardiothoracic Surgery, Papworth Hosp 1993

Panos, Anthony MD [T&CS] - **Spec Exp:** Cardiac Surgery-Adult; Transplant-Heart; Minimally Invasive Cardiac Surgery; **Hospital:** Jackson Meml Hosp; **Address:** Jackson Meml Hosp (R114), 1611 NW 12th Ave, ET3072, Miami, FL 33136; **Phone:** 305-585-5271; **Board Cert:** Thoracic Surgery 2004; **Med School:** Univ Toronto 1980; **Resid:** Surgery, Univ Toronto Affil Hosp 1987; Cardiovascular Surgery, Univ Toronto Affil Hosp 1990; **Fellow:** Thoracic Surgery, Toronto Genl Hosp 1985; Cardiovascular Surgery, St Michaels Hosp 1990; **Fac Appt:** Prof S, Univ Miami Sch Med

Pham, Si M MD [T&CS] - **Spec Exp:** Cardiothoracic Surgery; Transplant-Heart & Lung; **Hospital:** UHealth - Univ of Miami Hlth Sys, Jackson Meml Hosp; **Address:** Highland Professional Bldg, 1801 NW 9th Ave Fl 5, Miami, FL 33136; **Phone:** 305-355-5000; **Board Cert:** Surgery 2009; Thoracic & Cardiac Surgery 2011; Surgical Critical Care 2001; **Med School:** Univ Pittsburgh 1983; **Resid:** Surgery, Univ Pittsburgh Med Ctr 1989; **Fellow:** Cardiothoracic Surgery, Univ Pittsburgh Med Ctr 1992; **Fac Appt:** Prof S, Univ Miami Sch Med

Philpott, Jonathan M MD [T&CS] - **Spec Exp:** Cardiac Surgery; Atrial Fibrillation; Clinical Trials; **Hospital:** Sentara Norfolk Genl Hosp; **Address:** Mid-Atlantic Cardiothoracic Surgeons, Sentara Heart Hospital Fl 6, 600 Gresham Drive, Ste 8600, Norfolk, VA 23507; **Phone:** 757-388-6005; **Board Cert:** Surgery 2001; Surgical Critical Care 2002; Thoracic Surgery 2005; **Med School:** Eastern VA Med Sch 1994; **Resid:** Surgery, E Carolina Univ Affil Hosp 2000; **Fellow:** Thoracic Surgery, Hosp Univ Penn 2002; Med Coll VA-West Hosp 2004

Putnam Jr, Joe B MD [T&CS] - **Spec Exp:** Lung Cancer; Esophageal Cancer; Sarcoma-Soft Tissue; **Hospital:** Vanderbilt Univ Med Ctr (page 75), TN Valley Healthcare Sys-Nashville; **Address:** Vanderbilt Univ Med Ctr - Thoracic Surgery, 609 Oxford House, 1313 21st Ave S, Nashville, TN 37232-4682; **Phone:** 615-343-9202; **Board Cert:** Thoracic Surgery 2007; **Med School:** Univ NC Sch Med 1979; **Resid:** Surgery, Univ Rochester 1986; Thoracic Surgery, Univ Mich Med Ctr 1988; **Fellow:** Surgical Oncology, NCI/NIH-Surg Branch 1984; **Fac Appt:** Prof TS, Vanderbilt Univ

Quintessenza, James A MD [T&CS] - **Spec Exp:** Transplant-Heart; Coronary Artery Surgery; Cardiovascular Surgery; **Hospital:** All Children's Hosp; **Address:** 625 6th Ave S, Ste 475, St Petersburg, FL 33701; **Phone:** 727-767-6666; **Board Cert:** Thoracic Surgery 2007; **Med School:** Univ Fla Coll Med 1981; **Resid:** Surgery, Univ Florida Hosps 1986; **Fellow:** Thoracic Surgery, UCSD Medical Ctr 1988; **Fac Appt:** Assoc Clin Prof S, Univ S Fla Coll Med

Reed, Carolyn E MD [T&CS] - **Spec Exp:** Esophageal Cancer; Lung Cancer; **Hospital:** MUSC Med Ctr; **Address:** MUSC Ashley River Tower, 25 Courtenay Drive, Ste 7018, MSC 295, Charleston, SC 29425; **Phone:** 843-876-4845; **Board Cert:** Thoracic & Cardiac Surgery 2004; **Med School:** Univ Rochester 1977; **Resid:** Surgery, New York Hosp 1982; Thoracic Surgery, New York Hosp 1985; **Fellow:** Surgical Oncology, Meml Sloan Kettering Cancer Ctr 1983; **Fac Appt:** Prof S, Med Univ SC

Robinson, Lary A MD [T&CS] - **Spec Exp:** Lung Cancer; Mesothelioma; **Hospital:** H Lee Moffitt Cancer Ctr & Research Inst (page 59), Tampa Genl Hosp; **Address:** H Lee Moffitt Cancer Ctr, Div Thoracic Oncology, 12902 Magnolia Drive, Tampa, FL 33612-9497; **Phone:** 813-745-7282; **Board Cert:** Thoracic Surgery 2003; Surgery 2002; Surgical Critical Care 2000; **Med School:** Washington Univ, St Louis 1972; **Resid:** Surgery, Duke Univ Med Ctr 1974; Thoracic Surgery, Duke Univ Med Ctr 1981; **Fellow:** Cardiothoracic Surgery, St Thomas Hosp 1982; Cardiothoracic Surgery, Duke Univ Med Ctr 1983; **Fac Appt:** Prof S, Univ S Fla Coll Med

Rosenkranz, Eliot R MD [T&CS] - **Spec Exp:** Pediatric Cardiac Surgery; Transplant-Heart-Pediatric; Cardiac Surgery-Neonatal; Congenital Heart Surgery; **Hospital:** Jackson Meml Hosp, Univ of Miami Hosp; **Address:** Jackson Meml Hosp (R114), 1611 NW 12th Ave, ET3072, Miami, FL 33136-1005; **Phone:** 305-585-5271; **Board Cert:** Thoracic Surgery 2008; **Med School:** UCSD 1979; **Resid:** Surgery, UCLA Med Ctr 1985; **Fellow:** Cardiothoracic Surgery, UCLA Med Ctr 1987; **Fac Appt:** Prof S, Univ Miami Sch Med

Salerno, Tomas A MD [T&CS] - **Spec Exp:** Cardiothoracic Surgery; Heart Valve Surgery; Aortic Surgery; Coronary Artery Surgery; **Hospital:** Jackson Meml Hosp, Univ of Miami Hosp; **Address:** Jackson Meml Hosp (R114), 1611 NW 12th Ave, ET3072, Miami, FL 33136; **Phone:** 305-585-5271; **Board Cert:** Thoracic Surgery 2008; **Med School:** McGill Univ 1971; **Resid:** Surgery, Royal Victoria Hosp 1975; Cardiothoracic Surgery, Royal Victoria Hosp 1977; **Fac Appt:** Prof S, Univ Miami Sch Med

Savage, Edward B MD [T&CS] - **Spec Exp:** Heart Failure; Lung Cancer; Minimally Invasive Heart Valve Surgery; Mitral Valve Surgery; **Hospital:** Cleveland Clin - Weston (page 55); **Address:** Cleveland Clinic Florida, Div Cardiothoracic Surgery, 2950 Cleveland Clinic Blvd, Weston, FL 33331; **Phone:** 954-659-5320; **Board Cert:** Surgery 2004; Thoracic & Cardiac Surgery 2004; **Med School:** Yale Univ 1985; **Resid:** Surgery, Hosp Univ Penn 1992; Thoracic Surgery, Brigham & Womens Hosp 1994

Slaughter, Mark S MD [T&CS] - **Spec Exp:** Ventricular Assist Device (LVAD); Mitral Valve Surgery; Transplant-Heart; **Hospital:** Jewish Hosp Med Ctr (KY); **Address:** 201 Abraham Flexner Way, Ste 1200, Louisville, KY 40202; **Phone:** 502-583-8383; **Board Cert:** Surgery 2002; Thoracic & Cardiac Surgery 2003; **Med School:** Indiana Univ 1986; **Resid:** Surgery, Northwestern Meml Hosp 1992; **Fellow:** Thoracic Surgery, Univ Minnesota Affil Hosp 1994; **Fac Appt:** Prof T&CS, Univ Louisville Sch Med

Smith, Peter K MD [T&CS] - **Spec Exp:** Coronary Artery Surgery; Heart Valve Surgery; **Hospital:** Duke Univ Hosp, Durham VA Med Ctr; **Address:** Box 3442 Med Ctr, 8660 HAFS Bldg, Durham, NC 27710; **Phone:** 919-684-2890; **Board Cert:** Thoracic Surgery 2007; **Med School:** Duke Univ 1977; **Resid:** Surgery, Duke Univ Med Ctr 1984; Thoracic Surgery, Duke Univ Med Ctr 1987; **Fac Appt:** Prof S, Duke Univ

Staples, Edward D MD [T&CS] - **Spec Exp:** Transplant-Heart & Lung; Ventricular Assist Device (LVAD); **Hospital:** Malcolm Randall VA Med Ctr, Shands at Univ of FL; **Address:** 1601 SW Archer Rd, Gainesville, FL 32610; **Phone:** 352-376-1611; **Board Cert:** Thoracic Surgery 2004; Surgical Critical Care 2002; **Med School:** Univ S Fla Coll Med 1977; **Resid:** Surgery, Med Coll Va 1979; Surgery, Univ Hosp 1982; **Fellow:** Cardiothoracic Surgery, Univ Florida Affil Hosp 1984; **Fac Appt:** Assoc Prof S, Univ Fla Coll Med

Stowe, Cary MD [T&CS] - **Spec Exp:** Aortic Surgery; **Hospital:** Indian River Med Ctr; **Address:** 1040 37th Pl, Ste 101, Vero Beach, FL 32960; **Phone:** 772-563-4580; **Board Cert:** Thoracic Surgery 2008; Vascular Surgery 2008; **Med School:** Univ Alabama 1978; **Resid:** Surgery, Barnes Hosp 1982; **Fellow:** Vascular Surgery, Baylor Coll Med 1983; Cardiothoracic Surgery, Emory Univ Sch Med 1994

Thoracic & Cardiac Surgery

Tedder, Mark MD [T&CS] - **Spec Exp:** Ventricular Assist Device(LVAD); Congenital Heart Disease; Cardiac Surgery; **Hospital:** Saint Thomas Hosp - Nashville; **Address:** Cardiovascular Surgery Assocs, 4230 Harding Rd, Ste 430, Nashville, TN 37205; **Phone:** 615-385-4781; **Board Cert:** Thoracic Surgery 2007; **Med School:** Duke Univ 1988; **Resid:** Surgery, Duke Univ Med Ctr 1995; Cardiothoracic Surgery, Duke Univ Med Ctr 1997

Ungerleider, Ross M MD [T&CS] - **Spec Exp:** Pediatric Cardiac Surgery; Cardiac Surgery; Congenital Heart Surgery; **Hospital:** Wake Forest Baptist Med Ctr; **Address:** Dept of Cardiothoracic Surgery, Medical Ctr Blvd, Winston-Salem, NC 27157-1096; **Phone:** 336-716-2124; **Board Cert:** Thoracic Surgery 2007; Congenital Cardiac Surgery 2009; **Med School:** Rush Med Coll 1977; **Resid:** Surgery, Duke Univ Med Ctr 1987; **Fellow:** Cardiothoracic Surgery, Duke Univ Med Ctr 1989; Pediatric Cardiac Surgery, UCSF Med Ctr; **Fac Appt:** Prof

Weiman, Darryl S MD [T&CS] - **Spec Exp:** Cardiothoracic Surgery; Lung Cancer; Esophageal Surgery; **Hospital:** VA Med Ctr - Memphis; **Address:** VA Med Ctr, 1030 Jefferson Ave, Fl 3, rm CW353, Dept Surgery, Memphis, TN 38104; **Phone:** 901-577-7352; **Board Cert:** Surgery 2002; Thoracic & Cardiac Surgery 2010; **Med School:** St Louis Univ 1978; **Resid:** Surgery, Univ Chicago Pritzker Sch Med 1983; Thoracic Surgery, Univ Chicago Pritzker Sch Med 1984; **Fellow:** Cardiothoracic Surgery, Long Island Jewish Hosp 1991; **Fac Appt:** Prof S, Univ Tenn Coll Med

Zwischenberger, Joseph B MD [T&CS] - **Spec Exp:** Thoracic Cancers; Lung Cancer; Esophageal Cancer; Respiratory Failure; **Hospital:** Univ of Kentucky Albert B. Chandler Hosp; **Address:** UK HlthCare Chandler Med Ctr, 800 Rose St, rm MN-264, Lexington, KY 40536; **Phone:** 859-257-1000; **Board Cert:** Surgery 2002; Thoracic Surgery 2005; Surgical Critical Care 2008; **Med School:** Univ KY Coll Med 1977; **Resid:** Surgery, Univ Michigan Hosp 1984; Cardiothoracic Surgery, Univ Michigan Hosp 1985; **Fellow:** Cardiac Surgery, Natl Inst Hlth 1981; **Fac Appt:** Prof S, Univ KY Coll Med

Midwest

Baciewicz Jr, Frank A MD [T&CS] - **Spec Exp:** Esophageal Cancer; Lung Cancer; Minimally Invasive Thoracic Surgery; **Hospital:** Barbara Ann Karmanos Cancer Inst, Detroit Med Ctr; **Address:** Univ Surgeons, 4160 John R, Ste 615, Detroit, MI 48201; **Phone:** 800-527-6266; **Board Cert:** Thoracic & Cardiac Surgery 2005; Surgical Critical Care 2011; **Med School:** Univ VA Sch Med 1978; **Resid:** Surgery, Northwestern Univ Affil Hosps 1983; **Fellow:** Cardiothoracic Surgery, Univ Penn 1985; **Fac Appt:** Prof S, Wayne State Univ

Backer, Carl L MD [T&CS] - **Spec Exp:** Pediatric Cardiothoracic Surgery; Transplant-Heart; Tracheal Surgery; Congenital Heart Disease-Adult; **Hospital:** Lurie Chldn's Hosp-Chicago, Northwestern Meml Hosp; **Address:** 225 E Chicago Ave, Box 22, Chicago, IL 60611; **Phone:** 312-227-4030; **Board Cert:** Thoracic Surgery 2007; Congenital Cardiac Surgery 2009; **Med School:** Mayo Med Sch 1980; **Resid:** Surgery, Northwestern Meml Hosp 1985; **Fellow:** Cardiothoracic Surgery, Northwestern Meml Hosp 1987; Pediatric Cardiac Surgery, Chldns Meml Hosp 1988; **Fac Appt:** Prof S, Northwestern Univ

Bakhos, Mamdouh MD [T&CS] - **Spec Exp:** Mitral Valve Surgery; Minimally Invasive Cardiac Surgery; Transplant-Heart & Lung; **Hospital:** Loyola Univ Med Ctr, Adv Good Samaritan Hosp; **Address:** Loyola Univ, Dept Cardiothoracic Surgery, 2160 S First Ave, Bldg 110 - rm 6240, Maywood, IL 60153; **Phone:** 708-327-2503; **Board Cert:** Thoracic Surgery 2007; **Med School:** Syria 1971; **Resid:** Surgery, Huron Road Hosp 1976; **Fellow:** Thoracic Surgery, Loyola Univ Med Ctr 1978; **Fac Appt:** Prof TS, Loyola Univ-Stritch Sch Med

Brown, John W MD [T&CS] - **Spec Exp:** Cardiac Surgery-Neonatal & Pediatric; Transplant-Heart; Heart Valve Surgery; Congenital Heart Disease; **Hospital:** Riley Hosp for Children, IU Health University Hosp; **Address:** Indiana Univ Dept Surgery, 545 Barnhill Drive, EH 215, Indianapolis, IN 46202-5112; **Phone:** 317-274-7150; **Board Cert:** Thoracic Surgery 2007; Congenital Cardiac Surgery 2011; **Med School:** Indiana Univ 1970; **Resid:** Surgery, Univ Mich Med Ctr 1976; Cardiothoracic Surgery, Univ Mich Med Ctr 1978; **Fellow:** Cardiovascular Surgery, Natl Heart Lung-Blood Inst 1974; **Fac Appt:** Prof S, Indiana Univ

Cassivi, Stephen D MD [T&CS] - **Spec Exp:** Thoracic Surgery; Minimally Invasive Surgery; Transplant-Lung; Myasthenia Gravis; **Hospital:** Mayo Med Ctr & Clin - Rochester; **Address:** Mayo Clinic, 200 First St SW, Mayo Bldg Fl 12 - rm 12-55W, Rochester, MN 55905; **Phone:** 507-266-0911; **Board Cert:** Thoracic & Cardiac Surgery 2011; **Med School:** Univ Ottawa 1994; **Resid:** Surgery, Univ Toronto Hosps 2000; **Fellow:** Cardiothoracic Surgery, Barnes-Jewish Hosp 2002; **Fac Appt:** Assoc Prof TS, Mayo Med Sch

Damiano Jr, Ralph J MD [T&CS] - **Spec Exp:** Minimally Invasive Cardiac Surgery; Coronary Artery Surgery; Endoscopic Surgery; **Hospital:** Barnes-Jewish Hosp; **Address:** 660 S Euclid Ave, Campus Box 8234, St Louis, MO 63110; **Phone:** 314-362-7327; **Board Cert:** Thoracic Surgery 2002; **Med School:** Duke Univ 1980; **Resid:** Surgery, Duke Univ Med Ctr 1988; **Fellow:** Cardiothoracic Surgery, Duke Univ Med Ctr 1989; **Fac Appt:** Prof S, Washington Univ, St Louis

DeCamp Jr, Malcolm M MD [T&CS] - **Spec Exp:** Lung Surgery; Esophageal Surgery; Emphysema-Lung Volume Reduction; **Hospital:** Northwestern Meml Hosp; **Address:** Northwestern Div Thoracic Surgery, 676 N St Clair St, Ste 650, Chicago, IL 60611; **Phone:** 312-695-4630; **Board Cert:** Surgery 2001; Thoracic Surgery 2003; **Med School:** Univ Louisville Sch Med 1983; **Resid:** Surgery, Brighams & Womens Hosp 1986; Surgery, Brighams & Womens Hosp 1990; **Fellow:** Cardiac Surgery, Brighams & Womens Hosp 1993; **Fac Appt:** Prof S, Northwestern Univ

Deeb, G Michael MD [T&CS] - **Spec Exp:** Aortic Valve Disease; Aneurysm-Aortic; **Hospital:** Univ of Michigan Hosp; **Address:** U of M Cardiovascular Ctr, Fl 3, Recept C, 1500 E Med Ctr Drive, SPC 5864, Ann Arbor, MI 48109; **Phone:** 734-936-5851; **Board Cert:** Thoracic Surgery 2002; **Med School:** Univ Pittsburgh 1975; **Resid:** Surgery, Univ Pittsburgh Hosp 1979; **Fellow:** Thoracic & Cardiac Surgery, Univ Pittsburgh Hosp 1979; Chemosurgery, Univ Pittsburgh Hosp 1982; **Fac Appt:** Prof T&CS, Univ Mich Med Sch

Delius, Ralph MD [T&CS] - **Spec Exp:** Pediatric Cardiac Surgery; Congenital Heart Surgery; **Hospital:** Chldns Hosp of Michigan; **Address:** Chldns Hosp of Michigan, 3901 Beaubien Blvd, Detroit, MI 48201; **Phone:** 313-745-5538; **Board Cert:** Surgery 2001; Thoracic & Cardiac Surgery 2005; Congenital Cardiac Surgery 2011; **Med School:** UC Davis 1984; **Resid:** Surgery, Univ Michigan Hosp 1989; Cardiothoracic Surgery, Univ Iowa Hosp 1994; **Fellow:** Cardiothoracic Surgery, Univ Michigan Hosp 1990; Cardiac Surgery, Mass Genl Hosp 1992; **Fac Appt:** Assoc Prof S, Wayne State Univ

Deschamps, Claude MD [T&CS] - **Spec Exp:** Gastroesophageal Reflux Disease (GERD); Esophageal Cancer; Lung Cancer; **Hospital:** St. Mary's Hosp - Rochester MN (Mayo); **Address:** Mayo Clinic, Div Thoracic Surgery, 200 First St SW, Rochester, MN 55905; **Phone:** 507-284-8462; **Board Cert:** Surgery 2004; **Med School:** Univ Montreal 1979; **Resid:** Surgery, Univ Montreal Hosps 1984; Thoracic Surgery, Univ Montreal Hosps 1985; **Fellow:** Thoracic Surgery, Mayo Clinic 1987; **Fac Appt:** Prof S, Mayo Med Sch

Thoracic & Cardiac Surgery

Durham, Samuel J MD [T&CS] - **Spec Exp:** Cardiothoracic Surgery; **Hospital:** Lakeland Specialty Hosp; **Address:** Lakeshore Cardiothoracic Surgery, 2500 Niles Rd, Ste 6, St Joseph, MI 49085; **Phone:** 269-408-1660; **Board Cert:** Surgery 2011; Thoracic & Cardiac Surgery 2003; **Med School:** Harvard Med Sch 1983; **Resid:** Surgery, Univ Pittsburgh Med Ctr 1987; Thoracic Surgery, Univ Pittsburgh Med Ctr 1988; **Fellow:** Pediatric Surgery, Chldren's Hosp 1993; **Fac Appt:** Prof S, Ohio State Univ

Ferguson, Mark K MD [T&CS] - **Spec Exp:** Lung Cancer; Esophageal Cancer; Barrett's Esophagus; Minimally Invasive Surgery; **Hospital:** Univ of Chicago Med Ctr; **Address:** Univ Chicago Medical Ctr, 5841 S Maryland Ave, MC 5035, Chicago, IL 60637; **Phone:** 773-702-3551; **Board Cert:** Thoracic Surgery 2003; **Med School:** Univ Chicago-Pritzker Sch Med 1977; **Resid:** Surgery, Univ Chicago Hosps 1981; **Fellow:** Cardiothoracic Surgery, Univ Chicago Hosps 1984; **Fac Appt:** Prof S, Univ Chicago-Pritzker Sch Med

Galantowicz, Mark E MD [T&CS] - **Spec Exp:** Cardiothoracic Surgery; **Hospital:** Nationwide Chldn's Hosp; **Address:** 700 Children's Drive, Nationwide Chldns Hosp, Columbus, OH 43205; **Phone:** 614-722-3101; **Board Cert:** Thoracic Surgery 2004; Congenital Cardiac Surgery 2011; **Med School:** Cornell Univ 1987; **Resid:** Surgery, Columbia-Presby Med Ctr 1993; **Fellow:** Cardiothoracic Surgery, Columbia-Presby Med Ctr 1995; **Fac Appt:** Assoc Prof S, Ohio State Univ

Howington, John A MD [T&CS] - **Spec Exp:** Lung Cancer; Esophageal Cancer; Thymoma; Minimally Invasive Thoracic Surgery; **Hospital:** Evanston/North Shore Univ Hlth Sys, Highland Park/North Shore Univ Hlth Syst; **Address:** Evanston NorthShore Health System, 2650 Ridge Ave, Walgreen Bldg, Ste 3507, Evanston, IL 60201; **Phone:** 847-570-2868; **Board Cert:** Thoracic & Cardiac Surgery 2006; Surgery 2004; **Med School:** Univ Tenn Coll Med 1989; **Resid:** Surgery, Truman Med Ctr 1994; **Fellow:** Cardiothoracic Surgery, Vanderbilt Univ Med Ctr 1997; **Fac Appt:** Assoc Prof S, Univ Chicago-Pritzker Sch Med

Huddleston, Charles B MD [T&CS] - **Spec Exp:** Transplant-Lung-Pediatric; Transplant-Heart-Pediatric; Hypoplastic Left Heart Syndrome; **Hospital:** Cardinal Glennon Mem Children's Hosp, St. Louis Univ Hosp; **Address:** 1465 S Grand Blvd Fl 5 - rm 5730, St Louis, MO 63104; **Phone:** 314-268-4183; **Board Cert:** Thoracic Surgery 2007; **Med School:** Vanderbilt Univ 1978; **Resid:** Surgery, Vanderbilt Univ Hosp 1986; Cardiothoracic Surgery, Vanderbilt Univ Hosp 1988; **Fellow:** Pediatric Cardiothoracic Surgery, Hosp for Sick Chldn 1989; **Fac Appt:** Prof S, St Louis Univ

Iannettoni, Mark D MD [T&CS] - **Spec Exp:** Transplant-Lung; Lung Cancer; Esophageal Surgery; **Hospital:** Univ Iowa Hosp & Clinics; **Address:** Univ Iowa Hosp & Clinics, 200 Hawkins Drive, rm SE514GH, Iowa City, IA 52242; **Phone:** 319-356-1133; **Board Cert:** Surgery 2002; Thoracic Surgery 2002; **Med School:** SUNY Upstate Med Univ 1985; **Resid:** Surgery, SUNY Upstate Med Ctr 1991; Thoracic Surgery, Univ Mich Med Ctr 1993; **Fellow:** Thoracic Surgery, Univ Mich Med Sch 1994; **Fac Appt:** Prof T&CS, Univ Iowa Coll Med

Ilbawi, Michel N MD [T&CS] - **Spec Exp:** Pediatric Cardiac Surgery; Congenital Anomalies; Congenital Heart Disease; Congenital Heart Disease-Adult; **Hospital:** Adv Christ Med Ctr, Univ of IL Med Ctr at Chicago; **Address:** Hope Chldns Hosp at Adv Christ Med Ctr, 4440 W 95th St, Oak Lawn, IL 60453; **Phone:** 708-684-3029; **Board Cert:** Thoracic Surgery 2007; Congenital Cardiac Surgery 2009; **Med School:** Amer Univ Beirut 1971; **Resid:** Surgery, American Univ Hosp 1975; Thoracic Surgery, Univ Hosps 1977; **Fellow:** Thoracic Surgery, Chldns Meml Hosp 1978; **Fac Appt:** Clin Prof S, Univ IL Coll Med

Jeevanandam, Valluvan MD [T&CS] - **Spec Exp:** Minimally Invasive Heart Valve Surgery; Transplant-Heart; Artificial Heart Devices; **Hospital:** Univ of Chicago Med Ctr; **Address:** 5841 S Maryland Ave, MC 5040, Chicago, IL 60637-1483; **Phone:** 773-702-2500; **Board Cert:** Thoracic Surgery 2011; **Med School:** Columbia P&S 1984; **Resid:** Surgery, Columbia-Presby Med Ctr 1989; **Fellow:** Cardiothoracic Surgery, Columbia-Presby Med Ctr 1991; **Fac Appt:** Prof S, Univ Chicago-Pritzker Sch Med

Joyce, Lyle MD/PhD [T&CS] - **Spec Exp:** Cardiac Surgery-Adult; Minimally Invasive Cardiac Surgery; Heart Valve Surgery; **Hospital:** Mayo Med Ctr & Clin - Rochester; **Address:** Mayo Clin, Dept Cardiac Surg, 200 1st St SW, Rochester, MN 55905; **Phone:** 507-255-2000; **Board Cert:** Thoracic & Cardiac Surgery 2003; **Med School:** Baylor Coll Med 1973; **Resid:** Surgery, Univ Minn Hosp 1980; Cardiothoracic Surgery, Univ Utah Affil Hosps 1982; **Fac Appt:** Prof S, Mayo Med Sch

Liao, Kenneth K MD [T&CS] - **Spec Exp:** Minimally Invasive Surgery; Transplant-Heart; Transplant-Lung; Aneurysm-Thoracic Aortic; **Hospital:** Univ Minn Med Ctr, Fairview - Riverside Campus; **Address:** Univ Minn Med Ctr, Dept Surg, 420 Delaware St SE, MMC 207, Minneapolis, MN 55455; **Phone:** 612-625-3904; **Board Cert:** Surgery 2002; Thoracic Surgery 2003; **Med School:** China 1989; **Resid:** Surgery, Brookdale Univ Hosp 1999; Cardiothoracic Surgery, Univ Minn Hosp 2002; **Fellow:** Research, Albert Einstein Coll Med 1994; **Fac Appt:** Assoc Prof S, Univ Minn

Love, Robert B MD [T&CS] - **Spec Exp:** Transplant-Heart & Lung; Lung Cancer; Esophageal Cancer; Heart Valve Surgery; **Hospital:** Loyola Univ Med Ctr; **Address:** Loyola Univ Med Ctr, 2160 S First Ave Bldg 110 - rm 6243, Maywood, IL 60153; **Phone:** 708-327-2488; **Board Cert:** Surgery 2007; Thoracic & Cardiac Surgery 2010; Surgical Critical Care 2001; **Med School:** Rush Med Coll 1982; **Resid:** Surgery, Univ of Wisconsin Hosp 1988; Thoracic Surgery, Gloucestershire Royal Hosp 1989; **Fellow:** Cardiothoracic Surgery, Univ of Wisconsin Hosp 1991; **Fac Appt:** Prof TS, Loyola Univ-Stritch Sch Med

Lytle, Bruce W MD [T&CS] - **Spec Exp:** Heart Valve Surgery; Coronary Artery Surgery; Aortic Surgery; **Hospital:** Cleveland Clin (page 55); **Address:** Cleveland Clinic, Dept Thoracic Surgery, 9500 Euclid Ave, Desk J1-227, Cleveland, OH 44195; **Phone:** 216-444-6962; **Board Cert:** Thoracic & Cardiac Surgery 2007; **Med School:** Harvard Med Sch 1971; **Resid:** Surgery, Mass Genl Hsop 1975; Surgery, Shotley Bridge Hosp 1977; **Fellow:** Thoracic Surgery, Mass Genl Hosp 1979; **Fac Appt:** Prof TS, Cleveland Cl Coll Med/Case West Res

Mason, David P MD [T&CS] - **Spec Exp:** Minimally Invasive Thoracic Surgery; Lung Cancer; Mesothelioma; Transplant-Lung; **Hospital:** Cleveland Clin (page 55); **Address:** Cleveland Clinic, 9500 Euclid Ave, MC J4-1, Cleveland, OH 44195; **Phone:** 216-444-4053; **Board Cert:** Surgery 2011; Thoracic Surgery 2004; **Med School:** Columbia P&S 1994; **Resid:** Surgery, Brigham & Womens Hosp 2001; **Fellow:** Vascular Surgery, Univ Washington Med Ctr 1999; Thoracic Surgery, Brigham & Womens Hosp 2003

McCarthy, Patrick M MD [T&CS] - **Spec Exp:** Heart Valve Surgery; Coronary Artery Surgery; Ventricular Assist Device (LVAD); **Hospital:** Northwestern Meml Hosp; **Address:** Bluhm Cardiovascular Inst, 675 N St Clair St, Galter Bldg Fl 19 - Ste 100, Chicago, IL 60611-2968; **Phone:** 312-695-4965; **Board Cert:** Thoracic Surgery 2008; **Med School:** Loyola Univ-Stritch Sch Med 1980; **Resid:** Surgery, Mayo Clinic 1985; Thoracic Surgery, Mayo Clinic 1988; **Fellow:** Cardiopulmonary Transplant Surgery, Stanford Univ 1989; **Fac Appt:** Prof S, Northwestern Univ

Meyers, Bryan F MD [T&CS] - **Spec Exp:** Lung Cancer; Esophageal Cancer; Transplant-Lung; Emphysema-Lung Volume Reduction; **Hospital:** Barnes-Jewish Hosp, Barnes-Jewish West County Hosp; **Address:** 4921 Parkview Pl, Ste 8B, St Louis, MO 63110; **Phone:** 314-362-8598; **Board Cert:** Thoracic Surgery 2007; **Med School:** Univ Chicago-Pritzker Sch Med 1986; **Resid:** Surgery, Mass Genl Hosp 1996; **Fellow:** Cardiothoracic Surgery, Barnes Hosp-Wash Univ 1998; **Fac Appt:** Assoc Prof S, Washington Univ, St Louis

Thoracic & Cardiac Surgery

Moon, Marc R MD [T&CS] - **Spec Exp:** Aneurysm-Thoracic Aortic; Cardiothoracic Surgery; Mitral Valve Surgery; **Hospital:** Barnes-Jewish Hosp; **Address:** 660 S Euclid Ave, Box 8234, St Louis, MO 63110; **Phone:** 314-362-0993; **Board Cert:** Surgery 2005; Thoracic Surgery 2008; **Med School:** Wayne State Univ 1988; **Resid:** Surgery, Med Coll Wisc Affil Hosps 1995; Thoracic Surgery, Stanford Univ Hosp 1996; **Fac Appt:** Prof S, Washington Univ, St Louis

Naunheim, Keith S MD [T&CS] - **Spec Exp:** Lung Cancer; Esophageal Cancer; Chest Wall Tumors; Video Assisted Thoracic Surgery (VATS); **Hospital:** St. Louis Univ Hosp, SSM St Mary's Hlth Ctr - St Louis; **Address:** 3655 Vista Ave Fl 1, St Louis, MO 63110; **Phone:** 314-577-8360; **Board Cert:** Thoracic Surgery 2004; **Med School:** Univ Chicago-Pritzker Sch Med 1978; **Resid:** Surgery, Univ Chicago Hosp 1983; **Fellow:** Cardiothoracic Surgery, Univ Chicago Hosp 1985; **Fac Appt:** Prof TS, St Louis Univ

Orringer, Mark B MD [T&CS] - **Spec Exp:** Esophageal Cancer; Lung Cancer; Mediastinal Tumors; Lung Cancer; **Hospital:** Univ of Michigan Hosp; **Address:** Univ Mich, Taubman Ctr, 1500 E Med Ctr Drive, rm TC 2120, Box 5344, Ann Arbor, MI 48109; **Phone:** 734-936-4975; **Board Cert:** Surgery 1973; Thoracic Surgery 1974; **Med School:** Univ Pittsburgh 1967; **Resid:** Thoracic Surgery, Johns Hopkins Hosp 1973; **Fac Appt:** Prof S, Univ Mich Med Sch

Pagani, Francis D MD/PhD [T&CS] - **Spec Exp:** Transplant-Heart; Coronary Artery Surgery; Left Ventricular Assist Device (LVAD); **Hospital:** Univ of Michigan Hosp; **Address:** Univ Mich Med Ctr, 5144 Cardiovascular Ctr, 1500 E Med Ctr Drive, SPC 5864, Ann Arbor, MI 48109-5864; **Phone:** 734-647-2894; **Board Cert:** Surgery 2002; Thoracic Surgery 2004; **Med School:** Georgetown Univ 1986; **Resid:** Surgery, Georgetown Univ Med Ctr 1993; Thoracic Surgery, Univ Mich Hosp 1995; **Fellow:** Research, Univ Mass Med Ctr 1990; **Fac Appt:** Prof S, Univ Mich Med Sch

Patterson, G Alexander MD [T&CS] - **Spec Exp:** Lung Cancer; Esophageal Cancer; Transplant-Lung; Transplant-Heart & Lung; **Hospital:** Barnes-Jewish Hosp; **Address:** 660 S Euclid Ave, Box 8234, St Louis, MO 63110; **Phone:** 314-362-6025; **Board Cert:** Surgery 1978; Thoracic Surgery 1981; Vascular Surgery 1982; **Med School:** Canada 1974; **Resid:** Surgery, Queens Univ Med Ctr 1978; Vascular Surgery, Univ Toronto Med Ctr 1979; **Fellow:** Research, Toronto Genl Hosp 1981; Surgical Critical Care, Johns Hopkins Hosp 1982; **Fac Appt:** Prof S, Washington Univ, St Louis

Pochettino, Alberto B MD [T&CS] - **Spec Exp:** Aneurysm-Thoracic Aortic; Transplant-Lung; Left Ventricular Assist Device (LVAD); Heart Valve Surgery; **Hospital:** St. Mary's Hosp - Rochester MN (Mayo); **Address:** Mayo Clinic, 200 1st St SW, Rochester, MN 55905; **Phone:** 507-255-7066; **Board Cert:** Surgery 2005; Thoracic Surgery 2005; **Med School:** Northwestern Univ 1987; **Resid:** Surgery, SUNY-Upstate Med Ctr 1993; **Fellow:** Thoracic Surgery, Hosp Univ Penn 1995; Cardiopulmonary Transplant Surgery, Hosp Univ Penn 1997

Rice, Thomas W MD [T&CS] - **Spec Exp:** Esophageal Surgery; Minimally Invasive Thoracic Surgery; Lung Cancer; **Hospital:** Cleveland Clin (page 55); **Address:** Cleveland Clinic, 9500 Euclid Ave, Desk J4-1, Cleveland, OH 44195; **Phone:** 216-444-1921; **Board Cert:** Surgery 2004; Thoracic Surgery 2005; **Med School:** Univ Toronto 1978; **Resid:** Surgery, Univ Toronto Med Ctr 1983; Thoracic Surgery, Univ Toronto Med Ctr 1986; **Fellow:** Pulmonary Disease, UCSF Med Ctr 1984; **Fac Appt:** Prof S, Cleveland Cl Coll Med/Case West Res

Schaff, Hartzell MD [T&CS] - **Spec Exp:** Heart Valve Surgery; Congenital Heart Disease; Maze Procedure for Atrial Fibrillation; **Hospital:** St. Mary's Hosp - Rochester MN (Mayo); **Address:** Mayo Clin, Div Cardiovasc Surg, 200 First St SW, Rochester, MN 55905; **Phone:** 507-255-7068; **Board Cert:** Thoracic Surgery 2010; **Med School:** Univ Okla Coll Med 1973; **Resid:** Surgery, Johns Hopkins Hosp 1978; Thoracic Surgery, Johns Hopkins Hosp 1980; **Fellow:** Surgery, Johns Hopkins Hosp 1976; **Fac Appt:** Prof S, Mayo Med Sch

Smedira, Nicholas MD [T&CS] - **Spec Exp:** Transplant-Heart; Transplant-Lung; Ventricular Assist Device (LVAD); Aortic Surgery; **Hospital:** Cleveland Clin (page 55); **Address:** Cleveland Clin, Dept Cardiothoracic Surg, 9500 Euclid Ave, Desk J4-1, Cleveland, OH 44195; **Phone:** 216-445-7052; **Board Cert:** Thoracic & Cardiac Surgery 2003; **Med School:** Univ Rochester 1984; **Resid:** Surgery, UCSF Med Ctr 1991; Thoracic Surgery, UCSF Med Ctr 1994; **Fellow:** Cardiothoracic Surgery, UCSF Med Ctr 1994

Smith, John Michael MD [T&CS] - **Spec Exp:** Mitral Valve Robotic Surgery; **Hospital:** Good Samaritan Hosp - Cincinnati; **Address:** 4030 Smith Rd, Ste 300, Norwood, OH 45209; **Phone:** 513-421-3494; **Board Cert:** Surgery 2003; Thoracic Surgery 2006; **Med School:** Univ Louisville Sch Med 1989; **Resid:** Surgery, Good Samaritan Hosp 1994; **Fellow:** Cardiothoracic Surgery, Yale Univ Hosp 1996

Stuart, Richard S MD [T&CS] - **Spec Exp:** Cardiac Surgery; Cardiothoracic Surgery; Robotic Cardiac Surgery; **Hospital:** St. Luke's Hosp of Kansas City, N Kansas City Hosp; **Address:** St Luke's Hosp, MidAmerica Heart and Lung Inst, 4320 Wornall Rd Bldg 2 - Ste 50-11, Kansas City, MO 64111; **Phone:** 816-931-3312; **Board Cert:** Thoracic Surgery 2010; Surgical Critical Care 2003; **Med School:** Johns Hopkins Univ 1981; **Resid:** Surgery, Johns Hopkins Hosp 1986; **Fellow:** Cardiothoracic Surgery, Johns Hopkins Hosp 1989; **Fac Appt:** Clin Prof TS, Univ MO-Kansas City

Svensson, Lars G MD/PhD [T&CS] - **Spec Exp:** Aortic Surgery; Heart Valve Surgery-Percutaneous; Marfan's Syndrome; **Hospital:** Cleveland Clin (page 55); **Address:** Cleveland Clinic, 9500 Euclid Ave, Desk J4-1, Cleveland, OH 44195; **Phone:** 216-445-4813; **Med School:** South Africa 1978; **Resid:** Surgery, Johannesburg Hosp 1986; Cardiothoracic Surgery, Baylor Coll of Med 1991; **Fellow:** Cardiovascular Surgery, Cleveland Clinic 1987; Cardiovascular Surgery, Baylor Coll of Med 1989; **Fac Appt:** Prof S, Case West Res Univ

Turrentine, Mark W MD [T&CS] - **Spec Exp:** Cardiac Surgery-Pediatric; Transplant-Heart; Transplant-Lung; Congenital Heart Disease; **Hospital:** Riley Hosp for Children, IU Health University Hosp; **Address:** Indiana Univ Dept Surgery, 545 Barnhill Drive, EH 215, Indianapolis, IN 46202; **Phone:** 317-274-7150; **Board Cert:** Thoracic & Cardiac Surgery 2002; Congenital Cardiac Surgery 2011; **Med School:** Univ Kansas 1983; **Resid:** Surgery, Univ Kansas Med Ctr 1988; Cardiothoracic Surgery, Indiana Univ Med Ctr 1991; **Fellow:** Cardiothoracic Surgery, Texas Heart Inst 1986; Transplant Surgery, Indiana Univ Med Ctr 1989; **Fac Appt:** Prof S, Indiana Univ

Vigneswaran, Wickii MD [T&CS] - **Spec Exp:** Transplant-Lung; Thoracic Cancers; Mesothelioma; Hyperhidrosis-Palmar; **Hospital:** Univ of Chicago Med Ctr; **Address:** Univ Chicago Hosps, Lung Transplant Div, 5841 S Maryland Ave, MC 5040, Chicago, IL 60637; **Phone:** 773-795-1267; **Med School:** Sri Lanka 1978; **Resid:** Surgery, Royal Coll Surgeons 1983; Cardiothoracic Surgery, Royal Coll Surgeons 1990; **Fellow:** Cardiothoracic Transplant Surg, Mayo Clin 1994; **Fac Appt:** Prof S, Univ Chicago-Pritzker Sch Med

Walters, Henry L MD [T&CS] - **Spec Exp:** Pediatric Cardiac Surgery; Transplant-Heart-Pediatric; Cardiac Surgery-Neonatal; **Hospital:** Chldns Hosp of Michigan; **Address:** Chldns Hosp of Michigan, 3901 Beaubien Blvd, Detroit, MI 48201; **Phone:** 313-745-5538; **Board Cert:** Thoracic & Cardiac Surgery 2010; Congenital Cardiac Surgery 2009; **Med School:** Baylor Coll Med 1982; **Resid:** Surgery, Mass Genl Hosp 1988; **Fellow:** Pediatric Cardiothoracic Surgery, UAB Med Ctr 1992; **Fac Appt:** Prof S, Wayne State Univ

Weigel, Tracey L MD [T&CS] - **Spec Exp:** Esophageal Cancer; Lung Cancer; Mesothelioma; Graves' Disease; **Hospital:** Univ WI Hosp & Clins; **Address:** University of Wisconsin Hospital and Clinics, 600 Highland Ave, H4/316 CSC, Madison, WI 53792-7375; **Phone:** 608-265-0499; **Board Cert:** Surgery 2003; Thoracic Surgery 2006; **Med School:** Univ Rochester 1986; **Resid:** Surgery, Rhode Island Hosp 1993; **Fellow:** Surgical Oncology, Meml Sloan Kettering Cancer Ctr 1995; Cardiothoracic Surgery, Univ Wisconsin 1996; **Fac Appt:** Assoc Prof S, Univ Wisc

Thoracic & Cardiac Surgery

Ziemer, Gerhard MD/PhD [T&CS] - **Spec Exp:** Pediatric Cardiac Surgery; Neonatal & Infant Cardiac Surgery; Congenital Heart Disease; **Hospital:** Univ of Chicago Med Ctr; **Address:** Univ Chicago-Pediatric Cardiac Surgery, 5841 S Maryland Ave, MC 5040, Chicago, IL 60637; **Phone:** 773-702-2500; **Med School:** Germany 1978; **Resid:** Surgery, Hannover Med School Affil Hosp 1984; Cardiothoracic Surgery, Chldn's Hosp 1986; **Fellow:** Cardiothoracic Surgery, Hannover Med School Affil Hosp 1988; **Fac Appt:** Prof S, Univ Chicago-Pritzker Sch Med

Great Plains and Mountains

Bull, David A MD [T&CS] - **Spec Exp:** Cardiothoracic Surgery; Esophageal Cancer; **Hospital:** Univ Utah Hlth Care; **Address:** Univ Utah, Dept Cardiothoracic Surgery, 30 N 1900 East, Ste 3C127, Salt Lake City, UT 84132; **Phone:** 801-581-5311; **Board Cert:** Surgery 2008; Surgical Critical Care 2009; Vascular Surgery 2011; Thoracic Surgery 2004; **Med School:** UCSF 1985; **Resid:** Surgery, UCSF Medical Ctr 1987; Surgery, Univ Arizona Hosps 1990; **Fellow:** Vascular Surgery, Univ Arizona Hosps 1992; Cardiothoracic Surgery, Univ Arizona Hosps 1994; **Fac Appt:** Assoc Prof TS, Univ Utah

Campbell, David N MD [T&CS] - **Spec Exp:** Pediatric Cardiothoracic Surgery; Transplant-Heart-Pediatric; Transplant-Lung; Congenital Heart Surgery; **Hospital:** Chldn's Hosp - Aurora (CO), Univ of CO Hosp - Anschutz Inpatient Pav; **Address:** Childrens Hosp Cardiothoracic Surgery, 13123 E 16th Ave, Box 200, Aurora, CO 80045; **Phone:** 720-777-6624; **Board Cert:** Thoracic & Cardiac Surgery 2010; Surgical Critical Care 2000; Critical Care Medicine 2009; **Med School:** Rush Med Coll 1974; **Resid:** Surgery, Univ CO Med Ctr 1980; Cardiothoracic Surgery, Univ CO Med Ctr 1979; **Fellow:** Cardiothoracic Surgery, Chldn's Hosp 1981; **Fac Appt:** Prof S, Univ Colorado

Fullerton, David A MD [T&CS] - **Spec Exp:** Maze Procedure for Atrial Fibrillation; Ross Procedure for Aortic Valve Disease; Mitral Valve Surgery; Transplant-Heart & Lung; **Hospital:** Univ of CO Hosp - Anschutz Inpatient Pav, VA Eastern CO Health Care Sys-Denver; **Address:** Univ of Colorado, Cardiothoracic Surgery, 12631 E 17th Ave, rm 6602, MS C310, Aurora, CO 80045; **Phone:** 303-724-2798; **Board Cert:** Surgery 2007; Surgical Critical Care 2011; Thoracic Surgery 2011; **Med School:** Univ MO-Columbia Sch Med 1981; **Resid:** Surgery, Univ Wash Med Ctr 1987; Thoracic Surgery, Univ Colorado Hosp 1990; **Fac Appt:** Prof S, Univ Colorado

Guber, Myles S MD [T&CS] - **Spec Exp:** Minimally Invasive Heart Valve Surgery; Robotic Cardiac Surgery; Thoracic Surgery; **Hospital:** Porter Adventist Hosp; **Address:** Colorado Cardiovascular Surgical Assocs, 950 E Harvard Ave, Ste 550, Denver, CO 80210; **Phone:** 303-778-6527; **Board Cert:** Thoracic & Cardiac Surgery 2006; **Med School:** Northwestern Univ-Feinberg Sch Med 1980; **Resid:** Surgery, Louisiana State U Med Ctr 1985; **Fellow:** Thoracic & Cardiac Surgery, USC/Good SAmaritan Hosp 1987

Karwande, Shreekanth V MD [T&CS] - **Spec Exp:** Thoracic Cancers; Lung Cancer; Cardiac Surgery; **Hospital:** St. Mark's Hosp - Salt Lake City; **Address:** MountainStar Cardiovascular Surgery, 1160 E 3900 St S, Ste 3500, Ste 3500, Salt Lake City, UT 84124; **Phone:** 801-743-4750; **Board Cert:** Thoracic Surgery 2003; **Med School:** India 1973; **Resid:** Surgery, Erie Co Med Ctr 1981; Cardiothoracic Surgery, NY Hosp 1985; **Fellow:** Cardiothoracic Surgery, Meml Sloan Kettering Cancer Ctr

Mitchell, John D MD [T&CS] - **Spec Exp:** Lung Cancer; Esophageal Surgery; Transplant-Lung; Hyperhidrosis-Palmar; **Hospital:** Univ of CO Hosp - Anschutz Inpatient Pav, VA Eastern CO Health Care Sys-Denver; **Address:** Univ Colorado, Dept Cardiothoracic Surg, 12631 E 17th Ave, MS C310, Aurora, CO 80045; **Phone:** 303-724-2800; **Board Cert:** Surgery 2005; Thoracic Surgery 2007; **Med School:** Univ Mich Med Sch 1987; **Resid:** Surgery, Mass Genl Hosp 1994; Cardiothoracic Surgery, Mass Genl Hosp 1996; **Fac Appt:** Assoc Prof TS, Univ Colorado

Mitchell, Max B MD [T&CS] - **Spec Exp:** Congenital Heart Surgery; Heart Valve Surgery; Pediatric Cardiac Surgery; Transplant-Lung; **Hospital:** Chldn's Hosp - Aurora (CO), Univ of CO Hosp - Anschutz Inpatient Pav; **Address:** Childrens Hosp Cardiothoracic Surgery, 13123 E 16th Ave, B-200, Aurora, CO 80045; **Phone:** 720-777-6624; **Board Cert:** Surgery 2004; Thoracic Surgery 2007; Congenital Cardiac Surgery 2009; **Med School:** Geo Wash Univ 1988; **Resid:** Surgery, Univ Colorado Affil Hosp 1995; Cardiovascular Surgery, Univ Colorado Affil Hosp 1998; **Fellow:** Pediatric Cardiac Surgery, Royal Childrens Hosp 1999; **Fac Appt:** Assoc Prof S, Univ Colorado

Southwest

Aklog, Lishan MD [T&CS] - **Spec Exp:** Mitral Valve Surgery; Minimally Invasive Cardiac Surgery; Coronary Artery Surgery; Heart Failure; **Hospital:** St. Joseph's Hosp & Med Ctr - Phoenix; **Address:** Heart and Lung Institute, St Joseph's Hosp Med Ctr, 500 W Thomas Rd, Ste 500, Phoenix, AZ 85013-4224; **Phone:** 602-406-2996; **Board Cert:** Thoracic & Cardiac Surgery 2010; **Med School:** Harvard Med Sch 1989; **Resid:** Surgery, Brigham & Womens Hosp 1996; Cardiothoracic Surgery, Brigham & Womens Hosp 1998; **Fellow:** Cardiac Surgery, Harefield Hosp 1999; Cardiac Surgery, L'Hopital Broussais 1999

Calhoon, John H MD [T&CS] - **Spec Exp:** Transplant-Heart & Lung; Congenital Heart Surgery; Cardiac Surgery-Adult & Pediatric; **Hospital:** Univ Hlth Syst-San Antonio, Christus Santa Rosa Children's Hosp; **Address:** 7703 Floyd Curl Drive, Medical Bldg, MS 7841, San Antonio, TX 78229-3901; **Phone:** 210-567-2878; **Board Cert:** Surgery 2004; Thoracic Surgery 2007; **Med School:** Baylor Coll Med 1981; **Resid:** Surgery, Univ Hosp/Univ Texas HSC 1986; Univ Hosp/Univ Texas HSC 1988; **Fellow:** Pediatric Cardiac Surgery, Chldns Hosp/Harvard 1989; **Fac Appt:** Prof TS, Univ Tex, San Antonio

Caskey, Michael P MD [T&CS] - **Spec Exp:** Coronary Artery Surgery; Heart Valve Surgery; Maze Procedure for Atrial Fibrillation; Carotid Artery Surgery; **Hospital:** Banner Good Samaritan Regl Med Ctr - Phoenix; **Address:** Southwest Heart & Lung, 10930 N Tatum Blvd, Ste 103, Phoenix, AZ 85028; **Phone:** 602-263-7800; **Board Cert:** Thoracic & Cardiac Surgery 2003; **Med School:** Univ Tex Med Br, Galveston 1983; **Resid:** Surgery, Good Samaritan/VA Hosp 1988; Cardiovascular Surgery, Rush Presby-St Lukes Med Ctr 1990

Coselli, Joseph S MD [T&CS] - **Spec Exp:** Aneurysm-Abdominal & Thoracic Aortic; Marfan's Syndrome; Aortic Surgery; **Hospital:** St. Luke's Episcopal Hosp-Houston, Methodist Hosp - Houston; **Address:** 6770 Bertner St, Ste C350, Houston, TX 77030; **Phone:** 832-355-9910; **Board Cert:** Thoracic Surgery 2004; **Med School:** Univ Tex Med Br, Galveston 1977; **Resid:** Surgery, Baylor Affil Hosp 1982; Thoracic Surgery, Baylor Affil Hosp 1984; **Fac Appt:** Assoc Prof S, Baylor Coll Med

Diethrich, Edward B MD [T&CS] - **Spec Exp:** Vascular Surgery; Endovascular Surgery; Cardiovascular Surgery; **Hospital:** Arizona Heart Hosp; **Address:** Arizona Heart Foundation, 1910 E Thomas Rd, Ste 220, Phoenix, AZ 85016; **Phone:** 602-200-0437; **Board Cert:** Thoracic Surgery 1967; Surgery 1966; **Med School:** Univ Mich Med Sch 1960; **Resid:** Surgery, St Joseph Mercy Hosp 1964; **Fellow:** Cardiothoracic Surgery, Baylor Coll Med 1966; **Fac Appt:** Prof TS, Univ Ariz Coll Med

Echeverri, Luis G MD [T&CS] - **Spec Exp:** Cardiac Surgery; Aortic Surgery; Transplant-Heart; **Hospital:** Methodist Sugar Land Hosp, Meml Hermann SW Hosp; **Address:** 7737 Southwest Freeway, Ste 201, Houston, TX 77074; **Phone:** 713-776-3402; **Board Cert:** Surgery 2007; Thoracic Surgery 2010; **Med School:** Colombia 1982; **Resid:** Surgery, Univ Texas Med Ctr 1996; Cardiothoracic Surgery, Univ Arizona Med Ctr 2001; **Fellow:** Transplant Surgery, Univ Pittsburgh 1993; Cardiovascular Surgery, Texas Heart Inst 1998

Thoracic & Cardiac Surgery

Forbess, Joseph M MD [T&CS] - **Spec Exp:** Pediatric Cardiothoracic Surgery; Heart Valve Surgery-Pediatric; **Hospital:** Chldns Med Ctr of Dallas, UT Southwestern Med Ctr at Dallas; **Address:** Univ Texas SW Med Ctr, Div Ped Cardiothor Surg, 1935 Medical District Drive, Ste C3211, Dallas, TX 75235; **Phone:** 214-730-5437; **Board Cert:** Surgery 2008; **Med School:** Harvard Med Sch 1990; **Resid:** Surgery, Duke Univ Med Ctr 1997; Cardiothoracic Surgery, Duke Univ Med Ctr 1999; **Fellow:** Cardiac Surgery, Childrens Hosp 1994; **Fac Appt:** Assoc Prof TS, Univ Tex SW, Dallas

Fraser, Charles D MD [T&CS] - **Spec Exp:** Pediatric Cardiothoracic Surgery; Congenital Heart Surgery; **Hospital:** Texas Chldns Hosp; **Address:** Texas Chldns Hosp-Heart Ctr, 6621 Fannin St Fl 19, Houston, TX 77030-2399; **Phone:** 832-826-2030; **Board Cert:** Surgery 2010; Thoracic & Cardiac Surgery 2002; Congenital Cardiac Surgery 2009; **Med School:** Univ Tex Med Br, Galveston 1984; **Resid:** Surgery, Johns Hopkins Hosp 1990; Cardiovascular Surgery, Johns Hopkins Hosp 1993; **Fac Appt:** Prof S, Baylor Coll Med

Frazier Jr, O Howard MD [T&CS] - **Spec Exp:** Transplant-Heart; Lung Surgery; Artificial Heart Devices; **Hospital:** St. Luke's Episcopal Hosp-Houston, Texas Chldns Hosp; **Address:** Surgical Assocs-Texas Heart Institute, 6720 Bertner Ave, Ste C350, Houston, TX 77030; **Phone:** 832-355-4900; **Board Cert:** Surgery 1975; Thoracic & Cardiac Surgery 2005; **Med School:** Baylor Coll Med 1967; **Resid:** Surgery, Baylor Affil Hosp 1974; Thoracic Surgery, Texas Heart Inst 1976; **Fac Appt:** Prof S, Univ Tex, Houston

Harrell Jr, James E MD [T&CS] - **Spec Exp:** Transplant-Heart; Cardiac Surgery-Pediatric; **Hospital:** Covenant Children's Hosp; **Address:** 3606 21st St, Ste 103, Lubbock, TX 79410; **Phone:** 806-725-4425; **Board Cert:** Surgery 2006; Thoracic Surgery 2006; **Med School:** Baylor Coll Med 1978; **Resid:** Surgery, Univ Tex Hlth Scis Ctr 1984; Thoracic Surgery, Baylor Coll Med 1986; **Fellow:** Cardiovascular Surgery, Hosp Sick Chldn 1987

Jessen, Michael Erik MD [T&CS] - **Spec Exp:** Cardiac Surgery; Transplant-Heart; Aneurysm-Aortic; Heart Valve Surgery; **Hospital:** UT Southwestern Med Ctr at Dallas, Parkland Hlth & Hosp Sys; **Address:** 5323 Harry Hines Blvd, MS 8879, Dallas, TX 75390-8879; **Phone:** 214-645-7721; **Board Cert:** Surgery 2007; Thoracic Surgery 2011; **Med School:** Univ Manitoba 1981; **Resid:** Surgery, Univ Manitoba 1986; Thoracic Surgery, Duke Univ Med Ctr 1990; **Fellow:** Research, Duke Univ Med Ctr 1988; **Fac Appt:** Prof TS, Univ Tex SW, Dallas

Johnson, Scott B MD [T&CS] - **Spec Exp:** Thoracic Cancers; **Hospital:** Univ Hlth Syst-San Antonio; **Address:** UT Hlth-San Antonio, Cardiac Surgery, 7703 Floyd Curl Drive, MSC7841, San Antonio, TX 78229; **Phone:** 210-567-5615; **Board Cert:** Surgery 2010; Surgical Critical Care 2001; Thoracic Surgery 2004; **Med School:** Univ New Mexico 1987; **Resid:** Surgery, LAC-USC Hosp 1992; Surgery, UTHSC V Hosp 1995; **Fellow:** Cardiothoracic Surgery, LAC-USC Hosp 1993

Kernstine, Kemp H MD/PhD [T&CS] - **Spec Exp:** Lung Cancer; Esophageal Cancer; Tracheal Surgery; Esophageal Surgery; **Hospital:** UT Southwestern Med Ctr at Dallas; **Address:** UT SW Med Ctr, Cardiothoracic Surgery, 5323 Harry Hines Blvd, Dallas, TX 75390-8879; **Phone:** 214-645-7748; **Board Cert:** Thoracic Surgery 2004; Surgery 2001; **Med School:** Duke Univ 1982; **Resid:** Surgery, Univ Minn Med Ctr 1988; **Fellow:** Cardiothoracic Surgery, Brigham & Women's Hosp 1994; **Fac Appt:** Prof TS, Univ Tex SW, Dallas

Lanza, Louis MD [T&CS] - **Spec Exp:** Lung Cancer; Cardiothoracic Surgery; **Hospital:** Mayo Clinic - Phoenix; **Address:** Mayo Clinic Cardiothoracic Surgery, 5777 E Mayo Blvd, Phoenix, AZ 85054; **Phone:** 480-342-2270; **Board Cert:** Thoracic & Cardiac Surgery 2010; **Med School:** Loyola Univ-Stritch Sch Med 1981; **Resid:** Surgery, Univ Michigan Med Ctr 1988; Cardiovascular Surgery, Texas Heart Inst 1991; **Fellow:** Surgical Oncology, Natl Cancer Inst 1986; Thoracic Oncology, MD Anderson Cancer Ctr 1989

Mack, Michael J MD [T&CS] - **Spec Exp:** Transplant-Heart & Lung; Cardiac Surgery; Minimally Invasive Surgery; **Hospital:** Med City Dallas Hosp, Med Ctr of Plano; **Address:** 4716 Alliance Blvd, Pavilion 2, Ste 310, Plano, TX 75093; **Phone:** 972-596-6676; **Board Cert:** Internal Medicine 1976; Thoracic Surgery 2001; **Med School:** St Louis Univ 1973; **Resid:** Internal Medicine, Univ MN Hosp 1976; Surgery, Parkland Hosp 1980; **Fellow:** Thoracic Surgery, Parkland Hosp 1982

Ott, David A MD [T&CS] - **Spec Exp:** Heart Valve Surgery; Coronary Artery Surgery; Aneurysm-Abdominal Aortic; Carotid Artery Surgery; **Hospital:** St. Luke's Episcopal Hosp-Houston; **Address:** 1101 Bates Ave, Ste P-514, Houston, TX 77030-2607; **Phone:** 832-355-4900; **Board Cert:** Thoracic & Cardiac Surgery 2008; **Med School:** Baylor Coll Med 1972; **Resid:** Surgery, Baylor Coll Med 1976; Cardiothoracic Surgery, Tex Heart Inst 1978; **Fac Appt:** Clin Prof S, Baylor Coll Med

Reardon, Michael J MD [T&CS] - **Spec Exp:** Cardiac Tumors/Cancer; Heart Valve Surgery-Aortic; **Hospital:** Methodist Hosp - Houston, UT MD Anderson Cancer Ctr; **Address:** 6550 Fannin St, Ste 1401, Houston, TX 77030; **Phone:** 713-441-5200; **Board Cert:** Thoracic Surgery 2006; **Med School:** Baylor Coll Med 1978; **Resid:** Surgery, Baylor Affil Hosps 1983; Thoracic Surgery, Texas Heart Inst 1985; **Fac Appt:** Prof TS, Cornell Univ-Weill Med Coll

Rice, David C MD [T&CS] - **Spec Exp:** Mesothelioma; Thoracic Cancers; Minimally Invasive Surgery; **Hospital:** UT MD Anderson Cancer Ctr; **Address:** MD Anderson Cancer Ctr, 1515 Holcombe Blvd, Box 1489, Houston, TX 77030; **Phone:** 713-794-1477; **Board Cert:** Surgery 2002; Thoracic & Cardiac Surgery 2004; **Med School:** Ireland 1991; **Resid:** Surgery, Mayo Clinic 1998; Cardiothoracic Surgery, Baylor Affil Hosps 2001; **Fellow:** Thoracic Surgery, Mayo Clinic 1999

Roth, Jack MD [T&CS] - **Spec Exp:** Esophageal Cancer; Lung Cancer; Gene Therapy; **Hospital:** UT MD Anderson Cancer Ctr; **Address:** UT MD Anderson Cancer Ctr, Dept Thoracic & Cardiovasc Surg, 1515 Holcombe Blvd, Uni 1489, Houston, TX 77030-4000; **Phone:** 713-792-7664; **Board Cert:** Thoracic & Cardiac Surgery 2011; **Med School:** Johns Hopkins Univ 1971; **Resid:** Surgery, Johns Hopkins Hosp 1973; Thoracic Surgery, UCLA Med Ctr 1979; **Fellow:** Surgical Oncology, UCLA 1975; **Fac Appt:** Prof TS, Univ Tex, Houston

Safi, Hazim J MD [T&CS] - **Spec Exp:** Aneurysm-Abdominal Aortic; Aortic Surgery; Vascular Surgery; **Hospital:** Meml Hermann Hosp - Texas Med Ctr; **Address:** UT, Dept Cardiothoracic & Vascular Surg, 6400 Fannin St, Ste 2850, Houston, TX 77030; **Phone:** 713-500-5304; **Board Cert:** Vascular Surgery 2005; Thoracic Surgery 2007; **Med School:** Iraq 1970; **Resid:** Surgery, Baylor Affil Hosp 1980; Radiation Oncology, Baylor Affil Hosp 1981; **Fellow:** Thoracic Surgery, Baylor Coll Med 1983; **Fac Appt:** Prof S, Univ Tex, Houston

Smythe, W Roy MD [T&CS] - **Spec Exp:** Lung Cancer; Mesothelioma; **Hospital:** Scott & White Mem Hosp; **Address:** 2401 S 31st St, Temple, TX 76508; **Phone:** 254-724-5918; **Board Cert:** Surgery 2009; Thoracic & Cardiac Surgery 2010; **Med School:** Texas A&M Univ 1989; **Resid:** Surgery, Hosp Univ Penn 1996; **Fellow:** Cardiothoracic Surgery, Hosp Univ Penn 1998; Surgical Oncology, American Cancer Society 1996; **Fac Appt:** Asst Prof S, Univ Tex, Houston

Swisher, Stephen G MD [T&CS] - **Spec Exp:** Esophageal Cancer; Lung Cancer; Mesothelioma; Thoracic Cancers; **Hospital:** UT MD Anderson Cancer Ctr; **Address:** UT MD Anderson Cancer Ctr, Dept of Thoracic & Cardiovasc Surg, 1515 Holcombe Blvd, Unit 1489, Houston, TX 77030; **Phone:** 713-792-8659; **Board Cert:** Surgery 2002; Thoracic & Cardiac Surgery 2006; **Med School:** UCSD 1986; **Resid:** Surgery, UCLA Med Ctr 1993; **Fellow:** Surgical Oncology, UCLA Med Ctr 1990; Cardiothoracic Surgery, MD Anderson Canc Ctr 1996; **Fac Appt:** Prof TS, Univ Tex, Houston

Thoracic & Cardiac Surgery

Turner, William F MD [T&CS] - **Spec Exp:** Coronary Artery Surgery; Cardiac Surgery; **Hospital:** E TX Med Ctr-Tyler, Trinity Mother Frances Hosp; **Address:** 619 S Fleichel St, Ste 207, Tyler, TX 75701; **Phone:** 903-593-0900; **Board Cert:** Thoracic Surgery 2008; **Med School:** Baylor Coll Med 1981; **Resid:** Surgery, Baylor Coll Med 1987; Thoracic Surgery, Baylor Coll Med 1989

Walsh, Garrett L MD [T&CS] - **Spec Exp:** Esophageal Cancer; **Hospital:** UT MD Anderson Cancer Ctr; **Address:** UT MD Anderson Cancer Ctr, Dept of Thoracic & Cardiovasc Surg, 1515 Holcombe Blvd, Unit 1489, Houston, TX 77030; **Phone:** 713-792-6849; **Board Cert:** Surgery 2009; Thoracic & Cardiac Surgery 2009; **Med School:** Queens Univ 1983; **Resid:** Surgery, Royal Victoria Hosp-McGill 1988; Cardiovascular Surgery, McGill Univ Affil Hosp 1990; **Fac Appt:** Prof S, Univ Tex, Houston

West Coast and Pacific

Aldea, Gabriel S MD [T&CS] - **Spec Exp:** Thoracic Aortic Surgery; Heart Valve Surgery; Minimally Invasive Cardiac Surgery; **Hospital:** Univ Wash Med Ctr; **Address:** Univ Washington-Cardiothoracic Surgery, 1959 NE Pacific St, Box 356310, Seattle, WA 98195-6310; **Phone:** 206-221-3166; **Board Cert:** Thoracic Surgery 2010; **Med School:** Columbia P&S 1981; **Resid:** Surgery, NY Presby Hosp/Cornell 1986; Cardiothoracic Surgery, NY Presby Hosp/Cornell 1990; **Fellow:** Research, UCSF Affil Rsch Inst 1988; **Fac Appt:** Prof TS, Univ Wash

Bailey, Leonard L MD [T&CS] - **Spec Exp:** Cardiac Surgery-Pediatric; Congenital Heart Surgery; Transplant-Heart-Pediatric; **Hospital:** Loma Linda Chldns Hosp; **Address:** 11234 Anderson St, rm 1617, Loma Linda, CA 92354; **Phone:** 909-558-4200; **Board Cert:** Surgery 1975; Thoracic Surgery 2006; **Med School:** Loma Linda Univ 1969; **Resid:** Surgery, Loma Linda Univ Med Ctr 1973; Thoracic Surgery, Loma Linda Univ Med Ctr 1974; **Fellow:** Cardiovascular Surgery, Hosp Sick Chldn 1975; **Fac Appt:** Prof S, Loma Linda Univ

Bowdish, Michael E MD [T&CS] - **Spec Exp:** Thoracic Aortic Surgery; Aneurysm-Aortic; Left Ventricular Assist Device (LVAD); **Hospital:** Keck Med Ctr of USC (page 62); **Address:** USC Cardiovascular Thoracic Inst, 1520 San Pablo St, Ste 4300, Los Angeles, CA 90033; **Phone:** 323-442-5849; **Board Cert:** Surgery 2005; Thoracic & Cardiac Surgery 2009; **Med School:** Washington Univ, St Louis 1998; **Resid:** Surgery, USC Med Ctr 2005; Thoracic & Cardiac Surgery, NY Presby-Columbia Med Ctr 2008; **Fac Appt:** Asst Prof S, USC-Keck School of Medicine

Boyd, Walter Douglas MD [T&CS] - **Spec Exp:** Robotic Cardiac Surgery; Minimally Invasive Cardiac Surgery; Stem Cell Therapy & Biosurgery; Coronary Artery Surgery; **Hospital:** UC Davis Med Ctr; **Address:** 2221 Stockton Blvd, Cypres Bldg - rm 2112, Sacramento, CA 95817; **Phone:** 916-734-3861; **Med School:** Univ Ottawa 1984; **Resid:** Surgery, Ottawa Civic Hospital 1990; Cardiothoracic Surgery, Ottowa Civic Hospital 1992; **Fellow:** Transplantation/Mechanical Assist Devices, Ottawa Heart Inst 1995; **Fac Appt:** Prof S, UC Davis

Cameron, Robert B MD [T&CS] - **Spec Exp:** Lung Cancer; Mesothelioma; **Hospital:** UCLA Ronald Reagan Med Ctr; **Address:** UCLA Med Ctr, Dept Thoracic Surg, 10833 Le Conte Ave, rm 64-128CHS, Los Angeles, CA 90025; **Phone:** 310-470-8980; **Board Cert:** Surgery 2011; Thoracic Surgery 2005; **Med School:** UCLA 1984; **Resid:** Surgery, UCLA Med Ctr 1992; **Fellow:** Surgical Oncology, Natl Inst Hlth 1989; Cardiothoracic Surgery, NY Hosp/Cornell 1994

Cohen, Gordon MD/PhD [T&CS] - **Spec Exp:** Pediatric Cardiothoracic Surgery; Neonatal Surgery; Transplant-Heart-Pediatric; Heart Failure; **Hospital:** UCSF Med Ctr; **Address:** 513 Parnassus Ave, Ste S549, San Francisco, CA 94143; **Phone:** 415-476-3501; **Board Cert:** Thoracic & Cardiac Surgery 2010; **Med School:** Tulane Univ 1989; **Resid:** Surgery, UCLA Med Ctr 1996; Cardiothoracic Surgery, Univ Wash Med Ctr 1998; **Fellow:** Pediatric Cardiac Surgery, Great Ormond St Hosp for Chldn 1999; **Fac Appt:** Prof TS, Univ Wash

Cohen, Robbin G MD [T&CS] - **Spec Exp:** Minimally Invasive Surgery; Heart Valve Surgery; Thoracic Aortic Surgery; **Hospital:** Keck Med Ctr of USC (page 62), Huntington Memorial Hosp; **Address:** 1520 San Pueblo St, Ste 4300, Los Angeles, CA 90033; **Phone:** 323-442-5850; **Board Cert:** Thoracic Surgery 2008; **Med School:** Univ Colorado 1980; **Resid:** Surgery, Stanford Univ Med Ctr 1986; **Fellow:** Cardiothoracic Surgery, Stanford Univ Med Ctr 1989; **Fac Appt:** Assoc Prof TS, USC Sch Med

Dang, Michael H MD [T&CS] - **Spec Exp:** Cardiac Surgery; Peripheral Vascular Disease; Transplant-Heart; **Hospital:** Maui Meml Med Ctr; **Address:** Maui Heart and Vascular Clinic, 1849 Wili Pa Loop, Wailuku, HI 96793; **Phone:** 808-442-5667; **Board Cert:** Thoracic Surgery 2002; **Med School:** Univ Colorado 1968; **Resid:** Surgery, Baylor Univ Med Ctr 1976; Thoracic Surgery, Baylor Univ Med Ctr 1978

DeFilippi, Vincent J MD [T&CS] - **Spec Exp:** Minimally Invasive Cardiac Surgery; Mitral Valve Surgery; Maze Procedure for Atrial Fibrillation; Robotic Cardiac Surgery; **Hospital:** Salinas Valley Meml Hlthcare Systs, Stanford Univ Hosp & Clinics; **Address:** Stanford Univ at Salinas Valley, Cardiac Surgery Program, 212 San Jose St, Ste 301, Salinas, CA 93901; **Phone:** 831-759-3289; **Board Cert:** Thoracic Surgery 2005; **Med School:** Columbia P&S 1988; **Resid:** Surgery, Univ Chicago Hosps 1994; **Fellow:** Cardiothoracic Surgery, New York Hosp/Meml Sloan Kettering Cancer Ctr 1996; **Fac Appt:** Assoc Clin Prof TS, Stanford Univ

Grannis Jr, Frederic W MD [T&CS] - **Spec Exp:** Lung Cancer; Tobacco Abuse; Thoracic Cancers; Palliative Care; **Hospital:** City of Hope Natl Med Ctr, Methodist Hosp - Southern California; **Address:** Thor Surg-City of Hope Natl Med Ctr, 1500 E Duarte Rd, Duarte, CA 91010; **Phone:** 626-359-8111 x62669; **Board Cert:** Surgery 1975; Thoracic Surgery 2010; **Med School:** NY Med Coll 1969; **Resid:** Surgery, Mayo Clinic 1974; Thoracic Surgery, Mayo Clinic 1977; **Fac Appt:** Asst Clin Prof TS, UCSD

Gundry, Steven MD [T&CS] - **Spec Exp:** Cardiac Surgery-Adult & Pediatric; Cardiac Surgery-High Risk; Nutrition in Heart Disease; **Hospital:** Desert Regl Med Ctr, Eisenhower Med Ctr; **Address:** 555 E Tachevah Drive, 3West Bldg, Ste 103, Palm Springs, CA 92262; **Phone:** 760-323-5553; **Board Cert:** Thoracic Surgery 2005; **Med School:** Med Coll GA 1977; **Resid:** Surgery, Univ Michigan Hosps 1983; Thoracic Surgery, Univ Michigan Hosps 1985; **Fellow:** Pediatric Cardiac Surgery, Hosp-Sick Chldn 1986; **Fac Appt:** Clin Prof S, Loma Linda Univ

Handy Jr, John R MD [T&CS] - **Spec Exp:** Lung Cancer; Esophageal Cancer; Mesothelioma; Chest Wall Tumors; **Hospital:** Providence Portland Med Ctr; **Address:** Oregon Clinic-Cardiothoracic Surgery, 1111 NE 99th Ave, Ste 201, Portland, OR 97220; **Phone:** 503-963-3030; **Board Cert:** Surgery 2011; Thoracic Surgery 2001; **Med School:** Duke Univ 1983; **Resid:** Surgery, Brown Univ Hosp 1990; **Fellow:** Cardiothoracic Surgery, MUSC Med Ctr 1993

Hanley, Frank L MD [T&CS] - **Spec Exp:** Pediatric Thoracic Surgery; **Hospital:** Lucile Packard Chldn's Hosp, Chldns Hosp - Oakland; **Address:** 300 Pasteur Drive, FALK CVRB, MC 5407, Stanford, CA 94305-5407; **Phone:** 650-723-0190; **Board Cert:** Thoracic Surgery 2010; **Med School:** Tufts Univ 1978; **Resid:** Surgery, UCSF Med Ctr 1981; Cardiothoracic Surgery, UCSF Med Ctr 1988; **Fellow:** Research, UCSF Sch Med 1984; **Fac Appt:** Prof S, UCSF

Harken, Alden H MD [T&CS] - **Spec Exp:** Arrhythmias; Cardiac Surgery; Coronary Artery Surgery; **Hospital:** Alameda County Med Ctr-Highland Campus, UCSF Med Ctr; **Address:** UCSF East Bay Surgical Program, 1411 E 31st St, Oakland, CA 94602; **Phone:** 510-437-4091; **Board Cert:** Surgery 1990; Thoracic Surgery 2006; **Med School:** Case West Res Univ 1967; **Resid:** Surgery, Peter Bent Brigham Hosp 1970; Thoracic Surgery, Peter Bent Brigham Hosp 1973; **Fellow:** Cardiovascular Surgery, Boston Chldns Hosp 1971; **Fac Appt:** Prof S, UCSF

Thoracic & Cardiac Surgery

Jablons, David M MD [T&CS] - **Spec Exp:** Lung Cancer; Mesothelioma; Esophageal Surgery; **Hospital:** UCSF - Mt Zion Med Ctr; **Address:** UCSF Thoracic Surgery, 1600 Divisadero St Fl 4, San Francisco, CA 94115; **Phone:** 415-885-3882; **Board Cert:** Thoracic Surgery 2002; **Med School:** Albany Med Coll 1984; **Resid:** Surgery, New Eng Med Ctr-Tufts Univ 1986; Surgery, New Eng Med Ctr-Tufts Univ 1991; **Fellow:** Surgical Oncology, Natl Cancer Inst-NIH 1989; Cardiothoracic Surgery, New York Hosp-Cornell 1993; **Fac Appt:** Prof S, UCSF

Jamieson, Stuart W MD [T&CS] - **Spec Exp:** Pulmonary Embolism; Transplant-Heart & Lung; **Hospital:** UCSD Med Ctr; **Address:** UCSD Med Ctr, Div CTS, 9500 Gilman Drive, La Jolla, CA 92093-7892; **Phone:** 619-543-7777; **Med School:** England, UK 1971; **Resid:** Surgery 1975; **Fellow:** Cardiothoracic Surgery 1977; Cardiothoracic Surgery, Stanford Univ/American Heart Assoc 1980; **Fac Appt:** Prof S, UCSD

Laks, Hillel MD [T&CS] - **Spec Exp:** Congenital Heart Disease; Transplant-Heart; **Hospital:** UCLA Ronald Reagan Med Ctr; **Address:** UCLA Med Ctr, 10833 Le Conte Ave CHS Bldg, rm 62-215, Los Angeles, CA 90095-1741; **Phone:** 310-206-1837; **Board Cert:** Surgery 1975; Thoracic Surgery 2006; **Med School:** Africa 1965; **Resid:** Surgery, Peter Bent Brigham Hosp 1969; Thoracic Surgery, Peter Bent Brigham Hosp 1973; **Fac Appt:** Prof S, UCLA

Lamberti Jr, John J MD [T&CS] - **Spec Exp:** Pediatric Cardiac Surgery; Heart Valve Surgery; Congenital Heart Surgery; **Hospital:** Rady Children's Hosp - San Diego, UCSD Med Ctr; **Address:** 3030 Children's Way, Ste 202, MC 5078, San Diego, CA 92123-4227; **Phone:** 858-966-8030; **Board Cert:** Surgery 1973; Thoracic Surgery 1975; **Med School:** Univ Pittsburgh 1967; **Resid:** Surgery, Peter Bent Brigham Hosp 1972; Thoracic Surgery, Peter Bent Brigham Hosp 1973; **Fellow:** Pediatric Cardiac Surgery, Chldns Hosp 1974; **Fac Appt:** Prof S, UCSD

Merrick, Scot H MD [T&CS] - **Spec Exp:** Cardiac Surgery-Adult; Heart Valve Surgery; Coronary Revascularization; Congenital Heart Disease; **Hospital:** UCSF Med Ctr; **Address:** UCSF Med Ctr, Div Cardiothoracic Surg, 500 Parnassus Ave, Ste MU425, San Francisco, CA 94143-0118; **Phone:** 415-353-1606; **Board Cert:** Thoracic Surgery 2008; **Med School:** Univ Wash 1980; **Resid:** Surgery, UCSF Med Ctr 1985; **Fellow:** Cardiothoracic Surgery, UCSF Med Ctr 1987; **Fac Appt:** Assoc Prof S, UCSF

Miller, D Craig MD [T&CS] - **Spec Exp:** Thoracic Aortic Surgery; Mitral Valve Surgery; Aortic Surgery; Endovascular Surgery; **Hospital:** Stanford Univ Hosp & Clinics; **Address:** Stanford Univ Medical School, Dept Cardiovascular Surgery, 300 Pasteur Drive, Falk CVR Bldg, Stanford, CA 94305-5407; **Phone:** 650-725-3826; **Board Cert:** Thoracic Surgery 2008; **Med School:** Stanford Univ 1972; **Resid:** Thoracic & Cardiac Surgery, Standford Univ Med Ctr 1977; **Fac Appt:** Prof T&CS, Stanford Univ

Robbins, Robert C MD [T&CS] - **Spec Exp:** Transplant-Heart; Transplant-Lung; Cardiothoracic Surgery; **Hospital:** Stanford Univ Hosp & Clinics; **Address:** Stanford Cardiothoracic Surgery, 300 Pasteur Drive, Falk Research Bldg, 2nd Fl, Stanford, CA 94305-5407; **Phone:** 650-725-3828; **Board Cert:** Thoracic Surgery 2002; Surgery 2002; **Med School:** Univ Miss 1983; **Resid:** Surgery, Univ Miss Med Ctr 1988; **Fellow:** Thoracic Surgery, Stanford Univ Med Ctr 1991; **Fac Appt:** Prof TS, Stanford Univ

Shemin, Richard MD [T&CS] - **Spec Exp:** Minimally Invasive Cardiac Surgery; Heart Valve Surgery; Aneurysm-Thoracic Aortic; **Hospital:** UCLA Ronald Reagan Med Ctr; **Address:** 100 Medical Plaza, Ste 630E, Los Angeles, CA 90095; **Phone:** 310-206-8232; **Board Cert:** Thoracic Surgery 2002; **Med School:** Boston Univ 1974; **Resid:** Surgery, Brigham Hosp 1980; NYU Med Ctr 1982; **Fellow:** Cardiac Surgery, Natl Inst Hlth 1978; **Fac Appt:** Prof TS, UCLA-David Geffen Sch Med

Shrager, Joseph B MD [T&CS] - **Spec Exp:** Lung Cancer; Thymoma; Emphysema-Lung Volume Reduction; Chest Wall Tumors; **Hospital:** Stanford Univ Hosp & Clinics, VA Hlth Care Sys - Palo Alto; **Address:** Stanford Univ Medical Ctr, Falk Bldg, 300 Pasteur Drive, Fl 2 - rm CV207, MC 5407, Stanford, CA 94305-5407; **Phone:** 650-721-2086; **Board Cert:** Thoracic Surgery 2008; Surgery 2009; **Med School:** Harvard Med Sch 1988; **Resid:** Surgery, Hosp Univ Penn 1995; Thoracic Surgery, Mass Genl Hosp 1997; **Fac Appt:** Prof TS, Stanford Univ

Starnes, Vaughn A MD [T&CS] - **Spec Exp:** Transplant-Heart & Lung; Heart Valve Surgery; Ross Procedure for Aortic Valve Disease; Robotic Cardiac Surgery; **Hospital:** Keck Med Ctr of USC (page 62), Huntington Memorial Hosp; **Address:** USC Cardiothoracic Surgery, 1520 San Pablo St, Ste 4300, Los Angeles, CA 90033; **Phone:** 323-442-5849; **Board Cert:** Thoracic Surgery 2007; **Med School:** Univ NC Sch Med 1977; **Resid:** Surgery, Vanderbilt Univ Hosp 1984; Cardiovascular Surgery, Stanford Unv Hosp 1986; **Fellow:** Cardiothoracic Transplant Surg, Stanford Unv Hosp 1987; Pediatric Cardiac Surgery, Univ NC Hosp; **Fac Appt:** Prof TS, USC Sch Med

Thistlethwaite, Patricia A MD/PhD [T&CS] - **Spec Exp:** Cardiac Surgery; Lung Cancer; Cardiothoracic Surgery; **Hospital:** UCSD Med Ctr; **Address:** Sulpizio Cardiovascular Ctr, 9434 Medical Ctr Drive, San Diego, CA 92103; **Phone:** 619-543-7777; **Board Cert:** Surgery 2005; Thoracic Surgery 2007; **Med School:** Harvard Med Sch 1989; **Resid:** Surgery, Mass Genl Hosp 1994; **Fellow:** Cardiothoracic Surgery, Univ Pittsburgh Med Ctr 1997; **Fac Appt:** Prof S, UCSD

Trento, Alfredo MD [T&CS] - **Spec Exp:** Transplant-Heart; Cardiac Surgery; Pediatric Cardiac Surgery; Coronary Artery Surgery; **Hospital:** Cedars-Sinai Med Ctr; **Address:** Cedars-Sinai Med Ctr, Dept Thoracic Surg, 8700 Beverly Blvd,N Tower, Ste SCCT-2S03, Los Angeles, CA 90048; **Phone:** 310-423-3851; **Board Cert:** Thoracic Surgery 2005; **Med School:** Italy 1975; **Resid:** Surgery, Univ Mass Med Ctr 1982; Thoracic Surgery, Univ Pittsburgh Med Ctr 1985; **Fellow:** Cardiothoracic Surgery, Univ Mass Med Ctr 1982; **Fac Appt:** Prof S, UCLA

Vallieres, Eric MD [T&CS] - **Spec Exp:** Lung Cancer; Mesothelioma; Mediastinal Tumors; Thoracic Cancers; **Hospital:** Swedish Med Ctr-First Hill-Seattle; **Address:** 1101 Madison St, Ste 850, Seattle, WA 98104; **Phone:** 206-215-6800; **Board Cert:** Surgery 1988; Thoracic Surgery 1990; **Med School:** Canada 1982; **Resid:** Surgery, Univ Toronto Affil Hosp 1988; Thoracic Surgery, Univ Toronto Affil Hosp 1989; **Fellow:** Cardiovascular Surgery, Univ Montreal 1990

Verrier, Edward D MD [T&CS] - **Spec Exp:** Congenital Heart Disease-Adult; Heart Valve Surgery; Aortic Surgery; **Hospital:** Univ Wash Med Ctr, Northwest Hosp - Seattle; **Address:** University Washington Medical Ctr, 1959 NE Pacific St, Box 356310, Seattle, WA 98195-6310; **Phone:** 206-221-3166; **Board Cert:** Thoracic Surgery 2003; **Med School:** Tufts Univ 1974; **Resid:** Surgery, UCSF Med Ctr 1982; Thoracic Surgery, UCSF Med Ctr 1984; **Fellow:** Cardiac Surgery, UCSF Med Ctr 1980; **Fac Appt:** Prof TS, Univ Wash

Wells, Winfield J MD [T&CS] - **Spec Exp:** Tracheal Surgery-Pediatric; Congenital Heart Surgery; **Hospital:** Chldns Hosp - Los Angeles; **Address:** Chlds Hosp, Div Cardiothoracic Surgery, 4650 Sunset Blvd, MS 66, Los Angeles, CA 90027; **Phone:** 323-361-4148; **Board Cert:** Thoracic Surgery 2007; **Med School:** USC Sch Med 1970; **Resid:** Surgery, Columbia-Presby Med Ctr 1976; **Fac Appt:** Assoc Prof S, USC Sch Med

Wood, Douglas E MD [T&CS] - **Spec Exp:** Lung Cancer; Esophageal Cancer; Tracheal Surgery; Mesothelioma; **Hospital:** Univ Wash Med Ctr, Northwest Hosp - Seattle; **Address:** University of Washington, 1959 NE Pacific St, AA Bldg - rm 115, MS 356310, Seattle, WA 98195-6310; **Phone:** 206-685-3228; **Board Cert:** Surgery 2009; Thoracic Surgery 2011; **Med School:** Harvard Med Sch 1983; **Resid:** Surgery, Mass Genl Hosp 1989; **Fellow:** Surgical Critical Care, Mass Genl Hosp 1991; Cardiothoracic Surgery, Mass Genl Hosp 1991; **Fac Appt:** Prof TS, Univ Wash

THE MOUNT SINAI MEDICAL CENTER CARDIOTHORACIC SURGERY

One Gustave L. Levy Place
Fifth Avenue and 100th Street
New York, NY 10029-6574
Physician Referral: 1-800-MD-SINAI (637-4624)
www.mountsinai.org/heart
www.mitralvalverepair.org

THE DEPARTMENT OF CARDIOTHORACIC SURGERY at Mount Sinai is one of the nation's most prestigious programs. **In 2012, *U.S. News & World Report* ranked our cardiology and heart surgery service 10th in the country.** Cardiothoracic surgical patients benefit from an integrated and personalized care plan designed in coordination with expert cardiologists, anesthesiologists, perfusionists, and intensive care physicians. Mount Sinai is a quaternary referral center, meaning its surgeons often operate on the sickest and most complicated patients.

The Mitral Valve Repair Reference Center is one of the largest and most advanced in the nation. The superiority of mitral valve repair over replacement with a mechanical or bioprosthetic valve is now well established. Directed by David H. Adams, MD, Mount Sinai's Mitral Valve Repair Reference Center offers patients one of the highest percentages of successful valve repair in the world. In patients with mitral valve prolapse, our success rate in avoiding valve replacement approaches 100 percent. Our physicians are experts in mitral valve repair for patients with advanced cardiomyopathy. For patients who have associated atrial fibrillation, we offer the latest in concomitant arrhythmia surgery, including the MAZE procedure. Mitral valve repair with minimally invasive approaches is also performed when appropriate. Learn more about our Reference Center at www.mitralvalverepair.org.

The Cardiac Transplant and Assist Program, one of the largest in the nation, is under the direction of Anelechi Anyanwu, MD. We have been involved in the field of mechanical cardiac assistance from its inception, and have experience with most of the available FDA-approved devices. We have also played an active role in multi-institutional studies exploring permanent mechanical heart support.

Transcatheter Aortic Valve Replacement/Implantation (TAVR/TAVI) Program offers breakthrough treatment. Our physicians have been performing TAVR/TAVI for two years, with patients coming from around the world for this treatment. We were the first institution in the country to implant the Medtronic CoreValve Transcatheter Aortic Valve replacement device, and we are the first hospital in New York State able to implant both the Edwards Sapien Valve and the Medtronic CoreValve. These minimally invasive treatments spare patients from open-heart surgery and offer quicker recovery and return to daily activities. Our TAVR/TAVI program is led by Dr. David Adams, the National Co-Principal Investigator of the United States FDA pivotal trial of the Medtronic CoreValve Transcatheter Aortic Valve replacement device, and Dr. Samin Sharma, Director of Clinical Cardiology and Interventional Cardiology who, according to NYS Department of Health reports, has had the highest angioplasty success rate (lowest mortality less than 0.1 percent) for an interventional cardiologist in the state since 1994.

Pediatric and Congenital Cardiac Surgery Program achieves exceptional results. Led by Dr. Khanh Nguyen, patients from newborns to young adults are cared for in this program, which has achieved outstanding results with challenging problems by incorporating the most advanced techniques available. Part of only three active pediatric heart transplant centers in the state, our program also provides support for very sick hearts in infants and older children, using Extra-Corporeal Membrane Oxygenators (ECMO) or Ventricular Assist Devices (VAD). The care extended to the patient and family is supported by an outstanding multidisciplinary team. Superb post-operative care is provided in a dedicated Pediatric Cardiac Surgical Intensive Care Unit, under the direction of pediatric cardiologists, intensivists, and surgeons.

LEADING SURGEONS, UNPARALLELED POSSIBILITIES
The Department of Cardiothoracic Surgery at Mount Sinai is chaired by David H. Adams, MD, the Marie-Josée and Henry R. Kravis Professor. Dr. Adams is a world-renowned mitral repair surgeon. Anelechi Anyanwu, MD, leads one of the largest ventricular assist device and heart transplant centers in the country. He is also an expert in complex and re-operative valve surgery. Paul Stelzer, MD, is a specialist in aortic root surgery whose experience with the Ross procedure is unmatched, exceeding 20 years and 500 cases. These leaders work in concert with other members of Mount Sinai Heart, which is under the direction of world-renowned cardiologist Valentin Fuster, MD, PhD, to deliver unparalleled possibilities for patients with cardiovascular disease.

THE MOUNT SINAI MEDICAL CENTER
THORACIC SURGERY

One Gustave L. Levy Place
Fifth Avenue and 100th Street
New York, NY 10029-6574
Physician Referral: 1-800-MD-SINAI (637-4624)
www.mountsinai.org/thoracicsurgery

THORACIC SURGERY at The Mount Sinai Medical Center is known for its state-of-the-art surgery, multidisciplinary team approach to treatment, and commitment to compassionate patient care. Protocol-driven therapy ensures that Mount Sinai patients are given access to many clinical trials.

The Division of Thoracic Surgery at Mount Sinai engages in multidisciplinary collaboration, partnering with medical oncology, radiation oncology, pulmonary medicine, diagnostic and interventional radiology, gastroenterology, neurology, and anesthesiology, so patients can benefit from the insights of multiple experts across different specialties. This coordination among teams ensures seamless delivery of high-quality care to patients.

With an integrated approach to clinical care and research, our team of dedicated thoracic surgeons are experts in the treatment of all primary cancers of the chest, lung, esophagus, mediastinum, and airway, and all metastatic tumors of the chest. We also diagnose and treat patients who are affected by benign esophageal disorders such as gastroesophageal reflux disease, achalasia, and motility disorders.

Minimally Invasive Care: Minimally invasive interventions are preferred whenever possible, allowing less tissue damage, faster recovery time, and less scarring than open surgery. Mount Sinai's Division of Thoracic Surgery offers state-of-the-art assessment and treatment approaches, including thoroscopy, rigid and flexible bronchoscopy, and endoscopic laser resection in the diagnosis and management of thoracic conditions. The division has led the national trials for VATS (video-assisted thoracoscopic surgery) lobectomy, a procedure using three small incisions, which is now the surgical approach of choice, particularly for patients with early-stage lung cancer.

Personalized and Targeted Therapy: A unique part of our division is the integration and application of groundbreaking scientific research into the clinical care of our patients. These research efforts are being carried out in the Thoracic Surgery Translational Laboratory. Mount Sinai's thoracic surgeons and physician-scientists are conducting state-of-the-art translational thoracic research, including genomic analysis of tumors to better understand and predict behavior, in order to develop more directed, personalized, therapeutic approaches to treatment with novel targeted therapies.

Lung and Esophageal Cancer: Mount Sinai is New York City's leading center for comprehensive screening for lung and esophageal cancer, including CT scans for early detection, advanced endoscopic techniques, PET scans, and innovative MRI technology with ultrasensitive resolution. Our team is unique in our abilities to screen for cancers in people at risk, treat early cancers less invasively, and provide the most advanced protocol driven treatments available. Our approach to lung cancer care focuses on patients first, providing not only VATS and advanced minimally invasive techniques, but also an ability to treat advanced and challenging cases that require skills and expertise found in few other medical centers.

Mesothelioma: Irving J. Selikoff, MD, was the first to determine the association between mesothelioma and asbestos exposure. His tireless research efforts at Mount Sinai led to the Selikoff Center for Occupational and Environmental Medicine. This tradition of cutting-edge developments continues with Raja M. Flores' work using different modalities in the treatment of mesothelioma, such as the extrapleural pneumonectomy and pleurectomy (decortication) procedures. The Division of Thoracic Surgery is also currently involved in several ongoing studies with the goal of discovering new treatments for mesothelioma.

LEADING SURGEONS, PIONEERING RESEARCH

Led by Raja M. Flores, the Division of Thoracic Surgery is internationally recognized as a leader in thoracic surgery drawing patients from across the globe to seek our expertise.

Dr. Flores is a recognized leader in the treatment of mesothelioma and one of the first physicians in the world to use robotic surgery to treat lung and esophageal cancer. Dr. Flores established VATS lobectomy as the gold standard in the surgical treatment of lung cancer. He is one of the foremost educators of other surgeons about the VATS lobectomy.

Our award-winning physicians have consistently contributed to the evolution of this field through their efforts to bring about new technologies and therapies.

THORACIC SURGERY

About the Division of Thoracic Surgery
Thoracic Surgeons at NYU Langone Medical Center offer the most advanced diagnosis and treatment options available to patients for either benign or malignant lesions of the lung, esophagus, mediastinum and chest wall. All thoracic attending surgeons at the Medical Center are experts in minimally invasive, video-assisted thoracic surgery which minimizes patient discomfort and shortens recuperation time. We specialize in the following areas:

Airway Stenting
Patients experiencing trouble breathing may require stenting to maintain an open airway (windpipe). Treatment of primary and metastatic lung cancer often requires the use of hollow tubes (stents) to maintain an unobstructed airway. At NYU Langone, stent placement is performed in the operating room by an experienced team that includes a surgeon, anesthesiologist and nursing staff. The procedure can be performed through either rigid or flexible bronchoscopy using temporary (plastic) or more permanent (metal) stents. Post-operative patients are carefully monitored by a multidisciplinary team to ensure their comfort and care.

Minimally Invasive Thoracic Surgery
The Division of Thoracic Surgery offers a minimally invasive surgery program, incorporating both video-assisted and "open chest" techniques along with the newest methods for post-operative pain relief. The use of video-assisted equipment allows for a smaller incision without spreading the rib spaces, leading to greater patient comfort, a shorter recovery time and decreased length of stay for patients. Procedures offered include video-assisted thoracoscopy for biopsy with or without removal of a portion of the lungs, as well as repair of hiatal hernias and minimally invasive esophagectomy.

Pioneering Treatments
NYU Langone Medical Center continues to pioneer new treatments for the early detection of airway malignancies, diagnosis and treatment strategies for endobronchial abnormalities, investigation of non-surgical techniques for destruction of lung cancer nodules, and the use of stents (including replaceable stents) to relieve blockages of the windpipe and esophagus.

Research
NYU Langone is committed to state-of-the-art surgical management and development of novel treatment strategies through clinical trials. We also leverage the resources of the New York Thoracic Surgery Laboratory at Bellevue Hospital Center to search for genes and proteins in malignancies of the chest in order to develop novel targeted therapies.

Urology

A urologist manages benign and malignant medical and surgical disorders of the genitourinary system and the adrenal gland. This specialist has comprehensive knowledge of, and skills in, endoscopic, percutaneous and open surgery of congenital and acquired conditions of the urinary and reproductive systems and their contiguous structures.

Training Required: Five years

UROLOGY

New England

Albertsen, Peter C MD [U] - **Spec Exp:** Prostate Cancer; **Hospital:** Univ of Conn Hlth Ctr, John Dempsey Hosp; **Address:** 263 Farmington Ave, Dowling South Fl 2 - Ste 220, Farmington, CT 06030; **Phone:** 860-679-4100; **Board Cert:** Urology 2004; **Med School:** Columbia P&S 1978; **Resid:** Surgery, New England Deaconess Hosp 1980; Urology, Johns Hopkins Hosp 1984; **Fellow:** Preventive Medicine, Univ WI Affil Hosp 1990; **Fac Appt:** Prof U, Univ Conn

Babayan, Richard MD [U] - **Spec Exp:** Kidney Cancer; Prostate Cancer; **Hospital:** Boston Med Ctr; **Address:** Boston Med Ctr, Dept Urology, Shapiro Ctr Fl 3, 725 Albany St, Ste 3B, Boston, MA 02118; **Phone:** 617-638-8485; **Board Cert:** Urology 1982; **Med School:** Indiana Univ 1975; **Resid:** Surgery, Yale-New Haven Hosp 1977; Urology, Boston Univ Med Ctr 1980; **Fellow:** Urologic Oncology, Boston Univ Med Ctr 1982; **Fac Appt:** Prof U, Boston Univ

Bauer, Stuart B MD [U] - **Spec Exp:** Pediatric Urology; Neuro-Urology; Neurogenic Bladder; **Hospital:** Children's Hospital - Boston; **Address:** Chldns Hosp, Hunnewell-3, 300 Longwood Ave, Boston, MA 02115-6264; **Phone:** 617-355-7796; **Board Cert:** Urology 1977; **Med School:** Univ Rochester 1968; **Resid:** Urology, Tufts New Engl Med Ctr 1975; **Fac Appt:** Prof U, Harvard Med Sch

Caldamone, Anthony A MD [U] - **Spec Exp:** Pediatric Urology; **Hospital:** Rhode Island Hosp; **Address:** 2 Dudley St, Ste 185, Providence, RI 02905; **Phone:** 401-421-0710; **Board Cert:** Urology 1983; Pediatric Urology 2008; **Med School:** Brown Univ 1975; **Resid:** Urology, Strong Meml Hosp/Univ Rochester 1981; **Fellow:** Pediatric Urology, Childrens Hosp 1982; **Fac Appt:** Prof U, Brown Univ

Carpinito, Gennaro A MD [U] - **Spec Exp:** Kidney Cancer; Prostate Cancer; Testicular Cancer; Minimally Invasive Urologic Surgery; **Hospital:** Tufts Med Ctr; **Address:** Tufts Med Ctr, Div Urology, 800 Washington St, Box 142, Boston, MA 02111; **Phone:** 617-636-6317; **Board Cert:** Urology 1984; **Med School:** Boston Univ 1977; **Resid:** Urology, Boston Med Ctr 1982; **Fellow:** Urologic Oncology, Boston Univ 1984; **Fac Appt:** Prof U, Tufts Univ

Colberg, John W MD [U] - **Spec Exp:** Prostate Cancer; Bladder Cancer; Kidney Cancer; Testicular Cancer; **Hospital:** Yale-New Haven Hosp, Yale Med Group; **Address:** 20 York St, New Haven, CT 06510; **Phone:** 203-785-2815; **Board Cert:** Urology 2001; **Med School:** Washington Univ, St Louis 1985; **Resid:** Surgery, Yale-New Haven Hosp 1987; Urology, Yale-New Haven Hosp 1990; **Fac Appt:** Assoc Prof U, Yale Univ

Foster Jr, Harris E MD [U] - **Spec Exp:** Incontinence; Urodynamics; Voiding Dysfunction; Urology-Female; **Hospital:** Yale-New Haven Hosp, Yale Med Group; **Address:** 35 Park St, New Haven, CT 06520-8062; **Phone:** 203-200-4822; **Board Cert:** Urology 2012; **Med School:** Univ Miami Sch Med 1987; **Resid:** Surgery, Univ Michigan Med Ctr 1989; Urology, Univ Michigan Med Ctr 1992; **Fac Appt:** Prof U, Yale Univ

Gomery, Pablo MD [U] - **Spec Exp:** Neuro-Urology; Erectile Dysfunction; Voiding Dysfunction; Infertility-Male; **Hospital:** Mass Genl Hosp, Spaulding Rehab Hosp; **Address:** Mass Genl Hosp-Dept Urology, 55 Fruit St, GRB 1102, Boston, MA 02114; **Phone:** 617-726-8482; **Board Cert:** Urology 2010; **Med School:** Albert Einstein Coll Med 1974; **Resid:** Surgery, New England Deaconess Hosp 1977; Urology, Mass General Hosp 1980

Heney, Niall M MD [U] - **Spec Exp:** Urologic Cancer; Prostate Cancer; **Hospital:** Mass Genl Hosp; **Address:** Mass Genl Hosp, Dept Urology, 55 Fruit St, GRB 1102, Boston, MA 02114; **Phone:** 617-726-3011; **Board Cert:** Urology 1977; **Med School:** Ireland 1965; **Resid:** Urology, Regional Hosp 1972; Urology, Mass Genl Hosp 1976; **Fac Appt:** Prof U, Harvard Med Sch

Janeiro Jr, John J MD [U] - **Spec Exp:** Urologic Cancer; Kidney Stones; Vasectomy Reversal; **Hospital:** Southern NH Med Ctr, St. Joseph Hosp & Trauma Ctr; **Address:** Urology Center Southern New Hampshire, 17 Riverside St, Ste 201, Nashua, NH 03062; **Phone:** 603-883-1550; **Board Cert:** Urology 2008; **Med School:** Univ Mass Sch Med 1982; **Resid:** Urology, Lahey Clinic 1987; **Fellow:** Pediatric Urology, Childrens Hosp 1989

Kibel, Adam S MD [U] - **Spec Exp:** Prostate Cancer; Bladder Cancer; Kidney Cancer; Minimally Invasive Surgery; **Hospital:** Brigham and Women's Hosp (page 57), Dana-Farber Cancer Inst (page 57); **Address:** Brigham & Women's Hosp, Div of Urology, 45 Francis St, Boston, MA 02115; **Phone:** 617-732-6665; **Board Cert:** Urology 2009; **Med School:** Cornell Univ-Weill Med Coll 1991; **Resid:** Urology, Brigham & Women's Hosp 1997; **Fellow:** Urologic Oncology, Johns Hopkins Hosp 1999; **Fac Appt:** Prof U, Harvard Med Sch

Libertino, John A MD [U] - **Spec Exp:** Kidney Cancer; Prostate Cancer; Adrenal Tumors; **Hospital:** Lahey Clin; **Address:** Lahey Clinic, Dept Urology, 41 Mall Rd, Burlington, MA 01805-0001; **Phone:** 781-744-2511; **Board Cert:** Urology 1973; **Med School:** Georgetown Univ 1965; **Resid:** Surgery, Strong Meml Hosp 1967; Urology, Yale-New Haven Hosp 1970; **Fellow:** Urology, Yale-New Haven Hosp 1969; **Fac Appt:** Prof S, Harvard Med Sch

Loughlin, Kevin R MD [U] - **Spec Exp:** Prostate Cancer; Bladder Cancer; Penile Cancer; Incontinence-Female; **Hospital:** Brigham and Women's Hosp (page 57), Dana-Farber Cancer Inst (page 57); **Address:** 45 Francis St, ASBII-3, Boston, MA 02115; **Phone:** 617-732-6325; **Board Cert:** Urology 2004; **Med School:** NY Med Coll 1975; **Resid:** Pediatrics, New York Hosp 1978; Surgery, Bellevue Hosp Ctr 1979; **Fellow:** Urology, Brigham & Women's Hosp 1983; Urologic Oncology, Meml Sloan Kettering Cancer Ctr 1983; **Fac Appt:** Prof S, Harvard Med Sch

McDougal, W Scott MD [U] - **Spec Exp:** Penile Cancer; Prostate Cancer; Bladder Cancer; Urologic Cancer; **Hospital:** Mass Genl Hosp; **Address:** Mass Genl Hosp, 55 Fruit St, GRB Bldg, rm 1102, Boston, MA 02114; **Phone:** 617-726-3010; **Board Cert:** Surgery 1975; Urology 1992; **Med School:** Cornell Univ-Weill Med Coll 1968; **Resid:** Surgery, Univ Hosps Cleveland 1975; Urology, Univ Hosps Cleveland 1975; **Fellow:** Physiology, Yale Med Sch 1972; **Fac Appt:** Prof U, Harvard Med Sch

McGovern, Francis J MD [U] - **Spec Exp:** Prostate Cancer; Urologic Cancer; **Hospital:** Mass Genl Hosp; **Address:** 1 Hawthorne Pl, Ste 109, Boston, MA 02114; **Phone:** 617-726-3560; **Board Cert:** Urology 2009; **Med School:** Case West Res Univ 1983; **Resid:** Urology, Mass Genl Hosp 1989

O'Leary, Michael P MD [U] - **Spec Exp:** Sexual Dysfunction; Kidney Stones; Prostate Disease; **Hospital:** Brigham and Women's Hosp (page 57), Dana-Farber Cancer Inst (page 57); **Address:** Brigham & Women's Hosp, Div Urology, 45 Francis St, ASBII-3, Boston, MA 02115; **Phone:** 617-732-6398; **Board Cert:** Urology 2010; **Med School:** Geo Wash Univ 1980; **Resid:** Urology, Tufts New Eng Med Ctr 1982; Urology, Mass Genl Hosp 1986; **Fellow:** Urology, UCSF Med Ctr 1989; **Fac Appt:** Assoc Prof S, Harvard Med Sch

Urology

Oates, Robert D MD [U] - **Spec Exp:** Infertility-Male; Vasectomy Reversal; Reproductive Genetics; Congenital Absence of Vas Deferens; **Hospital:** Boston Med Ctr; **Address:** Boston Univ Med Ctr, Dept Urology, 725 Albany St Sharpiro Bldg - Ste 3B, Boston, MA 02118-2334; **Phone:** 617-638-8485; **Board Cert:** Urology 2010; **Med School:** Boston Univ 1982; **Resid:** Surgery, Boston Univ Hosp 1984; Urology, Boston Univ Hosp 1987; **Fellow:** Reproductive Medicine, Baylor Coll Med 1988; **Fac Appt:** Prof U, Boston Univ

Olumi, Aria F MD [U] - **Spec Exp:** Prostate Cancer; Testicular Cancer; Kidney Cancer; Bladder Cancer; **Hospital:** Mass Genl Hosp; **Address:** Mass General Urology Associates, 55 Fruit St, Ste YAW 7E, Boston, MA 02114; **Phone:** 617-643-0237; **Board Cert:** Urology 2012; **Med School:** Univ SC Sch Med 1992; **Resid:** Surgery, Brigham & Women's Hosp 1994; Urology, Brigham & Women's Hosp 2000; **Fellow:** Research, UCSF Affil Hosp 1998; **Fac Appt:** Assoc Prof S, Harvard Med Sch

Richie, Jerome P MD [U] - **Spec Exp:** Prostate Cancer; Testicular Cancer; Kidney Cancer; **Hospital:** Brigham and Women's Hosp (page 57), Dana-Farber Cancer Inst (page 57); **Address:** Brigham & Women's Hosp, 45 Francis St Fl 3 - Ste ASB2, Boston, MA 02115; **Phone:** 617-732-6325; **Board Cert:** Urology 2002; **Med School:** Univ Tex Med Br, Galveston 1969; **Resid:** Surgery, UCLA Med Ctr 1971; Urology, UCLA Med Ctr 1975; **Fac Appt:** Prof S, Harvard Med Sch

Sanda, Martin G MD [U] - **Spec Exp:** Prostate Cancer; Bladder Cancer; Kidney Cancer; Urologic Cancer; **Hospital:** Beth Israel Deaconess Med Ctr - Boston; **Address:** BIDMC-Dept of Urology, 330 Brookline Ave, Rabb 440, Boston, MA 02115; **Phone:** 617-735-2100; **Board Cert:** Urology 2007; **Med School:** Columbia P&S 1987; **Resid:** Surgery, Med Coll Virginia 1989; Urology, Johns Hopkins Hosp 1994; **Fellow:** Surgical Oncology, Natl Cancer Inst 1991; **Fac Appt:** Assoc Prof U, Harvard Med Sch

Sigman, Mark MD [U] - **Spec Exp:** Infertility-Male; Vasectomy Reversal; **Hospital:** Rhode Island Hosp; **Address:** 2 Dudley St, Ste 175, Providence, RI 02905-3247; **Phone:** 401-421-0710; **Board Cert:** Urology 2010; **Med School:** Univ Conn 1981; **Resid:** Surgery, Univ VA Med Ctr 1983; Urology, Univ VA Med Ctr 1987; **Fellow:** Male Reproduction, Baylor Coll Med 1989; **Fac Appt:** Assoc Prof U, Brown Univ

Singh, Dinesh MD [U] - **Spec Exp:** Laparoscopic Surgery; Robotic Surgery; Kidney Cancer; Prostate Cancer; **Hospital:** Yale-New Haven Hosp, Yale Med Group; **Address:** 35 Park St Fl 4, New Haven, CT 06519; **Phone:** 203-785-2815; **Board Cert:** Urology 2006; **Med School:** Columbia P&S 1997; **Resid:** Surgery, Brigham & Women's Hosp 1999; Urology, Harvard Med Sch Affil Hosp 2003; **Fellow:** Research, Dana Farber Cancer Inst 2001; Laparoscopic Surgery, Cleveland Clin 2004; **Fac Appt:** Asst Prof U, Yale Univ

Weiss, Robert M MD [U] - **Spec Exp:** Pediatric Urology; Testicular Cancer; Penile Cancer; Bladder Cancer; **Hospital:** Yale-New Haven Hosp, Yale Med Group; **Address:** 1 Long Wharf Drive, New Haven, CT 06511; **Phone:** 203-785-2815; **Board Cert:** Urology 1970; **Med School:** SUNY Downstate 1960; **Resid:** Surgery, Beth Israel Hosp 1962; Urology, Columbia Presby Hosp 1967; **Fellow:** Pharmacology, Columbia Presby Hosp 1965; **Fac Appt:** Prof U, Yale Univ

Mid Atlantic

Albala, David M MD [U] - **Spec Exp:** Prostate Cancer/Robotic Surgery; Kidney Stones; Laparoscopic Surgery; **Hospital:** Crouse Hosp, St. Joseph's Hosp Hlth Ctr; **Address:** Associated Medical Professionals, 1226 E Water St, Syracuse, NY 13210; **Phone:** 315-478-4185; **Board Cert:** Urology 2012; **Med School:** Mich State Univ 1983; **Resid:** Surgery, Dartmouth-Hitchcock Med Ctr 1985; Urology, Dartmouth-Hitchcock Med Ctr 1990; **Fellow:** Endourology, Wash Univ Med Ctr 1991

Alexander, Richard B MD [U] - **Spec Exp:** Prostate Disease; Prostate Cancer; **Hospital:** Univ of MD Med Ctr, Baltimore VA Med Ctr; **Address:** 29 S Greene St, Ste 500, Baltimore, MD 21201; **Phone:** 410-328-5109; **Board Cert:** Urology 2011; **Med School:** Johns Hopkins Univ 1981; **Resid:** Surgery, Vanderbilt Univ Affl Hosps 1983; Urology, Johns Hopkins Hosp 1988; **Fellow:** Cancer Immunology, Natl Cancer Inst 1989; **Fac Appt:** Prof U, Univ MD Sch Med

Bar-Chama, Natan MD [U] - **Spec Exp:** Infertility-Male; Erectile Dysfunction; Vasectomy Reversal; Varicocele Microsurgery; **Hospital:** Mount Sinai Med Ctr (page 64); **Address:** Center for Male Reproductive Health, 635 Madison Ave Fl 10, New York, NY 10022; **Phone:** 212-756-5777; **Board Cert:** Urology 2006; **Med School:** Albert Einstein Coll Med 1987; **Resid:** Urology, Montefiore Med Ctr 1993; **Fellow:** Male Infertility, Baylor Coll Med 1994; **Fac Appt:** Assoc Prof U, Mount Sinai Sch Med

Benson, Mitchell C MD [U] - **Spec Exp:** Prostate Cancer/Robotic Surgery; Bladder Cancer; Kidney Cancer; Continent Urinary Diversions; **Hospital:** NY-Presby/Columbia Univ Med Ctr, NY (page 66); **Address:** 161 Fort Washington Ave, Ste 1102, New York, NY 10032-3713; **Phone:** 212-305-5201; **Board Cert:** Urology 1984; **Med School:** Columbia P&S 1977; **Resid:** Surgery, Mount Sinai Med Ctr 1979; Urology, Columbia-Presby Hosp 1982; **Fellow:** Oncology, Johns Hopkins Hosp 1984; **Fac Appt:** Prof U, Columbia P&S

Blaivas, Jerry G MD [U] - **Spec Exp:** Uro-Gynecology; Urology-Female; Neurogenic Bladder; Incontinence after Prostate Cancer; **Hospital:** NY-Presby/Weill Cornell Med Ctr, NY (page 66), Lenox Hill Hosp (page 67); **Address:** 445 E 77th St, New York, NY 10075; **Phone:** 212-772-3900; **Board Cert:** Urology 1978; **Med School:** Tufts Univ 1968; **Resid:** Surgery, Boston Med Ctr 1971; Urology, New England Med Ctr 1976; **Fac Appt:** Clin Prof U, Cornell Univ-Weill Med Coll

Burnett II, Arthur L MD [U] - **Spec Exp:** Prostate Cancer; Erectile Dysfunction; **Hospital:** Johns Hopkins Hosp (page 61); **Address:** Brady Urological Inst, 601 N Caroline St Fl 4, Baltimore, MD 21287; **Phone:** 410-955-6100; **Board Cert:** Urology 2007; **Med School:** Johns Hopkins Univ 1988; **Resid:** Surgery, Johns Hopkins Hosp 1990; Urology, Johns Hopkins Hosp 1994; **Fac Appt:** Prof U, Johns Hopkins Univ

Canning, Douglas MD [U] - **Spec Exp:** Pediatric Urology; Hypospadias; **Hospital:** Chldns Hosp of Philadelphia; **Address:** Childrens Hosp, Div Urology, 34th St & Civic Ctr Blvd Wood Bldg Fl 3, Philadelphia, PA 19104; **Phone:** 215-590-2754; **Board Cert:** Urology 2010; Pediatric Urology 2008; **Med School:** Dartmouth Med Sch 1982; **Resid:** Urology, Naval Hosp 1987; **Fellow:** Pediatric Urology, Johns Hopkins Hosp 1988; **Fac Appt:** Prof U, Univ Pennsylvania

Carter, H Ballentine MD [U] - **Spec Exp:** Prostate Cancer; **Hospital:** Johns Hopkins Hosp (page 61); **Address:** Brady Urological Inst, 601 N Caroline St Fl 4, Baltimore, MD 21287; **Phone:** 410-955-6100; **Board Cert:** Urology 2010; **Med School:** Med Univ SC 1981; **Resid:** Surgery, New York Hosp 1983; Urology, New York Hosp 1987; **Fellow:** Research, Johns Hopkins Hosp 1989; **Fac Appt:** Prof U, Johns Hopkins Univ

Chen, David Y T MD [U] - **Spec Exp:** Kidney Cancer; Prostate Cancer; Robotic Surgery; Bladder Cancer; **Hospital:** Fox Chase Cancer Ctr (page 58); **Address:** Fox Chase Cancer Ctr, 333 Cottman Ave, Philadelphia, PA 19111; **Phone:** 215-728-2548; **Board Cert:** Urology 2006; **Med School:** Cornell Univ 1997; **Resid:** Urology, NY Presby-Cornell Med Ctr 2003; **Fellow:** Urologic Oncology, NY Presby-Cornell Med Ctr 2004; **Fac Appt:** Assoc Prof U, Temple Univ

Urology

Cohen, Jeffrey K MD [U] - **Spec Exp:** Urologic Cancer; Prostate Cancer; **Hospital:** Allegheny General Hosp, Canonsburg General Hospital; **Address:** Triangle Urological Group, 1307 Federal St, Ste 300, Pittsburgh, PA 15212-1757; **Phone:** 412-281-1757; **Board Cert:** Urology 2005; **Med School:** SUNY Upstate Med Univ 1979; **Resid:** Surgery, Univ Hosp 1981; Urology, Univ Hosp 1984; **Fellow:** Urologic Oncology, MD Anderson Cancer Ctr 1985; **Fac Appt:** Assoc Prof S, Drexel Univ Coll Med

Docimo, Steven G MD [U] - **Spec Exp:** Pediatric Urology; Minimally Invasive Surgery; Bladder Reconstruction; Voiding Dysfunction; **Hospital:** Chldns Hosp of Pittsburgh - UPMC; **Address:** Executive Suites Children's Hosp of Pittsburgh, Children's Hospital of Pittsburgh-UPMC, Pittsburgh, PA 15224; **Phone:** 412-692-7932; **Board Cert:** Urology 2008; Pediatric Urology 2008; **Med School:** Johns Hopkins Univ 1984; **Resid:** Surgery, Georgetown Univ Med Ctr 1986; Urology, Brigham & Womens Hosp 1990; **Fellow:** Pediatric Urology, Johns Hopkins 1994; Research, Childrens Hosp 1988; **Fac Appt:** Prof U, Univ Pittsburgh

Droller, Michael J MD [U] - **Spec Exp:** Urologic Cancer; Bladder Cancer; Prostate Cancer; Kidney Cancer; **Hospital:** Mount Sinai Med Ctr (page 64); **Address:** 5 E 98th St, Fl 6, Box 1272, New York, NY 10029-6501; **Phone:** 212-241-3868; **Board Cert:** Urology 2001; **Med School:** Harvard Med Sch 1968; **Resid:** Surgery, Peter Bent Brigham Hosp 1970; Urology, Stanford Univ Med Ctr 1976; **Fellow:** Immunology, Univ Stockholm 1977; **Fac Appt:** Prof U, Mount Sinai Sch Med

Fisch, Harry MD [U] - **Spec Exp:** Infertility-Male; Microsurgery; Vasectomy Reversal; **Hospital:** NY-Presby/Weill Cornell Med Ctr, NY (page 66), Lenox Hill Hosp (page 67); **Address:** 944 Park Ave, Ste 1C, New York, NY 10028; **Phone:** 212-879-0800; **Board Cert:** Urology 2010; **Med School:** Mount Sinai Sch Med 1983; **Resid:** Surgery, Montefiore Med Ctr 1985; Urology, Montefiore Med Ctr 1989; **Fac Appt:** Prof U, Columbia P&S

Gearhart, John P MD [U] - **Spec Exp:** Pediatric Urology; **Hospital:** Johns Hopkins Hosp (page 61); **Address:** Johns Hopkins Hospital, Brady Urological Institute, 600 N Wolfe St Marburg Bldg - Ste 146, Baltimore, MD 21287-2101; **Phone:** 410-955-5358; **Board Cert:** Urology 1982; **Med School:** Univ Louisville Sch Med 1975; **Resid:** Urology, Med Coll Georgia Hosp 1980; **Fellow:** Pediatric Urology, Alder Hey Chldns Hosp 1981; Pediatric Urology, Johns Hopkins Hosp 1985; **Fac Appt:** Prof U, Johns Hopkins Univ

Glassberg, Kenneth MD [U] - **Spec Exp:** Pediatric Urology; Genital Reconstruction; Varicocele in Adolescents; **Hospital:** Morgan Stanley Children's Hosp of NY-Presby, NY, NY-Presby/Columbia Univ Med Ctr, NY (page 66); **Address:** Morgan Stanley Chlds Hosp of NY-Presby, 3959 Broadway, rm 1117, New York, NY 10032; **Phone:** 212-305-9918; **Board Cert:** Urology 1977; Pediatric Urology 2009; **Med School:** SUNY Downstate 1968; **Resid:** Surgery, Montefiore Hosp Med Ctr 1972; Urology, Univ Hosp 1975; **Fellow:** Pediatric Urology, Adler Hey Chldns Hosp 1976; Pediatric Urology, Hosp For Sick Chldn 1976; **Fac Appt:** Prof U, Columbia P&S

Goldstein, Marc MD [U] - **Spec Exp:** Infertility-Male; Varicocele Microsurgery; Vasectomy & Vasectomy Reversal; Erectile Dysfunction; **Hospital:** NY-Presby/Weill Cornell Med Ctr, NY (page 66); **Address:** Cornell Inst for Reproductive Med, 525 E 68th St, Box 269, New York, NY 10065-4870; **Phone:** 212-746-5470; **Board Cert:** Urology 1982; **Med School:** SUNY Downstate 1972; **Resid:** Surgery, Columbia-Presby Med Ctr 1974; Urology, SUNY Downstate Med Ctr 1980; **Fellow:** Microsurgery, Rockefeller Univ 1982; Reproductive Medicine, Rockefeller Univ 1982; **Fac Appt:** Prof U, Cornell Univ-Weill Med Coll

Gomella, Leonard G MD [U] - **Spec Exp:** Prostate Cancer; Minimally Invasive Urologic Surgery; Urologic Cancer; **Hospital:** Thomas Jefferson Univ Hosp; **Address:** Thomas Jefferson Univ, 833 Chestnut St Fl 7 - Ste 703, Philadelphia, PA 19107-5001; **Phone:** 215-955-1000; **Board Cert:** Urology 2008; **Med School:** Univ KY Coll Med 1980; **Resid:** Surgery, Univ Kentucky Med Ctr 1982; Urology, Univ Kentucky Med Ctr 1986; **Fellow:** Urologic Oncology, Natl Cancer Inst 1988; **Fac Appt:** Prof U, Jefferson Med Coll

Grasso III, Michael MD [U] - **Spec Exp:** Urologic Cancer; Laparoscopic Surgery; Kidney Stones; Testicular Cancer; **Hospital:** Lenox Hill Hosp (page 67), Westchester Med Ctr; **Address:** 100 E 77 th St, East Bldg - Fl 4th, New York, NY 10075; **Phone:** 212-434-6300; **Board Cert:** Urology 2004; **Med School:** Jefferson Med Coll 1986; **Resid:** Surgery, Jefferson Univ Hosp 1988; Urology, Jefferson Univ Hosp 1992; **Fac Appt:** Prof U, NY Med Coll

Greenberg, Richard E MD [U] - **Spec Exp:** Prostate Cancer; Bladder Cancer; Kidney Cancer; Prostate Cancer/Robotic Surgery; **Hospital:** Fox Chase Cancer Ctr (page 58), Abington Mem Hosp; **Address:** Fox Chase Cancer Ctr, Div Urol-Dept Surg, 333 Cottman Ave, Philadelphia, PA 19111-2497; **Phone:** 215-728-5341; **Board Cert:** Urology 2004; **Med School:** Cornell Univ-Weill Med Coll 1976; **Resid:** Surgery, New York Hosp 1979; Urology, New York Hosp 1983; **Fac Appt:** Prof U, Temple Univ

Greenfield, Saul P MD [U] - **Spec Exp:** Pediatric Urology; Urinary Tract Infections; Neurogenic Bladder; Reconstructive Urologic Surgery; **Hospital:** Women & Chldn's Hosp of Buffalo, The; **Address:** Pediatric Urology of Western NY, 219 Bryant St, Buffalo, NY 14222; **Phone:** 716-878-7393; **Board Cert:** Urology 1984; Pediatric Urology 2008; **Med School:** Univ Pennsylvania 1977; **Resid:** Surgery, NYU Med Ctr 1979; Urology, Columbia-Presby Med Ctr 1982; **Fellow:** Pediatric Urology, Chldns Hosp Buffalo 1984; **Fac Appt:** Clin Prof U, SUNY Buffalo

Gribetz, Michael MD [U] - **Spec Exp:** Prostate Disease; Urology-Female; Sexual Dysfunction; Kidney Stones; **Hospital:** Mount Sinai Med Ctr (page 64); **Address:** 1155 Park Ave, New York, NY 10128-1209; **Phone:** 212-831-1300; **Board Cert:** Urology 1980; **Med School:** Albert Einstein Coll Med 1973; **Resid:** Surgery, Montefiore Med Ctr 1975; Urology, Mt Sinai Hosp 1978; **Fac Appt:** Asst Clin Prof U, Mount Sinai Sch Med

Hall, Simon J MD [U] - **Spec Exp:** Urologic Cancer; Minimally Invasive Urologic Surgery; Continent Urinary Diversions; Prostate Cancer; **Hospital:** Mount Sinai Med Ctr (page 64); **Address:** 5 E 98th St, Box 1272, New York, NY 10029; **Phone:** 212-241-4812; **Board Cert:** Urology 2009; **Med School:** Columbia P&S 1988; **Resid:** Surgery, Mt Sinai Med Ctr 1990; Urology, Boston Univ 1994; **Fellow:** Urology, Baylor Coll Med 1996; **Fac Appt:** Assoc Prof U, Mount Sinai Sch Med

Hensle, Terry MD [U] - **Spec Exp:** Pediatric Urology; Hypospadias; Urinary Reconstruction; Wilms' Tumor; **Hospital:** Hackensack Univ Med Ctr; **Address:** 699 Teaneck Rd, Ste 103, Teaneck, NJ 07616; **Phone:** 201-645-3362; **Board Cert:** Urology 1978; **Med School:** Cornell Univ-Weill Med Coll 1968; **Resid:** Surgery, Boston City Hosp 1973; Urology, Mass Genl Hosp 1976; **Fellow:** Pediatric Urology, Mass Genl Hosp 1977; Pediatric Urology, Great Ormond St Hosp 1978; **Fac Appt:** Prof U, Columbia P&S

Herr, Harry W MD [U] - **Spec Exp:** Bladder Cancer; Prostate Cancer; Testicular Cancer; **Hospital:** Meml Sloan-Kettering Cancer Ctr, NY-Presby/Weill Cornell Med Ctr, NY (page 66); **Address:** 1275 York Avenue, New York, NY 10021; **Phone:** 800-525-2225; **Board Cert:** Urology 1976; **Med School:** UCSF 1969; **Resid:** Urology, UC Irvine Med Ctr 1974; **Fellow:** Urology, Meml Sloan Kettering Cancer Ctr 1976; **Fac Appt:** Assoc Prof S, Cornell Univ-Weill Med Coll

Hrebinko Jr, Ronald L MD [U] - **Spec Exp:** Urinary Reconstruction; Kidney Cancer; Bladder Cancer; Testicular Cancer; **Hospital:** UPMC Presby, Pittsburgh, UPMC Shadyside; **Address:** Univ Pittsburgh Dept of Urology, Shadyside Medical Bldg, Ste 209, 5200 Centre Ave, Pittsburgh, PA 15232; **Phone:** 412-605-3022; **Board Cert:** Urology 2004; **Med School:** Univ Pittsburgh 1986; **Resid:** Urology, Univ Pittsburgh Med Ctr 1992; **Fellow:** Urologic Oncology, Roswell Park Cancer Ctr 1993; **Fac Appt:** Assoc Prof U, Univ Pittsburgh

Jackman, Stephen V MD [U] - **Spec Exp:** Prostate Cancer/Robotic Surgery; Kidney Cancer; Kidney Stones; Laparoscopic Surgery; **Hospital:** UPMC Shadyside, UPMC Presby, Pittsburgh; **Address:** 3471 Fifth Ave, Ste 700, Univ Pittsburgh Med Ctr,Urology Dept, Pittsburgh, PA 15213; **Phone:** 412-692-4095; **Board Cert:** Urology 2011; **Med School:** Yale Univ 1994; **Resid:** Urology, Johns Hopkins Hosp 2000; **Fac Appt:** Prof U, Univ Pittsburgh

Kane, Michael H MD [U] - **Spec Exp:** Brachytherapy; Prostate Cancer; Minimally Invasive Surgery; Incontinence after Prostate Cancer; **Hospital:** Sinai Hosp - Baltimore; **Address:** 113 Westminster Rd, Ste 104, Westminister, MD 21157; **Phone:** 443-821-3674; **Board Cert:** Urology 2005; **Med School:** Cornell Univ 1989; **Resid:** Urology, Mt Sinai Hosp 1995

Kaplan, Steven A MD [U] - **Spec Exp:** Urodynamics; Voiding Dysfunction; Incontinence after Prostate Cancer; Incontinence; **Hospital:** NY-Presby/Weill Cornell Med Ctr, NY (page 66); **Address:** 425 E 61 St, Fl 12, New York, NY 10065; **Phone:** 646-962-4811; **Board Cert:** Urology 2011; **Med School:** Mount Sinai Sch Med 1982; **Resid:** Surgery, Mount Sinai Hosp 1984; Urology, Columbia Presby Med Ctr 1988; **Fellow:** Urology, Columbia Presby Med Ctr 1990; **Fac Appt:** Prof U, Cornell Univ-Weill Med Coll

Katz, Aaron E MD [U] - **Spec Exp:** Prostate Cancer-Cryosurgery; Kidney Cancer-Cryosurgery; Complementary Medicine; Nutrition & Cancer Prevention; **Hospital:** Winthrop Univ Hosp; **Address:** 1401 Franklin Ave, Garden City, NY 11530; **Phone:** 516-535-1900; **Board Cert:** Urology 2006; **Med School:** NY Med Coll 1986; **Resid:** Urology, Maimonides Med Ctr 1992; **Fellow:** Urologic Oncology, Columbia Presby Med Ctr 1993; **Fac Appt:** Assoc Clin Prof U, Columbia P&S

Kavoussi, Louis R MD [U] - **Spec Exp:** Laparoscopic Surgery; Urologic Cancer; Prostate Cancer; Kidney Cancer; **Hospital:** Long Island Jewish Med Ctr (page 67), N Shore Univ Hosp (page 67); **Address:** Arthur Smith Institute for Urology, 450 Lakeville Rd, Ste M-41, New Hyde Park, NY 11042; **Phone:** 516-734-8558; **Board Cert:** Urology 2009; **Med School:** SUNY Buffalo 1983; **Resid:** Surgery, Barnes Jewish Hosp 1985; Urology, Barnes Jewish Hosp 1989; **Fac Appt:** Prof U, Hofstra N Shore-LIJ Sch Med

Kirschenbaum, Alexander M MD [U] - **Spec Exp:** Prostate Cancer; Bladder Cancer; Kidney Cancer; **Hospital:** Mount Sinai Med Ctr (page 64); **Address:** 229 E 79th St, Ste 1A, New York, NY 10075; **Phone:** 646-422-0926; **Board Cert:** Urology 2006; **Med School:** Mount Sinai Sch Med 1980; **Resid:** Surgery, Mt Sinai Hosp 1982; Urology, Mt Sinai Hosp 1985; **Fellow:** Urologic Oncology, Mt Sinai Hosp 1987; **Fac Appt:** Assoc Prof U, Mount Sinai Sch Med

Lanteri, Vincent J MD [U] - **Spec Exp:** Prostate Cancer/Robotic Surgery; Urologic Cancer; Minimally Invasive Urologic Surgery; **Hospital:** Hackensack Univ Med Ctr; **Address:** 255 W Spring Valley Ave, Ste 101, Maywood, NJ 07607; **Phone:** 201-487-8866; **Board Cert:** Urology 1982; **Med School:** Mexico 1974; **Resid:** Surgery, UMDNJ Med Ctr 1977; Urology, UMDNJ Med Ctr 1980; **Fellow:** Urologic Oncology, Roswell Park Cancer Inst 1981

Lepor, Herbert MD [U] - **Spec Exp:** Prostate Cancer; **Hospital:** NYU Langone Med Ctr (page 68); **Address:** 150 E 32nd St, Fl 2, NYU Urology Assocaites, New York, NY 10016; **Phone:** 646-825-6327; **Board Cert:** Urology 2006; **Med School:** Johns Hopkins Univ 1975; **Resid:** Urology, Johns Hopkins Hosp 1986; **Fac Appt:** Prof U, NYU Sch Med

Linsenmeyer, Todd A MD [U] - **Spec Exp:** Infertility-Male in Spinal Cord Injury; Voiding Dysfunction/Spinal Cord Injury; Urodynamics in Spinal Cord Injury; **Hospital:** Kessler Inst for Rehab - W Orange; **Address:** Kessler Inst Rehab, 1199 Pleasant Valley Way, West Orange, NJ 07052; **Phone:** 973-731-3900 x2274; **Board Cert:** Urology 2005; Physical Medicine & Rehabilitation 1990; Spinal Cord Injury Medicine 2002; **Med School:** Univ Hawaii JA Burns Sch Med 1979; **Resid:** Urology, Tripler AMC 1984; **Fellow:** Physical Medicine & Rehabilitation, Stanford Univ Hosp 1989; **Fac Appt:** Assoc Prof S, UMDNJ-NJ Med Sch, Newark

Loo, Marcus Hsieu-Hong MD [U] - **Spec Exp:** Prostate Disease; Kidney Stones; Voiding Dysfunction; Prostate Cancer; **Hospital:** NY-Presby/Weill Cornell Med Ctr, NY (page 66); **Address:** 254 Canal St, Ste 3001, New York, NY 10013-3501; **Phone:** 212-925-8388; **Board Cert:** Urology 2008; **Med School:** Cornell Univ-Weill Med Coll 1981; **Resid:** Surgery, NY Hosp-Cornell Med Ctr 1983; Urology, NY Hosp-Cornell Med Ctr 1988; **Fellow:** Urology, NY Hosp-Cornell Med Ctr 1984; **Fac Appt:** Clin Prof U, Cornell Univ-Weill Med Coll

Lowe, Franklin Charles MD [U] - **Spec Exp:** Prostate Disease; Complementary Medicine; Prostate Cancer; Kidney Stones; **Hospital:** St. Luke's - Roosevelt Hosp Ctr - Roosevelt Div (page 56), NY-Presby/Columbia Univ Med Ctr, NY (page 66); **Address:** 425 W 59th St, Ste 3A, New York, NY 10019-1104; **Phone:** 212-523-7790; **Board Cert:** Urology 2006; **Med School:** Columbia P&S 1979; **Resid:** Surgery, Johns Hopkins Hosp 1981; Urology, Johns Hopkins Hosp 1984; **Fac Appt:** Clin Prof U, Columbia P&S

Malkowicz, S Bruce MD [U] - **Spec Exp:** Prostate Cancer; Bladder Cancer; Kidney Cancer; Gene Therapy; **Hospital:** Hosp Univ Penn - UPHS (page 72); **Address:** Penn Urology, Perelman Center, 3400 Civic Center Blvd, 3 West, Philadelphia, PA 19104; **Phone:** 215-662-2891 x7330; **Board Cert:** Urology 2009; **Med School:** Univ Pennsylvania 1981; **Resid:** Surgery, Hosp Univ Penn 1983; Urology, Hosp Univ Penn 1987; **Fellow:** Urologic Oncology, USC Med Ctr 1998; Urologic Oncology, Hosp Univ Penn/Wistar Inst 1990; **Fac Appt:** Prof U, Univ Pennsylvania

McCullough, Andrew R MD [U] - **Spec Exp:** Erectile Dysfunction; Infertility-Male; Prostate Cancer; **Hospital:** Albany Med Ctr; **Address:** South Clinical Campus, 23 Hackett Blvd, Albany, NY 12208; **Phone:** 518-262-3341; **Board Cert:** Urology 2005; **Med School:** Univ MD Sch Med 1978; **Resid:** Urology, Johns Hopkins Hosp 1983; **Fellow:** Urologic Oncology, Johns Hopkins Hosp 1984; **Fac Appt:** Assoc Prof U, Albany Med Coll

Mohler, James L MD [U] - **Spec Exp:** Prostate Cancer; Robotic Surgery; **Hospital:** Roswell Park Cancer Inst; **Address:** Roswell Park Cancer Inst, Elm & Carlton Streets, Buffalo, NY 14263; **Phone:** 716-845-3159; **Board Cert:** Urology 2007; **Med School:** Med Coll GA 1980; **Resid:** Surgery, Univ Kentucky Med Ctr 1982; Urology, Univ Kentucky Med Ctr 1985; **Fellow:** Urologic Oncology, Johns Hopkins Hosp 1987; **Fac Appt:** Prof U, SUNY Buffalo

Mostwin, Jacek L MD/PhD [U] - **Spec Exp:** Prostate Cancer; **Hospital:** Johns Hopkins Hosp (page 61); **Address:** Brady Urological Inst, 601 N Caroline St Fl 4, Baltimore, MD 21287; **Phone:** 410-955-6100; **Board Cert:** Urology 2007; **Med School:** Univ MD Sch Med 1975; **Resid:** Surgery, Univ Michigan Med Ctr 1978; Urology, Johns Hopkins Hosp 1983; **Fac Appt:** Prof U, Johns Hopkins Univ

Mulhall, John P MD [U] - **Spec Exp:** Erectile Dysfunction; Peyronie's Disease; Penile Prostheses; Infertility-Male; **Hospital:** Meml Sloan-Kettering Cancer Ctr; **Address:** Kimmel Center, MSKCC, 353 E 68th St, Fl 5, New York, NY 10021; **Phone:** 646-422-4359; **Board Cert:** Urology 2008; **Med School:** Ireland 1985; **Resid:** Urology, Univ Conn Health Ctr 1995; **Fellow:** Urology, Boston Univ Med Ctr 1996; **Fac Appt:** Prof U, Cornell Univ-Weill Med Coll

Urology

Nagler, Harris M MD [U] - **Spec Exp:** Vasectomy Reversal; Infertility-Male; Varicocele Microsurgery; Erectile Dysfunction; **Hospital:** Beth Israel Med Ctr - Petrie Division (page 56); **Address:** Beth Israel Med Ctr, Dept Urology, 10 Union Square E, Ste 3A, New York, NY 10003-3314; **Phone:** 212-844-8700; **Board Cert:** Urology 1982; **Med School:** Temple Univ 1975; **Resid:** Urology, Columbia Presby Med Ctr 1980; **Fellow:** Reproductive Medicine, Columbia Presby Med Ctr 1981; **Fac Appt:** Prof U, Albert Einstein Coll Med

Naslund, Michael MD [U] - **Spec Exp:** Prostate Cancer; Prostate Disease; **Hospital:** Univ of MD Med Ctr; **Address:** UMMC-Maryland Prostate Ctr, 419 W Redwood St, Ste 320, Baltimore, MD 21201; **Phone:** 410-328-0800; **Board Cert:** Urology 2008; **Med School:** Johns Hopkins Univ 1981; **Resid:** Surgery, Johns Hopkins Hosp 1983; Urology, Johns Hopkins Hosp 1987; **Fac Appt:** Prof U, Univ MD Sch Med

Nelson, Joel B MD [U] - **Spec Exp:** Prostate Cancer; **Hospital:** UPMC Shadyside; **Address:** UPMC Shadyside Med Ctr, 5200 Centre Ave, Ste 209, Pittsburgh, PA 15232-1312; **Phone:** 412-605-3013; **Board Cert:** Urology 2008; **Med School:** Northwestern Univ 1988; **Resid:** Surgery, Northwestern MemL Hosp 1990; Urology, Northwestern Meml Hosp 1994; **Fellow:** Urology, Johns Hopkins Hosp; **Fac Appt:** Prof U, Univ Pittsburgh

Nitti, Victor MD [U] - **Spec Exp:** Urology-Female; Incontinence-Male & Female; Urodynamics; Voiding Dysfunction; **Hospital:** NYU Langone Med Ctr (page 68); **Address:** NYU Urology Assocs, 150 E 32nd St, 2nd Fl, New York, NY 10016; **Phone:** 646-825-6324; **Board Cert:** Urology 2002; **Med School:** UMDNJ-NJ Med Sch, Newark 1985; **Resid:** Surgery, Univ Hosp 1987; Urology, Univ Hosp 1991; **Fellow:** Female Urology, UCLA Med Ctr 1992; **Fac Appt:** Prof U, NYU Sch Med

Partin, Alan W MD/PhD [U] - **Spec Exp:** Prostate Cancer; Prostate Disease; **Hospital:** Johns Hopkins Hosp (page 61); **Address:** Brady Urological Inst, 601 N Caroline St Fl 4, Baltimore, MD 21287; **Phone:** 410-955-6100; **Board Cert:** Urology 2007; **Med School:** Johns Hopkins Univ 1989; **Resid:** Surgery, Johns Hopkins Hosp 1991; Urology, Johns Hopkins Hosp 1996; **Fac Appt:** Prof U, Johns Hopkins Univ

Poppas, Dix P MD [U] - **Spec Exp:** Genital Reconstruction-Pediatric; Robotic Surgery-Pediatric; Minimally Invasive Surgery-Pediatric; Pediatric Urology; **Hospital:** NY-Presby/Weill Cornell Med Ctr, NY (page 66); **Address:** Inst for Pediatric Urology, NY Presby Hosp-Weill Cornell, 525 E 68th St, rm F931, Box 94, New York, NY 10065; **Phone:** 212-746-5337; **Board Cert:** Urology 2008; Pediatric Urology 2008; **Med School:** Eastern VA Med Sch 1988; **Resid:** Urology, NY Hosp-Cornell Med Ctr 1994; **Fellow:** Pediatric Urology, Chldns Hosp Harvard Med Sch 1996; **Fac Appt:** Prof U, Cornell Univ-Weill Med Coll

Rushton Jr, H Gil MD [U] - **Spec Exp:** Pediatric Urology; Fetal Urology; Hypospadias; Hydronephrosis; **Hospital:** Chldns Natl Med Ctr; **Address:** Dept Urology, 111 Michigan Ave NW, Ste 400-W, Washington, DC 20010; **Phone:** 202-476-5042; **Board Cert:** Urology 2004; Pediatric Urology 2009; **Med School:** Univ SC Sch Med 1978; **Resid:** Urology, Univ SC Med Ctr 1983; **Fellow:** Pediatric Urology, Hosp Sick Chldn 1984; Pediatric Urology, Emory Chldns Hosp 1986; **Fac Appt:** Prof U, Geo Wash Univ

Sadeghi-Nejad, Hossein MD [U] - **Spec Exp:** Erectile Dysfunction; Peyronie's Disease; Prostate Disease; Infertility-Male; **Hospital:** Hackensack Univ Med Ctr, Univ Hosp-UMDNJ—Newark; **Address:** 20 Prospect Ave, rm 711, Hackensack, NJ 07601; **Phone:** 201-342-7977 x214; **Board Cert:** Urology 2009; **Med School:** McGill Univ 1989; **Resid:** Surgery, UCSF Med Ctr 1991; Urology, Boston Univ Med Ctr 1996; **Fellow:** Microsurgery, Boston Univ Med Ctr 1997; Reproductive Medicine, Boston Univ Med Ctr 1997; **Fac Appt:** Prof U, UMDNJ-NJ Med Sch, Newark

Samadi, David B MD [U] - **Spec Exp:** Prostate Cancer/Robotic Surgery; Kidney Cancer; Bladder Cancer; Urologic Cancer; **Hospital:** Mount Sinai Med Ctr (page 64); **Address:** 625 Madison Ave, Fl 2, New York, NY 10022; **Phone:** 212-241-8779; **Board Cert:** Urology 2004; **Med School:** SUNY Stony Brook 1994; **Resid:** Surgery, Montefiore Med Ctr 1996; Urology, Montefiore Med Ctr 2000; **Fellow:** Urologic Oncology, Meml Sloan Kettering Cancer Ctr 2001; Laparoscopic Surgery, Henri Mondor Hosp 2003; **Fac Appt:** Asst Prof U, Mount Sinai Sch Med

Sawczuk, Ihor S MD [U] - **Spec Exp:** Bladder Cancer; Kidney Cancer; Prostate Cancer/Robotic Surgery; Bladder Reconstruction; **Hospital:** Hackensack Univ Med Ctr, NY-Presby/Columbia Univ Med Ctr, NY (page 66); **Address:** Hackensack Univ Med Ctr, 360 Essex St, Ste 403, Hackensack, NJ 07601; **Phone:** 551-996-8090; **Board Cert:** Urology 2005; **Med School:** Med Coll PA Hahnemann 1979; **Resid:** Surgery, St Vincents Hosp 1981; Urology, Columbia-Presby Med Ctr 1984; **Fellow:** Urologic Oncology, Columbia-Presby Med Ctr 1986; **Fac Appt:** Prof U, Columbia P&S

Scardino, Peter T MD [U] - **Spec Exp:** Prostate Cancer; Bladder Cancer; Urologic Cancer; Urinary Reconstruction; **Hospital:** Meml Sloan-Kettering Cancer Ctr; **Address:** 1275 York Avenue, New York, NY 10065; **Phone:** 646-422-4329; **Board Cert:** Urology 1981; **Med School:** Duke Univ 1971; **Resid:** Surgery, Mass Genl Hosp 1973; Urology, UCLA Med Ctr 1979; **Fellow:** Urology, Natl Cancer Inst 1976; **Fac Appt:** Prof U, Cornell Univ-Weill Med Coll

Scherr, Douglas S MD [U] - **Spec Exp:** Prostate Cancer/Robotic Surgery; Bladder Cancer; Robotic Surgery; Testicular Cancer; **Hospital:** NY-Presby/Weill Cornell Med Ctr, NY (page 66); **Address:** Brady Urologic Health Ctr, 525 E 68th St Starr 900, New York, NY 10021; **Phone:** 212-746-5788; **Board Cert:** Urology 2003; **Med School:** Geo Wash Univ 1994; **Resid:** Urology, NY Hosp-Cornell Med Ctr 1999; **Fellow:** Urologic Oncology, Meml Sloan-Kettering Canc Ctr 2002; **Fac Appt:** Assoc Prof U, Cornell Univ-Weill Med Coll

Schlegel, Peter N MD [U] - **Spec Exp:** Prostate Cancer; Infertility-Male; **Hospital:** NY-Presby/Weill Cornell Med Ctr, NY (page 66), Hosp For Special Surgery (page 60); **Address:** Brady Urologic Health Ctr, 525 E 68th St Starr Bldg Fl 9 - Ste 900, New York, NY 10021-4870; **Phone:** 212-746-5491; **Board Cert:** Urology 2011; **Med School:** Univ Mass Sch Med 1983; **Resid:** Surgery, Johns Hopkins Hosp 1985; Urology, Johns Hopkins Hosp 1989; **Fellow:** Medical Oncology, Johns Hopkins Hosp 1987; Male Reproduction, NY Hosp-Cornell Med Ctr 1991; **Fac Appt:** Prof U, Cornell Univ-Weill Med Coll

Schoenberg, Mark P MD [U] - **Spec Exp:** Bladder Cancer; Urinary Reconstruction; **Hospital:** Johns Hopkins Hosp (page 61); **Address:** Brady Urological Inst, 601 N Caroline St Fl 4, Baltimore, MD 21287; **Phone:** 410-955-1039; **Board Cert:** Urology 2005; **Med School:** Univ Tex, Houston 1986; **Resid:** Surgery, Hosp U Penn 1988; Urologic Surgery, Hosp U Penn 1992; **Fellow:** Urologic Oncology, Brady Inst/Johns Hopkins 1994; **Fac Appt:** Prof U, Johns Hopkins Univ

Seftel, Allen D MD [U] - **Spec Exp:** Sexual Dysfunction; Infertility-Male; Prostate Disease; Peyronie's Disease; **Hospital:** Cooper Univ Hosp; **Address:** Cooper Univ Hosp, 3 Cooper Plaza, Ste 411, Camden, NJ 08103; **Phone:** 856-963-3577; **Board Cert:** Urology 2003; **Med School:** SUNY Downstate 1984; **Resid:** Urology, SUNY Downstate Med Ctr 1987; Urology, Univ Hosps-Case West Res 1990; **Fellow:** Reproductive Medicine, Boston Univ Med Ctr 1992; **Fac Appt:** Prof U

Shabsigh, Ridwan MD [U] - **Spec Exp:** Erectile Dysfunction; Hypogonadism; Clinical Trials; **Hospital:** Maimonides Med Ctr (page 63); **Address:** 3121 Ocean Ave, Brooklyn, NY 11235; **Phone:** 718-283-7746; **Board Cert:** Urology 2011; **Med School:** Syria 1976; **Resid:** Urology, Seepark Hosp 1983; Urology, Baylor Affil Hsop 1990; **Fellow:** Urology, Baylor Affil Hosp 1987; **Fac Appt:** Clin Prof U, Columbia P&S

Urology

Sheinfeld, Joel MD [U] - **Spec Exp:** Testicular Cancer; Fertility Preservation in Cancer; **Hospital:** Meml Sloan-Kettering Cancer Ctr; **Address:** 353 E 68th St, New York, NY 10065; **Phone:** 646-422-4311; **Board Cert:** Urology 2009; **Med School:** Univ Fla Coll Med 1981; **Resid:** Urology, Strong Meml Hosp 1986; **Fellow:** Urologic Oncology, Meml Sloan Kettering Cancer Ctr 1989; **Fac Appt:** Assoc Prof U, Cornell Univ-Weill Med Coll

Shenot, Patrick J MD [U] - **Spec Exp:** Voiding Dysfunction/Spinal Cord Injury; Voiding Dysfunction; Genitourinary Disorders; Incontinence; **Hospital:** Thomas Jefferson Univ Hosp, Magee Rehab Hosp; **Address:** 833 Chestnut St E, Ste 703, Philadelphia, PA 19107; **Phone:** 215-955-1000; **Board Cert:** Urology 2010; **Med School:** SUNY Stony Brook 1991; **Resid:** Surgery, Thos Jefferson Univ Hosp 1993; Urology, Thos Jefferson Univ Hosp 1997; **Fac Appt:** Asst Prof U, Thomas Jefferson Univ

Siegelbaum, Marc MD [U] - **Spec Exp:** Prostate Cancer; Laparoscopic Surgery; Kidney Cancer; Pediatric Urology; **Hospital:** St. Joseph Med Ctr; **Address:** Chesapeake Urology Assocs, 7505 Osler Drive, Ste 506, Towson, MD 21204; **Phone:** 410-296-0167; **Board Cert:** Urology 2009; **Med School:** Univ MD Sch Med 1982; **Resid:** Surgery, Sinai Hosp 1989; Urology, Temple Univ Hlth Sci Ctr 1991

Taneja, Samir S MD [U] - **Spec Exp:** Prostate Cancer; Kidney Cancer; Bladder Cancer; **Hospital:** NYU Langone Med Ctr (page 68); **Address:** NYU Urology Associates, 150 E 32nd St, Fl 2, New York, NY 10016-6024; **Phone:** 646-825-6321; **Board Cert:** Urology 2009; **Med School:** Northwestern Univ 1990; **Resid:** Urology, UCLA Med Ctr 1996; **Fellow:** Urologic Oncology, NYU Med Ctr 1998; **Fac Appt:** Prof U, NYU Sch Med

Tewari, Ashutosh K MD [U] - **Spec Exp:** Prostate Cancer/Robotic Surgery; **Hospital:** NY-Presby/Weill Cornell Med Ctr, NY (page 66); **Address:** Brady Urologic Health Center, 525 E 68th St, Starr 900, New York, NY 10021; **Phone:** 212-746-5638; **Board Cert:** Urology 2006; **Med School:** India 1984; **Resid:** Surgery, GSVM Medical College 1990; Urology, Henry Ford Hosp 2003; **Fellow:** Transplant Surgery, Liverpool Univ Med Ctr 1993; Urologic Oncology, Shands Healthcare 1995; **Fac Appt:** Assoc Prof U, Cornell Univ-Weill Med Coll

Trabulsi, Edouard J MD [U] - **Spec Exp:** Minimally Invasive Urologic Surgery; Urologic Cancer; Prostate Cancer; **Hospital:** Thomas Jefferson Univ Hosp; **Address:** 833 Chestnut St, Ste 703, Philadelphia, PA 19107; **Phone:** 215-955-1000; **Board Cert:** Urology 2005; **Med School:** SUNY Buffalo 1995; **Resid:** Surgery, Thomas Jefferson Univ Hosp 1997; Urology, Thomas Jefferson Univ Hosp 2001; **Fellow:** Urologic Oncology, Meml Sloan Kettering Cancer Ctr 2003; **Fac Appt:** Assoc Prof U, Thomas Jefferson Univ

Uzzo, Robert MD [U] - **Spec Exp:** Bladder Cancer; Prostate Cancer; Robotic Surgery; Minimally Invasive Urologic Surgery; **Hospital:** Fox Chase Cancer Ctr (page 58); **Address:** Fox Chase Cancer Ctr, 333 Cottman Ave, Philadelphia, PA 19111; **Phone:** 215-728-3501; **Board Cert:** Urology 2009; **Med School:** Cornell Univ-Weill Med Coll 1991; **Resid:** Surgery, New York Hosp-Cornell Med Ctr 1993; Urology, New York Hosp-Cornell Med Ctr 1997; **Fellow:** Urologic Oncology, Cleveland Clinic 1999; Renal Transplant, Cleveland Clinic 2000; **Fac Appt:** Assoc Prof S, Temple Univ

Van Arsdalen, Keith N MD [U] - **Spec Exp:** Infertility-Male; Varicocele Microsurgery; Urologic Cancer; Vasectomy Reversal; **Hospital:** Hosp Univ Penn - UPHS (page 72), Chldns Hosp of Philadelphia; **Address:** Penn Urology, 3400 Civic Ctr Blvd, Perelman Center Fl 3W, Philadelphia, PA 19104-4283; **Phone:** 215-662-2891; **Board Cert:** Urology 1984; **Med School:** Med Coll VA 1977; **Resid:** Surgery, Univ Maryland Hosp 1979; Urology, Med Coll Virginia 1982; **Fellow:** Urodynamics, Hosp Univ Penn 1983; **Fac Appt:** Prof U, Univ Pennsylvania

Vapnek, Jonathan M MD [U] - **Spec Exp:** Incontinence; Urology-Female; Neurogenic Bladder; Urodynamics; **Hospital:** Mount Sinai Med Ctr (page 64); **Address:** 229 E 79th St, Ste 1A, New York, NY 10075; **Phone:** 212-717-9500; **Board Cert:** Urology 2005; **Med School:** UCSD 1986; **Resid:** Surgery, UCSD Med Ctr 1988; Urology, UCSF Med Ctr 1992; **Fellow:** Neurourology, UC Davis Med Ctr 1993; **Fac Appt:** Assoc Clin Prof U, Mount Sinai Sch Med

Verghese, Mohan MD [U] - **Spec Exp:** Urologic Cancer; **Hospital:** Washington Hosp Ctr; **Address:** 110 Irving St NW, Ste 3B19, Washington, DC 20010; **Phone:** 202-877-3968; **Board Cert:** Urology 2005; **Med School:** India 1976; **Resid:** Surgery, Bay State Med Ctr 1980; Urology, Washington Hosp Ctr 1984; **Fellow:** Urologic Oncology, Roswell Park Meml Inst 1992

Walsh, Patrick MD [U] - **Spec Exp:** Prostate Cancer; **Hospital:** Johns Hopkins Hosp (page 61); **Address:** Brady Urological Inst, 601 N Caroline St Fl 4, Baltimore, MD 21287; **Phone:** 410-955-6100; **Board Cert:** Urology 1975; **Med School:** Case West Res Univ 1964; **Resid:** Surgery, Peter Bent Brigham Hosp/Chldns Hosp 1967; Urology, UCLA Med Ctr 1971; **Fellow:** Endocrinology, Harbor Genl Hosp 1970; **Fac Appt:** Prof U, Johns Hopkins Univ

Wein, Alan J MD/PhD [U] - **Spec Exp:** Prostate Cancer; Neuro-Urology; Urologic Cancer; Urodynamics; **Hospital:** Hosp Univ Penn - UPHS (page 72), Pennsylvania Hosp-UPHS (page 72); **Address:** Univ Penn Hlth Sys, Div Uro, Penn Med, 34th & Civic Ctr Blvd, Perelman Ctr, W Pavilion, Fl 3, Philadelphia, PA 19104-4283; **Phone:** 215-662-2891; **Board Cert:** Urology 1995; **Med School:** Univ Pennsylvania 1966; **Resid:** Surgery, Hosp Univ Penn 1968; Urology, Hosp Univ Penn 1972; **Fellow:** Urology, Hosp Univ Penn 1969; **Fac Appt:** Prof U, Univ Pennsylvania

Weiss, Robert E MD [U] - **Spec Exp:** Bladder Cancer; Kidney Cancer; Testicular Cancer; Robotic Surgery; **Hospital:** Robert Wood Johnson Univ Hosp - New Brunswick, Univ Med Ctr Princeton at Plainsboro; **Address:** 1 Robert Wood Johnson Pl Ste MB588, Dept Urology, New Brunswick, NJ 08901-1928; **Phone:** 732-235-7960; **Board Cert:** Urology 2004; **Med School:** NYU Sch Med 1985; **Resid:** Surgery, Mount Sinai Med Ctr 1987; Urology, Mount Sinai Med Ctr 1991; **Fellow:** Urologic Oncology, Meml Sloan Kettering Cancer Ctr 1994; **Fac Appt:** Assoc Prof U, UMDNJ-RW Johnson Med Sch

Yu, George W MD [U] - **Spec Exp:** Nutrition & Disease Prevention/Control; Nutrition & Cancer Prevention/Control; **Hospital:** G Washington Univ Hosp, Anne Arundel Med Ctr; **Address:** 122 Defense Hwy, Ste 224, Annapolis, MD 21401; **Phone:** 410-897-0540; **Board Cert:** Urology 1981; **Med School:** Tufts Univ 1973; **Resid:** Surgery, Brigham & Women's Hosp 1976; Urology, Johns Hopkins Hosp 1981; **Fac Appt:** Prof U, Geo Wash Univ

Southeast

Atala, Anthony MD [U] - **Spec Exp:** Pediatric Urology; Reconstructive Surgery; Hernia; Hypospadias; **Hospital:** Wake Forest Baptist Med Ctr; **Address:** Wake Forest Univ Baptist Med Ctr, Dept Urology, 140 Charlois Blvd, Winston-Salem, NC 27103; **Phone:** 336-716-4131; **Board Cert:** Urology 2008; Pediatric Urology 2008; **Med School:** Univ Louisville Sch Med 1985; **Resid:** Surgery, Univ Louisville Hosp 1987; Urology, Univ Louisville Hosp 1990; **Fellow:** Research, Boston Children's Hosp 1991; Pediatric Urology, Boston Children's Hosp 1992; **Fac Appt:** Prof U, Wake Forest Univ

Badlani, Gopal MD [U] - **Spec Exp:** Incontinence; Pelvic Organ Prolapse Repair; **Hospital:** Wake Forest Baptist Med Ctr; **Address:** Dept Urology-Reynolds Tower, Medical Ctr Blvd, Winston-Salem, NC 27157; **Phone:** 336-716-4131; **Board Cert:** Urology 1982; **Med School:** India 1973; **Resid:** Surgery, St Agnes Hosp 1977; Urology, LI Jewish Hosp 1980; **Fellow:** Urology, Baylor Med Ctr 1983; **Fac Appt:** Prof U, Wake Forest Univ

Urology

Balaji, K C MD [U] - **Spec Exp:** Prostate Cancer; Urologic Cancer; Robotic Surgery; Minimally Invasive Surgery; **Hospital:** Wake Forest Baptist Med Ctr; **Address:** Wake Forest Univ School of Medicine, Urology Clinic, 140 Charlois Blvd, Winston-Salem, NC 27103; **Phone:** 336-716-4131; **Board Cert:** Urology 2009; **Med School:** India 1986; **Resid:** Surgery, Lebanon Hosp Ctr 1993; Urology, Univ Mass Med Ctr 1997; **Fellow:** Urologic Oncology, Meml Sloan Kettering Cancer Ctr 1999; **Fac Appt:** Prof U, Wake Forest Univ

Beall, Michael E MD [U] - **Spec Exp:** Prostate Cancer; Testicular Cancer; Vasectomy Reversal; **Hospital:** Inova Fairfax Hosp, Reston Hosp Ctr; **Address:** Dominion Urological Consultants, 8503 Arlington Blvd, Ste 310, Fairfax, VA 22031; **Phone:** 703-208-4200; **Board Cert:** Urology 1979; **Med School:** Geo Wash Univ 1972; **Resid:** Urology, Geo Wash Univ Hosp 1977; **Fac Appt:** Assoc Clin Prof U, Geo Wash Univ

Brock III, John W MD [U] - **Spec Exp:** Pediatric Urology; Reconstructive Surgery; Bladder Exstrophy; Spina Bifida; **Hospital:** Vanderbilt Monroe Carrell Jr. Chldn's Hosp (page 75); **Address:** Vanderbilt Chldns Hosp, Div Ped Urology, 2200 Childrens Way, 4102 DOT, Nashville, TN 37232-9820; **Phone:** 615-936-1060; **Board Cert:** Urology 2008; Pediatric Urology 2008; **Med School:** Med Coll GA 1978; **Resid:** Urology, Vanderbilt Univ Med Ctr 1983; **Fac Appt:** Prof U, Vanderbilt Univ

Broderick, Gregory MD [U] - **Spec Exp:** Erectile Dysfunction; Voiding Dysfunction; Peyronie's Disease; **Hospital:** Mayo - Jacksonville; **Address:** Mayo Clinic, Dept Urology, 4500 San Pablo Rd, Jacksonville, FL 32224; **Phone:** 904-953-7330; **Board Cert:** Urology 2012; **Med School:** UCSF 1983; **Resid:** Surgery, UCSF Med Ctr 1985; Urology, UCSF Med Ctr 1988; **Fellow:** Neurourology, UC Davis Med Ctr 1990; **Fac Appt:** Prof U, Mayo Med Sch

Busby, J Erik MD [U] - **Spec Exp:** Prostate Cancer; Robotic Surgery; **Hospital:** Univ of Ala Hosp at Birmingham; **Address:** 1530 3rd Ave S, SOT 1105, Birmingham, AL 35294; **Phone:** 205-996-8765; **Board Cert:** Urology 2009; **Med School:** Med Univ SC 1998; **Resid:** Urology, UC Davis Hlth Ctr 2004; **Fellow:** Urologic Oncology, UT MD Anderson Cancer Ctr 2007; **Fac Appt:** Asst Prof S, Univ Alabama

Carson III, Culley C MD [U] - **Spec Exp:** Erectile Dysfunction; Kidney Stones; Peyronie's Disease; **Hospital:** NC Memorial Hosp - UNC, Durham Regional Hosp; **Address:** UNC, Urology Dept, 2113 Physicians Office Bldg, CB 7235, Chapel Hill, NC 27599-7235; **Phone:** 919-966-1315; **Board Cert:** Urology 1980; **Med School:** Geo Wash Univ 1971; **Resid:** Surgery, Dartmouth-Hitchcock Med Ctr 1973; Urology, Mayo Clinic 1978; **Fac Appt:** Prof U, Univ NC Sch Med

Chang, Sam S MD [U] - **Spec Exp:** Prostate Cancer; Bladder Cancer; Kidney Cancer; Testicular Cancer; **Hospital:** Vanderbilt Univ Med Ctr (page 75); **Address:** A1302 Vanderbilt University Med Ctr N, Nashville, TN 37232-2765; **Phone:** 615-322-2101; **Board Cert:** Urology 2010; **Med School:** Vanderbilt Univ 1992; **Resid:** Urology, Vanderbilt Univ Med Ctr 1998; **Fellow:** Urologic Oncology, Meml Sloan Kettering Cancer Ctr 1999; **Fac Appt:** Prof U, Vanderbilt Univ

Ciancio, Gaetano MD [U] - **Spec Exp:** Transplant-Kidney; Transplant-Pancreas; Kidney Cancer; **Hospital:** Jackson Meml Hosp, Univ of Miami Hosp; **Address:** 1801 NW 9th Ave Fl 5 - Ste 519, Miami, FL 33136; **Phone:** 305-355-5111; **Board Cert:** Urology 2005; **Med School:** Venezuela 1982; **Resid:** Surgery, Univ Miami/Jackson Meml Hosp 1989; Urology, Univ Miami/Jackson Meml Hosp 1993; **Fellow:** Transplant Surgery, Univ Miami/Jackson Meml Hosp 1995; **Fac Appt:** Prof U, Univ Miami Sch Med

Cookson, Michael S MD [U] - **Spec Exp:** Urologic Cancer; Bladder Cancer; Prostate Cancer; Testicular Cancer; **Hospital:** Vanderbilt Univ Med Ctr (page 75), Saint Thomas Hosp - Nashville; **Address:** Vanderbilt Univ Med Ctr, Urol Surg A1302 MCN, Nashville, TN 37232-2765; **Phone:** 615-322-2101; **Board Cert:** Urology 2006; **Med School:** Univ Okla Coll Med 1988; **Resid:** Urology, UTSA Med Ctr 1994; **Fellow:** Urologic Oncology, Meml Sloan-Kettering Cancer Ctr 1996; **Fac Appt:** Prof U, Vanderbilt Univ

Fraser Jr, Lionel B MD [U] - **Spec Exp:** Prostate Cancer; Incontinence after Prostate Cancer; Erectile Dysfunction; **Hospital:** Baptist Med Ctr-Jackson; **Address:** Metropolitan Urology, St Dominics West Med Tower, 971 Lakeland Drive, Ste 360, Jackson, MS 39216; **Phone:** 601-982-0982; **Board Cert:** Urology 2005; **Med School:** Univ Mich Med Sch 1977; **Resid:** Surgery, New England Deaconness Hosp 1979; **Fellow:** Urology, Brigham & Womens Hosp 1983

Greene, Graham MD [U] - **Spec Exp:** Urologic Cancer; **Hospital:** Lakeland Regl Med Ctr; **Address:** Lakeland Regl Cancer Ctr, 3525 Lakeland Hills Blvd, Lakeland, FL 33805; **Phone:** 863-603-6565; **Board Cert:** Urology 2007; **Med School:** Dalhousie Univ 1989; **Resid:** Urology, Victoria Genl Hosp 1994; **Fellow:** Urologic Oncology, M.D. Anderson Cancer Ctr 1997; **Fac Appt:** Assoc Prof

Hemal, Ashok K MD [U] - **Spec Exp:** Urologic Cancer; Robotic Surgery; Reconstructive Urologic Surgery; Laparoscopic Surgery; **Hospital:** Wake Forest Baptist Med Ctr; **Address:** Department of Urology, Medical Center Blvd, Winston-Salem, NC 27157; **Phone:** 336-716-5702; **Med School:** India 1981; **Resid:** Surgery, G R Med College 1985; Urology, Post Grad Inst Med Ed & Rsch 1988; **Fellow:** Robotic Surgery, Henry Ford Hosp; **Fac Appt:** Prof U, Wake Forest Univ

Irby III, Pierce B MD [U] - **Spec Exp:** Kidney Stones; Minimally Invasive Surgery; Vasectomy; **Hospital:** Carolinas Med Ctr, Presby Hosp - Charlotte; **Address:** McKay Urology, 1023 Edgehill Rd S, Charlotte, NC 28207; **Phone:** 704-355-8686; **Board Cert:** Urology 2003; **Med School:** Uniformed Srvs Univ, Bethesda 1983; **Resid:** Urology, Letterman Army Med Ctr 1990; **Fellow:** Endourology, UCSF Med Ctr 1992; **Fac Appt:** Assoc Clin Prof U, Univ NC Sch Med

Joseph, David B MD [U] - **Spec Exp:** Pediatric Urology; Urodynamics; Neuro-Urology; **Hospital:** Children's Hospital - Birmingham, Univ of Ala Hosp at Birmingham; **Address:** Childrens of Alabama, Dept of Urology, 1600 7th Ave S, Ste ACC-318, Birmingham, AL 35233; **Phone:** 205-638-9840; **Board Cert:** Urology 2005; Pediatric Urology 2008; **Med School:** Univ Wisc 1980; **Resid:** Urology, Univ Wisconsin Med Ctr 1985; **Fellow:** Pediatric Urology, Boston Childrens Hosp 1986; **Fac Appt:** Prof U, Univ Alabama

Keane, Thomas E MD [U] - **Spec Exp:** Urologic Cancer; Genitourinary Cancer; Prostate Cancer; Clinical Trials; **Hospital:** MUSC Med Ctr; **Address:** MUSC-Urology Dept, 96 Jonathan Lucas St, Ste CSB644, Charleston, SC 29425; **Phone:** 843-792-1666; **Board Cert:** Urology 2003; **Med School:** Ireland 1981; **Resid:** Urology, St Vincents Hosp 1986; Urology, N Tees Gen Hosp 1988; **Fellow:** Urology, Duke Univ Med Ctr 1993; **Fac Appt:** Prof U, Univ SC Sch Med

Kennelly, Michael J MD [U] - **Spec Exp:** Incontinence; Voiding Dysfunction; Pelvic Organ Prolapse Repair; Neurogenic Bladder; **Hospital:** Carolinas Med Ctr, Presby Hosp - Charlotte; **Address:** McKay Urology, 1023 Edgehill Rd S, Charlotte, NC 28207; **Phone:** 704-355-8686; **Board Cert:** Urology 2005; **Med School:** Univ Cincinnati 1989; **Resid:** Urology, Univ Mich Med Ctr 1994; **Fellow:** Neurology, UT Hlth Sci Ctr 1995; **Fac Appt:** Clin Prof U, Univ NC Sch Med

Kim, Edward D MD [U] - **Spec Exp:** Infertility-Male; Prostate Cancer; Bladder Cancer; **Hospital:** Univ of Tennesee Med Ctr; **Address:** University Urology, 1928 Alcoa Hwy, Ste 222, MS 37920, Med Office, B Bldg, Ste 222, Knoxville, TN 37920; **Phone:** 865-305-9254; **Board Cert:** Urology 2007; **Med School:** Northwestern Univ 1989; **Resid:** Urology, Northwestern Meml Hosp 1995; **Fellow:** Baylor Coll Med 1996; **Fac Appt:** Prof U, Univ Tenn Coll Med

Urology

Kirsch, Andrew J MD [U] - **Spec Exp:** Pediatric Urology; Urinary Reconstruction; Urinary Reflux/Obstruction; Bladder Exstrophy; **Hospital:** Chldns Hlthcare Atlanta @ Egleston, Chldns Hlthcare Atlanta @ Scottish Rite; **Address:** 5445 Meridian Mark Rd NE, Atlanta, GA 30342; **Phone:** 404-252-5206; **Board Cert:** Urology 2010; Pediatric Urology 2008; **Med School:** SUNY Downstate 1990; **Resid:** Surgery, Columbia Univ Affil Hosp 1992; Urology, Columbia Univ Affil Hosp 1996; **Fellow:** Pediatric Urology, Chldns Hosp 1998; **Fac Appt:** Clin Prof U, Emory Univ

Lloyd, L Keith MD [U] - **Spec Exp:** Erectile Dysfunction; Incontinence; Interstitial Cystitis; Neurogenic Bladder; **Hospital:** Univ of Ala Hosp at Birmingham; **Address:** UAB Urology, 1530 3rd Ave S, FOT 1105, Birmingham, AL 35294-3400; **Phone:** 205-975-0088; **Board Cert:** Urology 1976; **Med School:** Tulane Univ 1966; **Resid:** Urology, Tulane Univ Hosp 1974; **Fac Appt:** Prof U, Univ Alabama

Lockhart, Jorge L MD [U] - **Spec Exp:** Voiding Dysfunction; Bladder Cancer; Incontinence; Urinary Reconstruction; **Hospital:** Tampa Genl Hosp, H Lee Moffitt Cancer Ctr & Research Inst (page 59); **Address:** USF Dept Urology, 2 Tampa General Circle Fl 7, Tampa, FL 33606; **Phone:** 813-250-2213; **Board Cert:** Urology 1980; **Med School:** Uruguay 1973; **Resid:** Urology, Duke Univ Med Ctr 1977; **Fellow:** Urodynamics, Duke Univ Med Ctr 1978; **Fac Appt:** Prof S, Univ S Fla Coll Med

Lynne, Charles M MD [U] - **Spec Exp:** Infertility-Male in Spinal Cord Injury; Voiding Dysfunction/Spinal Cord Injury; Urodynamics; **Hospital:** Jackson Meml Hosp, Univ of Miami Hosp; **Address:** Professional Arts Ctr, 1150 NW 14 St, Ste 309, Miami, FL 33101; **Phone:** 305-243-6590; **Board Cert:** Urology 1974; **Med School:** Univ Miami Sch Med 1964; **Resid:** Urology, Univ Miami Affil Hosps 1971; **Fac Appt:** Prof U, Univ Miami Sch Med

McConnell, John D MD [U] - **Spec Exp:** Prostate Cancer; **Hospital:** Wake Forest Baptist Med Ctr; **Address:** Wake Forest Baptist Med Ctr, Medical Center Blvd, Winston-Salem, NC 27157; **Phone:** 336-716-3408; **Board Cert:** Urology 2004; **Med School:** Loyola Univ-Stritch Sch Med 1978; **Resid:** Surgery, Parkland Hosp 1980; Urology, Parkland Hosp 1984; **Fac Appt:** Prof U, Wake Forest Univ

Milam, Douglas F MD [U] - **Spec Exp:** Urodynamics; Voiding Dysfunction; Sexual Dysfunction; **Hospital:** Vanderbilt Univ Med Ctr (page 75); **Address:** Vanderbilt Dept Urologic Surgery, 1301 Med Ctr Drive N, Ste 3823, Nashville, TN 37232-2765; **Phone:** 615-322-2880; **Board Cert:** Urology 2003; **Med School:** W VA Univ 1986; **Resid:** Surgery, Univ Utah Hosps 1988; Urology, Univ Utah Hosps 1991; **Fac Appt:** Assoc Prof U, Vanderbilt Univ

Miller, Scott D MD [U] - **Spec Exp:** Robotic Surgery; Prostate Cancer/Robotic Surgery; Minimally Invasive Urologic Surgery; Reconstructive Surgery; **Hospital:** Northside Hosp; **Address:** Georgia Urology, 5670 Peachtree Dunwoody Rd, Ste 1250, Atlanta, GA 30342; **Phone:** 404-705-5201; **Board Cert:** Urology 2005; **Med School:** Med Coll GA 1990; **Resid:** Urology, Univ Kentucky Med Ctr 1995

Moul, Judd W MD [U] - **Spec Exp:** Prostate Cancer; Prostate Disease; Minimally Invasive Urologic Surgery; Clinical Trials; **Hospital:** Duke Univ Hosp, Durham VA Med Ctr; **Address:** Duke Univ Med Ctr, Duke South Bldg, rm 1573, Box 3707, Duke University Medical Center, Duke South Bldg, rm 1573, Box 3707, Durham, NC 27710; **Phone:** 919-684-5057; **Board Cert:** Urology 2008; **Med School:** Jefferson Med Coll 1982; **Resid:** Urology, Walter Reed Army Med Ctr 1987; **Fellow:** Urologic Oncology, Duke Univ Med Ctr 1989; **Fac Appt:** Prof S, Duke Univ

Patel, Vipul R MD [U] - **Spec Exp:** Prostate Cancer/Robotic Surgery; Kidney Cancer; **Hospital:** Florida Hosp Celebration Hlth; **Address:** 410 Celebration Pl, Ste 200, Celebration, FL 34747; **Phone:** 407-303-4673; **Board Cert:** Urology 2004; **Med School:** Baylor Coll Med 1995; **Resid:** Urology, Univ Miami; **Fellow:** Urologic Laparoscopic Surg-Endourology, Univ Miami

Patterson, Anthony L MD [U] - **Spec Exp:** Laparoscopic Surgery; Kidney Stones; **Hospital:** Univ of Tennesee Med Ctr; **Address:** UT Medical Group, 7945 Wolf River Blvd, Ste 350, Germantown, TN 38138-1733; **Phone:** 901-347-8350; **Board Cert:** Urology 2007; **Med School:** Univ Tenn Coll Med 1982; **Resid:** Surgery, Univ Tenn Med Ctr 1984; Urology, Univ Tenn Med Ctr 1987; **Fac Appt:** Assoc Prof U, Univ Tenn Coll Med

Penson, David F MD [U] - **Spec Exp:** Prostate Disease; Urologic Cancer; Bladder Cancer; Erectile Dysfunction; **Hospital:** Vanderbilt Univ Med Ctr (page 75); **Address:** 1301 Medical Ctr Drive, Ste 3823, Nashville, TN 37232; **Phone:** 615-322-2880; **Board Cert:** Urology 2009; **Med School:** Boston Univ 1991; **Resid:** Urology, UCLA Med Ctr 1997; **Fellow:** Urologic Oncology, Yale-New Haven Hosp 1999; **Fac Appt:** Prof U, Vanderbilt Univ

Pope IV, John C MD [U] - **Spec Exp:** Pediatric Urology; Kidney Stones; **Hospital:** Vanderbilt Monroe Carrell Jr. Chldn's Hosp (page 75); **Address:** Vanderbilt Chldns Hosp, Div Ped Urology, 2200 Children's Way, Ste 4102 DOT, Nashville, TN 37232; **Phone:** 615-936-1060; **Board Cert:** Urology 2008; Pediatric Urology 2008; **Med School:** Univ Tenn Coll Med 1989; **Resid:** Surgery, Vanderbilt Univ Med Ctr 1991; Urology, Vanderbilt Univ Med Ctr 1995; **Fellow:** Pediatric Urology, Indiana Univ Med Ctr 1997; **Fac Appt:** Assoc Prof U, Vanderbilt Univ

Pow-Sang, Julio M MD [U] - **Spec Exp:** Prostate Cancer; **Hospital:** H Lee Moffitt Cancer Ctr & Research Inst (page 59); **Address:** H Lee Moffitt Cancer Ctr, GU Clinic, 12902 Magnolia Drive, Tampa, FL 33612-9416; **Phone:** 813-972-8418; **Board Cert:** Urology 2011; **Med School:** Mexico 1978; **Resid:** Surgery, Univ Miami Sch Med 1983; Urology, Univ Miami Sch Med 1986; **Fellow:** Urologic Oncology, Univ Fla Coll Med 1987; **Fac Appt:** Prof S, Univ S Fla Coll Med

Preminger, Glenn M MD [U] - **Spec Exp:** Kidney Stones; **Hospital:** Duke Univ Hosp; **Address:** Box 3167 Med Ctr, Rm 1572D Duke South, White Zone, Durham, NC 27710; **Phone:** 919-681-5506; **Board Cert:** Urology 2003; **Med School:** NY Med Coll 1977; **Resid:** Surgery, N Carolina Meml Hosp 1979; Urology, N Carolina Meml Hosp 1983; **Fellow:** Urology, Univ Texas SW Med Ctr 1985; **Fac Appt:** Prof U, Duke Univ

Pruthi, Raj S MD [U] - **Spec Exp:** Urologic Cancer; Robotic Surgery; **Hospital:** NC Memorial Hosp - UNC; **Address:** UNC Dept Surgery, Urologic Surgery, 101 Manning Drive, Chapel Hill, NC 27599; **Phone:** 919-966-2571; **Board Cert:** Urology 2010; **Med School:** Duke Univ 1992; **Resid:** Surgery, Stanford Univ Hosp 1993; Urology, Stanford Univ Hosp 1998; **Fac Appt:** Prof U, Univ NC Sch Med

Robertson, Cary N MD [U] - **Spec Exp:** Prostate Cancer; Kidney Cancer; High Intensity Focused Ultrasound(HIFU); Testicular Cancer; **Hospital:** Duke Univ Hosp; **Address:** Duke Raleigh Hosp, 3480 Wake Forest Rd, Ste 506, Raleigh, NC 27609; **Phone:** 919-862-5600; **Board Cert:** Urology 2006; **Med School:** Tulane Univ 1977; **Resid:** Urology, Duke Univ Med Ctr 1985; **Fellow:** Urologic Oncology, Natl Inst Hlth 1987; **Fac Appt:** Assoc Prof U, Duke Univ

Rowland, Randall MD [U] - **Spec Exp:** Urologic Cancer; **Hospital:** Univ of Kentucky Albert B. Chandler Hosp; **Address:** Univ Kentucky Clin Dept Uro, Chandler Med Ctr, 800 Rose St, rm MS-283, Lexington, KY 40536-0001; **Phone:** 859-323-6677; **Board Cert:** Urology 1980; **Med School:** Northwestern Univ 1972; **Resid:** Urology, Northwestern Meml Hosp 1978; **Fellow:** Urology, Northwestern Meml Hosp 1977; **Fac Appt:** Prof U, Univ KY Coll Med

Sanders, William Holt MD [U] - **Spec Exp:** Prostate Cancer; Kidney Stones; Kidney Cancer; Vasectomy; **Hospital:** Northside Hosp; **Address:** 980 Johnson Ferry Rd NE, Ste 490, Atlanta, GA 30342-1767; **Phone:** 404-257-0133; **Board Cert:** Urology 2006; **Med School:** Emory Univ 1988; **Resid:** Surgery, Emory Affil Hosp 1990; Urology, Yale-New Haven Hosp 1993; **Fellow:** Urologic Oncology, Emory Univ Hosp 1994

Urology

Shaban, Stephen F MD [U] - **Spec Exp:** Infertility-Male; Congenital Absence of Vas Deferens; **Hospital:** Rex HlthCare, WakeMed-Raleigh Campus; **Address:** 2800 Blue Ridge Rd, Ste 405, Raleigh, NC 27607; **Phone:** 919-851-5482; **Board Cert:** Urology 2004; **Med School:** Mount Sinai Sch Med 1982; **Resid:** Urology, Univ S Fla 1987; **Fellow:** Male Reproduction, Baylor Coll Med 1988; **Fac Appt:** Prof U, Univ NC Sch Med

Smith, Joseph A MD [U] - **Spec Exp:** Prostate Cancer/Robotic Surgery; Bladder Cancer; Kidney Cancer; **Hospital:** Vanderbilt Univ Med Ctr (page 75); **Address:** Vanderbilt Univ Med Ctr, Dept Urology, A-1302 Medical Center North, Nashville, TN 37232-2765; **Phone:** 615-343-0234; **Board Cert:** Urology 2000; **Med School:** Univ Tenn Coll Med 1974; **Resid:** Surgery, Parkland Meml Hosp 1976; Urology, Univ Utah 1979; **Fellow:** Urologic Oncology, Meml Sloan Kettering Cancer Ctr 1980; **Fac Appt:** Prof U, Vanderbilt Univ

Soloway, Mark S MD [U] - **Spec Exp:** Bladder Cancer; Kidney Cancer; Prostate Cancer; Urologic Pathology; **Hospital:** Univ of Miami Hosp & Clins/Sylvester Comp Canc Ctr, Jackson Meml Hosp; **Address:** 1150 NW 14th St, Ste 309, Miami, FL 33136; **Phone:** 305-243-6596; **Board Cert:** Urology 1977; **Med School:** Case West Res Univ 1968; **Resid:** Surgery, Univ Hosps 1970; Urology, Univ Hosps 1975; **Fellow:** Surgery, Natl Cancer Inst 1972; **Fac Appt:** Prof U, Univ Miami Sch Med

Steers, William D MD [U] - **Spec Exp:** Incontinence; Erectile Dysfunction; Prostate Cancer/Robotic Surgery; **Hospital:** Univ of Virginia Health Sys; **Address:** UVA Hlth System, Dept Urology, PO Box 800422, Charlottesville, VA 22908-0422; **Phone:** 434-924-9107; **Board Cert:** Urology 2009; **Med School:** Med Coll OH 1980; **Resid:** Urology, Univ Tex Hlth Sci Ctr 1986; **Fellow:** Neurology, Univ Pittsburgh Med Ctr 1988; **Fac Appt:** Prof U, Univ VA Sch Med

Strup, Stephen E MD [U] - **Spec Exp:** Urologic Cancer; Minimally Invasive Urologic Surgery; Robotic Surgery; **Hospital:** Univ of Kentucky Albert B. Chandler Hosp; **Address:** Univ Kentucky Clin Dept Uro, Chandler Med Ctr, 800 Rose St, rm MS-283, Lexington, KY 40536-0001; **Phone:** 859-323-6679; **Board Cert:** Urology 2007; **Med School:** Indiana Univ 1988; **Resid:** Urology, Thomas Jefferson Univ Hosp 1994; **Fellow:** Urologic Oncology, National Cancer Inst 1996; **Fac Appt:** Prof S, Univ KY Coll Med

Su, Li-Ming MD [U] - **Spec Exp:** Prostate Cancer; Bladder Cancer; Testicular Cancer; **Hospital:** Shands at Univ of FL; **Address:** Shands at Univ Florida, Dept Urology, 1600 SW Archer Rd, Gainesville, FL 32610; **Phone:** 352-265-8282; **Board Cert:** Urology 2012; **Med School:** Cornell Univ-Weill Med Coll 1994; **Resid:** Surgery, NY Presby-Cornell Med Ctr 1996; Urology, NY Presby-Cornell Med Ctr 2000; **Fellow:** Robotic Surgery, Johns Hopkins Hosp 2001; **Fac Appt:** Prof U, Univ Fla Coll Med

Sutherland, Richard W MD [U] - **Spec Exp:** Pediatric Urology; **Hospital:** NC Memorial Hosp - UNC; **Address:** UNC-Chapel Hill, Div Urologic Surgery, 2113 Physicians Office Bldg, CB 7235, Chapel Hill, NC 27599-7235; **Phone:** 919-966-2573; **Board Cert:** Urology 2007; Pediatric Urology 2008; **Med School:** Oregon Hlth & Sci Univ 1989; **Resid:** Urology, Albany Med Ctr 1994; **Fellow:** Pediatric Urology, Baylor Coll Med 1996; **Fac Appt:** Assoc Prof U, Univ NC Sch Med

Teigland, Chris M MD [U] - **Spec Exp:** Prostate Cancer/Robotic Surgery; Kidney Cancer; Laparoscopic Surgery; **Hospital:** Carolinas Med Ctr; **Address:** Mckay Urology, 1023 Edgehill Rd S, Charlotte, NC 28207; **Phone:** 704-355-8686; **Board Cert:** Urology 2007; **Med School:** Duke Univ 1980; **Resid:** Surgery, Univ Utah Affil Hosps 1982; Urology, Univ Texas SW Med Ctr 1987; **Fac Appt:** Clin Prof U, Univ NC Sch Med

Terris, Martha K MD [U] - **Spec Exp:** Prostate Cancer; Brachytherapy; Urologic Cancer; Bladder Cancer; **Hospital:** Charlie Norwood VA Med Ctr - Augusta, Med Coll of GA Hosp and Clin (MCG Health Inc); **Address:** 950 15th St, Augusta, GA 30901; **Phone:** 706-733-0188; **Board Cert:** Urology 2007; **Med School:** Univ Miss 1986; **Resid:** Surgery, Duke Univ Med Ctr 1988; Urology, Stanford Univ Med Ctr 1995; **Fellow:** Ultrasound, Stanford Univ 1991; **Fac Appt:** Prof S, Med Coll GA

Wallen, Eric M MD [U] - **Spec Exp:** Laparoscopic Surgery; Prostate Cancer; Urologic Cancer; Robotic Surgery; **Hospital:** NC Memorial Hosp - UNC; **Address:** Div of Urologic Surgery, CB 7235, 2113 Physicians Office Bldg, 170 Manning Drive, Chapel Hill, NC 27599-7235; **Phone:** 919-966-8802; **Board Cert:** Urology 2010; **Med School:** UCLA 1994; **Resid:** Surgery, Stanford Univ Med Ctr 1996; Urology, Stanford Univ Med Ctr 2000; **Fac Appt:** Assoc Prof S, Univ NC Sch Med

Winfield, Howard N MD [U] - **Spec Exp:** Kidney Stones; Laparoscopic Surgery; Robotic Surgery; **Hospital:** DCH Reg Med Ctr; **Address:** W Alabama Urology Assoc, 701 University Blvd E, Ste 908, DCH Medical Tower 1, Tuscaloosa, AL 35401; **Phone:** 205-344-9393; **Board Cert:** Urology 2008; **Med School:** McGill Univ 1978; **Resid:** Urology, McGill Univ Tchg Hosp 1984; **Fellow:** Endourology, Washington Univ 1985; Endourology, UCLA 1986; **Fac Appt:** , Univ Iowa Coll Med

Midwest

Andriole Jr, Gerald L MD [U] - **Spec Exp:** Urologic Cancer; Prostate Cancer; Laparoscopic Surgery; **Hospital:** Barnes-Jewish Hosp, Barnes-Jewish West County Hosp; **Address:** Washington Univ School of Medicine, 4960 Children's Pl, Campus Box 8242, St Louis, MO 63110; **Phone:** 314-362-8212; **Board Cert:** Urology 2003; **Med School:** Jefferson Med Coll 1978; **Resid:** Surgery, Strong Meml Hosp 1980; Urology, Brigham & Womens Hosp 1983; **Fellow:** Urologic Oncology, NCI/NIH 1985; **Fac Appt:** Prof U, Washington Univ, St Louis

Bahnson, Robert Roy MD [U] - **Spec Exp:** Prostate Cancer; Bladder Cancer; Continent Urinary Diversions; **Hospital:** Ohio St Univ Med Ctr; **Address:** 915 Olentangy River Road, Ste 3100, Dept of Urology, 3142 Cramblett Med Ctr, Columbus, OH 43212; **Phone:** 614-293-3646; **Board Cert:** Urology 2006; **Med School:** Tufts Univ 1979; **Resid:** Surgery, Northwestern Meml Hosp 1981; Urology, Northwestern Meml Hosp 1985; **Fellow:** Urology, Northwestern Meml Hosp 1984; Research, Univ Pittsburgh 1991; **Fac Appt:** Prof U, Ohio State Univ

Bloom, David A MD [U] - **Spec Exp:** Pediatric Urology; Voiding Dysfunction; Genitourinary Reconstruction; Spina Bifida; **Hospital:** Univ of Michigan Hosp; **Address:** Univ Mich Hosp, Div Urology, 1500 E Med Ctr Dr, 3875 Taubman Ctr, Ann Arbor, MI 48109-5330; **Phone:** 734-232-4943; **Board Cert:** Urology 1982; Pediatric Urology 2008; **Med School:** SUNY Buffalo 1971; **Resid:** Surgery, UCLA Med Ctr 1976; Urology, UCLA Med Ctr 1980; **Fellow:** Pediatric Urology, Inst Urol-St Peters Hosp 1978; **Fac Appt:** Prof U, Univ Mich Med Sch

Bodner, Donald MD [U] - **Spec Exp:** Neuro-Urology; Spinal Cord Injury; **Hospital:** Univ Hosps Case Med Ctr (page 74); **Address:** Urologic Institute, 11100 Euclid Ave, MS LKS5046, Cleveland, OH 44106; **Phone:** 216-844-5503; **Board Cert:** Urology 2004; **Med School:** Indiana Univ 1979; **Resid:** Surgery, Case Western Reserve Univ Affil Hosp 1981; Urology, Case Western Reserve Univ Affil Hosp 1984

Brendler, Charles B MD [U] - **Spec Exp:** Prostate Cancer; **Hospital:** Evanston/North Shore Univ Hlth Sys; **Address:** NorthShore Univ HealthSystem, Dept of Surgery, 2650 Ridge Ave Walgreen Bldg - Ste 2507, Evanston, IL 60201; **Phone:** 847-657-5730; **Board Cert:** Urology 1981; **Med School:** Univ VA Sch Med 1974; **Resid:** Surgery, Duke Univ Med Ctr 1976; Urology, Duke Univ Med Ctr 1979; **Fellow:** Urologic Oncology, Univ Hosp Wales 1980; Urologic Oncology, Johns Hopkins Hosp 1982; **Fac Appt:** Clin Prof U, Univ Chicago-Pritzker Sch Med

Urology

Bushman, Wade MD [U] - **Spec Exp:** Neuro-Urology; Urodynamics; Urology-Female; **Hospital:** Univ WI Hosp & Clins; **Address:** Dept Urology, 600 Highland Ave, C52, Madison, WI 53792-3236; **Phone:** 608-263-4757; **Board Cert:** Urology 2006; **Med School:** Univ Chicago-Pritzker Sch Med 1986; **Resid:** Urology, Univ VA Med Ctr 1992; **Fac Appt:** Assoc Prof U, Univ Wisc

Cain, Mark P MD [U] - **Spec Exp:** Pediatric Urology; Hydronephrosis-Prenatal; Genitourinary Reconstruction; Incontinence; **Hospital:** Riley Hosp for Children, Peyton Manning Children's Hosp at St. Vincent; **Address:** 705 Riley Hospital for Children Barnhill Drive, Ste 4230, Indianapolis, IN 46202; **Phone:** 317-944-7439; **Board Cert:** Urology 2008; Pediatric Urology 2008; **Med School:** Oregon Hlth & Sci Univ 1987; **Resid:** Surgery, Albany Med Ctr 1989; Urology, Albany Med Ctr 1992; **Fellow:** Pediatric Urology, Mayo Clinic 1994; **Fac Appt:** Prof U, Indiana Univ

Campbell, Steven C MD/PhD [U] - **Spec Exp:** Kidney Cancer; Prostate Cancer; Bladder Cancer; **Hospital:** Cleveland Clin (page 55); **Address:** 9500 Euclid Ave, MS Q10-1, Glickman Urological & Kidney Inst, Cleveland, OH 44195; **Phone:** 216-444-5595; **Board Cert:** Urology 2008; **Med School:** Univ Chicago-Pritzker Sch Med 1989; **Resid:** Urology, Cleveland Clinic 1995; **Fellow:** Urology, Meml Sloan Kettering Cancer Ctr 1996; **Fac Appt:** Prof S, Cleveland Cl Coll Med/Case West Res

Catalona, William J MD [U] - **Spec Exp:** Prostate Cancer; Prostate Disease; **Hospital:** Northwestern Meml Hosp; **Address:** Northwestern Med Faculty Foundation, 675 N St Clair St, Ste 20-150, Chicago, IL 60611; **Phone:** 312-695-6126; **Board Cert:** Urology 1978; **Med School:** Yale Univ 1968; **Resid:** Surgery, UCSF Med Ctr 1970; Urology, Johns Hopkins Hosp 1976; **Fellow:** Surgical Oncology, Natl Cancer Inst 1972; **Fac Appt:** Prof U, Northwestern Univ

Chancellor, Michael B MD [U] - **Spec Exp:** Incontinence-Female; Urology-Female; Neuro-Urology; **Hospital:** Beaumont Hosp-Royal Oak; **Address:** William Beaumont Hosp, Urology, 3535 W 13 Mile Rd, Ste 404, Royal Oak, MI 48073; **Phone:** 248-551-3519; **Board Cert:** Urology 2010; **Med School:** Med Coll Wisc 1983; **Resid:** Surgery, Univ Michigan 1985; Urology, Univ Michigan 1988; **Fellow:** Neurourology, Columbia-Presby Med Ctr 1990; **Fac Appt:** Prof U, Univ Mich Med Sch

Coplen, Douglas E MD [U] - **Spec Exp:** Pediatric Urology; Urologic Cancer-Pediatric; Testicular Cancer-Pediatric; Fetal Urology; **Hospital:** St. Louis Chldns Hosp; **Address:** St Louis Children's Hosp, 4990 Children's Pl, Northwest Tower, Ste 1120, St Louis, MO 63110; **Phone:** 314-454-6034; **Board Cert:** Urology 2008; Pediatric Urology 2008; **Med School:** Indiana Univ 1985; **Resid:** Urology, Barnes Jewish Hosp 1992; **Fellow:** Pediatric Urology, Childrens Hosp 1994; **Fac Appt:** Asst Prof S, Washington Univ, St Louis

Donovan Jr, James F MD [U] - **Spec Exp:** Prostate Cancer/Robotic Surgery; Infertility-Male; Erectile Dysfunction; Kidney Cancer; **Hospital:** Univ Hosp - Cincinnati, Christ Hosp, The - Cincinnati; **Address:** Univ Cincinnati Med Ctr, Medical Arts Bldg, 222 Piedmont Ave, Ste 7000, Cincinnati, OH 45219; **Phone:** 513-475-8787; **Board Cert:** Urology 2009; **Med School:** Northwestern Univ 1978; **Resid:** Surgery, Northwestern Meml Hosp 1982; Urology, Northwestern Meml Hosp 1986; **Fellow:** Male Infertility, Baylor Coll Med 1986; **Fac Appt:** Prof U, Univ Cincinnati

Elder, Jack S MD [U] - **Spec Exp:** Pediatric Urology; Hypospadias; Urinary Reconstruction; Robotic Surgery; **Hospital:** Henry Ford- W Bloomfield Hosp, Chldns Hosp of Michigan; **Address:** 2799 W Grand Blvd, Fl K-9, Detroit, MI 48202; **Phone:** 313-916-7025; **Board Cert:** Urology 1984; Pediatric Urology 2009; **Med School:** Univ Okla Coll Med 1976; **Resid:** Surgery, Yale-New Haven Hosp 1978; Urology, Johns Hopkins Hosp 1982; **Fellow:** Pediatric Urology, Johns Hopkins Hosp 1982; Pediatric Urology, Chldns Hosp 1986; **Fac Appt:** Prof U, Case West Res Univ

Firlit, Casimir MD/PhD [U] - **Spec Exp:** Pediatric Urology; Genitourinary Reconstruction; Transplant-Kidney-Pediatric; **Hospital:** Cardinal Glennon Mem Children's Hosp; **Address:** Cardinal Glennon Chlds Hosp, 1465 S Grand Blvd, Fl 5, Glennon Hall, St Louis, MO 63104; **Phone:** 314-577-5334; **Board Cert:** Urology 1975; **Med School:** Loyola Univ-Stritch Sch Med 1965; **Resid:** Surgery, Hines VA Hosp 1970; Urology, Hines VA Hosp 1973; **Fellow:** Pediatric Urology, Chldns Meml Hosp 1974; **Fac Appt:** Prof U, St Louis Univ

Flanigan, Robert C MD [U] - **Spec Exp:** Urologic Cancer; Prostate Cancer; Kidney Cancer; Bladder Cancer; **Hospital:** Loyola Univ Med Ctr; **Address:** Loyola Univ Med-Fahey Bldg, 2160 S First Ave, rm 267, Maywood, IL 60153; **Phone:** 708-216-5100; **Board Cert:** Urology 2001; **Med School:** Case West Res Univ 1972; **Resid:** Surgery, Case West Univ Med Ctr 1978; Urology, Case West Univ Med Ctr 1978; **Fac Appt:** Prof U, Loyola Univ-Stritch Sch Med

Foster, Richard S MD [U] - **Spec Exp:** Testicular Cancer; Reconstructive Surgery; **Hospital:** IU Health University Hosp; **Address:** IU Health, Dept Urology, 535 Barnhill Drive, Ste 420, Indianapolis, IN 46202; **Phone:** 317-274-3458; **Board Cert:** Urology 2008; **Med School:** Indiana Univ 1980; **Resid:** Urology, Indiana Univ Hosp 1986; **Fac Appt:** Prof U, Indiana Univ

Gluckman, Gordon R MD [U] - **Spec Exp:** Prostate Cancer; Kidney Cancer; Minimally Invasive Urologic Surgery; Robotic Surgery; **Hospital:** Adv Luth Genl Hosp, Resurrection Med Ctr; **Address:** Northwest Suburban Urologists, 900 Rand Rd, Ste 120, Des Plaines, IL 60016; **Phone:** 847-823-3185; **Board Cert:** Urology 2006; **Med School:** Northwestern Univ 1989; **Resid:** Surgery, UCSF Med Ctr 1991; Urology, UCSF Med Ctr 1995; **Fac Appt:** Asst Clin Prof S, Ros Franklin Univ/Chicago Med Sch

Gujral, Saroj MD [U] - **Spec Exp:** Urologic Cancer; Urology-Female; **Hospital:** Albert Lea Med Ctr-Mayo Hlth Sys; **Address:** 404 W Fountain St, Albert Lea, MN 56007; **Phone:** 507-379-2130; **Board Cert:** Urology 1979; **Med School:** India 1970; **Resid:** Urology, Suburban Hosp 1978; Urology, Dalhousie Univ Med Ctrs

Jones, J Stephen MD [U] - **Spec Exp:** Prostate Cancer; **Hospital:** Cleveland Clin (page 55); **Address:** 9500 Euclid Ave, Glickman Urological & Kidney Inst, Cleveland, OH 44195; **Phone:** 216-839-3666; **Board Cert:** Urology 2012; **Med School:** Univ Ark 1986; **Resid:** Urology, Vanderbilt Univ Med Ctr 1993; **Fac Appt:** Prof S, Cleveland Cl Coll Med/Case West Res

Kaefer, Martin MD [U] - **Spec Exp:** Pediatric Urology; Reconstructive Surgery; Genitourinary Congenital Anomalies; Hydronephrosis-Prenatal; **Hospital:** Riley Hosp for Children, Franciscan St. Francis Hlth-Indianapolis; **Address:** IU Health - Pediatric Urology, 705 Riley Hospital Drive, rm 1210, Indianapolis, IN 46202; **Phone:** 317-944-8896; **Board Cert:** Urology 2010; Pediatric Urology 2008; **Med School:** Northwestern Univ 1989; **Resid:** Surgery, Indiana Univ Med Ctr 1991; Urology, Indiana Univ Med Ctr 1995; **Fellow:** Pediatric Urology, Childrens Hosp 1998; **Fac Appt:** Prof U, Indiana Univ

Kaouk, Jihad MD [U] - **Spec Exp:** Minimally Invasive Urologic Surgery; Robotic Surgery; Kidney Cancer; Bladder Cancer; **Hospital:** Cleveland Clin (page 55); **Address:** Cleveland Clinic, 9500 Euclid Ave, Cleveland, OH 44195; **Phone:** 216-444-2976; **Med School:** Lebanon 1993; **Resid:** Surgery, Amer Univ of Beirut Med Ctr 1996; Urology, Amer Univ of Beirut Med Ctr 1999; **Fellow:** Minimally Invasive Surgery, Cleveland Clinic 2001; Laparoscopic Surgery, Cleveland Clinic 2002; **Fac Appt:** Prof S, Cleveland Cl Coll Med/Case West Res

Kass, Evan J MD [U] - **Spec Exp:** Pediatric Urology; Hydronephrosis; Hypospadias; Varicocele in Adolescents; **Hospital:** Beaumont Hosp-Royal Oak; **Address:** 2221 Livernois Ave E, Ste 103, Troy, MI 48083; **Phone:** 248-519-0305; **Board Cert:** Urology 1978; Pediatric Urology 2009; **Med School:** SUNY Downstate 1968; **Resid:** Urology, Univ Mich Hosp 1976; **Fellow:** Pediatric Urology, Hosp for Sick Chldn 1978; **Fac Appt:** Assoc Prof U, Wayne State Univ

Klein, Eric A MD [U] - **Spec Exp:** Urologic Cancer; Testicular Cancer; Kidney Cancer; Prostate Cancer; **Hospital:** Cleveland Clin (page 55); **Address:** 9500 Euclid Ave, MS Q-10, Glickman Urologic and Kidney Institute, Cleveland, OH 44195-0001; **Phone:** 216-444-5591; **Board Cert:** Urology 2008; **Med School:** Univ Pittsburgh 1981; **Resid:** Urology, Cleveland Clinic Fdn 1986; **Fellow:** Urologic Oncology, Meml Sloan Kettering Canc Ctr 1989; **Fac Appt:** Prof S, Cleveland Cl Coll Med/Case West Res

Klutke, Carl G MD [U] - **Spec Exp:** Urology-Female; Incontinence; Urodynamics; **Hospital:** Barnes-Jewish Hosp; **Address:** 1040 N Mason Rd Bldg 1 - Ste 122, St Louis, MO 63141; **Phone:** 314-996-8060; **Board Cert:** Urology 2009; **Med School:** Univ Mich Med Sch 1983; **Resid:** Surgery, Henry Ford Hosp 1985; Urology, Henry Ford Hosp 1988; **Fellow:** Female Urology, UCLA Med Ctr 1989; **Fac Appt:** Assoc Prof S, Washington Univ, St Louis

Koch, Michael O MD [U] - **Spec Exp:** Prostate Cancer; Bladder Cancer; Robotic Surgery; Reconstructive Urologic Surgery; **Hospital:** IU Health University Hosp; **Address:** IU Health Physicians, Dept Urology, 535 Barnhill Drive, Ste 420, Indianapolis, IN 46202; **Phone:** 317-274-7338; **Board Cert:** Urology 2007; **Med School:** Dartmouth Med Sch 1981; **Resid:** Surgery, Dartmouth-Hitchcock Med Ctr 1983; Urology, Vanderbilt Univ Med Ctr 1987; **Fellow:** Surgical Research, Dartmouth Med Sch 1984; **Fac Appt:** Prof U, Indiana Univ

Kozlowski, James M MD [U] - **Spec Exp:** Prostate Cancer; Continent Urinary Diversions; Laparoscopic Surgery; **Hospital:** Northwestern Meml Hosp, Jesse Brown VA Med Ctr; **Address:** 675 N St Clair St, Fl 20 - rm 150, Chicago, IL 60611; **Phone:** 312-695-8146; **Board Cert:** Surgery 2004; Urology 1983; **Med School:** Northwestern Univ 1975; **Resid:** Surgery, McGaw Med Ctr 1979; Urology, McGaw Med Ctr 1982; **Fellow:** Research, NCI-Frederick Cancer Rsch 1984; **Fac Appt:** Assoc Prof U, Northwestern Univ

Lee, Cheryl T MD [U] - **Spec Exp:** Urologic Cancer; Bladder Cancer; **Hospital:** Univ of Michigan Hosp; **Address:** Univ of Michigan Cancer Ctr, 1500 E Medical Ctr Drive, Reception D LB1-229, Ann Arbor, MI 48109; **Phone:** 734-647-8903; **Board Cert:** Urology 2002; **Med School:** Albany Med Coll 1991; **Resid:** Urology, Albany Med Ctr; **Fellow:** Urologic Oncology, Meml Sloan Kettering Cancer Ctr 2000; **Fac Appt:** Assoc Prof U, Univ Mich Med Sch

Levine, Laurence A MD [U] - **Spec Exp:** Erectile Dysfunction; Infertility-Male; Peyronie's Disease; Prostate Cancer; **Hospital:** Rush Univ Med Ctr; **Address:** 1725 W Harrison St, Ste 352, Chicago, IL 60612; **Phone:** 312-563-5000; **Board Cert:** Urology 2009; **Med School:** Univ Colorado 1980; **Resid:** Surgery, Tufts-New Eng Med Ctr 1982; Urology, Brigham & Women's Hosp 1987; **Fac Appt:** Prof U, Rush Med Coll

McGuire, Edward J MD [U] - **Spec Exp:** Incontinence; Urology-Female; Neurogenic Bladder; Uro-Gynecology; **Hospital:** Univ of Michigan Hosp; **Address:** Univ Mich Med Ctr, Div Urology, 1500 E Med Ctr Drive, 3875 Taubman Ctr, Ann Arbor, MI 48109-5330; **Phone:** 734-232-4943; **Board Cert:** Urology 1975; **Med School:** Wayne State Univ 1965; **Resid:** Surgery, Yale-New Haven Hosp 1969; Urology, Yale-New Haven Hosp 1972; **Fac Appt:** Prof U, Univ Mich Med Sch

McVary, Kevin T MD [U] - **Spec Exp:** Prostate Cancer; Erectile Dysfunction; Prostate Disease; Minimally Invasive Surgery; **Hospital:** Northwestern Meml Hosp; **Address:** 675 N St Clair St, Fl 20 - rm 150, Chicago, IL 60611-4813; **Phone:** 312-695-8146; **Board Cert:** Urology 2010; **Med School:** Northwestern Univ 1983; **Resid:** Surgery, Northwestern Meml Hosp 1985; Urology, Northwestern Meml Hosp 1988; **Fellow:** Research, Northwestern Meml Hosp; **Fac Appt:** Prof U, Northwestern Univ

Menon, Mani MD [U] - **Spec Exp:** Prostate Cancer/Robotic Surgery; Transplant-Kidney; Urologic Cancer; **Hospital:** Henry Ford Hosp; **Address:** Henry Ford Hosp - Vattikuti Urology Inst, 2799 W Grand Blvd, Bldg K Fl 9, Detroit, MI 48202; **Phone:** 313-916-2066; **Board Cert:** Urology 1982; **Med School:** India 1969; **Resid:** Urology, Bryn Mawr Hosp 1974; Urology, Johns Hopkins Hosp 1980; **Fellow:** Transplant Surgery, Johns Hopkins Univ 1977; **Fac Appt:** Prof S, Univ Mass Sch Med

Mesrobian, Hrair-George O MD [U] - **Spec Exp:** Pediatric Urology; Bladder Exstrophy; Epispadias; **Hospital:** Chldns Hosp - Wisconsin; **Address:** 999 N 92nd St, Ste 330, Milwaukee, WI 53226; **Phone:** 414-266-3769; **Board Cert:** Urology 2005; Pediatric Urology 2008; **Med School:** Lebanon 1978; **Resid:** Surgery, SUNY Upstate Med Ctr 1980; Urology, UCSF Med Ctr 1983; **Fellow:** Pediatric Urology, Mayo Clinic 1984; **Fac Appt:** Prof U, Med Coll Wisc

Montague, Drogo K MD [U] - **Spec Exp:** Erectile Dysfunction; Genitourinary Prosthetics; Incontinence; Peyronie's Disease; **Hospital:** Cleveland Clin (page 55); **Address:** Glickmand Urological & Kidney Inst, Cleveland Clinic, 9500 Euclid Ave, Q10-1, Cleveland, OH 44195-5041; **Phone:** 216-444-5600; **Board Cert:** Urology 1995; **Med School:** Univ Mich Med Sch 1968; **Resid:** Surgery, Cleveland Clinic 1970; Urology, Cleveland Clinic 1973; **Fac Appt:** Prof U, Cleveland Cl Coll Med/Case West Res

Montie, James MD [U] - **Spec Exp:** Bladder Cancer; Prostate Cancer; Genitourinary Cancer; **Hospital:** Univ of Michigan Hosp; **Address:** UMH Cancer Ctr, Team 3, Reception D, Level B1-229, 1500 E Med Ctr Drive, Ann Arbor, MI 48109-5913; **Phone:** 734-647-8903; **Board Cert:** Urology 1978; **Med School:** Univ Mich Med Sch 1971; **Resid:** Urology, Cleveland Clinic Fdn 1976; **Fellow:** Urologic Oncology, Meml Sloan-Kettering Cancer Ctr 1979; **Fac Appt:** Prof U, Univ Mich Med Sch

Nehra, Ajay MD [U] - **Spec Exp:** Erectile Dysfunction; **Hospital:** Rush Univ Med Ctr; **Address:** Rush Univ Urology, Prof Bldg - Ste 762, 1725 W Harrison St, Chicago, IL 60612; **Phone:** 312-563-3447; **Board Cert:** Urology 2006; **Med School:** India 1984; **Resid:** Surgery, Boston Univ Med Ctr 1987; Urology, Maimonides Med Ctr 1993; **Fellow:** Female Urology, Boston Univ Sch Med 1989; Male Infertility, Boston Univ Sch Med 1995; **Fac Appt:** Prof U, Rush Med Coll

O'Donnell, Michael A MD [U] - **Spec Exp:** Bladder Cancer; Immunotherapy; Urologic Cancer; Ureter & Renal Pelvis Cancer; **Hospital:** Univ Iowa Hosp & Clinics; **Address:** Univ Iowa Hosp & Clin, Dept Urol, 200 Hawkins Drive RCP Bldg Fl 3, Iowa City, IA 52242-1089; **Phone:** 319-384-6040; **Board Cert:** Urology 2005; **Med School:** Duke Univ 1984; **Resid:** Surgery, Brigham & Womens Hosp 1987; Urology, Brigham & Womens Hosp 1991; **Fellow:** Urology, Brigham & Womens Hosp 1993; **Fac Appt:** Prof U, Univ Iowa Coll Med

Ohl, Dana MD [U] - **Spec Exp:** Infertility-Male; Erectile Dysfunction; **Hospital:** Univ of Michigan Hosp; **Address:** Univ Mich Med Ctr, Div Urology, 1500 E Med Ctr Drive, 3875 Taubman Ctr, Ann Arbor, MI 48109-5330; **Phone:** 734-232-4943; **Board Cert:** Urology 2008; **Med School:** Univ Mich Med Sch 1982; **Resid:** Urology, Univ Mich Hosps 1987; **Fac Appt:** Prof U, Univ Mich Med Sch

Rink, Richard C MD [U] - **Spec Exp:** Pediatric Urology; Reconstructive Urologic Surgery; Genital Reconstruction; Neurogenic Bladder; **Hospital:** Riley Hosp for Children, IU Health University Hosp; **Address:** IU Health - Pediatric Urology, 705 Riley Hospital Drive, Ste 1210, Indianapolis, IN 46202; **Phone:** 317-944-8896; **Board Cert:** Urology 2008; Pediatric Urology 2008; **Med School:** Indiana Univ 1978; **Resid:** Surgery, Emory Univ Med Ctr 1980; Urology, Indiana Univ Med Ctr 1984; **Fellow:** Pediatric Urology, Chldns Hosp-Harvard 1985; **Fac Appt:** Prof U, Indiana Univ

Ross, Lawrence S MD [U] - **Spec Exp:** Infertility-Male; Erectile Dysfunction; Prostate Disease; **Hospital:** Univ of IL Med Ctr at Chicago; **Address:** Univ Ctr of Urology, 60 E Delaware Pl, Ste 1420, Chicago, IL 60611; **Phone:** 312-440-5127; **Board Cert:** Urology 1974; **Med School:** Univ Chicago-Pritzker Sch Med 1965; **Resid:** Urology, Michael Reese Hosp 1970; **Fac Appt:** Prof U, Univ Chicago-Pritzker Sch Med

Sabanegh Jr, Edmund S MD [U] - **Spec Exp:** Infertility-Male; Microsurgery; Vasectomy; Vasectomy Reversal; **Hospital:** Cleveland Clin (page 55); **Address:** Cleveland Clinic-Urology, 9500 Euclid Ave, MC Q10-1, Cleveland, OH 44195; **Phone:** 216-444-5600; **Board Cert:** Urology 2012; **Med School:** Univ VA Sch Med 1985; **Resid:** Urology, Wilford Hall Med Ctr 1992; **Fellow:** Male Infertility, Cleveland Clinic 1994; **Fac Appt:** Assoc Prof U, Cleveland Cl Coll Med/Case West Res

Sandlow, Jay I MD [U] - **Spec Exp:** Infertility-Male; Varicocele Microsurgery; Vasectomy & Vasectomy Reversal; **Hospital:** Froedtert and Med Ctr of WI, St. Joseph's Hosp; **Address:** Med Coll of WI, Urology Dept, 9200 W Wisconsin Ave, Milwaukee, WI 53226-3522; **Phone:** 414-805-0805; **Board Cert:** Urology 2005; **Med School:** Rush Med Coll 1987; **Resid:** Urology, Univ Iowa Hosps 1993; **Fellow:** Infertility, Univ Iowa Hosps 1995; **Fac Appt:** Prof U, Med Coll Wisc

Schaeffer, Anthony MD [U] - **Spec Exp:** Interstitial Cystitis; Incontinence after Prostate Cancer; Urology-Female; Urinary Tract Infections; **Hospital:** Northwestern Meml Hosp; **Address:** 675 N St Clair St, Fl 20 - rm 150, Chicago, IL 60611; **Phone:** 312-695-8146; **Board Cert:** Urology 1978; **Med School:** Northwestern Univ 1968; **Resid:** Surgery, Northwestern Meml Hosp 1970; Urology, Stanford Med Ctr 1976; **Fac Appt:** Prof U, Northwestern Univ

See, William A MD [U] - **Spec Exp:** Prostate Cancer; Bladder Cancer; Testicular Cancer; **Hospital:** Froedtert and Med Ctr of WI; **Address:** Clnical Cancer Ctr-Urology Dept, 9200 W Wisconsin Ave, Milwaukee, WI 53226; **Phone:** 414-805-0805; **Board Cert:** Urology 2008; **Med School:** Univ Chicago-Pritzker Sch Med 1982; **Resid:** Urology, Univ Washington 1988; **Fellow:** Research, Natl Kidney Fdn/Univ Wash 1986; Research, Amer Fdn for Urol Dis/Univ Iowa 1990; **Fac Appt:** Prof U, Med Coll Wisc

Silber, Sherman J MD [U] - **Spec Exp:** Infertility-Male; Vasectomy Reversal; Infertility-IVF; Transplant-Ovarian Tissue; **Hospital:** St. Luke's Hosp - Chesterfield, MO; **Address:** St Luke's Hosp, 224 S Woods Mill Rd, Ste 730 S, Chesterfield, MO 63017-3451; **Phone:** 314-576-1400; **Board Cert:** Urology 1977; **Med School:** Univ Mich Med Sch 1966; **Resid:** Internal Medicine, PH Service Comm Corps 1969; Urology, Univ Michigan Hosp 1973; **Fellow:** Microsurgery, Univ Melbourne 1974

Steinberg, Gary D MD [U] - **Spec Exp:** Bladder Cancer; Kidney Cancer; Prostate Cancer; **Hospital:** Univ of Chicago Med Ctr; **Address:** Univ of Chicago Med Ctr, Div Urol, 5841 S Maryland Ave, rm J-653, MC 6038, Chicago, IL 60637-1447; **Phone:** 773-702-3080; **Board Cert:** Urology 2003; **Med School:** Univ Chicago-Pritzker Sch Med 1985; **Resid:** Surgery, Johns Hopkins Hosp 1987; Urology, Brady Urol Inst/Johns Hopkins 1991; **Fellow:** Clinical Oncology, Johns Hopkins Hosp 1989; **Fac Appt:** Prof U, Univ Chicago-Pritzker Sch Med

Sundaram, Chandru P MD [U] - **Spec Exp:** Kidney Cancer; Prostate Cancer; Adrenal Tumors; Polycystic Kidney Disease; **Hospital:** IU Health University Hosp; **Address:** 535 N Barnhill Drive, Ste 420, Indiana Cancer Pavilion, Dept. Of Urology, Indiana University School of Medicine, Indianapolis, IN 46202; **Phone:** 317-278-3098; **Board Cert:** Urology 2009; **Med School:** India 1985; **Resid:** Urology, Univ Minn Med Ctr 1997; **Fellow:** Endourology, Beth Israel Deaconess Med Ctr/Harvard Med Sch 1998; **Fac Appt:** Prof U, Indiana Univ

Wong, Carson MD [U] - **Spec Exp:** Laparoscopic Surgery; Endourology; Prostate Cancer/Robotic Surgery; Urinary Reconstruction; **Hospital:** Parma Community Genl Hosp, UH Ahuja Med Ctr (OH) (page 74); **Address:** 6900 Pearl Rd, Fl 2, Middleburgh Heights, OH 44130; **Phone:** 440-845-0414; **Board Cert:** Urology 2003; **Med School:** Univ Western Ontario 1995; **Resid:** Urology, McGill Univ Affil Hosps 2000; **Fellow:** Urologic Surgery, Univ Miami 2001; **Fac Appt:** U

Wood, David P MD [U] - **Spec Exp:** Genitourinary Cancer; Bladder Cancer; Prostate Cancer; Robotic Surgery; **Hospital:** Beaumont Hosp-Royal Oak; **Address:** Beaumont Physician Partners/Clin Faculty, 3711 W 13 Mile Rd, Royal Oak, MI 48073; **Phone:** 248-551-3519; **Board Cert:** Urology 2002; **Med School:** Univ Mich Med Sch 1983; **Resid:** Urology, Cleveland Clinic 1988; **Fellow:** Urologic Oncology, Meml Sloan-Kettering Cancer Ctr 1991; **Fac Appt:** Prof U, Univ Mich Med Sch

Zippe, Craig D MD [U] - **Spec Exp:** Prostate Cancer; Bladder Cancer; Kidney Cancer; **Hospital:** Univ Hosps Case Med Ctr (page 74), UH Richmond Med Ctr (page 74); **Address:** University Hospitals - Case Medical Ctr, 88 Center Rd, Ste 360, Bedford, OH 44146; **Phone:** 440-232-8955; **Board Cert:** Urology 2007; **Med School:** Rush Med Coll 1980; **Resid:** Surgery, Duke Univ Med Ctr 1983; Urology, Columbia Presby Med Ctr 1989; **Fellow:** Cancer Research, Rhode Island Hosp 1985; Urologic Oncology, Meml Sloan Kettering Cancer Ctr 1992; **Fac Appt:** Clin Prof U, Case West Res Univ

Great Plains and Mountains

Cartwright, Patrick C MD [U] - **Spec Exp:** Pediatric Urology; **Hospital:** Primary Children's Med Ctr, Univ Utah Hlth Care; **Address:** Primary Childrens Med Ctr, 100 N Mario Capecchi Drive, Ste 2200, Salt Lake City, UT 84113-1100; **Phone:** 801-662-5555; **Board Cert:** Urology 2010; Pediatric Urology 2010; **Med School:** Univ Tex SW, Dallas 1984; **Resid:** Urology, Univ Utah Affil Hosp 1989; **Fellow:** Pediatric Urology, Chldns Hosp 1990; **Fac Appt:** Prof S, Univ Utah

Childs, Stacy J MD [U] - **Spec Exp:** Voiding Dysfunction; Erectile Dysfunction; Prostate Cancer; Bladder Cancer; **Hospital:** Yampa Valley Med Ctr, Memorial Hosp - Craig; **Address:** 501 Anglers Drive, Ste 202, Steamboat Springs, CO 80487-8841; **Phone:** 970-871-9710; **Board Cert:** Urology 1979; **Med School:** Louisiana State U, New Orleans 1972; **Resid:** Urology, Carraway Meth Med Ctr 1977; **Fac Appt:** Clin Prof U, Univ Colorado

Crawford, E David MD [U] - **Spec Exp:** Prostate Cancer; Testicular Cancer; Bladder Cancer; **Hospital:** Univ of CO Hosp - Anschutz Inpatient Pav; **Address:** Univ CO Hosp, 1665 Aurora Ct, Anschutz Canc Pav, Ste 1004, MS F710, Aurora, CO 80045; **Phone:** 720-848-0170; **Board Cert:** Urology 1980; **Med School:** Univ Cincinnati 1973; **Resid:** Urology, Good Samaritan Hosp 1977; **Fellow:** Genitourinary Surgery, UCLA Med Ctr 1978; **Fac Appt:** Prof U, Univ Colorado

Davis, Bradley E MD [U] - **Spec Exp:** Prostate Cancer; Bladder Cancer; Kidney Cancer; Vasectomy Reversal; **Hospital:** Overland Pk Regl Med Ctr, Olathe Med Ctr; **Address:** 10550 Quivira Rd, Ste 105, Overland Park, KS 66215; **Phone:** 913-438-3833; **Board Cert:** Urology 2004; **Med School:** Univ Kansas 1986; **Resid:** Surgery, St Lukes Hosp 1991; Urology, Univ Kansas Med Ctr 1991; **Fellow:** Urologic Oncology, Meml Sloan-Kettering Cancer Ctr 1993; **Fac Appt:** Asst Clin Prof U, Univ Kansas

Griebling, Tomas L MD [U] - **Spec Exp:** Urology-Geriatric; Urology-Female; Incontinence; Reconstructive Surgery; **Hospital:** Univ of Kansas Hosp; **Address:** Univ Kansas Hosp-Urology Dept, 3901 Rainbow Blvd, MS 3106, Kansas City, KS 66160; **Phone:** 913-588-6147; **Board Cert:** Urology 2009; **Med School:** Univ Iowa Coll Med 1991; **Resid:** Urology, Univ Iowa Affil Hosp 1998; **Fellow:** Reconstructive Surgery, Univ Iowa Affil Hosp 2001; **Fac Appt:** Prof U, Univ Kansas

Urology

Lugg, James A MD [U] - **Spec Exp:** Prostate Cancer; Laparoscopic Surgery; Incontinence after Prostate Cancer; **Hospital:** Cheyenne Regl Med Ctr, Univ of CO Hosp - Anschutz Inpatient Pav; **Address:** 2301 House Ave, Ste 502, Cheyenne, WY 82001; **Phone:** 307-635-4131; **Board Cert:** Urology 2008; **Med School:** Northwestern Univ 1990; **Resid:** Urology, UCLA Med Ctr 1995; **Fac Appt:** Asst Prof U, Univ Colorado

Meacham, Randall B MD [U] - **Spec Exp:** Infertility-Male; Vasectomy Reversal; Sexual Dysfunction; **Hospital:** Univ of CO Hosp - Anschutz Inpatient Pav; **Address:** Univ CO, Dept Urology, 1635 Aurora Ct, Aurora, CO 80045; **Phone:** 720-848-1800; **Board Cert:** Urology 2002; **Med School:** Baylor Coll Med 1982; **Resid:** Surgery, Baylor Coll Med 1985; Urology, Baylor Coll Med 1989; **Fellow:** Urolithiasis, Baylor Coll Med 1984; Male Reproductive Medicine/Surgery, Baylor Coll Med 1990; **Fac Appt:** Prof U, Univ Colorado

Thrasher, J Brantley MD [U] - **Spec Exp:** Prostate Cancer; Reconstructive Urologic Surgery; **Hospital:** Univ of Kansas Hosp; **Address:** Univ Kansas Med Ctr, Dept Urology, 3901 Rainbow Blvd, MS 3016, Kansas City, KS 66160; **Phone:** 913-588-6146; **Board Cert:** Urology 2003; **Med School:** Med Univ SC 1986; **Resid:** Urology, Fitzsimons Army Med Ctr 1991; **Fellow:** Urologic Oncology, Duke Univ Med Ctr 1994; **Fac Appt:** Prof U, Univ Kansas

Southwest

Andrews, Paul E MD [U] - **Spec Exp:** Urologic Cancer; Minimally Invasive Urologic Surgery; Robotic Surgery; **Hospital:** Mayo Clinic - Phoenix; **Address:** Mayo Clinic-Urology, 5779 E Mayo Blvd, Phoenix, AZ 85054; **Phone:** 480-342-2951; **Board Cert:** Urology 2003; **Med School:** Texas Tech Univ 1987; **Resid:** Urology, Mayo Clinic 1993; **Fac Appt:** Prof U, Mayo Med Sch

Bans, Larry L MD [U] - **Spec Exp:** Prostate Cancer; Prostate Disease; Men's Health; **Hospital:** Banner Good Samaritan Regl Med Ctr - Phoenix; **Address:** Prostate Solutions of Arizona, 2525 E Arizona Biltmore Cir, Ste C236, Phoenix, AZ 85016; **Phone:** 602-426-9772; **Board Cert:** Urology 2004; **Med School:** Cornell Univ-Weill Med Coll 1978; **Resid:** Urology, Ind Univ Med Ctr 1983

Bardot, Stephen F MD [U] - **Spec Exp:** Urologic Cancer; Prostate Cancer; **Hospital:** Ochsner Med Ctr-New Orleans; **Address:** Ochsner Clinic, 1514 Jefferson Hwy Fl 4, Atrium 4 West, Dept Urology, New Orleans, LA 70121-2483; **Phone:** 504-842-4083; **Board Cert:** Urology 2002; **Med School:** Univ Kansas 1985; **Resid:** Surgery, St Luke's Hosp 1987; Urology, Kansas City Univ Med Ctr 1990; **Fellow:** Urologic Oncology, Cleveland Clinic 1991

Basler, Joseph W MD [U] - **Spec Exp:** Prostate Cancer; Urologic Cancer; Kidney Stones; **Hospital:** Audie L Murphy Meml Vets Hosp - San Antonio; **Address:** 7703 Floyd Curl Dr, MC-7845, San Antonio, TX 78229-3900; **Phone:** 210-567-5640; **Board Cert:** Urology 2011; **Med School:** Univ MO-Columbia Sch Med 1984; **Resid:** Surgery, Univ Missouri Affil Hosp 1986; Urology, Barnes Hosp/Wash Univ 1990; **Fac Appt:** Prof U, Univ Tex, San Antonio

Boone, Timothy B MD/PhD [U] - **Spec Exp:** Neuro-Urology; Urinary Reconstruction; Incontinence; **Hospital:** Methodist Hosp - Houston, St. Luke's Episcopal Hosp-Houston; **Address:** Scurlock Tower, 6560 Fannin St, Ste 2100, Houston, TX 77030-2769; **Phone:** 713-441-6455; **Board Cert:** Urology 2004; **Med School:** Univ Tex, Houston 1985; **Resid:** Surgery, Univ Tex SW Med Ctr 1987; Urology, Univ Tex SW Med Ctr 1991; **Fac Appt:** Prof U, Cornell Univ-Weill Med Coll

Buch, Jeffrey Phillip MD [U] - **Spec Exp:** Vasectomy Reversal; Infertility-Male; Sexual Dysfunction; **Hospital:** Baylor Univ Medical Ctr-Dallas; **Address:** Legacy Male Health Institute, 5616 Warren Pkwy, Ste 101, Frisco, TX 75034; **Phone:** 972-612-7131; **Board Cert:** Urology 2005; **Med School:** Univ Mich Med Sch 1980; **Resid:** Surgery, Albany Med Ctr 1982; Urology, Albany Med Ctr 1985; **Fellow:** Male Infertility, Baylor Coll Med 1987; Microsurgery, Baylor Coll Med 1987; **Fac Appt:** Assoc Clin Prof U, Univ Tex SW, Dallas

Culkin, Daniel J MD [U] - **Spec Exp:** Voiding Dysfunction; Interstitial Cystitis; Urologic Cancer; Laparoscopic Surgery; **Hospital:** OU Med Ctr; **Address:** OU Medical Ctr, Dept Urology, 825 NE 10th St, Ste 5400, Oklahoma City, OK 73104; **Phone:** 405-271-6452; **Board Cert:** Urology 2006; **Med School:** Creighton Univ 1979; **Resid:** Surgery, Loyola Univ Med Ctr 1981; Urology, Loyola Univ Med Ctr 1983; **Fellow:** Neurourology, Loyola Univ Med Ctr 1984; **Fac Appt:** Prof U, Univ Okla Coll Med

Ewalt, David H MD [U] - **Spec Exp:** Pediatric Urology; Hypospadias; Urinary Reconstruction; Neurogenic Bladder; **Hospital:** Chldns Med Ctr of Dallas, Med City Dallas Hosp; **Address:** 8315 Walnut Hill Lane, Ste 205, Dallas, TX 75231; **Phone:** 214-750-0808; **Board Cert:** Urology 2003; Pediatric Urology 2008; **Med School:** Univ Tex SW, Dallas 1984; **Resid:** Urology, Univ Texas SW Affil Hosps 1990; **Fellow:** Pediatric Urology, Chldns Hosp 1992

Gonzales, Edmond T MD [U] - **Spec Exp:** Pediatric Urology; **Hospital:** Texas Chldns Hosp; **Address:** Clinical Care Center, 6701 Fannin St, Ste 660, Houston, TX 77030; **Phone:** 832-822-3160; **Board Cert:** Urology 1975; Pediatric Urology 2008; **Med School:** Tulane Univ 1965; **Resid:** Surgery, Duke Univ Med Ctr 1968; Urology, Duke Univ Med Ctr 1972; **Fellow:** Pediatric Urology, Childrens Hosp; **Fac Appt:** Prof U, Baylor Coll Med

Grossman, H Barton MD [U] - **Spec Exp:** Bladder Cancer; **Hospital:** UT MD Anderson Cancer Ctr; **Address:** MD Anderson Cancer Ctr, Dept Urology, Unit 1373, 1515 Holcombe Blvd, Houston, TX 77030-4009; **Phone:** 713-792-3250; **Board Cert:** Urology 1979; **Med School:** Temple Univ 1970; **Resid:** Surgery, St Joseph Mercy Hosp 1974; Urology, Univ Michigan Med Ctr 1977; **Fellow:** Urologic Oncology, Meml Sloan Kettering Cancer Ctr 1979; **Fac Appt:** Clin Prof U, Univ Tex, Houston

Hellstrom, Wayne J MD [U] - **Spec Exp:** Infertility-Male; Erectile Dysfunction; Peyronie's Disease; Penile Prostheses; **Hospital:** Tulane Med Ctr; **Address:** Tulane Urology, 1415 Tulane Ave Fl 3, New Orleans, LA 70112; **Phone:** 504-988-5271; **Board Cert:** Urology 2007; **Med School:** McGill Univ 1981; **Resid:** Surgery, Montreal Genl/Royal Vistoria Hosp 1983; Urology, UCSF Med Ctr 1985; **Fellow:** Andrology, UC Davis Med Ctr 1988; **Fac Appt:** Prof U, Tulane Univ

Kadmon, Dov MD [U] - **Spec Exp:** Prostate Cancer; **Hospital:** St. Luke's Episcopal Hosp-Houston, Methodist Hosp - Houston; **Address:** Baylor Dept Urology, 6620 Main St, Ste 1325, Houston, TX 77030; **Phone:** 713-798-4001; **Board Cert:** Urology 1984; **Med School:** Israel 1970; **Resid:** Surgery, Barnes Jewish Hosp 1977; Urology, Barnes Jewish Hosp 1980; **Fellow:** Urology, Barnes Jewish Hosp 1982; **Fac Appt:** Prof U, Baylor Coll Med

Lerner, Seth P MD [U] - **Spec Exp:** Bladder Cancer; Testicular Cancer; Urinary Reconstruction; **Hospital:** St. Luke's Episcopal Hosp-Houston, Methodist Hosp - Houston; **Address:** 6620 Main St, Ste 1325, Houston, TX 77030; **Phone:** 713-798-4001; **Board Cert:** Urology 2012; **Med School:** Baylor Coll Med 1984; **Resid:** Surgery, Virginia Mason Hosp 1986; Urology, Baylor Affil Hosp 1990; **Fellow:** Urologic Oncology, LAC-USC Med Ctr 1992; **Fac Appt:** Prof U, Baylor Coll Med

Urology

Lipshultz, Larry I MD [U] - **Spec Exp:** Infertility-Male; Hormone Replacement-Male; Erectile Dysfunction; **Hospital:** St. Luke's Episcopal Hosp-Houston, Methodist Hosp - Houston; **Address:** 6224 Fannin St, O'Quinn Medical Twr, Ste 1700, MS 77030, Houston, TX 77030-2706; **Phone:** 713-798-4001; **Board Cert:** Urology 1977; **Med School:** Univ Pennsylvania 1968; **Resid:** Urology, Hosp Univ Penn 1975; **Fellow:** Reproductive Medicine, Univ Texas 1977; **Fac Appt:** Prof U, Baylor Coll Med

Miles, Brian J MD [U] - **Spec Exp:** Prostate Cancer; Urologic Cancer; Gene Therapy; **Hospital:** Methodist Hosp - Houston, St. Luke's Episcopal Hosp-Houston; **Address:** 6560 Fannin St, Ste 2100, Houston, TX 77030; **Phone:** 713-441-6455; **Board Cert:** Urology 1984; **Med School:** Univ Mich Med Sch 1974; **Resid:** Urology, Walter Reed Army Med Ctr 1982; **Fac Appt:** Clin Prof U, Baylor Coll Med

Pisters, Louis L MD [U] - **Spec Exp:** Prostate Cancer; Bladder Cancer; Genitourinary Cancer; Prostate Cancer/Robotic Surgery; **Hospital:** UT MD Anderson Cancer Ctr; **Address:** MD Anderson Cancer Ctr, Dept Urology, 1515 Holcombe Blvd, Unit 1373, Houston, TX 77030; **Phone:** 713-792-3250; **Board Cert:** Urology 2003; **Med School:** Univ Western Ontario 1986; **Resid:** Urology, Shands Hosp/Univ Florida 1991; **Fellow:** Urologic Oncology, MD Anderson Cancer Ctr 1993; **Fac Appt:** Assoc Prof U, Univ Tex, Houston

Roehrborn, Claus Georg MD [U] - **Spec Exp:** Prostate Cancer; Prostate Disease; Voiding Dysfunction; **Hospital:** UT Southwestern Med Ctr at Dallas, Parkland Hlth & Hosp Sys; **Address:** Professor and Chairman, Department of Urology at UT Southwestern Medical Center in Dallas, 5323 Harry Hines Blvd, Aston Bldg Fl 9 - Ste 110, Dallas, TX 75390-9110; **Phone:** 214-645-8765; **Board Cert:** Urology 2004; **Med School:** Germany 1980; **Resid:** Surgery, W Germany Army Hosp 1982; Urology, UT SW Med Ctr 1989; **Fellow:** Urology, Am Fdn Urol Dis 1991; **Fac Appt:** Prof U, Univ Tex SW, Dallas

Sagalowsky, Arthur I MD [U] - **Spec Exp:** Urologic Cancer; Transplant-Kidney; Testicular Cancer; Continent Urinary Diversions; **Hospital:** UT Southwestern Med Ctr at Dallas; **Address:** 5303 Harry Hines Blvd Fl 9 - Ste 110, Dallas, TX 75390-9110; **Phone:** 214-645-8765; **Board Cert:** Urology 1980; **Med School:** Indiana Univ 1973; **Resid:** Surgery, Indiana Univ Hosps 1975; Urology, Indiana Univ Hosps 1978; **Fellow:** Clinical Pharmacology, Univ Tex SW Med Ctr 1980; **Fac Appt:** Prof U, Univ Tex SW, Dallas

Slawin, Kevin M MD [U] - **Spec Exp:** Prostate Cancer; Prostate Cancer/Robotic Surgery; Prostate Disease; **Hospital:** Meml Hermann Hosp - Texas Med Ctr, Methodist Hosp - Houston; **Address:** Vanguard Urologic Inst, Meml Hermann Med Plaza, 6400 Fannin, Ste 2300, Houston, TX 77030; **Phone:** 713-366-7847; **Board Cert:** Urology 2005; **Med School:** Columbia P&S 1986; **Resid:** Surgery, Mt Sinai Med Ctr 1988; Urology, Columbia-Presby Hosp 1992; **Fellow:** Urologic Oncology, Baylor Coll Med 1994; **Fac Appt:** Clin Prof U, Baylor Coll Med

Strand, William R MD [U] - **Spec Exp:** Pediatric Urology; Laparoscopic Surgery; Hypospadias; Reconstructive Surgery; **Hospital:** Chldns Med Ctr of Dallas; **Address:** 4001 W 15th St Bldg 3 - Ste 300, Plano, TX 75093; **Phone:** 214-750-0808 x5400; **Board Cert:** Urology 2001; Pediatric Urology 2008; **Med School:** Mayo Med Sch 1983; **Resid:** Surgery, Naval Med Ctr 1984; Urology, Natl Naval Med Ctr 1988; **Fellow:** Pediatric Urology, Chldns Med Ctr of Dallas; **Fac Appt:** Assoc Prof U, Univ Tex SW, Dallas

Thompson Jr, Ian M MD [U] - **Spec Exp:** Prostate Cancer; Prostate Disease; **Hospital:** Univ Hlth Syst-San Antonio; **Address:** Univ Tex Hlth Scis Ctr, Dept Urol, 7703 Floyd Curl Drive, MC 7845, San Antonio, TX 78229; **Phone:** 210-567-5643; **Board Cert:** Urology 2005; **Med School:** Tulane Univ 1980; **Resid:** Urology, Brooke Army Med Ctr 1985; **Fellow:** Medical Oncology, Meml Sloan-Kettering Canc Ctr 1988; **Fac Appt:** Prof S, Univ Tex, San Antonio

Woo, Howard H MD [U] - **Spec Exp:** Pain-Pelvic; Voiding Dysfunction; Incontinence; Urology-Female; **Hospital:** Ochsner Med Ctr-New Orleans; **Address:** Ochsner Clinic, 1514 Jefferson Hwy, Dept Urology Fl 4, New Orleans, LA 70121; **Phone:** 504-842-4083; **Board Cert:** Urology 2006; **Med School:** Med Coll Wisc 1989; **Resid:** Surgery, UC Irvine Med Ctr 1991; Urology, Univ Colorado Affil Hosp 1995

West Coast and Pacific

Ahlering, Thomas E MD [U] - **Spec Exp:** Prostate Cancer/Robotic Surgery; **Hospital:** UC Irvine Med Ctr, VA Long Beach Hlthcare Sys; **Address:** UC Irvine Med Ctr, 333 City Blvd W, Ste 2100, Orange, CA 92868; **Phone:** 714-456-6068; **Board Cert:** Urology 2005; **Med School:** St Louis Univ 1979; **Resid:** Urology, LAC-USC Med Ctr 1984; **Fellow:** Urologic Oncology, USC-Norris Comp Cancer Ctr 1986; **Fac Appt:** Prof U, UC Irvine

Amling, Christopher L MD [U] - **Spec Exp:** Prostate Cancer/Robotic Surgery; Kidney Cancer; Bladder Cancer; Testicular Cancer; **Hospital:** OR Hlth & Sci Univ; **Address:** 3303 SW Bond Ave, MC CH10U, Portland, OR 97239; **Phone:** 503-346-1500; **Board Cert:** Urology 2008; **Med School:** Oregon Hlth & Sci Univ 1985; **Resid:** Urology, Duke Univ Med Ctr 1996; **Fellow:** Urologic Oncology, Mayo Clinic 1997; **Fac Appt:** Prof U, Univ Alabama

Baskin, Laurence S MD [U] - **Spec Exp:** Pediatric Urology; Hypospadias; **Hospital:** UCSF Med Ctr; **Address:** Urology Faculty Practice, 400 Parnassus Ave, Ste A-610, Box 0330, San Francisco, CA 94143-0330; **Phone:** 415-353-2200; **Board Cert:** Urology 2008; Pediatric Urology 2008; **Med School:** UCLA 1986; **Resid:** Urology, UCSF Med Ctr 1991; **Fellow:** Pediatric Urology, Chldns Hosp 1993; **Fac Appt:** Prof U, UCSF

Belldegrun, Arie S MD [U] - **Spec Exp:** Urologic Cancer; Gene Therapy; **Hospital:** UCLA Ronald Reagan Med Ctr; **Address:** 924 Westwood Blvd, Ste 1050, Los Angeles, CA 90024; **Phone:** 310-206-1434; **Board Cert:** Urology 2011; **Med School:** Israel 1974; **Resid:** Urology, Brigham and Women's Hosp 1985; **Fellow:** Urologic Oncology, Natl Cancer Inst, NIH 1988; **Fac Appt:** Prof U, UCLA

Boyd, Stuart D MD [U] - **Spec Exp:** Incontinence; Erectile Dysfunction; Urologic Cancer; **Hospital:** USC Norris Cancer Hosp (page 62), Keck Med Ctr of USC (page 62); **Address:** 1441 Eastlake Ave, Ste 7416, Los Angeles, CA 90089-9178; **Phone:** 323-865-3700; **Board Cert:** Urology 1984; **Med School:** UCLA 1975; **Resid:** Urology, UCLA Med Ctr 1982; **Fac Appt:** Prof U, USC Sch Med

Carroll, Peter R MD [U] - **Spec Exp:** Testicular Cancer; Prostate Cancer; Bladder Cancer; Bladder Reconstruction; **Hospital:** UCSF - Mt Zion Med Ctr; **Address:** UCSF Urologic Oncology Practice, 1600 Divisadero St Fl 3, San Francisco, CA 94115-1711; **Phone:** 415-353-7171; **Board Cert:** Urology 2006; **Med School:** Georgetown Univ 1979; **Resid:** Surgery, UCSF Med Ctr 1984; **Fellow:** Urology, Meml Sloan Kettering Cancer Ctr 1986; **Fac Appt:** Prof U, UCSF

Clayman, Ralph V MD [U] - **Spec Exp:** Kidney Stones; Kidney Cancer; Laparoscopic Surgery; Robotic Surgery; **Hospital:** UC Irvine Med Ctr; **Address:** UCI Med Ctr for Urological Care, 101 The City Drive S, Pavilion 3, Orange, CA 92868; **Phone:** 714-456-3330; **Board Cert:** Urology 2007; **Med School:** UCSD 1973; **Resid:** Urology, Univ Minn Med Ctr 1979; **Fac Appt:** Prof U, UC Irvine

Dalkin, Bruce MD [U] - **Spec Exp:** Urologic Cancer; Prostate Cancer; Bladder Cancer; Testicular Cancer; **Hospital:** Univ Wash Med Ctr; **Address:** Univ Washington-Dept Urology, 1959 NE Pacific St, Box 356510, Seattle, WA 98195; **Phone:** 206-598-4294; **Board Cert:** Urology 2002; **Med School:** Northwestern Univ 1985; **Resid:** Urology, Northwestern Meml Hosp 1991; **Fac Appt:** Prof U, Univ Wash

Daneshmand, Sia MD [U] - **Spec Exp:** Bladder Cancer; Testicular Cancer; Kidney Cancer; Testicular Cancer; **Hospital:** Keck Med Ctr of USC (page 62); **Address:** 1441 Eastlake Ave, Ste 7416, Los Angeles, CA 90089; **Phone:** 323-865-3700; **Board Cert:** Urology 2006; **Med School:** UC Davis 1996; **Resid:** Surgery, USC Med Ctr 1998; Urology, USC Med Ctr 2002; **Fellow:** Urologic Oncology, USC/Norris Comprehensive Cancer Ctr 2004; **Fac Appt:** Assoc Prof U, USC-Keck School of Medicine

Danoff, Dudley S MD [U] - **Spec Exp:** Prostate Cancer; Bladder Cancer; Erectile Dysfunction; **Hospital:** Cedars-Sinai Med Ctr; **Address:** 8635 W 3rd St, Ste 1 West, Los Angeles, CA 90048; **Phone:** 310-854-9898; **Board Cert:** Urology 1974; **Med School:** Yale Univ 1963; **Resid:** Urology, Yale-New Haven Hosp 1965; Urology, Columbia-Presby Med Ctr 1969

DeKernion, Jean B MD [U] - **Spec Exp:** Urologic Cancer; Kidney Cancer; Prostate Cancer; Prostate Disease; **Hospital:** UCLA Ronald Reagan Med Ctr; **Address:** 200 UCLA Medical Plaza Drive, Ste 140, Los Angeles, CA 90095-1738; **Phone:** 310-794-7700; **Board Cert:** Surgery 1973; Urology 1975; **Med School:** Louisiana State U, New Orleans 1965; **Resid:** Surgery, Univ Hosps-Case West Res 1967; Urology, Univ Hosps-Case West Res 1973; **Fellow:** Urologic Oncology, Natl Cancer Inst 1969; **Fac Appt:** Prof U, UCLA

Ellis, William J MD [U] - **Spec Exp:** Prostate Cancer/Robotic Surgery; Prostate Disease; Kidney Cancer; Urologic Cancer; **Hospital:** Univ Wash Med Ctr; **Address:** Univ Wash Med Ctr, Dept Urology, 1959 NE Pacific St, Box 356510, Seattle, WA 98195; **Phone:** 206-598-4294; **Board Cert:** Urology 2001; **Med School:** Johns Hopkins Univ 1985; **Resid:** Surgery, Northwestern Meml Hosp 1987; Urology, Northwestern Meml Hosp 1991; **Fac Appt:** Assoc Prof U, Univ Wash

Gill, Harcharan Singh MD [U] - **Spec Exp:** Urologic Cancer; Prostate Cancer; Prostate Disease; **Hospital:** Stanford Univ Hosp & Clinics; **Address:** 875 Blake Wilbur Drive, rm 2218, Palo Alto, CA 94305-5826; **Phone:** 650-725-5544; **Board Cert:** Urology 2004; **Med School:** Kenya 1977; **Resid:** Urology, Inst of Urology; Urology, Univ Hosp Penn 1991; **Fellow:** Urology, Univ Hosp Penn 1986; **Fac Appt:** Prof U, Stanford Univ

Gill, Inderbir Singh MD [U] - **Spec Exp:** Prostate Cancer; Kidney Cancer; Urologic Cancer; Minimally Invasive Urologic Surgery; **Hospital:** USC Norris Cancer Hosp (page 62); **Address:** USC/Norris Cancer Ctr, Dept Urology, 1441 Eastlake Ave, Ste 7416, Los Angeles, CA 90089; **Phone:** 323-865-3700; **Board Cert:** Urology 2008; **Med School:** India 1980; **Resid:** Surgery, Dayanand Med Coll & Hosp; Urology, Univ Kentucky Hosp 1993; **Fac Appt:** Prof U, Univ SC Sch Med

Ginsberg, David A MD [U] - **Spec Exp:** Incontinence; Urinary Reconstruction; Neuro-Urology; Neurogenic Bladder; **Hospital:** Keck Med Ctr of USC (page 62); **Address:** USC-Norris Cancer Ctr, 1441 Eastlake Ave, Ste 7416, Los Angeles, CA 90089; **Phone:** 323-865-3703; **Board Cert:** Urology 2008; **Med School:** USC Sch Med 1990; **Resid:** Surgery, LAC-USC Med Ctr 1992; Urology, LAc-USC Med Ctr 1996; **Fellow:** Reconstructive Surgery, UCLA Med Ctr 1997; **Fac Appt:** Assoc Clin Prof U, USC-Keck School of Medicine

Goldstein, Irwin MD [U] - **Spec Exp:** Sexual Dysfunction-Male & Female; Vulvar Pain; Erectile Dysfunction; Penile Microvascular Bypass Surgery; **Hospital:** Alvarado Hosp & Med Ctr, VA San Diego Hlthcre Sys; **Address:** San Diego Sexual Medicine, 5555 Reservoir Drive, Ste 300, San Diego, CA 92120; **Phone:** 619-265-8865; **Board Cert:** Urology 1982; **Med School:** McGill Univ 1975; **Resid:** Surgery, Boston Univ Med Ctr; Urology, Boston Univ Med Ctr 1980; **Fellow:** Urology, Boston Univ Med Ctr 1983; **Fac Appt:** Prof S, UCSD

Holden, Stuart MD [U] - **Spec Exp:** Kidney Cancer; **Hospital:** Cedars-Sinai Med Ctr; **Address:** 8635 W 3rd St, Ste 1 W, Los Angeles, CA 90048; **Phone:** 310-854-9898; **Board Cert:** Urology 1977; **Med School:** Cornell Univ-Weill Med Coll 1968; **Resid:** Surgery, NY Hosp-Cornell 1970; Urology, Emory Univ Hosp 1975; **Fellow:** Urology, Meml Sloan Kettering Cancer Ctr 1978

Kawachi, Mark H MD [U] - **Spec Exp:** Prostate Cancer/Robotic Surgery; Minimally Invasive Urologic Surgery; **Hospital:** City of Hope Natl Med Ctr; **Address:** Div Urologic Oncology, 1500 E Duarte Rd, Duarte, CA 91010-3012; **Phone:** 626-359-8111 x62655; **Board Cert:** Urology 2004; **Med School:** USC Sch Med 1979; **Resid:** Urology, USC Med Ctr 1984

Landman, Jaime MD [U] - **Spec Exp:** Minimally Invasive Urologic Surgery; Kidney Stones; Kidney Cancer; **Hospital:** UC Irvine Med Ctr; **Address:** 333 City Blvd W, Ste 2100, Orange, CA 92868; **Phone:** 714-456-3429; **Board Cert:** Urology 2003; **Med School:** Columbia P&S 1993; **Resid:** Urology, Mount Sinai Hosp 1999; **Fellow:** Urologic Laparoscopic Surg-Endourology, Wash Univ Med Ctr 2001; **Fac Appt:** Prof U, UC Irvine

Lange, Paul H MD [U] - **Spec Exp:** Prostate Cancer; **Hospital:** Univ Wash Med Ctr; **Address:** Univ Wash Med Ctr, Dept Urology, 1959 NE Pacific St, Box 356510, Seattle, WA 98195; **Phone:** 206-598-4294; **Board Cert:** Urology 2006; **Med School:** Washington Univ, St Louis 1967; **Resid:** Surgery, Duke Univ Med Ctr 1972; Urology, Univ Minn Med Ctr 1975; **Fellow:** Immunology, Univ Minn Med Ctr 1973; Research, Natl Inst Hlth 1970; **Fac Appt:** Prof U, Univ Wash

Lieskovsky, Gary MD [U] - **Spec Exp:** Prostate Cancer; **Hospital:** USC Norris Cancer Hosp (page 62), Keck Med Ctr of USC (page 62); **Address:** 1441 Eastlake Ave, Ste 7416, Los Angeles, CA 90089-0112; **Phone:** 323-865-3700; **Board Cert:** Urology 1980; **Med School:** Canada 1973; **Resid:** Urology, Univ Alberta Hosp 1978; **Fellow:** Urology, UCLA Med Ctr 1980; **Fac Appt:** Prof U, USC Sch Med

Lin, Daniel W MD [U] - **Spec Exp:** Bladder Cancer; **Hospital:** Univ Wash Med Ctr; **Address:** Urology Clinic at UWMC, 1959 NE Pacific St, Box 356158, Seattle, WA 98195; **Phone:** 206-598-4294; **Board Cert:** Urology 2003; **Med School:** Vanderbilt Univ 1994; **Resid:** Urology, Univ WA Med Ctr 2000; **Fellow:** Urologic Oncology, Meml Sloan-Kettering Canc Ctr 2001; **Fac Appt:** Assoc Prof U, Univ Wash

Marsh, Christopher L MD [U] - **Spec Exp:** Transplant-Kidney; Transplant-Pancreas; Transplant-Liver; Adrenal Surgery; **Hospital:** Scripps Green Hosp; **Address:** Scripps Clinic, 10666 N Torrey Pines Rd, MC N200, La Jolla, CA 92037; **Phone:** 858-554-4310; **Board Cert:** Urology 2006; **Med School:** Loma Linda Univ 1980; **Resid:** Urology, Loma Linda Univ Med Ctr 1986; **Fellow:** Transplant Surgery, Mayo Clinic 1987

McAninch, Jack W MD [U] - **Spec Exp:** Genitourinary Trauma; Genitourinary Reconstruction; **Hospital:** UCSF Med Ctr, San Francisco Genl Hosp; **Address:** San Francisco Genl Hosp, Dept Urology, 1001 Potrero Ave, Ste 3A20, San Francisco, CA 94110; **Phone:** 415-476-3372; **Board Cert:** Urology 1995; **Med School:** Univ Tex Med Br, Galveston 1964; **Resid:** Surgery, Darnall Army Hosp 1966; Urology, Letterman AMC 1969; **Fac Appt:** Prof U, UCSF

McClure, Robert D MD [U] - **Spec Exp:** Infertility-Male; **Address:** Seattle Reproductive Medicine, 1505 Westlake Ave N, Ste 400, Seattle, WA 98109; **Phone:** 206-301-5000; **Board Cert:** Urology 1979; **Med School:** Canada 1968; **Resid:** Urology, McGill Univ Hosp 1975; **Fellow:** Endocrinology, Univ Washington Med Ctr 1977

Merguerian, Paul A MD [U] - **Spec Exp:** Pediatric Urology; Bladder Exstrophy; Genital Reconstruction; Minimally Invasive Surgery; **Hospital:** Seattle Chldns Hosp; **Address:** Seattle Children's Hosp, W-7729-Urology, 4800 Sand Point Way NE, Seattle, WA 98105; **Phone:** 206-987-2509; **Board Cert:** Urology 2008; Pediatric Urology 2008; **Med School:** Israel 1980; **Resid:** Surgery, Strong Meml Hosp/Univ Rochester 1984; Urology, Strong Meml Hosp/Univ Rochester 1988; **Fellow:** Pediatric Urology, Hosp for Sick Chldn 1990; **Fac Appt:** Prof S, Dartmouth Med Sch

Porter, Christopher R MD [U] - **Spec Exp:** Urologic Cancer; Prostate Cancer; Testicular Cancer; Robotic Surgery; **Hospital:** Virginia Mason Med Ctr; **Address:** Virginia Mason Med Ctr, 1100 9th Ave, MS C7-URO, Seattle, WA 98101; **Phone:** 206-341-0560; **Board Cert:** Urology 2009; **Med School:** Rush Med Coll 1990; **Resid:** Urology, Brown Univ Affil Hosp 1997; **Fellow:** Urologic Oncology, Meml Sloan Kettering Canc Ctr 1999; **Fac Appt:** Assoc Clin Prof U, Univ Wash

Presti Jr, Joseph C MD [U] - **Spec Exp:** Prostate Cancer; Bladder Cancer; Kidney Cancer; Testicular Cancer; **Hospital:** Kaiser Permanente Oakland Med Ctr; **Address:** 280 W MacArthur Blvd, Oakland, CA 94611; **Phone:** 510-752-6796; **Board Cert:** Urology 2012; **Med School:** UC Irvine 1984; **Resid:** Surgery, UCSF Med Ctr 1986; Urology, UCSF Med Ctr 1989; **Fellow:** Urologic Oncology, Meml Sloan-Kettering Cancer Ctr 1992

Rajfer, Jacob MD [U] - **Spec Exp:** Erectile Dysfunction; Prostate Disease; Infertility-Male; **Hospital:** LAC - Harbor - UCLA Med Ctr, UCLA Ronald Reagan Med Ctr; **Address:** 1000 W Carson St, Dept of Urology, Torrance, CA 90502; **Phone:** 310-222-5189; **Board Cert:** Urology 1980; **Med School:** Northwestern Univ 1972; **Resid:** Surgery, St Josephs Hosp 1974; Urology, Johns Hopkins Hosp 1978; **Fellow:** Research, Johns Hopkins Hosp 1976; **Fac Appt:** Prof U, UCLA

Raz, Shlomo MD [U] - **Spec Exp:** Incontinence-Female; Urology-Female; **Hospital:** UCLA Ronald Reagan Med Ctr; **Address:** 200 Med Plaza Bldg 957366 - Ste 140, Los Angeles, CA 90095; **Phone:** 310-794-0206; **Board Cert:** Urology 1979; **Med School:** Uruguay 1962; **Resid:** Surgery, Hadassah Univ Hosp 1973; **Fellow:** Urology, UCLA Med Ctr 1975; **Fac Appt:** Prof U, UCLA

Sharlip, Ira D MD [U] - **Spec Exp:** Vasectomy Reversal; Erectile Dysfunction; Infertility-Male; **Hospital:** CA Pacific Med Ctr-Pacific Campus, UCSF Med Ctr; **Address:** 2100 Webster St, Ste 222, San Francisco, CA 94115-2376; **Phone:** 415-202-0250; **Board Cert:** Internal Medicine 1972; Urology 1977; **Med School:** Univ Pennsylvania 1965; **Resid:** Internal Medicine, Hosp Univ Penn 1967; Urology, UCSF Med Ctr 1975; **Fellow:** Urology, Middlesex Hosp 1976; **Fac Appt:** Clin Prof U, UCSF

Shortliffe, Linda D MD [U] - **Spec Exp:** Pediatric Urology; Hypospadias; Hydronephrosis; Vesicoureteral Reflux (VUR); **Hospital:** Lucile Packard Chldn's Hosp, Stanford Univ Hosp & Clinics; **Address:** Department of Urology S-287, SUMC MC:5118, 300 Pasteur Drive, Stanford, CA 94305-5118; **Phone:** 650-723-9779; **Board Cert:** Urology 2002; Pediatric Urology 2008; **Med School:** Stanford Univ 1975; **Resid:** Surgery, Tufts-New England Med Ctr 1977; Urology, Stanford Univ Med Ctr 1981; **Fellow:** Pediatric Urology, Chldn's Hosp 1987; **Fac Appt:** Prof U, Stanford Univ

Skinner, Eila C MD [U] - **Spec Exp:** Urologic Cancer; Genitourinary Disorders-Geriatric; Urinary Reconstruction; **Hospital:** USC Norris Cancer Hosp (page 62), Keck Med Ctr of USC (page 62); **Address:** USC-Keck Sch Med, Dept Urology, 1441 Eastlake Ave, Ste 7416, Los Angeles, CA 90089; **Phone:** 323-865-3700; **Board Cert:** Urology 2012; **Med School:** USC Sch Med 1983; **Resid:** Urology, LAC-USC Med Ctr 1988; **Fellow:** Urologic Oncology, LAC-USC Med Ctr 1990; **Fac Appt:** Assoc Prof U, USC Sch Med

Stoller, Marshall L MD [U] - **Spec Exp:** Laparoscopic Surgery; Kidney Stones; **Hospital:** UCSF Med Ctr; **Address:** Urology Faculty Practice, 400 Parnassus Ave, Ste A-610, San Francisco, CA 94145-0738; **Phone:** 415-353-2200; **Board Cert:** Urology 2009; **Med School:** Baylor Coll Med 1981; **Resid:** Surgery, UCSF Med Ctr 1983; Urology, UCSF Med Ctr 1987; **Fellow:** Urology, Prince Henry Hosp 1986; **Fac Appt:** Prof U, UCSF

Stone, Anthony R MD [U] - **Spec Exp:** Incontinence-Male & Female; Voiding Dysfunction; **Hospital:** UC Davis Med Ctr; **Address:** UC Davis Medical Group, 4860 Y St, Ste 2200, Sacramento, CA 95817-2214; **Phone:** 916-734-2222; **Board Cert:** Urology 2006; **Med School:** Scotland, UK 1972; **Resid:** Surgery, Stobhill Hosp 1978; Urology, Cardiff Royal Infirm 1983; **Fellow:** Urodynamics, Duke Univ Med Ctr 1986; **Fac Appt:** Prof U, UC Davis

Takayama, Thomas K MD [U] - **Spec Exp:** Urologic Cancer; Prostate Cancer; Robotic Surgery; Laparoscopic Surgery; **Hospital:** Overlake Hosp Med Ctr; **Address:** Washington Urology Associates, 1135 NE 116th Ave, Ste 620, Bellevue, WA 98004; **Phone:** 425-454-8016; **Board Cert:** Urology 2007; **Med School:** Tufts Univ 1985; **Resid:** Surgery, UMass Med Ctr 1987; Urology, Univ Washington Med Ctr 1993; **Fellow:** Urologic Oncology, Univ Washington Med Ctr 1996; **Fac Appt:** Assoc Prof U, Univ Wash

Turek, Paul J MD [U] - **Spec Exp:** Infertility-Male; Vasectomy Reversal; Microsurgery; Erectile Dysfunction; **Hospital:** CA Pacific Med Ctr-Pacific Campus, St. Francis Memorial Hosp; **Address:** 55 Francisco St, Ste 300, San Francisco, CA 94133; **Phone:** 415-392-3200; **Board Cert:** Urology 2005; **Med School:** Stanford Univ 1987; **Resid:** Surgery, Hosp Univ Penn 1989; Urology, Hosp Univ Penn 1993; **Fellow:** Microsurgery, Baylor Coll Med 1994; **Fac Appt:** Prof U, UCSF

Wilson, Timothy G MD [U] - **Spec Exp:** Prostate Cancer/Robotic Surgery; Minimally Invasive Urologic Surgery; Urinary Reconstruction; **Hospital:** City of Hope Natl Med Ctr; **Address:** Div Urologic Oncology, 1500 E Duarte Rd, Duarte, CA 91010; **Phone:** 626-359-8111 x62655; **Board Cert:** Urology 2001; **Med School:** Oregon Hlth & Sci Univ 1984; **Resid:** Urology, USC Med Ctr 1990; **Fellow:** Urologic Oncology, City Hosp Natl Med Ctr 1991; **Fac Appt:** Assoc Clin Prof U, USC Sch Med

Cleveland Clinic

Every life deserves world class care.

Urology

With nearly 70 physicians and scientists, Cleveland Clinic Glickman Urological & Kidney Institute's urology program is one of the world's largest and most comprehensive, and has been ranked #1 in the nation by *U.S. News & World Report*.

Urologic Cancer Treatment: We treat more than 1,000 prostate cancer patients annually utilizing a variety of surgical techniques, including robotic prostatectomy. We have the most experience in partial nephrectomy, with more than 3,000 performed to date and more than 1,200 performed using minimally invasive techniques.

Kidney Transplantation: Since the first kidney transplant at Cleveland Clinic in 1963, the program has performed more than 3,000 kidney transplants. Our surgeons pioneered the technique for removing donor kidneys through a single incision in the belly button.

Female Pelvic Health and Reconstructive Surgery: We treat women with genitourinary disorders, including urinary incontinence and pelvic organ prolapse.

Genitourinary Reconstruction: Our staff performs complex urethral reconstruction for stricture diseases using plastic surgery principles and completes about 60 procedures and 150 prosthetic surgeries annually.

Benign Prostatic Hyperplasia: We offer minimally invasive treatment options, including laser, microwave and radiofrequency therapies. Many of these options are performed on an outpatient basis with minimal catheterization.

Male Infertility: Comprehensive, individualized evaluation and treatment using state-of-the-art diagnostic procedures and microsurgical techniques.

Endourology and Stone Disease: We have treated more than 3,000 patients and have a success rate of greater than 90 percent with shock wave lithotripsy. Percutaneous kidney stone surgery is available for more complicated stone disease. On average, 900 procedures are performed each year.

Cleveland Clinic
Glickman Urological &
Kidney Institute
9500 Euclid Avenue
Cleveland, OH 44195

Offering Same-Day Appointments
Call 800.274.2009.

Treatment Guides
Cleveland Clinic has developed comprehensive treatment guides for many diseases and conditions. To download our free treatment guides, visit clevelandclinic.org/treatmentguides.

Online Medical Second Opinion
Call 216.444.3223 or
800.223.2273 ext. 43223 or
email eclevelandclinic@ccf.org.

Out-of-State Patients Assistance
Call 800.223.2273, ext. 55580 or
email medicalconcierge@ccf.org.

Visit Us At:
clevelandclinic.org

Follow Us On:
Facebook
www.facebook.com/clevelandclinic

Twitter
@ClevelandClinic

You Tube
www.youtube.com/clevelandclinic

Health Hub
health.clevelandclinic.org

UROLOGY

Urologists at NYU Langone Medical Center continue to pioneer in the surgical and medical treatment of urological disease and are recognized as a top urology program in the country by U.S. News and World Report.

Smilow Comprehensive Prostate Cancer Center
As part of the NCI-designated NYU Cancer Institute, the Center offers care by a team of uro-oncologic surgeons, radiation oncologists, oncologists, naturopathic doctors and radiologists.

Benign Prostatic Diseases
Innovative medical and surgical therapies for benign prostatic disease (as well as for prostatitis (the inflammation of the prostate gland), are offered.

Urological Diseases Center of Excellence
We are focused on discovering novel treatments for bladder and prostate cancer, while exploring how cancer markers can be used to determine how cancer treatments are working.

Female Urology and Incontinence
NYU Langone specializes in urological problems unique to women, including recurrent urinary tract infections, pelvic pain, prolapse and sexual dysfunction.

Latest Minimally Invasive Treatments
The Smilow Comprehensive Prostate Cancer Center, offers advances in prostate imaging and computer biopsy are providing valuable information about tumor location and growth to enable targeted treatment.

Male Sexual Health
Working in collaboration with NYU Langone's Fertility Center, urologists use the latest techniques to enable infertile couples to have children. Treatment is also offered to men suffering from erectile dysfunction and low testosterone.

Pediatric Urology and Reconstructive Surgery
Pediatric urologists focus on urinary system disorders in children from birth to early adults.

Robotic Urological Surgery
The Department's robotic surgery program includes prostate and kidney cancers, as well as female incontinence and urinary tract reconstruction.

Urologic Oncology
Because cancer treatment often requires a collaborative approach, urologists work closely with their colleagues at the NYU Cancer Institute to tailor treatments for each patient.

Vascular Surgery

a subspecialty of Surgery

A surgeon with expertise in the management of surgical disorders of the blood vessels, excluding the intercranial vessels or the heart.

Training Required: Five years in surgery *plus* additional training and examination.

VASCULAR SURGERY

New England

Belkin, Michael MD [VascS] - **Spec Exp:** Aneurysm; Arterial Bypass Surgery; Carotid Artery Surgery; **Hospital:** Brigham and Women's Hosp (page 57), Brigham and Women's Faulkner Hosp; **Address:** Brigham & Women's Hosp, Dept Vasc Surg, 75 Francis St Shapiro Bldg Fl 5, Boston, MA 02115; **Phone:** 857-307-1920; **Board Cert:** Vascular Surgery 2009; **Med School:** Univ Conn 1982; **Resid:** Surgery, Hartford Hosp 1987; **Fellow:** Vascular Surgery, Brigham & Women's Hosp 1989; **Fac Appt:** Assoc Prof S, Harvard Med Sch

Brewster, David C MD [VascS] - **Spec Exp:** Aneurysm-Abdominal Aortic; Endovascular Surgery; Angioplasty & Stent Placement; **Hospital:** Mass Genl Hosp, Newton - Wellesley Hosp; **Address:** Massachusetts General Hospital, 15 Parkman St, WAC 440, Boston, MA 02114; **Phone:** 617-726-3567; **Board Cert:** Surgery 1975; Vascular Surgery 2003; **Med School:** Columbia P&S 1967; **Resid:** Surgery, Mass Genl Hosp 1975; **Fellow:** Vascular Surgery, Mass Genl Hosp 1976; **Fac Appt:** Clin Prof S, Harvard Med Sch

Cambria, Richard P MD [VascS] - **Spec Exp:** Aneurysm-Abdominal Aortic; Cerebrovascular Disease; Renovascular Disease; Aortic Reconstruction; **Hospital:** Mass Genl Hosp, Newton - Wellesley Hosp; **Address:** Mass Genl Hosp, Dept Vascular Surgery, 15 Parkman St, WAC 440, Boston, MA 02114; **Phone:** 617-726-8278; **Board Cert:** Vascular Surgery 2006; **Med School:** Columbia P&S 1977; **Resid:** Surgery, Mass Genl Hosp 1978; **Fellow:** Vascular Surgery, Mass Genl Hosp 1984; **Fac Appt:** Prof S, Harvard Med Sch

Chaikof, Elliot L MD/PhD [VascS] - **Spec Exp:** Aneurysm-Aortic; Carotid Artery Disease; Peripheral Vascular Disease; Endovascular Surgery; **Hospital:** Beth Israel Deaconess Med Ctr - Boston; **Address:** BIDMC, Div Vascular Surgery, 110 Francis St NE, Ste 5B, Boston, MA 02215; **Phone:** 617-632-9959; **Board Cert:** Surgery 2002; Vascular Surgery 2003; **Med School:** Johns Hopkins Univ 1982; **Resid:** Surgery, Mass Genl Hosp 1985; Surgery, Mass Genl Hosp 1991; **Fellow:** Vascular Surgery, Emory Univ 1992; **Fac Appt:** Prof S, Harvard Med Sch

Cronenwett, Jack MD [VascS] - **Spec Exp:** Peripheral Vascular Disease; Aneurysm-Abdominal Aortic; Carotid Artery Surgery; **Hospital:** Dartmouth - Hitchcock Med Ctr, Mary Hitchcock Mem Hosp; **Address:** Dartmouth-Hitchcock Med Ctr, Sect Vascular Surgery, One Medical Center Drive, Lebanon, NH 03756; **Phone:** 603-650-8670; **Board Cert:** Vascular Surgery 2003; **Med School:** Stanford Univ 1973; **Resid:** Surgery, Univ Mich Hosp 1979; **Fellow:** Vascular Surgery, Univ Tenn Hosp 1980; **Fac Appt:** Prof S, Dartmouth Med Sch

Iafrati, Mark D MD [VascS] - **Spec Exp:** Endovascular Surgery; Vein Disorders; Wound Healing/Care; Hyperbaric Medicine; **Hospital:** Tufts Med Ctr, Steward Carney Hosp; **Address:** Tufts Medical Center, 800 Washington St, Box 259, Boston, MA 02111; **Phone:** 617-636-5019; **Board Cert:** Surgery 2005; Vascular Surgery 2005; **Med School:** Tufts Univ 1989; **Resid:** Surgery, Tufts New England Med Ctr 1995; **Fellow:** Vascular Surgery, Tufts New England Med Ctr 1997; **Fac Appt:** Assoc Prof S, Tufts Univ

Kwolek, Christopher J MD [VascS] - **Spec Exp:** Aneurysm-Abdominal & Thoracic Aortic; Endovascular Surgery; Carotid Artery Stent Placement; **Hospital:** Mass Genl Hosp, Newton - Wellesley Hosp; **Address:** Mass General Hospital, 15 Parkman St, Wang Bldg Fl 4, Boston, MA 02114; **Phone:** 617-724-6101; **Board Cert:** Surgery 2003; Vascular Surgery 2006; **Med School:** UCSF 1987; **Resid:** Surgery, New England Deaconess Hosp 1993; Vascular Surgery, Mass Genl Hosp 1995; **Fellow:** Endovascular Surgery, Arizona Heart Inst 1999; **Fac Appt:** Assoc Prof VascS, Harvard Med Sch

LaMuraglia, Glenn M MD [VascS] - **Spec Exp:** Carotid Body Tumors; Aneurysm-Aortic; Endovascular Surgery; Vascular Disease; **Hospital:** Mass Genl Hosp; **Address:** Mass Gen Hosp, Vascular Surgery, 55 Fruit St, Boston, MA 02114; **Phone:** 617-726-6997; **Board Cert:** Surgery 2004; Vascular Surgery 2007; **Med School:** Harvard Med Sch 1979; **Resid:** Surgery, Mass Genl Hosp 1985; Vascular Surgery, Mass Genl Hosp 1986; **Fac Appt:** Assoc Prof S, Harvard Med Sch

Mackey, William C MD [VascS] - **Spec Exp:** Carotid Artery Surgery; Aneurysm-Abdominal Aortic; Lower Limb Arterial Disease; **Hospital:** Tufts Med Ctr; **Address:** Tufts Medical Center, 800 Washington St, Box 1035, Boston, MA 02111; **Phone:** 617-636-5927; **Board Cert:** Surgery 2002; Vascular Surgery 2004; Surgical Critical Care 2007; **Med School:** Duke Univ 1977; **Resid:** Surgery, New York Hosp 1982; **Fellow:** Vascular Surgery, Tufts-New Eng Med Ctr 1984; **Fac Appt:** Prof S, Tufts Univ

Pomposelli, Frank B MD [VascS] - **Spec Exp:** Diabetic Leg/Foot; Aortic Surgery; Carotid Artery Disease; Endovascular Surgery; **Hospital:** Steward St Elizabeth's Med Ctr-Boston; **Address:** St. Elizabeth's Medical Center, Division of Vascular Surgery, 736 Cambridge St, CCP8, Brighton, MA 02135; **Phone:** 617-789-3309; **Board Cert:** Vascular Surgery 2008; **Med School:** Boston Univ 1979; **Resid:** Surgery, New England Deaconess Hosp 1986; **Fellow:** Peripheral Vascular Surgery, NYU Med Ctr 1987; **Fac Appt:** Prof S, Harvard Med Sch

Sumpio, Bauer E MD/PhD [VascS] - **Spec Exp:** Diabetic Leg/Foot; Endovascular Surgery; **Hospital:** Yale-New Haven Hosp, Yale Med Group; **Address:** Yale Univ School Medicine, Dept Surgery, 333 Cedar St, Box 208062, BB 204, New Haven, CT 06520; **Phone:** 203-785-6217; **Board Cert:** Vascular Surgery 2009; Surgery 2009; **Med School:** Cornell Univ-Weill Med Coll 1980; **Resid:** Surgery, Yale-New Haven Hosp 1986; **Fellow:** Vascular Surgery, Univ N Carolina Hosp 1987; **Fac Appt:** Prof S, Yale Univ

Mid Atlantic

Adelman, Mark MD [VascS] - **Spec Exp:** Carotid Artery Surgery; Aneurysm-Abdominal Aortic; Vein Disorders; Endovascular Surgery; **Hospital:** NYU Langone Med Ctr (page 68), Bellevue Hosp Ctr; **Address:** 530 1st Ave, Ste 6F, MS 10016, New York, NY 10016-6402; **Phone:** 212-263-7311; **Board Cert:** Surgery 1999; Vascular Surgery 2001; **Med School:** NYU Sch Med 1985; **Resid:** Surgery, NYU Med Ctr 1990; **Fellow:** Vascular Surgery, NYU Med Ctr 1991; **Fac Appt:** Prof VascS, NYU Sch Med

Atnip, Robert G MD [VascS] - **Spec Exp:** Aneurysm-Abdominal Aortic; Peripheral Vascular Disease; Carotid Artery Disease; Endovascular Surgery; **Hospital:** Penn State Milton S Hershey Med Ctr; **Address:** Hershey Med Ctr, Div Vascular Surg, 500 University Drive, MC H053, Hershey, PA 17033-0850; **Phone:** 717-531-4554; **Board Cert:** Surgery 2005; Vascular Surgery 2007; Surgical Critical Care 2010; **Med School:** Univ Alabama 1978; **Resid:** Surgery, Mass Genl Hosp 1984; **Fellow:** Vascular Surgery, Mass Genl Hosp 1985; **Fac Appt:** Prof S, Penn State Coll Med

Benckart, Daniel MD [VascS] - **Hospital:** Allegheny General Hosp; **Address:** Allegheny CVI1, 320 E North Ave, Pittsburgh, PA 15212; **Phone:** 412-359-8820; **Board Cert:** Thoracic Surgery 2004; Surgery 2003; Vascular Surgery 1999; **Med School:** Georgetown Univ 1977; **Resid:** Surgery, Vanderbilt Affil Hosp 1982; **Fellow:** Vascular Thoracic Surgery, NYU Med Ctr 1985; **Fac Appt:** Assoc Prof TS, Drexel Univ Coll Med

Vascular Surgery

Benvenisty, Alan I MD [VascS] - **Spec Exp:** Renovascular Disease; Aneurysm-Aortic; Endovascular Surgery; Minimally Invasive Vascular Surgery; **Hospital:** St. Luke's - Roosevelt Hosp Ctr - St Luke's Hosp (page 56), St. Luke's - Roosevelt Hosp Ctr - Roosevelt Div (page 56); **Address:** 1090 Amsterdam Ave Fl 12, New York, NY 10025; **Phone:** 212-523-4706; **Board Cert:** Surgery 2004; Vascular Surgery 2009; **Med School:** Columbia P&S 1978; **Resid:** Surgery, Columbia-Presby Med Ctr 1983; **Fellow:** Vascular Surgery, Columbia-Presby Med Ctr 1984; Transplant Surgery, Columbia-Presby Med Ctr 1984; **Fac Appt:** Clin Prof S, Columbia P&S

Brener, Bruce J MD [VascS] - **Spec Exp:** Endovascular Surgery; Minimally Invasive Vascular Surgery; Carotid Artery Surgery; Aneurysm-Aortic; **Hospital:** Newark Beth Israel Med Ctr, Saint Barnabas Med Ctr; **Address:** 200 S Orange Ave, Ste 109, Livingston, NJ 07039; **Phone:** 973-322-7233; **Board Cert:** Surgery 1972; Vascular Surgery 2005; **Med School:** Harvard Med Sch 1966; **Resid:** Surgery, Chldns Hosp Med Ctr 1968; Surgery, Peter Bent Brigham Hosp 1972; **Fellow:** Vascular Surgery, Mass Genl Hosp 1973; **Fac Appt:** Assoc Clin Prof S, Columbia P&S

Calligaro, Keith D MD [VascS] - **Spec Exp:** Aneurysm-Abdominal & Thoracic Aortic; Carotid Artery Disease; Lower Limb Arterial Disease; Aortic Stent Grafts; **Hospital:** Pennsylvania Hosp-UPHS (page 72); **Address:** 700 Spruce St, Ste 101, Philadelphia, PA 19106; **Phone:** 215-829-5000; **Board Cert:** Vascular Surgery 2008; **Med School:** UMDNJ-Rutgers Med Sch 1982; **Resid:** Surgery, Univ Hlth Sci/Chicago Med 1987; **Fellow:** Vascular Surgery, Montefiore Med Ctr/Albert Einstein 1989; **Fac Appt:** Clin Prof S, Univ Pennsylvania

Carpenter, Jeffrey P MD [VascS] - **Spec Exp:** Aneurysm-Abdominal & Thoracic Aortic; Carotid Artery Surgery; Endovascular Surgery; Peripheral Vascular Disease; **Hospital:** Cooper Univ Hosp; **Address:** 9 Centennial Blvd, Ste G, Voorhees, NJ 08043; **Phone:** 856-325-6516; **Board Cert:** Surgery 2001; Vascular Surgery 2010; **Med School:** Yale Univ 1986; **Resid:** Surgery, Hosp Univ Penn 1991; **Fellow:** Vascular Surgery, Hosp Univ Penn 1992; **Fac Appt:** Prof S

Criado, Frank J MD [VascS] - **Spec Exp:** Endovascular Surgery; Aneurysm-Abdominal & Thoracic Aortic; Carotid Artery Surgery; **Hospital:** Union Meml Hosp-Baltimore; **Address:** 3333 N Calvert St, Ste 570, Baltimore, MD 21218; **Phone:** 410-554-6400; **Board Cert:** Vascular Surgery 2008; **Med School:** Uruguay 1974; **Resid:** Surgery, Union Meml Hosp 1980; Vascular Surgery, Union Meml Hosp 1985; **Fellow:** Cardiovascular Surgery, Baylor Univ Med Ctr 1981

D'Ayala, Marcus D MD [VascS] - **Spec Exp:** Endovascular Surgery; Aneurysm-Abdominal Aortic; Carotid Artery Disease; Peripheral Vascular Disease; **Hospital:** New York Methodist Hosp; **Address:** NY Methodist Hospital, Dept Surgery, 506 Sixth St, Brooklyn, NY 11215; **Phone:** 718-780-3288; **Board Cert:** Surgery 2008; Vascular Surgery 2009; **Med School:** Univ Wisc 1992; **Resid:** Surgery, Montefiore Med Ctr 1997; **Fellow:** Vascular Surgery, Mt Sinai Med Ctr 1998; **Fac Appt:** Assoc Clin Prof S, Cornell Univ-Weill Med Coll

Darling III, R Clement MD [VascS] - **Spec Exp:** Aneurysm-Abdominal & Thoracic Aortic; Arterial Bypass Surgery; Carotid Artery Surgery; **Hospital:** Albany Med Ctr, St. Peter's Hosp - Albany; **Address:** Albany Med Ctr, Vascular Inst, 43 New Scotland Ave, MC 157, Albany, NY 12208; **Phone:** 518-262-5640; **Board Cert:** Surgery 1999; Vascular Surgery 2002; **Med School:** Univ Cincinnati 1984; **Resid:** Surgery, Beth Israel Deaconess Hosp 1989; **Fellow:** Vascular Surgery, Albany Med Ctr 1991; **Fac Appt:** Prof S, Albany Med Coll

Dougherty, Matthew J MD [VascS] - **Spec Exp:** Endovascular Stent Grafts; Aneurysm; **Hospital:** Pennsylvania Hosp-UPHS (page 72); **Address:** 700 Spruce St, Ste 101, Philadelphia, PA 19106; **Phone:** 215-829-5000; **Board Cert:** Vascular Surgery 2001; Surgery 1999; **Med School:** Harvard Med Sch 1984; **Resid:** Surgery, Mass Genl Hosp 1990; **Fellow:** Vascular Surgery, Mayo Clinic 1992; **Fac Appt:** Assoc Clin Prof S, Univ Pennsylvania

Fairman, Ronald M MD [VascS] - **Spec Exp:** Aneurysm-Aortic; Peripheral Vascular Disease; Carotid Artery Surgery; Aneurysm-Abdominal & Thoracic Aortic; **Hospital:** Hosp Univ Penn - UPHS (page 72); **Address:** Penn Heart & Vascular Center, Perelman Ctr for Advanced Medicine, 3400 Civic Center Blvd, Fl 2-East, Philadelphia, PA 19104; **Phone:** 215-615-4949; **Board Cert:** Vascular Surgery 2010; **Med School:** Thomas Jefferson Univ 1977; **Resid:** Surgery, Hosp Univ Penn 1983; **Fellow:** Vascular Surgery, Hosp Univ Penn 1984; **Fac Appt:** Prof S, Univ Pennsylvania

Fantini, Gary A MD [VascS] - **Spec Exp:** Spinal Access Surgery; **Hospital:** Hosp For Special Surgery (page 60), NY-Presby/Weill Cornell Med Ctr, NY (page 66); **Address:** 635 Madison Ave, Fl 7, New York, NY 10022; **Phone:** 212-317-4550; **Board Cert:** Surgery 2012; Vascular Surgery 2010; **Med School:** Albert Einstein Coll Med 1983; **Resid:** Surgery, NY Hosp-Cornell Med Ctr 1989; **Fellow:** Vascular Surgery, UCSF Med Ctr 1990; **Fac Appt:** Assoc Prof S, Cornell Univ-Weill Med Coll

Faries, Peter L MD [VascS] - **Spec Exp:** Aneurysm-Abdominal Aortic; Peripheral Vascular Disease; Renovascular Disease; Carotid Artery Surgery; **Hospital:** Mount Sinai Med Ctr (page 64); **Address:** 5 E 98th St, Ste 415, New York, NY 10029; **Phone:** 212-241-5386; **Board Cert:** Surgery 2008; Vascular Surgery 2009; **Med School:** Univ Pennsylvania 1992; **Resid:** Surgery, Montefiore Med Ctr 1998; **Fellow:** Vascular Surgery, Beth Israel Deaconess Med Ctr 2000; **Fac Appt:** Assoc Prof S, Cornell Univ-Weill Med Coll

Freischlag, Julie A MD [VascS] - **Spec Exp:** Aneurysm-Aortic; Carotid Artery Surgery; Thoracic Outlet Syndrome; **Hospital:** Johns Hopkins Hosp (page 61); **Address:** Johns Hopkins Hosp, Dept Surg, 720 Rutland Ave, Ross Bldg, Ste 759, Baltimore, MD 21205; **Phone:** 443-287-3497; **Board Cert:** Surgery 2005; Vascular Surgery 2005; **Med School:** Rush Med Coll 1980; **Resid:** Surgery, UCLA Medical Ctr 1986; **Fellow:** Vascular Surgery, UCLA Medical Ctr 1987; **Fac Appt:** Prof S, Johns Hopkins Univ

Golden, Michael A MD [VascS] - **Spec Exp:** Aneurysm; Endovascular Surgery; **Hospital:** Penn Presby Med Ctr - UPHS (page 72); **Address:** Penn Presbyterian Med Ctr, 51 N 39th St, Wright-Saunders, Ste 266, Philadelphia, PA 19104; **Phone:** 215-662-9660; **Board Cert:** Surgery 2007; Vascular Surgery 2010; **Med School:** Univ Pennsylvania 1981; **Resid:** Surgery, Brigham & Women's Hosp 1987; **Fellow:** Vascular Surgery, Brigham & Women's Hosp 1990; **Fac Appt:** Assoc Prof S, Univ Pennsylvania

Green, Richard M MD [VascS] - **Spec Exp:** Aneurysm-Abdominal Aortic; Carotid Artery Surgery; Percutaneous Vascular Interventions; **Hospital:** Lenox Hill Hosp (page 67); **Address:** 130 E 77th St, Fl 13, New York, NY 10075; **Phone:** 212-434-3420; **Board Cert:** Vascular Surgery 2003; **Med School:** Univ Rochester 1970; **Resid:** Surgery, Strong Meml Hosp 1976

Harrington, Elizabeth MD [VascS] - **Spec Exp:** Carotid Artery Surgery; Aneurysm-Aortic; Arterial Bypass Surgery-Leg; **Hospital:** Mount Sinai Med Ctr (page 64); **Address:** 2 E 93rd St, New York, NY 10128; **Phone:** 212-876-7400; **Board Cert:** Surgery 2009; Vascular Surgery 2006; **Med School:** NY Med Coll 1975; **Resid:** Surgery, Mt Sinai Hosp 1980; **Fellow:** Vascular Surgery, Mt Sinai Hosp 1981; **Fac Appt:** Assoc Prof VascS, Mount Sinai Sch Med

Makaroun, Michel S MD [VascS] - **Spec Exp:** Aneurysm-Aortic; Carotid Artery Disease; Endovascular Surgery; Peripheral Vascular Disease; **Hospital:** UPMC Shadyside, UPMC Presby, Pittsburgh; **Address:** Chrmn-Div Vascular Surg, Presby Univ Hosp, Ste A1011, 200 Lothrop St, Pittsburgh, PA 15213; **Phone:** 412-802-3333; **Board Cert:** Surgery 2004; Vascular Surgery 2009; **Med School:** Lebanon 1978; **Resid:** Surgery, American Univ Hosp 1980; Surgery, Univ Pittsburgh Med Ctr 1985; **Fac Appt:** Prof S, Univ Pittsburgh

Vascular Surgery

Marin, Michael L MD [VascS] - **Spec Exp:** Aneurysm-Aortic; Peripheral Vascular Disease; Limb Sparing Surgery; Endovascular Surgery; **Hospital:** Mount Sinai Med Ctr (page 64); **Address:** Mount Sinai Medical Ctr, 5 E 98th St, Box 1273, New York, NY 10029; **Phone:** 212-241-5315; **Board Cert:** Surgery 2011; **Med School:** Mount Sinai Sch Med 1984; **Resid:** Surgery, Columbia-Presby Med Ctr 1990; **Fellow:** Transplant Surgery, Columbia-Presby Med Ctr 1988; Vascular Surgery, Montefiore Med Ctr 1992; **Fac Appt:** Prof S, Mount Sinai Sch Med

McKinsey, James F MD [VascS] - **Spec Exp:** Aneurysm-Abdominal Aortic; Endovascular Surgery; Carotid Artery Surgery; **Hospital:** NY-Presby/Columbia Univ Med Ctr, NY (page 66); **Address:** NY Presby Hosp/Columbia U Med Ctr, Irving Pavilion Fl 5, 161 Fort Washington Ave, New York, NY 10032; **Phone:** 212-342-3255; **Board Cert:** Surgery 2001; Vascular Surgery 2003; **Med School:** Univ Fla Coll Med 1987; **Resid:** Surgery, Georgia Baptist Med Ctr 1992; **Fellow:** Vascular Surgery, Univ Chicago Hosps 1993; **Fac Appt:** Assoc Clin Prof S, Columbia P&S

Morrissey, Nicholas J MD [VascS] - **Spec Exp:** Minimally Invasive Vascular Surgery; Aneurysm-Abdominal & Thoracic Aortic; Carotid Artery Surgery; **Hospital:** NY-Presby/Columbia Univ Med Ctr, NY (page 66); **Address:** 161 Fort Washington Ave, Herbert Irving Pavilion, rm 538, New York, NY 10032; **Phone:** 212-342-2929; **Board Cert:** Surgery 2009; Vascular Surgery 2003; **Med School:** Univ Rochester 1992; **Resid:** Surgery, Strong Meml Hosp 1999; **Fellow:** Vascular Surgery, Mount Sinai Hosp 2001; **Fac Appt:** Assoc Prof S, Columbia P&S

Neville Jr, Richard F MD [VascS] - **Spec Exp:** Endovascular Surgery; Wound Healing/Care; **Hospital:** G Washington Univ Hosp, Inova Mt Vernon Hosp; **Address:** 2150 Pennsylvania Ave NW, Fl 6B, rm 407, PHC Bldg - Fl 4, Washington, DC 20037; **Phone:** 202-741-3210; **Board Cert:** Surgery 2000; Vascular Surgery 2002; **Med School:** Univ MD Sch Med 1983; **Resid:** Surgery, Georgetown Univ Hosp 1988; **Fellow:** Vascular Surgery, UMDNJ Affil Hosp 1991; **Fac Appt:** Assoc Prof S, Georgetown Univ

Perler, Bruce MD [VascS] - **Spec Exp:** Carotid Artery Surgery; Aneurysm; Arterial Bypass Surgery-Leg; **Hospital:** Johns Hopkins Hosp (page 61), Johns Hopkins Bayview Med Ctr (page 61); **Address:** Johns Hopkins Hosp, Dept Surgery, 600 N Wolfe St Harvey Bldg - Ste 611, Baltimore, MD 21287-8611; **Phone:** 410-955-2618; **Board Cert:** Vascular Surgery 2008; **Med School:** Duke Univ 1976; **Resid:** Surgery, Mass Genl Hosp 1981; **Fellow:** Vascular Surgery, Mass Genl Hosp 1982; **Fac Appt:** Prof S, Johns Hopkins Univ

Ricotta, John MD [VascS] - **Spec Exp:** Aneurysm; Carotid Artery Surgery; Vein Disorders; **Hospital:** Washington Hosp Ctr; **Address:** 110 Irving St NW, rm G253, Washington, DC 20010; **Phone:** 202-877-5133; **Board Cert:** Surgery 2004; Vascular Surgery 2003; **Med School:** Johns Hopkins Univ 1973; **Resid:** Surgery, Johns Hopkins Hosp 1977; **Fellow:** Vascular Surgery, Johns Hopkins Hosp 1979; **Fac Appt:** Prof S, Georgetown Univ

Riles, Thomas MD [VascS] - **Spec Exp:** Aneurysm-Aortic-Medical Management; Carotid Artery Medical Management; **Hospital:** NYU Langone Med Ctr (page 68); **Address:** NYU Med Ctr, Univ Vascular Assoc, 530 1st Ave, Ste 6F, New York, NY 10016; **Phone:** 212-263-6360; **Board Cert:** Vascular Surgery 2003; **Med School:** Baylor Coll Med 1969; **Resid:** Surgery, NYU Med Ctr 1976; **Fellow:** Vascular Surgery, NYU Med Ctr 1977; **Fac Appt:** Prof S, NYU Sch Med

Schneider, Darren B MD [VascS] - **Spec Exp:** Endovascular Surgery; Minimally Invasive Vascular Surgery; Aneurysm-Aortic; Peripheral Vascular Disease; **Hospital:** NY-Presby/Weill Cornell Med Ctr, NY (page 66); **Address:** Weill Cornell Dept Vascular Surgery, 525 E 68th St, New York, NY 10021; **Phone:** 212-746-5192; **Board Cert:** Surgery 2001; Vascular Surgery 2003; **Med School:** UCSD 1992; **Resid:** Surgery, UCSF Med Ctr 2000; **Fellow:** Interventional Radiology, UCSF Med Ctr 2001; Vascular Surgery, UCSF Med Ctr 2002; **Fac Appt:** Assoc Prof S, Cornell Univ-Weill Med Coll

Todd, George MD [VascS] - **Spec Exp:** Minimally Invasive Vascular Surgery; Aneurysm-Abdominal Aortic; Carotid Artery Surgery; **Hospital:** St. Luke's - Roosevelt Hosp Ctr - Roosevelt Div (page 56); **Address:** St Luke's-Roosevelt Hosp Ctr, Dept Surg, 1000 10th Ave, rm 5G77, New York, NY 10019; **Phone:** 212-523-7481; **Board Cert:** Surgery 2010; Vascular Surgery 2006; **Med School:** Penn State Coll Med 1974; **Resid:** Surgery, Columbia-Presby Med Ctr 1979; **Fellow:** Vascular Surgery, Columbia-Presby Med Ctr 1980; **Fac Appt:** Prof S, Columbia P&S

Southeast

Cherry Jr, Kenneth J MD [VascS] - **Spec Exp:** Vascular Reconstruction; Aortic Graft Infections; **Hospital:** Univ of Virginia Health Sys; **Address:** Univ Virginia Health System, PO Box 800679, Charlottesville, VA 22908-0679; **Phone:** 434-243-7052; **Board Cert:** Vascular Surgery 2004; **Med School:** Univ VA Sch Med 1974; **Resid:** Surgery, Univ Virginia Hosp 1980; Vascular Surgery, UCSF Med Ctr 1981; **Fac Appt:** Prof S, Univ VA Sch Med

Dattilo, Jeffery MD [VascS] - **Hospital:** Vanderbilt Univ Med Ctr (page 75), VA Tennessee Valley Healthcare System-Alvin C. Yor; **Address:** Vanderbilt University Medical Center, 1161 22nd Ave S, D-5237 Medical Center North, Nashville, TN 37232-2735; **Phone:** 615-322-2343; **Board Cert:** Surgery 2002; Vascular Surgery 2005; **Med School:** E Carolina Univ 1993; **Resid:** Surgery, Medical College of Virginia Hosp 2000; **Fellow:** Vascular Surgery, Mass Genl Hosp 2002; **Fac Appt:** Assoc Prof S, Vanderbilt Univ

Flynn, Timothy C MD [VascS] - **Spec Exp:** Peripheral Vascular Disease; Aortic Graft Infections; **Hospital:** Shands at Univ of FL; **Address:** 1600 SW Archer Rd, Box 100192, Gainesville, FL 32610-0286; **Phone:** 352-273-7520; **Board Cert:** Surgery 1999; Vascular Surgery 2008; Surgical Critical Care 1998; **Med School:** Baylor Coll Med 1974; **Resid:** Surgery, Univ Texas 1980; **Fac Appt:** Prof S, Univ Fla Coll Med

Hakaim, Albert G MD [VascS] - **Spec Exp:** Aneurysm-Abdominal Aortic; Endovascular Surgery; **Hospital:** Mayo - Jacksonville; **Address:** Mayo Clinic, Dept Vascular Surgery, 4500 San Pablo Rd, Ste 323N, Jacksonville, FL 32224; **Phone:** 904-953-2077; **Board Cert:** Surgery 2002; Vascular Surgery 2003; **Med School:** Ohio State Univ 1984; **Resid:** Surgery, Cleveland Clinic 1989; **Fellow:** Transplant Surgery, Boston Univ Hosp 1991; Vascular Surgery, Cleveland Clinic 1992; **Fac Appt:** Prof S, Mayo Med Sch

Hallett Jr, John W MD [VascS] - **Spec Exp:** Aneurysm-Abdominal Aortic; Carotid Artery Surgery; Thoracic Outlet Syndrome; **Hospital:** Roper Hosp; **Address:** Roper St Francis Heart & Vascular Ctr, 316 Calhoun St, Charleston, SC 29401; **Phone:** 843-720-5665; **Board Cert:** Vascular Surgery 2003; **Med School:** Duke Univ 1973; **Resid:** Surgery, Wilford Hall USAF Med Ctr 1978; **Fellow:** Vascular Surgery, Mass Genl Hosp-Harvard Med Sch 1979; **Fac Appt:** Assoc Clin Prof VascS, Med Univ SC

McCann, Richard L MD [VascS] - **Spec Exp:** Endovascular Surgery; **Hospital:** Duke Univ Hosp; **Address:** Duke Univ Med Ctr, Box 2990, Durham, NC 27710; **Phone:** 919-681-2406; **Board Cert:** Surgery 2003; Vascular Surgery 2006; **Med School:** Cornell Univ-Weill Med Coll 1974; **Resid:** Surgery, Duke Univ Med Ctr 1983; **Fac Appt:** Prof S, Duke Univ

Mitchell, Marc E MD [VascS] - **Spec Exp:** Renal Artery Stenosis; Carotid Artery Surgery; Aneurysm-Aortic; Peripheral Vascular Disease; **Hospital:** Univ Mississippi Med Ctr; **Address:** Univ Mississippi Med Ctr, Dept Surgery, 2500 N State St, Jackson, MS 39216; **Phone:** 601-984-5105; **Board Cert:** Surgery 2010; Surgical Critical Care 2005; Vascular Surgery 2007; **Med School:** Georgetown Univ 1984; **Resid:** Surgery, UCSF Med Ctr 1986; Surgery, Univ Mississippi Med Ctr 1991; **Fellow:** Cardiac Surgery, Natl Inst Hlth 1998; Vascular Surgery, Univ Penn 1997; **Fac Appt:** Prof S, Univ Miss

Vascular Surgery

Naslund, Thomas C MD [VascS] - **Spec Exp:** Endovascular Surgery; Aneurysm-Aortic; **Hospital:** Vanderbilt Univ Med Ctr (page 75); **Address:** Vanderbilt Univ Med Ctr, Div Vasc Surg, 1161 21st Ave S, D-5237 MCN, Nashville, TN 37232-2735; **Phone:** 615-322-2343; **Board Cert:** Vascular Surgery 2000; Surgery 1999; **Med School:** Vanderbilt Univ 1984; **Resid:** Surgery, Vanderbilt Univ Med Ctr 1990; **Fellow:** Vascular Surgery, Ochsner Med Fdn 1992; **Fac Appt:** Prof S, Vanderbilt Univ

Midwest

Acher, Charles W MD [VascS] - **Spec Exp:** Aneurysm-Abdominal & Thoracic Aortic; Cerebrovascular Disease; Endovascular Surgery; Limb Sparing Surgery; **Hospital:** Univ WI Hosp & Clins; **Address:** 451 Junction Rd, Madison, WI 53717; **Phone:** 608-265-4420; **Board Cert:** Vascular Surgery 2008; **Med School:** Indiana Univ 1973; **Resid:** Surgery, Univ Wisconsin Hosp 1978; **Fellow:** Peripheral Vascular Surgery, Gloucestershire Royal Hosp 1980; Vascular Surgery, Baylor Coll of Med 1983; **Fac Appt:** Prof S, Univ Wisc

Alexander, J Jeffrey MD [VascS] - **Spec Exp:** Peripheral Vascular Disease; Carotid Artery Disease; Dialysis Access; **Hospital:** MetroHealth Med Ctr; **Address:** MetroHealth Med Ctr, Heart/Vascular Dept, 2500 MetroHealth Drive, Ste H328, Cleveland, OH 44109-1998; **Phone:** 216-778-4811; **Board Cert:** Surgery 2002; Vascular Surgery 2006; **Med School:** Univ Pittsburgh 1978; **Resid:** Surgery, Univ Chicago Hosps 1983; **Fellow:** Vascular Surgery, Univ Chicago Hosps 1984; **Fac Appt:** Assoc Prof S, Case West Res Univ

Berguer, Ramon MD/PhD [VascS] - **Spec Exp:** Cerebrovascular Disease; Aortic & Visceral Artery Surgery; **Hospital:** Univ of Michigan Hosp; **Address:** Univ Michigan Dept Vascular Surg, 1500 E Medical Ctr Dr, SPC 5856, Ann Arbor, MI 48109; **Phone:** 888-287-1082; **Board Cert:** Surgery 1970; Vascular Surgery 2003; **Med School:** Spain 1963; **Resid:** Surgery, Henry Ford Hosp 1969; **Fellow:** Vascular Surgery, Henry Ford Hosp 1970; Vascular Surgery, Kings College Hosp; **Fac Appt:** Prof S, Univ Mich Med Sch

Clair, Daniel G MD [VascS] - **Spec Exp:** Carotid Artery Surgery; Aneurysm-Abdominal & Thoracic Aortic; Peripheral Vascular Disease; Endovascular Stent Grafts; **Hospital:** Cleveland Clin (page 55); **Address:** Cleveland Clinic, Dept Vascular Surgery, 9500 Euclid Ave, Desk H32, Cleveland, OH 44195; **Phone:** 216-444-3857; **Board Cert:** Surgery 2011; Vascular Surgery 2004; **Med School:** Univ VA Sch Med 1986; **Resid:** Surgery, Brigham & Women's Hosp 1992; **Fellow:** Oncology, Brigham & Women's Hosp 1991; Vascular Surgery, Brigham & Women's Hosp 1994

Comerota, Anthony J MD [VascS] - **Spec Exp:** Carotid Artery Disease; Gene Therapy; Aneurysm-Aortic; Peripheral Vascular Disease; **Hospital:** Toledo Hosp; **Address:** Jobst Vascular Ctr, 2109 Hughes Drive, Ste 400, Toledo, OH 43606; **Phone:** 419-291-2088; **Board Cert:** Vascular Surgery 2003; **Med School:** Temple Univ 1974; **Resid:** Surgery, Temple Univ Hosp 1978; **Fellow:** Vascular Surgery, Good Samaritan Hosp 1981; **Fac Appt:** Clin Prof S, Univ Mich Med Sch

Dalsing, Michael C MD [VascS] - **Spec Exp:** Peripheral Vascular Disease; Carotid Artery Disease; Aortic Reconstruction; Percutaneous Vascular Interventions; **Hospital:** IU Health Methodist Hosp, IU Health University Hosp; **Address:** 1801 N Senate Blvd, Indianapolis, IN 46202; **Phone:** 317-962-0280; **Board Cert:** Surgery 2002; Vascular Surgery 2003; Surgical Critical Care 2001; **Med School:** Med Coll Wisc 1978; **Resid:** Surgery, Indiana Univ Med Ctr 1983; **Fellow:** Vascular Surgery, Northwestern Univ Med Ctr 1984; **Fac Appt:** Prof S, Indiana Univ

Gloviczki, Peter MD [VascS] - **Spec Exp:** Aneurysm-Abdominal Aortic; Lower Limb Arterial Disease; Vein Disorders; **Hospital:** Mayo Med Ctr & Clin - Rochester; **Address:** Mayo Clin, Div Vasc Surg, 200 First St SW, Rochester, MN 55905-0001; **Phone:** 507-284-4652; **Board Cert:** Surgery 2010; Vascular Surgery 2008; **Med School:** Hungary 1972; **Resid:** Vascular Surgery, Semmelweis Med Sch 1980; Surgery, Mayo Clin 1987; **Fellow:** Vascular Surgery, Mayo Clin 1983; **Fac Appt:** Prof S, Mayo Med Sch

Greisler, Howard MD [VascS] - **Spec Exp:** Peripheral Vascular Disease; Aneurysm; Carotid Artery Disease; **Hospital:** Edward Hines, Jr. VA Hosp; **Address:** VA Hospital, 5000 S 5th Ave, Bldg 1, rm C417, Hines, IL 60141; **Phone:** 708-202-2036; **Board Cert:** Vascular Surgery 2003; **Med School:** Penn State Coll Med 1975; **Resid:** Surgery, Columbia Presby Med Ctr 1980; **Fellow:** Vascular Surgery, Columbia Presby Med Ctr 1981; **Fac Appt:** Prof S, Loyola Univ-Stritch Sch Med

Hodgson, Kim John MD [VascS] - **Spec Exp:** Aneurysm; Carotid Artery Surgery; Endovascular Surgery; **Hospital:** Memorial Med Ctr-Springfield, St. John's Hosp - Springfield; **Address:** 747 N Rutledge Fl 5, Box 19638, Springfield, IL 62702; **Phone:** 217-545-5555; **Board Cert:** Vascular Surgery 2005; **Med School:** Univ Pennsylvania 1981; **Resid:** Surgery, Albany Med Ctr 1986; **Fellow:** Vascular Surgery, Southern Ill Univ 1987; **Fac Appt:** Prof VascS, Southern IL Univ

Kazmers, Andris MD [VascS] - **Spec Exp:** Aneurysm-Abdominal & Thoracic Aortic; Carotid Artery Stent Placement; Angioplasty & Stent Placement; Endovascular Surgery; **Hospital:** Northern Michigan Hosp; **Address:** Petoskey Surgeons, 521 Monroe St, Petoskey, MI 49770; **Phone:** 231-487-1900; **Board Cert:** Vascular Surgery 2005; Surgery 2010; Surgical Critical Care 2010; **Med School:** Wayne State Univ 1976; **Resid:** Surgery, Univ Michigan Hosps 1982; **Fellow:** Vascular Surgery, Univ Michigan Hosps 1984

Kent, Kenneth C MD [VascS] - **Spec Exp:** Carotid Artery Surgery; Aneurysm-Abdominal Aortic; Lower Limb Arterial Disease; **Hospital:** Univ WI Hosp & Clins, Meriter Hosp; **Address:** Univ Wisconsin-Madison, Dept Surgery, H4/710D Clinical Sciences Ctr, 600 Highland Ave, Box 7375, Madison, WI 53792-7375; **Phone:** 608-265-8854; **Board Cert:** Surgery 2007; Vascular Surgery 2008; **Med School:** UCSF 1981; **Resid:** Surgery, UCSF Med Ctr 1986; **Fellow:** Vascular Surgery, Brigham & Women's Hosp 1988; **Fac Appt:** Prof S, Univ Wisc

McLafferty, Robert B MD [VascS] - **Spec Exp:** Minimally Invasive Vascular Surgery; Endovascular Stent Grafts; Carotid Artery Stent Placement; Aneurysm; **Hospital:** Memorial Med Ctr-Springfield, St. John's Hosp - Springfield; **Address:** SIU Surgical Clins, 421 N 9 St, Springfield, IL 62701; **Phone:** 217-545-5555; **Board Cert:** Surgery 2005; Vascular Surgery 2007; **Med School:** Univ VT Coll Med 1990; **Resid:** Surgery, Oregon Hlth Sci Ctr 1996; **Fellow:** Vascular Surgery, Oregon Hlth Sci Ctr 1998; **Fac Appt:** Prof VascS, Southern IL Univ

Pearce, William H MD [VascS] - **Spec Exp:** Aneurysm-Abdominal Aortic; Stroke; Peripheral Vascular Disease; **Hospital:** Northwestern Meml Hosp, Northwestern Lake Forest Hosp; **Address:** Galter Pavilion, 675 N St Clair St, Ste 19-100, Chicago, IL 60611-2647; **Phone:** 312-695-2714; **Board Cert:** Surgery 2010; Vascular Surgery 2003; **Med School:** Univ Colorado 1975; **Resid:** Surgery, Univ Co Hlth Sci Ctr 1981; **Fellow:** Vascular Surgery, Northwestern Meml Hosp 1982; **Fac Appt:** Prof S, Northwestern Univ

Sanchez, Luis A MD [VascS] - **Spec Exp:** Aneurysm-Abdominal & Thoracic Aortic; Endovascular Stent Grafts; Peripheral Vascular Disease; **Hospital:** Barnes-Jewish Hosp, Barnes-Jewish West County Hosp; **Address:** Washington Univ Sch Med, 660 S Euclid Ave, Box 8109, St Louis, MO 63110; **Phone:** 314-362-7408; **Board Cert:** Surgery 2004; Vascular Surgery 2003; **Med School:** Harvard Med Sch 1987; **Resid:** Surgery, Montefiore Med Ctr 1992; **Fellow:** Vascular Surgery, Montefiore Med Ctr 1994; **Fac Appt:** Prof VascS, Washington Univ, St Louis

Vascular Surgery

Shepard, Alexander D MD [VascS] - **Spec Exp:** Aneurysm-Aortic; Aortic Reconstruction; Vascular Surgery-Secondary; **Hospital:** Henry Ford Hosp; **Address:** 2799 W Grand Blvd, Ste K8, Detroit, MI 48202-2608; **Phone:** 313-916-3155; **Board Cert:** Surgery 2001; Vascular Surgery 2005; **Med School:** Johns Hopkins Univ 1976; **Resid:** Surgery, Johns Hopkins Hosp 1982; **Fellow:** Vascular Surgery, New England Med Ctr 1985; **Fac Appt:** Prof S, Wayne State Univ

Sicard, Gregorio A MD [VascS] - **Spec Exp:** Aneurysm-Abdominal Aortic; **Hospital:** Barnes-Jewish Hosp; **Address:** Washington Univ Sch Med, 660 S Euclid Ave, Box 8109, St Louis, MO 63110; **Phone:** 314-362-7841; **Board Cert:** Vascular Surgery 2002; **Med School:** Univ Puerto Rico 1972; **Resid:** Surgery, Barnes Hosp 1977; **Fellow:** Transplant Surgery, Wash Univ Hosp 1978; **Fac Appt:** Prof S, Washington Univ, St Louis

Stanley, James C MD [VascS] - **Spec Exp:** Peripheral Vascular Disease; Renovascular Disease; Aneurysm; **Hospital:** Univ of Michigan Hosp; **Address:** Univ Mich, Dept Vascular Surg, 1500 E Med Ctr Drive, CVC5167 SPC5167, Ann Arbor, MI 48109-5867; **Phone:** 734-936-5820; **Board Cert:** Surgery 1973; Vascular Surgery 2001; **Med School:** Univ Mich Med Sch 1964; **Resid:** Surgery, Univ Mich Med Ctr 1972; **Fac Appt:** Prof S, Univ Mich Med Sch

Great Plains and Mountains

Annest, Stephen J MD [VascS] - **Spec Exp:** Thoracic Outlet Syndrome; **Hospital:** Presby - St Luke's Med Ctr, Exempla Saint Jos. Hosp.-Denver; **Address:** Vascular Inst of The Rockies, 1601 E 19th Ave, Ste 3950, Denver, CO 80218; **Phone:** 303-539-0736; **Board Cert:** Surgery 2000; Vascular Surgery 2005; **Med School:** Univ Wash 1975; **Resid:** Surgery, Albany Med Ctr 1981; **Fellow:** Trauma, Albany Med Ctr 1980; Vascular Surgery, Baylor Univ Med Ctr 1982

Cooper, Michael A MD [VascS] - **Spec Exp:** Peripheral Vascular Disease; **Hospital:** Rose Med Ctr; **Address:** Colorado Cardiovascular Surgical Assocs, 4600 E Hale Pkwy, Ste 460, Denver, CO 80220; **Phone:** 303-388-7265; **Board Cert:** Surgery 2008; Vascular Surgery 2001; **Med School:** Univ Nebr Coll Med 1984; **Resid:** Surgery, Univ Kansas Med Ctr 1989; **Fellow:** Vascular Surgery, LSU Med Ctr 1992

Howard, Thomas C MD [VascS] - **Spec Exp:** Aortic Surgery; Aneurysm-Aortic; Carotid Artery Surgery; Lower Limb Arterial Disease; **Hospital:** Nebraska Med Ctr; **Address:** Surgery Ctr of the Heartland, 4242 Farnam St, Ste 490, Omaha, NE 68131; **Phone:** 402-552-3015; **Board Cert:** Surgery 1975; Vascular Surgery 2002; **Med School:** Yale Univ 1969; **Resid:** Surgery, Yale-New Haven Hosp 1974; **Fac Appt:** Assoc Prof S, Univ Nebr Coll Med

Weinstein, Eric S MD [VascS] - **Spec Exp:** Endovascular Surgery; Aneurysm-Abdominal Aortic; **Hospital:** Porter Adventist Hosp; **Address:** Colorado Cardiovascular Surgical Assocs, 950 E Harvard Ave, Ste 550, Denver, CO 80210; **Phone:** 303-778-6257; **Board Cert:** Vascular Surgery 2009; **Med School:** SUNY Buffalo 1981; **Resid:** Surgery, Case Western Reserve Univ 1988; **Fellow:** Research, Case Western Reserve Univ 1985; Vascular Surgery, UCSF Med Ctr 1999

Southwest

Blebea, John MD [VascS] - **Spec Exp:** Endovascular Surgery; Radiofrequency Tumor Ablation; **Address:** Univ OK Sch MedTulsa, Dept Surgery, 4502 E 41st St, Tulsa, OK 74135; **Phone:** 918-744-3523; **Board Cert:** Vascular Surgery 2000; **Med School:** Case West Res Univ 1982; **Resid:** Surgery, Georgetown Univ Hosp 1985; Vascular Surgery, UMDNJ 1986; **Fellow:** Vascular Surgery, Univ Rochester 1991; Endovascular Surgery, UPMC 2001; **Fac Appt:** Prof S, Case West Res Univ

Eidt, John F MD [VascS] - **Spec Exp:** Aneurysm-Abdominal Aortic; Carotid Artery Stent Placement; Endovascular Surgery; Peripheral Vascular Disease; **Hospital:** UAMS Med Ctr; **Address:** 4301 W Markham St, Slot 520-2, Little Rock, AR 72205; **Phone:** 501-686-6176; **Board Cert:** Surgery 2004; Vascular Surgery 2006; **Med School:** Univ Tex SW, Dallas 1981; **Resid:** Surgery, Brigham-Womens Hosp 1986; **Fellow:** Vascular Surgery, Univ Tex SW Med Ctr 1988; **Fac Appt:** Prof S, Univ Ark

Fowl, Richard J MD [VascS] - **Spec Exp:** Aneurysm-Aortic; Carotid Artery Surgery; Arterial Bypass Surgery-Leg; Endovascular Surgery; **Hospital:** Mayo Clinic - Phoenix; **Address:** Mayo Clinic, Dept Vascular Surgery, 5779 E Mayo Blvd, Phoenix, AZ 85054; **Phone:** 480-342-2868; **Board Cert:** Surgery 2011; Vascular Surgery 2004; **Med School:** Rush Med Coll 1978; **Resid:** Surgery, MCV Affil Hosp 1980; Surgery, Univ Iowa Med Ctr 1983; **Fellow:** Vascular Surgery, Mayo Clinic 1985; Endovascular Surgery, Cornell-Weill Med Coll 2004; **Fac Appt:** Prof S, Mayo Med Sch

Hollier, Larry H MD [VascS] - **Spec Exp:** Aortic Surgery; Carotid Artery Surgery; Endovascular Surgery; Aneurysm; **Hospital:** West Jefferson Med Ctr, LSU Interim Public Hosp; **Address:** 433 Bolivar St, Ste 815, New Orleans, LA 70112; **Phone:** 504-568-4800; **Board Cert:** Surgery 2007; Vascular Surgery 2001; **Med School:** Louisiana State U, New Orleans 1968; **Resid:** Surgery, Charity Hosp 1973; **Fellow:** Vascular Surgery, Baylor Med Ctr 1974; **Fac Appt:** Prof S, Louisiana State U, New Orleans

Kougias, Panagiotis MD [VascS] - **Spec Exp:** Vascular Reconstruction; Carotid Artery Surgery; Stroke; Endovascular Surgery; **Hospital:** St. Luke's Episcopal Hosp-Houston, DeBakey VA Med Ctr-Houston; **Address:** M DeBakey VA Med Ctr, 2002 Holcombe Blvd, Houston, TX 77030; **Phone:** 713-791-1414; **Board Cert:** Surgery 2005; Vascular Surgery 2007; **Med School:** Greece 1992; **Resid:** Surgery, E Tenn State Affil Hosp 2004; **Fellow:** Vascular Surgery, Baylor Coll Med 2006; **Fac Appt:** Asst Prof VascS, Baylor Coll Med

Lumsden, Alan B MD [VascS] - **Spec Exp:** Aortic Stent Grafts; Minimally Invasive Surgery; Vein Disorders; **Hospital:** Methodist Hosp - Houston; **Address:** 6550 Fannin St, Ste 1401, Smith Tower, Houston, TX 77030; **Phone:** 713-441-5200; **Board Cert:** Vascular Surgery 2002; **Med School:** Scotland, UK 1981; **Resid:** Surgery, Emory Univ Hosp 1987; **Fellow:** Vascular Surgery, Emory Univ Hosp 1989; **Fac Appt:** Prof VascS, Baylor Coll Med

Money, Samuel R MD [VascS] - **Spec Exp:** Aneurysm-Abdominal Aortic; Arterial Bypass Surgery-Leg; Endovascular Surgery; Aneurysm; **Hospital:** Mayo Clinic - Phoenix; **Address:** Mayo Clinic, Dept Vascular Surgery, 5779 E Mayo Blvd, Phoenix, AZ 85054; **Phone:** 480-342-2868; **Board Cert:** Surgery 2000; Vascular Surgery 2002; **Med School:** SUNY Downstate 1983; **Resid:** Surgery, Kings Co Med Ctr 1990; **Fellow:** Vascular Surgery, Ochsner Clinic 1993; **Fac Appt:** Prof S, Mayo Med Sch

West Coast and Pacific

Ahn, Sam S MD [VascS] - **Spec Exp:** Minimally Invasive Vascular Surgery; Endovascular Surgery; Thoracic Outlet Syndrome; Hyperhidrosis; **Hospital:** UCLA Ronald Reagan Med Ctr, St. John's Hlth Ctr, Santa Monica; **Address:** 1082 Glendon Ave, Los Angeles, CA 90024; **Phone:** 310-209-2011 x3; **Board Cert:** Surgery 2004; Vascular Surgery 2008; **Med School:** Univ Tex SW, Dallas 1978; **Resid:** Surgery, UCLA Med Ctr 1984; **Fellow:** Vascular Surgery, UCLA Med Ctr 1986; **Fac Appt:** Prof S, UCLA

Bandyk, Dennis F MD [VascS] - **Spec Exp:** Endovascular Stent Grafts; Lower Limb Arterial Disease; Thoracic Outlet Syndrome; **Hospital:** UCSD Med Ctr; **Address:** 9434 Medical Center Drive, MC 7241, La Jolla, CA 92037; **Phone:** 619-543-6980; **Board Cert:** Vascular Surgery 2001; **Med School:** Univ Mich Med Sch 1975; **Resid:** Surgery, Univ Wash Hosp 1980; **Fellow:** Vascular Surgery, Univ Wash Hosp 1981; **Fac Appt:** Prof S, Univ S Fla Coll Med

Flanigan, D Preston MD [VascS] - **Spec Exp:** Carotid Artery Surgery; Aneurysm; Vein Disorders; Minimally Invasive Surgery; **Hospital:** St. Joseph's Hosp - Orange; **Address:** 1140 W LaVeta Ave, Ste 850, Orange, CA 92868; **Phone:** 714-560-4450; **Board Cert:** Vascular Surgery 2011; **Med School:** Jefferson Med Coll 1972; **Resid:** Surgery, St Joseph-Mercy Hosp 1977; **Fellow:** Vascular Surgery, Northwest Med Ctr 1978; **Fac Appt:** Clin Prof S, UC Irvine

Gewertz, Bruce MD [VascS] - **Spec Exp:** Carotid Artery Surgery; Peripheral Vascular Disease; Aneurysm-Aortic; Renovascular Disease; **Hospital:** Cedars-Sinai Med Ctr; **Address:** 8700 Beverly Blvd, N Tower, Ste 8215, Los Angeles, CA 90048; **Phone:** 310-423-5884; **Board Cert:** Vascular Surgery 2002; **Med School:** Jefferson Med Coll 1972; **Resid:** Surgery, Univ Mich Hosp 1977; **Fac Appt:** Prof S, UCLA

Pevec, William C MD [VascS] - **Spec Exp:** Vascular Disease; Aortic Reconstruction; Endovascular Surgery; **Hospital:** UC Davis Med Ctr; **Address:** UC Davis Vascular Center, 4860 Y St, Ste 2100, Sacramento, CA 95817; **Phone:** 916-734-3800; **Board Cert:** Surgery 1999; Vascular Surgery 2001; **Med School:** Univ Cincinnati 1984; **Resid:** Surgery, Univ Pittsburgh Med Ctr 1990; **Fellow:** Vascular Surgery, Mass Genl Hosp 1992; **Fac Appt:** Prof VascS, UC Davis

Sobel, Michael MD [VascS] - **Spec Exp:** Vein Disorders; **Hospital:** Univ Wash Med Ctr, VA Puget Sound Hlth Care Sys; **Address:** East Side Specialty Center, 1700 116th Ave NE, Bellevue, WA 98004; **Phone:** 425-646-7777; **Board Cert:** Surgery 2002; Vascular Surgery 2008; **Med School:** Albert Einstein Coll Med 1975; **Resid:** Surgery, Beth Israel Hosp 1982; **Fellow:** Vascular Surgery, NYU Med Ctr 1983; **Fac Appt:** Prof VascS, Univ Wash

White, Rodney A MD [VascS] - **Spec Exp:** Aneurysm; Carotid Artery Surgery; Aortic Surgery-Complex; Endovascular Surgery; **Hospital:** LAC - Harbor - UCLA Med Ctr; **Address:** Harbor-UCLA Med Ctr, 1000 W Carson St, Box 11, Torrance, CA 90502; **Phone:** 310-222-2704; **Board Cert:** Vascular Surgery 2006; **Med School:** SUNY Upstate Med Univ 1974; **Resid:** Surgery, LAC-Harbor-UCLA Med Ctr 1979; **Fellow:** Vascular Surgery, LAC-Harbor-UCLA Med Ctr 1980; **Fac Appt:** Prof S, UCLA

Zarins, Christopher K MD [VascS] - **Spec Exp:** Carotid Artery Surgery; Aneurysm-Abdominal Aortic; Endovascular Surgery; **Hospital:** El Camino Hosp; **Address:** Stanford Univ Vascular Surgery, 300 Pasteur Drive, rm H-3600, MC 5642, Palo Alto, CA 94301; **Phone:** 650-725-5227; **Board Cert:** Surgery 1975; Vascular Surgery 2002; **Med School:** Johns Hopkins Univ 1968; **Resid:** Surgery, Univ Michigan Hosp 1974; **Fellow:** Surgery, Johns Hopkins Hosp 1972; **Fac Appt:** Prof Emeritus S, Stanford Univ

NYU Langone
MEDICAL CENTER

CARDIAC AND VASCULAR INSTITUTE
550 First Avenue *(at 31st Street)*
New York, NY 10016
www.NYULMC.org
Physician Referral: **888-7-NYU-MED** *(888-769-8633)*

VASCULAR SURGERY

Staffed by one of the largest vascular surgery teams in the country, NYU Langone Medical Center emphasizes both expert patient care and minimally invasive therapies. Physicians have extensive experience performing the most advanced procedures, including stents and angioplasty for carotid artery disease, aortic aneurysm repair and the repair and removal of blockages in arteries throughout the body. In addition to its expertise in arterial disease, NYU Langone is proud to offer one of the few academic Vein Centers in the United States. We specialize in the following areas:

Aortic Pathology
The Medical Center offers minimally invasive surgical solutions as well as treatments for complex aortic problems. Patients usually require no blood transfusions and are able to leave the hospital one or two days after surgery. We are also a training center for endovascular management of abdominal and thoracic aneurysms.

Carotid Artery Disease
NYU Langone remains a leader in both the screening for carotid disease and the prevention of stroke in patients being treated for carotid artery occlusive disease. Our physicians helped pioneer carotid endarterectomy as an open surgical procedure, and played a pivotal role in the development of carotid stenting.

Peripheral Arterial Disease
Vascular surgeons at the Medical Center draw on a wealth of experience in treating peripheral arterial disease (PAD). The team specializes in new and innovative technologies such as laser and "Silverhawk" atherectomy procedures, as well as cryoplasty. Additionally, we offer drug-eluting stents, which are coated with special medicines to prevent scar formation and reocclusion of the stent.

Vascular Screenings
Our physicians are committed to improving public awareness and understanding of vascular disease through preventative screenings. Vascular disease is among the leading causes of death in the U.S., yet is generally asymptomatic until a stroke or aneurysm occurs. Effective screening techniques include ultrasound scans of the aorta, ultrasound scans of the carotid arteries, and advanced blood pressure measurements.

Venous Disease
The Vein Center at NYU Langone is considered an authority in the minimally invasive treatment of venous disease. The Center treats patients with all forms of venous pathology, from venous insufficiency and varicose veins to occlusive disease and deep vein thrombosis.

Appendices

The Best in American Medicine
www.CastleConnolly.com

APPENDIX A:
Medical Boards

Introduction to ABMS and Osteopathic Specialties

The following pages contain descriptions of the "official" medical specialties, approved by the American Board of Medical Specialists (for M.D.s) or by the American Osteopathic Association (for D.O.s). These are important because they are the only specialties recognized by the official governing boards. There may be physicians who call themselves one kind of specialist or another, but they may not be certified by the "official" boards. There are, in fact, over 100 such "self-designated" boards, some simply groups of physicians interested in a given area of medicine with no qualifications for membership to other groups with very specific qualifications for membership.

It is important for the medical consumer to seek out physicians certified by the ABMS or AOA to assure their doctor has had the appropriate training and passed the board certification exam.

ABMS

The ABMS is an organization of ABMS Approved medical specialty boards. The mission of the ABMS is to maintain and improve the quality of medical care by assisting the Member Boards in their efforts to develop and utilize professional and educational standards for the evaluation and certification of physician specialists. The intent of certification of physicians is to provide assurance to the public that a physician specialist certified by a Member Board of the ABMS has successfully completed an approved educational program and evaluation process which includes an examination designed to assess the knowledge, skills, and experience required to provide quality patient care in that specialty. The ABMS serves to coordinate the activities of its Member Boards and to provide information to the public, the government, the profession and its Members concerning issues involving specialization and certification in medicine.

Following is a list of the addresses of the various medical specialty boards approved by the ABMS. Note that there are 24 board organizations for 25 medical specialties. Psychiatry and Neurology share the same board.

To find out if a physician is certified, consumers can call the individual boards which may charge a fee for the information, or they can contact the ABMS at (866) 275-2267 (no fee) or www.abms.org.

American Board of Allergy and Immunology

111 S Independence Mall E, Ste 701
Philadelphia, PA 19106
(215) 592-9466, (866) 264-5568

General Certification in Allergy and Immunology. Certifications awarded since 1989 are valid for 10 years. For those certified prior to 1989 there is no recertification requirement.

American Board of Anesthesiology

4208 Six Forks Rd, Ste 900
Raleigh, NC 27609-5735
(919) 745-2200

General Certification in Anesthesiology; with Special and Added Qualifications in Critical Care Medicine, Hospice & Palliative Medicine, Pain Medicine, Pediatric Anesthesiology and Sleep Medicine. Certifications awarded since 2000 are valid for 10 years.

American Board of Colon and Rectal Surgery

20600 Eureka Road, Suite 600
Taylor, MI 48180
(734) 282-9400

General Certification is in Colon and Rectal Surgery. Certifications awarded since 1990 are valid for 10 years.

American Board of Dermatology

Henry Ford Health System
1 Ford Place
Detroit, MI 48202-3450
(313) 874-1088

General Certification in Dermatology; with Special Qualifications Dermatopathology, and Pediatric Dermatology. Certifications awarded since 1991 are valid for 10 years.

American Board of Emergency Medicine

3000 Coolidge Road
East Lansing, MI 48823-6319
(517) 332-4800

General Certification in Emergency Medicine; with Special and Added Qualifications in Critical Care Medicine, Emergency Medical Services, Hospice & Palliative Medicine, Medical Toxicology, Pediatric Emergency Medicine, Sports Medicine and Undersea and Hyperbaric Medicine. Certifications awarded since 1980 are valid for 10 years

American Board of Family Medicine
1648 McGranthiana Pkwy, FL 5
Lexington, KY 40511
(859) 269-5626, (888) 995-5700

General Certification in Family Practice; with Added Qualifications in Adolescent
Medicine, Geriatric Medicine, Hospice & Palliative Medicine, Sleep Medicine and Sports
Medicine. Certifications awarded since 1970 are valid for 7 years.

American Board of Internal Medicine
510 Walnut Street, Suite 1700
Philadelphia, PA 19106-3699
(215) 446-3500, (800) 441-ABIM

General Certification in Internal Medicine; with Special Qualifications in Cardiovascular
Disease, Endocrinology, Diabetes and Metabolism, Gastroenterology, Hematology,
Infectious Disease, Medical Oncology, Nephrology, Pulmonary Disease, and
Rheumatology; and Added Qualifications in Advanced Heart Failure & Transplant
Cardiology, Adolescent Medicine, Clinical Cardiac Electrophysiology, Critical Care
Medicine, Geriatric Medicine, Hospice and Palliative Medicine, Interventional
Cardiology, Sleep Medicine, Sports Medicine and Transplant Hepatology. Certifications
awarded since 1990 are valid for 10 years.

American Board of Medical Genetics
9650 Rockville Pike
Bethesda, MD 20814-3998
(301) 634-7315

General Certification in Clinical Genetics (MD), Clinical Biochemical Genetics, Clinical
Cytogenetics and Clinical Molecular Genetics; with Added Qualifications in Medical
Biochemical Genetics and Molecular Genetic Pathology. Certifications awarded since
2002 are valid for 2 years.

American Board of Neurological Surgery
6550 Fannin Street, Suite 2139
Houston, TX 77030-2701
(713) 441-6015

General Certification in Neurological Surgery. Certifications awarded since 1999 are
valid for 10 years.

American Board of Nuclear Medicine
4555 Forest Park Boulevard, Suite 119
St. Louis, MO 63108
(314) 367-2225

General Certification in Nuclear Medicine. Certifications awarded since 1992 are valid for 10 years.

American Board of Obstetrics and Gynecology
2915 Vine Street, Suite 300
Dallas, TX 75204
(214) 871-1619

General Certification in Obstetrics and Gynecology; with Special Qualifications in Gynecologic Oncology, Maternal and Fetal Medicine, Reproductive Endocrinology/Infertility; and Added Qualifications in Critical Care Medicine, Female Pelvic Medicine and Reconstructive Surgery, and Hospice & Palliative Medicine. Certifications awarded since 1986 are valid for 6 years.

American Board of Ophthalmology
111 Presidential Boulevard, Suite 241
Bala Cynwyd, PA 19004-1075
(610) 664-1175

Certifications Awarded since 1992 are valid for 10 years. For those certified prior to 1992, there is no recertification requirement.

American Board of Orthopaedic Surgery
400 Silver Cedar Court
Chapel Hill, NC 27514
(919) 929-7103

General Certification in Orthopaedic Surgery; with Added Qualification in Hand Surgery; with Added Qualifications in Hand Surgery and Orthopaedic Sports Medicine. Certifications awarded since 1986 are valid for 10 years.

American Board of Otolaryngology
5615 Kirby Drive, Suite 600
Houston, TX 77005
(713) 850-0399

General Certification in Otolaryngology; with Added Qualifications in Neurotology, Pediatric Otolaryngology, Plastic Surgery within the Head and Neck and Sleep Medicine. Certifications awarded since 2002 are valid for 10 years.

American Board of Pathology
P.O. Box 25915
Tampa, FL 33622-5915
(813) 286-2444

General Certification in Anatomic and Clinical Pathology, Anatomic Pathology and Clinical Pathology; with Special Qualifications in Blood Banking/Transfusion Medicine, Chemical Pathology, Clinical Informatics, Dermatopathology, Forensic Pathology, Hematology, Medical Microbiology, Molecular Genetic Pathology, Neuropathology and Pediatric Pathology; and Added Qualifications in Cytopathology. Certifications awarded since 1997 are valid for 10 years.

American Board of Pediatrics
111 Silver Cedar Court
Chapel Hill, NC 27514-1651
(919) 929-0461

General Certification in Pediatrics; with Special Qualifications in Adolescent Medicine, Developmental-Behavioral Pediatrics, Neonatal-Perinatal Medicine, Pediatric Cardiology, Pediatric Critical Care Medicine, Pediatric Emergency Medicine, Pediatric Endocrinology, Pediatric Gastroenterology, Pediatric Hematology-Oncology, Pediatric Infectious Diseases, Pediatric Nephrology, Pediatric Pulmonology, and Pediatric Rheumatology; and Added Qualifications in Child Abuse Pediatrics, Medical Toxicology, Neurodevelopmental Disabilities, Pediatric Transplant Hepatology, Sleep Medicine and Sports Medicine. Certifications awarded since 1988 valid for 7 years.

American Board of Physical Medicine and Rehabilitation
3015 Allegro Park Lane, S.W.
Rochester, MN 55902-4139
(507) 282-1776

General Certification in Physical Medicine and Rehabilitation; with Special Qualifications in Brain Injury Medicine, Hospice & Palliative Medicine, Neuromuscular Medicine, Pain Medicine, Pediatric Rehabilitation Medicine, Spinal Cord Injury Medicine and Sports Medicine. Certifications awarded since 1993 are valid for 10 years.

American Board of Plastic Surgery
Seven Penn Center, Suite 400
1635 Market Street
Philadelphia, PA 19103
(215) 587-9322

General Certification in Plastic Surgery; with Added Qualifications in Hand Surgery and Plastic Surgery within the Head & Neck. Certifications awarded since 1995 are valid for a 10-year period.

American Board of Preventive Medicine
111 W Jackson, Ste 1110
Chicago, IL 60604
(312) 939-ABPM [2276]

General Certification in Aerospace Medicine, Occupational Medicine and Public Health and General Preventive Medicine; with Added Qualifications in Clinical Informatics, Undersea and Hyperbaric Medicine and Medical Toxicology. Certifications awarded since 1997 are valid for 10 years.

American Board of Psychiatry and Neurology
2150 E Lake Cook Rd, Ste 900
Buffalo Grove, IL 60089
(847) 229-6500

General Certification in Psychiatry, Neurology and Neurology with Special Qualification in Child Neurology; with Special Qualifications in Child and Adolescent Psychiatry, Epilepsy, Hospice & Palliative Medicine, Pain Medicine and Sleep Medicine; and Added Qualifications in Addiction Psychiatry, Brain Injury Medicine, Clinical Neurophysiology, Forensic Psychiatry, Geriatric Psychiatry, Neurodevelopmental Disabilities, Neuromuscular Medicine, Psychosomatic Medicine and Vascular Neurology . Certifications awarded since 1994 are valid for 10 years.

American Board of Radiology
5441 E. Williams Boulevard, Suite 200
Tucson, AZ 85711
(520) 790-2900

General Certification in Diagnostic Radiology, Medical Physics and Radiation Oncology; with Special Competency in Nuclear Radiology; and Added Qualifications in Hospice & Palliative Medicine, Neuroradiology, Nuclear Radiology, Pediatric Radiology and Vascular and Interventional Radiology. Radiological Physics is a non-clinical certification. Certificates are valid for 10 years.

American Board of Surgery
1617 John F. Kennedy Boulevard, Suite 860
Philadelphia, PA 19103-1847
(215) 568-4000

General Certification in Surgery and Vascular Surgery; with Special Qualifications in Pediatric Surgery and Surgery of the Hand; and Added Qualifications in Complex Surgical Oncology, Hospice & Palliative Medicine and Surgical Critical Care. Certifications awarded since 1976 are valid for 10 years.

American Board of Thoracic Surgery
633 North St. Clair Street, Suite 2320
Chicago, IL 60611
(312 202-5900

General Certification in Thoracic and Cardiac Surgery; with Special Qualifications in Congenital Cardiac Surgey. Certifications awarded since 1976 are valid for 10 years and Added Qualifications in Congenital Cardiac Surgery.

American Board of Urology
600 Peter Jefferson Pkwy, Ste 150
Charlottesville, VA 22911
(434) 979-0059

General Certification in Urology; with Special Qualifications in Pediatric Urology and Female Pelvic Medicine & Reconstructive Surgery. Certifications awarded as of 1985 are valid for 10 years with Special Qualifications in Pediatric Urology.

Osteopathic

The American Osteopathic Association (AOA) is a member association representing more than 78,000 osteopathic physicians (D.O.s). The AOA serves as the primary certifying body for D.O.s, and is the accrediting agency for all osetopathic medical colleges and health care facilities. The AOA's mission is to advance the philosophy and practice of osteopathic medicine by promoting excellence in education, research, and the delivery of quality, cost-effective healthcare within a distinct, unified profession. American Osteopathic Association 142 E Ontario Street Chicago, IL 60611.

Consumers may call the American Osteopathic Association at (800) 621-1773 or visit the website, www.osteopathic.org, for general certification information.

American Osteopathic Board of Anesthesiology

General certification in Anesthesiology; with Added Qualifications in Critical Care Medicine, and Pain Management. Certifications awarded since 2004 are valid for 10 years. For those certified prior to 2004 there is no recertification requirement.

American Osteopathic Board of Dermatology

General certification in Dermatology; with Added Qualifications in Dermatopathology and MOHS-Micrographic Surgery. Certifications awarded since 2004 are valid for 10 years.

American Osteopathic Board of Emergency Medicine

General certification in Emergency Medicine; with Added Qualifications in Emergency Medical Services, Medical Toxicology, and Sports Medicine. Certifications awarded since 1994 are valid for 10 years.

American Osteopathic Board of Family Physicians

General certification in Family Practice and Osteopathic Manipulative Treatment (OMT); with Added Qualifications in Adolescent Medicine, Geriatric Medicine, Sports Medicine, Hospice & Palliative Medicine, Sleep Medicine and Undersea & Hyperbaric Medicine. Certifications awarded since March 1,1997 are valid for 8 years.

American Osteopathic Board of Internal Medicine

General certification in Internal Medicine; with Special Qualifications in Allergy/Immunology, Cardiology, Endocrinology, Gastroenterology, Hematology, Infectious Disease, Nephrology, Oncology, Pulmonary Disease, Rheumatology; with Added Qualifications in Addiction Medicine, Critical Care Medicine, Clinical Cardiac Electrophysiology, Geriatric Medicine, Hospice & Palliative Medicine, Interventional Cardiology, Sleep Medicine, Sports Medicine and Undersea & Hyperbaric Medicine. Certifications awarded since 1993 are valid for 10 years.

American Osteopathic Board of Neurology and Psychiatry

General certification in Neurology and Psychiatry; with Special Qualifications in Child/Adolescent Psychiatry and Child/Adolescent Neurology; with Added Qualifications in Addiction Medicine, Geriatric Psychiatry, Hospice & Palliative Medicine, Neurophysiology and Sleep Medicine. Certifications awarded since 1995 are valid for 10 years.

American Osteopathic Board of Neuromusculoskeletal Medicine

(Formerly American Osteopathic Board of Special Proficiency in Osteopathic Manipulative Medicine)

General certification in Neuromusculoskeletal Medicine & Osteopathic Manipulative Medicine with Added Qualifications in Sports Medicine. Certifications awarded since 1995 are valid for 10 years. For those certified prior to 1995 there is no recertification requirement.

American Osteopathic Board of Nuclear Medicine

General certification in Nuclear Medicine. Certifications awarded since 1995 are valid for 10 years

American Osteopathic Board of Obstetrics and Gynecology

General certification in Obstetrics and Gynecology; with Special Qualifications in Gynecologic Oncology; Maternal and Fetal Medicine and Reproductive Endocrinology. Certifications awarded since June, 2002 are valid for 6 years.

American Osteopathic Board of Ophthalmology and Otolaryngology

General certification in Ophthalmology, Otolaryngolgy and Otolaryngology/Facial Plastic Surgery; with Added Qualifications in Otolaryngic Allergy and Sleep Medicine. Certifications awarded in Ophthalmology since 2000 are valid for 10 years. For those certified prior to 2000 there is no recertification requirement. Certifications awarded in Otolaryngology and/or Otolaryngology/Facial Plastic Surgery since 2002 are valid for 10 years.

American Osteopathic Board of Orthopaedic Surgery

General certification in Orthopaedic Surgery; with Added Qualifications in Hand Surgery. Certifications awarded since 1994 are valid for 10 years.

American Osteopathic Board of Pathology

General certification in Laboratory Medicine, Anatomic Pathology and Anatomic Pathology and Laboratory Medicine; with Special Qualifications in Forensic Pathology; and with Added Qualifications in Dermatopathology. Certifications awarded since 1995 are valid for 10 years.

American Osteopathic Board of Pediatrics

General certification in Pediatrics with Special Qualifications in Adolescent and Young Adult Medicine, Neonatology, Pediatric Allergy/Immunology and Pediatric Endocrinology; with Added Qualifications in Sports Medicine. Certifications awarded since 1995 valid for 7 years.

American Osteopathic Board of Physical Medicine and Rehabilitation Medicine

General certification in Physical Medicine and Rehabilitation; with Added Qualifications in Hospice & Palliative Medicine and Sports Medicine. Certifications awarded since 2004 are valid for 10 years.

American Osteopathic Board of Preventive Medicine

General certification in Preventive Medicine/Aerospace Medicine, Preventive Medicine/Occupational-Environmental Medicine and Preventive Medicine/Public Health; with Added Qualifications in Occupational Medicine and Undersea & Hyperbaric Medicine. Certifications awarded since 1994 are valid for 10 years.

American Osteopathic Board of Proctology

General certification in Proctology. Certifications awarded since 2004 are valid for 10 years.

Appendix A: Medical Boards

American Osteopathic Board of Radiology

General certification in Diagnostic Radiology and Radiation Oncology; with Added Qualifications in Angiography and Interventional Radiology, Diagnostic Ultrasound and Pediatric Radiology. Certifications awarded since 2002 are valid for 10 years.

American Osteopathic Board of Surgery

General certification in Surgery, Neurological Surgery, Plastic and Reconstructive Surgery, Thoracic Cardiovascular Surgery, Urological Surgery and General Vascular Surgery; with Added Qualifications in Surgical Critical Care. Certifications awarded since 1997 are valid for 10 years.

Appendix B:
Self-Designated Medical Specialties

This list of self-designated medical specialty groups was obtained from the American Board of Medical Specialties. However, it is important to point out that these groups are not recognized by the ABMS, the governing board for the recognized twenty-four medical specialty boards (listed in Appendix A).

The organizations listed below range from highly organized groups that are attempting to formalize training and certification in their field to informal groups interested in a particular aspect of medicine.

If you wish to obtain information from any of these groups you will have to do some detective work. Because so many are informal, the location, phone and mailing addresses change frequently, depending upon the person who is functioning as secretary or administrator.

The best way to track down one of these groups is to consult the doctor listings to find a doctor who has expressed a special interest in that field, and call his or her office. You might also call a nearby academic health center in the area to see if they have a faculty or staff member known to be involved in that particular medical interest. If that fails, take the same approach with your community hospital.

A

Abdominal Surgeons
Acupuncture Medicine
Addiction Medicine
Addictionology
Adolescent Psychiatry
Aesthetic Plastic Surgery
Alcoholism and Other Drug
 Dependencies (AMSAODD)
Algology (Chronic Pain)
Alternative Medicine
Ambulatory Anesthesia
Ambulatory Foot Surgery
Anesthesia
Arthroscopic Surgery
Arthroscopy (Board of North America)

B

Bariatric Medicine
Bionic Psychology
Bloodless Medicine & Surgery

C

Chelation Therapy
Chemical Dependence
Clinical Chemistry
Clinical Ecology
Clinical Medicine and Surgery
Clinical Neurology
Clinical Neurophysiology
Clinical Neurosurgery
Clinical Nutrition
Clinical Orthopaedic Surgery
Clinical Pharmacology
Clinical Polysomnography
Clinical Psychiatry
Clinical Psychology
Clinical Toxicology
Cosmetic Plastic Surgery
Cosmetic Surgery
Council of Non-Board Certified Physicians
Critical Care in Medicine & Surgery

D

Disability Analysis
Disability Evaluating Physicians

E

Electrodiagnostic Medicine
Electroencephalography
Electromyography & Electrodiagnosis
Environmental Medicine
Epidemiology (College)
Eye Surgery

F

Facial Cosmetic Surgery
Facial Plastic & Reconstructive Surgery
Family Practice, Certification
Forensic Examiners
Forensic Psychiatry
Forensic Toxicology

H

Hand Surgery
Head, Facial & Neck Pain & TMJ Orthopaedics
Health Physics
Homeopathic Physicians
Homeotherapeutics
Hypnotic Anesthesiology, National Board for

I

Independent Medical Examiners
Industrial Medicine & Surgery
Insurance Medicine
International Cosmetic & Plastic
 Facial Reconstructive Standards
Interventional Radiology

L

Laser Surgery
Law in Medicine
Longevity Medicine/Surgery

M

Malpractice Physicians
Maxillofacial Surgeons
Medical Accreditation (American Federation for)
Medical Hypnosis
Medical Laboratory Immunology
Medical-Legal Analysis of Medicine & Surgery
Medical Legal & Workers
 Comp. Medicine & Surgery
Medical-Legal Consultants
Medical Management
Medical Microbiology
Medical Preventics (Academy)
Medical Psychotherapists
Medical Toxicology
Microbiology (Medical Microbiology)
Military Medicine
Mohs Micrographic Surgery &
 Cutaneous Oncology

N

Neuroimaging
Neurologic & Orthopaedic Dental
 Medicine and Surgery
Neurological & Orthopaedic Medicine
Neurological & Orthopaedic Surgery
Neurological Microsurgery
Neurology
Neuromuscular Thermography
Neuro-Orthopaedic Dental Medicine
Neuro-Orthopaedic Electrodiagnosis
Neuro-Orthopaedic Laser Surgery
Neuro-Orthopaedic Psychiatry
Neuro-Orthopaedic Thoracic Medicine
Neurorehabilitation
Nutrition

O

Orthopaedic Medicine
Orthopaedic Microneurosurgery
Otorhinolaryngology

P

Pain Management (American Academy of)
Pain Management Specialties
Pain Medicine
Palliative Medicine
Percutaneous Diskectomy
Plastic Esthetic Surgeons
Prison Medicine
Professional Disability Consultants Psychiatric
 Medicine
Psychiatry (American National Board of)
Psychoanalysis (American Examining
 Board in)
Psychological Medicine (International)

Q

Quality Assurance & Utilization Review

R

Radiology & Medical Imaging
Rheumatologic Surgery
Rheumatological & Reconstructive Medicine
Ringside Medicine & Surgery

S

Skin Specialists
Sleep Medicine (Polysomnography)
Spinal Cord Injury
Spinal Surgery
Sports Medicine
Sports Medicine/Surgery

T

Toxicology
Trauma Surgery
Traumatologic Medicine & Surgery
Tropical Medicine

U

Ultrasound Technology
Urologic Allied Health Professionals
Urological Surgery

W

Weight Reduction Medicine

APPENDIX C:
Hospital Listings

The following is an alphabetical listing of all hospitals that have at least one Castle Connolly Top Doctor in this guide. Institutions listed in **Bold** are profiled in this Guide in association with Castle Connolly's *Partnership for Excellence* program. The abbreviations as they appear in the listings are in italics below. Due to the many changes taking place in the hospital industry, the names on this list may have changed subsequent to publication of this guide.

Abbott - Northwestern Hospital		(612) 863-4000
Abbott - Northwestern Hosp		
800 E 28th St	Minneapolis, MN 55407	MIDWEST
Abington Memorial Hospital		(215) 481-2000
Abington Mem Hosp		
1200 Old York Rd	Abington, PA 19001	MID ATLANTIC
Adventist Hinsdale Hospital		(630) 856-9000
Adventist Hinsdale Hosp		
120 N Oak St	Hinsdale, IL 60521	MIDWEST
Advocate Christ Medical Center		(708) 684-8000
Adv Christ Med Ctr		
4440 W 95th St	Oak Lawn, IL 60453	MIDWEST
Advocate Good Samaritan Hospital		(630) 275-5900
Adv Good Samaritan Hosp		
3815 Highland Ave	Downers Grove, IL 60515	MIDWEST
Advocate Illinois Masonic Medical Center		(773) 975-1600
Adv Illinois Masonic Med Ctr		
836 W Wellington Ave	Chicago, IL 60657-5147	MIDWEST
Advocate Lutheran General Hospital		(847) 723-2210
Adv Luth Genl Hosp		
1775 Dempster St	Park Ridge, IL 60068	MIDWEST
Akron Children's Hospital		(330) 543-1000
Akron Children's Hosp		
One Perkins Square	Akron, OH 44308	MIDWEST
Alamance Regional Med Ctr		(336) 538-7000
Alamance Regl Med Ctr		
1240 Huffman Mill Rd	Burlington, NC 27215	SOUTHEAST

Alameda County Medical Center-Highland Campus (510) 437-4800
Alameda County Med Ctr-Highland Campus
1411 E 31st St Oakland, CA 94602 WEST COAST AND PACIFIC

Albany Medical Center (518) 262-3125
Albany Med Ctr
43 New Scotland Ave Albany, NY 12208 MID ATLANTIC

Albert Einstein Medical Center (800) 346-7834
Albert Einstein Med Ctr
5501 Old York Rd Philadelphia, PA 19141 MID ATLANTIC

Albert Lea Medical Center-Mayo Health System (507) 373-2384
Albert Lea Med Ctr-Mayo Hlth Sys
404 W Fountain St Albert Lea, MN 56007 MIDWEST

Alegent Creighton University Medical Center (402) 449-4000
Alegent Creighton Univ Med Ctr
601 N 30th St Omaha, NE 68131-2197 GREAT PLAINS AND MOUNTAINS

Alexian Brothers Medical Center (847) 437-5500
Alexian Brothers Med Ctr
800 Biesterfield Rd Elk Grove Village, IL 60007 MIDWEST

All Children's Hospital (727) 898-7451
All Children's Hosp
501 6th St S St. Petersburg, FL 33701 SOUTHEAST

Allegheny General Hospital (412) 359-3131
Allegheny General Hosp
320 E. North Avenue Pittsburgh, PA 15212 MID ATLANTIC

Alta Bates Summit Medical Center-Alta Bates Campus (510) 204-4444
Alta Bates Summit Med Ctr-Alta Bates Campus
2450 Ashby Avenue Berkeley, CA 94705 WEST COAST AND PACIFIC

Alvarado Hospital & Medical Center (619) 287-3270
Alvarado Hosp & Med Ctr
6655 Alvarado Rd San Diego, CA 92120 WEST COAST AND PACIFIC

Ann & Robert H Lurie Children's Hospital of Chicago (312) 227-4000
Lurie Chldn's Hosp-Chicago
225 E Chicago Ave Chicago, IL 60611 MIDWEST

Anne Arundel Medical Center (443) 481-1000
Anne Arundel Med Ctr
2001 Medical Pkwy Annapolis, MD 21401 MID ATLANTIC

Aria Health- Torresdale Campus		(215) 612-4000
Aria Health- Torresdale		
Red Lion & Knights Rd	Philadelphia, PA 19114	MID ATLANTIC

Arizona Heart Hospital		(602) 532-1000
Arizona Heart Hosp		
1930 E Thomas Rd	Phoenix, AZ 85016	SOUTHWEST

Arkansas Children's Hospital		(501) 364-1100
Arkansas Chldns Hosp		
1 Children's Way	Little Rock, AR 72202	SOUTHWEST

Arthur G. James Cancer Hospital & Research Institute		(614) 293-3300
Arthur G James Cancer Hosp & Research Inst		
300 W 10th Ave, Ste 519	Columbus, OH 43210	MIDWEST

Atlanta Medical Center		(404) 265-4000
Atlanta Med Ctr		
303 Parkway Dr. NE	Atlanta, GA 30312	SOUTHEAST

Atlanta VA Medical Center		(404) 321-6111
Atlanta VA Med Ctr		
1670 Clairmont Rd	Decatur, GA 30033	SOUTHEAST

Audie L Murphy Memorial Veterans Hospital - San Antonio		(210) 617-5300
Audie L Murphy Meml Vets Hosp - San Antonio		
7400 Merton Minter Blvd	San Antonio, TX 78229	SOUTHWEST

Aultman Hospital		(330) 452-9911
Aultman Hosp		
2600 6th St SW	Canton, OH 44710-1799	MIDWEST

Austen Riggs Center		(413) 298-5511
Austen Riggs Ctr		
25 Main Street or PO Box 962	Stockbridge, MA 01262-0962	NEW ENGLAND

Banner Gateway Medical Center		(480) 543-2000
Banner Gateway Med Ctr		
1900 N Higley Rd	Gilbert, AZ 85234	SOUTHWEST

Banner Good Samaritan Regional Medical Center - Phoenix		(602) 839-2000
Banner Good Samaritan Regl Med Ctr - Phoenix		
1111 E McDowell Rd	Phoenix, AZ 85006	SOUTHWEST

Baptist Health System		(210) 297-9700
Baptist Hlth Sys		
615 Soledad	San Antonio, TX 78205	SOUTHWEST

Baptist Hospital - Nashville (615) 284-5555
Baptist Hosp - Nashville
2000 Church St Nashville, TN 37236 SOUTHEAST

Baptist Hospital - Pensacola (850) 434-4011
Baptist Hosp - Pensacola
1000 W Moreno St Pensacola, FL 32501 SOUTHEAST

Baptist Hospital of Miami (786) 596-1960
Baptist Hosp of Miami
8900 N Kendall Dr Miami, FL 33176 SOUTHEAST

Baptist Medical Center - San Antonio (210) 297-7000
Baptist Med Ctr - San Antonio
111 Dallas St San Antonio, TX 78205 SOUTHWEST

Baptist Medical Center-Jackson (601) 968-1000
Baptist Med Ctr-Jackson
1225 N State St Jackson, MS 39202 SOUTHEAST

Baptist Memorial Hospital-Memphis (901) 226-5000
Baptist Memorial Hospital-Memphis
6019 Walnut Grove Rd Memphis, TN 38120 SOUTHEAST

Barbara Ann Karmanos Cancer Institute (800) 527-6266
Barbara Ann Karmanos Cancer Inst
4100 John R Detroit, MI 48201 MIDWEST

Barnes-Jewish Hospital (314) 747-3000
Barnes-Jewish Hosp
One Barnes-Jewish Hospital Plaza St. Louis, MO 63110 MIDWEST

Barnes-Jewish West County Hospital (314) 996-8000
Barnes-Jewish West County Hosp
12634 Olive Blvd St. Louis, MO 63141 MIDWEST

Bascom Palmer Eye Institute (305) 326-6000
Bascom Palmer Eye Inst
900 NW 17 St Miami, FL 33136 SOUTHEAST

Baylor Institute for Rehabilitation (800) 422-9567
Baylor Inst for Rehabilitation
3505 Gaston Avenue Dallas, TX 75246 SOUTHWEST

Baylor Medical Center at Uptown (214) 443-3000
Baylor Med Cter at Uptown
2727 Lemmon Ave Dallas, TX 75204 SOUTHWEST

Baylor University Medical Center-Dallas (214) 820-0111
Baylor Univ Medical Ctr-Dallas
3500 Gaston Avenue Dallas, TX 75246 SOUTHWEST

Baystate Medical Center (413) 794-0000
Baystate Med Ctr
759 Chestnut Street Springfield, MA 01199 NEW ENGLAND

Beaumont Hospital-Royal Oak (248) 898-5000
Beaumont Hosp-Royal Oak
3601 W 13 Mile Rd Royal Oak, MI 48073 MIDWEST

Beaumont Hospital-Troy (248) 964-5000
Beaumont Hosp-Troy
44201 Dequindre Rd Troy, MI 48085 MIDWEST

Ben Taub General Hospital (713) 873-2000
Ben Taub Genl Hosp
1504 Taub Loop Houston, TX 77030 SOUTHWEST

Beth Israel Deaconess Medical Center - Boston (617) 667-7000
Beth Israel Deaconess Med Ctr - Boston
330 Brookline Ave Boston, MA 02215 NEW ENGLAND

Beth Israel Medical Center - Milton & Caroll Petrie Division (212) 420-2000
Beth Israel Med Ctr - Petrie Division
First Avenue at 16th Street New York, NY 10003 MID ATLANTIC

Bethesda North Hospital (513) 865-1111
Bethesda North Hosp
10500 Montgomery Rd Cincinnati, OH 45242-4415 MIDWEST

Boca Raton Regional Hospital (561) 955-7100
Boca Raton Regl Hosp
800 Meadows Road Boca Raton, FL 33486 SOUTHEAST

Bon Secours St Mary's Hospital (804) 285-2011
Bon Secours St Mary's Hosp
5801 Bremo Road Richmond, VA 23226 SOUTHEAST

Boston Medical Center (617) 638-8000
Boston Med Ctr
1 Boston Medical Center Pl Boston, MA 02118 NEW ENGLAND

Botsford Hospital (248) 471-8000
Botsford Hosp
28050 Grand River Ave Farmington Hills, MI 48336 MIDWEST

Boulder Community Hospital (303) 440-2273
Boulder Community Hospital
1100 Balsam Ave, Box 9019 Boulder, CO 80301-9019 GREAT PLAINS AND MOUNTAINS

Boys Town National Research Hospital (402) 498-6511
Boys Town Natl Rsch Hosp
555 N 30th St Omaha, NE 68131 GREAT PLAINS AND MOUNTAINS

Brenner Children's Hospital (336) 716-2011
Brenner Chldrn's Hosp
Medical Center Blvd Winston-Salem, NC 27157-1015 SOUTHEAST

Brigham and Women's Hospital (617) 732-5500
Brigham and Women's Hosp
75 Francis St Boston, MA 02115 NEW ENGLAND

Brooklyn Hospital Center-Downtown (718) 250-8000
Brooklyn Hosp Ctr-Downtown
121 DeKalb Avenue Brooklyn, NY 11201 MID ATLANTIC

Brookwood Medical Center (205) 877-1000
Brookwood Med Ctr
2010 Brookwood Medical Ctr Drive Birmingham, AL 35209-6804 SOUTHEAST

Broward Health Medical Center (954) 355-4400
Broward Hlth Med Ctr
1600 S Andrews Ave Fort Lauderdale, FL 33316 SOUTHEAST

Bryn Mawr Hospital (484) 337-3000
Bryn Mawr Hosp
130 S Bryn Mawr Ave Bryn Mawr, PA 19010-3143 MID ATLANTIC

Bucks Specialty Institute (215) 244-7400
Bucks Specialty Inst
3300 Tillman Drive Bensalem, PA 19020 MID ATLANTIC

Buffalo General Hospital (716) 859-5600
Buffalo General Hosp
100 High Street Buffalo, NY 14203 MID ATLANTIC

Burke Rehabilitation Hospital (914) 597-2500
Burke Rehab Hosp
785 Mamaroneck Avenue White Plains, NY 10605 MID ATLANTIC

Butler Hospital (401) 455-6200
Butler Hosp
345 Blackstone Blvd Providence, RI 02906 NEW ENGLAND

Cabell Huntington Hospital (304) 526-2000
Cabell Huntington Hosp
1340 Hal Greer Blvd Huntington, WV 25701-0195 MID ATLANTIC

California Pacific Medical Center - California Campus (415) 600-6000
CA Pacific Med Ctr - CA Campus
3700 California St San Francisco, CA 94114 WEST COAST AND PACIFIC

California Pacific Medical Center - Davies Campus (415) 600-6000
CA Pacific Med Ctr - Davies Campus
Castro at Duboce St San Francisco, CA 94114 WEST COAST AND PACIFIC

California Pacific Medical Center-Pacific Campus (415) 600-6000
CA Pacific Med Ctr-Pacific Campus
2333 Buchanan St, Box 7999 San Francisco, CA 94115 WEST COAST AND PACIFIC

Camden General Hospital (731) 584-6135
Camden Genl Hosp
175 Hospital St Camden, TN 38320 SOUTHEAST

Cape Cod Hospital (508) 771-1800
Cape Cod Hosp
27 Park St Hyannis, MA 02601-5203 NEW ENGLAND

Cardon Children's Medical Center (480) 412-5437
Cardon Children's Med Ctr
1400 S Dobson Rd Mesa, AZ 85202 SOUTHWEST

Carilion Roanoke Memorial Hospital (540) 981-7000
Carilion Roanoke Meml Hosp
1906 Belleview Ave, PO Box 13367 Roanoke, VA 24014 SOUTHEAST

Carle Foundation Hospital (217) 383-3311
Carle Foundation Hosp
611 W Park St Urbana, IL 61801 MIDWEST

Carolinas Medical Center (704) 355-2000
Carolinas Med Ctr
1000 Blythe Blvd, PO Box 32861 Charlotte, NC 28203-5871 SOUTHEAST

Carolinas Medical Center-University (704) 863-6000
Carolinas Med Ctr-Univ
8800 N Tryon St Charlotte, NC 28262 SOUTHEAST

Carolinas Specialty Hospital (704) 304-6450
Carolinas Specialty Hosp
2001 Vail Ave 7th Fl South Charlotte, NC 28207 SOUTHEAST

Carteret General Hospital (252) 808-6000
Carteret Genl Hosp
3500 Arendell St Morehead City, NC 28557 SOUTHEAST

Cedars-Sinai Medical Center (310) 423-3277
Cedars-Sinai Med Ctr
8700 Beverly Boulevard Los Angeles, CA 90048 WEST COAST AND PACIFIC

Centennial Medical Center (615) 342-1000
Centennial Med Ctr
2300 Patterson Street Nashville, TN 37203 SOUTHEAST

Central Baptist Hospital (859) 260-6100
Central Baptist Hosp
1740 Nicholasville Rd Lexington, KY 40503-1499 SOUTHEAST

Central DuPage Hospital (630) 933-1600
Central DuPage Hosp
25 N Winfield Rd Winfield, IL 60190 MIDWEST

Chandler Regional Medical Center (602) 963-4561
Chandler Regional Med Ctr
475 S Dobson Rd Chandler, AZ 85224-5695 SOUTHWEST

Charlie Norwood VA Medical Center - Augusta (706) 733-0188
Charlie Norwood VA Med Ctr - Augusta
One Freedom Way Augusta, GA 30904 SOUTHEAST

Chelsea Community Hospital (734) 593-6000
Chelsea Comm Hosp
775 S Main St Chelsea, MI 48118 MIDWEST

Chestnut Hill Hospital (212) 248-8200
Chestnut Hill Hosp
8835 Germantown Ave Philadelphia, PA 19118 MID ATLANTIC

Cheyenne Regional Medical Center (307) 634-2273
Cheyenne Regl Med Ctr
214 E 23rd St Cheyenne, WY 82001 GREAT PLAINS AND MOUNTAINS

Children's Healthcare of Atlanta at Egleston (404) 785-6000
Chldns Hlthcare Atlanta @ Egleston
1405 Clifton Rd NE Atlanta, GA 30322 SOUTHEAST

Children's Healthcare of Atlanta at Scottish Rite (404) 785-5252
Chldns Hlthcare Atlanta @ Scottish Rite
1001 Johnson Ferry Rd NE Atlanta, GA 30342 SOUTHEAST

Children's Hospital (804) 321-7474
Children's Hosp
2924 Brook Rd Richmond, VA 23220 SOUTHEAST

Children's Hospital - Aurora (Colorado) (720) 777-1234
Chldn's Hosp - Aurora (CO)
13123 E 16th Ave Aurora, CO 80045 GREAT PLAINS AND MOUNTAINS

Children's Hospital - Boston (617) 355-6000
Children's Hospital - Boston
300 Longwood Avenue Boston, MA 02115 NEW ENGLAND

Children's Hospital - Downtown Denver (720) 777-1360
Children's Hosp - Denver
1830 Franklin St Denver, CO 80218 GREAT PLAINS AND MOUNTAINS

Children's Hospital - Los Angeles (323) 660-2450
Chldns Hosp - Los Angeles
4650 Sunset Blvd Los Angeles, CA 90027 WEST COAST AND PACIFIC

Children's Hospital - New Orleans (504) 899-9511
Children's Hospital - New Orleans
200 Henry Clay Ave New Orleans, LA 70118 SOUTHWEST

Children's Hospital - Oakland (510) 428-3000
Chldns Hosp - Oakland
747 52nd St Oakland, CA 94609 WEST COAST AND PACIFIC

Children's Hospital - Omaha (402) 955-5400
Children's Hosp - Omaha
8200 Dodge St Omaha, NE 68114 GREAT PLAINS AND MOUNTAINS

Children's Hospital at OU Medical Center (405) 271-5437
Chldns Hosp OU Med Ctr
1200 Children's Ave Oklahoma City, OK 73104 SOUTHWEST

Children's Hospital at Shands/University of Florida (352) 265-0373
Children's Hosp at Shands/University of Florid
1600 SW Archer Road Gainesville, FL 32608 SOUTHEAST

Children's Hospital Central California (559) 353-3000
Chldns Hosp Central CA
9300 Valley Children's Pl Madera, CA 93638 WEST COAST AND PACIFIC

Children's Hospital of Alabama - Birmingham (205) 638-9100
Children's Hospital - Birmingham
1600 7th Ave South Birmingham, AL 35233 SOUTHEAST

Children's Hospital of Michigan (313) 745-5437
Chldns Hosp of Michigan
3901 Beaubian Blvd Detroit, MI 48201 MIDWEST

Children's Hospital of Orange County (714) 997-3000
Chldns Hosp Orange Co
455 S Main St Orange, CA 92868 WEST COAST AND PACIFIC

Children's Hospital of Philadelphia (215) 590-1000
Chldns Hosp of Philadelphia
34th St & Civic Center Blvd Philadelphia, PA 19104 MID ATLANTIC

Children's Hospital of Pittsburgh - UPMC (412) 692-5325
Chldns Hosp of Pittsburgh - UPMC
4401 Penn Ave Pittsburgh, PA 15224 MID ATLANTIC

Children's Hospital of the King's Daughters (757) 668-7000
Chldns Hosp of King's Daughters
601 Children's Ln Norfolk, VA 23507 SOUTHEAST

Children's Hospital of Wisconsin (414) 266-2000
Chldns Hosp - Wisconsin
9000 W Wisconsin Ave Milwaukee, WI 53226 MIDWEST

Children's Hospitals & Clinics of Minneapolis (612) 813-6000
Children's Hosps & Clinics of Minneapolis
2525 Chicago Ave Minneapolis, MN 55404 MIDWEST

Children's Medical Center of Dallas (214) 456-7000
Chldns Med Ctr of Dallas
1935 Medical District Drive Dallas, TX 75235 SOUTHWEST

Children's Memorial Hermann Hospital (713) 704-5437
Children's Meml Hermann Hosp
6411 Fannin St Houston, TX 77030 SOUTHWEST

Children's Mercy Hospitals & Clinics (816) 234-3000
Chldns Mercy Hosps & Clinics
2401 Gilham Rd Kansas City, MO 64108 MIDWEST

Children's National Medical Center - DC (202) 476-5000
Chldns Natl Med Ctr
111 Michigan Ave NW Washington, DC 20010 MID ATLANTIC

Christ Hospital, The - Cincinnati (513) 585-2000
Christ Hosp, The - Cincinnati
2139 Auburn Ave Cincinnati, OH 45219 MIDWEST

Christiana Hospital		(302) 733-1000
Christiana Hospital		
4755 Ogletown-Stanton Rd	Newark, DE 19718-0001	MID ATLANTIC
Christus Santa Rosa Children's Hospital		(210) 704-2011
Christus Santa Rosa Children's Hosp		
333 N Santa Rosa St	San Antonio, TX 78207	SOUTHWEST
Christus Santa Rosa Medical Center Hospital		(210) 705-6300
Christus Santa Rosa Med Ctr Hosp		
2827 Babcock Rd	San Antonio, TX 78229-6098	SOUTHWEST
Christus St Vincent Regional Medical Center-Santa Fe		(505) 983-3361
Christus St Vincent Reg Med Ctr-Santa Fe		
455 St Michaels Dr	Santa Fe, NM 87504-2107	SOUTHWEST
CHRISTUS St. Frances Cabrini Hospital		(318) 487-1122
CHRISTUS St. Frances Cabrini Hosp		
3330 Masonic Dr	Alexandria, LA 71301	SOUTHWEST
Cincinnati Children's Hospital Medical Center		(513) 636-4200
Cincinnati Chldns Hosp Med Ctr		
3333 Burnet Ave	Cincinnati, OH 45229-3039	MIDWEST
Cincinnati Shriners Hospital		(513) 872-6000
Cincinnati Shriners Hosp		
3229 Burnet Ave	Cincinnati, OH 45229-3095	MIDWEST
City of Hope National Medical Center		(626) 256-4673
City of Hope Natl Med Ctr		
1500 E Duarte Rd	Duarte, CA 91010	WEST COAST AND PACIFIC
Clara Maass Medical Center		(973) 450-2000
Clara Maass Med Ctr		
One Clara Maass Drive	Belleville, NJ 07109	MID ATLANTIC
Cleveland Clinic		(216) 444-2200
Cleveland Clin		
9500 Euclid Avenue	Cleveland, OH 44195	MIDWEST
Cleveland Clinic Florida - Weston		(954) 659-5000
Cleveland Clin - Weston		
2950 Cleveland Clinic Blvd	Weston, FL 33331	SOUTHEAST
Columbia Medical Center - Plano		(972) 596-6800
Columbia Med Ctr - Plano		
3901 West 15th Street	Plano, TX 75075	SOUTHWEST

Columbus Regional Medical Center (706) 571-1000
Columbus Regl Med Ctr
710 Center St Columbus, GA 31902 SOUTHEAST

Community Hospital East - Indianapolis (317) 355-5411
Commun Hosp E - Indianapolis
1500 N Ritter Ave Indianapolis, IN 46219 MIDWEST

Community Hospital of Monterey Peninsula (831) 624-5311
Comm Hosp of Monterey Pen
23625 Holman Hwy Monterey, CA 93940 WEST COAST AND PACIFIC

Community Memorial Hospital - Ventura (805) 652-5011
Comm Meml Hosp - Ventura
147 N Brent St Ventura, CA 93003 WEST COAST AND PACIFIC

Concord Hospital (603) 225-2711
Concord Hospital
250 Pleasant St Concord, NH 03301-2598 NEW ENGLAND

Connecticut Children's Medical Center (860) 545-9000
CT Chldns Med Ctr
282 Washington St Hartford, CT 06106 NEW ENGLAND

Connecticut Mental Health Center (203) 974-7300
Connecticut Mental Hlth Ctr
34 Park St New Haven, CT 06508-1842 NEW ENGLAND

Cook Children's Medical Center (682) 885-4000
Cook Chldns Med Ctr
801 7th Ave Fort Worth, TX 76104-2796 SOUTHWEST

Cooper University Hospital (856) 342-2000
Cooper Univ Hosp
1 Cooper Plaza Camden, NJ 08103 MID ATLANTIC

Covenant Children's Hospital (806) 725-0000
Covenant Children's Hosp
3610 21st St Lubbock, TX 79410 SOUTHWEST

Covenant Medical Center (319) 272-8000
Covenant Med Ctr
3421 W 9th St Waterloo, IA 50702-5499 MIDWEST

Crouse Hospital (315) 470-7111
Crouse Hosp
736 Irving Ave Syracuse, NY 13210-1607 MID ATLANTIC

Crozer - Chester Medical Center	(610) 447-2000	
Crozer - Chester Med Ctr		
One Medical Center Boulevard	Upland, PA 19013	MID ATLANTIC

CTCA at Eastern Regional Medical Center	(215) 537-7400	
CTCA at Eastern Regl Med Ctr		
1331 E Wyoming Ave	Philadelphia, PA 19124	MID ATLANTIC

CTCA at Midwestern Regional Medical Center	(847) 872-4561	
CTCA at Midwestern Reg Med Ctr		
2520 Elisha Ave	Zion, IL 60099	MIDWEST

CTCA at Southeastern Regional Medical Center	(770) 400-6000	
CTCA at Southeastern Regl Med Ctr		
600 Parkway North	Newnan, GA 30265	SOUTHEAST

CTCA at Western Regional Medical Center	(623) 207-3000	
CTCA at Western Regl Med Ctr		
14200 W Fillmore St	Goodyear, AZ 85338	SOUTHWEST

Dana-Farber Cancer Institute	(617) 632-3000	
Dana-Farber Cancer Inst		
450 Brookline Ave	Boston, MA 02215	NEW ENGLAND

Dartmouth - Hitchcock Medical Center	(603) 650-5000	
Dartmouth - Hitchcock Med Ctr		
1 Medical Center Dr	Lebanon, NH 03756-0002	NEW ENGLAND

DCH Regional Medical Center	(205) 759-7111	
DCH Reg Med Ctr		
809 University Blvd E	Tuscaloosa, AL 35401-2029	SOUTHEAST

Dell Children's Medical Center of Central Texas	(512) 324-0000	
Dell Children's Med Ctr of Central Texas		
4900 Mueller Blvd	Austin, TX 78723	SOUTHWEST

Denver Health Medical Center	(303) 436-6000	
Denver Health Med Ctr		
777 Bannock St	Denver, CO 80204	GREAT PLAINS AND MOUNTAINS

Desert Regional Medical Center	(760) 323-6511	
Desert Regl Med Ctr		
1150 N Indian Canyon Dr	Palm Springs, CA 92262	WEST COAST AND PACIFIC

Detroit Medical Center	(313) 578-3930	
Detroit Med Ctr		
3663 Woodward Ave, Ste 200	Detroit, MI 48201-2403	MIDWEST

DMC Surgery Hospital (248) 733-2200
DMC Surgery Hosp
30671 Stephenson Hwy Madison Heights, MI 48071 MIDWEST

Doctors' Hospital - Coral Gables (FL) (786) 308-3000
Doctors' Hosp - Coral Gables (FL)
5000 University Dr Coral Gables, FL 33146 SOUTHEAST

Doernbecher Children's Hospital/Oregon Health Science University (503) 494-8311
Doernbecher Chldns Hosp/OHSU
3181 SW Sam Jackson Park Rd Portland, OR 97239 WEST COAST AND PACIFIC

Duke University Hospital (919) 684-8111
· *Duke Univ Hosp*
2301 Erwin Rd, PO Box 3708 Durham, NC 27710 SOUTHEAST

Durham Regional Hospital (919) 470-4000
Durham Regional Hosp
3643 N Roxboro Rd Durham, NC 27704 SOUTHEAST

East Jefferson General Hospital (504) 454-4000
E Jefferson Genl Hosp
4200 Houma Blvd Metairie, LA 70006-2973 SOUTHWEST

East Texas Medical Center-Tyler (903) 597-0351
E TX Med Ctr-Tyler
1000 S Beckham Ave Tyler, TX 75701 SOUTHWEST

Edward Hines, Jr. VA Hospital (708) 202-3800
Edward Hines, Jr. VA Hosp
5000 South 5th Avenue Hines, IL 60141 MIDWEST

Edward Hospital (630) 527-3000
Edward Hosp
801 S Washington St Naperville, IL 60540 MIDWEST

Eisenhower Medical Center (760) 340-3911
Eisenhower Med Ctr
39000 Bob Hope Drive Rancho Mirage, CA 92270 WEST COAST AND PACIFIC

El Camino Hospital (650) 940-7000
El Camino Hosp
2500 Grant Road Mountain View, CA 94040 WEST COAST AND PACIFIC

El Paso Children's Hospital (915) 298-5444
El Paso Chldns Hosp
4845 Alameda Ave El Paso, TX 79905 SOUTHWEST

Elliot Hospital		(603) 669-5300
Elliot Hosp		
1 Elliot Way	Manchester, NH 03103	NEW ENGLAND
Elmhurst Hospital Center		(718) 334-4000
Elmhurst Hosp Ctr		
79-01 Broadway	Elmhurst, NY 11373	MID ATLANTIC
Emory University Hospital		(404) 712-2000
Emory Univ Hosp		
1364 Clifton Rd NE	Atlanta, GA 30322	SOUTHEAST
Emory University Hospital Midtown		(404) 686-4411
Emory Univ Hosp Midtown		
550 Peachtree St NE	Atlanta, GA 30308	SOUTHEAST
Englewood Hospital & Medical Center		(201) 894-3000
Englewood Hosp & Med Ctr		
350 Engle Street	Englewood, NJ 07631	MID ATLANTIC
Erie County Medical Center		(716) 898-3000
Erie County Med Ctr		
462 Grider St	Buffalo, NY 14215	MID ATLANTIC
Erlanger Medical Center		(423) 778-7000
Erlanger Med Ctr		
975 E 3rd St	Chattanooga, TN 37403	SOUTHEAST
Evanston Hospital		(847) 570-2000
Evanston Hosp		
2650 Ridge Ave	Evanston, IL 60201	MIDWEST
Evanston/North Shore University Health System		(847) 570-2000
Evanston/North Shore Univ Hlth Sys		
2650 Ridge Ave	Evanston, IL 60201	MIDWEST
Fairview Lakes Medical Center		(651) 982-7000
Fairview Lakes Med Ctr		
5200 Fairview Blvd	Wyoming, MN 55092	MIDWEST
Fairview Southdale Hospital		(952) 924-5000
Fairview Southdale Hosp		
6401 France Ave S	Edina, MN 55435-2199	MIDWEST
Fargo VA Medical Center		(701) 232-3241
Fargo VA Med Ctr		
2101 N Elm St	Fargo, ND 58102	GREAT PLAINS AND MOUNTAINS

Fletcher Allen Health Care-Medical Center Campus (802) 847-0000
Fletcher Allen Health Care- Med Ctr Campus
111 Colchester Ave Burlington, VT 05401 NEW ENGLAND

Floating Hospital for Children at Tufts Medical Center, The (617) 636-5000
Floating Hosp for Children at Tufts Med Ce
755 Washington St Boston, MA 02111 NEW ENGLAND

Florida Hospital - Celebration Health (407) 303-4000
Florida Hosp Celebration Hlth
400 Celebration Pl Celebration, FL 34747 SOUTHEAST

Florida Hospital - Orlando (407) 303-5600
Florida Hosp - Orlando
601 E Rollins St Orlando, FL 32803 SOUTHEAST

Florida Hospital-Tampa (813) 971-6000
Florida Hosp-Tampa
3100 E Fletcher Avenue Tampa, FL 33613 SOUTHEAST

Floyd Memorial Hospital & Health Services (812) 944-7701
Floyd Meml Hosp & Hlth Svcs
1850 State St New Albany, IN 47150-4997 MIDWEST

Forsyth Medical Center (336) 718-5000
Forsyth Med Ctr
3333 Silas Creek Pkwy Winston-Salem, NC 27103 SOUTHEAST

Four Winds Hospital (914) 763-8151
Four Winds Hosp
800 Cross River Road Katonah, NY 10536 MID ATLANTIC

Fox Chase Cancer Center (215) 728-6900
Fox Chase Cancer Ctr
333 Cottman Avenue Philadelphia, PA 19111 MID ATLANTIC

Franciscan St. Francis Health-Indianapolis (317) 528-5000
Franciscan St. Francis Hlth-Indianapolis
8111 S Emerson Ave Indianapolis, IN 46237 MIDWEST

Franklin Square Hospital (443) 777-7000
Franklin Square Hosp
9000 Franklin Square Drive Baltimore, MD 21237 MID ATLANTIC

Frazier Rehabilitation Institute (502) 582-7400
Frazier Rehab Inst
220 Abraham Flexner Way Louisville, KY 40202 SOUTHEAST

Frederick Memorial Hospital (301) 698-3300
Frederick Mem Hospital
400 West 7th Street Frederick, MD 21701 MID ATLANTIC

Froedtert & Medical Center of Wisconsin (414) 805-3000
Froedtert and Med Ctr of WI
9200 W Wisconsin Ave Milwaukee, WI 53226 MIDWEST

Gaston Memorial Hospital (704) 834-2000
Gaston Meml Hosp
2525 Court Dr Gastonia, NC 28054 SOUTHEAST

George Washington University Hospital (202) 715-4000
G Washington Univ Hosp
900 23rd St NW Washington, DC 20037 MID ATLANTIC

Georgetown University Hospital (202) 444-2000
Georgetown Univ Hosp
3800 Reservoir Rd NW Washington, DC 20007 MID ATLANTIC

Georgia Health Sciences Center (706) 721-0211
Georgia Hlth Sci Ctr
1120 15th Street Augusta, GA 30912 SOUTHEAST

Glenbrook Hospital-NorthShore University Health System (847) 657-5800
Glenbrook Hosp-NorthShore Univ Hlth Syst
2100 Pfingsten Rd Glenview, IL 60026 MIDWEST

Glendale Memorial Hospital & Health Center (818) 502-1900
Glendale Mem Hosp & Hlth Ctr
1420 S Central Ave Glendale, CA 91204-2594 WEST COAST AND PACIFIC

Good Samaritan Hosp - Cincinnati (513) 872-1400
Good Samaritan Hosp - Cincinnati
375 Dixmyth Ave Cincinnati, OH 45220 MIDWEST

Good Samaritan Hospital (443) 444-8000
Good Samaritan Hosp
5601 Loch Raven Blvd Baltimore, MD 21239 MID ATLANTIC

Good Samaritan Hospital - Los Angeles (213) 977-2121
Good Samaritan Hosp - LA
1225 Wilshire Boulevard Los Angeles, CA 90017 WEST COAST AND PACIFIC

Good Samaritan Medical Center - West Palm Beach (561) 655-5511
Good Sam Med Ctr - W Palm Beach
1309 N Flagler Dr West Palm Beach, FL 33401 SOUTHEAST

Gottlieb Memorial Hospital		(708) 681-3200
Gottlieb Meml Hosp		
701 W North Ave	Melrose Park, IL 60160	MIDWEST

Grady Health System		(404) 616-1000
Grady Hlth Sys		
80 Jesse Hill Jr SE	Atlanta, GA 30303	SOUTHEAST

Greater Baltimore Medical Center		(443) 849-2000
Greater Baltimore Med Ctr		
6701 N Charles St	Baltimore, MD 21204	MID ATLANTIC

Greenwich Hospital		(203) 863-3000
Greenwich Hosp		
Five Perryridge Road	Greenwich, CT 06830	NEW ENGLAND

H Lee Moffitt Cancer Center & Research Institute		(813) 745-4673
H Lee Moffitt Cancer Ctr & Research Inst		
12902 Magnolia Drive	Tampa, FL 33612-9497	SOUTHEAST

Hackensack University Medical Center		(551) 996-2000
Hackensack Univ Med Ctr		
30 Prospect Avenue	Hackensack, NJ 07601	MID ATLANTIC

Hahnemann University Hospital		(215) 762-7000
Hahnemann Univ Hosp		
Broad & Vine St	Philadelphia, PA 19102	MID ATLANTIC

Harborview Medical Center		(206) 744-3000
Harborview Med Ctr		
325 9th Ave	Seattle, WA 98104	WEST COAST AND PACIFIC

Harper University Hospital		(313) 745-8040
Harper Univ Hosp		
3990 John R St	Detroit, MI 48201-2097	MIDWEST

Harrison Medical Center		(360) 774-3911
Harrison Med Ctr		
2520 Cherry Ave	Bremerton, WA 98310-4270	WEST COAST AND PACIFIC

Hartford Hospital		(860) 545-5000
Hartford Hosp		
80 Seymour St	Hartford, CT 06102-5037	NEW ENGLAND

Healthsouth Lakeshore Rehabilitation Hospital		(205) 868-2000
Healthsouth Lakeshore Rehab Hosp		
3800 Ridgeway Drive	Birmingham, AL 35209	SOUTHEAST

Hennepin County Medical Center
Hennepin Cnty Med Ctr
701 Park Ave Minneapolis, MN 55415 (612) 873-3000 MIDWEST

Henrico Doctors Hospital
Henrico Doctors Hosp
1602 Skipwith Road Richmond, VA 23229 (804) 289-4500 SOUTHEAST

Henry Ford Hospital
Henry Ford Hosp
2799 W Grand Blvd Detroit, MI 48202 (313) 916-2600 MIDWEST

Henry Ford West Bloomfield Hospital
Henry Ford- W Bloomfield Hosp
6777 W Maple Rd West Bloomfield, MI 48322 (248) 661-4100 MIDWEST

Henry Mayo Newhall Memorial Hospital
Henry Mayo Newhall Memorial Hosp
23845 McBean Parkway Valencia, CA 91355 (661) 253-8000 WEST COAST AND PACIFIC

Highland Park Hospital - North Shore University Health System
Highland Park Hops-North Shore Univ Hlth Syst
777 Park Ave Highland Park, IL 60035 (847) 432-8000 MIDWEST

Hilton Head Regional Medical Center
Hilton Head Reg Med Ctr
25 Hospital Ctr Blvd Hilton Head, SC 29926 (843) 681-6122 SOUTHEAST

Hoag Hospital Irvine
Hoag Hosp Irvine
16200 Sand Canyon Ave Irvine, CA 92618 (949) 764-4624 WEST COAST AND PACIFIC

Hoag Memorial Hospital Presbyterian
Hoag Meml Hosp Presby
One Hoag Drive Newport Beach, CA 92663 (949) 645-8600 WEST COAST AND PACIFIC

Hollywood Presbyterian Medical Center
Hollywood Presby Med Ctr
1300 N Vermont Ave Los Angeles, CA 90027-6069 (213) 413-3000 WEST COAST AND PACIFIC

Holy Cross Hospital - Fort Lauderdale
Holy Cross Hosp - Fort Lauderdale
4725 N Federal Hwy Fort Lauderdale, FL 33308 (954) 771-8000 SOUTHEAST

Holy Cross Hospital - Silver Spring
Holy Cross Hospital - Silver Spring
1500 Forest Glen Road Silver Spring, MD 20910 (301) 754-7000 MID ATLANTIC

Hospital for Special Surgery　　　　　　　　　　　　　　(212) 606-1000
Hosp For Special Surgery
535 East 70th Street　　　　　　　New York, NY 10021　　　　　MID ATLANTIC

Hospital of Central CT at New Britain　　　　　　　　　　　(860) 224-5011
Hosp of Central CT at New Britain
100 Grand St　　　　　　　　　New Britain, CT 06050　　　　NEW ENGLAND

Hospital of the University of Pennsylvania - UPHS　　　　　(215) 662-4000
Hosp Univ Penn - UPHS
3400 Spruce Street　　　　　　　Philadelphia, PA 19104　　　MID ATLANTIC

Howard University Hospital　　　　　　　　　　　　　　　(202) 865-6100
Howard Univ Hosp
2041 Georgia Ave NW　　　　　　Washington, DC 20060　　　MID ATLANTIC

Hunter Holmes McGuire VA Medical Center - Richmond　　　(804) 675-5000
Hunter Holmes McGuire VA Med Ctr - Richmond
1201 Broad Rock Boulevard　　　　Richmond, VA 23249　　　　SOUTHEAST

Huntsville Hospital　　　　　　　　　　　　　　　　　　(256) 265-1000
Huntsville Hosp, The
101 Sivley Rd　　　　　　　　　Huntsville, AL 35801-4470　　SOUTHEAST

Hutzel Women's Hospital - Detroit　　　　　　　　　　　　(313) 745-7555
Hutzel Hosp - Detroit
3980 John R. Blvd　　　　　　　Detroit, MI 48201-2018　　　　MIDWEST

Indian River Medical Center　　　　　　　　　　　　　　(772) 567-4311
Indian River Med Ctr
1000 36th St　　　　　　　　　Vero Beach, FL 32960　　　　SOUTHEAST

Indiana University Health Methodist Hospital　　　　　　　(317) 962-2000
IU Health Methodist Hosp
1701 N Senate Blvd　　　　　　Indianapolis, IN 46202　　　　MIDWEST

Indiana University Health University Hospital　　　　　　　(317) 944-5000
IU Health University Hosp
550 N University Blvd　　　　　　Indianapolis, IN 46202　　　　MIDWEST

Ingalls Memorial Hospital　　　　　　　　　　　　　　　(708) 333-2300
Ingalls Meml Hosp
1 Ingalls Dr　　　　　　　　　Harvey, IL 60426　　　　　　MIDWEST

Inova Fair Oaks Hospital　　　　　　　　　　　　　　　(703) 391-3600
Inova Fair Oaks Hosp
3600 Joseph Siewick Dr　　　　　Fairfax, VA 22033　　　　　　SOUTHEAST

Inova Fairfax Hospital (703) 776-4001
Inova Fairfax Hosp
3300 Gallows Road Falls Church, VA 22042 SOUTHEAST

Inova Fairfax Hospital for Children (703) 776-4002
Inova Fairfax Hosp for Chldn
3300 Gallows Rd Fairfax, VA 22042 SOUTHEAST

INTEGRIS Baptist Medical Center - Oklahoma (405) 949-3011
INTEGRIS Baptist Med Ctr - OK
3300 NW Expressway Oklahoma City, OK 73112-9028 SOUTHWEST

Intermountain Medical Center (801) 507-7000
Intermountain Med Ctr
5121 S Cottonwood St Murray, UT 84157 GREAT PLAINS AND MOUNTAINS

Jackson Memorial Hospital (305) 585-1111
Jackson Meml Hosp
1611 NW 12th Ave Miami, FL 33136 SOUTHEAST

Jackson North Medical Center (305) 651-1100
Jackson N Med Ctr
160 NW 170 St North Miami Beach, FL 33169 SOUTHEAST

James J. Peters VA Medical Center-Bronx (718) 584-9000
James J. Peters VA Med Ctr-Bronx
130 W Kingsbridge Rd Bronx, NY 10468 MID ATLANTIC

Jeanes Hospital (215) 728-2000
Jeanes Hosp
7600 Central Ave Philadelphia, PA 19111 MID ATLANTIC

Jewish Hospital - Kenwood - Cincinnati (513) 686-3000
Jewish Hosp - Kenwood - Cincinnati
4777 E Galbraith Rd Cincinnati, OH 45236-2891 MIDWEST

Jewish Hospital - Louisville, KY (502) 587-4011
Jewish Hosp (KY)
200 Abraham Flexner Way Louisville, KY 40202 SOUTHEAST

JFK Medical Center - Atlantis (561) 965-7300
JFK Med Ctr - Atlantis
5301 S Congress Ave Atlantis, FL 33462 SOUTHEAST

JFK Medical Center - Edison (732) 321-7000
JFK Med Ctr - Edison
65 James St Edison, NJ 08818 MID ATLANTIC

Joe DiMaggio Children's Hospital		(954) 987-2000
Joe DiMaggio Chldns Hosp		
1005 Joe Dimaggio Drive	Hollywood, FL 33021	SOUTHEAST

John D. Dingell VA Medical Center, Detroit		(313) 562-1000
John D. Dingell VA Med Ctr, Detroit		
4646 John R. Street	Detroit, MI 48201	MIDWEST

Johns Hopkins Bayview Medical Center		(410) 550-0100
Johns Hopkins Bayview Med Ctr		
4940 Eastern Avenue	Baltimore, MD 21224	MID ATLANTIC

Johns Hopkins Hospital		(410) 955-5000
Johns Hopkins Hosp		
600 N Wolfe St	Baltimore, MD 21287	MID ATLANTIC

Kaiser Permanente Baldwin Park Medical Center		(626) 851-1011
Kaiser Permanente Baldwin Pk Med Ctr		
1011 Baldwin Park Blvd	Baldwin Park, CA 91706	WEST COAST AND PACIFIC

Kaiser Permanente Los Angeles Medical Center		(323) 783-4011
Kaiser Permanente LA Med Ctr		
1526 N Edgemont St	Los Angeles, CA 90027	WEST COAST AND PACIFIC

Kaiser Permanente Oakland Medical Center		(510) 752-1000
Kaiser Permanente Oakland Med Ctr		
280 West MacArthur Boulevard	Oakland, CA 94611	WEST COAST AND PACIFIC

Kaiser Permanente South San Francisco Medical Center		(650) 742-2000
Kaiser Permanente S San Francisco Med Ctr		
1200 El Camino Real	South San Francisco, CA 94080	WEST COAST AND PACIFIC

Kaiser Permanente Woodland Hills Medical Center		(818) 719-2000
Kaiser Permanente Woodland Hills Med Ctr		
5601 De Soto Ave	Woodland Hills, CA 91365	WEST COAST AND PACIFIC

Kalispell Regional Medical Center		(406) 752-5111
Kalispell Regl Med Ctr		
310 Sunnyview Ln	Kalispell, MT 59901-3199	GREAT PLAINS AND MOUNTAINS

Kapiolani Medical Center for Women & Children		(808) 983-6000
Kapiolani Med Ctr for Women & Chldn		
1319 Punahou St	Honolulu, HI 96826	WEST COAST AND PACIFIC

Keck Medical Center of USC		(323) 442-8500
Keck Med Ctr of USC		
1500 San Pablo St	Los Angeles, CA 90033	WEST COAST AND PACIFIC

Kenmore Mercy Hospital (845) 331-3131
Kenmore Mercy Hosp
2950 Elmwood Ave Kenmore, NY 14217 MID ATLANTIC

Kennedy Krieger Institute (443) 923-9200
Kennedy Krieger Inst
707 N Broadway Baltimore, MD 21205 MID ATLANTIC

Kessler Institute for Rehabilitation - West Orange (973) 731-3600
Kessler Inst for Rehab - W Orange
1199 Pleasant Valley Way West Orange, NJ 07052-1499 MID ATLANTIC

Kittitas Valley Community Hospital (509) 962-9841
Kittitas Valley Community Hosp
603 S Chestnut St Ellensburg, WA 98926 WEST COAST AND PACIFIC

Kootenai Medical Center (208) 666-2000
Kootenai Med Ctr
Kootenai Health Way Coeur d'Alene, ID 83814-2677 GREAT PLAINS AND MOUNTAINS

Kosair Children's Hospital (502) 629-6000
Kosair Chldn's Hosp
231 E Chestnut St Louisville, KY 40202 SOUTHEAST

La Grange Memorial Hospital (708) 245-9000
La Grange Meml Hosp
5101 S Willow Springs Rd La Grange, IL 60525 MIDWEST

LAC & USC Medical Center (323) 409-1000
LAC & USC Med Ctr
1200 N State St Los Angeles, CA 90033-4525 WEST COAST AND PACIFIC

LAC - Harbor - UCLA Medical Center (310) 222-2345
LAC - Harbor - UCLA Med Ctr
1000 W Carson St, Box 27 PO Box 2910 Torrance, CA 90502 WEST COAST AND PACIFIC

Lafayette General Medical Center (337) 289-7991
Lafayette Genl Med Ctr
1214 Coolidge Blvd Lafayette, LA 70503 SOUTHWEST

Lahey Clinic (781) 744-5100
Lahey Clin
41 Mall Road Burlington, MA 01805 NEW ENGLAND

Lakeland Regional Medical Center (863) 687-1100
Lakeland Regl Med Ctr
1324 Lakeland Hills Blvd Lakeland, FL 33805 SOUTHEAST

Lakeland Specialty Hospital	(269) 471-7761
Lakeland Specialty Hosp	
6418 Deans Hill Rd · Berrien Center, MI 49102	MIDWEST

Lancaster General Hospital	(717) 544-5511
Lancaster Genl Hosp	
555 N Duke St · Lancaster, PA 17602	MID ATLANTIC

Lankenau Hospital	(484) 476-2000
Lankenau Hosp	
100 Lancaster Ave · Wynnewood, PA 19096-3498	MID ATLANTIC

LDS Hospital	(801) 408-1100
LDS Hosp	
8th Ave & C St · Salt Lake City, UT 84143	GREAT PLAINS AND MOUNTAINS

Le Bonheur Children's Medical Center	(901) 287-5437
Le Bonheur Chldns Med Ctr	
50 N Dunlap · Memphis, TN 38103-2893	SOUTHEAST

Lee Memorial Health Systems	(239) 343-2000
Lee Memorial Hlth Systems	
2776 Cleveland Ave · Fort Myers, FL 33901	SOUTHEAST

Legacy Good Samaritan Medical Center	(503) 413-7711
Legacy Good Samaritan Med Ctr	
1015 NW 22nd Ave · Portland, OR 97210-3025	WEST COAST AND PACIFIC

Lenox Hill Hospital	(212) 434-2000
Lenox Hill Hosp	
100 East 77th Street · New York, NY 10021	MID ATLANTIC

Lenox Hill Hospital (Manhattan Eye, Ear & Throat Hosp)	(212) 838-9200
Lenox Hill Hosp (Manh Eye, Ear & Throat Hosp)	
210 East 64th Street · New York, NY 10021	MID ATLANTIC

Loma Linda Children's Hospital	(909) 558-8000
Loma Linda Chldns Hosp	
11234 Anderson St · Loma Linda, CA 92354	WEST COAST AND PACIFIC

Loma Linda University Medical Center	(909) 558-4000
Loma Linda Univ Med Ctr	
11234 Anderson St · Loma Linda, CA 92354	WEST COAST AND PACIFIC

Long Beach Memorial Medical Center	(562) 933-2000
Long Beach Meml Med Ctr	
2801 Atlantic Ave · Long Beach, CA 90806	WEST COAST AND PACIFIC

Long Island Jewish Medical Center (718) 470-7000
Long Island Jewish Med Ctr
270-05 76th Avenue New Hyde Park, NY 11040 MID ATLANTIC

Los Alamitos Medical Center (562) 598-1311
Los Alamitos Med Ctr
3751 Katella Ave Los Alamitos, CA 90720 WEST COAST AND PACIFIC

Louisiana State University Hospital (318) 675-5000
Louisiana State Univ Hosp
1501 Kings Highway P.O. Box 33932 Shreveport, LA 71130 SOUTHWEST

Loyola University Medical Center (708) 327-3627
Loyola Univ Med Ctr
2160 S 1st Ave Maywood, IL 60153 MIDWEST

Lucile Packard Children's Hospital (650) 497-8000
Lucile Packard Chldn's Hosp
725 Welch Rd Palo Alto, CA 94304 WEST COAST AND PACIFIC

Lutheran Medical Center - Cleveland (216) 696-4300
Lutheran Med Ctr - Cleveland
1730 W 25th St Cleveland, OH 44113 MIDWEST

Magee Rehabilitation Hospital (215) 587-3000
Magee Rehab Hosp
1513 Race St Philadelphia, PA 19102-1177 MID ATLANTIC

Magee-Womens Hospital of UPMC (412) 641-1000
Magee-Womens Hosp - UPMC
300 Halket Street Pittsburgh, PA 15213 MID ATLANTIC

Maimonides Medical Center (718) 283-6000
Maimonides Med Ctr
4802 Tenth Avenue Brooklyn, NY 11219 MID ATLANTIC

Maine Medical Center (207) 662-0111
Maine Med Ctr
22 Bramhall St Portland, ME 04102 NEW ENGLAND

Malcom Randall VA Medical Center (352) 376-1611
Malcom Randall VA Med Ctr
1601 SW Archer Rd Gainesville, FL 32608 SOUTHEAST

Maple Grove Hospital (763) 581-1000
Maple Grove Hosp
9875 Hospital Dr Maple Grove, MN 55369 MIDWEST

Marianjoy Rehabilitation Hospital (630) 462-4000
Marianjoy Rehab Hosp
26 W 171 Roosevelt Rd Wheaton, IL 60187 MIDWEST

Marin General Hospital (415) 925-7000
Marin Genl Hosp
250 Bon Air Rd Greenbrae, CA 94904 WEST COAST AND PACIFIC

Marina Del Rey Hospital (310) 823-8911
Marina Del Rey Hosp
4650 Lincoln Blvd Marina Del Rey, CA 90292 WEST COAST AND PACIFIC

Mary Bridge Children's Hospital & Health Center (253) 403-1000
Mary Bridge Chldns Hosp & Hlth Ctr
317 Martin Luther King Jr Way Tacoma, WA 98405 WEST COAST AND PACIFIC

Maryland General Hospital (410) 225-8000
Maryland Genl Hosp
827 Linden Ave Baltimore, MD 21201 MID ATLANTIC

Massachusetts Eye and Ear Infirmary (617) 523-7900
Mass Eye & Ear Infirmary
243 Charles Street Boston, MA 02114 NEW ENGLAND

Massachusetts General Hospital (617) 726-2000
Mass Genl Hosp
55 Fruit St Boston, MA 02114 NEW ENGLAND

Massachusetts Mental Health Center (617) 626-9300
MA Mental Hlth Ctr
180 Morton St Jamaica Plain, MA 02130 NEW ENGLAND

Mattel Children's Hospital at UCLA (310) 825-9111
Mattel Chldns Hosp at UCLA
10833 Le Conte Ave Los Angeles, CA 90095-1752 WEST COAST AND PACIFIC

Maui Memorial Medical Center (808) 244-9056
Maui Meml Med Ctr
221 Mahalani St Wailuku, HI 96793 WEST COAST AND PACIFIC

Mayo Clinic - Jacksonville, FL (904) 953-2000
Mayo - Jacksonville
4500 San Pablo Road Jacksonville, FL 32224 SOUTHEAST

Mayo Clinic - Phoenix (480) 515-6296
Mayo Clinic - Phoenix
5777 E Mayo Blvd Phoenix, AZ 85054 SOUTHWEST

Mayo Clinic - Rochester, MN (507) 284-2511
Mayo Med Ctr & Clin - Rochester
200 First St SW Rochester, MN 55905 MIDWEST

Mayo Clinic - Scottsdale (480) 301-8000
Mayo Clinic - Scottsdale
13400 E Shea Blvd Scottsdale, AZ 85259 SOUTHWEST

McLaren Flint (810) 342-2000
McLaren Flint
401 S. Ballenger Highway Flint, MI 48532 MIDWEST

McLean Hospital (617) 855-2000
McLean Hosp
115 Mill St Belmont, MA 02478 NEW ENGLAND

MD Anderson Cancer Center-Orlando (407) 648-3800
MD Anderson Cancer Ctr-Orlando
1400 S Orange Ave Orlando, FL 32806 SOUTHEAST

Meadowlands Hospital Medical Center (201) 392-3100
Meadowlands Hosp Med Ctr
55 Meadowland Parkway Secaucus, NJ 07096 MID ATLANTIC

Medical Center of Central Georgia (478) 633-1000
Med Ctr of Central GA
777 Hemlock Street Macon, GA 31201 SOUTHEAST

Medical City Dallas Hospital (972) 566-7000
Med City Dallas Hosp
7777 Forest Ln Dallas, TX 75230-2594 SOUTHWEST

Medical College of Virginia Hospitals (804) 828-9000
Med Coll of VA Hosp
1250 E Marshall St, Box 980510 Richmond, VA 23298 SOUTHEAST

Medical University of South Carolina Children's Hospital (843) 792-1414
MUSC Chldns Hosp
169 Ashley Ave Charleston, SC 29425 SOUTHEAST

Medical University of South Carolina Medical Center (843) 792-2300
MUSC Med Ctr
171 Ashley Ave Charleston, SC 29425 SOUTHEAST

MedStar Union Memorial Hospital (410) 554-2000
MedStar Union Meml Hosp
201 E University Pkwy Baltimore, MD 21218 MID ATLANTIC

Memorial Health University Medical Center - Savannah (912) 350-8000
Meml Hlth Univ Med Ctr - Savannah
4700 Waters Ave Savannah, GA 31404 SOUTHEAST

Memorial Hermann Hospital - Texas Medical Center (713) 704-4000
Meml Hermann Hosp - Texas Med Ctr
6411 Fannin Houston, TX 77030 SOUTHWEST

Memorial Medical Center-Springfield (217) 788-3000
Memorial Med Ctr-Springfield
701 N First St Springfield, IL 62781 MIDWEST

Memorial Regional Hospital (954) 987-2000
Meml Regl Hosp
3501 Johnson Street Hollywood, FL 33021 SOUTHEAST

Memorial Sloan-Kettering Cancer Center (212) 639-2000
Meml Sloan-Kettering Cancer Ctr
1275 York Avenue New York, NY 10021 MID ATLANTIC

Menninger Clinic (800) 351-9058
Menninger Clinic
12301 Main St Houston, TX 77035 SOUTHWEST

Mercy General Hospital - Sacramento (916) 453-4545
Mercy General Hosp - Sacramento
4001 J Street Sacramento, CA 95819 WEST COAST AND PACIFIC

Mercy Gilbert Medical Center (480) 728-8000
Mercy Gilbert Med Ctr
3555 S Val Vista Drive Gilbert, AZ 85297 SOUTHWEST

Mercy Health Center - Oklahoma City (405) 755-1515
Mercy Hlth Ctr - Oklahoma City
4300 W Memorial Dr Oklahoma City, OK 73120 SOUTHWEST

Mercy Hospital (305) 854-4400
Mercy Hosp
3663 S Miami Ave Miami, FL 33133 SOUTHEAST

Mercy Hospital - Coon Rapids (763) 236-6000
Mercy Hosp - Coon Rapids
4050 Coon Rapids Blvd Coon Rapids, MN 55433-2522 MIDWEST

Mercy Hospital - Fairfield (513) 870-7000
Mercy Hosp - Fairfield
3000 Mack Rd Fairfield, OH 45014 MIDWEST

Mercy Hospital - St Louis (314) 251-6000
Mercy Hosp - St Louis
615 S New Ballas Rd St Louis, MO 63141 MIDWEST

Mercy Medical Center - Baltimore (410) 332-9000
Mercy Med Ctr - Baltimore
345 St Paul Pl Baltimore, MD 21202 MID ATLANTIC

Methodist Hospital System (713) 790-3311
Methodist Hosp - Houston
6565 Fannin St Houston, TX 77030 SOUTHWEST

Methodist Hospital-Omaha (402) 354-4000
Methodist Hosp - Omaha
8303 Dodge St Omaha, NE 68114 GREAT PLAINS AND MOUNTAINS

Methodist Hospital-San Antonio (210) 575-4000
Methodist Hosp-San Antonio
7700 Floyd Curl Dr San Antonio, TX 78229 SOUTHWEST

Methodist Sugar Land Hospital (281) 274-7000
Methodist Sugar Land Hosp
16655 Southwest Freeway Sugar Land, TX 77479 SOUTHWEST

Methodist University Hospital - Memphis (901) 516-7000
Methodist Univ Hosp - Memphis
1265 Union Ave Memphis, TN 38104 SOUTHEAST

MetroHealth Medical Center (216) 778-7800
MetroHealth Med Ctr
2500 MetroHealth Drive Cleveland, OH 44109-1998 MIDWEST

Miami Children's Hospital (305) 666-6511
Miami Children's Hosp
3100 SW 62nd Ave Miami, FL 33155 SOUTHEAST

Michael E. DeBakey VA Medical Center - Houston (713) 791-1414
DeBakey VA Med Ctr-Houston
2002 Holcombe Blvd Houston, TX 77030-1414 SOUTHWEST

Michigan State University-Sparrow Hospital (517) 364-1000
Mich State Univ-Sparrow Hos
1215 E Michigan Ave, MS 0 Lansing, MI 48912 MIDWEST

Milford Hospital (203) 876-4000
Milford Hosp
300 Seaside Ave Milford, CT 06460 NEW ENGLAND

Mills-Peninsula Medical Center (650) 696-5400
Mills-Peninsula Med Ctr
1501 Trousdale Drive Burlingame, CA 94010 WEST COAST AND PACIFIC

Miriam Hospital (401) 793-2500
Miriam Hosp
164 Summit Avenue Providence, RI 02906-2894 NEW ENGLAND

Mission Hospital-Mission Viejo (949) 364-1400
Mission Hosp-Mission Viejo
27700 Medical Center Road Mission Viejo, CA 92691 WEST COAST AND PACIFIC

Missouri Baptist Medical Center (314) 996-5000
Missouri Baptist Med Ctr
3015 N Ballas Rd St Louis, MO 63131 MIDWEST

Mobile Infirmary Medical Center (251) 435-2400
Mobile Infirmary Med Ctr
5 Mobile Infirmary Circle Mobile, AL 36607-3513 SOUTHEAST

Montefiore Medical Center-Einstein Campus, NY (718) 904-2000
Montefiore Med Ctr-Einstein Campus, NY
1825 Eastchester Road Bronx, NY 10461 MID ATLANTIC

Montefiore Medical Center-Moses Campus, NY (718) 920-4321
Montefiore Med Ctr-Moses Campus, NY
111 East 210 Street Bronx, NY 10467 MID ATLANTIC

Montefiore Medical Center-Wakefield Campus, NY (718) 920-9000
Montefiore Med Ctr-Wakefield Campus, NY
600 E 233rd St Bronx, NY 10466 MID ATLANTIC

Morgan Stanley Children's Hospital of NewYork-Presbyterian, NY (212) 305-2500
Morgan Stanley Children's Hosp of NY-Presby, NY
622 W 168th St New York, NY 10032 MID ATLANTIC

Morristown Medical Center (973) 971-5000
Morristown Med Ctr
100 Madison Avenue Morristown, NJ 07960-6095 MID ATLANTIC

Moss Rehab Hospital (215) 663-6000
Moss Rehab Hosp
60 E Township Line Rd Elkins Park, PA 19027 MID ATLANTIC

Mott Children's Hospital (734) 936-4000
Mott Chldns Hosp
1500 E Medical Center Dr Ann Arbor, MI 48109 MIDWEST

Mount Auburn Hospital
(617) 492-3500
Mount Auburn Hosp
330 Mount Auburn St Cambridge, MA 02138 NEW ENGLAND

Mount Carmel West Hospital
(614) 234-5000
Mt Carmel W Hosp
793 W State St Columbus, OH 43085 MIDWEST

Mount Clemens Regional Medical Center
(586) 493-8000
Mount Clemens Regional Med Ctr
1000 Harrington Blvd Mount Clemens, MI 48043 MIDWEST

Mount Sinai Medical Center
(212) 241-6500
Mount Sinai Med Ctr
One Gustave L. Levy Pl New York, NY 10029 MID ATLANTIC

Mount Sinai Medical Center - Miami
(305) 674-2121
Mount Sinai Med Ctr - Miami
4300 Alton Rd Miami Beach, FL 33140 SOUTHEAST

Mountainview Hospital - Las Vegas
(702) 255-5000
Mountainview Hosp - Las Vegas
3100 N Tenaya Way Las Vegas, NV 89128 WEST COAST AND PACIFIC

Munroe Regional Medical Center
(352) 351-7200
Munroe Regional Med Ctr
1500 SW 1st Ave Ocala, FL 34471 SOUTHEAST

Nashville General Hospital at Meharry
(615) 341-4000
Nashville Genl Hosp
1818 Albion St Nashville, TN 37208 SOUTHEAST

National Institutes of Health - Clinical Center
(301) 496-4000
Natl Inst of Hlth - Clin Ctr
10 Center Drive Bethesda, MD 20892-0001 MID ATLANTIC

National Jewish Medical & Research Center
(303) 388-4461
Natl Jewish Med & Rsch Ctr
1400 Jackson St Denver, CO 80206-2762 GREAT PLAINS AND MOUNTAINS

National Rehabilitation Hospital
(202) 877-1000
Natl Rehab Hosp
102 Irving St NW Washington, DC 20010 MID ATLANTIC

Nationwide Children's Hospital
(614) 722-2000
Nationwide Chldn's Hosp
700 Children's Drive Columbus, OH 43205 MIDWEST

Nebraska Medical Center (402) 552-2000
Nebraska Med Ctr
4350 Dewey Ave Omaha, NE 68198 GREAT PLAINS AND MOUNTAINS

Nebraska Methodist Hospital (402) 354-4000
Nebraska Meth Hosp
8303 Dodge St Omaha, NE 68114 GREAT PLAINS AND MOUNTAINS

Nemours Children's Hospital - Orlando (407) 567-4000
Nemours Chldns Hosp - Orlando
13535 Nemours Pkwy Orlando, FL 32827 SOUTHEAST

Nemours/Alfred I. duPont Hospital for Children (302) 651-4000
Nemours/Alfred I. duPont Hosp for Chldn
1600 Rockland Rd Wilmington, DE 19803 MID ATLANTIC

New England Baptist Hospital (617) 754-5800
New England Bapt Hosp
125 Parker Hill Ave Boston, MA 02120 NEW ENGLAND

New Hanover Regional Medical Center (910) 343-7000
New Hanover Reg Med Ctr
2131 S 17th St Wilmington, NC 28401 SOUTHEAST

New York Eye & Ear Infirmary (212) 979-4000
New York Eye & Ear Infirm
310 East 14th Street New York, NY 10003 MID ATLANTIC

New York Hospital Queens (718) 670-2000
NY Hosp Queens
56-45 Main Street Flushing, NY 11355 MID ATLANTIC

New York Methodist Hospital (718) 780-3000
New York Methodist Hosp
506 Sixth Street Brooklyn, NY 11215 MID ATLANTIC

New York State Psychiatric Institute (212) 543-5000
NY State Psychiatric Inst
1051 Riverside Dr New York, NY 10032 MID ATLANTIC

Newark Beth Israel Medical Center (973) 926-7000
Newark Beth Israel Med Ctr
201 Lyons Ave Newark, NJ 07112 MID ATLANTIC

Newton - Wellesley Hospital (617) 243-6000
Newton - Wellesley Hosp
2014 Washington St Newton, MA 02462 NEW ENGLAND

NewYork-Presbyterian/Columbia University Medical Center, NY (212) 305-2500
NY-Presby/Columbia Univ Med Ctr, NY
622 W 168th St New York, NY 10032 MID ATLANTIC

NewYork-Presbyterian/Weill Cornell Medical Center, NY (212) 746-5454
NY-Presby/Weill Cornell Med Ctr, NY
525 E 68th St New York, NY 10021 MID ATLANTIC

North Carolina Memorial Hospital - UNC (919) 966-4131
NC Memorial Hosp - UNC
101 Manning Drive, Box 7600 Chapel Hill, NC 27514 SOUTHEAST

North Oaks Medical Center (985) 345-2700
North Oaks Med Ctr
15790 Paul Vega MD Dr Hammond, LA 70403 SOUTHWEST

North Shore Medical Center - Salem Hospital (978) 741-1200
N Shore Med Ctr - Salem Hosp
81 Highland Avenue Salem, MA 01970 NEW ENGLAND

North Shore University Hospital (516) 562-0100
N Shore Univ Hosp
300 Community Dr Manhasset, NY 11030 MID ATLANTIC

North Shore-LIJ Health System (516) 465-2600
NS-LIJ Hlth Sys
125 Community Drive Great Neck, NY 11021 MID ATLANTIC

Northern California Shriners Hospital (916) 453-2000
Northern CA Shriners Hosp
2425 Stockton Blvd Sacramento, CA 95817 WEST COAST AND PACIFIC

Northern Michigan Hospital (231) 487-4000
Northern Michigan Hosp
416 Connable Ave Petoskey, MI 49770 MIDWEST

Northern Nevada Medical Center (775) 331-7000
Northern Nevada Med Ctr
2375 E Prater Way Sparks, NV 89434-9644 WEST COAST AND PACIFIC

Northside Hospital - Atlanta (404) 851-8000
Northside Hosp
1000 Johnson Ferry Rd NE Atlanta, GA 30342 SOUTHEAST

Northwest Hospital - Seattle (206) 364-0500
Northwest Hosp - Seattle
1550 N 115th St Seattle, WA 98133-0806 WEST COAST AND PACIFIC

Northwest Medical Center		(954) 974-0400
Northwest Med Ctr		
2801 N State Rd 7	Margate, FL 33063	SOUTHEAST

Northwestern Memorial Hospital		(312) 926-2000
Northwestern Meml Hosp		
251 E Huron St	Chicago, IL 60611	MIDWEST

Norton Hospital		(502) 629-8000
Norton Hosp		
200 E Chestnut St	Louisville, KY 40202	SOUTHEAST

NYU Hospital for Joint Diseases		(212) 598-6000
NYU Hosp For Joint Diseases		
301 East 17th Street	New York, NY 10003	MID ATLANTIC

NYU Langone Medical Center		(212) 263-7300
NYU Langone Med Ctr		
550 First Avenue	New York, NY 10016	MID ATLANTIC

NYU Rusk Institute		(212) 263-1999
NYU Rusk Inst		
400 East 34th Street	New York, NY 10016	MID ATLANTIC

Ochsner Medical Center-Baton Rouge		(225) 752-2470
Ochsner Med Ctr-Baton Rouge		
17000 Medical Center Drive	Baton Rouge, LA 70816	SOUTHWEST

Ochsner Medical Center-Kenner		(504) 468-8600
Ochsner Med Ctr-Kenner		
180 W Esplanade Ave	Kenner, LA 70065-2467	SOUTHWEST

Ochsner Medical Center-New Orleans		(504) 842-3000
Ochsner Med Ctr-New Orleans		
1514 Jefferson Hwy	New Orleans, LA 70121	SOUTHWEST

Ohio State University Medical Center		(614) 293-8652
Ohio St Univ Med Ctr		
410 W 10th Avenue	Columbus, OH 43210	MIDWEST

OHSU Healthcare		(503) 494-8311
OHSU Hlthcare		
3181 SW Sam Jackson Park Rd	Portland, OR 97239	WEST COAST AND PACIFIC

Olathe Medical Center		(913) 791-4200
Olathe Med Ctr		
20333 W 151st St	Olathe, KS 66061-5352	GREAT PLAINS AND MOUNTAINS

Olive View-UCLA Medical Center　　　　　　　　　(818) 364-1555
Olive View-UCLA Med Ctr
14445 Olive View Dr　　　　　　　Sylmar, CA 91342　　　WEST COAST AND PACIFIC

Olympia Medical Center　　　　　　　　　　　　　(310) 657-5900
Olympia Med Ctr
5900 W Olympic Blvd　　　　　　　Los Angeles, CA 90036　WEST COAST AND PACIFIC

Oregon Health & Science University　　　　　　　(503) 494-8311
OR Hlth & Sci Univ
3181 SW Sam Jackson Park Rd　　　Portland, OR 97239-3098　WEST COAST AND
　　　　　　　　　　　　　　　　　　　　　　　　　　　　　PACIFIC

Orlando Regional Medical Center　　　　　　　　(321) 841-5111
Orlando Regl Med Ctr
1414 Kuhl Ave　　　　　　　　　　Orlando, FL 32806　　　SOUTHEAST

Orthopedic Specialty Hospital, The (TOSH)　　　(801) 314-4100
Ortho Spec Hosp, The (TOSH)
5848 Fashion Blvd　　　　　　　　Salt Lake City, UT 84107　GREAT PLAINS AND
　　　　　　　　　　　　　　　　　　　　　　　　　　　　　MOUNTAINS

OSF Saint Francis Medical Center　　　　　　　　(309) 655-2000
OSF Saint Francis Med Ctr
530 NE Glen Oak Ave　　　　　　　Peoria, IL 61637　　　　MIDWEST

OU Medical Center　　　　　　　　　　　　　　(405) 271-4700
OU Med Ctr
700 NE 13th St　　　　　　　　　　Oklahoma City, OK 73104-5098　SOUTHWEST

Our Lady of Lourdes Regional Medical Center - Lafayette　(337) 470-2000
Our Lady of Lourdes Reg Med Ctr - Lafayette
4801 Ambassador Caffery Pkwy　　Lafayette, LA 70508　　SOUTHWEST

Our Lady of the Lake Regional Medical Center　　(225) 765-6565
Our Lady of the Lake Regl Med Ctr
5000 Hennessy Blvd　　　　　　　Baton Rouge, LA 70808-4398　SOUTHWEST

Overlake Hospital Medical Center　　　　　　　　(425) 688-5000
Overlake Hosp Med Ctr
1035 116th Ave NE　　　　　　　Bellevue, WA 98004-4687　WEST COAST AND
　　　　　　　　　　　　　　　　　　　　　　　　　　　　　PACIFIC

Overland Park Regional Medical Center　　　　　(913) 541-5000
Overland Pk Regl Med Ctr
10500 Quivira Rd　　　　　　　　Overland Park, KS 66215　GREAT PLAINS AND
　　　　　　　　　　　　　　　　　　　　　　　　　　　　　MOUNTAINS

Palmetto Health Richland Memorial Hospital (803) 434-7000
Palmetto Health Richland Mem Hosp
5 Richland Medical Park Drive Columbia, SC 29203 SOUTHEAST

Paoli Hospital (484) 565-1000
Paoli Hosp
255 W Lancaster Ave Paoli, PA 19301-1792 MID ATLANTIC

Parkinson's Institute/Movement Disorders Treament Center, The (408) 734-2800
Parkinson's Inst/Movement Disorders Trmt Ctr, The
675 Almanor Ave Sunnyvale, CA 94085 WEST COAST AND PACIFIC

Parkland Health & Hospital System (214) 590-8000
Parkland Hlth & Hosp Sys
5201 Harry Hines Blvd Dallas, TX 75235 SOUTHWEST

Parma Community General Hospital (440) 743-3000
Parma Community Genl Hosp
7007 Powers Blvd Parma, OH 44129 MIDWEST

Penn Presbyterian Medical Center - UPHS (215) 662-8000
Penn Presby Med Ctr - UPHS
51 N 39th St Philadelphia, PA 19104 MID ATLANTIC

Penn State Children's Hospital (717) 531-8521
Penn State Chldns Hosp
500 University Dr Hershey, PA 17033 MID ATLANTIC

Penn State Milton S. Hershey Medical Center (717) 531-8521
Penn State Milton S Hershey Med Ctr
500 University Drive Hershey, PA 17033-0850 MID ATLANTIC

Pennsylvania Hospital - UPHS (215) 829-3000
Pennsylvania Hosp-UPHS
800 Spruce St, Ste 240 Philadelphia, PA 19107 MID ATLANTIC

Penrose Hospital (719) 776-5000
Penrose Hosp
2222 N Nevada Ave Colorado Springs, CO 80907 GREAT PLAINS AND
 MOUNTAINS

Peyton Manning Children's Hospital at St. Vincent (317) 338-2345
Peyton Manning Children's Hosp at St. Vincent
2001 W 86th St Indianapolis, IN 46260 MIDWEST

Philadelphia Shriners Hospital (215) 430-4000
Philadelphia Shriners Hosp
3551 N Broad St Philadelphia, PA 19140 MID ATLANTIC

Phillips Eye Institute (612) 775-8800
Phillips Eye Inst
2215 Park Ave S Minneapolis, MN 55404 MIDWEST

Phoenix Baptist Hospital & Medical Center (602) 249-0212
Phoenix Baptist Hosp & Med Ctr
2000 West Bethany Home Rd Phoenix, AZ 85015-2184 SOUTHWEST

Phoenix Children's Hospital (602) 933-1000
Phoenix Children's Hosp
1919 E Thomas Rd Phoenix, AZ 85106 SOUTHWEST

Physicians Regional Healthcare System-Pine Ridge (239) 348-4000
Physicians Regl Hlthcare Med Ctr-Pine Ridge
6101 Pine Ridge Rd Naples, FL 34119 SOUTHEAST

Piedmont Hospital (404) 605-5000
Piedmont Hosp
1968 Peachtree Rd NW Atlanta, GA 30309 SOUTHEAST

Pocono Medical Center (570) 421-4000
Pocono Med Ctr
206 E Brown St East Stroudsburg, PA 18301-3094 MID ATLANTIC

Porter Adventist Hospital (303) 778-1955
Porter Adventist Hosp
2525 S Downing St Denver, CO 80210-5876 GREAT PLAINS AND MOUNTAINS

Portsmouth Regional Hospital (603) 436-5110
Portsmouth Regl Hosp
333 Borthwick Ave Portsmouth, NH 03801-7002 NEW ENGLAND

Presbyterian - St Luke's Medical Center (303) 839-6000
Presby - St Luke's Med Ctr
1719 E 19th Ave Denver, CO 80218 GREAT PLAINS AND MOUNTAINS

Presbyterian Hospital - Charlotte (704) 384-4000
Presby Hosp - Charlotte
200 Hawthorne Ln Charlotte, NC 28204-2528 SOUTHEAST

Primary Children's Medical Center (801) 662-1000
Primary Children's Med Ctr
100 N Mario Capecchi Drive Salt Lake City, UT 84113-1100 GREAT PLAINS AND
MOUNTAINS

Providence Alaska Medical Center (907) 562-2211
Providence Alaska Med Ctr
3200 Providence Dr Anchorage, AK 99508-4615 WEST COAST AND
PACIFIC

Providence Hospital - Southfield (248) 849-3000
Providence Hosp - Southfield
16001 W Nine Mile Rd Southfield, MI 48075 MIDWEST

Providence Portland Medical Center (503) 215-1111
Providence Portland Med Ctr
4805 NE Glisan Portland, OR 97213-2967 WEST COAST AND PACIFIC

Providence Saint Joseph Medical Center (818) 843-5111
Providence St Joseph Med Ctr
501 S Buena Vista St Burbank, CA 91505 WEST COAST AND PACIFIC

Providence St Vincent Medical Center (503) 216-1234
Providence St Vincent Med Ctr
9205 SW Barnes Rd Portland, OR 97225-6622 WEST COAST AND PACIFIC

Queen's Medical Center - Honolulu (808) 538-9011
Queen's Med Ctr - Honolulu
1301 Punchbowl Street Honolulu, HI 96813 WEST COAST AND PACIFIC

Rady Children's Hospital - San Diego (858) 576-1700
Rady Children's Hosp - San Diego
3020 Children's Way San Diego, CA 92123 WEST COAST AND PACIFIC

Rancho Los Amigos National Rehabilitation Center (562) 401-7111
Rancho Los Amigos Natl Rehab Ctr
7601 East Imperial Highway Downey, CA 90242 WEST COAST AND PACIFIC

Randall Children's Hospital at Legacy Emanuel (503) 276-6500
Randall Chldns Hosp at Legacy
2801 Gantenbein Ave Portland, OR 97227 WEST COAST AND PACIFIC

Regional Medical Center - Memphis (901) 545-7100
Regional Med Ctr - Memphis
877 Jefferson Avenue Memphis, TN 38103 SOUTHEAST

Regions Hospital - St Paul (651) 254-3456
Regions Hosp - St Paul
640 Jackson Street St Paul, MN 55101 MIDWEST

Rehabilitation Institute of Chicago (312) 238-1000
Rehab Inst of Chicago
345 E. Superior Street Chicago, IL 60611 MIDWEST

Rehabilitation Institute of St. Louis (314) 658-3800
Rehab Inst St. Louis
4455 Duncan Ave St. Louis, MO 63110 MIDWEST

Reid Hospital & Health Care Services (765) 983-3000
Reid Hosp & Hlth Care Servs
1100 Reid Pkwy Richmond, IN 47374 MIDWEST

Renown Regional Medical Center (775) 982-4100
Renown Reg Med Ctr
1155 Mill St Reno, NV 89502 WEST COAST AND PACIFIC

Resnick Neuropsychiatric Hospital at UCLA (310) 825-0511
Resnick Neuropsychiatric Hosp at UCLA
760 Westwood Plaza Los Angeles, CA 90095 WEST COAST AND PACIFIC

Reston Hospital Center (703) 689-9000
Reston Hosp Ctr
1850 Town Center Pkwy Reston, VA 20190 SOUTHEAST

Resurrection Health Care Saint Joseph Hospital (773) 665-3000
Resurrection Hlth Care St Joseph Hosp
2900 N Lake Shore Dr Chicago, IL 60657 MIDWEST

Rex HealthCare (919) 784-3100
Rex HlthCare
4420 Lake Boone Trail Raleigh, NC 27607 SOUTHEAST

Rhode Island Hospital (401) 444-4000
Rhode Island Hosp
593 Eddy Street Providence, RI 02903-4923 NEW ENGLAND

Riddle Memorial Hospital (484) 227-9400
Riddle Meml Hosp
1068 W Baltimore Pike Media, PA 19063 MID ATLANTIC

Riley Hospital for Children (317) 944-5000
Riley Hosp for Children
705 Riley Hospital Drive Indianapolis, IN 46202 MIDWEST

Riverside Community Hospital (951) 788-3000
Riverside Comm Hosp
4445 Magnolia Avenue Riverside, CA 92501 WEST COAST AND PACIFIC

Riverview Medical Center (732) 741-2700
Riverview Med Ctr
1 Riverview Plaza Red Bank, NJ 07701 MID ATLANTIC

Robert Wood Johnson University Hospital - New Brunswick (732) 828-3000
Robert Wood Johnson Univ Hosp - New Brunswick
1 Robert Wood Johnson Pl New Brunswick, NJ 08903 MID ATLANTIC

Rochester General Hospital (585) 922-4000
Rochester Genl Hosp
1425 Portland Avenue Rochester, NY 14621 MID ATLANTIC

Rochester Methodist Hospital (507) 266-7890
Rochester Methodist Hosp
201 W Center St Rochester, MN 55902 MIDWEST

Roger Williams Medical Center (401) 456-2000
Roger Williams Med Ctr
825 Chalkstone Avenue Providence, RI 02908 NEW ENGLAND

Roper Hospital (843) 724-2000
Roper Hosp
316 Calhoun St Charleston, SC 29401 SOUTHEAST

Rose Medical Center (303) 320-2121
Rose Med Ctr
4567 E 9th Ave Denver, CO 80220-3941 GREAT PLAINS AND MOUNTAINS

Roswell Park Cancer Institute (716) 845-2300
Roswell Park Cancer Inst
Elm and Carlton Streets Buffalo, NY 14263 MID ATLANTIC

Ruby Memorial - WVU Hospital (304) 598-4000
Ruby Memorial - WVU Hosp
1 Medical Center Drive Morgantown, WV 26506 MID ATLANTIC

Rush University Medical Center (312) 942-5000
Rush Univ Med Ctr
1653 W Congress Pkwy Chicago, IL 60612-3833 MIDWEST

Sacred Heart Medical Center (541) 686-7300
Sacred Heart Med Ctr
1255 Hilyard St Eugene, OR 97440-3700 WEST COAST AND PACIFIC

Saint Barnabas Medical Center (973) 322-5000
Saint Barnabas Med Ctr
94 Old Short Hills Rd Livingston, NJ 07039-5672 MID ATLANTIC

Saint Francis Hospital - Memphis (901) 765-1000
St. Francis Hosp - Memphis
5959 Park Ave Memphis, TN 38119 SOUTHEAST

Saint John's Health Center (310) 829-5511
St. John's Hlth Ctr, Santa Monica
2121 Santa Monica Blvd Santa Monica, CA 90404 WEST COAST AND PACIFIC

Saint Joseph's Hospital - Atlanta (678) 843-7001
St. Joseph's Hosp - Atlanta
5665 Peachtree Dunwoody Rd NE Atlanta, GA 30342 SOUTHEAST

Saint Thomas Hospital - Nashville (615) 222-2111
Saint Thomas Hosp - Nashville
4220 Harding Road Nashville, TN 37205 SOUTHEAST

Salinas Valley Memorial Healthcare Systems (831) 757-4333
Salinas Valley Meml Hlthcare Systs
450 E Romie Ln Salinas, CA 93901 WEST COAST AND PACIFIC

Saline Memorial Hospital (501) 776-6000
Saline Meml Hosp
1 Medical Park Dr Benton, AR 72015 SOUTHWEST

Salt Lake Regional Medical Center (801) 350-4111
Salt Lake Regional Med Ctr
1050 E South Temple Salt Lake City, UT 84102 GREAT PLAINS AND MOUNTAINS

San Diego Hospice (619) 688-1600
San Diego Hospice
4311 3rd Ave San Diego, CA 92103-7499 WEST COAST AND PACIFIC

San Francisco General Hospital (415) 206-8000
San Francisco Genl Hosp
1001 Potrero Avenue San Francisco, CA 94110 WEST COAST AND PACIFIC

Sanford Medical Center Fargo (701) 234-2000
Sanford Med Ctr Fargo
801 Broadway Drive, PO Box 2010 Fargo, ND 58122 GREAT PLAINS AND MOUNTAINS

Sanford USD Medical Center (605) 333-1000
Sanford USD Med Ctr
1305 W 18th St Sioux Falls, SD 57117 GREAT PLAINS AND MOUNTAINS

Santa Barbara Cottage Hospital (805) 682-7111
Santa Barbara Cottage Hosp
400 W Pueblo St Santa Barbara, CA 93105 WEST COAST AND PACIFIC

Santa Monica - UCLA Medical Center and Orthopaedic Hospital (310) 319-4000
Santa Monica - UCLA Med Ctr & Ortho Hosp
1250 16th St Santa Monica, CA 90404 WEST COAST AND PACIFIC

Santa Rosa Memorial Hospital (747) 546-3210
Santa Rosa Meml Hosp
1165 Montgomery Drive Santa Rosa, CA 95405 WEST COAST AND PACIFIC

Sarasota Memorial Hospital (941) 917-9000
Sarasota Meml Hosp
1700 S Tamiami Trail Sarasota, FL 34239 SOUTHEAST

Schwab Rehabilitation Hospital (773) 522-2010
Schwab Rehab Hosp
1401 S. California Boulevard Chicago, IL 60608 MIDWEST

Scott & White Memorial Hospital (254) 724-2111
Scott & White Mem Hosp
2401 S 31st St Temple, TX 76508-0001 SOUTHWEST

Scottsdale Healthcare - Osborn (480) 882-4000
Scottsdale Hlthcare - Osborn
7400 E Osborn Rd Scottsdale, AZ 85251-6403 SOUTHWEST

Scottsdale Healthcare - Shea (480) 323-3000
Scottsdale Hlthcare - Shea
9003 E Shea Blvd Scottsdale, AZ 85260 SOUTHWEST

Scripps Green Hospital (858) 554-9100
Scripps Green Hosp
10666 N Torrey Pines Rd La Jolla, CA 92037 WEST COAST AND PACIFIC

Scripps Memorial Hospital - La Jolla (858) 626-4123
Scripps Meml Hosp - La Jolla
9888 Genesee Ave La Jolla, CA 92037 WEST COAST AND PACIFIC

Scripps Mercy Hospital & Medical Center (619) 294-8111
Scripps Mercy Hosp & Med Ctr
4077 Fifth Ave San Diego, CA 92103 WEST COAST AND PACIFIC

Seattle Children's Hospital (206) 987-2000
Seattle Chldns Hosp
4800 Sand Point Way NE Seattle, WA 98105 WEST COAST AND PACIFIC

Self Regional Healthcare (864) 725-4111
Self Regional Healthcare
1325 Spring St Greenwood, SC 29646 SOUTHEAST

Sentara Leigh Hospital (757) 261-6000
Sentara Leigh Hosp
830 Kempsville Rd Norfolk, VA 23502-3981 SOUTHEAST

Sentara Norfolk General Hospital (757) 388-3000
Sentara Norfolk Genl Hosp
600 Gresham Dr Norfolk, VA 23507 SOUTHEAST

Sentara Virginia Beach General Hospital		(757) 395-8000
Sentara VA Beach Genl Hosp		
1060 First Colonial Rd	Virginia Beach, VA 23454	SOUTHEAST

Sequoia Hospital		(650) 369-5811
Sequoia Hosp		
170 Alameda de las Pulgas	Redwood, CA 94062	WEST COAST AND PACIFIC

Shady Grove Adventist Hospital		(240) 826-6000
Shady Grove Adven Hosp		
9901 Medical Center Drive	Rockville, MD 20850	MID ATLANTIC

Shands at University of Florida		(352) 265-8000
Shands at Univ of FL		
1600 SW Archer Rd	Gainesville, FL 32610	SOUTHEAST

Shands Jacksonville Medical Center		(904) 244-0411
Shands Jacksonville Med Ctr		
655 W 8th St	Jacksonville, FL 32209	SOUTHEAST

Shawnee Mission Medical Center		(913) 676-2000
Shawnee Mission Med Ctr		
9100 W 74th St	Shawnee Mission, KS 66204	GREAT PLAINS AND MOUNTAINS

Shepherd Center - Atlanta		(404) 352-2020
Shepherd Ctr - Atlanta		
2020 Peachtree Rd NW	Atlanta, GA 30309-1402	SOUTHEAST

Sheppard Pratt Health System		(410) 938-3000
Sheppard Pratt Hlth Sys		
6501 N Charles St	Baltimore, MD 21285-6815	MID ATLANTIC

Sherman Hospital		(847) 742-9800
Sherman Hosp		
1425 N Randall Rd	Elgin, IL 60120	MIDWEST

Sibley Memorial Hospital		(202) 537-4000
Sibley Mem Hosp		
5255 Loughboro Road NW	Washington, DC 20016	MID ATLANTIC

Silver Hill Hospital		(203) 966-3561
Silver Hill Hosp		
208 Valley Rd	New Canaan, CT 06840-3899	NEW ENGLAND

Sinai Hospital - Baltimore		(410) 601-9000
Sinai Hosp - Baltimore		
2401 W Belvedere Ave	Baltimore, MD 21215	MID ATLANTIC

Sky Ridge Medical Center (720) 225-1000
Sky Ridge Med Ctr
10101 Ridge Gate Pkwy Lone Tree, CO 80124 GREAT PLAINS AND MOUNTAINS

South Miami Hospital (786) 662-4000
South Miami Hosp
6200 SW 73 St South Miami, FL 33143 SOUTHEAST

South Nassau Communities Hospital (516) 632-3000
South Nassau Comm Hosp
1 Healthy Way Oceanside, NY 11572 MID ATLANTIC

Southampton Hospital (631) 726-8200
Southampton Hosp
240 Meeting House Ln Southampton, NY 11968 MID ATLANTIC

Southern Arizona VA Health Care System - Tucson (520) 792-1450
Southern AZ VA Health Care Sys - Tucson
3601 S 6th Avenue Tucson, AZ 85723 SOUTHWEST

Southern Hills Hospital & Medical Center (702) 880-2100
Southern Hills Hosp & Med Ctr
9300 W Sunset Rd Las Vegas, NV 89148 WEST COAST AND PACIFIC

Southern New Hampshire Medical Center (603) 577-2000
Southern NH Med Ctr
8 Prospect St Nashua, NH 03061 NEW ENGLAND

Spaulding Rehabilitation Hospital (617) 573-7000
Spaulding Rehab Hosp
125 Nashua Street Boston, MA 02114 NEW ENGLAND

Spectrum Health - Blodgett Campus (616) 774-7444
Spectrum Hlth Blodgett Campus
1840 Wealthy St SE Grand Rapids, MI 49506 MIDWEST

Spectrum Health Butterworth Campus (616) 391-1774
Spectrum Hlth Butterworth Campus
100 Michigan St NE Grand Rapids, MI 49503 MIDWEST

SSM Cardinal Glennon Children's Hospital (314) 577-5600
SSM Cardinal Glennon Chldn's Hosp
1465 S Grand Blvd St Louis, MO 63104 MIDWEST

SSM St. Clare Health Ctr (636) 496-2000
SSM St. Clare Hlth Ctr
1015 Bowles Ave Fenton, MO 63026 MIDWEST

St. Alphonsus Regional Medical Center (208) 367-2121
St. Alphonsus Regl Med Ctr
1055 N Curtis Rd Boise, ID 83706-1370 GREAT PLAINS AND MOUNTAINS

St. Anthony Hospital - Oklahoma City (405) 272-7000
St. Anthony Hosp -Oklahoma City
1000 N Lee St Oklahoma City, OK 73102 SOUTHWEST

St. Anthony's Hospital - St Petersburg (727) 825-1100
St. Anthony's Hosp - St Petersburg
1200 7th Avenue North St Petersburg, FL 33705 SOUTHEAST

St. Charles Surgical Hospital (504) 529-6600
St. Charles Surgical Hosp
1717 St. Charles Ave New Orleans, LA 70130 SOUTHWEST

St. Christopher's Hospital for Children (215) 427-5000
St. Christopher's Hosp for Chldn
3601 A St Philadelphia, PA 19134 MID ATLANTIC

St. David's Medical Center (512) 476-7111
St. David's Med Ctr
919 E 32nd st Austin, TX 78705 SOUTHWEST

St. Elizabeth Healthcare-Edgewood (859) 301-2000
St. Elizabeth Hlthcare-Edgewood
1 Medical Village Dr Edgewood, KY 41017 SOUTHEAST

St. Francis Hospital & Medical Center (860) 714-4000
St. Francis Hosp & Med Ctr
114 Woodland St Hartford, CT 06105 NEW ENGLAND

St. Francis Hospital - Evanston (847) 316-4000
St. Francis Hosp - Evanston
355 Ridge Ave Evanston, IL 60202 MIDWEST

St. Francis Hospital - The Heart Center (516) 562-6000
St. Francis Hosp - The Heart Ctr
100 Port Washington Boulevard Roslyn, NY 11576 MID ATLANTIC

St. John's Hospital - Springfield (217) 544-6464
St. John's Hosp - Springfield
800 E Carpenter St Springfield, IL 62769 MIDWEST

St. John's Hospital-Maplewood MN (651) 232-7000
St. John's Hosp-Maplewood MN
1575 Beam Ave Maplewood, MN 55109 MIDWEST

St. John's Regional Medical Center (805) 988-2500
St. John's Regional Med Ctr
1600 N Rose Ave Oxnard, CA 93030 WEST COAST AND PACIFIC

St. Joseph Hospital (773) 665-3000
St. Joseph Hosp
2900 N Lake Shore Drive Chicago, IL 60657 MIDWEST

St. Joseph Hospital (360) 734-5400
St. Joseph Hosp - Bellingham
2901 Squalicum Pkwy Bellingham, WA 98225-1898 WEST COAST AND PACIFIC

St. Joseph Hospital & Trauma Center (603) 882-3000
St. Joseph Hosp & Trauma Ctr
172 Kinsley St Nashua, NH 03061 NEW ENGLAND

St. Joseph Medical Center (410) 337-1000
St. Joseph Med Ctr
7601 Osler Drive Baltimore, MD 21208 MID ATLANTIC

St. Joseph Medical Center - Tacoma (253) 426-4101
St. Joseph Med Ctr - Tacoma
1717 South J St Tacoma, WA 98405 WEST COAST AND PACIFIC

St. Joseph Mercy Hospital - Ann Arbor (734) 712-3456
St. Joseph Mercy Hosp - Ann Arbor
5301 McAuley Drive Ypsilanti, MI 48197 MIDWEST

St. Joseph Mercy Oakland Hospital (248) 858-3000
St. Joseph Mercy Oakland Hosp
44405 Woodward Ave Pontiac, MI 48341 MIDWEST

St. Joseph's Children's Hospital (813) 554-8500
St. Josephs Chldns Hosp
3001 W Dr Martin Luther King Jr Blvd Tampa, FL 33607 SOUTHEAST

St. Joseph's Hospital & Medical Center - Phoenix (602) 406-3000
St. Joseph's Hosp & Med Ctr - Phoenix
350 W Thomas Rd Phoenix, AZ 85013-4496 SOUTHWEST

St. Joseph's Hospital - Orange (714) 633-9111
St. Joseph's Hosp - Orange
1100 West Stewart Drive Orange, CA 92868 WEST COAST AND PACIFIC

St. Joseph's Hospital - Tampa (813) 870-4000
St. Joseph's Hosp - Tampa
3001 W Martin Luther King Jr Blvd Tampa, FL 33607 SOUTHEAST

St. Joseph's Hospital - Tucson		(520) 873-3000
St. Joseph's Hosp - Tucson		
350 N Wilmot Rd	Tucson, AZ 85711	SOUTHWEST
St. Joseph's Regional Medical Center - Paterson		(973) 754-2000
St. Joseph's Regl Med Ctr - Paterson		
703 Main St	Paterson, NJ 07503	MID ATLANTIC
St. Jude Children's Research Hospital		(901) 495-3300
St. Jude Children's Research Hosp		
262 Danny Thomas Pl	Memphis, TN 38105	SOUTHEAST
St. Louis Children's Hospital		(314) 454-6000
St. Louis Chldns Hosp		
One Children's Pl	St Louis, MO 63110	MIDWEST
St. Louis University Hospital		(314) 577-8000
St. Louis Univ Hosp		
3635 Vista at Grand Blvd	St Louis, MO 63110	MIDWEST
St. Luke's - Roosevelt Hospital Center - Roosevelt Division		(212) 523-4000
St. Luke's - Roosevelt Hosp Ctr - Roosevelt Div		
1000 Tenth Avenue	New York, NY 10019	MID ATLANTIC
St. Luke's - Roosevelt Hospital Center - St Luke's Hospital		(212) 523-4000
St. Luke's - Roosevelt Hosp Ctr - St Luke's Hosp		
1111 Amsterdam Ave	New York, NY 10025	MID ATLANTIC
St. Luke's Boise Medical Center		(208) 381-2222
St. Luke's Boise Med Ctr		
190 E Bannock St	Boise, ID 83712	GREAT PLAINS AND MOUNTAINS
St. Luke's Episcopal Hospital-Houston		(832) 355-1000
St. Luke's Episcopal Hosp-Houston		
6720 Bertner Avenue, PO Box 20269	Houston, TX 77030	SOUTHWEST
St. Luke's Hospital - Allentown Campus		(610) 628-8300
St. Luke's Hosp - Allentown		
1736 Hamilton St	Allentown, PA 18104	MID ATLANTIC
St. Luke's Hospital - Chesterfield, MO		(314) 434-1500
St. Luke's Hosp - Chesterfield, MO		
232 S Woods Mill Rd	Chesterfield, MO 63017	MIDWEST
St. Luke's Hospital - Duluth		(218) 249-5555
St. Luke's Hosp - Duluth		
915 E 1st St	Duluth, MN 55805-2193	MIDWEST

St. Luke's Hospital of Kansas City (816) 932-5100
St. Luke's Hosp of Kansas City
4401 Wornall Rd Kansas City, MO 64111 MIDWEST

St. Mark's Hospital - Salt Lake City (801) 268-7111
St. Mark's Hosp - Salt Lake City
1200 E. 3900 S Salt Lake City, UT 84124 GREAT PLAINS AND MOUNTAINS

St. Mary Medical Center - Long Beach (562) 491-9000
St. Mary Med Ctr - Long Beach
1050 Linden Ave Long Beach, CA 90813 WEST COAST AND PACIFIC

St. Mary's Hospital - Rochester, MN (Mayo Clinic) (507) 255-5123
St. Mary's Hosp - Rochester MN (Mayo)
1216 2nd St SW Rochester, MN 55902 MIDWEST

St. Mary's Medical Center - Huntington (304) 526-1234
St. Mary's Med Ctr - Huntington
2900 First Ave Huntington, WV 25702-1272 MID ATLANTIC

St. Mary's Medical Center - West Palm Beach (561) 844-6300
St. Mary's Med Ctr - W Palm Bch
901 45th St West Palm Beach, FL 33407 SOUTHEAST

St. Patrick Hospital & Health Sciences Center (406) 543-7271
St. Patrick Hospital - Missoula
500 W Broadway Missoula, MT 59802 GREAT PLAINS AND MOUNTAINS

St. Peter's Hospital - Albany (518) 525-1550
St. Peter's Hosp - Albany
315 S Manning Blvd Albany, NY 12208 MID ATLANTIC

St. Peter's University Hospital (732) 745-8600
St. Peter's Univ Hosp
254 Easton Ave New Brunswick, NJ 08901-1780 MID ATLANTIC

St. Rose Dominican Hospital - San Martin Campus (702) 492-8000
St. Rose Dom Hosp-San Martin
8280 W Warm Springs Rd Las Vegas, NV 89113 WEST COAST AND PACIFIC

St. Tammany Parish Hospital (985) 898-4000
St. Tammany Parish Hosp
1202 S Tyler St Covington, LA 70433 SOUTHWEST

St. Vincent Carmel Hospital (317) 582-7000
St. Vincent Carmel Hosp
13500 N Meridian St Carmel, IN 46032-1496 MIDWEST

St. Vincent Health System (501) 552-3000
St. Vincent Health System
2 St. Vincent Cir Little Rock, AR 72205 SOUTHWEST

St. Vincent Hospital - Green Bay (920) 433-0111
St. Vincent Hosp - Green Bay
835 S Van Buren St, P.O. Box 13508 Green Bay, WI 54307-3508 MIDWEST

St. Vincent Indianapolis Hospital (317) 338-2345
St. Vincent Indianapolis Hosp
2001 W 86th St Indianapolis, IN 46260-1991 MIDWEST

St. Vincent's Hospital - Birmingham (205) 939-7000
St. Vincent's Hosp - Birmingham
810 St. Vincent's Drive Birmingham, AL 35202-2407 SOUTHEAST

St. Vincent's Medical Center - Los Angeles (213) 484-7111
St. Vincent's Med Ctr - Los Angeles
2131 W 3rd St Los Angeles, CA 90057 WEST COAST AND PACIFIC

St. Vincent's Medical Center- Riverside (Jacksonville) (904) 308-7300
St. Vincent's Med Ctr - Riverside (Jacksonville)
1 Shircliff Way Jacksonville, FL 32204 SOUTHEAST

Stamford Hospital (203) 276-1000
Stamford Hosp
30 Shelburne Rd @ W Broad St, Box 9317 Stamford, CT 06904 NEW ENGLAND

Stanford University Hospital & Clinics (650) 723-4000
Stanford Univ Hosp & Clinics
300 Pasteur Dr Stanford, CA 94305 WEST COAST AND PACIFIC

Staten Island University Hospital - North (718) 226-9000
Staten Island Univ Hosp - North
475 Seaview Avenue Staten Island, NY 10305 MID ATLANTIC

Steven and Alexandra Cohen Children's Medical Center of New York (718) 470-3000
Steven & Alexandra Cohen Chldn's Med Ctr of NY
269-01 76th Ave New Hyde Park, NY 11040 MID ATLANTIC

Steward St. Elizabeth's Medical Center-Boston (617) 789-3000
Steward St Elizabeth's Med Ctr-Boston
736 Cambridge St Boston, MA 02135 NEW ENGLAND

Stony Brook University Medical Center (631) 444-4000
Stony Brook Univ Med Ctr
101 Nicolls Rd Stony Brook, NY 11794-8410 MID ATLANTIC

Suburban Hospital (301) 896-3100
Suburban Hosp
8600 Old Georgetown Rd Bethesda, MD 20814 MID ATLANTIC

Summerlin Hospital Medical Center (702) 233-7000
Summerlin Hosp Med Ctr
657 Town Center Drive Las Vegas, NV 89144 WEST COAST AND PACIFIC

Sunnyview Hospital & Rehabilitation Center (518) 382-4500
Sunnyview Hosp & Rehab Ctr
1270 Belmont Ave Schenectady, NY 12308-2198 MID ATLANTIC

Sunrise Hospital & Medical Center (702) 731-8000
Sunrise Hosp & Med Ctr
3186 Maryland Pkwy Las Vegas, NV 89109 WEST COAST AND PACIFIC

SUNY Downstate Medical Center (University Hospital of Brooklyn)- Central Brooklyn
 (718) 270-1000
SUNY Downstate Med Ctr (Univ Hosp of Bklyn)
450 Clarkson Ave Brooklyn, NY 11203 MID ATLANTIC

SUNY Downstate Medical Center (University Hospital of Brooklyn)-Long Island College Hospital
 (718) 780-1000
SUNY Downstate Med Ctr (Univ Hosp of Bklyn) - LICH
339 Hicks Street Brooklyn, NY 11201 MID ATLANTIC

SUNY Upstate Medical University Hospital (315) 464-5540
SUNY Upstate Med Univ Shos
750 E Adams Street Syracuse, NY 13210 MID ATLANTIC

Swedish Covenant Hospital (773) 878-8200
Swedish Covenant Hosp
5145 N California Ave Chicago, IL 60625 MIDWEST

Swedish Medical Center - Denver (303) 788-5000
Swedish Med Ctr - Denver
501 E Hamden Ave Englewood, CO 80110-2795 GREAT PLAINS AND
 MOUNTAINS

Swedish Medical Center-Cherry Hill Campus (206) 320-2000
Swedish Med Ctr-Cherry Hill Campus
500 17th Ave Seattle, WA 98122 WEST COAST AND PACIFIC

Swedish Medical Center-First Hill Campus - Seattle (206) 386-6000
Swedish Med Ctr-First Hill-Seattle
747 Broadway Seattle, WA 98122 WEST COAST AND PACIFIC

Tampa General Hospital (813) 844-7000
Tampa Genl Hosp
1 Tampa General Cir, PO Box 1289 Tampa, FL 33601 SOUTHEAST

Tanner Medical Center - Carrollton (770) 836-9666
Tanner Med Ctr
705 Dixie Street Carrollton, GA 30117 SOUTHEAST

Temple University Hospital (215) 707-2000
Temple Univ Hosp
3401 N Broad St Philadelphia, PA 19140-5189 MID ATLANTIC

Temple University Hospital-Episcopal Campus (215) 707-1200
Temple University Hosp-Episcopal Campus
100 E Lehigh Ave Philadelphia, PA 19125 MID ATLANTIC

Tennessee Valley Healthcare System - Nashville (615) 327-4751
TN Valley Healthcare Sys-Nashville
1310 24th Ave S Nashville, TN 37212 SOUTHEAST

Texas Children's Hospital (832) 824-1000
Texas Chldns Hosp
6621 Fannin St Houston, TX 77030 SOUTHWEST

Texas Health Presbyterian Hospital Dallas (214) 345-6789
TX Hlth Presby Hosp Dallas
8200 Walnut Hill Ln Dallas, TX 75231 SOUTHWEST

Texas Health Presbyterian Hospital Plano (972) 981-8000
TX Hlth Presby Hosp Plano
6200 West Parker Road Plano, TX 75093 SOUTHWEST

Texas Orthopedic Hospital (713) 799-8600
Texas Ortho Hosp
7401 S Main Houston, TX 77030 SOUTHWEST

Texas Scottish Rite Hospital for Children (214) 559-5000
Texas Scottish Rite Hosp for Chldn
2222 Welborn St Dallas, TX 75219 SOUTHWEST

Thomas Jefferson University Hospital (215) 955-6000
Thomas Jefferson Univ Hosp
111 S 11th St Philadelphia, PA 19107 MID ATLANTIC

TIRR Memorial Hermann (713) 799-5000
TIRR Meml Hermann
1333 Moursund Houston, TX 77030 SOUTHWEST

Toledo Hospital (419) 291-4000
Toledo Hosp
2142 N Cove Blvd Toledo, OH 43606 MIDWEST

Touro Infirmary (504) 897-7011
Touro Infirmary
1401 Foucher Street New Orleans, LA 70115 SOUTHWEST

Tucson Medical Center (520) 327-5461
Tucson Med Ctr
5301 E Grant Rd Tucson, AZ 85733-2195 SOUTHWEST

Tufts Medical Center (617) 636-5000
Tufts Med Ctr
800 Washington St Boston, MA 02111 NEW ENGLAND

Tulane Medical Center (504) 988-5800
Tulane Med Ctr
1415 Tulane Ave New Orleans, LA 70112 SOUTHWEST

Tulane-Lakeside Hospital (504) 988-5800
Tulane-Lakeside Hosp
4700 I-10 Service Rd Metairie, LA 70001 SOUTHWEST

UAB Highlands Hospital (205) 930-7000
UAB Highlands Hosp
1201 11th Ave S Birmingham, AL 35205-5299 SOUTHEAST

UAB Medical West (205) 481-7000
UAB Med West
995 9th Ave SW Bessemer, AL 35020 SOUTHEAST

UAB Spain Rehabilitation Center (205) 934-3450
UAB Spain Rehab Ctr
1717 6th Ave S Birmingham, AL 35249 SOUTHEAST

UCLA Ronald Reagan Medical Center (310) 825-9111
UCLA Ronald Reagan Med Ctr
757 Westwood Plaza Los Angeles, CA 90095 WEST COAST AND PACIFIC

UCSD Medical Center (858) 657-7000
UCSD Med Ctr
200 W Arbor Drive San Diego, CA 92103 WEST COAST AND PACIFIC

UCSD Thornton Hospital (858) 657-7000
UCSD Thornton Hosp
9300 Campus Point Drive La Jolla, CA 92037 WEST COAST AND PACIFIC

UCSF - Mount Zion Medical Center (415) 567-6600
UCSF - Mt Zion Med Ctr
1600 Divisadero St San Francisco, CA 94115 WEST COAST AND PACIFIC

UCSF Medical Center (415) 476-1000
UCSF Med Ctr
505 Parnassus Ave San Francisco, CA 94143 WEST COAST AND PACIFIC

UHealth - University of Miami Health System (305) 243-4000
UHealth - Univ of Miami Hlth Sys
1600 NW 10th Ave, Ste 1125 Miami, FL 33136 SOUTHEAST

UK HealthCare Good Samaritan Hospital (859) 226-7000
UK HealthCare Good Samaritan Hosp
310 S Limestone St Lexington, KY 40508 SOUTHEAST

UMass Memorial Medical Center (508) 334-1000
UMass Memorial Med Ctr
55 Lake Ave N Worcester, MA 01655 NEW ENGLAND

UMass Memorial Medical Center - University Campus (508) 334-1000
UMass Meml Med Ctr - Univ Campus
55 Lake Ave N Worcester, MA 01655-0002 NEW ENGLAND

United Hospital (651) 241-8000
United Hosp
333 N Smith Ave St Paul, MN 55102 MIDWEST

University Health System-San Antonio (210) 358-4000
Univ Hlth Syst-San Antonio
4502 Medical Dr San Antonio, TX 78229 SOUTHWEST

University Health Systems-Vidant Medical Center (252) 847-4100
Univ Hlth Sys-Vidant Med Ctr
2100 Stantonsburg Rd Greenville, NC 27835-6028 SOUTHEAST

University Hospital - Cincinnati (513) 584-1000
Univ Hosp - Cincinnati
234 Goodman St Cincinnati, OH 45219 MIDWEST

University Hospital - New Mexico (505) 272-2111
Univ Hosp - New Mexico
2211 Lomas Blvd NE Albuquerque, NM 87106 SOUTHWEST

University Hospital-UMDNJ-Newark (973) 972-4300
Univ Hosp-UMDNJ—Newark
150 Bergen St Newark, NJ 07103-2406 MID ATLANTIC

University Hospitals Case Medical Center (216) 844-1000
Univ Hosps Case Med Ctr
11100 Euclid Ave Cleveland, OH 44106 MIDWEST

University Hospitals Rainbow Babies & Children's Hospital (216) 844-3991
UH Rainbow Babies & Chldns Hosp
11100 Euclid Ave Cleveland, OH 44106 MIDWEST

University Medical Center of Princeton at Plainsboro (609) 853-7000
Univ Med Ctr Princeton at Plainsboro
One Plainsboro Rd Plainsboro, NJ 08536 MID ATLANTIC

University Medical Center of Southern Nevada - Las Vegas (702) 383-2000
Univ Med Ctr - Las Vegas
1800 W Charleston Blvd Las Vegas, NV 89102 WEST COAST AND PACIFIC

University Medical Center-Lubbock (806) 775-8200
Univ Med Ctr-Lubbock
602 Indiana Ave Lubbock, TX 79408 SOUTHWEST

University of Alabama Hospital at Birmingham (205) 934-4011
Univ of Ala Hosp at Birmingham
1802 6th Ave S Birmingham, AL 35249-6544 SOUTHEAST

University of Arizona Medical Center - South Campus (520) 874-2000
Univ Ariz Med Ctr-South Campus (Kino)
2800 E Ajo Way Tucson, AZ 85713 SOUTHWEST

University of Arizona Medical Center-University Campus (520) 694-0111
Univ Arizona Med Ctr-Univ Campus
1501 N Campbell Ave Tucson, AZ 85724-5128 SOUTHWEST

University of Arkansas for Medical Sciences Medical Center (501) 686-7000
UAMS Med Ctr
4301 W Markham St Little Rock, AR 72205 SOUTHWEST

University of California - Davis Medical Center (916) 734-2011
UC Davis Med Ctr
2315 Stockton Blvd Sacramento, CA 95817 WEST COAST AND PACIFIC

University of California - Irvine Medical Center (714) 456-7890
UC Irvine Med Ctr
101 The City Drive S Orange, CA 92868 WEST COAST AND PACIFIC

University of Chicago Comer Children's Hospital (773) 702-1000
Univ Chicago-Comer Chldn's Hosp
5721 S Maryland Ave Chicago, IL 60637 MIDWEST

University of Chicago Medical Center (773) 702-1000
Univ of Chicago Med Ctr
5841 S Maryland Ave Chicago, IL 60637 MIDWEST

University of Colorado Hospital-Anschutz Inpatient Pavilion (720) 848-4011
Univ of CO Hosp - Anschutz Inpatient Pav
12605 E 16th Ave Aurora, CO 80045 GREAT PLAINS AND MOUNTAINS

University of Connecticut Health Center - John Dempsey Hospital (860) 679-2000
Univ of Conn Hlth Ctr, John Dempsey Hosp
263 Farmington Ave Farmington, CT 06030 NEW ENGLAND

University of Illinois at Chicago Eye & Ear Infirmary (312) 996-6500
Univ of IL at Chicago Eye & Ear Infirm
1855 W Taylor St Chicago, IL 60612 MIDWEST

University of Illinois Medical Center at Chicago (312) 355-4000
Univ of IL Med Ctr at Chicago
1740 W Taylor St, Ste 1400 Chicago, IL 60612 MIDWEST

University of Iowa Hospitals and Clinics (319) 356-1616
Univ Iowa Hosp & Clinics
200 Hawkins Drive Iowa City, IA 52242 MIDWEST

University of Kansas Hospital (913) 588-5000
Univ of Kansas Hosp
3901 Rainbow Blvd Kansas City, KS 66160 GREAT PLAINS AND MOUNTAINS

University of Kentucky Albert B. Chandler Hospital (859) 323-5000
Univ of Kentucky Albert B. Chandler Hosp
800 Rose Street Lexington, KY 40536 SOUTHEAST

University of Louisville Hospital (502) 562-3000
Univ of Louisville Hosp
530 S Jackson St Louisville, KY 40202 SOUTHEAST

University of Maryland Medical Center (410) 328-8667
Univ of MD Med Ctr
22 S Greene St Baltimore, MD 21201 MID ATLANTIC

University of Miami Hosp & Clinics/Sylvester Comprehensive Cancer Cntr (305) 243-1000
Univ of Miami Hosp & Clins/Sylvester Comp Canc Ctr
1475 NW 12th Ave Miami, FL 33136 SOUTHEAST

University of Miami Hospital (305) 689-5000
Univ of Miami Hosp
1400 NW 12 Ave Miami, FL 33136 SOUTHEAST

University of Michigan Medical Center (734) 936-4000
Univ Michigan Med Ctr
1500 E Medical Center Dr Ann Arbor, MI 48109 MIDWEST

University of Minnesota Medical Center, Fairview - West Bank Campus		(612) 273-3000
Univ Minn Med Ctr, Fairview - West Bank Campus		
2450 Riverside Ave S	Minneapolis, MN 55454	MIDWEST
University of Mississippi Medical Center		(601) 984-1000
Univ Mississippi Med Ctr		
2500 N State St	Jackson, MS 39216	SOUTHEAST
University of Missouri Hospital		(573) 882-4141
Univ of Missouri Hosp		
1 Hospital Dr	Columbia, MO 65212	MIDWEST
University of Rochester Strong Memorial Hospital		(585) 275-2100
Univ of Rochester Strong Meml Hosp		
601 Elmwood Ave	Rochester, NY 14642	MID ATLANTIC
University of South Alabama Medical Center		(251) 471-7000
Univ of S AL Med Ctr		
2451 Fillingim St	Mobile, AL 36617	SOUTHEAST
University of Tennesee Medical Center		(865) 305-9000
Univ of Tennesee Med Ctr		
1924 Alcoa Hwy	Knoxville, TN 37920	SOUTHEAST
University of Texas Health Science Center at Tyler		(903) 877-7777
Univ of Texas Hlth Sci Ctr at Tyler		
11937 US Hwy 271	Tyler, TX 75708	SOUTHWEST
University of Texas MD Anderson Cancer Center		(713) 792-2121
UT MD Anderson Cancer Ctr		
1515 Holcombe Blvd	Houston, TX 77030-4095	SOUTHWEST
University of Toledo Medical Center		(419) 383-4000
Univ of Toledo Med Ctr		
3000 Arlington Ave	Toledo, OH 43614	MIDWEST
University of Utah Health Care		(801) 581-2121
Univ Utah Hlth Care		
50 N Medical Dr	Salt Lake City, UT 84132	GREAT PLAINS AND MOUNTAINS
University of Virginia Health System		(434) 924-0211
Univ of Virginia Health Sys		
1215 Lee Street	Charlottesville, VA 22903	SOUTHEAST
University of Washington Medical Center		(206) 598-3300
Univ Wash Med Ctr		
1959 NE Pacific St, PO Box 656355	Seattle, WA 98195	WEST COAST AND PACIFIC

University of Wisconsin Hospital & Clinics		(608) 263-6400
Univ WI Hosp & Clins		
600 Highland Avenue	Madison, WI 53792	MIDWEST

UPMC Hamot		(814) 877-6000
UPMC Hamot		
201 State Street	Erie, PA 16550-0001	MID ATLANTIC

UPMC Mercy		(412) 232-8111
UPMC Mercy, Pittsburgh		
1400 Locust Street	Pittsburgh, PA 15219	MID ATLANTIC

UPMC Montefiore		(412) 647-2345
UPMC Montefiore		
3459 Fifth Ave	Pittsburgh, PA 15213	MID ATLANTIC

UPMC Passavant-McCandless		(412) 367-6700
UPMC Passavant-McCandless		
9100 Babcock Blvd	Pittsburgh, PA 15237	MID ATLANTIC

UPMC Presbyterian		(412) 647-2345
UPMC Presby, Pittsburgh		
200 Lothrop St	Pittsburgh, PA 15213	MID ATLANTIC

UPMC Shadyside		(412) 623-2121
UPMC Shadyside		
5230 Centre Ave	Pittsburgh, PA 15232	MID ATLANTIC

UPMC South Side-Outpatient Center		(412) 488-5550
UPMC South Side-Out Pt Ctr		
2000 Mary St	Pittsburgh, PA 15203	MID ATLANTIC

UPMC St Margaret		(412) 784-4000
UPMC St Margaret		
815 Freeport Rd	Pittsburgh, PA 15215-3301	MID ATLANTIC

USC Norris Cancer Hospital		(323) 865-3000
USC Norris Cancer Hosp		
1441 Eastlake Ave	Los Angeles, CA 90033	WEST COAST AND PACIFIC

UT Medical Branch at Galveston(John Sealy Hospital)		(409) 772-1011
UT Med Br at Galveston(John Sealy Hosp)		
301 University Blvd	Galveston, TX 77555	SOUTHWEST

UT Southwestern Medical Center at Dallas		(214) 648-3111
UT Southwestern Med Ctr at Dallas		
5323 Harry Hines Blvd	Dallas, TX 75390	SOUTHWEST

VA Ann Arbor Healthcare System (734) 769-7100
VA Ann Arbor Healthcare Sys
2215 Fuller Rd Ann Arbor, MI 48105 MIDWEST

VA Connecticut Healthcare System-West Haven Campus (203) 932-5711
VA Conn Hlthcre Sys-W Haven Campus
950 Campbell Ave West Haven, CT 06516 NEW ENGLAND

VA Greater Los Angeles Healthcare System (310) 478-3711
VA Greater Los Angeles Hthecare Sys
11301 Wilshire Blvd Los Angeles, CA 90073 WEST COAST AND PACIFIC

VA Health Care System - Palo Alto (650) 493-5000
VA Hlth Care Sys - Palo Alto
3801 Miranda Ave Palo Alto, CA 94304 WEST COAST AND PACIFIC

VA Medical Center - Memphis (901) 523-8990
VA Med Ctr - Memphis
1030 Jefferson Ave Memphis, TN 38104 SOUTHEAST

VA Medical Center - Miami (305) 575-7000
VA Med Ctr - Miami
1201 NW 16th St Miami, FL 33125 SOUTHEAST

VA Medical Center - Portland (503) 220-8262
VA Medical Center - Portland
3710 SW US Veteran Hospital Rd, PO Box 1034 Portland, OR 97239 WEST COAST AND PACIFIC

VA Medical Center - San Francisco (415) 221-4810
VA Med Ctr - San Francisco
4150 Clement St San Francisco, CA 94121 WEST COAST AND PACIFIC

VA Medical Center - Washington, DC (202) 745-8000
VA Med Ctr - Washington
50 Irving St NW Washington, DC 20422 MID ATLANTIC

VA Puget Sound Health Care System (206) 762-1010
VA Puget Sound Hlth Care Sys
1660 S Columbian Way Seattle, WA 98108 WEST COAST AND PACIFIC

VA San Diego Healthcare System (858) 552-8585
VA San Diego Hlthcre Sys
3350 La Jolla Village Drive San Diego, CA 92161 WEST COAST AND PACIFIC

Vail Valley Medical Center (970) 476-2451
Vail Valley Med Ctr
181 W Meadow Dr Vail, CO 81657-5058 GREAT PLAINS AND MOUNTAINS

Valley Medical Center - Renton, WA (425) 228-3450
Valley Med Ctr-Renton, WA
404 S 43 St Renton, WA 98058-5010 WEST COAST AND PACIFIC

Vanderbilt Monroe Carrell Jr. Children's Hospital (615) 936-1000
Vanderbilt Monroe Carrell Jr. Chldn's Hosp
2200 Children's Way Nashville, TN 37232 SOUTHEAST

Vanderbilt University Medical Center (615) 322-5000
Vanderbilt Univ Med Ctr
1211 Medical Center Drive Nashville, TN 37232 SOUTHEAST

VCU Medical Center (804) 828-9000
VCU Med Ctr
1250 E Marshall St, PO Box 980510 Richmond, VA 23298 SOUTHEAST

Virginia Hospital Center - Arlington (703) 558-5000
Virginia Hosp Ctr - Arlington
1701 N George Mason Dr Arlington, VA 22205-3698 SOUTHEAST

Virginia Mason Medical Center (206) 223-6600
Virginia Mason Med Ctr
1100 Ninth Ave, Box 900 Seattle, WA 98111 WEST COAST AND PACIFIC

Waccamaw Community Hospital (843) 652-1000
Waccamaw Community Hosp
4070 Hwy 17 Bypass Murrells Inlet, SC 29576 SOUTHEAST

Wake Forest Baptist Medical Center (336) 716-2255
Wake Forest Baptist Med Ctr
Medical Center Blvd Winston-Salem, NC 27157-1015 SOUTHEAST

WakeMed Cary Hospital (919) 350-2300
WakeMed Cary
1900 Kildaire Farm Rd Cary, NC 27511-6616 SOUTHEAST

WakeMed-Raleigh Campus (919) 350-8000
WakeMed-Raleigh Campus
3000 New Bern Ave Raleigh, NC 27610 SOUTHEAST

Walter Reed National Military Medical Center (301) 295-4611
Walter Reed Natl Military Med Ctr
8901 Wisconsin Ave Bethesda, MD 20889-5600 MID ATLANTIC

Washington Hospital Center (202) 877-7000
Washington Hosp Ctr
110 Irving St NW Washington, DC 20010 MID ATLANTIC

Washington Hospital, The		(724) 225-7000
Washington Hosp, The		
155 Wilson Ave	Washington, PA 15301	MID ATLANTIC

Washington University Physicians		(314) 362-6828
Washington Univ Physicians		
4444 Forest Park Ave	St Louis, MO 63108	MIDWEST

Watauga Medical Center		(828) 262-4100
Watauga Med Ctr		
336 Deerfield Rd	Boone, NC 28607	SOUTHEAST

WellStar Windy Hill Hospital		(770) 644-1000
WellStar Windy Hill Hosp		
2540 Windy Hill Road	Marietta, GA 30067	SOUTHEAST

Wesley Woods Geriatric Hospital		(404) 728-6200
Wesley Woods Ger Hosp		
1821 Clifton Rd	Atlanta, GA 30329	SOUTHEAST

West Jefferson Medical Center		(504) 347-5511
West Jefferson Med Ctr		
1101 Medical Ctr Blvd	Marrero, LA 70072	SOUTHWEST

West Palm Hospital		(561) 842-6141
West Palm Hosp		
2201 45th St	West Palm Beach, FL 33407	SOUTHEAST

Westchester Medical Center		(914) 493-7000
Westchester Med Ctr		
95 Grasslands Road	Valhalla, NY 10595	MID ATLANTIC

Western Pennsylvania Hospital		(412) 578-5000
Western Penn Hosp		
4800 Friendship Avenue	Pittsburgh, PA 15224	MID ATLANTIC

Western Psychiatric Institute and Clinic-UPMC		(412) 624-1000
Western Psych Inst & Clin-UPMC		
3811 O'Hara St	Pittsburgh, PA 15213	MID ATLANTIC

White River Junction VA Medical Center		(802) 295-9363
White River Junction VA Med Ctr		
215 North Maine Street	White River Junction, VT 05009	NEW ENGLAND

Wills Eye Hospital		(215) 928-3000
Wills Eye Hosp		
840 Walnut St	Philadelphia, PA 19107-5598	MID ATLANTIC

Wilmington Hospital		(302) 733-1000
Wilmington Hosp		
501 W 14th St	Wilmington, DE 19801	MID ATLANTIC

Winthrop University Hospital		(516) 663-0333
Winthrop Univ Hosp		
259 1st St	Mineola, NY 11501	MID ATLANTIC

Wolfson Children's Hospital		(904) 202-8000
Wolfson Chldns Hosp		
800 Prudential Dr	Jacksonville, FL 32207	SOUTHEAST

Women & Infants Hospital of Rhode Island		(401) 274-1100
Women & Infants Hosp of RI		
101 Dudley Street	Providence, RI 02905	NEW ENGLAND

Women and Children's Hospital of Buffalo, The		(716) 878-7000
Women & Chldn's Hosp of Buffalo, The		
219 Bryant St	Buffalo, NY 14222	MID ATLANTIC

Yale-New Haven Hospital		(203) 688-4242
Yale-New Haven Hosp		
20 York St	New Haven, CT 06510	NEW ENGLAND

Yale-New Haven Hospital St Raphael Campus		(203) 789-3000
Yale-New Haven Hosp - St Raphael Campus		
1450 Chapel Street	New Haven, CT 06511	NEW ENGLAND

Yampa Valley Medical Center		(970) 879-1322
Yampa Valley Med Ctr		
1024 Central Park Dr	Steamboat Springs, CO 80487	GREAT PLAINS AND MOUNTAINS

Zucker Hillside Hospital		(718) 470-8100
Zucker Hillside Hosp		
75-59 263rd St	Glen Oaks, NY 11004	MID ATLANTIC

The Best in American Medicine
www.CastleConnolly.com

Appendix D:
Selected Resources

AMERICAN AMBULANCE ASSOCIATION (AAA)

The American Ambulance Association represents emergency and non-emergency medical transportation providers, advocating high quality pre-hospital care and keeping these providers aware of legislation and news that may affect them.

8400 West Park Drive, FL2
McLean, VA 22102

800-523-4447
703-610-9018
fax 703-610-0210
www.the-aaa.org/

AMERICA'S HEALTH INSURANCE PLANS (AHIP)

America's Health Insurance Plans is a national trade association representing nearly 1,300 member companies providing health benefits to more than 200 million Americans.

601 Pennsylvania Ave, NW
South Building Suite 500
Washington, DC 20004

202-778-3200
fax: 202-331-7487
www.ahip.org/

AMERICAN BOARD OF MEDICAL SPECIALTIES (ABMS)

The ABMS is the authoritative body for the recognition of medical specialties, coordinating 24 medical specialty boards (including 25 medical specialties) and providing information on the board certification of doctors.

222 N LaSalle, Ste 1500
Chicago, Illinois 60601

312-436-2600 or 866-ASK-ABMS
fax 847-328-3596
www.abms.org

AMERICAN HOSPITAL ASSOCIATION (AHA)

A national health advocacy organization, the AHA represents hospitals and healthcare networks in legislative and regulatory matters. In 1973 the AHA adopted the Patient Bill of Rights to help patients understand their rights and responsibilities.

155 N Wacker Drive
Chicago, IL 60606

800-424-4301 or 312-422-3000
fax 312-422-4796
www.aha.org/

325 7th St. NW
Washington, DC 20004

800-424-4301 or 202-638-1100
fax 202-626-2345

AMERICAN MEDICAL ASSOCIATION (AMA)

The AMA is an association that maintains information on physicians practicing throughout the nation. Healthcare consumers can use their database to check the location, licensing, education and specialty of many doctors in the United States.

515 North State Street
Chicago, IL 60654

800-621-8335
www.ama-assn.org/

CENTER FOR MEDICAL CONSUMERS

Provides volume and outcome data on certain medical procedures performed in New York state.

239 Thompson St.
New York, NY 10012

212-674-7105
fax 212-674-7100
centerformedicalconsumers@gmail.com
www.medicalconsumers.org

CENTERS FOR DISEASE CONTROL AND PREVENTION (CDC)

Part of the Department of Health and Human Services, the CDC's mission is to prevent and manage diseases and illnesses. Its Website contains information on a range of illnesses and the research being pursued to manage them. It also provides free faxed reports on disease risk and prevention in various parts of the world.

Public Inquiries/MASO
Mailstop E11
1600 Clifton Road
Atlanta, GA 30333

800-CDC-INFO
TTY: 888-232-6348

toll free number for international travelers 877 FYI-TRIP or 404-639-3534
fax information service for international travelers 888-232-3299
www.cdc.gov/netinfo.htm

THE CENTERWATCH CLINICAL TRIALS LISTING SERVICE

Profiles centers conducting clinical research by therapeutic area and geographic region, including more than 41,000 international industry and government-sponsored clinical trials and new FDA approved drug therapies, as well as 5,200 clinical trials that are actively recruiting patients.

10 Winthrop Square
Fl 5
Boston, MA 02110

617-948-5100
fax 617-948-5101
www.centerwatch.com

INTERNATIONAL ASSOCIATION FOR MEDICAL ASSISTANCE TO TRAVELLERS (IAMAT)

IAMAT is a non-profit organization that disseminates information on health and sanitary conditions worldwide. Membership is free but donations are appreciated. Members will receive a membership card making them eligible to access English speaking physicians all over the world. The organization also provides information on immunization requirements, malaria, and other tropical diseases, and sanitary and climactic conditions around the world. For information, send request in writing.

1623 Military Road #279
Niagra Falls, New York 14304-1745

716-754-4883
www.iamat.org

Joint Commission on Accreditation of Healthcare Organizations

The Joint Commission (JCAHO) is an independent, not-for-profit organization, which evaluates the quality and safety of care for nearly 17,000 health care organizations. To maintain and earn accreditation, organizations must have an extensive on-site review by a team of JCAHO health care professionals, at least once every three years. JCAHO is governed by a board that includes physicians, nurses, and consumers. JCAHO sets the standards by which health care quality is measured in America and around the world.

One Renaissance Boulevard
Oakbrook Terrace, IL 60181

630-792-5000
fax 630-792-5005
www.jcaho.org

Medic Alert Foundation

The Medic Alert Foundation (a non-profit organization) provides an "ID tag" engraved with personal medical facts, as well as a 24-hour emergency response center which can release additional personal medical details. Membership is $30/year (plus $9.95 initial setup fee) and members need to purchase the "ID tag" which sells for as low as $35.

2323 Colorado Avenue
Turlock, CA 95382

888-633-4298
Fax 209-669-2450
www.medicalert.org

Medline

A medical database including millions of medical references and abstracts from thousands of scientific and medical journals.

One Medline Place
Mundelein, Illinois 60060

1-800-MEDLINE (800-633-5463)
fax 1-800-351-1512
www.medline.com

The National Cancer Institute (NCI)

Part of the NIH, the NCI sponsors cancer clinical trials at more than 100 sites in the United States. Trials are carried out in major medical research centers, such as teaching hospitals, as well as in community hospitals, specialized medical clinics and even in doctors' offices.

Clinical Studies Support Center (CSSC)
6116 Executive Boulevard
Bethesda, MD 20892-8322

800-4-CANCER (800-422-6237)
www.nci.nih.gov
www.cancer.gov
cancergovstaff@mail.nih.gov

National Center for Complementary and Alternative Medicine Clearinghouse (NCCAMC)

The NCCAMC facilitates the evaluation of alternative medical treatment modalities to help determine their effectiveness and bring alternative medicine into mainstream medicine. This agency does not provide referrals.

9000 Rockville Pike
Bethesda, MD 20892

888-644-6226
fax 866-464-3616
www.nccam.nih.gov
info@nccam.nih.gov

NATIONAL CONSUMERS LEAGUE (NCL)

NCL is a private, nonprofit consumer advocacy organization. NCL strives to investigate, educate, and advocate on a variety of issues including healthcare. Membership is $20 annually, but individuals can also write to the organization for a list of publications that non-members can purchase.

1701 K Street, NW, Suite 1200
Washington, DC 20006

202-835-3323
fax 202-835-0747
www.nclnet.org
info@nclnet.org

THE NATIONAL INSTITUTES OF HEALTH (NIH)

An organization operated by the U.S. government, the NIH operates its own hospital at which the care provided is usually related to clinical studies its researchers are undertaking. Information about the Warren G. Magnuson Clinical Center is also available.

Patient Recruitment Referral Center
9000 Rockville Pike
Bethesda, MD 20892

212-346-5500
www.nih.gov
www.clinicaltrials.gov
nihinfo@od.nih.gov

NATIONAL INSURANCE INFORMATION INSTITUTE

The National Insurance Information Institute Helpline advises consumers on how to choose an insurance company or broker. It also offers an analysis of life insurance and assists in insurance complaints.

110 William St
New York, NY 10038

800-411-1222 or 301-496-4000
www.iii.org

THE PATIENT ADVOCATE FOUNDATION

A national non-profit organization that provides consultation, referrals and case management to patients to ensure that they are not denied access to healthcare, insurance coverage, employment and public assistance programs during an illness. In particular, the organization maintains comprehensive information on cancer treatment options that are available to consumers through a separate Web site: www.oncology.com.

421 Butler Farm Rd
Hampton, VA 23666

800-532-5274
fax 757-873-8999
www.patientadvocate.org/
help@patientadvocate.org

PEOPLE'S MEDICAL SOCIETY

The People's Medical Society, a nonprofit organization, is focused on educating the healthcare consumer about healthcare issues and medical rights. Their website provides information on useful books and publications as well as the latest healthcare developments.

P.O. Box 868
Allentown, PA 18105

610-770-1670
fax 610-770-0607
cbi@peoplesmed.org
www.peoplesmed.org

PERSONS UNITED LIMITING SUBSTANDARDS AND ERRORS IN HEALTHCARE (P.U.L.S.E.)
A support group for the survivors of medical malpractice and substandard healthcare, this nonprofit group also advocates patient education and patient-doctor communication.

PO Box 353
Wantagh NY 11793-0353

800-96-pulse (800-967-8573) or
516-579-4711
fax: 516-520-8105
www.PULSEamerica.org
www.PULSEofNY.org
pulse516@aol.com

Colorado Office

719-250-1286
PULSECOLO@YAHOO.COM

PUBLIC CITIZEN'S HEALTH AND RESEARCH GROUP
A non-profit organization, the Public Citizen's Group acts as a watchdog agency by advocating accountability and the open use of doctors' disciplinary backgrounds.

1600 20th Street NW
Washington, D.C. 20009

202-588-1000
www.citizen.org/hrg/

The Best in American Medicine
www.CastleConnolly.com

Appendix E:
Sources of Quality Data on Hospitals

U.S. NEWS AND WORLD REPORT

U.S. News & World Report has been the nation's leading source of information on hospital rankings since 1990. The Best Hospitals rankings evaluate medical centers on their competence in high-stakes situations. Their annual feature on Best Hospitals has become the standard in the field where rankings are concerned and is heavily anticipated and utilized by consumers and members of the health care profession. Castle Connolly teamed up with *U.S. News & World Report* in July 2011 to bring its listing of Top Doctors online to www.usnews.com/health in conjunction with the Top Hospitals rankings. There, consumers can search the full Castle Connolly database of nearly 30,000 Top Doctors across the nation.

WWW.WHYNOTTHEBEST.ORG

WhyNotTheBest.org was created and is maintained by The Commonwealth Fund, a private foundation working toward a high performance health system. It is a free resource for health care professionals and consumers interested in tracking performance on various measures of health care quality. It enables organizations to compare their performance against that of peer organizations, against a range of benchmarks and over a given period of time. Case studies and improvement tools spotlight successful improvement strategies of the nation's top performers. A regional map shows performance at the county, state and national levels. This site also includes process-of-care measures, patient satisfaction measures, readmission rates, mortality rates and average reimbursement rates. All of these performance measures are publicly reported on the Centers for Medicare and Medicaid Services website, Hospital Compare, and include data from nearly all U.S. hospitals.

THE LEAPFROG GROUP

The Leapfrog Group, http://www.leapfroggroup.org/cp, started in 1998 by a group of large employers. The Leapfrog Hospital Survey compares hospitals' performance on the national standards of safety, quality and efficiency - areas of healthcare that are most relevant to consumers. Hospitals that participate in The Leapfrog Hospital Survey achieve hospital-wide improvements that translate into saving millions of lives and cutting costs for hospitals and consumers. Leapfrog's survey results are later used to inform key employees on purchasing strategies.

HOSPITAL COMPARE

The Hospital Compare website was created through the efforts of the Centers for Medicare & Medicaid Services (CMS), an agency of the U.S. Department of Health and Human Services (DHHS), along with the Hospital Quality Alliance (HQA). The HQA was established to promote reporting on hospital quality of care. The HQA consists of organizations that represent consumers, hospitals, doctors and nurses, employers, accrediting organizations and Federal agencies. The information on this website can be used by patients requiring hospital care. This information helps the consumer and health care providers to compare the quality of care provided in participating hospitals. This information not only helps one to make good decisions about health care, but also encourages hospitals to improve the quality of the care that they provide to their communities. This website can be found at: http://www.hospitalcompare.hhs.gov/hospital-search.aspx or http://bit.ly/jdvCzW

Indices

Subject Index

A

Accessibility 18, 19

Admitting Privileges 14

Adverse Reactions 26, 31-33

Ambulatory Care Research Facility 34

American Board of Medical Specialties 5, 10, 41-42, 49-51

American Osteopathic Association 10

Areas of Clinical Study 34

Attendings 14

B

Bedside Manner 19

Benefits and Risks 32-33

Board Certification10-13, 37, 41, 51

Board Eligible 11

C

Cancer Trials 30

Clinical Cancer Centers 27

Clinical Research 2, 4, 25, 27-28, 33-35

Clinical Studies Support Center (CSSC) 35

Clinical Trials 25-28, 30-35

Closed Staffs 14

Comprehensive Cancer Centers 35

Continuing Medical Education (CME) 12

Control Group 28

Cosmetic Surgery 5, 7, 46

Council of Teaching Hospitals 3

Credentialing 14

D

Diplomates of the Board 11

Directory of Graduate Medical Education 10

Doctor-Patient Relationship 19

E

Experimental or Treatment Group 28

Experimental Procedures 30

F

Faculty Appointment 15, 37

Fellow xxix, xxx, 7, 37, 51

Fellowships 13

Follow-up Care 19, 34

Food and Drug Administration 29

Foreign Medical Graduates 9

Foreign Medical Schools 9

G

General Clinical Research Centers 34-35

Grandfathering 12

H

Health Insurance 18

Health Maintenance Organizations (HMO) 18, 27

Health Plan 5, 7, 18, 30-31

Hospital Appointment 2, 14-15

I

Inclusion Criteria 30

Informed Consent 29

Initial Consultation 21

Institutional Review Board 28

L

Laboratory Tests 31

Levels of Recognition 11

Liaison Committee for Medical Education 8

License Histories 4

Long-term Monitoring 19

M

Magnuson Clinical Center, see Warren Grant Magnuson Clinical Center 33-35

Maintenance Trials 31

Major Medical Centers 1-3, 14, 26

Malpractice Insurance 15

Mark O. Hatfield Clinical Research Center 34

Medical Affairs Office 5, 14

Medical College Admissions Tests 9

Medical History 21, 23, 31

Medical Records 21-23, 29, 34

Medical School 2-3, 8-11, 13, 15-16, 37, 49

Medical School Faculty 15

Medical Society Membership 15

N

National Cancer Institute (NCI) 26-27, 30-31, 35

National Institutes of Health (NIH) 25, 27, 33-35

Non-board Certified Doctors 11

O

Office and Practice Arrangements 18

Out-of-Network 18

P

Patient Recruitment and Public Liaison Office (PRPL) 34

Personal Chemistry 19

Placebo 28

Postgraduate Training 10

Prevention Trials 27

Primary Care 1, 3-4, 7, 8, 15, 18-19, 31, 42-44, 49

Private Insurance 29

Professional Reputation 13
Protocol 27-28, 30

R

Recertification 12, 50
Referral 3, 8, 14, 18, 35
Residency 2, 10-11, 16-17, 37, 49-50

S

Second Opinions 17-18
Selection Process 2
Self-Designated Medical Specialties 12
Side Effects 26-27, 32-33
Special Resources 25-26, 28, 30, 32, 34
Specialists 1-10, 12, 14-16, 18, 37, 41, 43, 49-51, 53
Specialties 3-6, 9-12, 14, 24, 38, 41-47, 49-51, 53
Standard Therapies 25
Subspecialties 1, 5-6, 10, 12-13, 15, 41-42, 49-50, 53

T

Therapeutic Approaches 1, 6, 25
Treatment Plan 21, 30
Treatment Studies 25, 30
Trust 19

U

United States Department of Health 33
United States Medical Licensing Exam 9

V

Veritas Medicine 26

W

Warren Grant Magnuson Clinical Center 33-35

Specialty & Special Expertise Index

This index lists the areas that the physicians listed in the Guide have identified as their "special expertise." They are specific elements of disease, procedures, techniques and treatments for which these physicians are best known and are referred patients. Each doctor's medical specialty is also included.

Spec	Name	St	Pg

A

Abdominal Imaging

Spec	Name	St	Pg
DR	Berland, L	AL	978
DR	Coakley, F	OR	982
DR	Dodd, G	CO	981
DR	Federle, M	CA	983
DR	Fishman, E	MD	975
DR	Grant, E	CA	983
DR	Levy, A	DC	976
DR	Megibow, A	NY	976
DR	Prince, M	NY	977
DR	Sivit, C	OH	981
DR	Weinreb, J	CT	973
DR	Zagoria, R	NC	980

Abdominal Wall Reconstruction

Spec	Name	St	Pg
PlS	Kuzon, W	MI	866
PlS	Seyfer, A	MD	858
PlS	Stahl, R	CT	851
S	Bellows, C	LA	1087
S	Deitch, E	NJ	1056
S	Fitzgibbons, R	NE	1085

Abdominoplasty

Spec	Name	St	Pg
PlS	Aly, A	CA	872
PlS	Davis, G	NC	861
PlS	Erdmann, D	NC	861
PlS	Eriksson, E	MA	850
PlS	Gallico, G	MA	850
PlS	Hunstad, J	NC	862
PlS	Lesavoy, M	CA	875
PlS	Markowitz, B	CA	875
PlS	Matarasso, A	NY	856
PlS	Nahabedian, M	DC	856
PlS	Ness, J	MN	867
PlS	Pitman, G	NY	857
PlS	Singh, N	MD	858

Abuse/Neglect

Spec	Name	St	Pg
AM	Diaz, A	NY	80
ChAP	Zeanah, C	LA	911
Ger	Lachs, M	NY	263

Achalasia

Spec	Name	St	Pg
Ge	Ravich, W	MD	237
Ge	Vaezi, M	TN	243

Acne

Spec	Name	St	Pg
D	Barbosa, V	IL	192
D	Eichenfield, L	CA	198
D	James, W	PA	187
D	Lowitt, M	MD	187
D	Lucky, A	OH	194

Acoustic Neuroma

Spec	Name	St	Pg
NS	Black, K	CA	495
NS	Eisenberg, H	MD	473
NS	Giannotta, S	CA	497
NS	Golfinos, J	NY	474
NS	Grubb, R	MO	487
NS	Gutin, P	NY	474
NS	Harsh, G	CA	497
NS	Judy, K	PA	475
NS	Martuza, R	MA	471
NS	Mayberg, M	WA	498
NS	Sisti, M	NY	479
NS	Stieg, P	NY	479
NS	Swaid, S	AL	484
NS	Thompson, B	MI	490
Oto	Arriaga, M	LA	681
Oto	Beatty, C	MN	673
Oto	Brackmann, D	CA	684
Oto	Driscoll, C	MN	674
Oto	Duckert, L	WA	684
Oto	Feghali, J	NY	659
Oto	Jenkins, H	CO	680
Oto	Kveton, J	CT	656
Oto	Lambert, P	SC	669
Oto	Linstrom, C	NY	662
Oto	Miyamoto, R	IN	676
Oto	Roland, J	NY	664
Oto	Rubinstein, J	WA	686
Oto	Shelton, C	UT	680
Oto	Telian, S	MI	678
Oto	Wackym, P	OR	687
Oto	Wazen, J	FL	672
Oto	Wiet, R	IL	678
RadRO	Loeffler, J	MA	947

Acromegaly

Spec	Name	St	Pg
EDM	Biller, B	MA	206
EDM	Katznelson, L	CA	223
EDM	Kennedy, L	OH	218
EDM	Klibanski, A	MA	207
EDM	Melmed, S	CA	223
Onc	Chang, S	CA	384

Acupuncture

Spec	Name	St	Pg
PM	Ngeow, J	NY	697

Spec	Name	St	Pg
PMR	Borg-Stein, J	MA	834
PMR	Dillard, J	NY	835

Acute Coronary Syndromes

Spec	Name	St	Pg
Cv	Eagle, K	MI	107
Cv	Rihal, C	MN	110
Cv	Williams, E	IN	112
IC	Bach, R	MO	130
IC	Gibson, C	MA	126
IC	Greene, R	CA	133
IC	Henry, T	MN	131
IC	Holmes, D	MN	131

ADD/ADHD

Spec	Name	St	Pg
ChAP	Abright, A	NY	907
ChAP	Alessi, N	MI	910
ChAP	Biederman, J	MA	906
ChAP	Bird, H	NY	907
ChAP	Bogrov, M	MD	908
ChAP	Boxer, G	MO	910
ChAP	Coffey, B	NY	908
ChAP	Dulcan, M	IL	910
ChAP	Hertzig, M	NY	908
ChAP	Heston, J	TN	910
ChAP	Hirsch, G	NY	908
ChAP	Hudziak, J	VT	906
ChAP	Koplewicz, H	NY	909
ChAP	Kwon, H	WA	912
ChAP	Leventhal, B	NY	909
ChAP	Martini, D	UT	911
ChAP	Rostain, A	PA	909
ChAP	Russell, A	CA	912
ChAP	Slomowitz, M	IL	911
ChAP	Spencer, T	MA	907
ChAP	Turecki, S	NY	909
ChAP	Wilens, T	MA	907
ChiN	Nass, R	NY	148
N	Finkel, M	FL	521
Ped	Burgess, D	NJ	726
Ped	Hershorin, E	FL	727
Ped	Jacob, M	IL	728
Ped	Roizen, N	OH	728
Psyc	Hoffman, D	CO	899
Psyc	Keepers, G	OR	901

ADD/PTSD

Spec	Name	St	Pg
Psyc	Manevitz, A	NY	893

Addiction Psychiatry

Spec	Name	St	Pg
AdP	Anton, R	SC	905
AdP	Ciraulo, D	MA	904
AdP	Collins, E	NY	904

Specialty & Special Expertise Index

Spec	Name	St	Pg
AdP	Frances, R	NY	904
AdP	Galanter, I	NY	904
AdP	Greenfield, S	MA	904
AdP	Howell, E	UT	905
AdP	Kampman, K	PA	904
AdP	Kleber, H	NY	905
AdP	Kosten, T	TX	906
AdP	Nitenson, N	MA	904
AdP	Schuckit, M	CA	906
AdP	Serota, R	PA	905
AdP	Stine, S	MI	905
AdP	Strain, E	MD	905
AdP	Walker, R	OR	906

Addiction/Substance Abuse

Spec	Name	St	Pg
AdP	Collins, E	NY	904
AdP	Frances, R	NY	904
AdP	Greenfield, S	MA	904
AdP	Howell, E	UT	905
AdP	Kampman, K	PA	904
AdP	Nitenson, N	MA	904
AdP	Serota, R	PA	905
AdP	Stine, S	MI	905
AdP	Strain, E	MD	905
AM	Adger, H	MD	80
ChAP	Deas, D	SC	910
ChAP	Wilens, T	MA	907
IM	Selwyn, P	NY	424
Psyc	Lawson, W	DC	893
Psyc	Rosenthal, R	NY	894
Psyc	Salloum, I	FL	896
Psyc	Strakowski, S	OH	898
Psyc	Weinstock, R	CA	903

Adolescent Behavior-High Risk

Spec	Name	St	Pg
AM	Ginsburg, K	PA	80
AM	Staggers, B	CA	82

Adolescent Gynecology

Spec	Name	St	Pg
AM	Diaz, A	NY	80
AM	Emans, S	MA	80
AM	Hergenroeder, A	TX	82
AM	Irwin, C	CA	82
AM	Kaplan, D	CO	81
AM	Kokotailo, P	WI	81
AM	Murray, P	WV	80
CG	Driscoll, D	PA	157
ObG	Greenfield, M	OH	561
ObG	Laufer, M	MA	556
ObG	Merritt, D	MO	562
RE	Ratts, V	MO	1014
RE	Sanfilippo, J	PA	1010

Adolescent Medicine

Spec	Name	St	Pg
AM	Adger, H	MD	80
AM	Adger, H	MD	80
AM	Anderson, M	CA	82
AM	Bermudez, O	CO	81
AM	Bravender, T	OH	81

Spec	Name	St	Pg
AM	Chambers, C	PA	80
AM	Diaz, A	NY	80
AM	Emans, S	MA	80
AM	Ginsburg, K	PA	80
AM	Hergenroeder, A	TX	82
AM	Irwin, C	CA	82
AM	Kaplan, D	CO	81
AM	Kokotailo, P	WI	81
AM	MacKenzie, R	CA	82
AM	Murray, P	WV	80
AM	Rudy, B	NY	80
AM	Sigel, E	CO	81
AM	Singh, N	MN	81
AM	Slap, G	PA	81
AM	Staggers, B	CA	82

Adolescent Psychiatry

Spec	Name	St	Pg
Psyc	Weinstock, R	CA	903

Adolescent Sports Medicine

Spec	Name	St	Pg
OrS	Curl, W	NC	628
OrS	Spindler, K	TN	631
SM	Metzl, J	NY	1041

Adrenal Cancer

Spec	Name	St	Pg
EDM	Hammer, G	MI	217
Onc	Oh, W	NY	347
Onc	Quinn, D	CA	389
PHO	Wolfe, L	NY	764
S	Lee, J	TX	1090
S	Solorzano, C	TN	1072
VIR	Wood, B	MD	994

Adrenal Disorders

Spec	Name	St	Pg
EDM	Bell, D	AL	213
EDM	Daniels, G	MA	207
EDM	Hammer, G	MI	217
EDM	Jacobs, T	NY	210
EDM	Kennedy, L	OH	218
EDM	Lechan, R	MA	208
EDM	Lipson, A	DC	211
EDM	Semenkovich, C	MO	219
EDM	Vance, M	VA	215
Nep	Blumenfeld, J	NY	457
Nep	Weiner, I	FL	460
PEn	New, M	NY	745
PEn	Oberfield, S	NY	745
PEn	Rivkees, S	FL	746

Adrenal Pathology

Spec	Name	St	Pg
Path	Weiss, L	CA	722

Adrenal Surgery

Spec	Name	St	Pg
S	Doherty, G	MA	1049
S	McHenry, C	OH	1079
S	Pachter, H	NY	1061
S	Prinz, R	IL	1081
S	Schlinkert, R	AZ	1092

Spec	Name	St	Pg
S	Weber, C	GA	1073
U	Marsh, C	CA	1177

Adrenal Tumors

Spec	Name	St	Pg
S	Angelos, P	IL	1074
S	Brunt, L	MO	1075
S	Butler, J	CA	1094
S	Duh, Q	CA	1095
S	Grant, C	MN	1077
S	Hanna, N	MD	1058
S	Hodin, R	MA	1049
S	Schulick, R	CO	1086
S	Udelsman, R	CT	1052
U	Libertino, J	MA	1149
U	Sundaram, C	IN	1170

Aggression Disorders

Spec	Name	St	Pg
ChAP	Steiner, H	CA	912

Aging

Spec	Name	St	Pg
Ger	Gambert, S	MD	263
Ger	Minaker, K	MA	262
OrS	Polly, D	MN	637

AIDS Related Cancers

Spec	Name	St	Pg
Hem	Levine, A	CA	326
Inf	Palefsky, J	CA	419
Inf	Polsky, B	NY	413
Onc	Aboulafia, D	WA	383
Onc	Abrams, D	CA	383
Onc	Ambinder, R	MD	334
Onc	Henry, D	PA	341
Onc	Kaplan, L	CA	387
Onc	Mitsuyasu, R	CA	388
Onc	Remick, S	WV	348
Onc	Volberding, P	CA	392
Onc	Von Roenn, J	IL	373
Psyc	Breitbart, W	NY	891

AIDS Related Lymphoma

Spec	Name	St	Pg
Onc	Morgan, D	TN	360

AIDS-Neurologic Complications

Spec	Name	St	Pg
N	Simpson, D	NY	517

AIDS/HIV

Spec	Name	St	Pg
AM	Rudy, B	NY	80
Ger	McCormick, W	WA	267
Hem	Levine, A	CA	326
IM	Fischl, M	FL	425
IM	Selwyn, P	NY	424
Inf	Ballon-Landa, G	CA	419
Inf	Bartlett, J	MD	410
Inf	Berkowitz, L	NY	410
Inf	Campbell, J	MO	416
Inf	Cancio, M	FL	414
Inf	Chaisson, R	MD	411
Inf	Cohn, S	IL	416

Spec	Name	St	Pg
Inf	Craven, D	MA	410
Inf	Daar, E	CA	419
Inf	Fichtenbaum, C	OH	416
Inf	Flaherty, J	IL	416
Inf	Flanigan, T	RI	410
Inf	Frank, I	PA	411
Inf	Gorensek, M	FL	415
Inf	Gumprecht, J	NY	411
Inf	Hammer, G	NY	411
Inf	Hammer, S	NY	411
Inf	Johnson, S	CO	418
Inf	Katner, H	GA	415
Inf	Keiser, P	TX	418
Inf	Kumar, P	DC	412
Inf	Louie, E	NY	412
Inf	Masur, H	MD	412
Inf	McGowan, J	NY	412
Inf	Mildvan, D	NY	412
Inf	O'Keefe, J	IL	416
Inf	Perlman, D	NY	412
Inf	Polsky, B	NY	413
Inf	Ratzan, K	FL	415
Inf	Richman, D	CA	419
Inf	Romagnoli, M	NY	413
Inf	Saag, M	AL	415
Inf	Salata, R	OH	417
Inf	Sax, P	MA	410
Inf	Scheld, W	VA	415
Inf	Schooley, R	CA	420
Inf	Siegel, M	WA	420
Inf	Squires, K	PA	413
Inf	Van Der Horst, C	NC	415
Inf	Wallach, F	NY	413
Inf	Wiviott, L	CA	420
Inf	Wormser, G	NY	413
Inf	Yancovitz, S	NY	414
N	Berger, J	KY	520
N	McArthur, J	MD	515
PA&I	Church, J	CA	733
PA&I	Shearer, W	TX	732
PInf	Andiman, W	CT	779
PInf	Bryson, Y	CA	784
PInf	Durbin, W	MA	780
PInf	Emmanuel, P	FL	781
PInf	Flynn, P	TN	782
PInf	Kleiman, M	IN	783
PInf	Kline, M	TX	784
PInf	McComsey, G	OH	783
PInf	McKinney, R	NC	782
PInf	Michaels, M	PA	781
PInf	Mitchell, C	FL	782
PInf	Petru, A	CA	785
PInf	Scott, G	FL	782
Pul	Hopewell, P	CA	939
Pul	Huang, L	CA	940

AIDS/HIV in Elderly

Inf	McGowan, J	NY	412

AIDS/HIV in Pregnancy

MF	Riley, L	MA	431

Spec	Name	St	Pg

AIDS/HIV in Women

Inf	Cohn, S	IL	416
Inf	Sha, B	IL	417
Inf	Squires, K	PA	413

AIDS/HIV Liaison Psychiatry

Psyc	Avery, E	TX	899

AIDS/HIV-Gastrointestinal Complications

Ge	Borum, M	DC	231
Ge	Dieterich, D	NY	232

Airway Disorders

A&I	Chandler, M	NY	84
A&I	Korenblat, P	MO	88
Oto	Hogikyan, N	MI	675
Oto	Patil, Y	OH	677
Oto	Zalzal, G	DC	667
PO	Arnold, J	OH	791
PO	Bower, C	AR	792
PO	Crockett, D	CA	793
PO	Darrow, D	VA	791
PO	Duncan, N	TX	792
PO	Friedman, E	TX	793
PO	Geller, K	CA	793
PO	Goldsmith, A	NY	789
PO	Holinger, L	IL	791
PO	Inglis, A	WA	793
PO	Miller, R	IL	792
PO	Myer, C	OH	792
PO	Richardson, M	OR	793
PO	Rosbe, K	CA	793
PO	Ward, R	NY	790
PPul	Sherman, J	VA	796
Pul	Burschtin, O	NY	924
Pul	Ernst, A	MA	922
Pul	Goldman, A	FL	931

Airway Reconstruction

Oto	Clark, K	OK	681
Oto	Couch, M	VT	655
Oto	Genden, E	NY	659
PO	Cotton, R	OH	791
PO	Parikh, S	WA	793

Albinism

Oph	Summers, C	MN	594

Alcohol Abuse

AdP	Anton, R	SC	905
AdP	Ciraulo, D	MA	904
AdP	Collins, E	NY	904
AdP	Galanter, I	NY	904
AdP	Greenfield, S	MA	904
AdP	Howell, E	UT	905
AdP	Kampman, K	PA	904
AdP	Kosten, T	TX	906

Spec	Name	St	Pg
AdP	Nitenson, N	MA	904
AdP	Schuckit, M	CA	906

Alcohol Abuse-Consultation

AdP	Walker, R	OR	906

Allergic Fungal Sinusitis

Oto	Kuhn, F	GA	669

Allergic Rhinitis

A&I	Henderson, W	WA	90
A&I	Sundy, J	NC	87
PA&I	Burks, A	NC	730

Allergy

A&I	Altman, L	WA	90
A&I	DeShazo, R	MS	86
A&I	Friedman, S	FL	86
A&I	Korenblat, P	MO	88
A&I	Li, J	MN	88
A&I	MacLean, J	MA	84
A&I	Montanaro, A	OR	90
A&I	Phillips, S	PA	85
A&I	Routes, J	WI	89
Oto	Corey, J	IL	674
PA&I	Gelfand, E	CO	732
PA&I	Lemanske, R	WI	731
PA&I	Schuberth, K	MD	730
PA&I	Sly, R	MD	730
PA&I	Wasserman, R	TX	732
PA&I	Wolf, R	IL	731
Pul	Sutherland, E	CO	937
Rhu	Gershwin, M	CA	1034

Allergy & Immunology

A&I	Altman, L	WA	90
A&I	Baker, J	MI	87
A&I	Ballas, Z	IA	87
A&I	Benenati, S	FL	86
A&I	Bernstein, D	OH	87
A&I	Bernstein, J	OH	88
A&I	Bonner, J	AL	86
A&I	Buchbinder, E	NY	84
A&I	Busse, W	WI	88
A&I	Castells, M	MA	84
A&I	Chandler, M	NY	84
A&I	Cunningham-Rundles, C	NY	84
A&I	DeShazo, R	MS	86
A&I	Ein, D	DC	85
A&I	Fishman, H	DC	85
A&I	Freeman, T	TX	89
A&I	Friedman, S	FL	86
A&I	Grammer, L	IL	88
A&I	Greenberger, P	IL	88
A&I	Gruchalla, R	TX	89
A&I	Henderson, W	WA	90
A&I	Jost, B	MO	88
A&I	Kaliner, M	MD	85

Specialty & Special Expertise Index

Spec	Name	St	Pg
A&I	Korenblat, P	MO	88
A&I	Ledford, D	FL	86
A&I	Lewis, J	AZ	89
A&I	Li, J	MN	88
A&I	Lieberman, P	TN	86
A&I	Lockey, R	FL	86
A&I	MacLean, J	MA	84
A&I	Markert, M	NC	87
A&I	Mazza, D	NY	85
A&I	Meltzer, E	CA	90
A&I	Metcalfe, D	MD	85
A&I	Montanaro, A	OR	90
A&I	Ostrom, N	CA	90
A&I	Pacin, M	FL	87
A&I	Phillips, S	PA	85
A&I	Routes, J	WI	89
A&I	Sanders, G	MI	89
A&I	Schubert, M	AZ	90
A&I	Shepherd, G	NY	85
A&I	Slankard, M	NY	85
A&I	Spector, S	CA	91
A&I	Sullivan, T	GA	87
A&I	Sundy, J	NC	87
A&I	Tamaroff, M	CA	91
A&I	Tillinghast, J	MO	89
A&I	Umetsu, D	MA	84
A&I	Wasserman, S	CA	91
A&I	Wong, D	AZ	90
A&I	Wong, J	MA	84
A&I	Wood, J	MO	89

Allergy up to age 50

PA&I	Bock, S	CO	732

Alopecia Areata

D	Duvic, M	TX	196

Alzheimer's Disease

Ger	Carr, D	MO	264
Ger	Gorbien, M	IL	265
Ger	Liem, P	AR	266
Ger	Morley, J	MO	265
Ger	Sachs, G	IN	265
GerPsy	Borson, S	WA	915
GerPsy	Burke, W	NE	914
GerPsy	Grossberg, G	MO	914
GerPsy	Kennedy, G	NY	913
GerPsy	Lyketsos, C	MD	913
GerPsy	Reisberg, B	NY	913
GerPsy	Rovner, B	PA	913
GerPsy	Small, G	CA	915
GerPsy	Streim, J	PA	913
GerPsy	Tune, L	GA	914
N	Ahern, G	AZ	532
N	Chui, H	CA	536
N	Cummings, J	NV	536
N	DeKosky, S	VA	520
N	Doody, R	TX	533
N	Farlow, M	IN	526
N	Feinberg, T	NY	511

Spec	Name	St	Pg
N	Filley, C	CO	531
N	Gilman, S	MI	526
N	Henderson, V	CA	537
N	Longo, F	CA	538
N	Marder, K	NY	515
N	Mayeux, R	NY	515
N	Mesulam, M	IL	528
N	Morris, J	MO	528
N	Petersen, R	MN	529
N	Relkin, N	NY	517
N	Sadowsky, C	FL	523
N	Zimmerman, E	NY	519
NRad	Drayer, B	NY	985
NS	Rezai, A	OH	489
Psyc	Arnold, S	PA	890
Psyc	Raskind, M	WA	902
Psyc	Weiner, M	TX	900

Amblyopia

Oph	Gallin, P	NY	574
Oph	Miller, J	AZ	597
Oph	Tychsen, L	MO	595
Oph	Warman, R	FL	587
Oph	Weiss, A	WA	604

Amblyopia & Vision Development

Oph	Burke, M	OH	589

Amniocentesis

MF	Genc, M	NY	432
MF	Grunebaum, A	NY	433
MF	McLaren, R	VA	435
MF	Nies, B	VA	435
MF	Philipson, E	OH	437
MF	Robinson, J	MA	431
MF	Strassner, H	IL	437

Amniotic Membrane Transplant

Oph	John, T	IL	590

Amputation Surgery

OrS	Pinzur, M	IL	637
OrS	Smith, D	WA	646

Amputee Rehabilitation

PMR	Esquenazi, A	PA	835
PMR	Gittler, M	IL	840
PMR	Kuiken, T	IL	841
PMR	Leonard, J	MI	841
PMR	Miknevich, M	PA	837
PMR	Munin, M	PA	837
PMR	Richter, E	CT	834
PMR	Volshteyn, O	MO	842
PMR	Wilson, A	TX	843

Amyloid Heart Disease

Cv	Follansbee, W	PA	98

Spec	Name	St	Pg
Cv	Young, J	OH	113

Amyloidosis

Hem	Comenzo, R	MA	310
Hem	Gertz, M	MN	319
H & PM	Davis, M	OH	407
Nep	Dember, L	PA	457
Onc	Stadtmauer, E	PA	350
Onc	Vescio, R	CA	392
Pul	Berk, J	MA	922

Amyloidosis/Joint Disease

Rhu	Gorevic, P	NY	1026

Amyotrophic Lateral Sclerosis (ALS)

N	Armon, C	MA	506
N	Barohn, R	KS	531
N	Cudkowicz, M	MA	507
N	Engel, W	CA	536
N	Feldman, E	MI	526
N	Glass, J	GA	521
N	Graves, M	CA	537
N	Harati, Y	TX	533
N	Jones, H	MA	507
N	Lacomis, D	PA	514
N	McCluskey, L	PA	515
N	Mitsumoto, H	NY	516
N	Newman, D	MI	528
N	Pascuzzi, R	IN	528
N	Roos, R	IL	529
N	Rutkove, S	MA	508
N	Shefner, J	NY	517
N	Sheikh, K	TX	534
N	Siddique, T	IL	530
N	Weiner, L	CA	539
N	Weiss, M	WA	539
N	Windebank, A	MN	530
N	Zimnowodzki, S	IL	531
PMR	Bach, J	NJ	835

Anal Cancer

CRS	Dietz, D	OH	173
CRS	Geisler, D	PA	170
CRS	Gorfine, S	NY	170
CRS	Nagle, D	MA	168
CRS	Welton, M	CA	178
DR	Coakley, F	OR	982
Onc	Berry, J	CA	384
Onc	Goldberg, R	OH	367

Anal Disorders & Reconstruction

CRS	Blatchford, G	NE	176
CRS	Gorfine, S	NY	170
CRS	Marcet, J	FL	172
CRS	Rafferty, J	OH	175

Spec	Name	St	Pg

Anal Sphincter Repair

Spec	Name	St	Pg
CRS	Coutsoftides, T	CA	177
CRS	Lowry, A	MN	174

Anaphylaxis

Spec	Name	St	Pg
A&I	Castells, M	MA	84
A&I	Greenberger, P	IL	88
A&I	Korenblat, P	MO	88
A&I	Lieberman, P	TN	86
A&I	Metcalfe, D	MD	85
A&I	Sullivan, T	GA	87
PA&I	Burks, A	NC	730
PA&I	Ownby, D	GA	731

Anemia

Spec	Name	St	Pg
Hem	Blinder, M	MO	318
Hem	Isola, L	NY	313
Hem	Raphael, B	NY	314
Hem	Soff, G	NY	315
Hem	Spivak, J	MD	315
Hem	Zuckerman, K	FL	318
PHO	Beyer, E	IL	769
PHO	Salvi, S	IL	773
PNep	Ault, B	TN	786

Anemia-Aplastic

Spec	Name	St	Pg
Hem	Maciejewski, J	OH	321
Hem	Mangan, K	PA	313
Hem	Schuster, M	NY	315
Onc	Antin, J	MA	327
Onc	Claxton, D	PA	336
Onc	Dang, C	PA	338
PHO	Boxer, L	MI	769
PHO	Camitta, B	WI	769
PHO	Guinan, E	MA	756
PHO	Wang, W	TN	769

Anemia-Cancer Related

Spec	Name	St	Pg
Hem	Rodgers, G	UT	322
Hem	Schiffman, F	RI	311
Hem	Wisch, N	NY	316

Anemias & Red Cell Disorders

Spec	Name	St	Pg
Hem	Telen, M	NC	318
PHO	Boxer, L	MI	769
PHO	Finklestein, J	CA	777
PHO	Thomas, G	OR	779

Aneurysm

Spec	Name	St	Pg
Cv	Braverman, A	MO	106
NRad	Hurst, R	PA	985
NRad	Pile-Spellman, J	NY	986
T&CS	Bolman, R	MA	1110
VascS	Belkin, M	MA	1184
VascS	Dougherty, M	PA	1186
VascS	Flanigan, D	CA	1194
VascS	Golden, M	PA	1187
VascS	Greisler, H	IL	1191

Spec	Name	St	Pg
VascS	Hodgson, K	IL	1191
VascS	Hollier, L	LA	1193
VascS	McLafferty, R	IL	1191
VascS	Money, S	AZ	1193
VascS	Perler, B	MD	1188
VascS	Ricotta, J	DC	1188
VascS	Stanley, J	MI	1192
VascS	White, R	CA	1194
VIR	Dake, M	CA	997

Aneurysm-Abdominal & Thoracic Aortic

Spec	Name	St	Pg
Cv	Krajcer, Z	TX	114
T&CS	Coselli, J	TX	1137
T&CS	Woo, Y	PA	1123
VascS	Acher, C	WI	1190
VascS	Calligaro, K	PA	1186
VascS	Carpenter, J	NJ	1186
VascS	Clair, D	OH	1190
VascS	Criado, F	MD	1186
VascS	Darling, R	NY	1186
VascS	Fairman, R	PA	1187
VascS	Kazmers, A	MI	1191
VascS	Kwolek, C	MA	1184
VascS	Morrissey, N	NY	1188
VascS	Sanchez, L	MO	1191

Aneurysm-Abdominal Aortic

Spec	Name	St	Pg
T&CS	Martin, T	FL	1126
T&CS	Ott, D	TX	1139
T&CS	Safi, H	TX	1139
VascS	Adelman, M	NY	1185
VascS	Atnip, R	PA	1185
VascS	Brewster, D	MA	1184
VascS	Cambria, R	MA	1184
VascS	Cronenwett, J	NH	1184
VascS	D'Ayala, M	NY	1186
VascS	Eidt, J	AR	1193
VascS	Faries, P	NY	1187
VascS	Gloviczki, P	MN	1191
VascS	Green, R	NY	1187
VascS	Hakaim, A	FL	1189
VascS	Hallett, J	SC	1189
VascS	Kent, K	WI	1191
VascS	Mackey, W	MA	1185
VascS	McKinsey, J	NY	1188
VascS	Money, S	AZ	1193
VascS	Pearce, W	IL	1191
VascS	Sicard, G	MO	1192
VascS	Todd, G	NY	1189
VascS	Weinstein, E	CO	1192
VascS	Zarins, C	CA	1194
VIR	Benenati, J	FL	994
VIR	Matsumoto, A	VA	995

Aneurysm-Aortic

Spec	Name	St	Pg
T&CS	Bowdish, M	CA	1140
T&CS	Bridges, C	NC	1124
T&CS	Deeb, G	MI	1131
T&CS	Girardi, L	NY	1116

Spec	Name	St	Pg
T&CS	Griffith, B	MD	1117
T&CS	Jessen, M	TX	1138
T&CS	Loulmet, D	NY	1119
T&CS	Stewart, A	NY	1122
VascS	Benvenisty, A	NY	1186
VascS	Brener, B	NJ	1186
VascS	Chaikof, E	MA	1184
VascS	Comerota, A	OH	1190
VascS	Fairman, R	PA	1187
VascS	Fowl, R	AZ	1193
VascS	Freischlag, J	MD	1187
VascS	Gewertz, B	CA	1194
VascS	Harrington, E	NY	1187
VascS	Howard, T	NE	1192
VascS	LaMuraglia, G	MA	1185
VascS	Makaroun, M	PA	1187
VascS	Marin, M	NY	1188
VascS	Mitchell, M	MS	1189
VascS	Naslund, T	TN	1190
VascS	Schneider, D	NY	1188
VascS	Shepard, A	MI	1192
VIR	Hovsepian, D	CA	998
VIR	Katzen, B	FL	994
VIR	Murphy, T	RI	992

Aneurysm-Aortic-Medical Management

Spec	Name	St	Pg
VascS	Riles, T	NY	1188

Aneurysm-Cerebral

Spec	Name	St	Pg
NRad	Berenstein, A	NY	985
NRad	Cross, D	MO	988
NRad	Dion, J	GA	987
NRad	Frei, D	CO	990
NRad	Grobelny, T	IL	988
NRad	Higashida, R	CA	991
NRad	Jensen, M	VA	987
NRad	Joseph, G	NC	987
NRad	Kallmes, D	MN	989
NRad	Larsen, D	CA	991
NRad	Masaryk, T	OH	989
NRad	Moran, C	MO	989
NRad	Morris, P	NC	987
NRad	Norbash, A	MA	984
NRad	Teitelbaum, G	CA	991
NRad	Vinuela, F	CA	991
NS	Barrow, D	GA	481
NS	Bederson, J	NY	472
NS	Dacey, R	MO	487
NS	Dempsey, R	WI	487
NS	Giannotta, S	CA	497
NS	Grady, M	PA	474
NS	Guthikonda, M	MI	488
NS	Harbaugh, R	PA	474
NS	Huang, J	MD	475
NS	Kim, D	TX	493
NS	Loftus, C	IL	488
NS	Martin, N	CA	498
NS	Moore, F	NJ	477
NS	Murali, R	NY	477
NS	Patel, A	NY	477

Specialty & Special Expertise Index

Spec	Name	St	Pg
NS	Riina, H	NY	478
NS	Rosenwasser, R	PA	478
NS	Sekhar, L	WA	498
NS	Selman, W	OH	490
NS	Shapiro, S	IN	490
NS	Solomon, R	NY	479
NS	Steinberg, G	CA	499
NS	Thompson, B	MI	490
VIR	Kumpe, D	CO	996

Aneurysm-Thoracic Aortic

Spec	Name	St	Pg
T&CS	Akins, C	MA	1110
T&CS	Elefteriades, J	CT	1110
T&CS	Liao, K	MN	1133
T&CS	Moon, M	MO	1134
T&CS	Pochettino, A	MN	1134
T&CS	Shemin, R	CA	1142
T&CS	Tranbaugh, R	NY	1122

Angelman Syndrome

Spec	Name	St	Pg
CG	Driscoll, D	FL	158
CG	Shoffner, J	GA	159

Angiogenesis

Spec	Name	St	Pg
IC	Ellis, S	OH	131
IC	Henry, T	MN	131
IC	Knopf, W	GA	130
IC	Perin, E	TX	132

Angiography-Coronary

Spec	Name	St	Pg
Cv	Klein, L	IL	109
IC	Moses, J	NY	127

Angioplasty

Spec	Name	St	Pg
Cv	Coppola, J	NY	97
Cv	Diver, D	CT	94
Cv	Ramee, S	LA	115
Cv	Weaver, W	MI	112
IC	Applegate, R	NC	129
IC	Feldman, T	IL	131
IC	Laham, R	MA	126
IC	Matar, F	FL	130
IC	Morris, D	GA	130

Angioplasty & Restenosis

Spec	Name	St	Pg
IC	Holmes, D	MN	131

Angioplasty & Stent Placement

Spec	Name	St	Pg
Cv	Edelen, J	CA	116
IC	Bailey, S	TX	132
IC	Chang, G	PA	127
IC	Dieter, R	IL	131
IC	Douglas, J	GA	129
IC	Ellis, S	OH	131
IC	Herrmann, H	PA	127
IC	Kandzari, D	GA	130
IC	Kleiman, N	TX	132
IC	Moses, J	NY	127

Spec	Name	St	Pg
IC	Pichard, A	DC	128
IC	Reddy, B	GA	130
IC	Reiner, J	DC	128
IC	Rosenfield, K	MA	126
IC	Shani, J	NY	129
IC	Sharma, S	NY	129
IC	Stone, G	NY	129
IC	Zelman, R	MA	127
VascS	Brewster, D	MA	1184
VascS	Kazmers, A	MI	1191
VIR	Kaufman, J	OR	998
VIR	McLean, G	PA	993

Angioplasty-Peripheral

Spec	Name	St	Pg
VIR	Smith, S	IL	996

Angioplasty-Pulmonary Artery

Spec	Name	St	Pg
PCd	Lock, J	MA	734

Ankle Reconstruction

Spec	Name	St	Pg
OrS	Levine, D	NY	621

Ankle Replacement & Revision

Spec	Name	St	Pg
OrS	Brage, M	WA	642
OrS	DeOrio, J	NC	628
OrS	Greisberg, J	NY	618
OrS	Nunley, J	NC	629
OrS	Sangeorzan, B	WA	645

Ankle Surgery

Spec	Name	St	Pg
SM	Paletta, G	MO	1043
SM	Scheller, A	MA	1040

Ankylosing Spondylitis

Spec	Name	St	Pg
Rhu	Bobrove, A	CA	1033
Rhu	Chang, R	IL	1030
Rhu	Hugenberg, S	IN	1031
Rhu	Kay, J	MA	1024
Rhu	Luthra, H	MN	1031

Anophthalmia

Spec	Name	St	Pg
Oph	Bernardino, C	CA	599
Oph	Tse, D	FL	586

Anorectal Disorders

Spec	Name	St	Pg
CRS	Abcarian, H	IL	173
CRS	Dietz, D	OH	173
CRS	Efron, J	MD	169
CRS	Eisenstat, T	NJ	169
CRS	Fry, R	PA	170
CRS	Heppell, J	AZ	177
CRS	Lederman, E	MO	174
CRS	Procaccino, J	NY	171
CRS	Schoetz, D	MA	169
CRS	Senagore, A	CA	178
CRS	Shah, N	RI	169
CRS	Shellito, P	MA	169

Spec	Name	St	Pg
CRS	Trudel, J	MN	175

Anorectal Malformations

Spec	Name	St	Pg
PS	Pena, A	OH	807
PS	Velcek, F	NY	804

Anorexia Nervosa-Severe

Spec	Name	St	Pg
IM	Mehler, P	CO	426

Anterior Segment Surgery

Spec	Name	St	Pg
Oph	Alward, W	IA	588
Oph	Caprioli, J	CA	599
Oph	Dhaliwal, D	PA	573
Oph	Page, T	MI	593
Oph	Samuelson, T	MN	594
Oph	Shamie, N	CA	604

Anterior Segment Trauma/Reconstruction

Spec	Name	St	Pg
Oph	Florakis, G	NY	574

Antibiotic Resistance

Spec	Name	St	Pg
Inf	Edmond, M	VA	414
Inf	Patterson, J	TX	418
Inf	Scheld, W	VA	415
PInf	Alexander, K	IL	782
PInf	Long, S	PA	781
PInf	McCracken, G	TX	784

Antiphospholipid Syndrome (APS)

Spec	Name	St	Pg
N	Hess, D	GA	522
Rhu	Belmont, H	NY	1025
Rhu	Petri, M	MD	1027
Rhu	Salmon, J	NY	1028

Anxiety & Depression

Spec	Name	St	Pg
AdP	Ciraulo, D	MA	904
AM	Singh, N	MN	81
ChAP	Bird, H	NY	907
ChAP	Slomowitz, M	IL	911
GerPsy	Stein, E	CA	915
Psyc	Bronheim, H	NY	891
Psyc	Sadock, V	NY	894

Anxiety & Mood Disorders

Spec	Name	St	Pg
AdP	Frances, R	NY	904
ChAP	Biederman, J	MA	906
ChAP	Hirsch, G	NY	908
ChAP	Koplewicz, H	NY	909
ChAP	Kwon, H	WA	912
Psyc	Appelbaum, P	NY	890
Psyc	Friedman, M	VT	888
Psyc	Levy, S	GA	896
Psyc	Locala, J	OH	898
Psyc	Price, L	RI	889
Psyc	Rosenthal, R	NY	894

Spec	Name	St	Pg
Psyc	Roy-Byrne, P	WA	902
Psyc	Schatzberg, A	CA	903
Psyc	Scott, C	PA	895
Psyc	Sussman, N	NY	895
Psyc	Thase, M	PA	895
Psyc	Wait, S	MD	895

Anxiety Disorders

Spec	Name	St	Pg
AM	Kaplan, D	CO	81
ChAP	Abright, A	NY	907
ChAP	Birmaher, B	PA	908
ChAP	Hagman, J	CO	911
ChAP	McKelvey, R	OR	912
ChAP	Riddle, M	MD	909
ChAP	Walkup, J	NY	909
Psyc	Bystritsky, A	CA	901
Psyc	Cohen, M	PA	891
Psyc	Eaton, J	DC	891
Psyc	Fyer, A	NY	892
Psyc	Hollander, E	NY	892
Psyc	McIntosh, J	UT	899
Psyc	Pi, E	CA	902
Psyc	Saxena, S	CA	903
Psyc	Stein, M	CA	903

Aortic & Visceral Artery Surgery

Spec	Name	St	Pg
VascS	Berguer, R	MI	1190

Aortic Diseases & Dissection

Spec	Name	St	Pg
Cv	Braverman, A	MO	106
Cv	Eagle, K	MI	107
Cv	O'Gara, P	MA	95
IC	Lasala, J	MO	131
IC	Schreiber, T	MI	131

Aortic Graft Infections

Spec	Name	St	Pg
VascS	Cherry, K	VA	1189
VascS	Flynn, T	FL	1189

Aortic Injuries

Spec	Name	St	Pg
S	Moore, E	CO	1085

Aortic Reconstruction

Spec	Name	St	Pg
VascS	Cambria, R	MA	1184
VascS	Dalsing, M	IN	1190
VascS	Pevec, W	CA	1194
VascS	Shepard, A	MI	1192

Aortic Stent Grafts

Spec	Name	St	Pg
VascS	Calligaro, K	PA	1186
VascS	Lumsden, A	TX	1193
VIR	Dake, M	CA	997

Aortic Surgery

Spec	Name	St	Pg
T&CS	Adams, D	NY	1113
T&CS	Bavaria, J	PA	1114
T&CS	Coselli, J	TX	1137
T&CS	DeRose, J	NY	1115
T&CS	Diehl, J	PA	1115
T&CS	Echeverri, L	TX	1137
T&CS	Graver, L	NY	1117
T&CS	Lazar, H	MA	1111
T&CS	Lytle, B	OH	1133
T&CS	Martin, T	FL	1126
T&CS	Miller, D	CA	1142
T&CS	Safi, H	TX	1139
T&CS	Salerno, T	FL	1129
T&CS	Sellke, F	RI	1112
T&CS	Smedira, N	OH	1135
T&CS	Stewart, A	NY	1122
T&CS	Stowe, C	FL	1129
T&CS	Svensson, L	OH	1135
T&CS	Verrier, E	WA	1143
T&CS	Warner, K	MA	1113
VascS	Hollier, L	LA	1193
VascS	Howard, T	NE	1192
VascS	Pomposelli, F	MA	1185

Aortic Surgery-Complex

Spec	Name	St	Pg
VascS	White, R	CA	1194

Aortic Valve Disease

Spec	Name	St	Pg
T&CS	Deeb, G	MI	1131

Aphasia

Spec	Name	St	Pg
N	Heilman, K	FL	521
N	Kirshner, H	TN	522
N	Mohr, J	NY	516

Apnea in Infants

Spec	Name	St	Pg
PPul	Givan, D	IN	796

Apnea/Robotic Surgery

Spec	Name	St	Pg
Oto	Thaler, E	PA	666

Appendix Cancer

Spec	Name	St	Pg
S	Bartlett, D	PA	1053
S	Mansfield, P	TX	1091
S	Sugarbaker, P	DC	1065

Arrhythmias

Spec	Name	St	Pg
CE	Anderson, M	IA	122
CE	Buxton, A	MA	118
CE	Callans, D	PA	119
CE	Cannom, D	CA	125
CE	Chinitz, L	NY	120
CE	Cohen, M	NY	120
CE	Curtis, A	NY	120
CE	DeLurgio, D	GA	121
CE	DiMarco, J	VA	121
CE	Donahue, J	OH	122
CE	Ellenbogen, K	VA	121
CE	Epstein, A	PA	120
CE	Epstein, L	MA	119
CE	Estes, N	MA	119
CE	Faddis, M	MO	123
CE	Gang, E	CA	125
CE	Gomes, J	NY	120
CE	Hammill, S	MN	123
CE	Higgins, S	CA	125
CE	Interian, A	FL	122
CE	Kay, G	AL	122
CE	Lerman, B	NY	120
CE	Levine, J	NY	121
CE	Lewkowiez, L	CO	124
CE	Lindsay, B	OH	123
CE	Link, M	MA	119
CE	Marchlinski, F	PA	121
CE	Mehta, D	NY	121
CE	Miller, J	IN	123
CE	Morady, F	MI	123
CE	Natale, A	TX	124
CE	Prystowsky, E	IN	123
CE	Ruskin, J	MA	119
CE	Schuger, C	MI	124
CE	Shen, W	AZ	124
CE	Sorrentino, R	GA	122
CE	Stevenson, W	MA	119
CE	Swerdlow, C	CA	125
CE	Tchou, P	OH	124
CE	Tomaselli, G	MD	121
CE	Waldo, A	OH	124
CE	Wang, P	CA	125
Cv	Abi-samra, F	LA	113
Cv	Anderson, J	UT	113
Cv	Benjamin, I	UT	113
Cv	Borzak, S	FL	103
Cv	Gliklich, J	NY	98
Cv	Myerburg, R	FL	104
Cv	Naccarelli, G	PA	100
Cv	Slater, W	NY	102
Cv	Volgman, A	IL	112
Cv	Waxman, H	PA	102
IC	Sacchi, T	NY	128
IC	Shorofsky, S	MD	129
PCd	Beerman, L	PA	734
PCd	Gillette, P	TX	740
PCd	Walsh, C	NY	736
PCd	Walsh, E	MA	734
PCd	Young, M	FL	738
T&CS	Chen, J	NY	1114
T&CS	Harken, A	CA	1141

Arrhythmias-Pediatric & Adult

Spec	Name	St	Pg
PCd	Fish, F	TN	737

Arterial & Venous Stents

Spec	Name	St	Pg
VIR	Keller, F	OR	998
VIR	Kumpe, D	CO	996

Arterial Bypass Surgery

Spec	Name	St	Pg
VascS	Belkin, M	MA	1184
VascS	Darling, R	NY	1186

Spec	Name	St	Pg

Arterial Bypass Surgery-Leg

Spec	Name	St	Pg
VascS	Fowl, R	AZ	1193
VascS	Harrington, E	NY	1187
VascS	Money, S	AZ	1193
VascS	Perler, B	MD	1188

Arterial Switch

PS	Quaegebeur, J	NY	804

Arteriovenous Malformations

N	Mohr, J	NY	516
NRad	Grobelny, T	IL	988
NRad	Morris, P	NC	987
NRad	Norbash, A	MA	984
NRad	Pile-Spellman, J	NY	986
NS	Diaz, F	MI	487
NS	Grady, M	PA	474
NS	Kim, D	TX	493
NS	Loftus, C	IL	488
NS	Morcos, J	FL	483
NS	Patel, A	NY	477
NS	Rosenwasser, R	PA	478
NS	Samson, D	TX	494
NS	Sekhar, L	WA	498
NS	Solomon, R	NY	479
NS	Steinberg, G	CA	499
VIR	Rilling, W	WI	996
VIR	Smith, S	IL	996

Arthritis

HS	Atkinson, R	HI	303
HS	Belsky, M	MA	294
HS	Carneiro, R	FL	298
HS	Friedman, D	FL	299
HS	Godzik, C	CA	304
HS	Greene, T	FL	299
HS	Hastings, H	IN	301
HS	Hunt, T	AL	299
HS	Imbriglia, J	PA	296
HS	Kulick, R	NY	296
HS	Lane, L	NY	296
HS	Light, T	IL	301
HS	Putnam, M	MN	302
HS	Raskin, K	NY	297
HS	Rayan, G	OK	303
OrS	Bronson, M	NY	615
OrS	Buly, R	NY	615
OrS	Deland, J	NY	616
OrS	Gladstone, J	NY	617
OrS	Goodman, S	CA	643
OrS	Gorab, R	CA	643
OrS	Jiranek, W	VA	629
OrS	Kraay, M	OH	635
OrS	Nunley, J	NC	629
OrS	Stuchin, S	NY	626
OrS	Thornhill, T	MA	613
OrS	Vail, T	CA	646
OrS	Wapner, K	PA	626
PRhu	Goldsmith, D	PA	799
PRhu	Lehman, T	NY	799

PRhu	Wilking, A	TX	801
Rhu	Allman, R	PA	1025
Rhu	Chang, R	IL	1030
Rhu	Fife, R	IN	1031
Rhu	Lipstate, J	LA	1033
Rhu	McAlindon, T	MA	1024
Rhu	Mease, P	WA	1034
Rhu	Schubert, R	DC	1028
Rhu	Sessoms, S	TX	1033
Rhu	Solitar, B	NY	1028
Rhu	Starz, T	PA	1028

Arthritis-Hip & Knee

OrS	Grelsamer, R	NY	618
OrS	Howe, K	CA	644

Arthritis-Knee

OrS	Leadbetter, W	MD	621

Arthritis-Septic

Inf	Bayer, A	CA	419

Arthroplasty Imaging

DR	Potter, H	NY	977

Arthroscopic Surgery

HS	Atkinson, R	HI	303
HS	Beredjiklian, P	PA	295
HS	Greene, T	FL	299
HS	Slutsky, D	CA	304
OrS	Bauman, P	NY	614
OrS	Bigliani, L	NY	614
OrS	Cooper, D	TX	640
OrS	Garrett, W	NC	628
OrS	Glashow, J	NY	618
OrS	Green, A	RI	611
OrS	Hausman, M	NY	618
OrS	Johnson, D	KY	629
OrS	Kelly, B	NY	621
OrS	Kocher, M	MA	612
OrS	Lock, T	MI	635
OrS	Millett, P	CO	639
OrS	Minas, T	MA	612
OrS	Nicholas, S	NY	623
OrS	Poehling, G	NC	630
OrS	Richmond, J	MA	612
OrS	Seltzer, D	AZ	641
OrS	Shelbourne, K	IN	637
OrS	Spindler, K	TN	631
OrS	Thomas, B	CA	646
OrS	Vo, P	FL	631
SM	Altchek, D	NY	1040
SM	Byrd, J	TN	1042
SM	Ciccotti, M	PA	1041
SM	Fronek, J	CA	1044
SM	Gill, T	MA	1040
SM	Hershman, E	NY	1041
SM	Ho, S	IL	1043
SM	Jones, D	LA	1044

SM	Levine, W	NY	1041
SM	Ma, C	CA	1044
SM	Mirzayan, R	CA	1044
SM	Nisonson, B	NY	1041
SM	Sennett, B	PA	1042
SM	Steiner, M	MA	1040
SM	Xerogeanes, J	GA	1043

Arthroscopic Surgery-Hip

OrS	Buly, R	NY	615
OrS	Kocher, M	MA	612
OrS	Mabrey, J	TX	641
OrS	McCarthy, J	OH	635
OrS	Padgett, D	NY	623
OrS	Philippon, M	CO	639
OrS	Westrich, G	NY	626
SM	Asnis, P	MA	1040

Arthroscopic Surgery-Knee

OrS	Bartolozzi, A	PA	614
OrS	Fulkerson, J	CT	611
OrS	Nuber, G	IL	636
OrS	Padgett, D	NY	623
OrS	Westrich, G	NY	626

Arthroscopic Surgery-Wrist

OrS	Goldner, R	NC	628

Artificial Heart Devices

T&CS	Frazier, O	TX	1138
T&CS	Jeevanandam, V	IL	1133
T&CS	Kormos, R	PA	1118
T&CS	Samuels, L	PA	1121

Arts in the Healing Process

Psyc	Avery, E	TX	899

Asbestos-related Lung Disease

OM	Harber, P	AZ	882
Pul	Rose, C	CO	937
T&CS	Krellenstein, D	NY	1118

Asherman's Syndrome

RE	Odem, R	MO	1014
RE	Walmer, D	NC	1012

Asperger's Syndrome

ChAP	Heston, J	TN	910
ChAP	Rostain, A	PA	909
Psyc	Brodkin, E	PA	891

Asthma

A&I	Altman, L	WA	90
A&I	Benenati, S	FL	86
A&I	Bernstein, D	OH	87
A&I	Bernstein, J	OH	88

Spec	Name	St	Pg
A&I	Bonner, J	AL	86
A&I	Busse, W	WI	88
A&I	Chandler, M	NY	84
A&I	Freeman, T	TX	89
A&I	Friedman, S	FL	86
A&I	Grammer, L	IL	88
A&I	Greenberger, P	IL	88
A&I	Henderson, W	WA	90
A&I	Korenblat, P	MO	88
A&I	Ledford, D	FL	86
A&I	Lewis, J	AZ	89
A&I	Li, J	MN	88
A&I	Lieberman, P	TN	86
A&I	MacLean, J	MA	84
A&I	Mazza, D	NY	85
A&I	Montanaro, A	OR	90
A&I	Pacin, M	FL	87
A&I	Routes, J	WI	89
A&I	Sanders, G	MI	89
A&I	Slankard, M	NY	85
A&I	Spector, S	CA	91
A&I	Sullivan, T	GA	87
A&I	Sundy, J	NC	87
A&I	Tamaroff, M	CA	91
A&I	Umetsu, D	MA	84
A&I	Wasserman, S	CA	91
A&I	Wong, J	MA	84
A&I	Wood, J	MO	89
PA&I	Bahna, S	LA	732
PA&I	Burks, A	NC	730
PA&I	Ehrlich, P	NY	729
PA&I	Gelfand, E	CO	732
PA&I	Kelly, C	VA	731
PA&I	Klein, R	RI	729
PA&I	Lemanske, R	WI	731
PA&I	Leung, D	CO	732
PA&I	Ownby, D	GA	731
PA&I	Pongracic, J	IL	731
PA&I	Schuberth, K	MD	730
PA&I	Sly, R	MD	730
PA&I	Spergel, J	PA	730
PA&I	Strunk, R	MO	731
PA&I	Wasserman, R	TX	732
PA&I	Wolf, R	IL	731
PA&I	Wood, R	MD	730
Ped	Jacob, M	IL	728
PPul	Dozor, A	NY	794
PPul	Gibson, R	WA	798
PPul	Givan, D	IN	796
PPul	Kattan, M	NY	794
PPul	Kim, Y	IN	797
PPul	Konstan, M	OH	797
PPul	Kurachek, S	MN	797
PPul	Lapey, A	MA	794
PPul	McCoy, K	OH	797
PPul	Morgan, W	AZ	797
PPul	Murphy, T	NC	796
PPul	Platzker, A	CA	798
PPul	Quittell, L	NY	795
PPul	Rubin, B	VA	796
PPul	Sherman, J	VA	796
PPul	Wall, M	OR	798

Spec	Name	St	Pg
Pul	Balk, R	IL	933
Pul	Boushey, H	CA	939
Pul	Brooks, S	FL	929
Pul	Burschtin, O	NY	924
Pul	Cooke, J	NY	925
Pul	Cooper, W	VA	930
Pul	Doherty, D	KY	930
Pul	Donohue, J	NC	930
Pul	Fanta, C	MA	922
Pul	Fulkerson, W	NC	930
Pul	Garrity, E	IL	933
Pul	Gerboth, G	AK	939
Pul	Grum, C	MI	933
Pul	Guidry, G	LA	938
Pul	Henke, D	NC	931
Pul	Irwin, R	MA	923
Pul	Jacoby, D	OR	940
Pul	Kaye, M	MN	934
Pul	King, T	CA	940
Pul	Lem, V	MO	934
Pul	Levin, D	OK	938
Pul	Libby, D	NY	926
Pul	Mahler, D	NH	923
Pul	Martin, R	CO	937
Pul	Matuschak, G	MO	935
Pul	Metersky, M	CT	923
Pul	Mosenifar, Z	CA	940
Pul	Nash, T	NY	926
Pul	Rizk, N	CA	940
Pul	Schwartz, D	CO	937
Pul	Silver, M	IL	935
Pul	Steinberg, H	NY	928
Pul	Thomashow, B	NY	928
Pul	Vaughey, E	VA	932
Pul	Villanueva, A	MA	924
Pul	Voelkel, N	VA	932
Pul	Wallace, J	CA	941
Pul	Wanner, A	FL	932
Pul	Weissler, J	TX	938
Pul	Wiedemann, H	OH	936

Asthma & Allergy

Spec	Name	St	Pg
A&I	Buchbinder, E	NY	84
A&I	Ein, D	DC	85
A&I	Fishman, H	DC	85
A&I	Gruchalla, R	TX	89
A&I	Kaliner, M	MD	85
A&I	Lockey, R	FL	86
A&I	Meltzer, E	CA	90
A&I	Ostrom, N	CA	90
A&I	Schubert, M	AZ	90
PA&I	Epstein, S	CA	733
PA&I	Fanous, Y	CA	733
PA&I	Skoner, D	PA	730
Pul	Wenzel, S	PA	929

Asthma & Chronic Lung Disease

Spec	Name	St	Pg
PPul	Loughlin, G	NY	795
PPul	Sallent, J	FL	796

Asthma up to age 50

Spec	Name	St	Pg
PA&I	Bock, S	CO	732

Ataxia

N	Gilman, S	MI	526
N	Reich, S	MD	517

Ataxia Telangiectasia

ChiN	Crawford, T	MD	147
PHO	Corey, S	IL	770
PHO	Sandlund, J	TN	768
PPul	Mcgrath-Morrow, S	MD	795

Atopic Dermatitis

D	Belsito, D	NY	184
D	Gottlieb, A	MA	183
D	Hanifin, J	OR	199
D	Paller, A	IL	195
D	Yan, A	PA	189
PA&I	Leung, D	CO	732
PA&I	Sampson, H	NY	729
PA&I	Sly, R	MD	730
PA&I	Spergel, J	PA	730

Atrial Fibrillation

CE	Asirvatham, S	MN	122
CE	Chinitz, L	NY	120
CE	DeLurgio, D	GA	121
CE	Gomes, J	NY	120
CE	Kay, G	AL	122
CE	Lerman, B	NY	120
CE	Levine, J	NY	121
CE	Lewkowiez, L	CO	124
CE	Mehta, D	NY	121
CE	Miller, J	IN	123
CE	Natale, A	TX	124
CE	Onufer, J	VA	122
CE	Prystowsky, E	IN	123
CE	Waldo, A	OH	124
CE	Wang, P	CA	125
CE	Wilber, D	IL	124
Cv	Abi-samra, F	LA	113
Cv	Halperin, J	NY	99
Cv	Tenenbaum, J	NY	102
Cv	Volgman, A	IL	112
Cv	Zusman, R	MA	96
T&CS	Philott, J	VA	1128

Atrial Septal Defect

IC	Chang, G	PA	127
IC	Herrmann, H	PA	127
PCd	Sommer, R	NY	736

Attachment Disorders

ChAP	Zeanah, C	LA	911

Specialty & Special Expertise Index

Spec	Name	St	Pg

Aural Atresia Repair
Oto	Kesser, B	VA	668

Autism
ChAP	Alessi, N	MI	910
ChAP	King, B	WA	912
ChAP	Leckman, J	CT	907
ChAP	Leventhal, B	NY	909
ChAP	Pomeroy, J	NY	909
ChAP	Rostain, A	PA	909
ChiN	Filipek, P	TX	152
ChiN	Kosofsky, B	NY	147
ChiN	Mandelbaum, D	RI	146
ChiN	Nass, R	NY	148
ChiN	Trauner, D	CA	154
NRad	Hunter, J	TX	990
Ped	Burgess, D	NJ	726
Ped	Roizen, N	OH	728
Ped	Walker, W	WA	729
PMR	Keen, M	IL	840
Psyc	Brodkin, E	PA	891
Psyc	Hollander, E	NY	892

Autism & Developmental Disorders
ChAP	McDougle, C	MA	907

Autism in Infants
ChiN	Filipek, P	TX	152

Autoimmune Disease
A&I	Busse, W	WI	88
A&I	Phillips, S	PA	85
D	Anhalt, G	MD	184
D	Werth, V	PA	189
D	Woodley, D	CA	200
Hem	Brodsky, R	MD	312
IM	Burt, R	IL	425
N	Adams, D	FL	519
N	Miller, A	NY	516
Ped	Infante, A	TX	728
Rhu	Gorevic, P	NY	1026
Rhu	Gourley, M	MD	1026
Rhu	Kimberly, R	AL	1030
Rhu	Mease, P	WA	1034
Rhu	Petri, M	MD	1027
Rhu	Sessoms, S	TX	1033
Rhu	Solomon, G	NY	1028
Rhu	Wener, M	WA	1034
Rhu	Wofsy, D	CA	1034

Autoimmune Liver Disease
Ge	Brown, R	NY	231
Ge	Raiford, D	TN	242
Ge	Vierling, J	TX	253

Autoimmune Lung Disease
Pul	Brown, K	CO	936

Spec	Name	St	Pg
Pul	Wenzel, S	PA	929

Autoimmune Rheumatic Disorders
Rhu	McAlindon, T	MA	1024

Autonomic Disorders
CE	Shen, W	AZ	124
Cv	Grubb, B	OH	108
PCd	Hanna, B	PA	735

B

Baha Implant
Oto	Young, N	IL	679

Balance Disorders
Ger	Studenski, S	PA	263
N	Hain, T	IL	526
Oto	Gianoli, G	LA	682
Oto	Hammerschlag, P	NY	660
Oto	Hoffman, R	NY	660
Oto	Kartush, J	MI	676

Barrett's Esophagus
Ge	Chang, K	CA	253
Ge	Cohen, J	NY	231
Ge	Eisen, G	OR	253
Ge	Estores, D	FL	240
Ge	Falk, G	PA	232
Ge	Fang, J	UT	249
Ge	Fleischer, D	AZ	252
Ge	Gerdes, H	NY	232
Ge	Gerson, L	CA	254
Ge	Ginsberg, G	PA	233
Ge	Greenwald, B	MD	233
Ge	Haber, G	NY	233
Ge	Infantolino, A	PA	234
Ge	Katz, P	PA	235
Ge	Lightdale, C	NY	236
Ge	Meiselman, M	IL	247
Ge	Pfau, P	WI	247
Ge	Ravich, W	MD	237
Ge	Reynolds, J	PA	238
Ge	Rothstein, R	NH	230
Ge	Savides, T	CA	255
Ge	Vargo, J	OH	248
Path	Montgomery, E	MD	710
S	Chand, B	IL	1075
S	Pellegrini, C	WA	1098
T&CS	Battafarano, R	MD	1114
T&CS	Ferguson, M	IL	1132

Bartter's Syndrome
Nep	Ellison, D	OR	465

Spec	Name	St	Pg

Beckwith-Wiedemann Syndrome
PlS	Napoli, J	DE	857

Behavioral Disorders
AM	Ginsburg, K	PA	80
ChAP	Boxer, G	MO	910
ChAP	King, B	WA	912
ChAP	Ponton, L	CA	912
Psyc	Reus, V	CA	902

Behavioral Neurology
N	Ahern, G	AZ	532
N	DeKosky, S	VA	520
N	Devinsky, O	NY	511
N	Heilman, K	FL	521
N	Kirshner, H	TN	522
Psyc	Neppe, V	WA	902

Behavioral Problems & Dementia
GerPsy	Grossberg, G	MO	914
GerPsy	Rovner, B	PA	913

Behcet's Syndrome
D	Fivenson, D	MI	193
D	Jorizzo, J	NC	191
Rhu	Spiera, H	NY	1028

Berger's Disease (IgA Nephropathy)
PNep	Wyatt, R	TN	786

Beryllium-induced Lung Disease
OM	Harber, P	AZ	882
Pul	Balmes, J	CA	939
Pul	Rossman, M	PA	927

Biliary Cancer
Onc	O'Reilly, E	NY	346
Onc	Patt, Y	NM	381
Onc	Posey, J	AL	361
Onc	Yen, Y	CA	392
S	Bouvet, M	CA	1093
S	Cameron, J	MD	1054
S	Drebin, J	PA	1056
S	Ellison, E	OH	1076
S	Heslin, M	AL	1069
S	Schulick, R	CO	1086
S	Warren, R	CA	1100
S	Yeo, C	PA	1066

Biliary Disease
Ge	Barnes, D	OH	244
Ge	Cunningham, J	AZ	251
Ge	Edmundowicz, S	MO	245
Ge	Freiman, H	NY	232

Spec	Name	St	Pg
Ge	Kowalski, T	PA	235
Ge	Lind, C	TN	241
Ge	Miskovitz, P	NY	236

Biliary Surgery

Spec	Name	St	Pg
PS	Meyers, R	UT	808
PS	Notrica, D	AZ	809
S	Ellison, E	OH	1076
S	Gower, R	AK	1096
S	Hebert, J	VT	1049
S	Levi, J	FL	1070
S	McAneny, D	MA	1051
S	Postier, R	OK	1091
S	Soper, N	IL	1083
S	Wood, R	TX	1093

Biochemical Genetics

Spec	Name	St	Pg
CG	Charrow, J	IL	160
CG	Craigen, W	TX	161
CG	Northrup, H	TX	162

Bioterrorism Preparedness

Spec	Name	St	Pg
Path	Walker, D	TX	719

Bipolar/Mood Disorders

Spec	Name	St	Pg
ChAP	Birmaher, B	PA	908
ChAP	Hirsch, G	NY	908
ChAP	Slomowitz, M	IL	911
ChAP	Wilens, T	MA	907
Psyc	Benes, F	MA	888
Psyc	Black, D	IA	897
Psyc	Bowden, C	IX	899
Psyc	Calabrese, J	OH	897
Psyc	Davidson, J	TX	899
Psyc	DePaulo, J	MD	891
Psyc	Hirschfeld, R	TX	900
Psyc	Kupfer, D	PA	893
Psyc	Lawson, W	DC	893
Psyc	Levy, S	GA	896
Psyc	McIntosh, J	UT	899
Psyc	Nurnberger, J	IN	898
Psyc	Price, L	RI	889
Psyc	Reus, V	CA	902
Psyc	Roy-Byrne, P	WA	902
Psyc	Salloum, I	FL	896
Psyc	Strakowski, S	OH	898
Psyc	Sussman, N	NY	895
Psyc	Weiner, R	NC	896
Psyc	Weisler, R	NC	896

Birth Defects

Spec	Name	St	Pg
CG	Carey, J	UT	161
CG	Desposito, F	NJ	157
CG	Holmes, L	MA	156
CG	Rosenbaum, K	DC	158
CG	Saul, R	SC	159
CG	Seaver, L	HI	163
CG	Stevenson, R	SC	159
Ped	Bull, M	IN	727

Spec	Name	St	Pg
PNep	Warady, B	MO	788

Birthmarks/Hemangiomas

Spec	Name	St	Pg
D	Alster, T	DC	184
D	Anderson, R	MA	182
D	Cunningham, B	CA	198
D	Orlow, S	NY	188
Oto	Waner, M	NY	666
PlS	Reinisch, J	CA	876
PlS	Zide, B	NY	860

Bladder Cancer

Spec	Name	St	Pg
Onc	Ahmann, F	AZ	376
Onc	Bajorin, D	NY	335
Onc	Dawson, N	DC	338
Onc	Dreicer, R	OH	367
Onc	Gelmann, F	NY	340
Onc	Godley, P	NC	357
Onc	Hussain, M	MI	368
Onc	Jonasch, E	TX	379
Onc	Levine, E	NY	344
Onc	Logothetis, C	TX	380
Onc	Nanus, D	NY	346
Onc	Petrylak, D	CT	331
Onc	Quinn, D	CA	389
Onc	Roth, B	MO	371
Onc	Scher, H	NY	348
Onc	Stadler, W	IL	372
Onc	Tagawa, S	NY	351
Onc	Vaughn, D	PA	351
Path	Amin, M	CA	719
Path	Bostwick, D	VA	713
Path	Cote, R	FL	713
Path	Epstein, J	MD	708
Path	Reuter, V	NY	711
Path	True, L	WA	722
RadRO	Fuss, M	OR	966
RadRO	Rotman, M	NY	952
U	Amling, C	OR	1175
U	Bahnson, R	OH	1165
U	Benson, M	NY	1151
U	Campbell, S	OH	1166
U	Carroll, P	CA	1175
U	Chang, S	TN	1160
U	Chen, D	PA	1151
U	Childs, S	CO	1171
U	Colberg, J	CT	1148
U	Cookson, M	TN	1161
U	Crawford, E	CO	1171
U	Dalkin, B	WA	1175
U	Daneshmand, S	CA	1176
U	Danoff, D	CA	1176
U	Davis, B	KS	1171
U	Droller, M	NY	1152
U	Flanigan, R	IL	1167
U	Greenberg, R	PA	1153
U	Grossman, H	TX	1173
U	Herr, H	NY	1153
U	Hrebinko, R	PA	1154
U	Kaouk, J	OH	1167
U	Kibel, A	MA	1149

Spec	Name	St	Pg
U	Kim, E	TN	1161
U	Kirschenbaum, A	NY	1154
U	Koch, M	IN	1168
U	Lee, C	MI	1168
U	Lerner, S	TX	1173
U	Lin, D	WA	1177
U	Lockhart, J	FL	1162
U	Loughlin, K	MA	1149
U	Malkowicz, S	PA	1155
U	McDougal, W	MA	1149
U	Montie, J	MI	1169
U	O'Donnell, M	IA	1169
U	Olumi, A	MA	1150
U	Penson, D	TN	1163
U	Pisters, L	TX	1174
U	Presti, J	CA	1178
U	Samadi, D	NY	1157
U	Sanda, M	MA	1150
U	Sawczuk, I	NJ	1157
U	Scardino, P	NY	1157
U	Scherr, D	NY	1157
U	Schoenberg, M	MD	1157
U	See, W	WI	1170
U	Smith, J	TN	1164
U	Soloway, M	FL	1164
U	Steinberg, G	IL	1170
U	Su, L	FL	1164
U	Taneja, S	NY	1158
U	Terris, M	GA	1165
U	Uzzo, R	PA	1158
U	Weiss, R	NJ	1159
U	Weiss, R	CT	1150
U	Wood, D	MI	1171
U	Zippe, C	OH	1171

Bladder Exstrophy

Spec	Name	St	Pg
U	Brock, J	TN	1160
U	Kirsch, A	GA	1162
U	Merguerian, P	WA	1178
U	Mesrobian, H	WI	1169

Bladder Reconstruction

Spec	Name	St	Pg
U	Carroll, P	CA	1175
U	Docimo, S	PA	1152
U	Sawczuk, I	NJ	1157

Blastomycosis

Spec	Name	St	Pg
PInf	Kleiman, M	IN	783

Bleeding/Coagulation Disorders

Spec	Name	St	Pg
Hem	Abrams, C	PA	311
Hem	Allen, S	NY	311
Hem	Baron, J	IL	318
Hem	Blinder, M	MO	318
Hem	Bockenstedt, P	MI	319
Hem	Cobos, E	TX	323
Hem	Cooper, B	TX	323
Hem	DeLoughery, T	OR	325

Specialty & Special Expertise Index

Spec	Name	St	Pg
Hem	Diuguid, D	NY	312
Hem	Kempin, S	NY	313
Hem	Kessler, C	DC	313
Hem	Leung, L	CA	326
Hem	Lin, W	TX	324
Hem	Linenberger, M	WA	326
Hem	Lyons, R	TX	324
Hem	Marks, P	CT	310
Hem	Ortel, T	NC	317
Hem	Palascak, J	OH	321
Hem	Rao, A	PA	314
Hem	Rodgers, G	UT	322
Hem	Schiffman, F	RI	311
Hem	Soff, G	NY	315
Hem	Strauss, J	TX	325
Hem	Streiff, M	MD	315
Onc	Attas, L	NJ	334
Onc	Bashevkin, M	NY	335
Onc	Rosove, M	CA	390
Onc	Silver, S	MI	372
Onc	Waintraub, S	NJ	352
Path	Chesney, C	TN	713
PHO	Beyer, E	IL	769
PHO	Bussel, J	NY	758
PHO	Castle, V	MI	770
PHO	Ducore, J	CA	777
PHO	Kobrinsky, N	ND	774
PHO	Kung, F	CA	778
PHO	Luchtman-Jones, L	DC	762
PHO	Marcus, J	NY	762
PHO	Parker, R	NY	763
PHO	Recht, M	OR	779
PHO	Ritchey, A	PA	763
PHO	Salvi, S	IL	773
PHO	Shapiro, A	IN	773
PHO	Thomas, G	OR	779
PHO	Valentino, L	IL	773
PHO	Weinblatt, M	NY	764
S	Wakefield, T	MI	1084

Blistering Diseases

D	Anhalt, G	MD	184
D	Fivenson, D	MI	193
D	Levy, M	TX	197
D	Shupack, J	NY	188
D	Stanley, J	PA	189
D	Werth, V	PA	189
D	Woodley, D	CA	200

Body Contouring

D	Grossman, M	NY	186
PlS	Cederna, P	MI	865
PlS	Evans, G	CA	873
PlS	Fisher, G	CA	873
PlS	Hardesty, R	CA	854
PlS	Hurwitz, D	PA	854
PlS	Mast, B	FL	862
PlS	Mustoe, T	IL	866
PlS	Romano, J	CA	876

Body Contouring after Weight Loss

PlS	Aly, A	CA	872
PlS	Edwards, M	NV	873
PlS	Erdmann, D	NC	861
PlS	Hammond, D	MI	865
PlS	Hunstad, J	NC	862
PlS	Kenkel, J	TX	870
PlS	Rappaport, N	TX	871
PlS	Smith, D	FL	863
PlS	Sood, R	IN	868
PlS	Young, V	MO	868

Body Dysmorphic Disorder (BDD)

Psyc	Bystritsky, A	CA	901
Psyc	Hollander, E	NY	892
Psyc	Phillips, K	RI	889
Psyc	Saxena, S	CA	903

Bone & Joint Pathology

Path	Rosenberg, A	FL	714
Path	Schiller, A	NY	711

Bone & Soft Tissue Pathology

Path	Brooks, J	PA	708
Path	Rubin, B	OH	716

Bone & Soft Tissue Tumors

HS	Athanasian, E	NY	295
OrS	Brien, E	CA	642
OrS	Bukata, S	NY	615
OrS	Cheng, E	MN	633
OrS	Friedlaender, G	CT	611
OrS	Joyce, M	OH	634
OrS	Lee, F	NY	621
OrS	McDonald, D	MO	635
OrS	O'Keefe, R	NY	623
OrS	Parsons, T	MI	636
OrS	Siegel, H	AL	630
OrS	Wurtz, L	IN	638
PHO	Ducore, J	CA	777

Bone Cancer

DR	Panicek, D	NY	976
Hem	Milhem, M	IA	321
OrS	Benevenia, J	NJ	614
OrS	Berrey, B	FL	627
OrS	Biermann, J	MI	632
OrS	Buckwalter, J	IA	633
OrS	Bukata, S	NY	615
OrS	Clohisy, D	MN	633
OrS	Dormans, J	PA	617
OrS	Frassica, F	MD	617
OrS	Gitelis, S	IL	633
OrS	Irwin, R	MI	634
OrS	Kelly, C	CO	639
OrS	Kneisl, J	NC	629

Spec	Name	St	Pg
OrS	Lane, J	NY	621
OrS	Les, K	MI	635
OrS	Mott, M	MI	636
OrS	O'Donnell, R	CA	645
OrS	Ready, J	MA	612
OrS	Sim, F	MN	637
OrS	Singer, D	HI	645
OrS	Wilkins, R	CO	640
PHO	Dome, J	DC	759
PHO	Loeb, D	MD	762
PHO	Schwartz, C	RI	757
PHO	Wexler, L	NY	764
PS	Morgan, W	TN	805
RadRO	Marcus, R	FL	955

Bone Densitometry

NuM	Dillehay, G	IL	550

Bone Disorders-Inherited

CG	Kronn, D	NY	157
CG	Weaver, D	IN	160

Bone Disorders-Metabolic

CG	Kronn, D	NY	157
DR	Dalinka, M	PA	974
DR	Gilsanz, V	CA	983
EDM	Bilezikian, J	NY	209
EDM	Bockman, R	NY	209
EDM	Clutter, W	MO	216
EDM	Dalkin, A	VA	214
EDM	Econs, M	IN	217
EDM	Holick, M	MA	207
EDM	Khosla, S	MN	218
EDM	Kronenberg, H	MA	207
EDM	LeBoff, M	MA	208
EDM	Orwoll, E	OR	223
EDM	Siris, E	NY	212
EDM	Watts, N	OH	219
Ger	Lyles, K	NC	264
Nep	Hruska, K	MO	461
Nep	Ott, S	WA	465
Nep	Stern, L	NY	458
OrS	Einhorn, T	MA	610
OrS	Kaplan, F	PA	620
OrS	Lane, J	NY	621
OrS	O'Keefe, R	NY	623
PEn	DiMeglio, L	IN	746
PEn	Gordon, C	RI	743
PEn	Levine, M	PA	744

Bone Infections

Inf	Nahass, R	NJ	412
Inf	Slama, T	IN	417
OrS	Anglen, J	IN	632
OrS	Browner, B	CT	610
OrS	Ebraheim, N	OH	633
OrS	Swiontkowski, M	MN	638
OrS	Wilkins, R	CO	640

Spec	Name	St	Pg

Bone Marrow & Stem Cell Transplant

Spec	Name	St	Pg
Hem	Yeager, A	AZ	325
Onc	Ball, E	CA	383
Onc	Lazarus, H	OH	369
Onc	Maloney, D	WA	388
Onc	Stadtmauer, E	PA	350
Onc	Waller, E	GA	363
PHO	Leung, W	TN	767
PHO	Matthay, K	CA	778

Bone Marrow Failure Disorders

Spec	Name	St	Pg
Onc	Dang, C	PA	338
Onc	Deeg, H	WA	385
PHO	Boxer, L	MI	769
PHO	Coccia, P	NE	774
PHO	Corey, S	IL	770
PHO	Hord, J	OH	771
PHO	Lipton, J	NY	762
PHO	Lipton, J	NY	762
PHO	Wang, W	TN	769

Bone Marrow Pathology

Spec	Name	St	Pg
Path	Arber, D	CA	719
Path	Foucar, M	NM	717
Path	Kurtin, P	MN	716
Path	Orazi, A	NY	710

Bone Marrow Transplant

Spec	Name	St	Pg
Hem	Adams, R	AZ	323
Hem	Ballen, K	MA	310
Hem	Barlogie, B	AR	323
Hem	Bigelow, C	MS	316
Hem	Brenner, M	TX	323
Hem	Champlin, R	TX	323
Hem	Cobos, E	TX	323
Hem	Copelan, E	OH	319
Hem	Di Persio, J	MO	319
Hem	Farag, S	IN	319
Hem	Filicko-O'Hara, J	PA	312
Hem	Forman, S	CA	325
Hem	Goldberg, J	PA	312
Hem	Gordon, L	IL	319
Hem	Isola, L	NY	313
Hem	Juckett, M	WI	320
Hem	Klingemann, H	MA	310
Hem	Larson, R	IL	320
Hem	Laughlin, M	VA	317
Hem	Linenberger, M	WA	326
Hem	Litzow, M	MN	320
Hem	Luger, S	PA	313
Hem	Mangan, K	PA	313
Hem	Maziarz, R	OR	326
Hem	McGlave, P	MN	321
Hem	Meehan, K	NH	310
Hem	Milhem, M	IA	321
Hem	Miller, K	MA	311
Hem	Munker, R	LA	324
Hem	Negrin, R	CA	326
Hem	Nimer, S	FL	317

Spec	Name	St	Pg
Hem	Porter, D	PA	314
Hem	Rowley, S	NJ	314
Hem	Schuster, M	NY	315
Hem	Schuster, S	PA	315
Hem	Snyder, D	CA	327
Hem	Solberg, L	FL	318
Hem	Spitzer, T	MA	311
Hem	Stiff, P	IL	322
Hem	Strair, R	NJ	315
Hem	Tallman, M	NY	316
Hem	Uberti, J	MI	322
Hem	Winter, J	IL	322
Hem	Yanovich, S	MD	316
Onc	Antin, J	MA	327
Onc	Appelbaum, F	WA	383
Onc	Armitage, J	NE	374
Onc	Bierman, P	NE	374
Onc	Bitran, J	IL	365
Onc	Bolwell, B	OH	365
Onc	Camoriano, J	AZ	378
Onc	Carabasi, M	PA	336
Onc	Chao, N	NC	355
Onc	Claxton, D	PA	336
Onc	Fay, J	TX	378
Onc	Flinn, I	TN	356
Onc	Flomenberg, N	PA	340
Onc	Freedman, A	MA	329
Onc	Hurd, D	NC	357
Onc	Jillella, A	GA	358
Onc	Kalaycio, M	OH	368
Onc	Kaminski, M	MI	369
Onc	Pohlman, B	OH	371
Onc	Press, O	WA	389
Onc	Shea, T	NC	362
Onc	Soiffer, R	MA	332
Onc	Vaughan, W	AL	363
Onc	Wingard, J	FL	364
PA&I	Cowan, M	CA	733
PA&I	Kamani, N	DC	729
PHO	Andrews, R	WA	776
PHO	Arceci, R	MD	758
PHO	Barredo, J	FL	765
PHO	Bertolone, S	KY	765
PHO	Cairo, M	NY	758
PHO	Camitta, B	WI	769
PHO	Carpenter, P	WA	776
PHO	Chen, A	MD	759
PHO	Coccia, P	NE	774
PHO	Cooper, L	TX	775
PHO	Davies, S	OH	770
PHO	Ferrara, J	MI	770
PHO	Garvin, J	NY	760
PHO	Graham, M	AZ	775
PHO	Grupp, S	PA	760
PHO	Guinan, E	MA	756
PHO	Haut, P	IN	771
PHO	Hayashi, R	MO	771
PHO	Horn, B	CA	777
PHO	Kapoor, N	CA	777
PHO	Kurtzberg, J	NC	767
PHO	Kushner, B	NY	761
PHO	Lipton, J	NY	762

Spec	Name	St	Pg
PHO	Loeb, D	MD	762
PHO	O'Reilly, R	NY	763
PHO	Olson, J	OR	778
PHO	Rosenthal, J	CA	779
PHO	Rubin, C	IL	773
PHO	Sakamoto, K	CA	779
PHO	Sandler, E	FL	768
PHO	Weinstein, H	MA	757

Bone Pathology

Path	Antonescu, C	NY	707
Path	Kahn, L	NY	709
Path	Mills, S	VA	713

Bone Tumors

Onc	Benedetto, P	FL	353
Onc	Forscher, C	CA	386
Onc	George, S	MA	329
Onc	Maki, R	NY	345
OrS	Aboulafia, A	MD	613
OrS	Conrad, E	WA	642
OrS	Eckardt, J	CA	643
OrS	Gebhardt, M	MA	611
OrS	Healey, J	NY	619
OrS	Henshaw, R	DC	619
OrS	Hornicek, F	MA	611
OrS	Kelly, C	CO	639
OrS	Kenan, S	NY	621
OrS	Lewis, V	TX	641
OrS	Malawer, M	MD	622
OrS	Mayerson, J	OH	635
OrS	Menendez, L	CA	644
OrS	Peabody, T	IL	636
OrS	Randall, R	UT	639
OrS	Scarborough, M	FL	630
OrS	Schmidt, R	PA	625
OrS	Schwartz, H	TN	630
OrS	Walling, A	FL	631
OrS	Ward, W	NC	631
OrS	Williams, R	TX	641
OrS	Wittig, J	NY	627
Path	Lucas, D	MI	716
Path	Schiller, A	NY	711
PHO	Aledo, A	NY	758
PHO	Harris, M	NJ	761
PHO	Hawkins, D	WA	777
PHO	Meyers, P	NY	762
PHO	Sandler, E	FL	768

Bone Tumors-Benign

OrS	Lee, F	NY	621

Bone Tumors-Metastatic

OrS	Buckwalter, J	IA	633
OrS	Hornicek, F	MA	611
OrS	Lee, F	NY	621
OrS	Schmidt, R	PA	625
OrS	Schwartz, H	TN	630
OrS	Siegel, H	AL	630

Specialty & Special Expertise Index

Spec	Name	St	Pg
RadRO	Meredith, R	AL	956

Bone/Joint Infections

Spec	Name	St	Pg
Inf	Brause, B	NY	411
Inf	Edmond, M	VA	414
Inf	Rao, N	PA	413
Inf	Romagnoli, M	NY	413
Inf	Schmitt, S	OH	417

Botox for Pain

Spec	Name	St	Pg
PM	Argoff, C	NY	696
PM	Ferrante, F	CA	702

Botox Therapy

Spec	Name	St	Pg
ChiN	Goldstein, E	GA	149
D	Avram, M	NY	184
D	Brandt, F	NY	185
D	Glogau, R	CA	199
D	Gordon, M	NY	186
N	Sethi, K	GA	523
N	Singer, C	FL	524
N	Stern, M	PA	518
Oph	Capo, H	FL	582
Oph	Carter, K	IA	589
Oph	McCann, J	UT	596
Oto	Blitzer, A	NY	658
Oto	Branham, G	MO	673
Oto	Sulica, R	NY	666
PM	Freitag, F	TX	701
PMR	Robinson, L	WA	844

Brachial Plexus Palsy

Spec	Name	St	Pg
HS	Bishop, A	MN	300
HS	Grossman, J	FL	299
HS	Hentz, V	CA	304
HS	Peljovich, A	GA	299
HS	Steinmann, S	MN	302
HS	Waters, P	MA	294
NS	Spinner, R	MN	490
PMR	Nelson, M	TX	843

Brachial Plexus Palsy-Pediatric

Spec	Name	St	Pg
HS	Kozin, S	PA	296
NS	Park, T	MO	489
NS	Piatt, J	DE	478

Brachytherapy

Spec	Name	St	Pg
RadRO	Anscher, M	VA	953
RadRO	Beitler, J	GA	953
RadRO	Ciezki, J	OH	959
RadRO	D'Amico, A	MA	946
RadRO	Ennis, R	NY	949
RadRO	Gejerman, G	NJ	950
RadRO	Grado, G	AZ	964
RadRO	Harrison, L	NY	950
RadRO	Henderson, R	FL	954
RadRO	Horwitz, E	PA	950
RadRO	Jhingran, A	TX	964

Spec	Name	St	Pg
RadRO	Kaplan, I	MA	946
RadRO	Koh, W	WA	966
RadRO	Kudrimoti, M	KY	954
RadRO	Lee, W	NC	955
RadRO	Malcolm, A	TN	955
RadRO	Medbery, C	OK	965
RadRO	Nori, D	NY	951
RadRO	Toonkel, L	FL	958
RadRO	Vicini, F	MI	962
RadRO	Vijayakumar, S	MS	958
RadRO	Zelefsky, M	NY	953
U	Kane, M	MD	1154
U	Terris, M	GA	1165

Brachytherapy & Theraspheres

Spec	Name	St	Pg
VIR	Coldwell, D	KY	994

Brain & Spinal Cord Tumors

Spec	Name	St	Pg
NS	Bederson, J	NY	472
NS	Berger, M	CA	495
NS	Brem, H	MD	472
NS	Carson, B	MD	473
NS	Harsh, G	CA	497
NS	Jallo, G	MD	475
NS	Kaufman, B	WI	488
NS	Kobrine, A	DC	476
NS	Laske, D	PA	476
NS	Malik, G	MI	488
NS	Moser, R	MA	471
NS	Naff, N	MD	477
NS	Olivi, A	MD	477
NS	Piepmeier, J	CT	471
NS	Reid, W	TN	484
NS	Robertson, J	TN	484
NS	Thompson, R	TN	485
Onc	Friedman, H	NC	356
PHO	Dunkel, I	NY	759
PHO	Kramer, K	NY	761
PHO	Lange, B	PA	762
RadRO	Kleinberg, L	MD	951
RadRO	Lewin, A	FL	955
RadRO	Marcus, R	FL	955

Brain & Spinal Malformations

Spec	Name	St	Pg
NS	Frim, D	IL	487

Brain & Spinal Surgery

Spec	Name	St	Pg
NS	Theodore, N	AZ	494

Brain & Spinal Tumors

Spec	Name	St	Pg
N	Newton, H	OH	528
NRad	Tenner, M	NY	986
NS	Bilsky, M	NY	472
NS	Caputy, A	DC	473
NS	Chen, C	NY	473
NS	Chen, T	CA	496
NS	Frim, D	IL	487
NS	Lang, F	TX	493
NS	Penar, P	VT	471

Spec	Name	St	Pg
NS	Sills, A	TN	484
NS	Swearingen, B	MA	471
RadRO	Flickinger, J	PA	949
RadRO	Hartford, A	NH	946
RadRO	Regine, W	MD	952
RadRO	Wara, W	CA	968

Brain & Spinal Tumors-Pediatric

Spec	Name	St	Pg
NS	Cohen, A	MA	470

Brain Development Abnormalities

Spec	Name	St	Pg
NRad	Barkovich, A	CA	990
NRad	Barnes, P	CA	990

Brain Imaging

Spec	Name	St	Pg
DR	Mountz, J	PA	976
NRad	Jarvik, J	WA	991
NRad	Osborn, A	UT	990

Brain Imaging-Pediatric

Spec	Name	St	Pg
NRad	Provenzale, J	NC	988

Brain Infections

Spec	Name	St	Pg
NuM	Alavi, A	PA	548
Path	Bollen, A	CA	719
PInf	Bradley, J	CA	784

Brain Injury

Spec	Name	St	Pg
ChAP	Martini, D	UT	911
ChiN	Griesemer, D	MA	146
ChiN	Ichord, R	PA	147
ChiN	Noetzel, M	MO	151
N	Fellus, J	NJ	511
N	Jordan, B	NY	512
N	Kelly, J	CO	531
NP	Davis, J	MA	446
NP	Delivoria-Papadopoulos, M	PA	447
NRad	Burdette, J	NC	987
NS	Adelson, P	AZ	492
NS	Carson, B	MD	473
NS	Wilberger, J	PA	480
PMR	Brown, A	MN	839
PS	Nance, M	PA	804

Brain Injury Rehabilitation

Spec	Name	St	Pg
N	Corbetta, M	MO	525
PMR	Bloch, R	MA	834
PMR	Flanagan, S	NY	836
PMR	Francisco, G	TX	842
PMR	Fried, G	PA	836
PMR	Glenn, M	MA	834
PMR	Ivanhoe, C	TX	843
PMR	Matthews, D	CO	842
PMR	Mayer, N	PA	837
PMR	Mysiw, W	OH	841
PMR	Ragnarsson, K	NY	837

Spec	Name	St	Pg
PMR	Richter, E	CT	834
PMR	Zafonte, R	MA	834

Brain Injury Rehabilitation-Pediatric

Spec	Name	St	Pg
PMR	Massagli, T	WA	844

Brain Injury-Neonatal

Spec	Name	St	Pg
NP	Anday, E	PA	446

Brain Injury-Pediatric

Spec	Name	St	Pg
NRad	Barnes, P	CA	990
NRad	Hunter, J	TX	990
NS	Ragheb, J	FL	483

Brain Injury-Traumatic

Spec	Name	St	Pg
N	Filley, C	CO	531
N	Kelly, J	CO	531
NS	Grady, M	PA	474
NS	Maroon, J	PA	477

Brain Malformations

Spec	Name	St	Pg
N	Kuzniecky, R	NY	513

Brain Mapping

Spec	Name	St	Pg
NRad	Faro, S	PA	985
NS	Silbergeld, D	WA	499

Brain Radiation Toxicity

Spec	Name	St	Pg
N	Rogers, L	OH	529

Brain Tumor Imaging

Spec	Name	St	Pg
NRad	Hesselink, J	CA	991
NRad	Koeller, K	MN	989
NRad	Loevner, L	PA	986
NRad	Murtagh, F	FL	988
NRad	Provenzale, J	NC	988

Brain Tumors

Spec	Name	St	Pg
ChiN	Allen, J	NY	147
ChiN	Cohen, B	OH	150
ChiN	Fisher, P	CA	153
ChiN	Keating, G	MN	150
ChiN	Packer, R	DC	148
ChiN	Phillips, P	PA	148
ChiN	Pomeroy, S	MA	146
DR	Elster, A	NC	979
N	Barger, G	MI	524
N	Batchelor, T	MA	506
N	Chamberlain, M	WA	535
N	Cloughesy, T	CA	536
N	DeAngelis, L	NY	510
N	Gilbert, M	TX	533
N	Glass, J	PA	512
N	Kunschner, L	PA	513
N	Laterra, J	MD	514

Spec	Name	St	Pg
N	Mikkelsen, T	MI	528
N	Moots, P	TN	522
N	Nabors, L	AL	523
N	Patchell, R	AZ	534
N	Posner, J	NY	516
N	Rogers, L	OH	529
N	Rosenfeld, S	OH	529
N	Schiff, D	VA	523
N	Taylor, L	MA	508
N	Vick, N	IL	530
N	Wen, P	MA	508
N	Yung, W	TX	535
NRad	Atlas, S	CA	990
NRad	Cha, S	CA	991
NRad	Dillon, W	CA	991
NRad	Faro, S	PA	985
NRad	Johnson, A	NC	987
NRad	Lis, E	NY	986
NRad	Maldjian, J	NC	987
NRad	Sze, G	CT	985
NRad	Vezina, L	DC	986
NS	Al-Mefty, O	MA	470
NS	Andrews, D	PA	472
NS	Apuzzo, M	CA	495
NS	Asher, A	NC	481
NS	Badie, B	CA	495
NS	Barnett, G	OH	486
NS	Black, K	CA	495
NS	Boop, F	TN	481
NS	Brem, S	PA	472
NS	Bruce, J	NY	473
NS	Chandler, J	IL	486
NS	Chandler, W	MI	487
NS	Cherny, W	ID	491
NS	Chiocca, E	OH	487
NS	Cosgrove, R	RI	470
NS	Dacey, R	MO	487
NS	Danielpour, M	CA	496
NS	David, C	MA	470
NS	Duhaime, A	MA	470
NS	Ellenbogen, R	WA	496
NS	Evans, J	PA	473
NS	Ewend, M	NC	481
NS	Fenstermaker, R	NY	474
NS	Friedman, A	NC	481
NS	Golfinos, J	NY	474
NS	Goumnerova, L	MA	470
NS	Greene, C	LA	492
NS	Grubb, R	MO	487
NS	Guthrie, B	AL	482
NS	Gutin, P	NY	474
NS	Hankinson, H	NM	492
NS	Heros, R	FL	482
NS	Hodes, J	KY	482
NS	Huang, J	MD	475
NS	Judy, K	PA	475
NS	Kim, D	TX	493
NS	Liau, L	CA	497
NS	Link, M	MN	488
NS	Linskey, M	CA	497
NS	Luken, M	IL	488
NS	Lunsford, L	PA	476

Spec	Name	St	Pg
NS	Mamelak, A	CA	498
NS	Markert, J	AL	483
NS	Martuza, R	MA	471
NS	McDermott, M	CA	498
NS	Meyer, F	MN	489
NS	Mickey, B	TX	494
NS	Moore, F	NJ	477
NS	Morcos, J	FL	483
NS	Myseros, J	VA	483
NS	Neuwelt, E	OR	498
NS	O'Rourke, D	PA	477
NS	Ojemann, J	WA	498
NS	Olson, J	GA	483
NS	Origitano, T	MT	491
NS	Ott, K	CA	498
NS	Patel, S	SC	483
NS	Pollack, I	PA	478
NS	Quigley, M	PA	478
NS	Raffel, C	OH	489
NS	Rich, K	MO	489
NS	Rigamonti, D	MD	478
NS	Rock, J	MI	489
NS	Rosenblum, M	MI	489
NS	Ruge, J	IL	490
NS	Ryken, T	IA	490
NS	Sampson, J	NC	484
NS	Sawaya, R	TX	494
NS	Schwartz, T	NY	478
NS	Sekhar, L	WA	498
NS	Sen, C	NY	478
NS	Shaffrey, M	VA	484
NS	Shapiro, S	IN	490
NS	Silbergeld, D	WA	499
NS	Sisti, M	NY	479
NS	Spencer, D	CT	471
NS	Spinner, R	MN	490
NS	Stieg, P	NY	479
NS	Sun, P	CA	499
NS	Sundaresan, N	NY	479
NS	Swaid, S	AL	484
NS	Tatter, S	NC	485
NS	Turtz, A	NJ	479
NS	Walker, M	UT	492
NS	Warnick, R	OH	491
NS	Weingart, J	MD	480
NS	Wharen, R	FL	485
NS	Yu, J	CA	499
NuM	Alavi, A	PA	548
Onc	Buckner, J	MN	365
Onc	Chang, S	CA	384
Onc	Fine, H	MD	339
Onc	Grossman, S	MD	341
Onc	Lacy, J	CT	331
Onc	Lesser, G	NC	358
Onc	McClay, E	CA	388
Onc	Peereboom, D	OH	370
Onc	Prados, M	CA	389
Onc	Von Burton, G	LA	382
Onc	Vredenburgh, J	NC	363
Onc	Ward, J	UT	376
Path	Bollen, A	CA	719
Path	Bruner, J	TX	717

Specialty & Special Expertise Index

Spec	Name	St	Pg
Path	Burger, P	MD	708
Path	De Masters, B	CO	717
Path	Jones, R	DC	709
Path	Mischel, P	CA	721
Path	Perry, A	CA	721
Path	Rosenblum, M	NY	711
Path	Zagzag, D	NY	712
PHO	Arndt, C	MN	769
PHO	Banerjee, A	CA	776
PHO	Berg, S	TX	775
PHO	Blaney, S	TX	775
PHO	Brecher, M	NY	758
PHO	Bruggers, C	UT	774
PHO	Cohen, K	MD	759
PHO	Ducore, J	CA	777
PHO	Dunkel, I	NY	759
PHO	Finlay, J	CA	777
PHO	Gajjar, A	TN	766
PHO	Garvin, J	NY	760
PHO	Geyer, J	WA	777
PHO	Gold, S	NC	766
PHO	Goldman, S	IL	771
PHO	Gururangan, S	NC	766
PHO	Halpern, S	NJ	760
PHO	Hetherington, M	MO	771
PHO	Hilden, J	CO	774
PHO	Horn, B	CA	777
PHO	Kieran, M	MA	757
PHO	Korones, D	NY	761
PHO	Kuttesch, J	PA	762
PHO	Manera, R	IL	772
PHO	Neuberg, R	SC	767
PHO	Nicholson, H	OR	778
PHO	Olshefski, R	OH	772
PHO	Plautz, G	OH	772
PHO	Puccetti, D	WI	772
PHO	Rood, B	DC	763
PHO	Rubin, C	IL	773
PHO	Russo, C	AL	768
PHO	van Hoff, J	NH	757
PHO	Wolff, J	MA	757
PMR	Stewart, P	AL	839
RadRO	Awan, A	IL	958
RadRO	Chakravarti, A	OH	959
RadRO	Cmelak, A	TN	954
RadRO	Crocker, I	GA	954
RadRO	Donahue, B	NY	949
RadRO	Fiveash, J	AL	954
RadRO	Goodman, R	NJ	950
RadRO	Hayman, J	MI	960
RadRO	Herman, T	OK	964
RadRO	Isaacson, S	NY	950
RadRO	Knisely, J	NY	951
RadRO	Kun, L	TN	954
RadRO	Larner, J	VA	955
RadRO	Larson, D	CA	967
RadRO	Movsas, B	MI	961
RadRO	Sandler, H	CA	968
RadRO	Schomberg, P	MN	962
RadRO	Seung, S	OR	968
RadRO	Shaw, E	NC	957
RadRO	St Clair, W	KY	957

Spec	Name	St	Pg
RadRO	Stea, B	AZ	965
RadRO	Werner-Wasik, M	PA	953

Brain Tumors & Hemifacial Spasms

NS	Harper, R	TX	493

Brain Tumors-Adult & Pediatric

NS	Kondziolka, D	PA	476
NS	Mapstone, T	OK	494
RadRO	Shrieve, D	UT	963
RadRO	Suh, J	OH	962
RadRO	Woo, S	KY	958

Brain Tumors-Benign

NS	Wilberger, J	PA	480
RadRO	Loeffler, J	MA	947

Brain Tumors-Complex

NS	Lang, F	TX	493

Brain Tumors-Metastatic

N	Phuphanich, S	CA	538
NS	Chen, T	CA	496
NS	Kondziolka, D	PA	476
NS	Laske, D	PA	476
NS	Olivi, A	MD	477
NS	Silbergeld, D	WA	499
Onc	Vredenburgh, J	NC	363
RadRO	Kleinberg, L	MD	951

Brain Tumors-Pediatric

N	Janss, A	GA	522
NS	Edwards, M	CA	496
NS	Feldstein, N	NY	474
NS	Sandberg, D	TX	494
NS	Selden, N	OR	499
NS	Souweidane, M	NY	479
NS	Sutton, L	PA	479
NS	Tomita, T	IL	490
NS	Wisoff, J	NY	480
RadRO	Merchant, T	TN	956
RadRO	Tarbell, N	MA	947

Brain Tumors-Recurrent

PHO	Kuttesch, J	PA	762

Brain/Spinal Cord Injury

PMR	Leslie, D	GA	839

Breast Augmentation

PlS	Aly, A	CA	872
PlS	Meltzer, T	AZ	871
PlS	Stadelmann, W	NH	851
PlS	Young, V	MO	868

Breast Cancer

Spec	Name	St	Pg
CG	Weitzel, J	CA	164
DR	Abbitt, P	FL	978
DR	Brem, R	DC	974
DR	Conant, E	PA	974
DR	Dershaw, D	NY	974
DR	Edelstein, B	NY	975
DR	Evers, K	PA	975
DR	Feig, S	CA	983
DR	Freimanis, R	NC	979
DR	Helvie, M	MI	980
DR	Hricak, H	NY	975
DR	Huynh, P	TX	982
DR	Lehman, C	WA	983
DR	Logan-Young, W	NY	976
DR	Mitnick, J	NY	976
DR	Monsees, B	MO	981
DR	Otto, P	TX	982
DR	Parikh, J	WA	983
DR	Roth, S	PA	977
DR	Stough, R	OK	982
DR	Ulissey, M	TX	982
DR	Weinreb, J	CT	973
GO	Braly, P	LA	287
GO	Chambers, S	AZ	287
GO	Fiorica, J	FL	281
GO	Kelley, J	PA	278
GO	Runowicz, C	FL	282
Hem	Flynn, P	MN	319
Hem	Schwartzberg, L	TN	317
Hem	Wisch, N	NY	316
NuM	Podoloff, D	TX	550
ObG	Goldman, M	CA	563
Onc	Abraham, J	WV	333
Onc	Albain, K	IL	364
Onc	Arteaga, C	TN	353
Onc	Arun, B	TX	377
Onc	Astrow, A	NY	334
Onc	Attas, L	NJ	334
Onc	Balducci, L	FL	353
Onc	Biggs, D	DE	335
Onc	Bitran, J	IL	365
Onc	Blackwell, K	NC	354
Onc	Brenin, C	VA	354
Onc	Brescia, F	SC	354
Onc	Brufsky, A	PA	335
Onc	Budd, G	OH	365
Onc	Burris, H	TN	354
Onc	Burstein, H	MA	328
Onc	Butler, W	SC	354
Onc	Buys, S	UT	374
Onc	Buzdar, A	TX	377
Onc	Camoriano, J	AZ	378
Onc	Carey, L	NC	355
Onc	Carlson, R	CA	384
Onc	Carpenter, J	AL	355
Onc	Celano, P	MD	336
Onc	Chabner, B	MA	328
Onc	Chang, J	TX	378
Onc	Chap, L	CA	384
Onc	Chew, H	CA	384

Specialty & Special Expertise Index

Spec	Name	St	Pg	Spec	Name	St	Pg	Spec	Name	St	Pg
Onc	Chitambar, C	WI	366	Onc	Morginstin, M	PA	345	Path	Chen, Y	CA	720
Onc	Chlebowski, R	CA	384	Onc	Mortimer, J	CA	388	Path	Connolly, J	MA	706
Onc	Cobleigh, M	IL	366	Onc	Muss, H	NC	360	Path	Cote, R	FL	713
Onc	Cohen, P	DC	337	Onc	Nabell, L	AL	360	Path	Hoda, S	NY	709
Onc	Cohen, S	NY	337	Onc	Nissenblatt, M	NJ	346	Path	Ljung, B	CA	721
Onc	Colon-Otero, G	FL	355	Onc	Northfelt, D	AZ	380	Path	Masood, S	FL	713
Onc	Come, S	MA	328	Onc	Norton, L	NY	346	Path	Mies, C	PA	710
Onc	Cowan, K	NE	375	Onc	O'Regan, R	GA	360	Path	Morrow, J	CT	707
Onc	Cristofanilli, M	PA	337	Onc	O'Shaughnessy, J	TX	380	Path	Patchefsky, A	PA	711
Onc	Daly, M	PA	337	Onc	Offit, K	NY	346	Path	Ross, J	NY	711
Onc	Dickler, M	NY	338	Onc	Olopade, O	IL	370	Path	Sahin, A	TX	718
Onc	Disis, M	WA	385	Onc	Oratz, R	NY	347	Path	Sanchez, M	NJ	711
Onc	Dizon, D	MA	328	Onc	Osborne, C	TX	381	Path	Schnitt, S	MA	707
Onc	Domchek, S	PA	338	Onc	Oster, M	NY	347	Path	Thor, A	CO	717
Onc	Doroshow, J	MD	338	Onc	Parker, B	CA	389	Path	Tornos, C	NY	712
Onc	Dutcher, J	NY	338	Onc	Pasmantier, M	NY	347	Path	Wilczynski, S	CA	722
Onc	Elias, A	CO	375	Onc	Pegram, M	CA	389	PlS	Collins, D	NH	850
Onc	Ellis, G	WA	385	Onc	Perez, E	FL	361	RadRO	Awan, A	IL	958
Onc	Ellis, M	MO	367	Onc	Raptis, G	NY	348	RadRO	Beitler, J	GA	953
Onc	Emens, L	MD	339	Onc	Robert, N	VA	361	RadRO	Buchholz, T	TX	963
Onc	Erban, J	MA	328	Onc	Romond, E	KY	361	RadRO	Chakravarthy, A	TN	954
Onc	Fabian, C	KS	375	Onc	Rosen, S	IL	371	RadRO	Donaldson, S	CA	965
Onc	Fitch, T	AZ	378	Onc	Rugo, H	CA	390	RadRO	Dritschilo, A	DC	949
Onc	Fox, K	PA	340	Onc	Russell, C	CA	390	RadRO	Ennis, R	NY	949
Onc	Fracasso, P	VA	356	Onc	Schnipper, L	MA	332	RadRO	Formenti, S	NY	949
Onc	Ganz, P	CA	386	Onc	Schuchter, L	PA	349	RadRO	Fowble, B	CA	966
Onc	Garber, J	MA	329	Onc	Schwartz, B	MN	372	RadRO	Freedman, G	PA	949
Onc	Gaynor, E	IL	367	Onc	Schwartz, M	FL	362	RadRO	Gaffney, D	UT	962
Onc	Geyer, C	TX	378	Onc	Shapiro, C	OH	372	RadRO	Goodman, R	NJ	950
Onc	Glaspy, J	CA	386	Onc	Shulman, L	MA	332	RadRO	Haffty, B	NJ	950
Onc	Glick, J	PA	340	Onc	Silverman, P	OH	372	RadRO	Halberg, F	CA	966
Onc	Goldstein, L	PA	340	Onc	Sledge, G	IN	372	RadRO	Halpern, H	IL	959
Onc	Gradishar, W	IL	368	Onc	Smith, T	MD	349	RadRO	Halyard, M	AZ	964
Onc	Graham, M	NC	357	Onc	Speyer, J	NY	349	RadRO	Hancock, S	CA	966
Onc	Gralow, J	WA	387	Onc	Stockdale, F	CA	391	RadRO	Harris, J	MA	946
Onc	Grana, G	NJ	341	Onc	Stone, J	FL	362	RadRO	Hayman, J	MI	960
Onc	Grossbard, M	NY	341	Onc	Stopeck, A	AZ	382	RadRO	Heimann, R	VT	946
Onc	Haley, B	TX	378	Onc	Strauss, G	MA	332	RadRO	Herman, T	OK	964
Onc	Hayes, D	MI	368	Onc	Strenger, R	RI	332	RadRO	Kachnic, L	MA	946
Onc	Hoffman, P	IL	368	Onc	Sutton, L	NC	363	RadRO	Kuske, R	AZ	964
Onc	Holland, J	NY	342	Onc	Swain, S	DC	350	RadRO	Lee, C	MN	960
Onc	Hollister, D	CT	330	Onc	Thigpen, J	MS	363	RadRO	Lewin, A	FL	955
Onc	Hortobagyi, G	TX	379	Onc	Tkaczuk, K	MD	351	RadRO	Macklis, R	OH	961
Onc	Hudis, C	NY	342	Onc	Toppmeyer, D	NJ	351	RadRO	Malcolm, A	TN	955
Onc	Hutchins, L	AR	379	Onc	Tripathy, D	CA	391	RadRO	Marks, L	NC	955
Onc	Ingle, J	MN	368	Onc	Urba, W	OR	392	RadRO	McCormick, B	NY	951
Onc	Isaacs, C	DC	343	Onc	Vahdat, L	NY	351	RadRO	Medbery, C	OK	965
Onc	Jahanzeb, M	FL	357	Onc	Valero, V	TX	382	RadRO	Mendenhall, N	FL	956
Onc	Kaufman, P	NH	330	Onc	Vinciguerra, V	NY	351	RadRO	Meredith, R	AL	956
Onc	Legare, R	RI	331	Onc	Von Burton, G	LA	382	RadRO	Morris, M	VA	956
Onc	Leighton, J	PA	344	Onc	Von Hoff, D	AZ	382	RadRO	Myerson, R	MO	961
Onc	Levine, E	NY	344	Onc	Von Roenn, J	IL	373	RadRO	Nicolaou, N	PA	951
Onc	Limentani, S	NC	359	Onc	Waintraub, S	NJ	352	RadRO	Nori, D	NY	951
Onc	Lippman, M	FL	359	Onc	Ward, J	UT	376	RadRO	Park, C	CA	967
Onc	Livingston, R	AZ	380	Onc	Weisberg, T	ME	333	RadRO	Pezner, R	CA	967
Onc	Loprinzi, C	MN	369	Onc	Wicha, M	MI	373	RadRO	Pierce, L	MI	961
Onc	Lyman, G	NC	359	Onc	Wierman, A	NV	392	RadRO	Porrazzo, M	DC	952
Onc	Makhoul, I	AR	380	Onc	Winer, E	MA	333	RadRO	Prosnitz, L	NC	956
Onc	Marcom, P	NC	359	Onc	Wolff, A	• MD	352	RadRO	Quivey, J	CA	967
Onc	Matulonis, U	MA	331	Onc	Yee, D	MN	374	RadRO	Rabinovitch, R	CO	963
Onc	Mintzer, D	PA	345	Path	Allred, D	MO	714	RadRO	Randolph-Jackson, P	DC	952
Onc	Moore, A	NY	345	Path	Bleiweiss, I	NY	708	RadRO	Recht, A	MA	947

Spec	Name	St	Pg
RadRO	Rose, C	CA	967
RadRO	Rosenman, J	NC	957
RadRO	Sailer, S	NC	957
RadRO	Shina, D	NM	965
RadRO	Small, W	IL	962
RadRO	Solin, L	PA	952
RadRO	Taghian, A	MA	947
RadRO	Toonkel, L	FL	958
RadRO	Vicini, F	MI	962
RadRO	Wazer, D	RI	947
RadRO	Weiss, M	PA	953
RadRO	Werner-Wasik, M	PA	953
RadRO	Wilson, J	WI	962
S	Alfonso, A	NY	1053
S	Ames, F	TX	1086
S	Axelrod, D	NY	1053
S	Babiera, G	TX	1087
S	Bear, H	VA	1067
S	Beauchamp, R	TN	1067
S	Beitsch, P	TX	1087
S	Bland, K	AL	1067
S	Boraas, M	PA	1054
S	Borgen, P	NY	1054
S	Brooks, A	PA	1054
S	Butler, J	CA	1094
S	Calvo, B	NC	1067
S	Chang, A	MI	1075
S	Chang, H	CA	1094
S	Cole, D	SC	1068
S	Crowe, J	OH	1075
S	Donohue, J	MN	1076
S	Dooley, W	OK	1087
S	Easter, D	CA	1095
S	Eberlein, T	MO	1076
S	Edge, S	NY	1056
S	Edney, J	NE	1085
S	Edwards, M	OH	1076
S	Eisenberg, B	NH	1049
S	Ellenhorn, J	CA	1095
S	Esserman, L	CA	1095
S	Estabrook, A	NY	1057
S	Euhus, D	TX	1088
S	Farrar, W	OH	1076
S	Feig, B	TX	1088
S	Finlayson, C	CO	1085
S	Frazier, T	PA	1057
S	Gabram, S	GA	1068
S	Giuliano, A	CA	1096
S	Goodson, W	CA	1096
S	Goulet, R	IN	1077
S	Grant, C	MN	1077
S	Grant, M	TX	1088
S	Gray, R	AZ	1088
S	Hanks, J	VA	1069
S	Herrmann, V	SC	1069
S	Hollingsworth, A	OK	1089
S	Hughes, K	MA	1050
S	Hunt, K	TX	1089
S	Iglehart, J	MA	1050
S	Johnson, R	PA	1059
S	Johnson Miller, D	IN	1078
S	Kavanah, M	MA	1050

Spec	Name	St	Pg
S	Kelley, M	TN	1069
S	Kim, J	OH	1078
S	Klimberg, V	AR	1090
S	Knudson, M	CA	1097
S	Krag, D	VT	1050
S	Krontiras, H	AL	1069
S	Lannin, D	CT	1050
S	Levine, E	NC	1070
S	Li, B	LA	1090
S	Mamounas, E	OH	1079
S	McGrath, P	KY	1070
S	McMasters, K	KY	1070
S	Morrow, M	NY	1060
S	Nathanson, S	MI	1080
S	Nelson, E	UT	1086
S	Newman, L	MI	1080
S	Nowak, E	NY	1061
S	O'Hea, B	NY	1061
S	Olson, J	MD	1061
S	Paz, I	CA	1098
S	Peterson, L	HI	1098
S	Pockaj, B	AZ	1091
S	Ponn, T	NH	1051
S	Roses, D	NY	1063
S	Ross, M	TX	1092
S	Sataloff, D	PA	1063
S	Sauter, E	ND	1086
S	Schnabel, F	NY	1063
S	Scott-Conner, C	IA	1082
S	Sener, S	CA	1099
S	Shapiro, R	NY	1064
S	Shenk, R	OH	1082
S	Sigurdson, E	PA	1064
S	Silverstein, M	CA	1100
S	Skinner, K	NY	1064
S	Smith, B	MA	1052
S	Stahl, D	OH	1083
S	Staren, E	AZ	1092
S	Stolier, A	LA	1092
S	Tafra, L	MD	1065
S	Tartter, P	NY	1065
S	Tchou, J	PA	1065
S	Tuttle, T	MN	1083
S	Urist, M	AL	1073
S	Van Zee, K	NY	1065
S	Walker, A	WI	1084
S	Wallace, A	CA	1100
S	Wapnir, I	CA	1100
S	Ward, B	CT	1052
S	Weigel, R	IA	1084
S	White, R	NC	1073
S	Whitworth, P	TN	1073
S	Willey, S	DC	1066
S	Winchester, D	IL	1084
S	Witt, I	IL	1084
S	Yeung, R	WA	1101
S	Zannis, V	AZ	1093

Breast Cancer & Surgery

Spec	Name	St	Pg
PlS	Fox, J	PA	854
S	Anderson, B	WA	1093

Spec	Name	St	Pg
S	Borgen, P	NY	1054
S	Brown, E	MI	1075
S	Byrd, D	WA	1094
S	Czerniecki, B	PA	1056
S	Graham, R	MA	1049
S	Julian, T	PA	1059
S	Karlan, S	CA	1096
S	Kaufman, C	WA	1097
S	Kirgan, D	NV	1097
S	Leeming, R	OH	1079
S	Leitch, A	TX	1090
S	Meric-Bernstam, F	TX	1091
S	Osborne, M	NY	1061
S	Simmons, R	NY	1064
S	Swistel, A	NY	1065
S	Thayer, S	MA	1052

Breast Cancer and Pregancy

Spec	Name	St	Pg
Onc	Livingston, R	AZ	380

Breast Cancer Genetics

Spec	Name	St	Pg
Onc	Buys, S	UT	374
Onc	Domchek, S	PA	338
Onc	Garber, J	MA	329
Onc	Graham, M	NC	357
Onc	Olopade, O	IL	370
S	Herrmann, V	SC	1069

Breast Cancer in Elderly

Spec	Name	St	Pg
S	Tartter, P	NY	1065

Breast Cancer Risk Assessment

Spec	Name	St	Pg
CG	Plon, S	TX	162
GO	Cain, J	MA	274
Onc	Buys, S	UT	374
Onc	Daly, M	PA	337
Onc	Domchek, S	PA	338
Onc	Fabian, C	KS	375
Onc	Isaacs, C	DC	343
Onc	Legare, R	RI	331
Onc	O'Regan, R	GA	360
Onc	Perez, E	FL	361
Onc	Stopeck, A	AZ	382
Path	Allred, D	MO	714
S	Hansen, N	IL	1077
S	Nathanson, S	MI	1080
S	Sauter, E	ND	1086
S	Tchou, J	PA	1065

Breast Cancer Vaccine Therapy

Spec	Name	St	Pg
Onc	Serody, J	NC	362

Breast Cancer-Early Detection

Spec	Name	St	Pg
RadRO	Berg, C	MD	948

Breast Cancer-High Risk Women

Spec	Name	St	Pg
RadRO	Berg, C	MD	948

Spec	Name	St	Pg
S	Estabrook, A	NY	1057
S	Gabram, S	GA	1068
S	Hansen, N	IL	1077
S	Hughes, K	MA	1050
S	Johnson Miller, D	IN	1078
S	Schnabel, F	NY	1063
S	Smith, B	MA	1052

Breast Cancer-Inflammatory

Onc	Cristofanilli, M	PA	337

Breast Cancer-Male

Onc	Hortobagyi, G	TX	379

Breast Cancer-Novel Therapies

Onc	Fleming, G	IL	367
Onc	Goldstein, L	PA	340
Onc	Pegram, M	CA	389
Onc	Rugo, H	CA	390
Onc	Vahdat, L	NY	351

Breast Cosmetic & Reconstructive Surgery

PlS	Ascherman, J	NY	852
PlS	Edwards, M	NV	873
PlS	Fox, J	PA	854
PlS	Hurwitz, D	PA	854
PlS	Koplin, L	CA	875
PlS	Leighton, W	AZ	871
PlS	Mast, B	FL	862
PlS	Noone, R	PA	857
PlS	Rappaport, N	TX	871
PlS	Sood, R	IN	868

Breast Disease

S	Axelrod, D	NY	1053
S	Boraas, M	PA	1054
S	Estabrook, A	NY	1057
S	Finlayson, C	CO	1085
S	Frazier, T	PA	1057
S	Gabram, S	GA	1068
S	Johnson, R	PA	1059
S	Kaufman, C	WA	1097
S	Leeming, R	OH	1079
S	Osborne, M	NY	1061
S	Sataloff, D	PA	1063
S	Tchou, J	PA	1065
S	Ward, B	CT	1052
S	Witt, T	IL	1084

Breast Imaging

DR	Abbitt, P	FL	978
DR	Bassett, L	CA	982
DR	Brem, R	DC	974
DR	Cardenosa, G	VA	978
DR	Conant, E	PA	974
DR	Dershaw, D	NY	974
DR	Feig, S	CA	983

DR	Freimanis, R	NC	979
DR	Helvie, M	MI	980
DR	Hricak, H	NY	975
DR	Jackson, V	IN	980
DR	Lehman, C	WA	983
DR	Otto, P	TX	982
DR	Parikh, J	WA	983
DR	Roth, S	PA	977
DR	Ulissey, M	TX	982

Breast Pathology

Path	Allred, D	MO	714
Path	Bleiweiss, I	NY	708
Path	Chen, Y	CA	720
Path	Connolly, J	MA	706
Path	Dahmoush, L	IA	715
Path	De Las Morenas, A	MA	706
Path	Ehya, H	PA	708
Path	Lage, J	SC	713
Path	Masood, S	FL	713
Path	Mies, C	PA	710
Path	Mills, S	VA	713
Path	Schnitt, S	MA	707
Path	Sewell, C	GA	714
Path	Sibley, R	CA	722

Breast Reconstruction

PlS	Allen, R	SC	860
PlS	Andersen, J	CA	873
PlS	Brandt, K	MO	865
PlS	Bucky, L	PA	853
PlS	Butler, C	TX	870
PlS	Coleman, J	IN	865
PlS	Colen, L	VA	861
PlS	Collins, D	NH	850
PlS	Cordeiro, P	NY	853
PlS	Da Lio, A	CA	873
PlS	Disa, J	NY	853
PlS	Fix, R	AL	861
PlS	Georgiade, G	NC	861
PlS	Grotting, J	AL	861
PlS	Hammond, D	MI	865
PlS	Hansen, J	OR	874
PlS	Hoffman, L	NY	854
PlS	Hultman, C	NC	862
PlS	Isik, F	WA	874
PlS	Jewell, M	OR	875
PlS	Leipziger, L	NY	855
PlS	Levine, J	NY	855
PlS	Loree, T	NY	855
PlS	Maxwell, G	TN	863
PlS	Mehrara, B	NY	856
PlS	Miller, M	OH	866
PlS	Olding, M	DC	857
PlS	Robb, G	TX	871
PlS	Rockwell, W	UT	869
PlS	Schusterman, M	TX	872
PlS	Serletti, J	PA	858
PlS	Sherman, R	CA	876
PlS	Slavin, S	MA	851
PlS	Slezak, S	MD	858

PlS	Smith, D	FL	863
PlS	Smith, P	FL	863
PlS	Stadelmann, W	NH	851
PlS	Stahl, R	CT	851
PlS	Sultan, M	NY	859
PlS	Ting, J	NY	859
PlS	Topham, N	PA	859
PlS	Vasconez, H	KY	864
PlS	Walton, R	IL	868
PlS	Wilkins, E	MI	868
PlS	Yetman, R	OH	868
PlS	Yuen, J	AR	872
S	Edington, H	PA	1057
S	Osborne, M	NY	1061
S	Patel, S	PA	1061
S	Wallace, A	CA	1100

Breast Reconstruction & Augmentation

PlS	Beasley, M	NC	860
PlS	Nahabedian, M	DC	856
PlS	Neumeister, M	IL	867

Breast Surgery

PlS	Carraway, J	VA	860
PlS	Constantian, M	NH	850
PlS	Gallico, G	MA	850
PlS	Puckett, C	MO	867
PlS	Wells, J	CA	877
S	Goulet, R	IN	1077
S	Gower, R	AK	1096
S	Grant, M	TX	1088
S	Herrmann, V	SC	1069
S	Lannin, D	CT	1050
S	Peterson, L	HI	1098
S	Stahl, D	OH	1083
S	Wapnir, I	CA	1100
S	Ward, B	CT	1052
S	Zannis, V	AZ	1093

Breathing Disorders

NP	Delivoria-Papadopoulos, M	PA	447
NP	Donn, S	MI	450
NP	Gewolb, I	MI	450
NP	Gross, I	CT	446
NP	Hendricks-Munoz, K	VA	449
NP	Lawson, E	MD	447
NP	Martin, R	OH	450
PPul	Green, T	IL	796
PPul	Keens, T	CA	798
PPul	Kemp, J	MO	796
PPul	Loughlin, G	NY	795
Pul	Mahler, D	NH	923

Bronchiectasis

Pul	Fanta, C	MA	922
Pul	Metersky, M	CT	923
Pul	O'Donnell, A	DC	927

Specialty & Special Expertise Index

Spec	Name	St	Pg
Pul	Tino, G	PA	928
Pul	Wenzel, S	PA	929

Bronchiolitis Obliterans

Pul	Stover-Pepe, D	NY	928

Bronchopulmonary Dysplasia

PPul	Mcgrath-Morrow, S	MD	795
PPul	Nielson, D	CA	798

Bronchoscopy

Pul	Maxfield, R	NY	926
Pul	Prakash, U	MN	935

Burn Care

PlS	Gottlieb, L	IL	865
PlS	Spence, R	MD	858
PMR	Sisung, C	IL	841
PS	Fallat, M	KY	805
PS	Foglia, R	TX	809
S	Bessey, P	NY	1053
S	Cairns, B	NC	1067
S	Deitch, E	NJ	1056
S	Demarest, G	NM	1087
S	Gamelli, R	IL	1077
S	Greenhalgh, D	CA	1096
S	Griswold, J	TX	1088
S	Haith, L	PA	1058
S	Hunt, J	TX	1089
S	Kagan, R	OH	1078
S	Lentz, C	NM	1090
S	Luterman, A	AL	1070
S	Meyer, A	NC	1070
S	Potenza, B	CA	1098
S	Ryan, C	MA	1051
S	Saffle, J	UT	1086
S	Winchell, R	ME	1052
S	Yurt, R	NY	1066

Burns-Reconstructive Plastic Surgery

PlS	Cederna, P	MI	865
PlS	Cruse, C	FL	861
PlS	Feldman, J	MA	850
PlS	Garner, W	CA	874
PlS	Glat, P	PA	854
PlS	Hultman, C	NC	862
PlS	Lee, R	IL	866
PlS	Leighton, W	AZ	871
PlS	Miller, T	CA	875
PlS	Molnar, J	NC	863
PlS	Orgill, D	MA	851
PlS	Rose, E	NY	858
PlS	Smith, D	FL	863
PlS	Sood, R	IN	868
PlS	Spence, R	MD	858

C

Calcium Disorders

EDM	Bergman, D	NY	209
EDM	Clutter, W	MO	216
EDM	Holick, M	MA	207
EDM	Jacobs, T	NY	210

Calcium Disorders in Newborn

PEn	Diamond, F	FL	745

Cancer Chemoembolization

VIR	Cohen, G	PA	993
VIR	Geschwind, J	MD	993
VIR	Mauro, M	NC	995
VIR	Salem, R	IL	996

Cancer Detection & Staging

NuM	Agress, H	NJ	548
NuM	Siegel, B	MO	550
NuM	Waxman, A	CA	551

Cancer Genetics

CG	Bale, A	CT	156
CG	Bialer, M	NY	157
CG	Gilbert, F	NY	157
Ge	Boland, C	TX	250
GO	Fields, A	DC	278
GO	Lancaster, J	FL	281
GO	Lu, K	TX	288
GO	Poliakoff, S	FL	282
Onc	Ford, J	CA	386
Onc	Grana, G	NJ	341
Onc	Marcom, P	NC	359
Onc	Offit, K	NY	346
PHO	Tomlinson, G	TX	776

Cancer Imaging

DR	Fishman, E	MD	975

Cancer Prevention

Ge	Kurtz, R	NY	235
Ge	Weinberg, D	PA	238
Onc	Alberts, D	AZ	377
Onc	Arun, B	TX	377
Onc	Daly, M	PA	337
Onc	Fitch, T	AZ	378
Onc	Grana, G	NJ	341
Onc	Lippman, S	CA	387
Onc	O'Regan, R	GA	360
Onc	Parnes, H	MD	347
Onc	Vinciguerra, V	NY	351
Pul	Unger, M	PA	929

Cancer Radiotherapy

VIR	Geschwind, J	MD	993

Spec	Name	St	Pg
VIR	Mauro, M	NC	995
VIR	Salem, R	IL	996
VIR	Wood, B	MD	994

Cancer Reconstruction

Oto	Alam, D	OH	672
PlS	Brandt, K	MO	865
PlS	Coleman, J	IN	865
PlS	Cruse, C	FL	861
PlS	Disa, J	NY	853
PlS	Evans, G	CA	873
PlS	Hansen, J	OR	874
PlS	Mehrara, B	NY	856
PlS	Menick, F	AZ	871
PlS	Miller, M	OH	866
PlS	Schusterman, M	TX	872
S	Swistel, A	NY	1065

Cancer Rehabilitation

PMR	Cheville, A	MN	839
PMR	DePompolo, R	MN	840
PMR	Gamble, G	IL	840
PMR	King, R	GA	838
PMR	Schwartz, L	PA	837
PMR	Stewart, P	AL	839
PMR	Stubblefield, M	NY	837

Cancer Risk Assessment

CG	Plon, S	TX	162
CG	Sutphen, R	FL	159
CRS	Stein, D	PA	171
Ge	Giardiello, F	MD	233
Ge	Weinberg, D	PA	238
Onc	Garber, J	MA	329
Onc	Grunberg, S	VT	330
Onc	Olopade, O	IL	370

Cancer Surgery

NS	Bailes, J	IL	485
PS	Chwals, W	MA	801
PS	Colombani, P	MD	802
PS	Davidoff, A	TN	805
PS	La Quaglia, M	NY	803
PS	Latchaw, L	NH	802
PS	Moss, R	OH	807
PS	Nuchtern, J	TX	809
PS	Rescorla, F	IN	807
PS	Rice, H	NC	805
PS	Ricketts, R	GA	806
PS	Shochat, S	TN	806
PS	Spigland, N	NY	804
S	Averbook, B	OH	1074
S	Billingsley, K	OR	1093
S	Bolton, J	LA	1087
S	Byrd, D	WA	1094
S	Chang, A	MI	1075
S	Chang, H	CA	1094
S	Daneker, G	GA	1068
S	Edge, S	NY	1056

Spec	Name	St	Pg
S	Edney, J	NE	1085
S	Ellenhorn, J	CA	1095
S	Gawande, A	MA	1049
S	Gray, R	AZ	1088
S	Kaufman, H	IL	1078
S	Kirgan, D	NV	1097
S	Krag, D	VT	1050
S	Krouse, R	AZ	1090
S	McCabe, D	AZ	1091
S	McGrath, P	KY	1070
S	Pockaj, B	AZ	1091
S	Postier, R	OK	1091
S	Roh, M	FL	1071
S	Salem, R	CT	1051
S	Schwartzentruber, D	IN	1082
S	Scott-Conner, C	IA	1082
S	Shapiro, R	NY	1064
S	Simeone, D	MI	1082
S	Sondak, V	FL	1072
S	Tuttle, T	MN	1083
S	Urist, M	AL	1073
S	Vetto, J	OR	1100

Cancer Survivors-Late Effects of Therapy

Spec	Name	St	Pg
ChiN	Keating, G	MN	150
H & PM	Friebert, S	OH	407
N	Janss, A	GA	522
Onc	Albain, K	IL	364
Onc	Dizon, D	MA	328
Onc	Ganz, P	CA	386
Onc	Garst, J	NC	356
Ped	Kleinerman, E	TX	728
Ped	Oeffinger, K	NY	727
PEn	Meacham, L	GA	746
PEn	Sklar, C	NY	745
PHO	Barredo, J	FL	765
PHO	Blatt, J	NC	765
PHO	Castellino, S	NC	765
PHO	Castle, V	MI	770
PHO	Diller, L	MA	756
PHO	Dreyer, Z	TX	775
PHO	Finklestein, J	CA	777
PHO	Friedman, D	TN	765
PHO	Gold, S	NC	766
PHO	Green, D	TN	766
PHO	Harris, M	NJ	761
PHO	Hayashi, R	MO	771
PHO	Hudson, M	TN	766
PHO	Marina, N	CA	778
PHO	Neglia, J	MN	772
PHO	Nicholson, H	OR	778
PHO	Plautz, G	OH	772
PHO	Puccetti, D	WI	772
PHO	Reaman, G	DC	763
PHO	Rosoff, P	NC	768
PHO	Russo, C	AL	768
PHO	Schwartz, C	RI	757
PHO	Shearer, P	MD	763
PHO	Tomlinson, G	TX	776
PHO	Vik, T	IN	773

Spec	Name	St	Pg
RadRO	Constine, L	NY	948
RadRO	Hancock, S	CA	966

Cancer-Hormonal Influences

Spec	Name	St	Pg
EDM	Earp, H	NC	214

Cancers-Rare & Unusual

Spec	Name	St	Pg
S	Neifeld, J	VA	1071

Capsule Endoscopy

Spec	Name	St	Pg
Ge	Cello, J	CA	253
Ge	Dea, S	CA	253
Ge	Gerson, L	CA	254
Ge	Kastenberg, D	PA	234
Ge	Leighton, J	AZ	252
Ge	Lewis, B	NY	235

Carcinoid Tumors

Spec	Name	St	Pg
Onc	Ahlgren, J	DC	333
Onc	Anthony, L	KY	353
Onc	Hande, K	TN	357
Onc	Kvols, L	FL	358
S	Choti, M	MD	1055
S	Wagman, L	CA	1100

Cardiac Catheterization

Spec	Name	St	Pg
Cv	Cabin, H	CT	94
Cv	Chizner, M	FL	103
Cv	Clements, S	GA	104
Cv	Coppola, J	NY	97
Cv	Corrigan, V	GA	104
Cv	Greenberg, M	NY	99
Cv	Kirshenbaum, J	MA	95
Cv	Phillips, H	NC	105
Cv	Rosenbush, S	IL	110
Cv	Schwartz, W	NY	101
Cv	Shlofmitz, R	NY	102
Cv	Waxman, H	PA	102
IC	Applegate, R	NC	129
IC	Bach, R	MO	130
IC	Bittl, J	FL	129
IC	Chang, G	PA	127
IC	Douglas, J	GA	129
IC	Feldman, M	TX	132
IC	Greene, R	CA	133
IC	Herrmann, H	PA	127
IC	Jacobs, A	MA	126
IC	Kimmelstiel, C	MA	126
IC	Lasala, J	MO	131
IC	Lee, J	PA	127
IC	Mahmud, E	CA	133
IC	Morris, D	GA	130
IC	Pichard, A	DC	128
IC	Sacchi, T	NY	128
IC	Shani, J	NY	129
IC	Whitlow, P	OH	132
IC	Williams, D	MA	126
PCd	Beekman, R	OH	738
PCd	Biancaniello, T	NY	734

Spec	Name	St	Pg
PCd	Cheatham, J	OH	738
PCd	Hanna, B	PA	735
PCd	Hoyer, M	IN	739
PCd	Lang, P	MA	733
PCd	Latson, L	FL	737
PCd	Lock, J	MA	734
PCd	Moskowitz, W	VA	737
PCd	Murphy, J	PA	735
PCd	Radtke, W	DE	735
PCd	Sommer, R	NY	736
PCd	Teitel, D	CA	741
PCd	Velvis, H	NY	736

Cardiac CT Angiography

Spec	Name	St	Pg
Cv	Poon, M	NY	101
Cv	Raff, G	MI	110
DR	Edelman, R	IL	980
DR	Zeman, R	DC	978
NuM	Ziffer, J	FL	550

Cardiac Effects in Cancer Therapy

Spec	Name	St	Pg
Onc	Speyer, J	NY	349

Cardiac Effects of Cancer/Cancer Therapy

Spec	Name	St	Pg
Cv	Steingart, R	NY	102
PCd	Steinherz, L	NY	736

Cardiac Effects of Chemotherapy

Spec	Name	St	Pg
Cv	Wells, G	NC	106

Cardiac Electrophysiology

Spec	Name	St	Pg
CE	Anderson, M	IA	122
CE	Asirvatham, S	MN	122
CE	Berger, R	MD	119
CE	Buxton, A	MA	118
CE	Callans, D	PA	119
CE	Cannom, D	CA	125
CE	Chinitz, L	NY	120
CE	Cohen, M	NY	120
CE	Curtis, A	NY	120
CE	DeLurgio, D	GA	121
CE	DiMarco, J	VA	121
CE	Donahue, J	OH	122
CE	Ellenbogen, K	VA	121
CE	Epstein, A	PA	120
CE	Epstein, L	MA	119
CE	Estes, N	MA	119
CE	Faddis, M	MO	123
CE	Feld, G	CA	125
CE	Gang, E	CA	125
CE	Gomes, J	NY	120
CE	Halperin, H	MD	120
CE	Hammill, S	MN	123
CE	Hayes, D	MN	123
CE	Higgins, S	CA	125
CE	Interian, A	FL	122

Specialty & Special Expertise Index

Spec	Name	St	Pg
CE	Kay, G	AL	122
CE	Lerman, B	NY	120
CE	Levine, J	NY	121
CE	Lewkowiez, L	CO	124
CE	Lindsay, B	OH	123
CE	Link, M	MA	119
CE	Love, C	OH	123
CE	Marchlinski, F	PA	121
CE	Mehta, D	NY	121
CE	Miller, J	IN	123
CE	Morady, F	MI	123
CE	Natale, A	TX	124
CE	Onufer, J	VA	122
CE	Prystowsky, E	IN	123
CE	Ruskin, J	MA	119
CE	Schuger, C	MI	124
CE	Shen, W	AZ	124
CE	Snyder, D	LA	125
CE	Sorrentino, R	GA	122
CE	Stevenson, W	MA	119
CE	Swerdlow, C	CA	125
CE	Tchou, P	OH	124
CE	Tomaselli, G	MD	121
CE	Waldo, A	OH	124
CE	Wang, P	CA	125
CE	Wilber, D	IL	124
Cv	Slater, W	NY	102
PCd	Fish, F	TN	737

Cardiac Imaging
Spec	Name	St	Pg
Cv	Budoff, M	CA	116
Cv	Cerqueira, M	OH	107
Cv	Kaul, S	OR	117
Cv	Poon, M	NY	101
DR	Bluemke, D	MD	974
DR	Fishman, E	MD	975
DR	Rubin, G	NC	979
NuM	Sandler, M	TN	549

Cardiac Intensive Care
Spec	Name	St	Pg
Cv	Nissen, S	OH	109
PCd	Hardin, J	IL	739

Cardiac MRI
Spec	Name	St	Pg
Cv	Anderson, J	UT	113
Cv	Raff, G	MI	110
DR	Edelman, R	IL	980
DR	Flamm, S	OH	980
PCd	Weinberg, P	PA	737

Cardiac Pathology
Spec	Name	St	Pg
Path	Roberts, W	TX	718

Cardiac Surgery
Spec	Name	St	Pg
T&CS	Athanasuleas, C	AL	1123
T&CS	Dang, M	HI	1141
T&CS	Echeverri, L	TX	1137
T&CS	Girardi, L	NY	1116
T&CS	Harken, A	CA	1141

Spec	Name	St	Pg
T&CS	Isom, O	NY	1117
T&CS	Jessen, M	TX	1138
T&CS	Karwande, S	UT	1136
T&CS	Kopf, G	CT	1111
T&CS	Mack, M	TX	1139
T&CS	Magovern, G	PA	1119
T&CS	Philpott, J	VA	1128
T&CS	Rosengart, T	NY	1121
T&CS	Singh, A	RI	1112
T&CS	Stuart, R	MO	1135
T&CS	Tedder, M	TN	1130
T&CS	Thistlethwaite, P	CA	1143
T&CS	Trento, A	CA	1143
T&CS	Turner, W	TX	1140
T&CS	Ungerleider, R	NC	1130
T&CS	Vlahakes, G	MA	1112

Cardiac Surgery-Adult
Spec	Name	St	Pg
T&CS	Conte, J	MD	1114
T&CS	Diehl, J	PA	1115
T&CS	Joyce, L	MN	1133
T&CS	Krieger, K	NY	1119
T&CS	Merrick, S	CA	1142
T&CS	Panos, A	FL	1128
T&CS	Rastegar, H	MA	1112

Cardiac Surgery-Adult & Pediatric
Spec	Name	St	Pg
T&CS	Calhoon, J	TX	1137
T&CS	Christian, K	TN	1124
T&CS	Drinkwater, D	TN	1125
T&CS	Gundry, S	CA	1141
T&CS	Kirklin, J	AL	1126
T&CS	Mullett, T	KY	1127
T&CS	Spray, T	PA	1122
T&CS	Warner, K	MA	1113

Cardiac Surgery-Geriatric
Spec	Name	St	Pg
T&CS	Edwards, N	NY	1115

Cardiac Surgery-High Risk
Spec	Name	St	Pg
T&CS	Furukawa, S	PA	1116
T&CS	Gundry, S	CA	1141

Cardiac Surgery-Neonatal
Spec	Name	St	Pg
T&CS	Bichell, D	TN	1123
T&CS	Rosenkranz, E	FL	1129
T&CS	Walters, H	MI	1135

Cardiac Surgery-Neonatal & Pediatric
Spec	Name	St	Pg
T&CS	Brown, J	IN	1131

Cardiac Surgery-Pediatric
Spec	Name	St	Pg
T&CS	Bailey, L	CA	1140
T&CS	Bichell, D	TN	1123
T&CS	Fontana, G	NY	1115
T&CS	Harrell, J	TX	1138

Spec	Name	St	Pg
T&CS	Turrentine, M	IN	1135

Cardiac Tumors, Myxomas
Spec	Name	St	Pg
T&CS	Grossi, E	NY	1117

Cardiac Tumors/Cancer
Spec	Name	St	Pg
T&CS	Reardon, M	TX	1139
T&CS	Sellke, F	RI	1112

Cardiomyopathy
Spec	Name	St	Pg
Cv	Bonow, R	IL	106
Cv	Elkayam, U	CA	116
Cv	Fonarow, G	CA	116
Cv	Manning, W	MA	95
Cv	Williams, E	IN	112
PCd	Driscoll, D	MN	739

Cardiomyopathy-Hypertrophic
Spec	Name	St	Pg
IC	Bach, R	MO	130

Cardiothoracic Surgery
Spec	Name	St	Pg
T&CS	Bains, M	NY	1114
T&CS	Bull, D	UT	1136
T&CS	Byrne, J	TN	1124
T&CS	Durham, S	MI	1132
T&CS	Galantowicz, M	OH	1132
T&CS	Girardi, L	NY	1116
T&CS	Glassford, D	TN	1125
T&CS	Lang, S	NY	1119
T&CS	Lanza, L	AZ	1138
T&CS	Martin, T	FL	1126
T&CS	Moon, M	MO	1134
T&CS	Oaks, T	NC	1128
T&CS	Pham, S	FL	1128
T&CS	Robbins, R	CA	1142
T&CS	Salerno, T	FL	1129
T&CS	Stuart, R	MO	1135
T&CS	Thistlethwaite, P	CA	1143
T&CS	Toyoda, Y	PA	1122
T&CS	Weiman, D	TN	1130

Cardiovascular Disease
Spec	Name	St	Pg
Cv	Abi-samra, F	LA	113
Cv	Alpert, J	AZ	113
Cv	Andersen, H	NY	96
Cv	Anderson, J	UT	113
Cv	Bairey, C	CA	116
Cv	Balady, G	MA	94
Cv	Ballantyne, C	TX	114
Cv	Bashore, T	NC	103
Cv	Bass, T	FL	103
Cv	Benjamin, I	UT	113
Cv	Blanchard, D	CA	116
Cv	Blumenthal, D	NY	96
Cv	Blumenthal, R	MD	97
Cv	Bonow, R	IL	106
Cv	Borer, J	NY	97
Cv	Borzak, S	FL	103

Specialty & Special Expertise Index

Spec	Name	St	Pg	Spec	Name	St	Pg	Spec	Name	St	Pg
Cv	Bourge, R	AL	103	Cv	Jaffe, A	MN	108	Cv	Sanborn, T	IL	111
Cv	Bove, A	PA	97	Cv	Jessup, M	PA	100	Cv	Saunders, E	MD	101
Cv	Braverman, A	MO	106	Cv	Johnson, A	CA	117	Cv	Schnittger, I	CA	118
Cv	Brozena, S	PA	97	Cv	Johnson, M	WI	109	Cv	Schulman, S	MD	101
Cv	Budoff, M	CA	116	Cv	Johnson, P	MA	94	Cv	Schwartz, A	NY	101
Cv	Burket, M	OH	106	Cv	Judelson, D	CA	117	Cv	Schwartz, W	NY	101
Cv	Byrd, B	TN	103	Cv	Katz, S	NY	100	Cv	Shah, P	CA	118
Cv	Cabin, H	CT	94	Cv	Kaul, S	OR	117	Cv	Shapiro, J	IL	111
Cv	Califf, R	NC	103	Cv	Kereiakes, D	OH	109	Cv	Shea, R	IN	111
Cv	Carabello, B	TX	114	Cv	Kirshenbaum, J	MA	95	Cv	Shlofmitz, R	NY	102
Cv	Catherwood, E	NH	94	Cv	Klein, L	IL	109	Cv	Silvestry, F	PA	102
Cv	Cerqueira, M	OH	107	Cv	Kobashigawa, J	CA	117	Cv	Simon, D	OH	111
Cv	Chaitman, B	MO	107	Cv	Konstam, M	MA	95	Cv	Skolnick, A	AK	118
Cv	Chizner, M	FL	103	Cv	Kostis, J	NJ	100	Cv	Slater, W	NY	102
Cv	Clements, S	GA	104	Cv	Krajcer, Z	TX	114	Cv	Smart, F	LA	115
Cv	Cohen, H	NY	97	Cv	Kuvin, J	MA	95	Cv	Smith, S	NC	106
Cv	Connolly, H	MN	107	Cv	Landzberg, J	NJ	100	Cv	Sorrentino, M	IL	111
Cv	Cooper, C	OH	107	Cv	Lewis, S	OR	117	Cv	Stainback, R	TX	115
Cv	Coppola, J	NY	97	Cv	Liang, B	CT	95	Cv	Stein, J	WI	111
Cv	Corrigan, V	GA	104	Cv	Lindenfeld, J	CO	113	Cv	Steingart, R	NY	102
Cv	Davidson, M	IL	107	Cv	Linton, M	TN	104	Cv	Stevenson, L	MA	96
Cv	DeNofrio, D	MA	94	Cv	Loscalzo, J	MA	95	Cv	Stewart, W	OH	111
Cv	Devereux, R	NY	97	Cv	Manning, W	MA	95	Cv	Tenenbaum, J	NY	102
Cv	Dichek, D	WA	116	Cv	Massin, E	TX	114	Cv	Thames, M	AZ	115
Cv	Diver, D	CT	94	Cv	Mather, P	PA	100	Cv	Tobis, J	CA	118
Cv	Eagle, K	MI	107	Cv	McPherson, D	TX	114	Cv	Topol, E	CA	118
Cv	Edelen, J	CA	116	Cv	Mehlman, D	IL	109	Cv	Vetrovec, G	VA	106
Cv	Edmundowicz, D	PA	97	Cv	Meller, J	NY	100	Cv	Vignola, P	NC	106
Cv	Eisen, H	PA	98	Cv	Moran, J	IL	109	Cv	Volgman, A	IL	112
Cv	Elkayam, U	CA	116	Cv	Myerburg, R	FL	104	Cv	von der Lohe, E	IN	112
Cv	Fintel, D	IL	107	Cv	Naccarelli, G	PA	100	Cv	Wagoner, L	OH	112
Cv	Fishbein, D	WA	116	Cv	Nagueh, S	TX	114	Cv	Walsh, M	IN	112
Cv	Follansbee, W	PA	98	Cv	Nishimura, R	MN	109	Cv	Waxman, H	PA	102
Cv	Fonarow, G	CA	116	Cv	Nissen, S	OH	109	Cv	Weaver, W	MI	112
Cv	Freeman, G	TX	114	Cv	Nocero, M	FL	105	Cv	Webb, G	OH	112
Cv	French, W	CA	117	Cv	O'Connell, J	GA	105	Cv	Weitz, H	PA	102
Cv	Friedman, S	NY	98	Cv	O'Connor, C	NC	105	Cv	Wells, G	NC	106
Cv	Fuster, V	NY	98	Cv	O'Gara, P	MA	95	Cv	Wilansky, S	AZ	115
Cv	Gandy, W	GA	104	Cv	O'Neill, W	MI	110	Cv	Wilkoff, B	OH	112
Cv	Gardin, J	NJ	98	Cv	Oparil, S	AL	105	Cv	Williams, E	IN	112
Cv	Geltman, E	MO	108	Cv	Parrillo, J	NJ	101	Cv	Williams, K	MI	113
Cv	Gibbons, R	MN	108	Cv	Pepine, C	FL	105	Cv	Young, J	OH	113
Cv	Gliklich, J	NY	98	Cv	Pfeffer, M	MA	95	Cv	Zoghbi, W	TX	115
Cv	Goldberg, N	NY	98	Cv	Phillips, H	NC	105	Cv	Zusman, R	MA	96
Cv	Goodman, D	NY	98	Cv	Phillips, R	MA	96	EDM	Eckel, R	CO	220
Cv	Gottdiener, J	MD	99	Cv	Poon, M	NY	101	Ger	Minaker, K	MA	262
Cv	Gottlieb, S	MD	99	Cv	Powers, E	SC	105	Ger	Wei, J	AR	266
Cv	Gould, K	TX	114	Cv	Quinones, M	TX	115				
Cv	Greenberg, M	NY	99	Cv	Raff, G	MI	110	**Cardiovascular Disease/Young Adult**			
Cv	Grubb, B	OH	108	Cv	Rahko, P	WI	110				
Cv	Halperin, J	NY	99	Cv	Ramee, S	LA	115	Cv	Blumenthal, R	MD	97
Cv	Hare, J	FL	104	Cv	Redberg, R	CA	118				
Cv	Harrison, J	NC	104	Cv	Reis, S	PA	101	**Cardiovascular Imaging**			
Cv	Hauptman, P	MO	108	Cv	Reiss, C	MO	110				
Cv	Hayes, S	MN	108	Cv	Rich, S	IL	110	Cv	Gandy, W	GA	104
Cv	Herling, I	PA	99	Cv	Ridker, P	MA	96	DR	Flamm, S	OH	980
Cv	Heroux, A	IL	108	Cv	Rihal, C	MN	110	DR	Rubin, G	NC	979
Cv	Horn, E	NY	99	Cv	Roberts, B	RI	96	DR	Thompson, B	IA	981
Cv	Hunt, S	CA	117	Cv	Rogers, J	NC	105	DR	White, R	OH	981
Cv	Hutter, A	MA	94	Cv	Rosenbush, S	IL	110	DR	Zeman, R	DC	978
Cv	Inra, L	NY	99	Cv	Russell, S	MD	101				
Cv	Iskandrian, A	AL	104	Cv	Safian, R	MI	110				

Specialty & Special Expertise Index

Spec	Name	St	Pg
Cardiovascular Interventional Radiology			
VIR	Gomes, A	CA	997
Cardiovascular Pathology			
Path	Fishbein, M	CA	720
Cardiovascular Surgery			
T&CS	Diethrich, E	AZ	1137
T&CS	Mayer, J	MA	1111
T&CS	Quintessenza, J	FL	1128
T&CS	Vander Salm, T	MA	1112
Carotid Artery Disease			
Cv	Krajcer, Z	TX	114
IC	Schreiber, T	MI	131
N	Goldstein, L	NC	521
VascS	Alexander, J	OH	1190
VascS	Atnip, R	PA	1185
VascS	Calligaro, K	PA	1186
VascS	Chaikof, E	MA	1184
VascS	Comerota, A	OH	1190
VascS	Dalsing, M	IN	1190
VascS	Greisler, H	IL	1191
VascS	Makaroun, M	PA	1187
VascS	Pomposelli, F	MA	1185
VIR	Katzen, B	FL	994
VIR	Matsumoto, A	VA	995
Carotid Artery Medical Management			
VascS	Riles, T	NY	1188
Carotid Artery Stent Placement			
Cv	Cohen, H	NY	97
Cv	Ramee, S	LA	115
Cv	Sanborn, T	IL	111
IC	Knopf, W	GA	130
IC	Mahmud, E	CA	133
IC	Petrossian, G	NY	128
IC	Reddy, B	GA	130
IC	Roubin, G	NY	128
NRad	Hurst, R	PA	985
NRad	Masaryk, T	OH	989
NRad	Moran, C	MO	989
NRad	Teitelbaum, G	CA	991
NRad	Tenner, M	NY	986
VascS	Eidt, J	AR	1193
VascS	Kazmers, A	MI	1191
VascS	Kwolek, C	MA	1184
VascS	McLafferty, R	IL	1191
Carotid Artery Surgery			
NS	David, C	MA	470
NS	Harbaugh, R	PA	474
NS	Loftus, C	IL	488
T&CS	Caskey, M	AZ	1137
T&CS	Ott, D	TX	1139

Spec	Name	St	Pg
VascS	Adelman, M	NY	1185
VascS	Belkin, M	MA	1184
VascS	Brener, B	NJ	1186
VascS	Carpenter, J	NJ	1186
VascS	Clair, D	OH	1190
VascS	Criado, F	MD	1186
VascS	Cronenwett, J	NH	1184
VascS	D'Ayala, M	NY	1186
VascS	Darling, R	NY	1186
VascS	Fairman, R	PA	1187
VascS	Faries, P	NY	1187
VascS	Flanigan, D	CA	1194
VascS	Fowl, R	AZ	1193
VascS	Freischlag, J	MD	1187
VascS	Gewertz, B	CA	1194
VascS	Green, R	NY	1187
VascS	Hallett, J	SC	1189
VascS	Harrington, E	NY	1187
VascS	Hodgson, K	IL	1191
VascS	Hollier, L	LA	1193
VascS	Howard, T	NE	1192
VascS	Kent, K	WI	1191
VascS	Kougias, P	TX	1193
VascS	Mackey, W	MA	1185
VascS	McKinsey, J	NY	1188
VascS	Mitchell, M	MS	1189
VascS	Morrissey, N	NY	1188
VascS	Perler, B	MD	1188
VascS	Ricotta, J	DC	1188
VascS	Todd, G	NY	1189
VascS	White, R	CA	1194
VascS	Zarins, C	CA	1194
Carotid Body Tumors			
VascS	LaMuraglia, G	MA	1185
Carpal Tunnel Syndrome			
HS	Abrams, R	CA	303
HS	Carneiro, R	FL	298
HS	Carroll, C	IL	300
HS	Cendales, L	GA	299
HS	Derman, G	IL	300
HS	Imbriglia, J	PA	296
HS	Kulick, R	NY	296
HS	Lane, L	NY	296
HS	Nagle, D	IL	302
HS	Raskin, K	NY	297
HS	Rosenwasser, M	NY	297
HS	Weiss, A	RI	294
NS	Taylon, C	NE	492
NS	Zager, E	PA	480
Cartilage Damage			
DR	Potter, H	NY	977
HS	Lee, W	MD	297
OrS	Anderson, L	CA	641
OrS	Brage, M	WA	642
OrS	Chu, C	PA	615
OrS	Gladstone, J	NY	617
OrS	Hungerford, M	MD	620

Spec	Name	St	Pg
OrS	Karas, S	GA	629
OrS	Mandelbaum, B	CA	644
OrS	Nuber, G	IL	636
OrS	O'Driscoll, S	MN	636
OrS	Zarins, B	MA	613
SM	Bush-Joseph, C	IL	1043
SM	Gambardella, R	CA	1044
SM	Ho, S	IL	1043
SM	Miniaci, A	OH	1043
SM	Rodeo, S	NY	1042
SM	Sennett, B	PA	1042
Cartilage Damage & Transplant			
OrS	Minas, T	MA	612
OrS	Plancher, K	NY	624
SM	Jones, D	LA	1044
SM	Williams, R	NY	1042
Castleman's Disease			
Onc	Camoriano, J	AZ	378
Onc	Sweetenham, J	NV	391
Cataract Surgery			
Oph	Afshari, N	NC	581
Oph	Alward, W	IA	588
Oph	Boxer Wachler, B	CA	599
Oph	Budenz, D	NC	582
Oph	Caprioli, J	CA	599
Oph	Crandall, A	UT	595
Oph	Cykiert, R	NY	572
Oph	Feder, R	IL	589
Oph	Forster, R	FL	583
Oph	Foster, C	MA	570
Oph	Gibralter, R	NY	574
Oph	Goldberg, D	NJ	574
Oph	Gorovoy, M	FL	583
Oph	Holland, E	OH	590
Oph	John, T	IL	590
Oph	Koch, D	TX	596
Oph	Lane, S	MN	591
Oph	Lichter, P	MI	591
Oph	Liebmann, J	NY	576
Oph	Lindstrom, R	MN	591
Oph	Mackool, R	NY	577
Oph	Magramm, I	NY	577
Oph	Maloney, R	CA	601
Oph	Masket, S	CA	602
Oph	McCulley, J	TX	597
Oph	Orlin, S	PA	578
Oph	Page, T	MI	593
Oph	Pepose, J	MO	593
Oph	Pflugfelder, S	TX	597
Oph	Robin, A	MD	579
Oph	Rosenberg, M	IL	594
Oph	Salz, J	CA	603
Oph	Samuelson, T	MN	594
Oph	Schein, O	MD	579
Oph	Schuman, J	PA	579
Oph	Seibel, B	CA	603
Oph	Serafano, D	CA	604

Spec	Name	St	Pg
Oph	Shamie, N	CA	604
Oph	Shingleton, B	MA	571
Oph	Solomon, K	SC	586
Oph	Stark, W	MD	580
Oph	Steinert, R	CA	604
Oph	Stulting, R	GA	586
Oph	Wallace, R	LA	598
Oph	Wang, M	TN	587
Oph	Waring, G	GA	587

Cataract Surgery Revision

Oph	Masket, S	CA	602

Cataract Surgery-Lens Implant

Oph	Cionni, R	UT	595
Oph	Culbertson, W	FL	582
Oph	Dodick, J	NY	573
Oph	Greenfield, D	FL	583
Oph	Lass, J	OH	591
Oph	Miller, K	CA	602
Oph	O'Brien, T	FL	585
Oph	Osher, R	OH	593
Oph	Page, T	MI	593
Oph	Parrish, R	FL	585
Oph	Perez, V	FL	586
Oph	Wright, K	CA	605

Cataract-Pediatric

Oph	Buckley, E	NC	582
Oph	Del Monte, M	MI	589
Oph	Hall, L	NY	575
Oph	Kerr, N	TN	584
Oph	Lambert, S	GA	584
Oph	Medow, N	NY	577
Oph	Plager, D	IN	593
Oph	Walton, D	MA	571
Oph	Wilson, M	SC	587

Catheter Ablation

CE	Berger, R	MD	119
CE	Donahue, J	OH	122
CE	Epstein, A	PA	120
CE	Halperin, H	MD	120
CE	Lerman, B	NY	120
CE	Miller, J	IN	123
CE	Onufer, J	VA	122
CE	Prystowsky, E	IN	123
CE	Shen, W	AZ	124
CE	Wilber, D	IL	124

Celiac Disease

Ge	Di Marino, A	PA	232
Ge	Elliott, D	IA	245
Ge	Forsmark, C	FL	240
Ge	Green, P	NY	233
Ge	Kastenberg, D	PA	234
Ge	Murray, J	MN	247
Ge	Semrad, C	IL	248
PGe	Baldridge, A	NJ	750

Spec	Name	St	Pg
PGe	Benkov, K	NY	750
PGe	Cohen, M	OH	752
PGe	Fasano, A	MD	750
PGe	Guandalini, S	IL	753
PGe	Hill, I	NC	752
PGe	Hoffenberg, E	CO	754
PGe	Leichtner, A	MA	749
PGe	Levy, J	NY	750
PGe	Snyder, J	DC	751

Central Nervous System Cancer

RadRO	Buatti, J	IA	959
RadRO	Markoe, A	FL	955
RadRO	Porrazzo, M	DC	952

Cerebral Palsy

ChiN	Brunstrom, J	MO	150
ChiN	Darras, B	MA	146
ChiN	Edgar, T	WI	150
ChiN	Goldstein, E	GA	149
ChiN	Noetzel, M	MO	151
ChiN	Volpe, J	MA	147
HS	Carlson, M	NY	295
HS	Peljovich, A	GA	299
OrS	Oppenheim, W	CA	645
OrS	Otsuka, N	NY	623
OrS	Sponseller, P	MD	625
OrS	Strongwater, A	NJ	626
Ped	Walker, W	WA	729
PMR	Alexander, J	NC	838
PMR	Matthews, D	CO	842
PMR	Webster, H	MA	834

Cerebral Palsy-Select Dorsal Rhizotomy

NS	Park, T	MO	489

Cerebrovascular Disease

N	Adams, H	IA	524
N	Albers, G	CA	535
N	Alexandrov, A	AL	519
N	Brown, R	MN	525
N	Burke, A	IL	525
N	Feldmann, E	MA	507
N	Fink, M	NY	511
N	Fisher, M	CA	536
N	Furie, K	RI	507
N	Greer, D	CT	507
N	Kasner, S	PA	512
N	Levine, S	NY	514
N	Logan, W	MO	527
N	Sila, C	OH	530
N	Wechsler, L	PA	518
N	Wityk, R	MD	519
NRad	Masaryk, T	OH	989
NRad	Pile-Spellman, J	NY	986
NS	Atkinson, J	MN	485
NS	Barrow, D	GA	481
NS	Hopkins, L	NY	475

Spec	Name	St	Pg
NS	Meyer, F	MN	489
NS	Samson, D	TX	494
NS	Sills, A	TN	484
VascS	Acher, C	WI	1190
VascS	Berguer, R	MI	1190
VascS	Cambria, R	MA	1184

Cerebrovascular Disease/Stroke

NRad	Frei, D	CO	990
NRad	Moran, C	MO	989
NRad	Rowley, H	WI	989

Cerebrovascular Malformations

NS	Riina, H	NY	478

Cerebrovascular Surgery

NS	Al-Mefty, O	MA	470
NS	Bailes, J	IL	485
NS	Dacey, R	MO	487
NS	David, C	MA	470
NS	Grady, M	PA	474
NS	Heros, R	FL	482
NS	Huang, J	MD	475
NS	Kim, D	TX	493
NS	Lemole, G	AZ	493
NS	Link, M	MN	488
NS	Loftus, C	IL	488
NS	Malik, G	MI	488
NS	Morcos, J	FL	483
NS	Rosenwasser, R	PA	478
NS	Spetzler, R	AZ	494
NS	Steinberg, G	CA	499
NS	Stieg, P	NY	479
NS	Wilson, J	NC	485
NS	Zager, E	PA	480

Cervical Cancer

GO	Abbas, F	MD	275
GO	Abu-Rustum, N	NY	276
GO	Berek, J	CA	289
GO	Berman, M	CA	289
GO	Boice, C	MD	276
GO	Burger, R	PA	276
GO	Caputo, T	NY	276
GO	Chi, D	NY	277
GO	DePriest, P	KY	280
GO	Di Saia, P	CA	289
GO	Dunton, C	PA	277
GO	Duska, L	VA	281
GO	Edwards, R	PA	277
GO	Finan, M	AL	281
GO	Fromm, G	TX	287
GO	Goff, B	WA	289
GO	Hatch, K	AZ	287
GO	Herzog, T	NY	278
GO	Horowitz, I	GA	281
GO	Husain, A	CA	290
GO	Johnston, C	MI	284

Specialty & Special Expertise Index

Spec	Name	St	Pg
GO	Kelley, J	PA	278
GO	King, S	PA	278
GO	Kline, R	LA	287
GO	Koulos, J	NY	278
GO	Levenback, C	TX	288
GO	Lin, J	DC	279
GO	Lucci, J	FL	282
GO	Lurain, J	IL	284
GO	Makhija, S	KY	282
GO	Moore, D	IN	284
GO	Muto, M	MA	275
GO	Pejovic, T	OR	290
GO	Penalver, M	FL	282
GO	Potkul, R	IL	285
GO	Rader, J	WI	285
GO	Remmenga, S	NE	286
GO	Rice, L	WI	285
GO	Rose, P	OH	285
GO	Rotmensch, J	IL	285
GO	Rubin, S	PA	279
GO	Runowicz, C	FL	282
GO	Rutherford, T	CT	275
GO	Schorge, J	MA	275
GO	Schwartz, P	CT	275
GO	Siller, B	TX	288
GO	Smith, D	IL	285
GO	Soisson, A	UT	286
GO	Valea, F	NC	283
GO	Van Nagell, J	KY	283
GO	Waggoner, S	OH	286
GO	Walker, J	OK	288
ObG	Argenta, P	MN	560
ObG	Lengyel, E	IL	561
Onc	Schilder, R	PA	349
Onc	Scudder, S	CA	390
Path	Cho, K	MI	715
Path	Gupta, P	PA	709
RadRO	Eifel, P	TX	964

Charcot Foot

OrS	Pinzur, M	IL	637

Chemical Exposure

A&I	Fishman, H	DC	85
OM	Gochfeld, M	NJ	882
Pul	Bascom, R	PA	924

Chemo-Radiation Combined Therapy

RadRO	Cooper, J	NY	948
RadRO	Formenti, S	NY	949
RadRO	Rich, T	VA	957

Chemoembolization & Tumor Ablation

VIR	Cho, K	MI	995
VIR	Darcy, M	MO	995
VIR	Gomes, A	CA	997
VIR	Weintraub, J	NY	994

Chest Diseases-Benign

T&CS	Nesbitt, J	TN	1127

Chest Pain-Non Cardiac

Ge	Rao, S	GA	242

Chest Radiology

DR	Black, W	NH	973
DR	Partain, C	TN	979

Chest Wall Deformities

PlS	Stahl, R	CT	851
PPul	Redding, G	WA	798
PS	Aiken, J	WI	806
PS	Black, C	TX	809
PS	Cass, D	TX	809
PS	Glick, P	NY	803
PS	Paidas, C	FL	805
PS	Shochat, S	TN	806
PS	Stylianos, S	NY	804
PS	Weber, T	IL	808

Chest Wall Reconstruction

PlS	Seyfer, A	MD	858
PlS	Stahl, R	CT	851
PlS	Yuen, J	AR	872

Chest Wall Tumors

T&CS	Cerfolio, R	AL	1124
T&CS	Handy, J	OR	1141
T&CS	Kiev, J	WV	1118
T&CS	Kucharczuk, J	PA	1119
T&CS	Marshall, M	DC	1120
T&CS	Naunheim, K	MO	1134
T&CS	Shrager, J	CA	1143
T&CS	Whyte, R	MA	1113

Chiari's Deformity

ChiN	Keating, G	MN	150
N	Kula, R	NY	513
NS	Ellenbogen, R	WA	496
NS	Feldstein, N	NY	474
NS	Frazee, J	CA	496
NS	Jallo, G	MD	475
NS	Luken, M	IL	488
NS	Oakes, W	AL	483
NS	Piatt, J	DE	478
NS	Selden, N	OR	499
NS	Shuer, L	CA	499
NS	Weingart, J	MD	480
NS	Wisoff, J	NY	480

Child & Adolescent Psychiatry

ChAP	Abright, A	NY	907
ChAP	Alessi, N	MI	910
ChAP	Biederman, J	MA	906
ChAP	Bird, H	NY	907

Spec	Name	St	Pg
ChAP	Birmaher, B	PA	908
ChAP	Bleiberg, E	TX	911
ChAP	Bogrov, M	MD	908
ChAP	Boxer, G	MO	910
ChAP	Brent, D	PA	908
ChAP	Campo, J	OH	910
ChAP	Coffey, B	NY	908
ChAP	Deas, D	SC	910
ChAP	Dulcan, M	IL	910
ChAP	Emslie, G	TX	911
ChAP	Foley, C	NY	908
ChAP	Fornari, V	NY	908
ChAP	Hagman, J	CO	911
ChAP	Hertzig, M	NY	908
ChAP	Herzog, D	MA	906
ChAP	Heston, J	TN	910
ChAP	Hirsch, G	NY	908
ChAP	Hudziak, J	VT	906
ChAP	King, B	WA	912
ChAP	Koplewicz, H	NY	909
ChAP	Kwon, H	WA	912
ChAP	Leckman, J	CT	907
ChAP	Leventhal, B	NY	909
ChAP	Luby, J	MO	911
ChAP	Martini, D	UT	911
ChAP	McCracken, J	CA	912
ChAP	McDougle, C	MA	907
ChAP	McKelvey, R	OR	912
ChAP	Pomeroy, J	NY	909
ChAP	Ponton, L	CA	912
ChAP	Rapoport, J	DC	909
ChAP	Riddle, M	MD	909
ChAP	Rostain, A	PA	909
ChAP	Russell, A	CA	912
ChAP	Sargent, A	MA	907
ChAP	Sexson, S	GA	910
ChAP	Slomowitz, M	IL	911
ChAP	Spencer, T	MA	907
ChAP	Steiner, H	CA	912
ChAP	Terr, L	CA	912
ChAP	Turecki, S	NY	909
ChAP	Walkup, J	NY	909
ChAP	Wamboldt, M	CO	911
ChAP	Wilens, T	MA	907
ChAP	Zeanah, C	LA	911

Child Abuse

Ped	Berkowitz, C	CA	728
Ped	Feldman, K	WA	728
Psyc	Vanderkolk, B	MA	890

Child Neurology

ChiN	Allen, J	NY	147
ChiN	Ashwal, S	CA	153
ChiN	Bale, J	UT	152
ChiN	Bergman, I	PA	147
ChiN	Bourgeois, B	MA	146
ChiN	Brunstrom, J	MO	150
ChiN	Cohen, B	OH	150
ChiN	Comi, A	MD	147
ChiN	Crawford, T	MD	147

Spec	Name	St	Pg
ChiN	Darras, B	MA	146
ChiN	De Vivo, D	NY	147
ChiN	Dure, L	AL	149
ChiN	Edgar, T	WI	150
ChiN	Epstein, L	IL	150
ChiN	Filipek, P	TX	152
ChiN	Finkel, R	FL	149
ChiN	Fisher, P	CA	153
ChiN	Goldstein, E	GA	149
ChiN	Gospe, S	WA	153
ChiN	Greenwood, R	NC	149
ChiN	Griesemer, D	MA	146
ChiN	Haas, R	CA	153
ChiN	Hershey, A	OH	150
ChiN	Holmes, G	NH	146
ChiN	Iannaccone, S	TX	152
ChiN	Ichord, R	PA	147
ChiN	Keating, G	MN	150
ChiN	Kosofsky, B	NY	147
ChiN	Kotagal, S	MN	150
ChiN	Kovnar, E	WI	151
ChiN	Lavenstein, B	VA	149
ChiN	Legido, A	PA	148
ChiN	Lott, I	CA	153
ChiN	Mandelbaum, D	RI	146
ChiN	Maytal, J	NY	148
ChiN	Mink, J	NY	148
ChiN	Mitchell, W	CA	153
ChiN	Nass, R	NY	148
ChiN	Noetzel, M	MO	151
ChiN	Packer, R	DC	148
ChiN	Patterson, M	MN	151
ChiN	Phillips, P	PA	148
ChiN	Pinter, J	OR	153
ChiN	Pomeroy, S	MA	146
ChiN	Riviello, J	NY	148
ChiN	Roddy, S	CA	153
ChiN	Rosser, T	CA	154
ChiN	Sankar, R	CA	154
ChiN	Santos, C	DC	148
ChiN	Scher, M	OH	151
ChiN	Sharp, G	AR	152
ChiN	Shaywitz, B	CT	146
ChiN	Shinnar, S	NY	149
ChiN	Sivaswamy, L	MI	151
ChiN	Tennison, M	NC	149
ChiN	Tonsgard, J	IL	151
ChiN	Trauner, D	CA	154
ChiN	Tuxhorn, I	OH	151
ChiN	Volpe, J	MA	147
ChiN	Wheless, J	TN	150
ChiN	Wiznitzer, M	OH	152
ChiN	Wyllie, E	OH	152
ChiN	Yamada, K	MO	152
ChiN	Zupanc, M	CA	154
N	Bebin, E	AL	520

Choanal Atresia

Spec	Name	St	Pg
PO	Ward, R	NY	790

Cholesteatoma

Spec	Name	St	Pg
Oto	Lambert, P	SC	669
Oto	Linstrom, C	NY	662
Oto	Parisier, S	NY	663
Oto	Young, N	IL	679
PO	McGill, T	MA	789

Cholesterol/Lipid Disorders

Spec	Name	St	Pg
Cv	Anderson, J	UT	113
Cv	Ballantyne, C	TX	114
Cv	Borzak, S	FL	103
Cv	Budoff, M	CA	116
Cv	Califf, R	NC	103
Cv	Davidson, M	IL	107
Cv	Edmundowicz, D	PA	97
Cv	Fintel, D	IL	107
Cv	French, W	CA	117
Cv	Gardin, J	NJ	98
Cv	Goodman, D	NY	98
Cv	Gould, K	TX	114
Cv	Hayes, S	MN	108
Cv	Herling, I	PA	99
Cv	Inra, L	NY	99
Cv	Judelson, D	CA	117
Cv	Kostis, J	NJ	100
Cv	Linton, M	TN	104
Cv	Moran, J	IL	109
Cv	Nissen, S	OH	109
Cv	Ridker, P	MA	96
Cv	Shah, P	CA	118
Cv	Stein, J	WI	111
Cv	Weaver, W	MI	112
Cv	Zusman, R	MA	96
EDM	Bell, D	AL	213
EDM	Blum, C	NY	209
EDM	Eckel, R	CO	220
EDM	Inzucchi, S	CT	207
EDM	Mazzone, T	IL	218
EDM	Semenkovich, C	MO	219
EDM	Seplowitz, A	NY	212
EDM	Sowers, J	MO	219
IM	Cushman, W	TN	425
IM	Rader, D	PA	424
PrM	Pearson, T	NY	883

Chronic Fatigue Syndrome

Spec	Name	St	Pg
Inf	Cunha, B	NY	411
Inf	Gorensek, M	FL	415
PInf	Krilov, L	NY	780

Chronic Fatigue-Elderly

Spec	Name	St	Pg
Ger	Ciocon, J	FL	263

Chronic Illness

Spec	Name	St	Pg
AM	Slap, G	PA	81
H & PM	Quill, T	NY	407
IM	Galland, L	NY	424

Chronic Lung Disease

Spec	Name	St	Pg
PPul	Kattan, M	NY	794
PPul	Platzker, A	CA	798

Chronic Lung Disease of Infancy

Spec	Name	St	Pg
PPul	Murphy, T	NC	796
PPul	Sallent, J	FL	796

Chronic Obstructive Lung Disease (COPD)

Spec	Name	St	Pg
PPul	Panitch, H	PA	795
Pul	Arcasoy, S	NY	924
Pul	Celli, B	MA	922
Pul	Christman, B	TN	930
Pul	Cooper, J	AL	930
Pul	Cooper, W	VA	930
Pul	Criner, G	PA	925
Pul	Deitz, J	PA	925
Pul	Doherty, D	KY	930
Pul	Donahoe, M	PA	925
Pul	Donohue, J	NC	930
Pul	Fanta, C	MA	922
Pul	Fletcher, E	IN	933
Pul	Fulkerson, W	NC	930
Pul	Guidry, G	LA	938
Pul	Hansen-Flaschen, J	PA	925
Pul	Haynes, J	AL	931
Pul	Henke, N	NC	931
Pul	Hyers, T	MO	934
Pul	Kaye, M	MN	934
Pul	Krowka, M	MN	934
Pul	Levin, D	OK	938
Pul	Libby, D	NY	926
Pul	Mahler, D	NH	923
Pul	Marini, J	MN	934
Pul	Martin, R	CO	937
Pul	Matuschak, G	MO	935
Pul	Mosenifar, Z	CA	940
Pul	Perret, P	LA	938
Pul	Rennard, S	NE	937
Pul	Rochester, C	CT	924
Pul	Sahn, S	SC	932
Pul	Silver, M	IL	935
Pul	Staton, G	GA	932
Pul	Sutherland, E	CO	937
Pul	Tapson, V	NC	932
Pul	Thomashow, B	NY	928
Pul	Tino, G	PA	928
Pul	Tobin, M	IL	936
Pul	Villanueva, A	MA	924

Cleft Palate/Lip

Spec	Name	St	Pg
CG	Saal, H	OH	160
Oto	Senders, C	CA	686
PlS	Ascherman, J	NY	852
PlS	Baker, S	DC	852
PlS	Bauer, B	IL	864
PlS	Billmire, D	OH	864
PlS	Boyajian, M	DC	852

Spec	Name	St	Pg
PlS	Bradley, J	CA	873
PlS	Dagum, A	NY	853
PlS	Georgiade, G	NC	861
PlS	Glat, P	PA	854
PlS	Gruss, J	WA	874
PlS	Hoffman, W	CA	874
PlS	Kane, A	TX	870
PlS	Kelly, K	TN	862
PlS	Kirschner, R	OH	865
PlS	Losee, J	PA	855
PlS	Low, D	PA	855
PlS	Mackay, D	PA	856
PlS	Magee, W	VA	862
PlS	Marsh, J	MO	866
PlS	Matthews, D	NC	862
PlS	Meara, J	MA	850
PlS	Mulliken, J	MA	851
PlS	Napoli, J	DE	857
PlS	Neumeister, M	IL	867
PlS	Patel, P	IL	867
PlS	Seyfer, A	MD	858
PlS	Stotland, M	NH	851
PlS	Vander Kolk, C	MD	860
PlS	Wells, J	CA	877
PlS	Yu, J	GA	864
PO	Haddad, J	NY	790

Clinical Genetics

Spec	Name	St	Pg
CG	Andersson, H	LA	161
CG	Anyane-Yeboa, K	NY	156
CG	Bale, A	CT	156
CG	Bartholomew, D	OH	160
CG	Bialer, M	NY	157
CG	Bianchi, D	MA	156
CG	Boles, R	CA	162
CG	Burton, B	IL	160
CG	Carey, J	UT	161
CG	Cassidy, S	CA	162
CG	Cederbaum, S	CA	162
CG	Charrow, J	IL	160
CG	Craigen, W	TX	161
CG	Cunniff, C	AZ	161
CG	Curry, C	CA	162
CG	Davis, J	NY	157
CG	Desnick, R	NY	157
CG	Desposito, F	NJ	157
CG	Driscoll, D	FL	158
CG	Driscoll, D	PA	157
CG	Falk, R	CA	162
CG	Gilbert, F	NY	157
CG	Graham, J	CA	162
CG	Grody, W	CA	163
CG	Holmes, L	MA	156
CG	Hoyme, H	SD	161
CG	Hudgins, L	CA	163
CG	Jayakar, P	FL	159
CG	Jonas, A	CA	163
CG	Jones, M	CA	163
CG	Korf, B	AL	159
CG	Kronn, D	NY	157
CG	Mahoney, M	CT	156

Spec	Name	St	Pg
CG	Marion, R	NY	158
CG	Morris, C	NV	163
CG	Mulvihill, J	OK	161
CG	Northrup, H	TX	162
CG	Nussbaum, R	CA	163
CG	Ostrer, H	NY	158
CG	Pauker, S	MA	156
CG	Pergament, E	IL	160
CG	Plon, S	TX	162
CG	Pyeritz, R	PA	158
CG	Randolph, L	CA	163
CG	Rosenbaum, K	DC	158
CG	Saal, H	OH	160
CG	Saul, R	SC	159
CG	Seashore, M	CT	156
CG	Seaver, L	HI	163
CG	Shapiro, L	NY	158
CG	Shoffner, J	GA	159
CG	Shulman, L	IL	160
CG	Stevenson, R	SC	159
CG	Sutphen, R	FL	159
CG	Ward, J	TN	159
CG	Weaver, D	IN	160
CG	Weitzel, J	CA	164
CG	Whelan, A	MO	161
CG	Wilcox, W	CA	164
CG	Zackai, E	PA	158

Clinical Neurophysiology

Spec	Name	St	Pg
N	Bertorini, T	TN	520

Clinical Trials

Spec	Name	St	Pg
AdP	Anton, R	SC	905
ChiN	Santos, C	DC	148
D	Bowen, G	UT	196
D	Gottlieb, A	MA	183
EDM	Ahmann, A	OR	221
EDM	Brillon, D	NY	209
EDM	Riddle, M	OR	224
Ge	Gish, R	CA	254
Ge	Greenwald, B	MD	233
Ge	Hanauer, S	IL	245
Ge	Okolo, P	MD	237
GO	Chan, J	CA	289
GO	Cornelison, T	MD	277
GO	Coukos, G	PA	277
GO	Creasman, W	SC	280
GO	De Geest, K	IA	283
GO	Edwards, R	PA	277
GO	Ghamande, S	GA	281
GO	Moore, D	IN	284
GO	Odunsi, A	NY	279
GO	Stehman, F	IN	286
GO	Teng, N	CA	291
Hem	Djulbegovic, B	FL	316
Hem	Flynn, P	MN	319
Hem	Grever, M	OH	320
Hem	Komrokji, R	FL	317
Hem	Kraut, E	OH	320
Hem	Maslak, P	NY	313
Hem	Nademanee, A	CA	326

Spec	Name	St	Pg
Hem	O'Donnell, M	CA	327
Hem	Slease, R	DE	315
Hem	Streiff, M	MD	315
IC	Gibson, C	MA	126
IC	Kandzari, D	GA	130
IM	Fischl, M	FL	425
Inf	Mildvan, D	NY	412
Inf	Saag, M	AL	415
N	Albers, G	CA	535
N	Chamberlain, M	WA	535
N	Cummings, J	NV	536
N	Janss, A	GA	522
N	Lipton, R	NY	514
N	Mitsumoto, H	NY	516
N	Newton, H	OH	528
N	Pennell, P	MA	508
N	Wolinsky, J	TX	535
NS	Brem, S	PA	472
NS	Markert, J	AL	483
NS	Sampson, J	NC	484
NS	Shaffrey, M	VA	484
NS	Yu, J	CA	499
Onc	Abbruzzese, J	TX	376
Onc	Abraham, J	WV	333
Onc	Advani, R	CA	383
Onc	Akerley, W	UT	374
Onc	Arun, B	TX	377
Onc	Berlin, J	TN	353
Onc	Bernard, S	NC	353
Onc	Birrer, M	MA	327
Onc	Blackwell, K	NC	354
Onc	Blobe, G	NC	354
Onc	Bunn, P	CO	374
Onc	Burris, H	TN	354
Onc	Butler, W	SC	354
Onc	Carducci, M	MD	336
Onc	Chang, J	TX	378
Onc	Chapman, P	NY	336
Onc	Chu, E	PA	336
Onc	Cohen, R	PA	337
Onc	Disis, M	WA	385
Onc	Ellis, G	WA	385
Onc	Ensminger, W	MI	367
Onc	Estey, E	WA	385
Onc	Ettinger, D	MD	339
Onc	Fine, R	NY	339
Onc	Flaherty, K	MA	329
Onc	Friedberg, J	NY	340
Onc	Geyer, C	TX	378
Onc	Gold, P	WA	386
Onc	Haas, N	PA	341
Onc	Hauke, R	NE	375
Onc	Herbst, R	CT	330
Onc	Holcombe, R	NY	342
Onc	Hortobagyi, G	TX	379
Onc	Hwu, P	TX	379
Onc	Jahanzeb, M	FL	357
Onc	Jurcic, J	NY	343
Onc	Kaminski, M	MI	369
Onc	Karp, J	MD	343
Onc	Kaufman, P	NH	330
Onc	Kohn, E	MD	343

Spec	Name	St	Pg
Onc	Kraft, A	SC	358
Onc	Limentani, S	NC	359
Onc	Marcom, P	NC	359
Onc	Mortimer, J	CA	388
Onc	O'Connor, O	NY	346
Onc	O'Regan, R	GA	360
Onc	Orlowski, R	TX	380
Onc	Perez, E	FL	361
Onc	Perry, D	DC	347
Onc	Pinto, H	CA	389
Onc	Ready, N	NC	361
Onc	Remick, S	WV	348
Onc	Robert-Vizcarrondo, F	AL	361
Onc	Schuchter, L	PA	349
Onc	Serody, J	NC	362
Onc	Sikic, B	CA	390
Onc	Sotomayor, E	FL	362
Onc	Triozzi, P	OH	373
Onc	Tripathy, D	CA	391
Onc	Trump, D	NY	351
Onc	Vahdat, L	NY	351
Onc	Wolchok, J	NY	352
Onc	Wolff, R	TX	383
Onc	Worden, F	MI	373
Oto	Weisman, R	CA	687
Path	Wilczynski, S	CA	722
PEn	DiMeglio, L	IN	746
PGe	Dubinsky, M	CA	755
PHO	Adamson, P	PA	758
PHO	Blaney, S	TX	775
PHO	Bruggers, C	UT	774
PHO	Croop, J	IN	770
PHO	Cunningham, J	IL	770
PHO	Goldman, S	IL	771
PHO	Halligan, G	PA	760
PHO	Jakacki, R	PA	761
PHO	Kreissman, S	NC	767
PHO	Maris, J	PA	762
PHO	Neuberg, R	SC	767
PHO	Razzouk, B	IN	773
PHO	Rheingold, S	PA	763
PHO	Ritchey, A	PA	763
PHO	Rosenthal, J	CA	779
PHO	Santana, V	TN	768
PHO	van Hoff, J	NH	757
PInf	Bryson, Y	CA	784
PInf	Edwards, K	TN	781
PInf	Flynn, P	TN	782
PPul	Borowitz, D	NY	794
Psyc	Mann, J	NY	893
Psyc	Weisler, R	NC	896
Pul	Brown, K	CO	936
RadRO	Blackstock, A	NC	953
RadRO	Bogart, J	NY	948
RadRO	Bradley, J	MO	958
RadRO	Kupelian, P	CA	966
RadRO	Le, Q	CA	967
RadRO	McGarry, R	KY	956
RadRO	Senzer, N	TX	965
RadRO	Willett, C	NC	958
Rhu	Wofsy, D	CA	1034
S	Averbook, B	OH	1074

Spec	Name	St	Pg
S	Geller, D	PA	1058
S	Julian, T	PA	1059
S	Leeming, R	OH	1079
S	Lowy, A	CA	1097
S	Meric-Bernstam, F	TX	1091
S	Olson, J	MD	1061
S	Ramanathan, R	PA	1062
S	Sauter, E	ND	1086
S	Willey, S	DC	1066
S	Yang, J	MD	1066
T&CS	Pass, H	NY	1120
T&CS	Philpott, J	VA	1128
U	Keane, T	SC	1161
U	Moul, J	NC	1162
U	Shabsigh, R	NY	1157

Clinical Trials Only

Spec	Name	St	Pg
IM	Gillman, M	MA	424
Onc	Arlen, P	MD	334
Onc	Gulley, J	MD	341

Clostridium Difficile Disease

Spec	Name	St	Pg
Ge	Brandt, L	NY	231
Ge	La Mont, J	MA	229
Ge	Surawicz, C	WA	255

Clotting Disorders in Pregnancy

Spec	Name	St	Pg
MF	Paidas, M	CT	431

Clubfoot

Spec	Name	St	Pg
OrS	Aronson, J	AR	640
OrS	Beaty, J	TN	627
OrS	Davidson, R	PA	616
OrS	Herzenberg, J	MD	619
OrS	Morcuende, J	IA	636

Clubfoot/Foot Deformities in Children

Spec	Name	St	Pg
OrS	Hyman, J	NY	620
OrS	Oppenheim, W	CA	645

Coarctation of the Aorta

Spec	Name	St	Pg
PCd	Hijazi, Z	IL	739
PCd	Moskowitz, W	VA	737

Cocaine Addiction

Spec	Name	St	Pg
AdP	Kampman, K	PA	904
AdP	Kleber, H	NY	905
AdP	Kosten, T	TX	906

Coccidioidomycosis

Spec	Name	St	Pg
Inf	Bayer, A	CA	419
Pul	Catanzaro, A	CA	939

Cochlear Implants

Spec	Name	St	Pg
Oto	Arriaga, M	LA	681

Spec	Name	St	Pg
Oto	Arts, H	MI	672
Oto	Balkany, T	FL	667
Oto	Beatty, C	MN	673
Oto	Driscoll, C	MN	674
Oto	Gantz, B	IA	675
Oto	Hammerschlag, P	NY	660
Oto	Haynes, D	TN	668
Oto	Hirsch, B	PA	660
Oto	Hoffman, R	NY	660
Oto	Jenkins, H	CO	680
Oto	Kang, D	NE	680
Oto	Kveton, J	CT	656
Oto	Linstrom, C	NY	662
Oto	Lustig, L	CA	685
Oto	Macias, J	AZ	682
Oto	Mattox, D	GA	669
Oto	Miyamoto, R	IN	676
Oto	O'Leary, M	CA	686
Oto	Parisier, S	NY	663
Oto	Pillsbury, H	NC	670
Oto	Roland, J	NY	664
Oto	Rubinstein, J	WA	686
Oto	Shelton, C	UT	680
Oto	Telian, S	MI	678
Oto	Telischi, F	FL	671
Oto	Tucci, D	NC	672
Oto	Wackym, P	OR	687
Oto	Wiet, R	IL	678
Oto	Young, N	IL	679
PO	Arjmand, E	OH	791
PO	Kazahaya, K	PA	790
PO	Lusk, R	NE	792
PO	Poe, D	MA	789
PO	Rosbe, K	CA	793

Cognitive Impairment-Mild

Spec	Name	St	Pg
Psyc	Arnold, S	PA	890

Cognitive Impairment/Mild

Spec	Name	St	Pg
N	Petersen, R	MN	529

Cognitive Loss in Aging

Spec	Name	St	Pg
Ger	Raji, M	TX	266
GerPsy	Reisberg, B	NY	913

Cognitive Psychotherapy

Spec	Name	St	Pg
ChAP	Alessi, N	MI	910
Psyc	Eisendrath, S	CA	901
Psyc	Gabbard, G	TX	900

Cognitive Rehabilitation

Spec	Name	St	Pg
PHO	Lange, B	PA	762

Collagen Vascular Diseases

Spec	Name	St	Pg
D	Falanga, V	RI	182

Colon & Rectal Cancer

Spec	Name	St	Pg
CRS	Beart, R	CA	177

Specialty & Special Expertise Index

Spec	Name	St	Pg
CRS	Beck, D	LA	176
CRS	Birnbaum, E	MO	173
CRS	Bleday, R	MA	168
CRS	Church, J	OH	173
CRS	Delaney, C	OH	173
CRS	Dietz, D	OH	173
CRS	Efron, J	MD	169
CRS	Fleshman, J	MO	173
CRS	Foley, E	WI	174
CRS	Fry, R	PA	170
CRS	Galandiuk, S	KY	172
CRS	Goldstein, S	PA	170
CRS	Golub, R	FL	172
CRS	Guillem, J	NY	170
CRS	Haas, E	TX	177
CRS	Harnsberger, J	NH	168
CRS	Heppell, J	AZ	177
CRS	Hicks, T	LA	177
CRS	Huber, P	TX	177
CRS	Hyman, N	VT	168
CRS	Kodner, I	MO	174
CRS	Lavery, I	OH	174
CRS	Lederman, E	MO	174
CRS	Longo, W	CT	168
CRS	Madoff, R	MN	174
CRS	Marcet, J	FL	172
CRS	Medich, D	PA	170
CRS	Milsom, J	NY	171
CRS	Mutch, M	MO	174
CRS	Nagle, D	MA	168
CRS	Nelson, H	MN	175
CRS	Nogueras, J	FL	172
CRS	Orkin, B	MA	168
CRS	Pello, M	NJ	171
CRS	Pemberton, J	MN	175
CRS	Procaccino, J	NY	171
CRS	Rafferty, J	OH	175
CRS	Ramamoorthy, S	CA	178
CRS	Read, T	MA	169
CRS	Roberts, P	MA	169
CRS	Sands, L	FL	172
CRS	Schoetz, D	MA	169
CRS	Senagore, A	CA	178
CRS	Shah, N	RI	169
CRS	Shellito, P	MA	169
CRS	Stamos, M	CA	178
CRS	Steinhagen, R	NY	171
CRS	Stryker, S	IL	175
CRS	Thorson, A	NE	176
CRS	Trudel, J	MN	175
CRS	Vernava, A	FL	172
CRS	Welton, M	CA	178
CRS	Wexner, S	FL	173
CRS	Whelan, R	NY	171
CRS	Wolff, B	MN	176
CRS	Worsey, M	CA	178
Ge	Cohen, L	NY	232
Ge	Itzkowitz, S	NY	234
Hem	Flynn, P	MN	319
Onc	Blobe, G	NC	354
Onc	Brenin, C	VA	354
Onc	Chabner, B	MA	328

Spec	Name	St	Pg
Onc	Chu, E	PA	336
Onc	Conry, R	AL	355
Onc	Engstrom, P	PA	339
Onc	Ford, J	CA	386
Onc	Goldberg, R	OH	367
Onc	Grem, J	NE	375
Onc	Hageboutros, A	NJ	341
Onc	Hochster, H	CT	330
Onc	Ilson, D	NY	342
Onc	Krishnamurthi, S	OH	369
Onc	Lacy, J	CT	331
Onc	Markowitz, S	OH	369
Onc	Mayer, R	MA	331
Onc	Messersmith, W	CO	376
Onc	Northfelt, D	AZ	380
Onc	O'Brien, T	OH	370
Onc	Patt, Y	NM	381
Onc	Saif, M	MA	332
Onc	Saltz, L	NY	348
Onc	Steen, P	ND	376
Onc	Venook, A	CA	392
Onc	Willson, J	TX	382
Onc	Wolff, R	TX	383
PS	La Quaglia, M	NY	803
RadRO	Minsky, B	TX	965
RadRO	Rich, T	VA	957
RadRO	Thomas, C	OR	968
S	Beauchamp, R	TN	1067
S	Cance, W	NY	1055
S	Curley, S	TX	1087
S	Cusack, J	MA	1048
S	Ellis, L	TX	1088
S	Howe, J	IA	1078
S	Newman, E	NY	1061
S	Paty, P	NY	1062
S	Shibata, D	FL	1072
S	Sigurdson, E	PA	1064
S	Sinanan, M	WA	1100
S	Tanabe, K	MA	1052
S	Weber, S	WI	1084

Colon & Rectal Cancer & Surgery

Spec	Name	St	Pg
CRS	Geisler, D	PA	170
CRS	Ludwig, K	WI	174
CRS	Mantyh, C	NC	172
CRS	Remzi, F	OH	175
CRS	Sokol, T	CA	178
CRS	Stein, D	PA	171
CRS	Varma, A	CA	178
CRS	Wise, P	MO	175
S	Lieberman, M	NY	1060
S	Schraut, W	PA	1064
S	Zinner, M	MA	1052

Colon & Rectal Cancer Detection

Spec	Name	St	Pg
Ge	Boland, C	TX	250
Ge	Butterly, L	NH	228
Ge	Early, D	MO	245
Ge	Farraye, F	MA	228

Spec	Name	St	Pg
Ge	Itzkowitz, S	NY	234
Ge	Kastenberg, D	PA	234
Ge	Levine, J	CO	250
Ge	Pochapin, M	NY	237
Ge	Rex, D	IN	247
Ge	Scudera, P	VA	242
Ge	Smoot, D	TN	243

Colon & Rectal Cancer Risk

Spec	Name	St	Pg
CG	Whelan, A	MO	161

Colon & Rectal Cancer-Familial Polyposis

Spec	Name	St	Pg
CRS	Church, J	OH	173
CRS	Mantyh, C	NC	172
CRS	Procaccino, J	NY	171
CRS	Vernava, A	FL	172
Ge	Burt, R	UT	249
Ge	Butterly, L	NH	228
Ge	Chung, D	MA	228
Ge	Giardiello, F	MD	233
Ge	Hoffman, B	SC	240
S	Skibber, J	TX	1092

Colon & Rectal Cancer-Hereditary

Spec	Name	St	Pg
CRS	Gearhart, S	MD	170
CRS	Guillem, J	NY	170
CRS	Wise, P	MO	175

Colon & Rectal Surgery

Spec	Name	St	Pg
CRS	Abcarian, H	IL	173
CRS	Bailey, H	TX	176
CRS	Beart, R	CA	177
CRS	Beck, D	LA	176
CRS	Beck, S	KY	171
CRS	Birnbaum, E	MO	173
CRS	Blatchford, G	NE	176
CRS	Bleday, R	MA	168
CRS	Chiu, Y	CA	177
CRS	Church, J	OH	173
CRS	Coutsoftides, T	CA	177
CRS	Delaney, C	OH	173
CRS	Dietz, D	OH	173
CRS	Efron, J	MD	169
CRS	Eisenstat, T	NJ	169
CRS	Fleshman, J	MO	173
CRS	Foley, E	WI	174
CRS	Fry, R	PA	170
CRS	Galandiuk, S	KY	172
CRS	Gearhart, S	MD	170
CRS	Geisler, D	PA	170
CRS	Goldstein, S	PA	170
CRS	Golub, R	FL	172
CRS	Gorfine, S	NY	170
CRS	Guillem, J	NY	170
CRS	Haas, E	TX	177
CRS	Hackford, A	MA	168
CRS	Harnsberger, J	NH	168

Spec	Name	St	Pg
CRS	Hartmann, R	FL	172
CRS	Heppell, J	AZ	177
CRS	Hicks, T	LA	177
CRS	Huber, P	TX	177
CRS	Hyman, N	VT	168
CRS	Kodner, I	MO	174
CRS	Lavery, I	OH	174
CRS	Lederman, E	MO	174
CRS	Lee, P	OR	177
CRS	Longo, W	CT	168
CRS	Lowry, A	MN	174
CRS	Ludwig, K	WI	174
CRS	Madoff, R	MN	174
CRS	Mantyh, C	NC	172
CRS	Marcet, J	FL	172
CRS	Medich, D	PA	170
CRS	Milsom, J	NY	171
CRS	Mutch, M	MO	174
CRS	Nagle, D	MA	168
CRS	Nelson, H	MN	175
CRS	Nogueras, J	FL	172
CRS	Orkin, B	MA	168
CRS	Pello, M	NJ	171
CRS	Pemberton, J	MN	175
CRS	Procaccino, J	NY	171
CRS	Rafferty, J	OH	175
CRS	Ramamoorthy, S	CA	178
CRS	Read, T	MA	169
CRS	Remzi, F	OH	175
CRS	Roberts, P	MA	169
CRS	Saclarides, T	IL	175
CRS	Sands, L	FL	172
CRS	Schatz, L	CO	176
CRS	Schoetz, D	MA	169
CRS	Senagore, A	CA	178
CRS	Shah, N	RI	169
CRS	Shellito, P	MA	169
CRS	Sokol, T	CA	178
CRS	Stamos, M	CA	178
CRS	Stein, D	PA	171
CRS	Steinhagen, R	NY	171
CRS	Stryker, S	IL	175
CRS	Thorson, A	NE	176
CRS	Trudel, J	MN	175
CRS	Varma, M	CA	178
CRS	Vernava, A	FL	172
CRS	Welton, M	CA	178
CRS	Wexner, S	FL	173
CRS	Whelan, R	NY	171
CRS	Williams, S	ID	176
CRS	Wise, P	MO	175
CRS	Wolff, B	MN	176
CRS	Wong, R	HI	178
CRS	Worsey, M	CA	178
PS	Pena, A	OH	807
S	Baker, C	VA	1066
S	Franklin, M	TX	1088
S	Hebert, J	VT	1049
S	Horvath, K	WA	1096
S	Howerton, R	NC	1069

Colon Cancer

Spec	Name	St	Pg
CRS	Blatchford, G	NE	176
CRS	Eisenstat, T	NJ	169
CRS	Hartmann, R	FL	172
Ge	Burt, R	UT	249
Ge	Giardiello, F	MD	233
Ge	Goldberg, M	IL	245
Ge	Raju, G	TX	252
Ge	Waye, J	NY	238
Onc	Benson, A	IL	364
Onc	De Simone, P	KY	356
Onc	Donehower, R	MD	338
Onc	Doroshow, J	MD	338
Onc	Holland, J	NY	342
Onc	Hollister, D	CT	330
Onc	Kemeny, N	NY	343
Onc	Makhoul, I	AR	380
Onc	Meropol, N	OH	370
Onc	Nissenblatt, M	NJ	346
Onc	Pasche, B	AL	361
Onc	Posey, J	AL	361
Onc	Ryan, D	MA	331
Path	Morrow, J	CT	707
RadRO	Smalley, S	KS	963
S	Ballantyne, G	GA	1066
S	Bentley, F	AR	1087
S	Bland, K	AL	1067
S	Calvo, B	NC	1067
S	Edye, M	NY	1057
S	Lillemoe, K	MA	1050
S	Mansfield, P	TX	1091
S	Michelassi, F	NY	1060
S	Ramanathan, R	PA	1062
S	Saha, S	MI	1081
S	Salky, B	NY	1063

Colon Cancer Screening

Spec	Name	St	Pg
Ge	Albert, M	DC	230
Ge	Aronchick, C	PA	230
Ge	Borum, M	DC	231
Ge	Brazer, S	NC	239
Ge	Proctor, D	CT	230
Ge	Yanda, R	GA	243

Colonoscopy

Spec	Name	St	Pg
Ge	Aronchick, C	PA	230
Ge	Butterly, L	NH	228
Ge	Cello, J	CA	253
Ge	Chung, D	MA	228
Ge	Cohen, J	NY	231
Ge	Feldman, E	CA	253
Ge	Green, P	NY	233
Ge	Hoops, T	PA	234
Ge	Levine, J	CO	250
Ge	Lipshutz, W	PA	236
Ge	Meiselman, M	IL	247
Ge	Ostroff, J	CA	255
Ge	Savides, T	CA	255
Ge	Siegel, C	NH	230
Ge	Waye, J	NY	238

Spec	Name	St	Pg
Ge	Weinberg, D	PA	238

Colostomy Avoidance

Spec	Name	St	Pg
CRS	Steinhagen, R	NY	171

Complementary Medicine

Spec	Name	St	Pg
Cv	Goodman, D	NY	98
EDM	Dobs, A	MD	210
Ger	Bloom, P	NY	262
GO	Granai, C	RI	274
IM	Cirigliano, M	PA	424
IM	Galland, L	NY	424
Onc	Abrams, D	CA	383
Onc	Axelrod, R	PA	335
Onc	Rugo, H	CA	390
Oph	Ritch, R	NY	579
Ped	Zeltzer, L	CA	729
PHO	Rheingold, S	PA	763
PHO	Sencer, S	MN	773
PMR	Dillard, J	NY	835
U	Katz, A	NY	1154
U	Lowe, F	NY	1155

Complex Diagnosis

Spec	Name	St	Pg
ChiN	Bergman, I	PA	147
D	Jorizzo, J	NC	191
IM	Cope, D	CA	426
PCd	Mahony, L	TX	740
Ped	Zitelli, B	PA	727

Complex Regional Pain Syndromes

Spec	Name	St	Pg
N	Oaklander, A	MA	508
PM	Audell, L	CA	702
PM	Baumann, P	GA	698
PM	Benzon, H	IL	699
PM	Gharibo, C	NY	697
PM	Jain, S	NY	697
PM	Prager, J	CA	703
PM	Rauck, R	NC	699
PM	Richman, D	NY	698
PM	Rosenquist, R	OH	700
PM	Weisman, S	WI	700

Concussion

Spec	Name	St	Pg
N	Jordan, B	NY	512
PMR	Herring, S	WA	843

Congenital Absence of Vas Deferens

Spec	Name	St	Pg
U	Oates, R	MA	1150
U	Shaban, S	NC	1164

Congenital Anomalies

Spec	Name	St	Pg
NS	Mapstone, T	OK	494
PS	Arensman, R	IL	806
PS	Chwals, W	MA	801
PS	Dillon, P	MO	807

Spec	Name	St	Pg
PS	Foglia, R	TX	809
PS	Grikscheit, T	CA	810
PS	Healey, P	WA	810
PS	Holterman, M	IL	807
PS	McGill, L	AZ	809
PS	Morgan, W	TN	805
PS	Moss, R	OH	807
PS	Nance, M	PA	804
PS	Reynolds, M	IL	808
PS	Sato, T	WI	808
PS	Spigland, N	NY	804
PS	Stylianos, S	NY	804
PS	Waldhausen, J	WA	811
T&CS	Ilbawi, M	IL	1132

Congenital Anomalies-Gastrointestinal

Spec	Name	St	Pg
PS	Alexander, F	NJ	802

Congenital Anomalies-Genitourinary

Spec	Name	St	Pg
PNep	Zilleruelo, G	FL	787

Congenital Anomalies-Gynecologic

Spec	Name	St	Pg
ObG	Laufer, M	MA	556
ObG	Merritt, D	MO	562
ObG	Pfeifer, S	PA	558

Congenital Anomalies-Limb

Spec	Name	St	Pg
CG	Hudgins, L	CA	163

Congenital Anomalies-Orthopaedic

Spec	Name	St	Pg
OrS	Pizzutillo, P	PA	624

Congenital Breast Anomalies

Spec	Name	St	Pg
PlS	Nichter, L	CA	875

Congenital Cranial Deformities

Spec	Name	St	Pg
NS	Luerssen, T	TX	493
NS	Sun, P	CA	499

Congenital Eye Disorders-Rare

Spec	Name	St	Pg
Oph	Masket, S	CA	602
Oph	Miller, K	CA	602

Congenital Fibrosis-Extraocular Muscles

Spec	Name	St	Pg
Oph	Hunter, D	MA	570

Congenital Hand Deformities

Spec	Name	St	Pg
HS	Godzik, C	CA	304
HS	Grossman, J	FL	299
HS	Kleinman, W	IN	301
HS	Kozin, S	PA	296

Spec	Name	St	Pg
HS	Mih, A	IN	301

Congenital Heart Disease

Spec	Name	St	Pg
Cv	Byrd, B	TN	103
Cv	Connolly, H	MN	107
Cv	Fuster, V	NY	98
Cv	Kuvin, J	MA	95
DR	Flamm, S	OH	980
IC	Bailey, S	TX	132
IC	Smalling, R	TX	132
PCCM	Easley, R	TX	742
PCd	Agarwala, B	IL	738
PCd	Bernstein, D	CA	740
PCd	Biancaniello, T	NY	734
PCd	Bierman, F	NY	734
PCd	Brenner, J	MD	734
PCd	Caldwell, R	IN	738
PCd	Cetta, F	MN	738
PCd	Cooper, R	NY	734
PCd	Dick, M	MI	738
PCd	Dreyer, W	TX	740
PCd	Epstein, M	FL	737
PCd	Feltes, T	OH	739
PCd	Hanna, B	PA	735
PCd	Hijazi, Z	IL	739
PCd	Mahony, L	TX	740
PCd	Newburger, J	MA	734
PCd	Pahl, E	IL	739
PCd	Parness, I	NY	735
PCd	Rocchini, A	MI	739
PCd	Rogers, J	TX	740
PCd	Rome, J	PA	736
PCd	Rychik, J	PA	736
PCd	Sommer, R	NY	736
PCd	Teitel, D	CA	741
PCd	Velvis, H	NY	736
PCd	Walsh, C	NY	736
PCd	Zahn, E	CA	741
T&CS	Brown, J	IN	1131
T&CS	Chen, J	NY	1114
T&CS	Del-Nido, P	MA	1110
T&CS	Ilbawi, M	IL	1132
T&CS	Jonas, R	DC	1118
T&CS	Kopf, G	CT	1111
T&CS	Laks, H	CA	1142
T&CS	Mavroudis, C	FL	1126
T&CS	Merrick, S	CA	1142
T&CS	Schaff, H	MN	1134
T&CS	Tedder, M	TN	1130
T&CS	Turrentine, M	IN	1135
T&CS	Ziemer, G	IL	1136

Congenital Heart Disease-Adult

Spec	Name	St	Pg
CE	Mehta, D	NY	121
Cv	Bashore, T	NC	103
Cv	Johnson, A	CA	117
Cv	McPherson, D	TX	114
Cv	Webb, G	OH	112
Cv	Wells, G	NC	106
IC	Carroll, J	CO	132
PCd	Cetta, F	MN	738

Spec	Name	St	Pg
PCd	Fish, F	TN	737
PCd	Hoyer, M	IN	739
T&CS	Backer, C	IL	1130
T&CS	Ilbawi, M	IL	1132
T&CS	Spray, T	PA	1122
T&CS	Verrier, E	WA	1143

Congenital Heart Disease-Adult & Child

Spec	Name	St	Pg
DR	White, R	OH	981
PCd	Beerman, L	PA	734
PCd	Bricker, J	TX	740
PCd	Cheatham, J	OH	738
PCd	Colvin, E	AL	737
PCd	Crosson, J	MD	735
PCd	Hardin, J	IL	739
PCd	Latson, L	FL	737
PCd	Moodie, D	TX	740
PCd	Moskowitz, W	VA	737
PCd	Radtke, W	DE	735

Congenital Heart Surgery

Spec	Name	St	Pg
PS	Bove, E	MI	807
T&CS	Bacha, E	NY	1114
T&CS	Bailey, L	CA	1140
T&CS	Bichell, D	TN	1123
T&CS	Burke, R	FL	1124
T&CS	Calhoon, J	TX	1137
T&CS	Campbell, D	CO	1136
T&CS	Christian, K	TN	1124
T&CS	Delius, R	MI	1131
T&CS	Drinkwater, D	TN	1125
T&CS	Fraser, C	TX	1138
T&CS	Gaynor, J	PA	1116
T&CS	Lamberti, J	CA	1142
T&CS	Mayer, J	MA	1111
T&CS	Mitchell, M	CO	1137
T&CS	Rosenkranz, E	FL	1129
T&CS	Ungerleider, R	NC	1130
T&CS	Warner, K	MA	1113
T&CS	Wells, W	CA	1143

Congenital Hemolytic Anemia

Spec	Name	St	Pg
PHO	Wolfe, L	NY	764

Congenital Hyperinsulinism

Spec	Name	St	Pg
PS	Adzick, N	PA	802

Congenital Infections

Spec	Name	St	Pg
PInf	Emmanuel, P	FL	781

Congenital Kidney Disease

Spec	Name	St	Pg
PNep	Fouser, L	WA	788

Congenital Limb Deformities

Spec	Name	St	Pg
HS	Peljovich, A	GA	299
HS	Rayan, G	OK	303

Spec	Name	St	Pg

Congenital Nervous System Malformations

NS	Ellenbogen, R	WA	496
NS	Greene, C	LA	492
NS	Myseros, J	VA	483

Congenital Neutropenia-Severe

PHO	Boxer, L	MI	769

Congenital Reproductive Anomalies

PS	Graziano, K	AZ	809

Congestive Heart Failure

Cv	Brozena, S	PA	97
Cv	Eisen, H	PA	98
Cv	Elkayam, U	CA	116
Cv	Fishbein, D	WA	116
Cv	Fonarow, G	CA	116
Cv	Geltman, E	MO	108
Cv	Jessup, M	PA	100
Cv	Johnson, A	CA	117
Cv	Johnson, M	WI	109
Cv	Kereiakes, D	OH	109
Cv	Kirshenbaum, J	MA	95
Cv	Kobashigawa, J	CA	117
Cv	Lewis, S	OR	117
Cv	Liang, B	CT	95
Cv	Lindenfeld, J	CO	113
Cv	Massin, E	TX	114
Cv	Moran, J	IL	109
Cv	O'Connell, J	GA	105
Cv	Rahko, P	WI	110
Cv	Reis, S	PA	101
Cv	Rogers, J	NC	105
Cv	Schwartz, W	NY	101
Cv	Smart, F	LA	115
Cv	Thames, M	AZ	115
Cv	Wagoner, L	OH	112
Cv	Walsh, M	IN	112
PCd	Mahony, L	TX	740

Conjoined Twins

NP	Muraskas, J	IL	451
PlS	Leighton, W	AZ	871
PS	Strauch, E	MD	804

Connective Tissue Disorders

CG	Cassidy, S	CA	162
D	Werth, V	PA	189
Rhu	Chatham, W	AL	1029
Rhu	Oddis, C	PA	1027
Rhu	Paget, S	NY	1027
Rhu	Silver, R	SC	1030

Constipation

CRS	Sokol, T	CA	178
Ge	Korsten, M	NY	235

Spec	Name	St	Pg
Ge	Rao, S	GA	242
Ge	Wald, A	WI	249
PGe	Bishop, W	IA	752

Contact Dermatitis

D	Belsito, D	NY	184
D	DeLeo, V	NY	186
D	Elmets, C	AL	190
D	James, W	PA	187
D	Sherertz, E	SC	192

Continent Urinary Diversions

U	Bahnson, R	OH	1165
U	Benson, M	NY	1151
U	Hall, S	NY	1153
U	Kozlowski, J	IL	1168
U	Sagalowsky, A	TX	1174

Cornea & External Eye Disease

Oph	Abbott, R	CA	598
Oph	Carlson, A	NC	582
Oph	Mannis, M	CA	602
Oph	Mondino, B	CA	602
Oph	Perez, V	FL	586

Cornea Transplant

Oph	Afshari, N	NC	581
Oph	Carlson, A	NC	582
Oph	Florakis, G	NY	574
Oph	Forster, R	FL	583
Oph	Gibralter, R	NY	574
Oph	Goldberg, D	NJ	574
Oph	Hersh, P	NJ	575
Oph	Maguire, L	MN	592
Oph	Manche, E	CA	602
Oph	McDonnell, P	MD	577
Oph	Perez, V	FL	586
Oph	Shamie, N	CA	604
Oph	Steinert, R	CA	604

Cornea Transplant & Artificial Cornea

Oph	Alfonso, E	FL	581
Oph	John, T	IL	590
Oph	Mannis, M	CA	602

Corneal & External Eye Disease

Oph	Culbertson, W	FL	582
Oph	Dhaliwal, D	PA	573
Oph	Irvine, J	CA	601
Oph	Lass, J	OH	591
Oph	Mathers, W	OR	602
Oph	McCulley, J	TX	597
Oph	O'Brien, T	FL	585
Oph	Pepose, J	MO	593

Corneal Disease

Oph	Durrie, D	KS	596

Spec	Name	St	Pg
Oph	Feder, R	IL	589
Oph	Florakis, G	NY	574
Oph	Foster, C	MA	570
Oph	Holland, E	OH	590
Oph	Krueger, R	OH	591
Oph	Lindstrom, R	MN	591
Oph	Mandel, E	NY	577
Oph	McDonnell, P	MD	577
Oph	Pflugfelder, S	TX	597
Oph	Rapuano, C	PA	579
Oph	Smith, R	CA	604
Oph	Solomon, K	SC	586
Oph	Steinert, R	CA	604
Oph	Wang, M	TN	587
Oph	Wilson, O	OH	595

Corneal Disease & Surgery

Oph	Alfonso, E	FL	581
Oph	Boxer Wachler, B	CA	599
Oph	Gibralter, R	NY	574
Oph	Katowitz, J	PA	576
Oph	Mackool, R	NY	577
Oph	Orlin, S	PA	578
Oph	Schein, O	MD	579
Oph	Updegraff, S	FL	587

Corneal Disease & Transplant

Oph	Cykiert, R	NY	572
Oph	Dana, R	MA	570
Oph	Gorovoy, M	FL	583
Oph	Stark, W	MD	580
Oph	Stulting, R	GA	586

Corneal Disease-Pediatric

Oph	Medow, N	NY	577

Coronary Angioplasty/Stents

CE	Cohen, M	NY	120
Cv	Chizner, M	FL	103
Cv	Kereiakes, D	OH	109
Cv	Konstam, M	MA	95
Cv	Rosenbush, S	IL	110
IC	Knopf, W	GA	130
IC	Lasala, J	MO	131
IC	Parikh, M	NY	128
IC	Petrossian, G	NY	128
IC	Roubin, G	NY	128
IC	Sacchi, T	NY	128
IC	Schreiber, T	MI	131
IC	Teirstein, P	CA	133

Coronary Artery Disease

Cv	Alpert, J	AZ	113
Cv	Bass, T	FL	103
Cv	Blumenthal, D	NY	96
Cv	Bonow, R	IL	106
Cv	Borzak, S	FL	103
Cv	Burket, M	OH	106
Cv	Califf, R	NC	103

Specialty & Special Expertise Index

Spec	Name	St	Pg
Cv	Cerqueira, M	OH	107
Cv	Chizner, M	FL	103
Cv	Dichek, D	WA	116
Cv	Diver, D	CT	94
Cv	Fintel, D	IL	107
Cv	French, W	CA	117
Cv	Fuster, V	NY	98
Cv	Inra, L	NY	99
Cv	Iskandrian, A	AL	104
Cv	Kaul, S	OR	117
Cv	Kirshenbaum, J	MA	95
Cv	Klein, L	IL	109
Cv	Kostis, J	NJ	100
Cv	Landzberg, J	NJ	100
Cv	Loscalzo, J	MA	95
Cv	Massin, E	TX	114
Cv	Mehlman, D	IL	109
Cv	Moran, J	IL	109
Cv	O'Gara, P	MA	95
Cv	Pepine, C	FL	105
Cv	Phillips, R	MA	96
Cv	Poon, M	NY	101
Cv	Powers, E	SC	105
Cv	Reiss, C	MO	110
Cv	Ridker, P	MA	96
Cv	Rihal, C	MN	110
Cv	Rosenbush, S	IL	110
Cv	Schwartz, W	NY	101
Cv	Shah, P	CA	118
Cv	Smith, S	NC	106
Cv	Stainback, R	TX	115
Cv	Tenenbaum, J	NY	102
Cv	Thames, M	AZ	115
Cv	Williams, E	IN	112
Cv	Williams, K	MI	113
Cv	Zusman, R	MA	96
IC	Bailey, S	TX	132
IC	Carroll, J	CO	132
IC	Douglas, J	GA	129
IC	Gray, W	NY	127
IC	Lasala, J	MO	131
IC	Smalling, R	TX	132
IC	Stone, G	NY	129
IC	Yeung, A	CA	133
NuM	Schelbert, H	CA	551

Coronary Artery Surgery

Spec	Name	St	Pg
T&CS	Acker, M	PA	1113
T&CS	Akins, C	MA	1110
T&CS	Aklog, L	AZ	1137
T&CS	Argenziano, M	NY	1113
T&CS	Boyd, W	CA	1140
T&CS	Caskey, M	AZ	1137
T&CS	Conte, J	MD	1114
T&CS	Damiano, R	MO	1131
T&CS	Fontana, G	NY	1115
T&CS	Galloway, A	NY	1116
T&CS	Graver, L	NY	1117
T&CS	Guyton, R	GA	1125
T&CS	Harken, A	CA	1141
T&CS	Isom, O	NY	1117
T&CS	Krieger, K	NY	1119
T&CS	Kron, I	VA	1126
T&CS	Lansman, S	NY	1119
T&CS	Lazar, H	MA	1111
T&CS	Lytle, B	OH	1133
T&CS	McCarthy, P	IL	1133
T&CS	McGiffin, D	AL	1126
T&CS	Morris, R	PA	1120
T&CS	Ott, D	TX	1139
T&CS	Pagani, F	MI	1134
T&CS	Quintessenza, J	FL	1128
T&CS	Salerno, T	FL	1129
T&CS	Sellke, F	RI	1112
T&CS	Smith, P	NC	1129
T&CS	Swistel, D	NY	1122
T&CS	Toyoda, Y	PA	1122
T&CS	Tranbaugh, R	NY	1122
T&CS	Trento, A	CA	1143
T&CS	Turner, W	TX	1140

Coronary Disease in Black Populations

Spec	Name	St	Pg
Cv	Saunders, E	MD	101

Coronary Revascularization

Spec	Name	St	Pg
T&CS	Merrick, S	CA	1142

Coronary Syndrome-Acute

Spec	Name	St	Pg
Cv	Klein, L	IL	109

Cosmetic & Reconstructive Surgery

Spec	Name	St	Pg
Oph	Ahmad, A	IL	588
PlS	Low, D	PA	855
PlS	Puckett, C	MO	867

Cosmetic & Reconstructive Surgery-Face

Spec	Name	St	Pg
Oto	Branham, G	MO	673
Oto	Graham, H	LA	682
Oto	Mangat, D	KY	669

Cosmetic Dermatology

Spec	Name	St	Pg
D	Arndt, K	MA	182
D	Avram, M	NY	184
D	Brandt, F	NY	185
D	Brody, H	GA	189
D	Crutchfield, C	MN	193
D	Dover, J	MA	182
D	Fewkes, J	MA	183
D	Fitzpatrick, R	CA	198
D	Geronemus, R	NY	186
D	Glogau, R	CA	199
D	Gordon, M	NY	186
D	Greenbaum, S	PA	186
D	Grimes, P	CA	199
D	Grossman, M	NY	186
D	Hanke, C	IN	193
D	Kilmer, S	CA	199
D	Lask, G	CA	199
D	Linder, J	AZ	197
D	Menter, M	TX	197
D	Neel, V	MA	184
D	Rigel, D	NY	188
D	Rubin, M	CA	200
D	Schultz, N	NY	188
D	Sobel, S	FL	192
D	Sokoloff, D	FL	192
D	Swanson, N	OR	200
D	Wheeland, R	AZ	198

Cosmetic Surgery

Spec	Name	St	Pg
D	Hruza, G	MO	193
D	Kriegel, D	NY	187
PlS	Ascherman, J	NY	852
PlS	Barone, C	TX	869
PlS	Grossman, J	CO	869
PlS	Hagan, K	TN	862
PlS	Hultman, C	NC	862
PlS	Isik, F	WA	874
PlS	Morgan, R	VA	863
PlS	Persing, J	CT	851
PlS	Serletti, J	PA	858
PlS	Taub, P	NY	859
PlS	Ting, J	NY	859
PlS	Tobin, G	KY	863
PlS	Vasconez, H	KY	864
PlS	Vogt, P	MN	868
PlS	Wilhelmi, B	KY	864
PlS	Wolfe, S	FL	864

Cosmetic Surgery-Breast

Spec	Name	St	Pg
PlS	Aston, S	NY	852
PlS	Barone, C	TX	869
PlS	Barton, F	TX	869
PlS	Bucky, L	PA	853
PlS	Burns, A	TX	870
PlS	Byrd, H	TX	870
PlS	Colen, L	VA	861
PlS	Da Lio, A	CA	873
PlS	Davis, G	NC	861
PlS	Dick, G	MD	853
PlS	Erdmann, D	NC	861
PlS	Eriksson, E	MA	850
PlS	Evans, G	CA	873
PlS	Fisher, G	CA	873
PlS	Fodor, P	CA	874
PlS	Grotting, J	AL	861
PlS	Hagan, K	TN	862
PlS	Hammond, D	MI	865
PlS	Hardesty, R	CA	874
PlS	Herman, C	PA	854
PlS	Hidalgo, D	NY	854
PlS	Horowitz, J	CA	874
PlS	Isik, F	WA	874
PlS	Jewell, M	OR	875
PlS	Kenkel, J	TX	870
PlS	Leaf, N	CA	875
PlS	Leipziger, L	NY	855

Specialty & Special Expertise Index

Spec	Name	St	Pg
PlS	Lesavoy, M	CA	875
PlS	Maxwell, G	TN	863
PlS	Medalie, D	OH	866
PlS	Metzinger, S	LA	871
PlS	Moses, M	LA	871
PlS	Mustoe, T	IL	866
PlS	Ness, J	MN	867
PlS	Nichter, L	CA	875
PlS	Paul, M	CA	876
PlS	Rand, R	WA	876
PlS	Romano, J	CA	876
PlS	Rosenberg, H	CA	876
PlS	Singer, R	CA	877
PlS	Slezak, S	MD	858
PlS	Stevens, W	CA	877
PlS	Sullivan, P	RI	851
PlS	Sultan, M	NY	859
PlS	Tebbetts, J	TX	872
PlS	Vander Kolk, C	MD	860
PlS	Wilcox, R	TX	872

Cosmetic Surgery-Eyes

Spec	Name	St	Pg
Oph	Stefanyszyn, M	PA	580

Cosmetic Surgery-Face

Spec	Name	St	Pg
Oto	Becker, F	FL	667
Oto	Denenberg, S	NE	680
Oto	Hopping, S	DC	660
Oto	Johnson, C	LA	682
Oto	Keller, G	CA	685
Oto	Larrabee, W	WA	685
Oto	Moe, K	WA	686
Oto	Papel, I	MD	663
Oto	Ries, W	TN	670
Oto	Spiegel, J	MA	657
Oto	Szachowicz, E	MN	678
Oto	Toriumi, D	IL	678
PlS	Baker, D	NY	852
PlS	Baker, S	DC	852
PlS	Bartlett, S	PA	852
PlS	Barton, F	TX	869
PlS	Bradley, J	CA	873
PlS	Bucky, L	PA	853
PlS	Burns, A	TX	870
PlS	Burstein, F	GA	860
PlS	Byrd, H	TX	870
PlS	Carraway, J	VA	860
PlS	Cederna, P	MI	865
PlS	Chiu, D	NY	853
PlS	Cohen, S	CA	873
PlS	Colen, L	VA	861
PlS	Constantian, M	NH	850
PlS	Da Lio, A	CA	873
PlS	Dick, G	MD	853
PlS	Dufresne, C	MD	854
PlS	Evans, G	CA	873
PlS	Fisher, G	CA	873
PlS	Fox, J	PA	854
PlS	Gregory, R	FL	861
PlS	Hamra, S	TX	870
PlS	Herman, C	PA	854

Spec	Name	St	Pg
PlS	Hester, T	GA	862
PlS	Hidalgo, D	NY	854
PlS	Hoffman, L	NY	854
PlS	Horowitz, J	CA	874
PlS	Hurwitz, D	PA	854
PlS	Imber, G	NY	854
PlS	Jewell, M	OR	875
PlS	Kenkel, J	TX	870
PlS	Koplin, L	CA	875
PlS	Little, J	DC	855
PlS	Mackay, D	PA	856
PlS	Manson, P	MD	856
PlS	Mast, B	FL	862
PlS	Matthews, D	NC	862
PlS	Maxwell, G	TN	863
PlS	McCarthy, J	NY	856
PlS	Metzinger, S	LA	871
PlS	Miller, T	CA	875
PlS	Moses, M	LA	871
PlS	Mustoe, T	IL	866
PlS	Nahabedian, M	DC	856
PlS	Ness, J	MN	867
PlS	Noone, R	PA	857
PlS	Ousterhout, D	CA	876
PlS	Papay, F	OH	867
PlS	Pitman, G	NY	857
PlS	Posnick, J	MD	857
PlS	Rand, R	WA	876
PlS	Rappaport, N	TX	871
PlS	Ristow, B	CA	876
PlS	Rohrich, R	TX	872
PlS	Rosenberg, H	CA	876
PlS	Siebert, J	WI	868
PlS	Singer, R	CA	877
PlS	Slavin, S	MA	851
PlS	Spinelli, H	NY	858
PlS	Staffenberg, D	NY	859
PlS	Stevens, W	CA	877
PlS	Sullivan, P	RI	851
PlS	Sultan, M	NY	859
PlS	Tabbal, N	NY	859
PlS	Thaller, S	FL	863
PlS	Thorne, C	NY	859
PlS	Vander Kolk, C	MD	860
PlS	Walton, R	IL	868
PlS	Wilcox, R	TX	872
PlS	Zins, J	OH	869

Cosmetic Surgery-Face & Body

Spec	Name	St	Pg
PlS	Aston, S	NY	852
PlS	Grotting, J	AL	861
PlS	Hardesty, R	CA	874
PlS	Markowitz, B	CA	875
PlS	Nichter, L	CA	875
PlS	Rose, E	NY	858

Cosmetic Surgery-Face & Breast

Spec	Name	St	Pg
PlS	Beals, S	AZ	870
PlS	Meltzer, T	AZ	871
PlS	Olding, M	DC	857
PlS	Price, G	MD	857

Spec	Name	St	Pg
PlS	Schusterman, M	TX	872
PlS	Singh, N	MD	858

Cosmetic Surgery-Face & Eyes

Spec	Name	St	Pg
Oph	Anderson, R	UT	595
Oph	McCann, R	UT	596
Oph	Putterman, A	IL	593
PlS	Leipziger, L	NY	855
PlS	Matarasso, A	NY	856

Cosmetic Surgery-Face & Neck

Spec	Name	St	Pg
Oto	Baker, S	MI	673
Oto	Gliklich, R	MA	655
PlS	Feldman, J	MA	850
PlS	Leaf, N	CA	875
PlS	Lesavoy, M	CA	875
PlS	Marten, T	CA	875
PlS	Paul, M	CA	876
PlS	Stuzin, J	FL	863

Cosmetic Surgery-Head & Neck

Spec	Name	St	Pg
PlS	Urata, M	CA	877

Cough

Spec	Name	St	Pg
Oto	Aviv, J	NY	657
Pul	Deitz, J	PA	925
Pul	Irwin, R	MA	923
Pul	Nash, T	NY	926

Cough-Chronic

Spec	Name	St	Pg
PO	Holinger, L	IL	791
PPul	Rubin, B	VA	796
PPul	Sherman, J	VA	796

Craniocervical Disorders

Spec	Name	St	Pg
NS	Menezes, A	IA	488

Craniofacial Disorders

Spec	Name	St	Pg
CG	Graham, J	CA	162
CG	Jones, M	CA	163
CG	Saal, H	OH	160

Craniofacial Surgery

Spec	Name	St	Pg
NS	Danielpour, M	CA	496
NS	Duhaime, A	MA	470
NS	Origitano, T	MT	491
NS	Pollack, I	PA	478
NS	Sklar, F	TX	494
Oto	Chowdhury, K	CO	679
PlS	Ascherman, J	NY	852
PlS	Barone, C	TX	869
PlS	Beals, S	AZ	870
PlS	Boyajian, M	DC	852
PlS	Buchman, S	MI	865
PlS	Deleyiannis, F	CO	869
PlS	Dufresne, C	MD	854
PlS	Glat, P	PA	854

Specialty & Special Expertise Index

Spec	Name	St	Pg
PlS	Hoffman, W	CA	874
PlS	Kane, A	TX	870
PlS	Kelly, K	TN	862
PlS	Kirschner, R	OH	865
PlS	Mackay, D	PA	856
PlS	Magee, W	VA	862
PlS	Ousterhout, D	CA	876
PlS	Patel, P	IL	867
PlS	Persing, J	CT	851
PlS	Polley, J	IL	867
PlS	Taub, P	NY	859
PlS	Thorne, C	NY	859
PlS	Yu, J	GA	864

Craniofacial Surgery-Pediatric

Spec	Name	St	Pg
PlS	Buchman, S	MI	865
PlS	Burstein, F	GA	860
PlS	Cohen, S	CA	873
PlS	McCarthy, J	NY	856
PlS	Meara, J	MA	850
PlS	Napoli, J	DE	857
PlS	Stotland, M	NH	851
PlS	Urata, M	CA	877

Craniofacial Surgery/Reconstruction

Spec	Name	St	Pg
NS	Walsh, J	LA	495
Oto	Costantino, P	NY	658
PlS	Baker, S	DC	852
PlS	Bartlett, S	PA	852
PlS	Cohen, S	CA	873
PlS	Losee, J	PA	855
PlS	Markowitz, B	CA	875
PlS	Marsh, J	MO	866
PlS	Matthews, D	NC	862
PlS	Papay, F	OH	867
PlS	Posnick, J	MD	857
PlS	Spinelli, H	NY	858
PlS	Staffenberg, D	NY	859
PlS	Tufaro, A	MD	860
PlS	Vander Kolk, C	MD	860
PlS	Vasconez, H	KY	864
PlS	Wolfe, S	FL	864

Craniosynostosis

Spec	Name	St	Pg
CG	Zackai, E	PA	158
NS	Dias, M	PA	473
NS	Jimenez, D	TX	493
NS	Shuer, L	CA	499

Cranofacial Surgery/Reconstruction

Spec	Name	St	Pg
PlS	Rodriguez, E	MD	857

Creutzfeldt-Jakob Disease (CJD)

Spec	Name	St	Pg
Path	Gambetti, P	OH	715

Critical Care

Spec	Name	St	Pg
Inf	Maki, D	WI	416
Inf	Masur, H	MD	412
MF	Besinger, R	IL	436
MF	Norwitz, E	MA	430
N	Becker, K	WA	535
N	Gress, D	VA	521
N	Suarez, J	TX	534
NP	Gross, I	CT	446
PCCM	Anand, K	TN	741
PCCM	Sarnaik, A	MI	742
PCCM	Thompson, A	PA	741
PM	Berde, C	MA	696
PPul	Kurachek, S	MN	797
PS	Gaines, B	PA	803
PS	Karrer, F	CO	808
PS	Reynolds, M	IL	808
PS	Tuggle, D	OK	810
Pul	Albertson, T	CA	938
Pul	Arroliga, A	TX	938
Pul	Bellamy, P	CA	939
Pul	Christman, B	TN	930
Pul	Cooke, J	NY	925
Pul	Criner, G	PA	925
Pul	Donahoe, M	PA	925
Pul	Gerboth, G	AK	939
Pul	Greenberg, H	NY	925
Pul	Hall, J	IL	933
Pul	Harman, E	FL	931
Pul	Heffner, J	OR	939
Pul	Ingbar, D	MN	934
Pul	Irwin, R	MA	923
Pul	Kaplan, J	KS	937
Pul	King, E	PA	926
Pul	LoRusso, T	VA	931
Pul	Marini, J	MN	934
Pul	Martinez, F	MI	934
Pul	Nelson, J	NY	926
Pul	O'Donnell, A	DC	927
Pul	Popovich, J	MI	935
Pul	Rizk, N	CA	940
Pul	Steiger, D	NY	928
Pul	Tharratt, R	CA	941
Pul	Vaughey, E	VA	932
Pul	Wheeler, A	TN	932
S	Barie, P	NY	1053
S	Buchman, T	GA	1067
S	Burke, P	MA	1048
S	Cioffi, W	RI	1048
S	Cohen, M	PA	1055
S	Cushing, B	ME	1048
S	Deitch, E	NJ	1056
S	Friese, R	AZ	1088
S	Gupta, R	NH	1049
S	Lentz, C	NM	1090
S	Luterman, A	AL	1070
S	McIntyre, R	CO	1085
S	Potenza, B	CA	1098
S	Rhee, P	AZ	1092
S	Weigelt, J	WI	1084
S	Winchell, R	ME	1052

Spec	Name	St	Pg
S	Yurt, R	NY	1066

Crohn's Disease

Spec	Name	St	Pg
CRS	Lederman, E	MO	174
CRS	Marcet, J	FL	172
CRS	Milsom, J	NY	171
CRS	Rafferty, J	OH	175
CRS	Roberts, P	MA	169
CRS	Vernava, A	FL	172
CRS	Welton, M	CA	178
CRS	Wolff, B	MN	176
Ge	Abreu, M	FL	239
Ge	Di Marino, A	PA	232
Ge	Hanauer, S	IL	245
Ge	Isaacs, K	NC	240
Ge	Lichtenstein, G	PA	236
Ge	Loftus, E	MN	247
Ge	Magun, A	NY	236
Ge	Plevy, S	NC	241
Ge	Sandborn, W	CA	255
Ge	Scherl, E	NY	238
Ge	Siegel, C	NH	230
Ge	Targan, S	CA	255
Ge	Young, R	NE	250
PGe	Baldassano, R	PA	750
PGe	Dubinsky, M	CA	755
PGe	Spivak, W	NY	751
S	Michelassi, F	NY	1060

Cross Cultural Psychiatry

Spec	Name	St	Pg
ChAP	McKelvey, R	OR	912
Psyc	Pi, E	CA	902

Cryoglobulinemia

Spec	Name	St	Pg
Rhu	Gorevic, P	NY	1026

CT Body Scan

Spec	Name	St	Pg
DR	Erasmus, J	TX	982
DR	Fishman, E	MD	975
DR	Megibow, A	NY	976
DR	Parsons, R	PA	977
DR	Weinreb, J	CT	973

CT Chest Scan

Spec	Name	St	Pg
DR	Black, W	NH	973

CT Colonography

Spec	Name	St	Pg
DR	Fidler, J	MN	980

CT Scan

Spec	Name	St	Pg
DR	Cohen, B	NY	974
DR	Yoon, S	NY	978
NuM	Agress, H	NJ	548
NuM	Freeman, L	NY	548

Cubital Tunnel Syndrome

Spec	Name	St	Pg
HS	Nagle, D	IL	302

Spec	Name	St	Pg

Cushing's Syndrome

Spec	Name	St	Pg
EDM	Biller, B	MA	206
EDM	Katznelson, L	CA	223
EDM	Thorner, M	VA	215
EDM	Weiss, R	IL	219
EDM	Young, I	NY	213
PEn	Levitsky, L	MA	743

Cutaneous Lymphoma

D	Belsito, D	NY	184
D	Bowen, G	UT	196
D	Cather, J	TX	196
D	Duvic, M	TX	196
D	Edelson, R	CT	182
D	Kim, Y	CA	199
D	Kupper, T	MA	183
D	Lebwohl, M	NY	187
D	Lessin, S	PA	187
D	Lim, H	MI	194
D	Olsen, E	NC	191
D	Ramsay, D	NY	188
D	Rook, A	PA	188
D	Shea, C	IL	195
D	Thiers, B	SC	192
D	Wheeland, R	AZ	198
D	Wood, G	WI	195
Onc	Kuzel, T	IL	369
Path	Le Boit, P	CA	721
RadRO	Hoppe, R	CA	966
RadRO	Wilson, L	CT	948

Cutaneous T-cell Lymphoma

D	Camisa, C	FL	190
D	Cather, J	TX	196
D	Rook, A	PA	188

Cystadenocarcinoma

S	Sugarbaker, P	DC	1065

Cystic Fibrosis

Inf	Huitt, G	CO	418
PA&I	Fanous, Y	CA	733
PGe	Baker, R	NY	750
PGe	Sokol, R	CO	754
PPul	Borowitz, D	NY	794
PPul	Dorkin, H	MA	794
PPul	Dovey, M	PA	794
PPul	Dozor, A	NY	794
PPul	Gibson, R	WA	798
PPul	Kattan, M	NY	794
PPul	Konstan, M	OH	797
PPul	Lapey, A	MA	794
PPul	McCoy, K	OH	797
PPul	Morgan, W	AZ	797
PPul	Murphy, T	NC	796
PPul	Nielson, D	CA	798
PPul	Orenstein, D	PA	795
PPul	Panitch, H	PA	795
PPul	Platzker, A	CA	798

PPul	Quittell, L	NY	795
PPul	Ramsey, B	WA	798
PPul	Rubin, B	VA	796
PPul	Tauber, D	PA	795
PPul	Wall, M	OR	798
PPul	Zeitlin, P	MD	795
Pul	Balk, R	IL	933
Pul	Garrity, E	IL	933
Pul	Grum, C	MI	933
Pul	Rosenbluth, D	MO	935
Pul	Simon, R	MI	935
Pul	Trulock, E	MO	936
Pul	Young, K	PA	929

Cystic Fibrosis Infection

PInf	Saiman, L	NY	781

Cytogenetic Disorders

CG	Hoyme, H	SD	161
CG	Zackai, E	PA	158

Cytopathology

Path	Cohen, M	UT	717
Path	Ehya, H	PA	708
Path	Nicosia, S	FL	714
Path	Silverman, J	PA	711

D

Dance Medicine

OrS	Padgett, D	NY	623

Dance/Ballet Injuries

SM	Metzl, J	NY	1041
SM	Micheli, L	MA	1040

Dance/Sports Medicine

OrS	Bauman, P	NY	614

Death & Dying

ChAP	Sexson, S	GA	910

Deep Brain Stimulation

N	Flaherty, A	MA	507
N	Vitek, J	MN	530
NS	Eisenberg, H	MD	473
NS	Kaplitt, M	NY	476
NS	Liker, M	CA	497
NS	Rezai, A	OH	489
NS	Whiting, D	PA	480

Defibrillaters

CE	Epstein, L	MA	119

Defibrillator Cable Extraction

CE	Epstein, L	MA	119
CE	Love, C	OH	123
Cv	Wilkoff, B	OH	112

Defibrillators

CE	Chinitz, L	NY	120
CE	Cohen, M	NY	120
CE	Curtis, A	NY	120
CE	DiMarco, J	VA	121
CE	Donahue, J	OH	122
CE	Ellenbogen, K	VA	121
CE	Epstein, A	PA	120
CE	Higgins, S	CA	125
CE	Lerman, B	NY	120
CE	Onufer, J	VA	122
CE	Schuger, C	MI	124
CE	Shen, W	AZ	124
CE	Sorrentino, R	GA	122
CE	Swerdlow, C	CA	125
CE	Wang, P	CA	125

Deformity Reconstruction

OrS	Helfet, D	NY	619
OrS	Strongwater, A	NJ	626

Delirium

Ger	Dyer, C	TX	266
Ger	Liem, P	AR	266

Dementia

Ger	Bloom, P	NY	262
Ger	Callahan, E	NY	262
Ger	Dyer, C	TX	266
Ger	Gorbien, M	IL	265
Ger	Greganti, M	NC	264
Ger	Liem, P	AR	266
Ger	McCormick, W	WA	267
Ger	Olson, J	IL	265
Ger	Palmer, R	VA	264
Ger	Tenover, J	CA	267
GerPsy	Borson, S	WA	915
GerPsy	Burke, W	NE	914
GerPsy	Greenwald, B	NY	913
GerPsy	Holroyd, S	VA	914
GerPsy	Kennedy, G	NY	913
GerPsy	Lyketsos, C	MD	913
GerPsy	Manepalli, J	MO	914
GerPsy	Mellow, A	MI	914
GerPsy	Reisberg, B	NY	913
GerPsy	Small, G	CA	915
GerPsy	Stein, E	CA	915
GerPsy	Tune, L	GA	914
N	Ahern, G	AZ	532
N	Chui, H	CA	536
N	DeKosky, S	VA	520
N	Feinberg, T	NY	511
N	Fellus, J	NJ	511
N	Foo, S	NY	511

Specialty & Special Expertise Index

Spec	Name	St	Pg
N	Gendelman, S	NY	512
N	Henderson, V	CA	537
N	Kieburtz, K	NY	513
N	Levine, D	NY	514
N	Marder, K	NY	515
N	Mayeux, R	NY	515
N	Mesulam, M	IL	528
N	Relkin, N	NY	517
N	Zimmerman, E	NY	519
Psyc	Arnold, S	PA	890
Psyc	Avery, E	TX	899
Psyc	Nelson, J	CA	902
Psyc	Weiner, M	TX	900

Demyelinating Neuropathy

Spec	Name	St	Pg
N	Lisak, R	MI	527

Depression

Spec	Name	St	Pg
AM	Kaplan, D	CO	81
ChAP	Emslie, G	TX	911
ChAP	Hagman, J	CO	911
ChAP	Heston, J	TN	910
ChAP	McKelvey, R	OR	912
Ger	Olson, J	IL	265
Ger	Tenover, J	CA	267
GerPsy	Burke, W	NE	914
GerPsy	Greenwald, B	NY	913
GerPsy	Grossberg, G	MO	914
GerPsy	Kennedy, G	NY	913
GerPsy	Kramer, B	CA	915
GerPsy	Lyketsos, C	MD	913
GerPsy	Manepalli, J	MO	914
GerPsy	Mellow, A	MI	914
GerPsy	Reisberg, B	NY	913
Psyc	Adler, D	MA	888
Psyc	Appelbaum, P	NY	890
Psyc	Avery, E	TX	899
Psyc	Canterbury, R	VA	895
Psyc	DePaulo, J	MD	891
Psyc	Eaton, J	DC	891
Psyc	Eisendrath, S	CA	901
Psyc	Giustra, L	GA	896
Psyc	Greden, J	MI	897
Psyc	Haque, W	TX	900
Psyc	Hirschfeld, R	TX	900
Psyc	Karasu, T	NY	892
Psyc	Leuchter, A	CA	901
Psyc	Levy, S	GA	896
Psyc	Marin, D	NY	894
Psyc	McIntosh, J	UT	899
Psyc	Nelson, J	CA	902
Psyc	Nurnberger, J	IN	898
Psyc	Price, L	RI	889
Psyc	Reus, V	CA	902
Psyc	Schatzberg, A	CA	903
Psyc	Thase, M	PA	895
Psyc	Weiner, R	NC	896
Psyc	Weisler, R	NC	896

Depression in Cardiovascular

Disease

Spec	Name	St	Pg
GerPsy	Veith, R	WA	915

Depression in the Elderly

Spec	Name	St	Pg
Psyc	Marin, D	NY	894
Psyc	Roose, S	NY	894

Depression-TMS Therapy

Spec	Name	St	Pg
Psyc	Manevitz, A	NY	893

Dermatofibrosarcoma Protruberans

Spec	Name	St	Pg
D	Bennett, R	CA	198
D	Russell, M	VA	192

Dermatologic Surgery

Spec	Name	St	Pg
D	Brody, H	GA	189
D	Eichler, C	FL	190
D	Fosko, S	MO	193
D	Krunic, A	IL	194
D	Maloney, M	MA	183
D	Otley, C	MN	194
D	Ratner, D	NY	188

Dermatology

Spec	Name	St	Pg
D	Alster, T	DC	184
D	Amonette, R	TN	189
D	Anderson, R	MA	182
D	Anhalt, G	MD	184
D	Arndt, K	MA	182
D	Arpey, C	MN	192
D	Avram, M	NY	184
D	Bailin, P	OH	192
D	Barbosa, V	IL	192
D	Bayliss, S	MO	192
D	Belsito, D	NY	184
D	Bennett, R	CA	198
D	Berg, D	WA	198
D	Bernstein, R	NY	185
D	Bickers, D	NY	185
D	Bolognia, J	CT	182
D	Bondi, E	PA	185
D	Bowen, G	UT	196
D	Brandt, F	NY	185
D	Braun, M	DC	185
D	Brodland, D	PA	185
D	Brody, H	GA	189
D	Brown, M	NY	185
D	Burton, C	NC	189
D	Butler, D	TX	196
D	Callen, J	KY	190
D	Camisa, C	FL	190
D	Carney, J	AR	196
D	Cather, J	TX	196
D	Cockerell, C	TX	196
D	Cohen, B	FL	190
D	Cohen, B	MD	185
D	Cook, J	NC	190

Spec	Name	St	Pg
D	Cornelius, L	MO	193
D	Cotsarelis, G	PA	185
D	Crutchfield, C	MN	193
D	Cunningham, B	CA	198
D	DeLeo, V	NY	186
D	Dover, J	MA	182
D	Dufresne, R	RI	182
D	Duvic, M	TX	196
D	Dzubow, L	PA	186
D	Edelson, R	CT	182
D	Eichenfield, L	CA	198
D	Eichler, C	FL	190
D	Elmets, C	AL	190
D	Falanga, V	RI	182
D	Fenske, N	FL	190
D	Fewkes, J	MA	183
D	Fitzpatrick, R	CA	198
D	Fivenson, D	MI	193
D	Flowers, F	FL	190
D	Fosko, S	MO	193
D	Franks, A	NY	186
D	Frieden, I	CA	198
D	Friedlander, S	CA	199
D	Garden, J	IL	193
D	Garrett, A	VA	190
D	Gellis, S	MA	183
D	Geronemus, R	NY	186
D	Gilchrest, B	MA	183
D	Glogau, R	CA	199
D	Gordon, M	NY	186
D	Gottlieb, A	MA	183
D	Green, H	FL	191
D	Greenbaum, S	PA	186
D	Greenway, H	CA	199
D	Grichnik, J	FL	191
D	Grimes, P	CA	199
D	Grossman, M	NY	186
D	Halpern, A	NY	186
D	Hanifin, J	OR	199
D	Hanke, C	IN	193
D	Hansen, R	AZ	197
D	Hruza, G	MO	193
D	James, W	PA	187
D	Johnson, T	MI	193
D	Johr, R	FL	191
D	Jorizzo, J	NC	191
D	Kalb, R	NY	187
D	Kane, K	MA	183
D	Kilmer, S	CA	199
D	Kim, Y	CA	199
D	Kirsner, R	FL	191
D	Koo, J	CA	199
D	Kress, D	PA	187
D	Kriegel, D	NY	187
D	Krueger, G	UT	196
D	Krunic, A	IL	194
D	Kupper, T	MA	183
D	Lask, G	CA	199
D	Lebwohl, M	NY	187
D	Leffell, D	CT	183
D	Leshin, B	NC	191
D	Lessin, S	PA	187

Spec	Name	St	Pg
D	Levy, M	TX	197
D	Lim, H	MI	194
D	Lim Quan, K	AZ	197
D	Linder, J	AZ	197
D	Liu, V	IA	194
D	Lowe, L	MI	194
D	Lowitt, M	MD	187
D	Lucky, A	OH	194
D	Maloney, M	MA	183
D	McMichael, A	NC	191
D	Menter, M	TX	197
D	Miller, S	MD	187
D	Mutasim, D	OH	194
D	Neel, V	MA	184
D	Neuburg, M	WI	194
D	Nghiem, P	WA	200
D	Nigra, T	DC	187
D	Nouri, K	FL	191
D	Olbricht, S	MA	184
D	Olsen, E	NC	191
D	Orengo, I	TX	197
D	Orlow, S	NY	188
D	Otley, C	MN	194
D	Paller, A	IL	195
D	Perone, J	TX	197
D	Pitts, J	AZ	197
D	Prioleau, P	NY	188
D	Ramsay, D	NY	188
D	Ratner, D	NY	188
D	Rhodes, A	IL	195
D	Richardson, T	CA	200
D	Rigel, D	NY	188
D	Rook, A	PA	188
D	Rubin, M	CA	200
D	Russell, M	VA	192
D	Schultz, N	NY	188
D	Shea, C	IL	195
D	Sherertz, E	SC	192
D	Shupack, J	NY	188
D	Sobel, S	FL	192
D	Sokoloff, D	FL	192
D	Sontheimer, R	UT	196
D	Soter, N	NY	189
D	Stanley, J	PA	189
D	Stern, R	MA	184
D	Swanson, N	OR	200
D	Swetter, S	CA	200
D	Taylor, R	TX	198
D	Thiers, B	SC	192
D	Treadwell, P	IN	195
D	Tsao, H	MA	184
D	Voorhees, J	MI	195
D	Werth, V	PA	189
D	Wheeland, R	AZ	198
D	Witman, P	OH	195
D	Wood, G	WI	195
D	Woodley, D	CA	200
D	Yan, A	PA	189
D	Zelickson, B	MN	195
D	Zitelli, J	PA	189

Spec	Name	St	Pg
Dermatomyositis			
D	Callen, J	KY	190
D	Franks, A	NY	186
D	Sontheimer, R	UT	196
PRhu	Ilowite, N	NY	799
PRhu	McCarthy, P	CT	799
PRhu	Myones, B	TX	801
PRhu	Schanberg, L	NC	800
PRhu	Sills, E	MD	800
PRhu	Wagner-Weiner, L	IL	800
PRhu	Wilking, A	TX	801
Rhu	Medsger, T	PA	1027
Rhu	Mitnick, H	NY	1027
Rhu	Oddis, C	PA	1027

Spec	Name	St	Pg
Dermatopathology			
D	Cockerell, C	TX	196
D	Flowers, F	FL	190
D	Lowe, L	MI	194
D	Mutasim, D	OH	194
Path	Bastian, B	CA	719
Path	Cochran, A	CA	720
Path	Gottlieb, G	MA	706
Path	Le Boit, P	CA	721
Path	Prieto, V	TX	718

Spec	Name	St	Pg
DES-Exposed Females			
RE	Haney, A	IL	1013

Spec	Name	St	Pg
Desmoid Tumors			
CRS	Church, J	OH	173
Onc	Maki, R	NY	345

Spec	Name	St	Pg
Developmental & Behavioral Disorders			
Ped	Burgess, D	NJ	726
Ped	Hofkosh, D	PA	726
Ped	Miller, K	MA	726
Ped	Rappaport, L	MA	726
Ped	Walker, W	WA	729

Spec	Name	St	Pg
Developmental & Mood Disorders			
Ped	Hershorin, E	FL	727

Spec	Name	St	Pg
Developmental Disorders			
AM	Slap, G	PA	81
CG	Cunniff, C	AZ	161
ChAP	Hertzig, M	NY	908
ChAP	King, B	WA	912
ChAP	Kwon, H	WA	912
ChAP	Pomeroy, J	NY	909
ChAP	Russell, A	CA	912
ChiN	Filipek, P	TX	152
ChiN	Kosofsky, B	NY	147
ChiN	Kovnar, E	WI	151
ChiN	Patterson, M	MN	151
N	Kuzniecky, R	NY	513

Spec	Name	St	Pg
Ped	Bull, M	IN	727
Ped	Hofkosh, D	PA	726
Ped	Palfrey, J	MA	726

Spec	Name	St	Pg
Diabetes			
EDM	Abrahamson, M	MA	206
EDM	Ahmann, A	OR	221
EDM	Akatsu, H	CA	222
EDM	Axelrod, L	MA	206
EDM	Barrett, E	VA	213
EDM	Beaser, R	MA	206
EDM	Bell, D	AL	213
EDM	Berkson, R	CA	222
EDM	Blum, C	NY	209
EDM	Brennan, M	MN	216
EDM	Brillon, D	NY	209
EDM	Broadstone, V	IN	216
EDM	Buse, J	NC	214
EDM	Clore, J	VA	214
EDM	Cohen, R	OH	216
EDM	Comi, R	NH	206
EDM	Cryer, P	MO	217
EDM	Cunningham, G	TX	220
EDM	D'Alessio, D	OH	217
EDM	Donner, T	MD	210
EDM	Eckel, R	CO	220
EDM	Edelman, S	CA	222
EDM	Ehrmann, D	IL	217
EDM	Emanuele, M	IL	217
EDM	Feinglos, M	NC	214
EDM	Fitzgerald, P	CA	222
EDM	Greene, L	NY	210
EDM	Herman, W	MI	217
EDM	Hirsch, I	WA	222
EDM	Inzucchi, S	CT	207
EDM	Ipp, E	CA	223
EDM	Kamdar, V	CA	223
EDM	Kennedy, L	OH	218
EDM	Klonoff, D	CA	223
EDM	Korytkowski, M	PA	211
EDM	Lash, R	MI	218
EDM	Lavis, V	TX	221
EDM	Lipson, A	DC	211
EDM	Mazzone, T	IL	218
EDM	McGill, J	MO	218
EDM	McMahon, M	MN	219
EDM	Nathan, D	MA	208
EDM	Nestler, J	VA	215
EDM	Ober, K	NC	215
EDM	Osei, K	OH	219
EDM	Ovalle, F	AL	215
EDM	Peters, A	CA	224
EDM	Philipson, L	IL	219
EDM	Powers, A	TN	215
EDM	Quinn, S	FL	215
EDM	Recker, R	NE	220
EDM	Riddle, M	OR	224
EDM	Rodbard, H	MD	211
EDM	Rubenfeld, S	TX	221
EDM	Rushakoff, R	CA	224
EDM	Schutta, M	PA	211

Spec	Name	St	Pg
EDM	Schwartz, S	PA	212
EDM	Semenkovich, C	MO	219
EDM	Seplowitz, A	NY	212
EDM	Shuldiner, A	MD	212
EDM	Skyler, J	FL	215
EDM	Smith, S	MN	219
EDM	Sowers, J	MO	219
EDM	Weissman, P	FL	216
EDM	Werner, P	IL	220
EDM	Wondisford, F	MD	213
EDM	Zimmerman, R	OH	220
Ger	Abrass, I	WA	266
Ger	Schwartz, R	CO	265
IM	Braunstein, S	NC	424
PEn	Allen, D	WI	746
PEn	Alter, C	PA	744
PEn	Arslanian, S	PA	744
PEn	Becker, D	PA	744
PEn	DiMeglio, L	IN	746
PEn	Foster, C	UT	748
PEn	Freemark, M	NC	746
PEn	Gitelman, S	CA	748
PEn	Klingensmith, G	CO	748
PEn	Levitsky, L	MA	743
PEn	Maclaren, N	NY	744
PEn	Menon, R	MI	747
PEn	Mirmira, R	IN	747
PEn	Norris, A	IA	747
PEn	Plotnick, L	MD	745
PEn	Rewers, M	CO	748
PEn	Rogers, D	OH	747
PEn	Rosenthal, S	CA	749
PEn	Silverstein, J	FL	746
PEn	Sperling, M	PA	745
PEn	Tamborlane, W	CT	744
PEn	White, N	MO	747
PEn	Wilson, D	CA	749
S	Hering, B	MN	1077
S	Oberholzer, J	IL	1080

Diabetes Clinical Trials

EDM	Korytkowski, M	PA	211

Diabetes in Minority Populations

EDM	Osei, K	OH	219

Diabetes in Pregnancy

EDM	Lash, R	MI	218
EDM	Seely, E	MA	208
IM	Gillman, M	MA	424
MF	Cohen, A	PA	432
MF	Landon, M	OH	436
MF	Landy, H	DC	433
MF	Moore, T	CA	440
MF	Norwitz, E	MA	430
MF	Plante, L	PA	433
MF	Socol, M	IL	437

Spec	Name	St	Pg

Diabetes in Women

EDM	Ovalle, F	AL	215
EDM	Seely, E	MA	208

Diabetes Prevention

EDM	Schutta, M	PA	211

Diabetes Surgery-Rubino's Procedure

S	Rubino, F	NY	1063

Diabetes-Amputation

OrS	Pinzur, M	IL	637

Diabetic Eye Disease/Retinopathy

Oph	Bressler, S	MD	572
Oph	Chang, S	NY	572
Oph	D'Amico, D	NY	573
Oph	Davis, J	FL	582
Oph	Del Priore, L	SC	582
Oph	Duker, J	MA	570
Oph	Edwards, P	MI	589
Oph	Flynn, H	FL	583
Oph	Friberg, T	PA	574
Oph	Fuchs, W	NY	574
Oph	Gentile, R	NY	574
Oph	Hariprasad, S	IL	590
Oph	Ho, A	PA	575
Oph	Humayun, M	CA	601
Oph	Lambert, H	TX	597
Oph	Maguire, J	PA	577
Oph	Meredith, T	NC	585
Oph	Muldoon, T	NY	578
Oph	Murray, T	FL	585
Oph	Nussbaum, J	GA	585
Oph	Olsen, T	GA	585
Oph	Petersen, M	OH	593
Oph	Rosenfeld, P	FL	586
Oph	Sadda, S	CA	603
Oph	Schachat, A	OH	594
Oph	Schiff, W	NY	579
Oph	Schwartz, S	CA	603
Oph	Shabto, U	NY	580
Oph	Sternberg, P	TN	586
Oph	Vander, J	PA	581
Oph	Walsh, J	NY	581
Oph	Yannuzzi, L	NY	581

Diabetic Kidney Disease

Nep	Johnston, J	PA	457
Nep	Kasinath, B	TX	463
Nep	Kobrin, S	PA	458
Nep	Lea, J	GA	460
Nep	Pohl, M	OH	462
Nep	Rodby, R	IL	462
Nep	Schreiber, M	OH	462
Nep	Schwartz, G	MN	462

Spec	Name	St	Pg
Nep	Seifter, J	MA	456
Nep	Toto, R	TX	464
Nep	Yee, J	MI	463

Diabetic Leg/Foot

EDM	Kamdar, V	CA	223
OrS	Weinfeld, S	NY	626
PlS	Attinger, C	DC	852
VascS	Pomposelli, F	MA	1185
VascS	Sumpio, B	CT	1185

Diabetic Vascular Disease Prevention

EDM	Barrett, E	VA	213

Diagnostic Problems

Ger	Greganti, M	NC	264
IM	Cope, D	CA	426
Inf	Nahass, R	NJ	412
Inf	Wormser, G	NY	413
N	Adams, D	FL	519
Ped	Gartner, J	DE	726
Pul	Hansen-Flaschen, J	PA	925
Pul	Harman, E	FL	931

Diagnostic Radiology

DR	Abbitt, P	FL	978
DR	Adler, R	NY	974
DR	Austin, J	NY	974
DR	Bahn, D	CA	982
DR	Bassett, L	CA	982
DR	Benson, C	MA	973
DR	Berland, L	AL	978
DR	Black, W	NH	973
DR	Bluemke, D	MD	974
DR	Brem, R	DC	974
DR	Cardenosa, G	VA	978
DR	Charboneau, J	MN	980
DR	Chiles, C	NC	979
DR	Coakley, F	OR	982
DR	Cohen, B	NY	974
DR	Cohen, H	TN	979
DR	Coleman, B	PA	974
DR	Conant, E	PA	974
DR	Dalinka, M	PA	974
DR	Dershaw, D	NY	974
DR	Dodd, G	CO	981
DR	Doubilet, P	MA	973
DR	Edelman, R	IL	980
DR	Edelstein, B	NY	975
DR	Elster, A	NC	979
DR	Erasmus, J	TX	982
DR	Evers, K	PA	975
DR	Federle, M	CA	983
DR	Feig, S	CA	983
DR	Fidler, J	MN	980
DR	Filly, R	CA	983
DR	Fishman, E	MD	975
DR	Flamm, S	OH	980

Spec	Name	St	Pg
DR	Freimanis, R	NC	979
DR	Fuhrman, C	PA	975
DR	Gefter, W	PA	975
DR	Gilsanz, V	CA	983
DR	Goodman, L	WI	980
DR	Grant, E	CA	983
DR	Helvie, M	MI	980
DR	Henschke, C	NY	975
DR	Holliday, R	NY	975
DR	Hricak, H	NY	975
DR	Hubbard, A	NE	981
DR	Huynh, P	TX	982
DR	Jackson, V	IN	980
DR	Jaramillo, D	PA	975
DR	Kanal, E	PA	976
DR	Kurtz, A	PA	976
DR	Lehman, C	WA	983
DR	Levy, A	DC	976
DR	Logan-Young, W	NY	976
DR	Mancuso, A	FL	979
DR	McCarthy, S	CT	973
DR	Megibow, A	NY	976
DR	Mirvis, S	MD	976
DR	Mitnick, J	NY	976
DR	Monsees, B	MO	981
DR	Mountz, J	PA	976
DR	Newman, J	MA	973
DR	Otto, P	TX	982
DR	Palmer, W	MA	973
DR	Panicek, D	NY	976
DR	Parikh, J	WA	983
DR	Parsons, R	PA	977
DR	Partain, C	TN	979
DR	Pathria, M	CA	983
DR	Patz, E	NC	979
DR	Pavlov, H	NY	977
DR	Potter, H	NY	977
DR	Prince, M	NY	977
DR	Rao, V	PA	977
DR	Reinus, W	PA	977
DR	Roth, S	PA	977
DR	Rubin, G	NC	979
DR	Shaw, D	WA	984
DR	Sivit, C	OH	981
DR	Stough, R	OK	982
DR	Swensen, S	MN	981
DR	Teal, J	DC	977
DR	Thompson, B	IA	981
DR	Thurmond, A	OR	984
DR	Ulissey, M	TX	982
DR	Weinreb, J	CT	973
DR	Wells, R	WI	981
DR	White, C	MD	978
DR	White, R	OH	981
DR	Wood, B	CA	984
DR	Yankelevitz, D	NY	978
DR	Yoon, S	NY	978
DR	Zagoria, R	NC	980
DR	Zeman, R	DC	978

Diagnostic Second Opinions

Spec	Name	St	Pg
Psyc	Eaton, J	DC	891

Dialectical Behavioral Therapy

Spec	Name	St	Pg
Psyc	Wait, S	MD	895

Dialysis Access

Spec	Name	St	Pg
S	Becker, Y	IL	1074
S	Lipkowitz, G	MA	1050
S	Stratta, R	NC	1073
VascS	Alexander, J	OH	1190
VIR	Aruny, J	CT	992
VIR	Denny, D	NJ	993

Dialysis Care

Spec	Name	St	Pg
Nep	Allon, M	AL	459
Nep	Bernardo, J	PA	457
Nep	Gaston, R	AL	459
Nep	King, A	CA	465
Nep	Kobrin, S	PA	458
Nep	Kraus, M	IN	461
Nep	Lea, J	GA	460
Nep	McCarthy, J	MN	461
Nep	Miller, B	MO	462
Nep	Schreiber, M	OH	462
Nep	Stern, L	NY	458
Nep	Swartz, R	MI	462
Nep	Toto, R	TX	464
Nep	Ward, D	CA	466
PNep	Brophy, P	IA	787
PNep	Conley, S	PA	785
PNep	Flynn, J	WA	788
PNep	Jabs, K	TN	786
PNep	Mendley, S	MD	786
PNep	Warady, B	MO	788

Diaphragm Pacing via Laparoscopy

Spec	Name	St	Pg
S	Onders, R	OH	1080

Diarrheal Diseases

Spec	Name	St	Pg
Ge	Farraye, F	MA	228
Ge	Pochapin, M	NY	237
Ge	Schiller, L	TX	252
Ge	Semrad, C	IL	248
Inf	Bakken, J	MN	416
Inf	DuPont, H	TX	418
PGe	Bishop, W	IA	752
PGe	Cohen, M	OH	752
PGe	Fasano, A	MD	750
PGe	Guandalini, S	IL	753
PGe	Hill, I	NC	752
PGe	Rhoads, J	TX	755
PInf	Kotloff, K	MD	780

DiGeorge Syndrome

Spec	Name	St	Pg
A&I	Markert, M	NC	87

Digestive Disorders

Spec	Name	St	Pg
Ge	Glombicki, A	TX	252
Ge	Owyang, C	MI	247
PGe	Guandalini, S	IL	753

Diplopia

Spec	Name	St	Pg
Oph	Magramm, I	NY	577

Disaster Preparedness

Spec	Name	St	Pg
PCCM	Fuhrman, B	TX	742
PrM	Hoffman, R	NY	883
Pul	Tharratt, R	CA	941

Disaster Psychiatry

Spec	Name	St	Pg
Psyc	Blumenfield, M	CA	900
Psyc	Pynoos, R	CA	902

Dissociative Disorders

Spec	Name	St	Pg
Psyc	Loewenstein, R	MD	893
Psyc	Wait, S	MD	895

Diverticulitis

Spec	Name	St	Pg
CRS	Lederman, E	MO	174
CRS	Ramamoorthy, S	CA	178
CRS	Read, T	MA	169
CRS	Roberts, P	MA	169
S	Edye, M	NY	1057

Diving Medicine

Spec	Name	St	Pg
Cv	Bove, A	PA	97

Dizziness

Spec	Name	St	Pg
N	Klein, P	NJ	513
Oto	Gianoli, G	LA	682
Oto	Goebel, J	MO	675

Down Syndrome

Spec	Name	St	Pg
CG	Marion, R	NY	158
CG	Pergament, E	IL	160
ChiN	Lott, I	CA	153
ChiN	Pinter, J	OR	153
Ped	Bull, M	IN	727
Ped	Roizen, N	OH	728
PHO	Rosoff, P	NC	768

Drug Abuse

Spec	Name	St	Pg
AdP	Galanter, I	NY	904
AdP	Kleber, H	NY	905

Drug Abuse-Consultation

Spec	Name	St	Pg
AdP	Walker, R	OR	906

Drug Allergy

Spec	Name	St	Pg
A&I	Bernstein, J	OH	88
A&I	Castells, M	MA	84

Spec	Name	St	Pg
A&I	Grammer, L	IL	88
A&I	Greenberger, P	IL	88
A&I	Gruchalla, R	TX	89
A&I	Jost, B	MO	88
A&I	Sullivan, T	GA	87
D	Stern, R	MA	184

Drug Development

Hem	Grever, M	OH	320
Hem	Kraut, E	OH	320
Onc	Daud, A	CA	385
Onc	Eckhardt, S	CO	375
Onc	Fine, R	NY	339
Onc	Hande, K	TN	357
Onc	Herbst, R	CT	330
Onc	Kaminski, M	MI	369
Onc	Kraft, A	SC	358
Onc	Markman, M	PA	345
Onc	Marshall, J	DC	345
Onc	O'Connor, O	NY	346
Onc	Peereboom, D	OH	370
Onc	Remick, S	WV	348
Onc	Robert-Vizcarrondo, F	AL	361
Onc	Schilder, R	PA	349
Onc	Schilsky, R	IL	372
Onc	Spriggs, D	NY	350
Onc	Wolff, A	MD	352
PHO	Adamson, P	PA	758
PHO	Blaney, S	TX	775
PHO	Furman, W	TN	765
PHO	Gajjar, A	TN	766
PHO	Kamen, B	NJ	761
PHO	Vik, T	IN	773

Drug Discovery

Onc	Belani, C	PA	335
Onc	Sosman, J	TN	362
Onc	Verschraegen, C	VT	333
Onc	Von Hoff, D	AZ	382

Drug Discovery & Development

Onc	Burris, H	TN	354
Onc	Carducci, M	MD	336
Onc	Cohen, R	PA	337
Onc	Doroshow, J	MD	338
Onc	Edelman, M	MD	339
Onc	Johnson, D	TX	379
Onc	Ratain, M	IL	371
Onc	Trump, D	NY	351
Onc	Wilding, G	WI	373
PHO	Berg, S	TX	775
PInf	Jacobs, R	AR	784

Drug Induced Lung Disease

Pul	Cooper, J	AL	930

Drug Sensitivity

PA&I	Sicherer, S	NY	730

Drug-Resistant Infections

PInf	Belcher, C	IN	782

Drugs & Aging

Ger	Flaherty, J	MO	265

Dry Eye Syndrome

Oph	Dana, R	MA	570
Oph	Kornmehl, E	MA	570

Dual Diagnosis

AdP	Strain, E	MD	905
ChAP	Deas, D	SC	910
Psyc	Lawson, W	DC	893
Psyc	Norman, K	CA	902
Psyc	Strakowski, S	OH	898

Dupuytren's Contracture

HS	Belsky, M	MA	294
HS	Carneiro, R	FL	298
HS	Carroll, C	IL	300
HS	Godzik, C	CA	304
OrS	Hotchkiss, R	NY	620

Dyskinesias

N	Goetz, C	IL	526

Dyslexia

ChiN	Shaywitz, B	CT	146

Dysmorphology

CG	Anyane-Yeboa, K	NY	156
CG	Graham, J	CA	162
CG	Hoyme, H	SD	161
CG	Jones, M	CA	163
CG	Northrup, H	TX	162
CG	Randolph, L	CA	163
CG	Seaver, L	HI	163
CG	Shapiro, L	NY	158
Ped	Jones, K	CA	728

Dystonia

ChiN	Mink, J	NY	148
N	Baser, S	PA	509
N	Bressman, S	NY	509
N	Lew, M	CA	537
N	Tanner, C	CA	539
NS	Baltuch, G	PA	472

Dystonia-Botox Therapy

N	Reich, S	MD	517

Ear Disorders/Surgery

Oto	Balkany, T	FL	667
Oto	Brackmann, D	CA	684
Oto	Caldarelli, D	IL	674
Oto	Feghali, J	NY	659
Oto	Gianoli, G	LA	682
Oto	Hoffman, R	NY	660
Oto	Jenkins, H	CO	680
Oto	Johnson, C	LA	682
Oto	Kang, D	NE	680
Oto	Kartush, J	MI	676
Oto	Kveton, J	CT	656
Oto	Lalwani, A	NY	662
Oto	Miyamoto, R	IN	676
Oto	Niparko, J	MD	663
Oto	Parisier, S	NY	663
Oto	Pillsbury, H	NC	670
Oto	Silverstein, H	FL	671
Oto	Telian, S	MI	678
Oto	Telischi, F	FL	671
Oto	Zalzal, G	DC	667
PO	Eavey, R	TN	791
PO	Miller, R	IL	792
PO	Poe, D	MA	789
PO	Rosenfeld, R	NY	790

Ear Infections

Oto	Hotaling, A	IL	675
Oto	Paparella, M	MN	677
Oto	Poole, M	GA	670
PInf	Wald, E	WI	783
PO	Casselbrant, M	PA	789
PO	Chan, K	CO	792
PO	Dolitsky, J	NY	789
PO	Haddad, J	NY	790
PO	Jones, J	NY	790
PO	Katz, R	OH	792

Ear Nose & Throat Imaging

DR	Rao, V	PA	977

Ear Reconstruction/Microtia

PlS	Bauer, B	IL	864
PlS	Reinisch, J	CA	876
PlS	Staffenberg, D	NY	859
PlS	Thorne, C	NY	859
PlS	Walton, R	IL	868
PO	Eavey, R	TN	791

Ear Reshaping (Otoplasty)

Oto	Farrior, E	FL	668
PlS	Kelly, K	TN	862

Ear Tumors

Oto	Jackler, R	CA	685
PO	Arnold, J	OH	791

E

Spec	Name	St	Pg

Ear, Nose & Throat Pathology
Spec	Name	St	Pg
Path	Mills, S	VA	713

Eating Disorders
Spec	Name	St	Pg
AM	Bermudez, O	CO	81
AM	Bravender, T	OH	81
AM	Hergenroeder, A	TX	82
AM	Irwin, C	CA	82
AM	MacKenzie, R	CA	82
AM	Sigel, E	CO	81
AM	Singh, N	MN	81
ChAP	Fornari, V	NY	908
ChAP	Hagman, J	CO	911
ChAP	Herzog, D	MA	906
ChAP	Ponton, L	CA	912
ChAP	Sargent, A	MA	907
ChAP	Steiner, H	CA	912
IM	Mehler, P	CO	426
Psyc	Brandt, H	MD	890
Psyc	Crow, S	MN	897
Psyc	Guarda, A	MD	892
Psyc	Jimerson, D	MA	889
Psyc	McCallum, K	MO	898
Psyc	Mitchell, J	ND	899
Psyc	Powers, P	FL	896
Psyc	Walsh, B	NY	895
Psyc	Weiner, K	CO	899
Psyc	Zerbe, K	OR	903

Eating Disorders/Obesity
Spec	Name	St	Pg
EDM	Eckel, R	CO	220
EDM	Jensen, M	MN	218
EDM	Shuldiner, A	MD	212
Psyc	Norman, K	CA	902

Echocardiography
Spec	Name	St	Pg
Cv	Blanchard, D	CA	116
Cv	Byrd, B	TN	103
Cv	Chaitman, B	MO	107
Cv	Clements, S	GA	104
Cv	Gandy, W	GA	104
Cv	Gardin, J	NJ	98
Cv	Goldberg, N	NY	98
Cv	Gottdiener, J	MD	99
Cv	Hayes, S	MN	108
Cv	Kaul, S	OR	117
Cv	Kuvin, J	MA	95
Cv	Manning, W	MA	95
Cv	McPherson, D	TX	114
Cv	Mehlman, D	IL	109
Cv	Nagueh, S	TX	114
Cv	Nishimura, R	MN	109
Cv	Quinones, M	TX	115
Cv	Rahko, P	WI	110
Cv	Redberg, R	CA	118
Cv	Schnittger, I	CA	118
Cv	Shapiro, J	IL	111
Cv	Shea, R	IN	111
Cv	Stein, J	WI	111
Cv	Stewart, W	OH	111
Cv	Wilansky, S	AZ	115
Cv	Zoghbi, W	TX	115
IC	Khawaja, S	GA	130
PCd	Bierman, F	NY	734
PCd	Caldwell, R	IN	738
PCd	Gewitz, M	NY	735
PCd	Lewin, M	WA	741
PCd	Minich, L	UT	739
PCd	Parness, I	NY	735
PCd	Rychik, J	PA	736

Echocardiography-Transesophageal
Spec	Name	St	Pg
Cv	McPherson, D	TX	114
Cv	Rahko, P	WI	110
Cv	Schnittger, I	CA	118
Cv	Shea, R	IN	111
Cv	Stainback, R	TX	115

Eczema
Spec	Name	St	Pg
A&I	Bernstein, J	OH	88
A&I	Mazza, D	NY	85
A&I	Umetsu, D	MA	84
D	Bayliss, S	MO	192
D	Crutchfield, C	MN	193
D	DeLeo, V	NY	186
D	Eichenfield, L	CA	198
D	Lowitt, M	MD	187
D	Menter, M	TX	197
D	Sherertz, E	SC	192
D	Shupack, J	NY	188
PA&I	Bahna, S	LA	732
PA&I	Sampson, H	NY	729
PA&I	Sicherer, S	NY	730

Ehlers-Danlos Syndrome
Spec	Name	St	Pg
CG	Davis, J	NY	157

Ehrlichiosis
Spec	Name	St	Pg
Inf	Auwaerter, P	MD	410
Inf	Bakken, J	MN	416

Elbow Reconstruction
Spec	Name	St	Pg
HS	Abrams, R	CA	303
HS	Baratz, M	PA	295
HS	Beredjiklian, P	PA	295
HS	Fischer, T	IN	300
HS	Hanel, D	WA	304
HS	Hastings, H	IN	301
HS	Mass, D	IL	301
OrS	Hausman, M	NY	618
OrS	Hotchkiss, R	NY	620
SM	Ciccotti, M	PA	1041

Elbow Replacement
Spec	Name	St	Pg
HS	Weiss, A	RI	294

Elbow Surgery
Spec	Name	St	Pg
HS	Badia, A	FL	298
HS	Belsky, M	MA	294
HS	Bozentka, D	PA	295
HS	Carroll, C	IL	300
HS	Cassidy, C	MA	294
HS	Cohen, M	IL	300
HS	Collins, E	TX	303
HS	Culp, R	PA	295
HS	Glickel, S	NY	296
HS	Graham, T	OH	301
HS	Raskin, K	NY	297
HS	Rosenwasser, M	NY	297
HS	Seitz, W	OH	302
HS	Sotereanos, D	PA	298
HS	Steinmann, S	MN	302
HS	Strauch, R	NY	298
OrS	Craig, E	NY	616
OrS	Endrizzi, D	ME	611
OrS	Goitz, H	MI	633
OrS	Green, A	RI	611
OrS	McCann, P	NY	622
OrS	O'Driscoll, S	MN	636
OrS	Plancher, K	NY	624
OrS	Ramsey, M	PA	624
OrS	Romeo, A	IL	637
OrS	Yamaguchi, K	MO	638
SM	Altchek, D	NY	1040
SM	Andrews, J	FL	1042

Elder Abuse
Spec	Name	St	Pg
Ger	Dyer, C	TX	266

Electrical Injury
Spec	Name	St	Pg
S	Cairns, B	NC	1067

Electrical Status Epilepticus Of Sleep
Spec	Name	St	Pg
ChiN	Riviello, J	NY	148

Electroconvulsive Therapy (ECT)
Spec	Name	St	Pg
GerPsy	Kramer, B	CA	915
Psyc	Weiner, R	NC	896

Electrodiagnosis
Spec	Name	St	Pg
N	Sirdofsky, M	DC	518
PMR	Aseff, J	DC	835
PMR	Clairmont, A	OH	839
PMR	Colachis, S	OH	839
PMR	Creamer, M	FL	838
PMR	Dumitru, D	TX	842
PMR	Feinberg, J	NY	836
PMR	Gater, D	VA	838
PMR	Haig, A	MI	840
PMR	Kevorkian, C	TX	843
PMR	King, J	TX	843
PMR	Leonard, J	MI	841
PMR	Mason, K	CO	842

Specialty & Special Expertise Index

Spec	Name	St	Pg
PMR	Miknevich, M	PA	837
PMR	Munin, M	PA	837
PMR	Munin, M	PA	837
PMR	Nelson, M	TX	843
PMR	Nobunaga, A	OH	841
PMR	Robinson, L	WA	844

Electromyography

N	Bertorini, T	TN	520
N	Busis, N	PA	510
N	Graves, M	CA	537
N	Josephson, D	IN	527
N	Kincaid, J	IN	527
N	Kurtzke, R	VA	522
N	Logigian, E	NY	515
N	Oh, S	AL	523
N	Pula, T	MD	516
N	Zimnowodzki, S	IL	531
PMR	Braddom, R	PA	835
PMR	La Ban, M	MI	841
PMR	Lutz, C	NY	836
PMR	Ma, D	NY	836
PMR	Robinson, L	WA	844

Electroretinograms (ERG)

Oph	Marmor, M	CA	602

Emphysema

Pul	Cooke, J	NY	925
Pul	Niederman, M	NY	926
Pul	Rennard, S	NE	937
Pul	Steinberg, H	NY	928
Pul	Tapson, V	NC	932
Pul	Thomashow, B	NY	928
Pul	Voelkel, N	VA	932
Pul	Wiedemann, H	OH	936

Emphysema & Asthma

Pul	Maxfield, R	NY	926

Emphysema-Lung Volume Reduction

Pul	Trulock, E	MO	936
T&CS	Cooper, J	PA	1114
T&CS	DeCamp, M	IL	1131
T&CS	Ginsburg, M	NY	1116
T&CS	Keenan, R	PA	1118
T&CS	Meyers, B	MO	1133
T&CS	Miller, D	GA	1127
T&CS	Shrager, J	CA	1143
T&CS	Sonett, J	NY	1121

Emphysema/Alpha-1 Antitrypsin Deficiency

Pul	Stoller, J	OH	936

Encephalitis

N	Roos, K	IN	529

Spec	Name	St	Pg
PMR	Evans, S	DC	835

Encephalocele

Oto	Linstrom, C	NY	662

Endocarditis

Inf	Corey, G	NC	414
Inf	Hartman, B	NY	411
Inf	Quagliarello, V	CT	410
Inf	Scheld, W	VA	415

Endocrine Cancers

EDM	Braunstein, G	CA	222
EDM	Clutter, W	MO	216
EDM	Kandeel, F	CA	223
EDM	Koch, C	MS	214
EDM	Lechan, R	MA	208
EDM	Sherman, S	TX	221
Path	Li Volsi, V	PA	710
PS	Skinner, M	TX	810
S	Calvo, B	NC	1067
S	Cance, W	NY	1055
S	Evans, D	WI	1076
S	Hanks, J	VA	1069
S	Moley, J	MO	1080
S	Olson, J	MD	1061
S	Solorzano, C	TN	1072
S	Sosa, J	CT	1052
S	Staren, E	AZ	1092

Endocrine Disorders

Ger	Abrass, I	WA	266

Endocrine Surgery

PS	Chwals, W	MA	801
S	Bouvet, M	CA	1093
S	Carty, S	PA	1055
S	Doherty, G	MA	1049
S	Duh, Q	CA	1095
S	Fahey, T	NY	1057
S	Farley, D	MN	1076
S	Fraker, D	PA	1057
S	Gawande, A	MA	1049
S	Hanks, J	VA	1069
S	Hodin, R	MA	1049
S	Howe, J	IA	1078
S	Kim, L	AR	1089
S	Livingston, E	TX	1090
S	McIntyre, R	CO	1085
S	Moore, F	MA	1051
S	Norton, J	CA	1098
S	Schlinkert, R	AZ	1092
S	Traynor, M	ND	1086
S	Udelsman, R	CT	1052
S	Weber, C	GA	1073
S	Weigel, R	IA	1084

Spec	Name	St	Pg

Endocrine Tumors

S	Carty, S	PA	1055
S	Lee, J	TX	1090
S	McAneny, D	MA	1051
S	Siperstein, A	OH	1082

Endocrinology

EDM	Recker, R	NE	220
Ger	Gambert, S	MD	263
Ger	Morley, J	MO	265

Endocrinology & Joint Disorders

Rhu	Lahita, R	NJ	1027

Endocrinology, Diabetes & Metabolism

EDM	Abrahamson, M	MA	206
EDM	Ahmann, A	OR	221
EDM	Ain, K	KY	213
EDM	Akatsu, H	CA	222
EDM	Axelrod, L	MA	206
EDM	Bahn, R	MN	216
EDM	Ball, D	MD	208
EDM	Barrett, E	VA	213
EDM	Beaser, R	MA	206
EDM	Bell, D	AL	213
EDM	Bergman, D	NY	209
EDM	Berkson, R	CA	222
EDM	Bhasin, S	MA	206
EDM	Bilezikian, J	NY	209
EDM	Biller, B	MA	206
EDM	Blum, C	NY	209
EDM	Bockman, R	NY	209
EDM	Braunstein, G	CA	222
EDM	Braverman, L	MA	206
EDM	Brennan, M	MN	216
EDM	Brillon, D	NY	209
EDM	Broadstone, V	IN	216
EDM	Burman, K	DC	209
EDM	Burmeister, L	MN	216
EDM	Buse, J	NC	214
EDM	Calvi, L	NY	209
EDM	Clore, J	VA	214
EDM	Clutter, W	MO	216
EDM	Cohen, R	OH	216
EDM	Comi, R	NH	206
EDM	Cooper, D	MD	210
EDM	Cryer, P	MO	217
EDM	Cunningham, G	TX	220
EDM	Cushing, G	MA	207
EDM	D'Alessio, D	OH	217
EDM	Dalkin, A	VA	214
EDM	Daniels, G	MA	207
EDM	Davies, T	NY	210
EDM	Dobs, A	MD	210
EDM	Donner, T	MD	210
EDM	Earp, H	NC	214
EDM	Eckel, R	CO	220
EDM	Econs, M	IN	217
EDM	Edelman, S	CA	222

Spec	Name	St	Pg
EDM	Ehrmann, D	IL	217
EDM	Emanuele, M	IL	217
EDM	Emanuele, N	IL	217
EDM	Feinglos, M	NC	214
EDM	Fitzgerald, P	CA	222
EDM	Gagel, R	TX	220
EDM	Goodman, N	FL	214
EDM	Greene, L	NY	210
EDM	Greenspan, S	PA	210
EDM	Hammer, G	MI	217
EDM	Heber, D	CA	222
EDM	Herman, W	MI	217
EDM	Hirsch, I	WA	222
EDM	Hoffman, A	CA	223
EDM	Holick, M	MA	207
EDM	Hsueh, W	TX	221
EDM	Inzucchi, S	CT	207
EDM	Ipp, E	CA	223
EDM	Jacobs, T	NY	210
EDM	Jensen, M	MN	218
EDM	Kahn, B	MA	207
EDM	Kamdar, V	CA	223
EDM	Kandeel, F	CA	223
EDM	Katznelson, L	CA	223
EDM	Kennedy, L	OH	218
EDM	Khosla, S	MN	218
EDM	Kleinberg, D	NY	210
EDM	Klibanski, A	MA	207
EDM	Klonoff, D	CA	223
EDM	Koch, C	MS	214
EDM	Kopp, P	IL	218
EDM	Korytkowski, M	PA	211
EDM	Kronenberg, H	MA	207
EDM	Ladenson, P	MD	211
EDM	Larsen, P	MA	207
EDM	Lash, R	MI	218
EDM	Lavis, V	TX	221
EDM	LeBoff, M	MA	208
EDM	Lechan, R	MA	208
EDM	Levine, R	NH	208
EDM	Lipson, A	DC	211
EDM	Mandel, S	PA	211
EDM	Marshall, J	VA	214
EDM	Mazzone, T	IL	218
EDM	McConnell, R	NY	211
EDM	McGill, J	MO	218
EDM	McMahon, M	MN	219
EDM	Melmed, S	CA	223
EDM	Nathan, D	MA	208
EDM	Nestler, J	VA	215
EDM	Ober, K	NC	215
EDM	Orwoll, E	OR	223
EDM	Osei, K	OH	219
EDM	Ovalle, F	AL	215
EDM	Pearce, E	MA	208
EDM	Peters, A	CA	224
EDM	Philipson, L	IL	219
EDM	Powers, A	TN	215
EDM	Quinn, S	FL	215
EDM	Recker, R	NE	220
EDM	Riddle, M	OR	224
EDM	Ridgway, E	CO	220

Spec	Name	St	Pg
EDM	Robbins, R	TX	221
EDM	Roberts, M	PA	211
EDM	Rodbard, H	MD	211
EDM	Ross, D	MA	208
EDM	Rubenfeld, S	TX	221
EDM	Rushakoff, R	CA	224
EDM	Schutta, M	PA	211
EDM	Schwartz, S	PA	212
EDM	Seely, E	MA	208
EDM	Semenkovich, C	MO	219
EDM	Seplowitz, A	NY	212
EDM	Sherman, S	TX	221
EDM	Shuldiner, A	MD	212
EDM	Singer, P	CA	224
EDM	Siris, E	NY	212
EDM	Skyler, J	FL	215
EDM	Smith, S	MN	219
EDM	Snyder, P	PA	212
EDM	Sowers, J	MO	219
EDM	Surks, M	NY	212
EDM	Swerdloff, R	CA	224
EDM	Thorner, M	VA	215
EDM	Tuttle, R	NY	212
EDM	Vance, M	VA	215
EDM	Waguespack, S	TX	221
EDM	Wartofsky, L	DC	213
EDM	Watts, N	OH	219
EDM	Weiss, R	IL	219
EDM	Weissman, P	FL	216
EDM	Werner, P	IL	220
EDM	Woeber, K	CA	224
EDM	Wondisford, F	MD	213
EDM	Xing, M	MD	213
EDM	Young, I	NY	213
EDM	Zimmerman, R	OH	220

Endometriosis

Spec	Name	St	Pg
GO	Fiorica, J	FL	281
GO	Magrina, J	AZ	288
ObG	Einarsson, J	MA	556
ObG	Filip, S	NC	559
ObG	Goldstein, M	NY	557
ObG	Jenkins, T	AL	559
ObG	Merritt, D	MO	562
ObG	Pfeifer, S	PA	558
ObG	Steege, J	NC	560
RE	Adamson, G	CA	1016
RE	Agarwal, S	CA	1016
RE	Carson, S	RI	1006
RE	Christman, G	MI	1012
RE	Clisham, P	LA	1015
RE	Coddington, C	MN	1013
RE	DeVane, G	FL	1011
RE	Diamond, M	MI	1013
RE	Dodds, W	MI	1013
RE	Durso, N	VA	1011
RE	Falcone, T	OH	1013
RE	Giudice, L	CA	1017
RE	Hornstein, M	MA	1006
RE	Huang, J	TX	1016
RE	Isaacson, K	MA	1007

Spec	Name	St	Pg
RE	Jacobs, L	IL	1013
RE	Johnson, J	MA	1007
RE	Luciano, A	CT	1007
RE	Marrs, R	CA	1017
RE	Miller, C	IL	1014
RE	Mukherjee, T	NY	1009
RE	Ory, S	FL	1012
RE	Petrozza, J	MA	1007
RE	Putman, J	TX	1016
RE	Ratts, V	MO	1014
RE	Schenken, R	TX	1016
RE	Schlaff, W	PA	1010
RE	Sondheimer, S	PA	1010
RE	Soules, M	WA	1018
RE	Surrey, E	CO	1015
RE	Van Voorhis, B	IA	1015
RE	Zinaman, M	MA	1007

Endometriosis-Adolescent

Spec	Name	St	Pg
ObG	Laufer, M	MA	556

Endometriosis-Intestine

Spec	Name	St	Pg
CRS	Bailey, H	TX	176

Endoscopic Sinus Surgery

Spec	Name	St	Pg
Oto	Bhattacharyya, N	MA	655
Oto	Close, L	NY	658
Oto	DiNardo, L	VA	668
Oto	Edelstein, D	NY	659
Oto	Fried, M	NY	659
Oto	Gold, S	NY	659
Oto	Jacobs, J	NY	661
Oto	Josephson, J	NY	661
Oto	Kingdom, T	CO	680
Oto	Kuhn, F	GA	669
Oto	Lawson, W	NY	662
Oto	Schaefer, S	NY	664
Oto	Schaitkin, B	PA	664
Oto	Senders, C	CA	686
Oto	Stankiewicz, J	IL	677

Endoscopic Strip Craniectomy

Spec	Name	St	Pg
NS	Jimenez, D	TX	493

Endoscopic Surgery

Spec	Name	St	Pg
NS	Evans, J	PA	473
NS	Jho, H	PA	475
NS	Martin, N	CA	498
NS	Souweidane, M	NY	479
Oto	Ossoff, R	TN	669
Oto	Samant, S	TN	671
Oto	Snyderman, C	PA	665
PS	Tracy, T	RI	802
RE	Goldberg, J	OH	1013
T&CS	Damiano, R	MO	1131

Endoscopic

Spec	Name	St	Pg
Surgery/Ventriculoscopy			
NS	Goumnerova, L	MA	470

Spec	Name	St	Pg
Endoscopic Therapies			
Ge	Early, D	MO	245
Ge	Haluszka, O	PA	233
Ge	Hoffman, B	SC	240
Ge	Lichtenstein, D	MA	229
Ge	Wilcox, C	AL	243

Spec	Name	St	Pg
Endoscopic Ultrasound			
Ge	Aslanian, H	CT	228
Ge	Canto, M	MD	231
Ge	Chang, K	CA	253
Ge	Das, A	AZ	251
Ge	Dea, S	CA	253
Ge	Early, D	MO	245
Ge	Faigel, D	AZ	251
Ge	Gerdes, H	NY	232
Ge	Ginsberg, G	PA	233
Ge	Gordon, S	NH	229
Ge	Greenwald, B	MD	233
Ge	Haber, G	NY	233
Ge	Haluszka, O	PA	233
Ge	Hawes, R	FL	240
Ge	Hoffman, B	SC	240
Ge	Infantolino, A	PA	234
Ge	Jonnalagadda, S	MO	246
Ge	Kantsevoy, S	MD	234
Ge	Kimmey, M	WA	254
Ge	Kowalski, T	PA	235
Ge	Lambiase, L	TN	241
Ge	Levy, M	MN	246
Ge	Lightdale, C	NY	236
Ge	Meiselman, M	IL	247
Ge	Mertz, H	TN	241
Ge	Pochapin, M	NY	237
Ge	Rex, D	IN	247
Ge	Savides, T	CA	255

Spec	Name	St	Pg
Endoscopy			
Ge	Albert, M	DC	230
Ge	Barkin, J	FL	239
Ge	Baron, T	MN	244
Ge	Butterly, L	NH	228
Ge	Canto, M	MD	231
Ge	Carr-Locke, D	NY	231
Ge	Cello, J	CA	253
Ge	Cohen, L	NY	232
Ge	Das, A	AZ	251
Ge	Dea, S	CA	253
Ge	Dieterich, D	NY	232
Ge	Edmundowicz, S	MO	245
Ge	Eisen, G	OR	253
Ge	Elliott, N	GA	240
Ge	Fang, J	UT	249
Ge	Farraye, F	MA	228
Ge	Fisher, R	CT	228
Ge	Forsmark, C	FL	240
Ge	Gerdes, H	NY	232

Spec	Name	St	Pg
Ge	Ginsberg, G	PA	233
Ge	Gostout, C	MN	245
Ge	Green, P	NY	233
Ge	Haber, G	NY	233
Ge	Hoops, T	PA	234
Ge	Kalloo, A	MD	234
Ge	Kelsey, P	MA	229
Ge	Kimmey, M	WA	254
Ge	Kochman, M	PA	235
Ge	Konicek, F	IL	246
Ge	Kurtz, R	NY	235
Ge	Lebwohl, O	NY	235
Ge	Lewis, B	NY	235
Ge	Magun, A	NY	236
Ge	Miskovitz, P	NY	236
Ge	Peikin, S	NJ	237
Ge	Petrini, J	CA	255
Ge	Pfau, P	WI	247
Ge	Proctor, D	CT	230
Ge	Reichelderfer, M	WI	247
Ge	Rex, D	IN	247
Ge	Rothstein, R	NH	230
Ge	Seidner, D	TN	242
Ge	Sherman, S	IN	248
Ge	Shike, M	NY	238
Ge	Vargo, J	OH	248
Ge	Waxman, I	IL	249
Ge	Waye, J	NY	238
Ge	Weinberg, D	PA	238
Ge	Weinstock, J	MA	230
Ge	Yanda, R	GA	243
ObG	Bradley, L	OH	560
Oto	Aviv, J	NY	657
PGe	Schwarz, S	NY	751
S	Marks, J	OH	1079
S	Ponsky, J	OH	1080

Spec	Name	St	Pg
Endourology			
U	Wong, C	OH	1171

Spec	Name	St	Pg
Endovascular Neurosurgery			
NRad	Morris, P	NC	987
NS	Patel, A	NY	477

Spec	Name	St	Pg
Endovascular Stent Grafts			
T&CS	Szeto, W	PA	1122
VascS	Bandyk, D	CA	1194
VascS	Clair, D	OH	1190
VascS	Dougherty, M	PA	1186
VascS	McLafferty, R	IL	1191
VascS	Sanchez, L	MO	1191
VIR	Dake, M	CA	997
VIR	Matsumoto, A	VA	995

Spec	Name	St	Pg
Endovascular Surgery			
NRad	Berenstein, A	NY	985
NRad	Hirsch, J	MA	984
NS	Hopkins, L	NY	475
T&CS	Diethrich, E	AZ	1137

Spec	Name	St	Pg
T&CS	Miller, D	CA	1142
VascS	Acher, C	WI	1190
VascS	Adelman, M	NY	1185
VascS	Ahn, S	CA	1193
VascS	Atnip, R	PA	1185
VascS	Benvenisty, A	NY	1186
VascS	Blebea, J	OK	1192
VascS	Brener, B	NJ	1186
VascS	Brewster, D	MA	1184
VascS	Carpenter, J	NJ	1186
VascS	Chaikof, E	MA	1184
VascS	Criado, F	MD	1186
VascS	D'Ayala, M	NY	1186
VascS	Eidt, J	AR	1193
VascS	Fowl, R	AZ	1193
VascS	Golden, M	PA	1187
VascS	Hakaim, A	FL	1189
VascS	Hodgson, K	IL	1191
VascS	Hollier, L	LA	1193
VascS	Iafrati, M	MA	1184
VascS	Kazmers, A	MI	1191
VascS	Kougias, P	TX	1193
VascS	Kwolek, C	MA	1184
VascS	LaMuraglia, G	MA	1185
VascS	Makaroun, M	PA	1187
VascS	Marin, M	NY	1188
VascS	McCann, R	NC	1189
VascS	McKinsey, J	NY	1188
VascS	Money, S	AZ	1193
VascS	Naslund, T	TN	1190
VascS	Neville, R	DC	1188
VascS	Pevec, W	CA	1194
VascS	Pomposelli, F	MA	1185
VascS	Schneider, D	NY	1188
VascS	Sumpio, B	CT	1185
VascS	Weinstein, E	CO	1192
VascS	White, R	CA	1194
VascS	Zarins, C	CA	1194

Spec	Name	St	Pg
Enteroscopy-Small Bowel			
Ge	Elliott, N	GA	240

Spec	Name	St	Pg
Environmental Health in Children			
OM	Landrigan, P	NY	882

Spec	Name	St	Pg
Environmental Medicine			
OM	Gochfeld, M	NJ	882
OM	Kipen, H	NJ	882
Pul	Bascom, R	PA	924

Spec	Name	St	Pg
Eosinophil Disorders			
A&I	Lewis, J	AZ	89

Spec	Name	St	Pg
Eosinophilic Esophagitis			
PA&I	Spergel, J	PA	730
PGe	Gupta, S	IN	753

Spec	Name	St	Pg
Epilepsy			
ChiN	Edgar, T	WI	150
ChiN	Greenwood, R	NC	149
ChiN	Legido, A	PA	148
ChiN	Pinter, J	OR	153
ChiN	Santos, C	DC	148
ChiN	Scher, M	OH	151
ChiN	Sharp, G	AR	152
ChiN	Tennison, M	NC	149
ChiN	Tuxhorn, I	OH	151
ChiN	Yamada, K	MO	152
ChiN	Zupanc, M	CA	154
N	Abou-Khalil, B	TN	519
N	Bebin, E	AL	520
N	Blum, A	RI	506
N	Brick, J	WV	510
N	DeGiorgio, C	CA	536
N	Devinsky, O	NY	511
N	Gross, P	MA	507
N	Heck, C	CA	537
N	Josephson, D	IN	527
N	Labiner, D	AZ	534
N	Luders, H	OH	527
N	Morrell, M	CA	538
N	Nicholl, J	LA	534
N	Oommen, K	TX	534
N	Sperling, M	PA	518
NRad	Faro, S	PA	985
NRad	Rowley, H	WI	989
NS	Asher, A	NC	481
NS	Bakay, R	IL	485
NS	Bingaman, W	OH	486
NS	Boop, F	TN	481
NS	Burchiel, K	OR	496
NS	Danielpour, M	CA	496
NS	Duhaime, A	MA	470
NS	Ewend, M	NC	481
NS	Goodman, R	NY	474
NS	Jallo, G	MD	475
NS	Liu, C	CA	497
NS	Mamelak, A	CA	498
NS	Meyer, F	MN	489
NS	Ojemann, J	WA	498
NS	Ragheb, J	FL	483
NS	Schwartz, T	NY	478
NS	Shuer, L	CA	499
NS	Walsh, J	LA	495
NS	Weiner, H	NY	480
NS	Wharen, R	FL	485
NS	Wilberger, J	PA	480
Ped	Vining, E	MD	727
Epilepsy in Pregnancy			
MF	Samuels, P	OH	437
N	Bergey, G	MD	509
N	Liporace, J	PA	514
N	Pennell, P	MA	508
N	Rubin, S	IL	530
Epilepsy in Tuberous Sclerosis			
ChiN	Riviello, J	NY	148
Epilepsy in Women			
N	Bergey, G	MD	509
N	Jobst, B	NH	507
N	Liporace, J	PA	514
N	Morrell, M	CA	538
N	Pennell, P	MA	508
Epilepsy/Seizure Disorders			
ChiN	Bourgeois, B	MA	146
ChiN	Gospe, S	WA	153
ChiN	Griesemer, D	MA	146
ChiN	Holmes, G	NH	146
ChiN	Kovnar, E	WI	151
ChiN	Mandelbaum, D	RI	146
ChiN	Maytal, J	NY	148
ChiN	Mitchell, W	CA	153
ChiN	Riviello, J	NY	148
ChiN	Sankar, R	CA	154
ChiN	Shinnar, S	NY	149
ChiN	Tonsgard, J	IL	151
ChiN	Wheless, J	TN	150
ChiN	Wyllie, E	OH	152
N	Armon, C	MA	506
N	Barkley, G	MI	525
N	Bergey, G	MD	509
N	Cole, A	MA	506
N	Ferrendelli, J	TX	533
N	Fisher, R	CA	537
N	French, J	NY	511
N	Hecox, K	WI	527
N	Jobst, B	NH	507
N	Krauss, G	MD	513
N	Krumholz, A	MD	513
N	Kuzniecky, R	NY	513
N	Labar, D	NY	514
N	Pedley, T	NY	516
N	Strom, L	CO	532
NS	Adelson, P	AZ	492
NS	Apuzzo, M	CA	495
NS	Baltuch, G	PA	472
NS	Bucholz, R	MO	486
NS	Caputy, A	DC	473
NS	Cosgrove, R	RI	470
NS	Eisenberg, H	MD	473
NS	Kestle, J	UT	491
NS	Madsen, J	MA	471
NS	Naff, N	MD	477
NS	Penar, P	VT	471
NS	Spencer, D	CT	471
Epispadias			
U	Mesrobian, H	WI	1169
Erectile Dysfunction			
EDM	Cunningham, G	TX	220
U	Bar-Chama, N	NY	1151
U	Boyd, S	CA	1175
U	Broderick, G	FL	1160
U	Burnett, A	MD	1151
U	Carson, C	NC	1160
U	Childs, S	CO	1171
U	Danoff, D	CA	1176
U	Donovan, J	OH	1166
U	Fraser, L	MS	1161
U	Goldstein, I	CA	1176
U	Goldstein, M	NY	1152
U	Gomery, P	MA	1148
U	Hellstrom, W	LA	1173
U	Levine, L	IL	1168
U	Lipshultz, L	TX	1174
U	Lloyd, L	AL	1162
U	McCullough, A	NY	1155
U	McVary, K	IL	1168
U	Montague, D	OH	1169
U	Mulhall, J	NY	1155
U	Nagler, H	NY	1156
U	Nehra, A	IL	1169
U	Ohl, D	MI	1169
U	Penson, D	TN	1163
U	Rajfer, J	CA	1178
U	Ross, L	IL	1170
U	Sadeghi-Nejad, H	NJ	1156
U	Shabsigh, R	NY	1157
U	Sharlip, I	CA	1178
U	Steers, W	VA	1164
U	Turek, P	CA	1179
Esophageal Cancer			
DR	Coakley, F	OR	982
Ge	Aslanian, H	CT	228
Ge	Estores, D	FL	240
Ge	Fleischer, D	AZ	252
Ge	Greenwald, B	MD	233
Onc	Adelstein, D	OH	364
Onc	Ajani, J	TX	377
Onc	Forastiere, A	MD	340
Onc	Fuchs, C	MA	329
Onc	Grem, J	NE	375
Onc	Ilson, D	NY	342
Onc	Loehrer, P	IN	369
Onc	Masters, G	DE	345
Onc	Reid, T	CA	390
Onc	Ross, H	AZ	381
Onc	Stoopler, M	NY	350
Onc	Sun, W	PA	350
Onc	Vokes, E	IL	373
Path	Goldblum, J	OH	715
Path	Odze, R	MA	707
RadRO	Bradley, J	MO	958
RadRO	Choi, N	MA	946
RadRO	Cox, J	TX	963
RadRO	Greenberger, J	PA	950
RadRO	Halpern, H	IL	959
RadRO	Kleinberg, L	MD	951
RadRO	Komaki, R	TX	964
RadRO	Konski, A	MI	960
RadRO	Martenson, J	MN	961

Spec	Name	St	Pg
RadRO	Minsky, B	TX	965
RadRO	Seung, S	OR	968
RadRO	Suntharalingam, M	MD	953
RadRO	Thomas, C	OR	968
RadRO	Videtic, G	OH	962
S	Aranha, G	IL	1074
S	August, D	NJ	1053
S	Beauchamp, R	TN	1067
S	Bolton, J	LA	1087
S	Brodsky, J	PA	1054
S	Cioffi, W	RI	1048
S	Karpeh, M	NY	1059
S	Levine, E	NC	1070
S	Livingstone, A	FL	1070
S	Paz, I	CA	1098
S	Pellegrini, C	WA	1098
S	Posner, M	IL	1081
S	Salo, J	NC	1071
S	Sutton, J	VT	1052
T&CS	Altorki, N	NY	1113
T&CS	Baciewicz, F	MI	1130
T&CS	Bains, M	NY	1114
T&CS	Brinckerhoff, L	MA	1110
T&CS	Bull, D	UT	1136
T&CS	Cerfolio, R	AL	1124
T&CS	D'Amico, T	NC	1125
T&CS	Demmy, T	NY	1115
T&CS	Deschamps, C	MN	1131
T&CS	Ferguson, M	IL	1132
T&CS	Fernando, H	MA	1111
T&CS	Flores, R	NY	1115
T&CS	Gaissert, H	MA	1111
T&CS	Handy, J	OR	1141
T&CS	Harpole, D	NC	1125
T&CS	Heitmiller, R	MD	1117
T&CS	Howington, J	IL	1132
T&CS	Jones, D	VA	1125
T&CS	Kaiser, L	PA	1118
T&CS	Keenan, R	PA	1118
T&CS	Keller, S	NY	1118
T&CS	Kernstine, K	TX	1138
T&CS	Kiernan, P	VA	1126
T&CS	Kiev, J	WV	1118
T&CS	Kucharczuk, J	PA	1119
T&CS	Landreneau, R	PA	1119
T&CS	Lau, C	VA	1126
T&CS	Love, R	IL	1133
T&CS	Marshall, M	DC	1120
T&CS	Mathisen, D	MA	1111
T&CS	Meyers, B	MO	1133
T&CS	Miller, D	GA	1127
T&CS	Moore, J	GA	1127
T&CS	Naunheim, K	MO	1134
T&CS	Nesbitt, J	TN	1127
T&CS	Ninan, M	TN	1128
T&CS	Orringer, M	MI	1134
T&CS	Park, B	NJ	1120
T&CS	Patterson, G	MO	1134
T&CS	Putnam, J	TN	1128
T&CS	Reed, C	SC	1128
T&CS	Roth, J	TX	1139
T&CS	Rusch, V	NY	1121
T&CS	Scott, W	PA	1121
T&CS	Soberman, M	MD	1121
T&CS	Sugarbaker, D	MA	1112
T&CS	Swanson, S	MA	1112
T&CS	Swisher, S	TX	1139
T&CS	Wain, J	MA	1112
T&CS	Walsh, G	TX	1140
T&CS	Watson, T	NY	1122
T&CS	Weigel, T	WI	1135
T&CS	Weksler, B	PA	1123
T&CS	Whyte, R	MA	1113
T&CS	Wood, D	WA	1143
T&CS	Wright, C	MA	1113
T&CS	Yang, S	MD	1123
T&CS	Zwischenberger, J	KY	1130

Esophageal Disorders

Ge	Benjamin, S	DC	231
Ge	Castell, D	SC	239
Ge	Cohen, L	NY	232
Ge	Di Marino, A	PA	232
Ge	Falk, G	PA	232
Ge	Fang, J	UT	249
Ge	Gerson, L	CA	254
Ge	Hoops, T	PA	234
Ge	Kahrilas, P	IL	246
Ge	Katz, P	PA	235
Ge	Koch, K	NC	241
Ge	Kotler, D	NY	235
Ge	Lipshutz, W	PA	236
Ge	Markowitz, D	NY	236
Ge	Mittal, R	CA	254
Ge	Murray, J	MN	247
Ge	Roth, B	CA	255
Ge	Vaezi, M	TN	243
PGe	Gunasekaran, T	IL	753
PGe	Spivak, W	NY	751
S	Richards, W	AL	1071
S	Sharp, K	TN	1072
S	Swanstrom, L	OR	1100
T&CS	Fernando, H	MA	1111

Esophageal Surgery

PS	Jennings, R	MA	801
S	Crookes, P	CA	1094
S	Dempsey, D	PA	1056
S	Hunter, J	OR	1096
S	Pellegrini, C	WA	1098
S	Peters, J	NY	1062
S	Reiner, M	NY	1063
S	Swanstrom, L	OR	1100
T&CS	Battafarano, R	MD	1114
T&CS	DeCamp, M	IL	1131
T&CS	Feins, R	NC	1125
T&CS	Iannettoni, M	IA	1132
T&CS	Jablons, D	CA	1142
T&CS	Kernstine, K	TX	1138
T&CS	Lazar, H	MA	1111
T&CS	Mitchell, J	CO	1136
T&CS	Mullett, T	KY	1127
T&CS	Rice, T	OH	1134

T&CS	Soberman, M	MD	1121
T&CS	Weiman, D	TN	1130

Esthesioneuroblastoma

Oto	Kennedy, D	PA	661
Oto	Olsen, K	MN	677

Ethics

Ger	Finucane, T	MD	263
H & PM	Arnold, R	PA	406
NP	Boyle, R	VA	449
NP	Holzman, I	NY	447
NP	Lemons, J	IN	450
NP	Meadow, W	IL	450
NP	Muraskas, J	IL	451
Onc	Brescia, F	SC	354
Onc	Levy, M	PA	344
Ped	Fost, N	WI	727
Ped	Lantos, J	MO	728
PHO	Morgan, E	IL	772
PHO	Santana, V	TN	768
S	Angelos, P	IL	1074

Ethics Issues in Neonatalogy

Ped	Lantos, J	MO	728

Ethnic Skin Disorders

D	Barbosa, V	IL	192
D	Grimes, P	CA	199
D	McMichael, A	NC	191

Ewing's Sarcoma

OrS	McDonald, D	MO	635
Path	Antonescu, C	NY	707
Ped	Kleinerman, E	TX	728
PHO	Hawkins, D	WA	777

Exercise Physiology

PCd	Driscoll, D	MN	739
PMR	Gater, D	VA	838
Rhu	Bunning, R	DC	1026

Eye Diseases-Hereditary

Oph	Drack, A	IA	589
Oph	Gorin, M	CA	600
Oph	Heckenlively, J	MI	590
Oph	Lewis, R	TX	597
Oph	Stone, E	IA	594
Oph	Summers, C	MN	594

Eye Growth/Development

Oph	Quinn, G	PA	578

Eye Infections

Oph	O'Brien, T	FL	585

Spec	Name	St	Pg

Eye Movement Disorders

Spec	Name	St	Pg
N	Lavin, P	TN	522

Eye Muscle Disorders

Oph	Choy, A	CA	600
Oph	Ellis, G	LA	596
Oph	Granet, D	CA	600
Oph	Hall, L	NY	575
Oph	Hunter, D	MA	570
Oph	McKeown, C	FL	584
Oph	Mills, M	PA	577
Oph	Nelson, L	PA	578
Oph	Wang, F	NY	581

Eye Muscle Surgery

Oph	Burke, M	OH	589
Oph	Koller, H	PA	576
Oph	Richard, J	OK	597
Oph	Rosenberg, M	IL	594

Eye Pathology

Oph	Rao, N	CA	603

Eye Tumors-Pediatric

Oph	Lueder, G	MO	592

Eye Tumors/Cancer

Oph	Abramson, D	NY	571
Oph	Albert, D	WI	588
Oph	Alward, W	IA	588
Oph	Augsburger, J	OH	588
Oph	Boxrud, C	CA	599
Oph	Char, D	CA	599
Oph	Drack, A	IA	589
Oph	Dutton, J	NC	583
Oph	Finger, P	NY	573
Oph	Haik, B	TN	584
Oph	Harbour, J	FL	584
Oph	Mieler, W	IL	592
Oph	Murphree, A	CA	602
Oph	Murray, T	FL	585
Oph	O'Brien, J	PA	578
Oph	Pulido, J	MN	593
Oph	Shields, J	PA	580
Oph	Soparkar, C	TX	598
Oph	Sternberg, P	TN	586
Oph	Wilson, D	OR	605
Oph	Wilson, M	TN	587
RadRO	Crocker, I	GA	954
RadRO	Markoe, A	FL	955
RadRO	McCormick, B	NY	951
RadRO	Quivey, J	CA	967
RadRO	Rotman, M	NY	952

Eyelid Cancer & Reconstruction

Oph	Cockerham, K	CA	600
Oph	Esmaeli-Azad, B	TX	596
Oph	Gigantelli, J	NE	596

Eyelid Cosmetic & Reconstructive Surgery

Oph	Ahmad, A	IL	588
Oph	Lisman, R	NY	576
Oph	Putterman, A	IL	593
Oph	Rubin, P	MA	571

Eyelid Problems/Ptosis/Blepharospasm

Oph	Anderson, R	UT	595

Eyelid Surgery

Oph	Baylis, H	CA	598
Oph	Cahill, K	OH	589
Oph	Carter, K	IA	589
Oph	Patrinely, J	FL	585
Oph	Stefanyszyn, M	PA	580
Oto	Larrabee, W	WA	685
PlS	Carraway, J	VA	860
PlS	Imber, G	NY	854
PlS	Miller, T	CA	875
PlS	Sanders, G	CA	876
PlS	Sullivan, P	RI	851
PlS	Tabbal, N	NY	859

Eyelid Surgery/Blepharoplasty

PlS	Leaf, N	CA	875
PlS	Metzinger, S	LA	871
PlS	Spinelli, H	NY	858

Eyelid Tumors/Cancer

Oph	Della Rocca, R	NY	573
Oph	Elner, V	MI	589
Oph	Yeatts, R	NC	587

Eyelid/Tear Duct Reconstruction

Oph	Cahill, K	OH	589
Oph	Lisman, R	NY	576
Oph	Mawn, L	TN	584

F

Fabry's Disease

CG	Wilcox, W	CA	164
N	Kolodny, E	NY	513
Nep	Thomas, C	IA	463

Facial Deformities/Reconstruction

PlS	Bentz, M	WI	864

Facial Feminization Surgery (FFS)

PlS	Ousterhout, D	CA	876

Facial Nerve Disorders

Oto	Bojrab, D	MI	673
Oto	Brackmann, D	CA	684
Oto	Hirsch, B	PA	660
Oto	Lalwani, A	NY	662
Oto	Roland, J	NY	664
Oto	Shelton, C	UT	680
Oto	Wax, M	OR	687
PlS	Manders, E	PA	856

Facial Paralysis

Oto	Hadlock, T	MA	656
Oto	Leonetti, J	IL	676
Oto	Pensak, M	OH	677
PlS	Sherman, R	CA	876

Facial Paralysis Reconstruction

PlS	Kuzon, W	MI	866
PlS	Rose, E	NY	858

Facial Plastic & Reconstructive Surgery

Oto	Gosselin, B	NH	655
Oto	Hayden, R	AZ	682
Oto	Marentette, L	MI	676
Oto	Moe, K	WA	686
Oto	Ries, W	TN	670
Oto	Shockley, W	NC	671
Oto	Teknos, T	OH	678
Oto	Wax, M	OR	687
Oto	Wong, B	CA	688
PlS	Bradley, J	CA	873
PlS	Cordeiro, P	NY	853
PlS	Eriksson, E	MA	850
PlS	Hunstad, J	NC	862
PlS	Leighton, W	AZ	871
PlS	Ristow, B	CA	876
PlS	Robb, G	TX	871
PlS	Rodriguez, E	MD	857
PlS	Rose, E	NY	858
PlS	Siebert, J	WI	868
PlS	Yu, J	GA	864

Facial Plastic Surgery

Oto	Epstein, J	FL	668
Oto	Farrior, E	FL	668
Oto	Hilger, P	MN	675
Oto	Pribitkin, E	PA	663
Oto	Quatela, V	NY	664
PlS	Ness, J	MN	867
PlS	Smith, P	FL	863

Facial Rejuvenation

D	Brody, H	GA	189

Specialty & Special Expertise Index

Spec	Name	St	Pg
D	DeLeo, V	NY	186
D	Garden, J	IL	193
D	Gordon, M	NY	186
D	Grossman, M	NY	186
D	Kilmer, S	CA	199
Oto	Graham, H	LA	682
PlS	Barton, F	TX	869
PlS	Beasley, M	NC	860
PlS	Burns, A	TX	870
PlS	Cederna, P	MI	865
PlS	Davis, G	NC	861
PlS	Dick, G	MD	853
PlS	Fodor, P	CA	874
PlS	Fox, J	PA	854
PlS	Gregory, R	FL	861
PlS	Hoffman, L	NY	854
PlS	Koplin, L	CA	875
PlS	Markowitz, B	CA	875
PlS	Marten, T	CA	875
PlS	Rand, R	WA	876
PlS	Rappaport, N	TX	871
PlS	Rohrich, R	TX	872
PlS	Romano, J	CA	876
PlS	Rosenberg, H	CA	876
PlS	Singh, N	MD	858
PlS	Stuzin, J	FL	863
PlS	Zins, J	OH	869

Facial Surgery-Chin & Lip

Spec	Name	St	Pg
PlS	Zide, B	NY	860

Facial Trauma/Fractures

Spec	Name	St	Pg
PlS	Baker, S	DC	852
PlS	Gruss, J	WA	874
PlS	Manson, P	MD	856
PlS	Matthews, D	NC	862

Facial Tumors

Spec	Name	St	Pg
PlS	Yu, J	GA	864

Falls in the Elderly

Spec	Name	St	Pg
Ger	Lipsitz, L	MA	262
Ger	Studenski, S	PA	263
Ger	Tinetti, M	CT	262

Family Therapy

Spec	Name	St	Pg
ChAP	Sargent, A	MA	907
Psyc	Liberman, R	CA	901

Fanconi Aplastic Anemia

Spec	Name	St	Pg
Ped	Berman, B	MI	727

Fanconi Syndrome

Spec	Name	St	Pg
PNep	Friedman, A	MN	787

Female Genital Cutting (FGC)

Education

Spec	Name	St	Pg
ObG	Nour, N	MA	556

Fertility in Cancer Survivors

Spec	Name	St	Pg
CG	Mulvihill, J	OK	161
PHO	Green, D	TN	766

Fertility Preservation in Cancer

Spec	Name	St	Pg
GO	Burnett, A	AR	287
GO	Del Priore, G	IN	284
GO	Fields, A	DC	278
GO	Gershenson, D	TX	287
Onc	Matulonis, U	MA	331
RE	Copperman, A	NY	1008
RE	Coutifaris, C	PA	1008
RE	Crowley, W	MA	1006
RE	Ginsburg, E	MA	1006
RE	Gracia, C	PA	1008
RE	Grazi, R	NY	1008
RE	Grifo, J	NY	1008
RE	Licciardi, F	NY	1009
RE	McGovern, P	NJ	1009
RE	Molo, M	IL	1014
RE	Noyes, N	NY	1009
RE	Patrizio, P	CT	1007
RE	Rosenwaks, Z	NY	1009
RE	Seifer, D	NY	1010
RE	Smikle, C	CA	1017
U	Sheinfeld, J	NY	1158

Fetal Abnormalities

Spec	Name	St	Pg
CG	Bianchi, D	MA	156
CG	Driscoll, D	PA	157
MF	Dooley, S	IL	436
MF	Genc, M	NY	432
MF	Robichaux, A	LA	439

Fetal Alcohol Syndrome

Spec	Name	St	Pg
CG	Cunniff, C	AZ	161
CG	Hoyme, H	SD	161
CG	Morris, C	NV	163
CG	Seaver, L	HI	163

Fetal Cardiology

Spec	Name	St	Pg
PCd	Lewin, M	WA	741
PCd	Rychik, J	PA	736

Fetal Diagnosis & Therapy

Spec	Name	St	Pg
MF	Blakemore, K	MD	431
MF	Copel, J	CT	430
MF	Goldberg, J	CA	440
MF	Koos, B	CA	440
MF	Moore, T	CA	440
MF	Treadwell, M	MI	437
MF	Wilkins-Haug, L	MA	431
ObG	Corteville, J	OH	560
ObG	Evans, M	NY	557

Fetal Echocardiography

Spec	Name	St	Pg
MF	Copel, J	CT	430
MF	Reed, K	AZ	439
MF	Robinson, J	MA	431
PCd	Biancaniello, T	NY	734
PCd	Bierman, F	NY	734
PCd	Colvin, E	AL	737
PCd	Crosson, J	MD	735
PCd	Parness, I	NY	735

Fetal Imaging

Spec	Name	St	Pg
DR	Hubbard, A	NE	981

Fetal Macrosomia

Spec	Name	St	Pg
MF	Benedetti, T	WA	439

Fetal MRI

Spec	Name	St	Pg
DR	Hubbard, A	NE	981

Fetal Neuroradiology

Spec	Name	St	Pg
NRad	Barnes, P	CA	990

Fetal Neurosurgery

Spec	Name	St	Pg
NS	Sutton, L	PA	479

Fetal Pathology

Spec	Name	St	Pg
Path	Faye-Petersen, O	AL	713

Fetal Surgery

Spec	Name	St	Pg
MF	Carr, S	RI	430
MF	Chmait, R	CA	440
MF	Robichaux, A	LA	439
MF	Wilkins-Haug, L	MA	431
ObG	De Lia, J	WI	561
PCd	Lock, J	MA	734
PS	Adzick, N	PA	802
PS	Albanese, C	CA	810
PS	Bond, S	KY	805
PS	Cass, D	TX	809
PS	Crombleholme, T	CO	808
PS	Farmer, D	CA	810
PS	Flake, A	PA	803
PS	Glick, P	NY	803
PS	Jennings, R	MA	801
PS	Krummel, T	CA	811
PS	Proctor, M	WA	811
PS	Tracy, T	RI	802

Fetal Surgical Imaging

Spec	Name	St	Pg
DR	Benson, C	MA	973

Fetal Therapy

Spec	Name	St	Pg
CG	Mahoney, M	CT	156
MF	Berkowitz, R	NY	431
MF	Cheng, E	WA	439
MF	Eddleman, K	NY	432

Spec	Name	St	Pg
MF	Mari, G	TN	435

Fetal Ultrasound

Spec	Name	St	Pg
MF	Parry, S	PA	433

Fetal Ultrasound/Obstetrical Imaging

Spec	Name	St	Pg
DR	Cohen, H	TN	979

Fetal Urology

Spec	Name	St	Pg
U	Coplen, D	MO	1166
U	Rushton, H	DC	1156

Fever in Returning Travelers

Spec	Name	St	Pg
Inf	Wallace, M	FL	415

Fevers of Unknown Origin

Spec	Name	St	Pg
Inf	Auwaerter, P	MD	410
Inf	Bartlett, J	MD	410
Inf	Cunha, B	NY	411
Inf	Trenholme, G	IL	417
PInf	Alexander, K	IL	782
PInf	McKinney, R	NC	782

Fevers-Periodic

Spec	Name	St	Pg
Ped	Infante, A	TX	728

Fibrodysplasia Ossificans Progressiv FOP

Spec	Name	St	Pg
OrS	Kaplan, F	PA	620

Fibromyalgia

Spec	Name	St	Pg
Rhu	Crofford, L	KY	1029
Rhu	Katz, R	IL	1031
Rhu	Rothenberg, R	MD	1028
Rhu	Solitar, B	NY	1028

Fine Needle Aspiration Biopsy

Spec	Name	St	Pg
Path	Ehya, H	PA	708
Path	Gupta, P	PA	709
Path	Ljung, B	CA	721
Path	Silverman, J	PA	711

Fluid/Electrolyte Balance

Spec	Name	St	Pg
Nep	Coe, F	IL	461
Nep	Gluck, S	CA	465
Nep	Olivero, J	TX	464
Nep	Weiner, I	FL	460

Food & Drug Allergy

Spec	Name	St	Pg
A&I	Buchbinder, E	NY	84
A&I	Shepherd, G	NY	85

Food Allergy

Spec	Name	St	Pg
A&I	Bonner, J	AL	86

Spec	Name	St	Pg
A&I	Castells, M	MA	84
A&I	Ein, D	DC	85
A&I	Slankard, M	NY	85
A&I	Umetsu, D	MA	84
PA&I	Bahna, S	LA	732
PA&I	Bock, S	CO	732
PA&I	Burks, A	NC	730
PA&I	Ehrlich, P	NY	729
PA&I	Epstein, S	CA	733
PA&I	Josephs, S	MD	729
PA&I	Leung, D	CO	732
PA&I	Ownby, D	GA	731
PA&I	Pongracic, J	IL	731
PA&I	Sampson, H	NY	729
PA&I	Sicherer, S	NY	730
PA&I	Spergel, J	PA	730
PA&I	Wasserman, R	TX	732
PA&I	Wood, R	MD	730
PPul	Lapey, A	MA	794

Food Allergy & Eczema

Spec	Name	St	Pg
A&I	Sanders, G	MI	89

Foodborne illnesses

Spec	Name	St	Pg
Inf	Lorber, B	PA	412

Foot & Ankle Surgery

Spec	Name	St	Pg
OrS	Bauman, P	NY	614
OrS	Brodsky, J	TX	640
OrS	Coughlin, M	ID	638
OrS	Deland, J	NY	616
OrS	DeOrio, J	NC	628
OrS	DiGiovanni, C	RI	610
OrS	Greisberg, J	NY	618
OrS	Levine, D	NY	621
OrS	Manoli, A	MI	635
OrS	Myerson, M	MD	622
OrS	Nunley, J	NC	629
OrS	Pinzur, M	IL	637
OrS	Saltzman, C	UT	639
OrS	Sangeorzan, B	WA	645
OrS	Smith, D	WA	646
OrS	Walling, A	FL	631
OrS	Wapner, K	PA	626
OrS	Weinfeld, S	NY	626
SM	Teitz, C	WA	1044

Foot & Ankle Surgery-Complex

Spec	Name	St	Pg
OrS	Brage, M	WA	642

Foot Deformities

Spec	Name	St	Pg
OrS	Davidson, R	PA	616
OrS	DeOrio, J	NC	628

Forensic Pathology

Spec	Name	St	Pg
Path	Mark, E	MA	706

Forensic Psychiatry

Spec	Name	St	Pg
AdP	Frances, R	NY	904
Psyc	Appelbaum, P	NY	890
Psyc	Eth, S	FL	895
Psyc	First, M	NY	892
Psyc	Greiner, C	NE	898
Psyc	Neppe, V	WA	902
Psyc	Wilson, D	FL	896

Fracture Deformities/Arm

Spec	Name	St	Pg
HS	Putnam, M	MN	302

Fractures

Spec	Name	St	Pg
HS	Melone, C	NY	297
HS	Wolfe, S	NY	298
OrS	Brage, M	WA	642

Fractures & Tendon Transfers

Spec	Name	St	Pg
HS	Abrams, R	CA	303
HS	Hastings, H	IN	301

Fractures in the Elderly

Spec	Name	St	Pg
OrS	Tornetta, P	MA	613

Fractures-Complex

Spec	Name	St	Pg
HS	Fischer, T	IN	300
OrS	Browner, B	CT	610
OrS	Buckwalter, J	IA	633
OrS	Tornetta, P	MA	613

Fractures-Complex & Non Union

Spec	Name	St	Pg
OrS	Anglen, J	IN	632
OrS	Ebraheim, N	OH	633
OrS	Friedlaender, G	CT	611
OrS	Helfet, D	NY	619
OrS	Joyce, M	OH	634
OrS	Lowenberg, D	CA	644
OrS	Muschler, G	OH	636
OrS	Rozbruch, S	NY	624
OrS	Webb, L	GA	631

Fractures-Non Union

Spec	Name	St	Pg
HS	Jupiter, J	MA	294
OrS	Browner, B	CT	610
OrS	Swiontkowski, M	MN	638
OrS	Wilkins, R	CO	640

Fractures-Pediatric

Spec	Name	St	Pg
OrS	Beaty, J	TN	627
OrS	Hyman, J	NY	620

Fractures-Stress

Spec	Name	St	Pg
OrS	Helfet, D	NY	619

Specialty & Special Expertise Index

Spec	Name	St	Pg		Spec	Name	St	Pg		Spec	Name	St	Pg
Frail Elderly					Ge	Brandt, L	NY	231		Ge	Goggins, M	MD	233
Ger	Callahan, E	NY	262		Ge	Brazer, S	NC	239		Ge	Goldberg, M	IL	245
Ger	Thomas, D	MO	265		Ge	Bresalier, R	TX	251		Ge	Gordon, S	NH	229
					Ge	Brown, K	MI	244		Ge	Gostout, C	MN	245
					Ge	Brown, R	NY	231		Ge	Green, P	NY	233
Frailty Syndrome					Ge	Bulat, R	LA	251		Ge	Greenwald, B	MD	233
Ger	Hanson, L	NC	264		Ge	Burt, R	UT	249		Ge	Haber, G	NY	233
Ger	Morley, J	MO	265		Ge	Butterly, L	NH	228		Ge	Haluszka, O	PA	233
PMR	De Lateur, B	MD	835		Ge	Canto, M	MD	231		Ge	Han, S	CA	254
					Ge	Carr-Locke, D	NY	231		Ge	Hanauer, S	IL	245
					Ge	Castell, D	SC	239		Ge	Hawes, R	FL	240
Frbromyalgia Syndrome (FMS)					Ge	Cello, J	CA	253		Ge	Herrine, S	PA	233
Psyc	Manevitz, A	NY	893		Ge	Chang, K	CA	253		Ge	Hoffman, B	SC	240
					Ge	Chari, S	MN	244		Ge	Hoops, T	PA	234
					Ge	Chey, W	MI	244		Ge	Hunter, E	ID	249
Fungal Infections					Ge	Chung, D	MA	228		Ge	Infantolino, A	PA	234
Inf	Edwards, J	CA	419		Ge	Chung, R	MA	228		Ge	Isaacs, K	NC	240
Inf	Galgiani, J	AZ	418		Ge	Cohen, J	NY	231		Ge	Itzkowitz, S	NY	234
Inf	O'Keefe, J	IL	416		Ge	Cohen, L	NY	232		Ge	Jacobson, I	NY	234
Inf	Patterson, T	TX	419		Ge	Cominelli, F	OH	244		Ge	Jensen, D	IL	246
Inf	Sepkowitz, K	NY	413		Ge	Crippin, J	MO	244		Ge	Jonnalagadda, S	MO	246
Inf	Sobel, J	MI	417		Ge	Cunningham, J	AZ	251		Ge	Kahrilas, P	IL	246
Inf	Van Der Horst, C	NC	415		Ge	Das, A	AZ	251		Ge	Kalloo, A	MD	234
PInf	Belcher, C	IN	782		Ge	Davis, G	TX	251		Ge	Kantsevoy, S	MD	234
PInf	Saiman, L	NY	781		Ge	Dea, S	CA	253		Ge	Kaplan, L	MA	229
					Ge	DeCross, A	NY	232		Ge	Kastenberg, D	PA	234
					Ge	DeVault, K	FL	239		Ge	Katz, P	PA	235
					Ge	Di Bisceglie, A	MO	244		Ge	Kelsey, P	MA	229
					Ge	Di Marino, A	PA	232		Ge	Kimmey, M	WA	254
G					Ge	Dienstag, J	MA	228		Ge	Koch, K	NC	241
					Ge	Dieterich, D	NY	232		Ge	Kochman, M	PA	235
					Ge	Drossman, D	NC	240		Ge	Konicek, F	IL	246
Gait Disorders					Ge	Early, D	MO	245		Ge	Korsten, M	NY	235
PMR	Kuiken, T	IL	841		Ge	Edmundowicz, S	MO	245		Ge	Kotler, D	NY	235
					Ge	Eisen, G	OR	253		Ge	Kowalski, T	PA	235
Gallbladder & Biliary Cancer					Ge	Elliott, D	IA	245		Ge	Kozarek, R	WA	254
RadRO	Rich, T	VA	957		Ge	Elliott, N	GA	240		Ge	Kurtz, R	NY	235
S	Hiotis, S	NY	1058		Ge	Ellis, J	CA	253		Ge	Kwo, P	IN	246
S	Jarnagin, W	NY	1058		Ge	Elta, G	MI	245		Ge	La Mont, J	MA	229
S	Pawlik, T	MD	1062		Ge	Estores, D	FL	240		Ge	La Russo, N	MN	246
S	Sielaff, T	MN	1082		Ge	Faigel, D	AZ	251		Ge	Lambiase, L	TN	241
S	Vauthey, J	TX	1092		Ge	Falk, G	PA	232		Ge	Lashner, B	OH	246
					Ge	Fallon, M	TX	251		Ge	Lebwohl, O	NY	235
Gastroenterology					Ge	Fang, J	UT	249		Ge	Leighton, J	AZ	252
Ge	Abreu, M	FL	239		Ge	Farraye, F	MA	228		Ge	Levine, J	CO	250
Ge	Al-Kawas, F	DC	230		Ge	Feldman, E	CA	253		Ge	Levy, M	MN	246
Ge	Albert, M	DC	230		Ge	Fennerty, M	OR	254		Ge	Lewis, B	NY	235
Ge	Anderson, K	TX	250		Ge	Fisher, R	PA	232		Ge	Lichtenstein, D	MA	229
Ge	Aronchick, C	PA	230		Ge	Fisher, R	CT	228		Ge	Lichtenstein, G	PA	236
Ge	Aslanian, H	CT	228		Ge	Fleischer, D	AZ	252		Ge	Liddle, R	NC	241
Ge	Bacon, B	MO	243		Ge	Forsmark, C	FL	240		Ge	Lightdale, C	NY	236
Ge	Baillie, J	NC	239		Ge	Freiman, H	NY	232		Ge	Lind, C	TN	241
Ge	Balart, L	LA	250		Ge	Fried, M	NC	240		Ge	Lipshutz, W	PA	236
Ge	Barkin, J	FL	239		Ge	Friedman, L	MA	229		Ge	Loftus, E	MN	247
Ge	Barnes, D	OH	244		Ge	Galati, J	TX	252		Ge	Loomba, R	CA	254
Ge	Baron, T	MN	244		Ge	Gerdes, H	NY	232		Ge	Lucey, M	WI	247
Ge	Bayless, T	MD	230		Ge	Gerson, L	CA	254		Ge	Magun, A	NY	236
Ge	Benjamin, S	DC	231		Ge	Gholam, P	OH	245		Ge	Markowitz, D	NY	236
Ge	Bloomer, J	AL	239		Ge	Giardiello, F	MD	233		Ge	Martin, P	FL	241
Ge	Boland, C	TX	250		Ge	Ginsberg, G	PA	233		Ge	Mason, J	MA	229
Ge	Borum, M	DC	231		Ge	Gish, R	CA	254		Ge	Mayer, L	NY	236
Ge	Boyer, T	AZ	251		Ge	Glombicki, A	TX	252		Ge	Meiselman, M	IL	247

Spec	Name	St	Pg	Spec	Name	St	Pg	Spec	Name	St	Pg
Ge	Mertz, H	TN	241	Ge	Vege, S	MN	249	S	Salky, B	NY	1063
Ge	Metz, D	PA	236	Ge	Vierling, J	TX	253	S	Soper, N	IL	1083
Ge	Miskovitz, P	NY	236	Ge	Wald, A	WI	249	S	Sweeney, J	GA	1073
Ge	Mittal, R	CA	254	Ge	Waxman, I	IL	249	T&CS	Deschamps, C	MN	1131
Ge	Munoz, S	PA	237	Ge	Waye, J	NY	238	T&CS	Watson, T	NY	1122
Ge	Murray, J	MN	247	Ge	Weinberg, D	PA	238				
Ge	Nunes, D	MA	229	Ge	Weinstock, J	MA	230	**Gastrointestinal Cancer**			
Ge	Okolo, P	MD	237	Ge	Wiesner, R	MN	249	CRS	Nelson, H	MN	175
Ge	Ostroff, J	CA	255	Ge	Wilcox, C	AL	243	Ge	Barkin, J	FL	239
Ge	Owyang, C	MI	247	Ge	Wolfe, M	OH	249	Ge	Bresalier, R	TX	251
Ge	Pasricha, P	MD	237	Ge	Yanda, R	GA	243	Ge	Chang, K	CA	253
Ge	Peikin, S	NJ	237	Ge	Young, R	NE	250	Ge	Cohen, J	NY	231
Ge	Petrini, J	CA	255	Ge	Younossi, Z	VA	243	Ge	Crippin, J	MO	244
Ge	Pezzone, M	PA	237	Ge	Zaman, A	OR	255	Ge	Das, A	AZ	251
Ge	Pfau, P	WI	247					Ge	Gerdes, H	NY	232
Ge	Plevy, S	NC	241	**Gastroesophageal Reflux Disease (GERD)**				Ge	Haluszka, O	PA	233
Ge	Pochapin, M	NY	237					Ge	Hoffman, B	SC	240
Ge	Poordad, F	TX	252	Ge	Benjamin, S	DC	231	Ge	Infantolino, A	PA	234
Ge	Porayko, M	TN	241	Ge	Brazer, S	NC	239	Ge	Kochman, M	PA	235
Ge	Proctor, D	CT	230	Ge	Castell, D	SC	239	Ge	Kurtz, R	NY	235
Ge	Raiford, D	TN	242	Ge	Chey, W	MI	244	Ge	Lebwohl, O	NY	235
Ge	Raju, G	TX	252	Ge	Cohen, L	NY	232	Ge	Lightdale, C	NY	236
Ge	Rao, S	GA	242	Ge	DeVault, K	FL	239	Ge	Okolo, P	MD	237
Ge	Ravich, W	MD	237	Ge	Di Marino, A	PA	232	Ge	Savides, T	CA	255
Ge	Reddy, K	PA	237	Ge	Feldman, E	CA	253	Ge	Shike, M	NY	238
Ge	Reichelderfer, M	WI	247	Ge	Fennerty, M	OR	254	Ge	Smoot, D	TN	243
Ge	Reuben, A	SC	242	Ge	Freiman, H	NY	232	Ge	Waxman, I	IL	249
Ge	Rex, D	IN	247	Ge	Gerson, L	CA	254	Onc	Abbruzzese, J	TX	376
Ge	Reynolds, J	PA	238	Ge	Katz, P	PA	235	Onc	Ahlgren, J	DC	333
Ge	Roth, B	CA	255	Ge	Levine, J	CO	250	Onc	Ajani, J	TX	377
Ge	Rothstein, R	NH	230	Ge	Lind, C	TN	241	Onc	Anthony, L	KY	353
Ge	Sandborn, W	CA	255	Ge	Lipshutz, W	PA	236	Onc	Back, A	WA	383
Ge	Sartor, R	NC	242	Ge	Markowitz, D	NY	236	Onc	Benedetto, P	FL	353
Ge	Savides, T	CA	255	Ge	Metz, D	PA	236	Onc	Benson, A	IL	364
Ge	Scherl, E	NY	238	Ge	Rao, S	GA	242	Onc	Berlin, J	TN	353
Ge	Schiano, T	NY	238	Ge	Ravich, W	MD	237	Onc	Bernard, S	NC	353
Ge	Schiff, E	FL	242	Ge	Reynolds, J	PA	238	Onc	Boston, B	TN	354
Ge	Schiller, L	TX	252	Ge	Roth, B	CA	255	Onc	Brescia, F	SC	354
Ge	Schulze, K	IA	248	Ge	Rothstein, R	NH	230	Onc	Chu, E	PA	336
Ge	Scudera, P	VA	242	Ge	Schulze, K	IA	248	Onc	Chung, K	SC	355
Ge	Seidner, D	TN	242	Ge	Shaker, R	WI	248	Onc	Crocenzi, T	OR	385
Ge	Semrad, C	IL	248	Ge	Vaezi, M	TN	243	Onc	Eckhardt, S	CO	375
Ge	Shah, R	CO	250	NP	Gewolb, I	MI	450	Onc	Engstrom, P	PA	339
Ge	Shaker, R	WI	248	PGe	Baker, R	NY	750	Onc	Ensminger, W	MI	367
Ge	Sherman, S	IN	248	PGe	Baker, S	NY	750	Onc	Fisher, G	CA	386
Ge	Shiffman, M	VA	242	PGe	Gunasekaran, T	IL	753	Onc	Ford, J	CA	386
Ge	Shike, M	NY	238	PGe	Gupta, S	IN	753	Onc	Fuchs, C	MA	329
Ge	Siegel, C	NH	230	PGe	Heyman, M	CA	755	Onc	Gaynor, E	IL	367
Ge	Silverman, W	IA	248	PGe	Levy, J	NY	750	Onc	George, S	MA	329
Ge	Slivka, A	PA	238	PGe	Mousa, H	OH	753	Onc	Glaspy, J	CA	386
Ge	Smoot, D	TN	243	PGe	Schwarz, S	NY	751	Onc	Gold, P	WA	386
Ge	Sorrell, M	NE	250	PGe	Snyder, J	DC	751	Onc	Goldberg, R	OH	367
Ge	Speeg, K	TX	252	PS	Foglia, R	TX	809	Onc	Grossbard, M	NY	341
Ge	Stump, D	TX	253	S	Ballantyne, G	GA	1066	Onc	Hageboutros, A	NJ	341
Ge	Surawicz, C	WA	255	S	Brunicardi, F	CA	1094	Onc	Hochster, H	CT	330
Ge	Targan, S	CA	255	S	Chand, B	IL	1075	Onc	Holcombe, R	NY	342
Ge	Te, H	IL	248	S	Crookes, P	CA	1094	Onc	Kane, M	CO	376
Ge	Tobias, H	NY	238	S	Dempsey, D	PA	1056	Onc	Kelsen, D	NY	343
Ge	Toskes, P	FL	243	S	Hunter, J	OR	1096	Onc	Kindler, H	IL	369
Ge	Tremaine, W	MN	248	S	Peters, J	NY	1062	Onc	Krishnamurthi, S	OH	369
Ge	Vaezi, M	TN	243	S	Rattner, D	MA	1051	Onc	Kvols, L	FL	358
Ge	Vargo, J	OH	248								

Spec	Name	St	Pg
Onc	Lacy, J	CT	331
Onc	Laheru, D	MD	344
Onc	Leighton, J	PA	344
Onc	Makhoul, I	AR	380
Onc	Marshall, J	DC	345
Onc	Mayer, R	MA	331
Onc	Meropol, N	OH	370
Onc	Messersmith, W	CO	376
Onc	Mintzer, D	PA	345
Onc	O'Brien, T	OH	370
Onc	Oster, M	NY	347
Onc	Pasche, B	AL	361
Onc	Patt, Y	NM	381
Onc	Perry, D	DC	347
Onc	Picozzi, V	WA	389
Onc	Posey, J	AL	361
Onc	Reid, T	CA	390
Onc	Ruggiero, J	NY	348
Onc	Ryan, D	MA	331
Onc	Schilsky, R	IL	372
Onc	Sun, W	PA	350
Onc	Taetle, R	AZ	382
Onc	Tempero, M	CA	391
Onc	Venook, A	CA	392
Onc	Vinciguerra, V	NY	351
Onc	Ward, J	UT	376
Onc	Weiner, L	DC	352
Onc	Weiss, G	VA	364
Onc	Willson, J	TX	382
Onc	Wolff, R	TX	383
Path	Chandrasoma, P	CA	720
Path	Crawford, J	NY	708
RadRO	Abrams, R	IL	958
RadRO	Blackstock, A	NC	953
RadRO	Chakravarthy, A	TN	954
RadRO	Crane, C	TX	963
RadRO	Donahue, B	NY	949
RadRO	Heimann, R	VT	946
RadRO	Kachnic, L	MA	946
RadRO	Koh, W	WA	966
RadRO	Konski, A	MI	960
RadRO	Landry, J	GA	955
RadRO	Lawrence, T	MI	960
RadRO	Lee, C	MN	960
RadRO	Martenson, J	MN	961
RadRO	Mendenhall, W	FL	956
RadRO	Minsky, B	TX	965
RadRO	Myerson, R	MO	961
RadRO	Randolph-Jackson, P	DC	952
RadRO	Regine, W	MD	952
RadRO	Rich, T	VA	957
RadRO	Shrieve, D	UT	963
RadRO	Small, W	IL	962
RadRO	Smalley, S	KS	963
RadRO	Tepper, J	NC	957
RadRO	Thomas, C	OR	968
RadRO	Wazer, D	RI	947
RadRO	Willett, C	NC	958
RadRO	Wolfson, A	FL	958
S	Bear, H	VA	1067
S	Beauchamp, R	TN	1067
S	Becker, J	MA	1048

Spec	Name	St	Pg
S	Bilchik, A	CA	1093
S	Brodsky, J	PA	1054
S	Chang, A	MI	1075
S	Cole, D	SC	1068
S	Cusack, J	MA	1048
S	Donohue, J	MN	1076
S	Drebin, J	PA	1056
S	Easter, D	CA	1095
S	Ellenhorn, J	CA	1095
S	Feig, B	TX	1088
S	Gibbs, J	NY	1058
S	Goodman, M	MA	1049
S	Graham, R	MA	1049
S	Greene, F	NC	1069
S	Heslin, M	AL	1069
S	Hoffman, J	PA	1058
S	Howe, J	IA	1078
S	Jackson, G	TX	1089
S	Karpeh, M	NY	1059
S	Kim, J	OH	1078
S	Krouse, R	AZ	1090
S	Li, B	LA	1090
S	Libutti, S	NY	1060
S	Lieberman, M	NY	1060
S	Lillemoe, K	MA	1050
S	Lowy, A	CA	1097
S	McCabe, D	AZ	1091
S	Michelassi, F	NY	1060
S	Moossa, A	CA	1097
S	Nagorney, D	MN	1080
S	Nakakura, E	CA	1097
S	Neifeld, J	VA	1071
S	Newman, E	NY	1061
S	Onders, R	OH	1080
S	Paty, P	NY	1062
S	Pawlik, T	MD	1062
S	Pisters, P	TX	1091
S	Posner, M	IL	1081
S	Reber, H	CA	1099
S	Salem, R	CT	1051
S	Salo, J	NC	1071
S	Sarr, M	MN	1081
S	Sasson, A	NE	1086
S	Shen, P	NC	1072
S	Sinanan, M	WA	1100
S	Tyler, D	NC	1073
S	Wagman, L	CA	1100
S	Warren, R	CA	1100
VIR	Mauro, M	NC	995
VIR	Weintraub, J	NY	994

Gastrointestinal Cancer & Rare Tumors

Spec	Name	St	Pg
Onc	Saltz, L	NY	348
S	Staley, C	GA	1072

Gastrointestinal Cancer & Surgery

Spec	Name	St	Pg
S	Alexander, H	MD	1053
S	Ashley, S	MA	1048
S	Behrns, K	FL	1067

Spec	Name	St	Pg
S	Curcillo, P	PA	1056
S	Duncan, M	MD	1056
S	Lee, K	PA	1059
S	Mahvi, D	IL	1079
S	McAneny, D	MA	1051
S	Nguyen, N	CA	1097
S	Norton, J	CA	1098
S	Pellegrini, C	WA	1098
S	Rattner, D	MA	1051
S	Sundaram, M	IL	1083
S	Talamonti, M	IL	1083
S	Thayer, S	MA	1052

Gastrointestinal Disorders

Spec	Name	St	Pg
NuM	Freeman, L	NY	548
PS	Dillon, P	MO	807

Gastrointestinal Disorders-Neonatal

Spec	Name	St	Pg
PGe	Thomas, D	CA	756

Gastrointestinal Functional Disorders

Spec	Name	St	Pg
Ge	Chey, W	MI	244
Ge	Drossman, D	NC	240
Ge	Fisher, R	PA	232
Ge	Schiller, L	TX	252
PGe	Di Lorenzo, C	OH	753
PGe	Mousa, H	OH	753

Gastrointestinal Imaging

Spec	Name	St	Pg
DR	Berland, L	AL	978
DR	Federle, M	CA	983
DR	Fidler, J	MN	980
DR	Megibow, A	NY	976

Gastrointestinal Metabolic Surgery

Spec	Name	St	Pg
S	Bessler, M	NY	1054
S	Chand, B	IL	1075
S	Rubino, F	NY	1063

Gastrointestinal Motility Disorders

Spec	Name	St	Pg
CRS	Sokol, T	CA	178
Ge	Benjamin, S	DC	231
Ge	Castell, D	SC	239
Ge	Chey, W	MI	244
Ge	Drossman, D	NC	240
Ge	Fisher, R	PA	232
Ge	Koch, K	NC	241
Ge	Korsten, M	NY	235
Ge	Lind, C	TN	241
Ge	Metz, D	PA	236
Ge	Mittal, R	CA	254
Ge	Owyang, C	MI	247
Ge	Pasricha, P	MD	237
Ge	Reynolds, J	PA	238

Spec	Name	St	Pg
Ge	Schiller, L	TX	252
Ge	Shaker, R	WI	248
Ge	Wald, A	WI	249
PGe	Di Lorenzo, C	OH	753
PGe	Mousa, H	OH	753
PS	Caty, M	CT	801
S	Sarr, M	MN	1081
S	Swanstrom, L	OR	1100

Gastrointestinal Pathology

Spec	Name	St	Pg
Path	Appelman, H	MI	714
Path	Bostwick, D	VA	713
Path	Chandrasoma, P	CA	720
Path	Crawford, J	NY	708
Path	Fogt, F	PA	709
Path	Goldblum, J	OH	715
Path	Greenson, J	MI	715
Path	Hamilton, S	TX	718
Path	Hruban, R	MD	709
Path	Klimstra, D	NY	710
Path	Montgomery, E	MD	710
Path	Odze, R	MA	707
Path	Petras, R	OH	716
Path	Rashid, A	TX	718
Path	Rutgers, J	CA	721
Path	Silverman, J	PA	711

Gastrointestinal Stromal Tumors

Spec	Name	St	Pg
Hem	Heinrich, M	OR	325
Onc	Maki, R	NY	345
Onc	von Mehren, M	PA	352
PHO	Wexler, L	NY	764
S	Zinner, M	MA	1052

Gastrointestinal Surgery

Spec	Name	St	Pg
CRS	Longo, W	CT	168
CRS	Schatz, L	CO	176
PS	Barksdale, E	OH	806
PS	Chen, M	AL	805
PS	Ginsburg, H	NY	803
PS	Gittes, G	PA	803
PS	Oldham, K	WI	807
PS	Rescorla, F	IN	807
PS	Ricketts, R	GA	806
PS	Schwartz, M	PA	804
PS	Warner, B	MO	808
S	Barie, P	NY	1053
S	Becker, J	MA	1048
S	Bellows, C	LA	1087
S	Brody, F	DC	1054
S	Brooks, D	MA	1048
S	Daneker, G	GA	1068
S	Dayton, M	NY	1056
S	Dempsey, D	PA	1056
S	Essner, R	CA	1095
S	Fitzgibbons, R	NE	1085
S	Galloway, J	GA	1068
S	Gawande, A	MA	1049
S	Greene, F	NC	1069
S	Horvath, K	WA	1096

Spec	Name	St	Pg
S	Hunter, J	OR	1096
S	Koruda, M	NC	1069
S	Livingston, E	TX	1090
S	MacDonald, K	NC	1070
S	Marks, J	OH	1079
S	Matthews, J	IL	1079
S	Mulvihill, S	UT	1085
S	Nowak, E	NY	1061
S	Pachter, H	NY	1061
S	Ponsky, J	OH	1080
S	Postier, R	OK	1091
S	Rege, R	TX	1091
S	Richards, W	AL	1071
S	Rogers, S	CA	1099
S	Rosemurgy, A	FL	1071
S	Rosen, M	OH	1081
S	Satava, R	WA	1099
S	Schirmer, B	VA	1072
S	Schlinkert, R	AZ	1092
S	Schraut, W	PA	1064
S	Sharp, K	TN	1072
S	Sinanan, M	WA	1100
S	Vickers, S	MN	1083
S	Walsh, R	OH	1084
S	Yeo, C	PA	1066

Gastroparesis

Spec	Name	St	Pg
Ge	Koch, K	NC	241
Ge	Pasricha, P	MD	237
Ge	Schulze, K	IA	248

Gaucher Disease

Spec	Name	St	Pg
CG	Desnick, R	NY	157
Hem	Allen, S	NY	311
N	Kolodny, E	NY	513
Onc	Attas, L	NJ	334

Gender Reassignment Surgery

Spec	Name	St	Pg
PlS	Alter, G	CA	872
PlS	Kuzon, W	MI	866
PlS	Medalie, D	OH	866
PlS	Meltzer, T	AZ	871
PlS	Ousterhout, D	CA	876

Gene Targeted Radiotherapy

Spec	Name	St	Pg
RadRO	Weichselbaum, R	IL	962

Gene Therapy

Spec	Name	St	Pg
Cv	Dichek, D	WA	116
GO	Chan, J	CA	289
GO	Lancaster, J	FL	281
Hem	Brenner, M	TX	323
Hem	Porter, D	PA	314
IC	Mahmud, E	CA	133
Onc	Hortobagyi, G	TX	379
Onc	Sotomayor, E	FL	362
PHO	Neuberg, R	SC	767
Pul	Sterman, D	PA	928
RadRO	Senzer, N	TX	965

Spec	Name	St	Pg
S	Hunt, K	TX	1089
T&CS	Roth, J	TX	1139
U	Belldegrun, A	CA	1175
U	Malkowicz, S	PA	1155
U	Miles, B	TX	1174
VascS	Comerota, A	OH	1190

Gene Therapy-Cardiac Angiogenesis

Spec	Name	St	Pg
Cv	Sanborn, T	IL	111
T&CS	Rosengart, T	NY	1121

Genetic Arrhythmias

Spec	Name	St	Pg
CE	Epstein, A	PA	120
Cv	Topol, E	CA	118

Genetic Disorders

Spec	Name	St	Pg
CG	Bartholomew, D	OH	160
CG	Cederbaum, S	CA	162
CG	Cunniff, C	AZ	161
CG	Desposito, F	NJ	157
CG	Grody, W	CA	163
CG	Mulvihill, J	OK	161
CG	Nussbaum, R	CA	163
CG	Ostrer, H	NY	158
CG	Sutphen, R	FL	159
CG	Weaver, D	IN	160
MF	Bahado-Singh, R	MI	435
MF	Cheng, E	WA	439
MF	Pridjian, G	LA	439
MF	Wapner, R	NY	434
MF	Wilkins-Haug, L	MA	431
Ped	Jones, K	CA	728
Ped	Morton, D	PA	727
RE	Rosenwaks, Z	NY	1009

Genetic Disorders-Blood

Spec	Name	St	Pg
PHO	Glader, B	CA	777

Genetic Disorders-Eye

Spec	Name	St	Pg
Oph	Kerr, N	TN	584

Genetic Disorders-Skin

Spec	Name	St	Pg
D	Levy, M	TX	197
D	Paller, A	IL	195
D	Yan, A	PA	189

Genetic Preimplantation Diagnosis

Spec	Name	St	Pg
CG	Pergament, E	IL	160

Genital Enhancement

Spec	Name	St	Pg
PlS	Alter, G	CA	872
PlS	Medalie, D	OH	866

Specialty & Special Expertise Index

Spec	Name	St	Pg
Genital Reconstruction			
U	Glassberg, K	NY	1152
U	Merguerian, P	WA	1178
U	Rink, R	IN	1169
Genital Reconstruction-Pediatric			
U	Poppas, D	NY	1156
Genitourinary Cancer			
DR	Parsons, R	PA	977
Onc	Bajorin, D	NY	335
Onc	Balducci, L	FL	353
Onc	Benedetto, P	FL	353
Onc	Boston, B	TN	354
Onc	Celano, P	MD	336
Onc	Clinton, S	OH	366
Onc	DiPaola, R	NJ	338
Onc	Ernstoff, M	NH	329
Onc	Glode, L	CO	375
Onc	Haas, N	PA	341
Onc	Higano, C	WA	387
Onc	Hogan, T	WV	342
Onc	Hudes, G	PA	342
Onc	Hussain, M	MI	368
Onc	Jonasch, E	TX	379
Onc	Kantoff, P	MA	330
Onc	Kucuk, O	GA	358
Onc	Loehrer, P	IN	369
Onc	Mathew, P	MA	331
Onc	Nanus, D	NY	346
Onc	Oh, W	NY	347
Onc	Perry, D	DC	347
Onc	Picozzi, V	WA	389
Onc	Scher, H	NY	348
Onc	Small, E	CA	391
Onc	Sweeney, C	MA	332
Onc	Taplin, M	MA	333
Onc	Trump, D	NY	351
Onc	Twardowski, P	CA	391
Onc	Vaughn, D	PA	351
Onc	Vogelzang, N	NV	392
Onc	Weiss, G	VA	364
Onc	Wilding, G	WI	373
Path	Wheeler, T	TX	719
RadRO	Ciezki, J	OH	959
RadRO	Forman, J	MI	959
RadRO	Kuban, D	TX	964
RadRO	Kupelian, P	CA	966
RadRO	Lee, A	TX	964
RadRO	Pollack, A	FL	956
RadRO	Roach, M	CA	967
RadRO	Russell, K	WA	968
RadRO	Sailer, S	NC	957
RadRO	Sandler, H	CA	968
RadRO	Schild, S	AZ	965
RadRO	Shrieve, D	UT	963
U	Keane, T	SC	1161
U	Montie, J	MI	1169
U	Pisters, L	TX	1174
U	Wood, D	MI	1171

Spec	Name	St	Pg
Genitourinary Congenital Anomalies			
U	Kaefer, M	IN	1167
Genitourinary Disorders			
U	Shenot, P	PA	1158
Genitourinary Disorders-Geriatric			
U	Skinner, E	CA	1178
Genitourinary Pathology			
Path	Amin, M	CA	719
Path	Reuter, V	NY	711
Path	Tomaszewski, J	NY	712
Genitourinary Prosthetics			
U	Montague, D	OH	1169
Genitourinary Radiology			
DR	Parsons, R	PA	977
DR	Zagoria, R	NC	980
Genitourinary Reconstruction			
PlS	Alter, G	CA	872
U	Bloom, D	MI	1165
U	Cain, M	IN	1166
U	Firlit, C	MO	1167
U	McAninch, J	CA	1177
Genitourinary Trauma			
U	McAninch, J	CA	1177
Geriatric Cardiology			
Cv	Gardin, J	NJ	98
Geriatric Endocrinology			
EDM	Axelrod, L	MA	206
Ger	Abrass, I	WA	266
Geriatric Functional Assessment			
Ger	Cooney, L	CT	262
Ger	Duthie, E	WI	264
Ger	Dyer, C	TX	266
Ger	Gorbien, M	IL	265
Ger	Palmer, R	VA	264
Ger	Reuben, D	CA	267
Ger	Supiano, M	UT	266
Ger	Tinetti, M	CT	262
Geriatric Medicine			
Ger	Abrass, I	WA	266
Ger	Allman, R	AL	263
Ger	Bloom, P	NY	262
Ger	Burton, J	MD	262

Spec	Name	St	Pg
Ger	Callahan, E	NY	262
Ger	Carr, D	MO	264
Ger	Ciocon, J	FL	263
Ger	Cooney, L	CT	262
Ger	Dale, L	MN	264
Ger	Duthie, E	WI	264
Ger	Dyer, C	TX	266
Ger	Finucane, T	MD	263
Ger	Flaherty, J	MO	265
Ger	Gambert, S	MD	263
Ger	Gorbien, M	IL	265
Ger	Greganti, M	NC	264
Ger	Hanson, L	NC	264
Ger	Lachs, M	NY	263
Ger	Liem, P	AR	266
Ger	Lipschitz, D	AR	266
Ger	Lipsitz, L	MA	262
Ger	Lyles, K	NC	264
Ger	McCormick, W	WA	267
Ger	Minaker, K	MA	262
Ger	Morley, J	MO	265
Ger	Olson, J	IL	265
Ger	Palmer, R	VA	264
Ger	Raji, M	TX	266
Ger	Resnick, N	PA	263
Ger	Reuben, D	CA	267
Ger	Sachs, G	IN	265
Ger	Schwartz, R	CO	265
Ger	Studenski, S	PA	263
Ger	Supiano, M	UT	266
Ger	Tenover, J	CA	267
Ger	Thomas, D	MO	265
Ger	Tinetti, M	CT	262
Ger	Wei, J	AR	266
Geriatric Neurology			
N	DeKosky, S	VA	520
N	Ferrendelli, J	TX	533
Geriatric Ophthalmology			
Oph	Sterns, G	NY	581
Geriatric Psychiatry			
GerPsy	Borson, S	WA	915
GerPsy	Burke, W	NE	914
GerPsy	Greenwald, B	NY	913
GerPsy	Grossberg, G	MO	914
GerPsy	Holroyd, S	VA	914
GerPsy	Kennedy, G	NY	913
GerPsy	Kramer, B	CA	915
GerPsy	Lyketsos, C	MD	913
GerPsy	Manepalli, J	MO	914
GerPsy	Mellow, A	MI	914
GerPsy	Reisberg, B	NY	913
GerPsy	Rovner, B	PA	913
GerPsy	Small, G	CA	915
GerPsy	Stein, E	CA	915
GerPsy	Streim, J	PA	913
GerPsy	Tune, L	GA	914
GerPsy	Veith, R	WA	915

Spec	Name	St	Pg
Psyc	Blazer, D	NC	895
Psyc	Ellison, J	MA	888
Psyc	Jenike, M	MA	889
Psyc	Marin, D	NY	894
Psyc	Nelson, J	CA	902
Psyc	Raskind, M	WA	902
Psyc	Roth, A	NY	894
Psyc	Weiner, M	TX	900

Geriatric Rehabilitation

Spec	Name	St	Pg
Ger	Allman, R	AL	263
PMR	Bloch, R	MA	834
PMR	Diamond, P	VA	838
PMR	Frost, F	OH	840
PMR	Miknevich, M	PA	837
PMR	Roth, E	IL	841

Germ Cell Tumors

Spec	Name	St	Pg
Onc	Margolin, K	WA	388
PHO	Marina, N	CA	778
PHO	Olson, T	GA	767
PS	Morgan, W	TN	805

Gestational Trophoblastic Disease

Spec	Name	St	Pg
GO	Burger, R	PA	276
GO	Curtin, J	NY	277
GO	Fromm, G	TX	287
GO	Giuntoli, R	MD	278
GO	Kohler, M	SC	281
GO	Lurain, J	IL	284
GO	Muntz, H	WA	290
GO	Plaxe, S	CA	290
GO	Soper, J	NC	283

Gitelman's Syndrome

Spec	Name	St	Pg
Nep	Ellison, D	OR	465

Glaucoma

Spec	Name	St	Pg
Oph	Alward, W	IA	588
Oph	Baerveldt, G	CA	598
Oph	Budenz, D	NC	582
Oph	Caprioli, J	CA	599
Oph	Crandall, A	UT	595
Oph	Gorovoy, M	FL	583
Oph	Greenfield, D	FL	583
Oph	Heuer, D	WI	590
Oph	Iwach, A	CA	601
Oph	Katz, L	PA	576
Oph	Kaufman, P	WI	590
Oph	Kwon, Y	IA	591
Oph	Lee, P	MI	591
Oph	Levin, A	PA	576
Oph	Lichter, P	MI	591
Oph	Liebmann, J	NY	576
Oph	Myers, J	PA	578
Oph	Parrish, R	FL	585
Oph	Quigley, H	MD	578
Oph	Ritch, R	NY	579

Spec	Name	St	Pg
Oph	Robin, A	MD	579
Oph	Samuelson, T	MN	594
Oph	Schuman, J	PA	579
Oph	Sergott, R	PA	580
Oph	Sherwood, M	FL	586
Oph	Shingleton, B	MA	571
Oph	Spaeth, G	PA	580
Oph	Tsai, J	CT	571
Oph	Vajaranant, T	IL	595
Oph	Wallace, R	LA	598
Oph	Weinreb, R	CA	604

Glaucoma-Pediatric

Spec	Name	St	Pg
Oph	Freedman, S	NC	583
Oph	Jaafar, M	DC	575
Oph	Medow, N	NY	577
Oph	Plager, D	IN	593
Oph	Traboulsi, E	OH	594
Oph	Walton, D	MA	571

Gliomas

Spec	Name	St	Pg
N	Batchelor, T	MA	506
N	Mikkelsen, T	MI	528
N	Rosenfeld, S	OH	529
N	Taylor, L	MA	508
NS	Chen, T	CA	496
NS	Friedman, A	NC	481
NS	Lang, F	TX	493
NS	Weingart, J	MD	480
Onc	Friedman, H	NC	356
Onc	Vredenburgh, J	NC	363
RadRO	Isaacson, S	NY	950

Glomerulonephritis

Spec	Name	St	Pg
IM	Holzman, L	PA	424
Nep	Appel, G	NY	456
Nep	Berns, J	PA	457
Nep	Bolton, W	VA	459
Nep	Cho, K	CA	465
Nep	Cohen, D	NY	457
Nep	Falk, R	NC	459
Nep	Kasinath, B	TX	463
Nep	Rodby, R	IL	462
Nep	Winston, J	NY	459
PNep	Andreoli, S	IN	787
PNep	Benfield, M	AL	786
PNep	Fouser, L	WA	788
PNep	Mendley, S	MD	786

Gorham-Stout Disease

Spec	Name	St	Pg
EDM	Watts, N	OH	219

Gout

Spec	Name	St	Pg
A&I	Sundy, J	NC	87
Rhu	Davis, W	LA	1032
Rhu	Fields, T	NY	1026
Rhu	Lawry, G	CA	1034
Rhu	Massarotti, E	MA	1024
Rhu	Weinstein, A	DC	1029

Spec	Name	St	Pg
Rhu	Wise, C	VA	1030

Graft vs Host Disease

Spec	Name	St	Pg
Hem	Brodsky, R	MD	312
Hem	Rowley, S	NJ	314
Hem	Yeager, A	AZ	325
Onc	Appelbaum, F	WA	383
Onc	Deeg, H	WA	385
Onc	Foss, F	CT	329
PGe	Molleston, J	IN	753
PHO	Carpenter, P	WA	776
PHO	Chen, A	MD	759
PHO	Ferrara, J	MI	770

Graves' Disease

Spec	Name	St	Pg
EDM	Bahn, R	MN	216
EDM	Burmeister, L	MN	216
EDM	Davies, T	NY	210
T&CS	Weigel, T	WI	1135

Graves' Disease-Eye

Spec	Name	St	Pg
EDM	Bahn, R	MN	216
Oto	Lanza, D	FL	669

Gravet Syndrome

Spec	Name	St	Pg
ChiN	Tuxhorn, I	OH	151

Growth Disorders

Spec	Name	St	Pg
PEn	Allen, D	WI	746
PEn	Alter, C	PA	744
PEn	DeLuca, F	PA	744
PEn	Diamond, F	FL	745
PEn	Freemark, M	NC	746
PEn	Garibaldi, L	PA	744
PEn	Geffner, M	CA	748
PEn	Levy, R	IL	747
PEn	Oberfield, S	NY	745
PEn	Plotnick, L	MD	745
PEn	Rivkees, S	FL	746
PEn	Wilson, D	CA	749
PNep	Friedman, A	MN	787

Growth Disorders in Childhood Cancer

Spec	Name	St	Pg
PEn	Meacham, L	GA	746
PEn	Sklar, C	NY	745
PEn	Zimmerman, D	IL	748

Growth Hormone Disorder-Adult

Spec	Name	St	Pg
EDM	Inzucchi, S	CT	207
EDM	Thorner, M	VA	215

Growth/Development Disorders

Spec	Name	St	Pg
PEn	Casella, S	NH	743
PEn	Eugster, E	IN	747
PEn	Foster, C	UT	748

Spec	Name	St	Pg
PEn	Kappy, M	CO	748
PEn	Levitsky, L	MA	743
PEn	Menon, R	MI	747
PEn	New, M	NY	745
PEn	Rogers, D	OH	747
PEn	Silverstein, J	FL	746
PEn	Sperling, M	PA	745
PEn	Zimmerman, D	IL	748

Guillain-Barre Syndrome

Spec	Name	St	Pg
N	Arnason, B	IL	524
N	Barohn, R	KS	531
N	Graves, M	CA	537
N	Ropper, A	MA	508

Gynecologic Cancer

Spec	Name	St	Pg
DR	McCarthy, S	CT	973
GO	Abbas, F	MD	275
GO	Alvarez, R	AL	280
GO	Barnes, W	DC	276
GO	Barter, J	MD	276
GO	Berkowitz, R	MA	274
GO	Berman, M	CA	289
GO	Boice, C	MD	276
GO	Brewer, M	CT	274
GO	Bristow, R	CA	289
GO	Burnett, A	AR	287
GO	Carlson, J	NJ	276
GO	Carney, M	HI	289
GO	Chambers, S	AZ	287
GO	Clarke-Pearson, D	NC	280
GO	Copeland, L	OH	283
GO	Cornelison, T	MD	277
GO	Cosin, J	DC	277
GO	Coukos, G	PA	277
GO	Currie, J	GA	280
GO	Davidson, S	CO	286
GO	DeMars, L	NH	274
GO	Di Saia, P	CA	289
GO	Dottino, P	NY	277
GO	Duska, L	VA	281
GO	Edwards, R	PA	277
GO	Fishman, D	NY	278
GO	Fowler, J	OH	284
GO	Giuntoli, R	MD	278
GO	Granai, C	RI	274
GO	Greer, B	WA	290
GO	Herzog, T	NY	278
GO	Karlan, B	CA	290
GO	Kelley, J	PA	278
GO	Kohler, M	SC	281
GO	Lentz, S	NC	282
GO	Levenback, C	TX	288
GO	Lin, J	DC	279
GO	Magrina, J	AZ	288
GO	Miller, D	TX	288
GO	Modesitt, S	VA	282
GO	Morgan, M	PA	279
GO	Mutch, D	MO	284
GO	Odunsi, A	NY	279
GO	Orr, J	FL	282

Spec	Name	St	Pg
GO	Penalver, M	FL	282
GO	Randall, T	PA	279
GO	Remmenga, S	NE	286
GO	Rotmensch, J	IL	285
GO	Singh, D	AZ	288
GO	Sood, A	TX	288
GO	Soper, J	NC	283
GO	Spann, C	GA	283
GO	Spirtos, N	NV	290
GO	Stehman, F	IN	286
GO	Tarraza, H	ME	275
ObG	Morgan, L	FL	559
Onc	Aghajanian, C	NY	333
Onc	Birrer, M	MA	327
Onc	Celano, P	MD	336
Onc	Dizon, D	MA	328
Onc	Fleming, G	IL	367
Onc	Fracasso, P	VA	356
Onc	Hochster, H	CT	330
Onc	Kohn, E	MD	343
Onc	Markman, M	PA	345
Onc	Matulonis, U	MA	331
Onc	McGuire, W	MD	345
Onc	Muggia, F	NY	346
Onc	Schilder, R	PA	349
Onc	Spriggs, D	NY	350
Onc	Thigpen, J	MS	363
Onc	Verschraegen, C	VT	333
Path	Li Volsi, V	PA	710
Path	Rutgers, J	CA	721
Path	Silva, E	TX	719
Path	Thor, A	CO	717
Path	Tornos, C	NY	712
Path	Wilczynski, S	CA	722
Path	Young, R	MA	707
RadRO	Gaffney, D	UT	962
RadRO	Grigsby, P	MO	959
RadRO	Halpern, H	IL	959
RadRO	Henderson, R	FL	954
RadRO	Jhingran, A	TX	964
RadRO	Jose, B	IN	960
RadRO	Kalnicki, S	NY	951
RadRO	Koh, W	WA	966
RadRO	Mendenhall, W	FL	956
RadRO	Mundt, A	CA	967
RadRO	Randall, M	KY	957
RadRO	Recht, A	MA	947
RadRO	Rotman, M	NY	952
RadRO	Russell, A	MA	947
RadRO	Schiff, P	NY	952
RadRO	Small, W	IL	962
RadRO	Wolfson, A	FL	958
S	Kavanah, M	MA	1050

Gynecologic Cancer Risk

Spec	Name	St	Pg
CG	Whelan, A	MO	161

Gynecologic Cancer-Rare

Spec	Name	St	Pg
GO	Brewer, M	CT	274
GO	Copeland, L	OH	283
GO	Creasman, W	SC	280

Spec	Name	St	Pg
GO	Pejovic, T	OR	290
GO	Rubin, S	PA	279

Gynecologic Imaging

Spec	Name	St	Pg
DR	Benson, C	MA	973
DR	Thurmond, A	OR	984

Gynecologic Oncology

Spec	Name	St	Pg
GO	Abbas, F	MD	275
GO	Abu-Rustum, N	NY	276
GO	Alvarez, R	AL	280
GO	Azodi, M	CT	274
GO	Barakat, R	NY	276
GO	Barnes, W	DC	276
GO	Barter, J	MD	276
GO	Berchuck, A	NC	280
GO	Berek, J	CA	289
GO	Berkowitz, R	MA	274
GO	Berman, M	CA	289
GO	Bicher, A	VA	280
GO	Bodurka, D	TX	286
GO	Boice, C	MD	276
GO	Borst, M	AZ	286
GO	Braly, P	LA	287
GO	Brewer, M	CT	274
GO	Bristow, R	CA	289
GO	Burger, R	PA	276
GO	Burke, T	TX	287
GO	Burnett, A	AR	287
GO	Cain, J	MA	274
GO	Caputo, T	NY	276
GO	Carlson, J	NJ	276
GO	Carney, M	HI	289
GO	Chambers, S	AZ	287
GO	Chan, J	CA	289
GO	Chi, D	NY	277
GO	Clarke-Pearson, D	NC	280
GO	Cliby, W	MN	283
GO	Copeland, L	OH	283
GO	Cornelison, T	MD	277
GO	Cosin, J	DC	277
GO	Coukos, G	PA	277
GO	Creasman, W	SC	280
GO	Currie, J	GA	280
GO	Curtin, J	NY	277
GO	Davidson, S	CO	286
GO	De Geest, K	IA	283
GO	Del Priore, G	IN	284
GO	DeMars, L	NH	274
GO	DePriest, P	KY	280
GO	Di Saia, P	CA	289
GO	Dottino, P	NY	277
GO	Dunton, C	PA	277
GO	Duska, L	VA	281
GO	Edwards, R	PA	277
GO	Fields, A	DC	278
GO	Finan, M	AL	281
GO	Fiorica, J	FL	281
GO	Fishman, D	NY	278
GO	Fowler, J	OH	284
GO	Fromm, G	TX	287

Spec	Name	St	Pg
GO	Gershenson, D	TX	287
GO	Ghamande, S	GA	281
GO	Giuntoli, R	MD	278
GO	Goff, B	WA	289
GO	Gostout, B	MN	284
GO	Granai, C	RI	274
GO	Greer, B	WA	290
GO	Hatch, K	AZ	287
GO	Havrilesky, L	NC	281
GO	Herzog, T	NY	278
GO	Horowitz, I	GA	281
GO	Husain, A	CA	290
GO	Johnston, C	MI	284
GO	Karlan, B	CA	290
GO	Kelley, J	PA	278
GO	King, S	PA	278
GO	Kline, R	LA	287
GO	Kohler, M	SC	281
GO	Koulos, J	NY	278
GO	Lancaster, J	FL	281
GO	Lele, S	NY	279
GO	Lentz, S	NC	282
GO	Levenback, C	TX	288
GO	Lin, J	DC	279
GO	Lu, K	TX	288
GO	Lucci, J	FL	282
GO	Lurain, J	IL	284
GO	Magrina, J	AZ	288
GO	Makhija, S	KY	282
GO	Miller, D	TX	288
GO	Modesitt, S	VA	282
GO	Moore, D	IN	284
GO	Morgan, M	PA	279
GO	Muntz, H	WA	290
GO	Mutch, D	MO	284
GO	Muto, M	MA	275
GO	Odunsi, A	NY	279
GO	Orr, J	FL	282
GO	Pejovic, T	OR	290
GO	Penalver, M	FL	282
GO	Plaxe, S	CA	290
GO	Poliakoff, S	FL	282
GO	Potkul, R	IL	285
GO	Rader, J	WI	285
GO	Randall, T	PA	279
GO	Remmenga, S	NE	286
GO	Reynolds, R	MI	285
GO	Rice, L	WI	285
GO	Rose, P	OH	285
GO	Rosenblum, N	PA	279
GO	Rotmensch, J	IL	285
GO	Rubin, S	PA	279
GO	Runowicz, C	FL	282
GO	Rutherford, T	CT	275
GO	Santin, A	CT	275
GO	Schink, J	IL	285
GO	Schorge, J	MA	275
GO	Schwartz, P	CT	275
GO	Siller, B	TX	288
GO	Singh, D	AZ	288
GO	Smith, D	IL	285
GO	Smith, L	CA	290

Spec	Name	St	Pg
GO	Soisson, A	UT	286
GO	Sood, A	TX	288
GO	Soper, J	NC	283
GO	Spann, C	GA	283
GO	Spirtos, N	NV	290
GO	Stehman, F	IN	286
GO	Stern, J	CA	291
GO	Tarraza, H	ME	275
GO	Teng, N	CA	291
GO	Valea, F	NC	283
GO	Van Nagell, J	KY	283
GO	Waggoner, S	OH	286
GO	Walker, J	OK	288

Gynecologic Pathology

ObG	Bartholomew, D	OH	560
Path	Balla, A	IL	715
Path	Bell, D	MN	715
Path	Cho, K	MI	715
Path	Dahmoush, L	IA	715
Path	De Las Morenas, A	MA	706
Path	Heller, D	NJ	709
Path	Kurman, R	MD	710
Path	Lage, J	SC	713
Path	Silva, E	TX	719
Path	Soslow, R	NY	711
Path	Ulbright, T	IN	716

Gynecologic Problems of Obesity

GO	Currie, J	GA	280

Gynecologic Surgery

ObG	De Cherney, A	MD	557
ObG	Parker, W	CA	563
ObG	Snyder, R	TX	563
ObG	Steege, J	NC	560

Gynecologic Surgery-Complex

GO	Carlson, J	NJ	276
GO	Chi, D	NY	277
GO	Clarke-Pearson, D	NC	280
GO	Dunton, C	PA	277
GO	Duska, L	VA	281
GO	Ghamande, S	GA	281
GO	Goff, B	WA	289
GO	Johnston, C	MI	284
GO	Kohler, M	SC	281
GO	Morgan, M	PA	279
GO	Muntz, H	WA	290
GO	Schwartz, P	CT	275
GO	Soper, J	NC	283
ObG	Eschenbach, D	WA	563

Gynecology in Cancer Patients

RE	Gracia, C	PA	1008

Gynecology Only

ObG	Carson, D	PA	557

Gynecology-African women only

ObG	Nour, N	MA	556

Gynecomastia

EDM	Rodbard, H	MD	211

H

Hair Loss

D	Barbosa, V	IL	192
D	Cohen, B	FL	190
D	Cotsarelis, G	PA	185
D	McMichael, A	NC	191
D	Nigra, T	DC	187
D	Olsen, E	NC	191

Hair Loss in Women

D	Bernstein, R	NY	185

Hair Restoration/Transplant

D	Avram, M	NY	184
D	Berg, D	WA	198
D	Bernstein, R	NY	185
D	Cohen, B	FL	190
D	Fitzpatrick, R	CA	198
Oto	Epstein, J	FL	668
Oto	Hopping, S	DC	660
S	Rassman, W	CA	1099

Hairy Cell Leukemia

Hem	Tallman, M	NY	316

Hand & Elbow Nerve Disorders

HS	Strauch, R	NY	298

Hand & Fingers Vascular Surgery

HS	Sampson, C	MA	294

Hand & Microvascular Surgery

HS	Chung, K	MI	300
PlS	Chiu, D	NY	853

Hand & Upper Extremity Surgery

HS	Abrams, R	CA	303
HS	Athanasian, E	NY	295
HS	Badia, A	FL	298

Specialty & Special Expertise Index

Spec	Name	St	Pg
HS	Bozentka, D	PA	295
HS	Brushart, T	MD	295
HS	Carlson, M	NY	295
HS	Cassidy, C	MA	294
HS	Chang, J	CA	304
HS	Collins, E	TX	303
HS	Culp, R	PA	295
HS	Eglseder, W	MD	296
HS	Goitz, R	PA	296
HS	Hentz, V	CA	304
HS	Kulick, R	NY	296
HS	Seitz, W	OH	302
HS	Sotereanos, D	PA	298

Hand & Upper Extremity Tumors

Spec	Name	St	Pg
HS	Athanasian, E	NY	295
HS	Szabo, R	CA	304
OrS	Singer, D	HI	645

Hand & Wrist Reconstrction

Spec	Name	St	Pg
OrS	Goldner, R	NC	628

Hand & Wrist Surgery

Spec	Name	St	Pg
HS	Beredjiklian, P	PA	295
HS	Carneiro, R	FL	298
HS	Glickel, S	NY	296
HS	Graham, T	OH	301
HS	Hunt, T	AL	299
HS	Meals, R	CA	304
HS	Stern, P	OH	302
HS	Strauch, R	NY	298
OrS	Goldner, R	NC	628

Hand Injuries

Spec	Name	St	Pg
HS	Sampson, C	MA	294
HS	Szabo, R	CA	304

Hand Injuries-Pediatric

Spec	Name	St	Pg
HS	Light, T	IL	301

Hand Reconstruction

Spec	Name	St	Pg
HS	Eglseder, W	MD	296
HS	Failla, J	MI	300
HS	Friedman, D	FL	299
HS	Hunt, T	AL	299
HS	Kleinman, W	IN	301
HS	Lane, L	NY	296
HS	Strauch, R	NY	298
HS	Weiland, A	NY	298
OrS	Hausman, M	NY	618
PlS	Yuen, J	AR	872

Hand Reconstruction-Pediatric

Spec	Name	St	Pg
HS	Ezaki, M	TX	303
HS	Jones, N	CA	304
HS	Mih, A	IN	301

Hand Surgery

Spec	Name	St	Pg
HS	Abrams, R	CA	303
HS	Athanasian, E	NY	295
HS	Atkinson, R	HI	303
HS	Badia, A	FL	298
HS	Baratz, M	PA	295
HS	Baratz, M	PA	295
HS	Belsky, M	MA	294
HS	Beredjiklian, P	PA	295
HS	Bishop, A	MN	300
HS	Bozentka, D	PA	295
HS	Breidenbach, W	AZ	303
HS	Brushart, T	MD	295
HS	Carlson, M	NY	295
HS	Carneiro, R	FL	298
HS	Carroll, C	IL	300
HS	Cassidy, C	MA	294
HS	Cendales, L	GA	299
HS	Chang, J	CA	304
HS	Chung, K	MI	300
HS	Cohen, M	IL	300
HS	Cohen, M	IL	300
HS	Collins, E	TX	303
HS	Culp, R	PA	295
HS	Derman, G	IL	300
HS	DeSilva, S	MI	300
HS	DeSilva, S	MI	300
HS	Eglseder, W	MD	296
HS	Ezaki, M	TX	303
HS	Failla, J	MI	300
HS	Failla, J	MI	300
HS	Fischer, T	IN	300
HS	Friedman, D	FL	299
HS	Gelberman, R	MO	301
HS	Glickel, S	NY	296
HS	Godzik, C	CA	304
HS	Goitz, R	PA	296
HS	Graham, T	OH	301
HS	Greene, T	FL	299
HS	Grossman, J	FL	299
HS	Grossman, J	FL	299
HS	Hanel, D	WA	304
HS	Hastings, H	IN	301
HS	Hentz, V	CA	304
HS	Hunt, T	AL	299
HS	Idler, R	CO	302
HS	Imbriglia, J	PA	296
HS	Jones, N	CA	304
HS	Jupiter, J	MA	294
HS	Jupiter, J	MA	294
HS	Kleinman, W	IN	301
HS	Koman, L	NC	299
HS	Kozin, S	PA	296
HS	Kozin, S	PA	296
HS	Kulick, R	NY	296
HS	Lane, L	NY	296
HS	Lee, W	MD	297
HS	Light, T	IL	301
HS	Lubahn, J	PA	297
HS	Mass, D	IL	301
HS	Meals, R	CA	304

Spec	Name	St	Pg
HS	Melone, C	NY	297
HS	Mih, A	IN	301
HS	Moneim, M	NM	303
HS	Nagle, D	IL	302
HS	Osterman, A	PA	297
HS	Peljovich, A	GA	299
HS	Putnam, M	MN	302
HS	Raphael, J	PA	297
HS	Raskin, K	NY	297
HS	Rayan, G	OK	303
HS	Rosenwasser, M	NY	297
HS	Sampson, C	MA	294
HS	Seitz, W	OH	302
HS	Slutsky, D	CA	304
HS	Sotereanos, D	PA	298
HS	Steinmann, S	MN	302
HS	Stern, P	OH	302
HS	Strauch, R	NY	298
HS	Szabo, R	CA	304
HS	Thoder, J	PA	298
HS	Trumble, T	WA	305
HS	Waters, P	MA	294
HS	Weiland, A	NY	298
HS	Weiss, A	RI	294
HS	Wolfe, S	NY	298
OrS	Hotchkiss, R	NY	620
OrS	Poehling, G	NC	630
OrS	Singer, D	HI	645
OrS	Stuchin, S	NY	626
PlS	Chang, B	PA	853
PlS	Dagum, A	NY	853
PlS	Erdmann, D	NC	861
PlS	Fix, R	AL	861
PlS	MacKinnon, S	MO	866
PlS	Molnar, J	NC	863
PlS	Morgan, R	VA	863
PlS	Neumeister, M	IL	867
PlS	Rockwell, W	UT	869
PlS	Sanger, J	WI	867
PlS	Wilhelmi, B	KY	864

Hand-Congenital Anomaly

Spec	Name	St	Pg
HS	Ezaki, M	TX	303
HS	Hanel, D	WA	304
HS	Light, T	IL	301
HS	Waters, P	MA	294

Hashimoto's Disease

Spec	Name	St	Pg
EDM	Burmeister, L	MN	216
EDM	Davies, T	NY	210

Head & Neck Autoimmune Disease

Spec	Name	St	Pg
Oto	Lebovics, R	NY	662

Head & Neck Cancer

Spec	Name	St	Pg
NRad	Loevner, L	PA	986
NRad	Sze, G	CT	985
Onc	Adelstein, D	OH	364

Spec	Name	St	Pg
Onc	Algazy, K	PA	334
Onc	Argiris, A	TX	377
Onc	Axelrod, R	PA	335
Onc	Brockstein, B	IL	365
Onc	Clark, J	IL	366
Onc	Cleary, J	WI	366
Onc	Cohen, R	PA	337
Onc	Cullen, K	MD	337
Onc	Dunphy, F	NC	356
Onc	Forastiere, A	MD	340
Onc	Glisson, B	TX	378
Onc	Grunberg, S	VT	330
Onc	Hong, W	TX	379
Onc	Kane, M	CO	376
Onc	Khuri, F	GA	358
Onc	Kies, M	TX	379
Onc	Langer, C	PA	344
Onc	Lippman, S	CA	387
Onc	Martins, R	WA	388
Onc	Mintzer, D	PA	345
Onc	Nabell, L	AL	360
Onc	Oster, M	NY	347
Onc	Pfister, D	NY	348
Onc	Pinto, H	CA	389
Onc	Posner, M	NY	348
Onc	Ready, N	NC	361
Onc	Shin, D	GA	362
Onc	Sidransky, D	MD	349
Onc	Troner, M	FL	363
Onc	Urba, S	MI	373
Onc	Vokes, E	IL	373
Onc	Worden, F	MI	373
Oto	Akervall, J	MI	672
Oto	Berke, G	CA	684
Oto	Bradford, C	MI	673
Oto	Browne, J	NC	667
Oto	Bumpous, J	KY	667
Oto	Burkey, B	OH	674
Oto	Califano, J	MD	658
Oto	Campbell, B	WI	674
Oto	Caruana, S	NY	658
Oto	Chalian, A	PA	658
Oto	Chowdhury, K	CO	679
Oto	Civantos, F	FL	667
Oto	Clayman, G	TX	681
Oto	Close, L	NY	658
Oto	Costantino, P	NY	658
Oto	Couch, M	VT	655
Oto	Davidson, B	DC	658
Oto	Day, T	SC	668
Oto	Deschler, D	MA	655
Oto	Diaz, E	TX	681
Oto	DiNardo, L	VA	668
Oto	Donald, P	CA	684
Oto	Donovan, D	TX	681
Oto	Eisele, D	MD	659
Oto	Fee, W	CA	684
Oto	Ferris, R	PA	659
Oto	Funk, G	IA	674
Oto	Goodwin, W	FL	668
Oto	Gosselin, B	NH	655
Oto	Grandis, J	PA	660
Oto	Grillone, G	MA	655
Oto	Har-El, G	NY	660
Oto	Hartig, G	WI	675
Oto	Haughey, B	MO	675
Oto	Hoffman, H	IA	675
Oto	Johnson, J	PA	661
Oto	Kaplan, M	CA	685
Oto	Koch, W	MD	661
Oto	Kraus, D	NY	662
Oto	Lavertu, P	OH	676
Oto	Leonetti, J	IL	676
Oto	Levine, P	VA	669
Oto	Lydiatt, D	NE	680
Oto	Lydiatt, W	NE	680
Oto	Myers, J	TX	683
Oto	Netterville, J	TN	669
Oto	Newkirk, K	DC	663
Oto	Nuss, D	LA	683
Oto	O'Malley, B	PA	663
Oto	Otto, R	TX	683
Oto	Ozer, E	OH	677
Oto	Pelzer, H	IL	677
Oto	Persky, M	NY	663
Oto	Rice, D	CA	686
Oto	Rosenthal, E	AL	670
Oto	Sasaki, C	CT	657
Oto	Schantz, S	NY	664
Oto	Siegel, G	IL	677
Oto	Singer, M	CA	687
Oto	Sinha, U	CA	687
Oto	Smith, R	NE	680
Oto	Snyderman, C	PA	665
Oto	Song, J	CO	681
Oto	Strome, S	MD	665
Oto	Suen, J	AR	683
Oto	Teknos, T	OH	678
Oto	Tufano, R	MD	666
Oto	Valentino, J	KY	672
Oto	Wang, S	CA	687
Oto	Weber, R	TX	683
Oto	Weinstein, G	PA	666
Oto	Weisman, R	CA	687
Oto	Weissler, M	NC	672
Oto	Weymuller, E	WA	687
Oto	Wolf, G	MI	678
Oto	Wong, R	NY	666
Oto	Yarbrough, W	CT	657
Oto	Yueh, B	MN	679
PlS	Loree, T	NY	855
PlS	Tufaro, A	MD	860
PMR	Schwartz, L	PA	837
PO	Crockett, D	CA	793
PO	Geller, K	CA	793
RadRO	Ang, K	TX	963
RadRO	Beitler, J	GA	953
RadRO	Brizel, D	NC	954
RadRO	Cooper, J	NY	948
RadRO	Eisbruch, A	MI	959
RadRO	Emami, B	IL	959
RadRO	Haffty, B	NJ	950
RadRO	Halyard, M	AZ	964
RadRO	Haraf, D	IL	960
RadRO	Harari, P	WI	960
RadRO	Harrison, L	NY	950
RadRO	Johnstone, P	IN	960
RadRO	Jose, B	IN	960
RadRO	Kalnicki, S	NY	951
RadRO	Kudrimoti, M	KY	954
RadRO	Laramore, G	WA	966
RadRO	Le, Q	CA	967
RadRO	Lee, C	MN	960
RadRO	Machtay, M	OH	961
RadRO	Mendenhall, W	FL	956
RadRO	Mittal, B	IL	961
RadRO	Morrison, W	TX	965
RadRO	Quivey, J	CA	967
RadRO	Sailer, S	NC	957
RadRO	Song, S	VA	957
RadRO	Streeter, O	DC	952
RadRO	Suntharalingam, M	MD	953
RadRO	Tripuraneni, P	CA	968
RadRO	Wilson, L	CT	948
RadRO	Zelefsky, M	NY	953
S	Flynn, M	KY	1068
S	Neifeld, J	VA	1071

Head & Neck Cancer & Surgery

Spec	Name	St	Pg
Oto	Andersen, P	OR	684
Oto	Blackwell, K	CA	684
Oto	Blair, E	IL	673
Oto	Futran, N	WA	685
Oto	Genden, E	NY	659
Oto	Goldenberg, D	PA	659
Oto	Hanna, E	TX	682
Oto	Hicks, W	NY	660
Oto	Keane, W	PA	661
Oto	Krespi, Y	NY	662
Oto	Kuhel, W	NY	662
Oto	Medina, J	OK	682
Oto	Miller, F	TX	683
Oto	Olsen, K	MN	677
Oto	Patil, Y	OH	677
Oto	Petruzzelli, G	GA	670
Oto	Pitman, K	MS	670
Oto	Samant, S	TN	671
Oto	Silverman, D	VT	657
Oto	Singh, B	NY	665
Oto	Spiegel, J	MA	657
Oto	Stenson, K	IL	678
Oto	Strome, M	NY	665
Oto	Urken, M	NY	666
Oto	Wilson, K	OH	678
Oto	Zeitels, S	MA	657
S	Jackson, G	TX	1089
S	Ridge, J	PA	1063
S	Saha, S	MI	1081
S	Shah, J	NY	1064

Head & Neck Cancer Reconstruction

Spec	Name	St	Pg
Oto	Futran, N	WA	685
Oto	Genden, E	NY	659

Spec	Name	St	Pg
Oto	Stenson, K	IL	678
Oto	Strome, M	NY	665
Oto	Urken, M	NY	666
Oto	Weisman, R	CA	687
PlS	Robb, G	TX	871
PlS	Yuen, J	AR	872

Head & Neck Imaging

Spec	Name	St	Pg
DR	Holliday, R	NY	975

Head & Neck Infectious Disease

Spec	Name	St	Pg
Oto	Lebovics, R	NY	662

Head & Neck Inflammatory Disorders

Spec	Name	St	Pg
Oto	Lebovics, R	NY	662

Head & Neck Pathology

Spec	Name	St	Pg
Path	Kahn, L	NY	709
Path	Wang, B	NY	712

Head & Neck Radiology

Spec	Name	St	Pg
DR	Mancuso, A	FL	979
NRad	Curtin, H	MA	984
NRad	Mukherji, S	MI	989
NRad	Osborn, A	UT	990
NRad	Zinreich, S	MD	986

Head & Neck Reconstruction

Spec	Name	St	Pg
Oto	Akervall, J	MI	672
Oto	Alam, D	OH	672
Oto	Blackwell, K	CA	684
Oto	Browne, J	NC	667
Oto	Bumpous, J	KY	667
Oto	Chalian, A	PA	658
Oto	Deschler, D	MA	655
Oto	Funk, G	IA	674
Oto	Gosselin, B	NH	655
Oto	Haughey, B	MO	675
Oto	Levine, P	VA	669
Oto	Picken, C	DC	663
Oto	Strome, S	MD	665
PlS	Andersen, J	CA	873
PlS	Deleyiannis, F	CO	869
PlS	Disa, J	NY	853
PlS	Miller, M	OH	866
PlS	Serletti, J	PA	858
PlS	Topham, N	PA	859
S	Patel, S	PA	1061

Head & Neck Surgery

Spec	Name	St	Pg
Oto	Baim, H	IL	672
Oto	Berke, G	CA	684
Oto	Hayden, R	AZ	682
Oto	Hilger, P	MN	675
Oto	Johnson, J	PA	661
Oto	Kaplan, M	CA	685

Spec	Name	St	Pg
Oto	Kim, D	MA	656
Oto	McMenomey, S	OR	686
Oto	Netterville, J	TN	669
Oto	Orloff, L	CA	686
Oto	Ozer, E	OH	677
Oto	Rebeiz, E	MA	657
Oto	Schaefer, S	NY	664
Oto	Schantz, S	NY	664
Oto	Shindo, M	OR	687
Oto	Singer, M	CA	687
Oto	Stewart, M	NY	665
Oto	Wackym, P	OR	687
Oto	Wang, S	CA	687
Oto	Weber, S	TX	683
Oto	Wong, B	CA	688
PlS	Coleman, J	IN	865
PO	Cotton, R	OH	791
PO	Drake, A	NC	791
PO	Duncan, N	TX	792
PO	Rosenfeld, R	NY	790
PO	Tunkel, D	MD	790
PS	Holterman, M	IL	807
PS	Rescorla, F	IN	807
S	Alfonso, A	NY	1053
S	Flynn, M	KY	1068

Head & Neck Trauma

Spec	Name	St	Pg
Oto	Funk, G	IA	674

Head & Neck Tumors

Spec	Name	St	Pg
Oto	Fried, M	NY	659
Oto	Kim, D	MA	656
PO	Cunningham, M	MA	789
PO	McGill, T	MA	789
PO	Myer, C	OH	792

Head & Neck Tumors Imaging

Spec	Name	St	Pg
DR	Rao, V	PA	977
NRad	Koeller, K	MN	989
NRad	Mukherji, S	MI	989

Head Injury

Spec	Name	St	Pg
NS	Zimmerman, C	ID	492
S	Britt, L	VA	1067

Headache

Spec	Name	St	Pg
ChiN	Goldstein, E	GA	149
ChiN	Hershey, A	OH	150
ChiN	Sankar, R	CA	154
ChiN	Shaywitz, B	CT	146
ChiN	Shinnar, S	NY	149
ChiN	Sivaswamy, L	MI	151
ChiN	Tennison, M	NC	149
N	Buchholz, D	MD	510
N	Charles, A	CA	536
N	Charney, J	NY	510
N	Corbett, J	MS	520
N	Couch, J	OK	532
N	Cutrer, F	MN	526

Spec	Name	St	Pg
N	Dodick, D	AZ	533
N	Finkel, A	NC	521
N	Foo, S	NY	511
N	Gendelman, S	NY	512
N	Klein, P	NJ	513
N	Lane, J	CO	532
N	Lavin, P	TN	522
N	Lipton, R	NY	514
N	Newman, L	NY	516
N	Petito, F	NY	516
N	Rothrock, J	NV	538
N	Sabo, T	CO	532
N	Saper, J	MI	530
N	Silberstein, S	PA	517
N	Swanson, J	MN	530
N	Weinberg, H	NY	519
NRad	Khandji, A	NY	985
PM	Argoff, C	NY	696
PM	Freitag, F	TX	701
PM	Loder, E	MA	696
PM	Robbins, L	IL	700
PM	Rosenquist, R	OH	700

Headache in Women

Spec	Name	St	Pg
N	Finkel, M	FL	521
N	Rubin, S	IL	530

Headache/Facial Pain

Spec	Name	St	Pg
PM	Racz, G	TX	701

Hearing & Balance Disorders

Spec	Name	St	Pg
Oto	Amedee, R	LA	681
Oto	Dornhoffer, J	AR	682
Oto	Harris, J	CA	685
Oto	Pensak, M	OH	677
Oto	Rauch, S	MA	656
Oto	Shelton, C	UT	680
Oto	Tucci, D	NC	672
Oto	Wazen, J	FL	672

Hearing Disorders

Spec	Name	St	Pg
Oto	Carey, J	MD	658
Oto	Feghali, J	NY	659
Oto	Goebel, J	MO	675
Oto	Haynes, D	TN	668
Oto	Paparella, M	MN	677
PO	Chan, K	CO	792
PO	Parikh, S	WA	793

Hearing Loss

Spec	Name	St	Pg
CG	Carey, J	UT	161
N	Hecox, K	WI	527
Oto	Arts, H	MI	672
Oto	Balkany, T	FL	667
Oto	Dornhoffer, J	AR	682
Oto	Farrior, J	FL	668
Oto	Gianoli, G	LA	682
Oto	Grundfast, K	MA	656
Oto	Hammerschlag, P	NY	660

Spec	Name	St	Pg
Oto	Kveton, J	CT	656
Oto	Lustig, L	CA	685
Oto	Macias, J	AZ	682
Oto	Mattox, D	GA	669
Oto	Parisier, S	NY	663
Oto	Rubinstein, J	WA	686
Oto	Telischi, F	FL	671
Oto	Wiet, R	IL	678
Oto	Young, N	IL	679
Oto	Yueh, B	MN	679
PO	Arjmand, E	OH	791
PO	Eavey, R	TN	791
PO	Goldsmith, A	NY	789
PO	Katz, R	OH	792

Heart Attack

Spec	Name	St	Pg
CE	Gomes, J	NY	120
Cv	Eagle, K	MI	107
Cv	Gibbons, R	MN	108
Cv	Myerburg, R	FL	104
Cv	Weaver, W	MI	112
IC	Holmes, D	MN	131

Heart Disease & Depression

Spec	Name	St	Pg
Cv	Jaffe, A	MN	108

Heart Disease in Athletes

Spec	Name	St	Pg
CE	Link, M	MA	119

Heart Disease in Cancer Patients

Spec	Name	St	Pg
Cv	Steingart, R	NY	102

Heart Disease in Diabetes Patients

Spec	Name	St	Pg
EDM	Hsueh, W	TX	221

Heart Disease in Down Syndrome

Spec	Name	St	Pg
PCd	Velvis, H	NY	736

Heart Disease in Pregnancy

Spec	Name	St	Pg
Cv	Connolly, H	MN	107
Cv	Elkayam, U	CA	116
Cv	Wells, G	NC	106
Cv	Wilansky, S	AZ	115
MF	Adam, K	TX	438
MF	Hibbard, J	IL	436
MF	Koos, B	CA	440

Heart Disease in Women

Spec	Name	St	Pg
Cv	Bairey, C	CA	116
Cv	Brozena, S	PA	97
Cv	Goldberg, N	NY	98
Cv	Hayes, S	MN	108
Cv	Johnson, P	MA	94
Cv	Judelson, D	CA	117

Spec	Name	St	Pg
Cv	Lewis, S	OR	117
Cv	Lindenfeld, J	CO	113
Cv	Oparil, S	AL	105
Cv	Pepine, C	FL	105
Cv	Redberg, R	CA	118
Cv	Reis, S	PA	101
Cv	Roberts, B	RI	96
Cv	Volgman, A	IL	112
Cv	von der Lohe, E	IN	112
Cv	Wagoner, L	OH	112
Cv	Walsh, M	IN	112
Cv	Wilansky, S	AZ	115
IC	Jacobs, A	MA	126

Heart Disease-Complex

Spec	Name	St	Pg
Cv	Horn, E	NY	99

Heart Failure

Spec	Name	St	Pg
CE	DeLurgio, D	GA	121
CE	Mehta, D	NY	121
CE	Sorrentino, R	GA	122
Cv	Borer, J	NY	97
Cv	Borzak, S	FL	103
Cv	Bourge, R	AL	103
Cv	Bove, A	PA	97
Cv	Califf, R	NC	103
Cv	DeNofrio, D	MA	94
Cv	French, W	CA	117
Cv	Gottlieb, S	MD	99
Cv	Hare, J	FL	104
Cv	Hauptman, P	MO	108
Cv	Heroux, A	IL	108
Cv	Horn, E	NY	99
Cv	Katz, S	NY	100
Cv	Konstam, M	MA	95
Cv	Landzberg, J	NJ	100
Cv	Mather, P	PA	100
Cv	Nagueh, S	TX	114
Cv	O'Connor, C	NC	105
Cv	Parrillo, J	NJ	101
Cv	Rich, S	IL	110
Cv	Rosenbush, S	IL	110
Cv	Russell, S	MD	101
Cv	Steingart, R	NY	102
Cv	Stevenson, L	MA	96
Cv	Young, J	OH	113
IC	Kimmelstiel, C	MA	126
PCd	Bernstein, D	CA	740
PCd	Gewitz, M	NY	735
PCd	Hsu, D	NY	735
PCd	Pahl, E	IL	739
PCd	Shaddy, R	PA	736
T&CS	Aklog, L	AZ	1137
T&CS	Athanasuleas, C	AL	1123
T&CS	Byrne, J	TN	1124
T&CS	Cohen, G	CA	1140
T&CS	Savage, E	FL	1129

Heart Failure & Ventricular

Spec	Name	St	Pg

Containment

Spec	Name	St	Pg
T&CS	Bolman, R	MA	1110
T&CS	Naka, Y	NY	1120

Heart Failure in Kidney Disease

Spec	Name	St	Pg
Nep	Schreiber, M	OH	462

Heart Laser Revascularization

Spec	Name	St	Pg
T&CS	Horvath, K	MD	1117

Heart Valve Disease

Spec	Name	St	Pg
Cv	Bashore, T	NC	103
Cv	Blumenthal, D	NY	96
Cv	Bonow, R	IL	106
Cv	Borer, J	NY	97
Cv	Braverman, A	MO	106
Cv	Byrd, B	TN	103
Cv	Carabello, B	TX	114
Cv	Clements, S	GA	104
Cv	Elkayam, U	CA	116
Cv	Fuster, V	NY	98
Cv	Gliklich, J	NY	98
Cv	Greenberg, M	NY	99
Cv	Harrison, J	NC	104
Cv	Herling, I	PA	99
Cv	Iskandrian, A	AL	104
Cv	Kobashigawa, J	CA	117
Cv	Landzberg, J	NJ	100
Cv	Manning, W	MA	95
Cv	McPherson, D	TX	114
Cv	Mehlman, D	IL	109
Cv	O'Gara, P	MA	95
Cv	O'Neill, W	MI	110
Cv	Phillips, R	MA	96
Cv	Powers, E	SC	105
Cv	Quinones, M	TX	115
Cv	Rahko, P	WI	110
Cv	Reiss, C	MO	110
Cv	Sanborn, T	IL	111
Cv	Shah, P	CA	118
Cv	Shea, R	IN	111
Cv	Silvestry, F	PA	102
Cv	Slater, W	NY	102
Cv	Stainback, R	TX	115
Cv	Stewart, W	OH	111
Cv	Tenenbaum, J	NY	102
Cv	Waxman, H	PA	102
Cv	Wells, G	NC	106
Cv	Wilansky, S	AZ	115
IC	Bailey, S	TX	132
IC	Carroll, J	CO	132
IC	Herrmann, H	PA	127
IC	Morris, D	GA	130
IC	Moses, J	NY	127
IC	Sharma, S	NY	129
IC	Smalling, R	TX	132
IC	Teirstein, P	CA	133
T&CS	Szeto, W	PA	1122

Specialty & Special Expertise Index

Spec	Name	St	Pg
Heart Valve Surgery			
PS	Quaegebeur, J	NY	804
T&CS	Acker, M	PA	1113
T&CS	Adams, D	NY	1113
T&CS	Akins, C	MA	1110
T&CS	Aldea, G	WA	1140
T&CS	Bavaria, J	PA	1114
T&CS	Bridges, C	NC	1124
T&CS	Brown, J	IN	1131
T&CS	Byrne, J	TN	1124
T&CS	Caskey, M	AZ	1137
T&CS	Chitwood, W	NC	1124
T&CS	Cohen, R	CA	1141
T&CS	Drinkwater, D	TN	1125
T&CS	Filsoufi, F	NY	1115
T&CS	Furukawa, S	PA	1116
T&CS	Graver, L	NY	1117
T&CS	Griffith, B	MD	1117
T&CS	Hargrove, W	PA	1117
T&CS	Hashim, S	CT	1111
T&CS	Horvath, K	MD	1117
T&CS	Isom, O	NY	1117
T&CS	Jessen, M	TX	1138
T&CS	Joyce, L	MN	1133
T&CS	Kanda, L	DC	1118
T&CS	Krieger, K	NY	1119
T&CS	Lamberti, J	CA	1142
T&CS	Lang, S	NY	1119
T&CS	Lansman, S	NY	1119
T&CS	Lazar, H	MA	1111
T&CS	Loulmet, D	NY	1119
T&CS	Love, R	IL	1133
T&CS	Lytle, B	OH	1133
T&CS	McCarthy, P	IL	1133
T&CS	McGiffin, D	AL	1126
T&CS	Merrick, S	CA	1142
T&CS	Mill, M	NC	1127
T&CS	Mitchell, M	CO	1137
T&CS	Murphy, D	GA	1127
T&CS	Ott, D	TX	1139
T&CS	Oz, M	NY	1120
T&CS	Pochettino, A	MN	1134
T&CS	Rastegar, H	MA	1112
T&CS	Salerno, T	FL	1129
T&CS	Schaff, H	MN	1134
T&CS	Sellke, F	RI	1112
T&CS	Shemin, R	CA	1142
T&CS	Smith, P	NC	1129
T&CS	Starnes, V	CA	1143
T&CS	Swistel, D	NY	1122
T&CS	Toyoda, Y	PA	1122
T&CS	Tranbaugh, R	NY	1122
T&CS	Verrier, E	WA	1143
T&CS	Warner, K	MA	1113
T&CS	Williams, M	NY	1123
Heart Valve Surgery-Aortic			
T&CS	Diehl, J	PA	1115
T&CS	Reardon, M	TX	1139
T&CS	Stewart, A	NY	1122

Spec	Name	St	Pg
Heart Valve Surgery-Mitral			
T&CS	Diehl, J	PA	1115
T&CS	Vander Salm, T	MA	1112
Heart Valve Surgery-Pediatric			
T&CS	Del-Nido, P	MA	1110
T&CS	Forbess, J	TX	1138
Heart Valve Surgery-Percutaneous			
T&CS	Guyton, R	GA	1125
T&CS	Svensson, L	OH	1135
Hemangiomas			
D	Cohen, B	MD	185
D	Frieden, I	CA	198
D	Friedlander, S	CA	199
D	Yan, A	PA	189
PO	Cunningham, M	MA	789
PO	McGill, T	MA	789
Hemangiomas/Birthmarks			
D	Bayliss, S	MO	192
PlS	Kane, A	TX	870
Hematologic Disorders			
PHO	Pendergrass, T	WA	778
PHO	Recht, M	OR	779
Hematologic Disorders in Cancer Patients			
Hem	Soff, G	NY	315
Hematologic Infections			
Inf	Slama, T	IN	417
Hematologic Malignancies			
Hem	Anderson, K	MA	310
Hem	Brodsky, R	MD	312
Hem	Cheson, B	DC	312
Hem	Di Persio, J	MO	319
Hem	Filicko-O'Hara, J	PA	312
Hem	Flynn, P	MN	319
Hem	Greer, J	TN	316
Hem	Grever, M	OH	320
Hem	Heinrich, M	OR	325
Hem	Kessler, C	DC	313
Hem	Kraut, E	OH	320
Hem	Lill, M	CA	326
Hem	Lin, W	TX	324
Hem	Maciejewski, J	OH	321
Hem	Mangan, K	PA	313
Hem	Millenson, M	PA	314
Hem	Mitchell, B	CA	326
Hem	Munker, R	LA	324
Hem	Nademanee, A	CA	326
Hem	Roodman, G	IN	321

Spec	Name	St	Pg
Hem	Schiffman, F	RI	311
Hem	Schuster, M	NY	315
Hem	Slease, R	DE	315
Hem	Sokol, L	FL	318
Onc	Advani, R	CA	383
Onc	Algazy, K	PA	334
Onc	Armitage, J	NE	374
Onc	Bashevkin, M	NY	335
Onc	Beatty, P	MT	374
Onc	Bergsagel, P	AZ	377
Onc	Bolwell, B	OH	365
Onc	Claxton, D	PA	336
Onc	Cohen, G	MD	336
Onc	Colon-Otero, G	FL	355
Onc	Druker, B	OR	385
Onc	Erban, J	MA	328
Onc	Gabrilove, J	NY	340
Onc	Mitsuyasu, R	CA	388
Onc	Morginstin, M	PA	345
Onc	Picozzi, V	WA	389
Onc	Rosen, S	IL	371
Onc	Rosove, M	CA	390
Onc	Shields, P	OH	372
Onc	Silver, S	MI	372
Onc	Strenger, R	RI	332
Onc	Taetle, R	AZ	382
Onc	Vaughan, W	AL	363
PHO	Hord, J	OH	771
PHO	Ritchey, A	PA	763
Hematology			
Hem	Abrams, C	PA	311
Hem	Adams, R	AZ	323
Hem	Adams-Graves, P	TN	316
Hem	Allen, S	NY	311
Hem	Anderson, K	MA	310
Hem	Baer, M	MD	312
Hem	Ballen, K	MA	310
Hem	Barlogie, B	AR	323
Hem	Baron, J	IL	318
Hem	Bigelow, C	MS	316
Hem	Blinder, M	MO	318
Hem	Bockenstedt, P	MI	319
Hem	Brenner, M	TX	323
Hem	Brodsky, R	MD	312
Hem	Byrd, J	OH	319
Hem	Champlin, R	TX	323
Hem	Cheson, B	DC	312
Hem	Cobos, E	TX	323
Hem	Comenzo, R	MA	310
Hem	Cooper, B	TX	323
Hem	Copelan, E	OH	319
Hem	Cortes, J	TX	323
Hem	Damon, L	CA	325
Hem	DeLoughery, T	OR	325
Hem	Di Persio, J	MO	319
Hem	Diuguid, D	NY	312
Hem	Djulbegovic, B	FL	316
Hem	Duffy, T	CT	310
Hem	Emanuel, P	AR	323
Hem	Farag, S	IN	319

Spec	Name	St	Pg
Hem	Filicko-O'Hara, J	PA	312
Hem	Flynn, P	MN	319
Hem	Fonseca, R	AZ	324
Hem	Forman, S	CA	325
Hem	Friedman, A	PA	312
Hem	Fruchtman, S	NY	312
Hem	Gertz, M	MN	319
Hem	Goldberg, J	PA	312
Hem	Gordon, L	IL	319
Hem	Greer, J	TN	316
Hem	Gregory, S	IL	320
Hem	Grever, M	OH	320
Hem	Habermann, T	MN	320
Hem	Heinrich, M	OR	325
Hem	Isola, L	NY	313
Hem	Juckett, M	WI	320
Hem	Kantarjian, H	TX	324
Hem	Keating, M	TX	324
Hem	Kempin, S	NY	313
Hem	Kessler, C	DC	313
Hem	Kipps, T	CA	325
Hem	Klingemann, H	MA	310
Hem	Komrokji, R	FL	317
Hem	Kraut, E	OH	320
Hem	Kuriakose, P	MI	320
Hem	Larson, R	IL	320
Hem	Laughlin, M	VA	317
Hem	Leung, L	CA	326
Hem	Levine, A	CA	326
Hem	Lill, M	CA	326
Hem	Lin, W	TX	324
Hem	Linenberger, M	WA	326
Hem	Litzow, M	MN	320
Hem	Luger, S	PA	313
Hem	Lyons, R	TX	324
Hem	Maciejewski, J	OH	321
Hem	Mangan, K	PA	313
Hem	Marks, P	CT	310
Hem	Marks, S	PA	313
Hem	Maslak, P	NY	313
Hem	Maziarz, R	OR	326
Hem	McGlave, P	MN	321
Hem	Mears, J	NY	313
Hem	Meehan, K	NH	310
Hem	Mesa, R	AZ	324
Hem	Milhem, M	IA	321
Hem	Millenson, M	PA	314
Hem	Miller, K	MA	311
Hem	Mitchell, B	CA	326
Hem	Munker, R	LA	324
Hem	Nademanee, A	CA	326
Hem	Nand, S	IL	321
Hem	Negrin, R	CA	326
Hem	Nimer, S	FL	317
Hem	O'Donnell, M	CA	327
Hem	Ortel, T	NC	317
Hem	Palascak, J	OH	321
Hem	Petersdorf, S	WA	327
Hem	Porcu, P	OH	321
Hem	Porter, D	PA	314
Hem	Powell, B	NC	317
Hem	Rai, K	NY	314

Spec	Name	St	Pg
Hem	Rao, A	PA	314
Hem	Raphael, B	NY	314
Hem	Rapoport, A	MD	314
Hem	Richardson, P	MA	311
Hem	Rodgers, G	UT	322
Hem	Roodman, G	IN	321
Hem	Rosenblatt, J	FL	317
Hem	Rowley, S	NJ	314
Hem	Savage, D	NY	314
Hem	Saven, A	CA	327
Hem	Schiffman, F	RI	311
Hem	Schiller, G	CA	327
Hem	Schuster, M	NY	315
Hem	Schuster, S	PA	315
Hem	Schwartzberg, L	TN	317
Hem	Singhal, S	IL	321
Hem	Slease, R	DE	315
Hem	Snyder, D	CA	327
Hem	Soff, G	NY	315
Hem	Sokol, L	FL	318
Hem	Solberg, L	FL	318
Hem	Spitzer, T	MA	311
Hem	Spivak, J	MD	315
Hem	Stewart, A	AZ	324
Hem	Stiff, P	IL	322
Hem	Stone, R	MA	311
Hem	Strair, R	NJ	315
Hem	Strauss, J	TX	325
Hem	Streiff, M	MD	315
Hem	Tallman, M	NY	316
Hem	Tefferi, A	MN	322
Hem	Telen, M	NC	318
Hem	Uberti, J	MI	322
Hem	Van Besien, K	IL	322
Hem	Vose, J	NE	322
Hem	Williams, M	VA	318
Hem	Winter, J	IL	322
Hem	Wisch, N	NY	316
Hem	Yanovich, S	MD	316
Hem	Yeager, A	AZ	325
Hem	Zuckerman, K	FL	318

Hematopathology

Spec	Name	St	Pg
Hem	Rodgers, G	UT	322
Path	Bagg, A	PA	708
Path	Banks, P	NC	713
Path	Behm, F	IL	715
Path	Chesney, C	TN	713
Path	Harris, N	MA	706
Path	Kinney, M	TX	718
Path	Morrow, J	CT	707
Path	Nathwani, B	CA	721
Path	Orazi, A	NY	710
Path	Swerdlow, S	PA	712
Path	Warnke, R	CA	722
Path	Weisenburger, D	NE	717
Path	Weiss, L	CA	722

Hemifacial Spasm

Spec	Name	St	Pg
NS	Sen, C	NY	478

Hemochromatosis

Spec	Name	St	Pg
PHO	Wolfe, L	NY	764

Hemolytic Uremic Syndrome

Spec	Name	St	Pg
PNep	Ault, B	TN	786
PNep	Kaplan, B	PA	785

Hemophagocytic Syndrome

Spec	Name	St	Pg
PHO	Morgan, E	IL	772

Hemophilia

Spec	Name	St	Pg
Hem	Kessler, C	DC	313
Hem	Marks, P	CT	310
Hem	Ortel, T	NC	317
Hem	Palascak, J	OH	321
Onc	Romond, E	KY	361
PHO	Buchanan, G	TX	775
PHO	Glader, B	CA	777
PHO	Halpern, S	NJ	760
PHO	Hoots, W	MD	761
PHO	Johnston, J	GA	766
PHO	Kobrinsky, N	ND	774
PHO	Kung, F	CA	778
PHO	Manco-Johnson, M	CO	774
PHO	Recht, M	OR	779
PHO	Shapiro, A	IN	773
PHO	Tebbi, C	FL	768
PHO	Valentino, L	IL	773

Hemophilia Related Disease

Spec	Name	St	Pg
OrS	Luck, J	CA	644

Hemorrhoids

Spec	Name	St	Pg
CRS	Eisenstat, T	NJ	169
CRS	Golub, R	FL	172
CRS	Gorfine, S	NY	170

Hepatic Iron Metabolism

Spec	Name	St	Pg
Ge	Bacon, B	MO	243

Hepatitis

Spec	Name	St	Pg
Ge	Barnes, D	OH	244
Ge	Boyer, T	AZ	251
Ge	Brown, R	NY	231
Ge	Davis, G	TX	251
Ge	Di Bisceglie, A	MO	244
Ge	Dienstag, J	MA	228
Ge	Dieterich, D	NY	232
Ge	Freiman, H	NY	232
Ge	Fried, M	NC	240
Ge	Gish, R	CA	254
Ge	Glombicki, A	TX	252
Ge	Hunter, E	ID	249
Ge	Jacobson, I	NY	234
Ge	Kotler, D	NY	235
Ge	Magun, A	NY	236
Ge	Martin, P	FL	241

Specialty & Special Expertise Index

Spec	Name	St	Pg
Ge	Munoz, S	PA	237
Ge	Nunes, D	MA	229
Ge	Reddy, K	PA	237
Ge	Schiano, T	NY	238
Ge	Sorrell, M	NE	250
Ge	Te, H	IL	248
Ge	Zaman, A	OR	255
PGe	Jonas, M	MA	749
PGe	Molleston, J	IN	753
PGe	Suchy, F	CO	755

Hepatitis B

Ge	Bloomer, J	AL	239

Hepatitis B & C

Ge	Han, S	CA	254
Ge	Kwo, P	IN	246
Ge	Poordad, F	TX	252
Ge	Tobias, H	NY	238
Ge	Vierling, J	TX	253
Inf	Nahass, R	NJ	412
PGe	Murray, K	WA	756
PGe	Schwarz, K	MD	751

Hepatitis B-Immune Response

Rhu	Cupps, T	DC	1026

Hepatitis C

Ge	Bacon, B	MO	243
Ge	Balart, L	LA	250
Ge	Brown, K	MI	244
Ge	Chung, R	MA	228
Ge	Di Bisceglie, A	MO	244
Ge	Fallon, M	TX	251
Ge	Galati, J	TX	252
Ge	Herrine, S	PA	233
Ge	Jacobson, I	NY	234
Ge	Jensen, D	IL	246
Ge	Schiff, E	FL	242
Ge	Shiffman, M	VA	242
Inf	Craven, D	MA	410

Hepatitis-Chronic

Ge	Porayko, M	TN	241
Ge	Scudera, P	VA	242

Hepatobiliary Surgery

PS	Tracy, T	RI	802
S	Adams, R	VA	1066
S	Billingsley, K	OR	1093
S	Cherqui, D	NY	1055
S	Colquhoun, S	CA	1094
S	Curley, S	TX	1087
S	Deziel, D	IL	1076
S	Eckhoff, D	AL	1068
S	Emond, J	NY	1057
S	Emre, S	CT	1049
S	Farley, D	MN	1076

S	Galloway, J	GA	1068
S	Hemming, A	CA	1096
S	Hoffman, J	PA	1058
S	Howerton, R	NC	1069
S	Jabbour, N	MA	1050
S	Jarnagin, W	NY	1058
S	Kendrick, M	MN	1078
S	Kinkhabwala, M	NY	1059
S	Knechtle, S	GA	1069
S	Lieberman, M	NY	1060
S	Moossa, A	CA	1097
S	Nagorney, D	MN	1080
S	Oberholzer, J	IL	1080
S	Philosophe, B	MD	1062
S	Reed, A	IA	1081
S	Reich, D	PA	1062
S	Reyes, J	WA	1099
S	Shaked, A	PA	1064
S	Teperman, L	NY	1065
S	Thayer, S	MA	1052
S	Vauthey, J	TX	1092
S	Walsh, R	OH	1084

Hepatopulmonary Syndrome

Pul	Krowka, M	MN	934

Hereditary Angioedema

A&I	Lockey, R	FL	86
A&I	Slankard, M	NY	85

Hereditary Cancer

CG	Grody, W	CA	163
CG	Ostrer, H	NY	158
CG	Plon, S	TX	162
CG	Shapiro, L	NY	158
CG	Sutphen, R	FL	159
CG	Weitzel, J	CA	164
CG	Whelan, A	MO	161
Ge	Boland, C	TX	250
Ge	Itzkowitz, S	NY	234
Onc	Markowitz, S	OH	369
Onc	Nissenblatt, M	NJ	346
Onc	Olopade, O	IL	370
Onc	Toppmeyer, D	NJ	351
S	Hughes, K	MA	1050

Hereditary Endocrine Cancers

EDM	Waguespack, S	TX	221

Hereditary Hemorrhagic Telangiectasia

CG	Pyeritz, R	PA	158
PHO	Valentino, L	IL	773
VIR	Trerotola, S	PA	994
VIR	White, R	CT	992

Hernia

PS	Aiken, J	WI	806

PS	Paidas, C	FL	805
PS	Velcek, F	NY	804
S	Baker, C	VA	1066
S	Barie, P	NY	1053
S	Brody, F	DC	1054
S	Brunt, L	MO	1075
S	Farley, D	MN	1076
S	Fitzgibbons, R	NE	1085
S	Greene, F	NC	1069
S	Meyers, W	PA	1060
S	Nowak, E	NY	1061
S	Pachter, H	NY	1061
S	Pomp, A	NY	1062
S	Rege, R	TX	1091
S	Reiner, M	NY	1063
S	Rosen, M	OH	1081
U	Atala, A	NC	1159

Hernia-Complex

S	Bellows, C	LA	1087
S	Livingston, E	TX	1090

Hernia-Sports

S	Brunt, L	MO	1075

Herpes Simplex

PInf	Bryson, Y	CA	784

Herpetic Neuralgia (Shingles)

PM	Audell, L	CA	702
PM	Raja, S	MD	697

Hidradenitis Suppurativa

D	Bennett, R	CA	198

High Intensity Focused Ultrasound(HIFU)

U	Robertson, C	NC	1163

Hip & Knee Reconstruction

OrS	Caillouette, J	CA	642
OrS	Einhorn, T	MA	610
OrS	McDonald, D	MO	635
OrS	Oakes, D	CA	645
OrS	Smith, E	MA	613

Hip & Knee Replacement

OrS	Blaha, J	MI	632
OrS	Bucholz, R	TX	640
OrS	Callaghan, J	IA	633
OrS	Copp, S	CA	642
OrS	Cornell, C	NY	616
OrS	Dorr, L	CA	643
OrS	Einhorn, T	MA	610
OrS	Finerman, G	CA	643
OrS	Luck, J	CA	644
OrS	Oakes, D	CA	645

Spec	Name	St	Pg
OrS	Padgett, D	NY	623
OrS	Ready, J	MA	612
OrS	Schmalzried, T	CA	645
OrS	Siegel, H	AL	630
OrS	Smith, E	MA	613
OrS	Stuchin, S	NY	626
OrS	Stulberg, S	IL	637
OrS	Thornhill, T	MA	613
OrS	Vail, T	CA	646
OrS	Wittig, J	NY	627
OrS	Wixson, R	IL	638

Hip & Knee Replacement in Bone Tumors

OrS	Healey, J	NY	619
OrS	Ready, J	MA	612

Hip Disorders & Dysplasia

OrS	Aronson, J	AR	640
OrS	Weinstein, S	IA	638

Hip Disorders-Pediatric

OrS	Herman, M	PA	619
OrS	McCarthy, J	OH	635
OrS	Roye, D	NY	624
OrS	Weinstein, S	IA	638

Hip Replacement

OrS	Brick, G	MA	610
OrS	Bronson, M	NY	615
OrS	Burke, D	MA	610
OrS	Gitelis, S	IL	633
OrS	Goldstein, W	IL	633
OrS	Gorab, R	CA	643
OrS	Howe, K	CA	644
OrS	Hume, E	PA	620
OrS	Jiranek, W	VA	629
OrS	Johnson, E	CA	644
OrS	Macaulay, W	NY	622
OrS	Muschler, G	OH	636
OrS	Reilly, D	MA	612
OrS	Rothman, R	PA	624
OrS	Salvati, E	NY	625
OrS	Sharkey, P	PA	625
OrS	Weiner, R	FL	631
OrS	Zuckerman, J	NY	627

Hip Replacement & Revision

OrS	Berry, D	MN	632
OrS	Buly, R	NY	615
OrS	Hungerford, M	MD	620
OrS	Jacobs, J	IL	634
OrS	Johanson, N	PA	620
OrS	Krackow, K	NY	621
OrS	Mabrey, J	TX	641
OrS	Parvizi, J	PA	623
OrS	Thomas, B	CA	646
OrS	Westrich, G	NY	626

Hip Replacement-Young Adults

OrS	Pellicci, P	NY	623

Hip Resurfacing

OrS	Oakes, D	CA	645
OrS	Pellicci, P	NY	623
OrS	Stuchin, S	NY	626
OrS	Thomas, B	CA	646
OrS	Vail, T	CA	646

Hip Surgery

OrS	Bono, J	MA	610
OrS	Crossett, L	PA	616
OrS	Garvin, K	NE	639
OrS	Hanssen, A	MN	634
OrS	Hozack, W	PA	620
OrS	Kelly, B	NY	621
SM	Byrd, J	TN	1042

Hirschsprung's Disease

PS	Doody, D	MA	801
PS	Notrica, D	AZ	809
PS	Proctor, M	WA	811
PS	Ricketts, R	GA	806
PS	Tracy, T	RI	802

Hirsutism

D	Olsen, E	NC	191

Histiocytoma

PHO	Arceci, R	MD	758
PHO	Nicholson, H	OR	778

Histoplasmosis

PInf	Belcher, C	IN	782
PInf	Christenson, J	IN	783
PInf	Kleiman, M	IN	783

HIV

Inf	Longworth, D	OH	416
Inf	Nahass, R	NJ	412
Inf	Schooley, R	CA	420
Inf	Wallace, M	FL	415

HIV & Blood Transfusions

Inf	Wallach, F	NY	413

HIV & Hepatitis co-infection

Inf	McGowan, J	NY	412

HIV and Lung Disease

PPul	Platzker, A	CA	798

HIV in Adolescents

AM	Rudy, B	NY	80

HIV in Pregnancy

Inf	Cohn, S	IL	416
Inf	McGowan, J	NY	412

HIV Related Kidney Disease

Nep	Winston, J	NY	459

Hives

A&I	Buchbinder, E	NY	84

Hodgkin's Disease Consultation

Onc	DeVita, V	CT	328

Hodgkin's Disease-Second Opinion

Onc	Canellos, G	MA	328

Hodgkin's Lymphoma

Hem	Emanuel, P	AR	323
Hem	Gordon, L	IL	319
Hem	Habermann, T	MN	320
Hem	Komrokji, R	FL	317
Hem	Slease, R	DE	315
Hem	Winter, J	IL	322
Onc	Ambinder, R	MD	334
Onc	Coleman, M	NY	337
Onc	Come, S	MA	328
Onc	Czuczman, M	NY	337
Onc	Fisher, R	NY	339
Onc	Friedberg, J	NY	340
Onc	Glick, J	PA	340
Onc	Goy, A	NJ	341
Onc	Hochberg, E	MA	330
Onc	Horwitz, S	NY	342
Onc	Lossos, I	FL	359
Onc	Moore, J	NC	360
Onc	Morgan, D	TN	360
Onc	O'Connor, O	NY	346
Onc	Smith, M	PA	349
PHO	Billett, A	MA	756
PHO	Brecher, M	NY	758
PHO	Chen, A	MD	759
PHO	Fallon, R	IN	770
PHO	Friedman, D	TN	765
PHO	Halpern, S	NJ	760
PHO	Hudson, M	TN	766
PHO	Hutchinson, R	MI	771
PHO	Keller, F	GA	766
PHO	Olson, J	OR	778
PHO	Schwartz, C	RI	757
PHO	Tebbi, C	FL	768
PHO	Weiner, M	NY	764
RadRO	Donaldson, S	CA	965
RadRO	Hoppe, R	CA	966
RadRO	Mendenhall, N	FL	956
RadRO	Nicolaou, N	PA	951
RadRO	Roberts, K	CT	947
RadRO	Yahalom, J	NY	953

Specialty & Special Expertise Index

Spec	Name	St	Pg
Hormonal Disorders			
EDM	Braunstein, G	CA	222
EDM	Dobs, A	MD	210
EDM	Goodman, N	FL	214
EDM	Korytkowski, M	PA	211
Ger	Schwartz, R	CO	265
ObG	Berga, S	NC	559
RE	Chang, R	CA	1017
RE	Dumesic, D	CA	1017
RE	Ory, S	FL	1012
RE	Richardson, M	KS	1015
RE	Winer, S	CA	1018
RE	Zacur, H	MD	1011
Hormone Replacement-Male			
U	Lipshultz, L	TX	1174
Hormone Secreting Tumors			
Ge	Liddle, R	NC	241
H & PMicine			
H & PM	Abrahm, J	MA	406
H & PM	Arnold, R	PA	406
H & PM	Block, S	MA	406
H & PM	Bricker, L	MI	407
H & PM	Davis, M	OH	407
H & PM	Ferris, F	CA	408
H & PM	Fine, R	TX	408
H & PM	Friebert, S	OH	407
H & PM	Jackson, V	MA	406
H & PM	Kutner, J	CO	407
H & PM	Pantilat, S	CA	408
H & PM	Portenoy, R	NY	406
H & PM	Quill, T	NY	407
H & PM	Ritchie, C	CA	408
H & PM	Santa-Emma, P	OH	407
H & PM	Selvaggi, K	MA	406
H & PM	Tulsky, J	NC	407
H & PM	Von Gunten, C	CA	408
H & PM	Weinstein, S	UT	408
Hospital Acquired Infections			
Inf	Ballon-Landa, G	CA	419
Inf	Craven, D	MA	410
Inf	Edmond, M	VA	414
Inf	Hammer, G	NY	411
Inf	Louie, E	NY	412
Inf	Patterson, J	TX	418
PInf	Baltimore, R	CT	779
HPV-Human Papilloma Virus			
GO	Soisson, A	UT	286
ObG	Hager, W	KY	559
Onc	Berry, J	CA	384
PInf	Alexander, K	IL	782
Human Granulocytic			

Spec	Name	St	Pg
Anaplasmosis			
Inf	Bakken, J	MN	416
Huntington's Disease			
ChiN	Dure, L	AL	149
N	Ashizawa, T	FL	520
N	Baser, S	PA	509
N	Kieburtz, K	NY	513
N	Longo, F	CA	538
N	Louis, E	NY	515
N	Marder, K	NY	515
N	Perlmutter, J	MO	528
N	Weiner, W	MD	519
N	Young, A	MA	509
Path	Gambetti, P	OH	715
Hydrocephalus			
NS	Bierbrauer, K	OH	486
NS	Bierbrauer, K	OH	486
NS	Dias, M	PA	473
NS	Frim, D	IL	487
NS	Kaplitt, M	NY	476
NS	Ojemann, J	WA	498
NS	Ruge, J	IL	490
NS	Sandberg, D	TX	494
NS	Sklar, F	TX	494
NS	Sutton, L	PA	479
NS	Tomita, T	IL	490
NS	Walker, M	UT	492
NS	Wisoff, J	NY	480
Ped	Walker, W	WA	729
Hydrocephalus-Adult			
NS	Goodman, R	NY	474
NS	Rigamonti, D	MD	478
Hydrocephalus-normal pressure			
N	Adams, D	FL	519
Hydronephrosis			
U	Kass, E	MI	1167
U	Rushton, H	DC	1156
U	Shortliffe, L	CA	1178
Hydronephrosis-Prenatal			
U	Cain, M	IN	1166
U	Kaefer, M	IN	1167
Hyperbaric Medicine			
S	Yurt, R	NY	1066
VascS	Iafrati, M	MA	1184
Hyperhidrosis			
VascS	Ahn, S	CA	1193

Spec	Name	St	Pg
Hyperhidrosis-Palmar			
T&CS	Cohen, N	MD	1114
T&CS	Keller, S	NY	1118
T&CS	Mitchell, J	CO	1136
T&CS	Nugent, W	NH	1111
T&CS	Vigneswaran, W	IL	1135
Hyperinsulinism			
PEn	Lustig, R	CA	749
Hyperinsulinism-Congenital			
PEn	Stanley, C	PA	745
Hypersensitivity Pneumonitis			
A&I	Greenberger, P	IL	88
Pul	Sharma, O	CA	941
Hypertension			
Cv	Ballantyne, C	TX	114
Cv	Blanchard, D	CA	116
Cv	Blumenthal, R	MD	97
Cv	Inra, L	NY	99
Cv	Judelson, D	CA	117
Cv	Kostis, J	NJ	100
Cv	Oparil, S	AL	105
Cv	Pepine, C	FL	105
Cv	Phillips, R	MA	96
Cv	Sorrentino, M	IL	111
Cv	Zusman, R	MA	96
EDM	Sowers, J	MO	219
Ge	Zaman, A	OR	255
Ger	Lipsitz, L	MA	262
Ger	Supiano, M	UT	266
IM	Bakris, G	IL	425
IM	Cushman, W	TN	425
IM	Fischbein, L	MO	425
IM	Mehler, P	CO	426
IM	Wright, J	OH	425
Nep	Ahmad, S	WA	464
Nep	August, P	NY	457
Nep	Bazari, H	MA	456
Nep	Berns, J	PA	457
Nep	Black, H	NY	457
Nep	Blumenfeld, J	NY	457
Nep	Coffman, T	NC	459
Nep	Ellison, D	OR	465
Nep	Fadem, S	TX	463
Nep	Gluck, S	CA	465
Nep	Johnston, J	PA	457
Nep	Josephson, M	IL	461
Nep	Kelepouris, E	PA	458
Nep	King, A	CA	465
Nep	Kobrin, S	PA	458
Nep	Mitch, W	TX	464
Nep	Olivero, J	TX	464
Nep	Perrone, R	MA	456
Nep	Piraino, B	PA	458
Nep	Pohl, M	OH	462
Nep	Rudnick, M	PA	458

Spec	Name	St	Pg
Nep	Schwartz, G	MN	462
Nep	Suki, W	TX	464
Nep	Textor, S	MN	462
Nep	Tolkoff-Rubin, N	MA	456
Nep	Yee, J	MI	463
PNep	Benfield, M	AL	786
PNep	Ellis, D	PA	785
PNep	Flynn, J	WA	788
PNep	Friedman, A	MN	787
PNep	Jabs, K	TN	786
PNep	Mendley, S	MD	786
PNep	Neiberger, R	FL	786

Hypertension in Children

PNep	Ettenger, R	CA	788
PNep	Fouser, L	WA	788

Hypertension in Obesity

PCd	Rocchini, A	MI	739

Hypertension in Pregnancy

MF	Genc, M	NY	432
MF	Hankins, G	TX	438
MF	Repke, J	PA	433
MF	Saade, G	TX	439
MF	Samuels, P	OH	437
Nep	August, P	NY	457

Hypertension-Complex

Cv	Saunders, E	MD	101
Nep	Lea, J	GA	460
Nep	Townsend, R	PA	458

Hypertension-Drug Resistent

Nep	Wilcox, C	DC	458

Hypertension-Renovascular

Nep	Wilcox, C	DC	458
VIR	Murphy, T	RI	992

Hypertension/Kidney Disease

Nep	August, P	NY	457
Nep	Toto, R	TX	464

Hyperthermia Treatment of Cancer

RadRO	Myerson, R	MO	961
RadRO	Prosnitz, L	NC	956

Hypertrophic Cardiomyopathy

PCd	Ackerman, M	MN	738
T&CS	Swistel, D	NY	1122

Hypnosis

Psyc	Spiegel, D	CA	903

Hypogammaglobulinemia

PA&I	Sleasman, J	FL	731

Hypoglycemia

EDM	Clore, J	VA	214
EDM	Comi, R	NH	206
EDM	Cryer, P	MO	217
EDM	Schutta, M	PA	211
PEn	Sperling, M	PA	745
PEn	Stanley, C	PA	745

Hypogonadism

EDM	Cunningham, G	TX	220
U	Shabsigh, R	NY	1157

Hypogonadism-Male

EDM	Dobs, A	MD	210

Hypoplastic Left Heart Syndrome

PS	Bove, E	MI	807
T&CS	Huddleston, C	MO	1132

Hypospadias

U	Atala, A	NC	1159
U	Baskin, L	CA	1175
U	Canning, D	PA	1151
U	Elder, J	MI	1166
U	Ewalt, D	TX	1173
U	Hensle, T	NJ	1153
U	Kass, E	MI	1167
U	Rushton, H	DC	1156
U	Shortliffe, L	CA	1178
U	Strand, W	TX	1174

Hypotension

Ger	Lipsitz, L	MA	262

Hypothalamic Dysfunction

EDM	Lechan, R	MA	208

Hysterectomy Alternatives

GO	Magrina, J	AZ	288
ObG	Filip, S	NC	559

Hysteroscopic Surgery

ObG	Bradley, L	OH	560
ObG	Jenkins, T	AL	559
ObG	Parker, W	CA	563
RE	Copperman, A	NY	1008
RE	Diamond, M	MI	1013
RE	Dumesic, D	CA	1017
RE	Falcone, T	OH	1013
RE	Grifo, J	NY	1008
RE	Grunfeld, L	NY	1008
RE	Hornstein, M	MA	1006
RE	Huang, J	TX	1016
RE	Stewart, E	MN	1014
RE	Yee, B	CA	1018

I

Immune Deficiencies-Primary

Inf	Segal, B	NY	413
Ped	Infante, A	TX	728

Immune Deficiency

A&I	Ein, D	DC	85
A&I	Lockey, R	FL	86
A&I	Tamaroff, M	CA	91
A&I	Umetsu, D	MA	84
A&I	Wong, J	MA	84
Inf	Van Der Horst, C	NC	415
PA&I	Fanous, Y	CA	733
PA&I	Gelfand, E	CO	732
PA&I	Lemanske, R	WI	731
PA&I	Shearer, W	TX	732
PA&I	Sullivan, K	PA	730
PA&I	Wolf, R	IL	731
PHO	Kapoor, N	CA	777
PRhu	Haines, K	NJ	799

Immune Deficiency-Skin Disorders

D	Edelson, R	CT	182
D	Jorizzo, J	NC	191
D	Mutasim, D	OH	194
D	Paller, A	IL	195
D	Rook, A	PA	188
D	Sontheimer, R	UT	196

Immune Deficiency-Thyroid

A&I	Baker, J	MI	87

Immunodeficiency Disorders

A&I	Cunningham-Rundles, C	NY	84
A&I	DeShazo, R	MS	86
A&I	Gruchalla, R	TX	89
A&I	Markert, M	NC	87
A&I	Montanaro, A	OR	90
A&I	Phillips, S	PA	85
A&I	Routes, J	WI	89
PA&I	Church, J	CA	733
PA&I	Cowan, M	CA	733
PA&I	Orange, J	TX	732
PA&I	Sleasman, J	FL	731
PA&I	Wasserman, R	TX	732
Rhu	Lahita, R	NJ	1027

Specialty & Special Expertise Index

Spec	Name	St	Pg
Immunopathology			
Path	Bhan, A	MA	706
Path	Tomaszewski, J	NY	712
Immunotherapy			
A&I	Cunningham-Rundles, C	NY	84
A&I	Sundy, J	NC	87
DR	Bahn, D	CA	982
GO	Giuntoli, R	MD	278
GO	Odunsi, A	NY	279
GO	Santin, A	CT	275
Hem	Maziarz, R	OR	326
Hem	Porcu, P	OH	321
IM	Fischl, M	FL	425
Nep	Ward, D	CA	466
Onc	Albertini, M	WI	364
Onc	Atkins, M	DC	334
Onc	Ball, E	CA	383
Onc	Chapman, P	NY	336
Onc	Emens, L	MD	339
Onc	Figlin, R	CA	386
Onc	Hwu, P	TX	379
Onc	Kirkwood, J	PA	343
Onc	Kwak, L	TX	379
Onc	Lynch, J	FL	359
Onc	Peace, D	IL	370
Onc	Pecora, A	NJ	347
Onc	Scheinberg, D	NY	348
Onc	Sosman, J	TN	362
Onc	von Mehren, M	PA	352
Onc	Weiner, G	IA	373
Onc	Weiner, L	DC	352
Onc	Wolchok, J	NY	352
PA&I	Kamani, N	DC	729
PHO	Chen, A	MD	759
PHO	Horn, B	CA	777
PHO	Kobrinsky, N	ND	774
PHO	Kushner, B	NY	761
PHO	Sondel, P	WI	773
S	Eberlein, T	MO	1076
S	Kaufman, H	IL	1078
S	Kim, J	OH	1078
S	Slingluff, C	VA	1072
S	White, R	NC	1073
S	Yang, J	MD	1066
U	O'Donnell, M	IA	1169
Imperforate Anus			
PS	Pena, A	OH	807
Impulse-Control Disorders			
Psyc	Burt, V	CA	900
Inborn Errors of Metabolism			
CG	Burton, B	IL	160
CG	Cederbaum, S	CA	162
CG	Ward, J	TN	159
CG	Wilcox, W	CA	164

Spec	Name	St	Pg
Incontinence			
Ger	Ciocon, J	FL	263
Ger	Resnick, N	PA	263
GO	Lentz, S	NC	282
ObG	Brodman, M	NY	557
ObG	De Lancey, J	MI	561
ObG	Hullfish, K	VA	559
ObG	Maynard, S	DC	558
ObG	Valaitis, S	IL	562
U	Badlani, G	NC	1159
U	Boone, T	TX	1172
U	Boyd, S	CA	1175
U	Cain, M	IN	1166
U	Foster, H	CT	1148
U	Ginsberg, D	CA	1176
U	Griebling, T	KS	1171
U	Kaplan, S	NY	1154
U	Kennelly, M	NC	1161
U	Klutke, C	MO	1168
U	Lloyd, L	AL	1162
U	Lockhart, J	FL	1162
U	McGuire, E	MI	1168
U	Montague, D	OH	1169
U	Shenot, P	PA	1158
U	Steers, W	VA	1164
U	Vapnek, J	NY	1159
U	Woo, H	LA	1175
Incontinence after Prostate Cancer			
U	Blaivas, J	NY	1151
U	Fraser, L	MS	1161
U	Kane, M	MD	1154
U	Kaplan, S	NY	1154
U	Lugg, J	WY	1172
U	Schaeffer, A	IL	1170
Incontinence-Fecal			
CRS	Abcarian, H	IL	173
CRS	Bailey, H	TX	176
CRS	Church, J	OH	173
CRS	Efron, J	MD	169
CRS	Gearhart, S	MD	170
CRS	Haas, E	TX	177
CRS	Ludwig, K	WI	174
CRS	Mantyh, C	NC	172
CRS	Nogueras, J	FL	172
CRS	Schoetz, D	MA	169
CRS	Sokol, T	CA	178
CRS	Thorson, A	NE	176
CRS	Wexner, S	FL	173
Ge	Rao, S	GA	242
Ge	Wald, A	WI	249
GO	Lentz, S	NC	282
S	Baker, C	VA	1066
Incontinence-Female			
ObG	Einarsson, J	MA	556
ObG	Karram, M	OH	561
ObG	Lucente, V	PA	557

Spec	Name	St	Pg
ObG	Walters, M	OH	562
U	Chancellor, M	MI	1166
U	Loughlin, K	MA	1149
U	Raz, S	CA	1178
Incontinence-Male & Female			
U	Nitti, V	NY	1156
U	Stone, A	CA	1179
Incontinence/Pelvic Floor Disorders			
CRS	Madoff, R	MN	174
CRS	Mutch, M	MO	174
CRS	Ramamoorthy, S	CA	178
Infant-Toddler Psychiatry			
ChAP	Zeanah, C	LA	911
Infection Control			
Inf	Galgiani, J	AZ	418
Inf	Wallach, F	NY	413
Infections in Cancer Patients			
Inf	Freifeld, A	NE	418
Inf	Polsky, B	NY	413
Inf	Segal, B	NY	413
Inf	Sepkowitz, K	NY	413
Inf	Siegel, M	WA	420
PHO	Siegel, S	CA	779
Infections in Immunocompromised Patients			
Inf	Cohen, M	NC	414
Inf	Cunha, B	NY	411
Inf	Edwards, J	CA	419
PInf	Alexander, K	IL	782
PInf	Emmanuel, P	FL	781
PInf	Flynn, P	TN	782
PInf	McComsey, G	OH	783
PInf	McKinney, R	NC	782
PInf	Michaels, M	PA	781
Infections in Int'l Adopted Children			
PInf	Krilov, L	NY	780
Infections in Pregnancy			
MF	Duff, W	FL	434
MF	Ismail, M	IL	436
MF	Parry, S	PA	433
ObG	Sweet, R	CA	563
Infections in Prosthetic Devices			
Inf	Brause, B	NY	411
Inf	Slama, T	IN	417

Spec	Name	St	Pg
Infections-CNS			
N	Gilden, D	CO	531
N	Simpson, D	NY	517
Infections-Congenital			
ChiN	Bale, J	UT	152
Infections-Emerging			
Path	Walker, D	TX	719
Infections-Neonatal			
MF	Ismail, M	IL	436
NP	Davis, J	MA	446
Infections-Neurologic			
ChiN	Bale, J	UT	152
N	Coyle, P	NY	510
N	Roos, K	IN	529
NS	Rosenblum, M	MI	489
Infections-Respiratory			
PInf	Krilov, L	NY	780
PInf	Meissner, H	MA	780
PInf	Wald, E	WI	783
Pul	Jacoby, D	OR	940
Pul	Niederman, M	NY	926
Infections-Surgical			
Inf	Gumprecht, J	NY	411
Inf	Hammer, G	NY	411
Inf	Hartman, B	NY	411
Inf	O'Keefe, J	IL	416
Infections-Transplant			
Inf	Alvarez-Elcoro, S	FL	414
Inf	Gorensek, M	FL	415
PInf	Green, M	PA	780
Infectious & Demyelinating Diseases			
N	Berger, J	KY	520
N	Cook, S	NJ	510
Infectious Diarrhea			
Ge	Surawicz, C	WA	255
Infectious Disease			
A&I	Bonner, J	AL	86
D	Friedlander, S	CA	199
IM	Fischl, M	FL	425
Inf	Alvarez-Elcoro, S	FL	414
Inf	Auwaerter, P	MD	410
Inf	Bakken, J	MN	416
Inf	Ballon-Landa, G	CA	419
Inf	Bartlett, J	MD	410

Spec	Name	St	Pg
Inf	Bayer, A	CA	419
Inf	Berkowitz, L	NY	410
Inf	Blumberg, H	GA	414
Inf	Brause, B	NY	411
Inf	Campbell, J	MO	416
Inf	Cancio, M	FL	414
Inf	Chaisson, R	MD	411
Inf	Cohen, M	NC	414
Inf	Cohn, S	IL	416
Inf	Corey, G	NC	414
Inf	Craven, D	MA	410
Inf	Cunha, B	NY	411
Inf	Daar, E	CA	419
Inf	DuPont, H	TX	418
Inf	Edmond, M	VA	414
Inf	Edwards, J	CA	419
Inf	Fichtenbaum, C	OH	416
Inf	Flaherty, J	IL	416
Inf	Flanigan, T	RI	410
Inf	Frank, I	PA	411
Inf	Freifeld, A	NE	418
Inf	Galgiani, J	AZ	418
Inf	Gorensek, M	FL	415
Inf	Gumprecht, J	NY	411
Inf	Hammer, G	NY	411
Inf	Hammer, S	NY	411
Inf	Hartman, B	NY	411
Inf	Huitt, G	CO	418
Inf	Johnson, S	CO	418
Inf	Katner, H	GA	415
Inf	Keiser, P	TX	418
Inf	Kumar, P	DC	412
Inf	Longworth, D	OH	416
Inf	Lorber, B	PA	412
Inf	Louie, E	NY	412
Inf	Luby, J	TX	418
Inf	Maki, D	WI	416
Inf	Masur, H	MD	412
Inf	McGowan, J	NY	412
Inf	Mildvan, D	NY	412
Inf	Mildvan, D	NY	412
Inf	Nahass, R	NJ	412
Inf	O'Keefe, J	IL	416
Inf	Palefsky, J	CA	419
Inf	Patterson, J	TX	418
Inf	Patterson, T	TX	418
Inf	Pearson, R	VA	415
Inf	Pearson, R	VA	415
Inf	Perlman, D	NY	412
Inf	Perlman, D	NY	412
Inf	Polsky, B	NY	413
Inf	Quagliarello, V	CT	410
Inf	Rao, N	PA	413
Inf	Ratzan, K	FL	415
Inf	Richman, D	CA	419
Inf	Romagnoli, M	NY	413
Inf	Saag, M	AL	415
Inf	Salata, R	OH	417
Inf	Sax, P	MA	410
Inf	Scheld, W	VA	415
Inf	Schmitt, S	OH	417
Inf	Schooley, R	CA	420

Spec	Name	St	Pg
Inf	Schooley, R	CA	420
Inf	Segal, B	NY	413
Inf	Sepkowitz, K	NY	413
Inf	Sha, B	IL	417
Inf	Siegel, M	WA	420
Inf	Slama, T	IN	417
Inf	Sobel, J	MI	417
Inf	Squires, K	PA	413
Inf	Tomford, J	OH	417
Inf	Trenholme, G	IL	417
Inf	Van Der Horst, C	NC	415
Inf	Wallace, M	FL	415
Inf	Wallace, R	TX	419
Inf	Wallach, F	NY	413
Inf	Wilson, W	MN	417
Inf	Wiviott, L	CA	420
Inf	Wormser, G	NY	413
Inf	Yancovitz, S	NY	414
MF	Andrews, W	AL	434
MF	Gibbs, R	CO	438
MF	Landers, D	MN	436
PA&I	Sleasman, J	FL	731
PInf	Kotloff, K	MD	780
PO	Harley, E	DC	790
Infectious Disease during Chemotherapy			
Inf	Freifeld, A	NE	418
Infectious Disease in Pregnancy			
MF	Riley, L	MA	431
ObG	Gonik, B	MI	561
Infectious Disease-Lung			
Pul	Campbell, G	MS	929
Pul	Hopewell, P	CA	939
Infectious Disease-Perinatal			
MF	Gravett, M	WA	440
PInf	Michaels, M	PA	781
Infectious Diseases-Gynecologic			
ObG	Hager, W	KY	559
ObG	Sweet, R	CA	563
ObG	Wiesenfeld, H	PA	558
Infectious Mononucleosis			
PInf	Andiman, W	CT	779
Infective Endocarditis			
Inf	Bayer, A	CA	419
Inf	Slama, T	IN	417
Infertility			
EDM	Goodman, N	FL	214
ObG	De Cherney, A	MD	557
ObG	Simon, J	DC	558

Specialty & Special Expertise Index

Spec	Name	St	Pg	Spec	Name	St	Pg	Spec	Name	St	Pg
ObG	Young, B	NY	558	RE	Goldberg, J	OH	1013	U	McCullough, A	NY	1155
RE	Adamson, G	CA	1016	RE	Grazi, R	NY	1008	U	Meacham, R	CO	1172
RE	Dodds, W	MI	1013	RE	Grunfeld, L	NY	1008	U	Mulhall, J	NY	1155
RE	Houmard, B	WA	1017	RE	Hill, J	NH	1006	U	Nagler, H	NY	1156
RE	Isaacson, K	MA	1007	RE	Hornstein, M	MA	1006	U	Oates, R	MA	1150
RE	Kutteh, W	TN	1012	RE	Huang, J	TX	1016	U	Ohl, D	MI	1169
RE	Licciardi, F	NY	1009	RE	Jacobs, L	IL	1013	U	Rajfer, J	CA	1178
RE	Luciano, A	CT	1007	RE	Johnson, J	MA	1007	U	Ross, L	IL	1170
RE	Milad, M	IL	1014	RE	Kazer, R	IL	1014	U	Sabanegh, E	OH	1170
RE	Odem, R	MO	1014	RE	Keltz, M	NY	1008	U	Sadeghi-Nejad, H	NJ	1156
RE	Sanfilippo, J	PA	1010	RE	Legro, R	PA	1009	U	Sandlow, J	WI	1170
RE	Schenken, R	TX	1016	RE	Licciardi, F	NY	1009	U	Schlegel, P	NY	1157
RE	Schlaff, W	PA	1010	RE	McClamrock, H	MD	1009	U	Seftel, A	NJ	1157
RE	Van Voorhis, B	IA	1015	RE	McGovern, P	NJ	1009	U	Shaban, S	NC	1164
RE	Weiss, G	NJ	1010	RE	Miller, C	IL	1014	U	Sharlip, I	CA	1178
RE	Wilson, E	TX	1016	RE	Moffitt, D	AZ	1016	U	Sigman, M	RI	1150
RE	Zinaman, M	MA	1007	RE	Molo, M	IL	1014	U	Silber, S	MO	1170
				RE	Mukherjee, T	NY	1009	U	Turek, P	CA	1179
				RE	Noyes, N	NY	1009	U	Van Arsdalen, K	PA	1158

Infertility in Cancer Patients

				RE	Ory, S	FL	1012
RE	Gracia, C	PA	1008	RE	Oskowitz, S	MA	1007

Infertility-Male in Spinal Cord Injury

		RE	Patrizio, P	CT	1007	U	Linsenmeyer, T	NJ	1155

Infertility-Advanced Maternal Age

				RE	Paulson, R	CA	1017	U	Lynne, C	FL	1162
RE	Paulson, R	CA	1017	RE	Petrozza, J	MA	1007				
RE	Seifer, D	NY	1010	RE	Putman, J	TX	1016				

Infertility/Genetics

				RE	Ratts, V	MO	1014	ObG	Simpson, J	FL	560
				RE	Rosenwaks, Z	NY	1009				

Infertility-Female

				RE	Sauer, M	NY	1010
ObG	Pfeifer, S	PA	558	RE	Seifer, D	NY	1010

Inflammation in Critical Illness

RE	Azziz, R	GA	1011	RE	Session, D	GA	1012	PCCM	Zimmerman, J	WA	743
RE	Blackwell, R	AL	1011	RE	Smikle, C	CA	1012				
RE	Carr, B	TX	1015	RE	Smith, Y	MI	1014				

Inflammatory Arthritis

RE	Dumesic, D	CA	1017	RE	Sondheimer, S	PA	1010	Rhu	Peng, S	WA	1034
RE	Haney, A	IL	1013	RE	Soules, M	WA	1018				
RE	Hill, J	NH	1006	RE	Steinkampf, M	AL	1012				

Inflammatory Arthritis-Consult

RE	Marrs, R	CA	1017	RE	Stewart, E	MN	1014	Rhu	Chang-Miller, A	AZ	1032
RE	Sondheimer, S	PA	1010	RE	Surrey, E	CO	1015				
				RE	Toth, T	MA	1007				

Inflammatory Bowel Disease

Infertility-IVF

				RE	Wallach, E	MD	1010	CRS	Abcarian, H	IL	173
				RE	Walmer, D	NC	1012	CRS	Bailey, H	TX	176
RE	Agarwal, S	CA	1016	RE	Widra, E	DC	1010	CRS	Beck, D	LA	176
RE	Barnes, R	IL	1012	RE	Winer, S	CA	1018	CRS	Coutsoftides, T	CA	177
RE	Bateman, B	VA	1011	RE	Yee, B	CA	1018	CRS	Efron, J	MD	169
RE	Brzyski, R	TX	1015	RE	Zacur, H	MD	1011	CRS	Eisenstat, T	NJ	169
RE	Buster, J	MA	1006	U	Silber, S	MO	1170	CRS	Fleshman, J	MO	173
RE	Carson, S	RI	1006					CRS	Goldstein, S	PA	170
RE	Cedars, M	CA	1017					CRS	Harnsberger, J	NH	168

Infertility-IVF Failure

RE	Christman, G	MI	1012					CRS	Hartmann, R	FL	172
RE	Clisham, P	LA	1015	ObG	Scher, J	NY	558	CRS	Heppell, J	AZ	177
RE	Coddington, C	MN	1013					CRS	Huber, P	TX	177
RE	Copperman, A	NY	1008					CRS	Hyman, N	VT	168

Infertility-Male

RE	Coutifaris, C	PA	1008					CRS	Lavery, I	OH	174
RE	DeVane, G	FL	1011	U	Bar-Chama, N	NY	1151	CRS	Longo, W	CT	168
RE	Diamond, M	MI	1013	U	Buch, J	TX	1173	CRS	Lowry, A	MN	174
RE	Dickey, R	LA	1015	U	Donovan, J	OH	1166	CRS	Madoff, R	MN	174
RE	Durso, N	VA	1011	U	Fisch, H	NY	1152	CRS	Milsom, J	NY	171
RE	Falcone, T	OH	1013	U	Goldstein, M	NY	1152	CRS	Mutch, M	MO	174
RE	Friedman, C	OH	1013	U	Gomery, P	MA	1148	CRS	Pello, M	NJ	171
RE	Fritz, M	NC	1011	U	Hellstrom, W	LA	1173				
RE	Ginsburg, E	MA	1006	U	Kim, E	TN	1161				
RE	Giudice, L	CA	1017	U	Levine, L	IL	1168				
				U	Lipshultz, L	TX	1174				
				U	McClure, R	WA	1177				

Spec	Name	St	Pg
CRS	Ramamoorthy, S	CA	178
CRS	Read, T	MA	169
CRS	Remzi, F	OH	175
CRS	Roberts, P	MA	169
CRS	Saclarides, T	IL	175
CRS	Shah, N	RI	169
CRS	Stamos, M	CA	178
CRS	Stein, D	PA	171
CRS	Stryker, S	IL	175
CRS	Varma, M	CA	178
CRS	Vernava, A	FL	172
CRS	Wise, P	MO	175
CRS	Wolff, B	MN	176
CRS	Worsey, M	CA	178
Ge	Abreu, M	FL	239
Ge	Albert, M	DC	230
Ge	Brandt, L	NY	231
Ge	Farraye, F	MA	228
Ge	Feldman, E	CA	253
Ge	Goldberg, M	IL	245
Ge	Hanauer, S	IL	245
Ge	Isaacs, K	NC	240
Ge	Itzkowitz, S	NY	234
Ge	Kimmey, M	WA	254
Ge	Kozarek, R	WA	254
Ge	La Mont, J	MA	229
Ge	Lashner, B	OH	246
Ge	Leighton, J	AZ	252
Ge	Lichtenstein, G	PA	236
Ge	Loftus, E	MN	247
Ge	Mason, J	MA	229
Ge	Mertz, H	TN	241
Ge	Pezzone, M	PA	237
Ge	Plevy, S	NC	241
Ge	Proctor, D	CT	230
Ge	Reichelderfer, M	WI	247
Ge	Rex, D	IN	247
Ge	Sartor, R	NC	242
Ge	Scherl, E	NY	238
Ge	Siegel, C	NH	230
Ge	Targan, S	CA	255
Ge	Weinstock, J	MA	230
Ge	Young, R	NE	250
PGe	Baldassano, R	PA	750
PGe	Baldridge, A	NJ	750
PGe	Bishop, W	IA	752
PGe	Christie, D	WA	755
PGe	Cohen, M	OH	752
PGe	Dubinsky, M	CA	755
PGe	Gunasekaran, T	IL	753
PGe	Hill, I	NC	752
PGe	Hoffenberg, E	CO	754
PGe	Leichtner, A	MA	749
PGe	Rhoads, J	TX	755
PGe	Rothbaum, R	MO	754
PGe	Schwarz, S	NY	751
PGe	Thomas, D	CA	756
PGe	Ulshen, M	NC	752
PS	Alexander, F	NJ	802
PS	Doody, D	MA	801
PS	Notrica, D	AZ	809
PS	Schwartz, M	PA	804

Spec	Name	St	Pg
PS	Shamberger, R	MA	802
S	Becker, J	MA	1048
S	Dayton, M	NY	1056
S	Hodin, R	MA	1049
S	Koruda, M	NC	1069
S	Schraut, W	PA	1064

Inflammatory Bowel Disease/Crohn's

Spec	Name	St	Pg
CRS	Birnbaum, E	MO	173
CRS	Delaney, C	OH	173
CRS	Galandiuk, S	KY	172
CRS	Gearhart, S	MD	170
CRS	Haas, E	TX	177
CRS	Kodner, I	MO	174
CRS	Medich, D	PA	170
CRS	Nogueras, J	FL	172
CRS	Pemberton, J	MN	175
CRS	Procaccino, J	NY	171
CRS	Schoetz, D	MA	169
CRS	Senagore, A	CA	178
CRS	Steinhagen, R	NY	171
CRS	Wexner, S	FL	173
Ge	Bayless, T	MD	230
Ge	Cominelli, F	OH	244
Ge	Elliott, D	IA	245
Ge	Fisher, R	CT	228
Ge	Konicek, F	IL	246
Ge	Lebwohl, O	NY	235
Ge	Lipshutz, W	PA	236
Ge	Mayer, L	NY	236
Ge	Roth, B	CA	255
Ge	Sandborn, W	CA	255
Ge	Tremaine, W	MN	248
PGe	Benkov, K	NY	750
PGe	Berman, J	IL	752
PGe	Heyman, M	CA	755
PGe	Kirschner, B	IL	753
PGe	Oliva-Hemker, M	MD	751
PGe	Wyllie, R	OH	754
PS	Dolgin, S	NY	803

Inflammatory Cytokines

Spec	Name	St	Pg
PHO	Ferrara, J	MI	770

Inflammatory Pulmonary Diseases

Spec	Name	St	Pg
Pul	Wenzel, S	PA	929

Inherited Disorders

Spec	Name	St	Pg
CG	Holmes, L	MA	156
CG	Jonas, A	CA	163
CG	Korf, B	AL	159
CG	Morris, C	NV	163
CG	Pyeritz, R	PA	158
CG	Weaver, D	IN	160
Hem	Rao, A	PA	314

Inherited Disorders of Nervous

Spec	Name	St	Pg
System			
N	Kolodny, E	NY	513

Inherited Metabolic Disorders

Spec	Name	St	Pg
CG	Andersson, H	LA	161
CG	Desnick, R	NY	157
CG	Seashore, M	CT	156
Nep	Hruska, K	MO	461

Insect Allergies

Spec	Name	St	Pg
A&I	Freeman, T	TX	89
A&I	Pacin, M	FL	87
A&I	Shepherd, G	NY	85

Intensity Modulated Radiotherapy (IMRT)

Spec	Name	St	Pg
RadRO	Chao, K	NY	948
RadRO	Cooper, J	NY	948
RadRO	Fuss, M	OR	966
RadRO	Gejerman, G	NJ	950
RadRO	Horwitz, E	PA	950
RadRO	Lee, W	NC	955
RadRO	Mundt, A	CA	967
RadRO	Quivey, J	CA	967
RadRO	Rose, C	CA	967
RadRO	Russell, A	MA	947
RadRO	St Clair, W	KY	957
RadRO	Wong, J	CA	968

Internal Medicine

Spec	Name	St	Pg
IM	Bakris, G	IL	425
IM	Bissell, D	CA	426
IM	Braunstein, S	NC	424
IM	Burt, R	IL	425
IM	Cirigliano, M	PA	424
IM	Cope, D	CA	426
IM	Cushman, W	TN	425
IM	Fischbein, L	MO	425
IM	Fischl, M	FL	425
IM	Galland, L	NY	424
IM	Gillman, M	MA	424
IM	Holzman, L	PA	424
IM	Mehler, P	CO	426
IM	Rabow, M	CA	426
IM	Rader, D	PA	424
IM	Selwyn, P	NY	424
IM	Tucker, R	AL	425
IM	Wright, J	OH	425

International Health

Spec	Name	St	Pg
GO	Granai, C	RI	274
Inf	Keiser, P	TX	418
PMR	Haig, A	MI	840
PrM	Cahill, J	NY	882
PrM	Cahill, K	NY	883

Interstitial Cystitis

Spec	Name	St	Pg
U	Culkin, D	OK	1173

Specialty & Special Expertise Index

Spec	Name	St	Pg
U	Lloyd, L	AL	1162
U	Schaeffer, A	IL	1170

Interstitial Lung Disease

Spec	Name	St	Pg
Path	Katzenstein, A	NY	710
Path	Travis, W	NY	712
PPul	Fan, L	CO	797
PPul	Redding, G	WA	798
Pul	Arcasoy, S	NY	924
Pul	Berk, J	MA	922
Pul	Brown, K	CO	936
Pul	Doherty, D	KY	930
Pul	Enelow, R	NH	922
Pul	Hansen-Flaschen, J	PA	925
Pul	King, T	CA	940
Pul	Kotloff, R	PA	926
Pul	Libby, D	NY	926
Pul	Loyd, J	TN	931
Pul	Lynch, J	CA	940
Pul	Mosenifar, Z	CA	940
Pul	Popovich, J	MI	935
Pul	Raghu, G	WA	940
Pul	Rossman, M	PA	927
Pul	Sahn, S	SC	932
Pul	Schwarz, M	CO	937
Pul	Sharma, O	CA	941
Pul	Staton, G	GA	932
Pul	Stover-Pepe, D	NY	928
Pul	Tino, G	PA	928
Pul	Weissler, J	TX	938

Interventional Cardiology

Spec	Name	St	Pg
Cv	Bass, T	FL	103
Cv	Cabin, H	CT	94
Cv	Cohen, H	NY	97
Cv	Cooper, C	OH	107
Cv	Corrigan, V	GA	104
Cv	Edelen, J	CA	116
Cv	Freeman, G	TX	114
Cv	French, W	CA	117
Cv	Greenberg, M	NY	99
Cv	Harrison, J	NC	104
Cv	Kereiakes, D	OH	109
Cv	Klein, L	IL	109
Cv	O'Neill, W	MI	110
Cv	Powers, E	SC	105
Cv	Ramee, S	LA	115
Cv	Rihal, C	MN	112
Cv	Safian, R	MI	110
Cv	Sanborn, T	IL	111
Cv	Shlofmitz, R	NY	102
Cv	Simon, D	OH	111
Cv	Tobis, J	CA	118
Cv	Vetrovec, G	VA	106
Cv	Vignola, P	NC	106
Cv	von der Lohe, E	IN	112
IC	Applegate, R	NC	129
IC	Bach, R	MO	130
IC	Bailey, S	TX	132
IC	Bittl, J	FL	129
IC	Carroll, J	CO	132

Spec	Name	St	Pg
IC	Chang, G	PA	127
IC	Dieter, R	IL	131
IC	Douglas, J	GA	129
IC	Ellis, S	OH	131
IC	Feldman, M	TX	132
IC	Feldman, T	IL	131
IC	Gibson, C	MA	126
IC	Gray, W	NY	127
IC	Greene, R	CA	133
IC	Henry, T	MN	131
IC	Herrmann, H	PA	127
IC	Holmes, D	MN	131
IC	Jacobs, A	MA	126
IC	Kandzari, D	GA	130
IC	Khawaja, S	GA	130
IC	Kimmelstiel, C	MA	126
IC	Kleiman, N	TX	132
IC	Knopf, W	GA	130
IC	Laham, R	MA	126
IC	Lasala, J	MO	131
IC	Lee, J	PA	127
IC	Leon, M	NY	127
IC	Mahmud, E	CA	133
IC	Matar, F	FL	130
IC	Morris, D	GA	130
IC	Moses, J	NY	127
IC	Palacios, I	MA	126
IC	Palacios, I	MA	126
IC	Parikh, M	NY	128
IC	Perin, E	TX	132
IC	Petrossian, G	NY	128
IC	Pichard, A	DC	128
IC	Reddy, B	GA	130
IC	Reiner, J	DC	128
IC	Resar, J	MD	128
IC	Rosenfield, K	MA	126
IC	Roubin, G	NY	128
IC	Sacchi, T	NY	128
IC	Schreiber, T	MI	131
IC	Shani, J	NY	129
IC	Sharma, S	NY	129
IC	Shorofsky, S	MD	129
IC	Smalling, R	TX	132
IC	Stone, G	NY	129
IC	Teirstein, P	CA	133
IC	Whitlow, P	OH	132
IC	Williams, D	MA	126
IC	Yeung, A	CA	133
IC	Zelman, R	MA	127
PCd	Beekman, R	OH	738
PCd	Biancaniello, T	NY	734
PCd	De Moor, M	MA	733
PCd	Hellenbrand, W	CT	733
PCd	Hijazi, Z	IL	739
PCd	Hsu, D	NY	735
PCd	Lang, P	MA	733
PCd	Latson, L	FL	737
PCd	Lock, J	MA	734
PCd	Murphy, J	PA	735
PCd	Perry, S	CA	741
PCd	Radtke, W	DE	735
PCd	Rocchini, A	MI	739

Spec	Name	St	Pg
PCd	Rome, J	PA	736
PCd	Velvis, H	NY	736
PCd	Zahn, E	CA	741
T&CS	Williams, M	NY	1123

Interventional Endoscopy

Spec	Name	St	Pg
Ge	Chang, K	CA	253
Ge	Infantolino, A	PA	234
Ge	Jonnalagadda, S	MO	246
Ge	Waxman, I	IL	249

Interventional Neuroradiology

Spec	Name	St	Pg
NRad	Berenstein, A	NY	985
NRad	Cross, D	MO	988
NRad	Dion, J	GA	987
NRad	Frei, D	CO	990
NRad	Grobelny, T	IL	988
NRad	Hirsch, J	MA	984
NRad	Hurst, R	PA	985
NRad	Jensen, M	VA	987
NRad	Larsen, D	CA	991
NRad	Mawad, M	TX	990
NRad	Moran, C	MO	989
NRad	Morris, P	NC	987
NRad	Norbash, A	MA	984
NRad	Orbach, D	MA	985
NRad	Pile-Spellman, J	NY	986
NRad	Teitelbaum, G	CA	991
NS	Amar, A	CA	495
NS	Patel, A	NY	477
VIR	Kumpe, D	CO	996
VIR	Yakes, W	CO	997

Interventional Pulmonology

Spec	Name	St	Pg
Pul	Ernst, A	MA	922
Pul	Kovitz, K	IL	934
Pul	Sterman, D	PA	928
Pul	Unger, M	PA	929

Interventional Radiology

Spec	Name	St	Pg
DR	Abbitt, P	FL	978
DR	Shaw, D	WA	984
DR	Teal, J	DC	977
DR	Yoon, S	NY	978
DR	Zagoria, R	NC	980
VIR	Lewis, C	GA	995

Intestinal Disorders

Spec	Name	St	Pg
PGe	Rhoads, J	TX	755
PGe	Squires, R	PA	751

Intestinal Parasites

Spec	Name	St	Pg
Ge	Elliott, D	IA	245

Intracranial Angioplasty & Stent

Spec	Name	St	Pg
NRad	Dion, J	GA	987
NRad	Higashida, R	CA	991
NRad	Hurst, R	PA	985

Spec	Name	St	Pg
NRad	Joseph, G	NC	987
NRad	Vinuela, F	CA	991

Intravascular Ultrasound
| Cv | Nissen, S | OH | 109 |
| IC | Reddy, B | GA | 130 |

Invasive Cardiology
| Cv | Smith, S | NC | 106 |
| IC | Bittl, J | FL | 129 |

Irritable Bowel Syndrome
Ge	Fang, J	UT	249
Ge	Feldman, E	CA	253
Ge	Mertz, H	TN	241
Ge	Pezzone, M	PA	237
Ge	Roth, B	CA	255
Ge	Tremaine, W	MN	248
Ge	Wald, A	WI	249
PGe	Levy, J	NY	750
PGe	Ulshen, M	NC	752

Ischemic Heart Disease
Cv	Jaffe, A	MN	108
Cv	Liang, B	CT	95
Cv	Reiss, C	MO	110
Cv	Silvestry, F	PA	102
Cv	Williams, E	IN	112

J

Jaw Tumors
| Path | Kahn, L | NY | 709 |

Joint Replacement
OrS	Bronson, M	NY	615
OrS	Caillouette, J	CA	642
OrS	Cornell, C	NY	616
OrS	Endrizzi, D	ME	611
OrS	Garvin, K	NE	639
OrS	Goodman, S	CA	643
OrS	Hozack, W	PA	620
OrS	Kraay, M	OH	635
OrS	Minas, T	MA	612
OrS	Pellicci, P	NY	623
OrS	Rothman, R	PA	624
OrS	Thornhill, T	MA	613
OrS	Vo, P	FL	631

Juvenile Arthritis
OrS	Johanson, N	PA	620
PRhu	Finkel, T	FL	800
PRhu	Goldsmith, D	PA	799
PRhu	Haines, K	NJ	799
PRhu	Ilowite, N	NY	799

Spec	Name	St	Pg
PRhu	Klein-Gitelman, M	IL	800
PRhu	McCarthy, P	CT	799
PRhu	Schanberg, L	NC	800
PRhu	Sherry, D	PA	799
PRhu	Sills, E	MD	800
PRhu	Wagner-Weiner, L	IL	800
PRhu	Warren, R	SC	800
Rhu	Albert, D	NH	1024

K

Kallmann's Syndrome
| RE | Crowley, W | MA | 1006 |

Kasabach-Merritt Syndrome (KMS)
| PHO | Bertolone, S | KY | 765 |

Kawasaki Disease
PCd	Bierman, F	NY	734
PCd	Cooper, R	NY	734
PCd	Gewitz, M	NY	735
PCd	Newburger, J	MA	734
PCd	Pahl, E	IL	739
PInf	Mason, W	CA	785
PInf	Meissner, H	MA	780
PInf	Shulman, S	IL	783
PRhu	Myones, B	TX	801

Keinbocks Disease
| HS | Slutsky, D | CA | 304 |

Keratoconus
Oph	Boxer Wachler, B	CA	599
Oph	Cykiert, R	NY	572
Oph	Florakis, G	NY	574
Oph	Hersh, P	NJ	575
Oph	Kornmehl, E	MA	570
Oph	Shamie, N	CA	604
Oph	Stulting, R	GA	586

Kidney Cancer
Onc	Antonia, S	FL	353
Onc	Atkins, M	DC	334
Onc	Biggs, D	DE	335
Onc	Clark, J	IL	366
Onc	Dawson, N	DC	338
Onc	Dreicer, R	OH	367
Onc	Dutcher, J	NY	338
Onc	Figlin, R	CA	386
Onc	Gelmann, E	NY	340
Onc	George, D	NC	356
Onc	Haas, N	PA	341
Onc	Hogan, T	WV	342
Onc	Hudes, G	PA	342

Spec	Name	St	Pg
Onc	Jonasch, E	TX	379
Onc	Kuzel, T	IL	369
Onc	Margolin, K	WA	388
Onc	Motzer, R	NY	346
Onc	Petrylak, D	CT	331
Onc	Quinn, D	CA	389
Onc	Samlowski, W	NV	390
Onc	Stadler, W	IL	372
Onc	Tagawa, S	NY	351
Onc	Thompson, J	WA	391
Onc	Vogelzang, N	NV	392
Onc	Wilding, G	WI	373
Path	Morrow, J	CT	707
PHO	Tomlinson, G	TX	776
S	Rosenberg, S	MD	1063
S	Schwartzentruber, D	IN	1082
S	Yang, J	MD	1066
U	Amling, C	OR	1175
U	Babayan, R	MA	1148
U	Benson, M	NY	1151
U	Campbell, S	OH	1166
U	Carpinito, G	MA	1148
U	Chang, S	TN	1160
U	Chen, D	PA	1151
U	Ciancio, G	FL	1160
U	Clayman, R	CA	1175
U	Colberg, J	CT	1148
U	Daneshmand, S	CA	1176
U	Davis, B	KS	1171
U	DeKernion, J	CA	1176
U	Donovan, J	OH	1166
U	Droller, M	NY	1152
U	Ellis, W	WA	1176
U	Flanigan, R	IL	1167
U	Gill, I	CA	1176
U	Gluckman, G	IL	1167
U	Greenberg, R	PA	1153
U	Holden, S	CA	1177
U	Hrebinko, R	PA	1154
U	Jackman, S	PA	1154
U	Kaouk, J	OH	1167
U	Kavoussi, L	NY	1154
U	Kibel, A	MA	1149
U	Kirschenbaum, A	NY	1154
U	Klein, E	OH	1168
U	Landman, J	CA	1177
U	Libertino, J	MA	1149
U	Malkowicz, S	PA	1155
U	Olumi, A	MA	1150
U	Patel, V	FL	1162
U	Presti, J	CA	1178
U	Richie, J	MA	1150
U	Robertson, C	NC	1163
U	Samadi, D	NY	1157
U	Sanda, M	MA	1150
U	Sanders, W	GA	1163
U	Sawczuk, I	NJ	1157
U	Siegelbaum, M	MD	1158
U	Singh, D	CT	1150
U	Smith, J	TN	1164
U	Soloway, M	FL	1164
U	Steinberg, G	IL	1170

Specialty & Special Expertise Index

Spec	Name	St	Pg
U	Sundaram, C	IN	1170
U	Taneja, S	NY	1158
U	Teigland, C	NC	1164
U	Weiss, R	NJ	1159
U	Zippe, C	OH	1171
VIR	McGahan, J	CA	998
VIR	Solomon, S	NY	993
VIR	Soulen, M	PA	994

Kidney Cancer-Cryosurgery

U	Katz, A	NY	1154

Kidney Disease

Spec	Name	St	Pg
IM	Bakris, G	IL	425
Nep	Bernardo, J	PA	457
Nep	Berns, J	PA	457
Nep	Butterly, D	NC	459
Nep	Cho, K	CA	465
Nep	Delmez, J	MO	461
Nep	Gaston, R	AL	459
Nep	Gluck, S	CA	465
Nep	Kliger, A	CT	456
Nep	Pohl, M	OH	462
Nep	Rudnick, M	PA	458
Nep	Venkat, K	MI	463
Nep	Weiner, I	FL	460
PNep	Chandar, J	FL	786
PNep	Ettenger, R	CA	788
PNep	Flynn, J	WA	788
PNep	McDonald, R	WA	788

Kidney Disease-Autoimmune

Nep	Helderman, J	TN	460
Nep	Salant, D	MA	456
PNep	Wyatt, R	TN	786

Kidney Disease-Chronic

Nep	Bolton, W	VA	459
Nep	Fadem, S	TX	463
Nep	King, A	CA	465
Nep	Kraus, M	IN	461
Nep	Lea, J	GA	460
Nep	Perrone, R	MA	456
Nep	Schwartz, G	MN	462
Nep	Townsend, R	PA	458
Nep	Winston, J	NY	459
Nep	Yee, J	MI	463
PNep	Cohn, R	IL	787
PNep	Warady, B	MO	788

Kidney Disease-Genetic

PNep	Kashtan, C	MN	787
PNep	Neiberger, R	FL	786

Kidney Disease-Geriatric

Nep	Kasiske, B	MN	461

Kidney Disease-Glomerular

Spec	Name	St	Pg
Nep	Bolton, W	VA	459
Nep	Helderman, J	TN	460
Nep	Rakowski, T	VA	460
Nep	Salant, D	MA	456

Kidney Disease-Metabolic

Nep	Kaysen, G	CA	465
Nep	Kliger, A	CT	456

Kidney Disease-Pediatric & Adult

Nep	Hruska, K	MO	461

Kidney Failure

Nep	Fadem, S	TX	463
Nep	Kobrin, S	PA	458
Nep	Mitch, W	TX	464
Nep	Piraino, B	PA	458
Nep	Swartz, R	MI	462
Nep	Winston, J	NY	459
PNep	Andreoli, S	IN	787
PNep	Ault, B	TN	786
PNep	Fouser, L	WA	788
PNep	Neiberger, R	FL	786

Kidney Failure-Acute

Nep	Bazari, H	MA	456
Nep	Kraus, M	IN	461
Nep	Okusa, M	VA	460
Nep	Olivero, J	TX	464
Nep	Perrone, R	MA	456
Nep	Rudnick, M	PA	458
Nep	Tolkoff-Rubin, N	MA	456
Nep	Toto, R	TX	464

Kidney Failure-Chronic

Nep	Ahmad, S	WA	464
Nep	Brennan, S	TX	463
Nep	Dember, L	PA	457
Nep	Kaysen, G	CA	465
Nep	McCarthy, J	MN	461
Nep	Miller, B	MO	462
Nep	Okusa, M	VA	460
Nep	Olivero, J	TX	464
Nep	Roth, D	FL	460
Nep	Seifter, J	MA	456
Nep	Stern, L	NY	458
Nep	Williams, G	NY	458
PNep	Andreoli, S	IN	787
PNep	Jabs, K	TN	786

Kidney Pathology

Path	Koss, M	CA	721
Path	Rennke, H	MA	707
Path	Sibley, R	CA	722
Path	Tomaszewski, J	NY	712

Kidney Stones

Spec	Name	St	Pg
Nep	Ahmad, S	WA	464
Nep	Brennan, S	TX	463
Nep	Coe, F	IL	461
Nep	Gluck, S	CA	465
Nep	Hruska, K	MO	461
Nep	Kelepouris, E	PA	458
Nep	Seifter, J	MA	456
Nep	Warnock, D	AL	460
Nep	Weiner, I	FL	460
PNep	Langman, C	IL	787
U	Albala, D	NY	1150
U	Basler, J	TX	1172
U	Carson, C	NC	1160
U	Clayman, R	CA	1175
U	Grasso, M	NY	1153
U	Gribetz, M	NY	1153
U	Irby, P	NC	1161
U	Jackman, S	PA	1154
U	Janeiro, J	NH	1149
U	Landman, J	CA	1177
U	Loo, M	NY	1155
U	Lowe, F	NY	1155
U	O'Leary, M	MA	1149
U	Patterson, A	TN	1163
U	Pope, J	TN	1163
U	Preminger, G	NC	1163
U	Sanders, W	GA	1163
U	Stoller, M	CA	1179
U	Winfield, H	AL	1165

Klippel-Trenaunay Syndrome

PCd	Driscoll, D	MN	739

Knee Cartilage/Meniscus Transplants

OrS	Anderson, L	CA	641
OrS	Miller, M	VA	629

Knee Injuries

OrS	Johnson, D	KY	629
OrS	Scott, W	NY	625
SM	Arendt, E	MN	1043
SM	Burke, C	PA	1041
SM	Fronek, J	CA	1044
SM	Gill, T	MA	1040
SM	Harner, C	PA	1041
SM	Hershman, E	NY	1041
SM	Levine, W	NY	1041
SM	Mirzayan, R	CA	1044
SM	Rodeo, S	NY	1042
SM	Steiner, M	MA	1040

Knee Injuries/ACL

OrS	Anderson, L	CA	641
OrS	Bach, B	IL	632
OrS	Chu, C	PA	615
OrS	Cooper, D	TX	640
OrS	Diduch, D	VA	628

Spec	Name	St	Pg
OrS	Fu, F	PA	617
OrS	Kaeding, C	OH	634
OrS	Mandelbaum, B	CA	644
OrS	Souryal, T	TX	641
OrS	Wickiewicz, T	NY	627
OrS	Zarins, B	MA	613
SM	Micheli, L	MA	1040
SM	Taft, T	NC	1042
SM	Williams, R	NY	1042
SM	Xerogeanes, J	GA	1043

Knee Injuries/ACL/Meniscus Tears

Spec	Name	St	Pg
OrS	Goitz, H	MI	633
OrS	Karas, S	GA	629

Knee Injuries/Ligament Surgery

Spec	Name	St	Pg
OrS	Hannafin, J	NY	618
OrS	Marx, R	NY	622
OrS	Warren, R	NY	626

Knee Ligament Reconstruction

Spec	Name	St	Pg
OrS	Bartolozzi, A	PA	614
OrS	Johnson, D	KY	629
OrS	Miller, M	VA	629
OrS	Shelbourne, K	IN	637
SM	Arendt, E	MN	1043
SM	Garth, W	AL	1042

Knee Reconstruction

Spec	Name	St	Pg
OrS	Garrett, W	NC	628
OrS	Grelsamer, R	NY	618
OrS	Krackow, K	NY	621
OrS	Kress, K	GA	629
OrS	Weiner, R	FL	631
SM	Bush-Joseph, C	IL	1043
SM	Ciccotti, M	PA	1041
SM	Miniaci, A	OH	1043

Knee Rehabilitation (Non-Surgical)

Spec	Name	St	Pg
OrS	Shelbourne, K	IN	637

Knee Replacement

Spec	Name	St	Pg
OrS	Brick, G	MA	610
OrS	Bronson, M	NY	615
OrS	Buly, R	NY	615
OrS	Burke, D	MA	610
OrS	Goldstein, W	IL	633
OrS	Gorab, R	CA	643
OrS	Haas, S	NY	618
OrS	Hume, E	PA	620
OrS	Jiranek, W	VA	629
OrS	Krackow, K	NY	621
OrS	Kress, K	GA	629
OrS	Macaulay, W	NY	622
OrS	Marx, R	NY	622
OrS	Muschler, G	OH	636

Spec	Name	St	Pg
OrS	Pellicci, P	NY	623
OrS	Reilly, D	MA	612
OrS	Rothman, R	PA	624
OrS	Salvati, E	NY	625
OrS	Scott, R	MA	612
OrS	Scott, W	NY	625
OrS	Sharkey, P	PA	625
OrS	Weiner, R	FL	631
OrS	Zuckerman, J	NY	627
SM	Nisonson, B	NY	1041

Knee Replacement & Revision

Spec	Name	St	Pg
OrS	Berry, D	MN	632
OrS	Booth, R	PA	615
OrS	Hungerford, M	MD	620
OrS	Jacobs, J	IL	634
OrS	Johanson, N	PA	620
OrS	Mabrey, J	TX	641
OrS	Parvizi, J	PA	623
OrS	Thomas, B	CA	646
OrS	Westrich, G	NY	626

Knee Surgery

Spec	Name	St	Pg
OrS	Bach, B	IL	632
OrS	Bauman, P	NY	614
OrS	Bono, J	MA	610
OrS	Crossett, L	PA	616
OrS	Elattrache, N	CA	643
OrS	Estwanik, J	NC	628
OrS	Garrett, W	NC	628
OrS	Garvin, K	NE	639
OrS	Glashow, J	NY	618
OrS	Haas, S	NY	618
OrS	Hanssen, A	MN	634
OrS	Heiden, E	UT	639
OrS	Hozack, W	PA	620
OrS	Johnson, C	MD	620
OrS	Jokl, P	CT	611
OrS	Kenter, K	OH	634
OrS	Richmond, J	MA	612
OrS	Rosenberg, T	UT	639
OrS	Shelbourne, K	IN	637
SM	Altchek, D	NY	1040
SM	Andrews, J	FL	1042
SM	Bradley, J	PA	1041
SM	Gambardella, R	CA	1044
SM	Hershman, E	NY	1041
SM	Ma, C	CA	1044
SM	Paletta, G	MO	1043
SM	Scheller, A	MA	1040
SM	Teitz, C	WA	1044
SM	Williams, R	NY	1042
SM	Xerogeanes, J	GA	1043

Knee-Microfracture Surgery

Spec	Name	St	Pg
OrS	Steadman, J	CO	639

Knee-Patella Problems

Spec	Name	St	Pg
OrS	Fulkerson, J	CT	611

Spec	Name	St	Pg
OrS	Gladstone, J	NY	617
OrS	Grelsamer, R	NY	618
OrS	Leadbetter, W	MD	621

L

Lacrimal Gland Disorders

Spec	Name	St	Pg
Oph	Gallin, P	NY	574
Oph	Kikkawa, D	CA	601
Oph	Tse, D	FL	586

Langerhans Cell Histiocytosis (LCH)

Spec	Name	St	Pg
Hem	Winter, J	IL	322
PHO	Razzouk, B	IN	773

Laparoscopic Abdominal Surgery

Spec	Name	St	Pg
S	Edye, M	NY	1057
S	Frantzides, C	IL	1077
S	Hunter, J	OR	1096
S	Petelin, J	KS	1086
S	Pomp, A	NY	1062
S	Salky, B	NY	1063
S	Satava, R	WA	1099
S	Shikora, S	MA	1051

Laparoscopic Surgery

Spec	Name	St	Pg
CRS	Coutsoftides, T	CA	177
CRS	Delaney, C	OH	173
CRS	Fleshman, J	MO	173
CRS	Goldstein, S	PA	170
CRS	Golub, R	FL	172
CRS	Haas, E	TX	177
CRS	Hartmann, R	FL	172
CRS	Kodner, I	MO	174
CRS	Milsom, J	NY	171
CRS	Nagle, D	MA	168
CRS	Nogueras, J	FL	172
CRS	Orkin, B	MA	168
CRS	Pello, M	NJ	171
CRS	Read, T	MA	169
CRS	Remzi, F	OH	175
CRS	Saclarides, T	IL	175
CRS	Senagore, A	CA	178
CRS	Stamos, M	CA	178
CRS	Stein, D	PA	171
CRS	Stryker, S	IL	175
CRS	Thorson, A	NE	176
CRS	Varma, M	CA	178
CRS	Wexner, S	FL	173
CRS	Whelan, R	NY	171
CRS	Wong, R	HI	178
GO	Azodi, M	CT	274
GO	Barakat, R	NY	276
GO	Barter, J	MD	276

Specialty & Special Expertise Index

Spec	Name	St	Pg
GO	Bicher, A	VA	280
GO	Burnett, A	AR	287
GO	Curtin, J	NY	277
GO	DeMars, L	NH	274
GO	Dottino, P	NY	277
GO	Fowler, J	OH	284
GO	Herzog, T	NY	278
GO	Horowitz, I	GA	281
GO	Morgan, M	PA	279
GO	Stern, J	CA	291
GO	Valea, F	NC	283
ObG	Argenta, P	MN	560
ObG	Brodman, M	NY	557
ObG	Goldstein, M	NY	557
ObG	Hager, W	KY	559
ObG	Parker, W	CA	563
ObG	Pfeifer, S	PA	558
ObG	Steege, J	NC	560
PS	Albanese, C	CA	810
PS	Caty, M	CT	801
PS	Nuchtern, J	TX	809
PS	Waldhausen, J	WA	811
RE	Adamson, G	CA	1016
RE	Carson, S	RI	1006
RE	Clisham, P	LA	1015
RE	Grifo, J	NY	1008
RE	Grunfeld, L	NY	1008
RE	Hornstein, M	MA	1006
RE	Smikle, C	CA	1017
RE	Yee, B	CA	1018
S	Ballantyne, G	GA	1066
S	Bessler, M	NY	1054
S	Bilchik, A	CA	1093
S	Blackstone, R	AZ	1087
S	Brody, F	DC	1054
S	Callery, M	MA	1048
S	Crookes, P	CA	1094
S	Daneker, G	GA	1068
S	Dempsey, D	PA	1056
S	Deziel, D	IL	1076
S	Doherty, G	MA	1049
S	Farley, D	MN	1076
S	Franklin, M	TX	1088
S	Frantzides, C	IL	1077
S	Fung, J	OH	1077
S	Geller, D	PA	1058
S	Howerton, R	NC	1069
S	Jackson, G	TX	1089
S	Kendrick, M	MN	1078
S	Marks, J	OH	1079
S	Melvin, W	OH	1079
S	Nguyen, N	CA	1097
S	Onders, R	OH	1080
S	Pappas, T	NC	1071
S	Phillips, E	CA	1098
S	Prinz, R	IL	1081
S	Rege, R	TX	1091
S	Reiner, M	NY	1063
S	Richards, W	AL	1071
S	Schirmer, B	VA	1072
S	Schlinkert, R	AZ	1092
S	Scott-Conner, C	IA	1082

Spec	Name	St	Pg
S	Sharp, K	TN	1072
S	Shibata, D	FL	1072
S	Siperstein, A	OH	1082
S	Soper, N	IL	1083
S	Sweeney, J	GA	1073
S	Unger, S	FL	1073
S	Wood, R	TX	1093
U	Albala, D	NY	1150
U	Andriole, G	MO	1165
U	Clayman, R	CA	1175
U	Culkin, D	OK	1173
U	Grasso, M	NY	1153
U	Hemal, A	NC	1161
U	Jackman, S	PA	1154
U	Kavoussi, L	NY	1154
U	Kozlowski, J	IL	1168
U	Lugg, J	WY	1172
U	Patterson, A	TN	1163
U	Siegelbaum, M	MD	1158
U	Singh, D	CT	1150
U	Stoller, M	CA	1179
U	Strand, W	TX	1174
U	Takayama, T	WA	1179
U	Teigland, C	NC	1164
U	Wallen, E	NC	1165
U	Winfield, H	AL	1165
U	Wong, C	OH	1171

Laparoscopic Surgery-Complex

Spec	Name	St	Pg
PS	Notrica, D	AZ	809

Laryngeal & Tracheal Disorders

Spec	Name	St	Pg
Oto	Burns, J	MA	655
Oto	Weissler, M	NC	672
Oto	Zalzal, G	DC	667

Laryngeal & Vocal Cord Surgery

Spec	Name	St	Pg
Oto	Burns, J	MA	655
Oto	Caldarelli, D	IL	674
Oto	Sulica, R	NY	666

Laryngeal & Voice Disorders

Spec	Name	St	Pg
Oto	Fried, M	NY	659

Laryngeal Cancer

Spec	Name	St	Pg
Onc	Pfister, D	NY	348
Oto	Andersen, P	OR	684
Oto	Courey, M	CA	684
Oto	Diaz, E	TX	681
Oto	Ferris, R	PA	659
Oto	Grillone, G	MA	655
Oto	Shapshay, S	NY	665
Oto	Strome, S	MD	665
Oto	Weinstein, G	PA	666
Oto	Wolf, G	MI	678
Oto	Woo, P	NY	666
Oto	Yoo, G	MI	679
Oto	Zeitels, S	MA	657

Spec	Name	St	Pg
S	Ridge, J	PA	1063

Laryngeal Cancer-Organ Preservation

Spec	Name	St	Pg
Oto	Diaz, E	TX	681
Oto	Rassekh, C	PA	664

Laryngeal Disorders

Spec	Name	St	Pg
Oto	Bastian, R	IL	673
Oto	Benninger, M	OH	673
Oto	Berke, G	CA	684
Oto	Courey, M	CA	684
Oto	Flint, P	OR	685
Oto	Ford, C	WI	674
Oto	Grillone, G	MA	655
Oto	Koufman, J	NY	661
Oto	Mirza, N	PA	662
Oto	Ossoff, R	TN	669
Oto	Sataloff, R	PA	664
Oto	Stasney, C	TX	683
Oto	Suen, J	AR	683
Oto	Woo, P	NY	666
PO	April, M	NY	789
PO	Tunkel, D	MD	790

Laser Surgery

Spec	Name	St	Pg
D	Anderson, R	MA	182
D	Cunningham, B	CA	198
D	Kriegel, D	NY	187
Oph	Mathers, W	OR	602
Oto	Caruana, S	NY	658
PlS	Kenkel, J	TX	870

Laser Vision Surgery

Spec	Name	St	Pg
Oph	Caster, A	CA	599
Oph	Clinch, T	MD	572
Oph	Dodick, J	NY	573
Oph	Gibralter, R	NY	574
Oph	Lane, S	MN	591
Oph	McCulley, J	TX	597
Oph	O'Brien, T	FL	585
Oph	Stulting, R	GA	586
Oph	Wang, M	TN	587

LASIK-Refractive Surgery

Spec	Name	St	Pg
Oph	Afshari, N	NC	581
Oph	Azar, D	IL	588
Oph	Boxer Wachler, B	CA	599
Oph	Carlson, A	NC	582
Oph	Caster, A	CA	599
Oph	Clinch, T	MD	572
Oph	Culbertson, W	FL	582
Oph	Cykiert, R	NY	572
Oph	Durrie, D	KS	596
Oph	Feder, R	IL	589
Oph	Goldberg, D	NJ	574
Oph	Gorovoy, M	FL	583
Oph	Hersh, P	NJ	575
Oph	Kornmehl, E	MA	570

Spec	Name	St	Pg
Oph	Mackool, R	NY	577
Oph	Maloney, R	CA	601
Oph	Manche, E	CA	602
Oph	Mandel, E	NY	577
Oph	Pepose, J	MO	593
Oph	Salz, J	CA	603
Oph	Serafano, D	CA	604
Oph	Updegraff, S	FL	587
Oph	Waring, G	GA	587
Oph	Wilson, S	OH	595

Latex Allergy

Spec	Name	St	Pg
A&I	Benenati, S	FL	86
PA&I	Ownby, D	GA	731
PA&I	Pongracic, J	IL	731

Learning Disorders

Spec	Name	St	Pg
ChiN	Nass, R	NY	148
ChiN	Shaywitz, B	CT	146
Ped	Hershorin, E	FL	727

Left Ventricular Assist Device (LVAD)

Spec	Name	St	Pg
T&CS	Bowdish, M	CA	1140
T&CS	Pagani, F	MI	1134
T&CS	Pochettino, A	MN	1134

Leg Ulcers

Spec	Name	St	Pg
D	Kirsner, R	FL	191

Lens Implants

Spec	Name	St	Pg
Oph	Goldberg, D	NJ	574
Oph	Pflugfelder, S	TX	597
Oph	Serafano, D	CA	604
Oph	Waring, G	GA	587

Lens Implants-Multifocal

Spec	Name	St	Pg
Oph	Mackool, R	NY	577
Oph	Solomon, K	SC	586

Lens Implants-Pediatric

Spec	Name	St	Pg
Oph	Wilson, M	SC	587

Leukemia

Spec	Name	St	Pg
Hem	Baer, M	MD	312
Hem	Ballen, K	MA	310
Hem	Bigelow, C	MS	316
Hem	Bockenstedt, P	MI	319
Hem	Cheson, B	DC	312
Hem	Cooper, B	TX	323
Hem	Copelan, E	OH	319
Hem	Cortes, J	TX	323
Hem	Damon, L	CA	325
Hem	Di Persio, J	MO	319
Hem	Duffy, T	CT	310
Hem	Emanuel, P	AR	323
Hem	Forman, S	CA	325

Spec	Name	St	Pg
Hem	Goldberg, J	PA	312
Hem	Gregory, S	IL	320
Hem	Grever, M	OH	320
Hem	Habermann, T	MN	320
Hem	Kantarjian, H	TX	324
Hem	Kempin, S	NY	313
Hem	Kipps, T	CA	325
Hem	Kraut, E	OH	320
Hem	Kuriakose, P	MI	320
Hem	Litzow, M	MN	320
Hem	Marks, P	CT	310
Hem	Marks, S	PA	313
Hem	Maslak, P	NY	313
Hem	Maziarz, R	OR	326
Hem	McGlave, P	MN	321
Hem	Mears, J	NY	313
Hem	Mesa, R	AZ	324
Hem	Miller, K	MA	311
Hem	Mitchell, B	CA	326
Hem	Nand, S	IL	321
Hem	Nimer, S	FL	317
Hem	O'Donnell, M	CA	327
Hem	Petersdorf, S	WA	327
Hem	Porter, D	PA	314
Hem	Powell, B	NC	317
Hem	Rai, K	NY	314
Hem	Raphael, B	NY	314
Hem	Rapoport, A	MD	314
Hem	Rosenblatt, J	FL	317
Hem	Saven, A	CA	327
Hem	Schiller, G	CA	327
Hem	Snyder, D	CA	327
Hem	Spitzer, T	MA	311
Hem	Spivak, J	MD	315
Hem	Stiff, P	IL	322
Hem	Stone, R	MA	311
Hem	Strair, R	NJ	315
Hem	Strauss, J	TX	325
Hem	Tallman, M	NY	316
Hem	Tefferi, A	MN	322
Hem	Williams, M	VA	318
Hem	Wisch, N	NY	316
Hem	Yeager, A	AZ	325
Hem	Zuckerman, K	FL	318
Onc	Chao, N	NC	355
Onc	Chitambar, C	WI	366
Onc	Claxton, D	PA	336
Onc	Dakhil, S	KS	375
Onc	Druker, B	OR	385
Onc	Estey, E	WA	385
Onc	Flinn, I	TN	356
Onc	Gabrilove, J	NY	340
Onc	Gerson, S	OH	367
Onc	Gockerman, J	NC	357
Onc	Golomb, H	IL	368
Onc	Hurd, D	NC	357
Onc	Jillella, A	GA	358
Onc	Jurcic, J	NY	343
Onc	Kalaycio, M	OH	368
Onc	Karp, J	MD	343
Onc	List, A	FL	359
Onc	Lossos, I	FL	359

Spec	Name	St	Pg
Onc	Moore, J	NC	360
Onc	O'Brien, S	TX	380
Onc	Orlowski, R	TX	380
Onc	Peterson, B	MN	370
Onc	Scheinberg, D	NY	348
Onc	Schiffer, C	MI	371
Onc	Shea, T	NC	362
Onc	Smith, M	PA	349
Onc	Soiffer, R	MA	332
Onc	Weiner, G	IA	373
Onc	Wetzler, M	NY	352
Onc	Wingard, J	FL	364
Path	Chang, K	CA	720
Path	Foucar, K	NM	717
Path	Kinney, M	TX	718
Path	Nathwani, B	CA	721
PHO	Aledo, A	NY	758
PHO	Altman, A	CT	756
PHO	Andrews, R	WA	776
PHO	Angiolillo, A	DC	758
PHO	Arceci, R	MD	758
PHO	Barredo, J	FL	765
PHO	Brecher, M	NY	758
PHO	Buchanan, G	TX	775
PHO	Cairo, M	NY	758
PHO	Camitta, B	WI	769
PHO	Carroll, W	NY	758
PHO	Castellino, S	NC	765
PHO	Corey, S	IL	770
PHO	Davies, S	OH	770
PHO	Felix, C	PA	759
PHO	Frantz, C	DE	759
PHO	Friedman, A	MD	760
PHO	Godder, K	VA	766
PHO	Gold, S	NC	766
PHO	Goldman, S	TX	775
PHO	Graham, M	AZ	775
PHO	Guarini, L	NY	760
PHO	Haut, P	IN	771
PHO	Hawkins, D	WA	777
PHO	Hayani, A	IL	771
PHO	Hayashi, R	MO	771
PHO	Homans, A	VT	757
PHO	Hutchinson, R	MI	771
PHO	Johnston, J	GA	766
PHO	Kamen, B	NJ	761
PHO	Keller, F	GA	766
PHO	Lange, B	PA	762
PHO	Luchtman-Jones, L	DC	762
PHO	Marcus, J	NY	762
PHO	Morgan, E	IL	772
PHO	Pui, C	TN	768
PHO	Razzouk, B	IN	773
PHO	Reaman, G	DC	763
PHO	Rheingold, S	PA	763
PHO	Ritchey, A	PA	763
PHO	Rosoff, P	NC	768
PHO	Sakamoto, K	CA	779
PHO	Sallan, S	MA	757
PHO	Sandler, E	FL	768
PHO	Small, D	MD	763
PHO	Tebbi, C	FL	768

Specialty & Special Expertise Index

Spec	Name	St	Pg
PHO	Vik, T	IN	773
PHO	Weiner, M	NY	764
PHO	Weinstein, H	MA	757
PHO	Winick, N	TX	776
PHO	Yaddanapudi, R	MI	774
PHO	York, T	MD	764

Leukemia & Lymphoma

Spec	Name	St	Pg
Hem	Allen, S	NY	311
Hem	Champlin, R	TX	323
Hem	Farag, S	IN	319
Hem	Filicko-O'Hara, J	PA	312
Hem	Friedman, A	PA	312
Hem	Greer, J	TN	316
Hem	Larson, R	IL	320
Hem	Linenberger, M	WA	326
Hem	Lyons, R	TX	324
Hem	Millenson, M	PA	314
Hem	Munker, R	LA	324
Hem	Solberg, L	FL	318
Onc	Aboulafia, D	WA	383
Onc	Ball, E	CA	383
Onc	Carabasi, M	PA	336
Onc	Coleman, M	NY	337
Onc	Fay, J	TX	378
Onc	Flomenberg, N	PA	340
Onc	Himelstein, A	DE	342
Onc	Hollister, D	CT	330
Onc	Lazarus, H	OH	369
Onc	Morgan, D	TN	360
Onc	Peace, D	IL	370
Onc	Petruska, P	MO	370
Onc	Rosen, S	IL	371
Onc	Silverman, L	NY	349
Onc	Stadtmauer, E	PA	350
Path	Bagg, A	PA	708
PHO	Coccia, P	NE	774
PHO	Halpern, S	NJ	760
PHO	Harris, M	NJ	761
PHO	Hilden, J	CO	774
PHO	Kung, F	CA	778
PHO	Manera, R	IL	772
PHO	Plautz, G	OH	772
PHO	Ribeiro, R	TN	768
PHO	Salvi, S	IL	773
PHO	Sandlund, J	TN	768
PHO	Siegel, S	CA	779
PHO	Steinherz, P	NY	764
PHO	Wechsler, D	NC	769
PHO	Weinblatt, M	NY	764

Leukemia in Down Syndrome

Spec	Name	St	Pg
PHO	Hilden, J	CO	774

Leukemia in Infants

Spec	Name	St	Pg
PHO	Dreyer, Z	TX	775
PHO	Felix, C	PA	759
PHO	Hilden, J	CO	774

Leukemia-Chronic Lymphocytic

Spec	Name	St	Pg
Hem	Byrd, J	OH	319
Hem	Keating, M	TX	324
Onc	Chanan-Khan, A	FL	355
Onc	Czuczman, M	NY	337

Leukemia-Chronic Myeloid

Spec	Name	St	Pg
Onc	Druker, B	OR	385
Onc	Wetzler, M	NY	352

Leukemia-Myeloid

Spec	Name	St	Pg
Hem	Komrokji, R	FL	317
Onc	Appelbaum, F	WA	383
Onc	Estey, E	WA	385

Leukoencephalopathy

Spec	Name	St	Pg
N	Filley, C	CO	531
Onc	Kesari, S	CA	387

Lichen Planus

Spec	Name	St	Pg
D	Camisa, C	FL	190

Liddle's Syndrome

Spec	Name	St	Pg
Nep	Warnock, D	AL	460

Ligament Reconstruction

Spec	Name	St	Pg
OrS	Hannafin, J	NY	618
OrS	Spindler, K	TN	631
SM	Asnis, P	MA	1040
SM	Hershman, E	NY	1041
SM	Mirzayan, R	CA	1044

Limb Deformities

Spec	Name	St	Pg
OrS	Aronson, J	AR	640
OrS	Davidson, R	PA	616
OrS	Feldman, D	NY	617
OrS	Gugenheim, J	TX	640
OrS	Herzenberg, J	MD	619
OrS	Lowenberg, D	CA	644
OrS	Paley, D	FL	630
OrS	Rozbruch, S	NY	624

Limb Lengthening

Spec	Name	St	Pg
OrS	Johnson, E	CA	644
OrS	Oppenheim, W	CA	645
OrS	Rozbruch, S	NY	624

Limb Lengthening (Ilizarov Procedure)

Spec	Name	St	Pg
OrS	Aronson, J	AR	640
OrS	Davidson, R	PA	616
OrS	Gugenheim, J	TX	640
OrS	Herzenberg, J	MD	619
OrS	Lowenberg, D	CA	644
OrS	Paley, D	FL	630

Limb Sparing Surgery

Spec	Name	St	Pg
OrS	Aboulafia, A	MD	613
OrS	Benevenia, J	NJ	614
OrS	Biermann, J	MI	632
OrS	Eckardt, J	CA	643
OrS	Gitelis, S	IL	633
OrS	Irwin, R	MI	634
OrS	Malawer, M	MD	622
OrS	Peabody, T	IL	636
OrS	Schmidt, R	PA	625
OrS	Smith, D	WA	646
OrS	Wurtz, L	IN	638
VascS	Acher, C	WI	1190
VascS	Marin, M	NY	1188

Limb Surgery/Reconstruction

Spec	Name	St	Pg
HS	Raphael, J	PA	297
OrS	Friedlaender, G	CT	611
OrS	Mayerson, J	OH	635
OrS	Rozbruch, S	NY	624
PlS	Attinger, C	DC	852
PlS	Sherman, R	CA	876

Liposuction

Spec	Name	St	Pg
PlS	Matarasso, A	NY	856
PlS	Pitman, G	NY	857
PlS	Sanders, G	CA	876
PlS	Tebbetts, J	TX	872

Liposuction & Body Contouring

Spec	Name	St	Pg
PlS	Aston, S	NY	852
PlS	Barton, F	TX	869
PlS	Beals, S	AZ	870
PlS	Beasley, M	NC	860
PlS	Bucky, L	PA	853
PlS	Byrd, H	TX	870
PlS	Da Lio, A	CA	873
PlS	Davis, G	NC	861
PlS	Dick, G	MD	853
PlS	Dufresne, C	MD	854
PlS	Edwards, M	NV	873
PlS	Fodor, P	CA	874
PlS	Gallico, G	MA	850
PlS	Gregory, R	FL	861
PlS	Grotting, J	AL	861
PlS	Hoffman, L	NY	854
PlS	Isik, F	WA	874
PlS	Jewell, M	OR	875
PlS	Koplin, L	CA	875
PlS	Leipziger, L	NY	855
PlS	Maxwell, G	TN	869
PlS	Medalie, D	OH	866
PlS	Moses, M	LA	871
PlS	Nichter, L	CA	875
PlS	Noone, R	PA	857
PlS	Olding, M	DC	857
PlS	Paul, M	CA	876
PlS	Price, G	MD	857
PlS	Rand, R	WA	876
PlS	Rohrich, R	TX	872

Spec	Name	St	Pg
PlS	Rosenberg, H	CA	876
PlS	Schusterman, M	TX	872
PlS	Singer, R	CA	877
PlS	Singh, N	MD	858
PlS	Slavin, S	MA	851
PlS	Stevens, W	CA	877
PlS	Sultan, M	NY	859
PlS	Wilcox, R	TX	872

Liver & Biliary Cancer

Spec	Name	St	Pg
S	Cioffi, W	RI	1048
S	Emond, J	NY	1057
S	Fong, Y	NY	1057
S	Fung, J	OH	1077
S	Jenkins, R	MA	1050
S	Kinkhabwala, M	NY	1059
S	Livingstone, A	FL	1070
S	Mulvihill, S	UT	1085
S	Newman, E	NY	1061
S	Pinson, C	TN	1071
S	Shen, P	NC	1072
S	Sinanan, M	WA	1100
S	Staley, C	GA	1072
S	Sundaram, M	IL	1083
S	Yeung, R	WA	1101

Liver & Biliary Disease

Spec	Name	St	Pg
Ge	Jacobson, I	NY	234
Ge	Jensen, D	IL	246
Ge	La Russo, N	MN	246
Ge	Tobias, H	NY	238

Liver & Biliary Imaging

Spec	Name	St	Pg
DR	Grant, E	CA	983

Liver & Biliary Surgery

Spec	Name	St	Pg
S	Chabot, J	NY	1055
S	Chapman, W	MO	1075
S	Cronin, D	WI	1075
S	Kinkhabwala, M	NY	1059
S	Matthews, J	IL	1079
S	Melvin, W	OH	1079
S	Meyers, W	PA	1060
S	Olthoff, K	PA	1061
S	Pinson, C	TN	1071
S	Salem, R	CT	1051
S	Selby, R	CA	1099
S	Sutton, J	VT	1052

Liver Cancer

Spec	Name	St	Pg
DR	Charboneau, J	MN	980
DR	Coakley, F	OR	982
DR	Dodd, G	CO	981
Ge	Brown, K	MI	244
Ge	Di Bisceglie, A	MO	244
Ge	Galati, J	TX	252
Ge	Gish, R	CA	254
Ge	Jensen, D	IL	246
Ge	Okolo, P	MD	237

Spec	Name	St	Pg
Ge	Porayko, M	TN	241
Ge	Shiffman, M	VA	242
Onc	Benson, A	IL	364
Onc	Berlin, J	TN	353
Onc	Ensminger, W	MI	367
Onc	Holcombe, R	NY	342
Onc	Kemeny, N	NY	343
Onc	Leighton, J	PA	344
Onc	O'Reilly, E	NY	346
Onc	Patt, Y	NM	381
Onc	Posey, J	AL	361
Onc	Reid, T	CA	390
Onc	Venook, A	CA	392
Onc	Weiner, L	DC	352
Onc	Yen, Y	CA	392
Path	Bhan, A	MA	706
Path	Greenson, J	MI	715
PHO	Furman, W	TN	765
PHO	Tomlinson, G	TX	776
PS	La Quaglia, M	NY	803
RadRO	Lawrence, T	MI	960
S	Abecassis, M	IL	1074
S	Abouljoud, M	MI	1074
S	Adams, R	VA	1066
S	Bartlett, D	PA	1053
S	Bolton, J	LA	1087
S	Brems, J	IL	1074
S	Busuttil, R	CA	1094
S	Callery, M	MA	1048
S	Cameron, J	MD	1054
S	Chapman, W	MO	1075
S	Cherqui, D	NY	1055
S	Colquhoun, S	CA	1094
S	Curley, S	TX	1087
S	Drebin, J	PA	1056
S	Eason, J	TN	1068
S	Emond, J	NY	1057
S	Emre, S	CT	1049
S	Fraker, D	PA	1057
S	Geller, D	PA	1058
S	Gibbs, J	NY	1058
S	Hemming, A	CA	1096
S	Hiotis, S	NY	1058
S	Hoffman, J	PA	1058
S	Jarnagin, W	NY	1058
S	Karpeh, M	NY	1059
S	Kendrick, M	MN	1078
S	Klein, A	CA	1097
S	Kuhn, J	TX	1090
S	Levi, J	FL	1070
S	Libutti, S	NY	1060
S	Mahvi, D	IL	1079
S	Marsh, J	PA	1060
S	McMasters, K	KY	1070
S	Millis, J	IL	1080
S	Nakakura, E	CA	1097
S	Nissen, N	CA	1098
S	Olthoff, K	PA	1061
S	Pawlik, T	MD	1062
S	Philosophe, B	MD	1062
S	Reich, D	PA	1062
S	Roh, M	FL	1071

Spec	Name	St	Pg
S	Salem, R	CT	1051
S	Sasson, A	NE	1086
S	Schulick, R	CO	1086
S	Selby, R	CA	1099
S	Sielaff, T	MN	1082
S	Sigurdson, E	PA	1064
S	Staren, E	AZ	1092
S	Talamonti, M	IL	1083
S	Tanabe, K	MA	1052
S	Teperman, L	NY	1065
S	Vauthey, J	TX	1092
S	Vickers, S	MN	1083
S	Wagman, L	CA	1100
S	Warren, R	CA	1100
S	Weber, S	WI	1084
S	Wood, R	TX	1093
S	Yeatman, T	FL	1073
S	Yeung, R	WA	1101
VIR	Brown, K	NY	992
VIR	Durham, J	CO	996
VIR	Goodwin, S	CA	997
VIR	Hicks, M	TX	997
VIR	McGahan, J	CA	998
VIR	Solomon, S	NY	993
VIR	Wood, B	MD	994

Liver Cancer-Metastatic

Spec	Name	St	Pg
S	Alexander, H	MD	1053
S	Choti, M	MD	1055

Liver Cancer/Chemoembolization

Spec	Name	St	Pg
VIR	Cohen, G	PA	993
VIR	Geschwind, J	MD	993
VIR	Hallisey, M	CT	992
VIR	Haskal, Z	MD	993
VIR	Rilling, W	WI	996
VIR	Salem, R	IL	996
VIR	Soulen, M	PA	994

Liver Cancer/Radioembolization

Spec	Name	St	Pg
VIR	Brown, D	PA	992

Liver Disease

Spec	Name	St	Pg
Ge	Anderson, K	TX	250
Ge	Bacon, B	MO	243
Ge	Balart, L	LA	250
Ge	Barnes, D	OH	244
Ge	Bloomer, J	AL	239
Ge	Borum, M	DC	231
Ge	Boyer, T	AZ	251
Ge	Brown, K	MI	244
Ge	Brown, K	NY	231
Ge	Chung, R	MA	228
Ge	Crippin, J	MO	244
Ge	Davis, G	TX	251
Ge	Dienstag, J	MA	228
Ge	Dieterich, D	NY	232

Specialty & Special Expertise Index

Spec	Name	St	Pg
Ge	Eisen, G	OR	253
Ge	Fallon, M	TX	251
Ge	Fried, M	NC	240
Ge	Friedman, L	MA	229
Ge	Galati, J	TX	252
Ge	Gholam, P	OH	245
Ge	Han, S	CA	254
Ge	Herrine, S	PA	233
Ge	Kaplan, L	MA	229
Ge	Konicek, F	IL	246
Ge	Korsten, M	NY	235
Ge	Kwo, P	IN	246
Ge	Lambiase, L	TN	241
Ge	Loomba, R	CA	254
Ge	Lucey, M	WI	247
Ge	Martin, P	FL	241
Ge	Miskovitz, P	NY	236
Ge	Munoz, S	PA	237
Ge	Nunes, D	MA	229
Ge	Poordad, F	TX	252
Ge	Porayko, M	TN	241
Ge	Reddy, K	PA	237
Ge	Reuben, A	SC	242
Ge	Schiano, T	NY	238
Ge	Schiff, E	FL	242
Ge	Shiffman, M	VA	242
Ge	Silverman, W	IA	248
Ge	Sorrell, M	NE	250
Ge	Te, H	IL	248
Ge	Tobias, H	NY	238
Ge	Vierling, J	TX	253
Ge	Younossi, Z	VA	243
Ge	Zaman, A	OR	255
PGe	Baker, S	NY	750
PGe	Benkov, K	NY	750
PGe	Bishop, W	IA	752
PGe	El-Youssef, M	MN	753
PGe	Hoffenberg, E	CO	754
PGe	Jonas, M	MA	749
PGe	McDiarmid, S	CA	756
PGe	Mittal, N	TX	755
PGe	Molleston, J	IN	753
PGe	Murray, K	WA	756
PGe	Narkewicz, M	CO	754
PGe	Novak, D	FL	752
PGe	Piccoli, D	PA	751
PGe	Schwarz, K	MD	751
PGe	Sokol, R	CO	754
PGe	Squires, R	PA	751
PGe	Suchy, F	CO	755
PGe	Ulshen, M	NC	752
PGe	Whitington, P	IL	754
S	Brems, J	IL	1074
S	Levi, S	FL	1070
S	Millis, J	IL	1080

Liver Failure

Ge	Crippin, J	MO	244
S	Klein, A	CA	1097

Liver Pathology

Path	Appelman, H	MI	714
Path	Bhan, A	MA	706
Path	Crawford, J	NY	708
Path	Demetris, A	PA	708
Path	Ferrell, L	CA	720
Path	Govindarajan, S	CA	720
Path	Greenson, J	MI	715
Path	Hamilton, S	TX	718
Path	Kanel, G	CA	721
Path	Norenberg, M	FL	714
Path	Odze, R	MA	707
Path	Rashid, A	TX	718
Path	Sibley, R	CA	722

Liver Surgery

PS	Karrer, F	CO	808
S	Abouljoud, M	MI	1074
S	Halff, G	TX	1089
S	Johnson, L	DC	1058
S	Schirmer, B	VA	1072

Liver Trauma

S	Moore, E	CO	1085

Liver Tumors

Ge	Sorrell, M	NE	250
S	Billingsley, K	OR	1093
VIR	Johnson, M	IN	995
VIR	Nemcek, A	IL	996

Long QT Interval Syndrome

CE	Waldo, A	OH	124
PCd	Ackerman, M	MN	738

Low Vision

Oph	Sterns, G	NY	581

Lower Limb Arterial Disease

VascS	Bandyk, D	CA	1194
VascS	Calligaro, K	PA	1186
VascS	Gloviczki, P	MN	1191
VascS	Howard, T	NE	1192
VascS	Kent, K	WI	1191
VascS	Mackey, W	MA	1185

Lower Limb Reconstruction

PlS	Attinger, C	DC	852
PlS	Wilkins, E	MI	868

Lower Limb Surgery in Children

OrS	McCarthy, J	OH	635

Lung Cancer

DR	Austin, J	NY	974
DR	Black, W	NH	973
DR	Chiles, C	NC	979
DR	Erasmus, J	TX	982
DR	Henschke, C	NY	975
DR	Patz, E	NC	979
DR	Swensen, S	MN	981
DR	Yankelevitz, D	NY	978
Hem	Schwartzberg, L	TN	317
Onc	Adelstein, D	OH	364
Onc	Aisner, J	NJ	334
Onc	Akerley, W	UT	374
Onc	Albain, K	IL	364
Onc	Algazy, K	PA	334
Onc	Antonia, S	FL	353
Onc	Argiris, A	TX	377
Onc	Axelrod, R	PA	335
Onc	Azzoli, C	NY	335
Onc	Belani, C	PA	335
Onc	Bitran, J	IL	365
Onc	Bonomi, P	IL	365
Onc	Bunn, P	CO	374
Onc	Butler, W	SC	354
Onc	Carbone, D	OH	365
Onc	Chachoua, A	NY	336
Onc	Chapman, R	MI	365
Onc	Clamon, G	IA	366
Onc	Cohen, R	PA	337
Onc	Cohen, S	NY	337
Onc	Conry, R	AL	355
Onc	Crawford, J	NC	355
Onc	Dowlati, A	OH	366
Onc	Dunphy, F	NC	356
Onc	Edelman, M	MD	339
Onc	Einhorn, L	IN	367
Onc	Ettinger, D	MD	339
Onc	Fossella, F	TX	378
Onc	Gandara, D	CA	386
Onc	Garst, J	NC	356
Onc	Glisson, B	TX	378
Onc	Golomb, H	IL	368
Onc	Greco, F	TN	357
Onc	Grunberg, S	VT	330
Onc	Hageboutros, A	NJ	341
Onc	Herbst, R	CT	330
Onc	Hoffman, P	IL	368
Onc	Holland, J	NY	342
Onc	Hollister, D	CT	330
Onc	Hong, W	TX	379
Onc	Jahanzeb, M	FL	357
Onc	Johnson, B	MA	330
Onc	Johnson, D	TX	379
Onc	Kalemkerian, G	MI	368
Onc	Kelly, K	CA	387
Onc	Khuri, F	GA	358
Onc	Kies, M	TX	379
Onc	Koczywas, M	CA	387
Onc	Kressel, B	DC	344
Onc	Kris, M	NY	344
Onc	Langer, C	PA	344
Onc	Lilenbaum, R	FL	358
Onc	Lippman, S	CA	387
Onc	Livingston, R	AZ	380
Onc	Lynch, J	FL	359

Spec	Name	St	Pg	Spec	Name	St	Pg	Spec	Name	St	Pg
Onc	Lynch, T	CT	331	RadRO	Cox, J	TX	963	T&CS	Kernstine, K	TX	1138
Onc	Martins, R	WA	388	RadRO	Emami, B	IL	959	T&CS	Kiernan, P	VA	1126
Onc	Masters, G	DE	345	RadRO	Greenberger, J	PA	950	T&CS	Kiev, J	WV	1118
Onc	Miller, A	NC	360	RadRO	Hahn, S	PA	950	T&CS	Krellenstein, D	NY	1118
Onc	Miller, D	KY	360	RadRO	Haraf, D	IL	960	T&CS	Kucharczuk, J	PA	1119
Onc	Natale, R	CA	388	RadRO	Hayman, J	MI	960	T&CS	Landreneau, R	PA	1119
Onc	Nissenblatt, M	NJ	346	RadRO	Heimann, R	VT	946	T&CS	Lanza, L	AZ	1138
Onc	Northfelt, D	AZ	380	RadRO	Jose, B	IN	960	T&CS	Lau, C	VA	1126
Onc	O'Brien, T	OH	370	RadRO	Kalnicki, S	NY	951	T&CS	Love, R	IL	1133
Onc	Pao, W	TN	360	RadRO	Komaki, R	TX	964	T&CS	Marshall, M	DC	1120
Onc	Pasmantier, M	NY	347	RadRO	Kudrimoti, M	KY	954	T&CS	Mason, D	OH	1133
Onc	Perry, D	DC	347	RadRO	Le, Q	CA	967	T&CS	Mathisen, D	MA	1111
Onc	Pisters, K	TX	381	RadRO	Lewin, A	FL	955	T&CS	Meyers, B	MO	1133
Onc	Ready, N	NC	361	RadRO	Marks, L	NC	955	T&CS	Miller, D	GA	1127
Onc	Robert-Vizcarrondo, F	AL	361	RadRO	McGarry, R	KY	956	T&CS	Mitchell, J	CO	1136
Onc	Ross, H	AZ	381	RadRO	Morris, M	VA	956	T&CS	Moore, J	GA	1127
Onc	Salgia, R	IL	371	RadRO	Movsas, B	MI	961	T&CS	Mullett, T	KY	1127
Onc	Sandler, A	OR	390	RadRO	Nori, D	NY	951	T&CS	Naunheim, K	MO	1134
Onc	Schiller, J	TX	381	RadRO	Randolph-Jackson, P	DC	952	T&CS	Nesbitt, J	TN	1127
Onc	Sherman, C	SC	362	RadRO	Roach, M	CA	967	T&CS	Nguyen, D	FL	1127
Onc	Shin, D	GA	362	RadRO	Rosenman, J	NC	957	T&CS	Ninan, M	TN	1128
Onc	Simon, G	TX	382	RadRO	Schiff, P	NY	952	T&CS	Oaks, T	NC	1128
Onc	Socinski, M	PA	349	RadRO	Schild, S	AZ	965	T&CS	Orringer, M	MI	1134
Onc	Steen, P	ND	376	RadRO	Seung, S	OR	968	T&CS	Orringer, M	MI	1134
Onc	Stone, J	FL	362	RadRO	Streeter, O	DC	952	T&CS	Park, B	NJ	1120
Onc	Stoopler, M	NY	350	RadRO	Suntharalingam, M	MD	953	T&CS	Pass, H	NY	1120
Onc	Strauss, G	MA	332	RadRO	Videtic, G	OH	962	T&CS	Patterson, G	MO	1134
Onc	Tester, W	PA	351	RadRO	Werner-Wasik, M	PA	953	T&CS	Pechet, T	PA	1120
Onc	Thigpen, J	MS	363	RadRO	Wilson, L	CT	948	T&CS	Pierson, R	MD	1120
Onc	Vinciguerra, V	NY	351	T&CS	Altorki, N	NY	1113	T&CS	Putnam, J	TN	1128
Onc	Vokes, E	IL	373	T&CS	Baciewicz, F	MI	1130	T&CS	Reed, C	SC	1128
Onc	Wierman, A	NV	392	T&CS	Bains, M	NY	1114	T&CS	Rice, T	OH	1134
Path	Cagle, P	TX	717	T&CS	Battafarano, R	MD	1114	T&CS	Robinson, L	FL	1129
Path	Hammar, S	WA	720	T&CS	Brinckerhoff, L	MA	1110	T&CS	Roth, J	TX	1139
Path	Katzenstein, A	NY	710	T&CS	Bueno, R	MA	1110	T&CS	Rusch, V	NY	1121
Path	Koss, M	CA	721	T&CS	Cameron, R	CA	1140	T&CS	Savage, E	FL	1129
Path	Leslie, K	AZ	718	T&CS	Cerfolio, R	AL	1124	T&CS	Scott, W	PA	1121
Path	Moran, C	TX	718	T&CS	Colson, Y	MA	1110	T&CS	Shrager, J	CA	1143
Path	Myers, J	MI	716	T&CS	D'Amico, T	NC	1125	T&CS	Smythe, W	TX	1139
Path	Travis, W	NY	712	T&CS	Demmy, T	NY	1115	T&CS	Soberman, M	MD	1121
Path	Yousem, S	PA	712	T&CS	Deschamps, C	MN	1131	T&CS	Swanson, S	MA	1112
Pul	Alberts, W	FL	929	T&CS	Downey, R	NY	1115	T&CS	Swisher, S	TX	1139
Pul	Cooke, J	NY	925	T&CS	Feins, R	NC	1125	T&CS	Thistlethwaite, P	CA	1143
Pul	Cooper, W	VA	930	T&CS	Ferguson, M	IL	1132	T&CS	Vallieres, E	WA	1143
Pul	Ernst, A	MA	922	T&CS	Fernando, H	MA	1111	T&CS	Wain, J	MA	1112
Pul	Garver, R	AL	930	T&CS	Flores, R	NY	1115	T&CS	Watson, T	NY	1122
Pul	Goldman, A	FL	931	T&CS	Friedberg, J	PA	1116	T&CS	Weigel, T	WI	1135
Pul	Guidry, G	LA	938	T&CS	Gaissert, H	MA	1111	T&CS	Weiman, D	TN	1130
Pul	Kern, J	CO	937	T&CS	Gharagozloo, F	DC	1116	T&CS	Weksler, B	PA	1123
Pul	King, E	PA	926	T&CS	Ginsburg, M	NY	1116	T&CS	Whyte, R	MA	1113
Pul	Libby, D	NY	926	T&CS	Grannis, F	CA	1141	T&CS	Wood, D	WA	1143
Pul	Maxfield, R	NY	926	T&CS	Handy, J	OR	1141	T&CS	Wright, C	MA	1113
Pul	Silver, M	IL	935	T&CS	Harpole, D	NC	1125	T&CS	Yang, S	MD	1123
Pul	Steinberg, H	NY	928	T&CS	Heitmiller, R	MD	1117	T&CS	Zwischenberger, J	KY	1130
Pul	Sterman, D	PA	928	T&CS	Howington, J	IL	1132	VIR	Hicks, M	TX	997
Pul	Unger, M	PA	929	T&CS	Iannettoni, M	IA	1132	VIR	Solomon, S	NY	993
RadRO	Beitler, J	GA	953	T&CS	Jablons, D	CA	1142				
RadRO	Blackstock, A	NC	953	T&CS	Jones, D	VA	1125				
RadRO	Bogart, J	NY	948	T&CS	Kaiser, L	PA	1118				
RadRO	Bradley, J	MO	958	T&CS	Karwande, S	UT	1136				
RadRO	Choi, N	MA	946	T&CS	Keenan, R	PA	1118				
RadRO	Choy, H	TX	963	T&CS	Keller, S	NY	1118				

Lung Cancer (advanced)

H & PM	Davis, M	OH	407
Onc	Azzoli, C	NY	335

Specialty & Special Expertise Index

Spec	Name	St	Pg
Lung Cancer in Women			
Pul	Unger, M	PA	929
Lung Disease			
DR	Goodman, L	WI	980
DR	Henschke, C	NY	975
DR	Swensen, S	MN	981
Pul	Enelow, R	NH	922
Pul	Garver, R	AL	930
Pul	Greenberg, H	NY	925
Pul	Martinez, F	MI	934
Pul	Popovich, J	MI	935
Pul	Shore, B	MO	935
Lung Disease in Newborns			
NP	Adams, J	TX	451
NP	Davidson, D	NY	447
NP	Davis, J	MA	446
NP	Dennery, P	PA	447
NP	Ehrenkranz, R	CT	446
NP	Frantz, I	MA	446
NP	Garcia-Prats, J	TX	452
NP	Holtzman, R	NC	449
NP	Kattwinkel, J	VA	449
NP	Perlman, J	NY	448
NP	Van Marter, L	MA	446
PS	Latchaw, L	NH	802
Lung Disease in Newborns-Genetic			
NP	Hamvas, A	MO	450
NP	Nogee, L	MD	448
NP	Whitsett, J	OH	451
Lung Disease-Complex			
Pul	Kotloff, R	PA	926
Lung Injuries-Inhalation Induced			
Pul	Boushey, H	CA	939
Pul	Brooks, S	FL	929
Lung Injuries-RSV related			
PPul	Sallent, J	FL	796
Lung Injury-Neonatal			
PPul	Mcgrath-Morrow, S	MD	795
Lung Injury/ARDS			
Pul	Balk, R	IL	933
Lung Pathology			
Path	Ehya, H	PA	708
Path	Gupta, P	PA	709
Path	Myers, J	MI	716

Spec	Name	St	Pg
Lung Pathology-Rare Tumors			
Path	Mark, E	MA	706
Lung Surgery			
T&CS	Cooper, J	PA	1114
T&CS	DeCamp, M	IL	1131
T&CS	Frazier, O	TX	1138
T&CS	Oaks, T	NC	1128
T&CS	Pechet, T	PA	1120
Lupus Nephritis			
Nep	Appel, G	NY	456
Nep	Falk, R	NC	459
Nep	Rodby, R	IL	462
Nep	Salant, D	MA	456
Nep	Suki, W	TX	464
Lupus/SLE			
D	Callen, J	KY	190
D	Fivenson, D	MI	193
D	Franks, A	NY	186
D	Sontheimer, R	UT	196
D	Werth, V	PA	189
PRhu	Finkel, T	FL	800
PRhu	Haines, K	NJ	799
PRhu	Ilowite, N	NY	799
PRhu	Klein-Gitelman, M	IL	800
PRhu	Lehman, T	NY	799
PRhu	McCarthy, P	CT	799
PRhu	Schanberg, L	NC	800
PRhu	Sherry, D	PA	799
PRhu	Sills, E	MD	800
PRhu	Wagner-Weiner, L	IL	800
PRhu	Warren, R	SC	800
PRhu	Wilking, A	TX	801
Rhu	Adams, E	IL	1030
Rhu	Allen, N	NC	1029
Rhu	Belmont, H	NY	1025
Rhu	Blume, R	NY	1025
Rhu	Bobrove, A	CA	1033
Rhu	Chatham, W	AL	1029
Rhu	Coblyn, J	MA	1024
Rhu	Crofford, L	KY	1029
Rhu	Curran, J	IL	1031
Rhu	Davis, W	LA	1032
Rhu	Ehresmann, G	CA	1033
Rhu	Gourley, M	MD	1026
Rhu	Katz, R	IL	1031
Rhu	Kimberly, R	AL	1030
Rhu	Lahita, R	NJ	1027
Rhu	Manzi, S	PA	1027
Rhu	Massarotti, E	MA	1024
Rhu	McCune, W	MI	1031
Rhu	Moder, K	MN	1032
Rhu	Moore, W	GA	1030
Rhu	Paget, S	NY	1027
Rhu	Peng, S	WA	1034
Rhu	Petri, M	MD	1027
Rhu	Polisson, R	MA	1024
Rhu	Rothenberg, R	MD	1028

Spec	Name	St	Pg
Rhu	Salmon, J	NY	1028
Rhu	Sessoms, S	TX	1033
Rhu	Spiera, H	NY	1028
Rhu	Steen, V	DC	1028
Rhu	Tsokos, G	MA	1025
Rhu	Wallace, D	CA	1034
Rhu	Weinstein, A	DC	1029
Rhu	Wener, M	WA	1034
Rhu	West, S	CO	1032
Rhu	Wofsy, D	CA	1034
Lupus/SLE in Menopause			
Rhu	Buyon, J	NY	1026
Lupus/SLE in Pregnancy			
MF	Druzin, M	CA	440
ObG	Witter, F	MD	558
Rhu	Buyon, J	NY	1026
Lupus/SLE in Women			
Rhu	Manzi, S	PA	1027
Lyme Disease			
Inf	Auwaerter, P	MD	410
Inf	Louie, E	NY	412
Inf	Perlman, D	NY	412
Inf	Wormser, G	NY	413
Inf	Yancovitz, S	NY	414
N	Coyle, P	NY	510
N	Logigian, E	NY	515
N	Petito, F	NY	516
PInf	Andiman, W	CT	779
PInf	Christenson, J	IN	783
PInf	Durbin, W	MA	780
PInf	Krilov, L	NY	780
PInf	Shapiro, E	CT	780
PRhu	Ilowite, N	NY	799
Rhu	Magid, S	NY	1027
Rhu	Schoen, R	CT	1024
Rhu	Shadick, N	MA	1025
Rhu	Simms, R	MA	1025
Rhu	Weinstein, A	DC	1029
Lyme Disease-Neuro Complications			
Psyc	Fallon, B	NY	892
Lymph Node Pathology			
Path	Arber, D	CA	719
Path	Cote, R	FL	713
Path	Foucar, M	NM	717
Path	Kurtin, P	MN	716
Path	Orazi, A	NY	710
Lymphangioleiomyomatosis(LAM)			
Pul	Ahya, V	PA	924
Pul	Kotloff, R	PA	926

Spec	Name	St	Pg
Pul	Lynch, J	CA	940

Lymphatic Malformations-Head & Neck

Spec	Name	St	Pg
PO	Friedman, E	TX	793
PO	McGill, T	MA	789
PO	Richardson, M	OR	793

Lymphedema

Spec	Name	St	Pg
Onc	Fox, K	PA	340
PMR	Cheville, A	MN	839
PMR	DePompolo, R	MN	840
PMR	Feldman, J	IL	840
PMR	Francis, K	NJ	836
PMR	Gamble, G	IL	840
PMR	King, R	GA	838
PMR	Richter, E	CT	834
PMR	Schwartz, L	PA	837
PMR	Stewart, P	AL	839
S	Sener, S	CA	1099

Lymphoma

Spec	Name	St	Pg
Hem	Baron, J	IL	318
Hem	Cooper, B	TX	323
Hem	Damon, L	CA	325
Hem	Djulbegovic, B	FL	316
Hem	Duffy, T	CT	310
Hem	Emanuel, P	AR	323
Hem	Forman, S	CA	325
Hem	Goldberg, J	PA	312
Hem	Gregory, S	IL	320
Hem	Habermann, T	MN	320
Hem	Kempin, S	NY	313
Hem	Levine, A	CA	326
Hem	Lill, M	CA	326
Hem	Marks, S	PA	313
Hem	Maziarz, R	OR	326
Hem	Mears, J	NY	313
Hem	Mitchell, B	CA	326
Hem	Nademanee, A	CA	326
Hem	Petersdorf, S	WA	327
Hem	Porcu, P	OH	321
Hem	Porter, D	PA	314
Hem	Rai, K	NY	314
Hem	Raphael, B	NY	314
Hem	Rapoport, A	MD	314
Hem	Rosenblatt, J	FL	317
Hem	Savage, D	NY	314
Hem	Saven, A	CA	327
Hem	Schuster, S	PA	315
Hem	Sokol, L	FL	318
Hem	Strair, R	NJ	315
Hem	Strauss, J	TX	325
Hem	Van Besien, K	IL	322
Hem	Vose, J	NE	322
Hem	Williams, M	VA	318
Hem	Wisch, N	NY	316
NuM	Dillehay, G	IL	550
Onc	Advani, R	CA	383
Onc	Ambinder, R	MD	334
Onc	Armitage, J	NE	374
Onc	Astrow, A	NY	334
Onc	Attas, L	NJ	334
Onc	Beatty, P	MT	374
Onc	Bierman, P	NE	374
Onc	Camoriano, J	AZ	378
Onc	Chao, N	NC	355
Onc	Chitambar, C	WI	366
Onc	Cohen, S	NY	337
Onc	Dakhil, S	KS	375
Onc	Dutcher, J	NY	338
Onc	Fisher, R	NY	339
Onc	Flinn, I	TN	356
Onc	Forero, A	AL	356
Onc	Freedman, A	MA	329
Onc	Friedberg, J	NY	340
Onc	Glaspy, J	CA	386
Onc	Gockerman, J	NC	357
Onc	Golomb, H	IL	368
Onc	Goy, A	NJ	341
Onc	Grossbard, M	NY	341
Onc	Hochberg, E	MA	330
Onc	Hurd, D	NC	357
Onc	Jillella, A	GA	358
Onc	Kaminski, M	MI	369
Onc	Kaplan, L	CA	387
Onc	Kwak, L	TX	379
Onc	Lossos, I	FL	359
Onc	Lynch, J	FL	359
Onc	Maloney, D	WA	388
Onc	Miller, T	AZ	380
Onc	O'Brien, S	TX	380
Onc	Offit, K	NY	346
Onc	Ozer, H	IL	370
Onc	Pusmantier, M	NY	347
Onc	Peterson, B	MN	370
Onc	Pohlman, B	OH	371
Onc	Press, O	WA	389
Onc	Romaguera, J	TX	381
Onc	Schiffer, C	MI	371
Onc	Schwartz, B	MN	372
Onc	Schwartz, M	FL	362
Onc	Serody, J	NC	362
Onc	Shea, T	NC	362
Onc	Smith, M	PA	349
Onc	Soiffer, R	MA	332
Onc	Sotomayor, E	FL	362
Onc	Straus, D	NY	350
Onc	Strenger, R	RI	332
Onc	Sweetenham, J	NV	391
Onc	Weiner, G	IA	373
Onc	Wierman, A	NV	392
Onc	Wilson, W	MD	352
Onc	Wingard, J	FL	364
Onc	Yunus, F	TN	364
Onc	Zelenetz, A	NY	352
Path	Banks, P	NC	713
Path	Chang, K	CA	720
Path	Harris, N	MA	706
Path	Kinney, M	TX	718
Path	Kurtin, P	MN	716
Path	Nathwani, B	CA	721
Path	Swerdlow, S	PA	712
Path	Warnke, R	CA	722
Path	Weisenburger, D	NE	717
Path	Weiss, L	CA	722
PHO	Aledo, A	NY	758
PHO	Andrews, R	WA	776
PHO	Angiolillo, A	DC	758
PHO	Blum, K	OH	769
PHO	Brecher, M	NY	758
PHO	Cairo, M	NY	758
PHO	Castellino, S	NC	765
PHO	Fallon, R	IN	770
PHO	Goldman, S	TX	775
PHO	Hayani, A	IL	771
PHO	Johnston, J	GA	766
PHO	Marcus, J	NY	762
PHO	Parker, R	NY	763
PHO	Pui, C	TN	768
PHO	Razzouk, B	IN	773
PHO	Reaman, G	DC	763
PHO	Small, D	MD	763
PHO	Weiner, M	NY	764
PHO	Weinstein, H	MA	757
RadRO	Abrams, R	IL	958
RadRO	Constine, L	NY	948
RadRO	Goodman, R	NJ	950
RadRO	Hoppe, R	CA	966
RadRO	Lee, C	MN	960
RadRO	Macklis, R	OH	961
RadRO	Markoe, A	FL	955
RadRO	McGarry, R	KY	956
RadRO	Mendenhall, N	FL	956
RadRO	Mittal, B	IL	961
RadRO	Nicolaou, N	PA	951
RadRO	Park, C	CA	967
RadRO	Prosnitz, L	NC	956
RadRO	Rabinovitch, R	CO	963
RadRO	Roberts, K	CT	947
RadRO	Russell, K	WA	968
RadRO	Song, S	VA	957
RadRO	Stea, B	AZ	965
RadRO	Tripuraneni, P	CA	968
RadRO	Yahalom, J	NY	953

Lymphoma Consultation

Spec	Name	St	Pg
Onc	DeVita, V	CT	328

Lymphoma, Cutaneous T Cell (CTCL)

Spec	Name	St	Pg
Onc	Foss, F	CT	329
Onc	Horwitz, S	NY	342

Lymphoma, Non-Hodgkin's

Spec	Name	St	Pg
Hem	Gordon, L	IL	319
Hem	Kipps, T	CA	325
Hem	Nand, S	IL	321
Hem	Porcu, P	OH	321
Hem	Stiff, P	IL	322
Hem	Winter, J	IL	322
NuM	Lamonica, D	NY	548

Spec	Name	St	Pg
NuM	Podoloff, D	TX	550
NuM	Wiseman, G	MN	550
Onc	Gerson, S	OH	367
Onc	Glick, J	PA	340
Onc	Horwitz, S	NY	342
Onc	Miller, T	AZ	380
Onc	Moore, J	NC	360
Onc	O'Connor, O	NY	346
Onc	Orlowski, R	TX	380
Onc	Pohlman, B	OH	371
PHO	Billett, A	MA	756
PHO	Blum, K	OH	769
PHO	Laver, J	TN	767
PHO	Park, J	WA	778
PHO	Sandlund, J	TN	768

Lymphoma-Cutaneous T Cell(CTCL)

Hem	Greer, J	TN	316

Lymphoma-Ocular (eye)

Oph	Gigantelli, J	NE	596

Lymphoma-Second Opinion

Onc	Canellos, G	MA	328

Lymphomas-Rare

Hem	Rosenblatt, J	FL	317
Onc	Lossos, I	FL	359
PHO	Blum, K	OH	769

Lymphomatoid Granulomatosis

Onc	Hochberg, E	MA	330

Lysosomal Disease

CG	Desnick, R	NY	157

Lysosomal Diseases

CG	Burton, B	IL	160
CG	Charrow, J	IL	160

M

Macular Degeneration

Oph	Blumenkranz, M	CA	599
Oph	Bressler, S	MD	572
Oph	Brown, G	PA	572
Oph	Brucker, A	PA	572
Oph	Davis, J	FL	582
Oph	Del Priore, L	SC	582
Oph	Edwards, P	MI	589
Oph	Friberg, T	PA	574
Oph	Gentile, R	NY	574
Oph	Gorin, M	CA	600

Spec	Name	St	Pg
Oph	Handa, J	MD	575
Oph	Hariprasad, S	IL	590
Oph	Ho, A	PA	575
Oph	Lambert, H	TX	597
Oph	Lewis, R	TX	597
Oph	Maguire, J	PA	577
Oph	Meredith, T	NC	585
Oph	Miller, J	MA	570
Oph	Murray, T	FL	585
Oph	Nussbaum, J	GA	585
Oph	Olsen, T	GA	585
Oph	Petersen, M	OH	593
Oph	Puliafito, C	CA	603
Oph	Sadda, S	CA	603
Oph	Schwartz, S	CA	603
Oph	Sternberg, P	TN	586
Oph	Vander, J	PA	581
Oph	Walsh, J	NY	581
Oph	Williams, G	MI	595

Macular Disease/Degeneration

Oph	Chang, S	NY	572
Oph	Flynn, H	FL	583
Oph	Fuchs, W	NY	574
Oph	Grossniklaus, H	GA	583
Oph	Mieler, W	IL	592
Oph	Muldoon, T	NY	578
Oph	Rosenfeld, P	FL	586
Oph	Schiff, W	NY	579
Oph	Shabto, U	NY	580
Oph	Yannuzzi, L	NY	581

Malabsorption Syndrome

Ge	Bayless, T	MD	230
Ge	Green, P	NY	233
Ge	Seidner, D	TN	242
Ge	Semrad, C	IL	248
Ge	Toskes, P	FL	243
PGe	Baker, R	NY	750
PGe	Hill, I	NC	752
PGe	Oliva-Hemker, M	MD	751

Malaria

Inf	Trenholme, G	IL	417
Inf	Wallace, M	FL	415

Mammography

DR	Dershaw, D	NY	974
DR	Evers, K	PA	975
DR	Helvie, M	MI	980
DR	Huynh, P	TX	982
DR	Lehman, C	WA	983
DR	Mitnick, J	NY	976
DR	Monsees, B	MO	981
DR	Parikh, J	WA	983
DR	Ulissey, M	TX	982

Mantle Cell Lymphoma

Hem	Williams, M	VA	318

Marfan's Syndrome

CG	Bialer, M	NY	157
CG	Burton, B	IL	160
CG	Davis, J	NY	157
CG	Marion, R	NY	158
CG	Pauker, S	MA	156
CG	Pyeritz, R	PA	158
Cv	Braverman, A	MO	106
Cv	Devereux, R	NY	97
PCd	Gelb, B	NY	735
PCd	Hardin, J	IL	739
PCd	Mahony, L	TX	740
PCd	Moodie, D	TX	740
T&CS	Coselli, J	TX	1137
T&CS	Girardi, L	NY	1116
T&CS	Svensson, L	OH	1135

Marital/Family/Sex Therapy

Psyc	Giustra, L	GA	896
Psyc	Manevitz, A	NY	893
Psyc	Sadock, V	NY	894

Mast Cell Diseases

A&I	Castells, M	MA	84
A&I	Lewis, J	AZ	89
A&I	Metcalfe, D	MD	85
Hem	Duffy, T	CT	310

Maternal & Fetal Medicine

MF	Abuhamad, A	VA	434
MF	Acker, D	MA	430
MF	Adam, K	TX	438
MF	Adashek, J	NV	439
MF	Andrews, W	AL	434
MF	Bahado-Singh, R	MI	435
MF	Baker, E	NH	430
MF	Bartelsmeyer, J	MO	435
MF	Benedetti, T	WA	439
MF	Berkowitz, R	NY	431
MF	Besinger, R	IL	436
MF	Blakemore, K	MD	431
MF	Caritis, S	PA	432
MF	Carr, S	RI	430
MF	Cheng, E	WA	439
MF	Chmait, R	CA	440
MF	Cohen, A	PA	432
MF	Copel, J	CT	430
MF	D'Alton, M	NY	432
MF	Dooley, S	IL	436
MF	Druzin, M	CA	440
MF	Duff, W	FL	434
MF	Dugoff, L	PA	432
MF	Eddleman, K	NY	432
MF	Ferguson, J	VA	434
MF	Fox, H	MD	432
MF	Genc, M	NY	432
MF	Gibbs, R	CO	438
MF	Goldberg, J	CA	440
MF	Grandis, A	NC	434
MF	Gravett, M	WA	440

Spec	Name	St	Pg
MF	Greene, M	MA	430
MF	Grunebaum, A	NY	433
MF	Hankins, G	TX	438
MF	Heffner, L	MA	430
MF	Heyl, P	KY	434
MF	Hibbard, J	IL	436
MF	Horsager, R	TX	438
MF	Hussey, M	IL	436
MF	Ismail, M	IL	436
MF	Johnson, T	MI	436
MF	Kelly, T	CA	440
MF	Koos, B	CA	440
MF	Kuller, J	NC	435
MF	Landers, D	MN	436
MF	Landon, M	OH	436
MF	Landy, H	DC	433
MF	Leslie, K	IA	437
MF	Macones, G	MO	437
MF	Mari, G	TN	435
MF	Mastrobattista, J	TX	438
MF	McLaren, R	VA	435
MF	Moore, T	CA	440
MF	Nies, B	VA	435
MF	Norwitz, E	MA	430
MF	Paidas, M	CT	431
MF	Parry, S	PA	433
MF	Philipson, E	OH	437
MF	Pinckert, T	MD	433
MF	Plante, L	PA	433
MF	Platt, L	CA	440
MF	Pridjian, G	LA	439
MF	Reed, K	AZ	439
MF	Repke, J	PA	433
MF	Riley, L	MA	431
MF	Robertson, P	CA	441
MF	Robichaux, A	LA	439
MF	Robinson, J	MA	431
MF	Saade, G	TX	439
MF	Samuels, P	OH	437
MF	Socol, M	IL	437
MF	Strassner, H	IL	437
MF	Tabsh, K	CA	441
MF	Thomas, R	PA	433
MF	Thorp, J	NC	435
MF	Tomich, P	NE	438
MF	Treadwell, M	MI	437
MF	Van Dorsten, J	SC	435
MF	Wapner, R	NY	434
MF	Wenstrom, K	RI	431
MF	Wilkins, I	IL	437
MF	Wilkins-Haug, L	MA	431
MF	Winn, H	MO	438
MF	Zalud, I	HI	441
ObG	Corteville, J	OH	560
ObG	Ordorica, S	NY	558

Maxillofacial & Craniofacial Surgery

Spec	Name	St	Pg
PlS	Gruss, J	WA	874

Maxillofacial Surgery

Spec	Name	St	Pg
Oto	Chowdhury, K	CO	679
PlS	Burstein, F	GA	860
PlS	Deleyiannis, F	CO	869
PlS	Napoli, J	DE	857
PlS	Papay, F	OH	867
PlS	Polley, J	IL	867
PlS	Posnick, J	MD	857
PlS	Taub, P	NY	859
PlS	Urata, M	CA	877
PlS	Wolfe, S	FL	864
PlS	Zins, J	OH	869

Maze Procedure for Atrial Fibrillation

Spec	Name	St	Pg
T&CS	Argenziano, M	NY	1113
T&CS	Bridges, C	NC	1124
T&CS	Caskey, M	AZ	1137
T&CS	DeFilippi, V	CA	1141
T&CS	Fullerton, D	CO	1136
T&CS	Hashim, S	CT	1111
T&CS	Schaff, H	MN	1134
T&CS	Vlahakes, G	MA	1112

McCune-Albright Syndrome

Spec	Name	St	Pg
EDM	Kopp, P	IL	218

Mechanical Ventilation

Spec	Name	St	Pg
PCCM	Thompson, A	PA	741
Pul	Celli, B	MA	922
Pul	Harman, E	FL	931
Pul	Marini, J	MN	934
Pul	Tobin, M	IL	936

Mediastinal Tumors

Spec	Name	St	Pg
Onc	Kris, M	NY	344
Path	Moran, C	TX	718
Path	Suster, S	WI	716
T&CS	Kaiser, L	PA	1118
T&CS	Keenan, R	PA	1118
T&CS	Keller, S	NY	1118
T&CS	Kiernan, P	VA	1126
T&CS	Kucharczuk, J	PA	1119
T&CS	Orringer, M	MI	1134
T&CS	Park, B	NJ	1120
T&CS	Scott, W	PA	1121
T&CS	Vallieres, E	WA	1143

Medical Oncology

Spec	Name	St	Pg
Onc	Abbruzzese, J	TX	376
Onc	Aboulafia, D	WA	383
Onc	Abraham, J	WV	333
Onc	Abrams, D	CA	383
Onc	Adelstein, D	OH	364
Onc	Advani, R	CA	383
Onc	Aghajanian, C	NY	333
Onc	Ahlgren, J	DC	333
Onc	Ahmann, F	AZ	376

Spec	Name	St	Pg
Onc	Aisner, J	NJ	334
Onc	Ajani, J	TX	377
Onc	Akerley, W	UT	374
Onc	Albain, K	IL	364
Onc	Albertini, M	WI	364
Onc	Alberts, D	AZ	377
Onc	Algazy, K	PA	334
Onc	Ambinder, R	MD	334
Onc	Anthony, L	KY	353
Onc	Antin, J	MA	327
Onc	Antonia, S	FL	353
Onc	Appelbaum, F	WA	383
Onc	Argiris, A	TX	377
Onc	Arlen, P	MD	334
Onc	Armitage, J	NE	374
Onc	Arteaga, C	TN	353
Onc	Arun, B	TX	377
Onc	Astrow, A	NY	334
Onc	Atkins, M	DC	334
Onc	Attas, L	NJ	334
Onc	Axelrod, R	PA	335
Onc	Azzoli, C	NY	335
Onc	Back, A	WA	383
Onc	Bajorin, D	NY	335
Onc	Balducci, L	FL	353
Onc	Ball, E	CA	383
Onc	Bashevkin, M	NY	335
Onc	Beatty, P	MT	374
Onc	Beer, T	OR	384
Onc	Belani, C	PA	335
Onc	Benedetto, P	FL	353
Onc	Benjamin, R	TX	377
Onc	Bensinger, W	WA	384
Onc	Benson, A	IL	364
Onc	Bergsagel, P	AZ	377
Onc	Berlin, J	TN	353
Onc	Bernard, S	NC	353
Onc	Berry, J	CA	384
Onc	Bierman, P	NE	374
Onc	Biggs, D	DE	335
Onc	Birrer, M	MA	327
Onc	Bitran, J	IL	365
Onc	Blackwell, K	NC	354
Onc	Blobe, G	NC	354
Onc	Bolger, G	AL	354
Onc	Bolwell, B	OH	365
Onc	Bonomi, P	IL	365
Onc	Bosl, G	NY	335
Onc	Boston, B	TN	354
Onc	Brenin, C	VA	354
Onc	Brescia, F	SC	354
Onc	Brockstein, B	IL	365
Onc	Bruera, E	TX	377
Onc	Brufsky, A	PA	335
Onc	Bubley, G	MA	328
Onc	Buckner, J	MN	365
Onc	Budd, G	OH	365
Onc	Bunn, P	CO	374
Onc	Burris, H	TN	354
Onc	Burstein, H	MA	328
Onc	Butler, W	SC	354
Onc	Buys, S	UT	374

Specialty & Special Expertise Index

Spec	Name	St	Pg
Onc	Buzdar, A	TX	377
Onc	Camoriano, J	AZ	378
Onc	Canellos, G	MA	328
Onc	Carabasi, M	PA	336
Onc	Carbone, D	OH	365
Onc	Carducci, M	MD	336
Onc	Carey, L	NC	355
Onc	Carlson, R	CA	384
Onc	Carpenter, J	AL	355
Onc	Celano, P	MD	336
Onc	Chabner, B	MA	328
Onc	Chachoua, A	NY	336
Onc	Chanan-Khan, A	FL	355
Onc	Chang, J	TX	378
Onc	Chang, S	CA	384
Onc	Chao, N	NC	355
Onc	Chap, L	CA	384
Onc	Chapman, P	NY	336
Onc	Chapman, R	MI	365
Onc	Chew, H	CA	384
Onc	Chitambar, C	WI	366
Onc	Chlebowski, R	CA	384
Onc	Chow, W	CA	385
Onc	Chu, E	PA	336
Onc	Chung, K	SC	355
Onc	Clamon, G	IA	366
Onc	Clark, J	IL	366
Onc	Claxton, D	PA	336
Onc	Cleary, J	WI	366
Onc	Clinton, S	OH	366
Onc	Cobleigh, M	IL	366
Onc	Cohen, G	MD	336
Onc	Cohen, P	DC	337
Onc	Cohen, R	PA	337
Onc	Cohen, S	NY	337
Onc	Coleman, M	NY	337
Onc	Colon-Otero, G	FL	355
Onc	Come, S	MA	328
Onc	Conry, R	AL	355
Onc	Cooney, K	MI	366
Onc	Cowan, K	NE	375
Onc	Crawford, J	NC	355
Onc	Cristofanilli, M	PA	337
Onc	Crocenzi, T	OR	385
Onc	Cullen, K	MD	337
Onc	Czuczman, M	NY	337
Onc	Dakhil, S	KS	375
Onc	Daly, M	PA	337
Onc	Dang, C	PA	338
Onc	Daud, A	CA	385
Onc	Dawson, N	DC	338
Onc	De Simone, P	KY	356
Onc	Deeg, H	WA	385
Onc	DeVita, V	CT	328
Onc	Dickler, M	NY	338
Onc	DiPaola, R	NJ	338
Onc	Disis, M	WA	385
Onc	Dizon, D	MA	328
Onc	Domchek, S	PA	338
Onc	Donehower, R	MD	338
Onc	Doroshow, J	MD	338
Onc	Dowlati, A	OH	366
Onc	Dreicer, R	OH	367
Onc	Druker, B	OR	385
Onc	Dunphy, F	NC	356
Onc	Dutcher, J	NY	338
Onc	Eckhardt, S	CO	375
Onc	Edelman, M	MD	339
Onc	Einhorn, L	IN	367
Onc	Eisenberger, M	MD	339
Onc	Elias, A	CO	375
Onc	Ellis, G	WA	385
Onc	Ellis, M	MO	367
Onc	Emens, L	MD	339
Onc	Engstrom, P	PA	339
Onc	Ensminger, W	MI	367
Onc	Erban, J	MA	328
Onc	Ernstoff, M	NH	329
Onc	Estey, E	WA	385
Onc	Ettinger, D	MD	339
Onc	Fabian, C	KS	375
Onc	Fay, J	TX	378
Onc	Figlin, R	CA	386
Onc	Fine, H	MD	339
Onc	Fine, R	NY	339
Onc	Fisher, G	CA	386
Onc	Fisher, R	NY	339
Onc	Fitch, T	AZ	378
Onc	Flaherty, K	MA	329
Onc	Fleming, G	IL	367
Onc	Flinn, I	TN	356
Onc	Flomenberg, N	PA	340
Onc	Forastiere, A	MD	340
Onc	Ford, J	CA	386
Onc	Forero, A	AL	356
Onc	Forscher, C	CA	386
Onc	Foss, F	CT	329
Onc	Fossella, F	TX	378
Onc	Fox, K	PA	340
Onc	Fracasso, P	VA	356
Onc	Freedman, A	MA	329
Onc	Friedberg, J	NY	340
Onc	Friedman, H	NC	356
Onc	Fuchs, C	MA	329
Onc	Gabrilove, J	NY	340
Onc	Gandara, D	CA	386
Onc	Ganz, P	CA	386
Onc	Garber, J	MA	329
Onc	Garnick, M	MA	329
Onc	Garst, J	NC	356
Onc	Gaynor, E	IL	367
Onc	Gelmann, E	NY	340
Onc	George, D	NC	356
Onc	George, S	MA	329
Onc	Gerson, S	OH	367
Onc	Geyer, C	TX	378
Onc	Glaspy, J	CA	386
Onc	Glick, J	PA	340
Onc	Glisson, B	TX	378
Onc	Glode, L	CO	375
Onc	Gockerman, J	NC	357
Onc	Godley, P	NC	357
Onc	Gold, P	WA	386
Onc	Goldberg, R	OH	367
Onc	Goldstein, L	PA	340
Onc	Golomb, H	IL	368
Onc	Goy, A	NJ	341
Onc	Gradishar, W	IL	368
Onc	Graham, M	NC	357
Onc	Gralow, J	WA	387
Onc	Grana, G	NJ	341
Onc	Greco, F	TN	357
Onc	Grem, J	NE	375
Onc	Grosh, W	VA	357
Onc	Grossbard, M	NY	341
Onc	Grossman, S	MD	341
Onc	Grunberg, S	VT	330
Onc	Gulley, J	MD	341
Onc	Haas, N	PA	341
Onc	Hageboutros, A	NJ	341
Onc	Haley, B	TX	378
Onc	Hande, K	TN	357
Onc	Hauke, R	NE	375
Onc	Hayes, D	MI	368
Onc	Henry, D	PA	341
Onc	Herbst, R	CT	330
Onc	Higano, C	WA	387
Onc	Himelstein, A	DE	341
Onc	Hochberg, E	MA	330
Onc	Hochster, H	CT	330
Onc	Hoffman, P	IL	368
Onc	Hogan, T	WV	342
Onc	Holcombe, R	NY	342
Onc	Holland, J	NY	342
Onc	Hollister, D	CT	330
Onc	Hong, W	TX	379
Onc	Hortobagyi, G	TX	379
Onc	Horwitz, S	NY	342
Onc	Hudes, G	PA	342
Onc	Hudis, C	NY	342
Onc	Hurd, D	NC	357
Onc	Hussain, M	MI	368
Onc	Hutchins, L	AR	379
Onc	Hwu, P	TX	379
Onc	Ilson, D	NY	342
Onc	Ingle, J	MN	368
Onc	Isaacs, C	DC	343
Onc	Jacobs, C	CA	387
Onc	Jahanzeb, M	FL	357
Onc	Jillella, A	GA	358
Onc	Johnson, B	MA	330
Onc	Johnson, D	TX	379
Onc	Jonasch, E	TX	379
Onc	Jurcic, J	NY	343
Onc	Kalaycio, M	OH	368
Onc	Kalemkerian, G	MI	368
Onc	Kaminski, M	MI	369
Onc	Kane, M	CO	376
Onc	Kantoff, P	MA	330
Onc	Kaplan, L	CA	387
Onc	Karp, J	MD	343
Onc	Kaufman, P	NH	330
Onc	Kelly, K	CA	387
Onc	Kelly, W	PA	343
Onc	Kelsen, D	NY	343
Onc	Kemeny, N	NY	343

Specialty & Special Expertise Index

Spec	Name	St	Pg	Spec	Name	St	Pg	Spec	Name	St	Pg
Onc	Kesari, S	CA	387	Onc	Mitsuyasu, R	CA	388	Onc	Reed, E	AL	361
Onc	Khuri, F	GA	358	Onc	Moore, A	NY	345	Onc	Reid, T	CA	390
Onc	Kies, M	TX	379	Onc	Moore, J	NC	360	Onc	Remick, S	WV	348
Onc	Kindler, H	IL	369	Onc	Morgan, D	TN	360	Onc	Richards, J	IL	371
Onc	Kirkwood, J	PA	343	Onc	Morginstin, M	PA	345	Onc	Robert, N	VA	361
Onc	Koczywas, M	CA	387	Onc	Mortimer, J	CA	388	Onc	Robert-Vizcarrondo, F	AL	361
Onc	Kohn, E	MD	343	Onc	Motzer, R	NY	346	Onc	Romaguera, J	TX	381
Onc	Kraft, A	SC	358	Onc	Muggia, F	NY	346	Onc	Romond, E	KY	361
Onc	Kressel, B	DC	344	Onc	Muss, H	NC	360	Onc	Rosen, S	IL	371
Onc	Kris, M	NY	344	Onc	Nabell, L	AL	360	Onc	Rosove, M	CA	390
Onc	Krishnamurthi, S	OH	369	Onc	Nanus, D	NY	346	Onc	Ross, H	AZ	381
Onc	Kucuk, O	GA	358	Onc	Natale, R	CA	388	Onc	Roth, B	MO	371
Onc	Kuzel, T	IL	369	Onc	Nissenblatt, M	NJ	346	Onc	Ruggiero, J	NY	348
Onc	Kvols, L	FL	358	Onc	Northfelt, D	AZ	380	Onc	Rugo, H	CA	390
Onc	Kwak, L	TX	379	Onc	Norton, L	NY	346	Onc	Russell, C	CA	390
Onc	Lacy, J	CT	331	Onc	O'Brien, S	TX	380	Onc	Ryan, D	MA	331
Onc	Laheru, D	MD	344	Onc	O'Brien, T	OH	370	Onc	Saif, M	MA	332
Onc	Langer, C	PA	344	Onc	O'Connor, O	NY	346	Onc	Saiki, J	NM	381
Onc	Lawson, D	GA	358	Onc	O'Day, S	CA	389	Onc	Salgia, R	IL	371
Onc	Lazarus, H	OH	369	Onc	O'Regan, R	GA	360	Onc	Saltz, L	NY	348
Onc	Legare, R	RI	331	Onc	O'Reilly, E	NY	346	Onc	Samlowski, W	NV	390
Onc	Leighton, J	PA	344	Onc	O'Shaughnessy, J	TX	380	Onc	Samuels, B	ID	376
Onc	Lesser, G	NC	358	Onc	Offit, K	NY	346	Onc	Sandler, A	OR	390
Onc	Levine, E	NY	344	Onc	Oh, W	NY	347	Onc	Scheinberg, D	NY	348
Onc	Levy, M	PA	344	Onc	Olopade, O	IL	370	Onc	Scher, H	NY	348
Onc	Lilenbaum, R	FL	358	Onc	Oratz, R	NY	347	Onc	Schiffer, C	MI	371
Onc	Lim, D	CA	387	Onc	Orlowski, R	TX	380	Onc	Schilder, R	PA	349
Onc	Limentani, S	NC	359	Onc	Osborne, C	TX	381	Onc	Schiller, J	TX	381
Onc	Lippman, M	FL	359	Onc	Oster, M	NY	347	Onc	Schilsky, R	IL	372
Onc	Lippman, S	CA	387	Onc	Ozer, H	IL	370	Onc	Schnipper, L	MA	332
Onc	List, A	FL	359	Onc	Pao, W	TN	360	Onc	Schuchter, L	PA	349
Onc	Livingston, R	AZ	380	Onc	Papadopoulos, N	TX	381	Onc	Schwartz, B	MN	372
Onc	Loehrer, P	IN	369	Onc	Parker, B	CA	389	Onc	Schwartz, M	FL	362
Onc	Logothetis, C	TX	380	Onc	Parnes, H	MD	347	Onc	Scudder, S	CA	390
Onc	Loprinzi, C	MN	369	Onc	Pasche, B	AL	361	Onc	Serody, J	NC	362
Onc	Lossos, I	FL	359	Onc	Pasmantier, M	NY	347	Onc	Shapiro, C	OH	372
Onc	Lyckholm, L	VA	359	Onc	Patel, S	TX	381	Onc	Shea, T	NC	362
Onc	Lyman, G	NC	359	Onc	Patt, Y	NM	381	Onc	Sherman, C	SC	362
Onc	Lynch, J	FL	359	Onc	Pavlick, A	NY	347	Onc	Shields, P	OH	372
Onc	Lynch, T	CT	331	Onc	Peace, D	IL	370	Onc	Shin, D	GA	362
Onc	Makhoul, I	AR	380	Onc	Pecora, A	NJ	347	Onc	Shulman, L	MA	332
Onc	Maki, R	NY	345	Onc	Peereboom, D	OH	370	Onc	Sidransky, D	MD	349
Onc	Maloney, D	WA	388	Onc	Pegram, M	CA	389	Onc	Sikic, B	CA	390
Onc	Marcom, P	NC	359	Onc	Perez, E	FL	361	Onc	Silver, S	MI	372
Onc	Margolin, K	WA	388	Onc	Perry, D	DC	347	Onc	Silverman, L	NY	349
Onc	Markman, M	PA	345	Onc	Peterson, B	MN	370	Onc	Silverman, P	OH	372
Onc	Markowitz, S	OH	369	Onc	Petruska, P	MO	370	Onc	Simon, G	TX	382
Onc	Marshall, J	DC	345	Onc	Petrylak, D	CT	331	Onc	Sledge, G	IN	372
Onc	Martins, R	WA	388	Onc	Pfister, D	NY	348	Onc	Small, E	CA	391
Onc	Masters, G	DE	345	Onc	Picozzi, V	WA	389	Onc	Smith, M	MA	332
Onc	Mathew, P	MA	331	Onc	Pienta, K	MI	371	Onc	Smith, M	PA	349
Onc	Matulonis, U	MA	331	Onc	Pinto, H	CA	389	Onc	Smith, T	MD	349
Onc	Mayer, R	MA	331	Onc	Pisters, K	TX	381	Onc	Socinski, M	PA	349
Onc	McClay, E	CA	388	Onc	Pohlman, B	OH	371	Onc	Soiffer, R	MA	332
Onc	McGuire, W	MD	345	Onc	Posey, J	AL	361	Onc	Sosman, J	TN	362
Onc	Meropol, N	OH	370	Onc	Posner, M	NY	348	Onc	Sotomayor, E	FL	362
Onc	Messersmith, W	CO	376	Onc	Prados, M	CA	389	Onc	Speyer, J	NY	349
Onc	Meyskens, F	CA	388	Onc	Press, O	WA	389	Onc	Spriggs, D	NY	350
Onc	Miller, A	NC	360	Onc	Quinn, D	CA	389	Onc	Staddon, A	PA	350
Onc	Miller, D	KY	360	Onc	Raptis, G	NY	348	Onc	Stadler, W	IL	372
Onc	Miller, T	AZ	380	Onc	Ratain, M	IL	371	Onc	Stadtmauer, E	PA	350
Onc	Mintzer, D	PA	345	Onc	Ready, N	NC	361	Onc	Steen, P	ND	376

Specialty & Special Expertise Index

Spec	Name	St	Pg	Spec	Name	St	Pg	Spec	Name	St	Pg
Onc	Stewart, F	WA	391	Onc	Wingard, J	FL	364	Onc	Grosh, W	VA	357
Onc	Stockdale, F	CA	391	Onc	Wolchok, J	NY	352	Onc	Hutchins, L	AR	379
Onc	Stone, J	FL	362	Onc	Wolff, A	MD	352	Onc	Hwu, P	TX	379
Onc	Stoopler, M	NY	350	Onc	Wolff, R	TX	383	Onc	Kirkwood, J	PA	343
Onc	Stopeck, A	AZ	382	Onc	Worden, F	MI	373	Onc	Kuzel, T	IL	369
Onc	Straus, D	NY	350	Onc	Yee, D	MN	374	Onc	Lawson, D	GA	358
Onc	Strauss, G	MA	332	Onc	Yen, Y	CA	392	Onc	Margolin, K	WA	388
Onc	Strenger, R	RI	332	Onc	Yunus, F	TN	364	Onc	McClay, E	CA	388
Onc	Sun, W	PA	350	Onc	Zelenetz, A	NY	352	Onc	Meyskens, F	CA	388
Onc	Sutton, L	NC	363					Onc	Miller, D	KY	360
Onc	Swain, S	DC	350					Onc	O'Day, S	CA	389
Onc	Sweeney, C	MA	332	**Medulloblastoma**				Onc	Papadopoulos, N	TX	381
Onc	Sweetenham, J	NV	391	NS	Raffel, C	OH	489	Onc	Pavlick, A	NY	347
Onc	Taetle, R	AZ	382	PHO	Gajjar, A	TN	766	Onc	Pecora, A	NJ	347
Onc	Tagawa, S	NY	351	PHO	O'Dorisio, M	IA	772	Onc	Richards, J	IL	371
Onc	Taplin, M	MA	333					Onc	Samlowski, W	NV	390
Onc	Tempero, M	CA	391					Onc	Schuchter, L	PA	349
Onc	Tester, W	PA	351	**Melanoma**				Onc	Sosman, J	TN	362
Onc	Thigpen, J	MS	363	D	Bolognia, J	CT	182	Onc	Strauss, G	MA	332
Onc	Thompson, J	WA	391	D	Bondi, E	PA	185	Onc	Thompson, J	WA	391
Onc	Tkaczuk, K	MD	351	D	Bowen, G	UT	196	Onc	Triozzi, P	OH	373
Onc	Toppmeyer, D	NJ	351	D	Brown, M	NY	185	Onc	von Mehren, M	PA	352
Onc	Torti, F	NC	363	D	Cornelius, L	MO	193	Onc	Weber, J	FL	363
Onc	Triozzi, P	OH	373	D	Fenske, N	FL	190	Onc	Weiss, G	VA	364
Onc	Tripathy, D	CA	391	D	Gellis, S	MA	183	Onc	Wolchok, J	NY	352
Onc	Troner, M	FL	363	D	Gilchrest, B	MA	183	Oto	Califano, J	MD	658
Onc	Trump, D	NY	351	D	Greenway, H	CA	199	Oto	Singer, M	CA	687
Onc	Twardowski, P	CA	391	D	Grichnik, J	FL	191	Path	Bastian, B	CA	719
Onc	Urba, S	MI	373	D	Halpern, A	NY	186	Path	Cochran, A	CA	720
Onc	Urba, W	OR	392	D	Johnson, T	MI	193	Path	Gottlieb, G	MA	706
Onc	Vahdat, L	NY	351	D	Johr, R	FL	191	Path	Prieto, V	TX	718
Onc	Valero, V	TX	382	D	Krunic, A	IL	194	PlS	Ariyan, S	CT	850
Onc	Varadhachary, G	TX	382	D	Kupper, T	MA	183	PlS	Chang, B	PA	853
Onc	Vaughan, W	AL	363	D	Leffell, D	CT	183	PlS	Yetman, R	OH	868
Onc	Vaughn, D	PA	351	D	Lowitt, M	MD	187	PlS	Zide, B	NY	860
Onc	Venook, A	CA	392	D	Miller, S	MD	187	RadRO	Wazer, D	RI	947
Onc	Verschraegen, C	VT	333	D	Orengo, I	TX	197	RadRO	Werner-Wasik, M	PA	953
Onc	Vescio, R	CA	392	D	Pitts, J	AZ	197	S	Averbook, B	OH	1074
Onc	Vinciguerra, V	NY	351	D	Prioleau, P	NY	188	S	Bear, H	VA	1067
Onc	Vogelzang, N	NV	392	D	Rhodes, A	IL	195	S	Brady, M	NY	1054
Onc	Vokes, E	IL	373	D	Rigel, D	NY	188	S	Brown, C	IL	1075
Onc	Volberding, P	CA	392	D	Shea, C	IL	195	S	Byrd, D	WA	1094
Onc	Von Burton, G	LA	382	D	Swetter, S	CA	200	S	Chang, A	MI	1075
Onc	Von Hoff, D	AZ	382	D	Taylor, R	TX	198	S	Coit, D	NY	1055
Onc	von Mehren, M	PA	352	D	Tsao, H	MA	184	S	Cusack, J	MA	1048
Onc	Von Roenn, J	IL	373	D	Wood, G	WI	195	S	Czerniecki, B	PA	1056
Onc	Vredenburgh, J	NC	363	D	Zitelli, J	PA	189	S	Dooley, W	OK	1087
Onc	Waintraub, S	NJ	352	Hem	Milhem, M	IA	321	S	Eberlein, T	MO	1076
Onc	Waller, E	GA	363	Onc	Albertini, M	WI	364	S	Edington, H	PA	1057
Onc	Ward, J	UT	376	Onc	Atkins, M	DC	334	S	Edney, J	NE	1085
Onc	Weber, J	FL	363	Onc	Biggs, D	DE	335	S	Edwards, M	OH	1076
Onc	Weiner, G	IA	373	Onc	Brockstein, B	IL	365	S	Eisenberg, B	NH	1049
Onc	Weiner, L	DC	352	Onc	Chapman, P	NY	336	S	Essner, R	CA	1095
Onc	Weisberg, T	ME	333	Onc	Chow, W	CA	385	S	Fraker, D	PA	1057
Onc	Weiss, G	VA	364	Onc	Clark, J	IL	366	S	Graham, R	MA	1049
Onc	Wetzler, M	NY	352	Onc	Cohen, G	MD	336	S	Gray, R	AZ	1088
Onc	Wicha, M	MI	373	Onc	Cohen, S	NY	337	S	Huth, J	TX	1089
Onc	Wierman, A	NV	392	Onc	Conry, R	AL	355	S	Johnson Miller, D	IN	1078
Onc	Wilding, G	WI	373	Onc	Daud, A	CA	385	S	Kaufman, H	IL	1078
Onc	Willson, J	TX	382	Onc	Dutcher, J	NY	338	S	Kavanah, M	MA	1050
Onc	Wilson, W	MD	352	Onc	Ernstoff, M	NH	329	S	Kelley, M	TN	1069
Onc	Winer, E	MA	333	Onc	Fay, J	TX	378	S	Kim, J	OH	1078
				Onc	Glaspy, J	CA	386				

Spec	Name	St	Pg
S	Krag, D	VT	1050
S	Kuhn, J	TX	1090
S	Lee, J	TX	1090
S	Leitch, A	TX	1090
S	Loggie, B	NE	1085
S	Mansfield, P	TX	1091
S	McCabe, D	AZ	1091
S	McMasters, K	KY	1070
S	Moley, J	MO	1080
S	Nathanson, S	MI	1080
S	Neifeld, J	VA	1071
S	Olson, J	MD	1061
S	Pockaj, B	AZ	1091
S	Rosenberg, S	MD	1063
S	Roses, D	NY	1063
S	Ross, M	TX	1092
S	Schwartzentruber, D	IN	1082
S	Sener, S	CA	1099
S	Shapiro, R	NY	1064
S	Shen, P	NC	1072
S	Shenk, R	OH	1082
S	Sigurdson, E	PA	1064
S	Slingluff, C	VA	1072
S	Sondak, V	FL	1072
S	Talamonti, M	IL	1083
S	Tanabe, K	MA	1052
S	Tyler, D	NC	1073
S	Tyler, D	NC	1073
S	Urist, M	AL	1073
S	Wallace, A	CA	1100
S	White, R	NC	1073
S	Yeung, R	WA	1101

Melanoma Early Detection/Prevention

D	Halpern, A	NY	186
D	Rhodes, A	IL	195
D	Schultz, N	NY	188
D	Swetter, S	CA	200

Melanoma Genetics

D	Tsao, H	MA	184

Melanoma Risk Assessment

D	Lessin, S	PA	187
D	Rhodes, A	IL	195

Melanoma-Advanced

Onc	Albertini, M	WI	364
Onc	Flaherty, K	MA	329
Onc	O'Day, S	CA	389

Melanoma-Choroidal (eye)

Oph	Abramson, D	NY	571
Oph	Augsburger, J	OH	588
Oph	Dutton, J	NC	583
Oph	Finger, P	NY	573
Oph	Grossniklaus, H	GA	583
Oph	Handa, J	MD	575

Oph	Harbour, J	FL	584
Oph	Schachat, A	OH	594
Oph	Shields, C	PA	580
Oph	Shields, J	PA	580
Oph	Wilson, M	TN	587
RadRO	Crocker, I	GA	954

Melanoma-Head & Neck

D	Fewkes, J	MA	183
Oto	Bradford, C	MI	673
Oto	Myers, J	TX	683
PlS	Stadelmann, W	NH	851

Memory Disorders

Ger	Ciocon, J	FL	263
Ger	Raji, M	TX	266
Ger	Sachs, G	IN	265
GerPsy	Borson, S	WA	915
GerPsy	Stein, E	CA	915
N	Doody, R	TX	533
N	Heilman, K	FL	521
N	Henderson, V	CA	537
N	Jordan, B	NY	512
N	Kelly, J	CO	531
N	Relkin, N	NY	517
N	Sadowsky, C	FL	523
N	Weinberg, H	NY	519
N	Zimmerman, E	NY	519
NRad	Murtagh, F	FL	988
Psyc	Arnold, S	PA	890
Psyc	Marin, D	NY	894
Psyc	Weiner, M	TX	900

Memory Loss

GerPsy	Small, G	CA	915

Men's Health

U	Bans, L	AZ	1172

Meniere's Disease

Oto	Arriaga, M	LA	681
Oto	Beatty, C	MN	673
Oto	Caldarelli, D	IL	674
Oto	Farrior, J	FL	668
Oto	Hammerschlag, P	NY	660
Oto	Harris, J	CA	685
Oto	Lambert, P	SC	669
Oto	Mattox, D	GA	669
Oto	Paparella, M	MN	677
Oto	Rauch, S	MA	656
Oto	Silverstein, H	FL	671
Oto	Wazen, J	FL	672

Meningioma

NS	Bederson, J	NY	472
NS	Bruce, J	NY	473
NS	Gutin, P	NY	474
NS	Krisht, A	AR	493

NS	Liu, C	CA	497
NS	McDermott, M	CA	498
NS	Olivi, A	MD	477
NS	Sisti, M	NY	479
RadRO	Loeffler, J	MA	947

Meningioma-Orbital (eye)

Oph	Cockerham, K	CA	600

Meningitis

Inf	Quagliarello, V	CT	410
Inf	Scheld, W	VA	415
PInf	Bradley, J	CA	784
PInf	Kaplan, S	TX	784
PInf	Kleiman, M	IN	783
PInf	McCracken, G	TX	784
PInf	Wald, E	WI	783

Menopause Problems

ObG	Filip, S	NC	559
ObG	Simon, J	DC	558
RE	Blackwell, R	AL	1011
RE	Fritz, M	NC	1011
RE	Johnson, J	MA	1007
RE	Luciano, A	CT	1007
RE	Richardson, M	KS	1015
RE	Smith, Y	MI	1014
RE	Weiss, G	NJ	1010

Menopause-Male

Ger	Morley, J	MO	265

Menstrual Disorders

AM	MacKenzie, R	CA	82
AM	Murray, P	WV	80
ObG	Berga, S	NC	559
ObG	Bradley, L	OH	560
ObG	Bradshaw, K	TX	563
RE	Chang, R	CA	1017
RE	Houmard, B	WA	1017
RE	Legro, R	PA	1009

Mental Retardation

CG	Davis, J	NY	157
CG	Falk, R	CA	162
CG	Graham, J	CA	162
CG	Stevenson, R	SC	159
ChAP	McDougle, C	MA	907
ChAP	Pomeroy, J	NY	909

Mercury Toxic Exposure

OM	Gochfeld, M	NJ	882

Merkel Cell Carcinoma

D	Nghiem, P	WA	200
Onc	Kelsen, D	NY	343
Onc	Pavlick, A	NY	347

Specialty & Special Expertise Index

Spec	Name	St	Pg
Onc	Samlowski, W	NV	390
PlS	Tufaro, A	MD	860
RadRO	Morrison, W	TX	965
S	Brady, M	NY	1054
S	Cusack, J	MA	1048

Mesothelioma

Spec	Name	St	Pg
Onc	Aisner, J	NJ	334
Onc	Bonomi, P	IL	365
Onc	Bunn, P	CO	374
Onc	Carbone, D	OH	365
Onc	Dakhil, S	KS	375
Onc	Ilson, D	NY	342
Onc	Johnson, B	MA	330
Onc	Johnson, B	MA	330
Onc	Kalemkerian, G	MI	368
Onc	Khuri, F	GA	358
Onc	Kindler, H	IL	369
Onc	Langer, C	PA	344
Onc	Martins, R	WA	388
Onc	Robert-Vizcarrondo, F	AL	361
Onc	Ross, H	AZ	381
Onc	Salgia, R	IL	371
Onc	Shin, D	GA	362
Onc	Simon, G	TX	382
Onc	Vogelzang, N	NV	392
Path	Cagle, P	TX	717
Path	Moran, C	TX	718
Pul	Sterman, D	PA	928
RadRO	Choi, N	MA	946
RadRO	Videtic, G	OH	962
S	Loggie, B	NE	1085
T&CS	Battafarano, R	MD	1114
T&CS	Bueno, R	MA	1110
T&CS	Cameron, R	CA	1140
T&CS	Colson, Y	MA	1110
T&CS	Flores, R	NY	1115
T&CS	Friedberg, J	PA	1116
T&CS	Handy, J	OR	1141
T&CS	Harpole, D	NC	1125
T&CS	Jablons, D	CA	1142
T&CS	Landreneau, R	PA	1119
T&CS	Mason, D	OH	1133
T&CS	Miller, D	GA	1127
T&CS	Pass, H	NY	1120
T&CS	Rice, D	TX	1139
T&CS	Robinson, L	FL	1129
T&CS	Rusch, V	NY	1121
T&CS	Smythe, W	TX	1139
T&CS	Sugarbaker, D	MA	1112
T&CS	Swisher, S	TX	1139
T&CS	Vallieres, E	WA	1143
T&CS	Vigneswaran, W	IL	1135
T&CS	Weigel, T	WI	1135
T&CS	Wood, D	WA	1143
T&CS	Yang, S	MD	1123

Metabolic Disorders

Spec	Name	St	Pg
ChiN	Ashwal, S	CA	153
ChiN	De Vivo, D	NY	147
ChiN	Patterson, M	MN	151

Spec	Name	St	Pg
EDM	Akatsu, H	CA	222
EDM	Cohen, R	OH	216
EDM	Dobs, A	MD	210
IM	Rader, D	PA	424

Metabolic Genetic Disorders

Spec	Name	St	Pg
CG	Bialer, M	NY	157
CG	Ward, J	TN	159

Metabolic Syndrome

Spec	Name	St	Pg
AM	Chambers, C	PA	80
Cv	Linton, M	TN	104
Cv	Reis, S	PA	101
EDM	Schwartz, S	PA	212
EDM	Thorner, M	VA	215
PEn	DeLuca, F	PA	744
PEn	Lustig, R	CA	749
PEn	Maclaren, N	NY	744

Metastatic Cancer

Spec	Name	St	Pg
S	Ellis, L	TX	1088

Microcystic Adnexal Carcinoma

Spec	Name	St	Pg
D	Russell, M	VA	192

Microdiscectomy

Spec	Name	St	Pg
NS	Chen, T	CA	496
NS	Haid, R	GA	482
NS	Maroon, J	PA	477
OrS	Boden, S	GA	628

Microscopic Colitis

Spec	Name	St	Pg
Ge	Bayless, T	MD	230
Ge	Loftus, E	MN	247

Microsurgery

Spec	Name	St	Pg
CRS	Orkin, B	MA	168
HS	Bishop, A	MN	300
HS	Cendales, L	GA	299
HS	Culp, R	PA	295
HS	Fischer, T	IN	300
HS	Friedman, D	FL	299
HS	Idler, R	CO	302
HS	Lubahn, J	PA	297
HS	Mih, A	IN	301
HS	Rayan, G	OK	303
HS	Slutsky, D	CA	304
HS	Stern, P	OH	302
NS	Barrow, D	GA	481
NS	Chen, C	NY	473
NS	Reid, W	TN	484
NS	Selman, W	OH	490
Oto	Strome, S	MD	665
PlS	Allen, R	SC	860
PlS	Andersen, J	CA	873
PlS	Brandt, K	MO	865
PlS	Chang, B	PA	853
PlS	Dagum, A	NY	853

Spec	Name	St	Pg
PlS	Disa, J	NY	853
PlS	Fix, R	AL	861
PlS	Levin, L	PA	855
PlS	Levine, J	NY	855
PlS	Low, D	PA	855
PlS	Mehrara, B	NY	856
PlS	Neumeister, M	IL	867
PlS	Rockwell, W	UT	869
PlS	Rodriguez, E	MD	857
PlS	Sanger, J	WI	867
PlS	Siebert, J	WI	868
PlS	Siemionow, M	OH	868
PlS	Topham, N	PA	859
PlS	Wilkins, E	MI	868
PlS	Yetman, R	OH	868
RE	Christman, G	MI	1012
RE	Goldberg, J	OH	1013
RE	Yee, B	CA	1018
U	Fisch, H	NY	1152
U	Sabanegh, E	OH	1170
U	Turek, P	CA	1179

Microvascular Surgery

Spec	Name	St	Pg
NS	Martin, N	CA	498
Oto	Blackwell, K	CA	684
Oto	Couch, M	VT	655
Oto	Hayden, R	AZ	682
Oto	Rosenthal, E	AL	670
Oto	Wax, M	OR	687

Migraine

Spec	Name	St	Pg
ChiN	Epstein, L	IL	150
ChiN	Hershey, A	OH	150
ChiN	Maytal, J	NY	148
ChiN	Nass, R	NY	148
ChiN	Sankar, R	CA	154
ChiN	Sivaswamy, L	MI	151
N	Buchholz, D	MD	510
N	Charles, A	CA	536
N	Cutrer, F	MN	526
N	Dodick, D	AZ	533
N	Finkel, A	NC	521
N	Lane, J	CO	532
N	Rothrock, J	NV	538
N	Sabo, T	CO	532
N	Saper, J	MI	530
N	Silberstein, S	PA	517
N	Swanson, J	MN	530
N	Wright, R	IL	531
PM	Loder, E	MA	696
PM	Robbins, L	IL	700

Migraine in Women

Spec	Name	St	Pg
N	Rubin, S	IL	530

Migraine-Chronic

Spec	Name	St	Pg
PM	Freitag, F	TX	701

Minimally Invasive Cardiac

Specialty & Special Expertise Index

Spec	Name	St	Pg
Surgery			
T&CS	Adams, D	NY	1113
T&CS	Aklog, L	AZ	1137
T&CS	Aldea, G	WA	1140
T&CS	Bacha, E	NY	1114
T&CS	Bakhos, M	IL	1130
T&CS	Bichell, D	TN	1123
T&CS	Boyd, W	CA	1140
T&CS	Bridges, C	NC	1124
T&CS	Chitwood, W	NC	1124
T&CS	Damiano, R	MO	1131
T&CS	DeFilippi, V	CA	1141
T&CS	DeRose, J	NY	1115
T&CS	Furukawa, S	PA	1116
T&CS	Grossi, E	NY	1117
T&CS	Guyton, R	GA	1125
T&CS	Hargrove, W	PA	1117
T&CS	Horvath, K	MD	1117
T&CS	Joyce, L	MN	1133
T&CS	Lang, S	NY	1119
T&CS	Loulmet, D	NY	1119
T&CS	Murphy, D	GA	1127
T&CS	Oz, M	NY	1120
T&CS	Panos, A	FL	1128
T&CS	Rastegar, H	MA	1112
T&CS	Shemin, R	CA	1142
T&CS	Smith, C	NY	1121
T&CS	Woo, Y	PA	1123
Minimally Invasive Esophageal Surgery			
T&CS	Bueno, R	MA	1110
Minimally Invasive Gynecologic Surgery			
RE	Haney, A	IL	1013
Minimally Invasive Heart Valve Surgery			
T&CS	Filsoufi, F	NY	1115
T&CS	Galloway, A	NY	1116
T&CS	Graver, L	NY	1117
T&CS	Guber, M	CO	1136
T&CS	Guy, T	PA	1117
T&CS	Jeevanandam, V	IL	1133
T&CS	Savage, E	FL	1129
Minimally Invasive Neurosurgery			
NS	Theodore, N	AZ	494
Minimally Invasive Spinal Surgery			
NRad	Hirsch, J	MA	984
NS	Branch, C	NC	481
NS	Bray, R	CA	496
NS	Brown, F	IL	486
NS	Fessler, R	IL	487
NS	Foley, K	TN	481
NS	Haid, R	GA	482
NS	Hartl, R	NY	475
NS	Kaiser, M	NY	475
NS	Levi, A	FL	482
NS	Maroon, J	PA	477
NS	Naff, N	MD	477
NS	Reid, W	TN	484
NS	Sekhon, L	NV	499
OrS	Cammisa, F	NY	615
OrS	Cappuccino, A	NY	615
OrS	Delamarter, R	CA	642
OrS	Garfin, S	CA	643
OrS	Goldstein, J	NY	618
OrS	Hecht, A	NY	619
OrS	Hilibrand, A	PA	619
OrS	Kim, C	CA	644
OrS	Riew, K	MO	637
Minimally Invasive Surgery			
CRS	Beck, D	LA	176
CRS	Geisler, D	PA	170
CRS	Wise, P	MO	175
GO	Carney, M	HI	289
GO	Fishman, D	NY	278
GO	Poliakoff, S	FL	282
GO	Schorge, J	MA	275
NS	Bauer, J	IL	486
NS	Caputy, A	DC	473
NS	Cohen, A	MA	470
NS	Ellenbogen, R	WA	496
NS	Jho, H	PA	475
NS	Lemole, G	AZ	493
NS	Sandberg, D	TX	494
NS	Schwartz, T	NY	478
NS	Souweidane, M	NY	479
ObG	Bartholomew, D	OH	560
ObG	Einarsson, J	MA	556
ObG	Famuyide, A	MN	561
ObG	Jenkins, T	AL	559
ObG	Maynard, S	DC	558
ObG	Visco, A	NC	560
ObG	Young, B	NY	558
OrS	Haas, S	NY	618
OrS	Jiranek, W	VA	629
OrS	Macaulay, W	NY	622
OrS	Sandhu, H	NY	625
OrS	Tornetta, P	MA	613
OrS	Vo, P	FL	631
OrS	Wetzel, F	PA	626
Oto	Akervall, J	MI	672
Oto	Kennedy, D	PA	661
Oto	Orloff, L	CA	686
Oto	Rosenthal, E	AL	670
PS	Barksdale, E	OH	806
PS	Black, C	TX	809
PS	Doody, D	MA	801
PS	Ford, H	CA	810
PS	Gaines, B	PA	803
PS	Holterman, M	IL	807
PS	Kane, T	DC	803
PS	Krummel, T	CA	811
PS	Lobe, T	CA	811
PS	Moss, R	OH	807
PS	Nakayama, D	GA	805
PS	Rodgers, B	VA	806
PS	Spigland, N	NY	804
PS	Voigt, R	MD	804
PS	Waldhausen, J	WA	811
RE	Falcone, T	OH	1013
RE	Isaacson, K	MA	1007
RE	Miller, C	IL	1014
RE	Petrozza, J	MA	1007
RE	Putman, J	TX	1016
RE	Sanfilippo, J	PA	1010
S	Bellows, C	LA	1087
S	Brodsky, J	PA	1054
S	Brooks, A	PA	1054
S	Brunt, L	MO	1075
S	Cherqui, D	NY	1055
S	Courcoulas, A	PA	1056
S	Curcillo, P	PA	1056
S	Duh, Q	CA	1095
S	Duncan, M	MD	1056
S	Fahey, T	NY	1057
S	Fitzgibbons, R	NE	1085
S	Frantzides, C	IL	1077
S	Horvath, K	WA	1096
S	Ikramuddin, S	MN	1078
S	Koruda, M	NC	1069
S	Lee, K	PA	1059
S	Morton, J	CA	1097
S	Nissen, N	CA	1098
S	Ponsky, J	OH	1080
S	Ramanathan, R	PA	1062
S	Rattner, D	MA	1051
S	Rogers, S	CA	1099
S	Rosemurgy, A	FL	1071
S	Rosen, M	OH	1081
S	Schauer, P	OH	1082
S	Schraut, W	PA	1064
S	Shibata, D	FL	1072
S	Simmons, R	NY	1064
S	Swanstrom, L	OR	1100
S	Sweeney, J	GA	1073
S	Tuttle, T	MN	1083
T&CS	Cassivi, S	MN	1131
T&CS	Cohen, N	MD	1114
T&CS	Cohen, R	CA	1141
T&CS	Del-Nido, P	MA	1110
T&CS	Ferguson, M	IL	1132
T&CS	Fontana, G	NY	1115
T&CS	Lazzaro, R	NY	1119
T&CS	Liao, K	MN	1133
T&CS	Mack, M	TX	1139
T&CS	Rice, D	TX	1139
T&CS	Rosengart, T	NY	1121
T&CS	Swistel, D	NY	1122
U	Balaji, K	NC	1160
U	Docimo, S	PA	1152
U	Irby, P	NC	1161
U	Kane, M	MD	1154
U	Kibel, A	MA	1149

Specialty & Special Expertise Index

Spec	Name	St	Pg
U	McVary, K	IL	1168
U	Merguerian, P	WA	1178
VascS	Flanigan, D	CA	1194
VascS	Lumsden, A	TX	1193

Minimally Invasive Surgery-Pediatric

Spec	Name	St	Pg
U	Poppas, D	NY	1156

Minimally Invasive Thoracic Surgery

Spec	Name	St	Pg
T&CS	Baciewicz, F	MI	1130
T&CS	Brinckerhoff, L	MA	1110
T&CS	Bueno, R	MA	1110
T&CS	Demmy, T	NY	1115
T&CS	Fernando, H	MA	1111
T&CS	Howington, J	IL	1132
T&CS	Jones, D	VA	1125
T&CS	Krellenstein, D	NY	1118
T&CS	Mason, D	OH	1133
T&CS	Nesbitt, J	TN	1127
T&CS	Nguyen, D	FL	1127
T&CS	Rice, T	OH	1134
T&CS	Sonett, J	NY	1121
T&CS	Weksler, B	PA	1123

Minimally Invasive Urologic Surgery

Spec	Name	St	Pg
U	Andrews, P	AZ	1172
U	Carpinito, G	MA	1148
U	Gill, I	CA	1176
U	Gluckman, G	IL	1167
U	Gomella, L	PA	1153
U	Hall, S	NY	1153
U	Kaouk, J	OH	1167
U	Kawachi, M	CA	1177
U	Landman, J	CA	1177
U	Lanteri, V	NJ	1154
U	Miller, S	GA	1162
U	Moul, J	NC	1162
U	Strup, S	KY	1164
U	Trabulsi, E	PA	1158
U	Uzzo, R	PA	1158
U	Wilson, T	CA	1179

Minimally Invasive Vascular Surgery

Spec	Name	St	Pg
VascS	Ahn, S	CA	1193
VascS	Benvenisty, A	NY	1186
VascS	Brener, B	NJ	1186
VascS	McLafferty, R	IL	1191
VascS	Morrissey, N	NY	1188
VascS	Schneider, D	NY	1188
VascS	Todd, G	NY	1189

Miscarriage-Recurrent

Spec	Name	St	Pg
MF	Druzin, M	CA	440
MF	Landy, H	DC	433
MF	Paidas, M	CT	431

Spec	Name	St	Pg
ObG	Ordorica, S	NY	558
ObG	Scher, J	NY	558
ObG	Young, B	NY	558
RE	Barnes, R	IL	1012
RE	DeVane, G	FL	1011
RE	Hill, J	NH	1006
RE	Houmard, B	WA	1017
RE	Kutteh, W	TN	1012
RE	Odem, R	MO	1014
RE	Ratts, V	MO	1014
RE	Walmer, D	NC	1012

Mitochondrial Disorders

Spec	Name	St	Pg
CG	Boles, R	CA	162
CG	Craigen, W	TX	161
CG	Shoffner, J	GA	159
ChiN	Cohen, B	OH	150
ChiN	Haas, R	CA	153
ChiN	Legido, A	PA	148

Mitral Valve Prolapse

Spec	Name	St	Pg
Cv	Andersen, H	NY	96

Mitral Valve Robotic Surgery

Spec	Name	St	Pg
T&CS	Hargrove, W	PA	1117
T&CS	Murphy, D	GA	1127
T&CS	Smith, J	OH	1135
T&CS	Woo, Y	PA	1123

Mitral Valve Surgery

Spec	Name	St	Pg
IC	Gray, W	NY	127
IC	Yeung, A	CA	133
T&CS	Adams, D	NY	1113
T&CS	Aklog, L	AZ	1137
T&CS	Bakhos, M	IL	1130
T&CS	Bolman, R	MA	1110
T&CS	Chitwood, W	NC	1124
T&CS	DeFilippi, V	CA	1141
T&CS	DeRose, J	NY	1115
T&CS	Filsoufi, F	NY	1115
T&CS	Fontana, G	NY	1115
T&CS	Fullerton, D	CO	1136
T&CS	Galloway, A	NY	1116
T&CS	Grossi, E	NY	1117
T&CS	Hashim, S	CT	1111
T&CS	Miller, D	CA	1142
T&CS	Moon, M	MO	1134
T&CS	Naka, Y	NY	1120
T&CS	Savage, E	FL	1129
T&CS	Slaughter, M	KY	1129
T&CS	Smith, C	NY	1121

Mobility Evaluation & Treatment

Spec	Name	St	Pg
Ger	Allman, R	AL	263
Ger	Cooney, L	CT	262
Ger	Studenski, S	PA	263
PMR	Esquenazi, A	PA	835

Mohs' Surgery

Spec	Name	St	Pg
D	Amonette, R	TN	189
D	Arpey, C	MN	192
D	Bailin, P	OH	192
D	Bennett, R	CA	198
D	Berg, D	WA	198
D	Bowen, G	UT	196
D	Braun, M	DC	185
D	Brodland, D	PA	185
D	Brown, M	NY	185
D	Carney, J	AR	196
D	Cook, J	NC	190
D	Dufresne, R	RI	182
D	Dzubow, L	PA	186
D	Fewkes, J	MA	183
D	Flowers, F	FL	190
D	Fosko, S	MO	193
D	Garrett, A	VA	190
D	Geronemus, R	NY	186
D	Glogau, R	CA	199
D	Green, H	FL	191
D	Greenbaum, S	PA	186
D	Greenway, H	CA	199
D	Hanke, C	IN	193
D	Hruza, G	MO	193
D	Johnson, T	MI	193
D	Kriegel, D	NY	187
D	Krunic, A	IL	194
D	Lask, G	CA	199
D	Leffell, D	CT	183
D	Leshin, B	NC	191
D	Lim Quan, K	AZ	197
D	Linder, J	AZ	197
D	Maloney, M	MA	183
D	Miller, S	MD	187
D	Neel, V	MA	184
D	Neuburg, M	WI	194
D	Nouri, K	FL	191
D	Olbricht, S	MA	184
D	Orengo, I	TX	197
D	Otley, C	MN	194
D	Perone, J	TX	197
D	Pitts, J	AZ	197
D	Prioleau, P	NY	188
D	Ratner, D	NY	188
D	Richardson, T	CA	200
D	Russell, M	VA	192
D	Swanson, N	OR	200
D	Taylor, R	TX	198
D	Wheeland, R	AZ	198
D	Zitelli, J	PA	189

Mood Disorders

Spec	Name	St	Pg
ChAP	Abright, A	NY	907
ChAP	Alessi, N	MI	910
ChAP	Bogrov, M	MD	908
ChAP	Boxer, G	MO	910
ChAP	Foley, C	NY	908
ChAP	Luby, J	MO	911
ChAP	Riddle, M	MD	909
GerPsy	Holroyd, S	VA	914

Spec	Name	St	Pg
GerPsy	Manepalli, J	MO	914
Psyc	Blazer, D	NC	895
Psyc	Gitlin, M	CA	901
Psyc	Hoffman, D	CO	899
Psyc	Janicak, P	IL	897
Psyc	Mann, J	NY	893
Psyc	Pi, E	CA	902

Motion Sickness

Spec	Name	St	Pg
N	Hain, T	IL	526

Motor Control Analysis

Spec	Name	St	Pg
PMR	Mayer, N	PA	837

Movement Disorders

Spec	Name	St	Pg
ChiN	Dure, L	AL	149
ChiN	Lavenstein, B	VA	149
ChiN	Mink, J	NY	148
ChiN	Noetzel, M	MO	151
N	Ahlskog, J	MN	524
N	Aminoff, M	CA	535
N	Ashizawa, T	FL	520
N	Azizi, S	PA	509
N	Baser, S	PA	509
N	Bressman, S	NY	509
N	Bruno, M	HI	535
N	Busis, N	PA	510
N	DeLong, M	GA	520
N	Fahn, S	NY	511
N	Flaherty, A	MA	507
N	Goetz, C	IL	526
N	Golbe, L	NJ	512
N	Hauser, R	FL	521
N	Hurtig, H	PA	512
N	Jankovic, J	TX	534
N	Langston, J	CA	537
N	Lew, M	CA	537
N	Maraganore, D	IL	528
N	Montgomery, E	AL	522
N	Nutt, J	OR	538
N	Olanow, C	NY	516
N	Perlmutter, J	MO	528
N	Reich, S	MD	517
N	Samii, A	WA	538
N	Sethi, K	GA	523
N	Shulman, L	MD	517
N	Singer, C	FL	524
N	Stern, M	PA	518
N	Tanner, C	CA	539
N	Tetrud, J	CA	539
N	Waters, C	NY	518
N	Watts, R	AL	524
N	Weiner, W	MD	519
N	Wooten, G	VA	524
N	Young, A	MA	509
NS	Baltuch, G	PA	472
NS	Burchiel, K	OR	496
NS	Hodes, J	KY	482
NS	Kondziolka, D	PA	476
NS	Lunsford, L	PA	476
NS	Nazzaro, J	KS	491
NS	Penar, P	VT	471
NS	Whiting, D	PA	480
PMR	Ivanhoe, C	TX	843

Movement Disorders-Botox Therapy

Spec	Name	St	Pg
N	Shulman, L	MD	517

Movement Disorders-Lower Limb

Spec	Name	St	Pg
N	Finkel, M	FL	521

MoyaMoya Disease

Spec	Name	St	Pg
N	Mohr, J	NY	516
NS	Harbaugh, R	PA	474
NS	Steinberg, G	CA	499
NS	Wilson, J	NC	485

MRI

Spec	Name	St	Pg
DR	Bluemke, D	MD	974
DR	Cohen, B	NY	974
DR	Dalinka, M	PA	974
DR	Edelman, R	IL	980
DR	Elster, A	NC	979
DR	Fidler, J	MN	980
DR	Kanal, E	PA	976
DR	Partain, C	TN	979
DR	Reinus, W	PA	977
DR	Weinreb, J	CT	973
DR	Yoon, S	NY	978
DR	Zagoria, R	NC	980
N	Kuzniecky, R	NY	513
NRad	Barkovich, A	CA	990
NRad	Burdette, J	NC	987
NRad	Johnson, A	NC	987
NRad	Khandji, A	NY	985
NRad	Modic, M	OH	989
NRad	Sze, G	CT	985
NRad	Thulborn, K	IL	989

MRI & CT of Brain & Spine

Spec	Name	St	Pg
NRad	Drayer, B	NY	985
NRad	Hesselink, J	CA	991

MRI Angiography

Spec	Name	St	Pg
DR	Prince, M	NY	977

MRI-Brain & Spine

Spec	Name	St	Pg
NRad	Atlas, S	CA	990

MRI-Breast

Spec	Name	St	Pg
DR	Evers, K	PA	975
DR	Lehman, C	WA	983
DR	Stough, R	OK	982

Mucositis

Spec	Name	St	Pg
RadRO	Martenson, J	MN	961

Muir-Torre Syndrome

Spec	Name	St	Pg
D	Olbricht, S	MA	184

Multiple Gestation

Spec	Name	St	Pg
MF	Abuhamad, A	VA	434
MF	Acker, D	MA	430
MF	Bartelsmeyer, J	MO	435
MF	Berkowitz, R	NY	431
MF	Carr, S	RI	430
MF	D'Alton, M	NY	432
MF	Dooley, S	IL	436
MF	Fox, H	MD	432
MF	Greene, M	MA	430
MF	Hussey, M	IL	436
MF	Landy, H	DC	433
MF	Socol, M	IL	437
MF	Thorp, J	NC	435
MF	Wapner, R	NY	434
MF	Wilkins, I	IL	437
MF	Winn, H	MO	438
NP	Muraskas, J	IL	451
ObG	Evans, M	NY	557
ObG	Witter, F	MD	558

Multiple Myeloma

Spec	Name	St	Pg
Hem	Allen, S	NY	311
Hem	Anderson, K	MA	310
Hem	Barlogie, B	AR	323
Hem	Copelan, E	OH	319
Hem	Djulbegovic, B	FL	316
Hem	Emanuel, P	AR	323
Hem	Farag, S	IN	319
Hem	Fonseca, R	AZ	324
Hem	Friedman, A	PA	312
Hem	Gertz, M	MN	319
Hem	Goldberg, J	PA	312
Hem	Gregory, S	IL	320
Hem	Linenberger, M	WA	326
Hem	Lyons, R	TX	324
Hem	Marks, S	PA	313
Hem	Mears, J	NY	313
Hem	Rai, K	NY	314
Hem	Raphael, B	NY	314
Hem	Rapoport, A	MD	314
Hem	Richardson, P	MA	311
Hem	Roodman, G	IN	321
Hem	Rosenblatt, J	FL	317
Hem	Savage, D	NY	314
Hem	Singhal, S	IL	321
Hem	Solberg, L	FL	318
Hem	Stewart, A	AZ	324
Hem	Strair, R	NJ	315
Hem	Williams, M	VA	318
NuM	Wiseman, G	MN	550
Onc	Aboulafia, D	WA	383
Onc	Ball, E	CA	383
Onc	Bensinger, W	WA	384

Spec	Name	St	Pg
Onc	Bergsagel, P	AZ	377
Onc	Chanan-Khan, A	FL	355
Onc	Coleman, M	NY	337
Onc	Czuczman, M	NY	337
Onc	Flinn, I	TN	356
Onc	Foss, F	CT	329
Onc	Gerson, S	OH	367
Onc	Jillella, A	GA	358
Onc	Kwak, L	TX	379
Onc	Lazarus, H	OH	369
Onc	O'Brien, T	OH	370
Onc	Orlowski, R	TX	380
Onc	Schiffer, C	MI	371
Onc	Silverman, L	NY	349
Onc	Smith, M	PA	349
Onc	Stadtmauer, E	PA	350
Onc	Straus, D	NY	350
Onc	Vescio, R	CA	392
Onc	Wingard, J	FL	364
Onc	Yunus, F	TN	364
OrS	Biermann, J	MI	632
RadRO	Meredith, R	AL	956
RadRO	Wong, J	CA	968
RadRO	Yahalom, J	NY	953

Multiple Sclerosis

N	Apatoff, B	NY	509
N	Arnason, B	IL	524
N	Berger, J	KY	520
N	Brooks, B	NC	520
N	Calabresi, P	MD	510
N	Cohen, J	OH	525
N	Cook, S	NJ	510
N	Corey-Bloom, J	CA	536
N	Coyle, P	NY	510
N	Elias, S	MI	526
N	Farlow, M	IN	526
N	Filley, C	CO	531
N	Frohman, E	TX	533
N	Galetta, S	PA	512
N	Gilden, D	CO	531
N	Gilman, S	MI	526
N	Goodin, D	CA	537
N	Hauser, S	CA	537
N	Lisak, R	MI	527
N	Lublin, F	NY	515
N	McArthur, J	MD	515
N	Miller, A	NY	516
N	Morgenlander, J	NC	522
N	Petito, F	NY	516
N	Pulst, S	UT	532
N	Reder, A	IL	529
N	Reed, N	OH	529
N	Roos, R	IL	529
N	Swerdlow, M	NY	518
N	Vas, G	NY	518
N	Vollmer, T	CO	532
N	Weiner, L	CA	539
N	Windebank, A	MN	530
N	Wolinsky, J	TX	535
PMR	Sliwa, J	IL	842

Multiple Sclerosis Imaging

NRad	Provenzale, J	NC	988

Multiple Sclerosis in Women

N	Rubin, S	IL	530

Multiple Sclerosis/Visual Disorders

N	Balcer, L	PA	509
N	Schatz, N	FL	523

Multisystem Disorders

Ped	Gartner, J	DE	726

Munchausen Syndrome

Psyc	Eisendrath, S	CA	901

Muscle Disorders

N	Busis, N	PA	510
N	Lacomis, D	PA	514

Muscle Pain-Stress Related

SM	Schechter, D	CA	1044

Muscular Dystrophy

ChiN	Crawford, T	MD	147
N	Amato, A	MA	506
N	Graves, M	CA	537
N	Siddique, T	IL	530
Path	Moore, S	IA	716
PMR	Webster, H	MA	834

Musculoskeletal Disorders

OrS	Herman, M	PA	619
PMR	Bloch, R	MA	834
PMR	Braddom, R	PA	835
PMR	Ma, D	NY	836
Rhu	Bunning, R	DC	1026
Rhu	Coblyn, J	MA	1024
Rhu	Hadler, N	NC	1029

Musculoskeletal Imaging

DR	Adler, R	NY	974
DR	Dalinka, M	PA	974
DR	Newman, J	MA	973
DR	Palmer, W	MA	973
DR	Palmer, W	MA	973
DR	Pathria, M	CA	983
DR	Pavlov, H	NY	977
DR	Potter, H	NY	977
DR	Reinus, W	PA	977

Musculoskeletal Infections

Inf	Wilson, W	MN	417
OrS	Menendez, L	CA	644

Spec	Name	St	Pg
OrS	Webb, L	GA	631

Musculoskeletal Injuries

PMR	Mason, K	CO	842
PMR	Press, J	IL	841

Musculoskeletal Injuries in Dancers

SM	Teitz, C	WA	1044

Musculoskeletal Tissue Banking

OrS	Joyce, M	OH	634

Musculoskeletal Tumor Imaging

DR	Panicek, D	NY	976

Musculoskeletal Tumors

OrS	Berrey, B	FL	627
OrS	Bos, G	WA	641
OrS	Bukata, S	NY	615
OrS	Gebhardt, M	MA	611
OrS	Henshaw, R	DC	619
OrS	Kneisl, J	NC	629
OrS	Luck, J	CA	644
OrS	Mayerson, J	OH	635
OrS	Menendez, L	CA	644
OrS	Mott, M	MI	636
OrS	Schwartz, H	TN	630

Muskuloskeletal Disorders

PMR	Herring, S	WA	843

Myasthenia Gravis

N	Arnason, B	IL	524
N	Ashizawa, T	FL	520
N	Barohn, R	KS	531
N	Elias, S	MI	526
N	Engel, W	CA	536
N	Harati, Y	TX	533
N	Jones, H	MA	507
N	Kula, R	NY	513
N	Lacomis, D	PA	514
N	Lisak, R	MI	527
N	Oh, S	AL	523
N	Pascuzzi, R	IN	528
N	Reder, A	IL	529
N	Swerdlow, M	NY	518
N	Vollmer, T	CO	532
N	Weiss, M	WA	539
N	Wright, R	IL	531
N	Zimnowodzki, S	IL	531
T&CS	Cassivi, S	MN	1131
T&CS	Kaiser, L	PA	1118

Mycobacterial Infections

Inf	Huitt, G	CO	418
Pul	Catanzaro, A	CA	939

Spec	Name	St	Pg
Pul	Iseman, M	CO	936
Pul	Nardell, E	MA	923

Mycosis Fungoides

Spec	Name	St	Pg
D	Lessin, S	PA	187
D	Rook, A	PA	188

Myelodysplastic Syndromes

Spec	Name	St	Pg
Hem	Baer, M	MD	312
Hem	Copelan, E	OH	319
Hem	Cortes, J	TX	323
Hem	Friedman, A	PA	312
Hem	Isola, L	NY	313
Hem	Komrokji, R	FL	317
Hem	Larson, R	IL	320
Hem	Luger, S	PA	313
Hem	Maslak, P	NY	313
Hem	Mesa, R	AZ	324
Hem	Miller, K	MA	311
Hem	Nand, S	IL	321
Hem	Nimer, S	FL	317
Hem	Petersdorf, S	WA	327
Hem	Powell, B	NC	317
Hem	Schuster, M	NY	315
Hem	Solberg, L	FL	318
Hem	Zuckerman, K	FL	318
Onc	Antin, J	MA	327
Onc	Deeg, H	WA	385
Onc	Estey, E	WA	385
Onc	Gabrilove, J	NY	340
Onc	Jurcic, J	NY	343
Onc	Karp, J	MD	343
Onc	List, A	FL	359
Onc	Pecora, A	NJ	347
Onc	Rosove, M	CA	390
Onc	Silverman, L	NY	349
Onc	Wetzler, M	NY	352
Path	Bagg, A	PA	708
PHO	Corey, S	IL	770

Myeloproliferative Disorders

Spec	Name	St	Pg
Hem	Baer, M	MD	312
Hem	Baron, J	IL	318
Hem	Cortes, J	TX	323
Hem	DeLoughery, T	OR	325
Hem	Djulbegovic, B	FL	316
Hem	Fruchtman, S	NY	312
Hem	Luger, S	PA	313
Hem	Mesa, R	AZ	324
Hem	Nand, S	IL	321
Hem	Snyder, D	CA	327
Hem	Spivak, J	MD	315
Hem	Tefferi, A	MN	322
Hem	Zuckerman, K	FL	318
Onc	Aboulafia, D	WA	383
Onc	Dang, C	PA	338
Onc	Deeg, H	WA	385
Onc	Gabrilove, J	NY	340
Onc	Rosove, M	CA	390
Onc	Silver, S	MI	372

Spec	Name	St	Pg
Onc	Wetzler, M	NY	352

N

Nail Surgery

Spec	Name	St	Pg
HS	Chung, K	MI	300

Narcolepsy

Spec	Name	St	Pg
Psyc	Doghramji, K	PA	891
Psyc	Kavey, N	NY	892

Nasal & Sinus Cancer & Surgery

Spec	Name	St	Pg
Oto	Andersen, P	OR	684
Oto	Krespi, Y	NY	662

Nasal & Sinus Disorders

Spec	Name	St	Pg
Oto	Benninger, M	OH	673
Oto	Caruana, S	NY	658
Oto	Corey, J	IL	674
Oto	Josephson, J	NY	661
Oto	Kern, R	IL	676
Oto	Kingdom, T	CO	680
Oto	Schley, W	NY	665
Oto	Siegel, G	IL	677
Oto	Sillers, M	AL	671
Oto	Stankiewicz, J	IL	677
Oto	Stewart, M	NY	665

Nasal & Sinus Surgery

Spec	Name	St	Pg
Oto	Blitzer, A	NY	658
Oto	Setzen, M	NY	665
Oto	Weber, S	TX	683

Nasal Allergy

Spec	Name	St	Pg
A&I	Benenati, S	FL	86
Oto	Hurst, M	WV	661
Oto	Senior, B	NC	671

Nasal Reconstruction

Spec	Name	St	Pg
Oto	Alam, D	OH	672
Oto	Edelstein, D	NY	659
Oto	Graham, H	LA	682
PlS	Menick, F	AZ	871
PlS	Miller, T	CA	875
PlS	Ristow, B	CA	876
PlS	Walton, R	IL	868

Nasal Surgery

Spec	Name	St	Pg
Oto	Bolger, W	FL	667
Oto	Branham, G	MO	673
Oto	Johnson, C	LA	682
Oto	Larrabee, W	WA	685

Natural Orifice Surgery (NOTES)

Spec	Name	St	Pg
S	Bessler, M	NY	1054
S	Curcillo, P	PA	1056
S	Marks, J	OH	1079
S	Rattner, D	MA	1051

Neck Masses

Spec	Name	St	Pg
Oto	Andersen, P	OR	684
Oto	Eisele, D	MD	659
Oto	Hotaling, A	IL	675
PO	April, M	NY	789
PO	Darrow, D	VA	791
PO	Dolitsky, J	NY	789
PO	Myer, C	OH	792
PO	Rosbe, K	CA	793

Necrotizing Enterocolitis

Spec	Name	St	Pg
NP	Holzman, I	NY	447
NP	La Gamma, E	NY	447
PS	Chwals, W	MA	801
PS	Grikscheit, T	CA	810

Neonatal & Infant Cardiac Surgery

Spec	Name	St	Pg
T&CS	Bacha, E	NY	1114
T&CS	Dabal, R	AL	1125
T&CS	Spray, T	PA	1122
T&CS	Ziemer, G	IL	1136

Neonatal Cardiology

Spec	Name	St	Pg
NP	Bucciarelli, R	FL	449
PCd	Gewitz, M	NY	735

Neonatal Cholestasis

Spec	Name	St	Pg
PGe	Suchy, F	CO	755

Neonatal Chronic Lung Disease (CLD)

Spec	Name	St	Pg
NP	Cole, F	MO	450
NP	Seidner, S	TX	452
NP	Van Marter, L	MA	446

Neonatal Critical Care

Spec	Name	St	Pg
NP	Bell, E	IA	450
NP	Gleason, C	WA	452
NP	Lawson, E	MD	447
NP	Perlman, J	NY	448
NP	Zach, T	NE	451

Neonatal Diabetes

Spec	Name	St	Pg
PEn	Sperling, M	PA	745

Neonatal Hemochromatosis

Spec	Name	St	Pg
NP	Bell, E	IA	450

Specialty & Special Expertise Index

Spec	Name	St	Pg
Neonatal Infections			
NP	La Gamma, E	NY	447
NP	Meadow, W	IL	450
NP	Polin, R	NY	448
PInf	Baker, C	TX	784
PInf	Baltimore, R	CT	779
PInf	Jacobs, R	AR	784
Neonatal Neurology			
ChiN	Legido, A	PA	148
ChiN	Mandelbaum, D	RI	146
ChiN	Scher, M	OH	151
ChiN	Volpe, J	MA	147
NP	Hendricks-Munoz, K	VA	449
NP	Perlman, J	NY	448
Neonatal Nutrition			
NP	Holzman, I	NY	447
Neonatal Pathology			
Path	Faye-Petersen, O	AL	713
Neonatal Surgery			
PS	Adzick, N	PA	802
PS	Black, C	TX	809
PS	Cass, D	TX	809
PS	Caty, M	CT	801
PS	Dolgin, S	NY	803
PS	Doody, D	MA	801
PS	Flake, A	PA	803
PS	Ginsburg, H	NY	803
PS	Glick, P	NY	803
PS	Grikscheit, T	CA	810
PS	Holterman, M	IL	807
PS	Jackson, R	AR	809
PS	Kane, T	DC	803
PS	Karrer, F	CO	808
PS	Latchaw, L	NH	802
PS	Nakayama, D	GA	805
PS	Nance, M	PA	804
PS	Oldham, K	WI	807
PS	Proctor, M	WA	811
PS	Rescorla, F	IN	807
PS	Rice, H	NC	805
PS	Ricketts, R	GA	806
PS	Rodgers, B	VA	806
PS	Sato, T	WI	808
PS	Schwartz, M	PA	804
PS	Strauch, E	MD	804
PS	Stylianos, S	NY	804
PS	Velcek, F	NY	804
PS	Voigt, R	MD	804
PS	Waldhausen, J	WA	811
PS	Warner, B	MO	808
PS	Weber, T	IL	808
T&CS	Cohen, G	CA	1140
Neonatal Surgery-			

Spec	Name	St	Pg
Gastrointestinal			
PS	Sawin, R	WA	811
Neonatal-Perinatal Medicine			
NP	Adams, J	TX	451
NP	Anday, E	PA	446
NP	Bancalari, E	FL	448
NP	Bell, E	IA	450
NP	Boyle, R	VA	449
NP	Bucciarelli, R	FL	449
NP	Cloherty, J	MA	446
NP	Cole, F	MO	450
NP	Davidson, D	NY	447
NP	Davis, J	MA	446
NP	Delivoria-Papadopoulos, M	PA	447
NP	Dennery, P	PA	447
NP	Dhanireddy, R	TN	449
NP	Donn, S	MI	450
NP	Ehrenkranz, R	CT	446
NP	Escobedo, M	OK	451
NP	Frantz, I	MA	446
NP	Garcia-Prats, J	TX	452
NP	Gewolb, I	MI	450
NP	Gleason, C	WA	452
NP	Gross, I	CT	446
NP	Hamvas, A	MO	450
NP	Hendricks-Munoz, K	VA	449
NP	Holtzman, R	NC	449
NP	Holzman, I	NY	447
NP	Hurt, H	PA	447
NP	Kattwinkel, J	VA	449
NP	La Gamma, E	NY	447
NP	Lawson, E	MD	447
NP	Lemons, J	IN	450
NP	Martin, R	OH	450
NP	Meadow, W	IL	450
NP	Milley, J	UT	451
NP	Muraskas, J	IL	451
NP	Nogee, L	MD	448
NP	Odom, M	TX	452
NP	Perlman, J	NY	448
NP	Polin, R	NY	448
NP	Seidner, S	TX	452
NP	Short, B	DC	448
NP	Silverman, G	PA	448
NP	Simmons, C	CA	452
NP	Steinhorn, R	CA	451
NP	Stevenson, D	CA	452
NP	Stiles, A	NC	449
NP	Van Marter, L	MA	446
NP	Watchko, J	PA	448
NP	Whitsett, J	OH	451
NP	Zach, T	NE	451
NP	Zubrow, A	PA	448
Neonatology			
NP	Bancalari, E	FL	448
NP	Boyle, R	VA	449
NP	Cloherty, J	MA	446

Spec	Name	St	Pg
NP	Delivoria-Papadopoulos, M	PA	447
NP	Dhanireddy, R	TN	449
NP	Escobedo, M	OK	451
NP	Holtzman, R	NC	449
NP	Hurt, H	PA	447
NP	Odom, M	TX	452
NP	Stevenson, D	CA	452
NP	Stiles, A	NC	449
NP	Zubrow, A	PA	448
Nephrogenic Systemic Fibrosis			
Rhu	Kay, J	MA	1024
Nephrology			
Nep	Ahmad, S	WA	464
Nep	Allon, M	AL	459
Nep	Appel, G	NY	456
Nep	August, P	NY	457
Nep	Bazari, H	MA	456
Nep	Bennett, W	OR	464
Nep	Bernardo, J	PA	457
Nep	Berns, J	PA	457
Nep	Black, H	NY	457
Nep	Blumenfeld, J	NY	457
Nep	Bolton, W	VA	459
Nep	Brennan, D	MO	461
Nep	Brennan, S	TX	463
Nep	Butterly, D	NC	459
Nep	Cho, K	CA	465
Nep	Coe, F	IL	461
Nep	Coffman, T	NC	459
Nep	Cohen, D	NY	457
Nep	Delmez, J	MO	461
Nep	Dember, L	PA	457
Nep	Ellison, D	OR	465
Nep	Fadem, S	TX	463
Nep	Falk, R	NC	459
Nep	Fulop, T	MS	459
Nep	Gaston, R	AL	459
Nep	Gluck, S	CA	465
Nep	Helderman, J	TN	460
Nep	Hruska, K	MO	461
Nep	Johnston, J	PA	457
Nep	Josephson, M	IL	461
Nep	Kasinath, B	TX	463
Nep	Kasiske, B	MN	461
Nep	Kaysen, G	CA	465
Nep	Kelepouris, E	PA	458
Nep	King, A	CA	465
Nep	Kliger, A	CT	456
Nep	Kobrin, S	PA	458
Nep	Kraus, M	IN	461
Nep	Lea, J	GA	460
Nep	McCarthy, J	MN	461
Nep	Miller, B	MO	462
Nep	Mitch, W	TX	464
Nep	Nolan, C	TX	464
Nep	Okusa, M	VA	460
Nep	Olivero, J	TX	464
Nep	Ott, S	WA	465

Spec	Name	St	Pg
Nep	Perrone, R	MA	456
Nep	Piraino, B	PA	458
Nep	Pohl, M	OH	462
Nep	Rakowski, T	VA	460
Nep	Riordan, J	CA	465
Nep	Rodby, R	IL	462
Nep	Roth, D	FL	460
Nep	Rudnick, M	PA	458
Nep	Salant, D	MA	456
Nep	Scandling, J	CA	465
Nep	Schreiber, M	OH	462
Nep	Schwartz, G	MN	462
Nep	Seifter, J	MA	456
Nep	Somerville, J	MN	462
Nep	Stern, L	NY	458
Nep	Suki, W	TX	464
Nep	Swartz, R	MI	462
Nep	Textor, S	MN	462
Nep	Thomas, C	IA	463
Nep	Tolkoff-Rubin, N	MA	456
Nep	Torres, V	MN	463
Nep	Toto, R	TX	464
Nep	Townsend, R	PA	458
Nep	Venkat, K	MI	463
Nep	Ward, D	CA	466
Nep	Warnock, D	AL	460
Nep	Weiner, I	FL	460
Nep	Wilcox, C	DC	458
Nep	Williams, G	NY	458
Nep	Winston, J	NY	459
Nep	Yee, J	MI	463

Nephrotic Syndrome

Nep	Appel, G	NY	456
Nep	Bazari, H	MA	456
Nep	Dember, L	PA	457
Nep	Okusa, M	VA	460
Nep	Warnock, D	AL	460
PNep	Benfield, M	AL	786
PNep	Cohn, R	IL	787
PNep	Harmon, W	MA	785
PNep	Zilleruelo, G	FL	787

Nerve Disorders/Surgery

HS	Atkinson, R	HI	303
HS	Derman, G	IL	300
HS	Jones, N	CA	304
HS	Putnam, M	MN	302
HS	Trumble, T	WA	305
HS	Wolfe, S	NY	298

Nerve Injuries

N	Oaklander, A	MA	508
N	Zimnowodzki, S	IL	531

Nerve Injuries/Surgery

PIS	Lee, R	IL	866

Nerve Surgery &

Spec	Name	St	Pg

Transplantation

NS	Belzberg, A	MD	472
NS	Freeman, T	FL	481
PlS	MacKinnon, S	MO	866

Nerve Tumors

NS	Belzberg, A	MD	472

Neuro-Endoscopy

NS	Frazee, J	CA	496
NS	Turtz, A	NJ	479

Neuro-Genetics

CG	Jayakar, P	FL	159
CG	Korf, B	AL	159
CG	Northrup, H	TX	162

Neuro-Immunology

N	Apatoff, B	NY	509
N	Becker, K	WA	535
N	Cohen, J	OH	525
N	Coyle, P	NY	510
N	Latov, N	NY	514

Neuro-Oncology

ChiN	Allen, J	NY	147
ChiN	Bergman, I	PA	147
ChiN	Fisher, P	CA	153
ChiN	Phillips, P	PA	148
ChiN	Pomeroy, S	MA	146
N	Barger, G	MI	524
N	Cascino, T	MN	525
N	Chamberlain, M	WA	535
N	Cloughesy, T	CA	536
N	DeAngelis, L	NY	510
N	Gilbert, M	TX	533
N	Glass, J	PA	512
N	Kunschner, L	PA	513
N	Laterra, J	MD	514
N	Moots, P	TN	522
N	Nabors, L	AL	523
N	Newton, H	OH	528
N	Patchell, R	AZ	534
N	Posner, J	NY	516
N	Rogers, L	OH	529
N	Rosenfeld, S	OH	529
N	Schiff, D	VA	523
N	Shapiro, W	AZ	534
N	Taylor, L	MA	508
N	Vick, N	IL	530
N	Wen, P	MA	508
N	Yung, W	TX	535
NRad	Murtagh, F	FL	988
NS	Bailes, J	IL	485
NS	Berger, M	CA	495
NS	Brem, S	PA	472
NS	Chandler, J	IL	486
NS	De Monte, F	TX	492

Spec	Name	St	Pg
NS	Evans, J	PA	473
NS	Liau, L	CA	497
NS	Lillehei, K	CO	491
NS	Neuwelt, E	OR	498
NS	O'Rourke, D	PA	477
NS	Olson, J	GA	483
NS	Park, T	MO	489
NS	Piepmeier, J	CT	471
NS	Pollack, I	PA	478
NS	Quigley, M	PA	478
NS	Rock, J	MI	489
NS	Rosenblum, M	MI	489
NS	Sundaresan, N	NY	479
NS	Thompson, R	TN	485
NS	Warnick, R	OH	491
Onc	Buckner, J	MN	365
Onc	Fine, H	MD	339
Onc	Friedman, H	NC	356
Onc	Grossman, S	MD	341
Onc	Kesari, S	CA	387
Onc	Lesser, G	NC	358
Onc	Lyckholm, L	VA	359
Onc	Peereboom, D	OH	370
Onc	Prados, M	CA	389
PHO	Blaney, S	TX	775
PHO	Gajjar, A	TN	766
PHO	Geyer, J	WA	777
PHO	Goldman, S	IL	771
PHO	Gururangan, S	NC	766
PHO	Jakacki, R	PA	761
PHO	Kieran, M	MA	757
PHO	Olson, J	OR	778
PHO	Puccetti, D	WI	772
PHO	Wolff, J	MA	757
RadRO	Flickinger, J	PA	949
RadRO	Isaacson, S	NY	950
RadRO	Larner, J	VA	955
RadRO	Larson, D	CA	967

Neuro-Ophthalmology

N	Balcer, L	PA	509
N	Corbett, J	MS	520
N	Frohman, E	TX	533
N	Galetta, S	PA	512
N	Gizzi, M	NJ	512
N	Goodwin, J	IL	526
N	Lavin, P	TN	522
N	Liu, G	PA	515
N	Newman, N	GA	523
N	Schatz, N	FL	523
Oph	Arnold, A	CA	598
Oph	Biousse, V	GA	582
Oph	Buckley, E	NC	582
Oph	Capo, H	FL	582
Oph	Cockerham, K	CA	600
Oph	Feldon, S	NY	573
Oph	Guy, J	FL	583
Oph	Hedges, T	MA	570
Oph	Krauss, H	CA	601
Oph	Kupersmith, M	NY	576
Oph	Lee, A	TX	597

Specialty & Special Expertise Index

Spec	Name	St	Pg
Oph	Mawn, L	TN	584
Oph	Miller, N	MD	577
Oph	Mizen, T	IL	592
Oph	Odel, J	NY	578
Oph	Rizzo, J	MA	571
Oph	Savino, P	CA	603
Oph	Schiffman, J	TX	598
Oph	Sergott, R	PA	580
Oph	Siatkowski, R	OK	598
Oph	Trobe, J	MI	594
Oph	Volpe, N	IL	595
Oph	Walton, D	MA	571

Neuro-Otology

Spec	Name	St	Pg
N	Hain, T	IL	526
N	Lavin, P	TN	522
Oto	Arts, H	MI	672
Oto	Balkany, T	FL	667
Oto	Carey, J	MD	658
Oto	Dornhoffer, J	AR	682
Oto	Feghali, J	NY	659
Oto	Gantz, B	IA	675
Oto	Harris, J	CA	685
Oto	Haynes, D	TN	668
Oto	Hirsch, B	PA	660
Oto	Holliday, M	MD	660
Oto	Jackler, R	CA	685
Oto	Jenkins, H	CO	680
Oto	Kesser, B	VA	668
Oto	Lambert, P	SC	669
Oto	Leonetti, J	IL	676
Oto	Macias, J	AZ	682
Oto	Mattox, D	GA	669
Oto	McKenna, M	MA	656
Oto	Miyamoto, R	IN	676
Oto	Niparko, J	MD	663
Oto	O'Leary, M	CA	686
Oto	Oghalai, J	CA	686
Oto	Paparella, M	MN	677
Oto	Pillsbury, H	NC	670
Oto	Rauch, S	MA	656
Oto	Roland, J	NY	664
Oto	Rubinstein, J	WA	686
Oto	Sataloff, R	PA	664
Oto	Telischi, F	FL	671
PO	Poe, D	MA	789

Neuro-Pathology

Spec	Name	St	Pg
N	Glass, J	GA	521
Path	Bollen, A	CA	719
Path	Bruner, J	TX	717
Path	Burger, P	MD	708
Path	Chandrasoma, P	CA	720
Path	De Masters, B	CO	717
Path	Gambetti, P	OH	715
Path	Jones, R	DC	709
Path	Mischel, P	CA	721
Path	Perry, A	CA	721
Path	Petito, C	FL	714
Psyc	Benes, F	MA	888

Neuro-Psychiatry

Spec	Name	St	Pg
GerPsy	Lyketsos, C	MD	913
N	Cummings, J	NV	536
N	Kent, T	TX	534
Psyc	Black, K	MO	897
Psyc	Fann, J	WA	901
Psyc	Keepers, G	OR	901
Psyc	Locala, J	OH	898
Psyc	Neppe, V	WA	902
Psyc	Wilson, D	FL	896

Neuro-Rehabilitation

Spec	Name	St	Pg
N	Corbetta, M	MO	525
N	Couch, J	OK	532
N	Fellus, J	NJ	511
N	Kirshner, H	TN	522
PMR	Currie, D	TX	842
PMR	Diamond, P	VA	838
PMR	Palmer, J	MD	837
PMR	Richter, E	CT	834

Neuro-Urology

Spec	Name	St	Pg
U	Bauer, S	MA	1148
U	Bodner, D	OH	1165
U	Boone, T	TX	1172
U	Bushman, W	WI	1166
U	Chancellor, M	MI	1166
U	Ginsberg, D	CA	1176
U	Gomery, P	MA	1148
U	Joseph, D	AL	1161
U	Wein, A	PA	1159

Neuroblastoma

Spec	Name	St	Pg
PHO	Blatt, J	NC	765
PHO	Castle, V	MI	770
PHO	Cheung, N	NY	759
PHO	Cohn, S	IL	770
PHO	Diller, L	MA	756
PHO	Frantz, C	DE	759
PHO	Furman, W	TN	765
PHO	Grupp, S	PA	760
PHO	Kramer, K	NY	761
PHO	Kreissman, S	NC	767
PHO	Kushner, B	NY	761
PHO	Maris, J	PA	762
PHO	Matthay, K	CA	778
PHO	O'Dorisio, M	IA	772
PHO	Park, J	WA	778
PHO	Sondel, P	WI	773
PHO	Vik, T	IN	773
PHO	Wechsler, D	NC	769
PS	Barksdale, E	OH	806
PS	Davidoff, A	TN	805
PS	La Quaglia, M	NY	803
PS	Morgan, W	TN	805
PS	Shamberger, R	MA	802

Neurocutaneous Disorders

Spec	Name	St	Pg
CG	Cassidy, S	CA	162

Spec	Name	St	Pg
ChiN	Rosser, T	CA	154

Neurodegenerative Disorders

Spec	Name	St	Pg
ChiN	Mitchell, W	CA	153
N	Farlow, M	IN	526
Path	Gambetti, P	OH	715

Neurodevelopmental Disabilities

Spec	Name	St	Pg
PMR	Keen, M	IL	840

Neuroendocrine Growth Disorders

Spec	Name	St	Pg
PEn	Oberfield, S	NY	745

Neuroendocrine Tumors

Spec	Name	St	Pg
EDM	Snyder, P	PA	212
Ge	Metz, D	PA	236
NS	Parent, A	MS	483
NS	Swearingen, B	MA	471
Onc	Ahlgren, J	DC	333
Onc	Ajani, J	TX	377
Onc	Anthony, L	KY	353
Onc	Engstrom, P	PA	339
Onc	Fine, R	NY	339
Onc	Goldberg, R	OH	367
Onc	Grosh, W	VA	357
Onc	Kane, M	CO	376
Onc	Kelsen, D	NY	343
Onc	Kvols, L	FL	358
Onc	Moore, J	NC	360
Onc	O'Reilly, E	NY	346
Onc	Saltz, L	NY	348
PHO	O'Dorisio, M	IA	772
S	Clark, O	CA	1094
S	Johnson Miller, D	IN	1078
S	Libutti, S	NY	1060
S	Sasson, A	NE	1086
S	Solorzano, C	TN	1072
S	Woltering, E	LA	1093

Neuroendocrinology

Spec	Name	St	Pg
EDM	Calvi, L	NY	209
EDM	Hoffman, A	CA	223
EDM	Kandeel, F	CA	223
EDM	Katznelson, L	CA	223
EDM	Kleinberg, D	NY	210
EDM	Marshall, J	VA	214
Ger	Minaker, K	MA	262
PEn	Lustig, R	CA	749
PEn	Rivkees, S	FL	746

Neurofibromatosis

Spec	Name	St	Pg
CG	Bialer, M	NY	157
CG	Carey, J	UT	161
CG	Charrow, J	IL	160
CG	Davis, J	NY	157
CG	Korf, B	AL	159

Spec	Name	St	Pg
CG	Mulvihill, J	OK	161
CG	Randolph, L	CA	163
CG	Saal, H	OH	160
CG	Saul, R	SC	159
ChiN	Allen, J	NY	147
ChiN	Greenwood, R	NC	149
ChiN	Packer, R	DC	148
ChiN	Phillips, P	PA	148
ChiN	Rosser, T	CA	154
N	Roos, K	IN	529
NRad	Vezina, L	DC	986

Neurogenetics

Spec	Name	St	Pg
CG	Shoffner, J	GA	159
ChiN	Patterson, M	MN	151
ChiN	Tennison, M	NC	149
N	Siddique, T	IL	530

Neurogenic Bladder

Spec	Name	St	Pg
PMR	Cardenas, D	FL	838
PMR	Fried, G	PA	836
U	Bauer, S	MA	1148
U	Blaivas, J	NY	1151
U	Ewalt, D	TX	1173
U	Ginsberg, D	CA	1176
U	Greenfield, S	NY	1153
U	Kennelly, M	NC	1161
U	Lloyd, L	AL	1162
U	McGuire, E	MI	1168
U	Rink, R	IN	1169
U	Vapnek, J	NY	1159

Neurologic Aspects of Systemic Disease

Spec	Name	St	Pg
N	Samuels, M	MA	508

Neurologic Complications of Cancer

Spec	Name	St	Pg
N	Moots, P	TN	522
N	Phuphanich, S	CA	538
N	Schiff, D	VA	523

Neurologic Imaging

Spec	Name	St	Pg
DR	Elster, A	NC	979
DR	Mountz, J	PA	976
N	Burke, A	IL	525
N	Corbetta, M	MO	525
NuM	Alavi, A	PA	548
NuM	Strashun, A	NY	549

Neurologic Rehabilitation

Spec	Name	St	Pg
N	Kelly, J	CO	531
PMR	Ahn, J	NY	834
PMR	Mason, K	CO	842
PMR	Roth, E	IL	841

Neurological Surgery

Spec	Name	St	Pg
NS	Adelson, P	AZ	492

Spec	Name	St	Pg
NS	Al-Mefty, O	MA	470
NS	Amar, A	CA	495
NS	Ames, C	CA	495
NS	Andrews, D	PA	472
NS	Apuzzo, M	CA	495
NS	Asher, A	NC	481
NS	Atkinson, J	MN	485
NS	Badie, B	CA	495
NS	Bailes, J	IL	485
NS	Bakay, R	IL	485
NS	Baltuch, G	PA	472
NS	Barnett, G	OH	486
NS	Barrow, D	GA	481
NS	Bauer, J	IL	486
NS	Bederson, J	NY	472
NS	Belzberg, A	MD	472
NS	Benzel, E	OH	486
NS	Berger, M	CA	495
NS	Bierbrauer, K	OH	486
NS	Bilsky, M	NY	472
NS	Bingaman, W	OH	486
NS	Black, K	CA	495
NS	Boggan, J	CA	496
NS	Boop, F	TN	481
NS	Borges, L	MA	470
NS	Branch, C	NC	481
NS	Bray, R	CA	496
NS	Brem, H	MD	472
NS	Brem, S	PA	472
NS	Brown, F	IL	486
NS	Bruce, J	NY	473
NS	Bucholz, R	MO	486
NS	Burchiel, K	OR	496
NS	Caputy, A	DC	473
NS	Carson, B	MD	473
NS	Chandler, J	IL	486
NS	Chandler, W	MI	487
NS	Chen, C	NY	473
NS	Chen, T	CA	496
NS	Cherny, W	ID	491
NS	Chiocca, E	OH	487
NS	Cohen, A	MA	470
NS	Cosgrove, R	RI	470
NS	Couldwell, W	UT	491
NS	Dacey, R	MO	487
NS	Danielpour, M	CA	496
NS	David, C	MA	470
NS	De Monte, F	TX	492
NS	Dempsey, R	WI	487
NS	Di Giacinto, G	NY	473
NS	Dias, M	PA	473
NS	Diaz, F	MI	487
NS	Duhaime, A	MA	470
NS	Edwards, M	CA	496
NS	Eisenberg, H	MD	473
NS	Ellenbogen, R	WA	496
NS	Evans, J	PA	473
NS	Ewend, M	NC	481
NS	Feldstein, N	NY	474
NS	Fenstermaker, R	NY	474
NS	Fessler, R	IL	487
NS	Foley, K	TN	481

Spec	Name	St	Pg
NS	Frazee, J	CA	496
NS	Freeman, T	FL	481
NS	Friedman, A	NC	481
NS	Frim, D	IL	487
NS	Giannotta, S	CA	497
NS	Gokaslan, Z	MD	474
NS	Golfinos, J	NY	474
NS	Goodman, R	NY	474
NS	Goumnerova, L	MA	470
NS	Grady, M	PA	474
NS	Green, B	FL	481
NS	Greene, C	LA	492
NS	Grubb, R	MO	487
NS	Gupta, N	CA	497
NS	Guthikonda, M	MI	488
NS	Guthrie, B	AL	482
NS	Gutin, P	NY	474
NS	Hadley, M	AL	482
NS	Haid, R	GA	482
NS	Hankinson, H	NM	492
NS	Harbaugh, R	PA	474
NS	Harper, R	TX	493
NS	Harrop, J	PA	475
NS	Harsh, G	CA	497
NS	Hartl, R	NY	475
NS	Heilman, C	MA	471
NS	Heros, R	FL	482
NS	Hodes, J	KY	482
NS	Hopkins, L	NY	475
NS	Huang, J	MD	475
NS	Jallo, G	MD	475
NS	Jho, H	PA	475
NS	Jimenez, D	TX	493
NS	Johnson, S	CO	491
NS	Judy, K	PA	475
NS	Kaiser, M	NY	475
NS	Kaplitt, M	NY	476
NS	Kaufman, B	WI	488
NS	Kestle, J	UT	491
NS	Khan, A	MD	476
NS	Kim, D	TX	493
NS	Kim, D	TX	493
NS	Kobrine, A	DC	476
NS	Kondziolka, D	PA	476
NS	Kotapka, M	PA	476
NS	Krisht, A	AR	493
NS	Kuntz, C	OH	488
NS	Landy, H	FL	482
NS	Lang, F	TX	493
NS	Laske, D	PA	476
NS	Lavyne, M	NY	476
NS	Lemole, G	AZ	493
NS	Levi, A	FL	482
NS	Levy, M	CA	497
NS	Liau, L	CA	497
NS	Liker, M	CA	497
NS	Lillehei, K	CO	491
NS	Link, M	MN	488
NS	Linskey, M	CA	497
NS	Liu, C	CA	497
NS	Loftus, C	IL	488
NS	Luerssen, T	TX	493

Specialty & Special Expertise Index

Spec	Name	St	Pg	Spec	Name	St	Pg	Spec	Name	St	Pg
NS	Luken, M	IL	488	NS	Selden, N	OR	499	N	Aminoff, M	CA	535
NS	Lunsford, L	PA	476	NS	Selman, W	OH	490	N	Apatoff, B	NY	509
NS	Madsen, J	MA	471	NS	Sen, C	NY	478	N	Armon, C	MA	506
NS	Malik, G	MI	488	NS	Shaffrey, C	VA	484	N	Arnason, B	IL	524
NS	Mamelak, A	CA	498	NS	Shaffrey, M	VA	484	N	Ashizawa, T	FL	520
NS	Mapstone, T	OK	494	NS	Shapiro, S	IN	490	N	Azizi, S	PA	509
NS	Markert, J	AL	483	NS	Shuer, L	CA	499	N	Balcer, L	PA	509
NS	Maroon, J	PA	477	NS	Silbergeld, D	WA	499	N	Barger, G	MI	524
NS	Martin, N	CA	498	NS	Sills, A	TN	484	N	Barkley, G	MI	525
NS	Martuza, R	MA	471	NS	Sisti, M	NY	479	N	Barohn, R	KS	531
NS	Mayberg, M	WA	498	NS	Sklar, F	TX	494	N	Baser, S	PA	509
NS	McCormick, P	NY	477	NS	Solomon, R	NY	479	N	Batchelor, T	MA	506
NS	McDermott, M	CA	498	NS	Souweidane, M	NY	479	N	Bebin, E	AL	520
NS	Menezes, A	IA	488	NS	Spencer, D	CT	471	N	Becker, K	WA	535
NS	Meyer, F	MN	489	NS	Spetzler, R	AZ	494	N	Bell, R	PA	509
NS	Mickey, B	TX	494	NS	Spinner, R	MN	490	N	Berger, J	KY	520
NS	Moore, F	NJ	477	NS	Steinberg, G	CA	499	N	Bergey, G	MD	509
NS	Morcos, J	FL	483	NS	Stieg, P	NY	479	N	Bernstein, R	IL	525
NS	Moser, R	MA	471	NS	Sun, P	CA	499	N	Bertorini, T	TN	520
NS	Murali, R	NY	477	NS	Sundaresan, N	NY	479	N	Blum, A	RI	506
NS	Myseros, J	VA	483	NS	Sutton, L	PA	479	N	Bressman, S	NY	509
NS	Naff, N	MD	477	NS	Swaid, S	AL	484	N	Brick, J	WV	510
NS	Nagib, M	MN	489	NS	Swearingen, B	MA	471	N	Broderick, J	OH	525
NS	Nazzaro, J	KS	491	NS	Tamargo, R	MD	479	N	Bromberg, M	UT	531
NS	Neuwelt, E	OR	498	NS	Tatter, S	NC	485	N	Brooks, B	NC	520
NS	O'Rourke, D	PA	477	NS	Taylon, C	NE	492	N	Brown, R	MN	525
NS	Oakes, W	AL	483	NS	Theodore, N	AZ	494	N	Bruno, M	HI	535
NS	Ojemann, J	WA	498	NS	Thompson, B	MI	490	N	Buchholz, D	MD	510
NS	Olivi, A	MD	477	NS	Thompson, R	TN	485	N	Burke, A	IL	525
NS	Olson, J	GA	483	NS	Tomita, T	IL	490	N	Busis, N	PA	510
NS	Origitano, T	MT	491	NS	Traynelis, V	IL	490	N	Calabresi, P	MD	510
NS	Ott, K	CA	498	NS	Turtz, A	NJ	479	N	Caplan, L	MA	506
NS	Parent, A	MS	483	NS	Van Loveren, H	FL	485	N	Cascino, T	MN	525
NS	Park, T	MO	489	NS	Walker, M	UT	492	N	Chamberlain, M	WA	535
NS	Patel, A	NY	477	NS	Walsh, J	LA	495	N	Charles, A	CA	536
NS	Patel, S	SC	483	NS	Warnick, R	OH	491	N	Charney, J	NY	510
NS	Penar, P	VT	471	NS	Weiner, H	NY	480	N	Chelimsky, T	WI	525
NS	Piatt, J	DE	478	NS	Weingart, J	MD	480	N	Chui, H	CA	536
NS	Piepmeier, J	CT	471	NS	Welch, W	PA	480	N	Cloughesy, T	CA	536
NS	Pollack, I	PA	478	NS	Wharen, R	FL	485	N	Cohen, J	OH	525
NS	Quigley, M	PA	478	NS	Whiting, D	PA	480	N	Cohen, J	NH	506
NS	Raffel, C	OH	489	NS	Wilberger, J	PA	480	N	Cole, A	MA	506
NS	Ragheb, J	FL	483	NS	Wilson, C	NC	485	N	Cook, S	NJ	510
NS	Reid, W	TN	484	NS	Wisoff, J	NY	480	N	Corbett, J	MS	520
NS	Rezai, A	OH	489	NS	Yonas, H	NM	495	N	Corbetta, M	MO	525
NS	Rich, K	MO	489	NS	Yu, J	CA	499	N	Corey-Bloom, J	CA	536
NS	Rigamonti, D	MD	478	NS	Zager, E	PA	480	N	Cornblath, D	MD	510
NS	Riina, H	NY	478	NS	Zimmerman, C	ID	492	N	Couch, J	OK	532
NS	Robertson, J	TN	484					N	Coull, B	AZ	533
NS	Rock, J	MI	489	**Neurology**				N	Coyle, P	NY	510
NS	Rodts, G	GA	484	N	Abou-Khalil, B	TN	519	N	Cudkowicz, M	MA	507
NS	Rosenblum, M	MI	489	N	Adams, D	FL	519	N	Cummings, J	NV	536
NS	Rosenwasser, R	PA	478	N	Adams, H	IA	524	N	Cutrer, F	MN	526
NS	Ruge, J	IL	490	N	Adams, R	SC	519	N	DeAngelis, L	NY	510
NS	Ryken, T	IA	490	N	Adornato, B	CA	535	N	DeGiorgio, C	CA	536
NS	Sampson, J	NC	484	N	Ahern, G	AZ	532	N	DeKosky, S	VA	520
NS	Samson, D	TX	494	N	Ahlskog, J	MN	524	N	DeLong, M	GA	520
NS	Sandberg, D	TX	494	N	Albers, G	CA	535	N	Devinsky, O	NY	511
NS	Sawaya, R	TX	494	N	Alberts, M	IL	524	N	Dewberry, R	MD	511
NS	Schwartz, T	NY	478	N	Alexandrov, A	AL	519	N	Dodick, D	AZ	533
NS	Sekhar, L	WA	498	N	Amato, A	MA	506	N	Doody, R	TX	533
NS	Sekhon, L	NV	499					N	Elias, S	MI	526

Spec	Name	St	Pg	Spec	Name	St	Pg	Spec	Name	St	Pg
N	Engel, W	CA	536	N	Kelly, J	CO	531	N	Oommen, K	TX	534
N	Engstrom, J	CA	536	N	Kent, T	TX	534	N	Pascuzzi, R	IN	528
N	Fahn, S	NY	511	N	Kieburtz, K	NY	513	N	Patchell, R	AZ	534
N	Farlow, M	IN	526	N	Kincaid, J	IN	527	N	Pedley, T	NY	516
N	Feinberg, T	NY	511	N	Kirshner, H	TN	522	N	Pennell, P	MA	508
N	Feldman, E	MI	526	N	Klein, P	NJ	513	N	Perlmutter, J	MO	528
N	Feldmann, E	MA	507	N	Kolodny, E	NY	513	N	Pestronk, A	MO	529
N	Fellus, J	NJ	511	N	Krauss, G	MD	513	N	Petersen, R	MN	529
N	Ferrendelli, J	TX	533	N	Krumholz, A	MD	513	N	Petito, F	NY	516
N	Filley, C	CO	531	N	Kula, R	NY	513	N	Phuphanich, S	CA	538
N	Fink, M	NY	511	N	Kunschner, L	PA	513	N	Posner, J	NY	516
N	Finkel, A	NC	521	N	Kurtzke, R	VA	522	N	Pula, T	MD	516
N	Finkel, M	FL	521	N	Kuzniecky, R	NY	513	N	Pulst, S	UT	532
N	Fisher, M	CA	536	N	Labar, D	NY	514	N	Reder, A	IL	529
N	Fisher, R	CA	537	N	Labiner, D	AZ	534	N	Reed, R	OH	529
N	Flaherty, A	MA	507	N	Lacomis, D	PA	514	N	Reich, S	MD	517
N	Foo, S	NY	511	N	Lane, J	CO	532	N	Relkin, N	NY	517
N	French, J	NY	511	N	Langston, J	CA	537	N	Richerson, G	IA	529
N	Frohman, E	TX	533	N	Laterra, J	MD	514	N	Ringel, S	CO	532
N	Furie, K	RI	507	N	Latov, N	NY	514	N	Rogers, L	OH	529
N	Furlan, A	OH	526	N	Lavin, P	TN	522	N	Roos, K	IN	529
N	Galetta, S	PA	512	N	Levine, D	NY	514	N	Roos, R	IL	529
N	Gendelman, S	NY	512	N	Levine, S	NY	514	N	Ropper, A	MA	508
N	Gilbert, M	TX	533	N	Lew, M	CA	537	N	Rosenbaum, R	OR	538
N	Gilden, D	CO	531	N	Lewis, R	MI	527	N	Rosenfeld, S	OH	529
N	Gilman, S	MI	526	N	Liporace, J	PA	514	N	Rothrock, J	NV	538
N	Gizzi, M	NJ	512	N	Lipton, R	NY	514	N	Rubin, S	IL	530
N	Glass, J	PA	512	N	Lisak, R	MI	527	N	Rutkove, S	MA	508
N	Glass, J	GA	521	N	Liu, G	PA	515	N	Sabo, T	CO	532
N	Goetz, C	IL	526	N	Logan, W	MO	527	N	Sacco, R	FL	523
N	Golbe, L	NJ	512	N	Logigian, E	NY	515	N	Sadowsky, C	FL	523
N	Goldstein, L	NC	521	N	Longo, F	CA	538	N	Sage, J	NJ	517
N	Goodin, D	CA	537	N	Louis, E	NY	515	N	Samii, A	WA	538
N	Goodwin, J	IL	526	N	Lublin, F	NY	515	N	Samuels, M	MA	508
N	Graves, M	CA	537	N	Luders, H	OH	527	N	Saper, C	MA	508
N	Greer, D	CT	507	N	Lutsep, H	OR	538	N	Saper, J	MI	530
N	Gress, D	VA	521	N	Maraganore, D	IL	528	N	Saver, J	CA	539
N	Gross, P	MA	507	N	Marder, K	NY	515	N	Schatz, N	FL	523
N	Grotta, J	TX	533	N	Mayeux, R	NY	515	N	Schiff, D	VA	523
N	Guilleminault, C	CA	537	N	McArthur, J	MD	515	N	Schwartzman, R	PA	517
N	Hain, T	IL	526	N	McCluskey, L	PA	515	N	Sethi, K	GA	523
N	Haley, E	VA	521	N	Mesulam, M	IL	528	N	Shapiro, W	AZ	534
N	Harati, Y	TX	533	N	Mikkelsen, T	MI	528	N	Shefner, J	NY	517
N	Hauser, R	FL	521	N	Miller, A	NY	516	N	Sheikh, K	TX	534
N	Hauser, S	CA	537	N	Mitsumoto, H	NY	516	N	Shulman, L	MD	517
N	Heck, C	CA	537	N	Mohr, J	NY	516	N	Siddique, T	IL	530
N	Hecox, K	WI	527	N	Montgomery, E	AL	522	N	Sila, C	OH	530
N	Heilman, K	FL	521	N	Moots, P	TN	522	N	Silberstein, S	PA	517
N	Henderson, V	CA	537	N	Morgenlander, J	NC	522	N	Simpson, D	NY	517
N	Hess, D	GA	522	N	Morrell, M	CA	538	N	Singer, C	FL	524
N	Hiesiger, E	NY	512	N	Morris, J	MO	528	N	Sirdofsky, M	DC	518
N	Homer, D	IL	527	N	Nabors, L	AL	523	N	Smith, W	CA	539
N	Hurtig, H	PA	512	N	Newman, D	MI	528	N	Sperling, M	PA	518
N	Jankovic, J	TX	534	N	Newman, L	NY	516	N	Stern, M	PA	518
N	Janss, A	GA	522	N	Newman, N	GA	523	N	Strom, L	CO	532
N	Jobst, B	NH	507	N	Newton, H	OH	528	N	Suarez, J	TX	534
N	Jones, H	MA	507	N	Nicholl, J	LA	534	N	Swanson, J	MN	530
N	Jordan, B	NY	512	N	Nolan, B	FL	523	N	Swerdlow, M	NY	518
N	Josephson, D	IN	527	N	Nutt, J	OR	538	N	Tanner, C	CA	539
N	Kase, C	MA	507	N	Oaklander, A	MA	508	N	Tayal, A	PA	518
N	Kasner, S	PA	512	N	Oh, S	AL	523	N	Taylor, L	MA	508
N	Katirji, B	OH	527	N	Olanow, C	NY	516	N	Tetrud, J	CA	539

Specialty & Special Expertise Index

Spec	Name	St	Pg
N	Vas, G	NY	518
N	Vick, N	IL	530
N	Vitek, J	MN	530
N	Vollmer, T	CO	532
N	Waters, C	NY	518
N	Watts, R	AL	524
N	Wechsler, L	PA	518
N	Weinberg, H	NY	519
N	Weiner, L	CA	539
N	Weiner, W	MD	519
N	Weiss, M	WA	539
N	Wen, P	MA	508
N	Windebank, A	MN	530
N	Wityk, R	MD	519
N	Wolinsky, J	TX	535
N	Wooten, G	VA	524
N	Wright, R	IL	531
N	Young, A	MA	509
N	Yung, W	TX	535
N	Zimmerman, E	NY	519
N	Zimnowodzki, S	IL	531

Neurometabolic Disorders

Spec	Name	St	Pg
ChiN	Cohen, B	OH	150
ChiN	Haas, R	CA	153

Neuromuscular Disorder & Vision Problems

Spec	Name	St	Pg
N	Goodwin, J	IL	526

Neuromuscular Disorders

Spec	Name	St	Pg
ChiN	Crawford, T	MD	147
ChiN	Darras, B	MA	146
ChiN	De Vivo, D	NY	147
ChiN	Edgar, T	WI	150
ChiN	Finkel, R	FL	149
ChiN	Goldstein, E	GA	149
ChiN	Gospe, S	WA	153
ChiN	Iannaccone, S	TX	152
ChiN	Lavenstein, B	VA	149
HS	Osterman, A	PA	297
N	Amato, A	MA	506
N	Bertorini, T	TN	520
N	Bromberg, M	UT	531
N	Brooks, B	NC	520
N	Busis, N	PA	510
N	Cohen, J	NH	506
N	Cudkowicz, M	MA	507
N	Engel, W	CA	536
N	Feldman, E	MI	526
N	Glass, J	GA	521
N	Harati, Y	TX	533
N	Jones, H	MA	507
N	Katirji, B	OH	527
N	Kincaid, J	IN	527
N	Kula, R	NY	513
N	Kurtzke, R	VA	522
N	Lacomis, D	PA	514
N	Lewis, R	MI	527
N	Logigian, E	NY	515

Spec	Name	St	Pg
N	Mitsumoto, H	NY	516
N	Morgenlander, J	NC	522
N	Newman, D	MI	528
N	Oh, S	AL	523
N	Pascuzzi, R	IN	528
N	Pestronk, A	MO	529
N	Ringel, S	CO	532
N	Roos, R	IL	529
N	Rosenbaum, R	OR	538
N	Rutkove, S	MA	508
N	Shefner, J	NY	517
N	Sheikh, K	TX	534
N	Simpson, D	NY	517
N	Sirdofsky, M	DC	518
N	Weinberg, H	NY	519
N	Weiss, M	WA	539
OrS	Otsuka, N	NY	623
OrS	Roye, D	NY	624
PMR	Bach, J	NJ	835
PMR	Ballard, P	DC	835
PMR	Kevorkian, C	TX	843
PMR	Kirschner, K	IL	840
PMR	La Ban, M	MI	841
PMR	Massagli, T	WA	844
PMR	Matthews, D	CO	842

Neuropathology

Spec	Name	St	Pg
Path	Moore, S	IA	716
Path	Rosenblum, M	NY	711
Path	Smith, T	MA	707
Path	Zagzag, D	NY	712

Neurophysiology

Spec	Name	St	Pg
ChiN	Kovnar, E	WI	151
ChiN	Tennison, M	NC	149
N	Abou-Khalil, B	TN	519
N	Pula, T	MD	516

Neuroradiology

Spec	Name	St	Pg
DR	Kanal, E	PA	976
DR	Mancuso, A	FL	979
DR	Teal, J	DC	977
DR	Yoon, S	NY	978
NRad	Atlas, S	CA	990
NRad	Ball, W	OH	988
NRad	Barkovich, A	CA	990
NRad	Barnes, P	CA	990
NRad	Berenstein, A	NY	985
NRad	Burdette, J	NC	987
NRad	Cha, S	CA	991
NRad	Cross, D	MO	988
NRad	Curtin, H	MA	984
NRad	Dillon, W	CA	991
NRad	Dion, J	GA	987
NRad	Drayer, B	NY	985
NRad	Faro, S	PA	985
NRad	Frei, D	CO	990
NRad	Grobelny, T	IL	988
NRad	Hackney, D	MA	984
NRad	Haughton, V	WI	988

Spec	Name	St	Pg
NRad	Hesselink, J	CA	991
NRad	Higashida, R	CA	991
NRad	Hirsch, J	MA	984
NRad	Hunter, J	TX	990
NRad	Hurst, R	PA	985
NRad	Jarvik, J	WA	991
NRad	Jensen, M	VA	987
NRad	Johnson, A	NC	987
NRad	Joseph, G	NC	987
NRad	Kallmes, D	MN	989
NRad	Khandji, A	NY	985
NRad	Koeller, K	MN	989
NRad	Larsen, D	CA	991
NRad	Lis, E	NY	986
NRad	Loevner, L	PA	986
NRad	Maldjian, J	NC	987
NRad	Masaryk, T	OH	989
NRad	Mawad, M	TX	990
NRad	Modic, M	OH	989
NRad	Moran, C	MO	989
NRad	Morris, P	NC	987
NRad	Mukherji, S	MI	989
NRad	Murtagh, F	FL	988
NRad	Norbash, A	MA	984
NRad	Orbach, D	MA	985
NRad	Osborn, A	UT	990
NRad	Pile-Spellman, J	NY	986
NRad	Provenzale, J	NC	988
NRad	Quencer, R	FL	988
NRad	Rowley, H	WI	989
NRad	Sze, G	CT	985
NRad	Teitelbaum, G	CA	991
NRad	Tenner, M	NY	986
NRad	Thulborn, K	IL	989
NRad	Vezina, L	DC	986
NRad	Vinuela, F	CA	991
NRad	Yousem, D	MD	986
NRad	Zimmerman, R	PA	986
NRad	Zinreich, S	MD	986
NS	Riina, H	NY	478

Neurosarcoidosis

Spec	Name	St	Pg
N	Corbett, J	MS	520

Neurotoxicology

Spec	Name	St	Pg
ChiN	Gospe, S	WA	153
N	Brooks, B	NC	520

Neurovascular Surgery

Spec	Name	St	Pg
NS	Rich, K	MO	489
NS	Thompson, B	MI	490
NS	Thompson, R	TN	485

Neutron Therapy for Advanced Cancer

Spec	Name	St	Pg
RadRO	Forman, J	MI	959
RadRO	Laramore, G	WA	966

Spec	Name	St	Pg

Nipple Sparing Mastectomy
S	Swistel, A	NY	1065
S	Tsangaris, T	MD	1065

Nocardia Infection
Inf	Wallace, R	TX	419

Non Tuberculous Mycobacteria
Inf	Wallace, R	TX	419

Non-Invasive Cardiology
Cv	Geltman, E	MO	108
Cv	Silvestry, F	PA	102

Noonan Syndrome
PCd	Gelb, B	NY	735

Nuclear Cardiology
Cv	Borer, J	NY	97
Cv	Bourge, R	AL	103
Cv	Cerqueira, M	OH	107
Cv	Chaitman, B	MO	107
Cv	Fintel, D	IL	107
Cv	Follansbee, W	PA	98
Cv	Gibbons, R	MN	108
Cv	Iskandrian, A	AL	104
Cv	Nocero, M	FL	105
Cv	Shea, R	IN	111
Cv	Skolnick, A	AK	118
Cv	Steingart, R	NY	102
Cv	Walsh, M	IN	112
Cv	Williams, K	MI	113
IC	Khawaja, S	GA	130
NuM	Dae, M	CA	551
NuM	Neumann, D	OH	550
NuM	Sanger, J	NY	549
NuM	Schelbert, H	CA	551
NuM	Strashun, A	NY	549
NuM	Ziffer, J	FL	550

Nuclear Endocrinology
NuM	Carrasquillo, J	NY	548
NuM	Sandler, M	TN	549

Nuclear Medicine
NuM	Agress, H	NJ	548
NuM	Alavi, A	PA	548
NuM	Alazraki, N	GA	549
NuM	Carrasquillo, J	NY	548
NuM	Dae, M	CA	551
NuM	Dillehay, G	IL	550
NuM	Freeman, L	NY	548
NuM	Goldsmith, S	NY	548
NuM	Klaas, V	WA	551
NuM	Lamonica, D	NY	548
NuM	Majd, M	DC	548
NuM	Neumann, D	OH	550

NuM	Neumann, R	MD	549
NuM	Pandit-Taskar, N	NY	549
NuM	Podoloff, D	TX	550
NuM	Sandler, M	TN	549
NuM	Sanger, J	NY	549
NuM	Schelbert, H	CA	551
NuM	Siegel, B	MO	550
NuM	Strashun, A	NY	549
NuM	Wahl, R	MD	549
NuM	Waxman, A	CA	551
NuM	Wiseman, G	MN	550
NuM	Ziffer, J	FL	550

Nuclear Oncology
NuM	Agress, H	NJ	548
NuM	Alazraki, N	GA	549
NuM	Freeman, L	NY	548
NuM	Neumann, D	OH	550
NuM	Sanger, J	NY	549

Nuclear Radiology
DR	Partain, C	TN	979
NuM	Klaas, V	WA	551

Nutrition
AM	Bravender, T	OH	81
AM	Singh, N	MN	81
EDM	Holick, M	MA	207
EDM	Jensen, M	MN	218
EDM	Kahn, B	MA	207
EDM	McMahon, M	MN	219
EDM	Osei, K	OH	219
Ge	Fisher, R	CT	228
Ge	Seidner, D	TN	242
Ge	Semrad, C	IL	248
Ge	Toskes, P	FL	243
Ger	Dale, L	MN	264
Ger	Lipschitz, D	AR	266
Ger	Thomas, D	MO	265
IM	Galland, L	NY	424
Nep	Mitch, W	TX	464
NP	Ehrenkranz, R	CT	446
NP	Escobedo, M	OK	451
NP	Lemons, J	IN	450
NP	Milley, J	UT	451
Ped	Jacob, M	IL	728
PEn	Ludwig, D	MA	743
PGe	Baker, R	NY	750
PGe	Baker, S	NY	750
PGe	Berman, J	IL	752
PGe	Black, D	TN	752
PGe	Fasano, A	MD	750
PGe	Gupta, S	IN	753
PGe	Heyman, M	CA	755
PGe	Kleinman, R	MA	749
PGe	Krebs, N	CO	754
PGe	Leichtner, A	MA	749
PGe	Novak, D	FL	752
PGe	Schwarz, S	NY	751
PGe	Sokol, R	CO	754

PGe	Spivak, W	NY	751
PGe	Vanderhoof, J	NE	755
PMR	Dillard, J	NY	835
PPul	Borowitz, D	NY	794
S	Bessey, P	NY	1053
S	Greenhalgh, D	CA	1096

Nutrition & AIDS
Ge	Kotler, D	NY	235

Nutrition & Cancer Prevention
EDM	Heber, D	CA	222
Ge	Kastenberg, D	PA	234
Ge	Mason, J	MA	229
Ge	Shike, M	NY	238
U	Katz, A	NY	1154

Nutrition & Cancer Prevention/Control
Onc	Clinton, S	OH	366
Onc	Kucuk, O	GA	358
S	Herrmann, V	SC	1069
U	Yu, G	MD	1159

Nutrition & Disease Prevention/Control
EDM	Heber, D	CA	222
IM	Gillman, M	MA	424
U	Yu, G	MD	1159

Nutrition & Obesity
EDM	Heber, D	CA	222

Nutrition in Acute Illness
Ge	Mason, J	MA	229

Nutrition in Autism
PGe	Levy, J	NY	750

Nutrition in Bowel Disorders
Ge	Fisher, R	CT	228
Ge	Mason, J	MA	229
Ge	Seidner, D	TN	242
PGe	Thomas, D	CA	756
PS	Barksdale, E	OH	806

Nutrition in Cancer Therapy
Onc	Kucuk, O	GA	358
Onc	Parker, B	CA	389

Nutrition in Heart Disease
T&CS	Gundry, S	CA	1141

Nystagmus
Oph	Demer, J	CA	600

Specialty & Special Expertise Index

Spec	Name	St	Pg
Oph	Granet, D	CA	600
Oph	Mitchell, P	CT	571

O

Obesity

AM	Bermudez, O	CO	81
EDM	Kahn, B	MA	207
Ge	Kaplan, L	MA	229
IM	Gillman, M	MA	424
PEn	Arslanian, S	PA	744
PEn	Diamond, F	FL	745
PEn	Ludwig, D	MA	743
PEn	Lustig, R	CA	749
PEn	Maclaren, N	NY	744
PEn	Silverstein, J	FL	746
PGe	Baker, S	NY	750
PGe	Black, D	TN	752
PGe	Gupta, S	IN	753
PGe	Krebs, N	CO	754
PGe	Novak, D	FL	752
PNep	Flynn, J	WA	788
Psyc	Crow, S	MN	897
RE	Jacobs, L	IL	1013

Obesity-Pediatric

CG	Driscoll, D	FL	158

Obesity/Bariatric Surgery

S	Ballantyne, G	GA	1066
S	Bessler, M	NY	1054
S	Blackstone, R	AZ	1087
S	Chand, B	IL	1075
S	Courcoulas, A	PA	1056
S	Crookes, P	CA	1094
S	Edye, M	NY	1057
S	Frantzides, C	IL	1077
S	Ikramuddin, S	MN	1078
S	Jayaseelan, N	TX	1089
S	Livingston, E	TX	1090
S	MacDonald, K	NC	1070
S	Morton, J	CA	1097
S	Nguyen, N	CA	1097
S	Phillips, E	CA	1098
S	Pomp, A	NY	1062
S	Posselt, A	CA	1098
S	Ramanathan, R	PA	1062
S	Richards, W	AL	1071
S	Rogers, S	CA	1099
S	Rubino, F	NY	1063
S	Sarr, M	MN	1081
S	Schauer, P	OH	1082
S	Shikora, S	MA	1051
S	Sweeney, J	GA	1073

Obsessive-Compulsive Disorder

ChAP	Coffey, B	NY	908
ChAP	Hudziak, J	VT	906
ChAP	Leckman, J	CT	907
ChAP	McCracken, J	CA	912
ChAP	McDougle, C	MA	907
ChAP	Rapoport, J	DC	909
Psyc	Black, D	IA	897
Psyc	Bystritsky, A	CA	901
Psyc	Davidson, J	TX	899
Psyc	Fallon, B	NY	892
Psyc	Greenberg, B	RI	888
Psyc	Hollander, E	NY	892
Psyc	Jenike, M	MA	889
Psyc	Phillips, K	RI	889
Psyc	Price, L	RI	889
Psyc	Rasmussen, S	RI	889
Psyc	Saxena, S	CA	903

Obstetric Pathology

Path	Lage, J	SC	713

Obstetric Ultrasound

DR	Benson, C	MA	973
DR	Doubilet, P	MA	973
DR	Filly, R	CA	983
DR	Kurtz, A	PA	976
MF	Bahado-Singh, R	MI	435
MF	Eddleman, K	NY	432
MF	Mari, G	TN	435
MF	Strassner, H	IL	437
MF	Zalud, I	HI	441
ObG	Corteville, J	OH	560

Obstetrics & Gynecology

ObG	Andersen, G	VA	559
ObG	Argenta, P	MN	560
ObG	Bader, T	PA	556
ObG	Bartholomew, D	OH	560
ObG	Berga, S	NC	559
ObG	Bradley, L	OH	560
ObG	Bradshaw, K	TX	563
ObG	Brodman, M	NY	557
ObG	Byrne, J	UT	562
ObG	Carson, D	PA	557
ObG	Cornella, J	AZ	563
ObG	Corteville, J	OH	560
ObG	Cramer, D	MA	556
ObG	De Cherney, A	MD	557
ObG	De Lancey, J	MI	561
ObG	De Lia, J	WI	561
ObG	Eckler, K	MA	556
ObG	Einarsson, J	MA	556
ObG	Eschenbach, D	WA	563
ObG	Evans, M	NY	557
ObG	Famuyide, A	MN	561
ObG	Filip, S	NC	559
ObG	Goldman, M	CA	563
ObG	Goldstein, M	NY	557
ObG	Gonik, B	MI	561

Spec	Name	St	Pg
ObG	Greenfield, M	OH	561
ObG	Hager, W	KY	559
ObG	Hale, D	IN	561
ObG	Hockstein, S	NY	557
ObG	Hullfish, K	VA	559
ObG	Iglesia, C	DC	557
ObG	Jenkins, T	AL	559
ObG	Karram, M	OH	561
ObG	King, A	ID	562
ObG	Laufer, M	MA	556
ObG	Lengyel, E	IL	561
ObG	Levine, E	IL	562
ObG	Lucente, V	PA	557
ObG	Maynard, S	DC	558
ObG	Merritt, D	MO	562
ObG	Morgan, L	FL	559
ObG	Myers, D	RI	556
ObG	Niebyl, J	IA	562
ObG	Nour, N	MA	556
ObG	Ordorica, S	NY	558
ObG	Parker, W	CA	563
ObG	Pfeifer, S	PA	558
ObG	Sanz, L	VA	559
ObG	Scher, J	NY	558
ObG	Simon, J	DC	558
ObG	Simpson, J	FL	560
ObG	Snyder, R	TX	563
ObG	Steege, J	NC	560
ObG	Sweet, R	CA	563
ObG	Valaitis, S	IL	562
ObG	Visco, A	NC	560
ObG	Walters, M	OH	562
ObG	Wiesenfeld, H	PA	558
ObG	Witter, F	MD	558
ObG	Young, B	NY	558

Occult Spinal Dysraphism (OSD)

NS	Oakes, W	AL	483

Occupational Asthma

A&I	Bernstein, D	OH	87
A&I	Bernstein, J	OH	88
OM	Harber, P	AZ	882
Pul	Sutherland, E	CO	937

Occupational Lung Disease

OM	Harber, P	AZ	882
OM	Kipen, H	NJ	882
Path	Mark, E	MA	706
Pul	Brooks, S	FL	929
Pul	Christiani, D	MA	922
Pul	Goldman, A	FL	931
Pul	Maxfield, R	NY	926
Pul	Redlich, C	CT	923
Pul	Rose, C	CO	937
Pul	Schwartz, D	CO	937
Pul	Shellito, J	LA	938

Specialty & Special Expertise Index

Spec	Name	St	Pg
Occupational Medicine			
OM	Gochfeld, M	NJ	882
OM	Harber, P	AZ	882
OM	Kipen, H	NJ	882
OM	Landrigan, P	NY	882
Pul	Bascom, R	PA	924
Pul	Hyers, T	MO	934
Occupational Musculoskeletal Disorders			
Rhu	Hadler, N	NC	1029
Occupational Skin Diseases			
D	Sherertz, E	SC	192
Oculoplastic & Orbital Surgery			
Oph	Ahmad, A	IL	588
Oph	Carter, K	IA	589
Oph	Choy, A	CA	600
Oph	Katowitz, J	PA	576
Oph	Kikkawa, D	CA	601
Oph	Lucarelli, M	WI	592
Oph	Ng, J	OR	603
Oph	Putterman, A	IL	593
Oph	Stefanyszyn, M	PA	580
PlS	Spinelli, H	NY	858
Oculoplastic Surgery			
Oph	Baylis, H	CA	598
Oph	Bernardino, C	CA	599
Oph	Boxrud, C	CA	599
Oph	Cahill, K	OH	589
Oph	Char, D	CA	599
Oph	Della Rocca, R	NY	573
Oph	Dutton, J	NC	583
Oph	Esmaeli-Azad, B	TX	596
Oph	Iliff, N	MD	575
Oph	Kidwell, E	DC	576
Oph	Kim, J	CA	601
Oph	Lisman, R	NY	576
Oph	Nerad, J	OH	592
Oph	Nunery, W	KY	585
Oph	Rubin, P	MA	571
Oph	Seiff, S	CA	604
Oph	Soparkar, C	TX	598
Oph	Tse, D	FL	586
Oph	Yeatts, R	NC	587
PlS	Carraway, J	VA	860
Ophthalmic Genetics			
Oph	Del Monte, M	MI	589
Oph	Edwards, P	MI	589
Oph	Levin, A	PA	576
Oph	Lewis, R	TX	597
Oph	Mets, M	IL	592
Oph	Murphree, A	CA	602

Spec	Name	St	Pg
Ophthalmic Pathology			
Oph	Albert, D	WI	588
Oph	Alfonso, E	FL	581
Oph	Eagle, R	PA	573
Oph	Grossniklaus, H	GA	583
Oph	Wilson, D	OR	605
Path	Fogt, F	PA	709
Ophthalmic Plastic Surgery			
Oph	Kikkawa, D	CA	601
Oph	Lucarelli, M	WI	592
Oph	Patrinely, J	FL	585
Ophthalmology			
Oph	Abbott, R	CA	598
Oph	Abrams, G	MI	587
Oph	Abramson, D	NY	571
Oph	Afshari, N	NC	581
Oph	Ahmad, A	IL	588
Oph	Albert, D	WI	588
Oph	Alfonso, E	FL	581
Oph	Alward, W	IA	588
Oph	Anderson, R	UT	595
Oph	Archer, S	MI	588
Oph	Arnold, A	CA	598
Oph	Augsburger, J	OH	588
Oph	Azar, D	IL	588
Oph	Azar, N	IL	588
Oph	Baerveldt, G	CA	598
Oph	Baker, J	MI	588
Oph	Baylis, H	CA	598
Oph	Bernardino, C	CA	599
Oph	Biousse, V	GA	582
Oph	Blumenkranz, M	CA	599
Oph	Borchert, M	CA	599
Oph	Boxer Wachler, B	CA	599
Oph	Boxrud, C	CA	599
Oph	Bressler, N	MD	571
Oph	Bressler, S	MD	572
Oph	Brown, G	PA	572
Oph	Brucker, A	PA	572
Oph	Buckley, E	NC	582
Oph	Budenz, D	NC	582
Oph	Burke, M	OH	589
Oph	Cahill, K	OH	589
Oph	Campochiaro, P	MD	572
Oph	Capo, H	FL	582
Oph	Caprioli, J	CA	599
Oph	Caputo, A	NJ	572
Oph	Carlson, A	NC	582
Oph	Carter, K	IA	589
Oph	Caster, A	CA	599
Oph	Chang, S	NY	572
Oph	Char, D	CA	599
Oph	Choy, A	CA	600
Oph	Cionni, R	UT	595
Oph	Clinch, T	MD	572
Oph	Cockerham, K	CA	600
Oph	Crandall, A	UT	595
Oph	Culbertson, W	FL	582

Spec	Name	St	Pg
Oph	Cykiert, R	NY	572
Oph	D'Amico, D	NY	573
Oph	Dana, R	MA	570
Oph	Davis, J	FL	582
Oph	Day, S	CA	600
Oph	De Juan, E	CA	600
Oph	Del Monte, M	MI	589
Oph	Del Priore, L	SC	582
Oph	Della Rocca, R	NY	573
Oph	Demer, J	CA	600
Oph	Dhaliwal, D	PA	573
Oph	Dodick, J	NY	573
Oph	Drack, A	IA	589
Oph	Duker, J	MA	570
Oph	Durrie, D	KS	596
Oph	Dutton, J	NC	583
Oph	Eagle, R	PA	573
Oph	Edwards, P	MI	589
Oph	Eggers, H	NY	573
Oph	Ellis, G	LA	596
Oph	Elner, V	MI	589
Oph	Esmaeli-Azad, B	TX	596
Oph	Eustis, H	LA	596
Oph	Feder, R	IL	589
Oph	Feldon, S	NY	573
Oph	Finger, P	NY	573
Oph	Fishman, G	IL	590
Oph	Florakis, G	NY	574
Oph	Flynn, H	FL	583
Oph	Forster, R	FL	583
Oph	Foster, C	MA	570
Oph	Freedman, S	NC	583
Oph	Freeman, W	CA	600
Oph	Friberg, T	PA	574
Oph	Fuchs, W	NY	574
Oph	Gallin, P	NY	574
Oph	Gentile, R	NY	574
Oph	Gibralter, R	NY	574
Oph	Gigantelli, J	NE	596
Oph	Goldberg, D	NJ	574
Oph	Gorin, M	CA	600
Oph	Gorovoy, M	FL	583
Oph	Granet, D	CA	600
Oph	Greenfield, D	FL	583
Oph	Greenwald, M	IL	590
Oph	Grossniklaus, H	GA	583
Oph	Guy, J	FL	583
Oph	Guyton, D	MD	574
Oph	Haik, B	TN	584
Oph	Hall, L	NY	575
Oph	Haller, J	PA	575
Oph	Handa, J	MD	575
Oph	Harbour, J	FL	584
Oph	Hariprasad, S	IL	590
Oph	Heckenlively, J	MI	590
Oph	Hedges, T	MA	570
Oph	Hersh, P	NJ	575
Oph	Hess, J	FL	584
Oph	Heuer, D	WI	590
Oph	Ho, A	PA	575
Oph	Hodapp, E	FL	584
Oph	Holland, E	OH	590

Specialty & Special Expertise Index

Spec	Name	St	Pg
Oph	Humayun, M	CA	601
Oph	Hunter, D	MA	570
Oph	Iliff, N	MD	575
Oph	Irvine, J	CA	601
Oph	Isenberg, S	CA	601
Oph	Iwach, A	CA	601
Oph	Jaafar, M	DC	575
Oph	Jabs, D	NY	575
Oph	John, T	IL	590
Oph	Katowitz, J	PA	576
Oph	Katz, L	PA	576
Oph	Kaufman, P	WI	590
Oph	Kerr, N	TN	584
Oph	Kidwell, E	DC	576
Oph	Kikkawa, D	CA	601
Oph	Kim, J	CA	601
Oph	Koch, D	TX	596
Oph	Koller, H	PA	576
Oph	Kornmehl, E	MA	570
Oph	Krauss, H	CA	601
Oph	Krueger, R	OH	591
Oph	Kupersmith, M	NY	576
Oph	Kushner, B	WI	591
Oph	Kwon, Y	IA	591
Oph	Lambert, H	TX	597
Oph	Lambert, S	GA	584
Oph	Lane, S	MN	591
Oph	Lass, J	OH	591
Oph	Lee, A	TX	597
Oph	Lee, P	MI	591
Oph	Levin, A	PA	576
Oph	Lewis, R	TX	597
Oph	Lichter, P	MI	591
Oph	Liebmann, J	NY	576
Oph	Lindstrom, R	MN	591
Oph	Lisman, R	NY	576
Oph	Lucarelli, M	WI	592
Oph	Lueder, G	MO	592
Oph	Mackool, R	NY	577
Oph	Magramm, I	NY	577
Oph	Maguire, J	PA	577
Oph	Maguire, L	MN	592
Oph	Maloney, R	CA	601
Oph	Manche, E	CA	602
Oph	Mandel, E	NY	577
Oph	Mannis, M	CA	602
Oph	Marmor, M	CA	602
Oph	Masket, S	CA	602
Oph	Mathers, W	OR	602
Oph	Mawn, L	TN	584
Oph	McCann, J	UT	596
Oph	McCulley, J	TX	597
Oph	McDonnell, P	MD	577
Oph	McKeown, C	FL	584
Oph	Medow, N	NY	577
Oph	Meredith, T	NC	585
Oph	Mets, M	IL	592
Oph	Mieler, W	IL	592
Oph	Miller, J	MA	570
Oph	Miller, J	AZ	597
Oph	Miller, K	CA	602
Oph	Miller, N	MD	577
Oph	Mills, M	PA	577
Oph	Mims, J	TX	597
Oph	Mitchell, P	CT	571
Oph	Mizen, T	IL	592
Oph	Mondino, B	CA	602
Oph	Muldoon, T	NY	578
Oph	Murphree, A	CA	602
Oph	Murray, T	FL	585
Oph	Myers, J	PA	578
Oph	Nelson, L	PA	578
Oph	Nerad, J	OH	592
Oph	Ng, J	OR	603
Oph	Nunery, W	KY	585
Oph	Nussbaum, J	GA	585
Oph	O'Brien, J	PA	578
Oph	O'Brien, T	FL	585
Oph	Odel, J	NY	578
Oph	Olitsky, S	MO	592
Oph	Olsen, T	GA	585
Oph	Orlin, S	PA	578
Oph	Osher, R	OH	593
Oph	Page, T	MI	593
Oph	Parrish, R	FL	585
Oph	Patrinely, J	FL	585
Oph	Paul, T	CA	603
Oph	Pepose, J	MO	593
Oph	Perez, V	FL	586
Oph	Petersen, M	OH	593
Oph	Pflugfelder, S	TX	597
Oph	Plager, D	IN	593
Oph	Pollard, Z	GA	586
Oph	Puliafito, C	CA	603
Oph	Pulido, J	MN	593
Oph	Putterman, A	IL	593
Oph	Quigley, H	MD	578
Oph	Quinn, G	PA	578
Oph	Rao, N	CA	603
Oph	Rapuano, C	PA	579
Oph	Regillo, C	PA	579
Oph	Reynolds, J	NY	579
Oph	Richard, J	OK	597
Oph	Ritch, R	NY	579
Oph	Rizzo, J	MA	571
Oph	Robin, A	MD	579
Oph	Rogers, G	OH	593
Oph	Rosenberg, M	IL	594
Oph	Rosenfeld, P	FL	586
Oph	Rubin, P	MA	571
Oph	Sadda, S	CA	603
Oph	Salz, J	CA	603
Oph	Samuelson, T	MN	594
Oph	Savino, P	CA	603
Oph	Schachat, A	OH	594
Oph	Schein, O	MD	579
Oph	Schiff, W	NY	579
Oph	Schiffman, J	TX	598
Oph	Schuman, J	PA	579
Oph	Schwartz, S	CA	603
Oph	Seibel, B	CA	603
Oph	Seiff, S	CA	604
Oph	Serafano, D	CA	604
Oph	Sergott, R	PA	580
Oph	Shabto, U	NY	580
Oph	Shamie, N	CA	604
Oph	Sherwood, M	FL	586
Oph	Shields, C	PA	580
Oph	Shields, J	PA	580
Oph	Shingleton, B	MA	571
Oph	Siatkowski, R	OK	598
Oph	Simon, J	NY	580
Oph	Smith, R	CA	604
Oph	Solomon, K	SC	586
Oph	Soparkar, C	TX	598
Oph	Spaeth, G	PA	580
Oph	Stark, W	MD	580
Oph	Stefanyszyn, M	PA	580
Oph	Steinert, R	CA	604
Oph	Sternberg, P	TN	586
Oph	Sterns, G	NY	581
Oph	Stone, E	IA	594
Oph	Stout, J	OR	604
Oph	Stulting, R	GA	586
Oph	Summers, C	MN	594
Oph	Traboulsi, E	OH	594
Oph	Trese, M	MI	594
Oph	Trobe, J	MI	594
Oph	Tsai, J	CT	571
Oph	Tse, D	FL	586
Oph	Tychsen, L	MO	595
Oph	Updegraff, S	FL	587
Oph	Vajaranant, T	IL	595
Oph	Vander, J	PA	581
Oph	Volpe, N	IL	595
Oph	Wallace, R	LA	598
Oph	Walsh, J	NY	581
Oph	Walton, D	MA	571
Oph	Wang, F	NY	581
Oph	Wang, M	TN	587
Oph	Waring, G	GA	587
Oph	Warman, R	FL	587
Oph	Weinreb, R	CA	604
Oph	Weiss, A	WA	604
Oph	Williams, G	MI	595
Oph	Wilson, D	OR	605
Oph	Wilson, M	SC	587
Oph	Wilson, M	TN	587
Oph	Wilson, S	OH	595
Oph	Wright, K	CA	605
Oph	Yannuzzi, L	NY	581
Oph	Yeatts, R	NC	587

Opiate Addiction

AdP	Howell, E	UT	905
AdP	Kampman, K	PA	904
AdP	Kleber, H	NY	905
AdP	Kosten, T	TX	906
AdP	Stine, S	MI	905
AdP	Strain, E	MD	905

Opsoclonus-Ataxia in Children

ChiN	Mitchell, W	CA	153

Spec	Name	St	Pg

Opthalmic Genetics

Spec	Name	St	Pg
Oph	Heckenlively, J	MI	590

Optic Nerve Disorders

Spec	Name	St	Pg
N	Galetta, S	PA	512
N	Goodwin, J	IL	526
N	Miller, A	NY	516
Oph	Biousse, V	GA	582
Oph	Borchert, M	CA	599
Oph	Lee, A	TX	597
Oph	Mizen, T	IL	592
Oph	Odel, J	NY	578
Oph	Sergott, R	PA	580
Oph	Trobe, J	MI	594

Optic Nerve Tumors

Spec	Name	St	Pg
Oph	Lee, A	TX	597

Oral Cancer

Spec	Name	St	Pg
Oto	Yoo, G	MI	679

Oral Dermatology

Spec	Name	St	Pg
D	Camisa, C	FL	190

Orbital & Eyelid Tumors/Cancer

Spec	Name	St	Pg
Oph	Anderson, R	UT	595
Oph	Esmaeli-Azad, B	TX	596
Oph	Iliff, N	MD	575
Oph	Lisman, R	NY	576
Oph	Rubin, P	MA	571
Oph	Soparkar, C	TX	598

Orbital Diseases

Spec	Name	St	Pg
Oph	Boxrud, C	CA	599
Oph	Haik, B	TN	584
Oph	McCann, J	UT	596
Oph	Miller, N	MD	577
Oph	Yeatts, R	NC	587

Orbital Surgery

Spec	Name	St	Pg
Oph	Bernardino, C	CA	599
Oph	Cahill, K	OH	589
Oph	Feldon, S	NY	573
Oph	Mawn, L	TN	584
Oph	Nunery, W	KY	585
Oph	Patrinely, J	FL	585

Orbital Tumors/Cancer

Spec	Name	St	Pg
Oph	Abramson, D	NY	571
Oph	Choy, A	CA	600
Oph	Cockerham, K	CA	600
Oph	Della Rocca, R	NY	573
Oph	Elner, V	MI	589
Oph	Finger, P	NY	573
Oph	Gigantelli, J	NE	596
Oph	Kim, J	CA	601

Spec	Name	St	Pg
Oph	Nerad, J	OH	592
Oph	Seiff, S	CA	604
Oph	Shields, C	PA	580
Oph	Tse, D	FL	586
Oph	Yeatts, R	NC	587
RadRO	Markoe, A	FL	955

Orthopaedic Imaging

Spec	Name	St	Pg
DR	Pavlov, H	NY	977

Orthopaedic Infectious Disease

Spec	Name	St	Pg
Inf	Flaherty, J	IL	416
Inf	Siegel, M	WA	420

Orthopaedic Surgery

Spec	Name	St	Pg
OrS	Abdu, W	NH	610
OrS	Aboulafia, A	MD	613
OrS	Agarwal, A	TX	640
OrS	Albert, T	PA	613
OrS	Albright, J	IA	631
OrS	An, H	IL	632
OrS	Anderson, L	CA	641
OrS	Anglen, J	IN	632
OrS	Archdeacon, M	OH	632
OrS	Aronson, J	AR	640
OrS	Bach, B	IL	632
OrS	Balderston, R	PA	614
OrS	Bartolozzi, A	PA	614
OrS	Bauman, P	NY	614
OrS	Beaty, J	TN	627
OrS	Benevenia, J	NJ	614
OrS	Berrey, B	FL	627
OrS	Berry, D	MN	632
OrS	Betz, R	PA	614
OrS	Biermann, J	MI	632
OrS	Bigliani, L	NY	614
OrS	Bitan, F	NY	614
OrS	Blaha, J	MI	632
OrS	Boachie-Adjei, O	NY	614
OrS	Boden, S	GA	628
OrS	Bono, J	MA	610
OrS	Booth, R	PA	615
OrS	Bos, G	WA	641
OrS	Brage, M	WA	642
OrS	Brick, G	MA	610
OrS	Bridwell, K	MO	632
OrS	Brien, E	CA	642
OrS	Brodsky, J	TX	640
OrS	Bronson, M	NY	615
OrS	Browner, B	CT	610
OrS	Bucholz, R	TX	640
OrS	Buckwalter, J	IA	633
OrS	Bukata, S	NY	615
OrS	Buly, R	NY	615
OrS	Burke, D	MA	610
OrS	Caillouette, J	CA	642
OrS	Callaghan, J	IA	633
OrS	Cammisa, F	NY	615
OrS	Cappuccino, A	NY	615
OrS	Carragee, E	CA	642

Spec	Name	St	Pg
OrS	Chapman, J	WA	642
OrS	Cheng, E	MN	633
OrS	Chu, C	PA	615
OrS	Clohisy, D	MN	633
OrS	Conrad, E	WA	642
OrS	Cooper, D	TX	640
OrS	Copp, S	CA	642
OrS	Cornell, C	NY	616
OrS	Coughlin, M	ID	638
OrS	Craig, E	NY	616
OrS	Crossett, L	PA	616
OrS	Curl, W	NC	628
OrS	Davidson, R	PA	616
OrS	Delahay, J	DC	616
OrS	Delamarter, R	CA	642
OrS	Deland, J	NY	616
OrS	DeOrio, J	NC	628
OrS	Diduch, D	VA	628
OrS	DiGiovanni, C	RI	610
OrS	Dillingham, M	CA	643
OrS	Dines, D	NY	616
OrS	Donaldson, W	PA	616
OrS	Dormans, J	PA	617
OrS	Dorr, L	CA	643
OrS	Ebraheim, N	OH	633
OrS	Eckardt, J	CA	643
OrS	Einhorn, T	MA	610
OrS	Eismont, F	FL	628
OrS	Elattrache, N	CA	643
OrS	Endrizzi, D	ME	611
OrS	Errico, T	NY	617
OrS	Estwanik, J	NC	628
OrS	Farmer, J	NY	617
OrS	Feldman, D	NY	617
OrS	Finerman, G	CA	643
OrS	Flatow, E	NY	617
OrS	Frassica, F	MD	617
OrS	Friedlaender, G	CT	611
OrS	Fu, F	PA	617
OrS	Fulkerson, J	CT	611
OrS	Garfin, S	CA	643
OrS	Garrett, W	NC	628
OrS	Garvin, K	NE	639
OrS	Gebhardt, M	MA	611
OrS	Gitelis, S	IL	633
OrS	Gladstone, J	NY	617
OrS	Glashow, J	NY	618
OrS	Goitz, H	MI	633
OrS	Goldner, R	NC	628
OrS	Goldstein, J	NY	618
OrS	Goldstein, W	IL	633
OrS	Goodman, S	CA	643
OrS	Gorab, R	CA	643
OrS	Graf, B	WI	634
OrS	Green, A	RI	611
OrS	Greisberg, J	NY	618
OrS	Grelsamer, R	NY	618
OrS	Gugenheim, J	TX	640
OrS	Haas, S	NY	618
OrS	Hannafin, J	NY	618
OrS	Hanssen, A	MN	634
OrS	Hausman, M	NY	618

Specialty & Special Expertise Index

Spec	Name	St	Pg	Spec	Name	St	Pg	Spec	Name	St	Pg
OrS	Healey, J	NY	619	OrS	McAfee, P	MD	622	OrS	Schuler, T	VA	630
OrS	Hecht, A	NY	619	OrS	McCance, S	NY	622	OrS	Schwab, F	NY	625
OrS	Heiden, E	UT	639	OrS	McCann, P	NY	622	OrS	Schwartz, H	TN	630
OrS	Helfet, D	NY	619	OrS	McCarthy, J	OH	635	OrS	Scott, R	MA	612
OrS	Henshaw, R	DC	619	OrS	McDonald, D	MO	635	OrS	Scott, W	NY	625
OrS	Herman, M	PA	619	OrS	McFarland, E	MD	622	OrS	Seltzer, D	AZ	641
OrS	Herzenberg, J	MD	619	OrS	Menendez, L	CA	644	OrS	Sharkey, P	PA	625
OrS	Hilibrand, A	PA	619	OrS	Miller, M	VA	629	OrS	Shelbourne, K	IN	637
OrS	Hochschuler, S	TX	640	OrS	Millett, P	CO	639	OrS	Siegel, H	AL	630
OrS	Hornicek, F	MA	611	OrS	Minas, T	MA	612	OrS	Sim, F	MN	637
OrS	Hotchkiss, R	NY	620	OrS	Morcuende, J	IA	636	OrS	Singer, D	HI	645
OrS	Howe, K	CA	644	OrS	Mott, M	MI	636	OrS	Smith, D	WA	646
OrS	Hozack, W	PA	620	OrS	Muschler, G	OH	636	OrS	Smith, E	MA	613
OrS	Hume, E	PA	620	OrS	Myerson, M	MD	622	OrS	Souryal, T	TX	641
OrS	Hungerford, M	MD	620	OrS	Nepola, J	IA	636	OrS	Spengler, D	TN	631
OrS	Hyman, J	NY	620	OrS	Neuwirth, M	NY	623	OrS	Spindler, K	TN	631
OrS	Iannotti, J	OH	634	OrS	Nicholas, S	NY	623	OrS	Spivak, J	NY	625
OrS	Irwin, R	MI	634	OrS	Nuber, G	IL	636	OrS	Sponseller, P	MD	625
OrS	Jacobs, J	IL	634	OrS	Nunley, J	NC	629	OrS	Steadman, J	CO	639
OrS	Jiranek, W	VA	629	OrS	O'Donnell, R	CA	645	OrS	Strongwater, A	NJ	626
OrS	Johanson, N	PA	620	OrS	O'Driscoll, S	MN	636	OrS	Stuchin, S	NY	626
OrS	Johnson, C	MD	620	OrS	O'Keefe, R	NY	623	OrS	Stulberg, S	IL	637
OrS	Johnson, D	KY	629	OrS	O'Leary, P	NY	623	OrS	Swiontkowski, M	MN	638
OrS	Johnson, E	CA	644	OrS	Oakes, D	CA	645	OrS	Thomas, B	CA	646
OrS	Jokl, P	CT	611	OrS	Oppenheim, W	CA	645	OrS	Thompson, G	OH	638
OrS	Joyce, M	OH	634	OrS	Otsuka, N	NY	623	OrS	Thornhill, T	MA	613
OrS	Kaeding, C	OH	634	OrS	Padgett, D	NY	623	OrS	Tolo, V	CA	646
OrS	Kaplan, F	PA	620	OrS	Paley, D	FL	630	OrS	Tornetta, P	MA	613
OrS	Karas, S	GA	629	OrS	Parsons, T	MI	636	OrS	Vaccaro, A	PA	626
OrS	Kasser, J	MA	611	OrS	Parvizi, J	PA	623	OrS	Vail, T	CA	646
OrS	Kelly, B	NY	621	OrS	Peabody, T	IL	636	OrS	Vo, P	FL	631
OrS	Kelly, C	CO	639	OrS	Pellicci, P	NY	623	OrS	Walling, A	FL	631
OrS	Kenan, S	NY	621	OrS	Peterson, D	AK	645	OrS	Wang, J	CA	646
OrS	Kenter, K	OH	634	OrS	Pettrone, F	VA	630	OrS	Wapner, K	PA	626
OrS	Kim, C	CA	644	OrS	Philippon, M	CO	639	OrS	Ward, W	NC	631
OrS	Kneisl, J	NC	629	OrS	Pinzur, M	IL	637	OrS	Warren, R	NY	626
OrS	Kocher, M	MA	612	OrS	Pizzutillo, P	PA	624	OrS	Watkins, R	CA	646
OrS	Kraay, M	OH	635	OrS	Plancher, K	NY	624	OrS	Webb, L	GA	631
OrS	Krackow, K	NY	621	OrS	Poehling, G	NC	630	OrS	Weiner, R	FL	631
OrS	Kress, K	GA	629	OrS	Polly, D	MN	637	OrS	Weinfeld, S	NY	626
OrS	Lane, J	NY	621	OrS	Rajacich, N	WA	645	OrS	Weinstein, J	NH	613
OrS	Lauerman, W	DC	621	OrS	Ramsey, M	PA	624	OrS	Weinstein, S	IA	638
OrS	Laurencin, C	CT	612	OrS	Randall, R	UT	639	OrS	Westrich, G	NY	626
OrS	Leadbetter, W	MD	621	OrS	Ready, J	MA	612	OrS	Wetzel, F	PA	626
OrS	Lebwohl, N	FL	629	OrS	Reilly, D	MA	612	OrS	Wickiewicz, T	NY	627
OrS	Lee, F	NY	621	OrS	Richardson, W	NC	630	OrS	Wiesel, S	DC	627
OrS	Lenke, L	MO	635	OrS	Richmond, J	MA	612	OrS	Wilkins, R	CO	640
OrS	Les, K	MI	635	OrS	Riew, K	MO	637	OrS	Williams, G	PA	627
OrS	Levine, D	NY	621	OrS	Rodosky, M	PA	624	OrS	Williams, R	TX	641
OrS	Lewis, V	TX	641	OrS	Romeo, A	IL	637	OrS	Wirth, M	TX	641
OrS	Lock, T	MI	635	OrS	Rosenberg, T	UT	639	OrS	Wittig, J	NY	627
OrS	Lowenberg, D	CA	644	OrS	Rothman, R	PA	624	OrS	Wixson, R	IL	638
OrS	Luck, J	CA	644	OrS	Roye, D	NY	624	OrS	Wurtz, L	IN	638
OrS	Mabrey, J	TX	641	OrS	Rozbruch, S	NY	624	OrS	Yamaguchi, K	MO	638
OrS	Macaulay, W	NY	622	OrS	Saltzman, C	UT	639	OrS	Yoo, J	OR	646
OrS	Malawer, M	MD	622	OrS	Salvati, E	NY	625	OrS	Zarins, B	MA	613
OrS	Mandelbaum, B	CA	644	OrS	Sandhu, H	NY	625	OrS	Zdeblick, T	WI	638
OrS	Manoli, A	MI	635	OrS	Sangeorzan, B	WA	645	OrS	Zuckerman, J	NY	627
OrS	Marsh, J	CT	612	OrS	Scarborough, M	FL	630				
OrS	Marx, R	NY	622	OrS	Schafer, M	IL	637		**Ostechondritis Dissecans (OCD)**		
OrS	Matsen, F	WA	644	OrS	Schmalzried, T	CA	645	SM	Micheli, L	MA	1040
OrS	Mayerson, J	OH	635	OrS	Schmidt, R	PA	625				

Spec	Name	St	Pg
Osteoarthritis			
Rhu	Fields, T	NY	1026
Rhu	Hochberg, M	MD	1026
Rhu	Hugenberg, S	IN	1031
Rhu	Magid, S	NY	1027
Rhu	O'Dell, J	NE	1032
Rhu	Shadick, N	MA	1025
Osteodystrophy			
PNep	Andreoli, S	IN	787
Osteomyelitis			
OrS	Browner, B	CT	610
OrS	Lowenberg, D	CA	644
OrS	Swiontkowski, M	MN	638
Osteonecrosis			
OrS	Einhorn, T	MA	610
OrS	Kelly, C	CO	639
OrS	Oakes, D	CA	645
OrS	Vail, T	CA	646
Osteopetrosis			
PHO	Coccia, P	NE	774
Osteoporosis			
EDM	Bergman, D	NY	209
EDM	Bilezikian, J	NY	209
EDM	Bockman, R	NY	209
EDM	Dalkin, A	VA	214
EDM	Econs, M	IN	217
EDM	Emanuele, M	IL	217
EDM	Greene, L	NY	210
EDM	Greenspan, S	PA	210
EDM	Holick, M	MA	207
EDM	Khosla, S	MN	218
EDM	Lash, R	MI	218
EDM	LeBoff, M	MA	208
EDM	Orwoll, E	OR	223
EDM	Recker, R	NE	220
EDM	Roberts, M	PA	211
EDM	Siris, E	NY	212
EDM	Watts, N	OH	219
EDM	Young, I	NY	213
Ger	Gambert, S	MD	263
Ger	Lyles, K	NC	264
Nep	Ott, S	WA	465
ObG	Simon, J	DC	558
PEn	DeLuca, F	PA	744
PEn	Levine, M	PA	744
RE	Luciano, A	CT	1007
Rhu	Hochberg, M	MD	1026
Rhu	Lindsey, S	LA	1033
Rhu	Lipstate, J	LA	1033
Rhu	Mease, P	WA	1034
Rhu	Mitnick, H	NY	1027
Rhu	Schoen, R	CT	1024
Rhu	West, S	CO	1032

Spec	Name	St	Pg
Osteoporosis in Men			
EDM	Greenspan, S	PA	210
EDM	Orwoll, E	OR	223
Osteoporosis Spine-Kyphoplasty			
NRad	Norbash, A	MA	984
OrS	Lane, J	NY	621
Osteoporosis Spine-Vertebroplasty			
NRad	Hirsch, J	MA	984
NRad	Jensen, M	VA	987
NRad	Kallmes, D	MN	989
VIR	Ketcham, D	MN	995
Osteoporosis-Juvenile			
PNep	Langman, C	IL	787
Otolaryngology			
Oto	Abaza, M	CO	679
Oto	Akervall, J	MI	672
Oto	Alam, D	OH	672
Oto	Amedee, R	LA	681
Oto	Andersen, P	OR	684
Oto	Arriaga, M	LA	681
Oto	Arts, H	MI	672
Oto	Aviv, J	NY	657
Oto	Baim, H	IL	672
Oto	Baker, S	MI	673
Oto	Balkany, T	FL	667
Oto	Bastian, R	IL	673
Oto	Beatty, C	MN	673
Oto	Becker, F	FL	667
Oto	Benninger, M	OH	673
Oto	Berke, G	CA	684
Oto	Bhattacharyya, N	MA	655
Oto	Blackwell, K	CA	684
Oto	Blair, E	IL	673
Oto	Blitzer, A	NY	658
Oto	Bojrab, D	MI	673
Oto	Bolger, W	FL	667
Oto	Brackmann, D	CA	684
Oto	Bradford, C	MI	673
Oto	Branham, G	MO	673
Oto	Browne, J	NC	667
Oto	Bumpous, J	KY	667
Oto	Burkey, B	OH	674
Oto	Burns, J	MA	655
Oto	Caldarelli, D	IL	674
Oto	Califano, J	MD	658
Oto	Campbell, B	WI	674
Oto	Carey, J	MD	658
Oto	Caruana, S	NY	658
Oto	Chalian, A	PA	658
Oto	Chowdhury, K	CO	679
Oto	Civantos, F	FL	667
Oto	Clark, K	OK	681
Oto	Clayman, G	TX	681
Oto	Close, L	NY	658

Spec	Name	St	Pg
Oto	Corey, J	IL	674
Oto	Costantino, P	NY	658
Oto	Couch, M	VT	655
Oto	Courey, M	CA	684
Oto	Davidson, B	DC	658
Oto	Day, T	SC	668
Oto	Denenberg, S	NE	680
Oto	Deschler, D	MA	655
Oto	Diaz, E	TX	681
Oto	DiNardo, L	VA	668
Oto	Donald, P	CA	684
Oto	Donovan, D	TX	681
Oto	Dornhoffer, J	AR	682
Oto	Driscoll, C	MN	674
Oto	Duckert, L	WA	684
Oto	Edelstein, D	NY	659
Oto	Eisele, D	MD	659
Oto	Epstein, J	FL	668
Oto	Farrior, E	FL	668
Oto	Farrior, J	FL	668
Oto	Fee, W	CA	684
Oto	Feghali, J	NY	659
Oto	Ferris, R	PA	659
Oto	Flint, P	OR	685
Oto	Ford, C	WI	674
Oto	Fried, M	NY	659
Oto	Friedman, M	IL	674
Oto	Funk, G	IA	674
Oto	Futran, N	WA	685
Oto	Gantz, B	IA	675
Oto	Genden, E	NY	659
Oto	Gianoli, G	LA	682
Oto	Gliklich, R	MA	655
Oto	Goebel, J	MO	675
Oto	Gold, S	NY	659
Oto	Goldenberg, D	PA	659
Oto	Goodwin, W	FL	668
Oto	Gosselin, B	NH	655
Oto	Graham, H	LA	682
Oto	Grandis, J	PA	660
Oto	Grillone, G	MA	655
Oto	Grundfast, K	MA	656
Oto	Hadlock, T	MA	656
Oto	Hammerschlag, P	NY	660
Oto	Hanna, E	TX	682
Oto	Har-El, G	NY	660
Oto	Harris, J	CA	685
Oto	Hartig, G	WI	675
Oto	Haughey, B	MO	675
Oto	Hayden, R	AZ	682
Oto	Haynes, D	TN	668
Oto	Hicks, W	NY	660
Oto	Hilger, P	MN	675
Oto	Hirsch, B	PA	660
Oto	Hoffman, H	IA	675
Oto	Hoffman, R	NY	660
Oto	Hogikyan, N	MI	675
Oto	Holliday, M	MD	660
Oto	Hopping, S	DC	660
Oto	Hotaling, A	IL	675
Oto	Hurst, M	WV	661
Oto	Jackler, R	CA	685

Specialty & Special Expertise Index

Spec	Name	St	Pg	Spec	Name	St	Pg	Spec	Name	St	Pg
Oto	Jacobs, J	NY	661	Oto	Paparella, M	MN	677	Oto	Teknos, T	OH	678
Oto	Jenkins, H	CO	680	Oto	Papel, I	MD	663	Oto	Telian, S	MI	678
Oto	Johnson, C	LA	682	Oto	Parisier, S	NY	663	Oto	Telischi, F	FL	671
Oto	Johnson, J	PA	661	Oto	Patil, Y	OH	677	Oto	Terris, D	GA	671
Oto	Jones, P	IL	676	Oto	Pelzer, H	IL	677	Oto	Thaler, E	PA	666
Oto	Josephson, J	NY	661	Oto	Pensak, M	OH	677	Oto	Toriumi, D	IL	678
Oto	Kang, D	NE	680	Oto	Persky, M	NY	663	Oto	Tucci, D	NC	672
Oto	Kaplan, M	CA	685	Oto	Peters, G	AL	670	Oto	Tufano, R	MD	666
Oto	Kartush, J	MI	676	Oto	Petruzzelli, G	GA	670	Oto	Urken, M	NY	666
Oto	Keane, W	PA	661	Oto	Piccirillo, J	MO	677	Oto	Valentino, J	KY	672
Oto	Keller, G	CA	685	Oto	Picken, C	DC	663	Oto	Vining, E	CT	657
Oto	Kennedy, D	PA	661	Oto	Pillsbury, H	NC	670	Oto	Wackym, P	OR	687
Oto	Kern, R	IL	676	Oto	Pitman, K	MS	670	Oto	Waner, M	NY	666
Oto	Kesser, B	VA	668	Oto	Poole, M	GA	670	Oto	Wang, S	CA	687
Oto	Kim, D	MA	656	Oto	Postma, G	GA	670	Oto	Wax, M	OR	687
Oto	Kingdom, T	CO	680	Oto	Pribitkin, E	PA	663	Oto	Wazen, J	FL	672
Oto	Koch, W	MD	661	Oto	Quatela, V	NY	664	Oto	Weber, R	TX	683
Oto	Koufman, J	NY	661	Oto	Randolph, G	MA	656	Oto	Weber, S	TX	683
Oto	Kraus, D	NY	662	Oto	Rassekh, C	PA	664	Oto	Weinstein, G	PA	666
Oto	Krespi, Y	NY	662	Oto	Rauch, S	MA	656	Oto	Weisman, R	CA	687
Oto	Kuhel, W	NY	662	Oto	Rebeiz, E	MA	657	Oto	Weissler, M	NC	672
Oto	Kuhn, F	GA	669	Oto	Rice, D	CA	686	Oto	Weymuller, E	WA	687
Oto	Kveton, J	CT	656	Oto	Ries, W	TN	670	Oto	Wiet, R	IL	678
Oto	Lalwani, A	NY	662	Oto	Roland, J	NY	664	Oto	Wilson, K	OH	678
Oto	Lambert, P	SC	669	Oto	Rosen, C	PA	664	Oto	Wolf, G	MI	678
Oto	Lanza, D	FL	669	Oto	Rosenthal, E	AL	670	Oto	Wong, B	CA	688
Oto	Larrabee, W	WA	685	Oto	Rubinstein, J	WA	686	Oto	Wong, R	NY	666
Oto	Lavertu, P	OH	676	Oto	Samant, S	TN	671	Oto	Woo, P	NY	666
Oto	Lawson, W	NY	662	Oto	Sasaki, C	CT	657	Oto	Woodson, B	WI	679
Oto	Lebovics, R	NY	662	Oto	Sataloff, R	PA	664	Oto	Woodson, G	IL	679
Oto	Leonetti, J	IL	676	Oto	Schaefer, S	NY	664	Oto	Yarbrough, W	CT	657
Oto	Levine, P	VA	669	Oto	Schaitkin, B	PA	664	Oto	Yoo, G	MI	679
Oto	Linstrom, C	NY	662	Oto	Schantz, S	NY	664	Oto	Young, N	IL	679
Oto	Lustig, L	CA	685	Oto	Schley, W	NY	665	Oto	Yueh, B	MN	679
Oto	Lydiatt, D	NE	680	Oto	Senders, C	CA	686	Oto	Zalzal, G	DC	667
Oto	Lydiatt, W	NE	680	Oto	Senior, B	NC	671	Oto	Zeitels, S	MA	657
Oto	Macias, J	AZ	682	Oto	Setzen, M	NY	665	Oto	Zwillenberg, S	PA	667
Oto	Mangat, D	KY	669	Oto	Shapshay, S	NY	665				
Oto	Marentette, L	MI	676	Oto	Shelton, C	UT	680	## Otology			
Oto	Mattox, D	GA	669	Oto	Shindo, M	OR	687	Oto	Farrior, J	FL	668
Oto	McKenna, M	MA	656	Oto	Shockley, W	NC	671	Oto	Haynes, D	TN	668
Oto	McMenomey, S	OR	686	Oto	Siegel, G	IL	677	Oto	Holliday, M	MD	660
Oto	Medina, J	OK	682	Oto	Sillers, M	AL	671	Oto	Macias, J	AZ	682
Oto	Metson, R	MA	656	Oto	Silverman, D	VT	657	Oto	McKenna, M	MA	656
Oto	Miller, F	TX	683	Oto	Silverstein, H	FL	671	Oto	Tucci, D	NC	672
Oto	Mirza, N	PA	662	Oto	Singer, M	CA	687	PO	Arnold, J	OH	791
Oto	Miyamoto, R	IN	676	Oto	Singh, B	NY	665	PO	Darrow, D	VA	791
Oto	Moe, K	WA	686	Oto	Sinha, U	CA	687	PO	Eavey, R	TN	791
Oto	Myers, J	TX	683	Oto	Smith, R	NE	680	PO	Kazahaya, K	PA	790
Oto	Naclerio, R	IL	676	Oto	Snyderman, C	PA	665	PO	Tunkel, D	MD	790
Oto	Netterville, J	TN	669	Oto	Song, J	CO	681				
Oto	Newkirk, K	DC	663	Oto	Spiegel, J	MA	657	## Otology & Neuro-Otology			
Oto	Niparko, J	MD	663	Oto	Stankiewicz, J	IL	677	Oto	Amedee, R	LA	681
Oto	Nuss, D	LA	683	Oto	Stasney, C	TX	683	Oto	Beatty, C	MN	673
Oto	O'Leary, M	CA	686	Oto	Stenson, K	IL	678	Oto	Bojrab, D	MI	673
Oto	O'Malley, B	PA	663	Oto	Stewart, M	NY	665	Oto	Duckert, L	WA	684
Oto	Oghalai, J	CA	686	Oto	Stringer, S	MS	671	Oto	Goebel, J	MO	675
Oto	Olsen, K	MN	677	Oto	Strome, M	NY	665	Oto	McMenomey, S	OR	686
Oto	Orloff, L	CA	686	Oto	Strome, S	MD	665				
Oto	Ossoff, R	TN	669	Oto	Suen, J	AR	683				
Oto	Otto, R	TX	683	Oto	Sulica, R	NY	666				
Oto	Ozer, E	OH	677	Oto	Szachowicz, E	MN	678				

Specialty & Special Expertise Index

Spec	Name	St	Pg

Otosclerosis/Stapedectomy

Spec	Name	St	Pg
Oto	Brackmann, D	CA	684
Oto	Duckert, L	WA	684
Oto	Farrior, J	FL	668
Oto	Wiet, R	IL	678

Ovarian Cancer

Spec	Name	St	Pg
CG	Plon, S	TX	162
CG	Shulman, L	IL	160
CG	Weitzel, J	CA	164
GO	Abbas, F	MD	275
GO	Abu-Rustum, N	NY	276
GO	Alvarez, R	AL	280
GO	Barakat, R	NY	276
GO	Barter, J	MD	276
GO	Berchuck, A	NC	280
GO	Berek, J	CA	289
GO	Bicher, A	VA	280
GO	Bodurka, D	TX	286
GO	Boice, C	MD	276
GO	Borst, M	AZ	286
GO	Braly, P	LA	287
GO	Brewer, M	CT	274
GO	Bristow, R	CA	289
GO	Burger, R	PA	276
GO	Cain, J	MA	274
GO	Caputo, T	NY	276
GO	Carlson, J	NJ	276
GO	Chambers, S	AZ	287
GO	Chan, J	CA	289
GO	Chi, D	NY	277
GO	Cliby, W	MN	283
GO	Copeland, L	OH	283
GO	Cornelison, T	MD	277
GO	Coukos, G	PA	277
GO	Creasman, W	SC	280
GO	Curtin, J	NY	277
GO	De Geest, K	IA	283
GO	Di Saia, P	CA	289
GO	Dunton, C	PA	277
GO	Duska, L	VA	281
GO	Edwards, R	PA	277
GO	Finan, M	AL	281
GO	Fromm, G	TX	287
GO	Ghamande, S	GA	281
GO	Giuntoli, R	MD	278
GO	Goff, B	WA	289
GO	Havrilesky, L	NC	281
GO	Herzog, T	NY	278
GO	Horowitz, I	GA	281
GO	Karlan, B	CA	290
GO	Kelley, J	PA	278
GO	King, S	PA	278
GO	Kline, R	LA	287
GO	Koulos, J	NY	278
GO	Lancaster, J	FL	281
GO	Lele, S	NY	279
GO	Lin, J	DC	279
GO	Lu, K	TX	288
GO	Lurain, J	IL	284
GO	Makhija, S	KY	282
GO	Modesitt, S	VA	282
GO	Moore, D	IN	284
GO	Muntz, H	WA	290
GO	Muto, M	MA	275
GO	Odunsi, A	NY	279
GO	Pejovic, T	OR	290
GO	Plaxe, S	CA	290
GO	Poliakoff, S	FL	282
GO	Potkul, R	IL	285
GO	Rader, J	WI	285
GO	Remmenga, S	NE	286
GO	Rice, L	WI	285
GO	Rose, P	OH	285
GO	Rosenblum, N	PA	279
GO	Rotmensch, J	IL	285
GO	Rubin, S	PA	279
GO	Runowicz, C	FL	282
GO	Rutherford, T	CT	275
GO	Santin, A	CT	275
GO	Schink, J	IL	285
GO	Schorge, J	MA	275
GO	Schwartz, P	CT	275
GO	Singh, D	AZ	288
GO	Smith, D	IL	285
GO	Smith, L	CA	290
GO	Sood, A	TX	288
GO	Spann, C	GA	283
GO	Spirtos, N	NV	290
GO	Teng, N	CA	291
GO	Van Nagell, J	KY	283
GO	Waggoner, S	OH	286
GO	Walker, J	OK	288
ObG	Argenta, P	MN	560
ObG	Cramer, D	MA	556
ObG	Lengyel, E	IL	561
Onc	Aghajanian, C	NY	333
Onc	Alberts, D	AZ	377
Onc	Astrow, A	NY	334
Onc	Birrer, M	MA	327
Onc	Colon-Otero, G	FL	355
Onc	Disis, M	WA	385
Onc	Fleming, G	IL	367
Onc	Kohn, E	MD	343
Onc	Markman, M	PA	345
Onc	Matulonis, U	MA	331
Onc	McGuire, W	MD	345
Onc	Pasmantier, M	NY	347
Onc	Reed, E	AL	361
Onc	Schilder, R	PA	349
Onc	Scudder, S	CA	390
Onc	Speyer, J	NY	349
Onc	Spriggs, D	NY	350
Onc	Verschraegen, C	VT	333
Path	Bell, D	MN	715
Path	Cho, K	MI	715
Path	Dubeau, L	CA	720
Path	Kurman, R	MD	710
Path	Nicosia, S	FL	714
Path	Tornos, C	NY	712
Path	Wilczynski, S	CA	722
Path	Young, R	MA	707
S	Hughes, K	MA	1050
S	Sugarbaker, P	DC	1065

Ovarian Cancer Risk Assessment

Spec	Name	St	Pg
Onc	Daly, M	PA	337

Ovarian Cancer-Early Detection

Spec	Name	St	Pg
GO	Azodi, M	CT	274
GO	Cain, J	MA	274
GO	DePriest, P	KY	280
GO	Fishman, D	NY	278
GO	Lu, K	TX	288
GO	Rutherford, T	CT	275
GO	Singh, D	AZ	288

Ovarian Cancer-High Risk

Spec	Name	St	Pg
ObG	Cramer, D	MA	556

Ovarian Failure

Spec	Name	St	Pg
ObG	Simpson, J	FL	560
RE	Legro, R	PA	1009

Ovarian Masses in Children/Adolescents

Spec	Name	St	Pg
PS	Dolgin, S	NY	803

Ovarian Rare & Borderline Tumors

Spec	Name	St	Pg
GO	Gershenson, D	TX	287

Oxalosis

Spec	Name	St	Pg
PNep	Langman, C	IL	787

P

Pacemakers

Spec	Name	St	Pg
CE	Callans, D	PA	119
CE	Chinitz, L	NY	120
CE	Cohen, M	NY	120
CE	Curtis, A	NY	120
CE	DiMarco, J	VA	121
CE	Ellenbogen, K	VA	121
CE	Epstein, L	MA	119
CE	Gomes, J	NY	120
CE	Halperin, H	MD	120
CE	Hammill, S	MN	123
CE	Hayes, D	MN	123
CE	Kay, G	AL	122
CE	Levine, J	NY	121
CE	Love, C	OH	123
CE	Marchlinski, F	PA	121
CE	Onufer, J	VA	122
CE	Sorrentino, R	GA	122
CE	Swerdlow, C	CA	125

Specialty & Special Expertise Index

Spec	Name	St	Pg
Cv	Myerburg, R	FL	104
Cv	Naccarelli, G	PA	100
PCd	Crosson, J	MD	735
PCd	Fish, F	TN	737

Paget's Disease of Bone

Spec	Name	St	Pg
EDM	Bergman, D	NY	209
EDM	Bockman, R	NY	209
EDM	Econs, M	IN	217
EDM	Siris, E	NY	212
EDM	Watts, N	OH	219
OrS	Bukata, S	NY	615
Rhu	Seton, M	MA	1025

Pain & Spasticity

Spec	Name	St	Pg
NS	Whiting, D	PA	480

Pain Care-Racial/Ethnic Disparities

Spec	Name	St	Pg
PM	Green, C	MI	699

Pain Management

Spec	Name	St	Pg
AdP	Howell, E	UT	905
DR	Palmer, W	MA	973
Ger	Bloom, P	NY	262
Ger	Finucane, T	MD	263
N	Schwartzman, R	PA	517
NS	Berger, M	CA	495
NS	Burchiel, K	OR	496
NS	Di Giacinto, G	NY	473
Onc	Levy, M	PA	344
PCCM	Anand, K	TN	741
Ped	Zeltzer, L	CA	729
PM	Argoff, C	NY	696
PM	Robbins, L	IL	700
PMR	Borg-Stein, J	MA	834
PMR	Creamer, M	FL	838
PMR	Dillard, J	NY	835
Pul	Shore, B	MO	935

Pain Management-Pediatric

Spec	Name	St	Pg
PM	Anghelescu, D	TN	698
PM	Berde, C	MA	696
PM	Koh, J	OR	702
PM	Vetter, T	AL	699
PM	Weisman, S	WI	700

Pain Medicine

Spec	Name	St	Pg
H & PM	Portenoy, R	NY	406
NS	Zimmerman, C	ID	492
PM	Abram, S	WI	699
PM	Anghelescu, D	TN	698
PM	Argoff, C	NY	696
PM	Audell, L	CA	702
PM	Ballantyne, J	WA	702
PM	Baumann, P	GA	698
PM	Benzon, H	IL	699
PM	Berde, C	MA	696

Spec	Name	St	Pg
PM	Burton, A	TX	701
PM	Christo, P	MD	696
PM	Cope, D	MD	696
PM	Covington, E	OH	699
PM	DeLeon, O	NY	697
PM	Diwan, S	NY	697
PM	Driver, L	TX	701
PM	Falco, F	DE	697
PM	Ferrante, F	CA	702
PM	Fine, P	UT	700
PM	Fishman, S	CA	702
PM	Fitzgibbon, D	WA	702
PM	Freitag, F	TX	701
PM	Fuller, N	CA	702
PM	Gharibo, C	NY	697
PM	Gobrial, W	FL	698
PM	Green, C	MI	699
PM	Hooten, W	MN	699
PM	Huntoon, M	TN	698
PM	Jain, S	NY	697
PM	Jasmin, L	CA	702
PM	Koh, J	OR	702
PM	Kreitzer, J	NY	697
PM	Loder, E	MA	696
PM	Macadaeg, K	IN	699
PM	Mackey, S	CA	703
PM	Mekhail, N	OH	700
PM	Ngeow, J	NY	697
PM	Noe, C	TX	701
PM	Peeters-Asdourian, C	MA	696
PM	Prager, J	CA	703
PM	Racz, G	TX	701
PM	Raja, S	MD	697
PM	Ramamurthy, S	TX	701
PM	Rauck, R	NC	699
PM	Richman, D	NY	698
PM	Robbins, L	IL	700
PM	Rosenquist, R	OH	700
PM	Rosner, H	CA	703
PM	Ross, E	MA	696
PM	Slatkin, N	CA	703
PM	Staats, P	NJ	698
PM	Suresh, S	IL	700
PM	Swarm, R	MO	700
PM	Vetter, T	AL	699
PM	Wallace, M	CA	703
PM	Walsh, N	TX	701
PM	Weinberger, M	NY	698
PM	Weisman, S	WI	700
PM	Wellington, J	IN	700

Pain-Abdominal Recurrent

Spec	Name	St	Pg
PGe	Gunasekaran, T	IL	753
PGe	Kirschner, B	IL	753

Pain-Abdominal/Functional

Spec	Name	St	Pg
Ge	Drossman, D	NC	240
Ge	Lambiase, L	TN	241

Pain-Acute

Spec	Name	St	Pg
PM	DeLeon, O	NY	697
PM	Swarm, R	MO	700

Pain-after Spinal Intervention

Spec	Name	St	Pg
PM	Diwan, S	NY	697
PM	Huntoon, M	TN	698
PM	Racz, G	TX	701
PM	Rosner, H	CA	703

Pain-Back

Spec	Name	St	Pg
N	Hiesiger, E	NY	512
NS	Bauer, J	IL	486
OrS	Lauerman, W	DC	621
OrS	Schwab, F	NY	625
OrS	Weinstein, J	NH	613
PM	Baumann, P	GA	698
PM	Benzon, H	IL	699
PM	Kreitzer, J	NY	697
PM	Ramamurthy, S	TX	701
PM	Rosenquist, R	OH	700
PM	Rosner, H	CA	703
PM	Staats, P	NJ	698
PM	Walsh, N	TX	701
PM	Weinberger, M	NY	698
PMR	Harris, D	TX	843
PMR	Kezar, L	AL	838
PMR	La Ban, M	MI	841
PMR	Press, J	IL	841
PMR	Sliwa, J	IL	842
Rhu	Hadler, N	NC	1029
SM	Schechter, D	CA	1044

Pain-Back & Neck

Spec	Name	St	Pg
PM	Ferrante, F	CA	702
PM	Gharibo, C	NY	697
PM	Mekhail, N	OH	700
PM	Noe, C	TX	701
PM	Richman, D	NY	698
PMR	Haig, A	MI	840
PMR	Ragnarsson, K	NY	837

Pain-Back & Shoulder

Spec	Name	St	Pg
N	Smith, W	CA	539

Pain-Back, Head & Neck

Spec	Name	St	Pg
PM	Racz, G	TX	701

Pain-Cancer

Spec	Name	St	Pg
H & PM	Abrahm, J	MA	406
H & PM	Portenoy, R	NY	406
H & PM	Selvaggi, K	MA	406
H & PM	Weinstein, S	UT	408
Onc	Grossman, S	MD	341
Onc	Levy, M	PA	344
PM	Anghelescu, D	TN	698
PM	Ballantyne, J	WA	702
PM	Benzon, H	IL	699

Spec	Name	St	Pg
PM	Burton, A	TX	701
PM	DeLeon, O	NY	697
PM	Diwan, S	NY	697
PM	Driver, L	TX	701
PM	Fine, P	UT	700
PM	Fishman, S	CA	702
PM	Fitzgibbon, D	WA	702
PM	Huntoon, M	TN	698
PM	Jain, S	NY	697
PM	Jasmin, L	CA	702
PM	Kreitzer, J	NY	697
PM	Mackey, S	CA	703
PM	Mekhail, N	OH	700
PM	Rauck, R	NC	699
PM	Slatkin, N	CA	703
PM	Staats, P	NJ	698
PM	Swarm, R	MO	700
PM	Wallace, M	CA	703
PM	Weinberger, M	NY	698
PM	Weisman, S	WI	700
PM	Wellington, J	IN	700
PMR	Cheville, A	MN	839
PMR	Stubblefield, M	NY	837
Psyc	Breitbart, W	NY	891
Psyc	Strouse, T	CA	903

Pain-Cancer, Spine

Spec	Name	St	Pg
N	Hiesiger, E	NY	512

Pain-Chronic

Spec	Name	St	Pg
NS	Brown, F	IL	486
NS	Cosgrove, R	RI	470
NS	Rezai, A	OH	489
PM	Ballantyne, J	WA	702
PM	Covington, E	OH	699
PM	DeLeon, O	NY	697
PM	Falco, F	DE	697
PM	Fine, P	UT	700
PM	Fishman, S	CA	702
PM	Gharibo, C	NY	697
PM	Mackey, S	CA	703
PM	Mekhail, N	OH	700
PM	Ramamurthy, S	TX	701
PM	Swarm, R	MO	700
PM	Vetter, T	AL	699
PM	Wallace, M	CA	703
PMR	King, J	TX	843
Psyc	Cohen, M	PA	891

Pain-Chronic after Head Injury

Spec	Name	St	Pg
N	Saper, J	MI	530

Pain-Chronic Pelvic

Spec	Name	St	Pg
RE	Petrozza, J	MA	1007

Pain-Facial

Spec	Name	St	Pg
N	Cutrer, F	MN	526
N	Finkel, A	NC	521
N	Kincaid, J	IN	527

Spec	Name	St	Pg
N	Newman, L	NY	516
NS	Patel, S	SC	483
PM	Rosenquist, R	OH	700

Pain-HIV patients

Spec	Name	St	Pg
H & PM	Arnold, R	PA	406

Pain-Interventional Techniques

Spec	Name	St	Pg
PM	Hooten, W	MN	699
PM	Macadaeg, K	IN	699

Pain-Inverventional Techniques

Spec	Name	St	Pg
PM	Argoff, C	NY	696

Pain-Low Back

Spec	Name	St	Pg
PM	Christo, P	MD	696
PMR	Braddom, R	PA	835
PMR	Lutz, C	NY	836
PMR	Lutz, G	NY	836

Pain-Lower Back (IDET Procedure)

Spec	Name	St	Pg
PMR	Lutz, C	NY	836

Pain-Lower Back (IDET procedure)

Spec	Name	St	Pg
PMR	Saal, J	CA	844

Pain-Musculoskeletal

Spec	Name	St	Pg
Ger	Ciocon, J	FL	263
PM	Diwan, S	NY	697
PMR	Schwartz, L	PA	837
PMR	Stubblefield, M	NY	837
PRhu	Sherry, D	PA	799

Pain-Musculoskeletal-Spine

Spec	Name	St	Pg
PM	Falco, F	DE	697

Pain-Musculoskeletal-Spine & Neck

Spec	Name	St	Pg
PM	Ngeow, J	NY	697

Pain-Neck

Spec	Name	St	Pg
PMR	Braddom, R	PA	835

Pain-Nerve Injury

Spec	Name	St	Pg
HS	Koman, L	NC	299

Pain-Neuropathic

Spec	Name	St	Pg
N	Moots, P	TN	522
N	Oaklander, A	MA	508
PM	Baumann, P	GA	698
PM	Benzon, H	IL	699
PM	Diwan, S	NY	697
PM	Ferrante, F	CA	702

Spec	Name	St	Pg
PM	Gharibo, C	NY	697
PM	Kreitzer, J	NY	697
PM	Mekhail, N	OH	700
PM	Ngeow, J	NY	697
PM	Raja, S	MD	697
PM	Wellington, J	IN	700
PMR	Stubblefield, M	NY	837

Pain-Pediatric

Spec	Name	St	Pg
PM	Wellington, J	IN	700

Pain-Pelvic

Spec	Name	St	Pg
Ge	Pezzone, M	PA	237
PM	Jain, S	NY	697
U	Woo, H	LA	1175

Pain-Pelvic & Perineal

Spec	Name	St	Pg
ObG	Steege, J	NC	560

Pain-Soft Tissue

Spec	Name	St	Pg
PMR	Aseff, J	DC	835

Pain-Spine

Spec	Name	St	Pg
N	Hiesiger, E	NY	512
PM	Christo, P	MD	696
PM	Macadaeg, K	IN	699
PM	Wellington, J	IN	700
PMR	Harris, D	TX	843
PMR	Kezar, L	AL	838
PMR	Lutz, C	NY	836

Palliative Care

Spec	Name	St	Pg
Ger	Allman, R	AL	263
Ger	Finucane, T	MD	263
Ger	Gorbien, M	IL	265
Ger	Hanson, L	NC	264
Ger	Sachs, G	IN	265
GerPsy	Manepalli, J	MO	914
H & PM	Abrahm, J	MA	406
H & PM	Arnold, R	PA	406
H & PM	Block, S	MA	406
H & PM	Bricker, L	MI	407
H & PM	Davis, M	OH	407
H & PM	Ferris, F	CA	408
H & PM	Fine, R	TX	408
H & PM	Friebert, S	OH	407
H & PM	Jackson, V	MA	406
H & PM	Kutner, J	CO	407
H & PM	Pantilat, S	CA	408
H & PM	Portenoy, R	NY	406
H & PM	Quill, T	NY	407
H & PM	Ritchie, C	CA	408
H & PM	Santa-Emma, P	OH	407
H & PM	Selvaggi, K	MA	406
H & PM	Tulsky, J	NC	407
H & PM	Von Gunten, C	CA	408
H & PM	Weinstein, S	UT	408
IM	Rabow, M	CA	426

Specialty & Special Expertise Index

Spec	Name	St	Pg
IM	Selwyn, P	NY	424
IM	Tucker, R	AL	425
N	Taylor, L	MA	508
Onc	Back, A	WA	383
Onc	Bernard, S	NC	353
Onc	Brescia, F	SC	354
Onc	Bruera, E	TX	377
Onc	Clamon, G	IA	366
Onc	Cleary, J	WI	366
Onc	Fitch, T	AZ	378
Onc	Himelstein, A	DE	342
Onc	Levy, M	PA	344
Onc	Lyckholm, L	VA	359
Onc	Markman, M	PA	345
Onc	Mintzer, D	PA	345
Onc	Smith, T	MD	349
Onc	Steen, P	ND	376
Onc	Sutton, L	NC	363
Onc	Von Roenn, J	IL	373
Onc	Worden, F·	MI	373
Ped	Lantos, J	MO	728
PHO	Godder, K	VA	766
PHO	Jakacki, R	PA	761
PHO	Kane, J	TX	776
PHO	Korones, D	NY	761
PHO	Morgan, E	IL	772
PHO	Russo, C	AL	768
PHO	Thomas, G	OR	779
PHO	Wolfe, L	NY	764
PM	Burton, A	TX	701
PM	Driver, L	TX	701
PM	Fine, P	UT	700
PM	Huntoon, M	TN	698
PM	Slatkin, N	CA	703
PM	Wallace, M	CA	703
PM	Weinberger, M	NY	698
Psyc	Breitbart, W	NY	891
Psyc	Strouse, T	CA	903
Psyc	Valentine, A	TX	900
Pul	Nelson, J	NY	926
Pul	Shore, B	MO	935
S	Hinshaw, D	MI	1078
S	Krouse, R	AZ	1090
T&CS	Grannis, F	CA	1141
T&CS	Pechet, T	PA	1120
VIR	Coldwell, D	KY	994

Palliative Care-Pediatric

Spec	Name	St	Pg
PM	Weisman, S	WI	700

Pancreatic & Biliary Disease

Spec	Name	St	Pg
Ge	Al-Kawas, F	DC	230
Ge	Barkin, J	FL	239
Ge	Carr-Locke, D	NY	231
Ge	Elta, G	MI	245
Ge	Faigel, D	AZ	251
Ge	Goldberg, M	IL	245
Ge	Gordon, S	NH	229
Ge	Kelsey, P	MA	229
Ge	Lichtenstein, D	MA	229
Ge	Meiselman, M	IL	247
Ge	Sherman, S	IN	248
Ge	Slivka, A	PA	238
Ge	Wilcox, C	AL	243

Pancreatic & Biliary Surgery

Spec	Name	St	Pg
S	Abecassis, M	IL	1074
S	Adams, R	VA	1066
S	Aranha, G	IL	1074
S	Dayton, M	NY	1056
S	Lillemoe, K	MA	1050
S	Prinz, R	IL	1081
S	Weber, S	WI	1084

Pancreatic Cancer

Spec	Name	St	Pg
Ge	Aslanian, H	CT	228
Ge	Cunningham, J	AZ	251
Ge	Edmundowicz, S	MO	245
Ge	Okolo, P	MD	237
Ge	Pochapin, M	NY	237
Ge	Slivka, A	PA	238
Ge	Waxman, I	IL	249
Onc	Abbruzzese, J	TX	376
Onc	Benedetto, P	FL	353
Onc	Benson, A	IL	364
Onc	Berlin, J	TN	353
Onc	Blobe, G	NC	354
Onc	Burris, H	TN	354
Onc	De Simone, P	KY	356
Onc	Donehower, R	MD	338
Onc	Fine, R	NY	339
Onc	Fisher, G	CA	386
Onc	Grem, J	NE	375
Onc	Holland, J	NY	342
Onc	Kindler, H	IL	369
Onc	Lacy, J	CT	331
Onc	Laheru, D	MD	344
Onc	Loehrer, P	IN	369
Onc	Meropol, N	OH	370
Onc	O'Reilly, E	NY	346
Onc	Picozzi, V	WA	389
Onc	Reid, T	CA	390
Onc	Ryan, D	MA	331
Onc	Saif, M	MA	332
Onc	Schilsky, R	IL	372
Onc	Sun, W	PA	350
Onc	Tempero, M	CA	391
Onc	Varadhachary, G	TX	382
Onc	Von Hoff, D	AZ	382
Onc	Wolff, R	TX	383
Path	Hruban, R	MD	709
RadRO	Konski, A	MI	960
RadRO	Lawrence, T	MI	960
RadRO	Minsky, B	TX	965
RadRO	Small, W	IL	962
RadRO	Weichselbaum, R	IL	962
S	Alexander, H	MD	1053
S	August, D	NJ	1053
S	Bartlett, D	PA	1053
S	Behrns, K	FL	1067
S	Bolton, J	LA	1087
S	Bouvet, M	CA	1093
S	Brems, J	IL	1074
S	Brodsky, J	PA	1054
S	Brunicardi, F	CA	1094
S	Callery, M	MA	1048
S	Cameron, J	MD	1054
S	Cance, W	NY	1055
S	Chabot, J	NY	1055
S	Choti, M	MD	1055
S	Coit, D	NY	1055
S	Colquhoun, S	CA	1094
S	Drebin, J	PA	1056
S	Ellison, E	OH	1076
S	Evans, D	WI	1076
S	Fahey, T	NY	1057
S	Fisher, W	TX	1088
S	Fong, Y	NY	1057
S	Gibbs, J	NY	1058
S	Hanna, N	MD	1058
S	Hemming, A	CA	1096
S	Heslin, M	AL	1069
S	Hiotis, S	NY	1058
S	Hoffman, J	PA	1058
S	Jarnagin, W	NY	1058
S	Jenkins, R	MA	1051
S	Karpeh, M	NY	1059
S	Kendrick, M	MN	1078
S	Leach, S	MD	1059
S	Lee, J	TX	1090
S	Lee, K	PA	1059
S	Levi, J	FL	1070
S	Lieberman, M	NY	1060
S	Lillemoe, K	MA	1050
S	Livingstone, A	FL	1070
S	Lowy, A	CA	1097
S	Mahvi, D	IL	1079
S	Marsh, J	PA	1060
S	McAneny, D	MA	1051
S	McFadden, D	CT	1051
S	Melvin, W	OH	1079
S	Moossa, A	CA	1097
S	Mulvihill, S	UT	1085
S	Nagorney, D	MN	1080
S	Nakakura, E	CA	1097
S	Nissen, N	CA	1098
S	Norton, J	CA	1098
S	Pachter, H	NY	1061
S	Pawlik, T	MD	1062
S	Pinson, C	TN	1071
S	Pisters, P	TX	1091
S	Posner, M	IL	1081
S	Postier, R	OK	1091
S	Reber, H	CA	1099
S	Rosemurgy, A	FL	1071
S	Sarr, M	MN	1081
S	Sasson, A	NE	1086
S	Schulick, R	CO	1086
S	Shen, P	NC	1072
S	Shenk, R	OH	1082
S	Sielaff, T	MN	1082
S	Simeone, D	MI	1082
S	Staley, C	GA	1072
S	Sundaram, M	IL	1083

Specialty & Special Expertise Index

Spec	Name	St	Pg
S	Sutton, J	VT	1052
S	Talamonti, M	IL	1083
S	Thayer, S	MA	1052
S	Tyler, D	NC	1073
S	Vickers, S	MN	1083
S	Walsh, R	OH	1084
S	Yeo, C	PA	1066
S	Zinner, M	MA	1052

Pancreatic Cancer(Familial)

Spec	Name	St	Pg
Ge	Chung, D	MA	228
Ge	Kurtz, R	NY	235

Pancreatic Cancer-Acinar Cell

Spec	Name	St	Pg
Onc	Colon-Otero, G	FL	355

Pancreatic Cancer-Early Detection

Spec	Name	St	Pg
Ge	Canto, M	MD	231
Ge	Goggins, M	MD	233

Pancreatic Disease

Spec	Name	St	Pg
Ge	Chari, S	MN	244
Ge	Edmundowicz, S	MO	245
Ge	Forsmark, C	FL	240
Ge	Hawes, R	FL	240
Ge	Jacobson, I	NY	234
Ge	Kalloo, A	MD	234
Ge	Kantsevoy, S	MD	234
Ge	Konicek, F	IL	246
Ge	Kowalski, T	PA	235
Ge	Kozarek, R	WA	254
Ge	Lambiase, L	TN	241
Ge	Liddle, R	NC	241
Ge	Ostroff, J	CA	255
Ge	Pasricha, P	MD	237
Ge	Toskes, P	FL	243
Ge	Vargo, J	OH	248
Ge	Vege, S	MN	249
PGe	Hoffenberg, E	CO	754

Pancreatic Endocrine Tumors

Spec	Name	St	Pg
Ge	Chung, D	MA	228
S	Yeo, C	PA	1066

Pancreatic Islet Cell Transplant

Spec	Name	St	Pg
EDM	Clore, J	VA	214
S	Brunicardi, F	CA	1094
S	Eckhoff, D	AL	1068
S	Fisher, J	CA	1095
S	Galloway, J	GA	1068
S	Hering, B	MN	1077
S	Kapur, S	NY	1059
S	Larsen, C	GA	1070
S	Markmann, J	MA	1051
S	Oberholzer, J	IL	1080
S	Posselt, A	CA	1098
S	Shapiro, R	PA	1064

Spec	Name	St	Pg
S	Weber, C	GA	1073

Pancreatic Surgery

Spec	Name	St	Pg
PS	Meyers, R	UT	808
S	Billingsley, K	OR	1093
S	Cameron, J	MD	1054
S	Chabot, J	NY	1055
S	Cronin, D	WI	1075
S	Daneker, G	GA	1068
S	Deziel, D	IL	1076
S	Galloway, J	GA	1068
S	Horvath, K	WA	1096
S	Howerton, R	NC	1069
S	Johnson, L	DC	1058
S	MacDonald, K	NC	1070
S	Matthews, J	IL	1079
S	Pappas, T	NC	1071
S	Reber, H	CA	1099
S	Reiner, M	NY	1063
S	Schirmer, B	VA	1072
S	Schulak, J	OH	1082
S	Sharp, K	TN	1072

Pancreatic/Biliary Endoscopy (ERCP)

Spec	Name	St	Pg
Ge	Baron, T	MN	244
Ge	Carr-Locke, D	NY	231
Ge	Cello, J	CA	253
Ge	Cohen, J	NY	231
Ge	Cunningham, J	AZ	251
Ge	Das, A	AZ	251
Ge	Dea, S	CA	253
Ge	Faigel, D	AZ	251
Ge	Forsmark, C	FL	240
Ge	Freiman, H	NY	232
Ge	Ginsberg, G	PA	233
Ge	Goldberg, M	IL	245
Ge	Gordon, S	NH	229
Ge	Haber, G	NY	233
Ge	Haluszka, O	PA	233
Ge	Hawes, R	FL	240
Ge	Kantsevoy, S	MD	234
Ge	Kimmey, M	WA	254
Ge	Kochman, M	PA	235
Ge	Kowalski, T	PA	235
Ge	Kozarek, R	WA	254
Ge	Ostroff, J	CA	255
Ge	Scudera, P	VA	242
Ge	Shaker, R	WI	248
Ge	Sherman, S	IN	248
Ge	Silverman, W	IA	248
Ge	Slivka, A	PA	238
Ge	Vargo, J	OH	248
Ge	Wilcox, C	AL	243
Ge	Yanda, R	GA	243

Pancreatic/Biliary Endoscopy(ERCP)

Spec	Name	St	Pg
Ge	Baillie, J	NC	239
Ge	Jonnalagadda, S	MO	246

Spec	Name	St	Pg
Ge	Levy, M	MN	246
Ge	Shah, R	CO	250

Panic Disorder

Spec	Name	St	Pg
GerPsy	Burke, W	NE	914
Psyc	Canterbury, R	VA	895
Psyc	Fyer, A	NY	892
Psyc	Haque, W	TX	900
Psyc	Roy-Byrne, P	WA	902
Psyc	Stein, M	CA	903

Pap Smear Abnormalities

Spec	Name	St	Pg
GO	DePriest, P	KY	280
ObG	Snyder, R	TX	563

Paraneoplastic Syndromes

Spec	Name	St	Pg
N	Posner, J	NY	516

Parapsoriasis

Spec	Name	St	Pg
D	Wood, G	WI	195

Parasitic Infections

Spec	Name	St	Pg
Inf	Hartman, B	NY	411
Inf	Pearson, R	VA	415
PrM	Cahill, J	NY	882
PrM	Cahill, K	NY	883

Parathyroid Cancer

Spec	Name	St	Pg
Oto	Kuhel, W	NY	662
Oto	Shindo, M	OR	687
Oto	Weber, S	TX	683
S	Clark, O	CA	1094
S	Roses, D	NY	1063
S	Sosa, J	CT	1052
S	Udelsman, R	CT	1052

Parathyroid Disease

Spec	Name	St	Pg
EDM	Daniels, G	MA	207
EDM	Econs, M	IN	217
EDM	Kopp, P	IL	218
EDM	Kronenberg, H	MA	207
Ger	Lyles, K	NC	264
NuM	Neumann, D	OH	550
Oto	Randolph, G	MA	656
Oto	Terris, D	GA	671

Parathyroid Disorders

Spec	Name	St	Pg
EDM	Bilezikian, J	NY	209
EDM	Bockman, R	NY	209
EDM	Emanuele, M	IL	217

Parathyroid Parathyroid Surgery

Spec	Name	St	Pg
S	Kim, L	AR	1089

Specialty & Special Expertise Index

Spec	Name	St	Pg
Parathyroid Surgery			
Oto	Keane, W	PA	661
Oto	Shindo, M	OR	687
Oto	Tufano, R	MD	666
S	Carty, S	PA	1055
S	Gosnell, J	CA	1096
S	McHenry, C	OH	1079
S	Norman, J	FL	1071
Parent Guidance in Parental Cancer			
Psyc	Rauch, P	MA	889
Parenting Issues			
AM	Adger, H	MD	80
ChAP	Boxer, G	MO	910
ChAP	Turecki, S	NY	909
Parkinson's Disease			
N	Ahlskog, J	MN	524
N	Aminoff, M	CA	535
N	Ashizawa, T	FL	520
N	Azizi, S	PA	509
N	Baser, S	PA	509
N	Bressman, S	NY	509
N	Bruno, M	HI	535
N	DeLong, M	GA	520
N	Fahn, S	NY	511
N	Flaherty, A	MA	507
N	Foo, S	NY	511
N	Gendelman, S	NY	512
N	Goetz, C	IL	526
N	Golbe, L	NJ	512
N	Hauser, R	FL	521
N	Hurtig, H	PA	512
N	Jankovic, J	TX	534
N	Kieburtz, K	NY	513
N	Langston, J	CA	537
N	Lew, M	CA	537
N	Maraganore, D	IL	528
N	Montgomery, E	AL	522
N	Nutt, J	OR	538
N	Olanow, C	NY	516
N	Perlmutter, J	MO	528
N	Pulst, S	UT	532
N	Reich, S	MD	517
N	Ropper, A	MA	508
N	Rosenbaum, R	OR	538
N	Sage, J	NJ	517
N	Samii, A	WA	538
N	Sethi, K	GA	523
N	Shulman, L	MD	517
N	Singer, C	FL	524
N	Stern, M	PA	518
N	Tanner, C	CA	539
N	Tetrud, J	CA	539
N	Waters, C	NY	518
N	Watts, R	AL	524
N	Weiner, W	MD	519
N	Wooten, G	VA	524

Spec	Name	St	Pg
N	Young, A	MA	509
NS	Baltuch, G	PA	472
NS	Freeman, T	FL	481
NS	Nazzaro, J	KS	491
NS	Rezai, A	OH	489
NS	Wharen, R	FL	485
Path	Norenberg, M	FL	714
Parkinson's Disease/Aging Brain			
NRad	Drayer, B	NY	985
Parkinson's Disease/Movement Disorders			
N	Gilman, S	MI	526
N	Louis, E	NY	515
N	Vitek, J	MN	530
NS	Bakay, R	IL	485
NS	Goodman, R	NY	474
NS	Guthrie, B	AL	482
NS	Kaplitt, M	NY	476
Parkinson's Disease/Visual Disorders			
N	Balcer, L	PA	509
Parotid Gland Tumors			
Oto	Alam, D	OH	672
Oto	Burkey, B	OH	674
Oto	Fee, W	CA	684
Oto	Johnson, J	PA	661
Paroxysmal Nocturnal Hemoglobinuria			
Hem	Mangan, K	PA	313
Patent Foramen Ovale			
PCd	Moskowitz, W	VA	737
Pathology			
Path	Allred, D	MO	714
Path	Amin, M	CA	719
Path	Antonescu, C	NY	707
Path	Appelman, H	MI	714
Path	Arber, D	CA	719
Path	Bagg, A	PA	708
Path	Balla, A	IL	715
Path	Banks, P	NC	713
Path	Bastian, B	CA	719
Path	Behm, F	IL	715
Path	Bell, D	MN	715
Path	Bhan, A	MA	706
Path	Bleiweiss, I	NY	708
Path	Bollen, A	CA	719
Path	Bostwick, D	VA	713
Path	Brooks, J	PA	708
Path	Bruner, J	TX	717
Path	Burger, P	MD	708

Spec	Name	St	Pg
Path	Cagle, P	TX	717
Path	Chandrasoma, P	CA	720
Path	Chang, K	CA	720
Path	Chen, Y	CA	720
Path	Chesney, C	TN	713
Path	Cho, K	MI	715
Path	Cochran, A	CA	720
Path	Cohen, M	UT	717
Path	Connolly, J	MA	706
Path	Cote, R	FL	713
Path	Crawford, J	NY	708
Path	Dahmoush, L	IA	715
Path	De Las Morenas, A	MA	706
Path	De Masters, B	CO	717
Path	Demetris, A	PA	708
Path	Dubeau, L	CA	720
Path	Ehya, H	PA	708
Path	Epstein, J	MD	708
Path	Faye-Petersen, O	AL	713
Path	Ferrell, L	CA	720
Path	Fishbein, M	CA	720
Path	Fletcher, C	MA	706
Path	Fogt, F	PA	709
Path	Foucar, M	NM	717
Path	Gambetti, P	OH	715
Path	Goldblum, J	OH	715
Path	Gottlieb, G	MA	706
Path	Govindarajan, S	CA	720
Path	Greenson, J	MI	715
Path	Gupta, P	PA	709
Path	Hamilton, S	TX	718
Path	Hammar, S	WA	720
Path	Harris, N	MA	706
Path	Heller, D	NJ	709
Path	Hoda, S	NY	709
Path	Hruban, R	MD	709
Path	Jones, R	DC	709
Path	Kahn, L	NY	709
Path	Kanel, G	CA	721
Path	Katzenstein, A	NY	710
Path	Kaufman, R	MA	706
Path	Kinney, M	TX	718
Path	Klimstra, D	NY	710
Path	Koss, M	CA	721
Path	Kurman, R	MD	710
Path	Kurtin, P	MN	716
Path	Lage, J	SC	713
Path	Le Boit, P	CA	721
Path	Leslie, K	AZ	718
Path	Li Volsi, V	PA	710
Path	Ljung, B	CA	721
Path	Lucas, D	MI	716
Path	Mark, E	MA	706
Path	Masood, S	FL	713
Path	Melamed, J	NY	710
Path	Mies, C	PA	710
Path	Mills, S	VA	713
Path	Mischel, P	CA	721
Path	Montgomery, E	MD	710
Path	Moore, S	IA	716
Path	Moran, C	TX	718
Path	Morrow, J	CT	707

Spec	Name	St	Pg
Path	Myers, J	MI	716
Path	Nathwani, B	CA	721
Path	Nicosia, S	FL	714
Path	Norenberg, M	FL	714
Path	O'Brien, M	MA	707
Path	Odze, R	MA	707
Path	Orazi, A	NY	710
Path	Patchefsky, A	PA	711
Path	Perry, A	CA	721
Path	Petito, C	FL	714
Path	Petras, R	OH	716
Path	Prieto, V	TX	718
Path	Rashid, A	TX	718
Path	Rennke, H	MA	707
Path	Reuter, V	NY	711
Path	Roberts, W	TX	718
Path	Rosenberg, A	FL	714
Path	Rosenblum, M	NY	711
Path	Ross, J	NY	711
Path	Rubin, B	OH	716
Path	Rutgers, J	CA	721
Path	Sahin, A	TX	718
Path	Sanchez, M	NJ	711
Path	Schiller, A	NY	711
Path	Schnitt, S	MA	707
Path	Sewell, C	GA	714
Path	Sibley, R	CA	722
Path	Silva, E	TX	719
Path	Silverman, J	PA	711
Path	Smith, T	MA	707
Path	Soslow, R	NY	711
Path	Suster, S	WI	716
Path	Swerdlow, S	PA	712
Path	Thor, A	CO	717
Path	Tomaszewski, J	NY	712
Path	Tornos, C	NY	712
Path	Travis, W	NY	712
Path	Triche, T	CA	722
Path	True, L	WA	722
Path	Ulbright, T	IN	716
Path	Walker, D	TX	719
Path	Wang, B	NY	712
Path	Warnke, R	CA	722
Path	Weisenburger, D	NE	717
Path	Weiss, L	CA	722
Path	Weiss, S	GA	714
Path	Wheeler, T	TX	719
Path	Wilczynski, S	CA	722
Path	Young, R	MA	707
Path	Yousem, S	PA	712
Path	Zagzag, D	NY	712

Pediatric & Adolescent Gynecology

Spec	Name	St	Pg
ObG	Bradshaw, K	TX	563
RE	Smith, Y	MI	1014
RE	Wilson, E	TX	1016

Pediatric & Adolescent Sports Medicine

Spec	Name	St	Pg
AM	Hergenroeder, A	TX	82

Pediatric & Adult Plastic Surgery

Spec	Name	St	Pg
PlS	Glat, P	PA	854

Pediatric Allergy & Immunology

Spec	Name	St	Pg
A&I	DeShazo, R	MS	86
A&I	Wong, D	AZ	90
PA&I	Bahna, S	LA	732
PA&I	Bock, S	CO	732
PA&I	Burks, A	NC	730
PA&I	Church, J	CA	733
PA&I	Cowan, M	CA	733
PA&I	Ehrlich, P	NY	729
PA&I	Epstein, S	CA	733
PA&I	Fanous, Y	CA	733
PA&I	Gelfund, E	CO	732
PA&I	Josephs, S	MD	729
PA&I	Kamani, N	DC	729
PA&I	Kelly, C	VA	731
PA&I	Klein, R	RI	729
PA&I	Lemanske, R	WI	731
PA&I	Leung, D	CO	732
PA&I	Orange, J	TX	732
PA&I	Ownby, D	GA	731
PA&I	Pongracic, J	IL	731
PA&I	Sampson, H	NY	729
PA&I	Schuberth, K	MD	730
PA&I	Shearer, W	TX	732
PA&I	Sicherer, S	NY	730
PA&I	Skoner, D	PA	730
PA&I	Sleasman, J	FL	731
PA&I	Sly, R	MD	730
PA&I	Spergel, J	PA	730
PA&I	Strunk, R	MO	731
PA&I	Sullivan, K	PA	730
PA&I	Wasserman, R	TX	732
PA&I	Wolf, R	IL	731
PA&I	Wood, R	MD	730

Pediatric Cancers

Spec	Name	St	Pg
Path	Triche, T	CA	722
PHO	Adamson, P	PA	758
PHO	Beyer, E	IL	769
PHO	Cohn, S	IL	770
PHO	Drachtman, R	NJ	759
PHO	Dunkel, I	NY	759
PHO	Frangoul, H	TN	765
PHO	Friedman, D	TN	765
PHO	Garvin, J	NY	760
PHO	Geyer, J	WA	777
PHO	Hord, J	OH	771
PHO	Kane, J	TX	776
PHO	Kobrinsky, N	ND	774
PHO	Korones, D	NY	761
PHO	Link, M	CA	778
PHO	Meyer, W	OK	776
PHO	Meyers, P	NY	762
PHO	Moscow, J	KY	767
PHO	Neuberg, R	SC	767
PHO	Park, J	WA	778

Spec	Name	St	Pg
PHO	Parker, R	NY	763
PHO	Pendergrass, T	WA	778
PHO	Sakamoto, K	CA	779
PHO	Sallan, S	MA	757
PHO	Sencer, S	MN	773
PHO	Sondel, P	WI	773
PHO	Steinherz, P	NY	764
PS	Bond, S	KY	805
PS	Dillon, P	MO	807
PS	Ehrlich, P	MI	807
PS	Farmer, D	CA	810
PS	Jackson, R	AR	809
PS	Paidas, C	FL	805
PS	Reynolds, M	IL	808
PS	Sawin, R	WA	811
PS	Shochat, S	TN	806
PS	Strauch, E	MD	804
PS	Warner, B	MO	808
RadRO	Constine, L	NY	948
RadRO	Donahue, B	NY	949
RadRO	Donaldson, S	CA	965
RadRO	Dritschilo, A	DC	949
RadRO	Fiveash, J	AL	954
RadRO	Kun, L	TN	954
RadRO	Marcus, J	FL	955
RadRO	Michalski, J	MO	961
RadRO	Roberts, K	CT	947
RadRO	Schomberg, P	MN	962
RadRO	Stea, B	AZ	965
RadRO	Wara, W	CA	968
RadRO	Woo, S	KY	958

Pediatric Cardiac Surgery

Spec	Name	St	Pg
PS	Jennings, R	MA	801
PS	Quaegebeur, J	NY	804
T&CS	Bacha, E	NY	1114
T&CS	Burke, R	FL	1124
T&CS	Dabal, R	AL	1125
T&CS	Delius, R	MI	1131
T&CS	Ilbawi, M	IL	1132
T&CS	Kanter, K	GA	1126
T&CS	Lamberti, J	CA	1142
T&CS	Mavroudis, C	FL	1126
T&CS	Mill, M	NC	1127
T&CS	Mitchell, M	CO	1137
T&CS	Rosenkranz, E	FL	1129
T&CS	Trento, A	CA	1143
T&CS	Ungerleider, R	NC	1130
T&CS	Walters, H	MI	1135
T&CS	Ziemer, G	IL	1136

Pediatric Cardic Surgery

Spec	Name	St	Pg
T&CS	Mayer, J	MA	1111

Pediatric Cardiology

Spec	Name	St	Pg
PCd	Ackerman, M	MN	738
PCd	Agarwala, B	IL	738
PCd	Beekman, R	OH	738
PCd	Beerman, L	PA	734
PCd	Bernstein, D	CA	740

Specialty & Special Expertise Index

Spec	Name	St	Pg
PCd	Biancaniello, T	NY	734
PCd	Bierman, F	NY	734
PCd	Brenner, J	MD	734
PCd	Bricker, J	TX	740
PCd	Caldwell, R	IN	738
PCd	Cetta, F	MN	738
PCd	Cheatham, J	OH	738
PCd	Colvin, E	AL	737
PCd	Cooper, R	NY	734
PCd	Crosson, J	MD	735
PCd	De Moor, M	MA	733
PCd	Dick, M	MI	738
PCd	Dreyer, W	TX	740
PCd	Driscoll, D	MN	739
PCd	Epstein, M	FL	737
PCd	Feltes, T	OH	739
PCd	Fish, F	TN	737
PCd	Fricker, F	FL	737
PCd	Gelb, B	NY	735
PCd	Gewitz, M	NY	735
PCd	Gillette, P	TX	740
PCd	Gullquist, S	VA	737
PCd	Hanna, B	PA	735
PCd	Hardin, J	IL	739
PCd	Hellenbrand, W	CT	733
PCd	Hijazi, Z	IL	739
PCd	Hoyer, M	IN	739
PCd	Hsu, D	NY	735
PCd	Lang, P	MA	733
PCd	Latson, L	FL	737
PCd	Lewin, M	WA	741
PCd	Lock, J	MA	734
PCd	Mahony, L	TX	740
PCd	Minich, L	UT	739
PCd	Moodie, D	TX	740
PCd	Moskowitz, W	VA	737
PCd	Murphy, J	PA	735
PCd	Newburger, J	MA	734
PCd	Pahl, E	IL	739
PCd	Parness, I	NY	735
PCd	Perry, S	CA	741
PCd	Radtke, W	DE	735
PCd	Rocchini, A	MI	739
PCd	Rogers, J	TX	740
PCd	Rome, J	PA	736
PCd	Rychik, J	PA	736
PCd	Shaddy, R	PA	736
PCd	Sherman, F	PA	736
PCd	Sommer, R	NY	736
PCd	Steinherz, L	NY	736
PCd	Teitel, D	CA	741
PCd	Velvis, H	NY	736
PCd	Walsh, C	NY	736
PCd	Walsh, E	MA	734
PCd	Weinberg, P	PA	737
PCd	Young, M	FL	738
PCd	Zahn, E	CA	741

Pediatric Cardiothoracic Surgery

Spec	Name	St	Pg
PS	Bove, E	MI	807

Spec	Name	St	Pg
PS	Colombani, P	MD	802
T&CS	Backer, C	IL	1130
T&CS	Campbell, D	CO	1136
T&CS	Chen, J	NY	1114
T&CS	Cohen, G	CA	1140
T&CS	Forbess, J	TX	1138
T&CS	Fraser, C	TX	1138
T&CS	Gaynor, J	PA	1116
T&CS	Jonas, R	DC	1118
T&CS	Kopf, G	CT	1111

Pediatric Clinical Genetics

Spec	Name	St	Pg
CG	Andersson, H	LA	161

Pediatric Critical Care Medicine

Spec	Name	St	Pg
PCCM	Anand, K	TN	741
PCCM	Dean, J	UT	742
PCCM	Easley, R	TX	742
PCCM	Fuhrman, B	TX	742
PCCM	Perez Fontan, J	TX	742
PCCM	Sarnaik, A	MI	742
PCCM	Schwarz, A	CA	743
PCCM	Sichting, K	IN	742
PCCM	Taylor, R	TX	742
PCCM	Thompson, A	PA	741
PCCM	Zimmerman, J	WA	743

Pediatric Dermatology

Spec	Name	St	Pg
D	Anderson, R	MA	182
D	Bayliss, S	MO	192
D	Cohen, B	MD	185
D	Cunningham, B	CA	198
D	Eichenfield, L	CA	198
D	Frieden, I	CA	198
D	Friedlander, S	CA	199
D	Gellis, S	MA	183
D	Hansen, R	AZ	197
D	Johr, R	FL	191
D	Kane, K	MA	183
D	Kress, D	PA	187
D	Levy, M	TX	197
D	Lucky, A	OH	194
D	Orlow, S	NY	188
D	Paller, A	IL	195
D	Rhodes, A	IL	195
D	Treadwell, P	IN	195
D	Witman, P	OH	195
D	Yan, A	PA	189

Pediatric Endocrinology

Spec	Name	St	Pg
PEn	Allen, D	WI	746
PEn	Alter, C	PA	744
PEn	Arslanian, S	PA	744
PEn	Becker, D	PA	744
PEn	Casella, S	NH	743
PEn	Cutler, L	OH	746
PEn	DeLuca, F	PA	744
PEn	Diamond, F	FL	745

Spec	Name	St	Pg
PEn	DiMeglio, L	IN	746
PEn	Eugster, E	IN	747
PEn	Foster, C	UT	748
PEn	Freemark, M	NC	746
PEn	Garibaldi, L	PA	744
PEn	Geffner, M	CA	748
PEn	Gitelman, S	CA	748
PEn	Gordon, C	RI	743
PEn	Gutai, J	MI	747
PEn	Kappy, M	CO	748
PEn	Klingensmith, G	CO	748
PEn	Levine, M	PA	744
PEn	Levitsky, L	MA	743
PEn	Levy, R	IL	747
PEn	Ludwig, D	MA	743
PEn	Lustig, R	CA	749
PEn	Maclaren, N	NY	744
PEn	Meacham, L	GA	746
PEn	Menon, R	MI	747
PEn	Mirmira, R	IN	747
PEn	New, M	NY	745
PEn	Norris, A	IA	747
PEn	Oberfield, S	NY	745
PEn	Plotnick, L	MD	745
PEn	Rewers, M	CO	748
PEn	Rivkees, S	FL	746
PEn	Rogers, D	OH	747
PEn	Rosenthal, S	CA	749
PEn	Silverstein, J	FL	746
PEn	Sklar, C	NY	745
PEn	Spack, N	MA	743
PEn	Sperling, M	PA	745
PEn	Stanley, C	PA	745
PEn	Tamborlane, W	CT	744
PEn	White, N	MO	747
PEn	Wilson, D	CA	749
PEn	Zimmerman, D	IL	748

Pediatric Eye Surgery-Ptosis

Spec	Name	St	Pg
Oph	Wright, K	CA	605

Pediatric Facial Plastic Surgery

Spec	Name	St	Pg
Oto	Waner, M	NY	666

Pediatric Gastroenterology

Spec	Name	St	Pg
PGe	Baker, R	NY	750
PGe	Baker, S	NY	750
PGe	Baldassano, R	PA	750
PGe	Baldridge, A	NJ	750
PGe	Benkov, K	NY	750
PGe	Berman, J	IL	752
PGe	Bishop, W	IA	752
PGe	Black, D	TN	752
PGe	Christie, D	WA	755
PGe	Cohen, M	OH	752
PGe	Di Lorenzo, C	OH	753
PGe	Dubinsky, M	CA	755
PGe	El-Youssef, M	MN	753
PGe	Fasano, A	MD	750
PGe	Guandalini, S	IL	753

Spec	Name	St	Pg
PGe	Gunasekaran, T	IL	753
PGe	Gupta, S	IN	753
PGe	Heyman, M	CA	755
PGe	Hill, I	NC	752
PGe	Hoffenberg, E	CO	754
PGe	Jonas, M	MA	749
PGe	Kirschner, B	IL	753
PGe	Kleinman, R	MA	749
PGe	Krebs, N	CO	754
PGe	Leichtner, A	MA	749
PGe	Levy, J	NY	750
PGe	McDiarmid, S	CA	756
PGe	Mittal, N	TX	755
PGe	Molleston, J	IN	753
PGe	Mousa, H	OH	753
PGe	Murray, K	WA	756
PGe	Narkewicz, M	CO	754
PGe	Novak, D	FL	752
PGe	Oliva-Hemker, M	MD	751
PGe	Piccoli, D	PA	751
PGe	Rhoads, J	TX	755
PGe	Rothbaum, R	MO	754
PGe	Schwarz, K	MD	751
PGe	Schwarz, S	NY	751
PGe	Snyder, J	DC	751
PGe	Sokol, R	CO	754
PGe	Spivak, W	NY	751
PGe	Squires, R	PA	751
PGe	Suchy, F	CO	755
PGe	Thomas, D	CA	756
PGe	Ulshen, M	NC	752
PGe	Vanderhoof, J	NE	755
PGe	Whitington, P	IL	754
PGe	Wyllie, R	OH	754

Pediatric Gastrointestinal Surgery

Spec	Name	St	Pg
CRS	Lavery, I	OH	174

Pediatric Glaucoma

Spec	Name	St	Pg
Oph	Hodapp, E	FL	584

Pediatric Gynecology

Spec	Name	St	Pg
AM	Emans, S	MA	80
ObG	Laufer, M	MA	556
ObG	Merritt, D	MO	562
PS	Velcek, F	NY	804
RE	Sanfilippo, J	PA	1010

Pediatric Hand Surgery

Spec	Name	St	Pg
HS	Chang, J	CA	304
HS	Hentz, V	CA	304
HS	Koman, L	NC	299
HS	Lee, W	MD	297
HS	Mih, A	IN	301
PlS	Bentz, M	WI	864
PlS	Sood, R	IN	868

Pediatric Hand/Arm Surgery

Spec	Name	St	Pg
HS	Carlson, M	NY	295

Pediatric Hematology-Oncology

Spec	Name	St	Pg
PHO	Abromowitch, M	NE	774
PHO	Adamson, P	PA	758
PHO	Albritton, K	TX	775
PHO	Aledo, A	NY	758
PHO	Altman, A	CT	756
PHO	Andrews, R	WA	776
PHO	Angiolillo, A	DC	758
PHO	Arceci, R	MD	758
PHO	Arndt, C	MN	769
PHO	Banerjee, A	CA	776
PHO	Barredo, J	FL	765
PHO	Berg, S	TX	775
PHO	Bertolone, S	KY	765
PHO	Beyer, E	IL	769
PHO	Billett, A	MA	756
PHO	Blaney, S	TX	775
PHO	Blatt, J	NC	765
PHO	Blum, K	OH	769
PHO	Boxer, L	MI	769
PHO	Brecher, M	NY	758
PHO	Bruggers, C	UT	774
PHO	Buchanan, G	TX	775
PHO	Bussel, J	NY	758
PHO	Cairo, M	NY	758
PHO	Camitta, B	WI	769
PHO	Carpenter, P	WA	776
PHO	Carroll, W	NY	758
PHO	Castellino, S	NC	765
PHO	Castle, V	MI	770
PHO	Chen, A	MD	759
PHO	Cheung, N	NY	759
PHO	Coccia, P	NE	774
PHO	Cohen, K	MD	759
PHO	Cohn, S	IL	770
PHO	Cooper, L	TX	775
PHO	Corey, S	IL	770
PHO	Croop, J	IN	770
PHO	Cunningham, J	IL	770
PHO	Davies, S	OH	770
PHO	Diller, L	MA	756
PHO	Dome, J	DC	759
PHO	Drachtman, R	NJ	759
PHO	Dreyer, Z	TX	775
PHO	Ducore, J	CA	777
PHO	Dunkel, I	NY	759
PHO	Fallon, R	IN	770
PHO	Felix, C	PA	759
PHO	Ferrara, J	MI	770
PHO	Finklestein, J	CA	777
PHO	Finlay, J	CA	777
PHO	Frangoul, H	TN	765
PHO	Frantz, C	DE	759
PHO	Friedman, A	MD	760
PHO	Friedman, D	TN	765
PHO	Furman, W	TN	765
PHO	Gajjar, A	TN	766
PHO	Garvin, J	NY	760

Spec	Name	St	Pg
PHO	Geyer, J	WA	777
PHO	Giardina, P	NY	760
PHO	Glader, B	CA	777
PHO	Godder, K	VA	766
PHO	Gold, S	NC	766
PHO	Goldman, S	TX	775
PHO	Goldman, S	IL	771
PHO	Graham, M	AZ	775
PHO	Green, D	TN	766
PHO	Greenberg, J	DC	760
PHO	Grupp, S	PA	760
PHO	Guarini, L	NY	760
PHO	Guinan, E	MA	756
PHO	Gururangan, S	NC	766
PHO	Halligan, G	PA	760
PHO	Halpern, S	NJ	760
PHO	Harris, M	NJ	761
PHO	Haut, P	IN	771
PHO	Hawkins, D	WA	777
PHO	Hayani, A	IL	771
PHO	Hayashi, R	MO	771
PHO	Helman, L	MD	761
PHO	Hetherington, M	MO	771
PHO	Hilden, J	CO	774
PHO	Homans, A	VT	757
PHO	Hoots, W	MD	761
PHO	Hord, J	OH	771
PHO	Horn, B	CA	777
PHO	Hudson, M	TN	766
PHO	Hutchinson, R	MI	771
PHO	Jakacki, R	PA	761
PHO	Johnston, J	GA	766
PHO	Kamen, B	NJ	761
PHO	Kane, J	TX	776
PHO	Kapoor, N	CA	777
PHO	Keller, F	GA	766
PHO	Kieran, M	MA	757
PHO	Kobrinsky, N	ND	774
PHO	Korones, D	NY	761
PHO	Kramer, K	NY	761
PHO	Kreissman, S	NC	767
PHO	Kung, F	CA	778
PHO	Kurtzberg, J	NC	767
PHO	Kushner, B	NY	761
PHO	Kuttesch, J	PA	762
PHO	Lange, B	PA	762
PHO	Laver, J	TN	767
PHO	Leung, W	TN	767
PHO	Link, M	CA	778
PHO	Lipton, J	NY	762
PHO	Loeb, D	MD	762
PHO	Luchtman-Jones, L	DC	762
PHO	Lusher, J	MI	771
PHO	Manco-Johnson, M	CO	774
PHO	Manera, R	IL	772
PHO	Marcus, J	NY	762
PHO	Marina, N	CA	778
PHO	Maris, J	PA	762
PHO	Matthay, K	CA	778
PHO	McLean, T	NC	767
PHO	Meyer, W	OK	776
PHO	Meyers, P	NY	762

Specialty & Special Expertise Index

Spec	Name	St	Pg
PHO	Morgan, E	IL	772
PHO	Moscow, J	KY	767
PHO	Neglia, J	MN	772
PHO	Neuberg, R	SC	767
PHO	Nicholson, H	OR	778
PHO	O'Dorisio, M	IA	772
PHO	O'Reilly, R	NY	763
PHO	Olshefski, R	OH	772
PHO	Olson, J	OR	778
PHO	Olson, T	GA	767
PHO	Park, J	WA	778
PHO	Parker, R	NY	763
PHO	Pendergrass, T	WA	778
PHO	Plautz, G	OH	772
PHO	Puccetti, D	WI	772
PHO	Pui, C	TN	768
PHO	Razzouk, B	IN	773
PHO	Reaman, G	DC	763
PHO	Recht, M	OR	779
PHO	Rheingold, S	PA	763
PHO	Ribeiro, R	TN	768
PHO	Ritchey, A	PA	763
PHO	Rood, B	DC	763
PHO	Rosenthal, J	CA	779
PHO	Rosoff, P	NC	768
PHO	Rubin, C	IL	773
PHO	Russo, C	AL	768
PHO	Sakamoto, K	CA	779
PHO	Sallan, S	MA	757
PHO	Salvi, S	IL	773
PHO	Sandler, E	FL	768
PHO	Sandlund, J	TN	768
PHO	Santana, V	TN	768
PHO	Schwartz, C	RI	757
PHO	Sencer, S	MN	773
PHO	Shapiro, A	IN	773
PHO	Shearer, P	MD	763
PHO	Siegel, S	CA	779
PHO	Small, D	MD	763
PHO	Sondel, P	WI	773
PHO	Steinherz, P	NY	764
PHO	Tebbi, C	FL	768
PHO	Thomas, G	OR	779
PHO	Tomlinson, G	TX	776
PHO	Valentino, L	IL	773
PHO	van Hoff, J	NH	757
PHO	Vik, T	IN	773
PHO	Wang, W	TN	769
PHO	Wechsler, D	NC	769
PHO	Weinblatt, M	NY	764
PHO	Weiner, M	NY	764
PHO	Weinstein, H	MA	757
PHO	Wexler, L	NY	764
PHO	Wiley, J	MD	764
PHO	Williams, J	AZ	776
PHO	Winick, N	TX	776
PHO	Wolfe, L	NY	764
PHO	Wolff, J	MA	757
PHO	Yaddanapudi, R	MI	774
PHO	York, T	MD	764

Pediatric Infectious Disease

Spec	Name	St	Pg
Inf	Gorensek, M	FL	415
PInf	Alexander, K	IL	782
PInf	Andiman, W	CT	779
PInf	Baker, C	TX	784
PInf	Baltimore, R	CT	779
PInf	Belcher, C	IN	782
PInf	Bell, L	PA	780
PInf	Bernstein, D	OH	783
PInf	Bradley, J	CA	784
PInf	Bryson, Y	CA	784
PInf	Christenson, J	IN	783
PInf	Demmler-Harrison, G	TX	784
PInf	Durbin, W	MA	780
PInf	Edwards, K	TN	781
PInf	Emmanuel, P	FL	781
PInf	Flynn, P	TN	782
PInf	Givner, L	NC	782
PInf	Green, M	PA	780
PInf	Ingram, D	NC	782
PInf	Jacobs, R	AR	784
PInf	Kaplan, S	TX	784
PInf	Kleiman, M	IN	783
PInf	Kline, M	TX	784
PInf	Kotloff, K	MD	780
PInf	Krilov, L	NY	780
PInf	Leonard, E	OH	783
PInf	Long, S	PA	781
PInf	Mason, W	CA	785
PInf	McComsey, G	OH	783
PInf	McCracken, G	TX	784
PInf	McKinney, R	NC	782
PInf	Meissner, H	MA	780
PInf	Michaels, M	PA	781
PInf	Mitchell, C	FL	782
PInf	Offit, P	PA	781
PInf	Petru, A	CA	785
PInf	Raszka, W	VT	780
PInf	Saiman, L	NY	781
PInf	Scott, G	FL	782
PInf	Shapiro, E	CT	780
PInf	Shulman, S	IL	783
PInf	Singh, N	DC	781
PInf	Wald, E	WI	783

Pediatric Nephrology

Spec	Name	St	Pg
PNep	Andreoli, S	IN	787
PNep	Ault, B	TN	786
PNep	Benfield, M	AL	786
PNep	Brophy, P	IA	787
PNep	Chandar, J	FL	786
PNep	Cohn, R	IL	787
PNep	Conley, S	PA	785
PNep	Ellis, D	PA	785
PNep	Ettenger, R	CA	788
PNep	Fivush, B	MD	785
PNep	Flynn, J	WA	788
PNep	Fouser, L	WA	788
PNep	Friedman, A	MN	787
PNep	Harmon, W	MA	785
PNep	Jabs, K	TN	786

Spec	Name	St	Pg
PNep	Jordan, S	CA	788
PNep	Kaplan, B	PA	785
PNep	Kashtan, C	MN	787
PNep	Langman, C	IL	787
PNep	McDonald, R	WA	788
PNep	Mendley, S	MD	786
PNep	Neiberger, R	FL	786
PNep	Roskes, S	MD	786
PNep	Warady, B	MO	788
PNep	Wyatt, R	TN	786
PNep	Zilleruelo, G	FL	787

Pediatric Neuro-Ophthalmology

Spec	Name	St	Pg
N	Liu, G	PA	515
Oph	Borchert, M	CA	599

Pediatric Neurology

Spec	Name	St	Pg
N	Hecox, K	WI	527
N	Kolodny, E	NY	513
Ped	Vining, E	MD	727

Pediatric Neuroradiology

Spec	Name	St	Pg
DR	Shaw, D	WA	984
NRad	Ball, W	OH	988
NRad	Barkovich, A	CA	990
NRad	Barnes, P	CA	990
NRad	Hunter, J	TX	990
NRad	Vezina, L	DC	986
NRad	Zimmerman, R	PA	986

Pediatric Neurosurgery

Spec	Name	St	Pg
NS	Adelson, P	AZ	492
NS	Bierbrauer, K	OH	486
NS	Boggan, J	CA	496
NS	Boop, F	TN	481
NS	Carson, B	MD	473
NS	Cherny, W	ID	491
NS	Cohen, A	MA	470
NS	Danielpour, M	CA	496
NS	Dias, M	PA	473
NS	Duhaime, A	MA	470
NS	Edwards, M	CA	496
NS	Ewend, M	NC	481
NS	Feldstein, N	NY	474
NS	Frim, D	IL	487
NS	Goumnerova, L	MA	470
NS	Greene, C	LA	492
NS	Gupta, N	CA	497
NS	Heilman, C	MA	471
NS	Jallo, G	MD	475
NS	Jimenez, D	TX	493
NS	Kaufman, B	WI	488
NS	Kestle, J	UT	491
NS	Lang, F	TX	493
NS	Levy, M	CA	497
NS	Luerssen, T	TX	493
NS	Madsen, J	MA	471
NS	Mapstone, T	OK	494
NS	Menezes, A	IA	488

Spec	Name	St	Pg
NS	Myseros, J	VA	483
NS	Nagib, M	MN	489
NS	Oakes, W	AL	483
NS	Ojemann, J	WA	498
NS	Parent, A	MS	483
NS	Park, T	MO	489
NS	Pollack, I	PA	478
NS	Raffel, C	OH	489
NS	Ragheb, J	FL	483
NS	Ruge, J	IL	490
NS	Sandberg, D	TX	494
NS	Selden, N	OR	499
NS	Shuer, L	CA	499
NS	Sklar, F	TX	494
NS	Souweidane, M	NY	479
NS	Sun, P	CA	499
NS	Tomita, T	IL	490
NS	Walker, M	UT	492
NS	Walsh, J	LA	495
NS	Weiner, H	NY	480
NS	Wisoff, J	NY	480
NS	Zager, E	PA	480

Pediatric Nuclear Medicine

NuM	Dae, M	CA	551
NuM	Majd, M	DC	548

Pediatric Ophthalmology

Oph	Archer, S	MI	588
Oph	Azar, N	IL	588
Oph	Baker, J	MI	588
Oph	Buckley, E	NC	582
Oph	Burke, M	OH	589
Oph	Capo, H	FL	582
Oph	Caputo, A	NJ	572
Oph	Day, S	CA	600
Oph	Del Monte, M	MI	589
Oph	Demer, J	CA	600
Oph	Drack, A	IA	589
Oph	Eggers, H	NY	573
Oph	Ellis, G	LA	596
Oph	Eustis, H	LA	596
Oph	Freedman, S	NC	583
Oph	Gallin, P	NY	574
Oph	Granet, D	CA	600
Oph	Greenwald, M	IL	590
Oph	Guyton, D	MD	574
Oph	Hall, L	NY	575
Oph	Hess, J	FL	584
Oph	Hunter, D	MA	570
Oph	Isenberg, S	CA	601
Oph	Jaafar, M	DC	575
Oph	Katowitz, J	PA	576
Oph	Kerr, N	TN	584
Oph	Koller, H	PA	576
Oph	Kushner, B	WI	591
Oph	Lambert, S	GA	584
Oph	Levin, A	PA	576
Oph	Lueder, G	MO	592
Oph	Magramm, I	NY	577
Oph	McKeown, C	FL	584

Spec	Name	St	Pg
Oph	Mets, M	IL	592
Oph	Miller, J	AZ	597
Oph	Mills, M	PA	577
Oph	Mims, J	TX	597
Oph	Mitchell, P	CT	571
Oph	Murphree, A	CA	602
Oph	Nelson, L	PA	578
Oph	Olitsky, S	MO	592
Oph	Paul, T	CA	603
Oph	Plager, D	IN	593
Oph	Pollard, Z	GA	586
Oph	Quinn, G	PA	578
Oph	Reynolds, J	NY	579
Oph	Richard, J	OK	597
Oph	Shields, C	PA	580
Oph	Shields, J	PA	580
Oph	Siatkowski, R	OK	598
Oph	Simon, J	NY	580
Oph	Traboulsi, E	OH	594
Oph	Tychsen, L	MO	595
Oph	Wang, F	NY	581
Oph	Warman, R	FL	587
Oph	Weiss, A	WA	604
Oph	Wilson, M	SC	587
Oph	Wright, K	CA	605

Pediatric Orthopaedic Cancers

OrS	O'Donnell, R	CA	645
OrS	Peabody, T	IL	636
OrS	Wurtz, L	IN	638

Pediatric Orthopaedic Surgery

OrS	Beaty, J	TN	627
OrS	Conrad, E	WA	642
OrS	Delahay, J	DC	616
OrS	Dormans, J	PA	617
OrS	Feldman, D	NY	617
OrS	Herman, M	PA	619
OrS	Herzenberg, J	MD	619
OrS	Hyman, J	NY	620
OrS	Kasser, J	MA	611
OrS	Kocher, M	MA	612
OrS	Lee, F	NY	621
OrS	Malawer, M	MD	622
OrS	Marsh, J	CT	612
OrS	McCarthy, J	OH	635
OrS	Morcuende, J	IA	636
OrS	Oppenheim, W	CA	645
OrS	Otsuka, N	NY	623
OrS	Paley, D	FL	630
OrS	Pizzutillo, P	PA	624
OrS	Rajacich, N	WA	645
OrS	Randall, R	UT	639
OrS	Roye, D	NY	624
OrS	Sponseller, P	MD	625
OrS	Strongwater, A	NJ	626
OrS	Thompson, G	OH	638
OrS	Tolo, V	CA	646

Pediatric Otolaryngology

Oto	Clark, K	OK	681
Oto	Grundfast, K	MA	656
Oto	Hotaling, A	IL	675
Oto	Jones, P	IL	676
Oto	Lalwani, A	NY	662
Oto	Naclerio, R	IL	676
Oto	Poole, M	GA	670
Oto	Senders, C	CA	686
Oto	Zwillenberg, S	PA	667
PO	April, M	NY	789
PO	Arjmand, E	OH	791
PO	Arnold, J	OH	791
PO	Bower, C	AR	792
PO	Casselbrant, M	PA	789
PO	Chan, K	CO	792
PO	Cotton, R	OH	791
PO	Crockett, D	CA	793
PO	Cunningham, M	MA	789
PO	Darrow, D	VA	791
PO	Dolitsky, J	NY	789
PO	Drake, A	NC	791
PO	Duncan, N	TX	792
PO	Eavey, R	TN	791
PO	Friedman, E	TX	793
PO	Geller, K	CA	793
PO	Goldsmith, A	NY	789
PO	Haddad, J	NY	790
PO	Harley, E	DC	790
PO	Holinger, L	IL	791
PO	Inglis, A	WA	793
PO	Jones, J	NY	790
PO	Katz, R	OH	792
PO	Kazahaya, K	PA	790
PO	Lusk, R	NE	792
PO	McGill, T	MA	789
PO	Miller, R	IL	792
PO	Myer, C	OH	792
PO	Parikh, S	WA	793
PO	Poe, D	MA	789
PO	Richardson, M	OR	793
PO	Rosbe, K	CA	793
PO	Rosenfeld, R	NY	790
PO	Tunkel, D	MD	790
PO	Ward, R	NY	790

Pediatric Pathology

Path	Faye-Petersen, O	AL	713
Path	Heller, D	NJ	709
Path	Triche, T	CA	722

Pediatric Plastic Surgery

PlS	Bartlett, S	PA	852
PlS	Beals, S	AZ	870
PlS	Bentz, M	WI	864
PlS	Boyajian, M	DC	852
PlS	Bradley, J	CA	873
PlS	Buchman, S	MI	865
PlS	Chang, B	PA	853
PlS	Coleman, J	IN	865

Specialty & Special Expertise Index

Spec	Name	St	Pg
PlS	Deleyiannis, F	CO	869
PlS	Gruss, J	WA	874
PlS	Hoffman, W	CA	874
PlS	Kane, A	TX	870
PlS	Kelly, K	TN	862
PlS	Losee, J	PA	855
PlS	Mackay, D	PA	856
PlS	Marsh, J	MO	866
PlS	Mulliken, J	MA	851
PlS	Papay, F	OH	867
PlS	Patel, P	IL	867
PlS	Polley, J	IL	867
PlS	Reinisch, J	CA	876
PlS	Staffenberg, D	NY	859
PlS	Stotland, M	NH	851
PlS	Taub, P	NY	859
PlS	Thaller, S	FL	863
PlS	Vasconez, H	KY	864

Pediatric Pulmonology

Spec	Name	St	Pg
PPul	Borowitz, D	NY	794
PPul	Cooper, D	CA	798
PPul	Dorkin, H	MA	794
PPul	Dovey, M	PA	794
PPul	Dozor, A	NY	794
PPul	Fan, L	CO	797
PPul	Gibson, R	WA	798
PPul	Givan, D	IN	796
PPul	Green, T	IL	796
PPul	Kattan, M	NY	794
PPul	Keens, T	CA	798
PPul	Kemp, J	MO	796
PPul	Kim, Y	IN	797
PPul	Konstan, M	OH	797
PPul	Kurachek, S	MN	797
PPul	Kurland, G	PA	794
PPul	Lapey, A	MA	794
PPul	Loughlin, G	NY	795
PPul	Marcus, C	PA	795
PPul	McCoy, K	OH	797
PPul	Mcgrath-Morrow, S	MD	795
PPul	Morgan, W	AZ	797
PPul	Murphy, T	NC	796
PPul	Nielson, D	CA	798
PPul	Orenstein, D	PA	795
PPul	Panitch, H	PA	795
PPul	Platzker, A	CA	798
PPul	Quittell, L	NY	795
PPul	Ramsey, B	WA	798
PPul	Redding, G	WA	798
PPul	Rubin, B	VA	796
PPul	Sallent, J	FL	796
PPul	Sherman, J	VA	796
PPul	Tauber, D	PA	795
PPul	Wall, M	OR	798
PPul	Warren, R	AR	797
PPul	Zeitlin, P	MD	795

Pediatric Radiology

Spec	Name	St	Pg
DR	Cohen, H	TN	979
DR	Gilsanz, V	CA	983

Spec	Name	St	Pg
DR	Hubbard, A	NE	981
DR	Jaramillo, D	PA	975
DR	Sivit, C	OH	981
DR	Wells, R	WI	981
DR	Wood, B	CA	984

Pediatric Rehabilitation

Spec	Name	St	Pg
PMR	Alexander, J	NC	838
PMR	Currie, D	TX	842
PMR	Evans, S	DC	835
PMR	Keen, M	IL	840
PMR	Massagli, T	WA	844
PMR	Matthews, D	CO	842
PMR	Nelson, M	TX	843
PMR	Webster, H	MA	834

Pediatric Rheumatology

Spec	Name	St	Pg
PRhu	Finkel, T	FL	800
PRhu	Goldsmith, D	PA	799
PRhu	Haines, K	NJ	799
PRhu	Ilowite, N	NY	799
PRhu	Klein-Gitelman, M	IL	800
PRhu	Lehman, T	NY	799
PRhu	McCarthy, P	CT	799
PRhu	Myones, B	TX	801
PRhu	Passo, M	SC	800
PRhu	Schanberg, L	NC	800
PRhu	Sherry, D	PA	799
PRhu	Sills, E	MD	800
PRhu	Wagner-Weiner, L	IL	800
PRhu	Warren, R	SC	800
PRhu	Wilking, A	TX	801
Rhu	Silver, R	SC	1030

Pediatric Sports Medicine

Spec	Name	St	Pg
OrS	Kocher, M	MA	612
SM	Micheli, L	MA	1040

Pediatric Surgery

Spec	Name	St	Pg
PS	Adzick, N	PA	802
PS	Aiken, J	WI	806
PS	Albanese, C	CA	810
PS	Alexander, F	NJ	802
PS	Andrews, W	MO	806
PS	Arensman, R	IL	806
PS	Barksdale, E	OH	806
PS	Black, C	TX	809
PS	Bond, S	KY	805
PS	Bove, E	MI	807
PS	Cass, D	TX	809
PS	Caty, M	CT	801
PS	Chen, M	AL	805
PS	Chwals, W	MA	801
PS	Colombani, P	MD	802
PS	Crombleholme, T	CO	808
PS	Davidoff, A	TN	805
PS	Dillon, P	MO	807
PS	Dolgin, S	NY	803
PS	Doody, D	MA	801

Spec	Name	St	Pg
PS	Ehrlich, P	MI	807
PS	Fallat, M	KY	805
PS	Farmer, D	CA	810
PS	Flake, A	PA	803
PS	Foglia, R	TX	809
PS	Ford, H	CA	810
PS	Gaines, B	PA	803
PS	Ginsburg, H	NY	803
PS	Gittes, G	PA	803
PS	Glick, P	NY	803
PS	Graziano, K	AZ	809
PS	Grikscheit, T	CA	810
PS	Healey, P	WA	810
PS	Hilfiker, M	CA	810
PS	Holterman, M	IL	807
PS	Jackson, R	AR	809
PS	Jennings, R	MA	801
PS	Kane, T	DC	803
PS	Karrer, F	CO	808
PS	Krummel, T	CA	811
PS	La Quaglia, M	NY	803
PS	Latchaw, L	NH	802
PS	Lillehei, C	MA	802
PS	Lobe, T	CA	811
PS	McGill, L	AZ	809
PS	Meyers, R	UT	808
PS	Morgan, W	TN	805
PS	Moss, R	OH	807
PS	Nakayama, D	GA	805
PS	Nance, M	PA	804
PS	Notrica, D	AZ	809
PS	Nuchtern, J	TX	809
PS	Oldham, K	WI	807
PS	Paidas, C	FL	805
PS	Pena, A	OH	807
PS	Proctor, M	WA	811
PS	Quaegebeur, J	NY	804
PS	Rescorla, F	IN	807
PS	Reynolds, M	IL	808
PS	Rice, H	NC	805
PS	Ricketts, R	GA	806
PS	Rodgers, B	VA	806
PS	Sato, T	WI	808
PS	Sawin, R	WA	811
PS	Schwartz, M	PA	804
PS	Shamberger, R	MA	802
PS	Shochat, S	TN	806
PS	Skinner, M	TX	810
PS	Spigland, N	NY	804
PS	Stein, J	CA	811
PS	Strauch, E	MD	804
PS	Stylianos, S	NY	804
PS	Tracy, T	RI	802
PS	Tuggle, D	OK	810
PS	Velcek, F	NY	804
PS	Voigt, R	MD	804
PS	Waldhausen, J	WA	811
PS	Warner, B	MO	808
PS	Weber, T	IL	808

Spec	Name	St	Pg
Pediatric Thoracic Surgery			
PS	Latchaw, L	NH	802
PS	Lillehei, C	MA	802
PS	Nuchtern, J	TX	809
PS	Oldham, K	WI	807
PS	Rodgers, B	VA	806
PS	Sawin, R	WA	811
PS	Spigland, N	NY	804
T&CS	Hanley, F	CA	1141
Pediatric Urology			
PS	Ginsburg, H	NY	803
PS	Lobe, T	CA	811
PS	Voigt, R	MD	804
U	Atala, A	NC	1159
U	Baskin, L	CA	1175
U	Bauer, S	MA	1148
U	Bloom, D	MI	1165
U	Brock, J	TN	1160
U	Cain, M	IN	1166
U	Caldamone, A	RI	1148
U	Canning, D	PA	1151
U	Cartwright, P	UT	1171
U	Coplen, D	MO	1166
U	Docimo, S	PA	1152
U	Elder, J	MI	1166
U	Ewalt, D	TX	1173
U	Firlit, C	MO	1167
U	Gearhart, J	MD	1152
U	Glassberg, K	NY	1152
U	Gonzales, E	TX	1173
U	Greenfield, S	NY	1153
U	Hensle, T	NJ	1153
U	Joseph, D	AL	1161
U	Kaefer, M	IN	1167
U	Kass, E	MI	1167
U	Kirsch, A	GA	1162
U	Merguerian, P	WA	1178
U	Mesrobian, H	WI	1169
U	Pope, J	TN	1163
U	Poppas, D	NY	1156
U	Rink, R	IN	1169
U	Rushton, H	DC	1156
U	Shortliffe, L	CA	1178
U	Siegelbaum, M	MD	1158
U	Strand, W	TX	1174
U	Sutherland, R	NC	1164
U	Weiss, R	CT	1150
Pediatrics			
Ped	Berkowitz, C	CA	728
Ped	Berlin, C	PA	726
Ped	Berman, B	MI	727
Ped	Bull, M	IN	727
Ped	Burgess, D	NJ	726
Ped	Feldman, K	WA	728
Ped	Fost, N	WI	727
Ped	Gartner, J	DE	726
Ped	Hershorin, E	FL	727
Ped	Hofkosh, D	PA	726

Spec	Name	St	Pg
Ped	Infante, A	TX	728
Ped	Jacob, M	IL	728
Ped	Jones, K	CA	728
Ped	Kleinerman, E	TX	728
Ped	Lantos, J	MO	728
Ped	Miller, K	MA	726
Ped	Morton, D	PA	727
Ped	Oeffinger, K	NY	727
Ped	Palfrey, J	MA	726
Ped	Rappaport, L	MA	726
Ped	Roizen, N	OH	728
Ped	Vining, E	MD	727
Ped	Walker, W	WA	729
Ped	Zeltzer, L	CA	729
Ped	Zitelli, B	PA	727
Pelvic & Acetabular Fractures			
OrS	Archdeacon, M	OH	632
OrS	Helfet, D	NY	619
OrS	Johnson, E	CA	644
OrS	Joyce, M	OH	634
OrS	Minas, T	MA	612
OrS	Webb, L	GA	631
Pelvic Congestion Syndrome			
VIR	Roberts, A	CA	998
VIR	Shlansky-Goldberg, R	PA	993
VIR	White, R	CT	992
Pelvic Floor Disorders			
CRS	Dietz, D	OH	173
CRS	Varma, M	CA	178
Pelvic Floor Reconstruction			
ObG	Hale, D	IN	561
ObG	Karram, M	OH	561
ObG	Lucente, V	PA	557
Pelvic Imaging			
DR	McCarthy, S	CT	973
Pelvic Organ Prolapse			
CRS	Birnbaum, E	MO	173
CRS	Ludwig, K	WI	174
Pelvic Organ Prolapse Repair			
GO	Hatch, K	AZ	287
ObG	Brodman, M	NY	557
ObG	De Lancey, J	MI	561
ObG	Einarsson, J	MA	556
ObG	Goldstein, M	NY	557
ObG	Hullfish, K	VA	559
ObG	Lucente, V	PA	557
ObG	Valaitis, S	IL	562
ObG	Visco, A	NC	560
ObG	Walters, M	OH	562
U	Badlani, G	NC	1159
U	Kennelly, M	NC	1161

Spec	Name	St	Pg
Pelvic Reconstruction			
GO	Currie, J	GA	280
GO	Fields, A	DC	278
GO	Fowler, J	OH	284
GO	Lentz, S	NC	282
GO	Mutch, D	MO	284
ObG	Cornella, J	AZ	563
ObG	Eckler, K	MA	556
ObG	Hullfish, K	VA	559
ObG	Sanz, L	VA	559
Pelvic Reconstruction After Cancer			
PlS	Tobin, G	KY	863
Pelvic Surgery			
S	Moore, E	CO	1085
Pelvic Surgery-Complex			
GO	Bodurka, D	TX	286
GO	Carney, M	HI	289
GO	Chan, J	CA	289
GO	Lele, S	NY	279
OrS	Schwartz, H	TN	630
Pelvic Tumors			
GO	Barnes, W	DC	276
GO	Penalver, M	FL	282
S	Paty, P	NY	1062
Pemphigus			
D	Anhalt, G	MD	184
D	Sobel, S	FL	192
D	Stanley, J	PA	189
D	Woodley, D	CA	200
Penile Cancer			
Onc	Godley, P	NC	357
RadRO	Anscher, M	VA	953
U	Loughlin, K	MA	1149
U	McDougal, W	MA	1149
U	Weiss, R	CT	1150
Penile Inversion Technique			
PlS	Meltzer, T	AZ	871
Penile Microvascular Bypass Surgery			
U	Goldstein, I	CA	1176
Penile Prostheses			
U	Hellstrom, W	LA	1173
U	Mulhall, J	NY	1155

Specialty & Special Expertise Index

Spec	Name	St	Pg
Peptic Acid Disorders			
Ge	Bresalier, R	TX	251
Ge	Chey, W	MI	244
Ge	Fisher, R	PA	232
Ge	Lichtenstein, D	MA	229
Ge	Metz, D	PA	236
Ge	Schulze, K	IA	248
Ge	Smoot, D	TN	243
Percutaneous ASD/PFO closure			
IC	Resar, J	MD	128
Percutaneous ASD/PFO Closure			
PCd	Rome, J	PA	736
Percutaneous Coronary Intervention			
IC	Knopf, W	GA	130
IC	Resar, J	MD	128
IC	Sacchi, T	NY	128
Percutaneous Valve Repair			
Cv	Silvestry, F	PA	102
IC	Gray, W	NY	127
IC	Resar, J	MD	128
IC	Shani, J	NY	129
Percutaneous Vascular Interventions			
Cv	Burket, M	OH	106
VascS	Dalsing, M	IN	1190
VascS	Green, R	NY	1187
Pericardial Disease			
Cv	Nishimura, R	MN	109
Perinatal Medicine			
MF	Ismail, M	IL	436
MF	Wapner, R	NY	434
PCCM	Sarnaik, A	MI	742
Perinatal Pathology			
Path	Faye-Petersen, O	AL	713
Path	Heller, D	NJ	709
Peripheral Nerve Disorders			
N	Sheikh, K	TX	534
NS	Belzberg, A	MD	472
NS	Levi, A	FL	482
NS	Zager, E	PA	480
Peripheral Nerve Surgery			
HS	Brushart, T	MD	295
HS	Chang, J	CA	304
HS	Gelberman, R	MO	301

Spec	Name	St	Pg
HS	Glickel, S	NY	296
HS	Greene, T	FL	299
HS	Grossman, J	FL	299
HS	Szabo, R	CA	304
NS	Chiocca, E	OH	487
NS	Kim, D	TX	493
NS	Kuntz, C	OH	488
NS	Lillehei, K	CO	491
NS	Spinner, R	MN	490
PlS	Chiu, D	NY	853
PlS	Ducic, I	DC	853
PlS	MacKinnon, S	MO	866
PlS	Siemionow, M	OH	868
Peripheral Neuropathy			
N	Adornato, B	CA	535
N	Amato, A	MA	506
N	Barohn, R	KS	531
N	Bromberg, M	UT	531
N	Cohen, J	NH	506
N	Cornblath, D	MD	510
N	Engel, W	CA	536
N	Engstrom, J	CA	536
N	Feldman, E	MI	526
N	Glass, J	GA	521
N	Jones, H	MA	507
N	Kincaid, J	IN	527
N	Latov, N	NY	514
N	Logigian, E	NY	515
N	Oaklander, A	MA	508
N	Pestronk, A	MO	529
N	Simpson, D	NY	517
N	Weiss, M	WA	539
N	Windebank, A	MN	530
PMR	Feinberg, J	NY	836
Peripheral Vascular Disease			
Cv	Burket, M	OH	106
Cv	Eagle, K	MI	107
Cv	Halperin, J	NY	99
Cv	Krajcer, Z	TX	114
Cv	Loscalzo, J	MA	95
IC	Dieter, R	IL	131
IC	Gray, W	NY	127
IC	Kandzari, D	GA	130
IC	Khawaja, S	GA	130
IC	Petrossian, G	NY	128
IC	Reddy, B	GA	130
IC	Roubin, G	NY	128
IC	Smalling, R	TX	132
S	Mannella, W	PA	1060
T&CS	Dang, M	HI	1141
VascS	Alexander, J	OH	1190
VascS	Atnip, R	PA	1185
VascS	Carpenter, J	NJ	1186
VascS	Chaikof, E	MA	1184
VascS	Clair, D	OH	1190
VascS	Comerota, A	OH	1190
VascS	Cooper, M	CO	1192
VascS	Cronenwett, J	NH	1184
VascS	D'Ayala, M	NY	1186

Spec	Name	St	Pg
VascS	Dalsing, M	IN	1190
VascS	Eidt, J	AR	1193
VascS	Fairman, R	PA	1187
VascS	Faries, P	NY	1187
VascS	Flynn, T	FL	1189
VascS	Gewertz, B	CA	1194
VascS	Greisler, H	IL	1191
VascS	Makaroun, M	PA	1187
VascS	Marin, M	NY	1188
VascS	Mitchell, M	MS	1189
VascS	Pearce, W	IL	1191
VascS	Sanchez, L	MO	1191
VascS	Schneider, D	NY	1188
VascS	Stanley, J	MI	1192
VIR	Benenati, J	FL	994
VIR	Cho, K	MI	995
VIR	Durham, J	CO	996
VIR	Hallisey, M	CT	992
VIR	Katzen, B	FL	994
Peritoneal Carcinomatosis			
S	Bartlett, D	PA	1053
S	Ellis, L	TX	1088
S	Goodman, M	MA	1049
S	Hanna, N	MD	1058
S	Kuhn, J	TX	1090
S	Levine, E	NC	1070
S	Lowy, A	CA	1097
S	Sugarbaker, P	DC	1065
Peritoneal Mucinous Carcinomatosis			
CRS	Guillem, J	NY	170
Personality Disorders			
ChAP	Bird, H	NY	907
ChAP	Bleiberg, E	TX	911
Psyc	Adler, D	MA	888
Psyc	Black, D	IA	897
Psyc	Cloninger, C	MO	897
Psyc	Gunderson, J	MA	888
Psyc	Karasu, T	NY	892
Psyc	McGlashan, T	CT	889
Psyc	Norman, K	CA	902
Personality Disorders-Borderline			
Psyc	Gabbard, G	TX	900
Psyc	Gunderson, J	MA	888
Personality Disorders-Clinical Trials			
Psyc	McGlashan, T	CT	889
PET Imaging			
Cv	Gould, K	TX	114
DR	Cohen, B	NY	974
DR	Erasmus, J	TX	982
DR	Patz, E	NC	979

Spec	Name	St	Pg
NuM	Agress, H	NJ	548
NuM	Carrasquillo, J	NY	548
NuM	Dillehay, G	IL	550
NuM	Freeman, L	NY	548
NuM	Goldsmith, S	NY	548
NuM	Pandit-Taskar, N	NY	548
NuM	Sandler, M	TN	549
NuM	Siegel, B	MO	550
NuM	Wahl, R	MD	549

PET Imaging-Brain

Spec	Name	St	Pg
NuM	Alavi, A	PA	548
NuM	Strashun, A	NY	549
NuM	Waxman, A	CA	551

PET Imaging-Breast

Spec	Name	St	Pg
NuM	Wahl, R	MD	549

Peyronie's Disease

Spec	Name	St	Pg
U	Broderick, G	FL	1160
U	Carson, C	NC	1160
U	Hellstrom, W	LA	1173
U	Levine, L	IL	1168
U	Montague, D	OH	1169
U	Mulhall, J	NY	1155
U	Sadeghi-Nejad, H	NJ	1156
U	Seftel, A	NJ	1157

Phenylketonuria (PKU)

Spec	Name	St	Pg
CG	Burton, B	IL	160
CG	Ward, J	TN	159
Ped	Berlin, C	PA	726

Pheochromocytoma

Spec	Name	St	Pg
EDM	Fitzgerald, P	CA	222
NuM	Neumann, D	OH	550
S	Angelos, P	IL	1074
S	Fahey, T	NY	1057

Photoaging

Spec	Name	St	Pg
D	Gilchrest, B	MA	183
D	Voorhees, J	MI	195

Photodynamic Therapy

Spec	Name	St	Pg
D	Bickers, D	NY	185
D	Elmets, C	AL	190
D	Grichnik, J	FL	191
D	Hanke, C	IN	193
RadRO	Hahn, S	PA	950

Photosensitive Skin Diseases

Spec	Name	St	Pg
D	DeLeo, V	NY	186
D	Koo, J	CA	199

Phototherapy

Spec	Name	St	Pg
D	Bickers, D	NY	185
D	Elmets, C	AL	190
D	Kalb, R	NY	187
D	Koo, J	CA	199
D	Lim, H	MI	194
D	Soter, N	NY	189
D	Stern, R	MA	184

Physical Medicine & Rehabilitation

Spec	Name	St	Pg
PMR	Ahn, J	NY	834
PMR	Alexander, J	NC	838
PMR	Aseff, J	DC	835
PMR	Bach, J	NJ	835
PMR	Ballard, P	DC	835
PMR	Bloch, R	MA	834
PMR	Borg-Stein, J	MA	834
PMR	Braddom, R	PA	835
PMR	Brown, A	MN	839
PMR	Cardenas, D	FL	838
PMR	Chen, D	IL	839
PMR	Cheville, A	MN	839
PMR	Clairmont, A	OH	839
PMR	Colachis, S	OH	839
PMR	Creamer, M	FL	838
PMR	Currie, D	TX	842
PMR	De Lateur, B	MD	835
PMR	DePompolo, R	MN	840
PMR	Diamond, P	VA	838
PMR	Dillard, J	NY	835
PMR	Dumitru, D	TX	842
PMR	Esquenazi, A	PA	835
PMR	Evans, S	DC	835
PMR	Feinberg, J	NY	836
PMR	Feldman, J	IL	840
PMR	Flanagan, S	NY	836
PMR	Francis, K	NJ	836
PMR	Francisco, G	TX	842
PMR	Fried, G	PA	836
PMR	Frost, F	OH	840
PMR	Gamble, G	IL	840
PMR	Gater, D	VA	838
PMR	Gittler, M	IL	840
PMR	Glenn, M	MA	834
PMR	Haig, A	MI	840
PMR	Harris, D	TX	843
PMR	Herring, S	WA	843
PMR	Ivanhoe, C	TX	843
PMR	Jackson, A	AL	838
PMR	Keen, M	IL	840
PMR	Kevorkian, C	TX	843
PMR	Kezar, L	AL	838
PMR	King, J	TX	843
PMR	King, R	GA	838
PMR	Kirschner, K	IL	840
PMR	Kirshblum, S	NJ	836
PMR	Kuiken, T	IL	841
PMR	La Ban, M	MI	841
PMR	Leonard, J	MI	841
PMR	Leslie, D	GA	839
PMR	Lutz, C	NY	836
PMR	Lutz, G	NY	836

Spec	Name	St	Pg
PMR	Ma, D	NY	836
PMR	Marino, R	PA	837
PMR	Mason, K	CO	842
PMR	Massagli, T	WA	844
PMR	Matthews, D	CO	842
PMR	Mayer, N	PA	837
PMR	McKinley, W	VA	839
PMR	Miknevich, M	PA	837
PMR	Munin, M	PA	837
PMR	Mysiw, W	OH	841
PMR	Nelson, M	TX	843
PMR	Nobunaga, A	OH	841
PMR	Palmer, J	MD	837
PMR	Press, J	IL	841
PMR	Ragnarsson, K	NY	837
PMR	Richter, E	CT	834
PMR	Robinson, L	WA	844
PMR	Roth, E	IL	841
PMR	Saal, J	CA	844
PMR	Schwartz, L	PA	837
PMR	Sisung, C	IL	841
PMR	Sliwa, J	IL	842
PMR	Stewart, P	AL	839
PMR	Stubblefield, M	NY	837
PMR	Volshteyn, O	MO	842
PMR	Webster, H	MA	834
PMR	Wilson, A	TX	843
PMR	Zafonte, R	MA	834

Pigmented Lesions

Spec	Name	St	Pg
D	Barbosa, V	IL	192
D	Gellis, S	MA	183
D	Grimes, P	CA	199
D	Johr, R	FL	191
D	McMichael, A	NC	191
D	Neuburg, M	WI	194
D	Shea, C	IL	195
PlS	Bauer, B	IL	864

Pilonidal Disease

Spec	Name	St	Pg
S	Buchman, T	GA	1067

Pineal Tumors

Spec	Name	St	Pg
NS	Black, K	CA	495

Pituitary Disorders

Spec	Name	St	Pg
EDM	Biller, B	MA	206
EDM	Calvi, L	NY	209
EDM	Comi, R	NH	206
EDM	Greene, L	NY	210
EDM	Hoffman, A	CA	223
EDM	Inzucchi, S	CT	207
EDM	Jacobs, T	NY	210
EDM	Katznelson, L	CA	223
EDM	Kennedy, L	OH	218
EDM	Kleinberg, D	NY	210
EDM	Klibanski, A	MA	207
EDM	Koch, C	MS	214
EDM	Kopp, P	IL	218

Specialty & Special Expertise Index

Spec	Name	St	Pg
EDM	Lechan, R	MA	208
EDM	Lipson, A	DC	211
EDM	Marshall, J	VA	214
EDM	Melmed, S	CA	223
EDM	Ridgway, E	CO	220
EDM	Robbins, R	TX	221
EDM	Singer, P	CA	224
EDM	Swerdloff, R	CA	224
EDM	Thorner, M	VA	215
EDM	Vance, M	VA	215
EDM	Weiss, R	IL	219
EDM	Young, I	NY	213
NRad	Khandji, A	NY	985
PEn	Geffner, M	CA	748
PEn	Levy, R	IL	747
PEn	Sklar, C	NY	745
RE	Crowley, W	MA	1006

Pituitary Surgery

Spec	Name	St	Pg
NS	Atkinson, J	MN	485
NS	Chandler, W	MI	487
NS	Mayberg, M	WA	498
NS	Rock, J	MI	489
NS	Selman, W	OH	490

Pituitary Tumors

Spec	Name	St	Pg
EDM	Fitzgerald, P	CA	222
EDM	Hoffman, A	CA	223
EDM	Melmed, S	CA	223
EDM	Robbins, R	TX	221
EDM	Snyder, P	PA	212
EDM	Waguespack, S	TX	221
NS	Bederson, J	NY	472
NS	Berger, M	CA	495
NS	Brem, H	MD	472
NS	Brem, S	PA	472
NS	Bruce, J	NY	473
NS	Couldwell, W	UT	491
NS	David, C	MA	470
NS	Ewend, M	NC	481
NS	Fenstermaker, R	NY	474
NS	Guthikonda, M	MI	488
NS	Harsh, G	CA	497
NS	Kotapka, M	PA	476
NS	Laske, D	PA	476
NS	Lillehei, K	CO	491
NS	Maroon, J	PA	477
NS	Meyer, F	MN	489
NS	Mickey, B	TX	494
NS	Murali, R	NY	477
NS	Origitano, T	MT	491
NS	Parent, A	MS	483
NS	Reid, W	TN	484
NS	Schwartz, T	NY	478
NS	Shapiro, S	IN	490
NS	Swaid, S	AL	484
NS	Swearingen, B	MA	471
NS	Tatter, S	NC	485
NS	Turtz, A	NJ	479
Onc	Chang, S	CA	384
Oto	O'Leary, M	CA	686

Spec	Name	St	Pg
Oto	Petruzzelli, G	GA	670
RE	Chang, R	CA	1017

Plasma Cell Disorders

Spec	Name	St	Pg
Hem	Barlogie, B	AR	323
Hem	Comenzo, R	MA	310
Hem	Gertz, M	MN	319
Hem	Gregory, S	IL	320

Plastic Bronchitis

Spec	Name	St	Pg
PPul	Rubin, B	VA	796

Plastic Surgery

Spec	Name	St	Pg
PlS	Allen, R	SC	860
PlS	Alter, G	CA	872
PlS	Aly, A	CA	872
PlS	Andersen, J	CA	873
PlS	Ariyan, S	CT	850
PlS	Ascherman, J	NY	852
PlS	Aston, S	NY	852
PlS	Attinger, C	DC	852
PlS	Baker, D	NY	852
PlS	Baker, S	DC	852
PlS	Barone, C	TX	869
PlS	Bartlett, S	PA	852
PlS	Barton, F	TX	869
PlS	Bauer, B	IL	864
PlS	Beals, S	AZ	870
PlS	Beasley, M	NC	860
PlS	Bentz, M	WI	864
PlS	Billmire, D	OH	864
PlS	Boyajian, M	DC	852
PlS	Bradley, J	CA	873
PlS	Brandt, K	MO	865
PlS	Buchman, S	MI	865
PlS	Bucky, L	PA	853
PlS	Burns, A	TX	870
PlS	Burstein, F	GA	860
PlS	Butler, C	TX	870
PlS	Byrd, H	TX	870
PlS	Carraway, J	VA	860
PlS	Cederna, P	MI	865
PlS	Chang, B	PA	853
PlS	Chiu, D	NY	853
PlS	Cohen, S	CA	873
PlS	Coleman, J	IN	865
PlS	Colen, L	VA	861
PlS	Collins, D	NH	850
PlS	Constantian, M	NH	850
PlS	Cordeiro, P	NY	853
PlS	Cruse, C	FL	861
PlS	Da Lio, A	CA	873
PlS	Dagum, A	NY	853
PlS	Daniel, R	CA	873
PlS	Davis, G	NC	861
PlS	Deleyiannis, F	CO	869
PlS	Dick, G	MD	853
PlS	Disa, J	NY	853
PlS	Ducic, I	DC	853
PlS	Dufresne, C	MD	854

Spec	Name	St	Pg
PlS	Edwards, M	NV	873
PlS	Erdmann, D	NC	861
PlS	Eriksson, E	MA	850
PlS	Evans, G	CA	873
PlS	Feldman, J	MA	850
PlS	Fisher, G	CA	873
PlS	Fix, R	AL	861
PlS	Fodor, P	CA	874
PlS	Fox, J	PA	854
PlS	Gallico, G	MA	850
PlS	Garner, W	CA	874
PlS	Georgiade, G	NC	861
PlS	Glat, P	PA	854
PlS	Gottlieb, L	IL	865
PlS	Gregory, R	FL	861
PlS	Grossman, J	CO	869
PlS	Grotting, J	AL	861
PlS	Gruss, J	WA	874
PlS	Hagan, K	TN	862
PlS	Hammond, D	MI	865
PlS	Hamra, S	TX	870
PlS	Hansen, J	OR	874
PlS	Hardesty, R	CA	874
PlS	Herman, C	PA	854
PlS	Hester, T	GA	862
PlS	Hidalgo, D	NY	854
PlS	Hoffman, L	NY	854
PlS	Hoffman, W	CA	874
PlS	Horowitz, J	CA	874
PlS	Hultman, C	NC	862
PlS	Hunstad, J	NC	862
PlS	Hurwitz, D	PA	854
PlS	Imber, G	NY	854
PlS	Isik, F	WA	874
PlS	Jewell, M	OR	875
PlS	Kane, A	TX	870
PlS	Kelly, K	TN	862
PlS	Kenkel, J	TX	870
PlS	Kirschner, R	OH	865
PlS	Koplin, L	CA	875
PlS	Kronowitz, S	TX	870
PlS	Kuzon, W	MI	866
PlS	Leaf, N	CA	875
PlS	Lee, R	IL	866
PlS	Leighton, W	AZ	871
PlS	Leipziger, L	NY	855
PlS	Lesavoy, M	CA	875
PlS	Levin, L	PA	855
PlS	Levine, J	NY	855
PlS	Little, J	DC	855
PlS	Loree, T	NY	855
PlS	Losee, J	PA	855
PlS	Low, D	PA	855
PlS	Mackay, D	PA	856
PlS	MacKinnon, S	MO	866
PlS	Magee, W	VA	862
PlS	Manders, E	PA	856
PlS	Manson, P	MD	856
PlS	Markowitz, B	CA	875
PlS	Marsh, J	MO	866
PlS	Marten, T	CA	875
PlS	Mast, B	FL	862

Spec	Name	St	Pg
PlS	Matarasso, A	NY	856
PlS	Matthews, D	NC	862
PlS	Maxwell, G	TN	863
PlS	McCarthy, J	NY	856
PlS	Meara, J	MA	850
PlS	Medalie, D	OH	866
PlS	Mehrara, B	NY	856
PlS	Meltzer, T	AZ	871
PlS	Menick, F	AZ	871
PlS	Metzinger, S	LA	871
PlS	Miller, M	OH	866
PlS	Miller, T	CA	875
PlS	Molnar, J	NC	863
PlS	Morgan, R	VA	863
PlS	Moses, M	LA	871
PlS	Mulliken, J	MA	851
PlS	Mustoe, T	IL	866
PlS	Nahabedian, M	DC	856
PlS	Napoli, J	DE	857
PlS	Ness, J	MN	867
PlS	Neumeister, M	IL	867
PlS	Nichter, L	CA	875
PlS	Noone, R	PA	857
PlS	Olding, M	DC	857
PlS	Orgill, D	MA	851
PlS	Ousterhout, D	CA	876
PlS	Papay, F	OH	867
PlS	Patel, P	IL	867
PlS	Paul, M	CA	876
PlS	Persing, J	CT	851
PlS	Pitman, G	NY	858
PlS	Polley, J	IL	867
PlS	Posnick, J	MD	857
PlS	Price, G	MD	857
PlS	Puckett, C	MO	867
PlS	Rand, R	WA	876
PlS	Rappaport, N	TX	871
PlS	Reinisch, J	CA	876
PlS	Ristow, B	CA	876
PlS	Robb, G	TX	871
PlS	Rockwell, W	UT	869
PlS	Rodriguez, E	MD	857
PlS	Rohrich, R	TX	872
PlS	Romano, J	CA	876
PlS	Rose, E	NY	858
PlS	Rosenberg, H	CA	876
PlS	Sanders, G	CA	876
PlS	Sanger, J	WI	867
PlS	Schusterman, M	TX	872
PlS	Serletti, J	PA	858
PlS	Seyfer, A	MD	858
PlS	Sherman, R	CA	876
PlS	Siebert, J	WI	868
PlS	Siemionow, M	OH	868
PlS	Singer, R	CA	877
PlS	Singh, N	MD	858
PlS	Slavin, S	MA	851
PlS	Slezak, S	MD	858
PlS	Smith, D	FL	863
PlS	Smith, P	FL	863
PlS	Sood, R	IN	868
PlS	Spence, R	MD	858

Spec	Name	St	Pg
PlS	Spinelli, H	NY	858
PlS	Stadelmann, W	NH	851
PlS	Staffenberg, D	NY	859
PlS	Stahl, R	CT	851
PlS	Stevens, W	CA	877
PlS	Stotland, M	NH	851
PlS	Stuzin, J	FL	863
PlS	Sullivan, P	RI	851
PlS	Sultan, M	NY	859
PlS	Tabbal, N	NY	859
PlS	Taub, P	NY	859
PlS	Tebbetts, J	TX	872
PlS	Thaller, S	FL	863
PlS	Thorne, C	NY	859
PlS	Ting, J	NY	859
PlS	Tobin, G	KY	863
PlS	Topham, N	PA	859
PlS	Tufaro, A	MD	860
PlS	Urata, M	CA	877
PlS	Vander Kolk, C	MD	860
PlS	Vasconez, H	KY	864
PlS	Vogt, P	MN	868
PlS	Walton, R	IL	868
PlS	Wells, J	CA	877
PlS	Wilcox, R	TX	872
PlS	Wilhelmi, B	KY	864
PlS	Wilkins, E	MI	868
PlS	Wolfe, S	FL	864
PlS	Yetman, R	OH	868
PlS	Young, V	MO	868
PlS	Yu, J	GA	864
PlS	Yuen, J	AR	872
PlS	Zide, B	NY	860
PlS	Zins, J	OH	869

Platelet Disorders

Spec	Name	St	Pg
Hem	DeLoughery, T	OR	325
Hem	Lyons, R	TX	324
Hem	Marks, P	CT	310
Hem	Rao, A	PA	314
PHO	Bussel, J	NY	758
PHO	Olson, T	GA	767
PHO	Parker, R	NY	763

Pleural Disease

Spec	Name	St	Pg
Pul	Light, R	TN	931
Pul	Sahn, S	SC	932
Pul	Villanueva, A	MA	924
T&CS	Friedberg, J	PA	1116

Pneumococcal Infections

Spec	Name	St	Pg
PInf	Kaplan, S	TX	784

Pneumoconiosis

Spec	Name	St	Pg
Pul	Rose, C	CO	937

Pneumocystis Carinii Pneumonia (PCP)

Spec	Name	St	Pg
Pul	Huang, L	CA	940

Pneumonia

Spec	Name	St	Pg
Inf	Craven, D	MA	410
Inf	Cunha, B	NY	411
Inf	Quagliarello, V	CT	410
PPul	Wall, M	OR	798
Pul	Guidry, G	LA	938
Pul	Nash, T	NY	926
Pul	Niederman, M	NY	926

Pneumonia-Recurrent

Spec	Name	St	Pg
PPul	Murphy, T	NC	796

POEMS Syndrome

Spec	Name	St	Pg
Hem	Comenzo, R	MA	310

Poison Control

Spec	Name	St	Pg
PrM	Hoffman, R	NY	883

Polycystic Kidney Disease

Spec	Name	St	Pg
Nep	Blumenfeld, J	NY	457
Nep	Perrone, R	MA	456
Nep	Rakowski, T	VA	460
Nep	Tolkoff-Rubin, N	MA	456
Nep	Torres, V	MN	463
PNep	Brophy, P	IA	787
PNep	Kaplan, B	PA	785
U	Sundaram, C	IN	1170

Polycystic Ovarian Syndrome

Spec	Name	St	Pg
EDM	Ehrmann, D	IL	217
EDM	Goodman, N	FL	214
EDM	Marshall, J	VA	214
EDM	Nestler, J	VA	215
RE	Azziz, R	GA	1011
RE	Barnes, R	IL	1012
RE	Brzyski, R	TX	1015
RE	Cedars, M	CA	1017
RE	Chang, R	CA	1017
RE	Coutifaris, C	PA	1008
RE	Diamond, M	MI	1013
RE	Dumesic, D	CA	1017
RE	Friedman, C	OH	1013
RE	Jacobs, L	IL	1013
RE	Kazer, R	IL	1014
RE	Legro, R	PA	1009
RE	Session, D	GA	1012
RE	Smith, Y	MI	1014
RE	Soules, M	WA	1018
RE	Walmer, D	NC	1012
RE	Wilson, E	TX	1016

Polycythemia Rubra Vera

Spec	Name	St	Pg
Hem	Fruchtman, S	NY	312
Hem	Spivak, J	MD	315
Hem	Streiff, M	MD	315

Specialty & Special Expertise Index

Spec	Name	St	Pg

Polymyalgia Rheumatica
Rhu	Magid, S	NY	1027

Polymyositis
Rhu	Curran, J	IL	1031
Rhu	Medsger, T	PA	1027
Rhu	Oddis, C	PA	1027
Rhu	Steen, V	DC	1028

Polypharmacology
Ger	Tenover, J	CA	267

Polypharmacology (Excess Medications)
Ger	Carr, D	MO	264

Porphyria
CG	Desnick, R	NY	157
Ge	Anderson, K	TX	250
Ge	Bloomer, J	AL	239
IM	Bissell, D	CA	426
Onc	Silver, S	MI	372

Portal Hypertension
S	Emre, S	CT	1049
S	Rosemurgy, A	FL	1071
VIR	Cohen, G	PA	993
VIR	Darcy, M	MO	995
VIR	Johnson, M	IN	995

Post Polio Syndrome
N	Pascuzzi, R	IN	528
PM	Walsh, N	TX	701

Post Polio Syndrome/Rehabilitation
PMR	Bach, J	NJ	835
PMR	Esquenazi, A	PA	835
PMR	Sliwa, J	IL	842

Post Traumatic Stress Disorder
ChAP	Fornari, V	NY	908
ChAP	Martini, D	UT	911
ChAP	Zeanah, C	LA	911
Psyc	Eth, S	FL	895
Psyc	Friedman, M	VT	888
Psyc	Greiner, C	NE	898
Psyc	Loewenstein, R	MD	893
Psyc	Pynoos, R	CA	902
Psyc	Raskind, M	WA	902
Psyc	Roy-Byrne, P	WA	902
Psyc	Spiegel, D	CA	903
Psyc	Stein, M	CA	903
Psyc	Vanderkolk, B	MA	890
Psyc	Wait, S	MD	895

Postpartum Depression
Psyc	Burt, V	CA	900

Power Doppler Imaging
DR	Adler, R	NY	974

Prader-Willi Syndrome
CG	Cassidy, S	CA	162
CG	Driscoll, D	FL	158
CG	Shoffner, J	GA	159
PEn	Freemark, M	NC	746

Praxis Functional Electrical Stim (FES)
OrS	Betz, R	PA	614

Pregnancy & Endocrine Disorders
EDM	Seely, E	MA	208

Pregnancy & Hematologic Abnormalities
MF	Berkowitz, R	NY	431
MF	Samuels, P	OH	437

Pregnancy Loss-Recurrent
RE	Keltz, M	NY	1008

Pregnancy-Advanced Maternal Age
MF	Heffner, L	MA	430

Pregnancy-African women only
ObG	Nour, N	MA	556

Pregnancy-High Risk
MF	Acker, D	MA	430
MF	Adam, K	TX	438
MF	Adashek, J	NV	439
MF	Bahado-Singh, R	MI	435
MF	Baker, E	NH	430
MF	Bartelsmeyer, J	MO	435
MF	Blakemore, K	MD	431
MF	Caritis, S	PA	432
MF	Cohen, A	PA	432
MF	Copel, J	CT	430
MF	D'Alton, M	NY	432
MF	Dooley, S	IL	436
MF	Duff, W	FL	434
MF	Dugoff, L	PA	432
MF	Eddleman, K	NY	432
MF	Ferguson, J	VA	434
MF	Fox, H	MD	432
MF	Genc, M	NY	432
MF	Grandis, A	NC	434
MF	Gravett, M	WA	440

MF	Greene, M	MA	430
MF	Grunebaum, A	NY	433
MF	Hankins, G	TX	438
MF	Heffner, L	MA	430
MF	Heyl, P	KY	434
MF	Hibbard, J	IL	436
MF	Ismail, M	IL	436
MF	Kelly, T	CA	440
MF	Koos, B	CA	440
MF	Landy, H	DC	433
MF	Macones, G	MO	437
MF	McLaren, R	VA	435
MF	Nies, B	VA	435
MF	Paidas, M	CT	431
MF	Parry, S	PA	433
MF	Philipson, E	OH	437
MF	Pinckert, T	MD	433
MF	Plante, L	PA	433
MF	Pridjian, G	LA	439
MF	Repke, J	PA	433
MF	Riley, L	MA	431
MF	Robertson, P	CA	441
MF	Robichaux, A	LA	439
MF	Saade, G	TX	439
MF	Strassner, H	IL	437
MF	Tabsh, K	CA	441
MF	Thomas, R	PA	433
MF	Tomich, P	NE	438
MF	Treadwell, M	MI	437
MF	Van Dorsten, J	SC	435
MF	Wenstrom, K	RI	431
MF	Wilkins-Haug, L	MA	431
MF	Winn, H	MO	438
MF	Zalud, I	HI	441
ObG	Bader, T	PA	556
ObG	Ordorica, S	NY	558
ObG	Scher, J	NY	558
ObG	Witter, F	MD	558

Preimplantation Genetic Diagnosis
RE	Grazi, R	NY	1008
RE	Grifo, J	NY	1008

Preiser's Disease
HS	Slutsky, D	CA	304

Premature Labor
MF	Besinger, R	IL	436
MF	Ferguson, J	VA	434
MF	Macones, G	MO	437
MF	Parry, S	PA	433
MF	Saade, G	TX	439
MF	Socol, M	IL	437
MF	Thorp, J	NC	435
MF	Wilkins, I	IL	437
ObG	Niebyl, J	IA	562

Prematurity Prevention

Spec	Name	St	Pg
MF	Adashek, J	NV	439
MF	Benedetti, T	WA	439
MF	Fox, H	MD	432
MF	Gravett, M	WA	440
MF	Norwitz, E	MA	430

Prematurity/Low Birth Weight Infants

Spec	Name	St	Pg
MF	Andrews, W	AL	434
MF	Gravett, M	WA	440
MF	Wilkins, I	IL	437
NP	Bell, E	IA	450
NP	Cole, F	MO	450
NP	Delivoria-Papadopoulos, M	PA	447
NP	Dhanireddy, R	TN	449
NP	Gleason, C	WA	452
NP	Holzman, I	NY	447
NP	La Gamma, E	NY	447
NP	Lawson, E	MD	447
NP	Muraskas, J	IL	451
NP	Perlman, J	NY	448

Prenatal Diagnosis

Spec	Name	St	Pg
CG	Anyane-Yeboa, K	NY	156
CG	Falk, R	CA	162
CG	Gilbert, F	NY	157
CG	Holmes, L	MA	156
CG	Hudgins, L	CA	163
CG	Mahoney, M	CT	156
CG	Pauker, S	MA	156
CG	Seaver, L	HI	163
CG	Shapiro, L	NY	158
CG	Shulman, L	IL	160
MF	Abuhamad, A	VA	434
MF	Adashek, J	NV	439
MF	Besinger, R	IL	436
MF	Cheng, E	WA	439
MF	Copel, J	CT	430
MF	D'Alton, M	NY	432
MF	Dugoff, L	PA	432
MF	Goldberg, J	CA	440
MF	Hibbard, J	IL	436
MF	Hussey, M	IL	436
MF	Johnson, T	MI	436
MF	Kuller, J	NC	435
MF	Mastrobattista, J	TX	438
MF	McLaren, R	VA	435
MF	Platt, L	CA	440
MF	Pridjian, G	LA	439
MF	Reed, K	AZ	439
MF	Robinson, J	MA	431
ObG	Byrne, J	UT	562
ObG	Gonik, B	MI	561
ObG	Simpson, J	FL	560

Prenatal Genetic Diagnosis

Spec	Name	St	Pg
CG	Bianchi, D	MA	156
CG	Driscoll, D	PA	157
CG	Falk, R	CA	162
CG	Pergament, E	IL	160
CG	Randolph, L	CA	163
ObG	Corteville, J	OH	560
RE	McClamrock, H	MD	1009

Prenatal Ultrasound

Spec	Name	St	Pg
MF	Abuhamad, A	VA	434
MF	Pridjian, G	LA	439
MF	Tomich, P	NE	438
MF	Wilkins, I	IL	437

Preventive Cardiology

Spec	Name	St	Pg
Cv	Andersen, H	NY	96
Cv	Bairey, C	CA	116
Cv	Balady, G	MA	94
Cv	Ballantyne, C	TX	114
Cv	Blumenthal, D	NY	96
Cv	Blumenthal, R	MD	97
Cv	Budoff, M	CA	116
Cv	Chizner, M	FL	103
Cv	Davidson, M	IL	107
Cv	Edmundowicz, D	PA	97
Cv	Fonarow, G	CA	116
Cv	Friedman, S	NY	98
Cv	Fuster, V	NY	98
Cv	Gandy, W	GA	104
Cv	Gardin, J	NJ	98
Cv	Goldberg, N	NY	98
Cv	Goodman, D	NY	98
Cv	Gould, K	TX	114
Cv	Hayes, S	MN	108
Cv	Herling, I	PA	99
Cv	Inra, L	NY	99
Cv	Kaul, S	OR	117
Cv	Kuvin, J	MA	95
Cv	Landzberg, J	NJ	100
Cv	Lewis, S	OR	117
Cv	Linton, M	TN	104
Cv	Redberg, R	CA	118
Cv	Reis, S	PA	101
Cv	Reiss, C	MO	110
Cv	Ridker, P	MA	96
Cv	Roberts, B	RI	96
Cv	Shah, P	CA	118
Cv	Shapiro, J	IL	111
Cv	Sorrentino, M	IL	111
Cv	Stein, J	WI	111
Cv	Volgman, A	IL	112
Cv	Weitz, H	PA	102
IM	Cushman, W	TN	425
IM	Rader, D	PA	424
PrM	Pearson, T	NY	883

Preventive Medicine

Spec	Name	St	Pg
Ger	Callahan, E	NY	262
Ger	Lipschitz, D	AR	266
IM	Braunstein, S	NC	424
IM	Cirigliano, M	PA	424
IM	Fischbein, L	MO	425

Spec	Name	St	Pg
ObG	Bradshaw, K	TX	563
ObG	Young, B	NY	558
PrM	Cahill, J	NY	882
PrM	Cahill, K	NY	883
PrM	Hoffman, R	NY	883
PrM	Pearson, T	NY	883
Rhu	Rothenberg, R	MD	1028

Prion Diseases

Spec	Name	St	Pg
N	Farlow, M	IN	526

PRK-Refractive Surgery

Spec	Name	St	Pg
Oph	Afshari, N	NC	581
Oph	Kornmehl, E	MA	570
Oph	Manche, E	CA	602
Oph	Mandel, E	NY	577
Oph	Wilson, S	OH	595

Progressive Osseous Heteroplasia POH

Spec	Name	St	Pg
OrS	Kaplan, F	PA	620

Progressive Supranuclear Palsy (PSP)

Spec	Name	St	Pg
N	Gizzi, M	NJ	512
N	Golbe, L	NJ	512
N	Weiner, W	MD	519

Prolactin Disorders

Spec	Name	St	Pg
EDM	Klibanski, A	MA	207
RE	Zacur, H	MD	1011

Prostate Cancer

Spec	Name	St	Pg
NuM	Podoloff, D	TX	550
Onc	Ahmann, F	AZ	376
Onc	Beer, T	OR	384
Onc	Bolger, G	AL	354
Onc	Boston, B	TN	354
Onc	Bubley, G	MA	328
Onc	Butler, W	SC	354
Onc	Clinton, S	OH	366
Onc	Dawson, N	DC	338
Onc	DiPaola, R	NJ	338
Onc	Donehower, R	MD	338
Onc	Dreicer, R	OH	367
Onc	Eisenberger, M	MD	339
Onc	Garnick, M	MA	329
Onc	Gaynor, E	IL	367
Onc	Gelmann, E	NY	340
Onc	George, D	NC	356
Onc	Glode, L	CO	375
Onc	Haas, N	PA	341
Onc	Hauke, R	NE	375
Onc	Higano, C	WA	387
Onc	Hudes, G	PA	342
Onc	Hussain, M	MI	368
Onc	Kantoff, P	MA	330
Onc	Kelly, W	PA	343

Spec	Name	St	Pg	Spec	Name	St	Pg	Spec	Name	St	Pg
Onc	Kraft, A	SC	358	RadRO	Medbery, C	OK	965	U	Hall, S	NY	1153
Onc	Kucuk, O	GA	358	RadRO	Mendenhall, N	FL	956	U	Heney, N	MA	1149
Onc	Levine, E	NY	344	RadRO	Michalski, J	MO	961	U	Herr, H	NY	1153
Onc	Logothetis, C	TX	380	RadRO	Movsas, B	MI	961	U	Jones, J	OH	1167
Onc	Mathew, P	MA	331	RadRO	Nori, D	NY	951	U	Kadmon, D	TX	1173
Onc	Motzer, R	NY	346	RadRO	Peschel, R	CT	947	U	Kane, M	MD	1154
Onc	Nanus, D	NY	346	RadRO	Pollack, A	FL	956	U	Kavoussi, L	NY	1154
Onc	Oh, W	NY	347	RadRO	Porrazzo, M	DC	952	U	Keane, T	SC	1161
Onc	Parnes, H	MD	347	RadRO	Roach, M	CA	967	U	Kibel, A	MA	1149
Onc	Peace, D	IL	370	RadRO	Rose, C	CA	967	U	Kim, E	TN	1161
Onc	Petrylak, D	CT	331	RadRO	Rosenman, J	NC	957	U	Kirschenbaum, A	NY	1154
Onc	Pienta, K	MI	371	RadRO	Rossi, C	CA	968	U	Klein, E	OH	1168
Onc	Reed, E	AL	361	RadRO	Rotman, M	NY	952	U	Koch, M	IN	1168
Onc	Roth, B	MO	371	RadRO	Russell, K	WA	968	U	Kozlowski, J	IL	1168
Onc	Scher, H	NY	348	RadRO	Sandler, H	CA	968	U	Lange, P	WA	1177
Onc	Schwartz, M	FL	362	RadRO	Schiff, P	NY	952	U	Lepor, H	NY	1154
Onc	Small, E	CA	391	RadRO	Schild, S	AZ	965	U	Levine, L	IL	1168
Onc	Smith, M	MA	332	RadRO	Stock, R	NY	952	U	Libertino, J	MA	1149
Onc	Stadler, W	IL	372	RadRO	Toonkel, L	FL	958	U	Lieskovsky, G	CA	1177
Onc	Sweeney, C	MA	332	RadRO	Tripuraneni, P	CA	968	U	Loo, M	NY	1155
Onc	Tagawa, S	NY	351	RadRO	Vicini, F	MI	962	U	Loughlin, K	MA	1149
Onc	Taplin, M	MA	333	RadRO	Vijayakumar, S	MS	958	U	Lowe, F	NY	1155
Onc	Tester, W	PA	351	RadRO	Wong, J	CA	968	U	Lugg, J	WY	1172
Onc	Torti, F	NC	363	RadRO	Zelefsky, M	NY	953	U	Malkowicz, S	PA	1155
Onc	Trump, D	NY	351	RadRO	Zietman, A	MA	948	U	McConnell, J	NC	1162
Onc	Vaughn, D	PA	351	U	Albertsen, P	CT	1148	U	McCullough, A	NY	1155
Onc	Vogelzang, N	NV	392	U	Alexander, R	MD	1151	U	McDougal, W	MA	1149
Onc	Wilding, G	WI	373	U	Andriole, G	MO	1165	U	McGovern, F	MA	1149
Path	Balla, A	IL	715	U	Babayan, R	MA	1148	U	McVary, K	IL	1168
Path	Bostwick, D	VA	713	U	Bahnson, R	OH	1165	U	Miles, B	TX	1174
Path	Epstein, J	MD	708	U	Balaji, K	NC	1160	U	Mohler, J	NY	1155
Path	Melamed, J	NY	710	U	Bans, L	AZ	1172	U	Montie, J	MI	1169
Path	Reuter, V	NY	711	U	Bardot, S	LA	1172	U	Mostwin, J	MD	1155
Path	Ross, J	NY	711	U	Basler, J	TX	1172	U	Moul, J	NC	1162
Path	True, L	WA	722	U	Beall, M	VA	1160	U	Naslund, M	MD	1156
RadRO	Anscher, M	VA	953	U	Brendler, C	IL	1165	U	Nelson, J	PA	1156
RadRO	Awan, A	IL	958	U	Burnett, A	MD	1151	U	Olumi, A	MA	1150
RadRO	Bogart, J	NY	948	U	Busby, J	AL	1160	U	Partin, A	MD	1156
RadRO	Ciezki, J	OH	959	U	Campbell, S	OH	1166	U	Pisters, L	TX	1174
RadRO	D'Amico, A	MA	946	U	Carpinito, G	MA	1148	U	Porter, C	WA	1178
RadRO	DeWeese, T	MD	949	U	Carroll, P	CA	1175	U	Pow-Sang, J	FL	1163
RadRO	Dicker, A	PA	949	U	Carter, H	MD	1151	U	Presti, J	CA	1178
RadRO	Dritschilo, A	DC	949	U	Catalona, W	IL	1166	U	Richie, J	MA	1150
RadRO	Ennis, R	NY	949	U	Chang, S	TN	1160	U	Robertson, C	NC	1163
RadRO	Forman, J	MI	959	U	Chen, D	PA	1151	U	Roehrborn, C	TX	1174
RadRO	Gejerman, G	NJ	950	U	Childs, S	CO	1171	U	Sanda, M	MA	1150
RadRO	Goodman, R	NJ	950	U	Cohen, J	PA	1152	U	Sanders, W	GA	1163
RadRO	Grado, G	AZ	964	U	Colberg, J	CT	1148	U	Scardino, P	NY	1157
RadRO	Hahn, S	PA	950	U	Cookson, M	TN	1161	U	Schlegel, P	NY	1157
RadRO	Hancock, S	CA	966	U	Crawford, E	CO	1171	U	See, W	WI	1170
RadRO	Haraf, D	IL	960	U	Dalkin, B	WA	1175	U	Siegelbaum, M	MD	1158
RadRO	Hartford, A	NH	946	U	Danoff, D	CA	1176	U	Singh, D	CT	1150
RadRO	Henderson, R	FL	954	U	Davis, B	KS	1171	U	Slawin, K	TX	1174
RadRO	Horwitz, E	PA	950	U	DeKernion, J	CA	1176	U	Soloway, M	FL	1164
RadRO	Johnstone, P	IN	960	U	Droller, M	NY	1152	U	Steinberg, G	IL	1170
RadRO	Jose, B	IN	960	U	Flanigan, R	IL	1167	U	Su, L	FL	1164
RadRO	Kalnicki, S	NY	951	U	Fraser, L	MS	1161	U	Sundaram, C	IN	1170
RadRO	Kaplan, I	MA	946	U	Gill, H	CA	1176	U	Takayama, T	WA	1179
RadRO	Kuettel, M	NY	951	U	Gill, I	CA	1176	U	Taneja, S	NY	1158
RadRO	Lee, A	TX	964	U	Gluckman, G	IL	1167	U	Terris, M	GA	1165
RadRO	Lee, W	NC	955	U	Gomella, L	PA	1153	U	Thompson, I	TX	1174
RadRO	Malcolm, A	TN	955	U	Greenberg, R	PA	1153	U	Thrasher, J	KS	1172

Spec	Name	St	Pg
U	Trabulsi, E	PA	1158
U	Uzzo, R	PA	1158
U	Wallen, E	NC	1165
U	Walsh, P	MD	1159
U	Wein, A	PA	1159
U	Wood, D	MI	1171
U	Zippe, C	OH	1171

Prostate Cancer (advanced)

Spec	Name	St	Pg
Onc	Godley, P	NC	357

Prostate Cancer-Cryosurgery

Spec	Name	St	Pg
DR	Bahn, D	CA	982
U	Katz, A	NY	1154

Prostate Cancer-MR Spectroscopy (MRSI)

Spec	Name	St	Pg
DR	Hricak, H	NY	975

Prostate Cancer-Vaccine Therapy

Spec	Name	St	Pg
Onc	Arlen, P	MD	334
Onc	Gulley, J	MD	341

Prostate Cancer/Robotic Surgery

Spec	Name	St	Pg
U	Ahlering, T	CA	1175
U	Albala, D	NY	1150
U	Amling, C	OR	1175
U	Benson, M	NY	1151
U	Donovan, J	OH	1166
U	Ellis, W	WA	1176
U	Greenberg, R	PA	1153
U	Jackman, S	PA	1154
U	Kawachi, M	CA	1177
U	Lanteri, V	NJ	1154
U	Menon, M	MI	1169
U	Miller, S	GA	1162
U	Patel, V	FL	1162
U	Pisters, L	TX	1174
U	Samadi, D	NY	1157
U	Sawczuk, I	NJ	1157
U	Scherr, D	NY	1157
U	Slawin, K	TX	1174
U	Smith, J	TN	1164
U	Steers, W	VA	1164
U	Teigland, C	NC	1164
U	Tewari, A	NY	1158
U	Wilson, T	CA	1179
U	Wong, C	OH	1171

Prostate Disease

Spec	Name	St	Pg
U	Alexander, R	MD	1151
U	Bans, L	AZ	1172
U	Catalona, W	IL	1166
U	DeKernion, J	CA	1176
U	Ellis, W	WA	1176
U	Gill, H	CA	1176

Spec	Name	St	Pg
U	Gribetz, M	NY	1153
U	Loo, M	NY	1155
U	Lowe, F	NY	1155
U	McVary, K	IL	1168
U	Moul, J	NC	1162
U	Naslund, M	MD	1156
U	O'Leary, M	MA	1149
U	Partin, A	MD	1156
U	Penson, D	TN	1163
U	Rajfer, J	CA	1178
U	Roehrborn, C	TX	1174
U	Ross, L	IL	1170
U	Sadeghi-Nejad, H	NJ	1156
U	Seftel, A	NJ	1157
U	Slawin, K	TX	1174
U	Thompson, I	TX	1174

Prosthesis Control

Spec	Name	St	Pg
PMR	Kuiken, T	IL	841

Proton Beam Therapy

Spec	Name	St	Pg
RadRO	DeLaney, T	MA	946
RadRO	Henderson, R	FL	954
RadRO	Johnstone, P	IN	960
RadRO	Lee, A	TX	964
RadRO	Marcus, R	FL	955
RadRO	Rossi, C	CA	968
RadRO	Russell, A	MA	947
RadRO	Tarbell, N	MA	947
RadRO	Woo, S	KY	958
RadRO	Zietman, A	MA	948

Pseudomembranous Colitis

Spec	Name	St	Pg
Inf	Bartlett, J	MD	410

Pseudomyxoma Peritonei

Spec	Name	St	Pg
S	Loggie, B	NE	1085

Pseudotumor Cerebri

Spec	Name	St	Pg
N	Adams, D	FL	519
N	Corbett, J	MS	520

Pseudoxanthoma Elasticum

Spec	Name	St	Pg
D	Lebwohl, M	NY	187
Oph	Fuchs, W	NY	574

Psoriasis

Spec	Name	St	Pg
D	Belsito, D	NY	184
D	Bickers, D	NY	185
D	Callen, J	KY	190
D	Camisa, C	FL	190
D	Cather, J	TX	196
D	Crutchfield, C	MN	193
D	Fenske, N	FL	190
D	Gottlieb, A	MA	183
D	Kalb, R	NY	187
D	Krueger, G	UT	196
D	Lebwohl, M	NY	187

Spec	Name	St	Pg
D	Menter, M	TX	197
D	Nigra, T	DC	187
D	Shupack, J	NY	188
D	Soter, N	NY	189
D	Stern, R	MA	184
D	Thiers, B	SC	192
D	Voorhees, J	MI	195
D	Woodley, D	CA	200

Psoriasis/Eczema

Spec	Name	St	Pg
D	Elmets, C	AL	190
D	Koo, J	CA	199
D	Orlow, S	NY	188

Psoriatic Arthritis

Spec	Name	St	Pg
D	Gottlieb, A	MA	183
Rhu	Bobrove, A	CA	1033
Rhu	Hugenberg, S	IN	1031
Rhu	Kay, J	MA	1024
Rhu	Massarotti, E	MA	1024
Rhu	Mitnick, H	NY	1027
Rhu	Pope, R	IL	1032
Rhu	Solomon, G	NY	1028

Psychiatric Barriers to Physical Rehab

Spec	Name	St	Pg
GerPsy	Streim, J	PA	913

Psychiatric Genetics

Spec	Name	St	Pg
Psyc	Nurnberger, J	IN	898

Psychiatric Rehabilitation

Spec	Name	St	Pg
Psyc	Liberman, R	CA	901

Psychiatry

Spec	Name	St	Pg
Psyc	Adler, D	MA	888
Psyc	Akhtar, S	PA	890
Psyc	Appelbaum, P	NY	890
Psyc	Arnold, S	PA	890
Psyc	Avery, E	TX	899
Psyc	Baile, W	TX	899
Psyc	Basch, S	NY	890
Psyc	Benes, F	MA	888
Psyc	Black, D	IA	897
Psyc	Black, K	MO	897
Psyc	Blazer, D	NC	895
Psyc	Blumenfield, M	CA	900
Psyc	Boronow, J	MD	890
Psyc	Bowden, C	TX	899
Psyc	Brandt, H	MD	890
Psyc	Breitbart, W	NY	891
Psyc	Brodkin, E	PA	891
Psyc	Bronheim, H	NY	891
Psyc	Burt, V	CA	900
Psyc	Buysse, D	PA	891
Psyc	Bystritsky, A	CA	901
Psyc	Calabrese, J	OH	897
Psyc	Canterbury, R	VA	895

Specialty & Special Expertise Index

Spec	Name	St	Pg
Psyc	Cloninger, C	MO	897
Psyc	Cohen, M	PA	891
Psyc	Crow, S	MN	897
Psyc	Davidson, J	TX	899
Psyc	DePaulo, J	MD	891
Psyc	Doghramji, K	PA	891
Psyc	Eaton, J	DC	891
Psyc	Eisendrath, S	CA	901
Psyc	Ellison, J	MA	888
Psyc	Eth, S	FL	895
Psyc	Fallon, B	NY	892
Psyc	Fann, J	WA	901
Psyc	First, M	NY	892
Psyc	Freedman, R	CO	898
Psyc	Friedman, B	CA	901
Psyc	Friedman, M	VT	888
Psyc	Fyer, A	NY	892
Psyc	Gabbard, G	TX	900
Psyc	Gitlin, M	CA	901
Psyc	Giustra, L	GA	896
Psyc	Goff, D	NY	892
Psyc	Greden, J	MI	897
Psyc	Greenberg, B	RI	888
Psyc	Greenberg, D	MA	888
Psyc	Greenberg, W	MA	888
Psyc	Greiner, C	NE	898
Psyc	Guarda, A	MD	892
Psyc	Gunderson, J	MA	888
Psyc	Haque, W	TX	900
Psyc	Hirschfeld, R	TX	900
Psyc	Hoffman, D	CO	899
Psyc	Hollander, E	NY	892
Psyc	Janicak, P	IL	897
Psyc	Jenike, M	MA	889
Psyc	Jimerson, D	MA	889
Psyc	Karasu, T	NY	892
Psyc	Kavey, N	NY	892
Psyc	Keepers, G	OR	901
Psyc	Klagsbrun, S	NY	893
Psyc	Klapheke, M	FL	896
Psyc	Krueger, R	NY	893
Psyc	Kunkel, E	PA	893
Psyc	Kupfer, D	PA	893
Psyc	Lawson, W	DC	893
Psyc	Leuchter, A	CA	901
Psyc	Levine, S	OH	897
Psyc	Levy, S	GA	896
Psyc	Liberman, R	CA	901
Psyc	Locala, J	OH	898
Psyc	Loewenstein, R	MD	893
Psyc	Manevitz, A	NY	893
Psyc	Mann, J	NY	893
Psyc	Marder, S	CA	901
Psyc	Marin, D	NY	894
Psyc	McCallum, K	MO	898
Psyc	McCann, M	MD	894
Psyc	McGlashan, T	CT	889
Psyc	McIntosh, J	UT	899
Psyc	Mitchell, J	ND	899
Psyc	Moench, L	UT	899
Psyc	Mohl, P	TX	900
Psyc	Nelson, J	CA	902
Psyc	Neppe, V	WA	902
Psyc	Norman, K	CA	902
Psyc	Nurnberger, J	IN	898
Psyc	Phillips, K	RI	889
Psyc	Pi, E	CA	902
Psyc	Powers, P	FL	896
Psyc	Price, L	RI	889
Psyc	Pynoos, R	CA	902
Psyc	Raskind, M	WA	902
Psyc	Rasmussen, S	RI	889
Psyc	Rauch, P	MA	889
Psyc	Reus, V	CA	902
Psyc	Riba, M	MI	898
Psyc	Roose, S	NY	894
Psyc	Rosenthal, N	MD	894
Psyc	Rosenthal, R	NY	894
Psyc	Rosse, R	DC	894
Psyc	Roth, A	NY	894
Psyc	Roy-Byrne, P	WA	902
Psyc	Sadock, V	NY	894
Psyc	Salloum, I	FL	896
Psyc	Salzman, C	MA	889
Psyc	Samberg, E	NY	894
Psyc	Saxena, S	CA	903
Psyc	Schatzberg, A	CA	903
Psyc	Scott, C	PA	895
Psyc	Shapiro, E	MA	889
Psyc	Spiegel, D	CA	903
Psyc	Stein, M	CA	903
Psyc	Strakowski, S	OH	898
Psyc	Strouse, T	CA	903
Psyc	Summergrad, P	MA	890
Psyc	Sussman, N	NY	895
Psyc	Thase, M	PA	895
Psyc	Valentine, A	TX	900
Psyc	Vanderkolk, B	MA	890
Psyc	Wait, S	MD	895
Psyc	Walsh, B	NY	895
Psyc	Weiner, K	CO	899
Psyc	Weiner, M	TX	900
Psyc	Weiner, R	NC	896
Psyc	Weinstock, R	CA	903
Psyc	Weisler, R	NC	896
Psyc	Wilson, D	FL	896
Psyc	Wooten, V	OH	898
Psyc	Zerbe, K	OR	903

Psychiatry in Body Image Awareness

Spec	Name	St	Pg
Psyc	Bronheim, H	NY	891

Psychiatry in Cancer

Spec	Name	St	Pg
H & PM	Block, S	MA	406
Psyc	Baile, W	TX	899
Psyc	Basch, S	NY	890
Psyc	Breitbart, W	NY	891
Psyc	Fann, J	WA	901
Psyc	Greenberg, D	MA	888
Psyc	Greiner, C	NE	898
Psyc	Klagsbrun, S	NY	893
Psyc	Kunkel, E	PA	893

Spec	Name	St	Pg
Psyc	Riba, M	MI	898
Psyc	Spiegel, D	CA	903
Psyc	Strouse, T	CA	903
Psyc	Valentine, A	TX	900

Psychiatry in Physical Illness

Spec	Name	St	Pg
ChAP	Campo, J	OH	910
ChAP	Herzog, D	MA	906
ChAP	Martini, D	UT	911
GerPsy	Borson, S	WA	915
GerPsy	Streim, J	PA	913
Psyc	Basch, S	NY	890
Psyc	Bronheim, H	NY	891
Psyc	Cohen, M	PA	891
Psyc	Fallon, B	NY	892
Psyc	Fann, J	WA	901
Psyc	Greiner, C	NE	898
Psyc	Kunkel, E	PA	893
Psyc	Locala, J	OH	898
Psyc	Rauch, P	MA	889
Psyc	Strouse, T	CA	903

Psychiatry in Pregnancy

Spec	Name	St	Pg
Psyc	Burt, V	CA	900

Psychiatry in Terminal Illness

Spec	Name	St	Pg
Psyc	Klagsbrun, S	NY	893

Psychiatry in Transplant Patients

Spec	Name	St	Pg
ChAP	Sexson, S	GA	910
Psyc	Locala, J	OH	898

Psychiatry of Prostate Cancer

Spec	Name	St	Pg
Psyc	Roth, A	NY	894

Psychoanalysis

Spec	Name	St	Pg
Psyc	Akhtar, S	PA	890
Psyc	Basch, S	NY	890
Psyc	Friedman, B	CA	901
Psyc	Gabbard, G	TX	900
Psyc	Klapheke, M	FL	896
Psyc	Samberg, E	NY	894
Psyc	Scott, C	PA	895
Psyc	Shapiro, E	MA	889
Psyc	Zerbe, K	OR	903

Psychodermatology

Spec	Name	St	Pg
D	Koo, J	CA	199

Psychopharmacology

Spec	Name	St	Pg
AdP	Ciraulo, D	MA	904
AdP	Kosten, T	TX	906
AdP	Schuckit, M	CA	906
ChAP	Biederman, J	MA	906
ChAP	Coffey, B	NY	908
ChAP	Hudziak, J	VT	906
ChAP	Koplewicz, H	NY	909

Spec	Name	St	Pg
ChAP	Leventhal, B	NY	909
ChAP	Riddle, M	MD	909
GerPsy	Tune, L	GA	914
PM	Robbins, L	IL	700
Psyc	Basch, S	NY	890
Psyc	Blumenfield, M	CA	900
Psyc	Bystritsky, A	CA	901
Psyc	First, M	NY	892
Psyc	Friedman, B	CA	901
Psyc	Friedman, M	VT	888
Psyc	Goff, D	NY	892
Psyc	Janicak, P	IL	897
Psyc	Loewenstein, R	MD	893
Psyc	Marder, S	CA	901
Psyc	Mohl, P	TX	900
Psyc	Nelson, J	CA	902
Psyc	Neppe, V	WA	902
Psyc	Pi, E	CA	902
Psyc	Reus, V	CA	902
Psyc	Salzman, C	MA	889
Psyc	Schatzberg, A	CA	903
Psyc	Sussman, N	NY	895
Psyc	Thase, M	PA	895
Psyc	Wilson, D	FL	896

Psychoses-Late Onset

Spec	Name	St	Pg
GerPsy	Holroyd, S	VA	914
GerPsy	Tune, L	GA	914

Psychosocial Support in Childhood Cancer

Spec	Name	St	Pg
PHO	Siegel, S	CA	779

Psychosomatic Disorders

Spec	Name	St	Pg
ChAP	Campo, J	OH	910
ChAP	Steiner, H	CA	912
Psyc	Blumenfield, M	CA	900
Psyc	Fallon, B	NY	892

Psychotherapy

Spec	Name	St	Pg
Psyc	Blumenfield, M	CA	900
Psyc	First, M	NY	892
Psyc	Giustra, L	GA	896
Psyc	Gunderson, J	MA	888
Psyc	Karasu, T	NY	892
Psyc	Mohl, P	TX	900
Psyc	Sadock, V	NY	894
Psyc	Salzman, C	MA	889

Psychotic Disorders

Spec	Name	St	Pg
Psyc	Black, D	IA	897
Psyc	Boronow, J	MD	890
Psyc	Janicak, P	IL	897
Psyc	Liberman, R	CA	901
Psyc	Strakowski, S	OH	898

Pubertal Disorders

Spec	Name	St	Pg
PEn	Allen, D	WI	746

Spec	Name	St	Pg
PEn	Alter, C	PA	744
PEn	Eugster, E	IN	747
PEn	Foster, C	UT	748
PEn	Freemark, M	NC	746
PEn	Garibaldi, L	PA	744
PEn	Geffner, M	CA	748
PEn	Kappy, M	CO	748
PEn	Plotnick, L	MD	745

Pulmonary Complications-Cancer Therapy

Spec	Name	St	Pg
PPul	Kim, Y	IN	797

Pulmonary Complications-Neurodisability

Spec	Name	St	Pg
PPul	Givan, D	IN	796
PPul	Warren, R	AR	797

Pulmonary Complications-Sickle Cell Dis

Spec	Name	St	Pg
PPul	Kim, Y	IN	797

Pulmonary Disease

Spec	Name	St	Pg
Pul	Ahya, V	PA	924
Pul	Alberts, W	FL	929
Pul	Albertson, T	CA	938
Pul	Antony, V	AL	929
Pul	Arcasoy, S	NY	924
Pul	Arroliga, A	TX	938
Pul	Auger, W	CA	939
Pul	Balk, R	IL	933
Pul	Balmes, J	CA	939
Pul	Bascom, R	PA	924
Pul	Bellamy, P	CA	939
Pul	Berk, J	MA	922
Pul	Bijwadia, J	MN	933
Pul	Boushey, H	CA	939
Pul	Brooks, S	FL	929
Pul	Brown, K	CO	936
Pul	Burschtin, O	NY	924
Pul	Campbell, G	MS	929
Pul	Catanzaro, A	CA	939
Pul	Celli, B	MA	922
Pul	Christiani, D	MA	922
Pul	Christie, J	PA	925
Pul	Christman, B	TN	930
Pul	Cooke, J	NY	925
Pul	Cooper, J	AL	930
Pul	Cooper, W	VA	930
Pul	Criner, G	PA	925
Pul	Deitz, J	PA	925
Pul	Doherty, D	KY	930
Pul	Donahoe, M	PA	925
Pul	Donohue, J	NC	930
Pul	Elliott, C	UT	936
Pul	Enelow, R	NH	922
Pul	Ernst, A	MA	922
Pul	Fahey, P	IL	933
Pul	Fanta, C	MA	922

Spec	Name	St	Pg
Pul	Fletcher, E	IN	933
Pul	Friedman, L	CT	923
Pul	Fulkerson, W	NC	930
Pul	Garrity, E	IL	933
Pul	Garver, R	AL	930
Pul	Gerboth, G	AK	939
Pul	Goldman, A	FL	931
Pul	Greenberg, H	NY	925
Pul	Grum, C	MI	933
Pul	Guidry, G	LA	938
Pul	Hall, J	IL	933
Pul	Hansen-Flaschen, J	PA	925
Pul	Harman, E	FL	931
Pul	Haynes, J	AL	931
Pul	Heffner, J	OR	939
Pul	Henke, D	NC	931
Pul	Hertz, M	MN	933
Pul	Hill, N	MA	923
Pul	Hopewell, P	CA	939
Pul	Huang, L	CA	940
Pul	Hyers, T	MO	934
Pul	Ingbar, D	MN	934
Pul	Irwin, R	MA	923
Pul	Iseman, M	CO	936
Pul	Jacoby, D	OR	940
Pul	Johnson, B	VA	931
Pul	Kaplan, J	KS	937
Pul	Kaye, M	MN	934
Pul	Kern, J	CO	937
Pul	King, E	PA	926
Pul	King, T	CA	940
Pul	Kotloff, R	PA	926
Pul	Kovitz, K	IL	934
Pul	Krowka, M	MN	934
Pul	Lem, V	MO	934
Pul	Levin, D	OK	938
Pul	Libby, D	NY	926
Pul	Light, R	TN	931
Pul	LoRusso, T	VA	931
Pul	Loyd, J	TN	931
Pul	Lynch, J	CA	940
Pul	Mahler, D	NH	923
Pul	Marini, J	MN	934
Pul	Martin, R	CO	937
Pul	Martinez, F	MI	934
Pul	Matuschak, G	MO	935
Pul	Maxfield, R	NY	926
Pul	Metersky, M	CT	923
Pul	Millman, R	RI	923
Pul	Mosenifar, Z	CA	940
Pul	Nardell, E	MA	923
Pul	Nash, T	NY	926
Pul	Nelson, J	NY	926
Pul	Niederman, M	NY	926
Pul	O'Donnell, A	DC	927
Pul	Pack, A	PA	927
Pul	Padilla, M	NY	927
Pul	Palevsky, H	PA	927
Pul	Patterson, J	OR	940
Pul	Perret, P	LA	938
Pul	Popovich, J	MI	935
Pul	Prakash, U	MN	935

Spec	Name	St	Pg
Pul	Raghu, G	WA	940
Pul	Redlich, C	CT	923
Pul	Rennard, S	NE	937
Pul	Rizk, N	CA	940
Pul	Rochester, C	CT	924
Pul	Rose, C	CO	937
Pul	Rosenbluth, D	MO	935
Pul	Rossman, M	PA	927
Pul	Rubin, L	CA	941
Pul	Sahn, S	SC	932
Pul	Schluger, N	NY	927
Pul	Schwab, R	PA	927
Pul	Schwartz, D	CO	937
Pul	Schwarz, M	CO	937
Pul	Sharma, O	CA	941
Pul	Shellito, J	LA	938
Pul	Shore, B	MO	935
Pul	Silver, M	IL	935
Pul	Simon, R	MI	935
Pul	Staton, G	GA	932
Pul	Steiger, D	NY	928
Pul	Steinberg, H	NY	928
Pul	Sterman, D	PA	928
Pul	Stoller, J	OH	936
Pul	Stover-Pepe, D	NY	928
Pul	Strollo, P	PA	928
Pul	Sutherland, E	CO	937
Pul	Tapson, V	NC	932
Pul	Tharratt, R	CA	941
Pul	Thomashow, B	NY	928
Pul	Tino, G	PA	928
Pul	Tobin, M	IL	936
Pul	Trulock, E	MO	936
Pul	Unger, M	PA	929
Pul	Vaughey, E	VA	932
Pul	Villanueva, A	MA	924
Pul	Voelkel, N	VA	932
Pul	Wallace, J	CA	941
Pul	Wanner, A	FL	932
Pul	Weissler, J	TX	938
Pul	Wenzel, S	PA	929
Pul	Wheeler, A	TN	932
Pul	White, D	MA	924
Pul	Wiedemann, H	OH	936
Pul	Wolfe, R	CA	941
Pul	Young, K	PA	929

Pulmonary Disease/Immunocompromised

Pul	Stover-Pepe, D	NY	928

Pulmonary Embolism

DR	Goodman, L	WI	980
Pul	Arcasoy, S	NY	924
Pul	Palevsky, H	PA	927
Pul	Popovich, J	MI	935
S	Wakefield, T	MI	1084
T&CS	Jamieson, S	CA	1142

Pulmonary Fibrosis

Pul	Bascom, R	PA	924
Pul	Berk, J	MA	922
Pul	Brown, K	CO	936
Pul	Criner, G	PA	925
Pul	Donohue, J	NC	930
Pul	Fulkerson, W	NC	930
Pul	King, T	CA	940
Pul	Loyd, J	TN	931
Pul	Lynch, J	CA	940
Pul	Padilla, M	NY	927
Pul	Raghu, G	WA	940
Pul	Rossman, M	PA	927
Pul	Sahn, S	SC	932
Pul	Schwartz, D	CO	937
Pul	Schwarz, M	CO	937
Pul	Staton, G	GA	932
Pul	Tino, G	PA	928

Pulmonary Hypertension

Cv	Bashore, T	NC	103
Cv	Bourge, R	AL	103
Cv	Horn, E	NY	99
Cv	Poon, M	NY	101
Cv	Rich, S	IL	110
Cv	Smart, F	LA	115
Cv	von der Lohe, E	IN	112
Cv	Wagoner, L	OH	112
NP	Steinhorn, R	CA	451
PCd	Hanna, B	PA	735
Pul	Arroliga, A	TX	938
Pul	Auger, W	CA	939
Pul	Criner, G	PA	925
Pul	Elliott, C	UT	936
Pul	Hertz, M	MN	933
Pul	Hill, N	MA	923
Pul	Krowka, M	MN	934
Pul	Loyd, J	TN	931
Pul	Mosenifar, Z	CA	940
Pul	Padilla, M	NY	927
Pul	Palevsky, H	PA	927
Pul	Rubin, L	CA	941
Pul	Steiger, D	NY	928
Pul	Steinberg, H	NY	928
Pul	Tapson, V	NC	932
Pul	Trulock, E	MO	936
Pul	Voelkel, N	VA	932

Pulmonary Hypertension of Newborn (PPHN)

NP	Donn, S	MI	450
NP	Seidner, S	TX	452
NP	Van Marter, L	MA	446

Pulmonary Infections

PPul	Gibson, R	WA	798
Pul	Ingbar, D	MN	934
Pul	Metersky, M	CT	923
Pul	Rizk, N	CA	940
Pul	Shellito, J	LA	938
Pul	Stover-Pepe, D	NY	928
Pul	Wallace, J	CA	941

Pulmonary Pathology

Path	Cagle, P	TX	717
Path	Fishbein, M	CA	720
Path	Hammar, S	WA	720
Path	Katzenstein, A	NY	710
Path	Klimstra, D	NY	710
Path	Koss, M	CA	721
Path	Leslie, K	AZ	718
Path	Mark, E	MA	706
Path	Patchefsky, A	PA	711
Path	Travis, W	NY	712
Path	Yousem, S	PA	712

Pulmonary Rehabilitation

PPul	Warren, R	AR	797

Pulmonary Vascular Disease

Pul	Garrity, E	IL	933
Pul	Palevsky, H	PA	927
Pul	Rubin, L	CA	941
Pul	Schwarz, M	CO	937

R

Radiation Oncology

RadRO	Abrams, R	IL	958
RadRO	Ang, K	TX	963
RadRO	Anscher, M	VA	953
RadRO	Awan, A	IL	958
RadRO	Beitler, J	GA	953
RadRO	Berg, C	MD	948
RadRO	Blackstock, A	NC	953
RadRO	Bogart, J	NY	948
RadRO	Bradley, J	MO	958
RadRO	Brizel, D	NC	954
RadRO	Buatti, J	IA	959
RadRO	Buchholz, T	TX	963
RadRO	Chakravarthy, A	TN	954
RadRO	Chakravarti, A	OH	959
RadRO	Chao, K	NY	948
RadRO	Choi, N	MA	946
RadRO	Choy, H	TX	963
RadRO	Ciezki, J	OH	959
RadRO	Cmelak, A	TN	954
RadRO	Constine, L	NY	948
RadRO	Cooper, J	NY	948
RadRO	Cox, J	TX	963
RadRO	Crane, C	TX	963
RadRO	Crocker, I	GA	954
RadRO	D'Amico, A	MA	946
RadRO	DeLaney, T	MA	946
RadRO	DeWeese, T	MD	949
RadRO	Dicker, A	PA	949

Spec	Name	St	Pg
RadRO	Donahue, B	NY	949
RadRO	Donaldson, S	CA	965
RadRO	Dritschilo, A	DC	949
RadRO	Eifel, P	TX	964
RadRO	Eisbruch, A	MI	959
RadRO	Emami, B	IL	959
RadRO	Ennis, R	NY	949
RadRO	Fiveash, J	AL	954
RadRO	Flickinger, J	PA	949
RadRO	Forman, J	MI	959
RadRO	Formenti, S	NY	949
RadRO	Fowble, B	CA	966
RadRO	Freedman, G	PA	949
RadRO	Fuss, M	OR	966
RadRO	Gaffney, D	UT	962
RadRO	Gejerman, G	NJ	950
RadRO	Goodman, R	NJ	950
RadRO	Grado, G	AZ	964
RadRO	Greenberger, J	PA	950
RadRO	Grigsby, P	MO	959
RadRO	Haffty, B	NJ	950
RadRO	Hahn, S	PA	950
RadRO	Halberg, F	CA	966
RadRO	Halpern, H	IL	959
RadRO	Halyard, M	AZ	964
RadRO	Hancock, S	CA	966
RadRO	Haraf, D	IL	960
RadRO	Harari, P	WI	960
RadRO	Harris, J	MA	946
RadRO	Harrison, L	NY	950
RadRO	Hartford, A	NH	946
RadRO	Hayman, J	MI	960
RadRO	Heimann, R	VT	946
RadRO	Henderson, R	FL	954
RadRO	Herman, T	OK	964
RadRO	Hoppe, R	CA	966
RadRO	Horwitz, E	PA	950
RadRO	Isaacson, S	NY	950
RadRO	Jhingran, A	TX	964
RadRO	Johnstone, P	IN	960
RadRO	Jose, B	IN	960
RadRO	Kachnic, L	MA	946
RadRO	Kalnicki, S	NY	951
RadRO	Kaplan, I	MA	946
RadRO	Kleinberg, L	MD	951
RadRO	Knisely, J	NY	951
RadRO	Koh, W	WA	966
RadRO	Komaki, R	TX	964
RadRO	Konski, A	MI	960
RadRO	Kuban, D	TX	964
RadRO	Kudrimoti, M	KY	954
RadRO	Kuettel, M	NY	951
RadRO	Kun, L	TN	954
RadRO	Kupelian, P	CA	966
RadRO	Kuske, R	AZ	964
RadRO	Landry, J	GA	955
RadRO	Laramore, G	WA	966
RadRO	Larner, J	VA	955
RadRO	Larson, D	CA	967
RadRO	Lawrence, T	MI	960
RadRO	Le, Q	CA	967
RadRO	Lee, A	TX	964

Spec	Name	St	Pg
RadRO	Lee, C	MN	960
RadRO	Lee, W	NC	955
RadRO	Lepanto, P	WV	951
RadRO	Lewin, A	FL	955
RadRO	Loeffler, J	MA	947
RadRO	Machtay, M	OH	961
RadRO	Macklis, R	OH	961
RadRO	Malcolm, A	TN	955
RadRO	Marcus, R	FL	955
RadRO	Markoe, A	FL	955
RadRO	Marks, L	NC	955
RadRO	Martenson, J	MN	961
RadRO	McCormick, B	NY	951
RadRO	McGarry, R	KY	956
RadRO	Medbery, C	OK	965
RadRO	Mendenhall, N	FL	956
RadRO	Mendenhall, W	FL	956
RadRO	Merchant, T	TN	956
RadRO	Meredith, R	AL	956
RadRO	Michalski, J	MO	961
RadRO	Minsky, B	TX	965
RadRO	Mittal, B	IL	961
RadRO	Morris, M	VA	956
RadRO	Morrison, W	TX	965
RadRO	Movsas, B	MI	961
RadRO	Mundt, A	CA	967
RadRO	Myerson, R	MO	961
RadRO	Nicolaou, N	PA	951
RadRO	Nori, D	NY	951
RadRO	Park, C	CA	967
RadRO	Peschel, R	CT	947
RadRO	Pezner, R	CA	967
RadRO	Pierce, L	MI	961
RadRO	Pollack, A	FL	956
RadRO	Porrazzo, M	DC	952
RadRO	Prosnitz, L	NC	956
RadRO	Quivey, J	CA	967
RadRO	Rabinovitch, R	CO	963
RadRO	Randall, M	KY	957
RadRO	Randolph-Jackson, P	DC	952
RadRO	Recht, A	MA	947
RadRO	Regine, W	MD	952
RadRO	Rich, T	VA	957
RadRO	Roach, M	CA	967
RadRO	Roberts, K	CT	947
RadRO	Rose, C	CA	967
RadRO	Rosenman, J	NC	957
RadRO	Rossi, C	CA	968
RadRO	Rotman, M	NY	952
RadRO	Russell, A	MA	947
RadRO	Russell, K	WA	968
RadRO	Sailer, S	NC	957
RadRO	Sandler, H	CA	968
RadRO	Schiff, P	NY	952
RadRO	Schild, S	AZ	965
RadRO	Schomberg, P	MN	962
RadRO	Senzer, N	TX	965
RadRO	Seung, S	OR	968
RadRO	Shaw, E	NC	957
RadRO	Shina, D	NM	965
RadRO	Shrieve, D	UT	963
RadRO	Small, W	IL	962

Spec	Name	St	Pg
RadRO	Smalley, S	KS	963
RadRO	Solin, L	PA	952
RadRO	Song, S	VA	957
RadRO	St Clair, W	KY	957
RadRO	Stea, B	AZ	965
RadRO	Stock, R	NY	952
RadRO	Streeter, O	DC	952
RadRO	Suh, J	OH	962
RadRO	Suntharalingam, M	MD	953
RadRO	Taghian, A	MA	947
RadRO	Tarbell, N	MA	947
RadRO	Tepper, J	NC	957
RadRO	Thomas, C	OR	968
RadRO	Toonkel, L	FL	958
RadRO	Tripuraneni, P	CA	968
RadRO	Vicini, F	MI	962
RadRO	Videtic, G	OH	962
RadRO	Vijayakumar, S	MS	958
RadRO	Wara, W	CA	968
RadRO	Wazer, D	RI	947
RadRO	Weichselbaum, R	IL	962
RadRO	Weiss, M	PA	953
RadRO	Werner-Wasik, M	PA	953
RadRO	Willett, C	NC	958
RadRO	Wilson, J	WI	962
RadRO	Wilson, L	CT	948
RadRO	Wolfson, A	FL	958
RadRO	Wong, J	CA	968
RadRO	Woo, S	KY	958
RadRO	Yahalom, J	NY	953
RadRO	Zelefsky, M	NY	953
RadRO	Zietman, A	MA	948

Radiation Therapy-Intraoperative

Spec	Name	St	Pg
RadRO	Harrison, L	NY	950

Radiofrequency Tumor Ablation

Spec	Name	St	Pg
DR	Charboneau, J	MN	980
S	Klimberg, V	AR	1090
T&CS	Cohen, N	MD	1114
VascS	Blebea, J	OK	1192
VIR	Brown, D	PA	992
VIR	Brown, K	NY	992
VIR	Coldwell, D	KY	994
VIR	Kay, D	LA	997
VIR	McGahan, J	CA	998
VIR	Nemcek, A	IL	996
VIR	Solomon, S	NY	993
VIR	Soulen, M	PA	994
VIR	Wood, B	MD	994

Radioimmunotherapy of Cancer

Spec	Name	St	Pg
NuM	Carrasquillo, J	NY	548
NuM	Pandit-Taskar, N	NY	549
NuM	Wahl, R	MD	549
NuM	Wiseman, G	MN	550
RadRO	Macklis, R	OH	961
RadRO	Wong, J	CA	968

Specialty & Special Expertise Index

Spec	Name	St	Pg
Radionuclide Therapy			
RadRO	Meredith, R	AL	956
Rare Disorders			
Ped	Morton, D	PA	727
Rare Genetic Disorders			
CG	Wilcox, W	CA	164
Rare Lung Disease-Pediatric			
PPul	Kim, Y	IN	797
Rare Skin Disorders			
D	Shupack, J	NY	188
Rasmussen's Syndrome			
N	Cole, A	MA	506
Ped	Vining, E	MD	727
Raynaud's Disease			
D	Franks, A	NY	186
Rhu	Clements, P	CA	1033
Rhu	Medsger, T	PA	1027
Rhu	Wigley, F	MD	1029
Reconstructive Microvascular Surgery			
HS	Hanel, D	WA	304
HS	Raphael, J	PA	297
HS	Steinmann, S	MN	302
OrS	Hausman, M	NY	618
Oto	Day, T	SC	668
Oto	Teknos, T	OH	678
Oto	Valentino, J	KY	672
PlS	Levin, L	PA	855
PlS	Molnar, J	NC	863
Reconstructive Plastic Surgery			
Oph	Lucarelli, M	WI	592
Oto	Toriumi, D	IL	678
PlS	Billmire, D	OH	864
PlS	Dagum, A	NY	853
PlS	Gottlieb, L	IL	865
PlS	Hultman, C	NC	862
PlS	Siemionow, M	OH	868
PlS	Thaller, S	FL	863
PlS	Tobin, G	KY	863
PlS	Wilhelmi, B	KY	864
PlS	Zide, B	NY	860
Reconstructive Surgery			
GO	Lele, S	NY	279
HS	Cendales, L	GA	299
HS	Chang, J	CA	304
HS	Chung, K	MI	300
HS	Lee, W	MD	297

Spec	Name	St	Pg
ObG	Hale, D	IN	561
Oph	Mawn, L	TN	584
Oph	Ng, J	OR	603
OrS	Agarwal, A	TX	640
OrS	Bos, G	WA	641
OrS	Burke, D	MA	610
OrS	Cheng, E	MN	633
OrS	Cooper, D	TX	640
OrS	Ebraheim, N	OH	633
OrS	Goodman, S	CA	643
OrS	Greisberg, J	NY	618
OrS	Kraay, M	OH	635
OrS	Macaulay, W	NY	622
OrS	Manoli, A	MI	635
OrS	Menendez, L	CA	644
OrS	O'Keefe, R	NY	623
OrS	Parsons, T	MI	636
OrS	Ward, W	NC	631
Oto	Baker, S	MI	673
Oto	Burkey, B	OH	674
Oto	Chalian, A	PA	658
Oto	Hicks, W	NY	660
Oto	Quatela, V	NY	664
Oto	Rosenthal, E	AL	670
Oto	Spiegel, J	MA	657
PlS	Bentz, M	WI	864
PlS	Cordeiro, P	NY	853
PlS	Ducic, I	DC	853
PlS	Dufresne, C	MD	854
PlS	Feldman, J	MA	850
PlS	Hagan, K	TN	862
PlS	Hardesty, R	CA	874
PlS	Hidalgo, D	NY	854
PlS	Hoffman, W	CA	874
PlS	Kronowitz, S	TX	870
PlS	Lee, R	IL	866
PlS	Lesavoy, M	CA	875
PlS	Loree, T	NY	855
PlS	MacKinnon, S	MO	866
PlS	Manson, P	MD	856
PlS	Sanger, J	WI	867
PlS	Serletti, J	PA	858
PlS	Seyfer, A	MD	858
PlS	Smith, D	FL	863
PS	Tuggle, D	OK	810
S	Edington, H	PA	1057
SM	Bradley, J	PA	1041
U	Atala, A	NC	1159
U	Brock, J	TN	1160
U	Foster, R	IN	1167
U	Griebling, T	KS	1171
U	Kaefer, M	IN	1167
U	Miller, S	GA	1162
U	Strand, W	TX	1174
Reconstructive Surgery-Complex			
OrS	Copp, S	CA	642
PlS	Brandt, K	MO	865
PlS	Patel, P	IL	867

Spec	Name	St	Pg
Reconstructive Surgery-Face			
Oto	Haughey, B	MO	675
Oto	Papel, I	MD	663
PlS	Baker, D	NY	852
PlS	Bartlett, S	PA	852
PlS	McCarthy, J	NY	856
PlS	Mehrara, B	NY	856
PlS	Menick, F	AZ	871
PlS	Smith, P	FL	863
Reconstructive Surgery-Skin			
D	Brodland, D	PA	185
D	Cook, J	NC	190
D	Swanson, N	OR	200
D	Zitelli, J	PA	189
Reconstructive Urologic Surgery			
U	Greenfield, S	NY	1153
U	Hemal, A	NC	1161
U	Koch, M	IN	1168
U	Rink, R	IN	1169
U	Thrasher, J	KS	1172
Rectal Cancer			
CRS	Gorfine, S	NY	170
Ge	Aslanian, H	CT	228
Onc	Kemeny, N	NY	343
RadRO	Konski, A	MI	960
RadRO	Tepper, J	NC	957
RadRO	Weichselbaum, R	IL	962
Rectal Cancer/Sphincter Preservation			
CRS	Abcarian, H	IL	173
CRS	Bailey, H	TX	176
CRS	Beart, R	CA	177
CRS	Delaney, C	OH	173
CRS	Fry, R	PA	170
CRS	Geisler, D	PA	170
CRS	Guillem, J	NY	170
CRS	Ludwig, K	WI	174
CRS	Mantyh, C	NC	172
CRS	Saclarides, T	IL	175
CRS	Stamos, M	CA	178
CRS	Thorson, A	NE	176
S	Skibber, J	TX	1092
Rectovaginal Fistula			
CRS	Birnbaum, E	MO	173
CRS	Hartmann, R	FL	172
CRS	Lowry, A	MN	174
CRS	Mutch, M	MO	174
Reflex Sympathetic Dystrophy (RSD)			
N	Reder, A	IL	529
N	Schwartzman, R	PA	517
PM	Audell, L	CA	702

Spec	Name	St	Pg
PM	Berde, C	MA	696
PM	Christo, P	MD	696
PM	Ferrante, F	CA	702
PM	Jain, S	NY	697
PM	Ngeow, J	NY	697
PM	Racz, G	TX	701
PM	Raja, S	MD	697
PM	Richman, D	NY	698
PM	Rosner, H	CA	703
PRhu	Sherry, D	PA	799

Refractive Surgery

Spec	Name	St	Pg
Oph	Cionni, R	UT	595
Oph	Dhaliwal, D	PA	573
Oph	Holland, E	OH	590
Oph	John, T	IL	590
Oph	Koch, D	TX	596
Oph	Krueger, R	OH	591
Oph	Lindstrom, R	MN	591
Oph	Maguire, L	MN	592
Oph	Maloney, R	CA	601
Oph	Mathers, W	OR	602
Oph	McDonnell, P	MD	577
Oph	Miller, K	CA	602
Oph	Orlin, S	PA	578
Oph	Page, T	MI	593
Oph	Pflugfelder, S	TX	597
Oph	Rapuano, C	PA	579
Oph	Rosenberg, M	IL	594
Oph	Samuelson, T	MN	594
Oph	Solomon, K	SC	586
Oph	Stark, W	MD	580
Oph	Steinert, R	CA	604
Oph	Updegraff, S	FL	587
Oph	Wallace, R	LA	598

Rehabilitation for Rheumatic Diseases

Spec	Name	St	Pg
Rhu	Ehresmann, G	CA	1033

Reiter's Syndrome

Spec	Name	St	Pg
Rhu	Solitar, B	NY	1028

Relapsing Polychondritis

Spec	Name	St	Pg
Oto	Lebovics, R	NY	662
Rhu	Luthra, H	MN	1031

Relationship Problems

Spec	Name	St	Pg
Psyc	Bronheim, H	NY	891
Psyc	Levine, S	OH	897

Renal Artery Stenosis

Spec	Name	St	Pg
IC	Dieter, R	IL	131
Nep	Textor, S	MN	462
Nep	Townsend, R	PA	458
VascS	Mitchell, M	MS	1189

Renal Replacement Therapy

Spec	Name	St	Pg
PNep	Chandar, J	FL	786

Renovascular Disease

Spec	Name	St	Pg
Cv	Ramee, S	LA	115
IC	Petrossian, G	NY	128
VascS	Benvenisty, A	NY	1186
VascS	Cambria, R	MA	1184
VascS	Faries, P	NY	1187
VascS	Gewertz, B	CA	1194
VascS	Stanley, J	MI	1192

Repetitive Motion Injuries

Spec	Name	St	Pg
HS	Derman, G	IL	300

Reproductive Endocrinology

Spec	Name	St	Pg
EDM	Bhasin, S	MA	206
EDM	Braunstein, G	CA	222
EDM	Goodman, N	FL	214
ObG	Berga, S	NC	559
ObG	De Cherney, A	MD	557
RE	Adamson, G	CA	1016
RE	Agarwal, S	CA	1016
RE	Azziz, R	GA	1011
RE	Barnes, R	IL	1012
RE	Bateman, B	VA	1011
RE	Blackwell, R	AL	1011
RE	Brzyski, R	TX	1015
RE	Buster, J	MA	1006
RE	Carr, B	TX	1015
RE	Carson, S	RI	1006
RE	Cedars, M	CA	1017
RE	Chang, R	CA	1017
RE	Christman, G	MI	1012
RE	Clisham, P	LA	1015
RE	Coddington, C	MN	1013
RE	Copperman, A	NY	1008
RE	Coutifaris, C	PA	1008
RE	Crowley, W	MA	1006
RE	DeVane, G	FL	1011
RE	Diamond, M	MI	1013
RE	Dickey, R	LA	1015
RE	Dodds, W	MI	1013
RE	Dumesic, D	CA	1017
RE	Durso, N	VA	1011
RE	Falcone, T	OH	1013
RE	Friedman, C	OH	1013
RE	Fritz, M	NC	1011
RE	Ginsburg, E	MA	1006
RE	Giudice, L	CA	1017
RE	Goldberg, J	OH	1013
RE	Gracia, C	PA	1008
RE	Grazi, R	NY	1008
RE	Grifo, J	NY	1008
RE	Grunfeld, L	NY	1008
RE	Haney, A	IL	1013
RE	Hill, J	NH	1006
RE	Hornstein, M	MA	1006
RE	Houmard, B	WA	1017
RE	Huang, J	TX	1016

Spec	Name	St	Pg
RE	Isaacson, K	MA	1007
RE	Jacobs, L	IL	1013
RE	Johnson, J	MA	1007
RE	Kazer, R	IL	1014
RE	Keltz, M	NY	1008
RE	Kutteh, W	TN	1012
RE	Legro, R	PA	1009
RE	Licciardi, F	NY	1009
RE	Luciano, A	CT	1007
RE	Marrs, R	CA	1017
RE	McClamrock, H	MD	1009
RE	McGovern, P	NJ	1009
RE	Milad, M	IL	1014
RE	Miller, C	IL	1014
RE	Moffitt, D	AZ	1016
RE	Molo, M	IL	1014
RE	Mukherjee, T	NY	1009
RE	Noyes, N	NY	1009
RE	Odem, R	MO	1014
RE	Ory, S	FL	1012
RE	Oskowitz, S	MA	1007
RE	Patrizio, P	CT	1007
RE	Paulson, R	CA	1017
RE	Petrozza, J	MA	1007
RE	Putman, J	TX	1016
RE	Ratts, V	MO	1014
RE	Richardson, M	KS	1015
RE	Rosenwaks, Z	NY	1009
RE	Sanfilippo, J	PA	1010
RE	Sauer, M	NY	1010
RE	Schenken, R	TX	1016
RE	Schlaff, W	PA	1010
RE	Seifer, D	NY	1010
RE	Session, D	GA	1012
RE	Smikle, C	CA	1017
RE	Smith, Y	MI	1014
RE	Sondheimer, S	PA	1010
RE	Soules, M	WA	1018
RE	Steinkampf, M	AL	1012
RE	Stewart, E	MN	1014
RE	Surrey, E	CO	1015
RE	Toth, T	MA	1007
RE	Van Voorhis, B	IA	1015
RE	Wallach, E	MD	1010
RE	Walmer, D	NC	1012
RE	Weiss, G	NJ	1010
RE	Widra, E	DC	1010
RE	Wilson, E	TX	1016
RE	Winer, S	CA	1018
RE	Yee, B	CA	1018
RE	Zacur, H	MD	1011
RE	Zinaman, M	MA	1007

Reproductive Endocrinology-Male

Spec	Name	St	Pg
EDM	Snyder, P	PA	212
EDM	Swerdloff, R	CA	224

Reproductive Genetics

Spec	Name	St	Pg
CG	Ward, J	TN	159
MF	Dugoff, L	PA	432

Specialty & Special Expertise Index

Spec	Name	St	Pg
MF	Eddleman, K	NY	432
MF	Wenstrom, K	RI	431
ObG	Byrne, J	UT	562
ObG	Evans, M	NY	557
U	Oates, R	MA	1150

Reproductive Surgery

RE	Azziz, R	GA	1011
RE	Buster, J	MA	1006
RE	Coddington, C	MN	1013
RE	Milad, M	IL	1014
RE	Moffitt, D	AZ	1016
RE	Noyes, N	NY	1009
RE	Odem, R	MO	1014
RE	Session, D	GA	1012

Respiratory Distress Syndrome (ARDS)

Pul	Arroliga, A	TX	938
Pul	Christman, B	TN	930
Pul	Donahoe, M	PA	925
Pul	Wheeler, A	TN	932
Pul	Wiedemann, H	OH	936

Respiratory Distress Syndrome (RDS)

NP	Cole, F	MO	450
NP	Donn, S	MI	450
NP	Lawson, E	MD	447
NP	Seidner, S	TX	452

Respiratory Failure

PCCM	Perez Fontan, J	TX	742
PCCM	Thompson, A	PA	741
PPul	Green, T	IL	796
Pul	Balk, R	IL	933
Pul	Celli, B	MA	922
Pul	Deitz, J	PA	925
Pul	Hall, J	IL	933
Pul	Heffner, J	OR	939
Pul	Ingbar, D	MN	934
Pul	Niederman, M	NY	926
Pul	Strollo, P	PA	928
Pul	Thomashow, B	NY	928
T&CS	Zwischenberger, J	KY	1130

Restless Legs Syndrome

N	Sethi, K	GA	523
Psyc	Doghramji, K	PA	891

Retina-Artificial

Oph	Del Priore, L	SC	582

Retina/Vitreous Surgery

Oph	Abrams, G	MI	587
Oph	Brucker, A	PA	572
Oph	Campochiaro, P	MD	572
Oph	Chang, S	NY	572

Spec	Name	St	Pg
Oph	Davis, J	FL	582
Oph	De Juan, E	CA	600
Oph	Flynn, H	FL	583
Oph	Gentile, R	NY	574
Oph	Haller, J	PA	575
Oph	Ho, A	PA	575
Oph	Humayun, M	CA	601
Oph	Lambert, H	TX	597
Oph	Meredith, T	NC	585
Oph	Mieler, W	IL	592
Oph	Muldoon, T	NY	578
Oph	Pulido, J	MN	593
Oph	Rosenfeld, P	FL	586
Oph	Schachat, A	OH	594
Oph	Sternberg, P	TN	586
Oph	Trese, M	MI	594
Oph	Yannuzzi, L	NY	581

Retinal Detachment

Oph	D'Amico, D	NY	573
Oph	Del Priore, L	SC	582
Oph	Hariprasad, S	IL	590
Oph	Olsen, T	GA	585
Oph	Petersen, M	OH	593
Oph	Rosenfeld, P	FL	586
Oph	Schiff, W	NY	579
Oph	Schwartz, S	CA	603
Oph	Shabto, U	NY	580

Retinal Disorders

Oph	Blumenkranz, M	CA	599
Oph	Bressler, N	MD	571
Oph	Bressler, S	MD	572
Oph	Brown, G	PA	572
Oph	Brucker, A	PA	572
Oph	Chang, S	NY	572
Oph	D'Amico, D	NY	573
Oph	Duker, J	MA	570
Oph	Edwards, P	MI	589
Oph	Friberg, T	PA	574
Oph	Fuchs, W	NY	574
Oph	Gentile, R	NY	574
Oph	Gorin, M	CA	600
Oph	Grossniklaus, H	GA	583
Oph	Haller, J	PA	575
Oph	Hariprasad, S	IL	590
Oph	Heckenlively, J	MI	590
Oph	Humayun, M	CA	601
Oph	Lewis, R	TX	597
Oph	Maguire, J	PA	577
Oph	Marmor, M	CA	602
Oph	Mets, M	IL	592
Oph	Miller, J	MA	570
Oph	Murray, T	FL	585
Oph	Odel, J	NY	578
Oph	Puliafito, C	CA	603
Oph	Regillo, C	PA	579
Oph	Schwartz, S	CA	603
Oph	Stone, E	IA	594
Oph	Vander, J	PA	581
Oph	Walsh, J	NY	581

Spec	Name	St	Pg
Oph	Williams, G	MI	595

Retinal Disorders-Inherited

Oph	Fishman, G	IL	590
Oph	Sadda, S	CA	603

Retinal Disorders-Pediatric

Oph	Duker, J	MA	570
Oph	Olsen, T	GA	585
Oph	Stout, J	OR	604
Oph	Trese, M	MI	594

Retinal Drug Toxicity

Oph	Marmor, M	CA	602

Retinal Dystrophies

Oph	Marmor, M	CA	602

Retinal Vascular Diseases

Oph	Brown, G	PA	572
Oph	Humayun, M	CA	601
Oph	Sadda, S	CA	603

Retinitis Pigmentosa

Oph	Fishman, G	IL	590

Retinoblastoma

Oph	Abramson, D	NY	571
Oph	Augsburger, J	OH	588
Oph	Finger, P	NY	573
Oph	Handa, J	MD	575
Oph	Harbour, J	FL	584
Oph	Lueder, G	MO	592
Oph	Murphree, A	CA	602
Oph	O'Brien, J	PA	578
Oph	Shields, C	PA	580
Oph	Shields, J	PA	580
Oph	Stout, J	OR	604
Oph	Wilson, M	TN	587
PHO	Dunkel, I	NY	759
PHO	Friedman, D	TN	765
PHO	Olson, T	GA	767
PHO	Pendergrass, T	WA	778
PHO	Rubin, C	IL	773

Retinopathy of Prematurity

NP	Hendricks-Munoz, K	VA	449
Oph	Freedman, S	NC	583
Oph	Nussbaum, J	GA	585
Oph	Reynolds, J	NY	579
Oph	Shabto, U	NY	580
Oph	Siatkowski, R	OK	598
Oph	Stout, J	OR	604

Retroperitoneal Fibrosis

Rhu	Solitar, B	NY	1028

Spec	Name	St	Pg

Rhabdomyosarcoma

PHO	Adamson, P	PA	758
PHO	Hawkins, D	WA	777
PHO	Wexler, L	NY	764

Rheumatic Diseases of Childhood

| PMR | Sisung, C | IL | 841 |

Rheumatic Heart Disease

| Cv | Follansbee, W | PA | 98 |
| PCd | Cooper, R | NY | 734 |

Rheumatoid Arthritis

PRhu	Lehman, T	NY	799
Rhu	Adams, E	IL	1030
Rhu	Belmont, H	NY	1025
Rhu	Blume, R	NY	1025
Rhu	Bobrove, A	CA	1033
Rhu	Bunning, R	DC	1026
Rhu	Chang, R	IL	1030
Rhu	Chatham, W	AL	1029
Rhu	Coblyn, J	MA	1024
Rhu	Crofford, L	KY	1029
Rhu	Curran, J	IL	1031
Rhu	Davis, W	LA	1032
Rhu	Ehresmann, G	CA	1033
Rhu	Fields, T	NY	1026
Rhu	Gershwin, M	CA	1034
Rhu	Hochberg, M	MD	1026
Rhu	Hugenberg, S	IN	1031
Rhu	Katz, R	IL	1031
Rhu	Kay, J	MA	1024
Rhu	Kimberly, R	AL	1030
Rhu	Lawry, G	CA	1034
Rhu	Lindsey, S	LA	1033
Rhu	Luthra, H	MN	1031
Rhu	Magid, S	NY	1027
Rhu	Massarotti, E	MA	1024
Rhu	McCune, W	MI	1031
Rhu	Mitnick, H	NY	1027
Rhu	Moder, K	MN	1032
Rhu	Moore, W	GA	1030
Rhu	O'Dell, J	NE	1032
Rhu	Paget, S	NY	1027
Rhu	Polisson, R	MA	1024
Rhu	Pope, R	IL	1032
Rhu	Rothenberg, R	MD	1028
Rhu	Salmon, J	NY	1028
Rhu	Schoen, R	CT	1024
Rhu	Shadick, N	MA	1025
Rhu	Simms, R	MA	1025
Rhu	Solomon, G	NY	1028
Rhu	Wallace, D	CA	1034
Rhu	Weinblatt, M	MA	1025
Rhu	Weinstein, A	DC	1029
Rhu	Wise, C	VA	1030
Rhu	Wofsy, D	CA	1034

Rheumatologic Dermatology

| D | Jorizzo, J | NC | 191 |

Rheumatologic Diseases of the Lung

| Pul | Steiger, D | NY | 928 |

Rheumatology

A&I	DeShazo, R	MS	86
Ger	Cooney, L	CT	262
Rhu	Adams, E	IL	1030
Rhu	Albert, D	NH	1024
Rhu	Allen, N	NC	1029
Rhu	Allman, R	PA	1025
Rhu	Belmont, H	NY	1025
Rhu	Blume, R	NY	1025
Rhu	Bobrove, A	CA	1033
Rhu	Brasington, R	MO	1030
Rhu	Bunning, R	DC	1026
Rhu	Buyon, J	NY	1026
Rhu	Chang, R	IL	1030
Rhu	Chang-Miller, A	AZ	1032
Rhu	Chatham, W	AL	1029
Rhu	Clements, P	CA	1033
Rhu	Coblyn, J	MA	1024
Rhu	Crofford, L	KY	1029
Rhu	Cupps, T	DC	1026
Rhu	Curran, J	IL	1031
Rhu	Davis, W	LA	1032
Rhu	Ehresmann, G	CA	1033
Rhu	Farber, M	NY	1026
Rhu	Fields, T	NY	1026
Rhu	Fife, R	IN	1031
Rhu	Gershwin, M	CA	1034
Rhu	Gorevic, P	NY	1026
Rhu	Gourley, M	MD	1026
Rhu	Hadler, N	NC	1029
Rhu	Hochberg, M	MD	1026
Rhu	Hugenberg, S	IN	1031
Rhu	Katz, R	IL	1031
Rhu	Kay, J	MA	1024
Rhu	Kimberly, R	AL	1030
Rhu	Lahita, R	NJ	1027
Rhu	Langford, C	OH	1031
Rhu	Lawry, G	CA	1034
Rhu	Lindsey, S	LA	1033
Rhu	Lipstate, J	LA	1033
Rhu	Luggen, M	OH	1031
Rhu	Luthra, H	MN	1031
Rhu	Magid, S	NY	1027
Rhu	Manzi, S	PA	1027
Rhu	Massarotti, E	MA	1024
Rhu	Mayes, M	TX	1033
Rhu	McAlindon, T	MA	1024
Rhu	McCune, W	MI	1031
Rhu	Mease, P	WA	1034
Rhu	Medsger, T	PA	1027
Rhu	Mitnick, H	NY	1027
Rhu	Moder, K	MN	1032
Rhu	Moore, W	GA	1030
Rhu	O'Dell, J	NE	1032
Rhu	Oddis, C	PA	1027
Rhu	Paget, S	NY	1027
Rhu	Peng, S	WA	1034
Rhu	Petri, M	MD	1027
Rhu	Plotz, P	MD	1028
Rhu	Polisson, R	MA	1024
Rhu	Pope, R	IL	1032
Rhu	Rothenberg, R	MD	1028
Rhu	Salmon, J	NY	1028
Rhu	Schoen, R	CT	1024
Rhu	Schubert, R	DC	1028
Rhu	Sergent, J	TN	1030
Rhu	Sessoms, S	TX	1033
Rhu	Seton, M	MA	1025
Rhu	Shadick, N	MA	1025
Rhu	Silver, R	SC	1030
Rhu	Simms, R	MA	1025
Rhu	Solitar, B	NY	1028
Rhu	Solomon, G	NY	1028
Rhu	Spiera, H	NY	1028
Rhu	Starz, T	PA	1028
Rhu	Steen, V	DC	1028
Rhu	Tsokos, G	MA	1025
Rhu	Vivino, F	PA	1029
Rhu	Wallace, D	CA	1034
Rhu	Warner, A	MO	1032
Rhu	Weinblatt, M	MA	1025
Rhu	Weinstein, A	DC	1029
Rhu	Wener, M	WA	1034
Rhu	West, S	CO	1032
Rhu	Wigley, F	MD	1029
Rhu	Wise, C	VA	1030
Rhu	Wofsy, D	CA	1034

Rhinitis

A&I	Buchbinder, E	NY	84
A&I	Busse, W	WI	88
A&I	Freeman, T	TX	89
A&I	Kaliner, M	MD	85
A&I	Lieberman, P	TN	86
A&I	Lockey, R	FL	86
A&I	Meltzer, E	CA	90
A&I	Pacin, M	FL	87
A&I	Sanders, G	MI	89
A&I	Tamaroff, M	CA	91
A&I	Wasserman, S	CA	91
Oto	Lanza, D	FL	669
Oto	Naclerio, R	IL	676
Oto	Stringer, S	MS	671
PA&I	Kelly, C	VA	731
PA&I	Skoner, D	PA	730

Rhinoplasty

Oto	Denenberg, S	NE	680
Oto	Edelstein, D	NY	659
Oto	Farrior, E	FL	668
Oto	Gliklich, R	MA	655
Oto	Larrabee, W	WA	685
Oto	Papel, I	MD	663
Oto	Pribitkin, E	PA	663

Specialty & Special Expertise Index

Spec	Name	St	Pg
Oto	Quatela, V	NY	664
Oto	Setzen, M	NY	665
Oto	Shockley, W	NC	671
Oto	Szachowicz, E	MN	678
Oto	Toriumi, D	IL	678
PlS	Aston, S	NY	852
PlS	Baker, D	NY	852
PlS	Barone, C	TX	869
PlS	Burstein, F	GA	860
PlS	Byrd, H	TX	870
PlS	Cohen, S	CA	873
PlS	Constantian, M	NH	850
PlS	Daniel, R	CA	873
PlS	Fisher, G	CA	873
PlS	Gallico, G	MA	850
PlS	Hamra, S	TX	870
PlS	Herman, P	PA	854
PlS	Hidalgo, D	NY	854
PlS	Hurwitz, D	PA	854
PlS	Matarasso, A	NY	856
PlS	Menick, F	AZ	871
PlS	Metzinger, S	LA	871
PlS	Moses, M	LA	871
PlS	Mustoe, T	IL	866
PlS	Ristow, B	CA	876
PlS	Rohrich, R	TX	872
PlS	Stuzin, J	FL	863
PlS	Sullivan, P	RI	851
PlS	Tabbal, N	NY	859
PlS	Tebbetts, J	TX	872
PlS	Thaller, S	FL	863
PlS	Thorne, C	NY	859
PlS	Zins, J	OH	869

Rhinoplasty Revision

Spec	Name	St	Pg
Oto	Josephson, J	NY	661
Oto	Kuhn, F	GA	669
PlS	Constantian, M	NH	850

Rhinosinusitis

Spec	Name	St	Pg
A&I	Bernstein, D	OH	87
A&I	Lewis, J	AZ	89
A&I	Wong, J	MA	84
Oto	Schaitkin, B	PA	664
Oto	Stankiewicz, J	IL	677

Rhinosinusitis & Asthma

Spec	Name	St	Pg
A&I	Shepherd, G	NY	85

Robotic Cardiac Surgery

Spec	Name	St	Pg
T&CS	Argenziano, M	NY	1113
T&CS	Boyd, W	CA	1140
T&CS	Brunsting, L	AL	1124
T&CS	Chitwood, W	NC	1124
T&CS	DeFilippi, V	CA	1141
T&CS	DeRose, J	NY	1115
T&CS	Filsoufi, F	NY	1115
T&CS	Guber, M	CO	1136
T&CS	Guy, T	PA	1117

Spec	Name	St	Pg
T&CS	Loulmet, D	NY	1119
T&CS	Smith, C	NY	1121
T&CS	Starnes, V	CA	1143
T&CS	Stuart, R	MO	1135
T&CS	Woo, Y	PA	1123

Robotic Hysterectomy

Spec	Name	St	Pg
ObG	Visco, A	NC	560

Robotic Surgery

Spec	Name	St	Pg
CRS	Orkin, B	MA	168
GO	Barakat, R	NY	276
GO	Cliby, W	MN	283
GO	Fields, A	DC	278
GO	Fowler, J	OH	284
GO	Magrina, J	AZ	288
GO	Moore, D	IN	284
GO	Muntz, H	WA	290
GO	Muto, M	MA	275
GO	Poliakoff, S	FL	282
GO	Potkul, R	IL	285
GO	Randall, T	PA	279
GO	Spann, C	GA	283
NS	Theodore, N	AZ	494
ObG	Bartholomew, D	OH	560
ObG	Cornella, J	AZ	563
ObG	Hale, D	IN	561
ObG	Sanz, L	VA	559
PS	Glick, P	NY	803
PS	Jackson, R	AR	809
PS	Jennings, R	MA	801
PS	Krummel, T	CA	811
PS	Lobe, T	CA	811
S	Newman, E	NY	1061
S	Ridge, J	PA	1063
T&CS	Del-Nido, P	MA	1110
T&CS	Feins, R	NC	1125
T&CS	Galloway, A	NY	1116
T&CS	Lazzaro, R	NY	1119
T&CS	Murphy, D	GA	1127
T&CS	Ninan, M	TN	1128
T&CS	Park, B	NJ	1120
T&CS	Pass, H	NY	1120
T&CS	Yang, S	MD	1123
U	Andrews, P	AZ	1172
U	Balaji, K	NC	1160
U	Busby, J	AL	1160
U	Chen, D	PA	1151
U	Clayman, R	CA	1175
U	Elder, J	MI	1166
U	Gluckman, G	IL	1167
U	Hemal, A	NC	1161
U	Kaouk, J	OH	1167
U	Koch, M	IN	1168
U	Miller, S	GA	1162
U	Mohler, J	NY	1155
U	Porter, C	WA	1178
U	Pruthi, R	NC	1163
U	Scherr, D	NY	1157
U	Singh, D	CT	1150
U	Strup, S	KY	1164

Spec	Name	St	Pg
U	Takayama, T	WA	1179
U	Uzzo, R	PA	1158
U	Wallen, E	NC	1165
U	Weiss, R	NJ	1159
U	Winfield, H	AL	1165
U	Wood, D	MI	1171

Robotic Surgery-Pediatric

Spec	Name	St	Pg
U	Poppas, D	NY	1156

Rocky Mountain Spotted Fever

Spec	Name	St	Pg
PInf	Givner, L	NC	782

Rosacea

Spec	Name	St	Pg
D	James, W	PA	187

Ross Procedure for Aortic Valve Disease

Spec	Name	St	Pg
T&CS	Fullerton, D	CO	1136
T&CS	Starnes, V	CA	1143

Rotator Cuff Surgery

Spec	Name	St	Pg
HS	Imbriglia, J	PA	296
OrS	Bigliani, L	NY	614
OrS	Diduch, D	VA	628
OrS	Endrizzi, D	ME	611
OrS	Flatow, E	NY	617
OrS	Goitz, H	MI	633
OrS	Green, A	RI	611
OrS	Iannotti, J	OH	634
OrS	Kaeding, C	OH	634
OrS	Matsen, F	WA	644
OrS	McFarland, E	MD	622
OrS	Nuber, G	IL	636
OrS	Richmond, J	MA	612
OrS	Rodosky, M	PA	624
OrS	Warren, R	NY	626
OrS	Wickiewicz, T	NY	627
OrS	Williams, G	PA	627
OrS	Yamaguchi, K	MO	638
OrS	Zarins, B	MA	613
OrS	Zuckerman, J	NY	627
SM	Asnis, P	MA	1040
SM	Bush-Joseph, C	IL	1043
SM	Fronek, J	CA	1044

Running Injuries

Spec	Name	St	Pg
SM	Metzl, J	NY	1041

S

Salivary Gland Tumors

Spec	Name	St	Pg
Onc	Martins, R	WA	388
Oto	Blair, E	IL	673
Oto	Ferris, R	PA	659

Spec	Name	St	Pg
Oto	Urken, M	NY	666
Oto	Weissler, M	NC	672
RadRO	Laramore, G	WA	966

Salivary Gland Tumors & Surgery

Spec	Name	St	Pg
Oto	Clayman, G	TX	681
Oto	Deschler, D	MA	655
Oto	Eisele, D	MD	659
Oto	Goldenberg, D	PA	659
Oto	Hoffman, H	IA	675
Oto	Lydiatt, W	NE	680
Oto	Olsen, K	MN	677
Oto	Rassekh, C	PA	664
Oto	Shockley, W	NC	671
Oto	Weber, R	TX	683
S	Shah, J	NY	1064

Sarcoidosis

Spec	Name	St	Pg
Pul	Donohue, J	NC	930
Pul	King, T	CA	940
Pul	Padilla, M	NY	927
Pul	Raghu, G	WA	940
Pul	Rose, C	CO	937
Pul	Rossman, M	PA	927
Pul	Sharma, O	CA	941
Pul	Staton, G	GA	932

Sarcoma

Spec	Name	St	Pg
Hem	Adams, R	AZ	323
Hem	Heinrich, M	OR	325
Hem	Milhem, M	IA	321
Onc	Benjamin, R	TX	377
Onc	Brockstein, B	IL	365
Onc	Chow, W	CA	385
Onc	Conry, R	AL	355
Onc	Ettinger, D	MD	339
Onc	Fitch, T	AZ	378
Onc	Grosh, W	VA	357
Onc	Hande, K	TN	357
Onc	Jacobs, C	CA	387
Onc	Kraft, A	SC	358
Onc	Meyskens, F	CA	388
Onc	Patel, S	TX	381
Onc	Samlowski, W	NV	390
Onc	Samuels, B	ID	376
Onc	Sandler, A	OR	390
Onc	Staddon, A	PA	350
Onc	Stewart, F	WA	391
Onc	Verschraegen, C	VT	333
Onc	Von Burton, G	LA	382
Onc	von Mehren, M	PA	352
OrS	Berrey, B	FL	627
OrS	Biermann, J	MI	632
OrS	Bos, G	WA	641
OrS	Healey, J	NY	619
OrS	Hornicek, F	MA	611
OrS	Malawer, M	MD	622
OrS	McDonald, D	MO	635
OrS	Scarborough, M	FL	630

Spec	Name	St	Pg
OrS	Sim, F	MN	637
OrS	Ward, W	NC	631
OrS	Wurtz, L	IN	638
Oto	Kraus, D	NY	662
Path	Brooks, J	PA	708
Path	Fletcher, C	MA	706
Path	Goldblum, J	OH	715
Path	Patchefsky, A	PA	711
Path	Rubin, B	OH	716
Path	Triche, T	CA	722
Path	Weiss, S	GA	714
PHO	Albritton, K	TX	775
PHO	Arndt, C	MN	769
PHO	Marina, N	CA	778
PHO	Meyer, W	OK	776
PHO	Meyers, P	NY	762
PHO	Olson, T	GA	767
PlS	Rockwell, W	UT	869
RadRO	Brizel, D	NC	954
RadRO	Constine, L	NY	948
RadRO	DeLaney, T	MA	946
RadRO	Donaldson, S	CA	965
RadRO	Hahn, S	PA	950
RadRO	Herman, T	OK	964
RadRO	Michalski, J	MO	961
RadRO	Pollack, A	FL	956
RadRO	Prosnitz, L	NC	956
RadRO	Tepper, J	NC	957
RadRO	Wara, W	CA	968
RadRO	Wolfson, A	FL	958
S	Brown, C	IL	1075
S	Dooley, W	OK	1087
S	Eilber, F	CA	1095
S	Eisenberg, B	NH	1049
S	Feig, B	TX	1088
S	Fraker, D	PA	1057
S	Leitch, A	TX	1090
S	Levine, E	NC	1070
S	Li, B	LA	1090
S	Nakakura, E	CA	1097
S	Nathanson, S	MI	1080
S	Pollock, R	TX	1091
S	Sondak, V	FL	1072
S	Weber, S	WI	1084
S	White, R	NC	1073

Sarcoma-Soft Tissue

Spec	Name	St	Pg
Onc	Chow, W	CA	385
Onc	Forscher, C	CA	386
Onc	George, S	MA	329
Onc	Maki, R	NY	345
Onc	Stockdale, F	CA	391
OrS	Benevenia, J	NJ	614
OrS	Healey, J	NY	619
OrS	Irwin, R	MI	634
OrS	Mayerson, J	OH	635
OrS	O'Donnell, R	CA	645
OrS	Randall, R	UT	639
OrS	Ready, J	MA	612
OrS	Schmidt, R	PA	625
OrS	Wittig, J	NY	627

Spec	Name	St	Pg
Path	Antonescu, C	NY	707
PHO	Wexler, L	NY	764
RadRO	Landry, J	GA	955
RadRO	Pezner, R	CA	967
S	August, D	NJ	1053
S	Brady, M	NY	1054
S	Hanna, N	MD	1058
S	Heslin, M	AL	1069
S	Hunt, K	TX	1089
S	Huth, J	TX	1089
S	Pisters, P	TX	1091
S	Singer, S	NY	1064
T&CS	Putnam, J	TN	1128

Scalp Disorders

Spec	Name	St	Pg
D	Cotsarelis, G	PA	185

Scar Revision

Spec	Name	St	Pg
D	Alster, T	DC	184
D	Lask, G	CA	199

Schizophrenia

Spec	Name	St	Pg
ChAP	Rapoport, J	DC	909
ChAP	Russell, A	CA	912
Psyc	Adler, D	MA	888
Psyc	Benes, F	MA	888
Psyc	Boronow, J	MD	890
Psyc	Davidson, J	TX	899
Psyc	Freedman, R	CO	898
Psyc	Goff, D	NY	892
Psyc	Hirschfeld, R	TX	900
Psyc	Liberman, R	CA	901
Psyc	Marder, S	CA	901
Psyc	McIntosh, J	UT	899
Psyc	Weiner, R	NC	896

Schizophrenia-Clinical Trials

Spec	Name	St	Pg
Psyc	McGlashan, T	CT	889

Schizophrenia-Early Detection/Treatment

Spec	Name	St	Pg
Psyc	McGlashan, T	CT	889

Scleroderma

Spec	Name	St	Pg
Cv	Follansbee, W	PA	98
D	Falanga, V	RI	182
D	Franks, A	NY	186
PRhu	Haines, K	NJ	799
PRhu	Lehman, T	NY	799
PRhu	Myones, B	TX	801
Rhu	Clements, P	CA	1033
Rhu	Ehresmann, G	CA	1033
Rhu	Mayes, M	TX	1033
Rhu	Medsger, T	PA	1027
Rhu	Peng, S	WA	1034
Rhu	Simms, R	MA	1025
Rhu	Spiera, H	NY	1028
Rhu	Steen, V	DC	1028

Specialty & Special Expertise Index

Spec	Name	St	Pg
Rhu	Wallace, D	CA	1034
Rhu	Wener, M	WA	1034
Rhu	Wigley, F	MD	1029

Scleroderma & Lung Disease

Spec	Name	St	Pg
Rhu	Silver, R	SC	1030

Scoliosis

Spec	Name	St	Pg
OrS	An, H	IL	632
OrS	Balderston, R	PA	614
OrS	Betz, R	PA	614
OrS	Boachie-Adjei, O	NY	614
OrS	Bridwell, K	MO	632
OrS	Cammisa, F	NY	615
OrS	Errico, T	NY	617
OrS	Feldman, D	NY	617
OrS	Goldstein, J	NY	618
OrS	Herman, M	PA	619
OrS	Hyman, J	NY	620
OrS	Kim, C	CA	644
OrS	Lauerman, W	DC	621
OrS	Lebwohl, N	FL	629
OrS	Lenke, L	MO	635
OrS	McAfee, P	MD	622
OrS	McCance, S	NY	622
OrS	Neuwirth, M	NY	623
OrS	Peterson, D	AK	645
OrS	Polly, D	MN	637
OrS	Roye, D	NY	624
OrS	Schafer, M	IL	637
OrS	Schwab, F	NY	625
OrS	Spivak, J	NY	625
OrS	Sponseller, P	MD	625
OrS	Thompson, G	OH	638
OrS	Tolo, V	CA	646
OrS	Weinstein, S	IA	638

Seizure Disorders

Spec	Name	St	Pg
N	Cloughesy, T	CA	536
N	DeGiorgio, C	CA	536
N	Labiner, D	AZ	534
N	Nicholl, J	LA	534

Seizure Disorders & Pregnancy

Spec	Name	St	Pg
MF	Greene, M	MA	430

Sentinel Node Surgery

Spec	Name	St	Pg
Oto	Pitman, K	MS	670
S	Czerniecki, B	PA	1056
S	Essner, R	CA	1095
S	Giuliano, A	CA	1096
S	Hansen, N	IL	1077
S	Klimberg, V	AR	1090
S	Krag, D	VT	1050
S	Nowak, E	NY	1061
S	O'Hea, B	NY	1061
S	Ross, M	TX	1092
S	Saha, S	MI	1081
S	Tartter, P	NY	1065

Sepsis

Spec	Name	St	Pg
PCCM	Zimmerman, J	WA	743
Pul	Christman, B	TN	930
Pul	Wheeler, A	TN	932
S	Buchman, T	GA	1067

Septic Shock

Spec	Name	St	Pg
Cv	Parrillo, J	NJ	101
PCCM	Zimmerman, J	WA	743

Sex Cord-Stromal Tumors

Spec	Name	St	Pg
GO	Gershenson, D	TX	287

Sex Development Disorders

Spec	Name	St	Pg
PEn	Eugster, E	IN	747

Sexual Addiction

Spec	Name	St	Pg
Psyc	First, M	NY	892

Sexual Anomalies

Spec	Name	St	Pg
PS	Graziano, K	AZ	809

Sexual Behavior-Compulsive

Spec	Name	St	Pg
Psyc	Krueger, R	NY	893

Sexual Differentiation Disorders

Spec	Name	St	Pg
CG	Cunniff, C	AZ	161

Sexual Dysfunction

Spec	Name	St	Pg
EDM	Bhasin, S	MA	206
ObG	Levine, E	IL	562
ObG	Simon, J	DC	558
Psyc	Levine, S	OH	897
Psyc	Sadock, V	NY	894
RE	Carson, S	RI	1006
U	Buch, J	TX	1173
U	Gribetz, M	NY	1153
U	Meacham, R	CO	1172
U	Milam, D	TN	1162
U	O'Leary, M	MA	1149
U	Seftel, A	NJ	1157

Sexual Dysfunction-Male & Female

Spec	Name	St	Pg
U	Goldstein, I	CA	1176

Sexual Health in Cancer Survivors

Spec	Name	St	Pg
Onc	Dizon, D	MA	328

Sexual Identity Issues

Spec	Name	St	Pg
Psyc	Eaton, J	DC	891
Psyc	Levine, S	OH	897

Sexually Transmitted Diseases

Spec	Name	St	Pg
AM	Chambers, C	PA	80
ObG	Hager, W	KY	559
ObG	Levine, E	IL	562
ObG	Sweet, R	CA	563
ObG	Wiesenfeld, H	PA	558
PInf	Kotloff, K	MD	780

Short Bowel Syndrome

Spec	Name	St	Pg
PGe	Heyman, M	CA	755
PGe	Mittal, N	TX	755
PGe	Vanderhoof, J	NE	755
PS	Grikscheit, T	CA	810
PS	Warner, B	MO	808
PS	Weber, T	IL	808

Shoulder & Elbow Surgery

Spec	Name	St	Pg
OrS	Elattrache, N	CA	643
OrS	Thornhill, T	MA	613
SM	Gambardella, R	CA	1044
SM	Levine, W	NY	1041
SM	Mirzayan, R	CA	1044
SM	Paletta, G	MO	1043

Shoulder & Knee Reconstruction

Spec	Name	St	Pg
OrS	Lock, T	MI	635

Shoulder & Knee Surgery

Spec	Name	St	Pg
OrS	Gladstone, J	NY	617
OrS	Laurencin, C	CT	612
OrS	Nicholas, S	NY	623
OrS	Pettrone, F	VA	630
SM	Ho, S	IL	1043
SM	Nisonson, B	NY	1041

Shoulder Arthroscopic Surgery

Spec	Name	St	Pg
OrS	Craig, E	NY	616
OrS	Flatow, E	NY	617
OrS	Fulkerson, J	CT	611
OrS	Hannafin, J	NY	618
OrS	Miller, M	VA	629
SM	Miniaci, A	OH	1043
SM	Williams, R	NY	1042

Shoulder Cartilage Implant

Spec	Name	St	Pg
OrS	Williams, G	PA	627

Shoulder Injuries

Spec	Name	St	Pg
OrS	Flatow, E	NY	617
OrS	Fu, F	PA	617
OrS	Kaeding, C	OH	634
OrS	Karas, S	GA	629
OrS	Richmond, J	MA	612
OrS	Zarins, B	MA	613
SM	Asnis, P	MA	1040
SM	Burke, C	PA	1041
SM	Fronek, J	CA	1044

Specialty & Special Expertise Index

Spec	Name	St	Pg
SM	Gill, T	MA	1040
SM	Steiner, M	MA	1040

Shoulder Problems-Complex

OrS	Romeo, A	IL	637

Shoulder Reconstruction

HS	Mass, D	IL	301
OrS	Diduch, D	VA	628
OrS	Kenter, K	OH	634
OrS	Nepola, J	IA	636
OrS	Nuber, G	IL	636
OrS	Romeo, A	IL	637
OrS	Williams, G	PA	627
SM	Ciccotti, M	PA	1041
SM	Garth, W	AL	1042
SM	Miniaci, A	OH	1043

Shoulder Replacement

OrS	Craig, E	NY	616
OrS	Dines, D	NY	616
OrS	Flatow, E	NY	617
OrS	Matsen, F	WA	644
OrS	Plancher, K	NY	624
OrS	Siegel, H	AL	630
OrS	Warren, R	NY	626
OrS	Williams, G	PA	627
OrS	Wirth, M	TX	641

Shoulder Surgery

HS	Badia, A	FL	298
HS	Carroll, C	IL	300
HS	Imbriglia, J	PA	296
HS	Seitz, W	OH	302
HS	Steinmann, S	MN	302
OrS	Bach, B	IL	632
OrS	Bartolozzi, A	PA	614
OrS	Bigliani, L	NY	614
OrS	Dines, D	NY	616
OrS	Endrizzi, D	ME	611
OrS	Glashow, J	NY	618
OrS	Green, A	RI	611
OrS	Iannotti, J	OH	634
OrS	Jokl, P	CT	611
OrS	Marx, R	NY	622
OrS	McCann, P	NY	622
OrS	McFarland, E	MD	622
OrS	Millett, P	CO	639
OrS	O'Driscoll, S	MN	636
OrS	Plancher, K	NY	624
OrS	Ramsey, M	PA	624
OrS	Rodosky, M	PA	624
OrS	Warren, R	NY	626
OrS	Wickiewicz, T	NY	627
OrS	Wirth, M	TX	641
OrS	Yamaguchi, K	MO	638
OrS	Zuckerman, J	NY	627
SM	Altchek, D	NY	1040
SM	Andrews, J	FL	1042

Spec	Name	St	Pg
SM	Bradley, J	PA	1041
SM	Ma, C	CA	1044
SM	Scheller, A	MA	1040
SM	Taft, T	NC	1042
SM	Xerogeanes, J	GA	1043

Shoulder Surgery-Complex

OrS	Seltzer, D	AZ	641

Shoulder Tumors

OrS	Wittig, J	NY	627

Sickle Cell Disease

Hem	Adams-Graves, P	TN	316
Hem	Bigelow, C	MS	316
Hem	Blinder, M	MO	318
Hem	Telen, M	NC	318
Ped	Berman, B	MI	727
PHO	Bertolone, S	KY	765
PHO	Buchanan, G	TX	775
PHO	Cunningham, J	IL	770
PHO	Drachtman, R	NJ	759
PHO	Guarini, L	NY	760
PHO	Hord, J	OH	771
PHO	Kung, F	CA	778
PHO	Sandler, E	FL	768
PHO	Tebbi, C	FL	768
PHO	Wang, W	TN	769
PHO	Weinblatt, M	NY	764

Sickle Cell Disease-Lung

Pul	Haynes, J	AL	931

Sinus Disorders

A&I	Benenati, S	FL	86
A&I	Chandler, M	NY	84
A&I	Ein, D	DC	85
A&I	Friedman, S	FL	86
A&I	Mazza, D	NY	85
A&I	Meltzer, E	CA	90
A&I	Schubert, M	AZ	90
A&I	Slankard, M	NY	85
A&I	Tamaroff, M	CA	91
A&I	Wasserman, S	CA	91
Oto	Baim, H	IL	672
Oto	Bhattacharyya, N	MA	655
Oto	Newkirk, K	DC	663
Oto	Poole, M	GA	670
PO	April, M	NY	789
PO	Arjmand, E	OH	791
PO	Cunningham, M	MA	789
PO	Darrow, D	VA	791
PO	Duncan, N	TX	792
PO	Haddad, J	NY	790
PO	Miller, R	IL	792
PO	Richardson, M	OR	793

Sinus Disorders/Surgery

Oto	Amedee, R	LA	681
Oto	Benninger, M	OH	673
Oto	Bolger, W	FL	667
Oto	Caldarelli, D	IL	674
Oto	Close, L	NY	658
Oto	DiNardo, L	VA	668
Oto	Fried, M	NY	659
Oto	Friedman, M	IL	674
Oto	Gold, S	NY	659
Oto	Jacobs, J	NY	661
Oto	Kennedy, D	PA	661
Oto	Kern, R	IL	676
Oto	Lanza, D	FL	669
Oto	Lawson, W	NY	662
Oto	Metson, R	MA	656
Oto	Naclerio, R	IL	676
Oto	Otto, R	TX	683
Oto	Piccirillo, J	MO	677
Oto	Picken, C	DC	663
Oto	Rebeiz, E	MA	657
Oto	Rice, D	CA	686
Oto	Schaefer, S	NY	664
Oto	Schaitkin, B	PA	664
Oto	Senior, B	NC	671
Oto	Sillers, M	AL	671
Oto	Thaler, E	PA	666
Oto	Vining, E	CT	657
Oto	Weymuller, E	WA	687
PO	Bower, C	AR	792
PO	Geller, K	CA	793
PO	Jones, J	NY	790
PO	Katz, R	OH	792
PO	Lusk, R	NE	792
PO	Parikh, S	WA	793
PO	Rosbe, K	CA	793
PO	Rosenfeld, R	NY	790
PO	Ward, R	NY	790

Sinus Surgery-Revision

Oto	Jacobs, J	NY	661

Sinus Tumors

Oto	Bolger, W	FL	667
Oto	Har-El, G	NY	660
Oto	Koch, W	MD	661
Oto	O'Malley, B	PA	663
Oto	Snyderman, C	PA	665
Oto	Vining, E	CT	657
Oto	Yoo, G	MI	679

Sinusitis

A&I	Altman, L	WA	90
A&I	Grammer, L	IL	88
A&I	Jost, B	MO	88
A&I	Kaliner, M	MD	85
PA&I	Kelly, C	VA	731
PO	Chan, K	CO	792

Specialty & Special Expertise Index

Spec	Name	St	Pg
Sjogren's Syndrome			
Rhu	Curran, J	IL	1031
Rhu	Pope, R	IL	1032
Rhu	Vivino, F	PA	1029
Rhu	Wise, C	VA	1030
Skeletal Dysplasia			
CG	Randolph, L	CA	163
CG	Wilcox, W	CA	164
Skin Cancer			
D	Amonette, R	TN	189
D	Arpey, C	MN	192
D	Bailin, P	OH	192
D	Bennett, R	CA	198
D	Berg, D	WA	198
D	Bickers, D	NY	185
D	Bolognia, J	CT	182
D	Bondi, E	PA	185
D	Braun, M	DC	185
D	Brodland, D	PA	185
D	Brown, M	NY	185
D	Butler, D	TX	196
D	Carney, J	AR	196
D	Cook, J	NC	190
D	Crutchfield, C	MN	193
D	Dufresne, R	RI	182
D	Duvic, M	TX	196
D	Dzubow, L	PA	186
D	Eichler, C	FL	190
D	Fenske, N	FL	190
D	Fosko, S	MO	193
D	Garrett, A	VA	190
D	Geronemus, R	NY	186
D	Gilchrest, B	MA	183
D	Green, H	FL	191
D	Greenbaum, S	PA	186
D	Greenway, H	CA	199
D	Grichnik, J	FL	191
D	Halpern, A	NY	186
D	Kim, Y	CA	199
D	Kriegel, D	NY	187
D	Krunic, A	IL	194
D	Kupper, T	MA	183
D	Lebwohl, M	NY	187
D	Leffell, D	CT	183
D	Leshin, B	NC	191
D	Lessin, S	PA	187
D	Lim, H	MI	194
D	Lim Quan, K	AZ	197
D	Linder, J	AZ	197
D	Lowe, L	MI	194
D	Lowitt, M	MD	187
D	Maloney, M	MA	183
D	McMichael, A	NC	191
D	Miller, S	MD	187
D	Neel, V	MA	184
D	Neuburg, M	WI	194
D	Nghiem, P	WA	200
D	Nigra, T	DC	187

Spec	Name	St	Pg
D	Nouri, K	FL	191
D	Olbricht, S	MA	184
D	Orengo, I	TX	197
D	Otley, C	MN	194
D	Pitts, J	AZ	197
D	Prioleau, P	NY	188
D	Ramsay, D	NY	188
D	Ratner, D	NY	188
D	Richardson, T	CA	200
D	Rigel, D	NY	188
D	Russell, M	VA	192
D	Sobel, S	FL	192
D	Sokoloff, D	FL	192
D	Stern, R	MA	184
D	Swanson, N	OR	200
D	Swetter, S	CA	200
D	Taylor, R	TX	198
D	Thiers, B	SC	192
D	Tsao, H	MA	184
D	Wood, G	WI	195
D	Zitelli, J	PA	189
Onc	Biggs, D	DE	335
Onc	Daud, A	CA	385
Onc	Ernstoff, M	NH	329
Onc	Pavlick, A	NY	347
Onc	Pfister, D	NY	348
Onc	Sosman, J	TN	362
Oto	Shockley, W	NC	671
Oto	Weber, R	TX	683
Path	Bastian, B	CA	719
Path	Le Boit, P	CA	721
Path	Prieto, V	TX	718
PlS	Manson, P	MD	856
RadRO	Cooper, J	NY	948
RadRO	Laramore, G	WA	966
RadRO	Machtay, M	OH	961
RadRO	Mittal, B	IL	961
RadRO	Morrison, W	TX	965
RadRO	Wilson, J	WI	962
S	Huth, J	TX	1089
S	Trisal, V	CA	1100
Skin Cancer in Transplant Patients			
D	Otley, C	MN	194
Skin Cancer Reconstruction			
PlS	Mast, B	FL	862
Skin Cancer-Head & Neck			
D	Fewkes, J	MA	183
Onc	Posner, M	NY	348
Oto	Bradford, C	MI	673
PlS	Tufaro, A	MD	860
Skin Cancer/Facial Reconstruction			
Oto	Papel, I	MD	663

Spec	Name	St	Pg
Skin Healing			
PlS	Garner, W	CA	874
Skin Laser Surgery			
D	Alster, T	DC	184
D	Arndt, K	MA	182
D	Arpey, C	MN	192
D	Avram, M	NY	184
D	Bailin, P	OH	192
D	Berg, D	WA	198
D	Burton, C	NC	189
D	Cohen, B	MD	185
D	Cook, J	NC	190
D	Dover, J	MA	182
D	Garden, J	IL	193
D	Geronemus, R	NY	186
D	Glogau, R	CA	199
D	Grossman, M	NY	186
D	Hanke, C	IN	193
D	Hruza, G	MO	193
D	Leffell, D	CT	183
D	Pitts, J	AZ	197
D	Rubin, M	CA	200
D	Schultz, N	NY	188
D	Sobel, S	FL	192
D	Wheeland, R	AZ	198
D	Zelickson, B	MN	195
Oto	Ries, W	TN	670
PlS	Gregory, R	FL	861
Skin Laser Surgery-Resurfacing			
D	Brody, H	GA	189
D	Fitzpatrick, R	CA	198
D	Kilmer, S	CA	199
D	Lask, G	CA	199
Oto	Branham, G	MO	673
Oto	Gliklich, R	MA	655
PlS	Stuzin, J	FL	863
PlS	Young, V	MO	868
Skin/Soft Tissue Infections			
Inf	Brause, B	NY	411
Inf	Edmond, M	VA	414
Skull Base Surgery			
NS	Al-Mefty, O	MA	470
NS	Bruce, J	NY	473
NS	Chandler, J	IL	486
NS	Chen, C	NY	473
NS	Couldwell, W	UT	491
NS	Eisenberg, H	MD	473
NS	Evans, J	PA	473
NS	Fenstermaker, R	NY	474
NS	Fessler, R	IL	487
NS	Golfinos, J	NY	474
NS	Heilman, C	MA	471
NS	Heros, R	FL	482
NS	Khan, A	MD	476
NS	Kotapka, M	PA	476

Spec	Name	St	Pg
NS	Krisht, A	AR	493
NS	Lemole, G	AZ	493
NS	Linskey, M	CA	497
NS	Martuza, R	MA	471
NS	Mickey, B	TX	494
NS	Murali, R	NY	477
NS	Nagib, M	MN	489
NS	Patel, S	SC	483
NS	Robertson, J	TN	484
NS	Rock, J	MI	489
NS	Stieg, P	NY	479
NS	Tamargo, R	MD	479
NS	Van Loveren, H	FL	485
NS	Wilson, J	NC	485
NS	Yonas, H	NM	495
Oto	Amedee, R	LA	681
Oto	Arriaga, M	LA	681
Oto	Browne, J	NC	667
Oto	Carey, J	MD	658
Oto	Civantos, F	FL	667
Oto	Close, L	NY	658
Oto	Day, T	SC	668
Oto	DiNardo, L	VA	668
Oto	Duckert, L	WA	684
Oto	Gantz, B	IA	675
Oto	Harris, J	CA	685
Oto	Holliday, M	MD	660
Oto	Jackler, R	CA	685
Oto	Kaplan, M	CA	685
Oto	Kingdom, T	CO	680
Oto	Lalwani, A	NY	662
Oto	McKenna, M	MA	656
Oto	Moe, K	WA	686
Oto	Rebeiz, E	MA	657
Oto	Samant, S	TN	671
Oto	Stringer, S	MS	671
Oto	Tucci, D	NC	672
Oto	Wazen, J	FL	672
PO	Kazahaya, K	PA	790

Skull Base Tumors

Spec	Name	St	Pg
NS	Bilsky, M	NY	472
NS	Brem, H	MD	472
NS	Chen, C	NY	473
NS	Couldwell, W	UT	491
NS	Friedman, A	NC	481
NS	Giannotta, S	CA	497
NS	Grubb, R	MO	487
NS	Guthikonda, M	MI	488
NS	Harsh, G	CA	497
NS	Judy, K	PA	475
NS	Link, M	MN	488
NS	Mayberg, M	WA	498
NS	McDermott, M	CA	498
NS	Olivi, A	MD	477
NS	Olson, J	GA	483
NS	Sekhar, L	WA	498
NS	Sen, C	NY	478
NS	Thompson, R	TN	485
Oto	Blair, E	IL	673
Oto	Bojrab, D	MI	673

Spec	Name	St	Pg
Oto	Califano, J	MD	658
Oto	Costantino, P	NY	658
Oto	Driscoll, C	MN	674
Oto	Har-El, G	NY	660
Oto	Hartig, G	WI	675
Oto	Hirsch, B	PA	660
Oto	Kraus, D	NY	662
Oto	Lanza, D	FL	669
Oto	Lavertu, P	OH	676
Oto	Levine, P	VA	669
Oto	Netterville, J	TN	669
Oto	O'Malley, B	PA	663
Oto	Olsen, K	MN	677
Oto	Pensak, M	OH	677
Oto	Persky, M	NY	663
Oto	Petruzzelli, G	GA	670
Oto	Rassekh, C	PA	664
Oto	Smith, R	NE	680
Oto	Song, J	CO	681
Oto	Vining, E	CT	657
RadRO	Machtay, M	OH	961
S	Shah, J	NY	1064

Skull Base Tumors & Surgery

Spec	Name	St	Pg
NS	Boggan, J	CA	496
NS	De Monte, F	TX	492
NS	Johnson, S	CO	491
NS	Liu, C	CA	497
NS	Morcos, J	FL	483
NS	Origitano, T	MT	491
NS	Spetzler, R	AZ	494
NS	Thompson, B	MI	490
Oto	Arts, H	MI	672
Oto	Chowdhury, K	CO	679
Oto	Donald, P	CA	684
Oto	Futran, N	WA	685
Oto	Hanna, E	TX	682
Oto	Kennedy, D	PA	661
Oto	Kim, D	MA	656
Oto	Leonetti, J	IL	676
Oto	Marentette, L	MI	676
Oto	McMenomey, S	OR	686
Oto	Nuss, D	LA	683
Oto	Snyderman, C	PA	665
Oto	Wax, M	OR	687

Skull-Base Tumors & Surgery

Spec	Name	St	Pg
Oto	O'Leary, M	CA	686

Sleep Apnea

Spec	Name	St	Pg
Oto	Bhattacharyya, N	MA	655
Oto	Josephson, J	NY	661
Oto	Shapshay, S	NY	665
PO	April, M	NY	789
PO	Goldsmith, A	NY	789

Sleep Disorders

Spec	Name	St	Pg
ChiN	Santos, C	DC	148
N	Gross, P	MA	507

Spec	Name	St	Pg
N	Strom, L	CO	532
Oto	Schley, W	NY	665
Oto	Senior, B	NC	671
PO	Dolitsky, J	NY	789
PPul	Gibson, R	WA	798
PPul	Kemp, J	MO	796
PPul	Redding, G	WA	798
PPul	Tauber, D	PA	795
Psyc	Buysse, D	PA	891
Psyc	Wooten, V	OH	898
Pul	King, E	PA	926

Sleep Disorders/Apnea

Spec	Name	St	Pg
ChiN	Kotagal, S	MN	150
N	Adornato, B	CA	535
N	Guilleminault, C	CA	537
N	Krumholz, A	MD	513
N	Nolan, B	FL	523
N	Saper, C	MA	508
Oto	Baim, H	IL	672
Oto	Edelstein, D	NY	659
Oto	Hotaling, A	IL	675
Oto	Hurst, M	WV	661
Oto	Krespi, Y	NY	662
Oto	Piccirillo, J	MO	677
Oto	Poole, M	GA	670
Oto	Senders, C	CA	686
Oto	Setzen, M	NY	665
Oto	Stewart, M	NY	665
Oto	Woodson, B	WI	679
PO	Bower, C	AR	792
PO	Lusk, R	NE	792
PPul	Givan, D	IN	796
PPul	Loughlin, G	NY	795
PPul	Marcus, C	PA	795
Psyc	Doghramji, K	PA	891
Psyc	Kavey, N	NY	892
Pul	Burschtin, O	NY	924
Pul	Fletcher, E	IN	933
Pul	Greenberg, H	NY	925
Pul	Johnson, B	VA	931
Pul	Kaplan, J	KS	937
Pul	LoRusso, T	VA	931
Pul	Millman, R	RI	923
Pul	Pack, A	PA	927
Pul	Patterson, J	OR	940
Pul	Schwab, R	PA	927
Pul	Strollo, P	PA	928
Pul	Vaughey, E	VA	932
Pul	Wallace, J	CA	941
Pul	White, D	MA	924

Sleep Disorders/Apnea/Snoring

Spec	Name	St	Pg
Oto	Friedman, M	IL	674
Oto	Johnson, J	PA	661

Sleep Medicine

Spec	Name	St	Pg
N	Armon, C	MA	506
Psyc	Kavey, N	NY	892

Specialty & Special Expertise Index

Spec	Name	St	Pg
Pul	Bijwadia, J	MN	933
Pul	O'Donnell, A	DC	927

Small Bowel Cancer

Spec	Name	St	Pg
S	Butler, J	CA	1094

Snoring/Sleep Apnea

Spec	Name	St	Pg
Oto	Graham, H	LA	682
Oto	Kern, R	IL	676
Oto	Krespi, Y	NY	662
Oto	Setzen, M	NY	665

Soft Tissue Pathology

Spec	Name	St	Pg
Path	Goldblum, J	OH	715
Path	Montgomery, E	MD	710
Path	Schiller, A	NY	711
Path	Weiss, S	GA	714

Soft Tissue Radiation Necrosis

Spec	Name	St	Pg
PMR	King, R	GA	838

Soft Tissue Radiation Necrosis-Breast

Spec	Name	St	Pg
PMR	King, R	GA	838

Soft Tissue Tumors

Spec	Name	St	Pg
DR	Panicek, D	NY	976
OrS	Aboulafia, A	MD	613
OrS	Berrey, B	FL	627
OrS	Eckardt, J	CA	643
OrS	Gitelis, S	IL	633
OrS	Hornicek, F	MA	611
OrS	Kelly, C	CO	639
OrS	Lewis, V	TX	641
OrS	Mott, M	MI	636
OrS	Peabody, T	IL	636
OrS	Walling, A	FL	631
OrS	Ward, W	NC	631
Path	Fletcher, C	MA	706
Path	Kahn, L	NY	709
Path	Lucas, D	MI	716

Solid Tumors

Spec	Name	St	Pg
Onc	Aisner, J	NJ	334
Onc	Bashevkin, M	NY	335
Onc	Kelly, W	PA	343
Onc	Petruska, P	MO	370
Onc	Ratain, M	IL	371
PHO	Berg, S	TX	775
PHO	Croop, J	IN	770
PHO	Dome, J	DC	759
PHO	Frantz, C	DE	759
PHO	Guarini, L	NY	760
PHO	Halligan, G	PA	760
PHO	Hayani, A	IL	771
PHO	Helman, L	MD	761
PHO	Kuttesch, J	PA	762
PHO	Marcus, J	NY	762

Spec	Name	St	Pg
PHO	Salvi, S	IL	773
PHO	Santana, V	TN	768
PHO	Siegel, S	CA	779
PHO	Williams, J	AZ	776
PS	Aiken, J	WI	806
PS	Alexander, F	NJ	802
RadRO	Donahue, B	NY	949
S	Loggie, B	NE	1085

Spasticity & Movement Disorders

Spec	Name	St	Pg
NS	Kaufman, B	WI	488
NS	Piatt, J	DE	478
NS	Walker, M	UT	492
PM	Jasmin, L	CA	702

Spasticity Management

Spec	Name	St	Pg
N	Siddique, T	IL	530
PMR	Ballard, P	DC	835
PMR	Clairmont, A	OH	839
PMR	Esquenazi, A	PA	835
PMR	Francisco, G	TX	842
PMR	Glenn, M	MA	834
PMR	Ivanhoe, C	TX	843
PMR	Keen, M	IL	840
PMR	Kirshblum, S	NJ	836
PMR	Marino, R	PA	837
PMR	Mayer, N	PA	837
PMR	Miknevich, M	PA	837
PMR	Munin, M	PA	837
PMR	Webster, H	MA	834

Special Health Care Needs (CSHCN)

Spec	Name	St	Pg
Ped	Palfrey, J	MA	726

Speech Disorders

Spec	Name	St	Pg
ChiN	Trauner, D	CA	154
N	Heilman, K	FL	521

Spina Bifida

Spec	Name	St	Pg
CG	Marion, R	NY	158
NS	Bierbrauer, K	OH	486
NS	Cherny, W	ID	491
NS	Dias, M	PA	473
NS	Selden, N	OR	499
PMR	Alexander, J	NC	838
PMR	Cardenas, D	FL	838
PS	Farmer, D	CA	810
U	Bloom, D	MI	1165
U	Brock, J	TN	1160

Spina Bifida-Adult

Spec	Name	St	Pg
PMR	Kirschner, K	IL	840

Spinal Access Surgery

Spec	Name	St	Pg
VascS	Fantini, G	NY	1187

Spinal Cord Disorders

Spec	Name	St	Pg
N	Engstrom, J	CA	536
N	Levine, D	NY	514
PM	Audell, L	CA	702

Spinal Cord Injury

Spec	Name	St	Pg
NRad	Faro, S	PA	985
NRad	Quencer, R	FL	988
NS	Adelson, P	AZ	492
NS	Harrop, J	PA	475
NS	Hodes, J	KY	482
NS	Levi, A	FL	482
NS	Shapiro, S	IN	490
OrS	Abdu, W	NH	610
OrS	Chapman, J	WA	642
OrS	Vaccaro, A	PA	626
OrS	Wang, J	CA	646
PMR	Ahn, J	NY	834
PMR	Ballard, P	DC	835
PMR	Bloch, R	MA	834
PMR	Cardenas, D	FL	838
PMR	Chen, D	IL	839
PMR	Colachis, S	OH	839
PMR	Creamer, M	FL	838
PMR	Fried, G	PA	836
PMR	Frost, F	OH	840
PMR	Gater, D	VA	838
PMR	Gittler, M	IL	840
PMR	Harris, D	TX	843
PMR	Jackson, A	AL	838
PMR	King, J	TX	843
PMR	Kirshblum, S	NJ	836
PMR	Marino, R	PA	837
PMR	McKinley, W	VA	839
PMR	Nobunaga, A	OH	841
PMR	Ragnarsson, K	NY	837
PMR	Volshteyn, O	MO	842
PMR	Zafonte, R	MA	834
U	Bodner, D	OH	1165

Spinal Cord Injury & Colonic Motility

Spec	Name	St	Pg
Ge	Korsten, M	NY	235

Spinal Cord Injury-Epidural Stimulation

Spec	Name	St	Pg
NS	Hodes, J	KY	482

Spinal Cord Injury-Pediatric

Spec	Name	St	Pg
HS	Kozin, S	PA	296
OrS	Betz, R	PA	614
PMR	Massagli, T	WA	844

Spinal Cord Stimulation

Spec	Name	St	Pg
PM	Christo, P	MD	696
PM	Jasmin, L	CA	702
PM	Rauck, R	NC	699

Spec	Name	St	Pg

Spinal Cord Surgery

Spec	Name	St	Pg
NS	Kobrine, A	DC	476

Spinal Cord Surgery-Pediatric

NS	Feldstein, N	NY	474

Spinal Cord Tumors

N	Schiff, D	VA	523
NRad	Lis, E	NY	986
NRad	Sze, G	CT	985
NS	Ames, C	CA	495
NS	Bilsky, M	NY	472
NS	Chiocca, E	OH	487
NS	Moore, F	NJ	477
NS	Quigley, M	PA	478
NS	Shaffrey, M	VA	484
Onc	Chang, S	CA	384
PHO	Gururangan, S	NC	766
PMR	Stewart, P	AL	839

Spinal Cord Tumors-Pediatric

NS	Ragheb, J	FL	483

Spinal Deformity

OrS	Albert, T	PA	613
OrS	Bitan, F	NY	614
OrS	Bridwell, K	MO	632
OrS	Lebwohl, N	FL	629
OrS	Lenke, L	MO	635
OrS	Richardson, W	NC	630
OrS	Schwab, F	NY	625
OrS	Weinstein, S	IA	638

Spinal Deformity-Pediatric

OrS	Betz, R	PA	614
OrS	Thompson, G	OH	638
OrS	Tolo, V	CA	646

Spinal Deformity-Pediatric & Adult

OrS	Lauerman, W	DC	621

Spinal Disc Replacement

NS	Haid, R	GA	482
NS	Hartl, R	NY	475
NS	Kaiser, M	NY	475
NS	Sekhon, L	NV	499
OrS	Balderston, R	PA	614
OrS	Bitan, F	NY	614
OrS	Boden, S	GA	628
OrS	Cammisa, F	NY	615
OrS	Cappuccino, A	NY	615
OrS	Carragee, E	CA	642
OrS	Delamarter, R	CA	642
OrS	Errico, T	NY	617
OrS	Goldstein, J	NY	618
OrS	McAfee, P	MD	622

Spinal Disorders

N	Swerdlow, M	NY	518
N	Weinberg, H	NY	519
NS	Chandler, J	IL	486
NS	Cosgrove, R	RI	470
NS	Huang, J	MD	475
NS	Kuntz, C	OH	488
NS	Lavyne, M	NY	476
NS	O'Rourke, D	PA	477
NS	Rigamonti, D	MD	478
NS	Weingart, J	MD	480
OrS	Abdu, W	NH	610
OrS	Boden, S	GA	628
OrS	Chapman, J	WA	642
PM	Baumann, P	GA	698
PM	Falco, F	DE	697
PM	Macadaeg, K	IN	699

Spinal Disorders-Degenerative

NS	Hadley, M	AL	482
NS	Sekhon, L	NV	499
NS	Sundaresan, N	NY	479
OrS	Bitan, F	NY	614
OrS	Farmer, J	NY	617

Spinal Imaging

NRad	Haughton, V	WI	988
NRad	Jarvik, J	WA	991
NRad	Modic, M	OH	989
NRad	Osborn, A	UT	990

Spinal Microdiscectomy

OrS	An, H	IL	632
OrS	Riew, K	MO	637

Spinal Muscular Atrophy (SMA)

ChiN	De Vivo, D	NY	147

Spinal Reconstructive Surgery

NS	Ames, C	CA	495
NS	Bilsky, M	NY	472
NS	Branch, C	NC	481
NS	Gokaslan, Z	MD	474
NS	Whiting, D	PA	480
OrS	Delamarter, R	CA	642
OrS	Lenke, L	MO	635
OrS	McAfee, P	MD	622

Spinal Rehabilitation

PMR	Borg-Stein, J	MA	834
PMR	Feinberg, J	NY	836
PMR	Harris, D	TX	843
PMR	Herring, S	WA	843
PMR	Lutz, G	NY	836

PMR	Saal, J	CA	844
SM	Saint-Phard, D	CO	1043

Spinal Surgery

NS	Bailes, J	IL	485
NS	Bauer, J	IL	486
NS	Belzberg, A	MD	472
NS	Benzel, E	OH	486
NS	Bingaman, W	OH	486
NS	Borges, L	MA	470
NS	Brown, F	IL	486
NS	Caputy, A	DC	473
NS	Di Giacinto, G	NY	473
NS	Diaz, F	MI	487
NS	Fessler, R	IL	487
NS	Foley, K	TN	481
NS	Frazee, J	CA	496
NS	Freeman, T	FL	481
NS	Green, B	FL	482
NS	Haid, R	GA	482
NS	Harper, R	TX	493
NS	Jho, H	PA	475
NS	Jimenez, D	TX	493
NS	Khan, A	MD	476
NS	Kim, D	TX	493
NS	Kobrine, A	DC	476
NS	Kotapka, M	PA	476
NS	Kuntz, C	OH	488
NS	Lavyne, M	NY	476
NS	Levi, A	FL	482
NS	Liker, M	CA	497
NS	Luken, M	IL	488
NS	McCormick, P	NY	477
NS	Moore, F	NJ	477
NS	Moser, R	MA	471
NS	Rodts, G	GA	484
NS	Rosenblum, M	MI	489
NS	Ryken, T	IA	490
NS	Sekhon, L	NV	499
NS	Shaffrey, C	VA	484
NS	Sundaresan, N	NY	479
NS	Swearingen, B	MA	471
NS	Traynelis, V	IL	490
NS	Turtz, A	NJ	479
NS	Welch, W	PA	480
NS	Wilson, J	NC	485
NS	Yu, J	CA	499
OrS	Abdu, W	NH	610
OrS	Albert, T	PA	613
OrS	An, H	IL	632
OrS	Balderston, R	PA	614
OrS	Boachie-Adjei, O	NY	614
OrS	Boden, S	GA	628
OrS	Brick, G	MA	610
OrS	Bridwell, K	MO	632
OrS	Cammisa, F	NY	615
OrS	Cappuccino, A	NY	615
OrS	Carragee, E	CA	642
OrS	Delamarter, R	CA	642
OrS	Donaldson, W	PA	616
OrS	Eismont, F	FL	628

Specialty & Special Expertise Index

Spec	Name	St	Pg
OrS	Errico, T	NY	617
OrS	Farmer, J	NY	617
OrS	Feldman, D	NY	617
OrS	Garfin, S	CA	643
OrS	Goldstein, J	NY	618
OrS	Hecht, A	NY	619
OrS	Hilibrand, A	PA	619
OrS	Hochschuler, S	TX	640
OrS	Kim, C	CA	644
OrS	Lauerman, W	DC	621
OrS	Lebwohl, N	FL	629
OrS	Lenke, L	MO	635
OrS	McCance, S	NY	622
OrS	Neuwirth, M	NY	623
OrS	O'Leary, P	NY	623
OrS	Peterson, D	AK	645
OrS	Polly, D	MN	637
OrS	Richardson, W	NC	630
OrS	Sandhu, H	NY	625
OrS	Schafer, M	IL	637
OrS	Schwab, F	NY	625
OrS	Spengler, D	TN	631
OrS	Spivak, J	NY	625
OrS	Vaccaro, A	PA	626
OrS	Wang, J	CA	646
OrS	Watkins, R	CA	646
OrS	Wetzel, F	PA	626
OrS	Wiesel, S	DC	627
OrS	Yoo, J	OR	646
OrS	Zdeblick, T	WI	638

Spinal Surgery-Cervical

Spec	Name	St	Pg
NS	Taylon, C	NE	492
OrS	Albert, T	PA	613
OrS	Hilibrand, A	PA	619
OrS	Kim, C	CA	644
OrS	Riew, K	MO	637
OrS	Schuler, T	VA	630

Spinal Surgery-Complex

Spec	Name	St	Pg
NS	Gokaslan, Z	MD	474
NS	Hadley, M	AL	482
NS	Hartl, R	NY	475
NS	Kaiser, M	NY	475
NS	Zimmerman, C	ID	492

Spinal Surgery-Low Back

Spec	Name	St	Pg
NS	Taylon, C	NE	492
OrS	Schuler, T	VA	630

Spinal Surgery-Neck

Spec	Name	St	Pg
OrS	Chapman, J	WA	642

Spinal Surgery-Pediatric

Spec	Name	St	Pg
NS	Menezes, A	IA	488
NS	Shaffrey, C	VA	484
OrS	Dormans, J	PA	617
OrS	Tolo, V	CA	646

Spinal Surgery-Pediatric & Adult

Spec	Name	St	Pg
OrS	Bitan, F	NY	614

Spinal Trauma

Spec	Name	St	Pg
NS	Ames, C	CA	495
NS	Harrop, J	PA	475
NS	Rodts, G	GA	484
OrS	Eismont, F	FL	628
OrS	Hilibrand, A	PA	619
OrS	Richardson, W	NC	630
OrS	Vaccaro, A	PA	626
OrS	Wang, J	CA	646

Spinal Tumor Imaging

Spec	Name	St	Pg
DR	Elster, A	NC	979
NRad	Koeller, K	MN	989
NRad	Loevner, L	PA	986
NRad	Murtagh, F	FL	988

Spinal Tumors

Spec	Name	St	Pg
ChiN	Keating, G	MN	150
N	Glass, J	PA	512
N	Patchell, R	AZ	534
N	Phuphanich, S	CA	538
NS	Black, K	CA	495
NS	Borges, L	MA	470
NS	Gokaslan, Z	MD	474
NS	Guthikonda, M	MI	488
NS	Harrop, J	PA	475
NS	Lavyne, M	NY	476
NS	Mamelak, A	CA	498
NS	McCormick, P	NY	477
NS	Rodts, G	GA	484
NS	Shaffrey, M	VA	484
NS	Yu, J	CA	499
OrS	Eismont, F	FL	628
OrS	Wang, J	CA	646
OrS	Weinstein, J	NH	613
PHO	Cohen, K	MD	759

Spine Imaging & Intervention

Spec	Name	St	Pg
NRad	Khandji, A	NY	985

Spleen Pathology

Spec	Name	St	Pg
Path	Arber, D	CA	719
Path	Orazi, A	NY	710

Spondylitis

Spec	Name	St	Pg
Rhu	Hadler, N	NC	1029

Spondyloarthritis-Consult

Spec	Name	St	Pg
Rhu	Chang-Miller, A	AZ	1032

Spondyloarthropathies

Spec	Name	St	Pg
PRhu	Schanberg, L	NC	800
Rhu	Adams, E	IL	1030

Sports Injuries

Spec	Name	St	Pg
HS	Belsky, M	MA	294
HS	Carlson, M	NY	295
HS	Friedman, D	FL	299
HS	Godzik, C	CA	304
HS	Graham, T	OH	301
HS	Lane, L	NY	296
HS	Rosenwasser, M	NY	297
SM	Schechter, D	CA	1044
SM	Scheller, A	MA	1040
SM	Sennett, B	PA	1042
SM	Teitz, C	WA	1044

Sports Injuries-Foot & Ankle

Spec	Name	St	Pg
OrS	DiGiovanni, C	RI	610
OrS	Nunley, J	NC	629

Sports Medicine

Spec	Name	St	Pg
Cv	Bove, A	PA	97
HS	Collins, E	TX	303
OrS	Albright, J	IA	631
OrS	Bach, B	IL	632
OrS	Bartolozzi, A	PA	614
OrS	Bigliani, L	NY	614
OrS	Callaghan, J	IA	633
OrS	Chu, C	PA	615
OrS	Cooper, D	TX	640
OrS	Craig, E	NY	616
OrS	Curl, W	NC	628
OrS	Deland, J	NY	616
OrS	Diduch, D	VA	628
OrS	Dillingham, M	CA	643
OrS	Dines, D	NY	616
OrS	Elattrache, N	CA	643
OrS	Finerman, G	CA	643
OrS	Fu, F	PA	617
OrS	Fulkerson, J	CT	611
OrS	Garrett, W	NC	628
OrS	Glashow, J	NY	618
OrS	Goitz, H	MI	633
OrS	Graf, B	WI	634
OrS	Grelsamer, R	NY	618
OrS	Heiden, E	UT	639
OrS	Johnson, D	KY	629
OrS	Jokl, P	CT	611
OrS	Kaeding, C	OH	634
OrS	Karas, S	GA	629
OrS	Kelly, B	NY	621
OrS	Kenter, K	OH	634
OrS	Kress, K	GA	629
OrS	Laurencin, C	CT	612
OrS	Lock, T	MI	635
OrS	Mandelbaum, B	CA	644
OrS	Marx, R	NY	622
OrS	McFarland, E	MD	622
OrS	Miller, M	VA	629
OrS	Millett, P	CO	639
OrS	Nicholas, S	NY	623
OrS	O'Driscoll, S	MN	636
OrS	Pettrone, F	VA	630

Specialty & Special Expertise Index

Spec	Name	St	Pg
OrS	Philippon, M	CO	639
OrS	Pizzutillo, P	PA	624
OrS	Poehling, G	NC	630
OrS	Ramsey, M	PA	624
OrS	Rodosky, M	PA	624
OrS	Romeo, A	IL	637
OrS	Rosenberg, T	UT	639
OrS	Schafer, I	IL	637
OrS	Scott, W	NY	625
OrS	Seltzer, D	AZ	641
OrS	Souryal, T	TX	641
OrS	Spindler, K	TN	631
OrS	Steadman, J	CO	639
OrS	Vo, P	FL	631
OrS	Wickiewicz, T	NY	627
PMR	Borg-Stein, J	MA	834
PMR	Feinberg, J	NY	836
PMR	Herring, S	WA	843
PMR	Lutz, G	NY	836
PMR	Press, J	IL	841
PMR	Saal, J	CA	844
SM	Altchek, D	NY	1040
SM	Andrews, J	FL	1042
SM	Arendt, E	MN	1043
SM	Arendt, E	MN	1043
SM	Asnis, P	MA	1040
SM	Bradley, J	PA	1041
SM	Burke, C	PA	1041
SM	Bush-Joseph, C	IL	1043
SM	Bush-Joseph, C	IL	1043
SM	Byrd, J	TN	1042
SM	Ciccotti, M	PA	1041
SM	Fronek, J	CA	1044
SM	Gambardella, R	CA	1044
SM	Garth, W	AL	1042
SM	Gill, T	MA	1040
SM	Harner, C	PA	1041
SM	Hershman, E	NY	1041
SM	Ho, S	IL	1043
SM	Jones, D	LA	1044
SM	Levine, W	NY	1041
SM	Ma, C	CA	1044
SM	Metzl, J	NY	1041
SM	Micheli, L	MA	1040
SM	Miniaci, A	OH	1043
SM	Mirzayan, R	CA	1044
SM	Nisonson, B	NY	1041
SM	Paletta, G	MO	1043
SM	Rodeo, S	NY	1042
SM	Saint-Phard, D	CO	1043
SM	Schechter, D	CA	1044
SM	Scheller, A	MA	1040
SM	Sennett, B	PA	1042
SM	Steiner, M	MA	1040
SM	Taft, T	NC	1042
SM	Taft, T	NC	1042
SM	Teitz, C	WA	1044
SM	Williams, R	NY	1042
SM	Xerogeanes, J	GA	1043

Sports Medicine Back Injuries

Spec	Name	St	Pg
OrS	Schuler, T	VA	630
OrS	Spivak, J	NY	625

Sports Medicine Radiology

DR	Palmer, W	MA	973
DR	Pavlov, H	NY	977

Sports Medicine-Women

OrS	Hannafin, J	NY	618
SM	Saint-Phard, D	CO	1043

Sports Neurology

N	Jordan, B	NY	512

Staphylococcal Infections

Inf	Corey, G	NC	414

Steatohepatitis

Ge	Raiford, D	TN	242

Stem Cell Therapy

N	Phuphanich, S	CA	538
Onc	Kesari, S	CA	387

Stem Cell Therapy & Biosurgery

T&CS	Boyd, W	CA	1140

Stem Cell Therapy in Heart Failure

Cv	Hare, J	FL	104
IC	Mahmud, E	CA	133
IC	Perin, E	TX	132

Stem Cell Transplant

Hem	Adams, R	AZ	323
Hem	Champlin, R	TX	323
Hem	Comenzo, R	MA	310
Hem	Damon, L	CA	325
Hem	Farag, S	IN	319
Hem	Greer, J	TN	316
Hem	Isola, L	NY	313
Hem	Klingemann, H	MA	310
Hem	Laughlin, M	VA	317
Hem	Lill, M	CA	326
Hem	Maciejewski, J	OH	321
Hem	Maslak, P	NY	313
Hem	Nimer, S	FL	317
Hem	Rowley, S	NJ	314
Hem	Savage, D	NY	314
Hem	Schwartzberg, L	TN	317
Hem	Slease, R	DE	315
Hem	Uberti, J	MI	322
Hem	Van Besien, K	IL	322
Onc	Antin, J	MA	327
Onc	Bensinger, W	WA	384

Onc	Carabasi, M	PA	336
Onc	Cohen, G	MD	336
Onc	Erban, J	MA	328
Onc	Flomenberg, N	PA	340
Onc	Foss, F	CT	329
Onc	Freedman, A	MA	329
Onc	Gerson, S	OH	367
Onc	Pecora, A	NJ	347
Onc	Soiffer, R	MA	332
Onc	Sweetenham, J	NV	391
Onc	Wicha, M	MI	373
PA&I	Kamani, N	DC	729
PHO	Arndt, C	MN	769
PHO	Barredo, J	FL	765
PHO	Cairo, M	NY	758
PHO	Cunningham, J	IL	770
PHO	Davies, S	OH	770
PHO	Fallon, R	IN	770
PHO	Frangoul, H	TN	765
PHO	Godder, K	VA	766
PHO	Goldman, S	TX	775
PHO	Graham, M	AZ	775
PHO	Grupp, S	PA	760
PHO	Haut, P	IN	771
PHO	Horn, B	CA	777
PHO	Kurtzberg, J	NC	767
PHO	Laver, J	TN	767
PHO	Link, M	CA	778
PHO	Lipton, J	NY	762
PHO	Sondel, P	WI	773

Stem Cell Transplant in Lupus/Crohn's

IM	Burt, R	IL	425

Stem Cell Transplant in MS

IM	Burt, R	IL	425

Stem Cell Transplant-Fetal

PA&I	Cowan, M	CA	733
PS	Flake, A	PA	803

Stem Cells in Orthopedics

OrS	Anderson, L	CA	641

Stereotactic Body Radiation Therapy

RadRO	Fuss, M	OR	966
RadRO	Kupelian, P	CA	966
RadRO	Suh, J	OH	962

Stereotactic Radiosurgery

NS	Andrews, D	PA	472
NS	Apuzzo, M	CA	495
NS	Asher, A	NC	481
NS	Bakay, R	IL	485
NS	Barnett, G	OH	486
NS	Branch, C	NC	481

Spec	Name	St	Pg
NS	Bucholz, R	MO	486
NS	Burchiel, K	OR	496
NS	Edwards, M	CA	496
NS	Fenstermaker, R	NY	474
NS	Golfinos, J	NY	474
NS	Guthrie, B	AL	482
NS	Kondziolka, D	PA	476
NS	Landy, H	FL	482
NS	Laske, D	PA	476
NS	Lemole, G	AZ	493
NS	Linskey, M	CA	497
NS	Liu, C	CA	497
NS	Lunsford, L	PA	476
NS	Markert, J	AL	483
NS	McDermott, M	CA	498
NS	Naff, N	MD	477
NS	Nazzaro, J	KS	491
NS	Ott, K	CA	498
NS	Penar, P	VT	471
NS	Rich, K	MO	489
NS	Robertson, J	TN	484
NS	Sills, A	TN	484
NS	Sisti, M	NY	479
NS	Swaid, S	AL	484
NS	Tatter, S	NC	485
Oto	McMenomey, S	OR	686
PM	Jasmin, L	CA	702
RadRO	Cmelak, A	TN	954
RadRO	Ennis, R	NY	949
RadRO	Fuss, M	OR	966
RadRO	Isaacson, S	NY	950
RadRO	Kleinberg, L	MD	951
RadRO	Knisely, J	NY	951
RadRO	Kupelian, P	CA	966
RadRO	Larson, D	CA	967
RadRO	Loeffler, J	MA	947
RadRO	McGarry, R	KY	956
RadRO	Medbery, C	OK	965
RadRO	Mendenhall, W	FL	956
RadRO	Movsas, B	MI	961
RadRO	Pezner, R	CA	967
RadRO	Porrazzo, M	DC	952
RadRO	Randall, M	KY	957
RadRO	Regine, W	MD	952
RadRO	Seung, S	OR	968
RadRO	Shaw, E	NC	957
RadRO	Stea, B	AZ	965
RadRO	Suh, J	OH	962
RadRO	Woo, S	KY	958

Stomach Cancer

Spec	Name	St	Pg
Onc	Ajani, J	TX	377
Onc	Grem, J	NE	375
RadRO	Hayman, J	MI	960
S	Aranha, G	IL	1074
S	August, D	NJ	1053
S	Coit, D	NY	1055
S	Donohue, J	MN	1076
S	Fong, Y	NY	1057
S	Gibbs, J	NY	1058
S	Hiotis, S	NY	1058

Spec	Name	St	Pg
S	Livingstone, A	FL	1070
S	Mansfield, P	TX	1091
S	Pockaj, B	AZ	1091
S	Shenk, R	OH	1082
S	Sundaram, M	IL	1083
S	Zinner, M	MA	1052

Strabismus

Spec	Name	St	Pg
Oph	Azar, N	IL	588
Oph	Buckley, E	NC	582
Oph	Burke, M	OH	589
Oph	Capo, H	FL	582
Oph	Caputo, A	NJ	572
Oph	Demer, J	CA	600
Oph	Drack, A	IA	589
Oph	Eustis, H	LA	596
Oph	Feldon, S	NY	573
Oph	Freedman, S	NC	583
Oph	Gallin, P	NY	574
Oph	Granet, D	CA	600
Oph	Guyton, D	MD	574
Oph	Hess, J	FL	584
Oph	Hunter, D	MA	570
Oph	Isenberg, S	CA	601
Oph	Kerr, N	TN	584
Oph	Koller, H	PA	576
Oph	Lambert, S	GA	584
Oph	Levin, A	PA	576
Oph	Magramm, I	NY	577
Oph	Mets, M	IL	592
Oph	Miller, J	AZ	597
Oph	Mills, M	PA	577
Oph	Mitchell, P	CT	571
Oph	Nelson, L	PA	578
Oph	Olitsky, S	MO	592
Oph	Plager, D	IN	593
Oph	Pollard, Z	GA	586
Oph	Reynolds, J	NY	579
Oph	Siatkowski, R	OK	598
Oph	Simon, J	NY	580
Oph	Tychsen, L	MO	595
Oph	Volpe, N	IL	595
Oph	Wang, F	NY	581
Oph	Weiss, A	WA	604
Oph	Wilson, M	SC	587

Strabismus-Adult & Pediatric

Spec	Name	St	Pg
Oph	Day, S	CA	600
Oph	Del Monte, M	MI	589
Oph	Eggers, H	NY	573
Oph	Hall, L	NY	575
Oph	Jaafar, M	DC	575
Oph	Kushner, B	WI	591
Oph	McKeown, C	FL	584
Oph	Mims, J	TX	597
Oph	Paul, T	CA	603
Oph	Rogers, G	OH	593
Oph	Warman, R	FL	587
Oph	Wright, K	CA	605

Streptococcal Infections

Spec	Name	St	Pg
PInf	Baker, C	TX	784
PInf	Givner, L	NC	782
PInf	Shulman, S	IL	783

Stress Management

Spec	Name	St	Pg
GerPsy	Stein, E	CA	915

Stroke

Spec	Name	St	Pg
ChiN	Kosofsky, B	NY	147
Cv	Stainback, R	TX	115
N	Adams, H	IA	524
N	Adams, R	SC	519
N	Adornato, B	CA	535
N	Albers, G	CA	535
N	Alexandrov, A	AL	519
N	Azizi, S	PA	509
N	Bell, R	PA	509
N	Broderick, J	OH	525
N	Brown, R	MN	525
N	Caplan, L	MA	506
N	Charney, J	NY	510
N	Chui, H	CA	536
N	Corbetta, M	MO	525
N	Couch, J	OK	532
N	Coull, B	AZ	533
N	Feldmann, E	MA	507
N	Fellus, J	NJ	511
N	Fink, M	NY	511
N	Fisher, M	CA	536
N	Foo, S	NY	511
N	Furie, K	RI	507
N	Furlan, A	OH	526
N	Gizzi, M	NJ	512
N	Gizzi, M	NJ	512
N	Goldstein, L	NC	521
N	Greer, D	CT	507
N	Gress, D	VA	521
N	Grotta, J	TX	533
N	Haley, E	VA	521
N	Hess, D	GA	522
N	Homer, D	IL	527
N	Josephson, D	IN	527
N	Kase, C	MA	507
N	Kasner, S	PA	512
N	Kent, T	TX	534
N	Kirshner, H	TN	522
N	Levine, D	NY	514
N	Levine, S	NY	514
N	Logan, W	MO	527
N	Mohr, J	NY	516
N	Morgenlander, J	NC	522
N	Reed, R	OH	529
N	Rothrock, J	NV	538
N	Sacco, R	FL	523
N	Saver, J	CA	539
N	Smith, W	CA	539
N	Suarez, J	TX	534
N	Tayal, A	PA	518
N	Vas, G	NY	518

Spec	Name	St	Pg
N	Vollmer, T	CO	532
N	Wechsler, L	PA	518
N	Wityk, R	MD	519
NRad	Cross, D	MO	988
NRad	Grobelny, T	IL	988
NRad	Hesselink, J	CA	991
NRad	Higashida, R	CA	991
NRad	Joseph, G	NC	987
NRad	Kallmes, D	MN	989
NRad	Larsen, D	CA	991
NRad	Maldjian, J	NC	987
NRad	Tenner, M	NY	986
NRad	Vinuela, F	CA	991
NS	Amar, A	CA	495
NS	Atkinson, J	MN	485
NS	Barrow, D	GA	481
NS	Dempsey, R	WI	487
NS	Hopkins, L	NY	475
NS	Riina, H	NY	478
NS	Selman, W	OH	490
NS	Yonas, H	NM	495
PMR	Brown, A	MN	839
VascS	Kougias, P	TX	1193
VascS	Pearce, W	IL	1191
VIR	Kumpe, D	CO	996

Stroke in Children

Spec	Name	St	Pg
ChiN	Ichord, R	PA	147
ChiN	Santos, C	DC	148
NRad	Orbach, D	MA	985

Stroke Prevention

Spec	Name	St	Pg
N	Lutsep, H	OR	538
N	Sacco, R	FL	523
N	Saver, J	CA	539
NRad	Larsen, D	CA	991
NS	Amar, A	CA	495

Stroke Rehabilitation

Spec	Name	St	Pg
PMR	Ahn, J	NY	834
PMR	Flanagan, S	NY	836
PMR	Francisco, G	TX	842
PMR	Frost, F	OH	840
PMR	Kevorkian, C	TX	843
PMR	King, J	TX	843
PMR	Palmer, J	MD	837
PMR	Roth, E	IL	841
PMR	Wilson, A	TX	843

Stroke-Neonatal

Spec	Name	St	Pg
NRad	Barkovich, A	CA	990

Stroke-Young Adults

Spec	Name	St	Pg
N	Becker, K	WA	535
N	Sila, C	OH	530

Stroke/Cerebrovascular

Disease

Spec	Name	St	Pg
N	Alberts, M	IL	524
N	Becker, K	WA	535
N	Bernstein, R	IL	525
N	Lutsep, H	OR	538

Sturge-Weber Syndrome

Spec	Name	St	Pg
ChiN	Comi, A	MD	147

Substance Abuse

Spec	Name	St	Pg
AdP	Schuckit, M	CA	906
AM	Kokotailo, P	WI	81
IM	Mehler, P	CO	426
Psyc	Canterbury, R	VA	895

Substance Abuse in ADHD Patients

Spec	Name	St	Pg
ChAP	Deas, D	SC	910

Substance Abuse-Consultation

Spec	Name	St	Pg
AdP	Walker, R	OR	906

Sudden Death Prevention

Spec	Name	St	Pg
CE	DeLurgio, D	GA	121
CE	Levine, J	NY	121
CE	Link, M	MA	119
CE	Tomaselli, G	MD	121
CE	Wilber, D	IL	124

Sudden Infant Death Syndrome (SIDS)

Spec	Name	St	Pg
NP	Kattwinkel, J	VA	449
PCd	Ackerman, M	MN	738
PCd	Walsh, C	NY	736
PPul	Keens, T	CA	798
PPul	Kemp, J	MO	796

Sudden Unexplained Death Syndrome (SUDS)

Spec	Name	St	Pg
PCd	Ackerman, M	MN	738

Suicide

Spec	Name	St	Pg
ChAP	Brent, D	PA	908
ChAP	McKelvey, R	OR	912
ChAP	Sargent, A	MA	907
Psyc	Hirschfeld, R	TX	900
Psyc	Mann, J	NY	893

Surfactant Biology

Spec	Name	St	Pg
NP	Cole, F	MO	450
NP	Donn, S	MI	450

Surgery

Spec	Name	St	Pg
S	Abecassis, M	IL	1074
S	Abouljoud, M	MI	1074

Spec	Name	St	Pg
S	Adams, R	VA	1066
S	Alexander, H	MD	1053
S	Alfonso, A	NY	1053
S	Ames, F	TX	1086
S	Anderson, B	WA	1093
S	Andreoni, K	FL	1066
S	Angelos, P	IL	1074
S	Aranha, G	IL	1074
S	Ascher, N	CA	1093
S	Ashley, S	MA	1048
S	August, D	NJ	1053
S	Averbook, B	OH	1074
S	Axelrod, D	NY	1053
S	Babiera, G	TX	1087
S	Baker, C	VA	1066
S	Ballantyne, G	GA	1066
S	Barie, P	NY	1053
S	Bartlett, D	PA	1053
S	Bartlett, S	MD	1053
S	Bear, H	VA	1067
S	Beauchamp, R	TN	1067
S	Becker, J	MA	1048
S	Becker, Y	IL	1074
S	Behrns, K	FL	1067
S	Beitsch, P	TX	1087
S	Bellows, C	LA	1087
S	Benedetti, E	IL	1074
S	Bentley, F	AR	1087
S	Bessey, P	NY	1053
S	Bessler, M	NY	1054
S	Bilchik, A	CA	1093
S	Billingsley, K	OR	1093
S	Blackstone, R	AZ	1087
S	Bland, K	AL	1067
S	Bolton, J	LA	1087
S	Boraas, M	PA	1054
S	Borgen, P	NY	1054
S	Bouvet, M	CA	1093
S	Brady, M	NY	1054
S	Brems, J	IL	1074
S	Britt, L	VA	1067
S	Brodsky, J	PA	1054
S	Brody, F	DC	1054
S	Bromberg, J	MD	1054
S	Brooks, A	PA	1054
S	Brooks, D	MA	1048
S	Brown, C	IL	1075
S	Brown, E	MI	1075
S	Brunicardi, F	CA	1094
S	Brunt, L	MO	1075
S	Buchman, T	GA	1067
S	Burke, P	MA	1048
S	Busuttil, R	CA	1094
S	Butler, J	CA	1094
S	Byrd, D	WA	1094
S	Cairns, B	NC	1067
S	Callery, M	MA	1048
S	Calvo, B	NC	1067
S	Cameron, J	MD	1054
S	Cance, W	NY	1055
S	Carty, S	PA	1055
S	Chabot, J	NY	1055

Specialty & Special Expertise Index

Spec	Name	St	Pg
S	Chand, B	IL	1075
S	Chang, A	MI	1075
S	Chang, H	CA	1094
S	Chapman, W	MO	1075
S	Cherqui, D	NY	1055
S	Choti, M	MD	1055
S	Cioffi, W	RI	1048
S	Clark, O	CA	1094
S	Cohen, M	PA	1055
S	Coit, D	NY	1055
S	Cole, D	SC	1068
S	Colquhoun, S	CA	1094
S	Conti, D	NY	1055
S	Cornwell, E	DC	1055
S	Courcoulas, A	PA	1056
S	Cronin, D	WI	1075
S	Crookes, P	CA	1094
S	Crowe, J	OH	1075
S	Curcillo, P	PA	1056
S	Curley, S	TX	1087
S	Cusack, J	MA	1048
S	Cushing, B	ME	1048
S	Czerniecki, B	PA	1056
S	Daneker, G	GA	1068
S	Dayton, M	NY	1056
S	Deitch, E	NJ	1056
S	Demarest, G	NM	1087
S	Dempsey, D	PA	1056
S	Deziel, D	IL	1076
S	Dixon, S	NV	1095
S	Doherty, G	MA	1049
S	Donohue, J	MN	1076
S	Dooley, W	OK	1087
S	Drebin, J	PA	1056
S	Duh, Q	CA	1095
S	Dulchavsky, S	MI	1076
S	Duncan, M	MD	1056
S	Eason, J	TN	1068
S	Easter, D	CA	1095
S	Eberlein, T	MO	1076
S	Eckhoff, D	AL	1068
S	Edge, S	NY	1056
S	Edington, H	PA	1057
S	Edney, J	NE	1085
S	Edwards, M	OH	1076
S	Edye, M	NY	1057
S	Eilber, F	CA	1095
S	Eisenberg, B	NH	1049
S	Ellenhorn, J	CA	1095
S	Ellis, L	TX	1088
S	Ellison, E	OH	1076
S	Emond, J	NY	1057
S	Emre, S	CT	1049
S	Esquivel, C	CA	1095
S	Esserman, L	CA	1095
S	Essner, R	CA	1095
S	Estabrook, A	NY	1057
S	Euhus, D	TX	1088
S	Evans, D	WI	1076
S	Fahey, T	NY	1057
S	Farley, D	MN	1076
S	Farrar, W	OH	1076

Spec	Name	St	Pg
S	Feig, B	TX	1088
S	Feliciano, D	GA	1068
S	Finlayson, C	CO	1085
S	Fisher, J	CA	1095
S	Fisher, W	TX	1088
S	Fitzgibbons, R	NE	1085
S	Flynn, M	KY	1068
S	Fong, Y	NY	1057
S	Fraker, D	PA	1057
S	Franklin, M	TX	1088
S	Frantzides, C	IL	1077
S	Frazier, T	PA	1057
S	Friese, R	AZ	1088
S	Fung, J	OH	1077
S	Gabram, S	GA	1068
S	Galloway, J	GA	1068
S	Gamelli, R	IL	1077
S	Gawande, A	MA	1049
S	Geller, D	PA	1058
S	Gibbs, J	NY	1058
S	Giuliano, A	CA	1096
S	Goodman, M	MA	1049
S	Goodson, W	CA	1096
S	Gosnell, J	CA	1096
S	Goulet, R	IN	1077
S	Gower, R	AK	1096
S	Graham, R	MA	1049
S	Grant, C	MN	1077
S	Grant, M	TX	1088
S	Gray, R	AZ	1088
S	Greene, F	NC	1069
S	Greenhalgh, D	CA	1096
S	Griswold, J	TX	1088
S	Gruber, S	MI	1077
S	Gupta, N	NH	1049
S	Haith, L	PA	1058
S	Halff, G	TX	1089
S	Hanks, J	VA	1069
S	Hanna, N	MD	1058
S	Hansen, N	IL	1077
S	Hebert, J	VT	1049
S	Hemming, A	CA	1096
S	Hering, B	MN	1077
S	Herrmann, V	SC	1069
S	Heslin, M	AL	1069
S	Hinshaw, D	MI	1078
S	Hiotis, S	NY	1058
S	Hodin, R	MA	1049
S	Hoffman, J	PA	1058
S	Holcomb, J	TX	1089
S	Hollingsworth, A	OK	1089
S	Horvath, K	WA	1096
S	Howe, J	IA	1078
S	Howerton, R	NC	1069
S	Hughes, K	MA	1050
S	Hunt, J	TX	1089
S	Hunt, K	TX	1089
S	Hunter, J	OR	1096
S	Huth, J	TX	1089
S	Iglehart, J	MA	1050
S	Ikramuddin, S	MN	1078
S	Jabbour, N	MA	1050

Spec	Name	St	Pg
S	Jackson, G	TX	1089
S	Jarnagin, W	NY	1058
S	Jayaseelan, N	TX	1089
S	Jenkins, R	MA	1050
S	Johnson, L	DC	1058
S	Johnson, R	PA	1059
S	Johnson Miller, D	IN	1078
S	Julian, T	PA	1059
S	Kagan, R	OH	1078
S	Kapur, S	NY	1059
S	Karlan, S	CA	1096
S	Karpeh, M	NY	1059
S	Kato, T	NY	1059
S	Kaufman, C	WA	1097
S	Kaufman, H	IL	1078
S	Kavanah, M	MA	1050
S	Kelley, M	TN	1069
S	Kendrick, M	MN	1078
S	Kim, J	OH	1078
S	Kim, L	AR	1089
S	Kinkhabwala, M	NY	1059
S	Kirgan, D	NV	1097
S	Klein, A	CA	1097
S	Klimberg, V	AR	1090
S	Knechtle, S	GA	1069
S	Knudson, M	CA	1097
S	Koruda, M	NC	1069
S	Krag, D	VT	1050
S	Krontiras, H	AL	1069
S	Krouse, R	AZ	1090
S	Kuhn, J	TX	1090
S	Lannin, D	CT	1050
S	Larsen, C	GA	1070
S	Leach, S	MD	1059
S	Lee, J	TX	1090
S	Lee, K	PA	1059
S	Leeming, R	OH	1079
S	Leitch, A	TX	1090
S	Lentz, C	NM	1090
S	Levi, J	FL	1070
S	Levine, E	NC	1070
S	Li, B	LA	1090
S	Libutti, S	NY	1060
S	Lieberman, M	NY	1060
S	Lillemoe, K	MA	1050
S	Lipkowitz, G	MA	1050
S	Livingston, E	TX	1090
S	Livingstone, A	FL	1070
S	Loggie, B	NE	1085
S	Lowy, A	CA	1097
S	Luterman, A	AL	1070
S	MacDonald, K	NC	1070
S	Mahvi, D	IL	1079
S	Mamounas, E	OH	1079
S	Mannella, W	PA	1060
S	Mansfield, P	TX	1091
S	Markmann, J	MA	1051
S	Marks, J	OH	1079
S	Marsh, J	PA	1060
S	Matas, A	MN	1079
S	Matthews, J	IL	1079
S	McAneny, D	MA	1051

Spec	Name	St	Pg	Spec	Name	St	Pg	Spec	Name	St	Pg
S	McCabe, D	AZ	1091	S	Posselt, A	CA	1098	S	Silverstein, M	CA	1100
S	McFadden, D	CT	1051	S	Postier, R	OK	1091	S	Simeone, D	MI	1082
S	McGrath, P	KY	1070	S	Potenza, B	CA	1098	S	Simmons, R	NY	1064
S	McHenry, C	OH	1079	S	Prinz, R	IL	1081	S	Sinanan, M	WA	1100
S	McIntyre, R	CO	1085	S	Ramanathan, R	PA	1062	S	Singer, S	NY	1064
S	McMasters, K	KY	1070	S	Rassman, W	CA	1099	S	Siperstein, A	OH	1082
S	Melvin, W	OH	1079	S	Rattner, D	MA	1051	S	Skibber, J	TX	1092
S	Meric-Bernstam, F	TX	1091	S	Reber, H	CA	1099	S	Skinner, K	NY	1064
S	Meyer, A	NC	1070	S	Reed, A	IA	1081	S	Slingluff, C	VA	1072
S	Meyers, W	PA	1060	S	Rege, R	TX	1091	S	Smith, B	MA	1052
S	Michelassi, F	NY	1060	S	Reich, D	PA	1062	S	Solorzano, C	TN	1072
S	Millis, J	IL	1080	S	Reiner, M	NY	1063	S	Sondak, V	FL	1072
S	Mistry, B	ND	1085	S	Renz, J	IL	1081	S	Soper, N	IL	1083
S	Moley, J	MO	1080	S	Reyes, J	WA	1099	S	Sosa, J	CT	1052
S	Montgomery, R	MD	1060	S	Rhee, P	AZ	1092	S	Stahl, D	OH	1083
S	Moore, E	CO	1085	S	Richards, W	AL	1071	S	Staley, C	GA	1072
S	Moore, F	MA	1051	S	Ridge, J	PA	1063	S	Staren, E	AZ	1092
S	Moossa, A	CA	1097	S	Roberts, J	CA	1099	S	Stewart, R	TX	1092
S	Morrow, M	NY	1060	S	Rogers, S	CA	1099	S	Stolier, A	LA	1092
S	Morton, J	CA	1097	S	Roh, M	FL	1071	S	Stratta, R	NC	1073
S	Mulvihill, S	UT	1085	S	Rosemurgy, A	FL	1071	S	Sugarbaker, P	DC	1065
S	Nagorney, D	MN	1080	S	Rosen, C	MN	1081	S	Sundaram, M	IL	1083
S	Nakakura, E	CA	1097	S	Rosen, M	OH	1081	S	Sutton, J	VT	1052
S	Nathanson, S	MI	1080	S	Rosenberg, S	MD	1063	S	Swanstrom, L	OR	1100
S	Neifeld, J	VA	1071	S	Roses, D	NY	1063	S	Sweeney, J	GA	1073
S	Nelson, E	UT	1086	S	Ross, M	TX	1092	S	Swistel, A	NY	1065
S	Newell, K	GA	1071	S	Rubino, F	NY	1063	S	Tafra, L	MD	1065
S	Newman, E	NY	1061	S	Ryan, C	MA	1051	S	Talamonti, M	IL	1083
S	Newman, L	MI	1080	S	Saffle, J	UT	1086	S	Tanabe, K	MA	1052
S	Nguyen, N	CA	1097	S	Saha, S	MI	1081	S	Tartter, P	NY	1065
S	Nissen, N	CA	1098	S	Salem, R	CT	1051	S	Tchou, J	PA	1065
S	Norman, J	FL	1071	S	Salky, B	NY	1063	S	Teperman, L	NY	1065
S	Norton, J	CA	1098	S	Salo, J	NC	1071	S	Thayer, S	MA	1052
S	Nowak, E	NY	1061	S	Sarr, M	MN	1081	S	Thistlethwaite, J	IL	1083
S	O'Hea, B	NY	1061	S	Sasson, A	NE	1086	S	Traynor, M	ND	1086
S	Oberholzer, J	IL	1080	S	Sataloff, D	PA	1063	S	Trisal, V	CA	1100
S	Olson, J	MD	1061	S	Satava, R	WA	1099	S	Tsangaris, T	MD	1065
S	Olthoff, K	PA	1061	S	Sauter, E	ND	1086	S	Tuttle, T	MN	1083
S	Onders, R	OH	1080	S	Scantlebury, V	DE	1063	S	Tyler, D	NC	1073
S	Osborne, M	NY	1061	S	Schaffer, R	CA	1099	S	Tzakis, A	OH	1083
S	Pachter, H	NY	1061	S	Schauer, P	OH	1082	S	Udelsman, R	CT	1052
S	Pappas, T	NC	1071	S	Schirmer, B	VA	1072	S	Unger, S	FL	1073
S	Patel, S	PA	1061	S	Schlinkert, R	AZ	1092	S	Urist, M	AL	1073
S	Paty, P	NY	1062	S	Schnabel, F	NY	1063	S	Van Zee, K	NY	1065
S	Pawlik, T	MD	1062	S	Schraut, W	PA	1064	S	Vauthey, J	TX	1092
S	Paz, I	CA	1098	S	Schulak, J	OH	1082	S	Vetto, J	OR	1100
S	Peitzman, A	PA	1062	S	Schulick, R	CO	1086	S	Vickers, S	MN	1083
S	Pellegrini, C	WA	1098	S	Schwartzentruber, D	IN	1082	S	Wagman, L	CA	1100
S	Perkins, J	WA	1098	S	Scott-Conner, C	IA	1082	S	Wakefield, T	MI	1084
S	Petelin, J	KS	1086	S	Selby, R	CA	1099	S	Walker, A	WI	1084
S	Peters, J	NY	1062	S	Sener, S	CA	1099	S	Wallace, A	CA	1100
S	Peterson, L	HI	1098	S	Shah, J	NY	1064	S	Walsh, R	OH	1084
S	Phillips, E	CA	1098	S	Shaked, A	PA	1064	S	Wapnir, I	CA	1100
S	Philosophe, B	MD	1062	S	Shapiro, R	NY	1064	S	Ward, B	CT	1052
S	Pinson, C	TN	1071	S	Shapiro, R	PA	1064	S	Warren, R	CA	1100
S	Pisters, P	TX	1091	S	Sharp, K	TN	1072	S	Weber, C	GA	1073
S	Pockaj, B	AZ	1091	S	Shen, P	NC	1072	S	Weber, S	WI	1084
S	Pollock, R	TX	1091	S	Shenk, R	OH	1082	S	Weigel, R	IA	1084
S	Pomp, A	NY	1062	S	Shibata, D	FL	1072	S	Weigelt, J	WI	1084
S	Ponn, T	NH	1051	S	Shikora, S	MA	1051	S	White, R	NC	1073
S	Ponsky, J	OH	1080	S	Sielaff, T	MN	1082	S	Whitworth, P	TN	1073
S	Posner, M	IL	1081	S	Sigurdson, E	PA	1064	S	Willey, S	DC	1066

Specialty & Special Expertise Index

Spec	Name	St	Pg
S	Winchell, R	ME	1052
S	Winchester, D	IL	1084
S	Witt, T	IL	1084
S	Woltering, E	LA	1093
S	Wood, R	TX	1093
S	Yang, J	MD	1066
S	Yeatman, T	FL	1073
S	Yeo, C	PA	1066
S	Yeung, R	WA	1101
S	Yurt, R	NY	1066
S	Zannis, V	AZ	1093
S	Zinner, M	MA	1052

Surgical Pathology

Path	Fletcher, C	MA	706
Path	Hoda, S	NY	709
Path	Leslie, K	AZ	718
Path	Lucas, D	MI	716
Path	Mills, S	VA	713
Path	Sewell, C	GA	714
Path	Silverman, J	PA	711
Path	Suster, S	WI	716
Path	Weiss, S	GA	714

Swallowing Disorders

Ge	Estores, D	FL	240
Ge	Falk, G	PA	232
Ge	Kahrilas, P	IL	246
Ge	Katz, P	PA	235
Ge	Lind, C	TN	241
Ge	Mittal, R	CA	254
Ge	Ravich, W	MD	237
Ge	Rothstein, R	NH	230
Ge	Shaker, R	WI	248
Ger	Finucane, T	MD	263
Oto	Abaza, M	CO	679
Oto	Aviv, J	NY	657
Oto	Bastian, R	IL	673
Oto	Blitzer, A	NY	658
Oto	Courey, M	CA	684
Oto	Hogikyan, N	MI	675
Oto	Mirza, N	PA	662
Oto	Pelzer, H	IL	677
Oto	Sasaki, C	CT	657
Oto	Sinha, U	CA	687
Oto	Song, J	CO	681
Oto	Strome, M	NY	665
Oto	Woodson, G	IL	679
PMR	Palmer, J	MD	837
PO	Holinger, L	IL	791
PPul	Loughlin, G	NY	795
PPul	Mcgrath-Morrow, S	MD	795

Swallowing Disorders-Botox Therapy

Ge	Pasricha, P	MD	237

Syncope

CE	Waldo, A	OH	124

Spec	Name	St	Pg
Ger	Lipsitz, L	MA	262
PCd	Crosson, J	MD	735
PCd	Young, M	FL	738

Syringomyelia & Spinal Cord Diseases

N	Kula, R	NY	513
N	Levine, D	NY	514
NS	Piatt, J	DE	478

T

Taste & Smell Disorders

Oto	Kern, R	IL	676

Tattoo Removal

D	Schultz, N	NY	188

Tear Duct Problems

Oph	Ahmad, A	IL	588
Oph	Pollard, Z	GA	586

Temperamentally Difficult Child

ChAP	Turecki, S	NY	909

Temporal Arteritis

Rhu	Allen, N	NC	1029

Tendon Surgery

HS	Derman, G	IL	300
HS	Gelberman, R	MO	301
HS	Greene, T	FL	299
HS	Jones, N	CA	304
HS	Kulick, R	NY	296
HS	Mass, D	IL	301
OrS	Wapner, K	PA	626

Testicular Cancer

Onc	Ahmann, F	AZ	376
Onc	Bajorin, D	NY	335
Onc	Bolger, G	AL	354
Onc	Bosl, G	NY	335
Onc	Dreicer, R	OH	367
Onc	Einhorn, L	IN	365
Onc	Godley, P	NC	357
Onc	Hauke, R	NE	375
Onc	Higano, C	WA	387
Onc	Hussain, M	MI	368
Onc	Jonasch, E	TX	379
Onc	Kantoff, P	MA	330
Onc	Levine, E	NY	344
Onc	Motzer, R	NY	346
Onc	Nanus, D	NY	346
Onc	Oh, W	NY	347

Spec	Name	St	Pg
Onc	Petrylak, D	CT	331
Onc	Quinn, D	CA	389
Onc	Roth, B	MO	371
Onc	Stadler, W	IL	372
Onc	Sweeney, C	MA	332
Onc	Vaughn, D	PA	351
Path	Reuter, V	NY	711
Path	Ulbright, T	IN	716
RadRO	Anscher, M	VA	953
RadRO	DeWeese, T	MD	949
RadRO	Peschel, R	CT	947
U	Amling, C	OR	1175
U	Beall, M	VA	1160
U	Carpinito, G	MA	1148
U	Carroll, P	CA	1175
U	Chang, S	TN	1160
U	Colberg, J	CT	1148
U	Cookson, M	TN	1161
U	Crawford, E	CO	1171
U	Dalkin, B	WA	1175
U	Daneshmand, S	CA	1176
U	Daneshmand, S	CA	1176
U	Foster, R	IN	1167
U	Grasso, M	NY	1153
U	Herr, H	NY	1153
U	Hrebinko, R	PA	1154
U	Klein, E	OH	1168
U	Lerner, S	TX	1173
U	Olumi, A	MA	1150
U	Porter, C	WA	1178
U	Presti, J	CA	1178
U	Richie, J	MA	1150
U	Robertson, C	NC	1163
U	Sagalowsky, A	TX	1174
U	Scherr, D	NY	1157
U	See, W	WI	1170
U	Sheinfeld, J	NY	1158
U	Su, L	FL	1164
U	Weiss, R	NJ	1159
U	Weiss, R	CT	1150

Testicular Cancer-Pediatric

U	Coplen, D	MO	1166

Tetanus

N	Reder, A	IL	529

Thalassemia

Ped	Berman, B	MI	727
PHO	Cunningham, J	IL	770
PHO	Giardina, P	NY	760
PHO	Weinblatt, M	NY	764

Thoracic & Cardiac Surgery

T&CS	Acker, M	PA	1113
T&CS	Adams, D	NY	1113
T&CS	Akins, C	MA	1110
T&CS	Aklog, L	AZ	1137
T&CS	Aldea, G	WA	1140

Spec	Name	St	Pg	Spec	Name	St	Pg	Spec	Name	St	Pg
T&CS	Altorki, N	NY	1113	T&CS	Filsoufi, F	NY	1115	T&CS	Kucharczuk, J	PA	1119
T&CS	Argenziano, M	NY	1113	T&CS	Flores, R	NY	1115	T&CS	Laks, H	CA	1142
T&CS	Athanasuleas, C	AL	1123	T&CS	Fontana, G	NY	1115	T&CS	Lamberti, J	CA	1142
T&CS	Bacha, E	NY	1114	T&CS	Forbess, J	TX	1138	T&CS	Landreneau, R	PA	1119
T&CS	Baciewicz, F	MI	1130	T&CS	Fraser, C	TX	1138	T&CS	Lang, S	NY	1119
T&CS	Backer, C	IL	1130	T&CS	Frazier, O	TX	1138	T&CS	Lansman, S	NY	1119
T&CS	Bailey, L	CA	1140	T&CS	Friedberg, J	PA	1116	T&CS	Lanza, L	AZ	1138
T&CS	Bains, M	NY	1114	T&CS	Fullerton, D	CO	1136	T&CS	Lau, C	VA	1126
T&CS	Bakhos, M	IL	1130	T&CS	Furukawa, S	PA	1116	T&CS	Lazar, H	MA	1111
T&CS	Battafarano, R	MD	1114	T&CS	Gaissert, H	MA	1111	T&CS	Lazzaro, R	NY	1119
T&CS	Bavaria, J	PA	1114	T&CS	Galantowicz, M	OH	1132	T&CS	Liao, K	MN	1133
T&CS	Bichell, D	TN	1123	T&CS	Galloway, A	NY	1116	T&CS	Loulmet, D	NY	1119
T&CS	Bolman, R	MA	1110	T&CS	Gaynor, J	PA	1116	T&CS	Love, R	IL	1133
T&CS	Bowdish, M	CA	1140	T&CS	Gharagozloo, F	DC	1116	T&CS	Lytle, B	OH	1133
T&CS	Boyd, W	CA	1140	T&CS	Ginsburg, M	NY	1116	T&CS	Mack, M	TX	1139
T&CS	Bridges, C	NC	1124	T&CS	Girardi, L	NY	1116	T&CS	Magovern, G	PA	1119
T&CS	Brinckerhoff, L	MA	1110	T&CS	Glassford, D	TN	1125	T&CS	Marshall, M	DC	1120
T&CS	Brown, J	IN	1131	T&CS	Grannis, F	CA	1141	T&CS	Martin, T	FL	1126
T&CS	Brunsting, L	AL	1124	T&CS	Graver, L	NY	1117	T&CS	Mason, D	OH	1133
T&CS	Bueno, R	MA	1110	T&CS	Griffith, B	MD	1117	T&CS	Mathisen, D	MA	1111
T&CS	Bull, D	UT	1136	T&CS	Grossi, E	NY	1117	T&CS	Mavroudis, C	FL	1126
T&CS	Burke, R	FL	1124	T&CS	Guber, M	CO	1136	T&CS	Mayer, J	MA	1111
T&CS	Byrne, J	TN	1124	T&CS	Gundry, S	CA	1141	T&CS	McCarthy, P	IL	1133
T&CS	Calhoon, J	TX	1137	T&CS	Guy, T	PA	1117	T&CS	McGiffin, D	AL	1126
T&CS	Cameron, R	CA	1140	T&CS	Guyton, R	GA	1125	T&CS	Merrick, S	CA	1142
T&CS	Campbell, D	CO	1136	T&CS	Handy, J	OR	1141	T&CS	Meyers, B	MO	1133
T&CS	Caskey, M	AZ	1137	T&CS	Hanley, F	CA	1141	T&CS	Mill, M	NC	1127
T&CS	Cassivi, S	MN	1131	T&CS	Hargrove, W	PA	1117	T&CS	Miller, D	CA	1142
T&CS	Cerfolio, R	AL	1124	T&CS	Harken, A	CA	1141	T&CS	Miller, D	GA	1127
T&CS	Chen, J	NY	1114	T&CS	Harpole, D	NC	1125	T&CS	Mitchell, J	CO	1136
T&CS	Chitwood, W	NC	1124	T&CS	Harrell, J	TX	1138	T&CS	Mitchell, M	CO	1137
T&CS	Christian, K	TN	1124	T&CS	Hashim, S	CT	1111	T&CS	Moon, M	MO	1134
T&CS	Cohen, G	CA	1140	T&CS	Heitmiller, R	MD	1117	T&CS	Moore, J	GA	1127
T&CS	Cohen, N	MD	1114	T&CS	Horvath, K	MD	1117	T&CS	Morris, R	PA	1120
T&CS	Cohen, R	CA	1141	T&CS	Howington, J	IL	1132	T&CS	Mullett, T	KY	1127
T&CS	Colson, Y	MA	1110	T&CS	Huddleston, C	MO	1132	T&CS	Murphy, D	GA	1127
T&CS	Conte, J	MD	1114	T&CS	Iannettoni, M	IA	1132	T&CS	Naka, Y	NY	1120
T&CS	Cooper, J	PA	1114	T&CS	Ilbawi, M	IL	1132	T&CS	Naunheim, K	MO	1134
T&CS	Coselli, J	TX	1137	T&CS	Isom, O	NY	1117	T&CS	Nesbitt, J	TN	1127
T&CS	D'Amico, T	NC	1125	T&CS	Jablons, D	CA	1142	T&CS	Nguyen, D	FL	1127
T&CS	Dabal, R	AL	1125	T&CS	Jamieson, S	CA	1142	T&CS	Ninan, M	TN	1128
T&CS	Damiano, R	MO	1131	T&CS	Jeevanandam, V	IL	1133	T&CS	Nugent, W	NH	1111
T&CS	Dang, M	HI	1141	T&CS	Jessen, M	TX	1138	T&CS	Oaks, T	NC	1128
T&CS	DeCamp, M	IL	1131	T&CS	Johnson, S	TX	1138	T&CS	Orringer, M	MI	1134
T&CS	Deeb, G	MI	1131	T&CS	Jonas, R	DC	1118	T&CS	Ott, D	TX	1139
T&CS	DeFilippi, V	CA	1141	T&CS	Jones, D	VA	1125	T&CS	Oz, M	NY	1120
T&CS	Del-Nido, P	MA	1110	T&CS	Joyce, L	MN	1133	T&CS	Pagani, F	MI	1134
T&CS	Delius, R	MI	1131	T&CS	Kaiser, L	PA	1118	T&CS	Panos, A	FL	1128
T&CS	Demmy, T	NY	1115	T&CS	Kanda, L	DC	1118	T&CS	Park, B	NJ	1120
T&CS	DeRose, J	NY	1115	T&CS	Kanter, K	GA	1126	T&CS	Pass, H	NY	1120
T&CS	Deschamps, C	MN	1131	T&CS	Karwande, S	UT	1136	T&CS	Patterson, G	MO	1134
T&CS	Diehl, J	PA	1115	T&CS	Keenan, R	PA	1118	T&CS	Pechet, T	PA	1120
T&CS	Diethrich, E	AZ	1137	T&CS	Keller, S	NY	1118	T&CS	Pham, S	FL	1128
T&CS	Downey, R	NY	1115	T&CS	Kernstine, K	TX	1138	T&CS	Philpott, J	VA	1128
T&CS	Drinkwater, D	TN	1125	T&CS	Kiernan, P	VA	1126	T&CS	Pierson, R	MD	1120
T&CS	Durham, S	MI	1132	T&CS	Kiev, J	WV	1118	T&CS	Pochettino, A	MN	1134
T&CS	Echeverri, L	TX	1137	T&CS	Kirklin, J	AL	1126	T&CS	Putnam, J	TN	1128
T&CS	Edwards, N	NY	1115	T&CS	Kopf, G	CT	1111	T&CS	Quintessenza, J	FL	1128
T&CS	Elefteriades, J	CT	1110	T&CS	Kormos, R	PA	1118	T&CS	Rastegar, H	MA	1112
T&CS	Feins, R	NC	1125	T&CS	Krellenstein, D	NY	1118	T&CS	Reardon, M	TX	1139
T&CS	Ferguson, M	IL	1132	T&CS	Krieger, K	NY	1119	T&CS	Reed, C	SC	1128
T&CS	Fernando, H	MA	1111	T&CS	Kron, I	VA	1126	T&CS	Rice, D	TX	1139

Specialty & Special Expertise Index

Spec	Name	St	Pg
T&CS	Rice, T	OH	1134
T&CS	Robbins, R	CA	1142
T&CS	Robinson, L	FL	1129
T&CS	Rosengart, T	NY	1121
T&CS	Rosenkranz, E	FL	1129
T&CS	Roth, J	TX	1139
T&CS	Rusch, V	NY	1121
T&CS	Safi, H	TX	1139
T&CS	Salerno, T	FL	1129
T&CS	Samuels, L	PA	1121
T&CS	Savage, E	FL	1129
T&CS	Schaff, H	MN	1134
T&CS	Scott, W	PA	1121
T&CS	Sellke, F	RI	1112
T&CS	Shemin, R	CA	1142
T&CS	Shrager, J	CA	1143
T&CS	Singh, A	RI	1112
T&CS	Slaughter, M	KY	1129
T&CS	Smedira, N	OH	1135
T&CS	Smith, C	NY	1121
T&CS	Smith, J	OH	1135
T&CS	Smith, P	NC	1129
T&CS	Smythe, W	TX	1139
T&CS	Soberman, M	MD	1121
T&CS	Sonett, J	NY	1121
T&CS	Spray, T	PA	1122
T&CS	Staples, E	FL	1129
T&CS	Starnes, V	CA	1143
T&CS	Stewart, A	NY	1122
T&CS	Stowe, C	FL	1129
T&CS	Stuart, R	MO	1135
T&CS	Sugarbaker, D	MA	1112
T&CS	Svensson, L	OH	1135
T&CS	Swanson, S	MA	1112
T&CS	Swisher, S	TX	1139
T&CS	Swistel, D	NY	1122
T&CS	Szeto, W	PA	1122
T&CS	Tedder, M	TN	1130
T&CS	Thistlethwaite, P	CA	1143
T&CS	Toyoda, Y	PA	1122
T&CS	Tranbaugh, R	NY	1122
T&CS	Trento, A	CA	1143
T&CS	Turner, W	TX	1140
T&CS	Turrentine, M	IN	1135
T&CS	Ungerleider, R	NC	1130
T&CS	Vallieres, E	WA	1143
T&CS	Vander Salm, T	MA	1134
T&CS	Verrier, E	WA	1143
T&CS	Vigneswaran, W	IL	1135
T&CS	Vlahakes, G	MA	1112
T&CS	Wain, J	MA	1112
T&CS	Walsh, G	TX	1140
T&CS	Walters, H	MI	1135
T&CS	Warner, K	MA	1113
T&CS	Watson, T	NY	1122
T&CS	Weigel, T	WI	1135
T&CS	Weiman, D	TN	1130
T&CS	Weksler, B	PA	1123
T&CS	Wells, W	CA	1143
T&CS	Whyte, R	MA	1113
T&CS	Williams, M	NY	1123
T&CS	Woo, Y	PA	1123

Spec	Name	St	Pg
T&CS	Wood, D	WA	1143
T&CS	Wright, C	MA	1113
T&CS	Yang, S	MD	1123
T&CS	Ziemer, G	IL	1136
T&CS	Zwischenberger, J	KY	1130

Thoracic Aortic Surgery

Spec	Name	St	Pg
S	Moore, E	CO	1085
T&CS	Aldea, G	WA	1140
T&CS	Bowdish, M	CA	1140
T&CS	Cohen, R	CA	1141
T&CS	Miller, D	CA	1142
T&CS	Szeto, W	PA	1122

Thoracic Cancers

Spec	Name	St	Pg
Onc	Chachoua, A	NY	336
Onc	Dowlati, A	OH	366
Onc	Edelman, M	MD	339
Onc	Garst, J	NC	356
Onc	Herbst, R	CT	330
Onc	Hong, W	TX	379
Onc	Johnson, B	MA	330
Onc	Kris, M	NY	344
Onc	Langer, C	PA	344
Onc	Lilenbaum, R	FL	358
Onc	Lynch, T	CT	331
Onc	Masters, G	DE	345
Onc	Pao, W	TN	360
Onc	Salgia, R	IL	371
Onc	Sherman, C	SC	362
Onc	Strauss, G	MA	332
RadRO	Bogart, J	NY	948
RadRO	Bradley, J	MO	958
RadRO	Cox, J	TX	963
RadRO	Kachnic, L	MA	946
RadRO	Le, Q	CA	967
T&CS	Altorki, N	NY	1113
T&CS	Colson, Y	MA	1110
T&CS	Demmy, T	NY	1115
T&CS	Downey, R	NY	1115
T&CS	Feins, R	NC	1125
T&CS	Friedberg, J	PA	1116
T&CS	Grannis, F	CA	1141
T&CS	Johnson, S	TX	1138
T&CS	Karwande, S	UT	1136
T&CS	Moore, J	GA	1127
T&CS	Nguyen, D	FL	1127
T&CS	Nugent, W	NH	1111
T&CS	Rice, D	TX	1139
T&CS	Soberman, M	MD	1121
T&CS	Sonett, J	NY	1121
T&CS	Swisher, S	TX	1139
T&CS	Vallieres, E	WA	1143
T&CS	Vigneswaran, W	IL	1135
T&CS	Zwischenberger, J	KY	1130

Thoracic Imaging

Spec	Name	St	Pg
DR	Fuhrman, C	PA	975
DR	Gefter, W	PA	975
DR	Goodman, L	WI	980

Spec	Name	St	Pg
DR	White, C	MD	978

Thoracic Insufficiency Syndrome

Spec	Name	St	Pg
PPul	Redding, G	WA	798

Thoracic Outlet Syndrome

Spec	Name	St	Pg
VascS	Ahn, S	CA	1193
VascS	Annest, S	CO	1192
VascS	Bandyk, D	CA	1194
VascS	Freischlag, J	MD	1187
VascS	Hallett, J	SC	1189

Thoracic Radiology

Spec	Name	St	Pg
DR	Austin, J	NY	974
DR	Chiles, C	NC	979
DR	Henschke, C	NY	975
DR	Patz, E	NC	979
DR	Rubin, G	NC	979
DR	Yankelevitz, D	NY	978

Thoracic Surgery

Spec	Name	St	Pg
PS	Caty, M	CT	801
T&CS	Cassivi, S	MN	1131
T&CS	Guber, M	CO	1136
T&CS	Lazzaro, R	NY	1119

Throat Disorders

Spec	Name	St	Pg
Oto	Sataloff, R	PA	664
Oto	Schley, W	NY	665
Oto	Silverman, D	VT	657

Thromboembolic Disorders

Spec	Name	St	Pg
Hem	Millenson, M	PA	314
Hem	Rao, A	PA	314
Pul	Auger, W	CA	939
Pul	Elliott, C	UT	936
Pul	Hyers, T	MO	934
Pul	Palevsky, H	PA	927
Pul	Steiger, D	NY	928
Pul	Tapson, V	NC	932

Thrombolytic Therapy

Spec	Name	St	Pg
N	Furlan, A	OH	526
VIR	Aruny, J	CT	992
VIR	Valji, K	WA	998

Thrombotic Disorders

Spec	Name	St	Pg
Hem	Abrams, C	PA	311
Hem	DeLoughery, T	OR	325
Hem	Kempin, S	NY	313
Hem	Ortel, T	NC	317
Hem	Palascak, J	OH	321
Hem	Soff, G	NY	315
Ped	Berman, B	MI	727
PHO	Buchanan, G	TX	775
PHO	Manco-Johnson, M	CO	774
PHO	Valentino, L	IL	773

Spec	Name	St	Pg
S	Wakefield, T	MI	1084

Thumb-Absence

Spec	Name	St	Pg
HS	Light, T	IL	301

Thymoma

Spec	Name	St	Pg
Onc	Aisner, J	NJ	334
Onc	Bonomi, P	IL	365
Onc	Bunn, P	CO	374
Onc	Carbone, D	OH	365
Onc	Kalemkerian, G	MI	368
Onc	Kris, M	NY	344
Onc	Loehrer, P	IN	369
Onc	Shin, D	GA	362
Onc	Simon, G	TX	382
RadRO	Cox, J	TX	963
RadRO	Komaki, R	TX	964
RadRO	Videtic, G	OH	962
T&CS	Gaissert, H	MA	1111
T&CS	Howington, J	IL	1132
T&CS	Marshall, M	DC	1120
T&CS	Shrager, J	CA	1143
T&CS	Weksler, B	PA	1123

Thyroid & Parathyroid Cancer & Surgery

Spec	Name	St	Pg
Oto	Bumpous, J	KY	667
Oto	Caruana, S	NY	658
Oto	Couch, M	VT	655
Oto	Ferris, R	PA	659
Oto	Genden, E	NY	659
Oto	Goldenberg, D	PA	659
Oto	Orloff, L	CA	686
Oto	Otto, R	TX	683
Oto	Patil, Y	OH	677
Oto	Peters, G	AL	670
Oto	Pitman, K	MS	670
Oto	Samant, S	TN	671
Oto	Urken, M	NY	666
Oto	Weber, R	TX	683
Oto	Weisman, R	CA	687
S	Angelos, P	IL	1074
S	Bland, K	AL	1067
S	Duh, Q	CA	1095
S	Edney, J	NE	1085
S	Grant, C	MN	1077
S	Siperstein, A	OH	1082
S	Solorzano, C	TN	1072

Thyroid & Parathyroid Surgery

Spec	Name	St	Pg
Oto	Blair, E	IL	673
Oto	Clayman, G	TX	681
Oto	Friedman, M	IL	674
Oto	Har-El, G	NY	660
Oto	Hayden, R	AZ	682
Oto	Kim, D	MA	656
Oto	Kraus, D	NY	662
S	Chabot, J	NY	1055
S	Flynn, M	KY	1068

Spec	Name	St	Pg
S	Jackson, G	TX	1089
S	Prinz, R	IL	1081
S	Shapiro, R	NY	1064
S	Traynor, M	ND	1086
S	Weber, C	GA	1073

Thyroid Cancer

Spec	Name	St	Pg
DR	Charboneau, J	MN	980
EDM	Ain, K	KY	213
EDM	Akatsu, H	CA	222
EDM	Ball, D	MD	208
EDM	Braunstein, G	CA	222
EDM	Burman, K	DC	209
EDM	Daniels, G	MA	207
EDM	Davies, T	NY	210
EDM	Gagel, R	TX	220
EDM	Kandeel, F	CA	223
EDM	Koch, C	MS	214
EDM	Kopp, P	IL	218
EDM	Ladenson, P	MD	211
EDM	Levine, R	NH	208
EDM	Mandel, S	PA	211
EDM	Ridgway, E	CO	220
EDM	Robbins, R	TX	221
EDM	Ross, D	MA	208
EDM	Rubenfeld, S	TX	221
EDM	Sherman, S	TX	221
EDM	Tuttle, R	NY	212
EDM	Waguespack, S	TX	221
EDM	Wartofsky, L	DC	213
EDM	Xing, M	MD	213
NRad	Loevner, L	PA	986
NuM	Dillehay, G	IL	550
NuM	Goldsmith, S	NY	548
NuM	Lamonica, D	NY	548
NuM	Pandit-Taskar, N	NY	549
NuM	Waxman, A	CA	551
NuM	Ziffer, J	FL	550
Onc	Grunberg, S	VT	330
Onc	Khuri, F	GA	358
Onc	Pfister, D	NY	348
Onc	Remick, S	WV	348
Oto	Browne, J	NC	667
Oto	Califano, J	MD	658
Oto	Chalian, A	PA	658
Oto	Eisele, D	MD	659
Oto	Fee, W	CA	684
Oto	Keane, W	PA	661
Oto	Kuhel, W	NY	662
Oto	Lavertu, P	OH	676
Oto	Lydiatt, W	NE	680
Oto	Persky, M	NY	663
Oto	Petruzzelli, G	GA	670
Oto	Randolph, G	MA	656
Oto	Schantz, S	NY	664
Oto	Singh, B	NY	665
Oto	Sinha, U	CA	687
Oto	Smith, R	NE	680
Oto	Suen, J	AR	683
Oto	Teknos, T	OH	678
Oto	Terris, D	GA	671

Spec	Name	St	Pg
Oto	Valentino, J	KY	672
Oto	Weber, S	TX	683
Oto	Wong, R	NY	666
Oto	Yoo, G	MI	679
Path	Li Volsi, V	PA	710
Path	Sanchez, M	NJ	711
Path	Suster, S	WI	716
Path	Wheeler, T	TX	719
PEn	Zimmerman, D	IL	748
PlS	Loree, T	NY	855
PS	Ehrlich, P	MI	807
PS	Skinner, M	TX	810
RadRO	Grigsby, P	MO	959
S	Alfonso, A	NY	1053
S	Butler, J	CA	1094
S	Byrd, D	WA	1094
S	Evans, D	WI	1076
S	Farrar, W	OH	1076
S	Giuliano, A	CA	1096
S	Graham, R	MA	1049
S	Hodin, R	MA	1049
S	Kim, L	AR	1089
S	Kuhn, J	TX	1090
S	Moore, F	MA	1051
S	Roses, D	NY	1063
S	Sener, S	CA	1099
S	Shah, J	NY	1064
S	Sosa, J	CT	1052
S	Udelsman, R	CT	1052

Thyroid Cancer & Surgery

Spec	Name	St	Pg
Oto	Clayman, G	TX	681
Oto	Shindo, M	OR	687
S	Clark, O	CA	1094
S	Gosnell, J	CA	1096
S	Hanks, J	VA	1069
S	Moley, J	MO	1080
S	Ridge, J	PA	1063

Thyroid Disease

Spec	Name	St	Pg
NuM	Ziffer, J	FL	550

Thyroid Disorders

Spec	Name	St	Pg
EDM	Ain, K	KY	213
EDM	Akatsu, H	CA	222
EDM	Bell, D	AL	213
EDM	Bergman, D	NY	209
EDM	Berkson, R	CA	222
EDM	Blum, C	NY	209
EDM	Braverman, L	MA	206
EDM	Brennan, M	MN	216
EDM	Brillon, D	NY	209
EDM	Burman, K	DC	209
EDM	Burmeister, L	MN	216
EDM	Comi, R	NH	206
EDM	Cooper, D	MD	210
EDM	Cushing, G	MA	207
EDM	Daniels, G	MA	207
EDM	Emanuele, M	IL	217
EDM	Feinglos, M	NC	214

Specialty & Special Expertise Index

Spec	Name	St	Pg
EDM	Fitzgerald, P	CA	222
EDM	Greene, L	NY	210
EDM	Jacobs, T	NY	210
EDM	Kamdar, V	CA	223
EDM	Ladenson, P	MD	211
EDM	Larsen, P	MA	207
EDM	Lash, R	MI	218
EDM	Levine, R	NH	208
EDM	Lipson, A	DC	211
EDM	Mandel, S	PA	211
EDM	McConnell, R	NY	211
EDM	McGill, J	MO	218
EDM	Pearce, E	MA	208
EDM	Powers, A	TN	215
EDM	Quinn, S	FL	215
EDM	Ridgway, E	CO	220
EDM	Ross, D	MA	208
EDM	Rubenfeld, S	TX	221
EDM	Schwartz, S	PA	212
EDM	Semenkovich, C	MO	219
EDM	Seplowitz, A	NY	212
EDM	Singer, P	CA	224
EDM	Surks, M	NY	212
EDM	Wartofsky, L	DC	213
EDM	Weiss, R	IL	219
EDM	Werner, P	IL	220
EDM	Woeber, K	CA	224
EDM	Xing, M	MD	213
EDM	Young, I	NY	213
NuM	Siegel, B	MO	550
NuM	Strashun, A	NY	549
Oto	Davidson, B	DC	658
Oto	Donovan, D	TX	681
Oto	Picken, C	DC	663
Oto	Pribitkin, E	PA	663
Oto	Randolph, G	MA	656
Oto	Tufano, R	MD	666
Path	De Las Morenas, A	MA	706
Path	Suster, S	WI	716
Path	Wheeler, T	TX	719
PEn	Alter, C	PA	744
PEn	Casella, S	NH	743
PEn	Geffner, M	CA	748
PEn	Kappy, M	CO	748
PEn	Levy, R	IL	747
PEn	Plotnick, L	MD	745
PEn	Rivkees, S	FL	746
PEn	Rogers, D	OH	747
PEn	Zimmerman, D	IL	748

Thyroid Disorders in Pregnancy

Spec	Name	St	Pg
EDM	Davies, T	NY	210
EDM	Mandel, S	PA	211
EDM	Seely, E	MA	208

Thyroid Eye Disease

Spec	Name	St	Pg
Oph	Bernardino, C	CA	599
Oph	Char, D	CA	599
Oph	Della Rocca, R	NY	573
Oph	Feldon, S	NY	573
Oph	Kikkawa, D	CA	601

Spec	Name	St	Pg
Oph	Lucarelli, M	WI	592
Oph	Miller, N	MD	577
Oph	Nunery, W	KY	585
Oph	Putterman, A	IL	593
Oph	Sergott, R	PA	580

Thyroid Surgery

Spec	Name	St	Pg
Oto	Campbell, B	WI	674
Oto	Hurst, M	WV	661
Oto	Terris, D	GA	671
Oto	Thaler, E	PA	666
PO	Kazahaya, K	PA	790
S	Britt, L	VA	1067
S	Doherty, G	MA	1049
S	Gower, R	AK	1096
S	McHenry, C	OH	1079

Thyroid Ultrasound

Spec	Name	St	Pg
DR	Benson, C	MA	973
DR	Grant, E	CA	983
EDM	Levine, R	NH	208
EDM	Mandel, S	PA	211
EDM	McConnell, R	NY	211

Tick-borne Diseases

Spec	Name	St	Pg
Inf	Auwaerter, P	MD	410
Inf	Bakken, J	MN	416
PInf	Saiman, L	NY	781

Tissue Banking

Spec	Name	St	Pg
OrS	Friedlaender, G	CT	611
PIS	Spence, R	MD	858

TMJ Imaging

Spec	Name	St	Pg
DR	Rao, V	PA	977

Tobacco Abuse

Spec	Name	St	Pg
Ger	Dale, L	MN	264
T&CS	Grannis, F	CA	1141

Toe-to-Hand Transfer

Spec	Name	St	Pg
HS	Jones, N	CA	304
PIS	Levin, L	PA	855

Tongue Cancer

Spec	Name	St	Pg
Oto	Diaz, E	TX	681
Oto	Myers, J	TX	683

Tonsil/Adenoid Disorders

Spec	Name	St	Pg
PO	Dolitsky, J	NY	789
PO	Miller, R	IL	792

Tourette's Syndrome

Spec	Name	St	Pg
ChAP	Coffey, B	NY	908
ChAP	Hirsch, G	NY	908
ChAP	Leckman, J	CT	907

Spec	Name	St	Pg
ChAP	McCracken, J	CA	912
ChAP	Rostain, A	PA	909
ChiN	Dure, L	AL	149
ChiN	Mink, J	NY	148
ChiN	Pinter, J	OR	153
ChiN	Roddy, S	CA	153
N	Bruno, M	HI	535
N	Couch, J	OK	532
N	Flaherty, A	MA	507
N	Jankovic, J	TX	534
N	Mesulam, M	IL	528
Ped	Berlin, C	PA	726
Psyc	Saxena, S	CA	903

Toxic Epidermal Neurolysis

Spec	Name	St	Pg
S	Ryan, C	MA	1051

Toxicology

Spec	Name	St	Pg
Pul	Albertson, T	CA	938
Pul	Tharratt, R	CA	941

Toxoplasmosis

Spec	Name	St	Pg
PInf	Bryson, Y	CA	784

Tracheal Stenosis

Spec	Name	St	Pg
Pul	Ernst, A	MA	922

Tracheal Surgery

Spec	Name	St	Pg
PO	Cotton, R	OH	791
T&CS	Backer, C	IL	1130
T&CS	Cerfolio, R	AL	1124
T&CS	Gaissert, H	MA	1111
T&CS	Kernstine, K	TX	1138
T&CS	Mathisen, D	MA	1111
T&CS	Wood, D	WA	1143
T&CS	Wright, C	MA	1113

Tracheal Surgery-Pediatric

Spec	Name	St	Pg
T&CS	Wells, W	CA	1143

Transfusion Free Surgery

Spec	Name	St	Pg
T&CS	Rosengart, T	NY	1121

Transfusion Medicine

Spec	Name	St	Pg
Hem	Telen, M	NC	318
Path	Kaufman, R	MA	706

Transgender Issues

Spec	Name	St	Pg
PEn	Spack, N	MA	743

Transpland Medicine-Pancreas

Spec	Name	St	Pg
Nep	Nolan, C	TX	464

Transplant Immunology

Spec	Name	St	Pg
PGe	McDiarmid, S	CA	756

Spec	Name	St	Pg
S	Knechtle, S	GA	1069
S	Larsen, C	GA	1070

Transplant Medicine - Heart

Spec	Name	St	Pg
Cv	Bourge, R	AL	103

Transplant Medicine - Liver

Spec	Name	St	Pg
PGe	Sokol, R	CO	754

Transplant Medicine-Bowel

Spec	Name	St	Pg
Ge	Schiano, T	NY	238
PGe	McDiarmid, S	CA	756

Transplant Medicine-Heart

Spec	Name	St	Pg
Cv	Brozena, S	PA	97
Cv	Corrigan, V	GA	104
Cv	DeNofrio, D	MA	94
Cv	Eisen, H	PA	98
Cv	Fishbein, D	WA	116
Cv	Fonarow, G	CA	116
Cv	Geltman, E	MO	108
Cv	Gottlieb, S	MD	99
Cv	Heroux, A	IL	108
Cv	Hunt, S	CA	117
Cv	Jessup, M	PA	100
Cv	Johnson, M	WI	109
Cv	Katz, S	NY	100
Cv	Kobashigawa, J	CA	117
Cv	Konstam, M	MA	95
Cv	Lindenfeld, J	CO	113
Cv	Massin, E	TX	114
Cv	Mather, P	PA	100
Cv	O'Connell, J	GA	105
Cv	Rogers, J	NC	105
Cv	Russell, S	MD	101
Cv	Smart, F	LA	115
Cv	Stevenson, L	MA	96
Cv	Wagoner, L	OH	112
Cv	Walsh, M	IN	112
Cv	Young, J	OH	113
PCd	Bernstein, D	CA	740
PCd	Bricker, J	TX	740
PCd	Caldwell, R	IN	738
PCd	Colvin, E	AL	737
PCd	Dreyer, W	TX	740
PCd	Fricker, F	FL	737
PCd	Hsu, D	NY	735
PCd	Pahl, E	IL	739
PCd	Shaddy, R	PA	736

Transplant Medicine-Heart & Lung

Spec	Name	St	Pg
Pul	Hertz, M	MN	933

Transplant Medicine-Kidney

Spec	Name	St	Pg
Nep	Bennett, W	OR	464
Nep	Brennan, D	MO	461
Nep	Brennan, S	TX	463
Nep	Butterly, D	NC	459
Nep	Coffman, T	NC	459
Nep	Cohen, D	NY	457
Nep	Gaston, R	AL	459
Nep	Helderman, J	TN	460
Nep	Josephson, M	IL	461
Nep	Kasiske, B	MN	461
Nep	Miller, B	MO	462
Nep	Nolan, C	TX	464
Nep	Roth, D	FL	460
Nep	Scandling, J	CA	465
Nep	Stern, L	NY	458
Nep	Suki, W	TX	464
Nep	Textor, S	MN	462
Nep	Thomas, C	IA	463
Nep	Tolkoff-Rubin, N	MA	456
Nep	Venkat, K	MI	463
Nep	Ward, D	CA	466
Nep	Williams, G	NY	458
PNep	Benfield, M	AL	786
PNep	Brophy, P	IA	787
PNep	Chandar, J	FL	786
PNep	Cohn, R	IL	787
PNep	Conley, S	PA	785
PNep	Ellis, D	PA	785
PNep	Ettenger, R	CA	788
PNep	Fivush, B	MD	785
PNep	Friedman, A	MN	787
PNep	Jabs, K	TN	786
PNep	Jordan, S	CA	788
PNep	Kashtan, C	MN	787
PNep	McDonald, R	WA	788
PNep	Mendley, S	MD	786
PNep	Warady, B	MO	788
PNep	Zilleruelo, G	FL	787

Transplant Medicine-Liver

Spec	Name	St	Pg
Ge	Barnes, D	OH	244
Ge	Bloomer, J	AL	239
Ge	Boyer, T	AZ	251
Ge	Brown, K	MI	244
Ge	Brown, R	NY	231
Ge	Chung, R	MA	228
Ge	Crippin, J	MO	244
Ge	Davis, G	TX	251
Ge	Dienstag, J	MA	228
Ge	Fried, M	NC	240
Ge	Galati, J	TX	252
Ge	Gholam, P	OH	245
Ge	Gish, R	CA	254
Ge	Glombicki, A	TX	252
Ge	Han, S	CA	254
Ge	Herrine, S	PA	233
Ge	Jensen, D	IL	246
Ge	Kwo, P	IN	246
Ge	La Russo, N	MN	246
Ge	Lucey, M	WI	247
Ge	Martin, P	FL	241
Ge	Munoz, S	PA	237
Ge	Poordad, F	TX	252
Ge	Porayko, M	TN	241
Ge	Raiford, D	TN	242
Ge	Reddy, K	PA	237
Ge	Schiano, T	NY	238
Ge	Shiffman, M	VA	242
Ge	Sorrell, M	NE	250
Ge	Speeg, K	TX	252
Ge	Te, H	IL	248
Ge	Vierling, J	TX	253
Ge	Wiesner, R	MN	249
PGe	Jonas, M	MA	749
PGe	Kleinman, R	MA	749
PGe	McDiarmid, S	CA	756
PGe	Mittal, N	TX	755
PGe	Molleston, J	IN	753
PGe	Narkewicz, M	CO	754
PGe	Schwarz, K	MD	751
PGe	Thomas, D	CA	756
PGe	Whitington, P	IL	754

Transplant Medicine-Lung

Spec	Name	St	Pg
PPul	Kurland, G	PA	794
Pul	Ahya, V	PA	924
Pul	Arcasoy, S	NY	924
Pul	Christie, J	PA	925
Pul	Garrity, E	IL	933
Pul	Hertz, M	MN	933
Pul	Kotloff, R	PA	926
Pul	Loyd, J	TN	931
Pul	Lynch, J	CA	940
Pul	Padilla, M	NY	927
Pul	Trulock, E	MO	936
Pul	Young, K	PA	929

Transplant Medicine-Pancreas

Spec	Name	St	Pg
Nep	Scandling, J	CA	465

Transplant Pathology

Spec	Name	St	Pg
Path	Demetris, A	PA	708
Path	Swerdlow, S	PA	712

Transplant Surgery

Spec	Name	St	Pg
S	Becker, Y	IL	1074
S	Jabbour, N	MA	1050
S	Johnson, L	DC	1058
S	Renz, J	IL	1081
S	Reyes, J	WA	1099
S	Shaked, A	PA	1064

Transplant Surgery-Pediatric

Spec	Name	St	Pg
PS	Chen, M	AL	805
PS	Healey, P	WA	810
PS	Paidas, C	FL	805
S	Cronin, D	WI	1075
S	Kato, T	NY	1059
S	Reyes, J	WA	1099
S	Thistlethwaite, J	IL	1083

Specialty & Special Expertise Index

Spec	Name	St	Pg
Transplant-Auto Transplantation			
S	Kato, T	NY	1059
Transplant-Bile Duct			
S	Rosen, C	MN	1081
Transplant-Bowel			
S	Benedetti, E	IL	1074
S	Tzakis, A	OH	1083
Transplant-Face			
PlS	Rodriguez, E	MD	857
PlS	Siemionow, M	OH	868
Transplant-Hand			
HS	Breidenbach, W	AZ	303
HS	Cendales, L	GA	299
HS	Lee, W	MD	297
PlS	Tobin, G	KY	863
Transplant-Heart			
T&CS	Acker, M	PA	1113
T&CS	Backer, C	IL	1130
T&CS	Brown, J	IN	1131
T&CS	Byrne, J	TN	1124
T&CS	Conte, J	MD	1114
T&CS	Dang, M	HI	1141
T&CS	Echeverri, L	TX	1137
T&CS	Edwards, N	NY	1115
T&CS	Elefteriades, J	CT	1110
T&CS	Frazier, O	TX	1138
T&CS	Gaynor, J	PA	1116
T&CS	Harrell, J	TX	1138
T&CS	Jeevanandam, V	IL	1133
T&CS	Jessen, M	TX	1138
T&CS	Kormos, R	PA	1118
T&CS	Kron, I	VA	1126
T&CS	Laks, H	CA	1142
T&CS	Lansman, S	NY	1119
T&CS	Liao, K	MN	1133
T&CS	Mayer, J	MA	1111
T&CS	Morris, R	PA	1120
T&CS	Oz, M	NY	1120
T&CS	Pagani, F	MI	1134
T&CS	Panos, A	FL	1128
T&CS	Pierson, R	MD	1120
T&CS	Quintessenza, J	FL	1128
T&CS	Robbins, R	CA	1142
T&CS	Samuels, L	PA	1121
T&CS	Slaughter, M	KY	1129
T&CS	Smedira, N	OH	1135
T&CS	Smith, C	NY	1121
T&CS	Toyoda, Y	PA	1122
T&CS	Trento, A	CA	1143
T&CS	Turrentine, M	IN	1135
T&CS	Vlahakes, G	MA	1112

Spec	Name	St	Pg
Transplant-Heart & Lung			
T&CS	Bakhos, M	IL	1130
T&CS	Bavaria, J	PA	1114
T&CS	Calhoon, J	TX	1137
T&CS	Fullerton, D	CO	1136
T&CS	Furukawa, S	PA	1116
T&CS	Griffith, B	MD	1117
T&CS	Jamieson, S	CA	1142
T&CS	Kirklin, J	AL	1126
T&CS	Love, R	IL	1133
T&CS	Mack, M	TX	1139
T&CS	Mavroudis, C	FL	1126
T&CS	Mill, M	NC	1127
T&CS	Mullett, T	KY	1127
T&CS	Naka, Y	NY	1120
T&CS	Patterson, G	MO	1134
T&CS	Pham, S	FL	1128
T&CS	Spray, T	PA	1122
T&CS	Staples, E	FL	1129
T&CS	Starnes, V	CA	1143
Transplant-Heart-Adult & Pediatric			
T&CS	Kirklin, J	AL	1126
T&CS	Mill, M	NC	1127
Transplant-Heart-Pediatric			
T&CS	Bailey, L	CA	1140
T&CS	Campbell, D	CO	1136
T&CS	Christian, K	TN	1124
T&CS	Cohen, G	CA	1140
T&CS	Huddleston, C	MO	1132
T&CS	Kanter, K	GA	1126
T&CS	Rosenkranz, E	FL	1129
T&CS	Walters, H	MI	1135
Transplant-Kidney			
PS	Andrews, W	MO	806
PS	Colombani, P	MD	802
PS	Healey, P	WA	810
PS	Schwartz, M	PA	804
S	Abecassis, M	IL	1074
S	Ascher, N	CA	1093
S	Bartlett, S	MD	1053
S	Becker, Y	IL	1074
S	Benedetti, E	IL	1074
S	Bentley, F	AR	1087
S	Bromberg, J	MD	1054
S	Conti, D	NY	1055
S	Eason, J	TN	1068
S	Eckhoff, D	AL	1068
S	Fisher, J	CA	1095
S	Fung, J	OH	1077
S	Gruber, S	MI	1077
S	Kapur, S	NY	1059
S	Knechtle, S	GA	1069
S	Larsen, C	GA	1070
S	Lipkowitz, G	MA	1050
S	Markmann, J	MA	1051
S	Matas, A	MN	1079

Spec	Name	St	Pg
S	Mistry, B	ND	1085
S	Montgomery, R	MD	1060
S	Newell, K	GA	1071
S	Perkins, J	WA	1098
S	Reed, A	IA	1081
S	Reich, D	PA	1062
S	Scantlebury, V	DE	1063
S	Schaffer, R	CA	1099
S	Shapiro, R	PA	1064
S	Stratta, R	NC	1073
S	Teperman, L	NY	1065
S	Thistlethwaite, J	IL	1083
U	Ciancio, G	FL	1160
U	Marsh, C	CA	1177
U	Menon, M	MI	1169
U	Sagalowsky, A	TX	1174
Transplant-Kidney-Adult & Pediatric			
S	Andreoni, K	FL	1066
S	Schulak, J	OH	1082
Transplant-Kidney-Pediatric			
U	Firlit, C	MO	1167
Transplant-Liver			
PS	Andrews, W	MO	806
PS	Colombani, P	MD	802
PS	Healey, P	WA	810
PS	Karrer, F	CO	808
PS	Meyers, R	UT	808
PS	Sawin, R	WA	811
S	Abecassis, M	IL	1074
S	Abouljoud, M	MI	1074
S	Ascher, N	CA	1093
S	Benedetti, E	IL	1074
S	Brems, J	IL	1074
S	Busuttil, R	CA	1094
S	Cherqui, D	NY	1055
S	Colquhoun, S	CA	1094
S	Cronin, D	WI	1075
S	Eckhoff, D	AL	1068
S	Emond, J	NY	1057
S	Fisher, J	CA	1095
S	Fung, J	OH	1077
S	Halff, G	TX	1089
S	Hemming, A	CA	1096
S	Jabbour, N	MA	1050
S	Jenkins, R	MA	1050
S	Kato, T	NY	1059
S	Kinkhabwala, M	NY	1059
S	Klein, A	CA	1097
S	Knechtle, S	GA	1069
S	Markmann, J	MA	1051
S	Marsh, J	PA	1060
S	Mistry, B	ND	1085
S	Nissen, N	CA	1098
S	Perkins, J	WA	1098
S	Philosophe, B	MD	1062
S	Pinson, C	TN	1071

Spec	Name	St	Pg
S	Posselt, A	CA	1098
S	Reed, A	IA	1081
S	Reich, D	PA	1062
S	Renz, J	IL	1081
S	Reyes, J	WA	1099
S	Roberts, J	CA	1099
S	Rosen, C	MN	1081
S	Schaffer, R	CA	1099
S	Shaked, A	PA	1064
S	Teperman, L	NY	1065
S	Thistlethwaite, J	IL	1083
S	Tzakis, A	OH	1083
S	Wood, R	TX	1093
U	Marsh, C	CA	1177

Transplant-Liver-Adult & Pediatric

Spec	Name	St	Pg
S	Andreoni, K	FL	1066
S	Chapman, W	MO	1075
S	Emre, S	CT	1049
S	Esquivel, C	CA	1095
S	Millis, J	IL	1080
S	Olthoff, K	PA	1061
S	Renz, J	IL	1081

Transplant-Lung

Spec	Name	St	Pg
Pul	Raghu, G	WA	940
T&CS	Campbell, D	CO	1136
T&CS	Cassivi, S	MN	1131
T&CS	Conte, J	MD	1114
T&CS	Cooper, J	PA	1114
T&CS	Ginsburg, M	NY	1116
T&CS	Iannettoni, M	IA	1132
T&CS	Lau, C	VA	1126
T&CS	Liao, K	MN	1133
T&CS	Mason, D	OH	1133
T&CS	McGiffin, D	AL	1126
T&CS	Meyers, B	MO	1133
T&CS	Mitchell, J	CO	1136
T&CS	Mitchell, J	CO	1137
T&CS	Ninan, M	TN	1128
T&CS	Patterson, G	MO	1134
T&CS	Pierson, R	MD	1120
T&CS	Pochettino, A	MN	1134
T&CS	Robbins, R	CA	1142
T&CS	Smedira, N	OH	1135
T&CS	Sonett, J	NY	1121
T&CS	Sugarbaker, D	MA	1112
T&CS	Turrentine, M	IN	1135
T&CS	Vigneswaran, W	IL	1135
T&CS	Wain, J	MA	1112

Transplant-Lung (Pathology)

Spec	Name	St	Pg
Path	Yousem, S	PA	712

Transplant-Lung-Pediatric

Spec	Name	St	Pg
T&CS	Huddleston, C	MO	1132
T&CS	Kanter, K	GA	1126

Transplant-Multi Organ

Spec	Name	St	Pg
S	Kato, T	NY	1059

Transplant-Ovarian Tissue

Spec	Name	St	Pg
U	Silber, S	MO	1170

Transplant-Pancreas

Spec	Name	St	Pg
S	Andreoni, K	FL	1066
S	Bartlett, S	MD	1053
S	Becker, Y	IL	1074
S	Benedetti, E	IL	1074
S	Bromberg, J	MD	1054
S	Fisher, J	CA	1095
S	Gruber, S	MI	1077
S	Kapur, S	NY	1059
S	Larsen, C	GA	1070
S	Markmann, J	MA	1051
S	Millis, J	IL	1080
S	Mistry, B	ND	1085
S	Newell, K	GA	1071
S	Oberholzer, J	IL	1080
S	Olthoff, K	PA	1061
S	Perkins, J	WA	1098
S	Philosophe, B	MD	1062
S	Posselt, A	CA	1098
S	Reed, A	IA	1081
S	Schaffer, R	CA	1099
S	Shapiro, R	PA	1064
S	Stratta, R	NC	1073
S	Thistlethwaite, J	IL	1083
U	Ciancio, G	FL	1160
U	Marsh, C	CA	1177

Transplant-Pancreas & Liver

Spec	Name	St	Pg
S	Eason, J	TN	1068
S	Schulak, J	OH	1082

Transplantation Psychiatry

Spec	Name	St	Pg
Psyc	Klapheke, M	FL	896

Transumbilical Breast Augmentation(TUBA)

Spec	Name	St	Pg
PlS	Horowitz, J	CA	874

Trauma

Spec	Name	St	Pg
HS	Eglseder, W	MD	296
HS	Hunt, T	AL	299
HS	Peljovich, A	GA	299
HS	Rosenwasser, M	NY	297
NS	Taylon, C	NE	492
NS	Zimmerman, C	ID	492
Oph	Mieler, W	IL	592
Oph	Ng, J	OR	603
OrS	Agarwal, A	TX	640
OrS	Anglen, J	IN	632
OrS	Archdeacon, M	OH	632
OrS	Cornell, C	NY	616
OrS	Delahay, J	DC	616

Spec	Name	St	Pg
OrS	Ebraheim, N	OH	633
OrS	Farmer, J	NY	617
OrS	Greisberg, J	NY	618
OrS	Johnson, E	CA	644
OrS	Nepola, J	IA	636
OrS	Otsuka, N	NY	623
OrS	Peterson, D	AK	645
OrS	Sangeorzan, B	WA	645
OrS	Seltzer, D	AZ	641
OrS	Smith, E	MA	613
OrS	Swiontkowski, M	MN	638
OrS	Tornetta, P	MA	613
OrS	Webb, L	GA	631
OrS	Weiner, R	FL	631
Oto	Stenson, K	IL	678
PS	Bond, S	KY	805
PS	Dillon, P	MO	807
PS	Fallat, M	KY	805
PS	Ford, H	CA	810
PS	Gaines, B	PA	803
PS	Nance, M	PA	804
PS	Reynolds, M	IL	808
PS	Stylianos, S	NY	804
PS	Tuggle, D	OK	810
S	Barie, P	NY	1053
S	Britt, L	VA	1067
S	Burke, P	MA	1048
S	Cioffi, W	RI	1048
S	Cohen, M	PA	1055
S	Cornwell, E	DC	1055
S	Cushing, B	ME	1048
S	Demarest, G	NM	1087
S	Dulchavsky, S	MI	1076
S	Feliciano, D	GA	1068
S	Friese, R	AZ	1088
S	Gupta, R	NH	1049
S	Holcomb, J	TX	1089
S	Hunt, J	TX	1089
S	Knudson, M	CA	1097
S	Lentz, C	NM	1090
S	McIntyre, R	CO	1085
S	Meyer, A	NC	1070
S	Peitzman, A	PA	1062
S	Rhee, P	AZ	1092
S	Stewart, R	TX	1092
S	Weigelt, J	WI	1084
S	Winchell, R	ME	1052

Trauma Neurology

Spec	Name	St	Pg
N	Finkel, M	FL	521

Trauma Psychiatry

Spec	Name	St	Pg
ChAP	Bleiberg, E	TX	911
ChAP	Fornari, V	NY	908
ChAP	Sargent, A	MA	907
ChAP	Steiner, H	CA	912
ChAP	Terr, L	CA	912
Psyc	Loewenstein, R	MD	893

Specialty & Special Expertise Index

Spec	Name	St	Pg
Trauma Radiology			
DR	Mirvis, S	MD	976
DR	Sivit, C	OH	981
Trauma Rehabilitation			
PM	Walsh, N	TX	701
PMR	Sisung, C	IL	841
Trauma-Reconstructive Plastic Surgery			
PlS	Lee, R	IL	866
Trauma-Upper & Lower Extremity			
HS	Cassidy, C	MA	294
Trauma/Critical Care			
S	Baker, C	VA	1066
S	Gamelli, R	IL	1077
S	Mistry, B	ND	1085
Travel Medicine			
Inf	Alvarez-Elcoro, S	FL	414
Inf	Ballon-Landa, G	CA	419
Inf	Corey, G	NC	414
Inf	DuPont, H	TX	418
Inf	Flaherty, J	IL	416
Inf	Gumprecht, J	NY	411
Inf	O'Keefe, J	IL	416
Inf	Pearson, R	VA	415
Inf	Perlman, D	NY	412
Inf	Rao, N	PA	413
Inf	Siegel, M	WA	420
Inf	Wallace, M	FL	415
PInf	Belcher, C	IN	782
PInf	Christenson, J	IN	783
PrM	Cahill, J	NY	882
Tremor			
N	Langston, J	CA	537
N	Tetrud, J	CA	539
Tremor & Dystonia			
N	Samii, A	WA	538
N	Vitek, J	MN	530
N	Wooten, G	VA	524
Tremor and Dystonia			
N	Louis, E	NY	515
Trigeminal Neuralgia			
NS	Carson, B	MD	473
NS	Goodman, R	NY	474
NS	Grubb, R	MO	487
NS	Kaplitt, M	NY	476
NS	Linskey, M	CA	497

Spec	Name	St	Pg
NS	Malik, G	MI	488
NS	Murali, R	NY	477
NS	Patel, S	SC	483
NS	Sen, C	NY	478
NS	Van Loveren, H	FL	485
NS	Yonas, H	NM	495
Trophoblastic Tumors			
GO	King, S	PA	278
Onc	Aghajanian, C	NY	333
Tropical Diseases			
Inf	Corey, G	NC	414
Inf	DuPont, H	TX	418
Inf	Pearson, R	VA	415
Inf	Rao, N	PA	413
Inf	Trenholme, G	IL	417
Path	Walker, D	TX	719
PrM	Cahill, J	NY	882
PrM	Cahill, K	NY	883
PrM	Cahill, K	NY	883
Tuberculosis			
Inf	Alvarez-Elcoro, S	FL	414
Inf	Blumberg, H	GA	414
Inf	Chaisson, R	MD	411
Inf	Huitt, G	CO	418
Inf	Sepkowitz, K	NY	413
PInf	Baltimore, R	CT	779
PInf	Saiman, L	NY	781
Pul	Catanzaro, A	CA	939
Pul	Friedman, L	CT	923
Pul	Hopewell, P	CA	939
Pul	Iseman, M	CO	936
Pul	Nardell, E	MA	923
Pul	Schluger, N	NY	927
Tuberous Breasts			
Onc	Stockdale, F	CA	391
PlS	Romano, J	CA	876
Tuberous Sclerosis			
ChiN	Rosser, T	CA	154
ChiN	Tonsgard, J	IL	151
N	Bebin, E	AL	520
N	Devinsky, O	NY	511
NS	Weiner, H	NY	480
Tumor Banking			
Path	Balla, A	IL	715
Tumor Banking-Brain			
Path	Zagzag, D	NY	712
Tumor Banking-Prostate			
Path	Melamed, J	NY	710

Spec	Name	St	Pg
Tumor Surgery			
PS	Aiken, J	WI	806
PS	Ginsburg, H	NY	803
PS	Meyers, R	UT	808
S	Crowe, J	OH	1075
Tumoral Calcinosis			
Ger	Lyles, K	NC	264
Tumors-Rare & Multiple			
S	Dooley, W	OK	1087
Turner Syndrome			
PEn	Eugster, E	IN	747
Twin to Twin Transfusion Syndrome (TTTS)			
CG	Bianchi, D	MA	156
MF	Abuhamad, A	VA	434
MF	Bahado-Singh, R	MI	435
MF	Carr, S	RI	430
MF	Chmait, R	CA	440
MF	Mari, G	TN	435
ObG	De Lia, J	WI	561
PS	Adzick, N	PA	802
PS	Albanese, C	CA	810
PS	Crombleholme, T	CO	808
PS	Farmer, D	CA	810

U

Spec	Name	St	Pg
Ulcerative Colitis			
CRS	Foley, E	WI	174
CRS	Fry, R	PA	170
CRS	Medich, D	PA	170
CRS	Rafferty, J	OH	175
CRS	Shellito, P	MA	169
CRS	Steinhagen, R	NY	171
CRS	Welton, M	CA	178
Ge	Abreu, M	FL	239
Ge	Albert, M	DC	230
Ge	Bayless, T	MD	230
Ge	Cominelli, F	OH	244
Ge	Hanauer, S	IL	245
Ge	Isaacs, K	NC	240
Ge	Lebwohl, O	NY	235
Ge	Leighton, J	AZ	252
Ge	Lichtenstein, G	PA	236
Ge	Loftus, E	MN	247
Ge	Magun, A	NY	236
Ge	Mayer, L	NY	236
Ge	Plevy, S	NC	241
Ge	Sandborn, W	CA	255
Ge	Scherl, E	NY	238
Ge	Siegel, C	NH	230

Specialty & Special Expertise Index

Spec	Name	St	Pg
Ge	Tremaine, W	MN	248
PGe	Baldassano, R	PA	750
PGe	Berman, J	IL	752
PGe	Dubinsky, M	CA	755
PGe	Kirschner, B	IL	753
PGe	Oliva-Hemker, M	MD	751
PGe	Spivak, W	NY	751
PGe	Wyllie, R	OH	754
PS	Dolgin, S	NY	803
S	Michelassi, F	NY	1060
S	Salky, B	NY	1063

Ultrasound

Spec	Name	St	Pg
DR	Abbitt, P	FL	978
DR	Adler, R	NY	974
DR	Bahn, D	CA	982
DR	Cohen, H	TN	979
DR	Coleman, B	PA	974
DR	Doubilet, P	MA	973
DR	Grant, E	CA	983
GO	Fishman, D	NY	278
MF	Baker, E	NH	430
MF	Blakemore, K	MD	431
MF	Dugoff, L	PA	432
MF	Ferguson, J	VA	434
MF	Hibbard, J	IL	436
MF	Mastrobattista, J	TX	438
MF	Platt, L	CA	440
MF	Reed, K	AZ	439
MF	Robinson, J	MA	431
MF	Treadwell, M	MI	437
ObG	Byrne, J	UT	562
ObG	Evans, M	NY	557
RE	Session, D	GA	1012

Unknown Primary Cancer

Spec	Name	St	Pg
Onc	Greco, F	TN	357
Onc	Hande, K	TN	357
Onc	Ilson, D	NY	342
Onc	Jacobs, C	CA	387
Onc	Kelsen, D	NY	343
Onc	Sikic, B	CA	390
Onc	Stewart, F	WA	391
Onc	Stoopler, M	NY	350
Onc	Varadhachary, G	TX	382
Onc	Ward, J	UT	376

Upper Extremity Surgery

Spec	Name	St	Pg
HS	Baratz, M	PA	295
HS	Idler, R	CO	302
HS	Osterman, A	PA	297

Upper Extremity Surgery-Pediatric

Spec	Name	St	Pg
HS	Kleinman, W	IN	301

Upper Extremity Trauma

Spec	Name	St	Pg
HS	Chung, K	MI	300
HS	Jupiter, J	MA	294
HS	Raphael, J	PA	297
HS	Trumble, T	WA	305
SM	Sennett, B	PA	1042

Ureter & Renal Pelvis Cancer

Spec	Name	St	Pg
U	O'Donnell, M	IA	1169

Urinary Reconstruction

Spec	Name	St	Pg
U	Boone, T	TX	1172
U	Elder, J	MI	1166
U	Ewalt, D	TX	1173
U	Ginsberg, D	CA	1176
U	Hensle, T	NJ	1153
U	Hrebinko, R	PA	1154
U	Kirsch, A	GA	1162
U	Lerner, S	TX	1173
U	Lockhart, J	FL	1162
U	Scardino, P	NY	1157
U	Schoenberg, M	MD	1157
U	Skinner, E	CA	1178
U	Wilson, T	CA	1179
U	Wong, C	OH	1171

Urinary Reflux/Obstruction

Spec	Name	St	Pg
U	Kirsch, A	GA	1162

Urinary Tract Infections

Spec	Name	St	Pg
Inf	Maki, D	WI	416
Inf	Sobel, J	MI	417
PInf	Wald, E	WI	783
PMR	Cardenas, D	FL	838
PNep	Ettenger, R	CA	788
U	Greenfield, S	NY	1153
U	Schaeffer, A	IL	1170

Urinary Tract Interventions

Spec	Name	St	Pg
VIR	Keller, F	OR	998

Uro-Gynecology

Spec	Name	St	Pg
GO	Hatch, K	AZ	287
GO	Morgan, M	PA	279
ObG	Brodman, M	NY	557
ObG	Cornella, J	AZ	563
ObG	De Lancey, J	MI	561
ObG	Eckler, K	MA	556
ObG	Hale, D	IN	561
ObG	Hullfish, K	VA	559
ObG	Iglesia, C	DC	557
ObG	Karram, M	OH	561
ObG	Lucente, V	PA	557
ObG	Myers, D	RI	556
ObG	Sanz, V	VA	559
ObG	Visco, A	NC	560
ObG	Walters, M	OH	562
U	Blaivas, J	NY	1151
U	McGuire, E	MI	1168

Urodynamics

Spec	Name	St	Pg
U	Bushman, W	WI	1166
U	Foster, H	CT	1148
U	Joseph, D	AL	1161
U	Kaplan, S	NY	1154
U	Klutke, C	MO	1168
U	Lynne, C	FL	1162
U	Milam, D	TN	1162
U	Nitti, V	NY	1156
U	Vapnek, J	NY	1159
U	Wein, A	PA	1159

Urodynamics in Spinal Cord Injury

Spec	Name	St	Pg
U	Linsenmeyer, T	NJ	1155

Urologic Cancer

Spec	Name	St	Pg
Onc	Carducci, M	MD	336
Onc	DiPaola, R	NJ	338
Onc	Einhorn, L	IN	367
Onc	Figlin, R	CA	386
Onc	Garnick, M	MA	329
Onc	Hauke, R	NE	375
Onc	Hogan, T	WV	342
Onc	Kelly, W	PA	343
Onc	Tagawa, S	NY	351
Onc	Torti, F	NC	363
Onc	Troner, M	FL	363
Path	Cohen, M	UT	717
Path	Ross, J	NY	711
RadRO	D'Amico, A	MA	946
RadRO	DeWeese, T	MD	949
RadRO	Dicker, A	PA	949
RadRO	Gejerman, G	NJ	950
RadRO	Nicolaou, N	PA	951
RadRO	St Clair, W	KY	957
RadRO	Stock, R	NY	952
RadRO	Zietman, A	MA	948
U	Andrews, P	AZ	1172
U	Andriole, G	MO	1165
U	Balaji, K	NC	1160
U	Bardot, S	LA	1172
U	Basler, J	TX	1172
U	Belldegrun, A	CA	1175
U	Boyd, S	CA	1175
U	Cohen, J	PA	1152
U	Cookson, M	TN	1161
U	Culkin, D	OK	1173
U	Dalkin, B	WA	1175
U	DeKernion, J	CA	1176
U	Droller, M	NY	1152
U	Ellis, W	WA	1176
U	Flanigan, R	IL	1167
U	Gill, H	CA	1176
U	Gill, I	CA	1176
U	Gomella, L	PA	1153
U	Grasso, M	NY	1153
U	Greene, G	FL	1161
U	Gujral, S	MN	1167
U	Hall, S	NY	1153

Specialty & Special Expertise Index

Spec	Name	St	Pg	Spec	Name	St	Pg	Spec	Name	St	Pg
U	Hemal, A	NC	1161	U	Beall, M	VA	1160	U	Gomella, L	PA	1153
U	Heney, N	MA	1149	U	Belldegrun, A	CA	1175	U	Gomery, P	MA	1148
U	Janeiro, J	NH	1149	U	Benson, M	NY	1151	U	Gonzales, E	TX	1173
U	Kavoussi, L	NY	1154	U	Blaivas, J	NY	1151	U	Grasso, M	NY	1153
U	Keane, T	SC	1161	U	Bloom, D	MI	1165	U	Greenberg, R	PA	1153
U	Klein, E	OH	1168	U	Bodner, D	OH	1165	U	Greene, G	FL	1161
U	Lanteri, V	NJ	1154	U	Boone, T	TX	1172	U	Greenfield, S	NY	1153
U	Lee, C	MI	1168	U	Boyd, S	CA	1175	U	Gribetz, M	NY	1153
U	McDougal, W	MA	1149	U	Brendler, C	IL	1165	U	Griebling, T	KS	1171
U	McGovern, F	MA	1149	U	Brock, J	TN	1160	U	Grossman, H	TX	1173
U	Menon, M	MI	1169	U	Broderick, G	FL	1160	U	Gujral, S	MN	1167
U	Miles, B	TX	1174	U	Buch, J	TX	1173	U	Hall, S	NY	1153
U	O'Donnell, M	IA	1169	U	Burnett, A	MD	1151	U	Hellstrom, W	LA	1173
U	Penson, D	TN	1163	U	Busby, J	AL	1160	U	Hemal, A	NC	1161
U	Porter, C	WA	1178	U	Bushman, W	WI	1166	U	Heney, N	MA	1149
U	Pruthi, R	NC	1163	U	Cain, M	IN	1166	U	Hensle, T	NJ	1153
U	Rowland, R	KY	1163	U	Caldamone, A	RI	1148	U	Herr, H	NY	1153
U	Sagalowsky, A	TX	1174	U	Campbell, S	OH	1166	U	Holden, S	CA	1177
U	Samadi, D	NY	1157	U	Canning, D	PA	1151	U	Hrebinko, R	PA	1154
U	Sanda, M	MA	1150	U	Carpinito, G	MA	1148	U	Irby, P	NC	1161
U	Scardino, P	NY	1157	U	Carroll, P	CA	1175	U	Jackman, S	PA	1154
U	Skinner, E	CA	1178	U	Carson, C	NC	1160	U	Janeiro, J	NH	1149
U	Strup, S	KY	1164	U	Carter, H	MD	1151	U	Jones, J	OH	1167
U	Takayama, T	WA	1179	U	Cartwright, P	UT	1171	U	Joseph, D	AL	1161
U	Terris, M	GA	1165	U	Catalona, W	IL	1166	U	Kadmon, D	TX	1173
U	Trabulsi, E	PA	1158	U	Chancellor, M	MI	1166	U	Kaefer, M	IN	1167
U	Van Arsdalen, K	PA	1158	U	Chang, S	TN	1160	U	Kane, M	MD	1154
U	Verghese, M	DC	1159	U	Chen, D	PA	1151	U	Kaouk, J	OH	1167
U	Wallen, E	NC	1165	U	Childs, S	CO	1171	U	Kaplan, S	NY	1154
U	Wein, A	PA	1159	U	Ciancio, G	FL	1160	U	Kass, E	MI	1167
				U	Clayman, R	CA	1175	U	Katz, A	NY	1154
				U	Cohen, J	PA	1152	U	Kavoussi, L	NY	1154

Urologic Cancer-Pediatric

Spec	Name	St	Pg
U	Coplen, D	MO	1166

Spec	Name	St	Pg	Spec	Name	St	Pg
U	Colberg, J	CT	1148	U	Kawachi, M	CA	1177
U	Cookson, M	TN	1161	U	Keane, T	SC	1161
U	Coplen, D	MO	1166	U	Kennelly, M	NC	1161
U	Crawford, E	CO	1171	U	Kibel, A	MA	1149
U	Culkin, D	OK	1173	U	Kim, E	TN	1161

Urologic Pathology

Spec	Name	St	Pg
Path	Bostwick, D	VA	713
Path	Dahmoush, L	IA	715
Path	Epstein, J	MD	708
Path	True, L	WA	722
U	Soloway, M	FL	1164

Spec	Name	St	Pg	Spec	Name	St	Pg
U	Dalkin, B	WA	1175	U	Kirsch, A	GA	1162
U	Daneshmand, S	CA	1176	U	Kirschenbaum, A	NY	1154
U	Danoff, D	CA	1176	U	Klein, E	OH	1168
U	Davis, B	KS	1171	U	Klutke, C	MO	1168
U	DeKernion, J	CA	1176	U	Koch, M	IN	1168
U	Docimo, S	PA	1152	U	Kozlowski, J	IL	1168
U	Donovan, J	OH	1166	U	Landman, J	CA	1177
U	Droller, M	NY	1152	U	Lange, P	WA	1177

Urology

Spec	Name	St	Pg	Spec	Name	St	Pg	Spec	Name	St	Pg
U	Ahlering, T	CA	1175	U	Elder, J	MI	1166	U	Lanteri, V	NJ	1154
U	Albala, D	NY	1150	U	Ellis, W	WA	1176	U	Lee, C	MI	1168
U	Albertsen, P	CT	1148	U	Ewalt, D	TX	1173	U	Lepor, H	NY	1154
U	Alexander, R	MD	1151	U	Firlit, C	MO	1167	U	Lerner, S	TX	1173
U	Amling, C	OR	1175	U	Fisch, H	NY	1152	U	Levine, L	IL	1168
U	Andrews, P	AZ	1172	U	Flanigan, R	IL	1167	U	Libertino, J	MA	1149
U	Andriole, G	MO	1165	U	Foster, H	CT	1148	U	Lieskovsky, G	CA	1177
U	Atala, A	NC	1159	U	Foster, R	IN	1167	U	Lin, D	WA	1177
U	Babayan, R	MA	1148	U	Fraser, L	MS	1161	U	Linsenmeyer, T	NJ	1155
U	Badlani, G	NC	1159	U	Gearhart, J	MD	1152	U	Lipshultz, L	TX	1174
U	Bahnson, R	OH	1165	U	Gill, H	CA	1176	U	Lloyd, L	AL	1162
U	Balaji, K	NC	1160	U	Gill, I	CA	1176	U	Lockhart, J	FL	1162
U	Bans, L	AZ	1172	U	Ginsberg, D	CA	1176	U	Loo, M	NY	1155
U	Bar-Chama, N	NY	1151	U	Glassberg, K	NY	1152	U	Loughlin, K	MA	1149
U	Bardot, S	LA	1172	U	Gluckman, G	IL	1167	U	Lowe, F	NY	1155
U	Baskin, L	CA	1175	U	Goldstein, I	CA	1176	U	Lugg, J	WY	1172
U	Basler, J	TX	1172	U	Goldstein, M	NY	1152	U	Lynne, C	FL	1162
U	Bauer, S	MA	1148								

Spec	Name	St	Pg		Spec	Name	St	Pg		Spec	Name	St	Pg
U	Malkowicz, S	PA	1155		U	Scardino, P	NY	1157		U	Gribetz, M	NY	1153
U	Marsh, C	CA	1177		U	Schaeffer, A	IL	1170		U	Griebling, T	KS	1171
U	McAninch, J	CA	1177		U	Scherr, D	NY	1157		U	Gujral, S	MN	1167
U	McClure, R	WA	1177		U	Schlegel, P	NY	1157		U	Klutke, C	MO	1168
U	McConnell, J	NC	1162		U	Schoenberg, M	MD	1157		U	McGuire, E	MI	1168
U	McCullough, A	NY	1155		U	See, W	WI	1170		U	Nitti, V	NY	1156
U	McDougal, W	MA	1149		U	Seftel, A	NJ	1157		U	Raz, S	CA	1178
U	McGovern, F	MA	1149		U	Shaban, S	NC	1164		U	Schaeffer, A	IL	1170
U	McGuire, E	MI	1168		U	Shabsigh, R	NY	1157		U	Vapnek, J	NY	1159
U	McVary, K	IL	1168		U	Sharlip, I	CA	1178		U	Woo, H	LA	1175
U	Meacham, R	CO	1172		U	Sheinfeld, J	NY	1158					
U	Menon, M	MI	1169		U	Shenot, P	PA	1158		**Urology-Geriatric**			
U	Merguerian, P	WA	1178		U	Shortliffe, L	CA	1178		U	Griebling, T	KS	1171
U	Mesrobian, H	WI	1169		U	Siegelbaum, M	MD	1158					
U	Milam, D	TN	1162		U	Sigman, M	RI	1150		**Urticaria**			
U	Miles, B	TX	1174		U	Silber, S	MO	1170		A&I	Altman, L	WA	90
U	Miller, S	GA	1162		U	Singh, D	CT	1150		A&I	Bonner, J	AL	86
U	Mohler, J	NY	1155		U	Skinner, E	CA	1178		A&I	MacLean, J	MA	84
U	Montague, D	OH	1169		U	Slawin, K	TX	1174		A&I	Shepherd, G	NY	85
U	Montie, J	MI	1169		U	Smith, J	TN	1164		A&I	Spector, S	CA	91
U	Mostwin, J	MD	1155		U	Soloway, M	FL	1164		A&I	Sullivan, T	GA	87
U	Moul, J	NC	1162		U	Steers, W	VA	1164		A&I	Wasserman, S	CA	91
U	Mulhall, J	NY	1155		U	Steinberg, G	IL	1170		A&I	Wong, J	MA	84
U	Nagler, H	NY	1156		U	Stoller, M	CA	1179		D	Soter, N	NY	189
U	Naslund, M	MD	1156		U	Stone, A	CA	1179					
U	Nehra, A	IL	1169		U	Strand, W	TX	1174		**Uterine Cancer**			
U	Nelson, J	PA	1156		U	Strup, S	KY	1164		GO	Abu-Rustum, N	NY	276
U	Nitti, V	NY	1156		U	Su, L	FL	1164		GO	Azodi, M	CT	274
U	O'Donnell, M	IA	1169		U	Sundaram, C	IN	1170		GO	Barakat, R	NY	276
U	O'Leary, M	MA	1149		U	Sutherland, R	NC	1164		GO	Berchuck, A	NC	280
U	Oates, R	MA	1150		U	Takayama, T	WA	1179		GO	Berek, J	CA	289
U	Ohl, D	MI	1169		U	Taneja, S	NY	1158		GO	Burger, R	PA	276
U	Olumi, A	MA	1150		U	Teigland, C	NC	1164		GO	Burke, T	TX	287
U	Partin, A	MD	1156		U	Terris, M	GA	1165		GO	Cain, J	MA	274
U	Patel, V	FL	1162		U	Tewari, A	NY	1158		GO	Caputo, T	NY	276
U	Patterson, A	TN	1163		U	Thompson, I	TX	1174		GO	Chi, D	NY	277
U	Penson, D	TN	1163		U	Thrasher, J	KS	1172		GO	Copeland, L	OH	283
U	Pisters, L	TX	1174		U	Trabulsi, E	PA	1158		GO	Creasman, W	SC	280
U	Pope, J	TN	1163		U	Turek, P	CA	1179		GO	Curtin, J	NY	277
U	Poppas, D	NY	1156		U	Uzzo, R	PA	1158		GO	De Geest, K	IA	283
U	Porter, C	WA	1178		U	Van Arsdalen, K	PA	1158		GO	Dunton, C	PA	277
U	Pow-Sang, J	FL	1163		U	Vapnek, J	NY	1159		GO	Finan, M	AL	281
U	Preminger, G	NC	1163		U	Verghese, M	DC	1159		GO	Fiorica, J	FL	281
U	Presti, J	CA	1178		U	Wallen, E	NC	1165		GO	Goff, B	WA	289
U	Pruthi, R	NC	1163		U	Walsh, P	MD	1159		GO	King, S	PA	278
U	Rajfer, J	CA	1178		U	Wein, A	PA	1159		GO	Kline, R	LA	287
U	Raz, S	CA	1178		U	Weiss, R	NJ	1159		GO	Koulos, J	NY	278
U	Richie, J	MA	1150		U	Weiss, R	CT	1150		GO	Lu, K	TX	288
U	Rink, R	IN	1169		U	Wilson, T	CA	1179		GO	Lurain, J	IL	284
U	Robertson, C	NC	1163		U	Winfield, H	AL	1165		GO	Makhija, S	KY	282
U	Roehrborn, C	TX	1174		U	Wong, C	OH	1171		GO	Pejovic, T	OR	290
U	Ross, L	IL	1170		U	Woo, H	LA	1175		GO	Plaxe, S	CA	290
U	Rowland, R	KY	1163		U	Wood, D	MI	1171		GO	Rader, J	WI	285
U	Rushton, H	DC	1156		U	Yu, G	MD	1159		GO	Rice, L	WI	285
U	Sabanegh, E	OH	1170		U	Zippe, C	OH	1171		GO	Rose, P	OH	285
U	Sadeghi-Nejad, H	NJ	1156							GO	Rosenblum, N	PA	279
U	Sagalowsky, A	TX	1174		**Urology-Female**					GO	Rotmensch, J	IL	285
U	Samadi, D	NY	1157		U	Blaivas, J	NY	1151		GO	Rubin, S	PA	279
U	Sanda, M	MA	1150		U	Bushman, W	WI	1166		GO	Rutherford, T	CT	275
U	Sanders, W	GA	1163		U	Chancellor, M	MI	1166		GO	Schorge, J	MA	275
U	Sandlow, J	WI	1170		U	Foster, H	CT	1148					
U	Sawczuk, I	NJ	1157										

Spec	Name	St	Pg
GO	Schwartz, P	CT	275
GO	Smith, L	CA	290
GO	Waggoner, S	OH	286
GO	Walker, J	OK	288
MF	Leslie, K	IA	437
Onc	Scudder, S	CA	390
Onc	Spriggs, D	NY	350
Path	Kurman, R	MD	710
RadRO	Eifel, P	TX	964

Uterine Cancer-Serous Carcinoma

GO	Gershenson, D	TX	287

Uterine Fibroid Embolization

VIR	Benenati, J	FL	994
VIR	Cohen, G	PA	993
VIR	Durham, J	CO	996
VIR	Hallisey, M	CT	992
VIR	Haskal, Z	MD	993
VIR	Hovsepian, D	CA	998
VIR	Johnson, M	IN	995
VIR	Kaufman, J	OR	998
VIR	Keller, F	OR	998
VIR	Ketcham, D	MN	995
VIR	McLean, G	PA	993
VIR	Murphy, T	RI	992
VIR	Rilling, W	WI	996
VIR	Shlansky-Goldberg, R	PA	993
VIR	Smith, S	IL	996
VIR	Trerotola, S	PA	994
VIR	Vogelzang, R	IL	996
VIR	Weintraub, J	NY	994
VIR	White, R	CT	992

Uterine Fibroids

ObG	Bradley, L	OH	560
ObG	Famuyide, A	MN	561
ObG	Filip, S	NC	559
ObG	Goldstein, M	NY	557
ObG	Hockstein, S	NY	557
ObG	Jenkins, T	AL	559
ObG	Parker, W	CA	563
RE	Christman, G	MI	1012
RE	Clisham, P	LA	1015
RE	Durso, N	VA	1011
RE	Huang, J	TX	1016
RE	Marrs, R	CA	1017
RE	Milad, M	IL	1014
RE	Miller, C	IL	1014
RE	Molo, M	IL	1014
RE	Mukherjee, T	NY	1009
RE	Ory, S	FL	1012
RE	Putman, J	TX	1016
RE	Stewart, E	MN	1014
RE	Van Voorhis, B	IA	1015
RE	Wallach, E	MD	1010
RE	Wilson, E	TX	1016
RE	Zacur, H	MD	1011
RE	Zinaman, M	MA	1007

Spec	Name	St	Pg
VIR	Denny, D	NJ	993
VIR	Goodwin, S	CA	997
VIR	Roberts, A	CA	998

Uveitis

Oph	Dana, R	MA	570
Oph	Davis, J	FL	582
Oph	Foster, C	MA	570
Oph	Jabs, D	NY	575
Oph	Perez, V	FL	586
Oph	Petersen, M	OH	593
Oph	Smith, R	CA	604

Uveitis/AIDS

Oph	Rao, N	CA	603

V

Vaccinations in Pregnancy

ObG	Gonik, B	MI	561

Vaccine Therapy

GO	Coukos, G	PA	277
Hem	Stiff, P	IL	322
Onc	Carducci, M	MD	336
Onc	Chapman, P	NY	336
Onc	Kwak, L	TX	379
Onc	Laheru, D	MD	344
Onc	Maloney, D	WA	388
Onc	Peace, D	IL	370
Onc	Scheinberg, D	NY	348
Onc	Small, E	CA	391
Onc	Sotomayor, E	FL	362
Onc	Triozzi, P	OH	373
Onc	Wolchok, J	NY	352
S	Cole, D	SC	1068
S	Huth, J	TX	1089
S	Kaufman, H	IL	1078
T&CS	Altorki, N	NY	1113

Vaccine Therapy-Clinical Trials Only

Onc	Arlen, P	MD	334
Onc	Gulley, J	MD	341

Vaccines

PInf	Baker, C	TX	784
PInf	Bernstein, D	OH	783
PInf	Demmler-Harrison, G	TX	784
PInf	Edwards, K	TN	781
PInf	Long, S	PA	781
PInf	Offit, P	PA	781
PInf	Shapiro, E	CT	780

Spec	Name	St	Pg

Vaginal Cancer

GO	Smith, L	CA	290
RadRO	Eifel, P	TX	964

Vaginal Reconstruction

ObG	Cornella, J	AZ	563
ObG	Sanz, L	VA	559
ObG	Walters, M	OH	562

Vaginal/Uterine Abnormalities

RE	DeVane, G	FL	1011
RE	Schlaff, W	PA	1010

Vaginitis

Inf	Sobel, J	MI	417
RE	Winer, S	CA	1018

Valley Fever

Inf	Galgiani, J	AZ	418

Varicocele Embolization

VIR	Johnson, M	IN	995
VIR	Ketcham, D	MN	995
VIR	Shlansky-Goldberg, R	PA	993
VIR	Smith, S	IL	996
VIR	Trerotola, S	PA	994
VIR	Vogelzang, R	IL	996
VIR	White, R	CT	992

Varicocele in Adolescents

U	Glassberg, K	NY	1152
U	Kass, E	MI	1167

Varicocele Microsurgery

U	Bar-Chama, N	NY	1151
U	Goldstein, M	NY	1152
U	Nagler, H	NY	1156
U	Sandlow, J	WI	1170
U	Van Arsdalen, K	PA	1158

Vascular & Interventional Radiology

VIR	Aruny, J	CT	992
VIR	Benenati, J	FL	994
VIR	Brown, D	PA	992
VIR	Brown, K	NY	992
VIR	Cho, K	MI	995
VIR	Cohen, G	PA	993
VIR	Coldwell, D	KY	994
VIR	Dake, M	CA	997
VIR	Darcy, M	MO	995
VIR	Denny, D	NJ	993
VIR	Durham, J	CO	996
VIR	Geschwind, J	MD	993
VIR	Gomes, A	CA	997
VIR	Goodwin, S	CA	997
VIR	Hallisey, M	CT	992

Spec	Name	St	Pg
VIR	Haskal, Z	MD	993
VIR	Hicks, M	TX	997
VIR	Hovsepian, D	CA	998
VIR	Johnson, M	IN	995
VIR	Katzen, B	FL	994
VIR	Kaufman, J	OR	998
VIR	Kay, D	LA	997
VIR	Keller, F	OR	998
VIR	Ketcham, D	MN	995
VIR	Kumpe, D	CO	996
VIR	Lewis, C	GA	995
VIR	Matsumoto, A	VA	995
VIR	Mauro, R	NC	995
VIR	McGahan, J	CA	998
VIR	McLean, G	PA	993
VIR	Murphy, T	RI	992
VIR	Nemcek, A	IL	996
VIR	Rilling, W	WI	996
VIR	Roberts, A	CA	998
VIR	Salem, R	IL	996
VIR	Shlansky-Goldberg, R	PA	993
VIR	Smith, S	IL	996
VIR	Solomon, S	NY	993
VIR	Soulen, M	PA	994
VIR	Trerotola, S	PA	994
VIR	Valji, K	WA	998
VIR	Vogelzang, R	IL	996
VIR	Weintraub, J	NY	994
VIR	White, R	CT	992
VIR	Wood, B	MD	994
VIR	Yakes, W	CO	997

Vascular Birthmarks

Spec	Name	St	Pg
D	Eichenfield, L	CA	198
D	Frieden, I	CA	198
D	Garden, J	IL	193
D	Levy, M	TX	197
D	Treadwell, P	IN	195
PlS	Bauer, B	IL	864
PlS	Burns, A	TX	870

Vascular Disease

Spec	Name	St	Pg
N	Roos, K	IN	529
VascS	LaMuraglia, G	MA	1185
VascS	Pevec, W	CA	1194
VIR	Aruny, J	CT	992
VIR	Dake, M	CA	997
VIR	Matsumoto, A	VA	995
VIR	Nemcek, A	IL	996
VIR	Roberts, A	CA	998

Vascular Disease-Upper Extremity

Spec	Name	St	Pg
HS	Koman, L	NC	299

Vascular Lesions of the CNS

Spec	Name	St	Pg
NRad	Masaryk, T	OH	989
NRad	Teitelbaum, G	CA	991

Vascular Lesions-Head & Neck

Spec	Name	St	Pg
Oto	Persky, M	NY	663
Oto	Suen, J	AR	683

Vascular Malformations

Spec	Name	St	Pg
CG	Graham, J	CA	162
D	Bayliss, S	MO	192
D	Cohen, B	MD	185
D	Friedlander, S	CA	199
NRad	Berenstein, A	NY	985
NRad	Orbach, D	MA	985
NS	Lunsford, L	PA	476
NS	Walsh, J	LA	495
Oto	Waner, M	NY	666
Oto	Wong, B	CA	688
PlS	Boyajian, M	DC	852
PlS	Low, D	PA	855
PlS	Mulliken, J	MA	851
PlS	Persing, J	CT	851
PO	Cunningham, M	MA	789
VIR	Cho, K	MI	995
VIR	Gomes, A	CA	997
VIR	Haskal, Z	MD	993
VIR	Hovsepian, D	CA	998
VIR	Vogelzang, R	IL	996
VIR	Weintraub, J	NY	994
VIR	Yakes, W	CO	997

Vascular Medicine

Spec	Name	St	Pg
IC	Dieter, R	IL	131
IC	Khawaja, S	GA	130

Vascular Neurology

Spec	Name	St	Pg
N	Armon, C	MA	506
N	Tayal, A	PA	518
NRad	Drayer, B	NY	985

Vascular Neurosurgery

Spec	Name	St	Pg
NS	Couldwell, W	UT	491
NS	Dempsey, R	WI	487
NS	Frazee, J	CA	496
NS	Krisht, A	AR	493
NS	Martin, N	CA	498
NS	Rigamonti, D	MD	478
NS	Samson, D	TX	494
NS	Tamargo, R	MD	479
NS	Yonas, H	NM	495

Vascular Reconstruction

Spec	Name	St	Pg
VascS	Cherry, K	VA	1189
VascS	Kougias, P	TX	1193

Vascular Surgery

Spec	Name	St	Pg
S	Mannella, W	PA	1060
S	Traynor, M	ND	1086
T&CS	Diethrich, E	AZ	1137
T&CS	Safi, H	TX	1139
VascS	Acher, C	WI	1190

Spec	Name	St	Pg
VascS	Adelman, M	NY	1185
VascS	Ahn, S	CA	1193
VascS	Alexander, J	OH	1190
VascS	Annest, S	CO	1192
VascS	Atnip, R	PA	1185
VascS	Bandyk, D	CA	1194
VascS	Belkin, M	MA	1184
VascS	Benckart, D	PA	1185
VascS	Benvenisty, A	NY	1186
VascS	Berguer, R	MI	1190
VascS	Blebea, J	OK	1192
VascS	Brener, B	NJ	1186
VascS	Brewster, D	MA	1184
VascS	Calligaro, K	PA	1186
VascS	Cambria, R	MA	1184
VascS	Carpenter, J	NJ	1186
VascS	Chaikof, E	MA	1184
VascS	Cherry, K	VA	1189
VascS	Clair, D	OH	1190
VascS	Comerota, A	OH	1190
VascS	Cooper, M	CO	1192
VascS	Criado, F	MD	1186
VascS	Cronenwett, J	NH	1184
VascS	D'Ayala, M	NY	1186
VascS	Dalsing, M	IN	1190
VascS	Darling, R	NY	1186
VascS	Dattilo, J	TN	1189
VascS	Dougherty, M	PA	1186
VascS	Eidt, J	AR	1193
VascS	Fairman, R	PA	1187
VascS	Fantini, G	NY	1187
VascS	Faries, P	NY	1187
VascS	Flanigan, D	CA	1194
VascS	Flynn, T	FL	1189
VascS	Fowl, R	AZ	1193
VascS	Freischlag, J	MD	1187
VascS	Gewertz, B	CA	1194
VascS	Gloviczki, P	MN	1191
VascS	Golden, M	PA	1187
VascS	Green, R	NY	1187
VascS	Greisler, H	IL	1191
VascS	Hakaim, A	FL	1189
VascS	Hallett, J	SC	1189
VascS	Harrington, E	NY	1187
VascS	Hodgson, K	IL	1191
VascS	Hollier, L	LA	1193
VascS	Howard, T	NE	1192
VascS	Iafrati, M	MA	1184
VascS	Kazmers, A	MI	1191
VascS	Kent, K	WI	1191
VascS	Kougias, P	TX	1193
VascS	Kwolek, C	MA	1184
VascS	LaMuraglia, G	MA	1185
VascS	Lumsden, A	TX	1193
VascS	Mackey, W	MA	1185
VascS	Makaroun, M	PA	1187
VascS	Marin, M	NY	1188
VascS	McCann, R	NC	1189
VascS	McKinsey, J	NY	1188
VascS	McLafferty, R	IL	1191
VascS	Mitchell, M	MS	1189
VascS	Money, S	AZ	1193

Specialty & Special Expertise Index

Spec	Name	St	Pg
VascS	Morrissey, N	NY	1188
VascS	Naslund, T	TN	1190
VascS	Neville, R	DC	1188
VascS	Pearce, W	IL	1191
VascS	Perler, B	MD	1188
VascS	Pevec, W	CA	1194
VascS	Pomposelli, F	MA	1185
VascS	Ricotta, J	DC	1188
VascS	Riles, T	NY	1188
VascS	Sanchez, L	MO	1191
VascS	Schneider, D	NY	1188
VascS	Shepard, A	MI	1192
VascS	Sicard, G	MO	1192
VascS	Sobel, M	WA	1194
VascS	Stanley, J	MI	1192
VascS	Sumpio, B	CT	1185
VascS	Todd, G	NY	1189
VascS	Weinstein, E	CO	1192
VascS	White, R	CA	1194
VascS	Zarins, C	CA	1194

Vascular Surgery-Secondary

Spec	Name	St	Pg
VascS	Shepard, A	MI	1192

Vasculitis

Spec	Name	St	Pg
D	Callen, J	KY	190
D	Soter, N	NY	189
N	Lisak, R	MI	527
Nep	Falk, R	NC	459
Nep	Salant, D	MA	456
PRhu	Finkel, T	FL	800
PRhu	Goldsmith, D	PA	799
PRhu	McCarthy, P	CT	799
PRhu	Myones, B	TX	801
PRhu	Sills, E	MD	800
PRhu	Wagner-Weiner, L	IL	800
Pul	Henke, D	NC	931
Rhu	Allen, N	NC	1029
Rhu	Blume, R	NY	1025
Rhu	Coblyn, J	MA	1024
Rhu	Cupps, T	DC	1026
Rhu	Katz, R	IL	1031
Rhu	Kimberly, R	AL	1030
Rhu	Lahita, R	NJ	1027
Rhu	Langford, C	OH	1031
Rhu	Lawry, G	CA	1034
Rhu	Paget, S	NY	1027
Rhu	Peng, S	WA	1034
Rhu	Sergent, J	TN	1030
Rhu	Spiera, H	NY	1028
Rhu	Wener, M	WA	1034
Rhu	West, S	CO	1032

Vasculitis of the Nervous System

Spec	Name	St	Pg
N	Vollmer, T	CO	532

Vasectomy

Spec	Name	St	Pg
U	Irby, P	NC	1161

Spec	Name	St	Pg
U	Sabanegh, E	OH	1170
U	Sanders, W	GA	1163

Vasectomy & Vasectomy Reversal

Spec	Name	St	Pg
U	Goldstein, M	NY	1152
U	Sandlow, J	WI	1170

Vasectomy Reversal

Spec	Name	St	Pg
U	Bar-Chama, N	NY	1151
U	Beall, M	VA	1160
U	Buch, J	TX	1173
U	Davis, B	KS	1171
U	Fisch, H	NY	1152
U	Janeiro, J	NH	1149
U	Meacham, R	CO	1172
U	Nagler, H	NY	1156
U	Oates, R	MA	1150
U	Sabanegh, E	OH	1170
U	Sharlip, I	CA	1178
U	Sigman, M	RI	1150
U	Silber, S	MO	1170
U	Turek, P	CA	1179
U	Van Arsdalen, K	PA	1158

Vein Disorders

Spec	Name	St	Pg
VascS	Adelman, M	NY	1185
VascS	Flanigan, D	CA	1194
VascS	Gloviczki, P	MN	1191
VascS	Iafrati, M	MA	1184
VascS	Lumsden, A	TX	1193
VascS	Ricotta, J	DC	1188
VascS	Sobel, M	WA	1194
VIR	Aruny, J	CT	992
VIR	Lewis, C	GA	995

Ventilation Management-Long Term

Spec	Name	St	Pg
PPul	Warren, R	AR	797

Ventricular Assist Device (LVAD)

Spec	Name	St	Pg
Cv	Horn, E	NY	99
Cv	O'Connell, J	GA	105
Cv	Smart, F	LA	115
Cv	Young, J	OH	113
T&CS	Acker, M	PA	1113
T&CS	Bolman, R	MA	1110
T&CS	Elefteriades, J	CT	1110
T&CS	Lansman, S	NY	1119
T&CS	Magovern, G	PA	1119
T&CS	McCarthy, P	IL	1133
T&CS	Morris, R	PA	1120
T&CS	Naka, Y	NY	1120
T&CS	Samuels, L	PA	1121
T&CS	Slaughter, M	KY	1129
T&CS	Smedira, N	OH	1135
T&CS	Staples, E	FL	1129

Ventricular Assist Device (VAD)

Spec	Name	St	Pg
T&CS	Szeto, W	PA	1122

Ventricular Assist Device(LVAD)

Spec	Name	St	Pg
T&CS	Tedder, M	TN	1130

Ventricular Septal Defect (Amplatzer R)

Spec	Name	St	Pg
PCd	Zahn, E	CA	741

Ventricular Tachycardia Ablation

Spec	Name	St	Pg
CE	Donahue, J	OH	122
CE	Lewkowiez, L	CO	124
CE	Link, M	MA	119

Vesicoureteral Reflux (VUR)

Spec	Name	St	Pg
U	Shortliffe, L	CA	1178

Video Assisted Thoracic Surgery (VATS)

Spec	Name	St	Pg
T&CS	Flores, R	NY	1115
T&CS	Gharagozloo, F	DC	1116
T&CS	Landreneau, R	PA	1119
T&CS	Naunheim, K	MO	1134
T&CS	Pechet, T	PA	1120
T&CS	Scott, W	PA	1121
T&CS	Swanson, S	MA	1112

Viral Infections

Spec	Name	St	Pg
Inf	Luby, J	TX	418
Inf	Polsky, B	NY	413
Inf	Van Der Horst, C	NC	415
PInf	Andiman, W	CT	779
PInf	Bernstein, D	OH	783
PInf	Christenson, J	IN	783
PInf	Demmler-Harrison, G	TX	784
PInf	Jacobs, R	AR	784
PInf	Mitchell, C	FL	782
Pul	Jacoby, D	OR	940

Vision-Unexplained Loss

Spec	Name	St	Pg
N	Schatz, N	FL	523
Oph	Borchert, M	CA	599

Visual Perception & Learning Disorders

Spec	Name	St	Pg
Oph	Koller, H	PA	576

Vitiligo

Spec	Name	St	Pg
D	Grimes, P	CA	199
D	Lim, H	MI	194
D	Nigra, T	DC	187

Spec	Name	St	Pg

Vocal Cord Disorders

Spec	Name	St	Pg
Oto	Donovan, D	TX	681
Oto	Hogikyan, N	MI	675
Oto	Mirza, N	PA	662
Oto	Netterville, J	TN	669
Oto	Ossoff, R	TN	669
Oto	Shapshay, S	NY	665
Oto	Stasney, C	TX	683
Oto	Stenson, K	IL	678
Oto	Sulica, R	NY	666
PO	Parikh, S	WA	793
Pul	Martin, R	CO	937

Vocal Cord Disorders-Botox Therapy

Spec	Name	St	Pg
Oto	Clark, K	OK	681

Voice after Laryngeal Cancer Surgery

Spec	Name	St	Pg
Oto	Deschler, D	MA	655

Voice Disorders

Spec	Name	St	Pg
Oto	Abaza, M	CO	679
Oto	Aviv, J	NY	657
Oto	Bastian, R	IL	673
Oto	Benninger, M	OH	673
Oto	Berke, G	CA	684
Oto	Blitzer, A	NY	658
Oto	Burns, J	MA	655
Oto	Clark, K	OK	681
Oto	Corey, J	IL	674
Oto	Donovan, D	TX	681
Oto	Flint, P	OR	685
Oto	Ford, C	WI	674
Oto	Grillone, G	MA	655
Oto	Hoffman, H	IA	675
Oto	Hogikyan, N	MI	675
Oto	Koufman, J	NY	661
Oto	Mirza, N	PA	662
Oto	Ossoff, R	TN	669
Oto	Postma, G	GA	670
Oto	Rosen, C	PA	664
Oto	Sasaki, C	CT	657
Oto	Sataloff, R	PA	664
Oto	Schley, W	NY	665
Oto	Silverman, D	VT	657
Oto	Sinha, U	CA	687
Oto	Stasney, C	TX	683
Oto	Strome, M	NY	665
Oto	Sulica, R	NY	666
Oto	Weissler, M	NC	672
Oto	Wilson, K	OH	678
Oto	Woo, P	NY	666
Oto	Woodson, G	IL	679
Oto	Zeitels, S	MA	657
PO	Goldsmith, A	NY	789
PO	Holinger, L	IL	791
PO	Inglis, A	WA	793

Voiding Dysfunction

Spec	Name	St	Pg
Ger	Resnick, N	PA	263
U	Bloom, D	MI	1165
U	Broderick, G	FL	1160
U	Childs, S	CO	1171
U	Culkin, D	OK	1173
U	Docimo, S	PA	1152
U	Foster, H	CT	1148
U	Gomery, P	MA	1148
U	Kaplan, S	NY	1154
U	Kennelly, M	NC	1161
U	Lockhart, J	FL	1162
U	Loo, M	NY	1155
U	Milam, D	TN	1162
U	Nitti, V	NY	1156
U	Roehrborn, C	TX	1174
U	Shenot, P	PA	1158
U	Stone, A	CA	1179
U	Woo, H	LA	1175

Voiding Dysfunction/Spinal Cord Injury

Spec	Name	St	Pg
U	Linsenmeyer, T	NJ	1155
U	Lynne, C	FL	1162
U	Shenot, P	PA	1158

Vomiting-Cyclic

Spec	Name	St	Pg
CG	Boles, R	CA	162
MF	Wapner, R	NY	434
ObG	Niebyl, J	IA	562

Von Hippel-Lindau Disease

Spec	Name	St	Pg
NS	Barnett, G	OH	486
NS	Olson, J	GA	483
S	Carty, S	PA	1055

Von Willebrand's Disease

Spec	Name	St	Pg
Hem	Bockenstedt, P	MI	319

Vulvar & Vaginal Cancer

Spec	Name	St	Pg
GO	Berek, J	CA	289
GO	Burke, T	TX	287
GO	Kline, R	LA	287
GO	Muto, M	MA	275
GO	Potkul, R	IL	285
GO	Santin, A	CT	275

Vulvar & Vaginal Disorders

Spec	Name	St	Pg
ObG	Eschenbach, D	WA	563
ObG	Levine, E	IL	562
ObG	Snyder, R	TX	563

Vulvar Disease/Cancer

Spec	Name	St	Pg
GO	Abu-Rustum, N	NY	276
GO	Caputo, T	NY	276
GO	Levenback, C	TX	288
GO	Modesitt, S	VA	282

Spec	Name	St	Pg
GO	Rosenblum, N	PA	279
GO	Smith, L	CA	290
GO	Stern, J	CA	291
RadRO	Eifel, P	TX	964

Vulvar Pain

Spec	Name	St	Pg
ObG	Levine, E	IL	562
U	Goldstein, I	CA	1176

W

Waldenstrom's Macroglobulinemia

Spec	Name	St	Pg
Hem	Gertz, M	MN	319
Onc	Coleman, M	NY	337
Onc	Czuczman, M	NY	337

Weaver Syndrome

Spec	Name	St	Pg
CG	Weaver, D	IN	160

Wegener's Granulomatosis

Spec	Name	St	Pg
Nep	Falk, R	NC	459
Rhu	Allen, N	NC	1029
Rhu	Belmont, H	NY	1025

Weight Management

Spec	Name	St	Pg
EDM	Broadstone, V	IN	216
Ge	Kaplan, L	MA	229
PEn	Wilson, D	CA	749
PGe	Krebs, N	CO	754

White Matter Disorders

Spec	Name	St	Pg
PMR	Evans, S	DC	835

Whooping Cough

Spec	Name	St	Pg
PInf	Long, S	PA	781

Williams Syndrome

Spec	Name	St	Pg
CG	Marion, R	NY	158
CG	Morris, C	NV	163

Wilms' Tumor

Spec	Name	St	Pg
PHO	Dome, J	DC	759
PHO	Green, D	TN	766
PHO	Plautz, G	OH	772
PHO	Steinherz, P	NY	764
PS	Ehrlich, P	MI	807
PS	Shamberger, R	MA	802
U	Hensle, T	NJ	1153

Wiskott-Aldrich Syndrome

Spec	Name	St	Pg
PHO	Bussel, J	NY	758

Specialty & Special Expertise Index

Spec	Name	St	Pg

Women & Addiction

| AdP | Greenfield, S | MA | 904 |

Women's Eye Health

| Oph | Vajaranant, T | IL | 595 |

Women's Health

Cv	Andersen, H	NY	96
Cv	Goldberg, N	NY	98
Cv	Johnson, P	MA	94
Ge	Borum, M	DC	231
GO	Husain, A	CA	290
IM	Cirigliano, M	PA	424
Inf	Cohn, S	IL	416
MF	Repke, J	PA	433
N	Liporace, J	PA	514
ObG	Argenta, P	MN	560
ObG	Bradshaw, K	TX	563
ObG	King, A	ID	562
ObG	Morgan, L	FL	559
ObG	Sweet, R	CA	563
Onc	Chlebowski, R	CA	384
RE	Blackwell, R	AL	1011
Rhu	Fife, R	IN	1031

Women's Health-Mental Health

| Psyc | Burt, V | CA | 900 |
| Psyc | Zerbe, K | OR | 903 |

Women's Health/Disabilities

| PMR | Kirschner, K | IL | 840 |

Women's Imaging

| DR | Edelstein, B | NY | 975 |
| DR | Thurmond, A | OR | 984 |

Wound Healing/Care

D	Arpey, C	MN	192
D	Falanga, V	RI	182
D	Fivenson, D	MI	193
D	Kirsner, R	FL	191
Ger	Thomas, D	MO	265
PlS	Attinger, C	DC	852
PlS	Garner, W	CA	874
PlS	Molnar, J	NC	863
PlS	Orgill, D	MA	851
S	Bessey, P	NY	1053
S	Buchman, T	GA	1067
S	Cairns, B	NC	1067
S	Dixon, S	NV	1095
S	Edington, H	PA	1057
S	Greenhalgh, D	CA	1096
S	Lentz, C	NM	1090
S	Luterman, A	AL	1070
S	Mannella, W	PA	1060
S	Ryan, C	MA	1051
S	Saffle, J	UT	1086
S	Yurt, R	NY	1066

Spec	Name	St	Pg
VascS	Iafrati, M	MA	1184
VascS	Neville, R	DC	1188

WPW Syndrome

| CE | Morady, F | MI | 123 |
| CE | Swerdlow, C | CA | 125 |

Wrist Reconstruction

| HS | Kleinman, W | IN | 301 |

Wrist Surgery

HS	Badia, A	FL	298
HS	Cohen, M	IL	300
HS	Hastings, H	IN	301
HS	Mass, D	IL	301
HS	Melone, C	NY	297
HS	Nagle, D	IL	302
HS	Osterman, A	PA	297
HS	Putnam, M	MN	302
HS	Seitz, W	OH	302
HS	Weiss, A	RI	294
HS	Wolfe, S	NY	298
OrS	Hotchkiss, R	NY	620

Wrist/Hand Injuries

HS	Collins, E	TX	303
HS	Graham, T	OH	301
HS	Raskin, K	NY	297
HS	Thoder, J	PA	298
HS	Weiland, A	NY	298

Z

Zenker Diverticulum

| Oto | Sasaki, C | CT | 657 |

Zollinger-Ellison Syndrome

| Ge | Wilcox, C | AL | 243 |

Alphabetical Listing of Doctors

Name	Specialty	Pg
A		
Abaza, Mona (CO)	Oto	679
Abbas, Fouad (MD)	GO	275
Abbitt, Patricia (FL)	DR	978
Abbott, Richard (CA)	Oph	598
Abbruzzese, James (TX)	Onc	376
Abcarian, Herand (IL)	CRS	173
Abdu, William (NH)	OrS	610
Abecassis, Michael (IL)	S	1074
Abi-samra, Freddy (LA)	Cv	113
Abou-Khalil, Bassel (TN)	N	519
Aboulafia, Albert (MD)	OrS	613
Aboulafia, David (WA)	Onc	383
Abouljoud, Marwan (MI)	S	1074
Abraham, Jame (WV)	Onc	333
Abrahamson, Martin (MA)	EDM	206
Abrahm, Janet (MA)	H & PM	406
Abram, Stephen (WI)	PM	699
Abrams, Charles (PA)	Hem	311
Abrams, Donald (CA)	Onc	383
Abrams, Gary (MI)	Oph	587
Abrams, Reid (CA)	HS	303
Abrams, Ross (IL)	RadRO	958
Abramson, David (NY)	Oph	571
Abrass, Itamar (WA)	Ger	266
Abreu, Maria (FL)	Ge	239
Abright, A Reese (NY)	ChAP	907
Abromowitch, Minnie (NE)	PHO	774
Abu-Rustum, Nadeem (NY)	GO	276
Abuhamad, Alfred (VA)	MF	434
Acher, Charles (WI)	VascS	1190
Acker, David (MA)	MF	430
Acker, Michael (PA)	T&CS	1113
Ackerman, Michael (MN)	PCd	738
Adam, Karolina (TX)	MF	438
Adams, David (FL)	N	519
Adams, David (NY)	T&CS	1113
Adams, Elaine (IL)	Rhu	1030
Adams, Harold (IA)	N	524
Adams, James (TX)	NP	451
Adams, Reid (VA)	S	1066
Adams, Robert (SC)	N	519
Adams, Roberta (AZ)	Hem	323
Adams-Graves, Patricia (TN)	Hem	316
Adamson, G David (CA)	RE	1016
Adamson, Peter (PA)	PHO	758
Adashek, Joseph (NV)	MF	439
Adelman, Mark (NY)	VascS	1185
Adelson, P David (AZ)	NS	492
Adelstein, David (OH)	Onc	364
Adger, Hoover (MD)	AM	80
Adler, David (MA)	Psyc	888
Adler, Ronald (NY)	DR	974
Adornato, Bruce (CA)	N	535
Advani, Ranjana (CA)	Onc	383
Adzick, N Scott (PA)	PS	802
Afshari, Natalie (NC)	Oph	581
Agarwal, Animesh (TX)	OrS	640
Agarwal, Sanjay (CA)	RE	1016
Agarwala, Brojendra (IL)	PCd	738
Aghajanian, Carol (NY)	Onc	333
Agress, Harry (NJ)	NuM	548
Ahern, Geoffrey (AZ)	N	532
Ahlering, Thomas (CA)	U	1175
Ahlgren, James (DC)	Onc	333
Ahlskog, J Eric (MN)	N	524
Ahmad, Amjad (IL)	Oph	588
Ahmad, Suhail (WA)	Nep	464
Ahmann, Andrew (OR)	EDM	221
Ahmann, Frederick (AZ)	Onc	376
Ahn, Jung (NY)	PMR	834
Ahn, Sam (CA)	VascS	1193
Ahya, Vivek (PA)	Pul	924
Aiken, John (WI)	PS	806
Ain, Kenneth (KY)	EDM	213
Aisner, Joseph (NJ)	Onc	334
Ajani, Jaffer (TX)	Onc	377
Akatsu, Haruko (CA)	EDM	222
Akerley, Wallace (UT)	Onc	374
Akervall, Jan (MI)	Oto	672
Akhtar, Salman (PA)	Psyc	890
Akins, Cary (MA)	T&CS	1110
Aklog, Lishan (AZ)	T&CS	1137
Al-Kawas, Firas (DC)	Ge	230
Al-Mefty, Ossama (MA)	NS	470
Alam, Daniel (OH)	Oto	672
Alavi, Abass (PA)	NuM	548

Alphabetical Listing of Doctors

Name	Specialty	Pg	Name	Specialty	Pg
Alazraki, Naomi (GA)	NuM	549	Altorki, Nasser (NY)	T&CS	1113
Albain, Kathy (IL)	Onc	364	Alvarez, Ronald (AL)	GO	280
Albala, David (NY)	U	1150	Alvarez-Elcoro, Salvador (FL)	Inf	414
Albanese, Craig (CA)	PS	810	Alward, Wallace (IA)	Oph	588
Albers, Gregory (CA)	N	535	Aly, Al Said (CA)	PlS	872
Albert, Daniel (WI)	Oph	588	Amar, Arun (CA)	NS	495
Albert, Daniel (NH)	Rhu	1024	Amato, Anthony (MA)	N	506
Albert, Michael (DC)	Ge	230	Ambinder, Richard (MD)	Onc	334
Albert, Todd (PA)	OrS	613	Amedee, Ronald (LA)	Oto	681
Albertini, Mark (WI)	Onc	364	Ames, Christopher (CA)	NS	495
Alberts, David (AZ)	Onc	377	Ames, Frederick (TX)	S	1086
Alberts, Mark (IL)	N	524	Amin, Mahul (CA)	Path	719
Alberts, W Michael (FL)	Pul	929	Aminoff, Michael (CA)	N	535
Albertsen, Peter (CT)	U	1148	Amling, Christopher (OR)	U	1175
Albertson, Timothy (CA)	Pul	938	Amonette, Rex (TN)	D	189
Albright, John (IA)	OrS	631	An, Howard (IL)	OrS	632
Albritton, Karen (TX)	PHO	775	Anand, Kanwaljeet (TN)	PCCM	741
Aldea, Gabriel (WA)	T&CS	1140	Anday, Endla (PA)	NP	446
Aledo, Alexander (NY)	PHO	758	Andersen, Glenna (VA)	ObG	559
Alessi, Norman (MI)	ChAP	910	Andersen, Holly (NY)	Cv	96
Alexander, Frederick (NJ)	PS	802	Andersen, James (CA)	PlS	873
Alexander, H Richard (MD)	S	1053	Andersen, Peter (OR)	Oto	684
Alexander, J Jeffrey (OH)	VascS	1190	Anderson, Benjamin (WA)	S	1093
Alexander, Joshua (NC)	PMR	838	Anderson, Jeffrey (UT)	Cv	113
Alexander, Kenneth (IL)	PInf	782	Anderson, Karl (TX)	Ge	250
Alexander, Richard (MD)	U	1151	Anderson, Kenneth (MA)	Hem	310
Alexandrov, Andrei (AL)	N	519	Anderson, Lesley (CA)	OrS	641
Alfonso, Antonio (NY)	S	1053	Anderson, Mark (IA)	CE	122
Alfonso, Eduardo (FL)	Oph	581	Anderson, Martin (CA)	AM	82
Algazy, Kenneth (PA)	Onc	334	Anderson, Richard (MA)	D	182
Allen, David (WI)	PEn	746	Anderson, Richard (UT)	Oph	595
Allen, Jeffrey (NY)	ChiN	147	Andersson, Hans (LA)	CG	161
Allen, Nancy (NC)	Rhu	1029	Andiman, Warren (CT)	PInf	779
Allen, Robert (SC)	PlS	860	Andreoli, Sharon (IN)	PNep	787
Allen, Steven (NY)	Hem	311	Andreoni, Kenneth (FL)	S	1066
Allman, Richard (PA)	Rhu	1025	Andrews, David (PA)	NS	472
Allman, Richard (AL)	Ger	263	Andrews, James (FL)	SM	1042
Allon, Michael (AL)	Nep	459	Andrews, Paul (AZ)	U	1172
Allred, D Craig (MO)	Path	714	Andrews, Robert (WA)	PHO	776
Alpert, Joseph (AZ)	Cv	113	Andrews, Walter (MO)	PS	806
Alster, Tina (DC)	D	184	Andrews, William (AL)	MF	434
Altchek, David (NY)	SM	1040	Andriole, Gerald (MO)	U	1165
Alter, Craig (PA)	PEn	744	Ang, Kie-Kian (TX)	RadRO	963
Alter, Gary (CA)	PlS	872	Angelos, Peter (IL)	S	1074
Altman, Arnold (CT)	PHO	756	Anghelescu, Doralina (TN)	PM	698
Altman, Leonard (WA)	A&I	90	Angiolillo, Anne (DC)	PHO	758

Name	Specialty	Pg	Name	Specialty	Pg
Anglen, Jeffrey (IN)	OrS	632	Arriaga, Moises (LA)	Oto	681
Anhalt, Grant (MD)	D	184	Arroliga, Alejandro (TX)	Pul	938
Annest, Stephen (CO)	VascS	1192	Arslanian, Silva (PA)	PEn	744
Anscher, Mitchell (VA)	RadRO	953	Arteaga, Carlos (TN)	Onc	353
Anthony, Lowell (KY)	Onc	353	Arts, H Alexander (MI)	Oto	672
Antin, Joseph (MA)	Onc	327	Arun, Banu (TX)	Onc	377
Anton, Raymond (SC)	AdP	905	Aruny, John (CT)	VIR	992
Antonescu, Cristina (NY)	Path	707	Ascher, Nancy (CA)	S	1093
Antonia, Scott (FL)	Onc	353	Ascherman, Jeffrey (NY)	PlS	852
Antony, Veena (AL)	Pul	929	Aseff, John (DC)	PMR	835
Anyane-Yeboa, Kwame (NY)	CG	156	Asher, Anthony (NC)	NS	481
Apatoff, Brian (NY)	N	509	Ashizawa, Tetsuo (FL)	N	520
Appel, Gerald (NY)	Nep	456	Ashley, Stanley (MA)	S	1048
Appelbaum, Frederick (WA)	Onc	383	Ashwal, Stephen (CA)	ChiN	153
Appelbaum, Paul (NY)	Psyc	890	Asirvatham, Samuel (MN)	CE	122
Appelman, Henry (MI)	Path	714	Aslanian, Harry (CT)	Ge	228
Applegate, Robert (NC)	IC	129	Asnis, Peter (MA)	SM	1040
April, Max (NY)	PO	789	Aston, Sherrell (NY)	PlS	852
Apuzzo, Michael (CA)	NS	495	Astrow, Alan (NY)	Onc	334
Aranha, Gerard (IL)	S	1074	Atala, Anthony (NC)	U	1159
Arber, Daniel (CA)	Path	719	Athanasian, Edward (NY)	HS	295
Arcasoy, Selim (NY)	Pul	924	Athanasuleas, Constantine (AL)	T&CS	1123
Arceci, Robert (MD)	PHO	758	Atkins, Michael (DC)	Onc	334
Archdeacon, Michael (OH)	OrS	632	Atkinson, John (MN)	NS	485
Archer, Steven (MI)	Oph	588	Atkinson, Robert (HI)	HS	303
Arendt, Elizabeth (MN)	SM	1043	Atlas, Scott (CA)	NRad	990
Arensman, Robert (IL)	PS	806	Atnip, Robert (PA)	VascS	1185
Argenta, Peter (MN)	ObG	560	Attas, Lewis (NJ)	Onc	334
Argenziano, Michael (NY)	T&CS	1113	Attinger, Christopher (DC)	PlS	852
Argiris, Athanassios (TX)	Onc	377	Audell, Laura (CA)	PM	702
Argoff, Charles (NY)	PM	696	Auger, William (CA)	Pul	939
Ariyan, Stephan (CT)	PlS	850	Augsburger, James (OH)	Oph	588
Arjmand, Ellis (OH)	PO	791	August, David (NJ)	S	1053
Arlen, Philip (MD)	Onc	334	August, Phyllis (NY)	Nep	457
Armitage, James (NE)	Onc	374	Ault, Bettina (TN)	PNep	786
Armon, Carmel (MA)	N	506	Austin, John (NY)	DR	974
Arnason, Barry (IL)	N	524	Auwaerter, Paul (MD)	Inf	410
Arndt, Carola (MN)	PHO	769	Averbook, Bruce (OH)	S	1074
Arndt, Kenneth (MA)	D	182	Avery, Eric (TX)	Psyc	899
Arnold, Anthony (CA)	Oph	598	Aviv, Jonathan (NY)	Oto	657
Arnold, James (OH)	PO	791	Avram, Marc (NY)	D	184
Arnold, Robert (PA)	H & PM	406	Awan, Azhar (IL)	RadRO	958
Arnold, Steven (PA)	Psyc	890	Axelrod, Deborah (NY)	S	1053
Aronchick, Craig (PA)	Ge	230	Axelrod, Lloyd (MA)	EDM	206
Aronson, James (AR)	OrS	640	Axelrod, Rita (PA)	Onc	335
Arpey, Christopher (MN)	D	192	Azar, Dimitri (IL)	Oph	588

Alphabetical Listing of Doctors

Name	Specialty	Pg	Name	Specialty	Pg
Azar, Nathalie (IL)	Oph	588	Baker, Emily (NH)	MF	430
Azizi, Sayed (PA)	N	509	Baker, James (MI)	A&I	87
Azodi, Masoud (CT)	GO	274	Baker, John (MI)	Oph	588
Azziz, Ricardo (GA)	RE	1011	Baker, Robert (NY)	PGe	750
Azzoli, Christopher (NY)	Onc	335	Baker, Shan (MI)	Oto	673
			Baker, Stephen (DC)	PlS	852
			Baker, Susan (NY)	PGe	750
			Bakhos, Mamdouh (IL)	T&CS	1130
B			Bakken, Johan (MN)	Inf	416
Babayan, Richard (MA)	U	1148	Bakris, George (IL)	IM	425
Babiera, Gildy (TX)	S	1087	Balady, Gary (MA)	Cv	94
Bach, Bernard (IL)	OrS	632	Balaji, K (NC)	U	1160
Bach, John (NJ)	PMR	835	Balart, Luis (LA)	Ge	250
Bach, Richard (MO)	IC	130	Balcer, Laura (PA)	N	509
Bacha, Emile (NY)	T&CS	1114	Baldassano, Robert (PA)	PGe	750
Baciewicz, Frank (MI)	T&CS	1130	Balderston, Richard (PA)	OrS	614
Back, Anthony (WA)	Onc	383	Baldridge, Alan (NJ)	PGe	750
Backer, Carl (IL)	T&CS	1130	Balducci, Lodovico (FL)	Onc	353
Bacon, Bruce (MO)	Ge	243	Bale, Allen (CT)	CG	156
Bader, Thomas (PA)	ObG	556	Bale, James (UT)	ChiN	152
Badia, Alejandro (FL)	HS	298	Balk, Robert (IL)	Pul	933
Badie, Behnam (CA)	NS	495	Balkany, Thomas (FL)	Oto	667
Badlani, Gopal (NC)	U	1159	Ball, Douglas (MD)	EDM	208
Baer, Maria (MD)	Hem	312	Ball, Edward (CA)	Onc	383
Baerveldt, George (CA)	Oph	598	Ball, William (OH)	NRad	988
Bagg, Adam (PA)	Path	708	Balla, Andre (IL)	Path	715
Bahado-Singh, Ray (MI)	MF	435	Ballantyne, Christie (TX)	Cv	114
Bahn, Duke (CA)	DR	982	Ballantyne, Garth (GA)	S	1066
Bahn, Rebecca (MN)	EDM	216	Ballantyne, Jane (WA)	PM	702
Bahna, Sami (LA)	PA&I	732	Ballard, Pamela (DC)	PMR	835
Bahnson, Robert (OH)	U	1165	Ballas, Zuhair (IA)	A&I	87
Baile, Walter (TX)	Psyc	899	Ballen, Karen (MA)	Hem	310
Bailes, Julian (IL)	NS	485	Ballon-Landa, Gonzalo (CA)	Inf	419
Bailey, H Randolph (TX)	CRS	176	Balmes, John (CA)	Pul	939
Bailey, Leonard (CA)	T&CS	1140	Baltimore, Robert (CT)	PInf	779
Bailey, Steven (TX)	IC	132	Baltuch, Gordon (PA)	NS	472
Bailin, Philip (OH)	D	192	Bancalari, Eduardo (FL)	NP	448
Baillie, John (NC)	Ge	239	Bandyk, Dennis (CA)	VascS	1194
Baim, Howard (IL)	Oto	672	Banerjee, Anuradha (CA)	PHO	776
Bains, Manjit (NY)	T&CS	1114	Banks, Peter (NC)	Path	713
Bairey, Cathleen Noel (CA)	Cv	116	Bans, Larry (AZ)	U	1172
Bajorin, Dean (NY)	Onc	335	Bar-Chama, Natan (NY)	U	1151
Bakay, Roy (IL)	NS	485	Barakat, Richard (NY)	GO	276
Baker, Carol (TX)	PInf	784	Baratz, Mark (PA)	HS	295
Baker, Christopher (VA)	S	1066	Barbosa, Victoria (IL)	D	192
Baker, Daniel (NY)	PlS	852	Bardot, Stephen (LA)	U	1172

Name	Specialty	Pg	Name	Specialty	Pg
Barger, Geoffrey (MI)	N	524	Bauman, Phillip (NY)	OrS	614
Barie, Philip (NY)	S	1053	Baumann, Patricia (GA)	PM	698
Barkin, Jamie (FL)	Ge	239	Bavaria, Joseph (PA)	T&CS	1114
Barkley, Gregory (MI)	N	525	Bayer, Arnold (CA)	Inf	419
Barkovich, A James (CA)	NRad	990	Bayless, Theodore (MD)	Ge	230
Barksdale, Edward (OH)	PS	806	Baylis, Henry (CA)	Oph	598
Barlogie, Bart (AR)	Hem	323	Bayliss, Susan (MO)	D	192
Barnes, David (OH)	Ge	244	Bazari, Hasan (MA)	Nep	456
Barnes, Patrick (CA)	NRad	990	Beall, Michael (VA)	U	1160
Barnes, Randall (IL)	RE	1012	Beals, Stephen (AZ)	PlS	870
Barnes, Willard (DC)	GO	276	Bear, Harry (VA)	S	1067
Barnett, Gene (OH)	NS	486	Beart, Robert (CA)	CRS	177
Barohn, Richard (KS)	N	531	Beaser, Richard (MA)	EDM	206
Baron, Joseph (IL)	Hem	318	Beasley, Michael (NC)	PlS	860
Baron, Todd (MN)	Ge	244	Beatty, Charles (MN)	Oto	673
Barone, Constance (TX)	PlS	869	Beatty, Patrick (MT)	Onc	374
Barredo, Julio (FL)	PHO	765	Beaty, James (TN)	OrS	627
Barrett, Eugene (VA)	EDM	213	Beauchamp, Robert (TN)	S	1067
Barrow, Daniel (GA)	NS	481	Bebin, E Martina (AL)	N	520
Bartelsmeyer, James (MO)	MF	435	Beck, David (LA)	CRS	176
Barter, James (MD)	GO	276	Beck, Sandra (KY)	CRS	171
Bartholomew, Deborah (OH)	ObG	560	Becker, Dorothy (PA)	PEn	744
Bartholomew, Dennis (OH)	CG	160	Becker, Ferdinand (FL)	Oto	667
Bartlett, David (PA)	S	1053	Becker, James (MA)	S	1048
Bartlett, John (MD)	Inf	410	Becker, Kyra (WA)	N	535
Bartlett, Scott (PA)	PlS	852	Becker, Yolanda (IL)	S	1074
Bartlett, Stephen (MD)	S	1053	Bederson, Joshua (NY)	NS	472
Bartolozzi, Arthur (PA)	OrS	614	Beekman, Robert (OH)	PCd	738
Barton, Fritz (TX)	PlS	869	Beer, Tomasz (OR)	Onc	384
Basch, Samuel (NY)	Psyc	890	Beerman, Lee (PA)	PCd	734
Bascom, Rebecca (PA)	Pul	924	Behm, Frederick (IL)	Path	715
Baser, Susan (PA)	N	509	Behrns, Kevin (FL)	S	1067
Bashevkin, Michael (NY)	Onc	335	Beitler, Jonathan (GA)	RadRO	953
Bashore, Thomas (NC)	Cv	103	Beitsch, Peter (TX)	S	1087
Baskin, Laurence (CA)	U	1175	Belani, Chandra (PA)	Onc	335
Basler, Joseph (TX)	U	1172	Belcher, Christopher (IN)	PInf	782
Bass, Theodore (FL)	Cv	103	Belkin, Michael (MA)	VascS	1184
Bassett, Lawrence (CA)	DR	982	Bell, David (AL)	EDM	213
Bastian, Boris (CA)	Path	719	Bell, Debra (MN)	Path	715
Bastian, Robert (IL)	Oto	673	Bell, Edward (IA)	NP	450
Batchelor, Tracy (MA)	N	506	Bell, Louis (PA)	PInf	780
Bateman, Bruce (VA)	RE	1011	Bell, Rodney (PA)	N	509
Battafarano, Richard (MD)	T&CS	1114	Bellamy, Paul (CA)	Pul	939
Bauer, Bruce (IL)	PlS	864	Belldegrun, Arie (CA)	U	1175
Bauer, Jerry (IL)	NS	486	Bellows, Charles (LA)	S	1087
Bauer, Stuart (MA)	U	1148	Belmont, H Michael (NY)	Rhu	1025

Alphabetical Listing of Doctors

Name	Specialty	Pg	Name	Specialty	Pg
Belsito, Donald (NY)	D	184	Berke, Gerald (CA)	Oto	684
Belsky, Mark (MA)	HS	294	Berkowitz, Carol (CA)	Ped	728
Belzberg, Allan (MD)	NS	472	Berkowitz, Leonard (NY)	Inf	410
Benckart, Daniel (PA)	VascS	1185	Berkowitz, Richard (NY)	MF	431
Benedetti, Enrico (IL)	S	1074	Berkowitz, Ross (MA)	GO	274
Benedetti, Thomas (WA)	MF	439	Berkson, Richard (CA)	EDM	222
Benedetto, Pasquale (FL)	Onc	353	Berland, Lincoln (AL)	DR	978
Benenati, James (FL)	VIR	994	Berlin, Cheston (PA)	Ped	726
Benenati, Susan (FL)	A&I	86	Berlin, Jordan (TN)	Onc	353
Benes, Francine (MA)	Psyc	888	Berman, Brian (MI)	Ped	727
Benevenia, Joseph (NJ)	OrS	614	Berman, James (IL)	PGe	752
Benfield, Mark (AL)	PNep	786	Berman, Michael (CA)	GO	289
Benjamin, Ivor (UT)	Cv	113	Bermudez, Ovidio (CO)	AM	81
Benjamin, Robert (TX)	Onc	377	Bernard, Stephen (NC)	Onc	353
Benjamin, Stanley (DC)	Ge	231	Bernardino, Carlo (CA)	Oph	599
Benkov, Keith (NY)	PGe	750	Bernardo, Jose (PA)	Nep	457
Bennett, Richard (CA)	D	198	Berns, Jeffrey (PA)	Nep	457
Bennett, William (OR)	Nep	464	Bernstein, Daniel (CA)	PCd	740
Benninger, Michael (OH)	Oto	673	Bernstein, David (OH)	PInf	783
Bensinger, William (WA)	Onc	384	Bernstein, David (OH)	A&I	87
Benson, Al (IL)	Onc	364	Bernstein, Jonathan (OH)	A&I	88
Benson, Carol (MA)	DR	973	Bernstein, Richard (IL)	N	525
Benson, Mitchell (NY)	U	1151	Bernstein, Robert (NY)	D	185
Bentley, Frederick (AR)	S	1087	Berrey, B Hudson (FL)	OrS	627
Bentz, Michael (WI)	PlS	864	Berry, Daniel (MN)	OrS	632
Benvenisty, Alan (NY)	VascS	1186	Berry, J Michael (CA)	Onc	384
Benzel, Edward (OH)	NS	486	Bertolone, Salvatore (KY)	PHO	765
Benzon, Honorio (IL)	PM	699	Bertorini, Tulio (TN)	N	520
Berchuck, Andrew (NC)	GO	280	Besinger, Richard (IL)	MF	436
Berde, Charles (MA)	PM	696	Bessey, Palmer (NY)	S	1053
Berediiklian, Pedro (PA)	HS	295	Bessler, Marc (NY)	S	1054
Berek, Jonathan (CA)	GO	289	Betz, Randal (PA)	OrS	614
Berenstein, Alejandro (NY)	NRad	985	Beyer, Eric (IL)	PHO	769
Berg, Christine (MD)	RadRO	948	Bhan, Atul (MA)	Path	706
Berg, Daniel (WA)	D	198	Bhasin, Shalender (MA)	EDM	206
Berg, Stacey (TX)	PHO	775	Bhattacharyya, Neil (MA)	Oto	655
Berga, Sarah (NC)	ObG	559	Bialer, Martin (NY)	CG	157
Berger, Joseph (KY)	N	520	Biancaniello, Thomas (NY)	PCd	734
Berger, Mitchel (CA)	NS	495	Bianchi, Diana (MA)	CG	156
Berger, Ronald (MD)	CE	119	Bichell, David (TN)	T&CS	1123
Bergey, Gregory (MD)	N	509	Bicher, Annette (VA)	GO	280
Bergman, Donald (NY)	EDM	209	Bickers, David (NY)	D	185
Bergman, Ira (PA)	ChiN	147	Biederman, Joseph (MA)	ChAP	906
Bergsagel, Peter (AZ)	Onc	377	Bierbrauer, Karin (OH)	NS	486
Berguer, Ramon (MI)	VascS	1190	Bierman, Fredrick (NY)	PCd	734
Berk, John (MA)	Pul	922	Bierman, Philip (NE)	Onc	374

Name	Specialty	Pg	Name	Specialty	Pg
Biermann, J Sybil (MI)	OrS	632	Blebea, John (OK)	VascS	1192
Bigelow, Carolyn (MS)	Hem	316	Bleday, Ronald (MA)	CRS	168
Biggs, David (DE)	Onc	335	Bleiberg, Efrain (TX)	ChAP	911
Bigliani, Louis (NY)	OrS	614	Bleiweiss, Ira (NY)	Path	708
Bijwadia, Jagdeep (MN)	Pul	933	Blinder, Morey (MO)	Hem	318
Bilchik, Anton (CA)	S	1093	Blitzer, Andrew (NY)	Oto	658
Bilezikian, John (NY)	EDM	209	Blobe, Gerard (NC)	Onc	354
Biller, Beverly (MA)	EDM	206	Bloch, Rina (MA)	PMR	834
Billett, Amy (MA)	PHO	756	Block, Susan (MA)	H & PM	406
Billingsley, Kevin (OR)	S	1093	Bloom, David (MI)	U	1165
Billmire, David (OH)	PlS	864	Bloom, Patricia (NY)	Ger	262
Bilsky, Mark (NY)	NS	472	Bloomer, Joseph (AL)	Ge	239
Bingaman, William (OH)	NS	486	Bluemke, David (MD)	DR	974
Biousse, Valerie (GA)	Oph	582	Blum, Andrew (RI)	N	506
Bird, Hector (NY)	ChAP	907	Blum, Conrad (NY)	EDM	209
Birmaher, Boris (PA)	ChAP	908	Blum, Kristie (OH)	PHO	769
Birnbaum, Elisa (MO)	CRS	173	Blumberg, Henry (GA)	Inf	414
Birrer, Michael (MA)	Onc	327	Blume, Ralph (NY)	Rhu	1025
Bishop, Allen (MN)	HS	300	Blumenfeld, Jon (NY)	Nep	457
Bishop, Warren (IA)	PGe	752	Blumenfield, Michael (CA)	Psyc	900
Bissell, Dwight (CA)	IM	426	Blumenkranz, Mark (CA)	Oph	599
Bitan, Fabien (NY)	OrS	614	Blumenthal, David (NY)	Cv	96
Bitran, Jacob (IL)	Onc	365	Blumenthal, Roger (MD)	Cv	97
Bittl, John (FL)	IC	129	Boachie-Adjei, Oheneba (NY)	OrS	614
Black, C Thomas (TX)	PS	809	Bobrove, Arthur (CA)	Rhu	1033
Black, Dennis (TN)	PGe	752	Bock, Samuel (CO)	PA&I	732
Black, Donald (IA)	Psyc	897	Bockenstedt, Paula (MI)	Hem	319
Black, Henry (NY)	Nep	457	Bockman, Richard (NY)	EDM	209
Black, Keith (CA)	NS	495	Boden, Scott (GA)	OrS	628
Black, Kevin (MO)	Psyc	897	Bodner, Donald (OH)	U	1165
Black, William (NH)	DR	973	Bodurka, Diane (TX)	GO	286
Blackstock, A William (NC)	RadRO	953	Bogart, Jeffrey (NY)	RadRO	948
Blackstone, Robin (AZ)	S	1087	Boggan, James (CA)	NS	496
Blackwell, Keith (CA)	Oto	684	Bogrov, Michael (MD)	ChAP	908
Blackwell, Kimberly (NC)	Onc	354	Boice, Charles (MD)	GO	276
Blackwell, Richard (AL)	RE	1011	Bojrab, Dennis (MI)	Oto	673
Blaha, John (MI)	OrS	632	Boland, Clement (TX)	Ge	250
Blair, Elizabeth (IL)	Oto	673	Boles, Richard (CA)	CG	162
Blaivas, Jerry (NY)	U	1151	Bolger, Graeme (AL)	Onc	354
Blakemore, Karin (MD)	MF	431	Bolger, William (FL)	Oto	667
Blanchard, Daniel (CA)	Cv	116	Bollen, Andrew (CA)	Path	719
Bland, Kirby (AL)	S	1067	Bolman, Ralph Morton (MA)	T&CS	1110
Blaney, Susan (TX)	PHO	775	Bolognia, Jean (CT)	D	182
Blatchford, Garnet (NE)	CRS	176	Bolton, John (LA)	S	1087
Blatt, Julie (NC)	PHO	765	Bolton, W Kline (VA)	Nep	459
Blazer, Dan (NC)	Psyc	895	Bolwell, Brian (OH)	Onc	365

Alphabetical Listing of Doctors

Name	Specialty	Pg	Name	Specialty	Pg
Bond, Sheldon (KY)	PS	805	Braddom, Randall (PA)	PMR	835
Bondi, Edward (PA)	D	185	Bradford, Carol (MI)	Oto	673
Bonner, James (AL)	A&I	86	Bradley, James (PA)	SM	1041
Bono, James (MA)	OrS	610	Bradley, James (CA)	PlS	873
Bonomi, Philip (IL)	Onc	365	Bradley, Jeffrey (MO)	RadRO	958
Bonow, Robert (IL)	Cv	106	Bradley, John (CA)	PInf	784
Boone, Timothy (TX)	U	1172	Bradley, Linda (OH)	ObG	560
Boop, Frederick (TN)	NS	481	Bradshaw, Karen (TX)	ObG	563
Booth, Robert (PA)	OrS	615	Brady, Mary (NY)	S	1054
Boraas, Marcia (PA)	S	1054	Brage, Michael (WA)	OrS	642
Borchert, Mark (CA)	Oph	599	Braly, Patricia (LA)	GO	287
Borer, Jeffrey (NY)	Cv	97	Branch, Charles (NC)	NS	481
Borg-Stein, Joanne (MA)	PMR	834	Brandt, Fredric (NY)	D	185
Borgen, Patrick (NY)	S	1054	Brandt, Harry (MD)	Psyc	890
Borges, Lawrence (MA)	NS	470	Brandt, Keith (MO)	PlS	865
Boronow, John (MD)	Psyc	890	Brandt, Lawrence (NY)	Ge	231
Borowitz, Drucy (NY)	PPul	794	Branham, Gregory (MO)	Oto	673
Borson, Soo (WA)	GerPsy	915	Brasington, Richard (MO)	Rhu	1030
Borst, Matthew (AZ)	GO	286	Braun, Martin (DC)	D	185
Borum, Marie (DC)	Ge	231	Braunstein, Glenn (CA)	EDM	222
Borzak, Steven (FL)	Cv	103	Braunstein, Seth (NC)	IM	424
Bos, Gary (WA)	OrS	641	Brause, Barry (NY)	Inf	411
Bosl, George (NY)	Onc	335	Bravender, Terrill (OH)	AM	81
Boston, Barry (TN)	Onc	354	Braverman, Alan (MO)	Cv	106
Bostwick, David (VA)	Path	713	Braverman, Lewis (MA)	EDM	206
Bourge, Robert (AL)	Cv	103	Bray, Robert (CA)	NS	496
Bourgeois, Blaise (MA)	ChiN	146	Brazer, Scott (NC)	Ge	239
Boushey, Homer (CA)	Pul	939	Brecher, Martin (NY)	PHO	758
Bouvet, Michael (CA)	S	1093	Breidenbach, Warren (AZ)	HS	303
Bove, Alfred (PA)	Cv	97	Breitbart, William (NY)	Psyc	891
Bove, Edward (MI)	PS	807	Brem, Henry (MD)	NS	472
Bowden, Charles (TX)	Psyc	899	Brem, Rachel (DC)	DR	974
Bowdish, Michael (CA)	T&CS	1140	Brem, Steven (PA)	NS	472
Bowen, Glen (UT)	D	196	Brems, John (IL)	S	1074
Bower, Charles (AR)	PO	792	Brendler, Charles (IL)	U	1165
Boxer, Gary (MO)	ChAP	910	Brener, Bruce (NJ)	VascS	1186
Boxer, Laurence (MI)	PHO	769	Brenin, Christiana (VA)	Onc	354
Boxer Wachler, Brian (CA)	Oph	599	Brennan, Daniel (MO)	Nep	461
Boxrud, Cynthia (CA)	Oph	599	Brennan, Michael (MN)	EDM	216
Boyajian, Michael (DC)	PlS	852	Brennan, Stephen (TX)	Nep	463
Boyd, Stuart (CA)	U	1175	Brenner, Joel (MD)	PCd	734
Boyd, Walter (CA)	T&CS	1140	Brenner, Malcolm (TX)	Hem	323
Boyer, Thomas (AZ)	Ge	251	Brent, David (PA)	ChAP	908
Boyle, Robert (VA)	NP	449	Bresalier, Robert (TX)	Ge	251
Bozentka, David (PA)	HS	295	Brescia, Frank (SC)	Onc	354
Brackmann, Derald (CA)	Oto	684	Bressler, Neil (MD)	Oph	571

Name	Specialty	Pg	Name	Specialty	Pg
Bressler, Susan (MD)	Oph	572	Brown, Karen (NY)	VIR	992
Bressman, Susan (NY)	N	509	Brown, Kevin (CO)	Pul	936
Brewer, Molly (CT)	GO	274	Brown, Kimberly (MI)	Ge	244
Brewster, David (MA)	VascS	1184	Brown, Marc (NY)	D	185
Brick, Gregory (MA)	OrS	610	Brown, Robert (MN)	N	525
Brick, John (WV)	N	510	Brown, Robert (NY)	Ge	231
Bricker, John (TX)	PCd	740	Browne, J Dale (NC)	Oto	667
Bricker, Leslie (MI)	H & PM	407	Browner, Bruce (CT)	OrS	610
Bridges, Charles (NC)	T&CS	1124	Brozena, Susan (PA)	Cv	97
Bridwell, Keith (MO)	OrS	632	Bruce, Jeffrey (NY)	NS	473
Brien, Earl (CA)	OrS	642	Brucker, Alexander (PA)	Oph	572
Brillon, David (NY)	EDM	209	Bruera, Eduardo (TX)	Onc	377
Brinckerhoff, Laurence (MA)	T&CS	1110	Brufsky, Adam (PA)	Onc	335
Bristow, Robert (CA)	GO	289	Bruggers, Carol (UT)	PHO	774
Britt, L D (VA)	S	1067	Bruner, Janet (TX)	Path	717
Brizel, David (NC)	RadRO	954	Brunicardi, F Charles (CA)	S	1094
Broadstone, Vasti Lima (IN)	EDM	216	Bruno, Michiko (HI)	N	535
Brock, John (TN)	U	1160	Brunsting, Louis (AL)	T&CS	1124
Brockstein, Bruce (IL)	Onc	365	Brunstrom, Janice (MO)	ChiN	150
Broderick, Gregory (FL)	U	1160	Brunt, L Michael (MO)	S	1075
Broderick, Joseph (OH)	N	525	Brushart, Thomas (MD)	HS	295
Brodkin, Edward (PA)	Psyc	891	Bryson, Yvonne (CA)	PInf	784
Brodland, David (PA)	D	185	Brzyski, Robert (TX)	RE	1015
Brodman, Michael (NY)	ObG	557	Buatti, John (IA)	RadRO	959
Brodsky, James (TX)	OrS	640	Bubley, Glenn (MA)	Onc	328
Brodsky, Jeffrey (PA)	S	1054	Bucciarelli, Richard (FL)	NP	449
Brodsky, Robert (MD)	Hem	312	Buch, Jeffrey (TX)	U	1173
Brody, Fred (DC)	S	1054	Buchanan, George (TX)	PHO	775
Brody, Harold (GA)	D	189	Buchbinder, Ellen (NY)	A&I	84
Bromberg, Jonathan (MD)	S	1054	Buchholz, David (MD)	N	510
Bromberg, Mark (UT)	N	531	Buchholz, Thomas (TX)	RadRO	963
Bronheim, Harold (NY)	Psyc	891	Buchman, Steven (MI)	PlS	865
Bronson, Michael (NY)	OrS	615	Buchman, Timothy (GA)	S	1067
Brooks, Ari (PA)	S	1054	Bucholz, Richard (MO)	NS	486
Brooks, Benjamin (NC)	N	520	Bucholz, Robert (TX)	OrS	640
Brooks, David (MA)	S	1048	Buckley, Edward (NC)	Oph	582
Brooks, John (PA)	Path	708	Buckner, Jan (MN)	Onc	365
Brooks, Stuart (FL)	Pul	929	Buckwalter, Joseph (IA)	OrS	633
Brophy, Patrick (IA)	PNep	787	Bucky, Louis (PA)	PlS	853
Brown, Allen (MN)	PMR	839	Budd, George (OH)	Onc	365
Brown, Charles (IL)	S	1075	Budenz, Donald (NC)	Oph	582
Brown, Daniel (PA)	VIR	992	Budoff, Matthew (CA)	Cv	116
Brown, Eric (MI)	S	1075	Bueno, Raphael (MA)	T&CS	1110
Brown, Frederick (IL)	NS	486	Bukata, Susan (NY)	OrS	615
Brown, Gary (PA)	Oph	572	Bulat, Robert (LA)	Ge	251
Brown, John (IN)	T&CS	1131	Bull, David (UT)	T&CS	1136

Alphabetical Listing of Doctors

Name	Specialty	Pg	Name	Specialty	Pg
Bull, Marilyn (IN)	Ped	727	Busuttil, Ronald (CA)	S	1094
Buly, Robert (NY)	OrS	615	Butler, Charles (TX)	PlS	870
Bumpous, Jeffrey (KY)	Oto	667	Butler, David (TX)	D	196
Bunn, Paul (CO)	Onc	374	Butler, John (CA)	S	1094
Bunning, Robert (DC)	Rhu	1026	Butler, William (SC)	Onc	354
Burchiel, Kim (OR)	NS	496	Butterly, David (NC)	Nep	459
Burdette, Jonathan (NC)	NRad	987	Butterly, Lynn (NH)	Ge	228
Burger, Peter (MD)	Path	708	Buxton, Alfred (MA)	CE	118
Burger, Robert (PA)	GO	276	Buyon, Jill (NY)	Rhu	1026
Burgess, David (NJ)	Ped	726	Buys, Saundra (UT)	Onc	374
Burke, Allan (IL)	N	525	Buysse, Daniel (PA)	Psyc	891
Burke, Charles (PA)	SM	1041	Buzdar, Aman (TX)	Onc	377
Burke, Dennis (MA)	OrS	610	Byrd, Benjamin (TN)	Cv	103
Burke, Miles (OH)	Oph	589	Byrd, David (WA)	S	1094
Burke, Peter (MA)	S	1048	Byrd, H Stephenson (TX)	PlS	870
Burke, Redmond (FL)	T&CS	1124	Byrd, J.W. (TN)	SM	1042
Burke, Thomas (TX)	GO	287	Byrd, John (OH)	Hem	319
Burke, William (NE)	GerPsy	914	Byrne, Janice (UT)	ObG	562
Burket, Mark (OH)	Cv	106	Byrne, John G (TN)	T&CS	1124
Burkey, Brian (OH)	Oto	674	Bystritsky, Alexander (CA)	Psyc	901
Burks, A Wesley (NC)	PA&I	730			
Burman, Kenneth (DC)	EDM	209			
Burmeister, Lynn (MN)	EDM	216			
Burnett, Alexander (AR)	GO	287			
Burnett, Arthur (MD)	U	1151	Cabin, Henry (CT)	Cv	94
Burns, A Jay (TX)	PlS	870	Cagle, Philip (TX)	Path	717
Burns, James (MA)	Oto	655	Cahill, John (NY)	PrM	882
Burris, Howard (TN)	Onc	354	Cahill, Kenneth (OH)	Oph	589
Burschtin, Omar (NY)	Pul	924	Cahill, Kevin (NY)	PrM	883
Burstein, Fernando (GA)	PlS	860	Caillouette, James (CA)	OrS	642
Burstein, Harold (MA)	Onc	328	Cain, Joanna (MA)	GO	274
Burt, Randall (UT)	Ge	249	Cain, Mark (IN)	U	1166
Burt, Richard (IL)	IM	425	Cairns, Bruce (NC)	S	1067
Burt, Vivien (CA)	Psyc	900	Cairo, Mitchell (NY)	PHO	758
Burton, Allen (TX)	PM	701	Calabrese, Joseph (OH)	Psyc	897
Burton, Barbara (IL)	CG	160	Calabresi, Peter (MD)	N	510
Burton, Claude (NC)	D	189	Caldamone, Anthony (RI)	U	1148
Burton, John (MD)	Ger	262	Caldarelli, David (IL)	Oto	674
Busby, J Erik (AL)	U	1160	Caldwell, Randall (IN)	PCd	738
Buse, John (NC)	EDM	214	Calhoon, John (TX)	T&CS	1137
Bush-Joseph, Charles (IL)	SM	1043	Califano, Joseph (MD)	Oto	658
Bushman, Wade (WI)	U	1166	Califf, Robert (NC)	Cv	103
Busis, Neil (PA)	N	510	Callaghan, John (IA)	OrS	633
Busse, William (WI)	A&I	88	Callahan, Eileen (NY)	Ger	262
Bussel, James (NY)	PHO	758	Callans, David (PA)	CE	119
Buster, John (MA)	RE	1006	Callen, Jeffrey (KY)	D	190

C

Name	Specialty	Pg	Name	Specialty	Pg
Callery, Mark (MA)	S	1048	Carneiro, Ronaldo (FL)	HS	298
Calligaro, Keith (PA)	VascS	1186	Carney, John (AR)	D	196
Calvi, Laura (NY)	EDM	209	Carney, Michael (HI)	GO	289
Calvo, Benjamin (NC)	S	1067	Carpenter, Jeffrey (NJ)	VascS	1186
Cambria, Richard (MA)	VascS	1184	Carpenter, John (AL)	Onc	355
Cameron, John (MD)	S	1054	Carpenter, Paul (WA)	PHO	776
Cameron, Robert (CA)	T&CS	1140	Carpinito, Gennaro (MA)	U	1148
Camisa, Charles (FL)	D	190	Carr, Bruce (TX)	RE	1015
Camitta, Bruce (WI)	PHO	769	Carr, David (MO)	Ger	264
Cammisa, Frank (NY)	OrS	615	Carr, Stephen (RI)	MF	430
Camoriano, John (AZ)	Onc	378	Carr-Locke, David (NY)	Ge	231
Campbell, Bruce (WI)	Oto	674	Carragee, Eugene (CA)	OrS	642
Campbell, David (CO)	T&CS	1136	Carrasquillo, Jorge (NY)	NuM	548
Campbell, G Douglas (MS)	Pul	929	Carraway, James (VA)	PlS	860
Campbell, J William (MO)	Inf	416	Carroll, Charles (IL)	HS	300
Campbell, Steven (OH)	U	1166	Carroll, John (CO)	IC	132
Campo, John (OH)	ChAP	910	Carroll, Peter (CA)	U	1175
Campochiaro, Peter (MD)	Oph	572	Carroll, William (NY)	PHO	758
Cance, William (NY)	S	1055	Carson, Benjamin (MD)	NS	473
Cancio, Margarita (FL)	Inf	414	Carson, Culley (NC)	U	1160
Canellos, George (MA)	Onc	328	Carson, Donald (PA)	ObG	557
Canning, Douglas (PA)	U	1151	Carson, Sandra (RI)	RE	1006
Cannom, David (CA)	CE	125	Carter, H Ballentine (MD)	U	1151
Canterbury, Randolph (VA)	Psyc	895	Carter, Keith (IA)	Oph	589
Canto, Marcia (MD)	Ge	231	Cartwright, Patrick (UT)	U	1171
Caplan, Louis (MA)	N	506	Carty, Sally (PA)	S	1055
Capo, Hilda (FL)	Oph	582	Caruana, Salvatore (NY)	Oto	658
Cappuccino, Andrew (NY)	OrS	615	Cascino, Terrence (MN)	N	525
Caprioli, Joseph (CA)	Oph	599	Casella, Samuel (NH)	PEn	743
Caputo, Anthony (NJ)	Oph	572	Caskey, Michael (AZ)	T&CS	1137
Caputo, Thomas (NY)	GO	276	Cass, Darrell (TX)	PS	809
Caputy, Anthony (DC)	NS	473	Casselbrant, Margaretha (PA)	PO	789
Carabasi, Matthew (PA)	Onc	336	Cassidy, Charles (MA)	HS	294
Carabello, Blase (TX)	Cv	114	Cassidy, Suzanne (CA)	CG	162
Carbone, David (OH)	Onc	365	Cassivi, Stephen (MN)	T&CS	1131
Cardenas, Diana (FL)	PMR	838	Castell, Donald (SC)	Ge	239
Cardenosa, Gilda (VA)	DR	978	Castellino, Sharon (NC)	PHO	765
Carducci, Michael (MD)	Onc	336	Castells, Maria (MA)	A&I	84
Carey, John (MD)	Oto	658	Caster, Andrew (CA)	Oph	599
Carey, John C (UT)	CG	161	Castle, Valerie (MI)	PHO	770
Carey, Lisa (NC)	Onc	355	Catalona, William (IL)	U	1166
Caritis, Steve (PA)	MF	432	Catanzaro, Antonino (CA)	Pul	939
Carlson, Alan (NC)	Oph	582	Cather, Jennifer (TX)	D	196
Carlson, John (NJ)	GO	276	Catherwood, Edward (NH)	Cv	94
Carlson, Michelle (NY)	HS	295	Caty, Michael (CT)	PS	801
Carlson, Robert (CA)	Onc	384	Cedars, Marcelle (CA)	RE	1017

Name	Specialty	Pg	Name	Specialty	Pg
Cederbaum, Stephen (CA)	CG	162	Chang-Miller, April (AZ)	Rhu	1032
Cederna, Paul (MI)	PlS	865	Chao, KS Clifford (NY)	RadRO	948
Celano, Paul (MD)	Onc	336	Chao, Nelson (NC)	Onc	355
Celli, Bartolome (MA)	Pul	922	Chap, Linnea (CA)	Onc	384
Cello, John (CA)	Ge	253	Chapman, Jens (WA)	OrS	642
Cendales, Linda (GA)	HS	299	Chapman, Paul (NY)	Onc	336
Cerfolio, Robert (AL)	T&CS	1124	Chapman, Robert (MI)	Onc	365
Cerqueira, Manuel (OH)	Cv	107	Chapman, William (MO)	S	1075
Cetta, Frank (MN)	PCd	738	Char, Devron (CA)	Oph	599
Cha, Soonmee (CA)	NRad	991	Charboneau, J William (MN)	DR	980
Chabner, Bruce (MA)	Onc	328	Chari, Suresh (MN)	Ge	244
Chabot, John (NY)	S	1055	Charles, Andrew (CA)	N	536
Chachoua, Abraham (NY)	Onc	336	Charney, Jonathan (NY)	N	510
Chaikof, Elliot (MA)	VascS	1184	Charrow, Joel (IL)	CG	160
Chaisson, Richard (MD)	Inf	411	Chatham, W (AL)	Rhu	1029
Chaitman, Bernard (MO)	Cv	107	Cheatham, John (OH)	PCd	738
Chakravarthy, Anuradha (TN)	RadRO	954	Chelimsky, Thomas (WI)	N	525
Chakravarti, Arnab (OH)	RadRO	959	Chen, Allen (MD)	PHO	759
Chalian, Ara (PA)	Oto	658	Chen, Chun (NY)	NS	473
Chamberlain, Marc (WA)	N	535	Chen, David (PA)	U	1151
Chambers, Christopher (PA)	AM	80	Chen, David (IL)	PMR	839
Chambers, Setsuko (AZ)	GO	287	Chen, Jonathan (NY)	T&CS	1114
Champlin, Richard (TX)	Hem	323	Chen, Mike (AL)	PS	805
Chan, John (CA)	GO	289	Chen, Thomas (CA)	NS	496
Chan, Kenny (CO)	PO	792	Chen, Yunn-Yi (CA)	Path	720
Chanan-Khan, Asher (FL)	Onc	355	Cheng, Edith (WA)	MF	439
Chancellor, Michael (MI)	U	1166	Cheng, Edward (MN)	OrS	633
Chand, Bipan (IL)	S	1075	Cherny, W Bruce (ID)	NS	491
Chandar, Jayanthi (FL)	PNep	786	Cherqui, Daniel (NY)	S	1055
Chandler, James (IL)	NS	486	Cherry, Kenneth (VA)	VascS	1189
Chandler, Michael (NY)	A&I	84	Chesney, Carolyn (TN)	Path	713
Chandler, William (MI)	NS	487	Cheson, Bruce (DC)	Hem	312
Chandrasoma, Parakrama (CA)	Path	720	Cheung, Nai-Kong V (NY)	PHO	759
Chang, Alfred (MI)	S	1075	Cheville, Andrea (MN)	PMR	839
Chang, Benjamin (PA)	PlS	853	Chew, Helen (CA)	Onc	384
Chang, Gene (PA)	IC	127	Chey, William (MI)	Ge	244
Chang, Helena (CA)	S	1094	Chi, Dennis (NY)	GO	277
Chang, James (CA)	HS	304	Childs, Stacy (CO)	U	1171
Chang, Jenny (TX)	Onc	378	Chiles, Caroline (NC)	DR	979
Chang, Karen (CA)	Path	720	Chinitz, Larry (NY)	CE	120
Chang, Kenneth (CA)	Ge	253	Chiocca, E Antonio (OH)	NS	487
Chang, R Jeffrey (CA)	RE	1017	Chitambar, Christopher (WI)	Onc	366
Chang, Rowland (IL)	Rhu	1030	Chitwood, W Randolph (NC)	T&CS	1124
Chang, Sam (TN)	U	1160	Chiu, David (NY)	PlS	853
Chang, Stanley (NY)	Oph	572	Chiu, Yanek (CA)	CRS	177
Chang, Susan (CA)	Onc	384	Chizner, Michael (FL)	Cv	103

Name	Specialty	Pg	Name	Specialty	Pg
Chlebowski, Rowan (CA)	Onc	384	Clayman, Gary (TX)	Oto	681
Chmait, Ramen (CA)	MF	440	Clayman, Ralph (CA)	U	1175
Cho, Kathleen (MI)	Path	715	Cleary, James (WI)	Onc	366
Cho, Kerry (CA)	Nep	465	Clements, Philip (CA)	Rhu	1033
Cho, Kyung (MI)	VIR	995	Clements, Stephen (GA)	Cv	104
Choi, Noah (MA)	RadRO	946	Cliby, William (MN)	GO	283
Choti, Michael (MD)	S	1055	Clinch, Thomas (MD)	Oph	572
Chow, Warren (CA)	Onc	385	Clinton, Steven (OH)	Onc	366
Chowdhury, Khalid (CO)	Oto	679	Clisham, P Ronald (LA)	RE	1015
Choy, Andrew (CA)	Oph	600	Cloherty, John (MA)	NP	446
Choy, Hak (TX)	RadRO	963	Clohisy, Denis (MN)	OrS	633
Christenson, John (IN)	PInf	783	Cloninger, C Robert (MO)	Psyc	897
Christian, Karla (TN)	T&CS	1124	Clore, John (VA)	EDM	214
Christiani, David (MA)	Pul	922	Close, Lanny (NY)	Oto	658
Christie, Dennis (WA)	PGe	755	Cloughesy, Timothy (CA)	N	536
Christie, Jason (PA)	Pul	925	Clutter, William (MO)	EDM	216
Christman, Brian (TN)	Pul	930	Cmelak, Anthony (TN)	RadRO	954
Christman, Gregory (MI)	RE	1012	Coakley, Fergus (OR)	DR	982
Christo, Paul (MD)	PM	696	Cobleigh, Melody (IL)	Onc	366
Chu, Constance (PA)	OrS	615	Coblyn, Jonathan (MA)	Rhu	1024
Chu, Edward (PA)	Onc	336	Cobos, Everardo (TX)	Hem	323
Chui, Helena (CA)	N	536	Coccia, Peter (NE)	PHO	774
Chung, Daniel (MA)	Ge	228	Cochran, Alistair (CA)	Path	720
Chung, Kevin (MI)	HS	300	Cockerell, Clay (TX)	D	196
Chung, Ki Young (SC)	Onc	355	Cockerham, Kimberly (CA)	Oph	600
Chung, Raymond (MA)	Ge	228	Coddington, Charles (MN)	RE	1013
Church, James (OH)	CRS	173	Coe, Fredric (IL)	Nep	461
Church, Joseph* (CA)	PA&I	733	Coffey, Barbara (NY)	ChAP	908
Chwals, Walter (MA)	PS	801	Coffman, Thomas (NC)	Nep	459
Ciancio, Gaetano (FL)	U	1160	Cohen, Alan (MA)	NS	470
Ciccotti, Michael (PA)	SM	1041	Cohen, Arnold (PA)	MF	432
Ciezki, Jay (OH)	RadRO	959	Cohen, Bernard (FL)	D	190
Ciocon, Jerry (FL)	Ger	263	Cohen, Bernard (MD)	D	185
Cioffi, William (RI)	S	1048	Cohen, Bruce (OH)	ChiN	150
Cionni, Robert (UT)	Oph	595	Cohen, Burton (NY)	DR	974
Ciraulo, Domenic (MA)	AdP	904	Cohen, David (NY)	Nep	457
Cirigliano, Michael (PA)	IM	424	Cohen, Gary (PA)	VIR	993
Civantos, Francisco (FL)	Oto	667	Cohen, Gary (MD)	Onc	336
Clair, Daniel (OH)	VascS	1190	Cohen, Gordon (CA)	T&CS	1140
Clairmont, Albert (OH)	PMR	839	Cohen, Harris L (TN)	DR	979
Clamon, Gerald (IA)	Onc	366	Cohen, Howard (NY)	Cv	97
Clark, Joseph (IL)	Onc	366	Cohen, Jeffrey (NH)	N	506
Clark, Keith (OK)	Oto	681	Cohen, Jeffrey (PA)	U	1152
Clark, Orlo (CA)	S	1094	Cohen, Jeffrey (OH)	N	525
Clarke-Pearson, Daniel (NC)	GO	280	Cohen, Jonathan (NY)	Ge	231
Claxton, David (PA)	Onc	336	Cohen, Kenneth (MD)	PHO	759

Alphabetical Listing of Doctors

Name	Specialty	Pg	Name	Specialty	Pg
Cohen, Lawrence (NY)	Ge	232	Connolly, James (MA)	Path	706
Cohen, Mark (IL)	HS	300	Conrad, E Chappie (WA)	OrS	642
Cohen, Martin (NY)	CE	120	Conry, Robert (AL)	Onc	355
Cohen, Michael (UT)	Path	717	Constantian, Mark (NH)	PlS	850
Cohen, Mitchell (OH)	PGe	752	Constine, Louis (NY)	RadRO	948
Cohen, Mitchell (PA)	Psyc	891	Conte, John (MD)	T&CS	1114
Cohen, Murray (PA)	S	1055	Conti, David (NY)	S	1055
Cohen, Myron (NC)	Inf	414	Cook, Jonathan (NC)	D	190
Cohen, Neri (MD)	T&CS	1114	Cook, Stuart (NJ)	N	510
Cohen, Philip (DC)	Onc	337	Cooke, Joseph (NY)	Pul	925
Cohen, Robbin (CA)	T&CS	1141	Cookson, Michael (TN)	U	1161
Cohen, Robert (OH)	EDM	216	Cooney, Kathleen (MI)	Onc	366
Cohen, Roger (PA)	Onc	337	Cooney, Leo (CT)	Ger	262
Cohen, Seymour (NY)	Onc	337	Cooper, Barry (TX)	Hem	323
Cohen, Steven (CA)	PlS	873	Cooper, Christopher (OH)	Cv	107
Cohn, Richard (IL)	PNep	787	Cooper, Dan (CA)	PPul	798
Cohn, Susan (IL)	PHO	770	Cooper, Daniel (TX)	OrS	640
Cohn, Susan (IL)	Inf	416	Cooper, David (MD)	EDM	210
Coit, Daniel (NY)	S	1055	Cooper, J Allen (AL)	Pul	930
Colachis, Samuel (OH)	PMR	839	Cooper, Jay (NY)	RadRO	948
Colberg, John (CT)	U	1148	Cooper, Joel (PA)	T&CS	1114
Coldwell, Douglas (KY)	VIR	994	Cooper, Laurence (TX)	PHO	775
Cole, Andrew (MA)	N	506	Cooper, Michael (CO)	VascS	1192
Cole, David (SC)	S	1068	Cooper, Rubin (NY)	PCd	734
Cole, Francis (MO)	NP	450	Cooper, William (VA)	Pul	930
Coleman, Beverly (PA)	DR	974	Cope, Dennis (CA)	IM	426
Coleman, John (IN)	PlS	865	Cope, Doris (MD)	PM	696
Coleman, Morton (NY)	Onc	337	Copel, Joshua (CT)	MF	430
Colen, Lawrence (VA)	PlS	861	Copelan, Edward (OH)	Hem	319
Collins, Dale (NH)	PlS	850	Copeland, Larry (OH)	GO	283
Collins, Eric (NY)	AdP	904	Coplen, Douglas (MO)	U	1166
Collins, Evan (TX)	HS	303	Copp, Steven (CA)	OrS	642
Colombani, Paul (MD)	PS	802	Copperman, Alan (NY)	RE	1008
Colon-Otero, Gerardo (FL)	Onc	355	Coppola, John (NY)	Cv	97
Colquhoun, Steven (CA)	S	1094	Corbett, James (MS)	N	520
Colson, Yolonda (MA)	T&CS	1110	Corbetta, Maurizio (MO)	N	525
Colvin, Edward (AL)	PCd	737	Cordeiro, Peter (NY)	PlS	853
Come, Steven (MA)	Onc	328	Corey, G Ralph (NC)	Inf	414
Comenzo, Raymond (MA)	Hem	310	Corey, Jacquelynne (IL)	Oto	674
Comerota, Anthony (OH)	VascS	1190	Corey, Seth (IL)	PHO	770
Comi, Anne (MD)	ChiN	147	Corey-Bloom, Jody (CA)	N	536
Comi, Richard (NH)	EDM	206	Cornblath, David (MD)	N	510
Cominelli, Fabio (OH)	Ge	244	Cornelison, Terri (MD)	GO	277
Conant, Emily (PA)	DR	974	Cornelius, Lynn (MO)	D	193
Conley, Susan (PA)	PNep	785	Cornell, Charles (NY)	OrS	616
Connolly, Heidi (MN)	Cv	107	Cornella, Jeffrey (AZ)	ObG	563

Name	Specialty	Pg	Name	Specialty	Pg
Cornwell, Edward (DC)	S	1055	Crombleholme, Timothy (CO)	PS	808
Corrigan, Victor (GA)	Cv	104	Cronenwett, Jack (NH)	VascS	1184
Cortes, Jorge (TX)	Hem	323	Cronin, David (WI)	S	1075
Corteville, Jane (OH)	ObG	560	Crookes, Peter (CA)	S	1094
Coselli, Joseph (TX)	T&CS	1137	Croop, James (IN)	PHO	770
Cosgrove, Rees (RI)	NS	470	Cross, DeWitte (MO)	NRad	988
Cosin, Jonathan (DC)	GO	277	Crossett, Lawrence (PA)	OrS	616
Costantino, Peter (NY)	Oto	658	Crosson, Jane (MD)	PCd	735
Cote, Richard (FL)	Path	713	Crow, Scott (MN)	Psyc	897
Cotsarelis, George (PA)	D	185	Crowe, Joseph (OH)	S	1075
Cotton, Robin (OH)	PO	791	Crowley, William (MA)	RE	1006
Couch, James (OK)	N	532	Cruse, C Wayne (FL)	PlS	861
Couch, Marion (VT)	Oto	655	Crutchfield, Charles (MN)	D	193
Coughlin, Michael (ID)	OrS	638	Cryer, Philip (MO)	EDM	217
Coukos, George (PA)	GO	277	Cudkowicz, Merit (MA)	N	507
Couldwell, William (UT)	NS	491	Culbertson, William (FL)	Oph	582
Coull, Bruce (AZ)	N	533	Culkin, Daniel (OK)	U	1173
Courcoulas, Anita (PA)	S	1056	Cullen, Kevin (MD)	Onc	337
Courey, Mark (CA)	Oto	684	Culp, Randall (PA)	HS	295
Coutifaris, Christos (PA)	RE	1008	Cummings, Jeffrey (NV)	N	536
Coutsoftides, Theodore (CA)	CRS	177	Cunha, Burke (NY)	Inf	411
Covington, Edward (OH)	PM	699	Cunniff, Christopher (AZ)	CG	161
Cowan, Kenneth (NE)	Onc	375	Cunningham, Bari (CA)	D	198
Cowan, Morton (CA)	PA&I	733	Cunningham, Glenn (TX)	EDM	220
Cox, James (TX)	RadRO	963	Cunningham, John (AZ)	Ge	251
Coyle, Patricia (NY)	N	510	Cunningham, John (IL)	PHO	770
Craig, Edward (NY)	OrS	616	Cunningham, Michael (MA)	PO	789
Craigen, William (TX)	CG	161	Cunningham-Rundles, Charlotte (NY)	A&I	
Cramer, Daniel (MA)	ObG	556	84		
Crandall, Alan (UT)	Oph	595	Cupps, Thomas (DC)	Rhu	1026
Crane, Christopher (TX)	RadRO	963	Curcillo, Paul (PA)	S	1056
Craven, Donald (MA)	Inf	410	Curl, Walton (NC)	OrS	628
Crawford, E David (CO)	U	1171	Curley, Steven (TX)	S	1087
Crawford, James (NY)	Path	708	Curran, James (IL)	Rhu	1031
Crawford, Jeffrey (NC)	Onc	355	Currie, Donald (TX)	PMR	842
Crawford, Thomas (MD)	ChiN	147	Currie, John (GA)	GO	280
Creamer, Michael (FL)	PMR	838	Curry, Cynthia (CA)	CG	162
Creasman, William (SC)	GO	280	Curtin, Hugh (MA)	NRad	984
Criado, Frank (MD)	VascS	1186	Curtin, John (NY)	GO	277
Criner, Gerard (PA)	Pul	925	Curtis, Anne (NY)	CE	120
Crippin, Jeffrey (MO)	Ge	244	Cusack, James (MA)	S	1048
Cristofanilli, Massimo (PA)	Onc	337	Cushing, Brad (ME)	S	1048
Crocenzi, Todd (OR)	Onc	385	Cushing, Gary (MA)	EDM	207
Crocker, Ian (GA)	RadRO	954	Cushman, William (TN)	IM	425
Crockett, Dennis (CA)	PO	793	Cutrer, F Michael (MN)	N	526
Crofford, Leslie (KY)	Rhu	1029	Cuttler, Leona (OH)	PEn	746

Alphabetical Listing of Doctors

Name	Specialty	Pg	Name	Specialty	Pg
Cykiert, Robert (NY)	Oph	572	David, Carlos (MA)	NS	470
Czerniecki, Brian (PA)	S	1056	Davidoff, Andrew (TN)	PS	805
Czuczman, Myron (NY)	Onc	337	Davidson, Bruce (DC)	Oto	658
			Davidson, Dennis (NY)	NP	447
			Davidson, Joyce (TX)	Psyc	899
			Davidson, Michael (IL)	Cv	107
D			Davidson, Richard (PA)	OrS	616
D'Alessio, David (OH)	EDM	217	Davidson, Susan (CO)	GO	286
D'Alton, Mary (NY)	MF	432	Davies, Stella (OH)	PHO	770
D'Amico, Anthony (MA)	RadRO	946	Davies, Terry (NY)	EDM	210
D'Amico, Donald (NY)	Oph	573	Davis, Bradley (KS)	U	1171
D'Amico, Thomas (NC)	T&CS	1125	Davis, Gary (TX)	Ge	251
D'Ayala, Marcus (NY)	VascS	1186	Davis, Glenn (NC)	PlS	861
Da Lio, Andrew (CA)	PlS	873	Davis, Janet (FL)	Oph	582
Daar, Eric (CA)	Inf	419	Davis, Jessica (NY)	CG	157
Dabal, Robert (AL)	T&CS	1125	Davis, Jonathan (MA)	NP	446
Dacey, Ralph (MO)	NS	487	Davis, Mellar (OH)	H & PM	407
Dae, Michael (CA)	NuM	551	Davis, William (LA)	Rhu	1032
Dagum, Alexander (NY)	PlS	853	Dawson, Nancy (DC)	Onc	338
Dahmoush, Laila (IA)	Path	715	Day, Susan (CA)	Oph	600
Dake, Michael (CA)	VIR	997	Day, Terry (SC)	Oto	668
Dakhil, Shaker (KS)	Onc	375	Dayton, Merril (NY)	S	1056
Dale, Lowell (MN)	Ger	264	De Cherney, Alan (MD)	ObG	557
Dalinka, Murray (PA)	DR	974	De Geest, Koen (IA)	GO	283
Dalkin, Alan (VA)	EDM	214	De Juan, Eugene (CA)	Oph	600
Dalkin, Bruce (WA)	U	1175	De Lancey, John (MI)	ObG	561
Dalsing, Michael (IN)	VascS	1190	De Las Morenas, Antonio (MA)	Path	706
Daly, Mary (PA)	Onc	337	De Lateur, Barbara (MD)	PMR	835
Damiano, Ralph (MO)	T&CS	1131	De Lia, Julian (WI)	ObG	561
Damon, Lloyd (CA)	Hem	325	De Masters, Bette (CO)	Path	717
Dana, Reza (MA)	Oph	570	De Monte, Franco (TX)	NS	492
Daneker, George (GA)	S	1068	De Moor, Michael (MA)	PCd	733
Daneshmand, Sia (CA)	U	1176	De Simone, Philip (KY)	Onc	356
Dang, Chi (PA)	Onc	338	De Vivo, Darryl (NY)	ChiN	147
Dang, Michael (HI)	T&CS	1141	Dea, Stanley (CA)	Ge	253
Daniel, Rollin (CA)	PlS	873	Dean, J. Michael (UT)	PCCM	742
Danielpour, Moise (CA)	NS	496	DeAngelis, Lisa (NY)	N	510
Daniels, Gilbert (MA)	EDM	207	Deas, Deborah (SC)	ChAP	910
Danoff, Dudley (CA)	U	1176	DeCamp, Malcolm (IL)	T&CS	1131
Darcy, Michael (MO)	VIR	995	DeCross, Arthur (NY)	Ge	232
Darling, R Clement (NY)	VascS	1186	Deeb, G Michael (MI)	T&CS	1131
Darras, Basil (MA)	ChiN	146	Deeg, H Joachim (WA)	Onc	385
Darrow, David (VA)	PO	791	DeFilippi, Vincent (CA)	T&CS	1141
Das, Ananya (AZ)	Ge	251	DeGiorgio, Christopher (CA)	N	536
Dattilo, Jeffery (TN)	VascS	1189	Deitch, Edwin (NJ)	S	1056
Daud, Adil (CA)	Onc	385	Deitz, Joel (PA)	Pul	925

Name	Specialty	Pg	Name	Specialty	Pg
DeKernion, Jean (CA)	U	1176	DeSilva, Stephen (MI)	HS	300
DeKosky, Steven (VA)	N	520	Desnick, Robert (NY)	CG	157
Del Monte, Monte (MI)	Oph	589	Desposito, Franklin (NJ)	CG	157
Del Priore, Giuseppe (IN)	GO	284	DeVane, Gary (FL)	RE	1011
Del Priore, Lucian (SC)	Oph	582	DeVault, Kenneth (FL)	Ge	239
Del-Nido, Pedro (MA)	T&CS	1110	Devereux, Richard (NY)	Cv	97
Delahay, John (DC)	OrS	616	Devinsky, Orrin (NY)	N	511
Delamarter, Rick (CA)	OrS	642	DeVita, Vincent (CT)	Onc	328
Deland, Jonathan (NY)	OrS	616	Dewberry, Robert (MD)	N	511
Delaney, Conor (OH)	CRS	173	DeWeese, Theodore (MD)	RadRO	949
DeLaney, Thomas (MA)	RadRO	946	Deziel, Daniel (IL)	S	1076
DeLeo, Vincent (NY)	D	186	Dhaliwal, Deepinder (PA)	Oph	573
DeLeon, Oscar (NY)	PM	697	Dhanireddy, Ramasubbareddy (TN)	NP	449
Deleyiannis, Frederic (CO)	PlS	869	Di Bisceglie, Adrian (MO)	Ge	244
Delius, Ralph (MI)	T&CS	1131	Di Giacinto, George (NY)	NS	473
Delivoria-Papadopoulos, Maria (PA)		NP	Di Lorenzo, Carlo (OH)	PGe	753
447			Di Marino, Anthony (PA)	Ge	232
Della Rocca, Robert (NY)	Oph	573	Di Persio, John (MO)	Hem	319
Delmez, James (MO)	Nep	461	Di Saia, Philip (CA)	GO	289
DeLong, Mahlon (GA)	N	520	Diamond, Frank (FL)	PEn	745
DeLoughery, Thomas (OR)	Hem	325	Diamond, Michael (MI)	RE	1013
DeLuca, Francesco (PA)	PEn	744	Diamond, Paul (VA)	PMR	838
DeLurgio, David (GA)	CE	121	Dias, Mark (PA)	NS	473
Demarest, Gerald (NM)	S	1087	Diaz, Angela (NY)	AM	80
DeMars, Leslie (NH)	GO	274	Diaz, Eduardo (TX)	Oto	681
Dember, Laura (PA)	Nep	457	Diaz, Fernando (MI)	NS	487
Demer, Joseph (CA)	Oph	600	Dichek, David (WA)	Cv	116
Demetris, Anthony (PA)	Path	708	Dick, Gregory (MD)	PlS	853
Demmler-Harrison, Gail (TX)	PInf	784	Dick, Macdonald (MI)	PCd	738
Demmy, Todd (NY)	T&CS	1115	Dicker, Adam (PA)	RadRO	949
Dempsey, Daniel (PA)	S	1056	Dickey, Richard (LA)	RE	1015
Dempsey, Robert (WI)	NS	487	Dickler, Maura (NY)	Onc	338
Denenberg, Steven (NE)	Oto	680	Diduch, David (VA)	OrS	628
Dennery, Phyllis (PA)	NP	447	Diehl, James (PA)	T&CS	1115
Denny, Donald (NJ)	VIR	993	Dienstag, Jules (MA)	Ge	228
DeNofrio, David (MA)	Cv	94	Dieter, Robert (IL)	IC	131
DeOrio, James (NC)	OrS	628	Dieterich, Douglas (NY)	Ge	232
DePaulo, J Raymond (MD)	Psyc	891	Diethrich, Edward (AZ)	T&CS	1137
DePompolo, Robert (MN)	PMR	840	Dietz, David (OH)	CRS	173
DePriest, Paul (KY)	GO	280	DiGiovanni, Christopher (RI)	OrS	610
Derman, Gordon (IL)	HS	300	Dillard, James (NY)	PMR	835
DeRose, Joseph (NY)	T&CS	1115	Dillehay, Gary (IL)	NuM	550
Dershaw, D David (NY)	DR	974	Diller, Lisa (MA)	PHO	756
Deschamps, Claude (MN)	T&CS	1131	Dillingham, Michael (CA)	OrS	643
Deschler, Daniel (MA)	Oto	655	Dillon, Patrick (MO)	PS	807
DeShazo, Richard (MS)	A&I	86	Dillon, William (CA)	NRad	991

Alphabetical Listing of Doctors

Name	Specialty	Pg	Name	Specialty	Pg
DiMarco, John (VA)	CE	121	Dornhoffer, John (AR)	Oto	682
DiMeglio, Linda (IN)	PEn	746	Doroshow, James (MD)	Onc	338
DiNardo, Laurence (VA)	Oto	668	Dorr, Lawrence (CA)	OrS	643
Dines, David (NY)	OrS	616	Dottino, Peter (NY)	GO	277
Dion, Jacques (GA)	NRad	987	Doubilet, Peter (MA)	DR	973
DiPaola, Robert (NJ)	Onc	338	Dougherty, Matthew (PA)	VascS	1186
Disa, Joseph (NY)	PlS	853	Douglas, John (GA)	IC	129
Disis, Mary (WA)	Onc	385	Dover, Jeffrey (MA)	D	182
Diuguid, David (NY)	Hem	312	Dovey, Mark (PA)	PPul	794
Diver, Daniel (CT)	Cv	94	Dowlati, Afshin (OH)	Onc	366
Diwan, Sudhir (NY)	PM	697	Downey, Robert (NY)	T&CS	1115
Dixon, Sherwood (NV)	S	1095	Dozor, Allen (NY)	PPul	794
Dizon, Don (MA)	Onc	328	Drachtman, Richard (NJ)	PHO	759
Djulbegovic, Benjamin (FL)	Hem	316	Drack, Arlene (IA)	Oph	589
Dobs, Adrian (MD)	EDM	210	Drake, Amelia (NC)	PO	791
Docimo, Steven (PA)	U	1152	Drayer, Burton (NY)	NRad	985
Dodd, Gerald (CO)	DR	981	Drebin, Jeffrey (PA)	S	1056
Dodds, William (MI)	RE	1013	Dreicer, Robert (OH)	Onc	367
Dodick, David (AZ)	N	533	Dreyer, William (TX)	PCd	740
Dodick, Jack (NY)	Oph	573	Dreyer, ZoAnn (TX)	PHO	775
Doghramji, Karl (PA)	Psyc	891	Drinkwater, Davis (TN)	T&CS	1125
Doherty, Dennis (KY)	Pul	930	Driscoll, Colin (MN)	Oto	674
Doherty, Gerard (MA)	S	1049	Driscoll, Daniel (FL)	CG	158
Dolgin, Stephen (NY)	PS	803	Driscoll, David (MN)	PCd	739
Dolitsky, Jay (NY)	PO	789	Driscoll, Deborah (PA)	CG	157
Domchek, Susan (PA)	Onc	338	Dritschilo, Anatoly (DC)	RadRO	949
Dome, Jeffrey (DC)	PHO	759	Driver, Larry (TX)	PM	701
Donahoe, Michael (PA)	Pul	925	Droller, Michael (NY)	U	1152
Donahue, Bernadine (NY)	RadRO	949	Drossman, Douglas (NC)	Ge	240
Donahue, J Kevin (OH)	CE	122	Druker, Brian (OR)	Onc	385
Donald, Paul (CA)	Oto	684	Druzin, Maurice (CA)	MF	440
Donaldson, Sarah (CA)	RadRO	965	Dubeau, Louis (CA)	Path	720
Donaldson, William (PA)	OrS	616	Dubinsky, Marla (CA)	PGe	755
Donehower, Ross (MD)	Onc	338	Ducic, Ivica (DC)	PlS	853
Donn, Steven (MI)	NP	450	Duckert, Larry (WA)	Oto	684
Donner, Thomas (MD)	EDM	210	Ducore, Jonathan (CA)	PHO	777
Donohue, James (NC)	Pul	930	Duff, William (FL)	MF	434
Donohue, John (MN)	S	1076	Duffy, Thomas (CT)	Hem	310
Donovan, Donald (TX)	Oto	681	Dufresne, Craig (MD)	PlS	854
Donovan, James (OH)	U	1166	Dufresne, Raymond (RI)	D	182
Doody, Daniel (MA)	PS	801	Dugoff, Lorraine (PA)	MF	432
Doody, Rachelle (TX)	N	533	Duh, Quan-Yang (CA)	S	1095
Dooley, Sharon (IL)	MF	436	Duhaime, Ann (MA)	NS	470
Dooley, William (OK)	S	1087	Duker, Jay (MA)	Oph	570
Dorkin, Henry (MA)	PPul	794	Dulcan, Mina (IL)	ChAP	910
Dormans, John (PA)	OrS	617	Dulchavsky, Scott (MI)	S	1076

Name	Specialty	Pg	Name	Specialty	Pg
Dumesic, Daniel (CA)	RE	1017	Edelman, Robert (IL)	DR	980
Dumitru, Daniel (TX)	PMR	842	Edelman, Steven (CA)	EDM	222
Duncan, Mark (MD)	S	1056	Edelson, Richard (CT)	D	182
Duncan, Newton (TX)	PO	792	Edelstein, Barbara (NY)	DR	975
Dunkel, Ira (NY)	PHO	759	Edelstein, David (NY)	Oto	659
Dunphy, Frank (NC)	Onc	356	Edgar, Terence (WI)	ChiN	150
Dunton, Charles (PA)	GO	277	Edge, Stephen (NY)	S	1056
DuPont, Herbert (TX)	Inf	418	Edington, Howard (PA)	S	1057
Durbin, William (MA)	PInf	780	Edmond, Michael (VA)	Inf	414
Dure, Leon (AL)	ChiN	149	Edmundowicz, Daniel (PA)	Cv	97
Durham, Janette (CO)	VIR	996	Edmundowicz, Steven (MO)	Ge	245
Durham, Samuel (MI)	T&CS	1132	Edney, James (NE)	S	1085
Durrie, Daniel (KS)	Oph	596	Edwards, John (CA)	Inf	419
Durso, Nancy (VA)	RE	1011	Edwards, Kathryn (TN)	PInf	781
Duska, Linda (VA)	GO	281	Edwards, Michael (OH)	S	1076
Dutcher, Janice (NY)	Onc	338	Edwards, Michael (CA)	NS	496
Duthie, Edmund (WI)	Ger	264	Edwards, Michael (NV)	PlS	873
Dutton, Jonathan (NC)	Oph	583	Edwards, Niloo (NY)	T&CS	1115
Duvic, Madeleine (TX)	D	196	Edwards, Paul (MI)	Oph	589
Dyer, Carmel (TX)	Ger	266	Edwards, Robert (PA)	GO	277
Dzubow, Leonard (PA)	D	186	Edye, Michael (NY)	S	1057
			Efron, Jonathan (MD)	CRS	169
			Eggers, Howard (NY)	Oph	573
E			Eglseder, W Andrew (MD)	HS	296
			Ehrenkranz, Richard (CT)	NP	446
Eagle, Kim (MI)	Cv	107	Ehresmann, Glenn (CA)	Rhu	1033
Eagle, Ralph (PA)	Oph	573	Ehrlich, Paul (NY)	PA&I	729
Early, Dayna (MO)	Ge	245	Ehrlich, Peter (MI)	PS	807
Earp, H Shelton (NC)	EDM	214	Ehrmann, David (IL)	EDM	217
Easley, Ronald (TX)	PCCM	742	Ehya, Hormoz (PA)	Path	708
Eason, James (TN)	S	1068	Eichenfield, Lawrence (CA)	D	198
Easter, David (CA)	S	1095	Eichler, Craig (FL)	D	190
Eaton, James (DC)	Psyc	891	Eidt, John (AR)	VascS	1193
Eavey, Roland (TN)	PO	791	Eifel, Patricia (TX)	RadRO	964
Eberlein, Timothy (MO)	S	1076	Eilber, Frederick (CA)	S	1095
Ebraheim, Nabil (OH)	OrS	633	Ein, Daniel (DC)	A&I	85
Echeverri, Luis (TX)	T&CS	1137	Einarsson, Jon (MA)	ObG	556
Eckardt, Jeffrey (CA)	OrS	643	Einhorn, Lawrence (IN)	Onc	367
Eckel, Robert (CO)	EDM	220	Einhorn, Thomas (MA)	OrS	610
Eckhardt, S Gail (CO)	Onc	375	Eisbruch, Avraham (MI)	RadRO	959
Eckhoff, Devin (AL)	S	1068	Eisele, David (MD)	Oto	659
Eckler, Kristen (MA)	ObG	556	Eisen, Glenn (OR)	Ge	253
Econs, Michael (IN)	EDM	217	Eisen, Howard (PA)	Cv	98
Eddleman, Keith (NY)	MF	432	Eisenberg, Burton (NH)	S	1049
Edelen, John (CA)	Cv	116	Eisenberg, Howard (MD)	NS	473
Edelman, Martin (MD)	Onc	339	Eisenberger, Mario (MD)	Onc	339

Alphabetical Listing of Doctors

Name	Specialty	Pg	Name	Specialty	Pg
Eisendrath, Stuart (CA)	Psyc	901	Ennis, Ronald (NY)	RadRO	949
Eisenstat, Theodore (NJ)	CRS	169	Ensminger, William (MI)	Onc	367
Eismont, Frank (FL)	OrS	628	Epstein, Andrew (PA)	CE	120
El-Youssef, Mounif (MN)	PGe	753	Epstein, Jeffrey (FL)	Oto	668
Elattrache, Neal (CA)	OrS	643	Epstein, Jonathan (MD)	Path	708
Elder, Jack (MI)	U	1166	Epstein, Laurence (MA)	CE	119
Elefteriades, John (CT)	T&CS	1110	Epstein, Leon (IL)	ChiN	150
Elias, Anthony (CO)	Onc	375	Epstein, Michael (FL)	PCd	737
Elias, Stanton (MI)	N	526	Epstein, Stuart (CA)	PA&I	733
Elkayam, Uri (CA)	Cv	116	Erasmus, Jeremy (TX)	DR	982
Ellenbogen, Kenneth (VA)	CE	121	Erban, John (MA)	Onc	328
Ellenbogen, Richard (WA)	NS	496	Erdmann, Detlev (NC)	PlS	861
Ellenhorn, Joshua (CA)	S	1095	Eriksson, Elof (MA)	PlS	850
Elliott, C. (UT)	Pul	936	Ernst, Armin (MA)	Pul	922
Elliott, David (IA)	Ge	245	Ernstoff, Marc (NH)	Onc	329
Elliott, Norman (GA)	Ge	240	Errico, Thomas (NY)	OrS	617
Ellis, Demetrius (PA)	PNep	785	Eschenbach, David (WA)	ObG	563
Ellis, George (LA)	Oph	596	Escobedo, Marilyn (OK)	NP	451
Ellis, Georgiana (WA)	Onc	385	Esmaeli-Azad, Bita (TX)	Oph	596
Ellis, Jonathan (CA)	Ge	253	Esquenazi, Alberto (PA)	PMR	835
Ellis, Lee (TX)	S	1088	Esquivel, Carlos (CA)	S	1095
Ellis, Matthew (MO)	Onc	367	Esserman, Laura (CA)	S	1095
Ellis, Stephen (OH)	IC	131	Essner, Richard (CA)	S	1095
Ellis, William (WA)	U	1176	Estabrook, Alison (NY)	S	1057
Ellison, David (OR)	Nep	465	Estes, N.A. Mark (MA)	CE	119
Ellison, E Christopher (OH)	S	1076	Estey, Elihu (WA)	Onc	385
Ellison, James (MA)	Psyc	888	Estores, David (FL)	Ge	240
Elmets, Craig (AL)	D	190	Estwanik, Joseph (NC)	OrS	628
Elner, Victor (MI)	Oph	589	Eth, Spencer (FL)	Psyc	895
Elster, Allen (NC)	DR	979	Ettenger, Robert (CA)	PNep	788
Elta, Grace (MI)	Ge	245	Ettinger, David (MD)	Onc	339
Emami, Bahman (IL)	RadRO	959	Eugster, Erica (IN)	PEn	747
Emans, Sarah (MA)	AM	80	Euhus, David (TX)	S	1088
Emanuel, Peter (AR)	Hem	323	Eustis, H Sprague (LA)	Oph	596
Emanuele, Mary Ann (IL)	EDM	217	Evans, Douglas (WI)	S	1076
Emanuele, Nicholas (IL)	EDM	217	Evans, Gregory (CA)	PlS	873
Emens, Leisha (MD)	Onc	339	Evans, James (PA)	NS	473
Emmanuel, Patricia (FL)	PInf	781	Evans, Mark (NY)	ObG	557
Emond, Jean (NY)	S	1057	Evans, Sarah (DC)	PMR	835
Emre, Sukru (CT)	S	1049	Evers, Kathryn (PA)	DR	975
Emslie, Graham (TX)	ChAP	911	Ewalt, David (TX)	U	1173
Endrizzi, Donald (ME)	OrS	611	Ewend, Matthew (NC)	NS	481
Enelow, Richard (NH)	Pul	922	Ezaki, Marybeth (TX)	HS	303
Engel, William King (CA)	N	536			
Engstrom, John (CA)	N	536			
Engstrom, Paul (PA)	Onc	339			

Name	Specialty	Pg
F		
Fabian, Carol (KS)	Onc	375
Faddis, Mitchell (MO)	CE	123
Fadem, Stephen (TX)	Nep	463
Fahey, Patrick (IL)	Pul	933
Fahey, Thomas (NY)	S	1057
Fahn, Stanley (NY)	N	511
Faigel, Douglas (AZ)	Ge	251
Failla, Joseph (MI)	HS	300
Fairman, Ronald (PA)	VascS	1187
Falanga, Vincent (RI)	D	182
Falco, Frank (DE)	PM	697
Falcone, Tommaso (OH)	RE	1013
Falk, Gary (PA)	Ge	232
Falk, Rena (CA)	CG	162
Falk, Ronald (NC)	Nep	459
Fallat, Mary (KY)	PS	805
Fallon, Brian (NY)	Psyc	892
Fallon, Michael (TX)	Ge	251
Fallon, Robert (IN)	PHO	770
Famuyide, Abimbola (MN)	ObG	561
Fan, Leland (CO)	PPul	797
Fang, John (UT)	Ge	249
Fann, Jesse (WA)	Psyc	901
Fanous, Yvonne (CA)	PA&I	733
Fanta, Christopher (MA)	Pul	922
Fantini, Gary (NY)	VascS	1187
Farag, Sherif (IN)	Hem	319
Farber, Martin (NY)	Rhu	1026
Faries, Peter (NY)	VascS	1187
Farley, David (MN)	S	1076
Farlow, Martin (IN)	N	526
Farmer, Diana (CA)	PS	810
Farmer, James (NY)	OrS	617
Faro, Scott (PA)	NRad	985
Farrar, William (OH)	S	1076
Farraye, Francis (MA)	Ge	228
Farrior, Edward (FL)	Oto	668
Farrior, Joseph (FL)	Oto	668
Fasano, Alessio (MD)	PGe	750
Fay, Joseph (TX)	Onc	378
Faye-Petersen, Ona (AL)	Path	713
Feder, Robert (IL)	Oph	589
Federle, Michael (CA)	DR	983
Fee, Willard (CA)	Oto	684

Name	Specialty	Pg
Feghali, Joseph (NY)	Oto	659
Feig, Barry (TX)	S	1088
Feig, Stephen (CA)	DR	983
Feinberg, Joseph (NY)	PMR	836
Feinberg, Todd (NY)	N	511
Feinglos, Mark (NC)	EDM	214
Feins, Richard (NC)	T&CS	1125
Feld, Gregory (CA)	CE	125
Feldman, David (NY)	OrS	617
Feldman, Edward (CA)	Ge	253
Feldman, Eva (MI)	N	526
Feldman, Joel (MA)	PlS	850
Feldman, Joseph (IL)	PMR	840
Feldman, Kenneth (WA)	Ped	728
Feldman, Marc (TX)	IC	132
Feldman, Ted (IL)	IC	131
Feldmann, Edward (MA)	N	507
Feldon, Steven (NY)	Oph	573
Feldstein, Neil (NY)	NS	474
Feliciano, David (GA)	S	1068
Felix, Carolyn (PA)	PHO	759
Fellus, Jonathan (NJ)	N	511
Feltes, Timothy (OH)	PCd	739
Fennerty, M Brian (OR)	Ge	254
Fenske, Neil (FL)	D	190
Fenstermaker, Robert (NY)	NS	474
Ferguson, James (VA)	MF	434
Ferguson, Mark (IL)	T&CS	1132
Fernando, Hiran (MA)	T&CS	1111
Ferrante, F Michael (CA)	PM	702
Ferrara, James (MI)	PHO	770
Ferrell, Linda (CA)	Path	720
Ferrendelli, James (TX)	N	533
Ferris, Frank (CA)	H & PM	408
Ferris, Robert (PA)	Oto	659
Fessler, Richard (IL)	NS	487
Fewkes, Jessica (MA)	D	183
Fichtenbaum, Carl (OH)	Inf	416
Fidler, Jeff (MN)	DR	980
Fields, Abbie (DC)	GO	278
Fields, Theodore (NY)	Rhu	1026
Fife, Rose (IN)	Rhu	1031
Figlin, Robert (CA)	Onc	386
Filicko-O'Hara, Joanne (PA)	Hem	312
Filip, Stanley (NC)	ObG	559
Filipek, Pauline (TX)	ChiN	152

Alphabetical Listing of Doctors

Name	Specialty	Pg	Name	Specialty	Pg
Filley, Christopher (CO)	N	531	Fitzgerald, Paul (CA)	EDM	222
Filly, Roy (CA)	DR	983	Fitzgibbon, Dermot (WA)	PM	702
Filsoufi, Farzan (NY)	T&CS	1115	Fitzgibbons, Robert (NE)	S	1085
Finan, Michael (AL)	GO	281	Fitzpatrick, Richard (CA)	D	198
Fine, Howard (MD)	Onc	339	Fiveash, John (AL)	RadRO	954
Fine, Perry (UT)	PM	700	Fivenson, David (MI)	D	193
Fine, Robert (TX)	H & PM	408	Fivush, Barbara (MD)	PNep	785
Fine, Robert (NY)	Onc	339	Fix, R Jobe (AL)	PlS	861
Finerman, Gerald (CA)	OrS	643	Flaherty, Alice (MA)	N	507
Finger, Paul (NY)	Oph	573	Flaherty, John (IL)	Inf	416
Fink, Matthew (NY)	N	511	Flaherty, Joseph (MO)	Ger	265
Finkel, Alan (NC)	N	521	Flaherty, Keith (MA)	Onc	329
Finkel, Michael (FL)	N	521	Flake, Alan (PA)	PS	803
Finkel, Richard (FL)	ChiN	149	Flamm, Scott (OH)	DR	980
Finkel, Terri (FL)	PRhu	800	Flanagan, Steven (NY)	PMR	836
Finklestein, Jerry (CA)	PHO	777	Flanigan, D Preston (CA)	VascS	1194
Finlay, Jonathan (CA)	PHO	777	Flanigan, Robert (IL)	U	1167
Finlayson, Christina (CO)	S	1085	Flanigan, Timothy (RI)	Inf	410
Fintel, Dan (IL)	Cv	107	Flatow, Evan (NY)	OrS	617
Finucane, Thomas (MD)	Ger	263	Fleischer, David (AZ)	Ge	252
Fiorica, James (FL)	GO	281	Fleming, Gini (IL)	Onc	367
Firlit, Casimir (MO)	U	1167	Fleshman, James (MO)	CRS	173
First, Michael (NY)	Psyc	892	Fletcher, Christopher (MA)	Path	706
Fisch, Harry (NY)	U	1152	Fletcher, Eugene (IN)	Pul	933
Fischbein, Lewis (MO)	IM	425	Flickinger, John (PA)	RadRO	949
Fischer, Thomas (IN)	HS	300	Flinn, Ian (TN)	Onc	356
Fischl, Margaret (FL)	IM	425	Flint, Paul (OR)	Oto	685
Fish, Frank (TN)	PCd	737	Flomenberg, Neal (PA)	Onc	340
Fishbein, Daniel (WA)	Cv	116	Florakis, George (NY)	Oph	574
Fishbein, Michael (CA)	Path	720	Flores, Raja (NY)	T&CS	1115
Fisher, Garth (CA)	PlS	873	Flowers, Franklin (FL)	D	190
Fisher, George (CA)	Onc	386	Flynn, Harry (FL)	Oph	583
Fisher, Jonathan (CA)	S	1095	Flynn, Joseph (WA)	PNep	788
Fisher, Mark (CA)	N	536	Flynn, Michael (KY)	S	1068
Fisher, Paul (CA)	ChiN	153	Flynn, Patricia (TN)	PInf	782
Fisher, Richard (NY)	Onc	339	Flynn, Patrick (MN)	Hem	319
Fisher, Robert (PA)	Ge	232	Flynn, Timothy (FL)	VascS	1189
Fisher, Robert (CA)	N	537	Fodor, Peter (CA)	PlS	874
Fisher, Rosemarie (CT)	Ge	228	Foglia, Robert (TX)	PS	809
Fisher, William (TX)	S	1088	Fogt, Franz (PA)	Path	709
Fishman, David (NY)	GO	278	Foley, Carmel (NY)	ChAP	908
Fishman, Elliot (MD)	DR	975	Foley, Eugene (WI)	CRS	174
Fishman, Gerald (IL)	Oph	590	Foley, Kevin (TN)	NS	481
Fishman, Henry (DC)	A&I	85	Follansbee, William (PA)	Cv	98
Fishman, Scott (CA)	PM	702	Fonarow, Gregg (CA)	Cv	116
Fitch, Tom (AZ)	Onc	378	Fong, Yuman (NY)	S	1057

Name	Specialty	Pg	Name	Specialty	Pg
Fonseca, Rafael (AZ)	Hem	324	Frassica, Frank (MD)	OrS	617
Fontana, Gregory (NY)	T&CS	1115	Frazee, John (CA)	NS	496
Foo, Sun-Hoo (NY)	N	511	Frazier, O Howard (TX)	T&CS	1138
Forastiere, Arlene (MD)	Onc	340	Frazier, Thomas (PA)	S	1057
Forbess, Joseph (TX)	T&CS	1138	Freedman, Arnold (MA)	Onc	329
Ford, Charles (WI)	Oto	674	Freedman, Gary (PA)	RadRO	949
Ford, Henri (CA)	PS	810	Freedman, Robert (CO)	Psyc	898
Ford, James (CA)	Onc	386	Freedman, Sharon (NC)	Oph	583
Forero, Andres (AL)	Onc	356	Freeman, Gregory (TX)	Cv	114
Forman, Jeffrey (MI)	RadRO	959	Freeman, Leonard (NY)	NuM	548
Forman, Stephen (CA)	Hem	325	Freeman, Theodore (TX)	A&I	89
Formenti, Silvia (NY)	RadRO	949	Freeman, Thomas (FL)	NS	481
Fornari, Victor (NY)	ChAP	908	Freeman, William (CA)	Oph	600
Forscher, Charles (CA)	Onc	386	Freemark, Michael (NC)	PEn	746
Forsmark, Christopher (FL)	Ge	240	Frei, Donald (CO)	NRad	990
Forster, Richard (FL)	Oph	583	Freifeld, Alison (NE)	Inf	418
Fosko, Scott (MO)	D	193	Freiman, Hal (NY)	Ge	232
Foss, Francine (CT)	Onc	329	Freimanis, Rita (NC)	DR	979
Fossella, Frank (TX)	Onc	378	Freischlag, Julie (MD)	VascS	1187
Fost, Norman (WI)	Ped	727	Freitag, Frederick (TX)	PM	701
Foster, C Stephen (MA)	Oph	570	French, Jacqueline (NY)	N	511
Foster, Carol (UT)	PEn	748	French, William (CA)	Cv	117
Foster, Harris (CT)	U	1148	Friberg, Thomas (PA)	Oph	574
Foster, Richard (IN)	U	1167	Fricker, Frederick (FL)	PCd	737
Foucar, M Kathryn (NM)	Path	717	Friebert, Sarah (OH)	H & PM	407
Fouser, Laurie (WA)	PNep	788	Fried, Guy (PA)	PMR	836
Fowble, Barbara (CA)	RadRO	966	Fried, Marvin (NY)	Oto	659
Fowl, Richard (AZ)	VascS	1193	Fried, Michael (NC)	Ge	240
Fowler, Jeffrey (OH)	GO	284	Friedberg, Jonathan (NY)	Onc	340
Fox, Harold (MD)	MF	432	Friedberg, Joseph (PA)	T&CS	1116
Fox, James (PA)	PlS	854	Frieden, Ilona (CA)	D	198
Fox, Kevin (PA)	Onc	340	Friedlaender, Gary (CT)	OrS	611
Fracasso, Paula (VA)	Onc	356	Friedlander, Sheila (CA)	D	199
Fraker, Douglas (PA)	S	1057	Friedman, Aaron (MN)	PNep	787
Frances, Richard (NY)	AdP	904	Friedman, Alan (MD)	PHO	760
Francis, Kathleen (NJ)	PMR	836	Friedman, Alan (PA)	Hem	312
Francisco, Gerard (TX)	PMR	842	Friedman, Allan (NC)	NS	481
Frangoul, Haydar (TN)	PHO	765	Friedman, Barry (CA)	Psyc	901
Frank, Ian (PA)	Inf	411	Friedman, Chad (OH)	RE	1013
Franklin, Morris (TX)	S	1088	Friedman, David (FL)	HS	299
Franks, Andrew (NY)	D	186	Friedman, Debra (TN)	PHO	765
Frantz, Christopher (DE)	PHO	759	Friedman, Ellen (TX)	PO	793
Frantz, Ivan (MA)	NP	446	Friedman, Henry (NC)	Onc	356
Frantzides, Constantine (IL)	S	1077	Friedman, Lawrence (MA)	Ge	229
Fraser, Charles (TX)	T&CS	1138	Friedman, Lloyd (CT)	Pul	923
Fraser, Lionel (MS)	U	1161	Friedman, Matthew (VT)	Psyc	888

Alphabetical Listing of Doctors

Name	Specialty	Pg	Name	Specialty	Pg
Friedman, Michael (IL)	Oto	674	Galantowicz, Mark (OH)	T&CS	1132
Friedman, Sanford (NY)	Cv	98	Galati, Joseph (TX)	Ge	252
Friedman, Stuart (FL)	A&I	86	Galetta, Steven (PA)	N	512
Friese, Randall (AZ)	S	1088	Galgiani, John (AZ)	Inf	418
Frim, David (IL)	NS	487	Galland, Leo (NY)	IM	424
Fritz, Marc (NC)	RE	1011	Gallico, G Gregory (MA)	PlS	850
Frohman, Elliot (TX)	N	533	Gallin, Pamela (NY)	Oph	574
Fromm, Geri-Lynn (TX)	GO	287	Galloway, Aubrey (NY)	T&CS	1116
Fronek, Jan (CA)	SM	1044	Galloway, John (GA)	S	1068
Frost, Frederick (OH)	PMR	840	Gambardella, Ralph (CA)	SM	1044
Fruchtman, Steven (NY)	Hem	312	Gambert, Steven (MD)	Ger	263
Fry, Robert (PA)	CRS	170	Gambetti, Pierluigi (OH)	Path	715
Fu, Freddie (PA)	OrS	617	Gamble, Gail (IL)	PMR	840
Fuchs, Charles (MA)	Onc	329	Gamelli, Richard (IL)	S	1077
Fuchs, Wayne (NY)	Oph	574	Gandara, David (CA)	Onc	386
Fuhrman, Bradley (TX)	PCCM	742	Gandy, Winston (GA)	Cv	104
Fuhrman, Carl (PA)	DR	975	Gang, Eli (CA)	CE	125
Fulkerson, John (CT)	OrS	611	Gantz, Bruce (IA)	Oto	675
Fulkerson, William (NC)	Pul	930	Ganz, Patricia (CA)	Onc	386
Fuller, Nicholas (CA)	PM	702	Garber, Judy (MA)	Onc	329
Fullerton, David (CO)	T&CS	1136	Garcia-Prats, Joseph (TX)	NP	452
Fulop, Tibor (MS)	Nep	459	Garden, Jerome (IL)	D	193
Fung, John (OH)	S	1077	Gardin, Julius (NJ)	Cv	98
Funk, Gerry (IA)	Oto	674	Garfin, Steven (CA)	OrS	643
Furie, Karen (RI)	N	507	Garibaldi, Luigi (PA)	PEn	744
Furlan, Anthony (OH)	N	526	Garner, Warren (CA)	PlS	874
Furman, Wayne (TN)	PHO	765	Garnick, Marc (MA)	Onc	329
Furukawa, Satoshi (PA)	T&CS	1116	Garrett, Algin (VA)	D	190
Fuss, Martin (OR)	RadRO	966	Garrett, William (NC)	OrS	628
Fuster, Valentin (NY)	Cv	98	Garrity, Edward (IL)	Pul	933
Futran, Neal (WA)	Oto	685	Garst, Jennifer (NC)	Onc	356
Fyer, Abby (NY)	Psyc	892	Garth, William (AL)	SM	1042
			Gartner, J Carlton (DE)	Ped	726
			Garver, Robert (AL)	Pul	930
			Garvin, James (NY)	PHO	760
G			Garvin, Kevin (NE)	OrS	639
			Gaston, Robert (AL)	Nep	459
Gabbard, Glen (TX)	Psyc	900	Gater, David (VA)	PMR	838
Gabram, Sheryl (GA)	S	1068	Gawande, Atul (MA)	S	1049
Gabrilove, Janice (NY)	Onc	340	Gaynor, Ellen (IL)	Onc	367
Gaffney, David (UT)	RadRO	962	Gaynor, J William (PA)	T&CS	1116
Gagel, Robert (TX)	EDM	220	Gearhart, John (MD)	U	1152
Gaines, Barbara (PA)	PS	803	Gearhart, Susan (MD)	CRS	170
Gaissert, Henning (MA)	T&CS	1111	Gebhardt, Mark (MA)	OrS	611
Gajjar, Amar (TN)	PHO	766	Geffner, Mitchell (CA)	PEn	748
Galandiuk, Susan (KY)	CRS	172	Gefter, Warren (PA)	DR	975
Galanter, I Marc (NY)	AdP	904			

Name	Specialty	Pg	Name	Specialty	Pg
Geisler, Daniel (PA)	CRS	170	Gilbert, Fred (NY)	CG	157
Gejerman, Glen (NJ)	RadRO	950	Gilbert, Mark (TX)	N	533
Gelb, Bruce (NY)	PCd	735	Gilchrest, Barbara (MA)	D	183
Gelberman, Richard (MO)	HS	301	Gilden, Donald (CO)	N	531
Gelfand, Erwin (CO)	PA&I	732	Gill, Harcharan (CA)	U	1176
Geller, David (PA)	S	1058	Gill, Inderbir (CA)	U	1176
Geller, Kenneth (CA)	PO	793	Gill, Thomas (MA)	SM	1040
Gellis, Stephen (MA)	D	183	Gillette, Paul (TX)	PCd	740
Gelmann, Edward (NY)	Onc	340	Gillman, Matthew (MA)	IM	424
Geltman, Edward (MO)	Cv	108	Gilman, Sid (MI)	N	526
Genc, Mehmet (NY)	MF	432	Gilsanz, Vicente (CA)	DR	983
Gendelman, Seymour (NY)	N	512	Ginsberg, David (CA)	U	1176
Genden, Eric (NY)	Oto	659	Ginsberg, Gregory (PA)	Ge	233
Gentile, Ronald (NY)	Oph	574	Ginsburg, Elizabeth (MA)	RE	1006
George, Daniel (NC)	Onc	356	Ginsburg, Howard (NY)	PS	803
George, Suzanne (MA)	Onc	329	Ginsburg, Kenneth (PA)	AM	80
Georgiade, Gregory (NC)	PlS	861	Ginsburg, Mark (NY)	T&CS	1116
Gerboth, Gregory (AK)	Pul	939	Girardi, Leonard (NY)	T&CS	1116
Gerdes, Hans (NY)	Ge	232	Gish, Robert (CA)	Ge	254
Geronemus, Roy (NY)	D	186	Gitelis, Steven (IL)	OrS	633
Gershenson, David (TX)	GO	287	Gitelman, Stephen (CA)	PEn	748
Gershwin, Merrill (CA)	Rhu	1034	Gitlin, Michael (CA)	Psyc	901
Gerson, Lauren (CA)	Ge	254	Gittes, George (PA)	PS	803
Gerson, Stanton (OH)	Onc	367	Gittler, Michelle (IL)	PMR	840
Gertz, Morie (MN)	Hem	319	Giudice, Linda (CA)	RE	1017
Geschwind, Jean-Francois (MD)	VIR	993	Giuliano, Armando (CA)	S	1096
Gewertz, Bruce (CA)	VascS	1194	Giuntoli, Robert (MD)	GO	278
Gewitz, Michael (NY)	PCd	735	Giustra, Lawrence (GA)	Psyc	896
Gewolb, Ira (MI)	NP	450	Givan, Deborah (IN)	PPul	796
Geyer, Charles (TX)	Onc	378	Givner, Laurence (NC)	PInf	782
Geyer, J Russell (WA)	PHO	777	Gizzi, Martin (NJ)	N	512
Ghamande, Sharad (GA)	GO	281	Glader, Bertil (CA)	PHO	777
Gharagozloo, Farid (DC)	T&CS	1116	Gladstone, James (NY)	OrS	617
Gharibo, Christopher (NY)	PM	697	Glashow, Jonathan (NY)	OrS	618
Gholam, Pierre (OH)	Ge	245	Glaspy, John (CA)	Onc	386
Giannotta, Steven (CA)	NS	497	Glass, Jon (PA)	N	512
Gianoli, Gerard (LA)	Oto	682	Glass, Jonathan (GA)	N	521
Giardiello, Francis (MD)	Ge	233	Glassberg, Kenneth (NY)	U	1152
Giardina, Patricia (NY)	PHO	760	Glassford, David (TN)	T&CS	1125
Gibbons, Raymond (MN)	Cv	108	Glat, Paul (PA)	PlS	854
Gibbs, John (NY)	S	1058	Gleason, Christine (WA)	NP	452
Gibbs, Ronald (CO)	MF	438	Glenn, Mel (MA)	PMR	834
Gibralter, Richard (NY)	Oph	574	Glick, John (PA)	Onc	340
Gibson, C Michael (MA)	IC	126	Glick, Philip (NY)	PS	803
Gibson, Ronald (WA)	PPul	798	Glickel, Steven (NY)	HS	296
Gigantelli, James (NE)	Oph	596	Gliklich, Jerry (NY)	Cv	98

Name	Specialty	Pg	Name	Specialty	Pg
Gliklich, Richard (MA)	Oto	655	Goldstein, Jeffrey (NY)	OrS	618
Glisson, Bonnie (TX)	Onc	378	Goldstein, Larry (NC)	N	521
Glode, L Michael (CO)	Onc	375	Goldstein, Lori (PA)	Onc	340
Glogau, Richard (CA)	D	199	Goldstein, Marc (NY)	U	1152
Glombicki, Alan (TX)	Ge	252	Goldstein, Martin (NY)	ObG	557
Gloviczki, Peter (MN)	VascS	1191	Goldstein, Scott (PA)	CRS	170
Gluck, Stephen (CA)	Nep	465	Goldstein, Wayne (IL)	OrS	633
Gluckman, Gordon (IL)	U	1167	Golfinos, John (NY)	NS	474
Gobrial, Wagih (FL)	PM	698	Golomb, Harvey (IL)	Onc	368
Gochfeld, Michael (NJ)	OM	882	Golub, Richard (FL)	CRS	172
Gockerman, Jon (NC)	Onc	357	Gomella, Leonard (PA)	U	1153
Godder, Kamar (VA)	PHO	766	Gomery, Pablo (MA)	U	1148
Godley, Paul (NC)	Onc	357	Gomes, Antoinette (CA)	VIR	997
Godzik, Cathleen (CA)	HS	304	Gomes, J Anthony (NY)	CE	120
Goebel, Joel (MO)	Oto	675	Gonik, Bernard (MI)	ObG	561
Goetz, Christopher (IL)	N	526	Gonzales, Edmond (TX)	U	1173
Goff, Barbara (WA)	GO	289	Goodin, Douglas (CA)	N	537
Goff, Donald (NY)	Psyc	892	Goodman, Dennis (NY)	Cv	98
Goggins, Michael (MD)	Ge	233	Goodman, Lawrence (WI)	DR	980
Goitz, Henry (MI)	OrS	633	Goodman, Martin (MA)	S	1049
Goitz, Robert (PA)	HS	296	Goodman, Neil (FL)	EDM	214
Gokaslan, Ziya (MD)	NS	474	Goodman, Robert (NJ)	RadRO	950
Golbe, Lawrence (NJ)	N	512	Goodman, Robert (NY)	NS	474
Gold, Philip (WA)	Onc	386	Goodman, Stuart (CA)	OrS	643
Gold, Scott (NY)	Oto	659	Goodson, William (CA)	S	1096
Gold, Stuart (NC)	PHO	766	Goodwin, James (IL)	N	526
Goldberg, Daniel (NJ)	Oph	574	Goodwin, Scott (CA)	VIR	997
Goldberg, Jack (PA)	Hem	312	Goodwin, W Jarrard (FL)	Oto	668
Goldberg, James (CA)	MF	440	Gorab, Robert (CA)	OrS	643
Goldberg, Jeffrey (OH)	RE	1013	Gorbien, Martin (IL)	Ger	265
Goldberg, Michael (IL)	Ge	245	Gordon, Catherine (RI)	PEn	743
Goldberg, Nieca (NY)	Cv	98	Gordon, Leo (IL)	Hem	319
Goldberg, Richard (OH)	Onc	367	Gordon, Marsha (NY)	D	186
Goldblum, John (OH)	Path	715	Gordon, Stuart (NH)	Ge	229
Golden, Michael (PA)	VascS	1187	Gorensek, Margaret (FL)	Inf	415
Goldenberg, David (PA)	Oto	659	Gorevic, Peter (NY)	Rhu	1026
Goldman, Allan (FL)	Pul	931	Gorfine, Stephen (NY)	CRS	170
Goldman, Mindy (CA)	ObG	563	Gorin, Michael (CA)	Oph	600
Goldman, Stanton (TX)	PHO	775	Gorovoy, Mark (FL)	Oph	583
Goldman, Stewart (IL)	PHO	771	Gosnell, Jessica (CA)	S	1096
Goldner, Richard (NC)	OrS	628	Gospe, Sidney (WA)	ChiN	153
Goldsmith, Ari (NY)	PO	789	Gosselin, Benoit (NH)	Oto	655
Goldsmith, Donald (PA)	PRhu	799	Gostout, Bobbie (MN)	GO	284
Goldsmith, Stanley (NY)	NuM	548	Gostout, Christopher (MN)	Ge	245
Goldstein, Edward (GA)	ChiN	149	Gottdiener, John (MD)	Cv	99
Goldstein, Irwin (CA)	U	1176	Gottlieb, Alice (MA)	D	183

Name	Specialty	Pg	Name	Specialty	Pg
Gottlieb, Geoffrey (MA)	Path	706	Green, Howard (FL)	D	191
Gottlieb, Lawrence (IL)	PlS	865	Green, Michael (PA)	PInf	780
Gottlieb, Stephen (MD)	Cv	99	Green, Peter (NY)	Ge	233
Gould, K Lance (TX)	Cv	114	Green, Richard (NY)	VascS	1187
Goulet, Robert (IN)	S	1077	Green, Thomas (IL)	PPul	796
Goumnerova, Liliana (MA)	NS	470	Greenbaum, Steven (PA)	D	186
Gourley, Mark (MD)	Rhu	1026	Greenberg, Benjamin (RI)	Psyc	888
Govindarajan, Sugantha (CA)	Path	720	Greenberg, Donna (MA)	Psyc	888
Gower, Roland (AK)	S	1096	Greenberg, Harly (NY)	Pul	925
Goy, Andre (NJ)	Onc	341	Greenberg, Jay (DC)	PHO	760
Gracia, Clarisa (PA)	RE	1008	Greenberg, Mark (NY)	Cv	99
Gradishar, William (IL)	Onc	368	Greenberg, Richard (PA)	U	1153
Grado, Gordon (AZ)	RadRO	964	Greenberg, William (MA)	Psyc	888
Grady, M Sean (PA)	NS	474	Greenberger, Joel (PA)	RadRO	950
Graf, Ben (WI)	OrS	634	Greenberger, Paul (IL)	A&I	88
Graham, H Devon (LA)	Oto	682	Greene, Clarence (LA)	NS	492
Graham, John (CA)	CG	162	Greene, Frederick (NC)	S	1069
Graham, Mark (NC)	Onc	357	Greene, Graham (FL)	U	1161
Graham, Michael (AZ)	PHO	775	Greene, Loren (NY)	EDM	210
Graham, Roger (MA)	S	1049	Greene, Michael (MA)	MF	430
Graham, Thomas (OH)	HS	301	Greene, Robert (CA)	IC	133
Gralow, Julie (WA)	Onc	387	Greene, Thomas (FL)	HS	299
Grammer, Leslie (IL)	A&I	88	Greenfield, David (FL)	Oph	583
Grana, Generosa (NJ)	Onc	341	Greenfield, Marjorie (OH)	ObG	561
Granai, Cornelius (RI)	GO	274	Greenfield, Saul (NY)	U	1153
Grandis, Arnold (NC)	MF	434	Greenfield, Shelly (MA)	AdP	904
Grandis, Jennifer (PA)	Oto	660	Greenhalgh, David (CA)	S	1096
Granet, David (CA)	Oph	600	Greenson, Joel (MI)	Path	715
Grannis, Frederic (CA)	T&CS	1141	Greenspan, Susan (PA)	EDM	210
Grant, Clive (MN)	S	1077	Greenwald, Blaine (NY)	GerPsy	913
Grant, Edward (CA)	DR	983	Greenwald, Bruce (MD)	Ge	233
Grant, Michael (TX)	S	1088	Greenwald, Mark (IL)	Oph	590
Grasso, Michael (NY)	U	1153	Greenway, Hubert (CA)	D	199
Graver, L Michael (NY)	T&CS	1117	Greenwood, Robert (NC)	ChiN	149
Graves, Michael (CA)	N	537	Greer, Benjamin (WA)	GO	290
Gravett, Michael (WA)	MF	440	Greer, David (CT)	N	507
Gray, Richard (AZ)	S	1088	Greer, John (TN)	Hem	316
Gray, William (NY)	IC	127	Greganti, Mac (NC)	Ger	264
Grazi, Richard (NY)	RE	1008	Gregory, Richard (FL)	PlS	861
Graziano, Kathleen (AZ)	PS	809	Gregory, Stephanie (IL)	Hem	320
Greco, F Anthony (TN)	Onc	357	Greiner, Carl (NE)	Psyc	898
Greden, John (MI)	Psyc	897	Greisberg, Justin (NY)	OrS	618
Green, Andrew (RI)	OrS	611	Greisler, Howard (IL)	VascS	1191
Green, Barth (FL)	NS	482	Grelsamer, Ronald (NY)	OrS	618
Green, Carmen (MI)	PM	699	Grem, Jean (NE)	Onc	375
Green, Daniel (TN)	PHO	766	Gress, Daryl (VA)	N	521

Alphabetical Listing of Doctors

Name	Specialty	Pg	Name	Specialty	Pg
Grever, Michael (OH)	Hem	320	Guilleminault, Christian (CA)	N	537
Gribetz, Michael (NY)	U	1153	Guinan, Eva (MA)	PHO	756
Grichnik, James (FL)	D	191	Gujral, Saroj (MN)	U	1167
Griebling, Tomas (KS)	U	1171	Gulley, James (MD)	Onc	341
Griesemer, David (MA)	ChiN	146	Gullquist, Scott (VA)	PCd	737
Griffith, Bartley (MD)	T&CS	1117	Gumprecht, Jeffrey (NY)	Inf	411
Grifo, James (NY)	RE	1008	Gunasekaran, T S (IL)	PGe	753
Grigsby, Perry (MO)	RadRO	959	Gunderson, John (MA)	Psyc	888
Grikscheit, Tracy (CA)	PS	810	Gundry, Steven (CA)	T&CS	1141
Grillone, Gregory (MA)	Oto	655	Gupta, Nalin (CA)	NS	497
Grimes, Pearl (CA)	D	199	Gupta, Prabodh (PA)	Path	709
Griswold, John (TX)	S	1088	Gupta, Rajan (NH)	S	1049
Grobelny, Thomas (IL)	NRad	988	Gupta, Sandeep (IN)	PGe	753
Grody, Wayne (CA)	CG	163	Gururangan, Sridharan (NC)	PHO	766
Grosh, William (VA)	Onc	357	Gutai, James (MI)	PEn	747
Gross, Ian (CT)	NP	446	Guthikonda, Murali (MI)	NS	488
Gross, Paul (MA)	N	507	Guthrie, Barton (AL)	NS	482
Grossbard, Michael (NY)	Onc	341	Gutin, Philip (NY)	NS	474
Grossberg, George (MO)	GerPsy	914	Guy, John (FL)	Oph	583
Grossi, Eugene (NY)	T&CS	1117	Guy, T Sloane (PA)	T&CS	1117
Grossman, H Barton (TX)	U	1173	Guyton, David (MD)	Oph	574
Grossman, John (CO)	PlS	869	Guyton, Robert (GA)	T&CS	1125
Grossman, John (FL)	HS	299			
Grossman, Melanie (NY)	D	186			
Grossman, Stuart (MD)	Onc	341			
Grossniklaus, Hans (GA)	Oph	583	# H		
Grotta, James (TX)	N	533	Haas, Eric (TX)	CRS	177
Grotting, James (AL)	PlS	861	Haas, Naomi (PA)	Onc	341
Grubb, Blair (OH)	Cv	108	Haas, Richard (CA)	ChiN	153
Grubb, Robert (MO)	NS	487	Haas, Steven (NY)	OrS	618
Gruber, Scott (MI)	S	1077	Haber, Gregory (NY)	Ge	233
Gruchalla, Rebecca (TX)	A&I	89	Habermann, Thomas (MN)	Hem	320
Grum, Cyril (MI)	Pul	933	Hackford, Alan (MA)	CRS	168
Grunberg, Steven (VT)	Onc	330	Hackney, David (MA)	NRad	984
Grundfast, Kenneth (MA)	Oto	656	Haddad, Joseph (NY)	PO	790
Grunebaum, Amos (NY)	MF	433	Hadler, Nortin (NC)	Rhu	1029
Grunfeld, Lawrence (NY)	RE	1008	Hadley, Mark (AL)	NS	482
Grupp, Stephan (PA)	PHO	760	Hadlock, Theresa (MA)	Oto	656
Gruss, Joseph (WA)	PlS	874	Haffty, Bruce (NJ)	RadRO	950
Guandalini, Stefano (IL)	PGe	753	Hagan, Kevin (TN)	PlS	862
Guarda, Angela (MD)	Psyc	892	Hageboutros, Alexandre (NJ)	Onc	341
Guarini, Ludovico (NY)	PHO	760	Hager, W David (KY)	ObG	559
Guber, Myles (CO)	T&CS	1136	Hagman, Jennifer (CO)	ChAP	911
Gugenheim, Joseph (TX)	OrS	640	Hahn, Stephen (PA)	RadRO	950
Guidry, George (LA)	Pul	938	Haid, Regis (GA)	NS	482
Guillem, Jose (NY)	CRS	170	Haig, Andrew (MI)	PMR	840

Name	Specialty	Pg	Name	Specialty	Pg
Haik, Barrett (TN)	Oph	584	Hanks, John (VA)	S	1069
Hain, Timothy (IL)	N	526	Hanley, Frank (CA)	T&CS	1141
Haines, Kathleen (NJ)	PRhu	799	Hanna, Brian (PA)	PCd	735
Haith, Linwood (PA)	S	1058	Hanna, Ehab (TX)	Oto	682
Hakaim, Albert (FL)	VascS	1189	Hanna, Nader (MD)	S	1058
Halberg, Francine (CA)	RadRO	966	Hannafin, Jo (NY)	OrS	618
Hale, Douglass (IN)	ObG	561	Hansen, Juliana (OR)	PlS	874
Haley, Barbara (TX)	Onc	378	Hansen, Nora (IL)	S	1077
Haley, Elliott (VA)	N	521	Hansen, Ronald (AZ)	D	197
Halff, Glenn (TX)	S	1089	Hansen-Flaschen, John (PA)	Pul	925
Hall, Jesse (IL)	Pul	933	Hanson, Laura (NC)	Ger	264
Hall, Lisabeth (NY)	Oph	575	Hanssen, Arlen (MN)	OrS	634
Hall, Simon (NY)	U	1153	Haque, Waheedul (TX)	Psyc	900
Haller, Julia (PA)	Oph	575	Har-El, Gady (NY)	Oto	660
Hallett, John (SC)	VascS	1189	Haraf, Daniel (IL)	RadRO	960
Halligan, Gregory (PA)	PHO	760	Harari, Paul (WI)	RadRO	960
Hallisey, Michael (CT)	VIR	992	Harati, Yadollah (TX)	N	533
Halperin, Henry (MD)	CE	120	Harbaugh, Robert (PA)	NS	474
Halperin, Jonathan (NY)	Cv	99	Harber, Philip (AZ)	OM	882
Halpern, Allan (NY)	D	186	Harbour, J William (FL)	Oph	584
Halpern, Howard (IL)	RadRO	959	Hardesty, Robert (CA)	PlS	874
Halpern, Steven (NJ)	PHO	760	Hardin, Joel (IL)	PCd	739
Haluszka, Oleh (PA)	Ge	233	Hare, Joshua (FL)	Cv	104
Halyard, Michele (AZ)	RadRO	964	Hargrove, W Clark (PA)	T&CS	1117
Hamilton, Stanley (TX)	Path	718	Hariprasad, Seenu (IL)	Oph	590
Hammar, Samuel (WA)	Path	720	Harken, Alden (CA)	T&CS	1141
Hammer, Gary (MI)	EDM	217	Harley, Earl (DC)	PO	790
Hammer, Glenn (NY)	Inf	411	Harman, Eloise (FL)	Pul	931
Hammer, Scott (NY)	Inf	411	Harmon, William (MA)	PNep	785
Hammerschlag, Paul (NY)	Oto	660	Harner, Christopher (PA)	SM	1041
Hammill, Stephen (MN)	CE	123	Harnsberger, Jeffrey (NH)	CRS	168
Hammond, Dennis (MI)	PlS	865	Harper, Richard (TX)	NS	493
Hamra, Sameer (TX)	PlS	870	Harpole, David (NC)	T&CS	1125
Hamvas, Aaron (MO)	NP	450	Harrell, James (TX)	T&CS	1138
Han, Steven-Huy (CA)	Ge	254	Harrington, Elizabeth (NY)	VascS	1187
Hanauer, Stephen (IL)	Ge	245	Harris, David (TX)	PMR	843
Hancock, Steven (CA)	RadRO	966	Harris, Jay (MA)	RadRO	946
Handa, James (MD)	Oph	575	Harris, Jeffrey (CA)	Oto	685
Hande, Kenneth (TN)	Onc	357	Harris, Michael (NJ)	PHO	761
Handy, John (OR)	T&CS	1141	Harris, Nancy (MA)	Path	706
Hanel, Douglas (WA)	HS	304	Harrison, J Kevin (NC)	Cv	104
Haney, Arthur (IL)	RE	1013	Harrison, Louis (NY)	RadRO	950
Hanifin, Jon (OR)	D	199	Harrop, James (PA)	NS	475
Hanke, C William (IN)	D	193	Harsh, Griffith (CA)	NS	497
Hankins, Gary (TX)	MF	438	Hartford, Alan (NH)	RadRO	946
Hankinson, Hal (NM)	NS	492	Hartig, Gregory (WI)	Oto	675

Alphabetical Listing of Doctors

Name	Specialty	Pg	Name	Specialty	Pg
Hartl, Roger (NY)	NS	475	Hellenbrand, William (CT)	PCd	733
Hartman, Barry (NY)	Inf	411	Heller, Debra (NJ)	Path	709
Hartmann, Rene (FL)	CRS	172	Hellstrom, Wayne (LA)	U	1173
Hashim, Sabet (CT)	T&CS	1111	Helman, Lee (MD)	PHO	761
Haskal, Ziv (MD)	VIR	993	Helvie, Mark (MI)	DR	980
Hastings, Hill (IN)	HS	301	Hemal, Ashok (NC)	U	1161
Hatch, Kenneth (AZ)	GO	287	Hemming, Alan (CA)	S	1096
Haughey, Bruce (MO)	Oto	675	Henderson, Randal (FL)	RadRO	954
Haughton, Victor (WI)	NRad	988	Henderson, Victor (CA)	N	537
Hauke, Ralph (NE)	Onc	375	Henderson, William (WA)	A&I	90
Hauptman, Paul (MO)	Cv	108	Hendricks-Munoz, Karen (VA)	NP	449
Hauser, Robert (FL)	N	521	Heney, Niall (MA)	U	1149
Hauser, Stephen (CA)	N	537	Henke, David (NC)	Pul	931
Hausman, Michael (NY)	OrS	618	Henry, David (PA)	Onc	341
Haut, Paul (IN)	PHO	771	Henry, Timothy (MN)	IC	131
Havrilesky, Laura (NC)	GO	281	Henschke, Claudia (NY)	DR	975
Hawes, Robert (FL)	Ge	240	Henshaw, Robert (DC)	OrS	619
Hawkins, Douglas (WA)	PHO	777	Hensle, Terry (NJ)	U	1153
Hayani, Ammar (IL)	PHO	771	Hentz, Vincent (CA)	HS	304
Hayashi, Robert (MO)	PHO	771	Heppell, Jacques (AZ)	CRS	177
Hayden, Richard (AZ)	Oto	682	Herbst, Roy (CT)	Onc	330
Hayes, Daniel (MI)	Onc	368	Hergenroeder, Albert (TX)	AM	82
Hayes, David (MN)	CE	123	Hering, Bernhard (MN)	S	1077
Hayes, Sharonne (MN)	Cv	108	Herling, Irving (PA)	Cv	99
Hayman, James (MI)	RadRO	960	Herman, Charles (PA)	PlS	854
Haynes, David (TN)	Oto	668	Herman, Martin (PA)	OrS	619
Haynes, Johnson (AL)	Pul	931	Herman, Terence (OK)	RadRO	964
Healey, John (NY)	OrS	619	Herman, William (MI)	EDM	217
Healey, Patrick (WA)	PS	810	Heros, Roberto (FL)	NS	482
Heber, David (CA)	EDM	222	Heroux, Alain (IL)	Cv	108
Hebert, James (VT)	S	1049	Herr, Harry (NY)	U	1153
Hecht, Andrew (NY)	OrS	619	Herrine, Steven (PA)	Ge	233
Heck, Christianne (CA)	N	537	Herring, Stanley (WA)	PMR	843
Heckenlively, John (MI)	Oph	590	Herrmann, Howard (PA)	IC	127
Hecox, Kurt (WI)	N	527	Herrmann, Virginia (SC)	S	1069
Hedges, Thomas (MA)	Oph	570	Hersh, Peter (NJ)	Oph	575
Heffner, John (OR)	Pul	939	Hershey, Andrew (OH)	ChiN	150
Heffner, Linda (MA)	MF	430	Hershman, Elliott (NY)	SM	1041
Heiden, Eric (UT)	OrS	639	Hershorin, Eugene (FL)	Ped	727
Heilman, Carl (MA)	NS	471	Hertz, Marshall (MN)	Pul	933
Heilman, Kenneth (FL)	N	521	Hertzig, Margaret (NY)	ChAP	908
Heimann, Ruth (VT)	RadRO	946	Herzenberg, John (MD)	OrS	619
Heinrich, Michael (OR)	Hem	325	Herzog, David (MA)	ChAP	906
Heitmiller, Richard (MD)	T&CS	1117	Herzog, Thomas (NY)	GO	278
Helderman, J Harold (TN)	Nep	460	Heslin, Martin (AL)	S	1069
Helfet, David (NY)	OrS	619	Hess, David (GA)	N	522

Name	Specialty	Pg	Name	Specialty	Pg
Hess, J Bruce (FL)	Oph	584	Hoffman, Andrew (CA)	EDM	223
Hesselink, John (CA)	NRad	991	Hoffman, Brenda (SC)	Ge	240
Hester, T Roderick (GA)	PlS	862	Hoffman, Daniel (CO)	Psyc	899
Heston, Jerry (TN)	ChAP	910	Hoffman, Henry (IA)	Oto	675
Hetherington, Maxine (MO)	PHO	771	Hoffman, John (PA)	S	1058
Heuer, Dale (WI)	Oph	590	Hoffman, Lloyd (NY)	PlS	854
Heyl, Peter (KY)	MF	434	Hoffman, Philip (IL)	Onc	368
Heyman, Melvin (CA)	PGe	755	Hoffman, Robert (NY)	PrM	883
Hibbard, Judith (IL)	MF	436	Hoffman, Ronald (NY)	Oto	660
Hicks, Marshall (TX)	VIR	997	Hoffman, William (CA)	PlS	874
Hicks, Terry (LA)	CRS	177	Hofkosh, Dena (PA)	Ped	726
Hicks, Wesley (NY)	Oto	660	Hogan, Thomas (WV)	Onc	342
Hidalgo, David (NY)	PlS	854	Hogikyan, Norman (MI)	Oto	675
Hiesiger, Emile (NY)	N	512	Holcomb, John (TX)	S	1089
Higano, Celestia (WA)	Onc	387	Holcombe, Randall (NY)	Onc	342
Higashida, Randall (CA)	NRad	991	Holden, Stuart (CA)	U	1177
Higgins, Steven (CA)	CE	125	Holick, Michael (MA)	EDM	207
Hijazi, Ziyad (IL)	PCd	739	Holinger, Lauren (IL)	PO	791
Hilden, Joanne (CO)	PHO	774	Holland, Edward (OH)	Oph	590
Hilfiker, Mary (CA)	PS	810	Holland, James (NY)	Onc	342
Hilger, Peter (MN)	Oto	675	Hollander, Eric (NY)	Psyc	892
Hilibrand, Alan (PA)	OrS	619	Holliday, Michael (MD)	Oto	660
Hill, Ivor (NC)	PGe	752	Holliday, Roy (NY)	DR	975
Hill, Joseph (NH)	RE	1006	Hollier, Larry (LA)	VascS	1193
Hill, Nicholas (MA)	Pul	923	Hollingsworth, Alan (OK)	S	1089
Himelstein, Andrew (DE)	Onc	342	Hollister, Dickerman (CT)	Onc	330
Hinshaw, Daniel (MI)	S	1078	Holmes, David (MN)	IC	131
Hiotis, Spiros (NY)	S	1058	Holmes, Gregory (NH)	ChiN	146
Hirsch, Barry (PA)	Oto	660	Holmes, Lewis (MA)	CG	156
Hirsch, Glenn (NY)	ChAP	908	Holroyd, Suzanne (VA)	GerPsy	914
Hirsch, Irl (WA)	EDM	222	Holterman, Mark (IL)	PS	807
Hirsch, Joshua (MA)	NRad	984	Holtzman, Ronald (NC)	NP	449
Hirschfeld, Robert (TX)	Psyc	900	Holzman, Ian (NY)	NP	447
Ho, Allen (PA)	Oph	575	Holzman, Lawrence (PA)	IM	424
Ho, Sherwin (IL)	SM	1043	Homans, Alan (VT)	PHO	757
Hochberg, Ephraim (MA)	Onc	330	Homer, Daniel (IL)	N	527
Hochberg, Marc (MD)	Rhu	1026	Hong, Waun (TX)	Onc	379
Hochschuler, Stephen (TX)	OrS	640	Hoops, Timothy (PA)	Ge	234
Hochster, Howard (CT)	Onc	330	Hooten, William (MN)	PM	699
Hockstein, Steven (NY)	ObG	557	Hoots, William (MD)	PHO	761
Hoda, Syed (NY)	Path	709	Hopewell, Philip (CA)	Pul	939
Hodapp, Elizabeth (FL)	Oph	584	Hopkins, L Nelson (NY)	NS	475
Hodes, Jonathan (KY)	NS	482	Hoppe, Richard (CA)	RadRO	966
Hodgson, Kim (IL)	VascS	1191	Hopping, Steven (DC)	Oto	660
Hodin, Richard (MA)	S	1049	Hord, Jeffrey (OH)	PHO	771
Hoffenberg, Edward (CO)	PGe	754	Horn, Biljana (CA)	PHO	777

Alphabetical Listing of Doctors

Name	Specialty	Pg	Name	Specialty	Pg
Horn, Evelyn (NY)	Cv	99	Hultman, C Scott (NC)	PlS	862
Hornicek, Francis (MA)	OrS	611	Humayun, Mark (CA)	Oph	601
Hornstein, Mark (MA)	RE	1006	Hume, Eric (PA)	OrS	620
Horowitz, Ira (GA)	GO	281	Hungerford, Marc (MD)	OrS	620
Horowitz, Jed (CA)	PlS	874	Hunstad, Joseph (NC)	PlS	862
Horsager, Robyn (TX)	MF	438	Hunt, John (TX)	S	1089
Hortobagyi, Gabriel (TX)	Onc	379	Hunt, Kelly (TX)	S	1089
Horvath, Karen (WA)	S	1096	Hunt, Sharon (CA)	Cv	117
Horvath, Keith (MD)	T&CS	1117	Hunt, Thomas (AL)	HS	299
Horwitz, Eric (PA)	RadRO	950	Hunter, David (MA)	Oph	570
Horwitz, Steven (NY)	Onc	342	Hunter, Ellen (ID)	Ge	249
Hotaling, Andrew (IL)	Oto	675	Hunter, Jill (TX)	NRad	990
Hotchkiss, Robert (NY)	OrS	620	Hunter, John (OR)	S	1096
Houmard, Brenda (WA)	RE	1017	Huntoon, Marc (TN)	PM	698
Hovsepian, David (CA)	VIR	998	Hurd, David (NC)	Onc	357
Howard, Thomas (NE)	VascS	1192	Hurst, Michael (WV)	Oto	661
Howe, James (IA)	S	1078	Hurst, Robert (PA)	NRad	985
Howe, Kevin (CA)	OrS	644	Hurt, Hallam (PA)	NP	447
Howell, Elizabeth (UT)	AdP	905	Hurtig, Howard (PA)	N	512
Howerton, Russell (NC)	S	1069	Hurwitz, Dennis (PA)	PlS	854
Howington, John (IL)	T&CS	1132	Husain, Amreen (CA)	GO	290
Hoyer, Mark (IN)	PCd	739	Hussain, Maha (MI)	Onc	368
Hoyme, H Eugene (SD)	CG	161	Hussey, Michael (IL)	MF	436
Hozack, William (PA)	OrS	620	Hutchins, Laura (AR)	Onc	379
Hrebinko, Ronald (PA)	U	1154	Hutchinson, Raymond (MI)	PHO	771
Hricak, Hedvig (NY)	DR	975	Huth, James (TX)	S	1089
Hruban, Ralph (MD)	Path	709	Hutter, Adolph (MA)	Cv	94
Hruska, Keith (MO)	Nep	461	Huynh, Phan (TX)	DR	982
Hruza, George (MO)	D	193	Hwu, Patrick (TX)	Onc	379
Hsu, Daphne (NY)	PCd	735	Hyers, Thomas (MO)	Pul	934
Hsueh, Willa (TX)	EDM	221	Hyman, Joshua (NY)	OrS	620
Huang, Jaou-Chen (TX)	RE	1016	Hyman, Neil (VT)	CRS	168
Huang, Judy (MD)	NS	475			
Huang, Laurence (CA)	Pul	940			
Hubbard, Anne (NE)	DR	981			
Huber, Philip (TX)	CRS	177	**I**		
Huddleston, Charles (MO)	T&CS	1132	Iafrati, Mark (MA)	VascS	1184
Hudes, Gary (PA)	Onc	342	Iannaccone, Susan (TX)	ChiN	152
Hudgins, Louanne (CA)	CG	163	Iannettoni, Mark (IA)	T&CS	1132
Hudis, Clifford (NY)	Onc	342	Iannotti, Joseph (OH)	OrS	634
Hudson, Melissa (TN)	PHO	766	Ichord, Rebecca (PA)	ChiN	147
Hudziak, James (VT)	ChAP	906	Idler, Richard (CO)	HS	302
Hugenberg, Steven (IN)	Rhu	1031	Iglehart, James (MA)	S	1050
Hughes, Kevin (MA)	S	1050	Iglesia, Cheryl (DC)	ObG	557
Huitt, Gwen (CO)	Inf	418	Ikramuddin, Sayeed (MN)	S	1078
Hullfish, Kathie (VA)	ObG	559	Ilbawi, Michel (IL)	T&CS	1132

Name	Specialty	Pg	Name	Specialty	Pg
Iliff, Nicholas (MD)	Oph	575	Jackson, Gilchrist (TX)	S	1089
Ilowite, Norman (NY)	PRhu	799	Jackson, Richard (AR)	PS	809
Ilson, David (NY)	Onc	342	Jackson, Valerie (IN)	DR	980
Imber, Gerald (NY)	PlS	854	Jackson, Vicki (MA)	H & PM	406
Imbriglia, Joseph (PA)	HS	296	Jacob, Molly (IL)	Ped	728
Infante, Anthony (TX)	Ped	728	Jacobs, Alice (MA)	IC	126
Infantolino, Anthony (PA)	Ge	234	Jacobs, Charlotte (CA)	Onc	387
Ingbar, David (MN)	Pul	934	Jacobs, Joseph (NY)	Oto	661
Ingle, James (MN)	Onc	368	Jacobs, Joshua (IL)	OrS	634
Inglis, Andrew (WA)	PO	793	Jacobs, Laurence (IL)	RE	1013
Ingram, David (NC)	PInf	782	Jacobs, Richard (AR)	PInf	784
Inra, Lawrence (NY)	Cv	99	Jacobs, Thomas (NY)	EDM	210
Interian, Alberto (FL)	CE	122	Jacobson, Ira (NY)	Ge	234
Inzucchi, Silvio (CT)	EDM	207	Jacoby, David (OR)	Pul	940
Ipp, Eli (CA)	EDM	223	Jaffe, Allan (MN)	Cv	108
Irby, Pierce (NC)	U	1161	Jahanzeb, Mohammad (FL)	Onc	357
Irvine, John (CA)	Oph	601	Jain, Subhash (NY)	PM	697
Irwin, Charles (CA)	AM	82	Jakacki, Regina (PA)	PHO	761
Irwin, Richard (MA)	Pul	923	Jallo, George (MD)	NS	475
Irwin, Ronald (MI)	OrS	634	James, William (PA)	D	187
Isaacs, Claudine (DC)	Onc	343	Jamieson, Stuart (CA)	T&CS	1142
Isaacs, Kim (NC)	Ge	240	Janeiro, John (NH)	U	1149
Isaacson, Keith (MA)	RE	1007	Janicak, Philip (IL)	Psyc	897
Isaacson, Steven (NY)	RadRO	950	Jankovic, Joseph (TX)	N	534
Iseman, Michael (CO)	Pul	936	Janss, Anna (GA)	N	522
Isenberg, Sherwin (CA)	Oph	601	Jaramillo, Diego (PA)	DR	975
Isik, F. (WA)	PlS	874	Jarnagin, William (NY)	S	1058
Iskandrian, Ami (AL)	Cv	104	Jarvik, Jeffrey (WA)	NRad	991
Ismail, Mahmoud (IL)	MF	436	Jasmin, Luc (CA)	PM	702
Isola, Luis (NY)	Hem	313	Jayakar, Parul (FL)	CG	159
Isom, O Wayne (NY)	T&CS	1117	Jayaseelan, Nirmal (TX)	S	1089
Itzkowitz, Steven (NY)	Ge	234	Jeevanandam, Valluvan (IL)	T&CS	1133
Ivanhoe, Cindy (TX)	PMR	843	Jenike, Michael (MA)	Psyc	889
Iwach, Andrew (CA)	Oph	601	Jenkins, Herman (CO)	Oto	680
			Jenkins, Roger (MA)	S	1050
			Jenkins, Todd (AL)	ObG	559
			Jennings, Russell (MA)	PS	801
J			Jensen, Donald (IL)	Ge	246
			Jensen, Mary (VA)	NRad	987
Jaafar, Mohamad (DC)	Oph	575	Jensen, Michael (MN)	EDM	218
Jabbour, Nicolas (MA)	S	1050	Jessen, Michael (TX)	T&CS	1138
Jablons, David (CA)	T&CS	1142	Jessup, Mariell (PA)	Cv	100
Jabs, Douglas (NY)	Oph	575	Jewell, Mark (OR)	PlS	875
Jabs, Kathy (TN)	PNep	786	Jhingran, Anuja (TX)	RadRO	964
Jackler, Robert (CA)	Oto	685	Jho, Hae-Dong (PA)	NS	475
Jackman, Stephen (PA)	U	1154	Jillella, Anand (GA)	Onc	358
Jackson, Amie (AL)	PMR	838			

Alphabetical Listing of Doctors

Name	Specialty	Pg	Name	Specialty	Pg
Jimenez, David (TX)	NS	493	Jones, Paul (IL)	Oto	676
Jimerson, David (MA)	Psyc	889	Jones, Robert (DC)	Path	709
Jiranek, William (VA)	OrS	629	Jonnalagadda, Sreenivasa (MO)	Ge	246
Jobst, Barbara (NH)	N	507	Jordan, Barry (NY)	N	512
Johanson, Norman (PA)	OrS	620	Jordan, Stanley (CA)	PNep	788
John, Thomas (IL)	Oph	590	Jorizzo, Joseph (NC)	D	191
Johnson, Allen (CA)	Cv	117	Jose, Baby (IN)	RadRO	960
Johnson, Annette (NC)	NRad	987	Joseph, David (AL)	U	1161
Johnson, Bruce (MA)	Onc	330	Joseph, Gregory (NC)	NRad	987
Johnson, Bruce (VA)	Pul	931	Josephs, Shelby (MD)	PA&I	729
Johnson, Calvin (LA)	Oto	682	Josephson, David (IN)	N	527
Johnson, Carl (MD)	OrS	620	Josephson, Jordan (NY)	Oto	661
Johnson, Darren (KY)	OrS	629	Josephson, Michelle (IL)	Nep	461
Johnson, David (TX)	Onc	379	Jost, Barbara (MO)	A&I	88
Johnson, Eric (CA)	OrS	644	Joyce, Lyle (MN)	T&CS	1133
Johnson, Jonas (PA)	Oto	661	Joyce, Michael (OH)	OrS	634
Johnson, Julia (MA)	RE	1007	Juckett, Mark (WI)	Hem	320
Johnson, Lynt (DC)	S	1058	Judelson, Debra (CA)	Cv	117
Johnson, Maryl (WI)	Cv	109	Judy, Kevin (PA)	NS	475
Johnson, Matthew (IN)	VIR	995	Julian, Thomas (PA)	S	1059
Johnson, Paula (MA)	Cv	94	Jupiter, Jesse (MA)	HS	294
Johnson, Ronald (PA)	S	1059	Jurcic, Joseph (NY)	Onc	343
Johnson, Scott (TX)	T&CS	1138			
Johnson, Stephen (CO)	NS	491			
Johnson, Steven (CO)	Inf	418	**K**		
Johnson, Timothy (MI)	D	193			
Johnson, Timothy (MI)	MF	436	Kachnic, Lisa (MA)	RadRO	946
Johnson Miller, Denise (IN)	S	1078	Kadmon, Dov (TX)	U	1173
Johnston, Carolyn (MI)	GO	284	Kaeding, Christopher (OH)	OrS	634
Johnston, J Martin (GA)	PHO	766	Kaefer, Martin (IN)	U	1167
Johnston, James (PA)	Nep	457	Kagan, Richard (OH)	S	1078
Johnstone, Peter (IN)	RadRO	960	Kahn, Barbara (MA)	EDM	207
Johr, Robert (FL)	D	191	Kahn, Leonard (NY)	Path	709
Jokl, Peter (CT)	OrS	611	Kahrilas, Peter (IL)	Ge	246
Jonas, Adam (CA)	CG	163	Kaiser, Larry (PA)	T&CS	1118
Jonas, Maureen (MA)	PGe	749	Kaiser, Michael (NY)	NS	475
Jonas, Richard (DC)	T&CS	1118	Kalaycio, Matt (OH)	Onc	368
Jonasch, Eric (TX)	Onc	379	Kalb, Robert (NY)	D	187
Jones, David (VA)	T&CS	1125	Kalemkerian, Gregory (MI)	Onc	368
Jones, Deryk (LA)	SM	1044	Kaliner, Michael (MD)	A&I	85
Jones, H Royden (MA)	N	507	Kallmes, David (MN)	NRad	989
Jones, J (OH)	U	1167	Kalloo, Anthony (MD)	Ge	234
Jones, Jacqueline (NY)	PO	790	Kalnicki, Shalom (NY)	RadRO	951
Jones, Kenneth (CA)	Ped	728	Kamani, Naynesh (DC)	PA&I	729
Jones, Marilyn (CA)	CG	163	Kamdar, Vikram (CA)	EDM	223
Jones, Neil (CA)	HS	304	Kamen, Barton (NJ)	PHO	761

Name	Specialty	Pg	Name	Specialty	Pg
Kaminski, Mark (MI)	Onc	369	Kasiske, Bertram (MN)	Nep	461
Kampman, Kyle (PA)	AdP	904	Kasner, Scott (PA)	N	512
Kanal, Emanuel (PA)	DR	976	Kass, Evan (MI)	U	1167
Kanda, Louis (DC)	T&CS	1118	Kasser, James (MA)	OrS	611
Kandeel, Fouad (CA)	EDM	223	Kastenberg, David (PA)	Ge	234
Kandzari, David (GA)	IC	130	Katirji, Bashar (OH)	N	527
Kane, Alex (TX)	PlS	870	Katner, Harold (GA)	Inf	415
Kane, Javier (TX)	PHO	776	Kato, Tomoaki (NY)	S	1059
Kane, Kay (MA)	D	183	Katowitz, James (PA)	Oph	576
Kane, Madeleine (CO)	Onc	376	Katz, Aaron (NY)	U	1154
Kane, Michael (MD)	U	1154	Katz, L Jay (PA)	Oph	576
Kane, Timothy (DC)	PS	803	Katz, Philip (PA)	Ge	235
Kanel, Gary (CA)	Path	721	Katz, Robert (OH)	PO	792
Kang, Dong-Kyoo (NE)	Oto	680	Katz, Robert (IL)	Rhu	1031
Kantarjian, Hagop (TX)	Hem	324	Katz, Stuart (NY)	Cv	100
Kanter, Kirk (GA)	T&CS	1126	Katzen, Barry (FL)	VIR	994
Kantoff, Philip (MA)	Onc	330	Katzenstein, Anna-Luise (NY)	Path	710
Kantsevoy, Sergey (MD)	Ge	234	Katznelson, Laurence (CA)	EDM	223
Kaouk, Jihad (OH)	U	1167	Kaufman, Bruce (WI)	NS	488
Kaplan, Bernard (PA)	PNep	785	Kaufman, Cary (WA)	S	1097
Kaplan, David (CO)	AM	81	Kaufman, Howard (IL)	S	1078
Kaplan, Frederick (PA)	OrS	620	Kaufman, John (OR)	VIR	998
Kaplan, Irving (MA)	RadRO	946	Kaufman, Paul (WI)	Oph	590
Kaplan, James (KS)	Pul	937	Kaufman, Peter (NH)	Onc	330
Kaplan, Lawrence (CA)	Onc	387	Kaufman, Richard (MA)	Path	706
Kaplan, Lee (MA)	Ge	229	Kaul, Sanjiv (OR)	Cv	117
Kaplan, Michael (CA)	Oto	685	Kavanah, Maureen (MA)	S	1050
Kaplan, Sheldon (TX)	PInf	784	Kavey, Neil (NY)	Psyc	892
Kaplan, Steven (NY)	U	1154	Kavoussi, Louis (NY)	U	1154
Kaplitt, Michael (NY)	NS	476	Kawachi, Mark (CA)	U	1177
Kapoor, Neena (CA)	PHO	777	Kay, Dennis (LA)	VIR	997
Kappy, Michael (CO)	PEn	748	Kay, G Neal (AL)	CE	122
Kapur, Sandip (NY)	S	1059	Kay, Jonathan (MA)	Rhu	1024
Karas, Spero (GA)	OrS	629	Kaye, Mitchell (MN)	Pul	934
Karasu, T Byram (NY)	Psyc	892	Kaysen, George (CA)	Nep	465
Karlan, Beth (CA)	GO	290	Kazahaya, Ken (PA)	PO	790
Karlan, Scott (CA)	S	1096	Kazer, Ralph (IL)	RE	1014
Karp, Judith (MD)	Onc	343	Kazmers, Andris (MI)	VascS	1191
Karpeh, Martin (NY)	S	1059	Keane, Thomas (SC)	U	1161
Karram, Mickey (OH)	ObG	561	Keane, William (PA)	Oto	661
Karrer, Frederick (CO)	PS	808	Keating, Gesina (MN)	ChiN	150
Kartush, Jack (MI)	Oto	676	Keating, Michael (TX)	Hem	324
Karwande, Shreekanth (UT)	T&CS	1136	Keen, Mary (IL)	PMR	840
Kase, Carlos (MA)	N	507	Keenan, Robert (PA)	T&CS	1118
Kashtan, Clifford (MN)	PNep	787			
Kasinath, Balakuntalam (TX)	Nep	463			

Alphabetical Listing of Doctors

Name	Specialty	Pg	Name	Specialty	Pg
Keens, Thomas (CA)	PPul	798	Khan, Agha (MD)	NS	476
Keepers, George (OR)	Psyc	901	Khandji, Alexander (NY)	NRad	985
Keiser, Philip (TX)	Inf	418	Khawaja, Shazib (GA)	IC	130
Kelepouris, Ellie (PA)	Nep	458	Khosla, Sundeep (MN)	EDM	218
Keller, Frank (GA)	PHO	766	Khuri, Fadlo (GA)	Onc	358
Keller, Frederick (OR)	VIR	998	Kibel, Adam (MA)	U	1149
Keller, Gregory (CA)	Oto	685	Kidwell, Earl (DC)	Oph	576
Keller, Steven (NY)	T&CS	1118	Kieburtz, Karl (NY)	N	513
Kelley, Joseph (PA)	GO	278	Kieran, Mark (MA)	PHO	757
Kelley, Mark (TN)	S	1069	Kiernan, Paul (VA)	T&CS	1126
Kelly, Bryan (NY)	OrS	621	Kies, Merrill (TX)	Onc	379
Kelly, Cynthia (VA)	PA&I	731	Kiev, Jonathan (WV)	T&CS	1118
Kelly, Cynthia (CO)	OrS	639	Kikkawa, Don (CA)	Oph	601
Kelly, James (CO)	N	531	Kilmer, Suzanne (CA)	D	199
Kelly, Karen (CA)	Onc	387	Kim, Choll (CA)	OrS	644
Kelly, Kevin (TN)	PlS	862	Kim, Daniel (MA)	Oto	656
Kelly, Thomas (CA)	MF	440	Kim, Daniel (TX)	NS	493
Kelly, W Kevin (PA)	Onc	343	Kim, Dong (TX)	NS	493
Kelsen, David (NY)	Onc	343	Kim, Edward (TN)	U	1161
Kelsey, Peter (MA)	Ge	229	Kim, Jonathan (CA)	Oph	601
Keltz, Martin (NY)	RE	1008	Kim, Julian (OH)	S	1078
Kemeny, Nancy (NY)	Onc	343	Kim, Lawrence (AR)	S	1089
Kemp, James (MO)	PPul	796	Kim, Youn (CA)	D	199
Kempin, Sanford (NY)	Hem	313	Kim, Young-Jee (IN)	PPul	797
Kenan, Samuel (NY)	OrS	621	Kimberly, Robert (AL)	Rhu	1030
Kendrick, Michael (MN)	S	1078	Kimmelstiel, Carey (MA)	IC	126
Kenkel, Jeffrey (TX)	PlS	870	Kimmey, Michael (WA)	Ge	254
Kennedy, David (PA)	Oto	661	Kincaid, John (IN)	N	527
Kennedy, Gary (NY)	GerPsy	913	Kindler, Hedy (IL)	Onc	369
Kennedy, Laurence (OH)	EDM	218	King, Aileen (ID)	ObG	562
Kennelly, Michael (NC)	U	1161	King, Andrew (CA)	Nep	465
Kent, Kenneth (WI)	VascS	1191	King, Bryan (WA)	ChAP	912
Kent, Thomas (TX)	N	534	King, Earl (PA)	Pul	926
Kenter, Keith (OH)	OrS	634	King, John (TX)	PMR	843
Kereiakes, Dean (OH)	Cv	109	King, Richard (GA)	PMR	838
Kern, Jeffrey (CO)	Pul	937	King, Stephanie (PA)	GO	278
Kern, Robert (IL)	Oto	676	King, Talmadge (CA)	Pul	940
Kernstine, Kemp (TX)	T&CS	1138	Kingdom, Todd (CO)	Oto	680
Kerr, Natalie (TN)	Oph	584	Kinkhabwala, Milan (NY)	S	1059
Kesari, Santosh (CA)	Onc	387	Kinney, Marsha (TX)	Path	718
Kesser, Bradley (VA)	Oto	668	Kipen, Howard (NJ)	OM	882
Kessler, Craig (DC)	Hem	313	Kipps, Thomas (CA)	Hem	325
Kestle, John RW (UT)	NS	491	Kirgan, Daniel (NV)	S	1097
Ketcham, Douglas (MN)	VIR	995	Kirklin, James (AL)	T&CS	1126
Kevorkian, Charles (TX)	PMR	843	Kirkwood, John (PA)	Onc	343
Kezar, Laura (AL)	PMR	838	Kirsch, Andrew (GA)	U	1162

Name	Specialty	Pg	Name	Specialty	Pg
Kirschenbaum, Alexander (NY)	U	1154	Koch, Kenneth (NC)	Ge	241
Kirschner, Barbara (IL)	PGe	753	Koch, Michael (IN)	U	1168
Kirschner, Kristi (IL)	PMR	840	Koch, Wayne (MD)	Oto	661
Kirschner, Richard (OH)	PlS	865	Kocher, Mininder (MA)	OrS	612
Kirshblum, Steven (NJ)	PMR	836	Kochman, Michael (PA)	Ge	235
Kirshenbaum, James (MA)	Cv	95	Koczywas, Marianna (CA)	Onc	387
Kirshner, Howard (TN)	N	522	Kodner, Ira (MO)	CRS	174
Kirsner, Robert (FL)	D	191	Koeller, Kelly (MN)	NRad	989
Klaas, Virginia (WA)	NuM	551	Koh, Jeffrey (OR)	PM	702
Klagsbrun, Samuel (NY)	Psyc	893	Koh, Wui-Jin (WA)	RadRO	966
Klapheke, Martin (FL)	Psyc	896	Kohler, Matthew (SC)	GO	281
Kleber, Herbert (NY)	AdP	905	Kohn, Elise (MD)	Onc	343
Kleiman, Martin (IN)	PInf	783	Kokotailo, Patricia (WI)	AM	81
Kleiman, Neal (TX)	IC	132	Koller, Harold (PA)	Oph	576
Klein, Andrew (CA)	S	1097	Kolodny, Edwin (NY)	N	513
Klein, Eric (OH)	U	1168	Komaki, Ritsuko (TX)	RadRO	964
Klein, Lloyd (IL)	Cv	109	Koman, L Andrew (NC)	HS	299
Klein, Patricia (NJ)	N	513	Komrokji, Rami (FL)	Hem	317
Klein, Robert (RI)	PA&I	729	Kondziolka, Douglas (PA)	NS	476
Klein-Gitelman, Marisa (IL)	PRhu	800	Konicek, Frank (IL)	Ge	246
Kleinberg, David (NY)	EDM	210	Konski, Andre (MI)	RadRO	960
Kleinberg, Lawrence (MD)	RadRO	951	Konstam, Marvin (MA)	Cv	95
Kleinerman, Eugenie (TX)	Ped	728	Konstan, Michael (OH)	PPul	797
Kleinman, Ronald (MA)	PGe	749	Koo, John (CA)	D	199
Kleinman, William (IN)	HS	301	Koos, Brian (CA)	MF	440
Klibanski, Anne (MA)	EDM	207	Kopf, Gary (CT)	T&CS	1111
Kliger, Alan (CT)	Nep	456	Koplewicz, Harold (NY)	ChAP	909
Klimberg, Vicki (AR)	S	1090	Koplin, Lawrence (CA)	PlS	875
Klimstra, David (NY)	Path	710	Kopp, Peter (IL)	EDM	218
Kline, Mark (TX)	PInf	784	Korenblat, Phillip (MO)	A&I	88
Kline, Richard (LA)	GO	287	Korf, Bruce (AL)	CG	159
Klingemann, Hans-Georg (MA)	Hem	310	Kormos, Robert (PA)	T&CS	1118
Klingensmith, Georgeanna (CO)	PEn	748	Kornmehl, Ernest (MA)	Oph	570
Klonoff, David (CA)	EDM	223	Korones, David (NY)	PHO	761
Klutke, Carl (MO)	U	1168	Korsten, Mark (NY)	Ge	235
Knechtle, Stuart (GA)	S	1069	Koruda, Mark (NC)	S	1069
Kneisl, Jeffrey (NC)	OrS	629	Korytkowski, Mary (PA)	EDM	211
Knisely, Jonathan (NY)	RadRO	951	Kosofsky, Barry (NY)	ChiN	147
Knopf, William (GA)	IC	130	Koss, Michael (CA)	Path	721
Knudson, Mary (CA)	S	1097	Kosten, Thomas (TX)	AdP	906
Kobashigawa, Jon (CA)	Cv	117	Kostis, John (NJ)	Cv	100
Kobrin, Sidney (PA)	Nep	458	Kotagal, Suresh (MN)	ChiN	150
Kobrine, Arthur (DC)	NS	476	Kotapka, Mark (PA)	NS	476
Kobrinsky, Nathan (ND)	PHO	774	Kotler, Donald (NY)	Ge	235
Koch, Christian (MS)	EDM	214	Kotloff, Karen (MD)	PInf	780
Koch, Douglas (TX)	Oph	596	Kotloff, Robert (PA)	Pul	926

Alphabetical Listing of Doctors

Name	Specialty	Pg	Name	Specialty	Pg
Koufman, Jamie (NY)	Oto	661	Krummel, Thomas (CA)	PS	811
Kougias, Panagiotis (TX)	VascS	1193	Krunic, Aleksandar (IL)	D	194
Koulos, John (NY)	GO	278	Kuban, Deborah (TX)	RadRO	964
Kovitz, Kevin (IL)	Pul	934	Kucharczuk, John (PA)	T&CS	1119
Kovnar, Edward (WI)	ChiN	151	Kucuk, Omer (GA)	Onc	358
Kowalski, Thomas (PA)	Ge	235	Kudrimoti, Mahesh (KY)	RadRO	954
Kozarek, Richard (WA)	Ge	254	Kuettel, Michael (NY)	RadRO	951
Kozin, Scott (PA)	HS	296	Kuhel, William (NY)	Oto	662
Kozlowski, James (IL)	U	1168	Kuhn, Frederick (GA)	Oto	669
Kraay, Matthew (OH)	OrS	635	Kuhn, Joseph (TX)	S	1090
Krackow, Kenneth (NY)	OrS	621	Kuiken, Todd (IL)	PMR	841
Kraft, Andrew (SC)	Onc	358	Kula, Roger (NY)	N	513
Krag, David (VT)	S	1050	Kulick, Roy (NY)	HS	296
Krajcer, Zvonimir (TX)	Cv	114	Kuller, Jeffrey (NC)	MF	435
Kramer, Barry (CA)	GerPsy	915	Kumar, Princy (DC)	Inf	412
Kramer, Kim (NY)	PHO	761	Kumpe, David (CO)	VIR	996
Kraus, Dennis (NY)	Oto	662	Kun, Larry (TN)	RadRO	954
Kraus, Michael (IN)	Nep	461	Kung, Faith (CA)	PHO	778
Krauss, Gregory (MD)	N	513	Kunkel, Elisabeth (PA)	Psyc	893
Krauss, Howard (CA)	Oph	601	Kunschner, Lara (PA)	N	513
Kraut, Eric (OH)	Hem	320	Kuntz, Charles (OH)	NS	488
Krebs, Nancy (CO)	PGe	754	Kupelian, Patrick (CA)	RadRO	966
Kreissman, Susan (NC)	PHO	767	Kupersmith, Mark (NY)	Oph	576
Kreitzer, Joel (NY)	PM	697	Kupfer, David (PA)	Psyc	893
Krellenstein, Daniel (NY)	T&CS	1118	Kupper, Thomas (MA)	D	183
Krespi, Yosef (NY)	Oto	662	Kurachek, Stephen (MN)	PPul	797
Kress, Douglas (PA)	D	187	Kuriakose, Philip (MI)	Hem	320
Kress, Kenneth (GA)	OrS	629	Kurland, Geoffrey (PA)	PPul	794
Kressel, Bruce (DC)	Onc	344	Kurman, Robert (MD)	Path	710
Kriegel, David (NY)	D	187	Kurtin, Paul (MN)	Path	716
Krieger, Karl (NY)	T&CS	1119	Kurtz, Alfred (PA)	DR	976
Krilov, Leonard (NY)	PInf	780	Kurtz, Robert (NY)	Ge	235
Kris, Mark (NY)	Onc	344	Kurtzberg, Joanne (NC)	PHO	767
Krishnamurthi, Smitha (OH)	Onc	369	Kurtzke, Robert (VA)	N	522
Krisht, Ali (AR)	NS	493	Kushner, Brian (NY)	PHO	761
Kron, Irving (VA)	T&CS	1126	Kushner, Burton (WI)	Oph	591
Kronenberg, Henry (MA)	EDM	207	Kuske, Robert (AZ)	RadRO	964
Kronn, David (NY)	CG	157	Kutner, Jean (CO)	H & PM	407
Kronowitz, Steven (TX)	PlS	870	Kutteh, William (TN)	RE	1012
Krontiras, Helen (AL)	S	1069	Kuttesch, John (PA)	PHO	762
Krouse, Robert (AZ)	S	1090	Kuvin, Jeffrey (MA)	Cv	95
Krowka, Michael (MN)	Pul	934	Kuzel, Timothy (IL)	Onc	369
Krueger, Gerald (UT)	D	196	Kuzniecky, Ruben (NY)	N	513
Krueger, Richard (NY)	Psyc	893	Kuzon, William (MI)	PlS	866
Krueger, Ronald (OH)	Oph	591	Kveton, John (CT)	Oto	656
Krumholz, Allan (MD)	N	513	Kvols, Larry (FL)	Onc	358

Name	Specialty	Pg	Name	Specialty	Pg
Kwak, Larry (TX)	Onc	379	Lane, Stephen (MN)	Oph	591
Kwo, Paul (IN)	Ge	246	Lang, Frederick (TX)	NS	493
Kwolek, Christopher (MA)	VascS	1184	Lang, Peter (MA)	PCd	733
Kwon, Hower (WA)	ChAP	912	Lang, Samuel (NY)	T&CS	1119
Kwon, Young (IA)	Oph	591	Lange, Beverly (PA)	PHO	762
			Lange, Paul (WA)	U	1177
			Langer, Corey (PA)	Onc	344
			Langford, Carol (OH)	Rhu	1031
L			Langman, Craig (IL)	PNep	787
La Ban, Myron (MI)	PMR	841	Langston, J William (CA)	N	537
La Gamma, Edmund (NY)	NP	447	Lannin, Donald (CT)	S	1050
La Mont, J Thomas (MA)	Ge	229	Lansman, Steven (NY)	T&CS	1119
La Quaglia, Michael (NY)	PS	803	Lanteri, Vincent (NJ)	U	1154
La Russo, Nicholas (MN)	Ge	246	Lantos, John (MO)	Ped	728
Labar, Douglas (NY)	N	514	Lanza, Donald (FL)	Oto	669
Labiner, David (AZ)	N	534	Lanza, Louis (AZ)	T&CS	1138
Lachs, Mark (NY)	Ger	263	Lapey, Allen (MA)	PPul	794
Lacomis, David (PA)	N	514	Laramore, George (WA)	RadRO	966
Lacy, Jill (CT)	Onc	331	Larner, James (VA)	RadRO	955
Ladenson, Paul (MD)	EDM	211	Larrabee, Wayne (WA)	Oto	685
Lage, Janice (SC)	Path	713	Larsen, Christian (GA)	S	1070
Laham, Roger (MA)	IC	126	Larsen, Donald (CA)	NRad	991
Laheru, Daniel (MD)	Onc	344	Larsen, Philip Reed (MA)	EDM	207
Lahita, Robert (NJ)	Rhu	1027	Larson, David (CA)	RadRO	967
Laks, Hillel (CA)	T&CS	1142	Larson, Richard (IL)	Hem	320
Lalwani, Anil (NY)	Oto	662	Lasala, John (MO)	IC	131
Lambert, H Michael (TX)	Oph	597	Lash, Robert (MI)	EDM	218
Lambert, Paul (SC)	Oto	669	Lashner, Bret (OH)	Ge	246
Lambert, Scott (GA)	Oph	584	Lask, Gary (CA)	D	199
Lamberti, John (CA)	T&CS	1142	Laske, Douglas (PA)	NS	476
Lambiase, Louis (TN)	Ge	241	Lass, Jonathan (OH)	Oph	591
Lamonica, Dominick (NY)	NuM	548	Latchaw, Laurie (NH)	PS	802
LaMuraglia, Glenn M (MA)	VascS	1185	Laterra, John (MD)	N	514
Lancaster, Johnathan (FL)	GO	281	Latov, Norman (NY)	N	514
Landers, Daniel (MN)	MF	436	Latson, Larry (FL)	PCd	737
Landman, Jaime (CA)	U	1177	Lau, Christine (VA)	T&CS	1126
Landon, Mark (OH)	MF	436	Lauerman, William (DC)	OrS	621
Landreneau, Rodney (PA)	T&CS	1119	Laufer, Marc (MA)	ObG	556
Landrigan, Philip (NY)	OM	882	Laughlin, Mary (VA)	Hem	317
Landry, Jerome (GA)	RadRO	955	Laurencin, Cato (CT)	OrS	612
Landy, Helain (DC)	MF	433	Lavenstein, Bennett (VA)	ChiN	149
Landy, Howard (FL)	NS	482	Laver, Joseph (TN)	PHO	767
Landzberg, Joel (NJ)	Cv	100	Lavertu, Pierre (OH)	Oto	676
Lane, Joseph (NY)	OrS	621	Lavery, Ian (OH)	CRS	174
Lane, Judy (CO)	N	532	Lavin, Patrick (TN)	N	522
Lane, Lewis (NY)	HS	296	Lavis, Victor (TX)	EDM	221

Alphabetical Listing of Doctors

Name	Specialty	Pg	Name	Specialty	Pg
Lavyne, Michael (NY)	NS	476	Leighton, John (PA)	Onc	344
Lawrence, Theodore (MI)	RadRO	960	Leighton, Jonathan (AZ)	Ge	252
Lawry, George (CA)	Rhu	1034	Leighton, William (AZ)	PlS	871
Lawson, David (GA)	Onc	358	Leipziger, Lyle (NY)	PlS	855
Lawson, Edward (MD)	NP	447	Leitch, A Marilyn (TX)	S	1090
Lawson, William (NY)	Oto	662	Lele, Shashikant (NY)	GO	279
Lawson, William (DC)	Psyc	893	Lem, Vincent (MO)	Pul	934
Lazar, Harold (MA)	T&CS	1111	Lemanske, Robert (WI)	PA&I	731
Lazarus, Hillard (OH)	Onc	369	Lemole, G Michael (AZ)	NS	493
Lazzaro, Richard (NY)	T&CS	1119	Lemons, James (IN)	NP	450
Le, Quynh-Thu Xuan (CA)	RadRO	967	Lengyel, Ernst (IL)	ObG	561
Le Boit, Philip (CA)	Path	721	Lenke, Lawrence (MO)	OrS	635
Lea, Janice (GA)	Nep	460	Lentz, Christopher (NM)	S	1090
Leach, Steven (MD)	S	1059	Lentz, Samuel (NC)	GO	282
Leadbetter, Wayne (MD)	OrS	621	Leon, Martin (NY)	IC	127
Leaf, Norman (CA)	PlS	875	Leonard, Ethan (OH)	PInf	783
LeBoff, Meryl (MA)	EDM	208	Leonard, James (MI)	PMR	841
Lebovics, Robert (NY)	Oto	662	Leonetti, John (IL)	Oto	676
Lebwohl, Mark (NY)	D	187	Lepanto, Philip (WV)	RadRO	951
Lebwohl, Nathan (FL)	OrS	629	Lepor, Herbert (NY)	U	1154
Lebwohl, Oscar (NY)	Ge	235	Lerman, Bruce (NY)	CE	120
Lechan, Ronald (MA)	EDM	208	Lerner, Seth (TX)	U	1173
Leckman, James (CT)	ChAP	907	Les, Kimberly (MI)	OrS	635
Lederman, Eric (MO)	CRS	174	Lesavoy, Malcolm (CA)	PlS	875
Ledford, Dennis (FL)	A&I	86	Leshin, Barry (NC)	D	191
Lee, Andrew (TX)	RadRO	964	Leslie, Donald (GA)	PMR	839
Lee, Andrew (TX)	Oph	597	Leslie, Kevin (AZ)	Path	718
Lee, Cheryl (MI)	U	1168	Leslie, Kimberly (IA)	MF	437
Lee, Chung (MN)	RadRO	960	Lesser, Glenn (NC)	Onc	358
Lee, Francis (NY)	OrS	621	Lessin, Stuart (PA)	D	187
Lee, Jeffrey (TX)	S	1090	Leuchter, Andrew (CA)	Psyc	901
Lee, Joon (PA)	IC	127	Leung, Donald (CO)	PA&I	732
Lee, Kenneth (PA)	S	1059	Leung, Lawrence (CA)	Hem	326
Lee, Patrick (OR)	CRS	177	Leung, Wing (TN)	PHO	767
Lee, Paul (MI)	Oph	591	Levenback, Charles (TX)	GO	288
Lee, Raphael (IL)	PlS	866	Leventhal, Bennett (NY)	ChAP	909
Lee, W P Andrew (MD)	HS	297	Levi, Allan (FL)	NS	482
Lee, W Robert (NC)	RadRO	955	Levi, Joe (FL)	S	1070
Leeming, Rosemary (OH)	S	1079	Levin, Alex (PA)	Oph	576
Leffell, David (CT)	D	183	Levin, David (OK)	Pul	938
Legare, Robert (RI)	Onc	331	Levin, Lawrence (PA)	PlS	855
Legido, Agustin (PA)	ChN	148	Levine, Alexandra (CA)	Hem	326
Legro, Richard (PA)	RE	1009	Levine, David (NY)	N	514
Lehman, Constance (WA)	DR	983	Levine, David (NY)	OrS	621
Lehman, Thomas (NY)	PRhu	799	Levine, Edward (NC)	S	1070
Leichtner, Alan (MA)	PGe	749	Levine, Elliot (IL)	ObG	562

Alphabetical Listing of Doctors

Name	Specialty	Pg	Name	Specialty	Pg
Levine, Ellis (NY)	Onc	344	Lieberman, Michael (NY)	S	1060
Levine, Joel (CO)	Ge	250	Lieberman, Phillip (TN)	A&I	86
Levine, Joseph (NY)	CE	121	Liebmann, Jeffrey (NY)	Oph	576
Levine, Joshua (NY)	PlS	855	Liem, Pham (AR)	Ger	266
Levine, Laurence (IL)	U	1168	Lieskovsky, Gary (CA)	U	1177
Levine, Michael (PA)	PEn	744	Light, Richard (TN)	Pul	931
Levine, Paul (VA)	Oto	669	Light, Terry (IL)	HS	301
Levine, Robert (NH)	EDM	208	Lightdale, Charles (NY)	Ge	236
Levine, Stephen (OH)	Psyc	897	Liker, Mark (CA)	NS	497
Levine, Steven (NY)	N	514	Lilenbaum, Rogerio (FL)	Onc	358
Levine, William (NY)	SM	1041	Lill, Michael (CA)	Hem	326
Levitsky, Lynne (MA)	PEn	743	Lillehei, Craig (MA)	PS	802
Levy, Angela (DC)	DR	976	Lillehei, Kevin (CO)	NS	491
Levy, Joseph (NY)	PGe	750	Lillemoe, Keith (MA)	S	1050
Levy, Michael (PA)	Onc	344	Lim, Dean Wee (CA)	Onc	387
Levy, Michael (MN)	Ge	246	Lim, Henry (MI)	D	194
Levy, Michael (CA)	NS	497	Lim Quan, Katherine (AZ)	D	197
Levy, Moise (TX)	D	197	Limentani, Steven (NC)	Onc	359
Levy, Richard (IL)	PEn	747	Lin, Daniel (WA)	U	1177
Levy, Steven (GA)	Psyc	896	Lin, Jeffrey (DC)	GO	279
Lew, Mark (CA)	N	537	Lin, Weei-Chin (TX)	Hem	324
Lewin, Alan (FL)	RadRO	955	Lind, Christopher (TN)	Ge	241
Lewin, Mark (WA)	PCd	741	Lindenfeld, JoAnn (CO)	Cv	113
Lewis, Blair (NY)	Ge	235	Linder, Jennifer (AZ)	D	197
Lewis, Curtis (GA)	VIR	995	Lindsay, Bruce (OH)	CE	123
Lewis, John (AZ)	A&I	89	Lindsey, Stephen (LA)	Rhu	1033
Lewis, Richard (TX)	Oph	597	Lindstrom, Richard (MN)	Oph	591
Lewis, Richard (MI)	N	527	Linenberger, Michael (WA)	Hem	326
Lewis, Sandra (OR)	Cv	117	Link, Mark (MA)	CE	119
Lewis, Valerae (TX)	OrS	641	Link, Michael (CA)	PHO	778
Lewkowiez, Laurent (CO)	CE	124	Link, Michael (MN)	NS	488
Li, Benjamin (LA)	S	1090	Linsenmeyer, Todd (NJ)	U	1155
Li, James Tung-Chieh (MN)	A&I	88	Linskey, Mark (CA)	NS	497
Li Volsi, Virginia (PA)	Path	710	Linstrom, Christopher (NY)	Oto	662
Liang, Bruce (CT)	Cv	95	Linton, MacRae (TN)	Cv	104
Liao, Kenneth (MN)	T&CS	1133	Lipkowitz, George (MA)	S	1050
Liau, Linda (CA)	NS	497	Liporace, Joyce (PA)	N	514
Libby, Daniel (NY)	Pul	926	Lippman, Marc (FL)	Onc	359
Liberman, Robert (CA)	Psyc	901	Lippman, Scott (CA)	Onc	387
Libertino, John (MA)	U	1149	Lipschitz, David (AR)	Ger	266
Libutti, Steven (NY)	S	1060	Lipshultz, Larry (TX)	U	1174
Licciardi, Frederick (NY)	RE	1009	Lipshutz, William (PA)	Ge	236
Lichtenstein, David (MA)	Ge	229	Lipsitz, Lewis (MA)	Ger	262
Lichtenstein, Gary (PA)	Ge	236	Lipson, Ace (DC)	EDM	211
Lichter, Paul (MI)	Oph	591	Lipstate, James (LA)	Rhu	1033
Liddle, Rodger (NC)	Ge	241	Lipton, Jeffrey (NY)	PHO	762

Alphabetical Listing of Doctors

Name	Specialty	Pg	Name	Specialty	Pg
Lipton, Richard (NY)	N	514	Lossos, Izidore (FL)	Onc	359
Lis, Eric (NY)	NRad	986	Lott, Ira (CA)	ChiN	153
Lisak, Robert (MI)	N	527	Loughlin, Gerald (NY)	PPul	795
Lisman, Richard (NY)	Oph	576	Loughlin, Kevin (MA)	U	1149
List, Alan (FL)	Onc	359	Louie, Eddie (NY)	Inf	412
Little, John (DC)	PlS	855	Louis, Elan (NY)	N	515
Litzow, Mark (MN)	Hem	320	Loulmet, Didier (NY)	T&CS	1119
Liu, Charles (CA)	NS	497	Love, Charles (OH)	CE	123
Liu, Grant (PA)	N	515	Love, Robert (IL)	T&CS	1133
Liu, Vincent (IA)	D	194	Low, David (PA)	PlS	855
Livingston, Edward (TX)	S	1090	Lowe, Franklin (NY)	U	1155
Livingston, Robert (AZ)	Onc	380	Lowe, Lori (MI)	D	194
Livingstone, Alan (FL)	S	1070	Lowenberg, David (CA)	OrS	644
Ljung, Britt-Marie (CA)	Path	721	Lowitt, Mark (MD)	D	187
Lloyd, L Keith (AL)	U	1162	Lowry, Ann (MN)	CRS	174
Lobe, Thom (CA)	PS	811	Lowy, Andrew (CA)	S	1097
Locala, Joseph (OH)	Psyc	898	Loyd, James (TN)	Pul	931
Lock, James (MA)	PCd	734	Lu, Karen (TX)	GO	288
Lock, Terrence (MI)	OrS	635	Lubahn, John (PA)	HS	297
Lockey, Richard (FL)	A&I	86	Lublin, Fred (NY)	N	515
Lockhart, Jorge (FL)	U	1162	Luby, James (TX)	Inf	418
Loder, Elizabeth (MA)	PM	696	Luby, Joan (MO)	ChAP	911
Loeb, David (MD)	PHO	762	Lucarelli, Mark (WI)	Oph	592
Loeffler, Jay (MA)	RadRO	947	Lucas, David (MI)	Path	716
Loehrer, Patrick (IN)	Onc	369	Lucci, Joseph (FL)	GO	282
Loevner, Laurie (PA)	NRad	986	Lucente, Vincent (PA)	ObG	557
Loewenstein, Richard (MD)	Psyc	893	Lucey, Michael (WI)	Ge	247
Loftus, Christopher (IL)	NS	488	Luchtman-Jones, Lori (DC)	PHO	762
Loftus, Edward (MN)	Ge	247	Luciano, Anthony (CT)	RE	1007
Logan, William (MO)	N	527	Luck, James (CA)	OrS	644
Logan-Young, Wende (NY)	DR	976	Lucky, Anne (OH)	D	194
Loggie, Brian (NE)	S	1085	Luders, Hans (OH)	N	527
Logigian, Eric (NY)	N	515	Ludwig, David (MA)	PEn	743
Logothetis, Christopher (TX)	Onc	380	Ludwig, Kirk (WI)	CRS	174
Long, Sarah (PA)	PInf	781	Lueder, Gregg (MO)	Oph	592
Longo, Frank (CA)	N	538	Luerssen, Thomas (TX)	NS	493
Longo, Walter (CT)	CRS	168	Luger, Selina (PA)	Hem	313
Longworth, David (OH)	Inf	416	Lugg, James (WY)	U	1172
Loo, Marcus (NY)	U	1155	Luggen, Michael (OH)	Rhu	1031
Loomba, Rohit (CA)	Ge	254	Luken, Martin (IL)	NS	488
Loprinzi, Charles (MN)	Onc	369	Lumsden, Alan (TX)	VascS	1193
Lorber, Bennett (PA)	Inf	412	Lunsford, L Dade (PA)	NS	476
Loree, Thom (NY)	PlS	855	Lurain, John (IL)	GO	284
LoRusso, Thomas (VA)	Pul	931	Lusher, Jeanne (MI)	PHO	771
Loscalzo, Joseph (MA)	Cv	95	Lusk, Rodney (NE)	PO	792
Losee, Joseph (PA)	PlS	855	Lustig, Lawrence (CA)	Oto	685

Name	Specialty	Pg		Name	Specialty	Pg
Lustig, Robert (CA)	PEn	749		Magovern, George (PA)	T&CS	1119
Luterman, Arnold (AL)	S	1070		Magramm, Irene (NY)	Oph	577
Luthra, Harvinder (MN)	Rhu	1031		Magrina, Javier (AZ)	GO	288
Lutsep, Helmi (OR)	N	538		Maguire, Joseph (PA)	Oph	577
Lutz, Christopher (NY)	PMR	836		Maguire, Leo (MN)	Oph	592
Lutz, Gregory (NY)	PMR	836		Magun, Arthur (NY)	Ge	236
Lyckholm, Laurel (VA)	Onc	359		Mahler, Donald (NH)	Pul	923
Lydiatt, Daniel (NE)	Oto	680		Mahmud, Ehtisham (CA)	IC	133
Lydiatt, William (NE)	Oto	680		Mahoney, Maurice (CT)	CG	156
Lyketsos, Constantine (MD)	GerPsy	913		Mahony, Lynn (TX)	PCd	740
Lyles, Kenneth (NC)	Ger	264		Mahvi, David (IL)	S	1079
Lyman, Gary (NC)	Onc	359		Majd, Massoud (DC)	NuM	548
Lynch, James (FL)	Onc	359		Makaroun, Michel (PA)	VascS	1187
Lynch, Joseph (CA)	Pul	940		Makhija, Sharmila (KY)	GO	282
Lynch, Thomas (CT)	Onc	331		Makhoul, Issam (AR)	Onc	380
Lynne, Charles (FL)	U	1162		Maki, Dennis (WI)	Inf	416
Lyons, Roger (TX)	Hem	324		Maki, Robert (NY)	Onc	345
Lytle, Bruce (OH)	T&CS	1133		Malawer, Martin (MD)	OrS	622
				Malcolm, Arnold (TN)	RadRO	955
				Maldjian, Joseph (NC)	NRad	987
				Malik, Ghaus (MI)	NS	488
M				Malkowicz, S Bruce (PA)	U	1155
Ma, C Benjamin (CA)	SM	1044		Maloney, David G (WA)	Onc	388
Ma, Dong (NY)	PMR	836		Maloney, Mary (MA)	D	183
Mabrey, Jay (TX)	OrS	641		Maloney, Robert (CA)	Oph	601
Macadaeg, Kevin (IN)	PM	699		Mamelak, Adam (CA)	NS	498
Macaulay, William (NY)	OrS	622		Mamounas, Eleftherios (OH)	S	1079
MacDonald, Kenneth (NC)	S	1070		Manche, Edward (CA)	Oph	602
Machtay, Mitchell (OH)	RadRO	961		Manco-Johnson, Marilyn (CO)	PHO	774
Macias, John (AZ)	Oto	682		Mancuso, Anthony (FL)	DR	979
Maciejewski, Jaroslaw (OH)	Hem	321		Mandel, Eric (NY)	Oph	577
Mack, Michael (TX)	T&CS	1139		Mandel, Susan (PA)	EDM	211
Mackay, Donald (PA)	PlS	856		Mandelbaum, Bert (CA)	OrS	644
MacKenzie, Richard (CA)	AM	82		Mandelbaum, David (RI)	ChiN	146
Mackey, Sean (CA)	PM	703		Manders, Ernest (PA)	PlS	856
Mackey, William (MA)	VascS	1185		Manepalli, Jothika (MO)	GerPsy	914
MacKinnon, Susan (MO)	PlS	866		Manera, Ricarchito (IL)	PHO	772
Macklis, Roger (OH)	RadRO	961		Manevitz, Alan (NY)	Psyc	893
Mackool, Richard (NY)	Oph	577		Mangan, Kenneth (PA)	Hem	313
Maclaren, Noel (NY)	PEn	744		Mangat, Devinder (KY)	Oto	669
MacLean, James (MA)	A&I	84		Mann, J John (NY)	Psyc	893
Macones, George (MO)	MF	437		Mannella, William (PA)	S	1060
Madoff, Robert (MN)	CRS	174		Manning, Warren (MA)	Cv	95
Madsen, Joseph (MA)	NS	471		Mannis, Mark (CA)	Oph	602
Magee, William (VA)	PlS	862		Manoli, Arthur (MI)	OrS	635
Magid, Steven (NY)	Rhu	1027		Mansfield, Paul (TX)	S	1091

Alphabetical Listing of Doctors

Name	Specialty	Pg	Name	Specialty	Pg
Manson, Paul (MD)	PIS	856	Marten, Timothy (CA)	PIS	875
Mantyh, Christopher (NC)	CRS	172	Martenson, James (MN)	RadRO	961
Manzi, Susan (PA)	Rhu	1027	Martin, Neil (CA)	NS	498
Mapstone, Timothy (OK)	NS	494	Martin, Paul (FL)	Ge	241
Maraganore, Demetrius (IL)	N	528	Martin, Richard (CO)	Pul	937
Marcet, Jorge (FL)	CRS	172	Martin, Richard (OH)	NP	450
Marchlinski, Francis (PA)	CE	121	Martin, Tomas (FL)	T&CS	1126
Marcom, Paul (NC)	Onc	359	Martinez, Fernando (MI)	Pul	934
Marcus, Carole (PA)	PPul	795	Martini, D Richard (UT)	ChAP	911
Marcus, Judith (NY)	PHO	762	Martins, Renato (WA)	Onc	388
Marcus, Robert (FL)	RadRO	955	Martuza, Robert (MA)	NS	471
Marder, Karen (NY)	N	515	Marx, Robert (NY)	OrS	622
Marder, Stephen (CA)	Psyc	901	Masaryk, Thomas (OH)	NRad	989
Marentette, Lawrence (MI)	Oto	676	Masket, Samuel (CA)	Oph	602
Margolin, Kim (WA)	Onc	388	Maslak, Peter (NY)	Hem	313
Mari, Giancarlo (TN)	MF	435	Mason, David (OH)	T&CS	1133
Marin, Deborah (NY)	Psyc	894	Mason, Joel (MA)	Ge	229
Marin, Michael (NY)	VascS	1188	Mason, Kristin (CO)	PMR	842
Marina, Neyssa (CA)	PHO	778	Mason, Wilbert (CA)	PInf	785
Marini, John (MN)	Pul	934	Masood, Shahla (FL)	Path	713
Marino, Ralph (PA)	PMR	837	Mass, Daniel (IL)	HS	301
Marion, Robert (NY)	CG	158	Massagli, Teresa (WA)	PMR	844
Maris, John (PA)	PHO	762	Massarotti, Elena (MA)	Rhu	1024
Mark, Eugene (MA)	Path	706	Massin, Edward (TX)	Cv	114
Markert, James (AL)	NS	483	Mast, Bruce (FL)	PIS	862
Markert, M Louise (NC)	A&I	87	Masters, Gregory (DE)	Onc	345
Markman, Maurie (PA)	Onc	345	Mastrobattista, Joan (TX)	MF	438
Markmann, James (MA)	S	1051	Masur, Henry (MD)	Inf	412
Markoe, Arnold (FL)	RadRO	955	Matar, Fadi (FL)	IC	130
Markowitz, Bernard (CA)	PIS	875	Matarasso, Alan (NY)	PIS	856
Markowitz, David (NY)	Ge	236	Matas, Arthur (MN)	S	1079
Markowitz, Sanford (OH)	Onc	369	Mather, Paul (PA)	Cv	100
Marks, Jeffrey (OH)	S	1079	Mathers, William (OR)	Oph	602
Marks, Lawrence (NC)	RadRO	955	Mathew, Paul (MA)	Onc	331
Marks, Peter (CT)	Hem	310	Mathisen, Douglas (MA)	T&CS	1111
Marks, Stanley (PA)	Hem	313	Matsen, Frederick (WA)	OrS	644
Marmor, Michael (CA)	Oph	602	Matsumoto, Alan (VA)	VIR	995
Maroon, Joseph (PA)	NS	477	Matthay, Katherine (CA)	PHO	778
Marrs, Richard (CA)	RE	1017	Matthews, David (NC)	PIS	862
Marsh, Christopher (CA)	U	1177	Matthews, Dennis (CO)	PMR	842
Marsh, James (PA)	S	1060	Matthews, Jeffrey (IL)	S	1079
Marsh, James (CT)	OrS	612	Mattox, Douglas (GA)	Oto	669
Marsh, Jeffrey (MO)	PIS	866	Matulonis, Ursula (MA)	Onc	331
Marshall, John (VA)	EDM	214	Matuschak, George (MO)	Pul	935
Marshall, John (DC)	Onc	345	Mauro, Matthew (NC)	VIR	995
Marshall, M Blair (DC)	T&CS	1120	Mavroudis, Constantine (FL)	T&CS	1126

Name	Specialty	Pg	Name	Specialty	Pg
Mawad, Michel (TX)	NRad	990	McCracken, George (TX)	PInf	784
Mawn, Louise (TN)	Oph	584	McCracken, James (CA)	ChAP	912
Maxfield, Roger (NY)	Pul	926	McCulley, James (TX)	Oph	597
Maxwell, G Patrick (TN)	PlS	863	McCullough, Andrew (NY)	U	1155
Mayberg, Marc (WA)	NS	498	McCune, W Joseph (MI)	Rhu	1031
Mayer, John (MA)	T&CS	1111	McDermott, Michael (CA)	NS	498
Mayer, Lloyd (NY)	Ge	236	McDiarmid, Suzanne (CA)	PGe	756
Mayer, Nathaniel (PA)	PMR	837	McDonald, Douglas (MO)	OrS	635
Mayer, Robert (MA)	Onc	331	McDonald, Ruth (WA)	PNep	788
Mayerson, Joel (OH)	OrS	635	McDonnell, Peter (MD)	Oph	577
Mayes, Maureen (TX)	Rhu	1033	McDougal, W Scott (MA)	U	1149
Mayeux, Richard (NY)	N	515	McDougle, Christopher (MA)	ChAP	907
Maynard, Steven (DC)	ObG	558	McFadden, David (CT)	S	1051
Maytal, Joseph (NY)	ChiN	148	McFarland, Edward (MD)	OrS	622
Maziarz, Richard (OR)	Hem	326	McGahan, John (CA)	VIR	998
Mazza, David (NY)	A&I	85	McGarry, Ronald (KY)	RadRO	956
Mazzone, Theodore (IL)	EDM	218	McGiffin, David (AL)	T&CS	1126
McAfee, Paul (MD)	OrS	622	McGill, Janet (MO)	EDM	218
McAlindon, Timothy (MA)	Rhu	1024	McGill, Leigh (AZ)	PS	809
McAneny, David (MA)	S	1051	McGill, Trevor (MA)	PO	789
McAninch, Jack (CA)	U	1177	McGlashan, Thomas (CT)	Psyc	889
McArthur, Justin (MD)	N	515	McGlave, Philip (MN)	Hem	321
McCabe, Daniel (AZ)	S	1091	McGovern, Francis (MA)	U	1149
McCallum, Kimberli (MO)	Psyc	898	McGovern, Peter (NJ)	RE	1009
McCance, Sean (NY)	OrS	622	McGowan, Joseph (NY)	Inf	412
McCann, John (UT)	Oph	596	McGrath, Patrick (KY)	S	1070
McCann, Merle (MD)	Psyc	894	Mcgrath-Morrow, Sharon (MD)	PPul	795
McCann, Peter (NY)	OrS	622	McGuire, Edward (MI)	U	1168
McCann, Richard (NC)	VascS	1189	McGuire, William (MD)	Onc	345
McCarthy, James (MN)	Nep.	461	McHenry, Christopher (OH)	S	1079
McCarthy, James (OH)	OrS	635	McIntosh, J Michael (UT)	Psyc	899
McCarthy, Joseph (NY)	PlS	856	McIntyre, Robert (CO)	S	1085
McCarthy, Patrick (IL)	T&CS	1133	McKelvey, Robert (OR)	ChAP	912
McCarthy, Paul (CT)	PRhu	799	McKenna, Michael (MA)	Oto	656
McCarthy, Shirley (CT)	DR	973	McKeown, Craig (FL)	Oph	584
McClamrock, Howard (MD)	RE	1009	McKinley, William (VA)	PMR	839
McClay, Edward (CA)	Onc	388	McKinney, Ross (NC)	PInf	782
McClure, Robert (WA)	U	1177	McKinsey, James (NY)	VascS	1188
McCluskey, Leo (PA)	N	515	McLafferty, Robert (IL)	VascS	1191
McComsey, Grace (OH)	PInf	783	McLaren, Rodney (VA)	MF	435
McConnell, John (NC)	U	1162	McLean, Gordon (PA)	VIR	993
McConnell, Robert (NY)	EDM	211	McLean, Thomas (NC)	PHO	767
McCormick, Beryl (NY)	RadRO	951	McMahon, M Molly (MN)	EDM	219
McCormick, Paul (NY)	NS	477	McMasters, Kelly (KY)	S	1070
McCormick, Wayne (WA)	Ger	267	McMenomey, Sean (OR)	Oto	686
McCoy, Karen (OH)	PPul	797	McMichael, Amy (NC)	D	191

Alphabetical Listing of Doctors

Name	Specialty	Pg	Name	Specialty	Pg
McPherson, David (TX)	Cv	114	Meropol, Neal (OH)	Onc	370
McVary, Kevin (IL)	U	1168	Merrick, Scot (CA)	T&CS	1142
Meacham, Lillian (GA)	PEn	746	Merritt, Diane (MO)	ObG	562
Meacham, Randall (CO)	U	1172	Mertz, Howard (TN)	Ge	241
Meadow, William (IL)	NP	450	Mesa, Ruben (AZ)	Hem	324
Meals, Roy (CA)	HS	304	Mesrobian, Hrair-George (WI)	U	1169
Meara, John (MA)	PlS	850	Messersmith, Wells (CO)	Onc	376
Mears, John Gregory (NY)	Hem	313	Mesulam, Marsel (IL)	N	528
Mease, Philip (WA)	Rhu	1034	Metcalfe, Dean (MD)	A&I	85
Medalie, Daniel (OH)	PlS	866	Metersky, Mark (CT)	Pul	923
Medbery, Clinton (OK)	RadRO	965	Mets, Marilyn (IL)	Oph	592
Medich, David (PA)	CRS	170	Metson, Ralph (MA)	Oto	656
Medina, Jesus (OK)	Oto	682	Metz, David (PA)	Ge	236
Medow, Norman (NY)	Oph	577	Metzinger, Stephen (LA)	PlS	871
Medsger, Thomas (PA)	Rhu	1027	Metzl, Jordan (NY)	SM	1041
Meehan, Kenneth (NH)	Hem	310	Meyer, Anthony (NC)	S	1070
Megibow, Alec (NY)	DR	976	Meyer, Fredric (MN)	NS	489
Mehler, Philip (CO)	IM	426	Meyer, William (OK)	PHO	776
Mehlman, David (IL)	Cv	109	Meyers, Bryan (MO)	T&CS	1133
Mehrara, Babak (NY)	PlS	856	Meyers, Paul (NY)	PHO	762
Mehta, Davendra (NY)	CE	121	Meyers, Rebecka (UT)	PS	808
Meiselman, Mick (IL)	Ge	247	Meyers, William (PA)	S	1060
Meissner, H Cody (MA)	PInf	780	Meyskens, Frank (CA)	Onc	388
Mekhail, Nagy (OH)	PM	700	Michaels, Marian (PA)	PInf	781
Melamed, Jonathan (NY)	Path	710	Michalski, Jeff (MO)	RadRO	961
Meller, Jose (NY)	Cv	100	Michelassi, Fabrizio (NY)	S	1060
Mellow, Alan (MI)	GerPsy	914	Micheli, Lyle (MA)	SM	1040
Melmed, Shlomo (CA)	EDM	223	Mickey, Bruce (TX)	NS	494
Melone, Charles (NY)	HS	297	Mieler, William (IL)	Oph	592
Meltzer, Eli (CA)	A&I	90	Mies, Carolyn (PA)	Path	710
Meltzer, Toby (AZ)	PlS	871	Mih, Alexander (IN)	HS	301
Melvin, W Scott (OH)	S	1079	Mikkelsen, Tom (MI)	N	528
Mendenhall, Nancy (FL)	RadRO	956	Miknevich, Mary Ann (PA)	PMR	837
Mendenhall, William (FL)	RadRO	956	Milad, Magdy (IL)	RE	1014
Mendley, Susan (MD)	PNep	786	Milam, Douglas (TN)	U	1162
Menendez, Lawrence (CA)	OrS	644	Mildvan, Donna (NY)	Inf	412
Menezes, Arnold (IA)	NS	488	Miles, Brian (TX)	U	1174
Menick, Frederick (AZ)	PlS	871	Milhem, Mohammed (IA)	Hem	321
Menon, Mani (MI)	U	1169	Mill, Michael (NC)	T&CS	1127
Menon, Ram (MI)	PEn	747	Millenson, Michael (PA)	Hem	314
Menter, M (TX)	D	197	Miller, Aaron (NY)	N	516
Merchant, Thomas (TN)	RadRO	956	Miller, Antonius (NC)	Onc	360
Meredith, Ruby (AL)	RadRO	956	Miller, Brent (MO)	Nep	462
Meredith, Travis (NC)	Oph	585	Miller, Charles (IL)	RE	1014
Merguerian, Paul (WA)	U	1178	Miller, D Craig (CA)	T&CS	1142
Meric-Bernstam, Funda (TX)	S	1091	Miller, Daniel (GA)	T&CS	1127

Name	Specialty	Pg	Name	Specialty	Pg
Miller, David (TX)	GO	288	Mitchell, Paul (CT)	Oph	571
Miller, Donald (KY)	Onc	360	Mitchell, Wendy (CA)	ChiN	153
Miller, Frank (TX)	Oto	683	Mitnick, Hal (NY)	Rhu	1027
Miller, Joan (MA)	Oph	570	Mitnick, Julie (NY)	DR	976
Miller, John (IN)	CE	123	Mitsumoto, Hiroshi (NY)	N	516
Miller, Joseph (AZ)	Oph	597	Mitsuyasu, Ronald (CA)	Onc	388
Miller, Karen (MA)	Ped	726	Mittal, Bharat (IL)	RadRO	961
Miller, Kenneth (MA)	Hem	311	Mittal, Naveen (TX)	PGe	755
Miller, Kevin (CA)	Oph	602	Mittal, Ravinder (CA)	Ge	254
Miller, Mark (VA)	OrS	629	Miyamoto, Richard (IN)	Oto	676
Miller, Michael (OH)	PlS	866	Mizen, Thomas (IL)	Oph	592
Miller, Neil (MD)	Oph	577	Moder, Kevin (MN)	Rhu	1032
Miller, Robert (IL)	PO	792	Modesitt, Susan (VA)	GO	282
Miller, Scott (GA)	U	1162	Modic, Michael (OH)	NRad	989
Miller, Stanley (MD)	D	187	Moe, Kristen (WA)	Oto	686
Miller, Thomas (AZ)	Onc	380	Moench, Louis (UT)	Psyc	899
Miller, Timothy (CA)	PlS	875	Moffitt, Drew (AZ)	RE	1016
Millett, Peter (CO)	OrS	639	Mohl, Paul (TX)	Psyc	900
Milley, J Ross (UT)	NP	451	Mohler, James (NY)	U	1155
Millis, J Michael (IL)	S	1080	Mohr, JP (NY)	N	516
Millman, Richard (RI)	Pul	923	Moley, Jeffrey (MO)	S	1080
Mills, Monte (PA)	Oph	577	Molleston, Jean (IN)	PGe	753
Mills, Stacey (VA)	Path	713	Molnar, Joseph (NC)	PlS	863
Milsom, Jeffrey (NY)	CRS	171	Molo, Mary (IL)	RE	1014
Mims, James (TX)	Oph	597	Mondino, Bartly (CA)	Oph	602
Minaker, Kenneth (MA)	Ger	262	Moneim, Moheb (NM)	HS	303
Minas, Tom (MA)	OrS	612	Money, Samuel (AZ)	VascS	1193
Miniaci, Anthony (OH)	SM	1043	Monsees, Barbara (MO)	DR	981
Minich, Lois (UT)	PCd	739	Montague, Drogo (OH)	U	1169
Mink, Jonathan (NY)	ChiN	148	Montanaro, Anthony (OR)	A&I	90
Minsky, Bruce (TX)	RadRO	965	Montgomery, Elizabeth (MD)	Path	710
Mintzer, David (PA)	Onc	345	Montgomery, Erwin (AL)	N	522
Mirmira, Raghu (IN)	PEn	747	Montgomery, Robert (MD)	S	1060
Mirvis, Stuart (MD)	DR	976	Montie, James (MI)	U	1169
Mirza, Natasha (PA)	Oto	662	Moodie, Douglas (TX)	PCd	740
Mirzayan, Raffy (CA)	SM	1044	Moon, Marc (MO)	T&CS	1134
Mischel, Paul (CA)	Path	721	Moore, Anne (NY)	Onc	345
Miskovitz, Paul (NY)	Ge	236	Moore, David (IN)	GO	284
Mistry, Bhargav (ND)	S	1085	Moore, Ernest (CO)	S	1085
Mitch, William (TX)	Nep	464	Moore, Francis (MA)	S	1051
Mitchell, Beverly (CA)	Hem	326	Moore, Frank (NJ)	NS	477
Mitchell, Charles (FL)	PInf	782	Moore, John (GA)	T&CS	1127
Mitchell, James (ND)	Psyc	899	Moore, Joseph (NC)	Onc	360
Mitchell, John (CO)	T&CS	1136	Moore, Steven (IA)	Path	716
Mitchell, Marc (MS)	VascS	1189	Moore, Thomas (CA)	MF	440
Mitchell, Max (CO)	T&CS	1137	Moore, Walter (GA)	Rhu	1030

Alphabetical Listing of Doctors

Name	Specialty	Pg	Name	Specialty	Pg
Moossa, AR (CA)	S	1097	Muggia, Franco (NY)	Onc	346
Moots, Paul (TN)	N	522	Mukherjee, Tanmoy (NY)	RE	1009
Morady, Fred (MI)	CE	123	Mukherji, Suresh (MI)	NRad	989
Moran, Cesar (TX)	Path	718	Muldoon, Thomas (NY)	Oph	578
Moran, Christopher (MO)	NRad	989	Mulhall, John (NY)	U	1155
Moran, John (IL)	Cv	109	Mullett, Timothy (KY)	T&CS	1127
Morcos, Jacques (FL)	NS	483	Mulliken, John (MA)	PlS	851
Morcuende, Jose (IA)	OrS	636	Mulvihill, John (OK)	CG	161
Morgan, David (TN)	Onc	360	Mulvihill, Sean (UT)	S	1085
Morgan, Elaine (IL)	PHO	772	Mundt, Arno (CA)	RadRO	967
Morgan, Linda (FL)	ObG	559	Munin, Michael (PA)	PMR	837
Morgan, Mark (PA)	GO	279	Munker, Reinhold (LA)	Hem	324
Morgan, Raymond (VA)	PlS	863	Munoz, Santiago (PA)	Ge	237
Morgan, Walter (TN)	PS	805	Muntz, Howard (WA)	GO	290
Morgan, Wayne (AZ)	PPul	797	Murali, Raj (NY)	NS	477
Morgenlander, Joel (NC)	N	522	Muraskas, Jonathan (IL)	NP	451
Morginstin, Mark (PA)	Onc	345	Murphree, A Linn (CA)	Oph	602
Morley, John (MO)	Ger	265	Murphy, Douglas (GA)	T&CS	1127
Morrell, Martha (CA)	N	538	Murphy, John (PA)	PCd	735
Morris, Colleen (NV)	CG	163	Murphy, Thomas (NC)	PPul	796
Morris, Douglas (GA)	IC	130	Murphy, Timothy (RI)	VIR	992
Morris, John (MO)	N	528	Murray, Joseph (MN)	Ge	247
Morris, Monica (VA)	RadRO	956	Murray, Karen (WA)	PGe	756
Morris, P Pearse (NC)	NRad	987	Murray, Pamela (WV)	AM	80
Morris, Rohinton (PA)	T&CS	1120	Murray, Timothy (FL)	Oph	585
Morrison, William (TX)	RadRO	965	Murtagh, F Reed (FL)	NRad	988
Morrissey, Nicholas (NY)	VascS	1188	Muschler, George (OH)	OrS	636
Morrow, Jon (CT)	Path	707	Muss, Hyman (NC)	Onc	360
Morrow, Monica (NY)	S	1060	Mustoe, Thomas (IL)	PlS	866
Mortimer, Joanne (CA)	Onc	388	Mutasim, Diya (OH)	D	194
Morton, D Holmes (PA)	Ped	727	Mutch, David (MO)	GO	284
Morton, John (CA)	S	1097	Mutch, Matthew (MO)	CRS	174
Moscow, Jeffrey (KY)	PHO	767	Muto, Michael (MA)	GO	275
Mosenifar, Zab (CA)	Pul	940	Myer, Charles (OH)	PO	792
Moser, Richard (MA)	NS	471	Myerburg, Robert (FL)	Cv	104
Moses, Jeffrey (NY)	IC	127	Myers, Deborah (RI)	ObG	556
Moses, Michael (LA)	PlS	871	Myers, Jeffrey (TX)	Oto	683
Moskowitz, William (VA)	PCd	737	Myers, Jeffrey (MI)	Path	716
Moss, R Lawrence (OH)	PS	807	Myers, Jonathan (PA)	Oph	578
Mostwin, Jacek (MD)	U	1155	Myerson, Mark (MD)	OrS	622
Mott, Michael (MI)	OrS	636	Myerson, Robert (MO)	RadRO	961
Motzer, Robert (NY)	Onc	346	Myones, Barry (TX)	PRhu	801
Moul, Judd (NC)	U	1162	Myseros, John (VA)	NS	483
Mountz, James (PA)	DR	976	Mysiw, W Jerry (OH)	PMR	841
Mousa, Hayat (OH)	PGe	753			
Movsas, Benjamin (MI)	RadRO	961			

Name	Specialty	Pg
N		
Nabell, Lisle (AL)	Onc	360
Nabors, L Burt (AL)	N	523
Naccarelli, Gerald (PA)	Cv	100
Naclerio, Robert (IL)	Oto	676
Nademanee, Auayporn (CA)	Hem	326
Naff, Neal (MD)	NS	477
Nagib, Mahmoud (MN)	NS	489
Nagle, Daniel (IL)	HS	302
Nagle, Deborah (MA)	CRS	168
Nagler, Harris (NY)	U	1156
Nagorney, David (MN)	S	1080
Nagueh, Sherif (TX)	Cv	114
Nahabedian, Maurice (DC)	PlS	856
Nahass, Ronald (NJ)	Inf	412
Naka, Yoshifumi (NY)	T&CS	1120
Nakakura, Eric (CA)	S	1097
Nakayama, Don (GA)	PS	805
Nance, Michael (PA)	PS	804
Nand, Sucha (IL)	Hem	321
Nanus, David (NY)	Onc	346
Napoli, Joseph (DE)	PlS	857
Nardell, Edward (MA)	Pul	923
Narkewicz, Michael (CO)	PGe	754
Nash, Thomas (NY)	Pul	926
Naslund, Michael (MD)	U	1156
Naslund, Thomas (TN)	VascS	1190
Nass, Ruth (NY)	ChiN	148
Natale, Andrea (TX)	CE	124
Natale, Ronald (CA)	Onc	388
Nathan, David (MA)	EDM	208
Nathanson, S David (MI)	S	1080
Nathwani, Bharat (CA)	Path	721
Naunheim, Keith (MO)	T&CS	1134
Nazzaro, Jules (KS)	NS	491
Neel, Victor (MA)	D	184
Neglia, Joseph (MN)	PHO	772
Negrin, Robert (CA)	Hem	326
Nehra, Ajay (IL)	U	1169
Neiberger, Richard (FL)	PNep	786
Neifeld, James (VA)	S	1071
Nelson, Edward (UT)	S	1086
Nelson, Heidi (MN)	CRS	175
Nelson, J Craig (CA)	Psyc	902
Nelson, Joel (PA)	U	1156
Nelson, Judith (NY)	Pul	926
Nelson, Leonard (PA)	Oph	578
Nelson, Maureen (TX)	PMR	843
Nemcek, Albert (IL)	VIR	996
Nepola, James (IA)	OrS	636
Neppe, Vernon (WA)	Psyc	902
Nerad, Jeffrey (OH)	Oph	592
Nesbitt, Jonathan (TN)	T&CS	1127
Ness, John (MN)	PlS	867
Nestler, John (VA)	EDM	215
Netterville, James (TN)	Oto	669
Neuberg, Ronnie (SC)	PHO	767
Neuburg, Marcelle (WI)	D	194
Neumann, Donald (OH)	NuM	550
Neumann, Ronald (MD)	NuM	549
Neumeister, Michael (IL)	PlS	867
Neuwelt, Edward (OR)	NS	498
Neuwirth, Michael (NY)	OrS	623
Neville, Richard (DC)	VascS	1188
New, Maria (NY)	PEn	745
Newburger, Jane (MA)	PCd	734
Newell, Kenneth (GA)	S	1071
Newkirk, Kenneth (DC)	Oto	663
Newman, Daniel (MI)	N	528
Newman, Elliot (NY)	S	1061
Newman, Joel (MA)	DR	973
Newman, Lawrence (NY)	N	516
Newman, Lisa (MI)	S	1080
Newman, Nancy (GA)	N	523
Newton, Herbert (OH)	N	528
Ng, John (OR)	Oph	603
Ngeow, Jeffrey (NY)	PM	697
Nghiem, Paul (WA)	D	200
Nguyen, Dao (FL)	T&CS	1127
Nguyen, Ninh (CA)	S	1097
Nicholas, Stephen (NY)	OrS	623
Nicholl, Jeffrey (LA)	N	534
Nicholson, H (OR)	PHO	778
Nichter, Larry (CA)	PlS	875
Nicolaou, Nicos (PA)	RadRO	951
Nicosia, Santo (FL)	Path	714
Niebyl, Jennifer (IA)	ObG	562
Niederman, Michael (NY)	Pul	926
Nielson, Dennis (CA)	PPul	798
Nies, Barbara (VA)	MF	435
Nigra, Thomas (DC)	D	187

Name	Specialty	Pg
Nimer, Stephen (FL)	Hem	317
Ninan, Mathew (TN)	T&CS	1128
Niparko, John (MD)	Oto	663
Nishimura, Rick (MN)	Cv	109
Nisonson, Barton (NY)	SM	1041
Nissen, Nicholas (CA)	S	1098
Nissen, Steven (OH)	Cv	109
Nissenblatt, Michael (NJ)	Onc	346
Nitenson, Nancy (MA)	AdP	904
Nitti, Victor (NY)	U	1156
Nobunaga, Austin (OH)	PMR	841
Nocero, Michael (FL)	Cv	105
Noe, Carl (TX)	PM	701
Noetzel, Michael (MO)	ChiN	151
Nogee, Lawrence (MD)	NP	448
Nogueras, Juan (FL)	CRS	172
Nolan, Bruce (FL)	N	523
Nolan, Charles (TX)	Nep	464
Noone, R Barrett (PA)	PlS	857
Norbash, Alexander (MA)	NRad	984
Norenberg, Michael (FL)	Path	714
Nori, Dattatreyudu (NY)	RadRO	951
Norman, James (FL)	S	1071
Norman, Kim (CA)	Psyc	902
Norris, Andrew (IA)	PEn	747
Northfelt, Donald (AZ)	Onc	380
Northrup, Hope (TX)	CG	162
Norton, Jeffrey (CA)	S	1098
Norton, Larry (NY)	Onc	346
Norwitz, Errol (MA)	MF	430
Notrica, David (AZ)	PS	809
Nour, Nawal (MA)	ObG	556
Nouri, Keyvan (FL)	D	191
Novak, Donald (FL)	PGe	752
Nowak, Eugene (NY)	S	1061
Noyes, Nicole (NY)	RE	1009
Nuber, Gordon (IL)	OrS	636
Nuchtern, Jed (TX)	PS	809
Nugent, William (NH)	T&CS	1111
Nunery, William (KY)	Oph	585
Nunes, David (MA)	Ge	229
Nunley, James (NC)	OrS	629
Nurnberger, John (IN)	Psyc	898
Nuss, Daniel (LA)	Oto	683
Nussbaum, Julian (GA)	Oph	585
Nussbaum, Robert (CA)	CG	163

Name	Specialty	Pg
Nutt, John (OR)	N	538

O

Name	Specialty	Pg
O'Brien, Joan (PA)	Oph	578
O'Brien, Michael (MA)	Path	707
O'Brien, Susan (TX)	Onc	380
O'Brien, Terrence (FL)	Oph	585
O'Brien, Timothy (OH)	Onc	370
O'Connell, John (GA)	Cv	105
O'Connor, Christopher (NC)	Cv	105
O'Connor, Owen (NY)	Onc	346
O'Day, Steven (CA)	Onc	389
O'Dell, James (NE)	Rhu	1032
O'Donnell, Anne (DC)	Pul	927
O'Donnell, Margaret (CA)	Hem	327
O'Donnell, Michael (IA)	U	1169
O'Donnell, Richard (CA)	OrS	645
O'Dorisio, M Sue (IA)	PHO	772
O'Driscoll, Shawn (MN)	OrS	636
O'Gara, Patrick (MA)	Cv	95
O'Hea, Brian (NY)	S	1061
O'Keefe, J Paul (IL)	Inf	416
O'Keefe, Regis (NY)	OrS	623
O'Leary, Michael (MA)	U	1149
O'Leary, Michael (CA)	Oto	686
O'Leary, Patrick (NY)	OrS	623
O'Malley, Bert (PA)	Oto	663
O'Neill, William (MI)	Cv	110
O'Regan, Ruth (GA)	Onc	360
O'Reilly, Eileen (NY)	Onc	346
O'Reilly, Richard (NY)	PHO	763
O'Rourke, Donald (PA)	NS	477
O'Shaughnessy, Joyce (TX)	Onc	380
Oakes, Daniel (CA)	OrS	645
Oakes, W Jerry (AL)	NS	483
Oaklander, Anne Louise (MA)	N	508
Oaks, Timothy (NC)	T&CS	1128
Oates, Robert (MA)	U	1150
Ober, K Patrick (NC)	EDM	215
Oberfield, Sharon (NY)	PEn	745
Oberholzer, Jose (IL)	S	1080
Oddis, Chester (PA)	Rhu	1027
Odel, Jeffrey (NY)	Oph	578
Odem, Randall (MO)	RE	1014

Name	Specialty	Pg	Name	Specialty	Pg
Odom, Michael (TX)	NP	452	Origitano, Thomas (MT)	NS	491
Odunsi, Adekunle (NY)	GO	279	Orkin, Bruce (MA)	CRS	168
Odze, Robert (MA)	Path	707	Orlin, Stephen (PA)	Oph	578
Oeffinger, Kevin (NY)	Ped	727	Orloff, Lisa (CA)	Oto	686
Offit, Kenneth (NY)	Onc	346	Orlow, Seth (NY)	D	188
Offit, Paul (PA)	PInf	781	Orlowski, Robert (TX)	Onc	380
Oghalai, John (CA)	Oto	686	Orr, James (FL)	GO	282
Oh, Shin (AL)	N	523	Orringer, Mark (MI)	T&CS	1134
Oh, William (NY)	Onc	347	Ortel, Thomas (NC)	Hem	317
Ohl, Dana (MI)	U	1169	Orwoll, Eric (OR)	EDM	223
Ojemann, Jeffrey (WA)	NS	498	Ory, Steven (FL)	RE	1012
Okolo, Patrick (MD)	Ge	237	Osborn, Anne (UT)	NRad	990
Okusa, Mark (VA)	Nep	460	Osborne, C (TX)	Onc	381
Olanow, C Warren (NY)	N	516	Osborne, Michael (NY)	S	1061
Olbricht, Suzanne (MA)	D	184	Osei, Kwame (OH)	EDM	219
Oldham, Keith (WI)	PS	807	Osher, Robert (OH)	Oph	593
Olding, Michael (DC)	PlS	857	Oskowitz, Selwyn (MA)	RE	1007
Olitsky, Scott (MO)	Oph	592	Ossoff, Robert (TN)	Oto	669
Oliva-Hemker, Maria (MD)	PGe	751	Oster, Martin (NY)	Onc	347
Olivero, Juan (TX)	Nep	464	Osterman, A Lee (PA)	HS	297
Olivi, Alessandro (MD)	NS	477	Ostrer, Harry (NY)	CG	158
Olopade, Olufunmilayo (IL)	Onc	370	Ostroff, James (CA)	Ge	255
Olsen, Elise (NC)	D	191	Ostrom, Nancy (CA)	A&I	90
Olsen, Kerry (MN)	Oto	677	Otley, Clark (MN)	D	194
Olsen, Timothy (GA)	Oph	585	Otsuka, Norman (NY)	OrS	623
Olshefski, Randal (OH)	PHO	772	Ott, David (TX)	T&CS	1139
Olson, Jack (IL)	Ger	265	Ott, Kenneth (CA)	NS	498
Olson, Janice (OR)	PHO	778	Ott, Susan (WA)	Nep	465
Olson, Jeffrey (GA)	NS	483	Otto, Pamela (TX)	DR	982
Olson, John (MD)	S	1061	Otto, Randal (TX)	Oto	683
Olson, Thomas (GA)	PHO	767	Ousterhout, Douglas (CA)	PlS	876
Olthoff, Kim (PA)	S	1061	Ovalle, Fernando (AL)	EDM	215
Olumi, Aria (MA)	U	1150	Ownby, Dennis (GA)	PA&I	731
Onders, Raymond (OH)	S	1080	Owyang, Chung (MI)	Ge	247
Onufer, John (VA)	CE	122	Oz, Mehmet (NY)	T&CS	1120
Oommen, Kalarickal (TX)	N	534	Ozer, Enver (OH)	Oto	677
Oparil, Suzanne (AL)	Cv	105	Ozer, Howard (IL)	Onc	370
Oppenheim, William (CA)	OrS	645			
Orange, Jordan (TX)	PA&I	732			
Oratz, Ruth (NY)	Onc	347			
Orazi, Attilio (NY)	Path	710	**P**		
Orbach, Darren (MA)	NRad	985			
Ordorica, Steven (NY)	ObG	558	Pachter, H Leon (NY)	S	1061
Orengo, Ida (TX)	D	197	Pacin, Michael (FL)	A&I	87
Orenstein, David (PA)	PPul	795	Pack, Allan (PA)	Pul	927
Orgill, Dennis (MA)	PlS	851	Packer, Roger (DC)	ChiN	148
			Padgett, Douglas (NY)	OrS	623

Alphabetical Listing of Doctors

Name	Specialty	Pg	Name	Specialty	Pg
Padilla, Maria (NY)	Pul	927	Parsons, Rosaleen (PA)	DR	977
Pagani, Francis (MI)	T&CS	1134	Parsons, Theodore (MI)	OrS	636
Page, Timothy (MI)	Oph	593	Partain, Clarence (TN)	DR	979
Paget, Stephen (NY)	Rhu	1027	Partin, Alan (MD)	U	1156
Pahl, Elfriede (IL)	PCd	739	Parvizi, Javad (PA)	OrS	623
Paidas, Charles (FL)	PS	805	Pasche, Boris (AL)	Onc	361
Paidas, Michael (CT)	MF	431	Pascuzzi, Robert (IN)	N	528
Palacios, Igor (MA)	IC	126	Pasmantier, Mark (NY)	Onc	347
Palascak, Joseph (OH)	Hem	321	Pasricha, P Jay (MD)	Ge	237
Palefsky, Joel (CA)	Inf	419	Pass, Harvey (NY)	T&CS	1120
Paletta, George (MO)	SM	1043	Passo, Murray (SC)	PRhu	800
Palevsky, Harold (PA)	Pul	927	Patchefsky, Arthur (PA)	Path	711
Paley, Dror (FL)	OrS	630	Patchell, Roy (AZ)	N	534
Palfrey, Judith (MA)	Ped	726	Patel, Aman (NY)	NS	477
Paller, Amy (IL)	D	195	Patel, Pravin (IL)	PlS	867
Palmer, Jeffrey (MD)	PMR	837	Patel, Sameer (PA)	S	1061
Palmer, Robert (VA)	Ger	264	Patel, Shreyaskumar (TX)	Onc	381
Palmer, William (MA)	DR	973	Patel, Sunil (SC)	NS	483
Pandit-Taskar, Neeta (NY)	NuM	549	Patel, Vipul (FL)	U	1162
Panicek, David (NY)	DR	976	Pathria, Mini (CA)	DR	983
Panitch, Howard (PA)	PPul	795	Patil, Yash (OH)	Oto	677
Panos, Anthony (FL)	T&CS	1128	Patrinely, James (FL)	Oph	585
Pantilat, Steven (CA)	H & PM	408	Patrizio, Pasquale (CT)	RE	1007
Pao, William (TN)	Onc	360	Patt, Yehuda (NM)	Onc	381
Papadopoulos, Nicholas (TX)	Onc	381	Patterson, Anthony (TN)	U	1163
Paparella, Michael (MN)	Oto	677	Patterson, G Alexander (MO)	T&CS	1134
Papay, Francis (OH)	PlS	867	Patterson, James (OR)	Pul	940
Papel, Ira (MD)	Oto	663	Patterson, Jan (TX)	Inf	418
Pappas, Theodore (NC)	S	1071	Patterson, Marc (MN)	ChiN	151
Parent, Andrew (MS)	NS	483	Patterson, Thomas (TX)	Inf	419
Parikh, Jay (WA)	DR	983	Paty, Philip (NY)	S	1062
Parikh, Manish (NY)	IC	128	Patz, Edward (NC)	DR	979
Parikh, Sanjay (WA)	PO	793	Pauker, Susan (MA)	CG	156
Parisier, Simon (NY)	Oto	663	Paul, Malcolm (CA)	PlS	876
Park, Bernard (NJ)	T&CS	1120	Paul, T Otis (CA)	Oph	603
Park, Catherine (CA)	RadRO	967	Paulson, Richard (CA)	RE	1017
Park, Julie (WA)	PHO	778	Pavlick, Anna (NY)	Onc	347
Park, Tae Sung (MO)	NS	489	Pavlov, Helene (NY)	DR	977
Parker, Barbara (CA)	Onc	389	Pawlik, Timothy (MD)	S	1062
Parker, Robert (NY)	PHO	763	Paz, Isaac (CA)	S	1098
Parker, William (CA)	ObG	563	Peabody, Terrance (IL)	OrS	636
Parnes, Howard (MD)	Onc	347	Peace, David (IL)	Onc	370
Parness, Ira (NY)	PCd	735	Pearce, Elizabeth (MA)	EDM	208
Parrillo, Joseph (NJ)	Cv	101	Pearce, William (IL)	VascS	1191
Parrish, Richard (FL)	Oph	585	Pearson, Richard (VA)	Inf	415
Parry, Samuel (PA)	MF	433	Pearson, Thomas (NY)	PrM	883

Name	Specialty	Pg	Name	Specialty	Pg
Pechet, Taine (PA)	T&CS	1120	Peters, Anne (CA)	EDM	224
Pecora, Andrew (NJ)	Onc	347	Peters, Glenn (AL)	Oto	670
Pedley, Timothy (NY)	N	516	Peters, Jeffrey (NY)	S	1062
Peereboom, David (OH)	Onc	370	Petersdorf, Stephen (WA)	Hem	327
Peeters-Asdourian, Christine (MA)	PM	696	Petersen, Michael (OH)	Oph	593
Pegram, Mark (CA)	Onc	389	Petersen, Ronald (MN)	N	529
Peikin, Steven (NJ)	Ge	237	Peterson, Bruce (MN)	Onc	370
Peitzman, Andrew (PA)	S	1062	Peterson, Davis (AK)	OrS	645
Pejovic, Tanja (OR)	GO	290	Peterson, Laura (HI)	S	1098
Peljovich, Allan (GA)	HS	299	Petito, Carol (FL)	Path	714
Pellegrini, Carlos (WA)	S	1098	Petito, Frank (NY)	N	516
Pellicci, Paul (NY)	OrS	623	Petras, Robert (OH)	Path	716
Pello, Mark (NJ)	CRS	171	Petri, Michelle (MD)	Rhu	1027
Pelzer, Harold (IL)	Oto	677	Petrini, John (CA)	Ge	255
Pemberton, John (MN)	CRS	175	Petrossian, George (NY)	IC	128
Pena, Alberto (OH)	PS	807	Petrozza, John (MA)	RE	1007
Penalver, Manuel (FL)	GO	282	Petru, Ann (CA)	PInf	785
Penar, Paul (VT)	NS	471	Petruska, Paul (MO)	Onc	370
Pendergrass, Thomas (WA)	PHO	778	Petruzzelli, Guy (GA)	Oto	670
Peng, Stanford (WA)	Rhu	1034	Petrylak, Daniel (CT)	Onc	331
Pennell, Page (MA)	N	508	Pettrone, Frank (VA)	OrS	630
Pensak, Myles (OH)	Oto	677	Pevec, William (CA)	VascS	1194
Penson, David (TN)	U	1163	Pezner, Richard (CA)	RadRO	967
Pepine, Carl (FL)	Cv	105	Pezzone, Michael (PA)	Ge	237
Pepose, Jay (MO)	Oph	593	Pfau, Patrick (WI)	Ge	247
Perez, Edith (FL)	Onc	361	Pfeffer, Marc (MA)	Cv	95
Perez, Victor (FL)	Oph	586	Pfeifer, Samantha (PA)	ObG	558
Perez Fontan, J Julio (TX)	PCCM	742	Pfister, David (NY)	Onc	348
Pergament, Eugene (IL)	CG	160	Pflugfelder, Stephen (TX)	Oph	597
Perin, Emerson (TX)	IC	132	Pham, Si (FL)	T&CS	1128
Perkins, James (WA)	S	1098	Philippon, Marc (CO)	OrS	639
Perler, Bruce (MD)	VascS	1188	Philipson, Elliot (OH)	MF	437
Perlman, David (NY)	Inf	412	Philipson, Louis (IL)	EDM	219
Perlman, Jeffrey (NY)	NP	448	Phillips, Edward (CA)	S	1098
Perlmutter, Joel (MO)	N	528	Phillips, Harry (NC)	Cv	105
Perone, Jennifer (TX)	D	197	Phillips, Katharine (RI)	Psyc	889
Perret, Philip (LA)	Pul	938	Phillips, Peter (PA)	ChiN	148
Perrone, Ronald (MA)	Nep	456	Phillips, Robert (MA)	Cv	96
Perry, Arie (CA)	Path	721	Phillips, S Michael (PA)	A&I	85
Perry, David (DC)	Onc	347	Philosophe, Benjamin (MD)	S	1062
Perry, Stanton (CA)	PCd	741	Philpott, Jonathan (VA)	T&CS	1128
Persing, John (CT)	PlS	851	Phuphanich, Surasak (CA)	N	538
Persky, Mark (NY)	Oto	663	Pi, Edmond (CA)	Psyc	902
Peschel, Richard (CT)	RadRO	947	Piatt, Joseph (DE)	NS	478
Pestronk, Alan (MO)	N	529	Piccirillo, Jay (MO)	Oto	677
Petelin, Joseph (KS)	S	1086	Piccoli, David (PA)	PGe	751

Alphabetical Listing of Doctors

Name	Specialty	Pg	Name	Specialty	Pg
Pichard, Augusto (DC)	IC	128	Pollard, Zane (GA)	Oph	586
Picken, Catherine (DC)	Oto	663	Polley, John (IL)	PlS	867
Picozzi, Vincent (WA)	Onc	389	Pollock, Raphael (TX)	S	1091
Pienta, Kenneth (MI)	Onc	371	Polly, David (MN)	OrS	637
Piepmeier, Joseph (CT)	NS	471	Polsky, Bruce (NY)	Inf	413
Pierce, Lori (MI)	RadRO	961	Pomeroy, John (NY)	ChAP	909
Pierson, Richard (MD)	T&CS	1120	Pomeroy, Scott (MA)	ChiN	146
Pile-Spellman, John (NY)	NRad	986	Pomp, Alfons (NY)	S	1062
Pillsbury, Harold (NC)	Oto	670	Pomposelli, Frank (MA)	VascS	1185
Pinckert, Thomas (MD)	MF	433	Pongracic, Jacqueline (IL)	PA&I	731
Pinson, C Wright (TN)	S	1071	Ponn, Teresa (NH)	S	1051
Pinter, Joseph (OR)	ChiN	153	Ponsky, Jeffrey (OH)	S	1080
Pinto, Harlan (CA)	Onc	389	Ponton, Lynn (CA)	ChAP	912
Pinzur, Michael (IL)	OrS	637	Poole, Michael (GA)	Oto	670
Piraino, Beth (PA)	Nep	458	Poon, Michael (NY)	Cv	101
Pisters, Katherine (TX)	Onc	381	Poordad, Fred (TX)	Ge	252
Pisters, Louis (TX)	U	1174	Pope, John (TN)	U	1163
Pisters, Peter (TX)	S	1091	Pope, Richard (IL)	Rhu	1032
Pitman, Gerald (NY)	PlS	857	Popovich, John (MI)	Pul	935
Pitman, Karen (MS)	Oto	670	Poppas, Dix (NY)	U	1156
Pitts, Jeanette (AZ)	D	197	Porayko, Michael (TN)	Ge	241
Pizzutillo, Peter (PA)	OrS	624	Porcu, Pierluigi (OH)	Hem	321
Plager, David (IN)	Oph	593	Porrazzo, Michael (DC)	RadRO	952
Plancher, Kevin (NY)	OrS	624	Portenoy, Russell (NY)	H & PM	406
Plante, Lauren (PA)	MF	433	Porter, Christopher (WA)	U	1178
Platt, Lawrence (CA)	MF	440	Porter, David (PA)	Hem	314
Platzker, Arnold (CA)	PPul	798	Posey, James (AL)	Onc	361
Plautz, Gregory (OH)	PHO	772	Posner, Jerome (NY)	N	516
Plaxe, Steven (CA)	GO	290	Posner, Marshall (NY)	Onc	348
Plevy, Scott (NC)	Ge	241	Posner, Mitchell (IL)	S	1081
Plon, Sharon (TX)	CG	162	Posnick, Jeffrey (MD)	PlS	857
Plotnick, Leslie (MD)	PEn	745	Posselt, Andrew (CA)	S	1098
Plotz, Paul (MD)	Rhu	1028	Postier, Russell (OK)	S	1091
Pochapin, Mark (NY)	Ge	237	Postma, Gregory (GA)	Oto	670
Pochettino, Alberto (MN)	T&CS	1134	Potenza, Bruce (CA)	S	1098
Pockaj, Barbara (AZ)	S	1091	Potkul, Ronald (IL)	GO	285
Podoloff, Donald (TX)	NuM	550	Potter, Hollis (NY)	DR	977
Poe, Dennis (MA)	PO	789	Pow-Sang, Julio (FL)	U	1163
Poehling, Gary (NC)	OrS	630	Powell, Bayard (NC)	Hem	317
Pohl, Marc (OH)	Nep	462	Powers, Alvin (TN)	EDM	215
Pohlman, Brad (OH)	Onc	371	Powers, Eric (SC)	Cv	105
Poliakoff, Steven (FL)	GO	282	Powers, Pauline (FL)	Psyc	896
Polin, Richard (NY)	NP	448	Prados, Michael (CA)	Onc	389
Polisson, Richard (MA)	Rhu	1024	Prager, Joshua (CA)	PM	703
Pollack, Alan (FL)	RadRO	956	Prakash, Udaya (MN)	Pul	935
Pollack, Ian (PA)	NS	478	Preminger, Glenn (NC)	U	1163

Name	Specialty	Pg	Name	Specialty	Pg
Press, Joel (IL)	PMR	841	Quintessenza, James (FL)	T&CS	1128
Press, Oliver (WA)	Onc	389	Quittell, Lynne (NY)	PPul	795
Presti, Joseph (CA)	U	1178	Quivey, Jeanne (CA)	RadRO	967
Pribitkin, Edmund (PA)	Oto	663			
Price, G Wesley (MD)	PlS	857			
Price, Lawrence (RI)	Psyc	889			
Pridjian, Gabriella (LA)	MF	439	# R		
Prieto, Victor (TX)	Path	718	Rabinovitch, Rachel (CO)	RadRO	963
Prince, Martin (NY)	DR	977	Rabow, Michael (CA)	IM	426
Prinz, Richard (IL)	S	1081	Racz, Gabor (TX)	PM	701
Prioleau, Philip (NY)	D	188	Rader, Daniel (PA)	IM	424
Procaccino, John (NY)	CRS	171	Rader, Janet (WI)	GO	285
Proctor, Deborah (CT)	Ge	230	Radtke, Wolfgang (DE)	PCd	735
Proctor, Monja (WA)	PS	811	Raff, Gilbert (MI)	Cv	110
Prosnitz, Leonard (NC)	RadRO	956	Raffel, Corey (OH)	NS	489
Provenzale, James (NC)	NRad	988	Rafferty, Janice (OH)	CRS	175
Pruthi, Raj (NC)	U	1163	Ragheb, John (FL)	NS	483
Prystowsky, Eric (IN)	CE	123	Raghu, Ganesh (WA)	Pul	940
Puccetti, Diane (WI)	PHO	772	Ragnarsson, Kristjan (NY)	PMR	837
Puckett, Charles (MO)	PlS	867	Rahko, Peter (WI)	Cv	110
Pui, Ching-Hon (TN)	PHO	768	Rai, Kanti (NY)	Hem	314
Pula, Thaddeus (MD)	N	516	Raiford, David (TN)	Ge	242
Puliafito, Carmen (CA)	Oph	603	Raja, Srinivasa (MD)	PM	697
Pulido, Jose (MN)	Oph	593	Rajacich, Nicholas (WA)	OrS	645
Pulst, Stefan (UT)	N	532	Rajfer, Jacob (CA)	U	1178
Putman, John (TX)	RE	1016	Raji, Mukaila (TX)	Ger	266
Putnam, Joe (TN)	T&CS	1128	Raju, Gottumukkala (TX)	Ge	252
Putnam, Matthew (MN)	HS	302	Rakowski, Thomas (VA)	Nep	460
Putterman, Allen (IL)	Oph	593	Ramamoorthy, Sonia (CA)	CRS	178
Pyeritz, Reed (PA)	CG	158	Ramamurthy, Somayaji (TX)	PM	701
Pynoos, Robert (CA)	Psyc	902	Ramanathan, Ramesh (PA)	S	1062
			Ramee, Stephen (LA)	Cv	115
			Ramsay, David (NY)	D	188
			Ramsey, Bonnie (WA)	PPul	798
# Q			Ramsey, Matthew (PA)	OrS	624
Quaegebeur, Jan (NY)	PS	804	Rand, Richard (WA)	PlS	876
Quagliarello, Vincent (CT)	Inf	410	Randall, Marcus (KY)	RadRO	957
Quatela, Vito (NY)	Oto	664	Randall, R Lor (UT)	OrS	639
Quencer, Robert (FL)	NRad	988	Randall, Thomas (PA)	GO	279
Quigley, Harry (MD)	Oph	578	Randolph, Gregory (MA)	Oto	656
Quigley, Matthew (PA)	NS	478	Randolph, Linda (CA)	CG	163
Quill, Timothy (NY)	H & PM	407	Randolph-Jackson, Pamela (DC)	RadRO	952
Quinn, David (CA)	Onc	389	Rao, A Koneti (PA)	Hem	314
Quinn, Graham (PA)	Oph	578	Rao, Nalini (PA)	Inf	413
Quinn, Suzanne (FL)	EDM	215	Rao, Narsing (CA)	Oph	603
Quinones, Miguel (TX)	Cv	115	Rao, Satish (GA)	Ge	242

Alphabetical Listing of Doctors

Name	Specialty	Pg	Name	Specialty	Pg
Rao, Vijay (PA)	DR	977	Reed, Carolyn (SC)	T&CS	1128
Raphael, Bruce (NY)	Hem	314	Reed, Eddie (AL)	Onc	361
Raphael, James (PA)	HS	297	Reed, Kathryn (AZ)	MF	439
Rapoport, Aaron (MD)	Hem	314	Reed, Robert (OH)	N	529
Rapoport, Judith (DC)	ChAP	909	Rege, Robert (TX)	S	1091
Rappaport, Leonard (MA)	Ped	726	Regillo, Carl (PA)	Oph	579
Rappaport, Norman (TX)	PlS	871	Regine, William (MD)	RadRO	952
Raptis, George (NY)	Onc	348	Reich, David (PA)	S	1062
Rapuano, Christopher (PA)	Oph	579	Reich, Stephen (MD)	N	517
Rashid, Asif (TX)	Path	718	Reichelderfer, Mark (WI)	Ge	247
Raskin, Keith (NY)	HS	297	Reid, Tony (CA)	Onc	390
Raskind, Murray (WA)	Psyc	902	Reid, William (TN)	NS	484
Rasmussen, Steven (RI)	Psyc	889	Reilly, Donald (MA)	OrS	612
Rassekh, Christopher (PA)	Oto	664	Reiner, Jonathan (DC)	IC	128
Rassman, William (CA)	S	1099	Reiner, Mark (NY)	S	1063
Rastegar, Hassan (MA)	T&CS	1112	Reinisch, John (CA)	PlS	876
Raszka, William (VT)	PInf	780	Reinus, William (PA)	DR	977
Ratain, Mark (IL)	Onc	371	Reis, Steven (PA)	Cv	101
Ratner, Desiree (NY)	D	188	Reisberg, Barry (NY)	GerPsy	913
Rattner, David (MA)	S	1051	Reiss, Craig (MO)	Cv	110
Ratts, Valerie (MO)	RE	1014	Relkin, Norman (NY)	N	517
Ratzan, Kenneth (FL)	Inf	415	Remick, Scot (WV)	Onc	348
Rauch, Paula (MA)	Psyc	889	Remmenga, Steven (NE)	GO	286
Rauch, Steven (MA)	Oto	656	Remzi, Feza (OH)	CRS	175
Rauck, Richard (NC)	PM	699	Rennard, Stephen (NE)	Pul	937
Ravich, William (MD)	Ge	237	Rennke, Helmut (MA)	Path	707
Rayan, Ghazi (OK)	HS	303	Renz, John (IL)	S	1081
Raz, Shlomo (CA)	U	1178	Repke, John (PA)	MF	433
Razzouk, Bassem (IN)	PHO	773	Resar, Jon (MD)	IC	128
Read, Thomas (MA)	CRS	169	Rescorla, Frederick (IN)	PS	807
Ready, John (MA)	OrS	612	Resnick, Neil (PA)	Ger	263
Ready, Neal (NC)	Onc	361	Reuben, Adrian (SC)	Ge	242
Reaman, Gregory (DC)	PHO	763	Reuben, David (CA)	Ger	267
Reardon, Michael (TX)	T&CS	1139	Reus, Victor (CA)	Psyc	902
Rebeiz, Elie (MA)	Oto	657	Reuter, Victor (NY)	Path	711
Reber, Howard (CA)	S	1099	Rewers, Marian (CO)	PEn	748
Recht, Abram (MA)	RadRO	947	Rex, Douglas (IN)	Ge	247
Recht, Michael (OR)	PHO	779	Reyes, Jorge (WA)	S	1099
Recker, Robert (NE)	EDM	220	Reynolds, James (PA)	Ge	238
Redberg, Rita (CA)	Cv	118	Reynolds, James (NY)	Oph	579
Redding, Gregory (WA)	PPul	798	Reynolds, Marleta (IL)	PS	808
Reddy, Bhagat (GA)	IC	130	Reynolds, R Kevin (MI)	GO	285
Reddy, K Rajender (PA)	Ge	237	Rezai, Ali (OH)	NS	489
Reder, Anthony (IL)	N	529	Rhee, Peter (AZ)	S	1092
Redlich, Carrie (CT)	Pul	923	Rheingold, Susan (PA)	PHO	763
Reed, Alan I (IA)	S	1081	Rhoads, J Marc (TX)	PGe	755

Name	Specialty	Pg	Name	Specialty	Pg
Rhodes, Arthur (IL)	D	195	Ritchey, A Kim (PA)	PHO	763
Riba, Michelle (MI)	Psyc	898	Ritchie, Christine (CA)	H & PM	408
Ribeiro, Raul (TN)	PHO	768	Riviello, James (NY)	ChiN	148
Rice, Dale (CA)	Oto	686	Rivkees, Scott (FL)	PEn	746
Rice, David (TX)	T&CS	1139	Rizk, Norman (CA)	Pul	940
Rice, Henry (NC)	PS	805	Rizzo, Joseph (MA)	Oph	571
Rice, Laurel (WI)	GO	285	Roach, Mack (CA)	RadRO	967
Rice, Thomas (OH)	T&CS	1134	Robb, Geoffrey (TX)	PlS	871
Rich, Keith (MO)	NS	489	Robbins, Larry (IL)	PM	700
Rich, Stuart (IL)	Cv	110	Robbins, Richard (TX)	EDM	221
Rich, Tyvin (VA)	RadRO	957	Robbins, Robert (CA)	T&CS	1142
Richard, James (OK)	Oph	597	Robert, Nicholas (VA)	Onc	361
Richards, Jon (IL)	Onc	371	Robert-Vizcarrondo, Francisco (AL)	Onc	361
Richards, William (AL)	S	1071	Roberts, Anne (CA)	VIR	998
Richardson, Marilyn (KS)	RE	1015	Roberts, Barbara (RI)	Cv	96
Richardson, Mark (OR)	PO	793	Roberts, John (CA)	S	1099
Richardson, Paul (MA)	Hem	311	Roberts, Kenneth (CT)	RadRO	947
Richardson, Timothy (CA)	D	200	Roberts, Michelle (PA)	EDM	211
Richardson, William (NC)	OrS	630	Roberts, Patricia (MA)	CRS	169
Richerson, George (IA)	N	529	Roberts, William (TX)	Path	718
Richie, Jerome (MA)	U	1150	Robertson, Cary (NC)	U	1163
Richman, Daniel (NY)	PM	698	Robertson, Jon (TN)	NS	484
Richman, Douglas (CA)	Inf	419	Robertson, Patricia (CA)	MF	441
Richmond, John (MA)	OrS	612	Robichaux, Alfred (LA)	MF	439
Richter, Edwin (CT)	PMR	834	Robin, Alan (MD)	Oph	579
Ricketts, Richard (GA)	PS	806	Robinson, Julian (MA)	MF	431
Ricotta, John (DC)	VascS	1188	Robinson, Lary (FL)	T&CS	1129
Riddle, Mark (MD)	ChAP	909	Robinson, Lawrence (WA)	PMR	844
Riddle, Matthew (OR)	EDM	224	Rocchini, Albert (MI)	PCd	739
Ridge, John (PA)	S	1063	Rochester, Carolyn (CT)	Pul	924
Ridgway, E (CO)	EDM	220	Rock, Jack (MI)	NS	489
Ridker, Paul (MA)	Cv	96	Rockwell, William (UT)	PlS	869
Ries, W Russell (TN)	Oto	670	Rodbard, Helena (MD)	EDM	211
Riew, K Daniel (MO)	OrS	637	Rodby, Roger (IL)	Nep	462
Rigamonti, Daniele (MD)	NS	478	Roddy, Sarah (CA)	ChiN	153
Rigel, Darrell (NY)	D	188	Rodeo, Scott (NY)	SM	1042
Rihal, Charanjit (MN)	Cv	110	Rodgers, Bradley (VA)	PS	806
Riina, Howard (NY)	NS	478	Rodgers, George (UT)	Hem	322
Riles, Thomas (NY)	VascS	1188	Rodosky, Mark (PA)	OrS	624
Riley, Laura (MA)	MF	431	Rodriguez, Eduardo (MD)	PlS	857
Rilling, William (WI)	VIR	996	Rodts, Gerald (GA)	NS	484
Ringel, Steven (CO)	N	532	Roehrborn, Claus (TX)	U	1174
Rink, Richard (IN)	U	1169	Rogers, Douglas (OH)	PEn	747
Riordan, John (CA)	Nep	465	Rogers, Gary (OH)	Oph	593
Ristow, Brunno (CA)	PlS	876	Rogers, James (TX)	PCd	740
Ritch, Robert (NY)	Oph	579	Rogers, Joseph (NC)	Cv	105

Name	Specialty	Pg	Name	Specialty	Pg
Rogers, Lisa (OH)	N	529	Rosengart, Todd (NY)	T&CS	1121
Rogers, Stanley (CA)	S	1099	Rosenkranz, Eliot (FL)	T&CS	1129
Roh, Mark (FL)	S	1071	Rosenman, Julian (NC)	RadRO	957
Rohrich, Rod (TX)	PlS	872	Rosenquist, Richard (OH)	PM	700
Roizen, Nancy Jean (OH)	Ped	728	Rosenthal, Eben (AL)	Oto	670
Roland, J Thomas (NY)	Oto	664	Rosenthal, Joseph (CA)	PHO	779
Romagnoli, Mario (NY)	Inf	413	Rosenthal, Norman (MD)	Psyc	894
Romaguera, Jorge (TX)	Onc	381	Rosenthal, Richard (NY)	Psyc	894
Romano, James (CA)	PlS	876	Rosenthal, Stephen (CA)	PEn	749
Rome, Jonathan (PA)	PCd	736	Rosenwaks, Zev (NY)	RE	1009
Romeo, Anthony (IL)	OrS	637	Rosenwasser, Melvin (NY)	HS	297
Romond, Edward (KY)	Onc	361	Rosenwasser, Robert (PA)	NS	478
Rood, Brian (DC)	PHO	763	Roses, Daniel (NY)	S	1063
Roodman, G David (IN)	Hem	321	Roskes, Saul (MD)	PNep	786
Rook, Alain (PA)	D	188	Rosner, Howard (CA)	PM	703
Roos, Karen (IN)	N	529	Rosoff, Philip (NC)	PHO	768
Roos, Raymond (IL)	N	529	Rosove, Michael (CA)	Onc	390
Roose, Steven (NY)	Psyc	894	Ross, Douglas (MA)	EDM	208
Ropper, Allan (MA)	N	508	Ross, Edgar (MA)	PM	696
Rosbe, Kristina (CA)	PO	793	Ross, Helen (AZ)	Onc	381
Rose, Cecile (CO)	Pul	937	Ross, Jeffrey (NY)	Path	711
Rose, Christopher (CA)	RadRO	967	Ross, Lawrence (IL)	U	1170
Rose, Elliott (NY)	PlS	858	Ross, Merrick (TX)	S	1092
Rose, Peter (OH)	GO	285	Rosse, Richard (DC)	Psyc	894
Rosemurgy, Alexander (FL)	S	1071	Rosser, Tena (CA)	ChiN	154
Rosen, Charles (MN)	S	1081	Rossi, Carl (CA)	RadRO	968
Rosen, Clark (PA)	Oto	664	Rossman, Milton (PA)	Pul	927
Rosen, Michael (OH)	S	1081	Rostain, Anthony (PA)	ChAP	909
Rosen, Steven (IL)	Onc	371	Roth, Andrew (NY)	Psyc	894
Rosenbaum, Kenneth (DC)	CG	158	Roth, Bennett (CA)	Ge	255
Rosenbaum, Richard (OR)	N	538	Roth, Bruce (MO)	Onc	371
Rosenberg, Andrew (FL)	Path	714	Roth, David (FL)	Nep	460
Rosenberg, Howard (CA)	PlS	876	Roth, Elliot (IL)	PMR	841
Rosenberg, Michael (IL)	Oph	594	Roth, Jack (TX)	T&CS	1139
Rosenberg, Steven (MD)	S	1063	Roth, Susan (PA)	DR	977
Rosenberg, Thomas (UT)	OrS	639	Rothbaum, Robert (MO)	PGe	754
Rosenblatt, Joseph (FL)	Hem	317	Rothenberg, Russell (MD)	Rhu	1028
Rosenblum, Marc (NY)	Path	711	Rothman, Richard (PA)	OrS	624
Rosenblum, Mark (MI)	NS	489	Rothrock, John (NV)	N	538
Rosenblum, Norman (PA)	GO	279	Rothstein, Richard (NH)	Ge	230
Rosenbluth, Daniel (MO)	Pul	935	Rotman, Marvin (NY)	RadRO	952
Rosenbush, Stuart (IL)	Cv	110	Rotmensch, Jacob (IL)	GO	285
Rosenfeld, Philip (FL)	Oph	586	Roubin, Gary (NY)	IC	128
Rosenfeld, Richard (NY)	PO	790	Routes, John (WI)	A&I	89
Rosenfeld, Steven (OH)	N	529	Rovner, Barry (PA)	GerPsy	913
Rosenfield, Kenneth (MA)	IC	126	Rowland, Randall (KY)	U	1163

Name	Specialty	Pg	Name	Specialty	Pg
Rowley, Howard (WI)	NRad	989	Saag, Michael (AL)	Inf	415
Rowley, Scott (NJ)	Hem	314	Saal, Howard (OH)	CG	160
Roy-Byrne, Peter (WA)	Psyc	902	Saal, Jeffrey (CA)	PMR	844
Roye, David (NY)	OrS	624	Sabanegh, Edmund (OH)	U	1170
Rozbruch, S Robert (NY)	OrS	624	Sabo, Tonia (CO)	N	532
Rubenfeld, Sheldon (TX)	EDM	221	Sacchi, Terrence (NY)	IC	128
Rubin, Brian (OH)	Path	716	Sacco, Ralph (FL)	N	523
Rubin, Bruce (VA)	PPul	796	Sachs, Greg (IN)	Ger	265
Rubin, Charles (IL)	PHO	773	Saclarides, Theodore (IL)	CRS	175
Rubin, Geoffrey (NC)	DR	979	Sadda, SriniVas (CA)	Oph	603
Rubin, Lewis (CA)	Pul	941	Sadeghi-Nejad, Hossein (NJ)	U	1156
Rubin, Mark (CA)	D	200	Sadock, Virginia (NY)	Psyc	894
Rubin, Peter (MA)	Oph	571	Sadowsky, Carl (FL)	N	523
Rubin, Stephen (PA)	GO	279	Saffle, Jeffrey (UT)	S	1086
Rubin, Susan (IL)	N	530	Safi, Hazim (TX)	T&CS	1139
Rubino, Francesco (NY)	S	1063	Safian, Robert (MI)	Cv	110
Rubinstein, Jay (WA)	Oto	686	Sagalowsky, Arthur (TX)	U	1174
Rudnick, Michael (PA)	Nep	458	Sage, Jacob (NJ)	N	517
Rudy, Bret (NY)	AM	80	Saha, Sukamal (MI)	S	1081
Ruge, John (IL)	NS	490	Sahin, Aysegul (TX)	Path	718
Ruggiero, Joseph (NY)	Onc	348	Sahn, Steven (SC)	Pul	932
Rugo, Hope (CA)	Onc	390	Saif, M Wasif (MA)	Onc	332
Runowicz, Carolyn (FL)	GO	282	Saiki, John (NM)	Onc	381
Rusch, Valerie (NY)	T&CS	1121	Sailer, Scott (NC)	RadRO	957
Rushakoff, Robert (CA)	EDM	224	Saiman, Lisa (NY)	PInf	781
Rushton, H Gil (DC)	U	1156	Saint-Phard, Deborah (CO)	SM	1043
Ruskin, Jeremy (MA)	CE	119	Sakamoto, Kathleen (CA)	PHO	779
Russell, Andrew (CA)	ChAP	912	Salant, David (MA)	Nep	456
Russell, Anthony (MA)	RadRO	947	Salata, Robert (OH)	Inf	417
Russell, Christy (CA)	Onc	390	Salem, Riad (IL)	VIR	996
Russell, Kenneth (WA)	RadRO	968	Salem, Ronald (CT)	S	1051
Russell, Mark (VA)	D	192	Salerno, Tomas (FL)	T&CS	1129
Russell, Stuart (MD)	Cv	101	Salgia, Ravi (IL)	Onc	371
Russo, Carolyn (AL)	PHO	768	Salky, Barry (NY)	S	1063
Rutgers, Joanne (CA)	Path	721	Sallan, Stephen (MA)	PHO	757
Rutherford, Thomas (CT)	GO	275	Sallent, Jorge (FL)	PPul	796
Rutkove, Seward (MA)	N	508	Salloum, Ihsan (FL)	Psyc	896
Ryan, Colleen (MA)	S	1051	Salmon, Jane (NY)	Rhu	1028
Ryan, David (MA)	Onc	331	Salo, Jonathan (NC)	S	1071
Rychik, Jack (PA)	PCd	736	Saltz, Leonard (NY)	Onc	348
Ryken, Timothy (IA)	NS	490	Saltzman, Charles (UT)	OrS	639
			Salvati, Eduardo (NY)	OrS	625
			Salvi, Sharad (IL)	PHO	773
			Salz, James (CA)	Oph	603
			Salzman, Carl (MA)	Psyc	889
			Samadi, David (NY)	U	1157

S

Name	Specialty	Pg
Saade, George (TX)	MF	439

Alphabetical Listing of Doctors

Name	Specialty	Pg	Name	Specialty	Pg
Samant, Sandeep (TN)	Oto	671	Sasaki, Clarence (CT)	Oto	657
Samberg, Eslee (NY)	Psyc	894	Sasson, Aaron (NE)	S	1086
Samii, Ali (WA)	N	538	Sataloff, Dahlia (PA)	S	1063
Samlowski, Wolfram (NV)	Onc	390	Sataloff, Robert (PA)	Oto	664
Sampson, Christian (MA)	HS	294	Satava, Richard (WA)	S	1099
Sampson, Hugh (NY)	PA&I	729	Sato, Thomas (WI)	PS	808
Sampson, John (NC)	NS	484	Sauer, Mark (NY)	RE	1010
Samson, Duke (TX)	NS	494	Saul, Robert (SC)	CG	159
Samuels, Brian (ID)	Onc	376	Saunders, Elijah (MD)	Cv	101
Samuels, Louis (PA)	T&CS	1121	Sauter, Edward (ND)	S	1086
Samuels, Martin (MA)	N	508	Savage, David (NY)	Hem	314
Samuels, Philip (OH)	MF	437	Savage, Edward (FL)	T&CS	1129
Samuelson, Thomas (MN)	Oph	594	Saven, Alan (CA)	Hem	327
Sanborn, Timothy (IL)	Cv	111	Saver, Jeffrey (CA)	N	539
Sanchez, Luis (MO)	VascS	1191	Savides, Thomas (CA)	Ge	255
Sanchez, Miguel (NJ)	Path	711	Savino, Peter (CA)	Oph	603
Sanda, Martin (MA)	U	1150	Sawaya, Raymond (TX)	NS	494
Sandberg, David (TX)	NS	494	Sawczuk, Ihor (NJ)	U	1157
Sandborn, William (CA)	Ge	255	Sawin, Robert (WA)	PS	811
Sanders, George (CA)	PlS	876	Sax, Paul (MA)	Inf	410
Sanders, Georgiana (MI)	A&I	89	Saxena, Sanjaya (CA)	Psyc	903
Sanders, William (GA)	U	1163	Scandling, John (CA)	Nep	465
Sandhu, Harvinder (NY)	OrS	625	Scantlebury, Velma (DE)	S	1063
Sandler, Alan (OR)	Onc	390	Scarborough, Mark (FL)	OrS	630
Sandler, Eric (FL)	PHO	768	Scardino, Peter (NY)	U	1157
Sandler, Howard (CA)	RadRO	968	Schachat, Andrew (OH)	Oph	594
Sandler, Martin (TN)	NuM	549	Schaefer, Steven (NY)	Oto	664
Sandlow, Jay (WI)	U	1170	Schaeffer, Anthony (IL)	U	1170
Sandlund, John (TN)	PHO	768	Schafer, Michael (IL)	OrS	637
Sands, Laurence (FL)	CRS	172	Schaff, Hartzell (MN)	T&CS	1134
Sanfilippo, Joseph (PA)	RE	1010	Schaffer, Randolph (CA)	S	1099
Sangeorzan, Bruce (WA)	OrS	645	Schaitkin, Barry (PA)	Oto	664
Sanger, James (WI)	PlS	867	Schanberg, Laura (NC)	PRhu	800
Sanger, Joseph (NY)	NuM	549	Schantz, Stimson (NY)	Oto	664
Sankar, Raman (CA)	ChiN	154	Schatz, Lisa (CO)	CRS	176
Santa-Emma, Philip (OH)	H & PM	407	Schatz, Norman (FL)	N	523
Santana, Victor (TN)	PHO	768	Schatzberg, Alan (CA)	Psyc	903
Santin, Alessandro (CT)	GO	275	Schauer, Philip (OH)	S	1082
Santos, Cesar (DC)	ChiN	148	Schechter, David (CA)	SM	1044
Sanz, Luis (VA)	ObG	559	Schein, Oliver (MD)	Oph	579
Saper, Clifford (MA)	N	508	Scheinberg, David (NY)	Onc	348
Saper, Joel (MI)	N	530	Schelbert, Heinrich (CA)	NuM	551
Sargent, Albert (MA)	ChAP	907	Scheld, W Michael (VA)	Inf	415
Sarnaik, Ashok (MI)	PCCM	742	Scheller, Arnold (MA)	SM	1040
Sarr, Michael (MN)	S	1081	Schenken, Robert (TX)	RE	1016
Sartor, Ryan (NC)	Ge	242	Scher, Howard (NY)	Onc	348

Name	Specialty	Pg	Name	Specialty	Pg
Scher, Jonathan (NY)	ObG	558	Schuchter, Lynn (PA)	Onc	349
Scher, Mark (OH)	ChiN	151	Schuckit, Marc (CA)	AdP	906
Scherl, Ellen (NY)	Ge	238	Schuger, Claudio (MI)	CE	124
Scherr, Douglas (NY)	U	1157	Schulak, James (OH)	S	1082
Schiano, Thomas (NY)	Ge	238	Schuler, Thomas (VA)	OrS	630
Schiff, David (VA)	N	523	Schulick, Richard (CO)	S	1086
Schiff, Eugene (FL)	Ge	242	Schulman, Steven (MD)	Cv	101
Schiff, Peter (NY)	RadRO	952	Schultz, Neal (NY)	D	188
Schiff, William (NY)	Oph	579	Schulze, Konrad (IA)	Ge	248
Schiffer, Charles (MI)	Onc	371	Schuman, Joel (PA)	Oph	579
Schiffman, Fred (RI)	Hem	311	Schuster, Michael (NY)	Hem	315
Schiffman, Jade (TX)	Oph	598	Schuster, Stephen (PA)	Hem	315
Schild, Steven (AZ)	RadRO	965	Schusterman, Mark (TX)	PlS	872
Schilder, Russell (PA)	Onc	349	Schutta, Mark (PA)	EDM	211
Schiller, Alan (NY)	Path	711	Schwab, Frank (NY)	OrS	625
Schiller, Gary (CA)	Hem	327	Schwab, Richard (PA)	Pul	927
Schiller, Joan (TX)	Onc	381	Schwartz, Allan (NY)	Cv	101
Schiller, Lawrence (TX)	Ge	252	Schwartz, Burton (MN)	Onc	372
Schilsky, Richard (IL)	Onc	372	Schwartz, Cindy (RI)	PHO	757
Schink, Julian (IL)	GO	285	Schwartz, David (CO)	Pul	937
Schirmer, Bruce (VA)	S	1072	Schwartz, Gary (MN)	Nep	462
Schlaff, William (PA)	RE	1010	Schwartz, Herbert (TN)	OrS	630
Schlegel, Peter (NY)	U	1157	Schwartz, L Matthew (PA)	PMR	837
Schley, W Shain (NY)	Oto	665	Schwartz, Marshall (PA)	PS	804
Schlinkert, Richard (AZ)	S	1092	Schwartz, Michael (FL)	Onc	362
Schluger, Neil (NY)	Pul	927	Schwartz, Peter (CT)	GO	275
Schmalzried, Thomas (CA)	OrS	645	Schwartz, Robert (CO)	Ger	265
Schmidt, Richard (PA)	OrS	625	Schwartz, Stanley (PA)	EDM	212
Schmitt, Steven (OH)	Inf	417	Schwartz, Steven (CA)	Oph	603
Schnabel, Freya (NY)	S	1063	Schwartz, Theodore (NY)	NS	478
Schneider, Darren (NY)	VascS	1188	Schwartz, William (NY)	Cv	101
Schnipper, Lowell (MA)	Onc	332	Schwartzberg, Lee (TN)	Hem	317
Schnitt, Stuart (MA)	Path	707	Schwartzentruber, Douglas (IN)	S	1082
Schnittger, Ingela (CA)	Cv	118	Schwartzman, Robert (PA)	N	517
Schoen, Robert (CT)	Rhu	1024	Schwarz, Adam (CA)	PCCM	743
Schoenberg, Mark (MD)	U	1157	Schwarz, Kathleen (MD)	PGe	751
Schoetz, David (MA)	CRS	169	Schwarz, Marvin (CO)	Pul	937
Schomberg, Paula (MN)	RadRO	962	Schwarz, Steven (NY)	PGe	751
Schooley, Robert (CA)	Inf	420	Scott, C Paul (PA)	Psyc	895
Schorge, John (MA)	GO	275	Scott, Gwendolyn (FL)	PInf	782
Schraut, Wolfgang (PA)	S	1064	Scott, Richard (MA)	OrS	612
Schreiber, Martin (OH)	Nep	462	Scott, W Norman (NY)	OrS	625
Schreiber, Theodore (MI)	IC	131	Scott, Walter (PA)	T&CS	1121
Schubert, Mark (AZ)	A&I	90	Scott-Conner, Carol (IA)	S	1082
Schubert, Richard (DC)	Rhu	1028	Scudder, Sidney (CA)	Onc	390
Schuberth, Kenneth (MD)	PA&I	730	Scudera, Peter (VA)	Ge	242

Alphabetical Listing of Doctors

Name	Specialty	Pg	Name	Specialty	Pg
Seashore, Margretta (CT)	CG	156	Sewell, C Whitaker (GA)	Path	714
Seaver, Laurie (HI)	CG	163	Sexson, Sandra (GA)	ChAP	910
See, William (WI)	U	1170	Seyfer, Alan (MD)	PlS	858
Seely, Ellen (MA)	EDM	208	Sha, Beverly (IL)	Inf	417
Seftel, Allen (NJ)	U	1157	Shaban, Stephen (NC)	U	1164
Segal, Brahm (NY)	Inf	413	Shabsigh, Ridwan (NY)	U	1157
Seibel, Barry (CA)	Oph	603	Shabto, Uri (NY)	Oph	580
Seidner, Douglas (TN)	Ge	242	Shaddy, Robert (PA)	PCd	736
Seidner, Steven (TX)	NP	452	Shadick, Nancy (MA)	Rhu	1025
Seifer, David (NY)	RE	1010	Shaffrey, Christopher (VA)	NS	484
Seiff, Stuart (CA)	Oph	604	Shaffrey, Mark (VA)	NS	484
Seifter, Julian (MA)	Nep	456	Shah, Jatin (NY)	S	1064
Seitz, William (OH)	HS	302	Shah, Nishit (RI)	CRS	169
Sekhar, Laligam (WA)	NS	498	Shah, Prediman (CA)	Cv	118
Sekhon, Lali (NV)	NS	499	Shah, Raj (CO)	Ge	250
Selby, Robert (CA)	S	1099	Shaked, Abraham (PA)	S	1064
Selden, Nathan (OR)	NS	499	Shaker, Reza (WI)	Ge	248
Sellke, Frank (RI)	T&CS	1112	Shamberger, Robert (MA)	PS	802
Selman, Warren (OH)	NS	490	Shamie, Neda (CA)	Oph	604
Seltzer, Dana (AZ)	OrS	641	Shani, Jacob (NY)	IC	129
Selvaggi, Kathy (MA)	H & PM	406	Shapiro, Amy (IN)	PHO	773
Selwyn, Peter (NY)	IM	424	Shapiro, Charles (OH)	Onc	372
Semenkovich, Clay (MO)	EDM	219	Shapiro, Edward (MA)	Psyc	889
Semrad, Carol (IL)	Ge	248	Shapiro, Eugene (CT)	PInf	780
Sen, Chandranath (NY)	NS	478	Shapiro, Jerrold (IL)	Cv	111
Senagore, Anthony (CA)	CRS	178	Shapiro, Lawrence (NY)	CG	158
Sencer, Susan (MN)	PHO	773	Shapiro, Richard (NY)	S	1064
Senders, Craig (CA)	Oto	686	Shapiro, Ron (PA)	S	1064
Sener, Stephen (CA)	S	1099	Shapiro, Scott (IN)	NS	490
Senior, Brent (NC)	Oto	671	Shapiro, William (AZ)	N	534
Sennett, Brian (PA)	SM	1042	Shapshay, Stanley (NY)	Oto	665
Senzer, Neil (TX)	RadRO	965	Sharkey, Peter (PA)	OrS	625
Sepkowitz, Kent (NY)	Inf	413	Sharlip, Ira (CA)	U	1178
Seplowitz, Alan (NY)	EDM	212	Sharma, Om Prakash (CA)	Pul	941
Serafano, Donald (CA)	Oph	604	Sharma, Samin (NY)	IC	129
Sergent, John (TN)	Rhu	1030	Sharp, Gregory (AR)	ChiN	152
Sergott, Robert (PA)	Oph	580	Sharp, Kenneth (TN)	S	1072
Serletti, Joseph (PA)	PlS	858	Shaw, Dennis (WA)	DR	984
Serody, Jonathan (NC)	Onc	362	Shaw, Edward (NC)	RadRO	957
Serota, Ronald (PA)	AdP	905	Shaywitz, Bennett (CT)	ChiN	146
Session, Donna (GA)	RE	1012	Shea, Christopher (IL)	D	195
Sessoms, Sandra (TX)	Rhu	1033	Shea, Richard (IN)	Cv	111
Sethi, Kapil (GA)	N	523	Shea, Thomas (NC)	Onc	362
Seton, Margaret (MA)	Rhu	1025	Shearer, Patricia (MD)	PHO	763
Setzen, Michael (NY)	Oto	665	Shearer, William (TX)	PA&I	732
Seung, Steven (OR)	RadRO	968	Shefner, Jeremy (NY)	N	517

Name	Specialty	Pg	Name	Specialty	Pg
Sheikh, Kazim (TX)	N	534	Shuldiner, Alan (MD)	EDM	212
Sheinfeld, Joel (NY)	U	1158	Shulman, Lawrence (MA)	Onc	332
Shelbourne, K Donald (IN)	OrS	637	Shulman, Lee (IL)	CG	160
Shellito, Judd (LA)	Pul	938	Shulman, Lisa (MD)	N	517
Shellito, Paul (MA)	CRS	169	Shulman, Stanford (IL)	PInf	783
Shelton, Clough (UT)	Oto	680	Shupack, Jerome (NY)	D	188
Shemin, Richard (CA)	T&CS	1142	Siatkowski, R Michael (OK)	Oph	598
Shen, Perry (NC)	S	1072	Sibley, Richard (CA)	Path	722
Shen, Win-Kuang (AZ)	CE	124	Sicard, Gregorio (MO)	VascS	1192
Shenk, Robert (OH)	S	1082	Sicherer, Scott (NY)	PA&I	730
Shenot, Patrick (PA)	U	1158	Sichting, Kay (IN)	PCCM	742
Shepard, Alexander (MI)	VascS	1192	Siddique, Teepu (IL)	N	530
Shepherd, Gillian (NY)	A&I	85	Sidransky, David (MD)	Onc	349
Sherertz, Elizabeth (SC)	D	192	Siebert, John (WI)	PlS	868
Sherman, Carol (SC)	Onc	362	Siegel, Barry (MO)	NuM	550
Sherman, Frederick (PA)	PCd	736	Siegel, Corey (NH)	Ge	230
Sherman, James (VA)	PPul	796	Siegel, Gordon (IL)	Oto	677
Sherman, Randolph (CA)	PlS	876	Siegel, Herrick (AL)	OrS	630
Sherman, Steven (TX)	EDM	221	Siegel, Martin (WA)	Inf	420
Sherman, Stuart (IN)	Ge	248	Siegel, Stuart (CA)	PHO	779
Sherry, David (PA)	PRhu	799	Siegelbaum, Marc (MD)	U	1158
Sherwood, Mark (FL)	Oph	586	Sielaff, Timothy (MN)	S	1082
Shibata, David (FL)	S	1072	Siemionow, Maria (OH)	PlS	868
Shields, Carol (PA)	Oph	580	Sigel, Eric (CO)	AM	81
Shields, Jerry (PA)	Oph	580	Sigman, Mark (RI)	U	1150
Shields, Peter (OH)	Onc	372	Sigurdson, Elin (PA)	S	1064
Shiffman, Mitchell (VA)	Ge	242	Sikic, Branimir (CA)	Onc	390
Shike, Moshe (NY)	Ge	238	Sila, Cathy (OH)	N	530
Shikora, Scott (MA)	S	1051	Silber, Sherman (MO)	U	1170
Shin, Dong Moon (GA)	Onc	362	Silbergeld, Daniel (WA)	NS	499
Shina, Donald (NM)	RadRO	965	Silberstein, Stephen (PA)	N	517
Shindo, Maisie (OR)	Oto	687	Siller, Barry (TX)	GO	288
Shingleton, Bradford (MA)	Oph	571	Sillers, Michael (AL)	Oto	671
Shinnar, Shlomo (NY)	ChiN	149	Sills, Allen (TN)	NS	484
Shlansky-Goldberg, Richard (PA)	VIR	993	Sills, Edward (MD)	PRhu	800
Shlofmitz, Richard (NY)	Cv	102	Silva, Elvio (TX)	Path	719
Shochat, Stephen (TN)	PS	806	Silver, Michael (IL)	Pul	935
Shockley, William (NC)	Oto	671	Silver, Richard (SC)	Rhu	1030
Shoffner, John (GA)	CG	159	Silver, Samuel (MI)	Onc	372
Shore, Bernard (MO)	Pul	935	Silverman, Damon (VT)	Oto	657
Shorofsky, Stephen (MD)	IC	129	Silverman, Gary (PA)	NP	448
Short, Billie (DC)	NP	448	Silverman, Jan (PA)	Path	711
Shortliffe, Linda (CA)	U	1178	Silverman, Lewis (NY)	Onc	349
Shrager, Joseph (CA)	T&CS	1143	Silverman, Paula (OH)	Onc	372
Shrieve, Dennis (UT)	RadRO	963	Silverman, William (IA)	Ge	248
Shuer, Lawrence (CA)	NS	499	Silverstein, Herbert (FL)	Oto	671

Alphabetical Listing of Doctors

Name	Specialty	Pg	Name	Specialty	Pg
Silverstein, Janet (FL)	PEn	746	Skyler, Jay (FL)	EDM	215
Silverstein, Melvin (CA)	S	1100	Slama, Thomas (IN)	Inf	417
Silvestry, Frank (PA)	Cv	102	Slankard, Marjorie (NY)	A&I	85
Sim, Franklin (MN)	OrS	637	Slap, Gail (PA)	AM	81
Simeone, Diane (MI)	S	1082	Slater, William (NY)	Cv	102
Simmons, Charles (CA)	NP	452	Slatkin, Neal (CA)	PM	703
Simmons, Rache (NY)	S	1064	Slaughter, Mark (KY)	T&CS	1129
Simms, Robert (MA)	Rhu	1025	Slavin, Sumner (MA)	PlS	851
Simon, Daniel (OH)	Cv	111	Slawin, Kevin (TX)	U	1174
Simon, George (TX)	Onc	382	Slease, Robert (DE)	Hem	315
Simon, James (DC)	ObG	558	Sleasman, John (FL)	PA&I	731
Simon, John (NY)	Oph	580	Sledge, George (IN)	Onc	372
Simon, Richard (MI)	Pul	935	Slezak, Sheri (MD)	PlS	858
Simpson, David (NY)	N	517	Slingluff, Craig (VA)	S	1072
Simpson, Joe (FL)	ObG	560	Slivka, Adam (PA)	Ge	238
Sinanan, Mika (WA)	S	1100	Sliwa, James (IL)	PMR	842
Singer, Carlos (FL)	N	524	Slomowitz, Marcia (IL)	ChAP	911
Singer, Daniel (HI)	OrS	645	Slutsky, David (CA)	HS	304
Singer, Mark (CA)	Oto	687	Sly, R Michael (MD)	PA&I	730
Singer, Peter (CA)	EDM	224	Small, Donald (MD)	PHO	763
Singer, Robert (CA)	PlS	877	Small, Eric (CA)	Onc	391
Singer, Samuel (NY)	S	1064	Small, Gary (CA)	GerPsy	915
Singh, Arun (RI)	T&CS	1112	Small, William (IL)	RadRO	962
Singh, Bhuvanesh (NY)	Oto	665	Smalley, Stephen (KS)	RadRO	963
Singh, Diljeet (AZ)	GO	288	Smalling, Richard (TX)	IC	132
Singh, Dinesh (CT)	U	1150	Smart, Frank (LA)	Cv	115
Singh, Nalini (DC)	PInf	781	Smedira, Nicholas (OH)	T&CS	1135
Singh, Navin (MD)	PlS	858	Smikle, Collin (CA)	RE	1017
Singh, Nimi (MN)	AM	81	Smith, Barbara (MA)	S	1052
Singhal, Seema (IL)	Hem	321	Smith, Craig (NY)	T&CS	1121
Sinha, Uttam (CA)	Oto	687	Smith, David (FL)	PlS	863
Siperstein, Allan (OH)	S	1082	Smith, Donna (IL)	GO	285
Sirdofsky, Michael (DC)	N	518	Smith, Douglas (WA)	OrS	646
Siris, Ethel (NY)	EDM	212	Smith, Eric (MA)	OrS	613
Sisti, Michael (NY)	NS	479	Smith, John (OH)	T&CS	1135
Sisung, Charles (IL)	PMR	841	Smith, Joseph (TN)	U	1164
Sivaswamy, Lalitha (MI)	ChiN	151	Smith, Lloyd (CA)	GO	290
Sivit, Carlos (OH)	DR	981	Smith, Matthew (MA)	Onc	332
Skibber, John (TX)	S	1092	Smith, Mitchell (PA)	Onc	349
Skinner, Eila (CA)	U	1178	Smith, Paul (FL)	PlS	863
Skinner, Kristin (NY)	S	1064	Smith, Peter (NC)	T&CS	1129
Skinner, Michael (TX)	PS	810	Smith, Ronald (CA)	Oph	604
Sklar, Charles (NY)	PEn	745	Smith, Russell (NE)	Oto	680
Sklar, Frederick (TX)	NS	494	Smith, Sidney (NC)	Cv	106
Skolnick, Alan (AK)	Cv	118	Smith, Steven (MN)	EDM	219
Skoner, David (PA)	PA&I	730	Smith, Steven (IL)	VIR	996

Name	Specialty	Pg	Name	Specialty	Pg
Smith, Thomas (MA)	Path	707	Soper, John (NC)	GO	283
Smith, Thomas (MD)	Onc	349	Soper, Nathaniel (IL)	S	1083
Smith, Wade (CA)	N	539	Sorrell, Michael (NE)	Ge	250
Smith, Yolanda (MI)	RE	1014	Sorrentino, Matthew (IL)	Cv	111
Smoot, Duane (TN)	Ge	243	Sorrentino, Robert (GA)	CE	122
Smythe, W Roy (TX)	T&CS	1139	Sosa, Julie (CT)	S	1052
Snyder, David (LA)	CE	125	Soslow, Robert (NY)	Path	711
Snyder, David (CA)	Hem	327	Sosman, Jeffrey (TN)	Onc	362
Snyder, John (DC)	PGe	751	Soter, Nicholas (NY)	D	189
Snyder, Peter (PA)	EDM	212	Sotereanos, Dean (PA)	HS	298
Snyder, Russell (TX)	ObG	563	Sotomayor, Eduardo (FL)	Onc	362
Snyderman, Carl (PA)	Oto	665	Soulen, Michael (PA)	VIR	994
Sobel, Jack (MI)	Inf	417	Soules, Michael (WA)	RE	1018
Sobel, Michael (WA)	VascS	1194	Souryal, Tarek (TX)	OrS	641
Sobel, Stuart (FL)	D	192	Souweidane, Mark (NY)	NS	479
Soberman, Mark (MD)	T&CS	1121	Sowers, James (MO)	EDM	219
Socinski, Mark (PA)	Onc	349	Spack, Norman (MA)	PEn	743
Socol, Michael (IL)	MF	437	Spaeth, George (PA)	Oph	580
Soff, Gerald (NY)	Hem	315	Spann, Cyril (GA)	GO	283
Soiffer, Robert (MA)	Onc	332	Spector, Sheldon (CA)	A&I	91
Soisson, Andrew (UT)	GO	286	Speeg, Kermit (TX)	Ge	252
Sokol, Lubomir (FL)	Hem	318	Spence, Robert (MD)	PlS	858
Sokol, Ronald (CO)	PGe	754	Spencer, Dennis (CT)	NS	471
Sokol, Thomas (CA)	CRS	178	Spencer, Thomas (MA)	ChAP	907
Sokoloff, Daniel (FL)	D	192	Spengler, Dan (TN)	OrS	631
Solberg, Lawrence (FL)	Hem	318	Spergel, Jonathan (PA)	PA&I	730
Solin, Lawrence (PA)	RadRO	952	Sperling, Mark (PA)	PEn	745
Solitar, Bruce (NY)	Rhu	1028	Sperling, Michael (PA)	N	518
Solomon, Gary (NY)	Rhu	1028	Spetzler, Robert (AZ)	NS	494
Solomon, Kerry (SC)	Oph	586	Speyer, James (NY)	Onc	349
Solomon, Robert (NY)	NS	479	Spiegel, David (CA)	Psyc	903
Solomon, Stephen (NY)	VIR	993	Spiegel, Jeffrey (MA)	Oto	657
Solorzano, Carmen (TN)	S	1072	Spiera, Harry (NY)	Rhu	1028
Soloway, Mark (FL)	U	1164	Spigland, Nitsana (NY)	PS	804
Somerville, James (MN)	Nep	462	Spindler, Kurt (TN)	OrS	631
Sommer, Robert (NY)	PCd	736	Spinelli, Henry (NY)	PlS	858
Sondak, Vernon (FL)	S	1072	Spinner, Robert (MN)	NS	490
Sondel, Paul (WI)	PHO	773	Spirtos, Nicola (NV)	GO	290
Sondheimer, Steven (PA)	RE	1010	Spitzer, Thomas (MA)	Hem	311
Sonett, Joshua (NY)	T&CS	1121	Spivak, Jeffrey (NY)	OrS	625
Song, John (CO)	Oto	681	Spivak, Jerry (MD)	Hem	315
Song, Shiyu (VA)	RadRO	957	Spivak, William (NY)	PGe	751
Sontheimer, Richard (UT)	D	196	Sponseller, Paul (MD)	OrS	625
Sood, Anil (TX)	GO	288	Spray, Thomas (PA)	T&CS	1122
Sood, Rajiv (IN)	PlS	868	Spriggs, David (NY)	Onc	350
Soparkar, Charles (TX)	Oph	598	Squires, Kathleen (PA)	Inf	413

Alphabetical Listing of Doctors

Name	Specialty	Pg	Name	Specialty	Pg
Squires, Robert (PA)	PGe	751	Steinhagen, Randolph (NY)	CRS	171
St Clair, William (KY)	RadRO	957	Steinherz, Laurel (NY)	PCd	736
Staats, Peter (NJ)	PM	698	Steinherz, Peter (NY)	PHO	764
Staddon, Arthur (PA)	Onc	350	Steinhorn, Robin (CA)	NP	451
Stadelmann, Wayne (NH)	PlS	851	Steinkampf, Michael (AL)	RE	1012
Stadler, Walter (IL)	Onc	372	Steinmann, Scott (MN)	HS	302
Stadtmauer, Edward (PA)	Onc	350	Stenson, Kerstin (IL)	Oto	678
Staffenberg, David (NY)	PlS	859	Sterman, Daniel (PA)	Pul	928
Staggers, Barbara (CA)	AM	82	Stern, Jeffrey (CA)	GO	291
Stahl, Donna (OH)	S	1083	Stern, Leonard (NY)	Nep	458
Stahl, Richard (CT)	PlS	851	Stern, Matthew (PA)	N	518
Stainback, Raymond (TX)	Cv	115	Stern, Peter (OH)	HS	302
Staley, Charles (GA)	S	1072	Stern, Robert (MA)	D	184
Stamos, Michael (CA)	CRS	178	Sternberg, Paul (TN)	Oph	586
Stankiewicz, James (IL)	Oto	677	Sterns, Gwen (NY)	Oph	581
Stanley, Charles (PA)	PEn	745	Stevens, W Grant (CA)	PlS	877
Stanley, James (MI)	VascS	1192	Stevenson, David (CA)	NP	452
Stanley, John (PA)	D	189	Stevenson, Lynne (MA)	Cv	96
Staples, Edward (FL)	T&CS	1129	Stevenson, Roger (SC)	CG	159
Staren, Edgar (AZ)	S	1092	Stevenson, William (MA)	CE	119
Stark, Walter (MD)	Oph	580	Stewart, A Keith (AZ)	Hem	324
Starnes, Vaughn (CA)	T&CS	1143	Stewart, Allan (NY)	T&CS	1122
Starz, Terence (PA)	Rhu	1028	Stewart, Elizabeth (MN)	RE	1014
Stasney, C Richard (TX)	Oto	683	Stewart, Forrest (WA)	Onc	391
Staton, Gerald (GA)	Pul	932	Stewart, Michael (NY)	Oto	665
Stea, Baldassarre (AZ)	RadRO	965	Stewart, Paula (AL)	PMR	839
Steadman, J Richard (CO)	OrS	639	Stewart, Ronald (TX)	S	1092
Steege, John (NC)	ObG	560	Stewart, William (OH)	Cv	111
Steen, Preston (ND)	Onc	376	Stieg, Philip (NY)	NS	479
Steen, Virginia (DC)	Rhu	1028	Stiff, Patrick (IL)	Hem	322
Steers, William (VA)	U	1164	Stiles, Alan (NC)	NP	449
Stefanyszyn, Mary (PA)	Oph	580	Stine, Susan (MI)	AdP	905
Stehman, Frederick (IN)	GO	286	Stock, Richard (NY)	RadRO	952
Steiger, David (NY)	Pul	928	Stockdale, Frank (CA)	Onc	391
Stein, David (PA)	CRS	171	Stolier, Alan (LA)	S	1092
Stein, Elliott (CA)	GerPsy	915	Stoller, James (OH)	Pul	936
Stein, James (CA)	PS	811	Stoller, Marshall (CA)	U	1179
Stein, James (WI)	Cv	111	Stone, Anthony (CA)	U	1179
Stein, Murray (CA)	Psyc	903	Stone, Edwin (IA)	Oph	594
Steinberg, Gary (CA)	NS	499	Stone, Gregg (NY)	IC	129
Steinberg, Gary (IL)	U	1170	Stone, Joel (FL)	Onc	362
Steinberg, Harry (NY)	Pul	928	Stone, Richard (MA)	Hem	311
Steiner, Hans (CA)	ChAP	912	Stoopler, Mark (NY)	Onc	350
Steiner, Mark (MA)	SM	1040	Stopeck, Alison (AZ)	Onc	382
Steinert, Roger (CA)	Oph	604	Stotland, Mitchell (NH)	PlS	851
Steingart, Richard (NY)	Cv	102	Stough, Rebecca (OK)	DR	982

Name	Specialty	Pg	Name	Specialty	Pg
Stout, J Timothy (OR)	Oph	604	Sulica, Radu Lucian (NY)	Oto	666
Stover-Pepe, Diane (NY)	Pul	928	Sullivan, Kathleen (PA)	PA&I	730
Stowe, Cary (FL)	T&CS	1129	Sullivan, Patrick (RI)	PlS	851
Strain, Eric (MD)	AdP	905	Sullivan, Timothy (GA)	A&I	87
Strair, Roger (NJ)	Hem	315	Sultan, Mark (NY)	PlS	859
Strakowski, Stephen (OH)	Psyc	898	Summergrad, Paul (MA)	Psyc	890
Strand, William (TX)	U	1174	Summers, C Gail (MN)	Oph	594
Strashun, Arnold (NY)	NuM	549	Sumpio, Bauer (CT)	VascS	1185
Strassner, Howard (IL)	MF	437	Sun, Peter (CA)	NS	499
Stratta, Robert (NC)	S	1073	Sun, Weijing (PA)	Onc	350
Strauch, Eric (MD)	PS	804	Sundaram, Chandru (IN)	U	1170
Strauch, Robert (NY)	HS	298	Sundaram, Magesh (IL)	S	1083
Straus, David (NY)	Onc	350	Sundaresan, Narayan (NY)	NS	479
Strauss, Gary (MA)	Onc	332	Sundy, John (NC)	A&I	87
Strauss, James (TX)	Hem	325	Suntharalingam, Mohan (MD)	RadRO	953
Streeter, Oscar (DC)	RadRO	952	Supiano, Mark (UT)	Ger	266
Streiff, Michael (MD)	Hem	315	Surawicz, Christina (WA)	Ge	255
Streim, Joel (PA)	GerPsy	913	Suresh, Santhanam (IL)	PM	700
Strenger, Rochelle (RI)	Onc	332	Surks, Martin (NY)	EDM	212
Stringer, Scott (MS)	Oto	671	Surrey, Eric (CO)	RE	1015
Strollo, Patrick (PA)	Pul	928	Sussman, Norman (NY)	Psyc	895
Strom, Laura (CO)	N	532	Suster, Saul (WI)	Path	716
Strome, Marshall (NY)	Oto	665	Sutherland, Everett (CO)	Pul	937
Strome, Scott (MD)	Oto	665	Sutherland, Richard (NC)	U	1164
Strongwater, Allan (NJ)	OrS	626	Sutphen, Rebecca (FL)	CG	159
Strouse, Thomas (CA)	Psyc	903	Sutton, John (VT)	S	1052
Strunk, Robert (MO)	PA&I	731	Sutton, Leslie (PA)	NS	479
Strup, Stephen (KY)	U	1164	Sutton, Linda (NC)	Onc	363
Stryker, Steven (IL)	CRS	175	Svensson, Lars (OH)	T&CS	1135
Stuart, Richard (MO)	T&CS	1135	Swaid, Swaid (AL)	NS	484
Stubblefield, Michael (NY)	PMR	837	Swain, Sandra (DC)	Onc	350
Stuchin, Steven (NY)	OrS	626	Swanson, Jerry (MN)	N	530
Studenski, Stephanie (PA)	Ger	263	Swanson, Neil (OR)	D	200
Stulberg, S David (IL)	OrS	637	Swanson, Scott (MA)	T&CS	1112
Stulting, R Doyle (GA)	Oph	586	Swanstrom, Lee (OR)	S	1100
Stump, David (TX)	Ge	253	Swarm, Robert (MO)	PM	700
Stuzin, James (FL)	PlS	863	Swartz, Richard (MI)	Nep	462
Stylianos, Steven (NY)	PS	804	Swearingen, Brooke (MA)	NS	471
Su, Li-Ming (FL)	U	1164	Sweeney, Christopher (MA)	Onc	332
Suarez, Jose (TX)	N	534	Sweeney, John (GA)	S	1073
Suchy, Frederick (CO)	PGe	755	Sweet, Richard (CA)	ObG	563
Suen, James (AR)	Oto	683	Sweetenham, John (NV)	Onc	391
Sugarbaker, David (MA)	T&CS	1112	Swensen, Stephen (MN)	DR	981
Sugarbaker, Paul (DC)	S	1065	Swerdloff, Ronald (CA)	EDM	224
Suh, John (OH)	RadRO	962	Swerdlow, Charles (CA)	CE	125
Suki, Wadi (TX)	Nep	464	Swerdlow, Michael (NY)	N	518

Alphabetical Listing of Doctors

Name	Specialty	Pg	Name	Specialty	Pg
Swerdlow, Steven (PA)	Path	712	Te, Helen (IL)	Ge	248
Swetter, Susan (CA)	D	200	Teal, James (DC)	DR	977
Swiontkowski, Marc (MN)	OrS	638	Tebbetts, John (TX)	PlS	872
Swisher, Stephen (TX)	T&CS	1139	Tebbi, Cameron (FL)	PHO	768
Swistel, Alexander (NY)	S	1065	Tedder, Mark (TN)	T&CS	1130
Swistel, Daniel (NY)	T&CS	1122	Tefferi, Ayalew (MN)	Hem	322
Szabo, Robert (CA)	HS	304	Teigland, Chris (NC)	U	1164
Szachowicz, Edward (MN)	Oto	678	Teirstein, Paul (CA)	IC	133
Sze, Gordon (CT)	NRad	985	Teitel, David (CA)	PCd	741
Szeto, Wilson (PA)	T&CS	1122	Teitelbaum, George (CA)	NRad	991
			Teitz, Carol (WA)	SM	1044
			Teknos, Theodoros (OH)	Oto	678
			Telen, Marilyn (NC)	Hem	318
# T			Telian, Steven (MI)	Oto	678
			Telischi, Fred (FL)	Oto	671
Tabbal, Nicolas (NY)	PlS	859	Tempero, Margaret (CA)	Onc	391
Tabsh, Khalil (CA)	MF	441	Tenenbaum, Joseph (NY)	Cv	102
Taetle, Raymond (AZ)	Onc	382	Teng, Nelson (CA)	GO	291
Tafra, Lorraine (MD)	S	1065	Tenner, Michael (NY)	NRad	986
Taft, Timothy (NC)	SM	1042	Tennison, Michael (NC)	ChiN	149
Tagawa, Scott (NY)	Onc	351	Tenover, Joyce (CA)	Ger	267
Taghian, Alphonse (MA)	RadRO	947	Teperman, Lewis (NY)	S	1065
Takayama, Thomas (WA)	U	1179	Tepper, Joel (NC)	RadRO	957
Talamonti, Mark (IL)	S	1083	Terr, Lenore (CA)	ChAP	912
Tallman, Martin (NY)	Hem	316	Terris, David (GA)	Oto	671
Tamargo, Rafael (MD)	NS	479	Terris, Martha (GA)	U	1165
Tamaroff, Marc (CA)	A&I	91	Tester, William (PA)	Onc	351
Tamborlane, William (CT)	PEn	744	Tetrud, James (CA)	N	539
Tanabe, Kenneth (MA)	S	1052	Tewari, Ashutosh (NY)	U	1158
Taneja, Samir (NY)	U	1158	Textor, Stephen (MN)	Nep	462
Tanner, Caroline (CA)	N	539	Thaler, Erica (PA)	Oto	666
Taplin, Mary-Ellen (MA)	Onc	333	Thaller, Seth (FL)	PlS	863
Tapson, Victor (NC)	Pul	932	Thames, Marc (AZ)	Cv	115
Tarbell, Nancy (MA)	RadRO	947	Tharratt, Robert (CA)	Pul	941
Targan, Stephan (CA)	Ge	255	Thase, Michael (PA)	Psyc	895
Tarraza, Hector (ME)	GO	275	Thayer, Sarah (MA)	S	1052
Tartter, Paul (NY)	S	1065	Theodore, Nicholas (AZ)	NS	494
Tatter, Stephen (NC)	NS	485	Thiers, Bruce (SC)	D	192
Taub, Peter (NY)	PlS	859	Thigpen, James (MS)	Onc	363
Tauber, Danna (PA)	PPul	795	Thistlethwaite, J Richard (IL)	S	1083
Tayal, Ashis (PA)	N	518	Thistlethwaite, Patricia (CA)	T&CS	1143
Taylon, Charles (NE)	NS	492	Thoder, Joseph (PA)	HS	298
Taylor, Lynne (MA)	N	508	Thomas, Bert (CA)	OrS	646
Taylor, R Stan (TX)	D	198	Thomas, Charles (OR)	RadRO	968
Taylor, Richard (TX)	PCCM	742	Thomas, Christie (IA)	Nep	463
Tchou, Julia (PA)	S	1065	Thomas, Dan (CA)	PGe	756
Tchou, Patrick (OH)	CE	124			

Alphabetical Listing of Doctors

Name	Specialty	Pg	Name	Specialty	Pg
Thomas, David (MO)	Ger	265	Torres, Vicente (MN)	Nep	463
Thomas, Gregory (OR)	PHO	779	Torti, Frank (NC)	Onc	363
Thomas, Ronald (PA)	MF	433	Toskes, Phillip (FL)	Ge	243
Thomashow, Byron (NY)	Pul	928	Toth, Thomas (MA)	RE	1007
Thompson, Ann Ellen (PA)	PCCM	741	Toto, Robert (TX)	Nep	464
Thompson, B Gregory (MI)	NS	490	Townsend, Raymond (PA)	Nep	458
Thompson, Brad (IA)	DR	981	Toyoda, Yoshiya (PA)	T&CS	1122
Thompson, George (OH)	OrS	638	Traboulsi, Elias (OH)	Oph	594
Thompson, Ian (TX)	U	1174	Trabulsi, Edouard (PA)	U	1158
Thompson, John (WA)	Onc	391	Tracy, Thomas (RI)	PS	802
Thompson, Reid (TN)	NS	485	Tranbaugh, Robert (NY)	T&CS	1122
Thor, Ann (CO)	Path	717	Trauner, Doris (CA)	ChiN	154
Thorne, Charles (NY)	PlS	859	Travis, William (NY)	Path	712
Thorner, Michael (VA)	EDM	215	Traynelis, Vincent (IL)	NS	490
Thornhill, Thomas (MA)	OrS	613	Traynor, Michael (ND)	S	1086
Thorp, John (NC)	MF	435	Treadwell, Marjorie (MI)	MF	437
Thorson, Alan (NE)	CRS	176	Treadwell, Patricia (IN)	D	195
Thrasher, J Brantley (KS)	U	1172	Tremaine, William (MN)	Ge	248
Thulborn, Keith (IL)	NRad	989	Trenholme, Gordon (IL)	Inf	417
Thurmond, Amy (OR)	DR	984	Trento, Alfredo (CA)	T&CS	1143
Tillinghast, Jeffrey (MO)	A&I	89	Trerotola, Scott (PA)	VIR	994
Tinetti, Mary (CT)	Ger	262	Trese, Michael (MI)	Oph	594
Ting, Jess (NY)	PlS	859	Triche, Timothy (CA)	Path	722
Tino, Gregory (PA)	Pul	928	Triozzi, Pierre (OH)	Onc	373
Tkaczuk, Katherine (MD)	Onc	351	Tripathy, Debasish (CA)	Onc	391
Tobias, Hillel (NY)	Ge	238	Tripuraneni, Prabhakar (CA)	RadRO	968
Tobin, Gordon (KY)	PlS	863	Trisal, Vijay (CA)	S	1100
Tobin, Martin (IL)	Pul	936	Trobe, Jonathan (MI)	Oph	594
Tobis, Jonathan (CA)	Cv	118	Troner, Michael (FL)	Onc	363
Todd, George (NY)	VascS	1189	Trudel, Judith (MN)	CRS	175
Tolkoff-Rubin, Nina (MA)	Nep	456	True, Lawrence (WA)	Path	722
Tolo, Vernon (CA)	OrS	646	Trulock, Elbert (MO)	Pul	936
Tomaselli, Gordon (MD)	CE	121	Trumble, Thomas (WA)	HS	305
Tomaszewski, John (NY)	Path	712	Trump, Donald (NY)	Onc	351
Tomford, J Walton (OH)	Inf	417	Tsai, James (CT)	Oph	571
Tomich, Paul (NE)	MF	438	Tsangaris, Theodore (MD)	S	1065
Tomita, Tadanori (IL)	NS	490	Tsao, Hensin (MA)	D	184
Tomlinson, Gail (TX)	PHO	776	Tse, David (FL)	Oph	586
Tonsgard, James (IL)	ChiN	151	Tsokos, George (MA)	Rhu	1025
Toonkel, Leonard (FL)	RadRO	958	Tucci, Debara (NC)	Oto	672
Topham, Neal (PA)	PlS	859	Tucker, Rodney (AL)	IM	425
Topol, Eric (CA)	Cv	118	Tufano, Ralph (MD)	Oto	666
Toppmeyer, Deborah (NJ)	Onc	351	Tufaro, Anthony (MD)	PlS	860
Toriumi, Dean (IL)	Oto	678	Tuggle, David (OK)	PS	810
Tornetta, Paul (MA)	OrS	613	Tulsky, James (NC)	H & PM	407
Tornos, Carmen (NY)	Path	712	Tune, Larry (GA)	GerPsy	914

Alphabetical Listing of Doctors

Name	Specialty	Pg	Name	Specialty	Pg
Tunkel, David (MD)	PO	790	Valentino, Leonard (IL)	PHO	773
Turecki, Stanley (NY)	ChAP	909	Valero, Vicente (TX)	Onc	382
Turek, Paul (CA)	U	1179	Valji, Karim (WA)	VIR	998
Turner, William (TX)	T&CS	1140	Vallieres, Eric (WA)	T&CS	1143
Turrentine, Mark (IN)	T&CS	1135	Van Arsdalen, Keith (PA)	U	1158
Turtz, Alan (NJ)	NS	479	Van Besien, Koen (IL)	Hem	322
Tuttle, R Michael (NY)	EDM	212	Van Der Horst, Charles (NC)	Inf	415
Tuttle, Todd (MN)	S	1083	Van Dorsten, J Peter (SC)	MF	435
Tuxhorn, Ingrid (OH)	ChiN	151	van Hoff, Jack (NH)	PHO	757
Twardowski, Przemyslaw (CA)	Onc	391	Van Loveren, Harry (FL)	NS	485
Tychsen, Lawrence (MO)	Oph	595	Van Marter, Linda (MA)	NP	446
Tyler, Douglas (NC)	S	1073	Van Nagell, John (KY)	GO	283
Tzakis, Andreas (OH)	S	1083	Van Voorhis, Bradley (IA)	RE	1015
			Van Zee, Kimberly (NY)	S	1065
			Vance, Mary Lee (VA)	EDM	215
			Vander, James (PA)	Oph	581
U			Vander Kolk, Craig (MD)	PlS	860
Uberti, Joseph (MI)	Hem	322	Vander Salm, Thomas (MA)	T&CS	1112
Udelsman, Robert (CT)	S	1052	Vanderhoof, Jon (NE)	PGe	755
Ulbright, Thomas (IN)	Path	716	Vanderkolk, Bessel (MA)	Psyc	890
Ulissey, Michael (TX)	DR	982	Vapnek, Jonathan (NY)	U	1159
Ulshen, Martin (NC)	PGe	752	Varadhachary, Gauri (TX)	Onc	382
Umetsu, Dale (MA)	A&I	84	Vargo, John (OH)	Ge	248
Unger, Michael (PA)	Pul	929	Varma, Madhulika (CA)	CRS	178
Unger, Stephen (FL)	S	1073	Vas, George (NY)	N	518
Ungerleider, Ross (NC)	T&CS	1130	Vasconez, Henry (KY)	PlS	864
Updegraff, Stephen (FL)	Oph	587	Vaughan, William (AL)	Onc	363
Urata, Mark (CA)	PlS	877	Vaughey, Ellen (VA)	Pul	932
Urba, Susan (MI)	Onc	373	Vaughn, David (PA)	Onc	351
Urba, Walter (OR)	Onc	392	Vauthey, Jean-Nicholas (TX)	S	1092
Urist, Marshall (AL)	S	1073	Vege, Santhi (MN)	Ge	249
Urken, Mark (NY)	Oto	666	Veith, Richard (WA)	GerPsy	915
Uzzo, Robert (PA)	U	1158	Velcek, Francisca (NY)	PS	804
			Velvis, Harmannus (NY)	PCd	736
			Venkat, K K (MI)	Nep	463
			Venook, Alan (CA)	Onc	392
V			Verghese, Mohan (DC)	U	1159
Vaccaro, Alexander (PA)	OrS	626	Vernava, Anthony (FL)	CRS	172
Vaezi, Michael (TN)	Ge	243	Verrier, Edward (WA)	T&CS	1143
Vahdat, Linda (NY)	Onc	351	Verschraegen, Claire (VT)	Onc	333
Vail, Thomas (CA)	OrS	646	Vescio, Robert (CA)	Onc	392
Vajaranant, Thasarat (IL)	Oph	595	Vetrovec, George (VA)	Cv	106
Valaitis, Sandra (IL)	ObG	562	Vetter, Thomas (AL)	PM	699
Valea, Fidel (NC)	GO	283	Vetto, John (OR)	S	1100
Valentine, Alan (TX)	Psyc	900	Vezina, L Gilbert (DC)	NRad	986
Valentino, Joseph (KY)	Oto	672	Vicini, Frank (MI)	RadRO	962

Name	Specialty	Pg	Name	Specialty	Pg
Vick, Nicholas (IL)	N	530	Wagner-Weiner, Linda (IL)	PRhu	800
Vickers, Selwyn (MN)	S	1083	Wagoner, Lynne (OH)	Cv	112
Videtic, Gregory (OH)	RadRO	962	Waguespack, Steven (TX)	EDM	221
Vierling, John (TX)	Ge	253	Wahl, Richard (MD)	NuM	549
Vigneswaran, Wickii (IL)	T&CS	1135	Wain, John (MA)	T&CS	1112
Vignola, Paul (NC)	Cv	106	Waintraub, Stanley (NJ)	Onc	352
Vijayakumar, Srinivasan (MS)	RadRO	958	Wait, Susan (MD)	Psyc	895
Vik, Terry (IN)	PHO	773	Wakefield, Thomas (MI)	S	1084
Villanueva, Andrew (MA)	Pul	924	Wald, Arnold (WI)	Ge	249
Vinciguerra, Vincent (NY)	Onc	351	Wald, Ellen (WI)	PInf	783
Vining, Eileen (MD)	Ped	727	Waldhausen, John HT (WA)	PS	811
Vining, Eugenia (CT)	Oto	657	Waldo, Albert (OH)	CE	124
Vinuela, Fernando (CA)	NRad	991	Walker, Alonzo (WI)	S	1084
Visco, Anthony (NC)	ObG	560	Walker, David (TX)	Path	719
Vitek, Jerrold (MN)	N	530	Walker, Joan (OK)	GO	288
Vivino, Frederick (PA)	Rhu	1029	Walker, Marion (UT)	NS	492
Vlahakes, Gus (MA)	T&CS	1112	Walker, R Dale (OR)	AdP	906
Vo, Phuc (FL)	OrS	631	Walker, William (WA)	Ped	729
Voelkel, Norbert (VA)	Pul	932	Walkup, John (NY)	ChAP	909
Vogelzang, Nicholas (NV)	Onc	392	Wall, Michael (OR)	PPul	798
Vogelzang, Robert (IL)	VIR	996	Wallace, Anne Marie (CA)	S	1100
Vogt, Peter (MN)	PlS	868	Wallace, Daniel (CA)	Rhu	1034
Voigt, Roger (MD)	PS	804	Wallace, Jeanne (CA)	Pul	941
Vokes, Everett (IL)	Onc	373	Wallace, Mark (FL)	Inf	415
Volberding, Paul (CA)	Onc	392	Wallace, Mark (CA)	PM	703
Volgman, Annabelle (IL)	Cv	112	Wallace, Richard (TX)	Inf	419
Vollmer, Timothy (CO)	N	532	Wallace, Robert (LA)	Oph	598
Volpe, Joseph (MA)	ChiN	147	Wallach, Edward (MD)	RE	1010
Volpe, Nicholas (IL)	Oph	595	Wallach, Frances (NY)	Inf	413
Volshteyn, Oksana (MO)	PMR	842	Wallen, Eric (NC)	U	1165
Von Burton, Gary (LA)	Onc	382	Waller, Edmund (GA)	Onc	363
von der Lohe, Elisabeth (IN)	Cv	112	Walling, Arthur (FL)	OrS	631
Von Gunten, Charles (CA)	H & PM	408	Walmer, David (NC)	RE	1012
Von Hoff, Daniel (AZ)	Onc	382	Walsh, B Timothy (NY)	Psyc	895
von Mehren, Margaret (PA)	Onc	352	Walsh, Christine (NY)	PCd	736
Von Roenn, Jamie (IL)	Onc	373	Walsh, Edward (MA)	PCd	734
Voorhees, John (MI)	D	195	Walsh, Garrett (TX)	T&CS	1140
Vose, Julie (NE)	Hem	322	Walsh, John (LA)	NS	495
Vredenburgh, James (NC)	Onc	363	Walsh, Joseph (NY)	Oph	581
			Walsh, Mary (IN)	Cv	112
			Walsh, Nicolas (TX)	PM	701
			Walsh, Patrick (MD)	U	1159
# W			Walsh, R Matthew (OH)	S	1084
Wackym, P Ashley (OR)	Oto	687	Walters, Henry (MI)	T&CS	1135
Waggoner, Steven (OH)	GO	286	Walters, Mark (OH)	ObG	562
Wagman, Lawrence (CA)	S	1100	Walton, David (MA)	Oph	571

Alphabetical Listing of Doctors

Name	Specialty	Pg	Name	Specialty	Pg
Walton, Robert (IL)	PlS	868	Waxman, Harvey (PA)	Cv	102
Wamboldt, Marianne (CO)	ChAP	911	Waxman, Irving (IL)	Ge	249
Waner, Milton (NY)	Oto	666	Waye, Jerome (NY)	Ge	238
Wang, Beverly (NY)	Path	712	Wazen, Jack (FL)	Oto	672
Wang, Frederick (NY)	Oph	581	Wazer, David (RI)	RadRO	947
Wang, Jeffrey (CA)	OrS	646	Weaver, David (IN)	CG	160
Wang, Ming (TN)	Oph	587	Weaver, W Douglas (MI)	Cv	112
Wang, Paul (CA)	CE	125	Webb, Gary (OH)	Cv	112
Wang, Steven (CA)	Oto	687	Webb, Lawrence (GA)	OrS	631
Wang, Winfred (TN)	PHO	769	Weber, Collin (GA)	S	1073
Wanner, Adam (FL)	Pul	932	Weber, Jeffrey (FL)	Onc	363
Wapner, Keith (PA)	OrS	626	Weber, Randal (TX)	Oto	683
Wapner, Ronald (NY)	MF	434	Weber, Samuel (TX)	Oto	683
Wapnir, Irene (CA)	S	1100	Weber, Sharon (WI)	S	1084
Wara, William (CA)	RadRO	968	Weber, Thomas (IL)	PS	808
Warady, Bradley (MO)	PNep	788	Webster, Harry (MA)	PMR	834
Ward, Barbara (CT)	S	1052	Wechsler, Daniel (NC)	PHO	769
Ward, David (CA)	Nep	466	Wechsler, Lawrence (PA)	N	518
Ward, Jewell (TN)	CG	159	Wei, Jeanne (AR)	Ger	266
Ward, John (UT)	Onc	376	Weichselbaum, Ralph (IL)	RadRO	962
Ward, Robert (NY)	PO	790	Weigel, Ronald (IA)	S	1084
Ward, William (NC)	OrS	631	Weigel, Tracey (WI)	T&CS	1135
Waring, George (GA)	Oph	587	Weigelt, John (WI)	S	1084
Warman, Roberto (FL)	Oph	587	Weiland, Andrew (NY)	HS	298
Warner, Ann (MO)	Rhu	1032	Weiman, Darryl (TN)	T&CS	1130
Warner, Brad (MO)	PS	808	Wein, Alan (PA)	U	1159
Warner, Kenneth (MA)	T&CS	1113	Weinberg, David (PA)	Ge	238
Warnick, Ronald (OH)	NS	491	Weinberg, Harold (NY)	N	519
Warnke, Roger (CA)	Path	722	Weinberg, Paul (PA)	PCd	737
Warnock, David (AL)	Nep	460	Weinberger, Michael (NY)	PM	698
Warren, Robert (SC)	PRhu	800	Weinblatt, Mark (NY)	PHO	764
Warren, Robert (AR)	PPul	797	Weinblatt, Michael (MA)	Rhu	1025
Warren, Robert (CA)	S	1100	Weiner, George (IA)	Onc	373
Warren, Russell (NY)	OrS	626	Weiner, Howard (NY)	NS	480
Wartofsky, Leonard (DC)	EDM	213	Weiner, I David (FL)	Nep	460
Wasserman, Richard (TX)	PA&I	732	Weiner, Kenneth (CO)	Psyc	899
Wasserman, Stephen (CA)	A&I	91	Weiner, Leslie (CA)	N	539
Watchko, Jon (PA)	NP	448	Weiner, Louis (DC)	Onc	352
Waters, Cheryl (NY)	N	518	Weiner, Michael (NY)	PHO	764
Waters, Peter (MA)	HS	294	Weiner, Myron (TX)	Psyc	900
Watkins, Robert (CA)	OrS	646	Weiner, Richard (NC)	Psyc	896
Watson, Thomas (NY)	T&CS	1122	Weiner, Richard (FL)	OrS	631
Watts, Nelson (OH)	EDM	219	Weiner, William (MD)	N	519
Watts, Ray (AL)	N	524	Weinfeld, Steven (NY)	OrS	626
Wax, Mark (OR)	Oto	687	Weingart, Jon (MD)	NS	480
Waxman, Alan (CA)	NuM	551	Weinreb, Jeffrey (CT)	DR	973

Name	Specialty	Pg	Name	Specialty	Pg
Weinreb, Robert (CA)	Oph	604	Werth, Victoria (PA)	D	189
Weinstein, Arthur (DC)	Rhu	1029	West, Sterling (CO)	Rhu	1032
Weinstein, Eric (CO)	VascS	1192	Westrich, Geoffrey (NY)	OrS	626
Weinstein, Gregory (PA)	Oto	666	Wetzel, F Todd (PA)	OrS	626
Weinstein, Howard (MA)	PHO	757	Wetzler, Meir (NY)	Onc	352
Weinstein, James (NH)	OrS	613	Wexler, Leonard (NY)	PHO	764
Weinstein, Sharon (UT)	H & PM	408	Wexner, Steven (FL)	CRS	173
Weinstein, Stuart (IA)	OrS	638	Weymuller, Ernest (WA)	Oto	687
Weinstock, Joel (MA)	Ge	230	Wharen, Robert (FL)	NS	485
Weinstock, Robert (CA)	Psyc	903	Wheeland, Ronald (AZ)	D	198
Weintraub, Joshua (NY)	VIR	994	Wheeler, Arthur (TN)	Pul	932
Weisberg, Tracey (ME)	Onc	333	Wheeler, Thomas (TX)	Path	719
Weisenburger, Dennis (NE)	Path	717	Whelan, Alison (MO)	CG	161
Weisler, Richard (NC)	Psyc	896	Whelan, Richard (NY)	CRS	171
Weisman, Robert (CA)	Oto	687	Wheless, James (TN)	ChiN	150
Weisman, Steven (WI)	PM	700	White, Charles (MD)	DR	978
Weiss, Arnold-Peter (RI)	HS	294	White, David (MA)	Pul	924
Weiss, Avery (WA)	Oph	604	White, Neil (MO)	PEn	747
Weiss, Geoffrey (VA)	Onc	364	White, Richard (OH)	DR	981
Weiss, Gerson (NJ)	RE	1010	White, Richard (NC)	S	1073
Weiss, Lawrence (CA)	Path	722	White, Robert (CT)	VIR	992
Weiss, Marisa (PA)	RadRO	953	White, Rodney (CA)	VascS	1194
Weiss, Michael (WA)	N	539	Whiting, Donald (PA)	NS	480
Weiss, Robert (NJ)	U	1159	Whitington, Peter (IL)	PGe	754
Weiss, Robert (CT)	U	1150	Whitlow, Patrick (OH)	IC	132
Weiss, Roy (IL)	EDM	219	Whitsett, Jeffrey (OH)	NP	451
Weiss, Sharon (GA)	Path	714	Whitworth, Pat (TN)	S	1073
Weissler, Jonathan (TX)	Pul	938	Whyte, Richard (MA)	T&CS	1113
Weissler, Mark (NC)	Oto	672	Wicha, Max (MI)	Onc	373
Weissman, Peter (FL)	EDM	216	Wickiewicz, Thomas (NY)	OrS	627
Weitz, Howard (PA)	Cv	102	Widra, Eric (DC)	RE	1010
Weitzel, Jeffrey (CA)	CG	164	Wiedemann, Herbert (OH)	Pul	936
Weksler, Benny (PA)	T&CS	1123	Wierman, Ann (NV)	Onc	392
Welch, William (PA)	NS	480	Wiesel, Sam (DC)	OrS	627
Wellington, Joshua (IN)	PM	700	Wiesenfeld, Harold (PA)	ObG	558
Wells, Gretchen (NC)	Cv	106	Wiesner, Russell (MN)	Ge	249
Wells, James (CA)	PlS	877	Wiet, Richard (IL)	Oto	678
Wells, Robert (WI)	DR	981	Wigley, Frederick (MD)	Rhu	1029
Wells, Winfield (CA)	T&CS	1143	Wilansky, Susan (AZ)	Cv	115
Welton, Mark (CA)	CRS	178	Wilber, David (IL)	CE	124
Wen, Patrick (MA)	N	508	Wilberger, James (PA)	NS	480
Wener, Mark (WA)	Rhu	1034	Wilcox, C Mel (AL)	Ge	243
Wenstrom, Katharine (RI)	MF	431	Wilcox, Christopher (DC)	Nep	458
Wenzel, Sally (PA)	Pul	929	Wilcox, Robert (TX)	PlS	872
Werner, Phillip (IL)	EDM	220	Wilcox, William (CA)	CG	164
Werner-Wasik, Maria (PA)	RadRO	953	Wilczynski, Sharon (CA)	Path	722

Alphabetical Listing of Doctors

Name	Specialty	Pg	Name	Specialty	Pg
Wilding, George (WI)	Onc	373	Wingard, John (FL)	Onc	364
Wilens, Timothy (MA)	ChAP	907	Winick, Naomi (TX)	PHO	776
Wiley, Joseph (MD)	PHO	764	Winn, Hung (MO)	MF	438
Wilhelmi, Bradon (KY)	PlS	864	Winston, Jonathan (NY)	Nep	459
Wilking, Andrew (TX)	PRhu	801	Winter, Jane (IL)	Hem	322
Wilkins, Edwin (MI)	PlS	868	Wirth, Michael (TX)	OrS	641
Wilkins, Isabelle (IL)	MF	437	Wisch, Nathaniel (NY)	Hem	316
Wilkins, Ross (CO)	OrS	640	Wise, Christopher (VA)	Rhu	1030
Wilkins-Haug, Louise (MA)	MF	431	Wise, Paul (MO)	CRS	175
Wilkoff, Bruce (OH)	Cv	112	Wiseman, Gregory (MN)	NuM	550
Willett, Christopher (NC)	RadRO	958	Wisoff, Jeffrey (NY)	NS	480
Willey, Shawna (DC)	S	1066	Witman, Patricia (OH)	D	195
Williams, David (MA)	IC	126	Witt, Thomas (IL)	S	1084
Williams, Eric (IN)	Cv	112	Witter, Frank (MD)	ObG	558
Williams, Gail (NY)	Nep	458	Wittig, James (NY)	OrS	627
Williams, George (MI)	Oph	595	Wityk, Robert (MD)	N	519
Williams, Gerald (PA)	OrS	627	Wiviott, Lory (CA)	Inf	420
Williams, James (AZ)	PHO	776	Wixson, Richard (IL)	OrS	638
Williams, Kim (MI)	Cv	113	Wiznitzer, Max (OH)	ChiN	152
Williams, Mathew (NY)	T&CS	1123	Woeber, Kenneth (CA)	EDM	224
Williams, Michael (VA)	Hem	318	Wofsy, David (CA)	Rhu	1034
Williams, Riley (NY)	SM	1042	Wolchok, Jedd (NY)	Onc	352
Williams, Ronald (TX)	OrS	641	Wolf, Gregory (MI)	Oto	678
Williams, Shauna (ID)	CRS	176	Wolf, Raoul (IL)	PA&I	731
Willson, James (TX)	Onc	382	Wolfe, Lawrence (NY)	PHO	764
Wilson, Amy (TX)	PMR	843	Wolfe, M Michael (OH)	Ge	249
Wilson, Daniel (FL)	Psyc	896	Wolfe, Robert (CA)	Pul	941
Wilson, Darrell (CA)	PEn	749	Wolfe, S Anthony (FL)	PlS	864
Wilson, David (OR)	Oph	605	Wolfe, Scott (NY)	HS	298
Wilson, Ellen (TX)	RE	1016	Wolff, Antonio (MD)	Onc	352
Wilson, J Frank (WI)	RadRO	962	Wolff, Bruce (MN)	CRS	176
Wilson, John (NC)	NS	485	Wolff, Johannes (MA)	PHO	757
Wilson, Keith (OH)	Oto	678	Wolff, Robert (TX)	Onc	383
Wilson, Lynn (CT)	RadRO	948	Wolfson, Aaron (FL)	RadRO	958
Wilson, Marion (SC)	Oph	587	Wolinsky, Jerry (TX)	N	535
Wilson, Matthew (TN)	Oph	587	Woltering, Eugene (LA)	S	1093
Wilson, Steven (OH)	Oph	595	Wondisford, Frederic (MD)	EDM	213
Wilson, Timothy (CA)	U	1179	Wong, Brian (CA)	Oto	688
Wilson, Walter (MN)	Inf	417	Wong, Carson (OH)	U	1171
Wilson, Wyndham (MD)	Onc	352	Wong, Duane (AZ)	A&I	90
Winchell, Robert (ME)	S	1052	Wong, Jeffrey (CA)	RadRO	968
Winchester, David (IL)	S	1084	Wong, Johnson (MA)	A&I	84
Windebank, Anthony (MN)	N	530	Wong, Richard (NY)	Oto	666
Winer, Eric (MA)	Onc	333	Wong, Ronald (HI)	CRS	178
Winer, Sharon (CA)	RE	1018	Woo, Howard (LA)	U	1175
Winfield, Howard (AL)	U	1165	Woo, Peak (NY)	Oto	666

Name	Specialty	Pg	Name	Specialty	Pg
Woo, Shiao (KY)	RadRO	958	Yankelevitz, David (NY)	DR	978
Woo, Y Joseph (PA)	T&CS	1123	Yannuzzi, Lawrence (NY)	Oph	581
Wood, Beverly (CA)	DR	984	Yanovich, Saul (MD)	Hem	316
Wood, Bradford (MD)	VIR	994	Yarbrough, Wendell (CT)	Oto	657
Wood, David (MI)	U	1171	Yeager, Andrew (AZ)	Hem	325
Wood, Douglas (WA)	T&CS	1143	Yeatman, Timothy (FL)	S	1073
Wood, Gary (WI)	D	195	Yeatts, R Patrick (NC)	Oph	587
Wood, John (MO)	A&I	89	Yee, Billy (CA)	RE	1018
Wood, R Patrick (TX)	S	1093	Yee, Douglas (MN)	Onc	374
Wood, Robert (MD)	PA&I	730	Yee, Jerry (MI)	Nep	463
Woodley, David (CA)	D	200	Yen, Yun (CA)	Onc	392
Woodson, B Tucker (WI)	Oto	679	Yeo, Charles (PA)	S	1066
Woodson, Gayle (IL)	Oto	679	Yetman, Randall (OH)	PlS	868
Wooten, George (VA)	N	524	Yeung, Alan (CA)	IC	133
Wooten, Virgil (OH)	Psyc	898	Yeung, Raymond (WA)	S	1101
Worden, Francis (MI)	Onc	373	Yonas, Howard (NM)	NS	495
Wormser, Gary (NY)	Inf	413	Yoo, George (MI)	Oto	679
Worsey, Michael (CA)	CRS	178	Yoo, Jung (OR)	OrS	646
Wright, Cameron (MA)	T&CS	1113	Yoon, Sydney (NY)	DR	978
Wright, Jackson (OH)	IM	425	York, Teresa (MD)	PHO	764
Wright, Kenneth (CA)	Oph	605	Young, Anne (MA)	N	509
Wright, Robert (IL)	N	531	Young, Bruce (NY)	ObG	558
Wurtz, L Daniel (IN)	OrS	638	Young, Iven (NY)	EDM	213
Wyatt, Robert (TN)	PNep	786	Young, James (OH)	Cv	113
Wyllie, Elaine (OH)	ChiN	152	Young, K Randall (PA)	Pul	929
Wyllie, Robert (OH)	PGe	754	Young, Ming-Lon (FL)	PCd	738
			Young, Nancy (IL)	Oto	679
			Young, Renee (NE)	Ge	250
			Young, Robert (MA)	Path	707
X			Young, V Leroy (MO)	PlS	868
Xerogeanes, John (GA)	SM	1043	Younossi, Zobair (VA)	Ge	243
Xing, Michael (MD)	EDM	213	Yousem, David (MD)	NRad	986
			Yousem, Samuel (PA)	Path	712
			Yu, George (MD)	U	1159
			Yu, Jack (GA)	PlS	864
Y			Yu, John (CA)	NS	499
			Yueh, Bevan (MN)	Oto	679
Yaddanapudi, Ravindranath (MI)	PHO	774	Yuen, James (AR)	PlS	872
Yahalom, Joachim (NY)	RadRO	953	Yung, WK Alfred (TX)	N	535
Yakes, Wayne (CO)	VIR	997	Yunus, Furhan (TN)	Onc	364
Yamada, Kelvin (MO)	ChiN	152	Yurt, Roger (NY)	S	1066
Yamaguchi, Ken (MO)	OrS	638			
Yan, Albert (PA)	D	189			
Yancovitz, Stanley (NY)	Inf	414			
Yanda, Randy (GA)	Ge	243	**Z**		
Yang, James (MD)	S	1066			
Yang, Stephen (MD)	T&CS	1123	Zach, Terence (NE)	NP	451

Alphabetical Listing of Doctors

Name	Specialty	Pg	Name	Specialty	Pg
Zackai, Elaine (PA)	CG	158	Zuckerman, Kenneth (FL)	Hem	318
Zacur, Howard (MD)	RE	1011	Zupanc, Mary (CA)	ChiN	154
Zafonte, Ross (MA)	PMR	834	Zusman, Randall (MA)	Cv	96
Zager, Eric (PA)	NS	480	Zwillenberg, Seth (PA)	Oto	667
Zagoria, Ronald (NC)	DR	980	Zwischenberger, Joseph (KY)	T&CS	1130
Zagzag, David (NY)	Path	712			
Zahn, Evan (CA)	PCd	741			
Zalud, Ivica (HI)	MF	441			
Zalzal, George (DC)	Oto	667			
Zaman, Atif (OR)	Ge	255			
Zannis, Victor (AZ)	S	1093			
Zarins, Bertram (MA)	OrS	613			
Zarins, Christopher (CA)	VascS	1194			
Zdeblick, Thomas (WI)	OrS	638			
Zeanah, Charles (LA)	ChAP	911			
Zeitels, Steven (MA)	Oto	657			
Zeitlin, Pamela (MD)	PPul	795			
Zelefsky, Michael (NY)	RadRO	953			
Zelenetz, Andrew (NY)	Onc	352			
Zelickson, Brian (MN)	D	195			
Zelman, Richard (MA)	IC	127			
Zeltzer, Lonnie (CA)	Ped	729			
Zeman, Robert (DC)	DR	978			
Zerbe, Kathryn (OR)	Psyc	903			
Zide, Barry (NY)	PlS	860			
Ziemer, Gerhard (IL)	T&CS	1136			
Zietman, Anthony (MA)	RadRO	948			
Ziffer, Jack (FL)	NuM	550			
Zilleruelo, Gaston (FL)	PNep	787			
Zimmerman, Christian (ID)	NS	492			
Zimmerman, Donald (IL)	PEn	748			
Zimmerman, Earl (NY)	N	519			
Zimmerman, Jerry (WA)	PCCM	743			
Zimmerman, Robert (PA)	NRad	986			
Zimmerman, Robert (OH)	EDM	220			
Zimnowodzki, Simon (IL)	N	531			
Zinaman, Michael (MA)	RE	1007			
Zinner, Michael (MA)	S	1052			
Zinreich, S James (MD)	NRad	986			
Zins, James (OH)	PlS	869			
Zippe, Craig (OH)	U	1171			
Zitelli, Basil (PA)	Ped	727			
Zitelli, John (PA)	D	189			
Zoghbi, William (TX)	Cv	115			
Zubrow, Alan (PA)	NP	448			
Zuckerman, Joseph (NY)	OrS	627			

Acknowledgments

The publishers would like to thank the entire staff for their many hours and days of intense and precise work on this guide in order to further its goal of assisting consumers in making the best healthcare choices.

Castle Connolly Executive Management:

Chairman	John K. Castle
President & CEO	John J. Connolly, Ed.D.
Vice President, Chief Medical & Research Officer	Jean Morgan, M.D.
Vice President, Chief Strategy & Operations Officer	William Liss-Levinson, Ph.D.

Vice President, Advertising	Mark McGinty
Senior Research & Healthcare Associate	Maryann Hynd, RN
Senior Research Associate & Book Production Manager	Sara Sezer

Research Coordinators

Terysia Browne
Tayler Chapman, DO
Neil Cohen
Catherine Hoffman-Freiria
Najette Miller
Yuliya Nagdimova
Zachary Preneta
Mariadiep Vu

Book Layout, Database Management	Russell Hodgson
Office Manager	Marcie Samartino
Manager, Client Relations	Hilary Knerr
Manager, Client Relations & Communications	Nicki Hughes
Account Specialist	Adam Akmal-Gonzalez
Project Manager	John Santa

We also would like to extend our gratitude to the American Board of Medical Specialties (ABMS) for allowing us to use excerpts, especially the descriptions of medical specialties and subspecialties, from the text of their publication "Which Medical Specialist for You?"

Other Publications from Castle Connolly Medical Ltd.:
America's Top Doctors® for Cancer; Top Doctors: New York Metro Area; Top Doctors: Chicago Metro Area; Top Doctors Southern California; Top Doctors Washington-Baltimore; Cancer Made Easier: New York—Metro Area, Eldercare and others...
Order online at http://www.castleconnolly.com/books

The Best in American Medicine
www.CastleConnolly.com

Corporate Membership for Corporations & Organizations

This service enables an employer to assist employees in identifying Top Doctors to care for themselves and their families. It is a low-cost, non-intrusive service that will result in better care and, ultimately, lower healthcare costs. For as low as a few dollars per year, employees can have complete access to the Castle Connolly website and database of Top Doctors who were nominated by their peers and screened by the Castle Connolly physician-led research team.

Instead of simply choosing a doctor's name from the phone book or a plan directory, the employee can compare physician names to the Castle Connolly database of 30,000 plus Top Doctors and select from among the best doctors in the country. This will result in overall better care, lower costs and improved morale. Once an employee logs on to the Castle Connolly database, valuable background information is available on every Top Doctor such as: medical school, board certifications, fellowships, hospital affiliations, residencies and much more, to allow them to make the best informed decision they can make when selecting a doctor.

Top Doctors can have an enormous impact. For patients and their families, the value of receiving first-class medical care is not measured in dollars – it is measured in quality and even length of life. Employers, however, can see the results in their bottom line. Faulty diagnoses and improper treatment take a toll in productivity and ripple out into higher workplace costs. No company should have to "make do" for weeks or months without a key employee or executive, when a Top Doctor may have solved the patient's problem quickly and efficiently. The effort to identify the best doctors from ordinary ones is justified by the money saved on incorrect treatments, unnecessary surgery and days lost from work.

The Corporate Membership is suited for employers of varying sizes and can also be of great value to professional, social, civic, fraternal and religious associations. Castle Connolly may also be able to adapt and tailor the presentation of the database to meet the specific corporate client's needs.

New Movers Program

The Castle Connolly New Movers Program is designed to alleviate that concern, or even fear, as well as the time-consuming struggle to identify the right – and best – doctors and hospitals in one's new community or region. The service can be provided on a family basis (those living in the household) or for a single client. The service includes identifying primary care physicians, including Pediatricians, OB/GYN's, Internists and Family Practitioners as well as other specialists that may be needed: for example, Ophthalmologists, Allergists, Endocrinologists, Surgeons or others as required.

Perhaps nothing is more challenging to a family that has relocated to a new community than finding appropriate healthcare resources, especially physicians. While they can turn to recommendations from new neighbors and friends, or select names from the phone book or a plan directory, that is hardly adequate, especially if there are special healthcare needs in the family.

A Castle Connolly Health Advisor will identify two or three recommendations for up to six different medical specialties. If, for some reason the client wishes to change doctors within two months, Castle Connolly will identify new physicians in the same specialty. After the selection process occurs, the Health Advisor will make an introductory phone call to the physician's office. This typically facilitates faster appointments.

Healthcare Solutions

Castle Connolly's Healthcare Solutions is designed to help your employees and their loved ones navigate through the healthcare system with less stress, faster service and better outcomes. It is a high touch service with a hands-on health advocate to serve as a guide and dedicated healthcare champion 24 hours a day, 7 days a week, 365 days a year. Why have your most valued employees, your most critical asset, spend their time -- and possibly company time –coping with difficult and complex medical issues they may know little about, when Castle Connolly's Healthcare Solutions professionals can resolve them quickly and expertly. With one phone call, your employees will gain priority access to a global network of best-in-class medical professionals, Castle Connolly Top Doctors™, and higher quality patient resources. Our professional staff coordinates the entire process to provide consistency and support during their time of need.

Services include, but are not limited to, the following:

» Identifying top physicians and hospitals (nationally)

» Identifying reputable non-physician providers, such as Dieticians, Physical and Occupational Therapists, etc.

» Facilitating second opinions

» Defining complex medical terminology and situations

» Providing a list of tailored questions to discuss with your medical team

» Conducting medical research on your health condition

» Navigating the healthcare system

» Assisting with medical record retrieval and/or arranging a medical record review

» Identifying and assisting with eldercare issues

» Coordinating a hospital transfer

» Arranging medical transport or evacuation for travelers

» Coordinating with the employers' other vendors for continuity of care

Healthcare Solutions can be made available to your organization as a specific number of cases during the course of the year with the option to obtain more, or as a yearly retainer. Organizations may opt to make this service available for all of their employees, or to select groups such as high level executives or partners.

For further information on Healthcare Solutions, Corporate Membership, New Movers, and Doctor-Patient Advisor Program, please contact:

Michael D. Wolf, Ph.D.
Executive Vice President
Castle Connolly Graduate Medical Publishing, Ltd.
212-644-9696
or
mwolf@ccgmp.com

The Best in American Medicine
www.CastleConnolly.com

Strategic Relationships

Castle Connolly Medical Ltd. has a number of strategic relationships that may be of interest to consumers and physicians.

U.S. News & World Report and Castle Connolly created a strategic collaboration that will bring the Castle Connolly Top Doctors® database to online visitors to the U.S. News website. The online database went live on http://health.usnews.com/top-doctors in mid-July 2011 and is linked with the U.S. News database of Best Hospitals. Consumers will be able to search the full database of Top Doctors across the nation, including all specialties and subspecialties. The detailed physician profiles, including designation of doctors affiliated with Castle Connolly's Partnership for Excellence hospital program, will be drawn from Castle Connolly's growing database of over 27,000 physicians currently accessible online at www.castleconnolly.com.

Vitals (www.vitals.com), an innovative online doctor review and comparison service from MDx Medical Inc., is the comprehensive source for vital information, peer evaluations and patient feedback on more than 700,000 doctors nationwide. Drawing upon prestigious information repositories, cutting-edge search and comparison technologies, and a robust patient feedback mechanism, Vitals has organized key information to help patients make an informed choice in their search for the right doctor. Castle Connolly and Vitals have a branding relationship in which those physicians who are Castle Connolly Top Doctors™ and appear on Vitals web sites have an icon indicating their status and recognition as a Castle Connolly Top Doctor.

In 2012, Castle Connolly will begin displaying insurance plans that are accepted by all physicians listed as Castle Connolly Top Doctors. An appointment scheduling feature will also appear on our site for those physicians who wish to participate in this feature. Additional information can be found at www.vitals.com.

Everyday Health, Inc. comprises some of the nation's leading online health information resources. With over 25 comprehensive health websites including www.EverydayHealth.com, www.Carepages.com, PDRHealth.com and www.WhatToExpect.com, information and knowledge is accessible on a wide range of health topics such as lifestyle offerings in pregnancy, diet and fitness to in-depth medical content for condition prevention and management.

In addition to their commitment to provide consumers with health solutions that span the health spectrum, they also provide a wide range of content and advertising-based services to healthcare entities including hospitals, physicians and other healthcare professionals. Castle Connolly has formed a strategic relationship with Everyday Health to offer one of these services in particular; Reputation Management Solutions.

More than 150 million people search listings and online healthcare directories each month making it imperative for physicians and hospitals to consistently update and manage their information on local directories, reviews sites and social networks. Understandably, this is, at times, an unfeasible commitment. Everyday Health's Reputation Management Solutions provides online visibility information which shows exactly where listings appear on the web, information across hundreds of directory sites, identifying and tips on how to respond to negative reviews and much more.

For more information, please contact our Manager of Client Relations at (212) 367-8400 Ext. 135.

Empowered Doctor is a media, news and marketing service. Empowered Doctor produces syndicated consumer health reports. Its video and text news stories appear on major media websites, including CBS. Empowered Doctor also provides marketing services to hospitals, clinics and individual physicians by generating visibility in online search and social media. Empowered Doctor's clients benefit from the company's efficient methodologies for generating new patient referrals.

For more information call 888-333-1027 or visit www.empowereddoctor.com

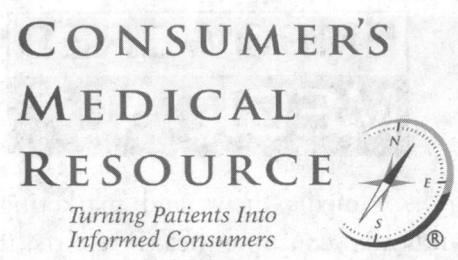

CONSUMER'S MEDICAL RESOURCE

*Turning Patients Into
Informed Consumers*

Consumer's Medical Resource was started in 1996 to offer high-quality, high-impact employee benefit programs to help employees and their dependents, and has been a pioneer in Medical Decision Support® services. CMR addresses all medical conditions at any point within the continuum of care, by providing personalized, evidence-based medical research, information, access to genuine, in-person second opinions and support services to employees who face serious, complicated, and chronic illness, or would like to become well-informed healthcare consumers.

Leveraging a state-of-the-art integrated model of web, phone, and print-based services, CMR enables employees to fully understand and evaluate their options so they can make the most informed medical decisions possible with their doctors. The company is privately held and currently provides services to more than 600,000 Americans, achieving extremely high levels of user and customer satisfaction, improved clinical quality outcomes, and generated excellent ROI.

Castle Connolly and CMR are working together to provide Castle Connolly's various corporate services to CMR client companies and their employees.

For more information, please visit: http://www.consumersmedical.com.

♥ sharecare

Sharecare is an interactive, social Q&A platform designed to greatly simplify the search for quality healthcare information and help consumers live their healthiest life. Sharecare has enlisted the nation's leading health experts, care providers, organizations, and brands to join the health and wellness conversation and empowering users with high-quality, relevant answers to their health questions from multiple expert perspectives and with interactive health and wellness tools to take action on what they've learned.

The website was launched in 2010 by Jeff Arnold, founder of WebMD, and Emmy–award winning host, Dr. Mehmet Oz, in partnership with Harpo Studios, Sony Pictures Television and Discovery Communications.

Castle Connolly teamed up with Sharecare in 2011. Dr. John Connolly, President and CEO of CCML, is one of the featured experts on Sharecare for healthcare choice questions. Find out more at www.sharecare.com

grandparents.com®
it's great to be grand.

Grandparents.com is dedicated to enhancing the lives of America's 70 million grandparents by fostering family connections, via child- and grandparent-friendly activities, travel ideas, compelling lifestyle features, expert advice, gift ideas, recipes, and more. Visitors have access to a range of tools, including groups, discussions, a homepage blog, photo sharing, and a Facebook page and Twitter feeds. Through the Grandparents.com Benefits Club, catering to America's 120 million grandparents, Boomers and seniors, members benefit from discounts and incentives they can use every day, in categories like gifts, clothes, and vitamins, plus exclusive opportunities to save on hotels, cruises, auto rentals, theme park trips, theatrical productions, and insurance. Grandparents can share their membership benefits with four extended family and household members. In 2010, Grandparents.com was ranked as the No. 3 website for seniors, boomers, and grandparents, following the U.S. Government and AARP. Castle Connolly provides access to its Top Doctors' database, its Doctor-Patient Advisor and New Movers programs for Grandparents.com members.

DrScore.com
PATIENTS SPEAK, DOCTORS LISTEN

Founded by Steven Feldman, M.D., DrScore.com is an interactive online survey site where patients can rate their physicians, as well as find a physician based on their service level preference.

The mission of DrScore.com is to improve medical care by giving patients a forum for rating their physician and by giving doctors an affordable, objective, non-intrusive means of documenting the quality of care that they provide. Visitors on Castle Connolly's website who are searching for "top doctors" have the option to also rate these and other physicians they have been to as patients, as well as to see if these physicians have been rated previously by other consumers on DrScore.com. Visitors to DrScore.com will be able to see if their doctors and/or other doctors are Castle Connolly "top doctors."

For more information, visit www.drscore.com.

The Good Works Health government-approved platform - www.goodworkshealth.com - offers physicians the opportunity to direct donations, based on the fair market value of their time, to charities of their choice in exchange for participation in educational programs.

Participating physicians can choose from more than a million approved charities to designate as the recipients of these donations. Good Works Health's unique platform reaches a growing community of medical professionals in many specialties that are motivated by the opportunity to do good works. Castle Connolly actively works with Good Works Health to promote these opportunities to its Castle Connolly Top Doctors®

LIFESTREAM MD

Castle Connolly Medical Ltd. has a strategic relationship with Castle Connolly LifeStream MD to provide a unique health advisory service designed for families and executives, especially those who travel regularly or may have more than one residence.

Each client is assigned a Castle Connolly LifeStream MD physician who is available to them by phone 24/7/365. A client call from anywhere in the world is answered promptly and the client is connected with their Castle Connolly LifeStream MD physician advisor.

The Castle Connolly LifeStream MD physician acts as a health manager assisting in navigation of an increasingly complex health care environment. The Castle Connolly LifeStream MD physician does not replace the member's primary physician or specialists, but provides additional independent counsel and services that provide security to our members either at home or while traveling.

In the United States, the Castle Connolly LifeStream MD physician will use the Castle Connolly database of Top Doctors to assure that the client is cared for in the best medical facilities by the top doctors. Assistance in securing timely appointments with specialists and records transfers is facilitated as needed. Outside of the United States, Castle Connolly LifeStream MD has an affiliation with International SOS, the world's largest and leading provider of travel medical assistance to assure the LifeStream MD member is cared for by the best doctors and hospitals available in that region or, if necessary, is transported to a place where that care is available.

The Best in American Medicine
www.CastleConnolly.com

National Physician of the Year Awards

Castle Connolly Medical Ltd. proudly hosted its seventh annual *National Physician of the Year Awards* on March 26, 2012 at The Pierre Hotel in New York City. It was a spectacular evening which allowed us to recognize both the outstanding honorees and the excellence of the many thousands of physicians throughout the nation.

The Genesis of the National Physician of the Year Award.

Each year we receive thousands of nominations from physicians and the medical leadership of major medical centers, specialty hospitals, teaching hospitals and regional and community medical centers across the United States as an integral part of our research, screening and selection process to identify *America's Top Doctors®*. The selected physicians, while spread across all fifty states and involved in more than 70 medical specialties and subspecialties, all share one distinguishing professional attribute: an unwavering dedication to their patients and to medicine as a whole. Each and every one of these outstanding medical professionals is a symbol of the clinical excellence that characterizes American medicine. In honor of these exemplary physicians, Castle Connolly Medical Ltd. has created the *National Physician of the Year Awards* to recognize the thousands of excellent, dedicated physicians across the United States. Our Medical Advisory Board selected the honorees from the hundreds nominated in a special nomination process conducted months before the event.

The honorees, Drs. Richard Edelson, Susan Mackinnon, and John M. Morton, are superb examples of excellence in clinical medical practice. In addition to these awards for Clinical Excellence, Castle Connolly Medical Ltd. honored Drs. Robert L. Brent and John G. Clarkson for their lifetime achievement in medicine. Ms. Marlo Thomas is a tireless fundraiser for St. Jude Children's Research Hospital and an exemplary recipient for the seventh National Health Leadership Award.

Each honoree received a beautiful and distinctive porcelain figurine created by the Boehm Porcelain Company exclusively for the National Physician of the Year Awards. The award features a golden caduceus, the symbol of the medical community, surrounded by a golden laurel wreath. Laurel wreaths were used by the ancients to crown and honor their leaders.

The caduceus and laurel rest upon a column accented by the signature Castle Connolly logo. By combining the caduceus and the laurel wreaths, the award embodies the excellence in medical achievement that the National Physician of the Year Awards celebrates each year.

2012 National Physician of the Year Awards Honorees

"Top Doctors Make a Difference ™"

For Clinical Excellence

Richard Edelson, M.D.
Aaron B. and Marguerite Lerner Professor
Chairman of the Department of Dermatology
Yale School of Medicine.

Susan Mackinnon, M.D.
Chief of Plastic and Reconstructive Surgery
Washington University School of Medicine

John M. Morton, M.D., M.P.H., F.A.C.S.
Associate Professor of Surgery
Stanford University
Chief of Minimally Invasive Surgery,
Director of Bariatric Surgery and Surgical Quality

For Lifetime Achievement

Robert L. Brent, M.D., Ph.D., D.Sc.
Distinguished Professor of Pediatrics, Radiology and Pathology
Louis and Bess Stein Professor of Pediatrics at the Jefferson Medical College
and the Nemours/Alfred I. DuPont Hospital for Children

John G. Clarkson, M.D.
Dean Emeritus and Professor of Ophthalmology
Anne Bates Leach Eye Hospital/Bascom Palmer Eye Institute
Department of Ophthalmology
Miller School of Medicine at the University of Miami

National Health Leadership

Marlo Thomas
National Outreach Director
St. Jude Children's Research Hospital

2011 National Physician of the Year Awards Honorees

"Doctors Make a Difference"

For Clinical Excellence

Armando E. Giuliano, M.D., FACS, FRCSED
Chief of Science and Medicine
John Wayne Cancer Institute at Saint John's Health Center,
Santa Monica, CA

O. Wayne Isom, M.D.
Chairman of the Dept. of Cardiothoracic Surgery
New York Presbyterian-Weill Cornell Medical College

David W. Kennedy, M.D.
Otorhinolaryngology Professor at the
University of Pennsylvania

For Lifetime Achievement

George P. Canellos, M.D.
Served as Founding Chief of Medical Oncology at
Dana-Farber Cancer Institute;

Matthew D. Davis, M.D.
University of Wisconsin Medical Center
Chair, UW Opthalmology

National Health Leadership

Evelyn H. Lauder
Chairman of The Breast Cancer Research Foundation®

Previous National Physician of the Year Award Honorees

2010

Clinical Excellence
John B. Buse, M.D., Ph.D.
Director of the Diabetes Care Center, Professor, Chief of the Division of
Endocrinology and Executive Associate Dean for Clinical Research,
University of North Carolina School of Medicine, Chapel Hill

Larry Norton, M.D.
Deputy Physician-in-Chief, Memorial Hospital, Memorial Sloan-Kettering
Cancer Center, for Breast Cancer Programs
Medical Director of the MSKCC's Breast and Imaging Center, Evelyn H.
Lauder Breast Center

Ching-Hon Pui, M.D.
Department Chair of Oncology, St. Jude Children's Research Hospital
Medical Director of the St. Jude International Outreach China Program,
holder of the Fahad Nassar Al-Rashid Chair of Leukemia Research

Lifetime Achievement
Basil I Hirschowitz, M.D.
Director, Gastroenterology Division, The University of Alabama
Receipient of the Kettering Medal from the General Motors Cancer
Foundation; Friedenwald Medal of the AGA; the Schindler Medal and the
Crystal Award for lifetime contributions to Endoscopy by the ASGE;
honorary doctorate of Gothenburg University; honorary fellow of the Royal
Society of Medicine

Leonard Apt, M.D.
Professor of Ophthalmology Emeritus; Director Emeritus and Founder of
the Division of Pediatric Opthalmology and Strabismus, and Co-Director of
UCLA's Center for Child Blindness

National Health Leadership
Alexandra Reeve Givens and Matthew Reeve
Trustees, The Christopher & Dana Reeve Foundation

2009

Clinical Excellence
Carol R. Bradford, M.D.,
Professor and Chair
Department of Otolaryngology
University of Michigan Medical System

Diane E. Meier, M.D.,
Director, Center to Advance Palliative Care
Mount Sinai School of Medicine

Judd W. Moul, M.D.,
Chief of Urology
Duke University Medical Center

Lifetime Achievement
Emil J. Freireich, M.D., D. Sc. (Hon.),
Ruth Harriet Ainsworth Chair, Distinguished Teaching Professor
Director, Special Medical Education Programs
Director, Adult Leukemia Research Program
The University of Texas M.D. Anderson Cancer Center

Thomas E. Starzl, M.D., Ph.D.
Professor of Surgery, Emeritus
Distinguished Service Professor
University of Pittsburgh Medical Center

National Health Leadership
Page Morton Black
Chairman of the Board, Parkinson's Disease Foundation

2008

Clinical Excellence
Robert W. Carlson, M.D.
Medical Oncology
Stanford University Medical Center

Stanley Chang, M.D.
Ophthalmology
New York-Presbyterian Hospital

L. Dade Lunsford, M.D.
Neurological Surgery
University of Pittsburgh Medical Center

Lifetime Achievement
Jacqueline A. Noonan, M.D.
Pediatric Cardiology
University of Kentucky Medical Center

Robert W. Schrier, M.D.
Nephrology
University of Colorado Health Sciences Center

National Health Leadership
Suzanne and Robert Wright
Vice-Chair of the Board, General Electric Company
Co-founders of Autism Speaks™

<u>2007</u>

Clinical Excellence
Delos M. Cosgrove, M.D.
Chairman, Board of Governors
CEO and President
The Cleveland Clinic

Joseph G. McCarthy, M.D.
Lawrence D. Bell Professor of Plastic Surgery
Director, The Institute of Reconstructive Plastic Surgery
NYU Medical Center

Patrick C. Walsh, M.D.
University Distinguished Service Professor and Director of Urology
The James Buchanan Brady Urological Institute
The Johns Hopkins Hospital

Lifetime Achievement
Maria Delivoria-Papadopoulos, M.D.
Director, The Neonatal Intensive Care Unit
St. Christopher's Hospital for Children;
Professor of Pediatrics, Physiology and Obstetrics/Gynecology
Drexel University College of Medicine

National Health Leadership
The Honorable Nancy G. Brinker
Founder of Susan G. Komen for the Cure
Former U.S. Ambassador to Hungary

2006

Clinical Excellence
Bart Barlogie, M.D., Ph.D.
Director, Myeloma Institute for Research Therapy
University of Arkansas for Medical Services

Marilyn J. Bull, M.D.
Morris Green Professor of Pediatrics
Riley Hospital for Children

Michael J. Zinner, M.D.
Moseley Professor of Surgery
Harvard Medical School
Surgeon-in-Chief, Brigham & Women's Hospital

Lifetime Achievement
Michael E. DeBakey, M.D.
Chancellor Emeritus, Baylor College of Medicine

National Health Leadership
Princess Yasmin Aga Khan
Honorary Vice Chair
Alzheimer's Association

Castle Connolly maintains Facebook, Twitter, LinkedIn and Sharecare accounts in an effort to keep consumers informed of the latest news not only regarding Castle Connolly Medical Ltd., its Top Doctors and Top Hospitals, but also reports on various health observances and events. A live Twitter feed can also be found on the homepage of www.castleconnolly.com.

Consumers who use our print guides, online database or refer to our regional magazine features can find up-to-date information about Castle Connolly, healthcare and medical news by logging onto these social networking sites:

www.facebook.com/TopDoctors

www.twitter.com/CastleConnolly

Blog - Ask America's Top Doctors™
www.castleconnolly.com/blog

http://linkd.in/mP4Lmb (case sensitive)

Do you have a story about a Castle Connolly Top Doctor or Top Hospital that you want to share? If so, please email a link to the article to:

Nicki Hughes
Manager, Client Relations & Communications
nhughes@castleconnolly.com

Castle Connolly has developed a website and online database – www.AmericasTopCosmeticDoctors.com – to enable consumers to search and identify top cosmetic specialists who have been nominated by their peers through an extensive selection process involving tens of thousands of American physicians. Nominated physicians' medical education, training, hospital appointments, disciplinary histories - and much more - are screened and reviewed by our physician-led research team. Those selected as top doctors may appear in a number of Castle Connolly guides/online databases, including www.AmericasTopCosmeticDoctors.com.

These doctors are specially trained in cosmetic procedures and spend the majority of their time in their medical practice doing cosmetic work. The Top Cosmetic Doctors whose profiles are included on this site are in one of only six medical specialties: Dermatology, Facial Plastic Surgery, Ophthalmology, Otolaryngology, Plastic Surgery or Surgery. The website also includes valuable information on how to select the right cosmetic doctor for you, as well as detailed information about some of the most common procedures.

For more information visit: www.AmericasTopCosmeticDoctors.com

Doctor-Patient Advisor for Individual Consumers

Doctor-Patient Advisor is a Castle Connolly Medical Ltd. service providing one-on-one consultations with a physician or nurse practitioner to individuals who have serious or complex medical problems or to anyone who feels he/she needs assistance finding the right physician for any purpose. Each client will receive personalized assistance in identifying the appropriate specialists for his/her condition, utilizing the Castle Connolly Medical Ltd. database of physicians and hospitals, as well as individual searches, to locate the best resources to meet the client's needs.

Fee: $375. For further information call (212) 367-8400 x 116.

Premium Membership at www.CastleConnolly.com

Reap the benefits of membership with Castle Connolly. Gain access to ALL online top doctor listings and get discounts on book purchases from our extensive catalog.

- Search among more than 28,000 Castle Connolly Top Doctor listings
- Search among select hospitals and centers of excellence
- Receive a 30% discount on all book purchases

Membership Levels:
- One year - $24.95
- Two years - $34.95

For more information visit: www.CastleConnolly.com/membership

Other Products From Castle Connolly

Castle Connolly Guides

Titles Include:

- *America's Top Doctors® for Cancer*
- *Top Doctors: New York Metro Area*

And Many More

To order other Castle Connolly guides at a 15% discount please visit
http://www.CastleConnolly.com/books
When ordering use discount code: **ATD12VAN**

Castle Connolly's Top Doctors Available Online

- Free Access to 20 -25% of Castle Connolly's Top Doctors
- Purchase Access to the entire database of more than 34,000 doctor profiles

http://www.castleconnolly.com/membership

Customer Feedback

We appreciate your comments regarding our guides. Please email us at
info@castleconnolly.com